Pathology of Infectious Diseases

Volume I

PATHOLOGY of INFECTIOUS DISEASES

VOLUME I

Editors

Daniel H. Connor, MD
Visiting Professor
Department of Pathology
Georgetown University School of Medicine
Washington, DC

Francis W. Chandler, DVM, PhD
Professor of Pathology
Department of Pathology
Medical College of Georgia
Augusta, Georgia

David A. Schwartz, MD, MS Hyg
Associate Professor of Pathology
Assistant Professor of Medicine (Infectious Diseases)
Emory University School of Medicine
Atlanta, Georgia

Herbert J. Manz, MD
Professor of Pathology
Department of Pathology
Georgetown University School of Medicine
Washington, DC

Ernest E. Lack, MD
Professor of Pathology
Department of Pathology
Georgetown University School of Medicine
Washington, DC

Assistant Editors

J. Kevin Baird, PhD
Lieutenant Commander
Medical Service Corps, United States Navy
and
Naval Medical Research Institute
Malaria Program
Rockville, Maryland

John P. Utz, MD
Professor Emeritus
Department of Medicine
Georgetown University School of Medicine
Washington, DC

APPLETON & LANGE
Stamford, Connecticut

97 98 99 00 01 / 10 9 8 7 6 5 4 3 2 1

Prentice Hall International (UK) Limited, *London*
Prentice Hall of Australia Pty. Limited, *Sydney*
Prentice Hall Canada, Inc., *Toronto*
Prentice Hall Hispanoamericana, S.A., *Mexico*
Prentice Hall of India Private Limited, *New Delhi*
Prentice Hall of Japan, Inc., *Tokyo*
Simon & Schuster Asia Pte. Ltd., *Singapore*
Editora Prentice Hall do Brasil Ltda., *Rio de Janeiro*
Prentice Hall, *Upper Saddle River, New Jersey*

Library of Congress Cataloging-in-Publication Data

Pathology of infectious diseases / [edited by] Daniel H. Connor . . .
[et al.].
p. cm.
ISBN 0-8385-1601-7 (case : alk. paper)
1. Communicable diseases—Diagnosis. 2. Diagnosis. Laboratory.
I. Connor, Daniel H. 1928– .
[DNLM: 1. Communicable Diseases—pathology WC 100P297 1997]
RC113.3.P36 1997
616.9′047—dc20
DNLM/DLC
for Library of Contgress 96-31452
CIP

Managing Editor, Development: Kathleen McCullough
Production Service: Spectrum Publisher Services, Mercedes Jackson
Designer: Mary Skudlarek

PRINTED IN HONG KONG

Note: Most of the magnifications stated in the figure legends are the original magnifications of the 35-mm transparencies or photographs.

ISBN 0-8385-1601-7
9 780838 516010 90000

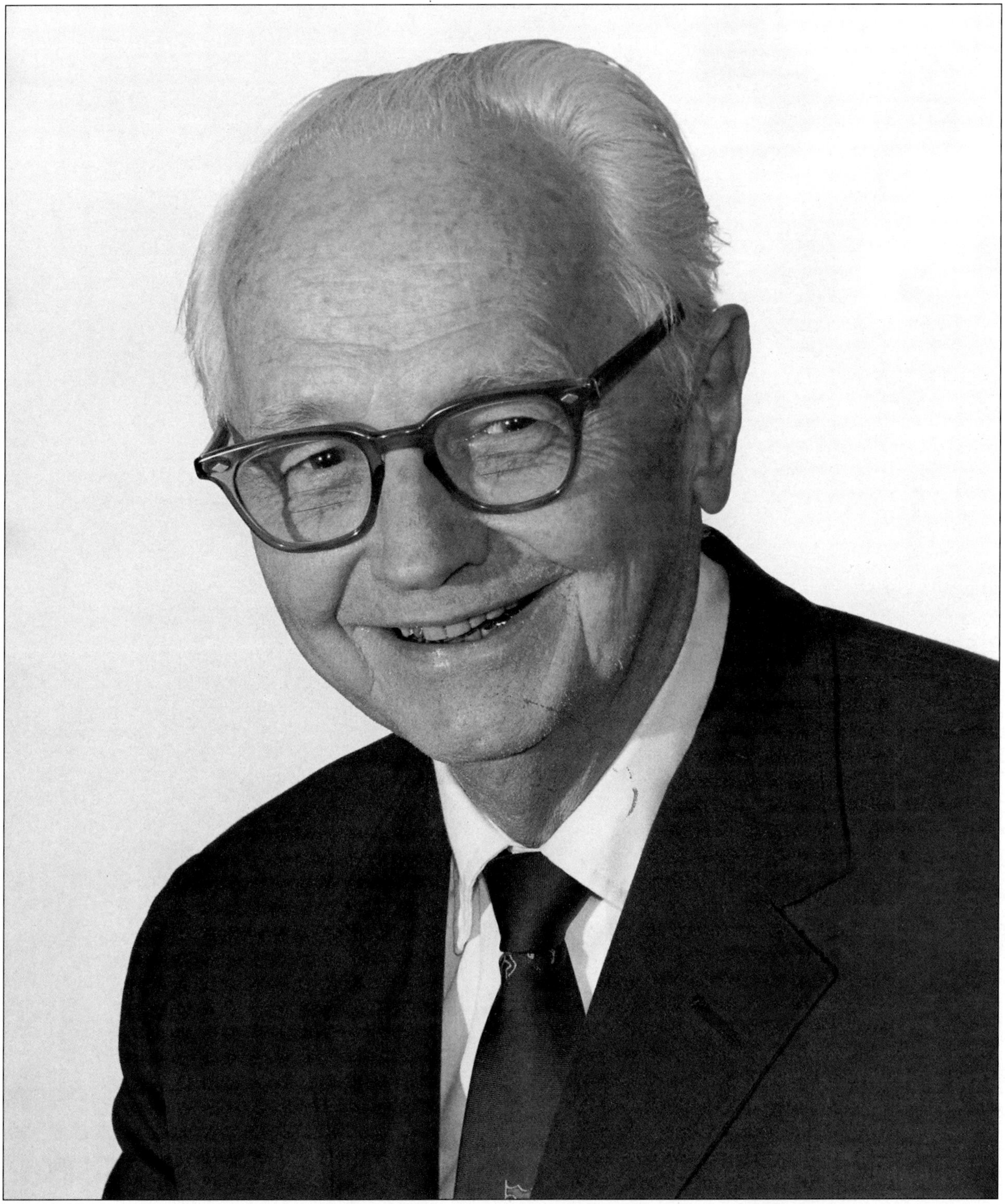

Dedicated to the memory of
Chapman H. Binford, AB, MD, DSc (Hon), DSc (Hon)
1900–1990

by those who worked with him and for him, to whom he was a trusted, selfless, and loyal friend; gifted teacher; dedicated medical scientist and leprologist; writer; editor; and, above all, devoted humanitarian.

Contents

Contributors

Carlos R. Abramowsky, MD
Director of Pediatric Pathology
and
Professor of Pathology
Emory University School of Medicine
Atlanta, Georgia

Masazumi Adachi, MD, ScD
Director of Laboratories
Kingsbrook Jewish Medical Center
Professor of Pathology
State University of New York, Health Science Center at Brooklyn
Brooklyn, New York

Ann M. Adams, PhD
Research Parasitologist
Seafood Products Research Center
United States Food and Drug Administration
Seattle District
Bothell, Washington

Masamichi Aikawa, MD
Professor
Institute of Medical Sciences
Tokai University
Kanagawa, Japan

Libero Ajello, PhD
Adjunct Professor
Ophthalmic Research Section
Emory Eye Center
Emory University School of Medicine
Atlanta, Georgia

Stephen D. Allen, MD
Professor of Pathology and Laboratory Medicine
and
Director
Division of Clinical Microbiology
Indiana University School of Medicine
Indianapolis, Indiana

Geoffrey Altschuler, MB, BS
Clinical Professor of Pathology
University of Oklahoma Health Sciences Center
and
Children's Hospital of Oklahoma
Oklahoma City, Oklahoma

Norio Azumi, MD, PhD
Medical Director
Molecular Diagnostic Laboratory
Georgetown University Medical Center
Professor of Pathology
Georgetown University School of Medicine
Washington, DC

J. Kevin Baird, PhD
Lieutenant Commander
Medical Service Corps, United States Navy
and
Naval Medical Research Institute
Malaria Program
Rockville, Maryland

John G. Banwell, MD
Attending Physician
Togus VA and Regional Medical Center
Adjunct Professor of Medicine
Case Western Reserve University School of Medicine
Cleveland, Ohio

Edwin Beckman, MD
Clinical Associate Professor of Pathology
Ochsner Medical Institutions
Tulane Medical School
New Orleans, Louisiana

Yanina Bednov, MD
Department of Pathology
Georgetown University School of Medicine
Washington, DC

William J. Bellini, MD
Chief
Measles Virus Section
Centers for Disease Control and Prevention
Atlanta, Georgia

Charles E. Binkley, BA
Medical Student
Georgetown University School of Medicine
Washington, DC

H. Braunstein, MD
Honorary Medical Staff
and
Retired Chairman
Department of Laboratories
San Bernardino County Medical Center
San Bernardino, California
Former Professor in Residence
Biomedical Sciences
University of California
Riverside, California

John Bryan, MD
Fellow in Pathology
George Washington University School of Medicine
Washington, DC

Alfred A. Buck, MD, DRPH
Professor of International Health, Molecular Biology, and Immunology
Johns Hopkins University
Baltimore, Maryland

James M. Burke, MD
Georgetown University School of Medicine
Washington, DC

Adam R. Burkey, MD
Research Fellow
Department of Neurosurgery
Georgetown University School of Medicine
Washington, DC

Joseph M. Campos, MD, PhD
Director
Microbiology Laboratory and Laboratory Informatics
Children's National Medical Center
Professor
Department of Pediatrics, Pathology and Microbiology/Immunology
George Washington University Medical Center
Washington, DC

Michael J. Carey, MD
Staff Pathologist (Resident)
University of Utah
Salt Lake City, Utah

Christopher L. Carroll, MD
Georgetown University School of Medicine
Washington, DC

Francis W. Chandler, DVM, PhD
Professor of Pathology
Department of Pathology
Medical College of Georgia
Augusta, Georgia

Clay J. Cockerell, MD
Director
Freeman–Cockerell Laboratories
and
Aston Dermatology Clinic
Associate Professor of Dermatopathology
and
Director
HIV Associated Skin Disease Clinic
University of Texas Southwestern Medical Center
Dallas, Texas

Daniel H. Connor, MD
Visiting Professor
Department of Pathology
Georgetown University School of Medicine
Washington, DC

Richard M. Conran, MD, PhD
Associate Professor of Pathology
Uniformed Services University of the Health Sciences
Bethesda, Maryland

James D. Cotelingam, MD
Captain
Medical Service Corps, United States Navy
Adjunct Professor of Pathology
Uniformed Services University of the Health Sciences
Bethesda, Maryland

John H. Cross, PhD
Professor of Tropical Public Health
Department of Preventive Medicine and Biometrics
Uniformed Services University of the Health Sciences
Bethesda, Maryland

Deborah Dean, MD, MPH
Assistant Professor
University of California at San Francisco School of Medicine
Francis I. Proctor Foundation
San Francisco, California

Ellen C. DeNigris, MD
Commander
Medical Service Corps, United States Navy
Assistant Professor of Pathology
Uniformed Services University of the Health Sciences
Bethesda, Maryland

William O. Dobbins III, MD
Professor Emeritus
Department of Medicine
University of Michigan Medical Center
Ann Arbor, Michigan

J. Stephen Dumler, MD
Director
Medical Microbiology Division
Johns Hopkins Hospital
Associate Professor of Pathology
Johns Hopkins School of Medicine
Baltimore, Maryland

Paul H. Duray, MD
Attending Surgical Pathologist
Warren G. Magnuson Clinical Center
Special Expert in Pathology
National Cancer Institute
National Institutes of Health
Bethesda, Maryland

Mark L. Eberhard, PhD
Division of Parasitic Diseases
National Center for Infectious Diseases
Centers for Disease Control and Prevention
Atlanta, Georgia

Isam A. Eltoum, MD, MRCPath
Fellow in Anatomic Pathology
University of Alabama at Birmingham
Birmingham, Alabama

Armando Filie, MD
Fellow in Cytology
George Washington University School of Medicine
Washington, DC

Sydney D. Finkelstein, MD
Associate Professor of Pathology
University of Pittsburgh Medical Center
Pittsburgh, Pennsylvania

James L. Fishback, MD
Associate Professor of Pathology
University of Kansas School of Medicine
Kansas City, Kansas

Nancy Fishback, MD, CDr, MC, USNR
Associate Professor of Pathology
Uniformed Services University of the Health Sciences
Bethesda, Maryland

Heather E. Fork, MD
Private Practice
Austin, Texas

Elie K. Fraiji, Jr., MD
Georgetown University School of Medicine
Washington, DC

J. K. Frenkel, MD, PhD
Professor Emeritus
University of Kansas
Lawrence, Kansas
Adjunct Professor
University of New Mexico
Santa Fe, New Mexico

David L. Fritz, DVM
Supervisor
Ultrastructural Pathology Group
US Army Medical Research Institute
of Infectious Diseases
Fort Detrick
Frederick, Maryland

Anthony A. Gal, MD
Staff Surgical Pathologist
Emory University Hospital
Associate Professor of Pathology
Emory University School of Medicine
Atlanta, Georgia

Monica V. E. Gallivan, MD
Associate Pathologist
Mount Vernon Hospital
Alexandria, Virginia

David L. Gang, MD
Chief
Anatomic Pathology
Baystate Medical Center
Springfield, Massachusetts
Professor of Pathology
Tufts University School of Medicine
Medford, Massachusetts

Fernando U. Garcia, MD
Director of Surgical Pathology
Allegheny University Hospital
Associate Professor of Pathology
Allegheny University School of Medicine—Center City
Philadelphia, Pennsylvania

David F. Garvin, MD
Director of Diagnostic Services
and
Professor of Pathology
Georgetown University School of Medicine
Washington, DC

Robert M. Genta, MD
Chief
Pathology and Laboratory Medicine
Veterans Affairs Medical Center
Professor of Medicine and Professor of Microbiology and Immunology
Baylor College of Medicine
Houston, Texas

Stanley J. Geyer, MD
Chairman
Department of Pathology and Laboratory Medicine
Western Pennsylvania Hospital
Clinical Professor of Pathology
University of Pittsburgh School of Medicine
Pittsburgh, Pennsylvania

Zachary D. Goodman, MD, PhD
Chief
Hepatic Pathology Division
Armed Forces Institute of Pathology
Washington, DC

M. Alba Greco, MD
Director of Pediatric Pathology
New York University–Bellevue Hospital
Associate Professor of Pathology
New York University Medical Center
New York, New York

H. G. Greenberg, MD
Professor of Medicine and Medical Investigation
Palo Alto Veterans Administration
Palo Alto, California
Stanford University Medical Center
Stanford, California

Thomas D. Griffin, MD
Johnson Griffin Dermatopathology Associates
Glenside, Pennsylvania

Max Grogl, PhD
United States Army Medical Research Unit
Brazil

Hans E. Grossniklaus, MD
F. Phinizy Calhoun Jr. Professor of Ophthalmic Pathology
and
Director
L. F. Montgomery Ophthalmic Laboratory
Emory University School of Medicine
Atlanta, Georgia

Robin Hampton, MD, PhD
Department of Pathology and Laboratory Medicine
Emory University School of Medicine
Atlanta, Georgia

Mark G. Hanly, MBChB, MRCPath, FCAP
Attending Pathologist
Medical College of Georgia Hospital and Clinics
Assistant Professor
Medical College of Georgia
Augusta, Georgia

Christian H. Hansen, MD
Resident Physician
Department of Pathology
Georgetown University Medical Center
Washington, DC

Abida K. Haque, MD
Professor and Director of Anatomic Pathology
University of Texas Medical Branch
Galveston, Texas

Phillip J. Harrity, MD
Staff Pathologist
Sinai Samaritan Medical Center
Clinical Assistant Professor of Pathology
Medical College of Wisconsin
Milwaukee, Wisconsin

Rod J. Hay, DM, FRCP, FRCPath
Professor of Cutaneous Medicine
and
Dean of the Institute of Dermatology
UMDS
Department of Dermatology
Guy's Hospital
London, England

Kurt F. Heim, MD, PhD
Senior Staff Fellow
Department of Transfusion Medicine
Clinical Center
National Institutes of Health
Bethesda, Maryland

Thomas K. Held, MD
Fellow in Hematology and Oncology
Humbolt University
Virchow Clinic
Berlin, Germany

Jeffrey F. Hines, MD
Staff Physician
Division of Gynecologic Oncology
Department of Obstetrics and Gynecology
Brooke Army Medical Center
San Antonio, Texas

Scott R. Hyde, PhD
Assistant Professor of Pathology
University of Oklahoma College of Medicine—Tulsa
Scientific Director of Perinatal Pathology and Diagnostic Molecular Biology
South Tulsa Pathology at Saint Francis Hospital
Tulsa, Oklahoma

Nancy K. Jaax, DVM
Colonel
United States Army
Chief
Pathology Division
United States Army Medical Research Institute of Infectious Diseases
Fort Detrick
Frederick, Maryland

Elaine S. Jaffe, MD
Chief
Hematopathology Section
Laboratory of Pathology
National Cancer Institute
National Institutes of Health
Bethesda, Maryland

A. Bennett Jenson, MD
Professor of Pathology
Georgetown University School of Medicine
Washington, DC

Jacqueline M. Junkins-Hopkins, MD
Johnson Griffin Dermatopathology Associates
Glenside, Pennsylvania

Juntra Karbwang, MD
Faculty of Tropical Medicine
Mahidol University
Bangkok, Thailand

David Katz, MD
Laboratory of Neuropathology
National Institute of Neurological Disorders and Stroke
Bethesda, Maryland

Kevin R. Kazacos, DVM, PhD
Director
Clinical Parasitology Laboratory
and
Professor of Parasitology
School of Veterinary Medicine
Purdue University
West Lafayette, Indiana

James W. Kazura, MD
Chief
Division of Georgraphic Medicine
and
Professor of Medicine and International Health
Case Western Reserve University School of Medicine
Cleveland, Ohio

James K. Kelly, MD
Chief
Anatomical Pathology
Greater Victoria Hospital Society
Victoria, British Columbia, Canada

Francisco A. Kerdel, MD
Professor of Clinical Dermatology
University of Miami
School of Medicine
Department of Dermatology
Cedars Medical Center
Miami, Florida

Mahmoud A. Khalifa, MD, PhD, FRCP(C)
Department of Pathology
General Hospital
Memorial University of Newfoundland
Saint John's, Newfoundland

Jung H. Kim, MD
Attending Physician
Yale–New Haven Hospital
Associate Professor
Section of Neuropathology
Yale University School of Medicine
New Haven, Connecticut

John M. Kissane, MD
Pathologist
Barnes–Jewish Hospital and Saint Louis Children's Hospital
Professor of Pathology and Pediatrics
Washington University School of Medicine
St. Louis, Missouri

Steven E. Kolker, MD
Resident in Pathology
University of California at San Francisco
San Francisco, California

Harry P. W. Kozakewich, MD
Associate Professor of Pathology
Children's Hospital
and
Harvard Medical School
Boston, Massachusetts

Princy N. Kumar, MD
Assistant Professor of Medicine
Division of Infectious Diseases
Georgetown University School of Medicine
Washington, DC

Ernest E. Lack, MD
Professor of Pathology
Department of Pathology
Georgetown University School of Medicine
Washington, DC

Elena R. Ladich, MD
Department of Pathology
Georgetown University School of Medicine
Washington, DC

Philip E. LeBoit, MD
Co-Director
Dermatopathology Service
and
Associate Professor of Clinical Pathology and Dermatology
University of California at San Francisco
San Francisco, California

Michael R. Lewin-Smith, MD
Department of Pathology
George Washington University Medical Center
Washington, DC

Lai Y. Lim, MT, ASCP
Department of Pathology
Georgetown University School of Medicine
Washington, DC

Alberto Thomaz Londero, MD
Emeritus Professor
Department of Microbiology
School of Medicine
Federal University of Santa Maria
Santa Maria, Brazil

Mario A. Luna, MD
Director
Autopsy Service
and
Professor of Pathology
University of Texas
M.D. Anderson Cancer Center
Houston, Texas

Bhagirath Majmudar, MD
Professor of Pathology
and
Associate Professor of Obstetrics and Gynecology
Emory University School of Medicine
Atlanta, Georgia

Elias E. Manuelidis, MD (Deceased)
Professor of Pathology
Yale University School of Medicine
New Haven, Connecticut

Laura Manuelidis, MD
Section of Neuropathology
Yale University School of Medicine
New Haven, Connecticut

Herbert J. Manz, MD
Professor of Pathology
Department of Pathology
Georgetown University School of Medicine
Washington, DC

Edith F. Marley, MD
Pathologist
Sunrise Hospital and Medical Center
and
Sunrise Children's Hospital Laboratory Consultants
Las Vegas, Nevada

Augusto Julio Martinez, MD
Professor of Pathology
Department of Gastrointestinal Sciences
University of Pittsburgh School of Medicine
Pittsburgh, Pennsylvania

M. Mathan, MD
Professor of Pathology
and
Head
Department of Gastrointestinal Sciences
Christian Medical College and Hospital
Tamil Nadu, India

Michael R. McGinnis, PhD
Professor of Pathology
University of Texas Medical Branch
Associate Director
WHO Collaborating Center for Tropical Diseases
Director
Medical Mycology Research Center
Galveston, Texas

Richard A. McPherson, MD
Chairman
Division of Clinical Pathology
Medical College of Virginia Hospitals
Professor of Pathology
Virginia Commonwealth University
Richmond, Virginia

Frederick A. Meier, MD
Chairman
Clinical and Anatomic Pathology
Alfred I. DuPont Institute
Wilmington, Delaware

Martin E. A. Mielke, MD
Associate Medical Director
Medical Microbiology and Infectious Diseases/Immunology
and
Associate Professor
Institute for Medical Microbiology
Free University (Berlin)
Berlin, Germany

James Patrick Mixon, MD
Department of Pathology
Emory University School of Medicine
Atlanta, Georgia

Elizabeth A. Montgomery, MD
Associate Professor of Pathology
Georgetown University School of Medicine
Washington, DC

Zuher M. Naib, MD
Professor Emeritus of Pathology
Emory University School of Medicine
Atlanta, Georgia

Kei-Ichiro Nakamura, MD
Department of Anatomy
Faculty of Medicine
Kyushu University
Fukuoka, Japan

Lydia Navarro-Román, MD
Humana Health Care Plans
San Antonio, Texas

Joseph T. Newsome, DVM
Staff Veterinarian
Research Resources Facility
Georgetown University School of Medicine
Washington, DC

Gregory Nikolaidis, MD
Resident in Pediatrics
Texas Children's Hospital
Baylor College of Medicine
Houston, Texas

Jerome T. O'Connell II, MD
Resident Physician
Department of Pathology
University of California at Los Angeles Medical Center
Los Angeles, California

Daniel P. O'Neill, MD
Resident Physician
California Pacific Medical Center
San Francisco, California

Jan Marc Orenstein, MD
Professor of Pathology
George Washington University Medical Center
Washington, DC

David A. Owen, MB, BCh, FRCPath, FRCP(C)
Head
Division of Anatomical Pathology
Vancouver Hospital and Health Sciences Centre
Professor of Pathology
University of British Columbia
Vancouver, British Columbia, Canada

Robert L. Owen, MD
Environmental Health Physician
Cell Biology and Aging Section
VA Medical Center
Professor of Medicine, Epidemiology, and Biostatistics
University of California at San Francisco
San Francisco, California

Philip E. S. Palmer, MD
Department of Radiology
University of California School of Medicine
Davis, California

Demosthenes Pappagianis, MD, PhD
Professor
Department of Medical Microbiology and Immunology
University of California School of Medicine
Davis, California

Robert R. Pascal, MD
Director
Division of Anatomic Pathology
Emory University Hospital
Profesor and Vice-Chairman
Department of Pathology and Laboratory Medicine
Emory University School of Medicine
Atlanta, Georgia

Claire M. Payne, PhD
Research Professor
Arizona Research Laboratories
Division of Biotechnology and Department of Microbiology and Immunology
University of Arizona College of Medicine
Tucson, Arizona

Gary R. Pearson, PhD
Professor
Department of Microbiology and Immunology
Georgetown University School of Medicine
Washington, DC

Philip E. Pellet, MD
Chief
Herpes Virus Section
Centers for Disease Control and Prevention
Atlanta, Georgia

Daniel P. Perl, MD
Director
Neuropathology Division
Mount Sinai Medical Center
Professor of Pathology
Mount Sinai School of Medicine
New York, New York

David H. Persing, MD
Director
Molecular Microbiology Laboratory
Mayo Clinic
Rochester, Minnesota

C. J. Peters, MD
Centers for Disease Control and Prevention
Atlanta, Georgia

Catherine P. Picken, MD
Assistant Professor
Department of Otolaryngology, Head and Neck Surgery
Georgetown University Medical Center
Washington, DC

Phillip F. Pierce, MD
Associate Professor of Medicine and Microbiology
Georgetown University Medical Center
Washington, DC

Duane Pinto, MD
Medical Resident
Beth Israel Hospital/Harvard Medical School
Boston, Massachusetts

Lisa G. Portnoy, DVM
Staff Veterinarian
Research Resources Facility
Georgetown University Medical Center
Instructor of Pathology
Georgetown University School of Medicine
Washington, DC

Ewald Pretner, MD
Staff Physician
Georgetown University Hospital
Washington, DC

David T. Purtilo, MD (Deceased)
Department of Pathology and Microbiology
University of Nebraska Medical Center
Omaha, Nebraska

John R. Rabbege, BS
Assistant Professor
Case Western Reserve University
Cleveland, Ohio

Evette Ramsay, MD
Resident Physician
Georgetown University School of Medicine
Washington, DC

Robert L. Rausch, DVM, PhD
Professor Emeritus
Department of Pathology
School of Public Health and Medicine
and
Department of Comparative Medicine
University of Washington School of Medicine
Seattle, Washington

Barbara S. Reisner, PhD
Associate Director
Clinical Microbiology Laboratory
and
Assistant Professor
Department of Pathology
University of Texas Medical Branch
Galveston, Texas

Gustavo C. Román, MD
Humana Health Care Plans
San Antonio, Texas

Theodore Rosen, MD
Chief of Dermatology
Houston VA Medical Center
Professor of Dermatology
Baylor College of Medicine
Houston, Texas

Marc K. Rosenblum, MD
Chief
Neuropathology and Autopsy Service
Memorial–Sloan Kettering Cancer Center
Associate Professor of Pathology
Cornell University Medical College
New York, New York

Leonard J. Rosenthal, PhD
Professor of Microbiology and Immunology
Georgetown University School of Medicine
Washington, DC

Heidrun Rotterdam, MD
Attending Pathologist
Columbia Presbyterian Medical Center
Professor of Clinical Pathology
College of Physicians and Surgeons of Columbia University
New York, New York

L. J. Saif, PhD
Professor of Virology and Immunology
Food Animal Health Research Program
Department of Veterinary Preventive Medicine
Ohio Agricultural Research and Development Center
Ohio State University
Wooster, Ohio

Nirmal K. Saini, MD
Acting Chief
Department of Anatomic Pathology
Pathologic Medicine Laboratory Service
Assistant Pathologist
George Washington University Medical Center
Washington, DC

Judy A. Sakanari, PhD
Assistant Adjunct Professor
University of California at San Francisco
San Francisco, California

Shukdeo Sankar, MD
Staff Physician
Whitman Walker Clinic and Max Robinson Center
Silver Spring, Maryland

Gerhard A. Schad, PhD
Department of Pathobiology
University of Pennsylvania School of Veterinary Medicine
Philadelphia, Pennsylvania

Stephen P. Schiffer, DVM, MS
Director
Research Resources Facility
and
Associate Professor of Cell Biology
Georgetown University School of Medicine
Washington, DC

David A. Schwartz, MD, MS Hyg
Associate Professor of Pathology
and
Assistant Professor of Medicine (Infectious Diseases)
Emory University School of Medicine
Research Scientist
National Center for Infectious Diseases
Centers for Disease Control and Prevention
Atlanta, Georgia

Christopher M. Seniw, MD
Resident Physician
Georgetown University Hospital
Washington, DC

John A. Shadduck, DVM
Texas A&M College of Veterinary Medicine
College Station, Texas

Robert J. Siegel, MD
Director
Pathology Laboratories
Crawford Long Hospital
Associate Professor
Department of Pathology and Laboratory Medicine
Emory University School of Medicine
Atlanta, Georgia

Bharatha Sinniah, MD
Professor and Chairman
Department of Parasitology
University of Malaya
Kuala Lumpur
Malaysia

Jerome H. Smith, MD
Pathologist
Autopsy Service
and
Professor of Pathology
University of Texas Medical Branch
Galveston, Texas

J. Thomas Stocker, MD
Professor of Pathology
Uniformed Services University of the Health Sciences
Bethesda, Maryland
Clinical Professor of Pathology
Georgetown University School of Medicine
Washington, DC

Melissa Conrad Stöppler, MD
Assistant Professor of Pathology
Georgetown University School of Medicine
Washington, DC

Alfonso J. Strano, MD, PhD
Director (Retired)
Microbiology Laboratory
Saint John's Hospital
Clinical Professor of Pathology
Southern Illinois University School of Medicine
Springfield, Illinois

Kimberly Studeman, MD
Resident Physician
Jackson Memorial Hospital
Miami, Florida

Ramiah Subramanian, MD
Medical Officer
United States Food and Drug Administration
Adjunct Associate Professor of Pathology
Georgetown University School of Medicine
Washington, DC

Tsieh Sun, MD
Director
Flow Cytometry Laboratory
VA Medical Center
Professor of Pathology
University of Colorado School of Medicine
Denver, Colorado

Donald E. Sweet, MD
Chairman
Department of Orthopedic Pathology
Armed Forces Institute of Pathology
Bethesda, Maryland

Bernard Tandler, PhD
Department of Geographical Medicine
Case Western Reserve University
Cleveland, Ohio

Van Q. Telford, DVM, MD
Medical Director
Department of Pathology
RHD Memorial Hospital
Dallas, Texas

Elizabeth R. Unger, MD, PhD
Associate Professor of Pathology
Emory University School of Medicine
Atlanta, Georgia

Matthias Unger, MD
Pathologist
Department of Pediatric Pathology and Placentology
Humbolt University
Virchow Clinic
Berlin, Germany

John P. Utz, MD
Professor Emeritus
Department of Medicine
Georgetown University School of Medicine
Washington, DC

Patrick J. Vaughan, MD
Department of Orthopedic Surgery
Medical College of Virginia
Richmond, Virginia

Phyllis R. Vezza, MD
Department of Pathology
Georgetown University School of Medicine
Washington, DC

Tuyethoa N. Vinh, MD
Department of Bone and Joint Pathology
Armed Forces Institute of Pathology
Washington, DC

Govinda S. Visvesvara, PhD
Parasitic Disease Branch
Centers for Disease Control and Prevention
Atlanta, Georgia

Franz von Lichtenberg, MD
Senior Pathologist
Brigham and Women's Hospital
Professor of Pathology Emeritus
Harvard Medical School
Boston, Massachusetts

David H. Walker, MD
Professor and Chairman
Department of Pathology
University of Texas Medical Branch
Director
WHO Collaborating Center for Tropical Diseases
Galveston, Texas

John C. Watts, MD
Chief
Surgical Pathology
William Beaumont Hospital
Associate Clinical Professor of Pathology
Wayne State University School of Medicine
Royal Oak, Michigan

A. Brian West, MB, FRCPath
Director of Surgical Pathology
and
Professor of Pathology
University of Texas Medical Branch
Galveston, Texas

Jacqueline A. Wieneke, MD
Resident in Pathology
Georgetown University Medical Center
Washington, DC

C. Mel Wilcox, MD
Director of Clinical Research
and
Associate Professor of Medicine
Division of Gastroenterology and Hepatology
University of Alabama at Birmingham
Birmingham, Alabama

Washington C. Winn, Jr., MD, MBA
Director
Clinical Microbiology Laboratory
Fletcher Allen Health Care
Professor of Pathology
University of Vermont College of Medicine
Burlington, Vermont

Edward J. Young, MD
Chief of Staff
VA Medical Center
Professor of Medicine
Baylor College of Medicine
Houston, Texas

Neal S. Young, MD
Chief
Clinical Service
Hematology Branch
National Institutes of Health
Bethesda, Maryland

David Zagzag, MD, PhD
Assistant Professor of Pathology
New York University Medical School
New York, New York

Sherif R. Zaki, MD
Chief
Molecular Pathology and Ultrastructural Activity
Centers for Disease Control and Prevention
Atlanta, Georgia

Introduction

Infectious diseases are the leading cause of death worldwide. In the United States, infectious diseases are the third leading cause of death. The World Health Organization estimates that approximately 17 million of the 52 million deaths (33%) worldwide in 1995 were caused by microbial agents. Infection with human immunodeficiency virus (HIV) is now the leading cause of death in the United States in persons between 25 and 44 years of age. In view of these facts, it is ironic that we are, in some ways, less prepared to address infectious diseases in the United States than we were in the mid-1960s.

As a result of improvements in sanitation and overall living conditions during the early part of the 20th century and the subsequent introduction of many vaccines and antibiotics, considerable complacency has developed regarding infectious diseases that many regarded as either preventable by immunization or treatable by antibiotics. The 1970s produced the beginning of a series of what, in retrospect, should have been loud wake-up calls regarding the challenges infectious diseases continue to pose domestically and globally. Rotaviral gastroenteritis, Lyme disease, legionnaires' disease, and toxic shock syndrome are a few of the infectious diseases first recognized during the 1970s. The most dramatic example of an emerging infectious disease, the acquired immunodeficiency syndrome (AIDS), was recognized in 1981, and hemorrhagic colitis caused by *Escherichia coli* O157:H7 was identified in 1982. The end of the 1980s saw the reemergence of measles and tuberculosis in the United States and the emergence of multiple drug resistance in *Mycobacterium tuberculosis* strains causing disease predominantly in persons infected with HIV.

Experiences with these and other emerging and reemerging diseases should have alerted physicians, microbiologists, researchers, public health officials, policy makers, and the public to the critical importance of ensuring the capacity to detect, respond to, and control these infections. In the fall of 1992, the Institute of Medicine (IOM) published a report entitled "Emerging Infections: Microbial Threats to Health in the United States." This report, developed under the leadership of Drs. Joshua Lederberg and Robert Shope, highlighted the complacency regarding emerging infections and identified the important factors in disease emergence and reemergence (changes in human demographics and behaviors, advances in technology and industry, economic development and changes in land use, increases in travel and commerce, microbial adaptation and change, and deterioration in the public health system at the local, state, national, and global levels). The IOM committee made 15 recommendations that stressed the need to improve surveillance and response capacity and also identified research issues and training priorities.

Since publication of this report, physicians, microbiologists, and public health officials have faced numerous challenges from microorganisms in the United States and abroad. Domestic challenges have included an interstate outbreak of hemorrhagic colitis caused by *E coli* O157:H7 associated with contaminated hamburger, a large waterborne disease outbreak of cryptosporidiosis associated with contaminated drinking water in Milwaukee, the outbreak of hantavirus pulmonary syndrome caused by a previously unrecognized hantavirus, the continued emergence of vancomycin-resistant enterococci and penicillin-resistant *Streptococcus pneumoniae*, and nationwide outbreaks of *Salmonella* serotype Enteritidis infection associated with contaminated ice cream and *Cyclospora* gastroenteritis associated with raspberries.

Internationally, a number of outbreaks have served as reminders that the world is a global village. Examples include plague in India and equine morbillivirus infection in Australia in 1994, Ebola hemorrhagic fever in Zaire and leptospirosis in Nicaragua in 1995, and a new variant of Creutzfeldt–Jakob disease (CJD) in the United Kingdom and a large outbreak of *E coli* O157:H7 hemorrhagic colitis in Japan in 1996. Each of these outbreaks illustrates the critical importance of adequate surveillance and response capacity, the critical role of the laboratory and the discipline of pathology in addressing emerging infections, and the global implications of a local problem.

The ability to address these emerging and reemerging microbial threats requires adequate surveillance and response capacity, ongoing research programs, strengthened prevention and control programs, and repair of the public health system at the local, state, national, and international levels. The discipline of pathology has played an important role in the recognition and characterization of the hantavirus pulmonary syndrome outbreak, diagnosis and subsequent prospective surveillance of Ebola hemorrhagic fever in Central Africa, identification of the etiologic agent in the leptospirosis outbreak in Nicaragua, and characterization of the variant form of CJD in the United Kingdom. Pathologists have also made vital contributions to recognition of opportunistic infections in HIV-infected and other immunodeficient patients. The chapters in this book clearly document the role of classic and modern molecular methods in assessing disease etiology and pathology of infectious diseases. The challenges that these diseases continue to pose demand a multidisciplinary approach and a supply of trained clinicians, microbiologists, pathologists, rodent and vector biologists, ecologists, behavioral scientists, and public health officials.

Future challenges are difficult to predict but certainly include more problems with antimicrobial-resistant infections, the threat of another influenza pandemic, the likelihood of increasing problems of dengue hemorrhagic fever, and the risk of urban yellow fever in the Western Hemisphere. The global HIV epidemic will put large numbers of people at risk for currently recognized and new opportunistic infections. The roles of hepatitis B virus in chronic liver disease and hepatocellular carcinoma, human papillomavirus in cervical cancer, and *Helicobacter pylori* infection in peptic ulcer disease and gastric cancer are now well established. It is likely that more chronic diseases will be found to have an infectious etiology. Pathologists clearly have an important role in the future in surveillance, diagnosis, and response to emerging and reemerging infections. This book should serve as a valuable source of information for them and for their colleagues in related disciplines.

James M. Hughes, MD
Assistant Surgeon General
Director, National Center for Infectious Diseases
Centers for Disease Control and Prevention
Atlanta, Georgia
September 1996

Foreword

We were all aware of the deaths of 34 people of legionnaires' disease in Philadelphia in 1976, of the 32 deaths by hantavirus infection in the southwestern United States in 1993, of the sudden outbreaks of Ebola virus in Africa in 1995, and, of course, of the worldwide spread of human immunodeficiency virus (HIV) and acquired immunodeficiency syndrome (AIDS). The intense drama of lethal infectious diseases has been highlighted in the mass media to focus public attention on microorganisms that threaten human health. A striking feature of the diseases mentioned is that every one of them was discovered only since the early 1970s and they were unknown when I studied microbiology in medical school. Moreover, during this relatively short time frame many other pathogenic human microbes have been discovered that cause diarrhea, hepatitis, arthritis, and leukemia. As if this were not enough, scourges of the past have begun to reemerge, and resistant strains of malaria, tuberculosis, *Escherichia coli,* and pneumococcus are taking hold.

Why are these epidemics happening now? The conquest and prevention of infectious diseases are arguably the greatest victories of medicine. The era of antibiotics and vaccines has brought under control such dread diseases as influenza, which killed more than half a million Americans in one season early in the 20th century, and smallpox, which has been eliminated altogether. Infectious diseases, however, remain a great threat to public health. Emerging and reemerging infections are being encountered for many reasons. Antibiotics themselves select for genetic changes and impart resistant phenotypes. Changes in society have a profound impact: population explosions, declining public health, and the efficient transmission of disease across geographic boundaries brought by modern day travel. The days have long past when the dying Duke of Gaunt could claim:

This fortress built by Nature herself
Against infection and the hand of war,
This blessed plot, this earth, this realm, this
England . . .

William Shakespeare (1564–1616), Richard II, II, i

Even then, infectious diseases still managed to spread through populations. Such plagues helped shape our species by inflicting severe selective pressures. Indeed, our genome carries the archeologic vestiges of past epidemics. These relics have left their imprint in the variable antibody genes of our immune system, in our blood types, and in our histocompatibility antigens. Humans and their microorganisms have been parallel evolutionary partners, and the human genome has molded a formidable immune system and tissue reaction in response to its microorganisms. This pattern of infection, disease, and the reshaping of the host response will inevitably continue.

For medicine to combat infectious disease requires great familiarity with it. This text, *Pathology of Infectious Diseases,* is a milestone toward that objective. Here we are taken into the diagnosis of human infectious disease as manifested by invasion of the organism, by its propagation, and by the ensuing host response. Detailed observations made by pathologists have been brought together in a single reference work that substantially encompasses the known infectious diseases that affect humankind. This comprehensive work underscores the principle that the microscope is still essential in revealing subtle clues linking a microorganism to a clinical disease process. Under the experienced leadership of Dr. Daniel H. Connor, together with Drs. Chandler, Schwartz, Manz, and Lack, the current body of knowledge of diagnostic pathology of human infectious disease has been assembled. Few could tackle the daunting task and credit is due to Dr. Connor and his colleagues for bringing this text to fruition. It is hoped that this special volume serves those who embark on the discovery, prevention, and treatment of the diseases described herein and the diseases that await discovery.

Jeffrey Cossman, MD
Chairman, Department of Pathology
Georgetown University School of Medicine
Washington, DC
August 1996

Preface

Winston Churchill said, "Writing a book is an adventure. At first it's a toy; then it becomes a mistress, then a master, and just when you become resigned to your servitude, you kill the monster and fling it about at the public."

This book, conceived in the fall of 1990, is the culmination of the efforts of many people, among whom we are most grateful to the contributing authors. As the saying goes, to accomplish a task, ask a busy person; this we did—repeatedly and persistently in our attempt to make the book comprehensive and timely. But 6 years is a long incubation period, and as a consequence, some authors updated their manuscripts once, twice, and even three times while awaiting publication—a reflection of the rapidly changing world of infectious diseases.

The idea of using quotations at the beginning of certain chapters started capriciously, almost as an afterthought, and at first were used only when they were pertinent to the subject—for instance, rabies (Chapter 30). But the quotations gained popularity with authors and editors, so our goal escalated to find one for each chapter. Dr. Sarah Frankel and Dr. Ann Marie Nelson, both at the US Armed Forces Institute of Pathology, furnished reference books that fueled our interest in pursuing quotations. And we took liberties. The chapter on clostridial infections (Chapter 54), for instance, was the vehicle for our favorite prose—President Lincoln's letter to Mrs. Lydia Bixby. How noble is such eloquence and humility! As Viscount Bryce has said of these four sentences, "I do not know where the nobility of self-sacrifice for a great cause, and the consolation which the thought of a sacrifice so made should bring, is set forth with such simple and pathetic beauty. Deep must be the fountains from which there issues so pure a stream." (Maybe one, or perhaps two, of Mrs. Bixby's sons died of a gas infection complicating a battlefield wound.) As our resources broadened, at least one quotation was selected for each chapter. This broader approach is best exemplified perhaps by Maxwell's equations used for Chapter 132 (Free-Living Amebic Infections). We hope the association of these equations and the subject need no explanation or justification. Finally, it seemed appropriate that Chapter 36 (Viral Infections by Human Herpesviruses 6, 7, and 8), which was completed on July 4, should have a quotation by Thomas Jefferson.

If there were stages of "toy" or "mistress" in the preparation of this book, they were fleeting. Now our "servitude" is over. We hope that this book will not be "flung about" but used regularly and with benefit by pathologists, clinicians, epidemiologists, veterinarians, and other medical scientists. We welcome helpful comments for any future editions. Our final prayer is that this century's great advances in medical science, including prevention, therapy, and technology, will become available soon to all people everywhere.

Daniel H. Connor, MD
Long Lake, Ontario, Canada
August 1996

Acknowledgments

Lorenz E. Zimmerman, MD, helped in many ways, reading some chapters and making his collection of pictures available. Evelma Jones at the Armed Forces Institute of Pathology located many of the illustrations. Cathy Cataldo typed, scanned, and mailed many manuscripts. We are especially grateful to the entire staff of the Georgetown University Dahlgren Memorial Medical Library, who were enormously helpful and always cheerful. Jeanne Larsen was never defeated by a remote or very old reference. Lilia Frilles, Alexandra Gomes, Terry Tobias, Tony Pasieka, Martha Cohn, and Brian Dobbs helped continuously with library work that sometimes seemed unending. Amanda Hall and Joni Douglass in Educational Media at Georgetown University School of Medicine helped produce many of the illustrations expertly and on time. We are grateful also to Carolyn James, Gloria Baptist, Patricia Jones, and Joan Edmondson of the Division of Media and Training Services, Public Health Practice Office, Centers for Disease Control and Prevention, Atlanta, Georgia, for assistance in obtaining some of the illustrative materials.

Pathology of Infectious Diseases

Volume I

PART I

General Considerations

CHAPTER 1

Approaches to the Pathologic Diagnosis of Infectious Diseases

Francis W. Chandler

There are three phases to treatment; diagnosis, diagnosis and diagnosis.

Sir William Osler (1849–1919)

Pathologists play a key role in recognizing infectious agents. In many instances, pathologists provide lifesaving answers with great speed, guide microbiologists in determining cause, and facilitate clinicians in patient management.[1] In addition, pathologists are in an excellent position to perceive new patterns of disease, and to detect and define emerging infections that represent newly recognized diseases (eg, AIDS, hantavirus pulmonary syndrome, legionnaires' disease). Ways in which surgical pathologists can contribute to the diagnosis of infectious diseases are listed in Table 1–1.

A definitive diagnosis of an infectious disease ideally is made by demonstrating the causative agent in tissues and exudates, and through culture and isolation. When microbiologic culture is not possible or when results are equivocal, pathologists should follow a systematic approach to detect and identify a suspected microorganism in a tissue specimen.[2] A schematic representation of such an approach, which emphasizes both traditional morphologic and novel molecular diagnostic methods, is presented in Figure 1–1. Although certain inflammatory patterns may suggest infection by a particular type of microbe, there are no absolute histologic criteria that permit an etiologic diagnosis based only on host response. Also, inflammatory patterns are usually atypical, paucireactive, and unreliable in patients with severe immune deficiencies (eg, AIDS). A causal agent first must be detected and then identified in tissue sections before a definitive histopathologic diagnosis can be made. In immunodeficient patients, the possibility of coexisting infection always should be considered, even when a single type of organism is abundant and quickly demonstrated.

Some microorganisms are morphologically distinctive and identified by direct microscopic examination with routine and special stains. For example, if typical forms of certain fungi and protozoans are observed in tissue sections, or if distinctive viral inclusion bodies are present, the organism can be named and the infection diagnosed. Many times, however, it is impossible to identify an infectious agent. Nevertheless, one can usually conclude that a particular type of microbe is present and then take steps to identify it. In addition to the special histologic and immunohistologic procedures outlined in Figure 1–1, the patient's history (including recent travels), clinical profile, and laboratory tests are important guidelines. In situ hybridization (ISH) and the polymerase chain reaction (PCR) can be done on formalin-fixed, paraffin-embedded specimens, and these frequently will enhance diagnostic specificity and sensitivity (see Chapters 3 and 4).

Several stains can be used to demonstrate infectious agents in tissue sections. Their applications are listed in Table 1–2. The two most important stains for screening are silver impregnation for bacteria and methenamine silver for fungi (Figure 1–1). Silver impregnation stains, such as the Steiner, Dieterle, and Warthin–Starry, demonstrate non-gram-reactive bacteria (eg, *Treponema pallidum, Borrelia burgdorferi,* the *Leptospira* spp, the *Bartonella* spp, *Calymmatobacterium granulomatis*). Silver impregnation procedures blacken all bacteria nonselectively and are excellent for demonstrating small, weakly gram-negative bacilli, such as the *Legionella* spp, *Francisella tularensis, Burkholderia pseudomallei* (formerly *Pseudomonas pseudomallei*), and *Helicobacter pylori.* The accretion of

TABLE 1–1. CONTRIBUTIONS OF SURGICAL PATHOLOGISTS TO THE DIAGNOSIS OF INFECTIOUS DISEASES

1. They provide a rapid morphologic diagnosis.
2. They establish the pathogenic significance of a cultural isolate.
3. They exclude infection from the differential diagnosis altogether by revealing another process that accounts for the clinical findings.
4. They establish a diagnosis when fresh tissue is not available for culture or when repeated cultures are negative.
5. They establish a diagnosis when morphology is the only reliable method available for certain diseases for which practical culture methods do not currently exist.

metallic silver on these bacteria coats them and makes them larger, often enabling their detection. Compared to Gram's stains, silver impregnation is more sensitive for small numbers of bacteria. Once detected, modified Gram's stains such as the Brown and Brenn (B&B), Brown–Hopps (B-H), and MacCallum–Goodpasture can be used to distinguish gram-positive and gram-negative bacteria, including the gram-positive actinomycetes of actinomycosis, nocardiosis, and actinomycotic mycetoma. The B-H stain is better for gram-negative bacteria and rickettsiae, and especially for weakly gram-negative bacilli when the basic fuchsin is increased from 0.1% to 1.0%.[3] The B&B stain is better for gram-positive bacteria.

In addition to being acid-fast, most *Mycobacterium* spp, particularly *M avium* complex, are periodic acid–Schiff (PAS)-positive, Gomori's (Grocott's) methenamine silver (GMS)-positive, and weakly gram-positive in paraffin sections. The *Nocardia* spp, *M leprae, L micdadei, L pneumophila* (rarely), and *Rhodococcus equi* are weakly acid fast and nonalcohol fast. Modified acid-fast stains, such as the Coates–Fite or Fite–Faraco, that use an aqueous solution of a weak acid for decolorization are required to stain these bacteria.

GMS or one of its more rapid variants is best for fungi because it provides good contrast for screening and it silvers fungal carcasses that do not always stain well with PAS and Gridley. When properly done, the GMS method eliminates nonspecific staining of normal tissues and necrotic debris, whereas the PAS and Gridley procedures do not. Also, the GMS stain is more sensitive because it demonstrates certain polysaccharide-rich nonfungal pathogens [eg, the causal agents of actinomycosis and nocardiosis, the *Mycobacterium* spp, nonfilamentous bacteria with polysaccharide capsules, cyst walls of *Pneumocystis carinii* and free-living soil amebae, algal cells (*Prototheca* spp and *Chlorella* spp), the spores of certain microsporidians, and the cytoplasmic granular inclusion bodies of cytomegalovirus]. As an all-purpose stain, it enables rapid screening of specimens from patients with acquired immunodeficiency syndrome (AIDS) and multiple infections.

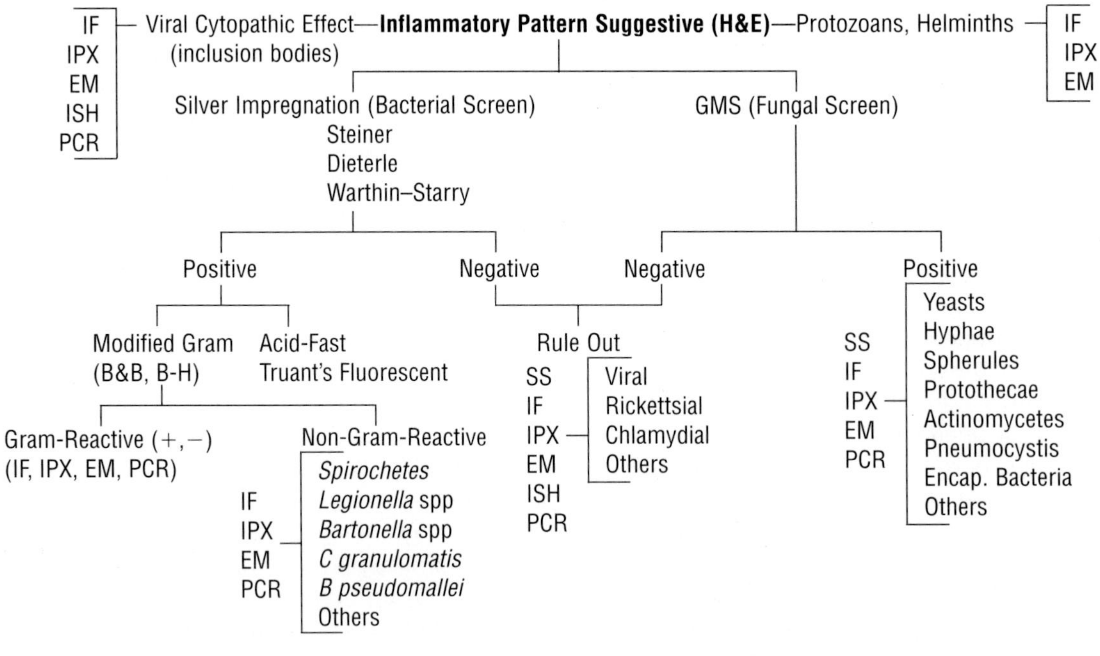

Figure 1–1. Schematic for the morphologic-molecular detection of infectious agents in fixed, paraffin-embedded tissue specimens. IF, immunofluorescence; IPX, immunoperoxidase; ISH, in situ hybridization; PCR, polymerase chain reaction; EM, electron microscopy; SS, special histologic stains; GMS, Gomori's methenamine silver; B&B, Brown and Brenn; B-H, Brown–Hopps.

TABLE 1–2. HISTOLOGIC STAINS FOR DEMONSTRATING INFECTIOUS AGENTS

Stains	Diagnostic Applications
Routine Hematoxylin-eosin (H&E)	Best stain to demonstrate overall tissue reaction; demonstrates viral inclusion bodies, protozoans, some bacteria and fungi, and Splendore–Hoeppli material that may border certain microorganisms; needed to detect dematiaceous (naturally pigmented) fungi
Viral inclusion body stains Lendrum's phloxine-tartrazine Attwood's phloxine-tartrazine Shorr's Masson's trichrome Bosch's and Schleifstein's methods for Negri bodies, and others	No stain is superior to H&E for detecting inclusion bodies; Masson's is especially useful for staining inclusion bodies of cytomegalovirus
Silver impregnation procedures Steiner Dieterle Warthin–Starry	Blacken all bacteria; required for non-gram-reactive bacteria (eg, spirochetes, *Bartonella* spp, *Calymmatobacterium granulomatis*); useful as a sensitive screen for weakly gram-negative bacteria (eg, *Legionella* spp, *Francisella tularensis, Burkholderia pseudomallei, Helicobacter pylori*)
Modified Gram stains for bacteria Brown and Brenn (B&B) Brown–Hopps (B-H) MacCallum–Goodpasture	Differentiate most gram-positive and gram-negative bacteria, and stain the actinomycetes and microsporidians gram-positive; B-H is best for gram-negative bacteria and rickettsiae; some fungi, especially blastoconidia of *Candida* spp and conidia of *Aspergillus* spp, are gram-positive
Acid-fast stains Ziehl–Neelsen Coates–Fite Fite–Faraco Truant's auramine rhodamine	Demonstrate *Mycobacterium* spp; Truant's has the highest sensitivity and therefore is useful for screening; Coates–Fite, Fite–Faraco, or other modified procedures are required for *M leprae, Nocardia* spp, *Rhodococcus equi,* and *Legionella micdadei,* all of which are weakly acid fast and not alcohol fast; some spores of *Nosema* spp, a microsporidian, are acid fast
Fungal stains Gomori's methenamine silver (GMS) Periodic acid–Schiff (PAS) reaction Gridley fungus	Useful for detecting and studying details of all fungi; GMS is best for screening and also stains actinomycetes, the cyst walls of *Pneumocystis carinii* and free-living amebas, certain encapsulated bacteria, mycobacteria, the intracytoplasmic granular inclusions of cytomegalovirus, and the spore coat of certain microsporidians; PAS stains the cytoplasm of *Entamoeba histolytica* trophozoites, the cyst walls of soil amebas, the polar granule of most microsporidians, and mycobacteria
Mucin stains Mayer's mucicarmine Southgate's mucicarmine Alcian blue Colloidal iron	Demonstrate mucoid capsule of *Cryptococcus neoformans,* thus differentiating this pleomorphic yeast-form fungus from others of similar size and shape; may also stain cell walls of *Blastomyces dermatitidis* and *Rhinosporidium seeberi*
Melanin stains Modified Fontana–Masson	Useful for staining the cell wall of *C neoformans,* which contains melanin-like substances; accentuates and confirms the presence of melanin in weakly pigmented agents of phaeohyphomycosis
Giemsa stains May–Grünwald Wolbach's Gaffney's	Demonstrate most protozoans, bacteria, rickettsiae, and chlamydiae; trophozoites and intracystic sporozoites of *P carinii;* and the intracytoplasmic kinetoplast and nucleus of leishmanias and amastigotes of *Trypanosoma cruzi;* Wolbach's stains these organisms more intensely
Connective tissue stains Wilder's reticulum Masson's trichrome Weber's modified trichrome Russell–Movat pentachrome	Wilder's stains kinetoplast of leishmanias and amastigotes of *T cruzi;* Masson's useful for demonstrating amebas, but offers little or no advantage if organisms cannot be seen in H&E-stained sections; Weber's trichrome useful for detecting microsporidial spores; Russell–Movat pentachrome excellent for studying morphology of nematodes, cestodes, and trematodes

Monoclonal antibodies or polyclonal antisera of proven sensitivity and specificity can be used for immunofluorescence or immunoenzymatic staining of infectious agents.[2,4,5] Immunohistologic staining can confirm a presumptive diagnosis, especially when fixed tissues only are available, and can identify a pathogen in contaminated specimens. The special histologic stains listed in Table 1–2 should be used before immunohistologic staining. This usually narrows the differential diagnosis, localizes the cause, and enables the pathologist to select the most appropriate immunologic reagents. For viral infections, immunohistologic techniques help when there are no inclusion bodies or when inclusion bodies are atypical. To enhance immunostaining of viral antigens, tissue sections can be digested with a proteolytic enzyme, such as a weak trypsin or pepsin solution, to "unmask" immunoreactive sites by freeing cross-linked antigen molecules.[4] Antigen retrieval by superheating of immersed tissue sections in a microwave oven or pressure cooker can also enhance immunostaining of certain infectious agents, especially viruses.[4,6,7] Because formalin fixation and paraffin embedment usually do not affect the antigenicity of bacteria, fungi, and protozoans, enzymatic digestion and antigen retrieval of tissue sections containing these microorganisms are often not necessary before immunohistologic staining.

The PCR and ISH are now used to identify microbial genes and their transcripts.[8–11] PCR, invented by Dr. Kary Mullis in 1983, is an exquisitely sensitive technique that employs in vitro, bidirectional, enzymatic synthesis and amplification of a defined deoxyribonucleic acid (DNA) sequence by repeated, automated cycles of heat denaturation, primer annealing, and thermostable DNA polymerase-mediated primer extension.[8,9] This technique results in an exponential increase in the number of template DNA sequences, and it can be used for the detection of virtually any pathogen for which even limited DNA or ribonucleic acid (RNA) sequencing is known and in which fresh or properly fixed, paraffinized infected tissue is available. Applications of PCR in infectious disease pathology include 1) rapid detection of specific microbial nucleic acid sequences in minute quantities (typically, PCR begins with picogram quantities of template DNA and yields nanogram quantities that can then be analyzed by conventional methods); 2) detection of agents that are difficult to cultivate or are noncultivatable; 3) detection of hazardous (highly pathogenic) agents; 4) detection of latent or dormant infections; 5) strain typing (viral, bacterial, fungal, protozoal); 6) detection of virulence and antimicrobial resistance determinants; and 7) phylogenetic classification of uncultured or unknown bacteria based on sequence analysis of the 16S ribosomal gene.[12,13] Because a large number of samples can be evaluated simultaneously, PCR is useful in investigating epidemics and in experimental studies on pathogenesis. The main disadvantage of PCR is that it cannot determine tissue localization of target nucleic acids. Another disadvantage is that PCR's exquisite sensitivity may result in false-positive reactions caused by "carryover" from previously amplified DNA (amplicon) or by contamination from true-positive specimens in close proximity within the laboratory.

Although not as sensitive as PCR, ISH combines the advantages of morphologic observation with molecular information at the level of defined nucleic acid sequences in intact tissues.[5,10] ISH has proven to be particularly useful for typing of human papillomaviruses in lesions of the genital tract, and for detecting and localizing nucleic acid sequences of viruses that are difficult or impossible to culture, that produce latent infections, or that do not produce characteristic inclusion bodies in hematoxylin-eosin (H&E)-stained tissue sections.[10,14] In contrast to other hybridization techniques (eg, Southern blot and dot blot), ISH enables the pathologist to identify directly the exact cell that contains the microbial DNA or RNA of interest in either frozen or fixed, deparaffinized tissue sections. The ISH procedure can be completed within 2–6 hours and, in addition to the hybridization reaction (signal), one can readily evaluate the tissue morphology by light microscopy using conventional counterstains. The advantages of colorimetric methods to detect hybridization include speed, simplicity, localization in tissue, elimination of hazardous radioisotopes, and potential for automation.[10,15] More recently, PCR amplification of DNA target sequences in intact tissue sections followed by detection of the amplified sequences by colorimetric ISH (PCR–ISH) has further increased sensitivity and extended research applications of these technologies.[16–19]

In conclusion, most infectious diseases can be accurately and rapidly diagnosed with experience, a battery of histologic and immunohistologic stains, and, when needed, novel molecular biologic techniques, by examining fixed, routinely processed tissues that contain the etiologic agent. Whenever possible, a histopathologic diagnosis should be confirmed by other complementary approaches, especially culture and serologic studies, that enhance the skills of the pathologist.

Modified and expanded from Chandler FW. Infectious disease pathology: morphologic and molecular approaches to diagnosis. (Editorial overview). *J Histotechnol.* 1995;18:183–186.

REFERENCES

1. Watts JC. Surgical pathology and the diagnosis of infectious diseases. *Am J Clin Pathol.* 1994;102:711–712. Editorial.
2. Chandler FW. Invasive microorganisms. In: Spicer SS, ed. *Histochemistry in Pathologic Diagnosis.* New York: Marcel Dekker; 1987:77–102.
3. Prophet EB, Mills B, Arrington JB, Sobin LH. *Laboratory Methods in Histotechnology.* Washington, DC: American Registry of Pathology, Armed Forces Institute of Pathology; 1992:221–222.
4. Cartun RW. Infectious disease. In: Taylor CR, Cote RJ, eds. *Immunomicroscopy: A Diagnostic Tool for the Surgical Pathologist.* 2nd ed. Philadelphia: WB Saunders; 1994: 401–415.
5. Yolken RH. Nucleic acids or immunoglobulins: which are the molecular probes of the future? *Mol Cell Probes.* 1988;2:87–96.

6. Shi S-R, Gu J, Kalra KL, Chen T, Cote RJ, Taylor CR. Antigen retrieval technique: novel approach to immunohistochemistry on routinely processed tissue sections. *Cell Vision.* 1995;2:6–22.
7. Chan JKC. Kitchen ideas in the immunohistochemistry laboratory? *Adv Anat Pathol.* 1995;2:1. Editorial.
8. Persing DH, Smith TF, Tenover FC, White TJ. *Diagnostic Molecular Microbiology: Principles and Applications.* Washington, DC: ASM Press; 1993.
9. Ehrlich GD, Greenberg SJ. *PCR-Based Diagnostics in Infectious Disease.* Boston: Blackwell Scientific; 1994.
10. Piper MA, Unger ER. *Nucleic Acid Probes. A Primer for Pathologists.* Chicago: ASCP Press; 1989.
11. Figueroa ME, Rasheed S. Molecular pathology and diagnosis of infectious diseases. *Am J Clin Pathol.* 1991;95 (suppl 1):S8–S21.
12. Relman DA, Loutit JS, Schmidt TM, et al. The agent of bacillary angiomatosis: an approach to the identification of uncultured pathogens. *N Engl J Med.* 1990;323: 1573–1580.
13. Relman DA, Falkow S. Identification of uncultured microorganisms: expanding the spectrum of characterized microbial pathogens. *Infect Agents Dis.* 1992;1:245–253.
14. Unger ER, Chandler FW, Chenggis ML, et al. Demonstration of human immunodeficiency virus by colorimetric in situ hybridization: a rapid technique for formalin-fixed paraffin-embedded material. *Mod Pathol.* 1989;2:200–204.
15. Unger ER, Brigati DJ, Chenggis ML, et al. Automation of in situ hybridization: application of the capillary action robotic workstation. *J Histotechnol.* 1988;11:253–258.
16. Bagasra O, Hauptman SP, Lischner HW, Sachs M, Pomerantz RJ. Detection of HIV-1 provirus in mononuclear cells by in situ PCR. *N Engl J Med.* 1992;326:1385–1391.
17. Nuovo GJ. *PCR In Situ Hybridization: Protocols and Applications.* 2nd ed. New York: Raven Press; 1994.
18. Bagasra O, Pomerantz RJ. In situ PCR: applications in the pathogenesis of diseases. *Cell Vision.* 1994;1:13–16.
19. Bagasra O, Seshamma T, Hansen J, Bobroski L, Pomerantz RJ. Application of in situ PCR methods in molecular biology: I. Details of methodology for general use. *Cell Vision.* 1994;1:324–335.

CHAPTER 2

Electron Microscopy in the Diagnosis of Infectious Diseases

Claire M. Payne

For most diagnoses all that is needed is an ounce of knowledge, an ounce of intelligence, and a pound of thoroughness!

Anonymous

Electron microscopy (EM) is an invaluable tool for studying the life cycle of infectious organisms and their specific cytopathic effects, and for understanding the pathogenesis of the infections they cause. The role of EM in detecting and identifying microbes, although well documented in the literature,[1–11] has been overshadowed by the development of other useful diagnostic techniques, such as cell culture, special stains, immunoassays, in situ hybridization, and polymerase chain reaction (PCR). There are, however, situations in which these other techniques cannot be used. For example, cell culture methods cannot be used if the infectious agents are fastidious (eg, gastrointestinal viruses), or if they are newly discovered pathogens and their in vitro culture conditions are not yet known (eg, outbreaks caused by previously undiscovered infectious agents). The histologic features of the microbe may not be pathognomonic by light microscopy, because the number of organisms may be sparse, the organisms may be partially degenerated (eg, the bacilli of Whipple's disease), they may be in unusual sites, or they may be obscured by other organisms. Special stains may be equivocal, especially if a biopsy submitted for diagnosis has been placed in a fixative whose components interfere with the chemistry of the staining reaction. Immunoassays, which rely on specific microbial antigens for detection, may be too specific and not detect microbial variants. In situ hybridization and PCR rely on the knowledge of characteristic gene sequences, which may not be known for some organisms. EM, however, is open-ended and is the best catchall technique that does not rely on any *a priori* suspicions of the possible etiologic agent. In addition to a diagnostic role, transmission EM may be valuable for proper therapy and prognosis and in avoiding additional and unnecessary invasive procedures for clinical workup, especially in neonates.

This chapter provides an overview of the instances in which EM is most helpful in the specific diagnosis of infectious diseases. An understanding of the ultrastructural and diagnostic features of certain viruses, bacteria, fungi, and protozoa, and their clinical settings, can have a significant impact on patient care. The myth that EM is no longer cost effective is dismantled by the end of this chapter. We discuss the critical role that pathologists have in assisting primary care physicians toward obtaining the most reliable and definitive diagnostic procedure for their patients.

VIRUSES

Viruses are below the resolution of the light microscope, so EM is especially useful in their identification. Because the diameter of most viruses is less than 0.1 μm, they can be most effectively seen in whole-mount, negatively contrasted (eg, phosphotungstic acid or ammonium molybdate) preparations.[12,13] In addition, most of the larger pathogenic viruses that infect humans, have characteristic surface features, so the whole-mount procedure can be definitive.[9,13]

Some viruses can also be readily characterized in epoxy-embedded, thin-sectioned tissue preparations, where characteristic ultrastructural features are used for identification. Evaluation of thin sections for viral particles should, however, only be left to the expert. Many cell organelles and inclusions have been misidentified as viral particles. These include nuclear pores, annulate lamellae, neurosecretory granules, coated vesicles, intrachromatinic granules, interchromatinic granules, vermicellar bodies, altered chromatin fibers, Cowdry type B inclusion bodies (accessory nucleoli), aggregates of glycogen particles or ribosomes, tubulovesicular structures (undulations of the endoplasmic reticulum), hemidesmosomes budding from the plasma membrane, multivesicular bodies, R-bodies and glycocalyceal bodies of the intestine, and Odland bodies of skin.

Several important virus groups are illustrated in this chapter and represent a cross-section of the clinical situations in which EM plays an important role in diagnosis.

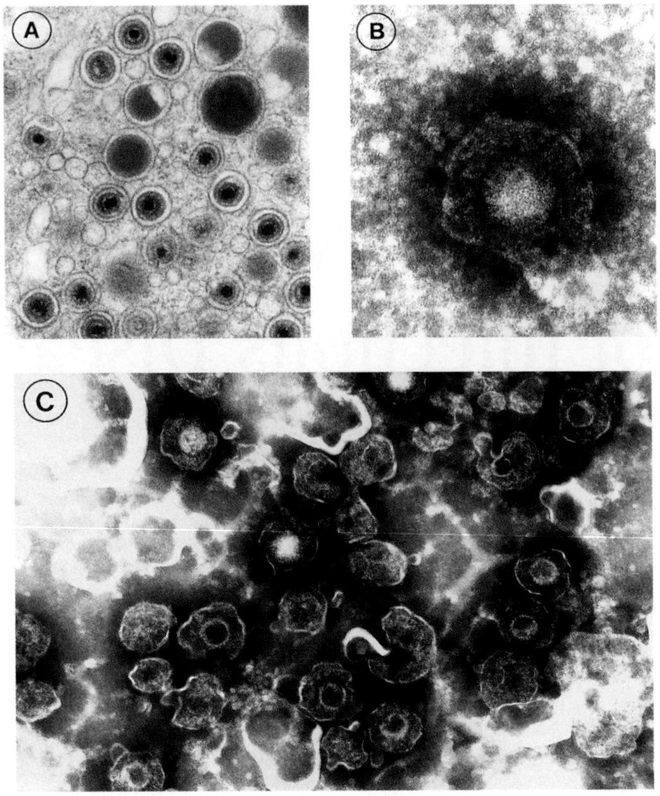

Figure 2–1. Electron micrographs of members of the herpesvirus group. (**A**) Intracytoplasmic cytomegaloviruses in a thin section of epoxy-embedded tissue. The viruses are contained within the cisternae of the endoplasmic reticulum. The electron-dense "nucleoid" is readily apparent (uranyl acetate, lead citrate counterstain). *(Photograph courtesy of Dr. Jan Orenstein, George Washington University Medical Center.)* (**B**) High-power electron micrograph of a herpes simplex virus negatively contrasted with phosphotungstic acid. The viral particle is enveloped in a host-derived membrane (whole-mount preparation, phosphotungstic acid stain). (**C**) Low-power electron micrograph of negatively contrasted herpesviruses obtained from the vesicle fluid of an immunodeficient patient. Note the high concentration of particles present in the vesicle fluid (whole-mount preparation, phosphotungstic acid stain).

Herpesviruses

The herpesvirus group includes herpes simplex virus type 1, herpes simplex virus type 2, varicella-zoster, cytomegalovirus (CMV), and Epstein–Barr virus. All members of the herpesvirus group have the same ultrastructural appearance by thin section (Figure 2–1, A) and negative contrast (Figure 2–1, B and C). The icosahedral nucleocapsid of the herpes virion measures 100 nm in diameter[9] and is enclosed within a complex envelope[14] derived from host cell membranes. The enveloped particles average 165 nm in diameter.[2] CMV can form both nuclear and cytoplasmic inclusions (Figure 2–1, A), whereas all of the other human herpesviruses form only intranuclear inclusions. Among the herpesviruses, the intracytoplasmic inclusion of CMV is the only one seen by light microscopy. The light microscopic appearance is due to collections of enveloped virions and excess envelope material. The large aggregates of herpesviruses within the nucleus are the ultrastructural counterpart to the Cowdry type A inclusion seen by light microscopy.[15] In the absence of large numbers of particles, Cowdry type A inclusions may be rare or absent,[16] and EM may offer a diagnosis of a herpesvirus. Antiviral drugs are most effective when given promptly.[17,18] For example, CMV from urine may take from 4 to 70 days to grow in tissue culture, whereas the diagnosis can be made within 4 hours by EM.[19,20]

Immunoelectron microscopy has been used to diagnose varicella-zoster virus rapidly in a complicated case of human infection by the T-cell lymphotropic virus type 1.[20] This directly influenced therapy, since the dose of acyclovir administered for varicella-zoster infection is twice that for herpes simplex virus infection.[21]

Neonatal herpesvirus infection is a severe and often fatal disease of newborns. Thousands of babies are born every day in the United States to women with genital herpes.[22] The infection is acquired most commonly during passage through the birth canal.[23] If the mother is in labor and has genital vesicles, EM of the vesicle fluid can render a diagnosis within 1 hour using the whole-mount, negative-contrast technique. This is possible because the number of easily identified herpesviruses in vesicle fluid is very high[9] (Figure 2–1, C). The physician may elect to perform a cesarean section, rather than risk the possibility of neonatal herpes infection.

Adenovirus

The diagnosis of adenovirus infection may be difficult by light microscopy because of the smudged nuclear changes that are in routine histopathologic sections.[1] In patients with acquired immunodeficiency syndrome (AIDS), adenovirus infection of the colorectum can be mistaken for CMV infection,[24] since adenovirus is an uncommon cause of intestinal illness in healthy, immunocompetent adults. If appropriate viral cultures have not been done, EM can show the characteristic features of the adenovirus group (Figure 2–2). Intranuclear aggregates of hexagonal adenovirus particles (60 to 70 nm in diameter) are readily observed in thin sections; some particles are arranged in paracrystalline or lattice arrays (Figure 2–2, A and B). Adenovirus should be considered in the differential diagnosis of chronic diarrhea in AIDS patients[24] and in viral gastroenteritis of infants and children.[5] The viral agents of gastroenteritis are discussed later.

The observation of adenoviruses using the whole-mount, negative-contrast preparation best illustrates the icosahedral structure on which virus geometry is based (Figure 2–2, C). Because adenoviruses have more capsomeres than herpesviruses (252 versus 162 capsomeres), the triangular facets of the 20-sided virion are more conspicuous than are those of herpesviruses [compare Figure 2–1, B (herpesvirus) with Figure 2–2, C (adenovirus)].

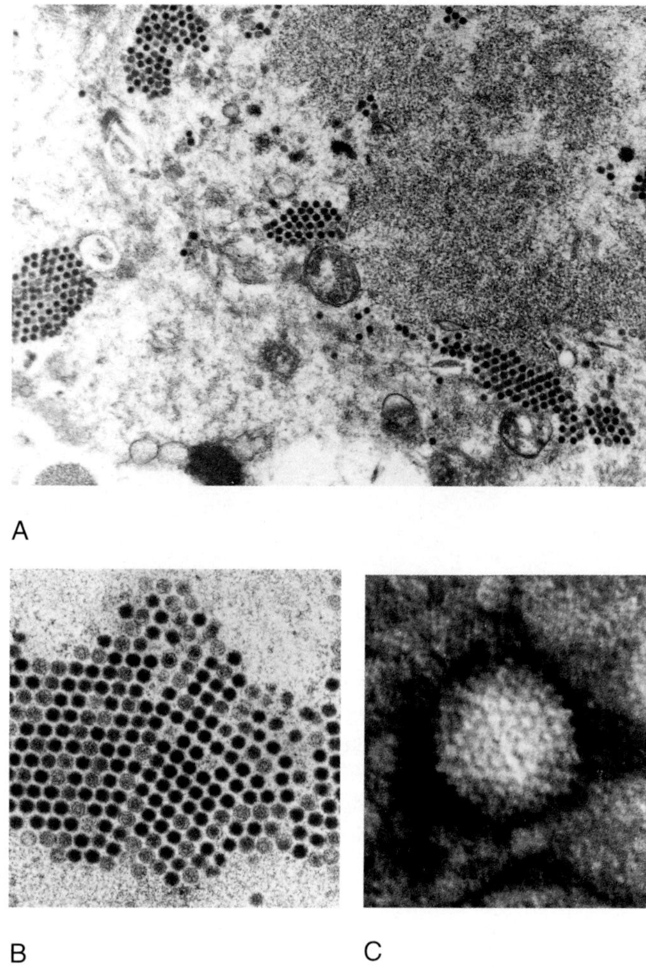

Figure 2–2. Electron micrographs of adenoviruses. (**A**) Adenoviruses in an epithelial cell from a patient with pneumonia. The cell is degenerating as evidenced by the breakdown of the nuclear envelope, loss of electron density of the chromatin, and cytoplasmic swelling. The nonenveloped adenoviruses can be seen to form paracrystalline or lattice arrays (thin section of epoxy-embedded tissue; uranyl acetate, lead citrate counterstain). *(Photograph courtesy of Dr. Francis W. Chandler, Medical College of Georgia.)* (**B**) Higher magnification of a paracrystalline array of adenoviruses (thin section of epoxy-embedded tissue; uranyl acetate, lead citrate). *(Photograph courtesy of Dr. Jan Orenstein, George Washington University Medical Center.)* (**C**) High magnification of an adenovirus negatively contrasted with phosphotungstic acid. Two of the 20 triangles that make up the facets of an icosahedron are readily seen. A single vertex capsomere (penton) is shared by five of the triangular facets. One side of each triangle is formed by one penton and five nonvertex capsomeres (hexons) (whole-mount preparation, phosphotungstic acid stain).

Papovavirus

This group includes the papillomaviruses, polyomaviruses, and vacuolating viruses, which range from 45 to 55 nm in diameter.[2] The papillomaviruses are large (55 nm) and cause warts. The polyoma–vacuolating viruses are smaller (45 nm) and cause systemic infections.[25] Although these DNA-containing particles have icosahedral symmetry, they contain only 72 capsomeres and, therefore, appear spherical (Figure 2–3, A). The capsomeres of the papovaviruses can be resolved in negatively contrasted preparations (Figure 2–3, B); however, they do not form straight rows and appear to be more randomly arranged when compared with adenovirus (Figure 2–2, C).

The two recognized human polyomaviruses are the JC virus and the BK virus. The JC virus causes progressive multifocal leukoencephalopathy[25–27] and the BK virus is associated with hemorrhagic cystitis in both immunodeficient[28] and immunocompetent[29] patients. Although kidney is a reservoir for latent papovavirus infection,[7] infection of renal tubular cells can be confused with infections by adenovirus and cytomegalovirus.[7] EM has proven most helpful in distinguishing papovavirus (Figure 2–3) from adenovirus (Figure 2–2) and herpesviruses (Figure 2–1).

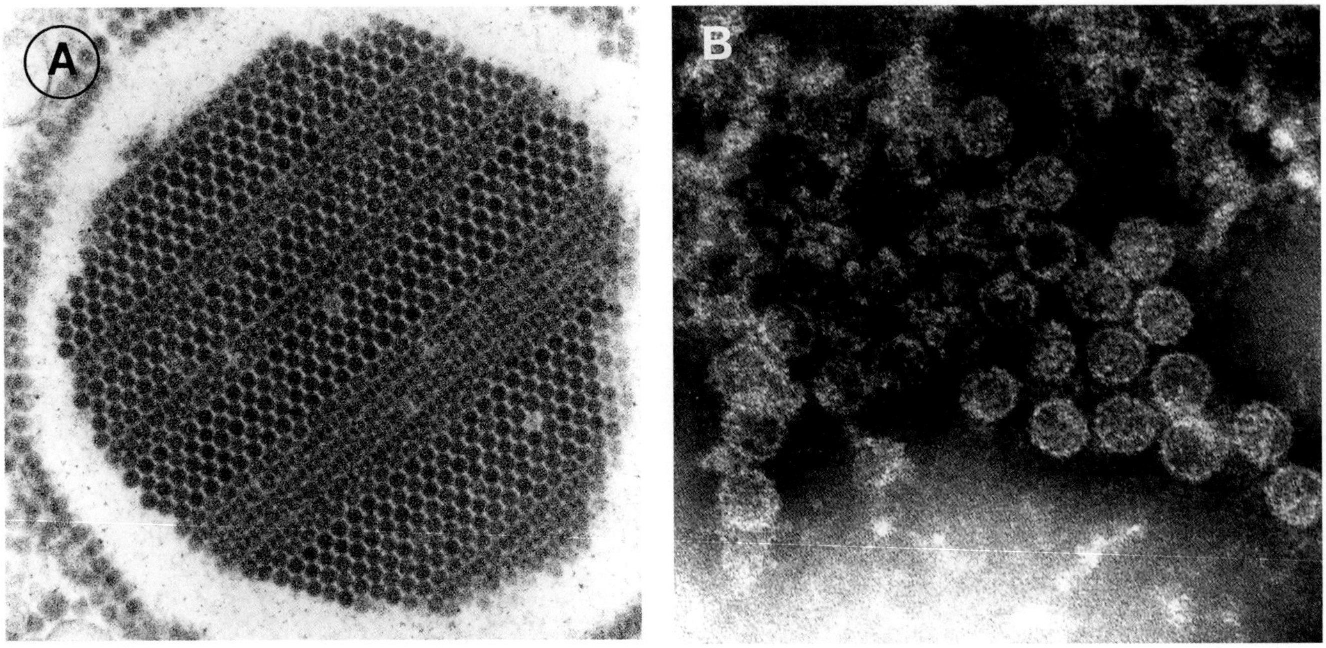

Figure 2–3. Electron micrographs of papovaviruses. (**A**) Pseudocrystalline array of spherical papovaviruses within cellular debris in the lumen of a renal tubule of a patient with AIDS and tubulointerstitial nephritis (autopsy material) (thin section of epoxy-embedded tissue; uranyl acetate, lead citrate counterstain). *(Reprinted by permission of the publisher from Orenstein JM. Ultrastructural pathology of human immunodeficiency virus infection. In:* Ultrastructural Pathology. *United Kingdom: Francis & Taylor Publishers; 1992;16:179–209.)* (**B**) Higher magnification of papovaviruses negatively contrasted with phosphotungstic acid. Note the circular appearance of the virions (whole-mount preparation, phosphotungstic acid stain).

Poxvirus

These DNA-containing viruses are large, oval and/or brick-shaped (Figure 2–4, A), and have a thread- or rope-like surface characteristic (Figure 2–4, B).[2,3] They are 140 to 260 nm wide and 220 to 450 nm long.[2] In thin sections, the poxviruses have a core, which appears as a cross-section of a flattened tube, and two opposing dense, oval, lateral bodies adjacent to the core (Figure 2–4, A).[2] EM was used many years ago to distinguish smallpox and chickenpox.[30,31] The large size and characteristic shape of the smallpox virus is easily distinguished from the smaller herpesvirus using the rapid whole-mount, negative-contrast technique. Although smallpox is no longer a threat, EM still provides a rapid diagnosis on vesicle fluid or skin scrapings obtained from patients infected with the vaccinia virus, *molluscum contagiosum* virus, paravaccinia virus (Milker's nodules), and the orf virus (contagious pustular dermatitis).[2]

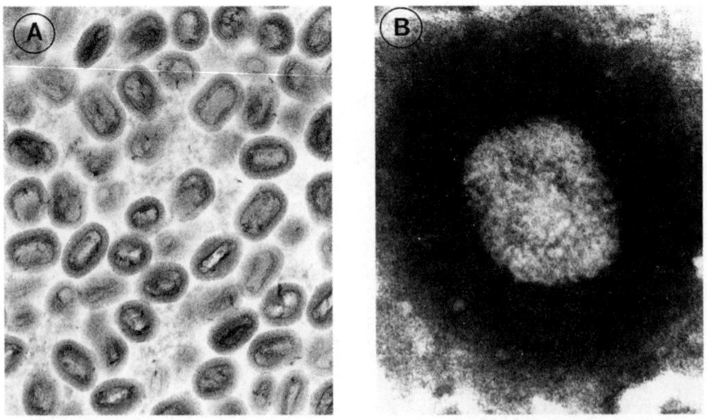

Figure 2–4. Electron micrographs of poxviruses. (**A**) Typical brick-shaped membrane-bound virions of molluscum contagiosum in a cytoplasmic vacuole of a squamous epithelial cell (thin section of epoxy-embedded tissue; uranyl acetate, lead citrate counterstain). *(Photograph courtesy of Dr. Jan Orenstein, George Washington University Medical Center.)* (**B**) High magnification of a brick-shaped poxvirus showing the threadlike surface appearance (whole-mount preparation, phosphotungstic acid stain).

Viral Agents of Gastroenteritis

Infectious diarrhea is a major cause of infant mortality in underdeveloped areas of the world and results in 5 to 18 million deaths annually.[6,32,33] Although it has

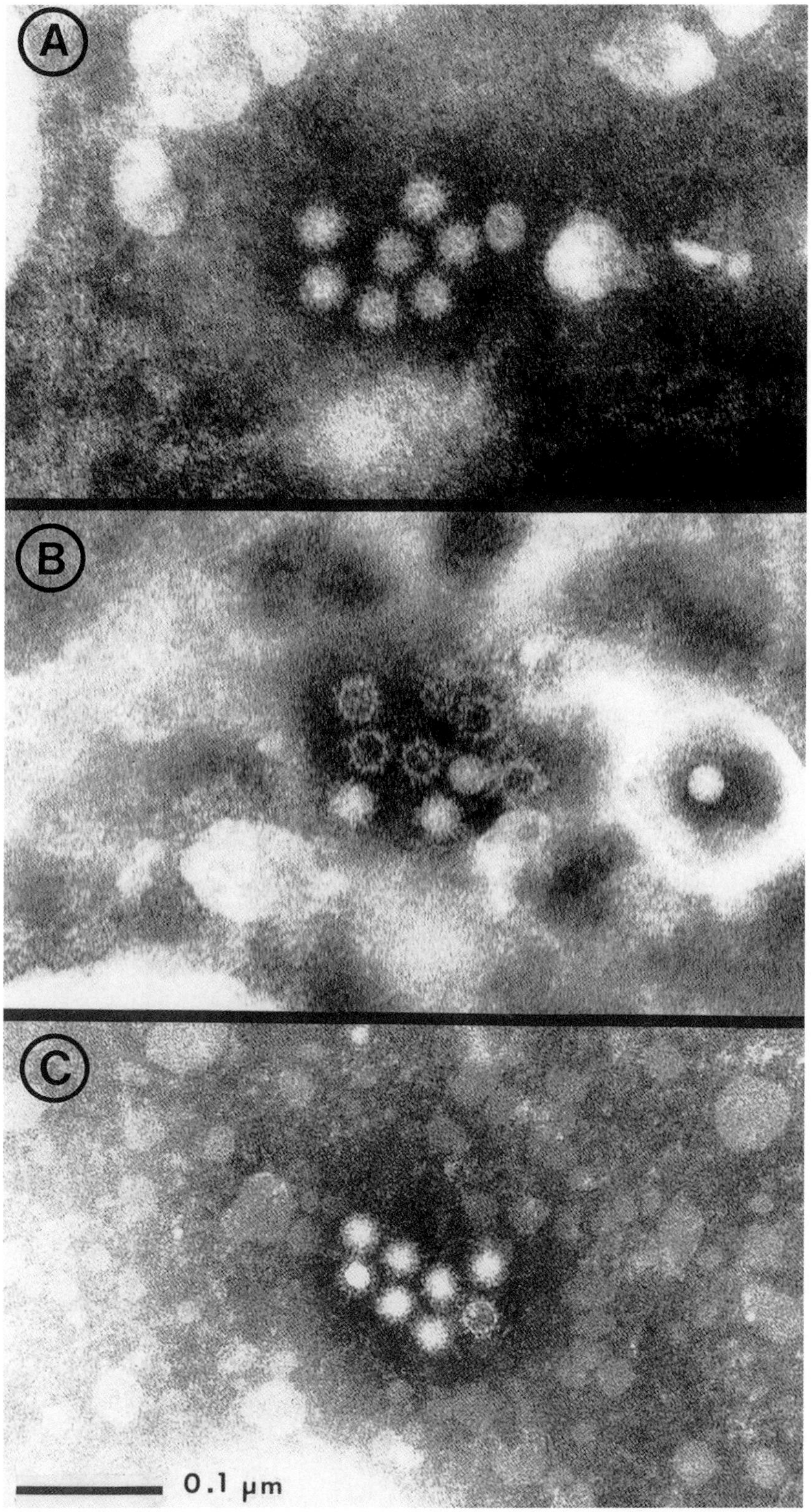

Figure 2–5. High-power electron micrographs of Norwalk-like agents photographed from stool specimens of three different patients with gastroenteritis. These small, round structured viruses all have spikelike projections, resulting in a feathery or fuzzy appearance typical of the Norwalk agent. The mean diameters of the viruses from the different stool specimens are different; the largest is in (**A**), the smallest in (**C**), and an intermediate diameter in (**B**) (whole-mount preparations, phosphotungstic acid stain).

been generally assumed that fatal diarrhea is restricted to developing countries, as many as 500 deaths per year occur in the United States.[8] Bacterial[34] and parasitic[35] pathogens together cause less than 50% of pediatric diarrheas.[36] In 1931, McLean first suspected a viral cause of nonbacterial gastroenteritis because of the seasonal incidence.[37] In 1947, Gordon et al[38] successfully transmitted epidemic gastroenteritis to human volunteers by oral administration of fecal filtrates. Although these studies implicated viruses, numerous attempts to grow the presumed viral pathogens using conventional cell and organ culture techniques were largely unsuccessful.[39] In 1972, however, Kapikian et al,[40] using immunoelectron microscopy, saw viral particles 27 nm in diameter that caused an outbreak of acute gastroenteritis in school children in Norwalk, Ohio. The Norwalk agent is a common cause of epidemics of diarrhea associated with contaminated drinking water and the consumption of raw oysters. Representative Norwalk-like agents are shown in Figure 2–5, A–C. The Norwalk-like agent has no distinctive pattern of capsomeres, but the tiny spikelike projections on the surface are characteristic.

Rotavirus is the most commonly diagnosed viral agent of acute gastroenteritis in childhood, accounting annually for an estimated 140 million infections, 1 million deaths in young children, and most hospital admissions for diarrhea in children under the age of 2.[6] Although children from 6 to 24 months of age are most commonly infected, younger infants can be affected[8] as can adults.[5,41] The classic rotavirus is 65 to 70 nm in diameter and has a characteristic wheellike appearance with "spokes" and surface "holes" created by a circular arrangement of capsomeres (Figure 2–6).

The viral agents of gastroenteritis are fastidious and cannot be grown routinely in tissue culture. EM remains the single most effective laboratory technique available to detect the diverse viral pathogens that cause gastroenteritis in humans.[42] Viral diarrhea is now well recognized, and numerous reviews and overviews of the ultrastructural findings have been published.[5,8,42–46] At least seven morphologically distinct viral or viral-like agents can be identified and include viruses based on icosahedral symmetry[45,47] (Figure 2–7, A–F) and the pleomorphic coronavirus-like or torovirus-like particles with a distinct surface fringe (Figures 2–8, 2–9, and 2–10). The small, round, featureless viruses belonging to the pico/parvovirus group are not believed to cause viral gastroenteritis in humans.

Immunoelectron microscopy has been used to aggregate viruses to increase the sensitivity of detection.[48] In one study in Arizona,[47] a large population of 30- to 54-nm particles, which resembled single-shelled rotaviruses by EM, were found in certain stool specimens. Single-shelled or "rough" rotavirus particles in

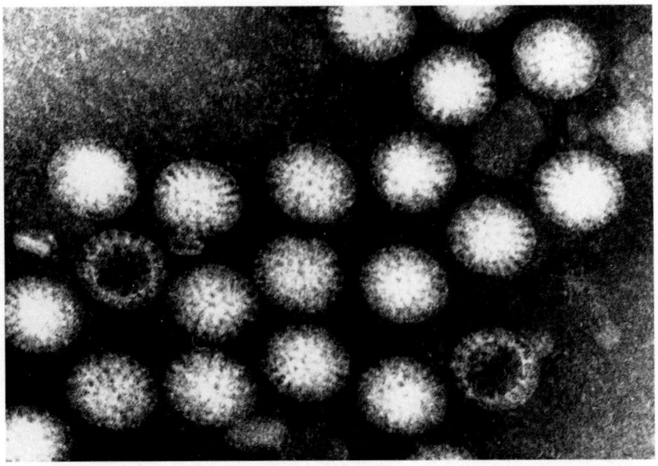

Figure 2–6. High-power electron micrograph of rotaviruses in a stool specimen of a child with gastroenteritis. The arrangement of the capsomeres resembles the spokes of a wheel, hence, the name "rotavirus" (Greek derivation: *rota* or "wheellike"). The particles shown here are double-shelled; the "rim" of the wheel is formed by the second shell, giving the particles a smooth appearance (whole-mount preparation, phosphotungstic acid stain).

the absence of the double-shelled "smooth" particles had not been previously described. Immunoelectron microscopy, using an antibody against human rotavirus, indicated that they were rotaviruses and not some other unidentified viral pathogen.

The exact classification and significance of the coronavirus-like[49,50] or torovirus-like particles[51,52] are still under investigation. It is clear that the pleomorphic fringed particles (Figure 2–8, A and B) are morphologically very different from classic respiratory coronaviruses, and bear a resemblance to the Berne virus of horses and the Breda virus of calves.[52] The Berne and Breda viruses are members of the torovirus group. The torovirus-like particles associated with diarrhea may be members of the coronavirus-like superfamily,[53,54] whose concept is based on evolution and phylogeny. Although some investigators believe these fringed particles to be nonspecific membranes, there are reasons to indicate that they are not nonspecific membranes simply shed into the stool: 1) naturally occurring "immune"-like aggregates can be seen in stools obtained from patients with either chronic diarrhea or during a period of convalescence (Figure 2–8, C); 2) the membranes of the particles tend to collapse onto the grid surface (Figure 2–9, A) and are not refractile, like that of nonspecific membranes (Figure 2–9, B); 3) they occur in large numbers in some samples to the exclusion of other debris usually found in stool (Figure 2–9, A); 4) there are budding forms; and 5) isolated particles from a patient with acute diarrhea are aggregated by convalescent serum from the same patient (Figure 2–10, A–C).

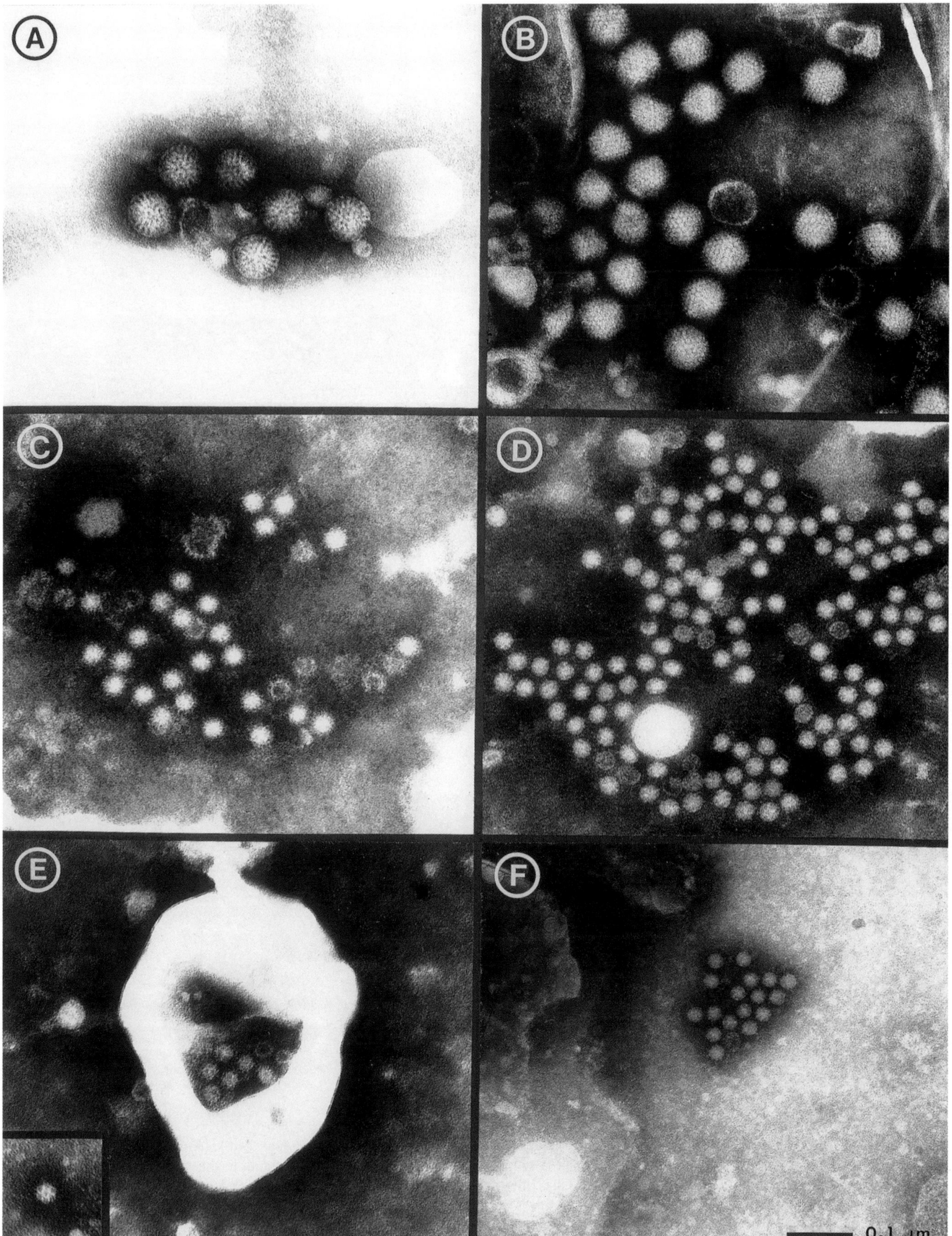

Figure 2–7. Composite of electron micrographs of enteric viruses displaying cubic symmetry (whole-mount preparation, phosphotungstic acid): (**A**) double-shelled rotavirus, (**B**) adenovirus, (**C**) Norwalk-like agent, (**D**) astrovirus, (**E**) calicivirus, and (**F**) picorna/parvovirus. *(Reprinted by permission of the publisher from Payne CM et al. An eight-year study of the viral agents of acute gastroenteritis in humans: ultrastructural observations and seasonal distribution with a major emphasis on coronavirus-like particles.* Diagn Microbiol Infect Dis. *1986;5:39–54.)*

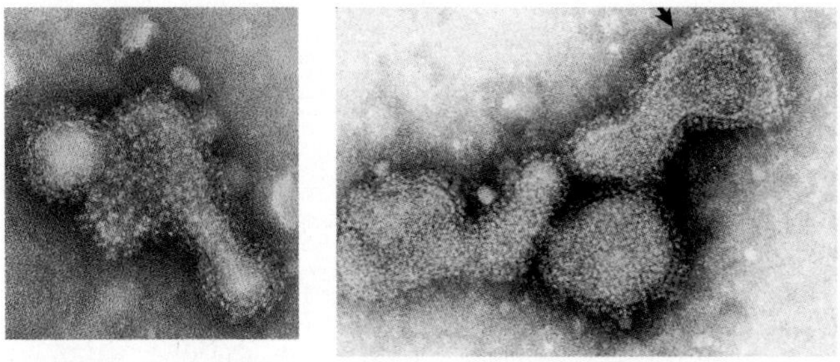

A B

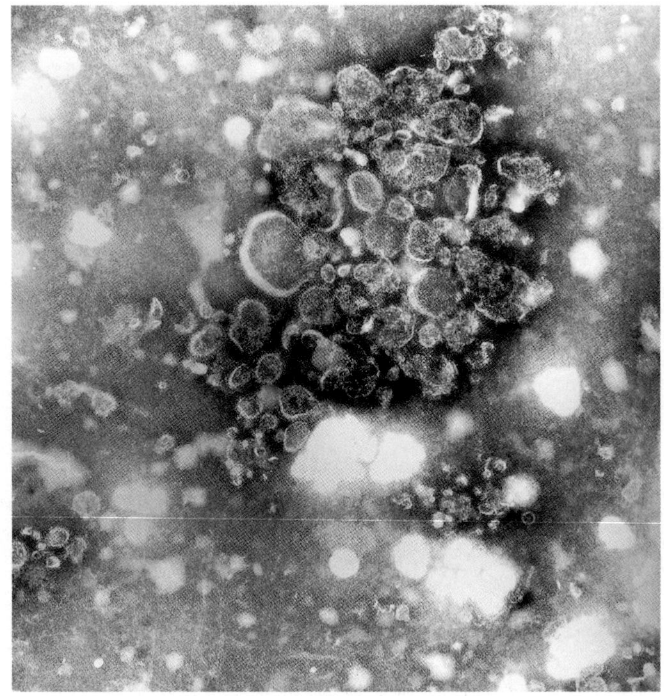

C

Figure 2–8. Electron micrographs of corona/torovirus-like particles in stool specimens of children with gastroenteritis (whole-mount preparations, phosphotungstic acid). (**A**) High magnification of a corona/torovirus-like particle. Note the irregular shape, thick fringe, and lack of penetration of stain into the particle's interior. *(Reprinted by permission of the publisher from Mortensen ML et al. Coronavirus-like particles in human gastrointestinal disease. Epidemiologic, clinical, and laboratory observations.* AJDC. *1985;139:928–934.)* (**B**) High magnification of a cluster of three corona/torovirus-like particles. One particle has a distinct electron-dense area *(arrow),* common in these particles. Whether this is pooling of the stain or the nucleic acid of the particle is not known. (**C**) Aggregates of pleomorphic, fringed particles in the stool of patients with chronic diarrhea. This may indicate a host immune response. *(B and C, reprinted by permission of the publisher from Payne CM et al. An eight-year study of the viral agents of acute gastroenteritis in humans: ultrastructural observations and seasonal distribution with a major emphasis on coronavirus-like particles.* Diagn Microbiol Infect Dis. *1986;5:39–54.)*

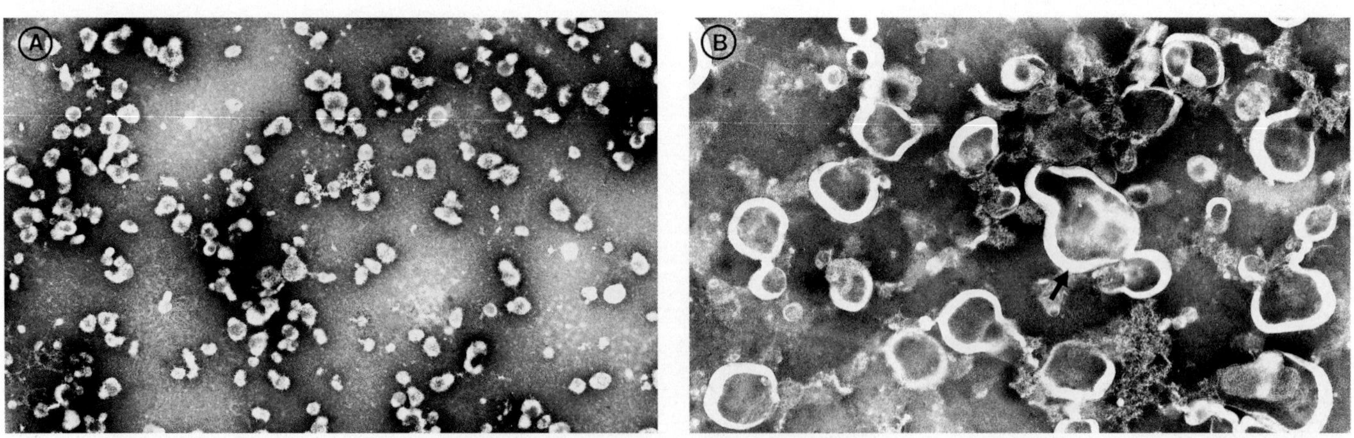

Figure 2–9. Low-power electron micrographs comparing a stool specimen containing a large number of corona/torovirus-like particles with nonspecific membranes (whole-mount preparation, phosphotungstic acid stain). (**A**) Corona/torovirus-like particles in the stool from a patient with gastroenteritis. The particles appear to collapse onto the surface of the grid, and a distinct "nucleoid" is in most of the particles. Note the absence of flagella and other debris common in stool specimens. (**B**) Nonspecific membrane profiles present in a stool specimen submitted for diagnosis. The membranes are elevated in part from the grid surface giving the profiles a refractile appearance *(arrow)* by electron microscopy. *(A and B, reprinted by permission of the publisher from Payne CM et al. An eight-year study of the viral agents of acute gastroenteritis in humans: ultrastructural observations and seasonal distributions with a major emphasis on coronavirus-like particles.* Diagn Microbiol Infect Dis. *1986;5:39–54.)*

EM proved invaluable in the identification of torovirus-like particles in the stools of symptomatic infants during an outbreak of gastrointestinal illness in a neonatal intensive care unit in 1979 in Tucson[55] and in 1994 in Phoenix. Because of its catchall nature, EM remains the method of choice for the diagnosis of viral gastroenteritis.

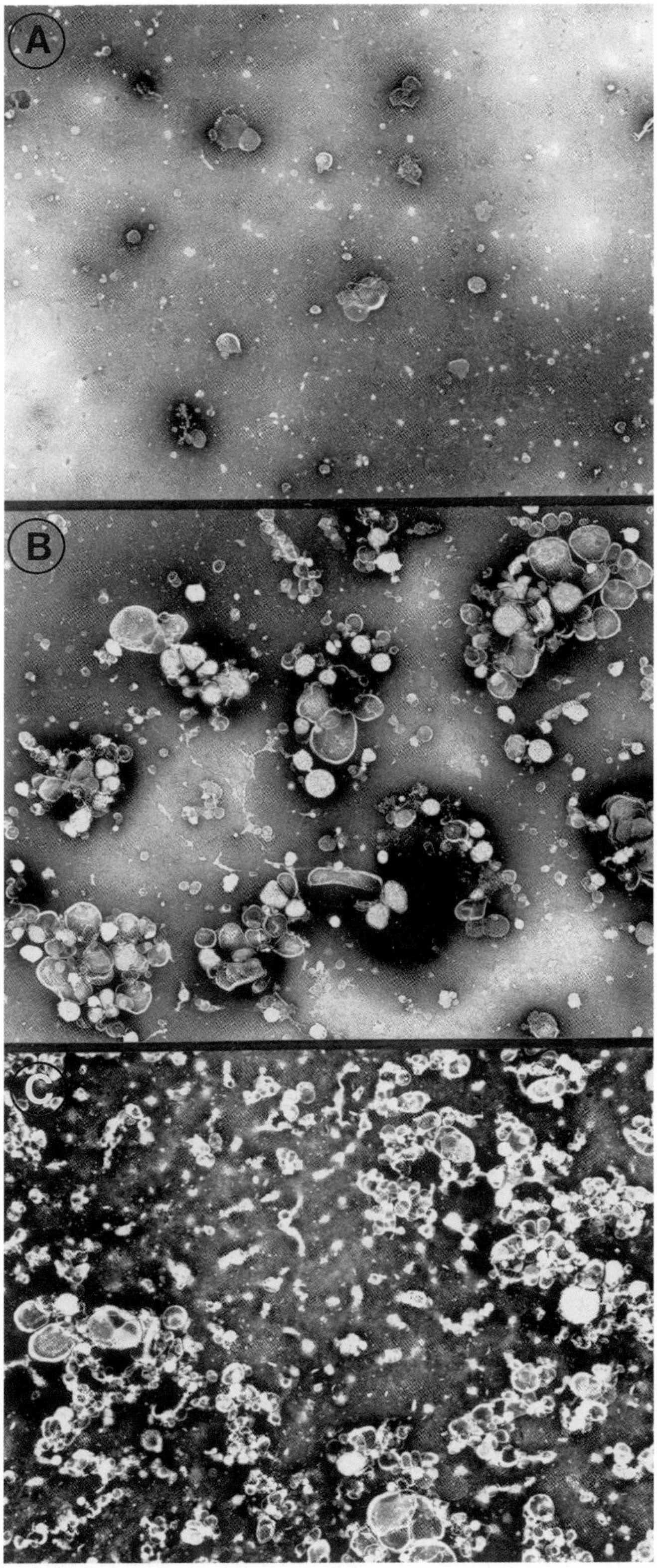

Figure 2–10. Immune electron micrographs of pleomorphic, enveloped, virus-like particles in stool obtained from an infant during an outbreak of gastrointestinal illness in a neonatal intensive care unit. The stool specimen was diluted 1 : 1 with 0.22% bovine serum albumin (**A**), mixed with a 1 : 8 dilution of convalescent-phase serum (day 25 after onset) from a symptomatic infant (**B**) and mixed 1 : 1 with undiluted convalescent-phase serum from the same symptomatic infant as in (**B**). Very little aggregation of viral particles is evident in (**A**), numerous small and large aggregates are in (**B**), and many more are in (**C**). *(Reprinted by permission of the publisher from Vaucher YE et al. Pleomorphic, enveloped, virus-like particles associated with gastrointestinal illness in neonates.* J Infect Dis. *1982;145:27–36.)*

Human Immunodeficiency Virus

In the spring of 1981, the Centers for Disease Control and Prevention (CDC) in Atlanta, Georgia, began to receive reports of Kaposi's sarcoma, *Pneumocystis carinii* pneumonia, and other opportunistic infections in homosexual men.[56] At first called gay-related immunodeficiency (GRID), CDC subsequently named the new disease acquired immunodeficiency syndrome (AIDS) and issued a working definition to be used in epidemiologic surveillance and clinical diagnosis. AIDS was characterized by Kaposi's sarcoma and/or life-threatening opportunistic infections in patients (<60 years old) for whom there was no recognized underlying cause for the immune deficiency.[56,57] The severity of the infection contrasted with the patient's prior appearance of good health.[58] Intense research during the next 2 years implicated the human immunodeficiency virus (HIV), a member of the family of T-cell lymphotropic retroviruses.

There is evidence that an immunosuppressive retrovirus existed in the United States before the late 1970s.[59–61] A 15-year-old, sexually active black male was admitted to St. Louis City Hospital in 1968 for extensive lymphedema of penis, scrotum, and lower limbs.[59] He had no history of travel outside of the Midwest, intravenous drug use, or blood transfusion. Over a 16-month clinical course his condition deteriorated and at autopsy there was widespread Kaposi's sarcoma of the aggressive, disseminated type. Western blots and antigen capture assays on serum and autopsy specimens frozen since 1969 disclosed that this teenager was infected with a virus closely related or identical to HIV type 1.[61]

Ultrastructural studies played an important role in AIDS research and helped to determine that HIV is a

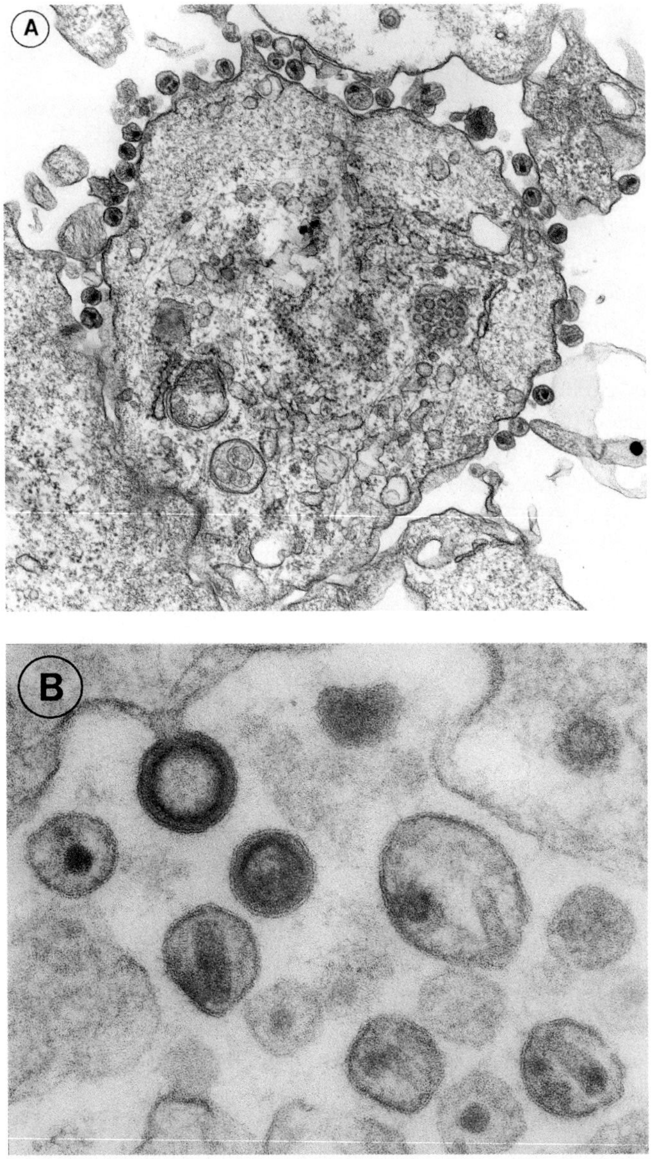

Figure 2–11. Electron micrographs of human immunodeficiency virus (HIV) (uranyl acetate, lead citrate counterstain). (**A**) HIV-1 particles, 100 to 130 nm in diameter, in culture of human peripheral blood mononuclear cells. Note the electron-dense truncated core within each viral particle. *(Photograph courtesy of Dr. Francis W. Chandler, Medical College of Georgia.)* (**B**) HIV particles in varying stages of morphogenesis in an intracytoplasmic vacuole in a macrophage infected with HIV in vitro. A late budding form, an apparently completed immature ring-shaped virion, a mature particle with its nucleoid cut in cross-section, and an aberrant particle can be seen. *(Reprinted by permission of the publisher from Orenstein JM. Ultrastructural pathology of human immunodeficiency virus infection. In:* Ultrastructural Pathology. *United Kingdom: Francis & Taylor Publishers; 1992;16:179–210.)*

member of the lentivirus family of retroviruses[62] (Figure 2–11, A). The initial search for the cause of AIDS in lymph nodes, lung, and peripheral blood samples was confounded by the fact that mononuclear cells, the harbingers of the replicating HIV particles, were few.[7] The visual identification of HIV was made in vitro after exposing cultured lymphocytes to the peripheral blood of AIDS patients[63] or lymph node tissue from a pre-AIDS patient.[64] The greatest number of HIV particles are in brain biopsy and autopsy specimens from patients with AIDS dementia complex, and autopsy specimens of spinal cord from patients with vacuolar myelopathy.[7] Care must be taken in the ultrastructural identification of HIV in patient specimens, so as not to confuse the particles with normal cellular structures or related retroviruses, such as human T lymphotropic virus type I (HTLV-I) and C-type particles.[7] It is most helpful to actually see the HIV particles in the process of budding (Figure 2–11, B), the *de novo* formation at the plasma membrane being characteristic of the lentiviruses.[7]

In addition to the identification of HIV, many other infectious agents have been detected in the tissues of AIDS patients. Knowledge of where EM can be most helpful in the identification of nonviral pathogens is addressed in the remainder of this chapter.

PARASITES OF THE SUBKINGDOM PROTOZOA

The prevalence of human parasitic diseases remains high throughout the world and claims more lives than do all the malignant neoplasms combined.[11] Parasites are members of two subkingdoms, the Protozoa (unicellular organisms) and the Metazoa (multicellular organisms including worms and insects). EM is most useful in the diagnosis of protozoan infections. Specific members of the subkingdom Protozoa may be underdiagnosed or misdiagnosed by light microscopy because of the following: The protozoans may appear as cellular debris,[11,65] they may be confused with leukocytes,[11] or the histologic features may not be pathognomonic. Occasionally, mucin droplets adhering to the microvillous surface of mucosal cells may resemble certain protozoans.[7] Although antisera for immunofluorescence and serologic studies are often used to diagnose parasitic infections, these tests are of little value in immunodeficient patients. The importance of EM in the diagnosis of some representative protozoans is discussed next.

Toxoplasma

The fine structure of the tachyzoites of this coccidial protozoan can be used to place the organism in the class Sporozoa. The organelles associated with host cell penetration,[65,66] such as the polar ring, conoid, rhoptries, and micronemes, are diagnostic of the group and have been reported in several patients with toxoplasmosis in which EM was essential for diagnosis.[67–70] In one case, more detailed ultrastructural examination demonstrated the method of multiplication, size (length and width of organisms at different stages), number of micronemes, and structure and location of the rhoptries, which enabled *Toxoplasma gondii* to be differentiated from closely related genera such as *Besnoitia, Sarcocystis,* and *Frenkelia.*[68] The unique combination of ultrastructural features of *Toxoplasma*—3 × 2 μm in size, few micronemes, nine rhoptries, an apical conoid, and a method of multiplication by endodyogeny (an internal budding process)—allowed for precise identification. A rapid and precise diagnosis of *Toxoplasma* encephalitis in a Haitian man with AIDS 24 hours after surgery allowed prompt treatment with pyrimethamine and sulfadiazine, and marked improvement neurologically within a week.[69]

Cryptosporidia

Cryptosporidia are coccidian protozoa of the class Sporozoa and undergo their complete life cycle in the intestine (Figures 2–12 and 2–13), although they may be in other sites.[71] Cryptosporidial infection has been described in more than 50 countries spanning six continents and involves both immunodeficient[72,73] and immunocompetent hosts. Like *Toxoplasma,* the trophozoites have a nucleus, mitochondria and endoplasmic reticulum, rhoptries, and micronemes, but contain a polar ring of microtubules instead of polar conoids.[71] Locomotion is thought to be accomplished by a form of flexing or gliding. Cryptosporidial organisms can be missed by light microscopy. The parasites are usually attached to the microvillous brush border of the epithelial cells. All stages in the development of the organism can be seen by EM in biopsy specimens (Figures 2–12 and 2–13).[11] The trophozoite (1.5 to 6.0 μm in diameter) takes up a pseudoexternal position. Although the trophozoite protrudes from the mucosal surface and appears to be externalized, EM clearly shows that it is in an intracellular parasitophorous vacuole[71,74] (Figures 2–12, A and B, and 2–13, A). The mature trophozoite undergoes schizogony (an asexual multiple budding process) producing eight merozoites and the mature schizont then releases the merozoites into the intestinal lumen (Figure 2–13, B). Merozoites then invade other epithelial cells and subsequently develop into trophozoites.[71]

Transmission EM has also been instrumental in correcting misdiagnoses of cryptosporidia.[7] Mucin droplets can adhere to the microvillous surface of the intestinal mucosal cells.[7] By light microscopy, therefore, attached mucin droplets may resemble cryptosporidia, which are in a similar location.[7]

Cyclospora

A newly identified intestinal pathogen of humans[75] has been classified as a coccidian protozoan of the genus *Cyclospora* based on ultrastructural features (Figure 2–14, A and B), in vitro sporulation, and excystation studies.[76,77] This protozoan is a cause of traveler's diarrhea.[78,79] Organisms that fit the description of *Cyclospora* have been identified in stool specimens from travelers returning to the United States or Great Britain from Haiti, Mexico, Guatemala, Puerto Rico, Morocco, Cambodia, Pakistan, India, and the Solomon

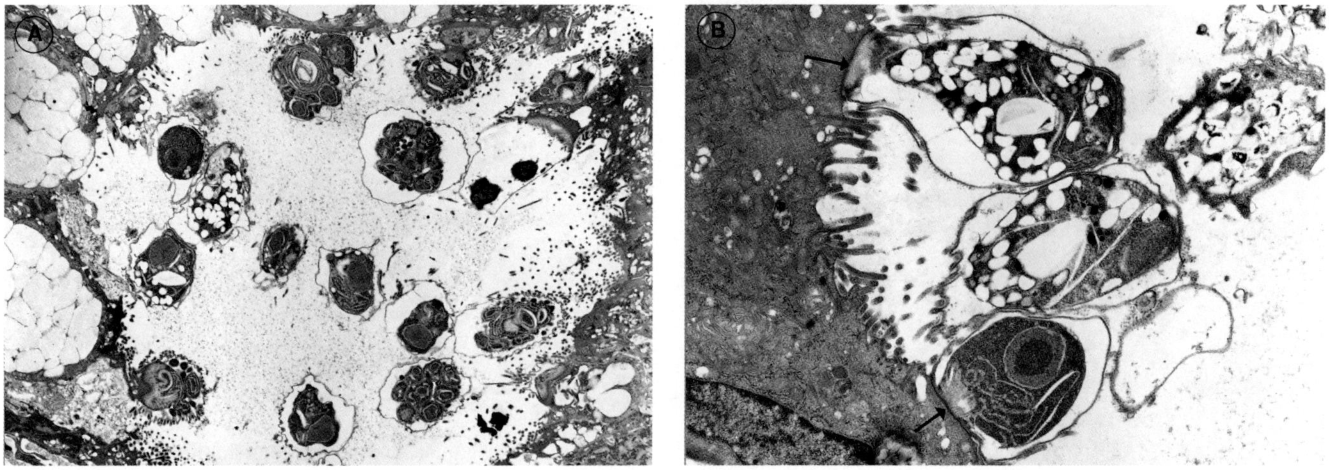

Figure 2–12. Electron micrographs of *Cryptosporidium* photographed from a colonic biopsy of a patient with AIDS (uranyl acetate, lead citrate counterstain). (**A**) *Cryptosporidium* in various stages of development in the lumen and on the surface of the colon. (**B**) Higher magnification of *Cryptosporidium* attached to the surface of the epithelial cells *(arrows)* but not invading them. *(Photographs courtesy of Dr. Micheline Federman, Deaconess Hospital, Harvard Medical School.)*

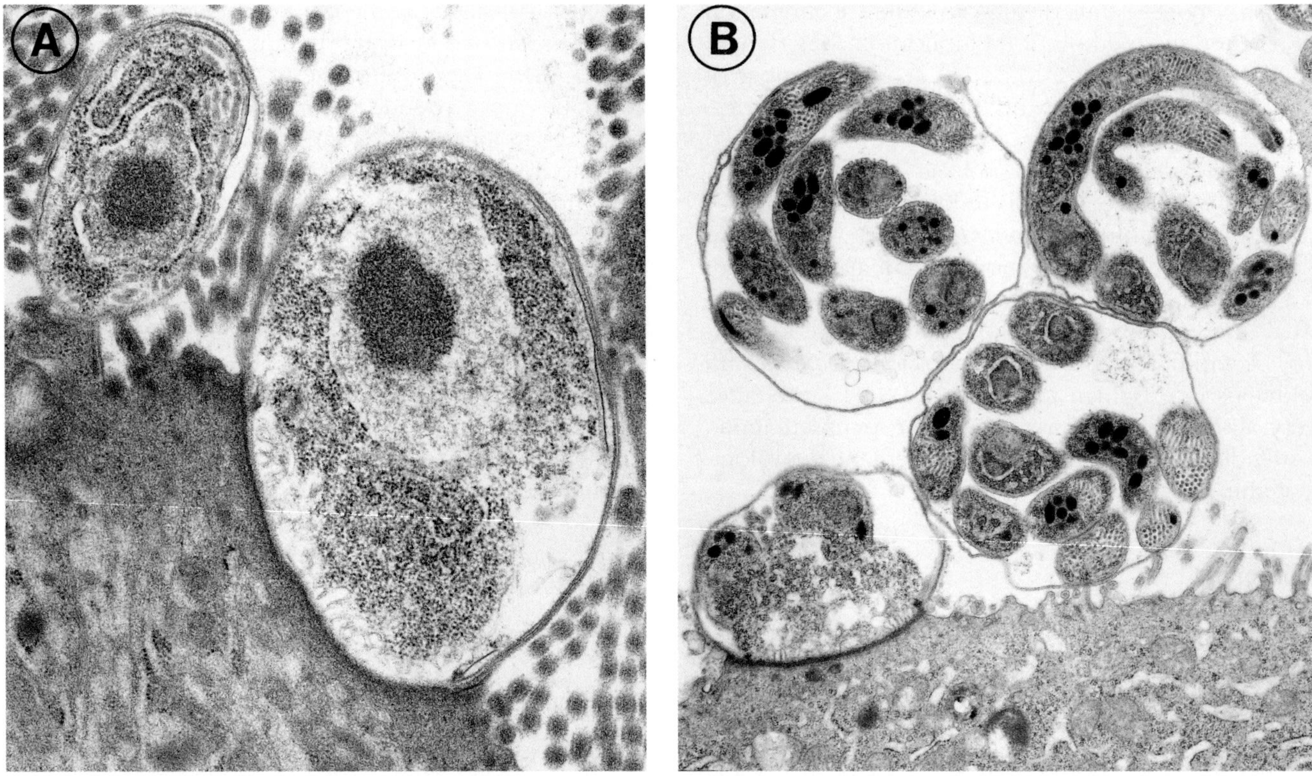

Figure 2–13. Electron micrographs of *Cryptosporidium* photographed from an intestinal biopsy of an immunodeficient patient (uranyl acetate, lead citrate counterstain). (**A**) Two trophozoites with nuclei, prominent nucleoli, and rough endoplasmic reticulum. One of the trophozoites is in an intracellular extracytoplasmic parasitophorous vacuole and shows its complicated feeding plaque. (**B**) Mature type I schizonts contain up to eight merozoites, which they release to infect more enterocytes. Short micronemes are within their anterior end. *(Photographs courtesy of Dr. Jan Orenstein, George Washington University Medical Center.)*

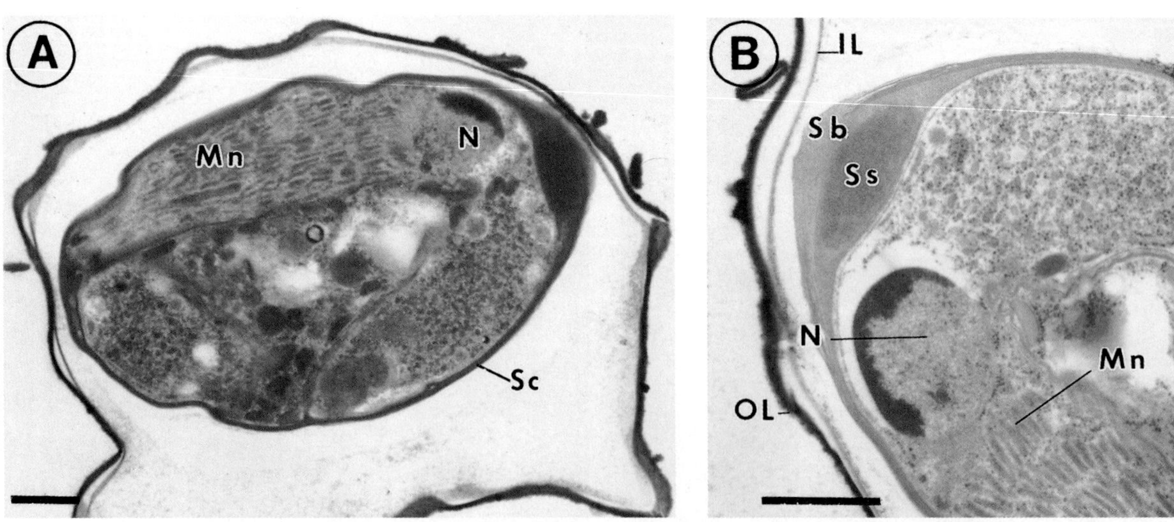

Figure 2–14. Electron micrographs of mature *C. cayetanenis* oocysts (uranyl acetate, lead citrate counterstain). (**A**) Ruptured oocyst with a cross-section of one sporocyst (Sc). Notice the anterior end of the sporozoite as well as the micronemes (Mn) and nucleus (N); bar = 1 μm. (**B**) High magnification of another sporocyst showing the Stieda body (Sb), Substieda body (Ss), micronemes (Mn), and nucleus (N). The inner layer (IL) and outer layer (OL) of the oocyst are also present; bar = 1 μm. *(Reprinted by permission of the publisher from Ortega YL et al. A new coccidian parasite (Apicomplexa: Eimeriidae) from humans.* J Parasitol. *1994;80:625–629.)*

Islands.[75] In a clinic in Haiti, *Cyclospora* were 11% of the enteric protozoa identified in more than 800 patients seropositive for HIV.[80] It is important to make this diagnosis, because the infection responds to trimethoprim–sulfamethoxazole.[80] These organisms resemble cryptosporidia in their morphologic features and in the diarrheal disease they cause.[76] Laboratory investigators should measure oocysts to distinguish *Cyclospora* from *Cryptosporidium,* because both genera stain avidly with the modified carbolfuchsin acid-fast stain.[75,81] The oocysts of *Cyclospora* are 8 to 10 μm in diameter and intermediate between those of *Cryptosporidia* and *Isospora,* hence the name "Big Crypto."[73,80] Another difference between *Cyclospora* and *Cryptosporidium* is that the latter are in parasitophorous vacuoles that protrude from the epithelial cell surface. These parasitophorous vacuoles containing cryptosporidial organisms are best observed by EM (Figures 2–12 and 2–13).

The taxonomic classification of *Cyclospora* eluded investigators between the years 1870 (first report) and 1993. The earlier electron microscopic studies did not reveal a nucleus, and the micronemes (organelles associated with host cell entry) were thought to represent the thylakoid membranes of chloroplasts; hence, the misclassification of this protozoan as a cyanobacterium (blue-green alga). The application of propane jet freezing and freeze substitution combined with EM allowed *Cyclospora* to be identified as a coccidian.[76,77] *Cyclospora* can now be considered as a fifth genus of coccidia and is readily distinguished from the other four (*Cryptosporidium, Isospora, Sarcocystis,* and *Toxoplasma*) on the basis of size, in vitro sporulation, excystation studies, and ultrastructural features.

Leishmania

Leishmaniasis is endemic in Asia, South America, Africa, and the Mediterranean, and travelers from other parts of the world may also acquire the disease.[82] Leishmania are transmitted by sandflies, and in general there are two types—cutaneous and visceral. There are a few records of human infections with lymph node enlargement alone. In two patients with enlarged cervical lymph nodes, whose disease manifested clinically as lymphoma and histologically as toxoplasmosis (granuloma formation),[82] a few macrophages contained small (1 to 2 μm) basophilic organisms in the cytoplasm. The differential diagnosis included toxoplasmosis, leishmaniasis, and histoplasmosis. Fungal stains excluded histoplasmosis. Although the size and shape of *Leishmania* and *Toxoplasma* are identical, the rod-shaped kinetoplast and target-shaped basal body, characteristics of flagellate protozoans, are features of leishmania. These findings suggest that leishmanial adenitis can remain unrecognized.[82] Biopsy specimens of lymph nodes showing only granulomatous lymphadenitis should be searched for leishmania by light microscopy and, if doubt persists, searched and studied by EM.

Giardia

This protozoan is a primitive eukaryote that is binucleate and contains abundant glycogen, free ribosomes, polysomes, and rough endoplasmic reticulum, but lacks mitochondria and a Golgi apparatus[83] (Figure 2–15). Giardia is the most commonly identified human intestinal parasite and occurs worldwide.[84] It is especially prevalent in children in developing countries.[85–87] The vast majority of children in rural Guatemala were infected with *Giardia* during the first 3 years of life. Giardiasis is frequently asymptomatic but may produce

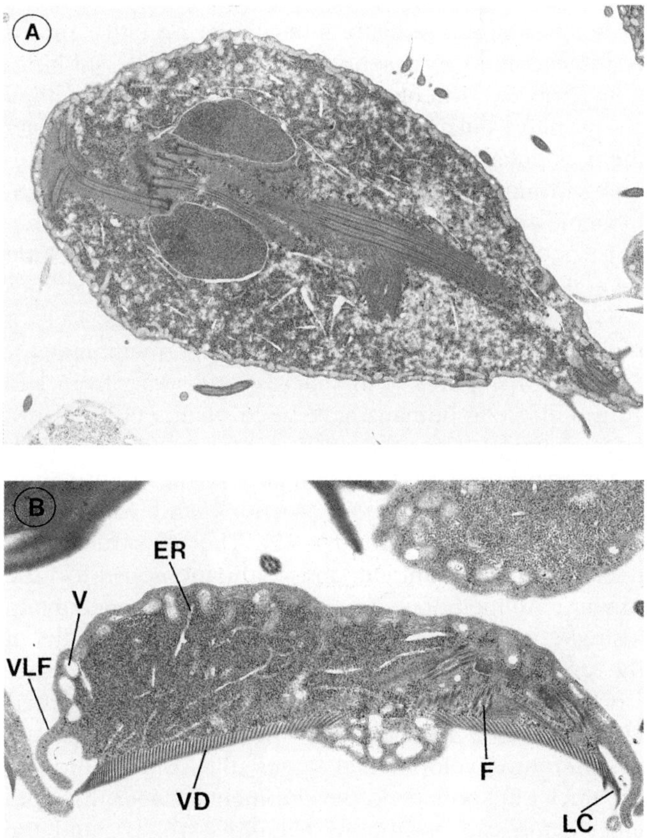

Figure 2–15. Electron micrographs of *Giardia lamblia* trophozoites (uranyl acetate, lead citrate counterstain). (**A**) The organism has a tadpole-like appearance in this plane. There are two nuclei, profiles of endoplasmic reticulum, longitudinal sections of flagella, vacuoles, and abundant glycogen (light areas within the cytoplasm). (**B**) Cross-section of a trophozoite showing the lateral crest (LC), ventrolateral flange (VLF), ventral disk (VD), vacuoles (V), endoplasmic reticulum (ER), and flagella (F). *(Photographs courtesy of Peggy Krasovich and Dr. Rod Adam, University of Arizona.)*

symptoms that range from acute gastroenteritis to those of malabsorption.[88] A definitive diagnosis can be made only by the detection of the cysts or trophozoites.[11] Light microscopic examination of stool specimens may be negative in 50% of cases.[88] It has been reported that the organisms may be overlooked because they resemble cellular debris.[88] By EM, characteristic features of this flagellated protozoan are easily discerned. The trophozoite contains two nuclei and abundant glycogen (Figure 2–15, A), eight kinetosomes, eight axonemes, and eight flagellae.[11] The ventral disk is striated and bounded on both sides by cytoplasmic folds (Figure 2–15, B). The two nuclei ("eyes") and overall shape of the trophozoite resemble a tadpole (Figure 2–15, A). A prompt diagnosis of giardiasis can result in effective treatment with a number of effective agents including the nitroimidazoles metronidazole and tinidiazole, quinacrine, and furazolidone.[89]

Microsporidia

Microsporidia are obligate intracellular primitive protozoans classified in a separate phylum of the subkingdom Protozoa, the Microspora.[90] Phylogenetically, they are primitive eukaryotes. The characteristics that classify them as eukaryotes are a nucleus with a nuclear envelope, an intracytoplasmic membrane system, and chromosome separation on mitotic spindles.[91] The characteristics that make them ancient protozoa include several prokaryotic features such as small ribosomes (70S) containing 16S and 23S ribosomal RNAs, lack of mitochondria, peroxisomes, and Golgi membranes.[91] Although the spores of the microsporidia vary from 1 to 12 μm, those in humans have been smaller (1 to 5 μm), necessitating EM for the analysis of structural details.[92] EM is considered the gold standard for the confirmation of microsporidia in tissue sections and for speciation[90,92] (Figures 2–16 and 2–17). The ultrastructure of microsporidia is unique and pathognomonic for the phylum. All members of the phylum Microspora contain a single polar tubule (part of the extrusion apparatus of the spores), which is diagnostic for the group. The specific ultrastructural features of the host–parasite interface (Figures 2–16 and 2–17), the size of the organism at different developmental stages, the configuration of the nuclei in spores and developmental stages, the specific features of sporogony (Figure 2–16, B), and the number and arrangement of the coils of the polar tubule in the spore allow most genera of microsporidia (eg, *Enterocytozoon, Septata, Encephalitozoon, Pleistophora, Nosema*) to be distinguished from each other.[7,91–97] For example, the spores of *Enterocytozoon bieneusi* have five to seven coils of polar tubules arranged in two rows (Figure 2–17, A), whereas those of *Septata intestinalis* have four to seven coils arranged in a single row (Figure 2–17, B).[90] All stages of *E bieneusi* develop in direct contact with the cytoplasm of the host cell (Figures 2–16, A, and 2–17, A), whereas the process of sporogony in *S intestinalis* occurs within a parasitophorous vacuole limited by a host-formed membrane (Figures 2–16, B and 2–17, B).[90,95–98] *Septata*

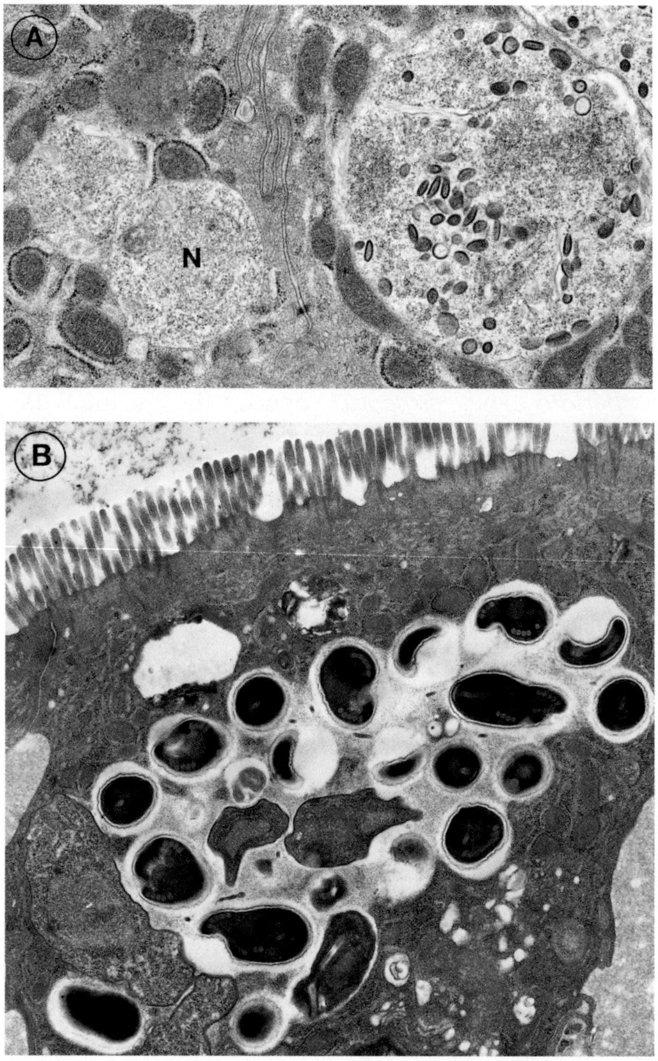

Figure 2–16. Electron micrographs comparing the host cell–parasite interface of two different species of microsporidia (uranyl acetate, lead citrate counterstain). (**A**) *Enterocytozoon bieneusi:* Lightly staining proliferative plasmodia containing abundant ribosomes in one enterocyte. One of the organisms contains a nucleus (N). Sporogonial plasmodia containing disklike polar tube precursors are in an adjacent enterocyte. *(Photograph courtesy of Dr. Jan Orenstein, George Washington University Medical Center.)* (**B**) *Septata intestinalis:* This microsporidian develops within a parasitophorous vacuole with honeycomb-like chambers. Note the various stages including meronts, sporoblasts, and electron-dense spores. *(Photograph courtesy of Dr. Micheline Federman, Deaconess Hospital, Harvard Medical School.)*

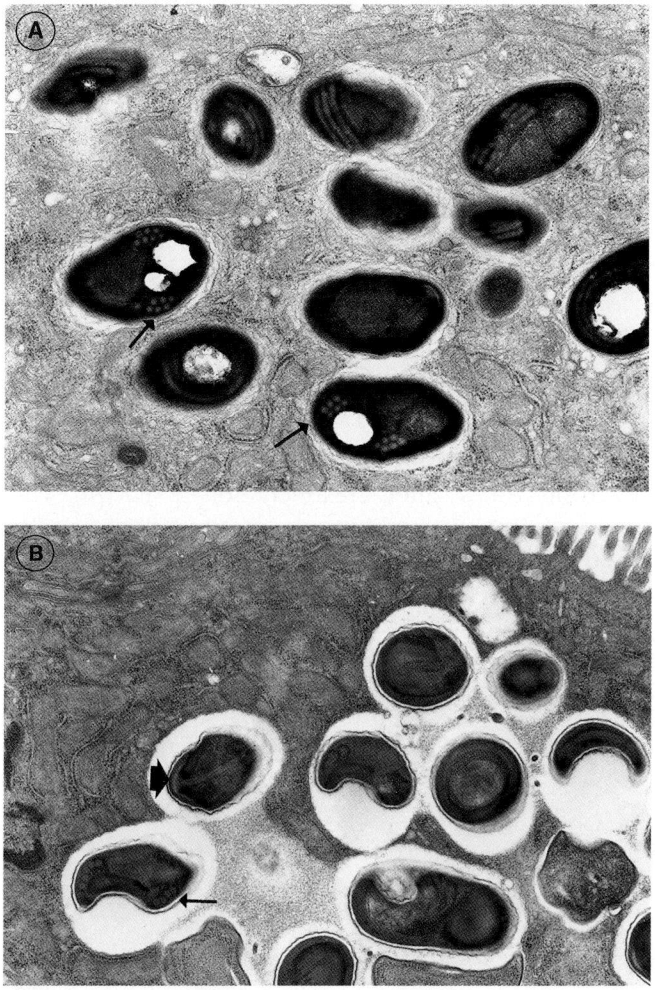

Figure 2–17. Higher magnification of electron micrographs of two different species of microsporidia to compare the arrangement of polar tube coils (uranyl acetate, lead citrate counterstain). (**A**) *Enterocytozoon bieneusi* spores with the characteristic double row of cross-sections of polar tube coil *(arrows).* (**B**) *Septata intestinalis* spores with the characteristic single row of cross-sections of the polar tube coil *(thin arrow)* and the anchoring disk *(thick arrow). (Photographs courtesy of Dr. Micheline Federman, Deaconess Hospital, Harvard Medical School.)*

intestinalis secretes a fibrillar network that surrounds the developing organisms, making the parasitophorous vacuole appear septate.

Microsporidia have gained increasing attention because they are opportunistic pathogens that cause significant morbidity in patients with AIDS.[73,92,95–100] Ultrastructural differentiation of spores of *E bieneusi* and *S intestinalis* in stool specimens may be important for patient care, because infection by *Septata* can be successfully treated with albendazole.[90,98] Patients with keratoconjunctivitis caused by *Encephalitozoon hellem* showed symptomatic improvement after topical application of fumagillin.[101]

The spectrum of clinically manifested microsporidial infections includes involvement of the intestine, eye (cornea and conjunctiva), muscle, and biliary tract. Systemic microsporidiosis is also in patients infected and not infected with HIV.[90,93] The mode of transmission is not known for all patients with microsporidial infection; animal reservoirs and contaminated ditch water have been implicated.[90] Because the host range of microsporidia is extensive, and more than 100 genera and almost 1000 species have been identified,[90] EM will continue to be valuable for diagnosis.

PARASITES OF UNCERTAIN TAXONOMY (*PNEUMOCYSTIS CARINII*)

Pneumocystosis is the most important opportunistic infection in AIDS patients, occurring in more than 80% of patients with the disease.[11,102–104] An outbreak of *P carinii* pneumonia was recently reported in a renal transplant unit among HIV-negative-immunodeficient patients.[105] A cluster of five patients occurred over a 3-month period in elderly patients without known predisposing factors.[106] *Pneumocystis carinii* is also the causative agent of a characteristic form of pneumonia seen in infants and children.[107] Pneumonia in these non-HIV-infected patients raises intriguing questions about host defense mechanisms, the possibility of different strains of *P carinii*, and nosocomial transmission of infection.[108]

Pneumocystis carinii is a unicellular organism without a definitely established taxonomic classification. That it is unicellular indicates that it may be a sporozoan of the toxoplasmid type[11] or a primitive fungus in which the mycelium is reduced to a unicellular state, but the ability to sporulate is preserved.[109] Historically it is thought to be protozoan because of its similar life cycle,[102,109] its susceptibility to antiprotozoal agents (eg, sulfonamide), and its poor response to antifungal agents, such as amphotericin B and the imidazoles. Ultrastructural, biochemical, and genetic analyses indicate that *P carinii* may be more closely related to fungi. *Pneumocystis carinii* differs from members of the Sarcodina group in not having a phagocytic apparatus, ameboid movement, etc; it differs from the Cnidospora in not having polar filaments and multinucleate plasmodia, and differs from the Sporozoa in not having a conoid (polar ring encircling a cylindrical, truncated cone), micronemes, rhoptries, and subpellicular tubules.[109] Certain ultrastructural features such as the appearance of the cell wall, complete lack of organelles of motility, and tightly interdigitating cytoplasmic membranes are consistent with a fungus.[109] Ribosomal RNA[110,111]; elastase enzymes; the genes for thymidylate synthetase, dihydrofolate reductase and mitochondrial proteins and antibody epitope[112] analysis also indicate a close relationship to fungi, especially the *Saccharomyces*. Biochemical analyses of the cyst walls indicate that they are rich in glucose (in the form of β-glucan). Zymolyase, a 1,3-β-glucanase, cleaves the cell wall and surface antigens of both fungi and *P carinii*.[113] The cyst wall sterols of *P carinii,* however, are based on cholesterol, as in mammals, and not on ergosterol, as in fungi.[102,114] These documented similarities of *P carinii* to fungi have stimulated efforts to culture *P carinii* on fungal mediums[115] and to develop the 1,3-β-glucan inhibitors of the echinocandin and papulocandin class of antifungal agents, as anti-*P carinii* drugs.[116]

Pneumocystis carinii cannot be readily identified in hematoxylin-eosin-stained sections,[11] but methenamine-silver nitrate stains the cysts of *Pneumocystis*.[11] Even with the silver stains, the histologic diagnosis may not be definitive. Some investigators recommend EM for a definitive diagnosis.[107] The ultrastructural features are distinctive (Figure 2–18). A conglomerate of cysts and thin-walled trophozoites (Figure 2–18, A) is the ultrastructural counterpart of the eosinophilic, frothy, exudative appearance on histologic sections.[117] Ultrastructural examination sometimes reveals many degenerate forms, which are not diagnostic by light microscopy. The cyst wall also shows a characteristic focal thickening by EM (Figure 2–18, B). Improved intracellular morphology was recently achieved using postfixation with osmium tetroxide and potassium ferrocyanide.[118] A marked improvement in staining of cell membranes, endoplasmic reticulum, nuclear membranes, and glycogen was observed.

EM was used also to demonstrate the persistence of trophozoites after treatment of *P carinii* with trimethoprim–sulfamethoxazole.[119] The failure of silver or other stains to detect the organisms may be related to the paucity of cysts after treatment and degeneration of the nuclei.[119] Newer fixation protocols for EM may allow physicians, in the future, to follow the effective-

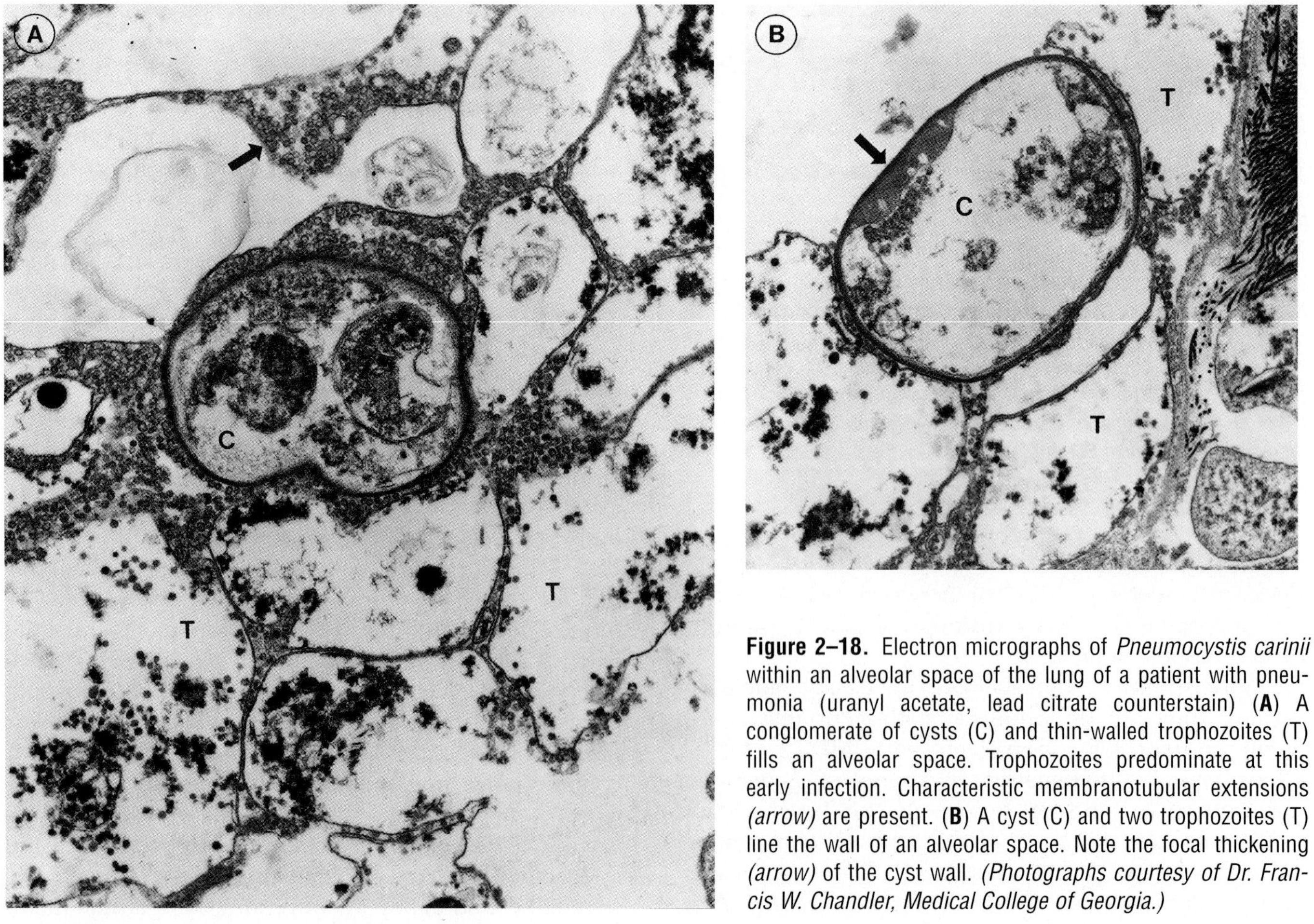

Figure 2–18. Electron micrographs of *Pneumocystis carinii* within an alveolar space of the lung of a patient with pneumonia (uranyl acetate, lead citrate counterstain) (**A**) A conglomerate of cysts (C) and thin-walled trophozoites (T) fills an alveolar space. Trophozoites predominate at this early infection. Characteristic membranotubular extensions *(arrow)* are present. (**B**) A cyst (C) and two trophozoites (T) line the wall of an alveolar space. Note the focal thickening *(arrow)* of the cyst wall. *(Photographs courtesy of Dr. Francis W. Chandler, Medical College of Georgia.)*

ness of antimicrobial agents against *P carinii* and to better tailor chemotherapy on an individual basis.

Bacterial Infections

Electron microscopic studies have elucidated the basic structure of the bacterial cell,[120] which has been correlated with its biologic functions and pathogenesis.[121] The bacterial cell has a simple structure characteristic of prokaryotes (Figures 2–19 through 2–23). There is no envelope around the nuclear material, and organelles such as mitochondria, endoplasmic reticulum, and Golgi structures are lacking.[10,120] Gram-positive bacteria can be distinguished from gram-negative bacteria on the basis of the ultrastructural features of the cell wall.[10] Gram-positive bacteria have a broad (12 to 30 nm), featureless layer of peptidoglycan underlain by a cytoplasmic membrane.[10,122] The cell wall of gram-negative bacteria is, however, multilayered[123] (Figures 2–21, D and 2–22, A). There is a cytoplasmic membrane covered

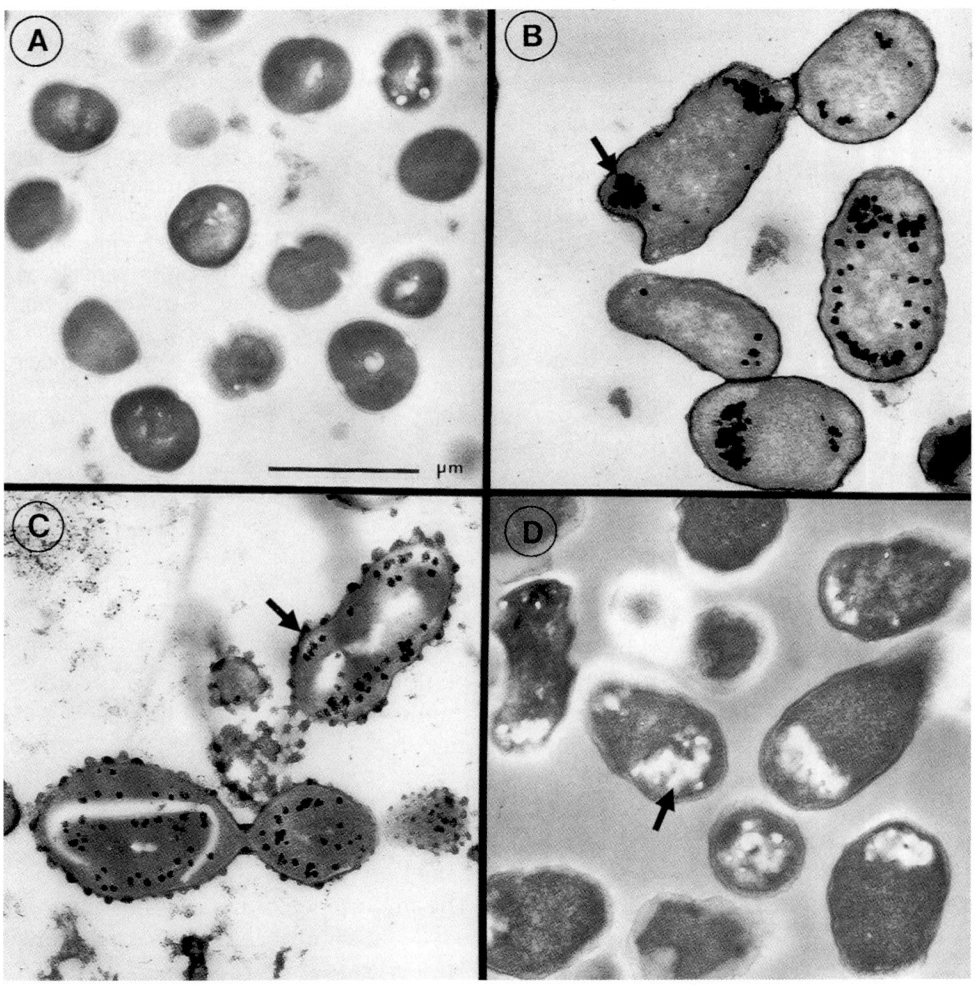

Figure 2–19. Electron micrographs of unrelated bacterial species stained by the PATCSP technique for polysaccharides. (**A**) *Staphylococcus aureus:* The cell wall is the extracellular electron-lucent structure surrounding the electron-dense cell cytoplasm. The cell membrane cannot be identified at this magnification. Note the lack of capsular material. (**B**) *Klebsiella:* Electron-dense capsular material with a smooth contour surrounds each organism. Large aggregates of intracellular glycogen particles are also present *(arrow)*. (**C**) *Streptococcus pneumoniae:* Electron-dense capsular material with a scalloped appearance *(arrow)* surrounds the two bacteria in the field. Punctate aggregates of intracellular glycogen are also present. (**D**) *Klebsiella* control: Same preparation as (**B**) except that the PATCSP procedure was run after omission of the oxidation step with periodic acid. No electron-dense capsular material surrounds the cells. The glycogen aggregates are now represented by clear areas in the cytoplasm *(arrow)*. *(Reprinted by permission of the publisher from Strohm H et al. Demonstration of* Bacteroides *capsules by light microscopy and ultrastructural cytochemistry.* Am J Clin Pathol. *1983;79: 591–597.)*

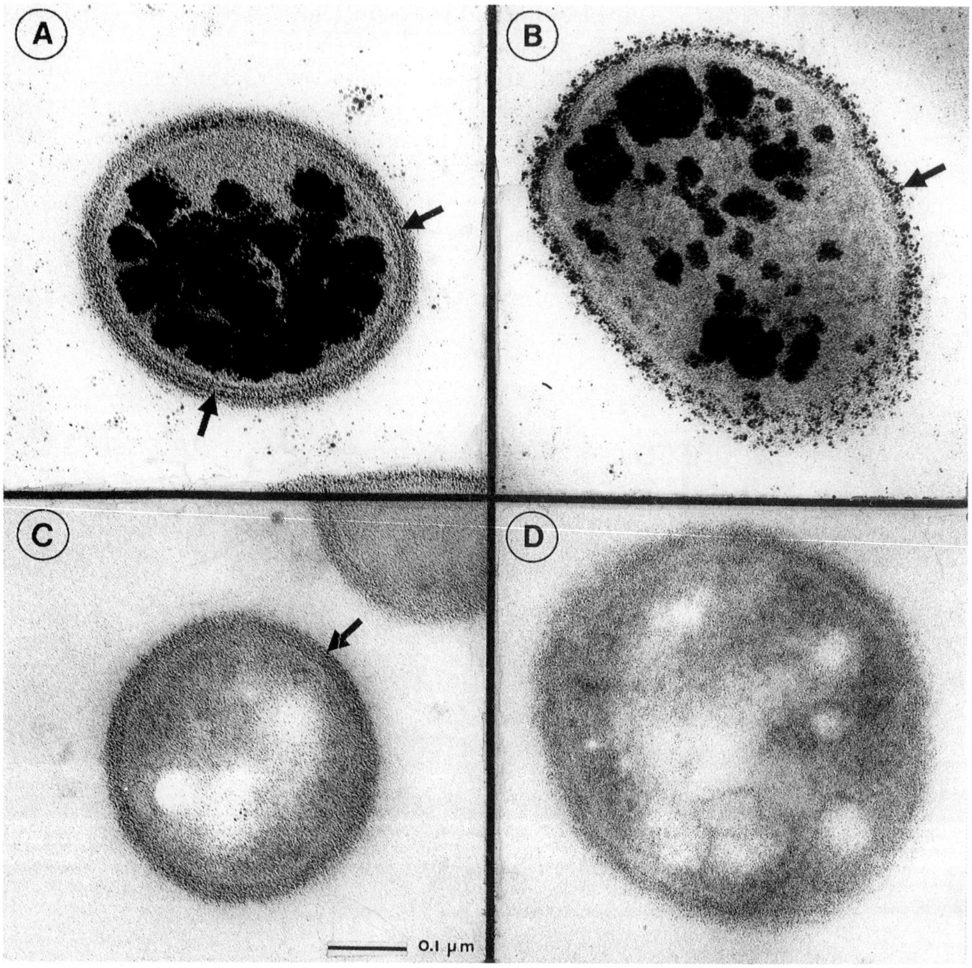

Figure 2–20. Electron micrographs of reference *Bacteroides* species stained by the PATCSP technique for polysaccharides. (**A**) *Bacteroides fragilis* (ATCC 23745): The electron-dense capsular material appears smooth and is external to the outer membrane of the cell wall *(arrows)*. Large lakes of intracellular glycogen fill the cytoplasm. (**B**) *Bacteroides vulgatus* (ATCC 8482): The electron-dense capsular material appears coarsely granular *(arrow)* and surrounds the cell. (**C**) *Bacteroides fragilis* control: Same preparation as (**A**) with omission of the oxidation step with periodic acid. (**D**) *Bacteroides vulgatus* control: Same preparation as (**B**) with omission of the oxidation step with periodic acid. *(Reprinted by permission of the publisher from Strohm H et al. Demonstration of* Bacteroides *capsules by light microscopy and ultrastructural cytochemistry.* Am J Clin Pathol. *1983; 79:591–597.)*

by a 3- to 5-nm peptidoglycan layer, followed by a relatively electron-transparent zone of varying thickness, and an outer membrane with specific receptor, barrier, transport, and antigenic properties.[10] In addition, there is a distinct polysaccharide-containing glycocalyx (capsule, slime layer) seen by EM[124] using the periodic acid thiocarbohydrazide silver proteinate (PATCSP) staining technique (Figures 2–19 through 2–21).[125]

Bacteria are readily identified in tissue sections by light microscopy because of their size (>0.2 μm in diameter), and those with capsules can usually be identified in India ink-stained wet mounts of whole organisms.[126] There are, however, several instances in which EM can help diagnose bacterial infections. These include the identification of small bacteria in tissue sections,[122,127] the distinction of a bacterial infection from neoplastic vascular proliferations,[128] the identification of bacteria similar to those causing cat-scratch disease,[7] the identification of capsular material negative by India ink preparations,[124] the identification of cell wall-deficient bacteria[129] including *Mycoplasma,*[7,130,131] the rapid identification of *Francisella tularensis* using immunoelectron microscopy,[132] the identification of bacteria as the causative agents of epidemic outbreaks of unknown cause (eg, legionnaires' disease), and in the monitoring of antibiotic treatment in Whipple's disease.[10,133–139]

Demonstration of Bacterial Capsules by Ultrastructural Cytochemical Methods

The importance of nonsporing anaerobic gram-negative bacilli in clinical infections has been well established. The *Bacteroides fragilis* group (BFG) is important because of its isolation from clinical infections and relative resistance to β-lactam antibiotics. The virulence of *B fragilis* has been attributed to the capsule identified by light and EM using ruthenium red staining.[140,141] Because narrow capsules (0.2 μm and less) cannot be distinguished from diffraction halos by light microscopy,[126] the increased resolution that the electron microscope provides has been helpful. Evidence for the presence of capsules in anaerobic gram-negative bacilli other than *B fragilis* has, however, been conflicting. Using the PATCSP staining procedure of Thiery[125] (Figures 2–19 through 2–21), it has become evident that

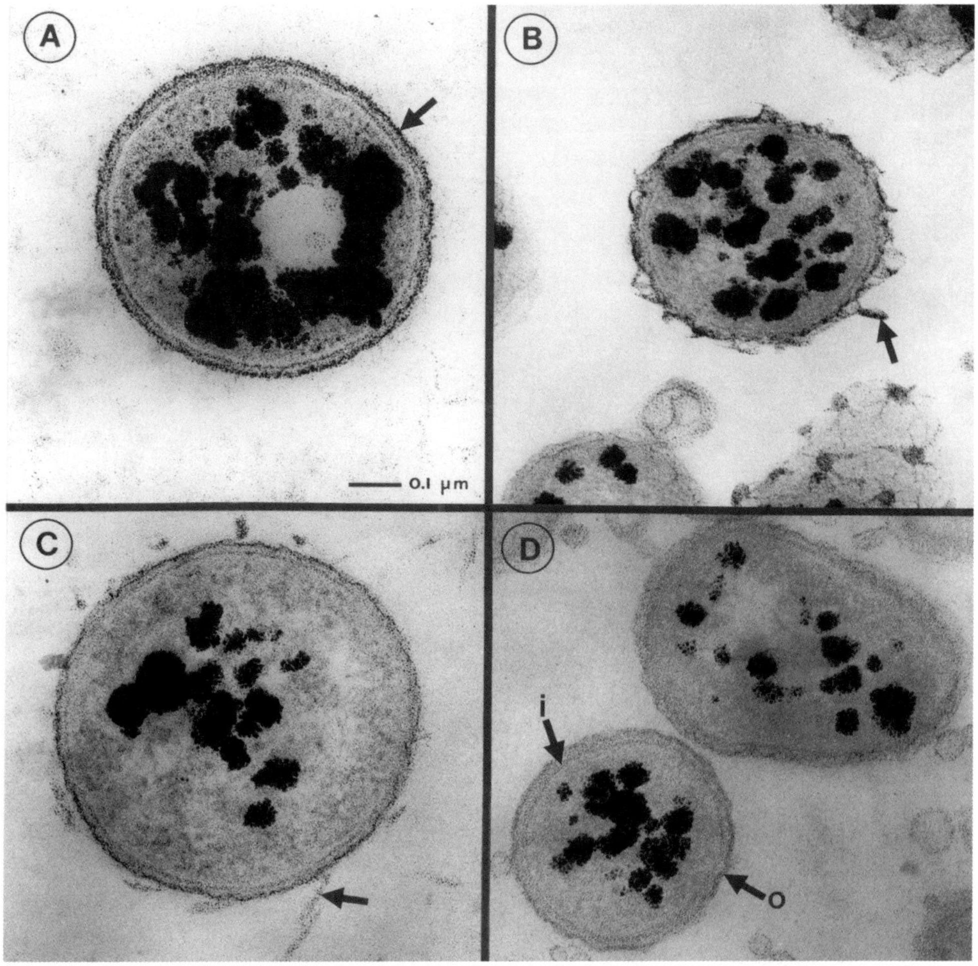

Figure 2–21. Electron micrographs of clinical *Bacteroides* isolates stained by the PATCSP technique. (**A**) *Bacteroides thetaiotaomicron:* The electron-dense capsular material appears finely granular *(arrow)* and surrounds the cell. Intracellular glycogen is also present. (**B**) *Bacteroides fragilis:* "Wispy" electron-dense capsular material surrounds the cell *(arrow).* (**C**) *Bacteroides thetaiotaomicron:* The electron-dense capsular material surrounds the cell and is of a "wispy" nature *(arrow).* (**D**) Non-*Bacteroides fragilis* group anaerobic gram-negative bacillus: No electron-dense capsular material can be seen surrounding the two bacterial profiles shown here. The inner (i) and outer (o) membranes are clearly evident. Although no capsular material is present, intracellular glycogen can still be seen. *(Reprinted by permission of the publisher from Strohm H et al. Demonstration of* Bacteroides *capsules by light microscopy and ultrastructural cytochemistry.* Am J Clin Pathol. *1983;79:591–597.)*

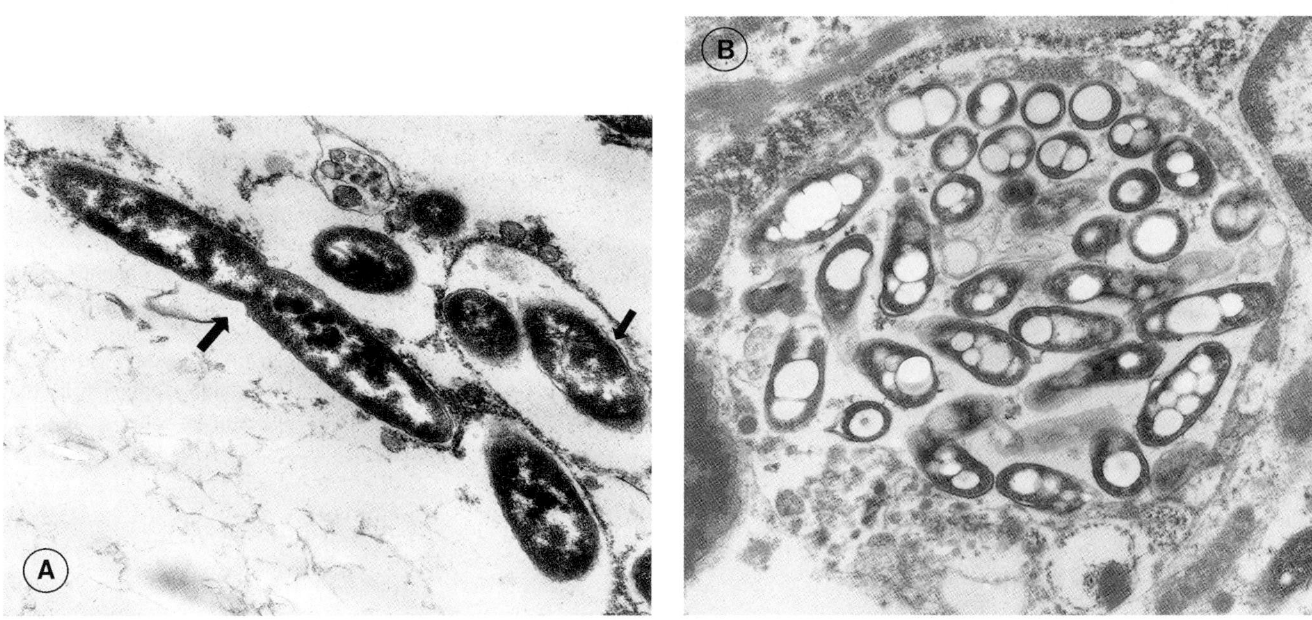

Figure 2–22. Electron micrographs of *Legionella pneumophila* cultured on the yolk sac membrane of embryonated hens' eggs (uranyl acetate, lead citrate counterstain). (**A**) Note the "pinching" division *(large arrow)* and the typical gram-negative cell wall *(small arrow).* The bacilli are within membrane-bound intracytoplasmic vacuoles. (**B**) A macrophage containing numerous vacuolated bacilli is shown. The membrane-enclosed, electron-lucent inclusions measure 30 to 200 nm in diameter and are morphologically suggestive of poly-β-hydroxybutyrate granules in sections. *(Photographs courtesy of Dr. Francis W. Chandler, Medical College of Georgia.)*

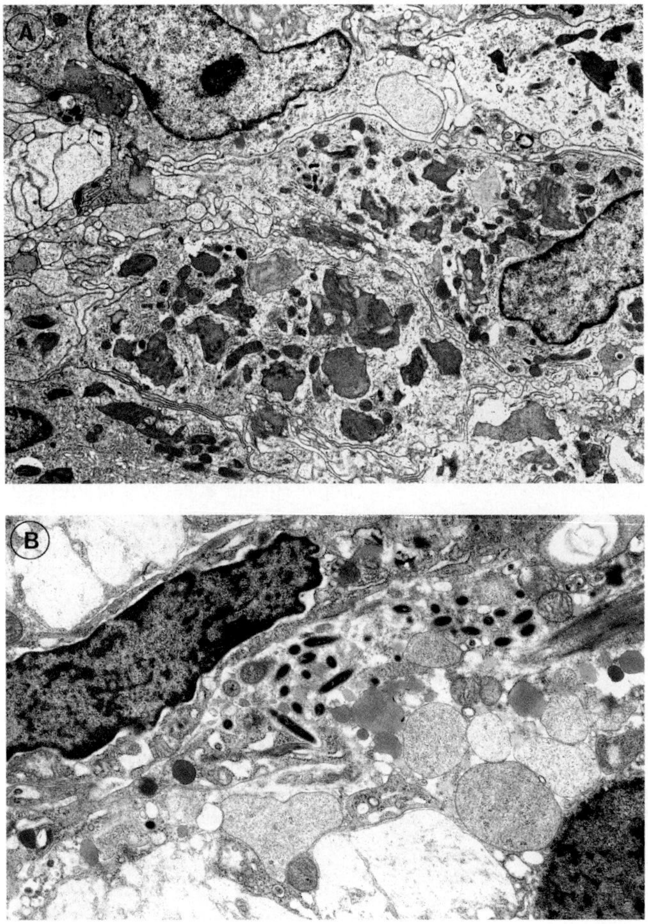

Figure 2–23. Low-power electron micrographs from a small intestinal biopsy of a patient with Whipple's disease (uranyl acetate, lead citrate counterstain). (**A**) Numerous electron-dense inclusions are within the phagolysosomes of macrophages within the lamina propria. These electron-dense inclusions are the cell wall remnants of the partially digested Whipple's bacteria. (**B**) Unphagocytosed Whipple's bacteria found within the lamina propria.

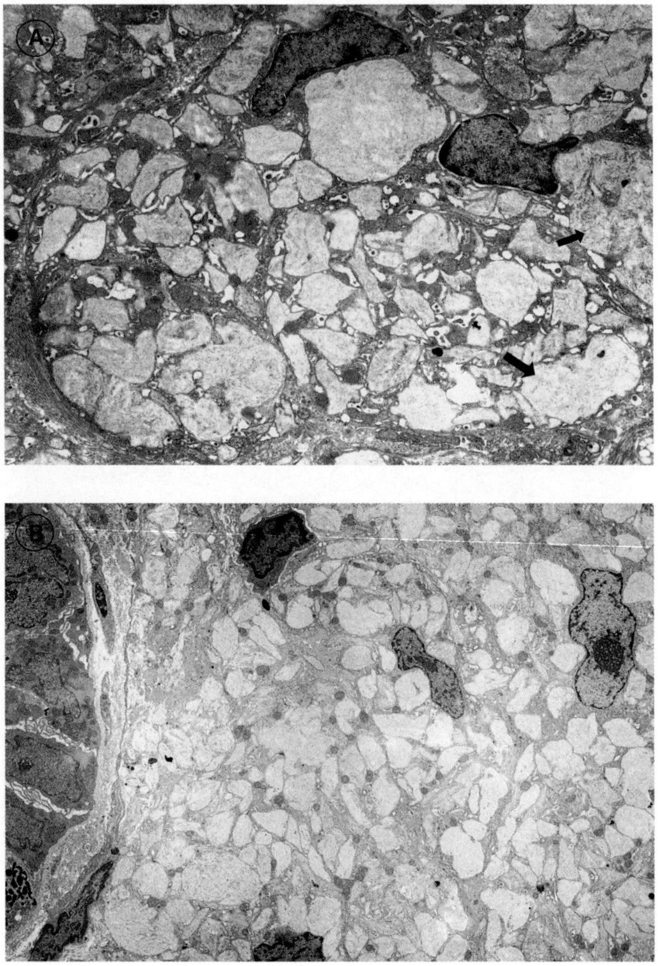

Figure 2–24. Low-power electron micrographs from small intestinal biopsies of the same patient shown in Figure 2–23 with Whipple's disease at two different times after antibiotic treatment (uranyl acetate, lead citrate counterstain). (**A**) Three months after antibiotic therapy: The cytoplasm of these macrophages is filled with phagolysosomes containing cell wall debris at different stages of digestion. The electron-lucent phagolysosome *(large arrow)* is at a more advanced stage of digestion compared with the phagolysosome *(smaller arrow)*. The contents of all of these phagolysosomes indicate a more advanced degree of digestion compared with those shown in Figure 2–23, A. (**B**) Ten months after antibiotic therapy: This biopsy was taken at a later time in antibiotic therapy compared with (**A**). The vast majority of the phagolysosomes in these macrophages are electron-lucent. This, coupled with the absence of new bacteria in the biopsy, indicates effective treatment.

other species of *Bacteroides* may possess capsular material (Figures 2–20, B, 2–21, A, and 2–21, C).[124] The advantage of the PATCSP staining process over that of ruthenium red is that with the PATCSP reaction, the identification of polysaccharide material is based on the presence of adjacent diol groups irrespective of charge, whereas ruthenium red reacts predominantly with acidic polysaccharides. Because the presence of a capsule is used as one criterion to determine virulence, the application of ultrastructural cytochemical techniques to clinical isolates may be useful for patient care.

Epidemic Outbreaks of Unknown Cause

The 58th annual convention of the American Legion's Pennsylvania Division was held at the Bellevue–Stratford Hotel in Philadelphia from July 21 to 24, 1976. Between July 22 and August 3, 149 of the conventioneers developed a puzzling illness characterized by fever, coughing, and pneumonia.[142] This was an unusual and explosive outbreak of pneumonia with no apparent cause. Because most of the conventioneers had returned home before becoming ill, it was not until

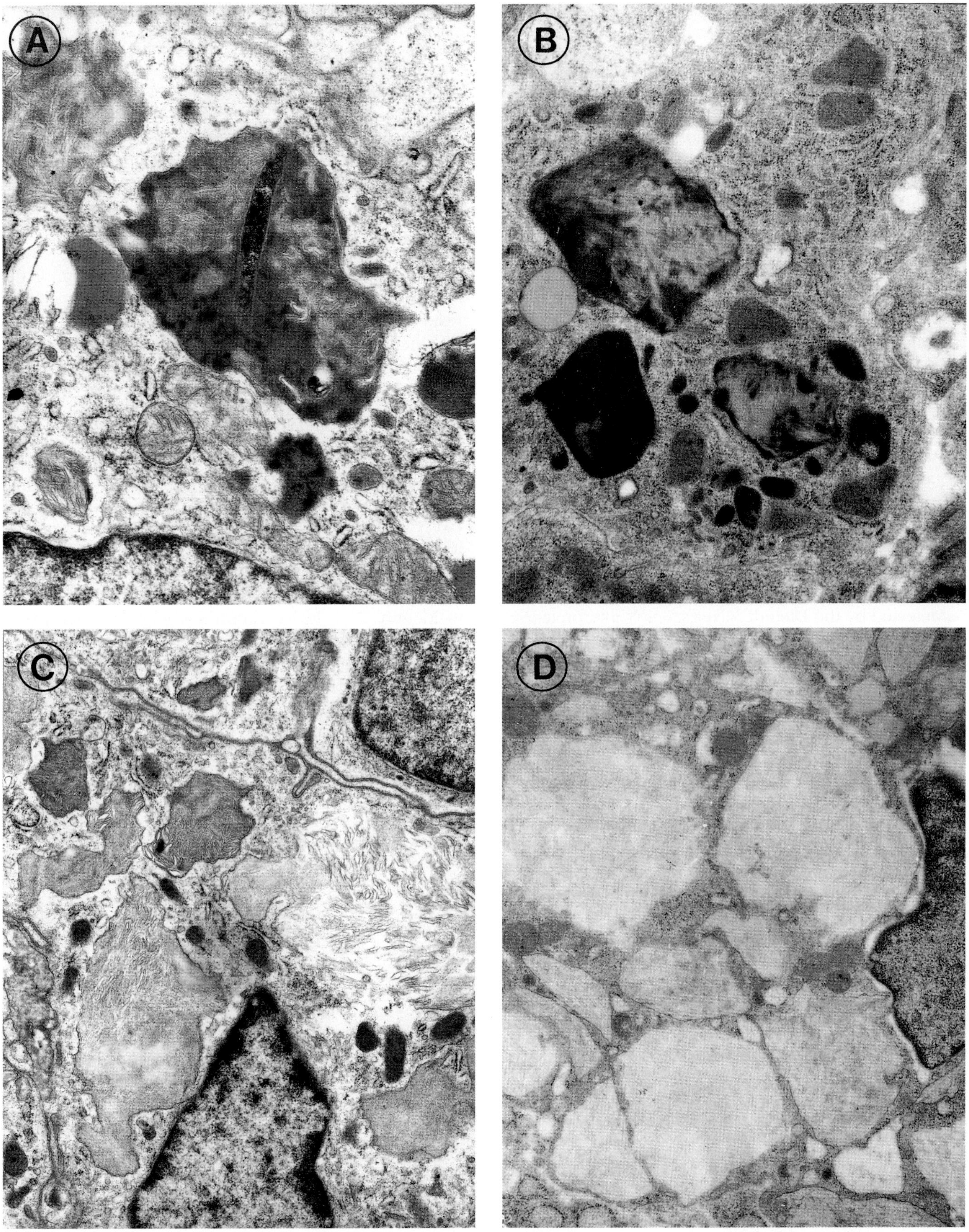

Figure 2–25. Higher magnification electron micrographs of the cytoplasm of intestinal macrophages indicating the progression in antibiotic treatment of Whipple's disease (same patient shown in Figures 2–23 and 2–24) (uranyl acetate, lead citrate counterstain). (**A**) Initial biopsy showing an electron-dense phagolysosome containing an intact Whipple's bacterium. (**B**) Initial biopsy showing electron-dense phagolysosomes and no intact bacterial cells in another macrophage. (**C**) After several months of antibiotic treatment, the substructure acquires a membranous appearance. (**D**) After 10 months of antibiotic treatment, the substructure of the vast majority of the phagolysosomes has a granulofibrillary appearance.

August 2 that reports to the Pennsylvania Department of Health made it clear that an epidemic had developed among those who attended the convention.[142] This started one of the largest and most complex investigations of an epidemic ever undertaken. The acute fibrinopurulent pneumonia of small air spaces, coined by the press as legionnaires' disease, was not, however, confined to the legionnaires. An additional 72 people, not at the convention, contracted the disease. All, however, had been in or near the Bellevue–Stratford Hotel. A total of 221 people became ill, and 34 of them died of pneumonia or complications of pneumonia.[142] The cooling towers for the air-conditioning system at the hotel were implicated in spreading the disease.

The clinical symptoms could have been caused by a variety of agents, including toxic substances and infectious organisms. Six months passed before the causative agent was discovered, and months after that the agent was identified as a previously unknown bacterium. EM helped to demonstrate that the infection was caused by bacteria (Figure 2–22).[143–146] The legionnaires' bacterium has a "pinching" division (Figure 2–22, A) and a multilayered wall typical of gram-negative bacteria (Figure 2–22, B). Although legionellae can be detected by the Dieterle silver stain,[142] interpretation is difficult.

Inhalation of aerosols, particularly from cooling towers, evaporative condensers, and air-conditioning systems, continues to be a mode of transmission of *Legionella pneumophila*.[147] Although modern techniques, such as PCR of *Legionella* DNA, can now be used to detect the organism in body fluids,[148] the catchall nature of EM remains critical in the detection of unknown organisms during sporadic outbreaks.

Whipple's Disease

In 1907, Whipple observed bacilli in a disorder of the intestine called intestinal lipodystrophy. Clinically, patients with this disorder presented with gastrointestinal blood loss and anemia. Because PAS-positive macrophages were in the lamina propria, the disorder was thought to be some form of storage disease,[10] and the bacteria were believed to be a consequence of the erosive changes associated with the disease. More than half a century later, the cause and pathogenesis of Whipple's disease were demonstrated by EM.[133–135,137] The ultrastructural correlate of the PAS-positive inclusions within the macrophages was determined to be undigested residues of the cell walls (Figures 2–23, A, 2–24, and 2–25) of Whipple's bacteria (Figures 2–23, B and 2–25, A). By EM, the bacteria can be observed free within the lamina propria (Figure 2–23, B) or within epithelial cells, neutrophils, and macrophages (Figure 2–25, A).

The reason for the lack of digestibility of the cell walls of Whipple's bacteria is unknown. A host enzyme may be lacking or perhaps it is some intrinsic property of the organism. Because the organism has defied attempts at culture, EM remains the best method of confirming the diagnosis. In addition, EM can be used to monitor the effectiveness of antibiotic treatment.[135,136,138] Before treatment, intact bacterial organisms are free in the lamina propria (Figure 2–23, B) or within phagolysosomes (Figure 2–25, A), and the macrophages are filled with the electron-dense cell wall residues (Figures 2–23, A, 2–25, A, and 2–25, B). After treatment with antibiotics, the ultrastructural appearance of the cell wall residues changes to membranous (Figure 2–25, C) and granulofibrillary (Figure 2–25, D) remnants within phagolysosomes.

CONCLUSION

EM can be used to identify many microorganisms, including viruses, protozoa, and bacteria. Because of its catchall nature, the electron microscope should be used as part of the armamentarium of laboratory procedures to identify any elusive causal agent of epidemics such as *Legionella* spp, HIV, and members of the coronavirus superfamily. In some instances, EM may be the most cost-effective diagnostic test and may also be used effectively to monitor therapy.

REFERENCES

1. Yunis EJ, Hashida Y, Haas JE. The role of electron microscopy in the identification of viruses in human disease. *Pathol Ann.* 1977;12(pt 1):311–330.
2. Yunis EJ, Agostini Jr. RM, and Atchison RW. An atlas of viral particles from human specimens. *Persp Pediatr Pathol.* 1978;4:387–429.
3. Doane FW. Virus morphology as an aid for rapid diagnosis. *Yale J Biol Med.* 1980;53:19–25.
4. Burns WA, Breitschneider A, Sobel H. Electron microscopy in diagnostic medicine. *Diagnostic Med.* March 1985:38–45.
5. Christensen ML. Human viral gastroenteritis. *Clin Microbiol Rev.* 1989;2:51–89.
6. Elliott EJ. Viral diarrhoeas in childhood. Electron microscopy has improved our understanding. *Brit Med J.* 1992;305:1111–1112.
7. Orenstein JM. Ultrastructural pathology of human immunodeficiency virus infection. *Ultrastructural Pathol.* 1992; 16:179–210.
8. Taterka JA, Cuff CF, Rubin DH. Viral gastrointestinal infections. *Gastroenterol Clin North Am.* 1992;21(2):303–330.
9. Madeley CR. The search for viruses by negative contrast. In: Papadimitriou JM, Henderson DW, Spagnolo DV, eds.

Diagnostic Ultrastructure of Non-Neoplastic Diseases. New York: Churchill Livingstone; 1992:chap 8.
10. Wills EF. Infectious agents: fungi, bacteria and viruses. In: Papadimitriou JM, Henderson DW, Spagnolo DV, eds. *Diagnostic Ultrastructure of Non-Neoplastic Diseases.* New York: Churchill Livingstone; 1992:chap 9.
11. Warton A. Diagnostic ultrastructure of human parasites. In: Papadimitriou JM, Henderson DW, Spagnolo DV, eds. *Diagnostic Ultrastructure of Non-Neoplastic Diseases.* New York: Churchill Livingstone; 1992:chap 10.
12. Anderson N, Doane FW. Agar diffusion method for negative staining of microbial suspensions in salt solutions. *Appl Microbiol.* 1972;24(3):495–496.
13. Madeley CR, Field AM. *Virus Morphology.* 2nd ed. Edinburgh: Churchill Livingstone; 1988.
14. Vernon SK, Lawrence WC, Long CA, Rubin BA, Sheffield JB. Morphological components of herpesvirus. IV. Ultrastructural features of the envelope and tegument. *J Ultrastructure Res.* 1982;81:163–171.
15. Fowler CB, Reed KD, Brannon RB. Intranuclear inclusions correlate with the ultrastructural detection of herpes-type virions in oral hairy leukoplakia. *Am J Surgical Pathol.* 1989;13(2):114–119.
16. White III CL, Taxy JB. Early morphologic diagnosis of herpes simplex virus encephalitis: advantages of electron microscopy and immunoperoxidase staining. *Human Pathol.* 1983;14:135–139.
17. Dunkle LM, Arvin AM, Whitley RJ, et al: A controlled trial of acyclovir for chickenpox in normal children. *N Engl J Med.* 1991;325:1539–1544.
18. Strauss SE, Ostrove JM, Inchauspe G, et al. Varicella-zoster virus infections. Biology, natural history, treatment and prevention. *Ann Internal Med.* 1988;108:221–237.
19. Henry C, Hartsock RJ, Kirk Z, and Behrer R. Detection of viruria in cytomegalovirus-infected infants by electron microscopy. *Am J Clin Pathol.* 1978;69:435–439.
20. Lee FK, Nahmias AJ, Stagno S. Rapid diagnosis of cytomegalovirus infection in infants by electron microscopy. *N Engl J Med.* 1978;299:1266–1270.
21. Folkers E, Vreeswijk J, Wagenaar F, Kapsenberg JG, Hulsebosch HJ, Oranje AP. Immunoelectron microscopy for rapid diagnosis of varicella-zoster virus in a complicated case of human T-cell lymphotropic virus type 1 infection. *J Clin Microbiol.* 1992;30:2487–2491.
22. Corey L. The diagnosis and treatment of genital herpes. *JAMA.* 1982;248:1041–1049.
23. Amstey MS. Management of pregnancy complicated by genital herpes virus infection. *Obstet Gynecol.* 1971; 37:515–519.
24. Janoff EN, Orenstein JM, Manischewitz JF, Smith PD. Adenovirus colitis in the acquired immunodeficiency syndrome. *Gastroenterology.* 1991;100:976–979.
25. Chaisson RE, Griffin DE. Progressive multifocal leukoencephalopathy in AIDS. *JAMA.* 1990;264:79–82.
26. Orenstein JM, Jannotta F. Human immunodeficiency virus and papovavirus infections in acquired immunodeficiency syndrome: an ultrastructural study of three cases. *Hum Pathol.* 1988;19:350–361.
27. ZuRhein G, Chou SM. Particles resembling papovaviruses in human cerebral demyelinating disease. *Science.* 1965; 148:1477–1479.
28. Arthur RR, Shah KV, Baust SJ, Santos GW, Saral R. Association of BK viruria with hemorrhagic cystitis in recipients of bone marrow transplant. *N Eng J Med.* 1986;315: 230–234.
29. Saitoh K, Koike N, Akiyama Y, Iwamura Y, Kimura H. Diagnosis of childhood cystitis by electron microscopy and PCR. *J Clin Pathol.* 1993;46:773–775.
30. Nagington J. Electron microscopy in differential diagnosis of poxvirus infections. *Brit Med J.* 1964;2:1499–1500.
31. Cruickshank JG, Bedson HS, Watson DH. Electron microscopy in the rapid diagnosis of smallpox. *Lancet.* 1966;2:527–530.
32. Kapikian AZ, Wyatt RG, Greenberg HB, et al. Approaches to immunization of infants and young children against gastroenteritis due to rotavirus. *Rev Infect Dis.* 1980; 2:459–469.
33. Wolf JL, Schreiber DS. Viral gastroenteritis. *Med Clin North Am.* 1982;66:575–595.
34. Sack RB. Human diarrheal disease caused by enterotoxigenic *Escherichia coli. Ann Rev Microbiol.* 1975;29:333–353.
35. Knight R. Giardiasis, isosporiasis and balantidiasis. *Clin Gastroenterol.* 1978;7:31–47.
36. Pickering LK, Evans DJ, Munoz O, et al. Prospective study of enteropathogens in children with diarrhea in Houston and Mexico. *J Pediatr.* 1978;93:383–388.
37. McLean CC. The periodic seasonal incidence of gastrointestinal symptoms complicating respiratory infections in childhood: seasonal gastroenteritis. *Southern Med J.* 1931;24:624–632.
38. Gordon I, Ingraham HS, Kerns RF. Transmission of epidemic gastroenteritis to human volunteers by oral administration of fecal filtrates. *J Exper Med.* 1947;86:409–422.
39. Wyatt RG, James WD. Methods of gastroenteritis virus culture in vivo and in vitro. In: Tyrrell DAJ, Kapikian AZ, eds. *Virus Infections of the Gastrointestinal Tract.* New York: Marcel Dekker; 1982:13–35.
40. Kapikian AZ, Wyatt RG, Dolin R, Thornhill TS, Kalica AR, Chanock RM. Visualization by immune electron microscopy of a 27-nm particle associated with acute infectious, non-bacterial gastroenteritis. *J Virol.* 1972;10:1075–1081.
41. Fang Z-Y, Ye Q, Ho M-S, et al. Investigation of an outbreak of adult diarrhea rotavirus in China. *J Infect Dis.* 1989;160:948–953.
42. Yong DCT, Peter JB. Using DEM to detect pediatric viral gastroenteritis. *Diagn Med.* Nov–Dec 1984:45–51.
43. Kjeldsberg E. Application of electron microscopy in viral diagnosis. *Pathol Res Practice.* 1980;167:3–21.
44. Blacklow NR, Cukor G. Viral gastroenteritis. *N Engl J Med.* 1981;304:397–406.
45. Payne CM, Ray CG, Borduin V, Minnich LL, Lebowitz MD. An eight-year study of the viral agents of acute gastroenteritis in humans: ultrastructural observations and seasonal distribution with a major emphasis on coronavirus-like particles. *Diagn Microbiol Infect Dis.* 1986;5:39–54.
46. Lew JF, Glass RI, Petric M, et al. Six-year retrospective surveillance of gastroenteritis viruses identified at ten elec-

tron microscopy centers in the United States and Canada. *Pediatr Infect Dis J.* 1990;9:709–714.
47. Payne CM, Ray CG, Yolken RH. The 30- to 54-nm rotavirus-like particles in gastroenteritis: incidence and antigenic relationship to rotavirus. *J Med Virol.* 1981; 7:299–313.
48. Berthiaume L, Alain R, McLaughlin B, Payment P, Trepanier P. Rapid detection of human viruses in faeces by a simple and routine immune electron microscopy technique. *J Gen Virol.* 1981;55:223–227.
49. Chany C, Moscovici O, Lebon, P, Rousset S. Association of coronavirus infection with neonatal necrotizing enterocolitis. *Pediatrics.* 1982;69:209–214.
50. Mortensen ML, Ray CG, Payne CM, Friedman AD, Minnich LL, Rousseau C. Coronaviruslike particles in human gastrointestinal disease. Epidemiologic, clinical, and laboratory observations. *Am J Dis Children.* 1985;139:928–934.
51. Koopmans M, Petric M, Glass RI, Monroe SS. Enzyme-linked immunosorbent assay reactivity of torovirus-like particles in fecal specimens from humans with diarrhea. *J Clin Microbiol.* 1993;31:2738–2744.
52. Beards CM, Brown DWG, Green J, Flewett TH. Preliminary characterisation of torovirus-like particles of humans: comparison with Berne virus of horses and Breda virus of calves. *J Med Virol.* 1986;20:67–78.
53. Snijder EJ, Horzinek MC, Spaan JM. The coronaviruslike superfamily. *Adv Exper Med Biol.* 1992;342:235–244.
54. Snijder EJ, Horzinek MC. Toroviruses: replication, evolution and comparison with other members of the coronavirus-like superfamily. *J Gen Virol.* 1993;74:2305–2316.
55. Vaucher YE, Ray CG, Minnich LL, Payne CM, Beck D, Lowe P. Pleomorphic, enveloped, virus-like particles associated with gastrointestinal illness in neonates. *J Infect Dis.* 1982;145:27–36.
56. Centers for Disease Control. Kaposi's sarcoma and pneumocystis pneumonia among homosexual men—New York City and California. *MMWR.* 1981;30:305–308.
57. Centers for Disease Control. Prevention of acquired immune deficiency syndrome (AIDS): report of inter-agency recommendations. *MMWR.* 1983;32:101–103.
58. Ioachim HL. Acquired immune deficiency disease after three years. The unsolved riddle. *Lab Invest.* 1984;51:1–6.
59. Elvin-Lewis M, Witte M, Witte C. Cole W, Davis J. Systemic chlamydial infection associated with generalized lymphedema and lymphangiosarcoma. *Lymphology.* 1973;6: 113–121.
60. Witte MH, Witte CL, Minnich LL, Finley PR. AIDS in 1968. *JAMA.* 1968;251:2657.
61. Garry RF, Witte MH, Gottlieb AA, et al. Documentation of an AIDS virus infection in the United States in 1968. *JAMA.* 1988;260:2085–2087.
62. Gonda M, Wong-Staal F, Gallo RC, Clements JE, Narayan O, Gilden RV. Sequence homology and morphologic similarity of HTLV-III and visna virus, a pathogenic lentivirus. *Science.* 1985;227:173–177.
63. Gallo RC, Sarin PS, Gelmann EP, et al. Isolation of human T-cell leukemia virus in acquired immune deficiency syndrome (AIDS). *Science.* 1983;220:865–867.
64. Barre-Sinoussi F, Chermann JC, Rey F, et al. Isolation of a T-lymphotropic retrovirus from a patient at risk for acquired immune deficiency syndrome (AIDS). *Science.* 1983;220:868–871.
65. Scholtyseck E, Mehlhorn H, Friedhoff K. The fine structure of the conoid of Sporozoa and related organisms. *Zeitschrift fur Parasitenkunde.* 1970;34:68–94.
66. Scholtyseck E, Mehlhorn H. Ultrastructural study of characteristic organelles (paired organelles, micronemes, micropores) of Sporozoa and related organisms. *Zeitschrift fur Parasitenkunde.* 1970;34:97–127.
67. Powell HC, Gibbs Jr CJ, Lorenzo AM, Lampert PW, Gajdusek DC. Toxoplasmosis of the central nervous system in the adult. Electron microscopic observations. *Acta Neuropathol. (Berlin)* 1978;41:211–216.
68. Sulzer AJ, Scholtyseck E, Callaway C, Smith MT, Huber TW. Diagnosis of toxoplasmosis by electron microscopic fine-structural analysis. *Am J Clin Pathol.* 1979;72:225–229.
69. Cerezo L, Alvarez M, Price G. Electron microscopic diagnosis of cerebral toxoplasmosis. *J Neurosurgery.* 1985; 63:470–472.
70. Tang TT, Harb JM, Dunne Jr WM, et al. Cerebral toxoplasmosis in an immunodeficient host. A precise and rapid diagnosis by electron microscopy. *Am J Clin Pathol.* 1986; 85:104–110.
71. Casemore DP, Sands RL, Curry A. Cryptosporidium species: a "new" human pathogen. *J Clin Pathol.* 1985; 38:1321–1336.
72. Godwin TA. Cryptosporidiosis in the acquired immunodeficiency syndrome: a study of 15 autopsy cases. *Hum Pathol.* 1991;22:1215–1224.
73. Mannheimer SB, Soave R. Protozoal infections in patients with AIDS. Cryptosporidiosis, isosporiasis, cyclosporiasis, and microsporidiosis. *Infect Dis Clin North Am.* 1994;8: 483–498.
74. Perrone TL, Dickersin GR. The intracellular location of cryptosporidia. *Hum Pathol.* 1983;14:1092–1093.
75. Wurz R. *Cyclospora:* a new identified intestinal pathogen of humans. *Clin Infect Dis.* 1994;18:620–623.
76. Ortega YR, Sterling CR, Gilman RH, Cama VA, Diaz F. Cyclospora species—a new protozoan pathogen of humans. *N Engl J Med.* 1993;328:1308–1312.
77. Ortega YR, Gilman RH, Sterling CR. A new coccidian parasite (Apicomplexa: Eimeriidae) from humans. *J Parasitol.* 1994;80:625–629.
78. Hoge CW, Schlim DR, Rajah R, et al. Epidemiology of diarrhoeal illness associated with coccidian-like organism among travellers and foreign residents in Nepal. *Lancet.* 1993;341:1175–1179.
79. Berlin OGW, Novak SM, Porschen RK, Long EG, Stelma GN, Schaeffer III FW. Recovery of *Cyclospora* organisms from patients with prolonged diarrhea. *Clin Infect Dis.* 1994;18:606–609.
80. Pape JW, Verdier R-I, Boncy M, Boncy J, Johnson Jr WD (*Cyclospora*) infection in adults infected with HIV. Clinical manifestations, treatment, and prophylaxis. *Ann Intern Med.* 1994;121:654–657.
81. Bronsdon MA. Rapid dimethyl sulfoxide-modified acid-fast stain of *Cryptosporidium* oocysts in stool specimens. *J Clin Microbiol.* 1984;19:952–953.

82. Daneshbod K. Localized lymphadenitis due to Leishmania simulating Toxoplasmosis. Value of electron microscopy for differentiation. *Am J Clin Pathol.* 1978;69:462–467.
83. Adam RD. The biology of *Giardia* spp (1991). *Microbiol Rev.* 1991;55:706–732.
84. Stevens DP. Selective primary health care; strategies for control of diseases in the developing world. XIX. Giardiasis. *Rev Infect Dis.* 1985;7:530–535.
85. Farthing MJG, Mata L, Urrutia JJ, Kronmal RA. Natural history of *Giardia* infection of infants and children in rural Guatemala and its impact on physical growth. *Am J Clin Nutrition.* 1986;43:395–405.
86. Gilman RH, Brown KH, Visvesvara GS, et al. Epidemiology and serology of *Giardia lamblia* in a developing country: Bangladesh. *Trans Royal Soc Trop Med Hyg.* 1985;79:469–473.
87. Mason PR, Patterson BA. Epidemiology of *Giardia lamblia* infection in children: cross-sectional and longitudinal studies in urban and rural communities in Zimbabwe. *Am J Trop Med Hyg.* 1987;37:277–282.
88. Klima M, Gyorkey P, Min K-W, Gyorkey F. Electron microscopy in the diagnosis of Giardiasis. *Arch Pathol Lab Med.* 1977;101:133–135.
89. Davidson RA. Issues in clinical parasitology: the treatment of giardiasis. *Am J Gastroenterol.* 1984;79:256–261.
90. Weber R, Bryan RT, Schwartz DA, Owen RL. Human microsporidial infections. *Clin Microbiol Rev.* 1994;7:426–461.
91. Canning EU, Hollister WS. Microsporidia of mammals—widespread pathogens or opportunistic curiosities? *Parasitol Today.* 1987;3:267–276.
92. Cali A. General microsporidian features and recent findings on AIDS isolates. *J Protozool.* 1991;38:625–630.
93. Margileth AM, Strano AJ, Chandra R, Neafie R, Blum M, McCully RM. Disseminated nosematosis in an immunologically compromised infant. *Arch Pathol.* 1973;95:145–150.
94. Pinnolis M, Egbert PR, Font RL, Winter FC. Nosematosis of the cornea. Case report, including electron microscopic studies. *Arch Ophthalmol.* 1981;99:1044–1047.
95. Cali A, Owen RL. Intracellular development of *Enterocytozoon,* a unique microsporidian found in the intestine of AIDS patients. *J Protozool.* 1990;37:145–155.
96. Orenstein JM. Microsporidiosis in the acquired immunodeficiency syndrome. *J Parasitol.* 1991;77:843–864.
97. Cali A, Orenstein JM, Kotler DP, Owen R. A comparison of two microsporidian parasites in enterocytes of AIDS patients with chronic diarrhea. *J Protozool.* 1991;38:96S–98S.
98. Molina J-M, Oksenhendler E, Beauvais B, et al. Disseminated microsporidiosis due to *Septata intestinalis* in patients with AIDS: clinical features and response to albendazole therapy. *J Infect Dis.* 1995;171:245–249.
99. Bartlett JG, Belitsos PC, Sears CL. AIDS enteropathy. *Clin Infect Dis.* 1992;15:726–735.
100. Asmuth DM, DeGirolami PC, Federman M, et al. Clinical features of microsporidiosis in patients with AIDS. *Clin Infect Dis.* 1994;18:819–825.
101. Diesenhouse MC, Wilson LA, Corrent GC, Visvesvara GS, Grossniklaus HE, Bryan RT. Treatment of microsporidial keratoconjunctivitis with topical fumagillin. *Am J Ophthalmol.* 1994;115:293–298.
102. Moe AA, Hardy WD. *Pneumocystis carinii* infection in the HIV-seropositive patient. *Infect Dis Clin North Am.* 1994;8:331–364.
103. Blaser MJ, Cohn DL. Opportunistic infections in patients with AIDS: clues to the epidemiology of AIDS and the relative virulence of pathogens. *Rev Infect Dis.* 1986;8:21–30.
104. Mills J. *Pneumocystis carinii* and *Toxoplasma gondii* infection in patients with AIDS. *Rev Infect Dis.* 1986;8:1001–1011.
105. Hennequin C, Page B, Roux P, Legendre C, Kreis H. Outbreak of *Pneumocystis carinii* pneumonia in a renal transplant unit. *Eur J Clin Microbiol Infect Dis.* 1995;14:122–126.
106. Jacobs JL, Libby DM, Winters RA, et al. A cluster of *Pneumocystis carinii* pneumonia in adults without predisposing illnesses. *N Engl J Med.* 1991;324:246–250.
107. Hasleton PS, Curry A, Rankin EM. *Pneumocystis carinii* pneumonia: a light microscopical and ultrastructural study. *J Clin Pathol.* 1981;34:1138–1146.
108. Walzer PD. *Pneumocystis carinii*—new clinical spectrum? *N Engl J Med.* 1991;324:263–265.
109. Haque A, Plattner SB, Cook RT, Hart MN. *Pneumocystis carinii.* Taxonomy as viewed by electron microscopy. *Am J Clin Pathol.* 1987;87:504–510.
110. Edman JC, Kovacs JA, Masur H, Santi DV, Elwood HJ, Sogin ML. Ribosomal RNA sequence shows *Pneumocystis carinii* to be a member of the fungi. *Nature.* 1988;334:519–522.
111. Stringer S, Stringer J, Blase M, Walzer P, Cushion M. *Pneumocystis carinii:* sequence from ribosomal RNA implies a close relationship with fungi. *Exper Parasitol.* 1989;68:450–461.
112. Lundgren B, Kovacs JA, Nelson NN, Stock F, Martinez A, Gill VJ. *Pneumocystis carinii* and specific fungi have a common epitope, identified by a monoclonal antibody. *J Clin Microbiol.* 1992;30:391–395.
113. De Stefano JA, Cushion MT, Puvanesarajah V, Walzer PD. Analysis of *Pneumocystis carinii* cyst wall. II. Sugar composition. *J Protozool.* 1990;37:436–441.
114. Walzer PD. *Pneumocystis carinii:* recent advances in basic biology and their clinical application. *AIDS.* 1993;7:1293–1305.
115. Cushion MT, Ebbets D. Growth and metabolism of *Pneumocystis carinii* in axenic culture. *J Clin Microbiol.* 1990;28:1385–1394.
116. Schmatz DM, Romancheck MA, Pittarelli LA, et al. Treatment of *Pneumocystis carinii* pneumonia with 1,3-beta-glucan synthesis inhibitors. *Proc Natl Acad Sci USA.* 1990;87:5950–5954.
117. Murry CE, Schmidt RA. Tissue invasion by *Pneumocystis carinii:* a possible cause of cavitary pneumonia and pneumothorax. *Hum Pathol.* 1992;23:1380–1387.
118. Goheen MP, Blumershine R, Bartlett MS, Hull MT, Smith JW. Improved intracellular morphology of *Pneumocystis carinii* from rat lung by postfixation with a mixture of

potassium ferrocyanide and osmium tetroxide. *Biotechnic Histochem.* 1992;67:140–148.

119. El-Sadr W, Sidhu G. Persistence of trophozoites after successful treatment of *Pneumocystis carinii* pneumonia. *Ann Intern Med.* 1986;105:889–890.
120. Costerton JW. The role of electron microscopy in the elucidation of bacterial structure and function. *Ann Rev Microbiol.* 1979;33:459–479.
121. Costerton JW, Irvin RT. The bacterial glycocalyx in nature and disease. *Ann Rev Microbiol.* 1981;35:299–324.
122. Kirk J. Diagnostic ultrastructure of *Listeria monocytogenes* in human central nervous tissue. *Ultrastructural Pathol.* 1993;17:583–592.
123. Costerton JW, Ingram JM, Cheng K-J. Structure and function of the cell envelope of gram-negative bacteria. *Bacteriol Rev.* 1974;38:87–110.
124. Strohm H, Payne CM, Ryan KJ. Demonstration of *Bacteroides* capsules by light microscopy and ultrastructural cytochemistry. *Am J Clin Pathol.* 1983;79:591–597.
125. Thiery JP. Mise en evidence des polysaccharides sur coupes fines en microscopic electronique. *J Microscopie.* 1967;6:987–1018.
126. Duguid JP. The demonstration of bacterial capsules and slime. *J Pathol Bacteriol.* 1951;63:673–685.
127. Orenstein JM, Kotler DP. Diarrheogenic bacterial enteritis in acquired immune deficiency syndrome: a light and electron microscopy study of 52 cases. *Hum Pathol.* 1995;26:481–492.
128. Schinella RA, Greco MA. Bacillary angiomatosis presenting as a soft-tissue tumor without skin involvement. *Hum Pathol.* 1990;21:567–569.
129. Piepkorn MW, Reichenbach DD. Infective endocarditis associated with cell wall-deficient bacteria. Electron microscopic findings in four cases. *Hum Pathol.* 1978;9:163–173.
130. Lo S-C, Dawson MS, Wong DM, et al. Identification of *Mycoplasma incognitus* infection in patients with AIDS: an immunohistochemical, in situ hybridization and ultrastructural study. *Am J Trop Med Hyg.* 1989;41:601–616.
131. Bauer FA, Wear DJ, Angritt P, Lo S-C. *Mycoplasma fermentans* (incognitus strain) infection in the kidneys of patients with acquired immunodeficiency syndrome and associated nephropathy: a light microscopic, immunohistochemical, and ultrastructural study. *Hum Pathol.* 1991;22:63–69.
132. Geisbert TW, Jahrling PB, Ezzell Jr JW. Use of immunoelectron microscopy to demonstrate *Francisella tularensis*. *J Clin Microbiol.* 1993;31:1936–1939.
133. Chears WC, Ashworth CT. Electron microscopic study of the intestinal mucosa in Whipple's disease. Demonstration of encapsulated bacilliform bodies in the lesion. *Gastroenterology.* 1961;41:129–138.
134. Yardley JH, Hendrix TR. Combined electron and light microscopy in Whipple's disease. *Bull Johns Hopkins Hosp.* 1961;109:80–98.
135. Ashworth CT, Douglas FC, Reynolds RC, Thomas PJ. Bacillus-like bodies in Whipple's disease; disappearance with clinical remission after antibiotic therapy. *Am J Med.* 1964;37:481–490.
136. Trier JS, Phelps PC, Eidelman S, Rubin CE. Whipple's disease: light and electron microscope correlation of jejunal mucosal histology with antibiotic treatment and clinical status. *Gastroenterology.* 1965;48:684–707.
137. Dobbins WO, Ruffin JM. A light- and electron-microscopic study of bacterial invasion in Whipple's disease. *Am J Pathol.* 1967;51:225–242.
138. Denholm RB, Mills PR, More IAR. Electron microscopy in the long term follow-up of Whipple's disease. Effect of antibiotics. *Am J Surgical Pathol.* 1981;5:507–516.
139. Dobbins III WO, Kawanishi H. Bacillary characteristics in Whipple's disease: an electron microscopic study. *Gastroenterology.* 1981;80:1468–1475.
140. Kasper DL. The polysaccharide capsule of *Bacteroides fragilis* subspecies fragilis: immunochemical and morphologic definition. *J Infect Dis.* 1976;133:79–87.
141. Kasper DL, Hayes ME, Reinap BG, Craft FO, Onderdonk AB, Polk BF. Isolation and identification of encapsulated strains of *Bacteroides fragilis*. *J Infect Dis.* 1977;136:75–81.
142. Fraser DW, McDade JE. Legionellosis. *Sci Am.* 1979;241:82–99.
143. Chandler FW, Hicklin MD, Blackmon JA. Demonstration of the agent of Legionnaire's disease in tissue. *N Engl J Med.* 1977;297:1218–1220.
144. Chandler FW, Blackmon JA, Hicklin MD, Cole RM, Callaway CS. Ultrastructure of the agent of Legionnaires' disease in the human lung. *Am J Clin Pathol.* 1979;71:43–50.
145. Chandler FW, Cole RM, Hicklin MD, Blackmon JA, Callaway CS. Ultrastructure of the Legionnaires' disease bacterium. *Ann Intern Med.* 1979;90:642–647.
146. Blackmon JA, Chandler FW, Cherry WB, et al. Review article. Legionellosis. *Am J Pathol.* 1981;103:429–465.
147. Breiman RF, Cozen W, Fields BS, et al. Role of air-sampling in an investigation of an outbreak of Legionnaires' disease associated with exposure to aerosols from an evaporative condenser. *J Infect Dis.* 1990;161:1257–1261.
148. Maiwald M, Schill M, Stockinger C, et al. Detection of *Legionella* DNA in human and guinea pig urine samples by the polymerase chain reaction. *Eur J Microbiol Infect Dis.* 1995;14:25–33.

CHAPTER 3

Immunohistochemistry and In Situ Hybridization Techniques in the Detection of Infectious Organisms

Norio Azumi

Art does not reproduce the visible; rather, it makes visible.

Paul Klee (1879–1940), Creative Credo

Make visible what, without you, might perhaps never have been seen.

Robert Bresson (b. 1907), Notes on the Cinematographer

INTRODUCTION

Confirming the diagnosis of a specific infectious disease continues to challenge pathologists and microbiologists alike. Traditionally, a diagnosis was made when the pathologist identified the infectious organism in a lesion and the microbiologist grew it in culture. When culture was not possible, however, the identification of the infectious agent fell solely on the shoulders of the anatomic pathologist who, by light microscopy and by special stains, was the mainstay in identifying infectious organisms in tissue sections.

Now, however, a new age has dawned in the diagnosis of infectious diseases: Antigen and DNA/RNA sequences specific to an infectious agent can be detected even from formalin-fixed paraffin-embedded sections using immunohistochemistry (IHC), in situ hybridization (ISH), and in situ polymerase chain reaction (PCR) techniques. These techniques have made it possible to identify specific infectious agents and their subtypes and simultaneously to observe tissue reaction. The advantages of these new techniques over conventional methods include high sensitivity and specificity with subtyping, reduced risk of exposure to laboratory personnel, promptness, and detection of organisms that are difficult or impossible to culture. The only limitation is the availability of specific antibodies and nucleic acid probes that detect the antigens and/or nucleic acid sequences of an infectious agent. A brief description of IHC and ISH techniques in tissue sections and their clinical application follows. The detection of specific DNA or RNA sequences can be also accomplished on extracted nucleic acids using PCR and ISH (see Chapter 4, Principles of Molecular Diagnostics).

OVERVIEW OF TECHNICAL ASPECTS

Immunofluorescence and Immunohistochemistry Methods

When an antibody that is specific to antigens (protein, polysaccharides) of a given organism (which is often called the primary antibody in modern multistep IHC) is applied to a tissue section, it attaches to the organism. The antibody, however, cannot be seen by light microscopy. Two major techniques make this antigen–antibody complex visible: IHC and immunofluorescence.

The most basic form of immunofluorescence uses a fluorescein compound, a such as fluorescein isothiocyanate or tetramethylrhodamin isothiocyanate, which are directly attached to the antibodies. Thus under a fluorescent microscope, the attached antibody (ie, where the organisms are present) emits visible light. Although this method is a simple one-step procedure, there are significant shortcomings: a low sensitivity, autofluorescence in formalin-fixed tissues, and poor visualization of surrounding tissue. Although this method still has limited use (eg, it is used to examine vaginal smears for trichomonads), IHC has largely replaced immunofluorescence.

There are many variations of the IHC technique, but the one used most widely that provides a high sensitivity without sacrificing specificity has three components: 1) a primary antibody, 2) a secondary or bridging antibody, and 3) a color developing system. The primary antibodies are specific to antigens and may be monoclonal or polyclonal. Monoclonal antibodies, when available, are usually preferred, because of the consistent quality and specific reactivity. Whereas polyclonal antibodies detect multiple, large epitopes, the monoclonal antibodies recognize a single, small epitope and when this epitope is masked or destroyed, a loss of reactivity will occur. A combination (a cocktail) of multiple monoclonal antibodies that recognize different epitopes of the same antigen and careful selection of specific clones that recognize fixation resistant epitopes and antigen retrieval all help to overcome this.

The secondary or bridging antibody is an antibody that reacts with the immunoglobulin species and class of the primary antibody. For example if the primary antibody is mouse IgG, then the secondary antibody is goat antibody against mouse IgG. Next, using the secondary antibody as a bridge, the color developing system must be localized. There are two main variations to do this. The first is the classic peroxidase–antiperoxidase (PAP) method. Here, the color developing system is composed of the third antibodies of the same immunoglobulin species and class as the primary antibody raised against peroxidase, which forms a PAP complex. The secondary antibody now can "bridge" the primary antibody and the PAP complex, thus peroxidase is linked to the primary antibody, which in turn is attached to the antigen (organisms). The same exact principle can be used in the alkaline phosphatase–antialkaline phosphatase method or with any enzyme.

The second, and more widely used, method is the avidin–biotin complex (ABC) method. In the ABC method, unique characteristics of biotin and avidin are exploited: 1) Biotin chemically binds to enzymes or antibodies readily (biotinylated enzyme or antibody), 2) avidin and biotin form strong and stable chemical bonds, and 3) avidin has excess biotin binding sites. Instead of using the third antibody, the secondary antibody and the enzyme are biotinylated. The biotinylated enzyme is mixed with avidin to form the ABC, which has unoccupied biotin biding sites in avidin. Thus when the secondary antibody and the ABC are layered consecutively, the enzyme is linked to the site of specific binding of the primary antibody. The last step in the color development system is the conversion of colorless chemicals to colored products with the help of the enzyme in the presence of an appropriate substrate. The most commonly used enzymes are peroxidase and alkaline phosphatase. Peroxidase is used with diaminobenzidine (DAB) (brown) or 3-amino-9-ethylcarbazole (AEC) (reddish brown) as chromogens and hydrogen peroxide as a substrate. Alkaline phosphatase is used with fast red TR (red) or fast blue BB (blue) as chromogens and naphthol AS-MX phosphate as a substrate. A DAB–peroxidase combination produces the most stable and permanent preparation.

The choice of method may be one of personal preference, but sometimes one method is better than the other. For example, the degree of interference from endogenous peroxidase and alkaline phosphatase in some normal tissues may vary depending on the IHC methods and types of tissues. Although most endogenous enzyme activities are abolished by formalin fixation and/or quenching using appropriate inhibitors, endogenous peroxidase activity in neutrophils, myeloid cells, and erythrocytes usually remains. Thus, when the IHC is performed on tissues with heavy inflammation and extensive hemorrhage or on bone marrow, alkaline–phosphatase may be a better choice. Another interference is due to abundant biotin in some normal tissues such as the liver. Although this is negligible in fixed tissues, the PAP method may yield better results than the ABC method when frozen sections are used. Finally, because most naturally occurring pigments such as melanin and hemosiderin are brown, they may interfere with the interpretation when DAB–peroxidase is used. Other enzyme and chromogen combinations that produced colors other than brown may be considered.

Antigens have multiple epitopes that can be detected by antibodies. However, fixation, especially with a cross-linking fixative such as formalin, may alter the epitopes to such a degree that they are not recognized by the antibodies. When tissue is fixed in cross-linking fixatives, pretreatment by proteolytic enzymes (enzyme digestion) such as trypsin, pepsin, and pronase may recover or "unmask" the epitopes. Alternatively, an antigen retrieval method using heat by microwave irradiation in citrate buffer achieves equivalent or better results and is now widely used in lieu of enzyme digestion. Because some antibodies detect epitopes that are not easily altered by fixation, the beneficial effects of antigen retrieval depend on the combination of antibodies and antigens (organisms). For example, commercially available antibodies to CMV, HIV, and *Pneumocystis carinii* require antigen retrieval or enzyme digestion.

In Situ Hybridization

ISH is very similar to IHC—IHC detects antigens using antibodies and ISH detects nucleic acid sequences using oligonucleotide probes. For example, an immediate-early antigen specific to CMV can be detected by the IHC and the DNA sequences that encode this protein by the ISH. The oligonucleotide probes used in ISH are complementary to the nucleic acid sequences of the organism through base-pairing. By choosing appropriate probes for either conserved or unique nucleic acid sequences, the ISH can be tailored to detect certain specific subtypes or larger related groups of organisms. An additional advantage over IHC or culture is that viral genomes can be detected even when complete viral particles are not produced and traditional cultures and IHC are negative. Although ISH may be performed on extracted nucleotides using gels and filters, ISH on tissue sections allows a pathologist to observe the location of the infectious organisms and tissue reaction to it.

The following is a brief description of the ISH technique on tissue sections. Chromosomal proteins, which cover strands of nucleic acids, must be removed by proteolytic digestion. Because the nucleic acids of infectious organisms including many viruses are "double stranded," they must be unraveled to a single strand by heating tissue sections to about 100°C for several minutes. Thus the nucleic acids strands are exposed, allowing them to combine with complementary nucleic acid probes. An oligonucleotide probe specific for an organism, which may be either labeled with radioactive isotopes or biotinylated, is then allowed to hybridize at 37°C for several hours. It is extremely important to maintain appropriate stringency conditions during the hybridization process to achieve the desired sensitivity and specificity. For example, with less stringent conditions, the probes may hybridize to similar but not completely complementary nucleic acid sequences. Autoradiography with radioactive probes or the color developing system identical to that used for the IHC with biotinylated probes are used to localize the signal. Because radioisotopes are cumbersome to use and lengthy exposure is usually necessary, biotinylated probes are most widely used for the detection of infectious organisms. Many commercially available probes are distributed in biotinylated forms as a kit, including washing buffers, with the stringency condition optimized. Although it is technically possible to amplify nucleic acid sequences by PCR in tissue sections (in situ PCR) and then to detect amplified nucleic acid sequences using the ISH technique, this method still remains investigational.

INDIVIDUAL ORGANISMS

Readers may wish to refer to the individual chapters in this book for the application of IHC and ISH techniques to a particular organism. The only limitations are the availability of specific antibodies or oligonucleotide probes and the preservation of epitopes or nucleic acids. No detailed discussion of the individual organisms is therefore necessary. However, some of the more important infectious organisms that a pathologist may encounter frequently are briefly discussed and selected references are also listed.

Cytomegalovirus

This virus contains double-stranded DNA. Commercially available antibodies usually detect fixation-resistant epitopes of immediate-early proteins, which require antigen retrieval for detection. These antibodies may be reactive intranuclearly before morphologically characteristic cytomegalic changes and intranuclear inclusions are formed. ISH will react with intracytoplasmic inclusions later in the infectious process (Figure 3–1, A). Commercially available DNA probes target the viral structural protein genes (late and immediate-early). Thus it is possible to detect proteins by IHC and the corresponding gene sequence by ISH (Figure 3–1, B) such as IE84 (protein) and *IE2* (gene), respectively. The sensitivity and specificity of IHC and ISH are better than light microscopic identification of inclusion bodies and compare favorably with culture and ISH using extracted DNA.

Herpes Simplex Virus

Like cytomegalovirus, herpes simplex virus (HSV 1 and 2) contains double-stranded DNA. The polyclonal antibodies raised against all the viral proteins are best in detecting herpesvirus in formalin-fixed paraffin-embedded sections (Figure 3–2). Because these polyclonal antibodies react with both type-specific and common antigens, there is some cross-reactivity of HSV 1 and 2. DNA probes are commercially available for the specific detection of HSV 1 and 2 that have a sensitivity equal to that of IHC.

JC Virus

JC virus also contains double-stranded DNA and causes progressive multifocal leukoencephalopathy (PML) in immunodeficient patients such as those infected with HIV. Because of the widespread use of stereotactic needle biopsy of the brain in patients with AIDS with sus-

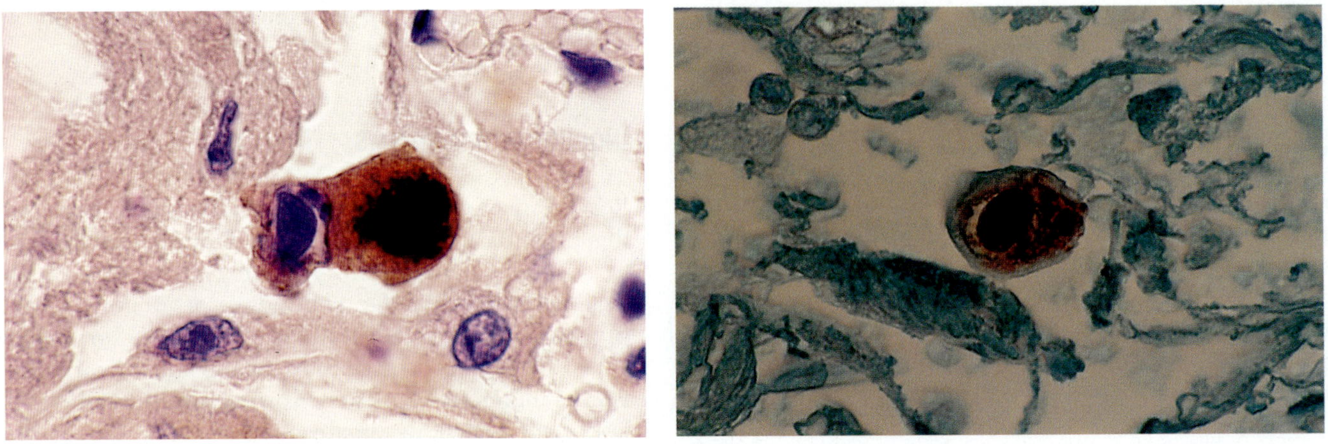

A B

Figure 3–1. Cytomegalovirus: The lung showing pneumonitis due to cytomegalovirus. Both intranuclear and intracytoplasmic inclusions are positive by (**A**) the immunoperoxidase and (**B**) in situ hybridization techniques.

pected encephalitis, pathologists often are confronted with different diagnostic possibilities including PML, herpetic, and toxoplasmic encephalitis. Although characteristic intranuclear inclusions and histologic changes are pathognomonic in some patients, the diagnosis may be difficult when there are only small tissue fragments or when typical inclusions are not found. Polyclonal antibodies raised against SV40 (simian polyomavirus) viral protein cross-react with JC virus (both are *Papovaviridae*) but do not react with herpesvirus and can be used for the diagnosis of PML. More specific detection of JC virus is possible using DNA probes to a subregion of the viral genome (early region *MAD1*) (Figure 3–3). Both IHC and ISH have about equal sensitivity when paraffin sections are used.

Human Papillomavirus

Although infection by human papillomavirus (HPV) is self-limited and most commonly causes "warts," it has become a widespread venereal disease in recent years and, more important, it is associated with epithelial dysplasia and carcinoma. More than 60 types of HPV are now recognized. HPV are tissue and site specific, and each produces a specific lesion. The "epidermodysplasia verruciformis" group, which includes types 6, 11, 16, 18, 31, 35, 42, 44, 45, 51, and 56, involves anogenital areas and is associated with dysplasia and carcinoma. Detection of only these types of HPV in biopsy specimens from the anogenital areas has practical benefit.

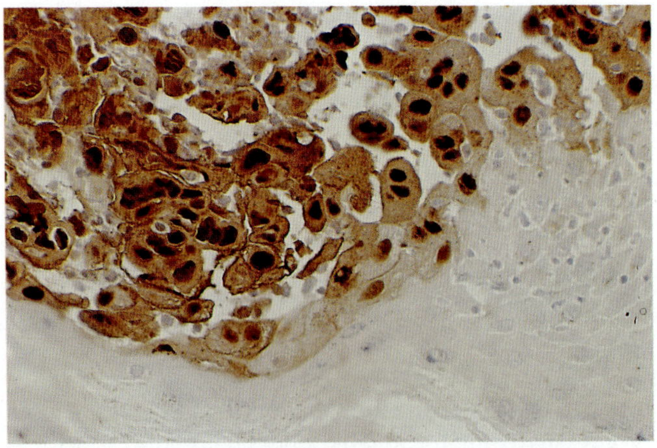

Figure 3–2. HSV 1: Skin with herpetic vesicles. Numerous intranuclear inclusion of herpesvirus type 1 (HSV 1) at the edge of the vesicle are noted (immunoperoxidase method).

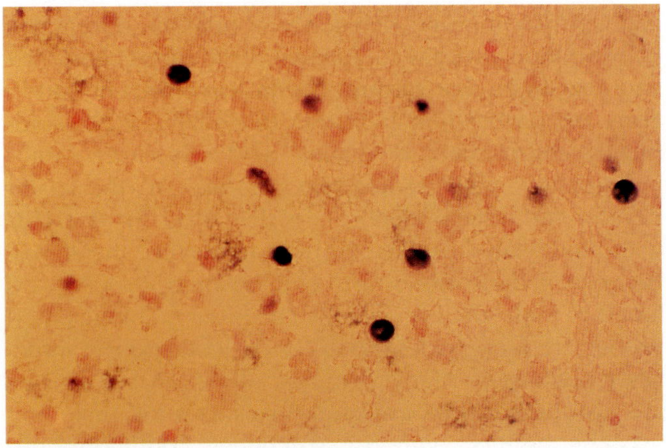

Figure 3–3. JC virus: Brain tissue with progressive multifocal leukoencephalitis. Many glial cells show intranuclear inclusion with a strong positive signal (in situ hybridization).

Unlike other viruses, the capsid protein of papillomavirus is highly conserved from species to species and from type to type. Polyclonal antibodies raised against capsid proteins, therefore, cross-react with all types of HPV and animal papillomaviruses as well. Another problem of the IHC method is that it only detects complete viral particles during productive infection (ie, HPV infection replicating complete viral particles). When viral DNA integrates itself into the human genome but becomes unproductive, a phenomenon associated with higher grade dysplasia and squamous cell carcinoma, IHC will not detect the HPV. Nevertheless, as a screening method or in patients with morphologically equivocal lesions, IHC may still be useful.

ISH can be tailored to detect individual types or a range of HPV types using single type-specific DNA probes or "cocktails" of DNA probes. HPV types 6, 11, 42, and 44 are associated with low oncogenic risk and HPV 16 and 18 with high oncogenic risk. The ISH method may not be able to detect HPV in higher grade dysplasia and squamous cell carcinoma because a copy number of HPV DNA may be small (as small as one copy per cell) and the estimated sensitivity of standard ISH is about 200 copies of HPV DNA per cell. An in situ PCR followed by ISH is reported to detect even one copy of an integrated viral genome. Controversy remains regarding whether IHC and ISH detection and typing of HPV are necessary for appropriate management of patients with HPV infection and dysplasia.

Toxoplasma

Identification of toxoplasma organisms by IHC has practical value in immunodeficient patients, especially in the brain lesions of AIDS patients and in myocardial biopsy specimens in patients with cardiac transplantation. Although cysts containing bradyzoites are readily identified by light microscopy, florid toxoplasma infections in immunodeficient patients often produce numerous tachyzoites without bradyzoites. In this situation, IHC helps to detect them. The wall of the cyst containing bradyzoites is composed of dead host or "nurse" cells and does not react with the antibodies (Figure 3–4).

Bacterial Infection

Although few bacteria and spirochetes have been studied using IHC, more and more antibodies are becoming commercially available. As a consequence, more bacterial organisms are being identified in formalin-fixed sections using IHC. However, several problems are associated with identification of the bacteria and spirochetes by IHC: 1) Many of the polyclonal antibodies may cross-react with similar or other organisms and 2) only part of the bacteria may react to antibodies. This second

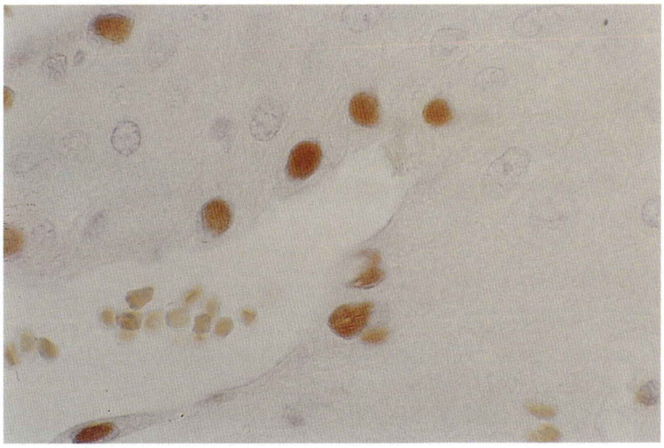

Figure 3–4. Toxoplasma: Placenta showing toxoplasmic infection. The content of the bradyzoites shows strong staining (immunoperoxidase method).

problem is further complicated by the coarse granular color products of many color developing systems used in IHC. This problem can be circumvented using the immunofluorescence technique. Sometimes, one can take advantage of the cross-reactivity; for example, it is possible to demonstrate *Helicobacter pylori* using antibodies to *Campylobacter* sp, which cross-react with *H pylori.*

SUGGESTED READINGS

The following are selected articles describing the detection of organisms using IHC and/or ISH.

Techniques

Naber SP. Molecular medicine. Molecular pathology—diagnosis of infectious disease. *N Engl J Med.* 1994:1212–1215.

Taylor CR, Cote RJ, eds. *Immunomicroscopy: A Diagnostic Tool for the Surgical Pathologist.* Philadelphia: WB Saunders; 1994.

Viruses

Adenovirus

Strickler JG, Singleton TP, Copenhaver CM, et al. Adenovirus in the gastrointestinal tracts of immunosuppressed patients. *Am J Clin Pathol.* 1992;97:555–558.

Cytomegalovirus

Arbustibi E, Grasso M, Diegoli M, et al. Histopathologic and molecular profile of human cytomegalovirus infections in patients with heart transplants. *Am J Clin Pathol.* 1992;98: 205–213.

Theise ND, Harber MM, Grimes MM. Detection of cytomegalovirus in lung allografts. Comparison of histologic and immunohistochemical findings. *Am J Clin Pathol.* 1991;96: 762–766.

Epstein–Barr Virus

Samoszuk M. Rapid detection of Epstein–Barr viral DNA by nonisotopic in situ hybridization. *Am J Clin Pathol.* 1001;96:448–453.

Hepatitis Virus

Davies SE, Lau JYN, O'Grady JG, et al. Evidence that hepatitis D virus needs hepatitis B virus to cause hepatocellular damage. *Am J Clin Pathol.* 1992;98:554–558.

Villari D, Pollicino T, Spinella S, et al. Hepatitis B e-antigen detection in formalin-fixed liver biopsy specimens. A tool to investigate wild-type and E-minus variant HBV infection. *Am J Clin Pathol.* 1995;103:136–140.

HIV Virus

Gosztonyi G, Artigas J, Lamperth L, Webster HD. Human immunodeficiency virus (HIV) distribution in HIV encephalitis: a study of 19 cases with combined use of in situ hybridization and immunocytochemistry. *J Neuropathol Exp Neurol.* 1994;53(5):521–534.

Human Papillomavirus

Duggan MA, Boras VF, Inoue M, McGregor SE, Robertson DI. Human papillomavirus DNA determination of anal condylomata, dysplasias, and squamous carcinomas with in situ hybridization. *Am J Clin Pathol.* 1989;92:16–21.

Gupta JW, Gupta PK, Rosenshein N, et al. Detection of human papillomavirus in cervical smears. A comparison of in situ hybridization, immunocytochemistry and cytopathology. *Acta Cytol.* 1987;31:387.

Kadish AS, Burk RD, Kress Y, et al. Human papillomaviruses of different types in precancerous lesions of the uterine cervix: histologic, immunocytochemical and ultrastructural studies. *Hum Pathol.* 1986;17:384.

Liang XM, Wieczorek RL, Koss LG. In situ hybridization with human papillomavirus using biotinylated DNA probes on archival cervical smears. *J Histochem Cytochem.* 1991;39: 771–775.

Lorimier P, Lamarcq L, Labat-Moleur F, Guillermet C, Bethier R, Stoebner P. Enhanced chemiluminescence: a high-sensitivity detection system for in situ hybridization and immunohistochemistry. *J Histochem Cytochem.* 1993;41: 1591–1597.

Nuovo GJ. *PCR In Situ Hybridization, Protocols and Applications.* New York: Raven Press; 1992.

Schadendorf D, Tiedemann K-H, Haas N, et al. Detection of human papillomaviruses in paraffin-embedded condylomata acuminata—comparison of immunohistochemistry, in situ hybridization, and polymerase chain reaction. *J Invest Dermatol.* 1991;97:549.

Wilbur DC, Reichman RC, Stoler MH. Detection of infection by human papillomavirus in genital condylomata. A comparison study using immunocytochemistry and in situ nucleic acid hybridization. *Am J Clin Pathol.* 1988;89:505.

Yang GC, Demopoulos RI, Chan W, Mittal KR. Superficial nuclear enlargement without koilocytosis as an expression of human papillomavirus infection of the uterine cervix: an in situ hybridization study. *Int J Gynecol Pathol.* 1992;11: 283–287.

Zehbe I, Rylander E, Strand A, Wilander E. Use of Probemix and OmniProbe biotinylated cDNA probes for detecting HPV infection in biopsy specimens from the genital tract. *J Clin Pathol.* 1993;46:437–440.

Influenza Virus

Kohama M, Cardenas JM, Seto JT. Immunoelectron microscopy study of the detection of the glycoproteins of influenza and Sendai viruses in infected cells by the immunoperoxidase method. *J Virol Methods.* 1981;3:293.

Luck PC, Helbig JH, Witzleb W. Immunofluroescent staining of influenza virus antigen in fixed and paraffin-embedded tissue of experimental infected hamsters. *Acta Histochem.* 1989;85:47.

Swenson PD, Kaplan MH. Rapid detection of influenza virus in cell culture by indirect immunoperoxidase staining with type-specific monoclonal antibodies. *Diagn Microbiol Infect Dis.* 1987;7:265.

JC Virus (Progressive Multifocal Leukoencephalopathy)

Aksamit AJ Jr. Nonradioactive in situ hybridization in progressive multifocal leukoencephalopathy. *Mayo Clin Proc.* 1993; 68(9):899–910.

Aksamit AJ, Gendelman HE, Orenstein JM, Pezeshkpour GH. AIDS-associated progressive multifocal leukoencephalopathy (PML): comparison to non-AIDS PML with in situ hybridization and immunohistochemistry. *Neurology.* 1990; 40:1073–1078.

Aksamit AJ, Sever JL, Major EO. Progressive multifocal leukoencephalopathy: JC virus detection by in situ hybridization compared with immunohistochemistry. *Neurology.* 1986; 36:499.

Hulette CM, Downey BT, Burger PC. Progressive multifocal leukoencephalopathy. Diagnosis by in situ hybridization with a biotinylated JC virus DNA probe using an automated Histomatic Code-On slide stainer. *Am J Surg Pathol.* 1991; 15:791–797.

Michalak WA, Cartun RW, Turner DO, et al. Immunocytochemical detection of papovavirus in progressive multifocal leukoencephalopathy (PML) with commercially available polyclonal antibody. *Mod Pathol.* 1989;2:63.

Mori M, Kurata H, Tajima M, Shimada H. JC virus detection by in situ hybridization in brain tissue from elderly patients. *Ann Neurol.* 1991;29:428–432.

Schmidbauer M, Budka H, Shah KV. Progressive multifocal leukoencephalopathy (PML) in AIDS and in the pre-AIDS era. A neuropathological comparison using immunocytochemistry and in situ DNA hybridization for virus detection. *Acta Neuropathol.* 1990;93:363.

Measles

Brown HR, Goller NL, Rudelli RD, Dymecki J, Wisniewski HM. Postmortem detection of measles virus in non-neural tissues in subacute sclerosing panencephalitis. *Ann Neurol.* 1989; 26:263–268.

McKenna MJ, Mills BG. Immunohistochemical evidence of measles virus in active otosclerosis. *Otolaryngol Head Neck Surg.* 1989;101:415.

McQuaid S, Allan GM. Detection protocols for biotinylated probes: optimization using multistep techniques. *J Histochem Cytochem.* 1992;40:569–574.

McQuaid S, Allen IV, McMahon J, Kirk J. Association of measles virus with neurofibrillary tangles in subacute sclerosing panencephalitis: a combined in situ hybridization and immunocytochemical investigation. *Neuropathol Appl Neurobiol.* 1994;20:103–110.

McQuaid S, Isserte S, Allan GM, Taylor MJ, Allen IV, Cosby SL. Use of immunocytochemistry and biotinylated in situ hybridization for detecting measles virus in central nervous system tissue. *J Clin Pathol.* 1990;43:329–333.

McQuaid S, Kirk J, Zhou AL, Allen IV. Measles virus infection of cells in perivascular infiltrates in the brain in subacute sclerosing panencephalitis: confirmation by non-radioactive in situ hybridization, immunocytochemistry and electron microscopy. *Acta Neuropathol (Berlin).* 1993;5:154–158.

Sata TS, Roth J, Zuber C, et al. Analysis of viral antigens in giant cells of measles pneumonia by immunoperoxidase method. *Virchows Arch A.* 1986;410:133.

Parvovirus

Frickenhofen N, Ablowitz JL, Safford M, et al. Persistent B19 parvovirus infection in patients infected with human immunodeficiency virus type 1 (HIV-1): a treatable cause of anemia in AIDS. *Ann Intern Med.* 1990;113:926.

Hassam S, Briner J, Tratschin JD, Siegl G, Heitz PU. In situ hybridization for the detection of human parvovirus B19 nucleic acid sequences in paraffin-embedded specimens. *Virchows Arch B Cell Pathol.* 1990;59:257–261.

Morey AL, Porter HJ, Keeling JW, Fleming KA. Non-isotopic in situ hybridization and immunophenotyping of infected cells in the investigation of human fetal parvovirus infection. *J Clin Pathol.* 1992;45:673–678.

Polyomavirus

Gerber MA, Shah KV, Thung SN, et al. Immunohistochemical demonstration of common antigens of polyomaviruses in routine histologic tissue sections of animals and man. *Am J Clin Pathol.* 1980;73:795.

Rabies Virus

Budka H, Popow-Kraupp T. Rabies and herpes simplex virus encephalitis. An immunohistological study on site and distribution of viral antigens. *Virchows Arch Pathol Anat.* 1981;390:353.

Respiratory Syncytial Virus

Cartun RW, Tahhan HR, Knibbs DR, et al. Immunocytochemical identification of respiratory syncytial virus (RSV) in formalin-fixed, paraffin-embedded tissue from immunocompromised hosts. *Mod Pathol.* 1989;2:15A.

Neilson KA, Yunis EJ. Demonstration of respiratory syncytial virus in an autopsy series. *Pediatr Pathol.* 1990;10:491–502.

Rift Valley Fever Virus

Arbrorio M, Hall WC. Diagnosis of a human case of Rift Valley fever by immunoperoxidase demonstration of antigen in fixed liver tissues. *Res Virol.* 1989;140:165.

Rotavirus

Graham DY, Estes MK. Comparison of methods for immunocytochemical detection of rotavirus infections. *Infect Immun.* 1979;26:686.

Varicella-Zoster Virus

Chretien F, Gray F, Lescs MC, et al. Acute varicella-zoster virus ventriculitis and meningo-myelo-radiculitis in acquired immunodeficiency syndrome. *Acta Neuropathol (Berlin).* 1993;86:659–665.

Horten B, Price RW, Jimenez D. Multifocal varicella-zoster virus leukoencephalitis temporally remote from herpes zoster. *Ann Neurol.* 1981;9:251.

Martin JR, Holt RK, Langston C, et al. Type-specific identification of herpes simplex and varicella-zoster virus antigen in autopsy tissues. *Hum Pathol.* 1991;22:75.

Morgello S, Block GA, Price RW, et al. Varicella-zoster virus leukoencephalitis and cerebral vasculopathy. *Arch Pathol Lab Med.* 1988;112:173.

Rummelt V, Wenkel H, Rummelt C, Jahn G, Meyer HJ, Naumann GO. Detection of varicella-zoster virus DNA and viral antigen in the late stage of bilateral acute retinal necrosis syndrome. *Arch Ophthalmol.* 1992;110:1132–1136.

Yellow Fever Virus

Monath TP, Ballinger ME, Miller BR, et al. Detection of yellow fever viral RNA by nucleic acid hybridization and viral antigen by immunocytochemistry in fixed human liver. *Am J Trop Med Hyg.* 1989;40:663.

Fungi

General

Moskowitz LB, Ganjei P, Cleary TJ, et al. Immunohistological identification of fungi in systemic and cutaneous mycoses. *Arch Pathol Lab Med.* 1986;110:433.

Aspergillus

Montone KT, Litzky LA. Rapid method for detection of *Aspergillus* 5S ribosmal RNA using a genus-specific oligonucleotide probe. *Am J Clin Pathol.* 1995;103:48–51.

Philips P, Weiner MH. Invasive aspergillosis diagnosed by immunohistochemistry with monoclonal and polyclonal reagents. *Hum Pathol.* 1987;18:1015.

Candida albicans

Monteagudo C, Marcilla A, Mormeneo S, et al. Specific immunohistochemical identification of *Candida albicans* in paraffin-embedded tissue with a new monoclonal antibody (1B12). *Am J Clin Pathol.* 1995;103:130–135.

Cryptococcus neoformans

Russel B, Beckett JH, Jacobs PH. Immunoperoxidase localization of *Sporothrix schenckii* and *Cryptococcus neoformans. Arch Dermatol.* 1979;115:433.

Histoplasma capsulatum

Klatt EC, Cosgrove M, Meyer PR. Rapid diagnosis of disseminated histoplasmosis in tissues. *Arch Pathol Lab Med.* 1986;110:1173–1175.

Sporothrix schenckii

Russel B, Beckett JH, Jacobs PH. Immunoperoxidase localization of *Sporothrix schenckii* and *Cryptococcus neoformans. Arch Dermatol.* 1979;115:433.

Trichophyton rubrum

Holden CA, Hay RJ, MacDonald DM. The antigenicity of *Trichophyton rubrum:* in situ studies by an immunoperoxidase technique in light and electron microscopy. *Acta Derm Venereol.* 1981;61:207.

Trichosporon beigelii

Kobayashi TK, Kotani S, Fujishita M, et al. Immunohistochemical identification of *Trichosporon beigelii* in histologic section by immunoperoxidase method. *Acta Cytol.* 1988;89:100.

Bacteria and Rickettsias

Bacteroides gingivalis

Saglie FR, Smith CT, Newman MG, et al. The presence of bacteria in the oral epithelium in periodontal disease. II. Immunohistochemical identification of bacteria. *J Periodontol.* 1986;57:492.

Borrelia burgdorferi (Lyme Disease)

Arrese-Estrada J, Melotte P, Hermanns JF, et al. Immunohistochemistry of *Borrelia*-type spirochetes. *Ann Derm Venereol.* 1991;118:277.

Cat Scratch Disease Bacillus

Min KW, Reed JA, Welch DF, Slater LN. Morphologically variable bacilli of cat scratch disease are identified by immunocytochemical labeling with antibodies to *Rochalimaea henselae. Am J Clin Pathol.* 1994;101:607–610.

Yu X, Raoult D. Monoclonal antibodies to Afipia felis—a putative agent of cat scratch disease. *Am J Clin Pathol.* 1994;101:603–606.

Chlamydia

Crum CP, Mitao M, Winkler B, et al. Localizing chlamydial infection in cervical biopsies with the immunoperoxidase technique. *Int J Gynecol Pathol.* 1984;3:191.

Shurbaji MS, Dumler JS, Gage WR, et al. Immunohistochemical detection of chlamydial antigens in association with cystitis. *Am J Pathol.* 1990;93:363.

Clostridium difficile

Qualman SJ, Petric M, Karmali MA, et al. *Clostridium difficile* invasion and toxin circulation in fatal pediatric pseudomembranous colitis. *Am J Clin Pathol.* 1990;94:410.

Coxiella burnetii (Q-Fever)

Raoult D, Laurent JC, Multillod M. Monoclonal antibodies to *Coxiella burnettii* for antigenic detection in cell cultures and in paraffin-embedded tissues. *Am J Clin Pathol.* 1994;101:318–320.

Escherichia coli

Park CH, Hixon DL, Morrison WL, Cook CB. Rapid diagnosis of enterohemorrhagic *Escherichia coli* O 157:H7 directly from fecal specimens using immunoflourescence stain. *Am J Clin Pathol.* 1994;101:91–94.

Qualman SJ, Gupta PK, Mendelsohn G. Intracellular *Escherichia coli* in urinary malakoplakia: a reservoir of infection and its therapeutic implications. *Am J Clin Pathol.* 1984; 81:35.

Haemophilus influenzae

Groeneveld K, van Alphen L, van Ketel RJ, et al. Nonculture detection of *Hemophilus influenzae* in sputum with monoclonal antibodies specific for outer membrane lipoprotein P6. *J Clin Microbiol.* 1989;27:2263.

Terpstra WJ, Groeneveld K, Eijk PP, et al. Comparison of two nonculture techniques for detection of *Hemophilus influenzae* in sputum. In situ hybridization and immunoperoxidase staining with monoclonal antibodies. *Chest.* 1988;94:126S.

Helicobacter pylori (Formerly Campylobacter pylori)

Barbosa AJA, Queroz DMM, Mendex EN, et al. Immunocytochemical identification of *Campylobacter pylori* in gastritis and correlation with culture. *Arch Pathol Lab Med.* 1988;112:523.

Cartun RW, Dryzmowski GA, Pedersen CA, et al. Immunocytochemical identification of *Helicobacter pylori* in formalin-fixed gastric biopsies. *Mod Pathol.* 1991;4:498.

Engstrand L, Pahlson C, Gustavsson S, et al. Monoclonal antibodies for rapid identification of *Campylobacter pyloridis. Lancet.* 1986;2:1402.

Hawtin PR, Stacey AR, Newell DG. Investigation of the structure and localization of the urease of *Helicobacter pylori* using monoclonal antibodies. *J Gen Microbiol.* 1990;136: 1995–2000.

Loffield RJLF, Strobberingh E, Flendrig JA, et al. *Helicobacter pylori* in gastric biopsy specimens. Comparison of culture, modified Giemsa stain, and immunohistochemistry. A retrospective study. *J Pathol.* 1991;165:69.

Listeria monocytogenes

McLauchlin J, Black A, Green HT, et al. Monoclonal antibodies show *Listeria monocytogenes* in necropsy tissue samples. *J Clin Pathol.* 1988;41:983.

Legionella pneumophila

Boyer JF, McWilliams E. Immunoperoxidase staining of *Legionella pneumophila*. *Histopathology.* 1982;6:191.

Fain JS, Bryan RN, Cheng L, et al. Rapid diagnosis of Legionella infection by a nonisotopic in situ hybridization method. *Am J Clin Pathol.* 1991;95:719–724.

Suffin SC, Kaufman AF, Whitaker B, et al. *Legionella pneumophila*. Identification in tissue sections by a new immunoenzymatic procedure. *Arch Pathol Lab Med.* 1980; 104:283.

Leptospira interrogans

Ferreira Alves VA, Regina Vianna M, Yasuda PH, et al. Detection of leptospiral antigen in the human liver and kidney using an immunoperoxidase staining procedure. *J Pathol.* 1987;151:125.

Mycobacteria

Barbolini G, Bisetti A, Colizzi V, et al. Immunohistologic analysis of mycobacterial antigens by monoclonal antibodies in tuberculosis and mycobacteriosis. *Hum Pathol.* 1989;20:1078.

Humphrey DM, Weiner MH. Mycobacterial antigen detection by immunohistochemistry in pulmonary tuberculosis. *Hum Pathol.* 1987;18:701.

Mshana RN, Humber DP, Harboe M, et al. Demonstration of mycobacterial antigens in nerve biopsies from leprosy patients using peroxidase–antiperoxidase immunoenzyme technique. *Clin Immunol Immunopathol.* 1983;29:359.

Pfaller MA. Application of new technology to the detection, identification, and antimicrobial susceptibility testing of mycobacteria. *Am J Clin Pathol.* 1994;101:329–337.

Wiley EL, Mulhollan TJ, Beck B, et al. Polyclonal antibodies raised against bacillus Calmette-Guerin, *Mycobacterium duvalii,* and *Mycobacterium paratuberculosis* used to detect mycobacteria in tissue with the use of immunohistochemical techniques. *Am J Clin Pathol.* 1990;94:307.

Mycoplasma

Chasey D, Woods SB. Detection of immunoperoxidase-labeled mycoplasmas in cell culture by light microscopy and electron microscopy. *J Med Microbiol.* 1984;17:23.

Lo S-C, Dawson MS, Wong DM, et al. Identification of *Mycoplasma incognitus* infection in patients with AIDS: an immunohistochemical, in situ hybridization and ultrastructural study. *Am J Trop Med Hyg.* 1989;41:601.

Lutsky I, Livni N, Mor N. Retrospective confirmation of mycoplasma infection by the immunoperoxidase technique. *Pathology.* 1986;18:390–392.

Neisseria gonorrhoeae

Cooper MD, McGraw PA, Melly MA. Localization of gonococcal lipopolysaccharide and its relationship to toxic damage in human fallopian tube mucosa. *Infect Immunol.* 1986;51:425.

Rickettsia rickettsii

Dumler JS, Gage WR, Pettis GL, et al. Rapid immunoperoxidase demonstration of *Rickettsia rickettsii* in fixed cutaneous specimens from patients with Rocky Mountain spotted fever. *Am J Clin Pathol.* 1990;93:410.

White WL, Patrick JD, Miller LR. Evaluation of immunoperoxidase techniques to detect *Rickettsia rikettsii* in fixed tissue sections. *Am J Clin Pathol.* 1994;101:747–752.

Staphylococci

Newbould MJ, Malam J, McIllmurray JM, et al. Immunohistologic localization of staphylococcal toxic shock syndrome toxin (TSST-1) antigen in sudden death syndrome. *J Clin Pathol.* 1989;42:935.

Streptococci

Andres T, MacPherson B. Identification of group B streptococci in tissue sections using the peroxidase-antiperoxidase method: a retrospective necropsy study. *J Clin Pathol.* 1980;33:1165.

Feldman RG, Law SM, Salisbury JR. Detection of group B streptococcal antigen in necropsy specimens using monoclonal antibody and immunoperoxidase staining. *J Clin Pathol.* 1986;39:223.

Hadfield TL, Neafie R, Lanoie LO. Tubo-ovarian abscess caused by *Streptococcus pneumoniae*. *Hum Pathol.* 1990; 21:1288.

Treponema pallidum

Beckett JH, Bigbee JW. Immunoperoxidase localization of *Treponema pallidum*. *Arch Pathol.* 1979;103:135.

Ohyama M, Itani Y, Tanaka Y, et al. Syphilitic placentitis: demonstration of *Treponema pallidum* by immunoperoxidase staining. *Virchows Arch A.* 1990;417:343.

Parasites

Cryptosporidium

Bonnin A, Petrella T, Dubremetz JF, et al. Histopathologic method for diagnosis of cryptosporidiosis using monoclonal antibodies. *Eur J Clin Microbiol Infect Dis.* 1990; 9:664–665.

McLauchlin J, Casemore DP, Harrison TG, et al. Identification of cryptosporidium oocytes by monoclonal antibody. *Lancet.* 1987;I:51.

Entamoeba histolytica

Kobayashi TK, Koretoh O, Kamachi M, et al. Cytologic demonstration of *Entamoeba histolytica* using immunoperoxidase techniques. Report of two cases. *Acta Cytol.* 1985;29:414.

Perez de Suarez E, Perez-Schael I, Perozo-Ruggeri G, et al. Immunocytochemical detection of *Entamoeba histolytica*. *Trans R Soc Trop Med Hyg.* 1987;81:624–626.

Fasciola hepatica

Demaree RS Jr, Hillyer GV. Immunoperoxidase localization of

Fasciola hepatica worm tegument antigens by electron microscopy. *Int J Parasitol.* 1982;12:179.

Leishmania

Azadeh B, Sells PG, Ejeckman GC et al. Localized *Leishmania* lymphadenitis. Immunohistochemical studies. *Am J Clin Pathol.* 1994;102:11–15.

Livni N, Abramowitz A, Lodner M, et al. Immunoperoxidase method of identification of *Leishmania* in routinely prepared histologic sections. *Virchows Arch A.* 1983;401:147.

Pneumocystis carinii

Amin MB, Mezger E, Zarbo RJ. Detection of *Pneumocystis carinii* comparative study of monoclonal antibody and sliver staining. *Am J Clin Pathol.* 1992;98:13–18.

Cartun RW, Lachman MF, Pedersen C, et al. Immunocytochemical identification of *Pneumocystis carinii* in formalin-fixed, paraffin-embedded tissues using monoclonal antibody "2G2." *Histotechnology.* 1990;13:117.

Cote RJ, Rosenblum M, Telzak EE, et al. Disseminated *Pneumocystis carinii* infection causing extrapulmonary organ failure: clinical, pathological and immunohistochemical analysis. *Mod Pathol.* 1990;3:25.

Homer KS, Wiley EL, Smith AL, et al. Monoclonal antibody to *Pneumocystis carinii* comparison with sliver stain in bronchial lavage specimens. *Am J Clin Pathol.* 1992; 97:619–624.

Linder J, Ye Y, Harrington DS, et al. Monoclonal antibodies marking T lymphocytes in paraffin-embedded tissue. *Am J Pathol.* 1987;127:1.

Walker AN, Garner RE, Horst MN. Immunocytochemical detection of chitin in *Pneumocystis carinii. Infect Immunol.* 1990;58:412.

Toxoplasma gondii

Conley FK, Jenkins KA, Remington JS. *Toxoplasma gondii* infection of the central nervous system: use of the peroxidase–antiperoxidase method to demonstrate *Toxoplasma* in formalin-fixed, paraffin-embedded tissue sections. *Hum Pathol.* 1981;12:690.

Warnke C, Tuazon CU, Kovacs A, et al. Toxoplasma encephalitis in patients with acquired immune deficiency syndrome: diagnosis and response to therapy. *Am J Trop Med Hyg.* 1987;36:509.

Trichomonas

Bennett BD, Bailey J, Gardner WA. Immunocytochemical identification of Trichomonads. *Arch Pathol Lab Med.* 1980;104:247.

O'Hara CM, Gardner WA, Bennet BD. Immunoperoxidase staining of *Trichomonas vaginalis* in cytology material. *Acta Cytol.* 1980;24:448.

CHAPTER 4

Principles of Molecular Diagnostics

Richard A. McPherson

The physician must look beyond the picture, now widely cherished, of the lonely, great-hearted doctor, bowed impotent beside the dying child. Modern transportation, modern methods of communication, and modern techniques of diagnosis and treatment have made that picture as obsolete as the village blacksmith at his charcoal forge.

William Dock (b. 1898)

MOLECULAR CHARACTERISTICS OF NUCLEIC ACIDS

Biochemical Properties of Nucleic Acids and Factors Affecting Hybridization

The capacity of nucleic acids to interact with one another is based on the complementarity of the nucleotide sequence in one strand to that in another strand.[1] Deoxyribonucleic acid (DNA) naturally occurs in the double-stranded state with perfect complementarity between the two strands. The polarity of strands of nucleic acid is conventionally defined according to the orientation of the phosphodiester bond from the fifth carbon on a (deoxy)ribose moiety to the third carbon on the adjacent (deoxy)ribose in the nucleic acid backbone of DNA or ribonucleic acid (RNA). The double helical structure of DNA is comprised of two antiparallel strands; one is directed from the 5′-end to the 3′-end, and the other is in the 3′ to 5′ direction. Interaction occurs between adenine (A) on one strand and thymidine (T) on the complementary strand through two shared hydrogen bonds; similarly cytosine (C) recognizes guanine (G) on different strands but through three hydrogen bonds.[2] Thus GC bonds are inherently more stable than are AT bonds between complementary strands. In RNA, uridine (U) occurs in place of thymidine, but otherwise serves the same functional purpose of binding to adenine. Other forces help to hold the two strands together in a helix, including a stabilization that results from stacking of the planar bases next to one another along the length of the molecule.

In addition to the complementary nature of the interaction between different strands of DNA with DNA or of DNA with RNA, self-complementarity can also occur in the same strand. In this configuration, a single strand of DNA or RNA may fold back on itself, giving rise to stems or loops depending on whether the self-complementary region are immediately adjacent to one another or flank other regions of noncomplementary sequences. This type of secondary structure is a regular finding in transfer RNA (tRNA) and ribosomal RNA (rRNA) because it stabilizes the otherwise single-stranded RNA, thereby protecting it from possible degradation by strand cuts. It also facilitates interaction with other molecules such as proteins and other nucleic acids because the secondary structure can impart unique physical characteristics. Messenger RNA (mRNA) can also contain self-complementarity, although the significance of secondary structure in mRNA is not clear. Self-complementarity in double-stranded DNA can probably arise anywhere it is encoded in the genes for tRNA, rRNA, or mRNA, and in other locations in noncoding regions. The result appears to be variations from the simple double helices of DNA in which stems may extend perpendicularly to the backbone of the DNA. These structural variations are thought to be in some form of thermal equilibrium with one another under normal physiologic conditions. These internal recognition phenomena could very well have to do with initiation and regulation of transcription, genome replication, etc. From a practical analytic standpoint, these alternate structures must be kept in mind when designing diagnostic assays because subtle variations may contribute significantly to the conditions under which reactions will proceed and to which nucleotide sequences are acceptable for use as targets.

The detection of molecules of DNA or RNA from viruses, bacteria, and other infectious agents is based on hybridization between a nucleic acid probe, which is generally constructed or synthesized for use as a reagent (and thus has a defined nucleotide sequence, which in turn defines its specificity of binding), and a target nucleic acid (unknown quantity of the analyte) in a clinical specimen. The general principle is that complementary strands may be separated by raising the temperature of a solution and thereby disrupting the hydrogen bonds holding the helix together. The absorbence of such a solution at 260 nm increases dramatically as double-stranded DNA breaks apart or melts into individual single strands at the melting temperature (T_m).[2] As the solution of separated DNA molecules is cooled, complementary strands once again bind to one another.[3] This process can also be accomplished at lower actual temperature by addition of chemicals such as formamide that also have the effect of causing duplexed DNA to melt.[4] When target DNA or RNA molecules are mixed with complementary probes under the melting (or denaturing conditions) and then placed under nondenaturing conditions, the probe sequences are able to hybridize with target molecules that may be present.

A hierarchy of relatedness between different organisms can be established by mixing double-stranded DNA isolated from each of two different organisms in the same solution, melting the DNA molecules by heat, and then observing the rate of reannealing (through optical absorbence at 260 nm) as the solution is cooled.[5] If the organisms are identical, reannealing will occur at its fastest rate. As the relatedness of the organisms diverges (ie, the nucleotide sequences differ), the longer the reannealing will take. By repeating this test sequentially on different pairs of organisms, a whole new taxonomy can be constructed. This process can be applied to DNA samples from viruses versus bacteria versus eukaryotes, etc.

The stability of a nucleic acid duplex is determined by several factors. Most significant is the degree of homology between strands. Under conditions of reduced stringency, annealing can proceed between strands that are not perfectly matched. However, the side effect of lowering stringency to allow duplex formation between partial but not necessarily complete matches is that binding may also occur in other undesired regions, thereby markedly altering the specificity of recognition between probe and target. This phenomenon may be exploited, for instance, when using a single probe to screen for the presence of any of several closely related viruses among whom serotype divergence corresponds to minor variation in nucleotide sequences.

Another factor determining strength of interaction is the relative content of GC (stronger) versus AT (weaker).[2] As a particular point, sequences with a high GC content and some degree of self-complementarity may never be suitable for use as probes or primers because they will almost certainly fold back on themselves before coming in contact with the desired target. The length of the probe may be important in applications such as in situ hybridization in which the probe must permeate physical barriers within fixed tissue sections before coming into contact with the target. In this instance, probes should be constructed to be in the size range of 200 to 500 nucleotides long.

In practice, it is usually necessary to evaluate and selectively set the conditions of hybridization according to each specific target nucleic acid and specimen type as required by sequence variability, secondary structures, and other idiosyncrasies of the organism and particular detection system. As a rule of thumb, it is useful to remember that duplexes between complementary strands of DNA and RNA are more stable than those between DNA and DNA.[6] Similarly RNA–RNA hybrids are even more stable. Thus the specificity of binding may be enhanced by using a more favorable combination of RNA and DNA as probe and target, which will permit more stringent washing steps in which nonspecific interactions are diminished.

Extraction, Electrophoresis, and Transfer Methods

Nucleic acids occur in association with proteins and lipids from membranes as they are packed within viral particles, within bacterial cells, etc. Consequently it is usually necessary to perform an extraction involving proteolytic digestion and treatment with phenol-chloroform-isoamyl alcohol followed by ethanol precipitation to purify and concentrate nucleic acids before analysis by methods in which an abundant amount of analyte is required.[7] For amplification methods in which only minute amounts of nucleic acid are likely to be present, extensive extraction may result in a substantial loss of signal and therefore the procedures are designed to liberate the nucleic acid target and make it accessible to the enzymatic reagents that will multiply it to amounts that are then detectable.

Large pieces of DNA may be difficult to analyze or manipulate. Instead, extracted DNA is frequently cleaved enzymatically to convert it to fragment sizes that are amenable to electrophoresis, transfer, and other actions. Restriction endonucleases are used for this purpose to generate reproducibly sized fragments.[8,9] Each restriction endonuclease (eg, *Eco*RI, *Bam*HI, *Hin*dIII) cuts double-stranded DNA at specific sites defined by the nucleotide sequence. These cut sites are generally palindromic, consisting of four, six, or eight defined nucleotides. These specific combinations of nucleotides occur randomly in large sequences, so the resulting fragments do not reflect functional units of DNA, but they are reproducible for a particular organism or strain of organism in which the DNA sequence is preserved (Figure 4–1).

Electrophoresis of nucleic acids is done in agarose gels generally about 1 cm thick and laid horizontally as submarine gels under an overlying buffer layer that helps to maintain constant temperature throughout the gel. By this means, the electrophoretic field is kept relatively free of distortion, and samples in wells across the gel migrate in register with one another.

Double-stranded nucleic acids can be visualized in gels by staining with ethidium bromide and illumination

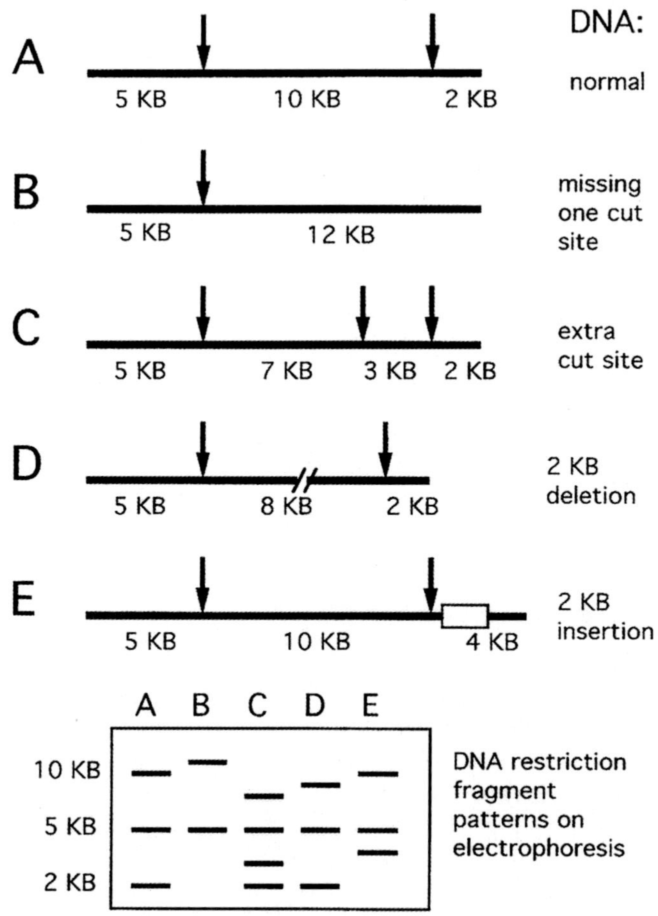

Figure 4–1. Different electrophoretic patterns obtained by restriction enzyme digestion (arrows represent enzyme cut sites) of DNA altered by mutation, insertion, or deletion.

with ultraviolet light. Ethidium bromide is a small planar molecule that intercalates into double-stranded regions of nucleic acids including self-complementary regions of RNA molecules. Ethidium bromide in solution does not fluoresce with ultraviolet light, but it does when bound to double-stranded nucleic acids. Thus ethidium bromide can be included in the gel buffer to allow visualization of the extent of migration during electrophoresis.

Typical agarose gels are useful for separating DNA fragments in the range of about 500 base pairs to roughly 20,000 base pairs. The upper range of fragment size resolution by standard methods is 50,000 base pairs. These fragments can then be seen as separate bands by ethidium bromide staining. This size range is almost always sufficient to resolve the several restriction fragments generated from viral genomes. However, genomes of bacteria and higher organisms are much larger, and so they yield too many individual fragments to be resolved by electrophoresis. Fragments of smaller sizes may be resolved by electrophoresis in polyacrylamide gels that have a tighter porosity and so limit the mobility of the smaller fragments. Very large fragments of DNA (>50,000 base pairs) may be electrophoresed under the special conditions of a pulsed field that permit resolution of very long molecules.[10,11] This application may be useful for examining very large fragments of yeast or bacterial DNA.[12–14] However, neither of these latter two methods is likely to have widespread clinical diagnostic application because of the special skills needed for performance. In fact, agarose gel electrophoresis is sufficiently complex to require special expertise and training. Because such electrophoresis may take several hours (or overnight) to perform, it is desirable to replace it in the future with a more automated method such as capillary electrophoresis using high-pressure-type separation systems.[15,16]

Electrophoresis results in nucleic acid fragments embedded throughout the thickness of a gel at the positions to which they migrated. For preparative isolation to individual fragments for other purposes (eg, cloning, reagents), ethidium bromide visualization can be used to cut out the gel section containing a desired fragment followed by extraction of the isolated fragment from the gel material. For analytic purposes, it is necessary to transfer the nucleic acids from within the thickness of a gel to the surface of a membrane where the fragments are accessible to hybridization with probes.[17] The transfer from a gel is usually done onto a membrane of either nitrocellulose or nylon (which is considerably more resilient to manipulations). Transfer can be done with flow movement of solvent perpendicularly to the gel surface directly in contact with the membrane. In this manner, a complete transfer should result of all nucleic acid fragments onto the membrane exactly in

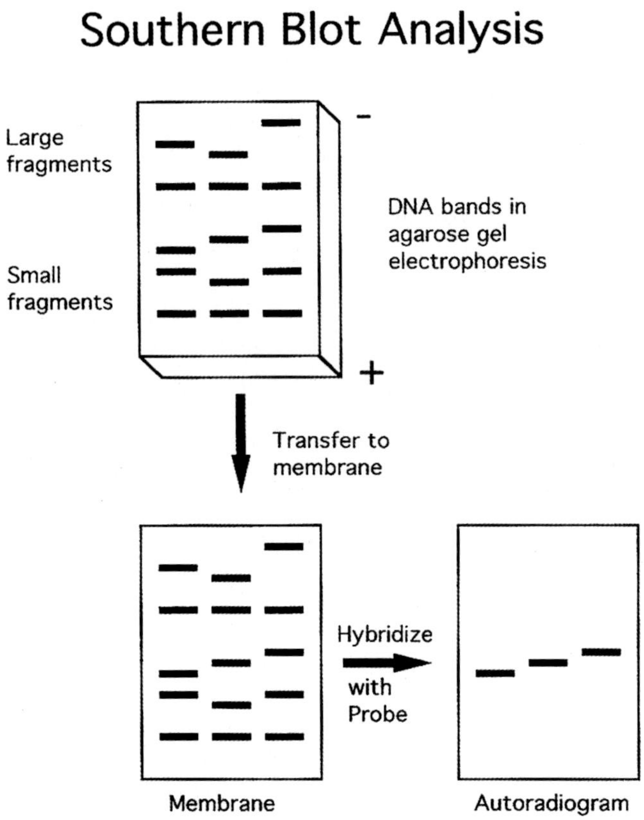

Figure 4–2. Outline of Southern blot analysis including electrophoresis of DNA fragments, transfer to membrane, and hybridization with probe.

register with their electrophoretic positions. The membrane is then soaked in a solution that permits hybridization of the nucleic acid fragments on its surface with a labeled probe. Following hybridization, the membrane is washed to remove unbound labeled probe, and it is exposed or developed to reveal locations to which the probe hybridized. When the nucleic acids subjected to electrophoresis, transfer, and probing are DNA, the process is termed Southern blot analysis (Figure 4–2).[18] When the nucleic acids being so tested are RNA, it is termed Northern blot analysis.[19] Similarly a Western blot consists of protein analysis by electrophoresis, transfer, and immunoprobing.

Nucleic Acid Labeling and Detection

The earliest methods of detecting reaction products of nucleic acid hybridization relied on radioactive labels. Typically probes have been labeled with ^{3}H, ^{14}C, ^{32}P, or ^{35}S, which are directly incorporated into the chemical structures of nucleic acids.[20] These isotopes require use of a scintillation counter or gamma counter or exposure to x-ray film for autoradiograms. Radioisotopes are widely used in research and for developing new assays because they are considered to be a gold standard for sensitivity, but their disadvantages (need for special detection equipment, short shelf-life, and disposal problems) make them less desirable than nonisotopic probe labels for clinical diagnostic assays.

Nonisotopic labeling of nucleic acids is accomplished by incorporation of chemical side groups into DNA precursors, which are in turn introduced into the probe molecules by enzymatic syntheses such as nick translation of previously purified DNA segments.[21] Biotin or digoxigenin can be used to label DNA by this means through spacer arms 10 or more carbon atoms long.[22–25] Placing the label molecule that far away from the DNA molecule allows detection to proceed with streptavidin (to biotin) or antibody (to digoxigenin) that are conjugated to indicator enzymes (such as alkaline phosphatase) without disturbing the hybridization of the probe target.[26] This type of enzymatic labeling has tremendous potential for in situ hybridization in tissue sections because it converts that technique to one that is compatible with conventional immunohistochemistry laboratories. But an even greater potential exists in establishing colorimetric assays to detect nucleic acids from infectious agents using automated instruments similar to many already in use for a multitude of serologic tests. Still another labeling refinement is one in which oligonucleotide probes are directly synthesized and can be end-labeled with a single nucleotide to which the indicator enzyme is already conjugated.[27] This type of labeling has the advantage of extraordinarily high levels of specific activities, because virtually every probe molecule can be labeled.

The final detection step for nonisotopic probes is accomplished by using an enzymatic substrate that is colorimetric or chemiluminescent.[28–30] In particular, chemiluminescence appears to have tremendous potential for low-level sensitivity as a recorder molecule for nucleic acid probes, especially for use on automated systems with defined reaction times and optical detection.[31]

DNA Sequencing

Nucleotide sequencing is performed on a single strand of a purified DNA fragment. Two general methods have been developed to generate the complete series of subfragments that correspond to the starting fragment, the fragment minus its end nucleotide, the fragment minus its last two nucleotides, the fragment minus the last three, etc. These subfragments, differing by one nucleotide each, can be resolved electrophoretically in polyacrylamide.[32]

The first method consists of a series of four chemical processes to break the original strand at nucleotide-specific sites.[33] The starting material is labeled at its other end with a radioisotope (usually ^{32}P), and the whole set of subfragments can then be identified by autoradiography.

A later enzymatic method promotes synthesis of DNA from the strand being sequenced with incorporation of the normal four deoxynucleosides plus one each of variant dideoxynucleosides, which are incorporated into the new strand but prevent it from elongating further.[34] This process is called *chain termination.* In a reaction solution to which have been added the four normal precursors plus a particular dideoxynucleoside (eg, dideoxyadenosine triphosphate, ddATP), an entire set of subfragments will be generated with termination at each different position of adenine in the sequence. Similar reactions are done individually with the other three dideoxynucleosides. The fragments may be radiolabeled to perform autoradiography following electrophoresis of each reaction in separate lanes. The sequence is then read at A, T, G, or C in turn, depending on which lane has a band when moving from the bottom to the top of the gel (Figure 4–3).

The enzymatic method has been further refined and automated by putting a different fluorescent label onto each of the four dideoxynucleosides so the reaction can be done in a single container instead of four. Electrophoretic separation can be read automatically by a mechanical scanner that identifies each individual fluorescent tag, thereby directly determining the DNA sequence in a single electrophoretic channel. This technique is applicable to sequencing large numbers of nucleotides with minimal operator interaction.

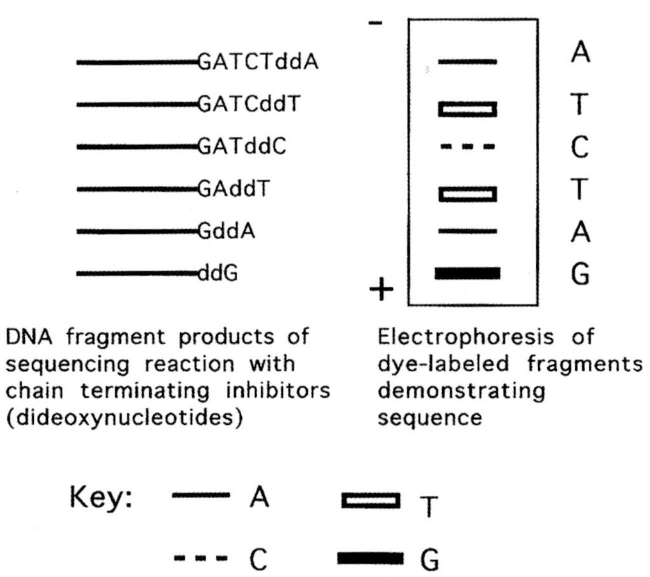

Figure 4–3. Products of DNA sequencing by dideoxynucleotide chain termination with fluorescent labeling and their electrophoretic resolution for automated DNA sequencing.

DIAGNOSTIC APPLICATIONS

Direct Hybridization Assays

In Solution

As developed in the early years of DNA techniques, hybridization can be performed in solution in which both target and labeled (usually radioisotopic) probes are dissolved. The presence of target is established by trapping of the probe in high-molecular-weight form or in double-stranded form. This technique requires physical separation of the hybridized from unhybridized probe before the detection step. This separation can be done by the traditional means of adding a suspension of hydroxylapatite, which binds double-stranded DNA. Other applications include solid phase binding to effect the separation. This method has been applied to detection of bacterial ribosomal RNA (which is present in multiple copies per bacterial cell) for mycoplasma, mycobacteria, and Legionella (Gen-Probe). It may also be useful for detecting other organisms present in high copy numbers.

Although on the surface the separation step may seem to be a minor issue, in fact it could very well be the single most important factor in automating the technology of nucleic acid testing. A direct comparison can be made with radioimmunoassays (RIA), which require separation of free from bound label. In contrast, enzyme immunoassays (EIA) have been developed in which there is no need to separate free from bound because those fractions have different enzymatic activities. Assays in which there is no need for separation are termed *homogeneous* whereas those with separation steps are termed *heterogeneous.* Homogeneous assays are inherently automatable and may be performed in minutes versus hours to days (cf, EIA versus RIA endocrine assays). Thus the future success of nucleic acid assays in large-scale testing rests heavily on whether they can be made homogeneous.

On Membranes

Nucleic acids extracted from samples can be directly attached to a solid phase membrane such as nitrocellulose or nylon.[35] Hybridization is then performed by soaking the membrane with the probe. Application of the samples can be done using devices with slots or as small spots or dots; hence, these assays are termed *slot blots* or *dot blots.* This type of direct blotting has the advantage over conventional culture techniques of speed of analysis, ability to detect nonviable organisms, and ability to detect noncultivable organisms. Direct blotting has been used to detect cytomegalovirus DNA,[36] human parvovirus DNA from bone marrow samples, and the presence of papillomavirus DNA in cervical biopsies.[37] However, a more widely used example has been quantitation of hepatitis B virus (HBV) DNA by dot blot. Because the concentration of HBV DNA in serum is the best indicator of viral replication in the liver, quantitative HBV DNA measurement has become an extremely important test for monitoring therapy of chronic hepatitis B with α-interferon. This assay has become a prototype for demonstrating many characteristics of dot blot techniques.

Quantitative DNA Assay

Quantitation of HBV DNA in serum is an excellent prototype for delineating the performance characteristics of assays that are intended to measure the amount of nucleic acid in a clinical specimen rather than just to detect the presence of an infectious agent. HBV is present in sufficiently abundant amounts in serum that direct measurement is feasible without amplification for clinical decision making. The HBV DNA is of course present within virion particles (Dane particles) in which HBV core proteins are complexed to the DNA and surrounded by a membrane lipid layer into which are inserted HBV surface antigen molecules. Thus to access the DNA for assay requires some form of denaturation (usually treatment with alkali) to break open the virions. The liberated DNA is subsequently trapped on solid support (eg, nylon membrane on the base of customized microtiter plate wells), hybridized with a labeled DNA probe usually consisting of the entire 3200-nucleotide-long genome, and the amount of bound probe is quantitated to indicate the concentration of HBV DNA in the original sample.[38]

A first consideration in setting up a quantitative assay in what materials to use for calibrators (standards). Dane particles representing complete virions may be obtained by buoyant density centrifugation of serum from infectious humans, but the yield of such virions is small, it would vary considerably between laboratories, and the long-term stability of such preparations is questionable. In addition, HBV DNA from virions is partly double stranded and partly single stranded with the relative proportions varying in a population of particles from a single patient's sample. Thus in natural infection, HBV DNA represents a somewhat fuzzy target.

For purposes of standardization, it is far easier to use recombinant HBV DNA that is obtained by conventional methods of cloning into a plasmid, propagation in bacterial cultures, and isolation by enzyme cleavage to remove the HBV DNA segment from the plasmid followed by preparative electrophoresis. The resulting cloned HBV DNA can be precisely and accurately quantitated by physical methods because it is made in such large amounts; it is then diluted to the concentrations used in the quantitative assay. This approach is now a very standard technique; however, it is deficient in at least two points: 1) The cloned DNA is not coated with HBV proteins and lipid membrane and so actual recovery of DNA from true virions is not reproduced in the treatment of standards, and 2) the cloned DNA is double stranded as opposed to the variable single-to-double-stranded DNA in natural HBV particles. Thus the most convenient standards are clearly a compromise between feasibility and ideal construction.

This type of standard preparation is likely to vary considerably between laboratories depending on a multitude of individual factors. However, interlaboratory standardization rests on having a single calibrator source that can be shared by all groups attempting to bring their assays into agreement. Present experience is that the results of HBV DNA quantitation may differ by as much as fivefold or more on the same sample measured with different assays. This type and magnitude of discrepancy is expected to occur with other quantitative nucleic acid assays until consensus samples are widely available for standardization.

One clear advantage that complete viral genomic testing has over measurement of antigen through immunoassay is that minor variations in the nucleotide sequence of the target are not likely to change detection and quantitation of the virus very much, whereas the corresponding differences in epitopes on the viral proteins may render them unrecognizable to antibody reagents. Thus nucleic acid testing clearly has a role to play in hepatitis diagnosis for cases in which the conventional serologic results may be ambiguous.

Although HBV DNA appears in serum early in the course of acute HBV infection, its measurement in acute hepatitis is not generally contributory because diagnosis is so readily accomplished by automated HBV antigen and antibody measurements.[39] Quantitation of HBV DNA is much more useful clinically for establishing infectivity in prolonged hepatitis B and in monitoring response to antiviral therapy.[40,41] Because of the widespread nature of chronic HBV infection and its potential for treatment with α-interferon, the assay for quantitation of HBV DNA in serum has become a staple of the molecular diagnostic laboratory. Concentration of HBV DNA is a better marker for early response to therapy and for early recurrence after treatment than are any of the HBV antigens or antibodies.[42]

One major limitation of dot blots is that nonspecific binding of probe to the membrane cannot be directly distinguished from true signal at very low levels.[43] One avenue to get around this dilemma is to perform a Southern blot analysis instead. If the hybridization signal appears in a discrete band(s) of expected size, it is probably the true target. If it is merely a blur extending over a wide range, it is more likely to represent nonspecific binding. Although the discriminating power of Southern blotting may be attractive, it comes at a high price of labor, equipment, and time compared to dot blotting, which can be semiautomated and can run multiple samples simultaneously in a 96-well microtiter plate format.

In Situ Hybridization

The principle of in situ hybridization is to probe tissue sections to demonstrate specific nucleic acids in infected cells.[44] The nature of the steps in the procedure are very similar to immunohistochemical staining. The differences have to do with pretreatment of sections with permeating agents such as proteases to open up the tissue matrix to diffusion of the probe and heating to denature the nucleic acids. Some of the reagents used in the hybridization reactions are also different. The power of in situ hybridization is its ability to identify specific infectious events on a cell-by-cell basis. Its weaknesses lie in requiring a relatively large copy number (usually hundreds) of DNA target molecules per cell, very stringent conditions for preservation of RNA targets, and the need to develop a different set of probe and hybridization parameters for virtually every infectious agent or gene under scrutiny. Examples of in situ hybridization are given in Chapter 3.

Restriction Fragment Sizing and Southern Blotting

Because restriction endonuclease cut sites occur randomly in genomic DNA, mutations may also occur within those sites with some probability. Furthermore, insertions and deletions of DNA can occur between the cut sites, giving rise to different fragment sizes from different strains of the same organism.[45] Within a single isolate, the fragment sizes are expected to remain relatively constant. A virus passed from one person to another should also retain the same fragment sizes. Thus in epidemiologic studies. the restriction length fragment sizes obtained from the DNA of the same species of isolate (eg, cytomegalovirus, herpes simplex virus) from different patients can be very discriminating as to whether a single organism has been passed from one patient to another or whether infections were acquired independently.[46]

Restriction digestion and electrophoresis may be done on larger amounts of purified DNA extracted from expanded pure cultures of isolates and then stained with ethidium bromide to yield the pattern of restriction fragments. Viruses with segmented RNA genomes can also be treated with electrophoresis and ethidium bromide staining to reveal characteristic fragment sizes (eg, rotavirus as extracted from stool samples). This type of analysis is generally limited to organisms with relatively small genomes to maintain a small number of restriction fragments (eg, 20 or fewer). Higher organisms such as bacteria with larger genomes yield so many restriction fragments that they overlap on electrophoresis in a nearly continuous blur of bands. Consequently, direct ethidium bromide staining of electrophoresed fragments is not particularly useful for bacteriology, and the need for large amounts of purified DNA also makes it inappropriate for routine viral identification.

To obviate this problem, Southern blot analysis can be used to examine selective microbial genes even in the presence of much larger amounts of DNA from unrelated organisms, including host human DNA such as what might arise from the presence of inflammatory cells in a clinical sample. Ribosomal genes have been used a great deal for classifying bacteria in this manner.[47] Of course, the ultimate analysis for microbial identification is complete nucleotide sequencing or sequencing of highly variable regions of specific genes within an infectious agent. Direct sequencing may also be necessary to identify particularly virulent variants of viral species such as HBV.[48–50]

DNA AMPLIFICATION METHODS

Methods for nucleic acid amplification are simplistically divided into two groups: the polymerase chain reaction (PCR) and other non-PCR methods that were invented later largely to avoid infringement on PCR patent rights for the development of alternative commercial applications.[51] The invention of PCR made possible amplification of defined sequences of DNA by a factor of 2 in each cycle of the reaction. Thus after 1 cycle, the number of copies is doubled; after 2 cycles, it is increased fourfold; after 10 cycles, it is increased by $2^{10} = 1024$; after 20 cycles, by more than 1 million; etc. Typical PCR assays utilize roughly 30 cycles, which theoretically should result in up to a billion-fold amplification. Thus, very small numbers of DNA molecules (even one) can theoretically be detected following multiple cycles of PCR. This property is very useful for infectious disease testing when even a single organism in a sample may be significant. Of course, PCR and other amplification methods have the advantage over culture that nucleic acids from nonviable organisms can be amplified and detected.

Polymerase Chain Reaction

In PCR, DNA synthesis is primed by oligonucleotides of defined sequence on either side of a region of DNA targeted for amplification (Figure 4–4).[52–54] The primers are usually about 20 nucleotides long, which confers a high degree of binding specificity since the probability is very low that such a sequence would occur randomly in DNA from another source. The end result of PCR is copies of the target sequence with the primers incorporated at each end. Detection of the reaction product

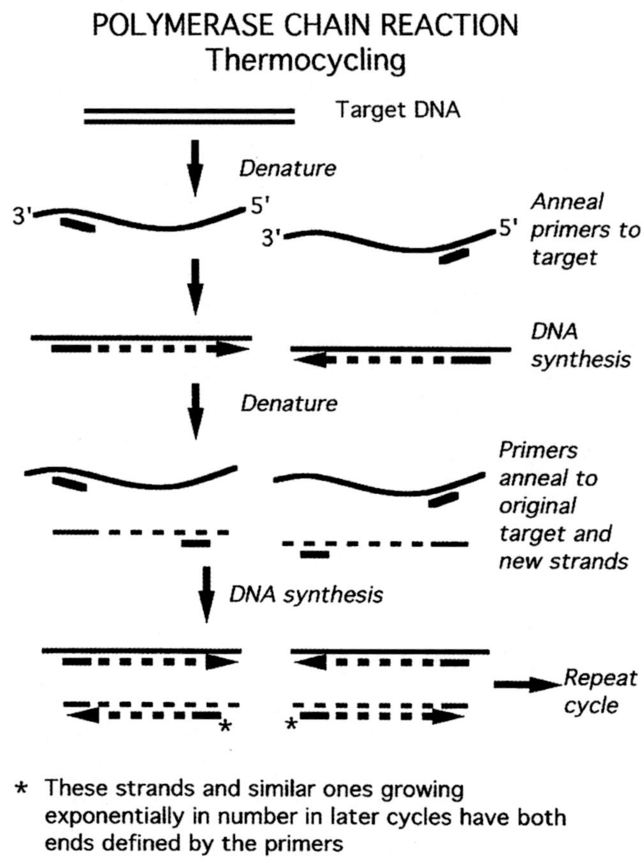

Figure 4–4. Polymerase chain reaction in which primers are used to initiate DNA synthesis catalyzed by *Taq* polymerase. Each cycle results in a twofold increase in the number of target DNA copies.

may be done by electrophoresis and ethidium bromide visualization of a DNA band of expected molecular size. Confirmation that the amplified sequence is indeed the one intended can be done by Southern blot analysis of that electrophoresis. Other applications utilize a 96-well microtiter plate format with colorimetric detection.

A single cycle of PCR consists of three temperature phases. The first is generally at about 94°C to denature DNA molecules into single strands. The second is cooler (50s to 60s degrees Celsius) allowing the primers to anneal to the single-stranded DNA targets. The third is slightly higher in temperature and permits enzymatic synthesis of DNA extending from the primer along the single-stranded DNA template (target). The reaction mixture contains target DNA (eg, sample) and primers plus abundant nucleotide precursors; *Taq* DNA polymerase, which is stable under wide fluctuations of temperature[55]; and a matrix of buffer with optimized concentrations of ions such as magnesium.[56] After each round of synthesis, the whole process is reiterated. The instrumentation required for PCR includes a thermocycler so that a sealed reaction vessel can be put in place and run through multiple cycles without further manipulation until amplification is completed and detection of products is performed.

As straightforward as PCR is, it must be practiced with strict attention to the avoidance of contamination between samples (ie, from positive to negative ones) and in particular from contamination of fresh unamplified samples with amplified products from previous reactions.[57] In practice, it is now recommended to prepare and seal samples for PCR in a clean preamplification room physically isolated (and with entrance through positive air pressure to keep out contaminants) from the amplification region where the thermocycler is located. After PCR is completed, the samples are opened for further analysis in a postamplification room (eg, at negative pressure to avoid expelling amplified products). Techniques for eliminating contamination in PCR have included chemical modification of the reaction product with an isopsoralen derivative (so-called PCR sterilization)[58] and light activation to prevent it from being further replicated.[59–61] The enzyme uracil DNA glycosylase may be used to remove uracil from reaction products that are then inactive as template (this method requires use of uracil instead of thymidine in the synthesis).[62,63] Direct illumination with ultraviolet light or gamma irradiation may also reduce the load of potential contamination.[64,65] No one, however, has yet devised a surefire technique to prevent contamination, thus pointing to a painstaking laboratory technique as essential for minimizing it. For infectious disease testing in which the mere presence of an organism may establish diagnosis, contamination from a laboratory environment may be extremely critical (eg, in locations where the organism being amplified by PCR has previously been cultured and copies of the genome may be floating in the room's dust). To overcome this potential difficulty, techniques such as nested PCR have been employed in which an initial reaction product with one set of primers is further amplified with an additional set of internal (nested) primers that should recognize the true target signal.[66]

PCR is poised to make a major impact on microbiologic testing.[67–73] A recent commercial application from Kodak utilizes a closed system for amplification continuing into hybridization and colorimetric detection for mycobacterial species. *Bordetella pertussis* is another bacterial pathogen examined by PCR in comparison with culture and serology.[74] Diagnosis of *Herpes simplex* may also be enhanced by PCR.[75] Of course, positive PCR results must be interpreted carefully as they may also be found in recovery phase when a patient is no longer infectious.[76,77]

Note that PCR is susceptible to some particular interfering substances that are likely to occur in clinical specimens.[78] These substances include heme and heparin and also anything that may introduce high concentrations of ions into the reaction mixture.[79–82] In addition, fixatives commonly used for preserving tissues may also inactivate *Taq* (especially the mercury in B5, which is frequently used for preserving lymph node morphology). However, amplifiable nucleic acids can be successfully and routinely extracted from sections of (neutral buffered) formalin-fixed, paraffin-embedded tissues.[83–87] Present efforts are also being directed at performing PCR within tissues or cells to enable localization of infectious agents to particular cells or cellular organelles identified histologically. This process is termed *in situ PCR*.[88,89]

Reverse Transcriptase PCR

PCR may also be employed to make copies from RNA molecules that have been converted to cDNA by reverse transcriptase. This methodology is generally referred to as *reverse transcriptase polymerase chain reaction* (RT–PCR). From knowledge of the number of amplification cycles and measurement of the amount of reaction product, it is also possible to estimate the quantity of starting target material. This application has been made with RT–PCR for quantitation of hepatitis C virus (HCV) RNA in serum.[90] HCV causes chronic hepatitis in a large percentage of cases, and it is now treated with α-interferon as is chronic HBV infection.[91,92] Quantitative RT–PCR for HCV RNA is an excellent prototype amplification assay for infectious disease testing.[93,94] Serologic assays for HCV antibodies are not useful for monitoring disease progress or response to antiviral therapy. Recent work comparing serum biochemical assays, RT–PCR, and liver biopsy indicate that RT–PCR has excellent correlation with disease activity.[95–98] Thus there is now a strong clinical demand to provide this assay.

RT–PCR uses relatively well conserved regions to amplify (eg, in the 5′-noncoding region and in the NS3 gene), because there is substantial variability in nucleotide sequences in the genes of different strains of HCV.[99–101] This variability is due to an inherent error rate of the viral polymerase in copying a single-stranded genome. Even more important is the question of whether quantitation of HCV RNA in serum is the proper assay to employ because the strain of HCV may shift in a patient during a course of interferon treatment, presumably due to the high rate of mutation.[102,103] Thus a more appropriate assay may be direct nucleotide sequencing of HCV genes to determine the strain and susceptibility of the virus at any particular time in a patient's course.[104] Of course, RT–PCR may always retain a place for early diagnosis of acute HCV infection before serologic response has developed.

Both PCR and RT–PCR have been used to detect a variety of organisms, including viruses and bacteria even from fecal material.[105–107] PCR remains something of a gold standard against which to judge other amplification methods.

Non-PCR Amplification Methods

A major driving force for inventing and promoting other amplification methods has been to offer alternative technologies with no patent infringement on PCR for commercial applications and to use cycle steps that are easy to automate, with detection of product also done in an automated manner.[108] There are several non-PCR amplifications now under development. Each one has its own patent priorities that are owned or licensed by different companies. It seems reasonable to expect that whatever methods succeed in the marketplace will do so because they can be automated to handle large numbers of samples with minimal operator intervention and that they will be at least equivalent to PCR in diagnostic power, but certainly should be better or faster than culture or antigen detection.

Ligase Chain Reaction

The process of ligase chain reaction (LCR) does not entail synthesis of strands of DNA but rather the joining together of oligonucleotide probes that have hybridized adjacent to one another on a target sequence of DNA (Figure 4–5).[109] If the target is not present, the probes will not come into alignment to be joined end to end to form a larger molecule by the reagent enzyme bacteriophage T4 ligase. The complete nucleotide sequence of the target DNA must be known to design and synthesize oligonucleotide probes that will hybridize successfully. Cycles are controlled by iterative heating and cooling to denature the target and newly formed product so that the probes can anneal to initiate another round of ligation. LCR now shows some promise for automation in commercial development by Abbott (Abbott Laboratories, Abbott Park, IL). In particular, applications have been made for *Listeria monocytogenes, Mycobacterium tuberculosis, Chlamydia trachomatis*, and *Neisseria gonorrhoeae*.[110]

Transcription-Mediated Amplification Systems

These methods utilize enzymes that normally are involved in DNA synthesis and RNA transcription. In self-sustained sequence replication (3SR), an RNA template is targeted by a probe that promotes complementary DNA strand synthesis by reverse transcriptase.[111–113] The RNA is then specifically degraded enzymatically. The single-stranded DNA copy is then made double stranded. Multiple copies of RNA are transcribed from that DNA product, and that RNA goes back into the previous cycle, ultimately making other DNA copies. This

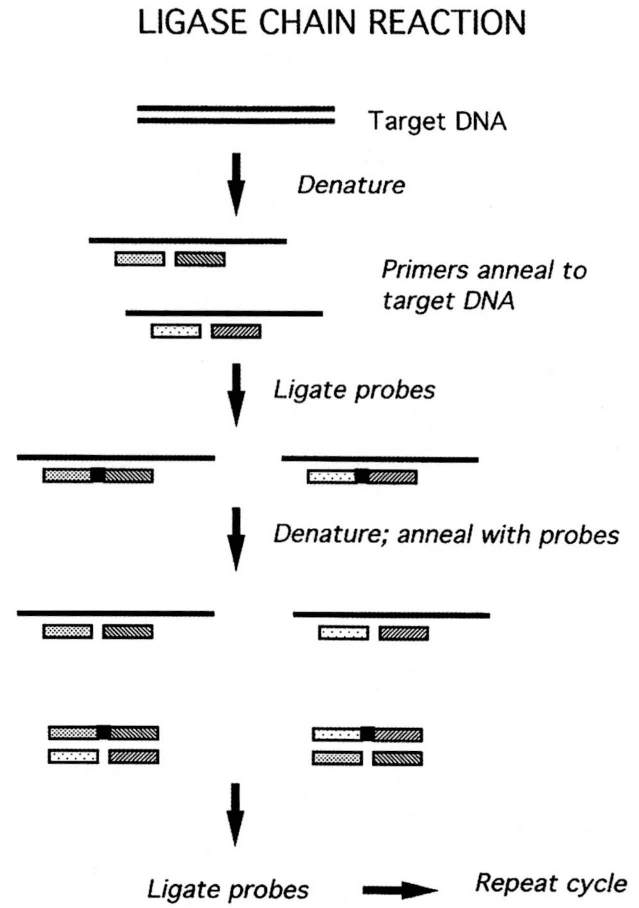

Figure 4–5. Ligase chain reaction in which probes are hybridized to adjacent positions on the target nucleic acid and then joined by T4 ligase. Each cycle of iteration results in a twofold increase in the number of ligated DNA copies.

process is isothermal without shift of temperature; therefore, the number of chemical reaction cycles is not known unless an internal standard is also amplified to determine the effective number of cycles for a given reaction mixture.

Gen-Probe rRNA Amplification System

This technique has been automated with applications under way for *M tuberculosis, C trachomatis,* and other organisms.[114–116] This isothermal process is autocatalytic and is a homogeneous system that does not require phase separation for detection. This is an important operational advantage because the assay is performed in a single reaction tube. The target is rRNA, which is present in thousands of copies per bacterium, thus theoretically making detection of a single microorganisms very feasible.

In the assay, rRNA is released from lysed bacteria and is made into a DNA copy (cDNA) with reverse transcriptase. This cDNA:RNA duplex is then used as template for transcription of multiple copies of RNA by T7 RNA polymerase. These new RNA molecules can in turn go through a cycle with reverse transcriptase to make another cDNA molecule. The principle of detection is hybridization protection in which acridium ester-labeled DNA probes bind to the amplified product. Unhybridized probe is decomposed chemically. The acridium ester is chemiluminescent while linked to the probe but not in degraded form. Thus chemiluminescent measurement yields direct detection of the product formed.

Qβ Replicase Amplification

This method relies on the RNA-dependent RNA polymerase of Qβ bacteriophage. Its specific RNA target is MDV-1 (for midivariant 1), which is incorporated into the probe, thereby focusing synthesis on the RNA of interest.[117] Million-fold to billion-fold amplifications are possible in minutes. This abundant level of synthesis makes it feasible to detect products colorimetrically.

Branched DNA Signal Amplification

This method amplifies the signal derived from hybridization reactions rather than amplifying the number of target molecules.[118–121] It is a nonisotopic technique that uses an enzyme-coupled probe. Target nucleic acid molecules are captured onto solid phase oligonucleotides through linking probes with defined sequence specificity. At the same time, branched DNA (bDNA) multimers participate by complementarity with linkers. Also binding to the bDNA (which has a multitude of sites, thereby giving rise to the amplification) are multiple enzyme-labeled probes that act in the final colorimetric detection step after washing away all the unbound probes. This method has succeeded in detecting down to 1000 copies of viral genome.

ASSAY PERFORMANCE

Nucleic acid-based diagnostic testing has evolved from research techniques that had great variability in performance between laboratories. That genesis has in some ways slowed down the introduction of standard clinical laboratory practices into nucleic acid testing. The requirement for Food and Drug Administration approval of commercial assays has certainly improved the prospects for incorporating standard aspects of calibration, quality control, proficiency testing, etc. Recent guidelines have also been issued for nucleic acid testing.[122]

Standardization

The availability of standard reference materials that may be exchanged among all participating laboratories is essential to establish uniform calibration. This need is particularly important for quantitative assays where the actual concentration of nucleic acid is important (eg, HBV or HCV in serum). However, even qualitative assays should be tested for sensitivity and specificity with authentically positive samples that can be exchanged with other users.

The issues of calibration are complicated by the difference between nucleic acids as they appear in viral particles (complexed with proteins and lipid membranes) versus the simple form of nucleic acids extracted and purified following cloning in plasmids and propagation in bacteria. Thus whatever material is used to standardize an assay should be translatable to native biological equivalents.

Quality Control

Both negative and positive materials should be used for assessing assay precision and determination of any assay drift or deviation. This control process is comparable to what is practiced in measuring many other biochemical analytes. However, amplification techniques introduce some special considerations. In particular, reactions with negative results may indicate that the sample tested had no target nucleic acid in it or that it could have had a true signal that was not amplified because an inhibitory substance was also present. Assessment of this possibility requires an internal quality control standard that is amplified in every specimen to demonstrate that each sample is usable. An example of this process is amplifying genes such as actin or globin that should be present in human genomic DNA extracts in genetic disease testing. For infectious agents, it may be necessary to introduce a control target with similar characteristics to the actual target; however, it must be constructed so that products from control and target can easily be distinguished.

Proficiency Testing

A periodic and independent check on calibration is achieved through use of proficiency survey testing in which aliquots of the same sample are sent as unknowns to participating laboratories. Compilation of all results allows an individual laboratory to assess its accuracy relative to other laboratories. The logistic problems of manufacturing biologically authentic samples that will be stable over long periods of time are considerable when dealing with nucleic acids. However, confidence in assay results is strengthened markedly by demonstration of good performance in comparison with peer laboratories.

REFERENCES

1. Watson JD, Crick FHC. Genetical implications of the structure of deoxyribonucleic acid. *Nature.* 1953; 171:964–967.
2. Keller GH. The probe-target interaction. In: Keller GH, Manak MM, eds. *DNA Probes.* 2nd ed. New York: Stockton Press; 1993:1–25.
3. Wetmur JG, Davidson N. Kinetics of renaturation of DNA. *J Molec Biol.* 1968;31:349–370.
4. Hamaguchi K, Geiduschek EP. The effect of electrolytes on the stability of the deoxyribonucleate helix. *J Am Chem Soc.* 1962;84:1329–1338.
5. McCarthy BJ, Bolton ET. An approach to the measurement of genetic relatedness among organisms. *Proc Natl Acad Sci USA.* 1963;50:156–164.
6. Nygaard AP, Hall BD. A method for the detection of RNA-DNA complexes. *J Molec Biol.* 1963;9:125–142.
7. Maniatis T, Fritsch EF, Sambrook J. Purification of nucleic acids. In: *Molecular Cloning: A Laboratory Manual.* Cold Spring Harbor, NY: Cold Spring Harbor Laboratory; 1982:458–462.
8. Nathans D, Smith HO. Restriction endonucleases in the analysis and restructuring of DNA molecules. *Ann Rev Biochem.* 1975;44:273–293.
9. Smith HO. Nucleotide sequence specificity of restriction endonucleases. *Science.* 1979;205:455–462.
10. Chu G, Vollrath D, Davis RW. Separation of large DNA molecules by contour-clamped homogeneous electric fields. *Science.* 1986;234:1582–1584.
11. Lai E, Birren BW, Clark SM, Simon MI, Hood L. Pulsed field gel electrophoresis. *BioTechniques.* 1989;7:34–42.
12. Miranda AG, Singh KV, Murray BE. DNA fingerprinting of *Entercoccus faecium* by pulsed-field gel electrophoresis may be a useful epidemiologic tool. *J Clin Microbiol.* 1991;29:2752–2757.
13. Vazquez JA, Beckley A, Sobel JD, Zervos MJ. Comparison of restriction enzyme analysis versus pulsed-field gradient gel electrophoresis as a typing system for *Candida albicans. J Clin Microbiol.* 1991;29:962–967.
14. Dembry LM, Vazquez JA, Zervos MJ. DNA analysis in the study of the epidemiology of nosocomial candidiasis. *Infect Contr Hosp Epidemiol.* 1994;15:48–53.
15. Katz ED, Dong MW. Rapid analysis and purification of polymerase chain reaction products by high-performance liquid chromatography. *BioTechniques.* 1990; 8:546–555.
16. Landers JP, Oda RP, Spelsberg TC, Nolan JA, Ulfelder KJ. Capillary electrophoresis: a powerful microanalytical

technique for biologically active molecules. *BioTechniques.* 1993;12:98–111.

17. Wahl GM, Stern M, Stark GR. Efficient transfer of large DNA fragments from agarose gels to diazobenzyloxymethyl-paper and rapid hybridization by using dextran sulfate. *Proc Natl Acad Sci USA.* 1979;76:3683–3687.
18. Southern EM. Detection of specific sequences among DNA fragments separated by gel electrophoresis. *J Molec Biol.* 1975;98:503–517.
19. Alwine JC, Kemp DJ, Stark GR. Method for detection of specific RNAs in agarose gels by transfer to diazobenzyloxymethyl paper and hybridization with DNA probes. *Proc Natl Acad Sci USA.* 1977;74:5350–5354.
20. Rigby PWS, Dieckman M, Rhodes C, Berg P. Labeling deoxyribonucleic acid to high specific activity in vitro by nick translation with DNA polymerase I. *J Molec Biol.* 1977;113:237–251.
21. Chu BCF, Wahl GM, Orgel LE. Derivatization of unprotected polynucleotides. *Nucleic Acids Res.* 1983;11: 6513–6529.
22. Chu BCF, Orgel LE. Detection of specific DNA sequences with short biotin-labeled probes. *DNA.* 1985;4:327–331.
23. Gebeychu G, Pao PY, SooChan P, Simms DA, Klevan L. Novel biotinylated nucleotide analogs for labeling and colorimetric detection of DNA. *Nucleic Acids Res.* 1987;15:4513–4534.
24. Keller GH, Cumming CU, Huang DP, Manak MM, Ting R. A chemical method for introducing haptens onto DNA probes. *Anal Biochem.* 1988;170:441–450.
25. Kessler C, Höltke H-J, Seibl R, Burg J, Mühlegger K. Nonradioactive labeling and detection of nucleic acids. 1. A novel DNA labeling and detection system based on digoxigenin:anti-digoxigenin ELISA principle (digoxigenin system). *Biol Chem Hoppe-Seyler.* 1990;371: 917–922.
26. Leary PM, Guerra CE, Lomeli H, Tussie-Luna I, Kramer FR. Rapid and sensitive colorimetric method for visualizing biotin-labeled DNA probes hybridized to DNA or RNA immobilized on nitrocellulose: bio-blots. *Proc Natl Acad Sci USA.* 1983;80:4045–4049.
27. Jablonski E, Moomaw EW, Tullis RH, Ruth JL. Preparation of oligodeoxynucleotide-alkaline phosphatase conjugates and their use as hybridization probes. *Nucleic Acids Res.* 1986;14;3015–3028.
28. Balaguer Térouanne B, Boussioux A-M, Nicolas J-C. Use of bioluminescence in nucleic acid hybridization reactions. *J Biolum Chemilum.* 1989;4:302–309.
29. Schaap AP, Akhavan H, Romano LJ. Chemiluminescent substrates for alkaline phosphatase: application to ultrasensitive enzyme-linked immunoassays and DNA probes. *Clin Chem.* 1989;35:1863–1864.
30. Nguyen NJ, McPherson RA. Cancer diagnosis. In: Keller GH, Manak MM, eds. *DNA Probes.* 2nd ed. New York: Stockton Press; 1993:483–523.
31. Nelson NC, Kacian DL. Chemiluminescent DNA probes: a comparison of the acridinium ester and dioxetane detection systems and their use in clinical diagnostic assays. *Clin Chim Acta.* 1990;194:73–90.
32. Rosenthal N. Fine structure of a gene—DNA sequencing. *N Engl J Med.* 1995;332:589–591.
33. Maxam A, Gilbert W. A new method for sequencing DNA. *Proc Natl Acad Sci USA.* 1977;74:560–564.
34. Sanger F, Nicklen S, Coulson AR. DNA sequencing with chain terminating inhibitors. *Proc Natl Acad Sci USA.* 1977;74:5463–5467.
35. Naber SP. Molecular pathology—diagnosis of infectious disease. *N Engl J Med.* 1994;331:1212–1215.
36. Buffone GJ, Demmler GJ, Schimbor CM, Yow MD. A hybridization assay for congenital cytomegalovirus infection. *J Clin Microbiol.* 1988;26:2184–2186.
37. Golts SP, Todd JA, Yang HL. A rapid DNA probe test for detecting HPV in biopsy specimens. *Am Clin Prod Rev.* December 1987:16–19.
38. Wen LT, Henneberger M, Nuyen N, McPherson RA. Quantitation of hepatitis B virus DNA in serum by ammonium sulfate precipitation and molecular hybridization. *J Clin Lab Anal.* 1994;8:44–50.
39. McPherson RA. Laboratory diagnosis of human hepatitis viruses. *J Clin Lab Anal.* 1994;8:369–377.
40. Lieberman HM, LaBrecque DR, Kew MC, Hadziyannis SJ, Shafritz DA. Detection of hepatitis B virus DNA directly in human serum by a simplified molecular hybridization test: comparison to HBeAg/anti-HBe status in HBsAg carriers. *Hepatology.* 1983;3:285–291.
41. Carloni G, Colloca S, Delfini C, Manzin A, Clementi M, Galibert F. Detection of HBV infectivity by spot hybridization in HBeAg-negative chronic carriers: HBV DNA in sera from asymptomatic and symptomatic subjects. *J Med Virol.* 1987;21:15–23.
42. Kuhns MC, McNamara AL, Perrillo RP, Cabal CM, Campbel CR. Quantitation of hepatitis B viral DNA by solution hybridization: comparison with DNA polymerase and hepatitis B e antigen during antiviral therapy. *J Med Virol.* 1989;27:274–281.
43. Walter E, Blum HE, Offensperger W-B, Zeschnigk C, Offensperger S, Gerok W. Spot-blot hybridization assay for the detection of hepatitis B virus DNA in serum: factors determining its sensitivity and specificity. *Hepatology.* 1987;7:557–562.
44. Abbondanzo SL, English CK, Kagan E, McPherson RA. Fatal adenovirus pneumonia in a newborn identified by electron microscopy and in situ hybridization. *Arch Pathol Lab Med.* 1989;113:1349–1353.
45. Mahayni R, Zervos M. The clinical laboratory's role in hospital infection control. *Lab Med.* 1994;25:642–647.
46. John JF. Molecular analysis of nosocomial epidemics. *Infect Dis Clin North Am.* 1989;3:683–700.
47. Yogev D, Halachmi D, Kenny GE, Razin S. Distinction of species and strains of mycoplasmas (mollicutes) by genomic DNA fingerprints with an rRNA gene probe. *J Clin Microbiol.* 1988;26:1198–1201.
48. Liang TJ, Hasegawa K, Rimon N, Wands JR, Ben-Porath E. A hepatitis B virus mutant associated with an epidemic of fulminant hepatitis. *N Engl J Med.* 1991; 423:1705–1709.
49. Ehata T, Omata M, Chang W-L, et al. Mutations in core nucleotide sequence of hepatitis B virus correlate with fulminant and severe hepatitis. *J Clin Invest.* 1993; 91:1206–1213.
50. Ehata T, Omata M, Yokosuka O, Hosoda K, Ohto M.

Variations in codons 84-101 in the core nucleotide sequence correlate with hepatocellular injury in chronic hepatitis B virus infection. *J Clin Invest.* 1992; 89:332–338.

51. Wolcott MJ. Advances in nucleic acid-based detection methods. *Clin Microbiol Rev.* 1992;5:370–386.
52. Mullis KB, Faloona FA. Specific synthesis of DNA in vitro via a polymerase-catalysed chain reaction. *Methods Enzymol.* 1987;155:335–350.
53. Saiki RK, Gelfand DH, Stoffel S, et al. Primer-directed enzymatic amplification of DNA with a thermostable DNA polymerase. *Science.* 1988;239:487–491.
54. Mullis KB. The unusual origin of the polymerase chain reaction. *Sci Am.* 1990;240:56–65.
55. Barany F. Genetic disease detection and DNA amplification using cloned thermostable ligase. *Proc Natl Acad Sci USA.* 1991;88:189–193.
56. Saiki RK. The design and optimization of the polymerase chain reaction. In: Erlich HA, ed. *PCR Technology: Principles and Applications for DNA Amplification.* New York: Stockton Press; 1989.
57. Kwok S, Higuchi R. Avoiding false positives with PCR. *Nature.* 1989;339:237–238.
58. Cimino GD, Metchette KC, Tessman JW, Hearst JE, Isaacs ST. Post-PCR sterilization: a method to control carryover contamination for the polymerase chain reaction. *Nucleic Acids Res.* 1991;19:99–107.
59. Isaacs ST, Tessman JW, Metchette KC, Hearst JE, Cimino GD. Post-PCR sterilization: development and application to an HIV-1 diagnostic assay. *Nucleic Acids Res.* 1991;19:109–116.
60. Aslanzadeh J. Application of hydroxylamine hydrochloride for post-PCR sterilization. *Ann Clin & Lab Sci.* 1992;22:280.
61. Prince AM, Andrus L. PCR: how to kill unwanted DNA. *BioTechniques.* 1992;12:358–360.
62. Longo MC, Berninger MS, Hartley JL. Use of uracil DNA glycosylase to control carryover contamination in polymerase chain reactions. *Gene.* 1990;93:125–128.
63. Thornton CG, Hartley JL, Rashtchian A. Utilizing uracil DNA glycosylase to control carryover contamination in PCR: characterization of residual UDG activity following thermal cycling. *BioTechniques.* 1992;13:180–182.
64. Fox JC, Ait-Khalid M, Webster A, Emery VC. Eliminating PCR contamination: is UV irradiation the answer? *J Virol Meth.* 1991;33:375–383.
65. Deragon J-M, Sinnett D, Mitchell G, Potier M, Labuda D. Use of γ irradiation to eliminate DNA contamination for PCR. *Nucleic Acids Res.* 1990;18:6149.
66. Porter-Jordan K, Rosenberg EL, Keiser J, et al. Nested polymerase chain reaction assay for the detection of cytomegalovirus overcomes false positives due to contamination with fragmented DNA. *J Med Virol.* 1990; 30:85–91.
67. Dale B, Dragon EA. Polymerase chain reaction in infectious disease diagnosis. *Lab Med.* 1994;25:637–641.
68. Bej AK, Mahbubani MH, Atlas RM. Detection of viable *Legionella pneumophila* in water by polymerase chain reaction. *Appl Environ Microbiol.* 1991;57:597–600.
69. Persing DH. Polymerase chain reactions: trenches to benches. *J Clin Microbiol.* 1991;29:1281–1285.
70. Shimizu H, McCarthy CA, Smaron MF, Burns JC. Polymerase chain reaction for detection of measles virus in clinical samples. *J Clin Microbiol.* 1993;31:1034–1039.
71. Jascjel G, Gaydos CA, Welsh LE, Quinn TC. Direct detection of *Chlamydia trachomatis* in urine specimens from symptomatic and asymptomatic men by using a rapid polymerase chain reaction assay. *J Clin Microbiol.* 1993;31:1209–1212.
72. Liebling MR, Nishio MJ, Rodriguez A, Sigal LH, Jin T, Louie JS. The polymerase chain reaction for the detection of *Borrelia burgdorferi* in human body fluids. *Arthritis Rheum.* 1993;36:665–675.
73. Kolk AHJ, Schuitema ARJ, Kuijper S, et al. Detection of *Mycobacterium tuberculosis* in clinical samples by using polymerase chain reaction and a nonradioactive detection system. *J Clin Microbiol.* 1992;30:2567–2575.
74. Grimprel E, Bégué P, Anjak I, Betsou F, Guiso N. Comparison of polymerase chain reaction, culture, and Western immunoblot serology for diagnosis of *Bordetella pertussis* infection. *J Clin Microbiol.* 1993;31:2745–2750.
75. Werner JC, Wiebrauk DL. Polymerase chain reaction for diagnosis of herpetic eye disease. *Lab Med.* 1994; 25:664–668.
76. Marcellin P, Martinot-Peignoux M, Loriot M-A, et al. Persistence of hepatitis B virus DNA demonstrated by polymerase chain reaction in serum and liver after loss of HBsAg induced by antiviral therapy. *Ann Intern Med.* 1990;112:227–228.
77. Lazizi Y, Pillot J. Delayed clearance of HBV-DNA detected by PCR in the absence of viral replication. *J Med Virol.* 1993;39:208–213.
78. Panaccio M, Good RT, Reed MB. A road map for PCR from clinical material. *J Clin Lab Anal.* 1994;8:315–322.
79. Beutler E, Gelbart E, Kuhl W. Interference of heparin with polymerase chain reactions. *BioTechniques.* 1990;9:166.
80. Weyant RS, Edmonds P, Swaminathan B. Effect of ionic and nonionic detergents on *Taq* polymerase. *BioTechniques.* 1990;9:308–309.
81. Khan G, Kangro HO, Coates PJ, Heath RB. Inhibitory effects of urine on the polymerase chain reaction for cytomegalovirus DNA. *J Clin Pathol.* 1991;44:360–365.
82. Yamaguchi Y, Hironaka T, Kajiwara M, Tateno E, Kita H, Hirai K. Increased sensitivity for detection of human cytomegalovirus in urine by removal of inhibitors for the polymerase chain reaction. *J Virol Meth.* 1992;37: 209–218.
83. Greer CE, Lund JK, Mano MM. PCR amplification from paraffin embedded tissues: recommendation on fixative for long-term storage and prospective studies. *PCR Meth Appl.* 1991;1:46–50.
84. Rogers BB, Alpert LC, Hine EA, Buffone GJ. Analysis of DNA in fresh and fixed tissue by the polymerase chain reaction. *Am J Pathol.* 1990;136:541–548.
85. Chen ML, Shien YS, Shim KS, Gerber MA. Comparative studies on the detection of hepatitis B virus DNA in frozen and paraffin sections by the polymerase chain reaction. *Mod Pathol.* 1991;4:555–558.

86. Class EC, Melchers WJ, van der Linden HC, Lindeman J, Quint WG. Human papillomavirus detection in paraffin-embedded cervical carcinomas and metastases of the carcinomas by the polymerase chain reaction. *Am J Pathol.* 1990;135:703–709.
87. Ben-Ezra J, Johnson DA, Rossi J, Cook N, Wu A. Effect of fixation on the amplification of nucleic acids from paraffin-embedded material by the polymerase chain reaction. *J Histochem Cytochem.* 1991;39:351–354.
88. Nuovo GJ. In situ detection of PCR-amplified DNA and cDNA. *Amplifications.* 1992;8:1–3.
89. Chiu K-P, Cohen S, Morris D, Jordan G. Intracellular amplification of proviral DNA in tissue sections using the polymerase chain reaction. *J Histochem Cytochem.* 1992;40:333–341.
90. Cuypers HTM, Bresters D, Winkel IN, et al. Storage conditions of blood samples and primer selection affect the yield of cDNA polymerase chain reaction products of hepatitis C virus. *J Clin Microbiol.* 1992;30:3220–3224.
91. Choo QL, Kuo G, Weiner AJ, Overby LR, Bradley DW, Houghton M. Isolation of a cDNA clone derived from a bloodborne non-A, non-B viral hepatitis genome. *Science.* 1989;244:359–362.
92. Cuthbert JA. Hepatitis C: progress and problems. *Clin Microbiol Rev.* 1994;7:505–532.
93. Brechot C. Polymerase chain reaction for the diagnosis of hepatitis B and C viral hepatitis. *J Hepatol.* 1993;17(suppl 3):S35–S41.
94. Cha T-A, Kolberg J, Irvine B, et al. Use of a signature nucleotide sequence of hepatitis C virus for detection of viral RNA in human serum and plasma. *J Clin Microbiol.* 1991;29:2528–2534.
95. Lau JYN, Davis GL, Kniffen J, et al. Significance of serum hepatitis C virus RNA levels in chronic hepatitis C. *Lancet.* 1993;1:2502–2504.
96. Yun Z-B, Lindh G, Weiland O, Johansson B, Sönnerborg A. Detection of hepatitis C virus (HCV) RNA by pcr related to HCV antibodies in serum and liver histology in Swedish blood donors. *J Med Virol.* 1993;39:57–61.
97. Kurosaki M, Enomoto N, Sato C, et al. Correlation of plama hepatitis C virus RNA levels with serum alanine aminotransferase in non-A, non-B chronic liver disease. *J Med Virol.* 1993;39:246–250.
98. Finkelstein SD, Sayegh R, Uchman S, Christensen S, Swalsky PA, Bodenheimer H. Disease activity of hepatitis C correlates with single-stage polymerase chain reaction detection of hepatitis C virus. *Am J Clin Pathol.* 1994;101:321–326.
99. Choo QL, Richman KH, Han JH, et al. Genetic organization and diversity of the hepatitis C virus. *Proc Natl Acad Sci USA.* 1991;88:2451–2455.
100. Hu K-Q, Yu C-H, Vierling JM. Direct detection of circulating hepatitis C virus RNA using probes from the 5′ untranslated region. *J Clin Invest.* 1992;89:2040–2045.
101. Okamoto M, Baba M, Kodama E, et al. Detection of hepatitis C virus genome in human serum by multi-targeted polymerase chain reaction. *J Med Virol.* 1993;41:6–10.
102. Huber KR, Knapp M, Bauer K. Subtyping hepatitis C virus. *Clin Chem.* 1995;41:319–320.
103. Cha TA, Beall E, Irvine B, et al. At least five related, but distinct, hepatitis C viral genotypes exist. *Proc Natl Acad Sci USA.* 1992;89:7144–7148.
104. Yoshioka K, Kakumu S, Wakita T, et al. Detection of hepatitis C virus by polymerase chain reaction and response to interferon-α therapy: relationship to genotypes of hepatitis C virus. *Hepatology.* 1992;16:293–299.
105. Glimaker M, Abebe A, Johansson B, Ehrnst A, Olcen P, Strannegard O. Detection of enteroviral RNA by polymerase chain reaction in faecal samples from patients with aseptic meningitis. *J Med Virol.* 1992;38:54–61.
106. Frankel G, Riley L, Giron JA, et al. Detection of *Shigella* in feces using DNA amplification. *J Infect Dis.* 1990; 161:1252–1256.
107. Olive DM. Detection of enterotoxigenic *Escherichia coli* after polymerase chain reaction. *J Clin Microbiol.* 1989; 27:1729–1734.
108. Barany F. The ligase chain reaction in a PCR world. *PCR Meth Appl.* 1991;1:5–16.
109. Backman K. Ligase chain reaction: diagnostic technology for the 1990s and beyond. *Clin Chem.* 1992;38:457–458.
110. Schachter J, Stamm WE, Quinn TC, Andrews WW, Burczak JD, Lee HH. Ligase chain reaction to detect *Chlamydia trachomatis* infection of the cervix. *J Clin Microbiol.* 1994;32:2540–2543.
111. Guatelli JC, Whitfield KM, Kwoh DY, Barringer KJ, Richman DD, Gingeras TR. Isothermal, in vitro amplification of nucleic acids by a multienzyme reaction modeled after retroviral replication. *Proc Natl Acad Sci USA.* 1990;87:1874–1878.
112. Gingeras TR, Prodanovich P, Latimer T, Guatelli JC, Richman DD, Barringer KJ. Use of self-sustained sequence replication amplification reaction to analyze and detect mutations in zidovudine-resistant human immunodeficiency virus. *J Infect Dis.* 1991;164:1066–1074.
113. Gingeras TR, Whitfield KM, Kwoh DY. Unique features of the self-sustained sequence replication (3SR) reaction in the in vitro amplification of nucleic acids. *Ann Biol Clin.* 1990;48:498–501.
114. Pokorski SJ, Vetter EA, Wollan PC, Cockerill FR III. Comparison of Gen-Probe group A streptococcus direct test with culture for diagnosing streptococcal pharyngitis. *J Clin Microbiol.* 1994;32:1440–1443.
115. Limberger RJ, Biega R, Evancoe A, McCarthy L, Slivienski L, Kirkwood M. Evaluation of culture and the Gen-Probe PACE 2 assay for detection of *Neisseria gonorrhoeae* and *Chlamydia trachomatis* in endocervical specimens transported to a state health laboratory. *J Clin Microbiol.* 1992;30:1162–1166.
116. Jonas V, Alden MJ, Curry JI, et al. Detection and identification of *Mycobacterium tuberculosis* directly from sputum sediments by amplification of rRNA. *J Clin Microbiol.* 1993;31:2410–2416.
117. Lizardi PM, Guerra CE, Lomeli H, Tussie-Luna I, Kramer FR. Exponential amplification of recombinant-RNA hybridization probes. *Bio/Technology.* 1988;6:1197–1202.

118. Urdea MS. Synthesis and characterization of branched DNA (bDNA) for the direct and quantitative detection of CMV, HBV, HCV, and HIV. *Clin Chem.* 1993;39:725–726.
119. Horn T, Urdea MS. Forks and combs and DNA: the synthesis of branched oligodeoxyribonucleotides. *Nucleic Acids Res.* 1989;17:6959–6967.
120. Urdea MS, Running JA, Horn T, Clyne J, Ku L, Warner BD. A novel method for the rapid detection of specific nucleotide sequences in crude biological samples without blotting or radioactivity: application to the analysis of hepatitis B virus in human serum. *Gene.* 1987; 61:253–264.
121. Urdea MS, Kolberg J, Clyne J, et al. Application of a rapid non-radioisotopic nucleic acid analysis system to the detection of sexually transmitted disease-causing organisms and their associated antimicrobial resistances. *Clin Chem.* 1989;35:1571–1575.
122. Molecular diagnostic methods for infectious diseases: proposed guidelines. National Committee for Clinical Laboratory Standards, Document MM3-P, March 1994; 14(4).

Part II

Viral Infections

CHAPTER 5

Adenoviruses

Washington C. Winn, Jr.

The natural dignity of our work, its unembarrassed kindness, its insight into life, its hold on science—for these privileges, and for all that they bring with them, up and up high over the top of the tree, the very heavens open, preaching thankfulness.

Stephen Paget (1855–1926)

DEFINITION

Adenoviruses are double-stranded DNA viruses divided into two genera: adenoviruses of mammals (mastadenoviruses) and aviadenoviruses of birds. Forty-seven serotypes of human adenoviruses, divided into four subgenera A–D, are now recognized. Types 43 through 47 were isolated only from patients with AIDS and were not in immunocompetent individuals.[1] Approximately half of the serotypes have been clearly associated with human disease.[2] A variety of age groups and organ systems is affected, and specific serotypes can often be associated with one or both parameters.

GEOGRAPHIC DISTRIBUTION

Adenoviruses are found worldwide. They are endogenous viruses of humans and were first isolated by Rowe from adenoidal tissue that was undergoing spontaneous degeneration in cell culture.[3] It has been estimated that 7% of respiratory tract infections in children are caused by adenoviruses.[4]

LIFE CYCLE, NATURAL HISTORY, AND EPIDEMIOLOGY

Adenoviruses replicate in the nucleus of infected cells, where the mature virions accumulate in masses as a crystalline array of polyhedral particles that can be seen with the light microscope as an intranuclear inclusion. Eventually, the mass of virions fills the nucleus, blurring the image of the nuclear membrane. The viruses are nonenveloped and are released to infect new cells by rupture of the infected cell.

The viruses remain latent in the lymphoepithelial tissue of the nasopharynx and other sites. Humans are the only hosts and most infections are sporadic, probably resulting from activation of endogenous viruses.[5] The potential for transmission by contaminated environmental vehicles is well illustrated by outbreaks of disease, often in closed populations of susceptible individuals.[6,7] A combination of ocular trauma and exposure to virus may increase the risk of keratoconjunctivitis.[7] Person-to-person transmission has been documented in families,[7] and may be a factor in epidemic disease among military recruits.[8,9] Severe pneumonia and systemic disease may occur in severely immunosuppressed patients, such as transplant patients.[5,10–13] Although not commonly infected, premature neonates are also at risk of fatal infection.[11]

MORPHOLOGY OF THE VIRUS

Adenoviruses are icosahedral, measuring approximately 70 nm in diameter (Figure 5–1). They consist of 252 capsomeres arranged with 12 capsomeres (hexons) on each side and one penton capsomere at each of 12 vertices. A fiber arises from each of the penton capsomeres. Neutralizing antibody is directed against the hexon antigens. As the virions are assembled in the

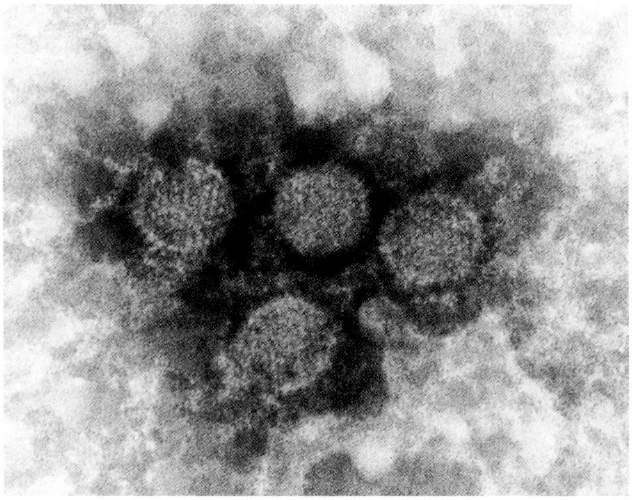

Figure 5–1. Adenovirus, type 1 virions released from infected WI-38 cells. The icosahedral virions appear spherical, and the individual capsomeres are outlined by the negative stain (phosphotungstic acid stain, ×274,000).

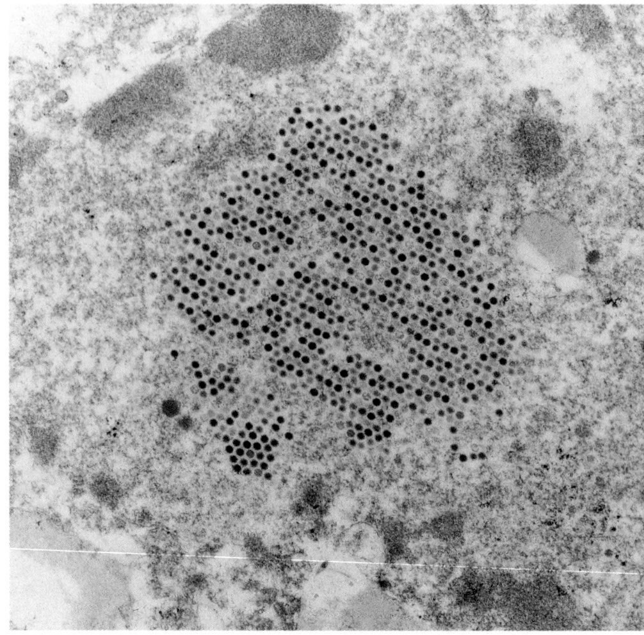

Figure 5–2. Individual adenovirus virions accumulate in the nucleus of an infected WI-38 cell. The icosahedral structure of the virions facilitates the packaging of the virions into a paracrystalline array (×32,000).

nucleus the icosahedral structure results in efficient packing of the particles to form a crystalline array (Figure 5–2).

CLINICAL FEATURES

Clinical disease caused by adenoviruses can be divided into three basic groups: respiratory infections, systemic infections, and gastroenteritis. Shortly after their discovery the viruses were named adenoidal–pharyngeal–conjunctival (APC) agents in recognition of common sites of infection. A variety of respiratory sites and combinations of sites may be affected by adenoviruses. As many as half of sporadic infections are asymptomatic.[4] Acute adenoviral pharyngitis may be accompanied by high fever and mimic streptococcal disease[14,15] or bacterial otitis media.[14,16] Tracheitis and lower respiratory infection are accompanied by fever, rhinorrhea, and sore throat (febrile catarrh). Cough and pulmonary infiltrates may also be present. Most infections are self-limited, but adenoviruses occasionally cause fatal pneumonia, particularly in military recruits and in immunodeficient patients. The most common serotypes isolated from adult patients with respiratory disease are 4 and 7.[2] Types 1, 2, 3, 5, 6, and 7 were statistically associated with respiratory tract disease in children.[4] Type 7 strains have been reported prominently from severe lower respiratory tract infection in infants and young children.[17,18] Other types, such as 3, 4, 8, 11, 21, 35, and intermediate strains, have been isolated from patients with fatal pneumonia.

Complications of adenovirus pneumonia include secondary bacterial infection,[19] hepatic and cerebral toxicity resembling Reye's syndrome,[20,21] coagulopathy including disseminated intravascular coagulation,[9,22] and infection of extrapulmonary organs, as discussed later. In addition, chronic pulmonary damage, including bronchiectasis can be demonstrated in many children years after the initial bout of adenoviral pneumonia.[23,24] Risk factors for chronic pulmonary disease include young age at the time of the pneumonia and a preceding "measles-like" illness.[25]

Pharyngoconjunctival fever is an adenoviral syndrome that afflicts children, often in small epidemics.[6,26] The disease is self-limited without involvement of the lower respiratory tract and without residual ocular damage. Type 3 strains are commonly isolated, and common sources, such as contaminated swimming pools, have been implicated as sources for the virus.[6]

Epidemic keratoconjunctivitis, first documented as "shipyard fever," is caused most commonly by type 8 adenovirus.[7] Types 19 and 37 have also been implicated in epidemic disease,[27,28] and other types may cause sporadic disease. Common sources for infection have been documented, and there is intrafamilial spread in approximately 10% of patients. The infection may be prolonged, and vision may be diminished during the keratitic phase. One patient, a medical house officer, developed acute conjunctivitis after caring for a immunocompetent patient who died of type 7A adenovirus pneumonia.[29]

A pertussis syndrome has been described in association with adenovirus infection, and cases have been reported in which there was no evidence of *Bordetella pertussis* infection, either by culture or by serology.[30] The difficulty of isolating *B pertussis* and the frequency of adenoviruses in normal children has made it difficult to establish a causal link between adenoviruses and whooping cough.

Gastroenteritis is a relatively new addition to the list of important adenovirus syndromes.[31,32] Although all serotypes may be in feces, clinical disease is associated primarily with types 40 and 41. Acute diarrhea, which is most common in young children and may occur in outbreaks, is watery and accompanied by fever. The infection is self-limited, but may persist for several weeks. It cannot be distinguished clinically from many other forms of viral gastroenteritis, but is not associated with the vomiting of rotavirus disease.

Respiratory serotypes of adenovirus, especially types 1, 2, 3, and 5, have been linked to intussusception, sometimes associated with a respiratory infection.[33] As with the pertussis syndrome, the etiologic role of the adenoviruses that may be isolated or visualized in tissue is not entirely clear. Serologic response to the isolated virus often cannot be demonstrated.

Extrarespiratory adenovirus infection is uncommon. It may complicate pneumonia, as the dominant clinical feature, or as part of disseminated infection in a severely immunodeficient patient.

Hemorrhagic cystitis in children, particularly young boys, may be caused by adenoviruses.[34] Types 11 and 21 have been isolated most frequently. The pathogenesis of the infection is unclear, and structural abnormalities of the lower urinary tract are not usually present. Tubulointerstitial nephritis, which appeared to derive from an ascending infection, has been described.[35]

Adenovirus infections of the central nervous system, which are uncommon, occur sporadically or as a part of epidemic respiratory disease. Meningitis and meningoencephalitis are not differentiated from other viral meningitides clinically or by examination of cerebrospinal fluid. In some infections it is not clear whether the neurologic disease represents direct viral infection or a postviral encephalitis.[36] Infections of other tissues, such as the myocardium or pericardium, may complicate respiratory infection.[37] Maculopapular rashes, sometimes resembling rubella, have been described as a manifestation of respiratory infection.[38]

Disseminated adenovirus disease usually occurs in the setting of severe immunosuppression[11,13,39,40] or in neonates.[41,42] Multiple organs may be involved, but a destructive hepatitis has figured prominently in the clinical presentation, especially in patients who have had organ transplants.[5,10,12] Disseminated infection may also occur rarely after adenoviral pneumonia in apparently healthy children.[22,43]

PATHOLOGY

Most adenoviral infections are self-limited, and there is little information on the lesions in the pharynx, eye, or urinary tract. Macroscopically, the lungs are congested and may be hyperinflated in children. Consolidated foci, which may be gray or red, are distributed throughout all lobes, but were concentrated in the posterior and lower lung zones in one report.[17] A lobar radiographic appearance has been described.[44] The bronchi may contain a mucoid, blood-tinged exudate, which occasionally appears purulent.[17]

The liver contains focal punched-out lesions, which may become confluent, without relationship to the portal tracts. Although the hepatic lesions were necrotic, the destruction was not as extensive as in herpetic hepatitis in one series of liver transplant patients.[12] At the other end of the spectrum there may be extensive hepatic necrosis, even producing the appearance of acute yellow atrophy.[11]

Microscopically, two patterns of reaction are seen in the lower respiratory tract.[17,45,46] The first is the pattern of diffuse alveolar damage, characterized by interstitial edema and inflammation, exudation of fluid into the air spaces, and hyaline membrane formation. The bronchiolar epithelium may show damage and regenerative change including metaplasia. The second pattern is a necrotizing lesion that may involve bronchi, bronchioles, and alveoli, accompanied by an intense infiltrate of neutrophils and macrophages (Figure 5–3). The inflammatory exudate may undergo karyorrhexis and karyolysis, producing an inflammatory exudate that suggests a bacterial process. Interstitial fibrosis, obliterative bronchiolitis, and bronchiectasis are potential sequelae of adenovirus infection.[47,48]

The hepatic lesions are characterized by necrosis of hepatocytes, which is focal, but may be very extensive or confluent. Characteristic intranuclear inclusions are usually evident (Figure 5–4).

Myocarditis has been described in a patient with virologically confirmed adenovirus pneumonia.[37] The myocardium was diffusely infiltrated with lymphocytes and plasma cells and fibers were fragmented, but inclusions were not demonstrated by light or electron microscopy. Rare fatal infections of the central nervous system are characterized by lymphocytic infiltration of meninges and perivascular spaces.[45] Little is known of the lesions of adenovirus gastroenteritis in humans. Murine adenovirus gastroenteritis causes mild cyto-

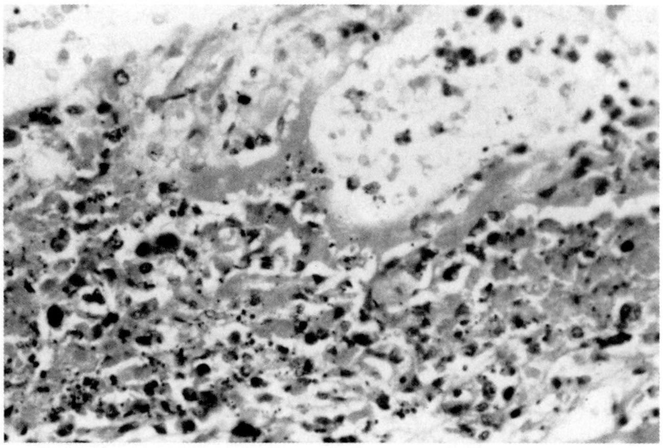

Figure 5–3. Adenovirus pneumonia. A necrotizing exudate with fibrin and karyorrhexis suggests the possibility of a bacterial process. The basophilic intranuclear inclusions and smudge cells must be differentiated from nonspecific degenerative changes (hematoxylin-eosin, ×250).

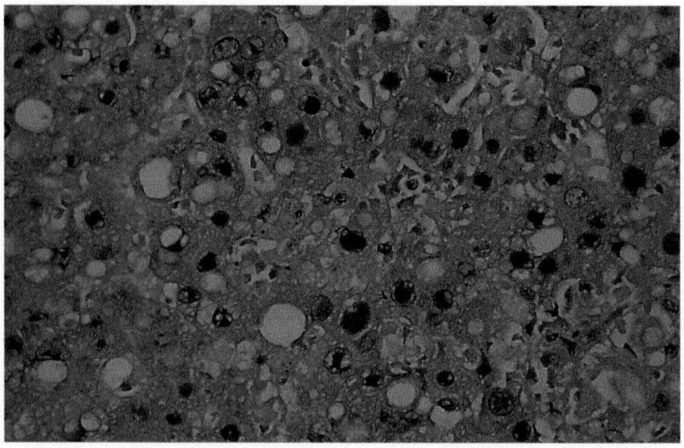

Figure 5–4. Adenovirus hepatitis. Multiple intranuclear inclusions in hepatocytes are concentrated at the edge of a necrotic lesion. The inclusions range from early stages with clearing around the inclusion and peripheral cellular chromatin to late stages when the nuclear membrane is distorted and blurred (smudge cells) (hematoxylin-eosin, ×250).

pathic effects and increased cellular extrusion from the ileal epithelium and large, bizarre, basophilic nuclei.[49]

The diagnostic lesion in adenovirus infections is an amphophilic or basophilic intranuclear inclusion (Figures 5–3 and 5–4), which has been demonstrated in vivo,[17,46] in cell culture, and in the explants of human tracheal epithelium.[50] The inclusions begin as small amphophilic inclusions that may be surrounded by an artifactual clearing with peripheralization of nuclear chromatin, resembling the inclusions of herpes simplex and varicella-zoster viruses. As the cellular infection progresses, the inclusion enlarges and becomes more basophilic, again with peripheralization and clumping of nuclear chromatin. Eventually, the outlines of the nuclear membrane are blurred by the mature inclusion, producing the characteristic smudge cell. There are no multinucleated giant cells. Inclusions may be in the areas of inflammation and necrosis, but are often most prominent around the edge of the lesions and in nonnecrotic tissue. Inclusions may be demonstrated by cytologic techniques as well as by histopathology. The phenomenon of ciliocytophora has been demonstrated cytologically in respiratory secretions from patients with adenovirus infection.[51]

ELECTRON MICROSCOPY

The characteristic inclusions can be demonstrated with the electron microscope if they are sufficiently plentiful.[52] The viral morphology is sufficiently distinctive to allow a diagnosis of adenovirus infection, although the type cannot be determined. The characteristic 70-nm virions appear round when viewed with the transmission microscope, but the icosahedral shape allows efficient packaging into a crystalline array. The mass of virions corresponds to the basophilic inclusion seen with the light microscope.

Enteric adenovirus infection was first diagnosed by demonstration of the virions in stool with the electron microscope. This technique does not distinguish between respiratory adenoviruses that are being excreted in the stool and enteric serotypes unless aggregation of the virions is accomplished by immunoelectron microscopy.[53]

DIFFERENTIAL DIAGNOSIS

In the lung the differential diagnosis consists of other causes of diffuse alveolar damage, including other viral infections. Other necrotizing viral infections and even bacterial infections are in the differential diagnosis of destructive lesions. Adenoviral hepatitis must be differentiated from other destructive, nonbacterial lesions, particularly those caused by herpes simplex virus. The differential diagnosis of the inclusions consists primarily of herpes simplex virus when the inclusion is young and amphophilic[54] and of cytomegalovirus in the older, basophilic inclusions.[55] Adenoviral smudge cells must be differentiated from basophilic reactive cells and nonspecific degenerative changes. The diagnosis is suggested by the mixture of young and old inclusions, the absence of cytomegaly and intracytoplasmic inclusions (cytomegalovirus), and the absence of multinucleated cells (herpes simplex virus). In the central nervous system, the primary differential is the intranuclear inclusion of JC virus in progressive multifocal leukoencephalopathy.

MOLECULAR DIAGNOSIS

The nature of the adenovirus inclusions can be established by immunoenzyme or immunofluorescence staining with monoclonal or polyclonal antisera. Pretreatment of tissue sections with trypsin facilitates the demonstration of adenovirus antigens in formalin-fixed tissues.[56] In situ hybridization has also been used to identify adenoviral antigens.[52] It is not clear whether these molecular techniques increase the sensitivity of detection of virus in comparison to detection of hematoxylin-eosin-stained sections, but they are useful for documenting the nature of inclusions that are of uncertain cause. Molecular methods have been most commonly employed for diagnosis of enteric adenovirus infection.[57,58]

CONFIRMATORY DIAGNOSIS

The definitive method for diagnosis of adenovirus infections is isolation of the virus in culture, after which serotyping can be done for epidemiologic purposes. Human embryonic kidney has traditionally been considered the most sensitive cell type for isolation of respiratory adenoviruses, but HEp-2 cells and A549 cells are also efficient hosts for adenoviral replication.[59] Cytopathic effect typically consists of rounded, clustered cells or a lattice appearance in the monolayer. Confirmation of adenovirus is most easily accomplished by immunofluorescence staining of the cell monolayer. Spin amplification of a virus followed by antigen detection reduces the detection time in cell culture,[60] but may not be practical in many laboratories.

Enteric adenoviruses do not replicate efficiently in conventional cell cultures. Graham 293 cells are often used for recovery of these serotypes,[61] but recently HEp-2 cells have been demonstrated to work well also.[62] Immunologic or molecular techniques for demonstration of types 40 or 41 are necessary to confirm the diagnosis.

Direct detection of adenoviruses in respiratory secretions can be used to provide an early diagnosis, but the technique is not sufficiently sensitive to substitute for culture.[63] Serologic diagnosis requires demonstration of IgM antibody or a fourfold increase in IgG antibody titer, and is therefore retrospective. An enzyme immunoassay, using hexon antigen, is more sensitive than the traditional complement fixation test.[64]

TREATMENT

There is no specific antiviral therapy for adenovirus infections, and the treatment is symptomatic and supportive.

REFERENCES

1. Hierholzer JC, Wigand R, Anderson LJ, Adrian T, Gold JWM. Adenoviruses from patients with AIDS: a plethora of serotypes and a description of five new serotypes of subgenus D (types 43–47). *J Infect Dis.* 1988;158:804–813.
2. Baum SG. Adenovirus. In: Mandell GL, Bennett JE, Dolin R, eds. *Principles and Practice of Infectious Diseases.* 4th ed. New York: Churchill Livingstone; 1995:1382–1387.
3. Rowe WP, Huebner RJ, Gillmore LK, et al. Isolation of a cytopathogenic agent from human adenoids undergoing spontaneous degeneration in tissue culture. *Proc Soc Exp Biol Med.* 1953;84:570.
4. Brandt CD, Kim HW, Vargosko AJ, et al. Infections in 18,000 infants and children in a controlled study of respiratory tract disease. I. Adenovirus pathogenicity in relation to serologic type and illness syndrome. *Am J Epidemiol.* 1969;90:484–500.
5. Shields AF, Hackman RC, Fife KH, Corey L, Meyers JD. Adenovirus infections in patients undergoing bone-marrow transplantation. *N Engl J Med.* 1985;312:529–533.
6. Centers for Disease Control and Prevention. Outbreak of pharyngoconjunctival fever at a summer camp—North Carolina, 1991. *MMWR.* 1992;41:342–344.
7. Sprague JB, Hierholzer JC, Currier RW II, Hattwick MAW, Smith MD. Epidemic keratoconjunctivitis. A severe industrial outbreak due to adenovirus type 8. *N Engl J Med.* 1973;289:1341–1346.
8. Dascomb HE, Hilleman MR. Clinical and laboratory studies in patients with respiratory disease caused by adenoviruses (RI-APC-ARD agents). *Am J Med.* 1956;21:161–174.
9. Dudding BA, Wagner SC, Zeller JA, Gmelich JT, French GR, Top FHJ. Fatal pneumonia associated with adenovirus type 7 in three military trainees. *N Engl J Med.* 1972; 286:1289–1292.
10. Varki NM, Bhuta S, Drake T, Porter DD. Adenovirus hepatitis in two successive liver transplants in a child. *Arch Pathol Lab Med.* 1990;114:106–109.
11. Zahradnik JM, Spencer MJ, Porter DD. Adenovirus infection in the immunocompromised patient. *Am J Med.* 1980;68:725–732.
12. Koneru B, Jaffe R, Esquivel CO, et al. Adenoviral infections in pediatric liver transplant recipients. *JAMA* 1987; 258:489–492.
13. Hierholzer JC. Adenoviruses in the immunocompromised host. *Clin Microbiol Rev.* 1992;5:262–274.
14. Ruuskanen O, Meurman O, Sarkkinen H. Adenoviral diseases in children: a study of 105 hospital cases. *Pediatrics.* 1985;76:79–83.
15. Ruuskanen O, Sarkkinen H, Meurman O, et al. Rapid diagnosis of adenoviral tonsillitis: a prospective clinical study. *J Pediatr.* 1984;104:725–728.

16. Sarkkinen H, Ruuskanen O, Meurman O, Puhakka H, Virolainen E, Eskola J. Identification of respiratory virus antigens in middle ear fluids of children with acute otitis media. *J Infect Dis.* 1985;151:444–448.
17. Becroft DM. Histopathology of fatal adenovirus infection of the respiratory tract in young children. *J Clin Pathol.* 1967;20:561–569.
18. Brown RS, Nogrady MB, Spence L, Wiglesworth FW. An outbreak of adenovirus type 7 infection in children in Montreal. *Can Med Assoc J.* 1973;108:434–439.
19. Ellenbogen C, Graybill JR, Silva J Jr, Homme PJ. Bacterial pneumonia complicating adenoviral pneumonia. *Am J Med.* 1974;56:169–178.
20. Morgan PN, Moses EB, Fody EP, Barron AL. Association of adenovirus type 16 with Reye's-syndrome-like illness and pneumonia. *South Med J.* 1984;77:827–830.
21. Ladisch S, Lovejoy FH, Hierholzer JC, et al. Extrapulmonary manifestations of adenovirus type 7 pneumonia simulating Reye syndrome and the possible role of an adenovirus toxin. *J Pediatr.* 1979;95:348–355.
22. Faden H, Gallagher M. Disseminated infection due to adenovirus type 4. *Clin Pediatr.* 1980;19:427–429.
23. Similä S, Linna O, Lanning P, Heikkinen E, Ala-Houhala M. Chronic lung damage caused by adenovirus type 7: a ten-year follow-up study. *Chest.* 1981;80:127–131.
24. Lang WR, Howden CW, Laws J, Burton JF. Bronchopneumonia with serious sequelae in children with evidence of adenovirus type 21 infection. *Br Med J.* 1969;1:73–79.
25. Sly PD, Soto-Quiros ME, Landau LI, Hudson I, Newton-John H. Factors predisposing to abnormal pulmonary function after adenovirus type 7 pneumonia. *Arch Dis Child.* 1984;59:935–939.
26. Payne SB, Grilli EA, Smith AJ, Hoskins TW. Investigation of an outbreak of adenovirus type 3 infection in a boys' boarding school. *J Hyg (Lond).* 1984;93:277–283.
27. Dawson CR, O'Day D, Vastine D. Adenovirus 19, a cause of epidemic keratoconjunctivitis, not acute hemorrhagic conjunctivitis. *N Engl J Med.* 1975;293,1:45–46.
28. Hierholzer JC, Guyer B, O'Day D, Schaffner W. Adenovirus type 19 keratoconjunctivitis. *N Engl J Med.* 1974; 290:1436.
29. Clinicopathologic Conference. Adult respiratory distress syndrome. *Am J Med.* 1971;50:521–529.
30. Connor JD. Evidence for an etiologic role of adenoviral infection in pertussis syndrome. *N Engl J Med.* 1970; 283:390–394.
31. Rodriguez WJ, Kim HW, Brandt CD, et al. Fecal adenoviruses from a longitudinal study of families in metropolitan Washington, D.C.: laboratory, clinical, and epidemiologic observations. *J Pediatr.* 1985;107:514–520.
32. Madeley CR. The emerging role of adenoviruses as inducers of gastroenteritis. *Pediatr Infect Dis.* 1986;5:S63–S74.
33. Porter HJ, Padfield, CJ, Peres LC, Hirschowitz L, Berry PJ. Adenovirus and intranuclear inclusions in appendices in intussusception. *J Clin Pathol.* 1993;46:154–158.
34. Numazaki Y, Kumasaka T, Yano N, et al. Further study on acute hemorrhagic cystitis due to adenovirus type 11. *N Engl J Med.* 1973;289:344–347.
35. Ito M, Hirabayashi N, Uno Y, et al. Necrotizing tubulinterstitial nephritis associated with adenovirus infection. *Hum Pathol.* 1991;22:1225–1231.
36. Similä S, Jouppila R, Salmi A, Pohjonen R. Encephalomeningitis in children associated with an adenovirus type 7 epidemic. *Acta Paediatr Scand.* 1970;59:310–316.
37. Henson D, Mufson MA. Myocarditis and pneumonitis with type 21 adenovirus infection. Association with fatal myocarditis and pneumonitis. *Am J Dis Child.* 1971;121:334–336.
38. Gutekunst RR, Heggie AD. Viremia and viruria in adenovirus infections. *N Engl J Med.* 1961;264:374–378.
39. Rodriguez FHJ, Liuzza GE, Gohd RH. Disseminated adenovirus serotype 31 infection in an immunocompromised host. *Am J Clin Pathol.* 1984;82:615–618.
40. Siegal FP, Dikman SH, Arayata RB, Bottone EJ. Fatal disseminated adenovirus 11 pneumonia in an agammaglobulinemic patient. *Am J Med.* 1981;71:1062–1067.
41. Green WR, Williams AW. Neonatal adenovirus pneumonia. *Arch Pathol Lab Med.* 1989;113:190–191.
42. Pinto A, Beck R, Jadavji T. Fatal neonatal pneumonia caused by adenovirus type 35. *Arch Pathol Lab Med.* 1992;116:95–99.
43. Benyesh-Melnick M, Rosenberg HS. The isolation of adenovirus type 7 from a fatal case of pneumonia and disseminated disease. *J Pediatr.* 1964;64:83–87.
44. Leers WD, Sarin MK, Kasupski GJ. Lobar pneumonia associated with adenovirus type 7. *Can Med Assoc J.* 1981; 125:1003–1004.
45. Chany C, Lepine P, Lelong M, Le-Tan-Vinh, Satge P, Virat J. Severe and fatal pneumonia in infants and young children associated with adenovirus infections. *Am J Hyg.* 1958;67:367–378.
46. Schonland M, Strong ML, Wesley A. Fatal adenovirus pneumonia: clinical and pathological features. *S Afr Med J.* 1976;50:1748–1751.
47. Becroft DM. Bronchiolitis obliterans, bronchiectasis, and other sequelae of adenovirus type 21 infection in young children. *J Clin Pathol.* 1971;24:72–82.
48. Kawai T, Fujiwara T, Aoyama Y, Aizawa Y, Yamada Y. Diffuse interstitial fibrosing pneumonitis and adenovirus infection. *Chest.* 1976;69:692–694.
49. Takeuchi A, Hashimoto K. Electron microscope study of experimental enteric adenovirus infection in mice. *Infect Immun.* 1976;13:569–580.
50. Craighead JE. Cytopathology of adenoviruses types 7 and 12 in human respiratory epithelium. *Lab Invest.* 1970; 22:553–557.
51. Naib ZM, Stewart JA, Dowdle WR, Casey HL, Marine WM, Nahmias AJ. Cytological features of viral respiratory tract infections. *Acta Cytol.* 1968;12:162–171.
52. Abbondanzo SL, English CK, Kagan E, McPherson RA. Fatal adenovirus pneumonia in a newborn identified by electron microscopy and in situ hybridization. *Arch Pathol Lab Med.* 1989;113:1349–1353.
53. Wood DJ, Bailey AS. Detection of adenovirus types 40 and 41 in stool specimens by immune electron microscopy. *J Med Virol.* 1987;21:191–199.

54. Myerowitz RL, Stalder H, Oxman MN, et al. Fatal disseminated adenovirus infection in a renal transplant recipient. *Am J Med.* 1975;59:591–598.
55. Landry ML, Fong CK, Neddermann K, Solomon L, Hsiung GD. Disseminated adenovirus infection in an immunocompromised host. Pitfalls in diagnosis. *Am J Med.* 1987;83:555–559.
56. Chandler FW, Gorelkin L. Immunofluorescence staining of adenovirus in fixed tissues pretreated with trypsin. *J Clin Microbiol.* 1983;17:371–373.
57. Niel C. Gomes SA, Leite JPG, Pereira HG. Direct detection and differentiation of fastidious and nonfastidious adenoviruses in stools by using a specific nonradioactive probe. *J Clin Microbiol.* 1986;24:785–789.
58. Herrmann JE, Perron-Henry DM, Blacklow NR. Antigen detection with monoclonal antibodies for the diagnosis of adenovirus gastroenteritis. *J Infect Dis.* 1987;155:1167–1171.
59. Koneman EW, Allen SD, Janda WM, Schreckenberger PC, Winn WC Jr. *Color Atlas and Textbook of Diagnostic Microbiology.* 4th ed. Philadelphia: JB Lippincott; 1992.
60. Espy MJ, Hierholzer JC, Smith TF. The effect of centrifugation on the rapid detection of adenovirus in shell vials. Am J Clin Pathol. 1987;88:358–360.
61. Brown M, Petric M. Evaluation of cell line 293 for virus isolation in routine viral diagnosis. *J Clin Microbiol.* 1986;23:704–708.
62. Perron-Henry DM, Herrmann JE, Blacklow NR. Isolation and propagation of enteric adenoviruses in HEp-2 cells. *J Clin Microbiol.* 1988;26:1445–1447.
63. Lehtomäki K, Julkunen I, Sandelin K, et al. Rapid diagnosis of respiratory adenovirus infections in young adult men. *J Clin Microbiol.* 1986;24:108–111.
64. Julkunen I, Lehtomäki K, Hovi T. Immunoglobulin class-specific serological responses to adenovirus in respiratory infections of young adult men. *J Clin Microbiol.* 1986; 24:112–115.

CHAPTER 6

Arboviral Encephalitides

Herbert J. Manz

The tick is a "blood-sucking acarid parasite of the suborder Ixodides, superfamily Ixodoidea." This vampire-like creature can have a soft or hard body—at least the latter doesn't leave a mess when you scratch at it. Among the varieties of tick is the adobe tick—this of course comes from tropical countries and lives chiefly on the inhabitants of mud huts. Then there is the Bandicoot tick—found only on coots that have learnt to walk too soon. Ticks find it easier to climb up bandy legs than straight ones. There is also the beady-legged winter horse tick—if your horse has beady eyes don't worry, only the legs count. Ticks also inhabit dogs. There are the American dog, British dog and brown dog ticks. When buying a dog make sure that it is oriental and has absolutely no brown hair.

Canad Med Assoc J 1979;121:323

INTRODUCTION AND CLASSIFICATION

As originally defined, the arboviruses (arthropod-borne) are actually a multifarious group of viruses (more than 350 species) sharing only the common feature of transmission by a variety of hematophagous arthropod vectors.[1–9] The designation, therefore, is functional and organizational—not taxonomic. Generically, four major clinical presentations characterize the arboviral diseases: 1) fever, 2) fever with rash, 3) hemorrhagic fever (and other systemic and organ/tissue dysfunction), and 4) encephalitis; in severe infections, there may be overlapping symptoms. Only a few viruses cause meningoencephalitis in humans; not every infected human develops encephalitis, so that asymptomatic infections exist, and, similar to seriously ill patients, infected humans develop humoral antibodies. The majority of these viruses is transmitted by mosquitoes, and a smaller number by ticks. Intrusion by man into a variety of natural habitats brings with it exposure to viral agents cycling in a complex relationship between natural, small, vertebrate animal reservoirs and arthropods. An essential cycle of viral replication must occur in the arthropod (the "extrinsic" incubation period) prior to transmission to the next host; transovarian infection occurs in certain arthropods. Man is an accidental and incidental host not necessary for maintenance of the cycles. Similarly, the horse is only an incidental host, but may serve a "sentinel," epidemiologic function just prior to human epidemics. Indeed, the horse has been falsely incriminated as essential in the transmission to humans, as implied in several arboviral encephalitides also bearing the official name "equine" (eg, eastern and western equine encephalitis, etc.).[10–12] Because many different ecological niches exist, which in turn depend on season, climatic variations, and fluctuating host and vector populations, it is not surprising that a variety of arboviral encephalitides have been discovered, varying in geographic distribution and annual incidence (ie, epidemics). Another common feature is their having an RNA genome. The viruses differ morphologically in structure, symmetry, possession of an envelope, and size (Table 6–1 and Figures 6–1 through 6–5).

As more viruses, vectors, and natural hosts were discovered and their human or veterinary diseases elu-

TABLE 6–1. GENERAL EPIDEMIOLOGY OF ARBOVIRAL ENCEPHALITIDES

Virus Group	Virus	Principal Vector(s)	Principal Reservoir(s)	Geographic Distribution
1. Alphavirus 60–65 nm; cubic symmetry; enveloped (Figs. 6–1 and 6–2)	EEE	*Culiseta melanura* *Aedes* sp	Passerine and marshland birds; domestic fowl	Atlantic and Gulf coasts of United States, Mexico, Panama
	WEE	*Culex tarsalis*	Wild birds: major reservoir, small wild mammals: minor reservoir	Western United States (especially central California), US and Canadian prairie states and provinces, Mexico
	VEE	*Mansonia titillans* *Aedes taeniorhynchus*	Small wild mammals; ? wild birds	Northern South America, Panama, Amazon basin
2. Flavivirus (Mosquito-borne) 37–60 nm; asymmetric; enveloped (Figs. 6–3 and 6–4)	St. LE	*C tarsalis* *C pipiens*	Wild birds; domestic fowl	Mississippi/Ohio river basin, Florida, Panama, Western United States
	JE	*C tritaeniorhynchus* other *Culex* sp *Aedes* sp	Wild birds; swine	Far East (India to Japan to Indonesia)
	MVE	*C annulirostris* other *Culex* sp *Aedes* sp	Wild aquatic birds (herons, egrets, pelicans)	Southeast and northwest Australia, New Guinea
3. Flavivirus (Tick-borne) 37–60 nm; asymmetric; enveloped	Far eastern (Russian spring-summer)	*Ixodes persulcatus* in Far East *I ricinus* (west of Urals)	Small mammals (rodents); wild birds	Siberia, far eastern Russia, eastern European Russia
	Central European	*I ricinus*	Mammals: (rodents); sheep, goats (domesticated)	Western European Russia, Central Europe, Scandinavia
	Louping Ill	*I ricinus*	Sheep	Scotland, Northern Ireland
	Powassan	*Ixodes* sp	Small mammals: squirrels, chipmunks	Ontario, Canada; northern United States
4. *Bunyaviridae* 90–100 nm; asymmetric; enveloped (Fig. 6–5)	California encephalitis serogroup	*A triseriatus* *Aedes* sp	Small mammals: rabbits, rodents, chipmunks, squirrels	Western and eastern United States, Canada, Siberia
5. Orbivirus 60–80 nm; cubic symmetry; naked	Colorado tick fever	*Dermocentor andersoni* other *Dermocentor* sp *Ixodes* sp	Small mammals: deer mice, ground squirrels, porcupines, coyotes	Northwestern United States, western Canada

Modified from references 2, 4–9, and 13.

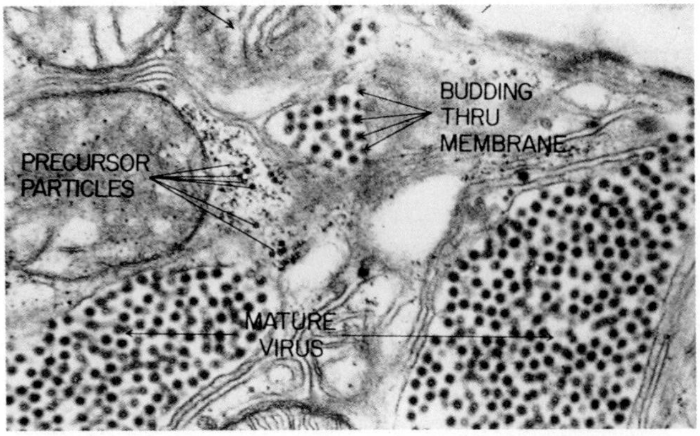

Figure 6–1. Eastern equine encephalitis (EEE) virus in mosquito (*Aedes triseriatus*) salivary gland cell. *(Photograph courtesy of the Centers for Disease Control and Prevention, Atlanta, Georgia;* ×50,000 approximately.)

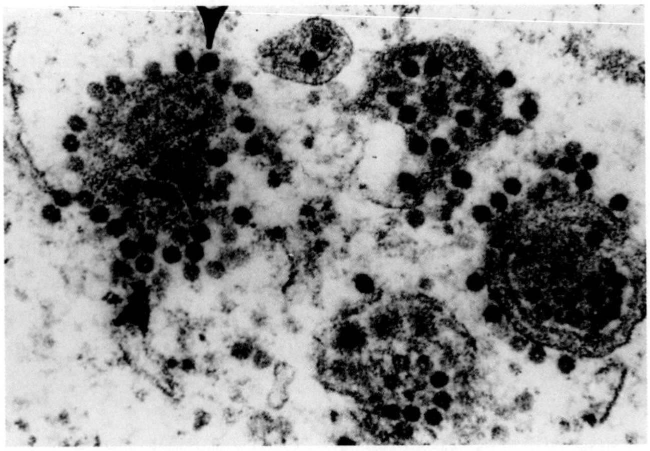

Figure 6–2. Eastern equine encephalitis (EEE) (*arrows*) in a human central nervous system. *(Photograph courtesy of the Centers for Disease Control and Prevention, Atlanta, Georgia;* ×120,000 approximately.)

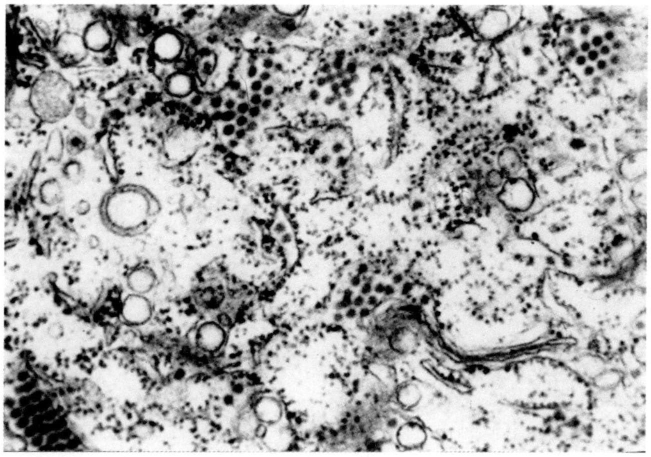

Figure 6–3. St. Louis encephalitis (St. LE) virus in a human central nervous system. *(Photograph courtesy of the Centers for Disease Control and Prevention, Atlanta, Georgia;* ×40,000 approximately.)

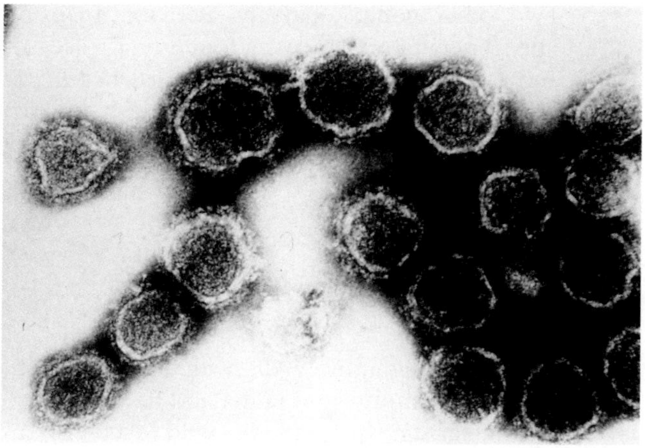

Figure 6–5. California equine encephalitis virus, negative staining. *(Photograph courtesy of the Centers for Disease Control and Prevention, Atlanta, Georgia;* ×100,000 approximately.)

cidated, the viruses were divided into groups based on serologic criteria, as follows:

I. Group A arboviruses, now classified as Alphaviruses of the family *Togaviridae*[6]:
   1) Western equine encephalitis (WEE) virus
   2) Eastern equine encephalitis (EEE) virus
   3) Venezuelan equine encephalitis (VEE) virus

II. Group B arboviruses, now classified as Flaviviruses of the family *Flaviviridae*[7]:
   1) St. Louis encephalitis (St. LE) virus
   2) Japanese B encephalitis (JBE) virus
   3) Murray Valley encephalitis (MVE) virus
   4) West Nile virus
   5) Ilheus virus

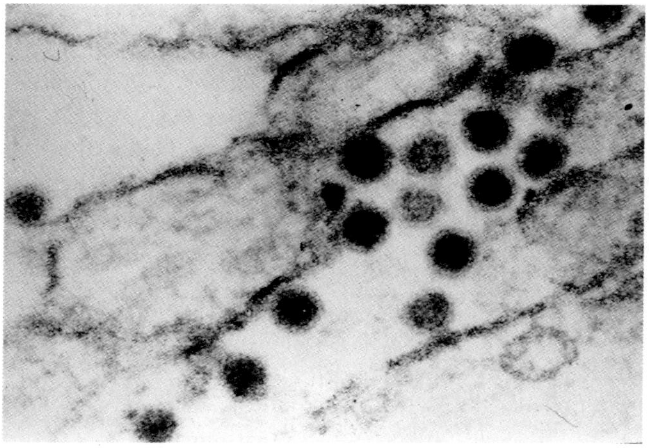

Figure 6–4. Viral particles of St. LE virus. *(Photograph courtesy of the Centers for Disease Control and Prevention, Atlanta, Georgia;* ×90,000 approximately.)

III. Tick-borne flaviviruses of the family *Flaviviridae*[7]:
   1) Far-eastern tick-borne encephalitis virus (formerly Russian spring-summer encephalitis [RSSE])
   2) Central European tick-borne encephalitis virus
   3) Kyasanur Forest disease virus
   4) Louping-ill virus
   5) Powassan virus
   6) Rociovirus

IV. California group (Bunyavirus of family *Bunyaviridae*)[8]:
   1) California encephalitis virus
      (a) La Crosse Virus
   2) Tahyna virus (of southern Central Europe)

V. Colorado tick fever virus (Orbivirus of the family *Reoviridae*).[9]

To provide a more complete overview of the relationship among the different arboviruses, many of which are described in relevant chapters of this text, the following thumbnail sketch is provided[6–9]:

1. The *Togaviridae* family also includes the genus Rubivirus, of which rubella is the only member.[6]
2. The Alphaviruses of the *Togaviridae* family also contain the extensive group associated with fever and polyarthritis (eg, Chikungunya, Ross River, and Sindbis viruses).[6]
3. Flaviviruses associated predominantly with fever/arthralgia/rash are related to the group B encephalitis arboviruses of the family *Flaviviridae* (eg, Yellow Fever, Dengue hemorrhagic fever, Kyasanur Forest disease, Omsk hemorrhagic fever).[7]
4. The *Bunyaviridae* family also incorporates, among others, the Hantaviruses.[8]

5. Two other genera, namely, Reovirus (causing upper respiratory and gastrointestinal disease) and Rotaviruses (causing severe diarrhea in infants and young children throughout the world) belong to the family *Reoviridae*.[9]

None of these latter agents is described in this chapter.

GENERAL EPIDEMIOLOGY

Generally, each geographic area, with its unique climate, surface topography, and fauna and flora, tends to have a characteristic "natural" or wild cycle of an arbovirus, a unique vector, and vertebrate host(s) (Table 6–1).[2–9,13] Thus, different mosquitoes or ticks are uniquely adapted to foster the replication of specific types of viruses and to feed on characteristic avian or mammalian victims, usually without appreciable harm to the vector or reservoir carrier by the transmitted virus. Also, the female mosquito is the biting and blood-sucking member; similarly, the reservoir must be in the viremic stage and have a sufficiently large viral burden to establish an infection in the arthropod. This extrinsic incubation period in the vector ranges from 4 to 15 days, during which period the vector apparently cannot transmit the virus to another vertebrate; thereafter, the vector remains infective for weeks or perhaps life. In some mosquitoes, vertical and transovarian passage of the virus (eg, California encephalitis virus, La Crosse stain, WEE virus) has been documented.[14,15] In temperate zones, where mosquitoes feed and breed during the summer season, human infections tend to occur in late summer and early fall, whereas tick-borne encephalitides have an earlier and longer season. In cold winter months, the virus probably persists in hibernating vectors (including nymphal ticks and mosquito larvae), vertebrate hosts (including hibernating rodents), and reptiles (especially snakes) and amphibia; periodic reintroduction of virus into an endemic area by migrating birds is less likely. In tropical and subtropical regions, the natural "wild" cycle between arthropod and vertebrate reservoir is not subjected to climatic and seasonal variations. With some of the tick-borne encephalitis viruses, milk and cheese of sheep and goats have been blamed as fomites.[16]

Finally, laboratory personnel in viral isolation and research laboratories are at risk of accidental infection with arboviruses by skin-penetrating injuries or viral aerosols.[17] Also, there may be the potential of transmission of arboviruses, specifically Colorado tick fever virus, by blood transfusions because of the incorporation of the virus in erythrocytes and its persistence for 3 to 4 months in a cell-associated viremia,[18,19] and of Japanese encephalitis virus in lymphocytes circulating in peripheral blood for as long as 8 months after the acute illness. Other arboviral encephalitides cause viremia in humans, but it is for a much shorter time and the viremia does not depend on circulating blood cell–virus interaction (eg, adherence or incorporation).[19,20] Transplacental and connatal/perinatal infections have also been reported,[20,21] although the risk of abortion and congenital malformations has not been adequately assessed.

GENERAL FEATURES OF CLINICAL PRESENTATION

With such a tremendously large number of viral agents and wide spectrum of clinical presentations in different epidemics and demographic groups, it is not surprising that a variety of clinical syndromes exist. In certain geographic areas and for certain arboviral infections, asymptomatic cases can be identified by serologic surveys following epidemics. Thus, for some of the arbovirus infections in the United States, the ratio of unrecognized or inapparent infections to those with clinical encephalitis is as follows: approximately 1000:1 for WEE in adults, but only 50:1 in children and 1:1 in infants in California[22]; 23:1 in an EEE epidemic in New Jersey;[23] and 806:1 in children versus 85:1 in the elderly for St. LE.[7] These data, of course, imply that infants are particularly susceptible to the full neurotropic potential of WEE virus and that the elderly are more severely affected by the St. LE virus. Analogously, there are different rates of infection between genders in different arboviral encephalitides; for instance, in tick-borne Far Eastern encephalitis, males outnumber females 5:1, because of the males' greater exposure to sylvan habitats in their occupations as lumbermen, hunters, and trappers. There is a similar male preponderance (2:1) for St. LE in rural western states, where *Culex tarsalis* is the principal vector; in the central and eastern states, however, there is a female predominance caused by "household" vectors, *Culex pipiens* and *Culex quinquefasciatus,* which tend to breed in urban and suburban environs. In this setting, the incidence and case-fatality rate are manifold higher in the elderly (older than 55 years) than the young; in southern US cities, the prevalence is higher in the African-American population residing in poorer, less sanitary wards.[7] In North America, a tabulation of those with arboviral encephalitides reported to the Centers for Disease Control and Prevention for the years 1955 to 1978 reveals a low of 45 in 1960 and a high of 2113 in 1975 (predominantly an epidemic of St. LE), with a mean of 290 per year, illustrating the wide range of incidence rates.[23]

In patients with mild meningoencephalitis or myelitis, there may be fever, headache, and a flulike illness and only slight, focal neurologic deficits or generalized symptoms of an inflammatory process in the central nervous system (CNS), such as neck stiffness.

Massive encephalitis sets on dramatically with high fever (to 105°F) and chills, headache and neck stiffness from elevated intracranial pressure and irritation of nerve roots, apathy, nausea, and vomiting. Altered states of consciousness include lethargy, confusion, drowsiness, stupor, irritability, disorientation, delirium, visual disturbances and photophobia, hallucinations, and coma. Infants and children tend to convulse. Depending on the particular component of the cerebral hemispheres, brainstem, or spinal cord involved, patients may also complain of dizziness or have dysphasia, hemiparesis, hyperreflexia, cerebellar ataxia, tremors, dystonic postures and choreoathetosis, sensory losses, flaccid paralysis of limb(s) (monoplegia, paraplegia, or tetraplegia), areflexia, and bladder and bowel dysfunction. Autonomic disturbances range from cardiac irregularities and fluctuations in blood pressure to respiratory abnormalities and disturbed patterns of sleep, particularly hypersomnia.[2–9,19,22,24]

In some of the arboviral encephalitides, generally tick-borne, (eg, Colorado tick fever and the Central European form of Far Eastern tick-borne encephalitis), there is a biphasic course.[7,9] After an incubation period of 7 to 14 days, the first phase is a days- or week-long grippelike illness of fever, pharyngitis, generalized myalgia, and headache related to viremia; there may then be an interim of 1 to 3 days of remission, followed abruptly by the more severely febrile second phase of meningitis, myelitis, and/or encephalitis, manifesting clinically as described previously, and caused by neural infection (so-called "saddle-backed" fever).[25] A somewhat unique clinical presentation with Japanese B virus encephalitis (JBE) is the Guillain-Barré syndrome.[26]

After 3 to 7 days, the high fever abates rapidly, with variably prompt recovery of neurologic deficits, unless the patient dies in the acute phase.

Although the majority of the arboviral encephalitides is nonfatal, the fatality rate differs in different epidemics. EEE appears to have the highest mortality rate, up to 75% of patients with encephalitis in some epidemics.[2,3,12] Among survivors of the various encephalitides, the virus is virtually always completely eliminated; nevertheless, the intra-erythrocytic location of the Colorado tick fever virus protects against circulating antibodies,[18] so that theoretically the virus could be transmitted by blood transfusions.[19] This elimination of virus applies particularly to the CNS; however, extensive damage to the CNS leaves variably severe, permanent neurologic deficits.[2–9] Again, some exceptions apply. The JBE virus may persist for prolonged periods of time in the cerebrospinal fluid (CSF) in occasional patients.[27] There is also a single report of chronic progressive encephalitis clinically and by brain biopsy, with elevated CSF antibodies to Far-eastern tick-borne encephalitis virus, but without isolation of the virus by culture[28]; however, a flavivirus (of the tick-borne complex) isolated from the CSF of a patient with amyotrophic lateral sclerosis induced myelitis and paresis of the legs in experimental animals.[29]

Neurologic deficits in survivors are, as a general paradigm, nonprogressive. Thus, patients may have reduced intellectual capacity, mental retardation, dementia, dysphasia, quadriplegia, hemiparesis, choreoathetosis and dystonic postures, psychologic and/or psychiatric abnormalities, and seizures. Auditory and visual impairment, ataxia and incoordination, hyperreflexia and spasticity, denervation muscular atrophy and hyporeflexia, impaired sphincter control, and somnolence are other manifestations.[2–9,12,30] Collectively, these residua demand considerable societal, economic, and medical costs.[12,31,32]

PATHOGENESIS

By definition, route of infection is by the bite of an arthropod into the skin (with rare exceptions, as indicated in the section on epidemiology). In many of these encephalitides, there is an initial replication of virus in lymph nodes followed by viremia, which permits dissemination, hematogenously, to the CNS.[33,34] Generally, plasma viremias tend to be cleared by immunoglobulin–viral complexes phagocytosed in the reticuloendothelial system. In cell-associated viremias (eg, Colorado tick fever virus incorporated within erythrocytes), the virus is protected from circulating, neutralizing antibodies.[18] The localization of virus in various parts of the CNS occurs across the cerebral capillary endothelial cell/astrocyte endfeet blood-brain barrier (BBB) or across fenestrated endothelial cells in CNS components without the usual BBB function (eg, choroid plexus, area postrema, etc.).[33–36] As a minor possible pathway, demonstrated in an experimental setting, such hematogenous dissemination is first to the peripheral nervous system, including the olfactory nerves, with a secondary, centripetal spread in or along axons into the CNS.[37] Breakdown of normal BBB function or enhanced neuroinvasiveness has been documented, in experimental settings, for cold stress,[38] and administration of lipopolysaccharide (bacterial endotoxin).[39]

Entry of the virus across the BBB may be by pinocytotic uptake and transport across endothelial cells, infection of endothelium and release of virus at the abluminal membrane, or transmigration of infected leukocytes.[33–36] Once in the parenchyma of the CNS, the virus attaches to specific cell surface receptors of certain neurons (and/or glial cells, less commonly), accounting at least in part for "neurotropism." These receptor molecules serve vital, regulatory, neuronal functions, which the virus uses surreptitiously to gain entry into the neuron.[34–36] Neurotropism is, in part, dependent on the immaturity of the CNS, at least for JBE virus.[40,41] The specific receptor molecules are known for a number of viruses (eg, CD4 T lymphocytes for human immunodeficiency virus, complement receptor for Epstein–Barr virus, and neurotransmitter receptors),[15] but not those for the arboviruses. There is even evidence that both susceptibility to and complications of infection with the La Crosse encephalitis virus (of the California encephalitis virus group) may have an immunogenetic component, as demonstrated by an association with certain histocompatibility antigens.[42] After the adsorption of the virus to the neuronal cell membrane, the virus enters the cell by endocytosis, or fusion and incorporation of the viral envelope with and into the cell membrane. During the "eclipse" phase, when viral particles cannot be recognized by ultrastructural study, the protective viral protein envelope is removed so that the viral nucleic acid is released and misappropriates the host cell's synthetic machinery for production of viral progeny—both the nucleic acid and the specific protein or glycoprotein envelope. Concurrently, the host cell's own metabolic pathways are disrupted, with variable functional impairments.[4,5,36]

As is well known for most infections, there is, in general, a dynamic interaction between host and infectious agent that is influenced by both host factors (age, immune status—including prior vaccination—underlying disease, immunosuppressive chemotherapy) and virus (type and strain, ie, attenuated or highly virulent, route of administration or acquisition and dose). The host's constitutive response to viral replication, cytolysis, and spread within the CNS is acute inflammation and a specific immune reaction. Various mediators of acute inflammation evoke hyperemia and emigration of circulating leukocytes.[43] Circulating and locally produced immunoglobulins[44,45] may inactivate cytocidally released virions but, unfortunately, may contribute to further cytolysis or cytodestruction by binding to virally infected cells via chemotaxis for neutrophils and monocytes. Immunosuppression by cyclophosphamide markedly enhanced invasiveness of viruses (WEE, VEE, and louping ill virus) as well as morbidity and mortality in monkeys.[46] However, the presence of autoantibodies to neuronal antigens in significant quantities in the CSF of patients with JBE was associated with a fatal outcome.[47] Various cytokines activate proliferation and migration of indigenous microglia and astrocytes.[43] In a mouse model of neuronal infection, the maturity of the neuron affects the outcome; thus, in immature neurons, the Sindbis virus (of the alphavirus group) induces neuronal death by apoptosis, whereas in mature neurons there is persistent infection, in part mediated by down-regulation of virus replication by the induction of antibodies to cell surface viral glycoproteins. Ultimately, virus may be cleared from the CNS unless virulent strains of the virus were used.[48] The humoral immune response is critical to the suppression of viral replication, as demonstrated in a severe combined immunodeficiency (SCID) mouse model with the administration of monoclonal antibody to the E2 envelope glycoprotein of the Sindbis virus.[49] The concurrent administration of specific antibody and an interferon inducer act synergistically to protect experimental animals, even when the alphavirus is already replicating in the CNS.[50]

GENERAL NEUROPATHOLOGIC ASPECTS

As a generalization, the encephalitides are accompanied simultaneously by leptomeningitis (ie, pleocytosis and elevated protein levels in the CSF) and histopathologically by chronic inflammatory cells in the subarachnoid space (Figure 6–6), including the perivascular (Virchow-Robin) spaces[2–9,36] (Figure 6–7). In assessing the degree of inflammation, topography, and quantity and quality of the neuropathologic inflammatory processes (Figures 6–8 and 6–9), the consensus of neuropathologists is that an etiologic diagnosis cannot be made, particularly because there is variation of the spatial distribution of lesions in different epidemics by the same virus. Likewise, the intensity of the inflammatory process and amount of necrosis (Figures 6–10 through 6–12) vary among different patients infected by the same agent.[2,3,51–57] Nevertheless, relatively unusual reaction patterns (when compared to the generic neuropathologic features of arboviral encephalitis) tend to characterize some of the diseases. Thus, in the tick-borne

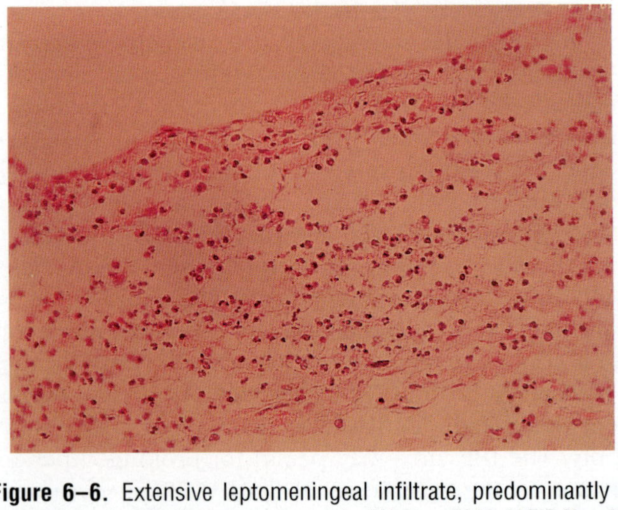

Figure 6–6. Extensive leptomeningeal infiltrate, predominantly of neutrophils, in EEE [hematoxylin-eosin (H&E) ×200]. (AFIP Neg 57-8220.)

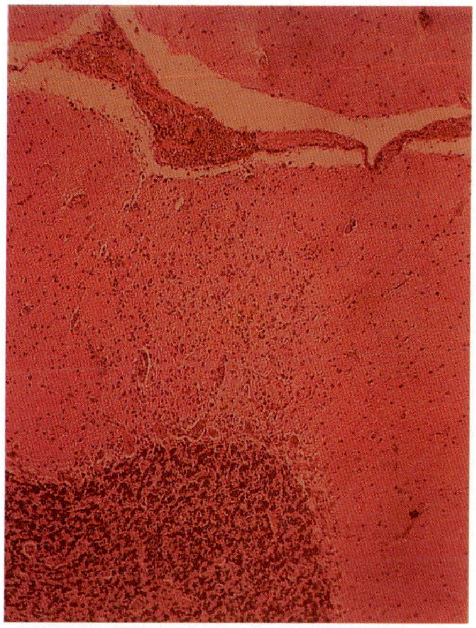

Figure 6–7. Inflammatory hemorrhagic infiltrate in the leptomeninges between the cerebellar folia, with extension along the perivascular (Virchow-Robin) spaces. There is also a brisk encephalitis, composed largely of monocytes/activated microglia, of the molecular layer outlining the dendritic arbor ("glial shrubs") of degenerating Purkinje cells; Tick-borne spring-summer encephalitis (H&E ×150). (AFIP Neg 11-6-3.)

encephalitides, bulbar encephalitis and myelitis resembling poliomyelitis are common.[29] Prominent neuronophagia in the spinal cord in acute infections, and massive mineralization, including brain stones as a late complication in survivors, have been present in JBE.[52] Severe EEE is characterized by focal and diffuse infil-

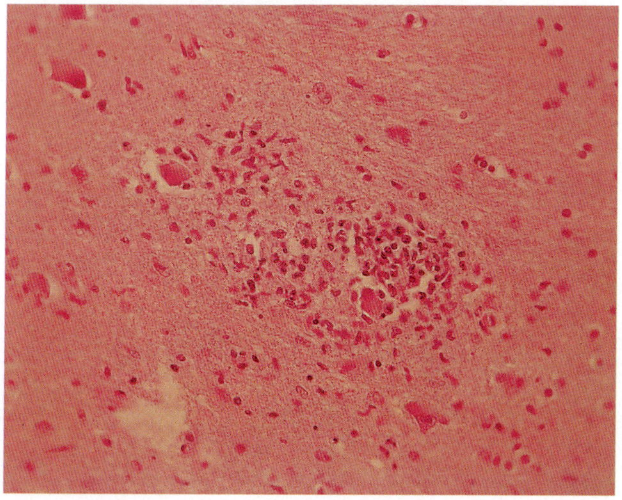

Figure 6–8. Microglial nodules and degenerated neurons with neuronophagia are evident in this case of Japanese B encephalitis (H&E ×150). (AFIP Neg 56-19048.)

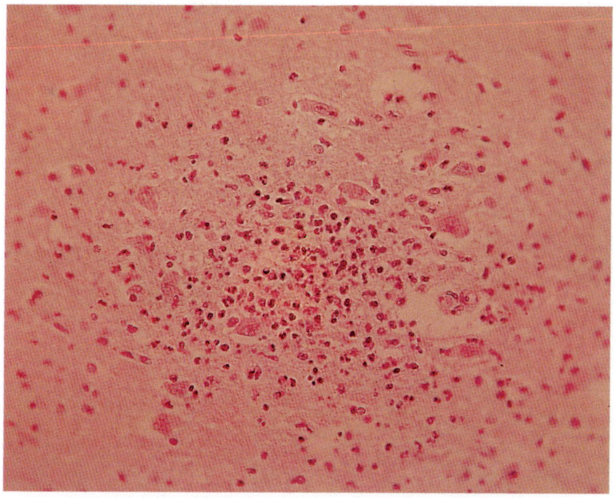

Figure 6–9. EEE encephalitis most pronounced in midbrain. Proliferated microglia, hematogenously derived monoctyes/macrophages, but particularly neutrophils, are striking features, together with neuronal necrosis (H&E ×250). (AFIP Neg 57-6073.)

trates and aggregates of neutrophils[55] (Figure 6–13) and a prominent vasculitis with fibrinoid necrosis and thrombi[2] (Figure 6–14).

PREVENTION AND CONTROL

On analysis of the simplistic schema of the natural cycle of virus/vector/host and the "unnatural" dissemination of arboviruses to humans and domesticated animals, simplistic methods of prevention might be anticipated. Thus, eradication of vector mosquitoes by destruction of their habitat (drainage of marshes and wetlands) has

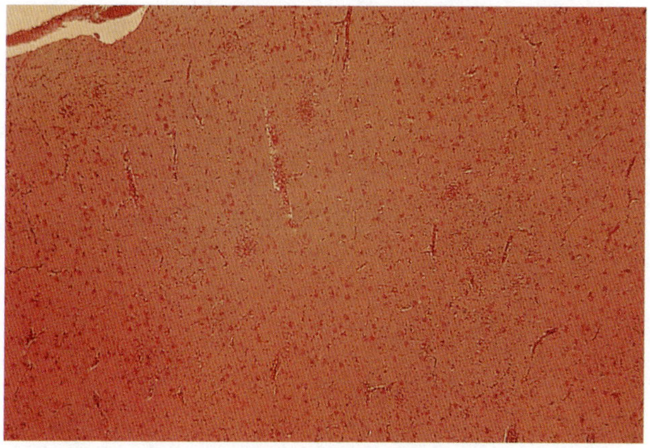

Figure 6–10. Diffuse leptomeningitis and encephalitis characterize this case of tick-borne (spring-summer) encephalitis. A multitude of microglial nodules is distributed throughout the cortex; the Virchow-Robin spaces contain an inflammatory cell infiltrate (H&E–van Gieson ×100). (AFIP Neg 56-1406.)

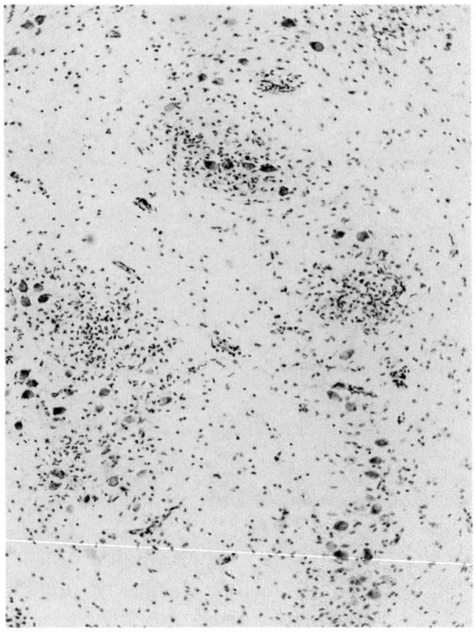

Figure 6–11. Multifocal neuronophagia and microglial nodules are in the inferior olivary nuclei in this patient with Central European tick-borne encephalitis (Cresyl-violet ×75). (AFIP Neg 64-2322.)

been modestly successful, but is now, in an era of environmental conservation, passé. Similarly, earlier practices of widespread spraying of insecticides have been unsatisfactory[58] because of the rapid restitution (from larvae) of a high population of mosquitoes, the emergence by natural selection of insecticide-resistant strains, and concern for upsetting the ecologic balance and damage to wildlife.

Prevention by vaccination exists for some of the arboviral encephalitides, particularly those with an endemic, high annual incidence, rather than those more apt to occur in sporadic epidemics. Thus, it has been well documented that a mouse brain–derived inactivated vaccine to JBE virus is very effective.[59,60] In spite of the potential for the development of postvaccinal encephalomyelitis (an autoimmune-mediated perivenular demyelination) or vaccine-caused encephalitis (a true viral infection by reversion of the inactivated virus to a more virulent strain), as documented with the use of other vaccines, these complications have not been reported. Vaccination of livestock is economically advantageous.

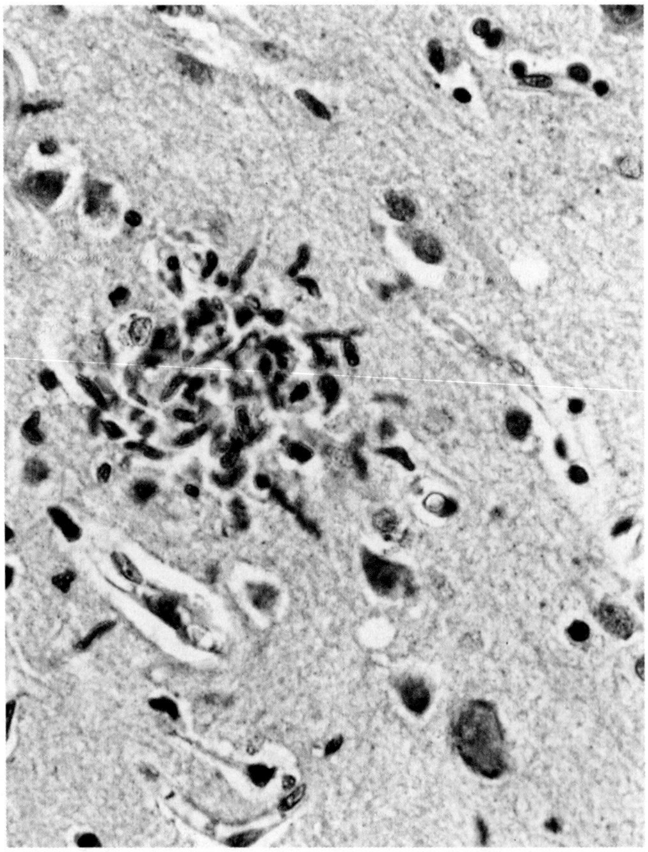

Figure 6–12. Typical microglial nodule composed of elongate, pleomorphic activated microglia and hematogenous monocytes/histiocytes in the cerebral cortex of patient with St. LE (H&E ×325). (AFIP Neg 64-2312.)

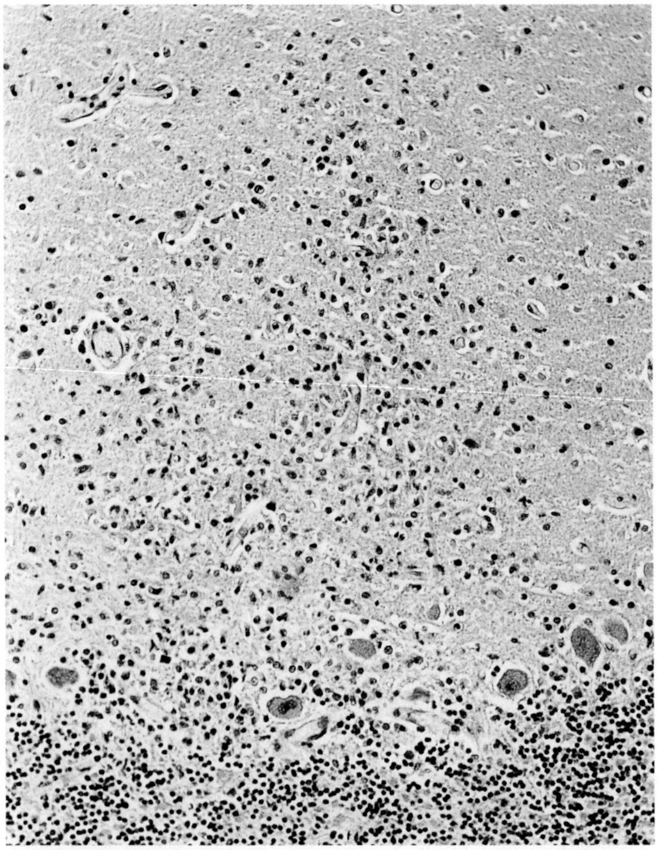

Figure 6–13. "Glial shrubbery" outlines the dendritic tree of degenerating and necrotic Purkinje cells in a case of EEE (H&E ×125). (AFIP Neg 64-2335.)

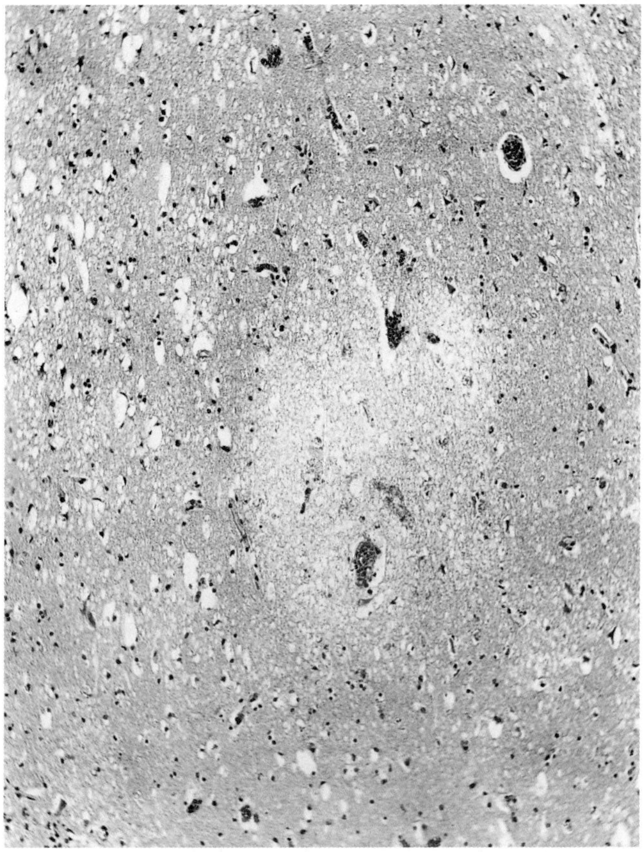

Figure 6–14. Area of rarefaction (infarction) necrosis around vessels with sludging of erythrocytes, in a larger area of acute cortical ischemia characterizes this case of fatal EEE (H&E ×100). (AFIP Neg 64-2332.)

EASTERN EQUINE ENCEPHALITIS

For illustrative and parochial reasons, EEE is discussed in more detail. First isolated in 1933 from the brain of a horse during an epizootic of equine encephalitis along the east coast of the United States, the virus was named Eastern Equine Encephalomyelitis virus to distinguish it from the virus of Western Equine Encephalomyelitis.[61,62] The first and one of the largest human epidemics (34 cases) was in Massachusetts in 1938,[63–67] with the majority (70%) in children younger than 10 years old. Mortality was high.[64,66,68] Since that time, epidemics have struck at irregular intervals in an area stretching from the Atlantic states to the Gulf of Mexico, as well as occasional infections in Michigan, upstate New York, and Ontario, Canada.[10,12,23,24,69,70] The natural cycle of the virus is maintained in coastal and intercoastal swamps and marshes (both salt and brackish) where the virus is passed among wild birds by the mosquito *Culiseta melanura*. When summer rains are exceptionally heavy,[69,70] the mosquito population explodes and disseminates the virus to peridomestic and domestic fowl (pheasants and chickens), which serve a "sentinel" function, allowing accurate predictions of fatal epizootics that have a major veterinary and economic impact, especially on horses.[10] Because *C melanura* rarely, if ever, bite humans, other mosquitoes, including *Aedes sollicitans*[71] and *Aedes albopictus* (an Asian import into the United States),[72] serve as "bridge" vectors by passing the virus to horses, swine,[73] and humans. In general, infections of domestic animals precede human infections by about 1 week. There are clinically inapparent infections detected serologically,[74] or mild infections with aseptic meningitis; unfortunately, however, most symptomatic infections of humans cause a very severe encephalitis. Following an epidemic in New Jersey in 1959, the ratio of those with inapparent infections to those with encephalitis was 23 : 1 overall. It was, however, much lower for children younger than 4 years of age (8 : 1) and much higher for adults in the 15- to 54-year age group (17 : 1 to 47 : 1), suggesting greater resistance to the virus by the adult CNS, rather than fewer bites by mosquitoes[75]; this contrasts with a ratio of 1000 : 1 for WEE in adults.[22] In that epidemic of EEE, 2.1% of the regional population had complement-fixing antibodies, with a gradient from a higher proportion positive near the coast to a much lower proportion further inland. Among household contacts of patients with encephalitis, the immune response was much higher still (7.3%).[76] This generally low rate of subclinical infection reflects the peculiar ecologic niche of the ornithophilic swamp mosquito, *C melanura*, with its preferred avian hosts, the passerine birds.

Among wild birds sampled in their natural habitats, there is a differential rate of susceptibility.[77–79] Fledglings, apparently, are bitten by *C melanura* and become infected.[78] The birds are amplifying hosts and are viremic for only a few days, then mount a brisk immune response without clinical manifestations; the antibody titer persists for the life of the bird. Depending on the type of antibody test and the ecologic niche of the bird, from 2% to 36% of the wild bird population may be infected.[79–81] The absence of symptoms, no doubt, depends on the failure of the virus to enter the CNS and replication of the virus must be extracerebral, probably in the liver.[77] Other birds, such as the whooping crane[82] and pheasants,[70,83] are much more vulnerable, but even these do not die of encephalitis; rather the virus is viscerotropic, not neurotropic as in humans and horses. Among penned pheasants, transmission may be bird-to-bird by pecking, oral secretions, or by inhalation, as well as by arthropod vectors.[83]

In the natural setting, only rare mosquitoes serve as vectors; thus from only 1 of 3881 mosquitoes (on average) was an equine encephalitis virus isolated.[84] In an experimental setting, however, permitting *C melanura* to feed on viremic chicks, a different perspective emerged: 92% of mosquitoes became infected with EEE and transmitted the virus with an 83% efficiency rate.[85] In the mosquito, the EEE virus is in the midgut, as determined by autoradiography, after permitting *C melanura* to feed on chicks injected with [3H] uridine-labelled EEEV.[86] A rapid reverse transcriptase/polymerase chain reaction assay is available to detect EEEV RNA in pooled mosquitoes or in avian tissues.[87] A similar technique has been used to detect other flaviviruses in human serum.[88] An enzyme immunoassay for IgM and IgG subclass antibodies to EEEV in sentinel chickens is another rapid diagnostic modality; antibodies developed within 2 to 4 days of injection.[89] Analogously, in humans a rapid and specific IgM detection method exists with very little cross-reactivity with other alphaviruses, because EEEV is a single species,[90] although it has 19 different antigenic variants.[91] These antibodies persist, presumably for life.[90] The 19 strains of EEEV are divided into 2 major antigenic types: 10 North American (NA-type) and 9 South American (SA-type).[91] There is much greater protein homogeneity in the NA-type viruses than in the SA-type,[92] in which there is a higher mutation rate; nevertheless, in spite of the structural protein differences, there is conservation of immunoreactive epitopes.[92] Nucleotide sequence analysis of the structural gene region of four NA EEEV strains revealed remarkable conservation between 1933 and 1985.[93] Similar oligonucleotide fingerprinting of EEEV, and assuming a stable low level of mutation, revealed the NA group to have diverged from the SA group approximately 1000 years ago; 2 SA subgroups diverged about 450 years ago.[94]

Among North American arboviral encephalitides, EEE carries the highest mortality rate (50% to 75%) in humans and survivors have the highest rate of complications.[2,3,12,66,68] Younger children and infants are particularly susceptible,[64,76] being prone to severe neurological deficits.[66,68] This suggests that the less mature brain may be especially vulnerable,[40,41,48] that the immune system may be less developed,[49] or that the inoculum of the mosquito is relatively greater in small children. Also known, however, is that different mosquitoes (even of the same species) inject viruses of varying numbers (by a factor of 100).[95] The greater virulence and neurotropism of EEEV are reflected in the more severe clinical manifestations, commonly ending in death or with profound neurologic, neuropsychiatric, and neurodevelopmental deficits in survivors, as well as in the extensively destructive neuropathologic features. A vasculitis with fibrin thrombi and fibrinoid necrosis is relatively common in brains at autopsy; similarly, a brisk neutrophilic reaction in brain tissue and in the subarachnoid space is also documented (Figures 6–6, 6–9, and 6–14).[2,55,64,66] The parenchymal and neuronal destruction as well as the inflammatory and vasculitic reaction are particularly prominent in basal ganglia and in the brainstem, although the cerebral cortex is not spared. In spite of, or perhaps because of, the rapid mounting of a brisk humoral immune response in fatal human cases, there are very marked inflammatory reaction, necrotizing encephalitis, neuronophagia, and vasculitis with fibrinoid necrosis and fibrin thrombi.

REFERENCES

1. Hammon WD, Reeves WC, Fray M. Mosquito vectors and inapparent animal reservoirs of St. Louis and Western equine encephalitis viruses. *Am J Public Health* 1943;33: 201–207.
2. Nieberg KC, Blumberg JM. Viral encephatitides. In: Minckler J, ed. *Pathology of the Nervous System.* Vol. 3. New York: McGraw-Hill; 1972:2279–2296.
3. Heffner RR Jr, Strano AJ. Arbovirus encephalitis. In: Binford CH, Connor DH, eds. *Pathology of Tropical and Extraordinary Diseases. An Atlas.* Vol 1. Washington, DC: Armed Forces Institute of Pathology; 1976:36–40.
4. Johnson RT. *Viral Infections of the Nervous System.* New York: Raven Press; 1982;105–119.
5. Leestma JE. Viral infections of the nervous system. In: Davis RL, Robertson DM, eds. *Textbook of Neuropathology.* 2nd ed. Baltimore: Williams & Wilkins; 1991;837–842; 844–849, 863–864.
6. Peters CJ, Dalrymple JM. Alphaviruses. In: Fields BN, Knipe DM, eds. *Fields' Virology.* 2nd ed. Vol. 2. New York: Raven Press; 1990;713–761.
7. Monath TP, Flaviviruses. In: Fields BN, Knipe DM, eds. *Fields' Virology.* 2nd ed. Vol. 1. New York: Raven Press; 1990;763–814.
8. Gonzalez-Scarano F and Nathanson N: Bunyaviruses. In: Fields BN and Knipe DM, eds, *Fields' Virology.* 2nd ed. Vol. 2. New York: Raven Press; 1990;1195–1228.
9. Knudson DL and Monath TP: Orbiviruses. In: Fields BN and Knipe DM, eds., *Fields' Virology.* 2nd ed. Vol 2. New York: Raven Press; 1990;1405–1433.
10. Dietz WH Jr, Galindo P, Johnson KM. Eastern Equine Encephalomyelitis in Panama: the epidemiology of the 1973 epizootic. *Am J Trop Med Hyg.* 1980;29:135–140.
11. Hollister AC Jr, Longshore WA, Dean BH, Stevens IM. The 1952 outbreak of encephalitis in California. Epidemiologic aspects. *Calif Med.* 1953;79:84–90.
12. Feemster RF. Equine encephalitis in Massachusetts. *N Engl J Med.* 1957;257:701–704.
13. Mitchell CF, Lvov SD, Savage HM, et al. Vector and host relationships of California serogroup viruses in western Siberia. *Am J Trop Med Hyg.* 1993;49:53–62.
14. Watts DM, Pantuwatana S, DeFoliart GR, Yuill TM, Thompson WH. Transovarial transmission of LaCrosse virus (California encephalitis group) in the mosquito, *Aedes triseriatus. Science.* 1973;182:1140–1141.
15. Fulhors CF, Hardy JL, Eldridge BF, Presser SB, Reeves WC. Natural vertical transmission of Western Equine Enceph-

alomyelitis virus in mosquitoes. *Science.* 1994;263: 676–678.
16. Gresikova M, Sekeyova M, Stupalova S, Necas S. Sheep milk–borne epidemic of tick-borne encephalitis in Slovakia. *Intervirology.* 1975;5:57–61.
17. The subcommittee on Arbovirus Laboratory Safety of the American Committee on Arthropod-Borne Viruses. Laboratory safety for arboviruses and certain other viruses of vertebrates. *Am J Trop Med Hyg.* 1980;29:1359–1381.
18. Emmons RW, Oshiro LS, Johnson HN, Lennette EH: Intraerythrocytic location of Colorado tick fever virus. *J Gen Virol.* 1987;17:185–195.
19. Philip RN, Casper EA, Cory J, Whitlock J. The potential for transmission of arboviruses by blood transfusion with particular reference to Colorado tick fever. In: Greenwalt J, Jamison GA, eds. *Transmissible Disease and Blood Transfusions.* New York: Grune and Stratton; 1975;175–196.
20. Chaturvedi UC, Mathur A, Chandra A, Das SK, Tandon HO, Singh UK. Transplacental infection with Japanese encephalitis virus. *J Infect Dis.* 1980;141:712–715.
21. Copps SC, Giddings LE. Transplacental transmission of Western Equine Encephalitis. *Pediatrics.* 1959;24:31–33.
22. Reeves WC, Hammon WM. Epidemiology of the arthropod-borne viral encephalitides in Kern County, California, 1943–1952. *Univ Calif Publ Publ Hlth.* 1962;4:1–257.
23. Monath TP. Arthropod-borne encephalitides in the Americas. *Bull Wld Hlth Organ.* 1979;57:513–533.
24. Altman R, Goldfield M, Sussman O. The impact of vector-borne viral diseases in the Middle Atlantic states. *Med Clin N Am.* 1967;51:661–671.
25. Silver HK, Meiklejohn G, Kempe CH: Colorado tick fever. *Amer J Dis Child.* 1961;101:56–61.
26. Ravi V, Taly AB, Shankar SK, et al. Association of Japanese encephalitis virus infection with Guillain–Barré syndrome in endemic areas of south India. *Acta Neurol Scand.* 1994;90:67–72.
27. Ravi V, Desai AS, Shenoy PK, Satishchandra P, Chandramuki A, Gourie-Devi M. Persistence of Japanese encephalitis virus in the human nervous system. *J Med Virol.* 1993;40:326–329.
28. Ogawa M, Okubo H, Tsuji Y, Yasui N, Someda K. Chronic progressive encephalitis occurring 13 years after Russian Spring-Summer Encephalitis. *J Neurol Sci.* 1973;19: 363–373.
29. Mueller WK, Schaltenbrand G. Attempts to reproduce amyotrophic lateral sclerosis in laboratory animals by inoculation of Schu virus isolated from a patient with apparent amyotrophic lateral sclerosis. *J Neurol.* 1979; 220:1–19.
30. Palmer RJ, Finley KH. Sequelae of encephalitis. Report of a study after the California epidemic. *Calif Med.* 1956;84: 98–100.
31. Earnest MP, Goolishian HA, Calverley JR, Hayes RO, Hill HR: Neurologic, intellectual, and psychologic sequelae following western encephalitis. *Neurology.* 1971;21: 969–974.
32. Froehlich H, Jarvis WR. Economic impact of diagnosis-related groups and severity of illness on reimbursement for central nervous system infections. *J Pediatr.* 1991;118: 693–697.
33. Mims CA. Aspects of the pathogenesis of virus diseases. *Bacter Rev.* 1964;28:30–71.
34. Johnson KP, Johnson RT. California encephalitis. II. Studies of experimental infection in the mouse. *J Neuropathol Exp Neurol.* 1968;27:390–400.
35. Pathak S, Webb HE: Possible mechanisms for the transport of Semliki Forest Virus into and within mouse brain. An electron-microscopic study. *J Neurol Sci.* 1974;23: 175–184.
36. Manz HJ. Pathology and pathogenesis of viral infections of the central nervous system. *Hum Pathol.* 1977;8:3–26.
37. Charles PC, Walters E, Margolis F, Johnston RE. Mechanism of neuroinvasion of Venezuelan equine encephalitis virus in the mouse. *Virology.* 1995;208:662–671.
38. Ben-Nathan D, Lustig S, Danenberg HD. Stress-induced neuroinvasiveness of a neurovirulent noninvasive Sindbis virus in cold or isolation subjected mice. *Life Sci.* 1991; 48:1493–1500.
39. Lustig S, Danenberg HD, Kafri Y, Kobiler D, Ben-Nathan D. Viral neuroinvasion and encephalitis induced by lipopolysaccharide and its mediators. *J Exp Med.* 1992; 176:707–712.
40. Ogata A, Nagashima K, Hall WW, Ishikawa M, Kimura-Kiroda J, Yasui K. Japanese encephalitis virus neurotropism is dependent on the degree of neuronal maturity. *J Virol.* 1991;65:880–886.
41. Tucker PC, Strauss EG, Kuhn RJ, Strauss JH, Griffin DE: Viral determinants of age-dependent virulence of Sindbis virus for mice. *J Virol.* 1993;67:4605–4610.
42. Case KL, West RM, Smith MG. Histocompatibility antigens and La Crosse encephalitis. *J Infect Dis.* 1993;168: 358–360.
43. Owens T, Renno T, Taupin V, Krakowski M. Inflammatory cytokines in the brain: does the CNS shape immune responses? *Immunol Today.* 1994;15:566–571.
44. Esiri MM, Gay D. Immunological and neuropathological significance of the Virchow-Robin space. *J Neurol Sci.* 1990;100:3–8.
45. Tyor WR, Griffin DE. Virus specificity and isotype expression of intraparenchymal antibody-secreting cells during Sindbis virus encephalitis in mice. *J Neuroimmunol.* 1993; 48:37–44.
46. Zlotnik I, Smith CEG, Grant DP, Peacock S. The effect of immunosuppression on viral encephalitis, with special reference to cyclophosphamide. *Br J Exp Path* 1970;51:434–439.
47. Desai A, Ravi V, Guru SC, et al. Detection of autoantibodies to neural antigens in the CSF of Japanese encephalitis patients and correlation of findings with the outcome. *J Neurol Sci.* 1994;122:109–116.
48. Griffin DE, Levine B, Ubol S, Hardwick JM. The effects of alphavirus infection on neurons. *Ann Neurol.* 1994; 35:S23–S27.
49. Levine B, Griffin DE. Persistence of viral RNA in mouse brains after recovery from acute alphavirus encephalitis. *J Virol* 1992;66:6429–6435.
50. Coppenhaver DH, Singh IP, Sarzotti M, Levy HB, Baron S. Treatment of intracerebral alphavirus infections in mice by a combination of specific antibodies and an interferon inducer. *Am J Trop Med Hyg.* 1995;52:34–40.

51. Weil A. Discussion. In: Scheinker IM. Histopathology of virus encephalitis. *J Neuropathol Exper Neurol.* 1948;7: 105–106.
52. Zimmerman H. Discussion. In: Scheinker IM. Histopathology of virus encephalitis. *J Neuropathol Exper Neurol* 1948;7:106.
53. Baker AB. Discussion. In: Scheinker IM. Histopathology of virus encephalitis. *J Neuropathol Exper Neurol.* 1948; 7:106.
54. Haymaker W. II Western Equine Encephalitis: Pathology. *Neurology.* 1958;8:861.
55. Haymaker W. III Eastern Equine Encephalitis: Pathology. *Neurology.* 1958;8:861–862.
56. Haymaker W. IV St. Louis Encephalitis: Pathology. *Neurology.* 1958;8:864.
57. Haymaker W. V Japanese Encephalitis: Pathology. *Neurology.* 1958;8:888.
58. Eldridge BF. Strategies for surveillance, prevention, and control of arbovirus diseases in western North America. *Am J Trop Med Hyg.* 1987;37(Suppl):77S–86S.
59. Igarashi A. Epidemiology and control of Japanese encephalitis. *World Health Stat Q.* 1992;45:299–305.
60. Hoke CH, Nisalak A, Sangawhipa N, et al. Protection against Japanese encephalitis by inactivated vaccines. *N Engl J Med.* 1988;319:608–614.
61. Ten Broeck C, Merrill MH. A serologic difference between eastern and western equine encephalomyelitis virus. *Proc Soc Exper Biol Med.* 1933;31:217–220.
62. Meyer KF, Haring CM, Howitt B. The etiology of epizootic encephalomyelitis of horses in the San Joaquin Valley. *Science.* 1931;74:227–228.
63. Fothergill LD, Dingle JH, Farber S, Connerly ML. Human encephalitis caused by the virus of the eastern variety of equine encephalomyelitis. *N Engl J Med.* 1938;219: 411–422.
64. Wesselhoeft C, Smith EC, Branch CF. Human encephalitis. Eight fatal cases, with four due to the virus of equine encephalomyelitis. *JAMA* 1938;111:1735–1741.
65. Feemster RF. Outbreak of encephalomyelitis in man due to eastern virus of equine encephalomyelitis. *Am J Pub Health.* 1938;28:1403–1410.
66. Farber S, Hill A, Connerly ML, Dingle JH. Encephalitis in infants and children caused by the virus of the eastern variety of equine encephalitis. *JAMA* 1940;114:1725–1731.
67. Webster LT, Wright FH. Recovery of eastern equine encephalomyelitis virus from brain tissue of human cases of encephalitis in Massachusetts. *Science.* 1938;88: 305–306.
68. Ayers JC, Feemster RF. The sequelae of eastern equine encephalomyelitis 1938 Massachusetts outbreak. *N Engl J Med.* 1949;240:960–962.
69. Letson GW, Bailey RE, Pearson J, Tsai TF. Eastern equine encephalitis (EEE): a description of the 1989 outbreak, recent epidemiologic trends, and the association of rainfall with EEE occurrence. *Am J Trop Med Hyg.* 1993;49: 677–685.
70. Hayes RO, Beadle LD, Hess AD, Sussman O, Bonese MJ. Entomological aspects of the 1959 outbreak of eastern encephalitis in New Jersey. *Am J Trop Med Hyg.* 1962; 11:115–121.
71. Freier JE. Eastern equine encephalomyelitis. *Lancet.* 1993; 342:1281–1282.
72. Mitchell CJ, Niebelski ML, Smith GC, et al. Isolation of eastern equine encephalitis virus from *Aedes albopictus* in Florida. *Science.* 1992;257:526–527.
73. Elvinger F, Liggett AD, Tang KN, et al. Eastern equine encephalomyelitis virus infection in swine. *J Am Vet Med Assoc.* 1994;205:1014–1016.
74. Clarke DH. Two nonfatal human infections with the virus of eastern encephalitis. *Am J Trop Med Hyg.* 1961;10: 67–70.
75. Goldfield M, Welsh JN, Taylor BF. The 1959 outbreak of eastern encephalitis in New Jersey. 5. The inapparent infection:disease ratio. *Am J Epidemiol.* 1968;87:32–38.
76. Goldfield M, Welsh JN, Taylor BF. The 1959 outbreak of eastern encephalitis in New Jersey. 4. CF reactivity following overt and inapparent infection. *Am J Epidemiol.* 1968;87:23–31.
77. Kissling RE, Chamberlain RW, Sikes RK, Edison ME. Studies on the North American arthropod-borne encephalitides. III. Eastern equine encephalitis in wild birds. *Am J Hyg.* 1954;60:251–265.
78. Dalrymple JM, Young OP, Eldridge BF, Russell PK. Ecology of arboviruses in a freshwater Maryland swamp. III. Vertebrate hosts. *Am J Epidemiol.* 1972;96:129–140.
79. Hayes RO, Daniels JB, Anderson KS, Parsons MA, Maxfield HK, LaMotte LC. Detection of eastern encephalitis virus and antibody in wild and domestic birds in Massachusetts. *Am J Hyg.* 1962;75:183–189.
80. McLean RG, Frier G, Parham GL, et al. Investigations of the vertebrate hosts of eastern equine encephalitis during an epizootic in Michigan, 1980. *Am J Trop Med Hyg.* 1985; 34:1190–1202.
81. Shope RE, de Andrade AHP, Bensabeth G, Causey OR, Humphrey PS. The epidemiology of EEE, WEE, SLE and Tralock viruses, with special references to birds, in a tropical rain forest near Belem, Brazil. *Am J Epidemiol.* 1966; 87:467–477.
82. Dein FJ, Carpenter JW, Clark GG, et al. Mortality of captive whooping cranes caused by eastern equine encephalitis virus. *J Am Vet Med Assoc.* 1986;189:1006–1010.
83. Holden P. Transmission of eastern equine encephalomyelitis in ring-necked pheasants. *Proc Soc Exper Biol Med.* 1955;88:607–610.
84. Saugstad ES, Dalrymple JM, Eldridge BF. Ecology of arboviruses in a Maryland freshwater swamp. I. Population dynamics and habitat distribution of potential mosquito vectors. *Am J Epidemiol.* 1972;96:114–122.
85. Howard JJ, Wallis RC. Infection and transmission of eastern equine encephalomyelitis virus with colonized *Culiseta melanura* (*Coquillet*). *Am J Trop Med Hyg.* 1974; 23:522–525.
86. Weaver SC, Scott TW, Lorenz LH, Repik PM. Detection of eastern equine encephalomyelitis virus deposition in *Culiseta melanura* following ingestion of radiolabeled virus in blood meals. *Am J Trop Med Hyg.* 1991;44: 250–259.
87. Vodkin MH, McLaughlin GL, Day JF, Shope RE, Novak RJ. A rapid diagnostic assay for eastern equine encephalomyelitis viral RNA. *Am J Trop Med Hyg.* 1993;49:772–776.

88. Chang GJ, Trent DW, Vorndam AV, Vergne E, Kinney RM, Mitchell CJ. An integrated target sequence and signal amplification assay reverse transcriptase-PCR-enzyme-linked immunosorbent assay, to detect and characterize flaviviruses. *J Clin Microbiol.* 1994;32:477–483.
89. Olson JG, Scott TW, Lorenz LH, Hubbard JL. Enzyme immunoassay for detection of antibodies against eastern equine encephalomyelitis virus in sentinel chickens. *J Clin Microbiol.* 1991;29:1457–1461.
90. Calisher CH, El-Kafrawi AO, Al-Deen MMI, et al. Complex specific immunoglobulin M antibody patterns in humans infected with alphaviruses. *J Clin Microbiol.* 1986;23: 155–159.
91. Casals J. Antigenic variants of eastern equine encephalitis virus. *J Exp Med.* 1964;119:547–565.
92. Striziki JM, Repik PM. Structural protein relationships among eastern equine encephalomyelitis viruses. *J Gen Virol.* 1994;75:2897–2909.
93. Weaver SC, Scott TW, Rico-Hess R. Molecular evolution of eastern equine encephalomyelitis virus in North America. *Virology.* 1991;182:774–784.
94. Weaver SC, Hagenbaugh A, Bellew LA, et al. Evolution of alphaviruses in the eastern equine encephalomyelitis complex. *J Virol.* 1994;68:158–169.
95. Chamberlain RW, Kissling RE, Sikes PK. Studies on the North American arthropod-borne encephalitides. VII. Estimation of amount of eastern equine encephalitis virus inoculated by *Aedes aegypti*. *Am J Hyg.* 1954;60:286–291.

CHAPTER 7

Coxsackieviruses

Sydney D. Finkelstein

Science, like art, music and poetry, tries to reduce chaos to the clarity and order of pure beauty.

Detlev W. Bronk, JAMA. 1965;191:991.

INTRODUCTION

The coxsackieviruses are small, single-stranded RNA viruses that have been subdivided into two major groups, A and B, each with their own shared common surface receptor.[1] First discovered and named for the site of initial isolation, Coxsackie, New York, in 1941, new forms continue to be identified and added, resulting in 29 serotypes of group A and 6 types of group B, as well as more recently identified forms that have been classified under the grouping of Enterovirus.[2] They are members of the Picornavirus group. Coxsackieviruses produce a wide range of human diseases, many with overlapping clinical features. Infections in suckling mice mimic many aspects of human disease and serve as research and clinical tools to study the pathobiology of coxsackievirus infection. In suckling mice, group A coxsackieviruses are characterized mainly, but not exclusively, by widespread necrotizing inflammation of skeletal muscle. Group B coxsackieviruses present a somewhat wider array of clinical disease, which most often includes encephalitis, focal myositis, and steatitis in suckling mice. Inoculation of specific coxsackievirus prototypes and related variants into specific strains of inbred mice mimics the human spectrum of differing organ involvement and also serves as a useful model to clarify human infections (Figures 7–1, 7–2, and 7–3). Although the specific aspects of their pathobiology have not been worked out as fully as other picornaviruses, experience has shown that their biology resembles closely that of polioviruses.

Coxsackieviruses have a worldwide distribution, with humans serving as the only natural reservoir.[3] They infect all ages and are even suspected to be an important cause of congenital malformation.[4,5] As with other picornaviruses, the vast majority of infections are either asymptomatic or characterized by mild nonspecific febrile illness. This is supported by the high rate of seropositivity in the adult population.[2,3]

As with enterovirus infection in general, initial portal of entry is the aerodigestive tract, with primary replication in the mucosal epithelial cells and their associated lymphoid tissue. Subsequent viremia carries the virus throughout the body where secondary sites of replication may lead to further viremia and dissemination. High titers of serum antibody are closely associated with elimination of the virus from the circulatory system. As described later, further tissue injury may ensue from immune-mediated tissue damage and/or persistent viral infection.

The mechanism for the broad spectrum of clinical disease syndromes produced by this group of viruses has remained a subject of intense investigation. The requirement for cell-specific surface receptors has been well demonstrated as a critical determinant of disease production in view of the close relationship between receptor number, viral tropism, and induction of disease under experimental and clinical conditions. Unlike poliovirus, the human gene encoding the coxsackievirus receptor has not yet been identified nor is its normal function known. Variant coxsackieviruses differing in disease activity compared to their parental strains have proved to be an important tool in understanding viral pathogenesis. Variants differing in their receptor tropism are closely associated with variations in disease production. As with other picornaviruses, modifying

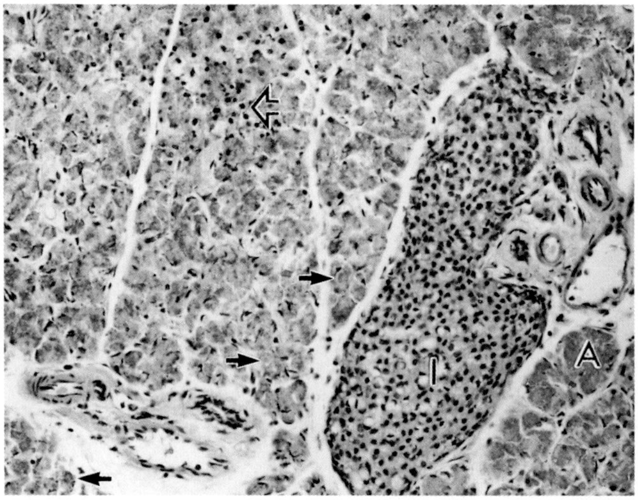

Figure 7–1. Experimental coxsackievirus infection of mice. Adult Balb/c mice were infected with Woodruff strain of group B coxsackievirus. Pancreas was harvested on day 2 postintraperitoneal inoculation. There is extensive coagulative necrosis of pancreas consistent with virologically mediated cell killing (*solid arrows*). Inflammatory cell infiltration (*open arrow*) is minimal. **A**, pancreatic acinar cells; **I**, islets of Langerhans (hematoxylin-eosin, ×250).

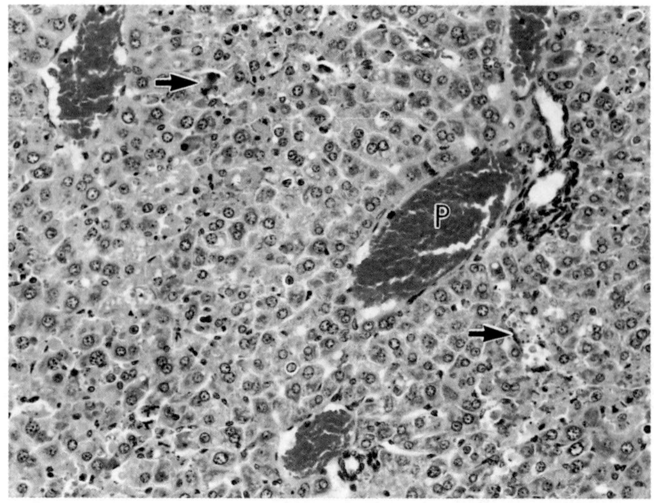

Figure 7–2. Experimental coxsackievirus infection of mice. Adult Balb/c mice were infected with Woodruff strain of group B coxsackievirus. Liver tissue was removed 4 days postintraperitoneal inoculation. The liver is undergoing coagulative necrosis that begins in the midzone of the lobule (*arrows*) and will extend to involve the entire lobule. The appearance, as with the pancreas, is consistent with virologically mediated cell killing. This strain of mouse dies soon from liver failure. **P**, portal vein branch (hematoxylin-eosin, ×250).

factors that affect disease production include duration and intensity of viremia, portal of entry, and extent of specific host immune response.[6]

In contrast to other members of the Picornavirus group, there are two aspects of pathobiology unique to coxsackieviruses. The first is the phenomenon of viral persistence, which has been best demonstrated in human cardiomyopathy.[7] In situ hybridization, using full and partial cDNA probes to the Coxsackievirus B genome on cardiac tissue derived from endocardial biopsies as well as from cardiac transplantation, has demonstrated persistent virus in patients with myocarditis as well as certain forms of chronic cardiomyopathy. The mechanism accounting for viral persistence is, however, unknown but subject to intense investigation.[7–9]

The second unique property associated with coxsackieviruses is the ability to incite significant autoimmune disease in certain hosts. Immune-mediated damage has been well demonstrated both experimentally and in human subjects with autoimmune diseases, such as myocarditis and glomerulonephritis.[3,6] Evidence for both antibody-mediated as well as cytolytic T-cell-mediated damage has been reported.[10,11] In murine models, infection with coxsackieviruses results in the production of antibodies capable of binding specifically to heart cells and exacerbating the inflammatory responses that result in cell damage. These circulating autoanti-

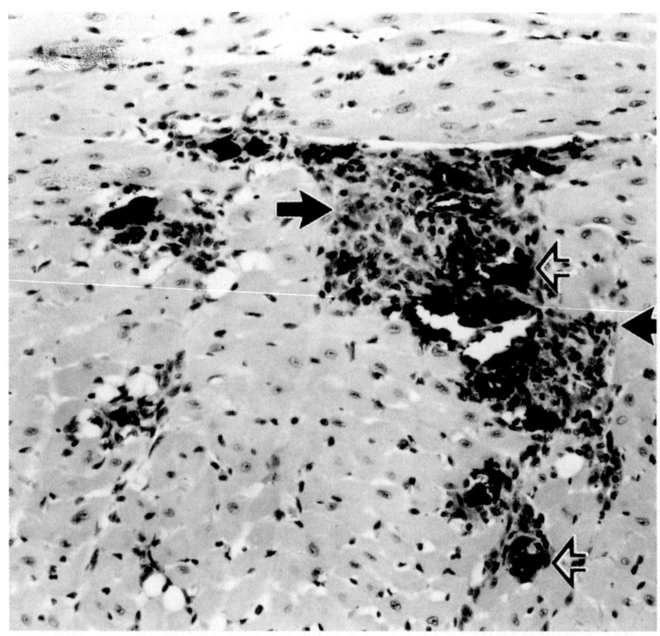

Figure 7–3. Experimental coxsackievirus infection. Adult HeJ mice were infected with Woodruff strain of group B coxsackievirus. Cardiac tissue obtained 14 days postintraperitoneal inoculation reveals combined cellular necrosis and dystrophic calcification (*open arrows*) together with an infiltrate of acute and chronic inflammatory cells (*solid arrows*). The latter has been proposed as supportive of immunologically mediated injury equivalent to that in human myocarditis and cardiomyopathy (hematoxylin-eosin, ×600).

bodies can be eluted from the hearts of myocarditis-susceptible mouse strains but not from strains resistant to the development of the disease. Furthermore, adoptive transfer of immunoregulatory cells has been shown to reproduce tissue damage. These and other studies support a growing body of data to suggest that in certain hosts coxsackievirus infection can be associated with the phenomenon of molecular mimicry that results in autoimmune tissue damage. The combination of persistent virus infection and autoimmunity may provide the basis for not just chronic heart failure but for many other diseases linked to coxsackievirus infection including diabetes mellitus, dermato/polymyositis (Figure 7–4), postviral fatigue syndrome, and renal disease. Some of these aspects are discussed later.

Myo/pericarditis is one of the best characterized and most intensively studied of the various coxsackievirus diseases. The disease usually follows a biphasic pattern, beginning as a mild nonspecific febrile illness. After a period of 2 to 3 weeks, the onset of cardiac involvement ensues, taking the form of chest pain, irregular rhythm, or even heart failure. Clinical evidence of pericardial involvement is usually found in the form of friction rub or electrocardiographic changes. The subsequent course is variable, spanning a range from complete recovery to fulminant disease and death. Recovery with residual cardiac injury of varying degrees usually occurs.

When available for examination, the acutely affected heart is usually enlarged and edematous with scattered petechial hemorrhages.[12] In long-standing disease, compensatory hypertrophy is present. Microscopically an interstitial mixed acute and chronic inflammation occurs associated with myocardial fiber necrosis in the acute stage of disease[13] (Figure 7–5). Chronically affected hearts have lymphohistiocytic interstitial inflammation with varying degrees of scarring. The extent of inflammation, myonecrosis, and scarring correlates with the clinical severity of injury.

None of the features just described is necessarily unique to coxsackievirus-induced myocardial disease. Given that coxsackievirus infection is the most common cause of virally induced heart disease, presumptive evidence of coxsackievirus can be made once other more easily identifiable microorganisms, such as fungi and parasites, are excluded. To confirm the diagnosis, however, demonstration of the organism is required. This can be done most readily by ultrastructural demonstration of the virus, which assumes the form of crystalline aggregates of particles approximately 30 nm in diameter. Unfortunately, this is successful only in a minority of patients, tending to be more common in fulminating acute infection. Chronic myocardial disease is usually negative for visible virus by electron microscopy.

High, moderate, and low association between coxsackievirus and organ damage can be made using criteria similar to those outlined for poliovirus infection (see Chapter 27, Polioviruses). Ideally, coxsackievirus should be isolated by culture from samples of heart tissue submitted fresh or sent frozen to the laboratory.

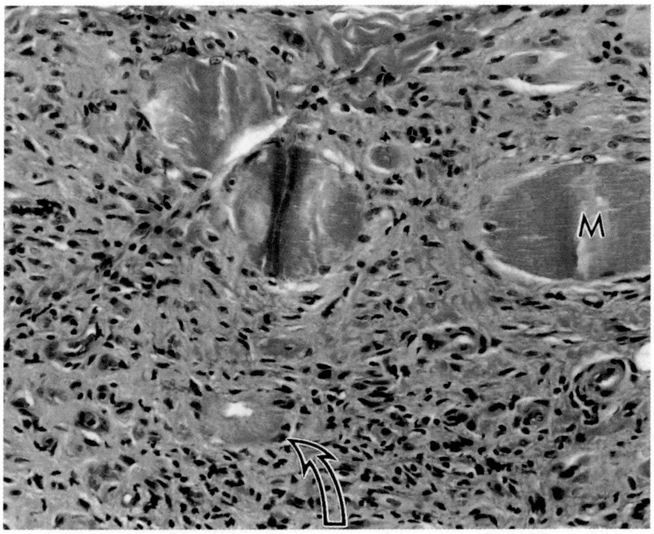

Figure 7–4. Human polymyositis. Extensive acute and chronic inflammation is seen and is associated with necrosis (*arrow*) of myofibers. Residual muscle fibers have undergone compensatory hypertrophy (**M**) (hematoxylin-eosin, ×400).

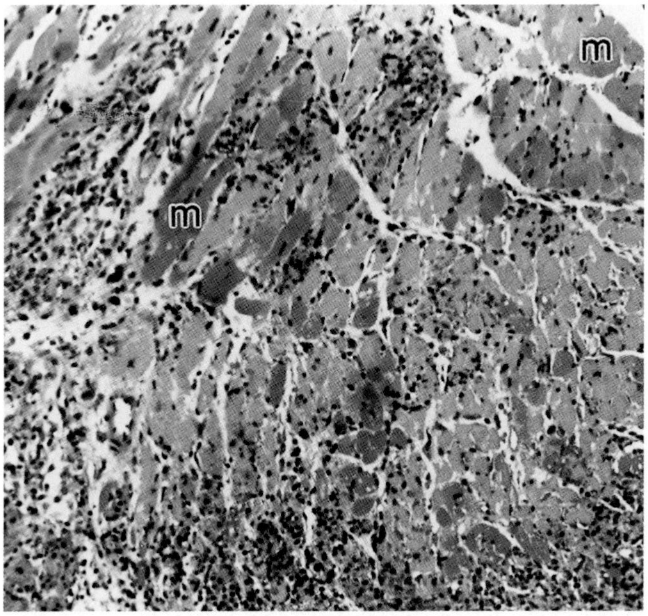

Figure 7–5. Human acute myocarditis. The heart reveals extensive interstitial inflammation associated with myocardial cell destruction (**m**). There was a rising titer to coxsackievirus group B (hematoxylin-eosin, ×250).

Alternatively, direct detection of the virus in diseased tissue can be made by immunohistochemical/immunofluorescent methods or by specific nucleic acid detection by in situ hybridization and/or polymerase chain reaction.[14–18] Antibodies are now available that are effective on paraffin-embedded tissue.[19] Parts or all of the coxsackievirus genome have been published for most strains and cDNA molecular detection probes can be engineered from a variety of repositories of the virus.[14,20] Complementary in situ hybridization probes are now available for both positive and negative strands of the virus.[17] The use of strand-specific probes to the negative replicative intermediary is especially noteworthy, because it provides a unique way to distinguish between quiescent and actively replicating virus. Viral isolation from blood, aerodigestive swabs, and stool together with demonstration of rising titer in paired sera constitute alternative methods for identifying likely coxsackievirus infection.

Encephalitis

Although viral meningitis is relatively commonly caused by coxsackieviruses, encephalitis is more unusual, but unfortunately more serious and even fatal (Figure 7–6). There is also often an associated infection involving other organs.[21]

AUTOIMMUNE DISEASE

Great interest has been raised in the role of coxsackievirus infection in a variety of autoimmune disorders. Elevated levels of antibodies to coxsackievirus have been found in patients with diabetes mellitus, glomerulonephritis, and chronic muscle diseases such as dermato/polymyositis[22] and postviral fatigue syndrome. There has been long-standing interest in the role of coxsackievirus infection as a causative agent for diabetes mellitus, particularly the juvenile form, given the frequency of infection in the younger age groups.[23–25] Additional support for a causative relationship between coxsackievirus infection and diabetes includes onset in fall and winter, consistent with the incidence of natural infection, as well as high levels of neutralizing antibody in affected patients compared to age-matched controls. Experimental models of murine infection have shown that tissue damage is not a requirement and that glucose intolerance can result from infection that produces islet cell dysfunction without inflammation or irreversible cell injury.[2,3] Demonstration of viral particles in chronically affected skeletal muscle provides support for the role of coxsackievirus infection as causally related to chronic fatigue syndrome with a pathogenesis based on a combination of persistent infection and related autoimmune-induced tissue injury.[26,27]

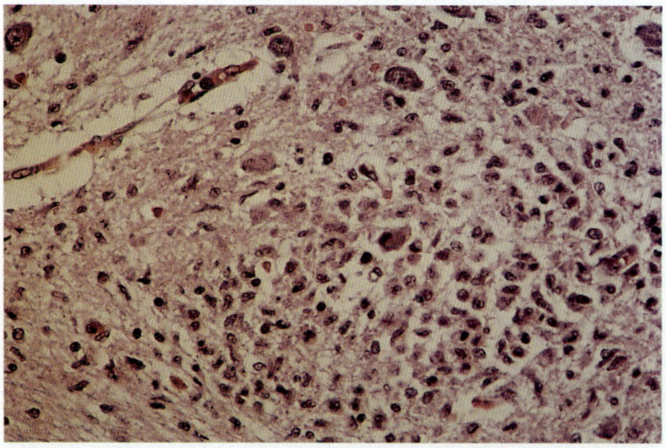

Figure 7–6. Human encephalitis. This infant had fatal viral myocarditis and encephalitis of brainstem caused by Coxsackievirus B2. Numerous macrophages are congregated in the inferior olive; several neurons are still evident (hematoxylin-eosin, ×250). *(Photograph courtesy of Herbert J. Manz, MD.)*

REFERENCES

1. Rueckert RR. Picornaviridae and their replication. In: Fields BN, Knipe DM, eds. *Virology.* New York: Raven Press; 1990:507–548.
2. Crowell RL, Landau BJ. Picornaviridae: enterovirus–coxsackieviruses. *CRC Clin Lab Sci Virol Rickettsiol.* 1978;1: 131–155.
3. Melnick JL. Enteroviruses: polioviruses, coxsackieviruses, echoviruses, and newer enteroviruses: In: Fields BN, Knipe DM, eds. *Virology.* New York: Raven Press; 1990: 549–606.
4. Gauntt CJ, Gudvangen RJ, Brans YW, Marlin AE. Coxsackievirus group B antibodies in the ventricular fluid of infants with severe anatomic defects of the central nervous system. *Pediatrics.* 1985;76:64–68.
5. Brown GC, Karvnas RS. Relationship of congenital anomalies and maternal infection with selected enteroviruses. *Am J Epidemiol.* 1972;95:207–217.
6. Levi G, Scalvini S, Volterrani M, et al. Coxsackie virus heart disease: 15 years after. *Euro Heart J.* 1988;9: 1303–1307.
7. Easton AJ, Eglin RP. The detection of coxsackievirus RNA in cardiac tissue by in situ hybridization. *J Gen Virol.* 1988;69:285–291.
8. Crowell RC, Finkelstein SD, Lee Hsu KH, et al. A murine model for coxsackievirus B3-induced acute myocardial necrosis for study of cellular receptor determinants of viral tropism. In: Schultheiss HP, ed. *New Concepts in Viral Heart Disease.* New York: Springer Verlag; 1988.
9. Bowles NE, Richardson PJ, Olsen EGJ, Archard LC. Detection of coxsackie B virus-specific RNA sequences in myocardial biopsy samples from patients with myocarditis and dilated cardiomyopathy. *Lancet.* 1986;1:1120.

10. Viral myocarditis—a tale of two diseases. *Lab Invest.* 1992;1:1–3. Editorial.
11. Landau BJ, Whittier PS, Finkelstein SD, et al. Induction of idiotypic virus resistance in adult inbred mice immunized with a variant of Coxsackievirus B3. *Microbiol Pathogenesis.* 1990;8:289–298.
12. Woodruff J. Viral myocarditis—a review. *Am J Pathol.* 1980;101:425.
13. Becker AE. Pathology of cardiomyopathies. In: Shaver JA, Brest AN, eds. *Cardiomyopathies: Clinical Presentation, Differential Diagnosis, and Management.* Philadelphia: FA Davis Company; 1988:9–31.
14. Kandolf R, Hofschneider PH. Molecular cloning of the genome of a cardiotropic Coxsackievirus B3 virus: full-length reverse-transcribed recombinant cDNA generates infectious virus in mammalian cells. *Proc Natl Acad Sci USA.* 1985;82:4818—4822.
15. Kandolf R, Ameis D, Kirschner P, et al. In situ detection of enteroviral genomes in myocardial cells by nucleic acid hybridization: an approach to the diagnosis of viral heart disease. *Proc Natl Acad Sci USA.* 1987;84:6272–6276.
16. Godeny EK, Gauntt CJ. In situ immune autoradiographic identification of cells in heart tissues of mice with coxsackievirus B3-induced myocarditis. *Am J Pathol.* 1987; 129:267.
17. Cova L, Kopecka H, Aymard M, Girard M. Use of cRNA probes for the detection of enteroviruses by molecular hybridization. *J Med Virol.* 1988;24:11–18.
18. Hohenadl C, Klingel K, Mertsching J, et al. Strand-specific detection of enteroviral RNA in myocardial tissue by an in situ hybridization. *Mol Cell Probes.* 1991;5:11–20.
19. Burch GE, Sun SC, Chu KC, Sohal RS, et al. Interstitial and coxsackievirus B myocarditis in infants and children: a comparative histologic and immunofluorescent study of 50 autopsied hearts. *JAMA.* 1968;203:1–8.
20. Kandolf R, Detlev A, Kirschner P, et al. In situ detection of enteroviral genomes in myocardial cells by nucleic acid hybridization: an approach to the diagnosis of viral heart disease. *Proc Natl Acad Sci USA.* 1987;84:6272.
21. Grist NR, Bell EJ, Assaad F. Enteroviruses in human disease. *Prog Med Virol.* 1978; 24:114–157.
22. Gyorkey F, Cabral GA, Gyorkey PK, et al. Coxsackie aggregates in muscle cells of a polymyositis patient. *Intervirology.* 1978;10:69–77.
23. Frank JA, Schmidt EV, Smith RE, Wilfert CM. Persistent infection of rat insulinoma cells with coxsackie B4 virus. *Arch Virol.* 1986;87:143.
24. Banatvala JE. Insulin-dependent (juvenile-onset, type 1) diabetes mellitus: Coxsackie B viruses revisited. *Prog Med Virol.* 1987;34:33–54.
25. Wagenknecht LE, Roseman JM, Herman WH. Increased incidence of insulin-dependent diabetes mellitus following an epidemic of Coxsackievirus B5. *Am J Epidemiol.* 1991;133:1024–1031.
26. Bowles NE, Dubowitz V, Sewry CA, et al. Dermatomyositis, polymyositis, and coxsackie-B-virus infections. *Lancet.* 1987;1:1104–1107.
27. Muir P, Nicholson F, Banatvala JE, Bingley PJ. Coxsackie B virus and postviral fatigue syndrome. *Br Med J.* 1991;302:658–659.

CHAPTER 8

Cytomegalovirus Infection

Ernest E. Lack, Francis W. Chandler, and Gary R. Pearson

To be astonished at anything is the first movement of the mind towards discovery.

Louis Pasteur (1822–1895)

DEFINITION

Cytomegalovirus (CMV) infection is caused by a member of the family *Herpesviridae,* which includes herpes simplex virus types 1 and 2, varicella-zoster virus (VZV), Epstein–Barr virus, and human herpesviruses types 6 and 7 (HV-6 and HV-7). Infection by CMV can be acquired before birth (congenital), at the time of delivery (perinatal), or later in life (postnatal).

EPIDEMIOLOGY

CMV has been detected in 0.5% to 2% of newborn infants[1,2] and is one of the most common congenital infections transmitted to the fetus in utero. Infants also can acquire infection at the time of delivery by exposure to CMV in the birth canal. Postnatal infections are acquired by close contact with anyone shedding the virus, usually by aerosolized oral secretions.[2] Among children attending day care centers, 20% to 70% of those who enter as young infants acquire CMV over a 1- to 2-year period.[2] CMV also can be transmitted from the infected child to the mother, and infection acquired by a pregnant woman can be transmitted to the fetus.[3] Transmission of primary CMV can occur in a variety of ways because the virus has been detected in body fluids including saliva, urine, breast milk, tears, stool, vaginal or cervical secretions, blood, and semen.[2] CMV can infect epithelium of epididymis, seminal vesicles, and uterine cervix, and can be sexually transmitted. The virus also can be transmitted by blood transfusion and by bone marrow or organ transplantation. Primary infection with CMV causes persistent or latent infection in the immunocompetent host, and endogenous reactivation of the virus can occur in response to different stimuli such as congenital or acquired defects of cellular immunity.

PATTERNS OF INFECTION

Infection with CMV is usually latent and asymptomatic in those with a normal immune system, and it can be detected retrospectively by seroepidemiologic studies.[4] When disease does occur in a patient with an intact immune system, it is usually transient, self-limited, and may resemble infectious mononucleosis with signs and symptoms that include myalgia, malaise, sore throat, headache, rash, and fever; there may be atypical lymphocytosis, and about 3% of patients develop jaundice.[1] Infection by CMV acquired in utero also may be asymptomatic; fewer than 5% of congenitally infected infants develop symptoms during the newborn period. Manifestations range from a mild self-limited illness to severe infection with jaundice, hepatosplenomegaly, encephalitis, and chorioretinitis. Infection may be fatal within the first few months of life, or the infant may survive with neurologic damage such as learning disabilities and hearing defects. Infection also can follow blood transfusions or cardiopulmonary bypass, and in these patients has been called "postperfusion syndrome." Donor leukocytes and donor organs also may transmit CMV, and antigenic stimulation by foreign antigens can sometimes activate endogenous latent infection by CMV in the recipient.[1]

Infection by CMV may be frequent and severe in children or adults with congenital or acquired defects of cellular immunity, underlying malignancy, immunosuppression due to steroid administration, and the acquired immunodeficiency syndrome (AIDS). Features of active disseminated CMV infection include fever, leukopenia, thrombocytopenia, petechiae, pneumonitis, hepatitis, chorioretinitis, adrenalitis, and encephalitis.[2] Infection by CMV in infants may be associated with a hemorrhagic–purpuric eruption, with mobile, blue-gray cutaneous lesions giving the affected infant an appearance likened to a "blueberry muffin" (Figure 8–1, A and B). An identical cutaneous eruption also has been reported with rubella.[5] Histologic studies have revealed extramedullary dermal erythropoiesis. The eruption may be transient or occur as a complication of disseminated, more severe infection.

UNUSUAL CLINICAL MANIFESTATIONS

Patients with active CMV infection who are symptomatic have clinical and laboratory manifestations that may be extremely variable. Some of the more unusual clinical manifestations occur in patients who are profoundly immunodeficient (eg, those with AIDS). Rare disseminated infections have been reported presenting with acalculous cholecystitis and acute pancreatitis.[6] Infection of the pancreas has been noted in immunodeficient patients, but only rarely does it cause clinical disease. In the setting of AIDS, there are several noteworthy but rare associations. Gastroenteritis and intestinal perforations have been reported to be caused by a severe form of CMV-related occlusive vasculitis.[7] Involvement of the peripheral and central nervous systems also has been reported in AIDS and includes a form of neurologic dysfunction characterized clinically as Guillain–Barré syndrome. A predominantly sensory, pseudotabetic syndrome and a sensorimotor polyradiculopathy are also caused by infection of particular subdivisions of the nervous system by CMV (Figure 8–2).[8,9]

The adrenal glands have received considerable attention as possible sites of endocrine disease in AIDS,[10] with CMV being the most common adrenotropic infectious agent. Of 164 autopsies of AIDS victims, 49% (n = 81) were actively infected with CMV, and the most common sites of infection included adrenals (75%), followed by lungs (58%), gastrointestinal tract (30%), central nervous system (20%), and retina (10%); 10% of the deaths in that study were attributed to infection by CMV, and two patients had Addison's disease.[11] Other studies have focused specifically on CMV adrenalitis in AIDS patients, in whom the incidence ranges from 42% to 55%.[12–15] When assessing the extent of adrenal necrosis, some studies have shown a relatively greater amount of necrosis within the medulla.[12,14] Other studies concluded that the extent of cortical necrosis was less than that usually associated with clinically overt adrenal cortical insufficiency (ie, 90%). The rapid adrenocorticotropic hormone (ACTH)-stimulation test may reveal subnormal cortisol responses in 5% to 10% of patients with AIDS, and some patients may be at risk for an adrenal crisis during episodes of severe illness, surgery, or trauma.[16] Some clinical manifestations in AIDS patients, however, can mimic those of adrenal cortical insufficiency such as nausea, vomiting, weight loss, and fatigue; findings more specific for adrenal involvement include postural

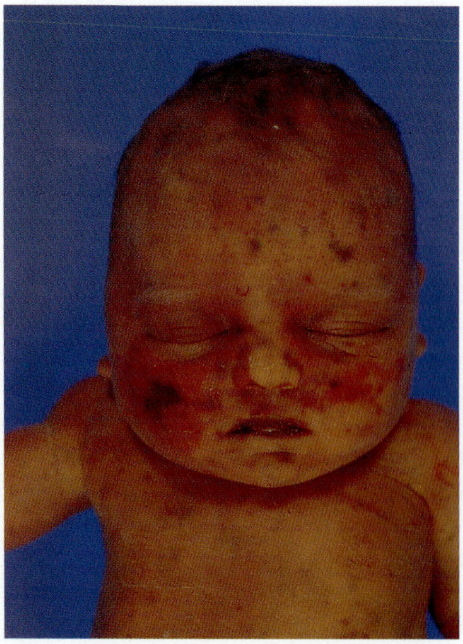

A

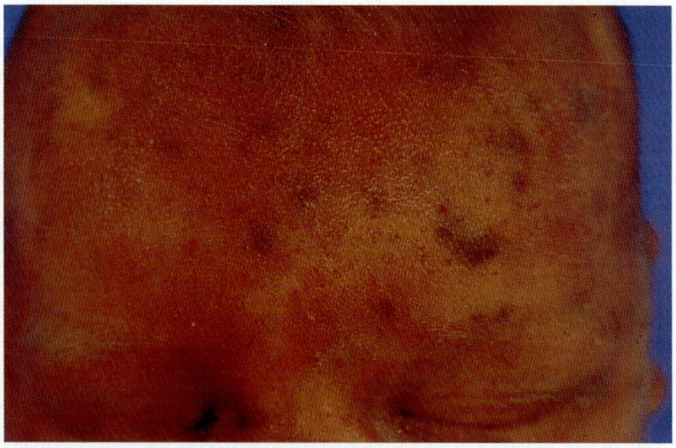

B

Figure 8–1. Newborn infant with fatal disseminated infection by CMV. (**A**) Numerous mobile cutaneous nodules involve trunk and face. (**B**) Closer view of blue-gray cutaneous nodules on forehead, which microscopically are foci of dermal erythropoiesis.

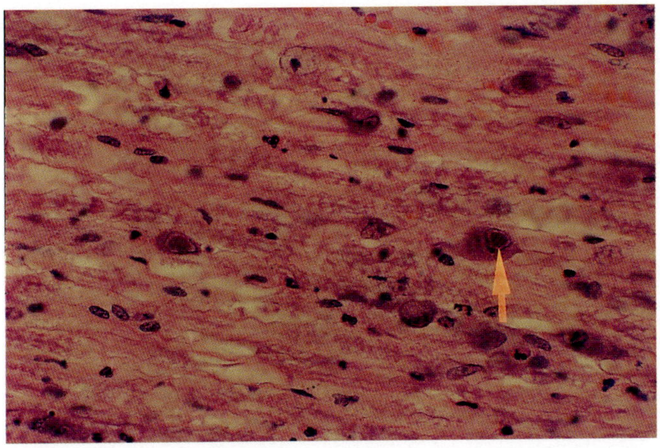

Figure 8–2. Disseminated CMV infection in an AIDS patient who had Guillain–Barré syndrome. At autopsy, there was extensive CMV neuritis involving the cauda equina. There are scattered areas of demyelination as well as conspicuous cells with typical viral cytopathic effect of CMV infection. Note intranuclear inclusion at tip of arrow (hematoxylin-eosin, ×100).

hypotension, hyponatremia, and hyperkalemia. Patients infected with human immunodeficiency virus (HIV) showed subnormal aldosterone and dehydroepiandrosterone secretions with normal cortisone production. Elevations of plasma ACTH in several patients, however, suggest that adrenal cortical capacity may become compromised when follow-up is sufficiently long.[17]

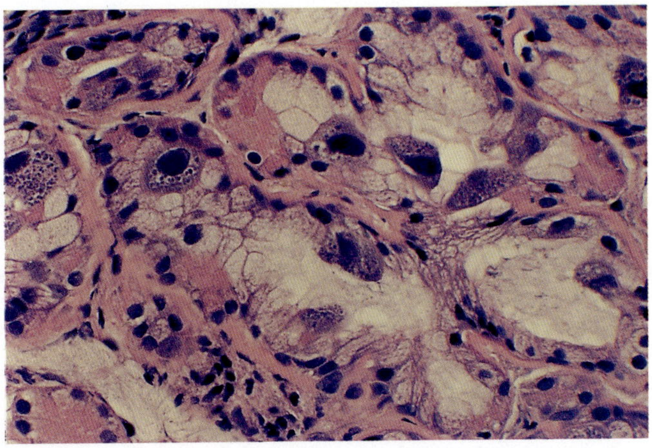

A

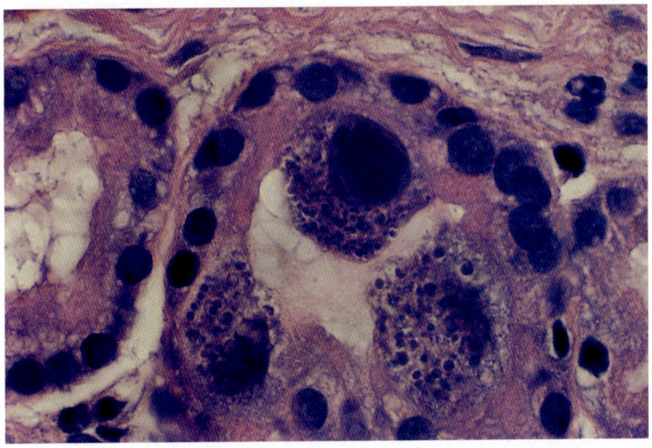

B

Figure 8–3. (**A**) Disseminated CMV infection in a young adult with AIDS. A biopsy specimen of paranasal sinus contains enlarged glandular epithelial cells with both intranuclear and intracytoplasmic inclusions characteristic of CMV (hematoxylin-eosin, ×400). (**B**) Higher magnification shows large intranuclear, deeply basophilic inclusion with smooth contours, a surrounding clear space, and margination of chromatin on the nuclear membrane. Near one pole is a small dotlike nucleolus. Other cells have multiple, granular, basophilic, intracytoplasmic inclusions (hematoxylin-eosin, ×400).

PATHOLOGY

The diagnostic hallmarks of active CMV infection include cytomegaly with both nuclear and cytoplasmic enlargement and characteristic intranuclear and intracytoplasmic inclusion bodies that are amphophilic to deeply basophilic. The single nuclear inclusion is characteristically round to oval with a smoothly contoured border. Often, the nucleolus is retained within the inclusion body. There is a clear zone or halo around the inclusion, and margination and condensation of chromatin on the inner aspect of the nuclear membrane. The cytomegalic changes may be recognized at relatively low magnification, permitting diagnosis (Figure 8–3, A). Fully developed intranuclear inclusions give little difficulty in diagnosis, but in earlier developmental stages the inclusion may be difficult to distinguish from other viral inclusions of the *Herpesviridae* family (ie, herpes simplex and VZV). The inclusion may be eosinophilic in some stages of development.[18] Configuration and size of the intranuclear inclusion also may vary depending on the plane of section. There may be a small, spherical or distorted nucleolus in or at the edge of the viral inclusion, which is often basophilic and may appear as an "accessory body" (Figure 8–3, B). Intracytoplasmic inclusions are multiple, and in early stages of development are small, basophilic, irregular, granular structures in the perinuclear area. Later, they increase in number and size (up to 3 μm) and migrate toward the cell membrane. Cytoplasmic inclusions coupled with a "megalic" change of the cytoplasm are valuable in diagnosis, even though the intranuclear inclusion may not be present in a particular plane of section as in Figure 8–3, B. The intranuclear inclusion usually has a symmetrical or asymmetrical clear halo (Fig-

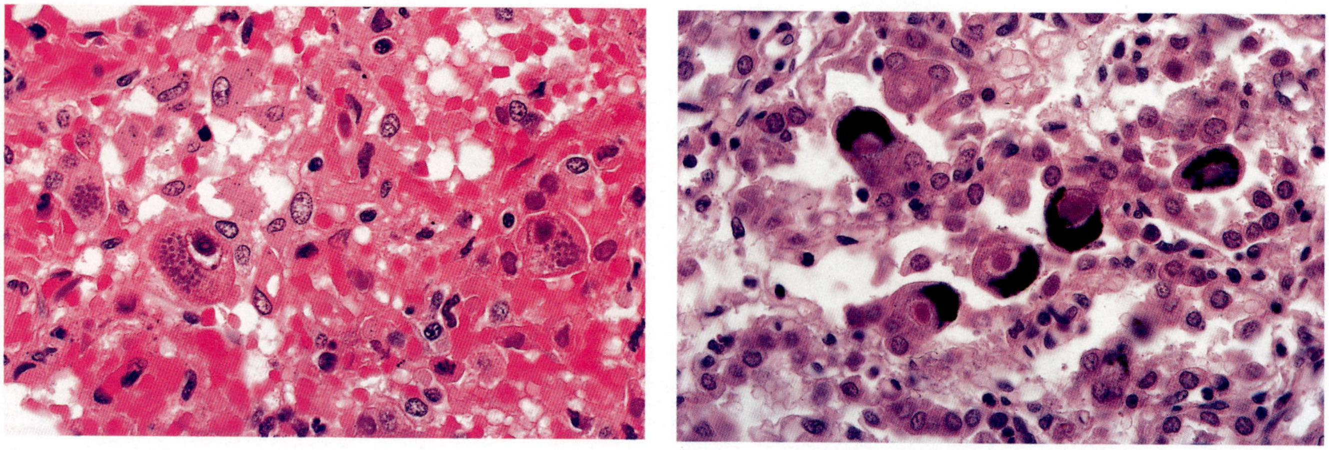

A B

Figure 8–4. (**A**) CMV pneumonitis. There is sparse mononuclear inflammation, and scattered alveolar lining cells have a characteristic viral cytopathic effect. Note prominent, granular, intracytoplasmic inclusions (hematoxylin-eosin, ×160) (**B**) CMV pneumonitis. Inclusion-bearing cells have blackened intracytoplasmic granules with silver staining. Intranuclear inclusions are not argyrophilic (Gomori's methenamine silver–hematoxylin-eosin, ×160).

ure 8–4, A). Intracytoplasmic inclusions are periodic acid–Schiff (PAS)-positive and also are vividly demonstrated as argyrophilic structures with Gomori's methanamine silver (GMS) silvering (Figure 8–4, B). Typical viral cytopathic effects can be in a variety of cells, including alveolar pneumocytes (Figure 8–4, A and B), endothelial cells (Figure 8–5, A),[19] fibroblasts, histiocytes, and exocrine and endocrine glandular epithelial cells (Figure 8–5, B). Table 8–1 summarizes the viral cytopathic effects caused by a variety of different viruses, including CMV.

After penetration of a susceptible cell by CMV, cellular function does not seem to be significantly impaired, and the cell may retain its viability despite continual shedding of virus for prolonged periods.[20] Latent infection can persist for years in the presence of a normal host immune response. Effective control requires intact cell-mediated immunity. Dominant factors influencing restriction of CMV gene expression and latency are not entirely known.[20] CMV vasculitis has been described with infection of vascular endothelium, and can lead to ischemia or necrosis with gastrointesti-

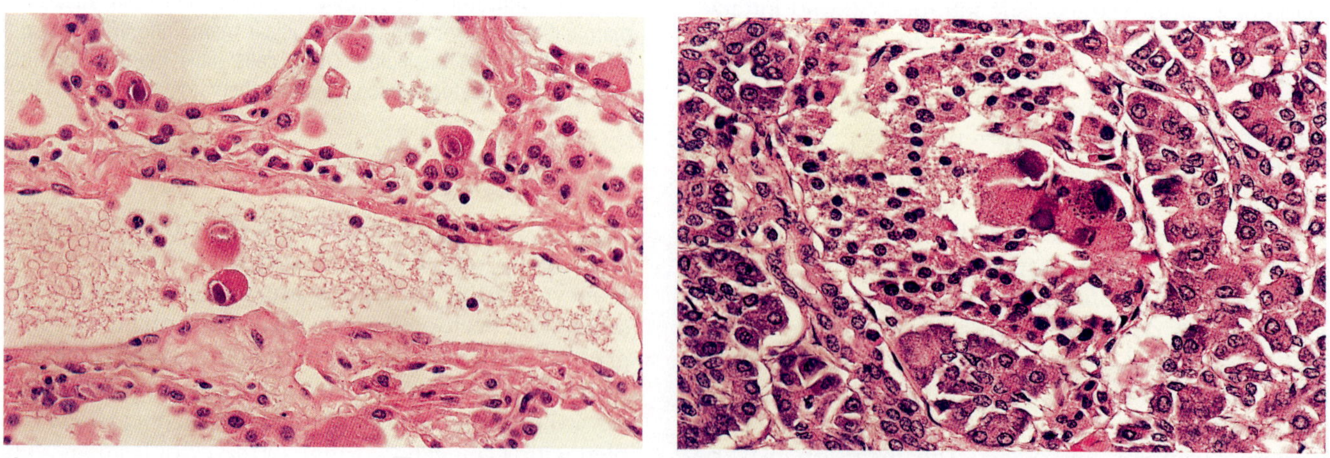

A B

Figure 8–5. (**A**) CMV pneumonitis. Several infected inclusion-bearing endothelial cells float freely in a vascular space (hematoxylin-eosin, ×100). (**B**) Disseminated CMV infection in a patient with AIDS. Typical viral cytopathic effect is seen in pancreatic islet cells (hematoxylin-eosin, ×100).

TABLE 8–1. COMPARISON OF TYPICAL CYTOPATHIC EFFECTS OF THREE HERPES-TYPE VIRUSES AND FIVE OTHER VIRUSES

Viruses	Intranuclear Inclusions (IN)	Intracytoplasmic Inclusions (IC)	Other Cytopathic Effects
Adenovirus	+	–	Early inclusions eosinophilic, finely granular, smaller, and herpes-like (Cowdry A); late inclusions deeply basophilic and larger, with nucleocytoplasmic blurring ("smudge cells")
Cytomegalovirus	+	+	Cytomegaly; nucleolus often retained; single, amphophilic IN (Cowdry A) inclusion. IC inclusions multiple, smaller, basophilic, GMS- and PAS-positive; IN inclusion formed early, IC inclusions later
Herpes simplex	+	–	Early inclusions amphophilic with "ground glass" appearance; late inclusions eosinophilic, homogeneous (Cowdy A), and surrounded by clear halo, with marginated chromatin; multinucleated syncytia (giant cells) and "molding"
Influenza	–	–	Inclusions are not produced
Measles	+	+	Multinucleated syncytia (giant cells); IN inclusions eosinophilic and herpes-like; IC inclusions pleomorphic, deeply eosinophilic, hyalinized, tallow-like
Parainfluenza	–	+[a]	Multinucleated syncytia (giant cells); IC inclusions, when present, pleomorphic, eosinophilic, and indistinct
Respiratory syncytial	–	+	Multinucleated syncytia (giant cells); multiple, discrete, smoothly contoured and deeply eosinophilic IC inclusions
Varicella-zoster	+	–	Similar to Herpes simplex

[a] Rarely observed. When present, usually seen in infections caused by types 2 and 3.

nal ulceration, pneumonitis, and cutaneous ulcers.[19] Diagnosis is possible in some patients by cytology. CMV pneumonitis, for example, has been diagnosed by examining bronchoalveolar lavage (BAL) fluid (Figure 8–6),[21] although the diagnosis of pneumocystis pneumonia by BAL is more common. This is probably because *Pneumocystis carinii* is typically intra-alveolar, whereas CMV-infected cells are attached to the alveolar lining and less apt to exfoliate during pulmonary lavage. Cytopathic effects may be in a wide range of cells in a variety of tissues and organs in the immunodeficient patient (eg, AIDS) (Figure 8–7). Identification of the virus may be difficult in early stages of development, but molecular techniques such as polymerase chain reaction (PCR) and in situ hybridization may help (Figure 8–8).

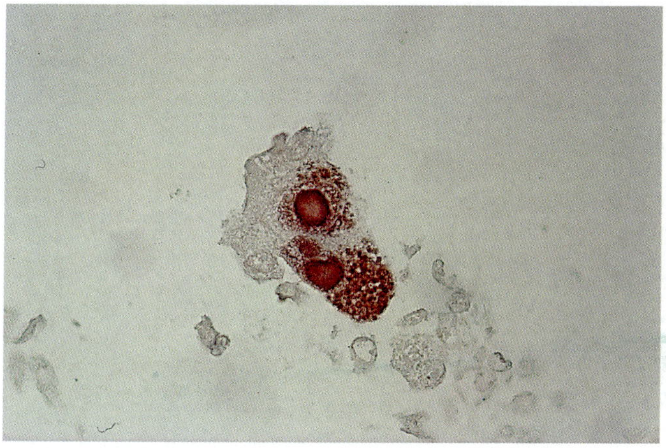

Figure 8–6. CMV pneumonitis in a patient with AIDS. In situ hybridization shows nuclear and cytoplasmic signal for CMV genome in two infected pneumocytes (×160).

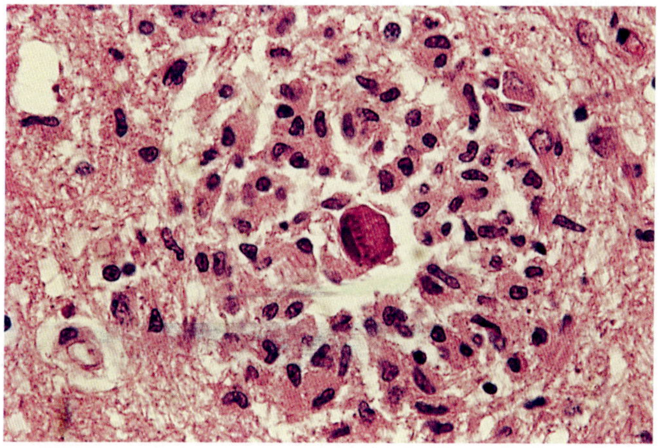

Figure 8–7. CMV encephalitis in a patient with AIDS. A CMV-infected neuron is near the center of a poorly defined aggregate of histiocytes (hematoxylin-eosin, ×100).

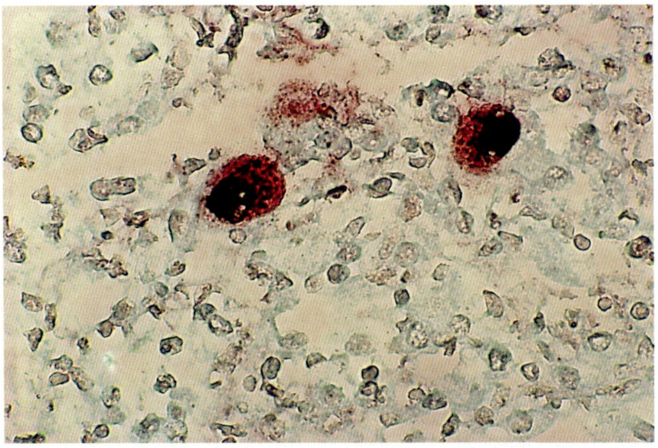

Figure 8–8. CMV pneumonitis. Two infected cells are detected by in situ hybridization (×400).

ULTRASTRUCTURAL FEATURES

The intranuclear inclusion at scanning magnification appears to be centrally placed with condensed filamentous or amorphous material separated from an intact nuclear membrane by a relatively clear zone or halo (Figure 8–9, A and B). In the cytoplasm, there may be aggregates of well-formed, mature virions with dense cores and multilayered envelopes. The virions are often numerous and appear to be free within the cytoplasm or contained within large, membrane-bound, cytoplasmic vacuoles. Complete CMV particles have a diameter of 120 to 200 nm and consist of an electron-dense core of double-stranded DNA, a capsid with icosahedral configuration, and a surrounding envelope. Viral replication occurs within the nucleus of the host cell (Figure 8–10), and a viral envelope forms as assembled nucleocapsids bud from the inner surface of the nuclear membrane or from cytoplasmic membranes.[2] The complex envelopment of CMV appears to involve successive coats derived from the nuclear membrane and from the endoplasmic reticulum or cytoplasmic vesicles.[22]

VIRAL ISOLATION IN VITRO

CMV can be detected in the cell cultures of human fibroblasts that best support growth for diagnosis.[2] The appearance and extent of cytopathogenic effect (CPE) depend on the amount of virus in the specimen; CPE may develop within 24 hours and progress rapidly to involve most of the monolayer if the viral titer is extremely high. Areas of CPE more commonly consist of enlarged, rounded, refractile cells appearing during the first week. In most laboratories, CMV isolates are identified solely on the basis of the characteristic CPE.[2] Suspected CMV can be confirmed by indirect immunofluorescence using commercially available monoclonal or polyclonal antibodies. The spin-amplification shell viral assay also can be used as a rapid method for the detection of CMV in clinical specimens and has proved to be a valuable adjunct to conventional viral isolation. It has the important features of being rapid, sensitive, and specific.[2]

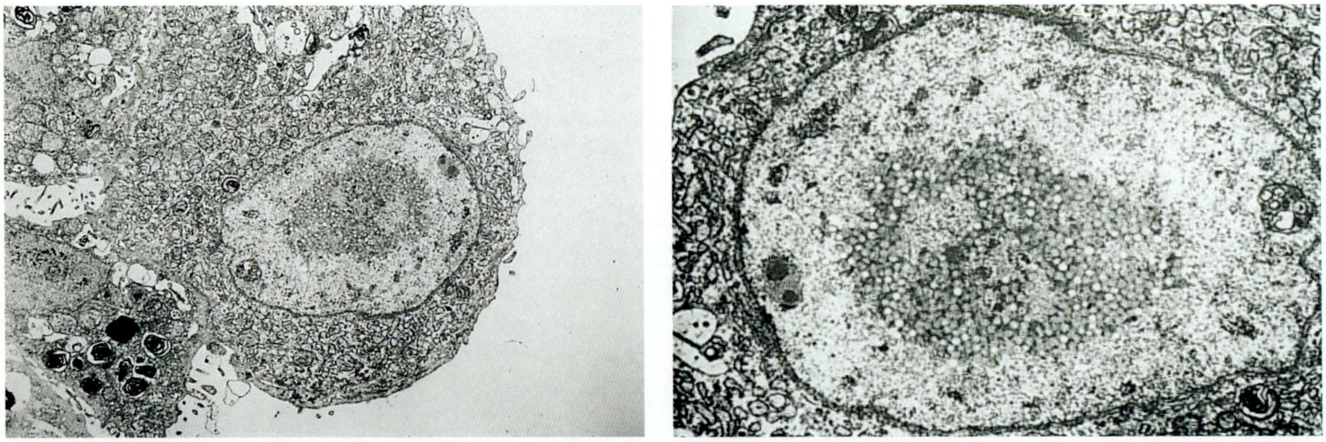

A B

Figure 8–9. (**A**) Transmission electron micrograph of CMV pneumonitis in an immunosuppressed infant. Cell is enlarged with well-defined intranuclear inclusion and peripheral clearing of nuclear chromatin (×1500). (**B**) Higher magnification of intranuclear inclusion shows numerous incomplete viral particles (uranyl acetate and lead citrate, ×10,000).

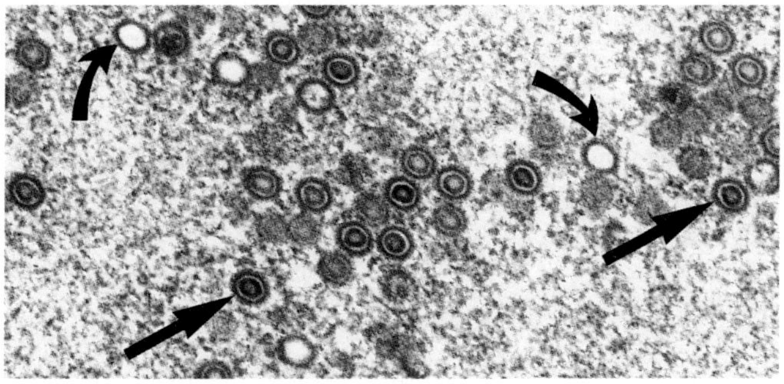

Figure 8–10. Transmission electron micrograph of intranuclear viral particles with intervening dispersed nuclear chromatin. Proviral forms (incomplete virions) consist of capsid and genetic core of viral DNA (*straight arrows*). Some capsids are empty (*curved arrows*) but most are complete. When capsids bud through the nuclear membrane, they obtain an electron-dense envelope and become complete virions, which are the infectious particles (uranyl acetate and lead citrate, ×50,000).

MODERN TECHNIQUES IN DIAGNOSIS

Because CMV can be detected by PCR assay and isolated from cultures of buffy coat cells, BAL, and other body fluids in the absence of clinical disease, direct demonstration of typical inclusion-bearing cells or of viral antigen and nucleic acid in clinical specimens is important to establish a definitive diagnosis of active CMV infection. A variety of sensitive methods is available for identifying and localizing CMV in tissue, including immunohistochemistry and in situ hybridization (Figure 8–8).[23–25] It has been the experience of the authors of this chapter that the diagnostic yield of immunohistochemistry using monoclonal antibodies to immediate early antigens is equal to or perhaps greater than that of in situ hybridization for active CMV infection. There also are a variety of serologic methods that can be used for diagnosis, including complement fixation tests, anticomplement immunofluorescence tests, a passive latex agglutination test, and enzyme immunoassays. Depending on the circumstances, seroconversion remains a reliable means for diagnosing primary infection, and screening of blood and organ donors and recipients may help prevent transmission to patients at high risk for severe disseminated infection.[2]

TREATMENT

Antiviral agents may be effective in treating severe CMV infection. Ganciclovir is a congener of acyclovir and has been used to treat and suppress serious infections. When the drug is discontinued, however, there is often progression or recurrence of disease.[26] Treatment has been associated with neutropenia (55%) and leukopenia (32%).[26] Foscarnet has a virostatic effect on CMV by inhibiting viral DNA polymerases. It has caused nephrotoxicity, but is otherwise well tolerated.[27]

OTHER HERPESVIRUSES

Human Herpesvirus Type 6

Since the late 1980s, two additional types of herpesviruses have been identified and designated HV-6 and HV-7. In 1986, HV-6 was first reported as a novel herpes B lymphotropic virus designated HBLV and was isolated from leukocytes in the peripheral blood of six patients, two of whom were seropositive for HIV.[28] Morphologically, the virus resembles other herpesviruses. A number of different strains of HV-6 have been identified, all closely related to one another, and restriction site polymorphisms within the genome can be used to differentiate isolates into two groups—HV-6A and HV-6B.[29,30] The main target cell for both strains is the T-lymphocyte.[31] HV-6 has been identified as the cause of exanthem subitum (roseola)[32] as well as an infection in infancy that resembles infectious mononucleosis.[33] Most HV-6 isolates from roseola and related febrile diseases have been HV-6B, with the exception of cultures from several patients from whom both variants were obtained.[30]

HV-6 differs from the other five herpesviruses by antigenic properties and failure to show homologous hybridization with nucleic acid sequences. Similarity of homologous sequences of base pairs in several studies has linked HV-6 most closely with human CMV.[34,35] A series of seroepidemiologic investigations suggests that infection with HV-6 is widespread in populations of apparently healthy adults and that the virus is typically acquired in early infancy. Seroconversion usually occurs between 1 and 3 years of age, with the seroprevalence ranging from 80% to 100% in adults under the age of 40, and somewhat lower levels (35%) between 62 and 88 years.[36] HV-6 can be isolated regularly from saliva, and oral shedding is probably a common means of transmission.[36]

HV-6 is associated with idiopathic pneumonitis in immunosuppressed patients following bone marrow transplantation[37]; this virus also has been associated with fatal pneumonitis in an immunodeficient infant.[38] Disseminated HV-6 infection also afflicts patients with AIDS.[39–41] Productive dual infection of human CD4+ T lymphocytes has been reported with HIV and HV-6,[42] so HV-6 might directly or indirectly deplete CD4+ T cells. It is difficult to be certain whether dissemination of HV-6 is merely an epiphenomenon of underlying immunodeficiency or indicates an active role of HV-6 in the pathogenesis of immune deficits associated with

AIDS.[39] There also are reports that HV-6 might play a role in retinitis in AIDS patients.[43] Herpes-like viral particles have been identified in cells of Kaposi's sarcoma and, using immunologic techniques, have been shown to be CMV[44]; in one patient, however, HV-6B and CMV were both identified.[45] Recent data suggest that HV-6 and CMV in AIDS-associated Kaposi's sarcoma most likely reflect disseminated viral infection, and although these viruses may be cofactors, they do not seem to be the only causative agents for the development of AIDS-associated Kaposi's sarcoma.[45] HV-6 also has been associated with chronic fatigue syndrome,[46] and more recently with multiple sclerosis (MS).[47] The association with MS is based on the expression of HV-6 antigens in the nuclei of oligodendrocytes from MS patients but not of controls. Another study reported HV-6 in oral carcinoma, suggesting that the virus acts as a cofactor with known carcinogens and could play a role on oncogenesis of oral carcinoma.[48]

Human Herpesvirus Type 7

The most recently described member of the *Herpesviridae* family is HV-7, isolated and characterized in 1990.[49] This virus has limited homology with HV-6, CMV, HSV, and VZV, with closest homology to CMV.[49,50] As with HV-6, the T lymphocyte appears to be the main target cell for this virus.[51] The role of HV-7 in human disease is largely unknown,[30] although there is evidence that HV-7 can cause exanthem subitum.[52] HV-7 has been isolated from circulating lymphocytes from an infant with a nonspecific febrile illness and no rash.[53] This virus also has been associated with chronic fatigue syndrome.[46] HV-7 has been isolated from the saliva of 75% of healthy adults, suggesting that it may be transmitted by contact with oral secretions.[30] A seroepidemiologic study by Wyatt et al concluded that primary infections with HV-7 occur later than with HV-6.[54] Current diagnostic tests for HV-7 employ a monoclonal antibody specific for HV-7, and PCR, which amplifies a DNA fragment specific for HV-7.

REFERENCES

1. Cohen JI, Corey GR. Cytomegalovirus infection in the normal host. *Medicine.* 1985;64:100–114.
2. Hodinka RL, Friedman HM. Human cytomegalovirus. In: Murray PR, Baron EJ, Pfaller MA, Tenover FC, Yolken RH, eds. *Manual of Clinical Microbiology.* 6th ed. Washington DC: AMS Press; 1995:884–894.
3. Pass RF, Little EA, Stagno S, Britt WJ, Alford CA. Young children as a probable source of maternal and congenital cytomegalovirus infection. *N Engl J Med.* 1987;316:1366–1370.
4. Jeffries DJ. The spectrum of cytomegalovirus infection and its management. *J Antimicrob Chemother.* 1989;23 (suppl E):1–10.
5. Brough AJ, Jones D, Page RH, Mizukami I. Dermal erythropoiesis in neonatal infants. A manifestation of intrauterine viral disease. *Pediatrics.* 1967;40:627–635.
6. Bigio EH, Hague AK. Disseminated cytomegalovirus infection presenting with acalculous cholecystitis and acute pancreatitis. *Arch Pathol Lab Med.* 1989;113:1287–1289.
7. Kyriazis AP, Mitra SK. Multiple cytomegalovirus-related intestinal perforations in patients with acquired immunodeficiency syndrome. Report of two cases and review of the literature. *Arch Pathol Lab Med.* 1992;116:495–499.
8. Budzilovich GN, Avitabile A, Niedt G, Aleksic SN, Rosenblum MK. Polyradiculopathy and sensory ganglionitis due to cytomegalovirus in acquired immune deficiency syndrome (AIDS). *Prog AIDS Pathol.* 1989;1:143–157.
9. Ropper AH. The Guillain–Barré syndrome. *N Engl J Med.* 1992;326:1130–1136.
10. Grinspoon SK, Bilezikian JP. HIV disease and the endocrine system. *N Engl J Med.* 1992;327:1360–1365.
11. Klatt EC, Shibata D. Cytomegalovirus infection in the acquired immunodeficiency syndrome. Clinical and autopsy findings. *Arch Pathol Lab Med.* 1988;112:540–544.
12. Glasgow BJ, Steinsapir KD, Anders K, Layfield LJ: Adrenal pathology in the acquired immune deficiency syndrome. *Am J Clin Pathol.* 1985;84:594–597.
13. Pulakhandam U, Dincsoy HP. Cytomegaloviral adrenalitis and adrenal insufficiency in AIDS. *Am J Clin Pathol.* 1990; 93:651–656.
14. Rotterdam H, Dembitzer F. The adrenal gland in AIDS. *Endocr Pathol.* 1993;4:4–14.
15. Chin B, Butany J, Kovacs K, Cheng Z. Cytomegalovirus adrenalitis in acquired immunodeficiency syndrome. *Endocr Pathol.* 1994;5:218–222.
16. Donovan DS, Dluhy RG. AIDS and its effect on the adrenal gland. *Endocrinologist.* 1991;1:227–232.
17. Findling JW, Buggy BP, Gilson IH, Brummitt CF, Bernstein BM, Raff H. Longitudinal evaluation of adrenocortical function in patients infected with the human immunodeficiency virus. *J Clin Endocrinol Metab.* 1994;79:1091–1096.
18. Strano AJ. Light microscopy of selected viral diseases (morphology of viral inclusion bodies). *Pathol Annu.* 1976;11:53–75.
19. Golden MP, Hammer SM, Wanke CA, Albrecht MA. Cytomegalovirus vasculitis. Case reports and review of the literature. *Medicine.* 1994;73:246–255.
20. Mocarski ES, Stinski MF. Persistence of the cytomegalovirus genome in human cells. *J Virol.* 1979;31:761–775.
21. Weiss RL, Snow GW, Schumann GE, Hammond ME. Diagnosis of cytomegalovirus pneumonitis on bronchoalveolar lavage fluid: comparison of cytology, immunofluorescence, and in-situ hybridization with viral isolation. *Diagn Cytopathol.* 1990;7:243–247.
22. Kasnic G Jr, Sayied A, Azar HA. Nuclear and cytoplasmic inclusions in disseminated cytomegalovirus infection. *Ultrastr Pathol.* 1982;3:229–235.
23. Jiwa M, Steinbergen RDM, Zwaan FE, Kluin PM, Raap AK, van der Ploeg M. Three sensitive methods for detection of

cytomegalovirus in lung tissue of patients with interstitial pneumonitis. *Am J Clin Pathol.* 1990;93:491–494.

24. Arbustini E, Grasso M, Diegoli M, et al. Histopathologic and molecular profile of human cytomegalovirus infections in patients with heart transplants. *Am J Clin Pathol.* 1992;98:205–213.
25. Nakamura Y, Sakuma S, Ohta Y, Kawano K, Hashimoto T. Detection of the human cytomegalovirus gene in placental chronic villitis by polymerase chain reaction. *Hum Pathol.* 1994;25:815–818.
26. Laskin OL, Cederberg DM, Mills J, Eror LJ, Mildvan D, Spector SA. Ganciclovir for the treatment and suppression of serious infections caused by cytomegalovirus. *Am J Med.* 1987;83:201–207.
27. Aschau J, Ringdén O, Ljungman P, Lönnqvist B, Ohlman S. Foscarnet for treatment of cytomegalovirus infections in bone marrow transplant recipients. *Scand J Infect Dis.* 1992;24:143–150.
28. Salahuddin SZ, Ablashi DV, Markham PD, et al. Isolation of a new virus, HBLV, in patients with lymphoproliferative disorders. *Science.* 1986;234:596–601.
29. Aubin J–T, Collandre H, Candotti D, et al. Several groups among human herpesvirus 6 strains can be distinguished by Southern blotting and polymerase chain reaction. *J Clin Microbiol.* 1991;29:367–372.
30. Stewart JA, Patton JL. Human herpesvirus 6 and other herpesviruses. In: Murray R, Baron EJ, Pfaller MA, Tenover FC, Yolken RH, eds. *Manual of Clinical Microbiology.* 6th ed. Washington, DC: AMS Press; 1995:911–917.
31. Steeper TA, Horwitz CA, Ablashi DV, et al. The spectrum of clinical and laboratory findings resulting from human herpesvirus-6 (HHV-6) in patients with mononucleosis-like illnesses not resulting from Epstein–Barr virus or cytomegalovirus. *Am J Clin Pathol.* 1990;93:776–783.
32. Yamanishi K, Okuno I, Shiraki K, et al. Identification of human herpesvirus-6 as a causal agent for exanthem subitum. *Lancet.* 1988;1:1065–1067.
33. Hanukoglu A, Somekh E. Infectious mononucleosis-like illness in an infant with acute herpesvirus 6 infection. *Pediatr Infect Dis J.* 1994;13:750–751.
34. Lawrence GL, Chee M, Craxton MA, Gompels UA, Honess RW, Barrell BG. Human herpesvirus 6 is closely related to human cytomegalovirus. *J Virol.* 1990;64:287–299.
35. Gompels UA, Nicholas J, Lawrence G, et al. The DNA sequence of human herpesvirus-6: structure, coding content, and genome evolution. *Virology.* 1995;209:29–51.
36. Levy JA, Greenspan D, Ferro F, Lennette ET. Frequent isolation of HHV-6 from saliva and high seroprevalence of the virus in the population. *Lancet.* 1990;335:1047–1050.
37. Cone RW, Hackman RC, Huang MLW, et al. Human herpesvirus 6 in lung tissue from patients with pneumonitis after bone marrow transplantation. *N Engl J Med.* 1993;329:156–161.
38. Knox KK, Pietryga D, Harrington DJ, Franciosi R, Carrigan DR. Progressive immunodeficiency and fatal pneumonitis associated with human herpesvirus 6 infection in an infant. *Clin Infect Dis.* 1995;20:406–413.
39. Corbellino M, Lusso P, Gallo RC, Porravicini C, Galli M, Moroni M. Disseminated human herpesvirus 6 infection in AIDS. *Lancet.* 1993;342:1242. Letter.
40. Knox KK, Carrigan DR. Disseminated active HHV-6 infection in patients with AIDS. *Lancet.* 1994:343:577–578.
41. Knox KK, Harrington DP, Carrigan DR. Fulminant human herpesvirus six encephalitis in a human immunodeficiency virus-infected infant. *J Med Virol.* 1995;45:288–292.
42. Lusso P, Ensoli B, Markham PD, et al. Productive dual infection in human CD4+ T lymphocytes by HIV-1 and HHV-6. *Nature.* 1989;337:370–373.
43. Qavi HB, Green MT, Pearson G, Ablashi D. Possible role of HHV-6 in the development of AIDS retinitis. *In Vivo.* 1994;8:527–532.
44. Ioachim HL, Dorsett B, Melamed J, Adsay V, Santagada EA. Cytomegalovirus, angiomatosis, and Kaposi's sarcoma: new observations of a debated relationship. *Mod Pathol.* 1992;5:169–178.
45. Kempf W, Adams V, Pfaltz M, et al. Human herpesvirus type 6 and cytomegalovirus in AIDS-associated Kaposi's sarcoma. No evidence for an etiological association. *Hum Pathol.* 1995;26:914–919.
46. Di Luca D, Zorzenon M, Miraudola P, Colle R, Botta GA, Cassai E. Human herpesvirus 6 and human herpesvirus 7 in chronic fatigue syndrome. *J Clin Microbiol.* 1995;33: 1660–1661.
47. Challoner PB, Smith KT, Parker JD, et al. Plaque-associated expression of human herpesvirus 6 in multiple sclerosis. *Proc Natl Acad Sci USA.* 1995;92:7440–7444.
48. Yadav M, Chandrashekran A, Vasudevan DM, Ablashi DV. Frequent detection of human herpesvirus 6 in oral carcinoma. *J Natl Cancer Inst.* 1994;86:1792–1794.
49. Frenkel N, Shirmer EC, Wyatt LS, et al. Isolation of a new herpesvirus from human CD4+ T cells. *Proc Natl Acad Sci USA.* 1990;87:748–752.
50. Berneman ZN, Ablashi DV, Li G, et al. Human herpesvirus 7 is a lymphotropic virus and is related to but significantly different from human herpesvirus 6 and human cytomegalovirus. *Proc Natl Acad Sci USA.* 1992;89:10552–10556.
51. Ablashi DV, Berneman ZN, Kramarsky B, Whitman J Jr, Asano Y, Pearson GR. Human herpesvirus-7 (HHV-7): current status. *Clin Diagn Virol.* 1995;4:1–13.
52. Ueda K, Miyazaki C, Okada K, et al. Human herpesvirus-6 (HHV-6): clinical and epidemiologic aspects of exanthem subitum. *Proc First Intl Herpesvirus Symp.*, Japan, Osaka, 1992, p. 18.
53. Partolani M, Cermelli C, Miraudola P, Di Luca D. Isolation of human herpesvirus 7 from an infant with febrile syndrome. *J Med Virol.* 1995;45:282–283.
54. Wyatt LS, Rodriguez WJ, Balachandran N, Frenkel N. Human herpesvirus-7: antigenic properties and prevalence in children and adults. *J Virol.* 1991;65:6260–6265.

CHAPTER 9

Echovirus Infection

Ernest E. Lack and David L. Gang

. . . the whole head is sick, and the whole heart faint.

Isaiah 1:5

The diseases which occur most frequently in rainy seasons are protracted fevers, fluxes of the bowels, mortifications, epilepsies, apoplexies, and quinsies; and in dry consumptive diseases, stranguries, and dysenteries.

Hippocrates (460–377 B.C.)

DEFINITION

Echovirus (enteric cytopathogenic human orphan virus) is an enterovirus in the family *Picornaviridae,* and is subdivided into 31 different serotypes. Among the different serotypes, echovirus 11 is most frequently associated with serious neonatal disease.

INTRODUCTION

The family *Picornaviridae* has been divided into five genera: aphtho-, cardio-, entero-, hepato-, and rhinoviruses based on physiochemical properties, pathogenicity, and also molecular characteristics.[1] The term *picorna* derives from *pico* ("very small") and RNA, which refers to the single-stranded nucleic acid component of the viruses. The echoviruses include 31 serotypes: 1 to 7, 9, 11 to 27, and 29 to 34. Echovirus 8 was deleted because it cross-reacts with echovirus 1: echovirus 10 was reclassified as reovirus type 1; and echovirus 28 was reclassified as rhinovirus type 1A.[2] The other enteroviruses include coxsackieviruses types A and B, polioviruses, and other enterovirus types. Some believe echoviruses 22 and 23 are closely related members of a distinct picornavirus group using nucleotide sequencing and hybridization analysis.[1,3]

EPIDEMIOLOGY

From 1970 through 1979 in the United States, 18,309 enteroviral agents were isolated from 18,152 patients, with 26% being under the age of 1 year and 56% under age 10 years.[4] The human alimentary tract is the natural habitat for these viruses. Overall, echoviruses were the most common enteroviral agents isolated (58%), with serotypes 9, 11, 4, 6, 7, and 3 in order of frequency.[4] Echovirus infections have a seasonal distribution, occurring most often in summer and early fall. Infection is usually asymptomatic, although in the neonatal age group it may cause serious and sometimes fatal disease. Transmission to the fetus may follow acute maternal infection in the last 1 or 2 weeks of pregnancy. The prevalence of echovirus infection among women of childbearing age or parturient women during community outbreaks has been estimated at 3% to 4%.[5,6] The virus can be isolated from oropharyngeal secretions, feces, vaginal secretions, and blood, and there is ample opportunity for exposure of the newborn before, during, and after parturition.

Variability in nucleotide sequence of the 5′ nontranslated regions (NTRs) of the viral genome can be utilized to rapidly identify enteroviral strains associated with particular outbreaks and distinguish them from other strains and serotypes. Identification of virus at the level of serotype is useful in epidemiologic investigation.[7] The epidemiologic features of infection by echovirus 22 differ from those of other enteroviruses. These differences include an association with diarrhea and respiratory disease in infants, more frequent predilection for children under the age of 1 year, and slightly different seasonal distribution. This has reinforced the view that echoviruses 22 and 23 may be distinct from the other major subgroup of echoviruses.[1,3,8] Echoviruses may be transmitted by direct contact with discharges from nose and throat or fecal material, including feces from pregnant women, newborn infants, and medical or paramedical contacts. Outbreaks of echovirus infection can occur in newborns in obstetrical wards or in nurseries, and the virus may spread through contaminated hands of staff members.[9] Activities strongly associated with nosocomial transmission include mouth care and gavage feedings. Infants at highest risk for secondary viral infection are those requiring the most intensive level of care and attention by nursing personnel.[6] As noted previously, echoviruses from a maternal infection may cross the placenta and infect the fetus.[5,6,9]

CLINICAL FEATURES

The incubation period for echovirus infection is usually 3 to 5 days with a range of 2 to 15 days. Signs and symptoms in the adult patient that suggest enteroviral infection include fever, myalgia, stiff neck, headache, cutaneous rash, and vesicular eruption on mucous membranes. Severe and fatal infections have been reported almost exclusively in newborns and young children, although severe infections have occasionally been seen in adults.[10] Echovirus infection is a common cause of viral encephalitis and meningitis in infants.[4] Hepatitis is frequently present in severe infections (Table 9–1). Echovirus occasionally causes paralysis and myocarditis, and infection in utero has rarely caused intrauterine death.[11] Other unusual manifestations of echovirus infection include orchitis, postviral fatigue syndrome,[12] and transient erythroblastopenia of childhood.[13] Although infection of the central nervous system is usually self-limited, there may be occasional neurologic sequelae, including porencephaly.[14] Serotypes of echovirus vary in their propensity for causing meningitis and encephalitis, ie, neurovirulence. The 5′ NTRs

TABLE 9–1. SUMMARY OF CLINICAL DATA IN FIVE FATAL NEONATAL ECHOVIRUS INFECTIONS

	Gestational Age (weeks)/Sex	Maternal History	Mode of Delivery	Onset of Illness (days)
Case 1	36/F	Fever, acute abdominal pain (1 day PTD)	Cesarean section	5
Case 2	39/F	Fever, abdominal cramps, diarrhea, rash (1 day PTD)	Vaginal	5
Case 3	33/M	Asymptomatic	Vaginal	6
Case 4	34/F	Fever, acute abdominal pain (1 day PTD)	Cesarean section	4
Case 5	35/M	Fever, abdominal pain, chills, (5 days PTD)	Vaginal	5

	Symptoms and Signs	Physical Findings	Course	Age at Death (days)
Case 1	Tachypnea, lethargy, respiratory distress	Hepatosplenomegaly, petechiae, jaundice	Hepatic failure, seizures, clinical sepsis, DIC	11
Case 2	Lethargy, poor feeding, acute cyanosis	Hepatomegaly, ascites	Clinical sepsis, DIC, renal failure, massive pulmonary hemorrhage	12
Case 3	Respiratory distress	Hepatomegaly, ascites	Repeated apnea, bradycardia, hypotension, clinical sepsis, DIC	12
Case 4	Lethargy, poor feeding	Hepatosplenomegaly, jaundice	Hepatic failure, renal failure, DIC	25
Case 5	Lethargy, poor feeding, fever	Hepatomegaly, jaundice	Hepatic failure, renal failure, DIC, ventricular hemorrhage	8

Abbreviations: PTD, prior to delivery; DIC, disseminated intravascular coagulation.

TABLE 9–2. SUMMARY OF POSTMORTEM FINDINGS IN FIVE FATAL ECHOVIRUS INFECTIONS

	Liver	Adrenal Glands	Kidneys	Heart	CNS	Lungs	Other
Case 1	Massive hemorrhagic necrosis	Massive hemorrhagic necrosis, calcification	Massive interstitial hemorrhage, acute tubular necrosis	Focal myocardial necrosis	Negative (examination limited to occipital lobe)	Massive intra-alveolar hemorrhage	Massive retroperitoneal hematoma
Case 2	Massive hemorrhagic necrosis with focal calcification	Massive hemorrhagic necrosis, calcification	Acute tubular necrosis	Massive myocarditis with myocardial necrosis and calcification	Essentially negative	Massive intra-alveolar hemorrhage	Massive retroperitoneal hematoma
Case 3	Massive hemorrhagic necrosis, mild diffuse acute and chronic inflammation	Hemorrhagic necrosis	Subcalyceal hemorrhage, fibrin thrombi in glomeruli	Fibrin deposition in small vessels, focal calcification	Cerebral hemorrhage	Focal pneumonitis, fibrin thrombi in small vessels	Fibrin thrombi in small vessels of various organs, retroperitoneal hemorrhage
Case 4	Necrosis, periportal fibrosis, chronic inflammation, bile duct proliferation, bile stasis	Small foci of necrosis, involution	Acute tubular necrosis	No lesions	No lesions	No lesions	—
Case 5	Massive hemorrhagic necrosis	Massive hemorrhagic necrosis	Marked papillary hemorrhage and necrosis	Mild myocarditis, focal hemorrhage	Subependymal and white matter necrosis	Fibrin thrombi in small vessels, patchy pneumonia	—

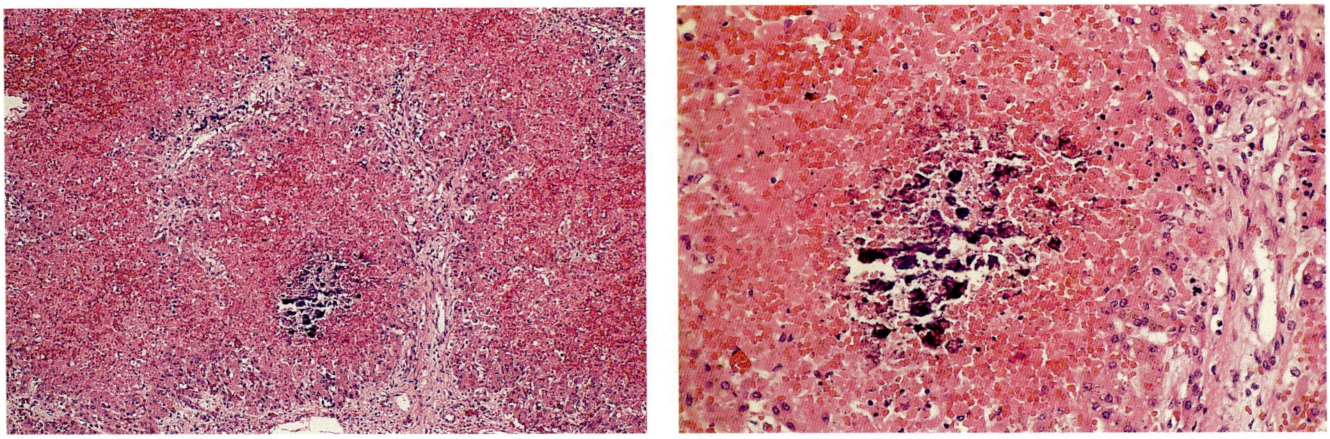

A B

Figure 9–1. Fatal neonatal echovirus 11 infection. (**A**) Hemorrhagic necrosis of hepatic parenchyma involving central and midzones (hematoxylin-eosin, ×100). (**B**) Confluent hemorrhagic necrosis of liver with dystrophic calcification. Note few intact hepatocytes adjacent to portal space (hematoxylin-eosin, ×200).

contain genomic factors necessary for replication, translation, and determinants of virulence. Echoviruses 4, 6, 9, 11, and 30 are neurovirulent and have been shown to be identical to the poliovirus in 18SrRNA binding sequence and the flanking conserved sequences, whereas less neurovirulent echoviruses showed variations in these regions.[15]

PATHOLOGY

Although neonatal and infantile echovirus infections are usually mild and self-limited, sporadic or epidemic outbreaks of severe illness can occur accompanied by occasional fatal outcome. In a study of five fatal infections of echovirus 11 in the Boston area in 1979, the postmortem findings were remarkably similar in all infants (Table 9–2).[16] The liver was severely damaged in all but one patient, with enlargement, red discoloration, and massive hemorrhagic necrosis of central and midlobular zones with relative sparing of periportal hepatocytes (Figure 9–1, A and B). In most patients, there was little if any cellular reaction. One child who survived for 25 days had periportal fibrosis with interlobular bridging necrosis, chronic inflammation, proliferation of the bile ducts, and bile stasis. Adrenal glands were hemorrhagic and resembled those of the Waterhouse–Friderichsen syndrome (Figure 9–2). Histologically, the adrenal glands had extensive areas of cortical necrosis with deposition of fibrin and cellular debris (Figure 9–3, A and B). Focal dystrophic calcification was noted in two autopsies. Two infants had myocarditis with small foci of myocardial calcifications (Figure 9–4). Small fibrin thrombi were in multiple organs, particularly liver and adrenal glands. No viral inclusions were recognized in any of the tissues examined by light microscopy. Ultrastructural study of liver in two autopsies revealed a few virus-like particles.

It is apparent that echovirus can infect a variety of cell types in different organs, and can lead to a wide variety of signs and symptoms. With regard to viral pathogenesis at the cellular level, several studies have identified receptor sites for attachment of echovirus to susceptible cells.[17–20] The integrin VLA-2 is a receptor

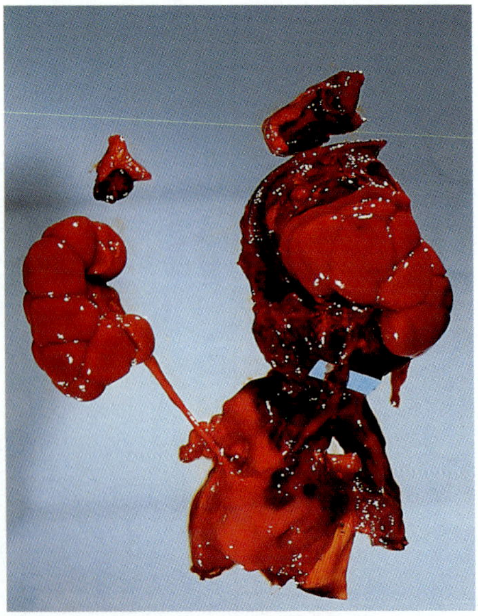

Figure 9–2. Fatal neonatal echovirus 11 infection in a 39-week-old infant. There is massive hemorrhage in both adrenal glands as well as a retroperitoneal hematoma. There was laboratory evidence of disseminated intravascular coagulation (DIC).

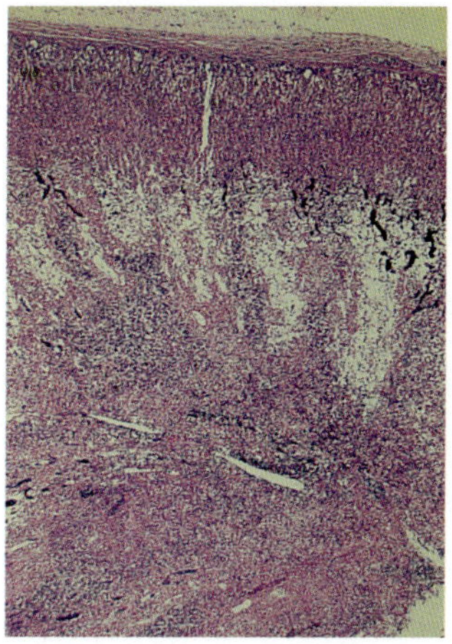

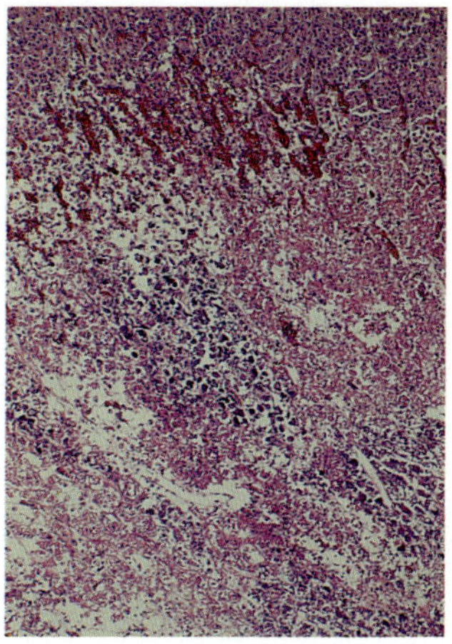

A B

Figure 9–3. Adrenal gland from an infant with fatal echovirus 11 infection and DIC. (**A**) There is extensive hemorrhagic necrosis of fetal cortex. Note serpiginous areas of dystrophic calcification (hematoxylin-eosin, ×40). (**B**) Extensive hemorrhagic necrosis of fetal cortex with spotty dystrophic calcification (hematoxylin-eosin, ×100).

for echovirus type 1. Integrins are adhesion receptors important in interactions between cells and extracellular matrix, and can mediate virus attachment, thus facilitating infection.[19] The α2 subunit of VLA-2 appears to be critical for infection by echoviruses 1 and 8, but other echovirus serotypes probably bind to other receptors.

DIAGNOSIS

Echovirus can be isolated in vitro and the differential susceptibility of various cell cultures has been used for presumptive grouping of viruses as well as polioviruses and coxsackieviruses A and B.[2] Common specimens for isolation are stool or rectal swab, throat swab, and cerebrospinal fluid. Echovirus induces distinctive or extensive cytopathic effect (CPE) in kidney cell lines of rhesus monkeys and also in RD cells (cell line from a human carcinoma). Certain strains of echovirus 11 induce extensive CPE in human kidney cell culture within a few hours of inoculation.[2] Final identification of a virus serotype within a group can be done by a neutralizing test using type-specific antiserum or immunofluorescence with available monoclonal antibodies. These procedures may be costly and time consuming, and may not be sufficiently sensitive. Polymerase chain reaction has been used also to detect and differentiate viruses in clinical specimens. The variability of nucleotide sequence in the 5′ NTRs can also be used to rapidly identify enteroviral strains at the serotype level. The diagnosis can also be made serologically on paired acute and convalescent sera, looking for a significant increase in antibody titer. Ultrastructural examination is seldom required for diagnosis. The virus is a small, 25- to 30-nm structure with icosahedral symmetry, 32 capsomeres, and a core of single-stranded RNA genome.

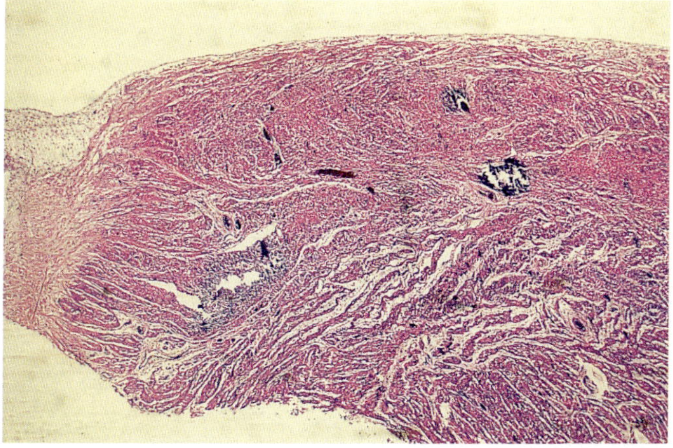

Figure 9–4. Fatal echovirus 11 infection. Small foci of myocardial necrosis with dystrophic calcification (hematoxylin-eosin, ×40).

TREATMENT

Treatment of patients with signs or symptoms of echovirus infection is usually supportive. In nurseries, rigorous handwashing is recommended to avoid outbreaks of infection by echovirus. An outbreak may dictate isolation and closure of a unit to new admissions. It has been shown that mothers of infants who subsequently developed severe echovirus disease had became ill during the last 5 days of pregnancy followed by raised specific maternal IgG antibodies. Maternal infection more than 5 to 7 days before delivery may induce maternal IgG antibodies that are transferred to and protect the fetus. Delivery should be delayed for 5 to 7 days in a woman in late pregnancy with signs or symptoms of enteroviral infection. Patients with echovirus infections have been treated with intravenous immunoglobulin, but a controlled trial for prevention of nosocomial transmission is needed to prove efficacy.[6] An infant with disseminated echovirus 11 infection was recently treated successfully by transfusion of maternal plasma.[21]

REFERENCES

1. Stanway G, Kalkkinen N, Roivainen M, et al. Molecular and biological characteristics of echovirus 22, a representative of a new picornavirus group. *J Virol.* 1994;68: 8232–8238.

2. Hsiung GD. Picornaviridae. In: Hsiung GD, Fang CKY, Landry ML, eds. *Hsiung's Diagnostic Virology.* 4th ed. New Haven: Yale University Press; 1994.
3. Auvinen P, Hyypiä T. Echoviruses include genetically distinct serotypes. *J Gen Virol.* 1990;71:2133–2139.
4. Moore M. Enteroviral disease in the United States, 1970–1979. *J Infect Dis.* 1982;146:103–108.
5. Modlin JF, Polk BF, Horton P, Etkind P, Crane E, Spiliotes A. Perinatal echovirus infection: risk of transmission during a community outbreak. *N Engl J Med.* 1981;305: 368–371.
6. Modlin JF. Echovirus infections of newborn infants. *Pediatr Infect Dis J.* 1988;7:311–312.
7. Drebot MA, Nguan CY, Campbell JJ, Lee SHS, Forward KR. Molecular epidemiology of enterovirus outbreaks in Canada during 1991–1992. Identification of echovirus 30 and Coxsackievirus B1 strains by amplicon sequencing. *J Med Virol.* 1994;44:340–347.
8. Ehrnst A, Eriksson M. Epidemiological features of type 22 echovirus infection. *Scand J Infect Dis.* 1993;25:275–281.
9. Magnius L, Sterner G, Enocksson E. Infections with echoviruses and coxsackieviruses in late pregnancy. *Scand J Infect Dis.* 1990;71(suppl):53–57.
10. Venkatoramani A, Zabaneh RI, Spech TJ, Gonzalez WR. Septic shock in an elderly patient: unusual presentation of echovirus infection. *South Med J.* 1993;86:1166–1167.
11. Johansson ME, Holmström S, Abebe A, et al. Intrauterine fetal death due to echovirus 11. *Scand J Infect Dis.* 1992; 24:381–385.
12. Steer RG. Echovirus 11 orchitis and postviral fatigue syndrome. *Med J Aust.* 1992;156:816. Letter.
13. Elian JC, Frappaz D, Pozzetto B, Freycon F. Transient erythroblastopenia of childhood presenting with echovirus 11 infection. *Acta Pediatr.* 1993;82:492–494.
14. Arron R, Naor N, Davidson S, Katz K, Mor C. Fatal outcome of neonatal echovirus 19 infection. *Pediatr Infect Dis J.* 1991;10:788–789.
15. Romero JR, Rotbart HA. Sequence analysis of the downstream 5′ nontranslated region of seven echoviruses with different neurovirulence phenotypes. *J Virol.* 1995;69: 1370–1375.
16. Mostoufizadeh M, Lack EE, Gang DC, Perez-Atayde AR, Driscoll SG. Postmortem manifestations of echovirus 11 sepsis in five newborn infants. *Hum Pathol.* 1983; 14:818–823.
17. Mbida AD, Gaudin OG, Sabido O, Pozzetto B, Le Bihan J-C. Monoclonal antibody specific for the cellular receptor of echoviruses. *Intervirology.* 1992;33:17–22.
18. Mbida AD, Pozzetto B, Gaudin OG, et al. A 44,000 glycoprotein is involved in the attachment of echovirus-11 onto susceptible cells. *Virology.* 1992;189:350–353.
19. Bergelson JM, Shepley MP, Chan BMC, Hemler ME, Finberg RW. Identification of the integrin VLA-2 as a receptor for echovirus 1. *Science.* 1992;225:1718–1720.
20. Bergelson JM, St. John N, Kawaguchi S, et al. Infection by echoviruses 1 and 8 depends on the α2 subunit of human VLA-2. *J Virol.* 1993;67:6847–6852.
21. Jantauseh BA, Luban NLC, Duffy L, Rodriguez WJ. Maternal plasma transfusion in the treatment of disseminated neonatal echovirus 11 infection. *Pediatr Infect Dis J.* 1995;14:154–155.

CHAPTER 10

Encephalomyocarditis Virus

Masazumi Adachi

It is the same thing which makes us mad or delirious, inspires us with dread or fear, whether by night or by day, brings sleeplessness, inopportune mistakes, aimless anxieties, absent-mindedness, and acts that are contrary to habit. These things that we suffer all come from the brain, where it is not healthy, but becomes abnormally hot, cold, moist, or dry.

Hippocrates (460–377? B.C.) The Sacred Disease, Section XVII (trans. W.H.S. Jones)

INTRODUCTION

Encephalomyocarditis (EMC) virus is in the family of picornaviruses and the genus of cardioviruses. The members of the genus include mengovirus, Maus Elberfeld (ME) virus, and Columbia SK virus. Several variants of the EMC virus have been reported (Table 10–1).[1–6] The A variant was obtained by serial passages of the wild strain [VR129, American Type Culture Collection (ATCC)] through the human astrocytoma (HTB-14) growing in nude rats.[1] The variants B (nondiabetogenic) and D (diabetogenic) were separated from the M variant.[2] The E (encephalotropic) and M (myocardiotropic) variants were selected from a naturally infected domestic pig (II38).[3] The variant F was originally isolated in Florida,[3] and the K variant was separated from the variant B and was lethal to mice at a very much lower dose (one plaque-forming unit).[4] The L variant, derived from the F variant, had been transmitted repeatedly in cultures of L cells.[3] The variant MM, originating from mouse brain,[4] is a good inducer of interferon (IFN), whereas the variant K induces little or no production of IFN.[4] The II38 variant was isolated from a domestic pig during an EMC virus outbreak in Panama.[5] The variant 221A is myotropic and produces myositis resembling polymyositis.[6] The EMC viruses are fatal to mice[7,8] and also to hamsters, cotton rats, guinea pigs, and pigs, whereas they produce only transient febrile reactions in rabbits and white rats.[7] Only rare cases of human infection with the virus have been reported.[9–13] The presence of neutralizing antibody titers to this virus in sera has been observed in 3% to 16% of the general population.[14,15]

PHYSICAL, CHEMICAL, AND BIOLOGICAL PROPERTIES

The virion of the EMC virus is 27 to 30 nm in diameter and consists of a capsid shell of 60 subunits, each of four proteins (VP1–VP4) arranged with icosahedral symmetry around a genome made up of single-strand RNA.[16] The molecular weights of these proteins range from 7 to 31 kd,[17,18] comparable to some picornaviral proteins (Table 10–2).[17,19–21] The virions are nonenveloped and are ether resistant. RNA replication involves the synthesis of a complementary RNA, which serves as a template for genomic RNA synthesis. The genomic RNA also serves as messenger RNA (mRNA), being translated into a polyprotein that is cleaved into all the viral proteins, including those proteins that serve as enzymes for specific cleavages. Replication and assembly take place in the cytoplasm, and the virus is released during cytolysis.

High-resolution three-dimensional x-ray crystallography suggests that the outer surfaces of the virus are formed of prominent protrusions surrounded by sub-

TABLE 10–1. VARIANTS OF ENCEPHALOMYOCARDITIS VIRUS

Variants	Ref.	Sources	Selections	Features
A	1	Wild (VR129: ATCC) strain	Serial passages through human astrocytoma	Oncolytic to astrocytoma cells
B	2	Variant M	Glucose tolerance tests	Nondiabetogenic
D	2	Variant M	Glucose tolerance tests	Diabetogenic
E	3	II38	Serial passages through mice brain	Neurotropic
F	3	Wild strain from mice in Florida	Original isolation	Natural infection in mice
K	4	Variant B	Glucose tolerance tests	Highly lethargic to mice
L	3	Variant F	Serial passages through L cells	Natural infection in mice
M	3	II38	Serial passages through mice hearts	Myocardiotropic
MM	4	Wild strain from mice	Original isolation	Natural infection in mice
II38	5	Wild strain from pigs in Panama	Original isolation	Natural infection in pigs
221A	6	Wild strain from mice	Original isolation	Natural infection in mice

surface depressions distributed around each icosahedral five axis of symmetry. These depressions, referred to as *pits* (cardiovirus), *canyons* (rhinovirus), or *valleys* (enterovirus), may function as the virus–cell attachment zones.[22] The virus agglutinates erythrocytes, which have glycophorin and show the major sialoglycoprotein in the surface membrane, serve as a viral receptor.[23]

LABORATORY DIAGNOSIS

Histologic studies are important in identifying involvement of tissues and in investigating the extent of infection in the body. The E variant shows major infection sites in the hippocampus and basal ganglia of mice (Figure 10–1).[7] Electron microscopic investigations show, in the infected cytoplasm, electron-dense viral particles arranged in parallel rows and crystalloids in tissues[7,8] and cultured cells (Figure 10–2).[24] Rapid determination of neutralizing antibodies can be made in cultured cell monolayers by inhibition of cytopathic effect by specific antibodies UM 21.1 (immunoglobulin G2B) and UM 21.2 (immunoglobulin G3) Figure 10–3).[25] The isolation of the EMC virus from fetal tissues and organs is performed on 10% homogenates of tissues prepared in 0.01 mol/L phosphate buffered saline (pH 7.4).[26] Aliquots (0.5 mL) of supernatant fluid are inoculated into the allantoic cavity of 11-day-old embryonating chicken eggs[27] and confluent cell monolayer.

TABLE 10–2. EMC VIRAL PROTEINS (DALTONS) AS COMPARED WITH SOME OTHER PICORNAVIRUSES[a]

Virus	Ref.	VP1	VP2	VP3	VP4
EMC	18	31,703	29,026	25,141	7,247
Polio	19	33,521	29,985	26,410	7,385
HRV14	20	32,381	28,503	26,195	7,178
FMD	21	23,267	24,669	24,323	8,480

[a] Modified from Rueckert[17] with permission.

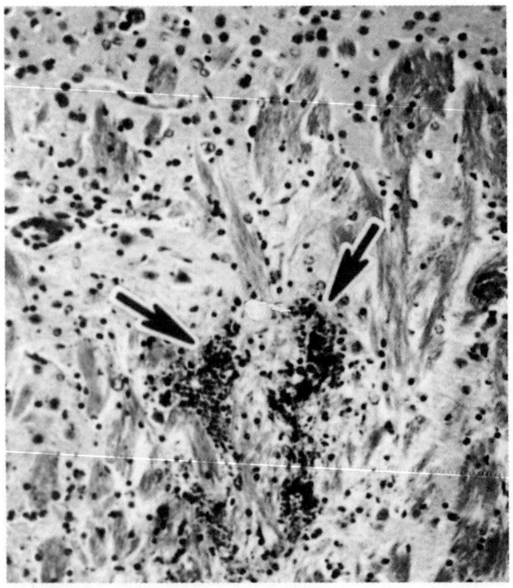

Figure 10–1. Basal ganglia of mouse killed the fifth day after injection of the E variant of the EMC virus. There are microscopic areas of necrosis containing basophilic material (*arrows*) mixed with microglial cells (hematoxylin-eosin, ×160). *(From Adachi et al[7] with permission.)*

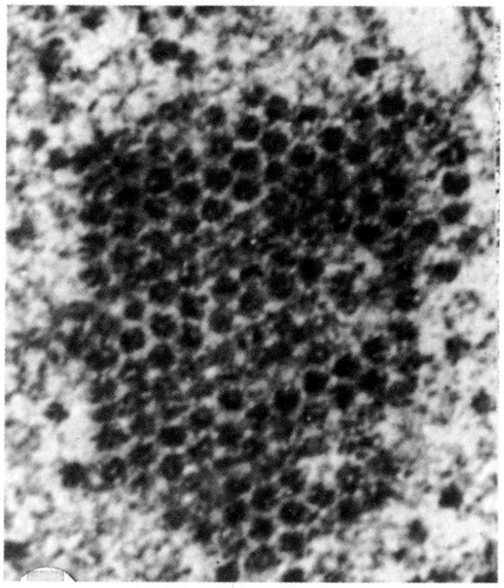

Figure 10–2. After 72 hours of incubation with the E variant of the EMC virus, the ultrastructure of the cultured cells from human fetal brain has a crystalloid pattern of aggregated particles (×126,000). *(From Adachi et al[24] with permission.)*

Continuous monkey kidney (Vero), baby hamster kidney (BHK-21), porcine kidney (PK-15), porcine fallopian tube (PFT), and swine testicle (ST) cell lines are used for virus isolation.[26,28–30] Cytopathogenic effects (CPEs) are observed only in the lungs and fetal (pool) tissues, with no evidence of viral replication in PK-15, PFT, and ST cell lines.[26] Viral purification is performed by differential and isopycnic ultracentrifugation in cesium chloride gradients.[29] Fractions of the continuous gradient corresponding to buoyant densities of 1.31 to 1.35 g/mL are used for rabbit immunization.[31] Specificity of the rabbit anti-EMC virus hyperimmune serum is confirmed by seroneutralization and indirect immunofluorescence.[30,32] Pathogenicity of the EMC virus isolates is investigated in mice.[26] CD-1 mice are inoculated intraperitoneally with 0.5 mL of infected cell culture supernatants (10^6 to 10^7 $TCID_{50}$/0.1 mL). One hundred percent mortality is observed within 48 hours postinoculation.[26]

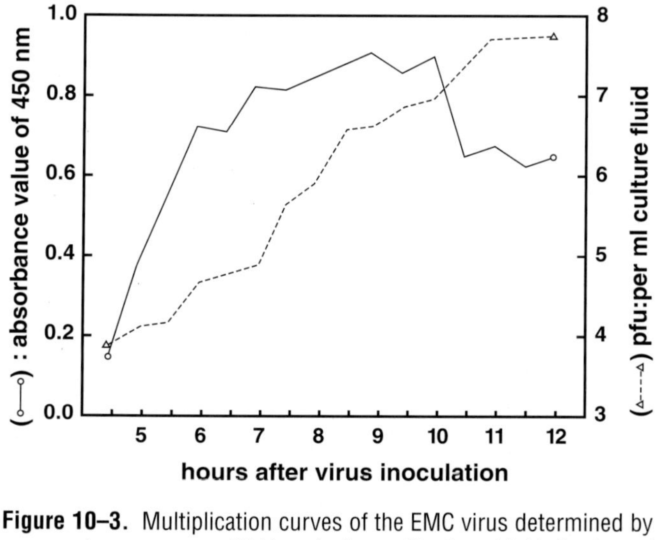

Figure 10–3. Multiplication curves of the EMC virus determined by enzyme immunoassay (EIA) and plaque titration. Multiplication of the virulent virus in L cells was simultaneously determined with EIA (O) and plaque titration (△). Mean (n = 3) absorbance values were given for each time point. Plaque titration was carried out with pooled (3 ×0.025 mL) supernatant fluids. *(From Vlaspolder et al[25] with permission.)*

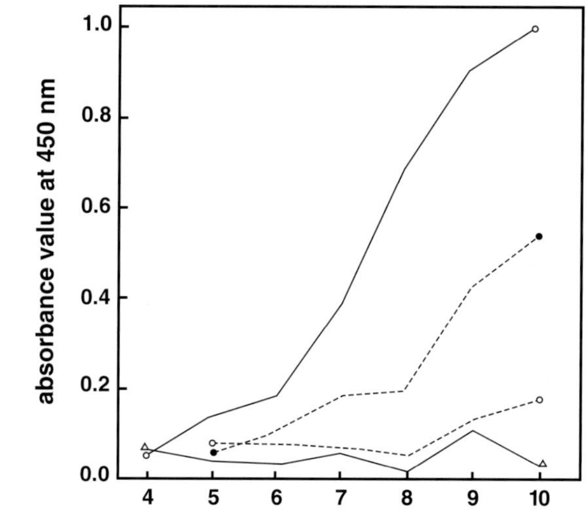

Figure 10–4. Multiplication curves of the EMC virus by EIA. The inhibitory effect of IFN L cells were preincubated for 2 hours at 37°C with either 1/150 (□) or 1/750 (●) dilutions of L-cell IFN before these cells were infected with the virulent virus at MOI of 10. Control L cells were preincubated with medium only, and thereafter these cells were infected (O) or not infected (△). At graded time intervals after virus inoculation, the L-cell monolayers were fixed, and subsequently EIA was performed with the horse radish peroxidase (HRPO)-labeled MAb UM 21.1. All points plotted are values for single measurements. *(From Vlaspolder et al[25] with permission.)*

TREATMENT

Prophylaxis and therapy of virulent EMC virus infection in mice were studied by IFN and enzyme-labeled virus-specific monoclonal antibodies.[26,33] Protective doses of these antibodies were injected intravenously in mice followed by intraperitoneal injection of the virus (10^4 LD_{50}) 3 hours later; full protection was obtained. L cells were preincubated for 20 hours at 37°C with IFN before these cells were infected with the virus. Multiplication of the virus is inhibited by IFN as early as 6 hours after the virus inoculation as compared with controls (Figure 10–4).[25]

ONCOLYTIC EFFECTS

Oncolytic effects of human tumors by the EMC virus have been reported[1,34–39]; the virus inhibits synthesis of host RNA and directs host cells to synthesize viral RNA.[40] Both in vivo (nude mice) and in vitro studies document this effect. Because the EMC virus usually is not seriously pathogenic in man and is tropic to neoplastic cells, this type of approach may be useful in the treatment of human tumors.

Acknowledgment. Mrs. Renee Brenner gave invaluable editorial assistance.

REFERENCES

1. Adachi M, Brooks SE, Stein MR, Hoffman LM. Establishment of a new variant of encephalomyocarditis (EMC-A) virus and its oncolytic effects on human astrocytoma in vitro and in nude rats. *J Neuropathol Exp Neurol.* 1991; 50:369.
2. Yoon JW, McClintock PR, Onodera T, Notkins AL. Virus-induced diabetes mellitus. XVIII. Inhibition by a non-diabetogenic variant of encephalomyocarditis virus. *J Exp Med.* 1980;152:878–892.
3. Craighead JE. Pathogenicity of the M and E variants of the encephalomyocarditis (EMC) virus. I. Myocardiotropic and neurotropic properties. *Am J Pathol.* 1966;48: 333–345.
4. Cerutis DR, Bruner RH, Thomas DC, Giron DJ. Tropism and histopathology of the D, B, K, and MM variants of encephalomyocarditis virus. *J Med Virol.* 1989;29:63–69.
5. Murnane TG, Craighead JE, Mondragon H, Shelokov A. Fatal disease of swine due to encephalomyocarditis virus. *Science.* 1960;131:498–499.
6. Cronin ME, Love LA, Miller FW, McClintock PR, Plotz PH. The natural history of encephalomyocarditis virus–induced myositis and myocarditis in mice. Viral persistence demonstrated by in situ hybridization. *J Exp Med.* 1988;168:1639–1648.
7. Adachi M, Volk BW, Tsai CY, Amsterdam D, Willmann KF. Light and electron microscopic studies of mouse CNS after subcutaneous administration of the E and M variants of the encephalomyocarditis virus. *Acta Neuropathol.* 1973; 25:169–178.
8. Adachi M, Volk BW, Amsterdam D, Brooks S, Tanapat P, Broome JD. Light and electron microscopic studies of "nude" mice CNS after subcutaneous administration of the E variant of the encephalomyocarditis (EMC) virus. *Acta Neuropathol.* 1977;37:89–93.
9. Smadel JF, Warren J. The virus of encephalomyocarditis and its apparent causation of disease in man. *J Clin Invest.* 1947;26:1197.
10. Koch F. Die encephalomyocarditis (EMC) und ihre Abgrenzung von der Poliomyelitis. *Z Kinderheilk.* 1950; 68:328–357.
11. Saphir O. Encephalomyocarditis. *Circulation.* 1952;6:843–850.
12. Jonkers AH. Serosurvey of encephalomyocarditis virus neutralizing antibodies in southern Louisiana and Peruvian Indian populations. *Am J Trop Med Hyg.* 1961;10: 593–598.
13. Meyer HM Jr, Johnson RT, Crawford IP, Dascomb HE, Rogers NG. Central nervous system syndromes of "viral" etiology. A study of 713 cases. *Am J Med.* 1960;29:334–347.
14. Jungeblut CW. Neutralization of Columbia SK and Yale SK virus by polioconvalescent and normal human sera. *Arch Pediatr.* 1950;67:519–530.
15. Barski G, Cornefert F. Position particulière des encéphalomyélites de type Mengo par rapport aux polymyélites. Répartition d'anticorps spécifiques chez certaines populations d'Afrique centrale et d'autres zones géographiques. *Bull World Health Organ.* 1957;17:991–999.
16. Putank JR, Philips BA. Picornaviral structure and assembly. *Microbiol Rev.* 1981;45:287–315.
17. Rueckert RR. Picornaviridae and their replication. In: Fields BN, Knipe DM, Chanock RM, et al, eds. *Fields Virology.* 2nd ed. New York: Raven Press; 1990:507–548.
18. Palmenberg AC, Kirby EM, Janda MR, et al. The nucleotide and deduced sequences of the encephalomyocarditis viral polyprotein coding region. *Nucleic Acids Res.* 1984;12:2969–2985.
19. Kitamura N, Semler BL, Rothberg PG, et al. Primary structure, gene organization and polypeptide expression of poliovirus RNA. *Nature (London).* 1981;291:547–553.
20. Callahan PL, Mizutani S, Colonno RJ. Molecular cloning and complete sequence determination of RNA genome of human rhinovirus type 14. *Proc Natl Acad Sci USA.* 1985;82:732–736.
21. Carroll AR, Rowlands DJ, Clarke BE. The complete nucleotide sequence of the RNA coding for the primary translation product of foot-and-mouth disease virus. *Nucleic Acids Res.* 1984;12:2461–2472.
22. Rossman MG, Palmenberg AC. Conservation of the putative receptor attachment site of picornaviruses. *Virology.* 1988;164:373–382.
23. Burness AT, Pardoe IU. A sialoglycopeptide from human erythrocytes with receptor-like properties for encephalomyocarditis and influenza viruses. *J Gen Virol.* 1983;64: 1137–1148.
24. Adachi M, Amsterdam D, Brooks SE, Volk BW. Ultrastructural alterations of tissue cultures from human fetal brain infected with the E variant of EMC virus. *Acta Neuropathol.* 1975;32:133–142.
25. Vlaspolder F, Harmsen T, van Veenendaal D, Kraaijeveld CA, Snippe H. Application of immunoassay of encephalomyocarditis virus in cell culture with enzyme-labeled virus-specific monoclonal antibodies for rapid detection of virus, neutralizing antibodies, and interferon. *J Clin Microbiol.* 1988;26:2593–2597.
26. Dea SA, Bilodeau R, Martineau GP. Isolation of encephalomyocarditis virus among stillborn and post-weaning pigs in Quebec. *Arch Virol.* 1991;17:121–128.
27. Morin M, Phaneuf JB, Sauvageau R, DiFranco E, Marsolais

G, Boudreault A. An epizootic of swine influenza in Quebec. *Can Vet J.* 1981;22:204–205.

28. Bouillant AMP, Dulac GC, Willis N, et al. Viral susceptibility of a cell line derived from the pig oviduct. *Can J Comp Med.* 1975;39:450–456.
29. Dea S, Elazhary MASY. Cultivation of a porcine adenovirus in porcine thyroid cell cultures. *Cornell Vet.* 1984;74:207–217.
30. Dea S, Vaillancourt J, Elazhary MASY, Martineau GP. Parvovirus-like particles associated with diarrhea in unweaned piglets. *Can J Comp Med.* 1985;49:343–345.
31. Dea S, Tijssen P. Identification of the structure proteins of turkey enteric coronavirus. *Arch Virol.* 1988;99:173–186.
32. Joo HS, Kim HS, Leman A. Detection of antibody to encephalomyocarditis virus in mummified or stillborn pigs. *Arch Virol.* 1988;100:131–134.
33. Vlaspolder F, Kraaijeveld CA, van Buuren R, Harmsen M, Benaissa-Trouw BJ, Snippe H. Prophylaxis and therapy of virulent encephalomyocarditis virus infection in mice by monoclonal antibodies. *Arch Virol.* 1988;98:123–130.
34. Adachi M, Brooks SE, Letizia L, Hoffman L, Schneck L. Destruction of human LMB-astrocytoma cells in-vitro and in-vivo mediated by the E variant of encephalomyocarditis virus (EMC-E). *J Neuropathol Exp Neurol.* 1982; 41:370.
35. Adachi M, Brooks SE, Letizia L, Hoffman LM, Schneck L. Destruction of human neuroblastoma cells in-vitro and in-vivo mediated by the E variant of encephalomyocarditis virus (EMC-E). *J Neuropathol Exp Neurol.* 1983;42:351.
36. Adachi M, Brooks SE, Stein MR, Hoffman LM, Schneck L. The effects on human retinoblastoma cells in-vitro and in-vivo after exposure to the E variant of encephalomyocarditis virus (EMC-E). *J Neuropathol Exp Neurol.* 1984;43:337.
37. Adachi M, Brooks SE, Rao C, Stein MR, Hoffman LM, Schneck L. Light and electron microscopic features of transformed human meningioma cells in-vitro infected by the M variant of encephalomyocarditis virus (EMC-M). *J Neuropathol Exp Neurol.* 1985;44:315.
38. Adachi M, Brooks SE, Stein MR, Hoffman LM, Schneck L. The effects on human carcinoma (CA) and sarcoma (SA) cells in-vitro after exposure to the E and M variants of encephalomyocarditis virus (EMC E and M). *Fed Proc.* 1986;45:956.
39. Adachi M. Experimental models and their treatment of some neurological disorders. Lipidosis and malignant tumors. *Neuropathology.* 1987;8:47–50.
40. Lawrence C, Thach RE. Encephalomyocarditis virus infection of mouse plasmacytoma cells. 1. Inhibition of cellular protein synthesis. *J Virol.* 1974;14:598–610.

CHAPTER 11

Epstein–Barr Virus and Human Diseases

*Elizabeth R. Unger and David T. Purtilo**

He (Denis Burkitt) left behind in Africa a store of good will, and I doubt whether there has ever been any doctor working in Africa who has either been better known or more loved.

Sir Ian W. J. McAdam in Mr. Burkitt and Africa, Bernard Glemser, World Publishing Company, Cleveland, 1970

INTRODUCTION

The virion of the Epstein–Barr virus (EBV) was originally identified by electron microscopy in a cultured cell line of African Burkitt's lymphoma.[1] Although originally identified in a lymphoma cell line, infectious mononucleosis (IM) was the first disease to be attributed to EBV infection. Since then EBV has been associated with several clinical entities, both benign and malignant.

EBV is an ubiquitous B lymphotropic herpesvirus with a seroprevalence in adults throughout the world of 80% to 90%. In common with other herpesviruses, EBV has both lytic (productive) and latent phases of infection. Most infections are latent and asymptomatic. Although virions are not produced during latency, latent infection is clearly not silent, as various viral proteins are identified, depending on the state of latency.[2] Latency is associated with immortalization of B lymphocytes and it is the latent state that is identified in EBV-associated malignancies. Host immune response plays a key role in determining the outcome of infection. New techniques expanding the range of clinical material that may be directly examined for viral genetic information and/or proteins suggest that the range of EBV-associated disease has not yet been fully defined.[3] An overview of the biology of EBV infection, host response, EBV-associated disease, and diagnostic methods is presented here.

BIOLOGY OF EPSTEIN–BARR VIRUS

EBV, herpesvirus 4, is an enveloped icosahedral virus with a linear double-stranded DNA genome of 172 kb. The genome consists of unique tandemly repeated DNA elements organized as TR (terminal repeat)–U(unique region)1–IR (internal repeat)1–U2–IR2–U3–IR3–U4–IR4–U5–TR.[4]

When the primary infection is in childhood it usually goes unnoticed, but when primary infection is delayed until adolescence or later IM results. The major route of transmission of EBV is through saliva, and oropharyngeal epithelial cells are the source of the infectious transmissible virus.[5] Virion envelope glycoprotein binds to the C3d component of complement (CR2) found on nearly all B lymphocytes.[6] Infection of mucosal B lymphocytes introduces the infection to the bloodstream where as many as 5% to 20% of B cells may become infected. EBV infection causes a polyclonal stimulation of B cells, which produce heterophile antibodies as well as antibodies directed against EBV proteins.

During the lytic (virus-productive) cycle, the synthesis and expression of EBV-determined nuclear antigen (EBNA) occurs several hours after infection and may be preceded or accompanied by the functional lymphocyte-detected membrane antigen (LYDMA).[7]

* Deceased.

Membrane antigen (MA) and early antigen (EA) expression follow. Next, viral DNA synthesis commences; finally, viral capsid antigen (VCA) is produced for the assembly and release of infectious virus particles.[8] Formation of episomal virus establishes a latent (nonproductive) infection in B lymphocytes, and approximately 10% of latently infected cells will become immortalized causing a permanent host–carrier state. Reentry of latently infected cells into the lytic cycle may cause reactivation of EBV infection. Recently two biotypes of EBV (types 1 and 2) have been identified that have significant differences in the *EBNA-2, EBNA-3A, -3B,* and *-3C* genes. The functional consequence of the protein differences in *EBNA-2* and *EBNA-3* is that type 1 is more efficient at immortalization than type 2.[9]

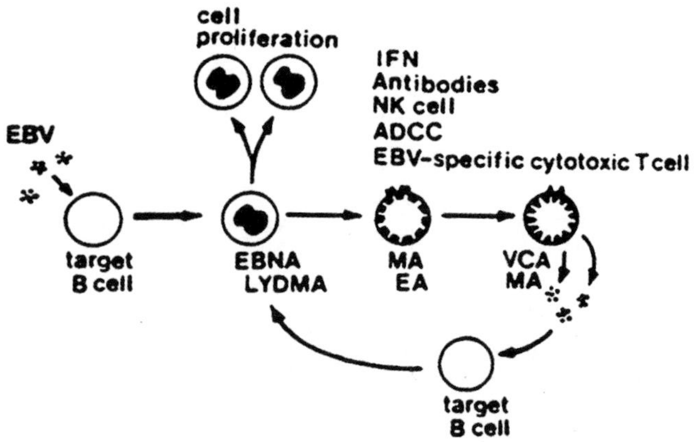

Figure 11–1. Diagram indicating immune events of EBV infection. EBV, Epstein–Barr virus; EBNA, EBV-determined nuclear antigen; LYDMA, lymphocyte-detected membrane antigen; MA, membrane antigen; EA, early antigen; VCA, viral capsid antigen; IFN, interferon; NK cell, natural killer cell; ADCC, antibody-dependent cell-mediated cytotoxicity. *(From Okano M, Thiele GM, David JR, Grierson HL, Purtilo DT. Epstein–Barr virus and human diseases: recent advances in diagnosis.* Clin Microbiol Rev. *1988;1:300–312. Published with permission of the American Society for Microbiology.)*

IMMUNE RESPONSE TO EPSTEIN–BARR INFECTION

The first line of defense comes from interferon liberated by virally infected B cells as well as those T cells responding to the virus.[10,11] Interferon controls EBV-induced B-cell lymphoproliferation by antiviral replication activity, antilymphocytic proliferative response, and boosting of natural killer (NK) cell activity.[10,12] NK cells do not require prior sensitization and memory to kill target cells. Interferon and NK cells act synergistically to protect against EBV. Cytotoxic T cells are the most important factor in controlling EBV-induced B-cell proliferation; however, activation of suppressor T cells by EBV impairs the normal T-cell response. The majority of the atypical lymphocytes in the peripheral blood during IM are suppressor T cells, and the T helper–suppressor ratio is reversed for an extended period of time.[13] Antibody-dependent cell-mediated cytotoxicity (ADCC) is an additional important immune response to EBV, as ADCC titers are prognostic in patients with Burkitt's lymphoma and nasopharyngeal carcinoma.[14] The normal immune events that follow EBV infection are shown in Figure 11–1.

Under normal circumstances antibody response to EBV is tightly regulated by the host immune system. The humoral response to primary EBV infection occurs rapidly, and most symptomatic patients show near peak titers of IgG and IgM to VCA when first examined. The IgG antibodies to VCA remain elevated, whereas IgM levels decrease and disappear 6 to 12 weeks after onset. Anti-EA-D (diffuse EA component) IgG antibodies develop transiently in some patients. Anti-EBNA IgG is absent during acute infection but is detected weeks to months later and persists for life. Anti-EA-R (restricted EA component) IgG antibodies are rarely in the acute phase of IM, but appear transiently during late convalescence, and some silent primary EBV infections in childhood, or more chronic infections of EBV, that is, Burkitt's lymphoma (BL). In general, reactivation of EBV infection is defined by finding serologically elevated antibody titers to VCA-IgG, EA-D (EA-R in patients with BL) and the preexistence of anti-EBNA IgG antibodies. A past EBV infection is identified by the

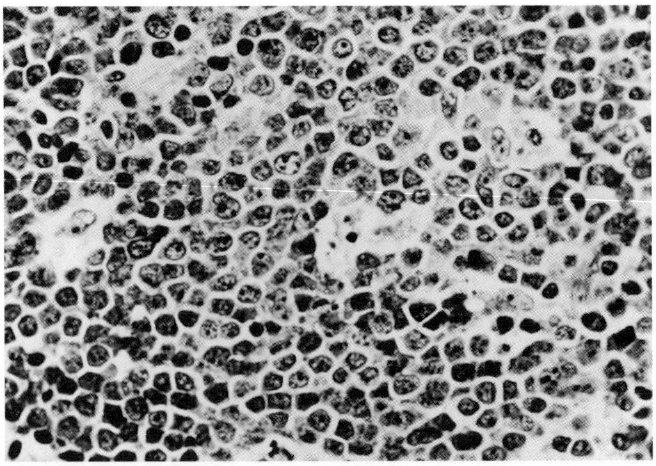

Figure 11–2. Histology of infectious mononucleosis, a benign lymphoproliferative disease caused by acute EBV infection. There is an absolute lymphocytosis in the peripheral blood. Phagocytic cells may closely resemble the "starry sky" pattern of BL (see Figure 11–6, A). The normal architecture of lymph nodes and spleen may be disturbed but not effaced by the many immunostimulated lymphocytes and lymph nodes. The normal immune responses of the host bring this infection under control.

absence of anti-VCA IgM antibodies and IgG antibodies against both VCA and EBNA.

Immunodeficient patients, especially children with a primary immunodeficiency, have either unusually low or high EBV antibody titers and a lack of antibody to EBNA.[10,15,16] A deficiency or dysfunction of immune surveillance against EBV infection permits productive cycles of viral replication, leading to production of EA, VCA antibodies. The lack of antibody to EBNA may be a consequence of decreased or absent immune T-cell function against EBV. In the absence of this cytotoxic response, EBNA is not released from the nuclear membrane of infected B cells and not accessible to stimulate antibody production.[15,17]

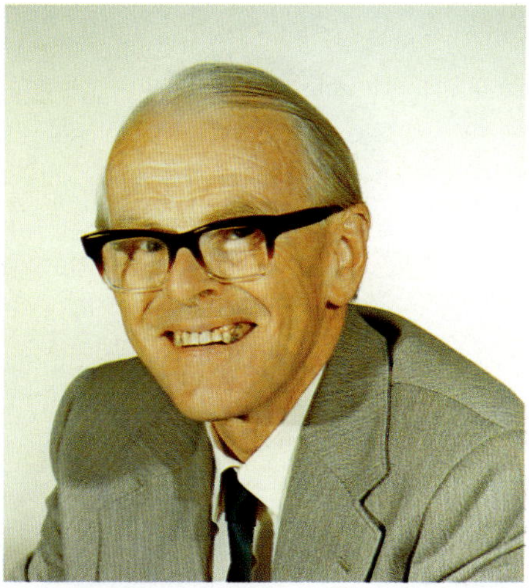

Figure 11–3. Denis Parsons Burkitt (1911–1993) taken during one of his lecture tours in the United States. *(Photograph by Daniel H. Connor, MD, 1973.)*

EBV-ASSOCIATED DISEASES

The spectrum of EBV-associated diseases including those in immunodeficient patients is discussed briefly. EBV in a lesion, of course, does not establish it as the etiologic agent for that lesion. EBV may be a secondary invader or an opportunistic infection.

Infectious Mononucleosis

As mentioned, when primary infection is delayed until age 10 to 30 years, there is symptomatic disease. The disease has an insidious onset and the typical patient with IM has sore throat, fever, fatigue, cervical lymphadenopathy, and splenomegaly.[18] There is lymphocytosis with a high percentage of atypical lymphocytes and heterophile antibodies. These signs and symptoms are caused by an immunological struggle between infected B cells and responding NK and T cells (Figure 11–2). Resolution generally is within a month, but fatigue sometimes persists.[18] Complications include hemolytic anemia, red cell aplasia, thrombocytopenia, virus-associated hemophagocytic syndrome, agranulocytosis, aplastic anemia, acquired agammaglobulinemia, and immune complex deposition in tissues. Other complications arise from the invasion of lymphocytes into the central and peripheral nervous systems leading to meningoencephalitis, transverse myelitis, Guillain–Barré syndrome, Bell's palsy, or cerebellar ataxia. There may be also fulminant hepatitis, arthritis, myocarditis, and nephritis.[18]

Burkitt's Lymphoma

In 1958, Denis Parsons Burkitt (Figure 11–3) described a disease now known as Burkitt's lymphoma. It was a malignant tumor of childhood involving jaw (Figure 11–4) and viscera (Figure 11–5) and later Burkitt noticed that the geographic distribution corresponded to areas of endemic malaria. The tumor is composed of a population of uniformly round lymphocytes with interspersed macrophages, giving a "starry sky" pattern (Figure 11–6). The pathologic features of this tumor are well described.[19] Tumors with identical features were subsequently identified in other areas—beyond the original geographic distribution—and these are referred to as nonendemic BL. Nonendemic BL tends to involve extranodal sites other than the jaw.

Approximately 98% of the endemic tumors contain EBV genome, whereas EBV is only identified in 20% of nonendemic tumors. The pathogenesis of endemic BL is currently attributed to impaired immune competence accompanying chronic malaria infection. The unchecked EBV infection causes sustained B-cell proliferation. These B cells are at increased risk for t(8,14) translocations, activating the *myc* oncogene and leading to neoplasia.

Other Lymphoid Malignancies

In contrast to the strong association of EBV with BL, the association of EBV with other lymphoid malignancies is more variable. In the United States, EBV is in 20% to 50% of Hodgkin's lymphomas (HL). The frequency of EBV detection apparently varies with the histologic subtype of HL and the age of the patient; the association may be stronger in other countries.[20–25]

EBV has also been identified in peripheral T-cell lymphomas[26–32]; the association appears particularly strong for nasal T-cell lymphomas and lymphomatoid granulomatosis. The role that EBV plays in the genesis of these lesions is still unclear. Detection of virus in the

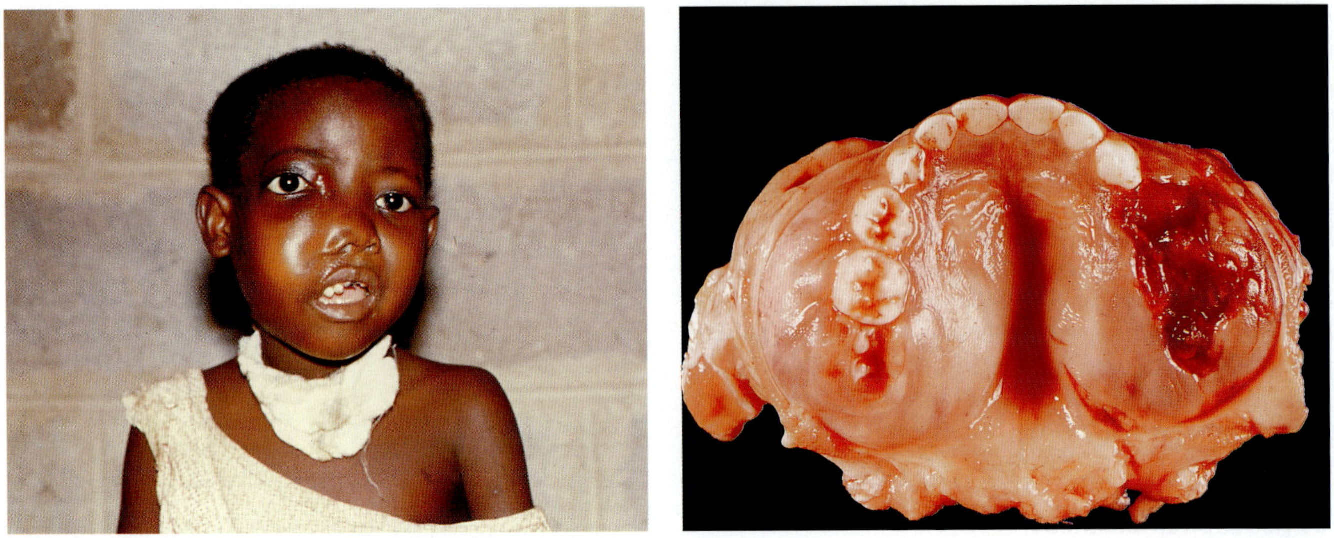

A B

Figure 11–4. (**A**) Young girl in eastern Zaire with BL of jaw. (**B**) BL of maxillae—removed at autopsy. The tumor is large; some of the teeth have loosened and dropped out. *(Photographs by Daniel H. Connor, MD, 1968 and 1962, respectively.)*

lesion does not prove a causal role and merely demonstrates a possible association. EBV is frequently detected in the lymphomas that develop in patients with acquired immunodeficiency syndrome (AIDS), both HL and non–Hodgkin's lymphomas (NHL).[33–37] Essentially, all AIDS-related primary central nervous system (CNS) lymphomas contain EBV genome.[38,39]

Nasopharyngeal Carcinoma

Nasopharyngeal carcinoma (NPC) of the undifferentiated type contains EBV genome nearly 100% of the time.[40] The tumor is derived from the epithelium of the nasopharynx and divided into keratinizing squamous cell carcinomas, nonkeratinizing carcinomas and undifferentiated (anaplastic) carcinomas according to the World Health Organization classification. There is often a dense lymphocytic infiltrate obscuring the epithelium and the tumor was once called a lymphoepithelioma (Figure 11–7). EBV is identified in the epithelial component of the tumor and is monoclonal, suggesting that the tumor is derived from one EBV-infected cell.

NPCs are predominantly in the male population of southern China where NPC is the most prevalent tumor in males, comprising about 20% of all cancers.[41] Genetic and certain cultural patterns predispose to the

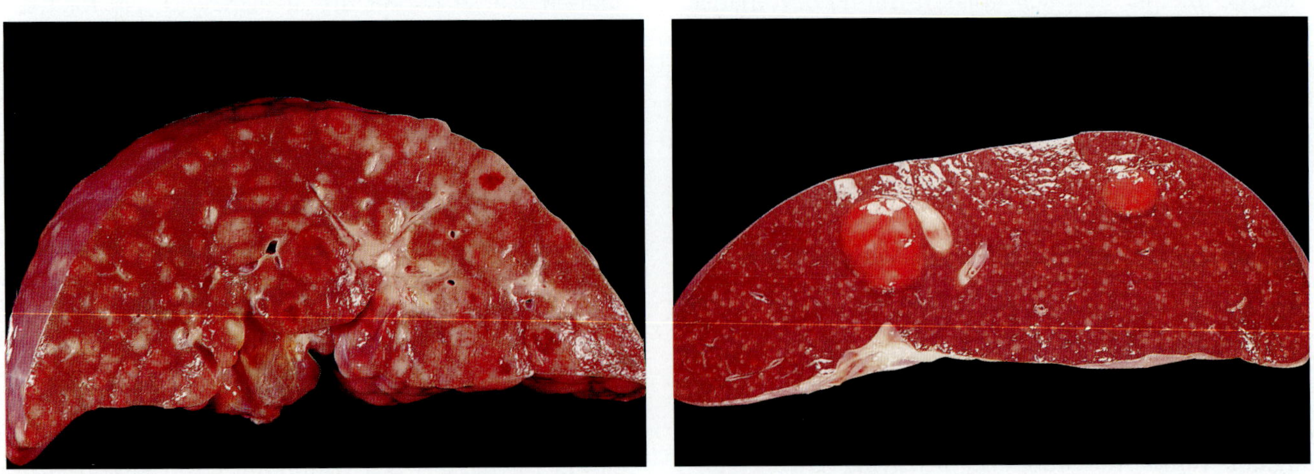

A B

Figure 11–5. (**A**) Multiple nodules of Burkitt's lymphoma in liver. (**B**) Two nodules of BL in spleen. *(Photographs by Daniel H. Connor, MD, 1962.)*

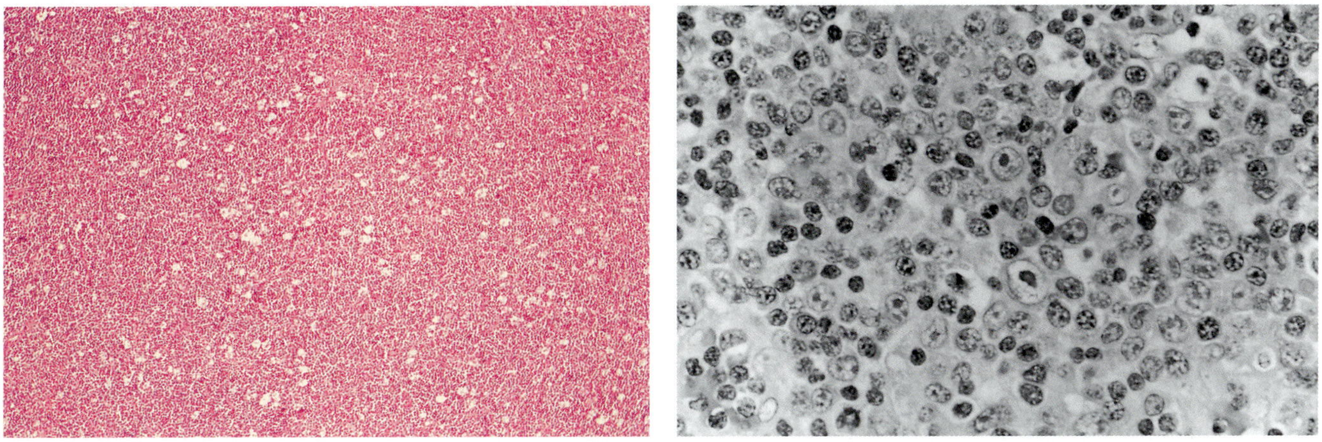

A B

Figure 11–6. (**A**) Patients with immunodeficiencies infected with EBV fail to control the B-cell proliferation. Sustained proliferation can lead to B-cell lymphomas, such as BL. Note the "starry sky" pattern. The clear spaces are macrophages. (**B**) A closer view of a BL. *(From Cohen SM et al Pivotal role of increased cell proliferation in human carcinogenesis.* Mod Pathol. *1991;4:371–378. Published with permission of the United States and Canadian Academy of Pathology, Inc.)*

tumor. Cantonese Chinese immigrants to the United States have a lower incidence in the second generation than their relatives in China, but the incidence remains higher than that of white Americans.[41] Eating salted fish containing appreciable quantities of nitrosodimethylamines and the use of *Euphorbiaceae* plant extracts in Chinese traditional medicine, which include phorbol esters, may induce replication of EBV. The etiologic association between the virus and the tumor is supported by finding elevated IgG and IgA antibodies against VCA and EA-D in these patients.

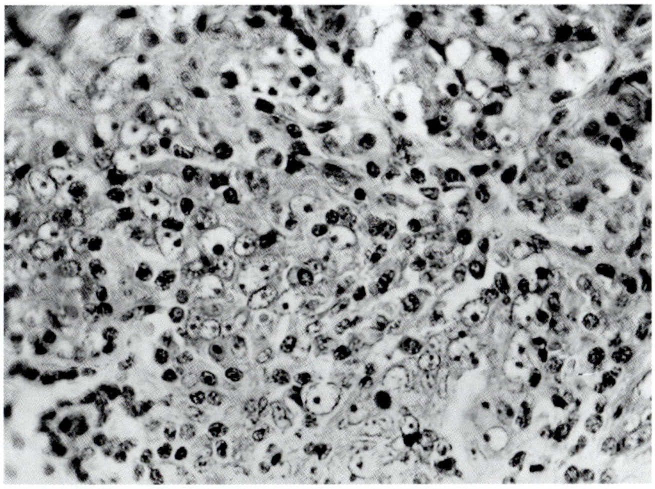

Figure 11–7. Nasopharyngeal carcinoma infiltrated with lymphoid cells. Cytoplasmic borders are indistinct, giving the impression of a syncytium. *(From Purtilo DT. Malignancies in the tropics. In: Binford CH, Connor DH, eds.* Pathology of Tropical and Extraordinary Diseases. *Washington, DC: Armed Forces Institute of Pathology; 1976:647–660. Published with permission of the Armed Forces Institute of Pathology.)*

Other Carcinomas

EBV is in carcinomas having lymphoepithelial-like features that are primary in sites other than the nasopharynx. These are lung (Figure 11–8)[42] and stomach.[35,43] EBV has also been in carcinomas of salivary gland,[44,45] thymic carcinoma,[46] and gastric adenocarcinoma.[47] The role of EBV in these tumors is being investigated.

Chronic Mononucleosis Syndrome

In 1948, Isaacs described IM lasting from months to years.[48] Several others have described a protracted illness usually preceded by IM, but with persistent fatigue, headaches, myalgia, lymphadenopathy, and low-grade fever.[49–53] This syndrome of unknown cause is interesting and confusing. It is not linked to EBV but many of the patients have EBV antibody profiles that suggest reactivation. Moreover, there is a lack of correlation between EBV antibody and chronic fatigue.[54]

X-Linked Lymphoproliferative Disease

Characteristics of X-linked lymphoproliferative disease (XLP) were described in 1975 in males of the Duncan family in whom the syndrome manifested as an inherited immunodeficiency with fatal or chronic IM, acquired hypogammaglobulinemia, or malignant lymphoma after infection with EBV.[55] The registry of XLP now contains records of more than 270 patients in 65 unrelated kindreds.[56] Because they fail to control B- and T-cell lymphoproliferative responses to EBV, espe-

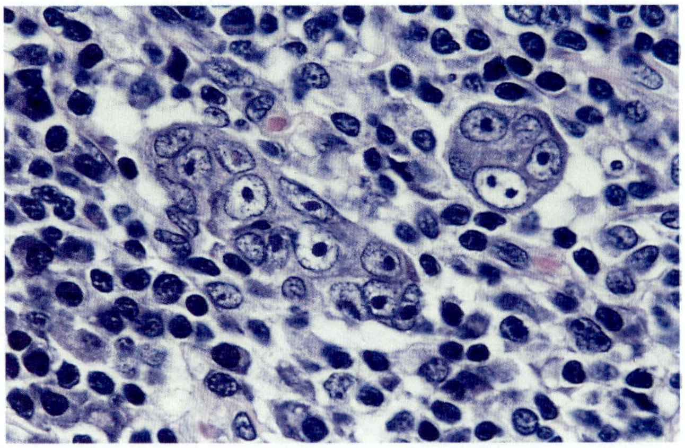

A

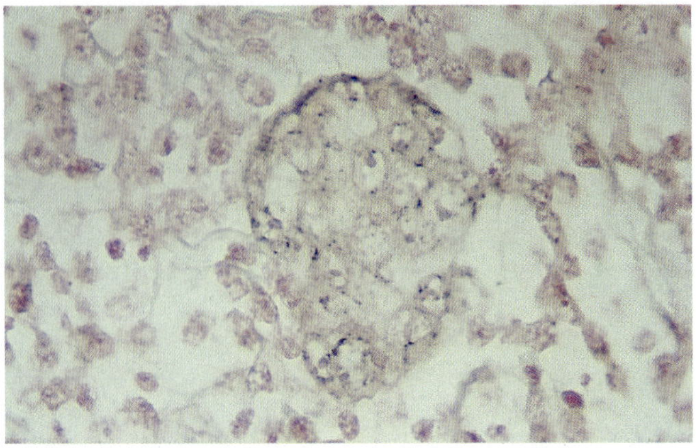

B

Figure 11–8. Lymphoepithelial-like carcinoma of lung. (**A**) Large malignant epithelial cells are surrounded by dense lymphoid infiltrates (hematoxylin-eosin, ×1000). (**B**) Demonstration of EBV genetic information by colorimetric in situ hybridization. Signal (dark blue-black color) is in nuclei of malignant epithelial cells [biotinylated probe against EBV genomic target (*Bam*HI W), avidin-alkaline phosphastase detection with BCIP/NBT substrate. Nuclear fast red counterstain, original magnification ×1000].

cially by cytotoxic T cells, NK cells, and suppressor T cells, two thirds of the male patients with XLP succumb to severe or fatal IM. Immunohistochemical studies of lesions in the liver and bone marrow reveal EBV-carrying B cells admixed with suppressor T cells and fewer numbers of NK cells.[56] These uncontrolled lymphoid cells cause fulminant hepatitis or the virus-associated hemophagocytic syndrome in bone marrow. In the one third of patients who survive primary EBV infection, excessive suppression of B cells by suppressor T cells leads to acquired hypogammaglobulinemia or agammaglobulinemia.[56] In contrast, about 20% of patients with sustained polyclonal B-cell proliferation evoked by EBV develop B-cell malignancy from molecular or cytogenetic alterations in a clone of cells.[57] Both t(8;14) and t(8;22) have been detected in two of the BL. About 85% of patients die by age 10 years and 100% by age 40 years.[56] Patients in early and late childhood (before infection with EBV) have subtle immune defects in response to tetanus and ΦX174 antigens.[58] In spite of these defects patients with XLP are not vulnerable to infectious agents other than EBV. The extensive and progressive immunologic defects in XLP are triggered by infection with EBV.

Ataxia-Telangiectasia and Other Primary Immunodeficiencies

Ataxia-telangiectasia (AT) is an autosomal recessive disorder characterized by progressive cerebellar ataxia, oculocutaneous telangiectasia, recurrent sinopulmonary infections, and a variable immunodeficiency, which is a progressive combined defect of T- and B-cell function.[59,60] Patients with AT are predisposed also to malignancies, mainly T-cell leukemia, B-cell lymphoma, Hodgkin's disease, and gastric adenocarcinoma. They have defective responses to EBV, often associated with increased IgG antibodies to VCA and EA-D, but low or nondetectable antibodies to EBNA. EBV-carrying lymphoproliferative diseases have been documented in patients with AT.[60,61]

Other patients with primary immune deficiency disorders, such as Wiskott–Aldrich syndrome, severe combined immunodeficiency, common variable immunodeficiency, and Chédiak–Higashi syndrome develop EBV-induced lymphoproliferative diseases.[62–65]

Post-Transplant Lymphoproliferative Disorders

EBV causes abnormal lymphoproliferative diseases in patients with kidney, heart, lung, liver, bone marrow, and thymic epithelium transplants.[64-66] Post-transplant lymphoproliferative disorder (PTLD) tends to be extranodal and frequently involves the gastrointestinal tract and central nervous system. It can be polyclonal, oligoclonal, or monoclonal[66] and transition from polyclonal to monoclonal B-cell proliferative lesions has been documented.[67] Withdrawal of immune suppression can cause regression of these tumors especially when the PTLD is polyclonal and involves the gut. Factors contributing to PTLD are iatrogenic impairment of immune surveillance, chronic antigenic stimulation from the allograft, or direct oncogenic effects of immunosuppressive drugs.[66] A three category classification of PTLD

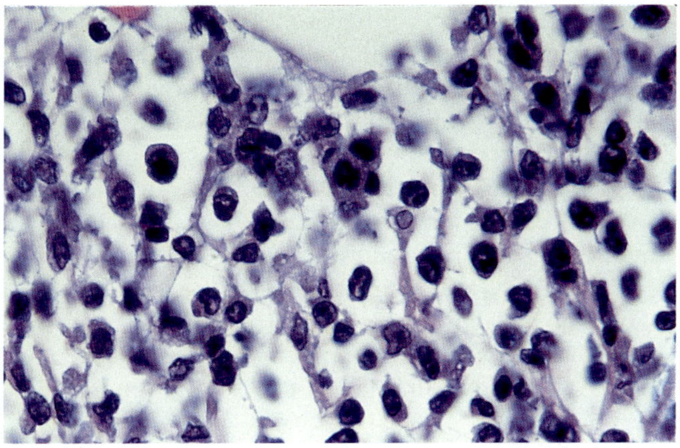

A

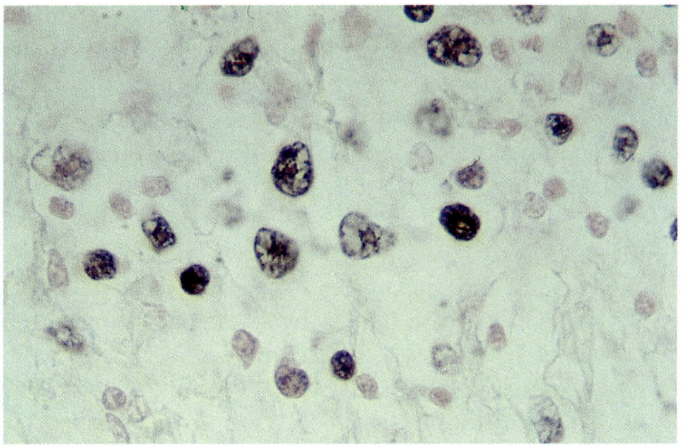

B

Figure 11–9. Post-transplant lymphoproliferative disorder. (**A**) Fatal PTLD after liver transplantation. Section taken at autopsy from one of multiple masses in the intestine showing markedly atypical lymphoid infiltrate (hemotoxylin-eosin, ×1000). (**B**) Demonstration of EBV by colorimetric in situ hybridization. Signal, dark blue-black color, is localized to nuclei [biotinylated probe directed against EBER (see Figure 11–11), avidin-alkaline phosphatase detection with BCIP/NBT substrate. Nuclear fast red counterstain, ×1000].

has been developed: 1) polymorphous diffuse B-cell hyperplasia characterized by invasive proliferation of B cells at various stages of development, 2) polymorphic B-cell lymphoma with confluent geographic necrosis and atypical immunoblastic cells (Figure 11–9), and 3) immunoblastic sarcoma.

Other Lesions in AIDS Patients

Hairy leukoplakia (Figure 11–10) is caused by productive EBV infection in the epithelium of the tongue of some homosexual males.[68] Children with AIDS develop lymphoid interstitial pneumonitis, which carries the EBV genome.[69]

DIAGNOSIS OF EPSTEIN–BARR VIRUS INFECTION

Serodiagnosis

Heterophile antibodies are detected during the acute phase of infection and may remain elevated during convalescence. These are IgM antibodies, agglutinate sheep or horse erythrocytes, and are detected with the Paul Bunnell, Davidsohn, or Monospot tests. A positive reaction is diagnostic of IM and is in the serum of approximately 85% of adult patients with IM.[18] Children younger than 4 years of age often fail to develop heterophile antibodies.[70] EBV-specific serodiagnostic tests are required to diagnose heterophile-antibody-negative patients of IM or IM-like illnesses. These tests are essential also for heterophile-antibody-positive patients with atypical manifestations, especially patients with lymphoproliferative lesions or immunodeficiency. In general, the interpretation of serological tests in patients with suspected EBV infection is based on the profile of antibody titers with a single serum specimen against a panel of four antigens: VCA, EA-D, EA-R, and EBNA. The antibodies to VCA, EA-D, and EA-R are measured

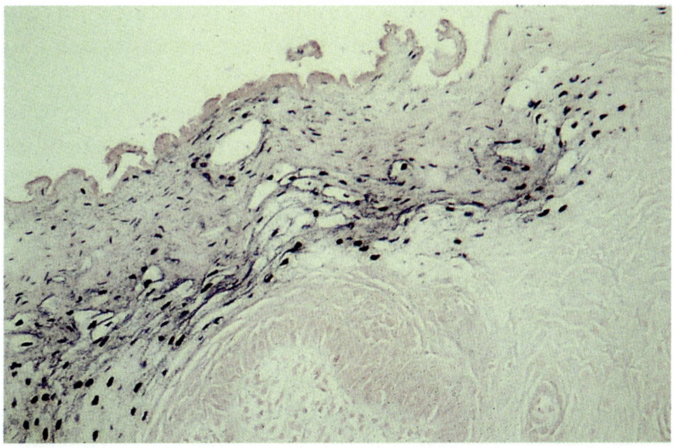

Figure 11–10. Oral "hairy" leukoplakia. Demonstration of EBV by colorimetric in situ hybridization. Signal, dark blue-black color, is localized to nuclei. Genomic probe must be used as target since EBV infection in oral leukoplakia is entirely productive. Hybridization reaction with EBER probe (see Figure 11–11 and text) is negative in these lesions [biotinylated probe against EBV genomic target (*Bam*HI W), avidin-alkaline phosphatase detection with BCIP/NBT substrate. Nuclear fast red counterstain, ×200].

by the indirect immunofluorescence (IDIF) assay; anti-EBNA antibodies must be measured by the anticomplement immunofluorescence (ACIF) method.[10,15,17,41] Enzyme-linked immunosorbent assays (ELISAs) have also been developed to detect antibodies specific for EBV-related antigens.[71] Serologic methods do not always correspond to the status of active EBV infection because they are indirect and depend on whether the patient has an intact immune system. For example, healthy individuals sometimes have elevated antibody titers without symptoms, whereas immunodeficient persons may develop disseminated EBV infection without the full spectrum of antibodies.[10,15]

Viral Isolation

Cocultivation of umbilical cord blood lymphocytes with specimens from a patient suspected of containing active EBV (eg, throat washings, peripheral blood lymphocytes, or cells from a lymphoproliferative lesion) may be done. If the assay is positive, EBV from the patient will immortalize cord blood lymphocytes. This kind of immortalization assay is not practical because of the narrow host range of EBV in vitro as well as the length and complexity of the assay. In addition, because type 2 virus is much less efficient at immortalization, it will be particularly underrepresented in these assays.

Detection of EBV in Tissues

Detection of EBV in tissue is important in establishing the association of EBV with lymphoproliferative disorders and malignancies. Diagnostic information regarding prognosis and treatment, however, is more dependent on accurate histopathologic classification of the lesion rather than on whether EBV is demonstrated; that is, therapy of a gastric carcinoma or Hodgkin's disease is not influenced by the presence or absence of EBV in the neoplasm. Sometimes the EBV is so characteristic of the lesion that identification of the virus may be useful as an adjunctive test when the diagnosis is based on limited clinical material. These situations include the diagnosis of nasopharyngeal carcinomas, differentiation of PTLD from rejection, and primary CNS lymphomas in the setting of immunosuppression. EBV is generally in a latent state in lymphomas, carcinomas, and PTLD. The extent of viral gene expression is limited and varies according to the state of latency.[2] EBNA-1 is the only antigen consistently expressed in all states of latency. EBNA may be detected by immunofluorescence but requires well-preserved fresh or frozen samples. To date, immunohistochemical techniques applicable to formalin-fixed paraffin-embedded sections have not been identified for EBNA. This problem limits the usefulness of immunohistochemistry as a screening tool for latent EBV in routine diagnostic samples. The limits of immunohistochemistry make molecular methods for the detection of EBV in clinical specimens attractive, and Southern blot hybridization, polymerase chain reaction, and in situ hybridization methods are all valid alternatives.[3,72]

Southern blot hybridization requires well-preserved fresh material for extraction of intact DNA. This method not only identifies the virus, but also when probing for viral terminal repeats, the clonality of the virus can be determined.[73–75] The Southern blot assay may also be used to differentiate between the two types of EBV based on differences in the EBNA-2 and EBNA-3 genes.

Polymerase chain reaction (PCR) assays have the advantage of improved sensitivity when compared to Southern blot assays. PCR may also be performed on very limited samples and fixed samples that cannot be assayed by Southern blot.[76–78] Both PCR and Southern blot assays, however, lose the morphologic context and cannot identify which cells contain the EBV genomes. Detection of EBV in neoplastic or cytologically atypical cells has a different implication than the detection of EBV in reactive lymphocytes surrounding the neoplasm. The first implicates EBV as active in the lesion, while the latter raises the possibility of asymptomatic latent infection.

For these reasons in situ hybridization assays have been particularly useful in the investigation of EBV-associated malignancies. Until recently, most EBV assays utilized a repetitive region of the EBV genome as the probe. This fragment, designated *Bam*HI W, is unique to EBV and is in multiple copies in the viral genome. Genomic DNA targets are stable to processing and resistant to ubiquitous RNases. The signal is in the nucleus and provides a rough guide to viral copy number. During latent infection, however, the number of viral copies per cell can be low, and many give a false-negative result.

Increased sensitivity may be achieved when products of genomic transcription are used as a target; for each genome, multiple mRNA copies may be synthesized, providing a natural biologic amplification of the target. The advantage of this amplification must be balanced by the extreme lability of mRNA. The discovery of two short transcripts in latently infected EBV cells of unknown function but high abundance has improved the sensitivity. These transcripts are products of RNA polymerase III, the polymerase that makes tRNA. They are referred to as *EBERs* (Epstein–Barr-encoded RNAs) and are approximately 170 bases. The EBERs are highly transcribed in latent EBV infection, more than 10^6 copies/cell, but not detected in purely productive infections. The combination of high copy number and high secondary structure results in an RNA target that is reliably present in routinely processed tissues. EBER tran-

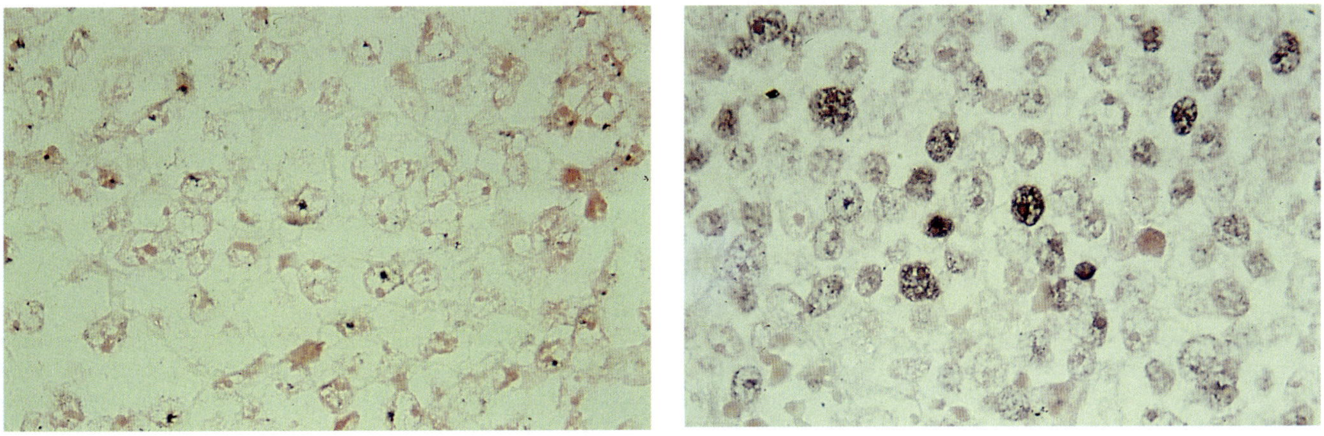

A B

Figure 11–11. Effect of probe selection on the sensitivity of in situ hybridization. Serial sections of the same formalin-fixed paraffin-embedded block of a post-transplantation lymphoproliferative disorder are hybridized for EBV genetic information. (Detection is with alkaline phosphatase and BCIP/NBT. Nuclear fast red counterstain, ×1000.) (**A**) Here the probe is directed against the repetitive *Bam*HI W genome target. Signal is visible as small nuclear dots. (**B**) Here the probe is directed against EBER-1, an RNA target that is highly transcribed in latent EBV infection. Signal is visible as diffuse nuclear stain with sparing of nucleolus. Except for the rare instances of purely productive EBV infection, in situ hybridization directed against EBER is more sensitive.

scripts are localized in the nucleus of infected cells. The difference in sensitivity between using the repetitive genomic region and EBER as a target is illustrated in Figure 11–11.

REFERENCES

1. Epstein MA, Achong BG, Barr YM. Virus particles in cultured lymphoblasts from Burkitt's lymphoma. *Lancet.* 1964;i:702–703.
2. Rowe M, Rowe DT, Gregory CD, et al. Differences in B cell growth phenotype reflect novel patterns of Epstein–Barr virus latent gene expression in Burkitt's lymphoma cells. *EMBO J.* 1987;6:2743–2751.
3. Ambinder RF, Mann RB. Detection and characterization of Epstein–Barr virus in clinical specimens. *Am J Pathol.* 1994;145:239–251.
4. Dambaugh TK, Hennessy S, Fennewald S, et al. The virus genome and its expression in latent infection In: Epstein MA, Achong BG, eds. *The Epstein–Barr Virus: Recent Advances.* London: W. Heinemann Medical Books; 1986:13.
5. Sixbey JW, Nedrud JG, Raab-Traub N, et al. Epstein–Barr virus replication in oropharyngeal epithelial cells. *N Engl J Med.* 1984;310:1225–1230.
6. Fingeroth JD, Weis JJ, Tedder TF, et al. Epstein–Barr virus receptor of human B lymphocytes is the C3d receptor CR2. *Proc Natl Acad Sci USA.* 1984;81:4510–4514.
7. Menezes J, Jondal M, Leibold W, et al. Epstein–Barr virus interactions with human lymphocyte subpopulations, virus adsorptions, kinetics of expression of Epstein–Barr virus-associated nuclear antigen, and lymphocyte transformation. *Infect Immun.* 1976;13:303–310.
8. Robinson JE, Miller G. Biology of lymphoid cells transformed by Epstein–Barr virus. In: Roizman B, ed. *The Herpesviruses.* New York: Plenum Press; 1982:151.
9. Cohen JI, Picchio GR, Mosier DE. Epstein–Barr virus nuclear protein 2 is a critical determinant for tumor growth in SCID mice and transformation in vitro. *J Virol.* 1992;66:7555–7559.
10. Purtilo DT. X-linked lymphoproliferative disease (XLP) as a model of Epstein–Barr virus-induced immunopathology. *Springer Semin Immunopathol.* 1991;13:181–197.
11. Thorley-Lawson DA. The transformation of adult but not newborn human lymphocytes by Epstein–Barr virus and phytohemagglutinin is inhibited by interferon: the early suppression by T cells of Epstein–Barr virus infection is mediated by interferon. *J Immunol.* 1981;126:829–833.
12. Zarling JM, Eskra L, Borden EC, et al. Activation of human natural killer cells cytotoxic for human leukemia cells by purified interferon. *J Immunol.* 1979;123:63–70.
13. Tosato G, Magrath J, Koski J, et al. Activation of suppressor T cells during Epstein–Barr-virus-induced infectious mononucleosis. *N Engl J Med.* 1979;301:1133–1137.
14. Pearson GR, Orr TW. Antibody-dependent lymphocyte cytotoxicity against cells expressing Epstein–Barr virus antigens. *J Natl Cancer Inst.* 1976;56:485–488.
15. Henle W, Henle G, Andersson J, et al. Antibody responses to Epstein–Barr virus-determined nuclear antigen (EBNA)-1 and EBNA-2 in acute and chronic Epstein–Barr virus infection. *Proc Natl Acad Sci USA.* 1987;84:570–574.
16. Purtilo DT, Stevenson M. Lymphotropic viruses as etiologic agents of lymphoma. *Hematol Oncol Clin North Am.* 1991;5:901–923.
17. Henle G, Henle W, Horwitz CA. Antibodies to Epstein–Barr virus-associated nuclear antigen in infectious mononucleosis. *J Infect Dis.* 1974;130:231–239.

18. Evans AS. Infectious mononucleosis and related syndrome. *Am J Med Sci.* 1978;276:325–339.
19. Linder J, Purtilo DT. Burkitt lymphoma. In: Purtilo DT, ed. *Immune Deficiency and Cancer: Epstein–Barr Virus and Lymphoproliferative Malignancies.* New York: Plenum Press; 1984:699.
20. Staal SP, Ambinder R, Beschorner WE, et al. A survey of Epstein–Barr virus DNA in lymphoid tissue: frequent detection in Hodgkin's disease. *Am J Clin Pathol.* 1989; 91:1–5.
21. Anagnostopoulos I, Herbst H, Niedobitek G, et al. Demonstration of monoclonal EBV genomes in Hodgkin's disease and Ki-1 positive anaplastic large cell lymphoma by combined Southern blot and in situ hybridization. *Blood.* 1989;74:810–816.
22. Ambinder RF, Browning PJ, Lorenzana I, et al. Epstein–Barr virus and childhood Hodgkin's disease in Honduras and the United States. *Blood.* 1993;81:462–467.
23. Chang KL, Albujar PF, Chen YY, et al. High prevalence of Epstein–Barr virus in the Reed–Sternberg cells of Hodgkin's disease occurring in Peru. *Blood.* 1993;81: 496–501.
24. Khan G, Norton AJ, Slavin G. Epstein–Barr virus in Hodgkin's disease—relationship to age and subtype. *Cancer.* 1993;71:3124–3129.
25. Jarrett RF, Gallagher A, Jones DB, et al. Detection of Epstein–Barr virus genomes in Hodgkin's disease: relation to age. *J Clin Pathol.* 1991;44:844–848.
26. Su I, Hsieh H, Lin K, et al. Aggressive peripheral T-cell lymphomas containing Epstein–Barr viral DNA: a clinicopathologic and molecular analysis. *Blood.* 1991;77: 799–808.
27. Harabuchi Y, Yamanaka N, Kataura A, et al. Epstein–Barr virus in nasal T-cell lymphomas in patients with lethal midline granuloma. *Lancet.* 1990;335:128–130.
28. Lee SH, Su IJ, Chen RL, et al. A pathologic study of childhood lymphoma in Taiwan with special reference to peripheral T-cell lymphoma and the association with Epstein–Barr viral infection. *Cancer.* 1991;68:1954–1962.
29. Tokunaga M, Imai S, Uemura Y, et al. Epstein–Barr virus in adult T-cell leukemia/lymphoma. *Am J Pathol.* 1993; 143:1263–1269.
30. Chen C, Sadler RH, Walling DM, et al. Epstein–Barr virus (EBV) gene expression in EBV-positive peripheral T-cell lymphomas. *J Virol.* 1993;67:6303–6308.
31. Borisch B, Henning I, Laeng RH, et al. Association of the subtype 2 of the Epstein–Barr virus with T-cell non-Hodgkin's lymphoma of the midline granuloma type. *Blood.* 1993;82:858–864.
32. Kanavaros P, Lescs MC, Briere J, et al. Nasal T-cell lymphoma: a clinicopathologic entity associated with peculiar phenotype and with Epstein–Barr virus. *Blood.* 1993; 81:2688–2695.
33. Guarner J, del Rio C, Hendrix L, et al. Composite Hodgkin's and non-Hodgkin's lymphoma in a patient with AIDS. In situ demonstration of Epstein–Barr virus. *Cancer.* 1990;66:796–800.
34. Guarner J, del Rio C, Carr D, et al. Non-Hodgkin's lymphomas in patients with HIV infection. Presence of Epstein–Barr virus by in-situ hybridization, clinical presentation and follow-up. *Cancer.* 1991;68:2460–2465.
35. Shibata D, Tokunaga M, Uemura Y, et al. Association of Epstein–Barr virus with undifferentiated gastric carcinomas with intense lymphoid infiltration. Lymphoepithelioma-like carcinoma. *Am J Pathol.* 1991;139:467–474.
36. Hamilton-Dutoit SJ, Rea D, Raphael M, et al. Epstein–Barr virus latent gene expression and tumor cell phenotype in AIDS-related non-Hodgkin's lymphoma. *Am J Pathol.* 1993;143:1072–1085.
37. Hamilton-Dutoit SJ, Pallesen G, Franzmann MB, et al. AIDS-related lymphoma: histopathology, immunophenotype, and association with Epstein–Barr virus as demonstrated by in situ nucleic acid hybridization. *Am J Pathol.* 1991;138:149–163.
38. Bashir RM, Harris NL, Hochberg FH, et al. Detection of Epstein–Barr virus in CNS lymphomas by in situ hybridization. *Neurology.* 1989;39:813–817.
39. MacMahon EME, Glass JD, Hayward SD, et al. Epstein–Barr virus in AIDS-related primary central nervous system lymphoma. *Lancet.* 1991;338:969–973.
40. zur Hausen H, Schulte-Holthausen H, Klein G, et al. EBV DNA in biopsies of Burkitt's tumors and anaplastic carcinoma of the nasopharynx. *Nature.* 1970;228:1056–1058.
41. De-The G. Epidemiology of Epstein–Barr virus and associated diseases in man. In: Roizman B, ed. *The Herpesviruses.* New York: Plenum Press; 1982:25.
42. Gal AA, Unger ER, Koss MN, et al. Detection of Epstein–Barr virus in lymphoepithelioma-like carcinoma of lung. *Mod Pathol.* 1991;4:264–268.
43. Oda K, Tamaru J, Takenouchi T, et al. Association of Epstein–Barr virus with gastric carcinoma with lymphoid stroma. *Am J Pathol.* 1993;143:1063–1071.
44. Hamilton-Dutoit SJ, Therkildsen MH, Nielsen NH, et al. Undifferentiated carcinoma of the salivary gland in Greenlandic Eskimos: demonstration of Epstein–Barr virus DNA by in situ nucleic acid hybridization. *Hum Pathol.* 1991; 22:811–815.
45. Raab-Traub N, Rajadurai P, Flynn K, et al. Epstein–Barr virus infection in carcinoma of the salivary gland. *J Virol.* 1991;65:7032–7036.
46. Mann RB, Wu T, Ling Y, et al. In situ localization of EBV in thymic carcinoma. *Mod Pathol.* 1992;5:363–366.
47. Tokunaga M, Land CE, Uemura Y, et al. Epstein–Barr virus in gastric carcinoma. *Am J Pathol.* 1993;143:1250–1254.
48. Isaacs R. Chronic infectious mononucleosis. *Blood.* 1948; 3:858–861.
49. DuBois RE, Seeley JK, Brus I, et al. Chronic mononucleosis syndrome. *Southern Med J.* 1984;77:1376.
50. Jones J, Ray C, Minnich L, et al. Evidence for active Epstein–Barr virus infection in patients with persistent unexplained illness: elevated anti-early antigen antibodies. *Ann Int Med.* 1985;102:1–6.
51. Komaroff A. The "chronic mononucleosis" syndrome. *Hosp Pract.* 1987;22:71–75.
52. Straus S, Tosato G, Armstrong G, et al. Persisting illness and fatigue in adults with evidence of Epstein–Barr virus infection. *Ann Int Med.* 1985;102:7–16.
53. Tobi M, Straus S. Chronic Epstein–Barr virus disease: a

workshop held by the National Institute of Allergy and Infectious Disease. *Ann Int Med.* 1985;103:951–953.

54. Holmes GP, Kaplan JE, Stewart JA, et al. A cluster of patients with a chronic mononucleosis-like syndrome: is Epstein–Barr virus the cause? *JAMA.* 1987;257:2297–2302.
55. Purtilo DT, Cassel CK, Yang JPS, et al. X-linked recessive progressive combined variable immunodeficiency (Duncan's disease). *Lancet.* 1975;i:935–940.
56. Grierson H, Purtilo DT: Epstein–Barr virus infections in males with the X-linked lymphoproliferative disorder. *Ann Int Med.* 1987;106:538–545.
57. Harrington DS, Weisenburger DD, Purtilo DT. Malignant lymphoma in the X-linked lymphoproliferative syndrome. *Cancer.* 1987;59:1419–1429.
58. Ochs HD, Sullivan JL, Wedgewood RJ, et al. X-linked lymphoproliferative syndrome: abnormal antibody response to bacteriophage ΦX174. In: Wedgwood R, Rosen F, eds. *Primary Immunodeficiency Disease.* New York: Alan R. Liss; 1983:321.
59. Border E. Ataxia telangiectasia: some historic, clinical and pathologic observations. In: Bergsma D, Good RA, Feinstad J, eds. *Immunodeficiency in Man and Animals.* Baltimore: Williams & Wilkins; 1975:255.
60. Okano M, Osato T, Koizumi S, et al. Epstein–Barr virus infection and oncogenesis in primary immunodeficiency. *AIDS Res.* 1986;1(suppl 2):5115–5119.
61. Saemundsen AK, Berkel AI, Henle W, et al. Epstein–Barr virus carrying lymphoma in a patient with ataxia telangiectasia. *Br Med J.* 1981;282:425–427.
62. Merino F, Klein G, Henle W, et al. Elevated antibody titers to Epstein–Barr virus and low natural killer cell activity in patients with Chédiak–Higashi syndrome. *Clin Immunol Immunopathol.* 1983;27:326–339.
63. Okano M, Mizuno F, Osato T, et al. Wiskott–Aldrich syndrome and Epstein–Barr virus-induced lymphoproliferation. *Lancet.* 1984;ii:933–934.
64. Reece ER, Gartner JG, Seemayer TA, et al. Epstein–Barr virus in a malignant lymphoproliferative disorder of B-cells occurring after thymic epithelial transplantation for combined immunodeficiency. *Cancer Res.* 1981;41:4243–4247.
65. Shearer WT, Ritz J, Finegold M, et al. Epstein–Barr virus-associated B-cell proliferations of diverse clonal origins after bone marrow transplantation in a 12-year-old patient with severe combined immunodeficiency. *N Engl J Med.* 1985;312:1151–1159.
66. Hanto DW, Frizzera G, Gajl-Peczalska KJ, et al. Epstein–Barr virus, immunodeficiency, and B cell lymphoproliferation. *Transplantation.* 1985;39:461–472.
67. Hanto DW, Gajl-Peczalska KJ, Kazimiera J, et al. Epstein–Barr virus (EBV) induced polyclonal and monoclonal B-cell lymphoproliferative diseases occurring after renal transplantation. *Ann Surg.* 1983;198:356–369.
68. Greenspan JS, Greenspan D, Lennette ET, et al. Replication of Epstein–Barr virus within the epithelial cells of oral "hairy" leukoplakia, an AIDS-associated lesion. *N Engl J Med.* 1985;313:1564–1571.
69. Joshi VV, Kauffman S, Oleske JM, et al. Polyclonal polymorphic B-cell lymphoproliferative disorder with prominent pulmonary involvement in children with acquired immune deficiency syndrome. *Cancer.* 1987;59:1455–1462.
70. Sumaya CV, Boswell RN, Ench E, et al. Epstein–Barr virus infectious mononucleosis in children. II. Heterophile antibody and viral-specific responses. *Pediatrics.* 1985;75:1011–1019.
71. Luka J, Chase RC, Pearson GR. A sensitive enzyme-linked immunosorbent assay (ELISA) against major EBV-associated antigens. I. Correlation between ELISA and immunofluorescence titers using purified antigens. *J Immunol Meth.* 1984;67:145–156.
72. Ambinder RF, Mann RB. Epstein–Barr-encoded RNA in situ hybridization: diagnostic applications. *Hum Pathol.* 1994;25:602–605.
73. Gulley ML, Raphael M, Lutz CT, et al. Epstein–Barr virus integration in human lymphomas and lymphoid cell lines. *Cancer.* 1992;70:185–191.
74. Katz BZ, Raab-Traub N, Miller G. Latent and replicating forms of Epstein–Barr virus DNA in lymphomas and lymphoproliferative diseases. *J Infect Dis.* 1989;160:589–597.
75. Gutierrez MI, Bhatia K, Magrath I. Replicative viral DNA in EBV-associated Burkitt's lymphoma biopsies. *Leukemia Res.* 1993;17:285–289.
76. Weiss LM, Chen YY, Liu XF, et al. Epstein–Barr virus and Hodgkin's disease: a correlative in situ hybridization and polymerase chain reaction study. *Am J Pathol.* 1991;139:1259–1265.
77. Ambinder RF, Lambe BC, Mann RB, et al. Oligonucleotides for polymerase chain reaction amplification and hybridization detection of Epstein–Barr virus DNA in clinical specimens. *Mol Cell Probes.* 1990;4:397–407.
78. Rogers BB, Alpert LC, Hine EA, et al. Analysis of DNA in fresh and fixed tissue by the polymerase chain reaction. *Am J Pathol.* 1990;136:541–548.

CHAPTER 12

Hantavirus-Associated Diseases

Sherif R. Zaki

This sickness doth infect
The very life-blood of our enterprise.

William Shakespeare (1564–1616), King Henry IV, Part I, Act III

INTRODUCTION

The isolation of the first recognized hantavirus (Hantaan virus), named for the river in South Korea, and its subsequent identification as the causative agent of hemorrhagic fever with renal syndrome (HFRS) was reported in 1978.[1] This relatively recent discovery belies the long history of hantaviral disease, probably first described by the Chinese as early as 960 A.D.[2] In the 1930s, Russian and Japanese physicians independently reported annual outbreaks of similar clinical syndromes named for different geographic localities where the outbreaks occurred.[3] A relatively milder form of the disease, now known as nephropathia epidemica, affected German and Finnish troops stationed in Lapland during World War I.[4] The disease gained global attention in the 1950s during the Korean conflict when thousands of United Nations military personnel contracted a hantaviral illness now known as Korean hemorrhagic fever. These diverse clinical syndromes all share various degrees of fever and renal involvement, with or without hemorrhagic manifestations, and are referred to collectively as HFRS in accordance with World Health Organization recommendations.[5] In the summer of 1993, the deaths of several previously healthy individuals caused by a rapidly progressive respiratory disease in the southwestern United States was causally linked to a previously unrecognized hantavirus. Clinically, the disease differs from HFRS in its pronounced pulmonary involvement and higher mortality rates and has become known as the hantavirus pulmonary syndrome (HPS).[6–9]

DEFINITION

Hantaviral diseases in humans are caused by a group of closely related, trisegmented, negative-sense RNA viruses of the genus *Hantavirus,* of the family *Bunyaviridae.*[10–12] The type and severity of disease depends largely on the serotype of the virus involved. Two classes of hantavirus-associated illnesses have been described: HFRS for disease in which the kidneys are primarily involved and HPS for disease in which the lungs are primarily affected.[8,13,14]

GEOGRAPHIC DISTRIBUTION AND EPIDEMIOLOGY

All recognized hantaviruses are zoonotic, and several distinct serotypes are distributed throughout the world (Table 12–1). Each hantavirus is maintained in nature by asymptomatic infection of rodents, and humans usually acquire the disease after inhalation of infectious rodent excreta or, in very rare instances, by the bites of rodents.[4,15,16] No human-to-human transmission or nosocomial outbreaks among health care workers have been documented. Epidemiologic studies of HFRS and HPS indicate that transmission is associated with exposure to rodents in and around the home, while performing agricultural activities, cleaning animal sheds, sleeping on the ground, and with certain occupations.[9,17–21] Natural population cycles of rodents, environmental factors, and certain human behaviors result in distinctive seasonal patterns of disease.[2]

TABLE 12–1. CHARACTERISTICS OF THE KNOWN HANTAVIRUSES

Virus	Geographic Region	Reservoir	Clinical Syndrome	Pathology	Mortality (%)
Hantaan	Asia	*Apodemus agrarius* (striped field mouse)	Severe HFRS	Renal	5–15
Dobrava	Balkans	*A flavivollis* (yellow-necked field mouse)	Severe HFRS	Renal	About 15[a]
Seoul	Worldwide	*Rattus norvegicus, R rattus*	Moderate HFRS	Renal	1
Puumala	Northern Europe	*Clethrionomys glareolus* (bank vole)	Mild HFRS (nephropathia epidemica)	Renal	1
Prospect Hill	United States	*Microtus pennsylvanicus* (meadow vole)	Unknown	Unknown	—
Sin Nombre	North America	*Peromyscus maniculatis* (deer mouse)	HPS	Pulmonary	52

[a] To date, although relatively few cases have been reported, the mortality rates appear to be even greater than in Asia. In one preliminary study, mortality rates of up to 35% have been reported.

As a group, hantaviral infections are worldwide, but different clinical syndromes are more or less confined to definite geographic areas and transmitted by one or more specific rodents (Table 12–1).[16,22,23] Hantaan (HTN) virus causes the most severe and often fatal form of HFRS, known as Korean hemorrhagic fever (KHF) in Korea and epidemic hemorrhagic fever in Japan and China. In the Balkan nations, another severe form of HFRS caused by the Dobrava (DOB) virus has been described. Seoul (SEO) virus, which is worldwide, causes a less severe form of the disease and has been diagnosed most frequently in Asia. Puumula (PUU) virus causes the mildest form of HFRS, namely nephropathia epidemica, in Scandinavia and Western Europe. Prospect Hill (PH) virus is indigenous to the United States, but has not been associated with human disease. Infections with Sin Nombre virus (SNV) and other closely related viruses have been recently linked to HPS, which, as noted previously, is a respiratory illness that follows a much more aggressive course with higher mortality rates than HFRS.[7–9,24–26]

MORPHOLOGY OF HANTAVIRUSES

Members of the genus *Hantavirus* have similar morphologic features.[3,27–29] Virus particles are 70 to 120 nm in diameter and generally appear spherical to oval, although pleomorphic forms may be seen. A lipid envelope containing glycoprotein spikes surrounds a core of the genome and its associated proteins (nucleocapsids) arranged in delicate tangles of filaments showing occasional granulation (Figure 12–1, A). Characteristic inclusion bodies in thin section electron microscopy (EM) and a unique grid-like pattern on negative-stain EM distinguish these viruses from other members of the family *Bunyaviridae* (Figure 12–1, B and C).[30,31]

CLINICAL FEATURES

The initial symptoms of HFRS and HPS are similar and resemble those in early phases of many other viral infections.[8,9,32–35] Fever, myalgias, headache, vomiting, weakness, and cough are common in early HFRS and HPS. In patients with HFRS, the febrile phase is followed by hypotension and oliguria. Hemorrhage, at least at the level of petechiae, occurs in at least one third of patients with HFRS due to PUU virus, whereas virtually all patients with HFRS associated with HTN virus have petechiae and most have severe hemostatic difficulties.[36,37] Renal involvement is in all patients with HFRS, and the clinical presentation ranges from a mild illness with minimal renal dysfunction to a more severe form with acute renal failure and shock. Recovery is usually complete, with no apparent long-term sequelae. Mortality rates for HFRS range from 1% to 15%, with shock and uremia being the main contributing causes of death, although pulmonary edema has been implicated in about 15% of patients.[38,39] Only HFRS patients who die during the later phases of renal failure typically show significant pulmonary edema. Severe pulmonary edema may be seen occasionally early in the course of HFRS, but therapeutic overhydration may be a factor in these patients.[33,34,40,41]

The clinical picture for HPS caused by infection with SNV is quite different from that for HFRS (Table 12–2).[8,9] The initial prodrome is followed by a rapidly

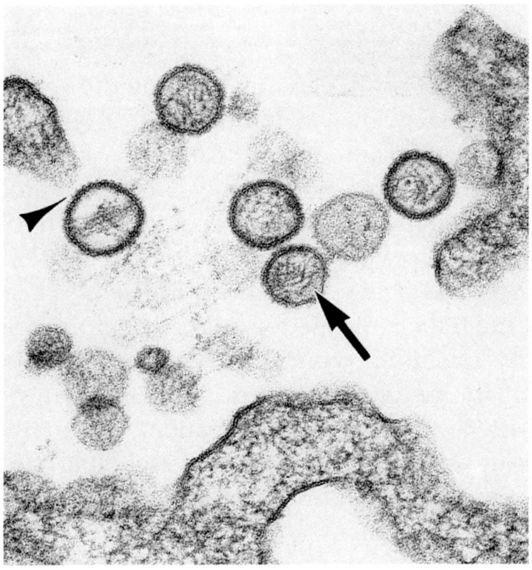

A

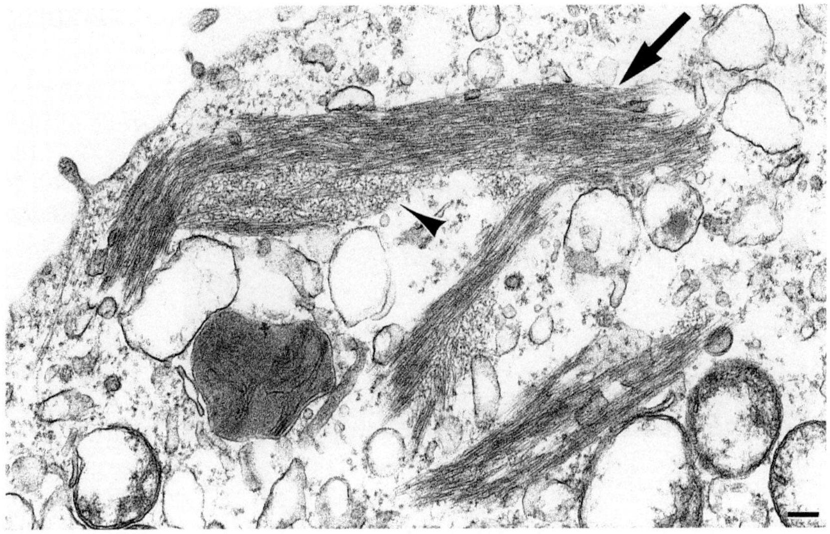

B

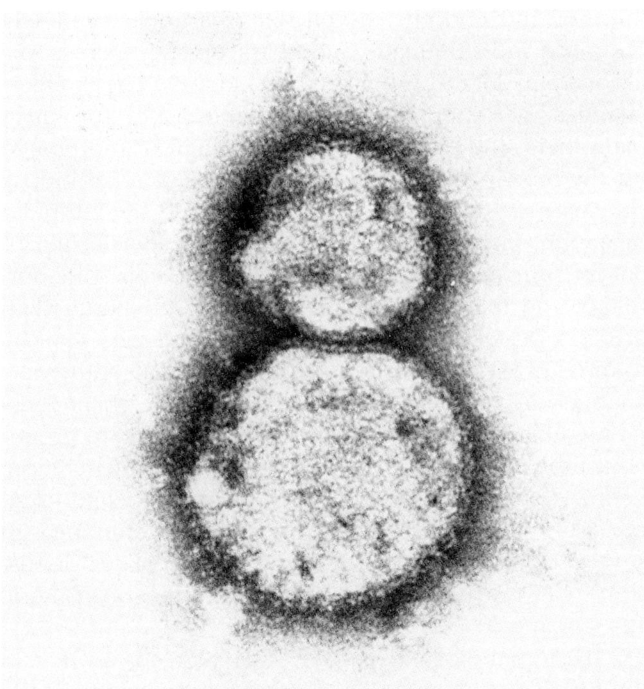

C

Figure 12–1. Sin Nombre virus (genus *Hantavirus*). (**A**) Virus as seen in thin section EM of Vero E6-infected cells. The envelope, which contains small surface spikes *(arrowhead),* surrounds a core containing nucleocapsids arranged in filaments *(arrow).* (**B**) Typical hantaviral inclusions in thin section EM of Vero E6-infected cells. Note both granular *(arrowhead)* and filamentous *(arrow)* forms of inclusions. (**C**) Characteristic grid-like pattern of hantavirus in negative stain EM. (Scale bars: A, B, C = 100 nm.) *(A and B photographs contributed by Cynthia Goldsmith and Dr. Charles Humphrey.)*

progressive pulmonary edema, respiratory insufficiency, and shock, with mortality rates exceeding 50%. The majority of deaths are within 2 days of hospitalization. Although chest radiographs may be normal early in HPS, interstitial edema develops in a majority of patients within 48 hours of admission (Figure 12–2, A and B).[42] Hemorrhages and peripheral signs of vasomotor instability, such as flushing, conjunctival injection, and periorbital edema as seen in HFRS, are extremely uncommon.[8,9]

Laboratory findings in hantavirus-associated illnesses include hemoconcentration, thrombocytopenia, leukocytosis with a left shift, and atypical lymphocytosis.[8,9,32,43] About 50% of patients with HPS can have proteinuria, but it is usually mild compared with the more severe proteinuria seen in most HFRS patients. Laboratory evidence of disseminated intravascular coagulation has been reported in both HFRS and HPS.[9,37]

TABLE 12–2. COMPARISON OF HFRS AND HPS

Characteristic	Hemorrhagic Fever with Renal Syndrome (HFRS)	Hanatavirus Pulmonary Syndrome (HPS)
Major target organ	Kidney	Lung
Secondary target organs	Lung, brain, liver	Kidney?, Heart?
First-phase clinical illness	Febrile	Febrile = "prodrome"
Second-phase clinical illness	Shock	Shock, pulmonary edema
Evolution of clinical illness	Oliguria, polyuria, convalescence	Recovery
Mortality	1–15%	52%

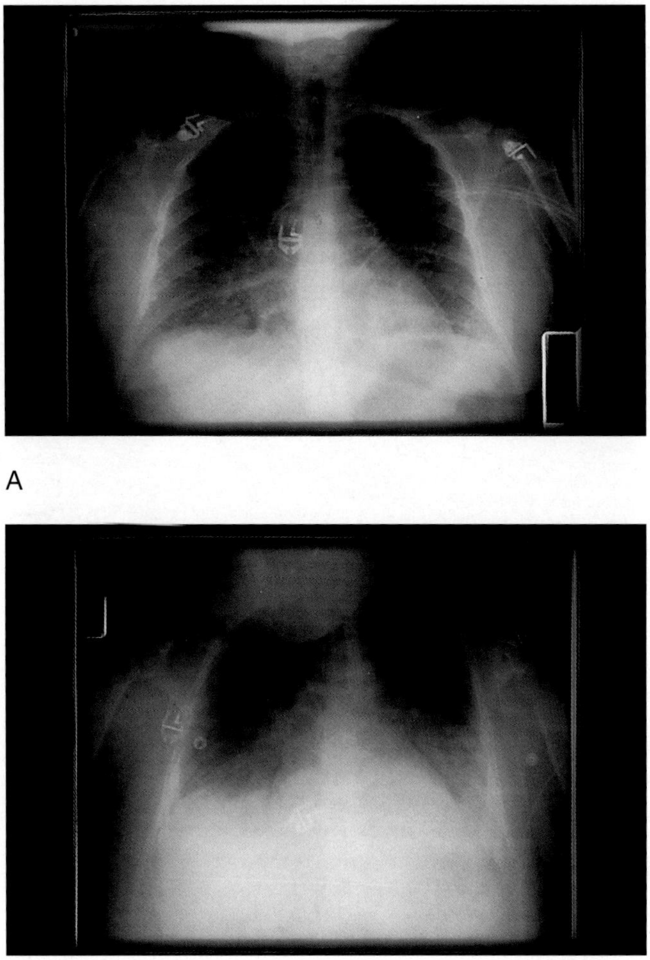

A

B

Figure 12–2. (**A**), (**B**) Serial radiographs obtained over 48 hours in a patient with hantavirus pulmonary syndrome. *(Photographs contributed by Dr. L. H. Ketai, University of New Mexico.)*

The onset of significant clinical symptoms in hantaviral infections is temporally associated with the emergence of a specific immune response, and hantaviral antigens have been detected in vascular endothelia of patients with fatal HPS and HFRS.[9,44] Thus, increased vascular permeability—the hallmark of the pathologic events of HPS and HFRS—most likely stems from endothelial damage and dysfunction. Because pulmonary edema is an uncommon feature in HFRS, the primary target organ appears to differ in the two syndromes, with the retroperitoneal compartment, including the kidneys, primarily involved in HFRS and the lungs in HPS. It is unclear how the shock in these infections relates to factors such as viral distribution and immunologic and pharmacologic mediators of capillary permeability.[9]

PATHOLOGY

The pathologic lesions of hantavirus-associated diseases are primarily vascular with variable degrees of generalized capillary dilatation and edema. Large quantities of protein-rich, gelatinous retroperitoneal edema fluid accumulate in the hypotensive phase of severe HFRS, whereas all patients with HPS have large bilateral pleural effusions and heavy edematous lungs.[40,45–47] In fatal Far Eastern HFRS, a distinctive triad of hemorrhagic necrosis of the junctional zone of the renal medulla, right atrium of the heart, and anterior pituitary can be seen (Figure 12–3, A and D).[40,41] In patients with HPS, hemorrhages are exceedingly rare, and ischemic necrotic lesions, except those attributed to shock, are not seen.[9,45]

Microscopically, morphologic changes of the endothelium are uncommon and, when present, consist of prominent and swollen endothelial cells. Vascular thrombi and endothelial cell necrosis are exceedingly rare. The most dramatic and characteristic microscopic lesions in HFRS involve the kidney. The mildest changes are in nephropathia epidemica (NE), for which pathologic studies have been relatively few and limited for the most part to serial examinations of renal biopsy specimens.[48–53] Common changes include slight tubular dilatation, interstitial edema, diffuse but sparse interstitial inflammatory infiltrate, interstitial medullary hemorrhage, and mild hypercellularity of the glomeruli (Figure 12–4). Occasional necrotic tubular cells can be found. In HTN-associated HFRS, the renal pathologic changes are more severe; in addition to the characteristic medullary hemorrhage and edema, there are prominent tubular lesions, including dilatation, degeneration, necrosis, and sloughing of the tubular epithelium (Figure 12–3, B and C).[40,41] An interstitial pneumonitis in severe HFRS, similar to that of HPS (see later discussion), can be seen also in some fatal infections (Figure 12–3, E and F).

Histopathologic changes of HPS occur mainly in the lung and spleen.[9,45] Microscopic examination of the lungs, in most patients, reveals a mild to moderate interstitial pneumonitis with variable degrees of congestion, edema, and mononuclear cell infiltration. The cellular infiltrate is a mixture of small and enlarged mononuclear cells with the appearance of immunoblasts. There are focal hyaline membranes, as well as extensive intra-alveolar edema, fibrin, and variable numbers of inflammatory cells (Figure 12–5, A and B). In typical infections, neutrophils are scanty and the respiratory epithelium is intact with no evidence of cellular debris, nuclear fragmentation, or type II pneumocyte hyperplasia. In fatal infections where patients survive longer than average, there are more characteristic and typical

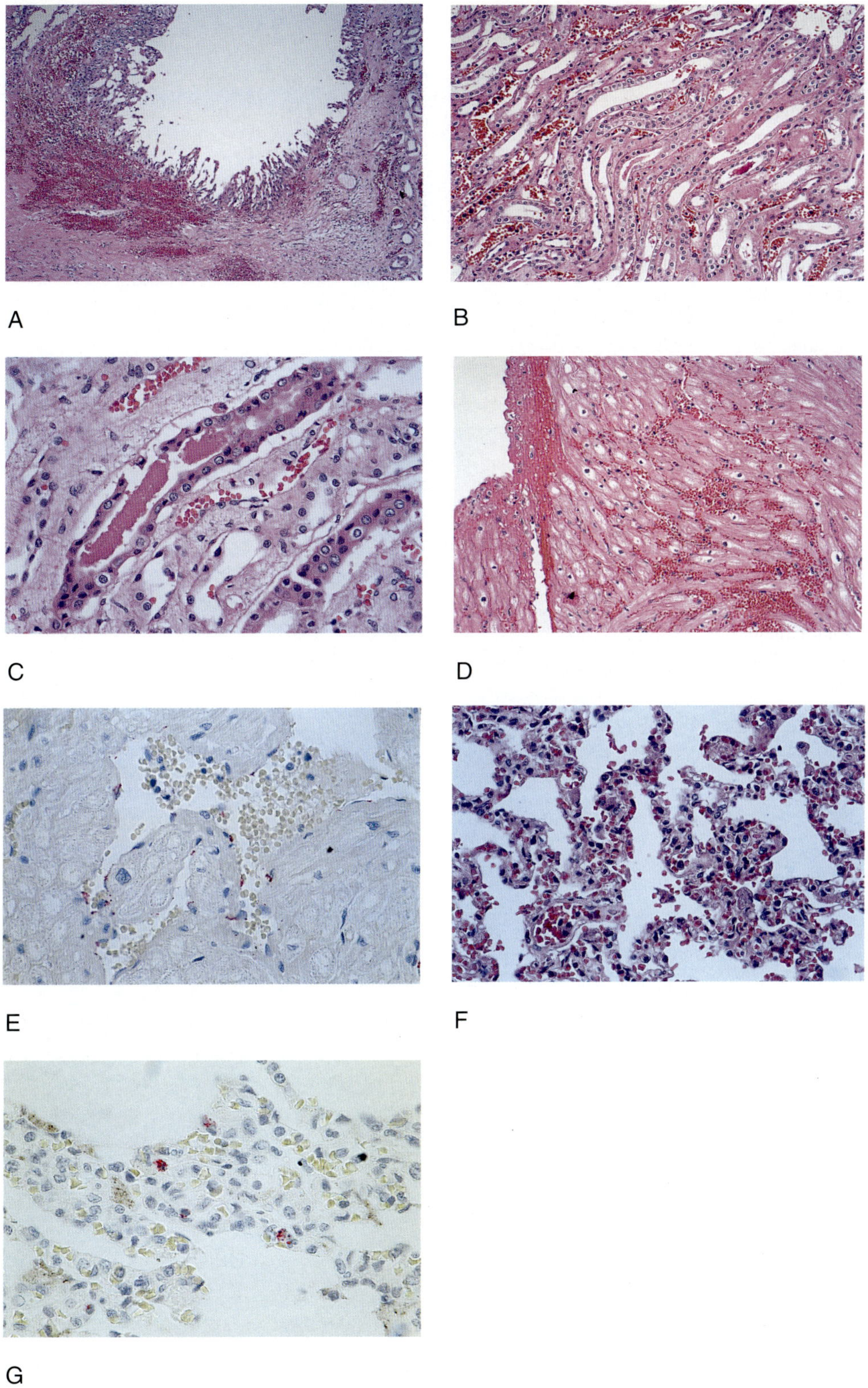

Figure 12–3. Severe hemorrhagic fever with renal syndrome (Korean hemorrhagic fever [KHF]). (**A**) Subepithelial hemorrhage and congestion in renal pelvis of patient with KHF. (**B**) Capillary congestion, patchy dilatation of tubules and slight interstitial edema in renal medulla. (**C**) High magnification showing interstitial edema and dilated tubules, one of which contains a cast with nuclear and cellular debris. Note variation in size, staining intensity, and location of nuclei within tubules. (**D**) Subendocardial hemorrhage and congestion in right atrium. (**E**) Several HTN antigen-positive endothelial cells lining the endocardium seen by immunohistochemistry (IHC). (**F**) Interstitial pneumonitis in KHF. Note thickening of alveolar septa by mononuclear cells and congested capillaries. (**G**) Focal staining of endothelial cells and macrophages in lung demonstrated by immunohistochemistry (hematoxylin-eosin, original magnifications: A, ×25; B, ×50; C, ×100; D, ×50; F, ×100; napthol fast red substrate with light hematoxylin counterstain, E, ×100; G ×158).

Figure 12–4. Mild hemorrhagic fever with renal syndrome (nephropathia epidemica). (**A**) Renal biopsy showing mild and patchy tubular dilatation, mild interstitial edema, focal inflammatory infiltrates, and occasional tubular casts. (**B**) Higher magnification showing slightly dilatated tubules with casts. The interstitium on the left is particularly loose, edematous, and contains a mononuclear cell infiltrate composed mainly of lymphocytes and plasma cells. (**C**) Glomerular capillaries in this biopsy specimen are slightly dilated, but there is no distinct proliferation of cells. The surrounding interstitium is slightly edematous. (**D**) Serial section of glomerulus in (**C**) showing immunostaining of PUU viral antigens in glomerular endothelium (hematoxylin-eosin, original magnifications: A, ×50; B, ×158; C, ×100; napthol fast red substrate with light hematoxylin counterstain, D, ×158).

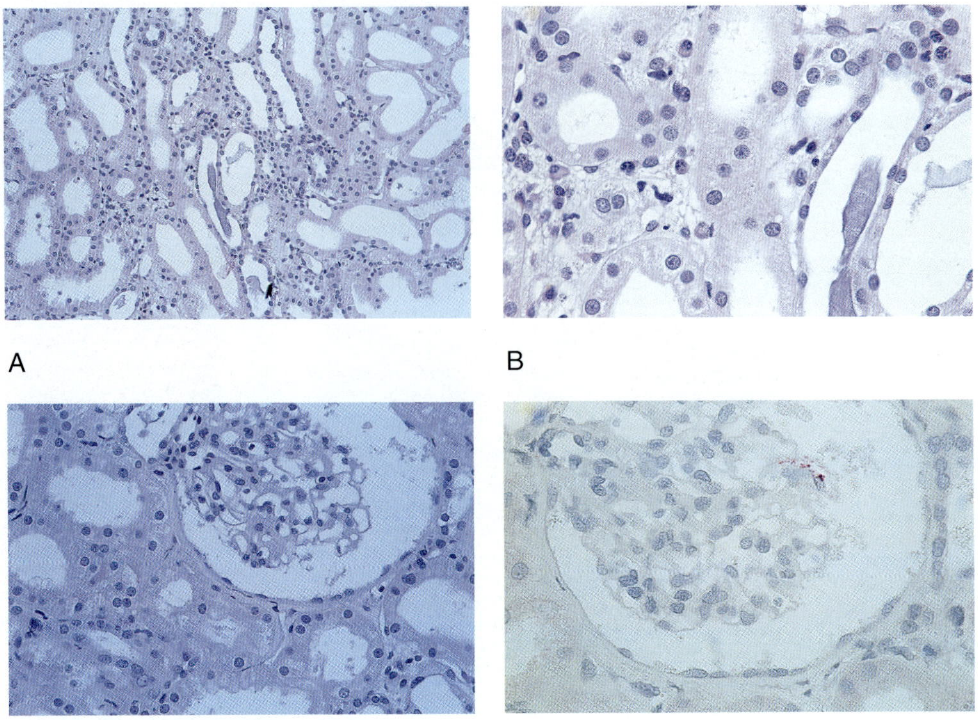

A B C D

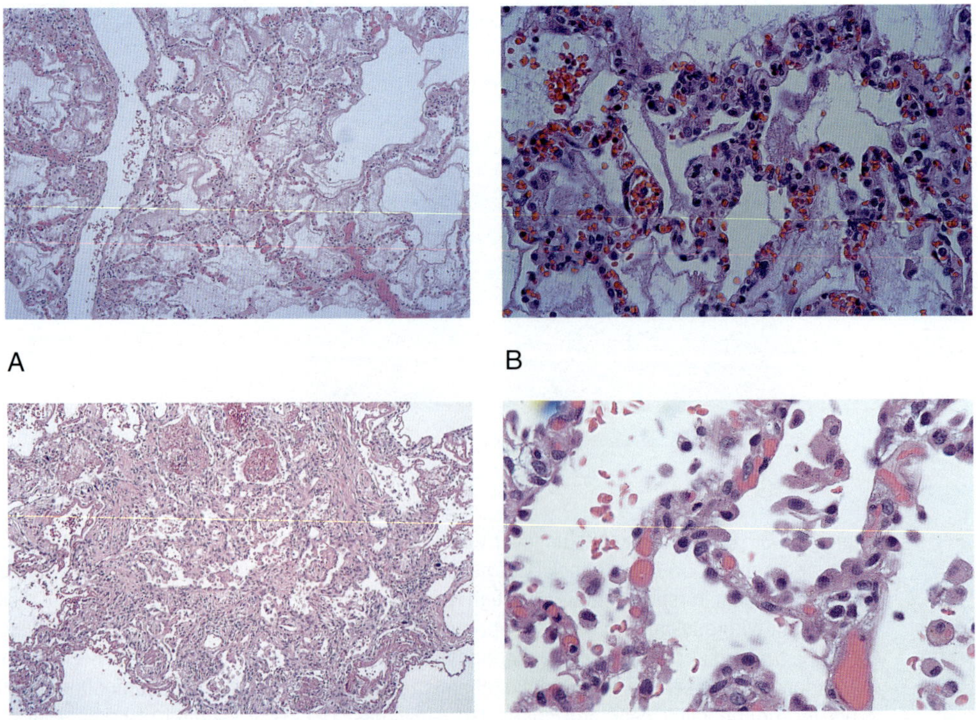

A B C D

Figure 12–5. Pulmonary histopathologic features of Hantavirus pulmonary syndrome (HPS). (**A**) Lung showing interstitial pneumonitis and intra-alveolar edema in typical case. (**B**) Higher magnification showing intra-alveolar fibrin deposits and mononuclear infiltrate. (**C**) Lung showing interstitial and alveolar fibrosis in an HPS patient who died on 19th day of illness. (**D**) Lung biopsy of an HPS patient who survived illness showing an alveolar septum with prominent type II pneumocyte proliferation (hematoxylin-eosin, original magnifications: A and C, ×25; B, ×100; D ×158).

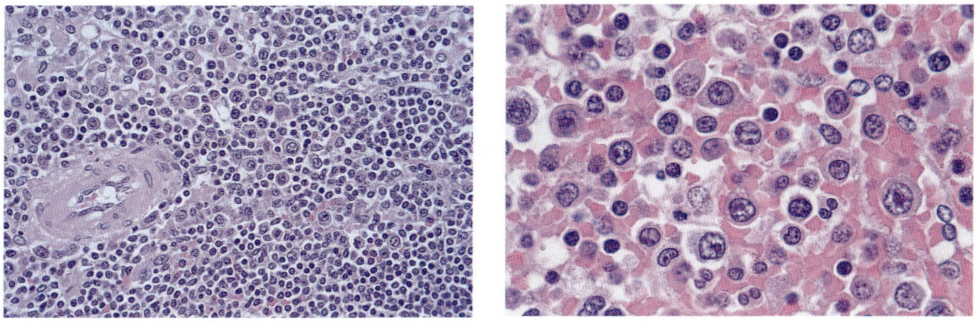

A B

Figure 12–6. Hantavirus pulmonary syndrome. (**A**) Spleen in which immunoblasts are seen in the periarteriolar sheath. (**B**) Higher magnification showing detailed features of immunoblasts. Note prominent nucleoli and high nuclear to cytoplasm ratio (hematoxylin-eosin, original magnifications: A, ×100; B, ×250).

histopathologic features of the exudative and proliferative stages of diffuse alveolar damage. Similar changes are observed in lung biopsies taken from patients who survive their illness. In these patients, proliferation of reparative type II pneumocytes, severe edematous and fibroblastic thickening of the alveolar septa with severe air space disorganization, and distortion of lung architecture can be seen (Figure 12–5, C and D). Other characteristic histopathologic findings in HPS include variable numbers of immunoblasts within red pulp and periarteriolar sheaths of the spleen and paracortex, within sinuses of lymph nodes, and in the peripheral blood (Figures 12–6 and 12–7). Similarly, large mononuclear cells can be in spleen, lymph nodes, blood, and hepatic portal triads in severe HFRS.[40,46]

Using immunohistochemistry (IHC), viral antigens are primarily in the endothelium of capillaries throughout various tissues in both HPS and HFRS (Figures 12–3, 12–4, and 12–8). In HPS, there are marked accumulations of hantaviral antigens in the pulmonary microvasculature and in follicular dendritic cells within the lymphoid follicles of spleen and lymph nodes.[9] In spite of extensive hantaviral IHC studies of patients, there is little evidence of cytopathic effect by electron microscopy. IHC of patients with HFRS also reveal hantaviral antigens in renal tubular epithelium. This suggests that acute renal failure, one of the primary clinical manifestations of HFRS, may be caused by direct viral infection of renal tubules. The absence of significant renal tubular staining in patients with HPS may explain why acute renal failure has not been a predominant finding in patients with HPS. Hantaviral nucleic acids can be localized also to endothelial and inflammatory cells in HPS tissues by using in situ hybridization (ISH) (Figure 12–9).

Electron microscope studies demonstrate infection of endothelial cells and macrophages in the lungs of patients with HPS.[9] The virus or virus-like particles in autopsy tissues are infrequent and difficult to identify because of the pleomorphism and also because of the deterioration of postmortem tissue (Figure 12–10). Typical hantaviral inclusions, however, are more frequent and their identity can be confirmed by immunolabeling (Figure 12–11). Similar inclusions are seen in epithelial cells of patients with HFRS and are thought to be ultrastructural markers of hantavirus-infected cells.[54–56]

DIAGNOSIS

HFRS should be considered in patients with fever and renal dysfunction or abdominal pain, especially among

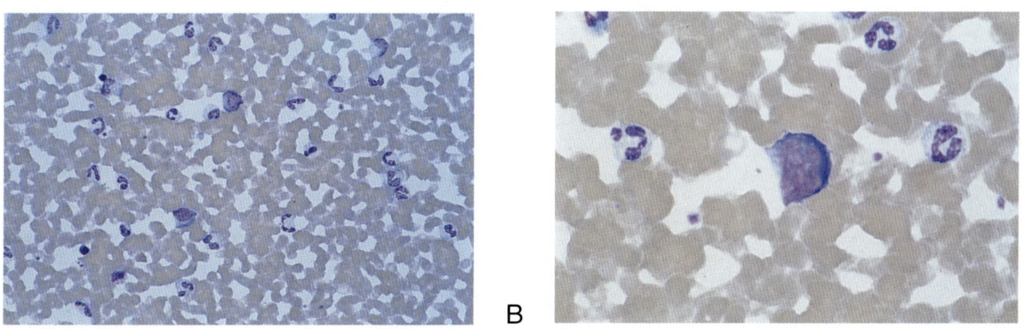

A B

Figure 12–7. Hantavirus pulmonary syndrome. (**A**) Peripheral blood smear showing marked hemoconcentration, leukocytosis with a left shift, thrombocytopenia, and circulating immunoblasts. (**B**) Immunoblast with deeply basophilic cytoplasm, high nuclear to cytoplasmic ratio, and prominent nucleoli as seen at higher magnification. Although characteristically seen in the spleen and peripheral blood, these cells can also be in the lung and lymph nodes of patients with HPS (Wright's stain, original magnifications: A, ×100; B, ×250).

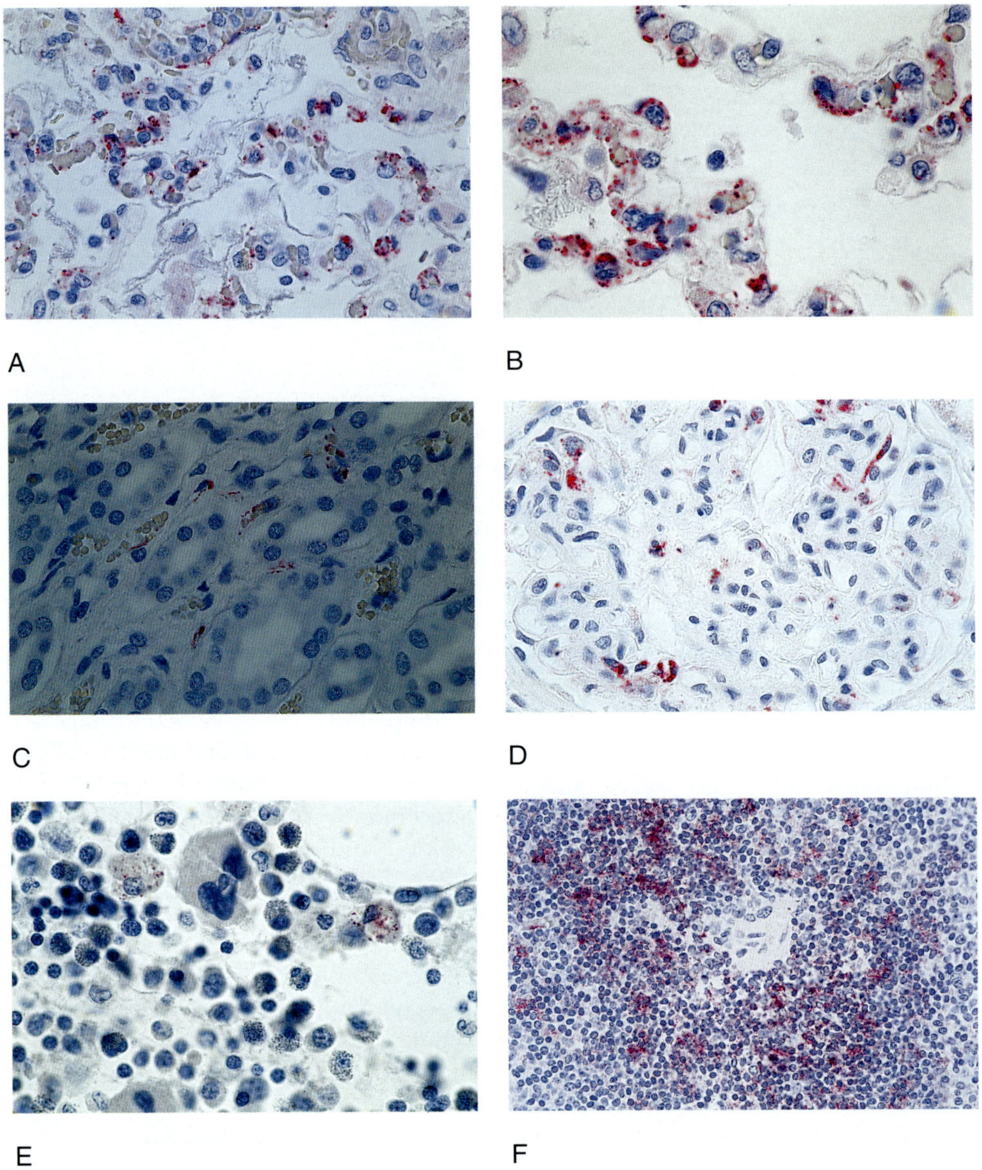

Figure 12–8. Hantavirus pulmonary syndrome. Immunostaining of hantaviral antigens in different organs as determined by IHC. (**A**) Low magnification of lung showing predominantly endothelial staining in pulmonary microvasculature. (**B**) High magnification showing fine granular immunostaining of SNV antigens along capillary walls. (**C**) Endothelial staining in interstitial capillaries of renal medulla. (**D**) SNV antigen immunostaining within renal glomerulus. (**E**) SNV antigen-positive macrophages in bone marrow. (**F**) Delicate reticular pattern of immuno staining of SNV antigens in lymphoid follicle of spleen (napthol fast red substrate with light hematoxylin counterstain, original magnifications: A, ×158; B, ×250; C and D, ×158; E, ×250; F, ×100).

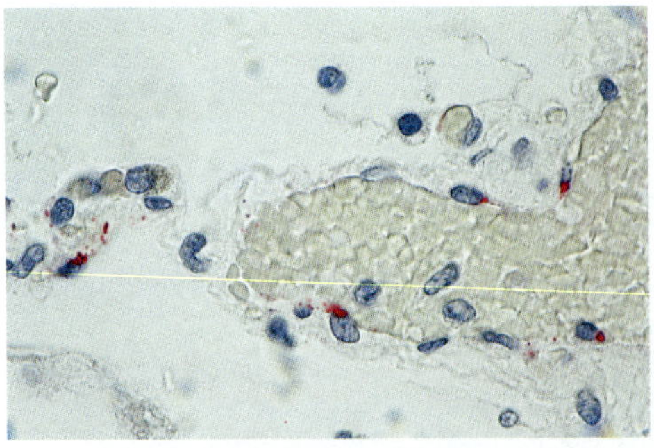

Figure 12–9. Hantavirus pulmonary syndrome. SNV-infected endothelial cells in lung by colorimetric in situ hybridization using digoxigenin-labeled probes (napthol fast red substrate with light hematoxylin counterstain, original magnification: ×250).

those living in, or traveling to, known HFRS-endemic areas. Diseases that can be confused with HFRS by clinical features include leptospirosis, rickettsial infections, and sepsis syndromes. The diagnosis of HPS should be suspected in patients with adult respiratory distress syndrome (ARDS) among previously healthy adults. The level of suspicion should be high when patients have been exposed to rodents in areas where *Peromyscus maniculatus* or other reservoirs of hantavirus are found, and when patients are from areas where other cases of HPS have been documented. Clinicians must distinguish HPS from other common acute respiratory illnesses such as pneumococcal pneumonia, influenza, and unexplained ARDS. Three clinical char-

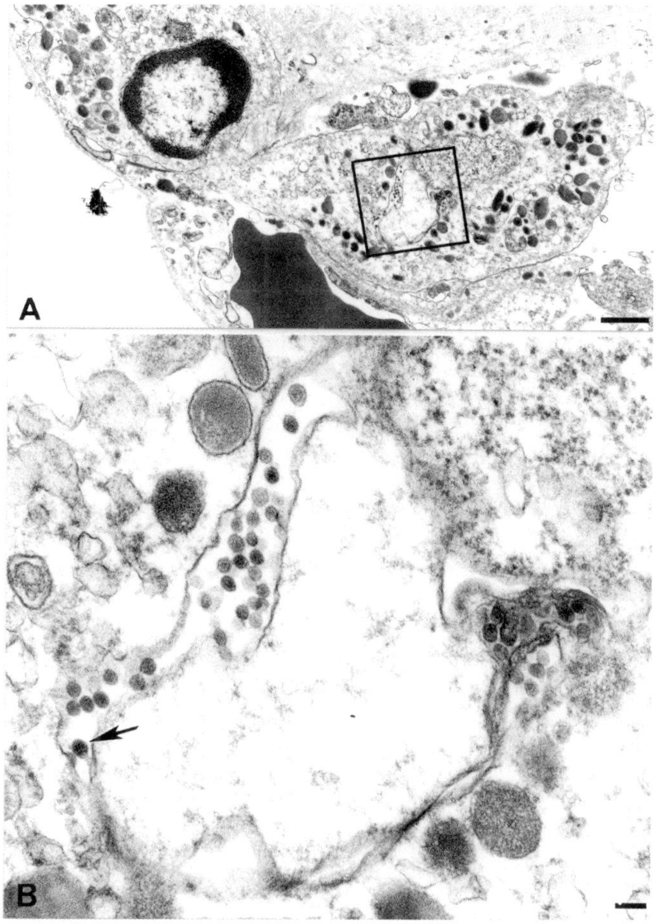

Figure 12–10. Hantavirus pulmonary syndrome. (**A**) Collection of viral-like particles in a pulmonary macrophage. (**B**) Higher magnification of boxed area showing several viral-like particles, including one budding particle *(arrow).* (Scale bars: A = 1 μm; B = 100 nm.) *(Photograph reproduced from Zaki et al*[9] *with permission of the* American Journal of Pathology.*)*

acteristics at admission (dizziness, nausea or vomiting, and absence of cough) and three initial laboratory abnormalities (low platelet count, low serum bicarbonate level, and elevated hematocrit level) are useful in identifying all patients with HPS and excluding HPS in at least 80% of patients with unexplained ARDS.[57] The diagnosis, suspected by history and clinical manifestations, can also be supported histopathologically. Although there is no single pathognomonic lesion that permits certain diagnosis, the overall pattern of lesions and hematologic findings may suggest the diagnosis.[9,45] Diseases that need to be distinguished pathologically from hantavirus-associated illnesses include a relatively large number of renal and pulmonary conditions, such as different viral, rickettsial, and bacterial infections, as well as various noninfectious diseases.

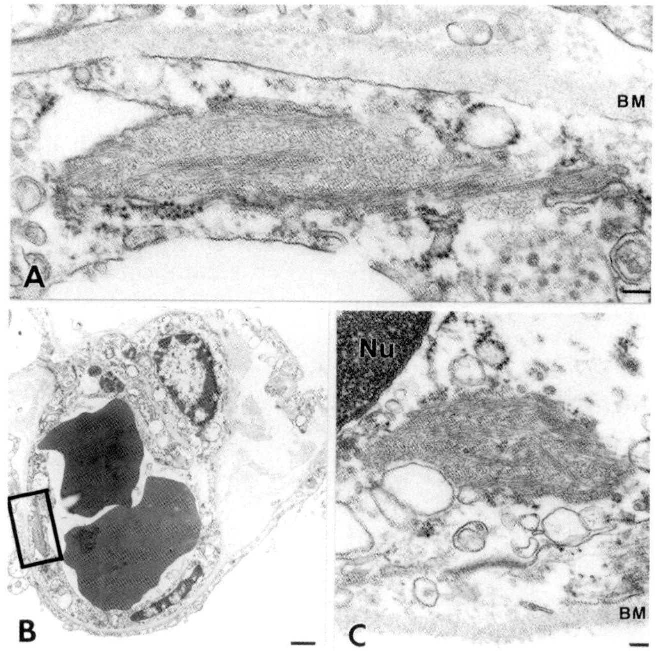

Figure 12–11. Hantavirus pulmonary syndrome. Typical hantaviral inclusions within the pulmonary microvasculature. (**A**) High magnification of boxed area in (**B**) showing a granulofilamentous inclusion within capillary endothelium. (**C**) Another hantaviral inclusion beside an endothelial cell nucleus. Inclusions are often associated with the Golgi and/or rough endoplasmic reticulum. BM, basement membrane; NU, nucleus. (Scale bars: A and C = 100 nm; B = 1 μm.) *(Photograph reproduced from Zaki et al*[9] *with permission of the* American Journal of Pathology.*)*

CONFIRMATIONAL TESTING

Isolation of hantaviruses in tissue cultures is difficult and requires a high level of biosafety. Virus-specific diagnosis and confirmation can be accomplished through serology, polymerase chain reaction (PCR) for hantavirus RNA, and/or IHC for hantaviral antigens.[9,58] Serologic testing can detect hantavirus-specific immunoglobulin M or rising titers of immunoglobulin G in patient sera and is considered the method of choice for laboratory confirmation of HFRS and HPS. Methods such as immunofluorescent assays and enzyme-linked immunosorbent assay (ELISA), which demonstrate specific antihantaviral antibodies, are currently used as rapid diagnostic tests, providing results within a few hours. PCR is aimed at detecting viral RNA in blood and tissues and has been extremely useful for diagnostic and epidemiologic purposes. Recently, synthetic hantaviral nucleocapsid proteins generated by reverse transcription PCR (RT–PCR) and recombinant DNA techniques and their application in serologic tests have improved the sensitivity and specificity of assays and overcome the problems of the availability of inactivated hantaviral antigens.[59,60] Detection of hantaviral RNA in formalin-fixed, paraffin-embedded archival tissue by RT–PCR is also feasible.[61] IHC testing of formalin-fixed tissues with specific monoclonal and polyclonal antibodies can be used to detect hantavirus antigens, and has been a sensitive method for laboratory confirmation of hantaviral infections.[9] IHC has a unique role in the diagnosis of HPS and HFRS when serum samples and frozen tissues are unavailable.[62,63]

TREATMENT AND PREVENTION

Management of patients with HPS or HFRS is often complex and phase specific. Supportive therapy, such as dialysis and circulatory and respiratory support, is the basis of treatment. Controlled studies suggest that ribavirin, a nucleoside analog, is effective in HTN infections if given early.[64,65] The efficacy of intravenous ribavirin for HPS is under investigation.[66] Preventive measures are aimed at decreasing the frequency of rodent–human contacts through environmental hygiene.[67,68]

REFERENCES

1. Lee H. Lee P, Johnson K. Isolation of the etiologic agent of Korean hemorrhagic fever. *J Infect Dis.* 1978;137(3): 298–308.
2. Lee HW. *Epidemiologic features of Korean hemorrhagic fever and research activities on this disease in the Republic of Korea.* Tokyo, Japan: WHO Working Group on Hemorrhagic Fever with Renal Syndrome; 1982.
3. Hung T. *Atlas of Hemorrhagic Fever with Renal Syndrome.* Beijing, China: Science Press; 1988.
4. McKee KT Jr, Leduc JW, Peters CJ. Hantaviruses. In: Belshe RB, ed. *Textbook of Human Virology.* 2nd ed. St. Louis, MO: Mosby; 1991:615–632.
5. World Health Organization. Hemorrhagic fever with renal syndrome: memorandum from a WHO meeting. *Bull WHO.* 1983;61:269–275.
6. Centers for Disease Control and Prevention. Outbreak of acute illness—southwestern United States, 1993. *MMWR.* 1993;42:421–424.
7. Nichol ST, Spiropoulou CF, Morzunov S, et al. Genetic identification of a hantavirus associated with an outbreak of acute respiratory illness. *Science.* 1993;262:914–917.
8. Duchin JS, Koster FT, Peters CJ, et al. Hantavirus pulmonary syndrome: a clinical description of 17 patients with a newly recognized disease. *N Engl J Med.* 1994; 330:949–955.
9. Zaki SR, Greer PW, Coffield LM, et al. Hantavirus pulmonary syndrome: pathogenesis of an emerging infectious disease. *Am J Pathol.* 1995;146:552–579.
10. Schmaljohn CS. Nucleotide sequence of the L genome segment of Hantaan virus. *Nucleic Acids Res.* 1990; 18:6728.
11. Schmaljohn CS, Dalrymple JM. Analysis of Hantaan virus RNA: evidence for a new genus of *Bunyaviridae. Virology.* 1983;131:482–491.
12. Xiao SY, Leduc JW, Chu YK, Schmaljohn CS. Phylogenetic analyses of virus isolates in the genus Hantavirus, family *Bunyaviridae. Virology.* 1994;198:205–217.
13. Lee HW. World Health Organization (WHO) Collaborating Center for Virus Reference and Research. In: Lee HW, Dalrymple JM, eds. *Manual of Hemorrhagic Fever with Renal Syndrome.* Seoul, Korea: Korea University; 1989:11–18.
14. Centers for Disease Control and Prevention. Update: hantavirus pulmonary syndrome—United States, 1993. *MMWR.* 1993;42:816–820.
15. Tsai TF. Hemorrhagic fever with renal syndrome: mode of transmission to humans. *Lab Anim Sci.* 1987;37:428–430.
16. Leduc JW. Epidemiology of Hantaan and related viruses. *Lab Anim Sci.* 1987;37:413–418.
17. Xu ZY, Guo CS, Wu YL, Zhang XW, Liu K. Epidemiological studies of hemorrhagic fever with renal syndrome: analysis of risk factors and mode of transmission. *J Infect Dis.* 1985;152:137–144.
18. Xu ZY, Tang YW, Kan LY, Tsai TF. Cats—source of protection or infection? A case-control study of hemorrhagic fever with renal syndrome. *Am J Epidemiol.* 1987;126: 942–948.
19. Ruo SL, Li YL, Tong Z, et al. Retrospective and prospective studies of hemorrhagic fever with renal syndrome in rural China. *J Infect Dis.* 1994;170:527–534.
20. Zeitz PS, Butler JC, Cheek JE, et al. A case-control study of hantavirus pulmonary syndrome during an outbreak in the southwestern United States. *J Infect Dis.* 1995;171: 864–870.
21. Armstrong LR, Zaki SR, Goldoft MJ, et al. Hantavirus pulmonary syndrome associated with entering or cleaning rarely used, rodent-infested structures. *J Infect Dis.* 1995; 172:1166.
22. Chu YK, Rossi C, Leduc JW, Lee HW, Schmaljohn CS, Dalrymple JM. Serological relationships among viruses in the Hantavirus genus, family *Bunyaviridae. Virology.* 1994; 198:196–204.
23. Childs JE, Ksiazek TG, Spiropoulou CF, et al. Serologic and genetic identification of *Peromyscus maniculatus* as the primary rodent reservoir for a new hantavirus in the southwestern United States. *J Infect Dis.* 1994;169: 1271–1280.
24. Rollin PE, Ksiazek TG, Elliott LH, et al. Isolation of Black Creek Canal virus, a new hantavirus from *Sigmodon hispidus* in Florida. *J Med Virol.* 1995;46:35–39.
25. Hjelle B, Krolikowski J, Torrez-Martinez N, Chavez-Giles F, Vanner C, Laposata E. Phylogenetically distinct hantavirus implicated in a case of hantavirus pulmonary syndrome in the northeastern United States. *J Med Virol.* 1995;46:21–27.
26. Khan AS, Spiropoulou CF, Morzunov S, et al. Fatal illness associated with a new hantavirus in Louisiana. *J Med Virol.* 1995;46:281–286.
27. Hung T, Chou Z, Zhao T, Xia S, Hang C. Morphology and morphogenesis of viruses of hemorrhagic fever with renal

syndrome (HFRS): some peculiar aspects of the morphogenesis of various strains of HFRS virus. *Intervirology.* 1985;23:97–108.
28. Goldsmith CS, Humphrey CD, Elliott LH, Zaki SR. Morphology of Muerto Canyon virus, causative agent of hantavirus pulmonary syndrome. In: Bailey GW, Garratt-Reed AJ, eds. *Proceedings Microscopy Society of America Fifty-Second Annual Meeting 1994.* San Francisco; 1994: 272–273.
29. Goldsmith CS, Elliott LH, Peters CJ, Zaki SR. Ultrastructural characteristics of Sin Nombre virus, causative agent of hantavirus pulmonary syndrome. *Arch Virol.* 1995;140: 2107–2122.
30. Martin ML, Lindsey-Regnery H, Sasso DR, McCormick JB, Palmer E. Distinction between *Bunyaviridae* genera by surface structure and comparison with Hantaan virus using negative stain electron microscopy. *Arch Virol.* 1985;86:17–28.
31. Humphrey CD, Goldsmith CS, Elliott L, Zaki SR. Identification of the pulmonary syndrome hantavirus by direct and colloidal gold immune electron microscopy. In: Bailey GW, Garratt-Reed AJ, eds. *Proceedings Microscopy Society of America Fifty-Second Annual Meeting.* San Francisco; 1994:274–275.
32. Powell GM. Hemorrhagic fever: a study of 300 cases. *Medicine.* 1954;33:97–153.
33. Swift W, Jr. Clinical aspects of the renal phase of epidemic hemorrhagic fever. *Ann Intern Med.* 1953;38:102–105.
34. Kim D. Clinical analysis of 111 fatal cases of epidemic hemorrhagic fever. *Am J Med.* 1965;39:218–220.
35. Lahdevirta J. Clinical features of HFRS in Scandinavia as compared with East Asia. *Scan J Infect Dis.* 1982;S36: 93–95.
36. Lahdevirta J. The minor problem of hemostatic impairment in nephropathia epidemica, the mild Scandinavian form of hemorrhagic fever with renal syndrome. *Rev Infect Dis.* 1989;11(S4):S860–S863.
37. Lee M, Kim B, Kim S, et al. Coagulopathy in hemorrhagic fever with renal syndrome (Korean hemorrhagic fever). *Rev Infect Dis.* 1989;11(S4):S877–S883.
38. Earle DP. Symposium on epidemic hemorrhagic fever. *Am J Med.* 1954;16:619–709.
39. Tsai TF. Hemorrhagic fever with renal syndrome: clinical aspects. *Lab Anim Sci.* 1987;37:419–427.
40. Lukes R. The pathology of thirty-nine fatal cases of epidemic hemorrhagic fever. *Am J Med.* 1954;16:639–650.
41. Steer A. Pathology of hemorrhagic fever: a comparison of the findings—1951 and 1952. *Am J Pathol.* 1955;31: 201–221.
42. Ketai LH, Williamson MR, Telepak RJ, et al. Hantavirus pulmonary syndrome: radiographic findings in 16 patients. *Radiology.* 1994;191:665–668.
43. Entwisle G, Hale E. Hemodynamic alterations in hemorrhagic fever. *Circulation.* 1957;15:414–425.
44. Kurata T, Sata T, Aoyama Y, et al. Systemic deposition of viral antigens in the vascular endothelia of hemorrhagic fever with renal syndrome. In: Kano K, Mori S, Sugisaki T, Torisu M, eds. *Cellular, Molecular and Genetic Approaches to Immunodiagnosis and Immunotherapy.* Tokyo, Japan: University of Tokyo Press; 1987:305–312.
45. Nolte KB, Feddersen RM, Foucar K, et al. Hantavirus pulmonary syndrome in the United States: pathologic description of a disease caused by a new agent. *Hum Pathol.* 1995;26:110–120.
46. Hullinghorst RL, Steer A. Pathology of epidemic hemorrhagic fever. *Ann Intern Med.* 1953;38:77–101.
47. Kessler W. Gross anatomic features found in 27 autopsies of epidemic hemorrhagic fever. *Ann Intern Med.* 1953; 38:73–76.
48. Collan Y, Mihatsch M, Lahdevirta J, Jokinen E, Romppanen T, Janunen E. Nephropathia epidemica: mild variant of hemorrhagic fever with renal syndrome. *Kidney Int.* 1991;40:S62–S71.
49. Lahdevirta J. Nephropathia epidemica in Finland. A clinical, histological, and epidemiological study. *Ann Clin Res.* 1971;3:1–154.
50. Lahdevirta J, Collan Y, Jokinen EJ, Hiltunen R. Renal sequelae to nephropathia epidemica. *Acta Pathol Microbiol Scand.* 1978;86:265–271.
51. Kuhlback B, Fortelius P, Tallgren CG. Renal histopathology in a case of nephropathia epidemica Myhrman. A study of successive biopsies. *Acta Pathol Microbiol Scand.* 1964;60:323–333.
52. Dimitrijevic J, Skataric V, Tomanovic S, et al. *Pathohistological findings in the kidney and liver in patients with haemorrhagic fever with renal syndrome (HFRS).* 3rd International Conference on HFRS and Hantaviruses 1995;68(Abstract).
53. Groen J, Bruijn JA, Gerding MN, Jordans JGM, Moll van Charante AW, Osterhaus ADME. *Histopathological findings and Puumalavirus antigen detection in kidney biopsies from patients with nephropathia epidemica.* 3rd International Conference on HFRS and Hantaviruses 1995;1:42. Abstract.
54. Hung T, Xia S, Chou Z, Gan S, Yanagihara R. Morphology and morphogenesis of viruses of hemorrhagic fever with renal syndrome: inclusion bodies—ultrastructural marker of hantavirus-infected cells. *Intervirology.* 1987;27:45–52.
55. Hung T, Zhou JY, Tang YM, Zhao TX, Baek LJ, Lee HW. Identification of Hantaan virus-related structures in kidneys of cadavers with haemorrhagic fever with renal syndrome. *Arch Virol.* 1992;122:187–199.
56. Kikuchi K, Imamura M, Ueno H, et al. An autopsy case of epidemic hemorrhagic fever (Korean hemorrhagic fever). *Sapporo Med J.* 1982;51:K17–K31.
57. Moolenaar RL, Dalton C, Lipman HB, et al. Clinical features that differentiate hantavirus pulmonary syndrome from three other acute respiratory illnesses. *Clin Infect Dis.* 1995;21:643–649.
58. Ksiazek TG, Peters CJ, Rollin PE, et al. Identification of a new North American hantavirus that causes acute pulmonary insufficiency. *Am J Trop Med Hyg.* 1995;52(2): 1017–1023.
59. Schmaljohn CS, Sugiyama K, Schmaljohn AL, et al. Baculovirus expression of the small genome segment of Hantaan virus and potential use of the expressed nucleocapsid protein as a diagnostic antigen. *J Gen Virol.* 1988; 69:777–786.
60. Feldmann H, Sanchez A, Morzunov S, et al. Utilization of autopsy RNA for the synthesis of the nucleocapsid antigen

of a newly recognized virus associated with hantavirus pulmonary syndrome. *Virus Res.* 1993;30:351–367.

61. Schwarz TF, Zaki SR, Morzunov S, Peters CJ, Nichol ST. Detection and sequence confirmation of Sin Nombre virus RNA in paraffin-embedded human tissues using one-step RT–PCR. *J Virol Meth.* 1995;51:349–356.
62. Zaki SR, Albers RC, Greer PW, et al. Retrospective diagnosis of a 1983 case of fatal hantavirus pulmonary syndrome. *Lancet.* 1994;343:1037–1038.
63. Zaki SR, Khan AS, Goodman RA, et al. Retrospective diagnosis of hantavirus pulmonary syndrome, 1978–1993: implications for emerging infectious disease. *Arch Pathol Lab Med.* 1995;120:134–139.
64. Andrei G, De Clercq E. Molecular approaches for the treatment of hemorrhagic fever virus infections. *Antiviral Res.* 1993;22:45–75.
65. Huggins J, Hsiang C, Cosgriff R, et al. Prospective, double-blind, concurrent, placebo-controlled clinical trial of intravenous ribavirin therapy of hemorrhagic fever with renal syndrome. *J Infect Dis.* 1991;164:1119–1127.
66. Chapman LE, Mertz G, Khan AS. Open label intravenous ribavirin for hantavirus pulmonary syndrome. In: *Abstracts of the 34th Interscience Conference on Antimicrobial Agents and Chemotherapy;* 1994:240. Abstract.
67. Centers for Disease Control and Prevention. Hantavirus infection—southwestern United States: interim recommendations for risk reduction. *MMWR.* 1993;42(RR-11): 1–12.
68. Centers for Disease Control and Prevention. Laboratory management of agents associated with hantavirus pulmonary syndrome: interim biosafety guidelines. *MMWR.* 1994;43(RR-7):1–7.

CHAPTER 13

Infection (Virus)-Associated Hemophagocytic Syndrome

Robert J. Siegel

And it is well to superintend the sick to make them well, to care for the healthy to keep them well, also to care for one's own self, so as to observe what is seemly.

Hippocrates (460–377 B.C.)

BACKGROUND

In 1939, Scott and Robb-Smith described histiocytic medullary reticulosis (HMR), a fatal disorder of adults characterized clinically by hepatosplenomegaly, fever, lymphadenopathy, and pancytopenia, and pathologically by "a systematized hyperplasia of histiocytes actively engaged in phagocytosis of erythrocytes."[1] Subsequently, the syndrome of familial hemophagocytic lymphohistiocytosis (FHL) was identified by Farquhar and Claireaux as a fatal familial disorder predominantly affecting infants, having many of the clinical features of HMR, with prominent hemophagocytosis by cytologically benign activated histiocytes.[2] Since then, a variety of hemophagocytic syndromes, involving either reactive or neoplastic proliferations of phagocytic cells, have been enumerated. Risdall et al[3] are credited with recognizing what they termed the virus-associated hemophagocytic syndrome, in which a generally favorable clinical course, presence of a viral infection, and absence of cytologic anaplasia of the proliferating cells allowed separation from the malignant conditions that may be associated with hemophagocytosis. Absence of family history and presence of infectious association were thought to separate this entity from FHL in infants, although this distinction may be arbitrary.[4] Because it is known now that nonviral infectious agents may be associated with the disorder, the term *infection (virus)-associated hemophagocytic syndrome (IAHS)* has been advocated and is used in this chapter.

CLINICAL FEATURES

IAHS usually presents as a severe, acute systemic illness, 2 to 6 weeks after a prodromal viral syndrome.[5] Commonly, underlying immunodeficiency, either congenital or acquired, is present (see later discussion). Typical findings are severe constitutional symptoms with high fever and hepatosplenomegaly. Laboratory evaluation discloses cytopenias, hepatic dysfunction, hypertriglyceridemia, and hypofibrinogenemia; evidence of true disseminated intravascular coagulation may or may not be present. Pleocytosis of spinal fluid is common also.

ASSOCIATED INFECTIOUS AGENTS

In the original group of 19 patients in the Risdall et al[3] series, cytomegalovirus was implicated in 10, Epstein–Barr virus (EBV) in 2, and adenovirus, herpes simplex, and varicella-zoster virus in 1 each. Subsequently, the syndrome has been associated with gram-negative bacteremia, tuberculosis, leishmaniasis, and fungal infection.[6] Several other organisms have been noted in case reports (eg, ehrlichiosis,[7] trichosporosis,[8] parvovirus B19)[9]; active disseminated infection seems to be the common clinical setting.[6]

RELATIONSHIP TO IMMUNODEFICIENCY

Fourteen of the 19 patients in the series of Risdall et al[3] were iatrogenically immunosuppressed, and IAHS subsequently has been noted in congenital and acquired immunodeficiency states including X-linked lymphoproliferative disorder (XLPD), Chédiak–Higashi syndrome, HIV infection, and following bone marrow transplantation.[10–13] Often, it is difficult to determine if the viral infection precedes or follows the immunodeficiency.[10] Immune defects have included lymphopenia, depressed proliferative response of lymphocytes to mitogens, decreased natural killer function, and decreased lymphocyte cytotoxicity to EBV-infected cells.[4,10]

An interesting association has been made between fatal infectious mononucleosis (IM) and IAHS. In a study of 52 cases of fatal IM, including both spontaneous cases and those associated with the XLPD, 80% had features of IAHS.[14] In these patients, a sequence of lymphoid hyperplasia, necrosis of bone marrow cells, lymphocyte depletion, and phagocytic histiocytic reaction was noted. The association of IAHS with this fatal disorder, as well as the high mortality of IAHS reported in children with immune deficiencies,[10] contrasts with the relatively benign course in the patients described by Risdall et al.[3] The reversibility of the immunodeficiency in the latter group may account for this disparity.[14]

PATHOLOGIC FINDINGS

The histologic feature present in all hemophagocytic syndromes is the widespread proliferation of histiocytic cells, which have engulfed formed elements of blood in their abundant cytoplasm, especially erythrocytes and platelets but also leukocytes (Figure 13–1). Cytologic features of the phagocytic cells are benign, and immunohistochemical and ultrastructural observations confirm their histiocytic nature.

The phagocytic cells are evident in bone marrow aspirate smears and trephine biopsy sections, although it has been noted that initial bone marrow examination is not infrequently negative.[4] Aside from the histiocytic proliferation, deposition of fibrin in bone marrow is said to be a distinctive feature.[4] A variable degree of lymphoid proliferation may be associated. Hypocellularity also may be seen, and there may be progression to marrow aplasia.[10]

Lymph nodes, which may be clinically enlarged, display generally intact architecture, and a histiocytic proliferation that has a prominent sinusoidal pattern (Figure 13–2). Lymphocyte depletion also has been described, and may represent a late manifestation of the syndrome. The generalized nature of the mononuclear–phagocyte system activation is evidenced by Kupffer cell and splenic macrophage proliferation.

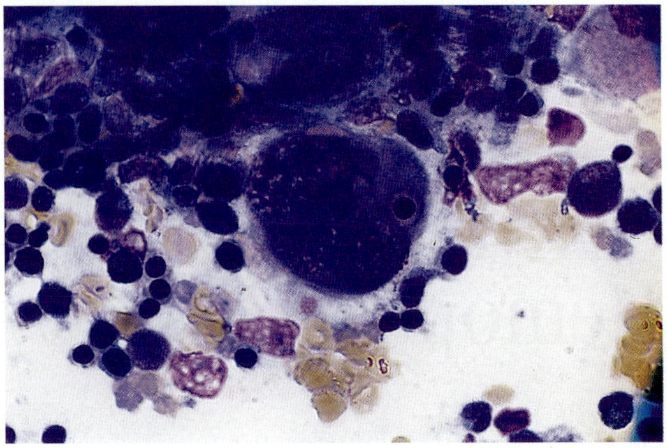

Figure 13–1. Smear of bone marrow aspirate showing hemophagocytosis in a large histiocytic cell *(center)* (×1000).

DIFFERENTIAL PATHOLOGIC DIAGNOSIS

Note that hemophagocytosis, particularly erythrophagocytosis, may be a nonspecific histiocytic reaction, and the diagnosis of a hemophagocytic syndrome requires clinicopathologic correlation (see Ref. 4 for proposed criteria). From the diagnostic histopathologic point of

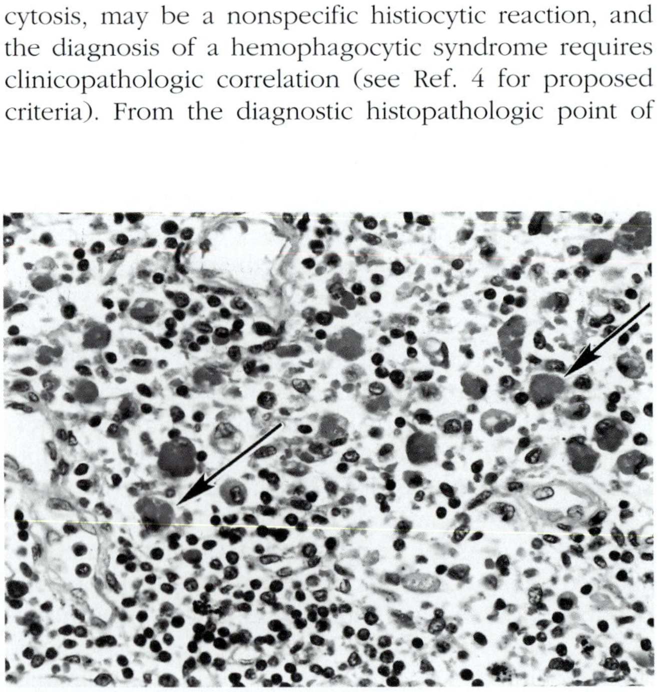

Figure 13–2. Lymph node sinuses contain numerous phagocytic histiocytes *(arrows),* each of which has engulfed multiple erythrocytes (×200).

view, the most important features are the cytologic appearance and phenotype of the phagocytic cells. If cytologically malignant, then a true histiocytic malignancy should be suspected; these are very rare. T-cell lymphomas, carcinomas, and other malignancies also may display hemophagocytosis. Immunohistochemical stains may be necessary to define the nature of the phagocytic cells.

If the phagocytic cells are cytologically benign histiocytes, and if features of a hemophagocytic syndrome are present, attention is then turned to the possibility of an infectious or familial association, and to the status of the immune system.

Another disorder to be considered in the differential diagnosis of lymph node hemophagocytosis is sinus histiocytosis with massive lymphadenopathy (Rosai–Dorfman disease).[15] The clinical presentation is of bilateral massive cervical lymphadenopathy especially in black children or young adults, who may have anemia but not leukopenia or thrombocytopenia. Lymph nodes display marked distention of sinuses by histiocytes exhibiting emperiopolesis, the intracytoplasmic accumulation of apparently undamaged hematopoietic cells. Nodal plasmacytosis and capsular fibrosis are additional features, and the histiocytic cells have a unique immunohistochemical phenotype (S-100 positive, CD1 negative).[16]

PATHOGENESIS

The pathogenesis of the hemophagocytic syndromes, including IAHS, has been theorized to involve unrestrained activation of the cellular immune system, with essentially all signs and symptoms attributable to the effects of cytokines.[4] This activation may be related to familial predisposition, infection, immune deficiency states, certain malignant neoplasms (particularly T-cell lymphoma), or some combination of risk factors.[4,17]

REFERENCES

1. Scott RB, Robb-Smith AHT. Histiocytic medullary reticulosis. *Lancet.* 1939;2:194–198.
2. Farquhar JW, Claireaux AE. Familial haemophagocytic reticulosis. *Arch Dis Child.* 1952;27:519–525.
3. Risdall RJ, McKenna RW, Nesbit ME, et al. Virus-associated hemophagocytic syndrome. A benign histiocytic proliferation distinct from malignant histiocytosis. *Cancer.* 1979; 44:993–1002.
4. Favara BE. Hemophagocytic lymphohistiocytosis: a hemophagocytic syndrome. *Semin Diagn Pathol.* 1992;9:63–74.
5. McKenna RW, Risdall RJ, Brunning RD. Virus associated hemophagocytic syndrome. *Hum Pathol.* 1981;12: 395–398.
6. Risdall RJ, Brunning RD, Hernandez JI, Gordon DH. Bacteria-associated hemophagocytic syndrome. *Cancer.* 1984; 54:2968–2972.
7. Abbott KC, Vukelja SJ, Smith CE, et al. Hemophagocytic syndrome: a cause of pancytopenia in human ehrlichiosis. *Am J Hematol.* 1991;38:230–234.
8. del Palacio A, Perez-Revilla A, Albanil R, Sotelo T, Kalter DC. Disseminated neonatal trichosporosis associated with the hemophagocytic syndrome. *Pediatr Infect Dis J.* 1990;9:520–522.
9. Boruchoff SE, Woda BA, Pihan GA, Durbin WA, Burstein D, Blacklow NR. Parvovirus B19-associated hemophagocytic syndrome. *Arch Intern Med.* 1990;150:897–898.
10. McClain K, Gehrz R, Grierson H, Purtilo D, Filipovich A. Virus-associated histiocytic proliferations in children. Frequent association with Epstein–Barr virus and congenital or acquired immunodeficiencies. *Am J Ped Hematol Oncol.* 1988;10:196–205.
11. Sasadeusz J, Buchanan M, Speed B. Reactive haemophagocytic syndrome in human immunodeficiency virus infection. *J Infect.* 1990;20:65–68.
12. Rubin CM, Burke BA, McKenna RW, et al. The accelerated phase of Chédiak–Higashi syndrome: an expression of the virus-associated hemophagocytic syndrome? *Cancer.* 1985;56:524–530.
13. Reardon DA, Roskos R, Hanson CA, Castle V. Virus-associated hemophagocytic syndrome following bone marrow transplantation. *Am J Pediatr Hematol Oncol.* 1991; 13:305–309.
14. Mroczek EC, Weisenburger DD, Lipscomb Grierson H, Markin R, Purtilo DT. Fatal infectious mononucleosis and virus-associated hemophagocytic syndrome. *Arch Pathol Lab Med.* 1987;111:530–535.
15. Rosai J, Dorfman RF. Sinus histiocytosis with massive lymphadenopathy: a pseudolymphomatous benign disorder. Analysis of 34 cases. *Cancer.* 1972;30:1174–1188.
16. Bonetti F, Chilosi M, Menestrina F, et al. Immunohistological analysis of Rosai–Dorfman histiocytosis. A disease of S-100+Cd1-histiocytes. *Virch Arch A.* 1987;411:129–135.
17. Fujiwara F, Hibi S, Imashuku S. Hypercytokinemia in hemophagocytic syndrome. *Am J Pediatr Hematol Oncol.* 1993;15:92–98.

Chapter 14

B Virus Infection (Infection by Cercopithecine Herpesvirus 1)

Stephen P. Schiffer

The mode of death is sadder than death itself.

Martial (1st century a.d.) Epigrams, XI.91

I confess freely to you, I could never look long upon a monkey, without very mortifying reflections.

Congreve, Letter to Dennis (1695)

DEFINITION AND HISTORIC OVERVIEW

Herpes B virus (Cercopithecine herpesvirus 1) is a zoonotic alphaherpesvirus enzootic in Asian monkeys of the genus *Macaca* (macaques), which includes rhesus and cynomolgus monkeys. Macaques infected with B virus usually develop a mild herpetic eruption of lips or oral structures followed by an asymptomatic latent infection. The medical importance of the virus comes from its virulence in humans in whom it causes almost invariably fatal ascending myelitis and encephalitis.

B virus was first recognized in 1932 when it killed a 29-year-old physician (Dr. W.B.) who had been bitten by a rhesus monkey as part of his polio research.[1] Since then there have been more than 30 reported human infections of B virus with 80% mortality.[2] Although the incidence of B virus infections in humans is very low, since 1987 there have been at least four deaths in the United States including the first cluster and documentation of human-to-human transmission.[3,4] These recent events have reestablished B virus as one of the most feared primate zoonoses for those who work with macaques or their tissues and fluids.

SYNONYMS

Several names have been given to B virus including *Herpesvirus simiae, Herpes simiae,* monkey B virus, and herpes B.[5] Based on its biologic and serologic relatedness, the Herpesvirus Study Group of the International Committee on Taxonomy of Viruses proposed the name Cercopithecine herpesvirus 1 (CHV-1) within the genus *Simplexvirus*, subfamily *Alphaherpesvirinae*, and family *Herpesviridae*.[6] For the purpose of this chapter, CHV-1 is referred to using the more familiar name, B virus (named "B" for Dr. W.B., the first recognized human infection).

GEOGRAPHIC DISTRIBUTION

Although B virus is indigenous to Asian macaques,[7] all documented human infections have been in developed countries, including the United States, Canada, and England. Recognizing that there must be frequent human–monkey exposure in Asian countries, some have suggested that the lack of human infections

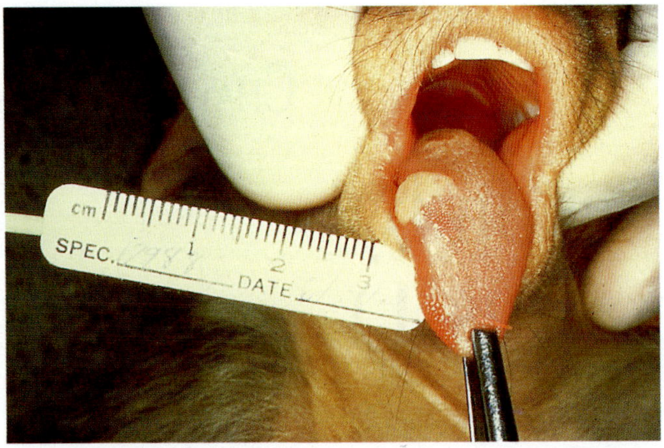

Figure 14–1. Lingual ulcer of a macaque infected with B virus. *(Photograph contributed by Dr. Jeffrey Roberts, California Regional Primate Research Center.)*

reported in these countries may reflect inadequate access to health care and diagnostic resources.[8]

LIFE CYCLE, NATURAL HISTORY, AND EPIDEMIOLOGY

The natural history of B virus infections in macaques resembles that of herpes simplex virus (HSV) in humans, in that the primary infection is followed by lifelong latency with the possibility of viral reactivation from the sensory ganglia.[7,9,10] Monkeys initially infected with B virus typically develop mild signs, including vesicles or ulcers of the tongue or lips (Figure 14–1).[5,7] Cutaneous ulcers and keratoconjunctivitis have also been described. Some monkeys may have no signs of infection. The neurotropic behavior of the B virus causes a latent infection in the monkey's trigeminal, lumbar, and/or sacral ganglia, with subsequent reactivation and shedding of virus in response to various stimuli.[5,9] B virus also may be in thoracic and abdominal viscera of infected macaques.[11] These tissues and primary cultures derived from them are potential hazards. Transmission between animals may be associated with fight wounds or transmission may be sexual.[9,10,12] Viral transmission from dam to offspring appears to be uncommon; newborn macaques may have maternal antibodies for up to 6 months of age.[13,14] Infection with seroconversion usually takes place at puberty when breeding within a group begins.[12] Seroconversion takes place 6 (IgM) to 12 (IgG) days postinfection.[15] The seroprevalence of B virus in macaque colonies may approach 100%,[9] although only about 2% of the animals may have clinically evident lesions.[7] Although shedding of virus from asymptomatic seropositive animals is uncommon,[13,16] B virus may be present in the oral, ocular, and genital secretions of macaques regardless of whether the animal has clinically evident lesions. Seronegative animals that were culture positive have also been described.[10,17] Immunosuppression in infected macaques may activate latent infections.[18]

Documented B virus infections of humans are rare, which indicates they are an uncommon result of macaque-related exposures.[19,20] Most reports have involved isolated cases, although recently two clusters have been described, involving four people in Florida and three in Michigan.[21] The highest risk of acquiring B virus from macaques is through the bite of an infected monkey with active lesions (Figure 14–2).[22] Contamination of broken skin or mucous membranes with oral, ocular, or genital secretions from an infected animal with or without active lesions is also dangerous[22] (Figure 14–3). One human infection following a needlestick injury has been reported.[23] Infection has followed exposure to infected monkey tissue cultures.[24] Aerosol transmission, although suspected, has not been confirmed.[25] Once infected, patients can shed virus from skin lesions, tears, saliva, urine, and feces.[4] The significance of viral shedding is that the first documented case of human-to-human transmission involved an animal handler who became infected when a rhesus monkey bit him on the forearm.[4] He developed herpetic lesions at the site and applied topical creams that his wife had also used on an area of contact dermatitis on her left ring finger. The husband subsequently died and the wife developed herpetic lesions at the ring finger site. When her lesions failed to resolve, a punch biopsy was done and B virus was isolated. She was treated with intravenous acyclovir and the skin lesions resolved

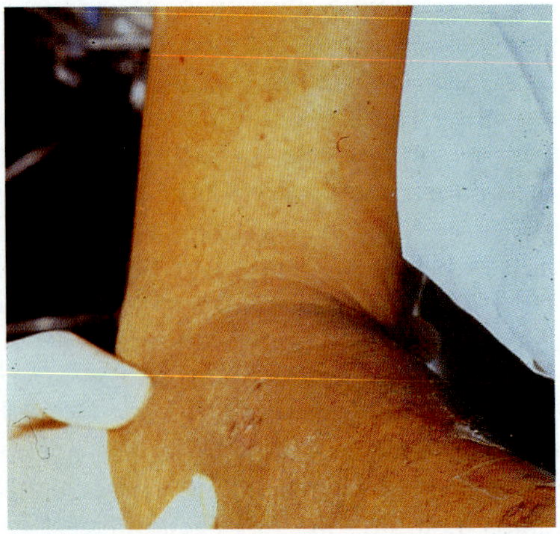

Figure 14–2. Healed bite wound of forearm that yielded B virus following punch biopsy. The patient subsequently died from B virus encephalomyelitis. *(Photograph contributed by Dr. Julia Hilliard, Southwest Foundation for Biomedical Research.)*

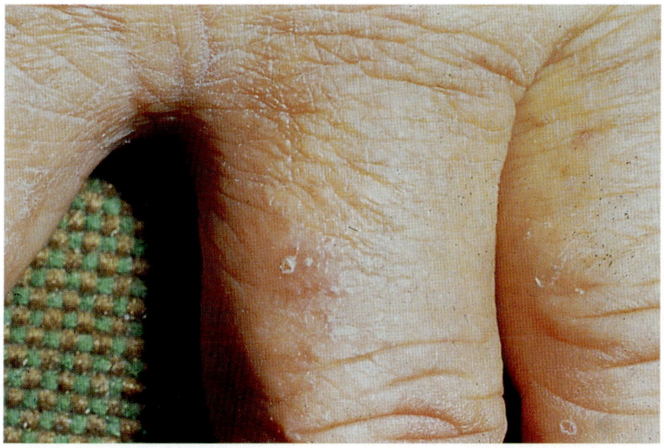

Figure 14–3. Healed finger lesion due to a cage scratch. B virus was isolated following a punch biopsy. *(Photograph contributed by Dr. Julia Hilliard, Southwest Foundation for Biomedical Research.)*

without further progression of disease. She was released with oral acyclovir. The possibility of human latent infections has been suggested by one patient, a virologist, who developed clinical signs 10 years after his last known exposure to monkeys.[26]

CHARACTERISTICS OF THE ORGANISM

The B virus morphologically, biologically, genetically, and antigenically resembles HSV.[7,8,27] B virus contains double-stranded DNA with a molecular weight of 107×10^6. Cross-hybridization has shown that HSV-1, HSV-2, and B virus form a closely related subgroup of primate herpesviruses.[28] B virus is unique among the herpesviruses in having the highest G + C content, rapid replication, and a broad host range in vivo and in vitro.[7] Extensive cross-reactivity for surface glycoprotein antigens has been shown between B virus and HSV-1 and HSV-2.[29] Interestingly, preexisting HSV titers in humans do not seem to be protective.[4] Although B virus isolates can be distinguished using restriction enzyme profiles depending on the species of macaque,[30] isolates cannot be divided into oral and genital types as are strains of HSV.[31] Fortunately, B virus is readily inactivated by formalin and heat, and cell-free virus is not likely to persist for long in the environment although the hazard must be recognized.[8,22]

CLINICAL FEATURES

The incubation period for symptomatic B virus infection is unknown.[4] Generally, symptoms occur within 1 month of exposure.[21,32,33] Initial symptoms typically are flulike and include fever, headache, nausea, and myalgia. Often these signs are accompanied by herpetiform vesicles or ulcers at the site of inoculation and by regional lymphadenopathy.[4,23] The site of exposure initially may be pruritic followed by numbness or paresthesia. In most patients, the disease progresses rapidly to the central nervous system (CNS), causing diplopia, photophobia, altered mentation, ascending flaccid paralysis, urinary retention, dysphagia, convulsions, and coma.[5] Respiratory arrest or encephalitis kills the patient.[23] Spinal taps have revealed increased pressure of cerebrospinal fluid (CSF).[5] Historically the few patients who survived B virus infections suffered serious neurologic sequelae. More recently, rapid diagnosis and antiviral drugs have saved patients from neurologic disease and death although evidence suggests that latent infections remain.[26]

PATHOLOGY

Lesions of the skin include herpetiform vesicles or ulcers at the site of infection (ie, bite, scratch, needlestick).[1,3,4,23,34,35] Some patients have had a hemorrhagic lymphadenopathy.[1] Within the CNS, there is a transverse/ascending myelitis and acute encephalitis.[36] The acute multifocal necrotizing encephalomyelitis may be associated with brainstem and spinal cord edema and hemorrhage (Figure 14–4).[1,5,36,37] Microscopically, the affected areas have meningeal infiltrates, perivascular cuffing, neuronal satellitosis and demyelination, focal edema, hemorrhage, and necrosis.[1,5,8] Focal necrosis of liver, spleen, lymph nodes, and adrenals also may be seen.[7] Ophthalmic lesions include necrotizing retinitis

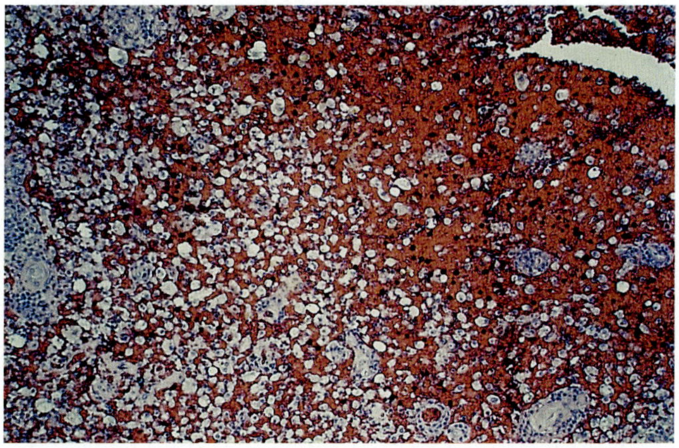

Figure 14–4. Section of C5-6 spinal cord from the patient in Figure 14–2. Tissue exhibits extensive hemorrhage and necrosis. *(Photograph contributed by Dr. Julia Hilliard, Southwest Foundation for Biomedical Research.)*

and panuveitis.[37] Intranuclear inclusion bodies have been reported.[5,36]

Electron micrographs reveal a typical herpesvirus consisting of an enveloped particle approximately 160 to 180 nm in diameter.[7,37] The B virion has an electron-dense toroid core with rotational symmetry. The loosely fitting envelope is studded with surface projections and tends to disintegrate easily.

Antemortem cytopathology for B virus infection has centered around vesicular lesions of the skin and abnormalities of CSF. Needle aspirates of herpetiform vesicles, ulcers, or scrapings from lesions typical of herpesvirus infections have revealed giant cells with distinct viral inclusions in Tzanck preparations.[3,4] CSF may have a lymphocytosis along with elevated levels of protein and glucose.[5]

DIAGNOSIS

Because virtually all victims of B virus infections have worked with nonhuman primates or their tissues, initial possibilities must include the zoonotic infections that involve the CNS (eg, rabies). When encephalomyelitis of unknown cause occurs, it is important to consider B virus if there is *any* history of association with macaques or their tissues.[2] The main differential diagnosis when evaluating tissues, however, is HSV encephalitis. One distinction is the tendency for B virus infections to involve the brainstem whereas HSV-1 infections characteristically have a temporal lobe predilection.[36]

CONFIRMATION

Confirmation of B virus infection ideally involves parallel serologic testing and viral isolation from both patient and suspect monkey. Follow-up samples should be obtained 14 to 21 days postexposure. Serologic testing for B virus is confused because immunologic epitopes of B virus are shared with HSV and other herpesviruses.[7,28,29,38] Antibodies to B virus are detected in about 50% of the general population irrespective of previous exposure to monkeys; these titers are probably a heterotypic response to HSV.[5,8] For this reason, laboratory testing for B virus infections in humans is now standardized but available in only a few licensed laboratories throughout the world.[33] Viral isolation can be done using swabs of skin wounds, conjunctiva, and pharynx.[4] Because B virus remains at the wound site for weeks,[8] skin biopsy has also been used for viral isolation.[21] If signs of CNS infection are evident, then CSF can also be used. Because of the hazardous nature of the virus, however, all viral isolation procedures should be done using strict biosafety precautions.[22] Methods for quicker diagnosis have been developed, including polymerase chain reaction,[2,27,39] restriction endonuclease digests,[4,30] and SDS–PAGE analysis of viral polypeptides.[8]

TREATMENT

So few patients have had B virus infections that no definitive treatment has been devised.[23] The most critical period for managing exposure to B virus is during the first few minutes postinjury when immediate wound cleansing with soap or detergent should be employed (or saline flush for conjunctival exposure).[3,33] The wound should be scrubbed thoroughly and irrigated for at least 15 to 20 minutes.[21] Thereafter, rapid diagnostic confirmation and therapy are of paramount importance if the replication of B virus is to be arrested before it invades the CNS.[8] Clinical experience and experimental evidence suggest that antiviral drugs such as acyclovir and ganciclovir can control infection.[8,33,40] Presumptive therapy with these drugs while awaiting test results is controversial but may be indicated for those individuals who are immunocompromised or develop signs consistent with infection.[21] It is generally believed that once the disease has progressed to encephalitis, the prognosis is extremely poor. Because discontinuation of drug therapy has resulted in viral shedding by surviving patients, lifelong antiviral therapy may be warranted.[8] Finally, although the risk of person-to-person transmission is low, patients and their fluids must be handled with proper precautions.[4,33]

PREVENTION

Although the risk of acquiring B virus infection from macaques appears to be very low, the consequences of symptomatic infection warrant preventive measures.[32,33] In general, unless a macaque is known to be free of B virus, all such primates should be presumed to be naturally infected. Because no vaccine for B virus is licensed, preventive efforts must center on reducing the risk of exposure.[17] Indeed, some fatal infections may have been consequences of failure to follow safety procedures.[4] The Centers for Disease Control and Prevention have developed extensive guidelines for handling monkeys and their tissues.[11,22,32,33] Each facility housing macaques should have a comprehensive occupational health program that addresses both the education and protection of personnel at risk, as well as written protocols detailing procedures to be followed in the event of an infection.[3,32,33] Because of the seriousness of infection with this virus, experienced medical personnel should be available for consultation to ensure prompt lifesaving treatment.

REFERENCES

1. Sabin AB, Wright AM. Acute ascending myelitis following a monkey bite with the isolation of a virus capable of reproducing the disease. *J Exp Med.* 1934;59:115–136.
2. Scinicariello F, Woodruff JE, Hilliard J. Identification by PCR of meningitis caused by herpes B virus. *Lancet.* 1993;341:1660–1661.
3. Centers for Disease Control and Prevention. B virus infection in humans—Pensacola, Florida. *MMWR.* 1987; 36:289–296.
4. Holmes GP, Hilliard JK, Klontz KC, et al. B virus (*Herpesvirus simiae*) infection in humans: epidemiologic investigation of a cluster. *Ann Intern Med.* 1990;112: 833–839.
5. Palmer AE. B virus, *Herpesvirus simiae*: historical perspective. *J Med Primat.* 1987;16:99–130.
6. Roizman B, Carmichael LE, Deinhardt F, et al. *Herpesviridae*—definition—provisional nomenclature, and taxonomy. *Intervirology.* 1981;16:201–217.
7. Ludwig H, Pauli G, Gelderblom H, et al. B virus (*Herpesvirus simiae*). In: Roizman B, ed. *The Herpesviruses.* New York: Plenum Press; 1983:2;385–428.
8. Weigler BJ. Biology of B virus in macaque and human hosts: a review. *Clin Infect Dis.* 1992;14:555–567.
9. Weigler BJ, Roberts JA, Hird DW, Lerche NW, Hilliard JK. A cross sectional survey for B virus antibody in a colony of group housed rhesus macaques. *Lab Anim Sci.* 1990;40:257–261.
10. Weigler BJ, Hird DW, Hilliard JK, et al. Epidemiology of cercopithecine herpesvirus 1 (B virus) infection and shedding in a large breeding cohort of rhesus monkeys. *J Infect Dis.* 1993;167:257–263.
11. Wells DL, Lipper SL, Hilliard JK, et al. *Herpesvirus simiae* contamination of primary rhesus monkey kidney cell cultures. CDC recommendations to minimize risks to laboratory personnel. *Diagn Microbiol Infect Dis.* 1989; 12:333–336.
12. Zwartouw T, MacArthur JA, Boulter EA, et al. Transmission of B virus infection between monkeys especially in relation to breeding colonies. *Lab Anim.* 1984;18:125–130.
13. Weir EC, Bhatt PN, Jacoby RO, Hilliard JK, Morgenstern S. Infrequent shedding and transmission of *Herpesvirus simiae* from seropositive macaques. *Lab Anim Sci.* 1993;43:541–544.
14. Simon MA, Daniel MD, Lee-Parritz D, King NW, Ringler DJ. Disseminated B virus infection in a cynomolgus monkey. *Lab Anim Sci.* 1993;43:545–550.
15. Lees DN, Baskerville A, Cropper LM, Brown DW. *Herpesvirus simiae* (B virus) antibody response and virus shedding in experimental primary infection of cynomolgus monkeys. *Lab Anim Sci.* 1991;41:360–364.
16. Whitley RJ. Cercopithecine herpesvirus 1 (B virus). In: Fields BN, Knipe DM, eds. *Virology.* 2nd ed. New York: Raven Press; 1990:2063–2075.
17. Ward JA, Hilliard JK. B virus-specific pathogen free (SPF) breeding colonies of macaques: issues, surveillance, and results in 1992. *Lab Anim Sci.* 1994;44:222–228.
18. Chellman GJ, Lukas VS, Eugui EM, et al. Activation of B virus (*Herpesvirus simiae*) in chronically immunosuppressed cynomolgus monkeys. *Lab Anim Sci.* 1992; 42:146–151.
19. Davidson WL, Hummeler K. B virus infection in man. *Ann NY Acad Sci.* 1960;85:970–979.
20. Kaplan JE. *Herpesvirus simiae* (B virus) infection in monkey handlers. *J Infect Dis.* 1988;157:1090. Letter.
21. Held JR. Infections caused by *Herpesvirus simiae* and other herpesviruses. In: Beran GW, ed. *Handbook of Zoonoses—Section B.* 2nd ed. Boca Raton, FL: CRC Press; 1994:505–507.
22. U.S. Department of Health and Human Services. *Biosafety in Microbiological and Biomedical Laboratories.* 3rd ed. HHS Publication No. CDC 93-8395. Washington, DC; 1993:108–109.
23. Artenstein AW, Hicks CB, Goodwin BS, Hilliard JK. Human infection with B virus following a needlestick injury. *Rev Infect Dis.* 1991;13:288–291.
24. Hummeler K, Davidson WL, Henle W, LaBoccetta AC, Ruch HG. Encephalomyelitis due to infection with *Herpesvirus simiae* (herpes B virus): a report of two fatal, laboratory-acquired cases. *N Engl J Med.* 1959;261:64–68.
25. Chappell WA. Animal infectivity of aerosols of monkey B virus. *Ann NY Acad Sci.* 1960;85:931–934.
26. Fierer J, Bazeley P, Braude AI. Herpes B virus encephalomyelitis presenting as ophthalmic zoster: a possible latent infection reactivated. *Ann Intern Med.* 1973;79:225–228.
27. Scinicariello F, Eberle R, Hilliard JK. Rapid detection of B virus (*Herpesvirus simiae*) DNA by polymerase chain reaction. *J Infect Dis.* 1993;168:747–750.
28. Hilliard JK, Black D, Eberle R. Simian alphaherpesviruses and their relation to the human herpes simplex viruses. *Arch Virol.* 1989;109:83–102.
29. Eberle R, Black D, Hilliard JK. Relatedness of glycoproteins expressed on the surface of simian herpesvirus virions and infected cells to specific HSV glycoproteins. *Arch Virol.* 1989;109:233–252.
30. Hilliard JK, Munoz RM, Lipper SI, Eberle R. Rapid identification of *Herpesvirus simiae* (B virus) DNA from clinical isolates in nonhuman primate colonies. *J Virol Meth.* 1986;13:55–62.
31. Wall LV, Zwartouw HT, Kelly DC. Discrimination between twenty isolates of *Herpesvirus simiae* (B virus) by restriction enzyme analysis of the viral genome. *Virus Res.* 1989;12:283–296.
32. Centers for Disease Control and Prevention. Guidelines for prevention of *Herpesvirus simiae* (B virus) infection in monkey handlers. *MMWR.* 1987;36:680–689.
33. Holmes GP, Chapman LE, Stewart JA, et al. Guidelines for the prevention and treatment of B-virus infection in exposed persons. *CID.* 1995;20:421–439.
34. Benson PM, Malane SL, Banks R, Hicks CB, Hilliard J. B virus (*Herpesvirus simiae*) and human infection. *Arch Dermatol.* 1989;125:1247–1248.
35. CDC. B virus infection in humans—Michigan. *MMWR.* 1989;38:453–454.
36. Esiri MM, Kennedy PGE. Virus diseases. In: Adams JH, Duchen LW, eds. *Greenfield's Neuropathology.* 5th ed. New York: Oxford University Press; 1992;335–399.
37. Nanda M, Curtin VT, Hilliard JK, Bernstein ND, Dix

RD. Ocular histopathologic findings in a case of human herpes B virus infection. *Arch Ophth.* 1990;108:713–716.

38. Norcott JP, Brown DW. Competitive radioimmunoassay to detect antibodies to herpes B virus and SA 8 virus. *J Clin Microbiol.* 1993;31:931–935.

39. Slomka MJ, Brown DW, Clewley JP, et al. Polymerase chain reaction for detection of *Herpesvirus simiae* (B virus) in clinical specimens. *Arch Virol.* 1993;131:89–99.

40. Zwartouw HT, Humphreys CR, Collins P. Oral chemotherapy of fatal B virus (*Herpesvirus simiae*) infection. *Antiviral Res.* 1989;11:275–283.

CHAPTER 15

Herpes Simplex Virus Infection

Mahmoud A. Khalifa and Ernest E. Lack

Throughout nature, infection without disease is the rule rather than the exception.

René J. Dubos (1901–1982), Man Adapting, Chapter VII

DEFINITION

Herpes simplex virus (HSV) (from *herpo* meaning "to creep") is a member of the family *Herpesviridae*. Other members of the *Herpesviridae* that can infect mankind are varicella-zoster virus, cytomegalovirus, Epstein–Barr virus, and human herpesvirus types 6 and 7. Some *Herpesviridae* infect other animals, eg, *Herpesvirus simiae,* which is a natural parasite of monkeys. Members of this family of viruses contain double-stranded DNA and are morphologically similar. HSV is divided into two variants, type 1 (HSV-1) and type 2 (HSV-2) and these have different epidemiologic, antigenic, and molecular properties.

NONDISSEMINATED HERPES SIMPLEX INFECTION

Clinical Features

Nearly all humans, at some time in their lives, become infected by one or more viruses of the family *Herpesviridae.* The vast majority of infections of HSV are either asymptomatic or cause mucosal or cutaneous lesions with minimal morbidity. HSV-1 usually infects nongenital sites (eg, gingivostomatitis) in a variety of locations. Primary infection results from exposure to cutaneous or mucosal lesions of a patient with HSV infection or with contaminated fomites. Person-to-person transmission is exemplified by wrestlers ("herpes gladiatorum") or patients who develop a herpetic whitlow (Figure 15–1), an infection of a finger that is frequently painful and may be seen in medical or dental personnel following exposure to HSV in a patient's mouth. Infections begin as small papules and progress to vesicles, which usually provoke little to no symptoms, but ulcerated lesions may be very painful in either HSV-1 [eg, herpetic esophagitis (Figure 15–2)] or HSV-2 infection. Herpetic pharyngitis caused by HSV-2 has been reported in male homosexuals. Localized herpetic lymphadenitis is an uncommon complication of HSV infection,[1,2] with well-circumscribed areas of necrosis containing cells with characteristic intranuclear inclusions. Herpetic encephalitis may be a severe and sometimes fatal illness. Extensive necrosis may occur, usually involving a temporal lobe, which can clinically mimic a neoplasm or abscess. Rapid confirmation of the diagnosis may permit prompt anti-HSV therapy and save the patient's life, although some patients have permanent neurologic disabilities. Porencephaly, hydranencephaly, and multicystic lesions of the brain can all be sequelae.[3]

HSV-2 involves primarily genital sites such as the penis (Figure 15–3), urethra, vulva, vagina, cervix (Figure 15–4), and rarely endometrium.[4] Latent endometrial infection can occur that can spread to the placenta, where infection usually is not accompanied by the characteristic intranuclear viral inclusions and cell death. For instance, the embryo or fetus can become infected without demonstrable placentitis.[5] Genital herpes is sexually transmitted and is increasingly recognized in the sexually active female. Following recovery there may be latent infection for years, even in the presence of circulating antibodies, with the virus lying dormant in dorsal root ganglia of nerves that innervate the cutaneous or mucosal site of primary infection. Recrudescence or reactivation of the virus may occur at a future time, and this may be triggered by a variety of factors

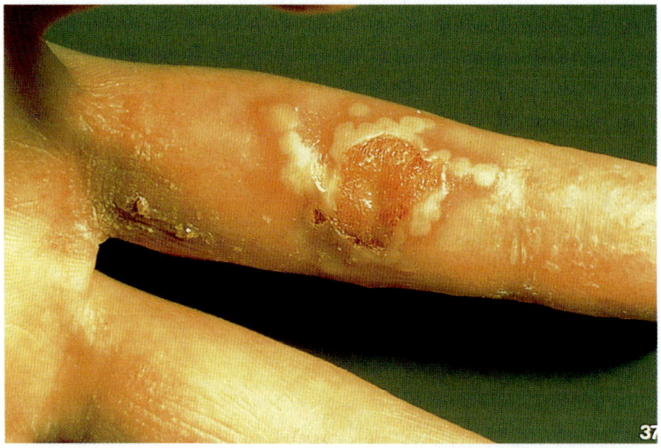

Figure 15–1. Herpetic whitlow. Lesion developed on the index finger of a nurse who had contact with a patient who had oral herpes simplex infection. Lesion is inflamed and ulcerated.

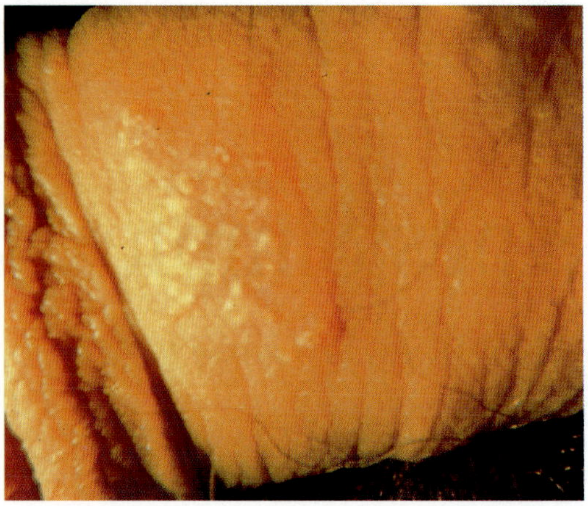

Figure 15–3. Herpes simplex infection of the penis. Small vesicles are closely grouped without ulceration or significant inflammation.

such as surgery, sunlight, fever, menstruation, emotional stress, or pregnancy.[6] Recurrent herpes infection often manifests as herpes labialis ("cold sore") at the mucocutaneous junction of lips or nose (Figure 15–5).

Pathology

The early herpetic lesion on skin or mucosal surface develops as small clusters of closely grouped vesicles (Figure 15–3), often with an erythematous base, and may progress to pustules, which become crusted and eventually heal without residue. Microscopically, the early intraepidermal or intramucosal vesicle shows separation and degeneration of epithelial cells with marked acantholysis and accumulation of intercellular proteinaceous fluid. Later there is a unilocular blister with intact roof of thinned epidermis (Figure 15–6, A). There is ballooning degeneration mainly at the base of vesicles. The ballooning degeneration is characterized by swelling of cells with homogenous eosinophilic cytoplasm and nucleomegaly with occasional multinucleated cells (Figure 15–6, B). The herpetic viral inclusion is a rounded, eosinophilic structure usually 3 to 8 μm in diameter and is often surrounded by a clear space or halo (Figure 15–6, C). There may be considerable variation in staining and shape of the viral inclusion (*vide infra*). Inflammatory cells may accumulate in the upper dermis and extend into the vesicle. When inflammation is severe and complicated by ulceration, the correct

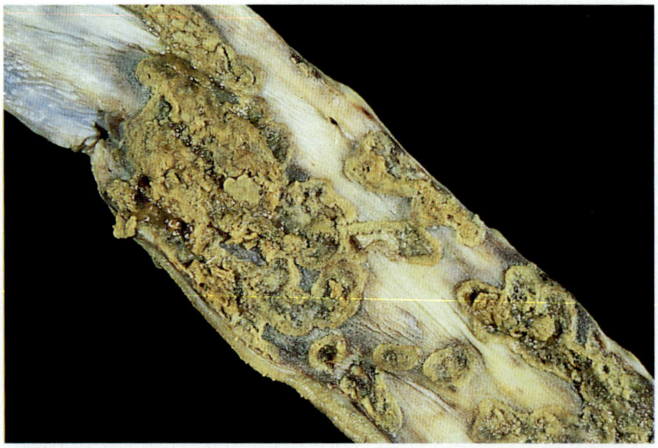

Figure 15–2. Extensive herpetic esophagitis in an adult patient at autopsy. Superficial mucosal ulcerations are partially covered by a fibrinopurulent exudate. *(Photograph courtesy of Manuel Marcial, MD)*

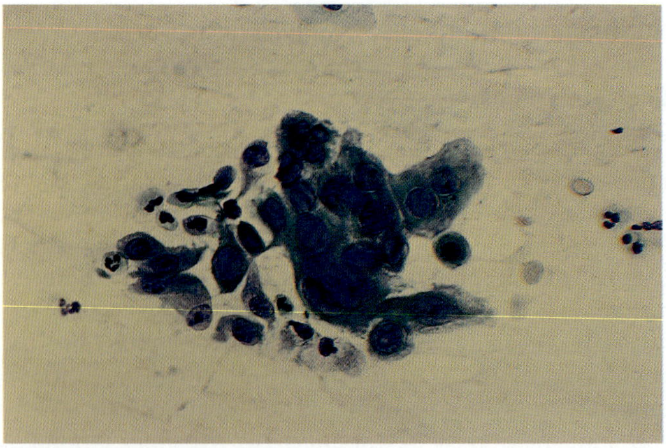

Figure 15–4. Herpes simplex infection of the cervix. Pap smear shows aggregate of multinucleated squamous cells with some molding and "ground glass" appearance of nuclei (papanicolaou stain, ×1000).

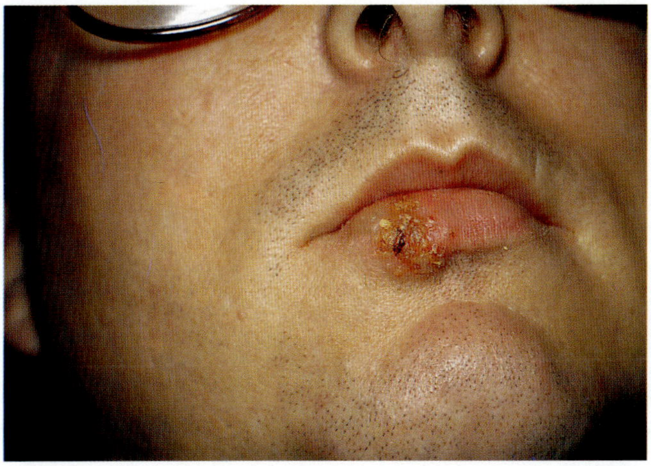

Figure 15–5. Reactivated herpes simplex infection of the upper lip in a male adult patient. Lesion is focally ulcerated with moist, irregular surface.

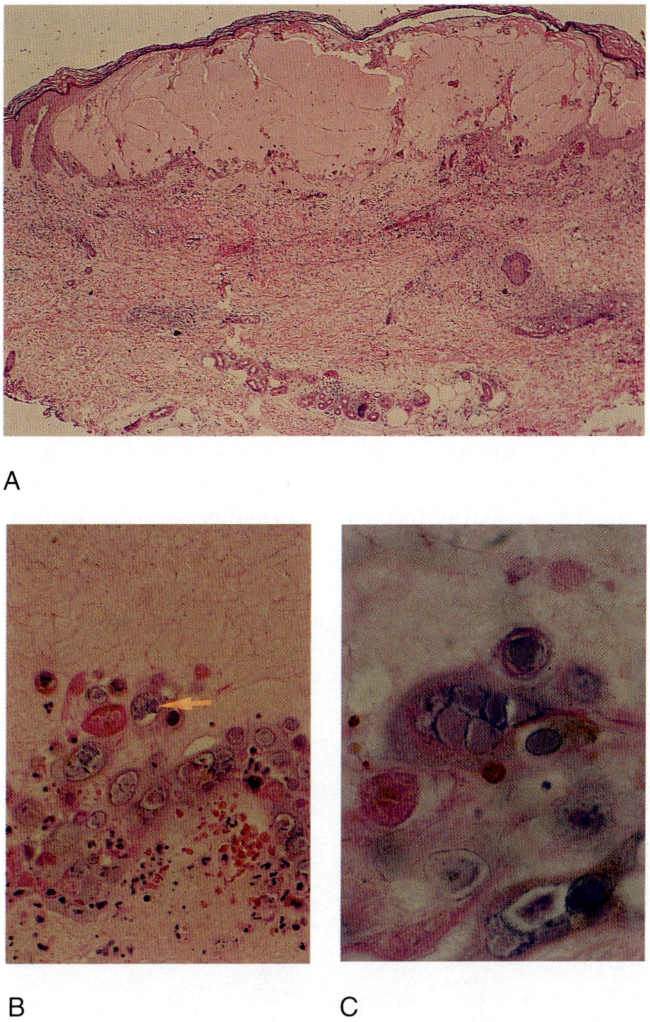

Figure 15–6. Herpes simplex infection of skin. (**A**) Unilocular vesicle shows much degeneration of keratinocytes along base. Roof of vesicle is intact (hematoxylin-eosin, ×40). (**B**) Ballooning degeneration of epidermal cells. Many nuclei have characteristic amphophilic to eosinophilic inclusions within nuclei *(arrow).* Some cells are multinucleated (hematoxylin-eosin, ×400). (**C**) Epidermal cells along base of intact vesicle show diagnostic viral cytopathic effect with amphophilic to eosinophilic intranuclear inclusions (hematoxylin-eosin, ×1000).

diagnosis may be obscured. If viral infection is suspected, biopsy of an early vesicle is desirable. Unroofing of intact vesicles may permit microscopic examination of stained smears (Tzanck preparation) for the diagnostic viral cytopathic effect of HSV.

The microscopic cytoarchitectural features of the vesicles produced by HSV are identical to those caused by varicella-zoster, but distinction is aided by clinical features as well as differences in antigenicity and growth characteristics in vitro. Herpetic encephalitis is probably a manifestation of reactivation of latent herpes infection. Neurons and astrocytic cells may be infected, but it may be very difficult to identify the virus without ancillary diagnostic techniques.

DISSEMINATED HERPES SIMPLEX INFECTION

Clinical Features

Disseminated herpes simplex in the newborn was first recognized by Hass in 1935, who referred to the process as hepatoadrenal necrosis.[7] Intranuclear viral inclusions of herpes had been recognized by Cowdry in 1934.[8] Although neonatal HSV infection may follow a relatively benign course, about half of the infants die. Most neonatal infections are caused by HSV-2, but about 20% are caused by HSV-1.[9] Disseminated HSV can develop in adult patients as a complication of underlying malignancy, malnutrition, burns, or states of deficient immunity including exogenous steroid administration and acquired immunodeficiency syndrome (AIDS). Disseminated HSV in immunodeficient adult patients is usually fatal in spite of antiviral therapy.[10] Rarely, cases of disseminated HSV have also been reported in ostensibly healthy patients.[11] Most infections in neonates are acquired from maternal HSV involving the genital tract, and transmission usually occurs during or shortly after parturition, with signs or symptoms of infection usually within the first 10 days of life (average age, 5 days).[9]

Infection can also develop from contact with penile vesicles from other individuals with active herpes infection, such as the mother's coital partner, resulting in contamination or infection of the birth canal. About 50% of infants die (average 6 days after onset), and 25% to 30% of survivors may have neurologic deficits, blindness, or both.[9]

Pathology

In disseminated herpes simplex infection viremia leads to involvement of various sites such as the liver, adrenal glands, oropharynx and esophagus, lung, brain, and eye. There may be distinctive punctuate areas of yellow-tan necrosis, usually 0.5 to 3 mm in diameter, with hyperemic rims, which on gross inspection might allow one to suspect strongly a viral cause (Figure 15–7, A and B). Visceral lesions often appear as "punched-out," well-demarcated zones of coagulative necrosis with little in the way of any inflammatory reaction (Figure 15–8, A); with hepatic involvement the necrotic foci are randomly distributed without any particular zone being affected. Sometimes necrotic foci may become confluent. The intranuclear viral inclusions may show some variation in shape and staining quality as conveyed in the detailed description of liver involvement and camera lucida drawings provided by Hass.[7] The inclusion may be amphophilic, homogeneous, or "glassy," and bordered by clumped chromatin (Cowdry type B inclusion) (Figure 15–8, B), or it may be deeply acidophilic, homogeneous, and centrally placed with a clear halo and peripheral condensation of chromatin (Cowdry type A inclusion) (Figure 15–9). The inclusion is greater than one half the diameter of the nucleus. During intranuclear replication of the virus, host DNA is involved in synthesizing protein for the viral particles, and the early inclusion body appears amphophilic. The viral nucleocapsid then acquires an envelope as it passes into the cytoplasm and becomes the complete infectious virus. Multinucleated cells are more likely to contain the amphophilic nuclear inclusions.[9] As the

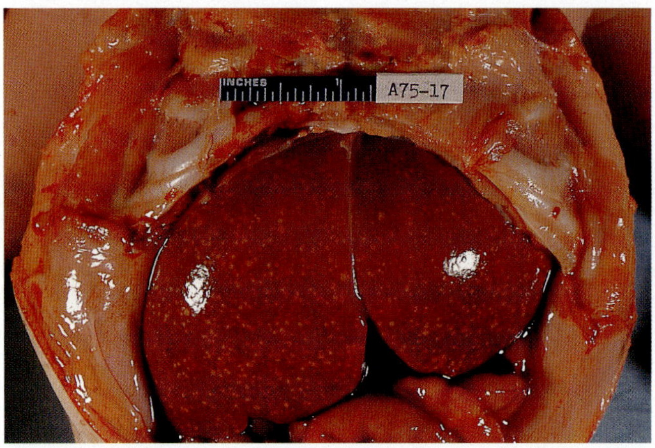

A

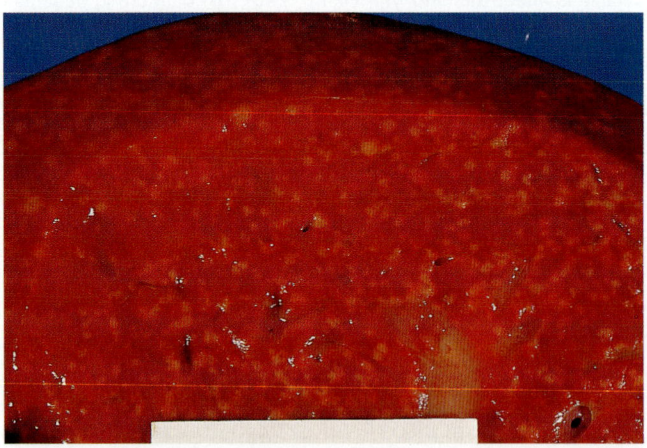

B

Figure 15–7. Fatal disseminated herpes simplex infection in a newborn. (**A**) Miliary foci of necrosis are evident beneath Glisson's capsule, which is smooth without evidence of wrinkling. (**B**) Cross-section of hepatic parenchyma [same case as (A)]. Punctuate areas of liver necrosis are pale yellow with hyperemic borders.

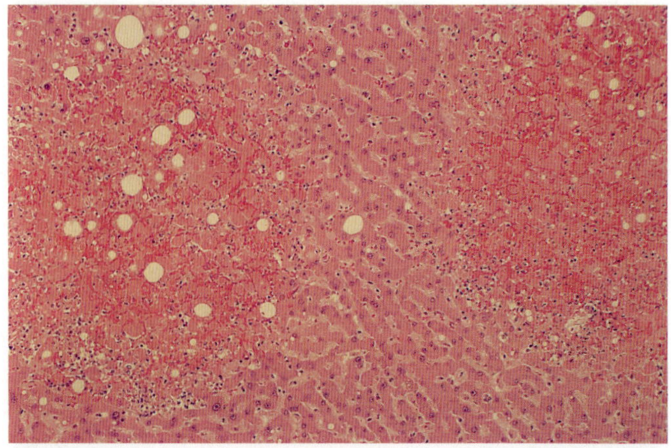

A

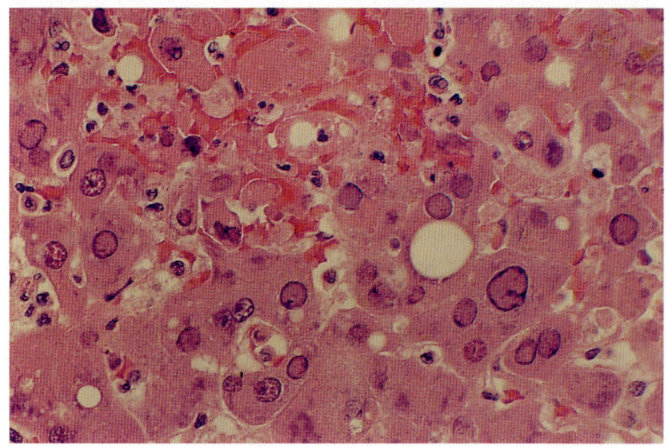

B

Figure 15–8. Liver in fatal disseminated herpes simplex infection in an adult. (**A**) Note rounded zones of coagulative necrosis with associated congestion. Viral inclusions were in hepatocytes bordering areas of necrosis (hematoxylin-eosin, ×40). (**B**) Numerous liver cells near necrotic zone have viral cytopathic effect of herpes infection (hematoxylin-eosin, ×400).

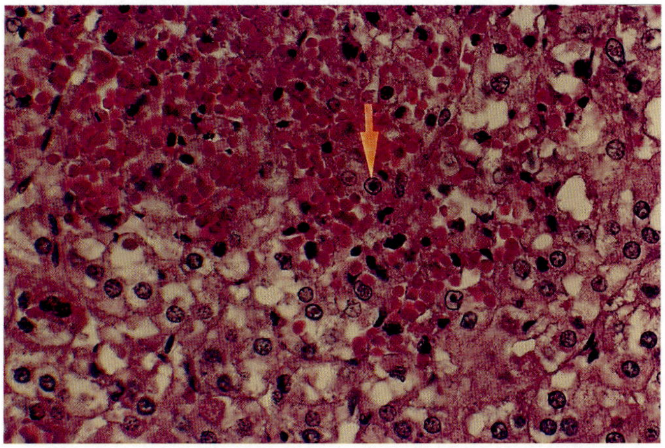

Figure 15–9. Adrenal gland in fatal disseminated herpes simplex infection. Note zone of coagulative necrosis and hemorrhage. Nucleus of occasional cortical cell at periphery *(arrow)* has Cowdry type A viral inclusion, which is deeply acidophilic and centrally placed with surrounding halo (hematoxylin-eosin, ×200).

viral DNA is encapsidated and egresses from the nucleus, the nuclear inclusion changes from amphophilic to eosinophilic, which reflects the excess viral capsid material synthesized by the nucleus.[12]

ANCILLARY DIAGNOSTIC TECHNIQUES

Herpes simplex virus infection can be diagnosed by ultrastructural study, but identification of the virus may be difficult due to sampling error (Figure 15–10). The intranuclear viral particle has a central core of double-stranded DNA 30 to 40 nm in diameter surrounded by a protein shell or capsid that measures approximately 100 nm (Figure 15–10, B). When the virus egresses from the nucleus, the capsid is enveloped by a lipid-rich portion of nuclear membrane with an intervening zone of glycoprotein-rich material, which completes the formation of the infectious viral particle or virion (150 to about 200 nm in diameter). The nucleocapsid (combined nucleic acid core and capsid) has icosahedral symmetry (20 equal triangular surfaces) with 162 capsomeres. Immunohistochemistry may provide a faster, more sensitive method for identification of the virus using monoclonal antibodies against HSV-1 versus

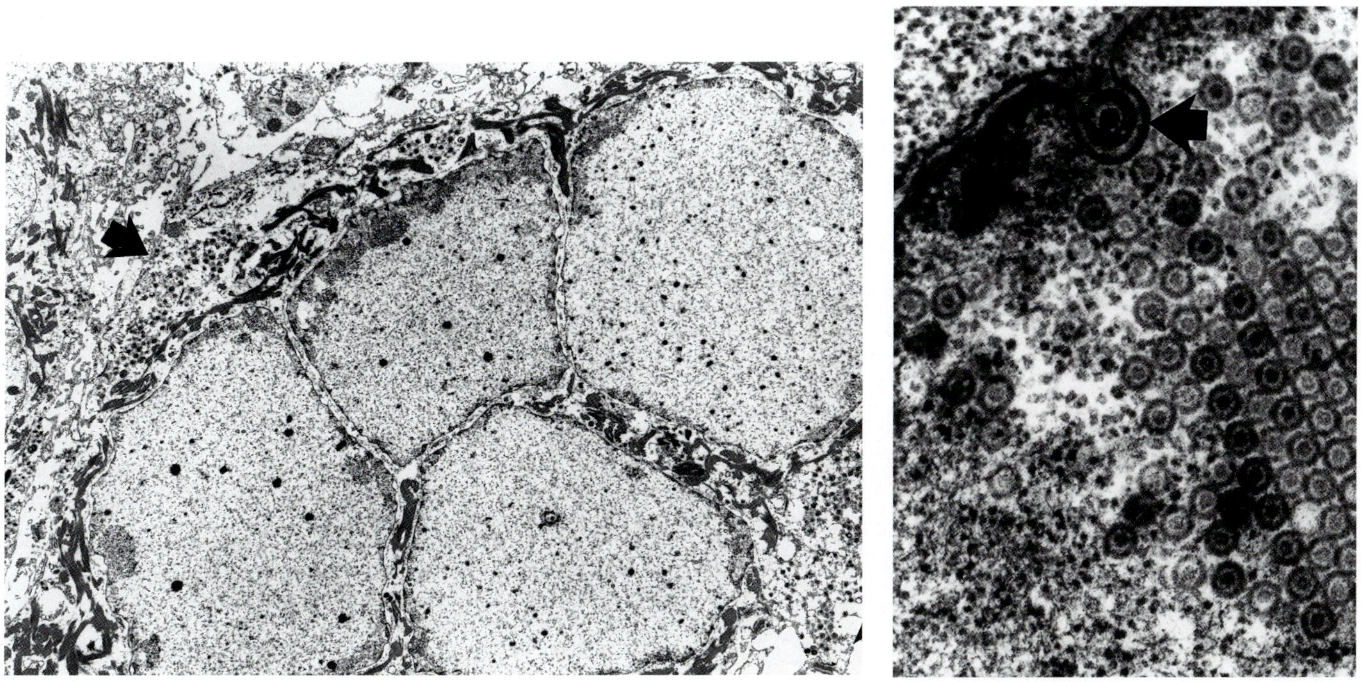

A B

Figure 15–10. Herpes simplex infection. (**A**) Infected multinucleated squamous cells show a relatively homogenous granular quality to nuclei ("ground glass" change) with peripheral aggregation of heterochromatin. Intact virions within cytoplasm are composed of a DNA core or genome, capsid, and envelope *(arrows)* (×20,000). (**B**) Numerous encapsidated viral particles with central DNA are present within nucleus of infected host cell and have characteristic symmetry. Note one virion with envelope being acquired from inner membrane of nucleus *(arrow)*. Herpes simplex virus particles with envelopes in cytoplasm have been found to be highly infectious (×75,000).

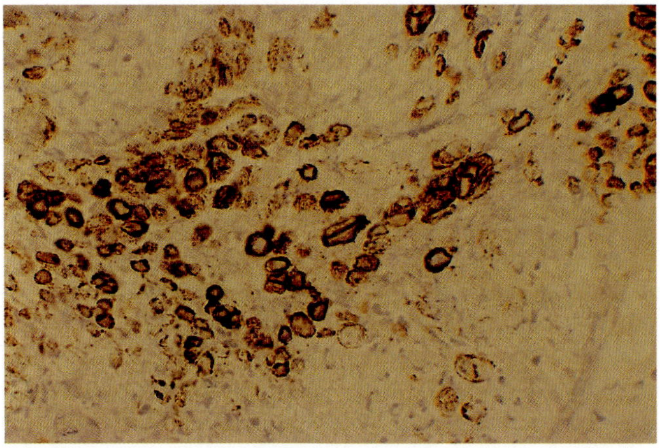

Figure 15–11. Herpes simplex infection of esophagus. Numerous cells are strongly immunostained for herpes antigen within cytoplasm (peroxidase antiperoxidase stain, ×200).

HSV-2 (Figure 15–11). Theoretically, antibodies directed against the envelope will show predominantly cytoplasmic staining, whereas antibody against the capsid will stain both nucleus and cytoplasm of the infected cell.

Other sensitive techniques have also been used such as polymerase chain reaction and in situ hybridization.[13,14] Immunohistochemistry and in situ hybridization were shown to be equally effective for detecting herpesvirus in paraffin sections.[15] The virus can be grown in tissue culture, but characteristic viral cytopathic effect may be delayed for several days (Figure 15–12).

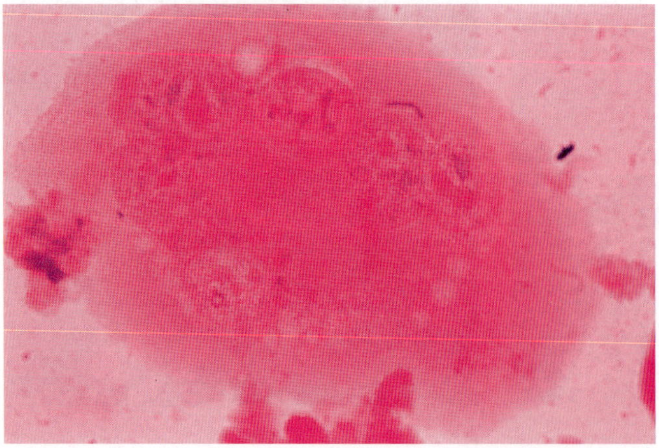

Figure 15–12. Characteristic cytopathic effect of tissue culture cells in vitro infected by herpes simplex virus. Culture was inoculated with specimen from newborn infant with fatal disseminated herpes simplex infection (hematoxylin-eosin stain, ×1000).

REFERENCES

1. Tamaru J, Mikata A, Horie H, et al. Herpes simplex lymphadenitis. *Am J Surg Pathol.* 1990;14:571–577.
2. Gaffey MJ, Ben-Ezra JM, Weiss LM. Herpes simplex lymphadenitis. *Am J Clin Pathol.* 1991;95:709–714.
3. Smith JB, Groover RV, Klass DW, Houser OW. Multicystic cerebral degeneration in neonatal herpes simplex virus encephalitis. *Am J Dis Child.* 1977;131:568–572.
4. Duncan DA, Varner RE, Mazur MT. Uterine herpes virus infection with multifocal necrotizing endometritis. *Hum Pathol.* 1989;20:1021–1024.
5. Schwartz DA, Caldwell E. Herpes simplex virus infection of the placenta. *Arch Pathol Lab Med.* 1991;115:1141–1144.
6. Melnick JL. The herpesvirus group. *Bull Pan Am Health Organ.* 1977;11:153–156.
7. Hass GM. Hepato-adrenal necrosis with intranuclear inclusion bodies. *Am J Pathol.* 1935;11:127–142.
8. Cowdry EV. The problem of intranuclear inclusions in virus diseases. *Arch Pathol.* 1934;18:527–542.
9. Singer DB. Pathology of neonatal herpes simplex virus infection. *Perspect Pediatr Pathol.* 1981;6:243–278.
10. Johnson JR, Egaas S, Gleaves CA, Hackman R, Bowden RA. Hepatitis due to herpes simplex virus in marrow-transplant recipients. *Clin Infect Dis.* 1992;14:38–45.
11. Rubin MH, Ward DM, Painter J. Fulminant hepatic failure caused by genital herpes in a healthy person. *JAMA.* 1985;253:1299–1301.
12. Robin ER, Jenson AB. Electron microscopic studies of animal viruses with emphasis on in vivo infections. *Prog Med Virol.* 1967;9:392–450.
13. Rogers BB, Josephson SL, Mak SK, Sweeney PJ. Polymerase chain reaction amplification of herpes simplex virus DNA from clinical samples. *Obstet Gynecol.* 1992;79:464–469.
14. Werner JC, Widebrauk DL. Polymerase chain reaction for diagnosis of herpetic eye disease. *Lab Med.* 1994;25:664–668.
15. Strickler JG, Manivel JC, Copenhaver CM, Kubic VL. Comparison of in situ hybridization and immunohistochemistry for detection of cytomegalovirus and herpes simplex virus. *Hum Pathol.* 1990;21:443–448.

CHAPTER 16

Human Immunodeficiency Virus Infection Cardiac Lesions

Phillip J. Harrity and Ramiah Subramanian

Art is long, and Time is fleeting,
And our hearts, though stout and brave,
Still, like muffled drums, are beating
Funeral marches to the grave.

Henry Wadsworth Longfellow (1807–1882), A Psalm of Life

. . . then I will do this to you: I will bring upon you sudden terror, wasting diseases and fever that will destroy your sight and drain away your life.

Leviticus 26:16

INTRODUCTION

The acquired immunodeficiency syndrome (AIDS) has increased tremendously in prevalence and importance worldwide. With AIDS, almost every organ and system in the body is involved. Here we discuss the direct and indirect effects of infection by the human immunodeficiency virus (HIV) on the heart.

Increased frequency of opportunistic infections such as *Pneumocystis carinii* and neoplasms such as Kaposi's sarcoma in homosexual men were associated with immunodeficiency.[1–3] Human immunodeficiency virus was subsequently found to cause profound immunosuppression. Cardiac changes were initially noted at autopsy in these patients and were not thought to have contributed to morbidity and mortality.[4–13] Retrospective and prospective echocardiographic studies revealed an increased incidence of cardiac abnormalities, with or without symptoms, in patients infected with HIV.[14–31] Further studies also disclosed a higher prevalence of cardiac dilatation, myocarditis, opportunistic infection, and neoplasms than was first reported.[32–66]

Anderson and Virmani[67] proposed a classification of cardiac abnormalities in patients infected with HIV, based on the heart layer affected. Their categories included pericardial, endocardial, and myocardial involvement, with HIV cardiomyopathy listed as a separate entity. Their classification, with minor modifications, has been followed in this chapter; primary myocardial involvement with HIV is subdivided into myocarditis and cardiomyopathy. Superimposed lesions including opportunistic infections and neoplasms involving the heart are discussed as secondary effects.

PRIMARY HIV-ASSOCIATED HEART DISEASE

Myocarditis in Patients with HIV

HIV-infected patients have left ventricular dysfunction or myocarditis (confirmed either by endomyocardial

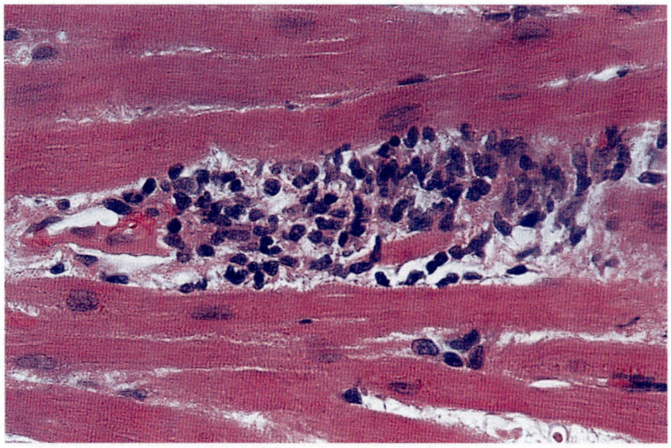

Figure 16–1. Endomyocardial biopsy with active myocarditis manifested by focal mononuclear cell infiltration and myocyte necrosis in a 38-year-old black female with AIDS. The patient had increasing dyspnea on exertion and congestive heart failure for 2 weeks. An echocardiogram revealed poor overall left ventricular function with a mildly dilated left ventricle and left atrium and preserved right ventricular function. There was mild pericardial effusion (hematoxylin-eosin, ×400). *(Photograph courtesy of Dr. Ahvie Herskowitz, Ischemia Research and Education Foundation, San Francisco, California.)*

biopsy or autopsy), with varying amounts of overlap.[14–22,25–27,30,32–34,68] A significant proportion of these patients had symptomatic ventricular dysfunction, mostly during the AIDS-positive portion of their illness, and some had myocarditis.

In general, the cause of the myocarditis may not be identifiable. Many viruses are cardiotropic.[69] An interstitial lymphocytic infiltrate, with or without associated myocyte injury, is the most common histologic finding in viral myocarditis (Figure 16–1). There may be other inflammatory cells, including neutrophils, eosinophils, and macrophages.[69,70] T lymphocytes predominate in the infiltrates, with variable numbers of B lymphocytes.[71] Herskowitz et al[68] noted a predominance of CD8+ T lymphocytes in HIV myocarditis. Idiopathic myocarditis in HIV-infected patients has been reviewed.[35–39,67,72] Its prevalence has varied from 0% to 60%.* This wide range may be a consequence of 1) inconsistencies in the pathologic definition of myocarditis, 2) variability of risk factors for HIV infection (intravenous drug abuse versus homosexual transmission), 3) stage of HIV disease studied (asymptomatic versus preterminal), and 4) nature of study design (eg, retrospective versus prospective analysis, clinical or pathologic).

Idiopathic Myocarditis

A distinction has been made between myocarditis of known cause and idiopathic myocarditis in some autopsy reports of HIV-infected patients.† Some of these investigators have separated Dallas criteria-positive myocarditis, with myocyte necrosis, from borderline myocarditis without necrosis.[73] In 165 of 958 patients (17%), there were lymphocytes in the interstices associated with necrosis of myofibers. In a further 98 patients (10%), there were interstitial lymphocytes but no necrosis.‡

Ten clinicopathologic studies have addressed the issue of idiopathic myocarditis in HIV-positive patients with cardiac symptoms. Histologic confirmation of myocarditis in these studies ranged from 4% to 100%.[15,18,24,28–31,33,56,68] In eight of these studies with 81 patients, 33 (41%) hearts had lymphocytic infiltrates with myocyte necrosis and 16 (20%) had lymphocytic interstitial infiltrates only.[18,24,28–30,33,56,68]

HIV Cardiomyopathy and Left Ventricular Dysfunction

Eleven to 54% of HIV-infected patients in nine clinicopathologic studies have had echocardiographic and radionuclide ventriculographic evidence of left ventricular dysfunction.[37] The relationship between left ventricular dysfunction, myocarditis, and cardiomyopathy has been investigated in clinicopathologic studies.[17–31,59,61,68,74–78] Twelve of these were prospective,[17–22,25,27,30,31,74,78] 10 had clearly stated follow-up periods,[17–20,23,24,27,30,31,74] and 6 commented on the potential reversibility of the ventricular dysfunction.[17,18,20,24,27,30]

Cardiomyopathy

The hearts of 107 patients with HIV were examined for cardiomyopathic changes at autopsy.[59,61,75,77] Five patients reported by Joshi et al[61] were pediatric patients. The remaining 102 patients were adults.[59,75,77] Approximately 60% of the adults had been intravenous drug abusers and 28% were homosexual. Segal and Factor[59] studied the hearts of 91 adult HIV-positive patients. Hypertrophy of myocardial cells and interstitial fibrosis—changes consistent with cardiomyopathy—were in 40% of patients overall and the relationship of these changes to known cardiac disease risk factors

* References 4–6, 9, 10, 14, 15, 18, 24, 28–31, 32–34, 40–66, 68.

† References 4–6, 9, 10, 32, 34, 35, 40–44, 46–55, 59–65.

‡ References 4–6, 9, 32, 34, 35, 40, 42, 43, 49, 50, 59–65.

(hypertension, diabetes, tobacco use, etc) was analyzed. The authors indicated that the histopathologic changes identified could have been accounted for by these cardiac risk factors.[59] Fourteen patients (13.1%) in the four studies were also noted to have myocarditis of varying causes.[59,61,75,77]

Cardiomyopathy and Left Ventricular Dysfunction

A total of 1069 HIV-infected patients were examined for ventricular dysfunction.[17–31,59,61,68,74–78] Overall, 45% were intravenous drug abusers, 36% were homosexuals, 11% contracted HIV by other means, and 8% were children. Tissue was examined in 8% (54 autopsy hearts and 37 biopsy specimens of endomyocardium). Approximately 22% of the adult patients had global left ventricular dysfunction; 1% had segmental motion abnormalities of the left ventricular wall; and 2% had global right ventricular dysfunction. In these studies, 48 (51.6%) of 93 patients with left ventricular dysfunction and 9 (52.9%) of 17 patients with right ventricular dysfunction reverted to normal during clinical follow-up.[17,18,20,24,27,30] Myocardial lymphocytic infiltrates with necrosis of myocytes were noted in 35 patients (38.5%); 24 (26.4%) had lymphocytic myocardial infiltrates without myocyte necrosis.

ISOLATION OF HIV

HIV has been isolated from the myocardium by various methods.[43,68,79–84] Rodriguez et al[79] separated human ventricular myocytes from interstitial myocardial dendritic-type cells by microdissection, before detection of HIV by nested polymerase chain reaction (PCR) amplification. HIV was isolated from the myocardium of five patients[79,83] in whom concomitant left ventricular dysfunction was noted. Two patients[79,84] had isolated right ventricular dilatation and dysfunction. Only one patient, in whom HIV was isolated from the myocardium, had focal myocarditis histologically.[82] There was no causal relation established between HIV in the myocardium, myocarditis, and left ventricular dysfunction in any of the patients.

SECONDARY HIV-ASSOCIATED HEART DISEASE

The most common cardiac diseases in patients with HIV are caused by immunosuppression rather than by the direct effects of HIV. These secondary diseases are classified by anatomic site (endocardial, myocardial, or pericardial) as well as by cause (infectious, drug-related, neoplastic, etc).

TABLE 16–1. COMPENDIUM OF REFERENCES

HIV-Related Pericardial Disease	
Pericardial effusion	(8,10,14,15,17,18,21–24,27–32,34,40,50,54, 55,58,68,76–77,83–100)
Pericarditis (with or without effusion)	
	Bacterial (24,88,92,94–96)
	Mycobacterial (9,14,29,41,87,89,93,94)
	Viral (14,85,86)
	Fungal (101,102)
	Not otherwise specified (9,25)
Neoplastic	Kaposi's sarcoma (4,6,9–12,14,31,34,40,62,65, 96–98,103)
	Lymphoma (10,13,14,66,91,99,100,104–110)
HIV-Related Myocardial Disease	
Myocarditis	(10,18,28,29,31,33,49,59,60,62,111)
	Bacterial (11,32,34,35)
	Viral (4,5,10,15,24,41–43,52,61,65,68)
	Fungal (4,5,10,14,30,32,34,35,41,42,47,68,111)
	Mycobacterial (10,32,41,66)
	Hypersensitivity (68)
	Rheumatic fever (48)
	Protozoal-parasitic (4,6,9,10,14,34,41,42,44,45, 50–52,54,55,57,58)
Neoplastic	Kaposi's Sarcoma (9,11,13,14,31,40,65)
	Lymphoma (10,66,99,100,104–106,108–110)
Other	Doxorubicin toxicity (15)
	TTP (112)
HIV-Related Endocardial Disease	
Endocarditis	(5–7,18,22,23,25,27–29,34,41,42,74)
	Infective (9,17,24,30,31,59,91)
	Bacterial (14,81,113–117)
	Fungal (111,118)
	Protozoal/parasitic (44)
	Nonbacterial thrombotic (4,8,10,40,119)
Neoplastic	Lymphoma (10,99,100,105,106)
	Kaposi's sarcoma (103)

Pericardial Disease

The most common cardiac manifestation associated with HIV infection overall is pericardial effusion.* Ten percent of patients with effusion had cardiac tamponade. The prevalence of pericardial effusions has ranged from 1% to 100%, with a mean of 25%. Pericardial effusions were in 28% of children.[18–24] References to other forms of pericardial disease are in Table 16–1.

* References 8, 10, 14, 15, 17, 18, 21–24, 27–32, 34, 40, 50, 54, 55, 58, 68, 76, 77, 83–100.

Myocardial Disease

Secondary myocardial diseases of known cause in HIV-infected patients are listed in Table 16–1. Cytomegalovirus (CMV) and *Toxoplasma gondii* were the most commonly isolated pathogens, involving approximately 2% and 4% of patients at autopsy, respectively. In clinicopathologic studies 2% had CMV myocarditis and 1% had toxoplasmosis. Other secondary myocardial diseases are summarized in Table 16–1.

Endocardial Disease

Secondary endocardial disease in HIV-infected patients manifests itself most commonly as infective or noninfective endocarditis (see Table 16–1). Involvement of endocardium by neoplasia (Kaposi's sarcoma and lymphoma) has been described (see Table 16–1). About 5% of HIV-infected children have had infective endocarditis.[18,24] The prevalence of endocarditis in adults was approximately 3%, equally divided between infective endocarditis and noninfective endocarditis. Other causes of endocardial disease are listed in Table 16–1.

Neoplastic Disease

Thirty studies have reported neoplastic involvement of heart in HIV infection—a total of 907 patients.† Seventeen of these studies are large cohorts, while others describe a single patient.‡ The major neoplasms identified in HIV-infected patients have been Kaposi's sarcoma and lymphomas. In 35 of the 40 patients (88%) with neoplasms, the pericardium and epicardium were involved. The myocardium was involved in 10 (25%). There was exclusive myocardial involvement in 3 patients. Kaposi's sarcoma involved the adventitia of epicardial coronary arteries in 12 patients (Figure 16–2). This involvement did not compromise myocardial perfusion.

Cardiac involvement by lymphoma has been reported in 28 patients (3% of the total population studied). Fourteen of these were of B cell, small noncleaved; 7 were large cell and large cell immunoblastic; and 1 was an apparent T-cell proliferative disorder. In 6 patients, the subtype of the lymphoma was not specified. (References are listed in Table 16–1.)

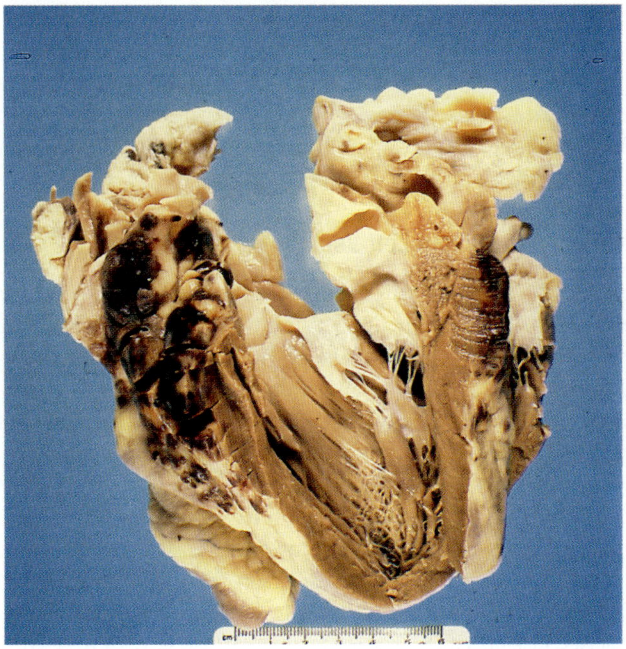

Figure 16–2. Kaposi's sarcoma involving the epicardium in a male homosexual AIDS patient. Kaposi's sarcoma extends over the anterior surface of the heart. The epicardial coronary arteries were surrounded by the neoplasm but the lumens were not narrowed.

CONCLUSIONS AND CAVEATS

Myocarditis in HIV Patients

Current views on idiopathic myocarditis propose an autoimmune pathogenesis, triggered by various insults, one of which could be viral infection—either latent or lytic—of myocardial cells.[120] There is also evidence that cytokines produced locally in the heart or circulating cytokines such as tumor necrosis factor-alpha and interleukin-6 may directly depress cardiac function.[120] In addition, the findings of Herskowitz et al[68] regarding increased MHC class I, but not class II, antigen expression in biopsy specimens of heart from HIV-positive patients with myocarditis further supports a virally induced immune-mediated cause. Although HIV infects various CD4 negative cells in culture[121,122] and can infect fetal cardiac cells in culture by way of cell surface Fc receptors,[68] these mechanisms have not been demonstrated in vivo. Proof of an autoimmune pathogenesis in general, and in HIV-infected patients in particular, is lacking and awaits definitive studies.

Although HIV has been isolated from myocardial cells as discussed earlier, no conclusive evidence exists that it is a direct cause of myocarditis. The assertion of Herskowitz et al,[68] that a slightly increased number of CD8+ myocardial interstitial lymphocytes represents myocarditis is an intriguing definition of myocarditis but not enough immunohistochemical T-cell subset studies have been performed to settle the matter. Intravenous drug abusers without HIV infection have myocarditis in which CD8+ T cells predominate.[123] Herskowitz et al[72] have also demonstrated nonlytic

† References 4–6, 8–14, 31, 34, 40, 42, 65, 66, 91, 96–100, 103–110.

‡ References 4–6, 8–10, 12, 14, 31, 34, 40, 42, 65, 91, 100, 107, 110.

CMV infection of myocytes in HIV patients as a possible cause of myocarditis and left ventricular dysfunction.

There are additional difficulties with HIV and myocarditis. First, not all authors agree on the definition of myocarditis. Second, there is a discrepancy between the rates of myocarditis in autopsy and clinicopathologic studies; the generally poor rate (mean 8.5%) of tissue examination in clinicopathologic studies makes their higher rates of myocarditis suspect. Third, many studies have not used advanced techniques for identification of the many possible cardiotropic viruses that may cause myocarditis in HIV-infected patients. A poor rate of tissue acquisition has greatly hindered such investigation.

HIV-Associated Left Ventricular Dysfunction and Cardiomyopathy

There can be little doubt that left and right ventricular dysfunction afflicts HIV-infected patients. The evidence suggests that HIV plays a direct role in left ventricular dysfunction, but does not conclusively establish such a role, nor is there proof that dysfunction can be necessarily equated with cardiomyopathy by the 1995 WHO/ISFC definition of cardiomyopathy.[124] The high rate of reversal of dysfunction noted in some and the low rate of tissue examination in many clinical studies are two reasons why such conclusions may be premature; additional prospective, long-term follow-up with better pathologic tissue correlation is needed for confirmation.

Acknowledgments. Ms. Judi Clark assisted in preparing the manuscript, Ms. Mary Jo Koenen assisted with the references, and Dr. Ahvie Herskowitz contributed the photomicrograph.

REFERENCES

1. Gottlieb MS, Schroff R, Schanker HM, et al. *Pneumocystis carinii* pneumonia and mucosal candidiasis in previously healthy homosexual men. *N Engl J Med.* 1981;305: 1425–1431.
2. *Pneumocystis* pneumonia: Los Angeles. *MMWR.* 1981;30: 250–252.
3. Hymes KB, Cheung TL, Green JB, et al. Kaposi's sarcoma in homosexual men: a report of eight cases. *Lancet.* 1981;2:598–600.
4. Guarda LA, Luna MA, Smith JL, Mansell PWA, Gyorkey F, Roca AN. Acquired immune deficiency syndrome: postmortem findings. *Am J Clin Pathol.* 1984;81:549–557.
5. Niedt GW, Schinella RA. Acquired immunodeficiency syndrome: clinicopathologic study of 56 autopsies. *Arch Pathol Lab Med.* 1985;109:727–734.
6. Reichert CM, O'Leary TJ, Levens DL, Simrell CR, Macher AM. Autopsy pathology in the acquired immune deficiency syndrome. *Am J Pathol.* 1983;112:357–382.
7. Hui AN, Koss MN, Meyer PR. Necropsy findings in acquired immunodeficiency syndrome: a comparison of premortem diagnoses with postmortem findings. *Hum Pathol.* 1984;15:670–676.
8. Fink L, Reichek N, St. John Sutton MG. Cardiac abnormalities in acquired immune deficiency syndrome. *Am J Cardiol.* 1984;54:1161–1163.
9. Roldan EO, Moskowitz L, Hensley GT. Pathology of the heart in acquired immunodeficiency syndrome. *Arch Pathol Lab Med.* 1987;111:943–946.
10. Klatt EC, Meyer PR. Pathology of the heart in acquired immunodeficiency syndrome (AIDS). *Arch Pathol Lab Med.* 1988;112:114.
11. Autran B, Gorin I, Leibowitch M, et al. AIDS in a Haitian woman with cardiac Kaposi's sarcoma and Whipple's disease. *Lancet.* 1983;ii:767–768.
12. Silver MA, Macher AM, Reichert CM, et al. Cardiac involvement by Kaposi's sarcoma in acquired immune deficiency syndrome (AIDS). *Am J Cardiol.* 1984;53: 983–985.
13. Guarner J, Byrnes RK, Chan WC, Birdsong G, Hertzler G, et al. Primary non-Hodgkin's lymphoma of the heart in two patients with the acquired immunodeficiency syndrome. *Arch Pathol Lab Med.* 1987;111:254–256.
14. Monseuz JJ, Kinney EL, Vittecoq D, et al. Comparison among acquired immune deficiency syndrome patients with and without clinical evidence of cardiac disease. *Am J Cardiol.* 1988;62:1311–1313.
15. Reilly JM, Cunnion RE, Anderson DW, et al. Frequency of myocarditis, left ventricular dysfunction and ventricular tachycardia in the acquired immune deficiency syndrome. *Am J Cardiol.* 1988;62:789–793.
16. Wu TC, Pizzomo MC, Hayward GS, et al. In situ detection of human cytomegalovirus immediate–early gene transcripts within cardiac myocytes of patients with HIV-associated cardiomyopathy. *AIDS* 1992;6:777–785.
17. Jacob AJ, Sutherland GR, Bird AG, et al. Myocardial dysfunction in patients infected with HIV: prevalence and risk factors. *Br Heart J.* 1992;68:549–553.
18. Lipshultz SE, Chanock S, Sanders SP, Colan SD, Perez-Atayde A, McIntosh K. Cardiovascular manifestations of human immunodeficiency virus infection in infants and children. *Am J Cardiol.* 1989;63:1489–1497.
19. Herskowitz A, Vlahov D, Willoughby SB, et al. Prevalence and incidence of left ventricular dysfunction in patients with human immunodeficiency virus infection. *Am J Cardiol.* 1993;71:955–958.
20. Herskowitz A, Willoughby SB, Vlahov D, Baughman KL, Ansari AA. Dilated heart muscle disease associated with HIV infection. *Eur Heart J.* 1995;16(suppl 0):50–55.
21. Levy WS, Simon GL, Rios JC, Ross AM. Prevalence of cardiac abnormalities in human immunodeficiency virus infection. *Am J Cardiol.* 1989;63:86–89.
22. Himelman RB, Chung WS, Chernoff DN, et al. Cardiac manifestations of human immunodeficiency virus infection: a two-dimensional echocardiographic study. *J Am Coll Cardiol.* 1989;13:1030–1036.
23. Kinney EL, Brafman D, Wright RJ. Echocardiographic find-

ings in patients with acquired immunodeficiency syndrome (AIDS) and AIDS-related complex (ARC). *Cathet Cardiovasc Diagn.* 1989;16:182–185.
24. Stewart JM, Kaul A, Gromisch DS, Reyes E, Woolf PK, Gowitz MH. Symptomatic cardiac dysfunction in children with human immunodeficiency virus infection. *Am Heart J.* 1989;117:140–144.
25. Raffanti SP, Chiaramida AJ, Sen P, Wright P, Middleton JR, Chiaramida S. Assessment of cardiac function in patients with acquired immunodeficiency syndrome. *Chest.* 1988;93:592–594.
26. Lipshultz SE, Orav EJ, Sanders SP, Rubin Hale A, McIntosh K, Colan SD. Cardiac structure and function in children with human immunodeficiency virus infection treated with Zidovudine. *N Engl J Med.* 1992;327:1260–1265.
27. Blanchard DG, Hagenhoff C, Chow LC, McCann HA, Dittrich HC. Reversibility of cardiac abnormalities in human immunodeficiency virus (HIV)-infected individuals: a serial echocardiographic study. *J Am Coll Cardiol.* 1991; 17:1270–1276.
28. Webb JG, Chan-Yan C, Kiess MC. Cardiac dysfunction associated with the acquired immunodeficiency syndrome (AIDS). *Clin Cardiol.* 1988;11:423–426.
29. Cohen IS, Anderson DW, Virmani R, et al. Congestive cardiomyopathy in association with the acquired immunodeficiency syndrome. *N Engl J Med.* 1986;315:628–630.
30. De Castro S, D'Amati G, Gallo P, et al. Frequency of development of acute global left ventricular dysfunction in human immunodeficiency virus infection. *J Am Coll Cardiol.* 1994;24:1018–1024.
31. Corallo S, Mutinelli MR, Moroni M, et al. Echocardiography detects myocardial damage in AIDS: prospective study in 102 patients. *Eur Heart J.* 1988;9:887–892.
32. Anderson DW, Virmani R, Reilly JM, et al. Prevalent myocarditis at necropsy in the acquired immunodeficiency syndrome. *J Am Coll Cardiol.* 1988;11:792–799.
33. Levy WS, Varghese PJ, Anderson DW, et al. Myocarditis diagnosed by endomyocardial biopsy in human immunodeficiency virus infection with cardiac dysfunction. *Am J Cardiol.* 1988;62:658–659.
34. Baroldi G, Corallo S, Moroni M, et al. Focal lymphocytic myocarditis in acquired immunodeficiency syndrome (AIDS): a correlative morphologic and clinical study in 26 consecutive fatal cases. *J Am Coll Cardiol.* 1988;12: 463–469.
35. Lewis W, Grody WW. AIDS and the heart: review and consideration of pathogenic mechanisms. *Cardiovasc Pathol.* 1992;1:53–64.
36. Francis CK. Cardiac involvement in AIDS. *Curr Probl Cardiol.* 1990;15:575–639.
37. McNulty CM. AIDS and the heart. In: Hurst JW, ed. *New Types of Cardiovascular Diseases: Topics in Clinical Cardiology.* New York: Igaku-Shoin; 1994:46–62.
38. Acierno LJ. Cardiac complications in acquired immunodeficiency syndrome (AIDS): a review. *J Am Coll Cardiol.* 1989;13:1144–1154.
39. Kaul S, Fishbein MC, Siegel RJ. Cardiac manifestations of acquired immune deficiency syndrome: a 1991 update. *Am Heart J.* 1991;122:535–554.
40. Lewis W. AIDS: cardiac findings from 115 autopsies. *Prog Cardiovasc Dis.* 1989;32:207–215.
41. Altieri PI, Lazala G, Torres JV, Climent C. Velez R. AIDS and the heart in the Caribbean: a silent entity. *Am J Cardiovasc Pathol.* 1992;4:25–30.
42. Fischer Hansen B. Pathology of the heart in AIDS: a study of 60 consecutive autopsies. *APMIS.* 1992;100:273–279.
43. Parravicini C, Baroldi G, Gaiera G, Lazzarin A. Phenotype of intramyocardial leukocytic infiltrates in acquired immunodeficiency syndrome (AIDS): a postmortem immunohistochemical study in 34 consecutive cases. *Mod Pathol.* 1991;4:559–565.
44. Ravalli S, Garcia RL, Vincent RA, Shein R. Disseminated *Pneumocystis carinii* infection in the acquired immunodeficiency syndrome. *NY State J Med.* 1990;90:155–157.
45. Rocha A, Oliveira de Meneses AC, Da Silva AM, et al. Pathology of patients with Chagas' disease and acquired immunodeficiency syndrome. *Am J Trop Med Hyg.* 1994;50(3):261–268.
46. Brady MT, Reiner CB, Singley C, Roberts WH III, Sneddon JM. Unexpected death in an infant with AIDS: disseminated cytomegalovirus infection with pancarditis. *Pediatr Pathol.* 1988;8:205–214.
47. Schonheyder H, Hoffman S, Elvang Jensen H, Fischer Hansen B, Franzmann MB. *Aspergillus fumigatus* fungaemia and myocarditis in a patient with acquired immunodeficiency syndrome. *APMIS.* 1992;100:605–608.
48. DiCarlo FJ, Anderson DW, Virmani R, et al. Rheumatic heart disease in a patient with acquired immunodeficiency syndrome. *Hum Pathol.* 1989;20:917–920.
49. Bharati S, Joshi VV, Connor EM, Oleske JM, Lev M. Conduction system in children with acquired immunodeficiency syndrome. *Chest.* 1989;96:406–413.
50. Hofman P, Drici MD, Gibelin P, Michiels JF, Thyss A. Prevalence of toxoplasma myocarditis in patients with the acquired immunodeficiency syndrome. *Br Heart J.* 1993; 70:376–381.
51. Jautzke G, Sell M, Thalmann U, et al. Extracerebral toxoplasmosis in AIDS: histological and immunohistological findings based on 80 autopsy cases. *Pathol Res Pract.* 1993;189:428–436.
52. Tolat D, Kim HS. Toxoplasmosis of the brain and heart: autopsy report of a patient with AIDS. *Texas Med.* 1989;85:40–42.
53. Hofman P, Bernard E, Michiels JF, Thyss A, LeFichoux Y, Loubiere R. Extracerebral toxoplasmosis in the acquired immunodeficiency syndrome (AIDS). *Pathol Res Pract.* 1993;189:894–901.
54. Adair OV, Randive N, Krasnow N. Isolated toxoplasma myocarditis in acquired immune deficiency syndrome. *Am Heart J.* 1989;118:856–857.
55. Mullins RJ, Bastian B, Sutherland DC. AIDS and the heart. *Aust NZ J Med.* 1988;18:809–811.
56. Beschorner WE, Baughman KL, Turnicky RP, et al. HIV-associated myocarditis: pathology and immunopathology. *Am J Pathol.* 1990;137(6):1365–1371.
57. Medlock MD, Tilleli JT, Pearl GS. Congenital cardiac toxoplasmosis in a newborn with acquired immunodeficiency syndrome. *Pediatr Infect Dis J.* 1990;9:129–132.

58. Scully RE, ed. Case 36-1992. Case records of the Massachusetts General Hospital. *N Engl J Med.* 1992;327: 790–799.
59. Segal BH, Factor SM. Myocardial risk factors other than human immunodeficiency virus infection may contribute to histologic cardiomyopathic changes in acquired immune deficiency syndrome. *Mod Pathol.* 1993;6:560–564.
60. van Hoeven KH, Segal BH, Factor SM. AIDS cardiomyopathy: first rule out other myocardial risk factors. *Int J Cardiol.* 1990;29:35–37.
61. Joshi VV, Gadol C, Connor E, Oleske JM, Mendelson J, Marin-Garcia J. Dilated cardiomyopathy in children with acquired immunodeficiency syndrome. *Hum Pathol.* 1988;19:69–73.
62. Baroldi G, Parravicini C, Gaiera G. Sudden cardiac death in a "silent" case of acquired immunodeficiency syndrome (AIDS). *G Ital Cardiol.* 1993;23:353–356.
63. Corallo S, Mutinelli, MR, Moroni M, Lazzarin A, Baroldi G. *Echocardiography Detects Cardiac Involvement in AIDS: Study in 70 Patients.* Third International Conference on AIDS; 1987; Washington, DC. Abstract 165:191.
64. Meyer PR, Klatt EC. AIDS and the heart. *Prog AIDS Pathol.* 1989;1:213–218.
65. Welch K, Finkbeiner W, Alpers CE, et al. Autopsy findings in the acquired immune deficiency syndrome. *JAMA.* 1984;252:1152–1159.
66. Constantino A, West TE, Gupta M, Loghmanee F. Primary cardiac lymphoma in a patient with acquired immune deficiency syndrome. *Cancer.* 1987;60:2801–2805.
67. Anderson DW, Virmani R. Emerging patterns of heart disease in human immunodeficiency virus infection. *Hum Pathol.* 1990;21:253–259.
68. Herskowitz A, Wu TC, Willoughby SB, et al. Myocarditis and cardiotropic viral infection associated with severe left ventricular dysfunction in late-stage infection with human immunodeficiency virus. *J Am Coll Cardiol.* 1994;24: 1025–1032.
69. Kereiakes DJ, Parmley WW. Myocarditis and cardiomyopathy. *Am Heart J.* 1984;108:1318–1326.
70. Edwards WD. Myocarditis and endomyocardial biopsy. *Cardiol Clin.* 1984;2:647–656.
71. Chow LH, Ye Y, Linder J, McManus BM. Phenotypic analysis of infiltrating cells in human myocarditis. An immunohistochemical study in paraffin-embedded tissue. *Arch Pathol Lab Med.* 1989;113:1357–1362.
72. Herskowitz A, Baughman KL. Effect of HIV infection on the heart. In: Braunwald E, ed. *Heart Disease: A Textbook of Cardiovascular Medicine.* Philadelphia: WB Saunders; 1994:1–10.
73. Aretz HT, Billingham ME, Edwards WD, et al. Myocarditis: a histopathologic definition and classification. *Am J Cardiovasc Pathol.* 1986:1:3–14.
74. Thuesen L, Moller A, Kristensen BO, Black F. Cardiac function in patients with human immunodeficiency virus infection and with no other active infections. *Dan Med Bull.* 1994;41:107–109.
75. Dworkin BM, Antonecchia PP, Smith F, et al. Reduced cardiac selenium content in the acquired immunodeficiency syndrome. *JPEN.* 1989;13:644–647.
76. Corboy JR, Fink L, Miller WT. Congestive cardiomyopathy in association with AIDS. *Radiology.* 1987;165:139–141.
77. Kaminski HJ, Katzman M, Wiest PM, et al. Cardiomyopathy associated with the acquired immune deficiency syndrome. *J AIDS.* 1988;1:105–110.
78. Jacob AJ, Sutherland GR, Bird AG, Brettle RP, Boon NA. Cardiac abnormalities associated with HIV infection. *Br Heart J.* 1991;66:77.
79. Rodriguez ER, Nasim S, Hsia J, et al. Cardiac myocytes and dendritic cells harbor human immunodeficiency virus in infected patients with and without cardiac dysfunction: detection by multiplex, nested, polymerase chain reaction in individually microdissected cells from right ventricular endomyocardial biopsy tissue. *Am J Cardiol.* 1991;68: 1511–1520.
80. Grody WW, Cheng L, Lewis W. Infection of the heart by the human immunodeficiency virus. *Am J Cardiol.* 1990; 66:203–206.
81. Flomenbaum M, Soeiro R, Udem SA, Kress Y, Factor SM. Proliferative membranopathy and human immunodeficiency virus in AIDS hearts. *J AIDS.* 1989;2:129–135.
82. Lipshultz SE, Fox CH, Perez-Atayde AR, et al. Identification of human immunodeficiency virus-1 RNA and DNA in the heart of a child with cardiovascular abnormalities and congenital acquired immune deficiency syndrome. *Am J Cardiol.* 1990;66:246–250.
83. Cenacchi G, Re MC, Furlini G, et al. Human immunodeficiency virus type 1 antigen detection in endomyocardial biopsy: an immunomorphological study. *Microbiologica.* 1990;13:145–149.
84. Calabrese LH, Proffitt MR, Yen-Lieberman B, Hobbs RE, Ratliff NB. Congestive cardiomyopathy and illness related to the acquired immunodeficiency syndrome (AIDS) associated with isolation of retrovirus from myocardium. *Ann Intern Med.* 1987;107:691–692.
85. Scott PJ, Conway SP, Da Costa P. Cardiac tamponade complicating cytomegalovirus pericarditis in a patient with AIDS. *J Infect.* 1990;20:92–93.
86. Freedberg RS, Gindea AJ, Dieterich DT, Greene JB. Herpes simplex pericarditis in AIDS. *NY State J Med.* 1987; 87:304–306.
87. Lin RY, Schwartz RA, Lambert WC. Cutaneous-pericardial tuberculous fistula in an immunocompromised host. *Int J Dermatol.* 1986;25:456–458.
88. Stechel RP, Cooper DJ, Greenspan J, Pizzarello RA, Tenenbaum MJ. Staphylococcal pericarditis in a homosexual patient with AIDS-related complex. *NY State J Med.* 1986;86:592–593.
89. D'Cruz IA, Sengupta EE, Abrahams C, Reddy HK, Turlapati RV. Cardiac involvement, including tuberculous pericardial effusion, complicating acquired immune deficiency syndrome. *Am Heart J.* 1986;112:1100–1101.
90. Cegielski JP, Ramaiya K, Lallinger GJ, Mtulia IA, Mbaga IM. Pericardial disease and human immunodeficiency virus in Dar es Salaam, Tanzania. *Lancet.* 1990;335:209–212.
91. Eisenberg MJ, Gordon AS, Schiller NB. HIV-associated pericardial effusions. *Chest.* 1992;102:956–958.
92. Karve MM, Murali MR, Shah HM, Phelps KR. Rapid evolution of cardiac tamponade due to bacterial pericarditis

in two patients with HIV-1 infection. *Chest.* 1992;101:1461–1463.
93. Woods GL, Goldsmith JC. Fatal pericarditis due to *Mycobacterium avium-intracellulare* in acquired immunodeficiency syndrome. *Chest.* 1989;95:1355–1357.
94. Turco M, Seneff M, McGrath BJ, Hsia J. Cardiac tamponade in the acquired immunodeficiency syndrome. *Am Heart J.* 1990;120:1467–1468.
95. Holtz HA, Lavery DP, Kapila R. Actinomycetales infection in the acquired immunodeficiency syndrome. *Ann Intern Med.* 1985;102:203–205.
96. Langer E, Mischke U, Stommer P, Harrer T, Stoll R. Kaposi-Sarkom mit Herzbeuteltamponade bei AIDS. *Dtsch Med Woch.* 1988;113:1187–1190.
97. Remick SC, Hoisington SA, Migliozzi JA. Epidemic Kaposi's sarcoma presenting with pleuropericarditis. *NY State J Med.* 1992;92:359–360.
98. Stotka JL, Good CB, Downer WR, Kapoor WN. Pericardial effusion and tamponade due to Kaposi's sarcoma in acquired immunodeficiency syndrome. *Chest.* 1989;95:1359–1361.
99. Goldfarb A, King CL, Rosenzweig BP, et al. Cardiac lymphoma in the acquired immunodeficiency syndrome. *Am Heart J.* 1989;118:1340–1344.
100. Gill PS, Chandraratna AN, Meyer PR, Levine AM. Malignant lymphoma: cardiac involvement at initial presentation. *J Clin Oncol.* 1987;5:216–224.
101. Zuger A, Louie E, Holzman RS, Simberkoff MS, Rahal JJ. Cryptococcal disease in patients with the acquired immunodeficiency syndrome. *Ann Intern Med.* 1986;104:234–240.
102. Schuster M, Valentine F, Holzman R. Cryptococcal pericarditis in an intravenous drug abuser. *J Infect Dis.* 1985;152:842.
103. Stiegman CK, Anderson DW, Macher AM, Sennesh JD, Virmani R. Fatal cardiac tamponade in acquired immunodeficiency syndrome with epicardial Kaposi's sarcoma. *Am Heart J.* 1988;116:1105–1107.
104. Wu AY, Faripour F, Cartun RW, et al. Identification of human immunodeficiency virus in the heart of a patient with acquired immunodeficiency syndrome. *Mod Pathol.* 1990;3:625–630.
105. Horowitz MD, Cox MM, Neibart RM, Blaker AM, Interian A Jr. Resection of right atrial lymphoma in a patient with AIDS. *Int J Cardiol.* 1992;34:139–142.
106. Balasubramanyam A, Waxman M, Kazal HL, Lee MH. Malignant lymphoma of the heart in acquired immune deficiency syndrome. *Chest.* 1986;90:243–246.
107. Ziegler JL, Bechstead JA, Volberding PA, et al. Non-Hodgkin's lymphoma in 90 homosexual men: relation to generalized lymphadenopathy and the acquired immune deficiency syndrome. *N Engl J Med.* 1984;311:565–570.
108. Kelsey RC, Saker A, Morgan M. Cardiac lymphoma in a patient with AIDS. *Ann Intern Med.* 1991;115:370–371.
109. Dalli E, Quesada A, Paya R. Cardiac involvement by non-Hodgkin's lymphoma in acquired immune deficiency syndrome. *Int J Cardiol.* 1990;26:223–225.
110. Ioachim HL, Cooper MC, Hellman GC. Lymphomas in men at high risk for acquired immune deficiency syndrome (AIDS): a study of 21 cases. *Cancer.* 1985;56:2831–2842.
111. Henochowicz S, Mustafa M, Lawrinson WE, Pistole M, Lindsay J Jr. Cardiac aspergillosis in acquired immune deficiency syndrome. *Am J Cardiol.* 1985;55:1239–1240.
112. Bell MD, Barnhart JS Jr, Martin JM. Thrombotic thrombocytopenic purpura causing sudden, unexpected death—a series of eight patients. *J Forensic Sci.* 1990;35:601–613.
113. Tunich PA, Lefkow P, Kronzon I. Aorta to right atrium fistula caused by endocarditis: diagnosis by color doppler echocardiography. *J Am Soc Echocardiogr.* 1989;2:53–55.
114. Bestetti RB, De C, Figueiredo JF, DaCosta JC. Salmonella tricuspid endocarditis in an intravenous drug abuser with human immunodeficiency virus infection. *Int J Cardiol.* 1991;30:361–362.
115. Serra W, Chioatto P, Totteri A, Aurier E, Botti G. Endocardite tricuspidale da *Stafilococco aureus* in AIDS. Discussione di un caso. *G Ital Cardiol.* 1988;18:240–242.
116. Pitchenik AE, Fishl MA, Dickinson GM, et al. Opportunistic infections and Kaposi's sarcoma among Haitians: evidence of a new acquired immunodeficiency state. *Ann Intern Med.* 1983;98:277–284.
117. Kinney EL, Monsuez JJ, Kitzis M, Vittecoq D. Treatment of AIDS-associated heart disease. *Angiology.* 1989;40:970–976.
118. Raffanti SP, Fyfe B, Carreiro S, Sharp SE, Hyma BA, Ratzan KR. Native valve endocarditis due to *Pseudallescheria boydii* in a patient with AIDS: case report and review. *Rev Infect Dis.* 1990;2:993–996.
119. Garcia I, Fainstein V, Rios A, et al. Nonbacterial thrombotic endocarditis in a male homosexual with Kaposi's sarcoma. *Arch Intern Med.* 1983;143:1243–1244.
120. Herskowitz A, Neumann DA, Ansari AA. Concepts of autoimmunity applied to idiopathic dilated cardiomyopathy. *J Am Coll Cardiol.* 1993;22:1385–1388.
121. Clapham PR, Weber JN, Whitby D, et al. Soluble CD4 blocks the infectivity of diverse strains of HIV and SIV for T cells and monocytes but not for brain and muscle cells. *Nature.* 1989;337:368–370.
122. Ikeuchi K, Kim S, Byrn RA, Goldring SR, Groopman JE. Infection of nonlymphoid cells by human immunodeficiency virus type 1 or type 2. *J Virol.* 1990;64:4226–4231.
123. Turnicky RP, Goodin J, Smialek JE, Herskowitz A, Beschorner WE. Incidental myocarditis with intravenous drug abuse: the pathology, immunopathology, and potential implications for human immunodeficiency virus-associated myocarditis. *Hum Pathol.* 1992;23:138–143.
124. Report of the 1995 WHO/ISFC task force on the definition and classification of cardiomyopathies. *Circulation.* 1995;93:841–842.

CHAPTER 17

Human Immunodeficiency Virus–Associated Lymphoid Disease

Robert J. Siegel

. . . And I made an autopsy in order to ascertain the cause of so peaceful a death, and found it proceeded from weakness through the failure of blood and of the artery that feeds the heart and the other lower members, which I found to be very parched and shrunk and withered . . . . The other autopsy was on a child of two years, and here I found everything the contrary to what it was in the case of the old man.

Leonardo da Vinci (1452–1519)

Lymphadenopathy was recognized as an important manifestation early in the acquired immunodeficiency syndrome (AIDS) epidemic. Numerous studies have defined histopathologic changes in lymph nodes in these patients, demonstrating the usefulness of lymph node biopsy in diagnosis of opportunistic infections and AIDS-associated neoplasms (Table 17–1). In addition, a progressive series of changes characteristic of, although not entirely specific for human immunodeficiency virus (HIV), may be in lymph nodes, mirroring the progression of disease and having implications for the immunopathogenesis of AIDS.

HIV-ASSOCIATED LYMPHADENOPATHY

In 1983, Brynes et al[1] described the histologic findings in lymph nodes from 24 homosexual and bisexual men who had persistent generalized lymphadenopathy. Most of these patients had a peculiar form of follicular hyperplasia, whereas 3 patients, who rapidly succumbed to opportunistic infections or malignant lymphoma, had an atypical pattern of lymphoid reaction. Since then, changes of HIV-associated lymphadenopathy (HIVL) have been well characterized, both morphologically and immunologically. Different classifications have been devised to encompass these changes, and anywhere from two[2] to six[3] separate patterns have been distinguished. The changes have been described in lymph nodes[2–5] as well as spleen.[6] Note that these changes represent a continuum, so that dividing the process into "stages" is arbitrary. Nevertheless, it is useful to consider the patterns at the two extremes of the spectrum to correspond to early (follicular hyperplasia, FH) and late (lymphoid depletion, LD) manifestations of HIV infection. An intermediate pattern reflects a varying degree of involution of follicles and hypervascular paracortical hyperplasia (follicular involution, FI).

Histologic Findings

In HIV-associated FH, large secondary follicles assume irregular and bizarre shapes (Figure 17–1). Mantle zones are intact at first, but later become attenuated, with the invagination of small lymphocytes into germinal centers. As FH and mantle zone attenuation progress, the large germinal centers tend to become indistinct (Figure 17–2). Continued intrusion of small lymphocytes into germinal centers, displacing clusters of follicular center cells, along with occasional associated hemorrhage, adds to the appearance of follicular disruption and fragmentation referred to as "follicle lysis" (Figure 17–3).[2]

Concomitant changes in the paracortex include hypervascularity and the proliferation of small lymphocytes, immunoblasts, and interdigitating reticulum cells

TABLE 17–1. LYMPH NODE FINDINGS IN HIV INFECTION

HIV-associated lymphadenopathy
Follicular hyperplasia
Follicular involution and mixed patterns
Lymphoid depletion
Castleman's disease-like changes
Neoplasms
Kaposi's sarcoma
Non-Hodgkin's lymphoma
Small noncleaved
Diffuse large cell
Large cell immunoblastic
Hodgkin's disease
Infections
Mycobacteria
Histoplasmosis
Cytomegalovirus
Toxoplasmosis
Bacillary angiomatosis

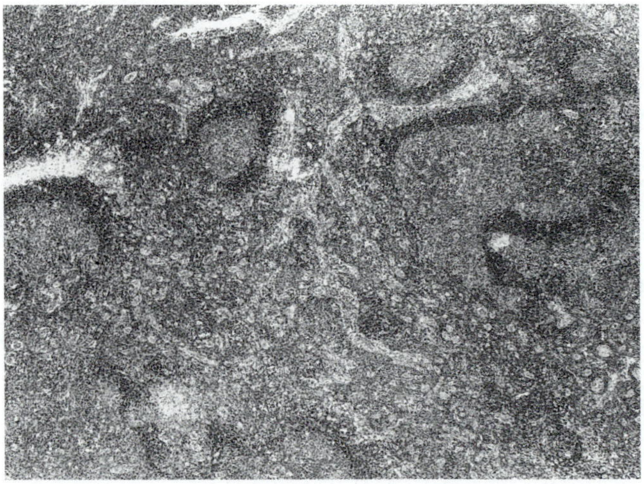

Figure 17–1. In HIV-associated florid follicular hyperplasia, numerous enlarged, irregularly shaped germinal centers are present (×20).

(Figure 17–4). Changes of dermatopathic lymphadenitis also have been described.[2] Multinucleated cells of lymphoid origin resembling the Warthin–Finkeldey giant cells of measles, and presumably representing HIV cytopathic effect,[2,7] are common (Figure 17–4). Groups of cells with moderate amounts of clear cytoplasm and slightly irregular lymphoid nuclei (monocytoid B lymphocytes) are adjacent to or within sinusoidal spaces (Figure 17–5). Sinuses otherwise are intact and often contain neutrophils.

The intermediate stage of HIVL (FI) is characterized by a reduction in size and cellular depletion of germinal centers. These become shrunken, hyalinized, and vascularized, leading to a "burnt-out" appearance (Figure 17–6). Tingeable body macrophages, abundant in the FH stage, are absent. The interfollicular tissue becomes increasingly vascularized and may show considerable paracortical hyperplasia before eventually becoming decreasingly cellular. Medullary plasmacytosis is common.

The LD pattern constitutes an "end stage" of HIVL. Previously reactive or involuted follicles are barely discernible as hyaline or vascularized scars. Macrophages and plasma cells predominate in a hypervascular stroma in which lymphocytes are markedly reduced in number (Figure 17–7). In some patients, the arborizing vascular proliferation, together with increased plasma cells and immunoblasts, closely mimics angioimmunoblastic lymphadenopathy.[3] The typical appearance of *Mycobacterium avium-intracellulare* complex (MAC) in lymph nodes, in which foamy *Mycobacteria*-filled histiocytes predominate, may be interpreted as a specific infection superimposed on the LD pattern (see later discussion).

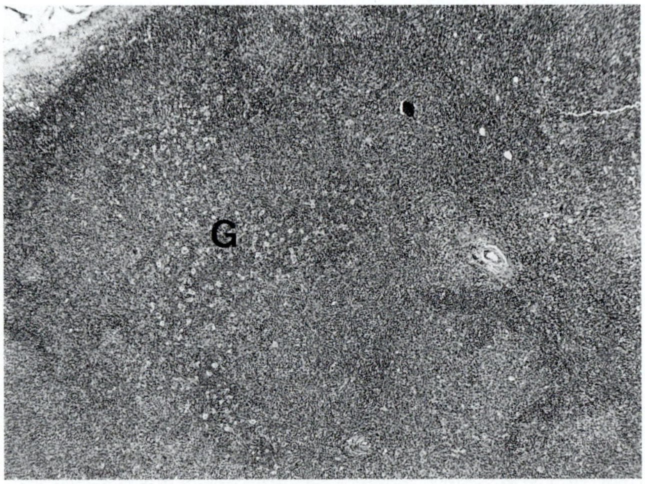

Figure 17–2. Hyperplastic germinal centers (G) are poorly demarcated from surrounding lymphoid tissue (×40).

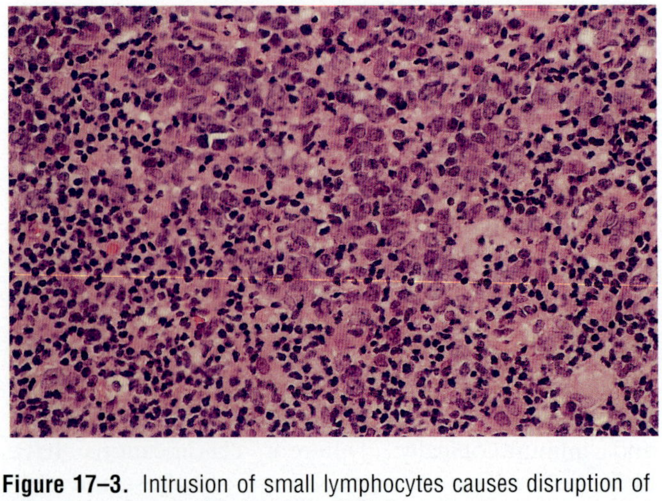

Figure 17–3. Intrusion of small lymphocytes causes disruption of follicular centers (follicle lysis) (×200).

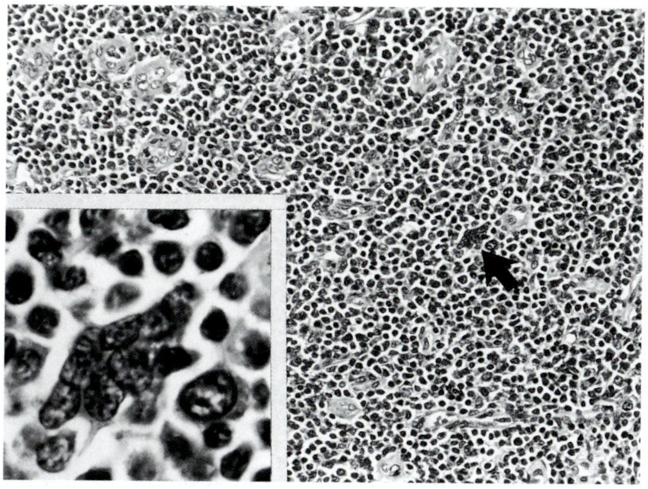

Figure 17–4. The paracortex displays diffuse hyperplasia with prominent vascularity and Warthin–Finkeldey giant cells (*arrow and inset*) (×200; inset, ×1000).

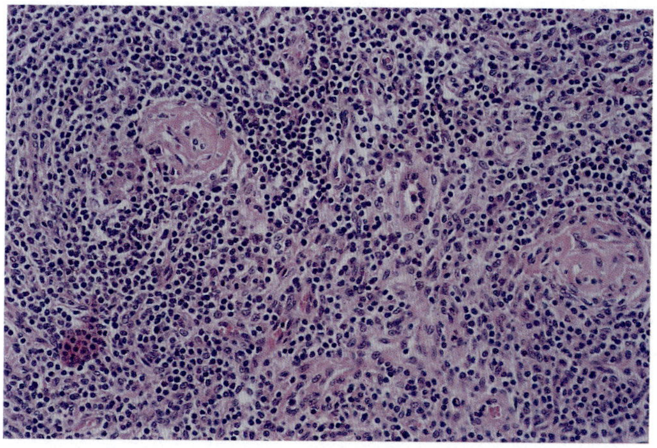

Figure 17–6. In the follicular involution stage of HIV-associated lymphadenopathy, "burnt-out" germinal centers are noted. In this example, the paracortex is becoming depleted of lymphocytes (×40).

In addition to the three basic patterns described, another lymphadenopathic change noted in HIV-infected patients resembles angiofollicular lymph node hyperplasia (Castleman's disease). In lymph nodes thus affected, germinal centers develop a peculiar "hyaline vascular" appearance characterized by a decrease in cellularity, prominent vascularity, and a surrounding concentric layering of small lymphocytes (Figure 17–8). Interfollicular tissue displays marked plasmacytosis. The importance of this pattern is the simultaneous presence or subsequent development of Kaposi's sarcoma in patients with these lymph node findings.[3,8,9]

Immunopathogenesis of Histologic Changes

Localization of HIV to lymph nodes presumably occurs early with initial viral dissemination in primary HIV infection.[10] As in other infections, the initial immune response leads to polyclonal activation of various immune effector cells, including B cells, T cells, and macrophages, manifested morphologically by the germinal center reaction.[10–12] The various cytokines produced by these activated cells probably play a role in maintaining the hyperplastic response.[13] The persistence (failure of clearance) of HIV leads to persistence

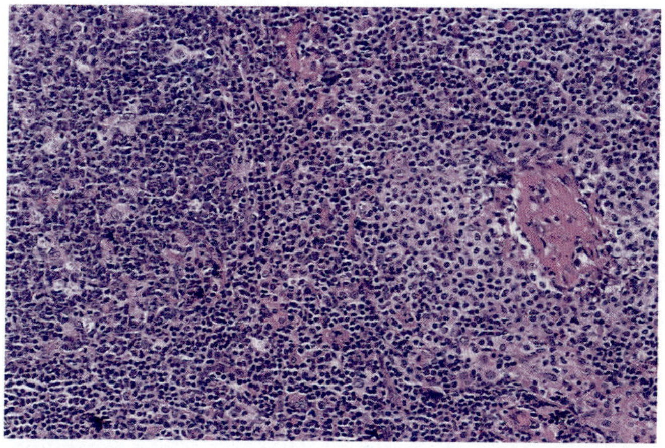

Figure 17–5. Monocytoid B lymphocytes (to right of center) are recognized by the pale appearance of their abundant cytoplasm (×200).

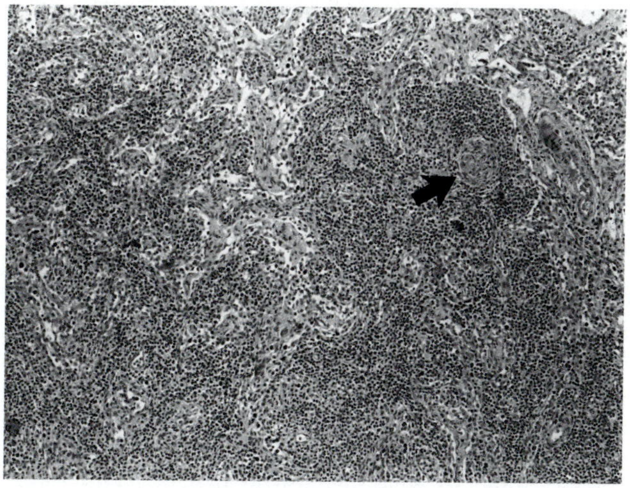

Figure 17–7. Lymphoid depleted pattern. This is a single remnant germinal center (*arrow*). Sinuses are prominent from depleted intervening lymphoid tissue (×100).

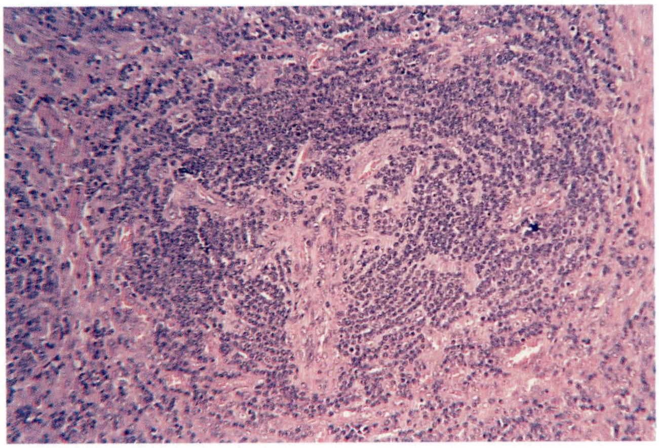

Figure 17–8. Castleman's disease-like changes consist of typical hyaline vascular germinal centers having penetrating blood vessels and "onion skin" layering of small lymphocytes (×100).

of the immune reaction. Trapping of HIV on the surface of follicular dendritic cells is potentiated by the expansion of this cell population as part of the early follicular hyperplasia.[10]

The small lymphocytes that invaginate the follicle, in follicle lysis, are of mixed phenotype, but include CD8+ cytotoxic/suppressor T cells, not a feature of non-HIV-related lymphoid hyperplasia.[11] Progressive disruption of the follicular dendritic reticulum cell network parallels morphologic disruption of the germinal center.[12] The progressive involution of germinal centers, with evolution from predominant FH to predominant FI patterns, mirrors a decline in CD4 count in peripheral blood and a redistribution of virus from lymph nodes to blood.[10] Destruction of the follicular dendritic cell network, with loss of the virus-trapping mechanism, is one factor favoring this redistribution.[10] In fact, HIV viral-mediated injury to these cells, which have an important role in maintaining the integrity of the germinal center and in antigen processing and presentation, may underlie many of the features of HIVL.[14]

In the paracortex, CD8+ T cells increase while CD4+ T cells decrease, leading to an inverted CD4:CD8 ratio as in peripheral blood. Later stages of HIVL are characterized immunologically by a progressive decline in follicular B cells, and continued inversion of the CD4:CD8 ratio primarily caused by the decline in number of interfollicular CD4+ T cells.[12]

In summary, the morphologic changes in lymph nodes have been interpreted as reflecting an immune response, initiated by and directed against HIV antigens and HIV-infected cells, leading at first to cellular proliferation and eventually to cytotoxic cellular destruction.[12]

Prognostic Significance of Patterns of HIVL

The correlation of histopathologic to clinical features in HIVL was intimated in early studies[1,15] and demonstrated subsequently. For example, in 79 patients with progressive generalized lymphadenopathy at risk for HIV infection, 58% of those with FH remained clinically stable and 42% progressed to AIDS, whereas of those with FI, 6% remained stable and 94% progressed to AIDS.[5] Similar observations have been made by others.[16,17] There is histologic progression between the various patterns: Progression from FH to mixed FH and FI to FI to LD occurred in 77% of sequential biopsies from 30 patients with HIV infection.[18] A close correlation between progressive histology and the development of opportunistic infection and systemic symptoms also was noted.[18] In addition, patients with AIDS whose lymph nodes displayed FH had a much longer survival time than those with FI or LD.

HIV-RELATED NEOPLASMS

Lymphadenopathic Kaposi's Sarcoma

Unlike the nonepidemic form of Kaposi's sarcoma (KS), which predated AIDS, most patients with AIDS-associated KS have involvement of viscera and skin, and up to 29% of patients may have visceral KS without cutaneous lesions.[19] Along with the gastrointestinal tract and lung, lymph nodes are a favored site of involvement.[19–21]

Histologically, KS in lymph nodes manifests the same vascular and spindle cell proliferation with extravasated erythrocytes and "eosinophilic globules" encountered in classic cutaneous KS (Figure 17–9). Involvement may be focal, with subcapsular or intrafollicular localization.[3] The differential diagnosis includes vascular transformation of lymph nodes sinuses as well as other vascular lesions of lymph nodes, a topic reviewed by Chan et al.[22] As mentioned previously, the finding of Castleman's disease-like changes in lymph nodes should prompt a search for associated lymphadenopathic KS.

Non-Hodgkin's Lymphoma

In the context of the known association between immunodeficiency and the development of malignant lymphoma, the fact that these neoplasms arise in patients with HIV infection is not surprising. Three large series, encompassing more than 250 patients, have established the spectrum of HIV-associated lymphoid neoplasia.[23–25] Compared to those that occur in the general population, HIV-related non-Hodgkin's lym-

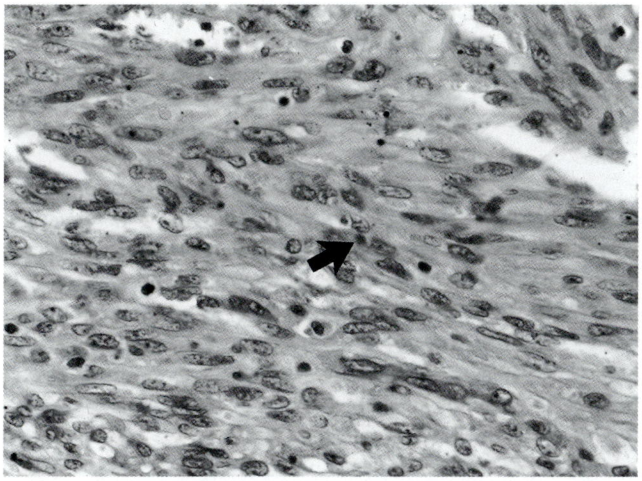

Figure 17–9. A proliferation of spindle cells, extravasated erythrocytes, and eosinophilic globules (*arrow*) characterize the histologic features of Kaposi's sarcoma (×400).

phomas (NHL) are notable for the high prevalence of diffuse aggressive histologic subtypes, the frequent presence of "B" symptoms (fever, weight loss), advanced disease at presentation, and occurrence in extranodal sites (central nervous system, gastrointestinal tract, bone marrow) including various "unusual" organs such as conjunctiva, skin, lungs, and heart (Figure 17–10).[23–26]

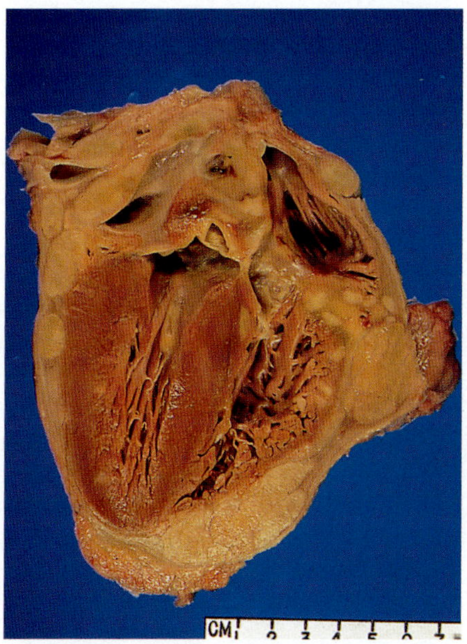

Figure 17–10. Malignant lymphoma of the heart in AIDS. Multiple confluent pericardial nodules distort the epicardial tissue and impinge on the myocardium.

Of the 231 patients with NHL in the three studies cited,[23–25] 60% had histologic subtypes considered high grade in the International Working Formulation (36% small noncleaved, 24% large cell immunoblastic) and 30% had diffuse large cell lymphoma of intermediate grade (Figure 17–11, A–C). Almost without exception, these lymphomas are of B-cell phenotype.

Evidence implicating Epstein–Barr virus (EBV) in the pathogenesis of NHL in HIV infection has emerged. Unlike most NHL in the general population, more than one third of those in HIV-infected individuals have EBV DNA sequences.[27,28] This virus also has been identified in lymph nodes from patients with HIVL, and its presence has been found to correlate with concurrent or subsequent development of NHL.[28]

Hodgkin's Disease

An association between HIV infection and Hodgkin's disease (HD) is less clear-cut. An increased incidence of HD is difficult to detect, because the age range of patients with AIDS overlaps that of HD in the general population. Nevertheless, certain differences between the two groups are apparent. Analogous to the presentation of HIV-associated NHL, HD in HIV-infected individuals is notable for the common presentation at an advanced stage (III and IV), a high frequency of systemic symptoms, and an aggressive course.[29,30]

INFECTIONS

A variety of opportunistic infections may be encountered in lymph node biopsies from HIV-infected individuals. These are not discussed in detail here because they are described in other chapters. Two infections with distinct features are described: MAC and bacillary angiomatosis (BA).

In MAC infection, the lymph node may be virtually replaced by histiocytes containing abundant foamy cytoplasm (Figure 17–12). Occasionally, these cells take on a spindly appearance, leading to a confusing histologic picture. Acid-fast stains demonstrate that the foaminess is caused by innumerable acid-fast bacilli (Figure 17–13). As mentioned previously, lymph nodes thus affected are considered to be a variant of the LD pattern of HIVL.

A peculiar cutaneous vascular proliferation distinct from KS, and associated with a cat scratchlike bacillus, has been recognized in HIV-infected patients.[31] The putative organism has been named *Rochalimaea henselae.*[32] This process, termed BA, may affect lymph nodes as well as other visceral organs.[33] Lymph node involvement is characterized by focal proliferation of capillary

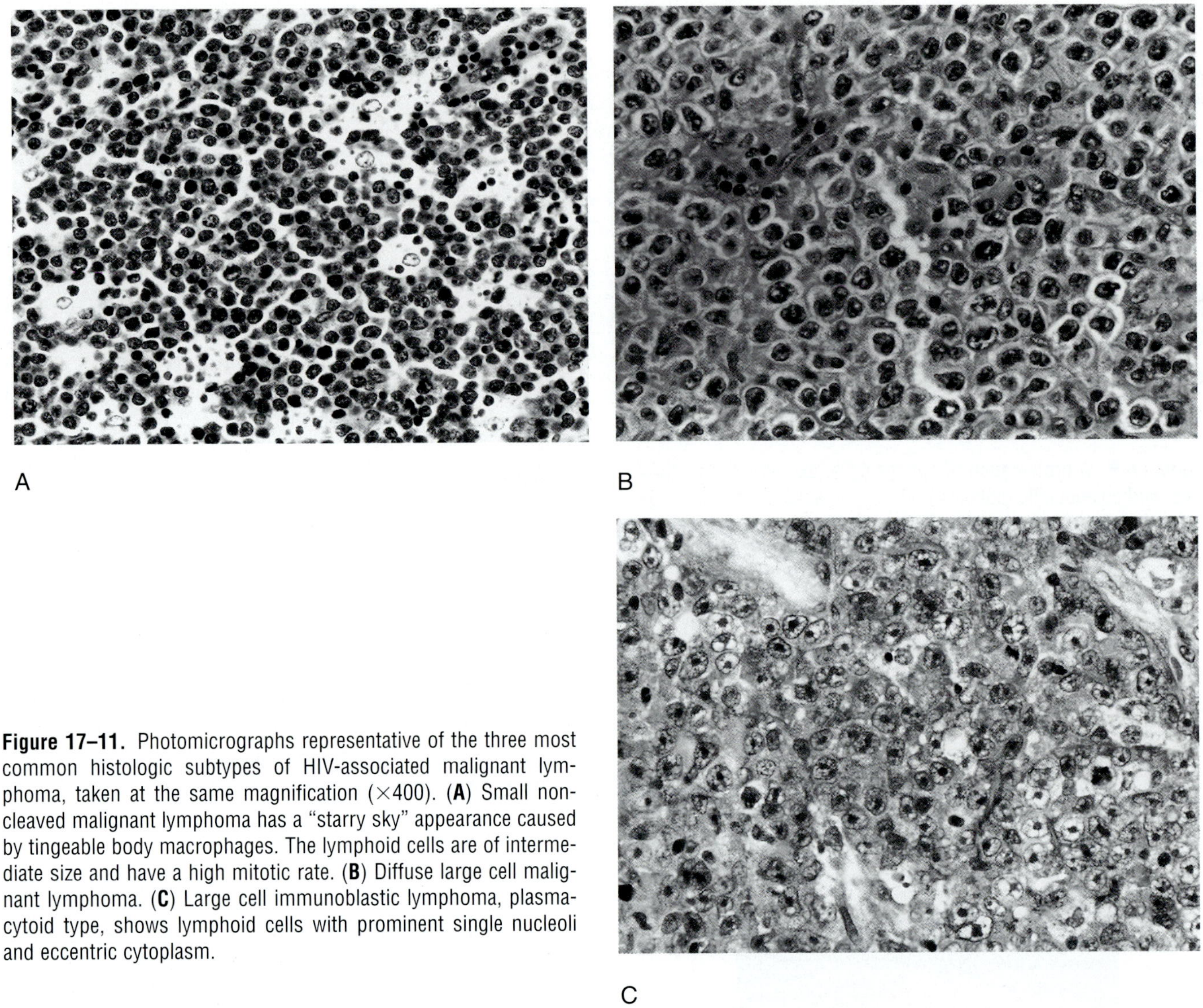

Figure 17–11. Photomicrographs representative of the three most common histologic subtypes of HIV-associated malignant lymphoma, taken at the same magnification (×400). (**A**) Small noncleaved malignant lymphoma has a "starry sky" appearance caused by tingeable body macrophages. The lymphoid cells are of intermediate size and have a high mitotic rate. (**B**) Diffuse large cell malignant lymphoma. (**C**) Large cell immunoblastic lymphoma, plasmacytoid type, shows lymphoid cells with prominent single nucleoli and eccentric cytoplasm.

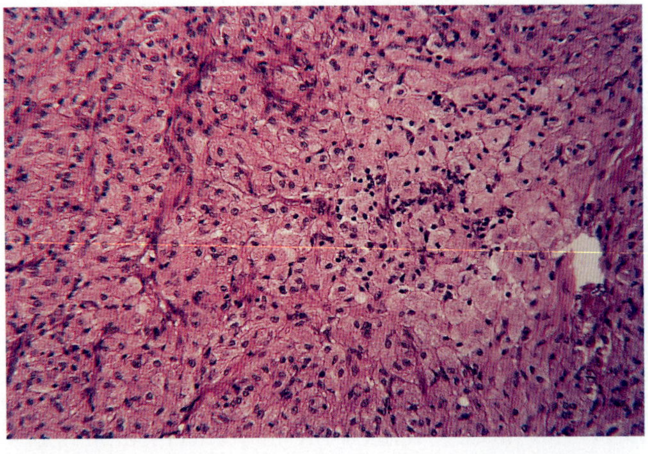

Figure 17–12. Lymph node in MAC infection shows depletion of lymphocytes and proliferation of histiocytes with abundant foamy cytoplasm (×200).

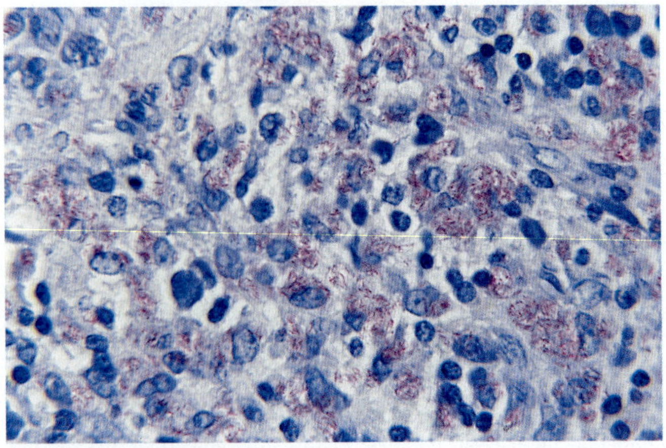

Figure 17–13. Acid-fast stain demonstrates numerous mycobacteria within histiocytic cells (×1000).

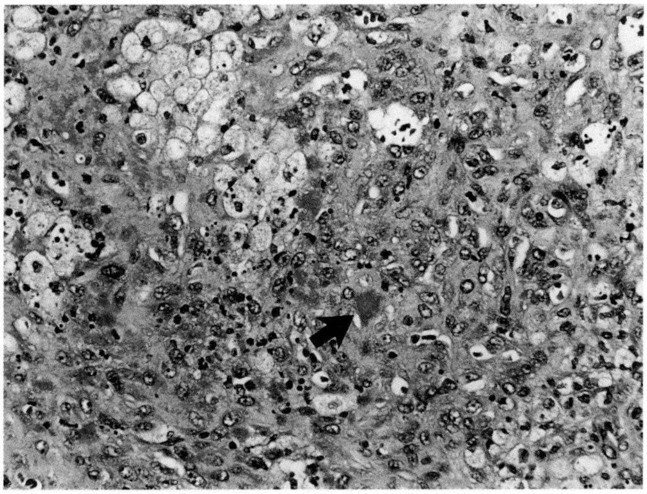

Figure 17–14. Features of bacillary angiomatosis in lymph node include vascular proliferation, foamy histiocytes (*upper left*), presence of neutrophils, and clumps of amorphous material representing aggregated organisms (*arrow*) (×200).

size vessels with plump endothelial cells, associated with the extracellular clumps of amorphous to granular eosinophilic material (Figure 17–14). There are collections of foamy histiocytes and neutrophils. A silver impregnation (Warthin–Starry) stain demonstrates that the extracellular material represents clumps of bacillary organisms (Figure 17–15). Recognition of this entity is important because antibiotic treatment can avert a fatal course.[33]

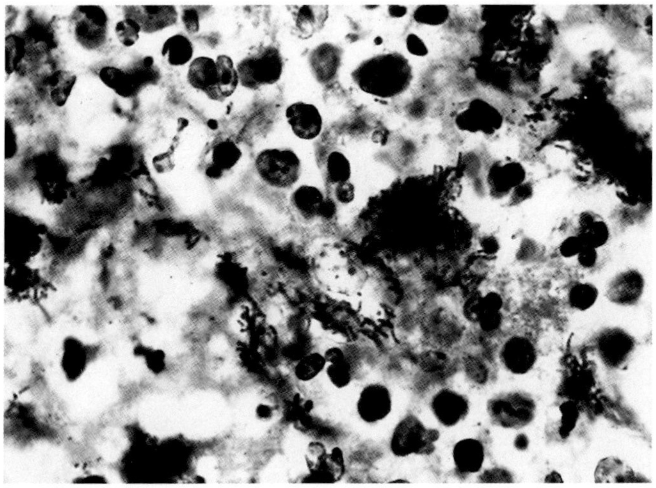

Figure 17–15. Warthin–Starry stain in bacillary angiomatosis reveals clumps of pleomorphic bacilli. (×1000).

REFERENCES

1. Brynes RK, Chan WC, Spira TJ, Ewing EP, Chandler FW. Value of lymph node biopsy in unexplained lymphadenopathy in homosexual men. *JAMA.* 1983;250:1313–1317.
2. Burns BF, Wood GS, Dorfman RF. The varied histopathology of lymphadenopathy in the homosexual male. *Am J Surg Pathol.* 1985;9:287–297.
3. Racz P, Tenner-Racz K, van Vloten F, et al. Classification of histopathological changes of lymph nodes in HIV-1 infection. *Antibiot Chemother.* 1991;43:201–213.
4. Ewing EP, Chandler FW, Spira TJ, Brynes RK, Chan WC. Primary lymph node pathology in AIDS and AIDS-related lymphadenopathy. *Arch Pathol Lab Med.* 1985;109: 977–981.
5. Ioachim HL, Cronin W, Roy M, Maya M. Persistent lymphadenopathies in people at high risk for HIV infection: clinicopathologic correlations and long-term follow-up in 79 cases. *Am J Clin Pathol.* 1990;93:208–218.
6. Falk S, Muller H, Stutte H. The spleen in acquired immunodeficiency syndrome (AIDS). *Pathol Res Pract.* 1988; 183:425–433.
7. Popovic M, Sarngadharan MG, Read E, Gallo RC. Detection, isolation and continuous production of cytopathic retroviruses (HTLV-III) from patients with AIDS and pre-AIDS. *Science.* 1984;224:497–500.
8. Harris NL. Hypervascular follicular hyperplasia and Kaposi's sarcoma in patients at risk for AIDS. *N Engl J Med.* 1984;310:462–463.
9. Lachant NA, Sun NCJ, Leong LA, Oseas RS, Prince HE. Multicentric angiofollicular lymph node hyperplasia (Castleman's disease) followed by Kaposi's sarcoma in two homosexual males with the acquired immunodeficiency syndrome (AIDS). *Am J Clin Pathol.* 1985;83:27–33.
10. Pantaleo G, Graziosi C, Demarest JF, et al. Role of lymphoid organs in the pathogenesis of human immunodeficiency virus (HIV) infection. *Immunol Rev.* 1994;140: 105–130.
11. Said JW. AIDS-related lymphadenopathies. *Sem Diagn Pathol.* 1988;5:365–375.
12. Muller H, Falk S. Schmidts HL, Stutte HJ. In situ immunophenotyping of lymphocytes/macrophages: grading of lymphadenopathy, staging and pathophysiology of HIV infection. *Res Virol.* 1990;141:171–184.
13. Boyle MJ, Berger MF, Tschuchnigg M, et al. Increased expression of interferon-gamma in hyperplastic lymph nodes from HIV-infected patients. *Clin Exp Immunol.* 1993;92:100–105.
14. Piris MA, Rivas C, Morente M, Rubio C, Martin C, Olivia H. Persistent and generalized lymphadenopathy: a lesion of follicular dendritic cells? *Am J Clin Pathol.* 1987;87: 716–724.
15. Davis JM, Mouradian J, Fernandez RD, Cunningham-Rundles S, Metroka CE. Acquired immune deficiency syndrome: a surgical perspective. *Arch Surg.* 1984;119:90–95.
16. Moresco L, Gipponi M, CaFiero F, et al. Role of diagnostic lymph node biopsies in 56 anti-HIV positive patients. *Cancer Detect Prev.* 1990;14:353–357.
17. Gerstoft J, Pallesen G, Mathiesen LR, Pedersen C, Gaub J, Lindhardt BO. The value of lymph node histology in

human immunodeficiency virus related persistent generalized lymphadenopathy. *APMIS.* 1989;suppl 8:24–27.

18. Chadburn A, Metrka C, Mouradian J. Progressive lymph node histology and its prognostic value in patients with acquired immunodeficiency syndrome and AIDS-related complex. *Hum Pathol.* 1989;20:579–587.
19. Lemlich G, Schwam L, Lebwohl M. Kaposi's sarcoma and acquired immunodeficiency syndrome: postmortem findings in twenty-four cases. *J Am Acad Dermatol.* 1987; 16:319–325.
20. Niedt GW, Schinella RA. Acquired immunodeficiency syndrome: clinicopathologic study of 56 autopsies. *Arch Pathol Lab Med.* 1985;109:727–734.
21. Welch K, Finkbeiner W, Alpers CE, et al. Autopsy findings in the acquired immune deficiency syndrome. *JAMA.* 1984;252:1152–1159.
22. Chan JK, Frizzera G, Fletcher CD, Rosai J. Primary vascular tumors of lymph nodes other than Kaposi's sarcoma. *Am J Surg Pathol.* 1992;16:335–350.
23. Ziegler JL, Beckstead JA, Volberding PA, et al. Non-Hodgkin's lymphoma in 90 homosexual men: relation to generalized lymphadenopathy and the acquired immunodeficiency syndrome. *N Engl J Med.* 1984;311:565–570.
24. Lowenthal DA, Strauss DJ, Campbell SW, Gold JWM, Clarkson BD, Koziner B. AIDS-related lymphoid neoplasia: the Memorial Hospital experience. *Cancer.* 1988; 61:2325–2337.
25. Knowles DM, Chamulak GA, Subar M et al. Lymphoid neoplasia associated with the acquired immunodeficiency syndrome (AIDS). *Ann Intern Med.* 1988;108:744–753.
26. Holladay A, Siegel R, Schwartz D. Cardiac malignant lymphoma in acquired immunodeficiency syndrome. *Cancer.* 1992;70:2203–2207.
27. Subar M, Neri A, Inghirami G, Knoles DM, Dalla-Favera R. Frequent *c-myc* oncogene activation and infrequent presence of Epstein–Barr virus genome in AIDS-associated lymphoma. *Blood.* 1988;72:667–671.
28. Shibata D, Weiss LM, Nathwani BN, Brynes RK, Levine AM. Epstein–Barr virus in benign lymph node biopsies from individuals infected with the human immunodeficiency virus is associated with concurrent or subsequent development of non-Hodgkin's lymphoma. *Blood.* 1991; 77:1527–1533.
29. Ree HJ, Strauchen JA, Khan AA, et al. Human immunodeficiency virus-associated Hodgkin's disease: clinicopathologic studies of 24 cases and preponderance of mixed cellularity type characterized by the occurrence of fibrohistiocytoid stromal cells. *Cancer.* 1991;67: 1614–1621.
30. Pelstring RJ, Zellmer RB, Sulak LE, Banks PM, Clare N. Hodgkin's disease in association with human immunodeficiency virus infection: pathologic and immunologic features. *Cancer.* 1991;67:1865–1873.
31. Milam MW, Balerdi MJ, Toney JF, Foulis PR, Milam CP, Behnke RH. Epithelioid angiomatosis secondary to disseminated cat scratch disease involving the bone marrow and skin in a patient with acquired immune deficiency syndrome: a case report. *Am J Med.* 1990;88:180–183.
32. Regnery RL, Anderson BE, Clarridge JE III, Rodriquez-Barradas MC, Jones DC, Carr JH. Characterization of a novel *Rochalimaea* species, *R. henselae* sp. nov., isolated from blood of a febrile, human immunodeficiency virus-positive patient. *J Clin Microbiol.* 1992;30:265–274.
33. Chan JKC, Lewin KJ, Lombard CM, Teitelbaum S, Dorfman RF. Histopathology of bacillary angiomatosis of lymph node. *Am J Surg Pathol.* 1991;15:430–437.

CHAPTER 18

Human Immunodeficiency Virus Infection Lesions in the Pediatric Age Group

M. Alba Greco and David Zagzag

But care and sorrow, and childbirth pain,
Left their traces on heart and brain.

John Greenleaf Whittier (1807–1892), Maud Muller

INTRODUCTION

Human immunodeficiency virus (HIV) infection is a multisystem disease affecting many organs in different ways.[1] Anatomic pathologists must be familiar with the broad and changing spectrum of morphologic alterations in pediatric HIV infection to be able to help in the evaluation of patients with acquired immunodeficiency syndrome (AIDS). Sometimes the anatomic pathologist will be the first to diagnose AIDS in a child. A high index of suspicion, ample sampling of tissue, and the application of a battery of histochemical, immunohistochemical, and molecular pathology techniques will lead to the specific, and correct, diagnosis.

Pediatric AIDS constitutes about 2% of the total reported cases of AIDS.[2] Because AIDS in children follows AIDS in women, it is important to note that women account for an increasing number and percentage of AIDS in adults.[3] Most women with AIDS are of reproductive age (84%), of ethnic minority (black 53%, Hispanic 21%), and live in metropolitan areas. The acquisition of HIV in women is most commonly associated with intravenous drug use and heterosexual intercourse with an infected partner.[3]

Nearly 90% of AIDS in children is from vertical transmission from an infected mother.[4,5] Although transmission is about 30%, the precise timing of the transmission is unknown. Definitions for early (in utero) and late (intrapartum) infections have been proposed on the basis of viral blood cultures and detection of HIV genome in infant cord and peripheral blood.[6] Many HIV-infected children die in the first year of life and most succumb before their fifth birthday. However, a longer survival time in children with perinatal infection and prolonged clinical latency has been reported.[7]

The pathologic manifestations of HIV infection in children are primary and secondary. The primary lesions are a direct cytopathic effect, especially on the lymphoreticular system and on the central nervous system (CNS), and the secondary manifestations are consequences of impaired cell-mediated immunity, autoimmune phenomena, opportunistic infections, and malignant tumors.

PERINATAL PATHOLOGY

Although HIV invades the infant through the placenta, only nonspecific pathologic features have been described in the placenta.[8–12] Placentomegaly is the only gross feature described in HIV-infected mothers.[13,14] Whether this is caused by HIV or by coexisting infections is not known. HIV-positive women are at risk for other sexually transmitted diseases such as syphilis, which is a well-known cause of placental hypertrophy.[15] Other infections affecting HIV-positive women may leave their marks on the placenta when these women become pregnant. Malaria and cryptococcosis of placenta in HIV-infected women have been reported[16,17] (Figure 18–1). Chorioamnionitis has been seen with high frequency in placentas of HIV-positive mothers. Studies by Jauniaux et al[13] and Chandwani et al[12] have demonstrated an incidence of chorioamnionitis of 43% and 62%, respectively, in seropositive women, as opposed to 20% and 26%, respectively, in control groups. Funisitis was associated with chorioamnionitis in these studies.[12,13] The significance of these findings and their relation to HIV infection is not known. No abnormalities of the villi are usually found in placentas of seropositive women.

In spite of the lack of pathologic findings, HIV antigens are in Hofbauer cells[18–21] and we and other researchers have detected viral antigens in trophoblastic cells.[11,12,19,21] Occasionally villous endothelial cells also contain HIV antigen.[11,19,21] HIV nucleic acids have been detected by in situ hybridization in trophoblastic cells,[11,12,21] and in macrophages and endothelial cells.[11,21] Backe et al[21] have identified viral antigens and nucleic acids in amniotic cells and maternal lymphocytes. Viral particles consistent with HIV have been reported in the syncytiotrophoblast, fibroblasts, and endothelial cells of villous capillaries.[13]

HIV antigen and nucleic acids in the villous macrophages is of particular interest in light of the role of monocytes in HIV infection. Villous macrophages express CD4,[22] the receptor needed for the HIV to enter cells. Once infected, these cells may enter the fetal circulation and infect fetal circulating cells or endothelial

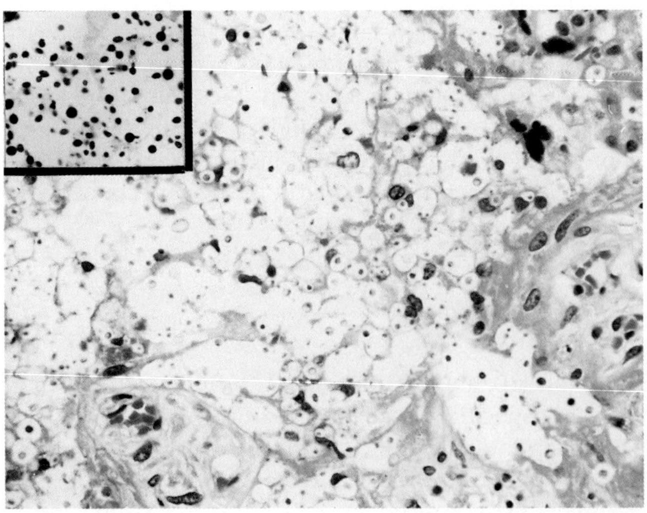

Figure 18–1. Placenta with cryptococci in the intervillous spaces (hematoxylin-eosin, ×40) *Inset:* The organisms are silvered with Grocott methenamine-silver stain (×40). *(Courtesy of Dr. C.R. Abramowsky, Department of Pathology, Emory University, Atlanta, Georgia.)*

cells. How the virus enters the villous cells via the trophoblastic layer is unknown. In vitro experiments, however, have demonstrated virions in endosomes and multivesicular bodies in the cytoplasm of trophoblastic cells and budding from the plasma membrane. These findings are consistent with an endocytosis-mediated mechanism of viral entry, and with trophoblastic cells supporting viral replication.[23] HIV-infected maternal lymphocytes may carry the virus to the syncytiotrophoblast.

OPPORTUNISTIC INFECTIONS

Opportunistic infections are seen at various times during the clinical course of HIV-infected children. Candidiasis is the most frequent opportunistic infection in children.[24] It begins as oral thrush in early infancy and may spread to the entire gastrointestinal tract (GIT). When invasive candidiasis is present, lungs, kidneys, heart, and brain may be affected.[25]

Pneumocystis carinii pneumonia (PCP) is the most frequent fatal opportunistic infection in the first year of life.[24,26] With early recognition and treatment there may be prolonged survival with atypical patterns, such as a cyst with necrosis and calcification (Figure 18–2, A and B).

The incidence of cytomegalovirus (CMV) infection at autopsy varies.[26] In the GIT, CMV causes ulcerations, transmural inflammation, perforation, strictures, pneumatosis, and ganglioneuronitis.[27,28] Pneumonia, encephalitis, hepatitis with giant cell transformation, and sialadenitis have all been described.[26,29,30] The pancreas may be focally involved. The viral inclusions may be atypical and require DNA probes or immunostaining to be identified.

Mycobacterium avium-intracellulare complex (MAC) may involve the mesenteric lymph nodes, GIT, spleen, liver, and bone marrow. Infection by MAC may affect the entire GIT and may cause malabsorption.[26,27,30]

Other infections such as tuberculosis, aspergillosis, cryptococcosis, cryptosporidiosis, histoplasmosis, herpes, adenovirus pneumonia, measles (Figure 18–3), and infection with the respiratory syncytial virus are common pathogens that afflict children with AIDS. Endemic infections may complicate the clinical course of HIV-infected patients in other parts of the world. In South America, for instance, Chagas' disease complicates AIDS in the pediatric age group.

LYMPHOPROLIFERATIVE SYNDROME

Twenty-five percent of children with AIDS develop a lymphoproliferative syndrome[24] characterized by gener-

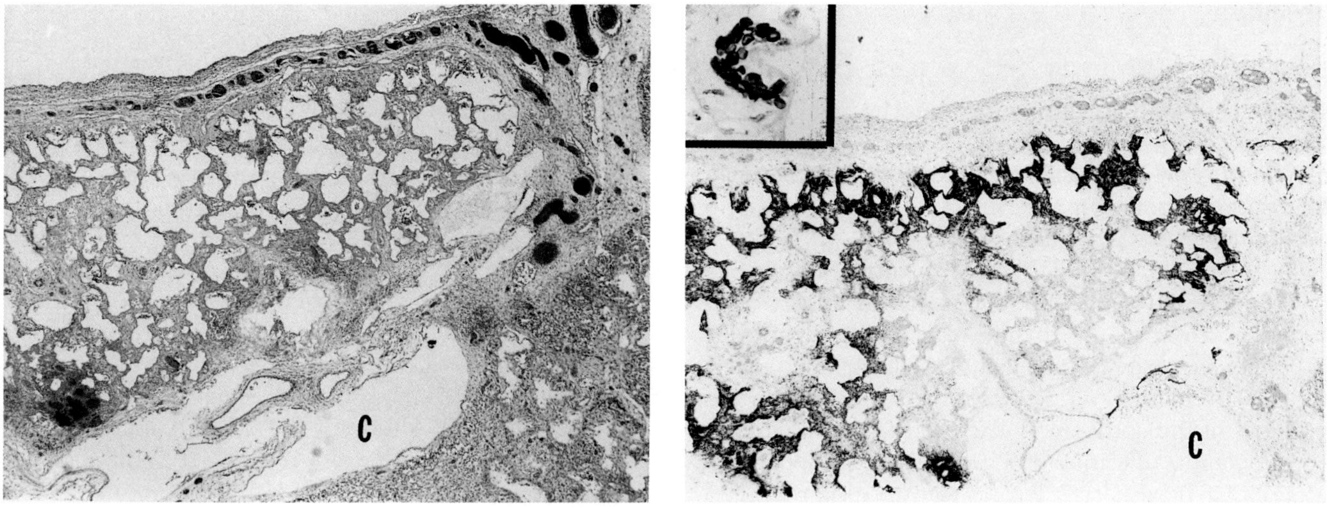

A B

Figure 18–2. (**A**) Lung with a cyst. (C) and subpleural necrosis with dilated air spaces (hematoxylin-eosin, ×80). (**B**) Same area of necrosis shown in part (**A**) showing dystrophic calcification (von Kossa's stain, ×80). *Inset: Pneumocystis carinii* are embedded in the calcified area (Gomori's methenamine-silver stain, ×2000).

alized lymphadenopathy and splenomegaly. There is proliferation of large lymphocytes and immunoblasts with hyperplastic follicles. Giant cells (polykaryocytes) are in HIV-infected lymphoid organs. Cell marker studies confirm that this is a polyclonal, polymorphic B-cell lymphoproliferation, which can progress to a lymphoma.[26] The lymphomas in pediatric AIDS appear in extranodal sites.

Symptomatic lymphoproliferative disease predominantly affects the lung, where nodular or diffuse interstitial infiltrates may be found. The process can surround airways and blood vessels or be in the interstitium.[26] The condition was first referred to as pulmonary lymphoid hyperplasia/lymphoid interstitial pneumonitis (PLH/LIP) complex. It is now believed that it is a systemic process in which lymphoid infiltrates may be in many other organs.[1,26,30] In lungs, this lesion represents bronchial-associated lymphoid tissue. Epstein–Barr viral DNA has been identified in some patients.[31] The salivary glands are often affected early in the disease and the patient appears to have chronic mumps.

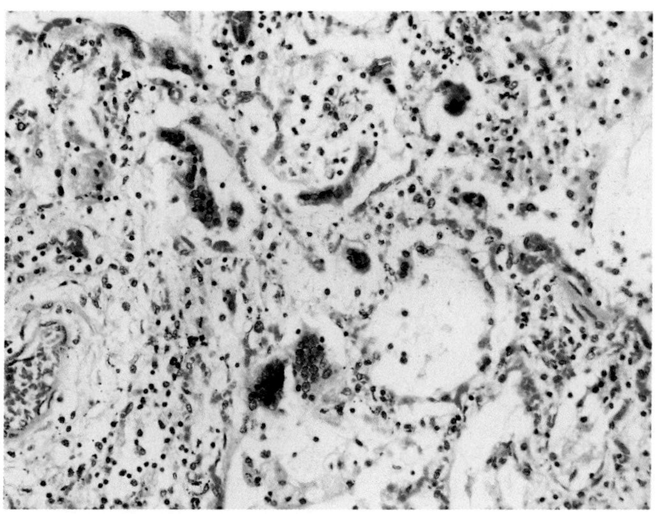

Figure 18–3. Measles giant cell pneumonia. The giant cells have viral inclusions in their nuclei (hematoxylin-eosin, ×40).

NEOPLASMS

Extranodal lymphoma, particularly of the CNS, may be seen in fewer than 5% of children with AIDS.[32] Histologically they are classified as large cell noncleaved, large cell immunoblastic, and small cell noncleaved Burkitt-like lymphoma. Cell marker studies have supported the B-cell origin of these lymphomas.[32] Non-Hodgkin's lymphomas in other organs such as lung[32] and liver[29] have been reported. Burkitt's lymphoma, affecting multiple organs, has also been seen in HIV-infected children.[33]

Kaposi's sarcoma (KS) is rare in children.[34] Vasoproliferative lesions have been observed in lymphoreticular organs and are thought to be a KS or Kaposoid lesion by some investigators.[35] Sarcomas such as gastrointestinal leiomyosarcoma and rhabdomyosarcoma of the biliary tract have been reported.[32,36,37]

THYMUS

The thymus is thought to be affected directly by HIV,[38,39] although an autoimmune mechanism has been suggested.[40] Because HIV has a selective ability to infect and replicate in cells that express CD4 antigen at their surface, both lymphocytes and epithelial cells of the thymus can be injured.

The weight of the thymus is almost always less than expected for age. In our series of 19 thymuses studied at autopsy, the thymic weight ranged from 4% to 75% of the expected weight. The major microscopic findings are marked reduction of the size of the lobules with loss of the corticomedullary demarcation, lymphocyte depletion of variable degree, and perilobular and intralobular fibrosis or sclerosis with focal fatty infiltration. Capillaries are prominent and perivascular sclerosis is frequent. The Hassall's corpuscles show a variable morphology. In some thymuses many normal corpuscles are still present but, for the most part, they are usually rudimentary, calcified, or cystic. The epithelial network is present and appears "naked" and densely packed. These cells are spindle-shaped or epithelioid with more abundant cytoplasm. Giant cells resembling the polykaryocytes are occasionally seen.[26] In addition, there may be epithelial giant cells that might represent a morphologic change induced by direct viral injury.[38] Cultured human thymic epithelium can be infected with HIV, resulting in the formation of giant cells.[38]

Thymic involution in AIDS appears to be more accelerated than in other infectious diseases of children.[26,41] Joshi has proposed that the HIV injures the normal thymus and that the type and severity of changes depend on the timing of the infection.[26] Immunohistochemistry and in situ hybridization have demonstrated viral antigens and viral RNA specific for HIV in thymic tissue.[38,41] Therefore, a direct mechanism of viral injury of the thymus may be important for the development of the immunodeficiency and the degree of damage may correlate with progression of the disease.

SPLEEN

Splenomegaly is a common clinical and autopsy finding in HIV-infected children. The spleen may be involved by opportunistic infections or lymphoproliferative disorders. The most common pathologic findings, however, are lymphoid depletion in both red and white pulp, disarray of the microarchitecture in both the B- and T-cell zones, and increased numbers of macrophages.[42,43] HIV-infected children quite often present with repeated bacterial infections,[44] very much like splenectomized or asplenic or functionally asplenic patients. These repeated infections are caused by encapsulated bacteria as in patients with low or no splenic activity. Functional hyposplenia has been described in HIV-infected adults and children.[45] Overwhelming infection caused death in 33 of 39 of our patients dying of AIDS. The most common infections were pneumonia, sepsis, meningitis, and abscesses of body cavities. *Streptococcus pneumoniae, Pseudomonas aeruginosa,* and *Escherichia coli* were the most common bacterial (nonmycobacterial) organisms cultured during life, whereas *P aeruginosa, Enterococcus* sp, *E coli,* and *Staphylococcus aureus* were most commonly isolated from postmortem specimens.[42,43]

Histologically, the spleen shows variable degrees of lymphocyte depletion, a decreased number of dendritic cells, and histiocytic proliferation. Other findings are plasmacytosis, immunoblastic proliferation, extramedullary hematopoiesis, increase in polymorphonuclear leukocytes, and giant cells (Warthin–Finkeldey type). Fibrosis and vascular changes such as sclerosis, calcification, and thrombosis can also be seen. In spite of the overwhelming number of positive bacterial cultures at autopsy, splenic bacterial abscesses are uncommon.[42] However, the spleen may be infected by MAC, *Candida* sp, and CMV. Primary lymphoma of the spleen is rare in children with AIDS. The spleen may be directly affected by HIV, because HIV RNA has been identified by in situ hybridization in splenic tissue of AIDS patients with thrombocytopenia.[46]

LYMPH NODE

Persistent generalized lymphadenopathy is common in children with HIV infection. The lymph nodes are enlarged with prominent lymphoid follicles and active germinal centers. Sinus histiocytosis may be present. HIV antigens and RNA have been found in the follicular dendritic cells in patients with AIDS.[47] The lymph nodes become small, depleted, fibrotic, and sclerotic as the disease progresses. Giant cells (polykaryocytes) can be in HIV-infected lymph nodes. They may be HIV-infected T lymphocytes.[48]

BONE MARROW

Anemia and thrombocytopenia are frequent in HIV-infected children. Bone marrow pathology, however, is not specific. The changes associated with HIV infection include hypercellularity, hypocellularity, myelodysplasia, plasmacytosis, histiocytosis, eosinophilia, megakaryocytic dysplasia, lymphoid hyperplasia, iron abnormalities, fibrosis, granulomas, and involvement by a variety of microorganisms and rare neoplasms. In children with HIV-related thrombocytopenia, the bone marrow aspirate shows an increased number of megakaryocytes, and large platelets are in the peripheral blood smear.[49]

LIVER

Liver disease in children with HIV infection causes hepatomegaly and elevation of enzymes. In biopsy specimens, the predominant features are chronic active hepatitis, portal lymphoplasmacytic infiltrate, and giant cell transformation of hepatocytes. In autopsy material, however, the changes are more nonspecific and include hepatocellular necrosis, mild portal mononuclear cell infiltrates, portal fibrosis, fatty degeneration of hepatocytes, and Kupffer's cell hyperplasia.[30,50] Some of these changes may be caused by a combination of factors such as malnutrition, drug toxicity, sepsis, and shock.

Chronic active hepatitis with predominance of cytotoxic/suppressor (T8) cells has been reported.[30] Giant cell transformation of hepatocytes is a nonspecific response of the liver cell to injury common in infants. These giant cells in the liver of HIV-infected children have been reported mainly in autopsy material,[29,30,50] but giant cell transformation has been encountered in liver biopsy specimens of HIV-infected children with the clinical syndrome of cholestasis and severe hepatitis in early infancy. This is associated with a poor outcome.[51,52] In some patients cholestatic hepatitis may be the initial presentation of HIV infection and may be an indicator disease for HIV infection in infants.[51] The liver shows giant hepatocytes intermixed with mononuclear inflammatory cells, cholestasis, and diffuse fibrosis (Figure 18–4). The pathogenesis of the giant cell transformation is unclear because no specific cause has been identified consistently by us or other investigators.[29,30,51] Some of the pathologic changes in the liver may be the result of an indirect effect mediated by other infected cells rather than a direct cytopathic effect of HIV. Immunohistochemical studies have demonstrated HIV antigens in Kupffer's cells[53,54] and lymphoid cells[53] in adults. Cao et al[54] have also demonstrated HIV mRNA in Kupffer's cells and viral antigen and viral RNA in occasional hepatocytes.

Opportunistic infections of the liver are less common in children than in adults, but CMV, adenovirus, and MAC are reported.[30,50] Two unusual features encountered were foreign body giant cells containing acid-fast bacilli and the pseudosarcomatous variant of MAC infection.[30,50] These nodules resembling "sarcomas" have been reported in lymph nodes of HIV-infected children[26] and are composed of histiocytes.[55]

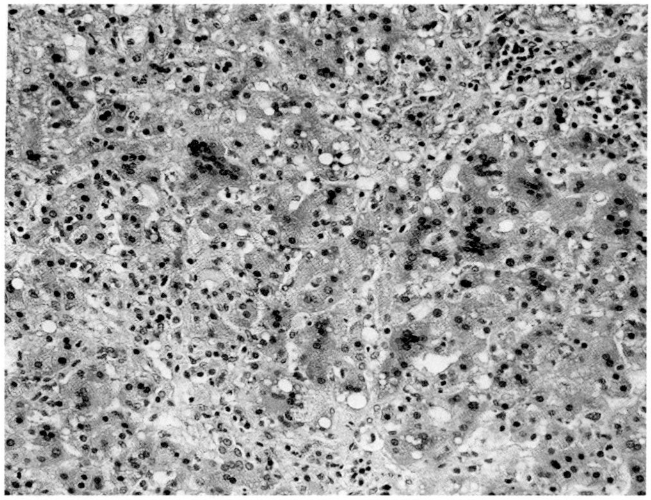

Figure 18–4. Liver showing giant cell transformation of the hepatocytes and chronic inflammation in a child who presented with cholestatic jaundice (hematoxylin-eosin, ×800).

GASTROINTESTINAL TRACT

HIV-infected children may have weight loss, diarrhea, bleeding, abdominal pain, and abdominal distention. The pathologic changes are variable and may be seen in any segment of the GIT. Organisms causing opportunistic infections commonly affect the GIT as local or systemic infections. The most common are *Candida*, CMV, MAC, *Cryptosporidium, Isospora, Salmonella,* and *Shigella.*[27,56] CMV can cause life-threatening complications and the primary lesion appears to be vasculitis.[57] Experience has shown the most common lesions to be necrotizing esophagitis and ulcers of stomach and intestines. A causal agent was identified in about half the lesions.[27,56] Necrotizing esophagitis can be associated with *Candida* and CMV. CMV colitis may cause transmural ulcers, which may perforate. In these patients, CMV inclusions are in endothelial cell, fibroblasts, smooth muscle cells, and macrophages. Thickening of the pylorus and duodenum, pneumatosis coli, and small bowel obstruction are also complications of CMV infection.[27,56]

MAC is in macrophages in the lamina propria with a diffuse distribution or forming aggregates. These children usually have persistent diarrhea and blunting of the villi. *Blastocystis hominis* and *Cryptosporidium* are other causes of diarrhea. Cryptosporidia adhere to the brush border of the epithelial cells of villi and crypts, and the degree of inflammation varies.

Some ulcers have no obvious cause (Figure 18–5). Whether they are caused by HIV or by an unidentified agent is not known. A vascular cause may be possible because intimal fibrosis and luminal narrowing of ves-

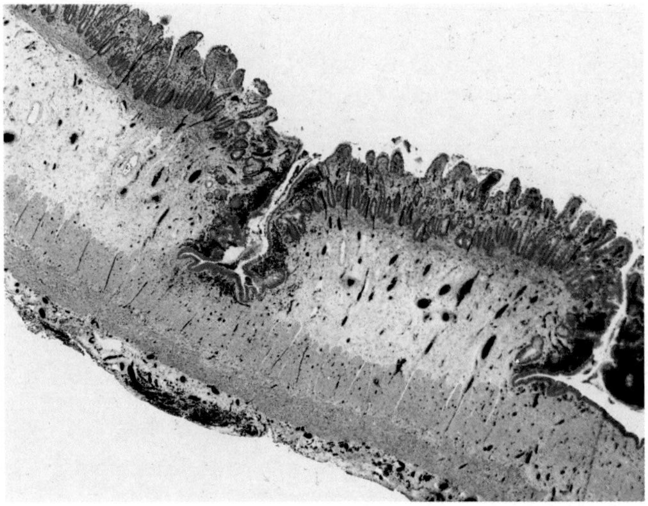

Figure 18–5. Small intestine showing an ulcer in a child who presented with GI bleeding (hematoxylin-eosin, ×80).

sels in the proximity of the ulcer have been seen.[27] The vasculopathy affecting the GIT may be similar to that described in other organs in children with AIDS.[26] Intestinal distention has been reported in children. Its cause is unclear, but we have encountered a child with CMV ganglioneuronitis of the intestinal plexuses who presented with diarrhea. CMV inclusions were only in the ganglion cells.[28] Perhaps this infection of the plexuses causes abnormal bowel function including distention and pain. When the biopsy is limited to the mucosa, viral inclusions in ganglion cells may be missed. HIV-associated enteropathy, characterized by a chronic inflammation of the small intestine, villous blunting or atrophy has been reported.[58] HIV genome or antigens have been in the intestinal epithelium or lymphoid aggregates in HIV-infected adults.[59] Nodular lymphoid infiltrates may be in the GIT but lymphoid depletion is more common. Miscellaneous lesions of the GIT include pneumatosis coli and aphthous ulcers of the cecum.

PANCREAS

Many of the pancreatic lesions in AIDS patients are not specific. These include inflammatory changes, steatonecrosis, fibrosis, ductular dilatation with inspissated secretion, hemorrhage, and thrombosis. Pancreatitis in AIDS patients may have a variety of causes including infectious agents, drugs, and circulatory disarrangement.[60,61] Drug toxicity affecting the islets with decreased number of beta cells and subsequent development of diabetes has been reported in an adult treated with Pentamidine.[62]

KIDNEY

The renal lesions seen in HIV infection are divided into two groups. One comprises the features of HIV-associated nephropathy (HIV-AN) and the other group has nonspecific changes. The lesion seen in the HIV-AN of pediatric AIDS has been described as focal glomerulosclerosis (FGS), mesangial hypercellularity (MH), immune complex glomerulonephritis (ICGN), and minimal change disease (MCD).[26,63–67] Of all these entities, FGS is most common in children and adults.[26,66] The specificity of some of these lesions has been questioned.[68] The renal functional abnormalities of the HIV-AN vary from proteinuria to renal failure, and although nephropathy may be one of the presenting clinical manifestations of pediatric AIDS, it is much less common than in adults.[63]

The incidence of HIV-AN in pediatric AIDS patients varies from 3% to 14%.[63,65] In our survey of 30 autopsies, 23% had glomerular abnormalities but only 13% had clinically evident renal disease.[69] The kidneys are usually enlarged in pediatric HIV infection. Glomerulomegaly, tubular dilatation, and inflammatory cell infiltrates may, in part, account for the nephromegaly. In any case, reduction in size or shrunken kidneys are not features of the HIV-AN.[67,69] The features typical of the FGS form of HIV-AN comprise sclerosis of glomeruli, segmental or global, microcystic dilatation of Bowman's space and renal tubules, enlarged visceral epithelial cells, patchy necrosis of tubular cells, protein casts, and interstitial inflammation (Figure 18–6). The MH variant of HIV-AN usually affects a smaller number of glomeruli, which show increased mesangial matrix and cells with minor tubulointerstitial changes. Studies by

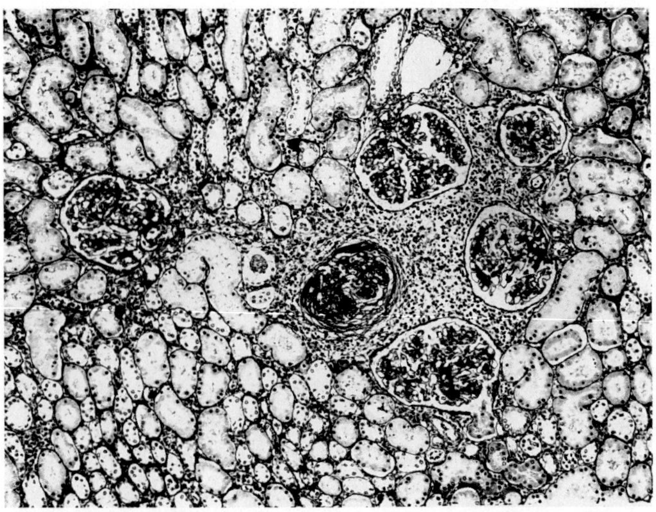

Figure 18–6. Kidney showing sclerotic glomeruli and interstitial lymphocytic infiltration (PAS silver methenamine stain, ×400).

immunofluorescence have documented IgG, IgM, and C3[63,65] with a coarse and irregular pattern, which argues against immune complex deposits. This has been corroborated by electron microscopic studies by us and others.[63,67,69] Tubuloreticular structures (24 nm in diameter) in the cytoplasm of glomeruloendothelial cells are almost always present in HIV-infected patients.

The pathogenesis of HIV-AN is controversial. Data suggesting a direct role of the HIV in AIDS-related FGS were reported by Cohen et al.[70] They demonstrated HIV nucleic acids and antigen in glomerular and tubular epithelial cells in adults with HIV-AN. Others, however, were unable to detect HIV proteins.[71,72] We had a similar experience in children with HIV-AN. We agree with Nadasdy et al[72] that the immunostaining in kidneys using archival material is largely nonspecific. The other variants of HIV-AN such as MH and ICGN may represent immunologic glomerular damage caused by altered immunofunction triggered by HIV because the CD4 receptor has been found in normal mesangial cells.[73]

Secondary nephrologic abnormalities in pediatric AIDS include those caused by fluid and electrolyte imbalances, hemodynamic factors, nephrotoxic substances, and opportunistic infections. Most of the time renal candidiasis and infection by CMV are in conjunction with disseminated diseases affecting multiple organs. Bacterial infections of kidney including MAC are rare in spite of a high frequency of multiple bacterial infections in these children.

CARDIOVASCULAR SYSTEM

Dilated cardiomyopathy, ventricular dysfunction, and pericardial effusion have been described in children with AIDS.[74] In some patients with inflammatory cells and myocytolysis, a diagnosis of myocarditis may be made. More often, the cardiac lesions are difficult to categorize.[75] There can be interstitial edema with reactive Anitschkow cells, fragmented hypertrophic myocardial fibers, and marantic endocarditis. HIV cardiomyopathy may be suspected but immunopathologic methods may be required to confirm and characterize this new entity.[76]

Fragmentation of the elastic lamina, intimal fibrosis, and mineralization of vessel walls occur in many organs and are described as HIV-related arteriopathy.[26] In the heart, small- and medium-size vessels, both in the conducting system and in surrounding myocardium, are involved.[26] The vasa vasorum of the great vessels can also be affected[77] (Figure 18–7). Pulmonary veno-occlusive disease and aneurysm of the coronary arteries and of cerebral arteries sometimes associated with vasculitis have been reported.[26] The pathogenesis of the HIV-related arteriopathy is not clear. Perhaps repeated viral, bacterial, or other infections damage elastic tissue.[25]

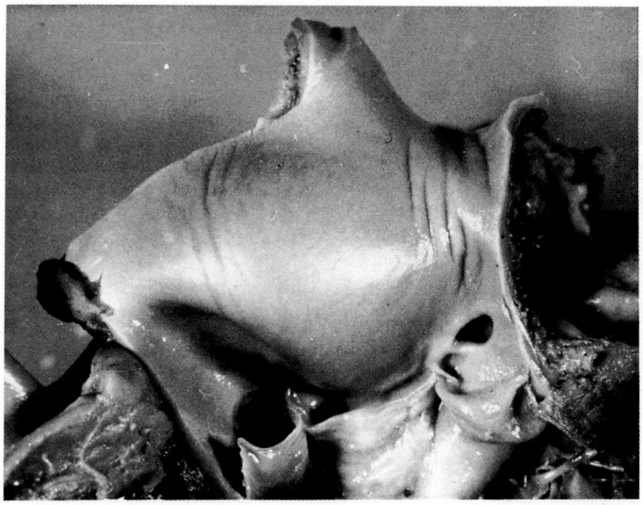

Figure 18–7. Ascending aorta showing wrinkling of the intima, mimicking, slightly, tree barking of syphilitic aortitis.

SKIN

The most common dermatologic manifestations in HIV-infected children are fungal and viral infections.[78] Persistent oral and diaper candidiasis are among the most frequently reported mucocutaneous manifestations. The herpes group is the most common viral infection. Infections with varicella-zoster usually cause severe problems because of the atypical presentation and rapid dissemination. Other viral agents and infections are *molluscum contagiosum,* multiple verruca vulgaris, and condylomata accuminata.[79] *S aureus* and pseudomonas infections have been reported in HIV-infected children. Unusual presentations of scabies are also seen in HIV-infected children.[79] Seborrheic dermatitis, ichthyosis, and xerosis are also common. Zinc deficiency may cause dermatosis such as acrodermatitis enteropathica.[79] Other cutaneous manifestations such as neoplastic disorders are much rarer in children. Two children with Kaposi's sarcoma primarily involving the skin have been reported.[80] In general, the severity of the cutaneous manifestations is closely associated to the degree of the T4 helper cell depletion and the lymphoproliferative responses.[79]

NERVOUS SYSTEM

HIV is neurotropic and the nervous system is one of the most seriously affected organs. Neurologic sequelae are frequent in children with AIDS.[81,82] The encephalopa-

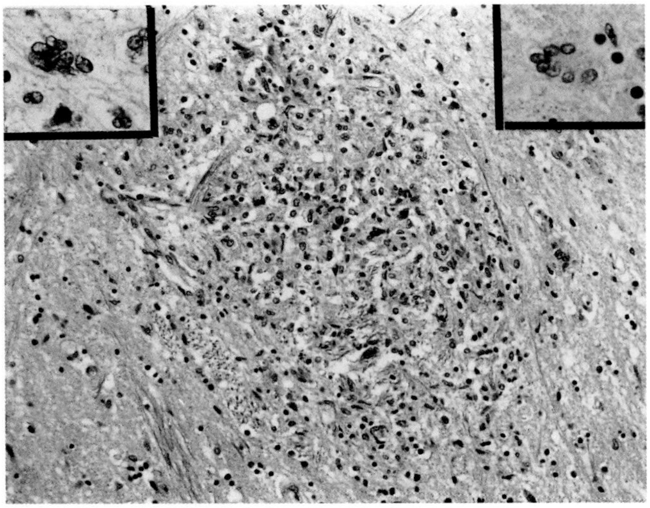

Figure 18–8. This microglial nodule also contains MGC (*insets*) (hematoxylin-eosin, ×400; *insets,* ×2000).

thy may be slowly progressive or fulminant. It occurs usually late in the disease, but can occasionally be the first manifestation of the HIV infection. It is characterized by low IQ, loss of developmental milestones, microcephaly, progressive weakness, and seizures. The latter are mainly in children with focal lesions such as vascular accidents and lymphomas.[83,84] We have, however, encountered seizures in terminally ill patients with no focal lesions. In these patients seizures may occur after cerebral ischemia. Neuroradiologic changes commonly include cerebral atrophy and hydrocephalus with dilatation of the subarachnoid space. Mineralization of basal ganglia and periventricular white matter is often present.

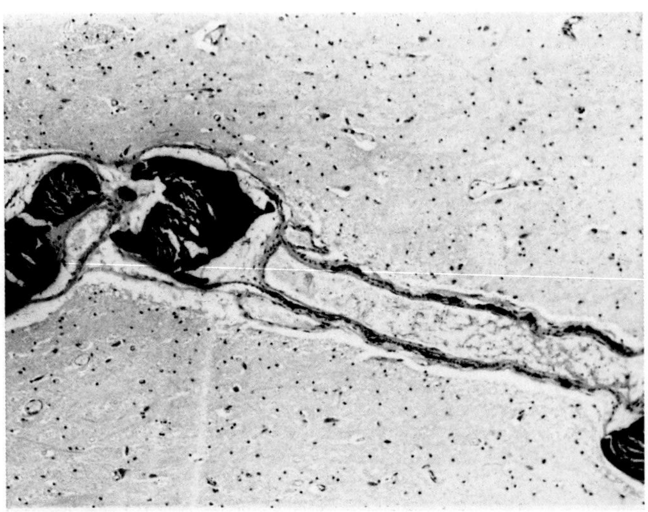

Figure 18–9. Siderocalcinosis of a blood vessel (hematoxylin-eosin, ×400).

Gross atrophy of the brain is common. In many of these children, the brain weighs less than expected for age. Histologic findings include multinucleated giant cells (MGC), microglial nodules (MGN), and siderocalcinosis of blood vessels. MGCs are frequently perivascular and in the white matter. They have crowded overlapping nuclei or nuclei located at the periphery of the cytoplasm (Figure 18–8). Their presence allows a diagnosis of HIV encephalopathy.[85] Electron microscopy, immunohistochemistry, in situ hybridization, and Southern blot have identified HIV particles, protein, or nucleic acids in their cytoplasm.[85,86] MGNs (Figure 18–8) are seen almost with the same frequency as MGC but they are not pathognomonic for HIV infection. Mineralization of blood vessels (Figure 18–9) is the most common histologic finding in HIV encephalopathy and corresponds to the deposition of calcium as well as of iron, a process described as siderocalcinosis. It is almost

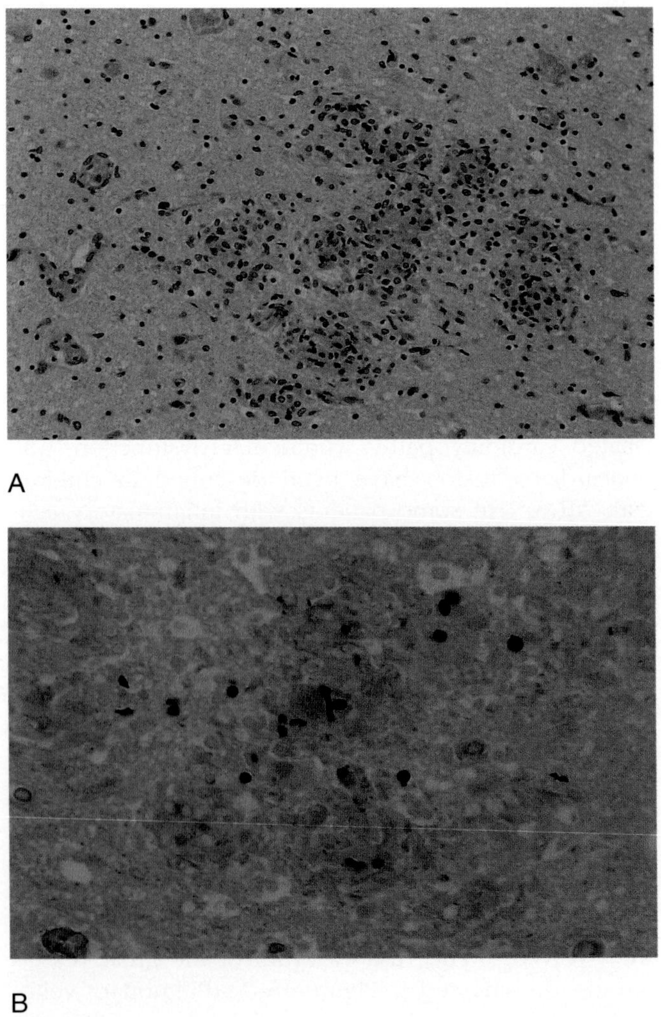

Figure 18–10. (**A**) Intraparenchymal granulomatous inflammation (hematoxylin-eosin, ×20). (**B**) Candidal organisms in the granulomas (Gomori's methenamine-silver stain, ×40).

always within the walls of vessels. The most common focal lesions in children are lymphomas[83] and vascular accidents.[84] Although rare when compared to adults with HIV infection, CNS lymphoma is the most common malignancy in pediatric AIDS.[83] They are mostly of the B-cell type and high grade.[83] Because children have been less exposed to a variety of infectious agents, opportunistic infections are less common than in adults. CNS infections usually occur in the setting of a systemic disease. In our experience candidiasis was the most frequent opportunistic infection of the CNS. In spite of the immunodepression of these patients, there may be both granulomatous and necrotizing lesions (Figure 18–10, A and B). We saw a single CMV infection. The cytomegalic inclusions were in circulating, endothelial, and choroid plexus cells and within MGN (Figure 18–11). We encountered a single case of disseminated MAC cerebral infection. The microorganisms were mainly within uninucleated and multinucleated histiocytic cells. These were preferentially distributed in the leptomeningeal and intraparenchymal perivascular spaces (Figure 18–12, A–C). Progressive multifocal leukoencephalopathy, a demyelinating disease caused by JC virus, is rare in children, with only four cases reported.[87] Other causes of active demyelination are also rare. Myelin pallor, spongiosis, and gliosis may be in white matter.[85] Because myelination is still occurring in many of these children, myelin abnormalities may represent delayed myelination rather than myelin loss.

Changes in the spinal cord include myelin abnormalities of the corticospinal tract in the lateral columns. Here also Wallerian degeneration, delayed myelination, or myelin injury are the three possible mechanisms.[88] We saw one patient with ascending necrotizing myelitis where no opportunistic infection could be demonstrated. There were typical HIV MGC at the edge of the

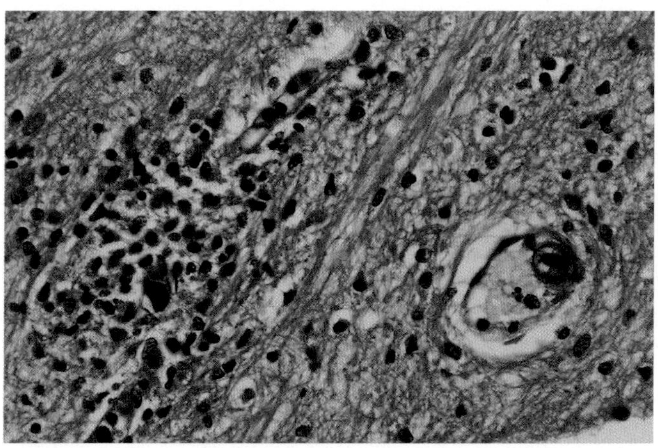

Figure 18–11. CMV infected cells are in both a vascular channel and within a microglial nodule (hematoxylin-eosin, ×40).

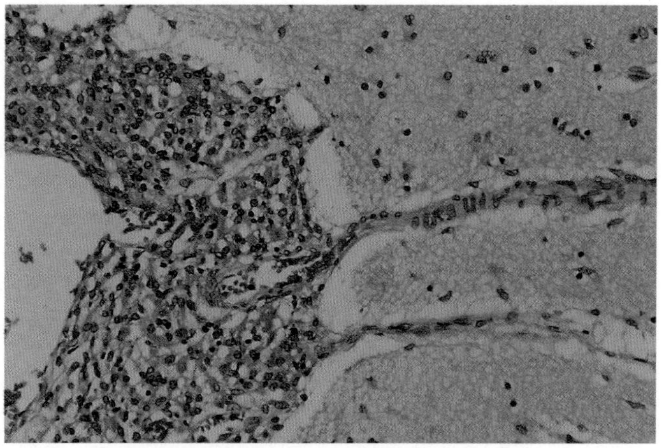

A

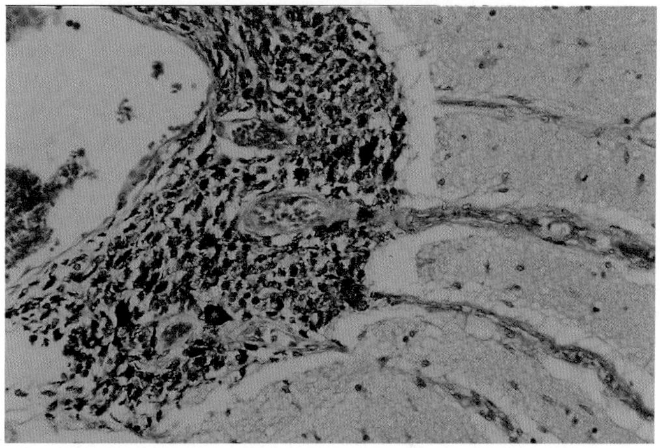

B

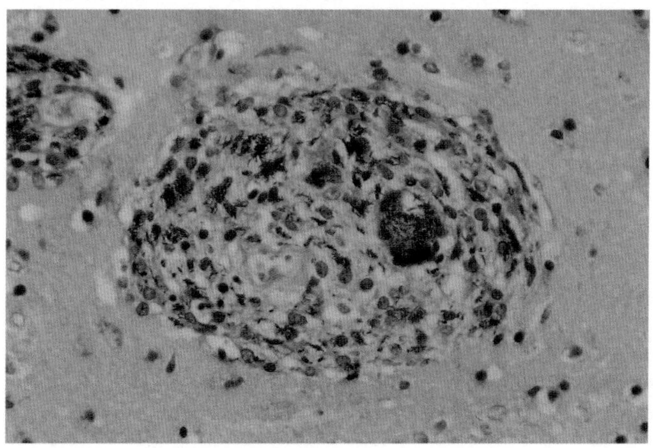

C

Figure 18–12. (**A**) Leptomeningeal perivascular histiocytic infiltrate in a child with disseminated infection by MAC (hematoxylin-eosin, ×20). (**B**) Matching section showing massive numbers of intracellular acid-fast bacilli (Ziehl–Neelsen acid-fast stain, ×20). (**C**) Intraparenchymal perivascular histiocytic infiltrate showing uninucleated and multinucleated cells containing acid-fast bacilli (Ziehl–Neelsen, ×40).

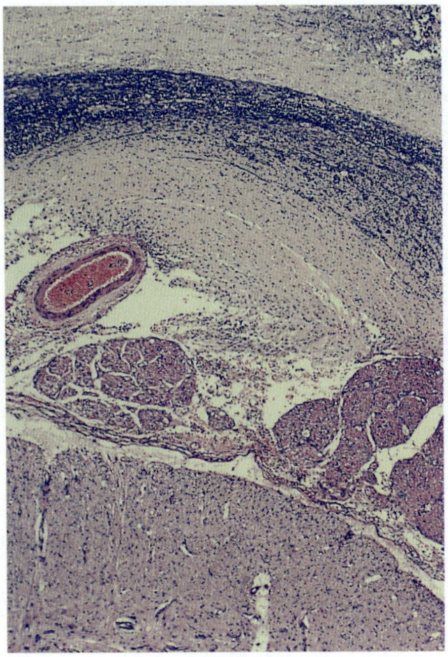

A

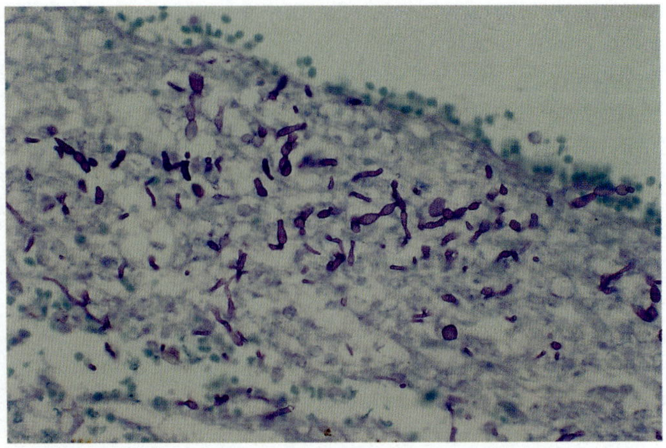

B

Figure 18–13. (**A**) Spinal subdural abscess in a child with disseminated candidiasis (hematoxylin-eosin, ×4 original magnification). (**B**) Candidal organisms at the edge of the suppuration (PAS stain, ×40).

necrosis. Opportunistic infections (Figure 18–13, A and B) and lymphomas can also be seen. Vacuolar myelopathy as seen in HIV-infected adults is rare in children.

The pathogenesis of the lesions in the CNS is not clear. Several hypotheses include direct cellular damage induced by HIV-1 gp 120 neuronal toxicity, immunologic-mediated damage, and indirect effect secondary to the production of cytokines, such as tumor necrosis factor alpha or interleukins, by microglial cells and/or astrocytes.[89–91]

TABLE 18–1. HIV PATHOLOGY

	Children	Adults
Thymus	++	+
CNS	++	+
OI	+	++
Bacterial infections	++	+
LIP/LP[a]	++	+/−
Lymphoma	+	++
KS	+	++
Arteriopathy	++	+/−
Cardiomyopathy	+	+
Progressive encephalopathy	++	+
Failure to thrive	++	−[b]
Lymphopenia	+	++
Hyperglobulinemia	++	+/−

[a]LIP/LP, lymphoid interstitial pneumonitis/lymphoproliferative syndrome.
[b]Wasting syndrome in adults.

CONCLUSION

HIV infection is a generalized disease affecting many organs. Some of the clinical and pathologic manifestations of HIV infection are thought to be directly related to the cytopathic effects of the virus and others are thought to be secondary. All the lesions described in children with AIDS occur in adults, but quantitative and qualitative differences emerge when both groups are compared (Table 18–1). These differences may be a reflection of the effects of the HIV on immature tissues. The diverse manifestations of HIV infection therefore may depend on viral load, time of infection, and host response.

Acknowledgment. The authors are grateful to Mrs. C. Lerro, Ms. J. Grecay, and Ms. M. Lynch for their assistance in preparing this manuscript, to the pathologists who contributed cases to the Pediatric AIDS Study Group, and to Drs. E. Kahn and V. Anderson for their continuous support.

REFERENCES

1. Anderson VM, Kahn E, Greco MA. Challenges in pediatric AIDS pathology. *Adv Pathol Lab Med.* 1993;6:313–343.
2. Centers for Disease Control and Prevention. *HIV/AIDS Surveillance Report.* October 1992;1–18.
3. Ellerbrock TV, Lieb V, Harrington PE, et al. Heterosexu-

ally transmitted human immunodeficiency virus infection among pregnant women in a rural Florida community. *N Engl J Med.* 1992;327:1704–1709.

4. Minkoff H, Nanda D, Menez R, et al. Pregnancies resulting in infants with acquired immunodeficiency syndrome or AIDS related complex: follow-up of mothers, children and subsequently born siblings. *Obstet Gynecol.* 1987; 69:288–291.
5. Gabiano C, Tovo PA, de Martino M, et al. Mother to child transmission of human immunodeficiency virus type 1: risk of infection and correlates of transmission. *Pediatrics.* 1992;90:369–374.
6. Bryson YJ, Luzuriaga K, Sullivan JL, et al. Proposed definitions for in utero versus intrapartum transmission of HIV-1. *N Engl J Med.* 1992;327:1246–1247.
7. Persaud D, Chandwani S, Rigaud M, et al. Delayed recognition of human immunodeficiency virus infection in preadolescent children. *Pediatrics.* 1992;90:688–691.
8. Lapointe N, Michaud J, Pekovic D, et al. Transplacental transmission of HTLV-III virus. *N Engl J Med.* 1985; 312:1325–1326.
9. Jovaisas E, Koch MA, Schafer A, et al. LAV/HTLV-III in 20-week fetus. *Lancet.* 1985;2:1129.
10. Sprecher S, Soumenkoff G, Puissant F, et al. Vertical transmission of HIV in 15-week fetus. *Lancet.* 1986;2:288–289.
11. Lewis SH, Reynolds-Kohler C, Fox HE, et al. HIV-1 in trophoblastic and villous Hofbauer cells, and haematological precursors in eight-week fetuses. *Lancet.* 1990;1:565–568.
12. Chandwani S, Greco MA, Mittal K, et al. Pathology and human immunodeficiency virus expression in placentas of seropositive women. *J Infect Dis.* 1991;163:1134–1138.
13. Jauniaux E, Nessman C, Imbert MC, et al. Morphological aspects of the placenta in HIV pregnancies. *Placenta.* 1989;9:633–642.
14. Page DV, Grady D, Ward S. The placental pathology of substance abuse. *Lab Invest.* 1989;60:69A.
15. Ricci JM, Fojaco RM, O'Sullivan MJ. Congenital syphilis: the University of Miami/Jackson Memorial Medical Center experience, 1986–1988. *Obstet Gynecol.* 1989;74:687–693.
16. Nelson AM, Firpo A, Kamenga M, Mullick FG, et al. Pediatric AIDS and perinatal HIV infection in Zaire: epidemiologic and pathologic findings. *Prog AIDS Pathol.* 1992; 3:1–34.
17. Kida M, Abramowsky CR, Santoscoy C. Cryptococcosis of the placenta in a woman with acquired immunodeficiency syndrome. *Hum Pathol.* 1989;20:920–921.
18. Brady K, Martin A, Page D, et al. Localization of human immunodeficiency virus in placental tissue. *Lab Invest.* 1989;60:69A.
19. Martin AW, Brady K, Smith SI, et al. Immunohistochemical localization of human immunodeficiency virus p24 antigen in placental tissue. *Hum Pathol.* 1992;23:411–414.
20. Mattern CFT, Murray K, Jensen A, et al. Localization of human immunodeficiency virus core antigen in term human placentas. *Pediatrics.* 1992;89:207–209.
21. Backe E, Jimenez E, Unger M, et al. Demonstration of HIV-1 infected cells in human placenta by in situ hybridization and immunostaining. *J Clin Pathol.* 1992;45: 871–874.
22. Goldstein J, Braverman M, Salafia C, et al. The phenotype of human placental macrophages and its variation with gestational age. *Am J Pathol.* 1988;133:648–659.
23. Douglas GC, Fry GN, Thirkill T, et al. Cell-mediated infection of human placental trophoblast with HIV in vitro. *AIDS Res Hum Retro.* 1991;7:735–740.
24. *AIDS Surveillance Update.* New York City Department of Health, Office of AIDS Surveillance. April 1992;1–23.
25. Leibovits E, Rigaud M, Chandwani S, et al. Disseminated fungal infections in children infected with human immunodeficiency virus. *Pediatr Infect Dis J.* 1991;10:888–894.
26. Joshi V. Pathology of acquired immunodeficiency syndrome (AIDS) in children. In: Joshi V, ed. *Pathology of AIDS and Other Manifestations of HIV Infection.* New York: Igaku-Shoin Publishers; 1990:239–269.
27. Kahn E, Greco MA, Daum F, et al. Pathology of the gastrointestinal tract in pediatric AIDS. *Surg Pathol* 1994; 5:239–252.
28. Anderson VM, Greco MA, Recalde AL, et al. Intestinal cytomegalovirus ganglioneuronitis in children with human immunodeficiency virus infection. *Pediatr Pathol.* 1990;10:167–174.
29. Jonas MM, Roldan EO, Lyons HJ, et al. Histopathologic features of the liver in pediatric acquired immune deficiency syndrome. *J Pediatr Gastroenterol Nutr.* 1989;9: 73–81.
30. Kahn E, Greco MA, Daum F, et al. Hepatic pathology in pediatric acquired immunodeficiency syndrome. *Hum Pathol.* 1991;22:1111–1119.
31. Andiman WA, Eastman R, Martin K, et al. Opportunistic lymphoproliferations associated with Epstein–Barr viral DNA in infants and children with AIDS. *Lancet.* 1985; 2:1390–1393.
32. DiCarlo FJ, Joshi VV, Oleske JM, et al. Neoplastic diseases in children with acquired immunodeficiency syndrome. *Prog AIDS Pathol.* 1990;2:163–185.
33. Young SA, Crocker DW. Burkitt's lymphoma in a child with AIDS. *Pediatr Pathol.* 1990;11:115–122.
34. Buck BE, Scott GB, Valdes-Dapena M, et al. Kaposi sarcoma in two infants with acquired immunodeficiency syndrome. *J Pediatr.* 1983;103:911–913.
35. Fojaco RM, Hemsley GT, Rodrigues MM, et al. AIDS in infants and children: an autopsy study of 77 cases in South Florida. *Prog AIDS Pathol.* (in press).
36. Ross JS, Del Rosario A, Bui HX, Sonbatti H, Solis O. Primary hepatic leiomyosarcoma in a child with acquired immunodeficiency syndrome. *Hum Pathol.* 1992;23: 69–72.
37. Van Hoeven KH, Factor SM, Kress Y, Woodruf JM. Visceral myogenic tumors. A manifestation of HIV infection in children. *Am J Surg Pathol.* 1993;17:1176–1181.
38. Baskin GB, Murphey-Corb M, Martin LN, et al. Thymus in simian immunodeficiency virus-infected Rhesus monkeys. *Lab Invest.* 1991;65:400–407.
39. Hays EF, Uittenbogaart CH, Brewer JC, et al. In vitro studies of HIV-1 expression in thymocytes from infants and children. *AIDS.* 1992;6:265–272.
40. Savino W, Dardenne M, Marche C, et al. Thymic epithelium in AIDS: an immunohistologic study. *Am J Pathol.* 1986;122:302–307.
41. Schuurman HJ, Krone WJA, Broekhuizen R, et al. The thy-

mus in acquired immune deficiency syndrome. Comparison with other types of immunodeficiency diseases, and presence of components of human immunodeficiency virus type 1. *Am J Pathol.* 1989;134:1329–1338.

42. Thomas PA, Anderson V, Mahnovski V, et al. Infections and the spleen in children with the acquired immunodeficiency syndrome: a possible morphologic model for functional asplenia. *Cell Vision J Analyt Morphol.* 1994; 1:208–217.
43. Thomas PA, Anderson VM, Greco MA. Systemic pathology in HIV infection and AIDS in children. The spleen. In: *Pediatric AIDS Fascicle.* Armed Forces Institute of Pathology (in press).
44. Krazinski DI, Borkowsky W, Bonk S, et al. Bacterial infections in human immunodeficiency virus infected children. *Pediatr Infect Dis J.* 1988;7:373–378.
45. Siddiqui AR. Functional hyposplenia in a child with the AIDS-related complex. *Clin Nucl Med.* 1988;13:840–841.
46. Prevot S, Fournier JG, Tardivel I. Detection by in situ hybridization of HIV 1 RNA in spleens of HIV 1 seropositive patients with thrombocytopenic purpura. *Pathol Res Pract.* 1989;185:187–193.
47. Parmentier HK, van Wichen D, Sie-Go DMDS, et al. HIV-1 infection and virus production in follicular dendritic cells in lymph nodes. *Am J Pathol.* 1990;137:247–251.
48. Kamel OW, LeBrun DP, Berry GJ, et al. Warthin–Finkeldey polykaryocytes demonstrate a T-cell immunophenotype. *Am J Clin Pathol.* 1992;97:179–183.
49. Karpatkin M. Thrombocytopenia in children infected by the human immunodeficiency virus. *Prog AIDS Pathol.* (in press).
50. Kahn E, Ishak KG. Hepatic pathology in pediatric AIDS. In: *Pediatric AIDS Fascicle.* Armed Forces Institute of Pathology (in press).
51. Persaud D, Bangaru B, Greco MA, et al. Cholestatic hepatitis in children infected with the human immunodeficiency virus. *Pediatr Infect Dis J.* 1993:12:492–498.
52. Witzleben CL, Marshall GS, Werner W, et al. HIV as cause of giant cell hepatitis. *Hum Pathol.* 1988;19:603–605.
53. Hoda SA, White JE, Gerber MA. Immunohistochemical studies of human immunodeficiency virus-1 in liver tissues of patients with AIDS. *Mod Pathol.* 1991;4:578–581.
54. Cao Y, Dieterich D, Thomas PA, et al. Identification and quantitation of HIV-1 in the liver of patients with AIDS. *AIDS.* 1992;6:65–70.
55. Bradwin M, Strauchen J, Jagirdar J. Sarcomatoid *M. avium intracellulare* infection (SMA II): evidence for monocytic histiocytic differentiation of spindle cells. *Lab Invest.* 1989;60:2A.
56. Kahn E. Gastrointestinal manifestations in pediatric AIDS. In: *Pediatric AIDS Fascicle.* Armed Forces Institute of Pathology (in press).
57. Roberts WH, Sneddon JM, Waldman J, et al. Cytomegalovirus infection of gastrointestinal endothelium demonstrated by simultaneous nucleic acid hybridization and immunohistochemistry. *Arch Pathol Lab Med.* 1989; 113:461–464.
58. McLoughlin LC, Nord KS, Joshi VV, et al. Severe gastrointestinal involvement in children with the acquired immunodeficiency syndrome. *J Pediatr Gastroenterol Nutr.* 1987;6:517–523.
59. Kotler DP, Reka S, Borcich A, et al. Detection, localization, and quantitation of HIV-associated antigens in intestinal biopsies from patients with HIV. *Am J Pathol.* 1991;139: 823–830.
60. Kahn E, Anderson VM, Greco MA, Magid M. Pancreatic disorders in pediatric acquired immune deficiency syndromy. *Hum Pathol.* 1995;26:765–770.
61. Kahn E, Moran CA, Anderson VM. Pancreatic disorders in pediatric AIDS. In: *Pediatric AIDS Fascicle.* Armed Forces Institute of Pathology (in press).
62. Hauser L, Sheehan P, Simpkins H. Pancreatic pathology in Pentamidine-induced diabetes in acquired immunodeficiency syndrome patients. *Hum Pathol.* 1991;22:926–929.
63. Connor E, Gupta S, Joshi V, et al. Acquired immunodeficiency syndrome-associated renal disease in children. *J Pediatr.* 1988;113:39–44.
64. Rousseau E, Russo P, Lapointe N, et al. Renal complications acquired immunodeficiency syndrome in children. *Am J Kid Dis.* 1989;11:48–50.
65. Strauss J, Abitol C, Zilleruelo G, et al. Renal disease in children with the acquired immunodeficiency syndrome. *N Engl J Med.* 1989;321:625–630.
66. D'Agati V, Shu JL, Carbone L, et al. Pathology of HIV-associated nephropathy: a detailed morphologic and comparative study. *Kidney Int.* 1989;35:1358–1370.
67. Cangiarella J, Feiner HD, Antonovych TT, Greco MA. Systemic pathology of HIV infection and AIDS in children. Urinary system. In: *Pediatric AIDS Fascicle.* Armed Forces Institute of Pathology (in press).
68. Foster S, Hawkins E, Hanson CG, Shearer W. Pathology of the kidney in childhood immunodeficiency: AIDS-related nephropathy is not unique. *Pediatr Pathol.* 1991; 11:63–74.
69. Feiner H, Horowitz L, Greco MA, et al. Renal disease in pediatric HIV infection. *Prog AIDS Pathol.* (in press).
70. Cohen P, Sun NCJ, Shapsak P, et al. Demonstration of human immunodeficiency virus in renal epithelium in HIV-associated nephropathy. *Mod Pathol.* 1989;2:125–128.
71. Barbiano di Belgiojoso G, Genderini A, Vago L, et al. Absence of HIV antigens in renal tissue from patients with HIV-associated nephropathy. *Nephrol Dial Transplant.* 1990;5:489.
72. Nadasdy T, Hanson-Painton O, Davis LD, et al. Conditions affecting the immunohistochemical detection of HIV in fixed and embedded renal and normal tissues. *Mod Pathol.* 1992;15:283.
73. Karlsson-Parra A, Dimeny E. HIV receptors (CD4 antigen) in normal human glomerular cells. *N Engl J Med.* 1989;320:741. Letter.
74. Lipshultz SE, Chanock S, Sander SP, et al. Cardiovascular manifestations of human immunodeficiency virus infection in infants and children. *Am J Cardiol.* 1989;63: 1489–1497.
75. Joshi VV, Gadol C, Connon E, et al. Dilated cardiomyopathy in children with acquired immunodeficiency syndrome: a pathologic study of five cases. *Hum Pathol.* 1988;19:69–73.

76. Lipshultz SE, Fox CH, Perez-Atayde AR, et al. Identification of human immunodeficiency virus-1 and DNA in the heart of a child with cardiovascular abnormalities and congenital acquired immune deficiency syndrome. *Am J Cardiol.* 1990;66:246–250.
77. Kabus D, Greco MA. Arteriopathy in children with AIDS: microscopic changes in the vasa vasorum with gross irregularities of aortic intima. *Pediatr Pathol.* 1991;11:793–795.
78. Straka BF, Whitaker DL, Morrison SH, et al. Cutaneous manifestations of the acquired immunodeficiency syndrome in children. *J Am Acad Dermatol.* 1988;18: 1089–1102.
79. Lim W, Sadick N, Gupta A, et al. Skin diseases in children with HIV infection and their association with degree of immunosuppression. *Int J Dermatol.* 1990;29:24–30.
80. Connor E, Baccon-Gibod L, Joshi V, et al. Cutaneous acquired immunodeficiency syndrome-associated Kaposi's sarcoma in pediatric patients. *Arch Dermatol.* 1990;126:791–793.
81. Epstein LG, Sharer LR, Goudsmit J, Neurological and neuropathological features of human immunodeficiency virus infection in children. *Ann Neurol.* 1988;23:S19–S23.
82. Belman AL, Diamond G, Dickson D, et al. Pediatric acquired immunodeficiency syndrome. Neurologic syndromes. *Am J Dis Child.* 1988;142:29–35.
83. Epstein LG, DiCarlo Jr. FJ, Hoshi VV, et al. Primary lymphoma of the central nervous system in children with acquired immunodeficiency syndrome. *Pediatrics.* 1988; 82:355–363.
84. Park YD, Belman AL, Dickson DW, et al. Stroke in pediatric acquired immunodeficiency syndrome. *Ann Neurol.* 1990;28:553–560.
85. Sharer LR, Epstein LG, Cho E-S, et al. Pathologic features of AIDS encephalopathy in children: evidence for LAV/HTLV-III infection of brain. *Hum Pathol.* 1986;17: 271–284.
86. Shaw GM, Harper ME, Hahn BH, et al. HTLV-III infection in brains of children and adults with AIDS encephalopathy. *Science.* 1985;227:177–182.
87. Berger JR, Scott G, Albrecht J, et al. Progressive multifocal leukoencephalopathy in HIV-1-infected children. *AIDS.* 1992;6:837–841.
88. Dickson DW, Belman AL, Kim TS, et al. Spinal cord pathology in pediatric acquired immunodeficiency syndrome. *Neurol.* 1989;39:227–235.
89. Tyor WR, Glass JD, Griffin JW, et al. Cytokine expression in the brain during the acquired immunodeficiency syndrome. *Ann Neurol.* 1992;31:349–360.
90. Aukrust P, Liabakk N-B, Muller F, et al. Serum levels of tumor necrosis factor-α (TNF-a) and soluble TNF receptors in human immunodeficiency virus type 1 infection—correlations to clinical, immunologic and virologic parameters. *J Infect Dis.* 1994;169:420–424.
91. Nuovo GJ, Galley F, MacConnell P, Braun A. In situ detection of polymerase chain reaction-amplified HIV-1 nucleic acids and tumor necrosis factor-α RNA in the central nervous system. *Am J Pathol.* 1994;144:659–666.

CHAPTER 19

Human Immunodeficiency Virus Infection Lesions of the Central Nervous System

Marc K. Rosenblum

And I will turn your feasts into mourning, and all your songs into lamentation; and I will bring up sackcloth upon all loins, and baldness upon every head; and I will make it as the mourning of an only son, and the end thereof as a bitter day.

Amos 8:10

O speculator concerning this machine of ours let it not distress you that you impart knowledge of it through another's death, but rejoice that our Creator has ordained the intellect to such excellence of perception.

Leonardo da Vinci (1452–1519), Quaderni d'Anatomia, Vol. II

INTRODUCTION

In the decade since its initial isolation from victims of the acquired immunodeficiency syndrome (AIDS), the human immunodeficiency virus type 1 (HIV-1) has come to be recognized as a highly neuroinvasive agent. The replication of this retrovirus in central nervous tissues is now known to produce histopathologic alterations unlike those associated with any other human pathogen and its damaging presence in the neuropil may be responsible for syndromes of progressive cognitive and motor dysfunction that rank among the most common and crippling manifestations of AIDS.[1,2] What follows is a discussion of central nervous system (CNS) infection by HIV-1, including a depiction of its unique neuropathologic features. The terminology and diagnostic criteria employed are those recommended in consensus proposals for a standardized clinical[3] and histomorphologic[4] nomenclature of HIV-1–associated neurologic diseases.

THE AGENT: MORPHOLOGY, TROPISMS, AND CYTOPATHIC EFFECTS

HIV-1 is a member of the Lentivirinae—from the Latin *lentus,* meaning "slow" or "lingering"—a subfamily of nontransforming retroviruses named for the protracted temporal evolution of the diseases with which its representatives are associated.[5,6] This taxonomy is predicated on the structural similarities of the agent's genome and patterns of genomic transcription to those of established lentiviruses,[7–11] shared cytopathic effects,[12,13] fine structural resemblances,[7,14–17] and unifying biologic properties that include, in addition to its encephalitogenic potential,[5,6] a tropism for the mono-

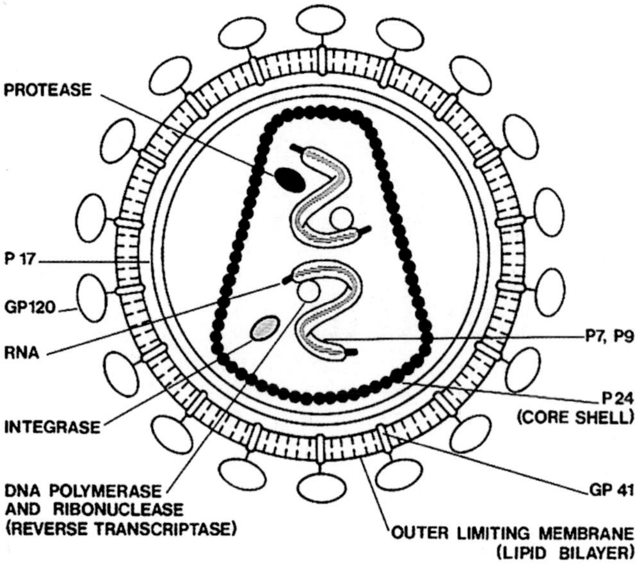

Figure 19–1. HIV-1. A schematic depiction based on immunoelectron microscopic localization of the agent's structural core proteins (P) and glycoproteins (GP), designated by their molecular weights in kilodaltons. See text for additional explanation. *(From Rosenblum[1] with permission.)*

cyte/macrophage.[6,18] Depicted schematically in Figure 19–1 and at the ultrastructural level in Figure 19–2, the mature HIV-1 virion consists of an inner formed "core" enveloped by a limiting membrane studded with glycoproteins. The core includes an electron-dense, cylindrical or bar-shaped nucleoid comprised of viral nucleic acids and enzymes integral to their processing, a tapering conical shell that encloses the nucleoid, and a capsid, anchored to the inner aspect of the envelope, for which a complex icosadeltahedral structure has been proposed.[19] HIV-1 assembly occurs in association with cell membranes, particles budding into the extracellular space from the plasmalemma or aggregating in membrane-delimited intracytoplasmic vacuoles derived from the Golgi apparatus or endoplasmic reticulum. Virions may also be found lying free in the cytoplasm of some infected cell types. The mature particle is spherical, averaging 100 to 120 nm in diameter, its nucleoid eccentrically positioned—a feature characteristic of the lentiviruses as a group.

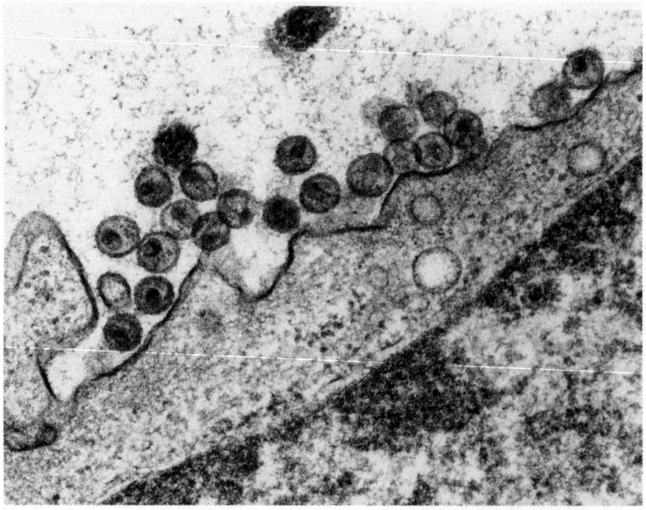

Figure 19–2. HIV-1. Note the eccentric location of the core density and tapered core shells visible in some of the mature particles, seen in apposition to the surface of an H9 lymphocyte (×70,000). *(Courtesy of M Meyenhofer and LR Sharer, MD, University of Medicine and Dentistry of New Jersey.)*

HIV-1 infection is initiated at the molecular level[20] principally by the high affinity binding of its 120-kilodalton (kd) envelope glycoprotein, gp120, to a 62-kd polypeptide, designated CD4, normally expressed on the surfaces of T helper lymphocytes, monocytes, Langerhan's, and follicular dendritic cells.[21] All are susceptible to HIV-1 infection. Autopsy studies (see later discussion) have not shown HIV-1 to be a truly neurotropic retrovirus (ie, one exhibiting a particular predilection for cells of neuroepithelial lineage), but a variety of laboratory observations have been invoked in theoretical support of resident CNS elements as potential targets of the agent. CD4-associated antigens[22] and gene transcripts encoding the receptor[22,23] have been detected in normal human brain tissue, whereas a number of reports describe the successful in vitro transmission of HIV-1 to cells derived from the nervous system and its associated neoplasms. These include astrocytes cultured from fetal brain and human gliomas of the astrocytic series,[24–31] a medulloblastoma line,[26] fibroblast-like cells derived from the choroid plexus,[32] and microglia.[33–35] Only a subset of susceptible cell lines in these studies could be shown to express CD4 or CD4 messenger RNA (mRNA). This, along with the failure of pretreatment with soluble recombinant CD4 or CD4-specific monoclonal antibodies to block viral transmission to some cells of neuroectodermal lineage, has been taken as evidence that HIV-1 exhibits a tropism for CNS elements not strictly circumscribed by the distribution of this surface determinant. Galactosyl ceramide and sulfatide, cell-surface glycolipids elaborated by oligodendroglia (among other cell types), have been proposed as alternative HIV-1 receptors on the strength of their ability to bind gp120 in vitro.[36] A novel gp120 binding site distinct from CD4 and galactosyl ceramide has been identified on the surface of human fetal astrocytes.[37]

In addition to figuring prominently in the penetration of target cells, the envelope glycoproteins of HIV-1 mediate the subsequent cytopathic effects of particular relevance to the neuropathology of cerebral retroviral infection (Figure 19–3). Typical of "productive" (as opposed to defective or latent) in vitro infec-

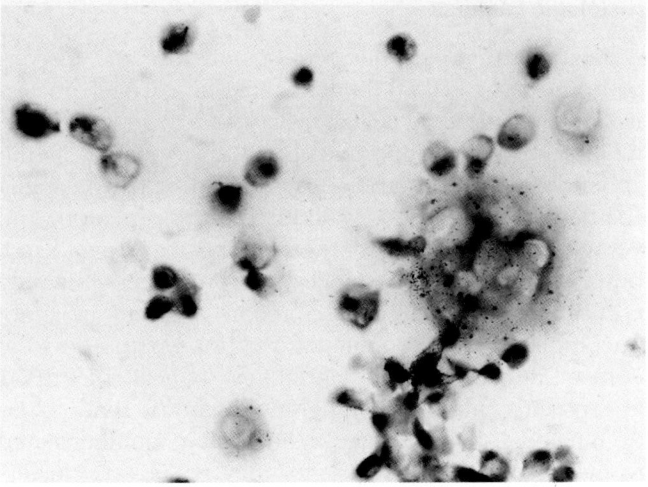

Figure 19–3. In vitro cytopathic effect of HIV-1. Seen here are cultured human macrophages exposed to HIV-1 (isolated from the brain of a patient with AIDS) and assayed for HIV-1–specific messenger RNA sequences by in situ hybridization and autoradiography using an ^{35}S-radiolabeled RNA probe. Multinucleated cells, such as the one present at right, are typical of HIV-1 in vitro and represent syncytia generated by cell fusion. The clustering of silver grains over this cell is indicative of its productive infection (Giemsa, ×400).

tion by HIV-1 and other lentiviruses is the formation of multinucleated cells.[12,13] These are generated by a process of plasmalemmal fusion[13,38] initiated as gp120 displayed on the surfaces of infected cells manifests its CD4-binding properties. Neighboring cells expressing the receptor are recruited, on contact, into progressively enlarging syncytia in which viral replication is amplified. As presently discussed, polykaryotes of similar appearance are a distinctive feature of this agent's replication in the nervous system and are critical to the histopathologic diagnosis of HIV-1 encephalitis.

INVASION OF THE CENTRAL NERVOUS SYSTEM

That the cerebrospinal fluid (CSF) is seeded early in the course of systemic HIV-1 infection, possibly during its acute viremic phase, is evident from viral isolation studies and assessments of intrathecal antibody responses to the agent.[39–43] The HIV-1 p24 core antigen has been detected within this compartment prior to seroconversion[44] and a seroconversion-associated aseptic meningitis[45,46] is thought to reflect an inflammatory reaction provoked by the local presence of the virus. The timing of neuroparenchymal penetration, however, is unresolved, as are the relative contributions of circulating CSF and blood to the propagation of CNS infection. Immunologic containment could account for the observation that the brains of HIV-1 seropositive individuals dying prior to the onset of AIDS generally exhibit little or no evidence of productive infection,[47–50] but may harbor HIV-1 proviral DNA.[51] The reported amplification of HIV-1–specific nucleic acid sequences from the brain of a patient dying 15 days after accidental intravenous infusion of a contaminated white blood cell preparation[52] suggests that invasion of the neuropil proper can follow close on primary infection. Experimental support for such a scenario includes the demonstration of viral replication in the brains of Rhesus macaques (*Macaca mulatta*) as early as 1 week following their intravenous inoculation with encephalitogenic strains of the closely related simian immunodeficiency virus (SIV).[53] The susceptibility of the developing nervous system to HIV-1 following its transplacental passage is underscored by recovery of the virus from fetal brain tissue.[54]

Whether HIV-1 penetrates the blood–brain barrier in free form or is ferried across by infected cells remains unsettled, but insights gleaned from the study of lentiviral encephalitides afflicting ruminants and subhuman primates suggest that the monocyte may play a critical role in this process. Levels of viral replication sufficiently restricted so as to preclude immune detection and clearance permit monocytes harboring agents such as the visna-maedi virus of sheep to act as "Trojan horses," seeding and persisting in target tissues that include the brain.[55,56] Monocyte-derived macrophages situated in the perivascular compartment appear, furthermore, to be the first demonstrably infected elements in experimental models of SIV encephalitis.[53] HIV-1 shares with these animal lentiviruses a tropism for the monocyte/macrophage.[18] The latter are relatively refractory to lysis by the agent, in contrast to T4 lymphocytes, and are able to support long-term infection at restricted levels of viral replication. Whereas T-cell infection is generally characterized by the assembly of HIV-1 in strict association with the plasmalemma and release of numerous particles from the cell surface, the monocyte/macrophage may sequester virions in membrane-bound intracytoplasmic vacuoles and suppress their subsequent exocytosis,[18,57] concealing its retroviral burden. Such cells constitute ideal vehicles for the covert dissemination and persistence of HIV-1 in the face of initially unimpaired immunologic responses and it would appear, in fact, that neuroinvasiveness is a property selectively associated with macrophage-adapted strains of the agent.[58]

THE NEUROPATHOLOGY OF HIV-1 ENCEPHALITIS

Macroscopic Features

The brain productively infected by HIV-1 may appear entirely unaltered on gross inspection but more com-

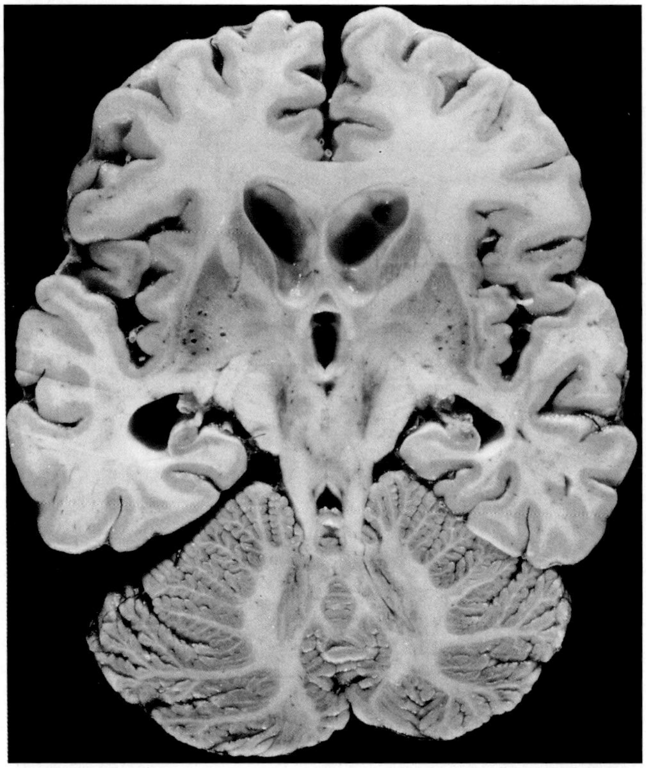

Figure 19–4. HIV-1–associated cerebral atrophy. This brain, from a profoundly demented adult with HIV-1 encephalitis, exhibits narrowing of the cortical ribbon, widened sulci, and ventricular dilatation indicative of diffuse brain injury and a loss of cerebral substance. As is typical in the absence of superimposed opportunistic infection or neoplasia, there are no focal lesions. *(From Rosenblum[1] with permission.)*

monly exhibits abnormalities indicative of diffuse injury (Figure 19–4). Modestly diminished brain weight, widened sulci, thinning of the cortical ribbon, and ventricular dilatation attest to a loss of cerebral substance in the vast majority of adult cases.[59] The centrum semiovale and corpus callosum may, in addition, evidence an indistinct gray mottling suggestive of a generalized white matter insult. Atrophy, often pronounced, is also characteristic of the infected child's brain.[60,61] The cortex may be grossly attenuated, the white matter shrunken and discolored, and the weight of the brain far short of that expected in this population. Unusually florid examples of HIV-1 encephalitis can exhibit focal necrotizing lesions of the cortex, white or central gray matter, but these are clearly exceptional. In the typical case, gross neuropathologic examination does not serve as a guide to targeted tissue sampling for detection of the agent. Furthermore, cerebral atrophy in the setting of AIDS is not strictly correlated with the demonstrable replication of HIV-1 in the brain, only a subset of such specimens exhibiting HIV-1 encephalitis on histologic study.

Histologic Features

A diagnosis that currently requires microscopic analysis of brain tissue, HIV-1 encephalitis[1,4,59–70] is characterized by loosely arrayed, often vasocentric inflammatory infiltrates scattered principally in the cerebral hemispheric white matter and corpus callosum, basal ganglia (particularly the globus pallidus), mesencephalon, and ventral pons. Any level of the neuraxis may be affected, but only occasional instances of florid, predominantly cortical involvement are on record[71,72] and it is not uncommon for the inflammatory process to shun the cortex altogether. The infiltrates typical of HIV-1 encephalitis, although nongranulomatous, tend to be dominated by macrophages, including multinucleated forms (Figure 19–5). The latter may present as clusters of overlapping, compressed, and molded nuclei virtually devoid of appreciable cytoplasm or assume the proportions and cytologic features of Touton- or Langhans'-type giant cells. Foamy cytoplasmic alterations indicative of lipid accumulation are common to both mononucleated and multinucleated variants, which may also contain intracytoplasmic pigments that include hemosiderin and lipofuscin. Lymphocytes are sparsely represented in most cases, particularly those of adult onset, although dense perivascular and intramural lymphoid infiltrates have been described as lending a "vasculitic" appearance to some examples of pediatric HIV-1 encephalitis.[61,73] CNS tissues surrounding loci of infection may evidence little reaction or exhibit varying degrees of rarefaction and astrogliosis.

The multinucleated cell is justly recognized as the hallmark of HIV-1 encephalitis. That such cells might represent markers of cerebral retroviral infection was first proposed[62] on the basis of their resemblance to the multinucleate syncytia generated by lentiviruses in vitro and their identification in brains shown to harbor the HIV-1 genome and proviral genomic sequences.[74] Although amitotic nuclear division has been posited to account for examples characterized by internuclear chromatin "bridges,"[75] most are believed to reflect cell fusion mediated in situ by HIV-1. These cells (and their mononuclear counterparts) contain HIV-1–specific nucleic acid sequences (Figure 19–6)[70,76–81] and express epitopes associated with the virus' structural core proteins and glycoproteins (Figure 19–7, A)[64,70,76,79,82–88] Electron microscopic studies[15,61,64,77,89–91] have confirmed that they are productively infected, harboring and releasing mature virions. Reported instances in which retroviral antigens and nucleic acids were present in abundance within brain tissues but multinucleated cells were not in evidence[79,84] indicate, however, that widespread productive cerebral infection can occur in the absence of cytopathic effects and suggest that some strains of HIV-1 may have limited capacity for inducing cell fusion.

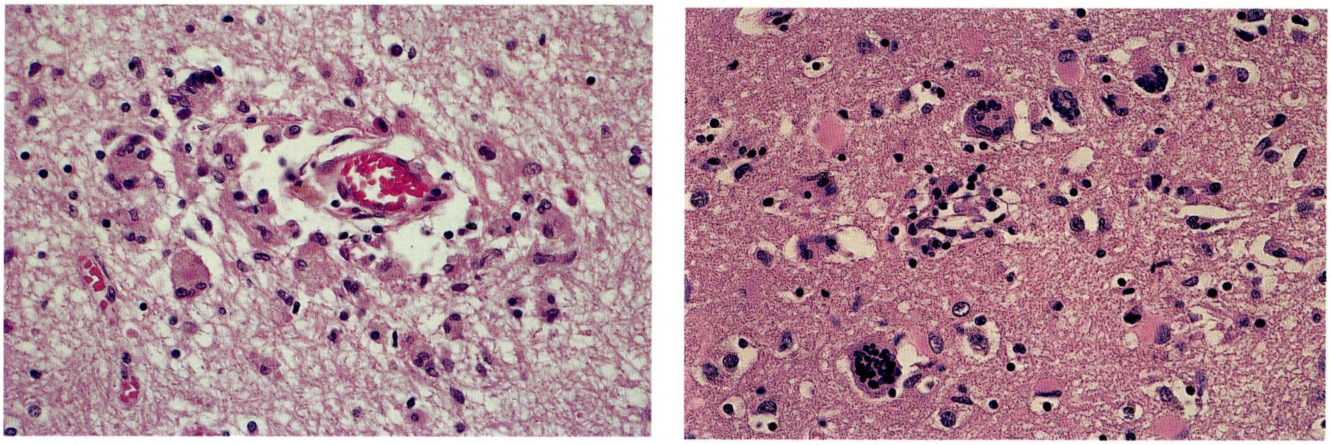

A B

Figure 19–5. HIV-1 encephalitis. Depicted in (**A**), taken from the deep cerebral white matter, is the most common histologic presentation of this retroviral encephalitis: a modest, nongranulomatous infiltrate of loosely aggregated inflammatory cells dominated by macrophages, including multinucleated forms. Note the perivascular distribution of the infiltrate and absence of necrosis or of striking alterations in the adjacent neuropil. The multinucleated elements that are an arresting feature of HIV-1 encephalitis and that are believed to represent in vivo counterparts of cells such as that pictured in Figure 19–3 are emphasized in (**B**), an example in which extensive infiltration of the white matter by HIV-1–infected macrophages was associated with the marked astrogliosis also depicted here (hematoxylin-eosin, **A**, ×100; **B**, ×250).

Although polykaryotic giant cells participate in a variety of granulomatous processes that potentially involve the brain (eg, mycoses, tuberculosis, sarcoidosis), no condition other than HIV-1 infection has been shown to evince disseminated, nongranulomatous cerebral infiltrates similar in their content of multinucleated elements and distribution to those under discussion. Consequently, investigators are in general agreement that the identification of such infiltrates suffices for a confident diagnosis of HIV-1 encephalitis.[4] Multinucleated cells may be encountered in other viral encephalitides, but these disorders exhibit distinctive morphologic alterations that should preclude their confusion with cerebral HIV-1 infection. Such elements may be visualized in the brains of immunosuppressed children, particularly leukemics, afflicted with a rare form of progressive measles encephalitis,[92] but in this setting are associated with conspicuous intranuclear inclusion bodies in neurons and oligodendroglia and may themselves exhibit nuclear cytopathic effects.

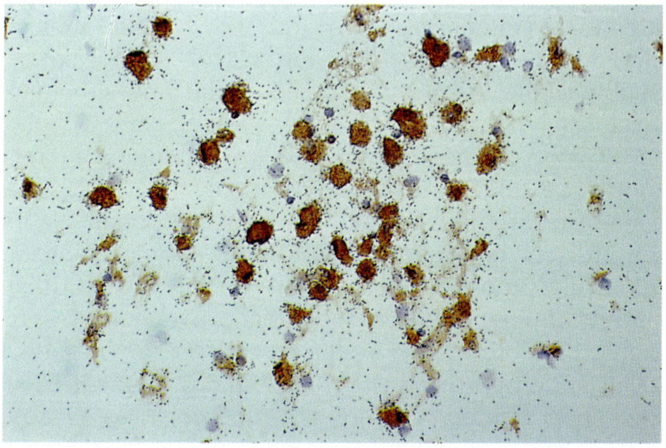

Figure 19–6. HIV-1 encephalitis. This focus of multinucleated cell encephalitis has been double labeled by lectin histochemistry for a macrophage/microglial marker (Ricinus communis agglutinin I) and in situ hybridization/autoradiography for HIV-1 mRNA expression employing an ^{35}S-radiolabeled RNA probe. The clustering of silver grains over and about cells stained by the lectin indicates that the inflammatory infiltrate is composed of macrophages/microglia that are productively infected by HIV-1 (hematoxylin counterstain ×100).

Multinucleated cells derived from astrocytes and the subependymal glia occur in some cases of florid, necrotizing encephalitis and ventriculitis caused by cytomegalovirus (CMV), although these contain the large intranuclear and cytoplasmic inclusions that typify CMV infection and do not bear any cytologic resemblance to the multinucleated macrophages of HIV-1 encephalitis.[93] This herpesvirus, however, deserves further consideration as the agent of a low-grade encephalomyelitis superficially similar to that associated with HIV-1 and commonly discovered at autopsy of immunocompromised patients, particularly victims of AIDS.[93] Cells exhibiting the cytopathic effects typical of the virus are often difficult to identify in this variant, characterized by disseminated "microglial" nodules composed of small lymphocytes and macrophages, but the cytoarchitectural features and topography of these

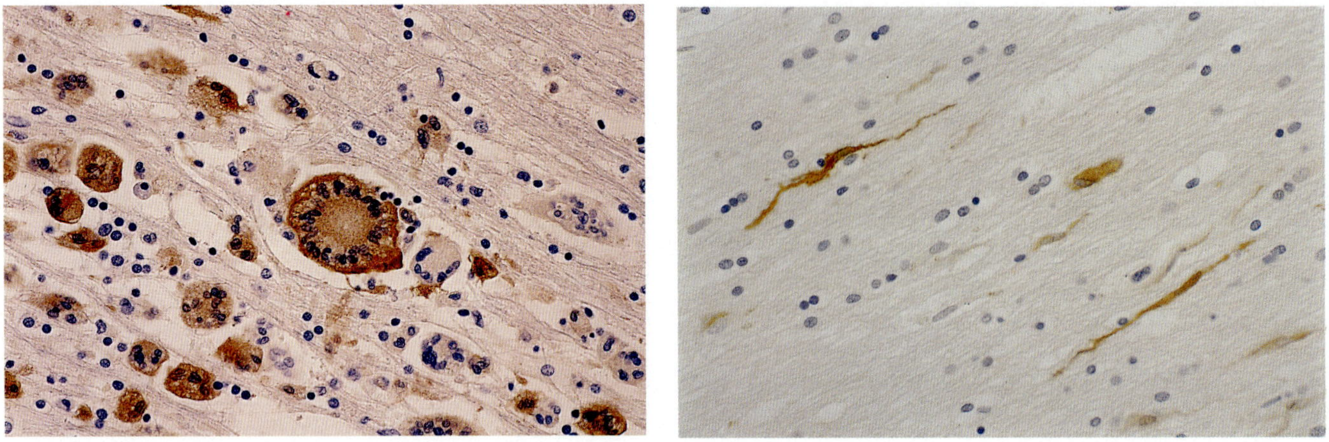

A B

Figure 19–7. HIV-1 encephalitis. As demonstrated here with a monoclonal antiserum to the agent's 41-kd transmembrane glycoprotein (gp41), the multinucleated cells characteristic of HIV-1 encephalitis (**A**) and a subset of process-bearing microglia (**B**) are productively infected and so express epitopes associated with structural components of the virion (anti-gp41 immunoperoxidase with hematoxylin counterstain, ×250).

inflammatory lesions should permit their ready distinction from the infiltrates provoked by HIV-1. More compact in structure than the loosely arranged cellular aggregates of HIV-1 encephalitis and devoid of multinucleated macrophages, these microglial nodules usually form as inflammatory elements converge on CMV-infected neurons and so are not typically vasocentric or situated in white matter, exhibiting, instead, a decided predilection for the cerebral cortex, basal ganglia, dentate, pontine, and inferior olivary nuclei.

Fine structural,[15,61,64,77,89,91] immunophenotypic,[34,64,76,77,79,85] and functional[57,94] analyses leave little doubt that the mononucleated and multinucleated cells bearing much of the cerebral retroviral burden in HIV-1 encephalitis are macrophages. Their vasocentric distribution is certainly consistent with the theory that circulating monocytes transport HIV-1 across the blood–brain barrier. Demonstrably infected cells distinguished by the conspicuous cytoplasmic processes, lectin, and immunohistochemical profiles of the microglia have also been depicted in autopsy studies of HIV-1 encephalitis (Figure 19–7, B)[1,79,85–88] and are believed by some to participate in the formation of multinucleated cells.[33,86,95–97] Whether these "dendritic" elements are infected in situ or represent the differentiated progeny of monocytes that enter the brain harboring the virus remains unresolved. Studies employing double-label methods (Figure 19–6)[1,76,77,79,85,87] for the definitive characterization of cells productively infected by HIV-1 in vivo have failed, for the most part, to support in vitro transmission data, cited earlier, which suggest a particular tropism of this retrovirus for neuroectodermal derivatives or to confirm the reported expression of HIV-1–specific structural antigens and nucleic acid sequences by astrocytes,[76,80,81,98,99] oligodendroglia,[80,99,100] and neurons.[76,80,101] Only rare published electron photomicrographs[89,91] depict HIV-1–type virions within what could be infected astrocytes, the ultrastructural identification of some particle-bearing cells as oligodendroglia[99] has been contested[102,103] and the agent has never been directly visualized within, or budding from, neurons, ependyma, or the epithelium of the choroid plexus. That cerebral endothelium is susceptible to HIV-1 has been suggested on the strength of immunohistochemical[76,98,104,105] and molecular probe[76,78] analyses but, again, not supported by double-label assay or confirmed at the fine structural level.

To the studies cited in the preceding paragraph should be added recent observations suggesting that central neuroepithelial cells, although not conducive to the efficient replication of HIV-1, do sustain latent or minimally productive forms of retroviral infection that smolder below the detectable by conventional assay methods. Noteworthy in this regard is the reported localization of proviral HIV-1 DNA and genomic RNA in low copy number to subsets of neurons, astrocytes, and, possibly, oligodendroglia by means of in situ gene amplification techniques.[106] Intriguing as well is evidence that reactive astrocytes in the brains of AIDS patients may express the agent's regulatory *nef* gene product, transcribed prior to such structural proteins as core p24 and envelope gp41. Overexpression of this gene would appear to be a marker for highly restricted astroglial infection both in autopsy tissues[107] and culture systems.[108]

HIV-1, then, may persist at low level in resident CNS elements of neuroepithelial derivation, but principally exploits macrophages and microglia for purposes of its intracerebral replication—a pattern of infection unique among human viral encephalitides. In light of these restricted tropisms, the frequent association of HIV-1 encephalitis with alterations indicative of generalized cerebral injury merits additional comment. Among the most arresting and common are manifestations of diffuse damage to the hemispheric white matter that include diminished staining intensity (accentuated in myelin preparations), astrocytosis, and spongy rarefaction.[1,59,64,65,73,85,109,110] Pronounced abnormalities of this sort may be exhibited by brains harboring only modest multinucleated cell infiltrates, a picture more degenerative than inflammatory in its histologic presentation and consequently designated as HIV-1 leukoencephalopathy by some neuropathologists.[4] Particularly striking in the deep centra semiovale, the observed pallor of the affected white matter reflects widespread myelin loss. Its pathogenesis, unknown at present, has not been shown to involve a reduction in oligodendrocyte numbers.[100] Some observers, however, have identified apoptic cells in the brains of HIV-1–infected patients that were thought to be oligodendroglia on morphologic grounds.[49]

Segregated under the term *diffuse poliodystrophy*[4,64] are similarly generalized, neurodegenerative-like alterations of cortical, central, and bulbar gray matter consisting of astrogliosis, microglial proliferation, and neuronal loss.[4,64,111] Quantitative morphometric studies suggest that neuronal depopulation of the cerebral cortex, although infrequently apprehended at the light microscopic level, is a regular feature of the HIV-1–infected brain.[112] Diminished synaptic density[113] and abnormalities of dendritic arborization[114,115] have also been detected in this setting. Finally, a variety of cerebrovascular lesions have been described in patients with AIDS,[116–126] by far the most common being mineralization of blood vessels in the basal ganglia and deep white matter.[61,70,126] The latter is particularly prevalent in the pediatric population. Abnormalities of the blood–brain barrier would appear to be frequent in the setting of AIDS and may contribute to white matter injury in these patients.[127,128]

These histologic indices of CNS injury obviously bear on the pathogenesis of AIDS-related cerebral atrophy and neurologic dysfunction, discussed later, but their relationship to the presence of HIV-1 in the neuropil is unclear. Diffuse subcortical gliosis and white matter damage, although especially pronounced in productively infected brains, may be encountered in the absence of overt HIV-1 encephalitis,[1,59,84,100,104] as may cortical neuronal loss[112] and diffuse poliodystrophy.[85] Such changes, then, do not constitute prima facie evidence of cerebral HIV-1 infection, the diagnosis of which requires, in the absence of multinucleated cell infiltrates, localization of the agent by immunohistochemical, fine structural, or molecular hybridization methods.[4] This is not, however, to exonerate occult retroviral infection of the brain as a possible cause of these insults. The role of HIV-1 in the evolution of cerebrovascular injury is similarly unsettled.

CLINICAL CORRELATES AND PATHOGENETIC CONSIDERATIONS

The groundbreaking studies that established HIV-1 as a neuroinvasive and encephalitogenic agent were prompted in large part by concern that retroviral infection of the CNS might be responsible for the distinctive AIDS-related neurologic syndromes currently designated as the HIV-1–associated cognitive/motor complex of adult-onset and progressive encephalopathy of childhood.[3] Recognized as AIDS-defining disorders,[129] these typically present in the late, symptomatic phase of systemic HIV-1 infection but are inexplicable as consequences of cerebral damage by conventional opportunists. Dominant manifestations of the pediatric syndrome include developmental regression or delay, pyramidal tract signs, and acquired microcephaly indicative of impaired brain growth.[60,130] Severe psychomotor retardation, pseudobulbar palsy, spasticity, and quadriparesis or plegia characterize its late stages. Afflicted adults exhibit disturbances of intellect and motor function that frequently evolve to frank dementia and significant gait impairment.[2,131] Some progress to a nearly vegetative, mute, and akinetic state.

The HIV-1–associated cognitive/motor complex and progressive encephalopathy of childhood have not yet submitted to a unifying etiologic or pathogenetic explication and remain clinically defined entities. Unresolved are their precise neuroanatomic and physiologic substrates as well as the function of cerebral HIV-1 infection in their evolution.[2] Especially problematic is the inconstant association of these disorders with conspicuous evidence of the agent's replication within the CNS.[83,84,104,132–134] While patients with advanced, crippling neurologic deficits are usually found, at autopsy, to suffer from widespread HIV-1 encephalitis, this is not invariably the case and the brains of those who are less severely, but unequivocally, impaired often contain few cells that can be shown to be productively infected.

It is conceivable that damaging bursts of viral replication within the nervous system are subsequently suppressed by immunologic mechanisms or that the agent is partially cleared from the brain due to the death of infected cells,[104,133] but the possibility must also be considered that HIV-1–associated neural injury is somehow initiated at highly restricted levels of local viral transcription or in the absence of cerebral infection altogether. HIV-1 encephalitis would, then, aggravate a process of tissue damage set into motion by systemic events (eg, the elaboration of circulating neurotoxins). That the presence of this agent in central nervous tissues may not suffice to cause cognitive impairment is further suggested by documented instances of HIV-1 encephalitis unattended by dementia.[84]

Although the mechanisms of HIV-1–associated cerebral injury remain wholly speculative, there is much experimental support for the notion that the virus need not penetrate neurons and glia in order to effect their dysfunction or death. Reviewed elsewhere,[2,58] the accumulated evidence includes demonstrations that cultured neural cell types resistant to infection may, nonetheless, be injured on exposure to subviral components of HIV-1, to HIV-1–infected monocytes, or to biologically active compounds generated in the course of macrophage–astrocyte interactions. The virus' transactivating protein (*tat*)[135] and 120-kd envelope glycoprotein (gp120)[136–138] have emerged from studies of this kind as potentially lethal neuronotoxins, the latter's effects involving calcium flux into neurons that is apparently mediated via action of the excitatory amino acid glutamate on neuronal *N*-methyl-D-aspartate (NMDA) receptors.[137,138] Arachidonic acid metabolites induced on binding of gp120 to monocytes[139] have been posited to play a critical role in HIV-1–associated neurotoxicity that may involve their ability to inhibit glutamate uptake systems normally used by neurons and astrocytes.[58,140] Behavioral retardation and widespread damage of cortical dendrites have been observed following administration of purified gp120 to neonatal rats,[141] and transgenic mice engineered to express gp120 within the CNS exhibit a spectrum of neuropathologic alterations—including astrocytosis, microglial activation, reduced synaptic density, and dendritic vacuolization—strikingly similar to changes commonly encountered in the brains of AIDS patients.[142] Noteworthy also is the reported correlation of the HIV-1–associated cognitive/motor complex with elevated CSF concentrations of the NMDA agonist quinolinic acid, an "excitotoxic" kynurenine pathway metabolite possibly derived from macrophages and microglia.[143,144]

HIV-1 may also inflict indirect injury on the CNS by inducing activated macrophages and microglia to elaborate neurotoxic monokines such as tumor necrosis factor alpha (TNF-α) and interleukin-1-beta (IL-1-β) that number among their effects "upregulation" of viral genomic transcription, damage to oligodendrocytes and myelin, alterations in neuronal function, and astrocytic proliferation.[58,144,145] Stimulated astrocytes may, in turn, amplify this insult by themselves producing TNF-α and by increasing monokine production via the modification of macrophage-derived leukotrienes and platelet activating factor.[58] Interactions of this sort have been invoked to explain observations of neuronal loss and astroglial hyperplasia, two prevalent AIDS-associated phenomena, in cultured neural tissues following exposure to supernatant fluids from cocultivated HIV-1–infected monocytes and astrocytes.[58,140,146] Similar findings have been documented in human fetal brain xenografts exposed to monocytes harboring the agent.[58,147]

Whether the diffuse cortical abnormalities, white matter alterations, microgliosis, and astrocytosis exhibited by the brains of encephalopathic AIDS patients actually reflect protracted exposure to pleiotropic cytokines and arachidonic acid metabolites is unknown, but their systemic and local elaboration constitutes an additional model of generalized cerebral injury "driven" by HIV-1 in the absence of neuronal or neuroglial infection. In one study, AIDS-associated dementia was found at autopsy to be more closely correlated with the magnitude of brain macrophage infiltration than with the actual retroviral burden as assessed by immunocytochemical assay.[84] Furthermore, elevated serum TNF-α levels have been correlated with severe manifestations of progressive encephalopathy in HIV-1–positive children[148] and increased concentrations of this monokine[149] and of eicosanoid arachidonic acid derivatives[150] noted in the CSF of neurologically impaired adults. TNF-α and IL-1-β expression have also been demonstrated within the brain tissues of autopsied AIDS patients.[106,151,152] Studies employing the reverse transcriptase polymerase chain reaction for intracerebral cytokine assay have documented significant local increases of TNF-α mRNA in samples derived from demented AIDS victims,[106,152] one group noting a concomitant decrease in mRNA encoding IL-4, a "downregulator" of macrophage activity.[152] Finally, mention should be made of the recent localization of IL-1-α and S100-β to macrophages/microglia and hyperplastic astrocytes, respectively, in postmortem cerebral tissues from HIV-1–seropositive patients.[153] The former, in addition to promoting astrocyte activation and proliferation, increases the synthesis of β-amyloid precursor proteins (β-APP), whereas the latter raises intraneuronal calcium levels and induces neurite extension. Intriguing is the observation that the cortical samples assayed in this study exhibited certain alterations resembling those of Alzheimer's disease, including the accumulation of β-APP immunoreaction product within neuronal perikarya and neurites and the presence within some neurons of neurofibrillary tangle-like structures labeled by a monoclonal antibody to an abnormally phosphorylated isoform of the Tau protein.

HIV-1 AND THE SPINAL CORD

As mentioned, the inflammatory lesions characteristic of productive HIV-1 infection are most commonly identified in the subcortical white matter and central gray, but multinucleated cell infiltrates of similar appearance and diagnostic significance may also be encountered at spinal levels of the central neuraxis and here qualify for the designation of HIV-1 myelitis.[4] Only rarely has selective involvement of the spinal cord been documented,[154] HIV-1 myelitis typically occurring in the patient with disseminated foci of cerebral infection as well (ie, encephalomyelitis).

Considerably more common than HIV-1 myelitis, and the leading cause of spinal cord dysfunction in the adult with AIDS, is the entity depicted in Figure 19–8 and termed vacuolar myelopathy.[155,156] This disorder is characterized by a process of intramyelinic vacuolization that lends a spongy appearance to the white matter of the spinal cord on microscopic examination. Astrogliosis and macrophage infiltration of varying magnitude are additional histologic features. As is the case in vitamin B_{12} deficiency–related subacute combined degeneration of the cord, which it greatly resembles, the brunt of the injury is typically borne by the lateral and posterior columns, a topography evident in some cases as pallor of these regions on gross examination and responsible for the progressive spastic paraparesis, ataxia, and incontinence associated with advanced lesions.

Vacuolar myelopathy has been posited by some investigators to result from the replication of HIV-1 in spinal cord tissues, but a number of discordant observations complicate this interpretation. Morphologically similar, if not identical, forms of spinal cord injury are known to result from noninfectious, metabolic, or toxic insults to the nervous system and have been documented in settings of immune dysregulation other than AIDS.[157] In addition to deficiencies of vitamin B_{12} and folic acid, prolonged exposure to nitrous oxide, hepatic cirrhosis, renal transplantation, and a variety of autoimmune and neoplastic diseases have been associated with vacuolar myelopathies of similar, if not identical, type. Furthermore, HIV-1 myelitis as defined earlier is generally unattended by diffuse vacuolar alterations, although the two processes may coexist on occasion. Particularly striking is the dissociation of HIV-1 myelitis and vacuolar myelopathy in children succumbing to AIDS.[158] Vacuolar myelopathy is exceedingly rare in this population, in spite of what appears to be a high incidence of productive spinal cord infection at autopsy.[73,158] Finally, attempts to demonstrate the local replication of the virus in affected cords have not been uniformly successful. Some workers have reported the

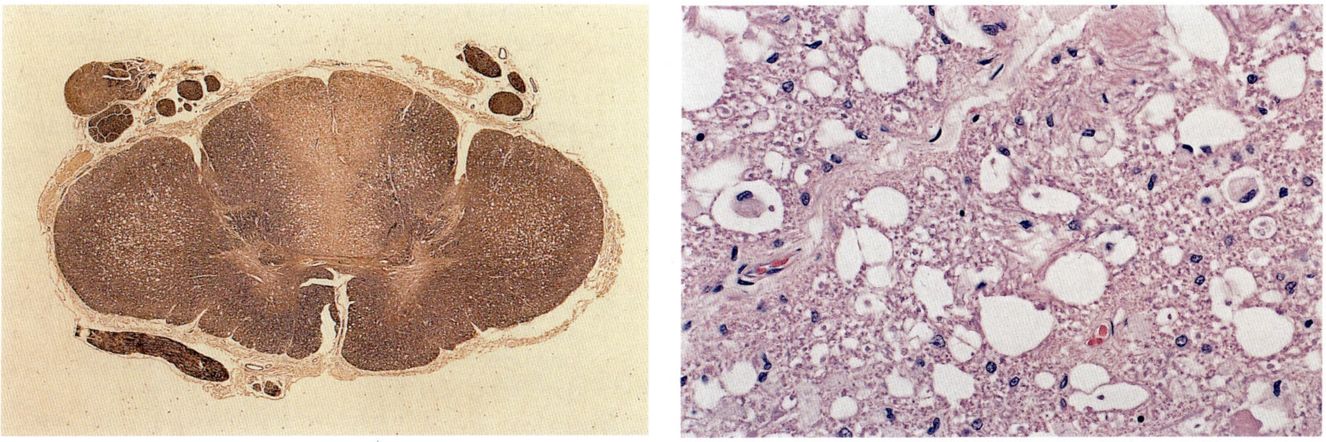

A B

Figure 19–8. Vacuolar myelopathy. (**A**) This whole-mount myelin preparation from the cervical spinal cord demonstrates extensive white matter vacuolization involving predominantly, although not exclusively, the lateral and posterior columns. This distribution is typical of AIDS-related vacuolar myelopathy. Note also the marked pallor of the median aspect of the posterior column. This reflects degeneration of the gracile tracts, another AIDS-associated spinal cord lesion. As shown here, the two processes may coexist (Weigert whole mount). (**B**) A more detailed view of the lateral column from this case emphasizes the vacuolar process that is the most common cause of spinal cord dysfunction in the HIV-1–infected adult. Note the sparse infiltrate of foamy macrophages, some within vacuolar spaces. As is usually the case, multinucleated cell infiltrates are not in evidence (hematoxylin-eosin, ×250).

consistent detection of HIV-1 in macrophages associated with the lesions of vacuolar myelopathy[85,159–161] and have found the severity of vacuolar change to correlate with the quantitative retroviral burden in the damaged white matter,[160] but most attempts to localize the agent have failed in spite of recourse to a variety of assay techniques.[162–167]

These discrepancies by no means exonerate HIV-1 as the cause of AIDS-related vacuolar myelopathy, but, for the present, preclude acceptance of this entity as a direct consequence of retroviral infection. Similar considerations apply to reports of vacuolar white matter change occurring at cerebral levels (ie, vacuolar leukoencephalopathy).[59,85,168] The precise role, if any, played by the local replication of HIV-1 in the pathogenesis of these disorders awaits clarification. As pointed out elsewhere,[167] disordered uptake and metabolism of vitamin B_{12} appear to be common in the setting of AIDS and remain suspect as pathogenetic factors in at least some cases of vacuolar myelopathy.

MISCELLANY

The interested reader is referred elsewhere for pathologic accounts of a variety of CNS lesions described in association with, but not definitively linked to, HIV-1 infection. These include reports of fulminant leukoencephalopathy,[169] spongiform encephalopathy,[170–172] an inflammatory, demyelinating disorder similar to (and possibly representing) multiple sclerosis,[173] and degeneration of the gracile tracts in patients with AIDS-related sensory neuropathy.[164,174] As illustrated in Figure 19–8, A, gracile tract degeneration and vacuolar myelopathy are commonly associated phenomena.

Acknowledgments. The author would like to extend his thanks to Kin Kong and Stephanie Alton, who supplied expert photographic assistance, and to Ellen Cohen and Tammy Son, who prepared the manuscript.

REFERENCES

1. Rosenblum MK. Infection of the central nervous system by the human immunodeficiency virus type 1: morphology and relation to syndromes of progressive encephalopathy and myelopathy in patients with AIDS. *Pathol Ann.* 1990;1:117–169.
2. Price RW, Perry SW, eds. *HIV, AIDS and the Brain.* New York: Raven Press; 1994.
3. Janssen RS, Cornblath DR, Epstein LG, et al. Nomenclature and research case definitions for neurologic manifestations of human immunodeficiency virus-type 1 (HIV-1) infection—report of a working group of the American Academy of Neurology AIDS Task Force. *Neurology.* 1991;41:778–785.
4. Budka H, Wiley CA, Kleihues P, et al. HIV-associated disease of the nervous system: review of nomenclature and proposal for neuropathology-based terminology. *Brain Pathol.* 1991;1:143–152.
5. Narayan O, Clements JE. Biology and pathogenesis of lentiviruses. *J Gen Virol.* 1989;70:1617–1639.
6. Haase AT. Pathogenesis of lentivirus infections. *Nature.* 1986;322:130–136.
7. Gonda MA, Wong-Staal F, Gallo RC, et al. Sequence homology and morphologic similarity of HTLV-III and visna virus, a pathogenic lentivirus. *Science.* 1985;227: 173–177.
8. Chiu IM, Yaniv A, Dahlberg JE, et al. Nucleotide sequence evidence for relationship of AIDS retrovirus to lentiviruses. *Nature.* 1985;317:366–368.
9. Sonigo P, Alizon M, Staskus K, et al. Nucleotide sequence of the visna lentivirus: relationship to the AIDS virus. *Cell.* 1985;42:369–382.
10. Stephens RM, Casey JW, Rice NR. Equine infectious anemia virus gag and pol genes: relatedness to visna and AIDS virus. *Science.* 1986;231:589–594.
11. Cullen BR. Regulation of HIV-1 gene expression. *FASEB J.* 1991;5:2361–2368.
12. Popovic M, Sarngadharan MG, Read E, Gallo RC. Detection, isolation and continuous production of cytopathic retroviruses (HTLV-III) from patients with AIDS and pre-AIDS. *Science.* 1984;224:497–500.
13. Lifson JD, Reyes GR, McGrath MS, et al. AIDS retrovirus induced cytopathology: giant cell formation and involvement of CD4 antigen. *Science.* 1986;232:1123–1127.
14. Munn RJ, Marx PA, Yamamoto JK, Gardner MB. Ultrastructural comparison of the retroviruses associated with human and simian acquired immunodeficiency syndromes. *Lab Invest.* 1985;53:194–199.
15. Meyenhofer MF, Epstein LG, Cho E-S, Sharer LR. Ultrastructural morphology and intracellular production of human immunodeficiency virus (HIV) in brain. *J Neuropathol Exp Neurol.* 1987;46:474–484.
16. Palmer E, Sporborg C, Harrison A, et al. Morphology and immunoelectron microscopy of AIDS virus. *Arch Virol.* 1985;85:189–196.
17. Gelderblom HR, Hausmann EHS, Ozel M, et al. Fine structure of human immunodeficiency virus (HIV) and immunolocalization of structural proteins. *Virology.* 1987;156:171–176.
18. Meltzer MS, Skillman DR, Gomatos PJ, et al. Role of mononuclear phagocytes in the pathogenesis of human immunodeficiency virus infection. *Annu Rev Immunol.* 1990;8;169–194.
19. Marx PA, Munn RJ, Joy KI. Computer emulation of thin section electron microscopy predicts an envelope-associated icosadeltahedral capsid for human immunodeficiency virus. *Lab Invest.* 1988;58:112–118.
20. Haseltine WA. Molecular biology of the human immunodeficiency virus type 1. *FASEB J.* 1991;5:2349–2360.
21. Sattentau OJ, Weiss RA. The CD4 antigen: physiological ligand and HIV receptor. *Cell.* 1988;52:631–633.

22. Funke I, Hahn A, Rieber EP, et al. The cellular receptor (CD4) of the human immunodeficiency virus is expressed on neurons and glial cells in human brain. *J Exp Med.* 1987;165:1230–1235.
23. Maddon PJ, Dalgleish AG, McDougal JS, et al. The T4 gene encodes the AIDS virus receptor and is expressed in the immune system and the brain. *Cell.* 1986;47:333–348.
24. Cheng-Mayer C, Rutka JT, Rosenblum ML, et al. Human immunodeficiency virus can productively infect cultured human glial cells. *Proc Natl Acad Sci USA.* 1987;84:3526–3530.
25. Christofinis G, Papadaki L, Sattentau Q, et al. HIV replicates in cultured human brain cells. *AIDS.* 1987;1:229–234.
26. Nath A, Hartloper V, Furer M, Fowke KR. Infection of human fetal astrocytes with HIV-1: viral tropism and the role of cell to cell contact in viral transmission. *J Neuropathol Exp Neurol.* 1995;54:320–330.
27. Mizrachi Y, Zeira M, Shahabuddin M, et al. Efficient binding, fusion and entry of HIV-1 into CD4-negative neural cells: a mechanism for neuropathogenesis in AIDS. *Bull Inst Pasteur.* 1991;89:81–96.
28. Dewhurst S, Sakai K, Bresser J, et al. Persistent productive infection of human glial cells by human immunodeficiency virus (HIV) and by infectious molecular clones of HIV. *J Virol.* 1987;61:3774–3782.
29. Brack-Werner R, Kleinschmidt A, Ludvigsen A, et al. Infection of human brain cells by HIV-1: restricted virus production in chronically infected human glial cell lines. *AIDS.* 1992;6:273–285.
30. Harouse JM, Kunsch C, Hartle HT, et al. CD4 independent infection of human neural cells by human immunodeficiency virus type 1. *J Virol.* 1989;63:2527–2533.
31. Clapham PR, Weber JN, Whitby D, et al. Soluble CD4 blocks the infectivity of diverse strains of HIV and SIV for T cells and monocytes but not for brain and muscle cells. *Nature.* 1989;337:368–370.
32. Harouse JM, Wroblewska Z, Laughlin MA, et al. Human choroid plexus cells can be latently infected with human immunodeficiency virus. *Ann Neurol.* 1989;25:406–411.
33. Watkins BA, Dorn HH, Kelly WB, et al. Specific tropism of HIV-1 for microglial cells in primary human brain cultures. *Science.* 1990;249:549–553.
34. Peudenier S, Hery C, Montagnier L, Tardieu M. Human microglial cells: characterization in cerebral tissue and in primary culture, and a study of their susceptibility to HIV-1 infection. *Ann Neurol.* 1991;29:152–161.
35. Sharpless NE, O'Brien WA, Verdin E, et al. Human immunodeficiency virus type 1 tropism for brain microglial cells is determined by a region of the env glycoprotein that also controls macrophage tropism. *J Virol.* 1992;66:2588–2593.
36. Bhat S, Spitalnik SL, Gonzalez-Scarano F, Silberberg DH. Galactosyl ceramide or a derivative is an essential component of the neural receptor for human immunodeficiency virus type 1 envelope glycoprotein gp 120. *Proc Natl Acad Sci USA.* 1991;88:7131–7134.
37. Ma M, Nath A, Geiger JD. Characterization of a novel binding site for the HIV-1 envelope glycoprotein on human fetal astrocytes. *J Virol.* 1994;68:6824–6828.
38. Lifson JD, Feinberg MB, Reyes GR, et al. Induction of CD4 dependent cell fusion by HTLV-III/LAV envelope glycoprotein. *Nature.* 1986;323:725–728.
39. McArthur JC, Cohen BA, Farzedegan H, et al. Cerebrospinal fluid abnormalities in homosexual men with and without neuropsychiatric findings. *Ann Neurol.* 1988;23(suppl):S34–S37.
40. Resnick L, Berger JR, Shapshak P, Tourtellotte WW. Early penetration of the blood–brain barrier by HIV-1. *Neurology.* 1988;38:9–14.
41. Goudsmit J, Wolters EC, Bakker M, et al. Intrathecal synthesis of antibodies to HTLV-III in patients without AIDS or AIDS-related complex. *Br Med J.* 1986;292:1231–1234.
42. Hollander H, Levy JA. Neurologic abnormalities and recovery of human immunodeficiency virus from cerebrospinal fluid. *Ann Intern Med.* 1987;106:692–695.
43. Chiodi F, Sonnerborg A, Albert J, et al. Human immunodeficiency virus infection of the brain. I. Virus isolation and detection of HIV specific antibodies in the cerebrospinal fluid of patients with varying clinical conditions. *J Neurol Sci.* 1988;85:245–257.
44. Goudsmit J, Paul DA, Lange JMA. Expression of human immunodeficiency virus antigen (HIV-Ag) in serum and cerebrospinal fluid during acute and chronic infection. *Lancet.* 1986;2:177–180.
45. Levy RL, Bredesen DE, Rosenblum ML. Neurological manifestations of the acquired immune deficiency syndrome (AIDS): experience at UCSF and review of the literature. *J Neurosurg.* 1985;62:475–495.
46. Hollander H, Stringari S. Human immunodeficiency virus-associated meningitis. Clinical course and correlations. *Am J Med.* 1987;83:813–816.
47. Esiri MM, Scaravilli F, Millard PR, Harcout-Webster JN. Neuropathology of HIV infection in hemophiliacs: comparative necropsy study. *Br Med J.* 1989;299:1312–1315.
48. Bell JE, Bursuttil A, Ironside JW, et al. Human immunodeficiency virus and the brain: investigation of virus load and neuropathologic changes in pre-AIDS subjects. *J Infect Dis.* 1993;168:818–824.
49. Gray F, Scaravilli F, Everall I, et al. Neuropathology of early HIV-1 infection. *Brain Pathol.* 1996;6:1–15.
50. Gray F, Lescs M-C, Keohane C, et al. Early brain changes in HIV infection: neuropathological study of 11 HIV-seropositive non-AIDS cases. *J Neuropathol Exp Neurol.* 1992;51:177–185.
51. Sinclair E, Gray F, Ciardi A, Scaravilli F. Immunohistochemical changes and PCR detection of HIV provirus DNA in brains of asymptomatic HIV-positive patients. *J Neuropathol Exp Neurol.* 1994;53:43–50.
52. Davis LE, Hjelle BL, Miller VE, et al. Early viral invasion of brain in iatrogenic human immunodeficiency virus infection. *Ann Neurol.* 1991;30:314–315. Abstract.
53. Chakrabarti L, Hurtrel M, Maire M-A, et al. Early viral replication in the brain of SIV-infected rhesus monkeys. *Am J Pathol.* 1991;139:1273–1280.
54. Jovaisas E, Koch MA, Schafer A, et al. LAV/HTLV-III in 20-week fetus. *Lancet.* 1985;2:1129.

55. Gendelman HE, Narayan O, Molineaux S, et al. Slow, persistent replication of lentiviruses: role of tissue macrophages and macrophage precursors in bone marrow. *Proc Natl Acad Sci USA.* 1985;82:7086–7090.
56. Peluso R, Haase A, Stowring L, et al. A Trojan Horse mechanism for the spread of visna virus in monocytes. *Virology.* 1985;147:231–236.
57. Orenstein JM, Meltzer MS, Phipps T, Gendelman HE. Cytoplasmic assembly and accumulation of human immunodeficiency virus types 1 and 2 in recombinant human colony stimulating factor-1 treated human monocytes: an ultrastructural study. *J Virol.* 1988;62:2578–2586.
58. Epstein LG, Gendelman HE. Human immunodeficiency virus type 1 infection of the nervous system: pathogenetic mechanisms. *Ann Neurol.* 1993;33:429–436.
59. Navia BA, Cho E-S, Petito CK, Price RW. The AIDS dementia complex. II. Neuropathology. *Ann Neurol.* 1986;19:525–535.
60. Epstein LG, Sharer LR. Neurology of human immunodeficiency virus infection in children. In: Rosenblum ML, Levy RM, Bredesen DE, eds. *AIDS and the Nervous System.* New York: Raven Press; 1988:79–101.
61. Sharer LR, Epstein LG, Cho E-S, et al. Pathologic features of AIDS encephalopathy in children: evidence for LAV/HTLV-III infection of brain. *Hum Pathol.* 1986;17: 271–284.
62. Sharer LR, Cho E-S, Epstein LG. Multinucleated giant cells and HTLV-III in AIDS encephalopathy. *Hum Pathol.* 1985;16:760.
63. Kato T, Hirano A, Llena JF, Dembitzer HM. Neuropathology of acquired immune deficiency syndrome (AIDS) in 53 autopsy cases with particular emphasis on microglial nodules and multinucleated cells. *Acta Neuropathol.* 1987;73:287–294.
64. Budka H, Costanzi G, Cristina S, et al. Brain pathology induced by infection with the human immunodeficiency virus (HIV). A histological, immunocytochemical and electron microscopical study of 100 autopsy cases. *Acta Neuropathol.* 1987;75:185–198.
65. Lang W, Miklossy J, Deruaz JP, et al. Neuropathology of the acquired immune deficiency syndrome (AIDS): a report of 135 consecutive autopsy cases from Switzerland. *Acta Neuropathol.* 1989;77:379–390.
66. Petito CK, Cho E-S, Lemann W, et al. Neuropathology of acquired immune deficiency syndrome (AIDS): an autopsy review. *J Neuropathol Exp Neurol.* 1986;45: 635–646.
67. Budka H. Multinucleated giant cells in brain: a hallmark of the acquired immune deficiency syndrome (AIDS). *Acta Neuropathol.* 1986;69:253–258.
68. Gray F, Gherardi R, Keohane C, et al. Pathology of the central nervous system in 40 cases of acquired immune deficiency syndrome (AIDS). *Neuropathol Appl Neurobiol.* 1988;14:365–380.
69. de la Monte SM, Ho DD, Schooley RT, et al. Subacute encephalomyelitis of AIDS and its relation to HTLV-III infection. *Neurology.* 1987;37:562–569.
70. Dickson DW, Belman AL, Park YD, et al. Central nervous system pathology in pediatric AIDS: an autopsy study. *Acta Pathol Microbiol Immunol Scand.* 1989;suppl 8: 40–57.
71. Giangaspero F, Scanabissi E, Baldacci MC, Betts CM. Massive neuronal destruction in human immunodeficiency virus (HIV) encephalitis—a clinicopathological study of a pediatric case. *Acta Neuropathol.* 1989; 78:662–665.
72. Clague CPT, Ostrowski MA, Deck JHN, et al. Severe diffuse necrotizing cortical encephalopathy in acquired immune deficiency syndrome (AIDS): an immunocytochemical and ultrastructural study. *J Neuropathol Exp Neurol.* 1988;47:346. Abstract.
73. Sharer LR. Pathology of HIV-1 infection of the central nervous system—a review. *J Neuropathol Exp Neurol.* 1992;51:3–11.
74. Shaw GM, Harper ME, Hahn BH, et al. HTLV-III infection in brains of children and adults with AIDS encephalopathy. *Science.* 1985;227:177–182.
75. Mizusawa H, Hirano A, Llena F. Nuclear bridges within multinucleated giant cells in subacute encephalitis of acquired immune deficiency syndrome (AIDS). *Acta Neuropathol.* 1988;76:166–169.
76. Wiley CA, Schrier RD, Nelson AJ, et al. Cellular localization of human immunodeficiency virus infection within the brains of acquired immune deficiency syndrome patients. *Proc Natl Acad Sci USA.* 1986;83:7089–7093.
77. Koenig S, Gendelman HE, Orenstein JM, et al. Detection of AIDS virus in macrophages in brain tissue from AIDS patients with encephalopathy. *Science.* 1986; 233:1089–1093.
78. Rostad SW, Sumi SM, Shaw C-M, et al. Human immunodeficiency virus (HIV) infection in brains with AIDS-related leukoencephalopathy. *AIDS Res Human Retrov.* 1987;3:363–373.
79. Vazeux R, Brousse N, Jarry A, et al. AIDS subacute encephalitis: identification of HIV-infected cells. *Am J Pathol.* 1987;126:403–410.
80. Stoler H, Eskin TA, Benn S, et al. Human T-lymphotropic virus type III infection of the central nervous system: a preliminary in situ analysis. *JAMA.* 1986;256:2360–2364.
81. Shapshak P, Sun NCJ, Resnick L, et al. The detection of HIV by in situ hybridization. *Mod Pathol.* 1990; 3:146–153.
82. Achim CL, Wang R, Miners DK, et al. Brain viral burden in HIV-infection. *J Neuropathol Exp Neurol.* 1994;53: 284–294.
83. Brew BJ, Rosenblum M, Cronin K, Price RW. AIDS dementia complex and HIV-1 brain infection: clinical-virological correlations. *Ann Neurol.* 1995;38:563–570.
84. Glass JD, Fedor H, Wesselingh SL, McArthur JC. Immunocytochemical quanitation of human immunodeficiency virus in the brain: correlations with dementia. *Ann Neurol.* 1995;38:755–762.
85. Budka H. Human immunodeficiency virus (HIV) envelope and core proteins in CNS tissues of patients with the acquired immune deficiency syndrome (AIDS). *Acta Neuropathol.* 1990;79:611–619.
86. Michaels J, Price RW, Rosenblum MK. Microglia in the giant cell encephalitis of acquired immune deficiency

syndrome: proliferation, infection and fusion. *Acta Neuropathol.* 1988;76:373–379.

87. Kure K, Lyman WD, Weidenheim KM, Dickson DW. Cellular localization of an HIV-1 antigen in subacute AIDS encephalitis using an improved double-labeling immunohistochemical method. *Am J Pathol.* 1990;136:1085–1092.
88. Kure K, Weidenheim KM, Lyman WD, Dickson DW. Morphology and distribution of HIV-1 gp41-positive microglia in subacute AIDS encephalitis: pattern of involvement resembling a multisystem degeneration. *Acta Neuropathol.* 1990;80:393–400.
89. Epstein LG, Sharer LR, Cho E-S, et al. HTLV-III/LAV-like retrovirus particles in the brains of patients with AIDS encephalopathy. *AIDS Res.* 1985;1:447–454.
90. Orenstein JM. Ultrastructural pathology of human immunodeficiency virus infection. *Ultrastruct Pathol.* 1992;16:179–210.
91. Mirra SS, del Rio C. The fine structure of acquired immunodeficiency syndrome encephalopathy. *Arch Pathol Lab Med.* 1989;113:858–865.
92. Esiri MM, Oppenheimer DR, Brownell B, Haire M. Distribution of measles antigen and immunoglobulin-containing cells in the CNS in subacute sclerosing panencephalitis (SSPE) and atypical measles encephalitis. *J Neurol Sci.* 1982;53:29–43.
93. Morgello S, Cho E-S, Nielsen S, et al. Cytomegalovirus encephalitis in patients with acquired immune deficiency syndrome: an autopsy study of 30 cases and a review of the literature. *Hum Pathol.* 1987;18:289–297.
94. Gartner S, Markovits P, Markovitz DM, et al. Virus isolation from and identification of HTLV-III/LAV-producing cells in brain tissue from a patient with AIDS. *JAMA.* 1986;256:2365–2371.
95. Dickson DW. Multinucleated giant cells in acquired immunodeficiency syndrome encephalopathy: origin from endogenous microglia? *Arch Pathol Lab Med.* 1986;110:967–968.
96. Brinkmann R, Schwinn A, Narayan O, et al. Human immunodeficiency virus infection in microglia: correlation between cells infected in the brain and cells cultured from infectious brain tissue. *Ann Neurol.* 1992;31:361–365.
97. Dickson DW, Lee SC, Hatch W, et al. Macrophages and microglia in HIV-related central nervous system neuropathology. In: Price RW, Perry SW, eds. *HIV, AIDS and the Brain.* New York: Raven; 1994:99–118.
98. Rhodes RH, Ward JM, Walker DL, Ross A. Progressive multifocal leukoencephalopathy and retroviral encephalitis in acquired immunodeficiency syndrome. *Arch Pathol Lab Med.* 1988;112:1207–1213.
99. Gyorkey F, Melnick JL, Gyorkey P. Human immunodeficiency virus in brain biopsies of patients with AIDS and progressive encephalopathy. *J Infect Dis.* 1987;155:870–876.
100. Esiri MM, Morris CS, Millard PR. Fate of oligodendrocytes in HIV-1 infection. *AIDS.* 1991;5:1081–1088.
101. Robert ME, Geraghty JJ, Miles SA, et al. Severe neuropathy in a patient with acquired immune deficiency syndrome (AIDS). Evidence for widespread cytomegalovirus infection of peripheral nerve and human immunodeficiency virus-like immunoreactivity of anterior horn cells. *Acta Neuropathol.* 1989;79:255–261.
102. Budka H, Lassmann H. Human immunodeficiency virus in glial cells? *J Infect Dis.* 1988;157:203. Letter.
103. Sharer LR, Prineas JW. Human immunodeficiency virus in glial cells, continued. *J Infect Dis.* 1988;157:204. Letter.
104. Wiley CA, Belman AL, Dickson DW, et al. Human immunodeficiency virus within the brains of children with AIDS. *Clin Neuropathol.* 1990;9:1–6.
105. Rhodes RH, Ward JM, Cowan RP, Moore PT. Immunohistochemical localization of human immunodeficiency viral antigens in formalin-fixed spinal cords with AIDS myelopathy. *Clin Neuropathol.* 1989;88:22–27.
106. Nuovo GJ, Gallery F, MacConnell P, Braun A. In situ detection of polymerase chain reaction-amplified HIV-1 nucleic acids and tumor necrosis factor-alpha RNA in the central nervous system. *Am J Pathol.* 1994;144:659–666.
107. Blumberg BM, Sharer LR, Saito Y, et al. Overexpression of HIV-1 nef as a marker for restricted infection of astrocytes in human CNS tissue. *J Cell Biochem.* 1993;17:96.
108. Kohleisen B, Neumann M, Hermann R, et al. Cellular localization of nef expressed in persistently HIV-infected low producer astrocytes. *AIDS.* 1992;6:1427–1436.
109. Kleihues P, Lang W, Burger PC, et al. Progressive diffuse leukoencephalopathy in patients with acquired immune deficiency syndrome. *Acta Neuropathol.* 1985;68:333–339.
110. Snider WD. Simpson DM, Nielsen SL, et al. Neurological complications of acquired immune deficiency syndrome: analysis of 50 patients. *Ann Neurol.* 1983;14:403–418.
111. Ciardi A, Sinclair E, Scaravilli F, et al. The involvement of the cerebral cortex in human immunodeficiency virus encephalopathy: a morphological and immunohistochemical study. *Acta Neuropathol.* 1990;81:51–59.
112. Everall I, Luthert P, Lantos P. A review of neuronal damage in human immunodeficiency virus infection: its assessment, possible mechanism and relationship to dementia. *J Neuropathol Exp Neurol.* 1993;52:561–566.
113. Wiley CA, Masliah E, Morey M, et al. Neocortical damage during HIV infection. *Ann Neurol.* 1991;29:651–657.
114. Masliah E, Ge N, Morey M, DeTeresa R, Terry RD, Wiley CA. Cortical dendritic pathology in human immunodeficiency virus encephalitis. *Lab Invest.* 1992;66:285–291.
115. Mervis RF, Boesel C, Rosenblum MK, Price RW. Abnormal neuronal morphology in the brain of an AIDS-infected child: a golgi study. *Proc Soc Neurosci.* 1987;13(2);1252. Abstract.
116. Rhodes RH. Histopathology of the central nervous system in the acquired immunodeficiency syndrome. *Hum Pathol.* 1987;18:636–643.
117. Mizusawa H, Hirano A, Llena JF, Shintaku M. Cerebrovascular lesions in acquired immune deficiency syndrome. *Acta Neuropathol.* 1988;76:451–457.
118. Vinters HV, Guerra WF, Eppolito L, Keith PE. Necrotizing vasculitis of the nervous system in a patient with AIDS-related complex. *Neuropathol Appl Neurobiol.* 1988;14:417–424.

119. Yankner BA, Skolnik PR, Shoukimas GM, et al. Cerebral granulomatous angiitis associated with isolation of human T-lymphotropic virus type III from the central nervous system. *Ann Neurol.* 1986;20:362–364.
120. Scaravilli F, Daniel SE, Harcourt-Webster N, Guiloff RJ. Chronic basal meningitis and vasculitis in acquired immune deficiency syndrome. A possible role for human immunodeficiency virus. *Arch Pathol Lab Med.* 1989;113: 192–195.
121. Cho E-S, Sharer LR, Peress NS, Little B. Intimal proliferation of leptomeningeal arteries and brain infarcts in subjects with AIDS. *J Neuropathol Exp Neurol.* 1987;46:385. Abstract.
122. Joshi VV, Pawel B, Connor E, et al. Arteriopathy in children with acquired immune deficiency syndrome. *Pediatric Pathol.* 1987;7:261–275.
123. Kure K, Park YD, Kim T-S, et al. Immunohistochemical localization of an HIV epitope in cerebral aneurysmal arteriopathy in pediatric acquired immune deficiency syndrome (AIDS). *Pediatric Pathol.* 1989;9:655–667.
124. Park YD, Belman AL, Kim T-S, et al. Stroke in pediatric acquired immunodeficiency syndrome. *Ann Neurol.* 1990;28:303–311.
125. Smith TW, DeGirolami U, Henin D, et al. Human immunodeficiency virus (HIV) leukoencephalopathy and the microcirculation. *J Neuropathol Exp Neurol.* 1990;49: 357–370.
126. Belman AL, Lantos G, Horoupian D, et al. AIDS: calcification of the basal ganglia in infants and children. *Neurology.* 1986;36:1192–1199.
127. Petito CK, Cash KS. Blood–brain abnormalities in the acquired immunodeficiency syndrome: immunohistochemical localization of serum proteins in post-mortem brain. *Ann Neurol.* 1992;32:658–666.
128. Power C, Kong P-A, Crawford TO, et al. Cerebral white matter changes in acquired immunodeficiency syndrome dementia: alterations of the blood–brain barrier. *Ann Neurol.* 1993;34:339–350.
129. Centers for Disease Control. Revision of the CDC surveillance case definition for acquired immunodeficiency syndrome. *MMWR.* 1987;36(suppl):1S–15S.
130. Belman AL, Diamond D, Dickson D, et al. Pediatric acquired immunodeficiency syndrome: neurologic syndromes. *Am J Dis Child.* 1988;142:29–35.
131. Navia BA, Jordan BO, Price RW. The AIDS dementia complex. I. Clinical features. *Ann Neurol.* 1986;19: 517–524.
132. Wiley CA, Achim C. Human immunodeficiency virus encephalitis is the pathological correlate of dementia in acquired immunodeficiency syndrome. *Ann Neurol.* 1994;36:673–676.
133. Vazeux R, Lacroix-Ciaudo C, Blanche S, et al. Low levels of human immunodeficiency virus replication in the brain tissue of children with severe acquired immunodeficiency syndrome encephalopathy. *Am J Pathol.* 1992;140:137–144.
134. Glass JD, Wesselingh SL, Selnes OA, McArthur JC. Clinical-neuropathologic correlation in HIV-associated dementia. *Neurology.* 1993;43:2230–2237.
135. Magnuson DSK, Knudsen BE, Geiger JD, et al. Human immunodeficiency virus type 1 tat activates non-*N*-methyl-D-aspartate excitatory amino acid receptors and causes neurotoxicity. *Ann Neurol.* 1995;37:373–380.
136. Lipton SA. HIV-related neurotoxicity. *Brain Pathol.* 1991;1:193–199.
137. Brenneman DE, Westbrook GL, Fitzgerald SP, et al. Neuronal cell killing by the envelope protein of HIV and its prevention by vasoactive intestinal peptide. *Nature.* 1988;335:639–642.
138. Lipton SA. Human immunodeficiency virus-infected macrophages, gp 120, and *N*-methyl-D-aspartate receptor-mediated neurotoxicity. *Ann Neurol.* 1993;33:227–228.
139. Wahl LM, Corcoran ML, Pyle SW, et al. Human immunodeficiency virus glycoprotein (gp 120) induction of monocyte arachidonic acid metabolites and interleukin 1. *Proc Natl Acad Sci USA.* 1989;86:621–625.
140. Genis P, Jett M, Bernton EW, et al. Cytokines and arachidonic acid metabolites produced during HIV-infected macrophage-astroglial interactions: implications for the neuropathogenesis of HIV disease. *J Exp Med.* 1992; 176:1703–1718.
141. Hill JM, Mervis RF, Avidor R, et al. HIV envelope protein-induced neuronal damage and retardation of behavioral development in rat neonates. *Brain Res.* 1993;603: 222–233.
142. Toggas SM, Masliah E, Rockenstein EM, et al. Central nervous system damage produced by expression of the HIV-1 coat protein gp 120 in transgenic mice. *Nature.* 1994;367:188–193.
143. Heyes MP, Brew BJ, Martin A, et al. Quinolinic acid in cerebrospinal fluid and serum in HIV-1 infection: relationship to clinical and neurological status. *Ann Neurol.* 1991;29:202–209.
144. Benveniste EN. Cytokine circuits in brain: implications for AIDS dementia complex. In: Price RW, Perry SW, eds. *HIV, AIDS and the Brain.* New York: Raven Press; 1994:71–88.
145. Wilt SG, Milward E, Zhou JM, et al. In vitro evidence for a dual role of tumor necrosis factor-alpha in human immunodeficiency virus type 1 encephalopathy. *Ann Neurol.* 1995;37:381–394.
146. Pulliam L, Herndier BG, Tang NM, McGrath MS. Human immunodeficiency virus-infected macrophages produce soluble factors that cause histological and neurochemical alterations in cultured human brains. *J Clin Invest.* 1991;87:503–512.
147. Cvetkovich TA, Lazar E, Blumberg BM, et al. Human immunodeficiency virus type 1 (HIV-1) infection of neural xenografts. *Proc Natl Acad Sci USA.* 1992;11:5162–5166.
148. Mintz M, Rapaport R, Oleske JM, et al. Elevated serum levels of tumor necrosis factor are associated with progressive encephalopathy in children with acquired immune deficiency syndrome. *Am J Dis Child.* 1989; 143:771–774.
149. Grimaldi LME, Martino GV, Franciotta DM, et al. Elevated alpha-tumor necrosis factor levels in spinal fluid from HIV-1 infected patients with central nervous system involvement. *Ann Neurol.* 1991;29:21–25.
150. Griffin DE, Wesselingh SL, McArthur JC. Elevated central

nervous system prostaglandins in human immunodeficiency virus-associated dementia. *Ann Neurol.* 1994;35: 592–597.

151. Tyor WR, Glass JD, Griffin JW, et al. Cytokine expression in the brain during the acquired immunodeficiency syndrome. *Ann Neurol.* 1992;31:349–360.
152. Wesselingh SL, Power C, Glass JD, et al. Intracerebral cytokine messenger RNA expression in acquired immunodeficiency syndrome dementia. *Ann Neurol.* 1993;33: 576–582.
153. Stanley LC, Mrak RE, Woody RC, et al. Glial cytokines as neuropathogenic factors in HIV-1 infection: pathogenic similarities to Alzheimer's disease. *J Neuropathol Exp Neurol.* 1994;53:231–238.
154. Geny C, Gherardi R, Boudes P, et al. Multifocal multinucleated giant cell myelitis in an AIDS patient. *Neuropathol Appl Neurobiol.* 1991;17:157–162.
155. Goldstick L, Mandybur TI, Bode R. Spinal cord degeneration in AIDS. *Neurology.* 1985;35:103–106.
156. Petito CK, Navia BA, Cho E-S, et al. Vacuolar myelopathy pathologically resembling subacute combined degeneration in patients with the acquired immune deficiency syndrome. *N Engl J Med.* 1985;312:874–879.
157. Kamin SS, Petito CK. Idiopathic myelopathies with white matter vacuolation in non-acquired immunodeficiency syndrome patients. *Hum Pathol.* 1991;22:816–824.
158. Sharer LR, Dowling PC, Michaels J, et al. Spinal cord disease in children with HIV-1 infection: a combined molecular biological and neuropathological study. *Neuropathol Appl Neurobiol.* 1990;16:317–331.
159. Eilbott DJ, Peress N, Burger H, et al. Human immunodeficiency virus type 1 in spinal cords of acquired immunodeficiency syndrome patients with myelopathy: expression and replication in macrophages. *Proc Natl Acad Sci USA.* 1989;86:3337–3341.
160. Weiser B, Peress N, La Neve B, et al. Human immunodeficiency virus type 1 expression in the central nervous system correlates directly with extent of disease. *Proc Natl Acad Sci USA.* 1990;87:3997–4001.
161. Rhodes RH, Ward JM, Cowan RP, Moore PT. Immunohistochemical localization of human immunodeficiency viral antigens in formalin-fixed cords with AIDS myelopathy. *Clin Neuropathol.* 1989;8:22–27.
162. Hénin D, Smith TW, DeGirolami U, et al. Neuropathology of the spinal cord in the acquired immunodeficiency syndrome. *Hum Pathol.* 1992;23:1106–1114.
163. Kure K, Llena JF, Lyman WD, et al. Human immunodeficiency virus-1 infection of the nervous system. *Hum Pathol.* 1991;22:700–710.
164. Scaravilli F, Sinclair E, Arango JC, et al. The pathology of the posterior root ganglia in AIDS and its relationship to the pallor of the gracile tract. *Acta Neuropathol.* 1991; 84:163–170.
165. Grafe MR, Wiley CA. Spinal cord and peripheral nerve pathology in AIDS: the roles of cytomegalovirus and human immunodeficiency virus. *Ann Neurol.* 1989;25: 561–566.
166. Rosenblum MK, Scheck AC, Cronin K, et al. Dissociation of AIDS-related vacuolar myelopathy and productive HIV-1 infection of the spinal cord. *Neurology.* 1989;39: 892–896.
167. Petito CK, Vecchio D, Chen Y-T. HIV antigen and DNA in AIDS spinal cords correlate with macrophage infiltration but not with vacuolar myelopathy. *J Neuropathol Exp Neurol.* 1994;53:86–94.
168. Schmidbauer M, Budka H, Okeda R, et al. Multifocal vacuolar leukoencephalopathy: a distinct HIV-associated lesion of the brain. *Neuropathol Appl Neurobiol.* 1990; 16:437–443.
169. Jones HR, Ho DD, Forgacs P, et al. Acute fulminating fatal leukoencephalopathy as the only manifestation of human immunodeficiency virus infection. *Ann Neurol.* 1988;23:519–522.
170. de la Monte SM, Moore T, Hedley-Whyte ET. Vacuolar encephalopathy of AIDS. *N Engl J Med.* 1986;315: 1549–1550. Letter.
171. Schwenk J, Cruz-Sanchez F, Gosztonyi G, Cervos-Navarro J. Spongiform encephalopathy in a patient with acquired immune deficiency syndrome (AIDS). *Acta Neuropathol.* 1987;74:389–392.
172. Artigas J, Niedobitek F, Grosse G, et al. Spongiform encephalopathy in AIDS dementia complex: report of five cases. *J AIDS.* 1989;2:374–381.
173. Berger JR, Sheremata WA, Resnick L, et al. Multiple sclerosis-like illness occurring with human immunodeficiency virus infection. *Neurology.* 1989;29:324–329.
174. Rance NE, McArthur JC, Cornblath DR, et al. Gracile tract degeneration in patients with sensory neuropathy and AIDS. *Neurology.* 1988;38:265–271.

CHAPTER 20

Human Papillomaviruses

Jeffrey F. Hines and A. Bennett Jenson

Why, you take your cat and go and get in the grave-yard 'long about midnight when somebody that was wicked has been buried; and when it's midnight a devil will come, or maybe two or three, but you can't see 'em, you can only hear something like the wind, or maybe hear 'em talk; and when they're taking that feller away, you heave your cat after 'em and say, 'Devil follow corpse, cat follow devil, warts follow cat, I'm done with ye!' That'll fetch any *wart.*

Samuel Langhorne Clemens (Mark Twain) (1835–1910), The Adventures of Tom Sawyer

INTRODUCTION

Papillomaviruses (PVs) cause a variety of proliferative lesions of cutaneous and mucosal surfaces such as the skin, oral cavity, larynx, and anogenital tract.[1] PV infections are ubiquitous in many vertebrate species including man. Each of the more than 60 types of human papillomavirus (HPV) has a particular anatomic preference or "tropism" to infect cutaneous, metaplastic, keratinizing, or nonkeratinizing squamous epithelium (Table 20–1).[2] Approximately two thirds of these infections are cutaneotropic and one third are mucosotropic. Cutaneotropic HPVs cause exophytic (verrucae vulgaris) and flat warts (verrucae plana). Mucosotropic HPVs are associated with latent infections as well as benign papillomas, which may progress to premalignant and malignant lesions, particularly of the uterine cervix. HPV infection of the anogenital tract is recognized as a sexually transmitted disease and plays a critical role in the development of more than 95% of malignant lesions of the cervix and its precursor lesions.[3–5] The oncogenic potential for these anogenital HPVs varies among types with HPV-16 and HPV-18 in the majority of cancers.

In this chapter, we summarize our current understanding of papillomavirus infection focusing on its molecular pathogenesis, epidemiology, and clinical syndromes. We also review recent advances in our understanding of anogenital HPVs and the prospect for new methods of detection, prevention, and treatment of HPV-associated disease.

HISTORICAL PERSPECTIVE

Warts have been described since antiquity in both humans and nonhumans. A viral cause for human warts was described in 1894 by Licht, who transmitted warts from his brother to himself by inoculation of material from a wart. In 1909, Cuiffo showed that warts were transmissible by cell-free extracts.[6] PVs were the first DNA carcinogenic viruses to be isolated and identified, when Shope and Hurst[7] described their studies with the cottontail rabbit papillomavirus (CRPV) in 1933. Studies during the next two decades demonstrated that warts containing CRPV were transmissible among rabbits and that they could progress to carcinoma. Electron microscopic studies in the 1940s and 1950s confirmed a viral cause for cutaneous warts.[8] Condyloma accuminatum has been recognized for years as a sexually transmitted disease, and in 1970 virus particles were identified in human genital warts.[9] Although the significance was not recognized at the time, the histologic link of HPV infection to cervical premalignancies came in the mid-1950s by Koss in his description of the koilocyte, a superficial squamous cell that reflects the cytopathic effect of PV infections.[10]

TABLE 20–1. CLINICOPATHOLOGIC GROUPING OF 67 HUMAN PAPILLOMAVIRUSES AND THE ONCOGENIC POTENTIAL OF THE LESIONS WITH WHICH THEY ARE FREQUENTLY ASSOCIATED

Group I: Cutaneotropic (Immunocompetent Host)	
1,4	Plantar warts (benign)
2, 26, 28, 29, 38, 49, 57, 60, 63, 65	Common warts (benign)
3, 10, 27	Flat warts (benign)
7	Butcher's warts (benign)
Group II: Cutaneotropic (Epidermodysplasia Verruciformis; Immunocompromised Host)	
5, 8	Macular lesions (highly malignant)
9, 12, 14, 15, 17, 19–25, 36, 37, 46–50	Macular or flat lesions (benign/ rarely malignant)
Group III: Mucosotropic	
13, 32	Focal epithelial hyperplasia (benign)
6, 11, 34, 39, 41–44	Condylomata, cervical intraepithelial neoplasia (low risk/benign)
30, 31, 33, 35, 51, 52, 58	Condylomata, cervical intraepithelial neoplasia, cervical cancer (intermediate risk/malignant)
16, 18, 45, 56	Cervical intraepithelial neoplasia, cervical cancer (highly malignant)
40, 53, 54, 55, 59, 61, 62 64, 66, 67	Condylomata, cervical intraepithelial, neoplasia, cervical cancer (risk pending evaluation)

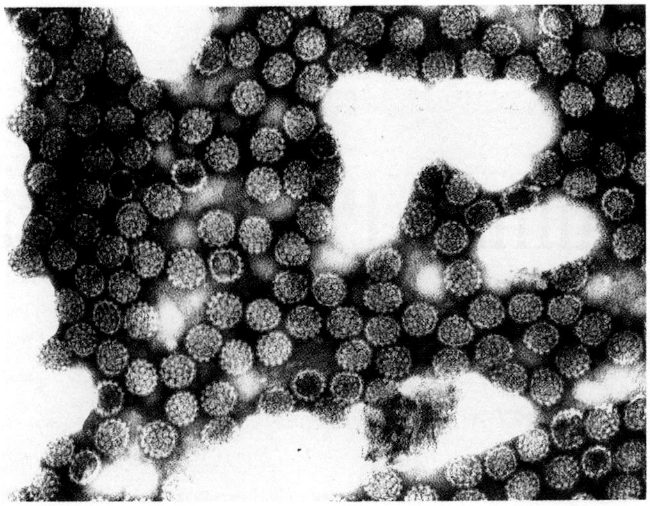

Figure 20–1. Electron micrograph of human papillomavirus particles isolated from a plantar wart (×300,000).

In spite of the wide distribution of PVs, studies on the biology of HPVs have been hampered by the inability to replicate the virus in cell culture. Recent advances in recombinant DNA technology have allowed molecular cloning and detailed biochemical analysis of the PV genome and immunologic analysis of its gene products. This has increased our understanding of the PVs.

STRUCTURE/GENETICS/MOLECULAR BIOLOGY

Papillomaviruses maintain remarkable similarity in their anatomic structure and genetic organization among all PVs. PV particles are 55 nm in diameter, consisting of 72 capsomers that form nonenveloped icosohedral-shaped virions (Figure 20–1).[11] They superficially resemble simian virus (SV) 40 and polyomaviruses, which contain 72 capsomers, but are only 45 nm in diameter. Although both are species of the papovavirus family, they are not related genetically or antigenically. The PV genome is organized as a closed, circular, doubled-stranded DNA molecule approximately 8000 base pairs long (Figure 20–2). Functionally, the PV genome can be divided into three regions: the "early" (E), "late" (L), and "long control regions" (LCRs) (Table 20–2). The early region encodes eight genes, which are responsible for viral DNA replication, transcriptional control, and cell transformation.[12] The E6 and E7 gene products are perhaps best studied among HPVs. Because of their interaction with tumor suppresser proteins p53 and pRb, respectively, they are designated as viral onco-

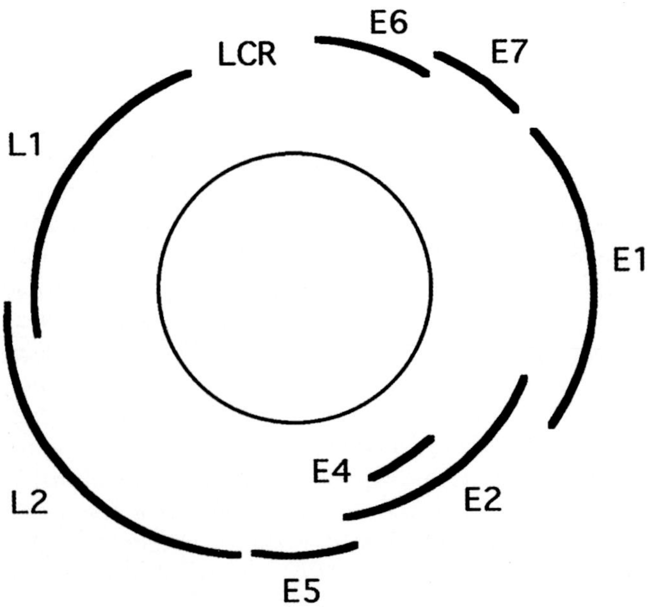

Figure 20–2. Genomic organization of HPVs. The circular genome for HPVs with early genes (E1–E7), late genes (L1 and L2), and a long control region (LCR) with promoter/enhancer elements is illustrated.

TABLE 20–2. PAPILLOMAVIRUS GENE FUNCTIONS

Open Reading Frame	Function
E1	Modulator of DNA replication
E2	Transcriptional regulation
E3	Unknown
E4	Cytoplasmic protein of productively infected cells
E5	Transformation
E6	Binding to p53, transformation
E7	Binding to pRb, transformation
E8	Replication, transcriptional regulation
L1	Major capsid protein
L2	Minor capsid protein

genes. This interaction is particularly evident in the highly oncogenic HPV types 16 and 18.[13] All genes or open reading frames (ORFs) are located on and transcribed from the same strand of DNA. The late region encodes the two structural proteins of the virion, L1 and L2, the major and minor capsid proteins, respectively. L1 and L2 are synthesized only in productive lesions (warts, condylomata) in terminally differentiated keratinocytes. The proteins are not expressed in transformed cells. The long control region contains the origin of DNA replication, transcriptional enhancer sequences, and several promoter elements for messenger RNA (mRNA) synthesis.[11]

CLASSIFICATION

Because of the similarities among the *pa*pillomaviruses, *po*lyomavirus of mice, and *va*cuolating virus of monkeys (SV 40), these viruses were grouped in 1962 as the *papovaviruses.*[14] Each papovavirus contains a genome of double-stranded DNA, lacks a lipid envelope, displays a slow growth cycle with replication in the host nucleus, produces latent and chronic infections, and is tumorgenic.

Among the HPVs, more than 60 different types have been described (Table 20–1).[2] Initial studies on typing HPV were performed on the basis of DNA homology. A new HPV type is defined as one in which the new HPV shares less than 50% DNA homology with known HPV types. Those viruses with more than 50% but less than 100% polynucleotide sequence homology are classified as subtypes.

The majority of classification of PVs is accomplished by genotyping using recombinant DNA rather than by serotyping like many other viruses. Currently, advances in molecular immunology have made it possible to consider serologic means for typing PVs.[15]

EPIDEMIOLOGY

The incidence and prevalence of HPV infection for the general population is unknown. Even in well-defined populations this is difficult to assess. Data on incidence and prevalence depend on many variables, which include the type and sensitivity of the diagnostic technique used to detect HPV infection, lifestyle of the group studied, the presence or absence of clinical infection, other cofactors that affect infection, and the natural history of the disease.

Flat or juvenile warts (verrucae plana) are primarily in young, school-age children. Common warts are most frequent in school-age and adolescent children.[16] Laryngeal condylomata are usually in preschool children and have a second peak in adult life.[17] Plantar warts are common in adolescents and young adults.[16] For anogenital disease, condylomata are common in young, sexually active men and women.[4] The association of HPV infection with cervical intraepithelial lesions and carcinomas is described later.

Numerous diagnostic techniques have been used and are being developed to detect HPV infection directly by genotyping or serotyping, or indirectly by phenotyping. Direct detection includes DNA hybridization (Southern blot, dot blot, in situ hybridization, capture hybridization), polymerase chain reaction (PCR), in situ PCR, Northern blotting, and serology. Indirect methods include exfoliative cytology, cervicography, and colposcopy with tissue histology.

PATHOGENESIS/IMMUNE RESPONSES

Cutaneotropic HPVs can be transmitted by direct and indirect contact. Similarly, mucosotropic HPVs are

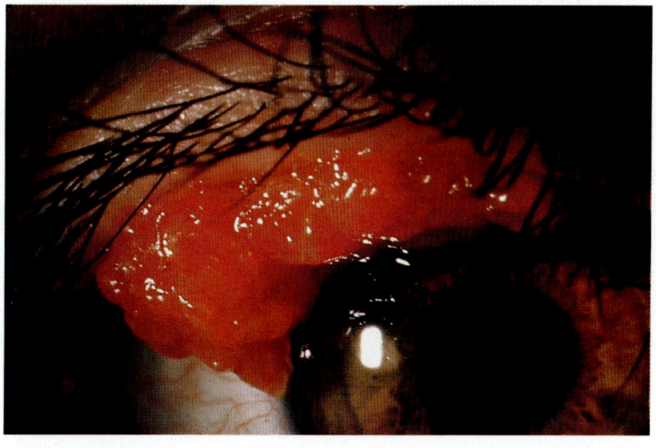

Figure 20–3. Recurrent conjunctival papillomatosis caused by HPV-11.

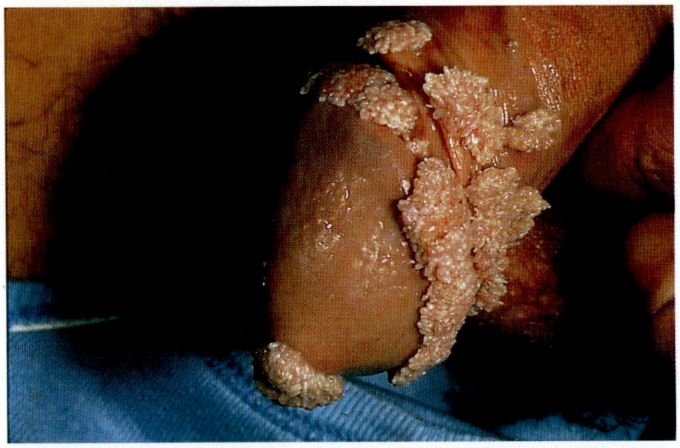

Figure 20–4. Extensive condylomata of penis caused by HPV-6.

easily transmissible. Infants, for instance, may contract HPV types, such as HPV-11, that cause naso-oral, conjunctival (Figure 20–3), laryngeal, and respiratory papillomatosis as they pass through the birth canal of mothers who have condylomata.[18] Anogenital warts are transmitted during coitus. This is supported by data that confirm the presence of similar HPV types on cervical and penile lesions (Figures 20–4, 20–5, and 20–6) in infected sexual partners.[19]

Several factors affect the rate of transmission of both cutaneotropic and mucosotropic HPVs. These include increased physical contact such as coitus with multiple partners, immunodeficient states, and pregnancy. These highly infectious viruses have relatively long incubation periods. Cutaneous warts usually appear at the site of inoculation within 1 to 3 months, but incubation periods as long as 20 months have been described.[16] Lesions caused by mucosotropic HPV types usually appear within 4 to 6 weeks in humans. The same incubation time is true for mucosotropic viruses that might infect the athymic nude mouse model.[20,21]

The host response to infection is similar for all HPV types. The three types of squamous epithelia (cutaneous–keratinized, mucosal–nonkeratinized, and metaplastic) are susceptible to HPV infection. Although infection may manifest itself differently for the HPV types, HPV infection begins in the basal layer of squamous epithelium. Presumably, virus from infected cells is released into epithelial breaks of the susceptible host.[22] We previously noted that PVs demonstrate tissue tropism for a particular type's anatomic site for infection. Equally important is the fact that HPVs can only replicate in the most differentiated keratinocytes.

After infection, three sequelae are possible. First, the HPV genome becomes stabilized as a nonintegrated episome and remains latent in the host without clinical or morphologic changes in the squamous epithelium. Second, an active infection is established with vegetative replication of HPVs, which induces the proliferation of squamous epithelia to become benign tumors (warts, papillomas). The expression of the early and late gene products accounts for the morphologic changes in the affected epithelium. Early gene expression causes cellular proliferation, which results in acanthosis. Late gene expression results in the production of the viral capsid proteins, which by electron microscopy and immunocytochemistry for genus-specific epitopes are evident only within the nuclei of the most terminally differentiated, superficial epithelial cells (keratinocytes). The HPV genome in latently infected cells and benign tumors is present in the nonintegrated, episomal form.

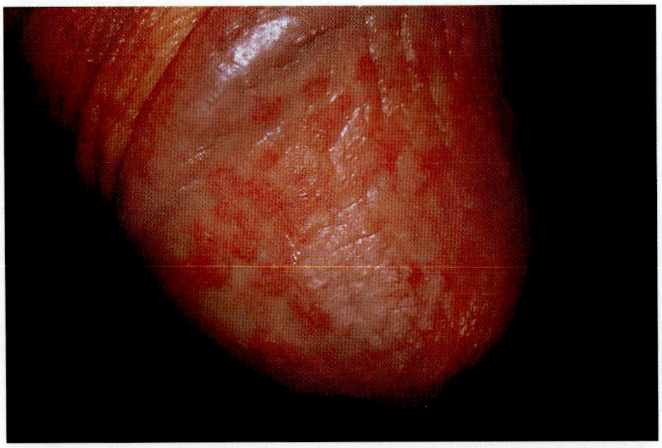

Figure 20–5. Glans penis with slightly discolored macules barely perceptible to the naked eye.

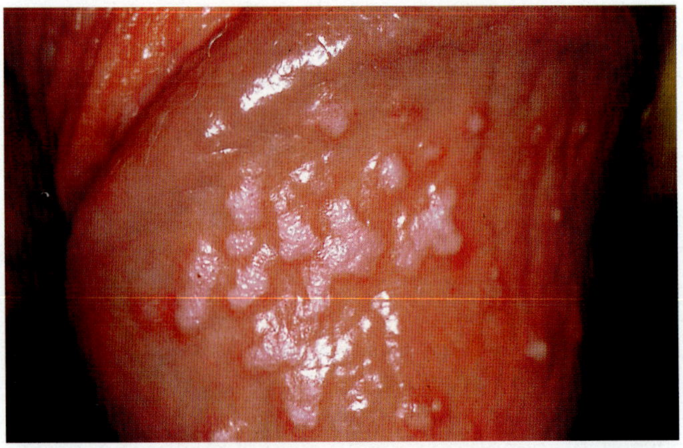

Figure 20–6. Topically applied acetic acid to the same glans penis, making the macules white and clearly visible. They are caused by HPV-16.

Viral capsid assembly in these productively infected, terminally differentiated keratinocytes causes degenerative changes in the nuclei and cytoplasm, which are classically recognized histologically as koilocytosis.[10] Third and finally, infection with certain HPV types has a high probability of being associated with dysplasias (6 and 11) or with malignancies (16 and 18). The HPV genome in the malignancies usually is not episomal but is integrated into the host genome at least 80% of the time. It has become evident that the viral E2 gene serves as the most significant site of integration into the host genome. With integration, the normal regulatory function of the E2 gene is interrupted. This appears to be critical for tumorigenesis. Specifically, this loss of regulation results in the overexpression of viral E6 and E7 oncoproteins.[23,24]

In vitro biologic assays have enabled investigators to study the transforming activity of cloned HPV DNA on primary and immortalized cells. Such assays have been used to evaluate the role of viral genes, which may be important in tumorigenesis. Assays of infected or transfected murine and human cells have been important tools in defining the role for E6 and E7 being necessary and sufficient for in vitro transformation.[25] Some of the cell lines produced by these assays are tumorigenic in nude mice alone; others require the cooperativity of the expressed *ras* oncogene to become tumorigenic. This tumorigenicity also appears to be dependent on the type of HPV DNA used.[26]

Immunologic responses to PV infection are probably an equally important aspect of host response to infection. Specifically, the persistence and spontaneous regression of lesions may be directly related to immune phenomena. For instance, patients with altered cellular immunity (immunosuppression, immunodeficient states, pregnancy) have a higher incidence of warts and condylomata.[27] In addition, patients with the congenitally acquired disease of impaired cellular immunity, epidermodysplasia verruciformis (EV), have associated warts and the rate of detection of HPV types 5 and 8 is high especially in warts that transform into squamous and basal cell carcinomas in areas exposed to sunlight.[28] Finally, HPV-associated cervical cancers that are metastatic frequently exhibit a reduction or total loss of expression of major histocompatibility complex (MHC) class I molecules. This suggests that downregulation of MHC class I molecules may help these cancers escape from cell-mediated immune surveillance.[29]

Humoral immune responses to PV infection have been quantified. Sera from animals and humans with a history of infection generally react positively by enzyme-linked immunosorbent assay with denatured PV capsid proteins.[30–32] Antibodies can also be detected in rabbit and murine species inoculated with intact HPV virions.[30,33] Humoral immunity appears to protect against HPV infection or the spread of infection. Recent advances in molecular biology have enabled investigators to synthesize recombinant virus-like particles (VLPs) and capsid proteins of PVs, which react with conformational-dependent, neutralizing antibodies.[15,34–36] This should allow for further investigation into the role that humoral immunity has in the natural history of papillomavirus infection.

CLINICAL SYNDROMES/CLINICAL PATHOLOGIC CORRELATION

Cutaneotropic HPV types cause a variety of warts with varied morphologies and oncogenicity (Table 20–1).[2] Verruca vulgaris is associated with HPV types 2, 26, 28, and 29. These warts are characteristically exophytic, have a crusty surface, and are benign. Verruca plantaris is associated with HPV types 1 and 4. These warts usually are singly on weight-bearing parts of the body and are benign. Flat (juvenile) warts are associated with HPV types 3, 10, and 27. They usually occur as multiple benign warts on the face, hands, and limbs. The final group of cutaneotropic HPVs cause macular warts in patients with EV. These include HPV types 5, 8, 9, 12, 14, 15, 17, 19, 20, 21, 22, 23, 24, 25, 36, 37, 46, 47, 48, 49, and 50. Types 5 and 8 are carcinogenic.[28]

Like the cutaneotropic viruses, the mucosotropic HPVs similarly display varied phenotypes. Several of the mucosotropic viruses are common to the naso-oral cavity, conjunctiva, larynx, and the respiratory tract (Table 20–1).[2] Focal epithelial hyperplasia associated with HPV types 13 and 32 has been described as multiple, flat to minimally elevated lesions of the oral cavity. Benign, pedunculated, singly occurring oral papillomas are the most common papilloma of the oral cavity. Laryngeal papillomas are most commonly associated with HPV-11. These benign exophytic papillomas are multiple in number and recur frequently. When extensive, they can cause airway obstruction. Malignant transformation has been described and in some patients may be related to radiation. The majority of extragenital mucosal HPV infections are caused by viruses that also infect the genital tract.[18]

The HPV types associated with anogenital infection have been the focus of much attention and research because of their obvious impact on women's health issues. Oriel and Almeida[9] in 1970 confirmed the sexual transmission of genital warts; 65% of sexual contacts displayed genital warts in approximately 6 weeks. Lorincz et al,[13] in an epidemiologic study of 2627 women, examined the prevalence of anogenital HPV infection among normal women and women with premalignant and invasive lesions using Southern blot hybridization. Moreover, the relative risk of oncogenic potential for 15 anogenital HPV types was defined for the association between the viral type and condylomatous, premalignant, and invasive lesions of the cervix. Three risk categories were thus defined. Low-risk HPV types (6, 11, 42, 43, and 44) were in approximately 20% of low-grade squamous intraepithelial lesions (LGSILs) but absent in all cancers. Intermediate-risk HPV types (31, 33, 35, 51, 52, and 58) were detected in 23% of high-grade squamous intraepithelial lesions (HGSILs) but in 10% of cancers. Finally, high-risk HPV types (16, 18, 45, and 56) were detected in 53% of HGSILs and in 74% of cancers. Adenocarcinomas of the cervix are usually caused by HPV-16 or HPV-18 and cause many rapidly developing carcinomas in young women.[13]

Anogenital HPV infections fall into three categories. Latent infections with no pathologically identifiable lesions comprise a large reservoir of virus and may be causal in transmission and autoinfection after activation by some cofactor. It is thought that 10% of sexually active individuals harbor HPV as latent infections.[37] Active infections are in up to 5% of sexually active women and appear as flat or exophytic condylomata of the cervix, vagina, or vulva. Condylomata (Figure 20–7) are usually associated with HPV-6 (Figure 20–8) and HPV-11. The condyloma sometimes persist for years, yet can regress spontaneously. Finally, HPV infection can be associated with squamous intraepithelial lesions and invasive cancers of the anogenital tract. Squamous intraepithelial lesions show characteristic disorderly, undifferentiated, proliferating basaloid and parabasaloid cells that occupy the lower one third of the epithelium for cervical intraepithelial neoplasia (CIN) I to full thickness involvement of the epithelium in CIN III lesions (Figure 20–9). Conversely, invasive cervical carcinomas extend beyond the basement membrane.

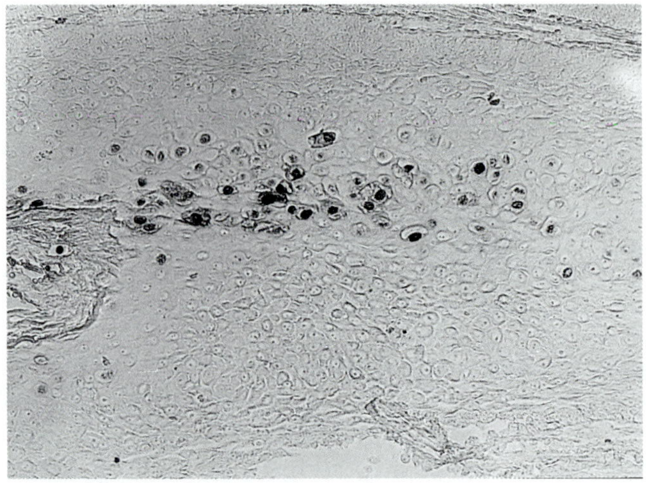

Figure 20–8. In situ hybridization detects infection of vulva by HPV-6, which causes condylomata. The intranuclear peroxidase shows the location of the HPV-6 DNA.

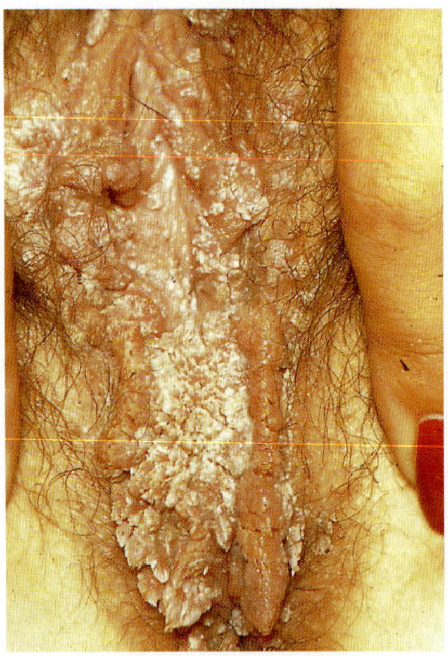

Figure 20–7. Extensive condylomata of vulva caused by HPV-6.

Cervical cancer is the best studied of the anogenital malignancies associated with HPV infection. In the United States, cervical cancer is the ninth most common malignancy in women preceded by breast, lung, colon, endometrium, ovary, pancreas, melanoma, and lymphoma. In 1993, there were an estimated 13,500 new cervical cancers in the United States and approximately 4400 deaths.[38] Worldwide, cervical cancer poses a significant public health problem causing some 500,000

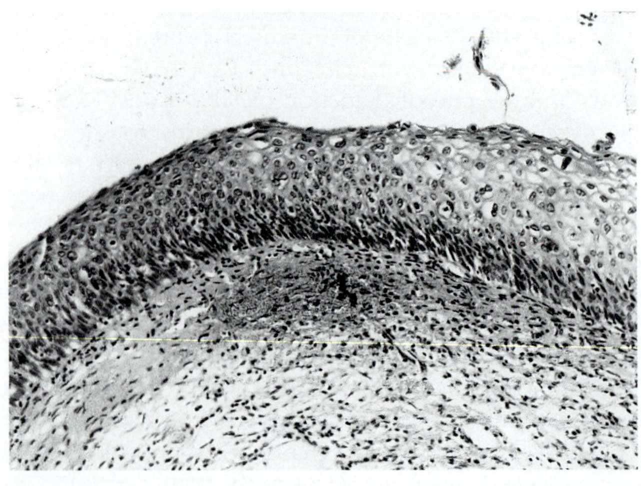

Figure 20–9. Cervical intraepithelial neoplasia. A continuum of CIN changes from CIN I on the right to CIN III on the left caused by HPV-16 (hematoxylin-eosin, ×100).

deaths each year.[6] Studies have documented the continuum of disease in its progression from squamous intraepithelial lesions to invasive carcinomas. This sequence of events and the rate of spontaneous regression has also been the focus of investigation. Sixteen percent of untreated mild dysplasias progress to CIS with a transit time ranging from 84 to 96 months. Approximately two thirds of these same mild dysplasias regress and 22% persist.[39] The majority of high grade lesions persist or progress. In two thirds of CIN III lesions, the transit time to invasive cancer is about 10 years.[40] Moreover, there is now substantial evidence to support a role for HPV infection in both premalignant and malignant cervical disease. Certainly, other factors are operative in the development of cervical cancer (ie, tobacco) but HPV appears to be necessary; eradication or protection against HPV infection would perhaps decrease the number of cervical cancers by 95%. Using sensitive PCR assays, HPV DNA can be detected in more than 95% of squamous and adenocarcinomas of the cervix.[41] This, combined with the odds ratio data for highly oncogenic HPV types ranging from 31 to 296 for the occurrence of cervical cancer, strongly supports the association of certain HPV infections with cervical disease.[13]

TABLE 20–3. THE BETHESDA SYSTEM (TBS) FOR REPORTING CERVICAL AND VAGINAL CYTOLOGIC DIAGNOSES

- Specimen adequacy
  - Identifying information and labeling
  - Clinical information
  - Cellular adequacy and preservation
  - Transformation zone/endocervical adequacy
- Descriptive diagnoses
  - Benign cellular changes
    - Infection (fungal, bacterial, viral, other)
    - Reactive changes (inflammation, atrophy, radiation, other)
  - Epithelial cell abnormalities
    - Squamous cell
      - Atypical squamous cells of undetermined significance
      - Low-grade squamous intraepithelial lesion (encompasses HPV infection and CIN I)
      - High-grade squamous intraepithelial lesion (encompasses CIN II, CIN III, CIS)
      - Squamous cell carcinoma
    - Glandular cell
      - Endometrial cells
      - Atypical glandular cells of undetermined significance
      - Endocervical adenocarcinoma
      - Endometrial adenocarcinoma
      - Extrauterine adenocarcinoma
      - Adenocarcinoma, NOS
  - Other malignant neoplasms

DETECTION

Molecular hybridization techniques are able to detect HPV genetic material in tissue and they can be modified depending on the state of the cells. Genetic material can be extracted from or identified in archival, formalin-fixed, and fresh cells and tissue. DNA hybridization tests such as Southern blotting, dot blotting, and in situ DNA hybridization (Figure 20–8) are available and allow for HPV detection and typing. Some kits approved by the Food and Drug Administration are commercially available (ie, Vira Type). Northern blotting, which detects mRNA, is used more often as a research tool.

PCR has become an extremely useful and powerful tool for detecting and typing HPV DNA. PCR has the advantage of being extremely sensitive but has the disadvantage of decreased specificity. It amplifies a single copy of viral DNA to tens of thousands of copies for qualitative and quantitative uses. Contamination is its only problem, which is, however, major in most laboratories.

Cytologic examination of exfoliated cells from the cervix (the Papanicolaou's smear, or Pap smear) has proven to be an effective screening method for premalignant and malignant lesions of the cervix. The traditional approach to the classification of the Pap smear was based on a numerical system that proved to be inadequate. In 1988, the National Cancer Institute convened a workshop charged with revising and standardizing cervical cytology. The result was a new classification designated the Bethesda system (Table 20–3). This classification has undergone revision and a simplified atlas was released in 1994.[42] Under the Bethesda system, premalignant lesions fall into three categories: *a*typical *s*quamous *c*ells of *u*ndetermined *s*ignificance (ASCUS), *l*ow-grade *s*quamous *i*ntraepithelial *l*esion (LSIL), and *h*igh-grade *s*quamous *i*ntraepithelial *l*esion (HSIL). HSILs include CIN II, CIN III, and CIS. These lesions obviously require confirmatory biopsy with subsequent ablative or excisional therapy. LSILs include CIN I and other HPV-associated lesions previously described as "condylomatous atypia" and "koilocytotic atypia." ASCUS are those abnormal cells that do not fit into LSIL or HSIL categories but display minor abnormalities previously described as atypical. "Undetermined significance" relates both the lack of a defined criteria for their description and the uncertain relationship of these cells to inflammation, HPV infection, cancer, or other conditions. Given the high prevalence of ASCUS and LSIL smears, cytology is not an effective triage tool in spite of its usefulness in screening. As a result, prospective studies are under way to address the issue of effective and efficient triage of ASCUS and LSIL smears. Some of these studies involve cervicography and HPV DNA testing as a part of the triage schema for screening.

Cervicography, photographs of the cervix taken at the time of pelvic examination after application of acetic acid to highlight abnormalities, is now available as an ancillary test to women with abnormal cervical cytology. The cervigrams are reviewed by experts whose diagnosis would determine if additional evaluation is indicated. Cervigrams, thus, may represent a complement to Pap smear screening and a low-cost alternative to colposcopy in defined circumstances.[43]

Colposcopy with directed biopsy for histologic confirmation of cervical lesions is the traditional means of diagnosing lesions that have exfoliated abnormal cells. Results of the colposcopic findings, in conjunction with tissue histology, direct additional therapy as indicated (Figure 20–10).

Serologic assays have been used to measure antibody response in patients to PV infection.[31,32] Correlation of these antibody reactivities with the presence of active and latent HPV infection, SIL, and cancer would be a true benefit of serologic testing. Until recently, development of such serologic assays has been hampered by the inability to propagate PVs in vitro, the inability to evaluate easily PV neutralization, and the very low levels of PV virions, characterized by the presence of viral structure proteins (Figure 20–11), in genital lesions. New methods of synthesizing recombinant PV capsid proteins and VLPs, which react with neutralizing and conformation-dependent antibodies, now provide a way to carry out seroepidemiologic studies of HPV infection and perhaps applications to serologic typing.[15,34–36,44]

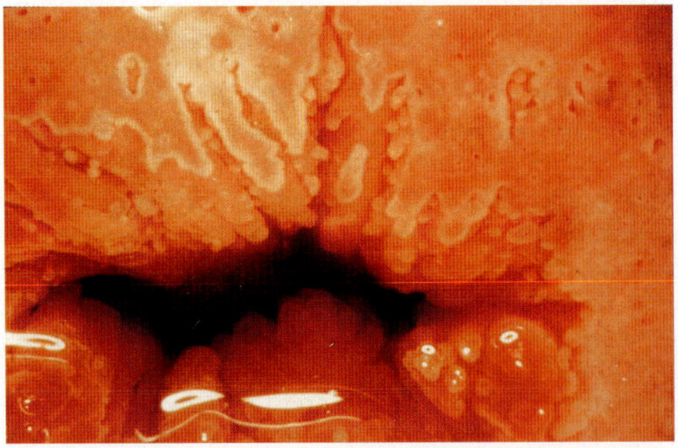

Figure 20–10. Colposcopic photograph of cervical transformation zone with diffusely scattered acetowhite staining, characteristic of HPV infection.

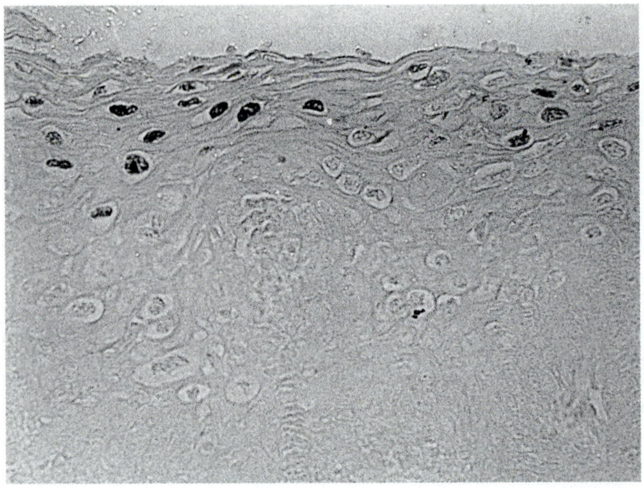

Figure 20–11. CIN I changes in cervix with localization of viral structure protein in nuclei of koilocytotic cells in the superficial layer.

TREATMENT

Cutaneous warts can be treated with a variety of destructive and surgical techniques. Typically, topical salicylic acid, glutaraldehyde, liquid nitrogen, podophyllin, laser ablation, and surgical excision are used with similar results. A large number recur regardless of the form of treatment.

Mucosal lesions of the conjunctiva, naso-oropharynx, larynx, and respiratory tract are treated similarly. The CO_2 laser has perhaps the best applicability to lesions in these anatomic locations. In addition, interferons have been used successfully to treat laryngeal papillomas.[45]

The treatment of invasive cervical cancer is not affected necessarily by HPV type. Until more information is available on the role that HPV types may have on tumor aggressiveness and recurrence, therapy for primary invasive cervical cancers limited to the cervix is with radiation therapy or radical surgery.

Treatment of HPV-associated anogenital tract lesions likewise consists of a variety of medical and surgical methods. Condylomata respond to topical podophyllin, bi- and trichloroacetic acid, CO_2 laser ablation, intralesional interferon injection, 5-fluorouracil, and surgical excision.[2] HSILs, after confirmatory biopsy, can be ablated or excised with cryosurgery, CO_2 laser, loop electrocautery excisional procedure (LEEP), or knife conization. As mentioned previously, there is controversy over the best triage scheme for ASCUS and LSIL smears. Each year approximately 2.5 million women are diagnosed with ASCUS and LSILs in the United States. The associated costs of colposcopic evaluations and interventions to remedy these lesions approaches $6 billion per annum.[46] It is increasingly evident that the cost and morbidity associated with diagnosis and treatment of these particular lesions have limited benefit to cancer prevention. The development of prospective trials is warranted to evaluate the efficacy of other triage strategies. Some of these trials involve the use of HPV testing and cervicography. At the present time, careful follow-up cytologic evaluation and/or colposcopic evaluation is indicated for these lesions.

FUTURE DIRECTIONS AND SUMMARY

Much epidemiologic, clinical, and scientific data has been collected supporting the role of HPV infection in the development of anogenital warts, SILs, and cancers. The future is likely to focus attention on new strategies for early detection, prevention, and treatment of HPV-associated lesions.

As we begin to understand more about the humoral immune response to HPV infection, the prospect for the development of a prophylactic vaccine against HPV infection can become a reality. Recombinantly synthesized PV capsid proteins and VLPs, which mimic the conformation of native virions and are reactive with conformation-dependent, neutralizing antibodies, may be the ideal reagents for a prophylactic protein vaccine.[15,34–36,44] Seroepidemiologic studies of HPV infections could be accomplished to determine which women are at risk for developing cervical cancers and, moreover, which women would most likely benefit from vaccination. It is believed that vaccines could save the lives of approximately 225,000 women worldwide.[46]

As we further elucidate the molecular and biological mechanisms by which HPVs and other factors act to transform epithelial cells, we can better target new treatment strategies. These strategies may be directed at altering humoral and cell-mediated immunity, at the expression of PV gene products, or perhaps at cofactors that work with PV gene products to affect transformation.

In summary, PVs are a ubiquitous group of viruses of varied oncogenic potential that cause infections of cutaneous and mucosal epithelia. The consequences of these infections, both benign and malignant, have a significant impact on society. Continued basic science and clinical research is needed to provide important information about mechanisms of carcinogenesis, natural history of infection, development of treatment and triage protocols, and for the development of novel ways of detection, treatment, and prevention.

REFERENCES

1. Pfister H. General introduction to papillomaviruses. In: Pfister F, ed. *Papillomaviruses and Human Cancer.* Boca Raton, Fla: CRC Press; 1990;1:2–10.
2. de Villiers E. Hybridization methods other than PCR: an update. In: Munoz N, Bosch FX, Shah KV, et al, eds. *Epidemiology of Cervical Cancer and Human Papillomaviruses.* Oxford, UK: Oxford University Press; 1992; 1:112–134.
3. Crum CP, Levine RU. Human papilloma virus infection and cervical neoplasia: new perspectives. *Int J Gynecol Pathol.* 1984;3:376–388.
4. Champion MJ. Clinical manifestations and natural history of genital human papillomavirus infection. *Obstet Gynecol Clin North Am.* 1987;14:363–388.
5. Syrjanen KJ. Biology of human papillomavirus infections and their role in squamous cell carcinogenesis. *Med Biol.* 1987;65:21–39.
6. Jenson AB, Lancaster WD. Association of human papillomavirus with benign, premalignant, and malignant anogenital lesions. In: Pfister F, ed. *Papillomaviruses and Human Cancer.* Boca Raton, Fla: CRC Press; 1990;1: 11–44.
7. Shope RE, Hurst EW. Infectious papillomatosis of rabbits; with a note on the histopathology. *J Exp Med.* 1933; 58:607–624.
8. Strauss MJ, Bunting H, Melnick JL. Virus-like particles and inclusion bodies in skin papillomas. *J Invest Dermatol.* 1949;15:433–444.
9. Oriel JD, Almeida JD. Demonstration of virus particles in human genital warts. *Br J Vener Dis.* 1970;46:37–42.
10. Koss LG, Durfee GR. Unusual patterns of squamous epithelium of the uterine cervix: cytologic and pathologic study of koilocytotic atypia. *Ann NY Acad Sci.* 1956; 63:1235.
11. Schlegel R. Papillomaviruses and human cancer. *Sem Virol.* 1990;1:297–306.
12. Yee C, Krishnan-Hewlett I, Baker CC, Schlegel R, Howley PM. Presence and expression of human papillomavirus sequences in human cervical carcinoma cell lines. *Am J Pathol.* 1985;119:361–366.
13. Lorincz AT, Reid R, Jenson AB, Greenberg MD, Lancaster WD, Kurman RJ. Human papillomavirus infection of the cervix: relative risk associations of 15 common anogenital types. *Obstet Gynecol.* 1992;3:328–337.
14. Melnick JL. Papova virus group. *Science.* 1962;135: 1128–1130.
15. Hines JF, Ghim SJ, Christensen ND, et al. Role of conformational epitopes expressed by human papillomavirus major capsid proteins in the serologic detection of infection and prophylactic vaccination. *Gynecol Oncol.* (in press).
16. Rowson KE, Mahy BW. Human papova virus. *Bacteriol Rev.* 1967;31:110–131.
17. Mounts P, Shah KV, Kashima H. Viral etiology of juvenile and adult onset squamous papilloma of the larynx. *Proc Natl Acad Sci USA.* 1982;79:5425–5429.

18. Hajek E. Contribution to the etiology of laryngeal papilloma in children. *J Laryngol Otol.* 1956;70:166.
19. Barrasso R, De Brux J, Croissant O, et al. High prevalence of papillomavirus-associated penile intraepithelial neoplasia in sexual partners of women with cervical intraepithelial neoplasia. *N Engl J Med.* 1987;317:916–923.
20. Oriel JD. Natural history of genital warts. *Br J Vener Dis.* 1971;47:1–13.
21. Kreider JW, Howlett MK, Leure-Dupree AE, et al. Laboratory production in vivo of infectious human papillomavirus type 11. *J Virol.* 1987;61:590–593.
22. Jenson AB, Kurman RJ, Lancaster WD. Tissue effects of and host response to human papillomavirus infection. *Obstet Gynecol Clin North Am.* 1987;14:397–406.
23. Cripe TP, Haugen TH, Turk JP, et al. Transcriptional regulation of the human papillomavirus-16 E6-E7 promotor by a keratinocyte-dependent enhancer, and by viral E2 trans-activator and repressor products: implications for carcinogenesis. *EMBO J.* 1987;6:3745–3753.
24. Matsukura T, Koi S, Sugase M. Both episomal and integrated forms of human papillomavirus type 16 are involved in invasive cancers. *Virology.* 1989;172:63–72.
25. Munger K, Phelps WC, Bubb V, Howley PM, Schlengel R. The E6 and E7 genes of human papillomavirus type 16 together are necessary and sufficient for transformation of primary human keratinocytes. *J Virol.* 1989;63:4417–4421.
26. Crook T, Storey A, Almond N, Osborn K, Crawford L. Human papillomavirus type 16 cooperates with activated *ras* and *fos* oncogenes in the hormone-dependent transformation of primary mouse cells. *Proc Natl Acad Sci USA.* 1988;85:8820–8824.
27. Reid TM, Fraser NG, Kernohan IR. Generalized warts and immunodeficiency. *Br J Dermatol.* 1976;95:559–564.
28. Jablonska S. Human papillomaviruses in skin carcinomas. In: Pfister F, ed. *Papillomaviruses and Human Cancer.* Boca Raton, Fla: CRC Press; 1990;1:45–71.
29. Connor ME, Stern PL. Loss of MHC class I expression in cervical carcinomas. *Int J Cancer.* 1990;46:1029–1035.
30. Jarrett WF, O'Neil BW, Gaukroger JM, Smith KT, Laird HM, Campo MS. Studies on vaccination against papillomaviruses: the immunity after infection and vaccination with bovine papillomaviruses of different types. *Vet Rec.* 1990;126:473–475.
31. Steele JC, Gallimore PH. Humoral assays of human sera of disrupted and non-disrupted epitopes of HPV type 1. *Virology.* 1990;174:388–398.
32. Bonnez W, DaRin C, Rose RC, Reichman RC. Use of human papillomavirus type 11 virions in an ELISA to detect specific antibodies in humans with condyloma acuminata. *J Gen Virol.* 1991;72:1343–1347.
33. Christensen ND, Kreider JW, Kan NC, DiAngelo SL. The open reading frame L2 of cotton tail rabbit papillomavirus contains antibody-inducing neutralizing epitopes. *Virology.* 1991;181:572–579.
34. Ghim SJ, Jenson AB, Schlegel R. HPV-1 L 1 protein expressed in cos cells displays conformational epitopes found on intact virions. *Virology.* 1992;190:548.
35. Kirnbauer R, Booy F, Cheng N, Lowy DR, Schiller JT. Papillomavirus L 1 major capsid protein self-assembles into virion-like particles that are highly immunogenic. *Proc Natl Acad Sci USA.* 1992;89:12180.
36. Zhou J, Sun XY, Stenzel DJ, Frazer IH. Expression of vaccinia recombinant HPV 16 L 1 and L 2 ORF proteins in epithelial cells is sufficient for assembly of HPV virion-like particles. *Virology.* 1991;185:251.
37. Ferenczy A, Mitao M, Nagai N. Latent papillomavirus infection and recurring genital warts. *N Engl J Med.* 1985;313:784–788.
38. *Cancer Facts and Figures.* American Cancer Society; 1993.
39. Nasiell K, Roger V, Nasiell M. Behavior of moderate cervical dysplasia during long term follow-up. *Obstet Gynecol.* 1986;67:665–669.
40. Richart RM. Causes and management of cervical intraepithelial neoplasia. *Cancer.* 1987;60:1951–1959.
41. Yoshikawa H, Kawana T, Kitagawa K. Detection and typing of multiple genital human papillomaviruses by DNA amplification with consensus primers. *Jpn J Cancer Res.* 1991;82:524–530.
42. Kurman RJ, Solomon D. *The Bethesda System for Reporting Cervical/Vaginal Cytologic Diagnoses.* New York: Springer-Verlag; 1994.
43. Tawa K, Forsythe A, Cove JK. A comparison of the papanicolaou smear and the cervigram: sensitivity, specificity, and cost analysis. *Obstet Gynecol.* 1988;71:229–235.
44. Hines JF, Ghim SJ, Christensen ND, et al. The expressed L1 proteins of HPV-1, HPV-6, and HPV-11 display type-specific epitopes with native conformation and reactivity with neutralizing and non-neutralizing antibodies. *Pathobiology* (in press).
45. Shah KV. Papillomavirus infections of the respiratory tract, the conjunctiva, and the oral cavity. In: Pfister F, ed. *Papillomaviruses and Human Cancer.* Boca Raton, Fla: CRC Press; 1990;1:73–90.
46. Bethesda Conference Workshop, 1993.

Chapter 21

Human T Lymphotropic Virus Type I

Lydia Navarro-Román, Gustavo C. Román, David Katz, and Elaine S. Jaffe

Thou know'st 'tis common; all that live must die,
Passing through nature to eternity.

William Shakespeare (1564–1616), Hamlet, I, ii, 72

DEFINITION

The retroviruses comprise a large group of RNA viruses characterized by the presence in the viral genome of a gene coding for the polymerase reverse transcriptase. This enzyme allows copying of viral RNA to DNA, which is then integrated into the genome of the host cell. In general, retroviruses have been associated with hematopoietic malignancies and with neurologic disorders in several animal species and, more recently, in humans. Retroviruses are classified in three subfamilies: oncoviruses, lentiviruses, and spumaviruses (or foamy viruses).[1] The human T lymphotropic virus type I (HTLV-I), the first human retrovirus to be isolated,[2] belongs to the subfamily *Oncovirinae* and is believed to cause adult T-cell leukemia/lymphoma (ATLL) and a chronic neurologic disorder currently called HTLV-I–associated myelopathy/tropical spastic paraparesis (HAM/TSP). Other conditions associated with HTLV-I infection include arthritis, pulmonary alveolitis, polymyositis, pseudoamyotrophic lateral sclerosis, and neuritis.[3] The second human retrovirus to be discovered, HTLV-II, was first isolated from a patient with hairy-cell leukemia[4] but has not been associated conclusively with a human hematopoietic malignancy. TSP[5] and cerebellar degeneration in Amerindians[6] have been reported to be linked to HTLV-II.

In addition to HTLV-I, this agent has also been named HTLVcr, human T-cell lymphotropic virus, adult T-cell leukemia virus (ATLV), human adult T-cell leukemia virus, human T-cell leukemia virus, and human T-cell leukemia/lymphoma virus.

GEOGRAPHIC DISTRIBUTION

The most striking feature of the geographic distribution of HTLV-I infection is the high prevalence of seropositivity among island populations. Seroprevalence increases with age and is usually highest in elderly women older than age 65.[7] Hyperendemic areas, ie, those where seroprevalence is higher than 15% in the normal population age 40 and older, have been reported in the Japanese islands of Kyushu, Shikoku, and Okinawa, as well as in Melanesia, particularly in Papua New Guinea, West New Guinea, Solomon Islands, and Vanuatu.[7,8] It has been estimated that 1.2 million carriers exist in Japan with a north to south gradient. Migrant Japanese populations in Brazil, Peru, Bolivia, and Hawaii also have high HTLV-I seroprevalence. In contrast, China and Korea have virtually no HTLV-I infection. Intermediate endemnicity has been reported in the Caribbean islands,[9,10] mainly Jamaica, Martinique, Haiti, St. Lucia, and Trinidad and Tobago, as well as in the Seychelles Islands in the Indian Ocean,[11] and Tumaco in the Pacific Ocean.[12] There are lower rates of HTLV-I infection in the continental United States, mainly among blacks in the Southeast,[13] and inland in Central and South America, predominantly in Panama, Colombia, Ecuador, Chile, and Brazil, as well as in sub-Saharan Africa. Seropositivity for HTLV-I among Amerindians[14] and among intravenous drug abusers in the United States and Europe is largely infection with HTLV-II.[15]

EPIDEMIOLOGY

It has been postulated that HTLV-I infection originated independently in Africa and Japan, and that HTLV-I has been present in Japan for more than 2000 years.[7] Simian T-lymphotropic viruses isolated from African green monkeys (AG-STLV) and from chimpanzees (CH-STLV) are very similar to HTLV-I. Persistence of HTLV-I among isolated insular populations indicates a pattern of infection characterized by high intrafamilial transmission mainly by maternal milk, and to a lesser degree by sexual contact. The following mechanisms of transmission have been described:

1. *Breast feeding:* Mother-to-child transmission via breast feeding is a major route in the persistence of endemic HTLV-I infection.[16] Efficiency of transmission from infected maternal milk ranges from 15% to 22%. Maternal milk has approximately 10^6 cells/mL, of which 10% are T lymphocytes. In carrier mothers, approximately 1% (10^3 cells/mL) of the T cells in breast milk are infected with HTLV-I. Measures to prevent breast feeding by infected mothers beyond the first trimester of life have resulted in decreased seroconversion of the offspring. In cases where infection is acquired perinatally, the incubation period for the development of leukemia or myelopathy is more than three decades. Intrauterine transmission during pregnancy has been demonstrated, but appears to occur with an efficiency of only 7%.[17]

2. *Sexual transmission:* Horizontal transmission occurs primarily from infected males to females, explaining in part the preponderance of the disease in older women married to carrier husbands with high antibody titers. In Japan, during a period of 10 years, the possibility of HTLV-I transmission from infected husband to wife was 61%, and from infected wife to husband only 0.4%.[18] Other sexual risk factors for HTLV-I transmission include male homosexual activity, contact with female prostitutes, history of venereal diseases, active syphilis, and more than 10 lifetime sexual partners.[19] In *de facto* polygamous societies such as those in Africa, the Seychelles, the Caribbean islands, and in the Pacific lowlands of Colombia, sexual transmission appears to be an important mechanism for maintaining HTLV-I endemia.

3. *Blood transfusion:* Seroconversion following blood transfusion was documented in 48% to 82% of seronegative recipients in Japan after receiving seropositive blood or blood components.[7] Seroconversion as a rule did not occur with the use of fresh-frozen plasma, indicating that transmission is mainly cell mediated. From 13% to 20% of patients with HAM/TSP have a previous history of blood transfusion.[20] The incubation period between blood transfusion and onset of neurologic symptoms is quite short: 2.5 years on average in Japan, and from 6 months to 8 years in Martinique. In endemic areas the likelihood of HTLV-I infection from this source is relatively high as 4% to 8% of all blood donors are asymptomatic but have antibodies to HTLV-I. These observations prompted the compulsory testing of all bloods for transfusion in Japan, Martinique, and the United States. A decrease in the incidence of HAM/TSP cases in Japan was documented following screening of blood donors for HTLV-I. In other countries with high HTLV-I seroprevalence, however, this remains a reservoir of infection. Needle sharing among drug addicts is another probable mechanism of transmission of HTLV-I.

VIROLOGICAL ASPECTS

HTLV-I is a type C retrovirus, subfamily *Oncovirinae*, with mature virions of 110 to 140 nm in diameter, characterized by a spherical, centrally located dense nucleoid, enveloped by a glycoprotein membrane with short spikes.[1] The core consists of a dimer of high-molecular-weight RNA subunits, nucleic acid binding proteins, Mg^{++}-dependent reverse transcriptase, and internal core proteins forming the capsid. The envelope, derived from the host cell, is a lipid bilayer to which are anchored both the smaller transmembrane viral protein (p20) and the larger outer membrane glycoprotein (gp46). The HTLV-I genome is similar to that of other retroviruses and contains open reading frames (ORFs) coding for the major structural proteins, *gag* (standing for *g*roup-specific *a*nti*g*en), *pol* (RNA-dependent DNA *pol*ymerase), and *env* (viral *env*elope) proteins.

The *gag*-encoded structural protein precursor is a 53-kd protein ($Pr53^{gag}$) composed of three individual proteins, p15, p24, and p19. The *pol* gene encodes for the protease enzyme reverse transcriptase. The *env* gene codes for an envelope glycoprotein precursor ranging in size from 61,000 to 68,000 d (gp61–68). This glycosylated precursor is cleaved into gp45, the outer envelope glycoprotein, and $p21^{env}$, the smaller transmembrane envelope nonglycosylated protein. The long terminal repeats (LTRs) are situated at the 5′ and 3′ ends of the genome. The U3 region contains regulatory sequences (promoters and enhancers), which activate viral transcription into messenger RNA. In addition, the HTLV-I genome possesses a unique region designated *pX*, between *env* and 3′LTR. The *pX* region codes for three nonstructural proteins named $p40^{tax}$, $p28^{rex}$, and $p21^{XIII}$. The $p40^{tax}$ protein is a transcriptional *trans*-activator for the HTLV-I LTR and for other cellular genes such as interleukin 2 (IL-2), IL-2 receptor alpha and beta chains, granulocyte macrophage colony-stimulating factors (GM-CSF), and lymphotoxins; $p28^{rex}$ is a post-transcriptional *trans*-regulatory protein for HTLV-I expression.

A high degree of immunologic cross-reactivity exists between the *gag* proteins and the reverse transcriptase of HTLV-I and HTLV-II; also, the *env* gene products of HTLV-I and HTLV-II are essentially identical. These two retroviruses are approximately 65% homologous at the nucleotide and amino acid level.[21] For these reasons, serologic assays, including enzyme-linked immunosorbent assay (ELISA), Western blot, and radioimmunoprecipitation (RIPA) are unable to distinguish between the antibody response to HTLV-I and II. HTLV-I/II separation is possible only by polymerase chain reaction (PCR) or by using synthetic peptides exclusively of HTLV-I or II.

LEUKEMOGENESIS

Epidemiologic studies have indicated that acquisition of infection shortly after birth is a risk factor for the development of leukemia, suggesting that a long latency period is required.[22] In contrast with HAM/TSP, no cases of ATLL have been reported following HTLV-I infection by blood transfusion. Other unknown factors, however, are probably also involved in leukemogenesis. Genetic predisposition to ATLL has been suggested by HLA studies in Japan. HTLV-I viral sequences appear to lack proto-oncogenes and random monoclonal viral integration occurs in different chromosomes.[23] Also, specific chromosomal abnormalities have not been observed in ATLL, suggesting that several oncogenes and suppressor genes may intervene in leukemogenesis. The *tax* gene may play an important role because *tax* proteins transactivate other viral and cellular promoters such as IL-2 and IL-2R, which are required to immortalize and transform cells in vitro. Ectopic production of GM-CSF under *tax* control may cause the eosinophilia seen in ATLL, as well as production of parathyroid hormone-related protein (PTHrP), an important factor in the typical hypercalcemia of ATLL. There is, however, only limited experimental evidence implicating *tax* directly in T-cell transformation. Interaction with other viral genes, such as *rex*, may be required.

ADULT T-CELL LEUKEMIA/LYMPHOMA

ATLL is a distinctive clinicopathologic entity and the first malignancy with documented viral cause in humans.[24] The disease is a T-cell form of non-Hodgkin's lymphoma with a post-thymic/mature T4+ cell phenotype. Only a small proportion of carriers (1 per 1500 to 2000) develops leukemia during their lifetime.[7] ATLL has peculiar epidemiologic features: There are geographic clusters, mainly in southwestern Japan and in the Caribbean where it usually begins in adulthood, affects both genders equally, and has a relatively short clinical course.[25] ATLL is classified into four clinical subtypes: acute, chronic, lymphoma, and smoldering.[25]

Acute ATLL

According to the reports from the T- and B-Cell Malignancy Study in Japan, and from experience at the National Cancer Institute (NCI) in the United States, the prototypic form of ATLL is characterized by late onset, with a mean of 56.3 years, and a male to female ratio of 1.2.[25,26] ATLL has an ethnic preponderance in Japanese from Kyushu and Okinawa, and blacks from the Caribbean and the southeastern United States. Cases in whites from Ecuador, Brazil, and Israel, and in an Aleutian from Alaska, however, have also been reported.[26] The disease begins with nonspecific symptoms such as abdominal pain, malaise, weakness, fever, cough, skin rash, and—in about 75% of patients—lymphadenopathy.[27] The principal clinical manifestations (Table 21–1) are leukemia, hepatosplenomegaly, skin lesions, lymphadenopathy, and invasion of lung. Hypercalcemia is typical, with or without lytic bone lesions; generalized increased uptake may be noted on radionucleotide scan. Hepatic failure and encephalopathy may be prominent. Involvement of cerebrospinal fluid and lym-

TABLE 21–1. CLINICAL MANIFESTATIONS OF ACUTE ADULT T-CELL LEUKEMIA[a]

Manifestation	At presentation (%)	During Course (%)
Leukemia	69	100
Lymphadenopathy	77	85
Hepatosplenomegaly	61	—[b]
Skin lesions	61	—
Hypercalcemia	75	83
Lytic bone lesions	38	—
Bone marrow infiltration	58	—
Stage IV	100	—

[a] From Jaffe.[26]

[b] —, not evaluated during clinical course.

phomatous meningitis are relatively frequent. Involvement of peripheral blood is common with circulating atypical lymphocytes demonstrating multilobed, pleomorphic nuclei (Figure 21–1). Anemia and thrombocytopenia are infrequent and mild and occur in the absence of bone marrow involvement by ATLL cells. Eosinophilia may be prominent. Most patients present with stage IV disease.[25–27]

Immunosuppression is common and is manifested by anergy on skin testing, impaired cellular and immune responses, and occurrence of opportunistic infections. Abnormalities of helper, killer, and suppressor T lymphocytes, and B-cell immunoglobulin synthesis have been reported. In spite of treatment with several forms of combination chemotherapy, the disease is aggressive and has a poor prognosis. The median survival is only 10 months.[25] Most deaths are caused by opportunistic infections, including *Pneumocystis carinii* pneumonia, cytomegalovirus infections, cryptococcal meningitis, fungal and bacterial sepsis, and strongyloidiasis.[25a]

Chronic ATLL

Patients with chronic leukemia have an absolute lymphocytosis, presence of abnormal T lymphocytes ($>3.5 \times 10^9$/L), increased lactate dehydrogenase (LDH) values up to twice the normal levels, and absence of hypercalcemia or bone involvement. Occasionally, these patients present with fever, skin lesions, pulmonary involvement, and slight lymphadenopathy.

Lymphoma Type of ATLL

Approximately 30% of patients present with prominent lymphadenopathy and tumors in skin and other organs, without overt involvement of peripheral blood. There is usually absence of hepatosplenomegaly, hypercalcemia, or increased LDH. The prognosis appears to be better than for ATLL, although these patients may evolve to acute leukemia. Lymphomatous presentations are more common in some endemic areas. For instance, in the Caribbean the lymphoma type of ATLL is more common than in Japan.

Smoldering ATLL

This clinical form is characterized mainly by long-lasting skin lesions such as erythema, papules, or nodules, infiltration of the skin by abnormal lymphocytes, and minimal involvement of peripheral blood by abnormal cells (0% to 2%). Some smoldering cases may have lymphocytic infiltrates of lung.[23] The disease evolves slowly but may develop into acute ATLL after several years. HTLV-I proviral DNA is monoclonally integrated in the abnormal T lymphocyte population in smoldering ATLL.[28] In contrast, HTLV-I is polyclonally integrated in healthy carriers. Table 21–2 summarizes the clinical

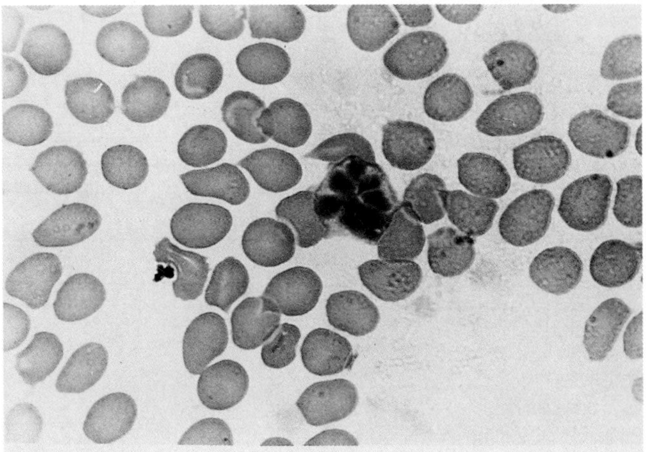

Figure 21–1. Abnormal circulating peripheral blood lymphocyte. Nucleus is markedly irregular, polylobated with condensed chromatin and moderately basophilic cytoplasm.

TABLE 21–2. CLASSIFICATION OF ADULT T-CELL LEUKEMIA/LYMPHOMA[a]

Category	Features
Acute leukemia	Frequent hepatosplenomegaly, lymphadenopathy, and skin infiltration. Common CNS involvement. Frequent "flower cells" in peripheral blood. Hypercalcemia, elevated LDH. Poor prognosis, death in months.
Chronic leukemia	Increased WBC count with T lymphocytosis, rare "flower cells." Pulmonary and skin disease. Some have slight lymphadenopathy, and hepatosplenomegaly. LDH up to twice normal. Absence of elevated Ca. Better survival of up to 5 years.
Lymphoma type	Predominant lymphadenopathy with absence of peripheral blood involvement; normal skin, liver, spleen, and LDH. Hypercalcemia may be observed. Progression to leukemia in some cases.
Smoldering type	Predominant cutaneous involvement. Rare involvement of lung and other tissues or organs. More than 5% abnormal T lymphocytes in peripheral blood. Normal lymphocyte count, Ca, LDH. Chronic disease for up to 10 years. May evolve to leukemia.

[a] Modified from the Japanese Lymphoma Study Group.[29]

classification of ATLL according to the Japanese Lymphoma Study Group.[29] A classification intended for epidemiological studies has been recently proposed.[29a]

PATHOLOGY

Peripheral Blood

Abnormal circulating cells are the hallmark of HTLV-I infection. Rare abnormal cells may be present in normal HTLV-I carriers and represent about 5% of the circulating lymphocytes in the smoldering type. The percentage of abnormal cells increases further in the chronic leukemia type and finally reaches the massive invasion of the peripheral blood characteristic of acute ATLL. The predominant abnormal circulating cell is a medium-size lymphocyte, with varying degrees of nuclear pleomorphism, polylobation and prominent nucleoli, thick nuclear membrane, and coarse chromatin. These cells are also known as *flower cells* (Figure 21–1). In the chronic type, in addition to flower cells, abnormal lymphocytes reminiscent of those of T-cell chronic lymphocytic leukemia (CLL-like cells) are present. In the smoldering type, and occasionally in carriers, there are a few abnormal circulating cells with coarse chromatin and slight indentation of nuclei.

Lymph Nodes

The histopathology of lymph nodes in ATLL is varied and there may be lymphomas of several histologic types (Table 21–3). In spite of the diversity, all cells are clonally related and are present in various proportions.[30] In the classic acute form of ATLL, involvement of lymph nodes is diffuse and the normal architecture is effaced with preservation of peripheral sinuses. Partially involved lymph nodes show a leukemic pattern of infiltration. The proliferating cells vary in both size and shape. The cells at the small end of the spectrum, so-called medium-size cells by the Japanese Lymphoma

TABLE 21–3. HISTOPATHOLOGY OF ADULT T-CELL LEUKEMIA/LYMPHOMA[a]

Type	NCI-USA (%)	Japan (%)
Small cell (WDL)[b]	0	2
Medium-size cell (PDL)	15	36
Mixed cell (MCT)	38	8
Large cell (HIST)	8	8
Large cell, immunoblastic (pleomorphic)	38	42
Other	0	3

[a] Modified from Jaffe et al.[30]
[b] JLSG classification. WDL, well-differentiated lymphocytic; PDL, poorly differentiated lymphocytic; MCT, mixed-cell type; HIST, histiocytic.

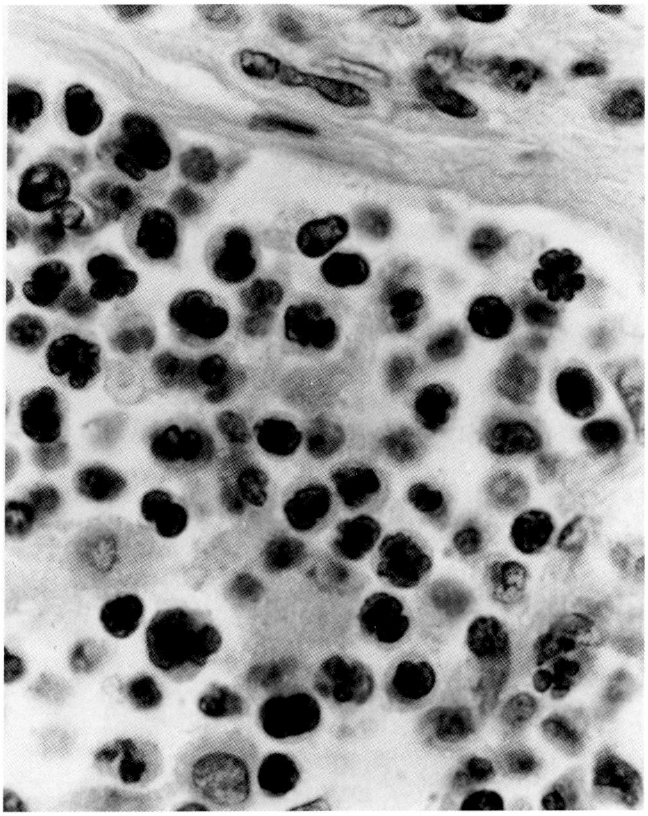

Figure 21–2. Medium-size cell type lymph node. Cells have pleomorphic irregular nuclei with condensed chromatin, and abundant pale cytoplasm.

Study Group (JLSG), are similar to those present in the peripheral blood and have markedly irregular and polylobated nuclear contours, condensed chromatin, and inconspicuous nucleoli (Figure 21–2). These cells predominate in the medium cell type but are present in different proportion in all the histologic variants. In the mixed cell type of the JLSG, large cells of varying size containing basophilic or amphophilic cytoplasm are found intermixed with the more abundant medium-size cells. In the large cell type there is diffuse involvement of the lymph node by cells of moderate size, with scant amount of cytoplasm. Nuclei are round to oval with dispersed chromatin and multiple small distinct nucleoli (Figure 21–3). Larger transformed cells, binucleated or multinucleated, and with prominent inclusion-like nucleoli resembling Reed–Sternberg cells, are occasionally present in the pleomorphic forms. Eosinophils are common.

Changes in lymph nodes associated with mild adenopathy have been reported in HTLV-I seropositive patients with infrequent atypical cells in the peripheral blood.[31] These lymph nodes had preserved nodal architecture, diffuse infiltration by small to medium lymphocytes (CD4+) and a few immunoblast-like cells in the

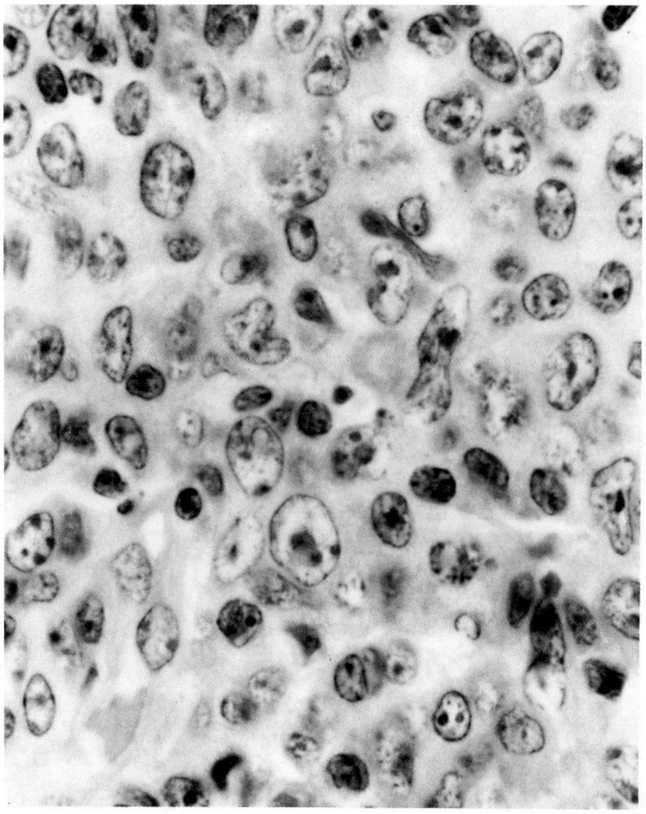

Figure 21–3. Malignant lymphoma, large cell type lymph node. Cells are relatively uniform in size with round to oval nuclei, nuclear contours, and multiple small nucleoli. Occasional lobulated cells are present.

enlarged paracortex, resembling changes of viral infection. Proviral DNA was detected in the lymph node by Southern blot, in situ hybridization, and PCR, but neither rearrangement nor deletion of T-cell receptors and immunoglobulin heavy chain genes was identified.[31] These changes may reflect an early reactive response to viral infection, prior to the development of malignancy.

Skin

Infiltration of skin by neoplastic cells is characteristic of ATLL. Skin lesions constitute a typical feature of the smoldering type, but are also in other forms such as acute ATLL. The most frequent finding in the skin is perivascular infiltration in the upper dermis by neoplastic pleomorphic cells, with epidermal compromise and formation of Pautrier microabscesses (Figure 21–4). Other reactive cells such as eosinophils and plasma cells are usually absent. The skin lesions are on occasion indistinguishable from those of mycosis fungoides/Sézary syndrome (MF/SS).[26,30]

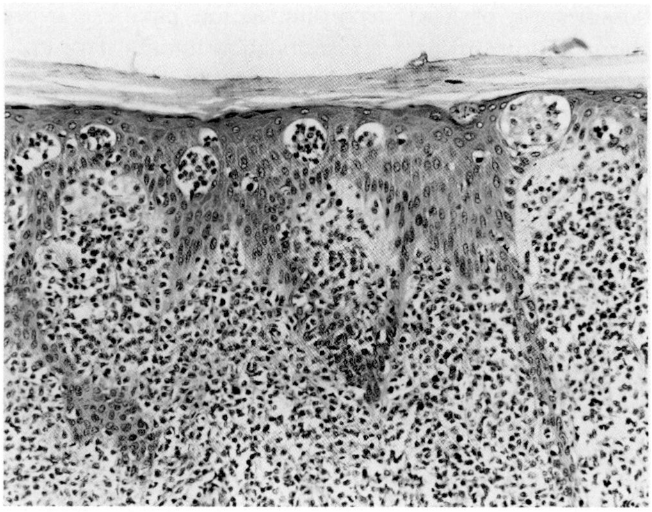

Figure 21–4. Skin. Cutaneous involvement in ATLL. Extensive dermal and epidermal lymphocytic infiltrate with Pautrier microabscesses.

BONE AND BONE MARROW

Neoplastic cells in bone marrow have been reported in 58% of patients at the NCI[26] and all presented in the leukemic stage. Bone marrow involvement was usually sparse, with rare cells dispersed among the normal marrow hematopoietic elements. Bone lesions in cases presenting with hypercalcemia consist of microcystic cortical degeneration with marked osteoclastic activity and bone remodeling (Figure 21–5). About 26% of all patients in Japan[25] and 75% in the United States[26,30] have hypercalcemia when first seen. Induction of PTHrP by the HTLV-I *trans*-activator from the *tax* gene product appears to be an important mechanism for production of hypercalcemia.[32,33]

NERVOUS SYSTEM

Neurologic Complications of ATLL

Leukemic cells in the cerebrospinal fluid (CSF) are frequent in acute ATLL. At autopsy the nervous system is involved in more than 60% of cases.[34] The most common finding is leukemic cell infiltration of the brain and the retina, accompanied in some cases by hemorrhage and necrosis. Disturbances of consciousness, confusion, and encephalopathy may also be caused by metabolic abnormalities, in particular hypercalcemia. Cytokines, such as tumor necrosis factor, lymphotoxin, and interleukins induced by expression of viral genes, may pro-

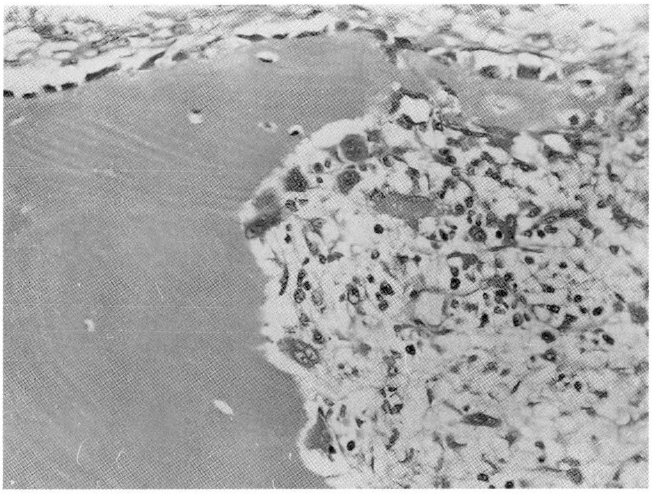

Figure 21–5. Bone marrow. Lytic bone lesion free of tumor with marked osteoclastic activity.

duce neurologic dysfunction. Meningoencephalitis from opportunistic infections, mainly cryptococcosis, is also common.[25a] Involvement of the peripheral nerves by leukemic infiltrates has been reported in more than 10% of fatal cases.

HTLV-I–Associated Myelopathy/Tropical Spastic Paraparesis

Tropical spastic paraparesis (TSP) is a chronic myelopathy prevalent in tropical regions.[35] TSP has been strongly linked to HTLV-I infection, not only in the Caribbean where this association was first demonstrated,[36] but also in other tropical regions, such as the Seychelles.[37] Additional evidence was the demonstration that most patients with "primary lateral sclerosis" in southwestern Japan actually had HTLV-I–associated myelopathy (HAM).[38] The two diseases are probably a single entity,[39] currently called HAM/TSP, defined as a chronic myelopathy characterized by the presence of anti–HTLV-I antibodies in serum and CSF. The lifetime risk of HAM/TSP has been calculated at one quarter of 1% among HTLV-I carriers.

The disease predominates in women with onset in late adult life, usually after 40 years of age.[40] HAM/TSP is characterized by a chronic and slowly progressive spastic paraparesis with back pain, impotence in males, spastic bladder, and sensory signs and symptoms, such as minimally decreased vibratory perception. Most patients have pyramidal tract signs, including spasticity, brisk knee reflexes, clonus, and Babinski's sign. Weakness of legs usually affects the proximal muscle groups causing a slow scissoring gait, with deliberate dragging and shuffling of the feet. The CSF usually has mildly increased protein and cells, and rare abnormal lymphocytes also.[36,38] The differential diagnosis of HAM/TSP includes the chronic progressive spinal form of multiple sclerosis (MS). In most patients, the clinical and laboratory findings permit the separation of the two diseases. In some patients with HAM/TSP, however, magnetic resonance imaging of brain reveals periventricular lesions whose pathologic basis is unknown,[41,42] although they could be chronic inflammatory infiltrates.[43] It has been clearly demonstrated, nonetheless, that HTLV-I does not cause MS.

The evidence that HTLV-I causes HAM/TSP includes the presence of IgG antibodies to HTLV-I in serum and CSF, usually in high titers,[36,38] detection of viral antigens and viral genome in peripheral and CSF lymphocytes,[44] or in central nervous system (CNS) autopsy tissue,[45,45a] and viral isolation from CSF lymphocytes. However, there has been no convincing morphologic demonstration of productive retroviral infection in the spinal cord of these patients.

The neuropathology of HAM/TSP is consistent with a chronic myelitis with degeneration of the white matter, particularly of the lateral columns (Figure 21–6),

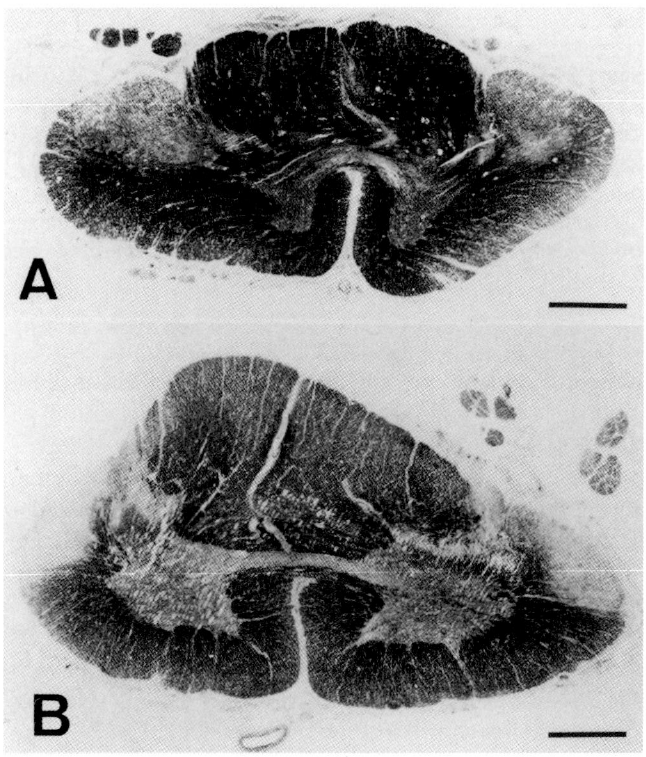

Figure 21–6. Spinal cord sections in patient with HAM/TSP showing symmetric degeneration of lateral columns. (**A**) Middle thoracic cord. (**B**) Lumbar cord (Klüver–Barrera stain; bar, 1 mm). *(Courtesy of Román, Vernant, and Osame.[3])*

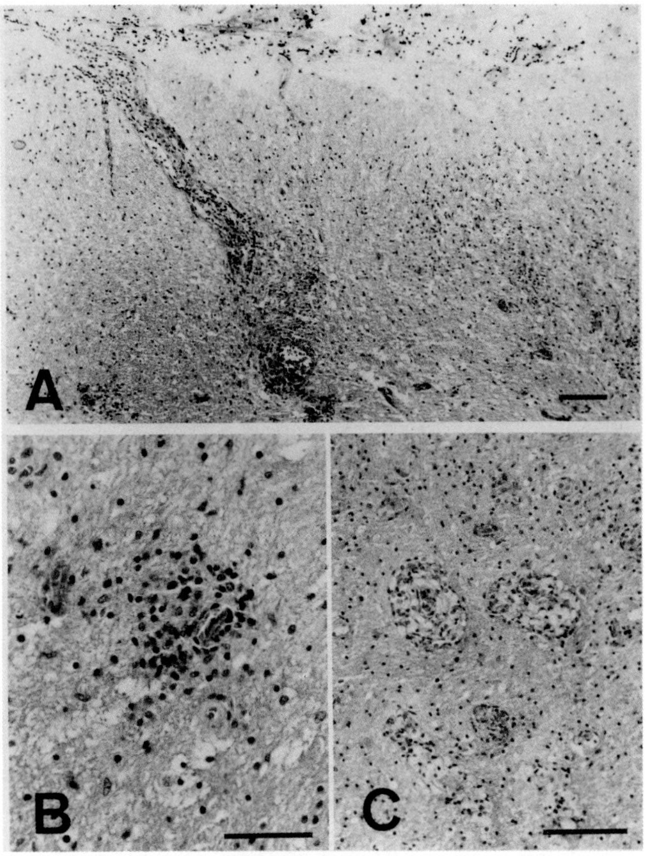

Figure 21–7. Microscopic appearance of spinal cord in HAM/TSP. (**A**) Inflammatory exudate in lumbar spinal cord and leptomeninges (hematoxylin-eosin, bar, 100 μm). (**B**) Perivascular and parenchymal mononuclear cell infiltration in lumbar spinal cord (hematoxylin-eosin; bar, 50 μm). (**C**) Perivascular accumulation of foamy macrophages in lateral columns of thoracic spinal cord (hematoxylin-eosin; bar, 100 μm). *(Courtesy of Román, Vernant, and Osame.[3])*

involving both axons and myelin, in combination with a chronic meningomyelitis and fibrous thickening of blood vessels.[45a,46] Additional features include leptomeningeal fibrosis and astrogliosis of the parenchyma, both presumably reactive (Figure 21–7). Perivascular inflammatory cell infiltrates may extend beyond the spinal cord to brain and cerebellum.[43,45a] Peripheral nerve involvement may occur.[46a] Mild inflammatory cell infiltrates may be around blood vessels but there is no vasculitis.[47] Patients have been described with HTLV-I–associated pseudoamyotrophic lateral sclerosis (pseudo-ALS) with atrophy and fasciculations of the tongue, small muscles of the hands, and other muscle groups.[48] An HTLV-I–associated inflammatory myopathy (polymyositis), with or without spastic paraparesis, has also been documented.[49,50,50a] A recent report of a child with congenital hydrocephalus, born to an HTLV-I–infected mother, suggests a potential for intrauterine infection of the nervous system.[51] TSP has been observed in patients dually infected with HIV-1 and HTLV-I[52] or with HIV-1 and HTLV-II,[53] requiring differentiation of the vacuolar myelopathy associated with the acquired immunodeficiency syndrome (AIDS), and raising issues of interaction between the human retroviruses.[54]

Other Lesions

Non-neurologic manifestations have been described in patients infected by HTLV-I, and these are often seen in association with HAM/TSP[3]: Pulmonary T-cell lymphocytic interstitial pneumonia and bronchoalveolar lymphocytosis have been reported in patients with HAM/TSP and among asymptomatic HTLV-I carriers in Martinique and Japan.[55] Pulmonary involvement may be subclinical, with normal chest x rays and computed tomography scans. Occasionally, mild interstitial pneumonitis is documented. Morphologically normal lymphocytes represent 20% of the cells in bronchial lavages, with an increased proportion of CD8+ and decreased CD4+ lymphocytes. Uveitis, arthropathy, Sjögren's or *sicca* syndrome, vasculitis, xerosis and ichthyoses, cryoglobulinemia, and monoclonal gammopathy have also been described.[3] The dual occurrence of HAM/TSP and ATLL remains exceptional.

HTLV-I in Mycosis Fungoides/Sézary Syndrome

Although patients with MF/SS are usually seronegative for HTLV-I antibodies, many studies suggest an association between MF/SS and HTLV or a related retrovirus. The cells lack the intact viral genome but using primers and probes specific for the *tax* region of HTLV I/II and the *pol* region of HTLV-I, approximately one third of patients are positive.[56] The lymphocytes are negative for reverse transcriptase and p24 protein, further evidence that intact virus is not present. These studies suggest a potential role for HTLV in MF/SS.[57]

DIAGNOSIS

Clinical Features

In the absence of identification of the virus, a working point score has been developed for the diagnosis of ATLL.[29a] This score uses routine clinical and laboratory data, immunophenotypic characterization of the tumor cells, and serologic data for HTLV-I antibodies. This approach should be useful in epidemiologic studies, where sophisticated laboratory analysis is not always possible. As noted earlier, ethnic differences do appear to have an impact on the clinical manifestations of HTLV-I.[58] Leukemia is much more common in individuals of Japanese ancestry than in patients of African-American descent with ATLL.

The HTLV-I virus has been isolated from peripheral lymphocytes of patients with ATLL, as well as from CSF lymphocytes of patients with HAM/TSP. Also, proviral DNA can be detected in peripheral blood and CSF lymphocytes by Southern blot hybridization, enzymatic DNA amplification, or PCR. More commonly, diagnosis is based on the demonstration of circulating antibodies by serologic techniques.

Serologic Diagnosis

As with any other viral infection, HTLV-I infection induces an immunologic response against a series of antigenic proteins. Screening for antibodies to HTLV-I/II is usually done with ELISA or particle agglutination assays.[59] Samples found to be repeatedly positive on the initial ELISA are confirmed by Western blot (WB), indirect immunofluorescent assay, or RIPA. A specimen is confirmed as HTLV I/II *positive* by the presence of antibodies to the core gene products (*gag* p24) and the envelope gene products (either *env* gp45 or gp61); *indeterminate*, when antibody to any viral gene product is found in either WB (p15, p19, p24, p33, gp45) or RIPA (p24, $p40^{tax}$, $Pr53^{gag}$, gp61); and *negative* if no antibodies to viral genes are observed on WB or RIPA. Further differentiation into HTLV-I or HTLV-II is possible by using synthetic envelope recombinant peptides (rgp46) or a common HTLV-I/II epitope purified recombinant transmembrane protein[60] or by PCR. The seroprevalence curve for HTLV-I increases progressively from 5% from birth to adolescence to about 35% to 50% among elderly women.[7]

Molecular Pathologic Diagnosis

Immunophenotypic Characteristics of ATLL

Typical ATLL cells have a mature helper T-cell surface phenotype with CD2, CD3, CD4, and CD5 being commonly expressed. CD7 is usually negative, CD8 and TCRδ1 lymphocytes are usually absent. High expression of the IL-2R alpha chain (p55 Tac protein) has been described and helps to differentiate ATLL from other peripheral T-cell lymphomas.[61] In addition to the usual CD+/CD8− phenotype, a minority of patients have aberrant expression of antigens and patients with CD4−/CD8− (double negative) and CD4+/CD8+ (double positive) have been described. During evolution of the disease, changes of cell surface antigen expression with deletions of CD3 and CD5 have also been described.[62]

Other Molecular Techniques

Demonstration of monoclonal or oligoclonal integration of HTLV-I provirus by the Southern blot technique provides definitive evidence of viral infection in cases of ATLL. This technique is applicable in patients where frozen tissue or cell suspensions are available for the extraction of high-molecular-weight genomic DNA. The use of the enzymatic in vitro amplification of DNA by PCR techniques allows the demonstration of proviral sequences in DNA extracted from tissues fixed in formalin and embedded in paraffin.[45a,63] Oligoprimers recognizing sequences corresponding to different regions of the viral genome, usually *pol, gag,* and *tax*, are used for this purpose. Amplification of at least two of the viral genes should be demonstrated. In situ hybridization techniques using DNA and RNA probes have been used experimentally to determine the presence of provirus in nervous tissues, muscle, lung, and other tissues.[64]

REFERENCES

1. Cann AJ, Chen ISY. Human T-cell leukemia virus types I and II. In: Fields BN, Knipe DR, eds. *Virology*. New York: Raven Press; 1990:1501–1527.
2. Poiesz BJ, Ruscetti FW, Gazdar AF, Bunn PA, Minna JD, Gallo RC. Detection and isolation of type C retrovirus particles from fresh and cultured lymphocytes in a patient with cutaneous T cell lymphoma. *Proc Natl Acad Sci USA*. 1980;77:7415–7419.
3. Román GC, Vernant J-C, Osame M, eds. *HTLV-I and the Nervous System*. New York: Alan Liss; 1989:93–609.
4. Kalyanaraman VS, Sarngadharan MG, Robert-Guroff M, Miyoshi M, Golde E, Gallo RC. A new subtype of human T-leukemia virus (HTLV-II) associated with a T cell variant of hairy cell leukemia. *Science*. 1982;218:571–573.
5. Jacobson S, Lehky T, Nishimura M, Robinson S, McFarlin DE, Dhib-Jalbut S. Isolation of HTLV-II from a patient with chronic, progressive neurologic disease clinically indistinguishable from HAM/TSP. *Ann Neurol*. 1993;33:392–396.
6. Hjelle B, Appenzeller O, Mills R. Chronic neurodegenerative disease associated with HTLV-II infection. *Lancet*. 1992;339:645–646.
7. Mueller N. The epidemiology of HTLV-I infection. *Cancer Causes Control*. 1991;2:37–52.
8. Yanagihara R, Ajdukiewicz AB, Garruto RM, et al. Human T-lymphotropic virus type I infection in the Solomon Islands. *Am J Trop Med Hyg*. 1991;44:122–130.
9. Blattner WA, Kalyanaraman VS, Robert-Guroff M, et al. The human type-C retrovirus, HTLV-I, in Blacks from the Caribbean region and relationship to adult T-cell leukemia/lymphoma. *Int J Cancer*. 1982;30:257–264.
10. Maloney EM, Murphy EL, Figueroa JP, et al. Human T-lymphotropic virus type I (HTLV-I) seroprevalence in Jamaica II. Geographic and ecologic determinants. *Am J Epidemiol*. 1991;133:1125–1134.
11. Lavanchy D, Bovet P, Hollanda J, Shamlaye CF, Burczak JD, Lee H. High seroprevalence of HTLV-I in the Seychelles. *Lancet*. 1991;337:248–249.

12. Trujillo JM, Concha M, Muñoz A, et al. Seroprevalence and cofactors of HTLV-I infection in Tumaco, Colombia. *AIDS Res Hum Retro.* 1992,8:651–657.
13. Blayney DW, Blattner WA, Robert-Guroff M, et al. The human T-cell leukemia/lymphoma virus in the southeastern United States. *JAMA.* 1983;250:1048–1052.
14. Gabbai AA, Bordin JO, Vieira-Filho JPB, et al. Selectivity of human T lymphotropic virus type-1 (HTLV-1) and HTLV-2 infection among different populations in Brazil. *Am J Trop Med Hyg.* 1993;49:664–671.
15. Lee H, Swanson P, Shorty VS, Zack JA, Rosenblatt JD, Chen ISY. High rate of HTLV-II infections in seropositive IV drug abusers in New Orleans. *Science.* 1989;244:471–475.
16. Hino S. Milk-borne transmission of HTLV-I as a major route in the endemic cycle. *Acta Paediatr Jpn.* 1989;31:428–435.
17. Fujino T, Fujiyoshi T, Yashiki S, Sonoda S, Otsuka H, Nagata Y. HTLV-I transmission from mother to fetus via placenta. *Lancet.* 1992;340:1157.
18. Kajiyama W, Kashiwagi S, Ikematsu H, Hayashi J, Nomura H, Okochi K. Intrafamilial transmission of adult T cell leukemia. *J Infect Dis.* 1986;154:851–857.
19. Murphy EL, Figueroa JP, Gibbs WN, et al. Sexual transmission of human T-lymphotropic virus. *Ann Intern Med.* 1989;111:555–560.
20. Osame M, Janssen R, Kubota H, et al. Nationwide survey of HTLV-I–associated myelopathy in Japan: association with blood transfusion. *Ann Neurol.* 1990;28:50–56.
21. Shimotohno K, Takahashi Y, Shimizu N, et al. Complete nucleotide sequence of an infectious clone of human T cell leukemia virus type II: an open reading frame for the protease gene. *Proc Natl Acad Sci USA.* 1985;82:3101–3105.
22. Yoshida M, Fujisawa J. Positive and negative regulation of HTLV-I gene expression and their role in leukemogenesis in ATL. In: Seiki M, Hinuma Y, Yoshida M, eds. *Advances in Adult T-cell Leukemia and HTLV-I Research.* Gann Monographs on Cancer Research No. 39. Tokyo: Japan Scientific Societies Press; 1992:217–236.
23. Takatsuki K, Hattori S, Hirayama Y, Yoshida M. Nonspecific integration of the HTLV-I provirus genome into adult T-cell leukemia cells. *Nature.* 1984;309:640–642.
24. Takatsuki K, Uchiyama T, Sagawa K, Yodoi J. Adult T-cell leukemia in Japan. In: Seno S, Takaku F, Irino S, eds. *Topics in Hematology.* Amsterdam: Excerpta Medica; 1977:73–77.
25. Shimoyama M, Takatsuki K, Araki K, and The Lymphoma Study Group (1984–1987): Major prognostic factors of patients with adult T-cell leukemia/lymphoma: a cooperative study. *Leukemia Res.* 1991;15:81–90.
25a. White JD, Zaknoen SL, Kasten-Sportes C, Navarro-Román L, Nelson DL, Waldman TA. Infectious complications and immunodeficiency in patients with HTLV-I-associated adult T-cell leukemia/lymphoma. *Cancer.* 1995;75:1598–1607.
26. Jaffe ES. Pathologic and clinical spectrum of post-thymic T-cell malignancies. *Cancer Invest.* 1984;2:413–426.
27. Kim JH, Durack DT. Manifestations of human T-lymphotropic virus type I infection. *Am J Med.* 1988;84:919–928.
28. Kinoshita K, Amagasaki T, Ikeda S, et al. Preleukemic state of adult T-cell leukemia: abnormal T lymphocytosis induced by human adult T-cell leukemia virus. *Blood.* 1985;66:120–127.
29. Shimoyama M, and members of The T-Lymphoma Study Group. Diagnostic criteria and classification of clinical subtypes of adult T-cell leukemia/lymphoma. *Br J Haematol.* 1991;79:428–439.
29a. Levine PH, Cleghorn F, Manns A, et al. Adult T-cell leukemia/lymphoma: a working point-score classification for epidemiological studies. *Int J Cancer.* 1994;59:491–493.
30. Jaffe ES, Cossman J, Blattner WA, et al. The pathologic spectrum of adult T-cell leukemia/lymphoma in the United States. *Am J Surg Pathol.* 1984;8:263–275.
31. Oshima K, Kikuchi M, Masuda Y, et al. Human T-cell leukemia virus type I associated lymphadenitis. *Cancer.* 1992;69:239–248.
32. Kiyokawa T, Yamaguchi K, Takeya M, et al. Hypercalcemia and osteoclast proliferation in adult T-cell leukemia. *Cancer.* 1987;59:1187–1191.
33. Watanabe T, Yamaguchi K, Takatsuki K, Osame M, Yoshida M. Constitutive expression of parathyroid hormone-related protein gene in human T-cell leukemia virus type I (HTLV-I) carriers and adult T-cell leukemia patients that can be *trans*-activated by HTLV-I *tax* gene. *J Exp Med.* 1990;172:759–765.
34. Román GC, Román LN, Osame M. Human T-lymphotropic virus type I neurotropism. *Prog Med Virol.* 1990;37:190–210.
35. Román GC, Spencer PS, Schoenberg BS, Tropical myeloneuropathies: the hidden endemias. *Neurology.* 1985;35:1158–1170.
36. Vernant JC, Maurs L, Gessain A, et al. Endemic tropical spastic paraparesis associated with human T-lymphotropic virus type I: a clinical and sero-epidemiological study of 25 cases. *Ann Neurol.* 1987;21:123–130.
37. Román GC, Schoenberg BS, Madden DL, et al. Human T-lymphotropic virus type I antibodies in the serum of patients with tropical spastic paraparesis in the Seychelles. *Arch Neurol.* 1987;44:605–607.
38. Osame M, Matsumoto M, Usuku K, et al. Chronic progressive myelopathy associated with elevated antibodies to human T-lymphotropic virus type I and adult T-cell leukemialike cells. *Ann Neurol.* 1987;21:117–122.
39. Román GC, Osame M. Identity of HTLV-I–associated tropical spastic paraparesis and HTLV-I–associated myelopathy. *Lancet.* 1988;i:651.
40. Román GC. Tropical spastic paraparesis and HTLV-I myelitis. In: McKendall RR, ed. *Handbook of Clinical Neurology: Viral Disease.* Amsterdam: Elsevier; 1989;56:525–542.
41. Mattson DN, McFarlin DE, Mora C, Zaninovic V. Central nervous system lesions detected by magnetic resonance imaging in an HTLV-I antibody positive symptomless individual. *Lancet.* 1987;ii:49.
42. Tournier-Lasserve E, Gout O, Gessain A, et al. HTLV-I,

brain abnormalities on magnetic resonance imaging, and relation with multiple sclerosis. *Lancet.* 1987;ii:49–50.

43. Smith CR, Dickson D, Samkoff L. Recurrent encephalopathy and seizures in a US native with HTLV-I–associated myelopathy/tropical spastic paraparesis. *Neurology.* 1992;42:658–661.
44. Bhagavati S, Ehrlich G, Kula RW, et al. Detection of human T-cell lymphoma/leukemia virus type I DNA and antigen in spinal fluid and blood of patients with chronic progressive myelopathy. *N Engl J Med.* 1988;318: 1141–1147.
45. Kira J, Itoyama Y, Koyanagi Y, et al. Presence of HTLV-I proviral DNA in central nervous system of patients with HTLV-I–associated myelopathy. *Ann Neurol.* 1992;31: 39–45.

45a. Navarro-Román L, Corbin D, Katz D, et al. Defective HTLV-I proviral DNA in spinal cord but absence in lymph node of a patient with concomitant tropical spastic paraparesis and Hodgkin's disease. *Human Pathol.* 1994;25:1101–1106.

46. Iwasaki Y. Pathology of chronic myelopathy associated with HTLV-I infection (HAM/TSP). *J Neurol Sci.* 1990; 96:103–123.

46a. Román GC. Tropical neuropathies. In: Hartung H-P, ed. *Peripheral Neuropathies: Part I.* Baillière's Clinical Neurology. London: Baillière Tindall; 1995;4:469–487.

47. Said G, Goulon-Goeau C, La Croix C, et al. Inflammatory lesions of peripheral nerve in a patient with human lymphotropic virus type-I–associated myelopathy. *Ann Neurol.* 1988;24:275–277.
48. Román GC, Vernant JC, Osame M. Motor neuron disease and HTLV-I infection. In: DeJong JMBV, ed. *Handbook of Clinical Neurology: Diseases of the Motor System.* 1991;59:447–457.
49. Morgan OS, Rodgers-Johnson P, Mora C, Char G. HTLV-I and polymyositis in Jamaica. *Lancet.* 1989;2:1184–1187.
50. Dalakas M, León-Monzón M, Illa I, Rodgers-Johnson P, Morgan O. Immunopathology of HTLV-I–associated polymyositis (HTLV-I-PM): studies in six patients. *Neurology.* 1992;42(suppl 3):301–302.

50a. Gabbai AA, Wiley CA, Oliveira ASB, et al. Skeletal muscle involvement in tropical spastic paraparesis/HTLV-I-associated myelopathy. *Muscle Nerve.* 1994;17:923–930.

51. Tohyama J, Kawahara H, Inagaki M, et al. Clinical and neuroradiologic findings of congenital hydrocephalus in an infant born to a mother with HTLV-I–associated myelopathy. *Neurology.* 1992;42:1406–1408.
52. Rosenblum MK, Brew BJ, Hahn B, et al. Human T-lymphotropic virus type-I–associated myelopathy in patients with the acquired immunodeficiency syndrome. *Hum Pathol.* 1992;23:513–519.
53. Berger JR, Svenningsson A, Najjanti S, Resnick L. Tropical spastic paraparesis-like illness occurring in a patient dually infected with HIV-1 and HTLV-II. *Neurology.* 1991;41:85–87.
54. Gessain A, Gout O. Chronic myelopathy associated with human T-lymphotropic virus type I (HTLV-I). *Ann Intern Med.* 1992;117:933–946.
55. Couderc LJ, Caubarrere I, Venet A, et al. Bronchoalveolar lymphocytosis in patients with tropical spastic paraparesis associated with human T-cell lymphotropic virus type I. *Ann Intern Med.* 1988;109:625–628.
56. Manca N, Piacentini E, Gelmi M, et al. Persistence of human T-cell lymphotropic virus type I (HTLV-I) sequences in peripheral blood mononuclear cells from patients with mycosis fungoides. *J Exp Med.* 1994;180: 1973–1978.
57. Hall WT. Human T-cell lymphotropic virus type I and cutaneous T-cell leukemia/lymphoma. *J Exp Med.* 1994; 180:1581–1585.
58. Levine PH, Manns A, Jaffe ES, et al. The effect of ethnic differences on the pattern of HTLV-I associated T-cell leukemia/lymphoma (HATL) in the United States. *Int J Cancer.* 1994;56:177–181.
59. Constantine NT, Callahan JD, Watts DM. *Retroviral Testing. Essentials for Quality Control and Laboratory Diagnosis.* Boca Raton, Fla: CRC Press; 1992:103–111.
60. Hadlock KG, Lipka J, Chow TP, Foung SKH, Reyes GR. Cloning and analysis of a recombinant antigen containing an epitope specific for human T-cell lymphotropic virus type II. *Blood.* 1992;79:2789–2796.
61. Waldmann TA. Human T-cell lymphotropic virus type I-associated adult T-cell leukemia. *JAMA.* 1995;273:735–737.
62. Kamihira S. Hemato-cytological aspects of adult T-cell leukemia. In: Seiki M, Hinuma Y, Yoshida M, eds. *Advances in Adult T-cell Leukemia and HTLV-I Research.* Gann Monographs on Cancer Research No. 39. Tokyo: Japan Scientific Societies Press; 1992:17–32.
63. Shibata D, Tokunaga M, Sasaki N, Nanba K. Detection of human T-cell leukemia virus type I proviral sequences from fixed tissues of seropositive patients. *Am J Clin Pathol.* 1991;95:536–539.
64. Higuchi I, Nerenberg M, Yoshimine K, et al. Failure to detect HTLV-I by in situ hybridization in the biopsied muscles of viral carriers with polymyositis. *Muscle Nerve.* 1992;15:43–47.

CHAPTER 22

Influenza and Parainfluenza Viruses

Washington C. Winn, Jr.

During the first great epidemic of influenza towards the end of the nineteenth century a London evening paper sent round a journalist-patient to all the great consultants of that day, and published their advice and prescriptions: a proceeding passionately denounced by the medical papers as a breach of confidence of these eminent physicians. The case was the same; but the prescriptions were different, and so was the advice.

George Bernard Shaw (1856–1950)

DEFINITION

The family *Myxoviridae* includes the two important influenza viruses, types A and B.[1] Influenza C virus is uncommonly associated with human infection, has not been classified, and is not considered further. Influenza viruses afflict numerous mammalian and avian species, but with rare exceptions these viruses do not cross species lines to infect humans. The major exception is the swine influenza virus, which has caused rare human infections,[2] and caused near panic and an ill-fated national immunization program in the mid-1970s.

The family *Paramyxoviridae* includes the four parainfluenza viruses, as well as measles, mumps, and respiratory syncytial viruses.[3,4] Important animal members of the family include canine distemper, Newcastle disease virus of fowl, Sendai virus of rodents, and simian virus 5.

GEOGRAPHIC DISTRIBUTION

All of these viruses are distributed throughout the world. They are equal opportunity pathogens, causing human misery without regard to race, religion, gender, age, or socioeconomic status. Attack rates and severity of disease for both groups of viruses, however, are greatest in infants,[5,6] and adults with chronic cardiopulmonary disease are also at increased risk of severe influenza infection.[7]

LIFE CYCLE AND EPIDEMIOLOGY

Influenza and parainfluenza viruses are single-stranded, helical RNA viruses that reproduce by budding from the cell surface (Figure 22–1). At the cell surface the virions collect a lipid envelope from the membrane of the host cell, into which several virus-specified proteins are inserted. Influenza viruses have a segmented genome, which facilitates reassortment among strains and allows transfer of genetic material among isolates from several mammalian species.[8] The two virus-specified surface proteins of pathogenetic and epidemiologic importance are the hemagglutinin and the neuraminidase spikes that protrude through the envelope. The hemagglutinin is essential for infection of cells in vitro and in vivo, is the most important antigenic determinant, and is commonly employed for detection of virus in cell cultures in the diagnostic virology laboratory. The function of neuraminidase is less clear, but it may involve destruction of protective cellular mucins or may facilitate the

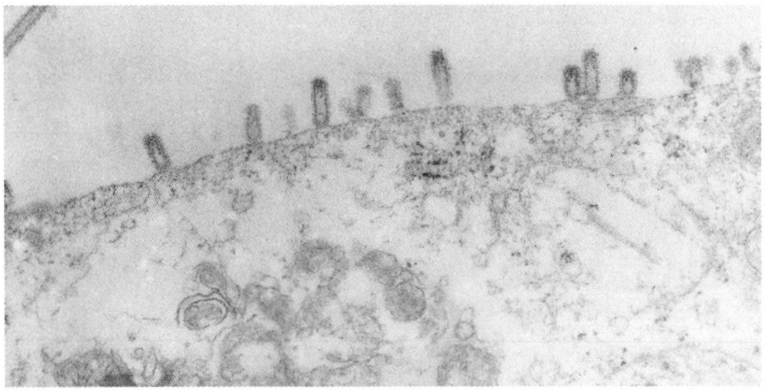

Figure 22–1. Virions of influenza A virus bud from the surface of an infected rhesus monkey kidney cell. After replication stages in the nucleus and cytoplasm, the final assembly of virions occurs at the cell membrane, which contributes the lipid envelope of the virus. The fuzzy border of the virions is produced by the hemagglutinin and neuraminidase spikes that are inserted into the envelope (original magnification, ×25,000).

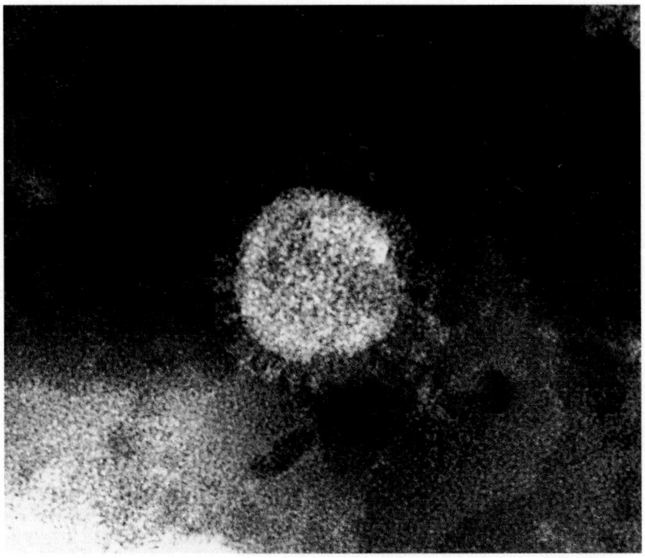

Figure 22–2. Influenza A virion. The helical RNA produces virions that vary from spherical to elongated. The fringe of hemagglutinin and neuraminidase spikes is evident around the periphery of the virion (phosphotungstic acid negative stain; original magnification, ×180,000).

budding of mature virions. Constant variation of the hemagglutinin and neuraminidase under the pressure of specific antibodies maintains a population of viruses capable of infecting mammalian hosts.[9] Substitution of a single amino acid in the hemagglutinin may render it unrecognizable by monoclonal antibodies and T lymphocytes.[10] The change may be gradual and incremental (antigenic drift) or dramatic and extensive (antigenic shift).[11,12] The parainfluenza viruses also contain two important surface glycoproteins: the HN (hemagglutinin–neuraminidase) and the F (fusion) protein, which participates in the entry of virions into the cell and results in syncytial formation in cell culture. There is antigenic variation of the parainfluenza viruses, but the extensive antigenic change in the influenza viruses does not occur.[3]

Most myxoviruses produce sporadic and epidemic disease primarily during the winter months, although infections may occur at any time of year.[13] Parainfluenza 3 virus infections show less pronounced seasonal predominance than is exhibited by the other viruses.[6] Epidemic disease is most commonly caused by the influenza viruses, because of the extensive antigenic variation that maintains a larger population of susceptible individuals. Traditionally a single strain of influenza virus A or B circulated, but in the past decade two predominant strains of influenza virus A have been in concurrent circulation, further complicating the job of vaccine manufacturers.[11]

MORPHOLOGY OF THE ORGANISM

The coiled, helical ribonucleoprotein is packaged in a round, oval, or elongated virion (Figure 22–2). The lipid coat that was contributed by the host cell contains the virus-specified glycoprotein antigens already described. Influenza viruses measure 80 to 120 nm in diameter, whereas parainfluenza viruses are somewhat larger and more pleomorphic, measuring 150 to 250 nm in diameter. When the virion is disrupted, long strands of the helical ribonucleoprotein may be released.[14]

CLINICAL DISEASE

Influenza viruses produce the influenza syndrome: a systemic illness characterized by fever, chills, myalgias, malaise, headache, and anorexia.[15–17] Confusion may be a prominent feature of the infection in the elderly patient. Respiratory symptoms, which include nasal discharge, sore throat, and a dry cough, may be overshadowed by systemic symptoms early in the infection and may be minimal in elderly individuals. Abrupt alterations in fever may result in shaking chills, suggesting bacterial infection, and the myalgia may be excruciating. Arthralgias may be present, but there is no arthritis. In children, cervical lymphadenopathy and croup may be prominent. Sore throats and otitis media may dominate the clinical picture.[18,19]

Differentiation of influenza A from bacterial sepsis may be difficult in the newborn infant.[20] "Gastric flu," which is a clinical reality, may be more common in children and in influenza B infections.[21,22] Disseminated intravascular coagulation has been reported as a complication of influenza A infection.[23]

The serious respiratory complications of influenza are primary influenza pneumonia and secondary bacterial infection, most commonly caused by *Haemophilus influenzae, Staphylococcus aureus,* and *Streptococcus pneumoniae.*[24] A bacterial cause was considered early in the century because of the prominence of *H influenzae,* but this bacterium has been less prominent in recent decades. Differentiation of primary viral pneumonia from secondary bacterial infection may be difficult on both clinical and pathologic grounds. Herpes simplex infection of the lower respiratory tract has also been described as a complication of influenza virus pneumonia.[25] Diffuse pulmonary fibrosis and reduced pulmonary function may be long-term sequelae.[26]

Systemic complications are infrequent, but well described. Myopathy has been demonstrated rarely[27] and rhabdomyolysis, even leading to myoglobinuria, has been described, particularly in children infected with influenza B virus. Influenza virus has been isolated from the lung or mycocardium of patients who died with myocarditis.[28,29] Guillain–Barré syndrome achieved international notoriety as a complication of the swine influenza immunization program in the 1970s, but Guillain–Barré syndrome occurs also after natural infection by many viruses. In children, especially those between 2 and 6 years of age, Reye's syndrome is a dreaded and often fatal complication. Influenza B virus is the most common cause of epidemic Reye's syndrome, but the syndrome may follow influenza A epidemics,[30,31] as well as sporadic viral infections. More recently, toxic shock syndrome has been described as an additional complication of secondary staphylococcal infections after influenza A infection.[32]

Parainfluenza viruses produce diverse respiratory infections, but extrapulmonary disease is much less common than with the influenza viruses. Disease is most commonly manifested by pharyngitis, conjunctivitis, and the common cold.[3,33] Disease is most common in children, but adult infection,[34] including fatal giant cell pneumonia,[35] has been described. Parainfluenza virus 3 causes the most severe disease, especially bronchiolitis, and is the only one of the parainfluenza viruses that commonly infects children younger than 6 months of age. Primary infections with type 3 virus are often febrile. Serious lower respiratory infections can be produced by any of the serotypes in immunosuppressed patients.[36–39] Primary viral otitis[18] may be caused by parainfluenza viruses, particularly type 3. Parainfluenza virus 4 is uncommon, usually mild, and not associated with particular clinical syndromes.[40] The association of virus type with clinical disease is summarized in Table 22–1. Parotitis and aseptic meningitis caused by parainfluenza virus 3 have been described.[41,42]

PATHOLOGY

The primary target for the myxoviruses is the respiratory epithelial cell from the nose to the air spaces. Influenza virus multiplies in explanted organ cultures of human nasal epithelium and destroys the monolayer, in contrast to rhinovirus, which multiplies in the epithelial cells without producing cytopathic changes.[43] Parainfluenza viruses 2 and 3 produce a characteristic cytopathic effect that includes syncytial cell formation.[44] Pathologic material is rarely examined in most human infections, however, and most of our information derives from study of the lung in fatal influenza pneumonia and infections with both types of virus in immunodeficient patients. Carson and colleagues[45] have demonstrated ultrastructural ciliary damage in nasal mucosal epithelium from patients who were undergoing viral infections, including influenza and parainfluenza disease.

The classic pathologic pattern elicited in influenza pneumonia is diffuse damage to the lining epithelium of the air spaces.[15–17,46] Although the changes may be diffusely distributed, they are focal in nature, often corresponding to lobular outlines.[46] Macroscopically, the lungs are congested, beefy, and firm (Figure 22–3). Later the air spaces may be prominently displayed, and interstitial fibrosis may further accentuate the architecture in those who survive the immediate period. There is an exudative response with accumulation of a fibrinous exudate in the air spaces and reactive changes in the alveolar lining cells. Hyaline membranes are fre-

TABLE 22–1. ASSOCIATION OF PARAINFLUENZA VIRUSES WITH CLINICAL DISEASE

Virus	Most Common Severe Clinical Disease	Less Common Severe Clinical Disease
Parainfluenza virus 1	Laryngotracheobronchitis (croup)	Bronchiolitis, pneumonia
Parainfluenza virus 2	Croup	Bronchiolitis, pneumonia
Parainfluenza virus 3	Bronchiolitis, pneumonia	Croup, parotitis, meningitis
Parainfluenza virus 4	None	None

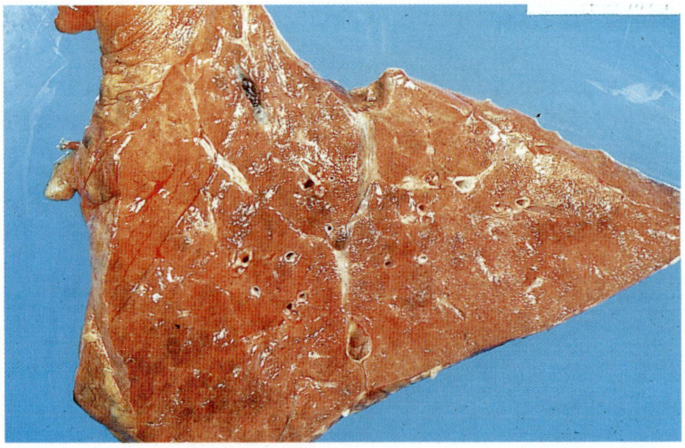

Figure 22–3. Fatal influenza A pneumonia in a pregnant woman. The lung demonstrates multiple areas of extensive consolidation, presenting a beefy appearance to the cut section. The cut edges of this unfixed section maintain their shape and contour.

quently apposed to the damaged epithelium (Figure 22–4). Thrombosis in small blood vessels has been noted in some reports. Erythrocytes are common in the exudate, but gross hemorrhage is uncommon. There may be neutrophils, and on occasion a concomitant necrotizing appearance may suggest bacterial pneumonia.[15,16] Necrotizing bronchitis, bronchiolitis, and alveolitis have been documented in an antemortem lung biopsy from a patient who had primary influenzal pneumonia,[47] as well as in autopsy tissue. Observers of epidemic disease have commented that it may be difficult to distinguish primary influenzal pneumonia from secondary staphylococcal infection pathologically, if the patient dies in the acute stages. Reactive changes in the alveoli and bronchioles may progress to hyperplasia and squamous metaplasia, a process that may begin in the first few days of infection (Figure 22–5). Interstitial fibrosis and obliterative bronchiolitis may be sequelae of the acute episode.[48]

The pathology of influenza pneumonia has been remarkably consistent, regardless of the type or strain of virus or the time and location of the infection. Investigators at Yale University were able to compare the histopathology of fatal infections from the Hong Kong influenza epidemic in the 1960s with material studied by Winternitz at that institution in the 1918 pandemic. The histologic changes were similar.[17] Limited descriptions of pneumonia produced by influenza B virus[49] and the swine strains of influenza A virus[50] conform to the classic pattern. A corollary of these observations is that the nature of the infecting virus cannot be distinguished by pathologic analysis.

Influenza myocarditis with interstitial lymphocytic inflammation and myocytolysis resembles other viral causes of myocarditis.[28,29] An epidemiologic study of forensic cases in which patients died suddenly with no documented explanation disclosed an increased frequency of influenza A pneumonia.[51] The phenomenon may, therefore, be more common than appreciated, but it is unlikely that overt myocarditis would be missed in the standard postmortem examination. A patient with myopathy associated with influenza B virus infection had focal muscle necrosis, but no inflammatory reaction on histologic examination. Ultrastructurally, there was segmental necrosis with glycogen depletion, mitochondrial abnormalities, and sarcolemmal necrosis, but without destruction of the basement membrane.[27]

The rare cases of fatal parainfluenza virus pneumonia, usually in immunodeficient patients, conform to

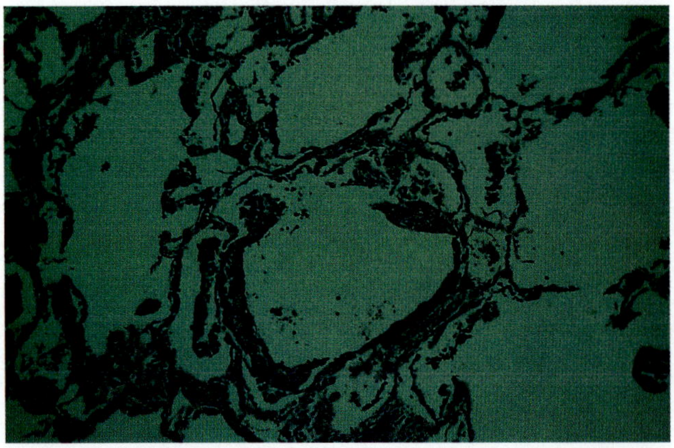

Figure 22–4. Influenza A pneumonia manifested by exudation of cells and proteinaceous fluid into the alveolar spaces. Prominent hyaline membranes are present (hematoxylin-eosin stain).

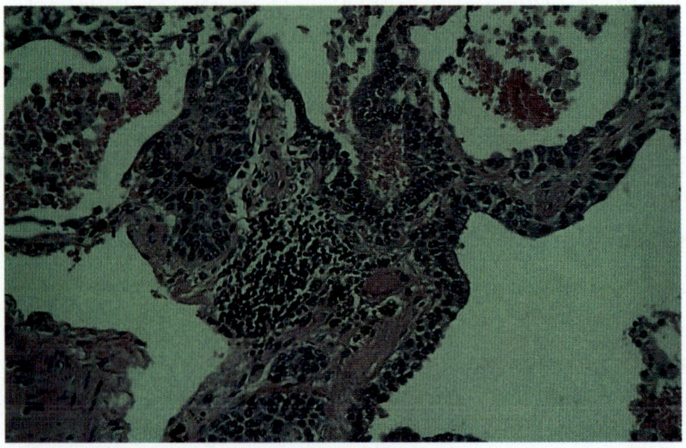

Figure 22–5. Influenza A pneumonia. The beginning of the healing phase is heralded by lymphocytic infiltration in the interstitium and squamous metaplasia of the bronchiolar epithelium. An active exudate remains in some of the air spaces (hematoxylin-eosin stain).

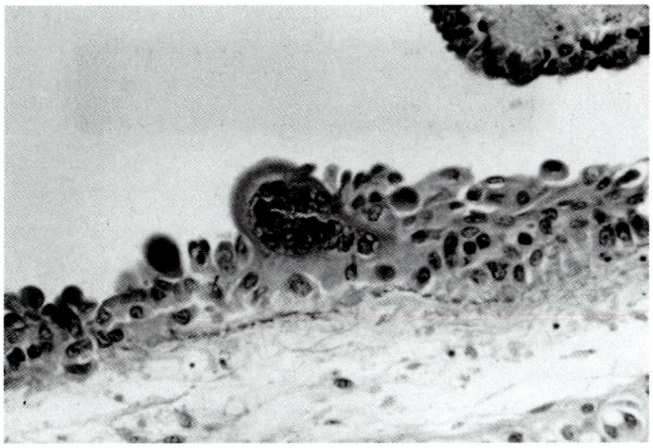

Figure 22–6. In vitro cytopathic effect of parainfluenza virus 3 in organ cultures of hamster tracheal epithelium. The virus has produced cytolytic effects, denuded the epithelium, and caused epithelial cell fusion to form syncytial giant cells (hematoxylin-eosin stain).

the description of influenza. The pathogen is most commonly parainfluenza virus 3, which may produce syncytial giant cells in vivo (Figure 22–6) as well as in vitro (Figure 22–7).[36,37] Parainfluenza virus 2 also may produce syncytial giant cells.[38] Cytologically, degenerative changes in ciliated epithelium, ciliocytophora, and small cytoplasmic inclusions may be present.[52]

Minimal data exist on the pathology of parainfluenza virus infections outside of the respiratory tract. An interesting report of syncytial hepatitis with paramyxoviral features in children and adults does not definitely link the disease with the paramyxoviruses.[53]

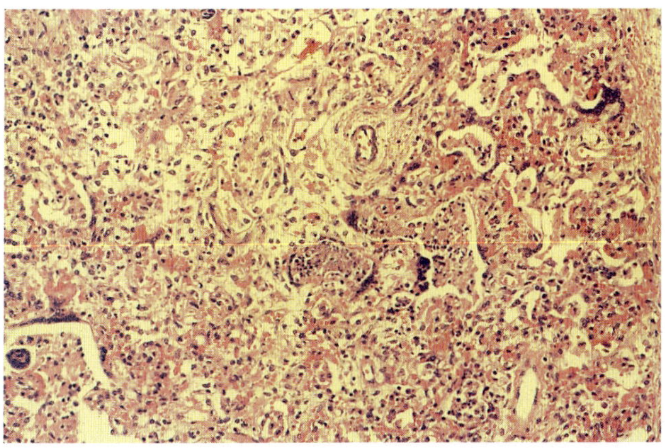

Figure 22–7. A mononuclear and proteinaceous exudate fills the air spaces of a child with fatal parainfluenza 3 virus pneumonia. Several syncytial giant cells stand out even at low power because of the density of the multiple nuclei. Intracytoplasmic inclusions were not evident (hematoxylin-eosin stain).

ULTRASTRUCTURE AND CYTOPATHOLOGY

Fibrillar intranuclear inclusions have been described in the respiratory epithelial cells of lungs infected by influenza A virus,[54] perhaps corresponding to the nuclear phase of replication by this virus, but inclusions are not seen with the light microscope. Damage to ciliated epithelium and ciliocytophora may be present, but there are no diagnostic cytopathologic changes.

DIFFERENTIAL DIAGNOSIS

The differential diagnosis of classic myxovirus pneumonia consists of the many other conditions that produce diffuse alveolar damage, including other viruses, other infectious agents (such as *Pneumocystis carinii*), oxygen toxicity, radiation damage, chemotherapy, and adult respiratory distress syndrome. The differential diagnosis of parainfluenza infections with syncytial cell formation includes measles, which usually produces intracytoplasmic inclusions with or without intranuclear inclusions, and respiratory syncytial virus, which may produce intracytoplasmic inclusions.

CONFIRMING DIAGNOSIS

The most important method for etiologic diagnosis of myxovirus infections is isolation of the virus in cell culture. Although influenza virus A grows well in the Madin–Darby cell line of canine kidney cells (MDCK) and parainfluenza viruses may be isolated in LLC-MK2 cells,[55] the most reliable cells are primary monkey kidney cultures, especially those obtained from rhesus monkeys. Influenza A, but not influenza B or parainfluenza viruses, can be isolated by inoculation of embryonated chicken eggs, but this method is not used frequently at present. Many strains of these viruses do not produce cytopathic effect in cell cultures, and they are best detected by hemadsorption of guinea pig erythrocytes onto the cell monolayer.[44]

Confirmation of the identity of the virus is most commonly accomplished by immunofluorescence of monolayers that have demonstrated cytopathic effect or positive hemadsorption. Spin amplification in shell vials followed by blind staining with a pool of fluoresceinated antibodies shorten the time to detection, and this technique may be useful when the prevalence of infections is high.[56] A positive result requires the application of multiple antisera to other shell vials or monolayers in conventional tubes.

Serologic diagnosis of myxovirus infections is retrospective and plays only a supportive role in the diagnostic armamentarium. Heterotypic responses make it impossible to pinpoint a parainfluenza etiology by serologic methods.[57]

MOLECULAR ASPECTS OF DIAGNOSIS

Direct detection of myxoviruses in clinical specimens has been accomplished by immunofluorescence and enzyme immunoassay, most successfully in nasopharyngeal aspirates or washings.[58] The sensitivity of these methods ranges from 20% to 80%. In comparison to respiratory syncytial virus, for which these approaches have been used widely, the lesser sensitivity, need for multiple reagents, and less compelling clinical implications have limited the application of immunoassay to influenza and parainfluenza viruses. From clinical and epidemiologic standpoints, the most important virus is influenza A. Enzyme immunoassays show promise for rapid diagnosis of this virus, for which immunofluorescence tests have low sensitivity. Molecular tools for detection of viral ribonucleic acid have not been extensively investigated.

THERAPY

Amantadine and rimantidine may be used to treat influenza A virus infections if applied early in the course, but they have been used most commonly as prophylactic therapy for high-risk patients, such as the elderly, in an epidemic situation.[59] There is no proven chemotherapy for influenza B and parainfluenza viruses. Prevention by yearly immunization programs is the primary strategy for control of influenza virus infections.[60]

REFERENCES

1. Betts RF. Influenza virus. In: Mandell GL, Bennett JE, Dolin R, eds. *Principles and Practice of Infectious Diseases*, 4th ed. New York: Churchill Livingstone; 1995: 1546–1567.
2. Gaydos JC, Hodder RA, Top FHJ, et al. Swine influenza A at Fort Dix, New Jersey (January–February 1976). I. Case finding and clinical study of cases. *J Infect Dis.* 1977;136: S356–S362.
3. Henrickson K, Ray R, Belshe R. Parainfluenza viruses. In: Mandell GL, Bennett JE, Dolin R, eds. *Principles and Practice of Infectious Diseases*, 4th ed. New York: Churchill Livingstone; 1995:1489–1496.
4. Vainiopää R, Hyypiä T. Biology of parainfluenza viruses. *Clin Microbiol Rev.* 1994;7:265–275.
5. Hall CE, Cooney MK, Fox JP. The Seattle virus watch. IV. Comparative epidemiologic observations of infections with influenza A and B viruses, 1965–1969, in families with young children. *Am J Epidemiol.* 1973;98:365–380.
6. Cooney MK, Fox JP, Hall CE. The Seattle virus watch. VI. Observations of infections with an illness due to parainfluenza, mumps, and respiratory syncytial viruses and *Mycoplasma pneumoniae*. *Am J Epidemiol.* 1975;101: 532–551.
7. Barker WH, Mullooly JP. Pneumonia and influenza deaths during epidemics: implications for prevention. *Arch Intern Med.* 1982;142:85–89.
8. Wright SM, Kawaoka Y, Sharp GB, Senne DA, Webster RG. Interspecies transmission and reassortment of influenza A viruses in pigs and turkeys in the United States. *Am J Epidemiol.* 1992;136:488–497.
9. Lambkin R, McLain L, Jones SE, Aldridge SL, Dimmock NJ. Neutralization escape mutants of type A influenza virus are readily selected by antisera from mice immunized with whole virus: a possible mechanism for antigenic drift. *J Gen Virol.* 1994;75:3493–3502.
10. Thomas DB, Skehel JJ, Mills KH, Graham CM. A single amino acid substitution in influenza hemagglutinin abrogates recognition by monoclonal antibody and a spectrum of subtype-specific L3T4+ T cell clones. *Eur J Immunol.* 1987;17:133–136.
11. Hope-Simpson RE, Golubev DB. A new concept of the epidemic process of influenza A virus. *Epidemiol Infect.* 1987;99:5–54.
12. Kendal AP. Epidemiologic implications of changes in the influenza virus genome. *Am J Med.* 1987;82:4–14.
13. Glezen WP, Payne AA, Snyder DN, Downs TD. Mortality and influenza. *J Infect Dis.* 1982;146:313–321.
14. Murphy FA, Coleman MT. Internal and surface structure of Hong Kong influenza virus. *Bull WHO.* 1969;41:703–704.
15. Martin CM, Kunin CM, Gottlieb LS, Barnes MW, Liu C, Finland M. Asian influenza A in Boston, 1957–1958. *Arch Intern Med.* 1959;103:515–542.
16. Oseasohn R, Adelson L, Kaji M. Clinicopathologic study of thirty-three fatal cases of Asian influenza. *N Engl J Med.* 1959;260:509–518.
17. Feldman PS, Cohan MA, Hierholzer WJJ. Fatal Hong Kong influenza: a clinical, microbiological and pathological analysis of nine cases. *Yale J Biol Med.* 1972:45:49–63.
18. Ruuskanen O, Arola M, Putto-Laurila A, et al. Acute otitis media and respiratory virus infections. *Pediatr Infect Dis J.* 1989;8:94–99.
19. Chonmaitree T, Howie VM, Truant AL. Presence of respiratory viruses in middle ear fluids and nasal wash specimens from children with acute otitis media. *Pediatrics.* 1986;77:698–702.
20. Dagan R, Hall CB. Influenza A virus infection imitating bacterial sepsis in early infancy. *Pediatr Infect Dis.* 1984;3:218–221.
21. Wright PF, Bryant JD, Karzon DT. Comparison of influenza B/Hong Kong virus infections among infants, children, and young adults. *J Infect Dis.* 1980;141:430–435.
22. Kerr AA, McQuillin J, Downham MA, Gardner PS. Gastric flu influenza B causing abdominal symptoms in children. *Lancet.* 1975;1:291–295.
23. Davison AM, Thomson D, Robson JS. Intravascular coagulation complicating influenza A virus infection. *Br Med J.* 1973;1:654–655.
24. Louria DB, Blumenfeld HL, Ellis JT, Kilbourne ED, Rogers

DE. Studies on influenza in the pandemic of 1957–1958. II. Pulmonary complications of influenza. *J Clin Invest.* 1959;38:213–265.

25. Klimek JJ, Lindenberg LB, Cole S, Ellison LH, Quintiliani R. Fatal case of influenza pneumonia with suprainfection by multiple bacteria and herpes simplex virus. *Am Rev Respir Dis.* 1976;113:683–688.
26. Winterbauer RH, Ludwig WR, Hammar SP. Clinical course, management, and long-term sequelae of respiratory failure due to influenza viral pneumonia. *Johns Hopkins Med J.* 1977;141:148–155.
27. Bove KE, Hilton PK, Partin J, Farrell MK. Morphology of acute myopathy associated with influenza B infection. *Pediatr Pathol.* 1983;1:51–66.
28. Finland M, Parker F, Jr., Barnes MW, Joliffe LS. Acute myocarditis in influenza A infections. Two cases of nonbacterial myocarditis, with isolation of virus from the lungs. *Am J Med Sci.* 1945;209:455–468.
29. Engblom E, Ekfors TO, Meurman OH, Toivanen A, Nikoskelainen J. Fatal influenza A myocarditis with isolation of virus from the myocardium. *Acta Med Scand.* 1983;213:75–78.
30. Hochberg FH, Nelson K, Janzen W. Influenza type B-related encephalopathy. The 1971 outbreak of Reye syndrome in Chicago. *JAMA.* 1975;231:817–821.
31. Ruben FL, Michaels RH. Reye syndrome with associated influenza A and B infection. *JAMA.* 1975;234:410–412.
32. MacDonald KL, Osterholm MT, Hedberg CW, et al. Toxic shock syndrome. A newly recognized complication of influenza and influenzalike illness. *JAMA.* 1987;257: 1053–1058.
33. Kapikian AZ, Bell JA, Mastrota FM, Huebner RJ, Wong DC, Chanock RM. An outbreak of parainfluenza 2 (croup-associated) virus infection. Association with acute undifferentiated febrile illness in children. *JAMA.* 1963;183:112–118.
34. Craighead JE, Shelokov A, Peralta PH, Vogel JE. Croup-associated virus infection in adults. Report of two cases. *N Engl J Med.* 1961;264:135–137.
35. Akizuki S, Nasu N, Setoguchi M, Yoshida S, Higuchi Y, Yamamoto S. Parainfluenza virus pneumonitis in an adult. *Arch Pathol Lab Med.* 1991;115:824–826.
36. Little BW, Tihen WS, Dickerman JD, Craighead JE. Giant cell pneumonia associated with parainfluenza virus type 3 infection. *Hum Pathol.* 1981;12:478–481.
37. Jarvis WR, Middleton PJ, Gelfand EW. Parainfluenza pneumonia in severe combined immunodeficiency disease. *J Pediatr.* 1979;94:423–425.
38. Karp D, Willis J, Wilfert CM. Parainfluenza virus II and the immunocompromised host. *Am J Dis Child.* 1974;127: 592–593.
39. Beard LJ, Robertson EF, Thong YH. Para-influenza pneumonia in DiGeorge syndrome two years after thymic epithelial transplantation. *Acta Paediatr Scand.* 1980; 69:403–406.
40. Rubin EE, Quennec P, McDonald JC. Infections due to parainfluenza virus type 4 in children. *Clin Infect Dis.* 1993;17:998–1002.
41. Zollar LM, Mufson MA. Acute parotitis associated with parainfluenza 3 virus infection. *Am J Dis Child.* 1970; 119:147–149.
42. Craver RD, Gohd RS, Sundin DR, Hierholzer JC. Isolation of parainfluenza virus type 3 from cerebrospinal fluid associated with aseptic meningitis. *Am J Clin Pathol.* 1993;99:705–707.
43. Winther B, Gwaltney JM, Hendley JO. Respiratory virus infection of monolayer cultures of human nasal epithelial cells. *Am Rev Respir Dis.* 1990;141:839–845.
44. Koneman EW, Allen SD, Janda WM, Schreckenberger PC, Winn WC, Jr. *Color Atlas and Textbook of Diagnostic Microbiology*, 4th ed. Philadelphia: JB Lippincott; 1992.
45. Carson JL, Collier AM, Hu SS. Acquired ciliary defects in nasal epithelium of children with acute viral upper respiratory infections. *N Engl J Med.* 1985;312:463–468.
46. Hers JFP, Masurel N, Mulder J. Bacteriology and histopathology of the respiratory tract and lungs in fatal Asian influenza. *Lancet.* 1958;Nov. 29:1141–1143.
47. Noble RL, Lillington GA, Kempson RL. Fatal diffuse influenzal pneumonia: premortem diagnosis by lung biopsy. *Chest.* 1973;63:644–646.
48. Laraya-Cuassay LR, DeForest A, Huff D, Lischner H, Huang NN. Chronic pulmonary complications of early influenza virus infection in children. *Am Rev Respir Dis.* 1977;116:617–625.
49. Hers JFP, Mulder J. Changes in the respiratory mucosa resulting from infection with influenza virus B. *J Pathol Bact.* 1957;73:565–568.
50. Smith TF, Burgert EOJ, Dowdle WR, Noble GR, Campbell RJ, Van SRE. Isolation of swine influenza virus from autopsy lung tissue of man. *N Engl J Med.* 1976;294: 708–710.
51. Drescher J, Zink P, Verhagen W, Flik J, Milbradt H. Recent influenza virus A infections in forensic cases of sudden unexplained death. *Arch Virol.* 1987;92:63–76.
52. Naib ZM, Stewart JA, Dowdle WR, Casey HL, Marine WM, Nahmias AJ. Cytological features of viral respiratory tract infections. *Acta Cytol.* 1968;12:162–171.
53. Phillips MJ, Blendis LM, Poucell S, et al. Syncytial giant-cell hepatitis. Sporadic hepatitis with distinctive pathological features, a severe clinical course, and paramyxoviral features. *N Engl J Med.* 1991;324:455–460.
54. Tamura H, Aronson BE. Intranuclear fibrillary inclusions in influenza pneumonia. *Arch Pathol Lab Med.* 1978;102: 252–257.
55. Frank AL, Couch RB, Griffis CA, Baxter BD. Comparison of different tissue cultures for isolation and quantitation of influenza and parainfluenza viruses. *J Clin Microbiol.* 1979;10:32–36.
56. Espy MJ, Smith TF, Harmon MW, Kendal AP. Rapid detection of influenza virus by shell vial assay with monoclonal antibodies. *J Clin Microbiol.* 1986;24:677–679.
57. Chanock RM, Wong DC, Huebner RJ, Bell JA. Serologic responses of individuals infected with parainfluenza viruses. *Am J Public Health.* 1960;50:1858–1865.
58. Wong DT, Welliver RC, Riddlesberger KR, Sun MS, Ogra PL. Rapid diagnosis of parainfluenza virus infection in children. *J Clin Microbiol.* 1982;16:164–167.
59. Douglas RG, Jr. Prophylaxis and treatment of influenza. *N Engl J Med.* 1990;322:443–450.
60. Fedson DS. Prevention and control of influenza in institutional settings. *Hosp Pract.* 1989;24:87–96.

CHAPTER 23

Lymphocytic Choriomeningitis Virus

Michael R. Lewin-Smith and Herbert J. Manz

The best laid schemes o' mice and men gang aft a-gley (oft go awry).

Robert Burns (1759–1796)

DEFINITION

Lymphocytic choriomeningitis is usually a self-limiting, acute, aseptic, viral meningitis caused by an RNA-virus of the family *Arenaviridae*, lymphocytic choriomeningitis virus (LCMV). LCMV was the first viral agent associated with aseptic meningitis to be identified, when in 1935 Rivers and Scott[1] reported the recovery of a filterable virus from the cerebrospinal fluid (CSF) of two patients suffering from a spontaneously resolving mononuclear cell (lymphocytic) meningitis. LCMV was subsequently demonstrated in 8% to 11% of "viral" central nervous system syndromes occurring in patients at one U.S. medical center between 1941 and 1958.[2]

ETIOLOGIC AGENT AND EPIDEMIOLOGY

LCMV is a member of the genus *Arenavirus* (by virtue of the ultrastructural appearance as "grains of sand"), which includes Lassa virus and Argentinean and Bolivian hemorrhagic fever viruses.[3] Although epidemiologic information is incomplete, LCMV appears to have a worldwide distribution.[4] While it was found early on that CSF from patients with active LCMV-associated meningitis syndromes could infect mice,[1] it also was soon recognized that infected domestic mice (*Mus musculus*) might be the source of human infections.[5] Indeed, although many mammals are infected, mice have been confirmed as the most important reservoir, and probably the only natural host for the virus. In a recent study from urban Baltimore, Maryland, where mice were trapped at various sites, 9% of mice were infected with LCMV, varying significantly from site to site (3.9% to 13.4%). The prevalence of LCMV antibodies in mice correlated significantly with estimates of mouse density at each location. It was suggested that this may result from contact or vertical transmission in mice "in conjunction with the highly structured social system of mice, which promotes inbreeding and limited dispersal."[6]

Transmission to humans is likely by inhalation of infected mouse excreta or possibly contamination of skin abrasions with infected mouse urine[7]; under natural conditions, the virus is not transmitted by arthropods nor is it transmitted from human to human; experimentally, however, the virus can be transmitted by mosquitoes. Although infections have been reported in every month of the year, the incidence is higher in winter. Incubation is 1 to 2 weeks. Antibodies to LCMV were present in the serum of 4.7% of 1141 patients visiting a sexually transmitted diseases clinic in Baltimore between 1986 and 1988. Prevalence increased with age. There was no significant statistical difference between seropositive and seronegative subjects with regard to frequency of rodent exposure.[8] The prevalence of serum antibodies has been demonstrated by enzyme-linked immunosorbent assay (ELISA) to be 5.1% (7 of 138) in healthy black women and 4.3% (2 of 46) of patients with all types of hepatitis or cirrhosis in Birmingham, Alabama. In the same study, none of 20 patients with non-A, non-B hepatitis, and 2.4% (2 of 82) of volunteers rejected from blood donation for high serum alanine aminotransferase in San Antonio, Texas, were seropositive for LCMV.[9] LCMV has been transmitted to hamsters, and humans involved in the pet trade have become infected.[10] Fatal outbreaks of viral disease documented in tamarins and marmosets in zoos probably have been caused by LCMV.[11]

PATHOGENESIS AND CLINICAL MANIFESTATIONS

The respiratory tract is the usual portal of entry, with the virus replicating in the respiratory epithelium. The clinical onset is an influenza-like syndrome. An initial viremia seeds all organs and tissues except the central nervous system (CNS); because the virus replicates in these non-neural tissues, however, a secondary viremia permits dissemination into the CNS. The spectrum of clinical disease associated with LCMV infection in humans is broad, ranging from a protracted flulike illness, to aseptic meningitis/encephalitis, to a fatal hemorrhagic syndrome.[2,12,13] A chronic meningitic picture also has been documented in mice[14] and humans.[15] In humans, a fatal infection of LCMV acquired from the mother "during the last stages of intrauterine life" has been reported.[16] There is evidence that prenatal infection leads to hydrocephalus.[17]

No outbreaks of LCMV were reported in the United States between 1974 and 1992, but in 1992 there was an outbreak of lymphocytic choriomeningitis in a research institute working with nude mice.[18] Ten percent of 82 employees at the institute had evidence of LCMV antibodies and seropositivity correlated with handling nude mice, cleaning their cages, and changing bedding and water.[18] This outbreak emphasizes the need for screening animals and their tumor cell lines for extraneous LCMV to avoid transmission to humans, as had been shown with infected hamsters in the 1970s.[10] Although infection by LCMV is uncommonly diagnosed and rarely reported in the United States,[10] sporadic infection in humans should not be overlooked.[19]

PATHOLOGY

LCMV is mainly restricted to the leptomeninges, which may appear cloudy from inflammation and leukocytic infiltration (Figure 23–1). Chronic leptomeningitis may cause hydrocephalus by obstructing the flow of CSF with leptomeningeal fibrosis and adhesions. In the rare patient with encephalitis caused by LCMV, neutrophils, lymphocytes, and histiocytes constitute the inflammatory cells in perivascular Virchow–Robin spaces (Figure 23–2) and multifocal parenchymal lesions. There may be parenchymal necrosis and hemorrhage, without the presence of inclusion bodies or glial nodules.[4] Neither the virus nor its replication appear to be cytotoxic; rather, the host immune response to virally infected cells mediates cell injury and death; initially, this

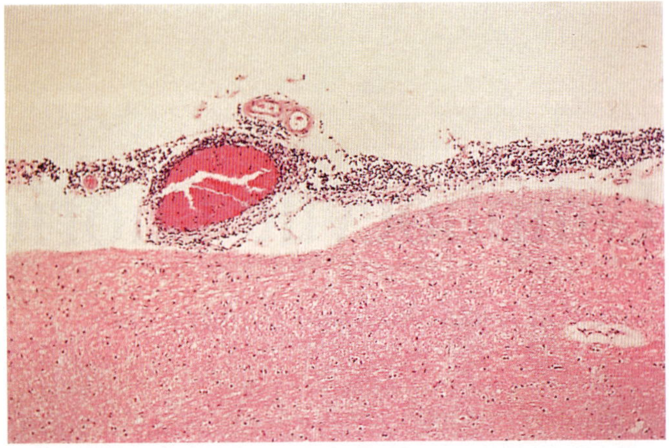

Figure 23–1. Human medulla oblongata. Leptomeningeal lymphocytic infiltrate caused by infection with the lymphocytic choriomeningitis virus (AFIP Neg 74-1305; ×42).

effect is produced by natural killer cells followed by cytotoxic T cells and their concomitant production of interferon.[20]

A thought-provoking mechanism of viral-induced neurologic disease, especially in chronic, persistent infections,[21] is the suppression of cellular "luxury functions," such as the neuronal ability to synthesize acetylcholine. Oldstone, Holmstoen, and Welsh,[22] for instance, illustrated that LCMV suppressed the acetylcholine synthesizing enzyme of cultured neuroblastoma cells. Similarly, in the mouse, persistent infection of the adenohypophyseal cells with LCMV suppressed the synthesis of growth hormone.[23]

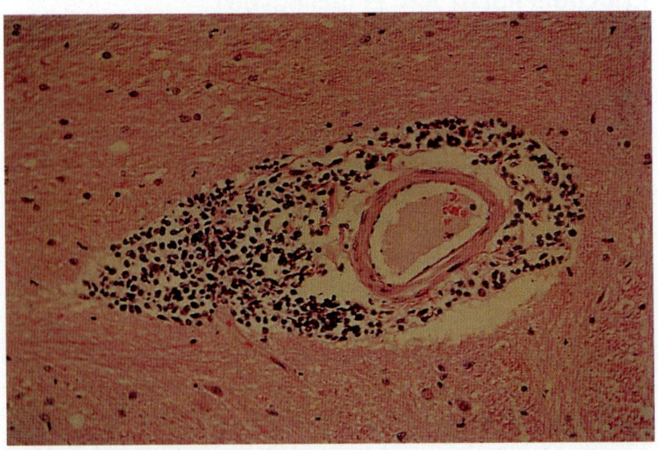

Figure 23–2. Human brain. Lymphocytic perivascular infiltrate caused by infection with the LCMV (AFIP Neg 74-1381; ×115).

DIAGNOSIS

The diagnosis in humans may be suggested by contact with mice or hamsters and is made by isolating the virus from blood or CSF early in the illness followed by seroconversion and/or appearance of IgM antibodies. Demonstration of virus or IgM antibodies in the CSF may also be diagnostic. A fourfold or greater rise in specific IgG titer indicates acute infection.[24] The main detection methods are indirect fluorescent antibody tests for antigen or cell culture for isolation of virus.[19] LCMV isolation in cell culture or laboratory animals requires laboratory biosafety level 3.[24] The most reliable method for LCMV isolation is considered to be intracranial inoculation of 3-week-old (weanling) mice.[25] An ELISA has been developed for detecting serum antibodies against LCMV.[9]

REFERENCES

1. Rivers TM, Scott TFM. Meningitis in man caused by a filterable virus. *Science.* 1935:81:439–440.
2. Meyer HM, Johnson RT, Crawford IP, Dascomb HE, Rogers NG. Central nervous system syndromes of "viral" etiology. *Am J Med.* 1960;29:334–347.
3. Ray GC, Minnich LL. Viruses, rickettsia and chlamydia. In: Henry JB, ed. *Clinical Diagnosis and Management by Laboratory Methods.* 18th ed. Philadelphia: WB Saunders; 1991;chap 47:1227, 1255.
4. Heffner RR, Strano AJ. Lymphocytic choriomeningitis. In: Binford CH, Connor DH, eds. *Pathology of Tropical and Extraordinary Diseases.* Washington, DC: Armed Forces Institute of Pathology; 1976;chap 8:47–48.
5. Armstrong C, Sweet LK. Lymphocytic choriomeningitis. Report of two cases with recovery of the virus from gray mice (*Mus musculus*) trapped in the two infected households. *Public Health Reports.* 1939;54:673–682.
6. Childs JE, Glass GE, Korch GW, Ksiazek TG, Leduc JW. Lymphocytic choriomeningitis virus infection and house mouse (*Mus musculus*) distribution in urban Baltimore. *Am J Trop Med Hyg.* 1992;47(1):27–34.
7. Skinner HH, Knight EH. Epidermal tissue as a primary site of replication of lymphocytic choriomeningitis virus in small experimental hosts. *J Hyg (London).* 1979;82:21–30.
8. Childs JE, Glass GE, Ksiazek TG, Rossi CA, Barrera Oro JG, Leduc JW. Human–rodent contact and infection with lymphocytic choriomeningitis and Seoul viruses in an inner-city population. *Am J Trop Med Hyg.* 1991;44(2): 117–121.
9. Stephensen CB, Blount SR, Lanford RE, et al. Prevalence of serum antibodies against lymphocytic choriomeningitis virus in selected populations from two U.S. cities. *J Med Virol.* 1992;38:27–31.
10. Gregg MB. Recent outbreaks of lymphocytic choriomeningitis in the United States of America. *Bull WHO.* 1975;52:549–553.
11. Stephenson CB, Jacob JR, Montali RJH, et al. Isolation of an arenavirus from a marmoset with callitrichid hepatitis and its serologic association with disease. *J Virol.* 1991; 65:3995–4000.
12. Warkel RL, Rinaldi CF, Bancroft WH, Cardiff RD, Holmes GE, Wilsnack RG. Fatal acute meningoencephalitis due to lymphocytic choriomeningitis virus. *Neurology.* 1973;23: 198–203.
13. Vanzee BE, Douglas RG, Betts RF, Bauman AW, Fraser DW, Hinman AK. Lymphocytic choriomeningitis in university hospital personnel: clinical features. *Am J Med.* 1975;58:803–809.
14. Traub E. Epidemiology of lymphocytic choriomeningitis in a mouse stock observed for four years. *J Exp Med.* 1939;69:801–817.
15. Baker AB. Chronic lymphocytic choriomeningitis. *J Neuropathol Exp Neurol.* 1947;6:253–264.
16. Komrower GM, Williams BL, Stones PB. Lymphocytic choriomeningitis in the newborn. *Lancet.* 1955;1:697–698.
17. Sheinbergas MM. Hydrocephalus due to prenatal infection with the lymphocytic choriomeningitis virus. *Infection.* 1976;4:185–191.
18. Dykewicz CA, Dato VM, Fisher-Hoch SP, et al. Lymphocytic choriomeningitis outbreak associated with nude mice in a research institute. *JAMA.* 1992;267(10): 1349–1353.
19. Jahrling PB, Peters CJ. Lymphocytic choriomeningitis virus, a neglected pathogen of man. *Arch Pathol Lab Med.* 1992;116:486–488.
20. Welsh RM, Doe WF. Cytotoxic cells induced during lymphocytic choriomeningitis virus infection of mice: natural killer cell activity in cultured spleen leukocytes concomitant with T-cell dependent immune interferon production. *Infection Immun.* 1980;30:473–483.
21. Gilden DH, Cole GA, Nathanson N. Immunopathogenesis of acute CNS disease produced by lymphocytic choriomeningitis virus. II. Adoptive immunization of virus carriers. *J Exp Med.* 1972;135:874–889.
22. Oldstone MBA, Holmstoen J, Welsh RM, Jr. Alterations of acetylcholine enzymes in neuroblastoma cells persistently infected with lymphocytic choriomeningitis virus. *J Cell Physiol.* 1977;91:459–472.
23. Oldstone MBA, Ahmed R, Byrne J, Buchmeier MJ, Riviere Y, Southern P. Virus and immune responses: lymphocytic choriomeningitis virus as a prototype model of viral pathogenesis. *Br Med Bull.* 1985;41:70–74.
24. Woods GL, Gutierrez Y, eds. Arenaviruses. In: Woods GL, Gutierrez Y, Walker DH, Purtilo DT, Shanley JD, eds. *Diagnostic Pathology of Infectious Diseases.* Philadelphia, Lea and Febiger; 1993; chap 20:141–143.
25. Jahrling PB. Arenaviruses and filoviruses. In: Lennette EH, ed., *Laboratory Diagnosis of Viral Infections,* 2nd ed. New York: Marcel Dekker; 1992;chap 13:281–317.

CHAPTER 24

Measles

Sherif R. Zaki and William J. Bellini

They wondered
If wheezles
Could turn
Into measles,
If sneezles
Would turn
Into mumps; . . .
All sorts of conditions
Of famous physicians
Came hurrying round
At a run. . . .
They expounded the reazles
For sneezles
And Wheezles,
The manner of measles
When new.
They said, "If he freezles
In draughts and in breezles,
Then PHTHEEZLES
May even ensue."

A. A. Milne (1882–1956), Now We Are Six

INTRODUCTION

Measles is believed to be a relatively new disease that emerged as humans began to live in towns and cities where population densities provided a sufficient number of susceptible people to maintain and transmit the virus. Rhazes of Baghdad, an Arab physician, is credited with the first known description of measles in the ninth century. Rhazes himself credits authors in the seventh century, for example, a Hebrew physician named El Yehudi, with the first clinical description of measles. Rhazes was able to distinguish measles (*hasbah*, Arabic for "eruption") from smallpox; the latter he considered less severe.[1]

Before the era of vaccination, measles was endemic in most populations worldwide. The disease would reach epidemic proportions depending on population size and density, birth rates, and other related factors. Major epidemics in the United States occurred about every 2 years and involved 3 to 4 million people. About 500,000 to 700,000 cases were reported annually.[2] The isolation of the measles virus in 1954[3] and subsequent development and use of live-attenuated vaccines in the early 1960s caused a precipitous decline of measles worldwide.[4] In spite of widespread distribution of the vaccine, measles is still common throughout the world, causing an estimated 40 million infections and more than 1 million infant deaths each year.

DEFINITION

Measles (rubeola) is an infectious, acute febrile viral illness characterized by upper respiratory tract symptoms, fever, and a maculopapular rash. The causative agent is an enveloped virus that contains a negative sense, single-strand RNA genome of 16,000 nucleotides. The virus is a member of the genus *Morbillivirus* of the family *Paramyxoviridae*.[5,6] Other human pathogens in this family include parainfluenza, mumps, and respiratory syncytial viruses.

GEOGRAPHIC DISTRIBUTION AND EPIDEMIOLOGY

Measles is a highly communicable disease of worldwide distribution. Before the introduction of measles vaccines, epidemics occurred about every 2 to 5 years when the percentage of nonimmune members of a population reached critical levels. Recently, epidemics have occurred in cycles of about 10 years. In small and isolated communities, measles circulation may cease altogether unless the virus is reintroduced. If introduced in nonimmune populations, the disease tends to be more severe and may infect more than 90% of the population.

Although still a significant problem in underdeveloped countries, measles infection became uncommon in the United States after the development and widespread use of an effective measles vaccine. However, a recrudescence of measles infection occurred in several large U.S. urban centers since the 1980s and was associated with reduced use of the vaccine among children and young adults. During the peak of this activity (ie, between 1989 and 1991), more than 50,000 infections and approximately 150 measles-associated deaths were reported.[7]

Measles virus is highly contagious and spread by aerosols and droplets from respiratory secretions of acute infections.[8–10] Less frequently, contaminated fomites transmit the virus. A person with acute measles is infective from just before onset of symptoms to defervescence. Most infections are in colder months. In developed countries, likely settings for exposure to measles virus are infectious disease clinics, pediatric emergency rooms, and physicians' offices.[11] Children are usually infected by 6 years of age, resulting in lifelong immunity. Almost all adults are immune. Clinical infection in children younger than 9 months of age is uncommon because of passive protection afforded the infant by the transfer of maternal antibodies. With the resurgence of measles in the United States, however, came the realization that most women of childbearing age acquired immunity to measles by vaccination and not by natural infection. Lower levels of maternal antibodies were transferred from an immunized mother to her infant; thus, in the United States there were a substantial number of infections in children younger than 1 year of age between 1989 and 1991.

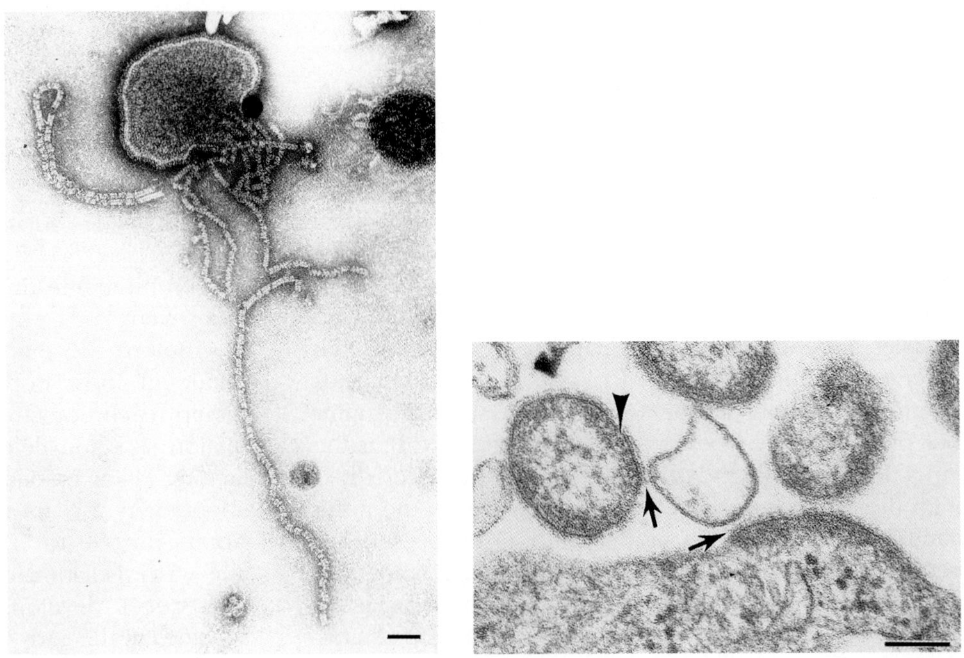

A B

Figure 24–1. (**A**) Distinctive structure of paramyxoviruses in negative stain electron microscope preparation. Free-lying nucleocapsids of parainfluenza virus with characteristic "herringbone" appearance. These structures are also within a particle that has been penetrated by stain. Note fine surface projections on surface of particle. *(Photomicrograph courtesy of Mary Lane Martin.)* (**B**) Measles virus (genus *Morbillivirus*). Virus in thin section electronmicrograph (EM) of Vero E6-infected cells. The envelope, which contains fine surface projections of the hemagglutinin (H) and fusion (F) glycoproteins (*arrows*), surrounds a core containing nucleocapsids (*arrowhead*) in cross-section (scale bars, 100 nm). *(Photomicrograph courtesy of Cynthia S. Goldsmith.)*

MORPHOLOGY OF MEASLES VIRUS

Measles virions are pleomorphic, generally spherical, enveloped particles between 120 and 250 nm in diameter. The virus is morphologically indistinguishable from other members of the *Paramyxoviridae* family when viewed by negative contrast electron microscopy (Figure 24–1, A).[12] A lipid envelope surrounds a helical nucleocapsid structure composed of RNA and protein. Two transmembrane glycoproteins, hemagglutinin (H) and fusion (F), are in the envelope and appear as surface projections (Figure 24–1, B). These proteins mediate viral attachment and fusion with respiratory epithelium. They are also believed to play a role in virus maturation through their interaction with the matrix (M) protein, which, in turn, is thought to interact with the nucleocapsid structure.

CLINICAL FEATURES

After an incubation period of about 1 to 2 weeks, the prodromal phase of measles begins with fever, rhinorrhea, cough, and conjunctivitis. Koplik's spots, which are small, irregular red spots with a bluish-white speck in the center, appear on the buccal mucosa in 50% to 90% of patients shortly before the onset of the rash. An erythematous maculopapular rash begins on the face 3 to 4 days after prodromal symptoms and usually spreads to the trunk and limbs (Figure 24–2). The symptoms gradually resolve, with the rash lasting approximately 6 days, fading in the same order as it appeared.

Although recovery is rapid and complete in most patients, complications can arise from continued and progressive virus replication, bacterial or viral superinfections, and/or an abnormal host–immune response.[10,13,14] The most common complications are secondary bacterial pneumonia and otitis media.[13] Other complications include febrile convulsions, encephalitis, liver function abnormalities, chronic diarrhea, and sinusitis. Several pulmonary and central nervous system (CNS) syndromes that are often fatal have been described (Table 24–1). About 1 of every 1000 patients dies, but the risk of death and other complications is increased in infants, adults, the malnourished, the immunodeficient, in those with underlying illnesses, and in countries whose populations are not immunized.[15–19] An example of the frequency of measles-associated complications can be shown with the recent resurgence of measles in the United States. Of 50,000 patients, 21% had one or more complications (diarrhea, 8%; otitis media, 6%; combination of giant cell pneumonia and secondary bacterial pneumonia, 6%; and encephalitis, 0.1%), 19% required hospitalization, and 0.3% died. The most frequent cause of death was pneumonia.

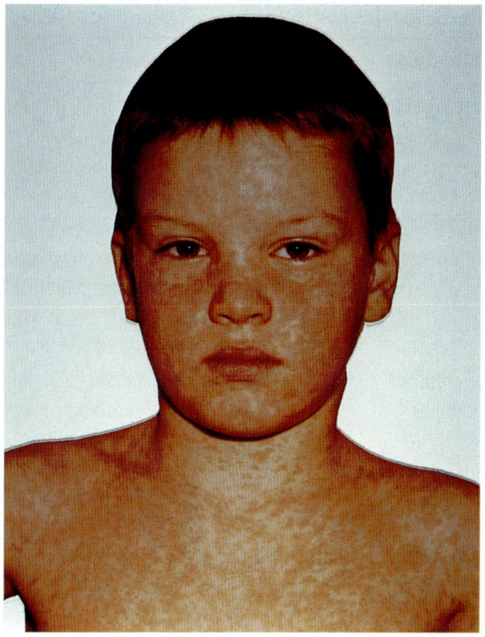

Figure 24–2. Measles on sixth day in a 6.5-year-old boy with fever, photophobia, coryza, and headache. In addition to the rash there is facial and periorbital edema, conjunctival injection, tearing, and tender cervical lymphadenopathy. The measles rash usually appears behind the ears and spreads rapidly to face, trunk, and limbs. *(Courtesy of Daniel H. Connor, MD, 1960.)*

PATHOGENESIS

The first step is attachment of the virus to surface receptors on respiratory epithelial cells. The receptor has been identified as the human membrane protein CD46, a member of the regulators of the complement activation gene cluster.[20] Adhesion and fusion of virus is mediated by both the H and F viral glycoproteins.[21] This is followed by local replication in respiratory mucosa and draining lymph nodes. Viremia follows, with dissemination throughout the reticuloendothelial system. Replication of virus at the secondarily infected sites causes lymphoid hyperplasia and characteristic reticuloendothelial multinucleated giant cells. A secondary viremia soon develops, with widespread dissemination of virus to different tissues by infected lymphocytes and monocytes. At this point, prodromal symptoms including cough, coryza, and conjunctivitis become more severe and replication of virus in the respiratory tract predisposes the patient to complications such as pneumonia and otitis media.

There are two types of multinucleated giant cells.[22,23] The "reticuloendothelial giant cell" (Warthin–Finkeldey) appears first during the incubation period and is in lymphoid tissues throughout the body (Figure 24–3). The second type is the "epithelial giant cell" and is in the epithelium of essentially every major organ (Figure 24–4). Infection of endothelial cells also appears to play an important role in the spread of infection.

TABLE 24–1. PULMONARY AND CNS COMPLICATIONS ASSOCIATED WITH MEASLES

Complications	Pathogenesis	Clinical Features	Pathologic Features
Pulmonary			
Secondary pneumonia	Secondary bacterial infection of damaged tissues; less commonly viral in origin.	As the rash fades, respiratory distress develops in association with persistence or recrudescence of fever; good prognosis if treated promptly.	Vary from an interstitial pneumonitis to that of secondary bacterial or viral pneumonia.
Giant cell pneumonia	Progressive measles replication; an opportunistic infection that rarely develops without an associated cell-mediated deficiency.	Severe and progressive pneumonia, usually without a rash; most cases fatal.	Measles virus in the characteristic multinucleated giant cells with both nuclear and cytoplasmic inclusions.
Atypical measles pneumonia	Atypical immune response in individuals previously vaccinated with inactivated vaccine; vaccine failed to induce immunity to fusion (F) surface glycoprotein responsible for spread of infection.	Pneumonia with segmental or lobar consolidation, hilar lymphadenopathy, and pleural effusions. Patients develop an atypical rash that frequently involves the feet and progresses proximally; generally self-limiting illness. The use of inactivated vaccine has been discontinued.	Little is known. Histologically, skin biopsy specimens show a combination of an Arthus reaction and delayed hypersensitivity.[59]
Central nervous system			
Acute postinfectious (allergic) encephalitis	Probably autoimmune demyelination.	Recrudescence of fever during convalescence from measles; headache, seizures, and changes in mental status; variable clinical course with mortality of about 10–20%; most survivors have neurologic sequelae.	Absence of virus, demyelination, necrosis, vascular injury, and hemorrhage.
Acute progressive measles (inclusion body) encephalitis	Progressive measles replication; an opportunistic infection which rarely develops without an associated cell-mediated deficiency.	Clinically extremely difficult to distinguish from acute postinfectious encephalitis; usually runs an acute or subacute fatal course.	Measles virus in neurons and glial cells, vascular cuffing, and perivenous demyelination.
Subacute sclerosing panencephalitis	Accumulation of certain mutations in genes encoding envelope proteins.	Long latent period (~6 years) after measles infection or vaccination; progressive mental retardation, motor dysfunction, seizures, coma, and uniformly fatal outcome within 1–2 years.	Measles virus in neurons and glial cells, vascular cuffing, gliosis, and demyelination.

The onset of the rash coincides temporally with the rise of serum antibody to measles virus. Interestingly, virus replication and giant cell formation cease with the appearance of rash. T-cell immunity is essential in clearing virus from lymphoid tissue and respiratory tract. Although children with congenital agammaglobulinemia respond normally to measles, patients with cell-mediated immunodeficiency develop giant cell pneumonia or encephalopathy but do not develop a rash.[15–18,24,25]

Immunity to the F surface glycoprotein is necessary to prevent the spread of measles infection.[26] An atypical measles syndrome characterized by pulmonary consolidation with pleural effusions and hilar lymphadenopathy develops in children exposed to the wild-type measles virus who had previously received the killed-measles virus vaccine.[27–29] Recipients of the formalin-inactivated vaccine have a good antibody response to the H protein, but antibodies to the functional region of the F protein and to the nucleoprotein are weak or absent. Perhaps the lack of a functional F antibody response plays a role in the spread of the virus.[30] Although formalin-fixed vaccines are no longer used, manufacturers involved in developing subunit vaccines for measles by using the F and H proteins must monitor for atypical measles, to ensure the safety of their products.

Subacute sclerosing panencephalitis (SSPE) occurs in patients who apparently have normal immune functions. Sequence evaluations of clones of the measles virus from brain specimens of SSPE patients have consistently shown an accumulation of mutations in the membrane protein genes (ie, the F, H, or M genes). These mutations are thought to account for the absence of viral budding at the cell surface in infected tissues of SSPE patients. This lack of budding would, in theory, enable the virus to escape immune surveillance and maintain a persistent and progressive infection.[31]

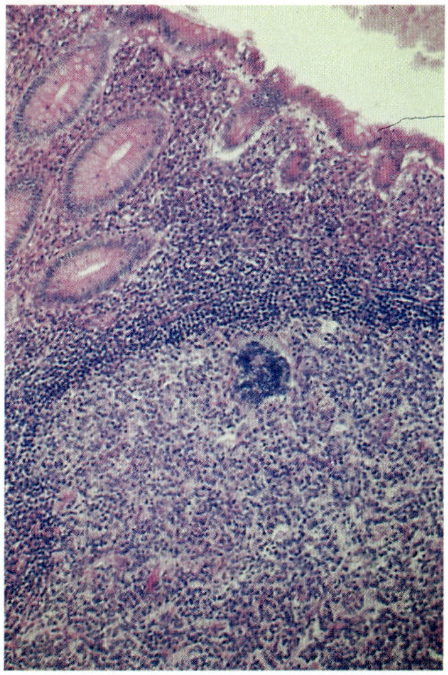

Figure 24–3. Section of vermiform appendix removed from a child during measles prodrome showing a very large Warthin–Finkeldey giant cell in the lymphoid tissue. The nuclei are prominent (hematoxylin-eosin, ×40). *(Courtesy of Ernest E. Lack, MD.)*

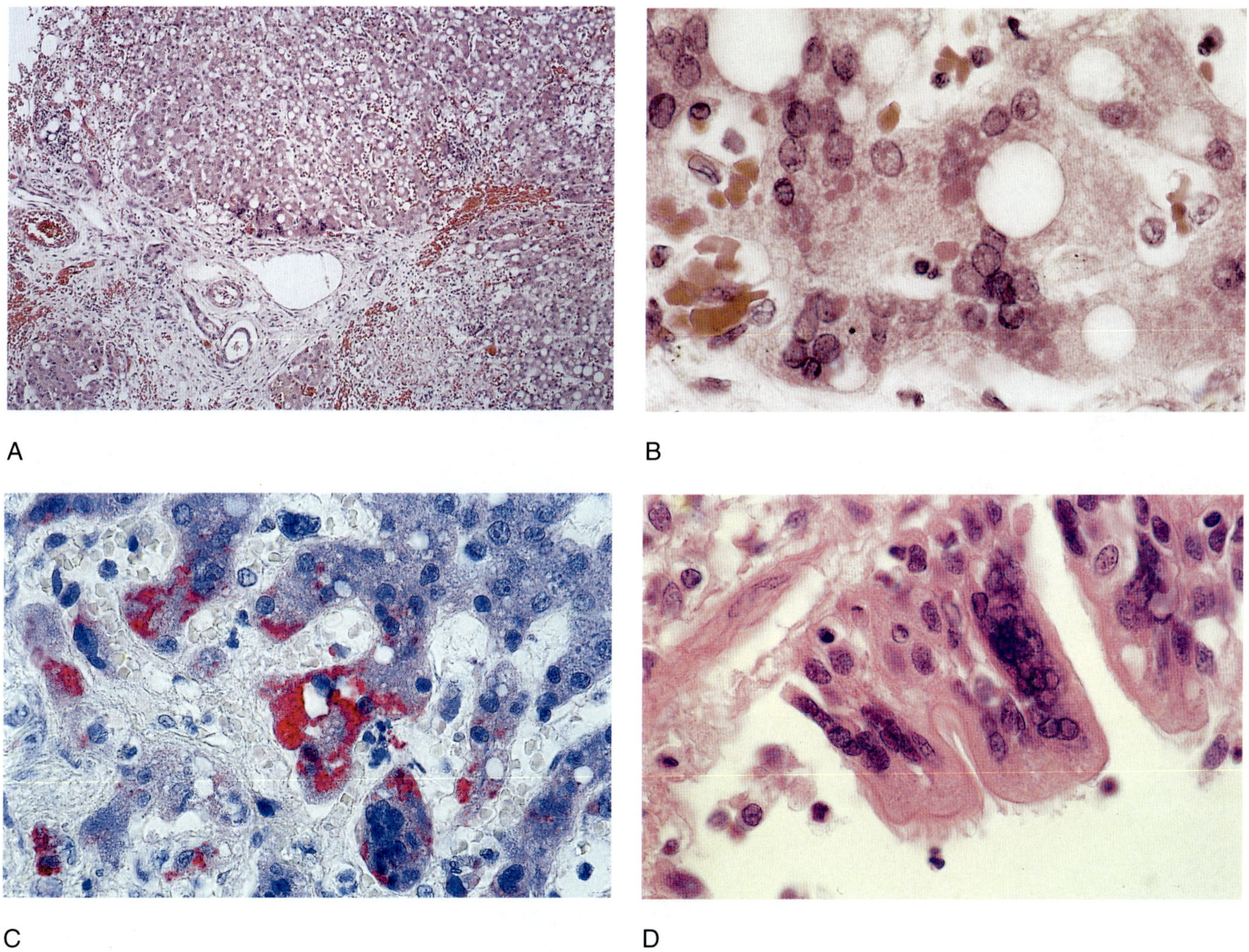

Figure 24–4. Multinucleated epithelial cells in measles. (**A**) Low-power photomicrograph of a liver showing focal areas of necrosis, leukocytic infiltration, and multinucleated giant cells (hematoxylin-eosin, ×25). (**B**) High-power photomicrograph of syncytial giant cells with eosinophilic, cytoplasmic, and nuclear inclusions (hematoxylin-eosin, ×250). (**C**) Measles antigens in the same hepatocytes as seen by immunohistochemistry (naphthol fast red substrate with light hematoxylin counterstain, ×158). (**D**) High-power photomicrograph of ciliated bronchiolar epithelial cells with characteristic measles inclusions (hematoxylin-eosin, ×250).

PATHOLOGY

The pathologic features of measles have been well described and several references containing detailed morphologic descriptions are recommended.[15,32–39] The typical morbilliform skin lesions, Koplik's spots, and measles lymphadenitis are seldom seen by the surgical pathologist as the clinical diagnosis usually is apparent. Histopathologic changes in the skin include mild congestion, edema, and a predominantly mononuclear infiltrate surrounding small vessels of the dermis, as well as other nonspecific features. Occasionally there are diagnostic multinucleated epithelial giant cells with eosinophilic cytoplasmic and nuclear inclusions.[37,40] Pathognomonic reticuloendothelial multinucleated giant cells (Warthin–Finkeldey) are in appendices from patients inadvertently operated on for acute appendicitis (Figure 24–3) before the emergence of diagnostic Koplik's spots and rash. Warthin–Finkeldey cells, which have been reported in various lymphoreticular tissues throughout the body, are typically large and contain from a few to up to 100 nuclei. These cells do not usually contain viral inclusions. The lymphoid tissues are typically hyperplastic, and the architecture is partially or totally obliterated by diffuse proliferation of immunoblasts.[41–43]

Patients with measles have a focal or generalized interstitial pneumonitis that resembles the pneumonia of many other viral infections. There are various degrees of peribronchial and interstitial mononuclear cell infiltrates, squamous metaplasia of bronchial epithelium, proliferation of type II pneumocyte alveolar lining cells, and intra-alveolar edema with or without mononuclear cell exudates and hyaline membranes (Figure 24–5). Secondary changes such as bacterial or viral superinfection or organizational changes may alter the appearance of the original lesions (Figure 24–6). The hallmark of the disease is the multinucleated epithelial giant cell (Figure 24–7). These cells, which are often numerous, are formed by fusion of bronchiolar or alveolar lining cells. In contrast to the reticuloendothelial giant cells, they generally contain characteristic nuclear and cytoplasmic inclusions. The intranuclear inclusions are homogenous, eosinophilic, more than one half the diameter of the nucleus, and surrounded by a slight indistinct halo. The cytoplasmic inclusions are deeply eosinophilic, vary in size, and some form large masses with a melted-tallow appearance. These

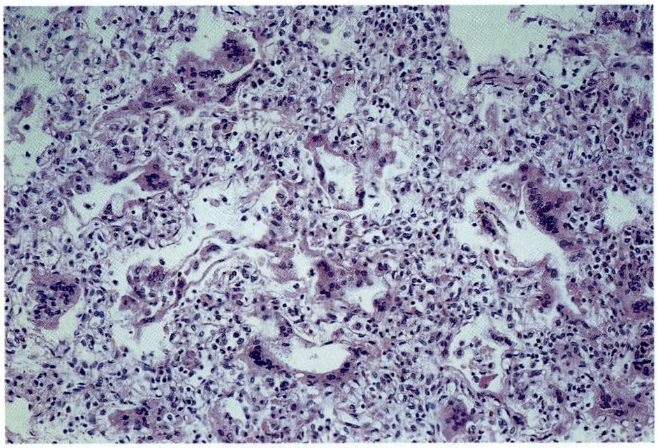

A

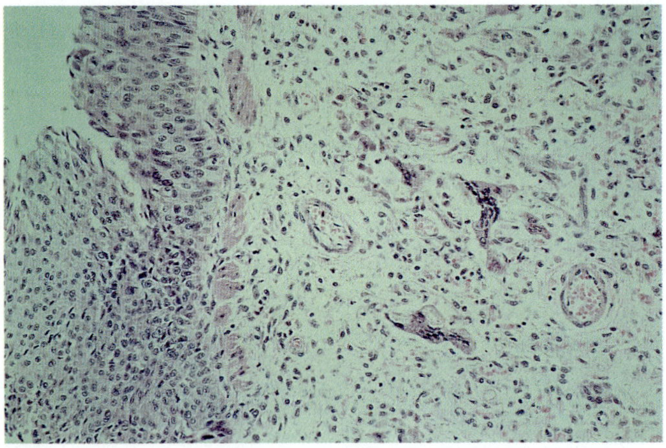

B

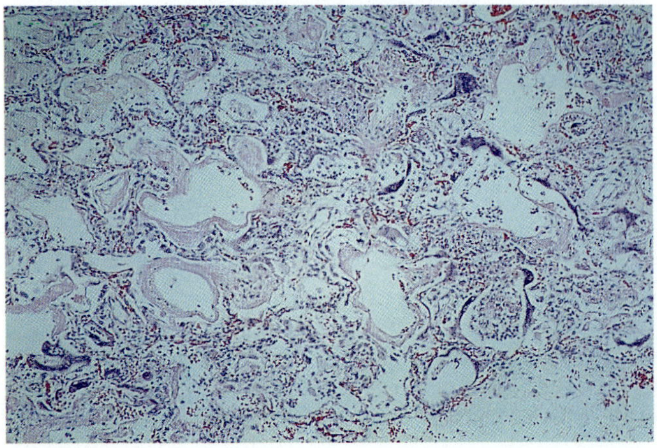

C

Figure 24–5. Measles pneumonia. (**A**) The classic features of interstitial pneumonitis of measles. The multinucleated giant cells are abundant and line the alveoli or lie free in alveolar spaces. (**B**) There is squamous metaplasia of the bronchiole and a few giant cells. (**C**) Diffuse alveolar damage and prominent hyaline membranes in a patient with measles pneumonia. Scattered multinucleated giant cells line some alveolar spaces (hematoxylin-eosin; A, ×50; B, ×50; C, ×25).

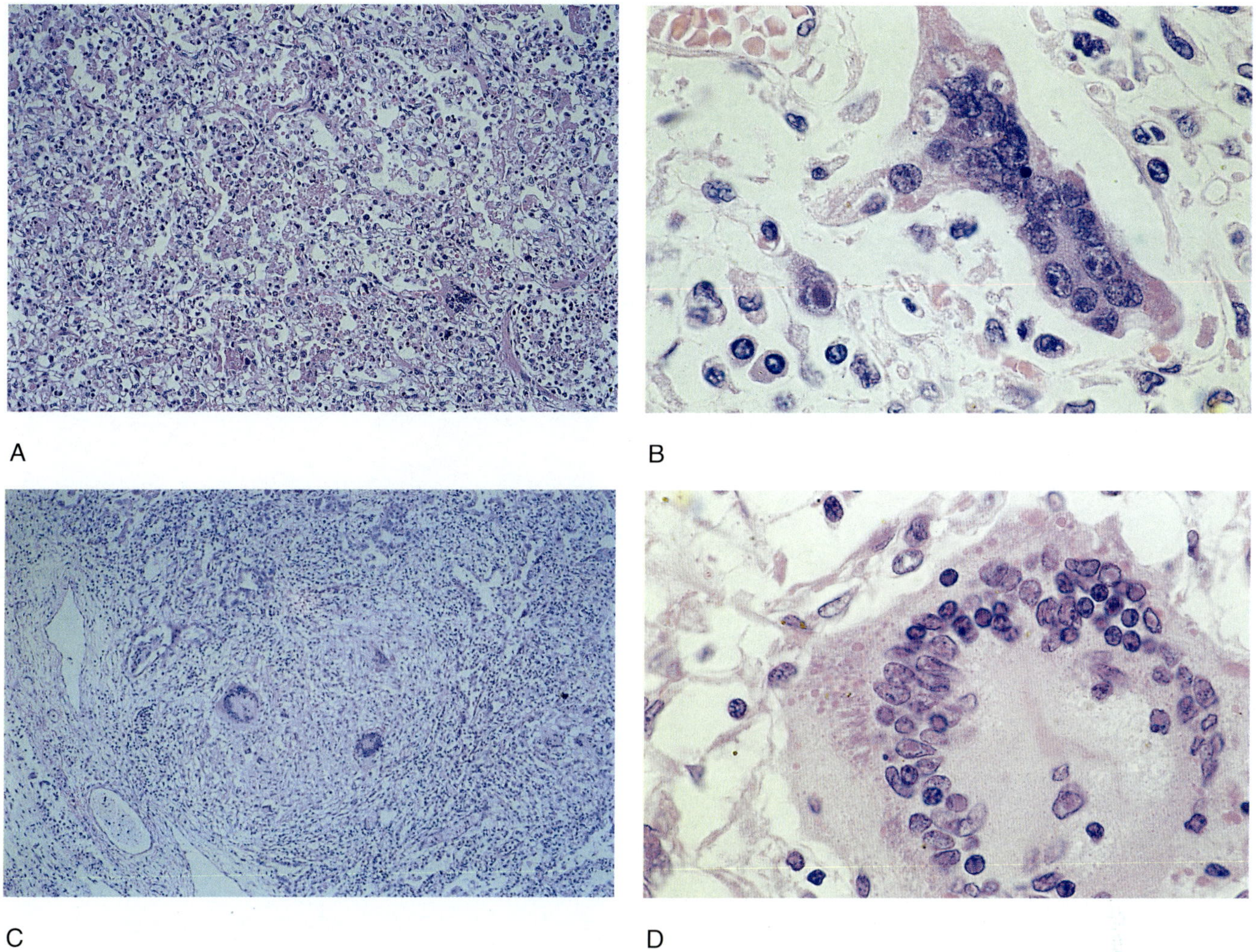

Figure 24–6. Measles pneumonia. (**A**) Measles pneumonia with secondary bacterial infection. Throughout the lung, the alveoli were filled with mixed inflammatory infiltrates, mainly neutrophils. Extensive search revealed rare multinucleated giant cells, but none contained viral inclusions. Diagnosis of measles pneumonia in this patient was accomplished through serologic testing. (**B**) Measles and cytomegalovirus pneumonia in a child with severe combined immunodeficiency. There is a large multinucleated measles giant cell and a cell with a basophilic cytomegalovirus intranuclear inclusion with a halo. (**C**) Low magnification of measles pneumonia showing an area with granuloma-like inflammatory reaction and giant cells. (**D**) Higher magnification of giant cell in part (C) showing characteristic cytoplasmic and intranuclear inclusions of measles (hematoxylin-eosin; A, ×50; B, ×250; C, ×25; D, ×250).

giant cells may undergo degenerative changes with progressive loss of cytoplasm, increasing basophilia, and shrinkage of nuclei. Measles virus in these giant cells may be demonstrated by immunofluorescent,[44,45] immunohistochemical (IHC),[16,46] and in situ hybridization (ISH) techniques (Figure 24–8).

SSPE shows the features of a subacute encephalitis (Figure 24–9). The meninges and perivascular spaces in the gray and white matter contain mononuclear cells. Focal changes scattered throughout the CNS include loss of neurons, hypertrophy of astrocytes, and microglial hyperplasia with gliosis. Viral inclusions are most frequently in nuclei of glial cells, but they are also in neurons and occasionally in the cytoplasm of infected cells. The infected nucleus is filled with an eosinophilic inclusion that compresses the chromatin against the nuclear membrane. Ultrastructurally, the nuclear inclusions seen by light microscopy are aggregates of measles virus nucleocapsids (Figure 24–10).

DIAGNOSIS

The diagnosis of typical measles usually can be made by clinical signs and symptoms. Causes of similar rashes, but without other features of measles, include rubella, dengue, infections by enteroviruses, and also drug reactions, especially to ampicillin. Measles should be in the differential diagnosis of unexplained pneumonia or encephalitis in those with immunodeficien-

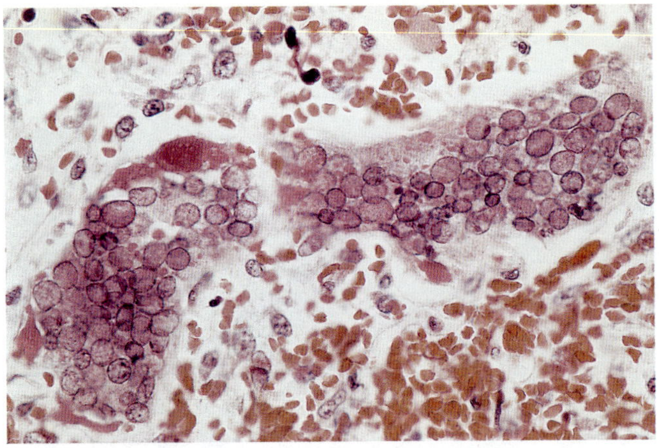

A

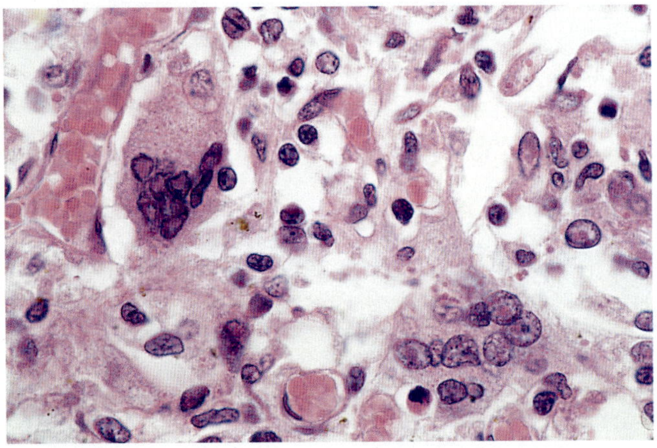

B

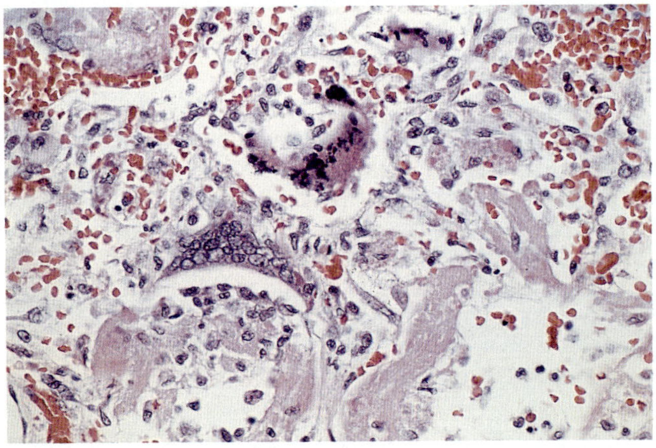

C

Figure 24–7. Histopathologic characteristics of viral inclusions in measles pneumonia. (**A**) Details of a multinucleated giant cell showing numerous eosinophilic cytoplasmic inclusions (hematoxylin-eosin, ×158). (**B**) Multinucleated measles giant cells with prominent eosinophilic intranuclear inclusions. The inclusions, which can sometimes be mistaken for those of herpes simplex virus, are separated from surrounding marginated chomatin by indistinct haloes (hematoxylin-eosin, ×250). (**C**) Degenerative changes in a multinucleated giant cell of measles (hematoxylin-eosin, ×100).

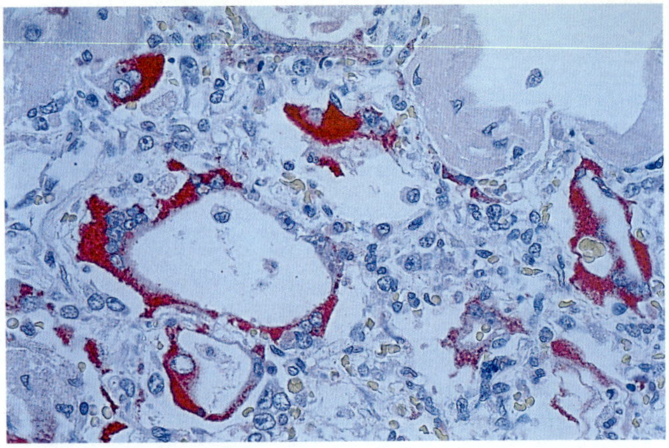

A

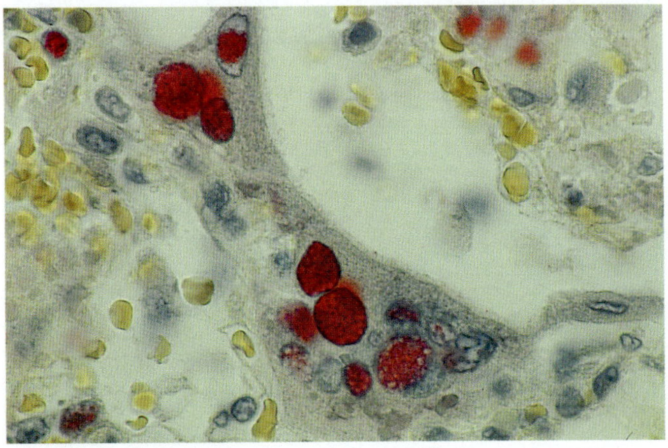

B

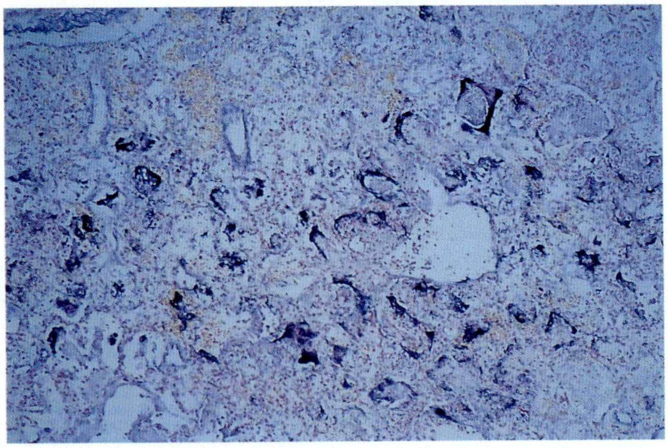

C

Figure 24–8. Immunohistochemistry and in situ hybridization in measles giant cell pneumonia. (**A**) Viral antigens in cytoplasm of giant cells by IHC staining. The multinucleated giant cells originate by fusion of infected alveolar lining epithelial cells. (**B**) Immunolocalization of viral antigens to nuclei of measles giant cell. The intranuclear inclusions of measles, which sometimes lack sharp circumscription (compare with Figure 24–7), are clearly shown (naphthol fast red substrate with light hematoxylin counterstain, A, ×100; B, ×250). (**C**) Low-power photomicrograph of lung containing numerous measles giant cells, demonstrated by colorimetric ISH using digoxigenin-labeled probes (NBT/BCIP substrate with nuclear fast red counterstain; ×25).

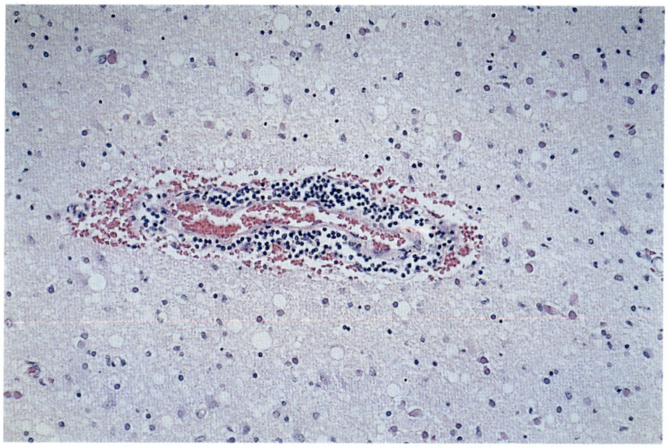

A

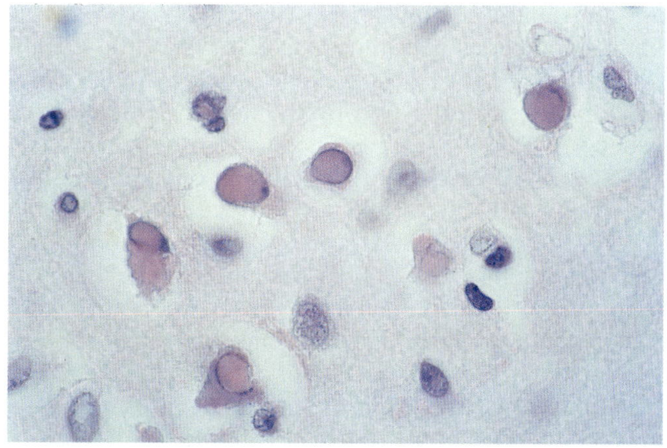

B

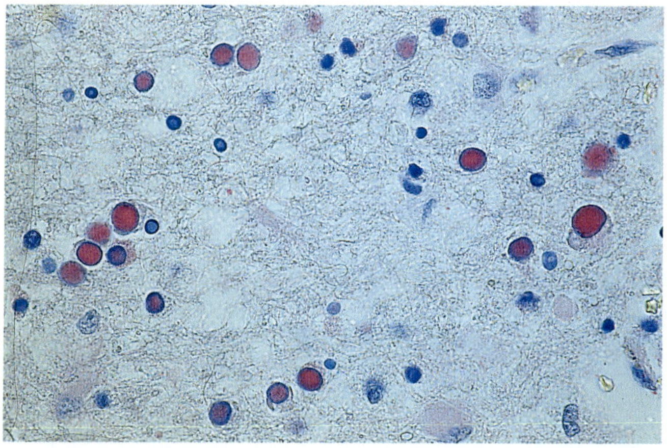

C

Figure 24–9. Subacute sclerosing panencephalitis (SSPE). (**A**) Perivascular lymphocytes and proliferation of microglia with gliosis. (**B**) Higher magnification showing multiple glial cells with hyalinized, intranuclear, eosinophilic inclusions with marginated chromatin (hematoxylin-eosin; A, ×50; B, ×250). (**C**) Confirmation and localization of measles antigens in same patient using immunohistochemistry (naphthol fast red substrate with light hematoxylin counterstain; ×158).

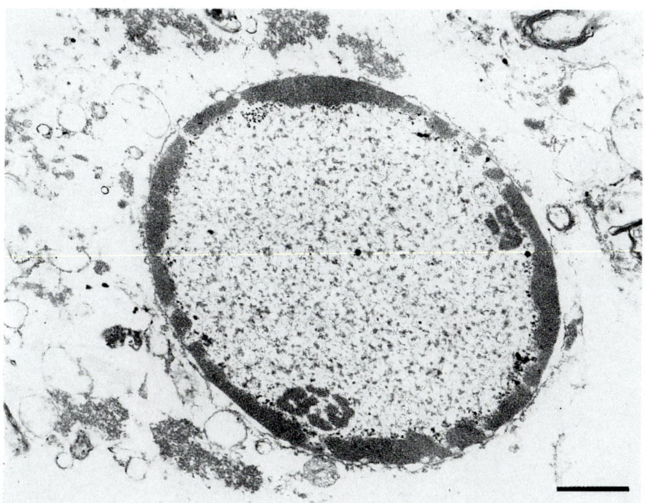

A

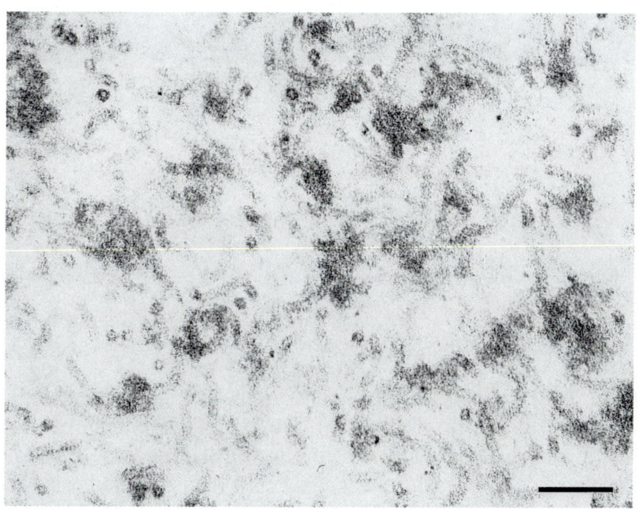

B

Figure 24–10. Subacute sclerosing panencephalitis (SSPE). (**A**) EM of part of a nucleus of a glial cell filled with numerous tubular nucleocapsids of measles virus. (**B**) Higher magnification showing longitudinal and cross-sectional profiles of measles nucleocapsids (scale bars: A, 1 μm; B, 100 nm). *(Electronmicrographs courtesy of Sylvia G. Whitfield.)*

cies. The differential diagnosis of SSPE should include other noninfectious and infectious diseases of the CNS, such as herpes, rubella, progressive multifocal leukoencephalopathy, and infection by the human immunodeficiency virus.

Typical measles giant cell pneumonia generally presents no difficulty for the surgical pathologist. Giant cells with both intranuclear and intracytoplasmic inclusions in a setting of interstitial pneumonitis are highly specific. Typical giant cells, however, are not in all measles pneumonia and their absence, therefore, does not exclude the diagnosis. Other viral and rickettsial agents may also cause similar interstitial pneumonitis, but without typical giant cells, and should be differentiated.[38] As previously noted, the histopathologic features of measles pneumonia can be variable, and secondary bacterial and viral infections may modify the changes, further complicating the diagnosis.[14,38] Other viral pathogens, such as respiratory syncytial virus,[47] parainfluenza,[48,49] varicella-zoster virus,[50] and a recently discovered equine morbillivirus,[51] as well as granulomatous diseases of the lung, may cause pneumonia with giant cells and also should be considered in the differential diagnosis. These clinical entities, however, can be separated by history, histopathologic features (Figure 24–11, A and B), and laboratory tests, including IHC assay (Figure 24–11, C).

The lymphadenitis that may develop after administration of live-attenuated vaccine should be differentiated from other viral lymphadenitides.[41–43,52,53] History of recent vaccination and Warthin–Finkeldey giant cells aid in this distinction. The intranuclear inclusions in the CNS of SSPE occasionally may be confused with those of herpes and other viral inclusions. In fact, the original observation of type A intranuclear inclusions in patients with SSPE led investigators initially to suspect a herpesvirus as the cause of SSPE. Electronmicroscopy, or preferably IHC[46,54,55] or ISH,[54,55] usually demonstrates the virus.

CONFIRMATION TESTING

Laboratory confirmation is useful to avoid possible confusion with other rash-causing illnesses. Diagnostic laboratory procedures consist of either direct detection of

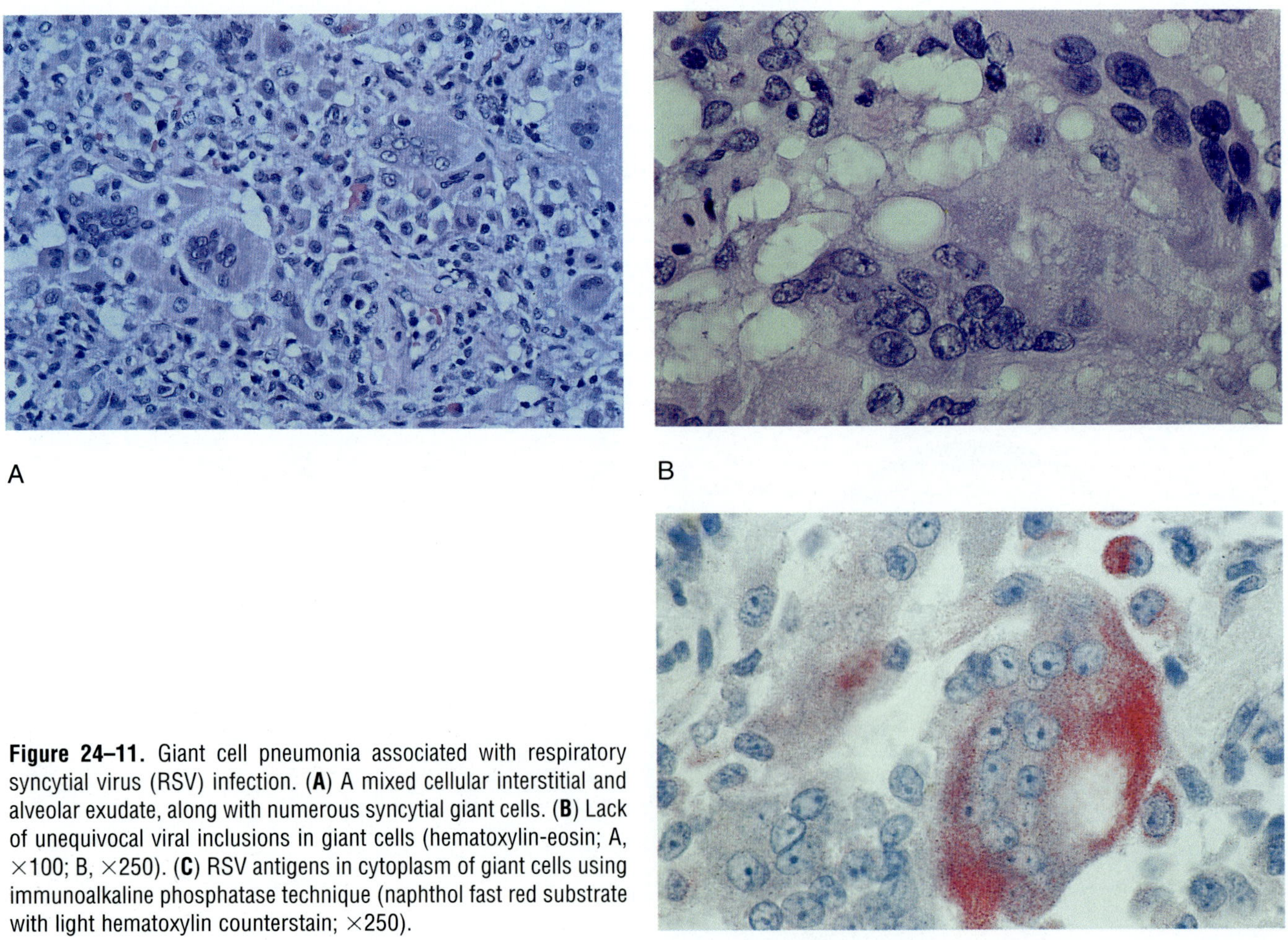

A B C

Figure 24–11. Giant cell pneumonia associated with respiratory syncytial virus (RSV) infection. (**A**) A mixed cellular interstitial and alveolar exudate, along with numerous syncytial giant cells. (**B**) Lack of unequivocal viral inclusions in giant cells (hematoxylin-eosin; A, ×100; B, ×250). (**C**) RSV antigens in cytoplasm of giant cells using immunoalkaline phosphatase technique (naphthol fast red substrate with light hematoxylin counterstain; ×250).

the virus or viral antigens, usually by indirect immunofluorescence or by serologic methods using hemagglutination inhibition, neutralization, or enzyme immunoassays. Specimens for serologic testing consist of acute and convalescent phase serum pairs. Antibody appears 1 to 2 days after onset of rash and titers peak approximately 2 weeks later. Alternatively, specific IgM antibody can be used to diagnose recent infection.[56]

IHC and ISH tests of formalin-fixed tissues with specific antibodies and nucleic acid probes are sensitive and specific for confirming measles. These methods have a unique role where archival tissues are the only specimens available. Electronmicroscopy may be useful, but as mentioned earlier, members of the paramyxovirus family have a similar microscopic appearance. Electronmicroscopic findings should therefore be interpreted in the context of other clinical, pathologic, and laboratory findings.

TREATMENT AND PREVENTION

Treatment is usually symptomatic. The most common complications, bacterial superinfections, should be treated promptly with appropriate antibiotics. Immune globulin, given within 6 days of exposure, can prevent or modify measles virus infection and is indicated for susceptible close contacts of measles patients who are at risk of developing severe illness. Measles vaccination may protect if given within 72 hours of exposure; however, it should not be given to women known to be pregnant or to women considering pregnancy in the next 3 months.

Measles vaccines are live-attenuated virus vaccines. Live-attenuated measles, mumps, and rubella vaccines generally are given as a combined vaccine at 15 months of age. Because the recent resurgence of measles in the United States was caused by a combination of failure to vaccinate and primary vaccine failure, a second dose of vaccine is now encouraged at school entry. For a discussion of the use of measles vaccines and immunoglobulin in preventing and treating measles, see the Centers for Disease Control and Prevention publication.[57]

Theoretically, measles virus should be readily eradicable. There is only a single serotype of the virus, and there is no animal reservoir in which the virus can persist. Almost every case is clinically identifiable and an effective, safe vaccine is available. Thus, widespread immunization sufficient to break the chain of transmission in developed as well as developing countries should eradicate the virus. In practice, the goal of eradication has been more difficult to achieve, and the consensus of opinion is that a new vaccine may be required.[58]

REFERENCES

1. Black FL. Measles. In: Evans AS, ed. *Viral Infections of Humans: Epidemiology and Control.* New York: Plenum; 1991:451–470.
2. Atkinson WL, Orenstein WA, Krugman S. The resurgence of measles in the United States, 1989–1990. *Annu Rev Med.* 1992;43:451–462.
3. Enders JF, Peebles TC, McCarthy K, Milovanovic M, Mitus A, Holloway A. Measles virus: a summary of experiments concerned with isolation, properties, and behavior. *Am J Public Health.* 1957;47:275–282.
4. Centers for Disease Control and Prevention. Measles—United States 1977–1980. *MMWR.* 1980;29:598.
5. Kingsbury DW. *Paramyxoviridae* and their replication. In: Fields BN, Knipe DM, eds. *Field's Virology,* 2nd ed. New York: Raven Press; 1990:945–962.
6. Kingsbury DW, Bratt MA, Choppin PW, et al. *Paramyxoviridae. Intervirology.* 1978;10:137–152.
7. Centers for Disease Control and Prevention. Measles surveillance—United States. *MMWR.* 1991;41(SS-6):1–7.
8. Babbott FL, Gordon JE. Modern measles. *Prog Med Sci.* 1954;228:334–361.
9. Goldberger J, Anderson JF. An experimental demonstration of the presence of the virus of measles in the mixed buccal and nasal secretions. *JAMA.* 1911;57:476–478.
10. Norrby E, Oxman MN. Measles virus. In: Fields BN, Knipe DM, eds. *Field's Virology,* 2nd ed. New York: Raven Press; 1990:1013–1043.
11. Centers for Disease Control and Prevention. Measles—Duval County, Florida, 1991–1992. *MMWR.* 1993;42:81–83.
12. Palmer E, Martin M. *Paramyxoviridae.* In: Palmer E, Martin M, eds. *Electron Microscopy in Viral Diagnosis.* Boca Raton, Fla: CRC Press; 1988:111–120.
13. Gremillion DH, Crawford GE. Measles pneumonia in young adults. An analysis of 106 cases. *Am J Med.* 1981; 71:539–542.
14. Kipps A, Kaschula ROC. Virus pneumonia following measles. A virological and histological study of autopsy material. *S Afr Med J.* 1976;50:1083–1088.
15. Breitfeld V, Hashida Y, Sherman FE, Odagiri K, Yunis EJ. Fatal measles infection in children with leukemia. *Lab Invest.* 1973;28:279–291.
16. Monafo WJ, Haslam DB, Roberts RL, Zaki SR, Bellini WJ, Coffin CM. Disseminated measles infection after vaccination in a child with a congenital immunodeficiency. *J Pediatr.* 1994;124:273–276.
17. Akhtar M, Young I. Measles giant cell pneumonia in an adult following long-term chemotherapy. *Arch Pathol.* 1973;96:145–148.
18. Archibald RWR, Weller RO, Meadow SR. Measles pneumonia and the nature of the inclusion-bearing giant cells: a light- and electron-microscope study. *J Pathol.* 1971;103: 27–40.
19. Christensen PE, Schmidt H, Bang HO, Anderson V, Jordal B, Jensen O. An epidemic of measles in southern Greenland, 1951. Measles in virgin soil. II. The epidemic proper. *Acta Med Scand.* 1953;144:430–449.
20. Naniche D, Varior-Krishnan G, Cervoni F, et al. Human membrane cofactor protein (CD46) acts as a cellular receptor for measles virus. *J Virol.* 1993;67:6025–6032.

21. Wild TF, Malvoisin E, Buckland R. Measles virus: both the haemagglutinin and fusion glycoproteins are required for fusion. *J Gen Virol.* 1991;72:439–442.
22. Robbins RC. Measles: clinical features. *Am J Dis Child.* 1962;103:266–273.
23. Sherman FE, Ruckle G. In vivo and in vitro cellular changes specific for measles. *Arch Pathol.* 1958;65:587–599.
24. Lewis MJ, Cameron AH, Shah KJ, Purdham DR, Mann JR. Giant-cell pneumonia caused by measles and methotrexate in childhood leukaemia in remission. *Br Med J.* 1978; 1:330–331.
25. Joliat G, Abetel G, Schlinder A, Kapanci Y. Measles giant cell pneumonia without rash in a case of lymphocytic lymphosarcoma. *Virchows Arch A Pathol Anat Histopathol.* 1973;358:215–224.
26. Merz DC, Scheid A, Choppin PW. The importance of antibodies to the fusion glycoprotein (f) of paramyxoviruses in the prevention of the spread of infection. *J Exp Med.* 1980;151:275–288.
27. Rauh LW, Schmidt R. Measles immunization with killed virus vaccine. *Am J Dis Child.* 1965;109:232.
28. Fulginiti VA, Eller JJ, Downie AW, Kempe CH. Altered reactivity to measles virus. Atypical measles in children previously immunized with inactivated measles virus vaccine. *JAMA.* 1967;202:1075–1080.
29. Laptook A, Wind E, Nussbaum M, Shenker IR. Pulmonary lesions in atypical measles. *Pediatrics.* 1978;62:42–46.
30. Norrby E, Enders-Ruckle G, ter Meulen V. Difference in the appearance of antibodies to structural components of measles virus after immunization with inactivated and live virus. *J Infect Dis.* 1975;132:262–269.
31. Baczko K. Lampe J, Liebert UG, et al. Clonal expansion of hypermutated measles virus in a SSPE brain. *Virology.* 1993;197:188–195.
32. Mallory FB, Medlar EM. The skin lesion in measles. *J Med Res.* 1920;41:327–348.
33. Strano AJ. Light microscopy of selected viral diseases (morphology of viral inclusion bodies). *Pathol Annu.* 1976;11:53–75.
34. Enders JF, McCarthy K, Mitus A, Cheatham WJ. Isolation of measles virus at autopsy in cases of giant-cell pneumonia without rash. *N Engl J Med.* 1959;261:875–881.
35. Radoycich GE, Zuppan CW, Weeks DA, Krous HF, Langston C. Patterns of measles pneumonitis. *Ped Pathol.* 1992;12:773–786.
36. Sobonya RE, Hiller FC, Pingleton W, Watanabe I. Fatal measles (rubeola) pneumonia in adults. *Arch Pathol Lab Med.* 1978;102:366–371.
37. Suringa DWR, Bank LJ, Ackerman B. Role of measles virus in skin lesions and Koplik's spots. *N Engl J Med.* 1970;283:1139–1142.
38. Strano AJ. Viral pneumonias (viral interstitial pneumonitis). In: Binford CH, Connor DH, eds. *Pathology of Tropical and Extraordinary Diseases.* Washington, DC: Armed Forces Institute of Pathology; 1976:57–64.
39. Becroft DM, Osborne DR. The lungs in fatal measles infection in childhood: pathological, radiological and immunological correlations. *Histopathology.* 1980;4:401–412.
40. Kimura A, Tosaka K, Nakao T. Measles rash. Light and electron microscopic study of skin eruptions. *Arch Virol.* 1975;47:295–307.
41. Allen MS, Talbot WH, McDonald RM. Atypical lymph-node hyperplasia after administration of attenuated, live measles vaccine. *N Engl J Med.* 1966;274:667–678.
42. Dorfman RF, Warnke R. Lymphadenopathy simulating the malignant lymphomas. *Hum Pathol.* 1974;5:519–550.
43. Stejskal J. Measles lymphadenopathy. *Ultrastruct Pathol.* 1980;1:234–247.
44. Koffler D. Giant cell pneumonia. Fluorescent antibody and histochemical studies on alveolar giant cells. *Arch Pathol.* 1964;78:267–273.
45. McQuillin J, Bell TM, Gardner PS, Downham PS. Application of immunofluorescence to a study of measles. *Arch Dis Child.* 1976;51:411–419.
46. Sata T, Kurata T, Aoyama Y, Sakaguchi M, Yamanouchi K, Takeda K. Analysis of viral antigens in giant cells of measles pneumonia by immunoperoxidase method. *Virchows Arch A Pathol Anat Histopathol.* 1986;410:133–138.
47. Delage G, Brochu P, Robillard L, Jasmin G, Joncas JH, Lapointe N. Giant cell pneumonia due to respiratory syncytial virus. *Arch Pathol Lab Med.* 1984;108:623–625.
48. Little BW, Tihen WS, Dickerman JD, Craighead JE. Giant cell pneumonia associated with parainfluenza virus type 3 infection. *Hum Pathol.* 1981;12:478–481.
49. Weintrub PS, Sullender WM, Lombard C, Link MP, Arvin A. Giant cell pneumonia caused by parainfluenza type 3 in a patient with acute myelomonocytic leukemia. *Arch Pathol Lab Med.* 1987;111:569–570.
50. Saito F, Yutani C, Imakita M, Ishibashi-Ueda H, Kanzaki T, Chiba Y. Giant cell pneumonia caused by varicella zoster virus in a neonate. *Arch Pathol Lab Med.* 1989;113: 201–203.
51. Murray K, Selleck P, Hooper P, et al. A morbillivirus that caused fatal disease in horses and humans. *Science.* 1995;268:94–97.
52. Allen MS, Talbot WH, McDonald R. Atypical lymph-node hyperplasia after administration of attenuated, live measles vaccine. *N Engl J Med.* 1966;274:677–678.
53. Dorfman RF, Herweg JC. Live, attenuated measles virus vaccine. Inguinal lymphadenopathy complicating administration. *JAMA.* 1966;198:230–231.
54. McQuaid S, Isserte S, Allan GM, Taylor MJ, Allen IV, Cosby SL. Use of immunocytochemistry and biotylinated in situ hybridization for detecting measles virus in central nervous system tissue. *J Clin Pathol.* 1990;43:329–333.
55. Kim TM, Brown HR, Lee SHS, et al. Delayed acute measles inclusion body encephalitis in a 9-year-old girl: ultrastructural, immunohistochemical, and in situ hybridization studies. *Mod Pathol.* 1992;5:348–352.
56. Hummel KB, Erdman DD, Heath HL, Bellini WJ. Baculovirus expression of the nucleoprotein of measles virus and the utility of the recombinant protein in diagnostic enzyme immunoassays. *J Clin Microbiol.* 1992;30: 2874–2880.
57. Centers for Disease Control and Prevention. Measles prevention: recommendations of the immunization practices advisory committee (ACIP). *MMWR.* 1989;38(suppl 9): 1–18.
58. Gellin BG, Katz SL. Measles: state of the art and future directions. *J Infect Dis.* 1994;170:S3–S14.
59. Annunziato D, Kaplan MH, Hall WW, et al. Atypical measles syndrome: pathologic and serologic findings. *Pediatrics.* 1982;70:203–209.

CHAPTER 25

Mumps

J. Thomas Stocker

O, that my face were not so full of O's!

William Shakespeare (1564–1616), Love's Labours Lost, V, II

DEFINITION

Mumps is an acute generalized viral infection of children and young adults by the mumps paramyxovirus. Mumps most often involves the parotid and other salivary glands where it causes diffuse interstitial edema, lymphocytic infiltrates, hemorrhage, and serofibrinous exudates.[1,2] Other manifestations include meningoencephalitis with neuronolysis and demyelination; orchitis with infarction, hyalinization, and fibrosis; pancreatitis, and deafness.

GEOGRAPHICAL DISTRIBUTION

Endemic throughout the world, mumps has seen a more than 95% decline in the United States following the introduction of live vaccine in 1967. A 99% decrease in the incidence of mumps (along with measles and rubella) was noted in Finland in 1992 following a comprehensive immunization program begun in 1982.[3] The incidence of mumps remains high, however, in countries without immunization programs.

EPIDEMIOLOGY

Mumps is spread from a human reservoir by airborne droplets, direct contact, fomites, and possibly by contact with urine of an infected person. The genders are equally affected. In countries with no immunization program, 85% of infections are in children younger than 15 years of age, although mumps is rarely seen in the first year of life due to the transplacental transfer of antibodies from mother to infant. However, mothers who develop mumps in the week before delivery may give birth to an infant with mumps or one who will develop the disease in the first week of life. Among nonimmunized adolescents and adults, there may be outbreaks in "closed populations" such as in military recruits, colleges, or the workplace. In the United States the annual incidence varied between 2982 and 12,848 cases in the 5-year period from 1984 to 1988.[4] Mumps is endemic throughout the year but most infections are in winter or early spring. Nearly one third of the infections will not develop clinical evidence of the disease.

The virus can be isolated from the saliva from 6 days before until 9 days after the first appearance of parotid gland swelling. Transmission of the virus may occur from 24 hours before appearance of the swelling to 3 days after the swelling subsides. Virus may be recovered from the urine up to 14 days after the onset of the clinical symptoms. Although second infections occasionally occur, lifelong immunity is usually conferred by immunization or by clinical or subclinical infection. Outbreaks, however, have been reported in even "highly vaccinated" (more than 95% of the population) school populations. Cheek et al[5] noted an 18% attack rate among 297 students in a high school in which 97% of the children had been vaccinated. Zimmerman et al[6] noted a fivefold increase of cases of mumps over a 3-year period in Switzerland, half of which were in vaccinated children. Complications including orchitis and meningitis were seen in 4% of cases.[6]

MORPHOLOGY OF THE MUMPS VIRUS

Mumps is caused by the mumps paramyxovirus, of which only one antigenic type is known. The virus contains a single-stranded, negative sense RNA surrounded by a helical nucleocapsid. Virions are pleomorphic with a roughly spherical shape, 85 to 300 nm in diameter. The nucleocapsid is surrounded by a three-layered lipid envelope. The outer layer contains two glycoproteins (the V and F antigens); one mediates neuraminidase and hemagglutinating activity, and the other facilitates lipid membrane fusion with the patient's cells. The internal layer contains the RNA protein NP, which is immunologically identical to the S antigen.[1,2,7,8] The hemagglutinating protein binds to sialic acid residues on host cells, initiating the infection, while the cell fusion protein fuses lipid bilayers, enabling penetration of the virus and cell-to-cell transfer of infection. The mumps virus can be cultured in a variety of cells, including embryonated chicken eggs and chicken embryo fibroblast tissue culture. Virus strains of wild viruses, laboratory strains, and vaccine strains can be separated and identified by polymerase chain reaction, nucleotide sequencing of the SH, F, and P genes, and determination of enzymatic activity of *N*-acetylneuraminidase.[9–12] In humans, the virus apparently enters through nose or mouth, replicates in the epithelium of the upper respiratory tract, then becomes bloodborne to seed the salivary glands and other organs.

TABLE 25–1. CLINICAL MANIFESTATIONS OF MUMPS

Organ	Manifestation
Parotid gland	Swelling, tenderness Pain elicited by tasting sour liquids Unilateral or bilateral
Submandibular gland	Swelling 10%–15% have only submandibular gland swelling
Central nervous system	Meningitis Fever, headache, lethargy Mild nuchal rigidity Encephalitis Seizures, focal neurologic signs Depressed levels of consciousness
Testes	Abrupt onset, fever, chills, nausea Vomiting, scrotal pain
Ovary	Pelvic pain, tenderness
Pancreas	Epigastric pain, tenderness Fever, chills, prostration
Heart	Nonspecific ST-T wave changes
Thyroid	Swelling, tenderness
Ear	Permanent or transient deafness Unilateral or bilateral
Kidney	Transient impaired concentrating ability
Joints	Migratory polyarthritis
Skin	Maculopapular erythematous rash

CLINICAL FEATURES

Although asymptomatic in about one third of patients, the mumps virus usually causes disease varying from a mild upper respiratory illness to severe multiorgan involvement (Table 25–1). The severity of the disease increases with age.[13] After an incubation period of 14 to 21 days (peak incidence of 17 to 18 days), mumps begins with symptoms of a nonspecific upper or lower respiratory illness. Prodromal manifestations, although infrequent, include fever, muscular pain, headache, and malaise. One to 2 days after the prodrome, the classic feature of enlargement of the parotid and other salivary glands begins. Either or both parotid glands may be involved with pain and swelling (Figures 25–1 and 25–2). The sequence begins with rapid swelling (in a matter of hours) between the posterior border of the mandible and the mastoid, extending in a series of crescents downward and forward, eventually pushing the ear lobe upward and outward. Edema of skin and soft tissue adds to the swollen appearance of the face. The submandibular gland also may be swollen, and, in 10% to 15% of patients, is involved in the absence of parotid gland swelling.

The central nervous system is involved in nearly half of mumps infections, usually as an asymptomatic pleocytosis in the cerebrospinal fluid. About 10% of patients develop symptoms of meningitis, only 40% to 50% of whom will have parotitis, making mumps one of the causes of "aseptic" meningitis in children and young adults. Postvaccination meningitis may also occur. Its incidence appears to be related to the degree of attenuation of the mumps virus vaccines. Currently used vaccines are essentially free of vaccine-strain–induced disease.[14]

Encephalitis occurs less frequently than meningitis and is more common in male patients. Clinical features include seizures, focal neurologic signs, and depressed levels of consciousness. Long-term sequelae are rare, although a chronic progressive encephalitis has been described as well as hydrocephalus.[15,16] The fatality rate for mumps meningoencephalitis is about 2%. Deafness—unilateral or bilateral, permanent or transient—may also occur.[17] Madle-Samardzija et al[18] noted hearing deficits in 46% of 237 patients, 71 of whom had parotitis and 166 had meningitis–meningoencephalitis. The loss was usually mild, and complete recovery occurred by 6 months; however, 2.53% of these patients had a total one-sided hearing loss. No correlation was

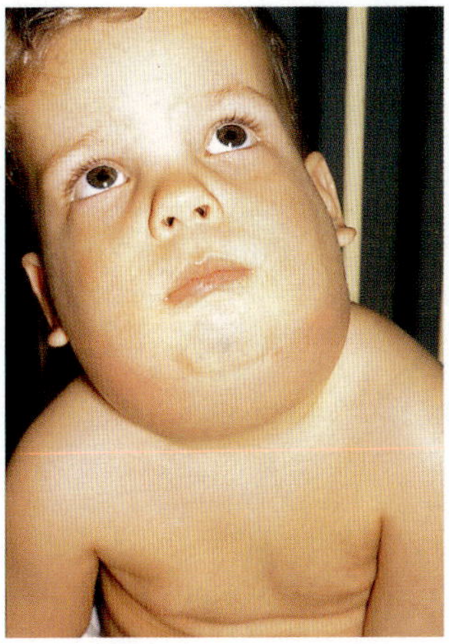

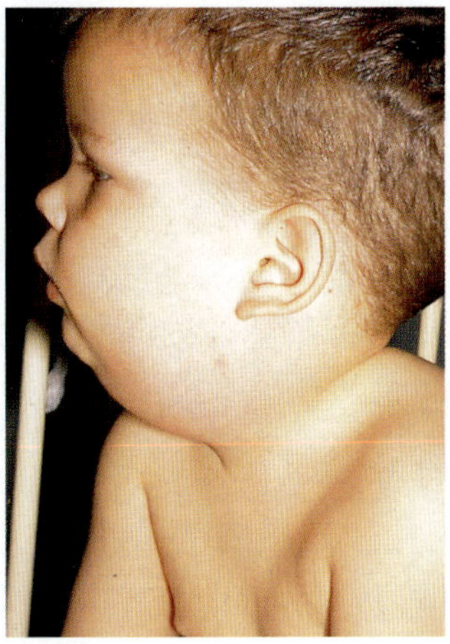

A B

Figure 25–1. (**A**) This 2.5-year-old boy developed a mild upper respiratory illness followed by unilateral, then bilateral, painful swelling of his neck. His younger sibling also developed mumps. *(Contributed by Melvin Museles, MD.)* (**B**) Same patient, same time, different view. *(Contributed by Melvin Museles, MD.)*

noted between the clinical manifestations and the degree of hearing loss.[18] Acute febrile polyneuritis (Guillain–Barré syndrome) following mumps has been noted rarely as it has in a variety of other viral infections, including varicella, measles, and infective hepatitis.[19]

Testicular and epididymal involvement occurs in nearly 20% of adult males with mumps, but is rare in childhood. Of those with mumps orchitis, bilateral involvement occurs in 15% to 25%. The orchitis follows the parotitis by 1 week and starts as an abrupt onset of fever, chills, nausea, headache, and lower abdominal pain, occasionally mimicking acute appendicitis. The testis is swollen and tender, with redness and edema of the skin adjacent to the testis. The infection subsides in 4 to 7 days and leads to testicular atrophy in 30% to 40% of patients. Impaired fertility is noted in 10% to 13%, but infertility is rare. Treatment of acute mumps orchitis with interferon-alfa-2 in postpubertal patients may prevent testicular atrophy and infertility.[20] In women, mastitis afflicts 7% to 30%, and about 5% have oophoritis. The ovary may be enlarged and tender, but subsequent infertility is rare.

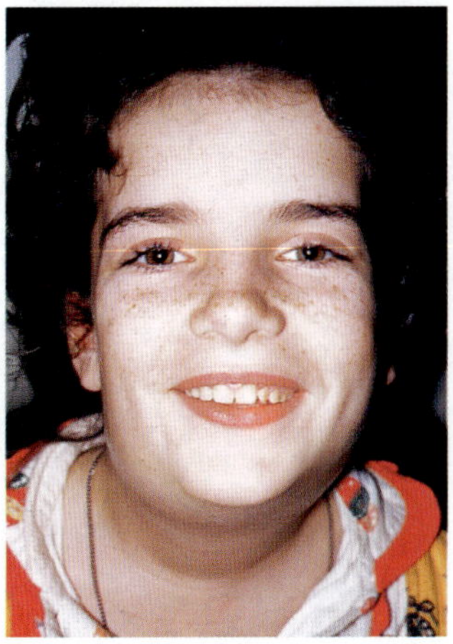

Figure 25–2. This 10-year-old girl has unilateral right-sided submaxillary swelling. *(Contributed by Melvin Museles, MD.)*

About 5% of patients have pancreatitis. At onset there is epigastric pain and tenderness, accompanied in severe infections by fever, chills, vomiting, and prostration. Mild or subclinical infections may be mistaken for gastroenteritis. Increased serum amylase is seen in patients with mumps, with and without pancreatic involvement.

Myocardial involvement presents as asymptomatic electrocardiographic changes (ST-T wave changes) in 15% of cases. Symptomatic myocardial or pericardial disease is rare. Arthritis and arthralgia may also be seen with mumps, beginning about 2 weeks after the onset of parotid gland swelling and lasting for up to 5 weeks, with recovery without residual joint damage.

Renal involvement takes the form of transient impaired urinary concentration, microscopic hematuria, or proteinuria in 60% of patients, but symptoms of renal involvement are rare. Ozen et al[21] described a 13-year-old boy with mumps who developed an acute hemolytic crisis (hemoglobin of 4.7 g/dL and reticulocyte count of 10.1%) with massive hemoglobinuria resulting in acute renal failure. The child's renal functions returned to normal in 10 days.

Infection during pregnancy is associated with an increased incidence of spontaneous abortion in the first trimester, but does not increase the risk of congenital malformations. Takano et al,[22] however, have noted the experimental development of Chiari type I malformation in the cerebellum of hamsters inoculated with mumps virus. Thrombocytopenia with fever and splenomegaly have also been noted in a newborn girl whose mother developed bilateral parotitis on the day of delivery. Severe respiratory distress also may complicate mumps in newborn infants.[23]

PATHOLOGY

The parotid gland in typical infections is grossly enlarged, and soft to moderately firm with areas of hemorrhage and focal necrosis. Necrotic debris may be expressed from ducts on the cut surface. Histologically, interstitial edema is prominent in the acute phase, and this is accompanied by a mild to moderate lymphocytic

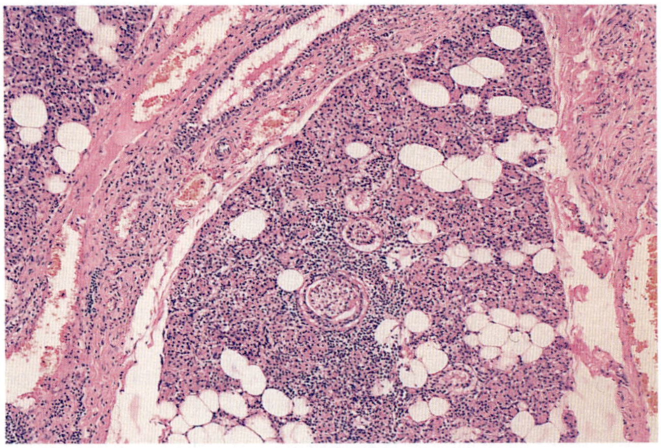

A

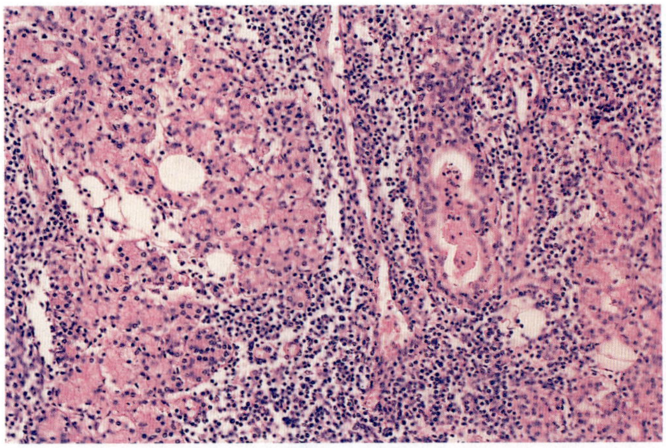

B

Figure 25–3. (**A**) The secretory and excretory ducts of the parotid gland are filled with inflammatory debris, which extends into the surrounding alveoli (hematoxylin-eosin, ×15). (**B**) The infiltrate of neutrophils and lymphocytes extends through the walls of the ducts (*right center*) into the surrounding interstitial spaces and alveoli lined by serous epithelial cells (hematoxylin-eosin, ×75).

infiltrate, hemorrhage, and a serofibrinous exudate. As the disease progresses, the glandular ducts undergo progressive epithelial necrosis and become filled with neutrophils and degenerated epithelial cells (Figure 25–3). The epithelial cells of the serous alveoli are relatively spared, but overflow of the inflammation from the ducts may be accompanied by interstitial edema. With resolution, the lymphocytic infiltrate subsides, the ductular epithelium regenerates, and the gland returns to normal. Similar changes occur in the submandibular and sublingual glands when they are involved. The multinucleated syncytial cells with intracytoplasmic eosinophilic inclusions noted in mumps-infected tissue cultures are not seen in histologic sections of infected glands.[24]

The testes display various degrees of gross edema and induration. The epididymis may be similarly involved but is rarely infected in the absence of testicular involvement (Figure 25–4). Histologically, the early changes consist of a mild to intense interstitial edema accompanied by a lymphocytic infiltrate. At this stage the spermatogenic cells may display few or no changes. As the inflammation increases, however, focal destruction of germinal epithelium occurs, but Leydig and Sertoli cells are spared. Resolution at this stage may leave little damage to the testes.[25] With more extensive reaction and compromise of the vascular supply, however, damage to the germinal epithelium and tubules may be significant, with necrosis and infarction leading to atrophy of the germinal epithelium, tubular hyalinization, and eventual fibrosis (Figure 25–5).

The cerebrospinal fluid in more than 50% of patients with mumps displays a lymphocytic pleocytosis and an elevated protein count regardless of whether there is clinical evidence of meningitis.[26] The pathology associated with mumps meningoencephalitis is rarely seen, because the vast majority of patients survive. When studied, however, there may be a perivascular mononuclear infiltrate in the leptomeninges, ependyma, and choroid plexus along with a generalized increase in microglial cells with sparing of neurons (Figure 25–6).[24] Herndon et al[27] have described an exfoliation of infected ependymal cells with reactive astrocytic proliferation and ependymal granulation at the site of ulceration. Stenosis of the aqueduct of Sylvius and foramen of Monro may be associated with obstructive hydrocephalus.[28–30] Hamdan et al[30]

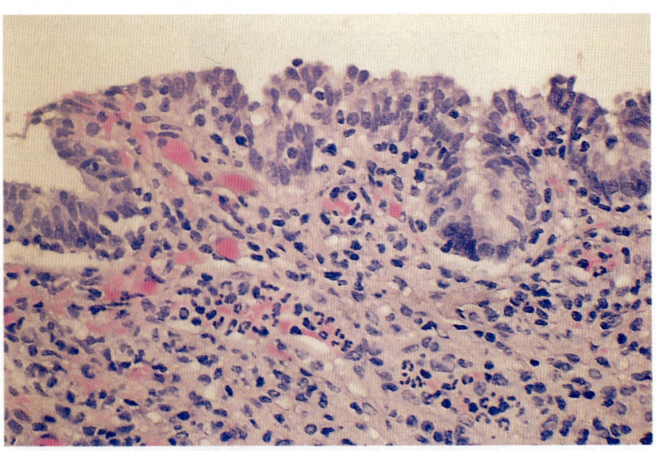

Figure 25–4. The epididymis in a 24-year-old man with mumps and painful scrotal swelling. There are neutrophils and lymphocytes throughout the pseudostratified columnar epithelium and underlying fibrovascular stroma (hematoxylin-eosin, ×100).

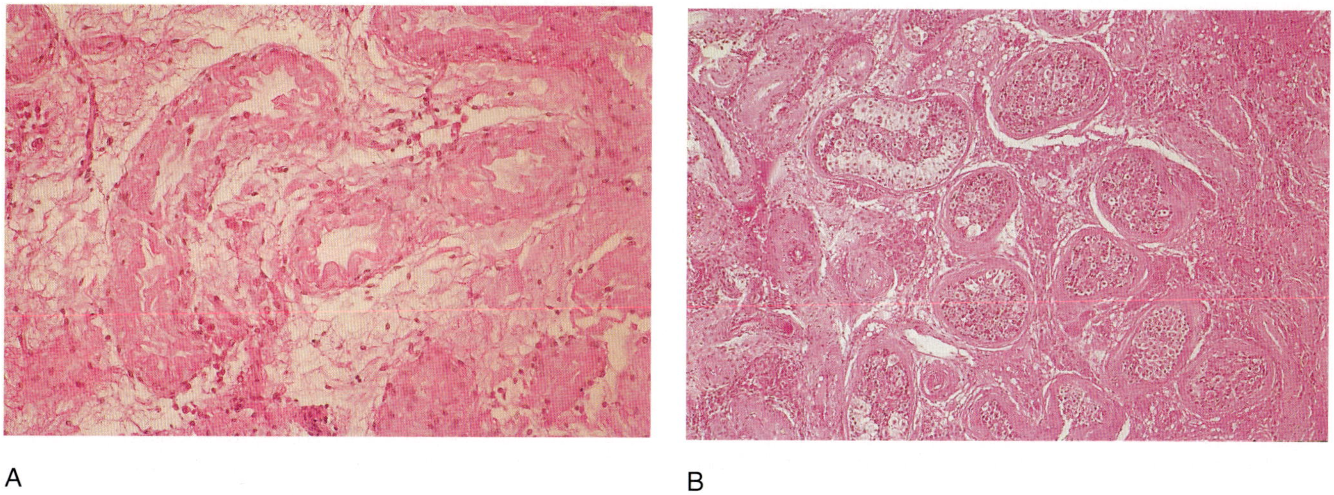

Figure 25–5. (A) Testis of a 27-year-old man who had had mumps orchitis at age 23. There is atrophy with hyalinization of the seminiferous tubules (hematoxylin-eosin, ×35). (B) In another area of testis of this same patient, there are foci of spermatogenesis in the seminiferous tubules (hematoxylin-eosin, ×35).

described subarachnoid hemorrhage in association with a mumps meningoencephalitis.

The pancreas shows similar changes to the parotid gland, with interstitial edema and obstruction of the ducts by neutrophils and necrotic debris.

DIFFERENTIAL DIAGNOSIS

The differential diagnosis includes the many causes of parotitis in children and adults, primarily infectious diseases. Other viruses that may infect the parotid gland include parainfluenza types 1 and 3, Coxsackieviruses A and B, echo virus, lymphocytic choriomeningitis, and influenza A. Viral cultures, serologic studies, or immunohistochemical stains may be helpful in identifying the specific viral agent. Acute suppurative parotitis may be caused by staphylococci, pneumococci, enteric gram-negative bacilli, streptococci, *Salmonella* sp, *Mycobacterium tuberculosis* sp, *Actinomyces* sp, and *Histoplasma capsulatum*, among others. Granulomas and abscesses are rare in mumps and would indicate that special stains including Gram's, acid-fast, and silver might be useful.

A variety of drugs may cause parotid enlargement. These include bromides, iodides, isoproterenol, phenothiazines, thiouracil, sulfixazole, phenylbutazone, beryllium, alpha-methyldopa, and heavy metals such as

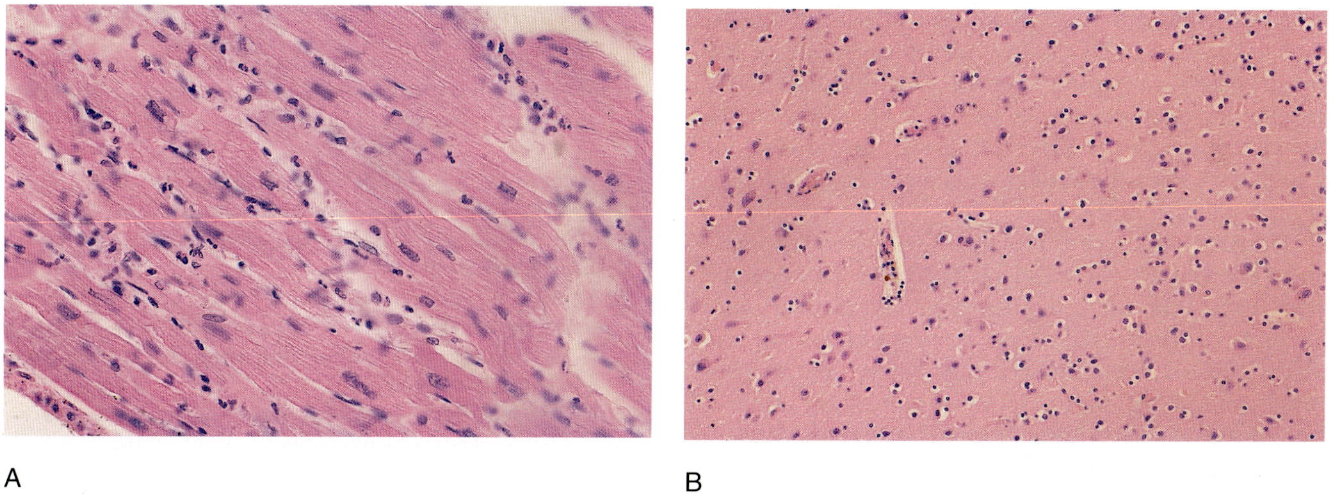

Figure 25–6. This 21-year-old man with headaches, fever, and bilateral mumps parotitis died suddenly. Sections of myocardium (A) revealed diffuse infiltrate of neutrophils and lymphocytes. (B) In the brain of the same patient there is diffuse meningoencephalitis characterized by lymphocytes surrounding vessels and extending into the neural tissue.

mercury and lead. Parotid enlargement may occur also from ductular obstruction as well as from benign and malignant tumors, including hemangioma, the most common salivary gland tumor in children. Systemic diseases leading to parotid enlargement include sarcoidosis, Waldenstrom macroglobulinemia, systemic lupus erythematosus, and Sjögren's syndrome. Metabolic disorders may also cause enlargement of the parotid; these include diabetes mellitus, alcoholism, cirrhosis, obesity, malnutrition, and uremia.

Scrotal enlargement may be caused by torsion of the testis (accompanied by pain and swelling), hydrocele, inguinal hernia, epididymitis from other infectious agents (e.g., *M. tuberculosis*), and a variety of germ- and nongerm-cell neoplasms including embryonal rhabdomyosarcoma, endodermal sinus tumor, lymphoma, embryonal sarcoma, teratoma, and seminoma.[31] The differential diagnosis of meningoencephalitis seen with mumps includes other viral causes of aseptic meningitis and encephalitis, which in the United States includes the enteroviruses, arboviruses, herpesviruses, and human immunodeficiency virus.[32]

DIAGNOSIS

The typical clinical findings of an acute generalized infection with nonsuppurative swelling and tenderness of the parotid glands is so characteristic of mumps and the illness is usually so mild that laboratory confirmation is seldom requested. When needed for the confirmation of the diagnosis, however, the virus can be readily recovered from saliva, urine, and cerebrospinal fluid (CSF), and has been isolated from breast milk and parotid gland blood.[7]

Saliva cultures may be obtained in the first 3 days of the illness by vigorously rubbing with a cotton swab moistened with buffered salt solution (BSS) the tonsils, oropharynx, and the area around the openings of the parotid gland (Stensen's ducts). Urine cultures, by clean-voided specimens, may be obtained as long as 14 days after the onset of illness. CSF may be positive for up to 9 days after the onset of clinically apparent central nervous system infection.

Monkey kidney cells are most often used for isolation of the mumps virus, which produces a cytopathic effect consisting of cell rounding and fusion with formation of giant cells. Viral hemagglutinins on the mumps-infected cell membranes allow a positive hemadsorption test with chicken or guinea pig erythrocytes. Hemadsorption inhibition tests, immunofluorescent staining, and neutralization tests may also be used.[7]

Serologic tests for mumps may be performed on acute- and convalescent-phase sera. Complement fixation tests for antibody to S and V antigens may be useful as a rapid diagnostic test in the first few days of the illness. A hemagglutination inhibition antibody appears within 4 days following the onset of symptoms and peaks about 1 week after onset. Antibodies in patient sera also may be detected with the neutralization test and the immunofluorescent antibody test. Test kits are available commercially for the latter test. Enzyme-linked immunosorbent assay (ELISA) is useful for detecting mumps-specific IgM and IgG antibody, with IgM detectable as early as 48 hours after onset. Immunofluorescent tests are available for detection of IgM, IgG, and IgA. Mumps-specific IgM also can be detected by a hemadsorption immunosorbent technique using microtiter wells coated with antihuman IgM, which is reacted with human serum, mumps agglutinin, and erythrocytes. If mumps-specific IgM is present, there is hemadsorption. Cross-reaction with parainfluenza viruses may confuse the diagnosis. Radioimmunoassay may also be used to detect mumps-specific immunoglobulins.[7]

TREATMENT

Treatment of patients with mumps is largely symptomatic and supportive, using analgesics to relieve the pain caused by the parotid gland swelling and antipyretics to reduce fever. Management of orchitis is also supportive, although Erpenbach noted prompt resolution of bilateral mumps orchitis with no evidence of testicular atrophy or oligospermia in four men treated with interferon-alpha-2B.[33] In patients with persistent vomiting from meningitis or pancreatitis, intravenous fluid may be necessary.

REFERENCES

1. Ray CG. Viruses of mumps and childhood exanthems. In: Sherris JC, ed. *Medical Microbiology. An Introduction to Infectious Diseases.* 2nd ed. New York: Elsevier;1992: 517–519.
2. Pomeroy C, Jordan MC. Mumps. In: Hoeprich PD, Jordan MC, Ronald AR, eds. *Infectious Diseases. A Treatise of Infectious Processes.* 5th ed. Philadelphia: JB Lippincott;1994:829–834.
3. Pertola H, Heinonen OP, Valle M, et al. The elimination of indigenous measles, mumps, and rubella from Finland by a 12-year, two-dose vaccination program. *N Engl J Med.* 1994;331:1397–1402.
4. Centers for Disease Control and Prevention. Summary of notifiable disease, United States. 1989. *MMRW.* 1989;38: 1–59.
5. Cheek JE, Baron R, Atlas H, Wilson DL, Crider Jr RD. Mumps outbreak in a highly vaccinated school population. *Arch Pediatr Adolesc Med.* 1995;149:774–778.

6. Zimmerman H, Matter HC, Kiener T. Mumps epidemiology in Switzerland: results from the Sentinella surveillance system 1986–1993. Sentinella Work Group. *Soz Praeventivmed.* 1995;40:80–92.
7. Kleiman MB. Mumps virus. In: Lennette EH, ed. *Laboratory Diagnosis of Viral Infections.* New York: Marcel Dekker; 1992:549–566.
8. Brunell PA. Mumps. In: Feigin RD, Cherry JD, eds. *Textbook of Pediatric Infectious Diseases.* 3rd ed. Philadelphia: WB Saunders; 1992:1610–1613.
9. Grubhoffer L, Hanova J, Otavova M. An attempt to analyze the functional difference between various mumps virus strains. *Acta Virol.* 1990;34:85–89.
10. Katayama K, Oya A, Tanabayashi K, et al. Differentiation of mumps vaccine strains from wild viruses by single-strand conformation polymorphism of the P gene. *Vaccine.* 1993;11:621–623.
11. Yamada A, Takeuchi K, Tanabayashi K, Hishiyama M, Sugiura A. Sequence variation of the P gene among mumps virus strains. *Virology.* 1989;172:374–376.
12. Kunkel U, Driesel G, Henning U, Gerike E, Willers H, Schreier E. Differentiation of vaccine and wild mumps viruses by polymerase chain reaction and nucleotide sequencing of the SH gene: brief report. *J Med Virol.* 1995;45:121–126.
13. Herzog C. Mumps epidemiology—worldwide. *Soz Praventivmed.* 1995;40:93–101.
14. Strohle A, Germann D. Mumps vaccines: virological basis. *Soz Praeventivmed.* 1995;40:102–109.
15. Haginoya K, Ike K, Iinuma K, et al. Chronic progressive mumps virus encephalitis in a child. *Lancet.* 1995;346:50. Letter.
16. Ogata H, Oka K, Mitsudome A. Hydrocephalus due to acute aqueductal stenosis following mumps infection: report of a case and review of the literature. *Brain Dev.* 1992;14:417–419.
17. Bang E, Kjaer I, Christensen L. Etiologic aspects and orthodontic treatment of unilateral localized arrested tooth-development combined with hearing loss. *Am J Orthod Dentofacial Orthop.* 1995;108:154–161.
18. Madle-Samardzija N, Dimic E, Topolac R, et al. Sensorineural impairment in the inner ear in epidemic parotitis. *Med Pregl.* 1993;46:357–360.
19. Murthy JM. Guillain–Barré syndrome following specific viral infections—an appraisal. *J Assoc Physicians India.* 1994;42:27–29.
20. Ruther U, Stilz S, Rohl E, et al. Successful interferon-alpha 2a therapy for a patient with acute mumps orchitis. *Eur Urol.* 1995;27:174–176.
21. Ozen S, Damarguc I, Besbas N, Saatci U, Kanra T, Gurgey A. A case of mumps with hemolytic crisis resulting in hemoglobinuria and acute renal failure. *J Med.* 1994;25:255–259.
22. Takano T, Uno M, Yamano T, Shimada M. Pathogenesis of cerebellar deformity in experimental Chiari type I malformation caused by mumps virus. *Acta Neuropathol.* 1994;87:168–173.
23. Lacour M, Maherzi M, Vienny H, Suter S. Thrombocytopenia in a case of neonatal mumps infection: evidence for further clinical presentations. *Eur J Pediatr.* 1993;152:739–741.
24. Baum SG, Litman N. Mumps virus. In: Mandell GL, Bennett JE, Dolin R, eds. *Principles and Practice of Infectious Disease.* New York: Churchill Livingstone; 1995:1496–1501.
25. Manson AL. Mumps orchitis. *Urology.* 1990;36:355–358.
26. Menkes JH. *Textbook of Child Neurology.* 5th ed. Baltimore: Williams and Wilkins; 1990:523–524.
27. Herndon RM, Johnson RT, Davis LE, Descalzi LR. Ependymitis in mumps virus meningitis, electron microscopical studies of cerebrospinal fluid. *Arch Neurol.* 1974;30:475–479.
28. Lahat E, Aladjem M, Schiffer J, Starinsky R. Hydrocephalus due to bilateral obstruction of the foramen of Monroe: a "possible" late complication of mumps encephalitis. *Clin Neurol Neurosurg.* 1993;95:151–154.
29. Takano T, Mekata Y, Yamano T, Shimada M. Early ependymal changes in experimental hydrocephalus after mumps virus inoculation in hamsters. *Acta Neuropathol.* 1993;85:521–525.
30. Hamdan H, Carrington D, Gledhill RF. Mumps virus meningoencephalitis complicated by subarachnoid haemorrhage. *J R Soc Med.* 1993;86:357–358.
31. Coffin CM, Dehner LP. The male reproductive system. In: Stocker JT, Dehner LP, eds. *Pediatric Pathology.* Philadelphia: JB Lippincott; 1992:905–918.
32. Dyken PR, Maertens P. Viral infections. In: Duckett S, ed. *Pediatric Neuropathology.* Baltimore: Williams and Wilkins; 1995:402–405.
33. Erpenbach KH. Systemic treatment with interferon-alpha 2B: an effective method to prevent sterility after bilateral mumps orchitis. *J Urol.* 1991;146:54–58.

CHAPTER 26

Parvovirus B19 Infection

Neal S. Young

A moment's insight is sometimes worth a life's experience.

Oliver Wendell Holmes (1809–1894)

DEFINITION

Parvoviruses cause a variety of animal diseases; in 1975, a pathogenic human parvovirus was discovered in the serum of a blood bank donor and named B19.[1] The *Parvoviridae* are characterized by their physical appearance (Figure 26–1) and genomic organization. All the virus's genetic information is contained in 5000 nucleotides of single-stranded DNA, which encodes two to three capsid proteins and one to two nonstructural proteins. B19 is a member of the Erythrovirus genus, which also includes genetically homologous and functionally similar simian viruses.[2] B19 parvovirus is also related to adeno-associated virus, another human (but apparently nonpathogenic) parvovirus that requires a second virus helper function for its replication. Canine parvovirus, feline panleucopenia virus, Aleutian disease virus, and porcine parvovirus are other autonomous members of the family, but these parvoviruses are species specific and do not infect humans. All the *Parvoviridae* require mitotically active cells for productive infection; parvovirus infection is cytotoxic, but under some circumstances virus can be latent in cells of tissue culture and patients.

EPIDEMIOLOGY

Stable genetic material and absence of a lipid envelope make parvoviruses resistant to heat and contribute to B19 parvovirus contagion. Infection is common and worldwide. As judged from the presence of specific IgG antibody to virus, about half the population acquires immunity to the virus in childhood, and the rate of seropositivity continues to rise with age. B19 parvovirus infection causes several distinct clinical syndromes (Table 26–1), but in most children and adults infection is probably asymptomatic.[3] In addition to these accepted parvovirus diseases, case reports of seroconversion associated with idiopathic thrombocytopenic purpura, agranulocytosis, and peripheral neuropathy suggest that the clinical spectrum of illness may not yet be defined from want of widely available clinical assays.

PATHOPHYSIOLOGY

Very high concentrations of virus in blood can be reached during acute infection, $\geq 10^{12}$ particles or genome copies per milliliter. Little virus is in urine or feces of inoculated volunteers, but virus is shed from the nasopharynx.[4] How the virus gains entry to the bloodstream of children or adults or traverses the placenta for uterine infection is unknown. The only known target cell of B19 parvovirus is in the bone marrow.[5] In the marrow, B19 parvovirus is highly tropic for late erythroid progenitor cells, the parental cells of circulating red blood cells (Figure 26–2). Erythroid tropism is determined by the cell receptor for virus, globoside, or red cell P antigen, which is on erythrocytes, megakaryocytes, and endothelial cells.[6] Virus replication within erythroid precursors is visible from DNA analysis, both for erythropoietic cells infected in vitro—marrow,[7] peripheral blood,[8] fetal liver,[9] and erythroleukemia cells[10]—and in marrow drawn from infected patients.[11] Infection in erythroid cells is efficient, each cell producing several thousand progeny viruses.[12] Although the virus does not replicate in other marrow cells, infection of megakaryocytes and limited expression of the

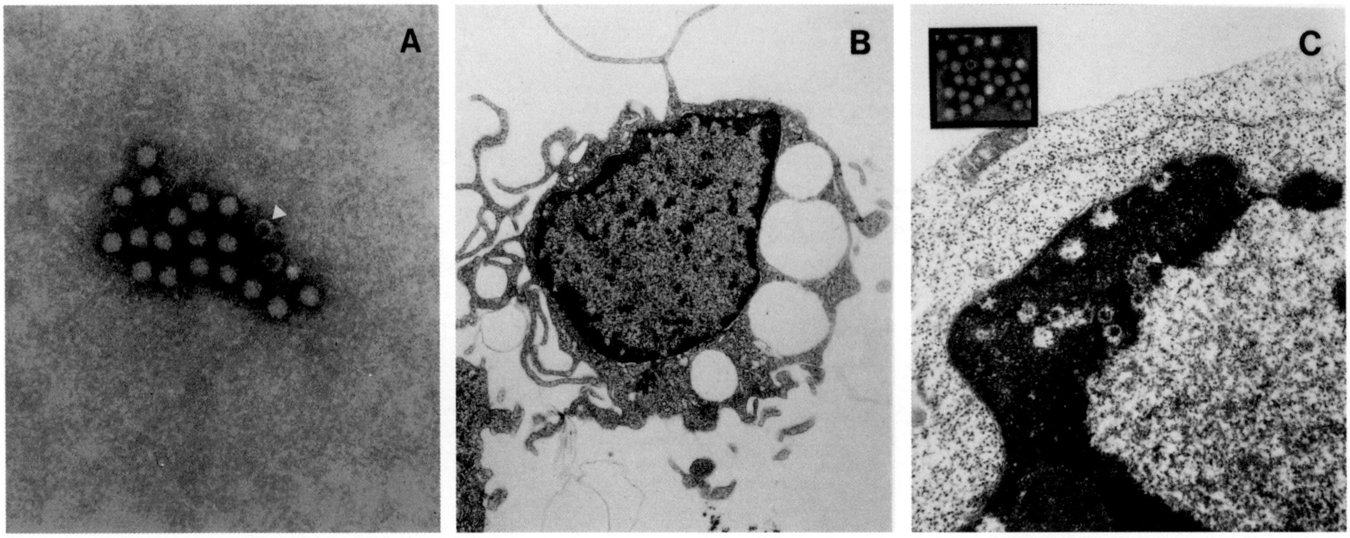

Figure 26–1. Electron microscopy. (**A**) Parvovirus in serum, showing characteristic small-size particles, about 25 nm in diameter, empty capsids (*arrowhead*), and icosahedral shape. *(Courtesy of Professor Y. E. Cossart.[45])* (**B**) Erythroid progenitor cell, infected in tissue culture, showing chromatin margination, vacuolization, and pseudopod formation.[46] (**C**) Virus in crystalline arrays within lacunae in the nucleus of an infected cell.

cytotoxic nonstructural viral protein could lead to thrombocytopenia.[13] In addition, the virus may be in tissue macrophages. In the immunologically competent host, virus infection is terminated with the production of neutralizing antibodies.[14,15]

CLINICAL FEATURES

The common manifestation of B19 parvovirus infection is fifth disease.[16] In children, fifth disease is a highly contagious but not very severe rash illness, with a characteristic lacy erythematous exanthem over the face ("slapped cheek"), trunk, and proximal portions of limbs; erythema may wax and wane for days or weeks, but the child is seldom febrile and may feel well. In adults, fifth disease often appears as a rheumatic syndrome, with arthralgia or arthritis mimicking rheumatoid arthritis. In a few patients, joint pains persist for months. Fifth disease is associated with the host's immune response to virus, not with viremia, in both experimental and natural infection. Although bone marrow is infected in normal individuals with parvovirus infection, this infection ordinarily has no clinical consequences.

TABLE 26–1. B19 PARVOVIRUS DISEASES

Syndrome	Infection	Host Character
Fifth disease	Acute	Normal children
Arthralgia/arthritis	Acute	Normal adults
Transient aplastic crisis	Acute	Underlying hemolysis
Acquired red cell aplasia	Chronic	Immunodeficiency
Congenital red cell aplasia	Chronic	Immunodeficiency
Hydrops fetalis	Chronic	Immunodeficiency
Vasculitis	?	?
Hemophagocytic syndrome	Acute	Immunodeficiency and normal children and adults
Paroxysmal cold hemoglobinuria	Postacute	Children

In persons with a high demand for red blood cell production, however, usually as a result of chronic hemolysis, interruption of erythropoiesis has more serious consequences. In these patients, acute parvovirus infection causes transient aplastic crisis, sudden appearance of anemia (as in compensated hereditary spherocytosis) or worsening of chronic anemia (as in sickle cell anemia).[5] Thrombocytopenia and/or leucopenia may also occur, but the anemia is responsible for morbidity, typically weakness and lassitude, and occasionally death from congestive heart failure. Aplastic crisis occurs during viremia and is transient because of the development of neutralizing antibodies. Red cell transfusions can be administered if indicated but otherwise no specific therapy is required.

In immunodeficient patients, neutralizing antibodies are not produced and parvovirus infection persists.[17] The clinical syndrome is that of pure red cell aplasia, and there are no associated symptoms of fifth disease

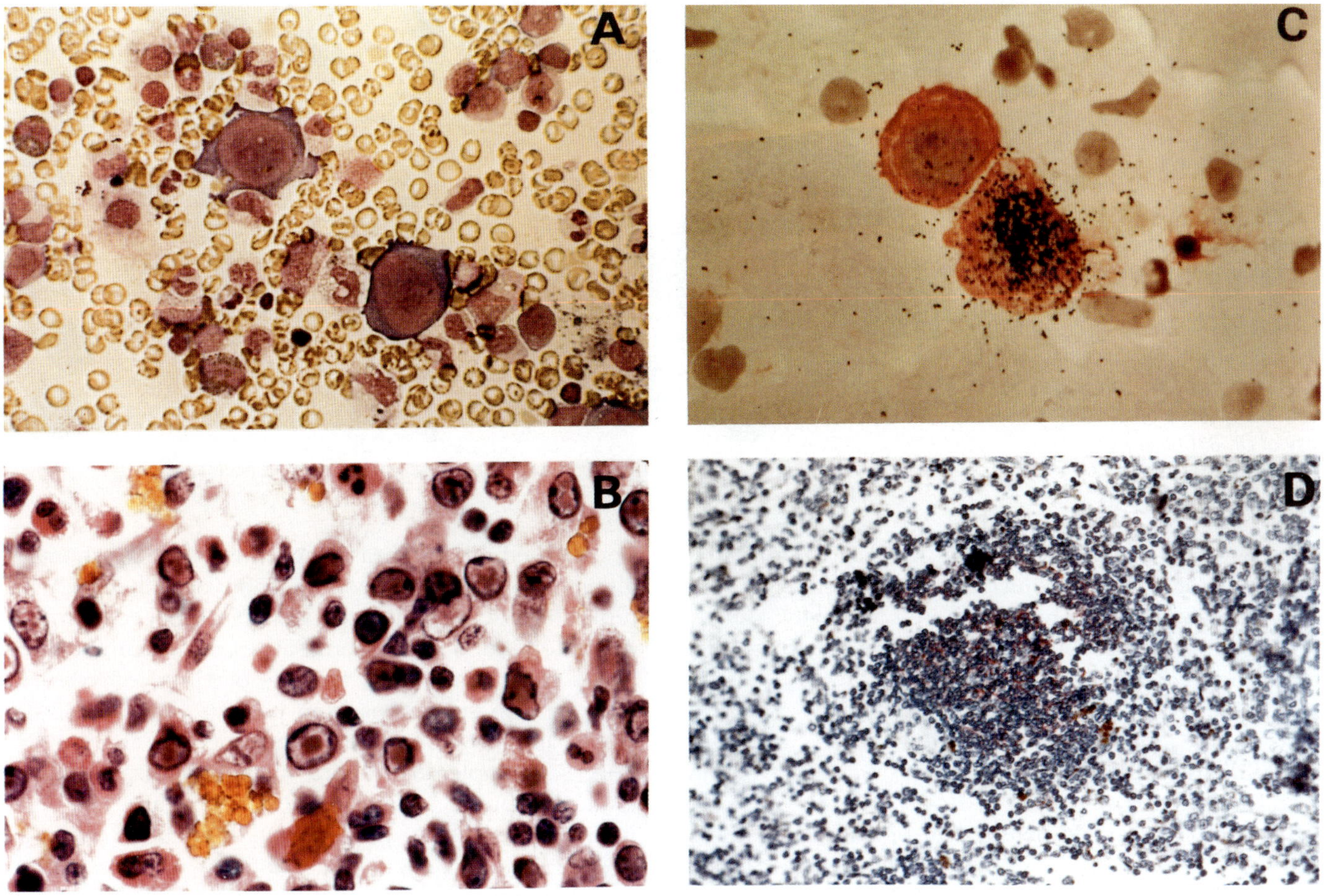

Figure 26–2. Light microscopy. (**A**) Giant pronormoblasts in an aspirate smear of bone marrow from a persistently infected patient; other erythroid precursor cells are absent. (**B**) Giant pronormoblast showing vacuoles and multiple nucleoli or nuclear inclusion bodies (**A** and **B** Wright's Giemsa stain). (**C**) Biopsy specimen of bone marrow from a persistently infected patient, also showing giant pronormoblasts and erythroid hypoplasia (hematoxylin-eosin).[11] (**D**) Giant pronormoblast showing capsid protein (immune enzyme reaction; red stain) and B19 parvovirus genetic material (in situ hybridization; overlying granules).

because immune complexes are not present. Persistent infection occurs in patients with congenital immunodeficiency, a suppressed immune system secondary to chemotherapy, and in the acquired immunodeficiency syndrome. Persistent infection can be cured[18] or ameliorated[19] by administration of commercial immunoglobulin.

Infection of pregnant women can occasionally lead to virus transmission to the fetus and either spontaneous abortion or birth of a stillborn infant[20–22] (Figure 26–3). Autopsies of hydropic fetuses have shown histologic cytopathic effects of virus, and B19 parvovirus was in many organs, especially liver, the site of erythropoiesis at midtrimester, and also spleen and myocardium.[23–29] Death is from heart failure. Hydrops has been diagnosed in utero and treated with intrauterine transfusion. Infants who survive hydrops may suffer congenital red cell aplasia or dysplasia.[30]

PATHOLOGY

Well-described pathologic changes in parvovirus infection have been restricted to hematopoietic organs. Parvovirus infection produces distinctive, perhaps pathognomonic, cytopathic effects in the host cell, the erythroid progenitor of marrow in the adult or liver in the fetus[31] (Figure 26–2). Cytotoxicity for the red cell precursor produces pure red cell aplasia, or an absence of morphologically recognizable erythroid cells in the bone marrow.

DIFFERENTIAL DIAGNOSIS

Fifth disease can be confused with measles and other childhood exanthems, but these would rarely offer pathologic specimens. Chronic red cell aplasia of the

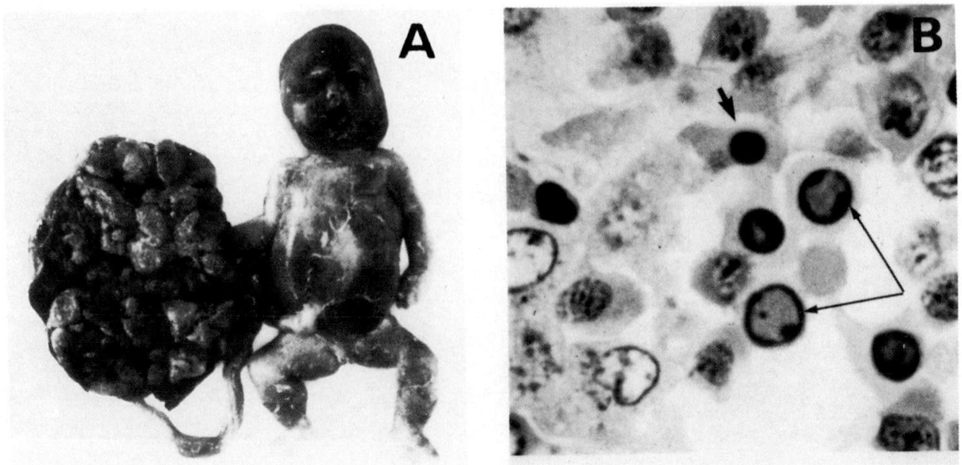

Figure 26–3. Hydrops fetalis. (**A**) A hydropic infant, infected with B19 parvovirus after midtrimester exposure of the mother.[23] *(Courtesy of Professor O.F. Caul.)* (**B**) Cytopathic effect in liver of a hydropic infant, showing large cell with marginated chromatin.[26] *(Courtesy of Dr. B. Cohen.)*

marrow can be associated with thymoma, "autoimmune" diseases, and chronic lymphocytic leukemia, or be termed idiopathic. Hydrops more commonly results from fetal–maternal blood group incompatability or severe α-thalassemia.

MOLECULAR DIAGNOSIS

B19 parvovirus can be detected in biopsy and pathologic specimens by a variety of techniques from immunology and molecular biology. The viral genome can be detected easily by hybridization techniques like dot or slot blot using specific DNA probes labeled radioactively[7,32] or with biotin[33] or digoxigenin.[34] A simple method for measuring virus based on hemagglutination also has been recently described.[35] Viral replication from single-stranded DNA proceeds through double-stranded DNA intermediates, which can be visualized by Southern blot analysis of virus cultivated in vitro[7] and in specimens from patients[11] (Figure 26–4). Gene amplification by the polymerase chain reaction,[36–38] simpler to employ than hybridization techniques, is prone to false-positive results and has been uniquely useful in rather limited circumstances, as described later. Genetic material also can be visualized in individual cells within pathologic specimens using in situ hybridization.[11,18] Virus capsid protein can be detected in individual cells by fluorescent or enzyme-linked methods using monoclonal antibodies to struc-

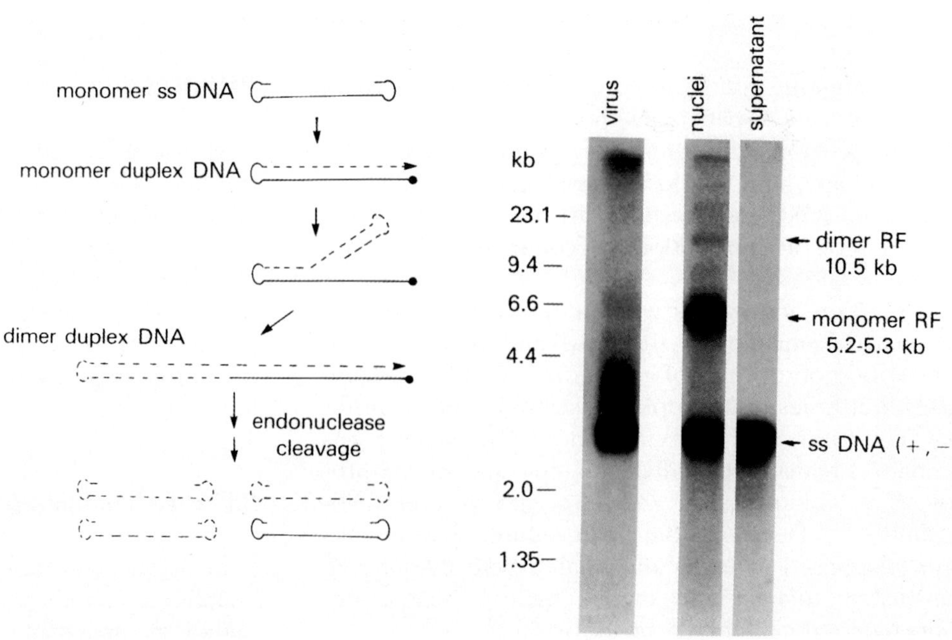

Figure 26–4. DNA analysis. Virus replication proceeds through double-stranded high-molecular-weight intermediates, as shown in the diagram on the left. This can be readily detected by Southern blot analysis, illustrated on the right.[7] Shown here is the pattern of serum virus and extracted DNA from cultures of infected marrow, but similar results can be obtained by analysis of infected tissues from patients.

tural proteins[39,40]; unfortunately, there is no similarly reliable method for nonstructural protein.

CLINICAL ASSAYS

Tissue culture of parvovirus is too specialized and laborious to be used as a clinical assay. Instead, specific antibody tests are used to confirm the diagnosis of infection, usually by capture immunoassays or enzyme-linked immunosorbent assay methods.[41–44] Antigen for these methods has been limited because of the scarcity of infected blood specimens; most workers now use engineered sources of viral protein, from bacteria, as synthetic peptides, and in baculovirus systems (which produce empty viral capsids). Such a large proportion of the adult population has been exposed to the virus that the presence of serum IgG is not useful diagnostically unless seroconversion can be documented in serial samples. IgG to virus may be present or absent in patients with persistent infection. IgM antibody is helpful, because it is found in convalescent-phase specimens for weeks after acute infection. In transient aplastic crisis and in persistent infection, viremia can be recognized as circulating viral particles (by immunoassay or electron microscopy) or viral DNA (by DNA hybridization), often in the absence of specific antibodies to virus. Two special circumstances occur in which B19 parvovirus may be especially occult: Virus may be detectable only by gene amplification in persistently infected immunodeficient patients who have remitted with immunoglobulin treatment,[19] and virus may be localized to the marrow and not circulate in infants with congenital parvovirus infection.[30]

CONCLUSION

B19 parvovirus has only recently entered into the medical literature and, even for those familiar with the virus, clinical diagnostic tests have not been generally available. For these reasons, the full spectrum of human parvovirus disease likely has not yet been defined. Pathologists should pursue the suspicion of parvovirus with adequate sample collection, storage, examination, and diagnostic tests.

REFERENCES

1. Young NS. Parvoviruses. In: Fields BM, Knipe DM, eds. *Virology*. 3rd ed. New York: Raven Press;1995.
2. O'Sullivan MG, Anderson DC, Fikes JD, et al. Identification of a novel simian parvovirus in cynomolgus monkeys with severe anemia: a paradigm of human B19 parvovirus infection. *J Clin Invest.* 1993;93:1571–1576.
3. Woolf AD, Campion GV, Chishick A, et al. Clinical manifestation of human parvovirus B19 in adults. *Arch Intern Med.* 1989;149:1153–1156.
4. Anderson MJ, Higgins PG, Davis LR, et al. Experimental parvoviral infection in humans. *J Infect Dis.* 1985;152:257–265.
5. Young N. Hematologic and hematopoietic consequences of B19 parvovirus infection. *Semin Hematol.* 1988;25: 159–172.
6. Brown KE, Anderson SM, Young NS. Erythrocyte P antigen: cellular receptor for B19 parvovirus. *Science.* 1993; 262:114–117.
7. Ozawa K, Kurtzman G, Young NS. Replication of the B19 parvovirus in human bone marrow cultures. *Science.* 1986;233:883–886.
8. Serke S, Schwarz TF, Baurmann H, et al. Productive infection of in vitro generated haemopoietic progenitor cells from normal human adult peripheral blood with parvovirus B19: studies by morphology, immunocytochemistry, flow-cytometry, and DNA-hybridization. *Br J Haematol.* 1991;79:6–13.
9. Brown KE, Mori J, Cohen BJ, Field AM. In vitro propagation of parvovirus B19 in primary foetal liver cultures. *J Gen Virol.* 1991;72(part 3):741–745.
10. Shimomura S, Komatsu N, Frickhofen N, Anderson S, Kajigaya S, Young NS. First continuous propagation of B19 parvovirus in a cell line. *Blood.* 1992;79:18–24.
11. Kurtzman G, Ozawa K, Hanson GR, Cohen B, Oseas R, Young N. Chronic bone marrow failure due to persistent B19 parvovirus infection. *N Engl J Med.* 1987;317:287–294.
12. Ozawa K, Kurtzman G, Young N. Productive infection by B19 parvovirus of human erythroid bone marrow cells in vitro. *Blood.* 1987;70:384–391.
13. Srivastava A, Bruno E, Briddell R, et al. Parvovirus B19-induced perturbation of human megakaryocytopoiesis in vitro. *Blood.* 1990;76:1997–2004.
14. Anderson MJ, Higgins PG, Davis LR, et al. Experimental parvoviral infection in humans. *J Infect Dis.* 1985;152: 257–265.
15. Kurtzman G, Cohen R, Field AM, Oseas R, Blaese RM, Young N. The immune response to B19 parvovirus infection and an antibody defect in persistent viral infection. *J Clin Invest.* 1989;84:1114–1123.
16. Anderson MJ, Cherry JD. Parvoviruses. In: Feigin RD, Cherry JD, eds. *Textbook of Pediatric Infectious Diseases*, 2nd ed. Philadelphia: WB Saunders; 1987:1646–1653.
17. Watari K, Asano S, Shirafuji N, et al. Serum granulocyte colony-stimulating factor levels in healthy volunteers and patients with various disorders as estimated by enzyme immunoassay. *Blood.* 1989;73:117–122.
18. Kurtzman JG, Frickhofen N, Kimball J, et al. Pure red cell aplasia of ten years' duration due to B19 parvovirus infection and its cure with immunoglobulin infusion. *N Engl J Med.* 1989;321:519–523.
19. Frickhofen N, Abkowitz J, Safford M, et al. Persistent parvovirus infection in patients infected with human immunodeficiency virus type 1 (HIV-1): a treatable cause of anemia in AIDS. *Ann Intern Med.* 1990;113:926–933.
20. Anderson LJ, Hurwitz ES. Human parvovirus B19 and pregnancy. *Clin Perinatol.* 1988;15:273–286.

21. Hall SM, Cohen BJ, Mortimer PP, et al. Prospective study of human parvovirus (B19) infection in pregnancy. *BMJ.* 1990;300:1166–1170.
22. Kinney JS, Anderson LJ, Farrar J, et al. Risk of adverse outcomes of pregnancy after human parvovirus B19 infection. *J Infect Dis.* 1988;157:663–667.
23. Caul OE, Usher JM, Burton AP. Intrauterine infection with human parvovirus B19: a light and electron microscopy study. *J Med Virol.* 1988;24:55–66.
24. Schwarz TF, Nerlich A, Hottentrager B, et al. Parvovirus B19 infection of the fetus. Histology and in situ hybridization. *Am J Clin Pathol.* 1991;96:121–126.
25. Clewley JP, Cohen BJ, Field AM. Detection of parvovirus B19 DNA, antigen, and particles in the human fetus. *J Med Virol.* 1987;23:367–376.
26. Anand A, Gray ES, Brown T, Clewley JP, Cohen BJ. Human parvovirus infection in pregnancy and hydrops fetalis. *N Engl J Med.* 1987;316:183–186.
27. Metzman R, Anand A, DeGiulio A, Knisely AS. Hepatic disease associated with intrauterine parvovirus B19 infection in a newborn premature infant. *J Pediatr Gastroenterol Nutr.* 1989;9:112–114.
28. Yagami K, Fukazawa T, Sugiyama Y, Fujii K. Pathogenesis of a newly isolated rat virus in newborn and juvenile rats. *Exp Anim.* 1991;40(3):349–356.
29. Nascimento JP, Hallam NF, Mori J, et al. Detection of B19 parvovirus in human fetal tissues by in situ hybridisation. *J Med Virol.* 1991;33:77–82.
30. Brown KE, Green SW, Antunez-de-Mayolo J, et al. Congenital anemia following transplacental B19 parvovirus infection. *Lancet.* 1994;343:895–896.
31. Young NS. B19 parvovirus. In: Young NS, ed. *Viruses and Bone Marrow.* New York: Marcel Dekker; 1993:75–117.
32. Mori J, Field AM, Clewley JP, Cohen BJ. Dot blot hybridization assay of B19 virus DNA in clinical specimens. *J Clin Microbiol.* 1989;27:459–464.
33. Cunningham AD, Pattison RJ, Craig KR. Detection of parvovirus DNA in human serum using biotinylated RNA hybridisation probes. *J Virol Meth.* 1988;19:279–288.
34. Zerbini M, Musiani M, Venturoli S, et al. Rapid screening for B19 parvovirus DNA in clinical specimens with a digoxigenin-labeled DNA hybridization probe. *J Clin Microbiol.* 1990;28:2496–2499.
35. Brown KE, Cohen BJ. Haemagglutination by parvovirus B19. *J Gen Virol.* 1992;73:2147–2149.
36. Frickhofen N, Young NS. A rapid method of sample preparation for detection of DNA viruses in human serum by polymerase chain reaction. *J Virol Meth.* 1991;45: 65–72.
37. Koch WC, Adler SP. Detection of human parvovirus B19 DNA by using the polymerase chain reaction. *J Clin Microbiol.* 1990;28:65–69.
38. Sevall JS. Detection of parvovirus B19 by dot-blot and polymerase chain reaction. *Mol Cell Probes.* 1990;4: 237–246.
39. Ozawa K, Young N. Characterization of capsid and noncapsid proteins of B19 parvovirus propagated in human erythroid bone marrow cell cultures. *J Virol.* 1987;61: 2627–2630.
40. Cotmore SF, McKie VC, Anderson LJ, Astell CR, Tattersall P. Identification of the major structural and nonstructural proteins encoded by human parvovirus B19 and mapping of their genes by procaryotic expression of isolated genomic fragments. *J Virol.* 1986;60:548–557.
41. Westmoreland D, Cohen BJ. Human parvovirus B19 infected fetal liver as a source of antigen for a radioimmunoassay for B19 specific IgM in clinical samples. *J Med Virol.* 1991;33:1–5.
42. Anderson LJ, Tsou C, Parker RA, et al. Detection of antibodies and antigens of human parvovirus B19 by enzyme-linked immunoabsorbent assays. *J Clin Microbiol.* 1986; 24:533–526.
43. Brown KE, Buckley MM, Cohen BJ, Samuel D. An amplified ELISA for the detection of parvovirus B19 IgM using monoclonal antibody to FITC. *J Virol Meth.* 1989;26: 189–198.
44. Erdman DD, Usher MJ, Tsou C, et al. Human parvovirus B19 specific IgG, IgA, and IgM antibodies and DNA in serum specimens from persons with erythema infectiosum. *J Med Virol.* 1991;35:110–115.
45. Cossart YE, Field AM, Cant B, et al. Parvovirus-like particles in human sera. *Lancet.* 1975;1:72–73.
46. Young NS, Harrison M, Moore JG, Mortimer PP, Humphries RK. Direct demonstration of the human parvovirus in erythroid progenitor cells infected in vitro. *J Clin Invest.* 1984;74:2024–2032.

CHAPTER 27

Polioviruses

Sydney D. Finkelstein

It is the province of knowledge to speak and it is the privilege of wisdom to listen.

Oliver Wendell Holmes (1809–1894)

Polioviruses are members of the enterovirus subgroup of picornaviruses and are small, single-stranded RNA viruses. The group, consisting of three distinct serotypes, A, B, and C, is best known for causing paralytic polio. They are also among the most intensively studied and characterized viruses and have been used in numerous studies to understand the mechanism of virologic cell injury.[1]

Polioviruses are small, 29 nm in diameter, icosahedral, nonenveloped viruses composed of a single-stranded positive, messenger active, RNA genome approximately 7500 base pairs long, in the form of a single continuous open reading frame with small noncoding regions at both ends.[2,3] The complete nucleic acid sequence of the RNA genome is known for each of the three distinct serotypes of polioviruses as well as their attenuated variants.[4–7] Translation of the virus yields a single, long polyprotein that is cleaved into individual structural and nonstructural proteins that direct all aspects of viral replication.[8,9] The three-dimensional structure of the virus has been determined using crystallographic methods.[10,11] This work has been essential in showing that the critical virus–host receptor attachment site is situated at the base of a canyon-like structure on the surface of the virus, enabling it to be relatively shielded from the host immune system.

Poliovirus-induced disease depends on specific organ and/or cell involvement that is determined by the presence or absence of specific host cell receptors for the virus.[12,13] Although the normal function of poliovirus receptor protein is not fully understood, it has been proved that the human gene responsible for making the poliovirus receptor is located on chromosome 19.[14–16] It has also been shown that this gene is a member of the immunoglobulin superfamily and that the protein may have properties enabling it to function as an extracellular binding protein or adhesion molecule.[16] As such, it normally may act to allow binding of extracellular growth factors or to participate in cell-to-cell interaction and cell adhesion. Upon attachment to the surface of the host cell, virus is internalized by endocytosis, it uncoats, and quickly begins translational and replicative activity. Host RNA and protein production is inhibited by complexing of host cap-binding protein with poliovirus protein 2A.[17] The resulting conditions favor synthesis of viral protein at the expense of the host, which also contributes to inability of the host cell to maintain plasma membrane integrity, important in ultimately leading to host cell death and cell lysis.[18]

The most significant pathogenic effect of poliovirus infection is invasion of motor neurons and proliferation within them, leading to paralysis. The degree of neurovirulence, defined as the ability of the virus to replicate and destroy cells in the central nervous system (CNS), has been studied intensively.[19] Comparison of differences in the genomic sequence between attenuated and parental neurovirulent strains has shown that attenuation can be due to a small number of base pair alterations leading to substitution of amino acids at critical points in the RNA virus.[20–23] For example, there are only 10 base pair differences in the 7441 genome length between the P3/Sabin attenuated variant and its P3/Leon neurovirulent parent. Recombinant technology, which has led to these observations, continues to play an important role in understanding the whole process of virus–host interaction.

Polioviruses are worldwide, with humans serving as the sole reservoir for the virus and the disease in the natural state.[3,24,25] Transmission is primarily by fecal–oral route and is therefore assisted by poor sanitation.

Upon entry into the host, poliovirus undergoes initial replication in the mucosal epithelial cells and adjacent lymphoid tissues of the gastrointestinal and upper respiratory tracts. Surface immunoglobulin production, particularly IgA, is important in limiting and controlling the extent of early viral infection. Primary viremia follows initial entry and local replication, allowing the virus access to all parts of the body including the CNS. Secondary sites of replication, mainly within the reticuloendothelial system, and ensuing secondary viremias are important in maintaining a high state of circulating virus, which assists further entry and infection of the CNS. Stimulation of host IgG and IgM production acts to diminish and eliminate the agent, serving as the primary mechanism to antagonize disease. Although the pattern of disease is based on specific tropism, which is in turn based on the presence or absence of receptors on susceptible cells, the severity of infection can be influenced greatly by the host's immune response. Factors that potentiate severity include young age, male gender, and increased physical activity. It is also important to realize that although the major pathway of poliovirus to the CNS is the hematogenous route, direct access by travel along neural pathways, once held to be the most important pathways, can occur as exemplified by paralytic disease following tonsillectomy. Direct access of the virus to the CNS under these circumstances provides the virus with a means to overcome host immune mechanisms rapidly and produce significant morbidity and potential mortality.

Poliovirus infection can take a number of well-characterized clinical forms. Asymptomatic infection is the most common, accounting for 90% to 96% of cases. Next most common is mild febrile illness, also called abortive poliomyelitis, which is 4% to 8% of infections. Approximately 4% of infections result in aseptic meningitis characterized usually as a biphasic disease starting with mild febrile illness, myalgia, and sore throat progressing to nuchal pain and rigidity. Confirmation requires isolation of the virus from the cerebrospinal fluid (CSF), which exhibits a moderate pleocytosis, initial mixed neutrophil–lymphocytic and then purely lymphocytic cellular reaction. The most serious result of poliovirus infection is paralytic disease, which is seen in 0.1% or less of cases.[2] Also taking the form of biphasic disease, virus enters the CNS where it selectively destroys motor nerve cells resulting in corresponding paralysis. The clinical and pathological features are described in more detail later. Finally, it has become increasingly recognized that recurrent onset of progressive muscular weakness can develop many years after infection and stabilization of motor deficits. Termed postpolio syndrome, the period of clinical latency is usually 25 to 30 years.[2] Also noted is a close relationship between prior poliovirus infection and subsequent development of amyotrophic lateral sclerosis, suggesting a causative relationship between the two,[26] but proof of a causative relationship has not been established.

The introduction initially of formalin-inactivated, killed poliovirus vaccine in the mid-1950s and then live attenuated poliovirus vaccine in the following decade has been one of the greatest success stories in the treatment of viral disease. Although the theoretical possibility exists that poliovirus disease can be eliminated, it nevertheless continues to be a significant cause of morbidity and mortality worldwide. The most important factor is the inability to provide access to the vaccine in segments of the world suffering political or social unrest. The World Health Organization reports 500,000 new cases of polio yearly, largely from parts of the Third World.[27] However, the disease should not be thought of as being solely limited to the Third World. There exists in the West a very small risk of vaccine-induced polio on the order of one case in 2.64 × 10,000,000 vaccine dosages. This should be regarded as most likely representing an underestimation of the actual frequency. In addition, socioeconomic and religious factors still result in small segments of the population not receiving adequate vaccination. There is also evidence that coexisting gastrointestinal viral infection can lead to ineffectiveness of the live vaccine due to viral interference that produces an inadequate specific antibody response.[28,29]

The clinical course of paralytic polio usually takes the form of a biphasic disease beginning with mild febrile illness, followed in 2 to 3 weeks by rapidly progressive muscle weakness. Muscle involvement is highly variable, but tends to be asymmetric and associated with flaccid paralysis consistent with loss of motor neurons. Three clinical patterns have been described: 1) spinal, consisting of asymmetric flaccid paralysis with intact sensation; 2) bulbar, involving motor deficits of swallowing, facial musculature, and respiratory function; and 3) encephalitic, the rarest form. As noted earlier, in recent years the renewed onset of muscle weakness in polio victims several decades after stabilization of motor deficits has been characterized as the postpolio syndrome.[2] Two forms have been described. Type 1 is in those with significant initial disease taking the form of progressive weakness in previously affected muscle groups. Type 2 postpolio disease appears to affect those with initially mild disease. These patients exhibit muscular weakness affecting a wider distribution of muscles, which is associated with histologic evidence of active myositis. The pathogenesis of this disorder is not known, but an autoimmune mechanism has been proposed. The reports of a higher incidence of amyotrophic lateral sclerosis in polio patients has raised the possibility that persistent virus may play a role.

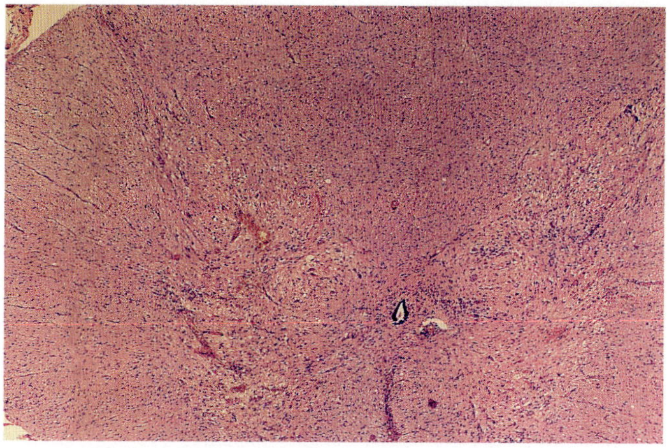

Figure 27–1. Cross section of spinal cord with inflammation of anterior and posterior grey horns (hematoxylin-eosin, ×10). *(Photograph by Ernest E. Lack, MD.)*

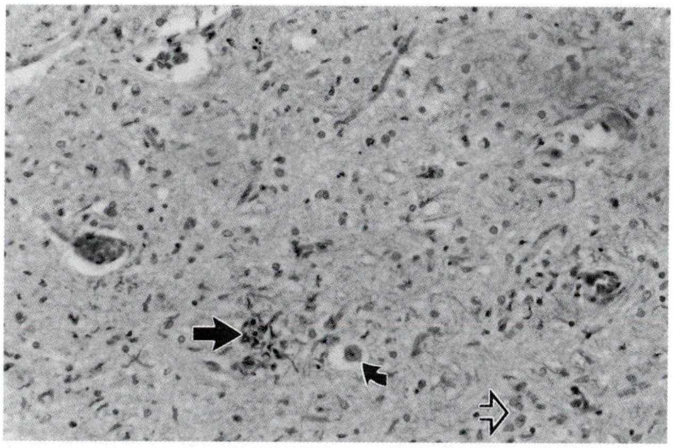

Figure 27–3. Human poliomyelitis, acute phase. Section from the anterior horn of the spinal cord reveals collections of microglial cells (*straight solid arrow*) removing cellular debris resulting from infection of motor nerve cells. There is a single residual motor neuron (*curved arrow*). There is evidence also of astrogliosis associated with depletion of neurons (*open arrow*) (hematoxylin-eosin, ×250).

Although isolation and culture of the virus from diseased spinal cords have not been accomplished, demonstration of the virus by immunohistochemical and in situ hybridization techniques in occasional reports has supported the contention of persistent infection.[30,31] Using poliovirus RNA probes and quantitative in situ hybridization, it has been possible to show that killing of neural cells is directly related to extent of viral replication.

Affected nervous tissue in paralytic polio shows a pattern of initially mixed and then chronic inflammation associated with destruction and loss of nerve cells. In the early phases of the illness there is inflammation with microglial nodules and neuronophagia (Figures 27–1 through 27–3). Infected nerve cells exhibit eosinophilic necrosis consistent with coagulative necrosis. Central chromatolysis may occasionally be seen during early stages of cell injury. Ultrastructurally, infected cells exhibit disorganization and disruption of cellular organelles in keeping with cell dissolution. Viral particles are not seen, although occasional reports have attested to the presence of a crystalline-type arrangement of small particles such as has been described for other picornavirus infections. Later in the disease, there are neuronal dropout (Figures 27–4 and 27–5) and reactive astrogliosis.

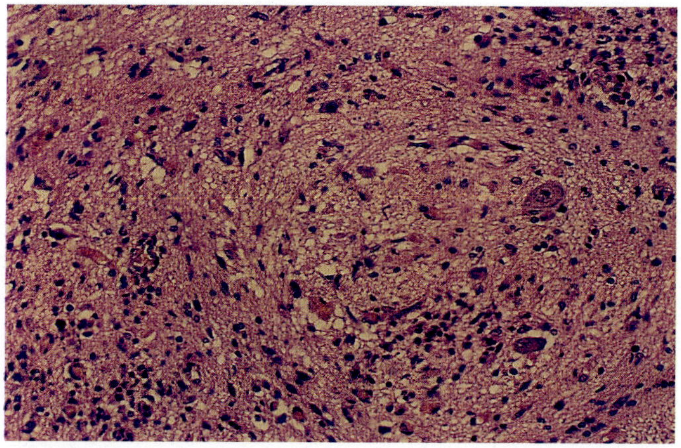

Figure 27–2. Anterior grey horn with neuronophagia, microglial nodules, diffuse myelitis, and one surviving anterior horn cell (hematoxylin-eosin, ×250). *(Photograph by Ernest E. Lack, MD.)*

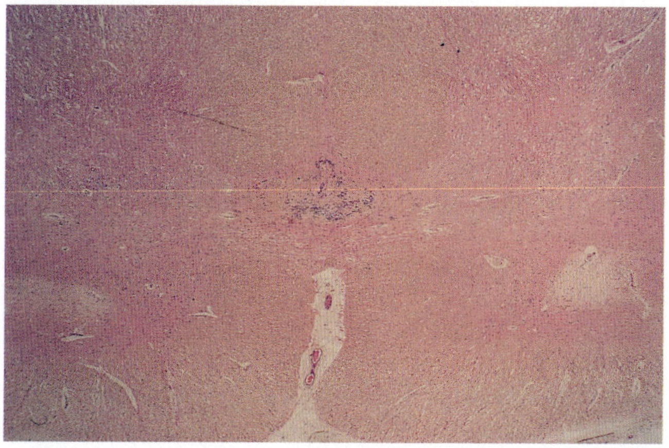

Figure 27–4. Cross section of cord of patient with poliomyelitis in the chronic, healed stage. The anterior horns show pallor and gliosis (hematoxylin-eosin, ×10). *(Photograph by Ernest E. Lack, MD.)*

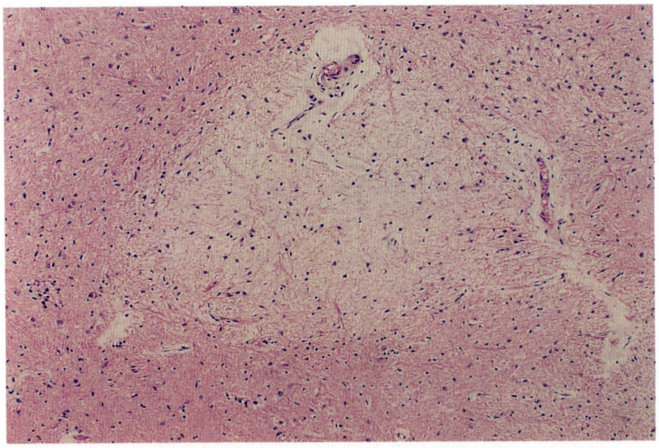

Figure 27–5. Higher magnifications of right anterior horn of Figure 27–4. There is complete neuronal dropout giving the anterior horn a loose hypocellular texture. There are a few lymphocytes around vessels and proliferation of astrocytes (hematoxylin-eosin, ×80). *(Photograph by Ernest E. Lack, MD.)*

Although the diagnosis of poliovirus can be strongly suspected on clinical grounds supported by typical histopathologic changes such as meningitis, encephalomyelitis, and neuronal cell necrosis, definitive diagnosis requires specific evidence of poliovirus presence. Such confirmation has been classified into highly associated, moderately associated, and lowly associated types.[2] High association requires recovery of poliovirus from diseased tissues or direct detection of specific poliovirus protein by immunohistochemical or immunofluorescent techniques or of poliovirus RNA by either in situ hybridization or nucleic acid amplification. Polyclonal antibodies for the virus are readily available for use on tissue sections. Although detection of nucleic acid is still experimental, the availability of the published full genome sequence of the virus should make nucleic acid detection feasible by a variety of molecular biological approaches.

Moderate association of poliovirus infection can be achieved by both isolating the virus from the throat, feces, or blood and by demonstrating a fourfold rise in paired serum titers obtained during active infection and in the convalescent period. A single blood determination of greater than 1:32 dilution of IgM specific poliovirus antibody may be used to accomplish the same purpose. When infection is suspected, therefore, it is best to secure viral cultures and serum promptly for subsequent testing. A low presumptive evidence of poliovirus infection may be achieved by either of the techniques outlined.

REFERENCES

1. Rueckert RR. Picornaviridae and their replication. In: Fields BN, Knipe DM, eds. *Virology.* New York: Raven Press; 1990:507–548.
2. Melnick JL. Enteroviruses: polioviruses, coxsackieviruses, echoviruses, and newer enteroviruses. In: Fields BN, Knipe DM, eds. *Virology,* 2nd ed. New York: Raven Press; 1990:549–606.
3. Crainic R, Couderc T, Martin A, Wychowski C, et al. An insight into poliovirus biology. *Adv Exp Med Biol.* 1989; 257:61–66.
4. Kitamura N, Semler B, Rothberg PG, et al. Primary structure, gene organization and polypeptide expression of poliovirus RNA. *Nature (Lond).* 1981;291:547–553.
5. Racaniello VR, Baltimore D. Molecular cloning of poliovirus cDNA and determination of the complete nucleotide sequence of the viral genome. *Proc Natl Acad Sci USA.* 1981;78:4887–4891.
6. Toyoda H, Kohara M, Kataoka Y, et al. Complete nucleotide sequences of all three poliovirus serotype genomes. Implication for genetic relationship, gene function and antigenic determinants. *J Mol Biol.* 1984;174:561–585.
7. Sarnow P, Jacobson SJ, Najita L. Poliovirus genetics. *Curr Top Microbiol Immunol.* 1990;161:155–188.
8. Sonenberg N. Poliovirus translation. *Curr Top Microbiol Immunol.* 1990;161:23–47.
9. Darnell JE, Levintow L. Poliovirus protein: source of amino acids and time course of synthesis. *J Biol Chem.* 1960;235:74–77.
10. Hogle JM. Preliminary studies of crystals on type 1 poliovirus. *J Mol Biol.* 1982;160:663–668.
11. Hogle JM, Chow M, Filman DJ. Three-dimensional structure of poliovirus at 2.9A resolution. *Science.* 1985;229: 1358–1365.
12. Crowell RL, Landau BJ. Receptors in the initiation of picornavirus infections. In: Fraenkel-Conrat H, Wagner RR, eds. *Comprehensive Virology.* New York: Plenum Press; 1983;18:1–42.
13. Ren R, Racaniello VR. Human poliovirus receptor gene expression and poliovirus tissue tropism in transgenic mice. *J Virol.* 1992;66:296–304.
14. Miller DA, Miller OJ, Dev VG, et al. Human chromosome 19 carries a poliovirus receptor gene. *Cell.* 1974;1: 167–173.
15. Couillin P, Huyghe F, Grisard MC, et al. Echovirus 6, 11, 19; coxsackie B3 sensitivities and poliovirus I, II, III sensitivities are on chromosome 19 respectively on l9qtr-ql33 and l9ql3l-ql33. *Cytogenet Cell Genet.* 1987;46:579–586.
16. Mendelsohn CL, Wimmer E, Racaniello VR. Cellular receptor for poliovirus: molecular cloning, nucleotide sequence and expression of a new member of the immunoglobulin superfamily. *Cell.* 1989;56:855–865.
17. Crawford N, Fire A, Samuels M, et al. Inhibition of transcription factor activity by poliovirus. *Cell.* 1981;27: 555–561.
18. Bablanian R, Eggers HJ, Tamm I. Studies on the mechanism of poliovirus-induced cell damage. II. The relation

between poliovirus growth and virus-induced morphological changes in cells. *Virology.* 1965;26:114–121.
19. Racaniello VR. Poliovirus neurovirulence. *Adv Virus Res.* 1988;34:217–246.
20. Nomoto A, Omata T, Toyoda H, et al. Complete nucleotide sequence of the attenuated poliovirus Sabin 1 strain genome. *Proc Natl Acad Sci USA.* 1982;79:5793–5797.
21. Evans DMA, Dunn G, Crowell RL, et al. Increased neurovirulence associated with a single nucleotide change in a noncoding region of the Sabin type 3 poliovaccine genome. *Nature (Lond).* 1985;314:548–550.
22. Svitkin YV, Pestova TV, Maslova SV, Agol VI. Point mutations modify the response of poliovirus RNA to a translation initiation factor: a comparison of neurovirulent and attenuated strains. *Virology.* 1988;166:394–404.
23. Chumakov KM, Norwood LP, Parker ML, et al. RNA sequence variants in live poliovirus vaccine and their relation to neurovirulence. *J Virol.* 1992;66:966–970.
24. Robbins FC. Poliomyelitis eradication: a continuing story. *FASEB J.* 1994;8:665–666.
25. Rico-Hesse R, Pallansch MA, Nottay BK, Kew OM. Geographic distribution of wild poliovirus type 1 genotypes. *Virology.* 1987;160:311–322.
26. Brahic M, Smith RA, Gibbs CJ, et al. Detection of picornavirus sequences in nervous tissue of amyotrophic lateral sclerosis and control patients. *Ann Neurol.* 1985;18:337–343.
27. Melnick JL. Vaccination against poliomyelitis: present possibilities and future prospects. *Am J Public Health.* 1988;78:304–305.
28. Kew OM, Nottay BK, Hatch MH, et al. Multiple genetic changes can occur in the oral poliovaccine upon replication in humans. *J Gen Virol.* 1981;56:337–347.
29. Nomoto A, Iizuka N, Kohara M, Arita M. Strategy for the construction of live picornavirus vaccines. *Vaccine.* 1988;6:134–137.
30. Petitjean J, Quibriac M, Freymuth F, Fuchs F. Specific detection of enteroviruses in clinical samples by molecular hybridization using poliovirus subgenomic riboprobes. *J Clin Microbiol.* 1990;28:307–311.
31. Yang CF, De L, Holloway BP, et al. Detection and identification of vaccine-related polioviruses by the polymerase chain reaction. *Virus Res.* 1991;20:157–179.

CHAPTER 28

Polyomaviruses and Progressive Multifocal Leukoencephalopathy

Sydney D. Finkelstein

All would live long but none would be old.

Proverb

Polyomaviruses are double-stranded DNA viruses, ubiquitous in nature, and capable of mammalian infection. Three species, SV40, JC, and BK viruses, are human pathogens.[1–3] Polyomaviruses first reached clinical importance in the mid- to late 1950s when millions of people were inadvertently exposed to SV40 virus from contaminated monkey kidney cell cultures used in the production of poliovirus vaccines.[2] This exposure is thought to have had no long-term effects. Progressive multifocal leukoencephalopathy (PML), an opportunistic infection of the central nervous system causing demyelination, was first described in 1958.[3] Suspected of being caused by a virus, SV40 and JC viruses were isolated from PML lesions in 1971.[4] All subsequent isolates have been of JC virus only.[5] Clinical disease attributed to BK virus, the remaining member of polyomavirus producing human disease, was first described in 1980.[3] Since then several reports of hemorrhagic cystitis and ureteral stenosis have been documented in renal allograft recipients[6] and cancer patients undergoing therapy.[7] Polyomaviruses continue to gain in clinical importance because of the greater use of immunosuppressive therapies[3] and as a result of the growing presence worldwide of human immunodeficiency virus (HIV) infection and acquired immunodeficiency syndrome (AIDS), an important predisposing cause for opportunistic infection.[8]

THE ORGANISM

Polyomaviruses contain a covalently closed, circular, double-stranded DNA genome 5000 base pairs in length.[2,9] Approximately 70% of the genomic sequence is identical in all member strains of virus. Transcription takes place in two stages, termed early and late, each occurring from separate strands of the DNA and in opposite directions from the point of origin of replication. The stage of early transcription, which proceeds immediately after viral uncoating in the host nucleus, yields the small (172 amino acids) and large (690 amino acids) T antigens, multifunctional proteins that initiate viral replication, activate and modulate specific host cell genes, and drive cellular transformation. The large T antigen, in particular, has been the subject of much investigation.[2,3,10] Located primarily in the host cell nucleus and to a lesser extent in the plasma membrane, it is capable of disturbing cell growth and differentiation, producing cell injury and death, and causing neoplastic transformation. The stage of late transcription leads to production of capsid proteins designated VP1, VP2, and VP3. VP1 is the most abundant, accounting for 75% of total capsid proteins.[11] VP1 has been shown to be responsible for cell tropism, viral attachment, and activation of specific host genes in anticipation of entry of virus into the cell.[11]

Polyomaviruses are entirely dependent on host enzymatic and synthetic machinery to carry out viral transcription and replication. Attachment of the virus to sialic acid-containing surface receptors leads to activation of host cell c-*myc* and c-*fos* genes designed to stimulate cell proliferation and prepare the cell for viral replication.[12–14] Virus enters the cell by endocytosis, uncoating directly in the nucleus.[15] T antigen, which directs early events of viral transcription and replication, binds to p53 and retinoblastoma gene products, further stimulating cell proliferation.[2] As a progressively greater share of host cell activity is channeled into use by the virus, late transcription occurs, leading to production of capsid proteins and infectious progeny. Release of mature virions results in cell death.

PATHOBIOLOGY

Polyomaviruses are believed to enter the host most commonly through the respiratory route as part of inapparent or mild upper respiratory tract infection. Initial viral replication most likely occurs in the respiratory tree. Viremia follows with generalized dissemination to secondary targets throughout the body. Initial contact with BK virus occurs during childhood, while that for JC virus takes place at a somewhat older age.[3] More than 75% of adults are seropositive for both of these viruses, providing strong support for reactivation of latent infection as the basis for adult disease.[16]

Cells susceptible to invasion by polyomaviruses undergo three types of infection. Lytic infection causes cytopathic death through the production and release of infectious progeny virus. This type of infection is exemplified by PML in which oligodendrocytes are destroyed by JC virus, manifesting as a demyelinating illness of the central nervous system (CNS). Abortive infection occurs in nonpermissive host cells, which can harbor residual viral particles in a state of latency. Latency for both JC and BK virus is believed to occur in renal tubular and transitional epithelial cells.[17,18] Abortive infection can also occur in B lymphocytes, which may serve as a vehicle for viral transport throughout the body to sites such as the CNS.[19] The third pattern of infection involves cell transformation. The mechanism of transformation is unclear, but likely involves latent infection followed by integration of coding regions for the T antigen and other parts of the viral genome into the host nucleus.[2,3] Human astrocytes can undergo infection with JC virus and, over time, neoplastic transformation, resulting in multifocal astrocytomas.[20,21]

Reactivation of latent infection represents a critical step in the pathogenesis of polyomavirus infection. A full understanding of the mechanism of reactivation is currently lacking, but it is known to be clearly linked to the development of immunodeficiency, either inherited or acquired.[22] As a major site for latent virus in the urinary lining cells, reactivation can be identified by spillage of replicating virus in the urine.[23] This has been demonstrated for a significant proportion of third trimester pregnant women who shed both JC and BK viruses.[23] Reactivation in this circumstance is thought to be related to relative immune depression of pregnancy.

Clinical disease usually follows a period of hematogenous dissemination in which the virus is carried through the bloodstream by infected carrier cells such as B lymphocytes.[24] The virus is transported into the brain tissue by these cells, which gain access to brain extracellular fluid via the Virchow–Robin perivascular spaces. A variety of techniques, including immunologic detection of viral proteins and in situ detection of viral nucleic acid, have clearly indicated that there is widespread exposure of the brain and that discrete lesions of PML arise from this generalized dissemination. JC virus is present in both the lesional and normal appearing brain tissue of PML patients as shown in Figure 28–1. This highly sensitive nucleic acid amplification reaction is used for viral detection, a finding consistent with initial widespread hematogenous dissemination of the organism early in infection.[24]

Active replication of the virus leads to much defective virus production as well as changes in genomic structure, which in turn can result in infectious progeny that exhibit differences in specific tissue tropism.[25] The severity of the disease is directly related to the degree of viral replication, which in turn correlates closely with the extent of depressed immune status. Long-term survival and remission following infection with polyomaviruses have been reported in patients experiencing a reversal in immune deficiency.

PROGRESSIVE MULTIFOCAL LEUKOENCEPHALOPATHY

Clinical

PML is a demyelinating disorder of the CNS due to cytopathic killing of oligodendrocytes infected with JC virus. PML is almost always an opportunistic infection, especially T-cell deficient states.[2,3] The degree of diminished immune status correlates with the aggressiveness of the disease. AIDS represents, at present, the most important predisposing cause of PML. It affects 3.8% of HIV-infected patients with AIDS, accounting for approximately 35% of total PML cases. Other predisposing conditions are allograft transplantation, hematopoietic malignancy and disseminated cancer, granulomatous disease including sarcoidosis and tuberculosis, and autoimmune states such as rheumatoid arthritis and systemic lupus erythematosus.[2,3]

PML tends to arise insidiously with signs of focal central nervous disease, the most common being limb weakness, visual loss, and/or cognitive dysfunc-

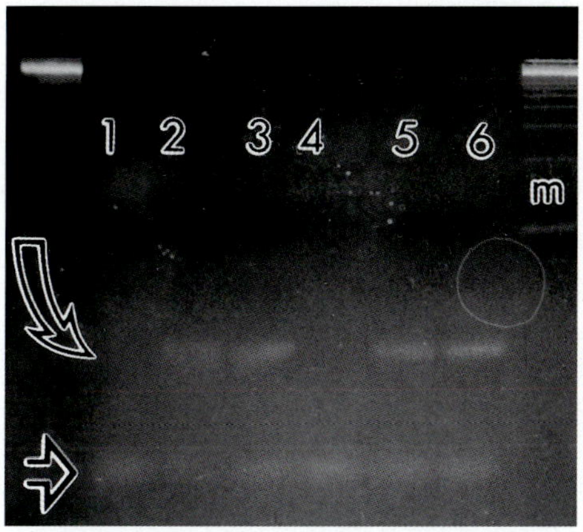

Figure 28–1. Detection of JC virus from formalin-fixed, paraffin-embedded tissue by polymerase chain reaction. Two samples from the same patient are used in duplicate together with negative controls (*lanes 1 and 4*). One sample (*lanes 2 and 3*) has been topographically taken from a histologic area of PML. The other sample (*lanes 5 and 6*) is from histologically normal-appearing area of the brain remote from the lesion. Specific amplification product (*curved arrow*) is detected in both samples, consistent with wide hematogenous dissemination of the virus to the CNS. Synthetic oligonucleotide probes are shown (*straight arrow*).

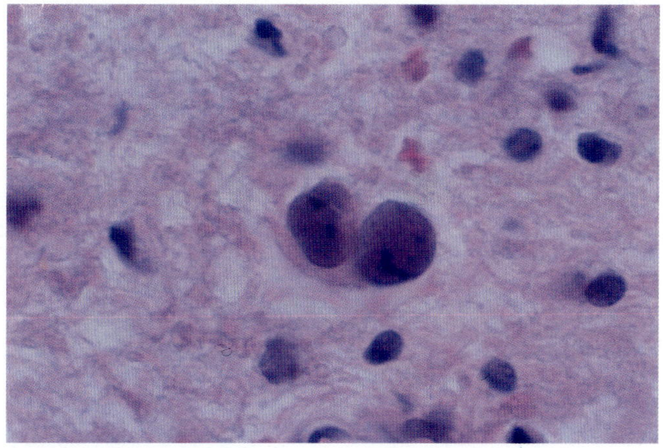

Figure 28–3. Biopsy specimen of white matter from patient with PML showing two enlarged homogeneous amphophilic oligodendroglial nuclei. This type of inclusion is characteristic of PML (hematoxylin-eosin, ×1000). *(Photograph courtesy of Herbert J. Manz.)*

tion.[26–28] Progression is usually relentless, with multifocal involvement of the CNS. Computed tomography (CT) and magnetic resonance imaging (MRI) are sensitive tools for detecting the lesions, which manifest as nonenhancing, low-density lesions free of mass effect on CT and high T2 signal on MRI, consistent with demyelination.[29,30] Serologic testing is in general not useful due to the high rate of seropositivity in the adult

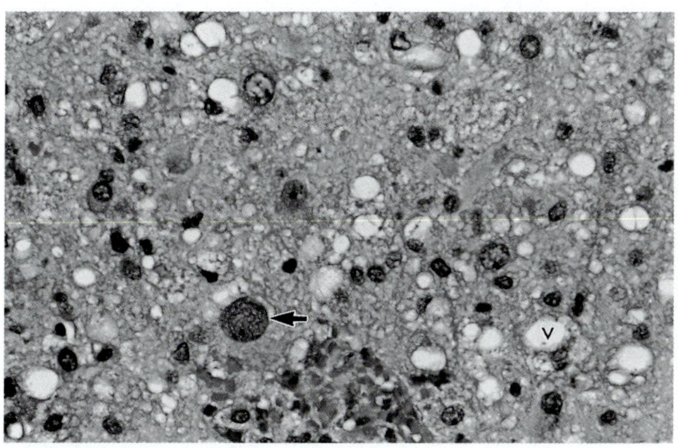

Figure 28–2. PML in a patient with AIDS. Section from the edge of a lesion reveals oligodendrocytes with nuclear enlargement and clearing typical of heavy viral loading of the celol (*arrow*). The white matter shows degeneration manifested by vacuolization (v) (hematoxylin-eosin, ×400).

population. Electroencephalographic and cerebrospinal fluid (CSF) alterations tend to be nonspecific.

The most reliable and definitive diagnostic test is brain biopsy, which reveals characteristic alterations on routine hematoxylin-eosin and myelin staining (Figures 28–2 and 28–3). Confirmation is then sought through the identification of polyomavirus by electron microscopy (Figures 28–4 through 28–6). Direct detection of the virus using immunologic detection systems (Figure 28–7) and nucleic acid hybridization strategies including polymerase chain reaction (Figure 28–1) are now in clinical use.

Average survival from the time of diagnosis is 3 to 6 months. Unfortunately, no specific antiviral agent exists at present. The most effective treatment strategy involves reversal of underlying immunosuppression. Positive responses to both HIV and JC virus infection have been reported in a patient with AIDS treated with AZT.[31,32] Anecdotal reports have attested to the efficacy of antiviral agents such as cytosine arabinoside; however, no large trial has been performed to prove its potential efficacy.[33]

Pathology

PML consists of multiple discrete foci of demyelination that expand centrifugally over time, tending to coalesce into large irregular lesions.[34] They can occur anywhere throughout the CNS (Figures 28–8 and 28–9), although favored sites include the junction of gray–white matter and the centrum semiovale of the cerebral hemispheres.[34] The areas of involvement on gross examination have a necrotic character, which is especially marked in HIV+ and other severely immunodeficient patients. Hemorrhage into the lesions and mass effect

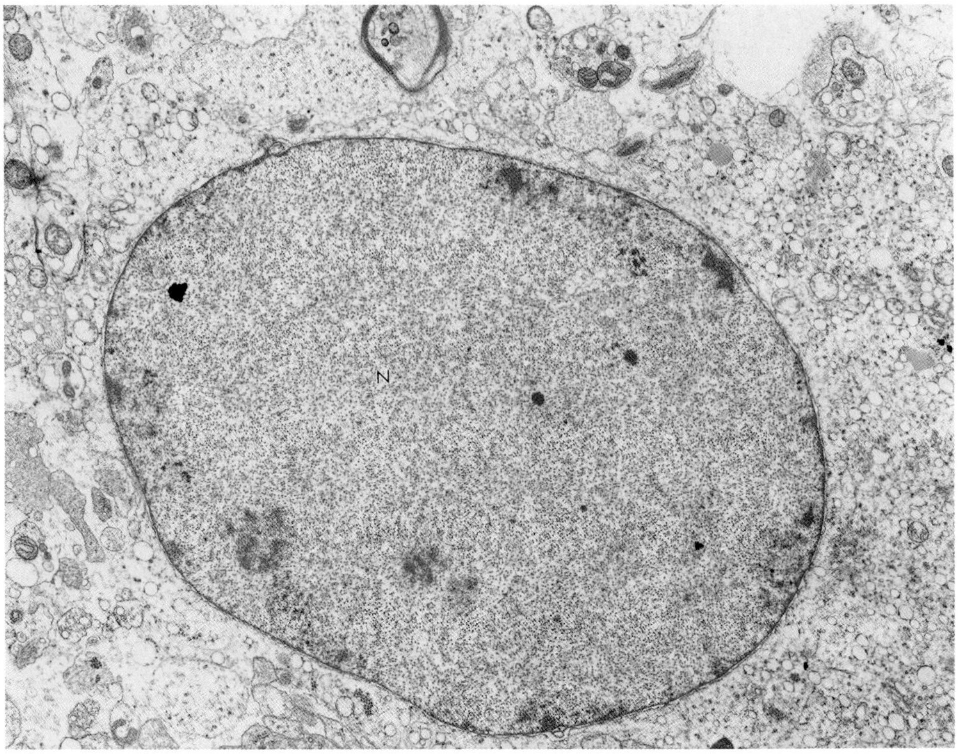

Figure 28–4. JC virus infected oligodendrocyte. Low-power electron micrograph reveals abundant amounts of virus in the nucleus (N) (modified Karnovsky's fixative, lead citrate/uranyl acetate, ×11,000).

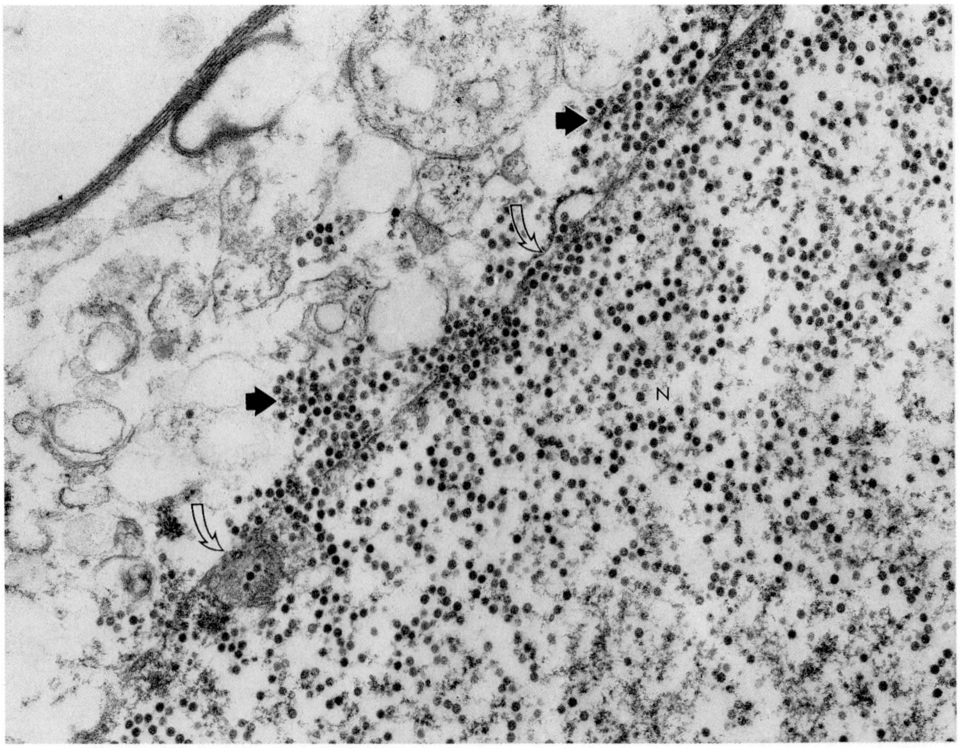

Figure 28–5. JC virus escaping (*solid arrows*) from the nucleus (N) of an infected cell. Nuclear membrane is shown (*curved arrows*). Escape of the virus from the nucleus heralds cytopathic destruction of the oligodendrocyte (modified Karnovsky's fixative, lead citrate/uranyl acetate, ×90,000).

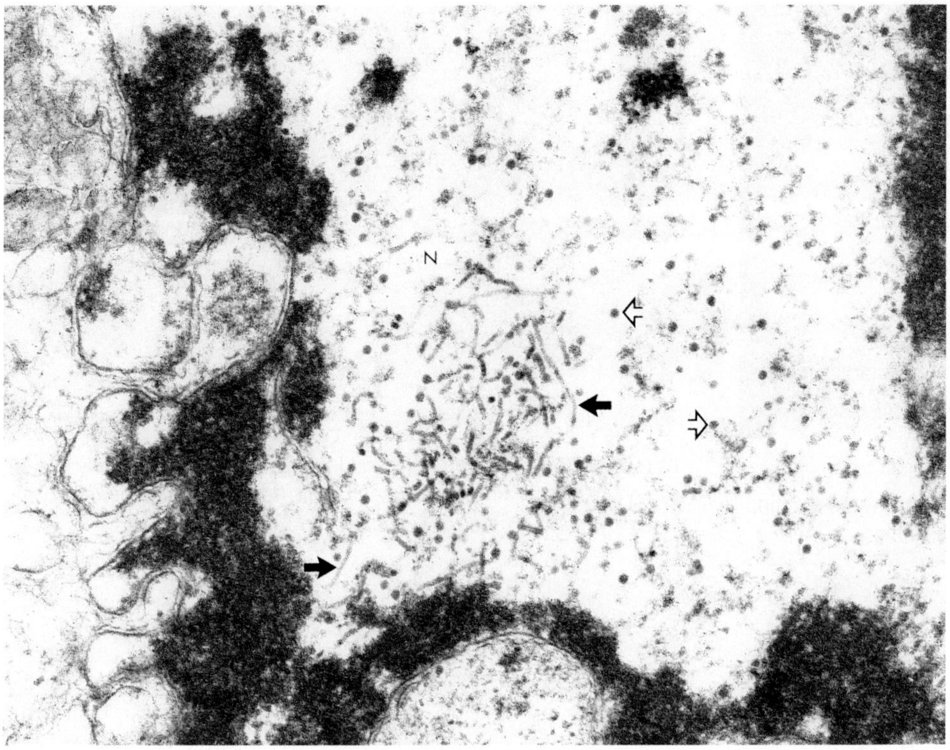

Figure 28–6. High magnification shows cross-sectional, dense, rounded outlines of the virus (*open arrows*) as well as the longitudinal filamentous cylindrical form (*solid arrows*). N, nucleus (modified Karnovsky's fixative, lead citrate/uranyl acetate, ×130,000).

are distinctly unusual and, when present, should raise doubt about the diagnosis.

The microscopic appearance is characteristic but depends on securing a site of actively involved brain tissue.[35] The most diagnostic area is the expanding peripheral edge of the lesion, which shows a variety of changes, including foamy macrophages engulfing myelin debris, sparse perivascular chronic inflammation, and infected oligodendrocytes (Figure 28–2),[35] which are most important for diagnosis and consist of two to three times enlarged oligodendrocytes with basophilic, water clear, chromatin-deficient nuclei (Figures 28–2 and 28–3). Their presence is required for presumptive diagnosis. Also characteristic of PML are enlarged, bizarre-appearing astrocytes with pleomorphic nuclei. They tend to be more numerous in the central and midzone areas of the lesions, but may be encountered at the edge as well. Their appearance may raise a suspicion for a neoplastic process, but their overall number and distribution are more in keeping with reactive, preoncogenic change. In rare circumstances, progression to solitary and multifocal gliomas has been reported in PML.

In rapidly evolving cases, the central regions may undergo necrosis and cavitation. Perivascular inflammation is usually sparse.[35] In those few patients exhibiting prolonged survival or remission, prominent perivascular inflammation was present, suggesting better host immune response. Note, however, that in AIDS patients perivascular inflammation can be prominent and ascribed to recruitment of HIV+ lymphocytes and macrophages into areas of myelin destruction. PML in AIDS tends to pursue a more necrotizing, fulminating clinical course.[36–39]

Demonstration of polyomavirus in affected brain tissue permits definitive diagnosis. Transmission electron microscopy of infected cells reveals crystalline arrays of 45-nm diameter icosahedral virions and fila-

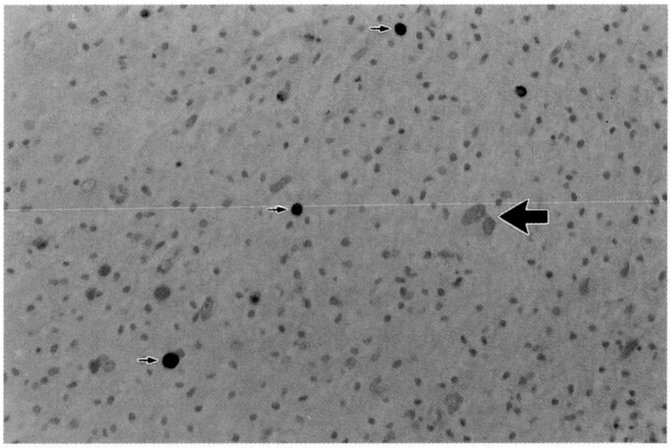

Figure 28–7. Immunohistochemical staining for JC virus in a lesion of PML. Infected nuclei stain brightly when viral content is high (*small arrows*). Note failure of nuclear staining of pleomorphic astrocytes (*large arrow*). These pleomorphic astrocytes also may contain virus (avidin-biotin horseradish peroxidase, ×250).

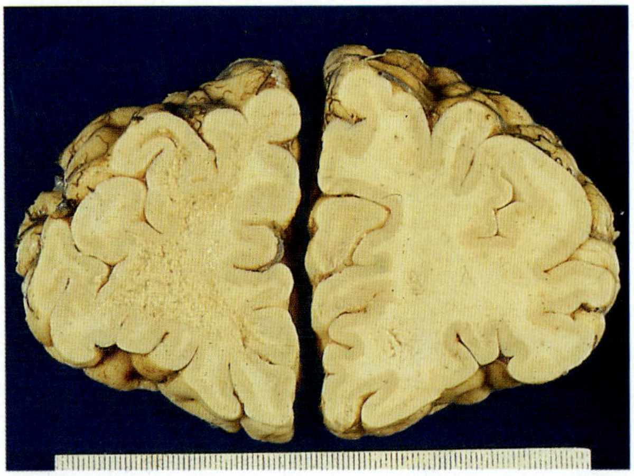

Figure 28–8. Coronal section of frontal lobes in a patient who developed PML after renal transplantation. There is destruction of white matter, more severe in the right hemisphere. *(Photograph courtesy of Herbert J. Manz.)*

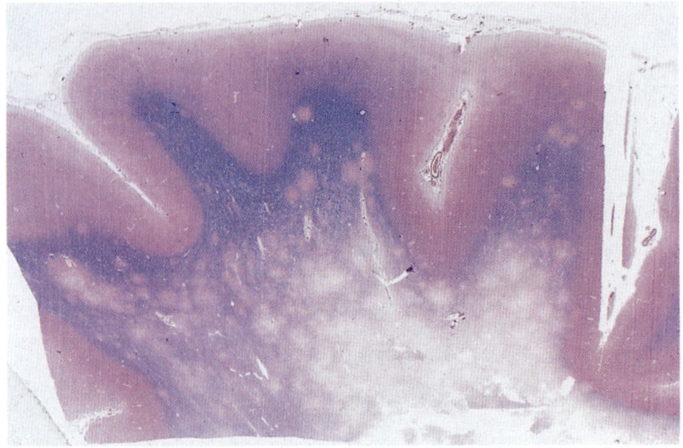

Figure 28–9. Section of frontal lobe with multiple, confluent foci of demyelination in centrum semiovale (luxol fast blue/hematoxylin-eosin, ×1). *(Photograph courtesy of Herbert J. Manz.)*

mentous rods (Figures 28–4 through 28–6). Immunologic detection of polyoma species-specific protein can be used diagnostically by both fluorescent and colorimetric means (Figure 28–7). Polyclonal and monoclonal antibodies to several polyomavirus proteins including the T antigens and capsid proteins are now readily available.[40] The distribution of immunopositive cells is generally wider in distribution than the demyelinative lesions, in keeping with dissemination via the hematogenous route.

Direct detection of viral DNA can be accomplished by a variety of methods, including in situ hybridization, Southern blot analysis, and polymerase chain reaction (PCR) (Figure 28–1).[41–47] In situ hybridization allows recognition of individual infected cells and in general parallels immunologic methods in sensitivity. Both techniques require a threshold of approximately 100 virions per cell as the lower limit of sensitivity. PCR, which can be performed on topographically selected sites from formalin-fixed tissue specimens as well as on urine and other infected material, is considered the most sensitive means of specific detection (Figure 28–1).

Failure to achieve diagnosis of PML can be attributed to several reasons,[48] the most common of which is a failure to obtain a representative sample of the lesion. This is especially so with needle biopsy of brain in which a diagnostic specimen is not obtained—a difficulty inherent in the technique. Preoperative clinical and radiologic correlation, selection of several alternative targets, and sampling directed at the edge of the lesion are useful guidelines. Sampling of the central regions is less valuable and runs the risk of overdiagnosis of bizarre glia as glioma. Overdiagnosis of PML is also possible, and the differential diagnosis should include other demyelinating conditions, infarction, and infection. It is prudent to delay definitive diagnosis until ultrastructural, immunologic, or nucleic acid hybridization studies secure the diagnosis.

BK VIRUS INFECTION

Clinical disease related to BK virus is less common than disease associated with JC virus. Reactivation of virus from latency in renal tubular and transitional epithelial cells with spillage into the urine is present in 30% of third trimester pregnancies. A majority of allograft transplant recipients shed virus in the urine. Clinical disease, however, is uncommon in these patients. Occasional reports of ureteral stenosis and hemorrhagic cystitis correlate with viral cytopathic effect of cells lining the urinary pathway.[49–51]

REFERENCES

1. Eckhart W. Polyomavirinae and their replication. In: Fields BN, Knipe DM, et al, eds. *Virology,* 2nd ed. New York: Raven Press, 1990:1593–1608.
2. Brady JN, Salzman NP. The papovaviridae: general properties of polyoma and SV40. In: Salzman NP, ed. *The Papovaviridae.* New York: Plenum Press; 1986;1:1–26.
3. Shah KV. Polyomaviruses. In: Fields BN, Knipe DM, et al, eds. *Virology,* 2nd ed. New York: Raven Press; 1990:1609–1624.
4. Padgett BL, Walker DL, ZuRhein GM, Eckroade RJ. Cultivation of papova-like virus from human brain with pro-

gressive multifocal leucoencephalopathy. *Lancet.* 1971;1:1257–1260.

5. Padgett BL, Rogers CM, Walker DL. JC virus, a human polyomavirus associated with progressive multifocal leukoencephalopathy: additional biological characteristics and antigenic relationships. *Infect Immun.* 1977;15:656–662.
6. Andrews CA, Shah KV, Daniel RW, et al. A serologic investigation of BK virus and JC virus infections in recipients of renal allografts. *J Infect Dis.* 1988;158:176–181.
7. Arthur RR, Shah KV, Baust SJ, et al. Association of BK viruria with hemorrhagic cystitis in recipients of bone marrow transplants. *N Engl J Med.* 1986;315:230–234.
8. Schmidbauer M, Budka H, Shah KV. Progressive multifocal leukoencephalopathy (PML) in AIDS and in the pre-AIDS era. *Acta Neuropathol.* 1990;80:375–380.
9. Kelly Jr TJ, Nathans D. The genome of simian virus 40. *Adv Virus Res.* 1977;21:85–173.
10. Trapp BD, Small JA, Pulley M, et al. Dysmyelination in transgenic mice containing JC virus early region. *Ann Neurol.* 1988;23:38–48.
11. Consigli RA, Griffith GR, Marriott SJ, Ludlow JW. Biochemical characterization of the polyoma-receptor interaction. In: Crowell RL, Lonberg-Holm K, eds. *Virus Attachment and Entry into Cells.* Washington, DC: American Society for Microbiology; 1986:44–53.
12. Rassoulzadegan M, Cowie A, Carr A, et al. The roles of individual polyoma virus early proteins in oncogenic transformation. *Nature.* 1982;300:713–718.
13. Zullo J, Stiles CD, Garcea RL. Regulation of c-*myc* and c-*fos* mRNA levels by polyomavirus: distinct roles for the capsid protein VP1 and the viral early proteins. *Proc Natl Acad Sci USA.* 1987;84:1210–1214.
14. Corallini A, Pagnani M, Caputo A, et al. Cooperation in oncogenesis between BK virus early region gene and the activated human c-Harvey *ras* oncogene. *J Gen Virol.* 1988;69:2671–2679.
15. Griffith GR, Consigli RA. Isolation and characterization of monopinocytotic vesicles containing polyomavirus from the cytoplasm of infected mouse kidney cells. *J Virol.* 1984;50:77–85.
16. Kahan A, Coleman D, Koss L. Activation of human polyomavirus infection—detection by cytologic technics. *Am J Clin Pathol.* 1980;74:326–332.
17. Dorries K, ter Muelen V. Progressive multifocal leukoencephalopathy: detection of papovavirus JC in kidney tissue. *J Med Virol.* 1983;11:307–317.
18. Chesters PM, Heritage J, McCance DJ. Persistence of DNA sequences of BK virus and JC virus in normal human tissues and in diseased tissues. *J Infect Dis.* 1983;47:676–684.
19. Houff SA, Major EO, Katz DA, et al. Involvement of JC virus-infected mononuclear cells from the bone marrow and spleen in the pathogenesis of progressive multifocal leukoencephalopathy. *N Engl J Med.* 1988;318:301–305.
20. Castaigne P, Rondot P, Escourolle R, et al. Leucoencephalopathie multifocale progressive et gliomes multiples. *Rev Neurol.* 1974;130:379–392.
21. Sima AAF, Finkelstein SD, McLachlan DR. Multiple malignant astrocytomas in a case of spontaneous progressive multifocal leukoencephalopathy. *Ann Neurol.* 1983;14:183–188.
22. Walker D, Padgett B. Progressive multifocal leukoencephalopathy. In: Fraenkel-Conrat H, Wagner RR, eds. *Comprehensive Virology.* New York: Plenum Press; 1983;18:161–193.
23. Coleman DV, Wolfendale MR, Daniel RA, et al. A prospective study of human polyomavirus infection in pregnancy. *J Infect Dis.* 1980;142:1–8.
24. Itoyama Y, deF Webster H, Sternberger NH, et al. Distribution of papovavirus, myelin-associated glycoprotein, and myelin basic protein in progressive multifocal leukoencephalopathy lesions. *Ann Neurol.* 1982;11:396–407.
25. Freund R, Calderone A, Dawe CJ, Benjamin TL. Polyomavirus tumor induction in mice: effects of polymorphisms of VP1 and large T antigen. *J Virol.* 1991;65:335–341.
26. Schlitt M, Morawetz RB, Bonnin J, et al. Progressive multifocal leukoencephalopathy: three patients diagnosed by brain biopsy, with prolonged survival in two. *Neurosurgery.* 1986;18:407–414.
27. Stoner GL, Walker DL, deF Webster H. Age distribution of progressive multifocal leukoencephalopathy. *Acta Neurol Scand.* 1988;78:307–312.
28. Elder GA, Sever JL. Neurologic disorders associated with AIDS retroviral infection. *Rev Infect Dis.* 1988;10:286–302.
29. Krupp LB, Lipton RB, Swerdlow ML, et al. Progressive multifocal leukoencephalopathy: clinical and radiographic features. *Ann Neurol.* 1985;17:344–349.
30. Mark AS, Atlas SW. Progressive multifocal leukoencephalopathy in patients with AIDS: appearance on MR images. *Radiology.* 1989;173:517–520.
31. Berger JR, Mucke L. Prolonged survival and partial recovery in AIDS-associated progressive multifocal leukoencephalopathy. *Neurology.* 1988;38:1060–1065.
32. Conway B, Halliday WC, Brunham RC. Human immunodeficiency virus-associated progressive multifocal leukoencephalopathy: apparent response to 3′-Azido-3′-deoxythymidine. *Rev Infect Dis.* 1990;12:479–482.
33. O'Riordan T, Daly PA, Hutchinson M, Shattock AG, Gardner SD. Progressive multifocal leukoencephalopathy—remission with cytarabine. *J Infect Dis.* 1990;20:51–54.
34. Richardson EP Jr, Webster HF. Progressive multifocal leukoencephalopathy: its pathological features. In: Sever JL, Madden DL, eds. *Polyomaviruses and Human Neurological Diseases.* New York: Liss; 1983:191.
35. Burger PC, Vogel FS. *Surgical Pathology of the Nervous System and Its Coverings.* 2nd ed. New York: John Wiley & Sons; 1982:195–203.
36. Gendelman HE, Phelps W, Feigenbaum L, et al. Transactivation of the human immunodeficiency virus long terminal repeat sequence by DNA viruses. *Proc Natl Acad Sci USA.* 1986;83:9759–9763.
37. Stoner GL, Ryschkewitsch CF, Walker DL, Webster H. JC papovavirus large tumor (T)-antigen expression in brain tissue of acquired immune deficiency syndrome (AIDS) and non-AIDS patients with progressive multifocal leukoencephalopathy. *Proc Natl Acad Sci USA.* 1986;83:2271–2275.
38. Rhodes RH, Ward JM, Walker DL, Ross AA. Progressive

multifocal leukoencephalopathy and retroviral encephalitis in acquired immunodeficiency syndrome. *Arch Pathol Lab Med.* 1988;112:1207–1213.

39. Vazeux R, Cumont M, Girard PM, et al. Severe encephalitis resulting from coinfections with HIV and JC virus. *Neurology.* 1990;40:944–948.
40. Hogan TF, Padgett BL, Walker DL, Borden EC, et al. Rapid detection and identification of JC virus and BK virus in human urine by using immuno-fluorescence microscopy. *J Clin Microbiol.* 1980;11:178–183.
41. Gerber MA, Shah KV, Thung SN, Zu Rhein GM. Immunohistochemical demonstration of common antigen of polyomaviruses in routine histologic tissue sections of animals and man. *Am J Clin Pathol.* 1980;73:794–797.
42. Aksamit AJ, Mourrain P, Sever JL, Major EO. Progressive multifocal leukoencephalopathy: investigation of three cases using in situ hybridization with JC virus biotinylated DNA probe. *Ann Neurol.* 1985;18:490–496.
43. Aksamit AJ, Sever JL, Major EO. Progressive multifocal leukoencephalopathy: JC virus detection by in situ hybridization compared with immunohistochemistry. *Neurology.* 1986;36:499–504.
44. Boerman RH, Arnoldus EPJ, Raap AK, et al. Diagnosis of progressive multifocal leucoencephalopathy by hybridisation techniques. *J Clin Pathol.* 1989;42:153–161.
45. Weber T, Turner RW, Frye S, et al. Specific diagnosis of progressive multifocal leukoencephalopathy by polymerase chain reaction. *J Infect Dis.* 1994;169:1138–1141.
46. Telenti A, Aksamit AJ, Proper J, Smith TF. Detection of JC virus DNA by polymerase chain reaction in patients with progressive multifocal leukoencephalopathy. *J Infect Dis.* 1990;162:858–861.
47. Phalen DN, Wilson VG, Graham DL. Polymerase chain reaction assay for avian polyomavirus. *J Clin Microbiol.* 1991;29:1030–1037.
48. Finkelstein SD. CT-guided stereotactic biopsy of brain tumors: pathologic considerations. *Am J Clin Oncol.* 1987;10:289–292.
49. Gardner SD, Mackenzie EFD, Smith C, Porter AA. Prospective study of the human polyomaviruses BK and JC and cytomegalovirus in renal transplant recipients. *J Clin Pathol.* 1984;37:578–586.
50. Schatzl HM, Sieger E, Jager G, et al. Detection by PCR of human polyomaviruses BK and JC in immunocompromised individuals and partial sequencing of control regions. *J Med Virol.* 1994;42:138–145.
51. Embrey JR, Silva FG, Helderman JH, et al. Long-term survival and late development of bladder cancer in renal transplant patient with progressive multifocal leukoencephalopathy. *J Urol.* 1988;139:580–581.

CHAPTER 29

Poxvirus Infections

Clay J. Cockerell

Morbid matter of various kinds, when absorbed into the system, may produce effects in some degree similar; but what renders the Cow Pox virus so extremely singular, is, that the person who has been thus affected is for ever after secure from the infection of the Small Pox; neither exposure to the variolous effluvia, nor the insertion of the matter into the skin, producing this distemper.

Edward Jenner (1749–1823)[1]

The execution date for the smallpox virus has been tentatively set for Friday, June 30, 1995.

David Brown[2]

DEFINITION

Poxvirus infections are caused by viruses of the family *Poxviridae.*

GEOGRAPHIC DISTRIBUTION

Poxviruses are distributed throughout the world, although some poxviruses infect specific animal reservoirs. Smallpox, one of the most devastating pestilences of human history, has been eradicated from the earth by immunization and enforced quarantine. Among the reasons this program succeeded are 1) immunization is effective, 2) humans do not become "carriers" of the virus, 3) smallpox virus has no animal reservoir, and 4) the strategy of "surveillance containment" was implemented whereby new infections are detected quickly, isolated, and all possible contacts vaccinated. In 1967, three endemic areas persisted—Asia (Bangladesh, India, Nepal, Pakistan, and Afghanistan), trans-Saharan Africa, and Indonesia. By August 1976, smallpox appeared to be confined to rural Ethiopia.[3] The last human infection was in 1977 in Merca, Somalia, and 2 years later the World Health Organization (WHO) declared the world free of smallpox—forever.

Many countries stopped vaccinating in 1980 (Figure 29–1). Smallpox virus, however, remains in two locations—at the Centers for Disease Control and Prevention in Atlanta, Georgia, and at the Moscow Institute for Viral Preparations. At both places the virus is sealed in deeply frozen vials and tightly secured. The debate over its fate continues.[2] Two late victims of the smallpox scourge were photographed in eastern Zaire in August 1968 (Figure 29–2, A and B). The WHO vaccination teams were in eastern Zaire at the time.

Molluscum contagiosum virus is worldwide. Monkeypox virus is endemic in Africa and Asia. Parapoxviruses infect domesticated animals including sheep, goats, and cattle, so in areas where these animals are herded the disease is endemic. Tanapox is endemic in the floodplain of the Tana River in Kenya and in other areas of Africa.

NATURAL HISTORY

Humans may be infected by a variety of these viruses, which often involve the skin. Humans may be infected

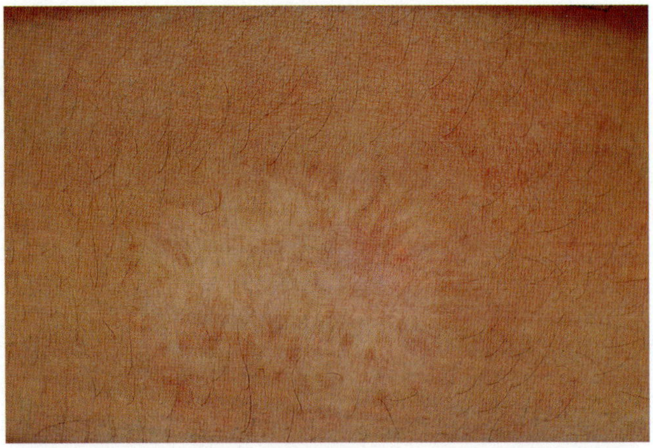

Figure 29–1. Smallpox vaccination scar on the skin of a 40-year-old Asian woman. Now rapidly disappearing from the human population, these scars are characteristically on the skin over the insertion of the deltoid muscle, depressed, hypopigmented, and have a stellate margin. *(Photograph by Daniel H. Connor, MD, 1995.)*

secondarily as with parapoxvirus infections. These include milker's nodule, orf, monkeypox, cowpox, and tanapox. In other infections, such as variola and molluscum contagiosum, humans are the primary host.

Poxviruses enter cells by endocytosis or by cell fusion. They then undergo uncoating after which there is transcription of viral genetic material producing infective virions.[4] The intracytoplasmic virions form inclusions, which can be visualized microscopically. Poxviruses induce growth factors as well as complement binding proteins.[5] Clinical disease is caused by these inflammatory mediators and by direct injury to the cell. In molluscum contagiosum, these inflammatory proteins probably are not induced to the same degree because inflammation in intact lesions is relatively minimal (vide infra). Intact virus is shed through the epidermis and spread over the skin, sometimes causing widespread lesions. This is especially true of molluscum contagiosum. Some poxviruses, such as variola, enter through the respiratory tract, spread to regional lymph nodes, then cause viremia and seed internal organs. Parapoxviruses are generally acquired by local inoculation producing localized lesions, although edema, lymphangitis, and lymphadenitis may develop. The reactions caused by poxviruses all show marked intracytoplasmic and/or intranuclear cytopathic effects with epidermal changes.

MORPHOLOGIC FEATURES OF THE ORGANISM

Poxviruses are complex double-stranded DNA viruses that are large in comparison to other viruses. They contain an envelope and generally have a somewhat rectangular or cylindrical appearance by electron microscopy (Figure 29–3).

CLINICAL MANIFESTATIONS

Skin lesions are a prominent feature of poxvirus infections. In general, there are papules or vesicles. Infection with the molluscum contagiosum virus gives rise to umbilicated translucent papules, usually in the groin or on the genitalia but they may be on any surface of the glabrous skin. The virus is spread by close contact, and is often transmitted sexually. The infection is eradicated by a cell-mediated response; therefore, it is frequently seen in patients with deficient cell-mediated immunity, especially those infected with human immunodeficiency virus (HIV) (Figure 29–4).[6,7] The virus tends to involve epithelium of the adnexa, causing an exoendo-

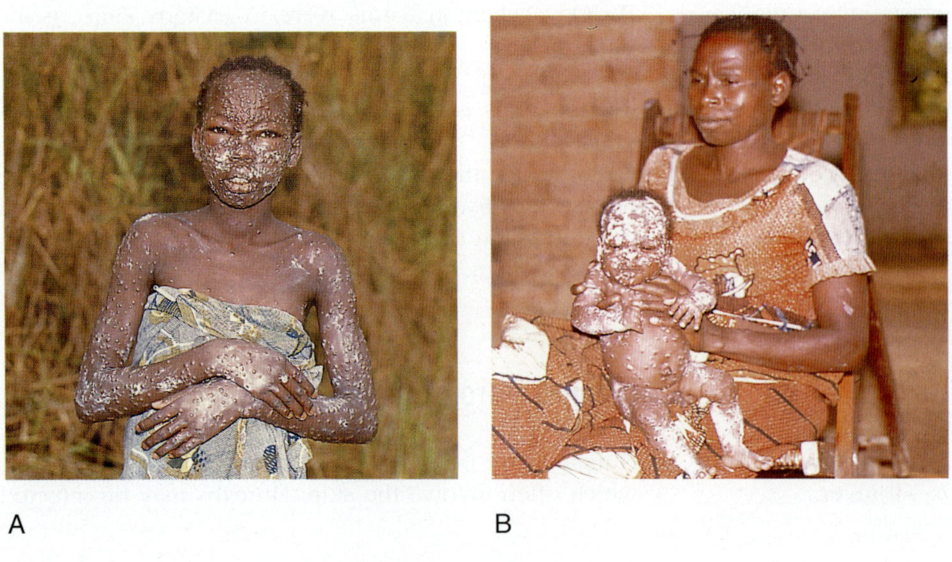

A B

Figure 29–2. African girl with smallpox (**A**) and an infant with smallpox (**B**). These photographs were taken in Oicha, eastern Zaire, in August 1968. WHO vaccination teams were in eastern Zaire at the time and brought smallpox in the region to an end. *(Photograph by Daniel H. Connor, MD, 1968.)*

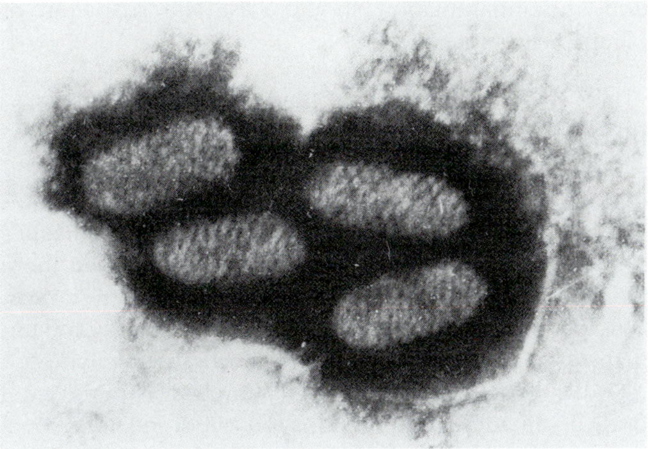

Figure 29–3. Ovoid-appearing structures characteristic of poxvirus. As depicted here, these DNA viruses are enveloped (electron microscope, original magnification ×115,000).

phytic papule with a central core.[8] Infection causes little acute inflammation, but when lesions rupture, there is often intense inflammation.[9]

Other poxvirus infections tend to produce a vesicular dermatitis associated with striking inflammation. Clinically, these are usually vesicles and bullae with erythema causing the clinical appearance of one or more boggy indurated plaques.[10,11] Lesions are usually near the hands as the virus is acquired by contact with contaminated fomites or infected animals (Figure 29–5). In time, lesions become crusted and eventually heal with minimal scarring.

HISTOPATHOLOGY

The most characteristic histologic feature of molluscum contagiosum infection is the intracytoplasmic purplish-to-red inclusion known as the molluscum body (Henderson–Patterson body). These often develop first in the epithelium of adnexal structures such as eccrine ducts and infundibula of hair follicles just above the basal cell layer, and appear as oval-shaped eosinophilic masses in the cytoplasm of keratinocytes. The developed lesion characteristically has a craterform indentation with intact epithelial borders, which corresponds to the umbilicated dome-shaped lesion noted clinically (Figure 29–6, A and B). The molluscum bodies increase in size and basophilia as infected cells pass upward. The nucleus characteristically is displaced and compressed peripherally (Figure 29–7).[12] Eventually, as molluscum bodies are released, the infected areas coalesce, causing the central umbilication.

Although little inflammation is evoked by the infection, trauma may rupture the lesions and cause acute inflammation.[9] On occasion, atypical lymphoid cells may resemble the Reed–Sternberg cells of Hodgkin's disease.[13] Deeply seated infections with prominent involvement of follicles may have one or more small cysts filled with molluscum bodies.

Parapoxvirus infections (orf, milker's nodule, tanapox) produce a characteristic ballooning degeneration of epidermal keratinocytes (a sign of the viral infection) associated with a very dense inflammatory cell infiltrate of lymphocytes, plasma cells, neutrophils, and eosinophils (Figures 29–8 through 29–10).[14] In early stages, intranuclear and intracytoplasmic eosinophilic

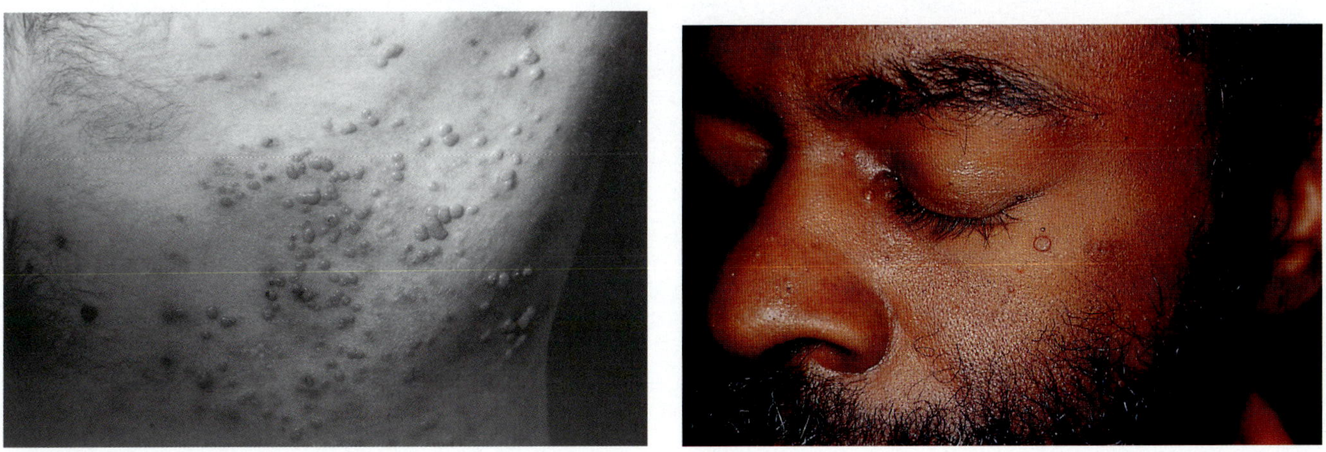

A B

Figure 29–4. (**A**) Molluscum contagiosum in a patient infected with HIV. The lesions are papular, multiple, widespread, translucent, and umbilicated—all features of molluscum contagiosum in immunodeficient patients. (**B**) Several papular lesions of molluscum contagiosum on the face of a patient with AIDS. The largest lesion (near the eye) is raised, fleshy, and slightly umbilicated.

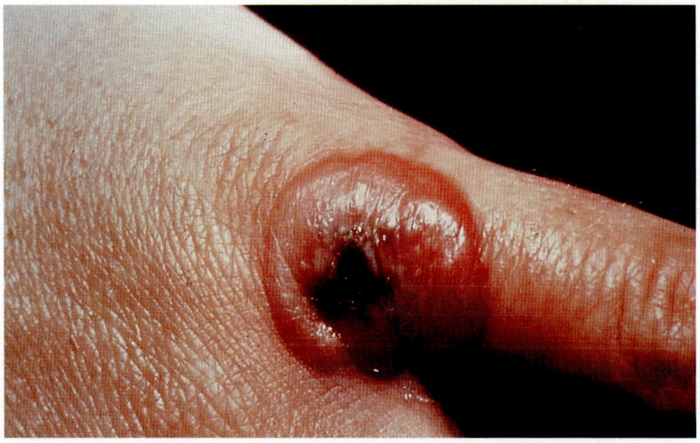

Figure 29–5. A boggy indurated plaque on the dorsal surface of the hand characteristic of orf, a parapoxvirus infection transmitted by sheep and goats.

inclusions are in the infected keratinocytes.[15] With increasing inflammation and epidermal necrosis, only marked ballooning, spongiosis, and an intense dermal inflammatory cell infiltrate can be appreciated (Figure 29–11). In time, the acute inflammation gradually gives way to granulation tissue and fibrosis. Marked epidermal hyperplasia associated with ballooning degeneration and inflammation should raise the suspicion of parapoxvirus infection.

DIFFERENTIAL PATHOLOGIC DIAGNOSIS

In molluscum contagiosum, the identification of molluscum bodies is pathognomonic. Difficulty in diagnosis may arise when there are few bodies or when there is an intense inflammatory cell infiltrate after trauma. This pattern may cause confusion with primary inflammatory dermatoses or even local cutaneous lymphoreticular neoplasia. A careful search for molluscum bodies, in additional sections or by doing additional biopsies, may be necessary to establish the diagnosis.

Parapoxvirus infections may share histologic features with other diseases that produce massive ballooning degeneration of keratinocytes such as blastomycosis-like pyoderma as well as acute reactions from topical irritants. Blastomycosis-like pyoderma may have similar changes of epidermal hyperplasia, but the degree of ballooning degeneration is minimal and there are no intracellular inclusions. Irritant reactions often have ballooning degeneration especially when there is maceration, but the degree of epidermal hyperplasia is less than that of poxvirus infections and, in general, no

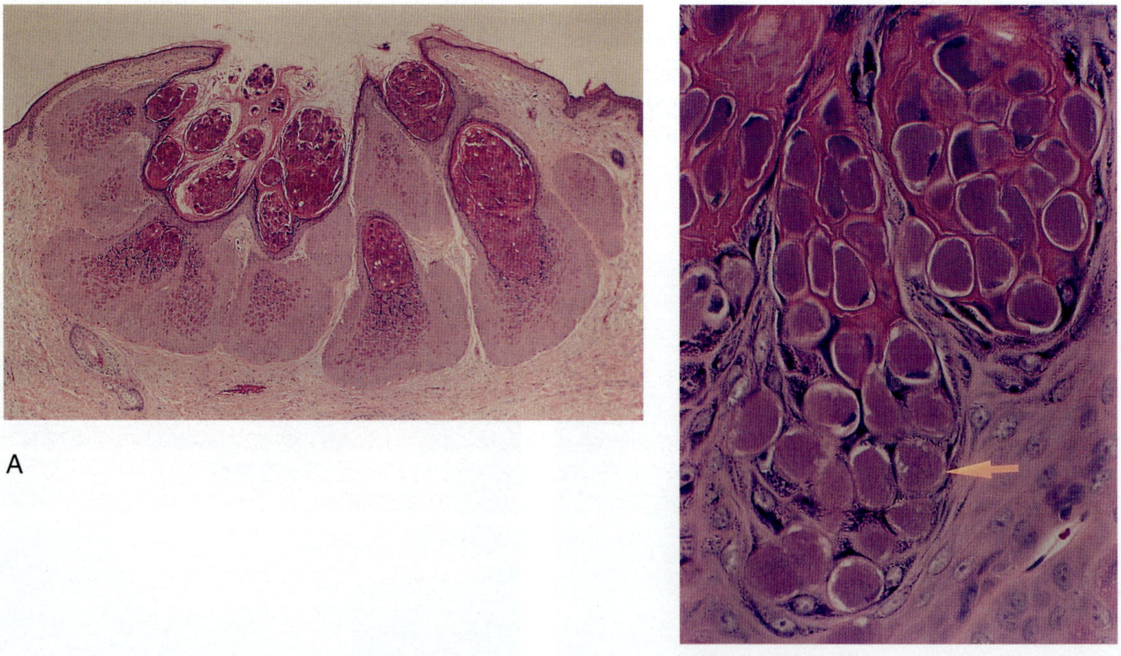

A

B

Figure 29–6. (**A**) *Molluscum contagiosum* of skin. The epithelium has a craterform indentation with inverted lobules of keratinocytes containing eosinophilic inclusions. The epithelium over the edge of the lesion is raised (hematoxylin-eosin, ×40). (**B**) Higher magnification showing viral inclusions (*arrow*). They have filled the cytoplasm, displaced the keratohyalin granules, and displaced and distorted the nucleus. The irregular, particulate substructure of the inclusion is apparent (hematoxylin-eosin, ×400).

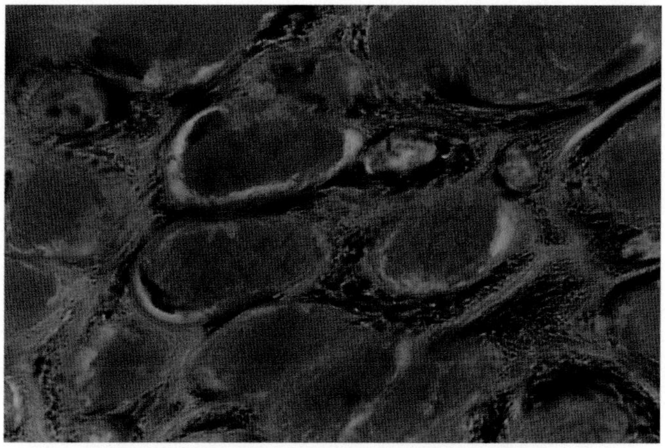

Figure 29–7. Higher magnification demonstrates the Henderson–Patterson bodies, which are intracytoplasmic viral particles. The nuclei of these infected cells is pushed to the side (hematoxylin-eosin, ×600).

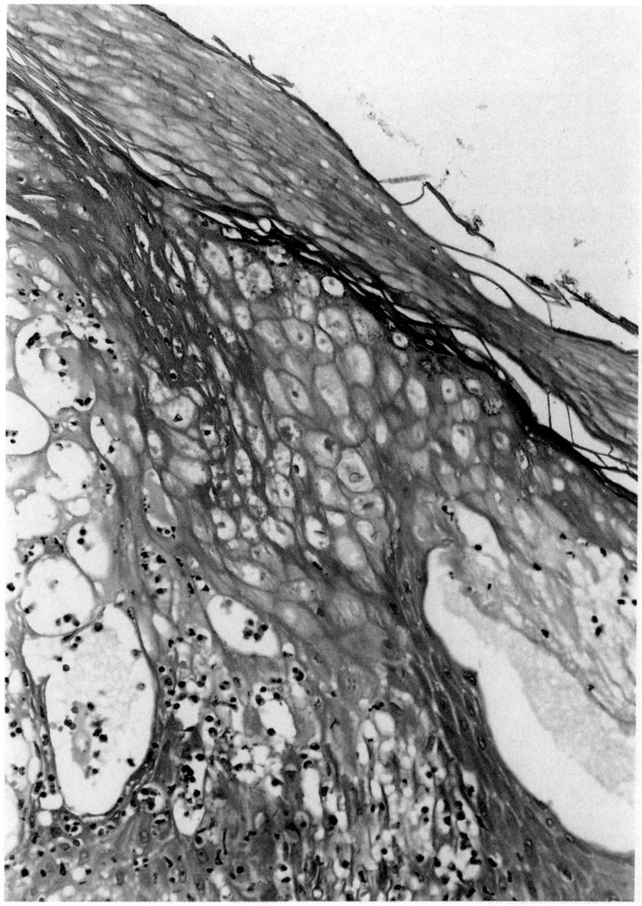

Figure 29–9. Higher magnification reveals spongiosis and ballooning degeneration in the epidermis. Note the inflammatory cells in spongiotic foci (hematoxylin-eosin, ×100).

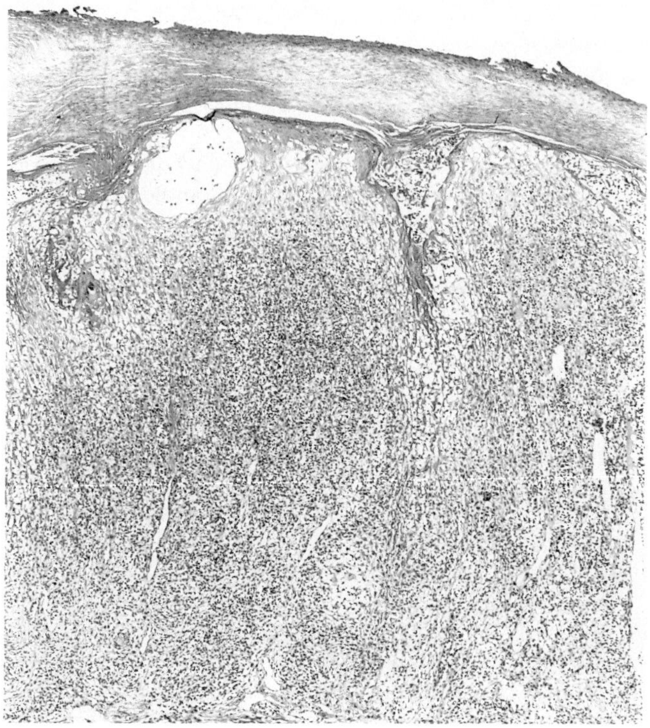

Figure 29–8. Parapoxvirus infection. Note the epithelial hyperplasia and the dense diffuse inflammatory cell infiltrate filling the dermis (hematoxylin-eosin, ×40).

multiloculated vesicles are formed. Finally, other diseases associated with ballooning degeneration such as deficiency diseases, ie, necrolytic migratory erythema and pellagra, may cause pallor and ballooning of the epidermis but there is little epidermal hyperplasia. Furthermore, ballooning is confined to the uppermost layers of epithelium and there are no intracytoplasmic inclusions.

MOLECULAR PATHOLOGIC DIAGNOSIS

In parapoxvirus infections when the diagnosis is difficult to confirm, electron microscopy may reveal intracytoplasmic viral particles.[16] Theoretically, polymerase chain reaction and in situ hybridization could be used for diagnosis, but because these infections are rare and self-limited these techniques have not been developed. Immunoperoxidase staining of orf using monoclonal antibody has recently revealed orf-specific labeling in 11 specimens, including some in which the diagnoses

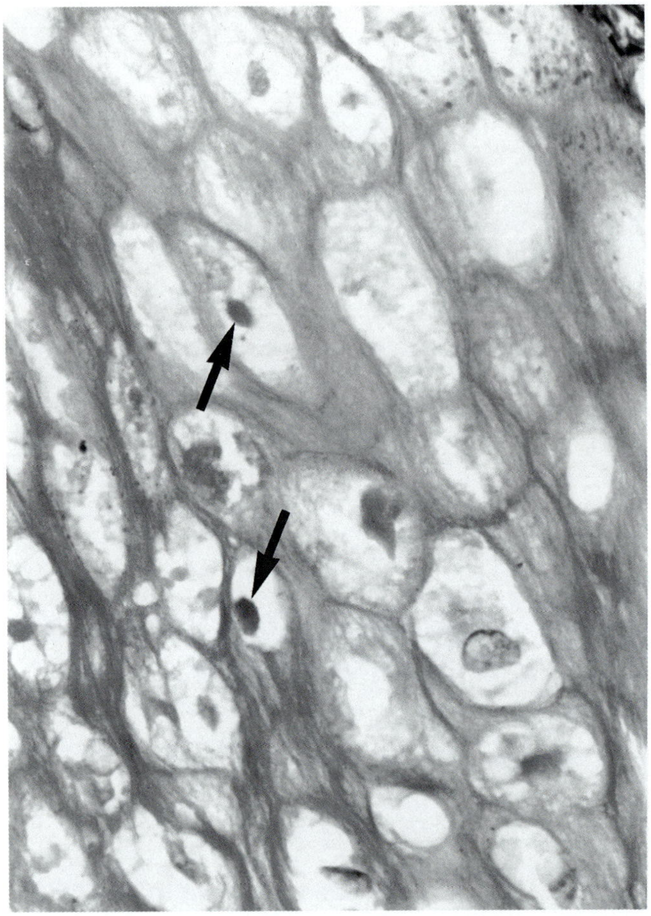

Figure 29–10. With further magnification, there is marked ballooning degeneration and intracytoplasmic eosinophilic inclusions, characteristic of the viral infection (hematoxylin-eosin, ×800).

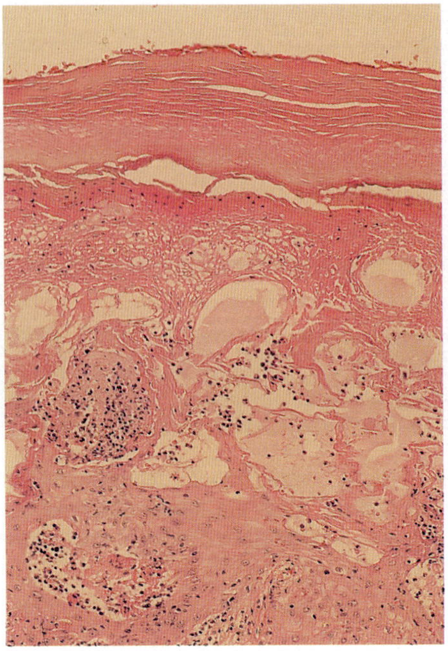

Figure 29–11. Late stage of milker's nodule, with marked spongiosis and vesicle formation in the epidermis (hematoxylin-eosin, ×200).

by routine light microscopy were equivocal.[16,17] This antibody, however, is not available commercially.

CONFIRMATIONAL TESTING AND DIAGNOSIS

Parapoxviruses grow in tissue cultures of various cell types including monkey kidney cells, human amnion cells, and human fibroblasts.[4] Rising antibody titers also may be used to confirm the diagnosis.[18]

REFERENCES

1. Jenner E. *An inquiry into the causes and effects of the variolae vaccinae, a disease discovered in some of the western counties of England, particularly Gloucestershire, and known by the name of the cow pox.* Second edition printed for the author by Sampson Low, London, 1880.
2. Brown D. Old enemy of mankind faces execution in June. *The Washington Post.* October 30, 1994:A3.
3. Henderson DA. The eradication of smallpox. *Sci Am.* 1976;235:25–33.
4. Moss B. In: Gorbach SL, Bartlett JG, Blacklow NR, eds. *Poxviruses in Infectious Diseases.* Philadelphia: WB Saunders; 1992;1365–1370.
5. Kotwal GJ, Moss B. Vaccinia virus encodes a secretory polypeptide structurally related to complement control proteins. *Nature.* 1988;335:176–179.
6. Katzman M, Carey JT, Elmets CA, et al. *Molluscum contagiosum* and the acquired immunodeficiency syndrome: clinical and immunological details of two cases. *Br J Dermatol.*
7. Cockerell CJ, Friedman-Kien AE. Skin manifestations of HIV infection. *Primary Care.* 1989;16:621.
8. Ive FA. Follicular *molluscum contagiosum*. *Br J Dermatol.* 1985;113:493–495.
9. Henao M, Freeman RG. Inflammatory *molluscum contagiosum.* Clinicopathological study of seven cases. *Arch Dermatol.* 1964;90:479–482.
10. Gill MJ, Arlette J, Buchan KA, et al. Human orf. *Arch Dermatol.* 1990;126:356–358.
11. Leavell UW Jr, Phillips IA. Milker's nodules. *Arch Dermatol.* 1975:111:1307–1311.
12. Lever WF, Schaumberg-Lever G, eds. *Histopathology of the Skin.* Philadelphia: JB Lippincott; 1983:407–409.
13. Kerl H, personal communication, 1989.
14. Ackerman AB. *Histologic Diagnosis of Inflammatory Skin Diseases.* Philadelphia: Lea and Febiger; 1978:508.

15. Evins S, Leavell UW Jr, Phillips LA. Intranuclear inclusions in milker's nodules. *Arch Dermatol.* 1971;103:91–93.
16. Nagington J. Electron microscopy in differential diagnosis of poxvirus infections. *Br Med J.* 1964;2:1499–1500.
17. Groves RW, Wilson-Jones E, MacDonald. Human orf: morphologic characteristics and immunohistochemical diagnosis. *J Cutan Pathol.* 1989;16:305. Abstract.
18. Hartmann AA, Buttner M, Stanka F, et al. Sero- und Immunodiagnostik bei Parapoxvirus-Infektion des Menschen *Hautarzt.* 1985;36:663–669.

CHAPTER 30

Rabies

Daniel P. Perl

When too little has been done for such a wound (bite of a mad animal), it usually gives rise to a fear of water which the Greeks call (hydrophobia). . . . In these cases there is very little hope for the sufferer. But still there is just one remedy, to throw the patient unawares into a water tank which he has not seen beforehand. If he cannot swim, let him sink under and drink, then lift him out; if he can swim, push him under at intervals so that he drinks his fill of water even against his will; for so his thirst and dread of water are removed at the same time. Yet this procedure incurs a further danger, that a spasm of sinews, provoked by the cold water, may carry off a weakened body. Lest this should happen, he must be taken straight from the tank and plunged into a bath of hot oil.

Celsus (25 B.C.–A.D. 50), De Medicina, Vol. 27 (trans. by W. G. Spencer)

. . . take heed of yonder dog!
Look when he fawns, he bites; and when he bites,
His venom tooth will rankle to the death:
Have not to do with him;
Sin, death, and hell, have set their marks on him . . .

William Shakespeare (1564–1616), King Richard III, I, iii

DEFINITION

Rabies is an acute viral disease of warm-blooded animals that is characterized by a prolonged incubation period followed by widespread involvement of the central nervous system (CNS). Typically rabies is transmitted through infected saliva by the bite of a rabid animal. Unless prevented by immunization within the incubation period, the disease is virtually fatal.

Rabies, known since antiquity, is also called *hydrophobia*, related to the distinctive dread of drinking, a common and prominent result of the acute phase of furious rabies. It is also known as *lyssa* (Greek for "madness").

GEOGRAPHIC DISTRIBUTION

Both wildlife and human rabies continue to be significant medical problems in many locations in the world. Worldwide, it is estimated that there are more than 50,000 human infections annually, most being in countries with a significant incidence of canine rabies. Animal rabies is much more frequent than human rabies, and dogs are the most commonly infected animal. Some regions of the world, however, have unique pockets of rabies involving other species. For example, in central Europe, the red fox is the predominant animal. In the United States, during the past several decades, raccoon rabies has spread northward up the Eastern seaboard, from northern Florida and Georgia to the Middle Atlantic states and more recently into southern New England.[1,2] Skunk rabies is widespread in the United States, particularly concentrated in the northern Plains states[3] and rabid bats have been identified in every state except Hawaii.

A number of island-bound populations have eliminated animal and human rabies by vaccinating dogs and by quarantining introduced animals. For example, Australia, Japan, Taiwan, New Zealand, and Great Britain are virtually free of rabies. Even in these locations, however, an infected traveler could reintroduce rabies because of the long incubation.

LIFE CYCLE/NATURAL HISTORY

It is generally believed that all examples of rabies, whether encountered in humans or in wildlife, represent the extension of the infection from one infected animal directly to another. In almost all instances, the infection is transmitted by the introduction of rabies virus in the saliva through a break in the skin. Rare examples of aerosol transmission of rabies have been documented,[4,5] but the exposure apparently must be massive. The viral inoculum initially stays within the site of the bite and in a short period of time (probably less than 1 or 2 days) enters into a dormant stage called "eclipse."[6,7] The eclipse period involves most of the incubation period, which in humans typically lasts from 3 to 12 weeks. At the end of this dormant phase there is a short period of local viral replication in muscle fibers within the wound site prior to invasion of the peripheral nervous system.[8,9] The virus is then carried up the axon of peripheral nerves that innervate the wound site. The virus is likely carried up the axoplasm by way of retrograde axoplasmic transport.[10,11] Once the virus arrives in the CNS there is extensive viral replication and spread throughout the neuraxis. The virus replicates primarily in neurons but glial cells are also invaded.[12,13] Soon after, there is extensive involvement of the CNS with centrifugal spread of the virus along the peripheral nerves. This is followed by viral replication in secretory organs, in particular, in the (acinar) salivary glands.[10,14,15] Changes in behavior are related, presumably, to involvement of limbic structures in the brain, causing aggressiveness and lack of fear of humans or other animals. This lack of fear with the high titers of virus in saliva is the diabolical combination that spreads the infection.

MORPHOLOGY OF THE ORGANISM

Rabies virus is classified within the rhabdovirus family (*rhabdo*, Greek for "rod-shaped") and is the prototype of the *Lyssavirus* genus.[16] It is a single-stranded RNA virus with a typical rhabdoviral bullet-shaped ultrastructure, with virions 75 nm in diameter and 180 nm long. The virions consist of a helically wound ribonuclear protein core, which is surrounded by a lipid envelope derived from the host cell membrane. The exterior of the virion is covered with 9- to 10-nm glycolipid spikelike protrusions.

CLINICAL FEATURES

The clinical manifestations of human rabies may be divided into five stages: incubation, prodrome, acute neurologic phase, coma, and death.

Incubation Period

The incubation period includes the time from initial exposure to the virus to the onset of symptoms in the prodromal phase. During this time the clinical features consist of the local damage of the initiating wound. The incubation period typically lasts from 30 to 90 days, although intervals from initial infection to onset may be as short as 9 days and as long as 1 year or more.[17,18] Bites on the head and neck have shorter incubation periods, but there are many exceptions,[18] and the incubation period for children also tends to be shorter. It is important to recognize that the wound typically will heal during the incubation period and, in the absence of a history of exposure to a rabid animal, the physician may be unable to document exposure.

Prodrome

The first symptoms may include nonspecific complaints such as malaise, generalized muscle aches, chills, abdominal pain, or fever. Accompanying neurologic features may also include headache, agitation, photophobia, and irritability. Pain, numbness, or paresthesias (burning, tingling, itching) in the region of the bite are common localizing symptoms. This may be related to entry and initial spread of virus into dorsal root ganglia and spinal cord. The prodrome is generally transitory, typically lasting 2 to 7 days.

Acute Neurologic Phase

The acute neurologic phase begins with the onset of severe objective neurologic signs and symptoms. For patients with hyperactivity, the term *furious rabies* is used, whereas patients with paralysis are called *paralytic* or *dumb rabies.*[17,19] Patients with furious rabies have severe anxiety, agitation, hallucinations, and other forms of hyperactive behavioral disturbance. Hydrophobia, characterized by choking, gagging, and laryngeal spasms, can be triggered by drinking liquids.

Sometimes the sight or the mere thought of liquids triggers an attack. Although characteristic of this phase, hydrophobia is noted in only 50% of patients. The mental status fluctuates, with periods of severe agitation interspersed with periods of lucidity and calm. As the illness progresses mental status deteriorates relentlessly, with increasing confusion progressing to stupor and eventually coma. In about 20% of patients a paralytic syndrome predominates, with progressive weakness and a flaccid paralysis of the limbs. In some patients the paralysis may be ascending in nature, mimicking Landry–Guillain–Barré syndrome.

Coma Phase

Coma may last for hours or days. Abnormal respiration, respiratory arrest, and death follow unless there is assisted ventilation. In addition, cardiac arrhythmias, EKG abnormalities, and cardiac arrest also may be noted.

Death

Without intensive nursing support and assisted ventilation, death comes usually within 7 days after the neurologic phase begins. With intensive care and support, patients may survive for 2 weeks or longer, but ultimately they die.[20,21] Only three nonfatal infections have been reported.[18,22,23]

PATHOLOGY

Gross Pathology

There are few gross changes in the brain. Mild cerebral edema with vascular congestion may be encountered; however, massive swelling with uncal and/or cerebellar tonsillar herniation are rare unless prolonged respiratory support has been given.

Light Microscopy, Including Special Stains

There are focal perivascular inflammatory cellular infiltrates, particularly in the upper brainstem, spinal cord, and thalamus (Figure 30–1). The cells that accumulate are mostly lymphocytes and monocytes, although plasma cells and even neutrophil cells may be present. The extent of inflammatory cell infiltrate varies and may be virtually absent. Focal microglial nodules (Babès nodules) also may be seen in areas of severe neuronal involvement, although neuronal destruction and neuronophagia are rare.

The most important diagnostic feature of rabies is the characteristic eosinophilic intracytoplasmic neuronal inclusion referred to as the *Negri body* (Figure 30–2). Negri bodies are best seen in the large pyramidal neurons of the Ammon's horn of the hippocampus (Figure 30–3) and in the Purkinje cells of the cerebellum. Using paraffin-embedded histologic examination, Negri bodies are identified in approximately 80% of cases[24] (Figure 30–4). Although earlier studies have emphasized the presence of a basophilic inner body (*Innerkörperchen*) for the identification of the Negri body (as opposed to the diagnostically less specific homogeneous inclusion called the *lyssa body*), electron microscopy has shown that most such inclusions also contain rabies viral particles.[12]

Electron Microscopy

Ultrastructurally, the Negri body consists of viral particles associated with a granular, electron-dense viral matrix. Two forms of Negri bodies are identified by electron microscopy.[12] One consists of a well-circumscribed, typically spherical aggregate of matrix surrounded by bullet-shaped rabies virions budding off the endoplasmic reticulum (Figure 30–5). These inclusions typically have an invagination introducing masses of

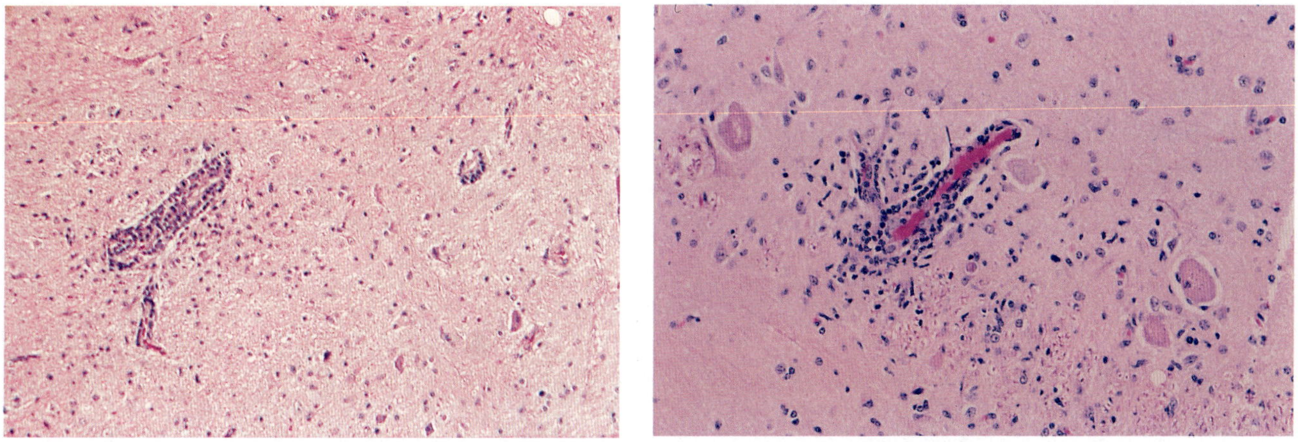

Figure 30–1. Micrographs of a brainstem experimentally infected with rabies virus that demonstrates perivascular chronic inflammatory cell infiltrates (hematoxylin-eosin, ×75, ×150).

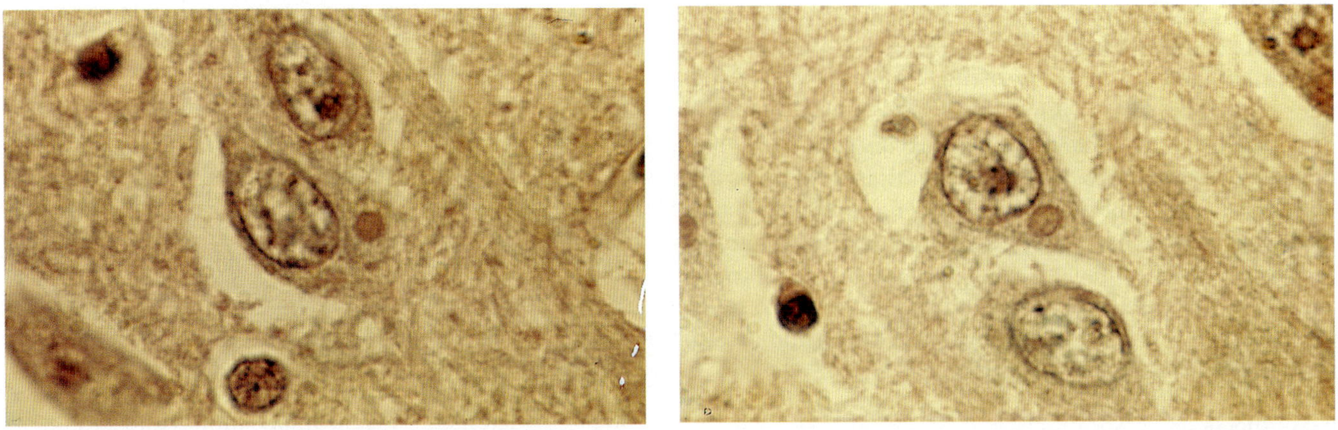

Figure 30–2. Micrographs showing pyramidal neurons containing prominent Negri bodies with inner body (*Innerkörperchen*) (hematoxylin-eosin, ×750).

virions into the central portion of the Negri body and forming what is visualized by light microscopy as the inner body. The second form of inclusion is primarily in the brainstem and cerebellum and is a more irregular mass of electron-dense matrix containing elongated tubular forms of the virus embedded within it (Figure 30–6). Typically, considerably more evidence of viral production is noted ultrastructurally than can be appreciated by light microscopy.

Differential Diagnosis

Rabies possesses such a distinctive pathologic picture that no other disorder resembles its histopathologic features. In some cases of rabies, however, Negri bodies may be inconspicuous and so few that finding histopathologic features that confirm the diagnosis may be extremely difficult. More frequently, particularly when a diagnosis of rabies has not been considered clinically, the relative paucity of perivascular infiltrates in some brains fails to remind the pathologist of the need to search for Negri bodies. The diagnosis, therefore, may be missed. In general, it is rather common for the diagnosis to be overlooked in nonendemic regions. Particular reasons for failure to consider the diagnosis include 1) the long incubation period in which the bite may have been forgotten and the resultant wound completely healed, and 2) the inability of the patient to provide a coherent history during the acute neurologic or coma phases of the illness. In nonendemic areas, it is not uncommon for the pathologist to be the first to diagnose rabies when unexpected death follows a rapid encephalopathic course. When this happens, many family members, acquaintances, and medical personnel who have been exposed to the patient may be required to have postexposure prophylaxis.[25]

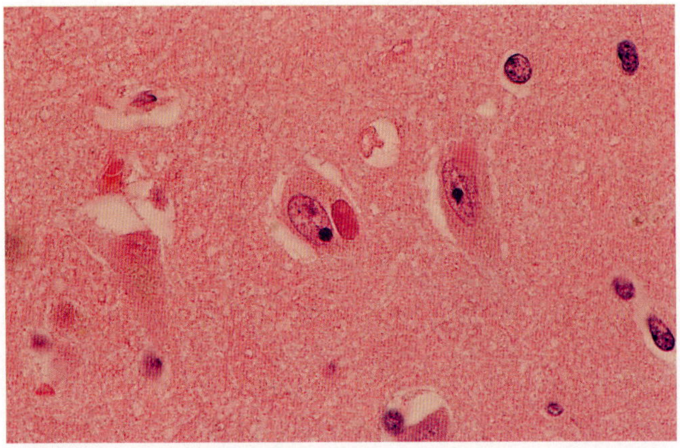

Figure 30–3. Micrograph of a pyramidal neuron of hippocampus containing a Negri body (hematoxylin-eosin, ×800).

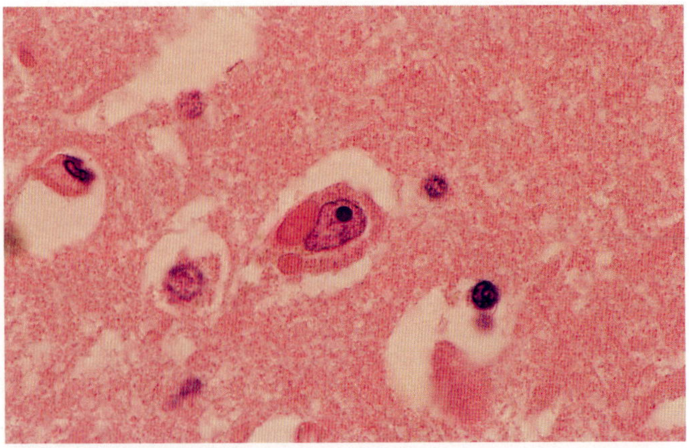

Figure 30–4. Micrograph of a pyramidal neuron of hippocampus containing two Negri bodies (hematoxylin-eosin, ×1000).

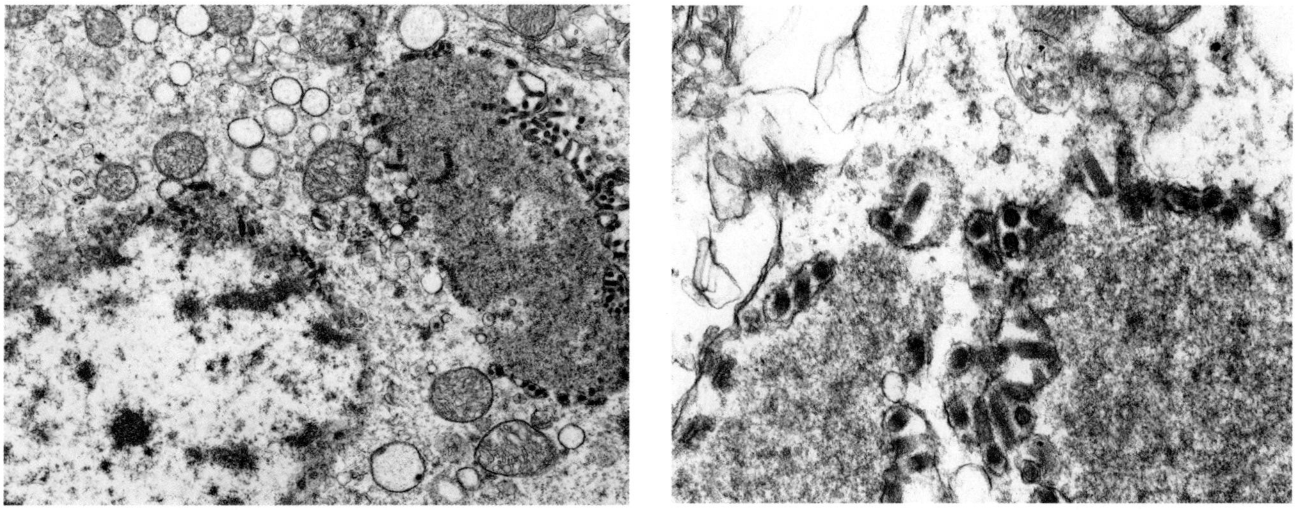

A B

Figure 30–5. (**A**) Electron micrograph of a neuron containing a Negri body with multiple bullet-shaped rabies virions at the periphery of the inclusion. (**B**) High-magnification electron micrograph demonstrating invagination of a Negri body filled with bullet-shaped rabies virions, some of which are budding off cellular membranes.

Diseases that can mimic acute furious rabies clinically include acute intermittent porphyria, tetanus, postrabies allergic encephalomyelitis, and other viral encephalitides. Paralytic rabies may be confused with poliomyelitis and Landry–Guillian–Barré syndrome.

Diagnosis (Molecular Aspects)

Rabies was one of the first viral infections in which fluorescent antibodies were used to establish a diagnosis.

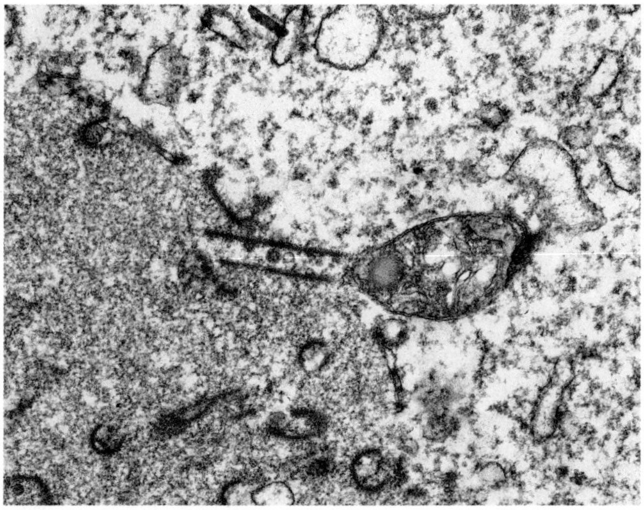

Figure 30–6. Electron micrograph of a portion of a Negri body containing elongated tubular forms of the rabies virus along with electron-dense granular viral matrix.

The technique generally uses freshly prepared smears of brain stained directly with fluorescein-tagged antibodies. These demonstrate brightly fluorescent masses of rabies viral antigen. High titers of neutralizing antibodies may mask fluorescent antibody staining. Paraffin embedding followed by trypsin pretreatment of histologic sections can increase sensitivity of the fluorescent antibody approach. Avidin-biotin techniques also enhance sensitivity. Other tissues and body fluids that may be examined for diagnostic purposes include corneal swabs and skin biopsy specimens (looking for rabies antigen in the neural plexus around hair follicles). Caution is advised with peripheral organs because false-negative results are common.

Confirming the Diagnosis

Rapid and accurate diagnosis of animal rabies is essential when humans have been exposed. Because of the urgency, the animal is killed and the brain subjected to immunofluorescent stains. Fluorescein-tagged antirabies hyperimmune serum is applied to smears of cerebral cortex, Ammon's horn of the hippocampus, cerebellum, midbrain, and lower brainstem. A positive reaction appears as particulate fluorescent positive intracytoplasmic masses. When the animal is a pet, quarantine and observation for 7 days is recommended. If the animal has no behavioral changes within 7 days, then the chances of transmission are negligible.

For viral isolation, mice are inoculated intracerebrally or by incubation of the inoculum in appropriate tissue culture systems, generally murine neuroblastoma cells. Mice inoculated with rabies virus become symptomatic within 5 to 12 days. Their brains are evaluated by immunofluorescent staining. Cultures in tissue cells become positive in 4 days. Fluorescent antibody studies reveal rabies viral antigen and, in spite of large amounts of viral particles, the cells do not show a cytopathogenic effect.

The diagnosis of rabies in humans can be confirmed also by demonstrating neutralizing antibodies in the serum of persons who have never been vaccinated against rabies. The patient's serum and the control serum are mixed with suspensions of mouse brain containing a standard titer of the CVS (challenge virus standard) strain of rabies virus. This mixture is then injected intracerebrally in mice. The viral neutralizing capacity of the patient's serum is then compared to that of the control serum.

TREATMENT

Once symptoms have begun, rabies is almost always fatal. Aggressive supportive nursing care and assisted ventilation have increased survival time, yet an invariably fatal course results. Aggressive assisted ventilation leads to massive cerebral edema and obliteration of the cerebral capillary bed followed by extensive autolytic changes—the "respirator brain." These changes may make it extremely difficult (or even impossible) for the pathologist to confirm the diagnosis. Immunization during the incubation period, primarily with human diploid cell vaccine, and by giving passive rabies immune globulin provide excellent protection when begun soon after exposure. The few examples of failure to protect from CNS infection generally involve delay in recognizing exposure to rabies virus.[26,27]

REFERENCES

1. Fishman HR, Grigor JK, Horman JT, Israel E. Epizootic of rabies in racoons in Maryland from 1981 to 1987. *J Am Vet Med Assoc* 1992;201:1883–1886.
2. Winkler WG, Jenkins SR. Raccoon rabies. In: Baer GM, ed. *The Natural History of Rabies.* Boca Raton, Fla: CRC Press; 1991:325–340.
3. Charlton KM, Webster WA, Casey GA. Skunk rabies. In: Baer GM, ed. *The Natural History of Rabies.* Boca Raton, Fla: CRC Press; 1991:307–324.
4. Conomy JP, Leibovitz A, McCombs W, Stinson J. Airborne rabies encephalitis: demonstration of rabies virus in the human central nervous system. *Neurology.* 1977;27:67–69.
5. Constantine DG, Emmons RW, Woodie JD. Rabies virus in nasal mucosa of naturally infected bats. *Science.* 1972; 175:1255–1256.
6. Baer GM, Cleary WF. A model in mice for the pathogenesis and treatment of rabies. *J Infect Dis.* 1972;125: 520–527.
7. Baer GM, Lentz TL. Rabies pathogenesis to the central nervous system. In: Baer GM, ed. *The Natural History of Rabies.* Boca Raton, Fla: CRC Press; 1991:105–120.
8. Murphy FA, Bauer S. Early street rabies virus infection in striated muscle and later progression to the central nervous system. *Intervirology.* 1974;3:256–268.
9. Murphy FA. Rabies pathogenesis. *Arch Virol.* 1977;54: 279–297.
10. Murphy FA, Bauer SP, Harrison AK, Winn WC. Comparative pathogenesis of rabies and rabies-like viruses, viral infection and transit from inoculation site to the central nervous system. *Lab Invest.* 1973;28:361–376.
11. Gillet JP, Dere P, Tsiang H. Axonal transport of rabies virus in the central nervous system of the rat. *J Neuropathol Exp Neurol.* 1986;45:619–634.
12. Perl DP, Good PF. The pathology of rabies in the central nervous system. In: Baer GM, ed. *The Natural History of Rabies.* Boca Raton, Fla: CRC Press; 1991:163–190.
13. Mrak RE, Young L. Rabies encephalitis in humans: pathology, pathogenesis and pathophysiology. *J Neuropathol Exp Neurol.* 1994;53:1–10.
14. Dierks RE, Murphy FA, Harrison AK. Extraneural rabies virus infection. Virus development in fox salivary gland. *Am J Pathol.* 1969;54:251–273.
15. Schneider LG. Spread of the virus from the central nervous system. In: Baer GM, ed. *The Natural History of Rabies.* Boca Raton, Fla: CRC Press; 1991:133–144.
16. Rupprecht CE, Dietzschold B, Wunner WH, Koprowski H. Antigenic relationships of lyssaviruses. In: Baer GM, ed. *The Natural History of Rabies.* Boca Raton, Fla.: CRC Press; 1991:69–100.
17. Hattwick MAW. Human rabies. *Pub Health Rev.* 1974;3:229–274.
18. Fishbein DB. Rabies in humans. In: Baer GM, ed. *The Natural History of Rabies.* Boca Raton, Fla.: CRC Press; 1991:519–550.
19. Chopra JS, Banerjee AK, Murthy JMK, Pal SR. Paralytic rabies: a clinico-pathologic study. *Brain.* 1980;103:789.
20. Warrell DA, Davidson NM, Pope HM, et al. Pathophysiologic studies in human rabies. *Am J Med.* 1976;60: 180–190.
21. Gode GR, Raju AV, Jayalakshmi TS, Kaul HL, Bhide NK. Intensive care in rabies therapy: clinical observations. *Lancet.* 1976;2:6.
22. Hattwick MAW, Weiss TT, Stechschulte J, et al. Recovery from rabies. A case report. *Ann Intern Med.* 1972; 76:931–942.
23. Porras C, Barboza JJ, Fuenzalida E, et al. Recovery from rabies in man. *Ann Intern Med.* 1976;85:44–48.
24. Dupont JR, Earle KM. Human rabies encephalitis. A study of forty-nine cases with a review of the literature. *Neurology.* 1965;15:1023–1034.
25. Helmick CG, Tauxe RV, Vernon AA. Is there a risk to contacts of patients with rabies? *Rev Infect Dis.* 1987;9: 511–518.
26. Johnson KP, Swoveland PT. Rabies. *Neurol Clin.* 1984;2:255–265.
27. Hemachudha T. Rabies. In: McKendall RR, ed. *Handbook of Clinical Neurology. Viral Disease.* New York: Elsevier Science; 1989;12(56):383–404.

CHAPTER 31

Respiratory Syncytial Virus

J. Thomas Stocker, Richard M. Conran, and Nancy Fishback

Man is neither unique nor central nor necessarily here to stay. But he is a product of circumstances special to the point of disbelief. . . . Change is the elixir of the human circumstance, and acceptance of challenge the way of our kind. We are bad-weather animals, disaster's fairest children. For the soundest of evolutionary reasons man appears at his best when times are worst.

Robert Ardrey (1908–1988), African Genesis

DEFINITION

Respiratory syncytial virus (RSV) causes upper then lower respiratory tract disease in infants and children throughout the world, with virtually everyone experiencing infection within the first few years of life. Mortality, fortunately, is very low in those with competent immune systems, but death from RSV is being identified with increasing frequency in those with organ transplants and in those infected with the human immunodeficiency virus (HIV). Infection with RSV causes pneumonia, bronchiolitis, tracheobronchitis, and occasionally otitis media (especially in infants and young children), and rarely causes meningitis, myelitis, and myocarditis.

GEOGRAPHIC DISTRIBUTION

RSV is a recognized pathogen worldwide. In children from both developing and developed countries, RSV has been identified as a cause of respiratory death.[1] In the United States, all geographic regions are affected. Gilchrist and colleagues[2] report no significant variation in onset of outbreaks among geographic regions, and they provide data suggesting that the RSV is present in communities throughout the year and that outbreaks in different regions of the country are independent of each other.[2]

Two distinct subgroups (A and B) of RSV have been identified. In the United States, RSV subgroup A accounts for approximately three fourths of isolates and is the dominant strain responsible for infections for most years.[3–5] Data suggest this pattern is present worldwide.

EPIDEMIOLOGY

RSV infection is usually self-limited, with most children exposed by age 2 years. Infection presents frequently as a common cold. Presentations with greater morbidity include laryngotracheobronchitis and pneumonia. In the neonate, approximately 50% of viral pneumonias are caused by RSV.[6] RSV is a frequent cause of winter outbreaks of acute respiratory infection, and, in the United States, it is estimated to cause 90,000 hospital admissions (1% to 2% of infected children) annually.[7–8] Approximately 50% of these admissions are for bronchiolitis and 25% for pneumonia. A systemic illness resembling sepsis is also recognized. RSV infection causes approximately 4500 respiratory deaths in infants and children in the United States annually.[5,9] In 1985, the cost of hospitalization for RSV-related disease was approximately $300 million.[5,8]

The majority of RSV infections in children in the United States are between November and April, with the peak incidence in January and February (Figure

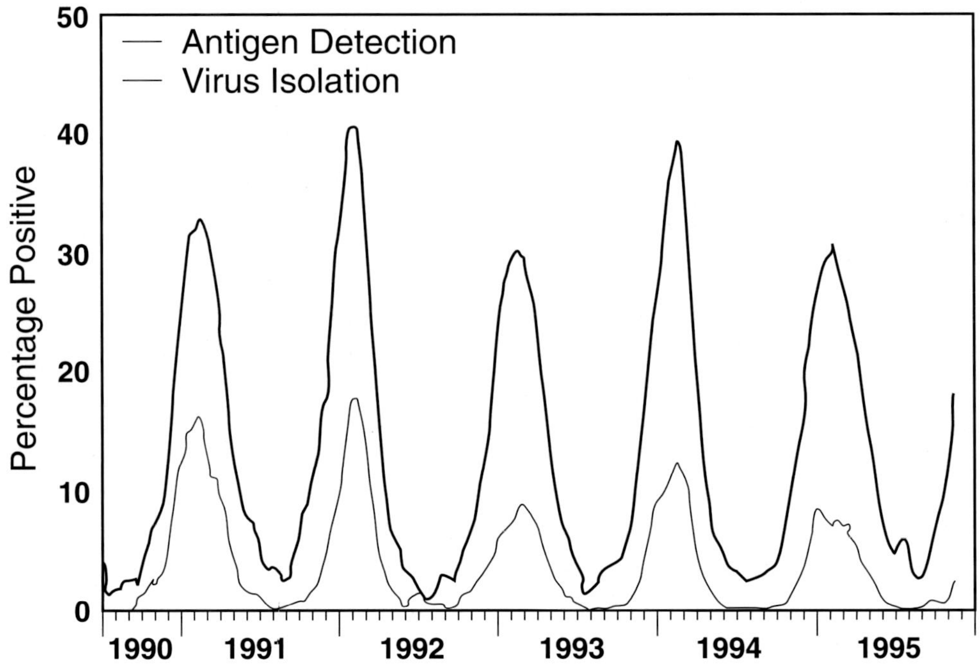

Figure 31–1. Percentages of specimens positive for respiratory syncytial virus, by method of confirmation and month for the United States, from July 1, 1990, through December 1, 1995 (laboratory-group mean, smoothed using a 5-week moving average) *(from Centers for Disease Control[9]).*

31–1), but isolated outbreaks during the summer have been reported.[2,10] Infection with RSV provides limited partial immunity. Reinfection is frequent; however, repeat infections are mild, usually consisting only of upper respiratory symptoms. Family members are the usual source of reinfection.[9] Breast-feeding provides the neonate with passive immunity.

DEMOGRAPHIC DATA

Clinically recognized RSV infection predominantly affects children less than 6 months of age, with a median age of 3 months.[11] Most infections are community acquired. Although the infants are otherwise healthy, there is usually a family history of illness. Nosocomial infections account for approximately 5% of RSV infections.[12] RSV infection in older children and in otherwise healthy adults has been reported in various settings. Thom and colleagues[10] described nine college students infected with RSV who presented to the university health clinic with respiratory infections. Infections were in summer, spring, and winter. A slight male predilection has been reported in hospitalized children (male:female 1.44:1).[11]

RISK FACTORS

Risk factors for acute respiratory infections are an immature or deficient immune system or environmental factors that promote excessive exposure to RSV. Hemming[1] lists age, prematurity, low birth weight, cardiopulmonary disease/bypass, congenital or acquired immune deficiency syndromes, malnutrition, overcrowding, increased exposure of a child to an infected host, environmental pollution (including secondhand smoke), and lack of breast-feeding as risk factors.[1] Male gender and a family history of asthma also have been reported as risk factors by LaVia and colleagues.[11] Approximately two thirds of hospitalized patients have at least one of these risk factors.[7] Infants with these underlying risk factors have greater morbidity, requiring lengthier hospitalizations. Hall and associates[3] report greater morbidity with subgroup A infections.

TRANSMISSION

Incubation is 4 to 8 days. Infection by aerosolized respiratory secretions is frequent. Equally important, because simple hand washing prevents the transmission, especially for nosocomial infections, is transmission of secretions from infected host by hand contamination to nasal and conjunctival mucosa.[13]

HIGH-RISK GROUPS

Most RSV infections are self-limited in children and young adults. Infants with underlying bronchopulmonary dysplasia, cystic fibrosis,[14] or congenital heart disease are at increased risk. A number of high-risk groups in children and adults have been identified. Children with congenital immune disorders, children or adults with acquired disorders such as acquired immunodeficiency syndrome (AIDS),[15,16] or patients with transplanted organs[17–19] have morbidity related to their underlying disease.

King and colleagues[15] found no difference in clinical symptoms between HIV-infected and non-HIV-infected children; however, prolonged shedding of virus is a public health factor in HIV-infected children. They report also that the median duration of viral shedding in HIV-infected children was 30 days compared to 6 days in non–HIV-infected children. Although treatment with ribavirin, a synthetic nucleoside analog approved for treatment of RSV since 1986, was effective in RSV infection in an adult patient with AIDS,[16] one child treated with ribavirin shed virus for 199 days.[15]

RSV is a significant pathogen in up to 3% of patients with bone marrow transplants.[19] In spite of treatment with ribavirin, Hertz and colleagues[20] reported that 50% of those with bone marrow transplants died of RSV pneumonia within a year after the transplant. A more recent study by Harrington and associates[18] reported that 58% of those with bone marrow transplants developed RSV pneumonia during an RSV outbreak. Of those patients who developed pneumonia, 78% died of their pneumonia. RSV pneumonia also has caused increased morbidity in those with solid organ transplants (kidney, liver).[17,19]

RSV infects and kills the elderly,[21] but because the clinical features of influenza and infection with RSV are similar, infection by RSV is underdiagnosed in the elderly. In a nursing home, Sorvillo and associates[22] reported 40% of the residents infected with RSV during an outbreak, with half of them with pneumonia and 20% dying of their infection. In an outbreak in a geriatric ward, Agius and associates[23] found 76% infected and 16% with serious complications.

NOSOCOMIAL INFECTIONS

In the hospital setting, RSV is probably spread by close contact between patients and healthcare workers.[12,13,24,25] Some investigators report that up to half of hospitalized children and healthcare workers on pediatric wards become infected during an RSV outbreak.[12,13,24] Experimental studies by Hall and Douglas[24] showed that 70% of healthy workers became infected with RSV when they contacted infected children. Also, 40% of workers became infected when they came in contact with the bedding of RSV-infected children.[12,13,24] Among adult patients in a combined pediatric–medical intensive care unit (ICU), RSV had infected 45% of intubated patients.[25] Significant morbidity and mortality has been reported with nosocomial infections involving hospitalized senior citizens. Contact-isolation procedures reduce nosocomial infections.

SUDDEN INFANT DEATH SYNDROME

Apnea is a recognized complication of RSV infection,[26,27] reported in up to 18% to 25% of hospitalized infants younger than 1 year of age. RSV infection as a cause of sudden infant death syndrome (SIDS) has been postulated. Isolation of RSV from infants dying of SIDS in Australia was reported in 26% (200 of 763) of infants compared to 18% in 56 age-matched controls who died predominantly from accidents. The incidence of RSV detection was greater (39%) in infants older than 3 months of age compared to infants younger than 3 months (14%).[28] Whether the RSV infection was incidental or related to the infant death is problematic. Although a number of cases administratively called SIDS are sudden death from RSV apnea, they would be reclassified when the cause is known.

MORPHOLOGY OF THE ORGANISM

The respiratory syncytial virus is a 120 to 300 nm, enveloped, single negative-strand RNA virus in the *Pneumovirus* genus within the *Paramyxoviridae* family. The viral envelope is described as thistle-like, with 12 nm spikes of glycoprotein 10 nm apart. An internal 13.5 nm nucleocapsid is helical with a 6.5 nm pitch.[29,30] The RSV genome encodes 10 quintessential viral proteins, including three (designated N, P, and L) associated with the nucleocapsid, four (F, G, M, and M2) with the envelope, two (NS1 and NS2) nonstructural proteins of the virion, and one (SH) that is virion associated. The F and G proteins appear to be associated with the infectivity of the virus, with the F protein initiating viral penetration through fusion of viral and cellular membranes. Replication of the virus occurs in the cytoplasm with RSV virions assembled at the cytoplasmic membranes. The two major groups of RSV, the A and B groups, differ primarily in the G protein.[3] Further subgrouping of these two groups has identified subgroups A1 through A5 and B1 through B4, which are determined by monoclonal antibodies.

RSV remains stable at body temperature for an hour; withstands acid medium poorly, and is deactivated by ether, chloroform, and a variety of detergents. Transmission is enhanced by warm room temperature and higher humidity, with the virus surviving for hours in the patient's secretions on nonporous surfaces. Infectivity decreases rapidly at 37°C after an hour with loss of 99% infectivity by 2 days.

CLINICAL FEATURES

The various clinical presentations of RSV are related to the age and premorbid condition of the host. In children younger than 3 years, the disease involves predominantly the lower respiratory tract. Whereas initial symptoms, including sneezing, pharyngitis, and cough, indicate an upper respiratory component, more than half of infected infants will develop signs of bronchiolitis and/or pneumonia. Fever, cough, and dyspnea are the most common findings in lower tract disease. The fever is usually low-grade and may be absent. Physical findings include retraction, tachypnea, wheezes, rales, and rhonchi.

Otitis media is found in 62% of children with group A infection and 75% of children with group B infection.[31] Bacterial coinfection may lead to chronic otitis media with effusion. Conversely, RSV was detected by polymerase chain reaction in 9.9% of the specimens collected from children undergoing myringotomy for chronic otitis media with effusion.[32]

The chest x ray in children with known RSV infection and clinical pneumonia or bronchiolitis may be normal in 20% to 50% of patients.[33–35] THe most common positive x-ray findings in young children with lower respiratory tract disease include hyperinflation, interstitial infiltrates, consolidation, and atelectasis. Unilateral right-sided hilar enlargement has been reported in one third of the patients.[36]

Hypoxemia is frequent in infants hospitalized with RSV. The desaturation may be profound and prolonged and does not always correlate with clinical indicators. Cyanosis is associated with hypoxemia, but hypoxemia may be found in infants who are not cyanotic.[37] Episodes of apnea occur in 20% of infants hospitalized for RSV infection and are more common in infants who were premature at birth and present in premature infants at a younger age.[26,27,38] These episodes are usually brief, nonobstructive, and occur during the first few days of illness, but there may be prolonged apnea requiring intubation and ventilation. Infants dying of SIDS have a higher incidence of RSV antigens than do infants the same age, raising the possibility that RSV infection in childhood may predispose to SIDS.[38] This has not been confirmed with a prospective study,[26] but the sample was small. Viral infections are not listed as relative risk factors for SIDS by the National Institute of Child Health and Human Development (NICHD) Cooperative Epidemiological Study.[39]

Hypercarbia is less common. Respiratory failure requiring mechanical ventilation occurs in less than 10% overall. Respiratory failure and death are more likely in infants with underlying disease, particularly congenital heart defects and bronchopulmonary dysplasia.[11,40] Infants who were premature at birth and infants who contracted RSV in the first 6 weeks of life were also at risk for respiratory complications. In older children and previously healthy adults, RSV infection may be asymptomatic. When symptoms are present, they tend to reflect upper respiratory tract involvement rather than lower. A prolonged cough, sinusitis, and otitis media are the most common manifestations. Up to 20% of patients develop reactive airways disease, which may persist for weeks after the illness.[29]

In the elderly, adults with underlying disease, such as chronic obstructive pulmonary disease (COPD) and in immunodeficient patients, the disease may involve both the upper and lower respiratory tracts. In one series upper respiratory symptoms, including sinusitis and otitis media, preceded fever and pulmonary infiltrates in the immunodeficient, with 36% mortality caused by viral infection.[17] RSV has been reported with AIDS and in patients undergoing organ transplants. Patients receiving bone marrow transplants are particularly at risk for RSV, often presenting with features of upper respiratory tract and sinus involvement as well as lung injury.[20] RSV has been documented in exacerbations of underlying obstructive airways disease, such as asthma, COPD, and bronchiectasis.

An association between RSV infection in early childhood and the subsequent development of asthma and atopy has been considered. An increased incidence of wheezing was found in children who had been hospitalized for RSV infection as infants,[41] but other studies indicate this tendency regresses with time.[42,43] Persistent viral infection has also been postulated as a factor in the pathogenesis of asthma and COPD[44]; however, RSV is known to complicate preexisting lung disease, and the relationship of viral infections to airways obstruction is not yet resolved.

Unusual presentations of RSV infection include arrhythmias, rash, and neurologic manifestations such as meningitis.[29] Shock and hypothermia may dominate the clinical picture, especially in very young infants and in the premature.[45]

PATHOLOGY

The pathologic changes of RSV are limited almost entirely to the lungs, and descriptions of these changes are derived almost exclusively from autopsy material.[46–48] Grossly, the lungs show areas of hyperinflation alternating with areas of consolidation and hemorrhage. Thick, mucoid material may be in larger bronchi and expressed from small bronchioles on the cut surface

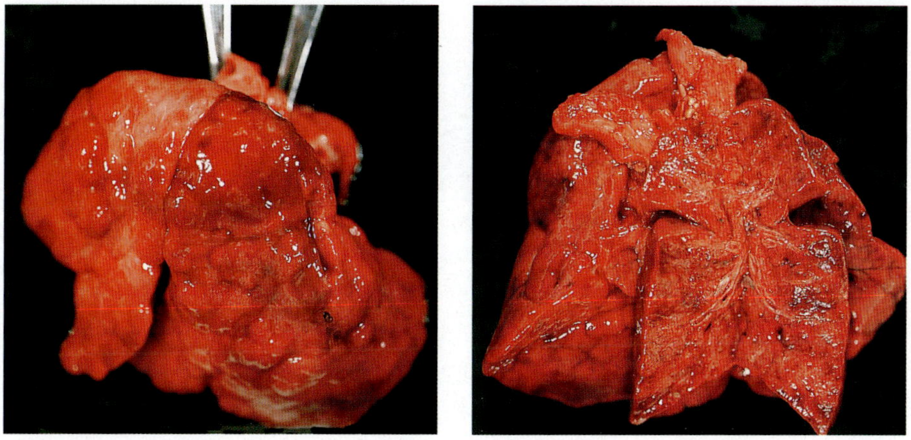

A B

Figure 31–2. (**A** and **B**) Lungs of a 4-month-old infant with bronchopulmonary dysplasia (BPD) who developed respiratory distress with a progressively worsening cough. Air-trapping was seen on chest x rays prior to death. The lungs display hyperinflation of acini typical of RSV and long-term "healed" BPD. On the cut surface (**B**), bronchi are partially occluded by mucoid material (see Figure 31–3). *(Photograph courtesy of Areta Kowal-Vern, MD, Loyola University Medical School, Chicago, Illinois.)*

(Figures 31–2 and 31–3). The hyperinflation noted on radiographs is caused by plugging of terminal and respiratory bronchioles with air trapping distal to the occluded areas. The material obstructing the bronchioles is composed of cellular debris of bronchial, bronchiolar, and alveolar epithelium mixed with mucus and inflammatory cells (Figures 31–4 and 31–5). The injury of the airway by RSV appears to begin as hyperplasia and squamous metaplasia of the epithelium, accompanied by desquamation of the epithelial cells (Figure 31–6). Large syncytial giant cells (from which RSV derives its name) are in and line alveolar spaces, but they may also be in bronchi and bronchioles. The alveolar involvement may be extensive, producing wide areas of consolidation also noted on radiographs.

Cytoplasmic inclusions, varying from 1 to 20 μm in diameter, are in bronchial, bronchiolar, and alveolar epithelium, syncytial giant cells, and sloughed intra-alveolar cells (Figure 31–7).[48] These globules, which stain with anti-RSV antibody, are often eosinophilic, homogeneous, and well defined in the paranuclear area, but they are granular and mildly basophilic when more peripheral (Figures 31–8 and 31–9). Clear "halos" may surround the smaller inclusions. Intranuclear inclusions have not been identified. In addition to the globules, staining for RSV displays cytoplasmic positivity in alveolar, bronchial, and bronchiolar epithelium; syncytial giant cells; and sloughed alveolar cells. The degree of staining in an alveolus varies from partial to total involvement. In bronchial and bronchiolar hyperplastic

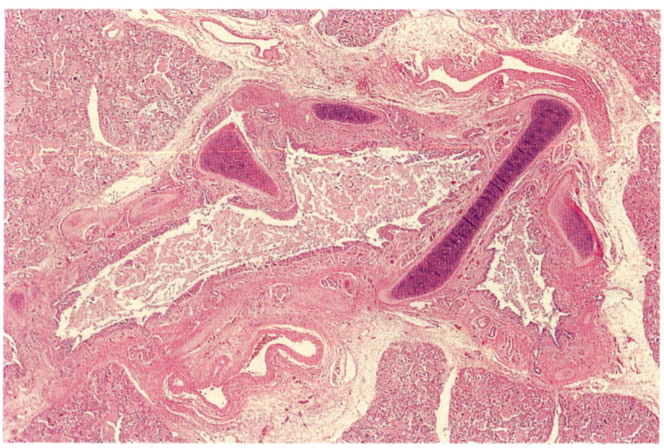

Figure 31–3. A bronchus near the hilum is filled with amorphus eosinophilic material (hematoxylin-eosin, ×15).

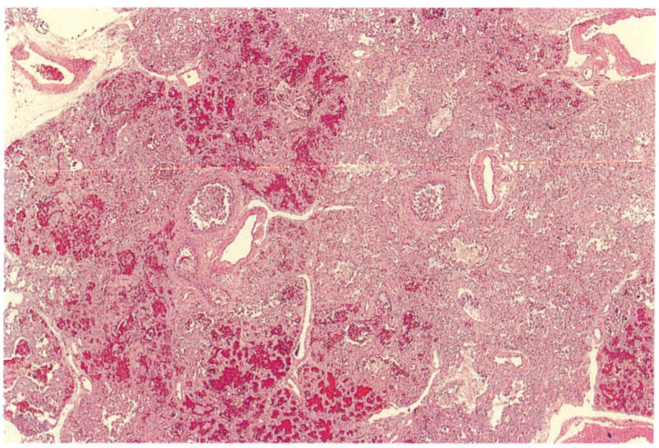

Figure 31–4. At low magnification, there are areas of alveolar hemorrhage and bronchioles and alveolar ducts filled with amorphous eosinophilic material (hematoxylin-eosin, ×10).

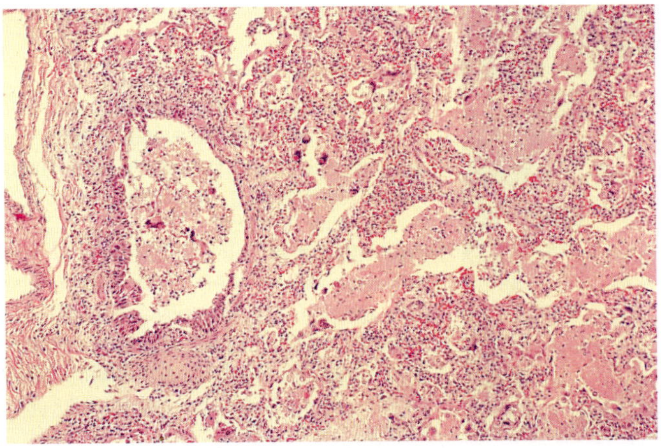

Figure 31–5. A small bronchus (*left*) and adjacent alveolar ducts are distended with amorphous material within which are numerous multinucleated giant cells (hematoxylin-eosin, ×25).

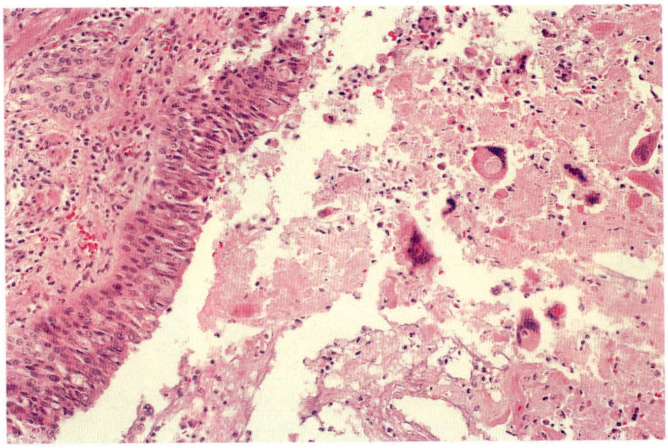

Figure 31–6. The epithelium of a bronchus is hyperplastic and focally necrotic (*top*). The material in the lumen consists of inflammatory cells, cellular debris, and multinucleated giant cells (hematoxylin-eosin, ×75).

epithelium, the staining is most intense in cells nearest the lumen.[48] A mild to moderate inflammatory infiltrate of mononuclear cells and neutrophils may also be in peribronchial, peribronchiolar, and interstitial tissue. A more severe acute bronchopneumonia may indicate a secondary bacterial infection.

Electron microscopy displays round to elongated profiles of the virus (Figure 31–10) 100 nm in diameter. Viral replication is in cytoplasmic sacs and seen as fuzzy "budding" from the membrane.

Rarely there may be adrenal hemorrhage and cytoplasmic inclusions of adrenal medullary and cortical cells similar to those in the bronchial epithelium. These were noted by Adams[46] in a 1947 epidemic of "virus pneumonitis with cytoplasmic inclusion bodies," thought to be RSV disease.

The peripheral blood may display a mild to moderate leukocytosis with a predominance of lymphocytes, many of which may be atypical or reactive. These lymphocytes are typically larger than normal circulating lymphocytes and have increased amounts of foamy cytoplasm. Nuclei may be multilobated and have indentations or grooves.[49] These changes are not specific for RSV and may be in a variety of childhood conditions,

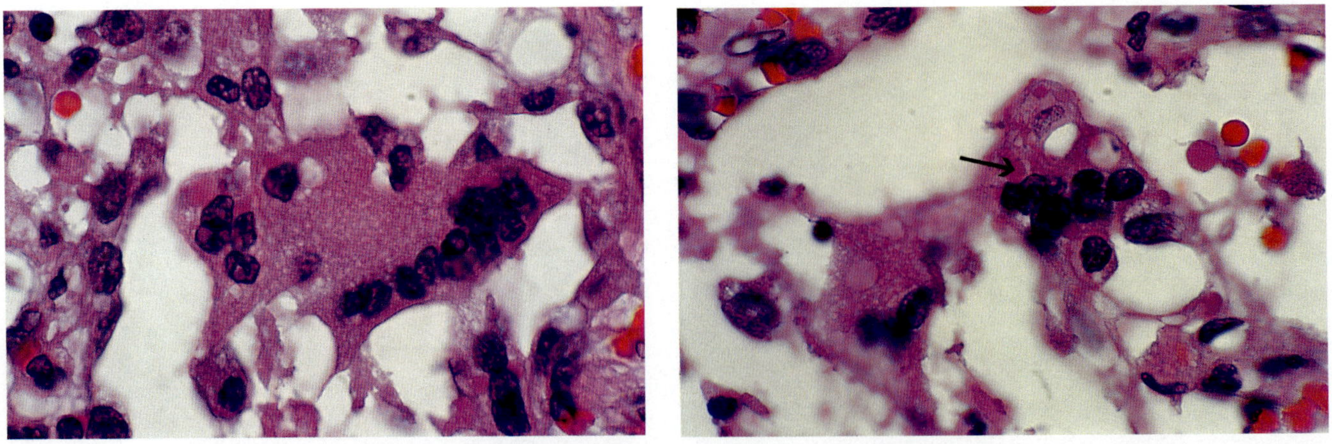

A

B

Figure 31–7. (**A** and **B**) Giant cells in the lumen of bronchi, bronchioles, and alveolar ducts contain many eccentrically placed slightly irregular nuclei with vesiculated nucleoplasm. The cytoplasm varies from granular to vesiculated and contains a number of perinuclear smooth eosinophilic globules. (**B**) A thin, clear "halo" surrounds a globule (*arrow*) (hematoxylin-eosin, ×200).

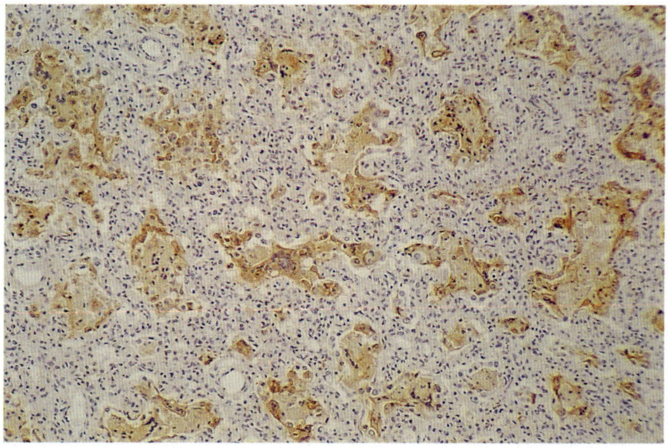

Figure 31–8. Immunoperoxidase staining for RSV displays diffuse positivity, not only of the giant cells but also of mononuclear cells and the amorphous material in bronchi, bronchioles, and alveolar ducts (RSV IP, ×50). *(Photograph courtesy of Tan Nguyen, MD, USUHS, Bethesda, Maryland.)*

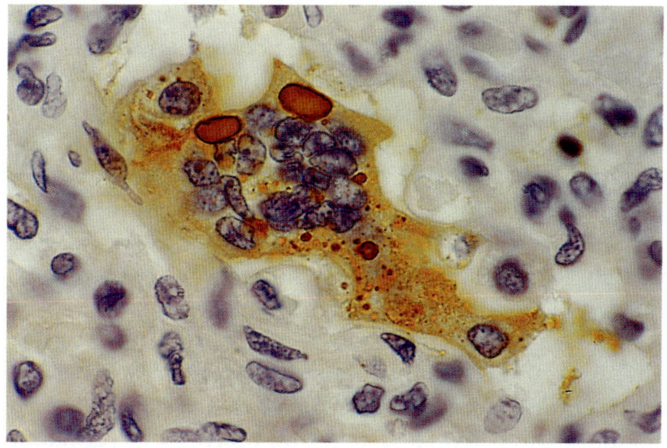

Figure 31–9. A multinucleated cell in an alveolar duct contains many intensely positive (for RSV) globules of varying size, including the perinuclear globules that correspond to those seen on hematoxylin-eosin (see Figure 31–6). Note also the diffuse staining of all of the cytoplasm of the cell (RSV IP, ×200).

including infectious mononucleosis, other viral infections, nonviral infections, and drug reactions. The reaction is thought to be caused by antigenic stimulation of the lymphocytes by the virus with subsequent transformation of the cells to produce antibodies or lymphokines.

DIAGNOSIS

The typical presentation of upper respiratory symptoms followed by pneumonia/bronchiolitis in a young child during community outbreaks strongly suggests the diagnosis. Laboratory confirmation may be obtained by a variety of methods. A detailed review of techniques is in *Laboratory Diagnosis of Viral Infections* (2nd ed.).[30] Nasopharyngeal aspirates or washes can be inoculated into cell cultures. The virus is labile, cannot be grown in embryonated eggs, and disappears in the first week of illness. Adequate specimens must be obtained early in the illness and inoculated promptly. Disadvantages of this technique include the need for strict handling and the time required to process the material.

For more rapid diagnosis, direct and indirect immunofluorescence for RSV antigens using commercially available sera can be done. These techniques also require an adequate specimen and there may be false-negative results with cross-reacting antigens. With adequate specimens and proper technique, the sensitivity and specificity of these procedures approach 85% to 95%.[30,43,50] Enzyme-linked immunosorbent assay (ELISA) using commercially available kits can also be performed on nasopharyngeal washings and aspirates. The sensitivity has been reported to be greater than 85%, and the technique can be performed on specimens that have been stored or shipped.[30,50]

TREATMENT

Treatment for lower respiratory tract involvement is supportive with attention to fluid replacement and supplemental oxygen if the pO_2 is less than 60 mm Hg.[43]

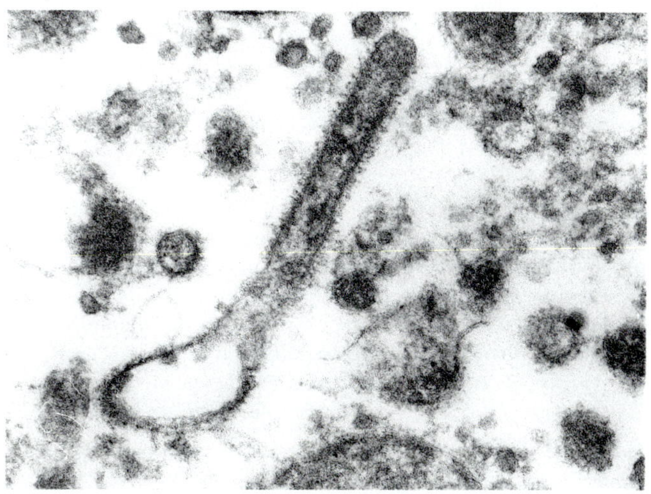

Figure 31–10. Elongate RSV particles in the cytoplasm of a giant cell measure approximately 100 nm in diameter and have a "fuzzy" border (×65,000). *(Photograph courtesy of Eduardo Yunis, MD, Children's Hospital of Pittsburgh, Pittsburgh, Pennsylvania.)*

If hypoxemia is persistent or severe, if apnea is prolonged, or if hypercarbia is significant, intubation and assisted ventilation should be considered. Although some infants seem to respond to bronchodilators, various studies have yielded conflicting and inconclusive results about their effectiveness. Ribavirin is recommended for children at high risk for complications and for infants who are severely ill.[51] Cystic fibrosis, congenital heart disease, bronchopulmonary dysplasia, immunodeficiency of AIDS, and other immunodeficiencies all predispose the infant to complications. Progressive hypoxemia and/or hypercarbia are indications of severity. Ribavirin is aerosolized into a tent, oxygen hood, or the delivery system of a mechanical ventilator for 3 to 7 days.[43,51] It is well tolerated and effective. Eye irritation has been reported in healthcare workers, and reports of teratogenicity in rats have led to the recommendation that pregnant women avoid direct contact with the aerosolized ribavirin.

Natural immunity to RSV is incomplete and short-lived, especially in the upper respiratory tract. Bronchiolitis and pneumonia rarely recur after an initial attack unless the patient is elderly or immunodeficient.[29,52] Human immunoglobulin with high titers of antibodies to RSV, administered intravenously, reduces the severity and incidence of RSV lower respiratory tract infection in high-risk children.[52–54]

REFERENCES

1. Hemming VG. Viral respiratory diseases in children: classification, etiology, epidemiology, and risk factors. *J Pediatr.* 1994;124:S13–S16.
2. Gilchrist S, Torok TJ, Gary HE, Alexander JP, Anderson LJ. National surveillance for respiratory syncytial virus, United States, 1985–1990. *J Infect Dis.* 1994;170:986–990.
3. Hall CB, Walsh EE, Schnabel KC, et al. Occurrence of groups A and B of respiratory syncytial virus over 15 years: associated epidemiologic and clinical characteristics in hospitalized and ambulatory children. *J Infect Dis.* 1990; 162:1283–1290.
4. Thomas E, Margach MJ, Orvell C, Morrison B, Wilson E. Respiratory syncytial virus subgroup B dominance during one winter season between 1987 and 1992 in Vancouver, Canada. *J Clin Microbiol.* 1994;32:238–242.
5. Heilman CA. Respiratory syncytial and parainfluenza viruses. *J Infect Dis.* 1990;161:402–406.
6. Abzug MJ, Beam AC, Gyorkos EA, Levin MJ. Viral pneumonia in the first month of life. *Pediatr Infect Dis J.* 1990;9:881–885.
7. Law BJ, De Carvalho V. Pediatric investigators collaborative network on infections in Canada. Respiratory syncytial virus infections in hospitalized Canadian children: regional differences in patient populations and management practices. *Pediatr Infect Dis J.* 1993;12:659–663.
8. Meissner HC. Economic impact of viral respiratory disease in children. *J Pediatr.* 1994;124:S17–S21.
9. Centers for Disease Control. Update: respiratory syncytial virus activity—United States, 1995–1996 season. *MMWR.* 1995;44:900–902.
10. Thom DH, Grayston JT, Wang S, Kuo C, Altman J. *Chlamydia pneumoniae* strain TWAR, *Mycoplasma pneumoniae,* and viral infections in acute respiratory disease in a university student health clinic population. *Am J Epidemiol.* 1990;132:248–256.
11. LaVia WV, Grant SW, Stutman HR, Marks MI. Clinical profile of pediatric patients hospitalized with respiratory syncytial virus infection. *Clinical Ped.* 1993;32:450–454.
12. Holladay RC, Campbell GD. Nosocomial viral pneumonia in the intensive care unit. *Clin Chest Med.* 1995;16: 121–133.
13. Hall CB. The nosocomial spread of respiratory syncytial viral infections. *Ann Rev Med.* 1983;34:311–319.
14. Abman SH, Ogle JW, Butler-Simon N, Rumack CM, Accurso FJ. Role of respiratory syncytial virus in early hospitalizations for respiratory distress of young infants with cystic fibrosis. *J Pediatr.* 1988;113:826–830.
15. King JC Jr, Burke AR, Clemens JD, et al. Respiratory syncytial virus illnesses in human immunodeficiency virus and noninfected children. *Pediatr Infect Dis J.* 1993;12: 733–739.
16. Sriskandan S, Shaunak S. Respiratory syncytial virus infection in an adult with AIDS. *Clin Infect Dis.* 1993;17:1065.
17. Englund JA, Sullivan CJ, Jordan MC, Dehner LP, Vercellotti GM, Balfour HH. Respiratory syncytial virus infection in immunodeficient adults. *Ann Int Med.* 1988;109:203–208.
18. Harrington RD, Hooton TM, Hackman RC, et al. An outbreak of respiratory syncytial virus in a bone marrow transplant center. *J Infect Dis.* 1992;165:987–993.
19. Sable CA, Hayden FG, Orthomyxoviral and paramyxoviral infections in transplant patients. *Infect Dis Clin NA.* 1995; 9:987–1003.
20. Hertz MI, Englund JA, Snover D, Bitterman PB, McGlave PB. Respiratory syncytial virus–induced acute lung injury in adult patients with bone marrow transplants: a clinical approach and review of the literature. *Medicine* (Baltimore). 1989;68:269–281.
21. Public Health Laboratory Service Communicable Disease Surveillance. Respiratory syncytial virus infection in the elderly, 1976–1982. *Br Med J.* 1983;287:1618–1619.
22. Sorvillo FJ, Huie SF, Strassburg MA, Butsumyo A, Shandera WX, Fannin SL. An outbreak of respiratory syncytial virus pneumonia in a nursing home for the elderly. *J Infect.* 1984;9:252–256.
23. Agius G, Dindinaud G, Biggar RJ, et al. An epidemic of respiratory syncytial virus in elderly people: clinical and serological findings. *J Med Virol.* 1990;30:117–127.
24. Hall CB, Douglas RG. Modes of transmission of respiratory syncytial virus. *J Pediatr.* 1981;99:100–103.
25. Guidry GG, Black-Payne CA, Payne DK, Jamison RM, George RB, Bocchini JA. Respiratory syncytial virus infection among intubated adults in a university medical intensive care unit. *Chest.* 1991;100:1377–1384.

26. Church NR, Anas NG, Hall CB, Brooks JG. Respiratory syncytial virus–related apnea in infants. *AJDC.* 1984;138: 247–250.
27. Anas N, Boettrich C, Hall CB, Brooks JG. The association of apnea and respiratory syncytial virus infection in infants. *J Pediatr.* 1982;101:65–68.
28. Williams AL, Uren EC, Bretherton L. Respiratory viruses and sudden infant death. *Br Med J.* 1984;288:1491–1493.
29. Hall CB, McCarthy CA. Respiratory syncytial virus. In: Mandell GL, Bennett JE, Dolin R, eds. *Principles and Practices of Infectious Diseases.* 4th ed. New York: Churchill Livingstone; 1995:1501–1519.
30. Hendry RM. Respiratory syncytial virus. In: Lennette EH, ed. *Laboratory Diagnosis of Viral Infections.* 2nd ed. New York: Marcel Dekker, Inc.; 1992:689–707.
31. Heikkinen T, Waris M, Ruuskanen O, Putto-Laurila A, Mertsola J. Incidence of acute otitis media associated with group A and B respiratory syncytial virus infections. *Acta Paediatr* (Norway). 1995;84:419–423.
32. Shaw CB, Obermyer N, Wetmore SJ, Spirou GA, Farr RW. Incidence of adenovirus and respiratory syncytial virus in chronic otitis media with effusion using the polymerase chain reaction. *Oto Larygol Head Neck Surg.* 1995;113: 234–241.
33. Penn CC, Liu C. Bronchiolitis following infection in adults and children. *Clin Chest Med.* 1993;14:645–654.
34. Friis B, Eiken M, Hornsleth A, Jensen A. Chest x-ray appearances in pneumonia and bronchiolitis. *Acta Paedriatr Scand.* 1990;79:219–225.
35. Melbye H, Berdal BP, Straume B, Russell H, Vorland L, Thacker WL. Pneumonia—a clinical or radiographic diagnosis? Etiology and clinical features of lower respiratory tract infection in adults in general practice. *Scand J Infect Dis* (Sweden). 1992;24:647–655.
36. Odita JC, Nwankwo M, Aghahowa JE. Hilar enlargement in respiratory syncytial virus pneumonia. *Eur J Radiol* (Germany). 1989;9:155–157.
37. Hall CB, Hall WJ, Speers DM. Clinical and physiological manifestations of bronchiolitis and pneumonia. *Am J Dis Child.* 1979;133:798–802.
38. Bruhn FW, Mokrohisky ST, McIntosh K. Apnea associated with respiratory syncytial virus infection in young infants. *J Pediatr.* 1977;90:382–386.
39. Valdes-Dapena M, McFeeley PA, Hoffman HJ, et al. *Histopathology Atlas for the Sudden Infant Death Syndrome.* Washington, DC: Armed Forces Institute of Pathology; 1993:1–22.
40. Wang EE, Law BJ, Stephens D. Pediatric Investigators Collaborative Network on Infections in Canada (PICNIC) prospective study of risk factors and outcomes in patients hospitalized with respiratory syncytial viral lower respiratory tract infection. *J Pediatr.* 1995;126:212–219.
41. Sigurs N, Bjarnason R, Sigurbergsson F, Kjellman B, Bjorksten B. Asthma and immunoglobulin E antibodies after respiratory syncytial virus bronchiolitis: a prospective cohort study with matched controls. *Pediatrics.* 1995;95: 500–505.
42. Welliver RC. RSV and chronic asthma. *Lancet.* 1995; 34:789–790.
43. Panitch HB, Callahan CW, Schidlow DV. Bronchiolitis in children. *Clin Chest Medicine.* 1993;14:715–731.
44. Hegele HG, Hayashi S, Hogg JC, Pare PD. Mechanisms of airway narrowing and hyperresponsiveness in viral respiratory tract infections. *J Respir Crit Car Med.* 1995;151: 1659–1665.
45. Njoku DB, Kliegman RM. Atypical extrapulmonary presentations of severe respiratory syncytial virus infection requiring intensive care. *Clin Ped.* 1993;32:455–460.
46. Adams JM. Primary virus infection with cytoplasmic inclusion bodies. Study of an epidemic involving thirty-two infants, with nine deaths. *JAMA.* 1947;116:925–933.
47. Adams JM, Imagawa DT, Zike K. Epidemic bronchiolitis and pneumonitis related to respiratory syncytial virus. *JAMA.* 1967;176:1037–1039.
48. Neilson KA, Yunis EJ. Demonstration of respiratory syncytial virus in an autopsy series. *Pediatr Pathol.* 1990;10: 491–502.
49. Murray JC, Gresil MV, Serabe BM, Harpel TL, Chinagumpala M, Mahoney DH Jr. Pathological case of the month. Peripheral blood "virocytes" associated with respiratory syncytial virus bronchiolitis. *Arch Pediatr Adolesc Med.* 1995;149:1033–1034.
50. Kellogg JA. Culture vs. direct antigen assays for detection of microbial pathogens from lower respiratory tract specimens suspected of containing the respiratory syncytial virus. *Arch Pathol Lab Med.* 1991;115:451–458.
51. Committee on Infectious Diseases. Use of ribavirin in the treatment of respiratory syncytial virus infection. *Pediatrics.* 1993;92:501–504.
52. Chanock RM, Parrott RH, Connors M, Collins PL, Murphy BR. Serious respiratory tract disease caused by respiratory syncytial virus: prospects for improved therapy and effective immunization. *Pediatrics.* 1992;90:137–143.
53. Groothius JR. Role of antibody and use of respiratory syncytial virus (RSV) immune globulin to prevent severe RSV disease in high-risk children. *J Pediatr.* 1994;124:S28–S32.
54. Levin MJ. Treatment and prevention options for respiratory syncytial virus infections. *J Pediatr.* 1994;124:S22–S26.

CHAPTER 32

Rotaviral Gastroenteritis

L. J. Saif and H. G. Greenberg

Men take diseases, one from another.
Therefore let men take heed of their company.

William Shakespeare (1564–1616), Henry IV, Part II

PATHOGENESIS OF GROUP A ROTAVIRUSES IN HUMANS

Rotaviruses are the single most important cause of severe dehydrating diarrhea in children. In spite of their global impact on public health, development of effective vaccines remains elusive.[1,2] Rotaviruses belong to at least seven distinct serogroups (A through G) based on antigenic relationships, with most serogroups possessing distinct genome electropherotypes of the 11 viral double-stranded RNA gene segments when analyzed by polyacrylamide gel electrophoresis.[3] Group A rotaviruses are the most common and widespread, infecting a variety of young animals, including human infants and children.[1,2] The pathogenicity of group A rotaviruses varies among different animal species and individual hosts, ranging from asymptomatic infections to severe and sometimes fatal diarrhea.[4,5] Variations in virulence exist among group A rotaviruses[6–8]; this aspect as well as the age and immune status of the host at infection and other multiple factors (dose, concurrent infections, nutritional status, etc) play a role in the broad spectrum of disease.[1–5]

Clinical infections with rotavirus are generally restricted to the young, occurring in infants and children in hospitals and who are primarily between 6 to 24 months of age.[2,5] Notable exceptions are the asymptomatic or mild infections of premature and newborn babies by group A rotavirus.[5,9] Genetic analysis of isolates from asymptomatic versus symptomatic neonates indicates that gene segment 4 is highly conserved among strains from asymptomatic infants, and that gene 4 product (VP4) may be related to virulence.[10,11] In addition, the widespread presence of transplacentally acquired maternal antibodies to rotavirus in newborns may moderate the severity of rotaviral infections in neonates as it does in colostrum-fed animals.[1,2,12,13]

Studies of the histopathologic changes in the small intestine of young children during acute rotaviral infection are limited.[14–19] Findings have varied from very limited to nondetectable abnormalities,[17,18] to mild alterations including broadening of the villi and mild cellular infiltration of the lamina propria, to severe changes with complete flattening of villi and heavy cellular infiltration.[14,16,19] Because most biopsy specimens from children have been obtained from relatively ill patients, it is not clear whether the findings reflect the spectrum of changes in milder illness. In addition, because virtually all human studies have involved small numbers of biopsy specimens taken only from the duodenum, the full spectrum of histopathologic changes is unclear.

There is also a paucity of studies directly investigating the mechanism of rotaviral-induced diarrhea in humans. Humans as well as pigs appear to develop lactose malabsorption during acute infection, and this osmotic load probably contributes to fluid loss.[18,20] Acute rotaviral infection alters intestinal absorption of some sugars[21] and decreases absorption of polyethylene glycol[22] but increases permeability to lactose.[23] At present, a unifying hypothesis that accounts for all the observed physiologic abnormalities in humans has not been presented. Rotavirus-induced pathologic and pathophysiologic changes in humans is limited, but much more information is available from a variety of animal species.

THE PATHOGENESIS OF GROUP A ROTAVIRUSES IN ANIMALS

Rotaviruses also are a leading cause of viral gastroenteritis in young animals, permitting detailed studies of viral pathogenesis in various animal models of rotaviral infection.[1–3] The histologic changes in the intestines of mice, pigs, calves, and lambs experimentally infected with group A rotaviruses have been reviewed.[1,2,4,5,24,25] In most infections, rotavirus was restricted to the villous epithelial cells of the small intestine, which exhibited a gradient of increasing susceptibility from crypts to villous tips.[1,2,4,5] In some species, however, rotaviruses infected sites in the colon but there were no colonic lesions.[8,26,27] Systemic infections as a result of viremia have been reported in some studies of infant mice infected with the epizootic diarrhea of infant mice (EDIM) strain of rotavirus.[28]

The general progression of events after rotaviral infection involves viral replication in the mature differentiated villous epithelium of the small intestine, rapidly leading to extensive destruction and desquamation of these cells and replacement by nondifferentiated cuboidal epithelial cells originating in the crypts.[4,5,24,25] Histologic lesions include degeneration, vacuolization, necrosis, and desquamation of infected villous cells leading to villous atrophy. Epithelia of adjacent villi may fuse. This is followed by hyperplasia of crypts and, in uncomplicated cases, regeneration of normal villi in a few days. Loss and fusion of the mature absorptive epithelial cells causes a malabsorptive, maldigestive diarrhea, often accompanied by dehydration and, in severe infections, death. Thus the mechanisms of fluid loss induced by rotaviruses relates to morphologic and functional damage of absorptive epithelial cells. This is accompanied by loss of enzymes responsible for digestion of disaccharides and loss of sodium, potassium, chloride, bicarbonate, and water, with ensuing acidosis and maldigestion/malabsorption of nutrients.[24,25,29,30] Undigested lactose further accentuates the osmotic loss of fluids.[18,20] Replacement of absorptive cells by enzymatically immature crypt cells that retain their secretory capacity causes further increased intestinal secretion.[4,5,24,25] Failure to treat those conditions by prompt administration of electrolytes may result in death in severely dehydrated children or animals.

The extent of epithelial cell damage varies among species and individuals reflecting differences in dose of rotavirus, virulence, host species, and host age and immune status.[1–9] In comparative studies of samples collected at different stages, there was only slight villous atrophy in pigs and calves examined in a few hours after the onset of diarrhea,[26,31–33] suggesting that the presence of villous atrophy was not a prerequisite for induction of diarrhea. Other more subtle histologic changes at this time (loss of cytoplasmic vacuolation in villous absorptive cells) may reflect the functional impairment of such cells contributing to the initiation of diarrhea. In the rotavirus-infected pigs, maximum villous atrophy was at about postinoculation hour (PIH) 60.[26,34] The severity of lesions varied in different species, with EDIM and lamb rotaviruses infecting the villous tips and producing no or slight atrophy,[8,25,35] but bovine and porcine rotaviruses infected the upper half or entire villus and induced pronounced villous atrophy.[26,33,34] In general, the distribution of morphologic lesions in the small intestine coincided closely with the localization of viral antigen detected by fluorescent antibodies (Figure 32–1).[26,27,33,34] In mice infected with EDIM, rotaviral antigens were first observed at postinoculation day (PID) 2, paralleling the appearance of diarrhea, and the infection persisted through PID 16.[27] Similarly, in pigs and lambs there was rotaviral antigen in villous epithelial cells between PIH 12 to 96.[8,26,31,32,34] The number of infected cells peaked early after inoculation (PIH 18 to 36) and then

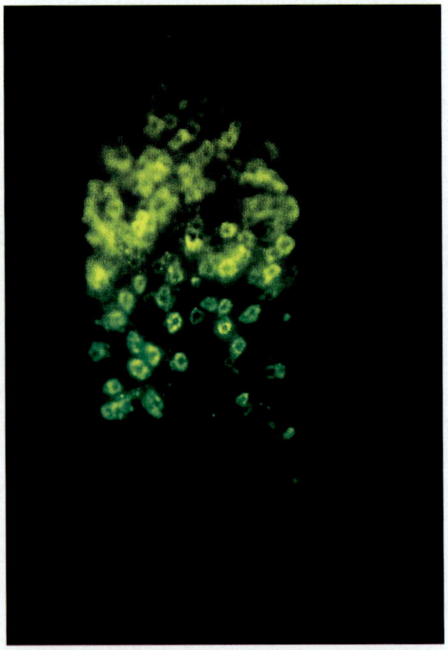

Figure 32–1. Immunofluorescent stain for group A rotavirus of an impression smear of a single small intestinal villus in the ileum of a gnotobiotic pig infected approximately 24 hours earlier with group A Wa human rotavirus. Infected enterocytes (bright green cytoplasmic fluorescence) are in the upper half of the villus (× 50).

decreased, coincident with the appearance of villous atrophy. Most rotaviral infections are transient and self-limiting because of the rapid loss of the susceptible, enzymatically differentiated absorptive cells and their replacement by crypt cells refractory to rotaviral infection.[33] The development of active mucosal immunity as early as PID 4 to 8 may further protect the newly differentiated epithelial cells from rotaviral infection.[36–38]

Variations in virulence also exist among rotaviral strains from the same species of host.[6–8] Several bovine group A rotaviruses were avirulent for gnotobiotic calves, although comparable amounts of virulent and avirulent rotaviruses were shed in feces.[6] Of particular interest was that group A rotaviruses associated with asymptomatic infection in children in India were serotypically similar (in G or P type) to serotypes common in cattle, suggesting the possibility of interspecies transmission of reassortant rotaviral strains attenuated for a heterologous host species.[39,40] However, other experimental infections of animals with rotaviral strains originating from heterologous host species has also led to clinical disease in the new host (refs. 13, 41, 42, and Saif, unpublished). This was demonstrated using bovine[41] and human[13,42] rotaviruses virulent for gnotobiotic pigs.

Studies of the effect of age on host susceptibility to clinical illness with rotavirus in mice and pigs suggest that the capacity of rotaviruses to induce diarrhea in suckling neonates but not adults may be related to the reduced quantity of rotavirus-binding receptors on villous epithelial cells in older animals.[43–45] Giving cortisone acetate to suckling mice induced partial premature intestinal maturation and led to a corresponding decreased susceptibility to group A rotaviral infection.[43] Another age-related factor that may directly influence host susceptibility to rotaviral infections is the rate of migration of intestinal epithelial cells. Epithelial cells proliferate in the crypts of the small intestine and become more enzymatically differentiated as they migrate to the tips of the villi, where they are shed into the lumen.[25] Absorptive epithelial cells regenerate more slowly in neonates and gnotobiotic animals than in older animals, and these slower migration rates also may contribute to the greater severity of rotaviral infections in younger hosts.[25]

THE PATHOGENESIS OF GROUP A HUMAN ROTAVIRUSES IN THE GNOTOBIOTIC PIG

Gnotobiotic pigs are a unique model for studying the pathogenesis of human rotaviral infections because gnotobiotic pigs have an extended period of susceptibility to infection and disease after inoculation with human rotaviral strains (refs. 13, 42, 46, 47, and Saif, unpublished). In addition, gnotobiotic pigs are born devoid of maternal antibodies (which they acquire postpartum only via colostrum uptake) and are maintained free of exposure to extraneous rotaviruses or other microbes in the gnotobiotic environment, thereby eliminating these factors as confounding variables in studies of human rotavirus pathogenesis.[13,42,46–48]

The pathogenesis of the Wa strain (G1[P8]) of virulent human rotavirus (pig-passaged infant stool) in gnotobiotic pigs has been investigated (refs. 13, 42, 46, 47, and Saif, unpublished), and it was found that clinical disease and morphologic lesions were similar, but the lesions were milder than those after infection of pigs with certain homologous strains of porcine rotaviruses.[26,31,32,46] Diarrhea developed in the orally inoculated pigs between PIH 13 and 48, and coincided with rotaviral antigen in the small intestine detected by immunofluorescence (Figure 32–1) and the onset of fecal shedding of rotavirus (PIH 24) detected by electron microscopy (Figure 32–2) or enzyme-linked immunosorbent assay (ELISA).[12] Diarrhea and viral antigen in the small intestine persisted through PIH 96 but were no longer detected by PID 7, although fecal shedding of rotavirus, detected by ELISA, was still evident in some pigs at this time.

Gross lesions in the infected pigs included thinned walls and distension of the small intestine by PIH 48 to 72. Histologic lesions at the onset of diarrhea (PIH 13) included lymphoreticular hyperplasia in the stroma of the tips of the villi of the small intestine and loss of normal villous absorptive cell vacuolation. Moderate to severe villous atrophy was in all regions of the small intestine by PIH 48 to 96 (Figure 32–3), but lesions were

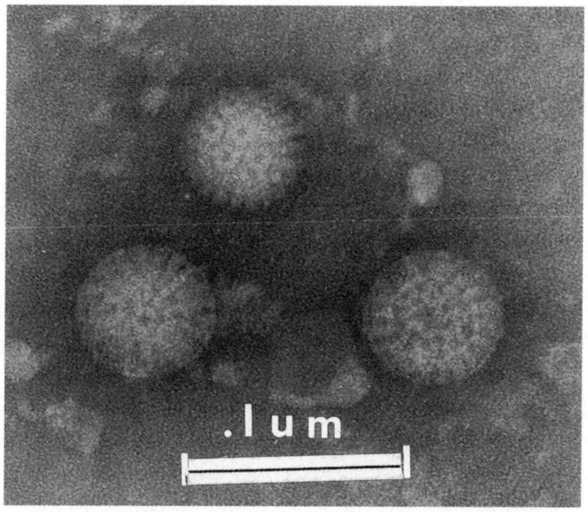

Figure 32–2. Negatively stained human group A rotavirus particles from the intestinal contents of an experimentally infected gnotobiotic pig.

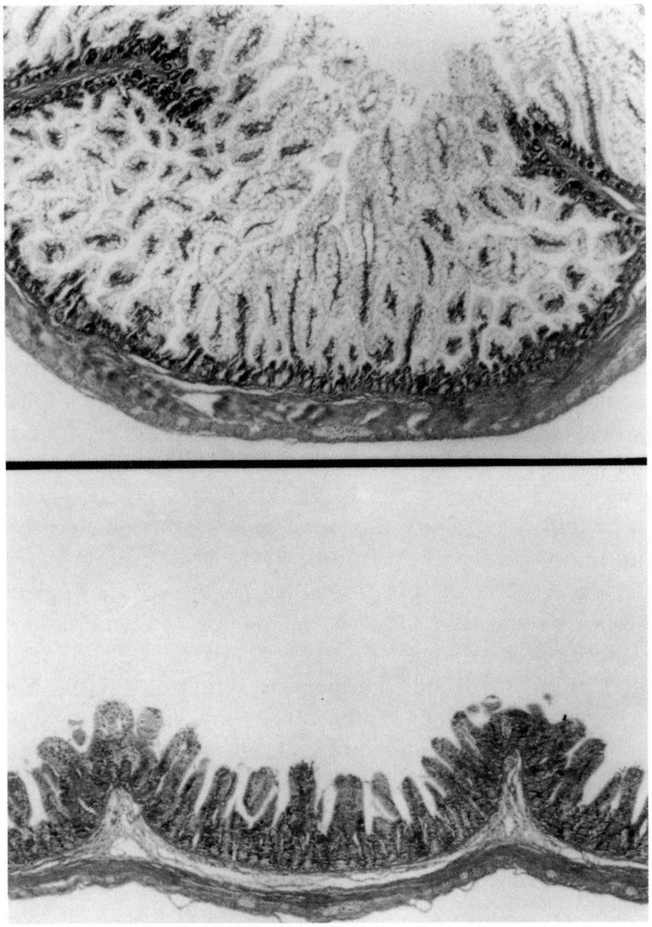

Figure 32–3. **(Top)** Jejunum from 8-day-old gnotobiotic pig showing normal mature vacuolated absorptive cells and villi (hematoxylin-eosin, ×10). **(Bottom)** Jejunum from 8-day-old gnotobiotic pig, inoculated by mouth 3 days earlier with a virulent human rotavirus (Wa strain). Note severe villous atrophy and early hyperplasia of crypts (hematoxylin-eosin, ×10). *(Courtesy of L. A. Ward.)*

most severe in the caudal region, and resolved by PID 7 concurrent with recovery from clinical disease. Hyperplasia of organized lymphoid structures in the small intestine and mesenteric lymph node was evident from PIH 48 through PID 7.

Thus the pathogenesis of human rotaviral infection in the gnotobiotic pig resembled that of homologous rotaviruses[26,29,31,32,34,46] and for rotaviral infections in other species[33,35] including the varying degrees of villous atrophy and lymphoreticular hyperplasia in duodenal and jejunal biopsy specimens from infants and children with rotaviral gastroenteritis.[14–19] Based on reported data from the gnotobiotic pig, the absence of histologic lesions in biopsy specimens of duodenum from humans or the lack of correlation between morphologic lesions and gastroenteritis[17,18] might be attributed to several factors. First, villous atrophy in the duodenum was less extensive and lesions persisted for a shorter time (PIH 24 to 48) than in the caudal small intestine, suggesting that examination of duodenal biopsies taken 48 hours or later after the onset of diarrhea may reveal no lesions. Second, the distribution of rotavirus-induced lesions was patchy, especially in the proximal small intestine, making it likely that such lesions could be missed in duodenal biopsies. In addition, host age, immune status, viral strain, and infectious dose likely play important roles in the distribution and severity of the lesions. Further research is needed to investigate the mechanism of rotavirus-induced diarrhea, particularly in the early stages before the appearance of pronounced cell damage culminating in villous atrophy. At present, human rotaviral infections are most rapidly and reliably diagnosed by ELISA,[2,11,13] cell culture immunofluorescence assays,[1–3,13] or immune electron microscopy[1–3] performed on stool samples collected from patients with acute diarrhea.

REFERENCES

1. Theil KW. Group A rotaviruses. In: Saif LJ, Theil KW, eds. *Viral Diarrheas of Man and Animals.* Boca Raton, Fla: CRC Press; 1990:35–72.
2. Kapikian A, Chanock R., eds. Rotavirus. In: B. Fields, ed. *Virology.* New York: Raven Press; 1990:1353–1403.
3. Saif LJ, Jiang BM. Nongroup A rotaviruses. In: Ramig RF, ed. *Rotaviruses, Current Topics in Microbiology and Immunology.* New York: Springer-Verlag; 1994;185: 339–371.
4. Saif LJ. Comparative aspects of enteric viral infections. In: Saif LJ, Theil KW, eds. *Viral Diarrheas of Man and Animals.* Boca Raton, Fla: CRC Press; 1990;2:9–34.
5. Greenberg HB, Clark HF, Offit PA. Rotavirus pathology and pathophysiology. In: Ramig RF, ed. *Rotaviruses, Current Topics in Microbiology and Immunology.* New York: Springer-Verlag; 1994;185:255–284.
6. Hall GA, Bridger JC, Parsons KR, Cook R. Variation in rotavirus virulence: a comparison of pathogenesis in calves between two rotaviruses of different virulence. *Vet Pathol.* 1993;30:223–233.
7. Castrucci G, Ferrari M, Frigeri F, et al. A study of cytopathic rotavirus strains isolated from calves with acute enteritis. *Comp Immun Microbiol Infect Dis.* 1983;6: 253–264.
8. Snodgrass DR, Angus KW, Gray EW. Rotavirus infection in lambs: pathogenesis and pathology. *Arch Virol.* 1977; 55:263–274.
9. Albert MJ, Unicomb LE, Barnes GL, Bishop RF. Cultivation and characterization of rotavirus strains infecting newborn babies in Melbourne, Australia, from 1975 to 1979. *J Clin Microbiol.* 1987;25:1635–1640.
10. Flores J, Midthun K, Hoshino Y, et al. Conservation of the fourth gene segment among rotaviruses recovered from asymptomatic newborn infants and its possible role in attenuation. *J Virol.* 1986;60:972–979.
11. Gorziglia M, Hoshino Y, Buckler-White A, et al. Conservation of amino acid sequence of vp8 and cleavage region of 84-kDa outer capsid protein among rotaviruses recov-

ered from asymptomatic neonatal infection. *Proc Natl Acad Sci USA.* 1986;83:7039–7043.
12. Saif L, Redman DR, Smith KL, Theil KW. Passive immunity to bovine rotavirus in newborn calves fed colostrum supplements from immunized or nonimmunized cows. *Infect Immun.* 1983;41:1118–1131.
13. Schaller JP, Saif LJ, Cordle CT, et al. Prevention of human rotavirus-induced diarrhea in gnotobiotic piglets using bovine antibody. *J Infect Dis.* 1992;165:623–630.
14. Barnes GL, Lownley RRW. Duodenal mucosal damage in 31 infants with gastroenteritis. *Arch Dis Child.* 1973; 48:343.
15. Bishop RF, Davidson GP, Holmes IH, Ruck BJ. Virus particles in epithelial cells of duodenal mucosa from children with acute non-bacteria gastroenteritis. *Lancet.* 1973; 11:1281.
16. Davidson GP, Barnes GI. Structural and functional abnormalities of the small intestine in infants and young children with rotaviral enteritis. *Acta Paediatr Scand.* 1979; 68:181–186.
17. Kohler VT, Erben U, Wiedersberg H, Bannert N. Histologische befunde der dunndarmschleimhaut bei rotaviralinfektionen im sauglings und kleinkindalter. *Kinderarztl Prax.* 1990;58:323–327.
18. Fiehring VC, Korting HJ, Jung G. Rotavirus and malabsorption. *Dt Z Verdau u Stoffwechselkr.* 1984;44:1–5.
19. Korting HJ, Fiehring C. Immunhistologischer Nachweis von Rotaviralantigen im Darmepithel von Kindern und Erwachsenen. *Arch Exp Vet Med.* 1983;37:159–162.
20. Hyams JS, Krause PJ, Gleason PA. Lactose malabsorption following rotavirus infection in young children. *J Pediatr.* 1981;99:916–918.
21. Mavrovichalis J, Evans N, McNeish AS, Bryden AS, Davies HA, Flewett TH. Intestinal damage in rotavirus and adenovirus gastroenteritis assessed by D-xylose malabsorption. *Arch Dis Child.* 1977;52:589–591.
22. Stintzing G, Johansen K, Magnusson KE, Svensson L, Sundqvist T. Intestinal permeability in small children during and after rotavirus diarrhoea assessed with different-size polyethylene glycols (PEG 400 and PEG 1000). *Acta Paediatr Scand.* 1986;75:1005–1009.
23. Noone C, Menzies IS, Banatvala JE, Scopes JW. Intestinal permeability and lactose hydrolysis in human rotaviral gastroenteritis assessed simultaneously by non-invasive differential sugar permeation. *Eur J Clin Invest.* 1986;16: 217–225.
24. Bachman PA, Hess RG. Comparative aspects of pathogenesis of immunity in animals. In: Tyrrell DAJ, Kapikian AZ, eds. *Viral Infections of the Gastrointestinal Tract.* New York: Marcel Dekker; 1985:361–397.
25. Moon HW. Pathophysiology of viral diarrhea. In: Kapikian AZ, ed. *Viral Infections of the Gastrointestinal Tract.* 2nd ed. New York: Marcel Dekker; 1994;27–52.
26. Theil KE, Bohl E, Cross R, Kohler E, Agnes A. Pathogenesis of porcine rotaviral infection in experimentally inoculated gnotobiotic pigs. *Am J Vet Res.* 1978;39:213–220.
27. Wilsnack RE, Blackwell JH, Parker JC. Identification of an agent of epizootic diarrhoea of infant mice by immunofluorescent and complement-fixation tests. *Am J Vet Res.* 1969;30:1195.
28. Adams WR, Kraft LJ. Epizootic diarrhea of infant mice: identification of the etiologic agent. *Science.* 1963;141: 359–360.
29. Davidson GP, Gall DG, Butler DG, Petric M, Hamilton JR. Human rotavirus gastroenteritis induced in conventional piglets: intestinal structure and transport. *J Clin Invest.* 1977;60:1402.
30. Woodard J, Chen W, Keku E, Liu S, Lecce J, Rhoads J. Altered jejunal potassium (Rb+) transport in piglet rotavirus enteritis. *Am Physio Soc.* 1993;265:G388–G393.
31. McAdaragh JP, Bergeland ME, Meyer RC, et al. Pathogenesis of rotaviral enteritis in gnotobiotic pigs: a microscopic study. *Am J Vet Res.* 1980;41:1572–1581.
32. Collins JE, Benfield DA, Duimstra JR. Comparative virulence of two porcine group A rotavirus isolates in gnotobiotic pigs. *Am J Vet Res.* 1989;50:827–835.
33. Mebus CA, Newman LE. Scanning electron, light and immunofluorescent microscopy of intestine of gnotobiotic calf infected with reovirus-like agent. *Am J Vet Res.* 1977; 38:553.
34. Pearson GR, McNulty MS. Pathologic changes in the small intestine of neonatal pigs infected with a pig reovirus-like agent (rotavirus). *J Comp Pathol.* 1977;87:363.
35. Adams WR, Kraft LM. Electron microscopic study of the intestinal epithelium of mice infected with the agent of epizootic diarrhea of infant mice (EDIM virus). *Am J Pathol.* 1967;51:39–60.
36. Chen W, Campbell T, VanCott J, Saif LJ. Enumeration of isotype-specific antibody secreting cells derived from gnotobiotic piglets inoculated with porcine rotavirus. *Vet Immunol Immunopath.* 1995;45:265–284.
37. Shaw R, Groene W, Mackow E, et al. VP4-specific intestinal antibody response to rotavirus in a murine model of heterotypic infection. *J Virol.* 1991;65:3052–3059.
38. Saif LJ. Development of nasal, fecal, and serum isotype-specific antibodies in calves challenged with bovine coronavirus or rotavirus. *Vet Immunol Immunopath.* 1987;17: 425–437.
39. Dunn SJ, Greenberg HB, Ward RL, et al. Serotype and genotypic characterization of human serotype 10 rotavirus for asymptomatic neonates. *J Clin Microbiol.* 1993;31: 165–169.
40. Das BK, Gentsch JR, Hoshino Y, et al. Characterization of the G serotypes and genogroup of New Delhi newborn rotavirus strain 116E. *Virology.* 1993;197:99–107.
41. Bridger JC, Brown JF. Antigenic and pathogenic relationships of three bovine rotaviruses and a porcine rotaviral. *J Gen Virol.* 1984;65:1151.
42. Wyatt RG, James WD, Bohl EH, et al. Human rotavirus type 2: cultivation in vitro. *Science.* 1980;207:189–191.
43. Wolf JL, Cukor G, Blacklow NR, Dambrauskas R, Trier JS. Susceptibility of mice to rotavirus infection: effects of age and administration of corticosteroids. *Infect Immun.* 1981; 33:565.
44. Riepenhoff-Talty M, Lee PC, Carmody PJ, Barrett HJ, Ogra PL. Age-dependent rotavirus–enterocyte interactions. *Proc Soc Exp Biol Med.* 1982;170:146.
45. Kirstein CG, Clare DA, Lecce JG. Development of resistance of enterocytes to rotavirus in neonatal, agammaglobulinemic piglets. *J Virol.* 1985;322:567.
46. Ward LA, Yuan L, Rosen BI, Saif LJ. Pathogenesis of an attenuated and a virulent strain of group A human

rotavirus in neonatal gnotobiotic pigs. *J Gen Virol.* 1996; 77:(July).

47. Saif LJ, Ward LA, Yuan L, Rosen BI, To TL. The gnotobiotic pig as a model for studies of disease pathogenesis and immunity to human rotavirus. *Arch Virol.* 1996 (in press).
48. Mehrazar K, Kim YB. Total parenteral nutrition in germfree colostrum-deprived neonatal miniature piglets: a unique model to study the ontogeny of the immune response. *J Parenter Enter Nutr.* 1988;12:563–568.

CHAPTER 33

Rubella (German Measles)

Carlos R. Abramowsky

The lay public have always held that congenital malformations have an extrinsic explanation—from being frightened by a dog to falling downstairs—and it will be strange if the influence of a mild illness in the first months of pregnancy accompanied by a rash, has escaped attention.

R. E. Hope-Simpson, Rubella and congenital malformations. Lancet. 1944.

INTRODUCTION

Rubella is caused by an RNA virus from the *Rubivirus* genus (family *Togaviridae*) where it stands as the only species.[1] The virus affects humans exclusively, in whom it causes two disease presentations: a benign exanthem in children 5 to 9 years old, and a potentially devastating congenital infection transmitted from the mother to the fetus through the placenta.

THE VIRUS

The virus contains at its genomic core a single strand of RNA (12 bp) enveloped by three glycosylated polypeptides (E1, E2, and C) associated with host-derived lipids. Of these glycoproteins, E1 is involved in the hemagglutination inhibition test. The protein envelope gives the virion an icosahedral shape with a spiked surface (Figures 33–1 and 33–2). The virus is sensitive to ultraviolet light (UV), visible light, extremes of pH, and common chemicals such as alcohol, ether, and formalin.[1]

EPIDEMIOLOGY

In contrast to other common childhood viral exanthems, rubella tends to appear in epidemics of 3- to 4-year cycles at 6- to 9-year intervals. The last epidemic, which proved to be very damaging, occurred in the mid-1960s. The advent of rubella vaccination seems to have aborted this natural history, except where prevention has been deficient.[1]

The traditional age group affected by this virus is the 5- to 9-year-old child; however, in the mid-1980s, largely unvaccinated patients older than 19 years constituted a significant proportion of the infected population. Vaccination, available since 1969, has targeted infants and women of reproductive age, with the consequent reduction of congenital rubella in the United States.[1,2]

TRANSMISSION

Congenital Rubella

In the 1964–1965 epidemic, there were about 20,000 cases of congenital infection, which can be contrasted to just a handful of patients per year in the late 1980s and 1990s. The virus is transmitted from mother to fetus preferentially in the first trimester, at the time when fetal organogenesis is most vulnerable. In the first 8 weeks of gestation in a group of infected pregnant women, 64% aborted or had infants with easily detectable anomalies.[3] The probability of the fetus suffering significant damage diminishes toward the middle of pregnancy and is negligible in the second half of pregnancy (weeks 20 to 40).[2]

A reasonable antibody titer to rubella confers lifelong immunity in both mother and fetus. In this, rubella differs from other congenital infections such as cytomegalovirus, in which fetal infection, albeit attenuated,

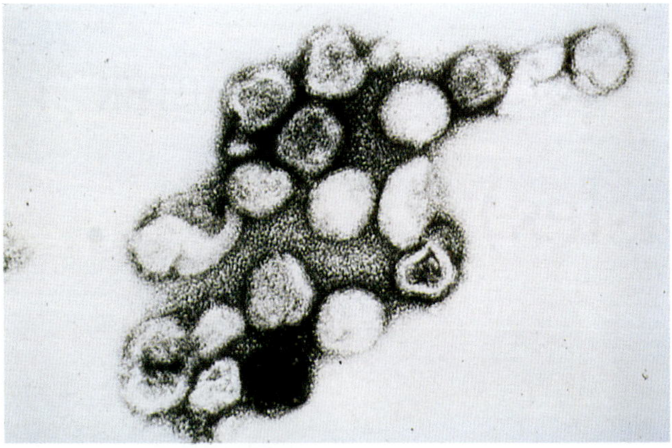

Figure 33–1. Rubella virions in an electron micrograph with $KMnO_4$ negative staining. The spiked envelope is characteristic of this icosahedral RNA virus (×120,000). *(Courtesy of Centers for Disease Control and Prevention.)*

can occur in spite of the presence of maternal immunity.[2]

Postnatal Rubella

In the postnatal individual, transmission of virus is by the respiratory route in droplets of nasopharyngeal secretions. From the respiratory sites the virus spreads through the circulation. The viral donor is deemed to be contagious 1 week before appearance of the exanthem to 2 weeks after. There is a widely differing ability either to transmit or be infected with the virus, which has been linked in several studies to human leukocyte antigen (HLA)-A1, -A8, -A28, and with blood type AB.[1]

CLINICAL ASPECTS

Postnatal Infection

The exanthem is not distinctive and needs to be distinguished from the rash caused by enteroviruses. Before its appearance, the patient suffers a prodromal illness including sore throat, nausea, anorexia, cough, and runny nose. There is no or a low fever. A few days later a characteristic lymphadenopathy in the postauricular region is noted (Figure 33–3), and 1 to 5 days later the rash appears. This is a fine maculopapular rash, which starts in the face and spreads centrifugally toward the trunk and limbs and lasts up to 3 days in most individuals (Figure 33–4). Infrequent complications include arthritis in multiple joints, encephalitis and other neurologic syndromes (Guillain–Barré), and thrombocytopenia.[1,4]

Congenital Infection

Congenital infection is characterized by its subacute or chronic character and is a prototype of viral-induced teratogenesis. As with other transplacental infections, the fetus suffers from growth retardation, which continues postnatally, probably because the virus remains

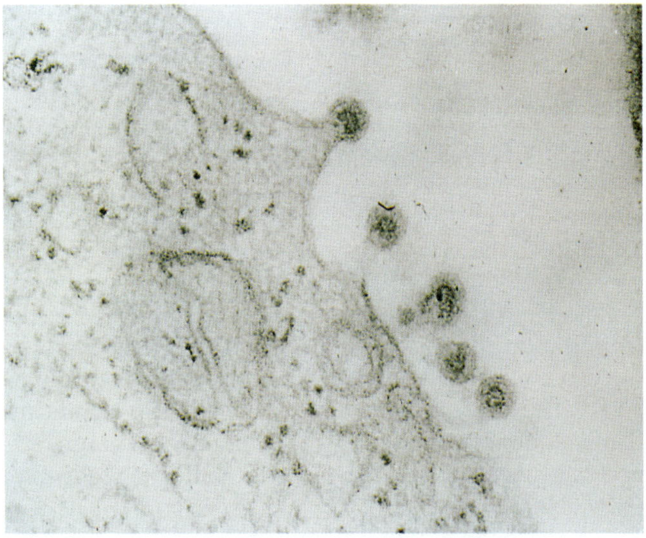

Figure 33–2. Rubella virions acquire their protein envelope as they bud off the cell surface (×80,000). *(Courtesy of Centers for Disease Control and Prevention.)*

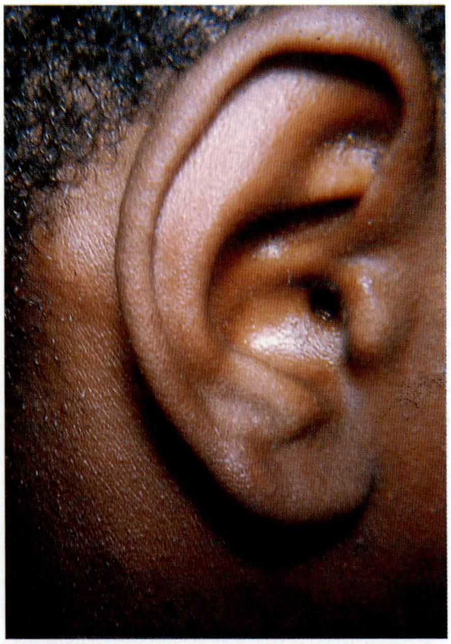

Figure 33–3. Retroauricular lymphadenopathy is one of the classic signs of postnatally acquired rubella infection. *(Courtesy of A. J. Nahmias, MD, Emory University.)*

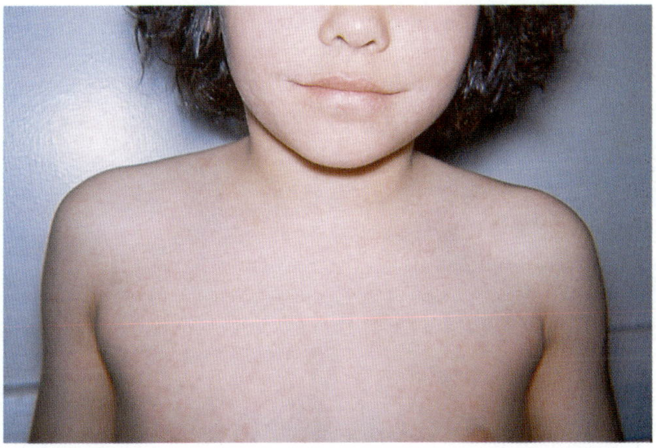

Figure 33–4. This infant with rubella has a diffuse macular rash, which started on the face and extended to trunk. *(Courtesy of A. J. Nahmias, MD, Emory University.)*

active as evidenced by its prolonged shedding in nasopharyngeal secretions.

As seen in similar infections described collectively as the TORCHS (Toxoplasmosis, Rubella, Cytomegalovirus, Herpes, Syphilis) group, the patients may have multiorgan involvement including myocarditis, hepatitis, hematologic cytopenia, meningoencephalitis, and visceromegaly.[5] Organs characteristically affected include the eyes with occurrence of cataracts (Figure 33–5) or a retinopathy and the hearing system with sensorineural deafness. Significant neurologic and sensorineural defects may persist throughout life.

Cardiac teratogenic effects are among the most characteristic of this virus and include patent ductus arteriosus, pulmonary artery or valvular stenosis, and supra-aortic stenosis.[1]

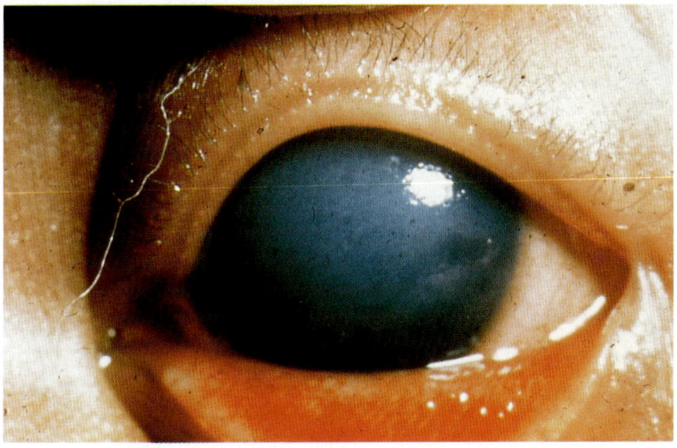

Figure 33–5. The white discoloration seen through the cornea is a cataract in a newborn with congenital rubella. *(Courtesy of Centers for Disease Control and Prevention.)*

IMMUNE RESPONSE AND DETECTION OF RUBELLA INFECTION

Most individuals respond effectively to this virus with a rise of IgM antibodies followed by IgG and IgA antibodies detectable 2 to 3 weeks after the infection. In the congenitally infected fetus, the antibody response is clouded by maternal IgG, which crosses the placenta and to which fetal antibodies may be added. The latter include IgM, IgG, and IgA. Because IgM and IgA are not maternal in origin, their measurement is the basis for most detection systems.[2]

Techniques have varied from hemagglutination inhibition, complement fixation, and more recently enzyme-linked immunosorbent assay (ELISA). After a peak in IgG antibody response, which lasts a few weeks, the titer settles at a lower level that persists for life. The initial response of fetal IgM disappears after a few months.[2]

Postnatally, some congenitally infected babies show a prolonged persistence of IgM antibodies for months if not years, and IgG titers tend to be much reduced in comparison to those of acquired rubella. These patients are considered tolerant to the virus and do not control it effectively. In these patients, rubella-specific cell-mediated immune responses also appear to be suppressed, and this may explain the prolonged viral shedding. In a few patients, IgM responses may not be detected in the newborn period, probably because the infection occurred immediately before delivery and the infant had not yet mustered an IgM antibody response.

PATHOLOGY OF RUBELLA

Postnatally Acquired Infection

Because this is essentially a benign disease, there are virtually no reliable histopathologic studies reported. A few older descriptions of cervical lymph nodes depict them as showing nonspecific hyperplasia and architectural effacement. After the 1964–1965 epidemic, a few reports on rubella encephalitis described cerebral swelling and nonspecific perivascular mononuclear cell infiltrates, features common to most viral encephalitides.[6]

Congenital Rubella

The congenital form of the infection occurs as the virus in maternal blood enters the placenta, where it makes its way to the fetal circulation and the fetus. The mechanisms whereby rubella virus (among others) penetrates and crosses the placental barrier are unknown. However, a barrier exists that seems to mature during gestation because maternal–fetal transmission rates of

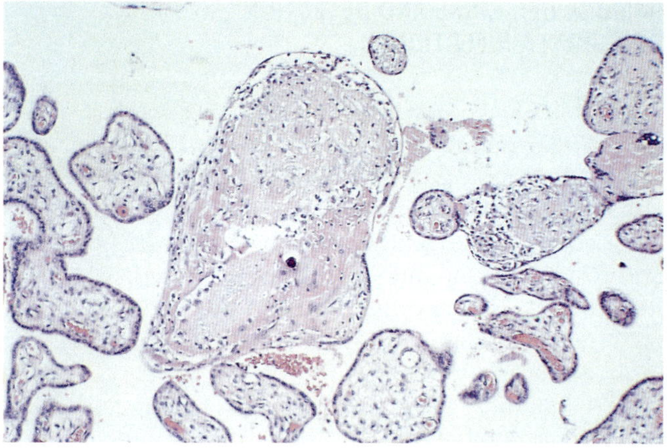

Figure 33–6. The micrograph shows a chronically inflamed placental villus from a woman infected with rubella during pregnancy. The baby had characteristic features of the congenital rubella syndrome (×100).

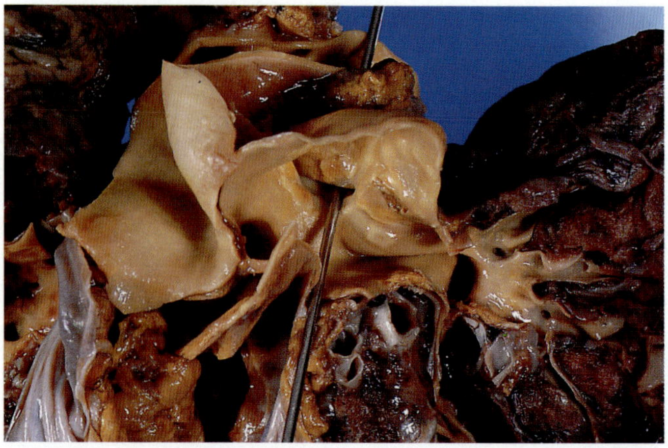

Figure 33–7. The metal probe is in a patent ductus arteriosus. This is a characteristic anomaly associated with the congenital rubella syndrome.

80% to 90% in the first trimester decrease markedly in the second half of pregnancy. Viral passage in the placenta elicits an inflammatory response within placental villi or villitis. These lesions are characterized by villous infiltration with mononuclear cells associated variably with necrosis or sclerosis of villous stroma[7,8] (Figure 33–6). In a large study, Driscoll also described vascular endothelial lesions.[9]

The pathology of congenital rubella has been well documented in many papers, particularly after the 1964–1965 epidemic.[10,11] The lesions can occur early in utero or shortly after birth, or later in life, becoming evident months or years later. From the originally described[12] classic triad of cataracts, deafness, and congenital heart disease, many other anomalies have been added to what is now called the *expanded rubella syndrome.* The probability of having a congenital defect ranges from 90% for infection in the first trimester to 25% for infection in the second trimester. A comprehensive list of lesions is published in Cherry's recent review.[1] From the pathologic standpoint, only the most common ones are discussed. In the initial reports, patent ductus arteriosus was the classic teratogenic cardiac lesion of congenital rubella (Figure 33–7). Subsequent studies have revealed also an increase in pulmonary stenosis involving the valve and the artery itself, often extending to peripheral intrapulmonary branches. Less frequent anomalies include atrial and ventricular septal defects, supravalvular coarctation of the aorta, and others. A peculiar fibrotic thickening of the intima, with narrowing of the vascular lumen, is seen in systemic and pulmonary vessels and heart valves (valvular sclerosis) and is characteristic of rubella (Figure 33–8).

Interstitial pneumonitis and peribronchiolitis with mononuclear cell infiltrates is also seen in congenital rubella along with other infections of the TORCH group (Figure 33–9). The liver may show necrosis or giant cell hepatitis with or without cholestasis. In later months or years a form of chronic liver disease with fibrosis or even frank cirrhosis may occur.[10,11]

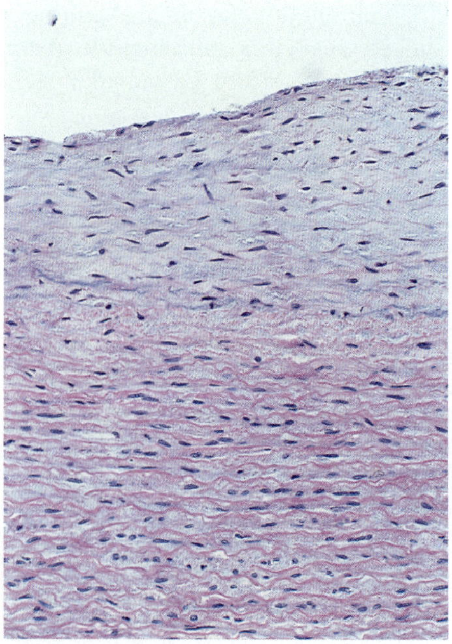

Figure 33–8. There is intimal fibrosis of aorta (shown here) and heart valves and peripheral pulmonary arteries in congenital rubella (×200).

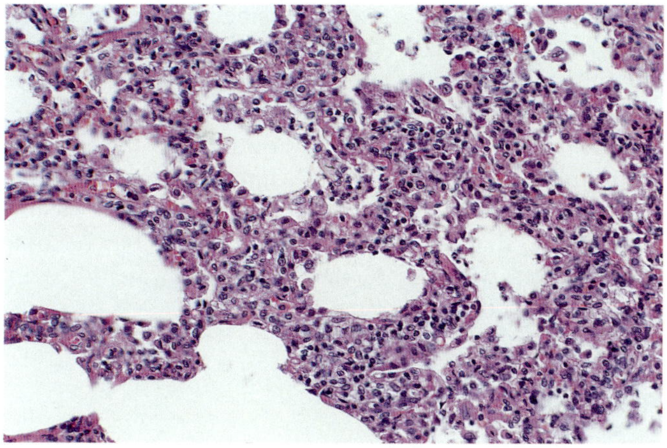

Figure 33–9. Pneumonitis with mononuclear inflammatory cells in the pulmonary interstitium is a feature of congenital rubella as it is with other congenital infections (×200).

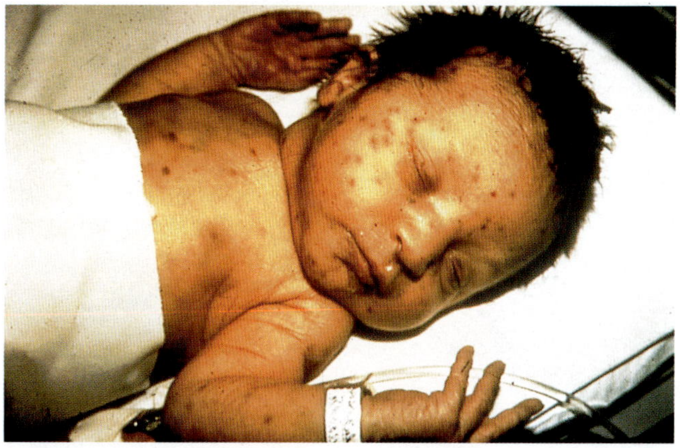

Figure 33–10. Infants with the congenital rubella syndrome present with characteristic dark red, slightly raised macules, which led to their designation "blueberry muffin babies." *(Courtesy of Centers for Disease Control and Prevention.)*

In the reticuloendothelial (hematopoietic or lymphoid) system the changes are variable and include hyperplasia and premature development of secondary germinal centers from viral antigenic stimulus. A few infants have a temporary rubella-induced immune unresponsiveness. These infants may have an inability to produce antibodies to virus and an inability to develop cellular immune responses, but pathologic descriptions in them are not available. In bone marrow and lymphoid organs there may be histiocytic proliferation and erythrophagocytosis. In patients with hemolytic anemia and thrombocytopenia, there may be marrow hyperplasia and extramedullary hematopoiesis.[10,11] Indeed, the characteristic macular dark red skin lesions that led to the designation "blueberry muffin baby," consist of dermal erythropoietic cell clusters[13] (Figures 33–10 and 33–11).

Major findings in the eye include microphthalmia, cataracts (Figure 33–5), sometimes with necrosis of the lens, inflammation or necrosis of the ciliary body, iridocyclitis, and retinitis[14] (Figure 33–12). Among the delayed manifestations of the congenital rubella syndrome the most serious are the sensorineural defects with involvement of hearing and neurologic functions. Pathologic studies of the hearing apparatus have shown chronic inflammatory lesions and fibrosis in the cochlea, within the organ of Corti and its surrounding structures[10,11] (Figure 33–13). In the central nervous system of affected patients, chronic meningeal inflammation, perivascular lymphocytic infiltrates, and gliosis are well described and can be seen in the white matter of the hippocampus and brainstem but not usually in the cerebellum. A characteristic lesion in chronic infections includes mineralization of cerebral arterioles[6,10,11] (Figure 33–14).

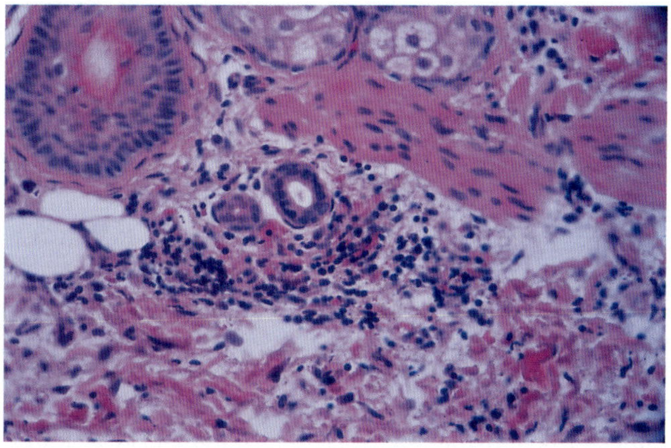

Figure 33–11. The skin lesions in congenital rubella consist of dermal infiltrates of erythropoietic cells as shown in this photomicrograph (×200).

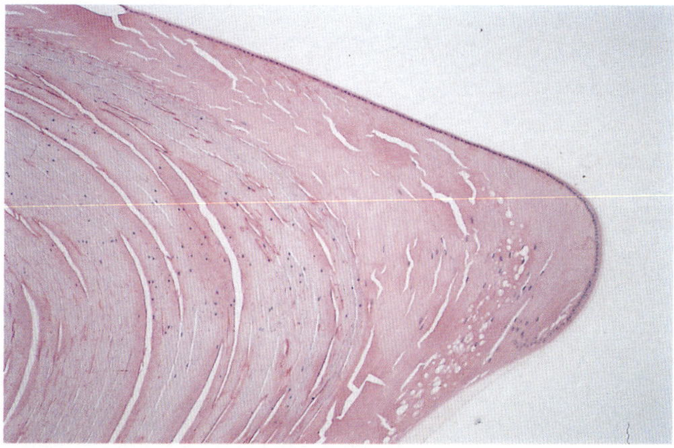

Figure 33–12. The compacted sclerotic fibers in the nuclear portion of the lens (the nuclear cataract) exhibit the persistence of cell nuclei, which is highly characteristic of congenital rubellar cataracts (×40). *(Contributed by H. Grossniklaus, MD, Emory University.)*

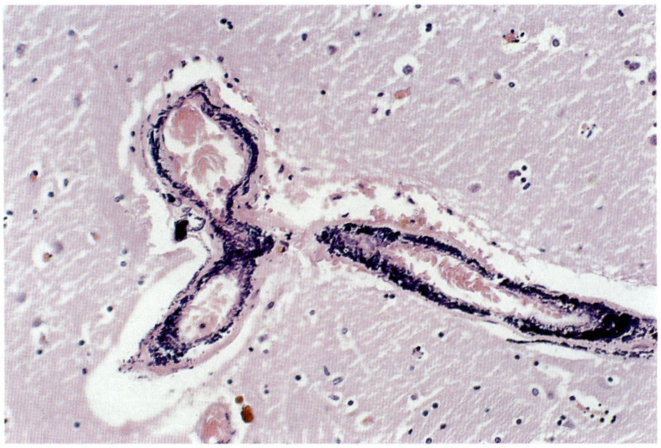

Figure 33–13. The photomicrograph shows chronic inflammation and fibrosis in internal ear structures of an infant with congenital rubella. This type of lesion accounts for the hearing defects in many of these patients (×200).

Bony changes in the metaphysis, reminiscent of congenital syphilis, with characteristic longitudinal radiologic striations are described in half the patients.[1] Less common pathologic abnormalities are seen in kidney: interstitial nephritis, pancreatic inflammation, biliary atresia, and thyroiditis.[10,11] Congenital rubella shares many clinical and pathologic features with other transplacentally transmitted viruses but is prominent because of the multisystemic devastation it causes. Its maternal–fetal transmission, preferentially in the first trimester when the uteroplacental circulation is barely established, differs from other organisms that are transmitted throughout gestation or in later trimesters.[5]

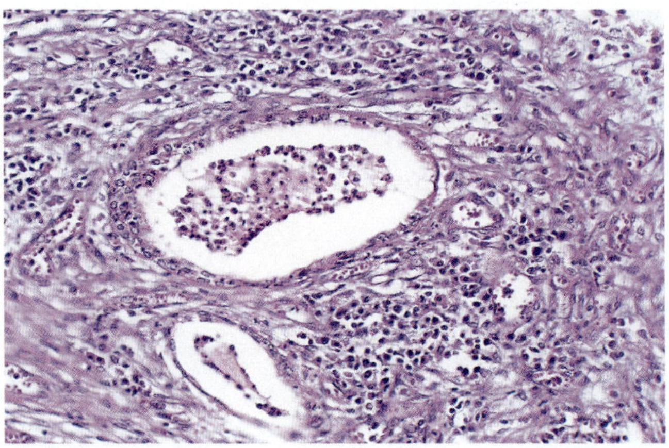

Figure 33–14. Mineralization of cerebral vessels with calcium and iron is common in patients with long-standing neurologic deficits (×100).

Of all microorganisms causing congenital infections, rubella stands out for its fetal and neonatal growth-stunting effects, its cell growth inhibitory effects, and its consistent teratogenic effects, which are probably caused by the first. Fortunately, this virus is also effectively stopped by a healthy maternal immune response whether naturally acquired or vaccine induced, so that this devastating syndrome has become a rarity, and will remain rare until public health complacency results in another epidemic.

REFERENCES

1. Cherry JD, Rubella. In: Feigin RD, Cherry JD, eds., *Textbook of Pediatric Infectious Diseases.* 3rd ed. Philadelphia: WB Saunders; 1992:1792–1817.
2. Cooper LZ, Preblud SR, Alford CA. Rubella. In: Remington J, Klein J, eds. *Infectious Diseases of the Fetus and Newborn.* Philadelphia: WB Saunders; 1995:268–295.
3. Peckham C. Congenital rubella in the UK before 1970. *Rev Infect Dis.* 1985;7(suppl 1):S11.
4. Heggie A. Pathogenesis of the rubella exanthem: distribution of rubella virus in the skin during rubella with and without rash. *J Infect Dis.* 1978;137:74–77.
5. Abramowsky CR, Nahmias AJ. Infections of the fetus & newborn. In: Reed GB, Claireaux AE, Cockburn F, eds. *Diseases of the Fetus and Newborn.* 2nd ed. London: Chapman & Hall; 1995:95–119.
6. Sherman E, Michaels RH, Kenny FM. Acute encephalopathy (encephalitis) complicating rubella. *JAMA.* 1965;192: 675–681.
7. Ornoy A, Segal S, Mishmi M, et al. Fetal and placental pathology in gestational rubella. *Am J Obstet Gynecol.* 1973;116:949–956.
8. Benirschke K, Kaufman P. *Pathology of the human placenta.* 3rd ed. New York: Springer-Verlag; 1995:587.
9. Driscoll SG. Histopathology of gestational rubella. *Am J Dis Child.* 1969;118:49.
10. Esterly R, Oppenheimer E. Intrauterine rubella infection. *Perspect Pediatr Pathol.* 1973;1:313–338.
11. Rosenberg HS, Esterly JR, Oppenheimer EH. Congenital rubella syndrome: the late effects and their relation to early lesions. *Perspect Pediatr Pathol.* 1981;8:183–202.
12. Gregg NM. Congenital cataract following german measles in the mother. *Trans Ophthalmol Soc Austr.* 1942;3:35–46.
13. Bayer WL, Sherman FE, Michaels RH, et al. Purpura in congenital and acquired rubella. *N Engl J Med.* 1965; 273:1362.
14. Boniuk M, Zimmerman LE. Ocular pathology in the rubella syndrome. *Arch Ophthalmol.* 1967;77:455–473.

CHAPTER 34

Transmissible Encephalopathies

Elias E. Manuelidis, Jung H. Kim, and Laura Manuelidis*

O Time, thou great devourer, and thou, envious Age, together you destroy all things; and, slowly gnawing with your teeth, you finally consume all things in lingering death!

Ovid (43 B.C.–A.D. 17?)

Transmissible encephalopathies (TEs) are caused by infectious viral-like agents that have not been defined on a molecular level. In humans, these agents cause dementia, most often accompanied by spongiform changes.

Creutzfeldt–Jakob disease (CJD), Gerstmann–Sträussler–Scheinker syndrome (GSS), and kuru are caused by similar infectious agents.[1,2] Although TEs generally affect older individuals, the recent transmission of infantile Alpers' disease[3] indicates an extended disease spectrum. Fatal familial insomnia (FFI),[4,5] characterized by insomnia, autonomic disturbance, motor dysfunction, and atrophy of selected thalamic nuclei, is a potential addition to the spectrum of this disease, but transmissibility of FFI has yet to be established. Scrapie of sheep, transmissible mink encephalopathy, chronic wasting disease of mule deer, elk, and white tigers, and bovine spongiform encephalopathy ("mad cow disease") represent comparable animal diseases that are caused by similar but distinct infectious agents. The successful transmission of human CJD to convenient small laboratory animals[6–8] opened the door for more detailed pathogenetic and molecular investigations of the human agent.

TEs are associated with a long incubation period and a fatal outcome. Thus they were initially classified with other "slow viral" diseases.[9] Because of some unusual resistance characteristics, the agent is sometimes called an "unconventional virus." The agent, in brain or brain homogenates, is relatively insensitive to germicidal chemicals and physical effects, including heat, ultraviolet irradiation, ionizing radiation, 70% ethanol, and formalin fixation. This poses a threat to laboratory personnel who deal routinely with human tissue.

The infectious TE agent(s), unlike most conventional viruses, does not induce any obvious inflammatory or immunologic reaction in the host. In tissue culture there are no cytopathic changes, but after passage in vitro there are transformed phenotypes.[10,11] Brain has the highest levels of infectivity, but the agent also is in the buffy coat of blood and in spleen cells.[12] Tissue cultures show relatively low titers of the agent and can lose infectivity on extended passage.[13–15]

Three major hypotheses have been advanced regarding the nature of the infectious agent: 1) a conventional virus, that is, a virus that contains a protected, agent-specific nucleic acid; 2) a prion, or an infectious host protein that contains fewer than 50 bases of nucleic acid; and 3) a virino,[16] in which a small agent-specific nucleic acid presumably is protected by a host-encoded protein. Prion protein and PrP are synonyms for a host protein that some consider the infectious agent[17]; Gp 34 is used to designate the full-length host glycoprotein prior to limited cleavage by proteinase K.[18] (For more detailed discussion of these hypotheses, see references 19–21.)

*Deceased.

CREUTZFELDT–JAKOB DISEASE

Definition

CJD is a rapidly progressive neurologic disease inducing profound dementia and eventual death, and is characterized microscopically by noninflammatory spongiform changes, neuronal loss, and gliosis in the gray structures of the central nervous system (CNS). The disease is transmissible to animals.

Jakob–Creutzfeldt disease, Jakob's disease (syndrome), and spongiform encephalomyelopathy are synonyms for CJD. Transmissible dementia, unconventional virus infection, unconventional virus disease, Prion disease, subacute spongiform encephalopathy, and subacute transmissible encephalopathy are all-inclusive synonyms for TEs. CJD cases also may be found in collections labeled as spastic pseudosclerosis, myoclonic dementia, subacute presenile polioencephalopathy, subacute progressive encephalopathy, subacute vascular encephalopathy, Nevin–Jones syndrome, Heidenhain's syndrome, and corticostriatospinal degeneration (see also ref. 22). Its geographic distribution is worldwide.

Epidemiology

CJD is a rare disease with an incidence of about one case per million persons per year. The true number of CJD cases may be much more than is apparent from neurologic disease.[20,23] About 10% of CJD cases have an autosomal dominant pattern of inheritance. A higher incidence of the disease has been noted in Libyan-born Jews in Israel[24] and in a rural area of Czechoslovakia.[25] In the latter case, there is a high proportion of cases with a mutation at codon 200 of the host encoded PrP (Gp 34) gene.[26]

Approximately 10% of CJD cases are associated with an autosomal dominant pattern of inheritance and are described as "familial" CJD. The incubation period in familial CJD appears to be between one and four decades, based on the evaluation of temporal and spatial separations between the affected parents and their children.[27] It is not clear whether this inheritance is due to genetic susceptibility to CJD infection or to some form of vertical transmission. However, no vertical transmission was demonstrable in rodent transmission experiments[28] or in human kuru.[29]

The natural mode of transmission is not known. In contrast, the iatrogenic transmission of CJD has been well documented, from a corneal transplant,[30] contaminated intracerebral electrodes,[31] dural grafts[32] and pituitary hormone therapy.[33] In the last instance incubation times to develop neurologic disease have been as long as 20 years after exposure to infectious material. Oral or parenteral hormone therapy presumably leads to viremia. The presence of viremia was demonstrated by successful transmission of CJD from buffy coat of blood in both experimental and human CJD.[12,34] Experimental transmission of CJD through corneal transplant was also successful.[35]

Eating scrapie-infected material probably leads to bloodstream infections via the gastrointestinal tract. Both transmissible mink encephalopathy and bovine spongiform encephalopathy ("mad cow disease") are believed to have been linked to the consumption of offals from scrapie-infected sheep.[36,37] Likewise, the high prevalence of CJD in Libyan Jews has been attributed to the dietary habit of eating eyeballs or lightly cooked sheep brains.[38,39] However, CJD cases have been reported in areas where scrapie does not exist, and vegetarians are known to be afflicted with the disease. (For further information, see the review on the epidemiology of CJD, reference 40.)

Clinical Features

Attempts have been made to subclassify CJD on a clinical basis, but these are of little value.[23,41] Female preponderance has been shown in some reports, but is not statistically different from that of the general population.[40] The highest incidence of this disease is seen in the sixth and seventh decades.

After a prodromal stage with vague personality changes, there may be alterations in higher cortical function, ataxic gait, visual disturbance, involuntary movement, dysphagia and/or dysarthria. Mental deterioration, including dementia, is the most common clinical manifestation, and is observed in almost all CJD cases. In general, mental deterioration is rapidly progressive. As the disease advances, clinical manifestations exhibited at the initial stage of the disease become progressively worse. In the final stage, patients become mute and unresponsive and enter a vegetative state. In the majority of cases, the entire clinical course typically lasts approximately 4 months before death occurs.[42] In approximately 5% to 10% of CJD cases, however, the clinical illness may last more than 2 years.

A variety of involuntary movements is common. Myoclonus occurs in more than 80% of CJD patients. Periodic sharp wave complexes, observed in most CJD patients, are an important and frequent EEG finding. This clinical triad (mental deterioration, myoclonus, and periodic sharp EEG complex) is noted in up to 75% of patients.

Pathology

Pathologic changes are limited to the CNS. In some cases, especially those with a prolonged clinical course, there may be gross atrophy of the brain. Atrophy of the brain is shown in a small number of the CJD cases, but

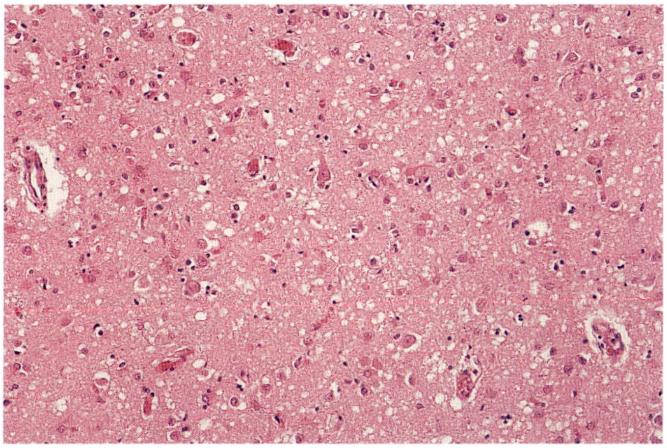

Figure 34–1. Cerebral cortex of a patient with terminal CJD, showing typical spongiform changes. There is some artefactual enlargement of perivascular and perineuronal spaces (hematoxylin-eosin, original magnification ×50).

is generally less severe than in typical Alzheimer's disease cases.

The three major histologic features of CJD are spongiform changes, gliosis, and neuronal loss.[23,43,44] There is no lymphocytic infiltrate in the CNS, in contrast to most viral encephalitides.

Spongiform changes are the most conspicuous light microscopic feature in CJD (Figure 34–1). Changes are generally restricted to the gray matter, including the cortex and subcortical gray structures. These changes are vacuoles in the neuropil, especially in dendritic processes.[43,44] Vacuoles, if abundant, have a tendency to form large, somewhat irregular, coalescent vacuoles. In some patients, spongiform changes take the form of rounded or polygonal empty spaces between a

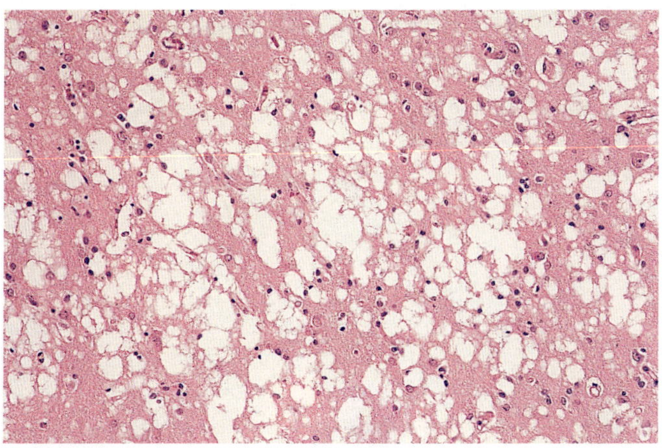

Figure 34–2. A severe form of spongiform changes ("spongiosis") in CJD. This extensive spongiform change is infrequent (hematoxylin-eosin, original magnification ×50).

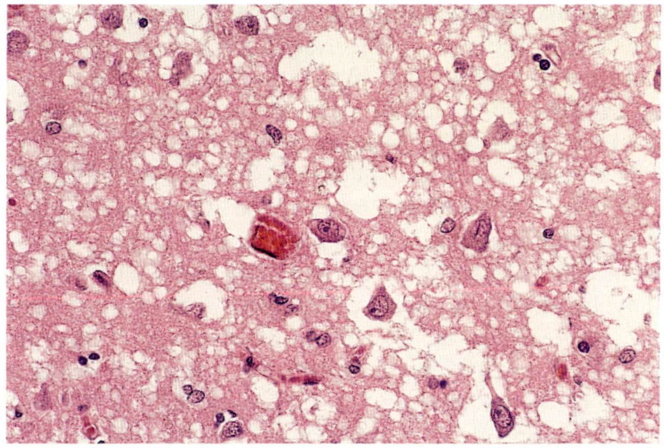

A

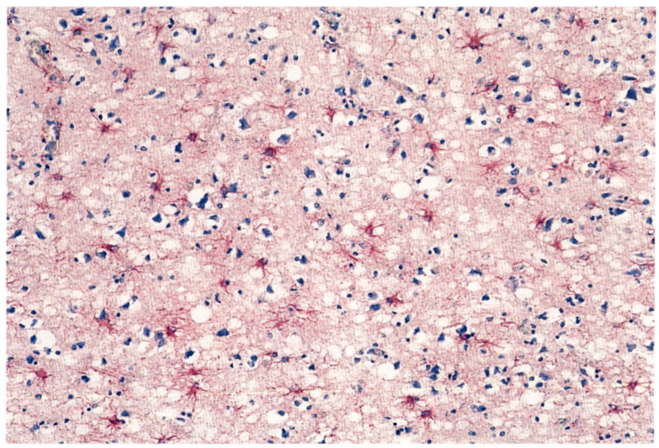

B

Figure 34–3. (**A**) A neuron near a vessel (near center of figure) has two intracytoplasmic vacuoles and the surrounding neuropil shows spongiform changes (hematoxylin-eosin, original magnification ×100). (**B**) Immunohistochemistry with GFAP antibody showing many reactive astrocytes with prominent spider leg–like tapering processes (red) (immunohistochemistry, ABC–alkaline phosphatase, original magnification ×50).

sievelike network of glial processes (Figure 34–2), for which the term "spongiosis" was suggested rather than "spongiform change."[45] Spongiform changes can be diffuse throughout various gray structures, but there are cases showing only patchy or focal spongiform changes. Another important diagnostic feature is vacuoles in the perikaryon of occasional neurons (Figure 34–3, A).

Spongiform changes in the white matter are more unusual. Vacuolization of white matter must be interpreted with caution, because it may represent the accumulation of nonspecific fluid caused by terminal metabolic or other derangements. The white matter commonly shows a diffuse proliferation of astrocytes, and myelin pallor. Interestingly, cases of transmissible

CJD in Asia characteristically have vacuolization in the white and the gray matter, and are known as "panencephalitic" CJD.[46] Changes in white matter and demyelination also can be seen in experimental CJD in selected mouse genotypes.[47]

Neuronal loss and gliosis are often found in CJD. The degree of neuronal loss can be subtle or obvious. If neuronal loss is severe, the neuropil is extremely pale from concomitant loss of neuronal processes. There may be scattered shrunken neurons, but similar neuronal alterations are present in a variety of conditions unrelated to CJD. Dark, shrunken neurons also are a common biopsy artifact.

Hypertrophy of reactive astrocytes can be seen in Figure 34–3, B. Although astrocytic hypertrophy can be caused by neuronal degeneration, the elevation of GFAP mRNA precedes the development of significant histologic changes in the brain of experimental animals.[48] Also, gliosis may be extensive in transmissible cases of CJD without spongiform changes.[49] Reactive astrocytes with enlarged, pale to semivesicular nuclei often display visible, tapering processes. Gemistocytic astrocytes can also be seen. Astrocytes usually show numerous glial filaments in their perikaryon as well as in their processes, which also show focal swellings and lucency.

Ten percent to 15% of patients with CJD also have neurofibrillary tangles, senile plaques, and granulovacuolar degeneration. These changes most likely reflect a normal aging phenomenon, because many CJD patients are elderly. Some reports on electron microscopy have noted viral-like structures, some of which have been interpreted as the infectious agent in CJD.[50–52] Several structures, however, appear to be artifacts,[23] and so far none has been identified in the most purified infectious preparations of CJD or scrapie.

Electron microscopic examination shows neuronal structures are severely damaged in both human and experimental CJD.[43,44,53] The neuronal perikaryoplasm may show focal or diffuse lucency. Regions of lucency can be seen within the normal perikaryoplasmic matrix. In general, there is a decreased number of subcellular organelles in the neuronal perikaryon. Dendrites and axons are focally or diffusely swollen (Figure 34–4). In affected neuronal processes, there is a drastic decrease or complete absence of subcellular organelles, except for some fluffy material and single or multilayered membrane-bound structures. The latter may derive from degenerating membranes of organelles, especially mitochondria, rough endoplasmic reticulum, and Golgi apparatus. Axons may have similar changes, and can be focally distended with nonspecific electron-dense bodies and intermediate filaments consistent with neurofilaments. The myelin sheath often shows focal splitting of its lamellae, and sometimes herniates into adjacent swollen dendrites. Both neurons and astrocytes contain an increased number of lysosomes.[43,44,54]

Abnormal fibrillar structures [scrapie-associated fibrils (SAF)] were initially found in detergent-extracted, negatively stained synaptosomal fractions of scrapie-infected mouse brain.[55] SAFs are composed of two to four twisted filaments of 4 to 6 nm in diameter, their

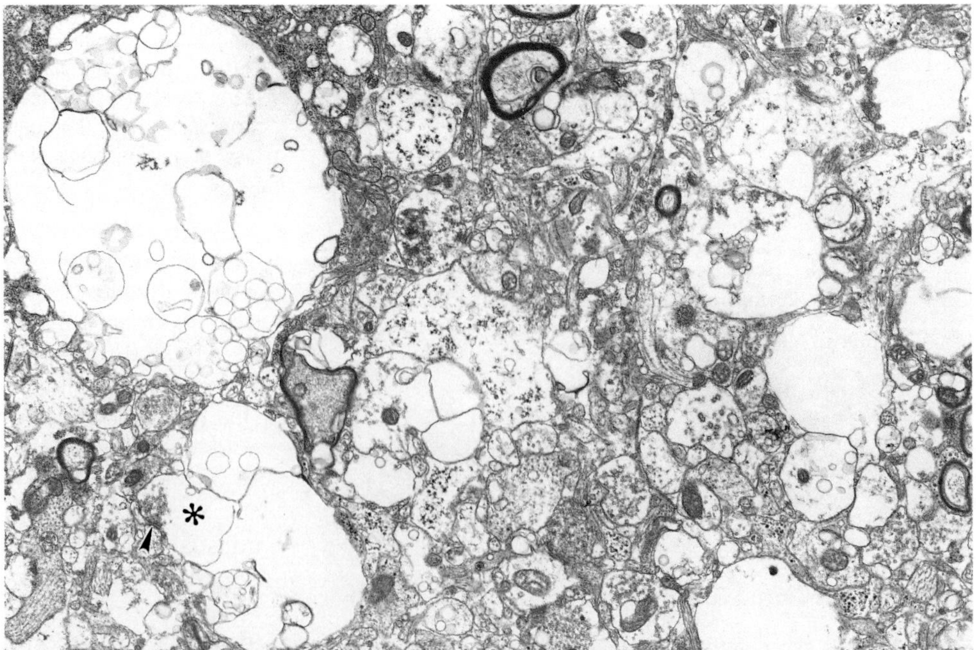

Figure 34–4. Distended vacuolar structures in this electron micrograph are swollen cellular processes. One distended process (*asterisk*) shows synaptic vesicles and a synaptic density (*arrowhead*), suggesting it is derived from an axon (×12,400).

length ranging from 50 to more than 500 nm. SAFs are also in biochemical preparations from human and experimental CJD.[18,56] In histologic specimens, extracellular plaques are apparent in human GSS, but not in most human CJD. These plaques are rich in Gp 34 ("prion" protein).

Diagnostic Significance of Spongiform Changes

Transmission of CJD to experimental animals has been reported using human biopsy material from suspected cases of CJD in which there were no significant pathologic findings.[45,49,57] Even a complete autopsy may not establish the diagnosis of CJD by histologic evaluation alone, because postmortem examination of a CJD brain may fail to disclose typical or significant spongiform changes.[43,45] A negative biopsy specimen or postmortem examination, therefore, cannot automatically exclude CJD. Nonetheless, spongiform changes in the cerebral gray structures are an important diagnostic feature in CJD,[23,45,46] even though they are sometimes difficult to distinguish from spongiform or vacuolar changes in unrelated metabolic diseases.

Although spongiform changes can be focal or relatively confined, absence of spongiform changes at autopsy may not be from incomplete sampling. "Collapse" of the original vacuoles may explain their absence.[58] Several experimental findings are pertinent. First, the route of infection can influence the degree of spongiform changes. In experimental CJD, inoculation of animals by peripheral routes produced minimal or inconspicuous spongiform changes.[43,53] Second, the titer and/or source of material were also important, because visceral tissue produced less florid changes than brain. Finally, significant spongiform changes occur only late in infection.[48,59,60] Similarly, PrP is seen only in a later stage of the disease, well after the infectious agent has increased to very high titers.[61,62]

Differential Diagnosis

"Vacuolar" changes in the brain can be caused by processing artifacts or by poor preservation of tissue. In such artefactual examples, there is often a pronounced irregular widening of the perivascular and pericellular space. Similar changes are common in cerebral edema from terminal metabolic, hypoxic, or other conditions. In addition, scattered coarse vacuoles are frequent in both white matter and gray structures. In contrast, vacuoles are generally limited to gray structures in CJD. Most importantly, discrete vacuoles are in the neuronal cytoplasm. Spongiform changes are also seen sometimes in acquired immunodeficiency syndrome[63,64] and in Alzheimer's disease.[65,66] This can present a diagnostic challenge to pathologists, because vacuolar changes in both diseases resemble those of TE by light and electron microscopy. In this situation, clinical and virologic data such as the delineation of PrP and SAF are helpful. In some cases, animal transmission is ultimately needed to demonstrate that a transmissible agent has caused the spongiform changes.

Molecular Pathologic Diagnosis

Tissue can be tested biochemically for abnormal sedimentation of Gp 34 in CJD-infected brain.[18,67] This change is only in late stages of experimental disease,[61] and aggregated pelleted material is resistant to limited digestion with proteinase K. When these conditions are properly controlled, the characteristic 27- to 29-kd PrP band[18,67] can be found in many, but not all, samples.[68] Thus, detection by Western blot of PrP and/or detection of SAF in such specimens, can help diagnostically. In such studies, poly- or monoclonal antibodies against PrP or synthetic Gp 34 peptides are used. In contrast with biochemical studies, immunohistochemistry with anti-PrP antibodies is less clear in a diagnostic setting because there are conflicting reports of its distribution in human and experimental TE. Because this protein is unusually expressed, it is sometimes difficult to resolve normal from pathologic staining. PrP immunostaining of neurons, neuropil, or glial cells has been seen with different methodologies. Also, particular antibodies may give different staining patterns.[69–73] It should be emphasized that PrP can be undetectable in material with a high titer of agent,[61,62] and thus transmission experiments are essential for a bona fide diagnosis. Routine histologic examination of biopsy or postmortem material, however, combined with typical clinical and EEG findings, usually renders a reasonably conclusive diagnosis.

GERSTMANN–STRÄUSSLER–SCHEINKER SYNDROME

Definition

Gerstmann–Sträussler–Scheinker syndrome is a progressive neurologic disorder, clinically characterized by cerebellar ataxia and dementia. Extracellular amyloid plaques are often in the cerebrum, brainstem, and/or cerebellum. In most patients there is a familial incidence with a pattern of autosomal dominant inheritance.

Synonyms include Gerstmann–Sträussler–Scheinker's disease, Gerstmann–Sträussler syndrome, and Sträussler's disease. In some instances, spinocerebellar ataxia with dementia and plaquelike deposits is used (see also all-inclusive synonyms for TE in the CJD section).

Geographic Distribution

Reported cases are almost exclusively from the northern hemisphere, including western Europe, Japan, and the United States, but the disorder is most likely worldwide.

Epidemiology

Familial GSS has been transmitted to animals.[74–76] Thus, GSS is considered a subtype of CJD. There are also sporadic cases of GSS, that is, with abundant plaques and the characteristic clinical picture (see later discussion). In familial GSS, some family members may have clinical features typical of CJD with rapid progression of the disease and myoclonus. In GSS, as in familial CJD, the combination of transmissibility and apparent inheritability presents an interesting problem. It is not known whether familial cases are caused by inheritance of genes that give an enhanced susceptibility to these agents, or if there is germline transmission of the infectious agent. In some GSS families, analysis of the host Gp 34 gene has revealed mutations at codons 102[77] or 117.[78] However, in experimental CJD, there is no evidence of maternal or germline-associated infection.[28]

Clinical Features

Cerebellar ataxia and unsteady gait are the most common initial manifestations. Dysarthria is another common feature. Reflexes in the lower limbs may be decreased or absent with positive extensor plantar responses. Mental deficiency may be mild at first, but eventually there is global dementia. Extrapyramidal rigidity, dysphagia, and weight loss may occur. Patients show diffuse symptoms and die after about 5 years. Typically, therefore, the clinical disease is longer than sporadic CJD. The average age at the time of death is 48 years.[75]

Pathology

Depending on the length of the clinical course, the brain may be grossly unremarkable or show a variable degree of atrophy. Histologically, spongiform change may not be prominent, and is in only about 65% of GSS,[75] in contrast to most patients with CJD. Variable degrees of neuronal loss and gliosis are also in the gray structures.

The most conspicuous histologic feature is amyloid plaques, most common in the cerebellar cortex. These are not typical of CJD. Plaques may also be in the cerebral cortex, deep gray structures, brainstem, and white matter.[75] Amyloid plaques assume several different forms. They usually have a large single amyloid core surrounded by a narrow rimlike halo ("kuru-like plaque") (Figure 34–5, A), sometimes encircled by "satellite" small cores. Another type of plaque has multiple small amyloid cores. The amyloid core of the GSS plaque has strong immunoreactivity with anti-PrP antisera (Figure 34–5, B). In other patients, there may be plaques without an amyloid core. Senile plaques with degenerating neurites also can be seen in some cases, but these may reflect unrelated changes of aging. Myelin pallor and demyelinization are frequent in the central white matter of the cerebrum, cerebellum, and various tracts.

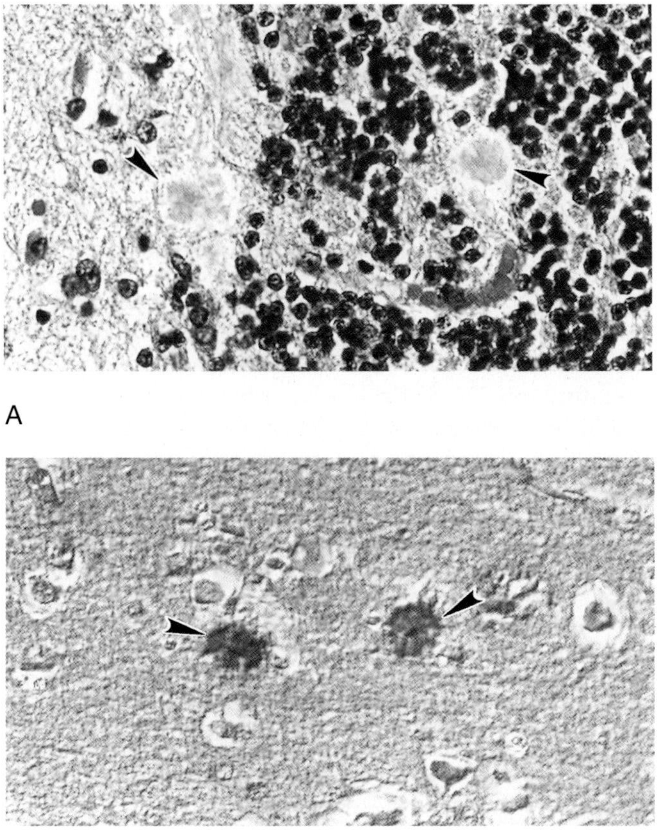

A

B

Figure 34–5. (**A**) Amyloid plaques (*arrowheads*) in the molecular layer of the cerebellar cortex of a GSS case (hematoxylin-eosin, original magnification ×50). (**B**) Strong immunopositivity with anti-PrP (Gp 34) antibody in a GSS amyloid plaque (*arrowheads*) (immunohistochemistry, ABC–DAB, original magnification ×100).

The amyloid core, by electronmicroscopy, is composed of mixed filamentous and osmiophilic amorphous deposits, or of radially arranged long bundles of 10-nm fibrils.[79]

Differential Pathologic Diagnosis

For spongiform changes, refer to the CJD section. GSS generally is distinguished from familial CJD by distinct and pathologic features: onset at an earlier age, a slow course, prominent cerebellar signs and symptoms, and characteristic amyloid plaques.

Molecular Pathologic Diagnosis

See CJD section for general comment.

Confirmational Testing and Diagnosis

See CJD section for general comment.

KURU

Kuru is confined to the Fore people in the Eastern Highlands of Papua New Guinea. Because the number of infections is dwindling, this disease should not pose a diagnostic problem for pathologists. The transmission of kuru is related to the practice of ritual cannibalism.[29] After cessation of this practice, incidence of kuru steadily declined.[29,80] Children born after the cessation of cannibalism have been free of kuru. The disease is clinically characterized by prominent cerebellar signs and mental impairment with eventual death. Pathologically, spongiform changes are in the cerebral gray structures and amyloid plaques ("kuru plaques") are in the cerebellum.[81,82] The plaque is composed mainly of a large amyloid core surrounded by a fine, fibrillar, rimlike, narrow halo.

ALPERS' DISEASE

Alpers' disease encompasses an etiologically heterogeneous group of disorders. There is progressive degeneration of gray structures with nonspecific swelling, and sometimes CJD-like spongiform changes.[3] Alpers' disease is also called spongy glioneuronal dystrophy, progressive cerebral poliodystrophy, and diffuse cortical sclerosis. The disease occurs early in life, often within the first 2 years, and severe generalized seizures are prominent. Although Alpers' original case showed only neuronal loss in the cortex and subcortical gray structures,[83] additional cases showed spongiform changes in the gray structures, similar to those seen in adult CJD. Because of this, some investigators suspected that Alpers' disease was a form of CJD.[84–86] The successful transmission of the disease from a 2.5-year-old girl to hamsters proves that at least some cases classified as Alpers' disease belong to the TE group; thus TEs are not limited to adults.[3]

Fatal familial insomnia has been transmitted experimentally,[87,88] but it is still uncertain if all "familial forms" of CJD are infectious.

REFERENCES

1. Gajdusek DC, Gibbs CJ Jr, and Alpers M. Experimental transmission of a kuru-like syndrome to chimpanzees. *Nature.* 1966;209:794–796.
2. Gibbs CJ Jr, Gajdusek DC, Asher DM, et al. Creutzfeldt–Jakob disease (spongiform encephalopathy): transmission to the chimpanzee. *Science.* 1968;161:388–389.
3. Manuelidis EE, Rorke LB. Transmission of Alpers' disease (chronic progressive encephalopathy) produces experimental Creutzfeldt–Jakob disease in hamsters. *Neurology.* 1989;39:615–621.
4. Lugaresi E, Medori R, Montagna P, et al. Fatal familial insomnia and dysautonimia with selective degeneration of thalamic nuclei. *N Engl J Med.* 1986;315:997–1003.
5. Manetto V, Medori R, Cortelli P, et al. Fatal familial insomnia: clinical and pathologic study of five new cases. *Neurology.* 1992;42:312–319.
6. Manuelidis EE. Transmission of Creutzfeldt–Jakob disease from man to guinea pig. *Science.* 1975;190:571–572.
7. Manuelidis EE, Angelo JN, Gorgacz EJ, Manuelidis L. Transmission of Creutzfeldt–Jakob disease to the Syrian hamster. *Lancet.* 1977;i:479.
8. Manuelidis EE, Gorgacz EJ, Manuelidis L. Transmission of Creutzfeldt–Jakob disease with scrapie-like syndromes to mice. *Nature.* 1978;271:778–779.
9. Sigurdsson B. Observations on three slow infections of sheep. *Br Vet J.* 1954;110:255, 307, 341.
10. Manuelidis EE, Fritch WW, Kim JH, Manuelidis L. Immortality of cell cultures derived from brains of mice and hamsters infected with Creutzfeldt–Jakob disease agent. *Proc Natl Acad Sci USA.* 1987;84:871–875.
11. Oleszak EL, Manuelidis L, Manuelidis EE. In vitro transformation elicited by Creutzfeldt–Jakob-infected brain material. *J Neuropathol Exp Neurol.* 1986;45:489–502.
12. Manuelidis EE, Gorgacz EJ, Manuelidis L. Viremia in experimental Creutzfeldt–Jakob disease. *Science.* 1978;200:1069–1071.
13. Race RE, Fadness LH, Cheseboro B. Characterization of scrapie infection in mouse neuroblastoma cells. *J Gen Virol.* 1987;68:1391–1399.
14. Rubenstein R, Scalici CL, Papini MC, Callahan SM, Carp RI. Further characterization of scrapie replication in PC12 cells. *J Gen Virol.* 1990;71:825–831.
15. Taraboulos A, Serban D, Prusiner SB. Scrapie prion proteins accumulate in the cytoplasm of persistently infected cultured cells. *J Cell Biol.* 1990;110:2117–2132.
16. Dickinson AG, Outram GW. The scrapie replication-site hypothesis and its implication for pathogenesis. In: Prusiner SG, Hadlow WJ, eds. *Slow Transmissible Diseases*

of the Nervous System. New York: Academic Press; 1979; 2:13–31.
17. Prusiner SB. Novel proteinaceous infectious particles cause scrapie. *Science.* 1982;216:136–144.
18. Manuelidis L, Valley S, Manuelidis EE. Specific protein associated with Creutzfeldt–Jakob disease and scrapie share antigenic and carbohydrate determinants. *Proc Natl Acad Sci USA.* 1985;82:4263–4267.
19. Manuelidis EE, Manuelidis L. Suggested links between different types of dementias: Creutzfeldt–Jakob disease, Alzheimer disease and retroviral CNS infections. *Alzheimer Dis Assoc Dis.* 1989;3:100–109.
20. Manuelidis L, Manuelidis EE. Creutzfeldt–Jakob disease and dementias. Mini-review. *Microbial Pathogenesis.* 1989; 7:157–164.
21. Manuelidis E, Manuelidis L. Transmissible encephalopathies. In: RG Webster, ed. *Encyclopedia of Virology.* New York: Academic Press; 1994:1361–1369.
22. Masters CL. Creutzfeldt–Jakob disease: its origins. *Alzheimer Dis. Assoc Dis.* 1989;3:46–51.
23. Manuelidis EE. Presidential address. Creutzfeldt–Jakob disease. *J Neuropathol Exp Neurol.* 1985;44:1–17.
24. Kahana E, Alter M, Braham J, Sofer D. Creutzfeldt–Jakob disease: focus among Libyan Jews in Israel. *Science.* 1974;183:90–91.
25. Ferak V, Kroupova Mayer V. Are population-genetic mechanisms responsible for clustering of cases of Creutzfeldt–Jakob disease? *Br Med J Clin Res.* 1981;282:521–522.
26. Goldfarb LG, Korczyn AD, Brown P, Chapman J, Gajdusek DC. Mutation in codon 200 of scrapie amyloid precursor gene linked to Creutzfeldt–Jakob disease in Sephardic Jews of Libyan and non-Libyan origin. *Lancet.* 1990; 336:637–638.
27. Masters CL, Gajdusek DC, Gibbs CJ Jr. The familial occurrence of Creutzfeldt–Jakob disease and Alzheimer's disease. *Brain.* 1981;104:535–558.
28. Manuelidis E, Manuelidis L. Experiments on maternal transmission of Creutzfeldt–Jakob disease in guinea pig. *Proc Soc Exp Biol Med.* 1979;160:233–236.
29. Gajdusek DC. Unconventional viruses and the origin and disappearance of kuru. *Science.* 1977;197:943–960.
30. Duffy P, Wolf J, Collins G, Devoe A, Streeten B, Cowen D. Possible person-to-person transmission of Creutzfeldt–Jakob disease. *N Engl J Med.* 1974;290:692–693.
31. Bernoulli CM, Siegfried J, Baumgartner G, et al. Danger of accidental person-to-person transmission of Creutzfeldt–Jakob disease. *Lancet.* 1977;1:478–479.
32. Prichard J, Thadani V, Kalb R, Manuelidis E, Hadler J. Rapidly progressive dementia in a patient who received a cadaveric dura mater graft. *MMWR.* 1987;36:49–55.
33. Brown P. Human growth hormone therapy and Creutzfeldt–Jakob disease: a drama in three acts. *Pediatrics.* 1988;81:85–92.
34. Manuelidis EE, Kim JH, Mericangas JR, Manuelidis L. Transmission to animals of Creutzfeldt–Jakob disease from human blood. *Lancet.* 1985;ii:896–897.
35. Manuelidis EE, Angelo JN, Gorgacz EJ, Kim JH, Manuelidis L. Experimental Creutzfeldt–Jakob disease transmitted via infected cornea. *N Engl J Med.* 1977;296:1334–1336.
36. Hartsough GR, Burger D. Encephalopathy of mink I. Epizootiologic and clinical observation. *J Infect Dis.* 1965; 115:387–392.
37. Wilesmith JW, Wells GAH. Bovine spongiform encephalopathy. *Curr Topics Microbiol Immunol.* 1991;172:21–38.
38. Goldberg H, Alter M, Kahana E. The Libyan Jewish focus of Creutzfeldt–Jakob disease: a search for the mode of natural transmission. In: Prusiner S, Hadlow WJ, eds. *Slow Transmissible Diseases of Nervous System.* New York: Academic Press; 1979;1:195–211.
39. Herzberg L, Herzberg BN, Gibbs CJ Jr, Sullivan W, Amyx H, Gajdusek DC. Creutzfeldt–Jakob disease: hypothesis for high incidence in Libyan Jews in Israel. *Science.* 1977; 186:848.
40. Brown P, Cathala F, Raubertas RF, Gajdusek C, Castaigne P. The epidemiology of Creutzfeldt–Jakob disease: conclusion of a 15-year investigation in France and review of the world literature. *Neurology.* 1987;37:895–904.
41. Masters CL, Gajdusek DC. The spectrum of Creutzfeldt–Jakob disease and the virus induced subacute spongiform encephalopathies. *Recent Adv Neuropathol.* 1982;2: 139–163.
42. Brown P, Cathala F, Castaigne P, Gajdusek C. Creutzfeldt–Jakob disease: clinical analysis of a consecutive series of 230 neuropathologically verified cases. *Ann Neurol.* 1986; 20:597–602.
43. Manuelidis EE, Manuelidis L. Clinical and morphological aspects of transmissible Creutzfeldt–Jakob disease. In: Zimmerman HM, ed. *Progress in Neuropathology.* New York: Raven Press; 1979:1–26.
44. Kim JH, Manuelidis EE. Pathology of human and experimental Creutzfeldt–Jakob disease. *Path. Ann.* 1983;18: 359–373.
45. Masters CL, Richardson EP Jr. Subacute spongiform encephalopathy (Creutzfeldt–Jakob disease). The nature and progression of spongiform change. *Brain.* 1978;101: 333–344.
46. Mizutani T, Okumura A, Oda M, Shiraki H. Panencephalitic type of Creutzfeldt–Jakob disease: primary involvement of the cerebral white matter. *J Neurol Neurosurg Psychiat.* 1981;44:103–115.
47. Manuelidis EE, Kim JH, Manuelidis L. Destructive white matter lesions in experimental Creutzfeldt–Jakob disease. In: Court LA, Dormont D, Brown P, Kinsbury DT, eds. *Unconventional Virus Diseases of the Central Nervous System.* Paris: Masson; 1989:221–230.
48. Manuelidis L, Tesin D, Sklaviadis T, Manuelidis EE. Astrocyte gene expression in Creutzfeldt–Jakob disease. *Proc Natl Acad Sci USA.* 1987;84:5937–5941.
49. Manuelidis EE, Manuelidis L, Pincus JH, Collins WF. Transmission from man to hamster of Cruetzfeldt–Jakob disease with clinical recovery. *Lancet.* 1978a;ii:40–42.
50. Bots GTAM, DeMan JCH, Verjaal A. Virus-like particles in brain tissue from two patients with Cruetzfeldt–Jakob disease. *Acta Neuropathol.* 1971;18:267–270.
51. Narang HK. Virus-like particles in Creutzfeldt–Jakob biopsy material. *Acta Neuropathol.* 1975;32:163–168.
52. Reyes JM, Hoenig EM. Intracellular spiral inclusion in cerebral cell processes in Creutzfeldt–Jakob disease. *J Neuropathol Exp Neurol.* 1981;40:1–8.
53. Manuelidis EE, Manuelidis L. Observations on Creutz-

feldt–Jakob disease propagated in small rodents. In: Prusiner S, Hadlow WJ, eds. *Slow Transmissible Diseases of the Nervous System.* New York: Academic Press;1979; 2:147–173.

54. Manuelidis EE, Gorgacz EJ, Manuelidis L. Interspecies transmission of Creutzfeldt–Jakob disease to Syrian hamsters with reference to clinical syndromes and strains of agent. *Proc Natl Acad Sci USA.* 1978;75:3432–3436.
55. Merz PA, Somerville RA, Wisniewski HM, Iqbal K. Abnormal fibrils from scrapie-infected brain. *Acta Neuropathol.* 1981;54:63–74.
56. Merz PA, Somerville RA, Wisniewski HM, Manuelidis L, Manuelidis EE. Scrapie-associated fibrils in Creutzfeldt–Jakob disease. *Nature.* 1983;306:474–476.
57. Kim JH, Lach B, Manuelidis EE. Creutzfeldt–Jakob disease with intranuclear vacuolar inclusions: a biopsy case of negative light microscopic finding and successful animal transmission. *Acta Neuropathol.* 1988;76:422–426.
58. Beck E, Daniel PM, Matthews WB, et al. Creutzfeldt–Jakob disease. The neuropathology of a transmission experiment. *Brain.* 1969;92:699–716.
59. Chandler RL. Ultrastructural observations on scrapie in the gerbil. *Res Vet Sci.* 1973;15:322–328.
60. Kim JH, Manuelidis EE. Serial ultrastructural study of experimental Creutzfeldt–Jakob disease in guinea pig. *Acta Neuropathol.* 1986;69:81–90.
61. Manuelidis L, Fritch W. Infectivity and host responses in Creutzfeldt–Jakob disease. *Virol.* 1996;216:46–59.
62. Xi YG, Ingrosso L, Ladogana A, Masullo C, Pocchiari M. Amphotericin B treatment dissociates in vivo replication of the scrapie agent from PrP accumulation. *Nature.* 1992; 356:598–601.
63. Artigas J, Niedobitek F, Grosse G, Heise W, Gosztonyi G. Spongiform encephalopathy in AIDS dementia complex: report of five cases. *J AIDS.* 1989;2:374–381.
64. Schwenk J, Cruz-Sanchez F, Gosztonyi G, Cervos-Navarro, J. Spongiform encephalopathy in a patient with acquired immune deficiency syndrome (AIDS). *Acta Neuropathol.* 1987;74:389–392.
65. Hansen LA, Masliah E, Terry RD, Mirra SS. A neuropathological subset of Alzheimer's disease with concomitant Lewy body disease and spongiform change. *Acta Neuropathol.* 1989;78:194–201.
66. Smith TW, Anwer U, De Girolami U, Drachman DA. Vacuolar changes in Alzheimer's disease. *Arch Neurol.* 1987; 44:1225–1228.
67. Manuelidis L, Manuelidis EE. Recent developments in scrapie and Creutzfeldt–Jakob disease. *Progr Med Virol.* 1986;33:78–98.
68. Brown P, Coker-Vann M, Pomeroy K, et al. Diagnosis of Creutzfeldt–Jakob disease by western blot identification of marker protein in human brain tissue. *N Engl J Med.* 1986;314:547–551.
69. Clinton J, Lantos PL, Rossor M, Mullan M, Roberts GW. Immunocytochemical confirmation of prion protein. *Lancet.* 1990;336:515.
70. DeArmond SJ, Mobley WC, DeMott DL, Barry RA, Beckstead JH, Prusiner SB. Changes in the localization of brain prion proteins during scrapie infection. *Neurology.* 1987; 37:1271–1280.
71. Muramoto T, Kitamoto T, Tateishi J, Goto I. The sequential development of abnormal prion protein accumulation in mice with Creutzfeldt–Jakob disease. *Am J Pathol.* 1992; 140:1411–1420.
72. Piccardo P, Safar J, Ceroni M, Gajdusek DC, Gibbs CJ Jr. Immunohistochemical localization of prion protein in spongiform encephalopathies and normal brain tissue. *Neurology.* 1990;40:518–522.
73. Diedrich JF, Bendheim PE, Kim YS, Carp RI, Haase AT. Scrapie-associated prion protein accumulates in astrocytes during scrapie infection. *Proc Natl Acad Sci USA.* 1991; 88:375–379.
74. Manuelidis EE, Kim JH, Manuelidis L. Serial transmission of Gerstmann–Sträussler–Scheinker disease to different strains of hamsters. In: *X Int. Cong. Neuropathol,* 1986, Stockholm, Sweden, p 187. Abstract.
75. Masters CL, Gajdusek DC, Gibbs CJ, Jr. Creutzfeldt–Jakob disease virus isolations from the Gerstmann–Sträussler syndrome. *Brain.* 1981;104:559–588.
76. Tateishi J, Sato Y, Nagara H, Boellaard JW. Experimental transmission of human subacute spongiform encephalopathy to small rodents. IV. Positive transmission from a typical case of Gerstmann–Sträussler-Scheinker's disease. *Acta Neuropathol.* 1984;64:85–88.
77. Hsiao K, Baker HF, Crow TJ, et al. Linkage of a prion protein missense variant to Gerstmann–Sträussler syndrome. *Nature.* 1989;338:342–345.
78. Tateishi J, Kitamoto T, Dohura K, et al. Immunochemical, molecular genetic, and transmission studies on a case of Gerstmann–Sträussler–Scheinker syndrome. *Neurology.* 1990;40:1578–1581.
79. Schlote W, Boellaard JW, Schumm F, Stöhr M. Gerstmann–Sträussler–Scheinker's disease. Electron microscopic observations on a brain biopsy. *Acta Neuropathol.* 1980;52: 203–211.
80. Alpers MP. Epidemiology and ecology of kuru. In: Prusiner S, Hadlow WJ, eds. *Slow Transmissible Diseases of the Nervous System.* New York: Academic Press; 1979; 1:67–90.
81. Beck E, Daniel PM. Kuru and Creutzfeldt–Jakob disease. Neuropathological lesions and their significance. In: Prusiner S, Hadlow WJ, eds. *Slow Transmissible Diseases of the Nervous System.* New York: Academic Press; 1979; 1:253–270.
82. Klatzo I, Gajdusek DC, Zigas V. Pathology of kuru. *Lab. Invest.* 1959;8:799–847.
83. Alpers BJ. Diffuse progressive degeneration of the gray matter of the cerebrum. *Arch Neurol Psychiatr.* 1931;25: 469–505.
84. Sandbank U, Chemke J. A case of infantile Jakob–Creutzfeldt disease. *Acta Neuropathol.* 1965;4:331–335.
85. Crompton MR. Alpers' disease—a variant of Creutzfeldt–Jakob disease and subacute spongiform encephalopathy? *Acta Neuropathol.* 1968;10:99–104.
86. Laurence KM, Cavanagh JB. Progressive degeneration of the cerebral cortex in infancy. *Brain.* 1968;91:261–280.
87. Tateishi J, et al. First experimental transmission of fatal familial insomnia. *Nature.* 1995;376:434–435.
88. Collinge J, et al. Transmission of fatal familial insomnia to laboratory animals. *Lancet.* 1995;346:569–570.

Chapter 35

Varicella-Zoster Virus Infection

Christian H. Hansen, Harry P. W. Kozakewich, and Ernest E. Lack

Eat no green apples or you'll droop,
Be careful not to get the croup,
Avoid the chicken pox and such
And don't fall out of windows much.

Edward Anthony (1895–?), Advice to small children

INTRODUCTION

The varicella-zoster virus (VZV, herpesvirus 3) causes two distinct clinical diseases: varicella (chickenpox) and herpes zoster (shingles). Although the clinical presentations of chickenpox and herpes zoster differ, a single virus causes both diseases. The clinical differences relate to host factors, such as previous exposure and immune competence. Primary infection, usually during childhood, causes varicella with a characteristic pruritic, papulovesicular exanthem. The virus then remains latent in sensory ganglia, where it may become reactivated, usually in adults, to cause herpes zoster, a painful vesicular rash over the corresponding sensory nerve distribution.

VIROLOGY

VZV is a ubiquitous virus, with humans being the only known hosts. The virus is morphologically similar to other herpesviruses, consisting of a spherical virion measuring approximately 200 nm. The virion contains an icosahedral capsid approximately 100 nm in diameter that encloses the viral genome. An amorphous protein layer, the tegument, surrounds the capsid. Function of the tegument includes regulation of viral and host transcription. Surrounding the tegument is an envelope consisting of lipoprotein derived from the nuclear membrane of the host that is acquired during viral shedding. The surface of the viral envelope displays numerous viral glycoprotein projections, which, along with the capsid proteins, are important antigenic stimuli for antibody production.[1]

The viral genome is linear, double-stranded DNA 125,000 base pairs long, which encodes approximately 80 proteins. The genome consists of two distinct regions, which have been designated the unique long and short regions; both of these regions are flanked by inverted repeat segments. During replication, the unique short region and its adjacent inverted repeat (short) region invert, allowing the creation of two isomers; also, inversion of the unique long region allows for four possible isomeric forms.[2] Genes encoding for several viral proteins, including thymidine kinase, DNA polymerase, and ribonucleotide reductase have been identified. Familiarity with the location and sequences of the base pairs of these genes has become important when applying molecular techniques (eg, polymerase chain reaction) to the diagnosis of VZV infection.

EPIDEMIOLOGY

VZV infection is worldwide and affects both genders equally, with no racial predilection. In Western countries, varicella predominantly affects children, although in tropical regions many patients become infected as adults. Varicella is highly contagious, with transmission through direct contact with mucocutaneous lesions or by inhalation of infectious respiratory droplets. Infection peaks during the winter and spring months, with declining incidence during the summer and fall.[3] In spite of being a reportable disease in the United States, patients with varicella are largely underreported, making interpretation of epidemiologic studies difficult. The estimated annual incidence, however, based on the reported number of cases, is between 135,000 and 220,000 (or 120 to 175 per 100,000 population).[3] Considerable differences have been observed between the reported annual incidence and the higher annual incidence estimated from independent surveys of clinical disease.[4] Varicella leads to an estimated 364,000 office visits to physicians annually and approximately 4000 hospitalizations each year.[5] Most patients are infected before age 15 years and the highest incidence is between age 5 and 9 years; less than 5% of primary infections in the United States are in adults.[3] Adult infections, however, are often more severe and have more frequent complications. Rarely, VZV infection may be fatal, with 50 to 120 deaths reported per year.[3]

Reactivation of latent VZV in patients who have had varicella causes herpes zoster. Immunodeficient patients are prone to primary or reactivation VZV infections[6]; an estimated 86% of those receiving bone marrow transplants, for example, develop VZV infection within 18 months.[7] In patients infected with the human immunodeficiency virus (HIV) infection, clinical VZV is evidence of progression to the acquired immunodeficiency syndrome (AIDS). In many patients, however, predisposing factors are not clearly identified.

Herpes zoster, unlike varicella, shows no seasonal variation, relating more to host immunologic factors than to transmissibility. Prevalence and incidence of herpes zoster in the adult population has been estimated to be 1.3 per 1000 per year.[6,8] Although herpes zoster may develop at any age, the incidence increases with advancing age. Occasionally, herpes zoster afflicts patients without a clinical history of varicella. These patients probably had subclinical varicella.

CLINICAL MANIFESTATIONS OF VARICELLA

The incubation period for varicella averages 14 days, with shorter incubation periods in immunodeficient hosts. Once infected there is acute viremia and hematogenous dissemination. In older children and adults, the typical rash is frequently preceded 2 to 3 days by a characteristic prodrome, which includes fever, chills, malaise, headache, backache, and anorexia. Occasionally, patients have sore throat and a dry, nonproductive cough. A transient scarlatiniform rash may appear just before or with the onset of the characteristic varicelliform rash.

The rash initially appears on the trunk, with subsequent spread to scalp, face, and limbs (centripetal distribution). The rash consists of crops of diffusely scattered maculopapular lesions 1 to 4 mm in diameter. The lesions progress from papules to vesicles filled with clear fluid on an erythematous skin base that has been classically described as a "dewdrop on a rose petal." Pruritus is often distressing during this vesicular stage. Within 8 to 12 hours, the vesicles become pustular and umbilicated, eventually becoming disrupted and crusted. Successive crops of vesicles appear over a 2- to 5-day period. It is characteristic to see groups of lesions in varying stages of progression within a given area. Because free virus is in the fluid, patients are infectious 24 to 48 hours before the rash until the time when all pustules have become crusted. Excoriation may leave shallow, pink, crater-like depressions and, if complicated by infection, there may be secondary scarring. Vesicles may develop also on mucous membranes in various sites, which often rupture rapidly, leaving multiple, small ulcerations.[9]

COMPLICATIONS OF VARICELLA

Although varicella in a normal child is limited usually to the characteristic eruption, there may be complicating bacterial infections of skin caused by *Staphylococcus aureus* and *Streptococcus pyogenes*. Rarely, there may be sepsis, toxic shock, hemolytic–uremic syndrome, gangrenous pneumonia, encephalitis, Reye's syndrome, and hepatitis.[10] Adults and immunodeficient patients are prone to varicella pneumonia; pregnant women are an important subgroup because varicella pneumonia may be fatal. Persistence of fever beyond the vesicular stage, onset of nonproductive cough, and continued eruption of skin may indicate varicella pneumonia. Although mild infections may improve in 5 to 7 days, respiratory failure may ensue. Overall mortality in adults ranges from 10% to 50%.[11,12] Approximately 25% of patients with varicella pneumonia develop complicating bacterial pneumonia and/or sepsis. Rare complications include myocarditis,[13] gastrointestinal hemorrhage,[14] gastritis,[15] acute retinal necrosis,[16] and arthritis.[17] Disseminated varicella can kill those who are immunodeficient (Figures 35–1 and 35–2). The advanced lesions of skin of some patients with disseminated varicella may resemble scalded skin (Figure 35–3). Complications in children differ in frequency with respect to age. Bacterial skin infections and pneumonia are most common in children younger than 5 years of age, whereas varicella encephalitis and Reye's syndrome become more common in patients between the ages of 5 and 14 years.

A number of conditions predispose patients to complications; this predisposition relates to inadequate cell-mediated immunity, with specific groups of patients being more susceptible than others. These groups most often include patients receiving bone marrow or organ

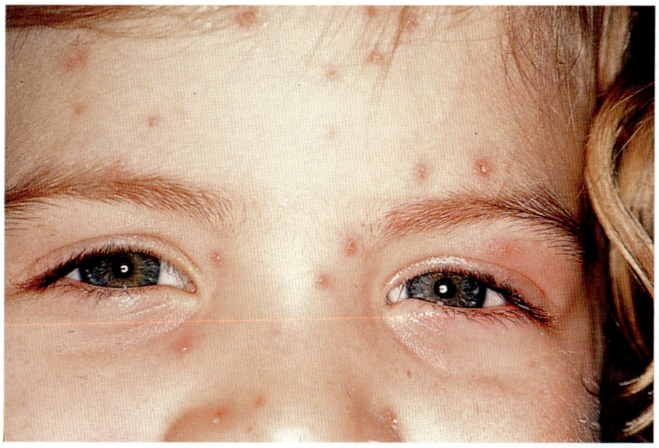

A

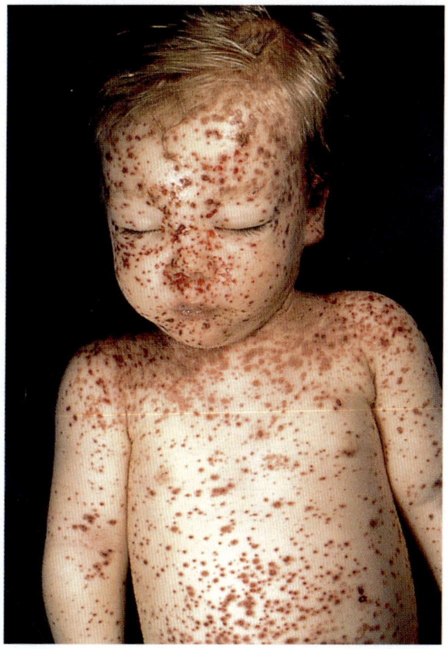

B

Figure 35–1. (**A**) Typical varicella (chickenpox) lesions in a 6-year-old girl with acute lymphoblastic leukemia (2 years in remission). The lesions are small vesicles with erythematous margins. A few days later, the varicella infection disseminated and she died. *(Contributed by G. Frederick Worsham, MD.)* (**B**) Disseminated varicella in a 10-month-old boy with agammaglobulinemia. The patient had three male siblings who died in infancy. He had been exposed to varicella in an older sister and developed a viral exanthem 8 days before death. Skin is extensively involved by punctate to confluent vesicles from 1 to 4 mm in diameter. At autopsy vesicles were in mucous membranes of mouth, gastrointestinal tract, liver, kidneys, lung, and spleen.

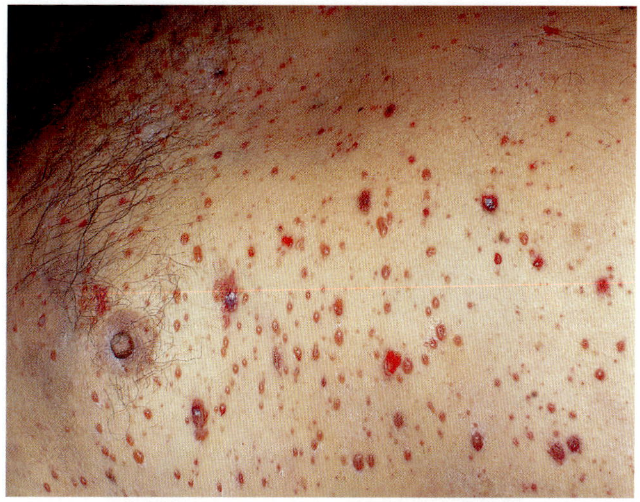

Figure 35–2. Fatal varicella in a 66-year-old man who had been treated with corticosteroids for chronic renal disease and was exposed to his grandchildren, who had chickenpox. His rash came up 3 days before admission and he died 6 days later. Before death he had thrombocytopenia and his blisters became bloody.

transplants, patients with malignancies (especially leukemias and lymphomas), patients receiving radiotherapy and/or chemotherapy, patients with AIDS, and those requiring immunosuppressive agents. Encephalitis following dissemination of VZV to the central nervous system (CNS) may cause acute cerebellar ataxia with nuchal rigidity, headache, nausea, vomiting, and tremors, and this is one of the more common serious complications of VZV infection. Cerebellar manifestations are more common in children, although adults typically display cerebral involvement with associated delirium, seizures, and coma. Cerebellar encephalitis usually resolves without serious sequelae, but the cerebral form often portends a more ominous course. Subclinical involvement of liver with elevated serum hepatic enzymes is common. Adults and children, however, are susceptible to VZV hepatitis, with immunodeficient patients at greatest risk. VZV hepatitis is also common in those who develop varicella pneumonia.[18] Reye's syndrome, usually seen in children, follows a viral infection—commonly influenza type B or VZV, and usually occurs 4 to 5 days after the onset of the varicella rash. Decreased activity of mitochondrial enzymes, including ornithine transcarbamylase and carbamylphosphate synthetase, may be important factors. Ingestion of salicylates during the acute viral illness increases the likelihood of Reye's syndrome, possibly related to synergistic activity with the virus, thereby inhibiting mitochondrial enzyme activity. Although the overall fatality rate is approximately 20%, patients with mild disease have a low death rate and few complica-

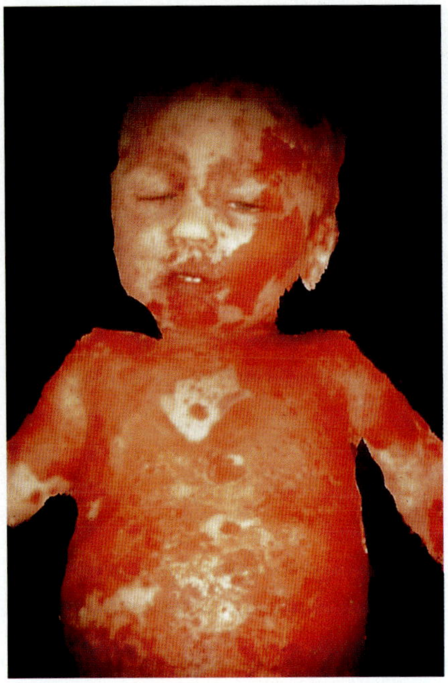

Figure 35–3. Disseminated varicella in a 10-month-old boy. There is extensive cutaneous involvement with confluent vesicular and crusted lesions over much of his body, especially trunk. Mucous membranes were also hemorrhagic and partially denuded.

tions. Thrombocytopenia has been associated with varicella although the exact cause is unknown.[19] Purpuric syndromes associated with varicella have been grouped into five distinct categories: febrile purpura, postinfectious purpura, anaphylactoid purpura, purpura fulminans, and malignant chickenpox with purpura.[20] Hemorrhagic complications of VZV may be fatal.

CONGENITAL VARICELLA

The risk of congenital anomalies in the fetus after maternal VZV infection is greatest during the first 20 weeks of gestation. At birth, infants are frequently small for their gestational age. Fetal infection may have a zosterlike dermatomal pattern and resolve with scarring. Neurologic abnormalities frequently correspond anatomically to the afflicted dermatome including limb paresis, microcephaly, Horner's syndrome, palsies of cranial nerves, and cortical atrophy. Dermatomal involvement may cause hypoplasia of a limb. Gastrointestinal and genitourinary anomalies relate to inadequate neural function, ie, gastroesophageal reflux and atonic bladder. Eye anomalies such as chorioretinitis, anisocoria, microphthalmia, and cataracts are frequent.[21–23] Fetal tissue obtained by chorionic villus sampling enables early diagnosis of fetal VZV infection. Extraction, amplification, and demonstration of VZV DNA from such samples, using the polymerase chain reaction (PCR) method, provides evidence of VZV infection.[24]

LATENT INFECTION

Most patients with varicella have no complications but during infection the virus infects sensory nerves and migrates to the sensory ganglia. VZV RNA has been demonstrated in neuronal and satellite cells within ganglia during the acute infection, although those with previous varicella continue to harbor latent VZV within the ganglia.[25] PCR has demonstrated the presence of VZV DNA within multiple sensory ganglia of seropositive patients at autopsy.[26] During latency, viral RNA is detectable primarily in ganglion cells. Involvement of non-neuronal satellite cells, which interface with multiple neurons, might allow the virus to involve large geographic areas during reactivation, eg, an entire dermatome.[25]

CLINICAL MANIFESTATIONS OF HERPES ZOSTER

Herpes zoster is preceded by a prodrome of pain, itching, burning, and paresthesias over a specific dermatome, hence the name *zoster* (Greek meaning "belt" or "girdle," *cingulum*, Latin for "girdle"). These symptoms may mimic a variety of other conditions, some serious, such as myocardial infarction, pleuritis, appendicitis, and cholecystitis. These symptoms precede the characteristic zoster eruption by 4 to 5 days. Occasionally, constitutional symptoms such as headache, fever, and malaise occur within the few days preceding onset. Rarely, patients may experience an acute segmental neuralgia without progressing to the eruptive phase, a phenomenon termed *zoster sine herpete*. Following the prodrome, vesicles erupt in a characteristic pattern, usually unilateral along a single dermatome; less commonly, more than one dermatome is involved. Herpes zoster most commonly involves the thoracic dermatomes (Figure 35–4A), followed by cranial nerve, lumbar, and sacral. In the cranial nerve distribution the ophthalmic branch of the trigeminal nerve is most commonly involved, followed by maxillary and mandibular branches.[6] At first there is an erythematous, maculopapular skin lesion confined to the distribution of a specific sensory nerve branch. Lesions may continue to develop within the dermatome over a period of 7 days and become vesicular within 24 hours. The vesi-

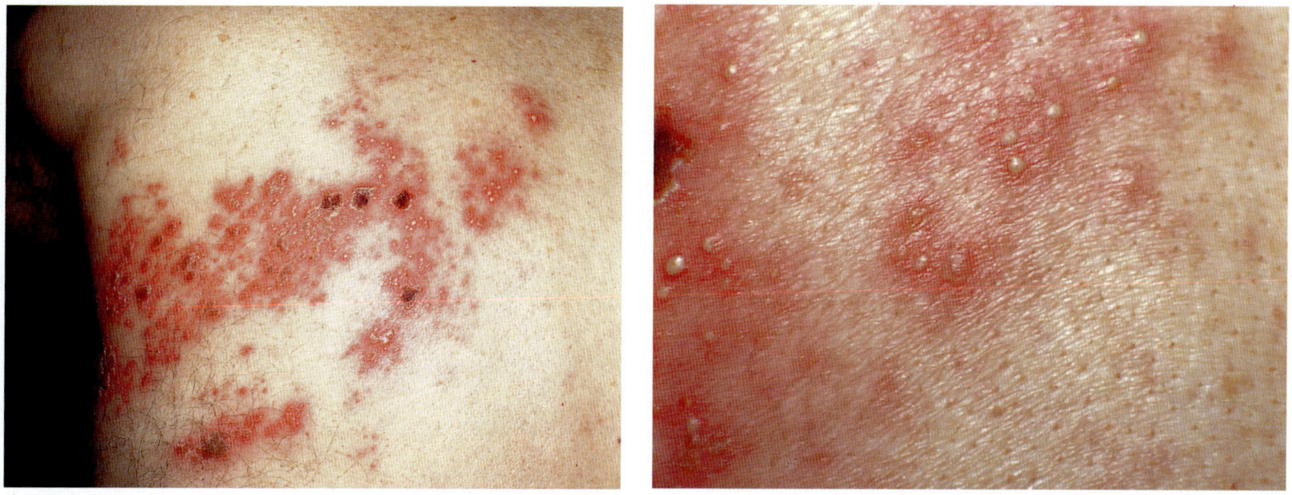

A B

Figure 35–4. (**A**) Herpes zoster on the thorax of a 76-year-old man. At first there was nothing but dull persistent pain over the left side of the chest; 48 hours after the onset of pain, a thorough study revealed no evidence of myocardial ischemia and the medical attendees were at a loss to explain the pain. The pain persisted, however, and 4 days later (6 days after the pain began) a red vesicular rash erupted on the left side of the chest extending from the sternum to the spine. At the time of the picture (11 days after the onset of pain and 5 days after onset of the eruption) the area was mottled bright red and covered with papulo-vesicles and several crusts. (**B**) Closer view of the lesion in **A** showing small pustular vesicles on an erythematous base. The fluid in the vesicles is clouded from an infiltrate of neutrophils. *(Photographs by Daniel H. Connor, MD, 1996)*

cles are clustered and vary in size. By the third day, the clear contents of the vesicles become cloudy, which is caused by the accumulation of neutrophils (Figure 35–4B). As in varicella, the pustules then become umbilicated followed by fluid resorption and crusting, and the lesions slough in 2 to 3 weeks (Figure 35–5). This eruptive phase may persist for longer periods in elderly, immunodeficient, or debilitated patients, and these patients may have more extensive inflammatory and occasionally hemorrhagic eruptions with possible secondary bacterial infection (Figure 35–6). Secondary infection may cause scarring, less frequently necrosis.[9]

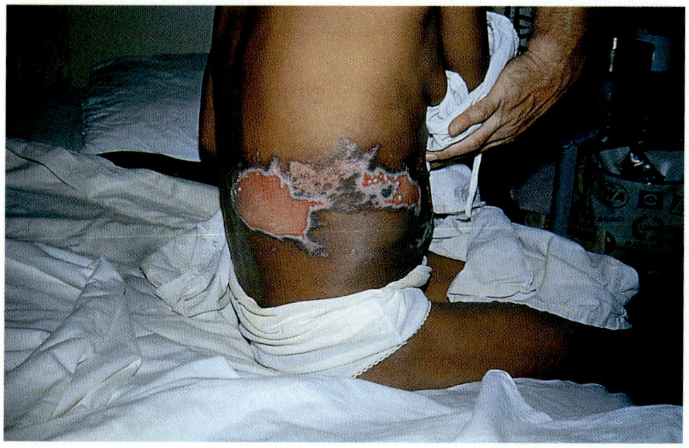

Figure 35–5. Later stage of herpes zoster in which vesicles have ruptured, leaving partially healing cutaneous ulcers with geographic borders of cutaneous hyperpigmentation.

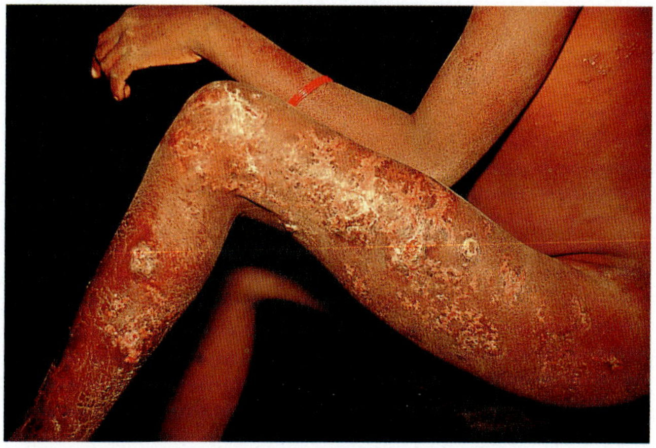

Figure 35–6. Late stage of herpes zoster with some areas of shallow cutaneous ulcers, scaling, and hyperpigmentation on the left lower limb. Some lesions became secondarily infected. *(By Daniel H. Connor, MD. 1976.)*

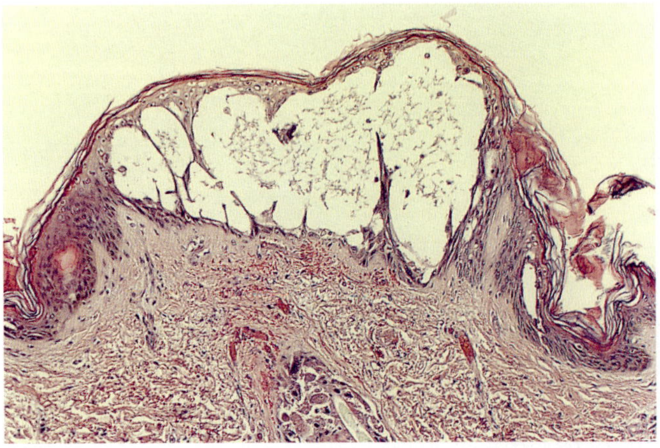

A

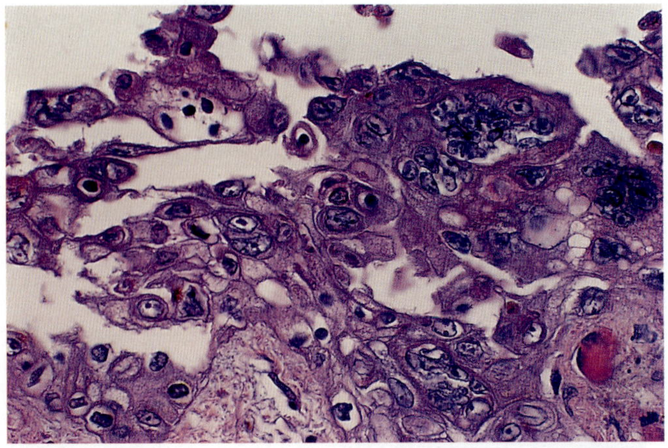

B

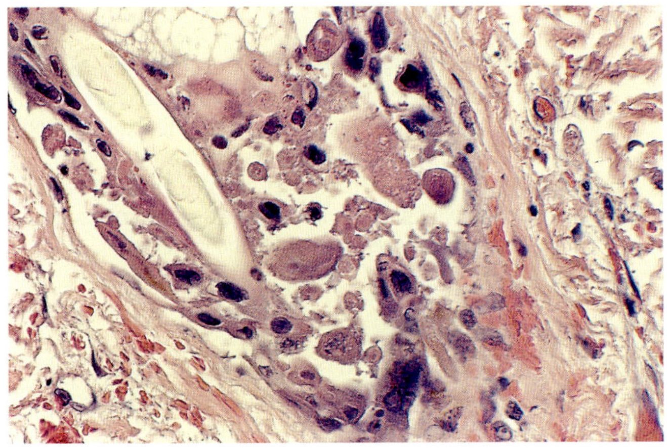

C

Figure 35–7. (**A**) Herpes zoster. Biopsy specimen shows intact intraepidermal vesicle with involvement of hair sheath in midlower portion of field. Note the marked acantholysis with pale proteinaceous material (hematoxylin-eosin, ×40). (**B**) Characteristic viral cytopathic effect in the same patient involving cells along the base and edge of vesicle as well as some detached cells. Some nuclei contain a well-defined viral inclusion, whereas other nuclei have smudged chromatin (hematoxylin-eosin, ×400). (**C**) Pilar unit beneath intact vesicle shows marked acantholysis with viral cytopathic effect of VZV infection (hematoxylin-eosin, ×400).

COMPLICATIONS OF HERPES ZOSTER

About 10% of patients have postherpetic neuralgia with pain and hyperesthesia over the afflicted dermatome following resolution of the eruption.[6] The pain can be excruciating, with insomnia and depression. Patients also may have paresthesias, anesthesia, and pruritus. Although spontaneous remission usually occurs within 6 months, the pain may persist for months to years. The incidence of postherpetic neuralgia increases with advancing age and is highest and generally persists for the longest periods in those with involvement of the trigeminal nerve.

About 20% of patients with ophthalmic herpes zoster may have ocular complications such as visual impairment, uveitis, keratitis, secondary glaucoma, cataract formation, iridocyclitis, panophthalmitis, canalicular scarring, and lid retraction.[6] The Ramsay Hunt syndrome is involvement of the geniculate ganglion and facial nerve by VZV, and is thus characterized by motor and sensory deficits such as unilateral loss of taste over the anterior two thirds of the tongue, auditory deficits, and unilateral facial weakness or paralysis. There may be a vesicular eruption over the tympanic membrane, external auditory canal, and auricle. Other less frequent complications include cutaneous scarring, pneumonia, neurologic motor deficits, meningoencephalitis, myelitis, granulomatous cerebral angiitis, and disseminated herpes zoster infection.[6,27]

DIAGNOSIS OF VARICELLA-ZOSTER

The majority of patients with VZV infection are diagnosed on clinical examination. A variety of methods, however, are available for detection of the virus and may aid in diagnosis when uncertainty exists. The Tzanck smear allows for rapid identification of epithelial cells infected with VZV. A vesicular or pustular lesion is ruptured and the fluid collected on a glass slide; in addition, the base and sides of the vesicle/pustule may be scraped with a sharp blade and the tissue is smeared onto a glass slide. The slides are air dried, stained with Giemsa or Diff-Quik, and examined for cells with intranuclear inclusion bodies and giant cells. The morphologic findings in Herpes simplex eruptions and VZV infection are indistinguishable, so diagnosis by Tzanck smear must be correlated with clinical features.[28]

HISTOPATHOLOGY

Skin lesions in varicella and in herpes zoster have similar histopathology and may be impossible to distinguish from cutaneous lesions of Herpes simplex infection. Hematogenous spread of the virus infects the endothelial cells of dermal capillaries followed by extension to epidermis causing intraepidermal vesicles (Figure 35–7, A–C). "Ballooning degeneration" of epithelial cells usually begins in the deeper layers of the epidermis and advances superficially, causing enlargement of epidermal cells with vacuolization of cytoplasm and loss of desmosomes. Most giant cells containing viral inclusions are at the base and within the walls of the vesicle. A viral inclusion is first recognized as a faintly basophilic intranuclear body with peripheral condensation of nuclear chromatin. Later, the inclusion becomes eosinophilic, more than one half the diameter of the nucleus, and has a clear zone between the inclusion and the condensed rim of nuclear chromatin. When the nucleus disintegrates, there may be inclusions within the cytoplasm. It is the combination of acantholysis, degeneration of epithelium, and increasing intercellular edema that causes the intraepidermal clear vesicle (Figure 35–7, B). Adnexal structures, such as hair follicles (Figure 35–7, C) and sebaceous glands may also be involved. Dermal capillaries are congested, causing the characteristic erythematous base.

In contrast to Herpes simplex infection, a leukocytoclastic vasculitis with occasional hemorrhage is in the dermis. Dermal endothelial cells are swollen and surrounded by an inflammatory cell infiltrate, mainly neutrophils and a few mononuclear cells. Erythrocytes may also be in the exudate. The vesicles become infiltrated with neutrophils and occasional mononuclear cells, changing the lesion from a vesicle to a pustule. Eventually, the fluid is resorbed and becomes crusted. With continued regeneration and growth of underlying epidermis, the crust sloughs.

There are several unusual cutaneous manifestations of VZV infection. Chronic lesions of herpes zoster in immunodeficient patients can become verrucous papules and plaques.[29] Other lesions, including granulomatous vasculitis,[30] cutaneous lymphoma,[31] and even Kaposi's sarcoma[32] have been described in affected dermatomes following resolution of vesicular lesions.

DORSAL ROOT GANGLIA

Involvement of dorsal root ganglia and sensory nerves produces distinctive histopathologic findings including inflammation of affected ganglion, adjacent nerve root, and posterior gray horn of spinal cord, degenerative change of sensory neuronal cells, necrosis, and thrombi in involved vessels. Changes in the corresponding anterior horn include central chromatolysis, neuronophagia, proliferation of microglia, and lymphocytic cuffing of blood vessels.[33,34] Infection of cranial nerves may cause brainstem involvement with necroinflammatory changes in blood vessels and infarction.[33] Changes of peripheral nerve are from destruction of ganglia and spinal cord. Wallerian degeneration is often in the posterior nerve roots and peripheral nerves. Less frequently, involvement of the anterior roots results from anterior horn infection.[34]

OTHER ORGANS

Disseminated VZV may involve a variety of organs. In the liver, for example, gross examination typically shows punctate, discrete foci of soft, yellow-white necrosis, often with a surrounding hemorrhagic rim (Figures 35–8, A and B) or the necrosis may be confluent (Figure 35–9). Zones of necrosis may become confluent. Microscopically, the necrosis is hemorrhagic with little or no inflammatory reaction. Eosinophilic inclusions are in adjacent hepatocytes (Figure 35–10). Intranuclear inclusions are in other organs including cells bordering punched out zones of necrosis and hemorrhage such as adrenal glands (Figure 35–11, A–C). These same changes can be seen in infected cells in vitro (Figure 35–12). Varicella of the placenta includes chronic villitis, granulomatous inflammation with giant cells, and viral inclusions.[35,36] These findings are important when attempting to predict fetal VZV infection after maternal infection during pregnancy.

IMMUNOHISTOCHEMISTRY AND POLYMERASE CHAIN REACTION

Monoclonal antibodies to antigens of VZV (eg, surface glycoproteins) are commercially available for identification of VZV in infected human tissue.[37] Specific identification of viral antigens using immunohistochemical methods is more specific than routine morphology, particularly in distinguishing infections caused by VZV from Herpes simplex virus. With the determination of the complete sequence of the VZV genome and subsequent localization of many viral genes, use of the PCR technique for amplification of VZV DNA has become possible. Primers have been developed that bind to specific viral gene sequences, creating a sensitive and specific assay for VZV infection.[24,38,39]

TREATMENT

Treatment of VZV infection in an immunocompetent host includes isolation from susceptible individuals until lesions have crusted, along with optional symptomatic treatment with antihistamines for pruritus and antipyret-

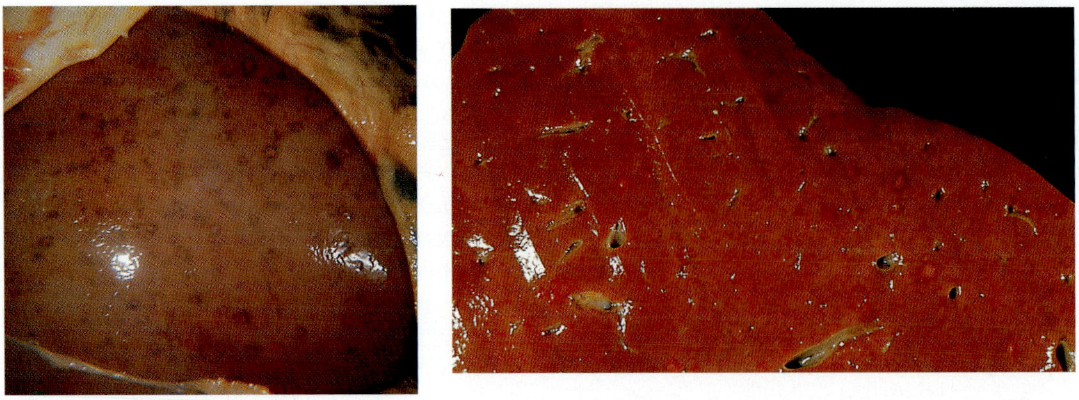

A B

Figure 35–8. (**A**) Disseminated VZV infection in a 7-year-old boy with chronic myelogenous leukemia. Capsular surface of the liver is studded with punctate lesions up to 3 mm in diameter. Many have a pale center and a hemorrhagic rim. (**B**) Liver, same patient, has numerous intraparenchymal foci of necrosis, which are discrete, soft, and yellow-white with congested or hemorrhagic borders.

ics for fever (acetominophen rather than aspirin to prevent Reye's syndrome). Antiviral therapy, however, is recommended for all immunodeficient patients and for immunocompetent patients with severe disease. Acyclovir, a chain-terminating purine nucleotide analog, acts selectively on infected cells and is usually given in high doses intravenously. VZV infections may be prevented or attenuated by giving varicella-zoster immune globulin (VZIG). Patients at high risk of complications should be treated with VZIG following exposure—including those who are immunodeficient, infants born to mothers with varicella less than 5 days before birth or within 2 days after delivery, and all premature infants. VZIG is given intramuscularly and if exposure persists, a repeat dose is given at 3 weeks.

Varicella-Zoster Virus Vaccine

A VZV vaccine (Varivax) is approved for clinical use. It is a live attenuated virus and is recommended for healthy children and adults without previous VZV infection. The vaccine is not recommended for children younger than 12 months of age, pregnant women, immunodeficient patients, and any who are hypersensi-

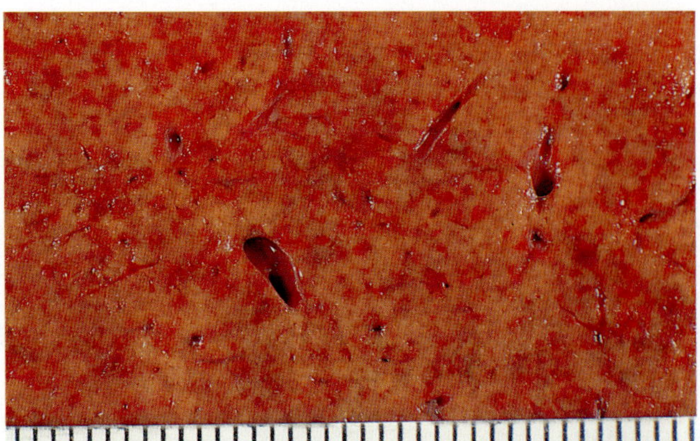

Figure 35–9. Liver in fatal VZV infection. There is extensive and confluent necrosis of parenchyma.

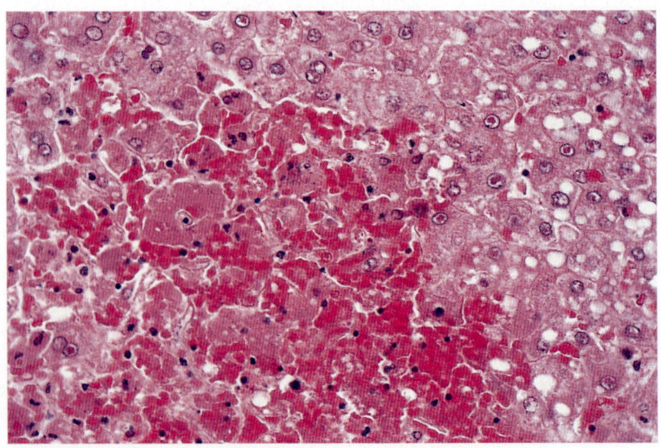

Figure 35–10. Disseminated VZV infection (same liver shown in Figure 35–8). Punched out area of hemorrhagic necrosis with several nuclei of hepatocytes containing well-defined eosinophilic inclusions with surrounding halos (hematoxylin-eosin, ×200).

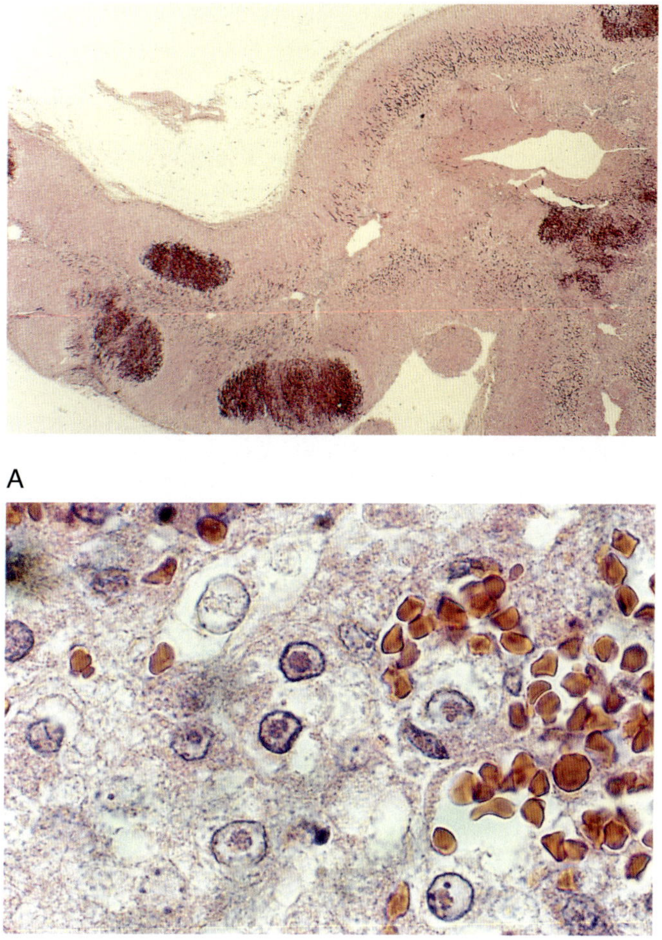

Figure 35–11. (**A**) Adrenal gland from an adult patient with disseminated VZV infection. Punched out areas of hemorrhagic necrosis involve mainly the cortex (hematoxylin-eosin, ×10). (**B**) Same case with a zone of hemorrhagic necrosis bordered by residual cortical cells (hematoxylin-eosin, ×100). (**C**) Higher magnification showing cortical cells with a single eosinophilic intranuclear (Cowdry type A) inclusion. The nuclear chromatin is condensed on the nuclear membrane (hematoxylin-eosin, ×1000).

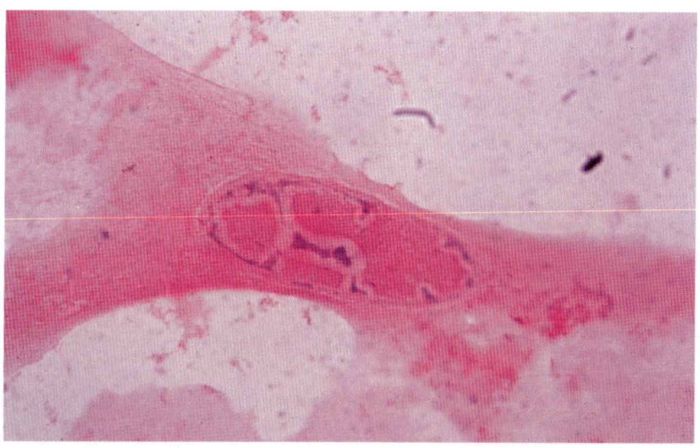

Figure 35–12. Cytopathic effect of tissue culture cells infected with VZV from a patient with disseminated chickenpox. Note the characteristic geographic eosinophilic intranuclear inclusion (hematoxylin-eosin, ×1000).

tive to nonactive components of the vaccine;[40] whether the vaccine should be given to those with leukemia awaits further study. Also undecided is whether VZV vaccine should be included as a standardized childhood vaccination. The VZV vaccine has been given with the measles, mumps, and rubella vaccines.[41,42] Although clinical trials have shown the vaccine to prevent or attenuate VZV infection, questions remain about proper dosage, persistence of long-term immunity, and about the hazards of shifting infection to the adult population. Continued research will provide answers to many of these questions.[40,41]

REFERENCES

1. Gelb LD. Varicella-zoster virus. In: Fields BN, Knipe DM, Chanock RM, et al, eds. *Virology*. New York: Raven Press; 1990:2011–2054.
2. Ostrove JM. Molecular biology of varicella zoster virus. *Adv Virus Res.* 1990;38:45–98.
3. Centers for Disease Control and Prevention. Summary of

notifiable diseases, United States 1993 *MMWR.* 1993; 42(53):
4. Finger R, Hughes JP, Meade BJ, Pelletier AR, Palmer CT. Age specific incidence of chickenpox. *Public Health Rep.* 1994;109(6):750–755.
5. Guess HA, Broughton DD, Melton LJ III, Kurland LT. Population-based studies of varicella complications. *Pediatrics.* 1986;78(suppl):723–727.
6. Ragozzino MW, Melton LJ III, Kurland LT, Chu CP, Perry HO. Population-based study of herpes zoster and its sequelae. *Medicine.* 1982;61(5):310–316.
7. Han CS, Miller W, Haake R, Weisdorf D. Varicella zoster infection after bone marrow transplantation: incidence, risk factors, and complications. *Bone Marrow Transplantation.* 1994;13:277–283.
8. Glynn C, Crockford G, Gavaghan D, Cardno P, Price D, Miller, J. Epidemiology of shingles. *J Royal Soc Med.* 1990; 83:617–619.
9. Oxman MN, Alani R. In: Fitzpatrick TB, Eisen AZ, Wolff K, Freedberg IM, Austen KF, eds. *Dermatology in General Medicine.* 4th ed. New York: McGraw-Hill; 1993:2543–2572.
10. Fleischer G, Henry W, McSorley M, Arbeter A, Plotkin S. Life-threatening complications of varicella. *Am J Dis Child.* 1981;135:896–899.
11. Triebwasser JH, Harris RE, Bryant RE, Rhoades ER. Varicella pneumonia in adults. *Medicine.* 1967;46:409–423.
12. Feldman S. Varicella-zoster virus pneumonitis. *Chest.* 1994;106(suppl 1):22S–27S.
13. Moore CM, Henry J, Benzing G III, Kaplan S. Varicella myocarditis. *Am J Dis Child.* 1969;118:899–902.
14. Sherman RA, Silva J Jr, Gandour-Edwards R. Fatal varicella in an adult: case report and review of gastrointestinal complications of chickenpox. *Rev Infect Dis.* 1991;13: 424–427.
15. Baker ÇJ, Gilsdorf JR, South MA, Singleton EB. Gastritis as a complication of varicella. *South Med J.* 1973;66:539–541.
16. Culbertson WW, Brod RD, Flynn HW Jr, et al. Chickenpox-associated acute retinal necrosis syndrome. *Ophthalmology.* 1991;98(11):1641–1645.
17. Baird RE, Daly P, Sawyer RH. Varicella arthritis diagnosed by polymerase chain reaction. *Ped Infect Dis J.* 1990; 10(12):950–952.
18. Patti ME, Selvaggi KJ, Kroboth FJ, Varicella hepatitis in the immunocompromised adult: a case report and review of the literature. *Am J Med.* 1990;88:77–80.
19. Espinoza C, Kuhn C. Viral infection of megakaryocytes in varicella with purpura. *Am J Clin Path.* 1974;61:203–208.
20. Maness DL, Rogers DY. Hemorrhagic complications of varicella. *Am Fam Phys.* 1987;35:151–155.
21. Alkalay AL, Pomerance JJ, Rimoin DL. Fetal varicella syndrome. *J Pediatr.* 1987;111:320–323.
22. Brunell PA. Fetal and neonatal varicella-zoster infections. *Sem Perinat.* 1983;7(1):47–56.
23. Brunell PA. Varicella in pregnancy, the fetus, and the newborn: problems in management. *J Infect Dis.* 1992;166 (suppl 1):S42–S47.
24. Isada NB, Paar DP, Johnson MP, et al. In utero diagnosis of congenital varicella zoster virus infection by chorionic villus sampling and polymerase chain reaction. *Am J Obstet Gynecol.* 1991;165:1727–1730.
25. Croen KD, Ostrove JM, Dragovic LJ, Straus SE: Patterns of gene expression and sites of latency in human nerve ganglia are different for varicella-zoster and herpes simplex viruses. *Proc Natl Acad Sci USA.* 1988;85: 9773–9777.
26. Mahalingham R, Wellish M, Wolf W, et al. Latent varicella-zoster viral DNA in human trigeminal and thoracic ganglia. *N Engl J Med.* 1990;323:627–631.
27. Cohen PR, Beltrani VP, Grossman ME. Disseminated herpes zoster in patients with human immunodeficiency virus infection. *Am J Med.* 1988;84:1076–1080.
28. Brodell RT, Helms SE, Devine M. Office dermatologic testing: the Tzanck preparation. *Am Fam Phys.* 1991;44(3): 857–860.
29. LeBoit PE, Limova M, Yen TS, Palefsky JM, White CR Jr, Berger TG. Chronic verrucous VZV infection in patients with the acquired immune deficiency syndrome (AIDS). *Am J Dermatopathol.* 1992;14:1–7.
30. Langenberg A, Yen TSB, LeBoit PE. Granulomatous vasculitis occurring after cutaneous herpes zoster despite absence of viral genome. *J Am Acad Dermatol.* 1991; 24:429–433.
31. Aloi FG, Appino A, Puiatt P. Lymphoplasmacytoid lymphoma arising in herpes zoster scars. *J Am Acad Dermatol.* 1990;22:130–131.
32. Niedt GW, Prioleau PG. Kaposi's sarcoma in a dermatome previously involved by herpes zoster. *J Am Acad Dermatol.* 1988;18:448–451.
33. Esiri MM, Kennedy PGE. In: Adams JH, Duchen LW, eds. *Greenfield's Neuropathology;* 5th ed. New York: Oxford University Press, 1992:352–355.
34. Richardson EP, DeGirolami U. *Pathology of the Peripheral Nerve. Major Problems in Pathology.* Philadelphia: WB Saunders; 1995; 32:38–44.
35. Robertson NJ, McKeever PA. Fetal and placental pathology in two cases of maternal varicella infection. *Pediatr Pathol.* 1992;12:545–550.
36. Qureshi F, Jacques SM. Maternal varicella during pregnancy: correlation of maternal history with fatal outcome and placental histopathology. *Mod Pathol.* 1995;8:6P.
37. Wroblewski Z, Devlin M, Reilly K, van Trieste H, Wellish M, Gilden DH. The production of varicella zoster virus antiserum in laboratory animals. *Arch Virol.* 1982;74: 233–238.
38. Koropchak CM, Graham G, Palmer J, et al. Investigation of varicella-zoster virus infection by polymerase chain reaction in the immunocompetent host with acute varicella. *J Infect Dis.* 1991;163:1016–1022.
39. Nahass GT, Goldstein BA, Zhu WY, Serfling U, Penneys NS, Leonardi CL. Comparison of Tzanck smear, viral culture, and DNA diagnostic methods in detection of herpes simplex and varicella-zoster infection. *JAMA.* 1992;268: 2541–2544.
40. Shelton D. Chickenpox vaccine promises protection, cost savings. *Am Med News.* April 3, 1995:5.
41. Gershon AA, La Russa P, Hardy I, Steinberg S, Silverstein S. Varicella vaccine: the American experience. *J Infect Dis.* 1992;166(suppl 1):S63–S68.
42. Brunell PA, Novelli VM, Lipton SV, Pollock B. Combined vaccine against measles, mumps, rubella, and varicella. *Pediatrics.* 1988;78:742–747.

CHAPTER 36

Viral Infections by Human Herpesviruses 6, 7, and 8

Philip E. Pellett

It rests now with ourselves alone to enjoy in peace and concord the blessings of self-government, so long denied to mankind: to show by example the sufficiency of human reason for the care of human affairs and that the will of the majority, the Natural law of every society, is the only sure guardian of the rights of man.

Thomas Jefferson (1743–1826)

INTRODUCTION

Four human herpesviruses were discovered since the mid-1980s: human herpesvirus 6 variant A (HHV-6A), human herpesvirus 6 variant B (HHV-6B), human herpesvirus 7 (HHV-7), and human herpesvirus 8 (HHV-8) (also known as Kaposi's sarcoma–associated herpesvirus, or KSHV). There is nothing to suggest that these are new viruses; all indications are that they have been part of human biology for eons. Their recent discovery was the product of new methods for propagating cells of the immune system and for detecting infectious agents in disease tissue. Only one of these recently discovered viruses has been linked to a disease that might be described as "new," that being HHV-8 and acquired immunodeficiency syndrome (AIDS)-associated Kaposi's sarcoma. HHV-6B has been clearly identified as the etiologic agent of a human disease (roseola infantum or exanthem subitum). More than 90% of the population has been infected with either or both HHV-6A and HHV-6B, more than 85% with HHV-7, and it is too soon to know how many have been infected with HHV-8. As with herpesviruses, these viruses likely infect their host for life. Both history and biology suggest that the clinical spectrum each infection by these viruses is broad and that each is linked with significant and specific clinical entities. It is only a matter of time and effort before these connections are made. The importance of this lies in 1) the possibility of using specific antiviral therapy or vaccines to treat or prevent diseases caused by these viruses, and 2) allowing correct diagnosis and treatment for diseases with symptoms that can be caused by more than one unrelated agent. As an example of this, primary infection with HHV-6B can cause roseola infantum [also known as exanthem subitum (ES) or sixth disease]. This disease of young children is characterized by a period of high fever followed by a rash. If an antibiotic is presumptively prescribed during the febrile (fever) period, the rash that is part of the normal course of roseola might be mistaken for a reaction to the antibiotic, and the child would be denied further use of the drug. Correct diagnosis of the cause of the rash would reduce the nonspecific use of antibiotics and keep that antibiotic in the arsenal of drugs available for that child.

HHV-6

HHV-6 was discovered by Dr. Zaki Salahuddin and coworkers[1] in the laboratory of Dr. Robert Gallo at the National Institutes of Health in 1986. Subsequent studies found that HHV-6 isolates form two groups of closely related, yet distinct viruses: HHV-6A and HHV-6B.[2] Nearly everyone has been infected by either or both of these viruses by the age of 4 years. An important aspect of the biology of these viruses is that they infect T lymphocytes. Because of their shared tropism for T cells, it is possible that HHV-6 and human immunodeficiency virus type 1 (HIV-1) interact during the development of AIDS. HHV-6 can induce changes in some lymphoid cells that permit HIV-1 infection.[3,4] In addition to peripheral blood T cells, HHV-6 is present in most normal brains.[5,6] In patients with multiple sclerosis (MS), HHV-6 is present in the plaque regions, with a cellular distribution different from that seen in normal brains[6]; the significance of this is being studied. The most clearly defined role for HHV-6 in disease is in the fever and rash syndromes related to ES that are associated with primary infection with HHV-6B. As many as 20% of febrile admissions to emergency departments for children between 6 and 12 months of age can be due to primary HHV-6 infections.[7] Such primary HHV-6 infections have been associated with significant disturbances of the central nervous system (CNS), including convulsions and encephalitis. HHV-6 infections may be important in immunodeficient patients, such as transplant recipients and AIDS patients, but the scope of HHV-6 activity in these situations has not been completely defined. The biology and molecular biology of HHV-6 have been reviewed elsewhere.[8,9]

Definition

HHV-6A and HHV-6B are members of the family *Herpesviridae,* subfamily *Betaherpesvirinae,* and genus *Roseolovirus.* HHV-6A and HHV-6B are readily distinguished by differences in growth properties, antigenicity, and nucleotide sequences, but are the most closely related pair of herpesviruses known.[2] Their next closest relatives are HHV-7 and human cytomegalovirus (HCMV). All of these viruses are members of the betaherpesvirus subfamily.

Synonyms

Initially, HHV-6 was named human B-lymphotropic virus (HBLV) because of an observed B-cell tropism[1]; the predominant T-cell tropism was described later and the name subsequently was changed to HHV-6 in accordance with standard herpesvirus nomenclature.

Geographic Distribution

HHV-6 is worldwide. In most populations, the seroprevalence exceeds 80% in adults, with some investigators finding nearly every specimen to be positive. In scattered populations, however, lower prevalence values have been observed. Current serologic methods do not discriminate between HHV-6A and HHV-6B; thus, the details of the geographic distribution of the variants are not known, but it is clear that both are widespread.

Life Cycle/Natural History/Epidemiology

HHV-6 DNA and infectious virus can be detected in saliva, which is a likely route for transmission. During primary infection, the virus replicates in CD4+ lymphocytes.[10] Viremia wanes with the rise in neutralizing antibody titer, and latent virus is later in macrophages and monocytes.[11] At some point, the virus takes up residence in the brain, with more than 80% of brains being polymerase chain reaction (PCR)-positive for the virus.[5,6] There may be other cellular repositories for latent or persistent virus.

HHV-6 infection normally is acquired very early in life, shortly after the waning of maternal antibody. By the age of 2 years nearly all children are seropositive. This suggests that the virus is a common inhabitant of the household environment. Primary infections that result in ES are caused by HHV-6B, and this variant is most associated with early acquisition. The average age of acquisition of HHV-6A has not been determined, and no disease has been associated with primary HHV-6A infection.

Morphology

HHV-6 has the morphologic features shared by other members of the herpesvirus family (Figure 36–1), including an electron-dense core that harbors the double-strand DNA genome of approximately 162 kb, a capsid of icosahedral symmetry, a tegument that appears in electron micrographs as an amorphous layer between the capsid and envelope, and the envelope, which is a cell-membrane–derived lipid bilayer studded with virally encoded glycoproteins and integral membrane proteins. In contrast with some herpesviruses, tegumented capsids frequently are in the cytoplasm of infected cells.[12,13]

Clinical Features

The spectrum of HHV-6 clinical associations is broad, but many of these associations have not met suggested standards for proof as causal agents.[14] The lack of proof may be a consequence of 1) the virus being a passenger in a disease or in diseased tissue, 2) simple insufficiency of time and effort necessary to complete a proof, 3) the small number of patients affected by some HHV-6–associated diseases, or 4) complexities in studying the association between a highly prevalent virus and diffusely defined diseases, such as chronic fatigue syndrome (CFS), or those with difficult-to-access affected tissues, such as MS. HHV-6B is a proved etiologic agent of ES and its variants[15]; other associations with diseases vary in their strength. The discussion of HHV-6 clinical features is broken into sections dealing with primary

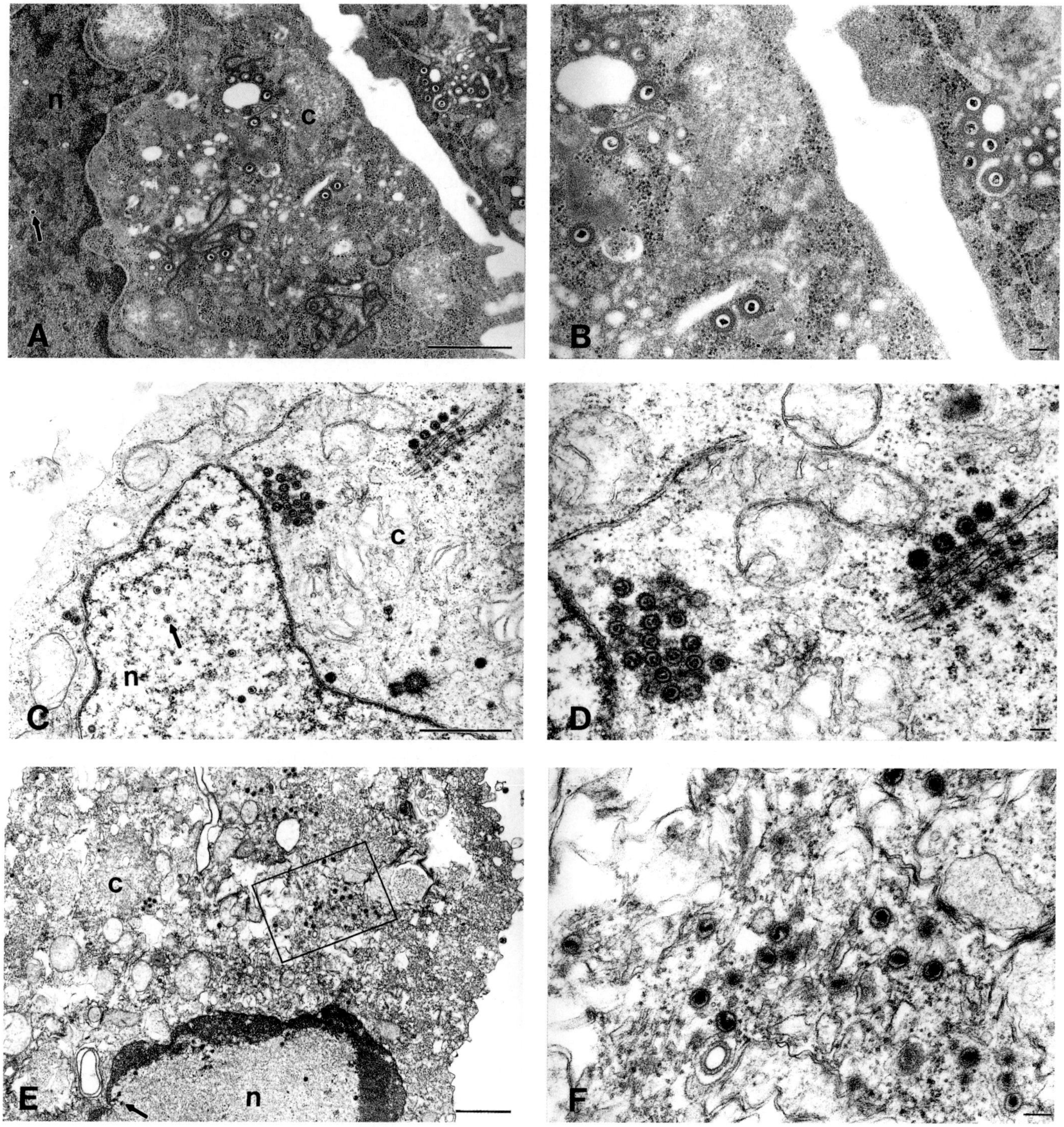

Figure 36–1. HHV-6, HHV-7, and HHV-8 ultrastructure. (**A**) Thin section electron micrograph of portions of adjacent HHV-6B(Z29)–infected lymphocytes. Virus particles are visible in the nucleus (n) (*arrow*) and cytoplasm (c). Nonenveloped capsids are in proximity of membranes of the Golgi apparatus and in association with strands of tegument-like material. (**B**) Enlargement of a portion of the cell shown in panel C showing virus particle structure. Note the thick teguments and absence of envelopes on the cytoplasmic particles that are not located within membrane-bounded structures. (**C**) Thin section electron micrograph of an HHV-7(SB)–infected lymphocyte. Naked capsids are present in the nucleus (*arrow*) and nonenveloped tegumented cytoplasmic particles are associated with annulate lamellae or are in clumps of tegument-like material. (**D**) Enlargement of a portion of the cell shown in **C**. HHV-6 and HHV-7 cytopathic effects and ultrastructure are essentially indistinguishable. (**E**) Thin section electron micrograph of an HHV-8–harboring body cavity–based lymphoma cell line (BCBL-1)[78] that was treated with a phorbol ester to induce lytic virus infection. Naked capsids (*arrow*) and marginated chromatin are present in the nucleus. Two enveloped extracellular virions are visible. (**F**) Enlargement of the boxed portion of **E** showing sparsely tegumented cytoplasmic particles. The scale bars represent 1 μm in **A**, **C**, and **E**, and 100 nm in **B**, **D**, and **F**. *(Courtesy of Cynthia Goldsmith and Jodi Black, Centers for Disease Control and Prevention.)*

infection, infection in immunodeficient patients, and illness associated with chronic infection. Clinical features of HHV-6 infection have been reviewed.[8,9]

Primary Infection

The vast majority of primary HHV-6 infections are in children younger than 2 years of age. The principal disease associated with primary infection is ES,[16] which is also known as roseola infantum, roseola, and sixth disease. Classic ES is characterized by a febrile (>39°C) period of 3 to 5 days followed by rapid defervescence and then an erythematous and macular or maculopapular rash of 1 to 3 days. Lymphocytosis and neutropenia are frequent during the exanthem, and the disease resolves without complication. HHV-6 viremia is at its maximum during the febrile phase, decreases rapidly with the onset of rash, and is eliminated when neutralizing antibodies appear. Perhaps 30% of children experience ES; primary HHV-6 infection in the remainder is either subclinical or associated with nonspecific symptoms. In addition to the classic presentation, primary HHV-6 infection has been associated with rash without fever, fever without rash, and a variety of other signs and symptoms. Febrile convulsions are not uncommon and other neurologic complications include bulging fontanels, encephalitis, meningitis, vomiting, irritability, and meningoencephalitis. Other severe manifestations of primary infection include fulminant hepatitis, intussusception, thrombocytopenic purpura, thrombocytopenia, hemophagocytic syndrome, and disseminated infection. Deaths have been associated with the more severe infections. Primary infection in adults can lead to more severe infection than is normally seen in children and includes prolonged lymphadenopathy, mononucleosis-like illness, and hepatitis. HHV-6 has been observed in the affected tissues of most cases of sinus histiocytosis with massive lymphadenopathy (Rosai–Dorfman disease).

Immunodeficient Patients

Herpesviruses are common opportunistic pathogens in immunodeficient patients. This is in large part a consequence of the high prevalence of most herpesviruses and the fact that once they have infected a host, they reside in the host for the remainder of the host's life. In an immunocompetent host the viruses normally are quiescent, and any periodic reactivations are quickly controlled by the immune system. During periods of immunosuppression, be they genetic, iatrogenic, or acquired, the endogenous herpesviruses may reactivate, and, in the absence of immune control, cause significant disease. HHV-6 activity has been detected in many patients who became immunodeficient either in conjunction with organ transplants or during AIDS. The precise role of HHV-6 in disease in these patients remains controversial,[8,17] but it seems likely that, in at least some of the instances in which the virus was found in proximity of diseased tissues and no other infectious agent was detected, the virus was involved in the pathologic process and was not merely a passenger.

HHV-6 activity has been observed following cardiac, hepatic, renal, and bone marrow transplantations, with renal and bone marrow recipients being the most thoroughly studied. In renal transplantation, HHV-6 antigens have been detected in distal tubular epithelial cells and in infiltrating interstitial lymphocytes,[18] and were detected more frequently in acute than in chronic rejection.[19] HHV-6 growth in vitro can be stimulated by the addition of anti-CD3 monoclonal antibodies.[20] Treatment of transplant recipients for rejection with either anti-CD3 or antilymphocyte globulin has been associated with HHV-6 activity in some studies.[8] HHV-6 is frequently active in bone marrow transplant recipients, and the activity has been associated with rash and graft-versus-host disease (GVHD), pneumonitis (Figure 36–2), sinusitis, febrile episodes, and graft failure. The difficulties of interpreting such associations are discussed in detail elsewhere.[8,17]

In addition to the fact that HHV-6 is a herpesvirus and herpesviruses cause disease in immunodeficient patients, the potential for an expanded role of HHV-6 in the progression of AIDS is suggested by the shared tropism of HIV-1 and HHV-6 for CD4+ lymphocytes. In vitro, HIV-1 and HHV-6 can each stimulate the other's replication, with consequent enhanced cytopathogenicity, although under some conditions there are inhibitory effects.[21,22] HHV-6 can activate HIV-1 to a lytic form in cell lines that harbor latent HIV-1.[23] Serologic studies have shed little light on whether HHV-6 and HIV-1 interact in vivo. The load of HHV-6 DNA in blood decreases as AIDS progresses, probably because of lymphocyte depletion. Nonetheless, HHV-6 DNA and antigens can be detected in lymph nodes of AIDS patients, and HHV-6 antigens are disseminated into many tissues and organs late in AIDS (Figure 36–3).[24,25] The contribution of such disseminated infections to the progression of disease is being studied. The role of HHV-6 in AIDS pneumonitis is controversial.[17,26]

Disease Associated with Chronic HHV-6 Infection

HHV-6 has been associated with three major types of chronic illness: malignancy, MS, and CFS.

HHV-6 and Malignancy. Several segments of the HHV-6 genome have the ability to transform cells in vitro to a tumorigenic phenotype. Many tissue specimens from every available tumor source have been assayed for HHV-6 DNA and antigens.[8,9] To summarize, HHV-6 DNA has been detected intermittently in tissues of non-Hodgkin's lymphoma, but there is no compelling evi-

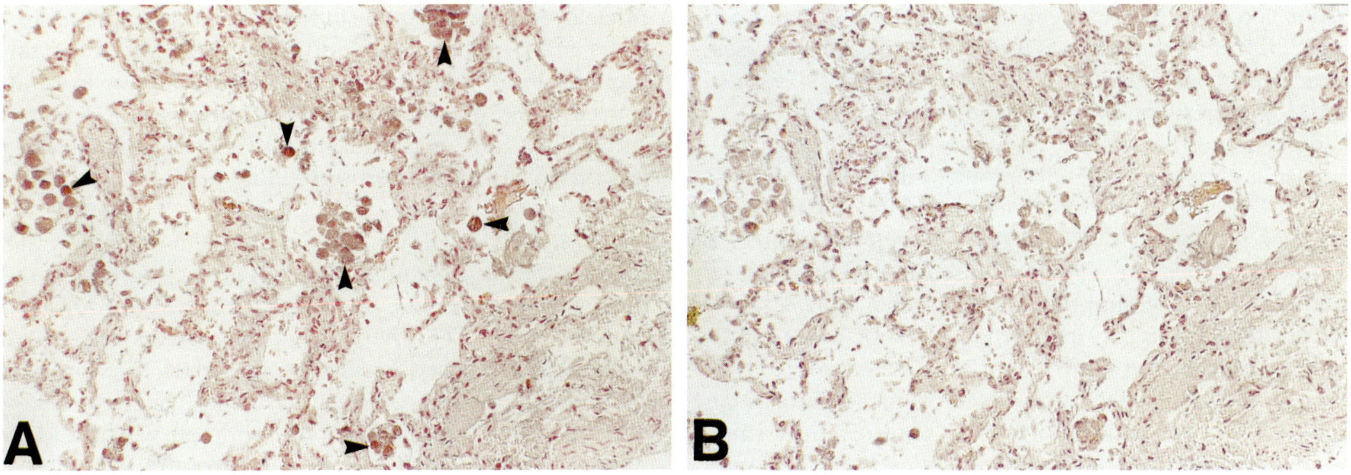

Figure 36–2. Immunohistochemical detection of HHV-6 infected cells in lung tissues from an autologous bone marrow transplant recipient with HHV-6 interstitial pneumonitis. (**A**) Tissue section stained with a rabbit hyperimmune serum specific for HHV-6 infected cells. Some of the infected cells present are noted (*arrowheads*). (**B**) Specificity control showing an adjacent serial section with HHV-6 specific hyperimmune serum after absorption with HHV-6 infected T lymphocytes (vector black enzyme substrate with nuclear fast red counterstain). *(Photographs contributed by Drs. K. K. Knox and D. R. Carrigan.)*

dence to suggest that the virus is causally related to these tumors. The association of HHV-6 with Hodgkin's disease (HD) is not so easily dismissed.[8,27] HHV-6 has been most closely associated with the nodular sclerosis HD subtype. In HD tissues, neoplastic cells (Reed–Sternberg, or RS cells) are relatively rare and frequently widely scattered. HHV-6 antigens have been identified in such cells; this association requires further study. Other associations between HHV-6 and malignancy include acute lymphocytic leukemia, $S100^{+}$ T-cell chronic lymphoproliferative disease, Kaposi's sarcoma, oral carcinoma, and cervical carcinoma. In all of these diseases, the suggestive preliminary studies require further work to define the role of the virus in the malignancy. For Kaposi's sarcoma and cervical carcinoma, which have been more clearly associated with other viruses, such studies will need to address the question of viral interactions.

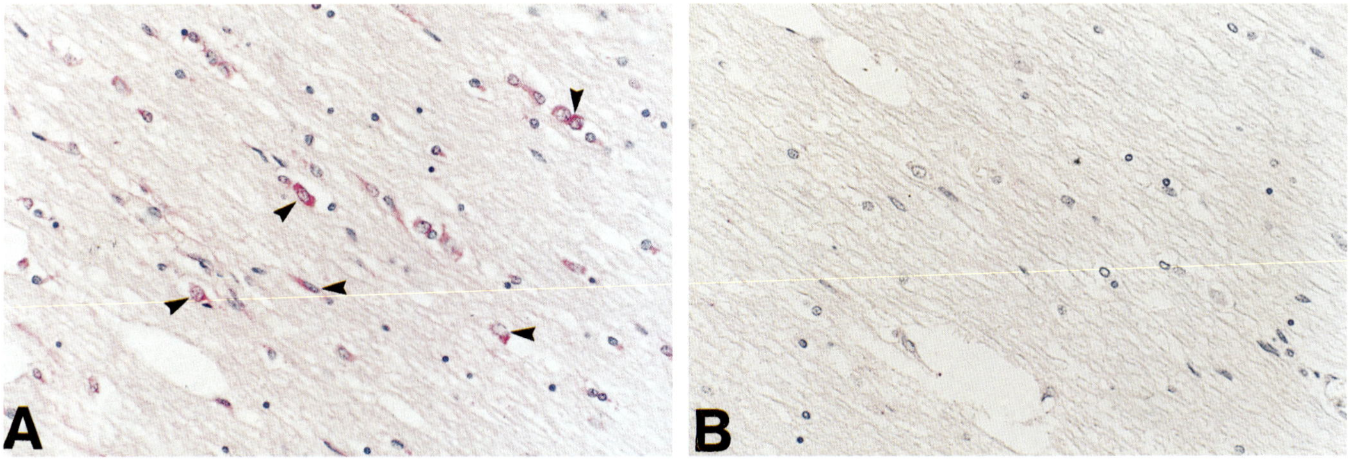

Figure 36–3. Immunohistochemical detection of HHV-6 infected cells in the white matter of the brain of an HIV-infected 9-year-old girl with HHV-6–associated leukoencephalopathy. (**A**) Numerous HHV-6 infected cells (*arrowheads*) within an area of active demyelination stained with a rabbit hyperimmune serum specific for HHV-6 infected cells. (**B**) Specificity control showing adjacent serial section of tissue after staining with preimmune serum from the rabbit used to produce the HHV-6 specific hyperimmune serum (vector red enzyme substrate with hematoxylin counterstain). *(Photographs contributed by Drs. K. K. Knox and D. R. Carrigan.)*

HHV-6 and MS. MS is a dymyelinating disease that most often affects young adults. Over the years, many viruses have been hypothesized to be the cause of MS, but on close scrutiny, preliminary suggestions have fallen aside. The current leading hypothesis suggests that the disease is caused by an autoimmune inflammatory reaction.[28] The argument for an involvement of HHV-6 in MS is as follows. HHV-6 can grow in cells of neuronal origin, is associated with CNS disease during primary infection and in immunodeficient patients, and is present in the brains of more than 80% of adults. MS patients have higher HHV-6 antibody titers than do controls, and HHV-6 DNA was detected in cerebrospinal fluid (CSF) of MS patients but not in controls. In normal brains, cytoplasmic HHV-6 antigens were found in gray matter neurons at low frequency.[6] In the brains of MS patients, the same monoclonal antibodies detected nuclear HHV-6 antigens in white matter oligodendrocytes of MS patients but not in controls, and the staining was more frequent near MS plaques than in uninvolved areas (Figure 36–4). These observations do not prove that HHV-6 is causally associated with MS, but are provocative and deserve follow-up.

HHV-6 and CFS. HHV-6 activity has been studied in CFS patients. Serologic studies have, in general, given equivocal results.[8] Higher average titers were found in patients with CFS than in matched controls in an immunoassay based on an expressed HHV-6 protein, p41.[29] Patients with other diseases, however, were not studied and a diagnostically useful cutoff was not identified. Interesting results have come from PCR studies of peripheral blood mononuclear cells (PBMC) from patients with CFS. Two groups have found that CFS

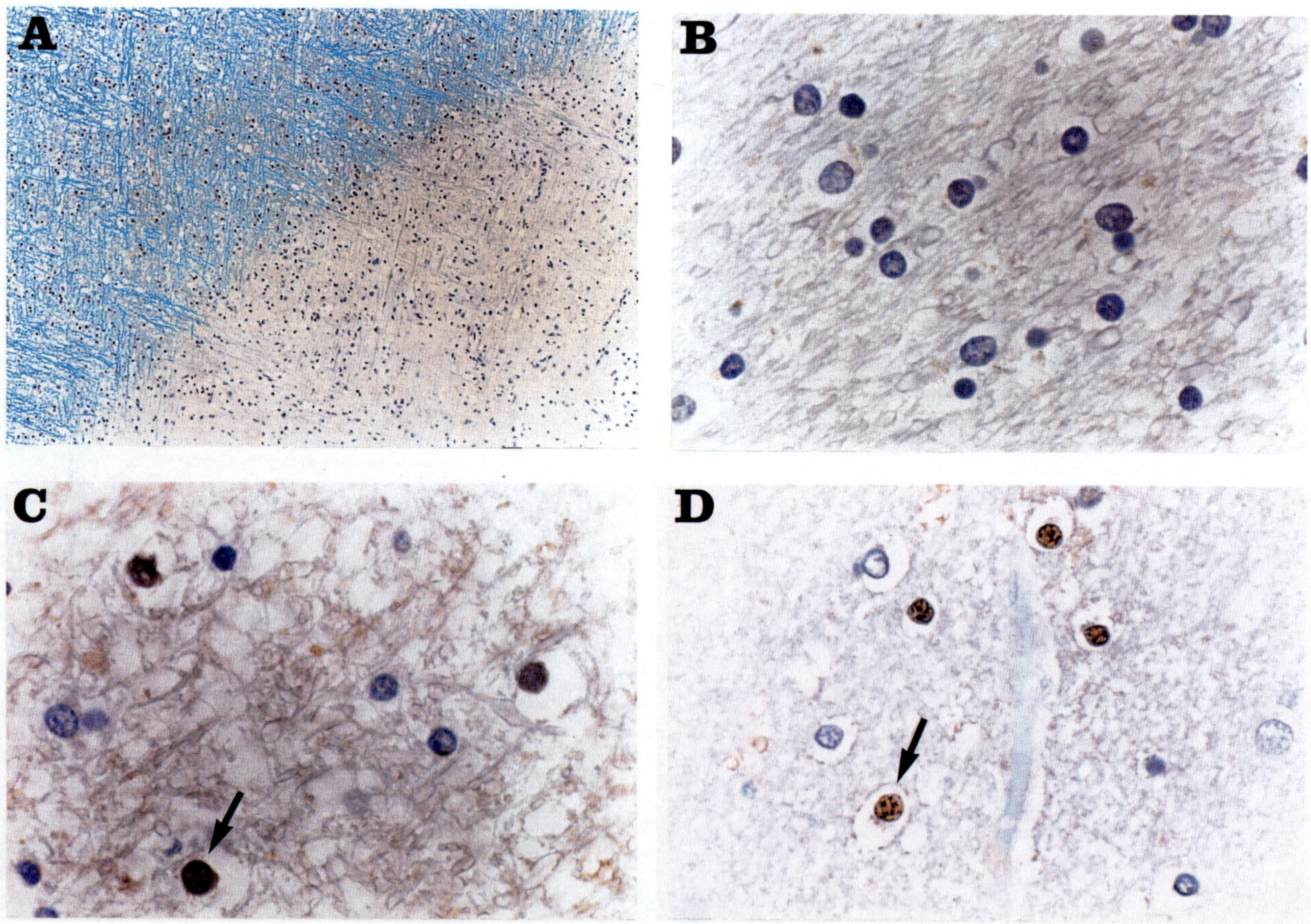

Figure 36–4. Immunocytochemical (ICC) localization of HHV-6 antigen in white matter from MS brain. (**A**) MS plaque stained for myelin with luxol fast blue (×25). Normal white matter is stained blue; the plaque is unstained. (**B–D**) Tissue stained with MAb to HHV-6B virion protein 101K, counterstained with hematoxylin (×250). (**B**) Normal white matter; oligodendrocytes are unstained. (**C**) MS plaque; nuclear staining of oligodendrocytes (*arrow*). (**D**) Focus of HHV-6 infection in apparently normal white matter from MS brain; nuclear staining of oligodendrocytes (*arrow*). *(Reprinted with permission from reference 6; photo courtesy of Peter Challoner.)*

patients were more likely than matched controls to be PCR positive for HHV-6A.[30,31] This is one of the few situations in which HHV-6A has been detected at a higher frequency than has HHV-6B (KS and pulmonary biopsies are the others), although less than one third of the CFS patients were positive for HHV-6A. The present evidence does not provide a compelling argument for a role for HHV-6 in CFS.

Pathology

Clinical manifestations associated with primary and chronic HHV-6 infection span a wide range. The overlap of these manifestations with those of illnesses that are either idiopathic or associated with other agents [eg, Epstein–Barr virus (EBV), HCMV, HHV-7, measles, and rubella] extends to the level of pathology. There is no identified clinical entity that can be diagnosed definitively as being HHV-6–associated without using HHV-6–specific assays and reagents (as discussed later, some patients with ES are associated with primary HHV-7 infection). This extends to the tissue level, where inflammation, inclusion bodies, syncytium, and necrosis are among the histologically observable features (Figures 36–2 and 36–5). In some patients, herpesvirus particles can be visualized by electron microscopy; this narrows the field of candidate organisms but does not implicate a specific herpesvirus.

Differential Diagnosis

HHV-6 should be considered in the differential diagnosis of febrile and/or exanthematous illness in children, particularly in those younger than 2 years of age. Approximately 50% of clinical diagnoses of measles or rubella that were not supported by laboratory results coincided with HHV-6 seroconversion.[32,33] Clinical features associated with primary HHV-6 infections that resulted in admission to a pediatric emergency department included fever (≥40°C), malaise or irritability, and inflamed tympanic membranes.[7] HHV-6 also should be considered in patients with lymphadenopathy who are EBV-negative and have a mononucleosis-like illness, including adults, as well as in patients with acute meningitis/encephalitis.[8,9]

In immunodeficient patients, HHV-6 should be considered in patients with pneumonitis, lymphadenopathy, rash and GVHD, acute renal transplant rejection, and bone marrow suppression in bone marrow transplant recipients.

Molecular Diagnosis

The standard array of molecular methods has been described for HHV-6, a limitation being their general lack of commercial availability. A complication in

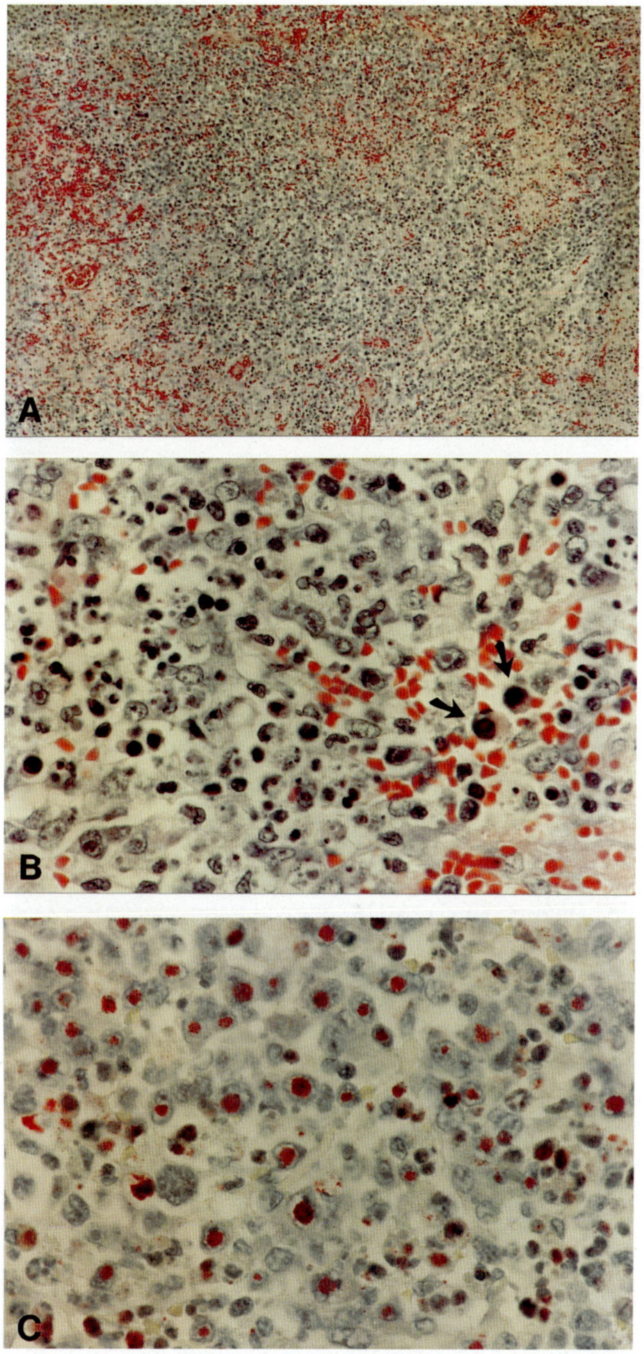

Figure 36–5. HHV-6 lymphadenitis. (**A**) A "punched out" central area of necrosis is seen surrounded by a peripheral transitional zone composed of granulation tissue [hematoxylin-eosin (H&E), × 125]. (**B**) High power magnification in the area of necrosis shows cells with intranuclear herpetic inclusions (*arrows*) interspersed with neutrophils and necrotic debris (H&E, ×900). (**C**) Area of necrosis probed for HHV-6 DNA by ISH (naphthol phosphate/fast red substrate with light hematoxylin counterstain, ×900). *(Courtesy of Sherif Zaki, Centers for Disease Control and Prevention).*

choosing molecular methods is that some reagents recognize both HHV-6A and HHV-6B, while others are variant-specific. For many purposes an initial screen with a cross-reactive assay followed by a variant-specific assay would be appropriate.

Plasmid clones suitable for use as probes for in situ or blot hybridization are available that span the HHV-6A and HHV-6B genomes.[34,35] Because of the close relationship between HHV-6A and HHV-6B, most plasmid clones efficiently cross-hybridize between the variants. Clones from the diploid portions of the genome offer the possibility of greater sensitivity. In situ hybridization methods have been used to study cases of encephalitis or encephalopathy,[36,37] Rosai–Dorfman syndrome,[38] and lymphadenitis (Figure 36–5).

PCR is widely used to study HHV-6; a host of primer combinations have been described. Well-characterized sets that allow for rapid variant discrimination are described.[26,39]

HHV-6 monoclonal antibodies are readily available. As with other reagents, some are variant-specific and some recognize both variants.[40,41] Monoclonal antibodies have been identified that react well in fixed-tissue sections[6,23,42] (Figure 36–4). Some of these antibodies are commercially available (Applied Biotechnologies, Inc., Columbia, MD; Chemicon International, Temecula, CA). Immunohistochemical analyses have proved useful in studying patients with encephalitis,[36,43] MS[6] (Figure 36–5), AIDS, demyelinating lesions[25] (Figure 36–3), chronic myelopathy,[44] renal transplant rejection,[19] pneumonitis[45,46,47] (Figure 36–2), and lymphadenopathy.[23]

Confirmational Diagnosis

Diagnosis of a pathologic involvement of HHV-6 in disease is seriously complicated by the high prevalence of the virus and its presence in the blood, saliva, and brains of healthy people. Even though HHV-6 can be detected in the blood of healthy people by PCR, virus is seldom cultured except during an active disease process such as ES or during posttransplant immunosuppression. Thus, positive viral cultures are strong indicators of viral activity. PCR positivity in plasma may be a surrogate marker for viremia.[48] Viral culture is usually performed by direct culture of phytohemagglutinin (PHA)-activated patient lymphocytes in the presence of interleukin-2 or by cocultivation with PHA-activated human umbilical cord blood lymphocytes, also in the presence of interleukin-2[49] (Figure 36–6). Some HHV-6 isolates have been adapted to grow in continuous T-cell lines, but initial passages normally replicate with very low efficiency in these cells; thus, they are not the best choice for diagnostic cultures.

An array of HHV-6 serodiagnostic methods has been described.[8,9] With respect to interpretation of HHV-6 serologic results, single serum specimens reveal little; given the prevalence of the virus, a positive result generally means that the patient is normal. Paired acute and convalescent specimens allow for comparison of antibody titers that may be indicative of viral activity. HHV-6 and HHV-7 are partially antigenically cross-reactive; thus, antigen adsorption steps are necessary to unambiguously differentiate HHV-6 from HHV-7 reactivity in immunofluorescent antibody (IFA) and enzyme linked immunosorbent assay (ELISA).[50] The major reactive HHV-6 protein in immunoblot assays (p100 or 101K)[26,51] is not cross-reactive with the major immunoreactive protein of HHV-7[50,52] and can serve as a sensitive and specific marker of HHV-6 infection. The utility of IgM assays is not clear, because as many as 5% of healthy adults are IgM seropositive at any given time.

Criteria to consider for diagnosing HHV-6 as the probable cause of a given pathologic state would include changes in status for relevant markers, consistency of the HHV-6 observations with other markers, the proximity of the HHV-6 activity to the affected tissues, and the absence of other agents.

Treatment

HHV-6 has greater in vitro susceptibility to ganciclovir and foscarnet than to acyclovir.[8,53] Although there have been several reports of the clinical use of ganciclovir, no controlled clinical trials have been reported. Transplant recipients with idiopathic pneumonitis, MS patients, and encephalitis patients are potential targets of HHV-6 antiviral therapy.[8]

HHV-7

HHV-7 was discovered in the laboratory of Dr. Niza Frenkel at the National Institutes of Health in 1990.[54] Much less is known about HHV-7 than about HHV-6. Within the herpesvirus family, HHV-6A and HHV-6B are genetically and biologically most closely related to HHV-7. Thus, HHV-7 also infects T lymphocytes. A difference is that HHV-7 uses the CD4 molecule as its cellular receptor[55]; the HHV-6 receptor has not been identified, but it is not CD4. The significance of this is that HIV-1 also uses CD4 as its receptor on T cells, thus the cell tropism of HHV-7 and HIV-1 might be even closer than that for HHV-6 and HIV-1. Further studies are needed to see whether this shared cell tropism has any effect on the course of AIDS. The clinical spectrum of HHV-7 is poorly defined, with primary HHV-7 infection being associated with some cases of roseola infantum and fever of unknown origin. The biology and molecular biology of HHV-7 have been reviewed.[56]

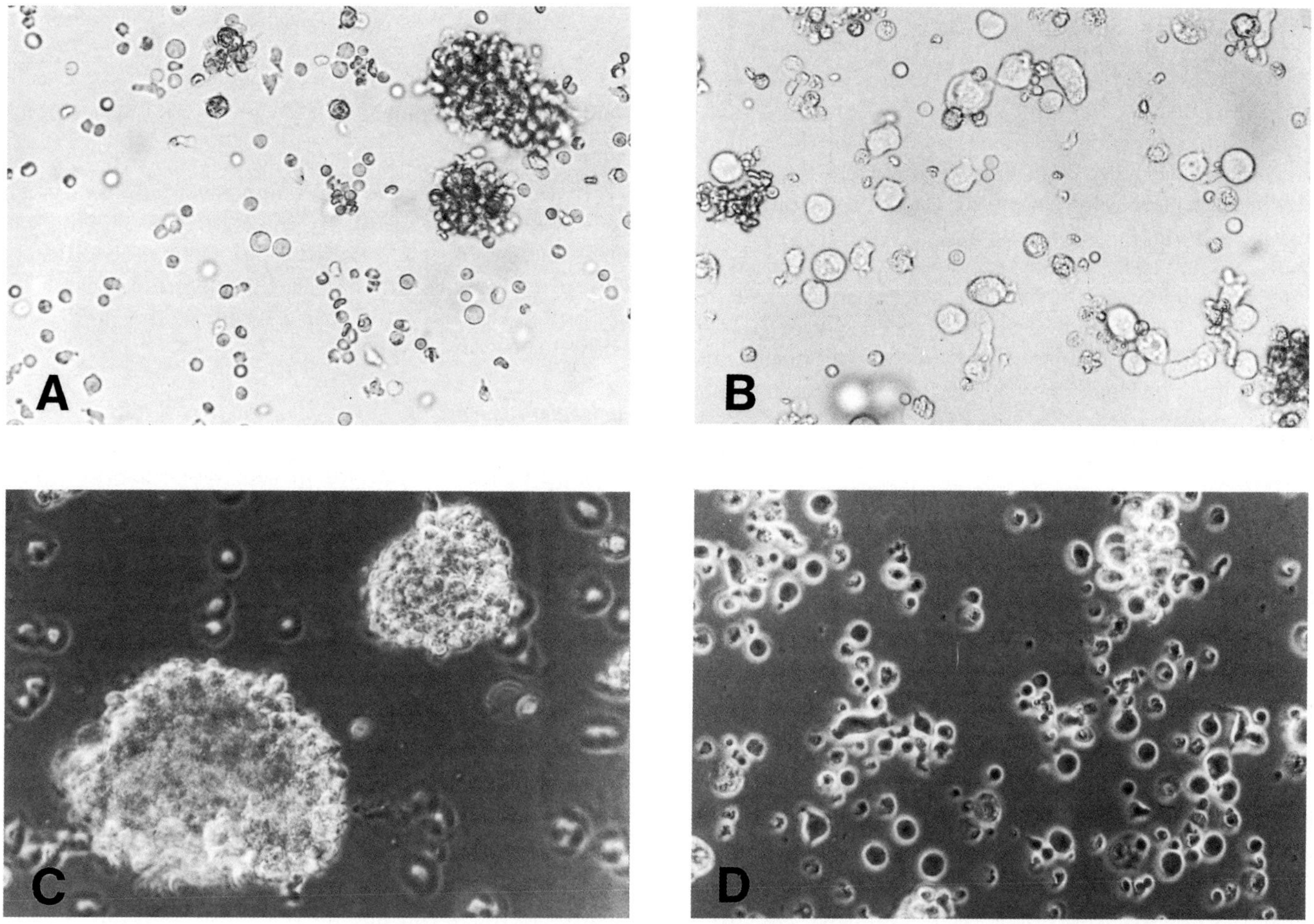

Figure 36–6. HHV-6 and HHV-7 cytopathic effects. (**A**) Uninfected human umbilical cord blood lymphocytes (CBL). The clumping is typical of healthy cultures (×40). (**B**) CBL infected with HHV-6B strain Z29. Infected cells are enlarged and refractile, and cell clumps have disaggregated (×40). (**C**) Uninfected CBL. As in **A**, the clumping is typical of healthy cultures (phase contrast, ×40). (**D**) CBL infected with HHV-7 strain SB. Infected cells are enlarged and refractile, and cell clumps have disaggregated (phase contrast, ×40). *(Courtesy of Jodi Black, Centers for Disease Control and Prevention.)*

Definition

HHV-7 is a member of the family *Herpesviridae,* subfamily *Betaherpesvirinae,* and genus *Roseolovirus.* Its closest relatives are HHV-6A and HHV-6B, followed by HCMV.

Geographic Distribution

Although not as well studied as HHV-6, all indications are that HHV-7 is widely distributed, with high seroprevalence observed in Japan, Brazil, Germany, Italy, the United Kingdom, and the United States.

Life Cycle/Natural History/Epidemiology

HHV-7 is a constitutive inhabitant of human saliva, with more than 75% of adults harboring infectious cell–free virus in their saliva at any given time.[57–59] Thus, it is likely that the major route of HHV-7 transmission is saliva. The details of primary HHV-7 infection are not well known. As mentioned previously, CD4 is a component of the HHV-7 receptor. The extent to which other molecules could serve as HHV-7 receptors in other cell types is not known. An important part of HHV-7 natural history is its interaction with HHV-6. HHV-7 is able to activate latent HHV-6 from peripheral blood lymphocytes.[54,60] How this contributes to pathology associated with either virus is not clear, but it has been hypothesized that the ES-like illnesses that have been described in association with primary HHV-7 infection may be reactivations of latent HHV-6.[56]

As with HHV-6, HHV-7 normally is acquired early in life, but most people acquire HHV-6 before HHV-7.[50,61,62] More than 80% of adults in some populations are HHV-7 seropositive. In contrast with HHV-6, more people experience their primary HHV-7 infection in late childhood and through the young adult years. It is likely that the clinical spectrum and severity of primary infection differs between these age groups. The differences in epidemiology between HHV-6 and HHV-7 are difficult to understand. Infectious HHV-6 is present in saliva at lower frequency than is HHV-7, yet HHV-6 is normally the first to be acquired. The slower climb of HHV-7 to near-universal prevalence is similarly difficult to rationalize. Prior infection with either HHV-6 or HHV-7 may modulate the course of primary infection with the other virus, because the viruses are immunologically partially cross-reactive.[50,61,63]

Morphology

HHV-7 shares the morphologic features of herpesviruses that were described for HHV-6[54,56,64] (Figure 36–1).

Clinical Features

HHV-7 prevalence in adults exceeds 80%, and nearly all seropositive adults constitutively secrete infectious virus in their saliva, indicating that HHV-7 establishes long-term latent or persistent infections. HHV-7 has not been extensively studied and the spectrum of HHV-7–associated disease has not been defined. This spectrum begins with primary infection and spans the range of diseases that might occur due to chronic disease or during immunosuppression.

Primary HHV-7 infections have been defined by seroconversion and by viral culture from patient PBMC. The relatively early age of acquisition of HHV-7 antibodies has led to study of acute diseases in young children. Primary HHV-7 infection is associated with a subset (approximately 10%) of ES cases that are clinically indistinguishable from HHV-6–associated ES.[65–68] Observations relating to HHV-7 activity have been reported on fewer than 100 patients; therefore, subtle differences in clinical profiles may not have been detectable. Consistent with in vitro results indicating that HHV-7 can reactivate HHV-6 from latency,[56] several children who had prior HHV-6–associated ES were culture-positive for both HHV-6 and HHV-7 during their HHV-7 conversion event.[65,66,68] Neurologic complications have been reported during illness associated with primary HHV-7 infection, including febrile convulsions and acute infantile hemiplegia.[67,69]

HCMV, HHV-6, and HHV-7 activities were monitored by PCR of PBMC from renal transplant recipients.[70] There was increased risk of development of cytomegalovirus (CMV)-disease when HCMV activity was concurrent with activity of either HHV-7 alone or HHV-7 plus HHV-6.

Pathology and Diagnosis

The pathology of HHV-7–associated disease has not been described. Differential diagnosis of illness associated with HHV-7 primary infection should include measles and rubella, because approximately 10% of clinical measles or rubella cases that were unable to be confirmed in the laboratory[32] were associated with HHV-7 seroconversions.

Molecular Diagnosis

DNA-based HHV-7 diagnostic tools include an HHV-7 plasmid probe suitable for in situ hybridization[58] (Figure 36–7), a set of PCR primers,[71] and a quantitative assay based on the PCR primers.[72]

Several monoclonal antibodies to HHV-7 have been described[59,65,73]; some of these cross-react with HHV-6 and some HHV-6 monoclonal antibodies cross-react with HHV-7.[58,61,73]

Confirmational Diagnosis

As with HHV-6, interpretation of HHV-7 diagnostic assays must take into account the high prevalence of HHV-7 and its presence in the blood and saliva of healthy people.

Some HHV-7 isolates have been adapted for growth in the T-cell line SupT1,[71] but the utility of this cell line for primary isolation has not been studied. Thus, PHA-activated primary human umbilical cord blood lymphocytes grown in the presence of IL-2 are the cells of choice for HHV-7 isolation (Figure 36–6). The ability of HHV-7 to activate latent HHV-6 makes adult peripheral blood lymphocytes less useful because of the possibility of outgrowth of endogenous HHV-6.

ELISA, IFA, syncytia-inhibition, and immunoblot assays have been described for detection of antibodies to HHV-7.[50,61,62,64,74] There is sufficient cross-reactivity with HHV-6 to cause confusion in some specimens, and antigen adsorption steps are needed to eliminate ambiguity in IFA and ELISA.[50] An HHV-7 encoded protein of 85 to 89 kDa apparent molecular weight is the most strongly reactive protein in immunoblots with human sera and is not cross-reactive with the major antigenic protein of HHV-6; thus, it appears to be a sensitive and specific serologic marker for HHV-7 infection.[50,52]

As with HHV-6, the criteria to consider for diagnosing HHV-7 as the probable cause of a given pathologic state include changes in status for relevant markers, consistency of the HHV-7 observations with other markers, the proximity of the HHV-7 activity to the affected tissues, and the absence of other agents.

Treatment

HHV-7 antiviral susceptibility has not been studied in detail, and clinical situations in which HHV-7 therapy would be indicated have not been defined. Preliminary results indicate that, in vitro, the virus is more susceptible to ganciclovir and foscarnet than to acyclovir[72]; (J. Black and P. Feorino, personal communication).

HHV-8

HHV-8 was discovered by Drs. Yuan Chang and Patrick Moore and coworkers at Columbia University in 1994.[75] Of the human herpesviruses, HHV-8 is most closely related to EBV and belongs in the gammaherpesvirus subfamily, other members of which have the ability to transform cells to a malignant phenotype. HHV-8 was

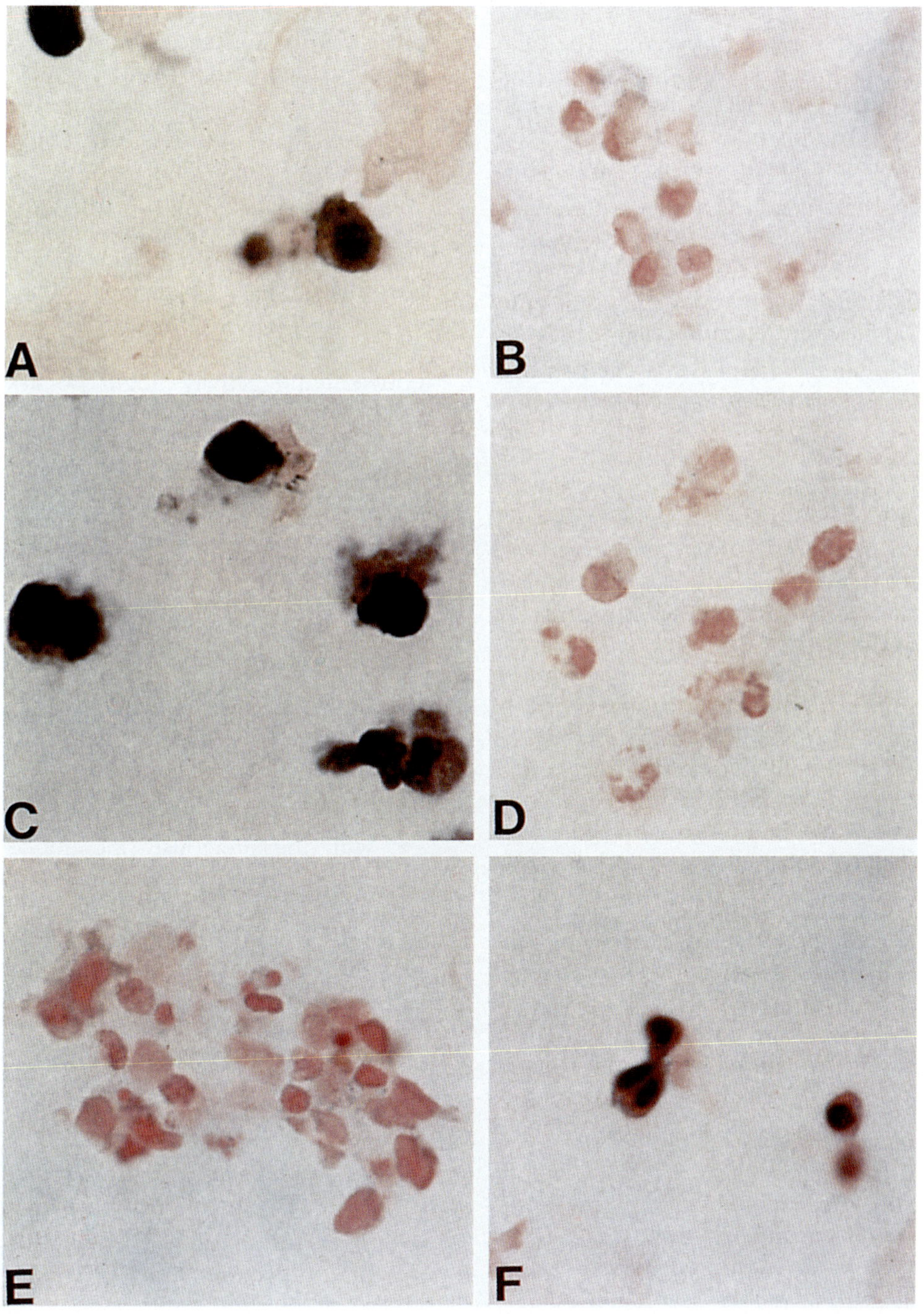

Figure 36–7. CBL infected with HHV-6A(U1102) (**A** and **B**), HHV-6B(Z29) (**C** and **D**), or HHV-7(SB) (**E** and **F**) were prepared for in situ hybridization as described in reference 58. **A, C,** and **E** were reacted with a cocktail of HHV-6 clones; **B, D,** and **E** were reacted with the HHV-7 clone pH7SB-268. *(Reprinted with permission from reference 58.)*

discovered in AIDS-associated Kaposi's sarcoma lesions and has subsequently been found in all forms of Kaposi's sarcoma as well as in other diseases with associated vascular hyperplasia, including multicentric Castleman's disease (MCD), angioimmunoblastic lymphadenopathy (AILD), and benign lymphadenopathies. In addition, HHV-8 has been associated specifically with a rare AIDS-associated lymphoma known as body cavity–based lymphoma (BCBL). Both HHV-8 and EBV are present in many BCBL, although HHV-8–positive/EBV-negative examples have been observed. The relative roles of the two viruses in the disease are not known. The identification of HHV-8 as the possible cause of Kaposi's sarcoma provides a route to treating the disease with antiviral therapy after drugs active against the virus are identified.

Definition

HHV-8 is a member of the family *Herpesviridae,* subfamily *Gammaherpesvirinae,* genus *Rhadinovirus.* Its closest relative is a simian herpesvirus, herpesvirus saimiri (HVS).[75,76] The most closely related human herpesvirus is EBV.

Synonyms

HHV-8 is also known as Kaposi's sarcoma–associated herpesvirus (KSHV).

Geographic Distribution

HHV-8 has been detected in Africa, Europe, North and South America, and Asia. Fine-grained descriptions of its distribution await development of reliable and simplified methods for measuring prevalence.

Life Cycle/Natural History/Epidemiology

Little is known of the HHV-8 life cycle. Based on its genetic similarity with HVS and EBV, it is anticipated that the virus can establish latency and in some manner immortalize cells. Some hints in this direction come from cell lines established from cases of BCBL. These cell lines have come in two major forms, one form in which both HHV-8 and EBV are present, and another that lacks EBV.[77–79] Viral DNA obtained from such cells has an apparent length of 270 kb,[76,80] which may represent dimers of the unit length HHV-8 genome. Transcription from the HHV-8 genome in BCBL cells is highly restricted, as would be expected for a latent infection. The phorbol ester 12-o-tetradecanoyl phorbol-13-acetate (TPA) can be used to induce the lytic cycle. After induction, much of the genome becomes transcriptionally active, viral DNA replicates to higher abundance, and intracellular and extracellular herpesvirus particles can be detected by electron microscopy.[78]

Two important and intertwined questions about HHV-8 epidemiology involve its prevalence and route(s) of transmission. Current evidence can be interpreted in two incompatible ways: 1) HHV-8 is a low-prevalence virus and a high percentage of people infected with HHV-8 develop KS, or 2) HHV-8 is at least moderately prevalent and additional factors are needed for KS. The divergent viewpoints on this subject are indicators that current diagnostic assays for HHV-8 have not been standardized and may be insensitive. Viral prevalence is commonly measured serologically; HHV-8 serology is in its infancy. Immunofluorescence and immunoblot assays detected HHV-8 antibodies in fewer than 70% of KS patients.[81] If KS is an extreme manifestation of HHV-8 disease, then the inability of the current generation of assays to detect HHV-8 antibodies in more than 30% of KS patients suggests that the assays are insufficiently sensitive to provide reliable estimates of viral prevalence in the general population, in which reduced viral activity might be associated with less intense immune stimulation.

PCR has been used to assess the tissue distribution of HHV-8 in various populations, and PCR results have been used to estimate HHV-8 prevalence in the absence of widely available and sensitive serologic methods. The limitations of PCR for this purpose are 1) the problem of what and how much of a tissue to sample, 2) the sensitivity of the PCR assay employed, and 3) the possibility of a false-positive result caused by PCR contamination. Thus, negative results can be due to any or all of the following: sampling a tissue the virus does not inhabit, sampling too little of a given tissue,[82] or employing an insensitive PCR assay. Positive results can be from PCR contamination.

With the previously mentioned caveats in mind and in anticipation that the interpretive boundaries and limitations of the present generation of HHV-8 diagnostic assays will be defined and surpassed, following is a summary of what is known about HHV-8 prevalence and tissue distribution.

As mentioned, serologic assays (IFA and immunoblot) have been developed based on cell lines that contain both EBV and HHV-8,[76,81] but they have not yet been applied to serosurveys of the general population.

Many body fluids and tissues have been screened by PCR for HHV-8 DNA, which has been detected most frequently in materials from KS patients, followed by HIV-1–infected patients without KS and transplant recipients. In KS patients, HHV-8 DNA has been detected in KS lesions, uninvolved skin, bronchoalveolar lavage (BAL) specimens from patients with pulmonary KS, PBMC, CD19-positive lymphocytes, bone marrow, sensory ganglia, prostate, and semen.[75,83–92]

Thus, in KS patients the virus is widely distributed in the body. HHV-8 DNA has been detected also in lymph nodes from patients with MCD.[93–96] Although many laboratories have reported negative results for detecting HHV-8 in materials obtained from healthy donors,[75,84,86,87,90,97] some laboratories, however, have reported detecting HHV-8 DNA in hyperplastic tonsils, prostate, kidney, cervical, and vulvar tissues as well as skin, foreskin, semen, and PBMC of healthy donors,[82,85,97,98] as well as in non-KS skin lesions of HIV-negative transplant recipients.[99] As described previously, there is an array of possible explanations for the discrepant results.

Detection of HHV-8 DNA in both male and female genital tissues and fluids suggests the possibility of sexual transmission, as well as transmission during birth. The latter possibility is consistent with observations made among a group of 100 Ugandan children with KS.[100] There were two major patterns of KS distribution, oro–facial and inguinal–genital, suggesting that the causative agent, possibly HHV-8, can be transmitted via mucosal routes, perhaps during birth or breastfeeding.

KS is prevalent in central and eastern Africa and in southeastern Europe; elevated incidence rates have been noted since the mid-1950s, much of the increase being associated with organ transplantation and AIDS.[100,101] The epidemiology of KS suggests an infectious and sexually transmissible cause; an agent other than HIV-1 was suggested to be involved in AIDS–KS, with oral–fecal contact being a risk factor.[101,102] The epidemiology of AIDS–KS suggests the recent spread of the KS agent in the human population, the movement of the agent closely tracking the spread of HIV-1, with the exception that KS is rarely transmitted by blood and even more rarely by blood products. Thus, KS is relatively rare in intravenous drug abusers and extremely rare in hemophiliacs, even though HHV-8 can be detected in the PBMC of KS patients. It is convenient to think that presence of HHV-8 corresponds to the probable development of KS,[87,90] but such a hypothesis does not account for the source of HHV-8 that is in transplant-associated KS and in the variety of tissues and fluids from HIV-negative persons described previously. It is probable that HHV-8 has at least moderate prevalence in the population, sufficient to act as a reservoir. The development of KS or any of the other diseases that might be caused by HHV-8 would be a consequence of any or all of the following: host factors, age, route of acquisition, and environmental factors. HHV-8 is an ancient virus[76]; this does not preclude recent introduction into humans, but that possibility seems remote given the narrow host range of most herpesviruses, especially gammaherpesviruses.

Morphology

In chemically induced cultures of the BCBL-1 cell line, the herpesvirus particles visible by electron microscopy have a diameter of approximately 100 nm and have the morphologic features expected of herpesviruses[78] (Figure 36–1).

Clinical Features

The major clinical associations for HHV-8 are all four forms of KS (classic or Mediterranean, African endemic, posttransplant, and AIDS-associated),[75,88,89,92,103] MCD,[93,95,96,104] angioimmunoblastic lymphadenopathy,[104] and BCBL.[77–79] HHV-8 has been detected in both HIV-positive and HIV-negative examples of each form, sometimes in association with other herpesviruses (EBV, HCMV, and HHV-6). In addition, in HIV-negative patients, HHV-8 has been detected in lymphadenopathies characterized by a predominantly follicular lesion, with giant germinal center hyperplasia and increased vascularity, resembling MCD.[104] As noted by Luppi and coworkers,[104] these HHV-8–associated lesions (except BCBL) share the property of vascular hyperplasia. Patients with MCD have increased likelihood of developing KS.[105] HHV-8 also has been detected in patients with follicular B-cell lymphoma associated with KS[106] and angiosarcoma in an HIV-negative patient.[107] The proximity of HHV-8 to diseased tissues is not of itself proof of cause; further study is required to determine whether the virus is present because of necessity or opportunity.

Pathology

KS

KS is a spindle-celled, vascular neoplasm that most often occurs in the skin, but can also affect mucosal, lymphoid, and visceral tissues. KS lesions are reddish-purple to brown, and early lesions can be difficult to recognize, sometimes resembling petechiae. Later, macules, papules, and nodules are common, sometimes simultaneously. Lesions can exceed several cm in diameter and eventually coalesce into larger masses. Histologically, KS lesions are characterized by proliferating spindle cells and vascular spaces lined with endothelial cells. Red blood cells can fill the vascular spaces and hemosiderin deposits are common. Late lesions may be predominantly angiomatous, spindle cell nodules, or mixed. Predisposing factors to KS include immune dysfunction, local inflammation, and previous trauma or infection (the Koebner phenomenon).[100]

By PCR–in situ hybridization, HHV-8 has been detected in both the spindle and endothelial cells that line the vascular spaces[108] (Figure 36–8). Transcripts of an HHV-8 structural gene have been detected in KS

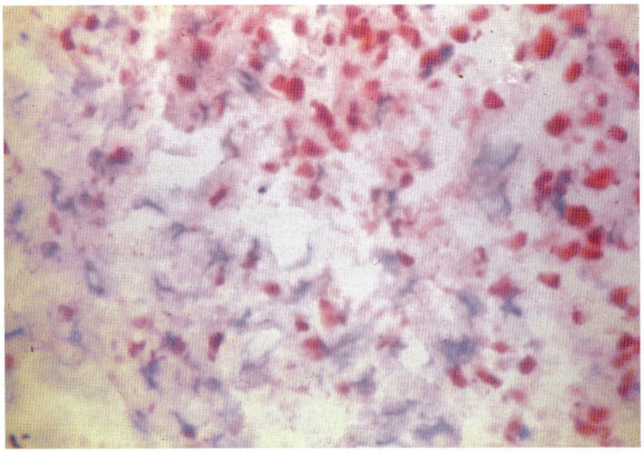

Figure 36–8. PCR–in situ hybridization of HHV-8 in a KS spindle cell nodule. The majority of spindle cells are positive for HHV-8. Methods used were as described in reference 108. *(Photograph courtesy of Chris Boshoff and Robin Weiss, Institute of Cancer Research.)*

lesions, suggesting that lytic viral replication may be taking place in at least a subset of cells.[103,109] This is consistent with sporadic reports dating back to 1972 of the visualization by electron microscopy of herpesvirus particles in cultured African KS cells[110] and in KS lesions.[111] Given the occasional detection of herpesviruses other than KS in KS lesions, immunoelectron microscopy is required to establish unequivocally the presence of HHV-8 virions in KS tissues.

The cellular biology of KS has been studied predominantly in cultured cells from specimens of KS. HHV-8 DNA has been detected by PCR only during early passages of such cells.[86,112] Cells cultured from KS lesions can have a spindle cell phenotype similar to a fibrocytic subset of the spindle cells that are present in KS lesions (positive for the fibroblastic antigen TE7 and smooth-muscle–specific alpha-actin, and negative for leukocytic and endothelial antigens).[113] It is possible that HHV-8–harboring or –susceptible cells are lost quickly and that the surviving selected cells do not represent the totality of cellular events in KS lesions.

Lymphadenopathies

MCD is defined as a plasma-cell type of Castleman's disease (an angiogenic, lymph node follicular hyperplasia) that presents as an idiopathic lymphoproliferative disease with multisystem involvement.[105] HHV-8 involvement in MCD has been studied by PCR of DNA extracted from biopsies, and the cellular localization of HHV-8 in MCD lesions has not been reported. HHV-8–associated AILDs have the histologic appearance of classic AILD.[104] As mentioned, HHV-8 DNA has been detected in HIV-negative patients in lymphadenopathies resembling MCD that are characterized by a predominantly follicular lesion, with giant germinal center hyperplasia and increased vascularity.[104]

BCBL

BCBL, also known as primary effusion lymphomas, are characterized by their confinement to body cavities, the absence of an identifiable tumor mass, clonal immunoglobulin rearrangements suggestive of a B-cell origin, an indeterminate immunophenotype, no c-*myc* rearrangements, complex karyotypes, and frequent presence of EBV.[77,79,114] HHV-8 DNA can be present at 40 to 80 genomes per cell, a much higher load than in KS lesions.[77,114]

Differential Diagnosis

Early lesions of KS are difficult to definitively identify histologically. In a series of 155 benign and malignant vascular lesions, only the 17 KS cases were positive for HHV-8 by PCR, indicating that PCR can be useful for differential diagnosis of early KS.[115] HHV-8–associated BCBL can be distinguished from other lymphomas by the criteria described previously. HHV-8 should be considered in the differential diagnosis of lymphadenopathies.

Diagnosis

The principal tool for diagnosis of HHV-8 in pathologic specimens has been PCR. Several primer sets have been described. The most commonly used set was described in the original paper on HHV-8.[75] It amplifies a 233 bp segment of a minor capsid protein. Nested primers that bracket this primer set as well as additional sets have been described.[84,85,90,98] In situ hybridization with a 25 bp oligomer, and IFA with AIDS–KS patient serum have been used to detect HHV-8 in cultured cells,[76] but these methods have not been applied to pathologic materials. Nonisotopic in situ hybridization with either a 918 bp cloned fragment of HHV-8 or a 30 bp oligomer were too insensitive to detect HHV-8 in KS biopsies; PCR–in situ hybridization was required[108] (Figure 36–8).

Conditions have not been identified for reliable culture of HHV-8 from clinical materials other than HHV-8–associated BCBL. Cultured cells obtained from KS biopsies have not proved useful for HHV-8 propagation. HHV-8 has been passaged to a limited extent from BCBL-derived cell lines into several cell lines and primary cell cultures, including CD19+ B-cells, but viral growth was at such a low level that PCR was needed to monitor the cultures.[76,80]

As mentioned previously, HHV-8 serology is in its infancy. IFA and immunoblot assays that employ antigens expressed in BCBL cell lines that are dually infected with HHV-8 and EBV have been described.[76,81]

As interpretation of such assays becomes more refined and more sensitive serologic assays are developed, they are likely to prove useful in confirming KS and for monitoring development of KS in at-risk patients.

Treatment

In one study, AIDS patients who for any reason received the drug foscarnet, which is active against other herpesviruses, developed KS less frequently than did others.[116] It remains to be determined whether this effect was due to activity of the drug on HHV-8.

REFERENCES

1. Salahuddin SZ, Ablashi DV, Markham PD, et al. Isolation of a new virus, HBLV, in patients with lymphoproliferative disorders. *Science.* 1986;234:596–601.
2. Ablashi D, Agut H, Berneman Z, et al. Human herpesvirus-6 strain groups: a nomenclature. *Arch Virol.* 1993;129:363–366.
3. Lusso P, De Maria A, Malnati M, et al. Induction of CD4 and susceptibility to HIV-1 infection in human CD8+ T lymphocytes by human herpesvirus 6. *Nature.* 1991; 349:533–535.
4. Lusso P, Garzino-Demo A, Crowley RW, Malnati MS. Infection of gamma/delta T lymphocytes by human herpesvirus 6: transcriptional induction of CD4 and susceptibility to HIV infection. *J Exp Med.* 1995;181:1303–1310.
5. Luppi M, Barozzi P, Maiorana A, Marasca R, Torelli G. Human herpesvirus 6 infection in normal human brain tissue. *J Infect Dis.* 1994;169:943–944.
6. Challoner PB, Smith KT, Parker JD, et al. Plaque-associated expression of human herpesvirus 6 in multiple sclerosis. *Proc Natl Acad Sci USA.* 1995;92:7440–7444.
7. Hall CB, Long CE, Schnabel KC, et al. Human herpesvirus-6 infection in children. A prospective study of complications and reactivation. *N Engl J Med.* 1994;331: 432–438.
8. Braun DK, Dominguez G, Pellett PE. Human herpesvirus 6. *Clin Microbiol Rev.* 1996; in press.
9. Pellett PE, Black JB. Human herpesvirus 6. In: Fields BN, Knipe DM, Howley PM, et al, eds. *Fields Virology.* Vol. 2. Philadelphia: Lippincott–Raven Publishers; 1996.
10. Takahashi K, Sonoda S, Higashi K, et al. Predominant CD4 T-lymphocyte tropism of human herpesvirus 6-related virus. *J Virol.* 1989;63:3161–3163.
11. Kondo K, Kondo T, Okuno T, Takahashi M, Yamanishi K. Latent human herpesvirus 6 infection of human monocytes/macrophages. *J Gen Virol.* 1991;72:1401–1408.
12. Roffman E, Albert JP, Goff JP, Frenkel N. Putative site for the acquisition of human herpesvirus 6 virion tegument. *J Virol.* 1990;64:6308–6313.
13. Nii S, Yoshida M, Uno F, Kurata T, Ikuta K, Yamanishi K. Replication of human herpesvirus 6 (HHV-6): morphological aspects. *Adv Exp Med Biol.* 1990;278:19–28.
14. Fredricks DN, Relman DA. Sequence-based identification of microbial pathogens: a reconsideration of Koch's postulates. *Clin Microbiol Rev.* 1996;9:18–33.
15. Griffiths P. Studies on the etiology of exanthema subitum (roseola infantum). *Rev Med Virol.* 1995;5:1–6.
16. Yamanishi K, Okuno T, Shiraki K, et al. Identification of human herpesvirus-6 as a causal agent for exanthem subitum. *Lancet.* 1988;1:1065–1067.
17. Cone RW, Huang ML, Hackman RC. Human herpesvirus 6 and pneumonia. *Leukemia & Lymphoma.* 1994;15: 235–241.
18. Okuno T, Higashi K, Shiraki K, et al. Human herpesvirus 6 infection in renal transplantation. *Transplantation.* 1990;49:519–522.
19. Hoshino K, Nishi T, Adachi H, et al. Human herpesvirus-6 infection in renal allografts: retrospective immunohistochemical study in Japanese recipients. *Transplant International.* 1995;8:169–173.
20. Kikuta H, Lu H, Tomizawa K, Matsumoto S. Enhancement of human herpesvirus 6 replication in adult human lymphocytes by monoclonal antibody of CD3. *J Infect Dis.* 1990;161:1085–1087.
21. Lusso P, Ensoli B, Markham PD, et al. Productive dual infection of human CD4+ T lymphocytes by HIV-1 and HHV-6. *Nature.* 1989;337:370–373.
22. Di Luca D, Secchiero P, Bovenzi P, et al. Reciprocal in vitro interactions between human herpesvirus-6 and HIV-1 Tat. *AIDS.* 1991;5:1095–1098.
23. Knox KK, Carrigan DR. Active HHV-6 infection in the lymph nodes of HIV infected patients: in vitro evidence that HHV-6 can break HIV latency. *J AIDS Hum Retrovirol.* 1996;11:370–378.
24. Knox KK, Carrigan DR. Disseminated active HHV-6 infections in patients with AIDS. *Lancet.* 1994;343: 577–578.
25. Knox KK, Carrigan DR. Active human herpesvirus (HHV-6) infection of the central nervous system in patients with AIDS. *J AIDS Hum Retrovirol.* 1995;9:69–73.
26. Cone RW, Huang M-LW, Hackman RC, Corey L. Coinfection with human herpesvirus 6 variants A and B in lung tissue. *J Clin Microbiol.* 1996;34:877–881.
27. Di Luca D, Dolcetti R, Mirandola P, et al. Human herpesvirus 6: a survey of presence and variant distribution in normal peripheral lymphocytes and lymphoproliferative disorders. *J Infect Dis.* 1994;170:211–215.
28. Steinman L. Multiple sclerosis: a coordinated immunological attack against myelin in the central nervous system. *Cell.* 1996;85:299–302.
29. Patnaik M, Komaroff AL, Conley E, Ojo-Amaize EA, Peter JB. Prevalence of IgM antibodies to human herpesvirus 6 early antigen (p41/38) in patients with chronic fatigue syndrome. *J Infect Dis.* 1995;172:1264–1267.
30. Di Luca D, Zorzenon M, Mirandola P, Colle R, Botta GA, Cassai E. Human herpesvirus 6 and human herpesvirus 7 in chronic fatigue syndrome. *J Clin Microbiol.* 1995;33: 1660–1661.
31. Yalcin S, Kuratsune H, Yamaguchi K, Kitani T, Yamanishi K. Prevalence of human herpesvirus 6 variants A and B in patients with chronic fatigue syndrome. *Microbiol Immunol.* 1994;38:587–590.
32. Black JB, Durigon E, Kite-Powell K, et al. HHV-6 and

HHV-7 seroconversion in children clinically diagnosed with measles or rubella. *Clin Infect Dis.* 1996; in press.
33. Tait DR, Ward KN, Brown DWG, Miller E. Measles and rubella misdiagnosed in infants as exanthem subitum (roseola infantum). *Brit Med J.* 1996;312:101–102.
34. Martin MED, Thomson BJ, Honess RW, et al. The genome of human herpesvirus 6: maps of unit-length and concatemeric genomes for nine restriction endonucleases. *J Gen Virol.* 1991;72:157–168.
35. Lindquester GJ, Inoue N, Allen RD, et al. Restriction endonuclease mapping and molecular cloning of the human herpesvirus 6 variant B strain Z29 genome. *Arch Virol.* 1996;141:367–379.
36. Drobyski WR, Knox KK, Majewski D, Carrigan DR. Fatal encephalitis due to variant B human herpesvirus-6 infection in a bone marrow–transplant recipient. *N Engl J Med.* 1994;330;1356–1360.
37. Saito Y, Sharer LR, Dewhurst S, Blumberg BM, Hall CB, Epstein LG. Cellular localization of human herpesvirus-6 in the brains of children with AIDS encephalopathy. *J Neurovirol.* 1995;1:30–39.
38. Levine PH, Jahan N, Murari P, Manak M, Jaffe ES. Detection of human herpesvirus 6 in tissues involved by sinus histiocytosis with massive lymphadenopathy (Rosai–Dorfman disease). *J Infect Dis.* 1992;166:291–295.
39. Yamamoto T, Mukai T, Kondo K, Yamanishi K. Variation of DNA sequence in immediate-early gene of human herpesvirus 6 and variant identification by PCR. *J Clin Microbiol.* 1994;32:473–476.
40. Foà-Tomasi L, Avitabile E, Campadelli-Fiume G. Selection of a monoclonal antibody specific for variant B human herpesvirus 6–infected mononuclear cells. *J Virol Methods.* 1995;51:289–296.
41. Ablashi DV, Balachandran N, Josephs SF, et al. Genomic polymorphism, growth properties, and immunologic variations in human herpesvirus-6 isolates. *Virology.* 1991;184:545–552.
42. Yamamoto M, Black JB, Stewart JA, Lopez C, Pellett PE. Identification of a nucleocapsid protein as a specific serological marker of human herpesvirus 6 infection. *J Clin Microbiol.* 1990;28:1957–1962.
43. Knox KK, Harrington DP, Carrigan DR. Fulminant human herpesvirus six encephalitis in a human immunodeficiency virus–infected infant. *J Med Virol.* 1995;45: 288–292.
44. MacKenzie IR, Carrigan DR, Wiley CA. Chronic myleopathy associated with human herpesvirus-6. *Neurology.* 1995;45:2015–2017.
45. Carrigan DR. Human herpesvirus-6 and bone marrow transplantation. In: Ablashi DV, Krueger GRF, Salahuddin SZ, eds. *Human Herpesvirus-6: Epidemiology, Molecular Biology, and Clinical Pathology.* Amsterdam: Elsevier; 1992.
46. Carrigan DR, Drobyski WR, Russler SK, Tapper MA, Knox KK, Ash RC. Interstitial pneumonitis associated with human herpesvirus-6 infection after marrow transplantation. *Lancet.* 1991;338:147–149.
47. Pitalia AK, Liu-Yin JA, Freemont AJ, Morris DJ, Fitzmaurice RJ. Immunohistological detection of human herpesvirus 6 in formalin-fixed, paraffin-embedded lung tissues. *J Med Virol.* 1993;41:103–107.
48. Secchiero P, Carrigan DR, Asano Y, et al. Detection of human herpesvirus 6 in plasma of children with primary infection and immunosuppressed patients by polymerase chain reaction. *J Infect Dis.* 1995;171:273–280.
49. Black JB, Sanderlin KC, Goldsmith CS, Gary HE, Lopez C, Pellett PE. Growth properties of human herpesvirus-6 strain Z29. *J Virol Methods.* 1989;26:133–145.
50. Black JB, Schwarz TF, Patton JL, et al. Evaluation of immunoassays for detection of antibodies to human herpesvirus 7. *Clin Diag Lab Immunol.* 1996;3:79–83.
51. Hashida T, Komura E, Yoshida M, et al. Hepatitis in association with human herpesvirus-7 infection. *Pediatrics.* 1995;96:783–785.
52. Foà-Tomasi L, Fiorilli MP, Avitabile E, Campadelli-Fiume G. Identification of an 85 kDa phosphoprotein as an immunodominant protein specific for human herpesvirus 7–infected cells. *J Gen Virol.* 1996;77:511–518.
53. Williams MV. HHV-6: response to antiviral agents. In: Ablashi DV, Krueger GRF, Salahuddin SZ, eds. *Human Herpesvirus-6: Epidemiology, Molecular Biology, and Clinical Pathology.* Amsterdam: Elsevier; 1992.
54. Frenkel N, Schirmer EC, Wyatt LS, et al. Isolation of a new herpesvirus from CD4+ T cells. *Proc Natl Acad Sci USA.* 1990;87:748–752.
55. Lusso P, Secchiero P, Crowley RW, Garzino-Demo A, Berneman ZN, Gallo RC. CD4 is a critical component of the receptor for human herpesvirus 7: interference with human immunodeficiency virus. *Proc Natl Acad Sci USA.* 1994;91:3872–3876.
56. Frenkel N, Roffman E. Human herpesvirus 7. In: Fields BN, Knipe DM, Howley PM, et al., eds. *Fields Virology.* Vol. 2. Philadelphia: Lippincott–Raven; 1996.
57. Wyatt LS, Frenkel N. Human herpesvirus 7 is a constitutive inhabitant of adult human saliva. *J Virol.* 1992;66: 3206–3209.
58. Black JB, Inoue N, Kite-Powell K, Zaki S, Pellett PE. Frequent isolation of human herpesvirus 7 from saliva. *Virus Res.* 1993;29:91–98.
59. Hidaka Y, Liu Y, Yamamoto M, et al. Frequent isolation of human herpesvirus 7 from saliva samples. *J Med Virol.* 1993;40:343–346.
60. Frenkel N, Wyatt LS. HHV-6 and HHV-7 as exogenous agents in human lymphocytes. *Dev Biol Stand.* 1992;76: 259–265.
61. Wyatt LS, Rodriguez WJ, Balachandran N, Frenkel N. Human herpesvirus 7: antigenic properties and prevalence in children and adults. *J Virol.* 1991;65:6260–6265.
62. Yoshikawa T, Asano Y, Kobayashi I, et al. Seroepidemiology of human herpesvirus 7 in healthy children and adults in Japan. *J Med Virol.* 1993;41:319–323.
63. Yasukawa M, Yakushijin Y, Furukawa M, Fujita S. Specificity analysis of human CD4+ T-cell clones directed against human herpesvirus 6 (HHV-6), HHV-7, and human cytomegalovirus. *J Virol.* 1993;67:6259–6264.

64. Secchiero P, Berneman ZN, Gallo RC, Lusso P. Biological and molecular characteristics of human herpesvirus 7: in vitro growth optimization and development of a syncytia inhibition test. *Virology.* 1994;202:506–512.
65. Tanaka K, Kondo T, Torigoe S, Okada S, Mukai T, Yamanishi K. Human herpesvirus 7: another causal agent for roseola (exanthem subitum). *J Pediatr.* 1994; 125:1–5.
66. Asano Y, Suga S, Yoshikawa T, Yazaki T, Uchikawa T. Clinical features and viral excretion in an infant with primary human herpesvirus 7 infection. *Pediatrics.* 1995;95: 187–190.
67. Torigoe S, Kumamoto T, Koide W, Taya K, Yamanishi K. Clinical manifestations associated with human herpesvirus 7 infection. *Arch Dis Child.* 1995;72:518–519.
68. Hidaka Y, Okada K, Kusuhara K, Miyazaki C, Tokugawa K, Ueda K. Exanthem subitum and human herpesvirus 7 infection. *Pediatr Infect Dis J.* 1994;13:1010–1011.
69. Portolani M, Cermelli C, Mirandola P, Di Luca D. Isolation of human herpesvirus 7 from an infant with febrile syndrome. *J Med Virol.* 1995;45:282–283.
70. Osman HKE, Peiris JSM, Taylor CE, Warwicker P, Jarrett RF, Madeley CR. "Cytomegalovirus disease" in renal allograft recipients: is human herpesvirus 7 a cofactor for disease progression? *J Med Virol.* 1996;48:295–301.
71. Berneman ZN, Ablashi DV, Li G, et al. Human herpesvirus 7 is a T-lymphotropic virus and is related to, but significantly different from, human herpesvirus 6 and human cytomegalovirus. *Proc Natl Acad Sci USA.* 1992; 89:10552–10556.
72. Seccherio P, Zella D, Crowley RW, Gallo RC, Lusso P. Quantitative PCR for human herpesviruses 6 and 7. *J Clin Microbiol.* 1995;33:2124–2130.
73. Foà-Tomasi L, Avitabile E, Ke L, Campadelli-Fiume G. Polyvalent and monoclonal antibodies identify major immunogenic proteins specific for human herpesvirus 7–infected cells and have weak cross-reactivity with human herpesvirus 6. *J Gen Virol.* 1994;75:2719–2727.
74. Clark DA, Freeland ML, Mackie LK, Jarrett RF, Onions DE. Prevalence of antibody to human herpesvirus 7 by age. *J Infect Dis.* 1993;168:251–252.
75. Chang Y, Cesarman E, Pessin MS, et al. Identification of herpesvirus-like DNA sequences in AIDS-associated Kaposi's sarcoma. *Science.* 1994;266:1865–1869.
76. Moore PS, Gao S-J, Dominguez G, et al. Primary characterization of a herpesvirus agent associated with Kaposi's sarcoma. *J Virol.* 1996;70:549–558.
77. Cesarman E, Chang Y, Moore PS, Said JW, Knowles DM. Kaposi's sarcoma–associated herpesvirus-like DNA sequences in AIDS-related body cavity–based lymphomas. *N Engl J Med.* 1995;332:1186–1191.
78. Renne R, Zhong W, Herndier B, et al. Lytic growth of Kaposi's sarcoma–associated herpesvirus (human herpesvirus 8) in culture. *Nature Med.* 1996;2:342–346.
79. Ansari MQ, Dawson DB, Nador R, et al. Primary body-cavity–based AIDS-related lymphomas. *Am J Clin Pathol.* 1996;105:221–229.
80. Mesri EA, Cesarman E, Arvanitakis L, et al. Human herpesvirus-8/Kaposi's sarcoma–associated herpesvirus is a new transmissible virus that infects B cells. *J Exp Med.* 1996;183:2385–2390.
81. Miller G, Rigsby MO, Heston L, et al. Antibodies to butyrate-inducible antigens of Kaposi's sarcoma–associated herpesvirus in patients with HIV-1 infection. *N Engl J Med.* 1996;334:1292–1297.
82. Bigoni B, Dolcetti R, de Lellis L, et al. Human herpesvirus 8 is present in the lymphoid system of healthy persons and can reactivate in the course of AIDS. *J Infect Dis.* 1996;173:542–549.
83. Corbellino M, Parravicini C, Aubin JT, Berti E. Kaposi's sarcoma and herpesvirus-like DNA sequences in sensory ganglia. *N Engl J Med.* 1996;334:1341–1342.
84. Corbellino M, Poirel L, Bestetti G, et al. Restricted tissue distribution of extralesional Kaposi's sarcoma–associated herpesvirus-like DNA sequences in AIDS patients with Kaposi's sarcoma. *AIDS Res Hum Retroviruses.* 1996;12: 651–657.
85. Monini P, de Lellis L, Fabris M, Rigolin F, Cassai E. Kaposi's sarcoma–associated herpesvirus DNA sequences in prostate tissue and human semen. *N Engl J Med.* 1996;334:1168–1172.
86. Ambroziak JA, Blackbourn DJ, Herndier BG, et al. Herpes-like sequences in HIV-infected and uninfected Kaposi's sarcoma patients. *Science.* 1995;268:582.
87. Whitby D, Howard MR, Tenant-Flowers M, et al. Detection of Kaposi sarcoma associated herpesvirus in peripheral blood of HIV-infected individuals and progression to Kaposi's sarcoma. *Lancet.* 1995;346:799–802.
88. Rady PL, Yen A, Martin RW III, Nedelcu I, Hughes TK, Tyring SK. Herpesvirus-like DNA sequences in classic Kaposi's sarcomas. *J Med Virol.* 1995;47:179–183.
89. de Lellis L, Fabris M, Cassai E, et al. Herpesvirus-like DNA sequences in non-AIDS Kaposi's sarcoma. *J Infect Dis.* 1995;172:1605–1607.
90. Moore PS, Kingsley LA, Holmberg SD, et al. Kaposi's sarcoma–associated herpesvirus infection prior to onset of Kaposi's sarcoma. *AIDS.* 1996;10:175–180.
91. Howard M, Brink N, Miller R, Tedder R. Association of human herpesvirus with pulmonary Kaposi's sarcoma. *Lancet.* 1995;346:712.
92. Noel JC. Kaposi's sarcoma and KSHV. *Lancet.* 1995;346: 1359.
93. Cesarman E, Knowles DM. Herpes-like DNA sequences, AIDS-related tumors, and Castleman's disease. *N Engl J Med.* 1995;333:799.
94. Soulier J, Grollet L, Oksenhendler E, et al. Kaposi's sarcoma–associated herpesvirus-like DNA sequences in multicentric Castleman's disease. *Blood.* 1995;86:1276–1280.
95. Gessain A, Sudaka A, Brière J, et al. Kaposi sarcoma–associated herpes-like virus (human herpesvirus type 8) DNA sequences in multicentric Castleman's disease: is there any relevant association in non-human immunodeficiency virus–infected patients? *Blood.* 1995;87: 414–416.
96. Corbellino M, Poirel L, Aubin JT, et al. The role of human

herpesvirus 8 and Epstein–Barr virus in the pathogenesis of giant lymph node hyperplasia (Castleman's disease). *Clin Infect Dis.* 1996;22:1120–1121.

97. Luppi M, Barozzi P, Maiorana A, et al. Frequency and distribution of herpesvirus-like DNA sequences (KSHV) in different stages of classic Kaposi's sarcoma and in normal tissues from an Italian population. *Int J Cancer.* 1996;66:427–431.
98. Lin J-C, Lin S-C, Mar E-C, et al. Is Kaposi's sarcoma–associated herpesvirus detectable in semen of HIV-infected homosexual men. *Lancet.* 1995;346:1601–1602.
99. Rady PL, Yen A, Rollefson JL, et al. Herpesvirus-like DNA sequences in non-Kaposi's sarcoma skin lesions of transplant patients. *Lancet.* 1995;345:1339–1340.
100. Ziegler JL, Katongole-Mbidde E. Kaposi's sarcoma in childhood: an analysis of 100 cases from Uganda and relationship to HIV infection. *Int J Cancer.* 1996;65: 200–203.
101. Levine AM. AIDS-related malignancies: the emerging epidemic. *J Natl Cancer Inst.* 1993;85:1382–1397.
102. Beral V, Peterman TA, Berkelman RL, Jaffe HW. Kaposi's sarcoma among persons with AIDS: a sexually transmitted infection? *Lancet.* 1990;335:123–128.
103. Huang YQ, Li JJ, Kaplan MH, et al. Human herpesvirus–like nucleic acid in various forms of Kaposi's sarcoma. Lancet. 1995;345:759–761.
104. Luppi M, Barozzi P, Maiorana A, et al. Human herpesvirus-8 DNA sequences in human immunodeficiency virus–negative angioimmunoblastic lymphadenopathy with giant germinal genter hyperplasia and increased cellularity. *Blood.* 1996;87:3903–3909.
105. Oksenhendler E, Duarte M, Soulier J, et al. Multicentric Castleman's disease in HIV infection: a clinical and pathological study of 20 patients. *AIDS.* 1996;10:61–67.
106. Robert C, Agbalika F, Blanc F, Dubertret L. HIV-negative patient with HHV-8 DNA follicular B-cell lymphoma associated with Kaposi's sarcoma. *Lancet.* 1996;347: 1042–1043.
107. Gyulai R, Kemeny L, Kiss M, Adám E, Nagy F, Dobozy A. Herpesvirus-like DNA sequence in angiosarcoma in a patient without HIV infection. *N Engl J Med.* 1996;334: 540–541.
108. Boshoff C, Schultz TF, Kennedy MM, et al. Kaposi's sarcoma–associated herpesvirus infects endothelial and spindle cells. *Nature Med.* 1995;1:1274–1278.
109. Moore PS, Chang Y. Detection of herpes-like DNA sequences in Kaposi's sarcoma in patients with and without HIV infection. *N Engl J Med.* 1995;332:1181–1185.
110. Giraldo G, Beth E, Haguenau F. Herpes-type virus particles in tissue culture of Kaposi's sarcoma from different geographic regions. *J Natl Cancer Inst.* 1972;49:1509–1526.
111. Ioachim HL. Kaposi's sarcoma and KSHV. *Lancet.* 1995;346:1360.
112. Lebbé C, de Crémoux P, Rybojad M, Costa da Cunha C, Morel P, Calvo F. Kaposi's sarcoma and new herpesvirus. *Lancet.* 1995;345:1180.
113. Kaaya EE, Parravicini C, Ordonez C, et al. Heterogeneity of spindle cells in Kaposi's sarcoma: comparison of cells in lesions and in culture. *J AIDS Hum Retrovirol.* 1995; 10:295–305.
114. Cesarman E, Moore PS, Rao PH, Inghirami G, Knowles DM, Chang Y. In vitro establishment and characterization of two acquired immunodeficiency syndrome–related lymphoma cell lines (BC-1 and BC-2) containing Kaposi's sarcoma–associated herpesvirus-like (KSHV) DNA sequences. *Blood.* 1995;86:2708–2714.
115. Jin Y-T, Tsai S-T, Yan J-J, Hsiao J-H, Lee Y-Y, Su I-J. Detection of Kaposi's sarcoma–associated herpesvirus-like sequence in vascular lesions: a reliable diagnostic marker for Kaposi's sarcoma. *Am J Clin Pathol.* 1996;105: 360–363.
116. Jones JL, Hanson DL, Chu SY, Ward JW, Jaffe HW. AIDS-associated Kaposi's sarcoma. *Science.* 1995;267:1078–1079.

CHAPTER 37

Viral Hemorrhagic Fevers

Sherif R. Zaki and C. J. Peters

Human destiny is bound to remain a gamble, because at some unpredictable time and in some unforseeable manner nature will strike back.

René J. Dubois (1901–1982)

INTRODUCTION

The combination of fever and hemorrhage can be caused by a diverse group of human pathogens, including viruses, rickettsiae, bacteria, protozoa, and fungi. However, the term hemorrhagic fever (HF) is usually reserved for systemic infections characterized by fever and hemorrhage caused by a special group of viruses transmitted to humans by arthropods and rodents. The syndrome was well described in the early part of this century by scientists in the Soviet Union dealing first with hemorrhagic fever with renal syndrome (HFRS) and later reinforced by their experience with outbreaks of Crimean Congo HF (CCHF), Central Asian HF (later shown to be CCHF), and Omsk HF.[1] These viruses persist in nature through zoonotic cycles, although dengue and sometimes yellow fever may be maintained by the bite of a mosquito intermediate.[2] With the exception of the dengue viruses, all of these agents have a degree of aerosol infectivity, necessitating special handling usually in biosafety level 4 facilities. Because these viruses are extremely virulent and associated with high mortality rates, they have gained public notoriety and are among the most threatening examples of what are commonly called emerging pathogens.

DEFINITION

Viral hemorrhagic fevers (VHFs) are febrile illnesses characterized by abnormal vascular regulation and vascular damage. They are caused by small, lipid-enveloped RNA viruses. The VHF syndrome, as well as pneumonia or other infectious disease syndromes, can be caused by a variety of viruses belonging to four different families (Table 37–1).

GEOGRAPHY AND EPIDEMIOLOGY

As a group, the VHFs are zoonotic and cause a somewhat similar syndrome. Infection is usually contracted from an arthropod or rodent; thus, the highest incidence and risk is among those traveling to or residing in rural settings. Notable exceptions include the occasional VHF in urban areas associated with reservoirs of Seoul virus (*Rattus norvegicus*), dengue viruses (*Aedes aegypti*), and urban yellow fever (*A aegypti*). Several of these VHFs can be spread from human to human and have been associated with nosocomial outbreaks among health care workers.

Hemorrhagic fever viruses are distributed worldwide, and the diseases they cause are traditionally named after the location where they were first described. The different viruses and associated HFs are more or less confined to distinct geographic areas (Table 37–1). Geographic patterns change, however, and introduction of an HF into a previously nonendemic area depends on multiple factors, including environmental conditions and air travel. For example, the Rift Valley fever virus was imported into Egypt and caused major epidemics there in 1977 and 1993.

MORPHOLOGIC FEATURES

The four families of viruses that cause HF syndrome differ in their genomic structure, replication strategy,

TABLE 37–1. GEOGRAPHY AND EPIDEMIOLOGY OF HEMORRHAGIC FEVER VIRUSES

Virus	Disease	Geography	Vector/Reservoir	Human Infection
Arenaviridae				
Junin	Argentine HF	Argentine pampas	Small field rodent, *Calomys musculinus*.	Infects agricultural workers disproportionately. Aerosol transmission to humans.
Machupo	Bolivian HF	Bolivia, Beni Province	Small field rodent, *C callosus*.	Rural residents and farmers main target; rodent can invade towns to cause epidemics. Aerosol transmission to humans.
Guanarito	Venezuelan HF	Venezuela, Portuguesa State	Chronic infection of field rodent, *Zygodontomys brevicauda*.	Rural residents in newly developed area in Venezuela with small farms.
Sabia	?	? rural area near Sao Paulo, Brazil	Presumably chronic infection of unidentified rodents.	Single infection in nature; little information on potential.
Lassa	Lassa fever	West Africa	Chronic infection of rodents of the genus *Mastomys*.	The reservoir rodent is very common in Africa and the disease is a major cause of severe febrile illness in West Africa. Spread to humans occurs by aerosols and by capturing the rodent for consumption, as well as person-to-person transmission. Lassa fever is the most commonly exported HF.
Bunyaviridae				
Rift Valley fever	Rift Valley fever	Sub-Saharan Africa	Vertical infection of floodwater *Aedes* mosquitoes. Epidemics occur from horizontal transmission by many different mosquito species between domestic animals, particularly sheep and cattle.	Humans acquire by mosquito bite; contact with blood of infected sheep, cattle, or goats; and aerosols generated from infected domestic animal blood. No interhuman transmission observed.
Crimean Congo HF	Crimean Congo HF	Africa, Middle East, Balkans, southern former Soviet Union, western China	Tick–mammal–tick infection. Vertical infection occurs in ticks. *Hyalomma* ticks are thought to be the natural reservoir but other genera may become infected and transmit.	Tick bite; squashing ticks; and exposure to aerosols or fomites from slaughtered cattle and sheep. (Domestic animals do not evidence illness but may become infected when transported to market or when held in pens for slaughter.) Nosocomial epidemics observed on numerous occasions.
Hantaan, Seoul, Puumala, and others	Hemorrhagic fever with renal syndrome (HFRS)	Worldwide, depending on rodent reservoir	Horizontal infection in a single rodent genus or species typical of the virus. Viruses associated with HFRS have been obtained from Muridae (subfamily Murinae) or from Avicolinae rodents	Aerosols from infected rodents. Some infections may be acquired from secondary aerosols or droplets from shed rodent excreta and secreta or from rodent bites. Interhuman transmission never documented.

(*continued*)

and morphologic features (Figure 37–1).[3] Arenaviruses, bunyaviruses, and filoviruses are negative-stranded, whereas flaviviruses are positive-stranded RNA viruses. All viruses have a lipid envelope that is acquired by budding at either the cell surface or the internal membranes. The size and shape of these viruses vary from relatively small (35 to 50 nm) uniform round particles, for the flaviviruses, to more pleomorphic, rod-shaped particles (measuring occasionally up to 15,000 nm) for the filoviruses.

CLINICAL FEATURES

VHFs typically begin as a febrile prodrome with myalgia occasionally accompanied by gastrointestinal disturbances. By the time medical attention is sought, patients usually have a severe, acute illness, with evidence of abnormal vascular regulation and vascular damage. Systemically, the abnormal vascular regulation manifests by mild hypotension in the early stages of the disease and by shock in more severe and advanced infections. Local

TABLE 37–1. (CONTINUED)

Virus	Disease	Geography	Vector/Reservoir	Human Infection
Bunyaviridae (continued)				
Sin Nombre, Black Creek Canal, Bayou, and others	Hantavirus pulmonary syndrome (HPS)	Americas	As for hantaviruses causing HFRS. All viruses associated with HPS have come from Muridae (subfamily Sigmodontinae) rodents, if the reservoir is known.	As for hantaviruses causing HFRS. Entering abandoned, closed buildings may be a particular risk in some settings.
Filoviridae				
Marburg, Ebola	Marburg HF Ebola HF	Africa, Philippines?	Unknown.	Infection of index case occurs by unknown route. Later spread among human or nonhuman primates by close contact with another case. Aerosol transmission suspected in some monkey infections.
Flaviridae				
Yellow fever	Yellow fever	Africa, South America	Mosquito–monkey–mosquito maintenance with occasional human infection when unvaccinated humans enter forest. Formerly large epidemics among humans with *Aedes aegypti* as mosquito vector.	Mosquito infection of humans entering forest and encountering infected sylvatic vector. Emergence of epidemics into African savannas using specific *Aedes* mosquito vectors. In cities or villages interhuman transmission by *A aegypti.* Fully developed cases are no longer viremic and direct interhuman transmission not believed to be a problem, although the virus is highly infectious (including aerosols) in the laboratory.
Dengue (Types 1–4)	Dengue HF, dengue shock syndrome (DHF/DSS)	Tropics and subtropics worldwide	Maintained by *Aedes aegypti*–human–*Aedes aegypti* transmission with frequent geographic transport of virus.	DHF/DSS is a problem only in areas where multiple dengue viruses are being transmitted. With the increased worldwide distribution of *A aegypti* and movement of dengue viruses in travelers, this zone is enlarging. The disease was first noted in Southeast Asia but is now common in the Americas and the Caribbean.
Kyasanur Forest disease (KFD)	KFD	Limited area of Mysore State, India	Tick–vertebrate–tick	Most infections occur from tick bite acquired in rural areas of the disease endemic zone. Monkey deaths may accompany increased virus activity.
Omsk HF (OHF)	OHF	Western Siberia	Poorly understood cycle involving ticks, voles, muskrats, and possibly waterborne transmission.	Few cases in recent years.
Middle Eastern flavivirus		Middle East?, Africa?	Unknown. Surmised to involve tick–domestic livestock–tick cycle by analogy to genetically related tick-borne flaviviruses	Transmitted to humans working in livestock-related occupations by unknown route.

vascular abnormalities usually are visible as conjunctival suffusion, flushing over the face and thorax, and various exanthems (Figure 37–2).[4] Vascular damage may be evident as capillary leakage in nondependent areas, such as periorbital edema, a propensity to develop pulmonary edema after fluid infusions, proteinuria, or by the presence of effusions in serous cavities.

Thrombocytopenia is characteristic and usually accompanied by hemorrhage, which may signal underlying vascular damage. The hemorrhage is usually petechial and common in skin and mucous membranes. In some VHFs, there may be remission of fever before recovery or progression to a more severe stage. Severe disease is usually accompanied by profuse bleeding, central nervous system disturbances, and frank shock. Some of the features of individual diseases are summarized in Table 37–2. Note that jaundice is a feature of yellow fever, but may also be a feature of severe Crimean Congo HF, Rift Valley fever, and filovirus HF. Renal insufficiency usually is proportional to the degree of shock, but in HFRS it dominates and is caused by primary renal lesions.

Hantavirus pulmonary syndrome (HPS) differs from the other diseases listed. The prodrome is terminated by the onset of pulmonary edema. Hypotension and shock may be problematic even if hypoxia is corrected. Although there is thrombocytopenia and abnormal partial thromboplastin time (PTT) is common, petechiae or bleeding occur in only a few patients.

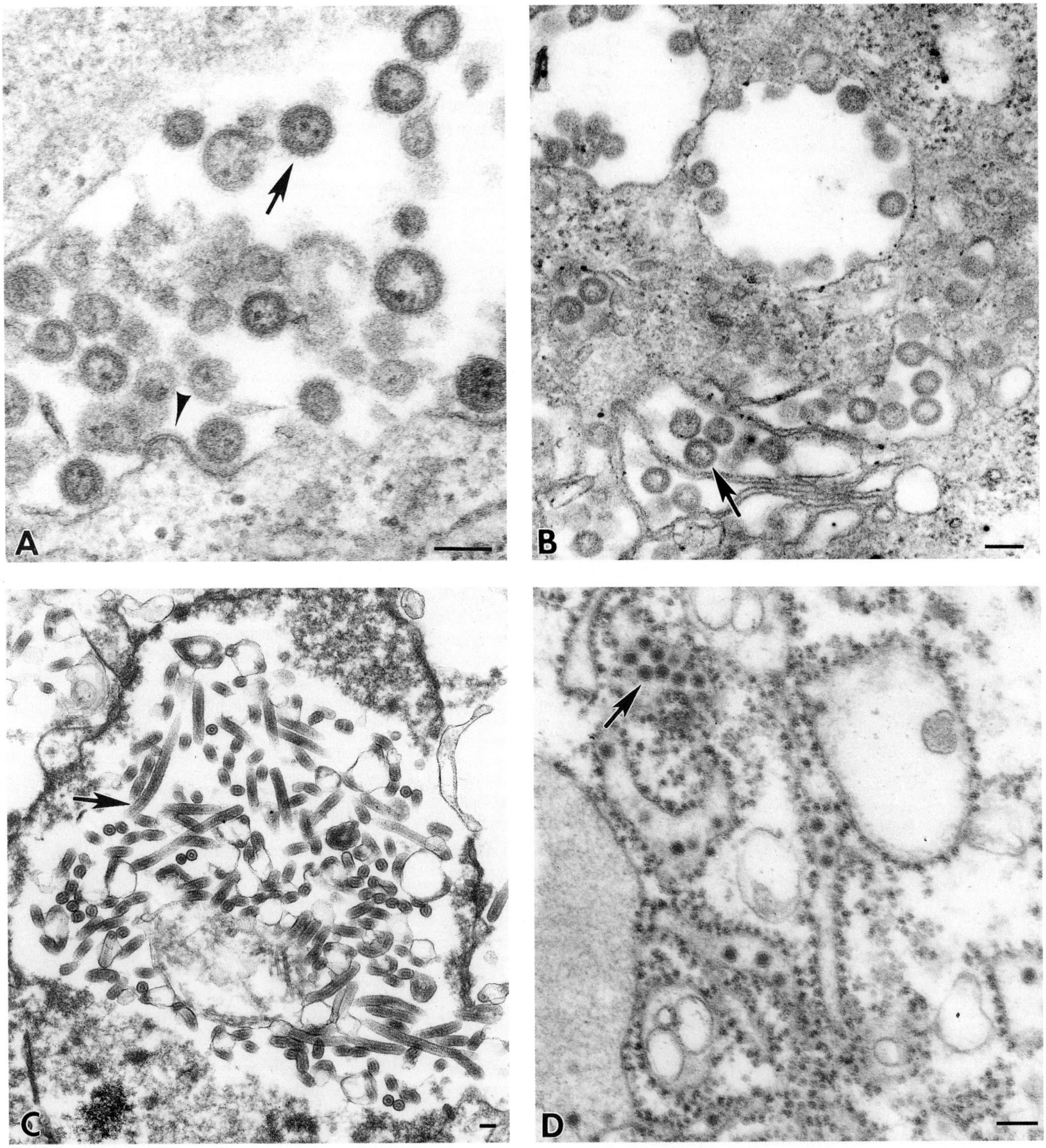

Figure 37–1. Ultrastructural characteristics of representative HF virus family members as seen in thin sections of tissue culture cells (**A, B, C**) and suckling mouse brain (**D**). (**A**) Machupo virus, an arenavirus, showing pleomorphic enveloped particles with internal ribosome-like granules. *(Contributed by F. A. Murphy, DVM.)* (**B**) Rift Valley fever virus, a member of the family Bunyaviridae, showing mostly spherical enveloped particles containing granular appearing viral nucleocapsids. *(Contributed by A. Harrison.)* (**C**) Ebola virus isolate, a filovirus, from 1995 Kikwit outbreak in Zaire, showing enveloped filamentous particles about 80 nm wide. Some filaments occasionally measure up to 15,000 nm long. *(Contributed by C. S. Goldsmith.)* (**D**) Yellow fever virus particles accumulating in dilated cisternae of rough endoplasmic reticulum of a liver cell. Flaviviruses measure 35 to 50 nm and have a dense core. *(Contributed by C. S. Goldsmith.) (Scale bars A–D, 100 nm.)*

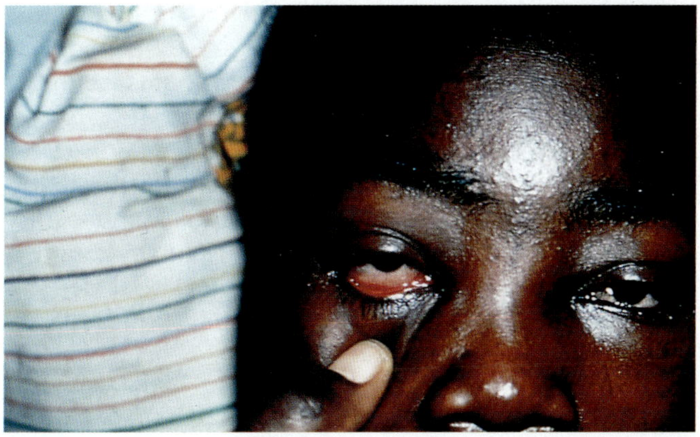

Figure 37–2 Patient with Lassa fever showing conjunctival injection and facial edema. *(Contributed by Mark H. Monson, MD, Curran Lutheran Hospital, Zorzor, Liberia.)*

Vascular and other major clinical manifestations also are largely confined to the thoracic cavity.

PATHOLOGY AND PATHOGENESIS

Although VHFs share many common pathologic features, the overall changes vary among the different diseases. The similar pathologic and immunopathologic findings in cases of VHF suggest that microvascular involvement and instability are important common pathogenetic pathways leading to shock and bleeding. Infection of macrophages and other cells of the mononuclear phagocytic system may play a critical role in the pathogenesis of VHF by secreting physiologically active

TABLE 37–2. CLINICAL FEATURES OF THE VIRAL HEMORRHAGIC FEVERS

Disease	Incubation (days)	Case : Infection Ratio	Case Fatality	Characteristic Features
Arenaviridae				
South American HFs	7–14	Most (>1/2) result in disease	15–30%	Typical cases have hypotension, shock, obvious bleeding, and neurologic symptoms such as dysarthria and intention tremor. Some cases have virtually pure neurologic syndrome.
Lassa fever	5–16	Mild infections probably common	~15%	Prostration and shock; fewer hemorrhagic or neurologic manifestations than South American HF except in severe cases. Less thrombocytopenia. Deafness develops in convalescence in 20%.
Bunyaviridae				
Rift Valley fever	2–5	~1%	~50%	Severe disease associated with bleeding, shock, anuria, icterus Encephalitis and retinal vasculitis also occur, but without overlap with HF syndrome.
Crimean Congo HF	3–12	20–100%	15–30%	Most severe bleeding and ecchymoses of all the HFs.
HFRS	9–35	>3/4 Hantaan, 1/20 Puumala	5–15% Hantaan, <1% Puumala	Febrile prodrome followed by shock and renal failure. Bleeding during fever, shock, and renal failure. Puumala infections similar course but much milder.
HPS	7–28[a]	Very high	40–50%	Febrile prodrome followed by acute pulmonary edema and shock.
Filoviridae				
Marburg or Ebola HF	3–16	High (particularly Zaire subtype of Ebola)	25–90%	Most severe of the HFs. Marked weight loss and prostration. Maculopapular rash common. Patients have had late sequelae (hepatitis, uveitis, orchitis) often with virus isolation from biopsy or aspiration.
Flaviviridae				
Yellow fever	3–6	80–95%	20%	Acute febrile period with defervescence accompanied in severe cases by jaundice, renal failure.
DHF/DSS	?[b]	0.007% of non-immune and 1% of heterologous immune	Probably <1%	High fever for 3–5 days with the development of shock lasting 1–2 days. DHF is not equated to DSS. DSS is the most dangerous manifestation and is due to an acute vascular leak. Attack rates, mortality quite variable with epidemic virus strain and surveillance.
KFD/OHF	3–8	Variable	0.5–9%	Typical biphasic disease with a febrile or hemorrhagic period often followed by CNS involvement. Similar to tick-borne encephalitis except hemorrhagic manifestations not characteristic of first phase of tick-borne encephalitis.

[a] Not known with certainty; estimated from available data.

[b] Uncomplicated dengue has an incubation of 3–15 days, but DHF/DSS may differ.

substances, including cytokines and other inflammatory mediators. However, the details of the pathogenesis of VHF are poorly understood,[5] and the differences observed among these diseases and the lack of significant anatomic lesions in some fatal infections emphasize the need for more comprehensive studies.

Common pathologic findings at autopsy include widespread petechial hemorrhages and ecchymoses of skin, mucous membranes, and internal organs. However, in many HF patients bleeding may be minimal or absent. Effusions, occasionally hemorrhagic, are also frequent. There may be widespread focal and sometimes massive necrosis in all organ systems and this is often ischemic in nature. Necrosis is usually most prominent in the liver and lymphoid tissues. In addition, the kidneys frequently show evidence of acute tubular necrosis secondary to shock. In some patients the necrosis is a consequence of direct viral cytopathic effect. Although lymphoid necrosis and depletion are the general rule, proliferative changes of lymphoid tissues may complicate some HFs, such as in hantavirus-related illnesses. Erythrophagocytosis is also common in the spleen, lymph nodes, and liver. A small number of patients have microvascular thrombosis, and it is possible that disseminated intravascular coagulation (DIC) is important in the pathogenesis of some of the different HFs but definitive hematologic studies and pathologic evidence at autopsy are often lacking. Common histopathologic changes in lung include various degrees of hemorrhage, interstitial pneumonitis, and diffuse alveolar damage.

A few excellent studies describe the pathologic features of certain HFs. With some diseases, however, little has been reported, mainly because of the risk of hemorrhage associated with biopsies and because of biosafety concerns during autopsy. Several of these references are listed in Table 37–3. The characteristic features that support the histopathologic diagnosis of the different VHFs are also summarized in Table 37–3. These features are not pathognomonic, and immuno-

TABLE 37–3. PATHOLOGIC FEATURES OF VIRAL HEMORRHAGIC FEVERS

Disease (references)	Pathologic Features[a]
Argentine HF (Refs. 14–17) Bolivian HF (Refs. 18–21) Venezuelan HF (Ref. 22) Lassa fever (Refs. 6–13)	Multifocal hepatocellular necrosis with minimal inflammatory response, interstitial pneumonitis, myocarditis, and lymphoid depletion. Extensive parenchymal cell and reticuloendothelial infection, more than morphologic lesions would suggest.
Rift Valley fever (RVF) (Refs. 39–42)	Widespread hepatocellular necrosis and hemorrhage, sometimes with midzonal distribution, minimal inflammatory response, DIC, lymphoid depletion, and encephalitis. RVF antigens in very few individual hepatocytes.
Crimean Congo HF (Refs. 36–38, 43)	Widespread hepatocellular necrosis and hemorrhage with minimal or no inflammatory cell response and lymphoid depletion. Hepatic and endothelial cell infection and damage.
Hemorrhagic fever with renal syndrome (Refs. 23–30)	Retroperitoneal edema in severe HFRS, mild to severe renal pathologic changes. Congestion and hemorrhagic necrosis of renal medulla, right atrium of the heart, and anterior pituitary. Extensive endothelial infection mainly in renal and cardiac microvasculature.
Hantavirus pulmonary syndrome (Refs. 31–35)	Large bilateral pleural effusions and heavy edematous lungs, mild to moderate interstitial pneumonitis, immunoblasts and atypical lymphocytes in lymphoid tissues and peripheral blood. Extensive infection of endothelial cells in pulmonary microvasculature.
Ebola HF (Refs. 48–60)	Extensive and disseminated infection and necrosis in major organs such as liver, spleen, lung, kidney, skin, and gonads. Extensive hepatocellular necrosis associated with formation of characteristic intracytoplasmic viral inclusions. Lymphoid depletion, microvascular infection, and injury.
Marburg HF (Refs. 44–47)	Similar to Ebola HF.
Yellow fever (Refs. 65,66,74,76)	Midzonal hepatocellular necrosis; minimal inflammatory response. Councilman bodies and microvesicular fatty change. Hepatocellular and Kupffer's cell infection.
Dengue HF/DSS (Refs. 67–72, 76)	Centrilobular and midzonal hepatocellular necrosis with minimal inflammatory response. Councilman bodies and microvesicular fatty change. Hyperplasia of mononuclear phagocytic cells in lymphoid tissues and atypical lymphocytes in peripheral blood. Widespread infection of mononuclear phagocytic and endothelial cells.
Kyasanur Forest disease (KFD) (Refs. 61–63)	Focal hepatocellular degeneration, fatty change, and necrosis. Pulmonary hemorrhage, depletion of Malpighian follicles, sinus histiocytosis, erythrophagocytosis, mild myocarditis, and encephalitis.
Omsk HF (Ref. 64)	Little known; scattered focal hemorrhage, interstitial pneumonia, and normal lymphoid tissues.

[a]These features represent the more characteristic pathologic findings in the different VHFs. More general findings seen to variable degrees in all HF are not listed in this table (see text).

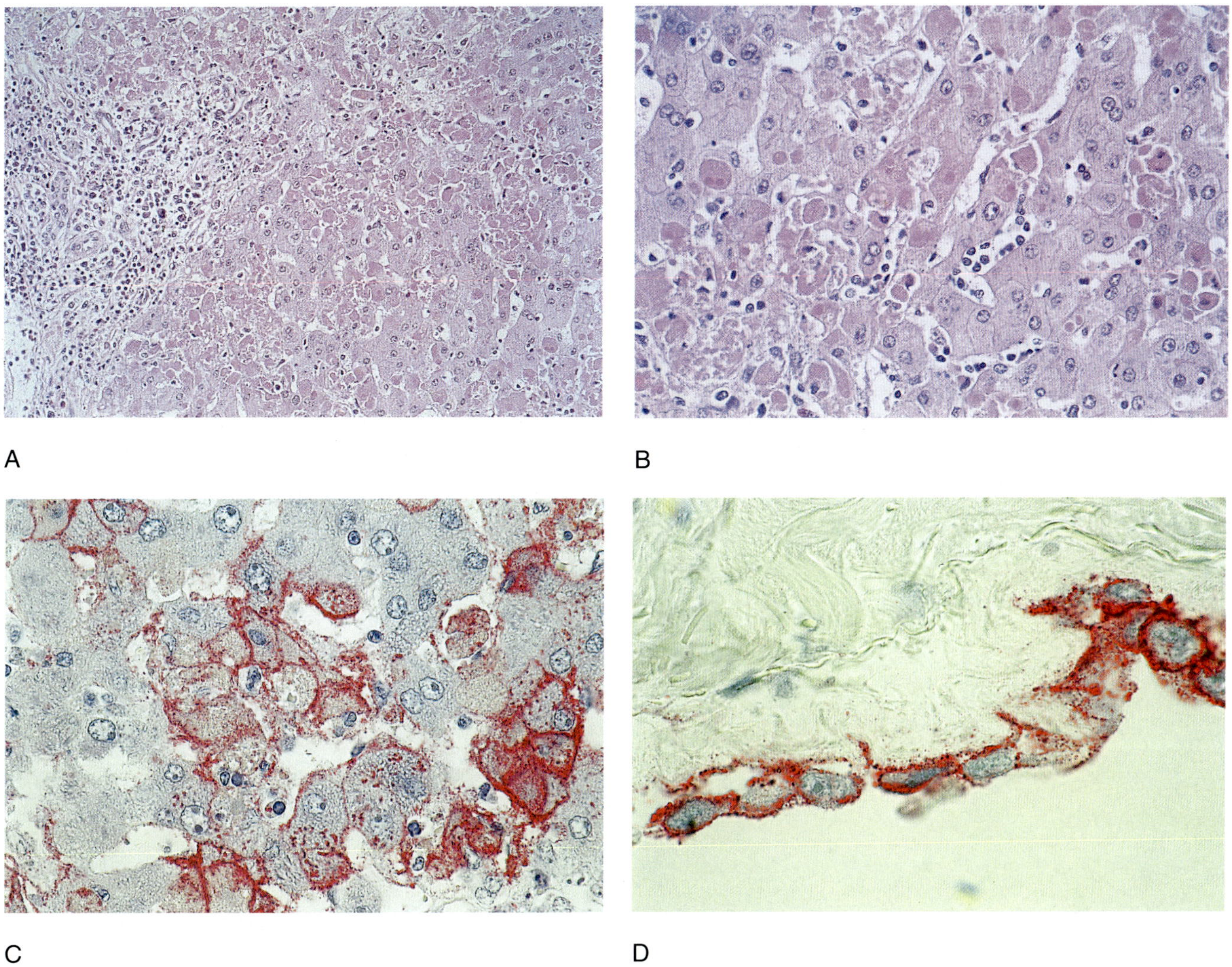

Figure 37–3. Lassa fever. (**A**) Hepatocellular necrosis and mononuclear cell infiltrates in portal tracts in fatal Lassa fever [hematoxylin-eosin (H&E), ×50]. (**B**) Higher magnification showing eosinophilic necrosis and Councilman bodies (H&E, ×100). (**C**) Using immunohistochemistry, abundant Lassa virus antigens are seen within cytoplasm of hepatocytes and sinusoidal lining cells (immunoalkaline phosphatase staining, naphthol fast red substrate with light hematoxylin counterstain, ×158). (**D**) Section of pleura showing immunostaining of Lassa virus antigens in mesothelial cells (immunoalkaline phosphatase staining, naphthol fast red substrate with light hematoxylin counterstain, ×250).

histochemistry and other laboratory tests are essential to confirm the diagnosis.

The histopathologic features in arenaviral infections, such as Lassa fever,[6–13] Argentine HF (AHF),[14–17] Bolivian HF (BHF),[18–21] and Venezuelan HF,[22] are strikingly similar (Figures 37–3 through 37–5). The most consistent microscopic feature is multifocal hepatocellular necrosis with cytoplasmic eosinophilia, Councilman bodies, nuclear pyknosis, and cytolysis. Inflammatory cell infiltrates and necrotic areas are usually mild and, when present, consist of neutrophils and mononuclear cells. Immunohistochemical studies demonstrate hepatocellular infection associated with focal necrosis (Figure 37–3, C). Extensive infection of macrophages and mesothelial cells lining several serosal surfaces is characteristic of arenavirus infections and helps explain serous effusions common in patients with these infections (Figure 37–3, D, and 37–5, B).[4,13] Other pathologic features include a mild interstitial pneumonitis and myocarditis, as well as infection and damage of reticuloendothelial tissues.

The pathologic features of hantavirus-associated diseases, namely, HFRS[23–30] and HPS,[31–35] were described in Chapter 12.[32] In CCHF[36–38] and Rift Valley

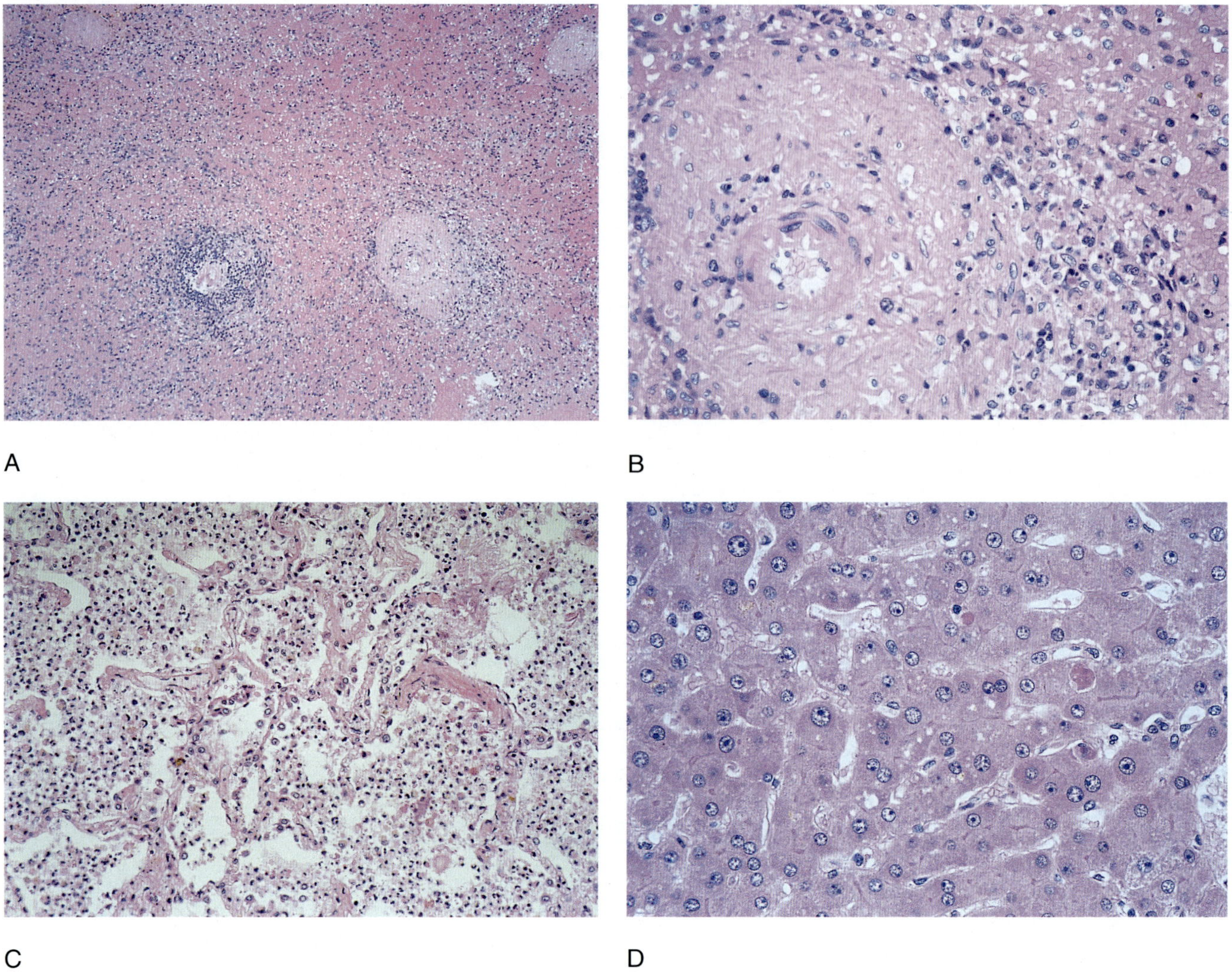

Figure 37–4. Argentine HF. (**A**) Low-magnification photomicrograph of spleen showing lymphocyte-depleted white pulp (H&E, ×25). (**B**) Higher magnification showing necrosis and karyorrhectic debris in periarteriolar sheath (H&E, ×100). (**C**) Lung of AHF with extensive intra-alveolar mixed inflammatory infiltrates, mainly neutrophils. Bacterial infection of lung may complicate over 50% of patients with fatal AHF (H&E, ×50). (**D**) Liver with focal acidophilic necrosis, sinusoidal dilatation, and microvesicular fatty change (H&E, ×100).

fever (RVF),[39–41] the main histopathologic lesions are in liver, spleen, and lung (Figures 37–6 and 37–7). Changes in liver resemble those in a number of VHFs and consist of widespread hepatocellular necrosis, usually midzonal in RVF, associated with variable degrees of hemorrhage and Councilman bodies. As in Lassa HF, the inflammatory cell response in necrotic areas is minimal or absent, and only a mild periportal mononuclear infiltrate is sometimes seen. Immunohistochemistry reveals focal infection of hepatocytes, Kupffer's cells, and sinusoidal lining cells (Figure 37–6, D).[42,43] The predominant features in lymphoid tissue include sinusoidal dilatation and generalized lymphoid depletion. Lungs may have interstitial pneumonitis and are usually congested with widespread intra-alveolar edema and hemorrhage. Rift Valley fever, in addition to typical features, may cause encephalitis and retinal lesions (Figure 37–7, B and C).

Among the VHFs the filoviruses cause the most widespread destructive lesions. The pathologic changes are similar in Marburg virus[44–47] and Ebola virus infections,[48–60] although the latter tends to be more severe. Necrosis is in many organs being maximal in liver, spleen, kidney, and gonads (Figure 37–8). The necrosis is both ischemic and related to cytopathic effect of the virus. The most characteristic changes are widespread

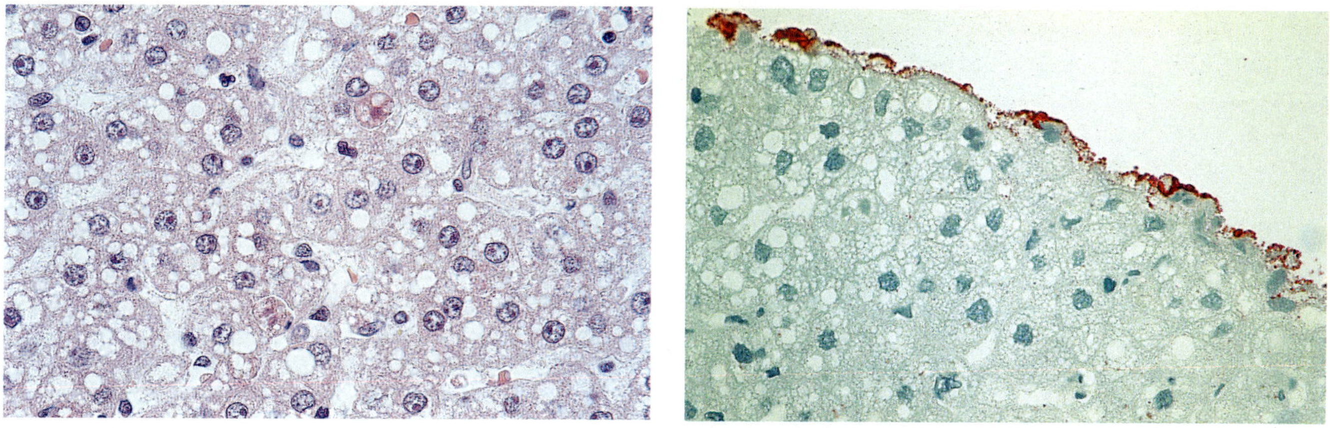

A B

Figure 37–5. Bolivian HF. (**A**) Focal hepatocellular necrosis and extensive microvesicular fatty change. Note numerous acidophilic bodies (H&E, ×158). (**B**) Immunohistochemical staining of Machupo viral antigens in serosal cells on surface of liver (immunoalkaline phosphatase staining, naphthol fast red substrate with light hematoxylin counterstain, ×158).

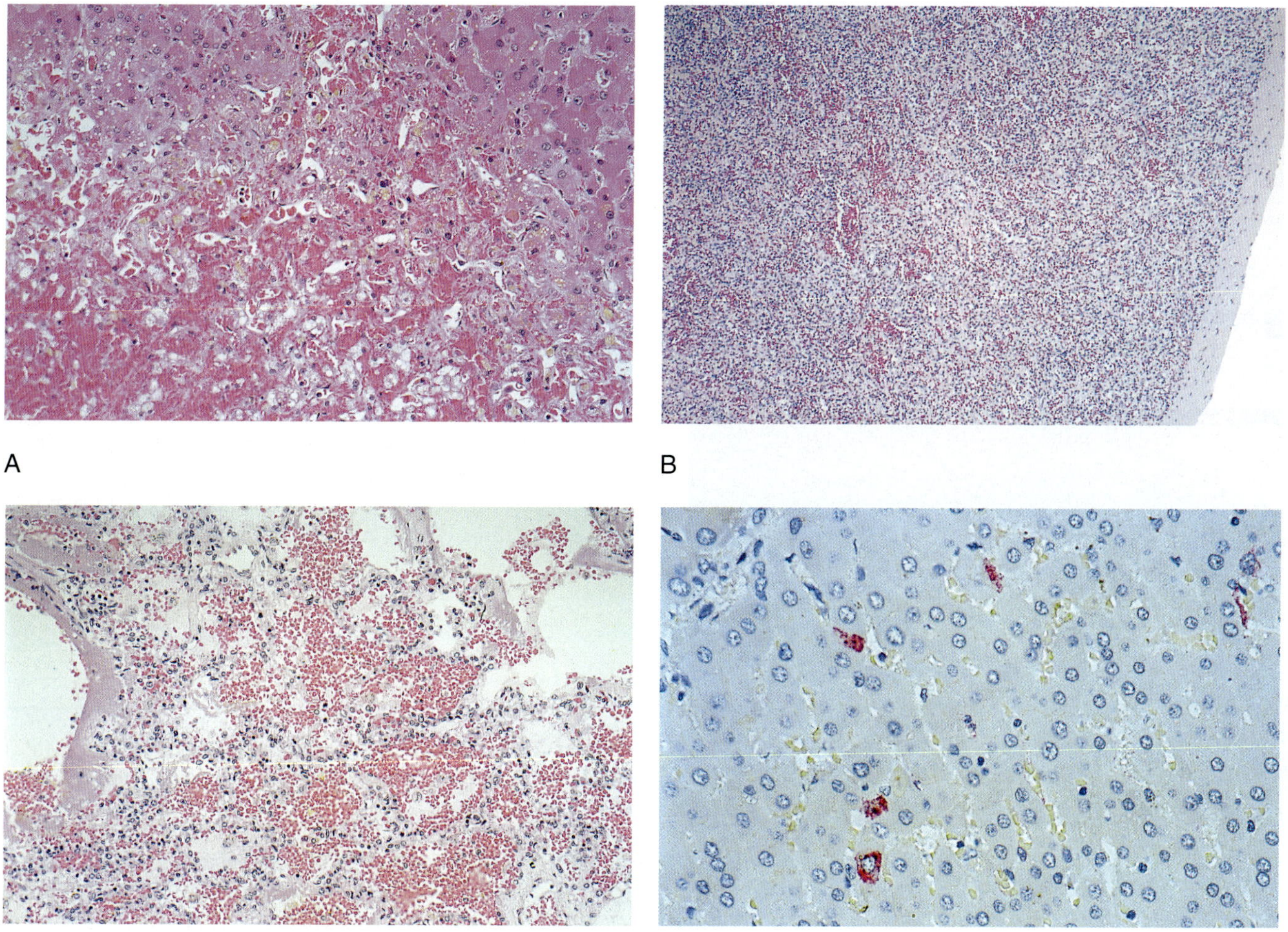

A B

C D

Figure 37–6. Crimean Congo HF. (**A**) Massive hemorrhage, focal necrosis, and effacement of hepatic architecture in typical CCHF case (H&E, ×50). (**B**) Necrosis of splenic red and white pulp with depleted lymphoid elements (H&E, ×25). (**C**) Massive intra-alveolar hemorrhage with hyaline membranes in fatal CCHF (H&E, ×50). (**D**) Focal presence of viral antigens in hepatocytes and sinusoidal lining cells in liver immunostained for CCHF (immunoalkaline phosphatase staining, naphthol fast red substrate with light hematoxylin counterstain, ×100).

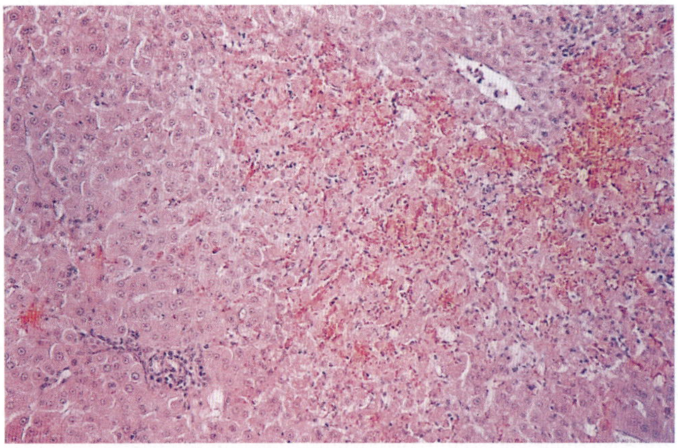

A

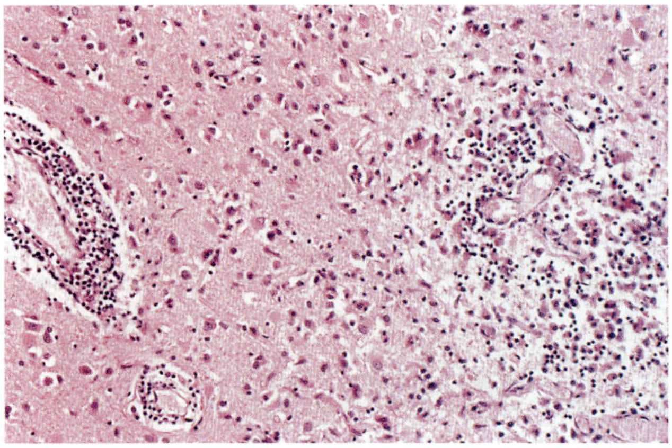

B

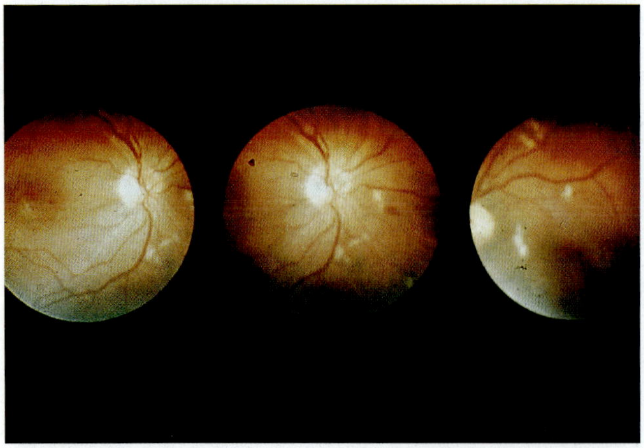

C

Figure 37–7. Rift Valley HF. (**A**) Focal hemorrhage and extensive necrosis in liver of a rhesus monkey fatally infected with Rift Valley fever virus (H&E, ×50). *(Contributed by T. Slone, DVM.)* (**B**) Perivascular mononuclear infiltrates and an area of focal necrosis in the cerebral cortex of a Rift Valley fever patient (H&E, ×50). (**C**) Retinal lesion of Rift Valley fever. *(Contributed by James Meegan, PhD.)*

hepatocellular necrosis, Councilman bodies, microvesicular fatty change, and Kupffer's cell hyperplasia (Figure 37–8, B). The portal tracts usually exhibit extensive karyorrhectic debris and a mononuclear inflammatory cell infiltrate. Characteristic intracytoplasmic viral inclusions are in hepatocytes (Figure 37–8, C). They are usually numerous, eosinophilic, and oval or filamentous, and ultrastructurally are aggregates of viral nucleocapsids (Figure 37–8, D and E). The viral inclusions and distribution of antigens can be confirmed and studied by immunohistochemistry (Figure 37–8, F).[58–60] There is extensive follicular necrosis of lymphoid tissues. There is edema of the myocardium but it is not associated with any appreciable inflammatory cell infiltrates. The lungs are usually hemorrhagic and have features of diffuse alveolar damage.

The descriptions of the pathology of Kyasanur Forest disease[61–63] and Omsk HF[64] are few, and the major findings are summarized in Table 37–3. Generally, microscopic appearances of fatal yellow fever[65,66] and dengue virus infections[67–72] are somewhat similar (Figures 37–9 and 37–10). The most consistent features are hepatocellular necrosis, Councilman bodies, and microvesicular fatty change. Although the acidophil or Councilman body is of diagnostic value in yellow fever,[73] it is not pathognomonic of yellow fever and can be seen in the different HFs as well as other hepatic diseases. In yellow fever the hepatic necrosis is extensive and midzonal, while in fatal dengue hemorrhagic fever (DHF/DSS) it is less severe and tends to be centrilobular or midzonal. In severe infections of both diseases, the necrosis may extend beyond the midzone, causing almost complete destruction of the lobule; a rim of intact hepatocytes, however, usually remains around the portal tracts and central veins. Follicular hyperplasia of spleen and lymph nodes can be seen in fatal dengue.

Figure 37–8. Ebola virus HF. (**A**) Low magnification of spleen with congestion and marked depletion of white pulp (H&E, ×50). (**B**) Liver showing hepatocellular necrosis, numerous Ebola viral inclusions, and dilated and congested sinusoids (H&E, ×100). (**C**) Higher magnification showing necrotic debris and hepatocytes containing typical intracytoplasmic, eosinophilic inclusions of Ebola virus (H&E, ×250). (**D**) Several Ebola viral inclusions (*arrows*) are in this thin-section electron micrograph of liver (scale bar 1 μm). (**E**) Higher magnification—the inclusions (*arrow*) consist of viral nucleocapsids seen mostly in longitudinal section (scale bar 1μm). (**F**) Massive viral burden can be seen in this section of liver immunostained for Ebola viral antigens. Antigens are in sinusoidal lining cells and hepatocytes (immunoalkaline phosphatase staining, naphthol fast red substrate with light hematoxylin counterstain, ×158).

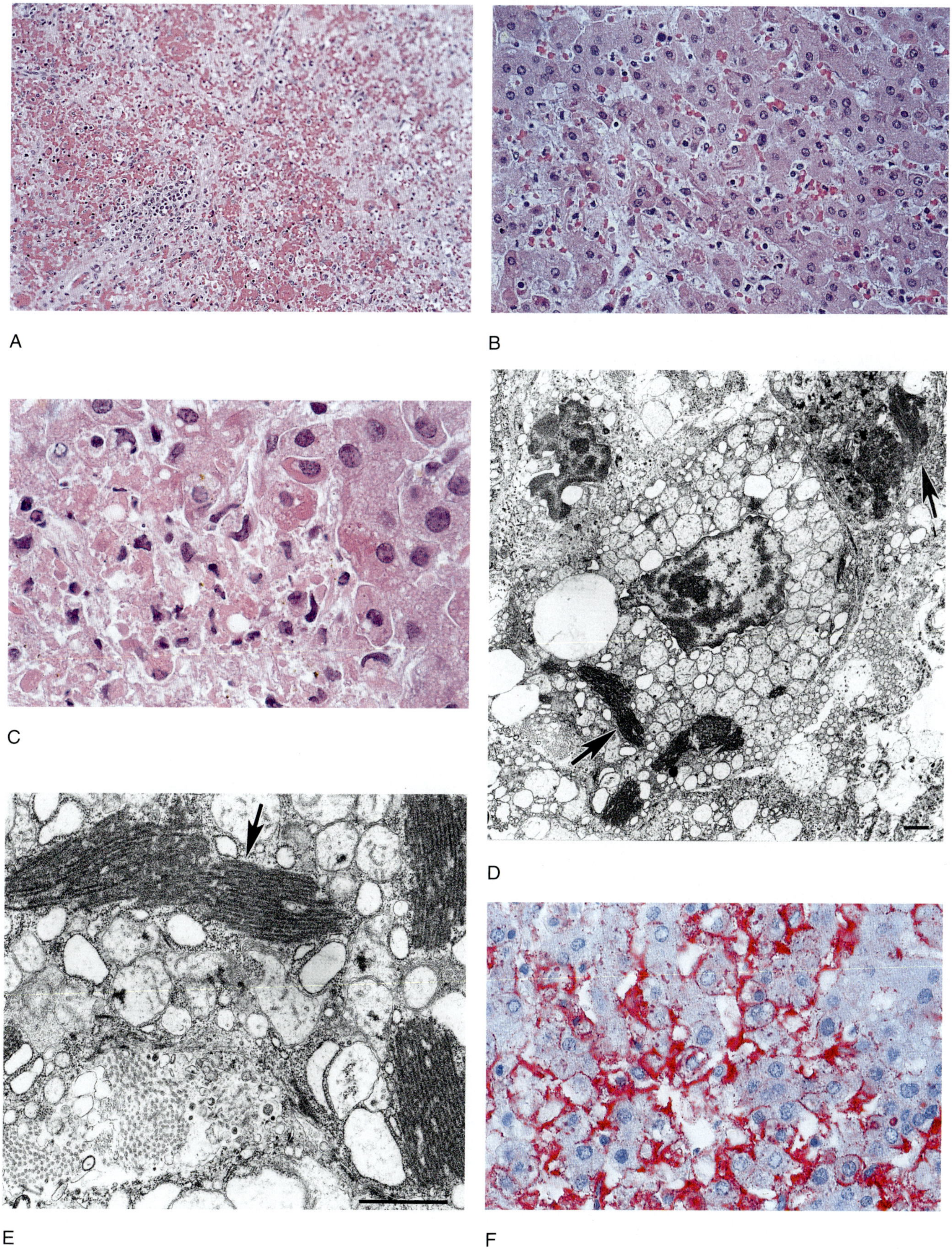
A
B
C
D
E
F

Otherwise, in both diseases, the histopathologic features in other organs are variable and resemble those of other VHFs. Immunohistochemistry is extremely valuable in providing a specific diagnosis and in differentiating these infections from other VHFs and diseases with similar histopathologic features, such as viral hepatitis and leptospirosis[74–76] (Figures 37–9 and 37–10).

DIAGNOSIS

The diagnosis of VHF should be suspected in any patient returning from an endemic area, particularly if there is travel to rural areas during the times of seasonal epidemics. There may be a history of exposure to the vector and exposure to ticks. Clinical features such as high fever, prostration, flushing, conjunctival injection, postural hypotension, and axillary petechiae may be present early in the course of the disease.

Laboratory findings may be helpful, although great care must be taken when handling potentially infectious blood and other body fluids according to guidelines for VHFs. Proteinuria is common or constant, depending on the disease. In hantavirus diseases, the white count is elevated or at least shows a left shift; atypical lymphocytes are usually present with thrombocytopenia. Thrombocytopenia is, in fact, characteristic of all

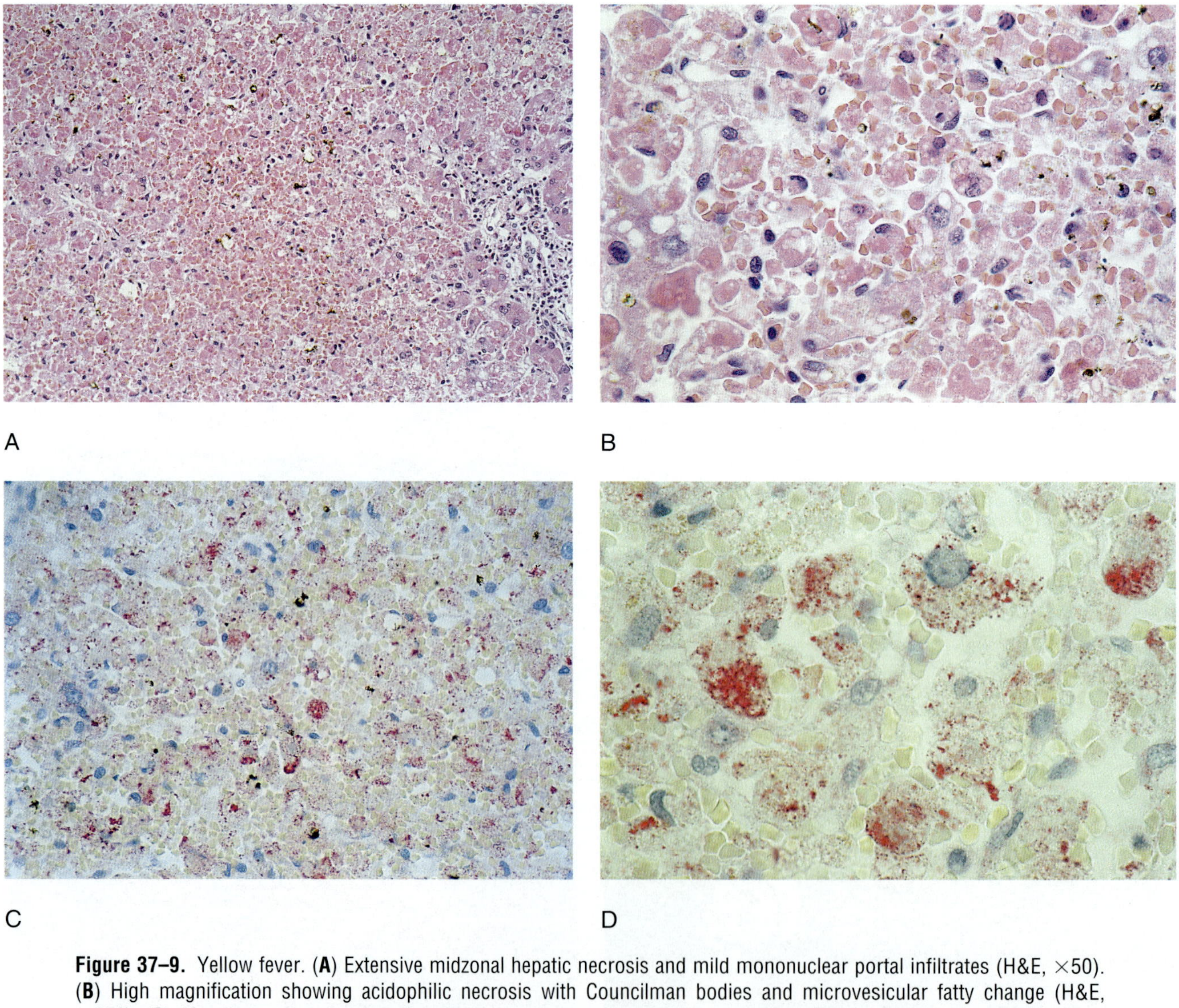

Figure 37–9. Yellow fever. (**A**) Extensive midzonal hepatic necrosis and mild mononuclear portal infiltrates (H&E, ×50). (**B**) High magnification showing acidophilic necrosis with Councilman bodies and microvesicular fatty change (H&E, ×158). (**C**) Abundant yellow fever viral antigens are in the midzone of the hepatic lobule in this immunohistochemical preparation (immunoalkaline phosphatase staining, antiflavivirus antibody, naphthol fast red substrate with light hematoxylin counterstain, ×100). (**D**) Higher magnification showing yellow fever viral antigens in hepatocytes and Kupffer's cells (immunoalkaline phosphatase staining, antiflavivirus antibody, naphthol fast red substrate with light hematoxylin counterstain, ×250).

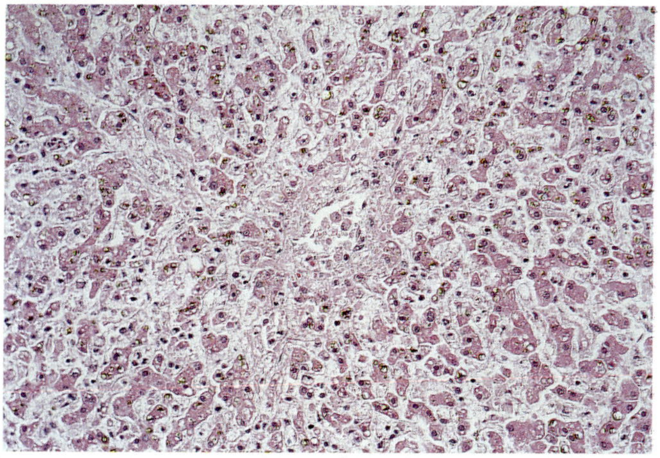

A

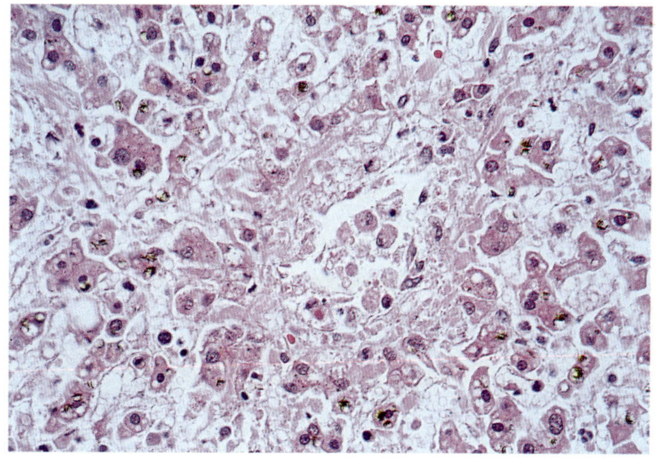

B

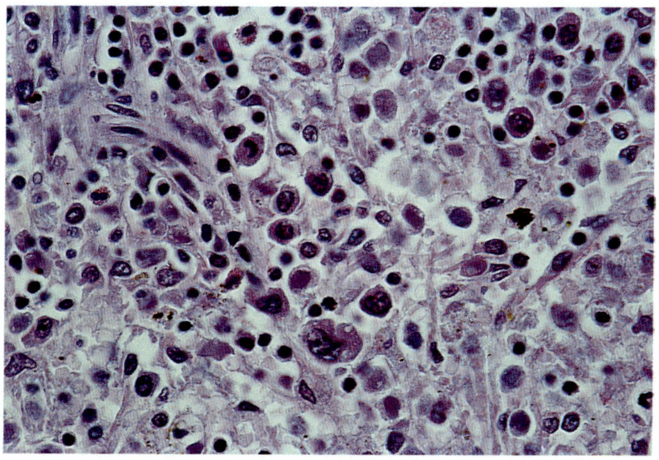

C

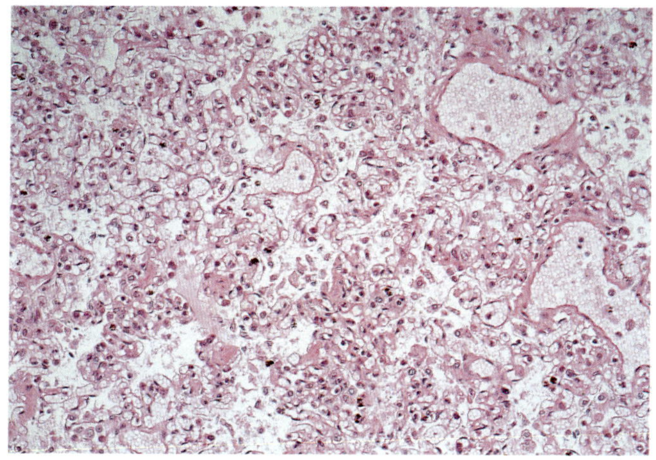

D

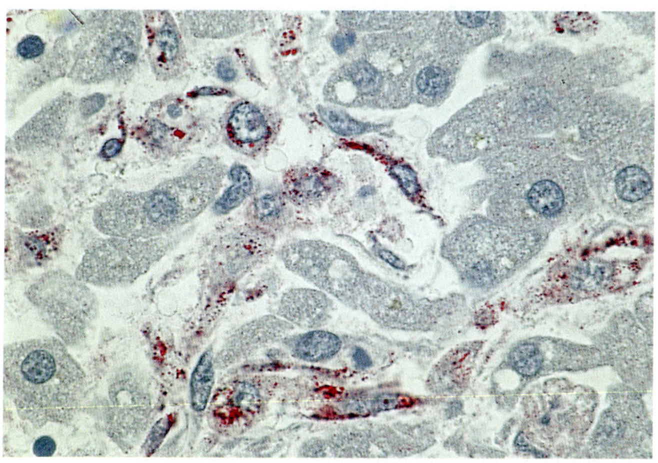

E

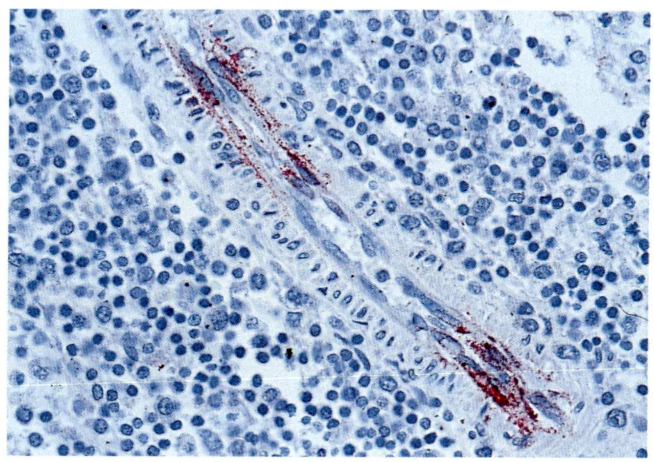

F

Figure 37–10. Dengue hemorrhagic fever. (**A**) Paracentral hepatic necrosis and sinusoidal congestion (H&E, ×50). (**B**) Higher magnification showing details of central area of hepatic lobule with a rim of intact hepatocytes around a central vein (H&E, ×100). (**C**) Numerous reactive mononuclear cells are in the spleen (H&E, ×158). (**D**) Lung with congestion and a mild mononuclear interstitial pneumonitis (H&E, ×50). (**E**) Immunostaining of liver showing viral antigens predominantly within Kupffer's cells. Hepatocytes are not stained (immunoalkaline phosphatase staining, anti-flavivirus antibody, Naphthol fast red substrate with light hematoxylin counterstain, ×250). (**F**) Immunostaining of dengue antigens within vascular endothelium of spleen (immunoalkaline phosphatase staining, anti-flavivirus antibody, Naphthol fast red substrate with light hematoxylin counterstain, ×100).

TABLE 37–4. DIAGNOSIS OF VIRAL HEMORRHAGIC FEVERS IN THE LABORATORY

Disease	Acute Serum Antigen ELISA	Acute Serum RT–PCR	Acute Serum Virus Isolation
Arenaviridae			
South American HF	Usually positive	Has been successfully applied	Usually positive
Lassa fever	Usually positive; if negative, IgM usually positive	Has been successfully applied; geographic variation in primers	Usually positive if patient still ill
Bunyaviridae			
Rift Valley fever	Positive in severe cases	Experimental	Readily isolated in first few days
Crimean Congo HF	Positive in severe cases	Useful; geographic variation in primers	Usually positive if patient ill
HFRS	Negative; IgM is test of choice	May be positive; primers must be carefully selected	Difficult to isolate
HPS	Negative; IgM is test of choice	Usually positive on clot first few days; primers must be carefully selected	Difficult to isolate
Filoviridae			
Marburg HF	Experimental	Experimental	Readily isolated
Ebola HF	Usually positive; IgM may be present	Positive	Most strains readily isolated
Flaviviridae			
Yellow fever	Variable; IgM is test of choice	Experimental	Readily isolated first 4 days
DHF/DSS	Variable; IgM is test of choice	Positive	Laborious; virus readily isolated if early specimens inoculated into mosquitoes
KFD/OHF	No experience	No experience	Usually isolated during the acute hemorrhagic phase

the HFs, with the exception of most Lassa fever patients, who nevertheless have dysfunctional platelets. Leukopenia is a constant feature of the South American HFs.

The major diseases that must be excluded are malaria, rickettsial diseases, leptospirosis, shigellosis, and typhoid, because all may mimic the HFs and all are treatable. Empiric treatment may be indicated for one or more of these infections. The usual differential diagnoses should be considered including regional diseases, such as trypanosomiasis, which may be associated with thrombocytopenia, and other medical conditions such as measles, lupus erythematosus, and hemolytic uremic syndrome.

The diagnosis of VHF, suspected by history and clinical manifestations, also can be supported histopathologically, and the overall pattern of histopathologic lesions may suggest a specific diagnosis. However, because the pathologic features of VHFs resemble other viral, rickettsial, and bacterial infections, an unequivocal diagnosis can be made only by laboratory tests such as immunohistochemistry and serology. The main pathologic differential diagnoses should include viral hepatitis, leptospirosis, malaria, and rickettsial infections.

CONFIRMATIONAL TESTING

Most of the VHFs can be diagnosed readily and rapidly from blood by a combination of detecting antigen by enzyme-linked immunosorbent assay (ELISA) and IgM ELISA. With most VHFs this combination of tests yields a diagnosis in virtually all patients within 24 to 48 hours of presentation; some patients with RVF and Crimean Congo HF—generally those with less severe disease—are exceptions. Some patients may require reverse transcriptase–polymerase chain reaction (RT–PCR) for enhanced sensitivity in mild or early infection or for genotyping (Table 37–4). Major obstacles to diagnosis are improperly collected specimens and delayed transport of samples to laboratories performing rapid, definitive tests.

Saliva, urine, and feces yield lesser numbers of viral isolates, but are worth testing in many patients because of the epidemiologic implications and to broaden the experience. Effusions are often good sources of virus in Lassa fever.

In convalescing patients, IgM can often be detected by ELISA for weeks or even a few months, but the duration has not been defined for substantial cohorts of

TABLE 37–5. PREVENTION AND TREATMENT OF VIRAL HEMORRHAGIC FEVERS

Disease	Prevention	Treatment
Argentine HF	Safe, effective vaccine used for high-risk residents of endemic area.	Infusion of convalescent plasma during first 8 days of illness reduces mortality from 15–30% to <1%.
Bolivian HF	Elimination of specific reservoir rodents from towns practical and effective. Sporadic cases due to exposure outside towns, person-to-person contact cannot be prevented.	Ribavirin likely to be effective and should be used in this and other arenavirus diseases unless alternative therapy available.
Lassa fever	None. Intensive village-based rodent control may reduce risk.	Ribavirin effective in reducing mortality; use in higher risk patients, eg, if AST>150.
Rift Valley fever	Vaccination of domestic livestock prevents epizootics/epidemics but not sporadic, endemic infections of humans. Human vaccine safe and effective but limited supply.	Ribavirin should be tried in HF patients based on studies in experimental animals.
Crimean Congo HF	Tick avoidance. No slaughter of acutely infected animals (healthy but viremic and therefore a threat). Barrier nursing of suspected patients.	Ribavirin should be used based on in vitro sensitivity and on uncontrolled South African experience.
HFRS	Rodent control and avoidance impractical in most cases. Investigational vaccines urgently need evaluation.	Early diagnosis and supportive care life saving. Ribavirin has positive effect during initial 4 days illness and should be used in Hantaan infection if available.
HPS	Rodent avoidance useful. Care should be taken before entering or cleaning closed buildings with rodent infestations.	Early diagnosis and supportive care potentially life saving. Avoidance of hypoxia and excessive hydration coupled with careful management of shock.
Ebola or Marburg HF	Barrier nursing and needle sterilization in African hospitals. Avoid close contact with suspicious patients. Careful evaluation of sick nonhuman primates.	None other than supportive, which may be of limited utility.
Yellow fever	Vaccine is probably the safest and most effective in the world. Control of *A aegypti* would eliminate urban transmission but sylvan transmission remains.	None other than supportive.
Dengue HF	Reduction of dengue transmission by *A aegypti* control. Currently investigational, vaccines will probably be available soon; possibly useful in travelers but unlikely to be a solution to hyperendemic dengue transmission that leads to dengue HF.	Supportive care effective and greatly reduces mortality.
Tick-borne flaviviruses	Avoidance of ticks. Post-exposure prophylaxis with specific IgG.	Supportive care.

patients. Paired sera tested by IgG ELISA or other serologic tests also may be useful.

Viruses can generally by isolated from organs at necropsy. Hantaviruses are an exception, possibly because they are difficult to cultivate. Immunohistochemistry (IHC) and in situ hybridization (ISH) done on formalin-fixed tissues with specific antibodies and nucleic acid probes are sensitive and specific for confirming the cause of the HF. These methods have a unique role when only archival tissues are available. Electron microscopy may have limited use as with filovirus infections.

TREATMENT AND PREVENTION

The HF viruses may pose a potential for nosocomial transmission and may be exotic to the region where patients are hospitalized. Thus special precautions must be taken. The topic has been hotly debated,[77–79] the biological basis for these concerns reviewed,[80] and guidelines established.[81,82]

Although no formal studies have been done, there is a strong clinical impression that patients with VHFs should not be moved, but admitted promptly to a local hospital. For instance in the 1950s when HFRS was common among U.S. troops in Korea, evacuation by helicopter was rapid and not traumatic—a great improvement over the usually long and traumatic journey by jeep or ambulance over rough roads.

Supportive care for bleeding, imbalance of fluid and electrolytes, shock, and hypoxia is recommended for any critically ill patient with VHF. These measures may be life saving for patients with DHF/DSS and contribute to survival of patients with most other HFs, but probably do not overcome the overwhelming viral replication and tissue damage of, for example, HF caused by Ebola (Zaire-subtype) infection. In general, fluid administration should be conservative because of the tendency to precipitate pulmonary edema and thus earlier use of cardiotonic and pressor drugs is indicated. In HPS, fluid management during hypotension or shock in the face of increased-permeability pulmonary edema is particularly difficult. Hypoxia may rapidly worsen in HPS and this should be planned while observing or transporting patients. The renal failure of HFRS and the severe hepatic involvement of yellow fever should be anticipated when treating patients with these infections.

The antiviral drug ribavirin is effective against arenaviruses in vitro and in animal models. There is good evidence for its efficacy in human Lassa fever, and these patients should receive intravenous ribavirin if their aspartate aminotransferase (AST) is >150 U/mL, indicating a severe course. The New World arenavirus HFs, also may respond to ribavirin, and it should be used in those patients. In the endemic zone, Argentine HF is routinely and successfully treated with adequate amounts of passive antibody infusion, but ribavirin is a reasonable alternative if convalescent-phase plasma is unavailable.

Ribavirin also has proven effective in HFs caused by bunyaviruses. Crimean Congo HF may respond to intravenous ribavirin and ribavirin should be used in these patients. Animals experimentally infected with Rift Valley fever virus respond to intravenous ribavirin, so it would be rational to use intravenous ribavirin for humans with severe RVF.

Vaccines are available for a few of the VHFs. Other preventive measures are aimed at avoiding and controlling rodents and arthropods (Table 37–5).

REFERENCES

1. Smorodintsev AA, Kazbintsev LI, Chudakov VG. *Virus Hemorrhagic Fevers.* Jerusalem: Israel Program for Scientific Translations; 1964:1–245.
2. Peters CJ, LeDuc JW. Viral hemorrhagic fevers: persistent problems, persistence in reservoirs. In: Mahy BWJ, Compans RW, eds. Chur, Switzerland: Harwood Academic Publishers; 1995;209–231.
3. Murphy FA. Virus taxonomy. In: Fields BN, Knipe DM, Howley PM, eds. *Field's Virology.* 3rd ed. Philadelphia: Lippincott-Raven; 1996:15–57.
4. Peters CJ, Zaki SR, Rollin PE. Viral hemorrhagic fevers. In: Mandell GL, ed. *Atlas of Infectious Diseases.* Vol. 8. Philadelphia: Current Medicine; 1997;10.1–10.26.
5. Peters CJ. Pathogenesis of viral hemorrhagic fevers. In: Nathanson N, Ahmed R, Gonzalez-Scarano F, et al, eds. *Viral Pathogenesis.* Philadelphia: Lippincott-Raven; 1996; 779–800.
6. Edington GM, White HA. The pathology of Lassa fever. *Trans R Soc Trop Med Hyg.* 1972;66:381–389.
7. Jahrling PB, Hesse RA, Eddy GA, Johnson KM, Callis RT, Stephen EL. Lassa virus infection of rhesus monkeys: pathogenesis and treatment with ribavirin. *J Infect Dis.* 1980;141:580–589.
8. McCormick JB, Walker DH, King IJ, et al. Lassa virus hepatitis: a study of fatal Lassa fever in humans. *Am J Trop Med Hyg.* 1986;35:401–407.
9. Walker DH, Johnson KM, Lange JV, Gardner JJ, Kiley MP, McCormick JB. Experimental infection of rhesus monkeys with Lassa virus and a closely related arenavirus, Mozambique virus. *J Infect Dis.* 1982;146:360–368.
10. Walker DH, McCormick JB, Johnson KM, et al. Pathologic and virologic study of fatal Lassa fever in man. *Am J Pathol.* 1982;107:349–356.
11. Winn WC, Walker DH. The pathology of human Lassa fever. *Bull WHO.* 1975;52:535–545.
12. Winn WC, Monath TP, Murphy FA, Whitfield SG. Lassa virus hepatitis. Observations on a fatal case from the 1972 Sierra Leone epidemic. *Arch Pathol.* 1975;99:599–604.
13. Shieh W, Greer PW, Ruo SL, Ksiazek TG, Peters CJ, Zaki SR. Lassa fever: immunohistochemical analysis of human tissues and pathogenetic implications. *Am J Pathol.* 1996 (in preparation).
14. Cossio P, Laguens R, Arana R, Segal A, Maiztegui J. Ultrastructural and immunohistochemical study of the human kidney in Argentine hemorrhagic fever. *Virchows Arch A Path Anat Histol.* 1975;368:1–9.
15. Elsner B, Schwarz E, Mando OC, Maiztegui J, Vilches A. Pathology of 12 fatal cases of Argentine hemorrhagic fever. *Am J Trop Med Hyg.* 1973;22:229–236.
16. Gonzalez PH, Cossio PM, Arana RM, Maiztegui JI, Laguens RP. Lymphatic tissue in Argentine hemorrhagic fever: pathologic features. *Arch Pathol Lab Med.* 1980;104: 250–254.
17. Maiztegui JI, Laguens RP, Cossio PM, et al. Ultrastructural and immunohistochemical studies in five cases of Argentine hemorrhagic fever. *J Infect Dis.* 1975;132:35–43.
18. Child PL, MacKenzie RB, Valverde LR, Johnson KM. Bolivian hemorrhagic fever. A pathologic description. *Arch Pathol.* 1967;83:434–445.
19. McLeod CG, Stookey JL, White JD, Eddy GA, Fry GA. Pathology of Bolivian hemorrhagic fever in the African green monkey. *Am J Trop Med Hyg.* 1978;27:822–826.
20. McLeod CG, Stookey JL, Eddy GA, Scott SK. Pathology of chronic Bolivian hemorrhagic fever in the rhesus monkey. *Am J Pathol.* 1976;84:211–224.
21. Terrell TG, Stookey JL, Eddy GA, Kastello MD. Pathology of Bolivian hemorrhagic fever in the rhesus monkey. *Am J Pathol.* 1973;73:477–494.
22. Salas R, de Manzione N, Tesh RB, et al. Venezuelan haemorrhagic fever. *Lancet.* 1991;338:1033–1036.
23. Kessler WH, Gross anatomic features found in 27 autopsies of epidemic hemorrhagic fever. *Ann Intern Med.* 1953;38:73–76.
24. Hullinghorst RL, Steer A. Pathology of epidemic hemorrhagic fever. *Ann Intern Med.* 1953;38:77–101.
25. Kikuchi K, Imamura M, Ueno H, et al. An autopsy case of epidemic hemorrhagic fever (Korean hemorrhagic fever). *Sapporo Med J.* 1982;51:K17–K31.
26. Lahdevirta J, Collan Y, Jokinen EJ, Hiltunen R. Renal sequelae to nephropathia epidemica. *Acta Pathol Microbiol Scand.* 1978;86:265–271.
27. Lahdevirta J. Nephropathia epidemica in Finland. A clinical, histological, and epidemiological study. *Ann Clin Res.* 1971;3:1–154.

28. Collan Y, Mihatsch M, Lahdevirta J, Jokinen E, Romppanen T, Janunen E. Nephropathia epidemica: mild variant of hemorrhagic fever with renal syndrome. *Kidney Int.* 1991;40:S62–S71.
29. Steer A. Pathology of hemorrhagic fever: a comparison of the findings—1951 and 1952. *Am J Pathol.* 1955;31: 201–221.
30. Lukes RJ. The pathology of thirty-nine fatal cases of epidemic hemorrhagic fever. *Am J Med.* 1954;16:639–650.
31. Zaki SR, Greer PW, Coffield LM, et al. Hantavirus pulmonary syndrome: pathogenesis of an emerging infectious disease. *Am J Pathol.* 1995;146:552–579.
32. Zaki SR. Hantavirus-associated diseases. In: Connor DH, Chandler FW, Schwartz DA, Manz HJ, Lack EE. eds. *The Pathology of Infectious Diseases.* Norwalk, Conn: Appleton and Lange; 1996.
33. Nolte KB, Feddersen RM, Foucar K, et al. Hantavirus pulmonary syndrome in the United States: pathologic description of a disease caused by a new agent. *Hum Pathol.* 1995;26:110–120.
34. Duchin JS, Koster FT, Peters CJ, et al. and Hantavirus Study Group. Hantavirus pulmonary syndrome: a clinical description of 17 patients with a newly recognized disease. *N Engl J Med.* 1994;330:949–955.
35. Zaki SR, Khan AS, Goodman RA, et al. Retrospective diagnosis of hantavirus pulmonary syndrome, 1978–1993: Implications for emerging infectious disease. *Arc Pathol Lab Med.* 1996;120:134–139.
36. Baskerville A, Satti AGO, Murphy FA, Simpson DIH. Congo-Crimean haemorrhagic fever in Dubai: histopathological studies. *J Clin Pathol.* 1981;34:871–874.
37. Suleiman MNEH, Musca-Baron JM, Harries JR, Satti AGO. Congo/Crimean haemorrhagic fever in Dubai. *Lancet.* 1980;2:939–941.
38. Joubert JR, King JB, Rossouw DJ, Cooper R. A nosocomial outbreak of Crimean-Congo haemorrhagic fever at Tygerberg Hospital. Part III. Clinical pathology and pathogenesis. *S Afr Med J.* 1985;68:722–728.
39. Abdel-Wahab KSE, El Baz LM, El Tayeb EM, Ossman MAM. Rift Valley fever virus infections in Egypt: pathological and virological findings in man. *Trans R Soc Trop Med Hyg.* 1978;72:392–396.
40. McGavran MH, Easterday BC. Rift Valley fever virus hepatitis. Light and electron microscopic studies in the mouse. *Am J Pathol.* 1963;42:587–607.
41. van Velden DJJ, Meyer JD, Olivier J, Gear JHS, McIntosh B. Rift Valley fever affecting humans in South Africa. A clinicopathological study. *S Afr Med J.* 1977;51:867–871,
42. Arborio M, Hall WC. Diagnosis of a human case of Rift Valley fever by immunoperoxidase demonstration of antigen in fixed liver tissue. *Res Virol.* 1989;140:165–168.
43. Burt FJ, Swanepoel R, Greer PW, Ksiazek TG, Peters CJ, Zaki SR. Immunohistochemical distribution of CCHF antigens in human tissues. *Arch Pathol Lab Med.* 1996; (in preparation).
44. Murphy FA, Simpson DIH, Whitfield SG, Zlotnik I, Carter GB. Marburg virus infection in monkeys. Ultrastructural studies. *Lab Invest.* 1971;24:279–291.
45. Kissling RE, Murphy FA, Henderson BE. Marburg virus. *Ann NY Acad Sci.* 1970;174:932–945.
46. Rippey JJ, Schepers NJ, Gear JHS. The pathology of Marburg virus disease. *S Afr Med J.* 1984;66:50–54.
47. Murphy FA, Simpson DIH, Whitfield SG, Zlotnik I, Carter GB. Marburg virus infection in monkeys. Ultrastructural studies. *Med Chir Dig.* 1972;1:325–332.
48. Fisher-Hoch SP, Brammer TL, Trappier SG, et al. Pathogenic potential of filoviruses: role of geographic origin of primate host and virus strain. *J Infect Dis.* 1992;166: 753–763.
49. Baskerville A, Bowen ETW, Platt GS, McArdell LB, Simpson DIH. The pathology of experimental Ebola virus infection in monkeys. *J Pathol.* 1978;125:131–138.
50. Geisberg TW, Jahrling PB, Hanes MA, Zack PM. Association of Ebola-related Reston virus particles and antigen with tissue lesions of monkeys imported to the United States. *J Comp Pathol.* 1992;106:137–152.
51. Murphy FA. Pathology of Ebola virus infection. In: Pattyn SR, ed. *Ebola Virus Haemorrhagic Fever.* Amsterdam: Elsevier/North-Holland Biomedical Press; 1978:43–59.
52. Baskerville A, Fisher-Hoch SP, Neild GH, Dowsett AB. Ultrastructural pathology of experimental Ebola haemorrhagic fever virus infection. *J Pathol.* 1985;147: 199–209.
53. International Study Team. Ebola haemorrhagic fever in Sudan, 1976. *Bull WHO.* 1978;56:247–270.
54. Dietrich M, Schumacher HH, Peters D, Knobloch J. Human pathology of Ebola (Maridi) virus infection in the Sudan. In: Pattyn SR, ed. *Ebola Virus Haemorrhagic Fever.* Amsterdam: Elsevier/North-Holland Biomedical Press; 1978:37–41.
55. Ellis DS, Simpson DIH, Francis DP, et al. Ultrastructure of Ebola virus particles in human liver. *J Clin Pathol.* 1978; 31:201–208.
56. Ryabchikova EI, Baranova SG, Tkachev VK, Grazhdantseva AA. Morphological changes in Ebola virus infection in guinea pigs. *Voprosy Virusologil.* 1993;4:176–179.
57. Pereboeva LA, Tkachev VK, Kolesnikova LV, Krendeleva LY, Ryabchikova EI, Smolina MP. Ultrastructural changes of guinea pig organs in sequential passages of Ebola virus. *Voprosy Virusologil.* 1993;4:179–182.
58. Jaax NJ, Davis KJ, Geisbert TJ, et al. Lethal experimental infection of rhesus monkeys with Ebola-Zaire (Mayinga) virus by the oral and conjunctival route of exposure. *Arch Pathol Lab Med.* 1996;120:140–155.
59. Zaki SR, Greer PW, Goldsmith CS, et al. Ebola virus hemorrhagic fever: pathologic, immunopathologic, and ultrastructural study. *Lab Invest.* 1996;74:133A. (Abstract).
60. Zaki SR, Greer PW, Coffield LM, et al. Outbreak of Ebola virus hemorrhagic fever, Kikwit, Zaire, 1995: pathologic, immunopathologic, and ultrastructural study. *Am J Pathol.* 1996 (in preparation).
61. Iyer CGS, Laxmana R, Work TH, Murthy DPN. Kyasanur Forest disease VI: pathological findings in three fatal human cases of Kyasanur Forest disease. *Ind J Med Sci.* 1959;13:1011–1022.
62. Iyer CGS, Work TH, Murthy DPN, Trapido H, Rajagopalan PK. Kyasanur Forest disease. VII. Pathological findings in monkeys, *Presbytis entellus* and *Macaca radiata,* found dead in the forest. *Ind J Med Res.* 1960;48:276–286.
63. Webb HE, Burston J. Clinical and pathological observations with special reference to the nervous system in

Macaca radiata infected with Kyasanur Forest disease virus. *Trans R Soc Trop Med Hyg.* 1966;60:325–331.

64. McCormick JB, Johnson KM. Viral hemorrhagic fevers. In: Warren KS, Mahmoud AAF, eds. *Tropical and Geographical Medicine.* New York: McGraw-Hill; 1984:676–697.
65. Vieira WT, Hayotto LC, de Lima CP, de Brito T. Histopathology of the human liver in yellow fever with special emphasis on the diagnostic role of the Councilman body. *Histopathology.* 1983;7:195–208.
66. Strano AJ. Yellow Fever. In: Binford CH, Connor DH, eds. *Pathology of Tropical and Extraordinary Diseases.* Washington, DC: Armed Forces Institute of Pathology; 1976:1–4.
67. Burke T. Dengue haemorrhagic fever: a pathological study. *Trans R Soc Trop Med Hyg.* 1968;62:682–691.
68. Boonpucknavig S, Boonpucknavig V, Bhamarapravati N, Nimmannitya S. Immunofluorescence study of skin rash in patients with dengue hemorrhagic fever. *Arch Pathol Lab Med.* 1979;103:463–466.
69. Boonpucknavig V, Bhamarapravati N, Boonpucknavig S, Futrakul P, Tanpaichitr P. Glomerular changes in dengue hemorrhagic fever. *Arch Pathol Lab Med.* 1976;100:206–212.
70. Bhamarapravati N, Tuchinda P, Boonpucknavig V. Pathology of Thailand haemorrhagic fever: a study of 100 autopsy cases. *Ann Trop Med Parasit.* 1967;61:500–510.
71. Fresh JW, Reyes V, Clarke EJ, Uylangco CV. Philippine hemorrhagic fever: a clinical, laboratory, and necropsy study. *J Lab Clin Med.* 1969;73:451–458.
72. Aung-Khin M, Khin MM, Thant-Zin M, Tin-U M. Changes in the tissues of the immune system in dengue haemorrhagic fever. *J Trop Med Hyg.* 1975;78:256–261.
73. Councilman WT. Report of Dr. William T. Councilman. In: Sternberg GM, ed. Report on etiology and prevention of yellow fever. US Marine Hospital Service Public Report Bulletin No. 2, 1980:151–159.
74. Hall WC, Crowell TP, Watts DM, et al. Demonstration of yellow fever and dengue antigens in formalin-fixed paraffin-embedded human liver by immunohistochemical analysis. *Am J Trop Med Hyg.* 1991;45:408–417.
75. Zaki SR. Leptospirosis associated with outbreak of acute febrile illness and pulmonary haemorrhage, Nicaragua, 1995. *Lancet.* 1996;347:535–536.
76. Shieh W, Ksiazek TG, Bethke FR, Greer PW, Zaki SR. Immunohistochemical diagnosis of flavivirus infection in paraffin-embedded human tissues. *Lab Invest.* 1996; 74:131A.
77. Bannister BA. Stringent precautions are advisable when caring for patients with viral hemorrhagic fevers. *Rev Med Virol.* 1993;3:3–6.
78. Fisher-Hoch SP. Stringent precautions are not advisable when caring for patients with viral haemorrhagic fevers. *Rev Med Virol.* 1993;3:7–13.
79. Peters CJ, Johnson ED, McKee KT, Jr. Filoviruses and management of viral hemorrhagic fevers. In: Belshe R, ed. *Textbook of Human Virology.* 2nd ed. St. Louis: Mosby Year Book; 1991:699–712.
80. Peters CJ, Jahrling PB, Khan AS. Management of patients infected with high-hazard viruses. *Arch Virol.* 1996 (in press).
81. Centers for Disease Control and Prevention. Management of patients with suspected viral hemorrhagic fever. *MMWR.* 1988;37:1–15.
82. Centers for Disease Control and Prevention. Update: management of patients with suspected viral hemorrhagic fever. *MMWR.* 1995;44:475–479.

CHAPTER 38

Viral Hepatitis

Zachary D. Goodman

For the King of Babylon stood at the parting of the way at the head of the two ways, to use divination: He made his arrows bright, he consulted with images, he looked in the liver.

Ezekiel 21:21

DEFINITIONS

Viral Hepatitis. This term is used for infection by any one of five viruses (Table 38–1) that are primarily hepatotropic. Excluded from this definition are systemic infections by viruses such as cytomegalovirus, Epstein–Barr, and hemorrhagic fever viruses even when they infect the liver.

Acute Hepatitis. This is a clinical syndrome characterized by abrupt onset of malaise, fatigue, nausea, vomiting, and right upper quadrant discomfort. Evidence of liver cell injury and necrosis includes release into the blood of intracellular hepatocellular enzymes, such as alanine aminotransferase (ALT) and aspartate aminotransferase (AST). Hepatocellular dysfunction usually includes inadequate excretion of bilirubin, so that within a few days the urine becomes dark (cola-colored), stools become light (clay-colored), and scleral icterus appears when the serum bilirubin rises to about 3 m/dL. Acute hepatitis usually runs its course over a few weeks with complete resolution.

Anicteric Hepatitis. Many patients infected with one of the hepatitis viruses have mild asymptomatic infections that can be detected only by demonstrating a rise in serum ALT activity and by documenting a seroconversion.

Fulminant Hepatitis. This is severe hepatitis, leading to liver failure and hepatic coma within 8 weeks. Typically there are high levels of serum aminotransferase activity (which may fall when there are no longer many viable hepatocytes) and a rising bilirubin. Most patients with fulminant hepatitis die unless they receive a liver transplant.

Cholestatic Hepatitis. This is acute hepatitis accompanied by deep jaundice and pruritus, simulating biliary obstruction. Recovery may be slow, and bilirubin may not return to normal for 2 to 6 months.

Chronic Hepatitis. This is persistent hepatocellular injury (lasting more than 6 months), as evidenced by elevated serum levels of intracellular enzymes such as ALT and AST. Chronic hepatitis is usually asymptomatic, but may be accompanied by chronic fatigue, nausea, anorexia, or upper abdominal pain.

Cirrhosis. This is end-stage liver disease, characterized by fibrosis and nodular regeneration with loss of normal hepatic acinar architecture and transformation of the entire liver into a distorted and scarred organ. Complications are those of portal hypertension, such as esophageal varices (which may result in fatal hemorrhage), ascites, splenomegaly, and edema, or of hepatocellular failure, such as hepatic encephalopathy, coagulopathy, and other consequences of inadequate functioning hepatic mass.

Hepatocellular Carcinoma. This is primary cancer of the liver in which the tumor cells resemble hepatocytes—a consequence of long-standing cirrhosis. The constant stimulus to regeneration presumably sets the stage for

TABLE 38–1. CHARACTERISTICS OF THE HEPATITIS VIRUSES

	Biologic	Clinical
Hepatitis A	Small RNA virus Similar to enteroviruses Fecal–oral transmission	Usually self-limited acute hepatitis Rarely cholestatic hepatitis, fulminant hepatitis
Hepatitis B	Small DNA virus Hepadnavirus Parenteral or sexual transmission	60% subclinical infection 30% acute hepatitis 1% fulminant hepatitis 10% chronic hepatitis
Hepatitis C	Small RNA virus Parenteral non-A, non-B hepatitis Related to Flaviviruses	Often subclinical Frequently chronic hepatitis (up to 75%)
Hepatitis D	Small RNA virus Coinfects with HBV Infects only those with HBsAg	More severe than HBV alone Frequently fulminant hepatitis
Hepatitis E	Epidemic (enteric) non-A, non-B hepatitis Fecal–oral transmission	Waterborne epidemics of cholestatic hepatitis in Asia and the tropics

mutations caused by chemicals, viral infection, and possibly other factors that lead to malignant neoplastic transformation.

THE VIRUSES: HEPATITIS A TO E

Biologic and Clinical Characteristics

Hepatitis A Virus

Hepatitis A virus (HAV) is a picornavirus (small RNA virus), a group that includes enteroviruses and rhinoviruses. The virus is 27 nanometers, nonenveloped, with a single serotype and only one immunodominant site. HAV is extremely infectious and highly stable under adverse conditions such as heat, drying, and acid. Consequently it is readily spread by the fecal–oral route through food or water with only minimal contamination necessary for transmission. Poor sanitation facilitates spread, so populations of developing countries are usually exposed during early childhood when the disease tends to be mild. In countries with good sanitation, the risk of infection comes later in life when infection tends to be more severe. HAV invades the gastrointestinal tract and then infects the liver, where it replicates in hepatocytes, but the virus is not cytopathic. Disease is produced when the host mounts an immune response. While the virus is replicating, viral particles are shed into the blood and the bile, thus excreted in feces, providing the opportunity for spread. Infection becomes apparent in 2 to 7 weeks (average 4 weeks) and coincides with the patient's immune response. Neutralizing antibody to hepatitis A antigen (anti-HAV) decreases production of virus and eliminates virus from the stool, but at the same time there is rising serum ALT, indicating necrosis of liver cells. During the acute phase of infection and immediately after recovery, the host produces IgM class anti-HAV. Thereafter, only IgG anti-HAV is found, but the antibody response confers lifelong immunity. Consequently, the diagnosis of acute hepatitis A is made by detecting IgM anti-HAV in the patient's serum.

Infection by HAV is a typical acute hepatitis. Severity varies, but about 70% of adults become jaundiced. Children younger than 2 years are usually asymptomatic, and severity tends to increase with age. Some patients have fulminant hepatitis, but this tends to be in those older than 50 years, and is rare with an incidence of less than 0.1%. Occasional patients relapse with what appears to be a new episode of hepatitis A 2 to 3 months after recovery. Rarely a patient will develop severe cholestatic jaundice that may persist for months, so-called "cholestatic hepatitis."

Hepatitis B Virus

Hepatitis B virus (HBV) is a 42-nanometer DNA virus. Similar hepatitis viruses infect woodchucks, ducks, prairie dogs, herons, and squirrels, and the name *hepadnaviruses* (hepatotropic DNA viruses) has been applied to this family. The complete HBV particle consists of a central core composed of the viral DNA (circular, partially double stranded) and the nucleocapsid hepatitis B core antigen (HBcAg) surrounded by a shell of the lipoprotein hepatitis B surface antigen (HBsAg). The viral genome is compact, consisting of only four genes, designated S, which produces HBsAg; C, which produces HBcAg and another protein called the *e* antigen (HBeAg); P, which produces a viral DNA polymerase; and X, which is thought to produce a trans-activating factor that regulates the level of viral replication. Several mutant forms of the virus have been identified, some of which have been associated with more severe liver disease.

Replication of HBV takes place predominantly in the liver, although other tissues also may be infected. Large quantities of HBsAg are produced and stored in hepatocytes and secreted into blood, possibly as a mechanism to induce immune tolerance in the host. HBcAg itself is not in blood but is there as part of the complete virion. HBeAg produced along with HBcAg, however, is secreted into the blood and indicates active production of virus and high infectivity. HBV is transmitted parenterally, although the route may not always be apparent. Blood transfusion, clotting factor concentrates for treating hemophilia, the sharing of needles by intravenous drug abusers, needle-stick injuries by medical workers, and any other direct contact with infected blood all transmit the virus. HBV is also in semen, vaginal mucus, and saliva, so sexual contact and maternal–infant transmission are routes of infection as well.

HBV has an incubation of 6 to 20 weeks (average 10 weeks), during which time the virus replicates in the liver. As with hepatitis A, infection is not apparent until the host mounts an immune response. HBsAg, HBeAg, and HBV DNA can all be detected in serum several weeks before symptoms begin, reaching peak titers at about the time illness begins. Antibodies to HBcAg (anti-HBc), initially of the IgM class, appear with the first prodromal symptoms and persist for several months, serving as a marker of acute infection. IgG anti-HBc appears later and persists for life. Antibodies to HBeAg (anti-HBe) appear after a few weeks, and antibodies to HBsAg (anti-HBs) during the convalescent phase. Some patients (approximately 15%) have symptoms that resemble serum sickness (arthralgias, fever, rash) associated with circulating immune complexes during the early stages. Most patients (approximately 60%) have only mild, often subclinical infections, seroconvert, and are unaware of the hepatitis. About 30% have a typical acute hepatitis with jaundice, then recover. Fewer than 1% have fulminant hepatitis with liver failure.

Overall about 10% of patients infected with HBV infection fail to mount an effective immune response, and these patients develop chronic infection. It is the mild, anicteric infections that are most likely to progress to chronic disease, and the state of the host immune system is of great importance in this regard. About 5% of adults but as many as 30% of infants and 90% of newborns infected with HBV develop chronic infection. Usually, chronic hepatitis is clinically silent but can be recognized by HBsAg in serum, with or without HBeAg, and by persistent elevations of serum AST and ALT, indicating ongoing hepatocellular injury. The course of chronic HBV infection varies. Some patients continue to produce HBsAg but remain healthy with no significant liver disease. Some clear the virus and recover after a number of years. An unknown number (25% to 50%), however, progress to cirrhosis over a course of years or decades, and hepatocellular carcinoma may be the terminal event. Immune-complex-mediated diseases may occur, also in the setting of chronic hepatitis B infection, although this is uncommon. Polyarteritis nodosa, other forms of vasculitis, membranous or membranoproliferative glomerulonephritis, and papular acrodermatitis have all been associated with chronic HBV infection.

Hepatitis C Virus

Hepatitis C virus (HCV) causes most of what was previously known as non-A, non-B hepatitis. HCV was detected in 1988 by modern techniques of molecular biology that bypassed traditional approaches. RNA fragments from the blood of a chimpanzee were used to synthesize complementary DNA, which was cloned in *Escherichia coli* and the gene products were tested against the serum of patients with chronic non-A, non-B hepatitis. After testing millions of clones, one was found to produce a peptide that reacted with antibodies in the patient's serum and thus could serve as a test for the virus. By isolation of overlapping clones, the entire 9400 nucleotide genome of the virus has been determined, and the functions of the viral genes are partially known. HCV is a single-stranded RNA virus with characteristics of a togavirus, distantly related to the flaviviruses, a group that includes yellow fever. The virus has structural genes that encode a nucleocapsid core and lipoprotein envelope as well as nonstructural genes that produce several enzymes with important roles in viral replication. Patients infected with HCV develop antibodies to these structural and nonstructural proteins (often not for several months after infection), but immunity does not result because there is rapid mutation of the virus. The envelope contains a hypervariable region where numerous mutations occur, producing what appears to be a successful strategy to foil the host immune system. This has produced a large number of HCV genotypes (or quasi species) throughout the world, some of which seem more virulent than others.

Parenteral exposure similar to that of HBV, whether through blood transfusion, intravenous drug abuse, or needle-stick injury, is the most widely recognized route of transmission of HCV. Sexual and perinatal transmission also probably occurs, but with lower efficiency than for HBV. Nevertheless, nearly 50% of patients who acquire HCV have no recognized risk factor or route of exposure. In spite of the similarity of HCV to some arboviruses, there are no epidemiologic data for an insect vector. In studies of post-transfusion hepatitis, HCV had an incubation of 6 to 8 weeks in most patients, with a range of 2 to 26 weeks. The events leading to the onset of disease are still unknown. Prospective studies of patients receiving blood transfusions have found that most have asymptomatic anicteric hepatitis detected only by daily measurements of the serum ALT. A few patients develop typical acute icteric hepatitis, but fulminant hepatitis from HCV is so rare that some dispute its existence.

The most serious consequence of HCV infection is the propensity for chronic liver disease. Between 50% and 80% of patients have persistent elevations of liver enzymes, and some investigators suggest that patients with HCV infection never completely eliminate the virus, providing a reservoir for transmission to other individuals. The ability of the virus to mutate rapidly allows it to escape immune surveillance. Chimpanzees that have recovered from experimentally induced HCV infection may be reinfected with other strains or even with the same strain of virus, indicating a lack of effective immunity. Anti-HCV antibodies are usually demonstrable within a few months of infection; however, although these are useful in diagnosis, they apparently play no role in pathogenesis or recovery.

The course of chronic hepatitis C is typically prolonged and fluctuating. Most patients remain asymptomatic, although a small minority complain of fatigue or malaise. Hepatic enzyme levels fluctuate widely, indicating alternating periods of quiescence and exacerbation. Antibodies to the virus do not bring about resolution, but may play a role in causing extrahepatic manifestations. Essential mixed cryoglobulinemia, vasculitis, glomerulonephritis, and a variety of autoimmune diseases have been associated with chronic HCV infection. About 20% of patients develop cirrhosis within a few years, but the true natural history of hepatitis C is not known as the disease may take many decades to unfold. Some patients die of end-stage liver disease, although others remain asymptomatic, even with established cirrhosis. Hepatocelluar carcinoma may be a terminal event, usually after long-standing cirrhosis.

Hepatitis D Virus

Hepatitis D virus (HDV), "delta agent," is a defective RNA virus that requires HBV as a helper. It is unique among animal viruses, but structurally resembles a class of plant pathogens called *viroids,* having a circular RNA genome smaller than any other animal RNA virus. HDV has a central core of HDV RNA and delta antigen protein surrounded by a shell of HBsAg, forming the infectious particle. Because HBsAg is required, HDV infects only those infected also with HBV. Those vaccinated against or recovered from infection by HBV cannot be infected with HDV. Modes of transmission appear to be similar to those for HBV. HDV infection occurs in two settings. Coinfection is said to occur when there is simultaneous infection with HBV and HDV. The HBV first infects the liver, providing the genetic coding for HBsAg. The HDV then uses the HBsAg for its own replication. Coinfection with HBV and HDV tends to be more severe than infection with HBV alone and carries a high risk of fulminant hepatitis. Superinfection is when a person with chronic HBV infection acquires HDV. This frequently exacerbates the underlying chronic hepatitis, or a previously stable patient may deteriorate. There may even be fulminant liver failure resembling coinfection. In coinfection, the patient has serologic markers of both acute HBV and acute HDV. The HBV infection produces a high (and usually rising) titer of IgM anti-HBc, while the coinfecting HDV induces a rising titer of anti-delta (often transiently). In superinfection, anti-HBc is present as a marker of the patient's chronic HBV infection, but this is of the IgG class, and the titer does not rise. The superinfecting HDV induces a rising titer of anti-delta more consistently than in coinfection. The combination of HBV and HDV usually causes a rapid progression to cirrhosis and its complications, but there does not appear to be a greater risk of hepatocellular carcinoma than with HBV alone.

Hepatitis E Virus

Hepatitis E virus (HEV) is a small RNA virus unrelated to the other hepatitis viruses. Electron microscopic and biophysical studies have suggested a structure similar to that of the *Calicivirus* family, although its exact classification is still uncertain. HEV has been documented in numerous outbreaks and epidemics in India and other parts of Asia as well as in Africa and Mexico, in parts of the world where most of the population is immune to HAV from early childhood. Infections in the United States and other developed countries have been in travelers to those underdeveloped areas. Many past epidemics of hepatitis in developing countries probably were caused by HEV. The pathogenesis of the disease is unknown, but there are many similarities to HAV infection. Like hepatitis A, HEV is spread almost exclusively by the fecal–oral route and is associated with poor sanitation, especially with contamination of water supplies. Also, HEV typically causes an acute, self-limited hepatitis, although in pregnant women infection is fatal in approximately 20%. Cholestatic hepatitis is frequent—more than 50% in some outbreaks. Chronic infection does not occur.

GEOGRAPHIC DISTRIBUTION

Hepatitis A occurs worldwide, but its expression varies from region to region depending on sanitary development. In the least developed countries of Asia, Africa, and Central and South America, infection is nearly universal in the first few years of life, but because infection is clinically silent in early childhood, symptomatic hepatitis A is not seen. In developed countries of western Europe and North America, most people are spared early infection, so there is a large unexposed population susceptible to infection and clinical disease when food or water becomes contaminated. Travelers to the Third World countries are at high risk. In countries that are partly but not highly developed, including eastern and southern Europe and parts of Asia, many become infected in late childhood or as adults, and most eventually contract the disease. These areas have the highest rates of clinically significant disease.

Hepatitis B occurs worldwide, but there are striking variations in its prevalence (Figure 38–1). In areas with high prevalence, such as China, Southeast Asia, and Southern Africa, 10% to 20% of the population are seropositive for HBsAg (so-called "carriers"), indicating chronic infection and serving as a reservoir for the virus. Nearly all other adults have antibodies to viral antigens, indicating past infection. In countries with moderate prevalence, such as Japan, Greece, and Italy, 2% to 5% of the population are carriers, whereas in areas of low prevalence, including northern Europe and the United States, the carrier rate is under 1%. In areas of high prevalence, HBV is a significant public health problem and is a leading cause of death from the complications of cirrhosis or hepatocellular carcinoma. In areas of low prevalence, HBV is still a significant cause of liver disease, causing 50% of acute hepatitis in the United States.

Hepatitis C is fairly uniform worldwide with a prevalence of 0.4% to 2.5% in blood donors of most countries. Some populations, however, are more heavily infected. In Japan there are localities with a prevalence of 16%, and more than 20% of some inner city groups in the United States have serologic evidence of infection.

Hepatitis D, in spite of its dependency on concurrent HBV infection, has a relatively low prevalence in some parts of the world such as East Asia, where HBV is common. Its greatest frequency is among HBsAg-positive people in northern South America, the Middle East, and parts of Africa (Figure 38–2). In these areas of high prevalence, more than 30% of carriers of HBsAg also have HDV. In South America, HDV caused many infections erroneously diagnosed as "yellow fever," as well as some mysterious diseases such as Labrea fever in Brazil and Santa Marta fever in Colombia. In many parts of the world with a low prevalence (less than 10% of HBsAg carriers), including North America and most of northern and western Europe, HDV tends to be a disease of HBV-positive drug addicts. Italy, where HDV was first discovered, and Greece, Central Asia, and parts of Africa and South America are intermediate in prevalence.

Hepatitis E (Figure 38–3) has caused a number of outbreaks, some of which were large epidemics. The first recognized was an epidemic of nearly 30,000 in Delhi, India, in 1955. Subsequent outbreaks have

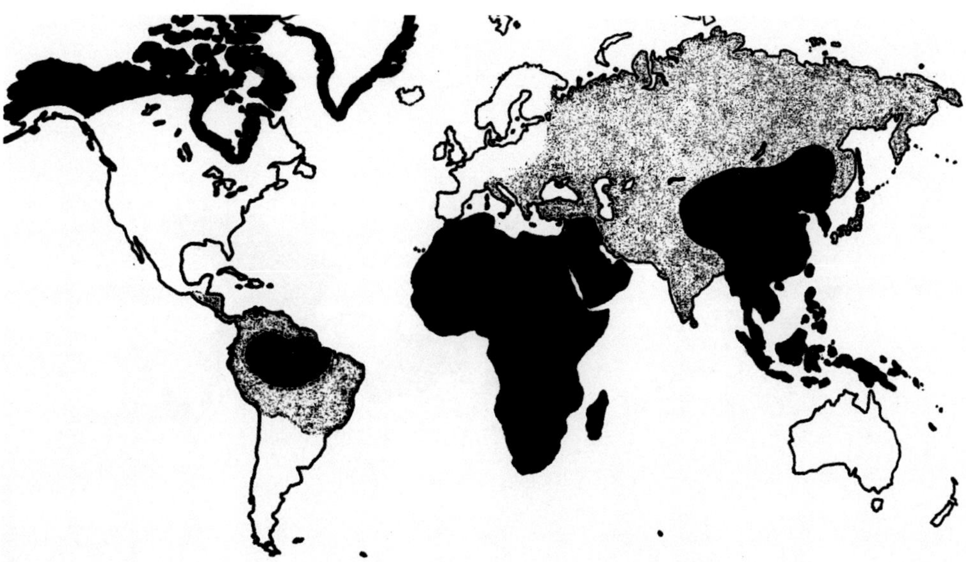

Figure 38–1. Distribution of hepatitis B. Areas with high (>8% of the population) prevalence of carriers of hepatitis B are black; areas with moderate prevalence (2% to 7%) are gray.

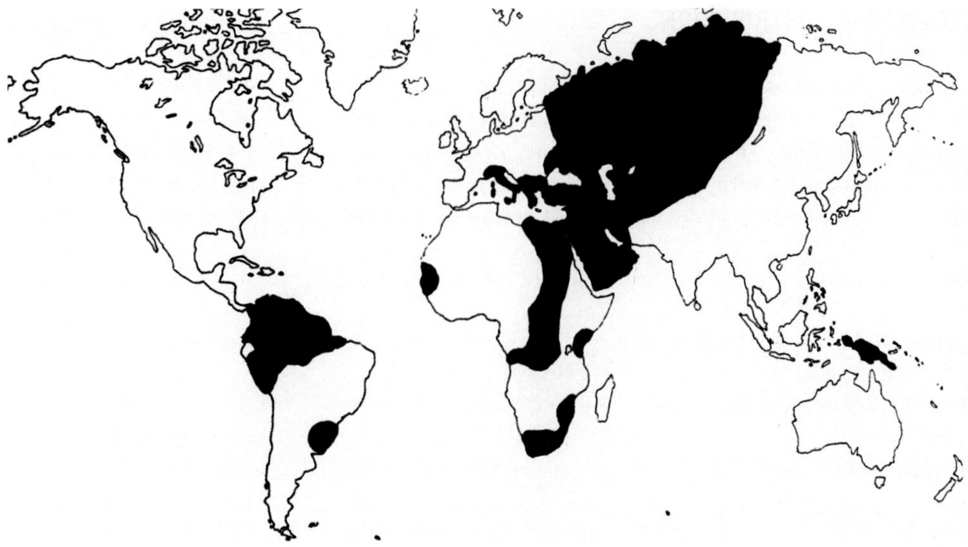

Figure 38–2. Distribution of hepatitis D. Countries known to have moderate (>10%) or high (>30%) rates of HDV infection of HBV carriers are black.

occurred in other parts of India and adjacent countries, Central and Southeast Asia, China, a number of countries in Africa, and in Mexico.

PATHOLOGY

Gross Pathology

Gross specimens of viral hepatitis are examined only when patients die or have liver transplants as lifesaving measures for severe hepatitis with liver failure or for end-stage cirrhosis.

Fulminant Hepatitis

The explanted or autopsy liver from a patient with fulminant hepatitis is typically small, flabby, and bile stained, the classic "acute yellow atrophy" as described by Rokitansky in the nineteenth century.

Cirrhosis

Cirrhotic livers may be large or small. The surface is bumpy and the entire liver may be distorted. It may also be bile stained, depending on the circumstances of the patient's terminal (or pretransplant) course. The left lobe frequently is enlarged. The liver is invariably firm from the diffuse scarring of cirrhosis. The cut surface consists of small, more or less spherical nodules. The size of the nodules is determined by the underlying disease and its duration. When most of the nodules are smaller than 3 mm, the cirrhosis is micronodular, and when most of the nodules are larger than 3 mm, the cirrhosis is macronodular. Occasionally cirrhotic livers

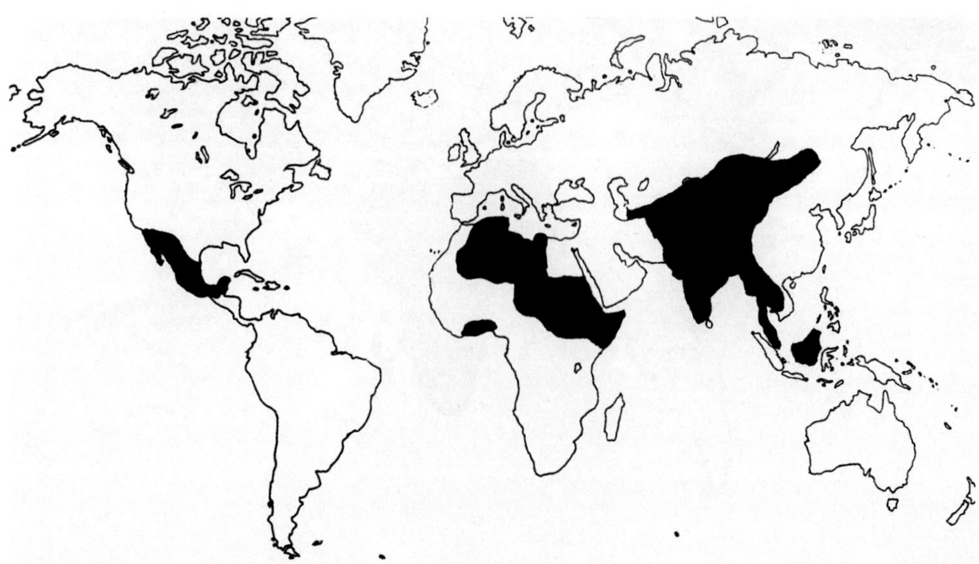

Figure 38–3. Distribution of hepatitis E. Countries in which outbreaks have been identified are black.

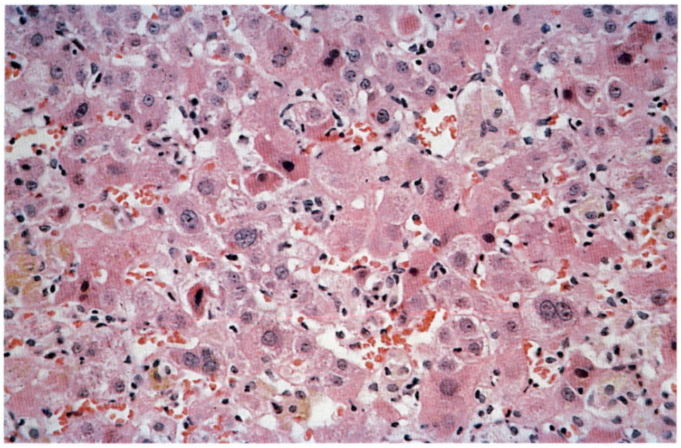

Figure 38–4. Acute viral hepatitis, moderately severe. There is lobular disarray with degeneration, apoptosis, and necrosis of liver cells, disruption of liver cell plates, hypertrophy of Kupffer cells, a predominantly lymphocytic inflammatory infiltrate, and regeneration of surviving liver cells.

contain distinctly larger nodules—up to 10 mm or more. These are called *macroregenerative nodules*.

Light Microscopy and Immunohistochemistry

Acute hepatitis, from infection by any of the hepatotropic viruses, causes liver cell injury and necrosis, both spotty and panacinar in distribution, and incites a characteristic response to that injury (Figures 38–4 and 38–5). The hepatocellular injury can take several forms, all representing the process and result of apoptosis or programmed death of hepatocytes. The best characterized form is acidophilic degeneration, in which hepatocytes shrink, losing intracellular water, and acquire a deeper color with acid dyes such as eosin. These hepatocytes may become angulated (rhomboid cells) or round, and their nuclei become pyknotic. The result is an acidophilic or apoptotic body. These bodies are fragments of cytoplasm or entire hepatocytes that have lost their nuclei and been extruded from the liver cell plates into the sinusoids, where they may be phagocytosed by Kupffer cells. Acidophilic bodies are scattered randomly throughout the acini, and their numbers reflect the severity of the hepatitis. Other liver cells undergo ballooning degeneration, in which the affected hepatocyte swells and loses its rectangular shape while the cytoplasm becomes pale and rarefied. Ballooning may be diffuse, but like acidophilic degeneration, it more often affects single cells or small groups of cells scattered randomly throughout the acinus. The result of ballooning is lysis of the cell, producing the lesion of focal (or "spotty") necrosis, which can be recognized as a small cluster of hypertrophied macrophages (Kupffer cells) and a few lymphocytes at the site of the dead and vanished hepatocyte. Hypertrophied Kupffer cells contain golden-brown lipofuscin pigment, which is positive with the periodic acid–Schiff (PAS) stain and represents the remnants of phagocytosed debris of the lysed cell. A reticulin stain reveals collapse or condensation of the supporting reticulin fibers caused by disruption of the cell plates at sites of necrosis. In severe infections there may be confluent necrosis of adjacent liver cells, most often in zone 3 of the acini, producing bridging necrosis. There is simultaneous regeneration of liver cells, recognized by enlargement of nuclei and nucleoli, mitoses and binucleation, and thickening of liver cell plates. Cholestasis may be prominent (cholestatic hepatitis), but this is uncommon. Fat may accumulate in liver cells. It is usually macrovesicular (rarely microvesicular) and mild.

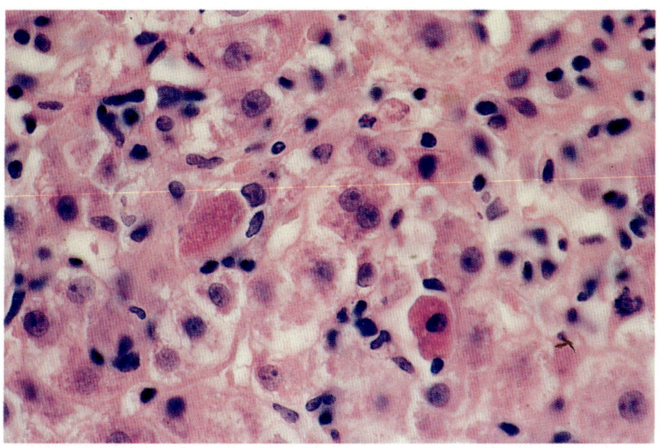

Figure 38–5. Acute viral hepatitis. Hepatocytes in various stages of apoptosis show ballooning and acidophilic degeneration and dropout. Lymphocytes are in contact with injured liver cells.

Injury and necrosis of liver cells is accompanied by inflammation. The Kupffer cells ingest debris of necrotic liver cells, becoming enlarged and engorged with lipofuscin, the indigestible residue of the dead hepatocytes. Other inflammatory cells, especially lymphocytes but sometimes plasma cells, eosinophils, and neutrophils, are in sinusoids and accumulate around degenerating and dead parenchymal cells. Some lymphocytes are in contact with hepatocytes and even within the cytoplasm of the injured cell. Presumably this reflects an immune-mediated attack on virally infected liver cells—the underlying mechanism of injury in viral hepatitis. Portal areas usually have increased numbers of inflammatory cells (predominantly lymphocytes and variable numbers of plasma cells, neutrophils, and eosinophils), but this tends to be commensurate with the degree of overall parenchymal injury, in contrast to chronic hepatitis, where the brunt of injury is portal. Some patients, however, especially those with hepatitis A and hepatitis C, have more exuberant portal inflammation with lymphoid aggregates and periportal necrosis, resembling the portal changes of chronic hepatitis. Bile ducts sometimes appear to be affected by the portal inflammatory infiltrate with injury of epithelial cells and occasionally disruption of the basement membrane.

The changes in a liver biopsy from a patient with acute hepatitis depend on the severity of the hepatitis and, in part, on the timing of the biopsy. The typical picture described here is seen in the early stages of clinical disease. As the disease runs its course, the acute hepatocellular injury becomes progressively less, and regeneration and repair are more prominent. During the resolving phase (1 to 3 months after onset of symptoms) there is little or no hepatocellular injury, but there are thickened cell plates with binucleate and multinucleate cells, indicating hepatic regeneration, as well as clusters of macrophages laden with lipofuscin and hemosiderin, evidence of cellular debris. At this stage intra-acinar inflammation abates, but portal inflammation increases, sometimes to the point of causing confusion with chronic hepatitis.

Variants of Acute Hepatitis

Acute cholestatic (cholangiolytic) hepatitis (Figure 38–6) is a combined hepatocellular–cholestatic injury. Histologically there is marked cholestasis with dilated canaliculi and pseudogland formation as well as hepatocellular degeneration, necrosis, and inflammation as in typical acute hepatitis. In some patients, cholangiolar proliferation with acute (neutrophilic) inflammation (acute cholangiolitis) may be prominent. Cholestatic hepatitis may resemble large duct biliary obstruction, and distinguishing the two may be difficult; recognition of the hepatitis-like hepatocellular injury is often the clue. Acute hepatitis of any cause may be cholestatic,

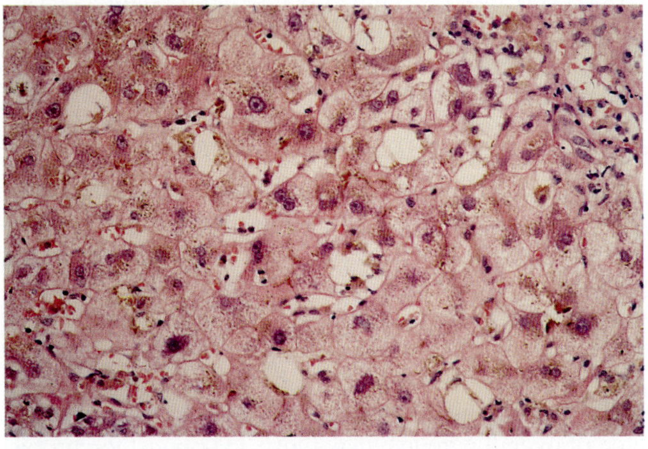

Figure 38–6. Cholestatic viral hepatitis. In addition to hepatocellular ballooning and lymphocytic infiltrate, there is cholestasis with bile pigment in hepatocytes and dilated bile canaliculi.

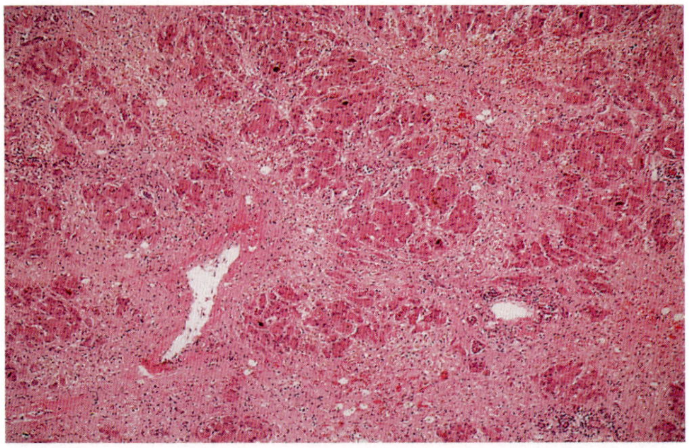

Figure 38–7. Acute viral hepatitis, severe, with submassive hepatic necrosis. There is confluent necrosis and dropout of most of the hepatocytes with collapse of the stroma. The few residual liver cells are regenerating, forming small nodules.

but drug-induced injury from some agents (eg, erythromycin, phenothiazines) is most frequent. Among the causes of viral hepatitis, HAV and HEV are most likely to cause a cholestatic hepatitis.

Acute hepatitis with submassive (confluent) necrosis (Figure 38–7) has all the features of typical acute hepatitis, but in addition shows necrosis and dropout of groups of adjacent hepatocytes, producing areas of collapsed stroma. This may take the form of bridging necrosis with portal-to-portal or portal-to-central linkage. The bridges are composed of collapsed reticulin, newly formed collagen fibers, hypertrophied Kupffer cells, and other inflammatory cells. The necrosis may be zonal, usually centrilobular involving acinar zones 2 and 3, but sometimes periportal, involving only zone 1 (especially in hepatitis A infection). The necrosis is described as multilobular or multiacinar when there is collapse of several adjacent lobules (or acini). If the patient survives the acute injury, there is usually regeneration from periportal regions that may become nodular with time, and may be confused with cirrhosis. A Masson stain, however, shows that the stroma between nodules has only early collagenization in the areas of collapse, and not the mature scars of cirrhosis.

Acute hepatitis with massive necrosis (fulminant hepatitis, acute yellow atrophy) is the most severe form of acute injury, with loss of all or nearly all hepatocytes and collapse of the supporting stroma, bringing the vascular structures and portal areas close together. Many engorged Kupffer cells filled with lipofuscin cling to the collapsed reticulin fibers, and terminal hepatic venules usually have prominent endophlebitis. Periportal areas show proliferation of ductules, which may be dilated and filled with inspissated bile. There are variable amounts of inflammation, usually with a predominance of lymphocytes, but sometimes with other inflammatory cell types.

Morphologic Clues to Etiology

Although morphologic features may suggest one virus over another (Table 38–2), serologic profiles and clinical history usually are necessary to confirm a diagnosis. Immunohistochemical techniques may be used to identify HDV but not the other viruses.

Hepatitis A tends to injure most severely the portal–periportal areas. There is relatively severe portal inflammation, often with plasma cells that seem more numerous than in acute hepatitis of other causes. There may be confluent necrosis in zone 1 with spillover of the portal inflammation into the parenchyma, causing piecemeal necrosis. There is spotty necrosis of zones 2 and 3 as well, but it may be impossible to distinguish acute hepatitis A from chronic hepatitis. Cholestasis also tends to be frequent in hepatitis A. Immunofluorescent staining of frozen sections sometimes demonstrates viral antigens, but this is seldom used in diagnosis.

Hepatitis B infection tends to look most like typical acute hepatitis with panacinar spotty necrosis. The injury in acinar zone 3 may be accentuated, producing zonal or bridging necrosis in severe infections. Viral antigens are destroyed by the host immune response and thus cannot be demonstrated in tissue sections.

Hepatitis C infection tends to look like typical acute hepatitis, but there is a greater tendency for fat to accumulate in liver cells. Some specimens have prominent acidophilic degeneration with angulated "rhomboid cells" and numerous acidophilic bodies. Others have numerous inflammatory cells in sinusoids, simulating infectious mononucleosis. In some, apparent injury of biliary epithelium produces a characteristic "hepatitis-associated bile duct lesion," in which lymphocytes and other inflammatory cells infiltrate and injure the epithelial cells but seldom completely destroy the duct. Portal lymphoid aggregates, resembling those in chronic hepatitis C, have been reported in acute infections caused by HCV, making the histologic distinction of acute from chronic hepatitis as difficult as in hepatitis A. Molecular techniques have yet to be used in acute hepatitis C.

Hepatitis D, as a coinfection or superinfection of hepatitis B, tends to cause a more severe hepatitis than other types with a high incidence of fulminant hepatitis and submassive or massive necrosis. Acidophilic bodies may be numerous. Routine immunohistochemistry is useful in acute hepatitis D, as delta antigen can be demonstrated in nuclei (Figure 38–8) in up to 80% of cases. Specimens from South America, where there are epidemics of fulminant delta hepatitis, often have prominent microvesicular fat accumulation in addition to hepatic necrosis. The combination of small droplet fat and acidophilic degeneration may produce a Councilman-like body as in yellow fever; many patients with hepatitis B plus D have probably been misdiagnosed as having yellow fever.

Hepatitis E produces cholestatic hepatitis in more than 50% of infections, although systematic studies have not been done recently. Bile-filled dilated canaliculi are frequent, producing a glandlike arrangement (so-called "pseudoglands"). Proliferation of ductules and acute inflammation (acute cholangiolitis) also can be prominent. HEV antigen has been demonstrated in tissue by immunofluorescence in experimental animals but has not been studied in humans.

TABLE 38–2. MORPHOLOGIC CLUES TO THE CAUSE OF ACUTE VIRAL HEPATITIS

Agent	Morphologic Clues
Hepatitis A	Heavy portal–periportal inflammation Plasma cells Cholestasis
Hepatitis B	Panacinar spotty necrosis, ± zone 3 accentuation
Hepatitis C	Fat (micro or macro) Many acidophilic bodies Mononucleosis-like sinusoidal infiltrates Bile duct injury Lymphoid aggregates
Hepatitis D	Microvesicular fat Many acidophilic bodies
Hepatitis E	Cholestasis Pseudoglands Ductular proliferation

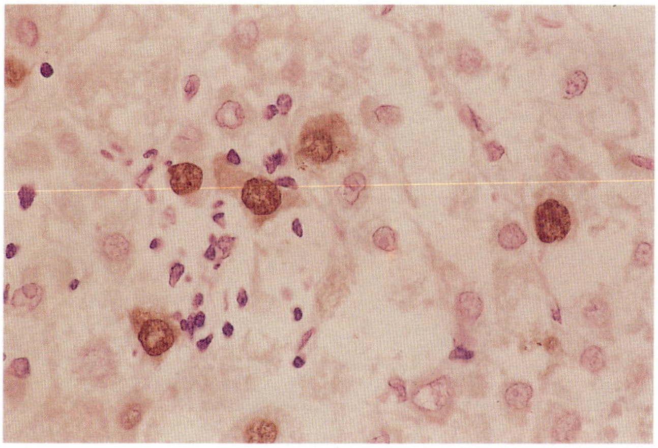

Figure 38–8. Acute hepatitis D. Delta antigen is in nuclei of hepatocytes (Immunoperoxidase staining with anti-delta as primary antibody).

Chronic Hepatitis

Chronic viral hepatitis can be caused by HBV, HCV, or HDV superimposed on HBV. Furthermore, HCV with HBV or with both HBV and HDV may infect high-risk populations such as intravenous drug abusers and hemophiliacs. In the United States, hepatitis C is by far the most common cause of chronic hepatitis, with approximately 85,000 new infections each year. In other countries (Figure 38–1), particularly in Africa and the Far East, chronic hepatitis B affects large segments of the population and is a major public health problem.

The type and severity of the disease produced by a chronic viral infection of the liver are products of the degree of continuing viral replication and the severity of the host immune response to the virus. In some patients there is little viral replication and only a mild response to the virus. These patients are usually asymptomatic and have minimal liver disease—so-called "healthy carriers." At the other extreme are those with active replication and an immune response that is brisk but not sufficient to eliminate the virus. Some of these progress to cirrhosis in a short time.

Morphologically chronic hepatitis, regardless of cause, has characteristic changes, present to a variable extent, in each patient. These include portal inflammation and injury, periportal injury in the form of piecemeal necrosis, spotty liver cell degeneration and necrosis with associated inflammation, and fibrosis. In all forms of chronic hepatitis the portal areas are infiltrated by lymphocytes and plasma cells to a greater degree than in acute hepatitis, and some have lymphoid aggregates or follicles with germinal centers (Figures 38–9 and 38–10). Bile ducts may appear to be injured and immersed by the infiltrate. As the disease progresses, the portal inflammation extends outward, injuring and destroying liver cells at the interface between parenchyma and connective tissue, so-called "piecemeal necrosis" (Figure 38–11). At one time the distinction between so-called chronic persistent hepatitis and chronic active hepatitis was made on the basis of whether a liver biopsy showed piecemeal necrosis, but this is no longer valid as follow-up studies have shown that some patients who initially have little or no piecemeal necrosis progress to end-stage cirrhosis over many years. In areas of piecemeal necrosis chronic inflammatory cells surround and invade injured hepatocytes, which undergo apoptosis and disappear, making room for more inflammatory cells to invade the acinus. The necroinflammatory changes are gradually succeeded by fibrosis, often best seen with a Masson or other collagen stain. Delicate collagen fibers form in areas of piecemeal necrosis and eventually condense into scars.

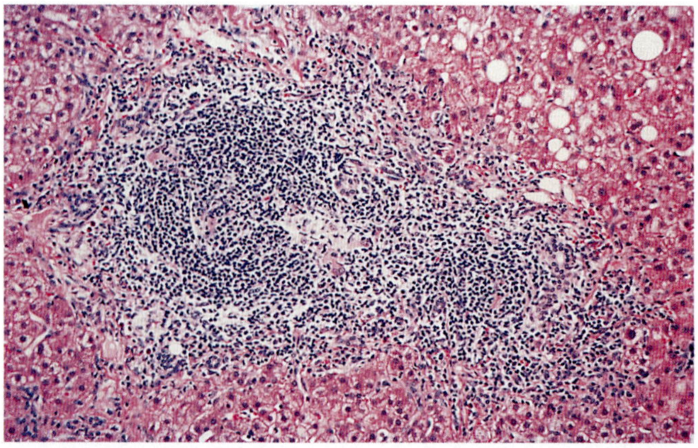

Figure 38–10. Chronic hepatitis C. There is chronic inflammation of this portal area with a lymphoid aggregate in the center. At the edges of the portal area, the interface between the parenchyma and portal connective tissue, inflammation spills into the acinus, destroying hepatocytes and expanding the portal tract by piecemeal necrosis.

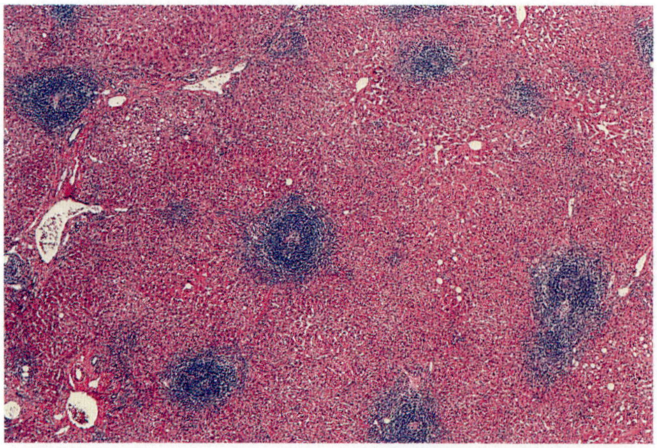

Figure 38–9. Chronic hepatitis C. There is chronic inflammation of the portal areas with lymphoid aggregates and follicles. In contrast to acute hepatitis, most of the injury is in the portal and periportal regions.

Most biopsies from patients with chronic hepatitis contain, in addition to piecemeal necrosis, intra-acinar necroinflammatory changes similar to those in acute hepatitis, but generally less severe. There is usually more intra-acinar injury when the biopsy is performed during an acute exacerbation of the chronic hepatitis. This may include an increase in spotty necrosis, ballooning degeneration, often most intense in zone 3, with dropout of hepatocytes and sometimes even confluent necrosis of whole zones of hepatic acini producing central-to-central or central-to-portal bridging necrosis and stromal collapse.

The histologic classification of chronic hepatitis has traditionally consisted of two major categories, chronic persistent hepatitis and chronic active hepatitis, even though there has always been dissatisfaction with these

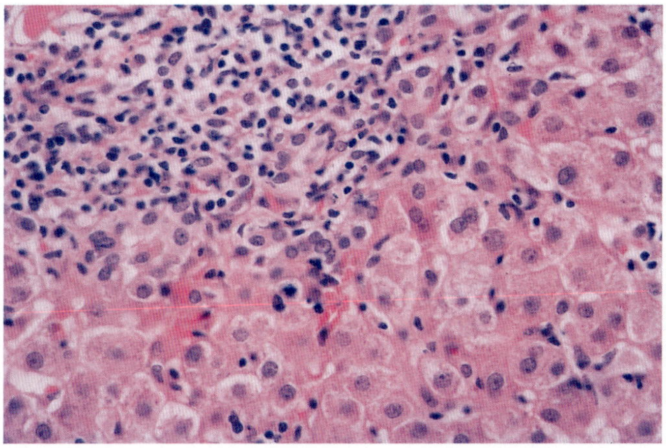

Figure 38–11. Piecemeal necrosis in chronic hepatitis. Lymphocytes emerge from the portal area and cause degeneration and dropout of hepatocytes. The limiting plate of the portal area is irregular and several degenerating liver cells are shrunken and eosinophilic.

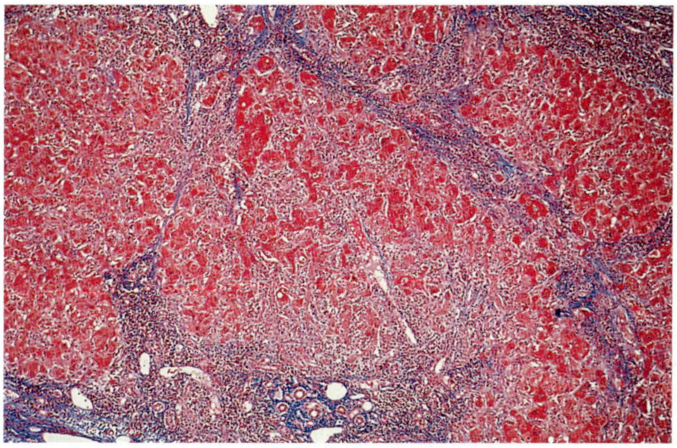

Figure 38–12. Fibrosis in chronic hepatitis. The Masson trichrome stain shows fibrous portal expansion with portal-to-portal bridging. New collagen fibers are in areas of piecemeal necrosis.

terms. Chronic hepatitis, in fact, is a spectrum of lesions from chronic persistent hepatitis at the mild end to severe chronic active hepatitis at the other end. Each point on the spectrum is a lesion with a slightly different rate of progression. Recent advances in understanding the causes and natural history of this type of liver disease have led to even greater dissatisfaction with these terms, and the prevailing current opinion is that the terms *chronic persistent hepatitis* and *chronic active hepatitis* as well as the equally poor but less widely used terms *chronic lobular hepatitis* and *chronic aggressive hepatitis* should be abandoned. In place of these terms, histopathologic diagnoses that incorporate pattern of injury, cause, and degree of injury should be used; for example, *chronic hepatitis B, mild activity,* or *chronic hepatitis C, moderately active with bridging fibrosis.*

Cirrhosis

The most serious consequence of chronic hepatitis is cirrhosis. Fibrous tissue is a nearly invariable part of chronic hepatitis, although the degree of fibrosis varies from patient to patient. Fibrosis is the progressive component of the disease, because scarring leads to architectural distortion and cirrhosis. Much of the fibrosis results from scarring that accompanies the progressive necroinflammation of piecemeal necrosis. As the disease progresses, portal-to-portal fibrous bridges are formed (Figure 38–12), filling zone 1 (periportal regions) between adjacent acini. There may also be formation of central-to-portal or central-to-central fibrous bridges that develop from superimposed episodes of necrosis involving zone 3 (so-called "passive septa"). In addition, there may be broad areas of fibrosis from healing of bouts of multiacinar necrosis. The scars contain elastic fibers as well as collagen fibers, and like scars in any tissue, these tend to contract. Contraction of the fibrous septa together with nodular regeneration of the surviving parenchyma produces architectural distortion, and when complete nodules have formed, the result is cirrhosis (Figure 38–13). When the necroinflammatory changes of piecemeal necrosis (now periseptal) continue unabated, terms such as *chronic hepatitis with cirrhosis* or *cirrhosis with active hepatitis* often are used.

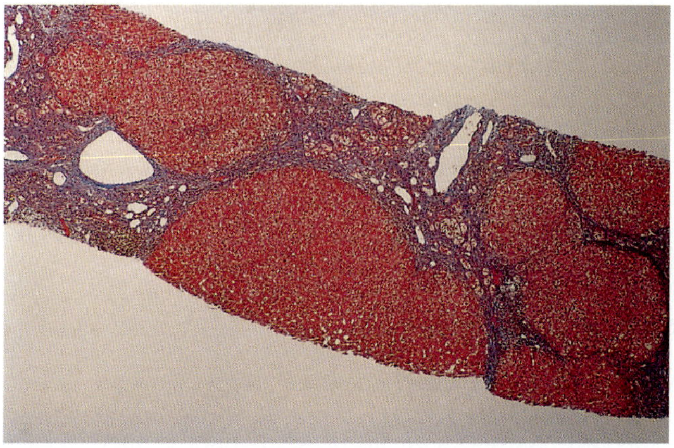

Figure 38–13. Cirrhosis in chronic hepatitis B (needle biopsy). The Masson trichrome stain shows cirrhotic nodules and portions of nodules separated by fibrous scars.

Hepatocellular Carcinoma

Hepatocellular carcinoma may develop in patients with long-standing chronic liver disease and is a frequent terminal event in patients with chronic viral hepatitis. This is one of the most common cancers worldwide, killing approximately one million persons each year, most in the Far East, sub-Saharan Africa, and in other parts of the world where hepatitis B is endemic. In the United States, hepatocellular carcinoma ranks as the 22nd most common cancer, with an annual incidence just below four cases per 100,000. It usually presents at an advanced stage and is nearly always fatal. Cirrhosis is the greatest risk factor for developing hepatocellular carcinoma, and perhaps most other causal factors actually operate by causing cirrhosis, which then causes carcinoma. In various parts of the world, 60% to 90% of hepatocellular carcinoma are in cirrhotic livers.

Chronic viral hepatitis is one of the most frequent antecedents of hepatocellular carcinoma. Several lines of evidence suggest a causal role for hepatitis B in the development of this tumor. Carriers of HBV are approximately 100 times more likely to develop hepatocellular carcinoma than noncarriers. DNA of hepatitis B virus integrates within the chromosomal DNA of non-neoplastic liver cells and tumor cells. Once integrated, the hepatitis B DNA may be rearranged, and it also may be associated with host chromosomal damage. Infection by hepatitis C also may play a causal role, especially in parts of the world where hepatitis B is less common. Furthermore, dual infections (HBV and HCV) may convey a greater risk of hepatocellular carcinoma than either alone. The risk of HDV is difficult to dissociate from the risk of the coinfecting hepatitis B.

Some cirrhotic livers contain putative precursor lesions, including various forms of liver cell dysplasia. Large cell dysplasia refers to hepatocytes that display nuclear changes resembling those of carcinoma. The nuclei are large, hyperchromatic, often irregular, and have one or more large or irregular nucleoli. The dysplastic cells, however, usually have abundant cytoplasm and are in non-neoplastic cords. Small cell dysplasia is a nodule of liver cells within a cirrhotic nodule. These dysplastic foci consist of smaller hepatocytes with more eosinophilia or more basophilia and with increased nuclear–cytoplasmic ratios and with increased numbers of nuclei per field.

Morphologic Clues to Cause

In chronic infection by hepatitis B, the virus is not effectively eliminated by the immune response, so viral antigens and genome may be demonstrable in tissue. The cytoplasm of cells containing large quantities of HBsAg has a uniformly finely granular appearance, the so-called "ground-glass cells" (Figure 38–14). These are scattered randomly and often in clusters. The number of ground-glass cells tends to be inversely related to the activity of the hepatitis, with most of the cells in livers with least active disease, whereas livers with the most activity tend to have the fewest ground-glass cells. Some stains, such as orcein and Victoria blue (Figure 38–15), react with HBsAg and are useful in identifying ground-glass cells, but these are now supplanted by the more sensitive immunoperoxidase stains. Hepatitis B surface antigen is demonstrated by routine immunostaining of paraffin-embedded tissue in 80% or more of specimens of chronic hepatitis B (Figure 38–16). Hepatitis B core antigen usually can be demonstrated immunohistochemically in nuclei and sometimes cytoplasm. Core antigen reflects active viral replication, and so the amount tends to be proportional to the activity of the hepatitis. Patients with recent acute exacerbations have the most core and will often have HBcAg in the cytoplasm of hepatocytes and in nuclei. Viral DNA also

TABLE 38–3. MORPHOLOGIC CLUES TO THE CAUSE OF CHRONIC VIRAL HEPATITIS

Agent	Morphologic Clues	Confirm with
Hepatitis B	Ground-glass hepatocytes	Orcein or other stain Immunoperoxidase for HBsAg, HBcAg
Hepatitis C	Fat, bile duct injury Portal lymphoid aggregates Talc (IV drug abuse)	Transfusion history Anti-HCV History of drug abuse
Hepatitis D		Immunoperoxidase for delta antigen Anti-delta

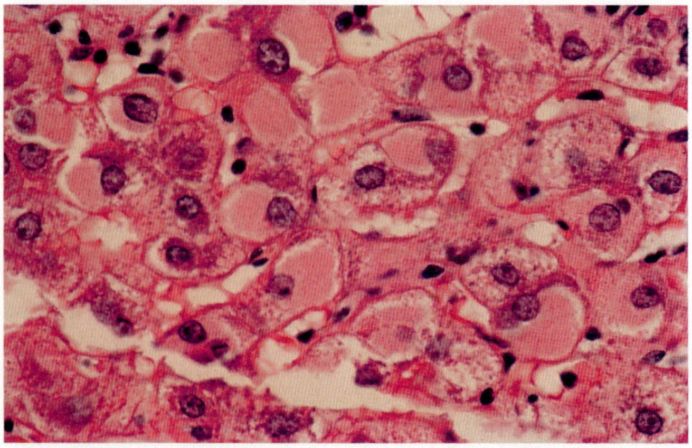

Figure 38–14. Chronic hepatitis B. Ground-glass hepatocytes containing large amounts of HBsAg have a uniformly eosinophilic cytoplasm.

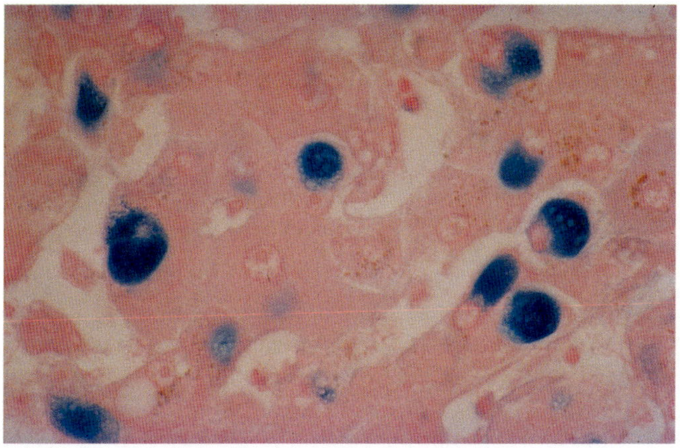

Figure 38–15. Chronic hepatitis B. Ground-glass cells stain with Victoria blue, confirming the presence of HBsAg.

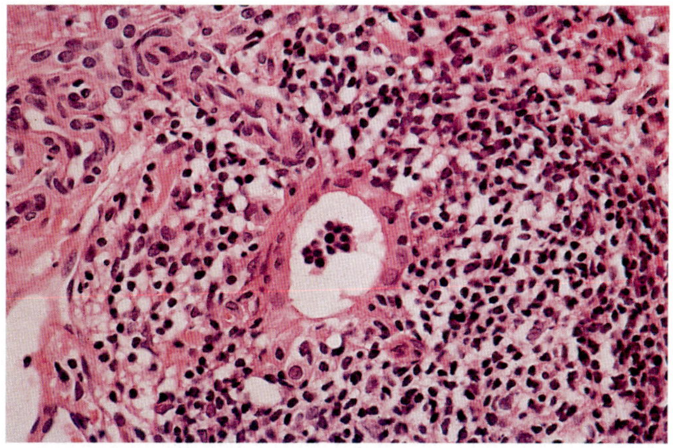

Figure 38–17. Chronic hepatitis C. This is a hepatitis-associated bile duct lesion showing epithelial injury and infiltration of the duct by portal inflammatory cells.

can be demonstrated by in situ hybridization, but this is generally used only in research laboratories.

Hepatitis D (delta) superimposed on hepatitis B tends to produce more severe disease than hepatitis B alone, but there are no features by light microscopy that specifically implicate hepatitis D. Delta antigen can nearly always be found in nuclei of hepatocytes by immunostaining and proves the presence of hepatitis D; HBsAg and/or HBcAg may be present as well.

Most patients with hepatitis C have a chronic infection lasting for decades, and liver biopsies usually show a mild to moderate chronic hepatitis. The severity, however, varies with periods of quiescence and exacerbation. Although histologic features in hepatitis C are not specific, discrete lymphoid aggregates in at least some portal areas are typical, and lymphoid follicles with germinal centers may be present as well. Lesions of bile ducts (Figure 38–17) are also typical, although not constant or specific. These show swelling, vacuolization, nuclear irregularity, and pseudostratification of epithelial cells of occasional interlobular bile ducts. The basement membrane may appear to be ruptured, and inflammatory cells infiltrate the duct, reminiscent of the "florid duct lesions" of primary biliary cirrhosis. The ductal lesions have been seen in all forms of hepatitis, but they are most common in chronic hepatitis C—about 25% of biopsies. Hepatitis C also has a greater tendency toward hepatocellular accumulation of fat than do other types of chronic hepatitis. Some fat is in about 50% to 75% of biopsies, and occasionally (less than 5%) the quantity of fat is impressive. When chronic hepatitis C is acquired as a consequence of IV drug use, Kupffer's cells and portal macrophages may contain birefringent talc crystals (an adulterant). HCV antigens and nucleic acids have been demonstrated in tissue, but even the most successful techniques fail in many patients, and most reports have used frozen sections, limiting the use for diagnosis.

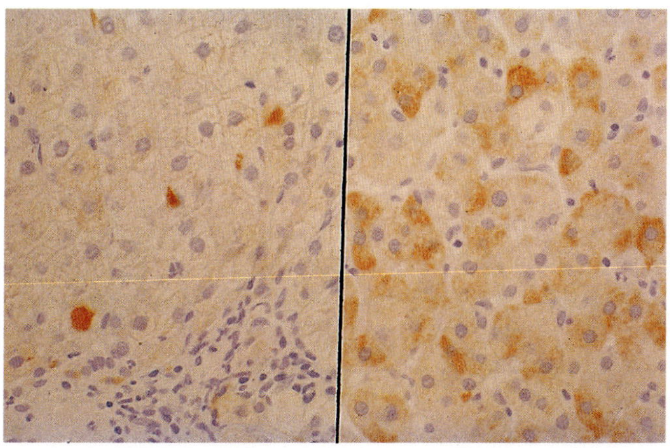

Figure 38–16. Chronic hepatitis B. Immunoperoxidase stain for HBsAg shows some areas with discrete and dark staining of the ground-glass cells (*left*), whereas other parts of the same liver show pale, diffuse, or membranous staining that would not be apparent with the Victoria blue or other histochemical techniques.

Differential Diagnosis

The differential diagnosis of acute and chronic viral hepatitis includes virtually all non-neoplastic liver diseases, a discussion of which is beyond the scope of this chapter. Some of the more important entities that may be confused with viral hepatitis clinically and pathologically are discussed next.

Other Viral Infections Most of these are readily distinguished from primary viral hepatitis on clinical and histologic grounds. Epstein–Barr virus (EBV) and cytomegalovirus (CMV) cause infectious mononucleosis in immunologically competent hosts. An acute hepatitis is part of the disease, but it differs from typical viral hepatitis in having less hepatocellular injury but a much greater sinusoidal inflammatory cell infiltrate (predominantly lymphocytes and plasma cells) producing a pattern of "Indian file" or "sinusoidal beading" and also hepatocellular regeneration with numerous mitoses. Viral inclusions are virtually never seen in CMV hepatitis. In immunocompromised individuals, however, CMV causes spotty necrosis, often with a neutrophilic inflammatory response, and typical intranuclear inclusions can be found. Adenovirus hepatitis is seen only in immunocompromised patients, in whom it can cause extensive necrosis and pleomorphic nuclear inclusions. Herpes simplex and herpes varicella-zoster rarely infect the livers of both normal and compromised hosts, producing patchy areas of coagulative necrosis that can become large and confluent with Cowdry type A herpetic nuclear inclusions around the edges of the necrotic lesions. Yellow fever and other viral hemorrhagic fevers cause a "salt-and-pepper" pattern of focal coagulative necrosis of liver cells, rather than the ballooning and focal necrosis of viral hepatitis.

Autoimmune hepatitis is, in general, the most severe type of chronic hepatitis, although like chronic viral hepatitis, there is much variability. Although this is a chronic disease that often leads to cirrhosis, it may have an acute clinical presentation and initial liver biopsies may show acute submassive hepatic necrosis, mimicking severe acute viral hepatitis. Biopsies may also show chronic hepatitis, usually quite severe, with areas of multiacinar necrosis and hepatocytic rosettes, or they may show cirrhosis with ongoing chronic hepatitis. A severe chronic hepatitis should suggest the diagnosis, but confirmation requires negative viral serology and laboratory evidence of autoimmunity, such as hypergammaglobulinemia and autoantibodies (antinuclear antibody, antismooth muscle antibody, etc).

Alcoholic liver disease may present with jaundice and hepatomegaly, causing it to be confused with viral hepatitis. Fat in a liver biopsy specimen should prompt a search for Mallory bodies (alcoholic hyalin) in zone 3 hepatocytes before making a diagnosis of viral hepatitis. Furthermore, a Masson stain usually shows some fibrosis around central veins, a feature that is typical of alcoholic hepatitis but not of viral hepatitis.

Mechanical biliary obstruction also can be confused with viral hepatitis clinically, especially with the cholestatic variant. Bile stasis without hepatocellular injury should prompt a search for features suggesting obstruction, such as acute cholangitis and bile infarcts, to avoid an erroneous diagnosis of viral hepatitis.

Chronic biliary tract diseases, such as the precirrhotic stages of primary biliary cirrhosis and primary sclerosing cholangitis, are usually associated with chronic portal inflammation and often with piecemeal and spotty parenchymal necrosis, causing them to be confused with chronic hepatitis. In these diseases, however, bile ducts are not merely injured but destroyed, so a search for ducts and for features of chronic cholestasis (periportal bile stasis, pseudoxanthomatous change, and ductular proliferation) must be done before making a diagnosis of chronic hepatitis.

Metabolic diseases, such as Wilson's disease and alpha-1-antitrypsin deficiency, can produce chronic inflammation and fibrosis leading to cirrhosis, and thus may be confused with chronic viral hepatitis. Stains for copper and the PAS stain to demonstrate the cytoplasmic globules of alpha-1-antitrypsin can help lead to the correct diagnosis. Wilson's disease also can present

TABLE 38–4. SEROLOGIC DIAGNOSIS OF VIRAL HEPATITIS

Virus	Test	Abbreviation	Interpretation of Positive Test
Hepatitis A	Antibody to hepatitis A virus	Anti-HAV	Acute or previous hepatitis A
	IgM class	IgM anti-HAV	Acute hepatitis A
	IgG class	IgG anti-HAV	Previous hepatitis A infection
Hepatitis B	Hepatitis B surface antigen	HBsAg	Acute or chronic hepatitis B
	Antibody to hepatitis B surface	Anti-HBs	Previous hepatitis B
	Antibody to hepatitis B core	Anti-HBc	Acute, chronic, or previous hepatitis B
	IgM class	IgM anti-HBc	Acute hepatitis B
	IgG class	IgG anti-HBc	Chronic or previous hepatitis B
	Hepatitis B e antigen	HBeAg	Acute or chronic hepatitis B with active viral replication and high infectivity
	Antibody to hepatitis B e antigen	Anti-HBe	Previous hepatitis B or chronic hepatitis B with little viral replication and low infectivity
Hepatitis C	Antibody to hepatitis C virus	Anti-HCV	Acute, chronic, or previous hepatitis C
	Hepatitis C RNA by PCR		Active hepatitis C replication
Hepatitis D	Antibody to delta antigen	Anti-delta	Acute, chronic, or previous hepatitis D
Hepatitis E	Antibody to hepatitis E antigen	Anti-HEV	Acute or previous hepatitis E

with acute hepatic necrosis, mimicking fulminant viral hepatitis. Patients with Wilson's disease are typically young, so this must be remembered in young patients with unexplained liver failure. Chemical studies of copper metabolism resolve the diagnosis.

Drug-induced injury can mimic virtually any type of liver disease, especially viral hepatitis. If the inflammatory infiltrate contains eosinophils or granulomas, or if the injury is severe with submassive or zonal necrosis, then drug-induced hepatitis is more likely than viral. Many cases of drug-induced injury are identical to viral hepatitis, however, so an accurate history of medications is essential to the evaluation of any patient with acute liver disease.

Serologic Diagnosis

The diagnosis of viral hepatitis is usually made or strongly suggested by a positive serology for one of the viruses. The most commonly used serologic tests are listed in Table 38–4.

SUGGESTED READINGS

Textbooks

Haubrich WS, Schaffner F, Berk JE, eds. *Bockus Gastroenterology,* 5th ed. Philadelphia: WB Saunders; 1995.

Kanel GC, Korula J. *Atlas of Liver Pathology.* Philadelphia: WB Saunders; 1992.

Lee RG. *Diagnostic Liver Pathology.* St. Louis: Mosby-Year Book; 1994.

Ludwig J. *Practical Liver Biopsy Interpretation.* Chicago: ASCP Press; 1992.

MacSween RNM, Anthony PP, Scheuer PJ, Burt AD, Portmann BC, eds. *Pathology of the Liver.* 3rd ed. Edinburgh: Churchill Livingstone; 1994.

Reubner BH, Montgomery CK, French SW. *Diagnostic Pathology of the Liver and Biliary Tract.* 2nd ed. New York: Hemisphere Publishing Corporation; 1991.

Scheuer PJ, Lefkowitch JH. *Liver Biopsy Interpretation.* 5th ed. London: WB Saunders; 1994.

Schiff L, Schiff ER, eds. *Diseases of the Liver.* 7th ed. Philadelphia: JB Lippincott; 1993.

Snover D. *Biopsy Diagnosis of Liver Disease.* Baltimore: Williams & Wilkins; 1992.

Zuckerman AJ, Thomas HC. *Viral Hepatitis: Scientific Basis and Clinical Management.* Edinburgh: Churchill Livingstone; 1993.

Hepatitis A

Abe H, Beninger PR, Ikejiri N, et al. Light microscopic findings of liver biopsy specimens from patients with hepatitis type A and comparison with type B. *Gastroenterology.* 1982; 83:938–947.

Lemon SM. Type A viral hepatitis. New developments in an old disease. *N Engl J Med.* 1985;313:1059–1067.

Taylor GM, Goldin RD, Karayiannis P, Thomas HC. In situ hybridization studies in hepatitis A infection. *Hepatology.* 1992;16:642–648.

Teixeira MR, Weller IVD, Murray A, et al. The pathology of hepatitis A in man. *Liver.* 1982;2:53–60.

Hepatitis B

Goodman ZD, Langloss JM, Bratthauer GL, Ishak KG. Immunohistochemical localization of hepatitis B surface antigen and hepatitis B core antigen in tissue sections. A source of false positive staining. *Am J Clin Pathol.* 1988; 89:533–537.

Houthoff HJ, Niermeijer P, Gips CH, et al. Hepatic morphologic findings and viral antigens in acute hepatitis B. A longitudinal study. *Virchows Arch A Path Anat Histol.* 1980; 389:153–166.

Hsu HC, Lai MY, Chen DS, et al. Correlation of hepatocyte HBsAg expression with virus replication and liver pathology. *Hepatology.* 1988;8:749–754.

Lindh G, Weiland O, Glaumann H. The application of a numerical scoring system for evaluating the histological outcome in patients with chronic hepatitis B followed in long term. *Hepatology.* 1988;8:98–103.

Mills CT, Lee E, Perrillo R. Relationship between histology, aminotransferase levels, and viral replication in chronic hepatitis B. *Gastroenterology.* 1990;99:519–524.

Naoumov NV, Daniels HM, Davison F, Eddleston ALWF, Alexander GJM, Williams R. Identification of hepatitis B virus-DNA in the liver by in situ hybridisation using a biotinylated probe. Relation to HBcAg expression and histology. *J Hepatol.* 1993;19:204–210.

Stocklin E, Gudat F, Krey G, et al. Delta antigen in hepatitis B: immunohistology of frozen and paraffin-embedded liver biopsies and relation to HBV infection. *Hepatology.* 1981;1:238–242.

Villari D, Raimondo G, Brancatelli S, Longo G, Rodino G, Smedile V. Histological features in liver biopsy specimens of patients with acute reactivation of chronic type B hepatitis. *Histopathology.* 1991;18:73–77.

Yoo JY, Howard R. Waggoner JG, Hoofnagle JH. Peroxidase-antiperoxidase detection of hepatitis B surface and core antigen in liver biopsy specimens from patients with chronic type B hepatitis. *J Med Virol.* 1987;23:273–281.

Hepatitis C

Blight K, Rowland R, Hall PD, et al. Immunohistochemical detection of the NS4 antigen of hepatitis C virus and its relation to histopathology. *Am J Pathol.* 1993;143:1568–1573.

Blight K, Trowbridge R, Rowland R, Gowans E. Detection of hepatitis C virus RNA by in situ hybridization. *Liver.* 1992; 12(special issue):286–289.

Choo QL, Kuo G, Weiner AJ, Overby LR, Bradley DW, Houghton M. Isolation of a cDNA clone derived from a blood-borne non-A, non-B viral hepatitis genome. *Science.* 1989;244:359–361.

DiBisceglie AM, Goodman ZD, Ishak KG, Hoofnagle JH, Melponder JJ, Alter HJ. Long-term clinical and histopathological follow-up of chronic post-transfusion hepatitis. *Hepatology.* 1991;14:969–974.

Dienes HP, Popper H, Arnold W, Lobeck H. Histologic observations in human hepatitis non-A, non-B. *Hepatology.* 1982; 2:562–571.

Gonzalez-Peralta RP, Fang JWS, Davis GL, et al. Optimization for the detection of hepatitis C virus antigens in the liver. *J Hepatol.* 1994;20:143–147.

Goodman ZD, Ishak KG. Histopathology of hepatitis C virus infection. *Sem Liv Dis.* 1995;15:70–81.

Kobayashi K, Hashimoto E, Ludwig J, Hisamitsu T, Obata H. Liver biopsy features of acute hepatitis C compared with hepatitis A, B, and non-A, non-B, non-C. *Liver.* 1993;13: 69–73.

Komminoth P, Adams V, Long AA, et al. Evaluation of methods for hepatitis C virus detection in archival liver biopsies. Comparison of histology, immunohistochemistry, reverse transcriptase polymerase chain reaction (RT PCR) and in situ RT-PCR. *Path Res Pract.* 1994;190:1017–1025.

Krawczynski K, Beach MJ, Bradley DW, et al. Hepatitis C antigen in hepatocytes: immunomorphologic detection and identification. *Gastroenterology.* 1992;103:622–629.

Kryger P, Christoffersen P. Light microscopic morphology of acute hepatitis non-A, non-B. A comparison with hepatitis type A and B. *Liver.* 1982;2:200–206.

Lefkowitch JH, Schiff ER, Davis GL, et al. Pathological diagnosis of chronic hepatitis C: a multicenter comparative study with chronic hepatitis B. *Gastroenterology.* 1993;104: 595–603.

Nuovo GJ, Lidonnici K, MacConnell P, Lane B. Intracellular localization of polymerase chain reaction (PCR)-amplified hepatitis C cDNA. *Am J Surg Pathol.* 1993;17:683–690.

Resnick RH, Koff R. Hepatitis C-related hepatocellular carcinoma: prevalence and significance. *Arch Intern Med.* 1993; 153:1672–1677.

Scheuer PJ, Ashrafzadeh P, Sherlock S, Brown D, Dusheiko GM. The pathology of hepatitis C. *Hepatology.* 1992;15: 567–571.

Schmidt M, Pirovino M, Altorfer J, Gudat F, Bianchi L. Acute hepatitis non-A, non-B; are there any specific light microscopic features? *Liver.* 1982;2:61–67.

Van der Poel CL, Cuypers HT, Reesink HW. Hepatitis C virus six years on. *Lancet.* 1994;344:1475–1479.

Van Doorn LJ. Molecular biology of the hepatitis C virus. *J Med Virol* 1994;43:345–356.

Vyberg M. The hepatitis-associated bile duct lesion. *Liver.* 1993;289–301.

Hepatitis D

Buitrago B, Popper H, Hadler SC, et al. Specific histologic features of Santa Marta hepatitis: a severe form of delta virus infection in northern South America. *Hepatology.* 1986;6: 1285–1291.

Govindarajan S, Chin KP, Redeker AG, Peters RL. Fulminant B viral hepatitis: role of delta agent. *Gastroenterology.* 1984; 86:1416–1420.

Govindarajan S, DeCock KM, Peters RL. Morphologic and immunohistochemical features of fulminant delta hepatitis. *Human Pathol.* 1985;16:262–267.

Govindarajan S, DeCock KM, Redeker AG. Natural course of delta superinfection in chronic hepatitis B virus-infected patients: histopathologic study with multiple liver biopsies. *Hepatology.* 1986;6:640–644.

Hoofnagle JH. Type D (delta) hepatitis. *JAMA.* 1989;261: 1321–1325.

Kanel GC, Govindarajan S, Peters RL. Chronic delta infection and liver biopsy changes in chronic active hepatitis B. *Ann Intern Med.* 1984;101:51–54.

Kojima T, Callea F, Desmyter J, Sakurai I, Desmet VJ. Immunolight and electron microscopic features of chronic hepatitis D. *Liver.* 1990;10:17–27.

Negro F, Baldi M, Bonino F, et al. Chronic HDV (hepatitis delta virus) hepatitis: intrahepatic expression of delta antigen, histologic activity and outcome of liver disease. *J Hepatol.* 1988;7:169–174.

Negro F, Baldi M, Brunetto MR, et al. The natural history of chronic delta hepatitis. *Hepatology.* 1986;6:1156.

Popper H, Thung SN, Gerber MA, et al. Histologic studies of severe delta agent infection in Venezuelan Indians. *Hepatology.* 1983;3:906–912.

Rizzetto M, Verme G, Recchia S, et al. Chronic hepatitis in carriers of hepatitis B surface antigen, with intrahepatic expression of the delta antigen. An active and progressive disease unresponsive to immunosuppressive treatment. *Ann Intern Med.* 1983;98:437–441.

Ryley NG, Heryet AR, Goldin R, Monjardino J, Saldanha J, Fleming KA. Coexpression of markers for hepatitis delta and hepatitis B viruses in human liver. *Histopathology.* 1992;20:331–337.

Verme G, Amoroso P, Lettieri G, et al. A histological study of hepatitis delta virus liver disease. *Hepatology.* 1986;6: 1303–1307.

Hepatitis E

Bradley DW, Krawczynski K, Cook EH, et al. Enterically transmitted non-A, non-B hepatitis: etiology of disease and laboratory studies in nonhuman primates. In: Zuckerman AJ, ed. *Viral Hepatitis and Liver Disease.* Edinburgh: AR Liss; 1988:138–147.

Gupta DN, Smetana HF. The histopathology of viral hepatitis as seen in the Delhi epidemics (1955–56). *Indian J Med Res.* 1957;45(suppl):101–113.

Morrow RH, Smetana HF, Sai FT, et al. Unusual features of viral hepatitis in Accra, Ghana. *Ann Intern Med.* 1968;68: 1250–1264.

Krawczynski K. Hepatitis E. *Hepatology.* 1993;17:932–941.

Wong DC, Purcell RH, Sreenivasan MA, et al. Epidemic and endemic hepatitis in India: evidence for non-A, non-B virus etiology. *Lancet.* 1980;2:876–879.

Chronic Hepatitis

Allaire GS, Goodman ZD, Ishak KG, Rabin L. Talc in liver tissue of intravenous drug abusers. A comparative study. *Am J Clin Pathol.* 1989;92:583–588.

Baptista A, Biarchi L, DeGroote J, et al. The diagnostic significance of periportal hepatic necrosis and inflammation. *Histopathology.* 1988;12:569–579.

Bianchi L. Liver biopsy interpretation in hepatitis. Part II: Histopathology and classification of acute and chronic viral hepatitis/differential diagnosis. *Path Res Pract.* 1983;178: 180–213.

Desmet VJ, Gerber M, Hoofnagle JH, Manns M, Scheuer PJ. Classification of chronic hepatitis: diagnosis, grading and staging. *Hepatology.* 1994;19:1513–1520.

Ishak KG: Chronic hepatitis: morphology and nomenclature. *Mod Pathol.* 1994;7:690–713.

Knodell RG, Ishak KG, Black WC, et al. Formulation and application of a numerical scoring system for assisting histological activity in asymptomatic chronic active hepatitis. *Hepatology.* 1981;1:431–435.

Popper H. Changing concepts of the evolution of chronic hepatitis and the role of piecemeal necrosis. *Hepatology.* 1983;3:758–762.

Scheuer PJ. Changing views on chronic hepatitis. *Histopathology.* 1986;10:1–4.

Scheuer PJ. Classification of chronic viral hepatitis: a need for reassessment. *J Hepatol.* 1991;13:372–374.

CHAPTER 39

Yellow Fever

Alfonso J. Strano

Many never walked on the foot path, but went into the middle of the streets, to avoid being infected in passing by houses wherein people had died. Acquaintances and friends avoided each other in the streets, and only signified their regard by a cold nod. The old custom of shaking hands fell into such general disuse, that many were affronted by even the offer of a hand.

Mathew Carey (1760–1839), A Short Account of the Malignant Fever Lately Prevalent in Philadelphia (1793)

DEFINITION

Yellow fever (YF) is an acute, febrile zoonosis of varying severity caused by a flavivirus. It is characterized by fever, bleeding, and hepatic and renal failure.

HISTORY/EPIDEMIOLOGY

For more than three and one-half centuries YF has been an important epidemic and endemic disease of tropical and subtropical South America and Africa within a band defined by the 12th latitudes north and south.[1–3] It was also a scourge of the Caribbean and port cities of North America and Europe and the first disease defined as being of viral etiology and arthropod-borne, the arthropod vector being *Aedes aegypti*. It is believed to have originated in Africa and been transported to the Western Hemisphere by personnel aboard sailing vessels. The vector cycle was perpetuated by breeding mosquitoes in the freshwater containers aboard ship.

It was Dr. Carlos Finlay of Havana, Cuba, who first proposed that YF is mosquito-borne; members of the U.S. YF Commission, Walter Reed, William Gorgas, and coworkers, confirmed Finlay's theory and developed programs of mosquito control that virtually eradicated YF from urban areas. In spite of these programs it was evident that endemic infections continued in the forested areas of the Western Hemisphere and the savanna and forest of Africa with occasional microepidemics in populated areas. Not until 1920, when the Rockefeller Foundation began its clinical efforts and basic research, was the sylvatic (jungle) cycle discovered.[4] The sylvatic cycle includes monkeys and other mammals as hosts and a variety of mosquitoes as vectors. The Rockefeller Foundation's program of vector control was highly successful in the Western Hemisphere, and therefore moved its programs to Africa. It was in Africa that the YF virus was finally isolated, and in 1937 a live attenuated vaccine 17-D was developed.[5]

In spite of this progress YF remains a public health problem in tropical areas with sporadic urban epidemics and migrating and recurring sylvatic cycles.[6–8] YF has never been reported in Asia.

The morphologic features of the YF 17-D virus are that it is a single-stranded RNA virus of 10,862 nucleotides, three structural proteins, C, M and E, and up to 12 nonstructural proteins. It is spherical, 40 to 50 nm in diameter and is inactivated by ether, bile salts, heat, or by incubation at 60°C for 10 minutes.[9]

CLINICAL MANIFESTATIONS

The incubation period is usually 3 to 6 days and in those persons with severe infections the onset is usually sudden, with high fever, chills, headache, and myalgia lasting 3 to 4 days. The second stage is dominated by hepatic and renal failure, hypotension, bradycardia, and bleeding tendencies. Ecchymoses and hemorrhage of the gums are common and gastric hemorrhage leads to black vomitus. Jaundice is usually mild or may be absent.[10]

Massive albuminuria, severe early jaundice, and marked prolongation of the prothrombin time with high levels of serum liver enzymes indicate a poor prognosis.[11,12] In fulminating infections, death may occur as early as the third or fourth day, although death on the sixth or seventh day is more common. After the tenth day renal failure is the usual cause of death. If the patient survives it is usually without sequelae, but pneumonia, parotitis, cutaneous infection, and renal abscesses may complicate recovery. The mortality has varied from 5% to 50%.

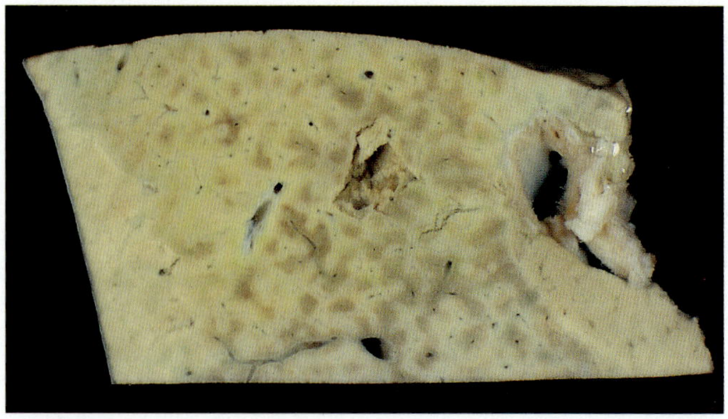

Figure 39–1. Fatal yellow fever in a patient from Trinidad with massive necrosis but without collapse of the hepatic architecture. Note the smooth capsule (AFIP Neg 78-9047).

PATHOLOGY

Gross Findings

As in the other viral hemorrhagic fevers, the gross features are nonspecific and usually include varying degrees of petechial hemorrhages of conjunctiva and mucous membranes and massive hemorrhages, icterus, degeneration of hepatocytes, and fatty metamorphosis of organs, especially heart and kidneys. The liver maintains its size and contour but is soft, friable, greasy, and yellowish (Figure 39–1). There may be gross evidence of necrosis.[3,13,14]

Microscopic Findings

The anatomic diagnosis of YF can be made with assurance from changes within the liver after the third and before the eighth day of illness. It becomes more difficult to make the diagnosis as the disease progresses. The three diagnostic hallmarks are midzonal necrosis, eosinophilic degeneration, and fatty metamorphosis.[3,13,14]

Midzonal Necrosis

The initial necrosis is focal and usually limited to the midzone. It may involve single liver cells or small groups of liver cells giving the pattern of necrosis a salt-and-pepper appearance (Figure 39–2). With more severe involvement, the midzone localization may be lost or obscured. Virtually complete necrosis of the lobule can pose a problem in differential diagnosis, but a single row of parenchymal cells usually surrounds the central veins and portal areas.[3,13,14]

Eosinophilic Degeneration

Sharply demarcated round to ovoid eosinophilic structures variously termed acidophilic, eosinophilic, Councilman, or Councilman-like bodies are characteristic but not pathognomonic.[15–17] Councilman bodies (Figure 39–3) originate as intracellular aggregates of altered cytoplasm (focal cytoplasmic degeneration) and stain intensely with eosin and wood stain scarlet (Movat). These aggregates may involve the entire cell or only a portion of it. As necrosis proceeds, the Councilman bodies or the entire necrotic cell shrink, detach from the surrounding hepatocyte or the remainder of its parent

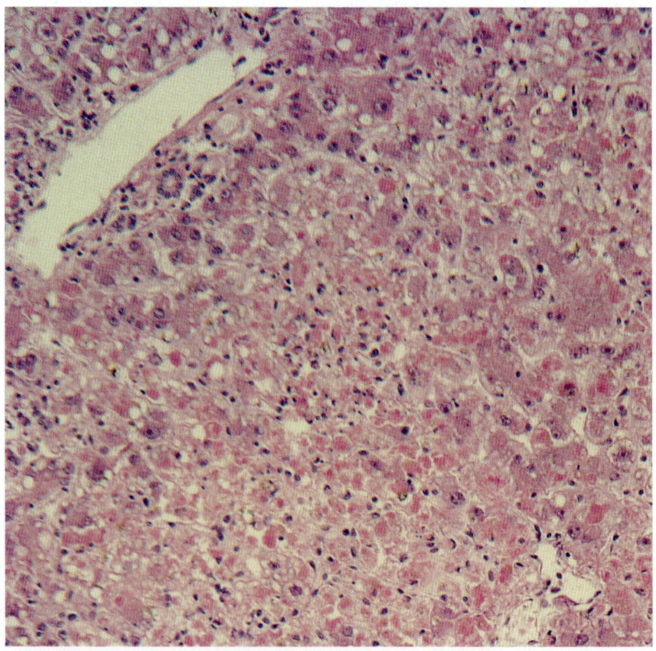

Figure 39–2. Liver. Same specimen shown in Figure 39–1. There is massive midzonal necrosis characterized by preservation of the lobular architecture and acidophilic bodies. The better preserved hepatocytes surround the portal tract and central vein and some have microvesicular fatty change (AFIP Neg 79-15395; hematoxylin-eosin, ×100).

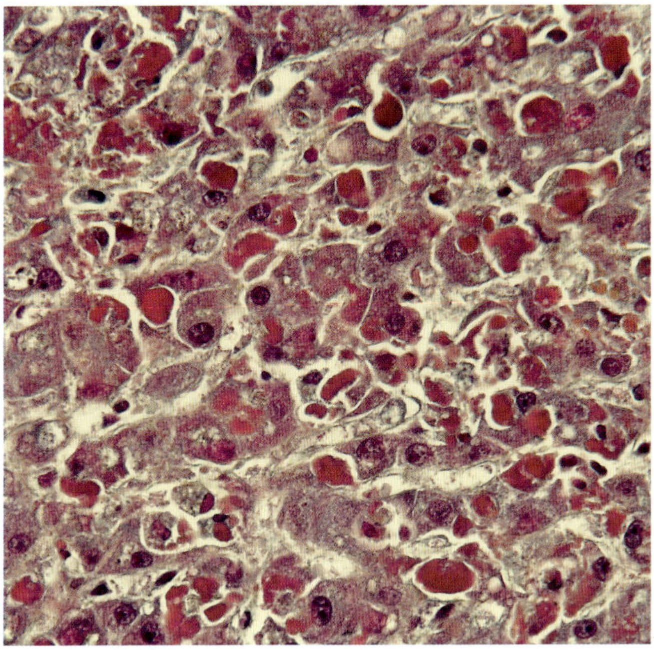

Figure 39–3. Liver. Multiple Councilman (acidophilic) bodies forming in the cytoplasm of hepatocytes. The more advanced Councilman bodies are in the sinusoids. There is microvesicular fatty change in the cytoplasm of hepatocytes (AFIP Neg 79-15410; Movat stain, ×200).

cell, and are extruded into the sinus, where they lie free or are phagocytosed by Kupffer's cells. The Councilman bodies may vary greatly in number and occasionally may be rare. Councilman bodies are not viral inclusion bodies.[17]

Fatty Metamorphosis

Lipid in the cytoplasm of the hepatocyte is a constant feature of YF and the diagnosis should not be made without it (Figures 39–4 and 39–5). The fatty change is

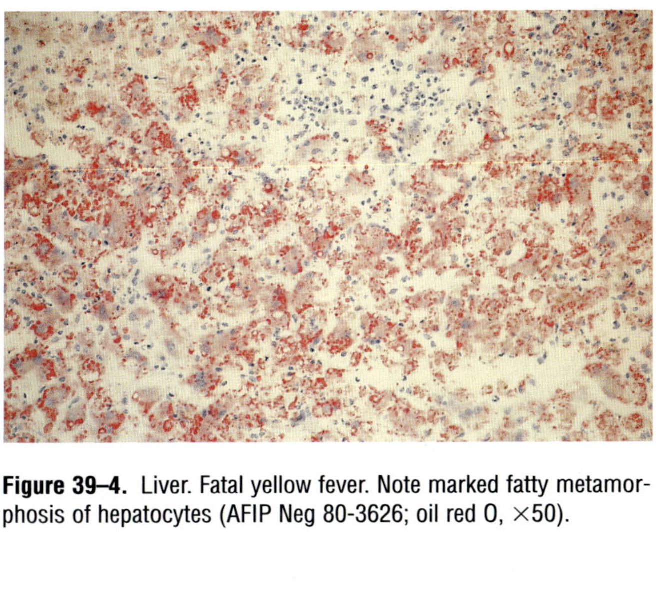

Figure 39–4. Liver. Fatal yellow fever. Note marked fatty metamorphosis of hepatocytes (AFIP Neg 80-3626; oil red O, ×50).

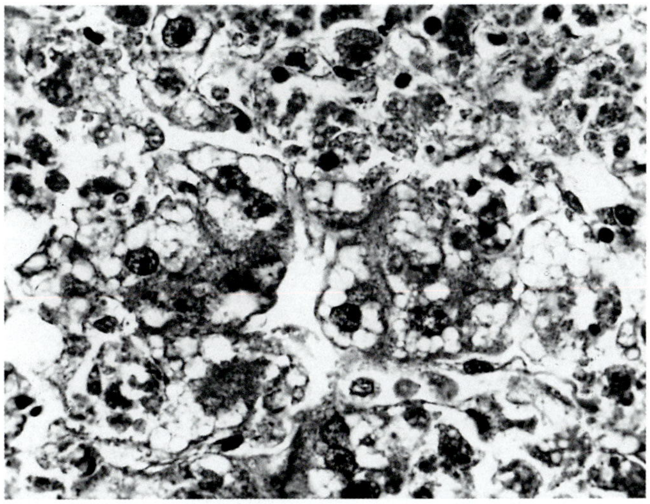

Figure 39–5. Liver. Fatty vacuolization of hepatocytes in the centrilobular zone (AFIP Neg 71-1983; hematoxylin-eosin, ×450).

multivacuolar and microvacuolar producing morula configurations, which are common in viral hepatic infections as compared to large vacuoles in livers with nutritional damage.[13,14,18] The extent of fatty change need not parallel the extent of necrosis or eosinophilic degeneration and may be in cells unaffected by these processes.

Other alterations include preservation of the hepatic reticulin network regardless of the extent of necrosis (Figure 39–6) and the striking paucity of an

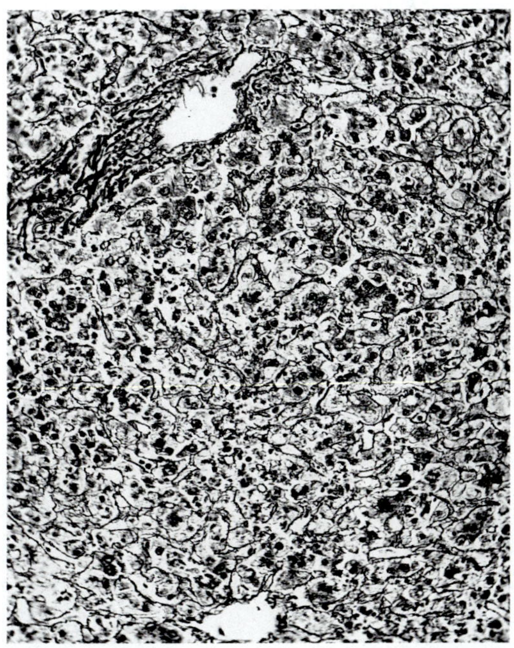

Figure 39–6. Liver. Intact reticular framework of a lobule with no significant fragmentation or collapse (portal tract at top and central vein at bottom) (AFIP Neg 71-1982; reticulum stain, ×115).

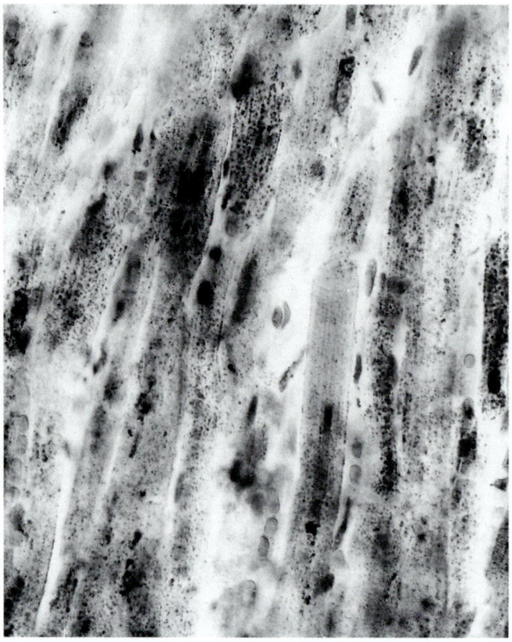

Figure 39–7. Heart. Fatty droplets in myofibers that are predominantly perinuclear (AFIP Neg N-43269; oil red O, ×45).

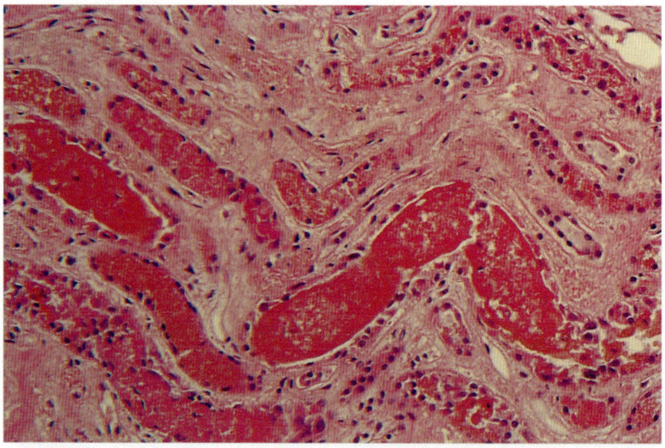

Figure 39–9. Kidney. Protein casts with slight bile staining and acute tubular necrosis (AFIP Neg 79-15409; hematoxylin-eosin, ×60).

inflammatory cell response. Small foci of histiocytes and more rarely neutrophils sometimes infiltrate the parenchyma near degenerating hepatocytes. Anything more than a minimal inflammatory cell response should raise doubts about the diagnosis of YF. If the patient dies between the seventh and tenth day, Torres bodies may be present.[19] These are amorphous masses within degenerating nuclei of hepatocytes. Villela bodies also may be seen at this time.[20] These are small, granular, yellow-to-ocher structures, scattered among the acidophilic bodies or within macrophages and Kupffer's cells. Although Torres and Villela bodies may be helpful, their inconsistency and lack of morphologic specificity limit their usefulness in diagnosis. Involvement of other organs in YF is reasonably common. The brain may be edematous and have petechial hemorrhages. The heart, as a rule, demonstrates moderate degeneration of myofibers and fatty metamorphosis (Figure 39–7). Kidneys have varying degrees of acute tubular necrosis and moderate to severe fatty change of tubular epithelium and protein casts (Figure 39–8 and 39–9).

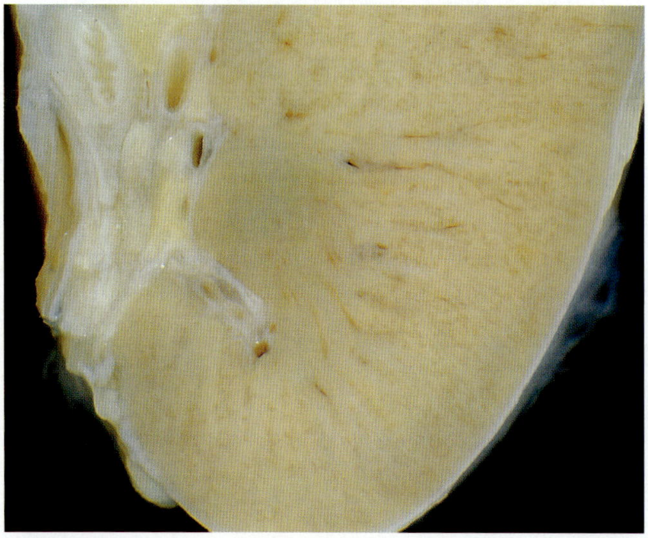

Figure 39–8. Kidney in fatal yellow fever showing bile discoloration (AFIP Neg 83-9637).

Electron microscopy has very little to offer in the diagnosis of YF. It enabled the definition of the Councilman body but failed to demonstrate other definitive features.

DIAGNOSIS

Clinical Diagnosis

The clinical features of YF are generally those of the hemorrhagic fever syndrome and cannot be separated definitively from other hemorrhagic fever syndromes.

Anatomic Diagnosis

YF cannot always be diagnosed by histopathologic means. The changes are most characteristic during the third to the seventh day of illness and difficulty may be encountered with specimens obtained late in the course of illness.[20] Generally, however, the characteristic combination of histopathologic features permits a fairly certain diagnosis. A comprehensive listing and definition of the most common entities from which YF must be differentiated and their defining characteristics are presented in the syllabus "Yellow fever and its differential histopathologic diagnosis" by Strano et al.[3]

Laboratory Diagnosis

Routine laboratory tests cannot confirm a diagnosis of YF. Their value is in assessing the prognosis of various organ failures and the extent of disseminated intravascular coagulopathy (DIC). A definitive diagnosis of YF can be made by isolating the virus or by demonstrating certain immunologic responses.[21–27] Viral isolation can be accomplished by the intracerebral inoculation of suckling mice or cell culture with infected material, ie, blood obtained during the first 4 days of illness or liver by the tenth day. The serologic diagnosis of YF can and is complicated by previous immunization and cross-reacting antibodies of other flaviviruses, such as occurs in many tropical areas. Generally the diagnosis can be made by complement fixation, hemagglutination inhibition, plaque reduction neutralization, immunofluorescence antibody test, and enzyme-linked immunosorbent assay. These procedures require specialized laboratories and trained personnel. For optimal results careful collection and handling of specimens are required. Also helpful is acute and convalescent serum, not always available in remote tropical areas.

PREVENTION AND TREATMENT

The success of vector control has virtually eradicated urban YF but the sylvatic cycle still poses a threat, as has been demonstrated periodically in Africa, South America, and the Caribbean.[4,6] Eradication of the sylvatic cycle does not seem possible; thus, prevention strategies are dependent on immunization with YF vaccines.[5,28–30]

The original 17-D vaccine is thermolabile, thus posing major problems in storage and delivery in the remote areas where it is needed most. The development of a thermostable 17-D vaccine is a major breakthrough and offers the best opportunity for the prevention of YF in remote tropical areas.

TREATMENT

The treatment of yellow fever has remained symptomatic and supportive because no specific antiviral therapy exists.

REFERENCES

1. Strode GK, ed. *Yellow Fever.* New York: McGraw Hill; 1951.
2. Scott HH. *A History of Tropical Medicine.* London: Edward Arnold; 1939;1:279–453.
3. Strano AJ, Dooley JR, Ishak KG. Yellow fever and its histopathologic differential diagnosis. Syllabus L15274. Washington, DC: American Registry of Pathology, AFIP; 1974.
4. Bres PL. A century of progress in combating yellow fever. *Bull WHO.* 1986;64:511–524.
5. Theiler M, Smith HH. Use of yellow fever virus modified by in vitro cultivation for human immunization. *J Exp Med.* 1937;65:787–800.
6. Present status of yellow fever; memorandum from a PAHO meeting. *Bull WHO.* 1986;64:511–524.
7. Resurgence of yellow fever. *World Health Forum.* 1993;14(1):91–92. News.
8. Loutan L, Robert CF, Raebar PA. Outbreak of yellow fever in Kenya: how doctors got the news. *Lancet.* 1993;17:341. Letter.
9. Rice CM, Lenches EM, Eddy SR, et al. Nucleotide sequence of yellow fever virus: implication for flavivirus gene expression and evaluation. *Science.* 1985;229:726–733.
10. Jones EM, Wilson DC. Clinical features of yellow fever cases at Van Christian Hospital during the 1969 epidemic on the Jos Plateau, Nigeria. *Bull WHO.* 1972;46:653–657.
11. Elton NW, Romero A. Clinical pathology of yellow fever. *Am J Clin Pathol.* 1955;25:135.
12. Trejos A, Romero A. Prothrombin levels in yellow fever. *Rev Biol Trop.* 1954;2:69–74.
13. Camain R, Labert D. Histopathologie desfaies amrils predeves post mortem et ponction biopsie hepatique. *Bull Who.* 1967;36:129–136.
14. Klotz O, Belt TH. The pathology of the liver in yellow fever. *Am J Pathol.* 1930;6:663–688.
15. Montenegro J. A cellula de Councilman–Rocha Lima no diagnostico da febre amarella humana. *Arg Hig Saude Publica.* 1939;5:17–27.
16. Biava C, Mukhlova-Montiel M. Electron microscopic observations on Councilman-like acidophilic bodies and other forms of acidophilic changes in human liver cells. *Am J Pathol.* 1965;46:775–802.
17. Child PL, Ruiz A. Acidophilic bodies: their chemical and physical nature in patients with Bolivian hemorrhagic fever. *Arch Pathol.* 1968;85:45–50.
18. Strano AJ. Labrea hepatitis. In: Binford CH, Connor DH, eds. *Pathology of Tropical and Extraordinary Diseases.* Washington, DC: AFIP; 1976.
19. Torres CM. Inclusions nucleaires acidophiles (degenerescence oxychromatique) dans le foi de Macacus rhesus inocule avec le virus Bresilien. *Compt Rend Soc Biol (Paris).* 1928;99:1344–1345.
20. Villela E. Histology of human yellow fever when death is delayed. *Arch Pathol.* 1941;31:665–669.
21. Monath TP, Croven RB, Muth DJ, et al. Limitations of the complement-fixation test for distinguishing naturally acquired from vaccine-induced yellow fever infection in

flavivirus-hyperendemic areas. *Am J Trop Med Hyg.* 1980; 29:624–634.
22. Monath TP, Hill LJ, Brown NV, et al. Sensitive and specific monoclonal immunoassay for detecting yellow fever virus in laboratory and clinical specimens. *J Clin Microbiol.* 1986;23:129–134.
23. Monath TP, Nystrom RR. Detection of yellow fever virus in serum by enzyme immunoassay. *Am J Trop Med Hyg.* 1984;33:151–157.
24. Casal J, Brown LV. Hemagglutination with arthropod-borne viruses. *Exp Med.* 1954;99:429–449.
25. Madrid AT, Porterfell JS. The flaviviruses (group B arbor viruses) a cross-neutralization study. *J Gen Virol.* 1974;23: 91–96.
26. Monath TP, Cropp CB, Muth DJ, Calisher CH. Indirect fluorescent antibody test for the diagnosis of yellow fever. *Roy Soc Trop Med Hyg.* 1981;75:282–286.
27. Calisher CH, Monath TP. *Togaviridae* and *Flaviviridae*: the alphaviruses and flaviviruses. In: Lennett EH, Halonen P, Murphy FA, eds. *Laboratory Diagnosis of Infectious Diseases. Principles and Practice.* New York: Springer-Verlag; 1988;2.
28. Rosenruieiz EC, Babione RW, Wisseman CL Jr. Immunological studies with group B arthropod-borne viruses. IV persistence of yellow fever antibodies following vaccination with 17D strain yellow fever vaccine. *Am J Trop Med Hyg.* 1963;12:230–235.
29. Center for Disease Control and Prevention. Yellow fever vaccine: recommendations of the immunization practices committee (APIC). *MMWR.* 1990:39.(No RR-6).
30. Roche JC, Jouan A, Brisan B. Comparative clinical study of a new 17D thermostable yellow fever vaccine. *Vaccine.* 1986;4:163–165.

Part III

Bacterial Infections

CHAPTER 40

Actinomycosis

Francis W. Chandler and Daniel H. Connor

The study of the causes of things must be preceded by the study of things caused.

Hughlings Jackson (1835–1911)

DEFINITION

Actinomycosis is a chronic bacterial infection that occurs sporadically throughout the world in humans and animals. Clinically and pathologically, actinomycosis is characterized by swelling, pain, draining sinuses, and a purulent discharge that contains yellow granules (compact bacterial aggregates) up to 3 mm in diameter.[1–3] Actinomycosis is not contagious, and the causal bacteria have never been isolated from soil, plants, or other natural habitats outside the body. The agents of actinomycosis are commensals of the mouth, throat, gastrointestinal tract, and vagina of apparently healthy people. The causal bacteria are thus endogenous and invade injured oral tissues, breaks in the intestinal mucosa, and sometimes other tissues when resistance is impaired. There is no increased incidence of actinomycosis in those with impaired immunity. Because actinomycosis is an endogenous infection, it is not classified under actinomycotic mycetoma (see Chapter 113), in spite of the fact that the causal agents commonly form granules in tissue.

ETIOLOGY

In the past, actinomycosis was included in textbooks of medical mycology, but now it is known that the causal organisms are anaerobic or microaerophilic filamentous bacteria in the order Actinomycetales. The most common agent of actinomycosis in humans is *Actinomyces israelii.* Other genera and species that cause actinomycosis in humans include *A naeslundii, A viscosus, Arachnia propionica,* and, rarely, *A odontolyticus, A bovis, A meyeri, Rothia dentocariosa,* and *Eubacterium nodatum.*[2–5] The principal agent of the disease in animals is *A bovis.* In tissue sections, all of these actinomycetes have identical morphologic and tinctorial features, ie, gram-positive, branched filaments about 1 μm in width. The agents of actinomycosis may occur as part of a mixed anaerobic infection, and recent experimental findings suggest that other bacteria enhance the pathogenicity of the actinomycetes.[6]

CLINICAL FEATURES

Most infections are either cervicofacial, thoracic, abdominal, or pelvic. Cervicofacial actinomycosis, or "lumpy jaw," is the most common form (Figure 40–1), and the disease may develop without antecedent injury to the oral mucosa.[2,7] Frequently, however, cervicofacial infection follows a dental extraction, or it may complicate dental caries, periodontal disease, or an accidental injury to the oral mucosa. Infected tissues are swollen, firm, and elastic, and as the disease progresses, abscesses and draining sinuses form. Serosanguineous to purulent exudates drain from the sinuses, and the exudates often contain actinomycotic "sulfur granules," named because of their yellow color, which resembles that of elemental sulfur. They are not, however, composed of sulfur as implied in some texts. Destructive osteomyelitis also may be present. If untreated, the infection may extend upward to involve sinuses, orbit, or cranial bones. The infection also may extend downward to the thorax and then disseminate to involve distant bones and joints, brain, spinal cord, and skin.

Thoracic actinomycosis usually is caused by aspiration of oropharyngeal contents, but it also may result from direct extension of a cervicofacial infection.[8–11] All

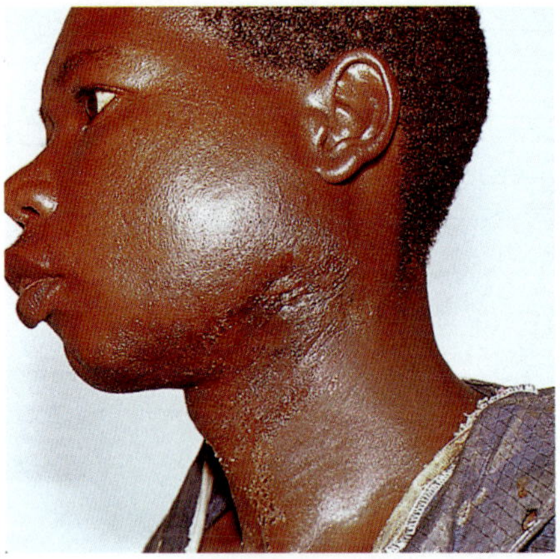

Figure 40–1. Cervicofacial actinomycosis, or "lumpy jaw." Note marked swelling and multiple openings of draining sinuses over the left mandible.

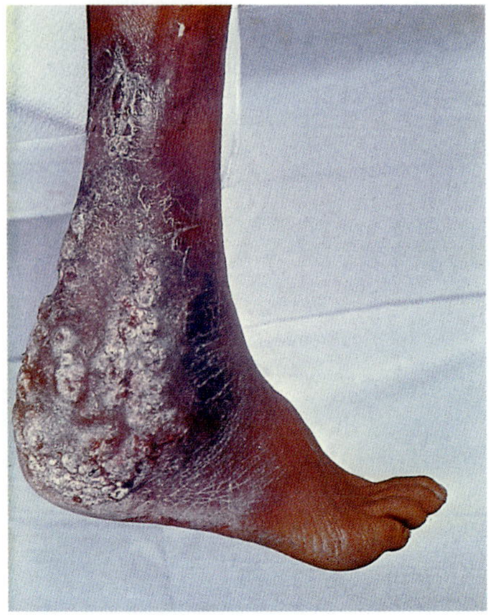

Figure 40–2. Actinomycosis of the lower leg and foot caused by *A bovis*. Note swelling, induration, and openings of draining sinuses.

tissues in the thorax are susceptible to infection, and symptoms of thoracic actinomycosis often suggest a malignancy.[12,13] Because the bacteria that cause actinomycosis are anaerobic and difficult to culture from the lung, pulmonary actinomycosis is usually diagnosed by histopathologic examination of biopsy specimens. Abdominal actinomycosis may result from direct extension of thoracic infection, but more commonly complicates a ruptured appendix or penetration of the actinomycete through the wall of the stomach or intestine.[2,14] Spread within the abdomen may involve the liver, kidneys, and other retroperitoneal structures, including vertebrae. Pelvic or genital actinomycosis may complicate neglected intrauterine devices.[15–18] Primary, localized actinomycosis has been reported in other sites, including limbs following human bites (Figure 40–2), and in lacrimal glands.[1–3]

PATHOLOGY

The usual reaction is suppurative, with abscesses that contain one or more spherical, oval, or scalloped actinomycotic granules bordered by refractile, intensely eosinophilic, clublike projections of Splendore–Hoeppli material (Figures 40–3 and 40–4).[4,19] Abscesses vary in size, may be solitary or multiple, and often interconnect via sinus tracts or open to a body surface or into a cavity. When very large, abscesses are often multilocular. Palisading epithelioid histiocytes and giant cells of both foreign body and Langhans types often surround the abscesses, and, in turn, are encapsulated by fibrosing granulation tissue. Macrophages that sometimes form the innermost portion of the wall surrounding an actinomycotic abscess may be numerous and have foamy cytoplasm because of their lipid content.

Actinomycotic granules range from 0.3 to 3 mm in diameter and, when large, can be seen with the naked eye when a stained tissue section is held up to the light. Granules also may be folded, chattered, fragmented, and even displaced from the center of an abscess during microtomy (Figure 40–5). Modified Gram stains such as the Brown–Brenn procedure reveal that each granule is composed of delicate, branched, gram-positive and often beaded filaments, about 1 μm in width, randomly embedded in an amorphous matrix of uncertain composition (Figures 40–6 and 40–7).[40,20,21] Beading of the filaments results from alternating regions of gram-positive and either gram-negative or nongram

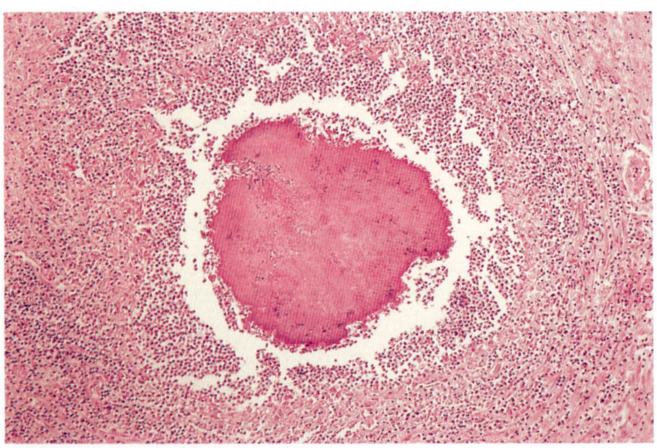

Figure 40–3. Abdominal actinomycosis caused by *A israelii*. A single, amphophilic granule is embedded in a hepatic abscess (hematoxylin-eosin, ×25).

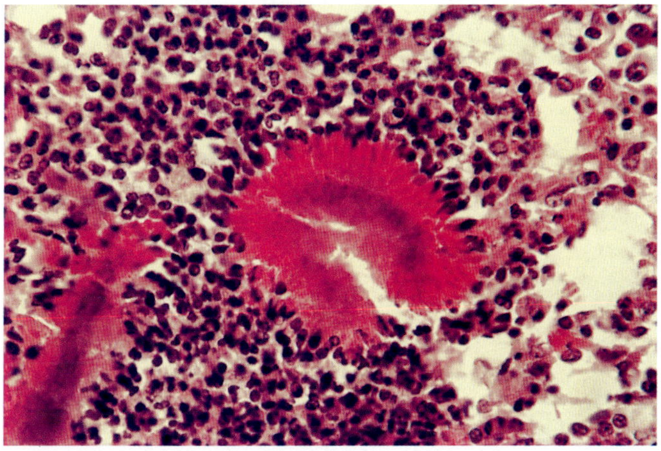

Figure 40–4. Cervicofacial actinomycosis caused by *A israelii.* An actinomycotic granule is surrounded by intensely eosinophilic, finger-like projections of Splendore–Hoeppli material. Although the entire granule is well stained, individual bacterial filaments are not visible (hematoxylin-eosin, ×250).

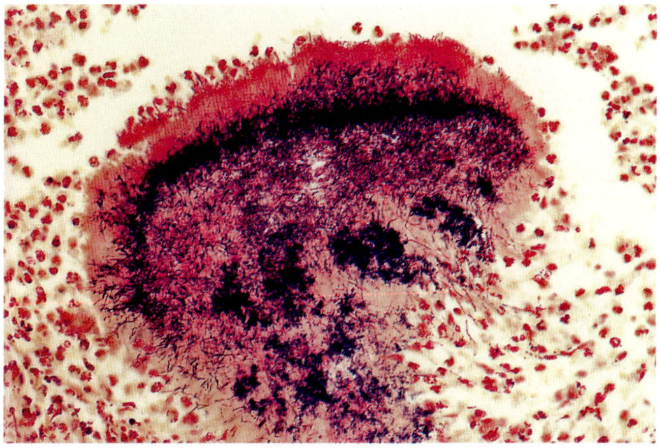

Figure 40–6. Abdominal actinomycosis caused by *A israelii.* Tangled, irregular aggregates of delicate, gram-positive filaments are embedded within the matrix of the granule (Brown–Brenn, ×150).

staining. The branches are usually at right angles (Figure 40–8). At the periphery of some granules, the filaments are radially oriented and covered with finger-like projections of Splendore–Hoeppli material, resulting in the older name of "ray fungus." Scattered bacillary and coccoid forms also may be detected within the granules (Figure 40–7). In hematoxylin-eosin (H&E)-stained tissue sections, entire amphophilic granules ensheathed by deeply eosinophilic, serrate Splendore–Hoeppli material and intimately surrounded by neutrophils are detected easily and represent the "sulfur granules" classically described in exudates of actinomycosis (Figure 40–9).[2,3] The individual bacterial filaments that form the basic structure of granules, however, are not visible and must be specially stained to be seen. Gomori's methenamine silver (GMS), silver impregnation (Steiner, Dieterle, or Warthin–Starry), and modified Gram stains clearly demonstrate actinomycetes in tissue sections and cytologic preparations (Figures 40–10 and 40–11); of these, the Brown–Brenn Gram stain has given the best results. H&E, Gridley, and periodic acid–Schiff (PAS) procedures do not stain the actinomycetes reliably. Unlike the *Nocardia* sp, filaments of the *Actinomyces* and related species are not even partially acid fast.[4,20]

In the serosanguineous to purulent exudates that drain from sinus tracts, actinomycotic ("sulfur") granules appear to the naked eye as soft, yellowish-brown to

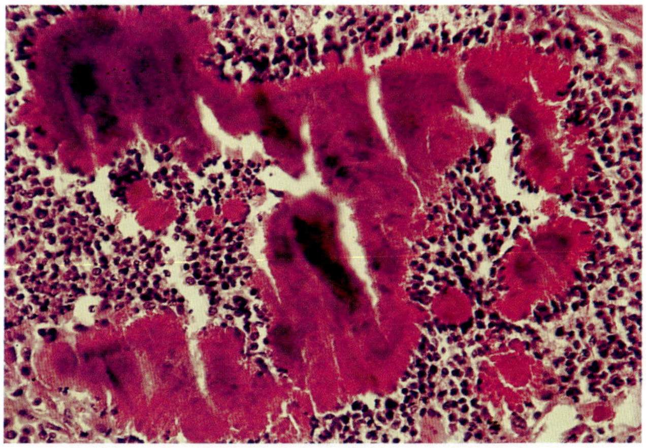

Figure 40–5. *Arachnia propionica* granule in thoracic actinomycosis. Because of its brittle, cement-like matrix, the granule has been fragmented and chattered during microtomy. Fragments of the granule are intimately surrounded by neutrophils (hematoxylin-eosin, ×160).

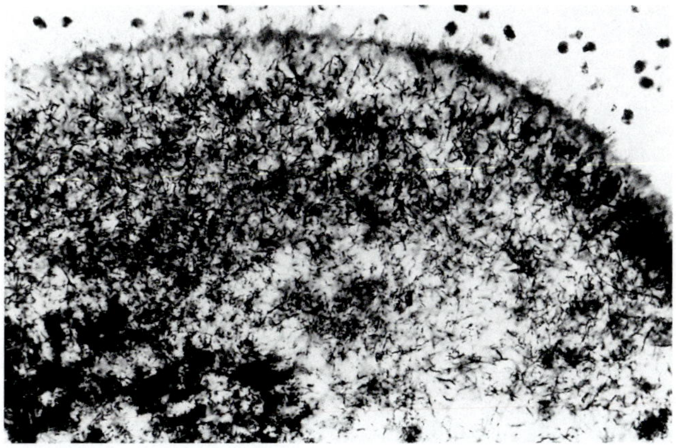

Figure 40–7. Abdominal actinomycosis. Delicate beaded filaments and coccobacillary forms, about 1 μm wide, are randomly oriented within the matrix of an *A israelii* granule (Brown–Brenn, ×480).

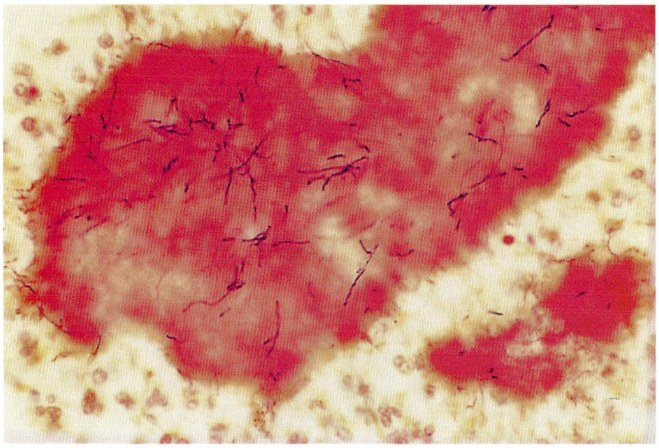

Figure 40–8. *Actinomyces israelii* granule. Bacterial filaments branch at approximately right angles and are randomly oriented within the dense, amorphous matrix of the granule (Brown–Brenn, ×250).

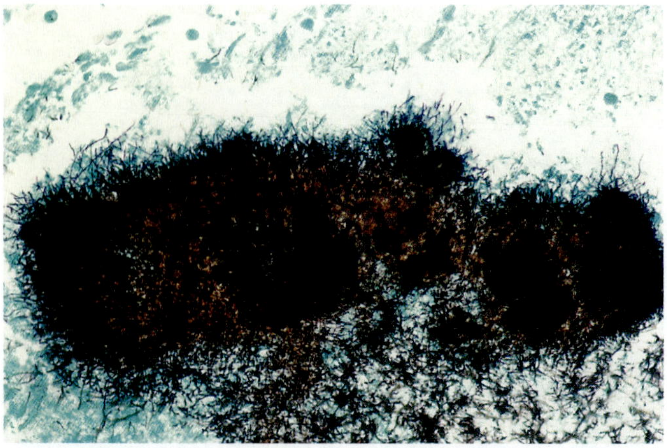

Figure 40–10. *Actinomyces israelii* granule in pelvic actinomycosis. Compact, tangled aggregates of delicate filaments and coccobacilli of this bacterium are strongly GMS positive and radiate at the periphery of the granule (GMS, ×50).

white, organized bacterial aggregates that range from 0.3 to 3.0 mm in diameter. The granules can be collected on gauze, crushed between two glass slides, and stained with Gram procedures to demonstrate individual bacterial filaments.

DIFFERENTIAL DIAGNOSIS

Two other infections resemble actinomycosis. These are botryomycosis and actinomycotic mycetoma caused by the *Nocardia* sp.[4] Botryomycosis is a misleading name because it is a chronic, localized bacterial infection that usually involves skin and soft tissues, and other tissues on rare occasions.[22,23] The bacteria may be cocci or bacilli, gram-positive or gram-negative, but are not filamentous. Like the actinomycetes, however, they form grains or granules that are often bordered by clublike projections of Splendore–Hoeppli material. Dissemination with visceral involvement is rare in botryomycosis. The bacteria that most commonly cause botryomycosis are *Staphylococcus aureus, Pseudomonas aeruginosa, Escherichia coli, Neisseria mucosa, Actinobacillus lignieresi,* and species in the genera *Streptococcus, Proteus, Bacillus,* and *Bacteroides.* In H&E-stained tissue sections, botryomycotic granules are indistinguishable from those of actinomycosis because individual bacteria within the granules are poorly delineated. The histopathologic diagnosis is established by demonstrating the causal agent within the granule, achieved with

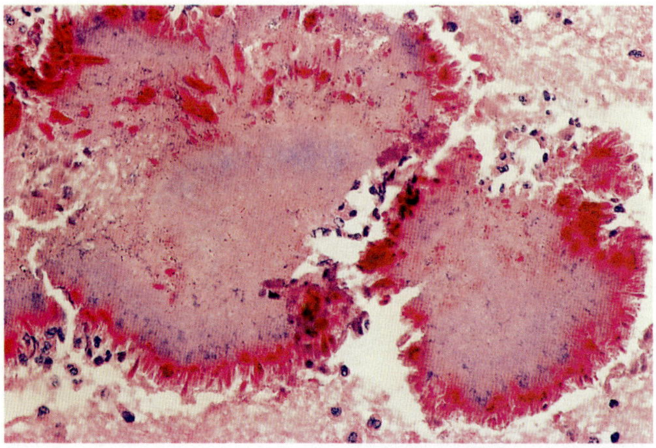

Figure 40–9. Thoracic actinomycosis. Individual amphophilic granules are ensheathed by deeply eosinophilic, serrate, Splendore–Hoeppli material. These are the "sulfur granules" classically described in exudates of actinomycosis (hematoxylin-eosin, ×50).

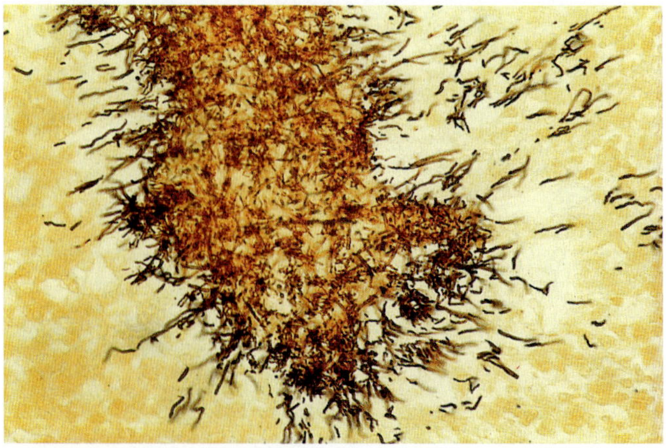

Figure 40–11. Pelvic actinomycosis caused by *A israelii.* Blackened bacterial filaments that branch at predominantly right angles are radially oriented at the periphery of the granule (Steiner silver impregnation, ×250).

modified Gram stains such as the Brown–Brenn or Brown–Hopps procedures. These stains demonstrate bacterial cocci and bacilli in botryomycosis in contrast to delicate, branched gram-positive filaments in actinomycosis. Culture, immunohistochemistry, or molecular methods are usually required for specific identification of the cause.

In tissue sections, the three pathogenic *Nocardia* sp—*N asteroides, N brasiliensis,* and *N otitidiscaviarum* (formerly *N caviae*)—appear as delicate, branched, and often beaded filaments that are gram-positive and morphologically similar to those of actinomycosis.[19,20] Unlike the agents of actinomycosis, however, the *Nocardia* sp are partially acid fast. This partial acid fastness can be demonstrated with modified acid-fast procedures that use an aqueous solution of a weak acid for decolorization. The term *nocardiosis* classically refers to a systemic infection with a primary pulmonary focus in which nocardial filaments do not form granules and are scattered throughout suppurative and necrotic exudates. Rarely, however, all three *Nocardia* sp also can cause actinomycotic mycetoma with granules that resemble those of actinomycosis in tissue sections stained with H&E, modified Gram, GMS, and silver impregnation procedures. Modified acid-fast stains are required to differentiate the nocardiae within the granules from the agents of actinomycosis. Both nocardiosis and actinomycotic mycetoma caused by the *Nocardia* sp are exogenous diseases, and infections are caused by nocardiae that are environmental saprophytes. The nocardiae are identified by culture followed by defining their physiologic and biochemical properties.

Granules formed by the *Actinomyces* sp and other agents of actinomycosis also must be distinguished from granules formed in eumycotic mycetomas caused by true fungi (see Chapter 113), because treatment of these two diseases is very different.[4,24] The granules of eumycotic mycetomas contain broad, septate hyphae and thick-walled, spherical chlamydoconidia, whereas the granules in actinomycosis contain compact aggregates of gram-positive filamentous bacteria. The granules in both diseases can be readily distinguished by using special stains for fungi and bacteria already described.

CONFIRMATIONAL TESTING AND DIAGNOSIS

The actinomycetes that cause actinomycosis can be specifically identified by isolating and characterizing them in culture.[2,3] Optimal growth is at 37°C on enriched, antibiotic-free media, where they form raised, whitish colonies that are either smooth or rough depending on the amount of filamentation. The more common agents of actinomycosis can be specifically identified by immunofluorescence of actinomycetes in exudates and in deparaffinized sections of formalin-fixed tissue (Figure 40–12).[25]

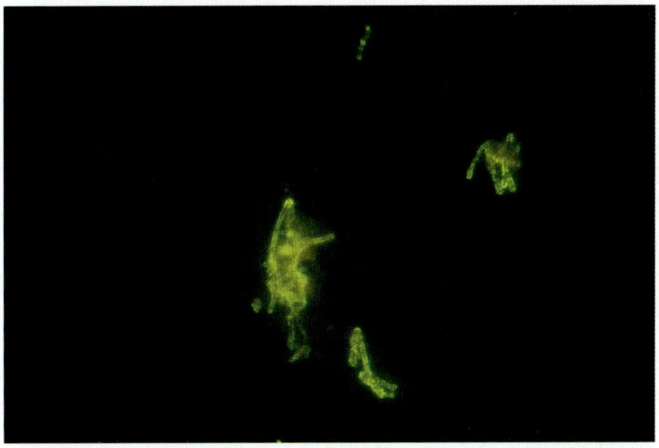

Figure 40–12. *Actinomyces israelii* in a cervical smear from a woman with pelvic actinomycosis. Individual, beaded, and branched filaments are brightly decorated with an immunofluorescence conjugate specific for this actinomycete (direct immunofluorescence, ×250).

TREATMENT

Penicillins given in high doses are the drugs of choice. To prevent relapse, the patient is treated for 6 weeks with penicillin, followed by tetracycline for up to 12 months.[26,27] Other antibiotics are effective in patients allergic to penicillins. Surgical drainage and excision, when indicated, are also important in treating actinomycosis.[28]

REFERENCES

1. Brown JR. Human actinomycosis: a study of 181 subjects. *Hum Pathol.* 1973;4:319–330.
2. Peabody JW, Seabury JH. Actinomycosis and nocardiosis. *J Chronic Dis.* 1975;5:374–403.
3. Causey WA. Actinomycosis. In: *Handbook of Clinical Neurology, Vol 35. Infections of the Nervous System, Part III.* Amsterdam: North Holland Publishing; 1978:383–394.
4. Chandler FW, Watts JC. *Pathologic Diagnosis of Fungal Infections.* Chicago: ASCP Press; 1987:265–271.
5. Hill GB. *Eubacterium nodatum* mimics *Actinomyces* in intrauterine device-associated infections and other settings within the female genital tract. *Obstet Gynecol.* 1992;79:534–538.
6. Jordan HV, Kelly DM, Heeley JD. Enhancement of experimental actinomycosis in mice by *Eikenella corroidens. Infect Immun.* 1984;46:367–371.
7. Kanya KJ. Cervico-facial actinomycosis (a case report). *J Oral Med.* 1985;40:166–167.

8. Suzuki JB, Delisle AL. Pulmonary actinomycosis of periodontal origin. *J Periodontol.* 1984;55:581–584.
9. Balikian JP, Cheng TH, Costello P, Herman PG. Pulmonary actinomycosis. A report of three cases. *Radiology.* 1978; 128:613–616.
10. Dicpinigaitis PV, Bleiweiss IJ, Krellenstein DJ, Halton KP, Teirstein AS. Primary endobronchial actinomycosis is association with foreign body aspiration. *Chest.* 1992; 101:283–285.
11. Kwong JS, Muller NL, Godwin JD, Aberle D, Grymaloski MR. Thoracic actinomycosis: CT findings in eight patients. *Radiology.* 1992;183:189–192.
12. Wright EP, Holmberg K, Houston J, et al. Pulmonary actinomycosis simulating a bronchial neoplasm. *J Infect.* 1983;6:179–181.
13. Ariel I, Breuer R, Kamal NS, et al. Endobronchial actinomycosis simulating bronchogenic carcinoma. Diagnosis by bronchial biopsy. *Chest.* 1991;99:493–495.
14. Berardi RS. Abdominal actinomycosis. *Surg Gynecol Obstet.* 1979;149:257–266.
15. Bhagavan BS, Gupta PK. Genital actinomycosis and intrauterine contraceptive devices. *Hum Pathol.* 1978;9: 567–578.
16. Gupta PK. Intrauterine contraceptive devices: vaginal cytology, pathologic changes and clinical implications. *Acta Cytol.* 1982;26:571–613.
17. Nayar M, Chandra M, Chitraratha K, Das SK, Chowdhary GR. Incidence of actinomycetes infection in women using intrauterine contraceptive devices. *Acta Cytol.* 1985;29: 111–116.
18. Muller-Holzner E, Ruth NR, Abfalter E, et al. IUD-associated pelvic actinomycosis: a report of five cases. *Int J Gynecol Pathol.* 1995;14:70–74.
19. Oddó D, González S. Actinomycosis and nocardiosis: a morphologic study of 17 cases. *Path Res Pract.* 1986;181: 320–326.
20. Robboy SJ, Vickery AL. Tinctorial and morphologic properties distinguishing actinomycosis and nocardiosis. *N Engl J Med.* 1970;282:593–596.
21. Hotchi M, Schwarz J. Characterization of actinomycotic granules by architecture and staining methods. *Arch Pathol.* 1972;93:392–400.
22. Greenblatt M, Heredia R, Rubenstein L, Alpert S. Bacterial pseudomycosis ("botryomycosis"). *Am J Clin Pathol.* 1964; 41:188–193.
23. Hacker P. Botryomycosis review. *Int J Dermatol.* 1983; 22:455–458.
24. Winslow DJ. Mycetoma. In: Baker RD et al, eds. *The Pathologic Anatomy of Mycoses. Human Infection with Fungi, Actinomycetes and Algae.* New York: Springer-Verlag; 1971:589–613.
25. Happonen RP, Viander M. Comparison of fluorescent antibody technique and conventional staining methods in diagnosis of cervicofacial actinomycosis. *J Oral Pathol.* 1982;11:417–425.
26. Weese WC, Smith IM. A study of 57 cases of actinomycosis over a 36-year period. A diagnostic "failure" with good prognosis after treatment. *Arch Intern Med.* 1975;135: 1562–1568.
27. Bennhoff DF. Actinomycosis: diagnostic and therapeutic considerations and a review of 32 cases. *Laryngoscope.* 1984;94:1198–1217.
28. Harris LF, Kakani PR, Selah CE. Actinomycosis. Surgical aspects. *Am Surg.* 1985;51:262–264.

Chapter 41

Anthrax

Nancy K. Jaax and David L. Fritz

Infectious Disease is one of the few genuine adventures left in the world.

Hans Zinsser (1878–1940), Rats, Lice and History

DEFINITIONS AND HISTORICAL BACKGROUND

Anthrax is a zoonotic disease caused by the bacterium *Bacillus anthracis.* Although anthrax is primarily a disease of herbivores (cows, horses, sheep, goats), *B anthracis* infects humans and other mammals. There is tremendous variability in the susceptibility of various animals to infection. Carnivores and carrion eaters resist infection, whereas sheep and goats are susceptible.[1] Humans are infected by contact with infected animals or animal products.

Few other diseases are as rich in historical background, or have had such a profound impact on the development of microbiology. Anthrax has been recognized for centuries, and descriptions of disease consistent with anthrax were reported in early Hebrew, Greek, and Roman records. In Europe, from the seventeenth to the nineteenth century, anthrax caused many human deaths, as well as enormous losses of domestic livestock. Fundamental concepts of bacterial infection and immunity stemmed from Koch's and Pasteur's studies of *B anthracis* in the 1800s. These concepts included the development of Koch's postulates for infectious agents, and the development of an attenuated bacterial vaccine by Pasteur and coworkers.[2]

Anthrax has many synonyms including charbon, milzbrand, black bain, woolsorter's disease, ragpicker's disease, tanner's disease, and Siberian or splenic fever, and is a classic occupational disease. It occurs most frequently in agricultural workers exposed to infected animals or in industrial workers who handle spore-contaminated hides and wool fibers in hide processing and textile plants. With improved wool- and hide-handling procedures that reduce and inactivate spores, and vaccination of livestock and workers, human anthrax in the Western world has become rare. In developing countries, epidemics in humans usually occur during concurrent epizootics in susceptible animals. One of the largest epidemics on record was in Zimbabwe in the early 1980s. In that epidemic, more than 6000 people were infected.[3] The other notable outbreak occurred in 1979 in Sverdlovsk, Russia, where more than 60 people died from inhalation anthrax. The actual number of deaths in the Sverdlovsk outbreak has never been established because official information was suppressed by the former USSR.[4] This outbreak was initially reported in 1980 to have resulted from cutaneous exposure and ingestion of contaminated meat; autopsy findings, however, were consistent with aerosol exposure.[5] International attention was drawn to the Sverdlovsk epidemic because it may have been caused by accidental release of infectious anthrax spores from a military facility in the district where most of the patients lived.[5–7]

GEOGRAPHIC DISTRIBUTION

Anthrax is worldwide, with the highest incidence in tropical and subtropical climates. Parts of Africa, Asia, southern Europe, Australia, and North and South America are subject to repeated outbreaks of anthrax in populations of domestic and wild animals.[2] Alkaline soil with high levels of organic matter and poor drainage combined with alternating rain and drought promote sporulation and subsequent multiplication of *B anthracis* in the soil. In the United States, endemic areas are found where soils are high in calcium and nitrogen and have a periodic abundance of water. Animals are infected primarily by ingestion of vegetation contaminated by spores or spore-laden soil associated with plant roots, but other modes of infection also occur. Rainwater can carry anthrax spores from contaminated soil into low-lying water holes, where they settle to the bottom. During subsequent drought when the water levels are low, animals are infected by drinking the residual water heavily contaminated with spores.[2] During periods of heavy rainfall in poorly drained areas, spores may be leached from the soil or suspended in puddles and ingested by animals.[2] Flies feeding on infected carcasses may pass intact spores in feces deposited on leaves and foliage, which are then consumed by herbivores, or they may infect animals directly through the feeding activity of blood sucking.[2] Significant outbreaks in nonendemic areas are usually related to those who handle contaminated imported hides or wool; or, in the case of animals, by ingesting contaminated food products used to make animal rations.[8]

MORPHOLOGY AND CHARACTERISTICS OF THE ORGANISM

Bacillus anthracis is a large, gram-positive, aerobic, nonmotile, spore-forming bacillus that cannot easily be differentiated morphologically from *B cereus* or *B thuringiensis*. On solid culture media, *B anthracis* forms large, raised, granular colonies with irregular borders frequently referred to as "medusa head" or "comet tails." In mammalian hosts, bacilli are in pairs or short chains, but in smears from agar colonies there are long chains of large, rod-shaped organisms 1 to 1.25 by 3 to 5 microns, typically referred to as "boxcar" or "bamboo rod" in appearance. In vivo, as well as under certain culture conditions, virulent strains produce a capsule of poly-D-glutamic acid.[9] The vegetative form of the organism is not as hardy as the spore form, and is quickly destroyed by autolytic enzymes and putrefactive organisms in a degenerating animal carcass. Sporulation is inhibited by elevated carbon dioxide within the carcass, but occurs rapidly if the carcass is opened and the organism is exposed to the lower atmospheric levels of carbon dioxide. Anthrax spores resist destruction, and can persist for many years in soil.

CLINICAL FEATURES OF ANTHRAX

Anthrax is usually classified as cutaneous, gastrointestinal, or inhalational. Septicemic anthrax with bacteremia, toxemia, and associated secondary manifestations may follow any mode of infection, but is rare in cutaneous anthrax and usual with inhalational or gastrointestinal anthrax. When it occurs, septicemic anthrax develops in two phases. First, there is establishment of infection, multiplication of the organism, and dissemination. If multiplication of the organism is not controlled, the second phase of overwhelming septicemia and toxemia develops suddenly.

Cutaneous Anthrax

Approximately 95% of all reported human anthrax is cutaneous.[10,11] The classic cutaneous lesion of anthrax occurs in man, swine, rabbits, and horses. Lesions usually occur where spores come into contact with abraded skin, because the spores will not actually penetrate intact skin. Although not a major source of infection, anthrax can also be transmitted by biting flies that have fed on the carcasses of animals that died of anthrax.[12] The cutaneous lesion first is macular, and becomes papular within 48 hours. A pruritic vesicle develops, with the surrounding tissue appearing dark blue to black. The vesicle ruptures and produces the diagnostically significant black eschar (Figure 41–1). The eschar has been likened to a piece of coal in appearance, hence the name anthrax (*anthrax* is Greek for "coal"). Infections are usually self-limiting and relatively painless, but treatment is recommended. Treatment with penicillin sterilizes the localized lesion within 24 hours, and retraction and healing follow within 2 to 3 weeks. If penicillin is delayed or not administered, bacteria can establish and proliferate. An extensive localized reaction consisting of cellulitis and regional lymphadenopathy is often referred to as "malignant edema."[13] If left

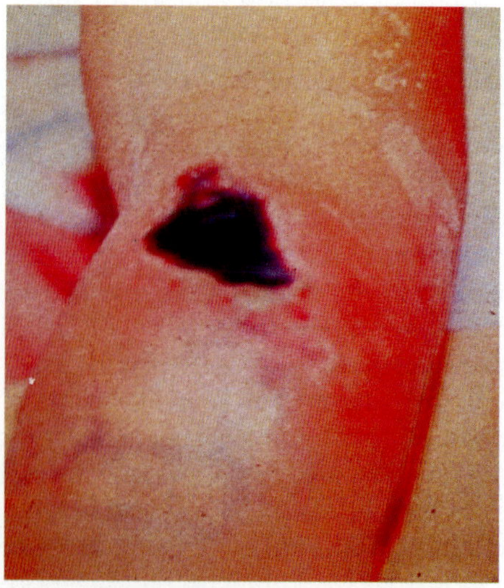

Figure 41–1. Typical cutaneous lesion of anthrax. *(Photograph courtesy of Dr. Arnold Kaufman, Centers for Disease Control, Atlanta, Georgia.)*

untreated, the disease can progress to systemic infection, toxemia, and death.[9]

Gastrointestinal Anthrax

Primary gastrointestinal anthrax in humans is extremely rare and has never been reported in the United States. Monkeys are relatively resistant to high doses of orally administered spores, as are carnivores, suggesting that a preexistent lesion or condition might be necessary to establish infection. Malnutrition has been considered a predisposing factor as well.[13] The majority of reported outbreaks of enteric anthrax have been in Africa and southeastern Asia, where cultural and religious beliefs have precluded detailed studies[7]; 10 cases have been published, however.[14–16] The gastrointestinal form usually presents either as a localized oropharyngeal lesion (probably resulting from colonization of organisms in a mucosal lesion) or as a severe systemic disease, with a localized primary lesion that is usually solitary in terminal ileum or cecum.[5] In the localized oropharyngeal form, ingested organisms gain entrance to the submucosal tissues through oral or oropharyngeal tissue, probably a consequence of abrasions or penetrations caused by spore-contaminated, high-roughage foodstuffs. Localized ulcers, cervical and submandibular lymphadenopathy, and regional edema are common sequelae. Patients with gastrointestinal anthrax present with nausea, vomiting, anorexia, and fever accompanied by abdominal pain. In the septicemic phase, hematemesis and bloody diarrhea may also develop, with shock and death.

Inhalational Anthrax

Inhalational anthrax frequently is referred to as woolsorter's disease, because it was recognized to be an occupational hazard of factory workers who handled contaminated wool or hides. Disinfecting wool and hides and vaccinating workers have controlled occupational anthrax. Natural outbreaks of inhalational anthrax have occurred rarely in this century. Only 18 cases were reported in the United States from 1900 to 1980.[17] Inhalational anthrax is rapidly progressive and usually fatal. Onset is 1 to 5 days after inhaling spores, and is characterized by fever, myalgia, and nonproductive cough suggesting bronchitis or influenza. There is neutrophilia with a left shift, and dramatic depression of blood oxygen levels. Severe respiratory distress develops suddenly, with stridor, dyspnea, and cyanosis. Radiographically, there frequently is a characteristic expansion of the mediastinal space by edema (Figure 41–2).[13] Shock frequently develops, and death usually occurs within 24 to 48 hours of onset.

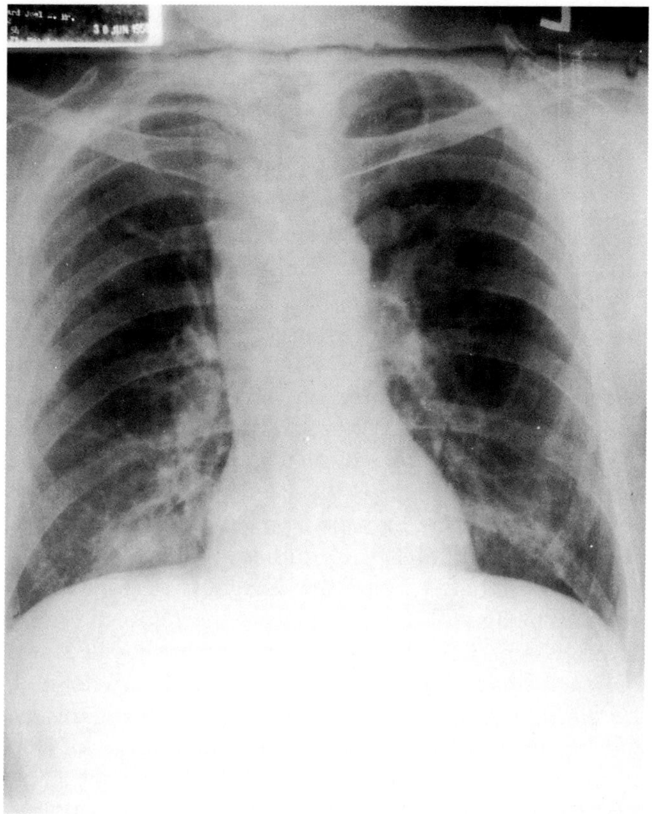

Figure 41–2. Chest radiograph of a patient with acute inhalational anthrax. Note the characteristic increased density and expansion of the mediastinal space by edema.

PATHOGENESIS

The anthrax bacillus possesses three primary, plasmid-encoded virulence factors. The capsule, composed of a high-molecular-weight polypeptide, poly-D-glutamic acid,[18] is encoded by the pX02 plasmid.[19] The capsule acts as a virulence factor by virtue of its negative charge, which physically inhibits phagocytosis of the vegetative bacilli.[20] Virulent strains also produce two exotoxins composed of three separate proteins termed *protective antigen, edema factor,* and *lethal factor.* Edema toxin is composed of edema factor, a calmodulin-dependent adenylate cyclase, and protective antigen. Lethal toxin is composed of two proteins, lethal factor and protective antigen. Both toxins are encoded by the pX01 plasmid.[21] The proteins are individually nontoxic, but act in binary combinations to produce two distinct toxic responses, edema and death.[21] The toxins are thought to increase host susceptibility to infection through their effect on both neutrophils and macrophages.[22–24] Anthrax edema factor, by increasing intracellular cyclic adenosine monophosphate (cAMP), inhibits neutrophil phagocytosis and oxidative processes.[22] The anthrax lethal toxin is cytolytic for macrophages at high concentrations[23] and causes release of tumor necrosis factor (TNF) and interleukin 1 (IL-1) at lower concentrations.[24] Both TNF and IL-1 can induce severe changes in endothelial cells.[25–27] Recent experiments in mice passively immunized against IL-1 suggest that shock and death from anthrax result primarily from the effects of high levels of cytokines, principally IL-1, produced by macrophages that have been stimulated by the anthrax lethal toxin.[24] Further definitive studies in experimental models measuring cytokine levels and using cytokine antagonists are required to assess the role of IL-1, TNF, and other cytokines in the pathogenesis of the disease process. As a result of the combined virulence factors, there is localized proliferation of the organism and tissue damage from reaction to the components of anthrax toxin. Studies by Ross[28] demonstrated that inhaled spores are phagocytosed by alveolar macrophages and transported to the regional lymph nodes, where they germinate to vegetative bacilli. Once the macrophages of the lymph nodes are overwhelmed, the efferent lymphatics become laden with organisms, and bacilli enter the blood, where they are picked up by the reticuloendothelial system (RES). It is only after the RES capacity of the body is overwhelmed that large numbers of the organisms appear in the blood and are distributed throughout the body. The massive numbers of organisms present in the blood at death (approximately 1×10^9/mL) are a classic feature of the disease. At the point of bacteremia and sepsis, the number of bacilli increases logarithmically, doubling every 48 minutes until the terminal level (which appears to be host specific) is reached.[29] Ross also demonstrated that not all spores germinate immediately, but may remain dormant for extended periods. It is this phenomenon that accounts for the recurrence of clinical anthrax septicemia if antibiotics are only used for short periods of time and then discontinued without administration of protective vaccine.[30]

Gross Pathology

The hallmark lesions of anthrax are hemorrhage and edema. In patients with localized cutaneous anthrax without the septicemic phase, hemorrhage and edema are usually limited to the tissue adjacent to the site of inoculation and the regional lymph node. The characteristic "malignant pustule" and relatively painless eschar are probably diagnostic when coupled with a history of exposure (Figure 41–1).

Except for the site of initial entry and the mediastinal edema in patients with respiratory exposure, the nature and distribution of the lesions of septicemic anthrax are virtually identical regardless of route of infection. The severe, localized primary necrotizing and hemorrhagic lesion at the portal of entry is considered specific enough to establish the mode of infection in humans,[5] although that distinction is not as clear in rhesus monkeys infected experimentally by aerosol.[30a] The severe localized reaction is caused by the toxin produced by the initially localized bacteria. The bacteria tend to colonize areas of lung or gastrointestinal (GI) tract that have lesions from other causes. Examples include parasitic nodules, neoplasms, or foci of chronic active inflammation. A focal lesion that resembles an abscess then forms, and direct dissemination of the organism to the bloodstream without transport through the lymphatics is possible. The infection appears to bypass thoracic or mesenteric nodes, and an overwhelming infection of the spleen develops.[31]

The largest and most complete pathologic study of inhalational anthrax in humans is the study of 42 Sverdlovsk cases published by Abramova et al.[5] Their findings were consistent with earlier reports of human cases of inhalational anthrax[17,32] and also with published experimental studies in nonhuman primates.[30a,31,33] The study by Abramova et al revealed that inhalational anthrax was characterized by hemorrhagic thoracic lymphadenitis and hemorrhagic mediastinitis in all 42 patients. The mediastinal tissue was a translucent, edematous mass and had a gelatinous consistency. Eleven patients had a focus of primary pulmonary anthrax (focal hemorrhagic necrotizing pneumonia). Manifestations of hematogenous spread of *B anthracis* included serohemorrhagic and hemorrhagic leptomeningitis (21 patients), hematogenous spread to the submucosa of the GI tract (39 patients), and mesenteric lymphadenitis (9 patients) (Figure 41–3). The hemorrhagic meningitis is striking (Figure 41–4), and is often referred to as a "cardinal's cap" because of the bright color and location of the hemorrhage.[7] Edema of the mediastinum, pleural effusions, and enlarged, hemorrhagic lymph nodes were consistent findings; the lesions were compatible with increased vascular permeability caused by the anthrax toxins. Similar lesions occur experimentally in nonhuman primates, confirming the relevance of the experimental model.[30,31]

LIGHT MICROSCOPY INCLUDING SPECIAL STAINS

Light microscopy reveals hemorrhage, edema, necrosis, fibrin deposition, a variable degree of inflammatory cell infiltrate, mostly neutrophils, and profound bacillemia. There is pronounced lymphoid necrosis with sinus histiocytosis and variable hemorrhage in the lymph nodes (Figure 41–5). Splenic lesions are characterized by lym-

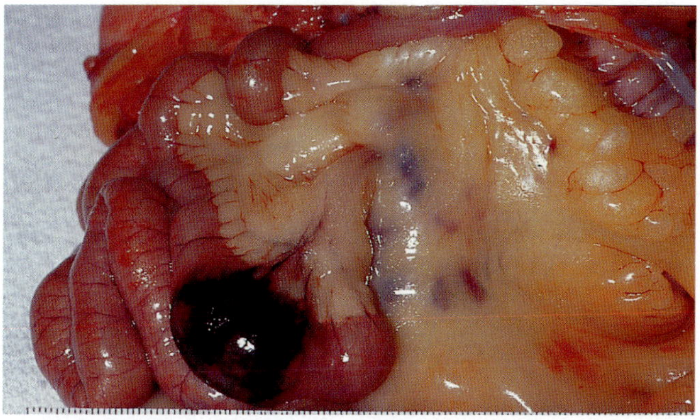

Figure 41–3. Small intestine and mesentery from a monkey given a lethal dose of *B anthracis* by inhalation. A hemorrhagic infarct in one segment of the intestine is accompanied by multifocal small ecchymotic serosal hemorrhages. Several hemorrhagic mesenteric lymph nodes can be seen through the mesenteric adipose tissue.

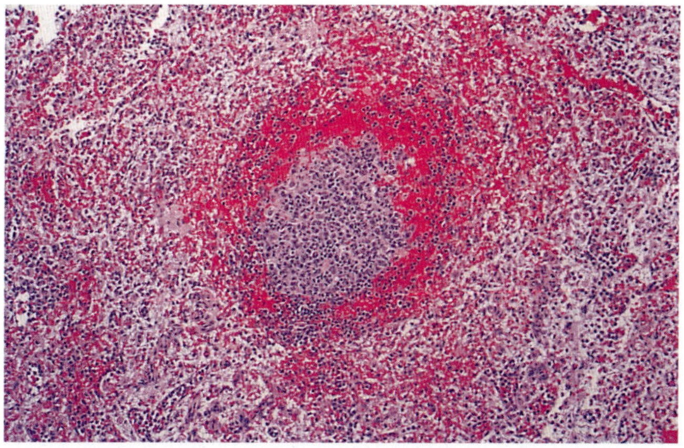

Figure 41–5. Spleen from a monkey given a lethal dose of *B anthracis* by inhalation. In the white pulp, there is lymphoid depletion of the periarteriolar lymphoid sheath and marked hemorrhage in the marginal zone (hematoxylin-eosin, ×50).

phoid necrosis, depletion of the splenic white pulp, and acute, fibrinopurulent necrosis. The hemorrhagic meningitis is characterized by hemorrhage, fibrinopurulent inflammation, and bacilli in and around blood vessels. In aerosol-exposed rhesus monkeys, the initial lesions are pulmonary edema and hemorrhage and acute pneumonia (Figure 41–6); necrotizing vasculitis in the walls of small cerebral blood vessels, hemorrhage in the neuropil (Figures 41–7 and 41–8), and disseminated intravascular coagulation may also occur. Blood films, touch preparations, and tissues all reveal a myriad of typically shaped ("boxcar" or "bamboo rod"), encapsulated gram-positive bacilli (Figure 41–9).

Immunocytochemistry using monoclonal antibody to the polysaccharide cell wall provides specific identification of the organism.[34] Success with this technique requires some degradation of the capsule because this allows the antibody access to the cell wall. Degradation proceeds quickly, however, and by 72 hours false-negatives are not a problem (Figure 41–10).

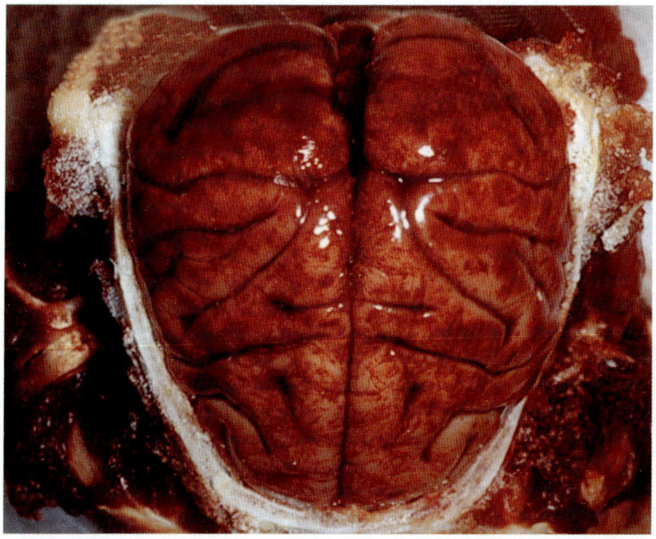

Figure 41–4. Dorsal surface of the brain of a monkey given a lethal dose of *B anthracis* by inhalation. Note the striking perivascular hemorrhage most prominent in the sulci, extending over the surface of the brain.

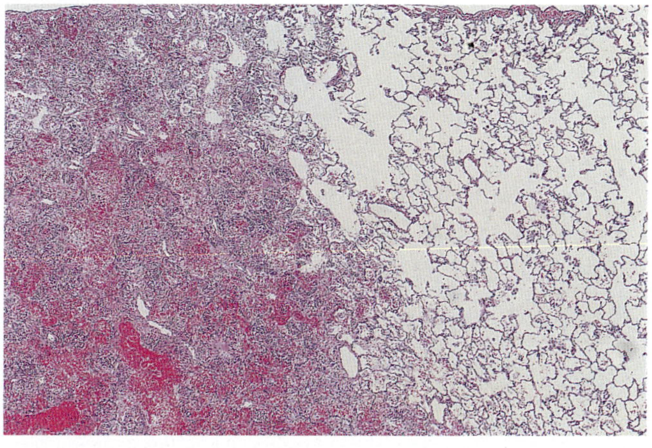

Figure 41–6. Lung from a monkey given a lethal dose of *B anthracis* by inhalation. The right half of the lung field is normal in contrast to the left half, in which there is moderate, suppurative, hemorrhagic pneumonia. Myriad bacilli, present in most alveoli, are not discernible at this low magnification (hematoxylin-eosin, ×25).

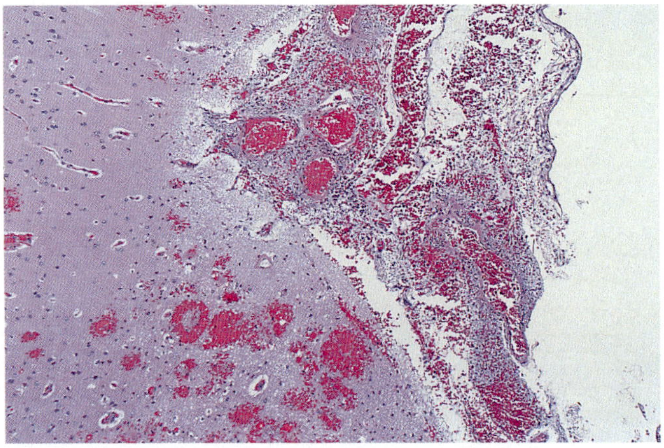

Figure 41–7. Cerebral cortex and overlying meninges from a monkey given a lethal dose of *B anthracis* by inhalation. Note the multifocal parencyhmal hemorrhages of the cortex. The meninges are moderately thickened mostly by myriad bacilli, and to a lesser degree by leukocytes and hemorrhage (not seen at this low magnification) (hematoxylin-eosin, ×50).

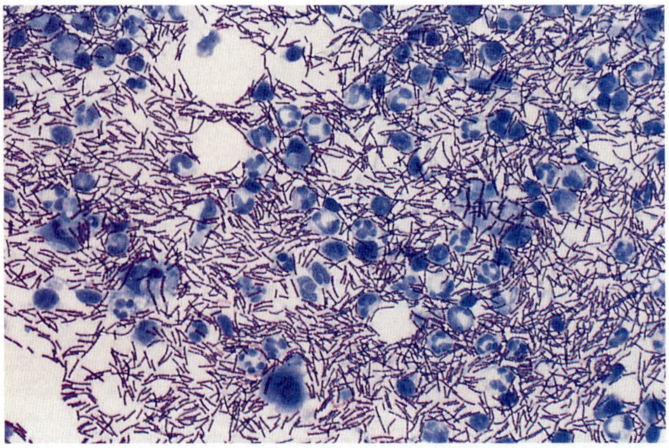

Figure 41–9. Impression smear from the tracheobronchial lymph node of a monkey given a lethal dose of *B anthracis* by inhalation. Myriad magenta-stained bacilli occur individually and in chains along with scattered blue-stained leukocytes (Wright–Giemsa, ×100).

ELECTRON MICROSCOPY

Electron microscopic findings indicate that the mononuclear phagocytic system of the spleen clears and degrades bacilli. As bacillemia levels increase, splenic neutrophils increase in number and become more active in phagocytosing bacilli than are macrophages. In nonhuman primates, transmission electron microscopy (TEM) reveals that extracellular bacilli in spleens are nearly always surrounded by an electron-lucent zone, presumed to be the capsule (Figure 41–11). This zone is not observed in intracellular bacilli. The lack of a distinct osmiophilic capsule as reported by Shakhbanov[35] is not surprising given the severe necrotizing and suppurative process present in the tissue. In spite of many phagocytes, phagocytosed bacilli are few.

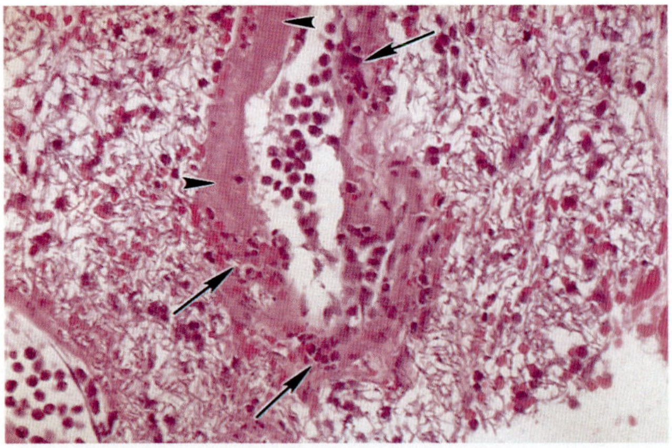

Figure 41–8. In the media of this meningeal arteriole from the cerebrum of a monkey given a lethal dose of *B anthracis* by inhalation, there are scattered, small aggregates of leukocytes (mostly neutrophils) with occasional erythrocytes. Note the segment of medial fibrinoid change in the media. Myriad bacilli accompanied by mild, acute inflammatory cell infiltrate are present in the meninges surrounding the arteriole (hematoxylin-eosin, ×100).

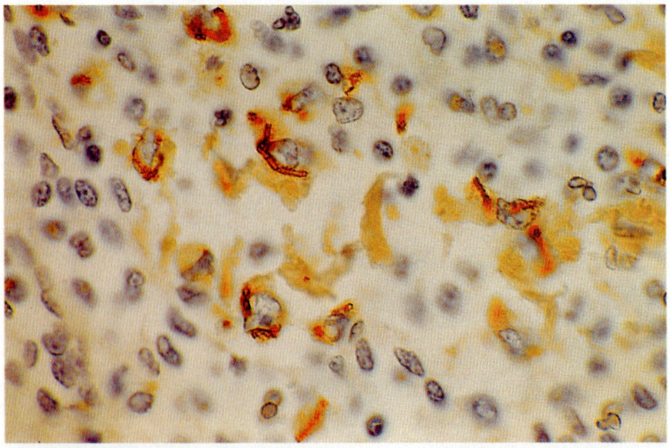

Figure 41–10. Splenic red pulp from a monkey given a lethal dose of *B anthracis* by inhalation demonstrating positive staining with monoclonal antibody EAII-6G6 against cell wall polysaccharide of *B anthracis*. Whole and fragmented bacilli are in the cytoplasm of splenic macrophages, although extracellular bacilli are not evident (immunoperoxidase, ×250).

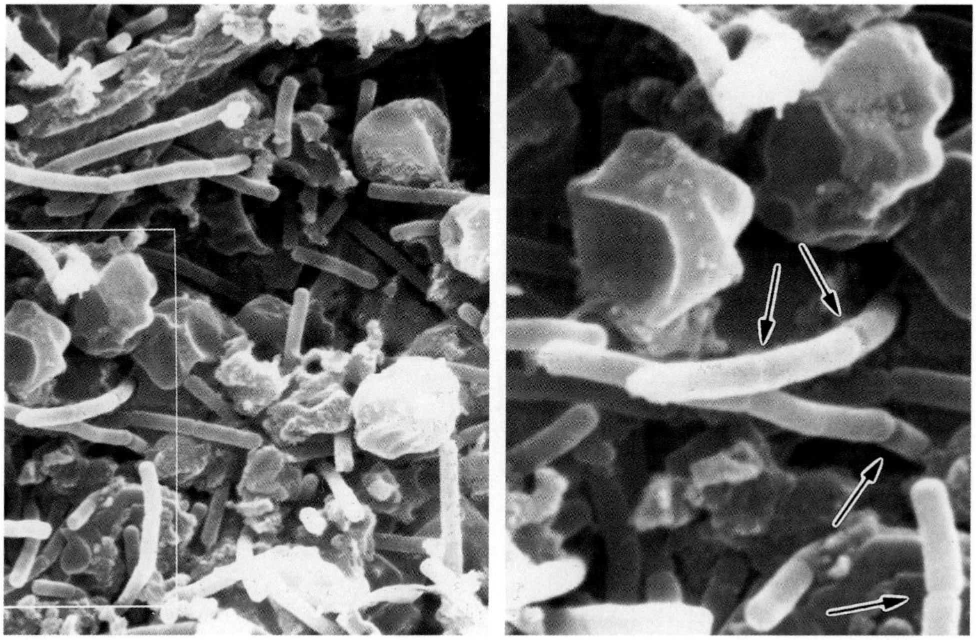

Figure 41–11. (*Left*) Splenic red pulp from a monkey given a lethal dose of *B anthracis* by inhalation. Admixed with erythrocytes are myriad bacilli, many of which are in long chains (×1175). (*Right*) At a higher magnification, distinct constrictions (*arrows*) along the chain demarcate transverse septa, which separate bacilli (×2720).

Immunostaining of encapsulated extracellular bacilli is poor, probably because the capsular polysaccharide prevents antibody from reaching the cell wall (Figures 41–12 and 41–13).

DIFFERENTIAL DIAGNOSIS

The critical step in diagnosis is to obtain a history. Anthrax without exposure to infected animals or animal products is exceedingly rare. In patients with a cutaneous lesion only, acute staphylococcal cellulitis may be mistaken for a malignant anthrax pustule; a history and Gram stain of the exudate differentiate these two. In patients with systemic disease and a cutaneous lesion, other infections must be considered, such as tularemia, plague, cat scratch disease, rat bite fever, and sporotrichosis. In patients with inhalational anthrax, the characteristic widening of the mediastinum by edema (on chest radiograph) favors a diagnosis of anthrax.

DIAGNOSIS

A presumptive clinical diagnosis is made by history, clinical signs, and gram-positive bacilli on smears of blood; or at autopsy by impression smears of spleen and lymph node (Figure 41–9). Definitive diagnosis in active infections is based on culture, and identification of *B anthracis*. The morphology of the organism coupled with the presence of a capsule and spore formation, its colony appearance,[36] tests for pathogenicity in laboratory animals,[37] presence of antibody [detected by enzyme-linked immunosorbent assay or indirect hemagglutination assay (IHA)] to protective antigen or lethal toxin in the patient's blood, and demonstration of the components of the anthrax lethal toxin in vitro [protective antigen (PA) and lethal factor][21] have all been used.

Immunocytochemistry performed with monoclonal antibody against cell wall galactose-*N*-acetylglucosamine polysaccharide, which is essentially unique to *B anthracis,* has been performed successfully on cultures, impression smears, and tissue sections of autopsy material.[34,38]

TREATMENT

Successful treatment requires an understanding of the pathogenesis. It is advantageous to think of treatment in two phases, one to protect against multiplication of the organism, and the other to protect against the effects of the anthrax toxins if there is septicemia. Prompt therapy when anthrax is suspected is important. Delaying treatment for definitive laboratory results can be fatal, particularly in patients with inhalational exposure. Experimental studies demonstrate that once a critical level of bacteremia is reached, eradicating *B anthracis* will not prevent a fatal toxemia.[20] Penicillin is the antibiotic of choice, although other antibiotics (doxycycline and ciprofloxacin) are effective if penicillin is contraindicated. In septicemic anthrax, supportive therapy for shock is also necessary. Toxins in the pathogenesis of anthrax suggest a regimen of antiserum for patients

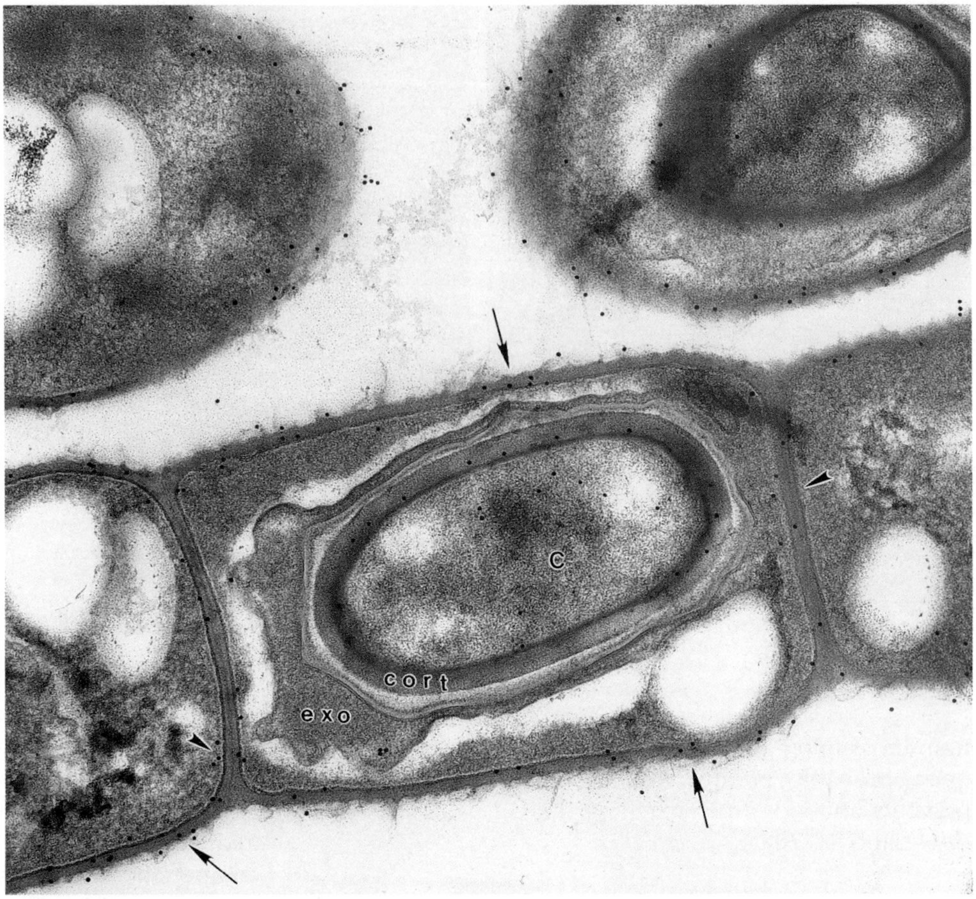

Figure 41–12. Sporangium and spore from a culture of *B anthracis* treated with monoclonal antibody EAII-6G6 conjugated with 10-nm immunogold. In the spore, the core (C), cortex (cort), and exopsporium (exo) are immunolabeled, whereas only the cell wall (*arrows*) and transverse septum (*arrowheads*) of the sporangium and adjacent vegetative cells are labeled (×28,500).

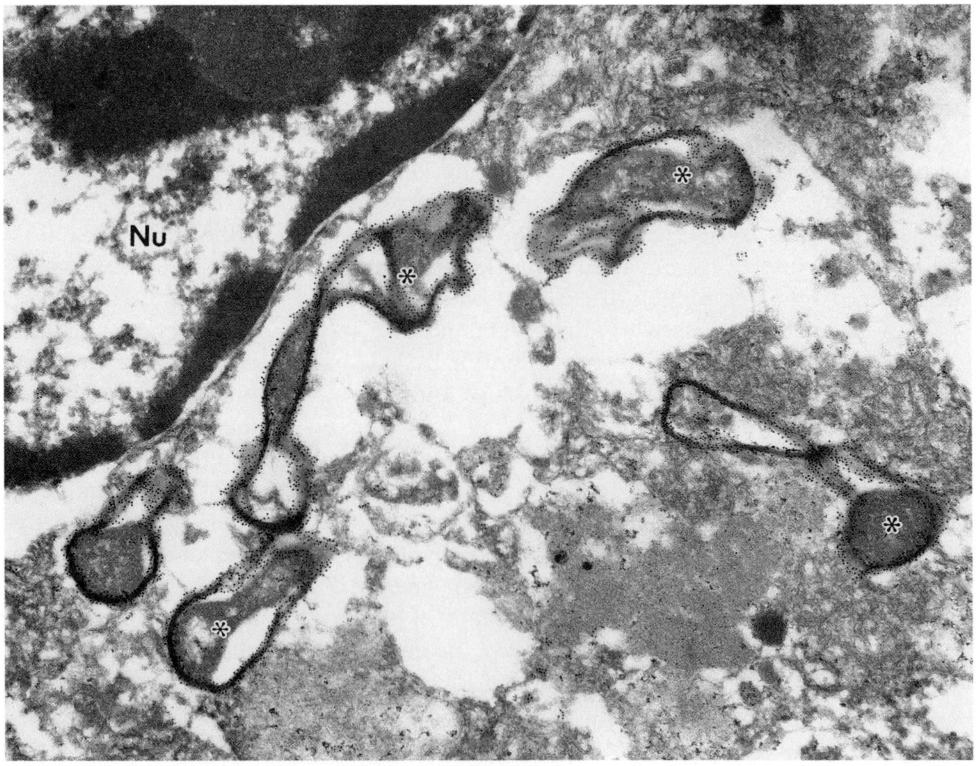

Figure 41–13. Medullary sinus macrophage in the tracheobronchial lymph node of a monkey given a lethal dose of *B anthracis* by inhalation. This tissue has been treated with monoclonal antibody EAII-6G6 conjugated with 10-nm immunogold. Note contorted profiles (*asterisks*) of degraded intracellular bacilli whose cell wall polysaccharide is labeled with gold particles. The cell nucleus (Nu) with prominent nucleolus is in the upper left (×10,000).

with septicemic anthrax,[39] but currently there is no product available for human use. In patients with known exposure, prophylactic penicillin should be given immediately, coupled with vaccination to prevent latent infection.[6] It is necessary to maintain the regimen long enough to allow sporulation of residual spores. Studies by Henderson[30] showed that up to 20% of inhaled anthrax spores were still in the lungs of primates 42 days after exposure. Although treatment with penicillin for 5 or 10 days (beginning day 1 after aerosol exposure of monkeys) was protective during antibiotic therapy, the animals died when the antibiotic was stopped.[30] The study by Friedlander et al[33] supported this finding. One primate, for instance, died 58 days after the antibiotic therapy was stopped. Furthermore, these animals failed to develop an immune response, and did not survive a second aerosol exposure. Successful long-term survival requires prolonged antibiotic treatment and vaccination.

PROPHYLAXIS

In most countries, livestock populations at risk are immunized annually with commercial vaccines composed of viable spores of *B anthracis.* Sterne strain, a nonencapsulated toxigenic variant that is safe and efficacious.[40] In contrast, the currently licensed human anthrax vaccine supplied by the Michigan Department of Public Health is prepared from culture supernatants of an avirulent strain of *B anthracis,* and is composed primarily of protective antigen.[40] Vaccination is recommended for occupationally at-risk individuals, including laboratory workers who work with the agent. This vaccine has been given to more than 20,000 people since it was licensed in 1971. Current field data estimate its effectiveness at 90% in protecting workers in woolen mills. Recent experimental studies support this conclusion (Friedlander et al, to be published).

REFERENCES

1. Lincoln RE, Walker JS, Klein F, Haines BW. Anthrax. *Ad Vet Sci.* 1964;9:327–368.
2. Ezzell JW, Wilhelmsen CL. *Bacillus anthracis.* In: Gyles CL, Thoen CO, eds. *Pathogenesis of Bacterial Infections in Animals.* Ames: Iowa State University Press; 1993:36–43.
3. Davies JC. A major epidemic of anthrax in Zimbabwe. *Cent Afr J Med* 1982:12:291–298.
4. Wade N. Death at Sverdlovsk: a critical diagnosis. *Science.* 1981;209:1501–1502.
5. Abramova FA, Grinberg LM, Yampolskaya OV, Walker DH. Pathology of inhalation anthrax in 42 cases from the Sverdlovsk outbreak of 1979. *Proc Natl Acad Sci USA.* 1993;90:2291–2294.
6. Knudson G. Treatment of anthrax in man: history and current concepts. *Mil Med.* 1986;151:71–76.
7. Walker DH, Yampolska O, Grinberg LM. Death at Sverdlovsk: What have we learned? *Am J Pathol.* 1994;144:1135–1141.
8. Spears HN. Anthrax. *Vet Rec.* 1959;71:637–643.
9. Rees HB Jr., Martin DD, Smithe MA. *Anthrax.* In: Balows A, Hausler WJ Jr, Ohashi M, Turano A, eds. *Laboratory Diagnosis of Infectious Diseases: Principles and Practice.* New York: Springer-Verlag; 1988;1:57–68.
10. Parvizpour D. Human anthrax in Iran: an epidemiological study of 468 cases. *Int J Zoonoses.* 1978;5:69–74.
11. Taylor JP, Dimmit DC, Ezzell JW, Whitford H. Indigenous human cutaneous anthrax in Texas. *South Med J.* 1993; 86:1–4.
12. Sen SK, Minett FC. Experiments on the transmission of anthrax through flies. *Ind J Vet Sci An Husb.* 1944;14: 149–158.
13. Dutz W, Kohout E. Anthrax. *Pathol Annu.* 1971;6:209–248.
14. Bhat P, Mohan DN, Srinivasa H. Intestinal anthrax with bacteriological investigations. *J Infect Dis.* 1985;152: 1357–1358.
15. Nalin D, Begum S, Sahunja R, et al. Survival of a patient with intestinal anthrax. *Am J Med.* 1977;62:130–132.
16. Jena GP. Intestinal anthrax in man, a case report. *Cent Afr J Med.* 1980;26:253–254.
17. Brachman PS. Inhalation anthrax. *Ann New York Acad of Sci.* 1980;353:83–93.
18. Record BR, Wallis RG. Physicochemical examination of polyglutamic acid from *Bacillus anthracis* grown in vivo. *Biochem J.* 1956;63:443–447.
19. Uchida I, Sekizaki T, Hashimoto K, Terakado N. Association of the encapsulation of *Bacillus anthracis* with a 60 megadalton plasmid. *J Gen Micro.* 1985;131:363–367.
20. Keppie J, Smith H, Harris-Smith PW. The chemical basis of virulence of *Bacillus anthracis*: The role of the terminal bacteremia in death of guinea pigs from anthrax. *Brit J Exp Pathol.* 1955;36:323–335.
21. Leppla SH, Ivins BE, Ezzell JW Jr. *Anthrax toxin.* In: Lieve L, ed. *Microbiology 1985.* Washington, DC: American Society for Microbiology; 1985:666.
22. O'Brien J, Friedlander A, Dreier T, Ezzell J, Leppla S. Effects of anthrax toxin components on human neutrophils. *Infect Immun.* 1985;47:306–310.
23. Friedlander AM. Macrophages are sensitive to anthrax lethal toxin through an acid-dependent process. *J Biol Chem.* 1986;261:7123–7126.
24. Hanna PC, Acosta D, Collier RJ. On the role of macrophages in anthrax. *Proc Natl Acad Sci USA.* 1993;90:10198–10201.
25. Libby P, Ordovas JM, Auger KR, Robbins AH, Birinyi LK, Dinarello CA. Endotoxin and tumor necrosis factor induce interleukin-1 gene expression in adult human vascular endothelial cells. *An J Pathol.* 1986;124:179–185.
26. Nawroth PP, Bank I, Handley D, Cassimeris J, Chess L, Stern D. Tumor necrosis factor/cachectin interacts with endothelial cell receptors to induce release of interleukin 1. *J Exp Med.* 1986;163:1363–1375.
27. Sato N, Goto T, Haranaka K, et al. Actions of tumor

necrosis factor on cultured vascular endothelial cells: morphologic modulation, growth inhibition, and cytotoxicity. *J Natl Cancer Inst.* 1986;76:1113–1121.

28. Ross JM. The pathogenesis of anthrax following the administration of spores by the respiratory route. *J Pathol Bacteriol.* 1957;73:485–494.
29. Lincoln RE, Hodges DR, Klein F, et al. Role of the lymphatics in the pathogenesis of anthrax. *J Infect Dis.* 1965;115:481–494.
30. Henderson DW, Peacock S, Belton FC. Observations on the prophylaxis of experimental pulmonary anthrax in the monkey. *J Hyg.* 1956;54:28–36.

30a. Fritz DL, Jaax NK, Lawrence WB, et al. Pathology of experimental inhalation of anthrax in the rhesus monkey. *Lab Invest.* 1995;73:691–702.

31. Gleiser CA, Berdjis CC, Hartman HA, Gochenour WS. Pathology of experimental respiratory anthrax in Macaca mulatta. *Br J Exp Pathol.* 1963;44:416–426.
32. Albrink WS, Brooks SM, Biron RE, Kopel M. Human inhalation anthrax: a report of three fatal cases. *Am J Pathol.* 1960;36:457–468.
33. Friedlander AM, Welkos SL, Pitt MLM, et al. Postexposure prophylaxis against experimental inhalation anthrax. *J Infect Dis.* 1993;167:1239–1242.
34. Ezzell JW, Abshire TG, Little SF, Lidgerding BC, Brown C. Identification of *Bacillus anthracis* by using monoclonal antibody to cell wall galactose-*N*-acetylglucosamine polysaccharide. *J Clin Microbiol.* 1990;28:223–231.
35. Shakhbanov AA. Ultrastructure of *Bacillus anthracis* and *Bacillus cereus*. *Zh Mikrobiol Epidemiol Immunobiol.* 1975;6:92–96.
36. Doyle RJ, Keller KF, Ezzell JW. *Bacillus.* In: Lennette EH, Balows WJ, Hausler WJ Jr, Shadomy HJ, eds. *Manual of Clinical Microbiology.* 4th ed. Washington, DC: American Society for Microbiology; 1985:211–215.
37. Brown ER, Moody MD, Treece EL, Smith CW. Differential diagnosis of *Bacillus cereus, Bacillus anthracis,* and *Bacillus cereus* var. Mycoides. *J Bact.* 1958;75:499–509.
38. McGee ED, Fritz DL, Ezzell JW, Newcomb HL, Brown RJ, Jaax NK. Anthrax in a dog. *Vet Pathol.* 1994;31:471–473.
39. Belton FC, Strange RE. Studies on a protective antigen produced in vitro from *Bacillus anthracis:* Medium and methods of production. *Br J Exper Pathol.* 1954;37: 144–152.
40. Ezzell JW Jr, Abshire TG. Immunological analysis of cell-associated antigens of *Bacillus anthracis. Infect Immun.* 1988;56(349):349–356.

CHAPTER 42

Bacillary Angiomatosis

Philip E. LeBoit

A disease known is half cured.

Proverb

DEFINITION

Bacillary angiomatosis (BA) is a reactive vascular proliferation caused by bacilli of the genus *Bartonella* (formerly *Rochalimaea*), specifically *B henselae* and *B quintana*. BA was initially described in the skin, but can occur in a variety of viscera or as septicemia.[1] The tissue reaction varies from organ to organ; in some sites fibrosis can be prominent, and in the liver and spleen peliosis is the usual response.[2] First reports were in patients infected with the human immunodeficiency virus (HIV); infections were subsequently identified in other immunocompromised patients, such as those receiving cytotoxic chemotherapy, and later in some apparently immunocompetent patients as well.[3,4]

SYNONYMS

Synonyms for BA include epithelioid angiomatosis (so named because of the morphology of the endothelial cells in many patients),[5] and bacillary ailuronosis (derived from the Greek word for "cat," because of the putative identity of *B henselae* with the cat scratch bacillus). Some reports of BA have appeared under the heading of cutaneous or disseminated cat scratch disease. Most conventional cat scratch disease appears to be caused by one of the agents of BA, *B henselae,* but some may be caused by an unrelated pathogen, *Afipia felis.*[6]

GEOGRAPHIC DISTRIBUTION

The geographic distribution of BA is unclear. Reports from both North and South America, from Africa, from Europe, and a few from Asia reveal that its occurrence largely parallels that of HIV infection. Because domestic cats, (cat fleas), and ticks appear to be major reservoirs of *B henselae,* the prevalence of this organism in them and the carriage of bacilli by other insects needs to be studied. The occurrence of BA in a hunter who skinned a squirrel raises the possibility that *B henselae* has mammalian hosts other than man.[7]

NATURAL HISTORY AND EPIDEMIOLOGY

BA is at least in part a zoonosis, because one of its agents, *B henselae,* is harbored by both cats and their fleas.[8] Immunocompromised patients who own cats, especially kittens (defined as cats younger than 1 year in age), and have been licked, bitten, or scratched by a cat seem to have an increased incidence of BA, as evidenced by a case-controlled study. The cat flea *Ctenocephalides felis* is a proposed vector for transmission to humans. *Bartonella henselae* has been isolated from the blood of cats belonging to patients with BA, and by the polymerase chain reaction (PCR) from their fleas. The length of time of bacteremia in cats who carry *B henselae* and whether such factors as infection with feline leukemia virus prolong bacteremia are unknown.[9] Although some BA is caused by *B quintana,* the louse *Pediculus humanus,* which transmits the same agent in trench fever, does not seem to play a role in BA. Tick bites have been implicated in bacteremia caused by *B henselae.*[7] Ticks are reservoirs of *B quintana* in outbreaks of trench fever. The species of ticks that can host *B henselae* and their distribution are not known. Other reported animal hosts of agents causing BA include a parakeet and a pet rat.[10,11]

Human-to-human transmission has not been documented in BA, and reservoirs other than cats and their

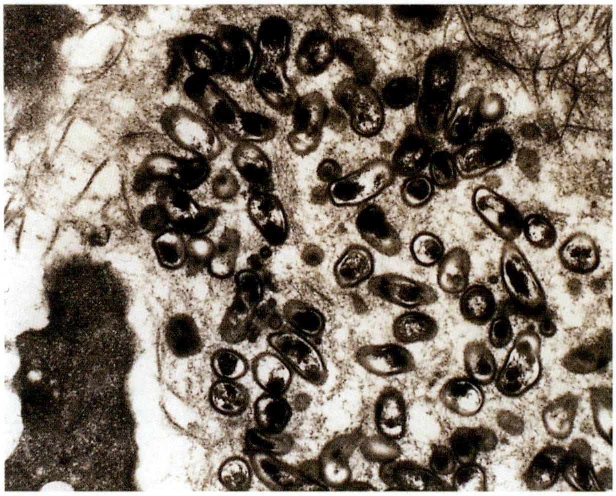

Figure 42–1. Bacillary angiomatosis of skin. Cluster of bacilli in interstitial tissue (electron microscopy).

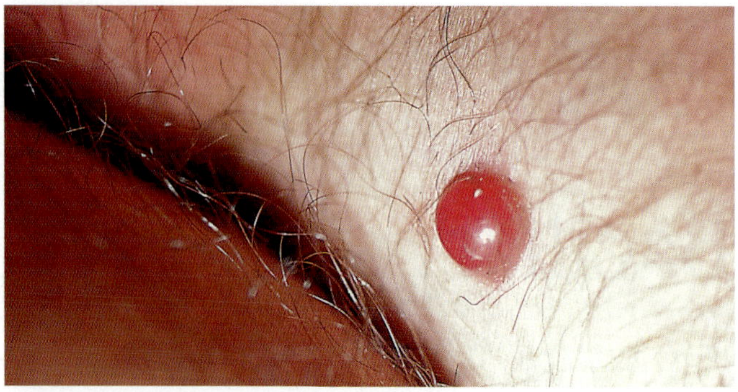

Figure 42–2. A cherry-red papule of cutaneous BA. Although this is characteristic, lesions of Kaposi's sarcoma and pyogenic granuloma can have an identical appearance.

fleas are unknown. Conventional cat scratch disease, which seems in many patients to be caused by *B henselae,* sometimes develops after splinter wounds and dog bites or scratches, implying that BA could also be similarly transmitted.

MORPHOLOGIC FEATURES OF THE ORGANISM

Both agents of BA, *B henselae* and *B quintana,* are small (approximately 1 μm wide, 3 μm long) coccobacilli with a trilaminar cell wall visible by electron microscopic examination (Figure 42–1). The organisms occur in profusion in the tissue infiltrates of BA, where they form extracellular clusters.[12]

CLINICAL FEATURES

Bacillary angiomatosis has now been reported to affect almost every organ system, but cutaneous lesions are most common. These lesions can be few or many, small or large, and occur with or without systemic disease. Papules (raised, rounded lesions less than 1 cm in diameter) and nodules (similarly shaped lesions of more than 1 cm in diameter) of BA range from skin colored to pink to deep red or purple, with intact, smooth, or ulcerated surfaces (Figure 42–2). Collarettes of scale often surround papules and nodules of BA. Subcutaneous rounded masses of BA are generally skin colored (Figure 42–3).

The number and distribution of lesions of cutaneous BA appear to reflect the degree of immunosuppression and the route of infection. Patients with less compromised immunity and a clear history of traumatic inoculation often have only a few lesions, or a single one at the site of entry. Patients with overwhelming infection can be covered with myriad lesions, which shows a propensity to involve mucocutaneous junctions.

BA can present as a subcutaneous mass, mimicking a soft tissue neoplasm when cutaneous lesions are absent.[13,14] Erosion of underlying bone can occur, as can osteolytic bone lesions.[15]

Lymph nodes involved by BA are often markedly enlarged and can be affected in the absence of other lesions, or can accompany visceral peliosis.[16,17]

Any mucosal surface can be the site of BA. Prior to the recognition of BA as an infection treatable by antibiotics, widespread mucosal lesions developed in patients with overwhelming infection.[5] Endobronchial, tracheal, and esophageal lesions can be life threatening.[18,19]

In addition to abdominal fullness, bacillary peliosis hepatis can cause elevated transaminase levels with a normal or slightly elevated bilirubin.[2] Splenic and hepatic peliosis may cause catastrophic intra-abdominal hemorrhage if a vascular space ruptures. Splenic peliosis often causes pancytopenia.

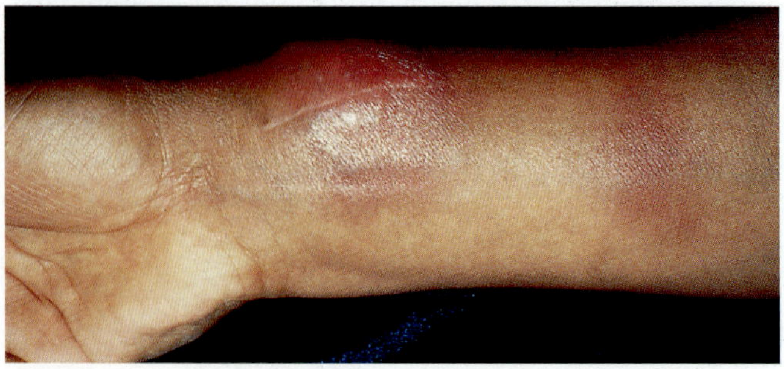

Figure 42–3. Subcutaneous BA. Unlike more superficial lesions, deep lesions are skin colored. The scar is an attempted incision and drainage.

Ophthalmic involvement is a newly recognized complication of BA.[20] Loss of visual acuity can be accompanied by retinal lesions, macular exudates, and optic nerve head swelling. The diagnosis can be difficult if cutaneous lesions of BA are absent, and rest largely on serologic studies. Conjunctival BA can also occur.[21] Conventional cat scratch disease can be complicated by Parinaud's oculoglandular syndrome, which consists of preauricular lymphadenopathy and conjunctivitis on the side of a cat scratch. The conjunctival lesions are granulomatous, but some patients suffering from this complication of cat scratch disease have had conjunctival BA rather than conventional cat scratch disease.[12] Many of the patients with ophthalmic BA are immunocompetent, suggesting that intraocular inoculation of organisms does not require an immune deficit.[20,21]

Patients with intracerebral BA can present with headache, seizures, cranial nerve dysfunction, psychiatric symptoms, and blindness.[1,22,23] Antibodies to *B henselae* are more prevalent in patients with AIDS and neurologic symptoms than in those without such symptoms.[22]

Systemic symptoms caused by BA may be difficult to distinguish from other causes of immune deficiencies, particularly those with advanced acquired immunodeficiency syndrome (AIDS). For instance, most patients with BA and HIV infection have fewer than 100 T cells/mm^3. Septicemia, fever, malaise, visual impairment, bone pain, stridor, dysphagia, and other signs can be the result of widespread infection. Bacteremia with *B henselae* can develop in the absence of tissue infiltrates of BA.[7,24,25]

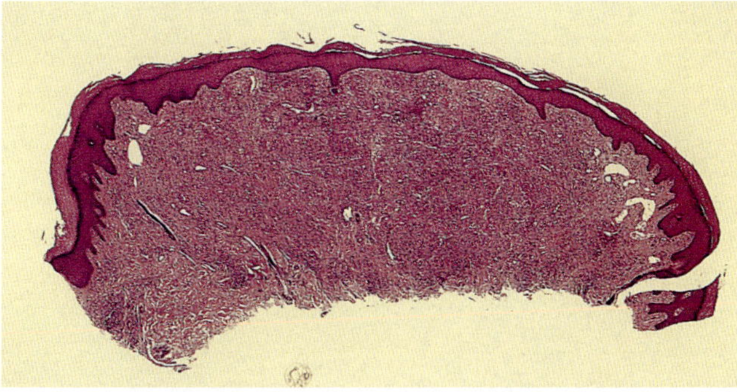

A

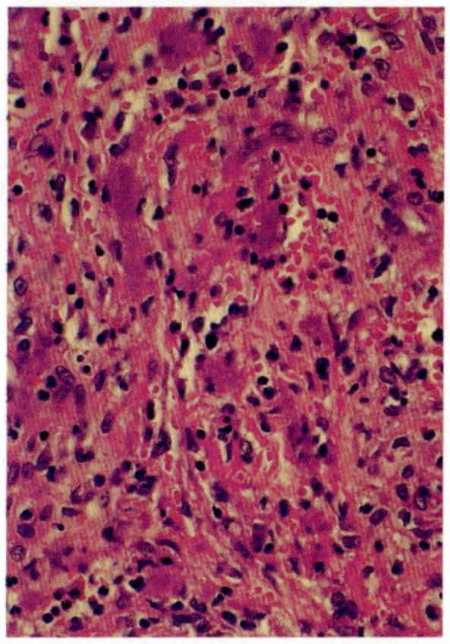

B

Figure 42–4. (**A**) A pedunculated superficial cutaneous lesion of BA. The contour resembles that of pyogenic granuloma. (**B**) Higher magnification reveals clumps of purplish-staining organisms and a few neutrophils in apposition to them.

PATHOLOGY

Gross Pathology

The macroscopic appearance of cutaneous lesions was described earlier. Lymph nodes affected by BA are enlarged, with red–brown or punctate red areas.[17] Splenic peliosis may cause massive enlargement with pink or red nodules, or small blood-filled cystic spaces.[26] Hepatic involvement can cause marked enlargement, blood-filled spaces, and pale mucoid nodules, either adjoining the spaces or separately.[2] Cerebral masses of BA have not yet been described in autopsy specimens, but have been documented by imaging studies and by biopsy.

Microscopic Pathology

Cutaneous lesions of BA were the first to be described and are the most familiar to pathologists. There are well-circumscribed rounded areas of vascular proliferation, situated in the superficial or deep dermis, or both. Superficial dermal lesions are often pedunculated and encompassed by epithelial collarettes, and have edematous stroma (Figure 42–4). The areas of vascular proliferation feature small, rounded vessels with variably protuberant endothelial cells, in which nuclei can be cuboidal and vesicular, with prominent nucleoli. Especially in deep dermal lesions, the proliferation can have a compact appearance, and the lumina of vessels can be inapparent. A reticulin stain reveals small, rounded vascular profiles in such foci. Interspersed between vessels are macrophages, dermal dendrocytes, and solitary polygonal or spindle-shaped endothelial cells. The isolated appearance of these cells is most likely the result of tangential sectioning of vessels. The causative bacilli are evident as purplish or amphophilic granular clusters, the exact hue depending on the way that the hematoxylin-eosin stain is balanced. These colonies are extracellular, and are often surrounded by neutrophils and nuclear dust derived from neutrophils (Figure 42–5). Bacilli and neutrophils are decreased in number

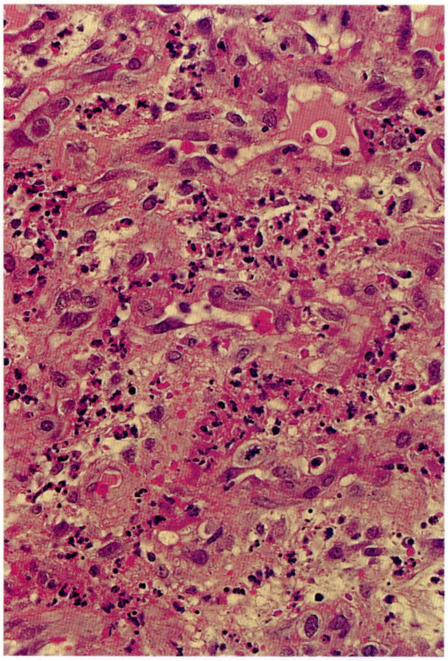

Figure 42–5. Cutaneous BA in which many fragmented neutrophils largely obscure the organisms. Note the swollen protruding endothelial cells.

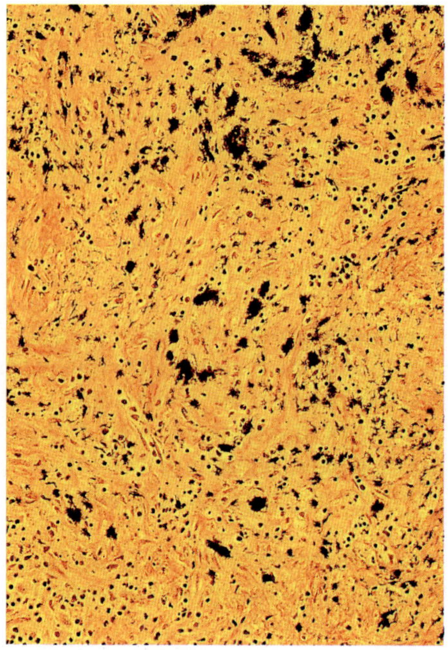

Figure 42–7. A Warthin–Starry–stained section showing clusters of bacilli in a spleen with BA. Single bacilli are at the edges of some of the clusters.

in partially treated lesions, in which macrophages may predominate[27] (Figure 42–6).

The bacilli are best demonstrated by silver stains such as the Warthin–Starry, Steiner, or Dieterle methods (Figure 42–7). Gomori's methenamine silver method is

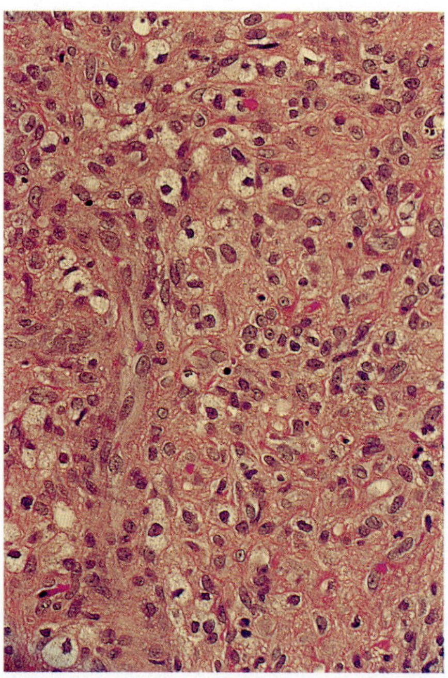

Figure 42–6. From a patient treated for BA: A solid appearance is imparted by swollen endothelial cells, fibrosis, and macrophages.

ineffectual in showing them, as are periodic acid–Schiff, acid-fast, and modified Gram's stains. Many laboratories have difficulty using the Warthin–Starry stain to confirm the diagnosis of BA. The organisms stain best with this method at pH 3.2. The glassware used for the stain should be acid washed. A procedure using the microwave oven is particularly effective. Pathologists evaluating Warthin–Starry–stained sections can use the staining of nuclei within the same section as a control. Properly stained sections have a thin deposit of silver around nuclei, with punctate deposits marking nucleoli, and occasionally nucleolar organizing regions can be discerned. If the nuclei of cells in the background are invisible, a negative staining result cannot be trusted. Some laboratories have used the Giemsa stain successfully rather than silver-based methods.[28] Because silver methods deposit metallic silver on bacteria, the bacilli appear larger than when stained by the Geimsa method. With Giemsa staining, the bacilli appear short and purple against a background of pink collagen. Although technically much simpler than silver stains, North American laboratories do not perform Giemsa stains as well as those in other areas in which the method is routinely performed for the evaluation of lymphoproliferative diseases; the Giemsa stain has not been as reliable as a properly performed Warthin–Starry stain.

BA in lymph nodes can cause effacement of nodal architecture. Organisms are often more abundant than in cutaneous lesions, although neutrophils can be

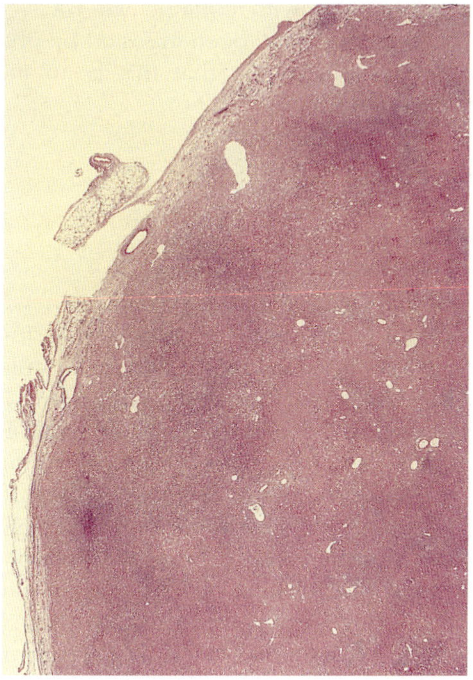

A

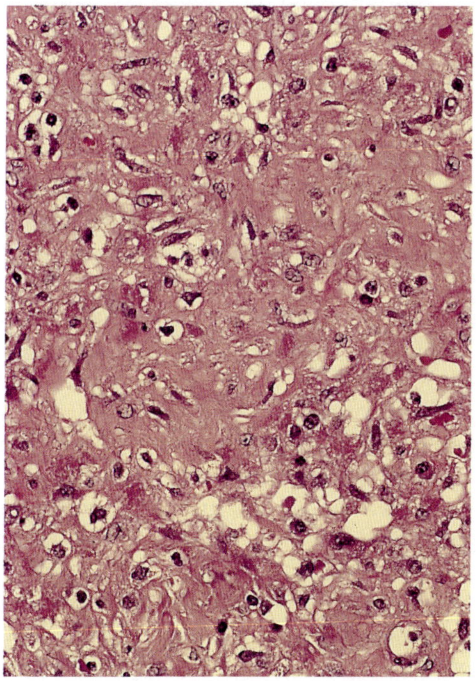

B

Figure 42–8. (**A**) This lymph node with BA is almost completely effaced. (**B**) On higher magnification, there is only scant inflammatory response, as is the case in many visceral infiltrates of BA. Clusters of organisms are intensely eosinophilic.

scant.[17] In one patient, granulomas containing only a few organisms were alongside vascular channels separating large colonies of bacilli[1] (Figure 42–8).

BA in most other viscera shows features similar to those in cutaneous lesions or in nodes. Occasional lesions are largely sclerotic, with little vascular proliferation, especially in the spleen (Figure 42–9).[4] Clusters of organisms with a few neutrophils and scant dust may be the only histologic clues to the diagnosis.

Although lymphocytes and plasma cells are important components of the host response to *B bacilliformis* in lesions of verruga peruana, in most organs neutrophils are the predominant cell in the host response of BA. The conjunctiva, which normally contains abundant lymphoid tissue, appears to be an exception. In one patient with conjunctival BA, large lymphocytes with irregular nuclear contours were in a biopsy specimen, a finding that could potentially cause confusion with lymphoma, which also has an increased incidence in immunocompromised patients.[21]

Peliosis hepatis and peliosis splenis caused by *B henselae* and *B quintana* feature rounded spaces filled with blood and lined by an attenuated endothelium. These are often surrounded by myxoid stroma containing clusters of bacilli, a few neutrophils with scant nuclear dust, and sometimes foamy macrophages[2] (Figure 42–10). The peliotic reaction in the spleen is sometimes associated with endothelial proliferation resembling that of BA in other organs. Splenic sinusoids surrounding the vasoproliferative nodules can be dilated and have protuberant endothelial cells.[26]

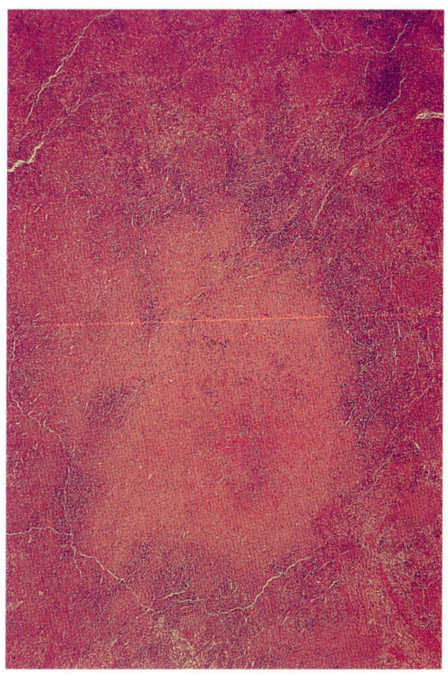

Figure 42–9. Spleen with a fibrotic reaction to infection by *B henselae*.

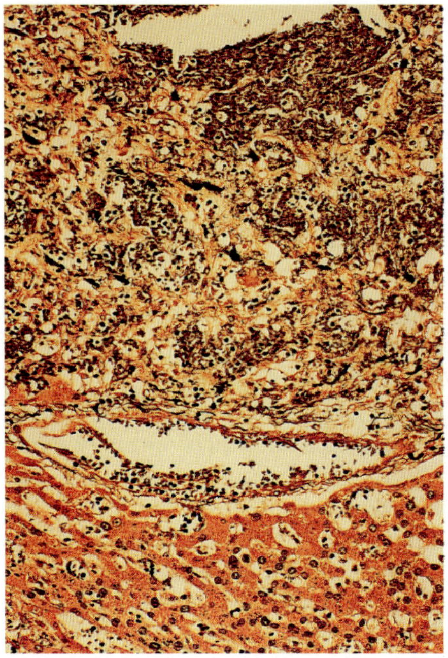

Figure 42–10. A Warthin–Starry–stained section of bacillary peliosis hepatis with parenchyma at the bottom, and a blood-filled space at the top. The erythrocytes have some deposition of silver on their membranes. There are clusters of bacilli in a zone of myxoid stroma separating the two.

Other pathologic processes can also be present in tissue affected by BA, especially in immunosuppressed patients. Cytomegalovirus, atypical mycobacteria, a variety of fungi, and Kaposi's sarcoma are the most common concurrent findings.[29,30]

Cytopathology

Only a few fine-needle aspirates have been performed on patients with BA, mostly from cutaneous lesions. The most remarkable features are neutrophils and neutrophilic nuclear dust, and the absence of clusters of spindled cells as seen in Kaposi's sarcoma.

ULTRASTRUCTURAL FEATURES

Electron microscopic examination of BA has been done mostly to confirm the presence of bacteria, as sometimes the Warthin–Starry procedure can cause artifacts that mimic organisms. Other notable features include the presence of Weibel–Palade bodies in the cytoplasm of endothelial cells, intercellular lumina between closely apposed endothelial cells, and the extracellular distribution of the bacilli in most organs.[12,31] In some patients with peliosis hepatis, organisms are in Kupffer's cells as well as extracellular.[16] Single bacilli were in pericytes in one patient with conjunctival BA.[21] The cell walls of bacteria that have been ingested by phagocytes are often intact, suggesting that this is an ineffective mode of bacterial killing.[21]

DIFFERENTIAL DIAGNOSIS

The differential diagnosis of BA varies somewhat from organ to organ. The superficial cutaneous lesions of BA resemble pyogenic granuloma, a benign vascular proliferation that has been more rationally termed lobular capillary hemangioma, clinically and pathologically. Both lesions can present as smooth surfaced red papules or nodules, with epithelial collarettes, and there is a rare disseminated form of pyogenic granuloma that can mimic BA in patients with widely distributed lesions. Pathologically, both vascular proliferations can be surrounded by epithelial collarettes, have an attenuated and sometimes ulcerated epidermis, and project above the surface of surrounding skin. An important clue to the diagnosis of pyogenic granuloma, visible at scanning magnification is the separation of its vessels into lobules by bands of fibrosis; this is not a feature of BA. In pyogenic granuloma, but not in BA, the central vessel in each group often has an ectatic jaggedly shaped lumen. Whereas neutrophils are in ulcerated lesions of pyogenic granuloma, they diminish in number away from the ulcer; however, in BA they are diffusely distributed throughout and there is abundant nuclear debris. Colonies of bacteria reside on the surface of ulcerated lesions of pyogenic granuloma, although they are present interstitially throughout lesions of BA.

Angiolymphoid hyperplasia with eosinophilia, or epithelioid hemangioma, can resemble BA clinically and shares with many cases epithelioid endothelial cells. Eosinophils are uncommon in BA, and neutrophils are rare in angiolymphoid hyperplasia with eosinophilia. Many lesions of angiolymphoid hyperplasia with eosinophilia have several muscular vessels nearby, thought to be evidence of an arteriovenous shunt; such vessels are absent from BA. The cytoplasm of endothelial cells in angiolymphoid hyperplasia is often deeply eosinophilic; that of BA is palely eosinophilic by comparison. Intracytoplasmic vacuoles, which are conspicuous in angiolymphoid hyperplasia with eosinophilia, epithelioid hemangioendothelioma, and spindle cell hemangioendothelioma, are absent in BA.

Kaposi's sarcoma (KS) is much more common than BA in patients infected with HIV, and can be clinically indistinguishable. Although BA does not cause patches (flat areas of discoloration of the skin), papules and nodules of KS and BA can so closely resemble each other that clinicians who have seen dozens of patients with BA cannot distinguish the two. Microscopically the proliferations are distinctively different. The endothelial proliferation in BA is not centered around preexisting structures as are early lesions of KS, and its vascular channels are rounded rather than slitlike or jagged. Eosinophilic globules, a hallmark of KS, are rare in BA. Although KS features lymphocytes and plasma cells, BA has infiltrates of neutrophils. The endothelial cells of KS are not as protrusive as those of BA frequently are. The purplish granular-appearing colonies of bacteria found in BA are, of course, absent from KS. Just as BA can coexist with other infections in the same patient or even in the same tissue sample, BA and KS can occur together in a similar fashion.[32,33]

Conventional bartonellosis, or Carrión's disease, is caused by *B bacilliformis.* It is endemic in the highlands of the Andes, where it is transmitted by the sandfly *Lutzomyia.* It has an acute form with a febrile hemolytic illness—Oroya fever, and a chronic form in which cutaneous vascular lesions—verruga peruana (Peruvian warts)—develop. These lesions resemble BA histologically, but differ in that colonies of organisms (termed *Rocha–Lima bodies*) are fewer. Whether the bacilli are intracellular or extracellular is disputed. Some organisms appear to lie within phagolysosomes, others in labyrinthine cisterns formed by invaginations of the cell membrane, and others lie extracellularly.[34] Rocha–Lima bodies appear to be intracytoplasmic by light microscopy, but may actually comprise bacteria within cisterns. Lymphocytes and plasma cells, rather than neutrophils and leukocytoclastic debris, are typical of verruga peruana. Verruga peruana can have unusual histologic features, including a spindle cell form that has to date not been reported with BA.[35] The staining pattern of the bacillus is similar, although *B bacilliformis* stains with Giemsa as well as with appropriate silver stains.

Nodal BA must be distinguished from the entities mentioned here, and also from vascular transformation of lymph node sinuses. The latter condition affects only nodal sinusoids, unlike BA, and lacks an inflammatory component. The endothelial cells are not as protrusive.[17] Nodal hemangiomas also lack the latter features, and may have thrombi in vascular lumina.

Bacillary peliosis hepatis and splenis can resemble peliosis not caused by infection. The presence of myxoid stroma adjacent to the peliotic spaces favors BA, and bacteria are often visible in hematoxylin-eosin stained sections.

Erythema elevatum diutinum is an unusual form of cutaneous vasculitis that appears to be increased in incidence in patients with HIV disease.[36] Although early lesions show largely the changes of a small vessel leukocytoclastic vasculitis, later lesions are markedly fibrotic. Neutrophils and nuclear dust can abound in both, and vessels can increase in number. Because of these findings, the condition can be confused with BA. The clinical lesions of erythema elevatum diutinum differ from those of BA by their strikingly symmetrical distribution, and location on the extensor surfaces of acral skin. Endothelial cells are not remarkably prominent, and the neutrophilic infiltrate is centered around vessels rather than around clumps of organisms, as in BA.

MOLECULAR AND IMMUNOPATHOLOGIC DIAGNOSIS

The agent of BA was identified by molecular biologic methods prior to its culture. In 1990, Relman and colleagues reported on their sequencing of the 16S RNA gene fragment from specimens of BA. 16S RNA is in all bacteria, but has unique sequences in each organism. They used PCR to amplify enough 16S RNA to sequence it.[37] The results placed the agent of BA in close proximity to *B quintana* and *B bacilliformis,* among the α-proteobacteria. Sequencing of 16S RNA from the agent of BA, *B henselae,* once that agent was cultured, established that it was identical to Relman's sequence. Some BA have been caused by *B quintana,* the agent of trench fever, rather than *B henselae.* The two organisms appear to differ in only a small secondary structure in their 16S RNA gene.[38] PCR of fresh or paraffin-embedded tissue can be used to confirm the presence of either agent of BA.

Although in situ hybridization to detect the causative bacilli has not been explored, staining with a polyclonal antibody to *B henselae* can be used to confirm the diagnosis.[39] The immune serum stains *B quintana* weakly, but is not reactive with lesions of KS or with other organisms that are silver positive but do not take conventional stains for organisms. Some cat scratch disease caused by *Afipia felis* also do not stain.

The presence of genomic material from the Epstein–Barr virus in endothelial cells and macrophages in BA suggests that it has a role in its pathogenesis.[40] Only one study of two cases, both of which contained the virus, has been documented, and there are no reports of staining for Epstein–Barr viral latent membrane proteins to date.

Several studies have examined immunohistochemical findings in the tissue reaction to the agents of BA. Unlike those of KS, the endothelial cells of BA express factor VIII related antigen, and bind with B9H9 even after formalin fixation and paraffin embedding.[41] Mature vessels in both conditions stain for CD34[42] In some "solid-appearing" infiltrates of BA, it seems evident that cells other than endothelial ones contribute to the infiltrates. Factor XIIIa positive dermal dendrocytes are scattered throughout many lesions of BA.[43] Dermal dendrocytes are dendritic cells that ordinarily are distributed around vessels in both the superficial and deep dermis, as well as interstitially. Macrophages, identified by Mac 387 or CD68 also contribute to densely cellular lesions. Pericytes, which stain with a variety of antisera to actin, appear to be a minor cellular population in BA.

CONFIRMATIONAL TESTING AND DIAGNOSIS

The diagnosis of BA can be confirmed by conventional histopathologic examination supplemented with either special stains or electron microscopy. Only when the tissue reaction is atypical, or there is bacteremia without evident tissue involvement, or a specimen cannot be obtained is there need for recourse to other methods to establish a diagnosis.

Isolation of *B henselae* and *B quintana* from the blood can be accomplished by the blood centrifugation–lysis method.[10] Direct plating of homogenized tissue onto heart infusion agar containing 5% rabbit blood without antibiotics is often successful.[44] The incubation conditions are high humidity with 5% CO_2 for at least 4 weeks. Although the two causative organisms differ in their 16S RNA sequences by only a few base pairs, they can be differentiated by the morphology of their colonies on agar plates.

PCR also can be used to confirm the presence of *B henselae* or *B quintana*. Because the technique is labor intensive and the diagnosis of BA can be made with certainty by other means, it is most applicable to research studies.

Serologic studies by indirect immunofluorescence also can be used to confirm the diagnosis of BA.[22,45] The identification of *B quintana* can be confused by serologic cross reactivity with *Chlamydia pneumoniae* and possibly *Coxiella burnetii*.[46] Pulsed gel electrophoresis can also be used to differentiate between strains of the same species of *Bartonella*.[47]

TREATMENT

BA responds readily to a variety of antibiotics, including erythromycin, tetracycline and its derivatives, clarithromycin, and azithromycin. The resolution of lesions may take many weeks, especially in immunocompromised patients.

REFERENCES

1. LeBoit PE. The expanding spectrum of a new disease, bacillary angiomatosis. *Arch Dermatol.* 1990;126:808–811. Comment.
2. Perkocha LA, Geaghan SM, Yen TS, et al. Clinical and pathological features of bacillary peliosis hepatis in association with human immunodeficiency virus infection *N Engl J Med.* 1990;323:1581–1586. See comments.
3. Myers SA, Prose NS, Garcia JA, Wilson KH, Dunsmore KP, Kamino H. Bacillary angiomatosis in a child undergoing chemotherapy. *J Pediatr.* 1992;121:574–578.
4. Tappero JW, Koehler JE, Berger TG, et al. Bacillary angiomatosis and bacillary splenitis in immunocompetent adults. *Ann Intern Med.* 1993;118:363–365. See comments.
5. Cockerell CJ, Webster GF, Whitlow MA, Friedman-Kien AE. Epithelioid angiomatosis: a distinct vascular disorder in patients with the acquired immunodeficiency syndrome or AIDS-related complex. *Lancet.* 1987;2:654–656.
6. Brenner DJ, Hollis DG, Moss CW, et al. Proposal of *Afipia gen. nov.,* with *Afipia felis sp. nova.* (formerly the cat scratch disease bacillus), *Afipia clevelandensis sp. nov.* (formerly the Cleveland Clinic Foundation strain), *Afipia broomeae sp. nov.,* and three unnamed genospecies. *J Clin Microbiol.* 1991;29:2450–2460.
7. Lucey D, Dolan MJ, Moss CW, et al. Relapsing illness due to *Rochalimaea henselae* in immunocompetent hosts. Implication for therapy and new epidemiologic associations. *Clin Infect Dis.* 1992;14:683–688.
8. Koehler JE, Glaser CA, Tappero JW. *Rochalimaea henselae* infection. A new zoonosis with the domestic cat as reservoir. *JAMA.* 1994;271:531–535. See comments.
9. Groves MG, Harrington KS. *Rochalimaea henselae* infections: newly recognized zoonoses transmitted by domestic cats. *J Am Vet Med Assoc.* 1994;204:267–271.
10. Koehler JE, Quinn FD, Berger TG, LeBoit PE, Tappero JW. Isolation of *Rochalimaea* species from cutaneous and osseous lesions of bacillary angiomatosis. *N Engl J Med.* 1992;327:1625–1631. See comments.
11. Cockerell CJ, Bergstresser PR, Myrie-Williams C, Tierno PM. Bacillary epithelioid angiomatosis occurring in an immunocompetent individual *Arch Dermatol.* 1990;126: 787–790. See comments.
12. LeBoit PE, Berger TM, Egbert BM, et al. Epithelioid haemangioma-like vascular proliferation in AIDS: manifestation of cat scratch disease bacillus infection? *Lancet.* 1988; i:960–963.
13. Schinella RA, Greco MA. Bacillary angiomatosis presenting as a soft-tissue tumor without skin involvement. *Hum Pathol.* 1990;21:567–569.
14. Herts BR, Rafii M, Spiegel G. Soft-tissue and osseous lesions caused by bacillary angiomatosis: unusual manifestations of cat-scratch fever in patients with AIDS. *AJR Am J Roentgenol.* 1991;157:1249–1251.
15. Baron AL, Steinbach LS, LeBoit PE, Mills CM, Gee JH, Berger TG. Osteolytic lesions and bacillary angiomatosis in HIV infection: radiologic differentiation from AIDS-related Kaposi sarcoma. *Radiology.* 1990;177:77–81.
16. Leong SS, Cazen RA, Yu GS, LeFevre L, Carson JW. Abdominal visceral peliosis associated with bacillary angiomatosis. Ultrastructural evidence of endothelial destruction by bacilli. *Arch Pathol Lab Med.* 1992;116: 866–871.
17. Chan JK, Lewin KJ, Lombard CM, Teitelbaum S, Dorfman RF. Histopathology of bacillary angiomatosis of lymph node. *Am J Surg Pathol.* 1991;15:430–437.

18. Foltzer MA, Guiney WB Jr, Wager GC, Alpern HD. Bronchopulmonary bacillary angiomatosis. *Chest.* 1993;104:973–975.
19. Slater LN, Min KW. Polypoid endobronchial lesions. A manifestation of bacillary angiomatosis. *Chest.* 1992;102:972–974.
20. Golnik KC, Marotto ME, Fanous MM, et al. Ophthalmic manifestations of *Rochalimaea* species *Am J Ophthalmol.* 1994;118:145–151. See comments.
21. Lee WR, Chawla JC, Reid R. Bacillary angiomatosis of the conjunctiva. *Am J Ophthalmol.* 1994;118:152–157. See comments.
22. Schwartzman WA, Patnaik M, Barka NE, Peter JB. *Rochalimaea* antibodies in HIV-associated neurologic disease. *Neurology.* 1994;44:1312–1316.
23. Spach DH, Panther LA, Thorning DR, Dunn JE, Plorde JJ, Miller RA. Intracerebral bacillary angiomatosis in a patient infected with human immunodeficiency virus. *Ann Intern Med.* 1992;116:740–742. See comments.
24. Regnery RL, Anderson BE, Claridge III JE, Rodriguez-Barradas MC, Jones DC, Carr JH. Characterization of a novel *Rochalimaea* species, *R. henselae sp. nov.,* isolated from blood of a febrile, human immunodeficiency virus-positive patient. *J Clin Microbiol.* 1992;30:265–274.
25. Welch DF, Pickett DA, Slater LN, Steigerwalt AG, Brenner DJ. *Rochalimaea henselae sp. nov.,* a cause of septicemia, bacillary angiomatosis, and parenchymal bacillary peliosis. *J Clin Microbiol.* 1992;30:275–280.
26. Mulvany NJ, Billson VR. Bacillary angiomatosis of the spleen. *Pathology.* 1993;25:398–401.
27. LeBoit PE, Berger TG, Egbert BM, Beckstead JH, Yen TS, Stoler MH. Bacillary angiomatosis. The histopathology and differential diagnosis of a pseudoneoplastic infection in patients with human immunodeficiency virus disease. *Am J Surg Pathol.* 1989;13:909–920.
28. Tsang WY, Chan JK, Wong CS. Giemsa stain for histological diagnosis of bacillary angiomatosis. *Histopathology.* 1992;21:299. Letter.
29. Lopez-Elzaurdia C, Fraga J, Sols M, Burgos E, Sanchez Garcia M, Garcia-Diez A. Bacillary angiomatosis associated with cytomegalovirus infection in a patient with AIDS. *Br J Dermatol.* 1991;125:175–177.
30. Sagerman PM, Relman DA, Niroomand F, Niedt GW. Localization of *Mycobacterium avium-intracellulare* within a skin lesion of bacillary angiomatosis in a patient with AIDS. *Diagn Mol Pathol.* 1992;1:212–216.
31. Kostianovsky M, Greco MA. Angiogenic process in bacillary angiomatosis. *Ultrastruct Pathol.* 1994;18:349–355.
32. Steeper TA, Rosenstein H, Weiser J, Inampudi S, Snover DC. Bacillary epithelioid angiomatosis involving the liver, spleen, and skin in an AIDS patient with concurrent Kaposi's sarcoma. *Am J Clin Pathol.* 1992;97:713–718.
33. Berger TG, Tappero JW, Kaymen A, LeBoit PE. Bacillary (epithelioid) angiomatosis and concurrent Kaposi's sarcoma in acquired immunodeficiency syndrome. *Arch Dermatol.* 1989;125:1543–1547.
34. Arias-Stella J, Lieberman PH, Erlandson RA, Arias-Stella Jr. J. Histology, immunochemistry, and ultrastructure of the verruga in Carrion's disease. *Am J Surg Pathol.* 1986;10:595–610.
35. Arias-Stella J, Lieberman PH, Garcia-Caceres U, et al. Verruga peruana mimicking neoplasms. *Am J Dermatopathol.* 1987;9:279–291.
36. LeBoit PE, Cockerell CJ. Nodular lesions of erythema elevatum diutinum in patients infected with the human immunodeficiency virus. *J Am Acad Dermatol.* 1993;28:919–922.
37. Relman DA, Loutit JS, Schmidt TM, Falkow S, Tompkins LS. The agent of bacillary angiomatosis. An approach to the identification of uncultured pathogens. *N Engl J Med.* 1990;323:1573–1580. See comments.
38. Relman DA, Lepp PW, Sadler KN, Schmidt TM. Phylogenetic relationships among the agent of bacillary angiomatosis, *Bartonella bacilliformis,* and other alphaproteobacteria. *Mol Microbiol.* 1992;6:1801–1807.
39. Reed JA, Brigati DJ, Flynn SD, et al. Immunocytochemical identification of *Rochalimaea henselae* in bacillary (epithelioid) angiomatosis, parenchymal bacillary peliosis, and persistent fever with bacteremia. *Am J Surg Pathol.* 1992;16:650–657.
40. Guarner J, Unger ER. Association of Epstein–Barr virus in epithelioid angiomatosis of AIDS patients. *Am J Surg Pathol.* 1990;14:956–960.
41. Kostianovsky M, Lamy Y, Greco MA. Immunohistochemical and electron microscopic profiles of cutaneous Kaposi's sarcoma and bacillary angiomatosis. *Ultrastruct Pathol.* 1992;16:629–640.
42. Suster S, Wong TY. On the discriminatory value of anti-HPCA-1 (CD-34) in the differential diagnosis of benign and malignant cutaneous vascular proliferations. *Am J Dermatopathol.* 1994;16:355–363.
43. Arrese Estrada J, Pierard GE. Dendrocytes in verruga peruana and bacillary angiomatosis. *Dermatology.* 1992;184:22–25.
44. Koehler JE, Tappero JW. Bacillary angiomatosis and bacillary peliosis in patients infected with human immunodeficiency virus. *Clin Infect Dis.* 1993;17:612–624.
45. Slater LN, Coody DW, Woolridge LK. Welch DF. Murine antibody responses distinguish *Rochalimaea henselae* from *Rochalimaea quintana. J Clin Microbiol.* 1992;30:1722–1727.
46. Relman DA. Has trench fever returned? *N Engl J Med.* 1995;332:463–464.
47. Maurin M, Roux V, Stein A, Ferrier F, Viraben R, Raoult D. Isolation and characterization by immunofluorescence, sodium dodecyl sulfate-polyacrylamide gel electrophoresis, western blot, restriction fragment length polymorphism-PCR, 16S rRNA gene sequencing, and pulsed-field gel electrophoresis of *Rochalimaea quintana* from a patient with bacillary angiomatosis. *J Clin Microbiol.* 1994;32(5):1166–1171.

CHAPTER 43

Bacillus cereus Infection

Edith F. Marley and Nirmal K. Saini

. . . man is a thickened node in the web of a universe of forces which, ever repetitively and ever anew, flow in and out of him; he is part of an ecology that involves plants, animals, climate, soil, and all kinds of radiant forces and chemicals.

Abraham Myerson (1881–1948), in the foreword to Speaking of Man

DEFINITION

Members of the genus *Bacillus* are aerobic or facultatively anaerobic, spore-forming, gram-positive or gram-variable bacilli.[1] *Bacillus anthracis,* the causative agent of anthrax, is best known. Of the nonanthrax species, *B cereus* is well known as a cause of toxin-mediated food poisoning. *Bacillus* species are ubiquitous in nature and have usually been considered contaminants when isolated from clinical specimens. Increasingly these species, primarily *B cereus,* are being reported as pathogens, particularly in the immunocompromised, in neonates, and in patients with indwelling lines, shunts, or prostheses. Intravenous drug abusers are at risk from contaminated heroin and from the paraphernalia of injection.[2–6]

EPIDEMIOLOGY

Bacillus organisms are usually found in decaying organic matter, soil, dust, and water. They may be found in raw, dried, or processed foods, particularly previously or partially cooked rice. Some species are part of the normal intestinal flora of humans.[7] They are commonly isolated from superficial skin lesions. The ubiquitous distribution of *B cereus* in nature and in the hospital environment[8] warrants its consideration when gram-positive bacilli are recovered from an immunodeficient patient with suspected sepsis. Assessing the significance of laboratory isolates of *Bacillus* species requires careful clinical evaluation.

CLINICAL MANIFESTATIONS

Clinical infections with *B cereus* can be separated into gastrointestinal (GI) and non-GI; the latter may be either localized or systemic.[6] *Bacillus cereus* food poisoning is characterized by either toxin-induced emetic or diarrheagenic syndromes. Non-GI disease is further divided into five groups: 1) local infections, frequently ocular and wound infections; 2) bacteremia and septicemia; 3) infections of the central nervous system, usually shunt- or trauma-associated; 4) respiratory infections; and 5) endocarditis.

Other *Bacillus* species, such as *B subtilis* and *B sphaericus* have been implicated in non-GI infections,[7] although the epidemiology and pathogenicity of these species remain obscure.

PATHOLOGY

Local infections present primarily as postsurgical (often orthopedic) or traumatic wound, burn, or ocular infections. Primary cutaneous infection usually presents as a single necrotic bulla. The large bacilli of *B cereus* may be mistaken for *Clostridium* species. Deep severe infections, necrotizing fasciitis, and osteomyelitis may occur. *Bacillus cereus* is a major cause of severe keratitis, endophalmitis, and panophthalmitis; these infections may be caused by trauma, contaminated contact lens solutions, or by hematogenous spread (Figure 43–1). The classic ophthalmic lesion is a corneal ring abscess accompanied by periorbital edema, retinal hemorrhage, and perivasculitis.

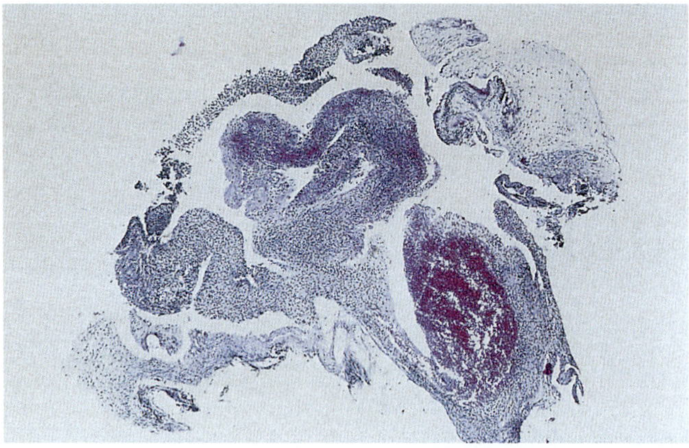

Figure 43–1. Tissue excised from the site of a scleral laceration; prolapsed infected intraocular tissue, mainly vitreous and some retina (hematoxylin-eosin, ×4). *(Photograph courtesy of Dr. Andrew Ferry, Medical College of Virginia, Richmond, Virginia.)*

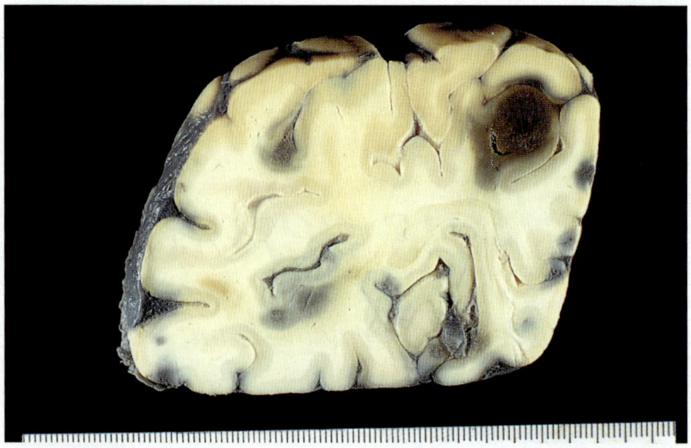

Figure 43–2. Cerebrum with multiple hemorrhagic, necrotic lesions at the gray–white junction with associated subarachnoid hemorrhage.

Systemic disease is almost always associated with a portal of entry. The majority of clinically significant infections causing septicemia have occurred in intravenous drug abusers, in patients receiving hemodialysis, or with indwelling catheter lines. Neonates and patients with underlying malignancies also are at risk. Ocular and pulmonary infections, rhabdomyolysis, abscesses, and endocarditis may be sequelae of bacteremia. Dissemination from gastrointestinal infection generally is not believed to occur. Fatal bacteremia developed after acute gastroenteritis in a leukemic patient in Japan.[2] Mucosal ulcerations with colonies of gram-positive bacilli were in the stomach and colon, suggesting possible dissemination from a GI source.

Bacillus meningitis and encephalitis have been reported in both adults and children, frequently associated with recent surgery, ventricular shunts, or following spinal anesthesia. Brain abscesses may occur. Extensive subarachnoid hemorrhage may be associated with multiple necrotic lesions primarily located at the gray–white junction, a result of hematogenous spread[3] (Figures 43–2 and 43–3). Ischemic tissue damage may result from infective vasculitis. In neutropenic patients there may be little to no inflammatory response.

Pneumonia, necrotizing pneumonitis, abscesses, and pleuritis can occur in at-risk groups. Endocarditis caused by *B cereus* has been associated with intravenous drug use (predominately tricuspid valve involvement) or underlying valvular disease.

PATHOGENESIS

Bacillus cereus produces several toxins, including an emetic and a diarrheal toxin produced during exponential growth on enhanced media. Proteases, phospholipases, hemolysins, and a necrotizing enterotoxin are associated with severe disease.[6] Phospholipase C catalyzes hydrolysis of membrane phospholipids. Molecular studies have shown that the tandemly encoded activities, phospholipase C and sphinomyelinase, constitute a biologically functional cytolytic determinant of *B cereus* termed *cereolysin AB*.[9] Hemolysin BL is a unique tripartite hemolysin that also mediates vascular permeability, implicating it as enterotoxigenic.[10] Hemolysin and phospholipase are associated with local infections, particularly ocular infections, and may help to initiate systemic disease.[6] Release of lysosomal enzymes from neutrophils may contribute to tissue damage. Lesions caused by *B cereus* tend to be necrotizing.[2–4] Tissue findings, hemorrhage, and coagulative necrosis may in part be caused by ischemic damage as a consequence of septic vasculitis and thrombosis. There may be either vascular invasion or bacterial microthrombi.

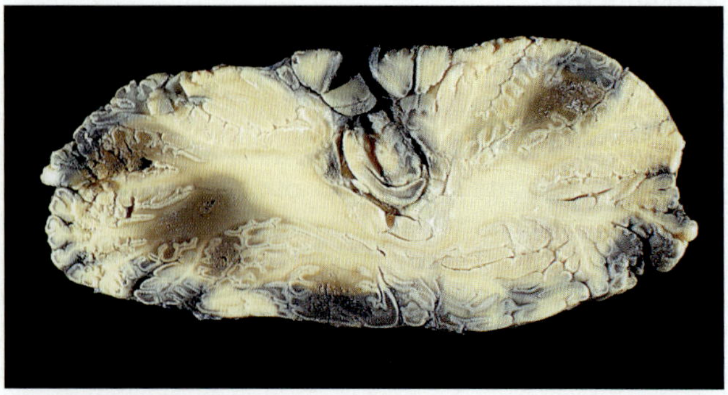

Figure 43–3. Cerebellum with bilateral, similar, hemorrhagic necrotic lesions.

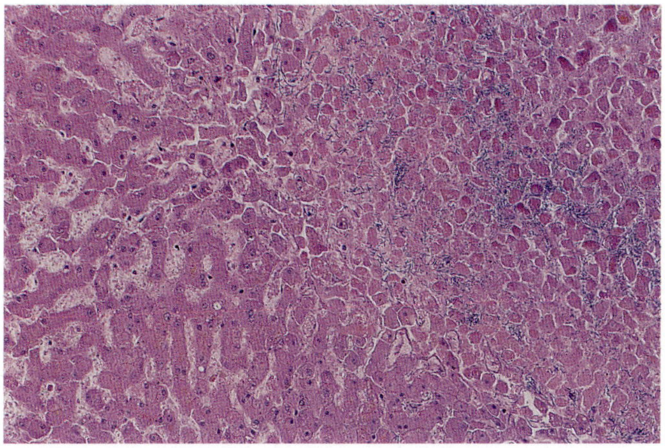

Figure 43–4. Section of liver showing focus of necrosis with abundant hematoxylin staining bacilli (hematoxylin-eosin, ×50).

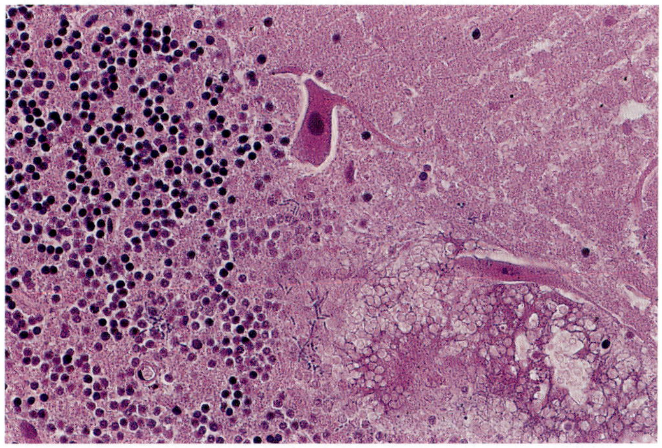

Figure 43–6. Higher magnification with hematoxylin staining bacilli at the edge of necrotic tissue. Residual Purkinje cell and small cells of the granular layer are present (hematoxylin-eosin, ×100).

DIAGNOSIS

Vasculitis, coagulative necrosis, and hemorrhage are usually evident in histologic sections. In hematoxylin-eosin–stained tissue sections *B cereus* is usually present as clusters of large bacilli in areas of necrosis that stain with hematoxylin (Figures 43–4 through 43–6). Their gram positivity can be verified by a tissue gram stain such as the Brown–Brenn stain (Figure 43–7). *Bacillus cereus* also has been found to be consistently periodic acid–Schiff positive after diastase digestion in human tissue.[11] For confirmation, infected blood or tissue can be cultured on nutrient or blood agar. In general, *B cereus* is motile, hemolytic on blood agar, penicillin resistant, and resistant to bacteriophage gamma, distinguishing it from *B anthracis*.[6] Serologic studies for flagellar antigens and recombinant DNA techniques for plasmid analysis can be used for strain identification.

TREATMENT

Although non-GI disease caused by *B cereus* is not common, delay in appropriate treatment may cause significant morbidity and mortality in central nervous system or systemic disease. *Bacillus cereus* is resistant to β-lactam antibiotics. These include the third-generation cephalosporins, which are often used initially to treat febrile neutropenic patients prior to identification of a specific organism. Removal of any foreign body, such

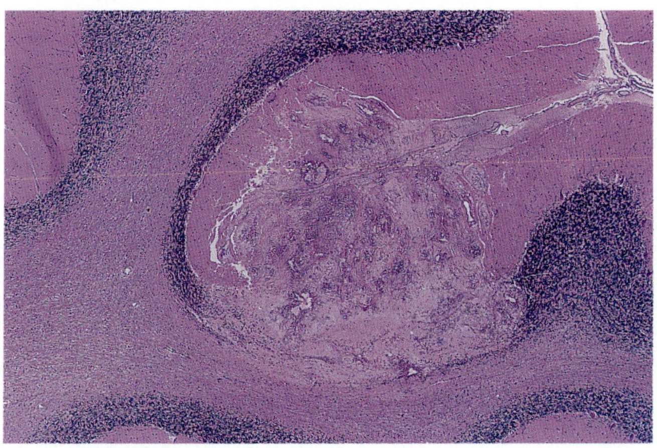

Figure 43–5. Section of cerebellar cortex with microscopic focus of necrosis (hematoxylin-eosin, ×10).

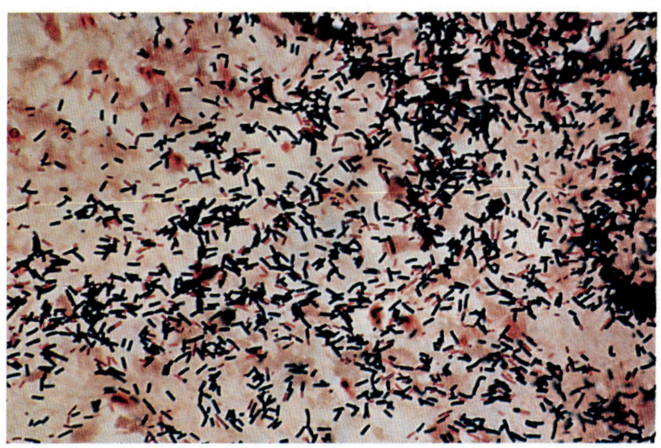

Figure 43–7. Brown–Brenn stain for bacteria in tissue excised from site of a scleral laceration. There are abundant gram-positive bacilli (Brown–Brenn, ×1000). *(Photograph courtesy of Dr. Andrew Ferry, Medical College of Virginia, Richmond, Virginia.)*

as an intravascular catheter and therapy with vancomycin or clindamycin, with or without gentamicin, is appropriate for patients with suspected *Bacillus* infections who are seriously ill.[7]

REFERENCES

1. Konenman EW. The aerobic gram-positive bacilli. In: Konenman EW, Allen SD, Janda WM, et al, eds. *Diagnostic Microbiology.* Philadelphia: JB Lippincott; 1992:467–518.
2. Funada H, Uotani C, Machi T, et al. *Bacillus cereus* bacteremia in an adult with acute leukemia. *Jpn J Clin Oncol.* 1988;18:69–74.
3. Marley EF, Saini NK, Venkatraman C, Orenstein JM: Fatal *Bacillus cereus* meningoencephalitis in an adult with acute myelogenous leukemia. *S Med J.* 1995;88:969–972.
4. Jenson HB, Levy SR, Duncan C, et al. Treatment of multiple brain abscesses caused by *Bacillus cereus. Pediatr Infect Dis J.* 1989;8:795–798.
5. Weisse ME, Bass JW, Jarrett RV, et al. Nonanthrax *Bacillus* infections of the central nervous system. *Pediatr Infect Dis J.* 1991;10:243–246.
6. Drobniewski FA. *Bacillus cereus* and related species. *Clin Microbiol Rev.* 1993;6:324–338.
7. Tuazon CU. Other *Bacillus* species. In: Mandell GL, Douglas RG Jr, Bennett JE, eds. *Principles and Practice of Infectious Diseases.* New York: Churchill Livingstone; 1985:1595–1599.
8. Bryce EA, Smith JA, Tweeddale M, et al. Dissemination of *Bacillus cereus* in an intensive care unit. *Infect Control Hosp Epidemiol.* 1993;14:459–462.
9. Gilmore MS, Cruz-Rodz AL, Leimeister-Wachter M, et al. A *Bacillus cereus* cytolytic determinant, cerolysin AB, which comprises the phospholipase C and sphinomyelinase genes: nucleotide sequence and genetic linkage. *J Bacteriol.* 1989;171:744–753.
10. Beecher DJ, Macmillan JD. Characterization of the components of hemolysin BL from *Bacillus cereus. Infect Immun.* 1991;59:1778–1784.
11. Khavari PA, Bolognia JL, Eisen R, et al. Periodic acid–Schiff–positive organisms in primary cutaneous *Bacillus cereus* infection. Case report and an investigation of the periodic acid–Schiff staining properties of bacteria. *Arch Dermatol.* 1991;127:543–546.

CHAPTER 44

Bacterial Diarrheas and Dysenteries

James K. Kelly and David A. Owen

'Tis now the very witching time of night,
When church yards yawn and hell itself breathes out
Contagion to this world.

William Shakespeare (1564–1616)

SALMONELLAE

Salmonellae are unencapsulated, motile, gram-negative bacilli that ferment dextrose but not lactose. Serotyping by somatic O and flagellar H antigens is a valuable epidemiologic tool.[1] *Salmonella* serotypes are referred to as species for convenience (eg, *Salmonella* bioserotype typhimurium is referred to as *Salmonella typhimurium*). Humans are the only host to *S typhi* and there is no animal or other reservoir for this organism. Chronic carriers of typhoid bacilli harbor the organism in the gallbladder, usually in association with gallstones. Other salmonellae are primarily animal pathogens, with humans as an occasional host (eg, *S cholerae-suis* preferentially infects pigs). The majority of salmonellae (eg, *S typhimurium* and *S enteritidis*) are not host adapted and infect humans and animals. Human salmonellosis expresses one of four clinical pictures: 1) the asymptomatic carrier state, 2) gastroenteritis, 3) enteric fever, and 4) septicemia with foci of metastatic suppuration.[2]

Typhoid (enteric) fever may be caused by *S typhi* and *S enteritidis*, serotypes paratyphi A or B. These organisms are endemic where safe water and sanitation are lacking, and small numbers of infections continue in developed nations as well. *Salmonella typhi* is transmitted through contaminated food or water and outbreaks often are traced to chronic carriers, usually older women who carry the infection in the gallbladder. The incubation period is 9 to 14 days. In affluent countries, most infections are acquired by foreign travel.[3] Nontyphoid salmonellae are an important public health problem in affluent countries, where organisms are transmitted in eggs, poultry meat, and dairy products. Patients with hypochlorhydria have increased susceptibility to infection. Nosocomial infection can be a problem. *Salmonella enteritidis* infections are increasing worldwide, with eggs as the main source.[4]

Pathogenesis

Experimentally, within 12 hours of ingestion, salmonellae cause the microvilli on the enterocytes to elongate, to become bulbous, and to disintegrate, allowing the bacteria to adhere to the cell membrane and invaginate it until they are enclosed in a vacuole in the cytoplasm[5,6] (Figure 44–1). Within 24 hours after ingestion, salmonellae have crossed the abluminal cell membrane into the lamina propria and are endocytosed by macrophages. Salmonellae can multiply within intracellular vacuoles. Virulent strains subsequently migrate to lymph nodes, enter the bloodstream, disseminate through the body, and multiply further in phagocytic cells of the reticuloendothelial system including liver, spleen, and bone marrow. Nontyphoid salmonellae remain localized in the mucosa unless the host is immunocompromised or the organism is of unusual virulence. Salmonellae are preferentially transported across the membranous enterocytes (M cells) into the gut-associated lymphoid tissue. Mucosal invasion evokes an acute inflammatory response (edema, congestion, and neutrophils) in the ileum and colon.[7,8]

Most virulence factors are encoded in the bacterial genome. They include a heat shock protein that binds the bacterium to intestinal mucus,[9] a protein that binds to the epidermal growth factor receptor on enterocytes,[10] and the *inv*E gene product, a homolog of

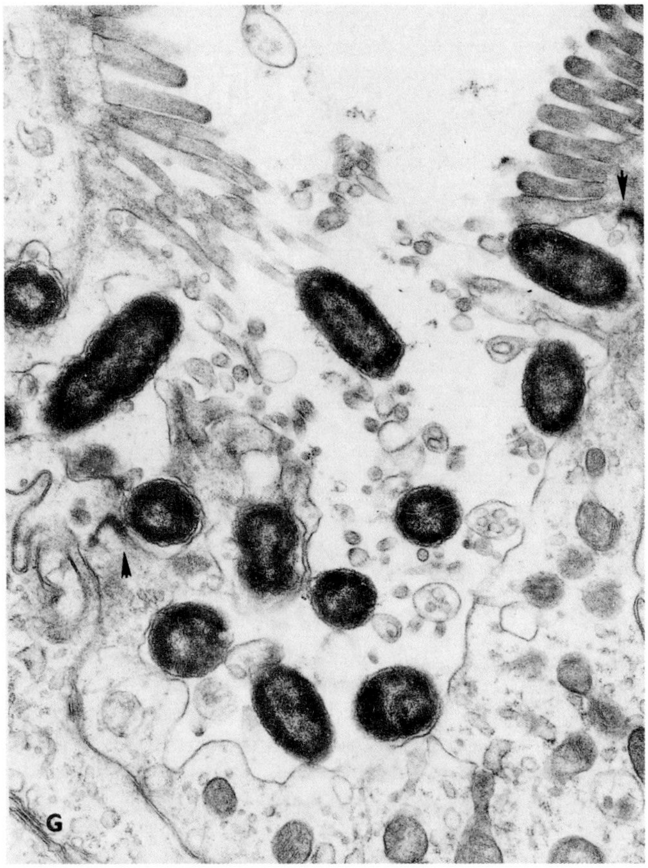

Figure 44–1. Ileum of guinea pig. The microvilli are disrupted, and bacteria adhere to the surface membrane and are being endocytosed into the enterocyte. Arrows indicate desmosomes (AFIP Neg 75-2050-3).

Yersinia outer membrane protein, that assists penetration into the enterocyte.[11] Immunoglobulin A antibodies to *Salmonella* surface antigen prevent adherence to and invasion of the epithelial cells.[12] Many strains of *Salmonella* carry a large plasmid that encodes a virulence-associated region that is not required for adherence or invasion of epithelial cells, but permits intracellular survival, proliferation, and ultimately dissemination.[2]

The mechanisms by which salmonellae cause diarrhea are under active investigation. Salmonellae mediate fluid secretion in ileal loops in the absence of mucosal damage[13] and the enteric nerves mediate the fluid secretory response.[14] Various serotypes produce enterotoxins that may promote diarrhea,[1] and neutrophil infiltration of the mucosa induces diarrhea.

Clinical Features

Typhoid fever is a severe systemic infection that presents with malaise, headache, constipation, and a progressive, stepwise rise in fever over several days. A rose-spot rash develops on the abdomen, and there is leukopenia with a relative lymphocytosis. The fever stabilizes at its maximum for about 1 week, then declines progressively but with fluctuations over the following week. In the second or third week the stools are of low volume, watery, and of "pea-soup" consistency. Ulceration of Peyer's patches may cause massive hemorrhage or perforation; however, these complications develop in less than 1% of patients.[15–17] In the preantibiotic era, other complications encountered included bronchitis and pneumonia, hepatitis, myocarditis, meningitis, encephalopathy, parotitis, arthritis, orchitis, or osteomyelitis,[15] complications are still reported rarely. Perforated typhoid enteritis carries a high mortality from overwhelming sepsis.[18] The gold standard for diagnosis is culture of *S typhi* from blood, stools, or urine. Blood culture is positive in the active stage of infection in about 90% of patients; stool and urine cultures are positive late in the infection. Urine cultures often are positive late in the course. The Widal serologic test is unreliable. New enzyme-linked immunosorbent assay (ELISA) tests and rapid antigen detection methods are being developed to meet the need for inexpensive and reliable diagnosis of disease in underdeveloped countries.[19] Chloramphenicol was the drug of choice for typhoid fever until drug-resistant strains emerged and it was superseded by amoxycillin and trimethoprim–sulfamethoxazole. Strains resistant to all three drugs emerged in Asia in 1992, and the fluoroquinolone ciprofloxacin has become the drug of choice for both sensitive and resistant strains. Because fluoroquinolones damage cartilage in growing animals,[20] pediatricians have reservations about their use in children, and third-generation cephalosporins (especially cephtriaxone) are the alternatives.[20,21] In patients with severe toxemia, a course of high-dose dexamethasone may be lifesaving.[22] Intestinal hemorrhage is treated by transfusion; perforation is treated by laparotomy and oversewing. The friable ileum is easily perforated during handling at laparotomy, and segmental resection may be required.[16]

Nontyphoid salmonellae cause nausea, vomiting, fever, abdominal pain, and diarrhea in 8 to 48 hours of ingesting contaminated food. Diarrhea is usually watery and self-limited, lasting 7 to 10 days, but occasional infections are severe, with bloody diarrhea and, rarely, toxic dilatation. Stool culture is required for diagnosis. Endoscopy shows patchy erythema, exudation, and sometimes diffuse erythema and ulceration that can resemble ulcerative colitis. To complicate matters, patients with inflammatory bowel disease are susceptible to intercurrent *Salmonella* infection, and infection can cause relapse of colitis. Biopsy features that favor ulcerative colitis are crypt architectural distortion, basal plasmacytosis, and basal cryptitis, whereas edema and a predominantly superficial neutrophil infiltrate favor infection. Fluid and electrolytes are the mainstay of treatment, and antibiotic treatment is not beneficial in the absence of septicemia or persistent symptoms.[23] When antibiotics are required and in "high-risk" patients who are immunosuppressed, have endovascular prostheses, or debilitating diseases, ciprofloxacin is the drug of choice.[20] When the distinction between ulcerative colitis and salmonellosis is unclear, antibiotics and corticosteroids are given, and a further biopsy of the rectum after 6 weeks will usually confirm the diagnosis.[20]

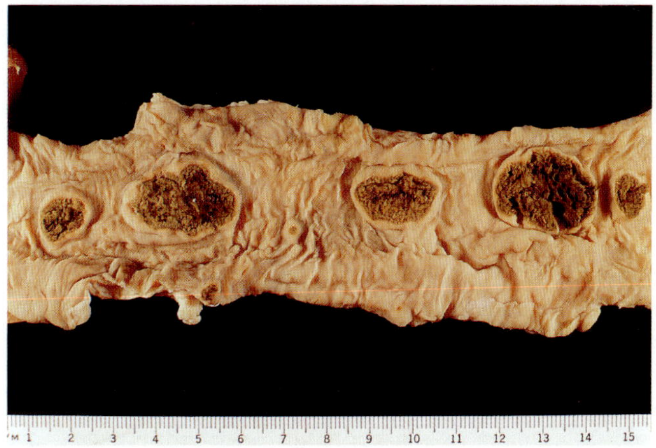

Figure 44–3. Terminal ileum from patient with fatal typhoid fever. The entire surface of the Peyer's patches is necrotic, centrally ulcerated, and hemorrhagic. *(Specimen from Zaire courtesy of Jerome H. Smith, MD, photograph by Daniel H. Connor, MD, 1974).*

Pathology

The pathology of typhoid fever affects primarily the intestinal lymphoid tissue of the ileum, appendix, and colon, and is traditionally described as four sequential stages, each lasting about 1 week: hyperplasia, necrosis, ulceration, and healing.[15,24–28] Microscopically, the predominant cell type in the lesions of typhoid is the monocyte–macrophage. The neutrophil is inconspicuous.[24,25] Hyperplasia develops during the incubation period and the onset of fever. The Peyer's patches become enlarged, elevated, and hyperemic. The mucosa is intact but may show foci of neutrophilic cryptitis. The germinal centers, mantle zones, and interfollicular areas are progressively infiltrated by macrophages that show erythrophagocytosis and tingible bodies and that ultimately obliterate the lymphoid follicles. Plasma cells and immunoblasts also are increased and the infiltrate extends into the submucosa. Lymphatics at the margin of the patch are dilated and contain immunoblasts, lymphocytes, and monocytes.

The necrotic stage corresponds roughly to the phase of maximal fever. Necrosis begins as localized foci in a Peyer's patch and with fibrinous exudation in the mucosa around it (Figures 44–2 through 44–4). Necrosis may progress to involve virtually the entire patch and the overlying mucosa (Figure 44–3).[24,25] The ulceration stage supervenes when the necrotic tissue has sloughed and corresponds roughly to the phase of lysis of fever. The ulcer base usually lies on the muscularis propria but occasionally penetrates through it. Because the ulcers are in Peyer's patches, they are oval and longitudinal, and located on the antimesenteric border of the terminal ileum. Microscopically, variable proportions of the Peyer's patches remain viable. Underlying deep ulcers is a fibrinous exudate on the

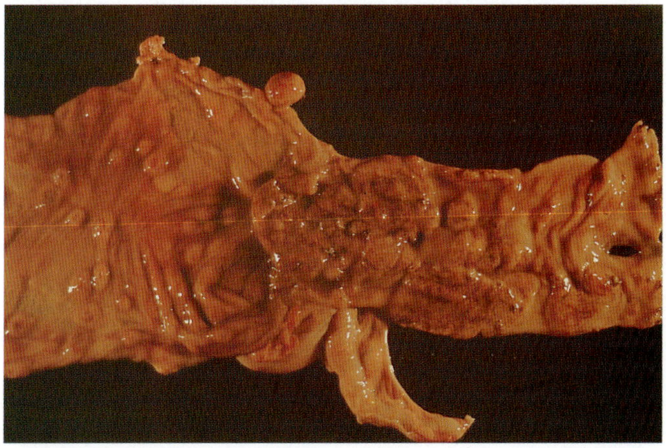

Figure 44–2. Terminal ileum and cecum. The Peyer's patches are enlarged, elevated, hemorrhagic, and necrotic. The solitary lymphoid follicles of the colon are enlarged, pale, and have a central hemorrhagic dimple (AFIP Neg 62-4724-1).

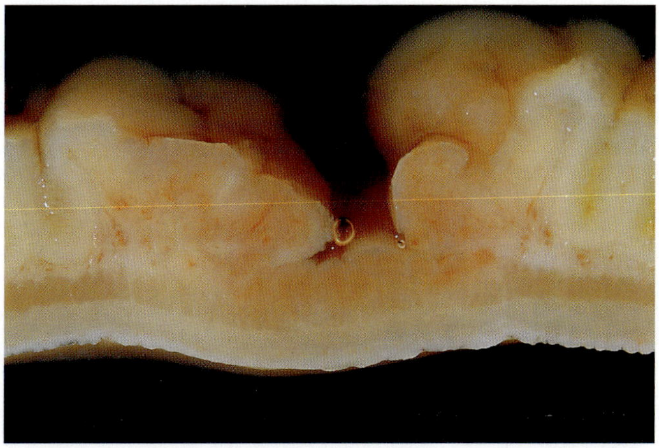

Figure 44–4. Cross section of an ulcerated Peyer's patch in terminal ileum of typhoid fever. The ulcer, although small, goes to the muscularis mucosae. *(Specimen contributed by Ronald C. Tolls, MD, photograph by Daniel H. Connor, MD, 1974).*

peritoneal surface, and at surgery, the bowel wall is friable and easily perforated at sites of ulceration. There is minimal infiltration of neutrophils throughout. In the healing stage, the ulcers are covered by a thin layer of granulation tissue and a single layer of intestinal epithelium. Healing is rapid and generally is not characterized by fibrosis or stricture.

Mesenteric lymph nodes have a similar reaction pattern. They become greatly enlarged from distension of the sinusoids by macrophages that show erythrophagocytosis and, later, foci of necrosis.[17,24] The inflammatory reaction may extend beyond the nodes into the adipose tissue.[24] Typhoid nodules, granulomatoid aggregates of macrophages and lymphocytes, are in the liver, spleen, bone marrow, kidney, testis, and salivary gland[25] (Figure 44–5). The spleen is enlarged up to 500 to 1000 g, soft, and easily ruptured, and the red pulp contains typhoid nodules.[25] The liver is enlarged and shows typhoid nodules, enlarged Kupffer's cells, foci of hepatocytic necrosis, microabscesses, and sinusoidal dilatation. The kidneys show typhoid nodules and sometimes swelling and degeneration of the cells of the proximal convoluted tubules, or an immune complex glomerulonephritis. The heart may be dilated and show focal necrosis or fatty change of myocardial cells. Skeletal muscle may show Zenker's degeneration, a focal necrosis of muscle fibers that lose striations and become hypereosinophilic and hyalinized. Deep venous thrombosis is a well-recognized complication. Typhoid osteomyelitis is rare except in those patients with sickle cell anemia.[29] The gallbladder may show chronic follicular cholecystitis.

Nontyphoid salmonellae cause acute infectious ileocolitis indistinguishable from other infectious colitides.[30,31] The changes are self-limited, and the mucosa returns to normal in about 2 weeks. In infections with persistent diarrhea, there may be distortion, branching, and dilatation of crypts, making distinction from idiopathic ulcerative colitis difficult.[32,33]

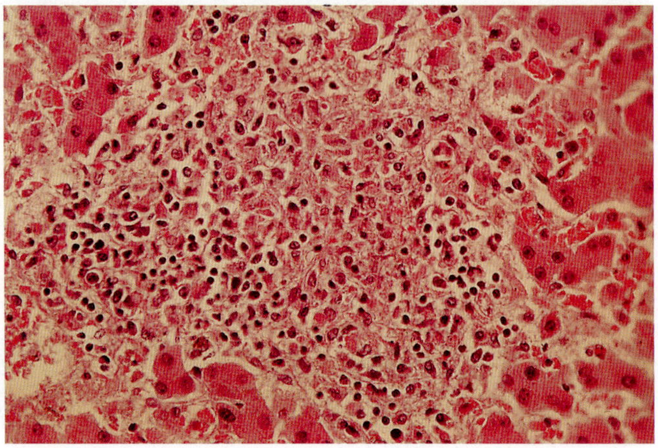

Figure 44–5. A granulomatoid aggregate in liver. The lesion is sharply defined and comprised of macrophages, most of which have the suggestion of an epithelioid configuration. Scattered lymphocytes and plasma cells also are present (AFIP Neg 72-4603).

CAMPYLOBACTERS

Campylobacters are small, curved (S-shaped or comma-shaped), motile, gram-negative, microaerophilic bacteria that have a single polar flagellum. *Campylobacter jejuni* is the main group associated with diarrhea, and is a major cause of infectious diarrhea worldwide, accounting for about 5% of all diarrheal illnesses in Western countries. It was the development of specific selective media by Butzler et al[34] in 1973 and by Skirrow[35] in 1977 that revealed the prevalence and importance of *C jejuni* as a cause of infectious diarrhea. The second main group of campylobacters, *C fetus,* causes opportunistic infections. A third group, including *C cinaedi, C fennelliae, C laridis,* and *C coli,* is associated with diarrhea, abdominal cramps, hematochezia, and proctocolitis, and these organisms are transmitted among homosexual men by anilingus.[36,37]

Campylobacter jejuni is a component of the normal bowel flora of many wild and domestic birds and has been isolated from farm animals. It is transmitted by the fecal–oral route, by poultry and uncooked meats, by pets (especially sick dogs), by unpasteurized milk, and by water contaminated with animal excreta.[38] Age-specific incidence is highest in children younger than 5 years, but older children and adults also can be affected. Infants are protected by breast milk that contains antibodies to campylobacter flagellin.[39] Most infections are sporadic, but large outbreaks attributed to common sources have been reported.[38] Travelers to Third World countries are at increased risk. The incubation period is 2 to 5 days and the median period of excretion of organisms during convalescence is 2 to 3 weeks when untreated. On the Indian subcontinent, up to 40% of healthy children younger than 2 years of age may excrete *C jejuni* at any one time, and isolation rates are not higher in children with diarrhea than from children who are healthy.[40]

Pathogenesis

Studies of volunteer and clinical human infections have shown that as few as 100 campylobacter organisms ingested in milk can cause disease.[41,42] The mucus is colonized and traversed rapidly by the spiral and oscillatory movements of the flagella.[42] In animal models and in some patients, invasion of colonic epithelium can be demonstrated and although bacteremia has been reported, it is rarely found when sought systematically. Invasion of cell lines can involve either a microtubule-dependent or a microfilament-dependent pathway.[43,44]

Some strains of *C jejuni* produce a heat-labile enterotoxin resembling cholera toxin but in much lower quantities than toxigenic *Escherichia coli* or *Vibrio cholerae*,[45] however, the toxin was not detectable in experimentally infected rabbit ileal loops.[46] A heat-labile cytolethal distending toxin is produced by about 40% of isolates, but the significance of the toxin is uncertain.[47] *Campylobacter jejuni* produces superoxide dismutase, a protection against superoxide radicals that assists intracellular survival.[48] Host-derived mediators of secretion involved in diarrhea include prostaglandin E2 and protein kinase C.[49,50]

Clinical Features

The onset of diarrhea is preceded by a period of fever and malaise of up to 24 hours, or, exceptionally, up to 4 days. Diarrhea begins gradually or explosively and is watery and offensive, but many patients are more distressed by the severe abdominal pain than the diarrhea. Occasionally, appendicitis or mesenteric adenitis is diagnosed in infected children. Fecal incontinence may be a problem but tenesmus is not. The illness lasts from a few days to 3 weeks.[34,35,51–54] Most infections are self-limited and last less than 1 week, but some patients relapse or have a prolonged illness. One patient with myeloproliferative disorder developed toxic megacolon[55] and one child with ill-defined immunosuppression developed fatal enterocolitis.[56] Rarely, pseudomembranous colitis and massive lower gastrointestinal hemorrhage have been described.[54]

Pathology

Human data are limited mainly to the colon, which endoscopically displays erythema and friability of variable extent and severity, and sometimes aphthoid ulcers.[57] The histologic features are indistinguishable from other bacterial infectious colitides caused by organisms such as *Salmonella* or *Shigella*[58,59] and include edema of the lamina propria, neutrophil infiltration with cryptitis, crypt abscesses, capillary congestion, and preservation of the crypt architecture.[59] Campylobacter colitis can complicate inflammatory bowel disease and cause flare-up or relapse.

SHIGELLAE

Shigellae are nonmotile, gram-negative bacilli that are closely related to *E coli* but do not ferment lactose. The genus *Shigella* includes four species: *Sh dysenteriae, Sh flexneri, Sh boydii,* and *Sh sonnei.* The predominant species are now *Sh flexneri* and *Sh sonnei.* For unknown reasons, *Sh dysenteriae*-1 has declined in incidence since the early part of the 20th century but is still an important pathogen. *Shigella boydii* is mainly encountered in India and Bangladesh.[60] Shigellosis is endemic in tropical and subtropical underdeveloped parts of Africa, Southern Asia, and Central America, which lack water treatment and sanitation. Seasonal peaks and periodic regional epidemics occur and cause significant morbidity and mortality.[61–64]

Epidemiology and Pathogenesis

The majority of patients are children younger than 5 years,[65] although breast-fed infants younger than 6 months of age are spared because of the passive immunity from breast milk. *Shigella* is transmitted by the fecal–oral route, and the infecting dose may be a very small number of bacteria, unlike *Salmonella* or *E coli,* which require millions of organisms.[66] Although acid-sensitive in vitro, *Shigella* appears resistant to gastric acid in vivo and hypochlorhydric patients have not been reported to have increased susceptibility.

Shigellae can invade epithelial cells, make a potent cytotoxin (Shiga toxin), and can kill macrophages.[67] The relative contribution of each of these virulence factors has not been defined. Experimentally, in the rhesus monkey, the earliest manifestation of infection is watery diarrhea caused by fluid secretion of the proximal jejunum combined with an absorption defect in the colon.[68] Later the organisms invade the colonic epithelial cells, producing the dysenteric phase. *Shigella dysenteriae*-1 produces a thousand-fold more Shiga toxin than other species.[69] Shiga toxin is composed of one enzymatic A subunit and five receptor-binding B subunits. The intestinal receptor is the glycolipid Gb_3. After binding to the receptor, the A subunit is internalized and, through a complex series of steps, inhibits protein synthesis and causes cell death. It may be absorbed and detected in blood, and is the putative cause of the hemolytic uremic syndrome. Interleukin-1-beta may induce Shiga toxin sensitivity in endothelial cells and contribute to the development of hemolytic uremic syndrome (HUS).[70]

Shigellae are endocytosed by M cells or by ordinary enterocytes.[71] Within the membrane-bound endocytotic vesicle, the shigellae digest the membrane, escape into the cytoplasm, and spread to adjacent epithelial cells.[72–75] *Shigella flexneri* enters cell monolayers almost exclusively from the basolateral aspect, suggesting that after initially invading through the facilitation of M cells, they may spread from cell to cell through the basal aspect, avoiding the apical defensive barriers.[76] The epithelial ulceration that typifies shigellosis thus may be caused by destruction of epithelial cells by bacterial invasion through the basal (abluminal) membrane. Transmigration of neutrophils may allow invasion of mucosa by opening the paracellular pathway (cell junctions) to invasive microorganisms.[77] Once in the lamina propria, shigellae kill the resident macrophages in great numbers by apoptosis.[67] The genes required for cell invasion and macrophage killing are located on a 220-kb plasmid.

Pathology

The extent of involvement of the colon is variable, and subtotal involvement is most common.[78–80] In the initial stage the disease is continuous, then becomes patchy during the recovery stage.[79] The earliest endoscopic abnormality is mucosal edema appearing as swollen, pale mucosa lacking a normal vascular pattern and compromising the lumen in severe infections.[79] Ulcers appear next, and are usually small, discrete, star-shaped, sometimes serpiginous, and uncommonly linear or aphthoid. The mucosa around ulcers then becomes friable with punctate discrete mucosal hemorrhages, which are the sole remaining change once the clinical disease has settled.[79]

In most fatal infections the entire colon and terminal ileum are involved (Figure 44–6); rarely the rectosigmoid alone is affected.[78,81] The most common mucosal lesions in fatal infections are erythema and edema, with superficial ulceration in 40%, pseudomembranes in 20%, and a granular mucosa from lymphoid hyperplasia in 8%[81] (Figure 44–6). *Shigella dysenteriae*-1 sometimes produces a pseudomembranous colitis.[82,83]

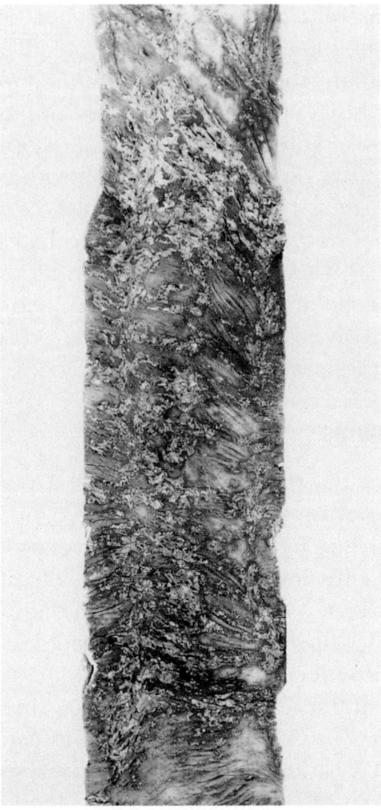

Figure 44–6. Colon of fatal human shigellosis. The entire colon is involved and there is extensive superficial ulceration, pseudomembranous exudation, and mucosal congestion and hemorrhage (AFIP Neg 39126).

Changes in mucosal biopsy specimens are most severe in the rectum and include edema, capillary congestion, swelling of endothelial cells, focal hemorrhages, crypt hyperplasia, depletion of goblet cells, margination and infiltration of neutrophils, and micro-ulcers with associated purulent exudate.[84,85] Specialized epithelial cells over lymphoid follicles are the first to be damaged.[84] Crypt abscesses and capillary thrombi are common. Patients biopsied late in the course and a high proportion of those at autopsy show dilatation and branching of crypts.[85]

Other organ disease found at autopsy commonly includes pneumonia and fatty liver but, only rarely, adult respiratory distress syndrome. Systemic complications include septicemia, hypokalemia, hyponatremia, hypoglycemia, leukemoid reaction, malnutrition, and opportunistic infections.

Clinical Features

Shigella dystenteriae-1 is the most virulent *Shigella,* causing classic dysentery with considerable mortality. Classic dysentery begins with fever, abdominal cramps, and watery diarrhea, and progresses within hours to intense abdominal pain and tenesmus, accompanied by frequent, bloody, mucoid, low-volume stools. Straining at stool may cause rectal prolapse. Fever can reach 39°C or higher and is unresponsive to antipyretic agents. There can be toxic dilatation of the colon, and plain radiographs of abdomen display ulceration with surviving mucosal islands. The colon may perforate and cause fecal peritonitis, which carries up to 50 percent mortality.[86] Death usually is associated with severe ulcerating colitis, with complications such as severe malnutrition with profound hypoproteinemia and immunodeficiency, pneumonia (caused by other organisms), septicemia, hyponatremia, hypokalemia, and hypoglycemia.[78,81] Protein-energy malnutrition is a strong risk factor for *Shigella* bacteremia, and infants younger than 1 year are most often affected.[87] Other complications include seizures, neurologic manifestations, and HUS.[82] The last two complications may be caused by systemic shiga toxemia. HUS is the triad of microangiopathic hemolytic anemia, thrombocytopenia, and renal failure. It is a self-limited condition if the patient survives the acute renal failure, and occurs almost exclusively with *Sh dysenteriae*-1. The renal pathology consists of thrombosis of glomerular capillaries and afferent arterioles together with endothelial swelling. Patients with HUS often display pseudomembranous colitis.[62]

Malnourished children fail to develop fever and, in spite of antibiotic therapy, may develop chronic colitis lasting weeks or months with persistently positive stool cultures. This chronic infection exacerbates malnutrition and is itself life-threatening. The terminal event is often secondary bacteremia or pneumonia.[60] Recent epidemics of shigellosis in children in Bangladesh and Central America have had fatality rates of 7%.[61,62]

Shigella flexneri is less virulent than *Sh dysenteriae* and causes diarrhea or dysentery. *Shigella sonnei* infections usually are moderately severe and associated with severe cramping, abdominal pain, fever, prostration, and low-volume stools with blood and mucus. They are self-limited, but may take 1 week or more to resolve.

Treatment

The cornerstone of treatment is antibiotic therapy with either ampicillin or trimethoprim–sulfamethoxazole, but bacterial resistance is a major problem. Fluoroquinolones are becoming the drugs of choice, especially in returning travelers. Nalidixic acid is also effective in most resistant infections. In infants, supportive care mainly consists of maintaining nutrition, because dehydration is not a major problem in classic dysentery.

REFERENCES

Salmonella

1. Candy DCA, Stephen J. *Salmonella.* In: Farthing MJG, Keusch GT, eds. *Enteric Infection, Mechanisms, Manifestations and Management.* London: Chapman and Hall; 1989:289–298.
2. Fang FC, Fierer J. Human infection with *Salmonella dublin. Medicine.* 1991;70:198–207.
3. Ryan CA, Hargrett-Bean NT, Blake PA. *Salmonella typhi* infections in the United States, 1975–1984: increasing role of foreign travel. *Rev Infect Dis.* 1989;2:1–8.
4. Rodrigue DC, Tauxe RV, Rowe B. International increase in *Salmonella enteritidis*: a new pandemic? *Epidemiol Infect.* 1990;105:21–27.
5. Takeuchi A. Electron microscopic studies of experimental *Salmonella* infection. I. Penetration into the intestinal epithelium by *Salmonella typhimurium. Am J Pathol.* 1967;50:109–136.
6. Takeuchi A. Electron microscope observations on penetration of the gut epithelial barrier by *Salmonella typhimurium.* In: Schlessinger D, ed. *Microbiology.* Washington, DC: ASM Publications; 1975:174–181.
7. Rout WR, Formal SB, Dammin GJ, Gianella RA. Pathophysiology of *Salmonella* diarrhea in the rhesus monkey: intestinal transport, morphological and bacteriological studies. *Gastroenterology.* 1974;67:59–70.
8. Wallis TS, Hawker RJH, Candy DCA, et al. Quantitation of the leukocyte influx into rabbit ileal loops induced by strains of *Salmonella typhimurium* of different virulence. *J Med Microbiol.* 1989;30:149–156.
9. Ensgraber M, Loos M. A 66-kilodalton heat shock protein of *Salmonella typhimurium* is responsible for binding of the bacterium to intestinal mucus. *Infect Immun.* 1992; 60:3072–3078.
10. Galan JE, Pace J, Hayman MJ. Involvement of the epidermal growth factor receptor in the invasion of cultured mammalian cells by *Salmonella typhimurium. Nature.* 1992;357:588–589.
11. Ginocchio C, Pace J, Galan JE. Identification and molecular characterization of a *Salmonella typhimurium* gene involved in triggering the internalization of salmonellae into cultured epithelial cells. *Proc Natl Acad Sci USA.* 1992;89:5976–5980.
12. Michetti P, Porta N, Mahan MJ, et al. Monoclonal immunoglobulin A prevents adherence and invasion of polarized epithelial cell monolayers by *Salmonella typhimurium. Gastroenterology.* 1994;107:915–923.
13. Wallis TS, Starkey WG, Stephen J, Haddon SJ, Osborne MP, Candy DCA. The nature and role of mucosal damage in relation to *Salmonella typhimurium*-induced fluid secretion in the rabbit ileum. *J Med Microbiol.* 1986; 22:39–49.
14. Brunsson I. Enteric nerves mediate the fluid secretory response due to *Salmonella typhimurium* R5 infection in the rat small intestine. *Acta Physiol Scand.* 1987;85: 787–617.
15. Huckstep RL. Pathology. In: Huckstep RL, ed. *Typhoid Fever and Other Salmonella Infections.* New York: Churchill Livingstone; 1962:35–43.
16. Archampong EQ. Operative treatment of typhoid perforation of the bowel. *Br Med J.* 1969;3:273–276.
17. Strate RW, Bannayan GA. Typhoid fever causing massive lower gastrointestinal hemorrhage. *JAMA.* 1976;236: 1979–1980.
18. Meier DE, Imediegwu OO, Tarpley JL. Perforated typhoid enteritis: operative experience with 108 cases. *Am J Surg.* 1989;157:423–427.
19. Quiroga T, Goycoolea M, Tagle R, Gonzales F, Rodriguez L, Villarroel L. Diagnosis of typhoid fever by two serologic methods: enzyme-linked immunosorbent assay of antilipopolysaccharide of *Salmonella typhi* antibodies and Widal test. *Diagn Microbiol Infect Dis.* 1992;15:651–656.
20. Mandal BK. *Salmonella typhi* and other salmonellas. *Gut.* 1994;35:726–728.
21. Coovadia YM, Gathiram V, Bhamjee A, et al. An outbreak of multiresistant *Salmonella typhi* in South Africa. *Q J Med.* 1992;298:91–100.
22. Levine MM. Typhoid fever and enteric fever. In: *Current Therapy in Infectious Disease—2.* New York: Decker; 1986:173–175.
23. Geddes AM. "I have been back from holiday for a week and still have diarrhea." *Br Med J.* 1983;286:513.
24. Mallory FB. A histological study of typhoid fever. *J Exp Med.* 1898;3:611–638.
25. Smith JH. Typhoid fever. In: Binford CH, Connor DH, eds. *Pathology of Tropical and Extraordinary Diseases.* Washington, DC: Armed Forces Institute of Pathology; 1976: 123–129.
26. Rubin RH, Weinstein L. Pathology and pathophysiology of *Salmonella* infection. In: *Salmonellosis, Microbiologic,*

Pathologic and Clinical Features. New York: Stratton; 1977:25–35.
27. Hepps K, Sutton FM, Goodgame RW. Multiple left-sided colon ulcers due to typhoid fever. *Gastrointest Endoscopy.* 1991;37:479–480.
28. Gonzales A, Vargas V, Guarner L, Accarino A, Guardia J. Toxic megacolon in typhoid fever. *Arch Intern Med.* 1985;145:2120.
29. Hendrickse RG, Collard P. *Salmonella* osteitis in Nigerian children. *Lancet.* 1960;1:80–82.
30. Day DW, Mandal BK, Morson BC. The rectal biopsy appearances in *Salmonella* colitis. *Histopathology.* 1978;2: 117–131.
31. McGovern VJ, Slavutin LJ. Pathology of *Salmonella* colitis. *Am J Surg Pathol.* 1979;3:483–490.
32. Boyd JF. Pathology of the alimentary tract in *Salmonella typhimurium* food-borne infection. *Gut.* 1985;26:935–944.
33. Sachdev HP, Chadha V, Malhotra V, Verghese A, Puri RK. Rectal histopathology in endemic *Shigella* and *Salmonella* diarrhea. *J Pediatr Gastroenterol Nutr.* 1993;16:33–38.

Campylobacter

34. Butzler JP, Dekeyser P, Detrain M, Dehaen F. Related vibrios in stools. *J Pediatr.* 1973;82:493–495.
35. Skirrow MB. Campylobacter enteritis: a "new" disease. *Br Med J.* 1977;2:9–11.
36. Quinn TC, Goodell SE, Fennell C, et al. Infections with *Campylobacter jejuni* and *Campylobacter*-like organisms in homosexual men. *Ann Intern Med.* 1984;101:187–192.
37. Totten PA, Fennell CL, Tenover FC, et al. *Campylobacter cinaedi* (sp. nov.) and *Campylobacter fennelliae* (sp. nov.): two new *Campylobacter* species associated with enteric disease in homosexual men. *J Infect Dis.* 1985;151: 131–139.
38. Riordan T, Humphrey TJ, Fowles A. A point source outbreak of campylobacter infection related to bird-pecked milk. *Epidemiol Infect.* 1993;110:261–265.
39. Nachamkin I, Fischer SH, Yang XH, Benitez O, Cravioto A. Immunoglobulin A antibodies directed against *Campylobacter jejuni* flagellin present in breast-milk. *Epidemiol Infect.* 1994;112:359–365.
40. Black RE, Levine MM, Clements ML, Hughes TP, Blaser MJ. Experimental *Campylobacter jejuni* infection in humans. *J Infect Dis.* 1988;157:472–479.
41. Robinson DA. Infective dose of *Campylobacter jejuni* in milk. *Br Med J.* 1981;282:1584.
42. Lee A, O'Rourke JL, Barrington PJ, Trust TJ. Mucus colonization as a determinant of pathogenicity in intestinal infection by *Campylobacter jejuni:* a mouse cecal model. *Infect Immun.* 1986;51:536–546.
43. Oelschlaeger TA, Guerry P, Kopecko DJ. Unusual microtubule-dependent endocytosis mechanisms triggered by *Campylobacter jejuni* and *Citrobacter freundii. PNAS.* 1993;90:6884–6888.
44. Konkel ME, Mead DJ, Hayes SF, Cieplak W. Translocation of *Campylobacter jejuni* across human polarized epithelial cell monolayer cultures. *J Infect Dis.* 1992;166: 308–315.
45. Klipstein FA, Engert RF. Immunological relationship of the B subunits of *Campylobacter jejuni* and *Escherichia coli* heat-labile enterotoxins. *Infect Immun.* 1985;48:629–633.
46. Everest PH, Goossens H, Sibbons P, et al. Pathological changes in the rabbit ileal loop model caused by *Campylobacter jejuni* from human colitis. *J Med Microbiol.* 1993; 38:316–321.
47. Johnson WM, Lior H. A new heat-labile cytolethal distending toxin (CLDT) produced by *Campylobacter* spp. *Microbial Pathogenesis.* 1988;4:115–126.
48. Pesci EC, Cottle DL, Pickett CL. Genetic, enzymatic, and pathogenic studies of the iron superoxide dismutase of *Campylobacter jejuni. Infect Immun.* 1994;62:2687–2694.
49. Everest PH, Cole AT, Hawkey CJ, et al. Roles of leukotriene B4, prostaglandin E2, and cyclic AMP in *Campylobacter jejuni*-induced intestinal fluid secretion. *Infect Immun.* 1993;61:4885–4887.
50. Kaur R, Ganguly NK, Kumar L, Walia BN. Studies on the pathophysiological mechanism of *Campylobacter jejuni*-induced fluid secretion in rat ileum. *FEMS Microbiol Lett.* 1993;111:327–330.
51. Pai CH, Sorger S, Lackman L, Sinai RE, Marks MI. *Campylobacter* gastroenteritis in children. *J Pediatr.* 1979;94: 589–591.
52. Karmali MA, Fleming PC. *Campylobacter* enteritis in children. *J Pediatr.* 1979;94:527–533.
53. Blaser MJ, Reller LB. *Campylobacter* enteritis. *N Engl J Med.* 1981;305:1444–1452.
54. Blaser MJ, Berkowitz ID, LaForce FM, et al. *Campylobacter* enteritis: clinical and epidemiologic features. *Ann Intern Med.* 1979;91:179–185.
55. Kalkay MN, Ayanian ZS, Lehaf EA, Baldi A. Campylobacter-induced toxic megacolon. *Am J Gastroenterol.* 1983; 78:557–559.
56. Coffin CM, L'Heureaux P, Dehner LP. Campylobacter-associated enterocolitis in childhood: report of a fatal case. *Am J Clin Pathol.* 1982;78:117–123.
57. Bentley D, Lynn J, Laws JW. Campylobacter colitis with intestinal aphthous ulceration mimicking obstruction. *Br Med J.* 1985;291:634.
58. Lambert ME, Schofield PF, Ironside AG, Mandal BK. Campylobacter colitis. *Br Med J.* 1989;i:857–859.
59. Price AB, Jewkes J, Sanderson PJ. Acute diarrhoea: Campylobacter colitis and the role of rectal biopsy. *J Clin Pathol.* 1979;32:990–997.

Shigella

60. Keusch GT, Bennish M. Shigella. In: Farthing MJG, Keusch GT, eds. *Enteric Infection: Mechanisms, Manifestations and Management.* Boston: Chapman and Hall; 1989: 265–282.
61. Gangarosa EJ, Peter DR, Math LJ, et al. Epidemic Shiga bacillus dysentery in central America. II. Epidemiologic studies in 1969. *J Infect Dis.* 1970;122:181–190.
62. Rahaman MM, Khan MM, Aziz KMS, Islam MS, Kibriya AKMG. An outbreak of dysentery caused by *Shigella dysenteriae* type 1 on a coral island in the bay of Bengal. *J Infect Dis.* 1975;132:15–19.
63. Mata LJ, Caceres A, Torres MF. Epidemic shiga dysentery in central America. *Lancet.* 1971;1:600–601.

64. Parsonnet J, Greene KD, Gerber AR, et al. *Shigella dysenteriae* type 1 infections in US travellers to Mexico, 1988. *Lancet.* 1989;ii:543–545.
65. Blaser MJ, Pollard RA, Feldman RA. *Shigella* infections in the United States 1974–1980. *J Infect Dis.* 1983;147: 771–775.
66. Keusch GT. Shigellosis. In: Evans AS, Feldman H, eds. *Bacterial Infections in Humans.* New York: Plenum Press; 1982:487–509.
67. Zychlinsky A, Prevost MC, Sansonetti PJ. *Shigella flexneri* induces apoptosis in infected macrophages. *Nature.* 1992;358:167–169.
68. Rout WR, Formal SB, Gianella RA, Dammin GJ. Pathophysiology of *Shigella* diarrhea in the rhesus monkey: intestinal transport, morphological and bacteriological studies. *Gastroenterology.* 1975;68:270–278.
69. Bartlett AV, Prado D, Cleary TG, Pickering LK. Production of Shiga toxin and other cytotoxins by serogroups of *Shigella. J Infect Dis.* 1986;154:996–1002.
70. Kaye SA, Louise CB, Boyd B, Lingwood CA, Obrig TG. Shiga toxin-associated hemolytic uremic syndrome: interleukin-1 beta enhancement of Shiga toxin cytotoxicity toward human vascular endothelial cells in vitro. *Infect Immun.* 1993;61:3886–3891.
71. Wassef JS, Keren DF, Mailloux JL. Role of M cells in initial antigen uptake and in ulcer formation in the rabbit intestinal loop model of shigellosis. *Infect Immun.* 1989; 57:858–863.
72. Formal SB, Hale TL, Sansonetti PJ. Invasive enteric pathogens. *Rev Infect Dis.* 1983;5:5702–5707.
73. Clerc P, Ryter A, Mounier J, Sansonetti PJ. Plasmid-mediated early killing of eucaryotic cells by *Shigella flexneri* as studied by infection of J774 macrophages. *Infect Immun.* 1987;55:521–527.
74. Sansonetti PJ, Ryter A, Clerc P, Maurelli AT, Mounier J. Multiplication of *Shigella flexneri* within HeLa cells: lysis of the phagocytic vacuole and plasmid-mediated contact hemolysis. *Infect Immun.* 1986;51:461–469.
75. Bernardini ML, Mounier J, d'Hauteville H, Coquis-Rondon M, Sansonetti PJ. Identification of icsA, a plasmid locus of *Shigella flexneri* that governs bacterial intra- and intercellular spread through interaction with F-actin. *PNAS.* 1989;86:3867–3871.
76. Mounier J, Vasselon T, Hellio R, Lesourd M, Sansonetti PJ. *Shigella flexneri* enters human colonic Caco-2 epithelial cells through the basolateral pole. *Infect Immun.* 1992; 60:237–248.
77. Perdomo JJ, Gounon P, Sansonetti PJ. Polymorphonuclear leukocyte transmigration promotes invasion of colonic epithelial monolayer by *Shigella flexneri. J Clin Invest.* 1993;93:633–643.
78. Islam MM, Azad AK, Bardhan PK, Raqib R, Islam D. Pathology of shigellosis and its complications. *Histopathology.* 1994;24:65–71.
79. Khuroo MS, Mahajan R, Zargar SA, et al. The colon in shigellosis: serial colonoscopic appearances in *Shigella dysenteriae* 1. *Endoscopy.* 1990;22:35–38.
80. Speelman P, Kabir I, Moyenul I. Distribution and spread of colonic lesions in shigellosis: A colonoscopic study. *J Infect Dis.* 1984;150:899–903.
81. Butler T, Dunn D, Dahms B, Islam M. Causes of death and the histopathologic findings in fatal shigellosis. *Pediatr Infect Dis J.* 1989;8:767–772.
82. Raghupathy P, Date A, Shastry JCM, Sudarsanam A, Jadhav M. Hemolytic-uremic syndrome complicating shigella dysentery in south Indian children. *Br Med J.* 1978;1: 1518–1521.
83. Kelber M, Ament ME. *Shigella dysenteriae* 1: A forgotten cause of pseudomembranous colitis. *J Pediatr* 1976;89: 595–596.
84. Mathan MM, Mathan VI. Morphology of rectal mucosa of patients with shigellosis. *Rev Infect Dis.* 1991;13(suppl 4): S314–S318.
85. Anand BS, Malhotra V, Bhattacharya SK, et al. Rectal histology in acute bacillary dysentery. *Gastroenterology.* 1986;90:654–660.
86. Azad MAK, Islam M, Butler T. Colonic perforation in *Shigella dysenteriae* 1 infection. *Pediatr Infect Dis.* 1986; 5:103–104.
87. Struelens MJ, Patte D, Kabir I, et al. Shigella septicemia: prevalence, presentation, risk factors, and outcome. *J Infect Dis.* 1985;152:784–790.

CHAPTER 45

Bartonellosis—Infection by *Bartonella bacilliformis*

Elizabeth A. Montgomery and Fernando U. Garcia

There are many kinds of slavery and many kinds of freedom. But reading is still the path.

Carl Sagan (1934–), The Demon Haunted World

DEFINITION

Human bartonellosis is a biphasic bacterial infection caused by *Bartonella bacilliformis.* There is a phase in the blood and a phase in tissue. Human pathogens closely related to *B bacilliformis* include *B henselae* (formerly *Rochalimaea henselae*) and *B elizabethae* (formerly *R elizabethae*), as well as *B quintana* (formerly *Rickettsia quintana*) and are described in other chapters. By nucleic acid hybridization, there is greater than 40% homology between *B bacilliformis* and the *Rochalimeae* sp. Carrión's disease, Oroya fever, verruga peruana, and la verruga are synonyms.

HISTORICAL ASPECTS

During the construction of a railway between Lima and La Oroya, Peru, between 1869 and 1873, 7000 workers died of a febrile illness, which came to be known as Oroya fever,[1] also called Carrión's disease, after Daniel A. Carrión, a medical student who established the relationship between the febrile condition (Oroya fever) and the cutaneous nodules, called "verruga peruana." In 1885, after inoculating himself with blood from a cutaneous lesion of a patient, Carrión became febrile and died.[2] In endemic areas, the term *la verruga* is used to encompass both manifestations of this biphasic disease.

GEOGRAPHIC DISTRIBUTION

Human bartonellosis is limited to a defined region that bridges the Colombian, Ecuadorian, and Peruvian Andes (Figure 45–1). This region extends from southern Colombia (5°N) to mid-Peru (13°S). Here it afflicts those on both the eastern and western slopes of the Andes between the 1000- and 3000-meter elevations. The endemic areas are further defined by the distribution of the nocturnal vector sandfly, *Lutzomyia verrucarum,* for within the endemic regions reproduction of the fly is favored by climatic conditions. The most important geographic site of bartonellosis is the Santa River basin in the department of Huaraz, Peru. The Santa River runs from south to north, between two parallel chains of mountains, at an average altitude of 2500 meters above sea level, turning abruptly west, perforating the mountains through a steep canyon, and emptying into the Pacific Ocean. The narrow valley along the river, together with several subsidiaries forms an area of approximately 500 square kilometers where bartonellosis has been endemic since pre-Colombian times. Each year during the rainy season (January through March), bartonellosis increases and then diminishes during winter. Below Chincha (13°S), 200 kilometers south of Lima, not a single infection has been identified, but Allison et al[3] identified bartonellosis in a pre-Inca mummy in the Nazca region, 100 kilometers south of Chincha. Thus bartonellosis had a wider range in pre-

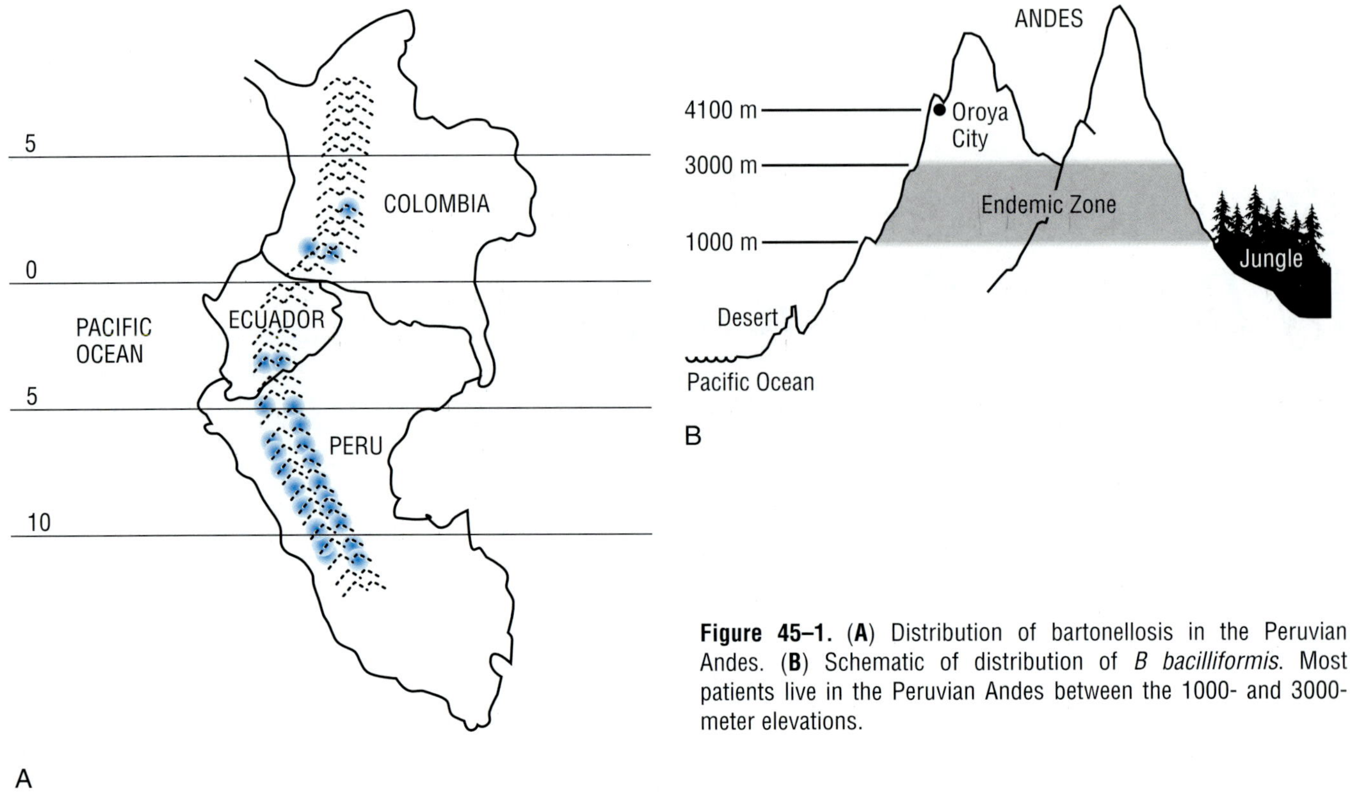

Figure 45–1. (**A**) Distribution of bartonellosis in the Peruvian Andes. (**B**) Schematic of distribution of *B bacilliformis.* Most patients live in the Peruvian Andes between the 1000- and 3000-meter elevations.

Inca times, or perhaps the body had been carried to and buried in Nazca. In recent years several outbreaks of bartonellosis have been reported throughout the northern part of Peru, as well as in Ecuador and in Colombia.[4]

LIFE CYCLE, NATURAL HISTORY, AND EPIDEMIOLOGY

As noted, bartonellosis is transmitted from person to person by *Lutzomyia (Phlebotomus) verrucarum,* a nocturnal sandfly that proliferates in small humid caves and holes in the endemic area. Humans are the only known reservoir for *B bacilliformis.* The bacteria are in the vector's biting apparatus. *Lutzomyia verrucarum* reproduces during the rainy season (January through March) and inoculates the bacteria while feeding. Unknown, however, is the location of the bacteria during incubation. Natives of endemic areas probably have repeated transient bacteremias to maintain a pool of infected sandflies, because humans in the endemic areas are the only known reservoirs of *B bacilliformis.* Attempts to identify *B bacilliformis* in local plants and animals and attempts to infect local fauna have not been successful. In fact, the only experimental animal in which the disease has been produced is the Macaca rhesus, a monkey alien to Peru.[5] The only plant study was performed some years ago by Herrer.[6] The culture media used for this study, however, was for *B bacilliformis,* not media appropriate for phytobacteria, which may be in the latex of native plants.

After incubation of about 3 weeks (range, 3 weeks to 2 months), those without prior tolerance become febrile and have an acute, severe, hemolytic anemia, caused by parasitization of virtually 100% of circulating erythrocytes by *B bacilliformis.* Some erythrocytes contain multiple bacilli. Then the bacillus invades the reticuloendothelial system and hepatosplenomegaly and lymphadenopathy follow. In the preantibiotic era, the mortality at this stage was approximately 40%; the current figure is about 8%.[7] A tissue phase, which signals improvement, appears about 2 months after the hematic phase and is characterized by verruga peruana nodules mostly on face and limbs. These nodules may reappear from time to time in natives of endemic areas. In these areas, where more than 60% of asymptomatic individuals have antibodies to *B bacilliformis,* infections may follow an abbreviated course and, as noted earlier, healthy natives can harbor the bacillus.[7,8] This latter group presumably is the natural reservoir.[1]

MORPHOLOGY AND BIOLOGIC CHARACTERISTICS OF THE ORGANISM

Bartonella bacilliformis is a hemotropic, mobile, pleomorphic, gram-negative flagellated coccoid bacterium that elaborates an angiogenesis factor in vitro.[9] This angiogenesis factor and other similarities to *B henselae*[10,11] strongly suggest parallels between bartonellosis and bacillary angiomatosis (Chapter 42).[12–17] *Bartonella bacilliformis* penetrates cells by pouching into the cytoplasmic membrane with a rotatory movement.[18] In addition, *B bacilliformis* produces an extracellular protein that deforms erythrocytes.[19] The flagella are also crucial for invading erythrocytes.[20]

Bartonella bacilliformis belongs to the newly formed genus *Bartonella* and, as noted, other members of this genus are *B quintana, B henselae,* and *B elizabethae.*[11] The members of this genus and the diseases they cause have received little attention because the bacilli are grown with great difficulty. Furthermore, bartonellosis is a sharply limited remote disease of the Andean hinterland. New molecular techniques such as polymerase chain reaction (PCR), however, have 1) enabled identification of these organisms in immunodeficient patients, 2) enabled isolation and characterization of new members of the genus, and 3) focused attention on the members of this genus and the diseases they cause. *Bartonella* species require more than 7 days of incubation and cannot be detected by routine culture methods. *Bartonella* species grow best on solid or semisolid media and do not produce sufficient turbidity nor convert sufficient substrate to CO_2 to be detected by standard blood culture systems. Freshly prepared heart infusion agar containing 5% or 10% defibrinated rabbit or horse blood has been used. *Bartonella bacilliformis* grows under humid microaerophilic conditions, and optimally at 25 to 30°C, in contrast to 37°C for other members of the genus. It is catalase positive and possesses unique fatty acids. PCR technology has been developed for detecting *B bacilliformis* in cultures, in blood, and in formalin-fixed tissues.[21]

CLINICAL FEATURES

As briefly outlined earlier, after the bite of the infected fly, the infection has two phases.[1,4,8,22–24] The first is hematogenous, and varies in severity. Some natives to the endemic zones have positive blood cultures without any clinical findings for weeks. Among children in the endemic area, the cutaneous phase may erupt without a clinically apparent hematic phase,[1,4,8,22–24] presumably a consequence of passive immunity from their mothers. Those who are not native to the endemic areas or natives with low immunity to *B bacilliformis* develop severe disease after inoculation of organisms by the sandfly. The host–bacteria interactions during the incubation period have not been fully studied, but perhaps the bacteria proliferate in endothelial cells of regional lymph nodes or dermal venules close to the bite.[25,26] Subsequently, bacteria are released into the blood where, by a process of forced endocytosis, they penetrate and deform the walls of red blood cells. This deformation is caused by a factor produced by the bacteria.[19] Almost 100% of circulating erythrocytes are parasitized by the bacteria and each can simultaneously harbor several organisms (Figure 45–2). During this phase patients have fever, malaise, pallor, hepatosplenomegaly, and lymphadenopathy.

The reticuloendothelial cells within the liver, spleen, bone marrow, and lymph nodes phagocytize infected red cells, leading to a hemolytic type of anemia without intravascular hemolysis. Coombs' test is negative and specific antibodies are not markedly elevated. Glomerulonephritis and other inflammatory conditions attributable to immune complex deposits, however, are not complications of bartonellosis.

The acute anemia of the hematic phase is among the most severe types of anemia known.[27,7] In a matter of a few days the red cell count can drop to close to 1 million or even less. At this stage the enlarged liver, spleen, bone marrow, and lymph nodes contain histiocytes laden with *B bacilliformis.* At the peak of the phagocytic phase, there is evidence of immunodepression. For example, skin tests for tuberculosis as well as serologic tests become negative. Many years ago, Pedro

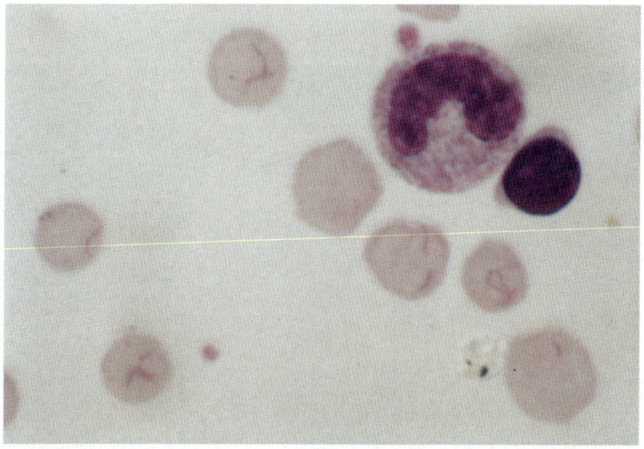

Figure 45–2. Hematic phase of bartonellosis (Oroya fever). Blood film showing erythrocytes parasitized with numerous *Bartonella* organisms. Gram characteristics are not apparent on Giemsa-stained preparations. *Bartonella bacilliformis* is gram-negative (Giemsa, ×1350).

Weiss demonstrated a state of "anergy" at this point in the natural history of bartonellosis.[2] Because of this induced immunodeficiency, miliary tuberculosis, *Salmonella* septicemia (or septicemia caused by other intestinal bacteria), generalized toxoplasmosis, histoplasmosis, and other infections frequently complicate the hematic phase.[27] Before the era of antibiotics, these secondary infections were the major cause of death, with infections by Salmonellae being most common. The mechanisms of the immunosuppression have not been elucidated. A "blockade" of the reticuloendothelial system by bacteria of the genus *Bartonella* has been postulated. Patrucco demonstrated inversion of the helper/suppressor T-cell ratio at the end of the hematic phase, which suggests a cell-mediated mechanism.[28]

The second phase (cutaneous phase) generally follows the hematic episode. Natives regard it as the curative sign (Figure 45–3). The cutaneous/tissue phase may also develop after an ill-defined stage with headaches and pain in bones and joints. Generally, the cutaneous nodules herald a relief of symptoms. In a good proportion of patients, however, the cutaneous nodules appear in those who were previously asymptomatic.

The significance of these cutaneous angioblastic nodules remains obscure. The bacilli in the cutaneous nodules elaborate in angiogenic factor that stimulates in vitro proliferation of human endothelial cells, hence the comparison between bartonellosis and bacillary angiomatosis (see Chapter 42). In contrast to bacillary angiomatosis, verruga peruana does not involve internal organs. Verruga peruana nodules are self-limiting; they heal without scars unless superinfected, and develop regardless of the antibiotic treatment given during the hematic phase.

GROSS PATHOLOGY

Lesions of verruga peruana usually appear weeks to several months after the acute stage and are an eruption of cutaneous nodules. The eruption is of limited duration and the mortality in this phase is very low. The verrugas develop and regress in stages so that growth and regression may coexist. This is a chronic stage and it may last from 2 months to 2 years after the primary infection. These skin lesions have three distinct appearances, which have been designated as miliary, nodular, and mular. Overall, the nodules of all stages are red and have loosely marginated cut surfaces (Figure 45–4).

Miliary Type

Lesions of the miliary type are small (less than 1 cm), superficial, and usually symmetrically distributed on the lower limbs, upper limbs, face, and even conjunctiva (Figure 45–5). This predilection for the dermis of the cooler parts of the body probably reflects the organism's optimal growth at 25 to 27°C. The color of the nodules ranges from vivid red to purple, and the overlying skin is shiny and tense. The verrugas are firm and painless. Occasionally, they involve the oral, ocular, or nasal mucosa. Nodules in the urinary bladder have been reported. Regression begins after maximum development. The epidermis over the verruga exfoliates followed by ulceration and hemorrhage. As noted, however, there are no scars in uncomplicated cases.

Nodular Type

Nodular-type lesions (Figure 45–3) can reach several centimeters in diameter and extend deeply into the sub-

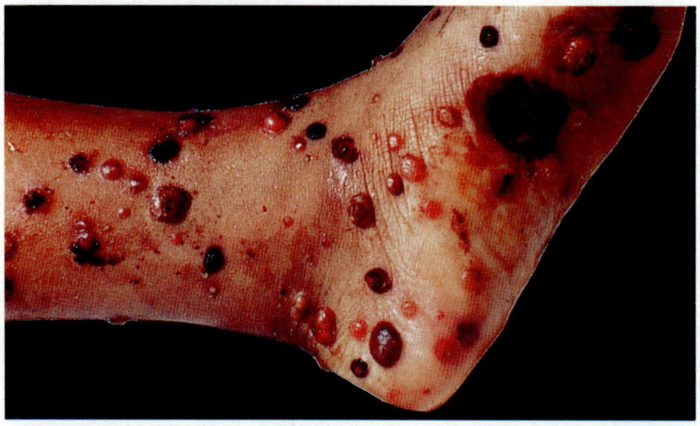

Figure 45–3. Verruga peruana, nodular form. These nodules are characteristic of the tissue phase of bartonellosis and typically herald the patient's recovery from the life-threatening hematic phase. *(Contributed by I. Biaggioni, MD.)*

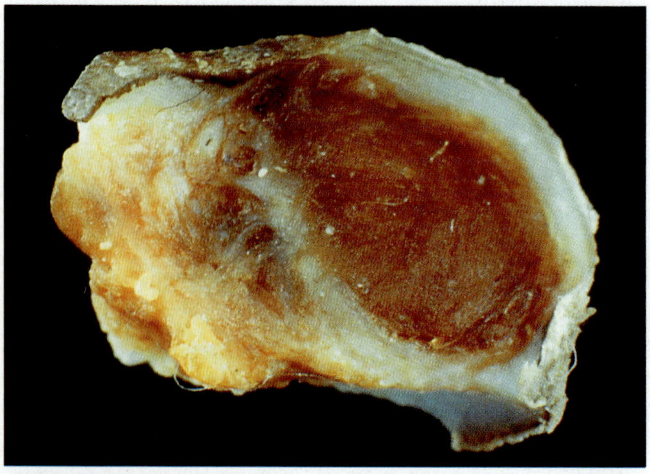

Figure 45–4. Cut surface of a nodular verruga. Note the beefy red color of the lesion.

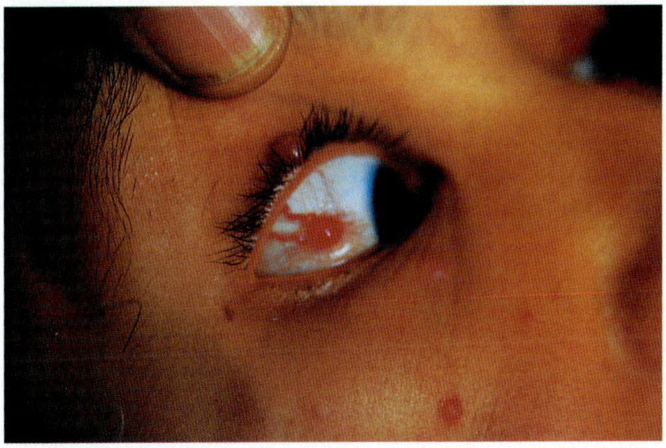

Figure 45–5. Verruga peruana of the conjunctiva of a pregnant woman. *(Contributed by U. Garcia-Caceres.)*

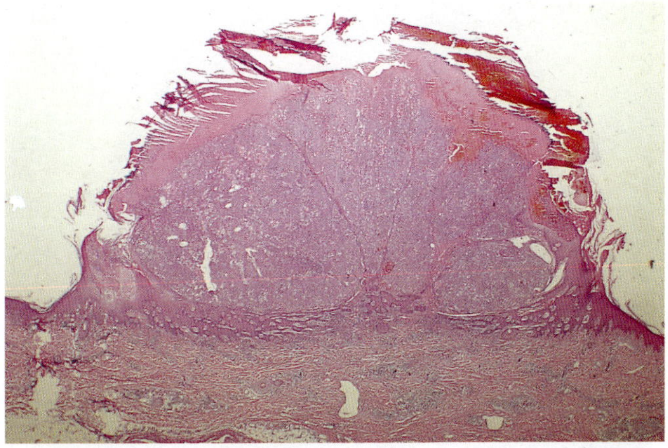

Figure 45–6. Verruga peruana, nodular form. Healed lesions typically leave unblemished skin, but ulceration or secondary infections may sometimes cause scarring [hematoxylin-eosin (H&E), ×4].

cutaneous tissue. They are less numerous than miliary nodules but follow a similar course. They are more prone to ulceration and hyperkeratosis. Scarring is more frequent, presumably a result of superinfection.

Mular Type

This is the least frequent presentation of verruga peruana. The lesion is a single large verruga, usually more than 5 cm across, and most commonly on the face or limbs. It is usually ulcerated and more painful. Typically, it leaves a scar.

LIGHT MICROSCOPY, INCLUDING SPECIAL STAINS

All verruga lesions, regardless of their macroscopic appearance, contain vasoformative elements, commonly mixed with inflammatory cells, and typically arranged in a multinodular or lobulated pattern (Figure 45–6).[29–32] Superficial nodules may be polypoid and, when accompanied by well-formed vessels with patent lumina, may suggest a pyogenic granuloma or a lesion of bacillary angiomatosis. Lesions that arise in less distensible tissues may exhibit more solid mitotically active "angioblastic" growth, suggesting neoplasm[29] (Figure 45–7) that also can have a predominantly spindle morphology.[30] All of these lesions are identified and unified by the presence of plump atypical endothelial (verruga) cells. Depending on the stage of the lesions, lymphocytes and plasma cells or neutrophils with microabscesses may dominate. Also there may be fibrin, cellular necrosis, and fibrosclerosis. Rocha–Lima inclusions, which may be fleeting, help confirm the diagnosis (Figure 45–8). These are intracytoplasmic inclusions in endothelial cells, first described by Rocha–Lima and best seen when tissues are fixed in buffered neutral formalin, embedded in glycol methacrylate, and stained with Giemsa.[30] Similar inclusions have been reproduced in vitro. They are large phagosomes in endothelial cells containing many degenerating bacteria.[26] They also are lightly silvered with the Warthin–Starry technique. When inclusions are not present, the diagnosis rests on clinicopathologic correlation, the presence of plump atypical endothelial cells and small interstitial clusters of silvered (blackened) bacteria using the Warthin–Starry technique.

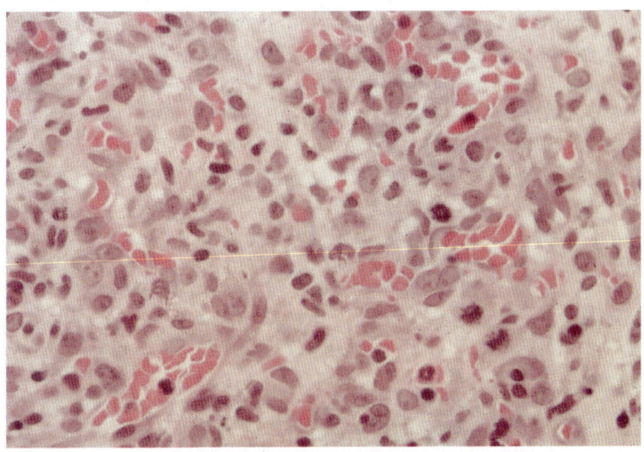

Figure 45–7. High magnification of the lesion in Figure 45–6. In this field there is a relatively solid proliferation of endothelial cells. Despite the plump appearance of the proliferating cells and the presence of mitoses, the lesion is lobulated (see Figure 45–6), an important feature in support of a benign process (H&E, ×500).

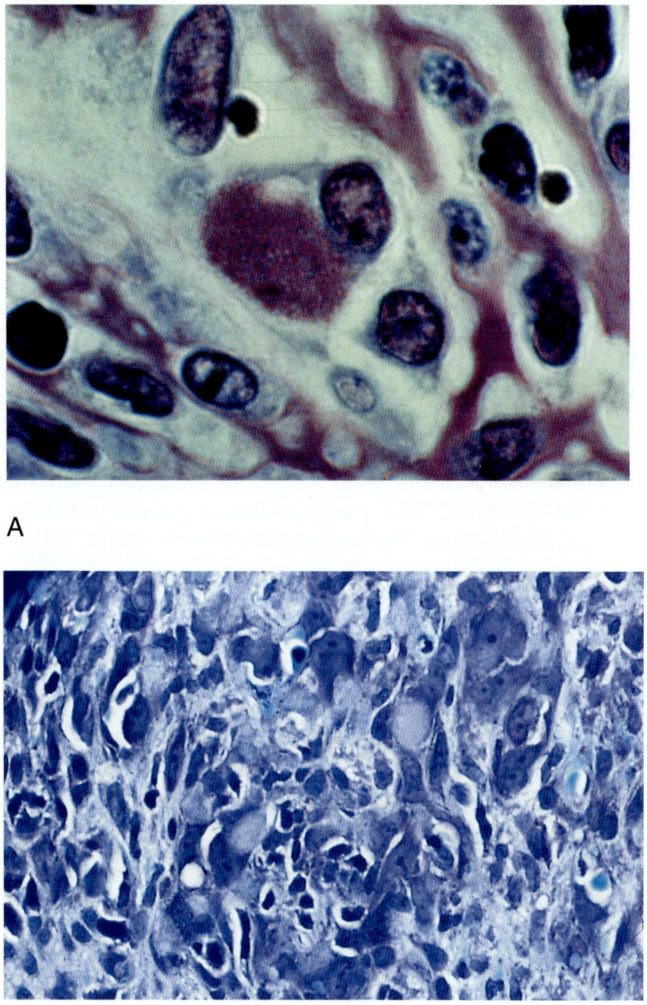

A

B

Figure 45–8. (**A**) Rocha–Lima inclusion, seen in tissue embedded in glycol methacrylate. These are endothelial phagocytic cells, which may contain bacteria, extracellular matrix components, or both (Giemsa, ×850). *(Contributed by J. Arias-Stella Sr., MD.)* (**B**) Rocha–Lima inclusion, seen in tissue embedded in paraffin and stained with Giemsa (×350). Note the pale staining in thicker sections. *(Contributed by J. Arias-Stella Sr., MD.)*

Regressing lesions contain a predominance of lymphocytes and histiocytic cells, which could presumably be mistaken for a lymphoproliferative disorder, a distinction addressed by lack of clonality.

ELECTRON MICROSCOPY

Ultrastructurally, *B bacilliformis* is in the extracellular space apposed to vessels and in the interstitium between proliferating endothelial cells (Figure 45–9). The inclusions seen by light microscopy correspond to endothelial phagocytic cells demonstrating rudimentary cell junctions and few lysozymes. Cell surface invaginations in these cells produce interanastomosing channels with vacuoles containing bacteria and/or components of extracellular matrix. Regressed lesions lack organisms on ultrastructural studies.[29,33]

DIFFERENTIAL DIAGNOSIS

The nodular type of verruga may resemble pyogenic granuloma and bacillary angiomatosis. Since bartonellosis is, for all practical purposes, restricted to a limited geographic locale, this differential diagnosis does not arise frequently. Although pyogenic granulomas (lobular capillary hemangiomas) resemble verruga peruana, in their deeper aspects, they consist of a lobulated proliferation of well-formed vascular channels that are of progressively smaller caliber at the periphery of individual lobules, and there is little inflammation in the deeper parts of the lesions. The lobules are separated by loose fibromyxoid stroma. Of course, the term "pyogenic granuloma" is an etiologic and pathologic misnomer that has been retained over time. An infectious cause for pyogenic granulomas has been largely disproved and most believe they represent an exaggerated form of vascular hyperplasia or a variant of capillary hemangioma. The most common sites are gingiva, fingers, lips, face, and tongue, a distribution that differs from that of verruga peruana, which more commonly affects the limbs.

Bacillary angiomatosis should be at the forefront of the differential diagnosis when evaluating vascular proliferations in immunodeficient patients, particularly those infected with the human immunodeficiency virus (HIV). Bacillary angiomatosis, a relatively new disease, is caused in most patients by *B henselae.* Unlike the lesions of verruga peruana, bacillary angiomatosis may involve internal organs. The lesions of bacillary angiomatosis contain a lobulated proliferation of capillary-sized vessels set in a background of microabscesses, leukocytoclastic debris, and amorphous granular amphophilic material teeming with clumps of bacteria best seen with the Warthin–Starry silver impregnation technique (at pH 4.0). Distinction between bacillary angiomatosis and verruga peruana is readily accomplished by attention to clinical history and by the presence of extracellular bacterial masses.

When endothelial cell proliferation dominates, the differential diagnosis of verruga peruana could include carcinoma, malignant melanoma, epithelioid hemangioendothelioma, a vascular neoplasm classified as a "borderline" malignant lesion by the World Health

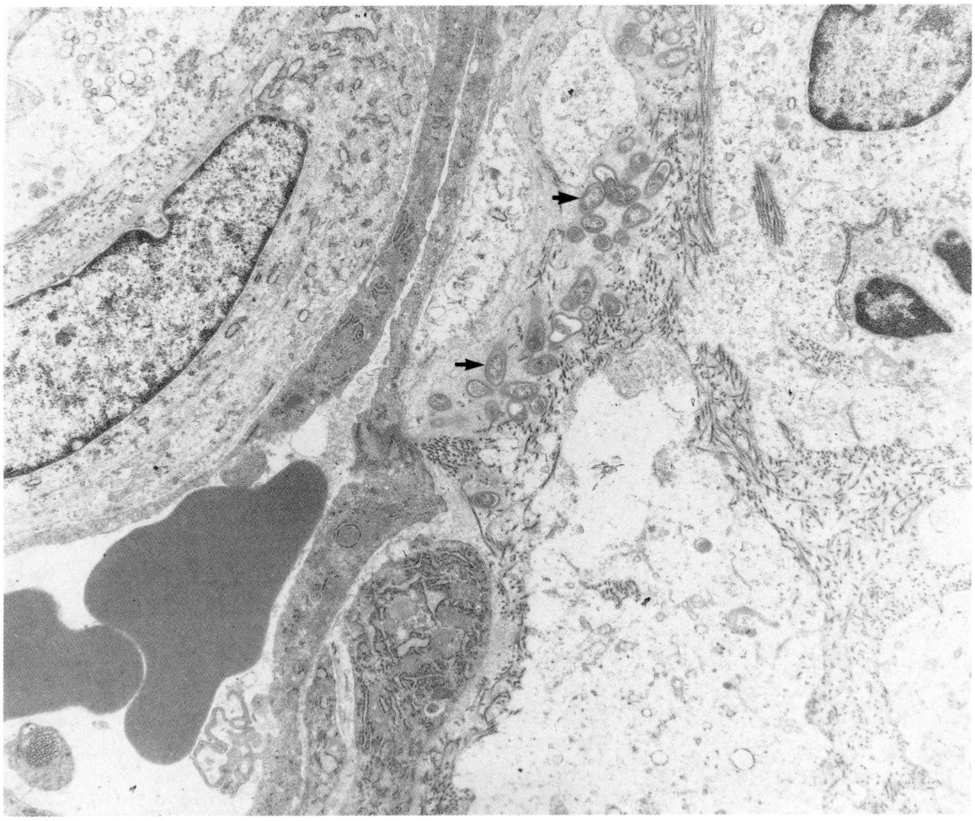

Figure 45–9. Electron micrograph of skin showing groups of bacteria in interstitium (*arrows*) next to a capilary, suggesting hematogenous spread. The number of bacteria is small, never reaching the number in bacillary angiomatosis (×3130).

Organization, or Kaposi's sarcoma. Identifying bacilli or Rocha–Lima inclusions is the most reliable way to arrive at a definitive diagnosis. Since bacilli or inclusions may be fleeting, a high index of suspicion based on clinical features is essential. A selected panel of immunohistochemical studies excludes carcinoma and melanoma since the former reacts with antibodies directed against epithelial antigens and the proliferating cells of the latter typically express S-100 protein or stain with HMB-45 antibody, and verruga peruana lesions express only endothelial and dermal dendrocytic markers. Distinction between verruga peruana and epithelioid hemangioendothelioma is on morphologic grounds. Epithelioid hemangioendotheliomas lack a lobulated growth pattern and are usually infiltrative, typically have minimal inflammation, are commonly deep lesions, and contain cells with intracytoplasmic lumina in a chondrohyaline matrix. Kaposi's sarcoma differs by having a different epidemiologic presentation, and frequently has abundant hyaline globules, which are erythrophagolysosomes in varying stages of disintegration, and an infiltrative growth pattern rather than a lobulated one. Extravasated erythrocytes, hemosiderin, endothelial cell apoptosis, and a plasma cell rather than neutrophilic inflammatory infiltrate are all characteristics of Kaposi's sarcoma. It also has a proclivity for internal organs, which is absent in verruga peruana. Distinguishing features of verruga peruana, bacillary angiomatosis, and Kaposi's sarcoma and listed in Table 45–1.

TREATMENT

Treatment of Oroya fever has evolved little since the late 1940s and early 1950s. Chloramphenicol, first reported by Krumdiek in 1949,[23] remains the standard therapy. Typically, patients defervesce within 24 hours after treatment and undergo a prompt reticulocyte response. Furthermore, chloramphenicol also acts against the salmonellosis that frequently ensues.[24] In a more recent report of an outbreak in Shumpillan, a remote Andean village, the fatality rate for those receiving no antibiotic was 88%, whereas 10 acutely ill individuals given chloramphenicol survived and were healthy 2 months after treatment.[4] Although other antibiotics might be effective, there has been little room for experimentation during outbreaks of this rare life-threatening illness.

TABLE 45–1. DISTINGUISHING FEATURES OF VERRUGA PERUANA, BACILLARY ANGIOMATOSIS, AND KAPOSI'S SARCOMA

	Verruga Peruana	Bacillary Angiomatosis	Kaposi's Sarcoma
Distribution	Face and limbs	Skin surfaces, lymph nodes, and internal organs	Skin surfaces, lymph nodes, and internal organs
Microabscesses	Absent	Present	Absent
Extracellular bacterial masses	Absent	Present	Absent
Intracellular inclusions	Present	Absent	Absent
Interstitial acute inflammation	Present	Present	Absent
Hyaline globules	Present (rare)	Absent	Present

Acknowledgments. Dr. Peter L. McEvoy, Walter Reed Army Medical Center, reviewed this manuscript and made helpful suggestions. Dr. Uriel Garcia-Caceres, University Peruana Cayetano Heredia, also made helpful suggestions.

REFERENCES

1. Howe C. Carrión's disease: immunologic studies. *Arch Intern Med.* 1943;72:147–167.
2. Garcia-Caceres U, Garcia FU. Bartonellosis. An immunodepressive disease and the life of Daniel Alcides Carrión. *Am J Clin Pathol.* 1991;95(suppl 1):S51–S59.
3. Allison MJ, Pezzia A, Gerszten E, Mendoza D. A case of Carrión's disease associated with human sacrifice from Huari culture of southern Peru. *Am J Phys Anthropol.* 1985;41:295–300.
4. Gray GC, Johnson AA, Thornton SA, et al. An epidemic of oroya fever in the Peruvian Andes. *Am J Trop Med Hyg.* 1990;42:215–221.
5. Noguchi H III. The behaviour of *Bartonella bacilliformis* in *Macacus rhesus*. *J Exp Med.* 1926;44:697–703.
6. Herrer A. Carrión's disease. I. Studies on plants claimed to be reservoirs of *Bartonella bacilliformis*. *Am J Trop Med.* 1953;2:637–643.
7. Maguina-Vargas CP. Estudio clinico de 145 casos de bartonellosis en el Hospital Nacional Cayetano Heredia: 1969–1992. Doctoral thesis, Universidad Peruana Cayetano Heredia, 1992.
8. Herrer A. Carrión's disease. II. Presence of *Bartonella bacilliformis* in the peripheral blood of patients with the benign form. *Am J Trop Med Hyg.* 1953;2:645–649.
9. Garcia FU, Wojta J, Broadley KN, et al. *Bartonella bacilliformis* stimulates endothelial cells in vitro and is angiogenic in vivo. *Am J Pathol.* 1990;136:1125–1135.
10. O'Connor SP, Dorsch M, Steigerwalt AG, et al. 16S rRNA sequences of *Bartonella bacilliformis* and cat scratch disease bacillus reveal phylogenetic relationships with the alpha-2 subgroup of the class Protobacteria. *J Clin Microbiol.* 1991;29:2144–2150.
11. Brenner DJ, O'Connor SP, Winkler HH, Steigerwalt AG. Proprosals to unify the genera *Bartonella* and *Rochalimaea,* with descriptions of *Bartonella quintana* comb nov, *Bartonella vinsonii* comb nov, *Bartonella henselae* comb nov, and *Bartonella elizabethae* comb nov, and to remove the family Bartonellaceae from the order Rickettsiales. *Int J System Bacteriol.* 1993;43:777–786.
12. Stoler MH, Bonfiglio TA, Steigbigel RT. An atypical subcutaneous infection associated with acquired immune deficiency syndrome. *Am J Clin Pathol.* 1983;80:714–718.
13. LeBoit PE, Berger TG, Egbert BM, et al. Bacillary angiomatosis. The histopathology and differential diagnosis of a pseudoneoplastic infection in patients with human immunodeficiency virus disease. *Am J Surg Pathol.* 1989; 13:909–920.
14. Cockerel CJ, LeBoit PE. Bacillary angiomatosis: a newly characterized, pseudoneoplastic, infectious, cutaneous vascular disorder. *J Am Acad Dermatol.* 1990;22:501–512.
15. Relman DA, Loutit JS, Schmidt TM, et al. The agent of bacillary angiomatosis: an approach to the identification of uncultured pathogens. *N Engl J Med.* 1990;323: 1573–1580.
16. Relman DA, Falkow S, LeBoit PE, et al. The organism causing bacillary angiomatosis, peliosis hepatis, and fever and bacteremia in immunocompromised patients. *N Engl J Med.* 1991;324:1514. Letter.
17. Reed JA, Brigati DJ, Flynn SD, et al. Immunocytochemical identification of *Rochalimea henselae* in bacillary (epithelioid) angiomatosis, parenchymal bacillary peliosis, and persistent fever with bacteremia. *Am J Surg Pathol.* 1992; 16:650–657.
18. Benson LA, Kar K, McLaughlin G, Ihler GM. Entry of *Bartonella bacilliformis* into erythrocytes. *Infect Immun.* 1986;54:347–353.
19. Mernaugh G, Ihler GM. Deformation factor: an extracellular protein synthesized by *Bartonella bacilliformis* that deforms erythrocyte membranes. *Infect Immun.* 1992;60: 937–943.
20. Scherer DC, DeBuron-Connors I, Minnick MF. Characterization of *Bartonella bacilliformis* flagella and effect of antiflagellin antibodies on invasion of human erythrocytes. *Infect Immun.* 1993;61:4962–4971.
21. Maass M, Schreiber M, Knobloch J. Detection of *Bartonella bacilliformis* in cultures, blood and formalin preserved skin biopsies by use of the polymerase chain reaction. *Trop Med Parasitol.* 1992;43:191–194.

22. Delgado LM. El brote de verruga en la vejiga. *Rev Med Peruana.* 1935;7:91–93.
23. Krumdiek CF. La enfermedad de Carrión o verruga peruana en el nino. *Anales de la Fac de Med de Lima.* 1949; 32:4.
24. Urteaga O, Payne EH. Treatment of the acute febrile phase of Carrión's disease with chloramphenicol. *Am J Trop Med Hyg.* 1955;4:507–511.
25. McGinnis Hill E, Raji A, Valenzuela MS, Garcia FU, Hoover R. Adhesion to and invasion of cultured human cells by *Bartonella bacilliformis. Infect Immun.* 1992;60; 4051–4058.
26. Garcia FU, Wojta J, Hoover RL. Interactions between live *Bartonella bacilliformis* and endothelial cells. *J Infect Dis.* 1992;165:1138–1141.
27. Weinman D. Infectious anemia due to Bartonella and related red cell parasites. *Trans Am Phylo Soc.* 1944;33: 243–287.
28. Patrucco R. Enfermedad de Carrión. Estudio de inmunidad humoral y celular. *Rev Hosp Ctr Sanidad Fuerzas Policiales.* 1985;2:15–22.
29. Arias-Stella J, Lieberman PH, Erlandson RA, Arias-Stella Jr J. Histology, immunochemistry and ultrastructure of the verruga in Carrión's disease. *Am J Surg Pathol.* 1986;10: 595–610.
30. Arias-Stella J, Lieberman PH, Garcia-Caceres U, Erlandson RA, Kruger H, Arias-Stella J Jr. Verruga peruana mimicking malignant neoplasms. *Am J Dermatopathol.* 1987;9: 279–291.
31. Arrese Estrada J, Greimers R, Maguina-Vargas CP, Pierard GE. Nuclear planimetry and DNA flow cytometry of verruga peruana. *Anat Quant Cytol Histol.* 1992;14:354–358.
32. Arrese Estrada J, Pierard GE. Dendrocytes in verruga peruana and bacillary angiomatosis. *Dermatology.* 1992; 184:22–25.
33. Recavarren S, Lumbreras H. Pathogenesis of the verruga in Carrión disease. *Am J Pathol.* 1986;10:595–610.

CHAPTER 46

Botryomycosis

Francis W. Chandler and John C. Watts

As fester'd members rot but by degree,
Till bones and flesh and sinews fall away, . . .

William Shakespeare (1564–1616), Henry VIII, II

DEFINITION

Botryomycosis (Greek, *botrys,* like a bunch of grapes) is a chronic localized and progressive pseudomycosis caused by certain nonfilamentous bacteria.[1–4] The causative agents are usually gram-positive cocci and, less commonly, gram-negative bacilli. Infection is more frequently confined to the skin and soft tissues, but also can involve viscera.[5–8] In infected tissues, the bacteria characteristically form large, organized aggregates known as grains or granules, the diagnostic hallmark of botryomycosis.[1,9] Clinically, botryomycosis mimics actinomycosis (Chapter 40) and mycetoma (Chapter 113).[5,10] A synonym is bacterial pseudomycosis.

EPIDEMIOLOGY

Botryomycosis is sporadic and worldwide. The male to female ratio is approximately 3:2, and the ages of patients have ranged from 9 months to 80 years.[11] Since the initial description of botryomycosis in a human by Opie in 1913,[12] more than 80 cases have been reported in the literature. The bacterium most frequently isolated has been *Staphylococcus aureus.* Other bacteria cultured from botryomycotic granules include *Pseudomonas aeruginosa, Escherichia coli, Actinobacillus lignieresi, Neisseria mucosa,* and species belonging to the genera *Bacillus, Bacteroides, Proteus,* and *Streptococcus.*[1–4,8,13]

CLINICAL FEATURES

Based on the anatomic sites of involvement, there are two clinical forms of botryomycosis: integumentary (skin and soft tissues) and visceral.[1,2,14] Patients typically present with the integumentary form characterized by an indurated subcutaneous nodule with sinus tracts that open to the skin (Figure 46–1, A). Granules that may be visible with the naked eye are found in the purulent exudate that drains from the sinuses, in curettings, and in sections of infected tissue. The granules are spherical or lobulated, 0.2 to 2.0 mm in diameter, and are soft, yellow or white, organized bacterial aggregates that are microcolonies (Figure 46–1, B).[1,9] Exposed surfaces such as hands, feet, and head are most often involved, and some infections follow local trauma or penetrating injury.[2,15,16] Hematogenous or lymphatic dissemination is rare, but infection often spreads locally to involve contiguous skeletal muscle and bone. In chronic infections, severe fibrosis and destructive osteomyelitis can result in tumefaction and deformity. Visceral botryomycosis is rare and usually develops without associated integumentary infection.[6–8,17–19] Organs most frequently involved include lung, liver, heart, brain, prostate gland, and kidney. When lung is involved, infection can be either primary or, rarely, secondary.[20,21]

PATHOGENESIS

The pathogenesis of granule formation in botryomycosis is not entirely understood. Brunken et al[11] postulated that either defective host resistance or infection by bacteria with attenuated virulence may be key factors in persistence and aggregation of bacteria in botryomycosis. Whatever the underlying cause, the bacterial pathogens are not killed in tissue by host defenses. There have been several reports of botryomycosis in

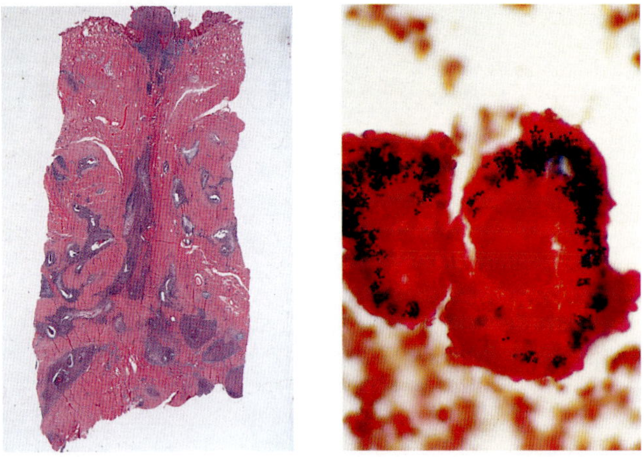

A B

Figure 46–1. (**A**) Botryomycosis of skin and subcutaneous tissue of shoulder. Note multiple interconnecting abscesses that drain into a central sinus tract that erupts onto the surface of the skin through a nodule of granulation tissue [hematoxylin-eosin (H&E), ×1.3]. *(Contributed by Daniel H. Connor, MD.)* (**B**) Granule in one of the abscesses shown in part (**A**). The bacteria form a microcolony, are gram-positive cocci, and are embedded in a dense amorphous coagulum (Brown–Hopps tissue Gram stain, ×200).

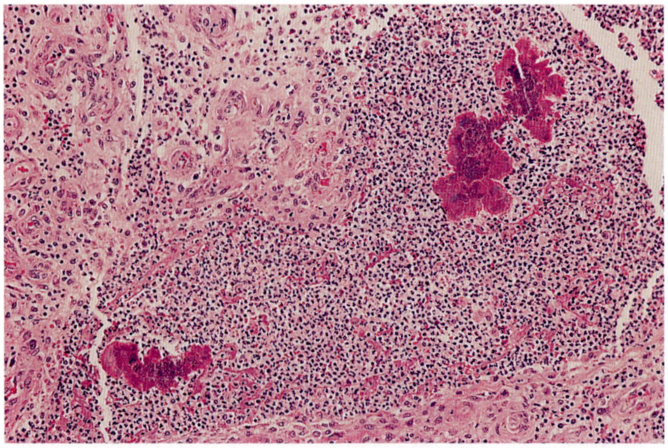

Figure 46–2. Integumentary botryomycosis. A subcutaneous abscess contains three bacterial granules and is surrounded by inflammatory granulation tissue. At this magnification, the granules are best recognized by their hematoxylinophilic centers and prominent, peripheral mantles of eosinophilic Splendore–Hoeppli material (H&E, ×40).

immunodeficient patients, including those with chronic granulomatous disease,[8,21] immunoglobulin deficiencies,[13] and the acquired immunodeficiency syndrome (AIDS).[22] Botryomycosis also has been reported in patients with abnormal functions of their neutrophils,[11,21] and as a complication of cystic fibrosis,[23] diabetes mellitus,[7,20] and extensive follicular mucinosis.[24] Most cases of primary pulmonary botryomycosis have been in children with cystic fibrosis.[20,23]

In one patient with AIDS and botryomycosis,[22] granules composed of gram-positive cocci were demonstrated in the purulent exudate draining from an anal fistula and ischiorectal abscesses. The authors postulated that the bacteria were able to survive, replicate, and aggregate within the cytoplasm of giant cells, followed by extrusion of granules into extracellular spaces, because of defects in intracellular killing of organisms by the mononuclear phagocyte system. The defects were thought to be caused by failure in induction of control of macrophage activity by T-helper lymphocytes.

PATHOLOGY

The abscesses are surrounded by epithelioid histiocytes, giant cells, and granulation tissue with fibrous scarring, and they contain one or more spherical to lobulated granules (Figures 46–2 and 46–3). Abscesses are often interconnected by sinus tracts, both of which contain abundant intact neutrophils that may adhere to the surface of a granule (Figures 46–1, B, 46–4, and 46–5). Eosinophils rarely infiltrate the inflamed tissue.

Bacteria that form botryomycotic granules are usually hematoxylinophilic, and they are embedded in an amorphous eosinophilic to amphophilic matrix or ground substance (Figure 46–5). Immunofluorescence has shown that each bacterium within the granule is surrounded by abundant immunoglobulin that glues the bacteria together.[3,22] Entire granules are often ensheathed by intensely eosinophilic, radiating, finger-like

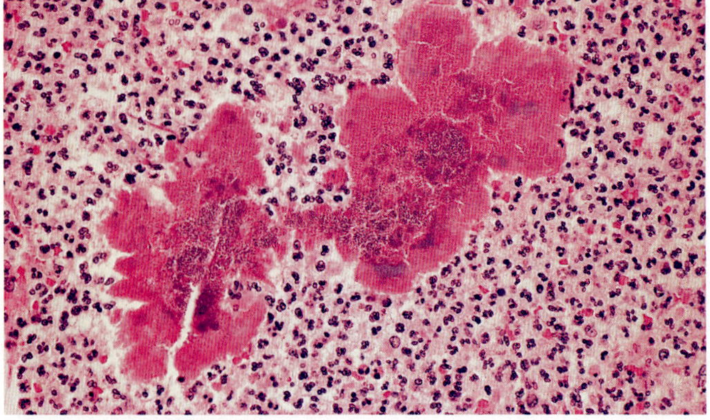

Figure 46–3. Botryomycosis caused by *S aureus*. Two botryomycotic granules are surrounded by an acute suppurative inflammatory reaction. Each granule is composed of compact, finely granular, and hematoxylinophilic bacterial cocci, and is ensheathed by abundant, eosinophilic, Splendore–Hoeppli material (H&E, ×100).

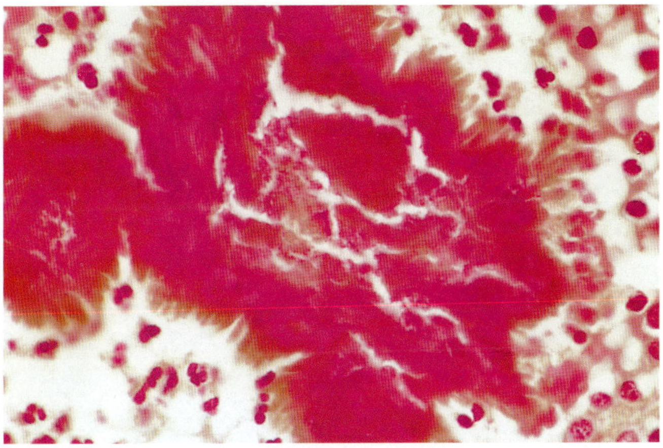

Figure 46–4. Botryomycosis caused by *P aeruginosa.* A granule composed of compact, gram-negative bacilli is located within an inflammatory sinus tract and ensheathed by gram-negative, radiating projections of Splendore–Hoeppli material. Neutrophils intimately adhere to the surface of the granule (Brown–Hopps, ×250).

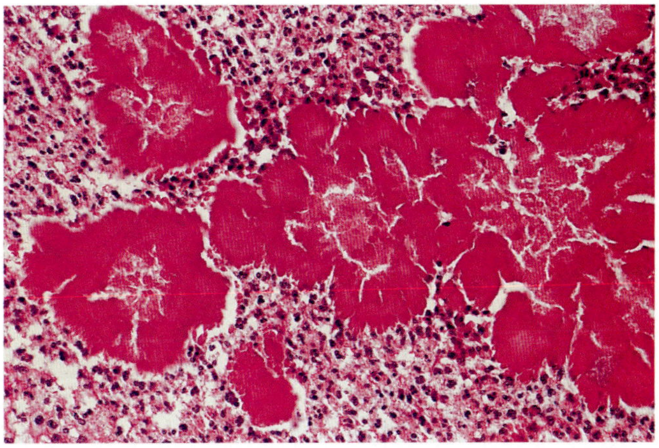

Figure 46–6. *Pseudomonas* botryomycosis. A subcutaneous abscess contains lobulated, bacterial granules surrounded by radiating, broad, finger-like projections of intensely eosinophilic Splendore–Hoeppli material. Aggregated bacteria within the centers of the granules are not readily visible at this magnification (H&E, ×100).

projections of Splendore–Hoeppli material (Figure 46–6). Although the granules are easily detected in H&E stained tissue sections, individual bacteria within the granules are difficult to resolve, even with an oil-immersion objective (Figure 46–5). The morphologic and tinctorial features of the bacteria that form the granules are best demonstrated with modified Gram stains, such as Brown–Brenn (best for gram-positive bacteria) or Brown–Hopps (best for gram-negative bacteria); Splendore–Hoeppli material at the periphery of the granule is gram-negative[9] (Figure 46–7). When these stains are used, bacteria are readily delineated within the granule, where they are often arranged in small, grapelike clusters (Figure 46–8). Foreign materials such as splinters and slivers, presumed to have been introduced with the bacteria by traumatic implantation, also may be detected within or near the granules[9] (Figure 46–9). Giant cells within or at the periphery of an abscess sometimes contain individual and clustered bacteria.

In botryomycotic granules, gram-positive bacteria that were nonviable prior to fixation of the specimen

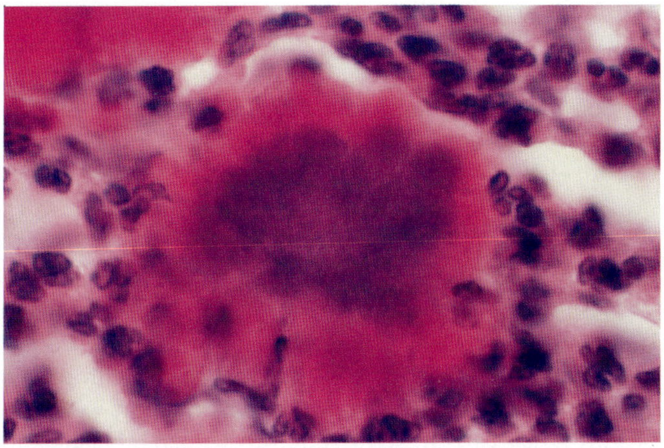

Figure 46–5. Integumentary botryomycosis caused by *S aureus.* The small bacterial granule consists of aggregated, hematoxylinophilic cocci surrounded by brightly eosinophilic Splendore–Hoeppli material. Abundant neutrophils adhere to the surface of the granule. Individual cocci that form the granule are difficult to resolve, even with an oil-immersion objective (H&E, ×500).

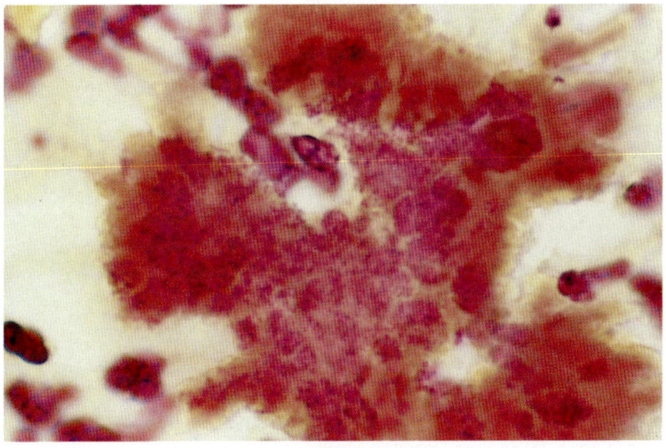

Figure 46–7. *Pseudomonas* botryomycosis. Numerous, compact, gram-negative bacilli that form the granule are visible under an oil-immersion objective. The peripheral Splendore–Hoeppli material is also gram-negative (Brown–Brenn, ×500).

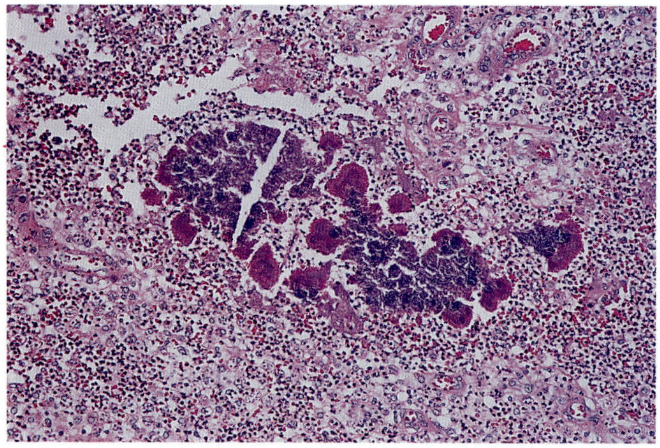

Figure 46–8. Botryomycosis involving the scrotum. A subcutaneous abscess contains a prominent bacterial granule. Note that the hematoxylinophilic bacteria within the granule are arranged in small, grapelike clusters. A peripheral mantle of eosinophilic, Splendore–Hoeppli material is readily visible, even at low magnification (H&E, ×40).

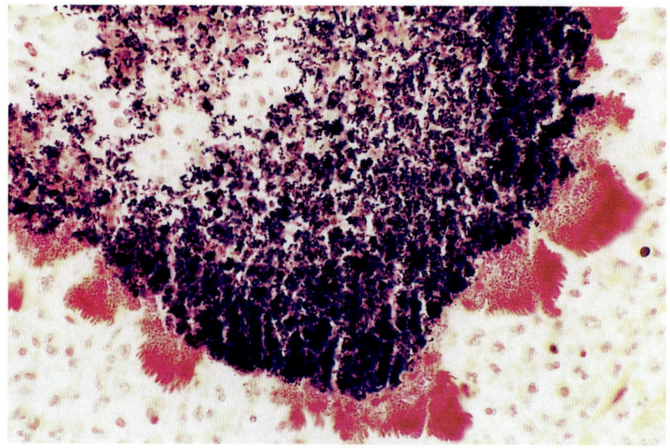

Figure 46–10. Botryomycosis caused by *S aureus*. The center of a large granule is composed of typical, compact, gram-positive cocci. Nonviable staphylococci near the periphery of the granule are refractile and either gram-negative or non-gram-reactive (Brown–Brenn, ×160).

will sometimes swell, be refractile, and gram-negative or non-gram-reactive[9] (Figure 46–10). This is true particularly at the periphery of large granules from patients who had received antibiotic therapy. When this occurs, any of the silver impregnation stains (Steiner, Dieterle, Warthin–Starry) blacken all bacteria nonselectively and are excellent for demonstrating degenerated, non–gram-reactive organisms. Once bacteria are demonstrated, a presumptive histopathologic diagnosis can be confirmed by culture or, if appropriate antibodies are available, by immunohistochemistry.[25] Although one grain usually contains a single type of bacterium, occasionally there may be mixed nonfilamentous bacteria and these may contribute to the pathogenesis of the disease.[9]

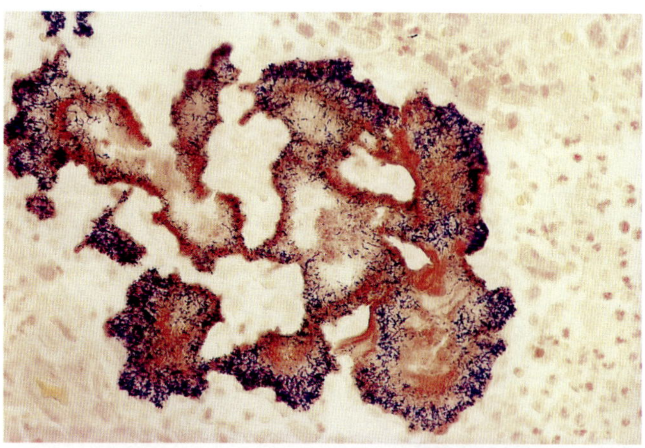

Figure 46–9. Staphylococcal botryomycosis. A perirectal abscess contains a large, lobulated granule composed of abundant gram-positive cocci and pigmented fecal material. Examination with the oil-immersion objective also revealed gram-negative bacilli in the granule (Brown–Brenn, ×100).

DIFFERENTIAL DIAGNOSIS

In H&E-stained sections, granules of botryomycosis usually cannot be distinguished from actinomycosis and actinomycotic mycetoma.[9,10] The host response is also similar in each of these infections, and their respective granules are commonly bordered by radiating clubs of Splendore–Hoeppli material. The three different types of granules can be readily differentiated when appropriate histologic stains are used for the infectious agents. Careful examination at high magnification is necessary to determine the morphologic and tinctorial features of the bacteria.

CONFIRMATIONAL TESTING AND DIAGNOSIS

Histopathologic or cytologic evaluation and culture are needed to distinguish botryomycosis from actinomycosis and actinomycotic mycetoma. Granules in exudates or curettings can be retrieved with forceps, washed in sterile physiologic saline, pressed under a coverslip or between two glass microscope slides, Gram-stained, and examined microscopically. Other washed granules can be inoculated onto culture media, or processed for routine histopathology. When attempting to culture the causal agent, botryomycotic granules should be crushed before inoculation. If only fixed tissues are available, immunohistologic identification of bacteria in deparaffinized sections using species-specific antibodies is a valuable adjunctive tool for diagnosis.[25]

TREATMENT

Selected antibiotics can sometimes be used effectively to treat patients with botryomycosis. Chronic infections, however, do not usually respond to antibiotic therapy alone. Adjunctive surgery combined with prolonged intravenous antibiotics is almost always needed to eradicate the infection.

REFERENCES

1. Winslow DJ. Botryomycosis. *Am J Pathol.* 1959;35: 153–167.
2. Greenblatt M, Heredia R, Rubenstein L, Alpert S. Bacterial pseudomycosis ("botryomycosis"). *Am J Clin Pathol.* 1964;41:188–193.
3. Martin-Pasqual A, Perez AG. Botryomycosis. *Dermatologica.* 1975;51:302–308.
4. Hacker P. Botryomycosis review. *Int J Dermatol.* 1983;22: 455–458.
5. Picou K, Batres E, Jarratt M. Botryomycosis. A bacterial cause of mycetoma. *Arch Dermatol.* 1979;115:609–610.
6. Winslow DJ, Chamblin SA. Disseminated visceral botryomycosis. Report of a fatal case probably caused by *Pseudomonas aeruginosa. Am J Clin Pathol.* 1960;33:43–47.
7. Leibowitz MR, Asvat MS, Kalla AA, Wing G. Extensive botryomycosis in a patient with diabetes and chronic active hepatitis. *Arch Dermatol.* 1981;117:739–742.
8. Washburn RG, Bryan CS, DiSalvo AF, et al. Visceral botryomycosis caused by *Neisseria mucosa* in a patient with chronic granulomatous disease. *J Infect Dis.* 1985;151: 563–564.
9. Chandler FW, Watts JC. *Pathologic Diagnosis of Fungal Infections.* Chicago: ASCP Press; 1987:273–277.
10. Neuhauser EBD. Actinomycosis and botryomycosis. *Postgrad Med.* 1970;48:59–61.
11. Brunken RC, Lichon-Chao N, van den Broeck H. Immunologic abnormalities in botryomycosis. *J Am Acad Dermatol.* 1983;9:428–434.
12. Opie EL. Human botryomycosis of the liver. *Arch Intern Med.* 1913;11:425–439.
13. Bishop GF, Greer KE, Horwitz DA. *Pseudomonas* botryomycosis. *Arch Dermatol.* 1976;112:1568–1570.
14. Auger C. Human actinobacillary and staphylococcic actinophytosis. *Am J Clin Pathol.* 1948;18:645–652.
15. Olmstead M, Finn M. Botryomycosis in pierced ears. *Arch Dermatol.* 1982;118:925–927.
16. Green EG, Schwartz JN. Bacterial pseudomycosis (botryomycosis) in an otherwise normal child. *South Med J.* 1984;77:396–399.
17. Richmond I, Mene A. Renal botryomycosis. *Histopathology.* 1992;20:67–69.
18. Omar T, Cooper K. Botryomycosis of the liver. *Histopathology.* 1995;27:71–73.
19. Wu WQ, Catteneu EA, Lasi A, Halde C. Botryomycosis: first report of human brain involvement. *South Med J.* 1978;71:1530–1533.
20. Speir WA, Mitchener JW, Galloway RF. Primary pulmonary botryomycosis. *Chest.* 1971;60:92–93.
21. Paz HL, Little BJ, Ball WC, Winkelstein JA. Primary pulmonary botryomycosis. A manifestation of chronic granulomatous disease. *Chest.* 1992;101:1160–1162.
22. Toth IR, Kazal HL. Botryomycosis in acquired immunodeficiency syndrome. *Arch Pathol Lab Med.* 1987;111: 246–249.
23. Katznelsen D, Vawter GF, Foley GE, Shwachman H. Botryomycosis, a complication of cystic fibrosis. *J Pediatr.* 1964;65:525–539.
24. Harman RRM, English MP, Halford M, et al. Botryomycosis. A complication of extensive follicular mucinosis. *Br J Dermatol.* 1980;102:215–222.
25. Cartun RW. Immunohistochemistry of infectious diseases. *J Histotechnol.* 1995;18:195–202.

CHAPTER 47

Brucellosis

Edward J. Young

Anyone who lives on milk, being still an infant, is not acquainted with the teaching about righteousness.

Hebrews 5:13

A good cow may have an ill calf.
An ill cow may have a good calf.

Scottish Proverbs

DEFINITION

Brucellosis (undulant fever, Mediterranean fever, Malta fever) is a zoonosis caused by bacteria belonging to the genus *Brucella.* Humans are accidental hosts, acquiring the disease by direct contact with infected animals or by ingesting contaminated milk or milk products. The spectrum of human illness ranges from subclinical to chronic, but the disease rarely is fatal.

GEOGRAPHIC DISTRIBUTION

Brucellosis, although worldwide, is especially prevalent in the Mediterranean basin, the Arabian peninsula, the Indian subcontinent, Mexico, and in parts of Central America, South America, and Africa. In the United States, human brucellosis is rare, with fewer than 100 infections reported to the Centers for Disease Control and Prevention in each of the years from 1992 through 1995.

EPIDEMIOLOGY AND NATURAL HISTORY

Virtually all human infections are traced to direct or indirect contact with animals. Traditionally the risk of contracting brucellosis was greatest among ranchers, veterinarians, workers in abattoirs, and laboratory personnel; however, recent studies in Texas[1] and in California[2] indicate that transmission of *B melitensis* is principally foodborne, involving unpasteurized goat cheese. Identification of the species or biovars of *Brucella* recovered from humans can be a clue to the source of infection. *Brucella abortus* is usually of bovine origin, whereas *B melitensis* generally comes from goats or sheep. *Brucella suis* biovar 1 is limited to swine in North and South America; *B suis* biovar 2 is confined mainly to Europe, and *B suis* biovar 4 is restricted to Arctic caribou and reindeer. *Brucella canis* is a pathogen of dogs and is the least common cause of human infection.

MORPHOLOGY AND ULTRASTRUCTURE

The brucellae are small, gram-negative coccobacilli that lack flagella, endospores, or a capsule. The ultrastructure is similar to the enterobacteria, with a cell envelope consisting of an outer layer of lipopolysaccharide protein. The surface polysaccharide of smooth (S) strains consists of a homopolymer of *N*-formyl perosamine (4-formamido-4,6-dideoxy-D-mannose). The lipid components are in close proximity to the peptidoglycan layer, which forms the major part of the cell wall. Matrix and porin proteins penetrate the peptidoglycan at irregular intervals and are partially exposed at the cell surface. The results of DNA–DNA hybridization reveal a high degree of relatedness between all of the *Brucella* nomen species. Restriction endonuclease analysis shows differences in base sequences between species and strains. DNA–RNA hybridization suggests a relationship between *Brucella* and the genera *Agrobacterium, Phyllobacterium,* and *Rhizobium,* which are plant pathogens.

CLINICAL FEATURES

The bacteria invade through the alimentary tract, lungs, conjunctivae, and abrasions of the skin. The nutritional and immune status of the host, the route of inoculation, the species of *Brucella,* and the size of the inoculum may each be important variables in determining whether infection occurs. Regardless of the route of infection, organisms localize in tissues of the reticuloendothelial system, and involvement of the lymph nodes, spleen, liver, and bone marrow are common. The incubation time is variable, but symptoms usually occur within 3 to 4 weeks of exposure. The onset can be insidious or abrupt. The disease is characterized by a multitude of nonspecific symptoms, including fever, chills, profuse (often malodorous) sweats, body aches, anorexia, lethargy, fatigue, mental inattention, and depression. Often there is a paucity of abnormal physical findings.[3]

PATHOLOGY

Heart and Blood Vessels

Endocarditis is the most common fatal complication, occurring in from less than 1% to 3% of patients.[4] Before effective antimicrobial chemotherapy and surgery to replace infected heart valves, brucella endocarditis was nearly always fatal.[5] The aortic valve is involved more commonly than the mitral valve, and aneurysms or abscesses of the sinus of Valsalva are especially common (Figure 47–1). Mycotic aneurysms of the ventricle, brain, aorta, and other arteries have been reported. Histologic examination of the myocardium often reveals focal collections of mononuclear cells, and rarely granulomas. Disseminated intravascular coagulation (DIC) with splenic and renal infarcts is common. Pericarditis can accompany endocarditis or can be the principal manifestation. Rapid techniques to isolate brucella from blood, combined with two-dimensional echocardiography, have improved the ability to diagnose endocarditis, and medical and surgical therapies have improved the outcome.[5,6]

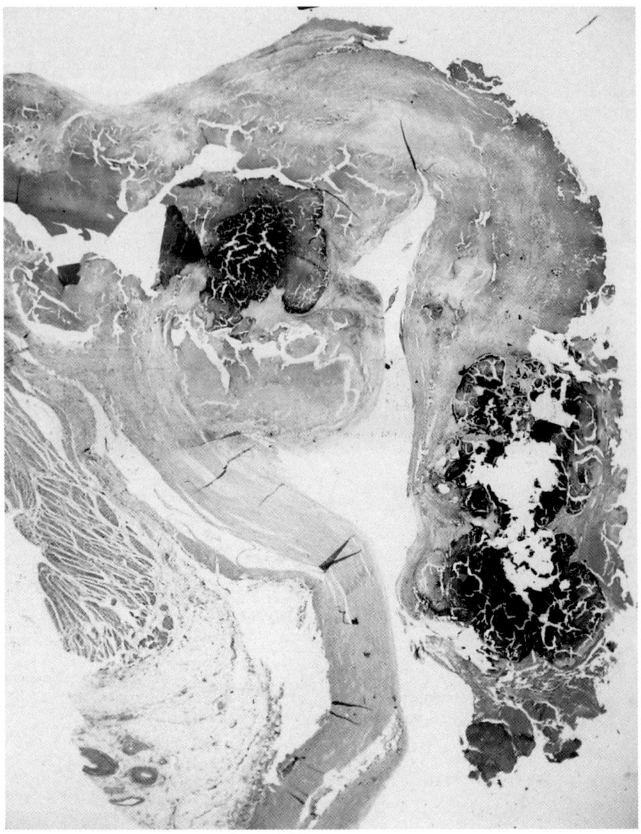

Figure 47–1. Aortic valve (*B abortus*); partially calcified, deformed valve of infective endocarditis (AFIP Neg 73-904; ×6.5).

Neurobrucellosis

Direct invasion of the nervous system in brucellosis is rare, occurring in less than 5% of patients. A variety of neurologic syndromes have been described, including meningitis, encephalitis, radiculoneuritis, myelitis, cerebral mycotic aneurysm, and peripheral neuropathy.[7] *Brucella* meningitis can be acute or chronic; in the latter, psychiatric manifestations are common.[8] Analysis of cerebrospinal fluid (CSF) reveals elevated protein, a lymphocytic pleocytosis, and, in some patients, hypoglycorrhachia. Organisms are rarely seen by Gram's stain, and cultures of CSF yield growth in less than 25%. Most patients have specific antibodies in serum. Oligoclonal IgG in CSF suggests intrathecal antibody production. Although the infection usually spreads hematogenously, brucella spondylitis has been reported to extend into the CSF.[9] Histologic findings in neurobrucellosis include leptomeningitis, adhesive arachnoiditis, vasculitis, and leukoencephalitis (Figure 47–2).

Liver and Biliary Tract

Although hepatomegaly is reported in only 30% to 60% of patients and liver function tests can be normal, the liver is probably always involved in brucellosis, even if

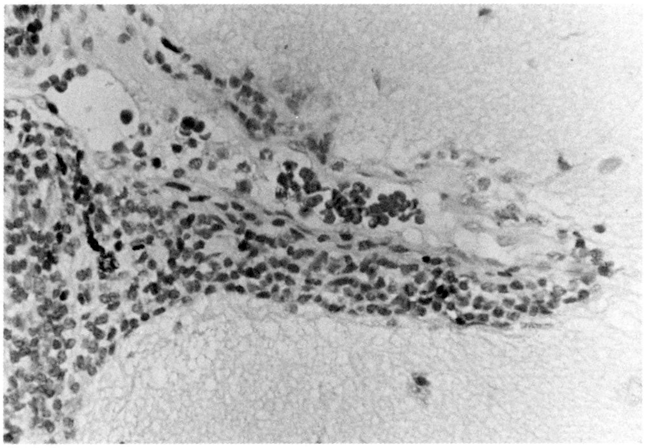

Figure 47–2. Meningeal biopsy (*B suis*) showing infiltrate of lymphocytes and plasma cells and small amount of hemosiderin (hematoxylin-eosin, original magnification ×350). *(Photograph courtesy of T. Satterwhite.)*

only transiently. A variety of hepatic lesions have been described, including noncaseating granulomas, which are indistinguishable from sarcoidosis.[10] In addition, nonspecific hepatitis without granulomas has been reported, notably when infection is caused by *B melitensis*.[11] Chronic suppurative lesions of the liver, often with calcification, have been described in infections caused by *B suis*. The spectrum of hepatic lesions caused by *B melitensis* is illustrated in Figures 47–3 and 47–4. In spite of the extent of hepatic injury, cirrhosis resulting from brucella hepatitis is rare. Another complication is acute cholecystitis, in which the mucosa of the gallbladder is infiltrated with inflammatory cells or granulomas.

Bones and Joints

Osteoarticular complications occur in 20% to 40% of patients with brucellosis.[12] Sacroiliitis is reported to be the most common lesion, followed by arthropathy involving the hips, knees, and other joints. Spondylitis of the lumbar spine is common and is diagnosed by bone scan, computed tomography or nuclear magnetic resonance scan.[13] Osteomyelitis can involve the long bones but is most common in the vertebrae, where it resembles spinal tuberculosis. Both suppurative and reactive arthritis have been described. Synovial fluid contains a mononuclear cell pleocytosis, elevated protein, and normal concentrations of glucose. Cultures of joint fluid yield brucellae in about 50% of patients. Biopsy specimens of synovial tissue reveal a nonspecific proliferative synovitis with neovascularization, chronic inflammation, and occasionally granulomas. The rate of recovery of brucellae from bone marrow is said to be greater than from blood.[14] Granulomas are detected in bone marrow in up to 75% of patients[15]; however, they are usually small and have indistinct borders (Figure 47–5). Occasionally there is an increase in histiocytes, which may show erythrophagocytosis.[16]

Spleen and Lymph Nodes

As with the liver, the spleen is probably always involved in brucellosis. Splenomegaly is reported in 20% to 40% of patients. Among the pathologic changes are nodular lymphoid hyperplasia, increased numbers

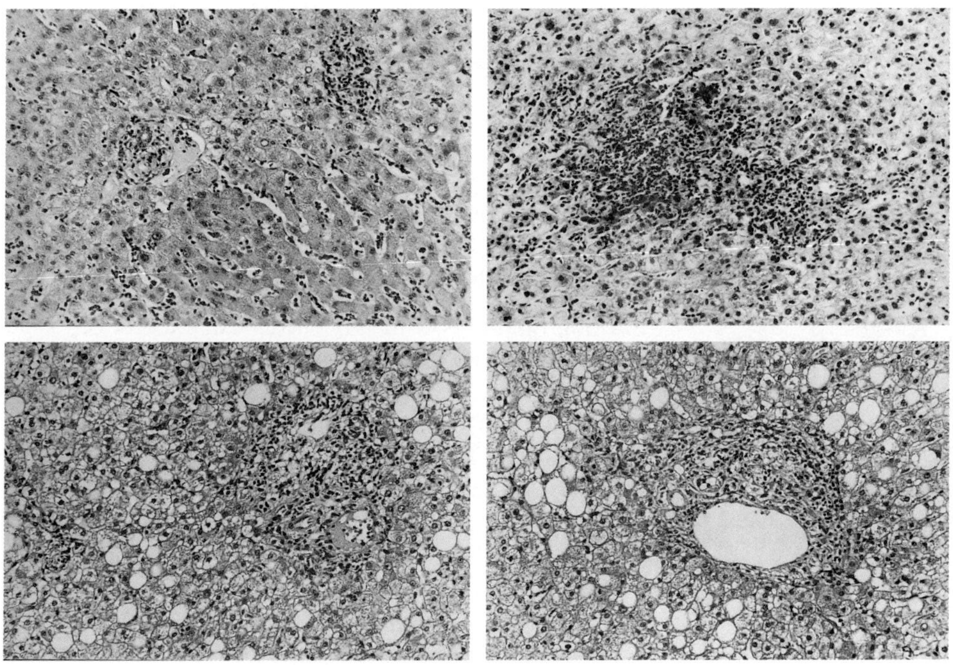

Figure 47–3. The spectrum of hepatic lesions (*B melitensis*). (*Upper left*) There are small aggregates of mononuclear cells within portal triads and around individual foci of hepatocellular necrosis. (*Upper right*) There are larger and more conspicuous aggregates obscuring the portal structures and expanding into adjacent liver parenchyma in a fashion indistinguishable from active hepatitis. (*Lower left and right*) Aggregates of inflammatory cells that include histiocytes form loose granulomas. These may be in portal triads (*lower left*) or adjacent to central veins (*lower right*) (hematoxylin-eosin, original magnification ×200).

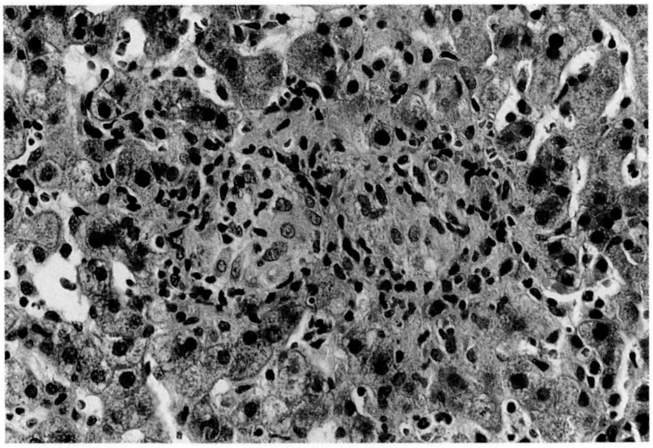

Figure 47–4. The spectrum of hepatic lesions (*B melitensis*) continued. There are two small granulomas comprised of epithelioid cells and histiocytes in the parenchyma. Small discrete granulomas such as these may be more common in infections caused by *B abortus* (hematoxylin-eosin, ×400).

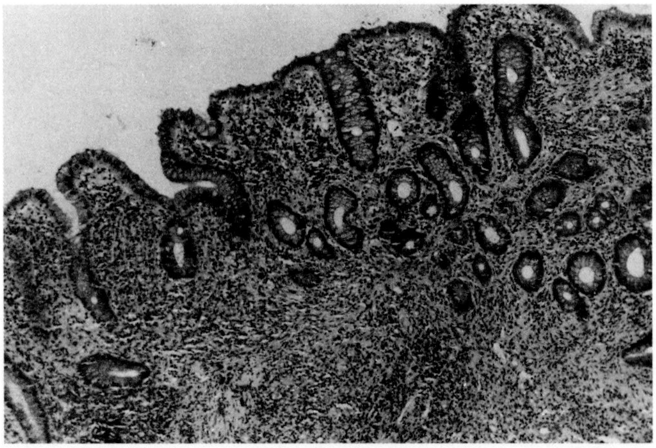

Figure 47–6. Colon (*B melitensis*) showing distortion of the colonic mucosa with irregular size, shape, and distribution of crypts. Dense inflammatory infiltrate in the lamina propria (hematoxylin-eosin, original magnification ×80). *(Photograph courtesy of E. Stermer, Am J Gastroenterol. 1991;86:918.)*

of macrophages, and, occasionally, small granulomas.[17] Partially calcified splenic granulomas, notably those caused by *B suis,* have on rare occasions appeared many years after the original infection. Similarly, lymphadenopathy is a common finding, and suppurative lymphadenitis caused by *B suis* has been reported.

Lungs

Airborne transmission of brucellosis is suspected and is especially common in abattoirs.[18] Respiratory tract manifestations of brucellosis, nevertheless, are rare, and most diagnoses have been made by abnormal chest roentgenograms in patients with serologic or bacteriologic evidence of systemic infection. Rarely have brucellae been identified in stains or cultures of sputum. Granulomas of the lung caused by brucella can, by x ray, resemble bronchogenic carcinoma.[19]

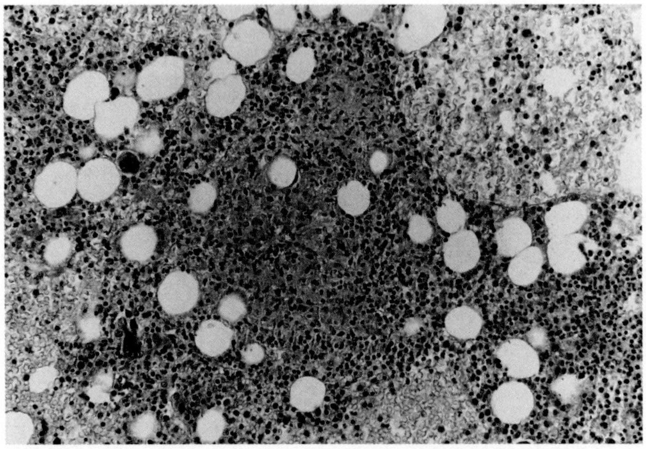

Figure 47–5. Bone marrow (*B melitensis*) showing coalesced epithelioid cell granulomas surrounded by a thin rim of lymphocytes (hematoxylin-eosin, original magnification ×200).

Gastrointestinal Tract

Brucellosis, like typhoid fever, is an enteric fever in which systemic symptoms usually predominate over gastrointestinal complaints. Nevertheless, anorexia, nausea, vomiting, abdominal pain, diarrhea, or constipation are common complaints. Autopsy studies from the preantibiotic era described hyperemia of the intestinal mucosa, but ulcerations of Peyer's patches was said to be less common than in typhoid fever.[20] Evidence of ileocecal involvement by *B melitensis* has been documented radiographically and by endoscopic biopsy. Microscopic examination of the ileocecal valve reveals shallow erosions bordered by granulation tissue infiltrated by lymphocytes and histiocytes (Figure 47–6).[21,22]

Genitourinary Tract

Although patients with brucellosis can excrete brucellae in their urine, renal involvement is uncommon. Chronic pyelonephritis characterized by infiltrates of lymphocytes and occasionally granulomas can mimic renal tuberculosis (Figures 47–7 and 47–8). Glomerulonephritis, believed to be of immune complex origin, can complicate brucella endocarditis. In addition, rare cases of focal glomerulonephritis have been reported in which mesangial deposits of IgA were found. Orchitis is reported in up to 20% of men with brucellosis. The testes or epididymis are infiltrated with lymphocytes

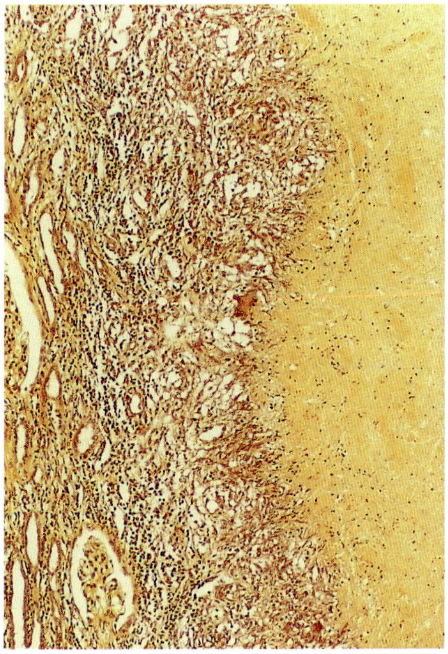

Figure 47–7. Caseating granuloma, caused by *B abortus,* in the kidney of a Midwestern cattle farmer. The granuloma is sharply circumscribed. Langhans giant cells and epithelioid cells, some of which are pallisaded, surround the caseating central area. A narrow band of viable kidney around the necrotic center contains lymphocytes (Brown–Hopps tissue gram stain, ×200). *(Courtesy of Daniel H. Connor, MD, and Ernest E. Lack, MD.)*

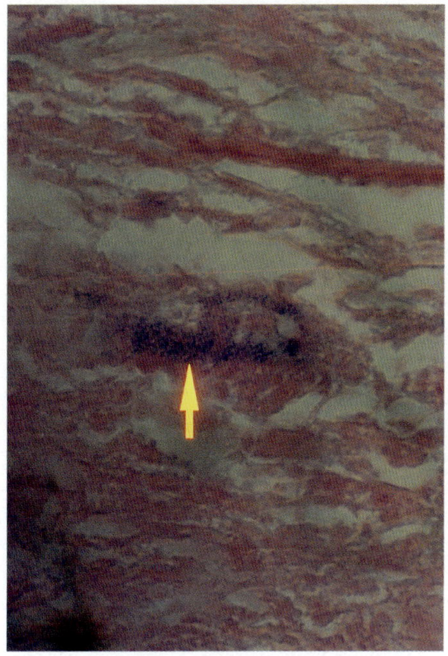

Figure 47–8. Same granuloma shown in Figure 47–7; a rare attempt to demonstrate *Brucella* organisms in tissue sections. There are a few scattered clusters of faintly stained coccobacilli in the caseating area (*arrow*) (Giemsa stain, ×1000). *(Courtesy of Daniel H. Connor, MD, and Ernest E. Lack, MD.)*

and plasma cells, and there is atrophy of the seminiferous tubules. In women, rare cases of salpingitis, cervicitis, and pelvic abscesses have been reported. Although brucellosis can cause abortion, there is little evidence that the incidence is higher than with other bacteremic infections.

Laboratory Diagnosis

A definitive diagnosis is made by recovering brucellae from blood or other tissues. In the absence of bacteriologic confirmation, a presumptive diagnosis is made by demonstrating high or rising titers of specific antibodies in the serum. A variety of serologic methods have been applied to brucellosis, but the serum agglutination test (SAT) is most widely used.[23] The SAT measures the total quantity of agglutinating antibodies (IgM, IgG, and IgA). Because low titers of IgM antibodies can persist for months to years after infection, the presence of IgG agglutinins correlates best with active infection. To differentiate between IgM and IgG antibodies, the SAT is performed with the addition of 0.05 mol/L 2-mercaptoethanol (2ME), which renders IgM antibodies nonagglutinable. Regardless of the method, serologic tests for brucellosis should be performed with standardized antigens and using appropriate controls. In addition, serum samples should always be diluted beyond 1:320 in order to avoid a prozone reaction. Although no single titer is always diagnostic, the majority of patients with active infection have titers higher than 160. The interpretation of brucella serologic tests must be correlated with the history, other clinical data, and epidemiologic information.

REFERENCES

1. Taylor PM, Perdue JN. The changing epidemiology of human brucellosis in Texas, 1977–1986. *Am J Epidemiol.* 1989;130:160–165.
2. Chomel BB, DeBess EE, Mangiamele DM, et al. Changing trends in the epidemiology of human brucellosis in California from 1973 to 1992: a shift toward foodborne transmission. *J Infect Dis.* 1994;170:1216–1223.
3. Young EJ. Human brucellosis. *Rev Infect Dis.* 1983; 5:821–842.
4. Peery TM, Belter LF. Brucellosis and heart disease. II. Fatal brucellosis: a review of the literature and report of new cases. *Am J Pathol.* 1960;36:673–697.
5. Jacobs F, Abramowicz D, Vereerstraeten P, LeClerc JL, Zech F, Thys JP. Brucella endocarditis: the role of combined medical and surgical treatment. *Rev Infect Dis.* 1990; 12:740–744.

6. Al-Harthi SS. The morbidity and mortality pattern of *Brucella* endocarditis. *Intern J Cardiol.* 1989;25:321–324.
7. Bouza E, Garcia de la Torre M, Parras F, Guerrero A, Rodriquez-Creixems M, Gobernado J. Brucellar meningitis. *Rev Infect Dis.* 1987;9:810–822.
8. Mousa ARM, Koshy T, Araj GF, et al. Brucella meningitis: presentation, diagnosis and treatment. A prospective study of ten cases. *Quart J Med.* 1986;60:873–885.
9. McLean DR, Russell N, Khan MY. Neurobrucellosis: clinical and therapeutic features. *Clin Infect Dis.* 1992;15: 582–590.
10. Spink WW, Hoffbauer FW, Walker WW, Green RA. Histopathology of the liver in human brucellosis. *J Lab Clin Med.* 1949;34:40–58.
11. Young EJ. *Brucella melitensis* hepatitis: the absence of granulomas. *Ann Intern Med.* 1979;91:414–415.
12. Gotuzzo E, Alarcon GS, Bocanegra TS, et al. Articular involvement in human brucellosis: a retrospective analysis of 304 cases. *Sem Arthritis Rheum.* 1982;12:245–255.
13. Ariza J, Gudiol F, Valverde J, et al. Brucellar spondylitis: a detailed analysis based on current findings. *Rev Infect Dis.* 1985;7:656–664.
14. Gotuzzo E. Carrillo C, Guerra J, Llosa L. An evaluation of diagnostic methods for brucellosis: the value of bone marrow cultures. *J Infect Dis.* 1986;153:122–125.
15. Sundberg D, Spink WW. The histopathology of lesions in the bone marrow of patients having active brucellosis. *Blood.* 1947;(special issue 1)7–32.
16. Martin-Moreno S, Soto-Guzman O, Bernaldo-de-Quiros J, Reverte-Cejudo D, Bascones-Casas C. Pancytopenia due to hemo-phagocytosis in patients with brucellosis: a report of four cases. *J Infect Dis.* 1983;147:445–449.
17. Hunt AC, Bothwell PW. Histologic findings in human brucellosis. *J Clin Pathol.* 1967;20:267–272.
18. Kaufmann AF, Fox MD, Boyce JM, et al. Airborne spread of brucellosis. *Ann NY Acad Sci.* 1980;353:105–114.
19. Lubani MM, Lulu AR, Araj GF, Khateeb MI, Qurtom MAF, Dudin KI. Pulmonary brucellosis. *Quart J Med.* 1989;71: 319–324.
20. Sharp WB. Pathology of undulant fever. *Arch Pathol.* 1934;18:72–108.
21. Jorens PG, Michielsen PP, Van den Enden EJ, et al. A rare cause of colitis: *Brucella melitensis*. *Dis Colon Rectum.* 1991;34:194–196.
22. Stermer E, Levy N, Potasman I, Jaffe M, Boss J. Brucellosis as a cause of severe colitis. *Am J Gastroenterol.* 1991;86: 917–919.
23. Young EJ. Serologic diagnosis of human brucellosis: analysis of 214 cases by agglutination tests and review of the literature. *Rev Infect Dis.* 1991;13:359–372.

CHAPTER 48

Buruli Ulcer—Infection with *Mycobacterium ulcerans*

Michael J. Carey and Daniel H. Connor

Ugliness is a point of view; an ulcer is wonderful to a pathologist.

Austin O'Malley

DEFINITION AND SYNONYMS

Mycobacterium ulcerans is an acid-fast bacillus that grows optimally at 32°C and infects the skin and subcutaneous tissue of humans. The typical ulcer is an indolent, essentially painless, necrotizing ulcer. Synonyms include Buruli ulcer (Uganda), Searle's ulcer and Bairnsdale ulcer (Australia), and Kakerifu ulcer and Toro ulcer (Zaire).

EPIDEMIOLOGY

Infection by *M ulcerans* was first described as a disease in the Bairnsdale district in Australia in 1948, although Sir Albert Cook may have described the disease in Africa in 1897. Infection by *M ulcerans* has been identified in Australia,[1] Benin, Bolivia, Cameroon, Congo (Brazzaville), Gabon,[2] Ghana, Ivory Coast, Liberia,[3] Malaysia, Mexico, New Guinea,[4] Nigeria,[5] Sri Lanka, Uganda, Republic of Zaire, and probably also in Angola, Peru, northern Sumatra, and Mozambique (Figure 48–1). Two cases reported from Kiribati,[6] in the Pacific, were atypical clinically and pathologically had neither the characteristic fat necrosis nor acid-fast bacilli. They are probably not infection by *M ulcerans.* Mayman has postulated that the endemic areas share a common origin, the ancient southern land mass Gondwana, which plate tectonics subsequently separated into India, Australia, New Guinea, Africa, South America, and Antarctica, with *M ulcerans* now spanning these separate land masses.[7,8] Those afflicted tend to live in swampy lowlands and in river valleys that drain rain forests. In Uganda, patients live along the course of the Victoria Nile, in Zaire they live in isolated swamps along the Zaire River and its major tributaries, and in New Guinea they live along the Kamusi River. Most of these areas are sparsely populated. Contagion is unlikely, although in Benin a high rate of infection among closely related patients was described.[9] There is no convincing evidence that an insect transmits or harbors *M ulcerans.* Because single lesions predominate, most investigators believe that the organism enters through the skin.

The opinion that infection follows percutaneous inoculation is supported by the observation that infections have developed at sites of hypodermic injections and other penetrating traumas. All types of penetrating trauma in endemic areas are therefore suspect, and Meyers et al[10] have described Buruli ulcers arising at the site of trauma. In Uganda, grasses used in thatching have been studied as possible vehicles for *M ulcerans,* but without conclusive results. As with other mycobacteria, *M ulcerans* survives exposure to ultraviolet light only briefly, so an open reservoir such as vegetation seems unlikely. Most lesions occur on the lower limbs, however, so exposure to soil and vegetation could be a causal factor. Because some endemic areas parallel slow moving rivers, some researchers believe the reservoir is in or near open water. Many patients, however, never contact river water directly.

Koala bears of Australia acquire the infection in nature and are thus reservoirs for *M ulcerans,* but no other aquatic or land animals are known to be naturally

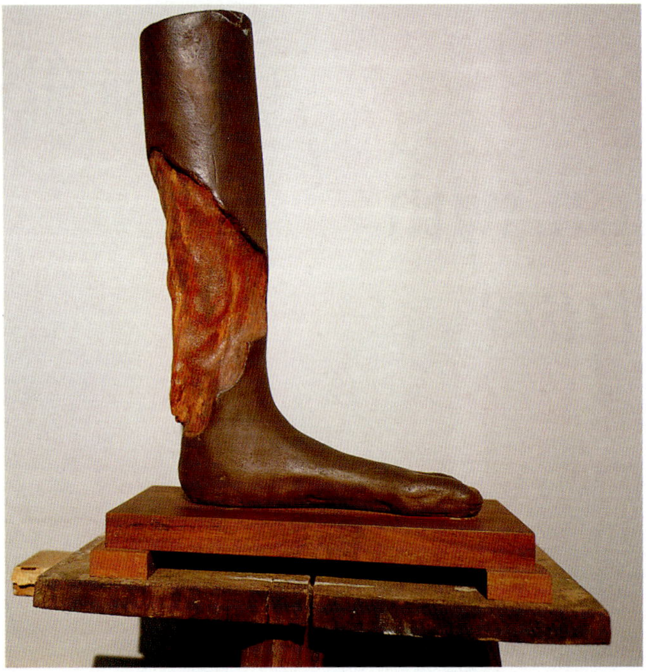

Figure 48–1. Model of a Buruli ulcer in the medical museum, Lorenzo Marques, Mozambique. This museum was developed under the supervision of the late Professor Emanuel Prâtes. Several models of chronic cutaneous ulcers were in his museum. They were undiagnosed and all characteristic of Buruli ulcer. *(Photograph courtesy of Daniel H. Connor, MD, 1964.)*

infected.[11] A study conducted in the Ivory Coast suggests a link between endemic progression of *M ulcerans* and increasing numbers of Tilapia, a freshwater fish that could serve as a reservoir.[12] Snakes also have been implicated as reservoirs. One report describes disseminated osteomyelitis developing after a snakebite,[13] probably a consequence of contamination by *M ulcerans* of the venomous wound.

Persons of all age groups may be infected, but graphs show a peak incidence in the second and third decades of life. Children younger than 15 years of age are most commonly affected, with no overall sex difference in most studies.[14] The incidence and prevalence are unknown, but in one endemic area along the Victoria Nile almost 10% of recently settled refugees became infected over a period of about 2 years. Generally, however, endemic areas tend to be sparsely populated so that the total number of those exposed is small. Recent reports have suggested an increasing incidence in West Africa. A study in the Daloa region of the Ivory Coast,[15] for instance, shows a threefold increase between 1987 and 1991, with a local prevalence as high as 16.3% Proximity to the Lobos River correlates with increased risk.

More frequent infection of the right arm and leg tends to implicate handedness, or some related activity, but swimming and fishing in the Lobos river did not increase risk. Long trousers were protective, especially against infection of legs. Rate was highest at 10 to 14 years of age (143 per 1000) with no gender difference. Little is known of the epidemiology in the Americas, but as data develop, a comparison with other endemic areas will probably yield further clues to other reservoirs of *M ulcerans* and to the mechanism of its transmission.

CLINICAL FEATURES

The first sign is a slowly enlarging, hard, circumscribed, movable mass in the subcutaneous tissue (Figure 48–2). The nodule is not painful, tender, red, or swollen, but the overlying skin itches. As the mass enlarges, a blister develops, breaks when scratched, then forms an ulcer. The ulcer gradually expands and deepens. X-ray examination may reveal mineralization (Figures 48–3 through 48–5). The perimeter of the developed ulcer is usually scalloped, sometimes widely undermined, and the base is partly or completely covered by a white necrotic

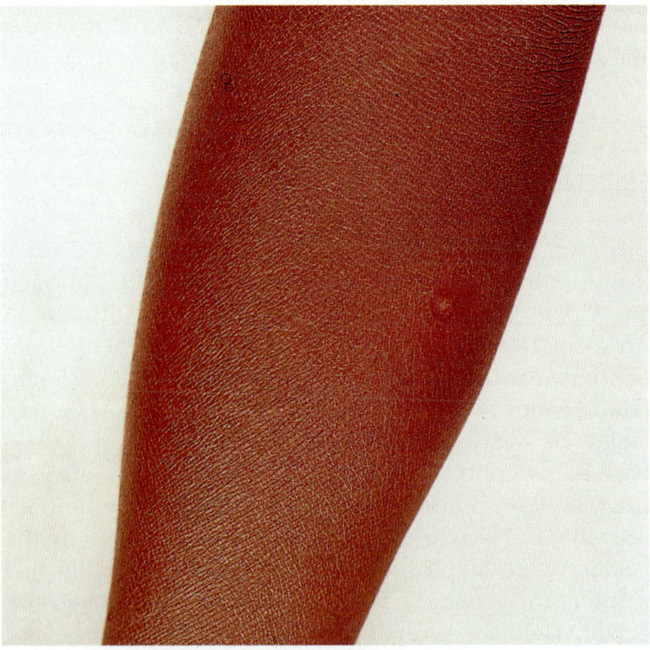

Figure 48–2. Swelling of the mid forearm in a 9-year-old Ugandan youth. The swelling was a 3- × 5-cm area of induration. A small blister is beginning to form over the center of the induration. The blister itched. *(Photograph courtesy of Daniel H. Connor, MD, 1963.)*

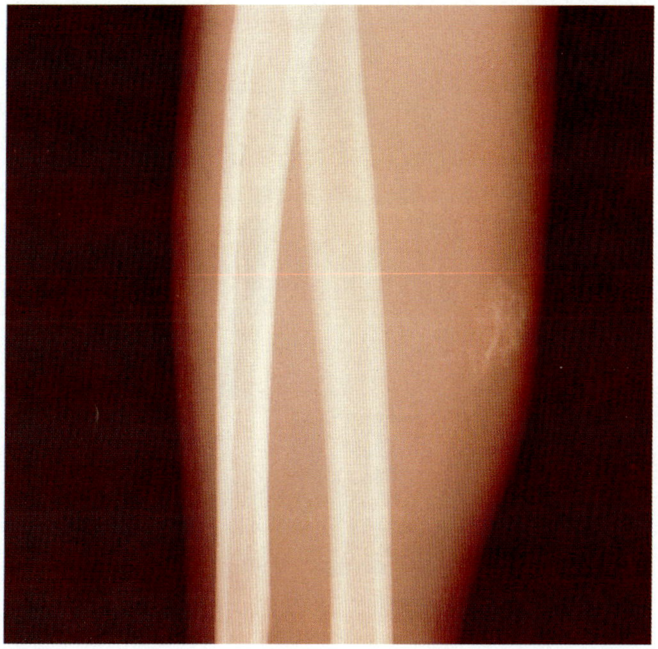

Figure 48–3. X-ray of the forearm shown in Figure 48–2. There are mineral deposits in the area of induration (AFIP Neg 65-3139.).

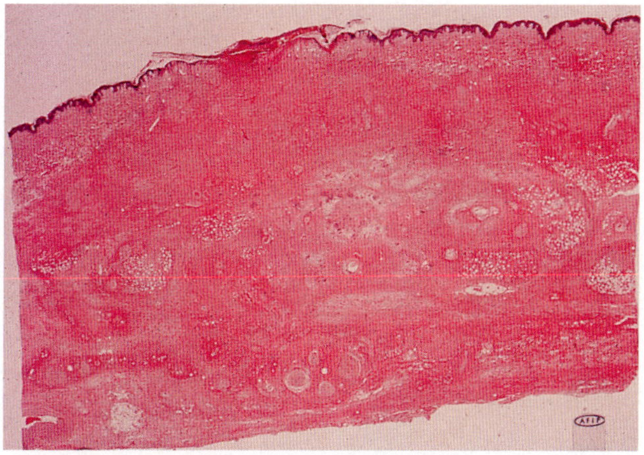

Figure 48–4. Section of the lesion shown in Figures 48–2 and 48–3. Mineralization is not conspicuous, but the necrosis of the dermis is characteristic of infection by *M ulcerans*. Somatic nuclei are lost as is the capillary circulation. A ghost outline of the tissue remains. Ghosts of vessels, nerves, collagen, fat cells, and lobules can be identified (AFIP Neg 65-1411; hematoxylin-eosin, ×4).

coagulum (Figure 48–6). As the ulcer enlarges, the surrounding skin becomes edematous. Even when ulcers are large (Figures 48–7 and 48–8), patients feel well, remain active, have no fever, malaise, or lymphadenopathy, and have no leukocytosis. The uncomplicated ulcer is not malodorous, and secondary bacterial infection is usually not a problem. Desquamation and hyperpigmentation of the skin around the advancing edge of the ulcer may be prominent. Most ulcers are on the limbs, frequently over major joints, but about 10% are on the trunk (Figure 48–9). The palms and soles are spared, and the face and scalp are only rarely involved. Sometimes ulcers remain small and inconspicuous while infection spreads widely in the subcutaneous tissues. For example, even if not ulcerated, the skin over a wide area may be detached from fascia (Figure 48–10). Ulcers may persist for months or years, but eventually tend to heal even if modern medical care is not available (Figure 48–11). Healing usually begins at the proximal or upper margin and may progress across the base of the ulcer, while there is extension of the ulcer at the distal or dependent margin. The result is a broad, depressed scar (Figure 48–12). Complications are common. Some patients develop contraction deformity and lymphedema, and in other patients gradual extension has prompted amputation.

PATHOGENESIS AND PATHOLOGY

Sections through skin and subcutaneous adipose tissue reveal yellow or yellowish-gray areas of opaque necrosis in dermis, lower dermis, and panniculus. Microscopically, the early, nonulcerated lesions are circum-

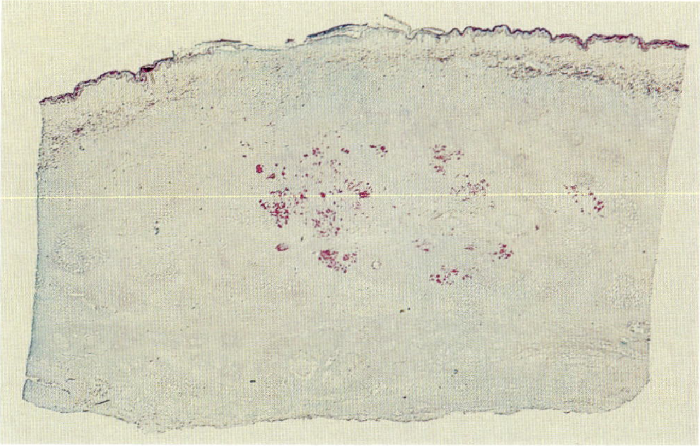

Figure 48–5. A parallel section of the section shown in Figure 48–4. Clusters of acid-fast bacilli are localized in the center of the necrosis. The perimeter of the necrotic zone is free of organisms (Ziehl–Neelsen stain, ×4).

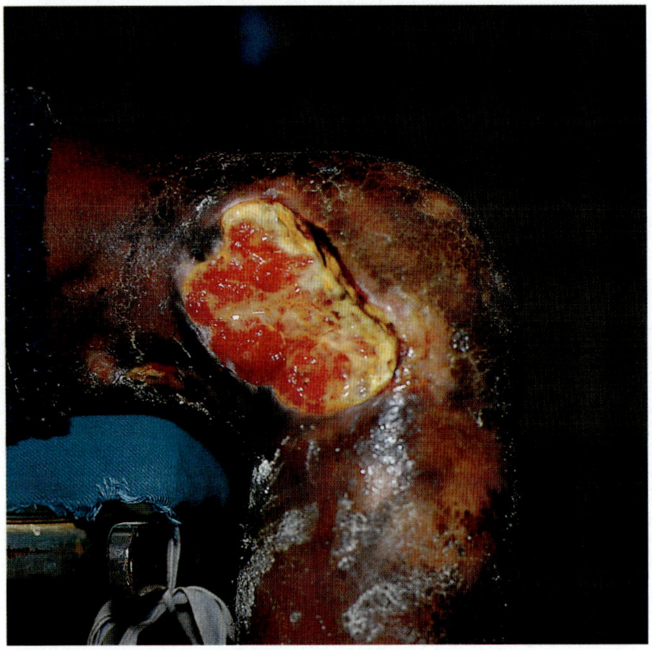

Figure 48–6. An 8-year-old boy from Fasawolu, Liberia, with a Buruli ulcer on the lateral aspect of his right knee. The edges are scalloped and undermined, and part of the base is covered with a yellow coagulum. His knee was frozen at 90 degrees flexion. *(Photograph courtesy of Daniel H. Connor, MD, 1978.)*

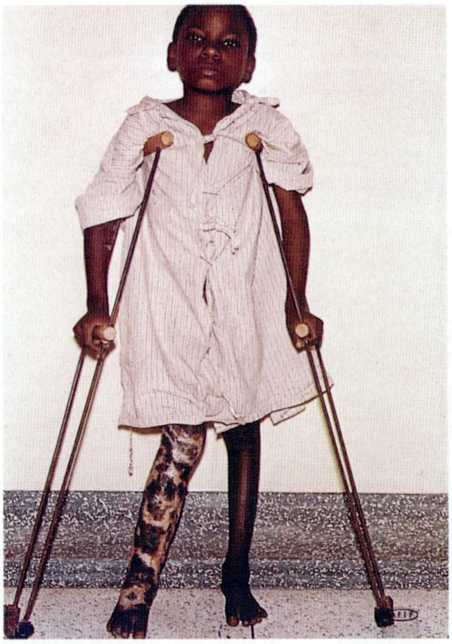

Figure 48–8. The same patient shown in Figure 48–7, 7 months after coming to Mulago Hospital. He left the hospital with his mother 1 month later. He had no recurrence. *(Photograph courtesy of Daniel H. Connor, MD, 1963.)*

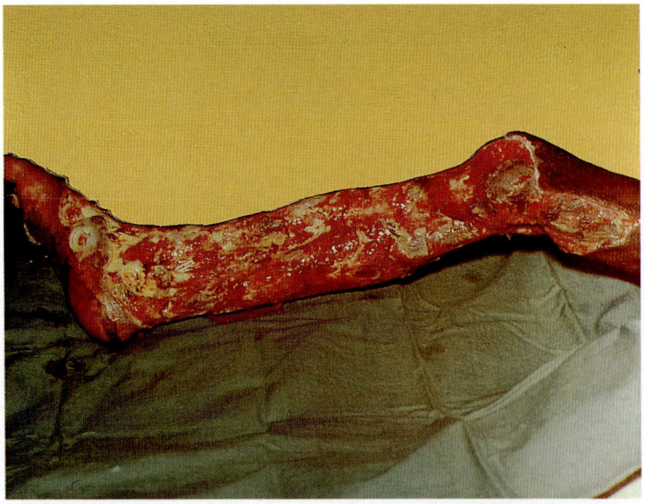

Figure 48–7. Very large ulcer on the leg of a 7-year-old Ugandan youth. He walked many miles to Mulago Hospital, Kampala, with his mother. He had no fever, malaise, or lymphadenopathy. The lesion was treated by repeated debridements and grafting, and healed in 7 months. *(Photograph courtesy of Daniel H. Connor, MD, 1963.)*

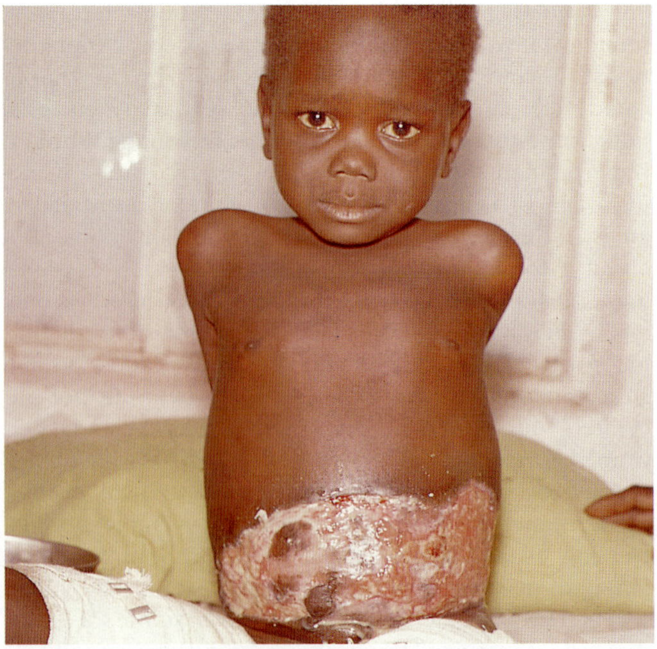

Figure 48–9. A 6-year-old Ugandan boy from the West Nile district, with a Buruli ulcer on the abdomen. This ulcer has been debrided and grafted. The margin is hyperpigmented. *(Patient of Ted Williams, MD, and Peter Williams, MD, Kuluva Hospital. Photograph courtesy of Daniel H. Connor, MD, 1963.)*

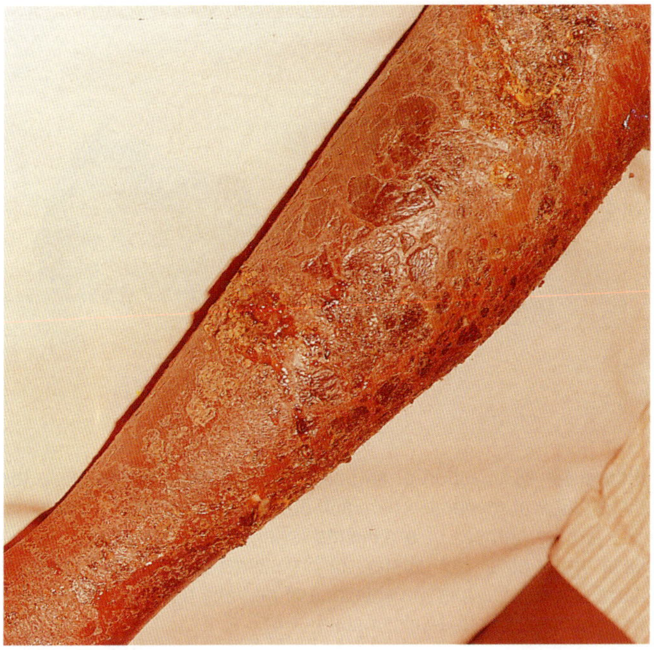

Figure 48–10. This patient's infection has spread subcutaneously to involve the entire leg. The overlying skin is scaly, but without a significant ulcer. *(Photograph courtesy of Daniel H. Connor, MD, 1963.)*

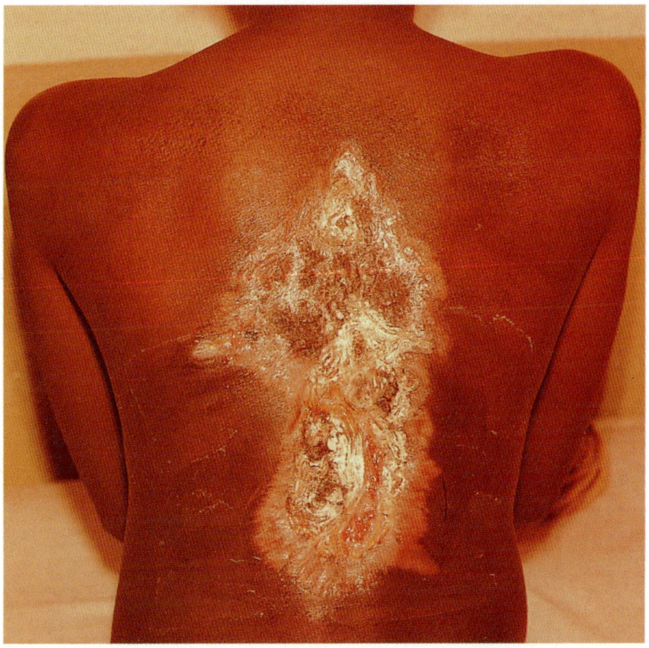

Figure 48–11. Without modern medical care, healing is protracted. This ulcer, untreated for 3 years, is shown when almost completely healed. *(Photograph courtesy of Daniel H. Connor, MD, 1963.)*

scribed foci of necrosis with acid-fast bacilli centered in the area of necrosis (Figures 48–4 and 48–5). These early lesions are symmetrical and involve contiguous structures in the deep dermis, panniculus, and deep fascia. Necrosis and bacteria spread peripherally, with necrosis extending beyond the bacteria. There is tissue edema of the dermis at the viable margin, but inflammatory cells are inconspicuous with only a few scattered lymphocytes, histiocytes, and eosinophils around the perimeter of the necrotic tissue. As the necrosis advances, cells lose their nuclei but retain their outlines for several weeks to several months. This "ghost outline" of previously viable cells and tissue is a characteristic feature. The authors of this chapter have not seen typical caseation necrosis described in the Australian cases.[16] Fibrin accumulates in the necrotic tissue, especially in and between the ghosts of dead fat cells. The capillary circulation is destroyed. Larger vessels are involved as well, but even if their walls become necrotic, most maintain the lumens and pass blood. Although the lumens of some vessels of the deep dermis are obliterated, a pattern identifiable as ischemic necrosis has not been reported. Furthermore, the necrosis around clusters of bacilli in early, nonulcerated lesions is characteristic of the necrosis seen in all stages of infection. The necrosis may spread to the muscle and deep fascia and, rarely, to bone. Mineralized foci are in areas of necrosis. Clumps and masses of acid-fast bacilli are in the necrotic sloughs of the ulcer bed and are concentrated in a deep plane in the necrotic fat (Figure 48–13). Bacilli in some clumps are long and tightly aligned, giving the clump a wavy appearance. As the necrosis spreads superficially, dermal papillae swell and the rete ridges may elongate. The epidermis becomes spongiotic and separates above the basal layer before sloughing.

As the ulcer enlarges, the margin becomes more deeply undermined. The flap may be undermined for 10 to 15 cm (Figure 48–14). A granulomatous reaction in the margin of the ulcer precedes healing and may indicate an improving host response, or it could mean macrophages and their derivatives are able to survive waning concentrations of *M ulcerans* toxin at the perimeter. Healing and exacerbation may alternate for months. Staging of infection is being promoted. In stage 1, a subcutaneous nodule is present; in stage 2, cellulitis develops; in stage 3, there is ulceration; and in stage 4, there is scar formation. Patients may have lesions of different stages simultaneously.[9]

The African lesions studied suggest that necrosis is caused by a mycobacterial exotoxin because the extensive necrosis extends symmetrically beyond the clusters of bacilli. The possibility of a mycobacterial toxin was stated in a clinic–pathologic study by Connor and Lunn.[17] Furthermore, toxic products have been identified in cultures of *M ulcerans*.[18] In vitro the toxin suppresses both T and B lymphocytes, and this may explain the lack of a granulomatous response and the

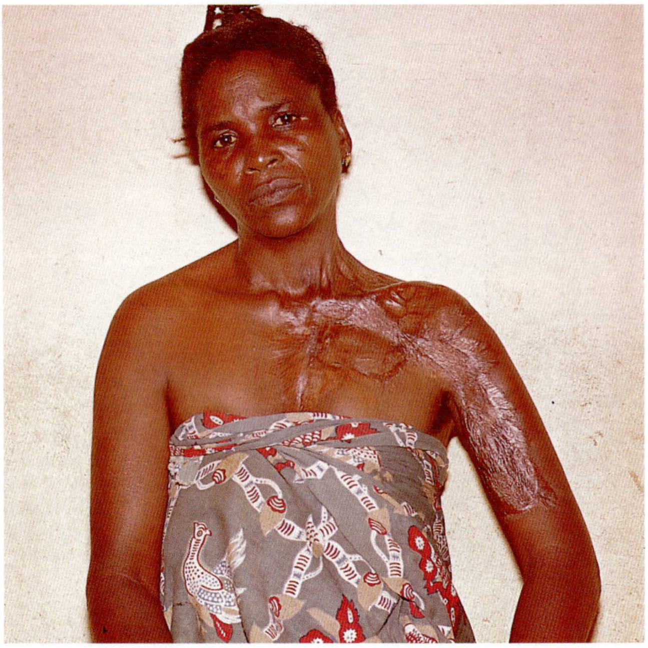

Figure 48–12. Healed Buruli ulcers often appear as depressed scars, which resemble healed third-degree burns. *(Patient of Wayne M. Meyers, MD. Photograph courtesy of Daniel H. Connor, MD, 1968.)*

lack of lymphadenopathy.[19] A simpler explanation would be that the toxin destroys all somatic cells on contact. Filtrates of *M ulcerans* have a therapeutic effect as an antitumor agent in mice.[20]

TREATMENT AND PREVENTION

Because ulcers tend to develop on exposed skin, wearing long trousers, boots, and long-sleeved shirts near water and vegetation may be protective. Vaccination with bacille Calmette-Guérin may confer some limited short-term immunity and may limit the duration of the ulcer.[14] Smaller lesions, especially those not yet ulcerated, can be cured by en bloc excision. Rifampin and streptomycin frequently are effective in preulcerative and early ulcerative stages. Larger lesions are debrided, widely excised, and skin grafted, preserving viable tissue. Recurrent foci of infection then are excised and regrafted when recognized. Heat therapy has proved beneficial when the entire lesion can be warmed continuously to about 40°C under a cradle or in a heated jacket. The higher temperature may act by inhibiting multiplication of *M ulcerans,* by improving local cell-mediated immunity, by stimulating granulation tissue, or perhaps by all three mechanisms.[21] Hyperbaric oxygen has shown efficacy as a treatment in trials with mice.[22] Limbs should not be amputated except in those patients where secondary infection is life-threatening.

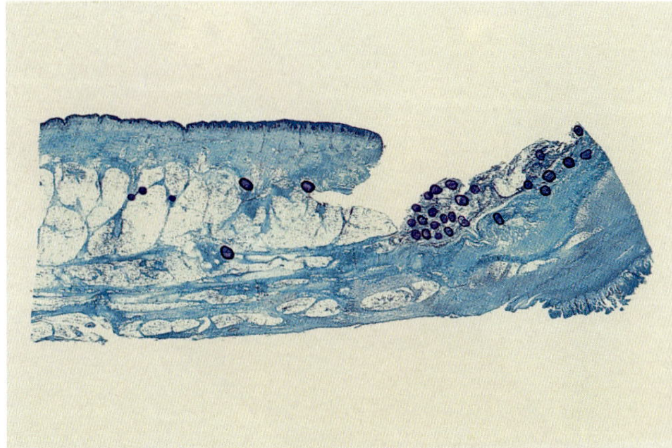

Figure 48–13. Section of an undermined Buruli ulcer to show the distribution of mycobacteria. Each dot marks a focus of organisms. The largest number of organisms is in the necrotic slough in the base of the ulcer, but clusters of organisms are beneath the intact dermis and epidermis. An envelope of necrotic tissue surrounds the mycobacteria (Ziehl–Neelsen stain, ×4).

DIAGNOSIS AND DIFFERENTIAL DIAGNOSIS

Smears of necrotic tissue of the base and undermined edge of the ulcer, stained by the Ziehl–Neelsen technique, reveal large numbers of acid-fast bacilli. A biopsy specimen taken deeply enough to include necrotic fat, which contains acid-fast bacilli, also confirms the diagnosis. Clusters of acid-fast bacilli within tissue showing the characteristic features of Buruli necrosis is diagnostic. Culture of the organism usually requires 6 to 8 weeks, so is not practical for clinical diagnosis. Analysis

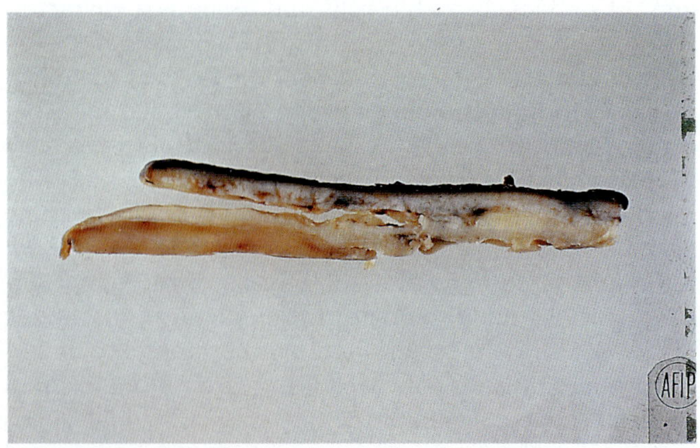

Figure 48–14. Vertical section of an ulcer margin. An opaque necrotic coagulum covers the base. The flap is undermined for 4 cm. *(Photograph courtesy of Daniel H. Connor, MD, 1968.)*

of mycocerosate waxes by gas chromotography–mass spectrometry techniques can identify *M ulcerans* directly in infected tissue, without prior cultivation,[23,24] and DNA amplification also has been used for specific identification of *M ulcerans*.[13] Three conditions are known to resemble ulcers caused by *M ulcerans:* 1) Tropical phagedenic ulcer, the most common cutaneous ulcer in some parts of the tropics, is distinguished by its putrid odor, its intense pain in the early stages, its location below the knee, its hard, raised margin (which is not undermined), the absence of acid-fast bacilli in the exudate, and the presence of fuso-spirochetal organisms; 2) ulcers developing in patients with kwashiorkor or marasmus usually are associated with other signs of malnutrition, including characteristic "flaky paint" dermatitis; these ulcers may contain a mixed flora but do not contain acid-fast bacilli; 3) spreading necrosis and ulceration caused by venomous insects, scorpions, and other animals may resemble *M ulcerans* infections. Usually there is a clear-cut history of a bite or sting, and there may be a mixed bacterial growth throughout the necrotic tissues. Rapid healing with antibiotics and failure to find acid-fast bacilli are features that help distinguish ulcers caused by venoms.

REFERENCES

1. Bryson AM. *Mycobacterium ulcerans* in Australia. *Med J Aust.* 1975;2:887.
2. Burchard GD, Bierther M. Buruli ulcer: clinical pathological study of 23 patients in Lambarene, Gabon. *Trop Med Parasitol.* 1986;37:1–8.
3. Monson MH, Gibson DW, Connor DH, Kappes R, Hienz HA. *Mycobacterium ulcerans* in Liberia: a clinicopathologic study of 6 patients with Buruli ulcer. *Acta Trop.* 1984;41:165–172.
4. Reid IS. *Mycobacterium ulcerans* infection: a report of 13 cases at the Port Moresby General Hospital, Papua. *Med J Aust.* 1967;1:427–431.
5. Oluwasanmi JO, Solankee TF, Olurin EO, Itayemi SO, Alabi GO, Lucas AO. *Mycobacterium ulcerans* (Buruli) skin ulceration in Nigeria. *Am J Trop Med Hyg.* 1976;25: 122–128.
6. Christie M. Suspected *Mycobacterium ulcerans* disease in Kiribati. *Med J Aust.* 1987;146:600–604.
7. Hayman J. *Mycobacterium ulcerans*: an infection from Jurassic time? *Lancet.* 1984;2:1015–1016.
8. Seevanayagam S, Hayman J. *Mycobacterium ulcerans* infection; Is the "Bairnsdale ulcer" also a Ceylonese disease? *Ceylon Med J.* 1992;37:125–127.
9. Muelder K, Nourou A. Buruli ulcer in Benin. *Lancet.* 1990; 336:1109–1111.
10. Myers WM, Shelly WM, Connor DH, et al. Human *Mycobacterium ulcerans* infections developing at sites of trauma to skin. *Am J Trop Med Hyg.* 1974;23:919.
11. Mitchell PJ, McOrist S, Bilney R. Epidemiology of *Mycobacterium ulcerans* infection in koalas (*Phascolarctos cinereus*) on Raymond Island, southeastern Australia. *J Wildl Dis.* July 23, 1987;386–390.
12. Darie H, Le Guyadec T, Touze JE. Aspects epidemiologiques et cliniques de l'ulcere de Buruli en Cote-d'Ivoire. A propos de 124 observations recentes. *Bull Soc Pathol Exot.* 1993;86:272–276.
13. Hofer M, Hirschel B, Kirschner P, et al. Brief report: disseminated osteomyelitis from *Mycobacterium ulcerans* after a snakebite. *N Engl J Med.* 1993;328:1007–1009.
14. Amofah GK, Sayoe-Moses C, Adjei-Acquah C, Frimpong EH. Epidemiology of Buruli ulcer in Amansie West district, Ghana. *Trans Roy Soc Trop Med Hyg.* 1993;87:644–654.
15. Marston BJ, Diallo MO, Horsburgh CR Jr, et al. Emergence of Buruli ulcer disease in the Daloa region of Cote d'Ivoire. *Am J Trop Med Hyg.* 1995;52:219–224.
16. Hayman J. Out of Africa: observations on the histopathology of *Mycobacterium ulcerans* infection. *J Clin Pathol.* 1993;46:5–9.
17. Connor DH, Lunn HF. Buruli ulceration. A clinicopathologic study of 38 Ugandans with *Mycobacterium ulcerans* ulceration. *Arch Pathol.* 1966;81:183–199.
18. Hockmeyer WT, Krieg RE, Reich M, Johnson RD. Further characterization of *Mycobacterium ulcerans* toxins. *Infect Immun.* 1978;21:124–128.
19. Pimsler M, Sponsler TA, Meyers WM. Immunosuppressive properties of the soluble toxin from *Mycobacterium ulcerans. J Infect Dis.* 1988;157:577–580.
20. Heggers JP, Robson MC, Yetter JF, Kreig RE Jr, Jennings PB. Tumoricidal effects of *Mycobacterium ulcerans* toxin on murine adenocarcinoma (C3HBA). *J Surg Oncol.* 1979;11:161–169.
21. Meyers WM, Shelly WM, Connor DH. Heat treatment of *Mycobacterium ulcerans* infections without surgical excision. *Am J Trop Med Hyg.* 1974;23:924.
22. Krieg RE, Wolcott JH, Confer A. Treatment of *Mycobacterium ulcerans* infection by hyperbaric oxygenation. *Aviat Space Environ Med.* 1975;46:1241–1245.
23. Minnikin DE, Besra GS, Bolton RC, et al. Identification of the leprosy bacillus and related mycobacteria by analysis of mycocerosate profiles. *Ann Soc Belg Med Trop.* 1993;73: 25–34.
24. Daffe M, Laneele MA, Roussel J, Asselineau C. Lipides specifiques de *Mycobacterium ulcerans. Ann Microbiol.* 1984;135:191–201.

CHAPTER 49

Cat Scratch Disease

Clay J. Cockerell and Daniel H. Connor

Those who'll play with cats must expect to be scratched.

Miguel de Cervantes (1547–1616)

DEFINITION AND GEOGRAPHY

Cat scratch disease (CSD) is a zoonotic infection caused by any one of a group of recently defined rickettsial microorganisms of the α-2 subgroup of α-proteobacteria, specifically *Bartonella* (formerly *Rochalimaea*) *henselae*.[1] Some infections may be caused by related organisms, including *Afipia felis* and *B quintana,* the cause of trench fever.[2,3] CSD is worldwide and most common in autumn and winter, and found especially in dwellings where cats are kept as pets.

HISTORY

The first recognition of CSD was apparently in 1931 by Professor Robert Debré at the University of Paris.[4] The patient, a 10-year-old boy with multiple cat scratches on his forearms, had draining epitrochlear lymphadenitis. At first Debré thought the boy had tuberculous lymphadenitis but the tuberculin test was nonreactive, the fistula had developed more quickly than is usual for tuberculous lymphadenitis, all bacteriologic studies were fruitless, and the lesions healed in several weeks—too quickly for tuberculosis. Thus Debré concluded that the lesion was not tuberculosis but probably related, in some way, to the scratches of the patient's pet kittens.[4]

In 1932 Professor Lee Foshay, a microbiologist at the University of Cincinnati, recognized an ulceroglandular disease that followed the scratches of cats and called it "cat fever."[5] A lifelong student of tularemia, Foshay originally recognized these patients as a subgroup of tularemia. In 1945, Franklin M. Hangar and Harry M. Rose, members of the Department of Medicine at the College of Physicians and Surgeons of Columbia University in New York City, developed a skin test using pus aspirated from Hangar's swollen, fluctuant, tender, infraclavicular lymph node. Rose sterilized and diluted the pus, then injected some into Hangar's skin. An intense "tuberculin-like" reaction developed and, later, this same material produced reactions in some of Foshay's patients. Hanger is thus the first patient to have had a positive skin test for CSD. Debré, after visiting Foshay in Cincinnati in 1947, began similar studies in Paris and published in 1950.[6,7] Pierre Mollaret, a Parisian pathologist working independently of Debré, collected specimens, did serologic studies, transmitted the disease to a volunteer and to monkeys, and described the histopathologic lesions in the lymph nodes.[8–11]

In the early 1950s Worth B. Daniels and Frank G. MacMurray, colleagues widely known for their scholarship and dynamic teaching, published series of 60 patients[5] and 160 patients[12] describing the epidemiologic setting, the variation in clinicopathologic features, and the results of skin testing. The large numbers of patients and records they were able to collect and study alerted medical communities in the United States and abroad to the fact that CSD was not a rare disease. By word of mouth it became known also that they would supply antigen to patients with suspected CSD. In fact they supplied antigen for "maybe 2000" patients.[4]

For the next 30 years the cause of CSD was presumed to be viral or perhaps related to the "lymphogranuloma venereum-psittacosis group of organisms." It seems paradoxical now that the name "cat scratch disease" was frequently modified to "non-bacterial lymphadenitis" on title pages and in indices.[5]

The first recognition of the bacterial cause of CSD was in February 1981 at the Armed Forces Institute of Pathology. The infectious disease group there saw, in Warthin–Starry stained sections, clusters of bacilli in the necrotizing lesions of an enlarged supraclavicular lymph node removed from an 11-year-old girl from Columbia, Maryland. This and subsequent lymph nodes from patients with typical CSD revealed that the bacilli, although coated with silver in early lesions (using silver impregnation techniques), were invisible with routine stains and were virtually invisible with the usual special stains used to demonstrate bacteria. The bacilli they saw, however, were convincing because they were 1) in the tissue, 2) intracellular, 3) limited to the lesions and concentrated in the centers of the lesions, 4) abundant in early lesions, but 5) increasingly scarce to vanishing as the lesions resolved. Binford's postulates for the recognition of an infectious agent were thus met,[13] and subsequently bacilli were identified in lymph nodes of 29 of 34 patients with lymphadenitis characteristic of CSD.[14] A gram-negative bacillus was cultured from 10 of 19 patients[15] and named *Afipia felis.*[2] Now, however, there is increasingly convincing evidence that *Bartonella henselae,* the cause of bacillary angiomatosis, is the major cause of CSD.[16–19] Furthermore, *B henselae* has been isolated from the blood of cats and kittens as well as from their fleas, confirming that both CSD and bacillary angiomatosis are zoonoses.[19,20]

At present, the organisms and the spectrum of syndromes they cause are confusing. Why, for instance, does *B henselae* cause CSD in one patient and bacillary angiomatosis in another? Apparently the difference is not entirely explained by the patient's immune status. Why does bacillary angiomatosis respond to antibiotics and CSD usually not, and why does *B quintana* cause trench fever in some and CSD in others?[21] Perhaps answers will come soon in this rapidly advancing field.

NATURAL HISTORY

Infection usually follows a bite, scratch, or other penetrating injury by a kitten or cat. Most infections are in children and young adults between 3 and 21 years,[22] although all ages are affected. In one study, 87% of 1200 patients were 18 years or under.[23] Cats and kittens are the source of the organism for most patients and the wound of the scratch is the portal of entry. Interestingly, cats that infect humans are rarely ill. This has recently been corroborated by the finding of *Bartonella* sp and antibodies directed to them in the blood of cats implicated in human infections.[24] Some infections cannot be traced to cats and these organisms may be from soil or possibly from an ectoparasite. As noted, *B henselae* and *B quintana* have both been identified in cat fleas.

Clinically, there is usually a "primary" lesion at the site of inoculation with lymphadenopathy 3 weeks to 3 months after inoculation.[25] Lesions heal in several weeks to several months. CSD is not contagious and it is rare for more than one family member to be affected at a time. Subclinical infections are frequent, ie, up to 18% of families of patients and 23% in veterinarians.[26] Antibiotics are generally not required but ciprofloxacin may be effective.[27] Following CSD, patients develop both humoral and cell-mediated immune responses to the microorganisms.[22]

FEATURES OF THE CAUSATIVE MICROORGANISMS

The causative organisms are weakly gram-negative coccobacilli, approximately 0.2 μm by 1 to 2.5 μm. By electron microscopy the cell wall is characteristic of a gram-negative bacillus (Figure 49–1).[23] Bartonellae are small, gram-negative bacilli assigned to the family Rickettsiaceae.[1] In addition to CSD, *B quintana* and *B henselae* are associated with bacillary angiomatosis, bacillary peliosis hepatitis, and bacteremia.[28] *Bartonella*

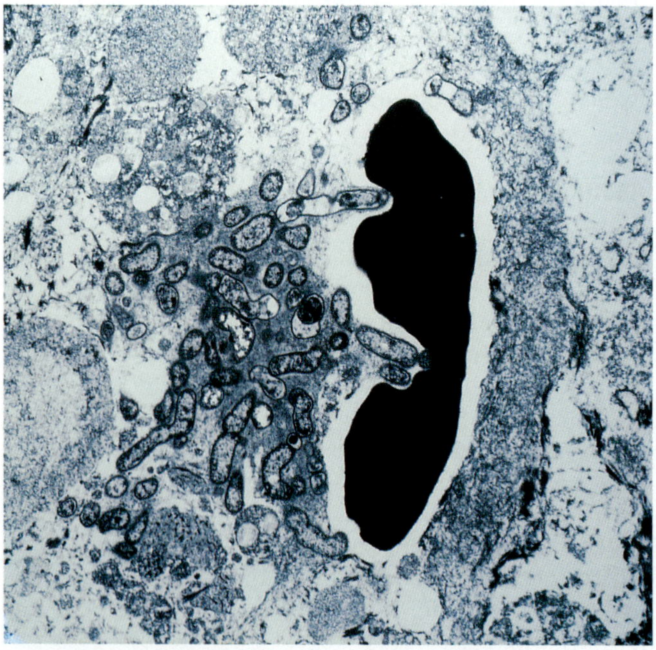

Figure 49–1. Electron micrograph showing CSD bacilli. They are concentrated in the wall of a small vessel, have pushed into the lumen, and indented an erythrocyte (AFIP Neg; transmission electron micrograph, ×6500).

elizabethae has been isolated from the blood of one immunocompetent patient with endocarditis.[29] Other members of the α-2 subgroup of the α-proteobacteria include other Rickettsiae, Ehrlichiae, and *B bacilliformis* and *A felis,* the only non-*Bartonella* organism that has been associated with CSD.[30–34] *Bartonella* and *Afipia* species grow extracellularly, whereas Rickettsiae and Ehrlichiae grow intracellularly.

Bartonella henselae is a small, slightly curved, lightly staining gram-negative bacillus that grows best in a microaerophilic environment.[35] It is 0.5 μm by 1 to 2 μm. A ratchety twitching motility has been described that alternates from clockwise to counterclockwise. In vitro the colonies are typically white and invaginate the agar.[23,36] The organism is oxidase-, catalase-, and urease-negative and is susceptible in vitro to erythromycin, macrolides, tetracyclines, chloramphenicol, fluoroquinolones, rifampin, aminoglycosides, and trimethoprim–sulfamethoxazole.[23,36] Clusters of subpolar flagellae have been demonstrated by electron microscopy.

Bartonella quintana is an aerobic, gram-negative, nonmotile bacillus 0.3 μm to 0.5 μm wide by 1 to 1.7 μm long. Colonies are small, round, mucoid, and translucent. Antimicrobial susceptibilities are similar to those of *B henselae.*[37,38] *Afipia felis* is an aerobic, gram-negative, motile bacillus 0.3 to 0.7 μm by 1 to 2 μm, similar to *Bartonella* organisms. Colonies are small but often whitish and less fastidious than *Bartonella* sp.

CLINICAL FEATURES

The characteristic clinical syndrome consists of an initial lesion that develops at the site where the organisms are

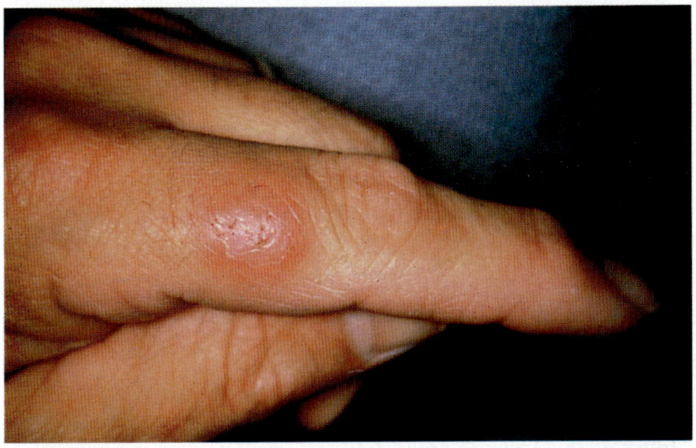

Figure 49–2. Primary lesion of CSD, at the site of inoculation on the left index finger. The lesion is a localized, erythematous, scaling, and weeping papule. This is followed by epitrochlear lymphadenopathy but lymphangitis is not a feature (AFIP Neg 83-9603).

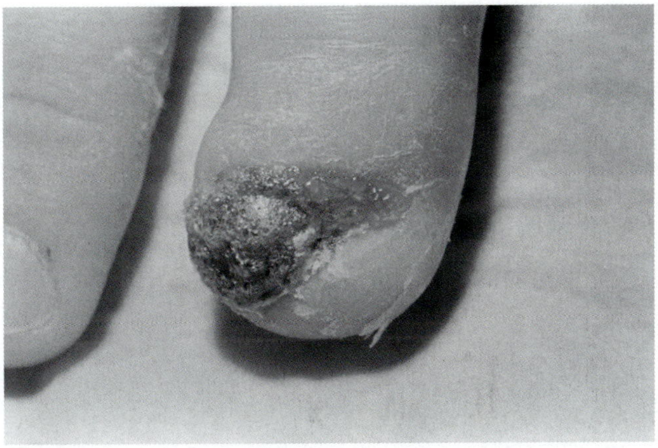

Figure 49–3. Primary lesion in another patient. There is localized scaling, ulceration, and suppuration. *(Contributed by Richard Johnson.)*

introduced—the primary cutaneous lesion—followed by enlargement of regional lymph nodes.[25] Primary lesions develop 3 to 5 days after the scratch or bite of the kitten or cat and are solitary, or rarely multiple, papules or papulopustules (Figures 49–2 and 49–3).[39] Lesions may become vesicular and crusted in 2 to 3 days. The primary lesion may go unnoticed or it may persist and be slightly painful or, rarely, there may be no primary lesion. Usually the primary lesion regresses spontaneously in less than 2 weeks and leaves a small scar in up to 90% of patients. Symptoms in the primary stage are usually mild, although approximately 60% of patients have fever lasting for a few days to 2 weeks.[39] Lymphadenopathy develops in virtually all patients, usually 1 to 2 weeks after the primary lesion appears. The affected node or nodes are those that drain the primary lesion. In contrast to some other infections associated with regional lymphadenopathy, there is no apparent lymphangitis. Lymphadenopathy involves only one node in 85% of patients, although multiple nodes are occasionally involved. Bilateral lymphadenopathy is rare and usually a consequence of separate inoculations or a single inoculation near the midline. Affected nodes are large, tender, and occasionally drain to the surface. The lymphadenopathy regresses without treatment in a few weeks or regression may be delayed for several months. Persistent or recurrent enlargement is uncommon.[39] Some patients have low-grade fever, headache, and malaise.

Although CSD is usually confined to skin and regional lymph nodes, there may be other complications. Occasionally, primary inoculation is on a mucosal surface or conjunctiva and does not require injury.[40] In this situation, there is granulation tissue and a granulo-

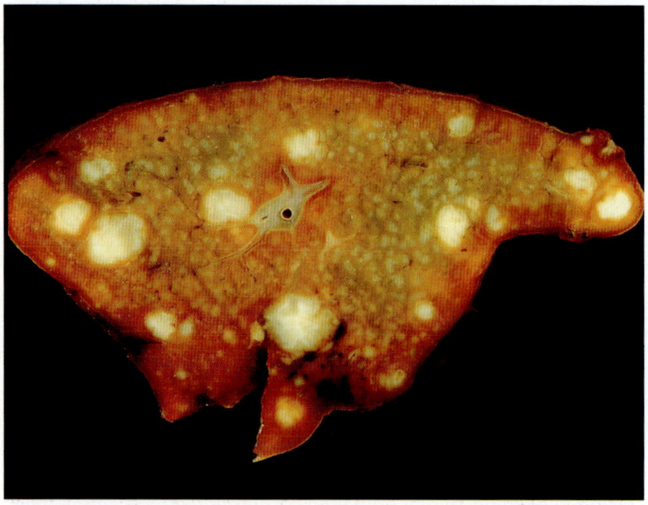

Figure 49–4. Cut surface of the spleen of a patient with disseminated CSD. The white foci are pyogranulomatous foci. *(By Daniel H. Connor, MD, 1986.)*

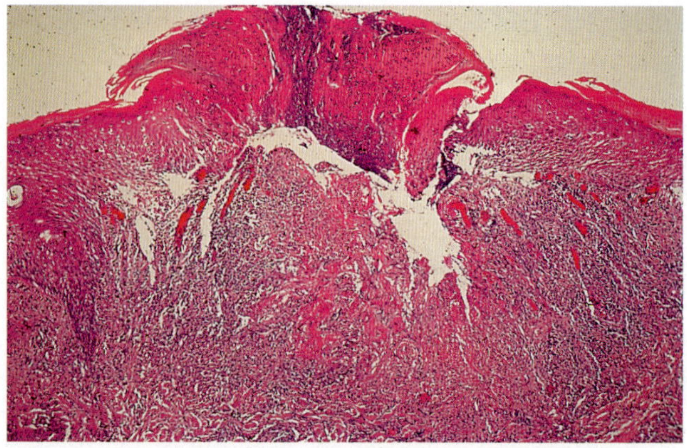

Figure 49–5. Biopsy specimen of a primary site. The epidermis is necrotic and crusted. The underlying dermis is hyperemic and infiltrated with lymphocytes, plasma cells, and macrophages [AFIP Neg, 1983; hematoxylin-eosin (H&E), ×7.2].

matous conjunctivitis that is usually painless and associated with an enlarged preauricular lymph node. CSD is one cause of the oculoglandular syndrome of Parinaud.

Unusual complications of CSD are morbilliform eruptions, urticaria, thrombocytopenic purpura, erythema nodosum, erythema multiforme, and erythema marginatum. Each of these has been associated with CSD, and they tend to be more frequent when infection is severe or when there are systemic complications. These include sepsis, arthritis, osteolytic lesions, visceral lymphadenopathy, central and peripheral nervous system disease, pneumonia, granulomatous hepatitis[25,41–43] and splenomegaly (Figure 49–4), which develops in up to 12% of patients.[23]

Even in those with systemic complications, most infections resolve without treatment. Recently, however, therapy with ciprofloxacin has been shown to hasten recovery.[38] Patients have increased numbers of circulating neutrophils and slight elevation of sedimentation rate. No other significant abnormalities are noted in uncomplicated infections, although with hepatic involvement, hepatocellular enzymes may be elevated.

PATHOLOGY

The primary cutaneous lesion is characterized by epidermal hyperplasia and a dermal inflammatory infiltrate consisting of neutrophils surrounded by histiocytes in palisaded array.[15] In the primary lesion shown in Figure 49–5 collagen fibers in the upper dermis are degenerating and there is necrosis of epidermis, forming an eschar. Capillaries around the central area of necrosis are dilated and congested. Silver impregnation silvers the organisms (Figure 49–6). In lymph nodes the process is at first necrotizing, then suppurative, and before healing, both suppurative and granulomatous. In the acute stage lymph nodes are soft, swollen, and have foci of necrosis on their cut surfaces (Figure 49–7). Microscopically early lesions are degeneration foci containing swollen tortuous capillaries, which have a pink

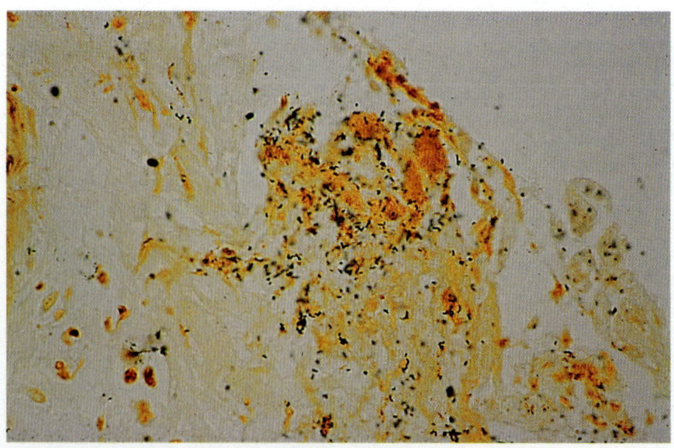

Figure 49–6. Silver impregnation stain of the lesion in Figure 49–5 reveals many bacilli in the upper dermis and in the crusted portion of the lesion. Colloidal silver coats the bacilli, making them opaque (black) and larger than normal. (AFIP Neg, 1983; Warthin–Starry, ×180).

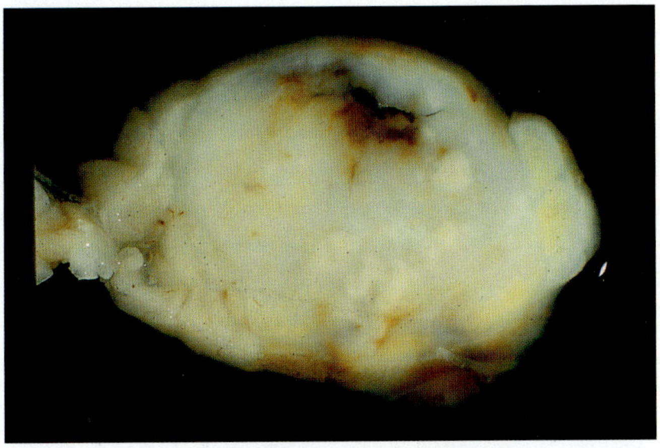

Figure 49–7. Lymph node from patient with CSD. The node is soft and swollen, making it almost spherical. The capsule is thickened and there are foci of necrosis, mainly in the outer cortex, that are opaque and yellow (gross, ×1.5). *(By Daniel H. Connor, MD.)*

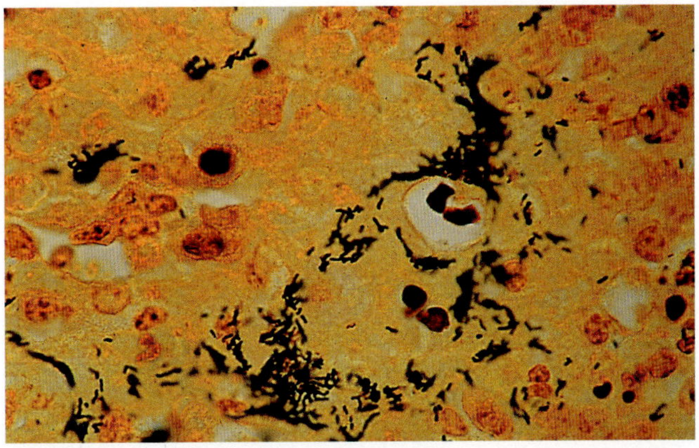

Figure 49–9. Cat scratch lymphadenitis—from the same lymph node shown in Figures 49–7 and 49–8. Note the causal bacilli in the walls of the swollen capillaries, almost outlining them, and in adjacent surrounding tissue (AFIP Neg, 1981; Warthin–Starry, ×290).

hyaline appearance (Figure 49–8). Silver impregnation done on these early lesions usually reveals the causal bacilli packed in the walls of the swollen capillaries and in adjacent cortex (Figure 49–9). Eosinophils and plasma cells may be in the interstices. As the foci of suppuration grow they coalesce to form stellate abscesses (Figure 49–10), which become surrounded by histiocytes, epithelioid cells, and occasional giant cells (Figure 49–11).[15,44,45] If immune mechanisms fail to check the infection at this stage, expanding suppuration and continuing coalescence of abscesses rupture through the capsule of the node and onto the surface

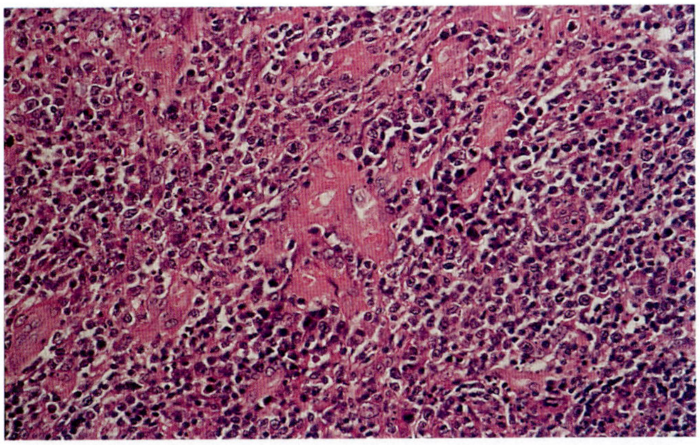

Figure 49–8. Section of the node in Figure 49–7 revealing early changes of CSD lymphadenitis. The early lesions are, as shown here, tortuous capillaries with swollen walls and surrounded by neutrophils. Early lesions are multiple and frequently in the subcapsular cortex near the termination of the afferent lymphatics. Silver impregnation stains done on early lesions reveal the causal bacilli in the walls of swollen capillaries and in adjacent tissue (AFIP Neg, 1981; H&E, ×72).

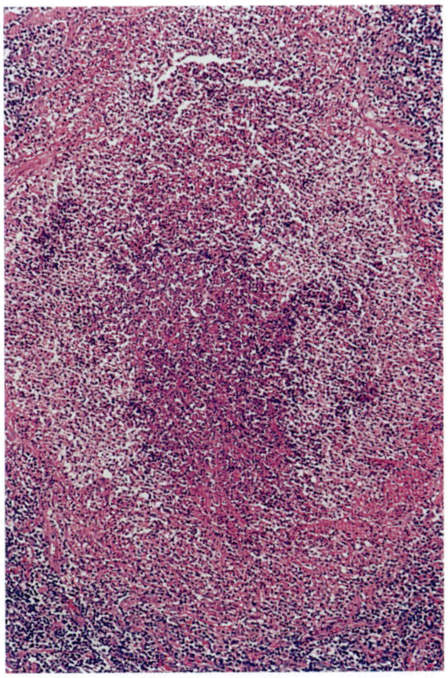

Figure 49–10. Small foci of suppuration have coalesced to form an abscess, which is beginning to have a stellate outline. Macrophages and epithelioid cells have collected around the abscess (H&E, ×28).

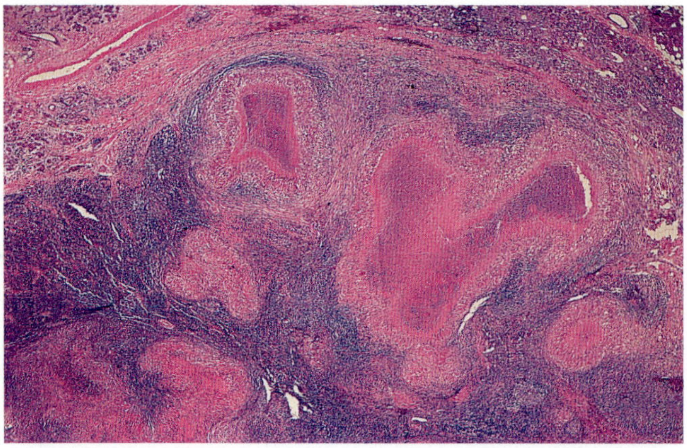

Figure 49–11. A later lesion in which the stellate pyogranulomatous lesions are clearly defined. If the lesions continue to expand, they will continue to coalesce and then rupture through the capsule of the node to reach the surface of the skin (AFIP Neg, December 1984; H&E, ×7.2).

of the skin (Figure 49–12). By now bacilli have lost their orientation in and around small vessels but bacilli still may be identified in areas of suppuration (Figure 49–13). Eventually the suppurative component becomes less conspicuous, leaving a granulomatous perimeter and central caseation (Figure 49–14). The caseous centers, however, unlike the centers of tuberculous lesions, rarely calcify.

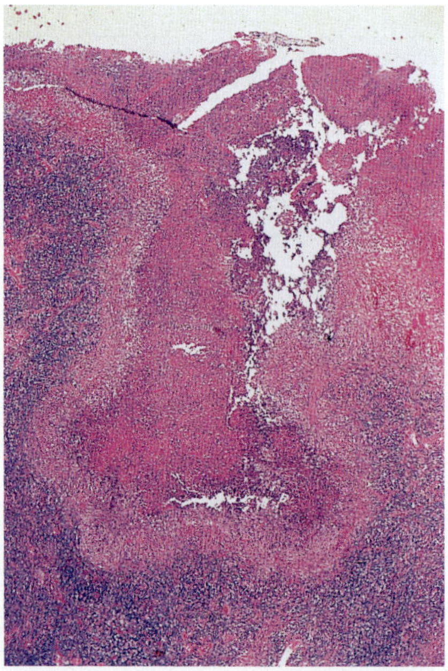

Figure 49–12. Here the necrosis extended through the capsule and onto the skin (not shown). When the granulomatous component is well developed, as it is here, the bacilli are few, frequently fragmented, imperfectly silvered, and usually mistaken for artifactual debris, if they are seen (H&E, ×7.2).

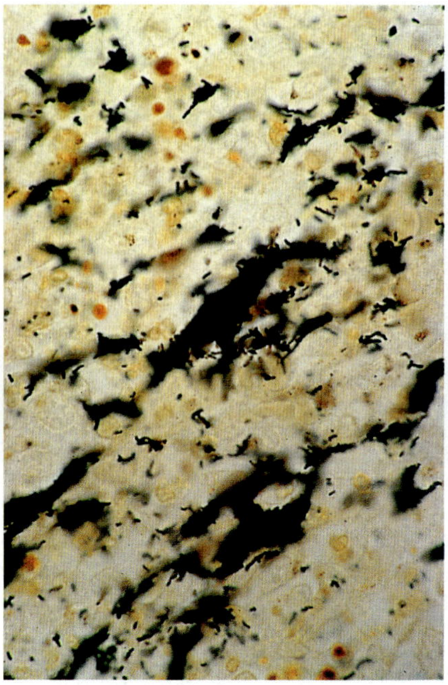

Figure 49–13. The center of a stellate abscess in a lymph node from a patient with CSD. There are many bacilli. The causal bacteria, at this stage, are numerous but not defining small blood vessels as in early lesions. Here the bacilli are bunched and scattered but limited to areas of necrosis (Warthin–Starry, ×290).

DIFFERENTIAL PATHOLOGICAL DIAGNOSIS

The differential diagnosis of local cutaneous lesions includes other forms of local suppurative inflammatory reactions such as ruptured folliculitis and localized staphylococcal infections. Histologic sections of skin lesions in the acute suppurative phase usually reveal discrete or clustered silvered (opaque) bacilli in the necrotic skin as already described. Bacilli in lymph nodes may be quite striking in early lesions but as the lesions become granulomatous the bacilli are sharply decreased and often the few that remain are fragmented and distorted to the point where they resemble debris, making it impossible to be certain of their identity. (It is perhaps not surprising, therefore, that the cause of CSD went unrecognized for 50 years.) When the granulomatous reaction develops, the differential diagnosis may include other forms of granulomatous disease, such as infections by atypical mycobacteria, deep fungal infections and even noninfectious granulomatous processes. The degree of epidermal hyperplasia and the absence of intraepidermal abscesses, as well as sections specially stained for microorganisms, aid in distinguishing deep fungal infections from atypical mycobacterial

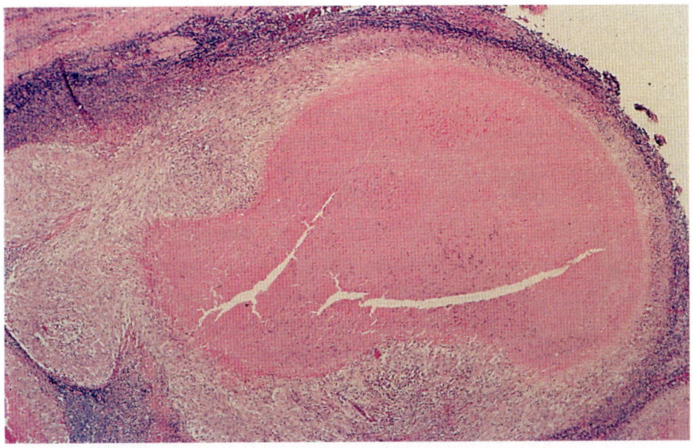

Figure 49–14. Resolving lesion of CSD in a lymph node. The center now resembles caseation necrosis—an eosinophilic coagulum surrounded by a granulomatous layer. Helpful in distinguishing CSD from tuberculosis is the lack of mineral in the areas of caseation. Areas of caseation in tuberculosis and histoplasmosis, however, almost always contain mineral. Lesions of lymphogranuloma venereum, brucellosis, syphilis (gumma), and tularemia may resemble closely the lesions of CSD (H&E, ×11.5).

infections. Stellate abscesses, characteristic of CSD, are characteristic also of lymphogranuloma venereum as well as other rare infections including tularemia and brucellosis. Most helpful in diagnosing CSD is the clinical setting and less helpful is the demonstration of the bacilli by silver impregnation and by culture.

MOLECULAR DIAGNOSIS

DNA primers have been developed for use with the polymerase chain reaction for evaluation of CSD.[2,46] Although this is primarily a research technique, this may be done when the diagnosis is otherwise uncertain. In addition, hyperimmune rabbit serum or serum from patients with documented CSD has been used to develop an indirect immunoperoxidase stain that may demonstrate organisms in tissue sections.[47]

CONFIRMATIONAL TESTING AND DIAGNOSIS

Skin testing, with CSD antigen made of pus aspirated from lymph nodes of lesions of CSD, may be done. A positive reaction is induration and erythema in the skin at the site of injection.[22] Now, however, this test is mainly of historical interest and is not used routinely. Antibody titers may be determined also in selective infections. Finally, recent reports have demonstrated that the organism may be cultured using brain–heart infusion biphasic medium at 32° and 37°C. Organisms may also grow on brain–heart infusion agar after incubation at 32°C.[26]

REFERENCES

1. Brenner DJ, O'Connor SP, Winkler HH, Steigerwalt AG. Proposals to unify the genera *Bartonella* and *Rochalimaea,* with descriptions of *Bartonella quintana* comb nov, *Bartonella vinsonii* comb nov, *Bartonella henselae* comb nov, and *Bartonella elizabethae* comb nov, and to remove the family Bartonellaceae from the order *Rickettsiales. Int J Syst Bacteriol.* 1993;43:777–786.
2. Brenner DJ, Hollis DG, Moss CW, et al. Proposal of *Afipia,* gen nov, with *Afipia felis,* sp nov (formerly the cat scratch disease bacillus), *Afipia clevelandensis,* sp nov (formerly the Cleveland Clinic Foundation strain), *Afipia broomeae,* sp nov, and three unnamed genospecies. *J Clin Microbiol.* 1991;29:2450–2460.
3. Welch DF, Pickett DA, Slater LN, et al. *Rochalimaea henselae* sp nov, a cause of septicemia, bacillary angiomatosis, and parenchymal bacillary peliosis. *J Clin Microbiol.* 1992;30:275–280.
4. Carithers HA. Cat scratch disease: Notes on history. *Am J Dis Child.* 1970;119:200–203.
5. Daniels WB, MacMurray FB. Cat scratch disease; nonbacterial regional lymphadenitis: a report of 60 cases. *Ann Intern Med.* 1952;37:697–713.
6. Debré R, Lamy M, Jammet ML, Costil L, Mozziconacci P. La maladie des griffes de chat. *Semaine d hôp Paris.* 1950; 26:1895–1904.
7. Debré R. La maladie des griffes de chat. *Marseille méd.* 1950;87:375–378.
8. Mollaret P, Reilly J, Bastin R, Tournier P. Sur une adénopathie régionale subaigu' et spontanément curable, avec intradermo-réaction et lésions ganglionnaires particulières. *Bull et mêm Soc méd d hôp de Paris.* 1950;66: 424–449.
9. Mollaret P, Reilly J, Bastin R, Tournier P. Documentation nouvelle sur l'adénopathie régionale subaigu' et spontanément curable, décrite en 1950: la lympho-réticulose bénigne d'inoculation. *Presse méd.* 1950;58:1353–1355.
10. Mollaret P, Reilly J, Bastin R, Tournier P. I. Lymphoréticulose bénigne d'inoculation et démonstration de l'inoculabilité au singe. *Bull et mêm Soc méd d hôp de Paris.* 1951;67:687–693.
11. Mollaret P, Reilly J, Bastin R, Tournier P. II. Lymphoréticulose bénigne d'inoculation et caractérisation du virus par sérologie et colorations. *Bull et mêm Soc méd d hôp de Paris.* 1951;67:693–702.
12. Daniels WB, MacMurray FB. Cat scratch disease; report of one hundred and sixty cases. *JAMA.* 1954;154:1247–1251.
13. Nelson AM, Sledzik PS, Mullick FG. The Army Medical Museum/Armed Forces Institute of Pathology and Emerging Infections. From camp fevers and diarrhea during the American Civil War in the 1860s to global molecular epidemiology and pathology in the 1990s. *Arch Pathol Lab Med.* 1996;120:129–133.

14. Wear DJ, Margileth AM, Hadfield TL, et al. Cat-scratch disease: a bacterial infection. *Science.* 1983;221:1403–1405.
15. English CK, Wear DJ, Margileth AM, et al. Cat-scratch disease. Isolation and culture of the bacterial agent. *JAMA.* 1988;259:1347–1352.
16. Regnery RL, Olson JG, Perkins BA, Bibb W. Serological response to *Rochalimaea henselae* antigen in suspected cat-scratch disease. *Lancet.* 1992;339:1443–1445.
17. Perkins BA, Swaminanthan B, Jackson LA, et al. *N Engl J Med.* 1992;327:1599–1600. Letter.
18. Dolan MJ, Wong JT, Regnery RL, et al. Syndrome of *Rochalimaea henselae* adenitis suggesting cat scratch disease. *Ann Intern Med.* 1993;118:331–336.
19. Koeler JE, Glaser CA, Tappero JW. *Rochalimaea henselae* infection: a new zoonosis with domestic cat as reservoir. *JAMA.* 1994;271:531–535.
20. Demers DM, Bass JW, Vincent JM, et al. Cat scratch disease in Hawaii: etiological and seroepidemiological studies. *J Pediatr.* 1995;127:23–26.
21. Tompkins DC, Steigbigel RT. *Rochalimaea's* role in cat scratch disease and bacillary angiomatosis. *Ann Intern Med.* 1993;118:388–390. Editorial.
22. Hadfield TL. Cat scratch disease. In: Gorbach SL, Bartlett JG, Blacklow NR, eds. *Infectious Diseases.* Philadelphia: WB Saunders; 1992:1318–1323.
23. Carithers HA. Cat scratch disease. An overview based on a study of 1200 patients. *Am J Dis Child.* 1985;139: 1124–1133.
24. Hall AV, Roberts CM, Maurice PD, McLean KA, Shousha S. Cat-scratch disease in patient with AIDS: atypical skin manifestation. *Lancet.* 1988;2:453–454.
25. Margileth AM. Antiobiotic therapy for cat-scratch disease: clinical study of therapeutic outcome in 268 patients and a review of the literature. *Pediatr Infect Dis J.* 1992;11: 474–478.
26. Holley HP Jr. Successful treatment of cat-scratch disease with ciprofloxacin. *JAMA.* 1991;265:1563–1565.
27. Regnery R, Martin M, Olson J. Naturally occurring *"Rochalimaea henselae"* infection in domestic cat. *Lancet.* 1992;340:557–558.
28. Birtles RJ, Harrison TG, Taylor AG. The causative agent of bacillary angiomatosis. *N Engl J Med.* 1991;325:1447–1448.
29. Relman DA, Lepp PW, Sadler KN, Schmidt TM. Phylogenetic relationships among the agent of bacillary angiomatosis, *Bartonella bacilliformis,* and other alpha proteobacteria. *Mol Microbiol.* 1992;6:1801–1807.
30. Brenner DJ, O'Connor SP, Hollis DG, Weaver RE, Steigerwalt AG. Molecular characterization and proposal of neotype strain for *Bartonella bacilliformis. J Clin Microbiol.* 1991;29:1299–1302.
31. Cockerell CJ, Tierno PM. Friedman-Kien AE, Kim KS. Clinical, histologic, microbiologic, and biochemical characterization of the causative agent of bacillary (epithelioid) angiomatosis: a rickettsial illness with features of bartonellosis. *J Invest Dermatol.* 1991;97:812–817.
32. Regnery RL, Anderson BE, Clarridge JE III, Rodriguez-Barradas MC, Jones DC, Carr JH. Characterization of a novel *Rochalimaea* species, *R henselae* sp nov, isolated from blood of a febrile, human immunodeficiency virus-positive patient. *J Clin Microbiol.* 1992;30:265–274.
33. Koehler JE, Quinn FD, Berger TG, LeBoit PE, Tappero JW. Isolation of *Rochalimaea* species from cutaneous and osseous lesions of bacillary angiomatosis. *N Engl J Med.* 1992;327:1625–1631.
34. Maurin M, Raoult D. In vitro antibiotic susceptibility of *Rochalimaea* isolates of the three species *R quintana, R vinsonii,* and the novel species *R henselae.* In: Program and abstracts of the 32nd general meeting of the American Society for Microbiology. Washington, DC: American Society for Microbiology; 1992:229. Abstract 710.
35. Weiss E, Moulder JW. Order 1. Rickettsiales Gieszczkiewicz 1939,25[AL]. In: Kreig NR, Holt JG, eds. *Bergey's Manual of Systematic Bacteriology.* Baltimore: Williams and Wilkins; 1984:687–728.
36. Loftus MJ, Sweeney G, Goldberg MH. Parinaud oculoglandular syndrome and cat scratch fever. *J Oral Surg.* 1938:218–220.
37. Delahoussaye PM. Osborne BM. Cat scratch disease presenting as abdominal visceral granulomas. *J Infect Dis.* 1990;161:71–78.
38. Margileth AM, Wear DJ, English CK. Systemic cat scratch disease: report of 23 patients with prolonged or recurrent severe bacterial infection. *J Infect Dis.* 1987;155:390–402.
39. Johnson WT, Helwig EB. Cat-scratch disease: histopathologic changes in the skin. *Arch Dermatol.* 1969;100: 148–154.
40. Caputo R, Ackerman AB, Sison-Torre EQ. Cat scratch disease. In: Dhillon I, Hirsch E, Tang S, eds. *Pediatric Dermatology and Dermatopathology.* Philadelphia: Lea and Febiger; 1990:305–316.
41. Lever WF, Schaumberg-Lever G. Bacterial diseases. In: *Histopathology of the Skin.* 7th ed. Philadelphia: JB Lippincott; 1990:345.
42. O'Conner SP, Dorsch M, Steigerwalt AG et al. 16S rRNA sequences of *Bartonella bacilliformis* and cat scratch disease bacillus reveal phylogenetic relationships with the alpha-2 subgroup of the class *Proteobacteria. J Clin Microbiol.* 1991;29:2144–2150.
43. LeBoit PE, Berger TG, Egbert BM, et al. Epithelioid haemangioma-like vascular proliferation in AIDS: manifestation of cat scratch disease bacillus infection. *Lancet.* 1988;i:960–963.
44. Adal KA, Cockerell CJ, Petri WA Jr. Cat scratch disease, bacillary angiomatosis, and other infections due to *Rochalimaea. N Engl J Med.* 1994;330:1509–1515.
45. Daly JS, Worthington MG, Brenner DJ, et al. *Rochalimaea elizabethae* sp nov isolated from a patient with endocarditis. *J Clin Microbiol.* 1993;31:872–881.
46. Relman DA, Loutit JS, Schmidt TM, Falkow S, Tompkins LS. The agent of bacillary angiomatosis: an approach to the identification of uncultured pathogens. *N Engl J Med.* 1990;323:1573–1580.
47. Birtles RJ, Harrison TG, Fry NK, Saunders NA, Taylor AG. Taxonomic considerations of *Bartonella bacilliformis* based on phylogenetic and phenotypic characteristics. *FEMS Microbiol Lett.* 1991;67:187–191.

CHAPTER 50

Chancroid

Gregory Nikolaidis and Theodore Rosen

The pains of love be sweeter far
Than all the other pleasures are.

Dreyden, Tyranic Love, Act IV, Scene I

DEFINITION

Chancroid (or "soft chancre") is a sexually transmitted disease caused by the gram-negative bacillus *Haemophilus ducreyi.* This fastidious organism was first identified by Ducrey in 1889,[1] but was not cultured successfully until 1897.[2] Chancroid is characterized by tender, nonindurated ulcers that have a ragged, undermined border. The ulcers may be single or multiple, and are usually on the penis, vulva, or cervix.[3–6] More than half of the patients have an associated unilateral or bilateral inguinal lymphadenitis.[6,7]

EPIDEMIOLOGY

Outbreaks of chancroid erupt at intervals throughout the world. In tropical countries, such as Kenya and Thailand, chancroid is among the most common diseases transmitted sexually.[8,9] In the United States, however, chancroid is uncommon and typically arises in the context of an epidemic. There have been several large outbreaks since 1980. Most of these have been in large cities such as New York, Boston, Miami, Dallas, and Houston.[4,10–12] The disease is now considered to be endemic in South Florida and in New York City.[13] Chancroid is often spread by prostitutes in the United States, and therefore heterosexual men account for 80% of infections.[4,12–14]

CLINICAL FEATURES

After an incubation period of 2 to 11 days, a tender papule arises at the site of inoculation. The papule becomes pustular and ruptures to form an irregularly shaped ulcer with undermined edges and an erythematous halo.[15] The ulcers are soft, tender, and may infect apposing areas of skin by autoinoculation.[3,7] These ulcers are most common on the penis in men (Figures 50–1 and 50–2) and on the vulva in women.[3–6] In 50% of the patients, inguinal adenopathy develops in the first week of disease.[6,7] The adenopathy is tender, and if untreated often becomes suppurative (bubo).

PATHOLOGY

Biopsy of a chancroid ulcer shows a distinctive triple zone of inflammation (Figure 50–3).[12,16–18] The superficial layer is comprised of fibrin, necrotic tissue, neutrophils, and red blood cells. The middle zone is wide and contains proliferating vessels with swollen endothelial cells. At the junction with the superficial zone, these vessels are occluded and occasionally thrombosed. The deep zone merges with the middle zone and has a dense lymphocytic and plasma cell infiltrate. The identification of these three zones has a 90% accuracy rate in diagnosing chancroid.[17,18]

Tissue sections may be stained with Giemsa, gram, hematoxylin-eosin, pyronine, or methylene blue to demonstrate the zones of inflammation. *Haemophilus ducreyi,* however, are rarely identified in tissue sections[17] but are more readily demonstrated in pus aspirated from the undermined edge of an ulcer or from a bubo.[19]

Tissue sections studied by electron microscopy reveal coccobacilli in groups and aggregates in the interstitial space. They appear as rods about 1.3 μm

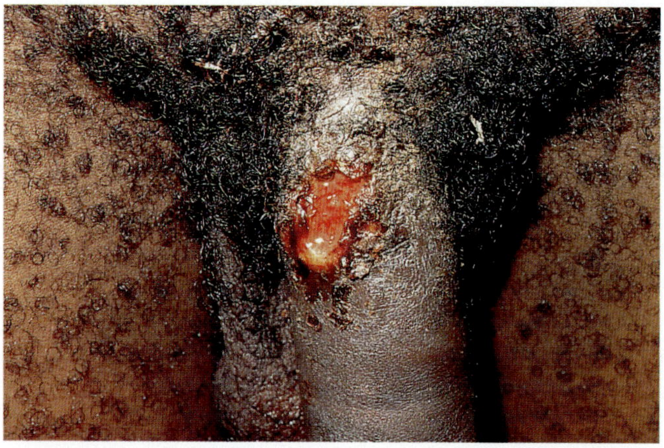

Figure 50–1. An acute, early ulcer of chancroid on the shaft of the penis with striking inguinal lymphadenopathy.

long and 0.5 μm wide with rounded ends. Only rarely are bacilli identified in phagosomes of macrophages.

DIAGNOSIS

When tissue sections reveal the characteristic three zones but no organisms, the definitive diagnosis of chancroid is made by in vitro culture. Diagnosis based solely on the shape and reaction in the ulcer may prove erroneous, because clinical variants exist and mixed infections are common.[20–22] Gram staining and silver staining of the margin of the ulcer or of the exudate aspirated from the ulcer reveals gram-negative coccobacilli in chains with a clustering that has been described as having a "school of fish" appearance (Figure 50–4).[23] The bacilli usually are extracellular and surrounded by neutrophils. Gram staining of the ulcer exudate, nevertheless, has a sensitivity of only 50%.[17] Other diagnostic techniques are no longer used. The autoinoculation technique was stopped for ethical reasons,

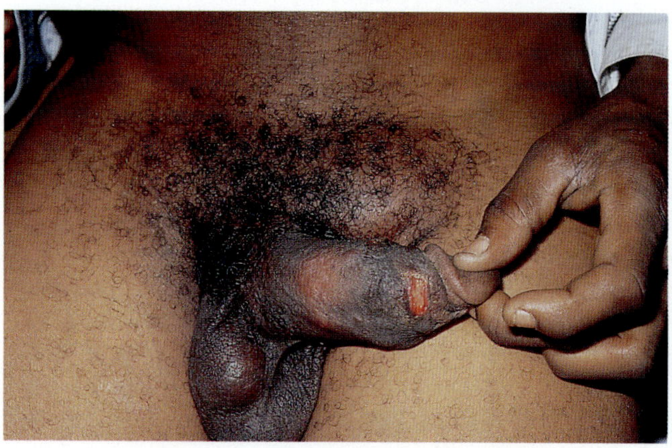

Figure 50–2. Healing chancroid of foreskin.

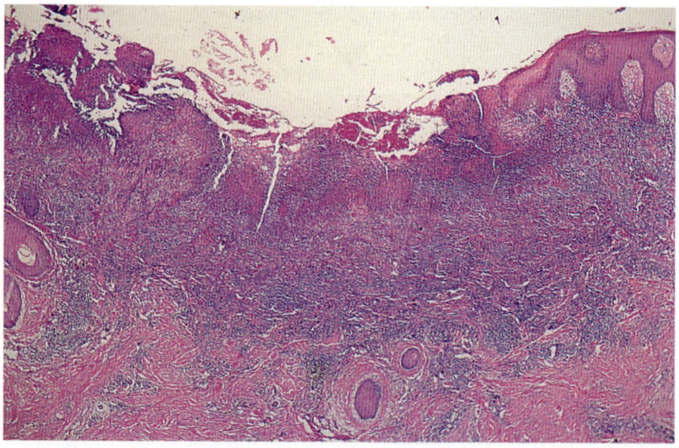

Figure 50–3. Chancroid of anal skin showing the characteristic three layers of reaction: 1) a superficial necrotic layer comprised of neutrophils, fibrin, necrotic tissue, and red blood cells, 2) a middle zone containing proliferating vessels, and 3) a deep zone containing lymphocytes and plasma cells (hematoxylin-eosin, ×7.5).

and the Ito-Reenstierne test is no longer available. Biopsies are rarely done on genital ulcers because they are painful, and often unable to be performed in clinics for sexually transmitted diseases.

Numerous advances have been made in the diagnosis by culture since Ducrey's first isolation. In 1920, Teague and Diebert[24] reported positive cultures in 140 of 270 infections using a heat-inactivated rabbit's blood medium. Diagnosis of chancroid, however, was tedious and complicated by contaminants before the 1970s. In 1978, Hammond and coworkers[25] used a selective medium of chocolate agar and vancomycin with rabbit's blood and recovered *H ducreyi* from 8 of 16 genital ulcers. Sotteneck et al[26] improved the sensitivity of this

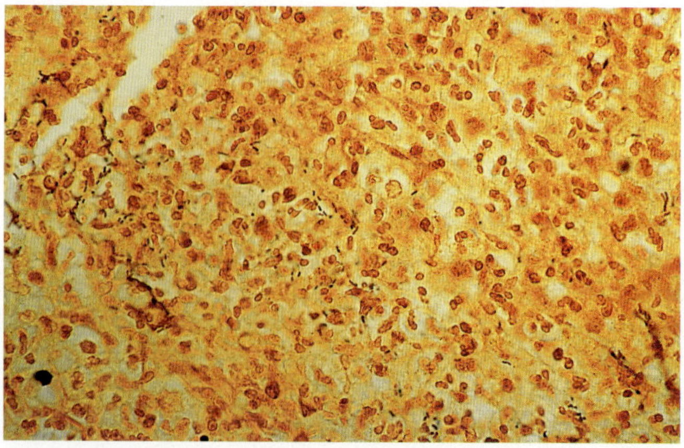

Figure 50–4. Necrotic exudate in the floor of a chancroid ulcer. The bacilli are coated with a colloid of metallic silver and thus appear thicker than they do when stained with simple dyes. The clustering of the bacilli, sometimes in parallel rows, has been described as a "school of fish." There is clustering and some parallel arrangement of the bacilli here (Warthin–Starry, ×650).

medium to 70% by adding 10% fetal bovine serum. In 1984, Nsanze et al[27] recovered 81% by using a biplate of gonococcal base agar with 2% bovine hemoglobin and 5% fetal calf serum and a Mueller–Hinton–based agar with 5% chocolatized horse blood. Other investigators have reported similar results using this protocol.[28,29]

Newer and more rapid methods of diagnosis have emerged since the 1980s. Dot immunobinding and enzyme immunoassays have been developed, but have limited sensitivity.[30,31] Recently, an immunofluorescent monoclonal antibody test has been reported to be 93% sensitive in detecting *H ducreyi*.[32] Future diagnostic techniques most likely will include the detection of bacterial DNA through radiolabeled probes or by polymerase chain reaction.[33,34]

TREATMENT

Currently the Centers for Disease Control and Prevention recommend that patients with chancroid be treated with oral erythromycin, 500 mgm four times a day for 7 days, or a single dose of ceftriaxone, 250 mgm injected intramuscularly. A single-dose therapy with 1.0 g azithromycin has been recently approved as an alternative treatment.

REFERENCES

1. Morse SA. Chancroid and *Haemophilus ducreyi*. *Clin Microbiol Rev.* 1989;2:137–157.
2. Davis L. Observations on the distribution and culture of the chancroid bacillus. *J Med Res.* 1903;9:401–414.
3. Faro S. Lymphogranuloma venerum, chancroid and granuloma inguinale. *Obstet Gynecol Clin North Am.* 1989; 16:517–530.
4. Jones C, Rosen T, Clarridge J, et al. Chancroid: results from an outbreak in Houston, Texas. *South Med J.* 1990; 83:1384–1389.
5. Kraus SJ. Diagnosis and management of acute genital ulcers in sexually active patients. *Sem Dermatol.* 1990;9: 160–166.
6. Schmid GP. Approach to the patient with genital ulcer disease. *Med Clin North Am.* 1990;74:1559–1572.
7. Margolis RJ, Hood AF. Chancroid: diagnosis and treatment. *J Am Acad Dermatol.* 1982;6:493–499.
8. Plummer FA, Nsanze H, Karasira P, et al. Epidemiology of chancroid and *Haemophilus ducreyi* in Nairobi, Kenya. *Lancet.* 1983;2:1293–1295.
9. Taylor DN, Duangman C, Suvongse C, et al. The role of *Haemophilus ducreyi* in penile ulcers in Bangkok, Thailand. *Sex Trans Dis.* 1984;11:148–151.
10. Centers for Disease Control. Sexually transmitted disease statistics. Atlanta, GA 1982;134:37–38.
11. Centers for Disease Control. Chancroid—Massachusetts. *MMWR.* 1985;34:711–718.
12. McCarley ME, Cruz PD, Sontheimer RD. Chancroid: clinical variants and other findings from an epidemic in Dallas County. *J Am Acad Dermatol.* 1988;19:330–337.
13. Ronald AR, Plummer FA. Chancroid and granuloma inguinale. *Sex Trans Dis.* 1989;9:535–543.
14. Schulte JM, Matrich FA, Schmid A. Chancroid in the United States, 1981–1990. *MMWR.* 1992;41:57–61.
15. Flumara NJ, Rothman K, Tran S. The diagnosis and treatment of chancroid. *J Am Acad Dermatol.* 1986;15:939–943.
16. Freinkel AL. Histological aspects of sexually transmitted genital lesions. *Histopathology.* 1987;11:819–831.
17. Heyman A, Beeson PB, Sheldon WH. Diagnosis of chancroid. *JAMA.* 1945;129:935–938.
18. Sheldon WH, Heyman A. Studies on chancroid: observations on the histology with evaluation of biopsy as a diagnostic procedure. *Am J Pathol.* 1946;32:415–422.
19. Lever WF. *Histopathology of the Skin.* Philadelphia: Lippincott; 1983.
20. Sturn AW, Stolting GJ, Cormare RH, et al. Clinical and microbiological evaluation of 46 episodes of genital ulceration. *Genitourin Med.* 1987;63:98–101.
21. Nsanze H, Fast MV, D'Costa JL, et al. Genital ulcers in Kenya. *Br J Ven Dis.* 1981;57378–381.
22. Salzman RS, Kraus SJ, Miller RG, et al. Chancroid ulcers that are not chancroid. *Arch Dermatol.* 1984;120:636–639.
23. Joseph AK, Rosen T. Laboratory techniques used in the diagnosis of chancroid, granuloma inguinale, and lymphogranuloma venereum. *Dermatol Clin.* 1994;12:1–8.
24. Teague O, Diebert O. The value of the cultural method in the diagnosis of chancroid. *J Urol.* 1920;4:543–550.
25. Hammond GW, Lian CJ, Wilt JC, et al. Comparison of specimen collection and laboratory techniques for isolation of *Haemophilus ducreyi*. *J Clin Microbiol.* 1978;7: 739–743.
26. Sotteneck FO, Biddle JW, Kraus SJ, et al. Isolation and identification of *Haemophilus ducreyi* in a clinical study. *J Clin Microbiol.* 1980;12:170–174.
27. Nsanze H, Plummer FA, Maggwa AB, et al. Comparison of media for the primary isolation of *Haemophilus ducreyi*. *Sex Transm Dis.* 1984;11:6–9.
28. Dylewski J, Nsanze H, Maithe G, et al. Laboratory diagnosis of *Haemophilus ducreyi*. *Diagn Microbiol Infect Dis.* 1986;4:241–245.
29. Lubwama SW, Plummer FA, Nidnaya-Achola J, et al. Isolation and identification of *Haemophilus ducreyi* in a clinical laboratory. *J Med Microbiol.* 1986;22:175–178.
30. Schalla WO, Sanders LL, Schmidt G, et al. Use of dot immunobinding and immunofluorescence assays to investigate clinically suspected chancroid. *J Infect Dis.* 1986; 153:879–887.
31. Museyi K, Van Dyck E, Vervoort T, et al. Use of an enzyme immunoassay to detect serum IgG antibodies to *Haemophilus ducreyi*. *J Infect Dis.* 1988;157:1039–1043.
32. Karim QN, Finn GY, Easmon CSF, et al. Rapid diagnosis of *Haemophilus ducreyi* in clinical and experimental infections using monoclonal antibody. *Genitourin Med.* 1989;65:361–365.
33. Parsons LM, Shayegani M, Waring AL, et al. DNA probes for the identification of *Haemophilus ducreyi*. *J Clin Microbiol.* 1989;27:1441–1445.
34. Jones C, Rosen T. Cultural diagnosis of chancroid. *Arch Dermatol.* 1991;127:1823–1827.

CHAPTER 51

Chlamydial Infections

Chlamydia trachomatis

Deborah Dean

One-half of the troubles of this life can be traced to saying yes too quickly and not saying no soon enough.

Josh Billings (1818–1885)

CLASSIFICATION

Chlamydia trachomatis is one of the three currently recognized species of *Chlamydia*. These organisms comprise a single order, Chlamydiales, a single family, Chlamydiaceae, and one genus, *Chlamydia*. *Chlamydia* have historically been named *Bedsonia* or *Miyangawanella*. The other two species of the genus are *Chlamydia psittaci* and *Chlamydia pneumoniae*. Recently, a new agent has been isolated from sheep and cattle that appears to be closely related to *Chlamydia*. Although this agent was proposed as *Chlamydia pecorum* in 1992,[1] additional analyses are required before classifying this agent as the fourth species of the genus. *Chlamydia trachomatis* is made up of three biovars: trachoma, lymphogranuloma venereum (LGV), and mouse pneumonitis. With the exception of the mouse pneumonitis biovar, *C trachomatis* infects only humans. The human biovars and their strains have 87% to 99% DNA homology with each other, yet display only 30% homology with the mouse pneumonitis biovar. *Chlamydia trachomatis* is responsible for both ocular and genital tract infections. These infections are caused by one or more serovars, which are classified serologically. The basis for this serotyping is the antigenic variation of the major outer membrane protein (MOMP) of the organism. The serovars can be grouped by antigenic relatedness as follows: Serogroup B (serovars B, Ba, D, Da, E, and L2); intermediate serogroup (serovars F and G); and serogroup C (serovars A, C, H, I, Ia, J, K, L1, and L3). The serovars A through K have historically been referred to as trachoma-inclusion conjunctivitis agents, or TRIC. Serovars A, B, Ba, and C are considered the agents of trachoma, a chronic inflammatory disease of the eye (see the "Trachoma" section of this chapter). Some B, Ba, and C serovars along with serovars D through K, Da, and Ia cause oculogenitourinary and genitoanorectal infections in humans. Although these serovars have been the mainstay for classifying the organism, a new system has been developed that is based on the MOMP gene (*omp1*) of *C trachomatis* and is referred to as *omp1* genotyping.[2,3] This new system of typing is evolving and will be of great importance for determining the association of chlamydiae with specific diseases, for evaluating the pathogenesis of these diseases, and for transmission studies in sexually transmitted disease (STD) and trachoma populations.

INTRODUCTION AND HISTORY

The identification of *C trachomatis* as a cause of genital tract infections was delayed until smear and culture methods became available for detecting *Neisseria gonorrhoeae* (GC). Once GC was excluded as the cause of urethritis, ophthalmia neonatorum, and cervicitis, there were suspicions that a unique infectious agent caused these diseases. In 1907, Halberstaedter and Prowazek were the first to see the typical intracytoplasmic inclusions of *Chlamydia* in conjunctival scrapings from an orangutan infected with material from a human with trachoma. Subsequently, similar inclusions were seen in scrapings from an infant with inclusion blenorrhea and in the genital tract of a mother and the urethra of a father with an infant who had ophthalmia neonatorum.[4] Although *C psittaci* was isolated in 1929 and LGV was isolated in 1935, the trachoma agent was not isolated until the 1950s, in part because it failed to infect mice. T'ang et al[5] successfully propagated this agent using embryonized hens' yolk sacs. Two years later, in 1959, a genital strain of *C trachomatis* was finally isolated.

In spite of the successful isolation of ocular and genital strains of chlamydiae, the delay of up to 6 weeks for definitive identification of the organism hampered progress in the biology of chlamydiae and the diseases they caused. Thus, it was a major breakthrough when in 1965 Gordon and Quan[6] developed a tissue culture system that provided results within 48 to 72 hours. In a subsequent series of studies using this technique, up to 50% of men with nongonococcal urethritis were found to infected with *C trachomatis*.[7] Tissue culture paved the way for the identification of the organism from a number of different anatomic sites, providing information on the spectrum of diseases associated with *C trachomatis*. In 1970, Wang and Grayston[8] introduced a technique for immunotyping *C trachomatis*, allowing for the identification of serovars. Since the early 1970s, *C trachomatis* has become associated with an increasing number of clinical syndromes, largely due to improved and more widely used culture techniques along with the use of newer commercial diagnostics, such as the direct fluorescent antibody (DFA) test, enzyme linked immunosorbent assay (ELISA), and DNA-based technologies, such as nucleic acid hybridization probes, the ligase chain reaction (LCR), and the polymerase chain reaction (PCR).

The natural history of infections of the genital tract by *C trachomatis* is not well understood. What little is known comes from trachoma research and a few studies of treated and untreated adults.[9,10] Chlamydiae elicit an immune response that facilitates the resolution of infection in most patients. Chronic asymptomatic and persistent infections of the conjunctival and genital mucosa, however, are common and not easily recognized by distinguishing clinical criteria. Chronic infections may persist for months, and this increases the potential for transmission and sequelae. Furthermore, chlamydial DNA and viable organisms have been recovered from the fallopian tubes of women with tubal infertility.[11,12] Currently we know that up to 80% of women and 30% of men are asymptomatic,[13] yet it is unclear if chlamydiae can establish a chronic latent focus of infection in the genital tract that can be reactivated by immune or other stimuli. A recurrence of *C trachomatis* respiratory infections has been reported following immunosuppressive treatment,[14] and similar findings have also been reported for trachoma patients following topical steroid treatment.[15]

EPIDEMIOLOGY

Chlamydia trachomatis infections of the genital tract have been recognized within the last decade as the most common STD in the developed world, and may be equally common in the developing world. In the United States, the incidence of infection is estimated at 4 million cases per year, with an annual cost of more than $2.4 billion dollars.[16] Chlamydial genital infections and their sequelae in women account for approximately 80% of this cost. A large number of studies have focused on the prevalence of, and risk factors for, infection among women of all age groups, but relatively few studies have addressed similar problems in men, although this is an area of expanding research. The highest prevalence rates of infection are among sexually active adolescent women, exceeding 10%,[16] and for women attending STD clinics where rates are 15% to 19%.[17,18] Screening of women attending family planning clinics has revealed a rate of 6% to 13%, with the lowest infection rates for women examined at university (5% to 10%) and prenatal clinics (4% to 8%).[13] There are few data for women seen in private practice or primary care settings.

Clinical signs associated with but not pathognomonic of chlamydial infections include cervicitis with friable mucosa, mucopurulent discharge, and/or effacement of the squamocolumnar junction.[13] The majority of genital infections in women is subclinical and non-acute. This is substantiated by recent studies demonstrating viable organisms in the endometrium and salpinx of asymptomatic women.[19] Although pelvic inflammatory disease (PID) can be self-limiting, in many patients luminal fallopian tube and paratubal scarring leads to the sequelae of ectopic pregnancies, tubal infertility, and chronic pelvic pain. Epidemiologic analyses of ectopic pregnancies have found that prior chlamydial infections of the fallopian tubes and ectopic pregnancies are associated.[20] Furthermore, progression of disease is associated also with an immunopathogenic response that follows repeat infections.[21] Thus, asymptomatic and repeat *C trachomatis* infections probably cause more severe subclinical inflammation and tubal damage than other organisms.[22]

Demographic characteristics reveal that young age (<25 years) is the strongest and most consistent factor associated with chlamydial STDs among women.[13] This may be caused in part by the higher prevalence of cervical ectopy in young women, and this increases the number of cells susceptible to infection. Indeed, cervical ectopy may predispose to increased shedding of the organism.[23] This ectopy may also explain the higher risk of PID in this age group.[24] In older women, risk factors include lower socioeconomic status, African-American race, nulliparity, and single marital status.[13] Other factors associated with chlamydial infections include concurrent infection with GC and multiple or new sex partners.[13] In both age groups, sexual intercourse with a man with chlamydial urethritis increases the risk of infection by more than 30%.[24]

The epidemiology of *C trachomatis* infections in men is less clear. The highest prevalence rates are in men attending STD clinics (15% to 20%).[13] Up to 13% of young men coming to adolescent clinics are also infected.[13] Overall, asymptomatic infections occur in 4% to 30% of men.[25–27] Although youth, multiple sex partners, and concurrent infection with or without a history of GC infection are considered risk factors for chlamydial infections, more comprehensive studies are required to address these problems. Those who are heterosexual, nonwhite, and under 20 years of age, however, have a consistently higher prevalence rate of infection.[25]

There are very few data on the efficacy of transmission of *C trachomatis. Chlamydia trachomatis,* however, is considered to be less easily transmitted than GC. Barrier contraceptives, including the cervical cap, diaphragm, and condoms, appear to protect against infection and thus decrease the risk of transmission. Although a few studies present evidence for an increased risk of infection with birth control pills,[28] this is not conclusive.[13] Most studies that attempt to address transmission are limited by the difficulty in enrolling partners, differential sensitivity of culture and other diagnostic tests for detecting chlamydiae, and selection bias. From data on couples with discordant infections, women transmitted chlamydiae to their male partners 32% of the time, whereas men transmitted chlamydiae to their female partners 40% of the time.[29] The premise for these numbers was an estimation of the average frequency of intercourse per couple. This may, however, overestimate the risk of transmission for a single act of intercourse.[13] For adolescents, the frequency of intercourse, regardless of the number of partners, is strongly associated with chlamydial infections.[30] Some studies have shown a 45% to 65% rate of infection for female partners of infected males and a rate of 25% to 45% for male partners of infected women.[31–33] This apparent increase in transmission to females may actually represent an inability to diagnose all infections in men appropriately, as sampling the urethra may be biased, because this is an invasive and less accepted procedure unless there is active, symptomatic disease. Also the tests used for diagnosis, such as tissue culture, may be less sensitive for detecting chlamydiae in men than in women. This theory was supported by a recent paper that compared culture versus PCR as a diagnostic tool for determining transmission rates in a heterosexual population. PCR revealed not only a higher rate of positive samples for chlamydiae but equal rates of transmission to partners for either men or women.[34] Coinfection with GC may also affect transmission. Women who are infected with GC are more likely to have a concurrent infection with *C trachomatis;* indeed, a higher titer of infectious chlamydial organisms is usually present in those who are infected with both. Furthermore, recurrence rates for chlamydial infections with the same serovar are higher among patients with GC and chlamydiae than among those infected by *C trachomatis* alone.[35] Finally, the role of core groups in the maintenance and transmission of chlamydial infections is unclear. Currently, these groups do not appear to be as important for chlamydial transmission as they are for GC.[36] This may in part be explained by the already high prevalence of chlamydiae in high-risk populations. If there is a decline in chlamydial rates, however, core groups may become a critical factor in facilitating transmission.

MORPHOLOGY AND DEVELOPMENTAL CELL CYCLE

Chlamydia are prokaryotes. Until the 1960s, *Chlamydia* were considered viruses because of their small size and the difficulty encountered with their in vitro propagation. However, they are now classified as bacteria because they contain ribosomes; divide by binary fission; are inhibited by antibacterial drugs; and are morphologically, metabolically, and structurally similar to gram-negative bacteria. They express outer membrane and lipopolysaccharide proteins that are functionally analogous to those in *E coli. Chlamydia* have a unique biphasic developmental cell cycle that distinguishes them from all other obligate intracellular pathogens. The infectious form of the organism is the elementary body (EB). The EB is metabolically inert but contains both ATP and inactive ATPase.[37] It possesses a rigid, almost spore-like outer membrane composed of disulfide cross-linking of cysteine residues on MOMP and between MOMP and two cysteine-rich outer membrane proteins of 12 and 60 kilodaltons (kD), respectively. The structural integrity of this membrane allows the EB to survive for short periods outside the host cell, but the precise time it remains viable is unknown. The developmental cell cycle of chlamydiae is initiated when the EB comes in contact with the cell surface of epithelial cells. There is evidence that this initial binding to host cells is facilitated by divalent cations and polycations.[21] Alternatively, attachment may proceed using heparin sulfate as a bridge between receptors on its surface and the host cell.[38] *Chlamydiae* may attach by a common but as yet unknown receptor. This is suggested because chlamydial attachment is inhibited by competing heterologous serovars.[39] Although the MOMP has been considered an adhesion protein in this process, this has not been definitively determined.

Receptor-mediated endocytosis is the primary mechanism of uptake for the EB[40]; however, pinocytosis and phagocytosis do occur, the latter by a microfilament-dependent mechanism. Once the endophagosome or inclusion body, as it is called, has formed, there is ineffective host lysosomal fusion that permits intracellular survival of the organism. The developmental cycle appears to be regulated by transcription because there are a number of different genes that have been identified as promoters, and mRNA has been described that appears to be life-cycle specific.[9] Within 6 to 8 hours, the 200 to 350 nm EB differentiates into a metabolically active reticulate body (RB) of 800 to 1000 nm by cleavage of the disulfide bonds and synthesis of new proteins. During this process, ATPase is activated by reducing agents.[41] Essential host cell metabolites, including high-energy phosphate compounds,[37] are transported across the endophagosome membrane and along with the stores of ATP and activated ATPase, provide the energy for RB replication that takes place by binary fission (Figure 51–1). The inclusion body expands with replication products and glycogen and displaces the nucleus to one end of the cell (Figure 51–2). The RBs condense back down into EBs by compaction of chromatin into an electron dense nucleoid and by the formation of disulfide bonds, creating once again the rigid outer membrane structure. The number of new infectious units produced is from 100 to more than 1000 per cell.[42] At the completion of the cell cycle, the host cell is either lysed by rupture of the inclusion body or the cell expels the inclusion body via a process similar to exocytosis, thereby releasing the infectious EBs. The completion of one cell cycle in tissue culture requires 48 to 72 hours, depending on the serovar.

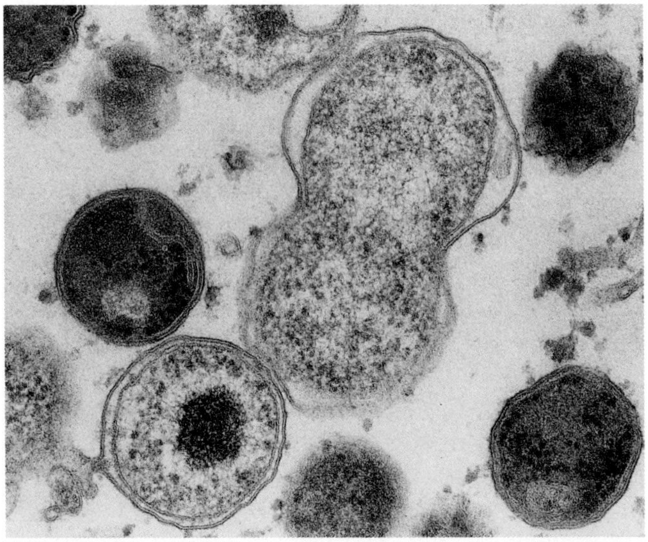

Figure 51–1. High magnification of part of a *C trachomatis* inclusion showing a dividing reticulate body, two elementary bodies (EB), and an intermediate form with its typical nucleoid. The EBs contain glycogen, which appears as a light haze among the electron dense body (×78,000). *(Photograph courtesy of Barbara Nichols, PhD, San Francisco, California.)*

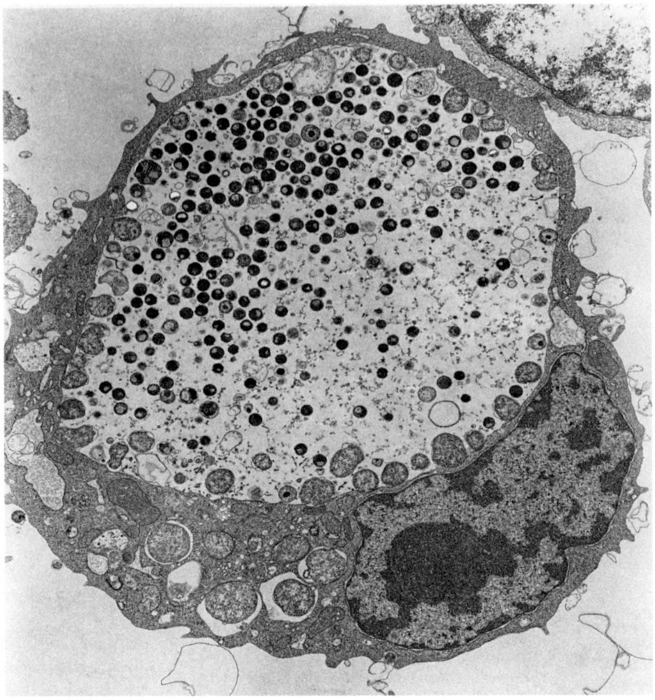

Figure 51–2. Electron micrograph of an inclusion containing *C trachomatis* cultured for 40 hours in L929 cells, showing EBs, intermediate forms, and reticulate bodies. Most of the reticulate bodies are at the periphery of the inclusion (×7500). *(Photograph courtesy of Mary Louise Chiappino, San Francisco, California.)*

As noted, the EB contains a unique outer membrane protein (MOMP) with lipopolysaccharide (LPS) components. Some determinants in the LPS are genus-specific. MOMP is the most abundant and immunogenic surface protein and has an approximate mass of 40 kD, which differs by serovar. This protein contains serovar-, serogroup-, species-, and genus-specific epitopes. There are four variable segments of MOMP, designed VS1–4; VS1, VS2, and VS4 are surface-exposed epitopes. VS3 does not share this property with the other variable segments, but it does contain two T-cell determinants that can elicit T-cell help for antibody pro-

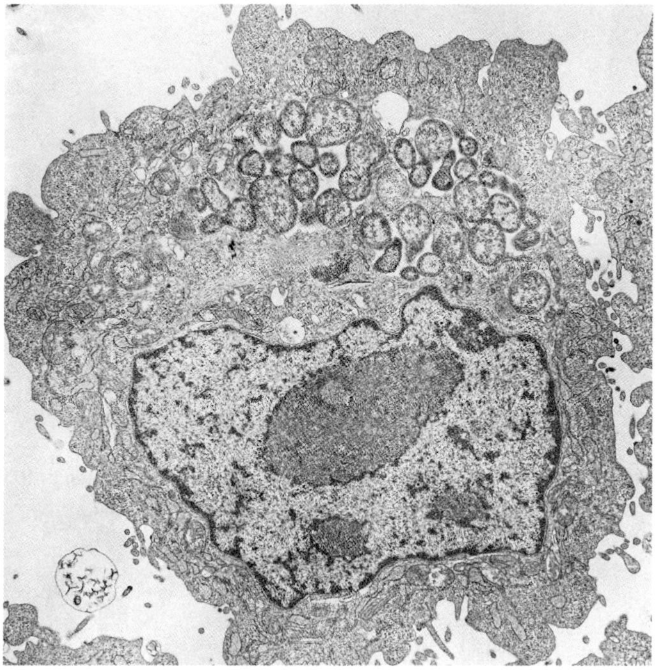

Figure 51–3. Electron micrograph of inclusions containing *C psittaci* in an L929 cell 24 hours after inoculation. Note that the several separate inclusions all contain reticulate bodies (×8400). *(Photograph courtesy of Barbara Nichols, PhD, San Francisco, California.)*

duction directed at protective antigens on MOMP.[43] MOMP is expressed throughout the life cycle, whereas the 12 kD and 60 kD outer membrane proteins are expressed late in development at a time when the RB is condensing back into an infectious EB.[21]

The three species of chlamydiae differ by inclusion morphology, metabolism, host cell preference, antigenic determinants, and antimicrobial susceptibility. The morphology of the EBs for both *C psittaci* and *C trachomatis* is almost identical, whereas for *C pneumoniae* it appears pear-shaped with a larger periplasmic space. The RBs are morphologically the same for all species. When cells are infected with more than one *C trachomatis* EB, the inclusion bodies tend to fuse to form one or, at most, two bodies. For *C psittaci* and *C pneumoniae*, multiple small inclusions can be visualized for each infecting EB. These inclusions can be quite variable in shape, especially for *C psittaci* (Figure 51–3). Only *C trachomatis* accumulates gylcogen, which can be identified by staining with iodine. The three species share antigenic determinants in the LPS. However, primary serovar-, subspecies-, and species-specific epitopes are in the MOMP. All species are susceptible to tetracyclines, whereas all *C trachomatis* and few *C psittaci* strains are susceptible to sulfonamides. Only *C trachomatis* and *C psittaci* contain a 7.5 kB plasmid. There is considerable sequence variation in the plasmid between these species, but little variation among serovars of *C trachomatis.* Although the function of this extrachromosomal material is not known, it may play a role in replication[44]; yet some strains of *C trachomatis* lack this plasmid and can still be propagated in tissue culture.[45]

CLINICAL FEATURES

The syndromes attributed to chlamydiae most closely resemble GC infection in terms of the sites of infection; predilection for columnar and transitional epithelium; and capacity for producing extensive inflammation, epithelial ulceration, and scarring.[10] The known sites of infection include the urethra, epididymis, endocervix, endometrium, salpinx, adnexae (including the ovaries), Bartholin's duct, perihepatic region, and rectum. The presumptive sites include the vagina in postmenopausal women,[46] the peritoneum,[47] and the prostate, for which a definitive diagnosis is difficult because material obtained after massaging the prostate passes through a potentially infected urethra.

The cervix and urethra are the primary sites of chlamydial infection in women. Effacement of the squamocolumnar junction, seen in many young women, including those on birth control pills, predisposes to infection. The presentation of chlamydial infections in women can mimic GC infection, be nonspecific, produce few symptoms, or be completely asymptomatic and quite insidious. Only 30% of these women present with symptoms, which include vaginal bleeding or spotting and discharge. In the latter case, other causal agents may be responsible and should be considered in the diagnostic workup. Although chlamydiae cannot infect the squamous epithelium of the vagina in adults, a vaginal infection in a girl may signal a chlamydial infection of the transitional epithelium that is present until puberty. The signs of cervical infection are friability, increased erythema, edema, and/or a discharge from the cervical os that may be clear or purulent. However, women may also have a normal appearing cervix. Colposcopy usually reveals a follicular cervicitis with some degree of ectopy and erythema (Figure 51–4).[48] Other symptoms include dysuria, pelvic pain, dyspareunia, and/or abdominal pain. The latter symptoms suggest progression of infection to endometrium, salpinx, or pelvic space.

There is some evidence that chlamydial infections of cervix enhance the acquisition and transmission of HIV. In vitro, chlamydiae recruited neutrophils and interacted with them to increase HIV replication.[49] Of the few in vivo studies, one case-control study showed a significant odds ratio with narrow confidence interval

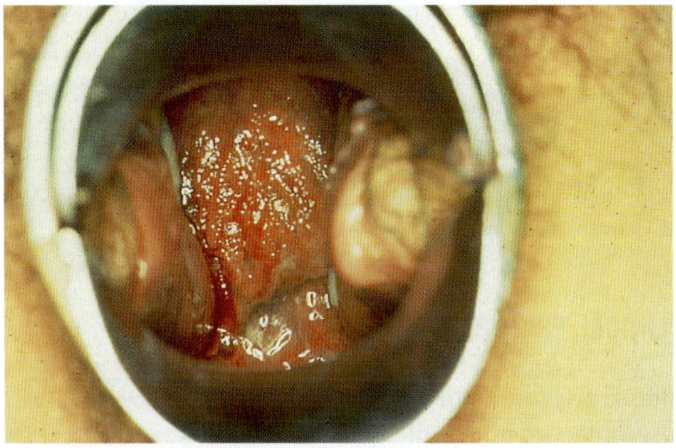

Figure 51–4. Chlamydial cervicitis with granulation tissue of the zone of transformation. *(Photograph courtesy of David A. Schwartz, MD.)*

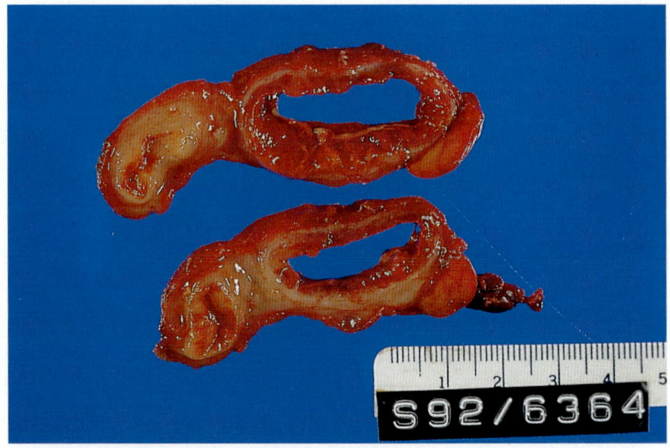

Figure 51–5. Patient with chronic salpingitis and obstruction of the distal portion of the tube caused by infection with *C trachomatis.* *(Photograph courtesy of David A. Schwartz, MD.)*

for HIV seroconversion among female prostitutes infected with *C trachomatis.*[50] In another study of high risk women, a significantly higher *C trachomatis* prevalence rate was noted for HIV-positive asymptomatic women than both HIV-negative women and controls with unknown HIV status.[51] These results were independent of CD4+, CD8+, and total lymphocyte counts. Although more definitive data are required, if chlamydiae do increase the risk of HIV infection, this would offer an important incentive for enhanced screening for, and treatment of, chlamydial infections as a public health control measure for the spread of HIV.

Urethritis caused by *C trachomatis* has become increasingly prevalent in the last decade. It is believed to cause the acute urethral syndrome that is defined as dysuria, and frequency with fewer than 10^5 organisms per milliliter of urine. Some women with this syndrome also may have frank pyuria. Chlamydial urethritis is now the most common pathogen causing nonenteric urethritis in university women who present with dysuria, urgency, and/or frequency.[52] These symptoms are usually more gradual in onset and of longer duration than those caused by enteric pathogens. Frequently there is a history of a new sex partner or multiple sexual contacts. Chlamydiae have also been isolated from women with acute bartholinitis, but many of these women are coinfected with GC.

PID is one of the most common and serious sequelae of *C trachomatis* genital infections. PID includes endometritis with or without salpingitis, pelvic peritonitis, periappendicitis, and perihepatitis. PID caused by chlamydiae tends to have a more chronic and subacute course than do infections with GC. The proportion of women with mucocervicitis who have endometritis is about 40%; however, only 8% of women with endocervicitis develop salpingitis.[9] The symptoms of PID have a broad range and include mild to severe pelvic and/or lower abdominal pain, fatigue, and/or mild to severe prostration. Infected women may also be asymptomatic, during which time the organism may continue to spread and produce inflammation. This can lead to abscess, fibrosis, pelvic scarring, and adhesions with subsequent tubal occlusion. These outcomes may be facilitated by recurrent or persistent infection. Laparoscopy may reveal inflammation and fibrous adhesions or scarring of fallopian tubes (Figure 51–5) and peritoneum. The signs of chlamydial PID include fever, cervical motion tenderness, adnexal tenderness, or adnexal mass as in those with ovarian abscess (Figure 51–6). The long-term sequelae of PID are chronic pelvic pain, tubal infertility, and ectopic pregnancy. These reproductive consequences are more likely among women with chlamydial PID than in women with gonococcal PID. The severity of infection and number of episodes of infection increase the risk for tubal infertility.[53] Serologic data indicating prior chlamydial infection have also been strongly associated with both tubal infertility (Figure 51–7) and ectopic pregnancy.[9] In addition, viable chlamydial organisms and chlamydial antigens and DNA have been recovered from the damaged fallopian tubes of infertile women.[11,12] Yet less than half of these women have a history of symptomatic PID. Thus, tubal infertility may be the first sign of chlamydial infection. There is some recent evidence that tubal scarring may also be induced by a hypersensitivity reaction to chlamydial heat shock protein (hsp) 60[54]; however, additional research is required in this area.

Fitz-Hugh–Curtis syndrome is an uncommon complication of chlamydial PID. This syndrome occurs when the organism tracks retroperitoneally to the liver, producing inflammation of the liver capsule and perihepatic area (Figure 51–8). Unlike chlamydial cervicitis,

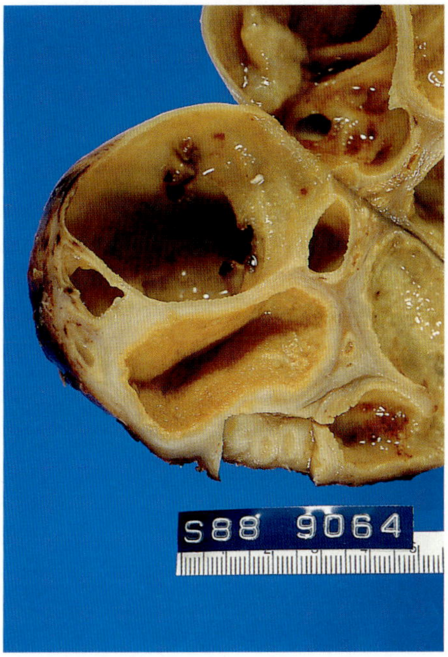

Figure 51–6. Gross photograph of a chlamydial abscess of the ovary. *(Photograph courtesy of David A. Schwartz, MD.)*

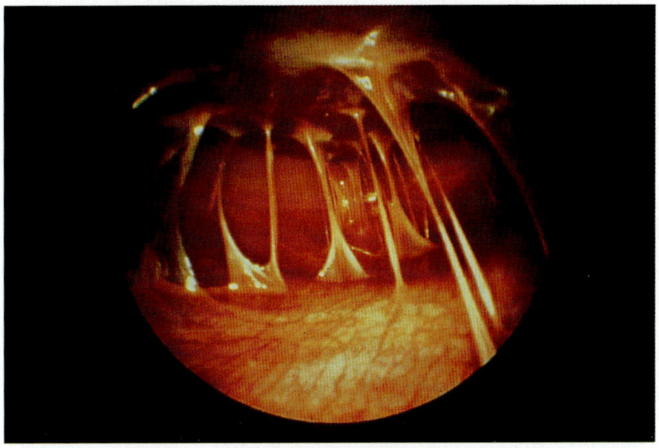

Figure 51–8. Patient with Fitz-Hugh–Curtis syndrome and "violin string" adhesions seen through the laparoscope. *(Photograph reprinted with permission from Stephen Morse, MD, Centers for Disease Control, Atlanta, Georgia.)*

urethritis, or PID, this infection is almost always symptomatic, with patients presenting with right upper quadrant pain, fever, prostration, nausea, and occasionally jaundice. These patients may have no prior or current history of PID or symptoms suggesting infection. Cultures of genitalia usually produce no growth in these patients.

For men, urethritis is the most common clinical feature of infection by *C trachomatis*. Approximately 50% of symptomatic nongonococcal infections and more than 50% of postgonococcal urethritis are caused by chlamydiae.[13] Patients treated for GC infection but who develop postgonococcal urethritis are frequently infected with chlamydiae. Currently, chlamydiae coinfect 20% of patients with GC urethritis. Although approximately 30% of men are asymptomatic, the most frequent symptoms are urethral discharge, itching, and dysuria. The onset of symptoms is less acute and more prolonged than for GC infection. This may reflect in part the longer incubation period of chlamydiae, which is 7 to 14 days, compared with 4 days for GC. The common signs of infection are a clear, gray, or whitish discharge that may be apparent only in the morning before urination. Less often, patients present with a purulent discharge. However, the clinical presentation of chlamydial urethritis cannot be reliably distinguished from GC infection. The association of chlamydiae with prostatitis is unclear. Recently, a number of men with abacterial prostatitis were examined by ultrasound and biopsy.[55] Although inflammatory cells were noted, chlamydiae were not detected in any samples. Thus, there is no convincing evidence that chlamydiae cause prostatitis.

Heterosexual men under age 35 years are at increased risk for developing epididymitis, which usually presents as a unilateral infection with localized pain and, rarely, fever, although the infection can be clinically indolent. An enlarged spermatic cord and erythema of overlying scrotum may be present (Figure 51–9). In addition, an epididymal "tumor" may form.[56] During the acute phase of infection, oligospermia has been reported[57]; however, it is unclear if this has a lasting effect on fertility, as one testicle usually remains unaffected.

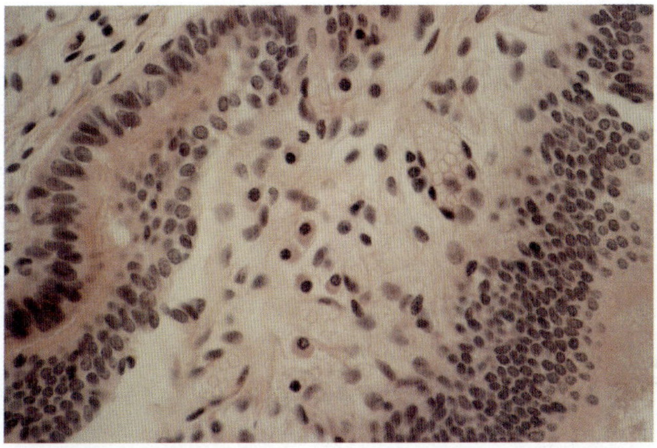

Figure 51–7. Human fallopian tube containing a few plasma cells. This patient has a history of chlamydial infection and continues to be seropositive (hematoxylin-eosin ×400). *(Photograph courtesy of Dorothy Patton, PhD, Seattle, Washington.)*

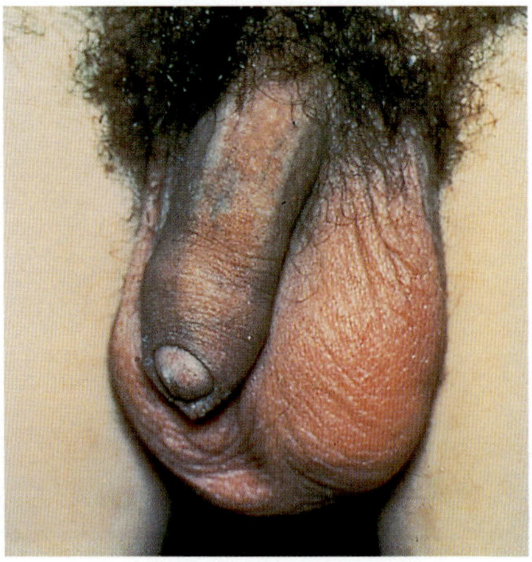

Figure 51–9. Patient with *C trachomatis* epididymitis with unilateral scrotal erythema and edema. *(Photograph reprinted with permission of Stephen Morse, MD, Centers for Disease Control, Atlanta, Georgia.)*

Chlamydial proctitis and proctocolitis is more common among homosexual men, although it can occur in infants and heterosexual adults.[58] The serovars most frequently associated with these diseases are D through K and the LGV serovars L1–3. Direct inoculation through anal intercourse is the most common route of spread in both men and women. The non-LGV serovars may produce an asymptomatic infection or mild disease consisting of rectal pain, abdominal pain, mucopurulent discharge, bleeding, tenesmus, diarrhea, and, rarely, ulceration. The LGV serovars tend to produce severe proctitis with ulceration and proctocolitis.

Chlamydia sp cause inclusion conjunctivitis in adults (Figure 51–10). This clinical syndrome is sometimes referred to as paratrachoma. Approximately 50% of those with inclusion conjunctivitis have a genital tract infection caused by chlamydiae[59]; however, only 1% of patients with chlamydial STDs have ocular infections.[59] The mode of transmission is presumed to be autoinoculation from the genital tract or direct inoculation from an infected partner. For the remaining 50%, it is unclear how the organism is transmitted. It may be that eye-to-hand-to-eye contact in adults is more common than currently suspected. There also are a few infections from accidental ocular inoculation from infected infants and from genital material during surgery.[60] There is also evidence that *C pneumoniae* and *C psittaci* cause a proportion of these infections.[61,62] *C pneumoniae* may colonize the upper respiratory tract and nasal pharynx, providing a reservoir for ocular infection. *C psittaci* is a common pathogen in birds as well as mammals; thus, close contact with infected pets may predispose to infection (Figure 51–11).[61] Inclusion conjunctivitis is usually a unilateral infection that presents with a foreign-body sensation. Patients tend to have conjunctival suffusion and follicles with or without a discharge that may be serous, mucoid, or, rarely, mucopurulent. Ipsilateral periauricular lymphadenopathy is an uncommon finding in these patients. With progression of infection, patients may develop keratitis or pannus, which is characterized as an infiltration of vessels onto the surface of the cornea. At this stage, the clinical findings are indistinguishable from trachoma. Rarely, the infection is complicated by anterior uveitis. More commonly, the infection spreads to cause otitis media.[63] With appropriate treatment, there is usually complete resolution of the disease. Some patients who are not treated, however, may develop chronic infections and conjunctival scarring, which is similar to the scarring seen in trachoma.

Inclusion conjunctivitis in infants is distinct from inclusion conjunctivitis in adults. This syndrome is

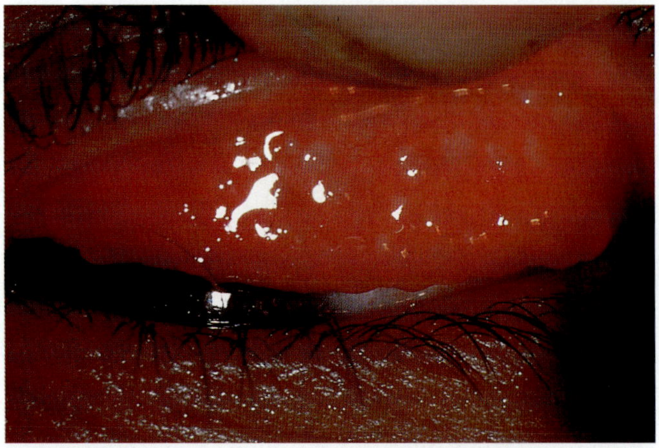

Figure 51–10. Patient with unilateral follicular conjunctivitis caused by autoinoculation from the genital tract. Note the cobblestone appearance of the upper tarsus from lymphoid follicles.

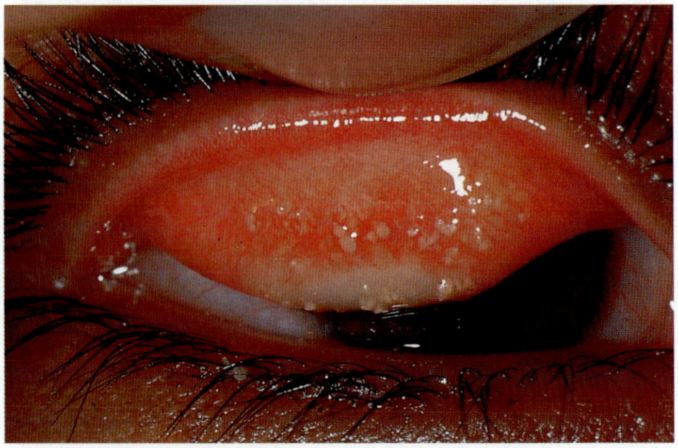

Figure 51–11. Unilateral chronic follicular conjunctivitis by infection with *C psittaci* in an adult woman who is a bird breeder.

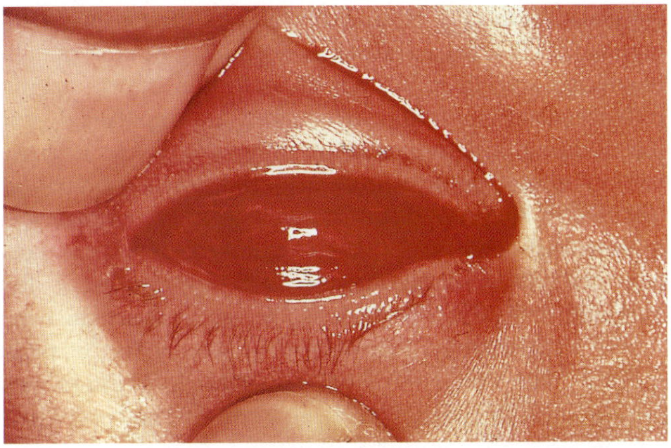

Figure 51–12. Ophthalmia neonatorum caused by *C trachomatis* in an infant. *(Photograph reprinted with permission from Stephen Morse, MD, Centers for Disease Control, Atlanta, Georgia.)*

referred to as ophthalmia neonatorum or inclusion blennorrhea and occurs 1 to 3 weeks after birth (Figure 51–12). Infants acquire infection during passage through an infected birth canal, from infected caregivers by hand-to-eye contact, or occasionally by perinatal infection from rupture of the placenta before delivery. Although 60% of infants born to infected mothers have serologic evidence of chlamydial infections, at most only 44% develop ophthalmia neonatorum.[64] The incubation period is from 5 days to 6 weeks. Prophylaxis at birth with topical tetracyclines or erythromycin does not appear to prevent these infections. Infants present with a serous or mucoid discharge and only rarely follicles, as the conjunctiva does not develop a lymphoid layer until about 6 weeks of age. The infection can progress to a purulent discharge with hyperemia and bleeding. Most infections, however, resolve without treatment. Mild or subclinical infections may persist and can lead to conjunctival scarring with corneal ulceration years later. Ophthalmia neonatorum is often associated with rhinitis in both genders or with vulvovaginitis in the female.[9] Another complication of opthalmia neonatorum is infant pneumonitis, which can occur as early as 2 weeks or as late as 6 months after the initial infection, and is the most common cause of infant pneumonitis in the United States. Approximately 50% of infants with pneumonitis have had conjunctivitis and more than 50% have had otitis media.[65] Infants present with nasal obstruction and discharge, a staccato cough, and tachypnea, and, on chest x ray, they have bilateral interstitial infiltrates. Frequently, they have elevated IgM antibodies to *C trachomatis,* and *C trachomatis* can be isolated from the nasopharynx. Although infant pneumonitis can be life threatening, most infections are presumed to be mild. However, the late sequelae are small airway and obstructive airways disease. Because *C trachomatis* can stay in the nasopharynx, urogenital tract, and rectum for approximately 3 years after birth, it may be impossible to distinguish infection acquired at birth from infection acquired from sexual abuse.[66]

Chlamydial STDs have been recognized as the major cause for reactive arthritis. The onset of the arthritis occurs concurrently or 7 to 20 days postinfection. Reactive arthritis is one of three clinical features that make up Reiter's syndrome. The other two are urethritis and conjunctivitis, iritis, or uveitis (Figure 51–13). Each can be chronic or recurrent. This type of arthritis is immune-mediated and does not appear to be a response to the organism in the joint, although this is controversial. An unconfirmed study has found chlamydiae in the synovia of patients with chlamydial urethritis.[67] Electron microscopy and immunocytochemical studies of synovial membranes have demonstrated organisms similar to chlamydiae,[68] but hybridization and amplification of chlamydial DNA have yielded variable results. Men with reactive arthritis and chlamydial urethritis have responded symptomatically to antichlamydial treatment in contrast to men with other infectious diseases. Furthermore, a similar treatment regimen showed a reduction in recurrent arthritis in men with Reiter's syndrome compared with penicillin treatment alone.[9] Taken together, these data suggest that chlamydiae may reside in some form in the synovial tissue of men with sexually reactive arthritis; further research is required to clarify this issue. Among men presenting with acute arthritis, approximately 70% will have concomitant chlamydial urethritis. Only 1% of men with nongonococcal urethritis (NGU), however, develop reactive arthritis, and 30% of these will have Reiter's syndrome.[9] Patients with Reiter's syndrome have antichlamydial antibodies as well as antibodies to chlamydial hsp60 in both sera and synovial fluid.[69]

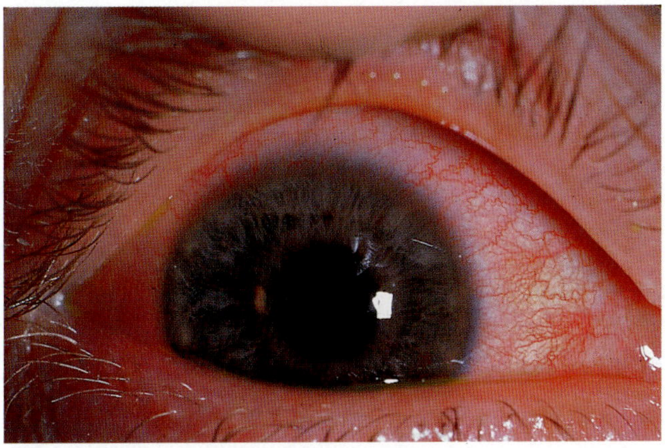

Figure 51–13. Iridocyclitis in a patient with recurrent Reiter's syndrome.

Thus, immune complexes or chlamydial proteins or both may play a direct role in the pathogenesis of this disease.

PATHOLOGY

The lesions of chlamydial infections are frequently indistinguishable from those of other pathogens, but herein an attempt is made to clarify specific versus nonspecific findings for each one of the urogenital infections caused by *C trachomatis*.

C trachomatis infects the columnar epithelial cells of the endocervix and upper genital tract of women and, in prepubescent girls, the transitional cell epithelium of the vagina. Epithelial cells of the urethra, rectum, and conjunctiva in both genders, as well as columnar cells in the infant bronchi, are also prime targets for infection. The nasopharynx, Bartholin's duct, and epididymis are additional sites of infection. The initial infection is characterized by an infiltration of neutrophils, and as infection progresses the tissue is invaded by macrophages, lymphocytes, plasma cells, and, less frequently, eosinophils, unless the site is the infant lung.[9]

Changes in chlamydial cervicitis and urethritis are remarkably similar to those of GC (Figure 51–14). Colposcopic findings of chlamydial cervicitis reveal extensive inflammation at the transition zone in approximately 45% of these infections.[70] Increased surface vascularity, immature metaplasia, papillary formation, and hypertrophic follicles are also features. These latter findings occur later in the infection and are characteristic of, but not pathognomonic for, *C trachomatis*. On cytology there may be metaplastic and endocervical cell atypias.[71] With progression of the infection, the histopathologic manifestations include a dense stromal inflammation with plasma cells, intraepithelial and intraluminal inflammation or microabscesses, necrosis of epithelium or ulceration, and well-formed lymphoid follicles of macrophages and transformed lymphocytes in germinal centers.[70,72] The epithelium overlying these lymphoid follicles frequently becomes thin or is lost altogether. Rarely do these follicles become necrotic. Active inflammation can persist for weeks and possibly months, with extension to the endometrium and salpinx in untreated or partially treated women. The cervix usually heals with complete resolution. In some patients, infection in the cervix resolves while infection of the upper genital tract progresses. The changes of the upper genital tract are similar to those of the cervix. Acute versus chronic endometritis or salpingitis can be differentiated by cell type. An infiltrate of neutrophils in the tubal lumen and stroma represents acute infection (Figure 51–15). In some patients, the tubal epithelium is ulcerated in focal areas. The fallopian tubes are almost always infected bilaterally, and as the illness progresses, the ampulla of the tubes can become dilated by fusing of fimbriae from an organizing exudate.[73] This purulent exudate frequently extends from the involved serosa to the pelvic walls and includes the ovaries. Tubo-ovarian abscesses can be extensive involving the walls of the fallopian tube, uterus, and broad ligament on the affected side (Figure 51–6). After about 10 to 14 days the infection becomes chronic, with infiltration of plasma cells, macrophages, and lymphocytes (Figure 51–16, A and B). Numerous cytotoxic T cells are in the mucosa and submucosa, which may facilitate an immu-

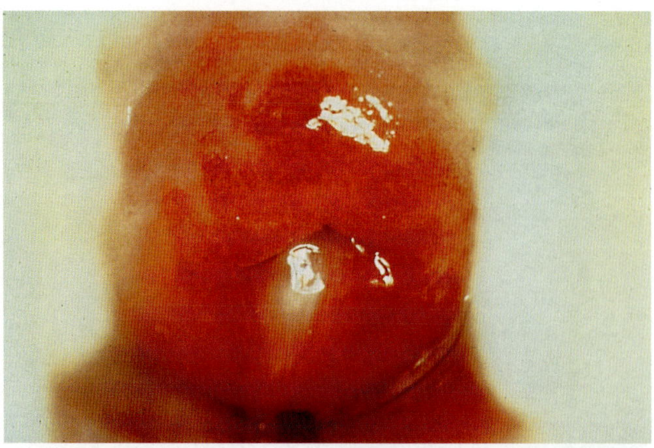

Figure 51–14. Colposcopic exam of a cervix infected with *C trachomatis*. Note the erythema and the mucopurulent discharge coming from the cervical os. *(Photograph reprinted with permission of Stephen Morse, MD, Centers for Disease Control, Atlanta, Georgia.)*

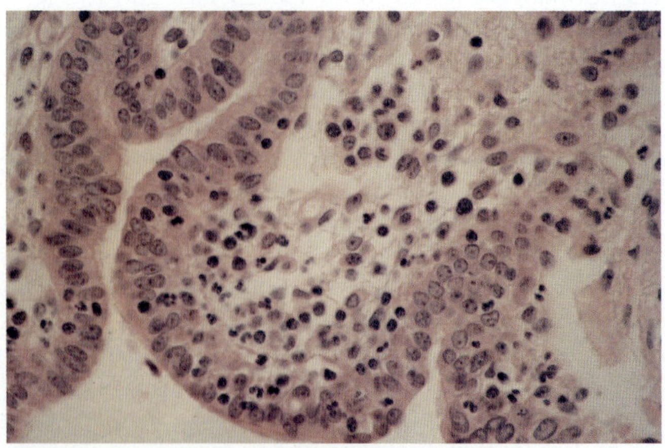

Figure 51–15. Acute salpingitis in human fallopian tube. Note the extensive infiltrate of neutrophils in the submucosa (hematoxylin-eosin ×400). *(Photograph courtesy of Dorothy Patton, PhD, Seattle, Washington.)*

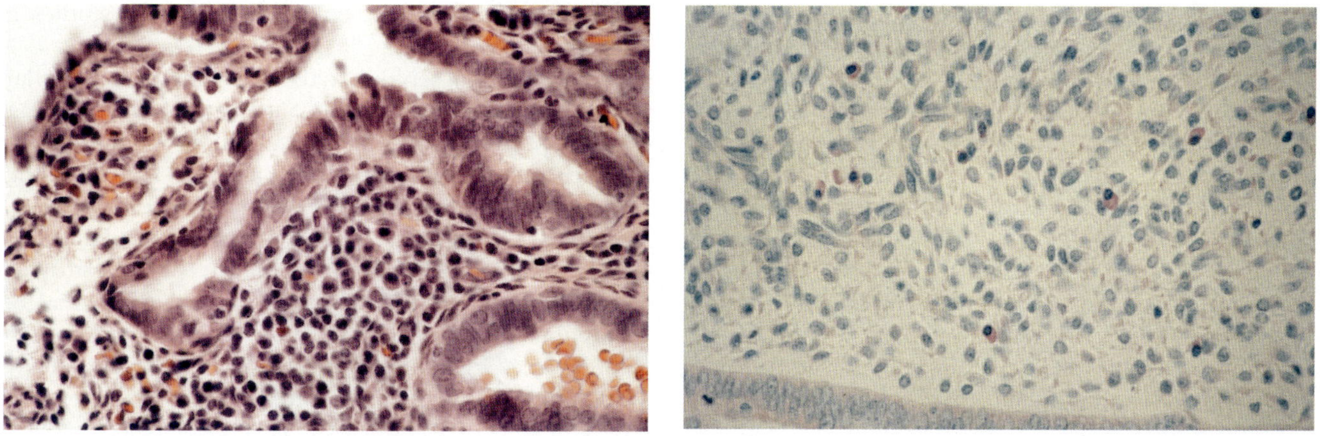

A B

Figure 51–16. (**A**) Section of fallopian tube from a patient with a history of postinfectious tubal disease who is seropositive for *C trachomatis*. The submucosa contains an inflammatory infiltrate consisting of mononuclear cells and plasma cells (hematoxylin-eosin, ×400). *(Photograph courtesy of Dorothy Patton, PhD, Seattle, Washington.)* (**B**) Methyl green-pyronine stain of endometrial tissue from the same lesion shown in (A). Note the plasma cells in the stromal tissues beneath the epithelium (×400). *(Photograph courtesy of Dorothy Patton, PhD, Seattle, Washington.)*

nopathologenic mechanism for tissue damage and subsequent scarring.[72] In some patients, plasma cells may be few and difficult to distinguish from stromal granulocytes. The spindle-cell change in the stroma also suggests chronic infection. As the exudate organizes, fibrosis and adhesions become more apparent, and these adhesions can actually take on a multiglandular structure as the tubal plicae form adhesions in different regions of the tube.[73] This is called "follicular salpingitis." Plasma cells in the endometrium or salpinx with or without lymphoid follicles support a presumptive diagnosis of chlamydial PID.

Chlamydia contain surface proteins that elicit short-term humor immunity. This immunity prevents reinfection with homologous but not heterologus strains for a few months. The organism also has surface proteins that induce a protective or hypersensitivity reaction that can lead to tissue damage, and this may be facilitated by repeat infection. Animal models of chlamydial infections of the genital tract have revealed that repeat or recurrent infections, unlike primary infection, enhance and accelerate inflammation.[74,75] The outcome in these infections is extensive scarring, adhesions, and tubal obstruction. Specific serovars or genotypes of the organism may also contribute to other diseases. Recent research using *omp1* genotyping has revealed variants of serovar F that appear to be more virulent and produce upper genital tract infections. Significantly, F genotype variants caused symptomatic PID with histopathologic changes on endometrial biopsies compared with nonvariant F genotypes that produce mild or asymptomatic infections in the lower genital tract.[3] There is evidence that chlamydial hsp60 may also play a role in this response because it has a high sequence homology with hsps from a number of other pathogens that cause chronic infections.[76,77] There is some recent evidence that tubal scarring may be induced by a hypersensitivity reaction in direct response to hsp60.[54] In in vitro studies, hsp60 is overproduced in response to interferon-γ—a cytokine that is made in response to chlamydial infection.[78] Interferon effectively inhibits the replication of the organism by depleting the amino acid tryptophan, which is essential for chlamydial growth. Once the interferon is removed, however, the organism becomes fully functional. This is one potential mechanism for persistent infections that could explain the chronic inflammation and scarring in infected patients. Antibody responses to chlamydial hsp60 are significantly higher in women with tubal infertility and ectopic pregnancies than in unaffected women. Human antibodies to chlamydial hsp60 have also been found to react with a similar hsp in humans.[79,80] In addition, antibodies elicited in response to certain epitopes on the hsps have been implicated in autoimmune reactions.[81] Thus, some degree of autoimmunity may explain in part the sequelae of chronic infections of the endometrium, salpinx, synovia, and conjunctiva.

Bartholinitis is an acute or chronic infection of the Bartholin's duct. Chlamydiae can produce an acute infection, with dilation of the duct after a progressive infiltration with neutrophils. A chronic infection can also develop with cyst formation. In the absence of acute symptoms and inflammation, however, malignancy must be excluded. Much of the bartholinitis is caused by concurrent infections with chlamydiae and GC. Appropriate treatment usually resolves the infection completely.

Proctitis caused by non-LGV serovars of chlamydiae is mild and frequently asymptomatic. When symptomatic, there is usually some mucosal edema and erythema. Small ulcers may form and heal by fibrosis, but strictures do not form. There is a nonspecific inflammation with eosinophils.

Chlamydial inclusion conjunctivitis in both infants and adults is a benign and sometimes suppurative infection that can last for 3 to 12 months. Within the first 2 weeks of infection, the conjunctiva becomes hyperemic and edematous. A monocyte-rich purulent exudate and conjunctival friability are prominent in infants during this time. In adults, the discharge is serous to mucopurulent, and, after approximately 2 weeks, an infiltrate of lymphocytes with follicles and superficial keratitis are apparent. The follicles are most prominent on the lower tarsal conjunctiva, but the upper tarsal conjunctiva may also be involved (Figure 51–10). With chronic infection, the follicles may be less prominent. Infants rarely develop lymphoid follicles. Epithelial keratitis, subepithelial opacities, and marginal and central infiltrates are characteristics of corneal involvement in both infants and adults. Pannus formation is uncommon and consists of a superficial invasion of the cornea by vessels. The marked progression of disease seen in trachoma patients versus those with inclusion conjunctivitis is in part explained by the infecting serovar. The rare scarring in infant and adult inclusion conjunctivitis may be caused by chronic infection from inadequate or no treatment or repeat infection where the source of infection is a host reservoir, such as the nasopharynx in the infant or the urogenitoanal tract in the adult. In addition, inappropriate treatment with topical steroids can produce a severe protracted keratoconjunctivitis with subsequent conjunctival scarring. The corneal scarring in trachoma is not a feature of inclusion conjunctivitis.

Because the neonatal lung can be infected with a number of different pathogens, the features of infant pneumonitis caused by *C trachomatis* remain unclear. With intracellular replication and spread of *C trachomatis* in the respiratory tract, infants develop some combination of alveolar pneumonia, interstitial pneumonia, and bronchiolitis. The interstitial infiltrates are plasma cells, neutrophils, lymphocytes, and monocytes with a remarkable preponderance of eosinophils.[9]

The urethra in the male patient is susceptible to invasive *C trachomatis* and may develop similar histopathologic and cytological changes to those in the cervix. Histologic examination of mucosa and spongiosum tissue in men with *C trachomatis* infection revealed subepithelial lymphocytes and plasma cells with occasional granulocytes.[82] Two of these patients had strictures of unknown cause, suggesting that *C trachomatis* plays a role, but more extensive studies are required.

Chlamydial epididymitis is an intrascrotal inflammatory infection that occurs after spread of the organism from infected urethral tissue, although spread from the prostate is also possible. In acute infection, there are chlamydial inclusions in ductal epithelial cells. The lumen of the duct frequently contains neutrophils. Occasionally, abscesses may form and destroy the ducts. Squamous metaplasia is rare in chlamydial epididymitis but must be distinguished from squamous cell carcinoma. In a recent study, six cases of chlamydial epididymitis were described.[56] All had severe epididymitis with periductal and intraepithelial proliferation. Two had squamous metaplasia. In the periductal region, the inflammatory cells were lymphocytes, plasma cells, and nonfoamy histiocytes, whereas lymphocytes and neutrophils were prominent in the epithelium. One patient had lymphoepithelial complexes that consisted of dense intraepithelial infiltrates of lymphocytes. Microabscesses of less than 3 mm were in five of the patients in areas where there was minimal destruction of ducts. These findings were distinct from the histopathologic features of epididymitis from bacterial pathogens in which abscesses and tissue destruction were common. Xanthogranulomatous reactions were typical during the resolution phase of the disease.

There is still controversy about the presence of chlamydial organisms in the synovial tissue or the synovial space in reactive arthritis. Therefore, the pathology of chlamydial-related arthritis is difficult to define. Some reports describe the use of DNA- or RNA-hybridization probes or PCR techniques to detect chlamydial RNA or DNA in synovial tissues. Some studies have shown inflammatory cell infiltrates with proliferation of the synovia on biopsy specimens in relation to positive hybridization tests. These findings, however, are nonspecific, and further research is required to determine the true association of chlamydial organisms with synovitis. Reactive arthritis in chlamydial infections also may be triggered by a T-lymphocyte immune response to chlamydial antigens.

The EB is a spheroid particle that can be visualized by a fluorescent-labeled monoclonal antibody that is either species-specific for the MOMP of *C trachomatis* or genus-specific for the LPS. The EBs appear as extracellular round, apple-green fluorescing particles on a background of epithelial cells that are counterstained with Evan's blue (Figure 51–17). A lack of epithelial cells renders the specimen nonreadable. EBs are frequently obtained from swabbing of actively infected sites, including endocervix, urethra, infant and adult conjunctiva, nasopharynx, and rectum. EBs from biopsy specimens of acutely infected endometrium or salpinx, however, can be visualized only by electron microscopy (EM). On EM, the EB has a dense central mass, a glyco-

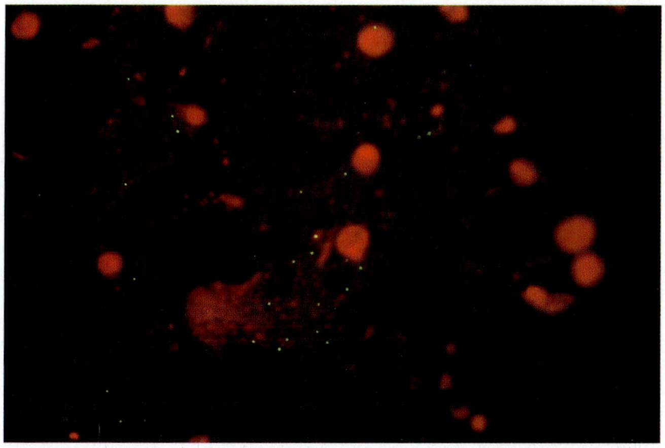

Figure 51–17. Fluorescein-conjugated monoclonal antibody detects the EBs in a cervical smear from a patient with a serovar F infection. The EB are apple green, fluorescing, round, extracellular particles.

gen haze, a trilaminar membrane, and a cell wall that appears to have in-foldings (Figure 51–1). The typical intracytoplasmic inclusions of chlamydiae can be seen in scrapings of adult and infant conjunctivae and from smears of the other sites. Most nonconjunctival smears however, are stained for EBs. For conjunctival scrapings, there are four available staining techniques to visualize the inclusion: Giemsa, iodine, fluorescein, or peroxidase-labeled monoclonal antibodies. Giemsa staining reveals a granular and less dense inclusion that is smaller and more compact in the early stage of the cell cycle. Thus, the inclusion varies in size, as do the features, depending on the stage of development. The inclusion is basophilic, with the EBs staining reddish purple and the RBs staining deep blue in contrast to the dark red host cell. The inclusion can be mistaken for other bacteria, goblet cells, keratin, eosinophilic granules, or pigment granules.[83] Giemsa stains are usually reserved for infant conjunctivitis as they are highly sensitive for detecting chlamydiae in this age group. The inclusion bodies can also be identified with Jones or Lugol's iodine, which stains the glycogen-containing inclusion a dark red in contrast to the yellow background (Figure 51–18). This stain, however, is rarely used to detect chlamydiae because it is insensitive. Fluorescein-conjugated monoclonal antibodies are available also to detect inclusions in tissue culture. These impart a bright green fluorescing color to the inclusion in contrast to the dark red nucleus and cell cytoplasm (Figure 51–19, A and B). Peroxidase-conjugated stains are also available.

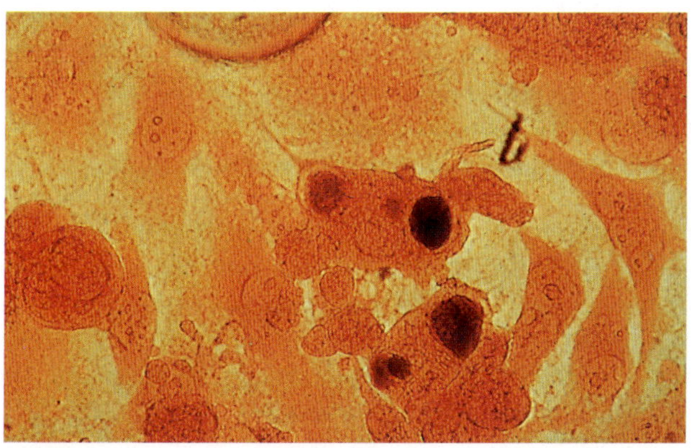

Figure 51–18. Iodine stain of a tissue culture specimen from a patient with *C trachomatis* infection showing the darkly stained glycogen-containing inclusion. *(Photograph courtesy of the Centers for Disease Control, Atlanta, Georgia.)*

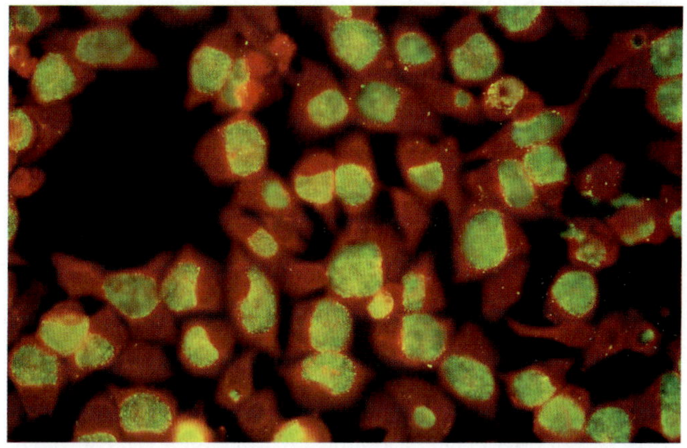

A

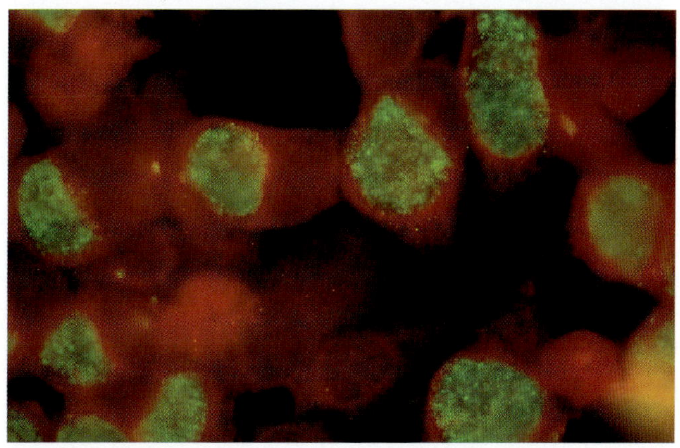

B

Figure 51–19. (**A**) Fluorescent-conjugated monoclonal antibody detects inclusions of *C trachomatis* in a monolayer of McCoy cells. The inclusion appears as a fluorescing body within the cytoplasmic membrane. This patient was infected with serovar D (×400). (**B**) Fluorescent-conjugated monoclonal antibody staining of *C trachomatis* inclusions in a monolayer of McCoy cells. The inclusion appears as a fluorescing body within the cytoplasmic membrane. (This is the same patient as in [A].) (×1000)

Inclusions in biopsy material can be appreciated by two methods: EM and immunohistochemistry. Both techniques are confined to research laboratories. On EM, the inclusion body appears as an intracellular body with an indistinct cell membrane (Figure 51–2). The inclusion varies in size and intra-inclusion components depending on the developmental stage. Early in development there are EBs transforming into RBs; later, there is a predominance of RBs, dividing RBs, intermediate bodies, and nonspecific material (Figure 51–2). Late findings include small RBs and numerous EBs. Immunohistochemical staining can be performed on frozen sections, formalin fixed tissue, and on paraffin-embedded sections. There are now a number of commercial polyclonal and monoclonal antibodies that are genus-specific and some that are species-specific for *C trachomatis.* None of these antibodies, however, can distinguish the serovars.

DIAGNOSIS

Since the mid-1980s, significant advances in diagnostic techniques for chlamydiae have broadened our understanding of the spectrum of genital diseases caused by this organism. Yet, tissue culture using mammalian cell lines has remained the gold standard. The newer non-culture tests include DFA, ELISA, DNA hybridization or probe assays, and commercial PCR and LCR tests. Because chlamydiae are obligate intracellular pathogens, collection of specimens becomes particularly critical if laboratories are to have confidence in the results. Thus, the main objective has been to obtain infected epithelial cells from the conjunctiva, urethra, endocervix, nasopharynx, or rectum for these different tests. However, the future of chlamydial diagnostics will be noninvasive tests that are rapid and sensitive for asymptomatic and symptomatic patients in the low and high prevalence populations.

TISSUE CULTURE

The techniques for cell culture have improved significantly since the 1970s, yet remain only 70% to 90% sensitive with a 100% specificity, depending on the laboratory. Although there are many more university and public health laboratories in the country with facilities for culturing chlamydial tissue, cell culture is infrequently the test of choice because it is expensive, requires considerable technical expertise, and takes 3 to 7 days. This delay has an impact on healthcare professionals who are trying to provide appropriate and rapid treatment for symptomatic and asymptomatic patients as well as the patients' sexual contacts. This delay also impedes behavioral interventions that often carry the most impact at the time of the first clinic visit, when patients are symptomatic or worried about their contacts.[13]

Specimens for tissue culture must be transported to 4°C in special media and inoculated on appropriate monolayers within 24 hours. Alternatively, the specimens can be stored at −80°C; however, there will be some loss of viability over time even at this temperature. Species- or genus-specific fluorescein-conjugated monoclonal antibodies are used routinely to detect the inclusion at 48 or 72 hours. Alternatively, the sample may be passaged blindly before staining with the monoclonal antibody; however, large numbers of EBs can induce a dose-dependent cytotoxicity.

Cell culture is the test of choice for endocervical specimens from symptomatic and asymptomatic women, vaginal samples from prepubescent girls, urethral and rectal samples from both sexes, and nasopharyngeal samples from infants. It is also the test of choice in low prevalence populations and in the case of sexual abuse.[16]

ANTIGEN DETECTION TESTS

The DFA test has a unique advantage over tissue culture in that the quality of the specimen can be determined. The patient's sample is applied directly to a slide and all the cellular elements can be visualized under light microscopy. Adequate specimens contain epithelial cells. Two different fluorescein-conjugated monoclonal antibodies are employed in DFA, one of which detects the MOMP of *C trachomatis* and is thus species-specific; the other is genus-specific and reacts with the LPS. In high prevalence populations, DFA has a sensitivity of 70% to 90% and a specificity of 96% to 99% compared with culture of cervical and symptomatic male urethral samples. These rates vary in moderate to low prevalence populations, in different age groups, and among those with different risk factors for STDs.[13] There is also variation in results depending on the laboratory performing the test and the quality of the specimens.

DFA is recommended for specimens of cervix from low and high prevalence populations, for urethral specimens from symptomatic adolescent and young adult men in high prevalence populations, for conjunctival samples from infants, and for samples of rectum.[13] The latter samples, however, must be performed in a reference laboratory. The DFA test can be used in low prevalence populations, but must be confirmed.

ELISA is similar to DFA in that chlamydial antigens are the target for detection. In this assay, polyclonal or monoclonal antibodies directed against the LPS are conjugated with an enzyme that reacts with substrate to produce a color change if chlamydiae are present. A spectrophotometer is used for detection. Confirmatory testing is required for the ELISA tests. Most kits contain a blocking antibody that binds to the chlamydial LPS; if an aliquot of the same specimen that was positive is rerun with the blocking antibody, it should give a negative result. If not, the test would be a false positive and the reactivity would be presumed to be against the LPS of other bacteria present in the vagina or urinary tract.

The sensitivities and specificities for the ELISA tests are similar to those for DFA. ELISA is also recommended in the same clinical situations as DFA, with confirmation required in low prevalence populations. ELISA, however, can be used for urine samples from symptomatic young men, but not for samples from the rectum.[13]

NUCLEIC ACID BASED TECHNIQUES

Hybridization probes were the first nucleic acid test to be developed for chlamydiae. They are species-specific for *C trachomatis*. The probes, however, cannot determine whether there is active infection as for culture or for DFA and ELISA where the presence of EBs are presumed to indicate active infection. The probe is composed of DNA that hybridizes with a complementary strand of chlamydial ribosomal RNA. Luminescing complexes are detected by a luminometer as a digital representation of the intensity of the output. The sensitivity and specificity of the probes are similar to those for the ELISA test, and they can be used in similar clinical situations.[13] Probes should not be used on urine samples from men.

Since 1991, two additional commercial nucleic acid tests, the LCR and the PCR, have been developed and approved by the Food and Drug Administration. Both are based on detection of a segment of the chlamydial plasmid that is present in *C trachomatis* and *C psittaci*. The LCR relies on hybridization of four probes to the DNA template and amplification of the probe to provide a signal that is recorded by a luminometer. In contrast, for PCR, the actual chlamydial DNA is amplified, hybridized to a specific probe, and detected by a spectrophotometer. The sensitivities and specificities of both are excellent and, in some studies, higher than DFA and culture. Both tests can be used reliably to detect chlamydiae in endocervical specimens and in urine and urethral samples from symptomatic and asymptomatic males. LCR can be used also for female urine samples. However, the interpretation of a positive test in an asymptomatic patient in a low prevalence population is difficult, as this may represent residual DNA and not active infection.[13]

SEROLOGY

There are two serologic tests available to detect chlamydiae: the complement fixation test (CF) and the microimmunofluorescence test (MIF). Both tests are nonspecific for chlamydiae as there is cross-reactivity among serovars and species in the MIF test, and chlamydial antibodies can remain in the host for many years. In addition, these tests are not routinely available in clinical laboratories. The CF test uses genus-specific chlamydial antigens, whereas the MIF test uses EBs from each of 15 representative serovars and those from *C pneumoniae* and *C psittaci*. Sera of patients in serial dilutions are reacted against these antigens and a fluorescein-conjugated anti-human IgM or IgG antibody is then used to detect the positive antibody antigen complex. The CF test is indicated for LGV in that a single negative serum excludes this diagnosis. The MIF test using IgM antibodies is indicated for infant pneumonitis, and a fourfold rise in antibody titers from acute to convalescent phase provides a presumptive diagnosis for LGV.

OTHER TESTS

The leukocyte esterase test (LET) is a marker for urinary tract infection but does not identify the causal organism(s). LET is a dipstick test that detects enzymes released by neutrophils. It has been used effectively as a screening test for adolescent boys with a sensitivity of 46% to 100% and specificity of 83% to 100%.[13] Further testing in women and older men is required before it can be recommended in this setting.

Neutrophils also can be used as diagnostic markers for urethritis or cystitis. Four or more neutrophils per high power field on a Gram's stain of endourethral material confirm urethritis. More than 10 neutrophils per high power field in a first catch urine are also highly suggestive of urethritis in adolescent men. These findings are diagnostic for nongonococcal urethritis when GC fails to grow or is not demonstrated on Gram's stain. A presumptive diagnosis of mucopurulent cervicitis can be made when more than 10 neutrophils are present per high power field of cervical smears. Swabbing of the cervix with these results is referred to as a positive swab test.

CONFIRMATORY TESTING

Confirmatory testing is required for nonculture methods of diagnosis. Ideally, two samples for chlamydiae testing would be available, whereby a completely different test could be run on the second paired sample to confirm the first test; however, this is rarely the case and impractical in the clinical setting. A second approach would be to use remnant material from the first test. The second test should differ from the first and should detect chlamydial antigen or DNA. The use of a blocking antibody for confirming the ELISA test is available; however, this is not as good as repeating the test with an alternate diagnostic test. Additional studies are required to determine the best confirmatory test for each nonculture test used. Unfortunately, a lack of confirmation does not rule out infection.

REFERENCES

1. Fukushi H, Hirai K. Proposal of *Chlamydia pecorum* sp. nov. for *Chlamydia* strains derived from ruminants. *Intern J Sys Bacteriol.* 1992;42:306–308.
2. Dean D, Schachter J, Dawson CR, Stephens RS. Comparison of the major outer membrane protein variant sequence regions of B/Ba isolates: a molecular epidemiologic approach to *Chlamydia trachomatis* infections. *J Infect Dis.* 1992;166:383–392.
3. Dean D, Odens E, Bolan G. Padian N, Schachter J. Major outer membrane protein variants of *Chlamydia trachomatis* are associated with severe genital tract infections and histopathology in San Francisco. *J Infect Dis.* 1995;172:1013–1022.
4. Lindner K. Augenoblennorrhoe, Einschlussblennorrhoe and Trachoma. *Graefe's Arch Clin Exp Ophthalmol.* 1911; 78:380–389.
5. T'ang FF, et al. Trachoma virus in chick embryo. *Natl. Med J China.* 1957;43:81–89.
6. Gordon FB, Quan AL. Isolation of the trachoma agent in cell culture. *Proc Soc Exp Bio Med.* 1965;118:354–359.
7. Darougar S, Jones BR, Kinnison JR, et al. Chlamydial infection: advances in the diagnostic isolation of *Chlamydia,* including TRIC agent, from the eye, genital tract and rectum. *Brit J Vener Dis.* 1972;48:416–420.
8. Wang SP, Grayston JT. Immunologic relationship between genital TRIC, lymphogranuloma venereum, and related organisms in a new microtiter indirect immunofluorescence test. *Am J Ophthalmol.* 1970;70:367–374.
9. Jones RB. Chlamydial diseases. In: Mandell GL, Bennett JE, Dolin R, eds. *Principles and Practice of Infectious Diseases.* New York: Churchill Livingstone; 1995:1676–1693.
10. Stamm WE, Holmes KK. *Chlamydia trachomatis* infections of the adult. In: Holmes KK, Mardh P-A, Sparling PF, et al., eds. *Sexually Transmitted Diseases.* 2nd ed. New York: McGraw-Hill; 1990:181–193.
11. Campbell LA, Patton DL, Moore DE, et al. Detection of *Chlamydia trachomatis* deoxyribonucleic acid in women with tubal infertility. *Fertil Steril.* 1993;59:45–50.
12. Shepard MK, Jones RB. Recovery of *Chlamydia trachomatis* from endometrial and fallopian tube biopsies in women with infertility of tubal origin. *Fertil Steril.* 1989; 52:232–238.
13. Weinstock H, Dean D, Bolan G. *Chlamydia trachomatis* infections. In: Cohen MS, Hook III EW, Hitchcock PJ, eds. *Infectious Disease Clinics of North America: Sexually Transmitted Diseases in the AIDS era: Part II.* Philadelphia: W.B. Saunders Company; 1995:797–820.
14. Ito JI, Comess KA, Alexander ER, et al. Pneumonia due to *Chlamydia trachomatis* in an immunocompromised adult. *N Engl J Med.* 1982;307:95–98.
15. Ormsby HL, Thompson GA, Cousineau GG, Lloyd LA, Hassard J. Topical therapy in inclusion conjunctivitis. *Am J Ophthalmol.* 1952;35:1811–1814.
16. Centers for Disease Control and Prevention. Recommendations for the prevention and management of *Chlamydia trachomatis* infections. *MMWR.* 1993;42(RR–12):1–36.
17. Kent GP, Harrison HR, Berman SM. Screening for *Chlamydia trachomatis* infection in a sexually transmitted disease clinic: comparison of diagnostic tests with clinical and historical risk factors. *Sex Transm Dis.* 1988;15:51–57.
18. Magder LS, Harrison HR, Ehret JM, et al. Factors related to genital *Chlamydia trachomatis* and its diagnosis by culture in a sexually transmitted disease clinic. *Am J Epidemiol.* 1988;28:298–308.
19. Jones RB, Mammel JB, Shepard MK, Fisher RR. Recovery of *Chlamydia trachomatis* from the endometrium of women at risk for chlamydial infections. *Am J Obstet Gynecol.* 1986;155:35–39.
20. Westrom L, Bengtsson LPH, Mardh P-A. Incidence, trends, and risks of ectopic pregnancy in a population of women. *Br Med J.* 1981;282:15–19.
21. Morrison RP, Manning DS, Caldwell HD. Immunology of *Chlamydia trachomatis* infections: Immunoprotective and immunopathogenetic responses. In: Gallin JI, Fauci AS, Quinn TC, eds. *Advances in Host Defense Mechanisms, Vol. 8, Sexually Transmitted Diseases.* New York: Raven Press; 1992;57–84.
22. Wolner-Hanssen P, Kiviat NB, Holmes KK. Atypical pelvic inflammatory disease: Subacute, chronic, or subclinical upper genital tract infection in women. In: Holmes KK, Märdu P-A, Sparling PF, et al, eds. *Sexually Transmitted Diseases.* 2nd ed. New York: McGraw-Hill; 1990:615–620.
23. Barnes RC, Katz BP, Batteiger B, et al. Quantitative culture of endocervical *Chlamydia trachomatis.* J Clin Microbiol. 1990;28:774–780.
24. Cates W Jr, Wasserheit JN. Genital chlamydial infections: Epidemiology and reproductive sequelae. *Am J Obstet Gynecol.* 1991;164:1771–1781.
25. Karam GH, Martin DH, Flotte TR, et al. Asymptomatic *Chlamydia trachomatis* infections among sexually active men. *J Infect Dis.* 1986;154:900–903.
26. McNagny SE, Parker RM, Zenilman JM, et al. Urinary leukocyte esterase test. A screening method for the detection of asymptomatic chlamydial and gonococcal infections in men. *J Infect Dis.* 1992;165:573–576.
27. Stamm WE, Koutsky LA, Beneditti JK, et al. *Chlamydia trachomatis* urethral infections in men. Prevalence, risk factors, and clinical manifestations. *Ann Intern Med.* 1984; 100:47–51.
28. Cottingham J, Hunter D. *Chlamydia trachomatis* and oral contraceptive use: a quantitative review. *Genitourinary Med.* 1992;68:209–216.
29. Katz BP. Estimating transmission probabilities for chlamydial infection. *Stat Med.* 1992;11:565–757.
30. Blythe MJ, Katz BP, Orr DP, et al. Historical and clinical

factors associated with *Chlamydia trachomatis* genitourinary infection in female adolescents. *J Pediatr.* 1988;112: 1000–1004.

31. Ramstedt K, Forssman L, Giesecke J, Johannisson G. Epidemiologic characteristics of two different populations of women with *C trachomatis* infection and their male partners. *Sex Transm Dis.* 1991;18:205–210.
32. Lycke I, Lowhagen GB, Hallhagen G, Johannisson G, Ramstedt K. The risk of transmission of genital *C trachomatis* infections in less than that of genital *Neisseria gonorrhoeae* infection. *Sex Transm Dis.* 1980;7:6–10.
33. Viscidi RP, Bobo L, Hook EW, Quinn TC. Transmission of *Chlamydia trachomatis* among sex partners assessed by polymerase chain reaction. *J Infect Dis.* 1993;168:488–492.
34. Quinn TC, Gaydos C, Welsh L, et al. Reassessment of *Chlamydia trachomatis* transmission by polymerase chain reaction among 460 sexual partners. In: Orfila J, Byrne GI, Chernesky MA, et al, eds. *Chlamydial Infections.* Bologna, Italy: Societa Editrice Esculapio; 1994:21–24.
35. Batteiger BE, Fraiz J, Newhall WJ, Katz BP, Jones RB. Association of recurrent chlamydial infection with gonorrhea. *J Infect Dis.* 1989;159:661–669.
36. Brunham RC, Plummer FA. A general model of sexually transmitted disease epidemiology and its implications for control. *Med Clin N Amer.* 1990;74:1339–1352.
37. Tipples G, McClarty G. The obligate intracellular bacterium *Chlamydia trachomatis* is auxotrophic for three of the four ribonucleoside triphosphates. *Mol Microbiol.* 1993;8:1105–1114.
38. Zhang JP, Stephens RS. Mechanism of *C trachomatis* attachment to eukaryotic host cells. *Cell.* 1992;69:861–869.
39. Vretou E, Goswami PC, Bose SK. Adherence of multiple serovars of *Chlamydia trachomatis* to a common receptor on HeLa and McCoy cells is mediated by thermolabile proteins. *J Gen Microbiol.* 1989;135:3229–3237.
40. Wyrick PB, Choong J, Davis CH, et al. Entry of genital *Chlamydia trachomatis* into polarized human epithelial cells. *Infect Immun.* 1989;57:2378–2389.
41. Peeling R, Peeling J, Brunham R. High-resolution ^{31}P nuclear magnetic resonance study of *Chlamydia trachomatis:* induction of ATPase activity in elementary bodies. *Infect Immun.* 1989;57:3338–3344.
42. Moulder JW. Interaction of chlamydiae and host cells in vitro. *Microbiol Rev.* 1991;55:143–190.
43. Su H, Morrison RP, Watkins NG, Caldwell HD. Identification and characterization of T helper cell epitopes of the major outer membrane protein of *Chlamydia trachomatis. J Exp Med.* 1990;172:203.
44. Hatt C, Ward ME, Clarke IN. Analysis of the entire nucleotide sequence of the cryptic plasmid of *Chlamydia trachomatis* serovar L1. Evidence for involvement in DNA replication. *Nucleic Acids Res.* 1988;16:4053–4067.
45. Peterson EM, Markoff BA, Schachter J, et al. The 7.5-kb plasmid present in *Chlamydia trachomatis* is not essential for the growth of this microorganism. *Plasmid.* 1990;23: 144–148.
46. Goldmeier D, Ridgway GL, Oriel JO. Chlamydial vulvovaginitis in a post menopausal woman. *Lancet.* 1981;2: 476–477. Letter.
47. Lannigan R, Hardy G, Tanton R, Marrie TJ. *Chlamydia trachomatis* peritonitis and ascites following appendectomy. *Can Med Assoc J.* 1980;123:295–296.
48. Dunlop EMC, Garner A, Darougar S, et al. Colposcopy, biopsy, and cytology results in women with chlamydial cervicitis. *Genitourin Med.* 1989;65:22–31.
49. Ho JL, He S, Hu A, et al. Neutrophils from human immunodeficiency virus (HIV)-seronegative donors induce HIV replication from HIV-infected patients' mononuclear cells and cell lines: an in vitro model of HIV transmission facilitated by *Chlamydia trachomatis. J Exp Med.* 1995;181; 1493–1505.
50. Laga M, Manoka A, Kivuvu M, et al. Non-ulcerative sexually transmitted diseases as risk factors for HIV-1 transmission in women: results from a cohort study. *AIDS.* 1993;7:95–102.
51. Spinillo A, Gorini G, Regazzetti A, et al. Asymptomatic genitourinary *Chlamydia trachomatis* infection in women seropositive for HIV infection. *Obstet Gyn.* 1994;83: 1005–1010.
52. Stamm WE. Diagnosis of *Chlamydia trachomatis* genitourinary infections. *Ann Intern Med.* 1988;108:710–717.
53. Westrom L, Joesoef R, Reynolds G, et al. Pelvic inflammatory disease and fertility: a cohort study of 1,844 women with laparoscopically verified disease and 657 control women with normal laparoscopic results. *Sex Transm Dis.* 1992;19:185–192.
54. Wagar EA, Schachter J, Bavoil P, et al. Differential human serologic response to two 60,000 molecular weight *Chlamydia trachomatis* antigens. *J Infect Dis.* 1990;162: 922–927.
55. Doble A, Thomas BJ, Walker MM, Hams JR, Witherow RO, Taylor-Robinson D. The role of *Chlamydia trachomatis* in chronic abacterial prostatitis: a study utilizing ultrasound guided biopsy. *J Urol.* 1989;141:332–333.
56. Hori S, Tsutsumi Y. Histological differentiation between chlamydial and bacterial epididymitis. *Human Pathol.* 1995;26:402–407.
57. Berger RE, Alexander ER, Harnisch JP, et al. Etiology, manifestations, and therapy of acute epididymitis: prospective study of 50 cases. *J Urol.* 1979;121:750–754.
58. Schachter J, Grossman M, Holt J, et al. Infection with *Chlamydia trachomatis:* involvement of multiple anatomic sites in neonates. *J Infect Dis.* 1979;139:232–234.
59. Ronnerstam R, Persson K, Hansson H, et al. Prevalence of chlamydial eye infection in patients attending an eye clinic, a VD clinic, and in healthy persons. *Br J Ophthalmol* 1985;69:385–388.
60. Thygeson P, Stone W. Epidemiology of inclusion conjunctivitis. *Arch Ophthalmol* 1942;27:91–122.
61. Dean D, Shama A, Schachter J, Dawson CR. Molecular identification of an avian strain of *Chlamydia psittaci* causing severe keratoconjunctivitis in a bird fancier. *Clin Infect Dis.* 1995;20:1179–1185.
62. Lietman T, Dawson C, Dean D. Follicular conjunctivitis caused by non-trachomatis chlamydial species. *Invest Ophthalmol Vis Sci* (abstract 4706) 1995;S1016.
63. Dawson CR, Schachter J. TRIC agent infections of the eye and genital tract. *Am J Ophthalmol.* 1971;63:1288–1298.
64. Harrison HR, Alexander ER. Chlamydial infections in infants and children. In: Holmes KK, Mardh P-A, Sparling

PF, et al, eds. *Sexually Transmitted Diseases.* 2nd ed. New York: McGraw-Hill; 1990:811–820.

65. Tipple MA, Beem MO, Saxon EM. Clinical characteristics of the afebrile pneumonia associated with *Chlamydia trachomatis* infection in infants less than six months of age. *Pediatrics.* 1979;63:192–197.
66. Shahmanesh M. Problems with non-gonococcal urethritis. *Int J STD AIDS.* 1994;5:390–399. Editorial.
67. Schachter J. Isolation of bedsoniae from human arthritis and abortion issues. *Am J Ophthalmol.* 1967;63(Suppl): 1082–1086.
68. Rahman MU, Hudson AP, Schumacher HR Jr. *Chlamydia* and Reiter's syndrome (reactive arthritis). *Rheum Dis Clin North Am.* 1992;18:67–79.
69. Inman RD, Morrison RP. Immunoblot analysis of reactivity to chlamydial 57kD heat shock protein in Reiter's syndrome. *Arthritis Rheum.* 1990;33:S26. Abstract.
70. Paavonen J, Meyer B, Vesterinen E, Saksela E. Colposcopic and histological findings in cervical chlamydial infections. *Lancet.* 1980;2:320.
71. Kiviat NB, Paavonen JA, Brockway J, et al. Cytologic manifestations of cervical and vaginal infections. I. Epithelial and inflammatory cellular changes. *JAMA.* 1985;253: 989–996.
72. Kiviat NB, Paavonen JA, Wolner-Hanssen P, et al. Histopathology of endocervical infection caused by *Chlamydia trachomatis, Herpes simplex* virus, *Trichomonas vaginalis,* and *Neisseria gonorrhoeae. Hum Pathol.* 1990;21:831–837.
73. Walker DH, Dumler JS. Rickettsial and *Chlamydial* diseases. In: Damjanov I, Linder J, eds. *Anderson's Pathology.* 10th ed. St. Louis: Mosby-Year Book; 1996:866–885.
74. Patton DL. Immunopathology and histopathology of experimental chlamydial salpingitis. *Rev Infect Dis.* 1985;7: 746–753.
75. Patton DL, Wolner-Hanssen P, Cosgrove SJ, Holmes KK. The effects of *Chlamydia trachomatis* on the female reproductive tract of the *Macaca nemestrina* after a single tubal challenge following repeated cervical inoculations. *Obstet Gynecol.* 1990;76:643–650.
76. Morrison RP, Belland RP, Lyng K, Caldwell HD. Chlamydial disease pathogenesis. The 57-kD chlamydial hypersensitivity antigen is a stress response protein. *J Exp Med.* 1989;169:663–675.
77. Danilitton SL, MacLean IW, Peeling R, Winston S, Brunham RC. The 75-kilodalton protein of *Chlamydia trachomatis:* a member of the heat shock protein 70 family? *Infect Immun.* 1990;58:189–196.
78. Beatty WL, Byrne GI, Morrison RP. Morphologic and antigenic characterization of interferon-gamma mediated persistent *Chlamydia trachomatis* infection in vitro. *Proc Natl Acad Sci USA.* 1993;90:1–5.
79. Cerrone MC, Ma JJ, Stephens RS. Cloning and sequence of the gene for heat shock protein 60 from *Chlamydia trachomatis* and immunological reactivity of the protein. *Infect Immun.* 1991;59:79–90.
80. Yi Y, Zhong G, Brunham RC. Continuous B-cell epitopes in *Chlamydia trachomatis* heat shock protein 60. *Infect Immun.* 1993;61:1117–1120.
81. Lamb JR, Young DB. T cell recognition of stress proteins. A link between infectious and autoimmune disease. *Mol Biol Med.* 1990;7:311–321.
82. Barbagli G, Azzaro F, Menchi I, Amorosi A, Selli C. Bacteriologic, histologic and ultrasonographic findings in strictures recurring after urethrotomy. A preliminary study. *Scand J Urol Nephrol.* 1995;29:193–195.
83. Yoneda C, Dawson CR, Daghfous T, et al. Cytology as a guide to the presence of chlamydial inclusions in Giemsa-stained conjunctival smears. *Br J Ophthalmol.* 1975;59: 116–124.

Lymphogranuloma Venereum

David A. Schwartz

Do not trifle with love.

Alfred de Musset (1810–1857).

For my loins are filled with a loathsome disease:
and there is no soundness in my flesh.

Psalms 41:8

CLASSIFICATION

Lymphogranuloma venereum (LGV) is one of several sexually transmitted diseases caused by *Chlamydia trachomatis*. It is also known as tropical, strumous, or climatic bubo; Durand-Nicolas-Favre disease; poradenitis inguinalis; or lymphogranuloma inguinale. The disease is usually caused by one of three invasive LGV biovar strains of *C trachomatis* serotypes L1, L2, or L3, but other strains have been isolated from patients with clinical symptoms consistent with genitoanorectal LGV.[1–4]

INTRODUCTION

Throughout history LGV has been confused with other sexually transmitted diseases. This confusion was partially from failure to recognize the common etiologic agent of the varied clinical manifestations of LGV, which were often described as discrete clinicopathologic entities. For example, the buboes of LGV were confused with those of chancroid, and LGV-associated adenopathy was believed to result from syphilis or Herpes simplex virus infections. LGV was probably mentioned in ancient medical texts and was described by John Hunter in 1786.[5,6] It was not until 1913, however, that Durand, Nicolas, and Favre established the infection as a distinct clinical and pathologic entity. Phylactos determined a common cause of LGV and climatic bubo in 1922, and Frei developed the skin test for LGV that bears his name in 1925. *C trachomatis* was first identified in 1907 by Halberstaedtler and Prowazek in conjunctival scrapings from a patient with trachoma. In 1935, *C trachomatis* was identified as the chlamydial agent of LGV when it was cultivated in embryonated eggs, permitting the manufacture of standardized antigen for the Frei skin test and serodiagnostic tests.

LGV is a chronic disease with a variety of acute and late manifestations. The disease has three stages of infection similar to syphilis, of which the primary lesion is a small and inconspicuous genital papule or herpetiform ulcer that is short-lived and produces few symptoms. The secondary stage is characterized by acute lymphadenitis with buboes (termed the inguinal syndrome, but not to be confused with granuloma inguinale) and/or acute hemorrhagic proctitis (the anogenitorectal syndrome) as well as fever and other systemic signs of infection. Although most patients recover without further sequelae after the secondary phase of infection, a minority of those infected develop signs of third stage infection, including genital ulcers, fistulas, rectal strictures, and genital elephantiasis ("esthiomene").

EPIDEMIOLOGY

LGV is a sexually transmitted disease that occurs sporadically in North America, Europe, Australia, and most of Asia and South America. It is endemic in India, east and west Africa, the Caribbean, and parts of Southeast Asia and South America. The prevalence of LGV is not known because few countries require reporting, and it is frequently confused with other infections. Much of the reported data on prevalence are based on screening with the Frei skin test or results of serology, neither of which is specific for LGV. Since 1950, no European nation has reported more than a few dozen infections annually.[7] In contrast, a single municipal clinic in Ethiopia reports several thousand infections annually. As with other sexually transmitted diseases, LGV is more common in urban than rural areas, and sexual promiscuity and low socioeconomic status are risk factors. Many of the reported infections from nonendemic areas are in travelers, sailors, and military personnel who acquire the infection while in endemic areas.[8]

In the United States, LGV is rare. Of the many millions who have chlamydial disease in the United States, fewer than 600 cases of LGV are reported annually.[4] In many of these, however, the diagnosis is based on low-titer complement fixation. LGV is most common in homosexual men and presents as proctitis.[2] The most common LGV serovar isolated in the United States is L2, but recently five additional patients from the United States were infected with the rare LGV serovar L1, all of whom were homosexual men with symptomatic proctitis.[9]

Acute LGV has its peak incidence in the third decade and is much more frequently reported in men than in women, with a ratio of 5:1 or greater. Because early symptomatic infection is less common in women and diagnosis may be delayed, late complications such as hyperplasia, ulceration and hypertrophy of genitalia (esthiomene), and rectal strictures are reported more frequently in women than in men.

Chlamydia cannot penetrate intact skin or mucous membranes, and it is believed that the agent probably enters the body through minute breaks in the skin. Although the frequency of infection following exposure is not known, the disease is not believed to be as contagious as gonorrhea. Because the endocervix is the most common site of infection in women and may remain infected for months, LGV may be acquired by the fetus during transit through the birth canal.

MORPHOLOGY AND LIFE CYCLE

The cause of LGV, *C trachomatis,* is a small gram-negative bacterium with a limited metabolic capability that restricts its growth to an intracellular environment of parasitized cells. The life cycle of *C trachomatis* has three stages: 1) the infective particles known as elementary particles penetrate the host cell; 2) they develop within the cytoplasm into a reticulate body, a metabolically active form that exists intracellularly only and subsequently undergoes division by binary fission; and 3) the reticulate bodies transform into elementary bodies that are released from the host cell by exocytosis.

CLINICAL FEATURES

The primary lesion of LGV develops after an incubation period of 3 to 12 days or longer and may take four forms—a papule, a shallow ulcer or erosion, a small herpetiform lesion, or nonspecific urethritis. The most common site of occurrence in men is the coronal sulcus, followed by the frenum, prepuce, penis, urethra, glans, and scrotum (Figures 51–20 and 51–21). In women, the lesion is most common on the posterior vaginal wall, the fourchette, the posterior lip of the cervix, and the vulva. Primary lesions of LGV in men can be associated with a cordlike lymphangitis of the dorsal penis and a large, painful lymphangial nodule, termed a "bubonulus." These bubonuli can rupture, creating draining sinuses of the urethra and deforming scars of the penis. In women, LGV cervicitis can extend locally, resulting in perimetritis and salpingitis.

The secondary stage occurs days to months (average: 10 to 30 days) after the primary lesion. There is lymphadenopathy of inguinal lymph nodes accompanied by such systemic symptoms as fever, chills, anorexia, headache, meningismus, myalgias, and arthalgias. Changes in laboratory findings include leukocytosis, elevated erythrocyte sedimentation rate, abnormal liver function tests, and hypergammaglobulinemia. The inguinal bubo begins as a firm, slightly painful and gradually enlarging mass that is unilateral in two thirds of patients (Figure 51–22). Within 1 to 2 weeks, the bubo becomes more tender and fluctuant, and the overlying skin become livid. The bubo ruptures in about one third of patients, and this relieves the pain and fever (Figure 51–23). Numerous sinus tracts form after rupture, which drain thick pus for up to several months.

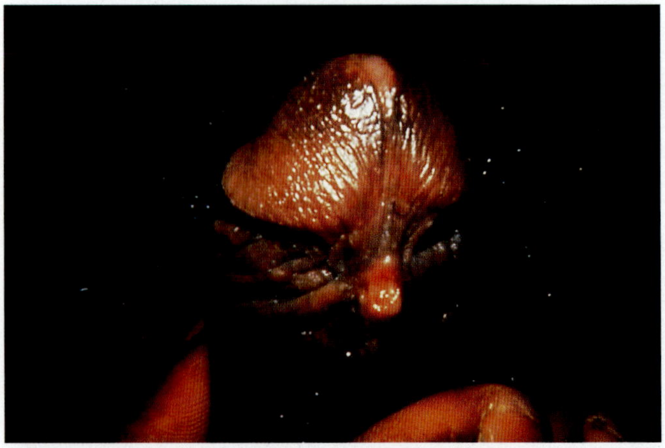

Figure 51–20. Primary lesions of LGV on the penis. There is a small ulcer of the frenum with associated edema and erythema. *(Photograph courtesy of the Centers for Disease Control and Prevention, Atlanta, Georgia.)*

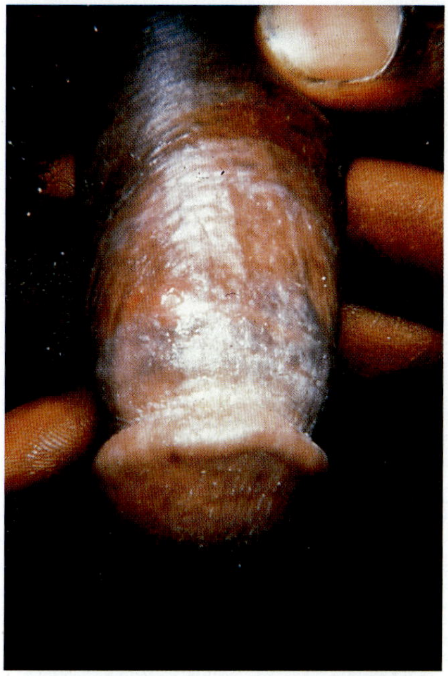

Figure 51–21. Primary lesions of LGV on the penis. There is a tiny ulcer on the penile shaft with surrounding erythema. *(Photograph courtesy of the Centers for Disease Control and Prevention, Atlanta, Georgia.)*

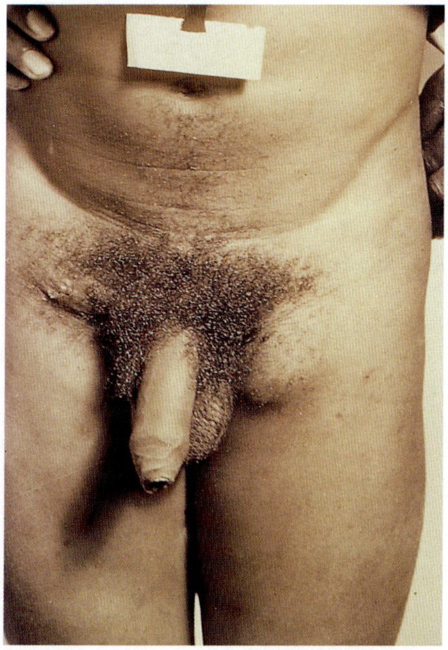

Figure 51–22. Bilateral inguinal lymphadenopathy (buboes) in a man with LGV. The right bubo is draining (AFIP Neg 74-9546).

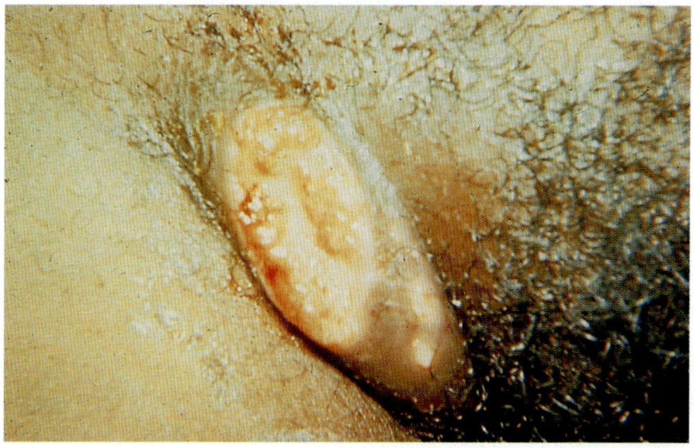

Figure 51–23. Ulcerated inguinal bubo in a patient with secondary LGV. *(Photograph courtesy of the Centers for Disease Control and Prevention, Atlanta, Georgia.)*

Healing of the inguinal bubo usually predicts the end of disease in men, but relapse of buboes can occur in up to 20% of untreated patients. Those buboes that do not rupture undergo slow involution and form nonsuppurative inguinal masses (Figure 51–24). In approximately 20% of patients, the femoral lymph nodes are also affected and are separated from the enlarged inguinal lymph nodes by Poupart's ligament, forming the "groove sign" (Figures 51–25 and 51–26). An important subacute manifestation of LGV is the anogenitorectal syndrome, which includes proctocolitis, perirectal abscesses, ischiorectal and rectovaginal fistulas, anal fistulas, and rectal stricture (Figure 51–27).

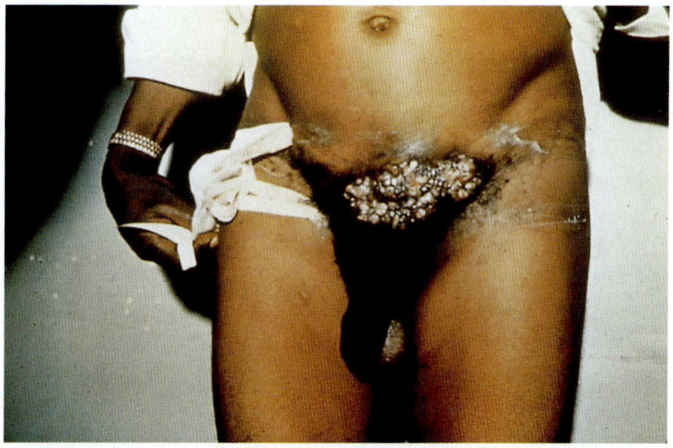

Figure 51–24. These inguinal buboes have formed large masses in a patient with chronic LGV. *(Photograph courtesy of the Centers for Disease Control and Prevention, Atlanta, Georgia.)*

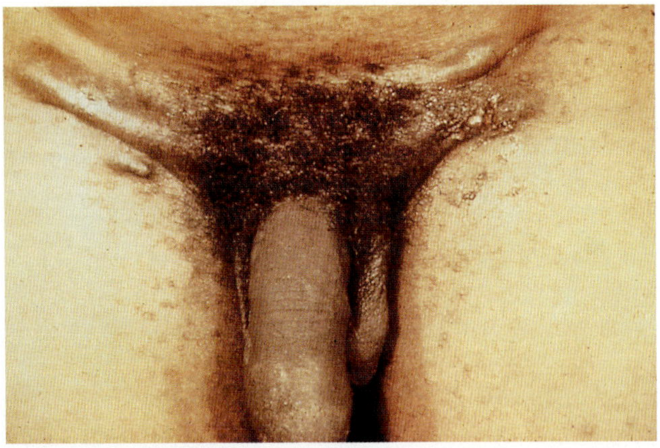

Figure 51–25. "Groove sign" in a man with LGV. Although this sign is often said to be pathognomonic for LGV, it is infrequent in LGV and may be produced by other conditions. *(Photograph courtesy of the Centers for Disease Control and Prevention, Atlanta, Georgia.)*

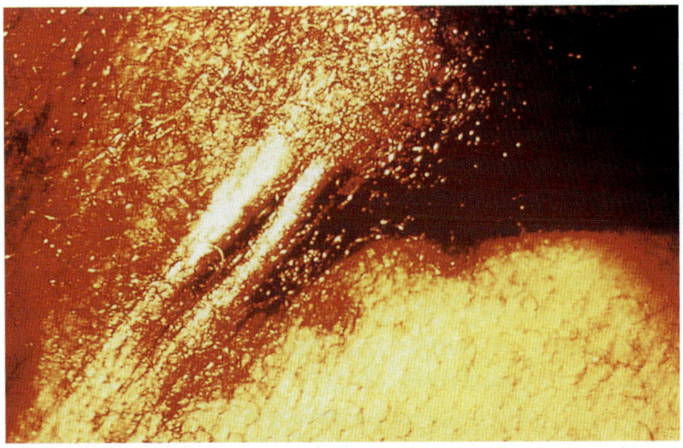

Figure 51–26. Close-up of the "groove sign." *(Photograph courtesy of the Centers for Disease Control and Prevention, Atlanta, Georgia.)*

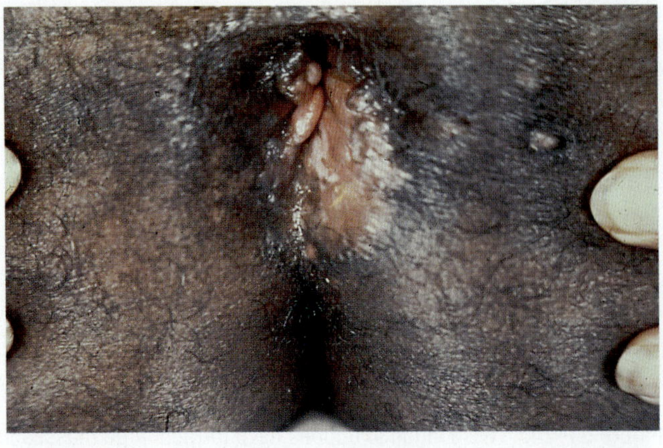

Figure 51–27. Anal stricture from a patient with anogenitorectal syndrome of LGV. *(Photograph courtesy of the Centers for Disease Control and Prevention, Atlanta, Georgia.)*

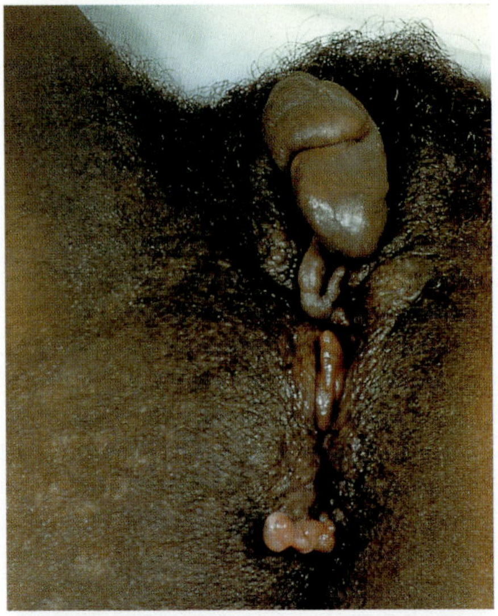

Figure 51–28. Early enlargement of female genitalia (elephantiasis) caused by chronic LGV. *(Photograph courtesy of the Centers for Disease Control and Prevention, Atlanta, Georgia.)*

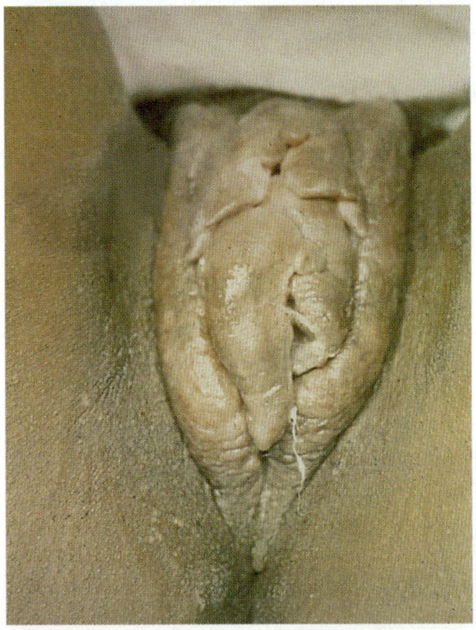

Figure 51–29. Late stage female genital elephantiasis, or esthiomene, caused by LGV. *(Photograph courtesy of the Centers for Disease Control and Prevention, Atlanta, Georgia.)*

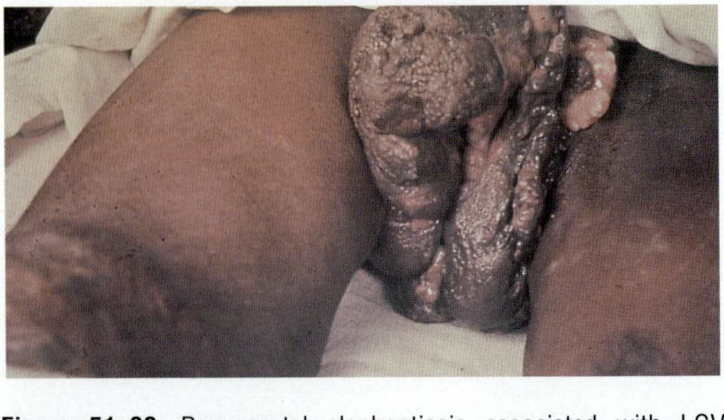

Figure 51–30. Penoscrotal elephantiasis associated with LGV. *(Photograph courtesy of the Centers for Disease Control and Prevention, Atlanta, Georgia.)*

Esthiomene is a term derived from the Greek word for "eating away" and is used to describe LGV of the lymphatics of the scrotum, penis, or vulva. The chronic progressive lymphangitis, edema, and sclerosing fibrosis of the subcutaneous structures of these tissues can cause dramatic induration and enlargement (elephantiasis) of the affected parts. Ulceration may occur that is at first superficial but later becomes destructive. Most patients with esthiomene are women, and the chronic ulcerations are most common on the external surface of the labia majora, genitocrural folds, and lateral regions of the perineum (Figures 51–28 and 51–29). Other clinical complications of LGV include papillary growths on the urethral meatus in women, penoscrotal elephantiasis (Figure 51–30), follicular conjunctivitis, and growth of smooth pedunculated perianal lesions ("lymphorrhoids").

PATHOLOGY

Although the histologic features of LGV may suggest LGV in patients with an appropriate clinical history, the lesions are nonspecific and similar microscopic findings may occur in other infections. In the initial stages of infection, a small epidermal vesicle or papule forms that promptly bursts, ulcerates, and oozes pus. A thin layer of fibrin and neutrophils covers the ulcer, and beneath the ulcer is a mixed inflammatory cell infiltrate that is composed of neutrophils, mononuclear cells, and, occasionally, giant cells. The histologic differential diagnosis of the primary lesion includes pyogenic abscesses; the inoculation site of cat scratch disease; and such other causes of genital ulceration as syphilis, trauma, aphthous ulcers, and postherpetic ulcers. In healing lesions, there may be edema and fibrosis at the periphery. Biopsy of late skin lesions of LGV reveals the nonspecific findings of dilated lymphatic vessels, chronic lymphedema with fibrosis, and pseudoepitheliomatous hyperplasia.[10,11,12]

LGV is predominantly a disease of lymph nodes, and it is these structures that have the most characteristic microscopic lesions (Figures 51–31 and 51–32). The underlying pathologic process is a combination of thrombolymphangitis and perilymphangitis, with subsequent spread of the inflammatory process into surrounding soft tissues. The lymphangitis consists of endothelial proliferation in the lymphatic vessels lining lymph nodes. The nodes draining the primary site enlarge rapidly from follicular lymphoid hyperplasia. Simultaneously, small discrete foci of necrosis form that are surrounded by densely packed endothelial cells. These areas attract neutrophils and coalesce into microabscesses with a stellate outline. These stellate microabscesses are frequently surrounded by a zone of palisaded epithelioid cells, macrophages, lymphocytes, and, occasionally, giant cells. As infection persists, the capsule of the lymph node thickens with fibrous tissue. Eventually, the neutrophils vanish and the central area becomes homogenous and eosinophilic, resembling caseation necrosis. Fibrosis and granulation tissue surround the lesion, and its contour changes from stellate

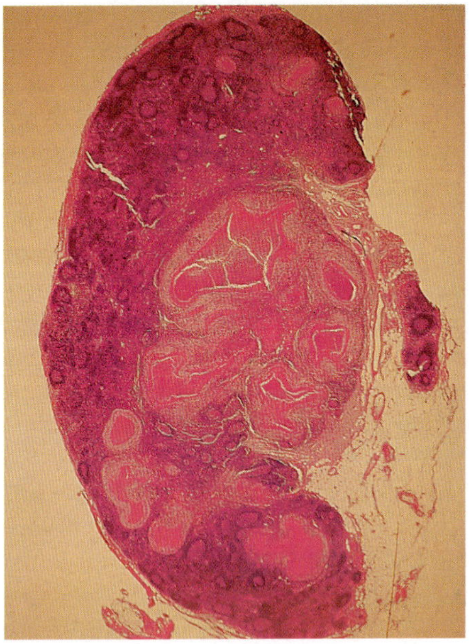

Figure 51–31. Lymph node from a patient with LGV. This low magnification photomicrograph demonstrates late-stage microabscesses and effacement of normal nodal architecture. The lesions are now large and have begun to lose their stellate outlines (hematoxylin-eosin, ×7.5, AFIP Neg 74-14602).

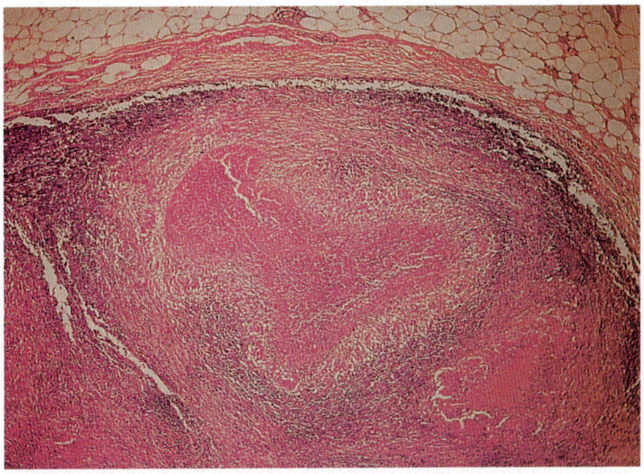

Figure 51–32. Characteristic early stellate abscess in lymph node of a patient with LGV. There is central necrosis containing neutrophils and necrotic debris, surrounded by palisading epithelioid cells and macrophages, and a broad zone of lymphocytes and plasma cells (hematoxylin-eosin, ×50, AFIP Neg 72-1434).

to spherical. Although the necrotic centers of these lesions are paucicellular and eosinophilic, unlike true caseation necrosis mineral deposits are not usually a feature. Inflammation joins the adjacent lymph nodes together by periadenitis, which, with progression, can rupture the lymph node, causing fistulas, abscesses, or sinus tracts.[5,7,10] The active phase of inflammation can persist for weeks to months before subsiding. Because healing of LGV is by fibrosis, the normal structure of the lymph nodes may be altered, causing obstruction of subcutaneous and submucous lymph vessels. The chronic edema and sclerosing fibrosis that result can cause induration and enlargement of the affected tissues.

The histological findings of LGV proctocolitis resemble the changes of inflammatory bowel disease. The colonic lesions of LGV have a distal left-sided predominance, in contrast to the usual right-sided predominance with rectal sparing in Crohn's disease. The important histopathologic findings of LGV of the large intestine includes follicular lymphohistiocytic and plasmacellular infiltrates in the submucosa, muscularis propria, and serosa; neuromatous hyperplasia in the myenteric and submucosal plexuses; and extensive thickening and fibrosis of the bowel wall. Although the lesions of LGV in the large intestine may be patchy, focal, or discontinuous, there is a distinct gradation in severity of inflammation and fibrosis from proximal to distal. The rectum is uniformly involved, whereas more proximal portions of colon are generally spared severe inflammation.[13] The rectal strictures of LGV may be mistaken for cancer as well as tuberculosis, actinomycosis, and schistosomiasis. Mucosal biopsies are frequently performed to establish the diagnosis.

Rarely, organisms enter the bloodstream and involve unusual sites. LGV has caused meningoencephalitis[14]; chronic cholecystitis[15]; and fibrous perihepatic (patients with Fitz-Hugh–Curtis syndrome), abdominal, and pelvic adhesions.[7] Supraclavicular lymphadenitis with mediastinal lymphadenopathy and pericarditis have also been described.[16] Primary infections of the mouth and pharynx from oral–genital contact can cause lesions of these mucosae, as well as lymphadenitis of the submaxillary or submandibular lymph nodes.[17]

Chlamydial inclusions are most easily demonstrated in smears and biopsy specimens of infected tissues during the early phases of infection by using Giemsa stain or fluorescent antibodies.[7,18] With Giemsa staining, the elementary bodies appear purple in contrast to the blue cytoplasm. Fully formed inclusions are compact perinuclear masses that stain dark purple. Unfortunately, Giemsa staining for detection of chlamydial organisms lacks adequate sensitivity and specificity. Although immunofluorescent antibodies are available to detect *C trachomatis* in formalin-fixed tissue sections, they are not specific for the serovars that cause LGV.[19]

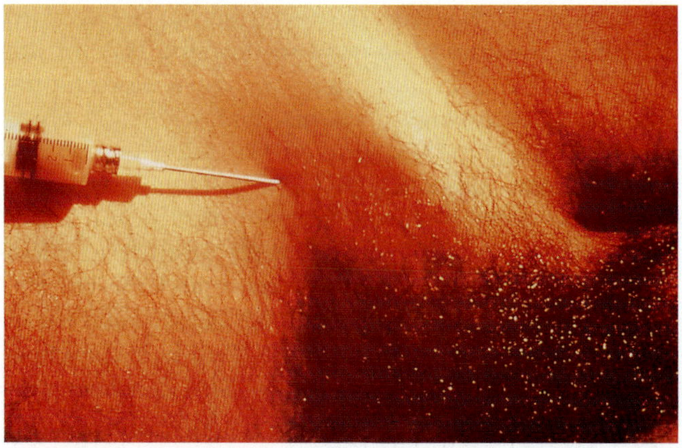

Figure 51–33. Needle aspiration of inguinal bubo being performed on a patient with suspected LGV. Culture is positive in approximately one third of these specimens. *(Photograph courtesy of the Centers for Disease Control and Prevention, Atlanta, Georgia.)*

DIAGNOSIS

The diagnosis of LGV is ideally made by the isolation of an LGV serovar from a bubo; ulcer; or from infected rectum, cervix, or urethra. Unfortunately, aspirates from buboes are culture positive in only 30% of suspected lesions (Figure 51–33). A complement fixation (CF) test with a fourfold increase in titer, or a single titer of 1:64 or higher is very suggestive of LGV. The microimmunofluorescent (Micro-IF) test is more sensitive than CF, although the Micro-IF test cross-reacts with other non-LGV chlamydial serovars. The lesions in biopsy specimens of lymph nodes can be highly suggestive of LGV in the appropriate clinical setting and when other causes of inguinal adenopathy (eg, chancroid, granuloma inguinale, syphilis) are excluded.

REFERENCES

1. Schacter J, Barnes R. Infections caused by *Chlamydia trachomatis*. In: Morse SA, Moreland AA, Holmes KK, eds. *Atlas of Sexually Transmitted Diseases and AIDS*. 2nd ed. New York: Mosby-Wolfe; 1996:65–86.
2. Bowie WR, Holmes KK. *Chlamydia trachomatis* (trachoma, perinatal infections, lymphogranuloma venereum, and other genital infections). In: Mandell GL, Bennett JE, Dolin R, eds. *Principles and Practice of Infectious Diseases*. 4th ed. New York: Churchill Livingstone; 1995: 1684–1685.
3. Maccato M. Lymphogranuloma venereum, chancroid, and granuloma inguinale. In: Pastorek JG II, ed. *Obstetric and*

Gynecologic Infectious Disease. New York: Raven Press; 1994:609–616.

4. Ronald AR, Alfa MJ. Chancroid, lymphogranuloma venereum, and granuloma inguinale. In: Gorbach SL, Bartlett JG, Blacklow NR, eds. *Infectious Diseases.* Philadelphia: WB Saunders; 1992:845–852.
5. Schachter J, Osoba AO. Lymphogranuloma venereum. *Br Med Bull.* 1983;39:151–154.
6. Hammerschlat MR. Lymphogranuloma venereum. In: Felman YM, ed. *Sexually Transmitted Diseases.* New York: Churchill Livingston; 1986:93.
7. Perine PL, Osoba AO. Lymphogranuloma venereum. In: Holes KK, Mårdh P-E, Sparling PF, Weisner PJ, eds. *Sexually Transmitted Diseases.* 2nd ed. New York: McGraw-Hill; 1990:195–204.
8. Abrams AJ. Lymphogranuloma venereum. *JAMA.* 1968; 205:199–202.
9. Bauwens JE, Lampe MF, Suchland RJ, Wong K. Stamm WE. Infection with *Chlamydia trachomatis* lymphogranuloma venereum serovar L1 in homosexual men with proctitis: molecular analysis of an unusual case cluster. *Clin Infect Dis.* 1995;20:576–581.
10. Smith EB, Custer RP. The histopathology of lymphogranuloma venereum. *J Urol.* 1950;63:546–548.
11. Jerden MS. Chlamydial infections. In: Farmer ER, Hood AF, eds. *Pathology of the Skin.* Norwalk, CT: Appleton and Lange; 1990:334–337.
12. Sheldon WH, Heyman A. Lymphogranuloma venereum. *Am J Pathol.* 1947;23:653–664.
13. de la Monte SM, Hutchins GM. Follicular proctocolitis and neuromatous hyperplasia with lymphogranuloma venereum. *Hum Pathol.* 1985;16:1025–1032.
14. Sabin AB, Aring CD. Meningoencephalitis in man caused by the virus of lymphogranuloma venereum. *JAMA.* 1942; 120:1376.
15. Coutts WE. Contribution to the knowledge of lymphogranulomatosis venereum as a general disease. *J Trop Med Hyg.* 1936;39:13.
16. Sheldon WH, et al. Lymphogranuloma venereum of supraclavicular lymph nodes with mediastinal lymphadenopathy and pericarditis. *Am J Med.* 1948;5:320.
17. Thorsteinsson SB, Musher DM, Min KW, et al. Lymphogranuloma venereum: a cause of cervical lymphadenopathy. *JAMA.* 1936;235:1882.
18. Paavonen J. Chlamydial infections: microbiological, clinical and diagnostic aspects. *Med Biol.* 1979;57:152.
19. Klotz SA, Drutz DJ, Tam MR, Reed KH. Hemorrhagic proctitis due to lymphogranuloma venereum serogroup L2. Diagnosis by fluorescent monoclonal antibody. *N Engl J Med.* 1983;308:1563–1565.

Trachoma

Deborah Dean

Let there be sight to heal the soul of man.

Sanskrit proverb

I will lead the blind by ways they have not known, along unfamiliar paths I will guide them; I will turn darkness into light before them and make the rough places smooth. These are the things I will do; I will not foresake them.

Isaiah 42:16

Great crowds came to him, bringing the lame, the blind, the crippled, the mute and many others, and laid them at his feet; and he healed them.

Matthew 15:30

CLASSIFICATION

Trachoma is a chronic infection of the eye caused by *Chlamydia trachomatis. Chlamydia trachomatis* is one of the three known species of *Chlamydia,* the other two being *Chlamydia pneumoniae* and *Chlamydia psittaci.* Each can be differentiated based on glycogen production, antibiotic susceptibilities, and, less specifically, morphology of the inclusion. There are three biologic variants that make up *C trachomatis.* They include the biovars that cause trachoma, lymphogranuloma venereum (LGV), and mouse pneumonitis. The trachoma and LGV biovars are confined to humans; no zoonotic hosts have been identified. The trachoma biovar represents subtypes of the organism that cause both sexually transmitted diseases and trachoma. These subtypes are serologically classified into 18 different serovars. The serotyping designations are based on monoclonal and polyclonal recognition of epitopes on the major outer membrane protein (MOMP) of the organism. Additional serovars may exist but these have yet to be fully characterized. The serovars causing trachoma are A, B, Ba, and C, and have been referred to as the trachoma agent. However, some B and Ba serovars are noted to infect the human genital tract and vary in *omp1,* which is the gene that encodes for MOMP. A new typing system is being developed that is based on *omp1* and is referred to as *omp1* genotyping.[1] *Omp1* genotyping may supplant serotyping in certain clinical settings. For example, in endemic or hyperendemic trachoma populations, few serovars but many distinct genotypes predominate. Thus, the identification and study of genotypes in these populations could significantly facilitate transmission studies and aid in vaccine development

INTRODUCTION

Although the agent of trachoma was not recognized until the 20th century, the disease has been well described since antiquity. The first report was from China in the 27th century BC, where a treatment for trichiasis was described. Later there was mention of a conjunctival disease similar to trachoma in the Ebers Papyrus from Egypt that dates to 1800 BC. In the first century BC the name trachoma appeared, which meant "rough swelling" in Greek. Trachoma was also reported by Galen in 61 AD and in numerous descriptions in medieval writings. The disease was disseminated to Europe by crusaders returning from the Middle East during the Middle Ages. Not until the Napoleonic era, however, did trachoma become a significant blinding disease of epidemic proportions among French and

English military and civilian populations. Subsequently, 19th century ophthalmology textbooks were filled with descriptions of conjunctival follicles, superficial corneal vascularization, and scarring.[2]

The intracellular inclusions of trachoma were identified by Halberstaedter and von Prowazek in 1907. In the 1920s, these inclusions were believed to cause trachoma, in spite of the controversy that trachoma may be due to another bacterial agent termed *Bacterium granulosis*.[3] The agent of trachoma was not cultivated until 1957, although *C psittaci* and LGV had been isolated more than 20 years earlier. Copper sulfate solutions or crystals were the initial treatments for trachoma. The subsequent introduction of sulfonamides and their systemic use in Native American Indian populations led to a decline in the prevalence, and, in many tribes, trachoma was eradicated by 1942.[4] Since World War II, most European and other developed countries have had a dramatic decline in prevalence rates, largely from improved sanitation, personal hygiene, and control programs. Subsequently, the tetracyclines and erythromycins led to topical treatment studies by the World Health Organization (WHO) of populations in trachoma endemic areas. Although continuous and intermittent topical treatment regimens were efficacious in reducing prevalence, these results were short-lived. In fact, systemic therapy with sulfonamides or tetracyclines had more consistent and longer term success.[5] Sulfonamides are rarely used today as chlamydiae can develop resistance to these drugs. Newer macrolides such as azithromycin may prove to be appropriate for the treatment of trachoma, especially in children, because systemic tetracycline treatment is contraindicated. To date, however, there are limited data on their efficacy, and recurrence of infection may limit their usefulness.

The last decade has provided an enhanced understanding of the clinical, microbiologic, and immunologic characteristics of trachoma. In addition, a new and simplified grading system for clinical trachoma has provided insights into the clinical epidemiology of the disease, including risk factors and disease prevalence. The pathogenesis of trachoma, however, remains unclear, and the development of vaccines proceeds slowly.

EPIDEMIOLOGY

Trachoma is the leading cause of preventable blindness in the world. It is worldwide and prevails in North and sub-Saharan Africa; the Middle East; the Northern Indian subcontinent; Southeast Asia; and pockets of Australia, the South Pacific Islands, and North, Central, and South America.[6] More than 500 million people worldwide are afflicted. Of these, 100 million have severe visual deficits and 9 million are blind. By the year 2020, those with blinding disease are projected to reach 12 million.[7] Trachoma is endemic or hyperendemic in these communities where blinding or nonblinding disease may be the outcome. The epidemiologic patterns tend to be based on the degree of endemicity within the community. In hyperendemic communities, there is a high load of infectious organisms with frequent reinfection, high prevalence rates of disease among children, and conjunctival scarring that occurs at different rates and severity in most age groups. Many of those with scarring develop trichiasis and entropion, which can lead to corneal abrasion, bacterial superinfections, and blindness. In endemic communities, the disease can take two forms. In one form, the overall infection rate in the village is low, but a small number of families are heavily infected, which provides a nidus for repeat infection. The sequelae in these families are similar to those mentioned previously. In the other form, onset is delayed and few develop blindness, but the overall infection rate in the community may be moderate or high.[2,8]

The prevalence of active trachoma varies from 25% to 65%.[9] These findings are based on culture and antigen detection; however, not all those with clinically active trachoma can be confirmed by diagnostic tests. In Tanzania, 43% of patients with trachomatous follicles (TF) and 23% of those with intense trachoma (TI) were negative for chlamydiae.[10] There are a number of explanations for this: The diagnostic tests have limited sensitivity; there may be sampling errors; other pathogens may mimic the inflammatory findings of trachoma; and autoimmunity may play a role in these findings. Furthermore, the conjunctiva can remain inflamed for 6 to 9 weeks following treatment,[11] during which time it would be unlikely to detect chlamydiae. In studies in The Gambia, the problem of clinical disease without demonstrable chlamydial infection has been addressed by examining and testing household members every 2 weeks.[9] A new infection could be detected 2 weeks before the development of inflammatory changes. Detectable organisms were present for an additional 2 to 6 weeks, whereas clinical disease persisted for up to 30 weeks in children. In adults, the duration of clinical disease averaged only 2 weeks. Thus, it appears that the time of sampling is one critical factor in determining the cause of the disease. Additional studies in other trachoma endemic regions of the world are required to confirm these findings.

The rates of documented infection for clinically inactive disease range from 5% to 24%.[10–14] In one study in Tanzania, 24% of the children who had no evidence for clinical disease were positive for *C trachomatis* by polymerase chain reaction (PCR).[12]

Those at greatest risk are children younger than 10 years. Most children are infected by age 2, with a steady decline in prevalence after age 5. However, adolescent and adult women of childbearing age or female caregivers continue to have rates of active infection that range from 5% to 10%.[10–14] These are most likely repeat infections from infected children. Adult women also tend to have more severe disease and sequelae than men; recurrent infections in these women are believed to be an important factor. Because children compose more than 50% of the population in these communities, they are the primary reservoir of the organism. Eye-to-hand-to-eye contact is probably the most common model of transmission; however, reservoirs within the host, including the nasopharynx and rectum, may be sources of reinfection of the ocular mucosa.[14]

The intensity of disease in children varies considerably, but, for any one child, this intensity can be quite stable at different times in spite of appropriate treatment. This phenomenon was previously thought to be a result of environmental factors, but this is now thought to be a combination of factors including the environment, individual host immune responses, and, possibly, the genetic make-up of the host. Progression of disease to conjunctival scarring and trichiasis or entropion is more frequent in adults who had moderate or severe disease in childhood. The duration of inflammation is also believed to be important in the development of these sequelae; however, these may not become manifest for 10 to 40 years after the initial childhood infection.[15] Thus, blindness caused by trachoma is less common in young adults than in older adults. Furthermore, dry eyes in older patients with trichiasis or entropion may predispose the cornea to abrasion and bacterial superinfection.

Risk factors for trachoma are crowding, poverty, children in the household, more than one child per sleeping room, lack of water use or lack of water, and poor personal hygiene.[10,16] Flies may be an important vector for transmission in Africa. In one report, a child's ocular secretions were stained with fluorescein. Subsequently, fluorescein was detected on the legs and bodies of flies in the study household and in the eyes of children in the same family within 15 to 30 minutes.[17] It is unclear, however, what size inoculum can be carried on flies and whether this is sufficient to cause infection. In addition, chlamydiae are obligate intracellular pathogens that may not survive long outside the host. Coinfection with other bacteria may also be a risk factor for trachoma. In many endemic areas, especially Africa, there are seasonal outbreaks of bacterial conjunctivitis. Furthermore, most children are colonized with pathogenic and nonpathogenic organisms that may contribute to trachoma and severity of disease when the microbial balance is tipped toward infection. A previous study in Tunisia reported a higher prevalence of bacterial coinfection only in those with moderate to severe trachoma.[2] Bacterial coinfection may also enhance conjunctival and corneal inflammation, which may lead to conjunctival scarring and superficial corneal vascularization.[18] This is an area of research that has been ignored since the mid 1980s but is important in understanding the pathogenesis of trachoma.

MORPHOLOGY AND LIFE CYCLE

Chlamydia resemble gram-negative bacteria in morphology, metabolism, and structure; however, they are obligate intracellular parasites as they require nutrients from the host cell for replication. The infectious particle of the organism is the spore-like elementary body (EB), which is metabolically inert. The EB attaches to susceptible epithelial cells either by cations or heparin sulfate mediated binding or via a receptor mechanism or both, and is subsequently taken up into a phagosome. Lysosomal fusion with the endophagosome or inclusion body is inhibited, which allows for the intracellular survival of the organism. The EB is transformed into a reticulate body (RB) within a few hours. The RB is the metabolically active form of the organism and is incapable of survival outside the host cell. Nutrients and essential amino acids are transported across the inclusion membrane and replication proceeds by binary fission. Within 48 to 72 hours, the RBs condense back down into infectious EBs. The EBs are released from the cell by one of two possible mechanisms: rupture of the inclusion body or extrusion of the intact inclusions by a process similar to exocytosis.

CLINICAL FEATURES

Trachoma is defined as a chronic follicular conjunctivitis that has persisted for at least 15 days. Early in the disease it is characterized by a follicular conjunctivitis that is indistinguishable from that caused by *C trachomatis* sexually transmitted serovars or *C. psittaci* or *C pneumoniae* strains.[19] Later, it becomes a cicatricial conjunctivitis with superficial corneal vascularization. The onset of trachoma can be acute or insidious. Patients with trachoma may present with a foreign body sensation. The entire upper tarsal conjunctiva typically is involved and contains lymphoid follicles that occur in the subconjuctival epithelium (Figure 51–34). These follicles appear as clear, yellowish, or gray-white avascular lesions that are 0.2 to 2 mm in diameter.[2] Inflammatory infiltrates (papillary hypertrophy) with conjunctival thickening can be present. In children younger than 2 years, the papillary changes may be the only indication of trachoma as follicle formation is less common in this age group. In addition, the infection may go unnoticed in

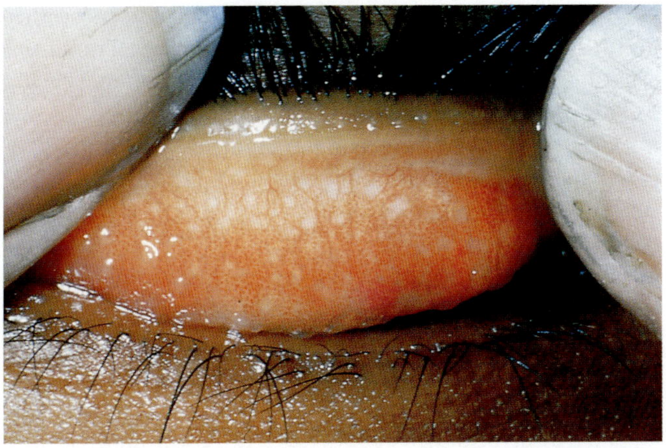

Figure 51–34. Chronic follicular conjunctivitis in a young woman. She has intense trachoma in the upper tarsus (TI), numerous lymphoid follicles (F3), and pronounced papillary hypertrophy (P3).

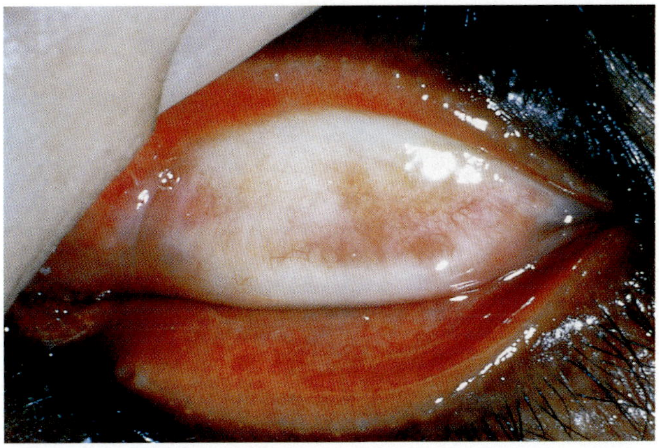

Figure 51–36. Older Nepali woman with severe conjunctival scarring that is starting to distort the upper lid.

young infants who may become a nidus of infection for spread to other children in the family. The intensity of these inflammatory infiltrates tends to increase in children up to 6 to 8 years. The corneal involvement of the disease includes punctate epithelial erosions that usually occur in the upper half of the cornea, although they can be found at any location on the cornea. Shallow peripheral ulcers and anterior infiltrates of stroma are also common. These infiltrates can range in size from those that require a slit lamp to see to those with frank ulceration. Lymphoid follicles at the limbus are a characteristic feature of trachoma that lead to the formation of Herbert's pits (Figure 51–35). Pannus may also develop and is composed of superficial corneal vessels with cellular infiltrates (Figure 51–35). Pannus is most prominent at the superior limbal margin, but it can occur at any point along the limbal margin and does not progress to the point where vision is disturbed.

In the later stages of trachoma, fine linear or stellate scars appear across the conjunctivae that may progress to a broader band of scars or synechiae in more severe infections (Figure 51–36). Children may have these scars by age 4 years (Figure 51–37). As the scarring progresses, the upper tarsus becomes distorted, leading to trichiasis (inward turning eyelashes) (Figure 51–38) and entropion (inward displacement of the margin of the eyelid). These inturned eyelashes can produce corneal abrasions that become superinfected with bacteria; the abrasions heal by scarring. Thus, varying degrees of corneal opacification develop and cause

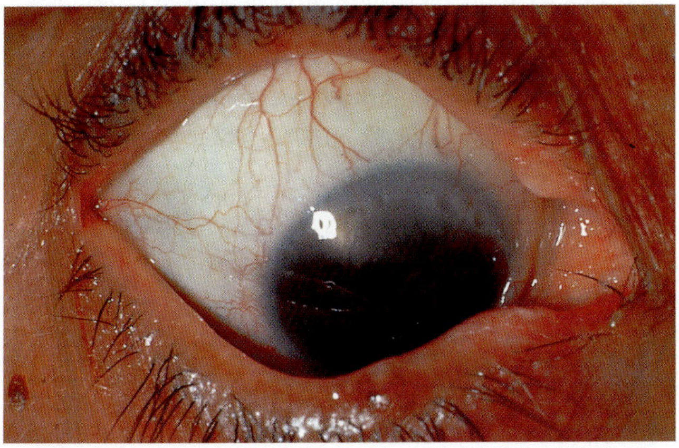

Figure 51–35. Superficial corneal vascularization (pannus) in an Egyptian adult at the superior cornea. Herbert's pits are at the corneal–limbal junction. *(Photograph courtesy of Dr. Chandler R. Dawson, San Francisco, California.)*

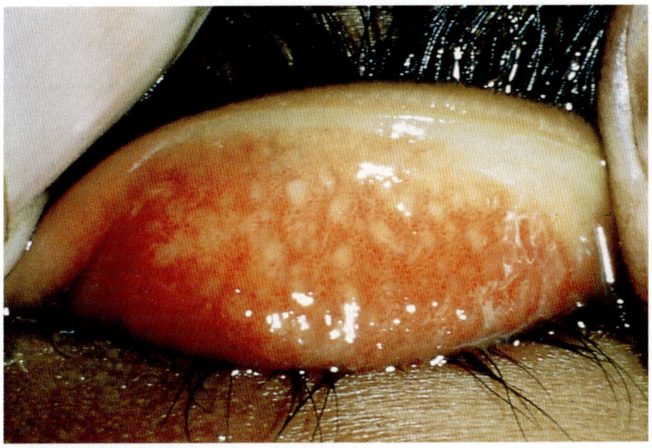

Figure 51–37. Follicular conjunctivitis in a Nepali child with trachoma. The upper tarsus has intense trachoma (TI) with more than five lymphoid follicles (F3), pronounced papillary hypertrophy (P3), and fine scattered scars (C1).

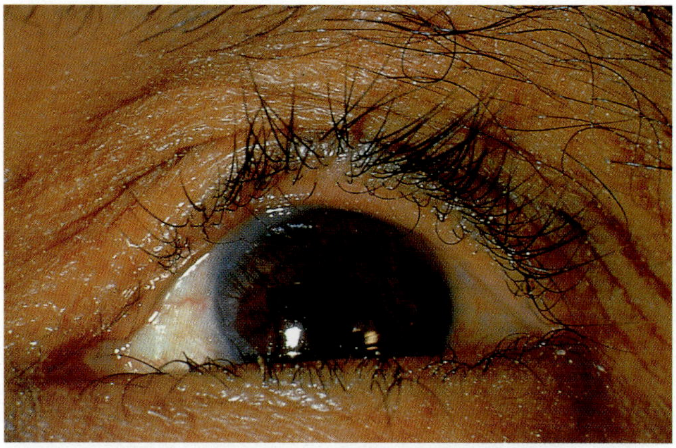

Figure 51–38. Trichiasis in an Egyptian adult. *(Photograph courtesy of Dr. Chandler R. Dawson, San Francisco, California.)*

visual deficits or blindness. In addition, the entire lid may become distorted, which can prevent apposition of the lids and subsequent exposure keratitis (or trauma). Stenosis of the lacrimal duct is a late complication of scarring. This may cause a dry eye syndrome, which in turn contributes to the development of corneal abrasions. Because the sequelae of conjunctival scarring usually do not appear until adulthood, most blindness that occurs is in adults and the elderly.

Although trachoma is one disease that causes a chronic follicular conjunctivitis, there are other conditions that meet the definition of this disease. The differential diagnoses include folliculosis; toxic follicular conjunctivitis caused by cosmetics, drugs, or molluscum contagiosum; other bacteria; inclusion conjunctivitis from sexually transmitted chlamydial organisms; inclusion conjunctivitis caused by other species of *Chlamydia*[19]; Axenfeld's chronic follicular conjunctivitis; chronic follicular keratoconjunctivitis of Thygeson; Parinaud's oculoglandular syndrome; or Vernal catarrh.[2] The common bacterial pathogens that cause chronic follicular conjunctivitis are *Haemophilus influenzae, H aegyptius, Moraxella* sp, *Neisseria meningitidis, N gnorrhoeae,* and *Streptococcus pneumoniae.* In regions where trachoma is suspected, the detection of chlamydiae in the population suggests that this is the cause even when there may be concurrent outbreaks of bacterial or viral conjunctivitis.

PATHOLOGY

In the early stages of trachoma, the conjunctival epithelium and subepithelium are infiltrated with neutrophils. The conjunctiva is bound down to the tarsal plate and, at these sites, raised villous processes develop and form papillae.[20] Within the center of each papilla is a vascular tuft. In addition, there are bands or folds of epithelium that surround and separate the papillae. The entire conjunctiva can become thickened from increasing inflammatory cell infiltrates and dilated vessels of the papillae. With time, the cellular infiltrate becomes lymphocytic, involving the submucosa and occasionally the underlying connective tissue. The lymphocytes form follicles that lack germinal centers. As the disease progresses, some lymphoid follicles form germinal centers that are composed of an outer layer of lymphocytes and a more central layer of macrophages with a few B and T cell lymphocytes.[21–23] The macrophages may assist in presentation of antigen to T cells that are then capable of a harmful immune response. The germinal center is displaced to the surface of the follicle, which distinguishes it from the follicle of a typical lymph node. These follicles are in the conjunctival mucosa (Figure 51–37), the subepithelium, and the underlying connective tissue. A dense infiltrate of lymphocytes is frequently between these follicles. These lymphocytes include both CD4+ and CD8+ cell types.[22] Macrophages, in addition to the germinal centers, may be in the conjunctival epithelium. In contrast, plasma cells may be throughout the epithelium and subepithelium and are most indicative of chronic infection. The conjunctival epithelium overlying the follicles is infiltrated with lymphocytes and can be quite thin. In addition, there may be disruption of the surface membrane of goblet cells and flattening of microvilli that are part of the normal absorptive surface of the epithelium.[23] This may break down the normal defense mechanism of the epithelium. This histopathologic structure resembles the Peyer's patch of the small intestine.

As the disease advances, the follicles can become necrotic and surrounded by connective tissue, which invariably leads to scarring.[20,24] There may be posttrachomatous degeneration characterized by epithelial-lined cysts within the epithelium (Figure 51–39). These cysts are trapped islands of epithelium that separate the raised papillae. Trichiasis is a late sequela of scarring (Figure 51–38), and results from a gradual contraction of the superficial and deep scars that are close to the margin of the lid.

Follicles also may develop on the cornea. These follicles form at the scleral–corneal border and do not ulcerate or induce fibrosis. Thus, they heal without scarring. The follicles do, however, cause Herbert's pits, which are points of depression at the limbus (Figure 51–35).[25] These are the only pathognomonic feature of trachoma. The cornea is also susceptible to pannus formation, which is a superficial vascularization of this tissue (Figure 51–35). Pannus is almost exclusively limited to the limbal margin. It occurs predominantly at the superior limbal border but may occur at the inferior limbus or any point along this corneal margin.

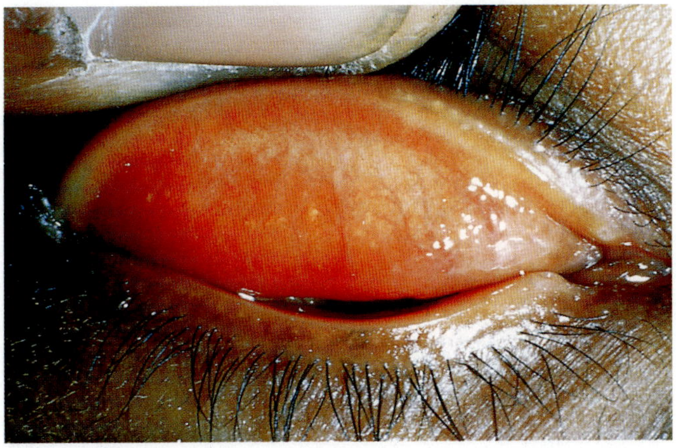

Figure 51–39. Conjunctival scarring and posttrachomatous degeneration in a 50-year-old Nepali woman.

The immunopathogenesis of trachoma is not well understood. During early human vaccine trials and subsequent research in nonhuman primate models, immunity to *C trachomatis* appeared to be serovar-specific, short-lived, and dose-dependent.[26–28] Both humoral and T-cell dependent responses appear to be important in this process. Repeat infection with chlamydiae is also a major factor for severe sequelae. Repeated infections with the same or different serovars of *C trachomatis* are thought to be common in children. This concept was based on a 10-year study of 32 households in Taiwan, where many of the children had numerous infections.[26] Interestingly, early vaccine studies in Taiwan demonstrated hypersensitivity reactions among children who later became infected with local serovars.[27] Furthermore, in the monkey model of trachoma, only monkeys that had been repeatedly infected or immunologically stimulated before infection with an early vaccine developed pannus and conjunctival scarring.[28] These findings have been corroborated in other animals[29,30] and suggest that progression of disease is associated with an immunopathogenic response following repeated infections. As children become adolescents and adults, there is a continuous decrease in the prevalence of active disease and the severity of clinical findings. A number of adults, especially those older than 25 years, will have *C trachomatis* antigens in their conjunctivae and only about 10% will have clinically active disease[31,32]; however, it is usually possible to isolate the organism from only 1% of these patients. In addition, antigen-positive adults are more likely to develop progressive scarring. Secretory immunoglobulin A (sIgA) antibodies are not usually at mucosal sites in the absence of antigenic stimulation. In one study conducted in The Gambia, 43% of adults with inactive disease and scarring had chlamydial antigens and sIgA antibodies.[31] Furthermore, only 7% of the adults with no clinical disease living in low prevalence communities for chlamydiae had sIgA antibodies, compared with 41% living in an area of high prevalence. In addition, IgG antibodies in tears were significantly correlated with those who were antigen positive and not with those who were antigen negative, suggesting real yet inapparent infection.[31]

The pathogenesis of trachoma may also be related to the ability of the organism to evade host immune responses. If the surface antigens mutate slightly, chlamydiae may be able to infect or persist in the host at a time when the patient would be immune to the homologous strain (from which the mutant was derived). This is suggested by a study in which isolates from a trachoma endemic region of Tunisia were sequenced over a 3-year period.[1] In one village, serovars B and Ba persisted but varied at the gene and MOMP level to reveal 15 of 23 mutants of serovar B or Ba. During the same 3-year period, these mutants shifted but were still closely related to the prototype serovars in the community. New immunologic variants, however, were identified in this trachoma endemic area.[33] Similar work in The Gambia has also shown significant mutations with subtle shifts in genotypes and surface antigens during a 6-month period.[34] Host immune response to specific chlamydial proteins may predispose also to more severe disease. Conjunctival inflammation in the host occurs within 24 hours in response to infectious EBs. This is not true for inactivated EBs, MOMP, or LPS. There is another protein, however, that is a homologue to the 60 kD GroEl heat shock protein (hsp) of *E coli* that may also cause an inflammatory response in the conjunctiva.[35] This chlamydial hsp60 is surface exposed and elicits a significant humoral immune response in patients with severe trachoma and in those with tubal infertility and ectopic pregnancies.[35,36] Studies in vitro have shown that chlamydiae can develop into a latent form in response to treatment with penicillin and to immune mediators such as gamma interferon and tumor necrosis factor. Some of these "latent" infections produced an increase in chlamydial hsp60 expression,[37] which has been associated with immunopathogenic responses in both conjunctival[35,38] and fallopian tissues. Thus, latent forms of chlamydiae that produce antigen may be widely present among adults who are culture negative and have clinically inapparent infection. This may be a source of reinfection or spread of infection when environmental conditions favor the transformation of the latent form into an infectious one. In the mouse, the immune response to chlamydial hsp60 is genetically restricted, which may explain in part the diversity in severity of trachoma within a population.[39] Some autoimmunity may be involved also. A late inflammatory response in patients with trichiasis was found in one study in which there was a predominance of T and B cells[40]; however, low-grade chlamydial infection, persistent infection, reexposure, or sequestration of the organism in the subconjunctiva may also explain apparent late inflammation. Alternatively, depressed cell-mediated immunity may limit the host's ability to clear organisms,[41] thus leading to persistent infection, low-grade inflammation, and severe scarring of conjunctiva. Currently, the pathogenesis of trachoma is thought to be related to a severe and prolonged inflammatory response, deleterious host immune responses, and repeat infections during childhood.

The typical intracellular inclusion bodies of *C trachomatis* can be visualized by Giemsa or iodine staining of conjunctival smears, fluorescent-conjugated monoclonal antibody staining of tissue culture specimens inoculated with conjunctival material, or immunohistochemical staining of frozen or paraffin embedded tissue. Conjunctival swabbings are applied to a glass slide, fixed with methanol, and then stained, or swabbings can be placed in chlamydiae transport media that is then inoculated onto a monolayer of cells in tissue culture. Rarely, conjunctival tissue may be available after repair of trichiasis or entropion, which can be analyzed immunohistochemically. In Giemsa stains, the inclusion body is an intracytoplasmic, hypodense body with a basophilic stippled pattern (Figure 51–40). Giemsa stained inclusions, however, can be confused with keratin, nuclear extrusions, goblet cells, eosinophilic granules, pigment granules, and other bacteria.[42] Jones' or Lugol's iodine stains the glycogen containing inclusion of *C trachomatis*. It imparts a dark yellow-brown color to the inclusion, but is infrequently used because it is insensitive. Fluorescein-conjugated antibodies are used to detect inclusions in cell culture. This imparts apple-green color to the inclusion body that stands out against the dark red cells counterstained with Evans blue (Figure 51–41). Peroxidase-conjugated monoclonal antibodies are also available to detect chlamydial inclusions but are less frequently used. Commercial polyclonal and monoclonal antibodies also are available to detect chlamydial inclusions immunohistochemically. They can be used on frozen or paraffin embedded tissues and are *Chlamydia* species- or genus-specific.

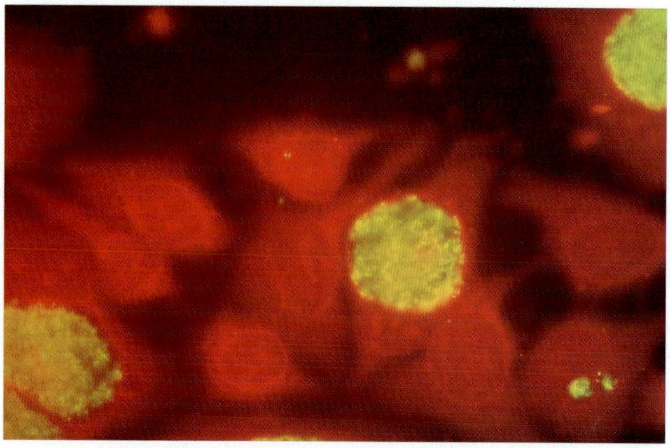

Figure 51–41. Immunofluorescence detects chlamydial inclusion bodies in a monolayer of McCoy cells infected from a conjunctival specimen of a Nepali child with trachoma (×1000).

The EBs of *C trachomatis* can be visualized by staining conjunctival smears with fluorescein-conjugated antibodies (Figure 51–42). There are two types of antibodies available. One is species-specific and recognizes the MOMP of *C trachomatis*. The other is genus-specific and recognizes the LPS of *Chlamydia*. The cytologic appearance of the EB is an extracellular, round, fluorescing apple-green particle; however, the

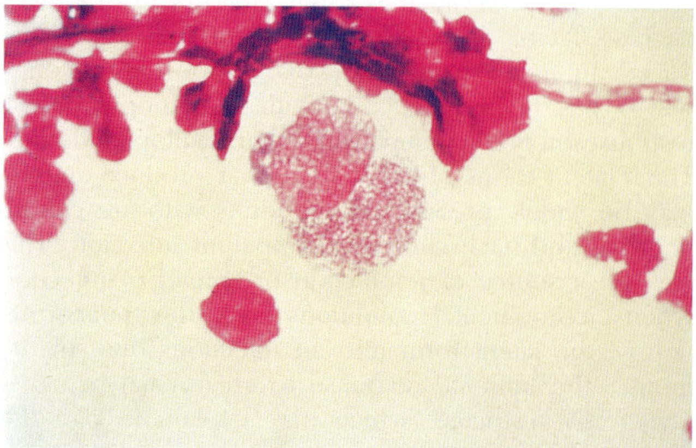

Figure 51–40. Giemsa stained conjunctival smear from a child with trachoma. The inclusion body has a slightly basophilic, granular, appearance. *(Photograph courtesy of Dr. Chandler R. Dawson, San Francisco, California.)*

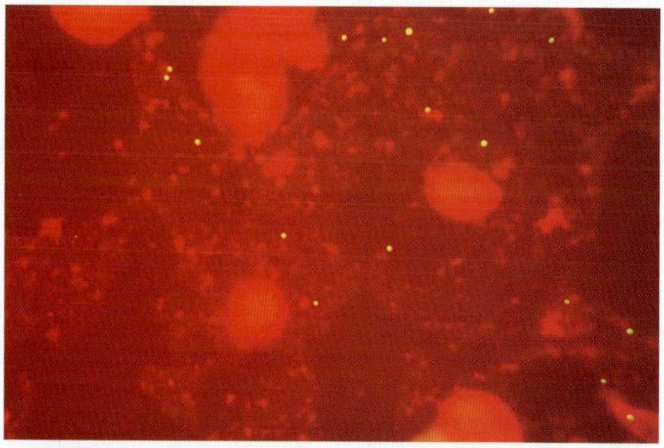

Figure 51–42. Immunofluorescence detects EBs by DFA; conjunctival smear from a Nepali child with trachoma (×400).

EB can easily be confused with nonspecific fluorescence that occurs even with appropriate preparation of the slides. Thus, technical expertise is critical for interpreting the results.

DIAGNOSIS

The clinical features of trachoma can be used for a presumptive diagnosis. WHO developed a modified trachoma grading scale for primary healthcare workers.[43] This system has, however, also been used by researchers in the field. The grading system simplifies the previous WHO and MacCallan classification systems[6] and has helped to clarify the prevalence, risk factors, and epidemiology of trachoma.[9] The modified grading retains certain features of the more extensive system; for example, the degree of inflammatory intensity (TF, TI), the progression of disease to trichiasis (TT), and certain scarring sequelae (CO). It does not, however, describe mild follicular conjunctivitis or the degree of conjunctival scarring that is important for predicting the complications of the disease.[9] The following is the simplified WHO grading scale[43]:

- TF: Trachoma follicles—Five or more follicles in the central upper tarsal conjunctiva
- TI: Intense trachoma—Diffuse infiltration of the upper tarsal conjunctiva that obscures the deep tarsal vessels over 50% or more of the tarsal surface
- TS: Trachomatous scarring of the conjunctiva
- TT: Trichiasis (inturned eyelashes) that touch the eye
- CO: Corneal opacity that impairs vision
- Active trachoma: Presence of TF or TI
- Intense trachoma: Presence of TI
- Cicatricial trachoma: Presence of TS
- Healed trachoma: TS without TF or TI

Important indicators for trachoma in a community are at least two of the following for each subject examined[6]:

1. Follicles in the upper tarsal conjunctiva
2. Limbal follicles or their sequelae, Herbert's pits
3. Typical conjunctival scarring
4. Vascular pannus more extensive at the superior limbus

Herbert's pits are the only pathognomonic finding; their presence in a community is highly indicative of trachoma. Direct detection of chlamydiae with the appropriate clinical findings confirms the presence of endemic or hyperendemic trachoma.

The options for the diagnosis of *C trachomatis* ocular infections include Giemsa, iodine, or DFA staining of conjunctival smears; nucleic acid hybridization probe test of conjunctival smears or swabs; culture of conjunctival swabs; EIA or ELISA test of conjunctival swabs; or commercial PCR or LCR tests of conjunctival swabs. The Giemsa stain is relatively cheap and easy to perform, especially in developing countries. Thus, it can be used to screen in areas where trachoma is suspected or known to exist in endemic or hyperendemic form. Technical expertise is required, however, and the overall sensitivity of this test is not very good (approximately 60%). Giemsa stained conjunctival smears should first be inspected to be sure the specimen is adequate. Separated epithelial cells and neutrophils, or other cells including lymphocytes, macrophages, Leber, and plasma cells, denote an adequate specimen and suggest chlamydial infection. These smears can also be used to evaluate the degree of inflammation and to look for bacterial superinfections.[2] The Giemsa stain detects the inclusion body within an infected cell; it imparts a basophilic, stippled appearance to the inclusion that contrasts with the dense, dark blue to purple cell (Figure 51–40). The staining of the inclusion, however, must be differentiated from other entities that can give a similar appearance (see previous pathology section). Lugol's or Jones' iodine also stain the inclusion body. This test is similar to the Giemsa stains in that the sensitivity is poor (approximately 30% to 40%) and it should be used only in hyperendemic regions. With the DFA test, the quality of the smear can also be assessed. The monoclonal antibodies used in this test are either species-specific, reacting with the MOMP of *C trachomatis,* or genus-specific, reacting with the LPS of *Chlamydia.* Either antibody stains the EBs a fluorescing, apple-green color (Figure 51–42). The EBs are extracellular round dots on the slide and can be confused with debris; therefore, technical expertise is required. This test is more sensitive than Giemsa or iodine stains (approximately 80% to 90%). Commercial hybridization probes are also available to detect chlamydial DNA. These are designed to hybridize with complementary strands of chlamydial plasmid or *omp1* DNA from a smear that has been applied to filter paper or extracted from a conjunctival swab. The sensitivity of these tests ranges from approximately 70% to 90%.

Tissue culture is still the gold standard for the detection of *C trachomatis,* but it has limited sensitivity in endemic and hyperendemic communities—up to 90%.[44] This may be from delayed culture (facilities may be lacking in developing countries). Thus, specimens must be stored at −70°C and transported to a laboratory for cell culture. *Chlamydiae* lose viability on freezing, and some strains, especially serovar C, are difficult to propagate. Cell culture is expensive and requires technical expertise. Results are usually available within 48 to 72 hours, although a first or second passage can increase the number of positive samples but delay the reporting time by 3 to 7 days.[44] Species- and genus-specific monoclonal antibodies are available for detecting chlamydial inclusions. They appear as fluorescing, intracytoplasmic inclusions that are round to ovoid or sometimes irregular (Figure 51–41).

Commercial EIA or ELISA tests employ polyclonal or monoclonal antibodies to detect the EB. These antibodies are directed against the LPS of *Chlamydia* and are conjugated with an enzyme that reacts with substrate to produce a color change, the detection of which requires a spectrophotometer. The sensitivity of this test (70% to 85%) is not as good as for DFA, probe, or culture, and it also requires technical expertise to perform. The kits, however, contain a confirmatory test with a blocking antibody that binds to the chlamydial LPS. When the sample is rerun with the blocking antibody, the test should be negative if the positive result was caused by *Chlamydia*. If not, the antibodies are most likely reacting with bacterial LPS.

The most recent tests developed for detecting *Chlamydia* are commercial PCR and LCR tests. These relay on the annealing of DNA primers with a complementary strand of DNA from the chlamydial plasmid that is in *C trachomatis* and *C psittaci*. The LCR test amplifies a signal generated by the hybridization of primers to the plasmid template. For the PCR test, the actual plasmid DNA is amplified and a hybridization assay detects the amplified product. This product is then identified by a spectrophotometer. To date, however, these tests have not been used in endemic regions and, therefore, have not been approved for ocular specimens. The sensitivities and specificities of these tests in trachoma settings are probably similar to those in STD populations. Commercial immunohistochemical polyclonal and monoclonal antibodies are also available to detect chlamydial inclusion bodies. They can be used on frozen and paraffin embedded tissue and are *Chlamydia* species- or genus-specific.

The two serologic tests available to detect chlamydiae are the microimmunofluorescent test (MIF) and the complement fixation test (CF), both of which are available only in reference laboratories. The MIF test uses EBs from each serovar and those from *C pneumoniae* and *C psittaci* as antigens in the assay. In contrast, the CF test employs a group-reactive chlamydial antigen, the LPS. Serial dilutions of patient sera or tears are reacted against the antigens, and a fluorescein-conjugated antihuman IgM or IgG antibody is then used to detect antibody–antigen binding. Neither test is specific for chlamydiae, however, and thus they cannot be used to diagnose active infection. The reason for this is that patient antibodies may cross-react with different *C trachomatis* serovars and between species. In addition, antibody responses may represent a previous sexually transmitted infection of chlamydiae and not an ocular infection.

REFERENCES

1. Dean D, Schachter J, Dawson C, Stephens RS. Comparison of the major outer membrane protein sequence variant regions of B/Ba isolates: a molecular epidemiologic approach to *Chlamydia trachomatis* infections. *J Infect Dis.* 1992;166:383–392.
2. Schachter J, Dawson CR. Trachoma. In: *Human Chlamydial Infections.* Littleton, MA: PSG Publishing; 1978: 63–96.
3. Noguchi H. The etiology of trachoma. *J Exp Med.* 1928; 48:1–53.
4. Forster WG, McGibony JR. Trachoma. *Am J Ophthalmol.* 1944;27:1107–1117.
5. Dawson CR, Hanna L. A resume of experience in controlled trials with topical and systemic tetracycline and systemic sulfonamide. *Ophthalmol Dig.* 1971;33:30–36.
6. Dawson CR, Jones BR, Tarizzo ML. *Guide to Trachoma Control.* Geneva: World Health Organization; 1981:7–56.
7. Schachter J, Dawson CR. The epidemiology of trachoma predicts more blindness in the future. *Scand J Infect Dis.* 1990;69(Suppl):55–62.
8. Assaad FA, Sundaresan T, Maxwell-Lyons F. The household pattern of trachoma in Taiwan. *Bull WHO.* 1971;44: 605–615.
9. Dawson CR. Trachoma and other chlamydial eye diseases. In: Orfila J, Byrne GI, Chernesky MA, et al, eds. *Chlamydial Infections.* Bologna, Italy: Societa Editrice Esculapio; 1994;277–287.
10. Taylor HR, Rapoza PA, West S, et al. The epidemiology of infection in trachoma. *Invest Ophthalmol Vis Sci.* 1989;30: 1823–1833.
11. West S, Munoz B, Bobo L, et al. Non-ocular chlamydia infection and risk of ocular reinfection after mass treatment in a trachoma endemic area. *Invest Ophthalmol Vis Sci.* 1993;34:3194–3198.
12. Bobo L, Munoz B, Viscidi R, et al. Diagnosis of *Chlamydia trachomatis* eye infection in Tanzania by polymerase chain reaction/enzyme immunoassay. *Lancet.* 1991;338: 847–850.
13. Dean D, Palmer L, Pant CR, Courtright P, Falkow S. Use of a *Chlamydia trachomatis* DNA probe for detection of ocular chlamydiae. *J Clin Microbiol.* 1989;27:1062–1067.
14. Malaty R, Zaki S, Said ME, et al. Extraocular infections in children in areas with endemic trachoma. *J Inf Dis.* 1981; 143:853.
15. Kupka K, Nizetic B, Reinhards J. Sampling studies of epidemiology and control of trachoma in Southern Morocco. *Bull WHO.* 1968;39:547–561.
16. Brechner RJ, West S, Lynch M. Trachoma and flies. Individual and environmental risk factors. *Arch Ophthalmol.* 1992;110:687–689.
17. Jones BR. Prevention of blindness from trachoma. *Trans Ophthalmol Soc UK.* 1975;95:16–33.
18. Dawson CR, Whitcher JP, Lyon C, Schachter J. Response to treatment in ocular chlamydial infections (trachoma

and inclusion conjunctivitis): Analogies with nongonococcal urethritis. In: Hobson D, Holmes KK, eds. *Nongonococcal urethritis.* Washington, DC: American Society of Microbiology; 1977:135–139.

19. Dean D, Shama A, Schachter J, Dawson CR. Molecular identification of an avian strain of *Chlamydia psittaci* causing severe keratoconjunctivitis in a bird fancier. *Clin Infect Dis.* 1995;20:1179–1185.
20. Badir G, Wilson RP, Maxwell-Lyons F. The histopathology of trachoma. *Bull Egypt Ophthalmol Soc.* 1953;46:129.
21. Cosgrove PA, Patton DL, Kuo C-C, et al. Experimentally induced ocular chlamydial infection in infant pig-tailed macaques. *Invest Ophthalmol Vis Sci.* 1989;30:995–1003.
22. el-Assar AM, Van den Oord JJ, Geboes K, et al. Immunopathology of trachomatous conjunctivitis. *Br J Ophthalmol.* 1989;73:276–282.
23. Patton DL, Taylor HR. The histopathology of experimental trachoma: ultrastructural changes in the conjunctival epithelium. *J Infect Dis.* 1986;153:870–878.
24. Duke-Elder S. Diseases of the outer eye. Part 1. In: *System of Ophthalmology, Vol VIII.* London: Henry Kingston; 1965;578–596.
25. Dawson CR, Juster R, Marx R, et al. Limbal disease in trachoma and other ocular chlamydial infections: risk factor for corneal vascularization. *Eye.* 1989;3:204–209.
26. Grayston JT, Wang SP, Yeh LJ, Kuo CC. Importance of reinfection in the pathogenesis of trachoma. *Rev Infec Dis.* 1985;7:717–725.
27. Grayston JT, Woolridge RL, Wang SP. Trachoma vaccine studies on Taiwan. *Ann NY Acad Sci.* 1962;98:352–366.
28. Wang S-P, Grayston JT, Alexander ER. Trachoma vaccine studies in monkeys. *Am J Ophthalmol.* 1967;63:1615–1630.
29. Monnickendam MA, Darougar S, Treharne JD, Tilbury AM. Development of chronic conjunctivitis with scarring and pannus, resembling trachoma in guinea pigs. *Br J Ophthalmol.* 1980;64:284–290.
30. Taylor HR, Johnson SL, Prendergast RA, Schachter J, Dawson CR, Silverstein AM. An animal model of trachoma. II. The importance of reinfection. *Invest Ophthalmic Vis Sci.* 1982;23:506–515.
31. Ward M, Bailey R, Lesley A, Kajbaf M, Robertson J, Mabey D. Persisting inapparent chlamydial infection in a trachoma endemic community in The Gambia. *Scand J Infect Dis.* 1990;69(Suppl):137–148.
32. Mabey DCW, Bailey RL, Ward ME, Whittle HC. A longitudinal study of trachoma in a Gambian village: implications concerning the pathogenesis of chlamydial infection. *Epidemiol Infect.* 1992;108:343–351.
33. Dean D. Molecular characterization of new *Chlamydia trachomatis* serological variants from a trachoma endemic region of Africa. In: Orfila J, Byrne GI, Chernesky M, et al, eds. *Chlamydial Infections.* Bologna: Societa Editrice Esculapio; 1994:259–262.
34. Hayes LJ, Pecharatana S, Bailey RL, et al. Extent and kinetics of genetic change in the omp1 gene of *Chlamydia trachomatis* in two villages with endemic trachoma. *J Infect Dis.* 1995;172:268–272.
35. Morrison RP, Lyung K, Caldwell HD. Chlamydial disease pathogens: ocular delayed hypersensitivity elicited by a genus specific 57 kD protein. *J Exp Med.* 1989;169: 663–675.
36. Bierly J, Dawson CR, Jones M, Stephens RS. Serological evaluation for 60,000 molecular weight heat shock protein (HSP 60) in patients with trachoma. *Invest Ophthalmol Vis Sci.* 1992;33:848.
37. Beatty WL, Byrne GI, Morrison RP. Morphologic and antigenic characterization of interferon gamma mediated persistent *Chlamydia trachomatis* in vitro. *Proc Natl Acad Sci USA.* 1993;90:3998–4002.
38. Taylor HR, Maclean IW, Brunham RC, Pal S, Whittum-Hudson J. *Chlamydial* heat shock proteins and trachoma. *Infect Immun.* 1990;58:3061–3063.
39. Zhong G, Brunham RC. Antibody responses to the chlamydial heat shock proteins HSP 60 and HSP 70 are H-2 linked. *Infect Immun.* 1990;6:3143–3149.
40. Reacher MH, Pier J, Rapoza PA, et al. T cells and trachoma. Their role in cicatricial disease. *Ophthalmology.* 1991;98:334–341.
41. Holland MJ, Bailey RL, Hayes LJ, Whittle HC, Mabey DCW. Conjunctival scarring in trachoma is associated with depressed cell-mediated immune responses to chlamydial antigens. *J Infect Dis.* 1993;168:1528–1531.
42. Yoneda C, et al. Cytology as a guide to the presence of chlamydial inclusions in Giemsa-stained conjunctival smears. *Brit J Ophthalmol.* 1975;59:116–124.
43. Thylefors B, Dawson CR, Jones BR, Taylor HR, West SK. A simple system for the assessment of trachoma and its complications. *Bull WHO.* 1987;65:477–483.
44. Dean D, Pant CR, O'Hanley P. Improved sensitivity of a modified polymerase chain reaction amplified DNA probe in comparison with serial tissue culture passage for detection of *Chlamydia trachomatis* in conjunctival specimens from Nepal. *Diag Microbiol Infect Dis.* 1989;12:133–137.

CHAPTER 52

Cholera

John G. Banwell, James K. Kelly, David A. Owen, and M. Mathan

Diseases crucify the soul of man, attenuate our bodies, dry them, wither them, shrivel them up like old apples, . . .

Robert Burton (1577–1640)

We can pray over the cholera victim, or we can give her 500 milligrams of tetracycline every 12 hours. (There is still a religion, Christian Science, that denies the germ theory of disease; if prayer fails, the faithful would rather see their children die than give them antibiotics.)

Carl Sagan (b. 1934)

DEFINITION

Cholera is caused by cholera toxin-producing strains of the O group of *Vibrio cholerae* bacteria. The disease has been of major significance worldwide for many centuries and has attracted attention through its ability to bring about epidemics of diarrhea severe enough to result in dehydration and circulatory collapse in adults and children with severe mortality if left untreated. Until the 1980s, mortality from the disease was often 70% to 80%; since then, effective rehydration therapy has reduced mortality to less than 1%. Cholera has been endemic in West Bengal and Bangladesh since recorded time and many pandemics originated there. The El Tor biotype emerged in Indonesia in 1961 and has caused several outbreaks and epidemics, most recently in South America.[1] In 1992 a relative of the El Tor strain, *V cholerae* O139, appeared as the first non-O1 serotype to cause epidemic diarrhea in India and Bangladesh. Vibrios are rod-shaped, curved, gram-negative bacteria that exhibit vibrating motility in fresh, wet stools. *Vibrio cholerae* O1 is most rapidly identified by darkfield examination of stool and is confirmed by nullifying vibrio motility with cholera-specific antiserum.[2] Vibrios give a positive oxidase reaction and grow on salt-containing selective media such as thiosulfate citrate bile salts sucrose agar. Toxigenic and nontoxigenic strains are identified by a cholera toxin DNA probe.[3]

EPIDEMIOLOGY

Vibrio cholerae, like other vibrios, inhabits marine or estuarine niches where they colonize chitinaceous and nonchitinaceous organisms, including copepods and other plankton. Dormant, viable *V cholerae* can persist in noncultivable but infectious forms in aquatic environments and is apparently protected from gastric acid by association with chitin.[4] Cholera is transmitted by the fecal–oral route and through contaminated water, infected shellfish, or person-to-person contact. An inoculum of $>10^8$ organisms is required to cause diarrhea in volunteers, although hypochlorhydria allows infection with a dose as low as 1000 organisms,[4] and tropical hypochlorhydria, a condition that is poorly understood, may be a predisposing factor to infection. People with blood group O are at greater risk than those with other blood groups.[5] In endemic areas, cholera is a disease of children. In nonendemic areas, people of all ages are at risk.

PATHOGENESIS

In volunteer studies, a clinical syndrome identical to cholera can be produced by ingestion of cholera toxin or infectious organisms.[3] Once it has entered the gastrointestinal tract and successfully passed the acid peptic gastric barrier, the organism adheres to and multiplies on the mucosa of the small intestine (Figure 52–1). At this site it elaborates a protein enterotoxin—cholera toxin. The toxin is composed of A and B subunits. The B subunit binds the toxin to GM_1 ganglioside receptors on the brush border membrane of the mucosal cells. Subsequently, a subcomponent of the A fragment, A_1, crosses the intestinal cell membrane, where it mediates chloride secretion and inhibition of sodium chloride absorption through stimulation of cyclic adenosine monophosphate (cAMP). The severe iso-osmotic diarrhea of cholera is mainly a consequence of cholera toxin, which indirectly provokes chloride secretion by the small bowel crypt cells. Toxin coregulating pili are produced coordinately with toxin, and these pili are colonization factors.[6] Cholera toxin (CT) cannot be the sole cause of diarrhea since nontoxigenic strains of *V cholerae* O1 also induce diarrhea[4] that has been linked to a heat-labile enterotoxin that alters the configuration of tight junctions, called zonula occludens toxin (ZOT).[7] Recent experiments indicate that CT causes release of 5-hydroxytryptamine from enterochromaffin cells.[8] CT stimulates mucosal afferent neurons that synapse through the myenteric plexus and to a lesser extent through the submucosal plexus of the enteric nervous system.[9,10] These CT-induced neuronal impulses may stimulate crypt cells to secrete chloride and evoke intestinal secretion.

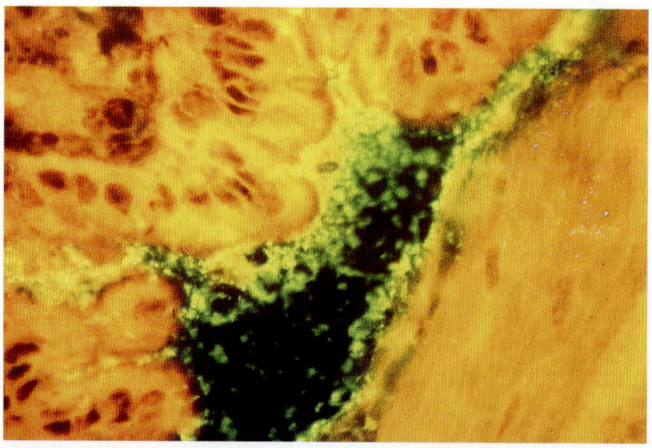

Figure 52–1. The vibrios are light green and form a layer on the surface of the small intestine. At no time during the course of infection is the wall of the intestine invaded (fluorescein-labeled antiserum, ×1040).

CLINICAL FEATURES

Most patients develop acute, mild to moderate watery diarrhea, but those with severe infections have extreme diarrhea, with outputs of stool that can exceed 1 L/hour in adults. The stools resemble rice water due to their content of mucoprotein. Fever is usually absent. There may be vomiting at the onset of the diarrhea. Dehydration and hypovolemia may develop within hours. The dehydration causes weakness, hypotension, tachycardia, and decreased skin turgor. Treatment consists of replacing lost fluid and electrolytes by the oral route if the patients are conscious, otherwise intravenous methods must be used. Several antibiotics that are active against *V cholerae* O1[1] decrease the duration and severity of diarrhea.

PATHOLOGY

Small bowel biopsy specimens of human cholera reveal no abnormality of mucosa on routine light microscopy.[11,12] Endoscopic biopsy samples obtained from those with early cholera diarrhea, however, have revealed ultrastructural changes.[13] Widening of intercellular spaces and alteration of apical junctional complexes were evident in villi of the epithelial cells. In crypt epithelium, blebbing of the microvillous border and mitochondrial changes was prominent (Figures 52–2, A and B, and 52–3, A and B). Degranulation of argentaffin cells, mucosal mast cells, and eosinophils was observed. Others have reported similar findings.[14]

At autopsy, victims of cholera are dehydrated with wrinkled skin, sunken eyes, and sunken cheeks. The lungs are red but dry. Patients treated by intravenous fluid may have congestion and edema of lungs.[15] In patients dying early in the course of the disease, the small bowel may be full of fluid that has a reddish tinge and contains floating mucus. Intussusception may occur in dehydrated patients. The serosa is excessively sticky. The intestinal fluid may also be gray, almost odorless, and contain floating membranes of autolysed bowel mucosa. The detached epithelium was originally believed to be an intravital occurrence, but endoscopic small bowel biopsy studies have failed to reveal any significant abnormality of the mucosa or significant differences from those of patients with other nonspecific

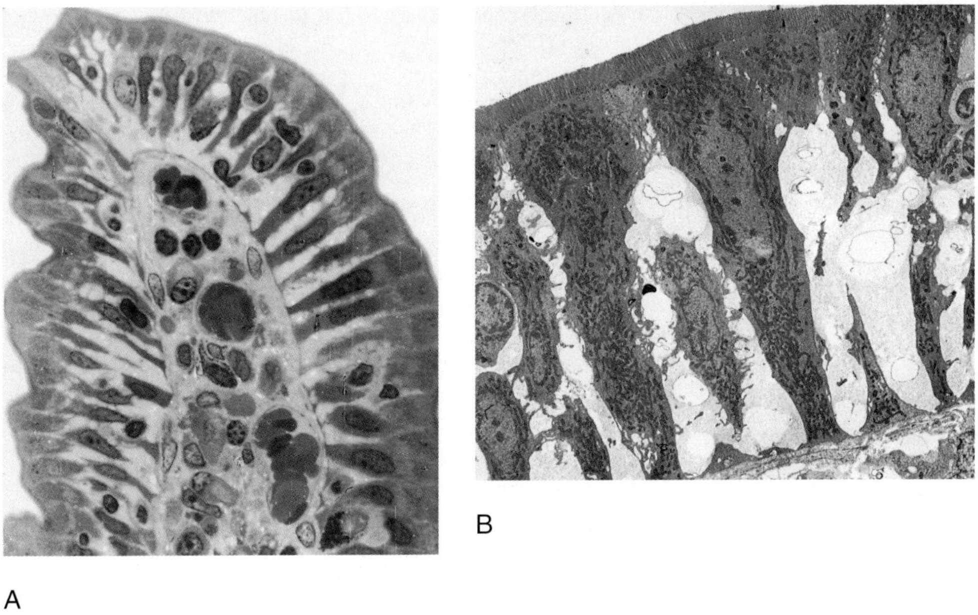

Figure 52–2. Patient with cholera. (**A**) The upper third of the villi have wide intercellular spaces more prominent toward the base of the cells. The blood vessels in the lamina propria are congested (×850). *(From Mathan,[13] with permission.)* (**B**) Electron micrograph of normal enterocytes from the upper third of the villi with widened intercellular spaces (×2600). *(From Mathan,[13] with permission.)*

diarrheal diseases or of normal people.[12] In those dying rapidly, the kidneys show no external abnormality, but in those dying after a protracted illness, the kidneys are enlarged and hyperemic with small hemorrhages and sometimes wedge-shaped infarcts. In patients with postcholeric uremia there may be tubular necrosis and fatty change or cortical ischemia.[13] The large intestine typically is empty. Mesenteric lymph nodes usually are moderately enlarged. The liver may be reduced in size and show fatty change.[15]

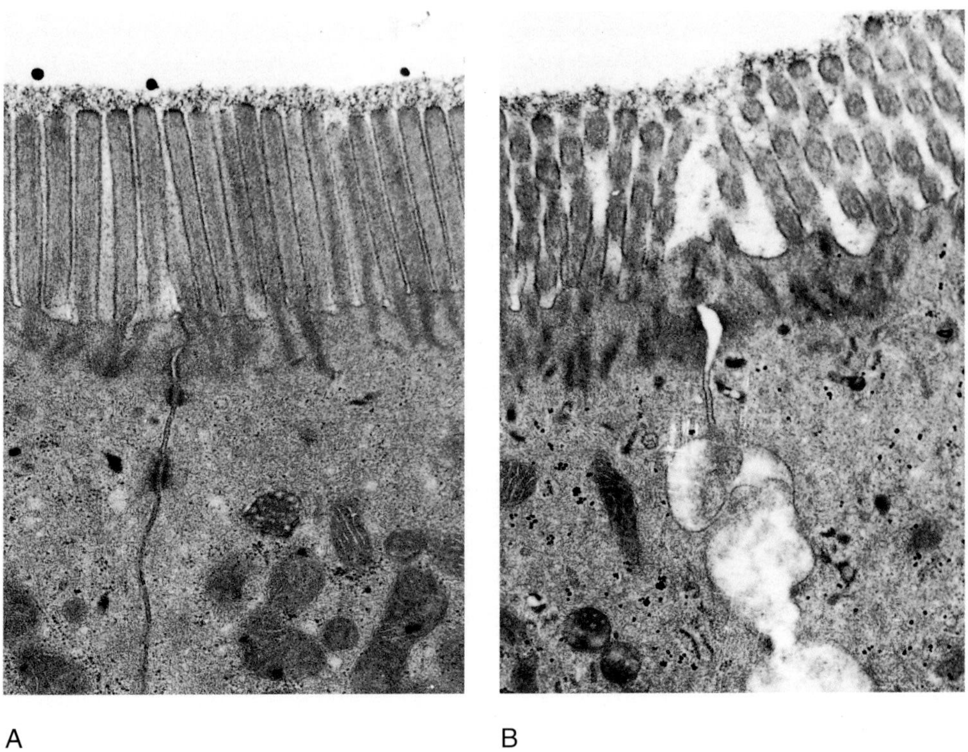

Figure 52–3. (**A**) Normal apical junctional complex of enterocytes of the upper third of villi from a control subject (×25,000). *(From Pollitzer,[15] with permission.)* (**B**) In a patient with cholera, the zonula occludens appears rounded and the zonula adherens is widened with condensation of actin filaments. The intercellular space is widened (×25,000). *(From Mathan,[13] with permission.)*

REFERENCES

1. Glass RI, Libel M, Brandling-Bennett AD. Epidemic cholera in the Americas. *Science.* 1992;256:1524–1525.
2. Benenson AS, Islam MG, Greenough WB III. Rapid identification of *Vibrio cholerae* by darkfield microscopy. *Bull WHO.* 1964;30:827.
3. Nalin DR. Cholera and severe toxigenic diarrheas. *Gut.* 1994;35:145–149.
4. Levine MM, Kaper GB, Black RE, Clements ML. New knowledge on pathogenesis of bacterial enteric infections as applied to vaccine development. *Microbiol Rev.* 1983;47:510–550.
5. Glass RI, Holmgren J, Haley CE, et al. Predisposition for cholera of individuals with O blood group: possible evolutionary significance. *Am J Epidemiol.* 1985;121:791–796.
6. Taylor RK, Miller VL, Furlong DB, Mekalanos JJ. Use of PhoA gene fusions to identify a plus colonization factor coordinately regulated with cholera toxin. *PNAS.* 1987;84: 2833–2837.
7. Fasano A, Baudry B, Pumplin DW, et al. *Vibrio cholerae* produces a second enterotoxin which affects intestinal tight junctions. *PNAS.* 1991;88:5242–5246.
8. Cassuto J, Jodal M, Lundgren O. The effect of nicotinic and muscarinic receptor blockade in cholera toxin–induced intestinal secretion in rats and cats. *Acta Physiol Scand.* 1982;114:573–577.
9. Jodal M, Holmgren S, Lundgren O, Sjoquist A. Involvement of the myenteric plexus in the cholera toxin–induced net fluid secretion in the rat small intestine. *Gastroenterology.* 1993;105:1286–1293.
10. Nilson O, Cassuto J, Larsson PA, et al. 5-Hydroxytryptamine and cholera secretion: a histochemical and physiologic study. *Gut.* 1983;24:542–548.
11. Sprinz H, Sribhibhadh R, Gangarosa EJ, Benyajati C, Kundel D, Halstead S. Biopsy of small bowel of Thai people. *Am J Clin Pathol.* 1962;36:43–51.
12. Gangarosa EJ, Beisel WR, Benyajati C, Sprinz H, Piyaratn P. The nature of the gastrointestinal lesion in Asiatic cholera and its relation to pathogenesis: a biopsy study. *Am J Trop Med Hyg.* 1960;9:125–135.
13. Mathan M, Chandy G, Mathan VI. Ultrastructural changes in the upper small intestinal mucosa in patients with cholera. *Gastroenterology.* 1995;109:422–430.
14. Asakura H, Tsuchiya M, Watanabe Y, et al. Electron microscopic study of the jejunal mucosa in human cholera. *Gut.* 1974;15:531–544.
15. Pollitzer. Cholera. World Health Organization, Monograph 43. Geneva. 1959:461–487.

CHAPTER 53

Citrobacter Infections

David A. Schwartz

. . . At first the infant,
Mewling and puking in the nurse's arms.

. . . Last scene of all,
That ends this strange eventful history,
Is second childishness and mere oblivion,
Sans teeth, sans eyes, sans taste, sans everything.

William Shakespeare (1564–1616), As You Like It, III, I

INTRODUCTION

Citrobacter is a genus comprised of enteric gram-negative rod-shaped bacilli belonging to the family Enterobacteriaceae, tribe Citrobactereae. All members of the family Enterobacteriaceae are widely distributed in soil and on plants, and also colonize the gastrointestinal tract of humans and animals. *Citrobacter* sp have been associated with a variety of human diseases, including urinary tract infections, osteomyelitis, diarrhea, neonatal sepsis and meningitis, and invasive infections in those with immunodeficiencies. Now *Citrobacter* are recognized with increasing frequency to cause human disease.[1]

CLASSIFICATION

Although the genus *Citrobacter* was originally placed in the tribe Salmonelleae on the basis of biochemical similarities, the genus is currently placed in the tribe Citrobactereae.[2] There are three species of *Citrobacter: C diversus, C freundii,* and *C amalonaticus.* Previous designations of *Citrobacter* isolates include *Levinea amalonatica* (*C amalonaticus*), *C koseri* (*C diversus*), and *Colobactrum freundii* and *Escherichia freundii* (*C freundii*). The *Citrobacter* sp share many structural and antigenic features with other members of the family Enterobacteriaceae, including a complex cell wall composed of murein, lipoprotein, phospholipid, protein, and lipopolysaccharide arranged in layers.

HISTORY

Werkman and Gillen suggested the term *Citrobacter* in 1931 for "citrate-positive coliaerogenes intermediates," which were isolated from stool.[3] *Citrobacter* was first implicated as a cause of gastroenteritis in an outbreak of mild disease in 1946.[4] Human disease caused by *Citrobacter* was first established in 1960 when two patients had meningitis caused by *C freundii.*[5] From 1970 to 1979, *Citrobacter* was recognized as a significant cause of central nervous system infection when 69 patients with *Citrobacter* meningitis were reported in one study,[6] and 4% of cases of neonatal meningitis in the First Neonatal Meningitis Cooperative Study Group were found to be caused by *Citrobacter* sp.[7]

EPIDEMIOLOGY

The epidemiologic risk factors for infection by *Citrobacter* sp differ between two major groups of patients who develop disease—neonates and debilitated or immunodeficient adults. *Citrobacter diversus* is the most frequently isolated species from neonatal *Citrobacter* meningitis. Most *Citrobacter* meningitis in the United

States is reported from the southern states; biotype d or serotype O2 and O1 are the most common strains of *C diversus* identified.[6] Most neonatal meningitis caused by *Citrobacter* is sporadic, but clusters of patients with *Citrobacter* meningitis have been reported. When *Citrobacter* is introduced into the nursery, it colonizes up to 79% of infants.[8] In one neonate who developed sepsis and meningitis, the infant's mother was the source of infection.[9] In a nursery outbreak of *C diversus*, bacteria were isolated more frequently from the umbilicus than from the infants' stools, suggesting that the infection was spread from umbilicus to umbilicus by contaminated hands of the nursing staff.[10] *Citrobacter* is an unusual pathogen in children after the first several months of life.

Citrobacter sp cause a wide spectrum of disease in immunodeficient or debilitated adult patients. Most isolates of *Citrobacter* from this age group are from patients with secondary infection or colonization, and are of no clinical significance. In these patients, the urinary tract is the most common source of isolation of *Citrobacter* sp: 5% to 12% of bacterial isolates from urinary tract infections are *Citrobacter* sp. Sputum is the second most common clinical source of *Citrobacter* sp.[11]

CLINICAL FEATURES

Citrobacter is an important cause of neonatal meningitis, with fever, lethargy, poor feeding, irritability, vomiting, seizures, jaundice, and a bulging fontanelle being the most common presenting signs. Eighty-five percent of neonatal infections have a mean age of onset of 7 days, while the remainder are after 3 weeks of age.[6] Infection and surgical manipulation of colonized umbilical cord stumps have preceded *Citrobacter* bacteremia and meningitis.[10] A complication of *Citrobacter* meningitis is brain abscess—three quarters being intracerebral abscesses (Figure 53–1).[6] Concurrent with an episode of meningitis, 35% of patients also have *Citrobacter* isolated from blood.[6]

In adult patients, *Citrobacter* has caused nosocomial infections, especially involving the urinary and respiratory tracts of debilitated patients.[1,12] *Citrobacter diversus* has been isolated from a perinephric abscess in a diabetic with a transplanted kidney.[13] *Citrobacter* is also associated with nosocomial bacteremias and endocarditis,[14] the former often polymicrobial with a high mortality rate. Although *Citrobacter* occasionally has been incriminated as a cause of gastrointestinal disease, the frequent isolation of this organism from stool of asymptomatic patients makes it difficult to assess a causal relationship. *Citrobacter freundii* has been described as a cause of peritonitis in debilitated adults with liver disease or pancreatitis. The organism has also been associated with acute appendicitis in an otherwise healthy adult.[15] Infections of bone and soft tissues by *Citrobacter* can also occur. In one study of adult patients, 3% of *Citrobacter* pathogens were isolated from joints or bone.[15] A 3-year-old child treated with

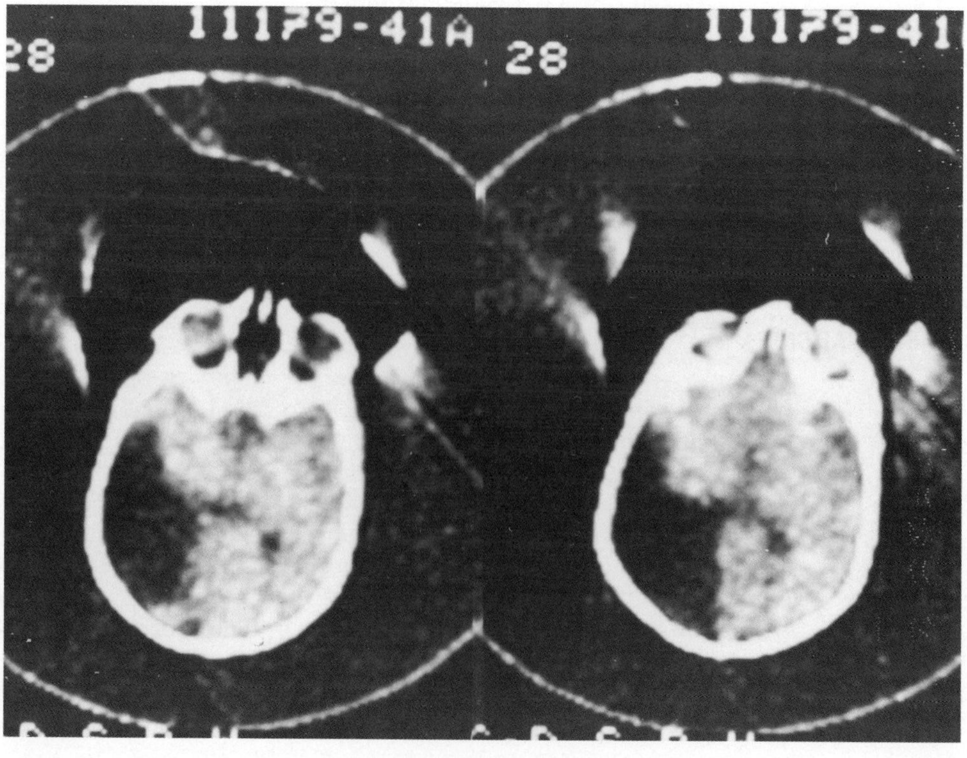

Figure 53–1. Computerized axial tomogram showing right intracerebral abscess. Microbiologic cultures from this abscess were positive for *C diversus*.

multiple antibiotics and corticosteroids developed *Citrobacter* osteomyelitis of multiple sites of the lower limbs.

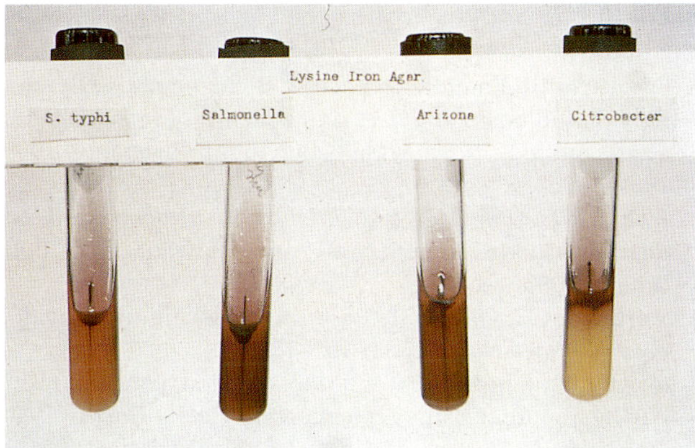

Figure 53–3. *Citrobacter freundii* reaction on lysine iron agar. The purple slant and yellow butt indicate fermentation of glucose.

PATHOLOGY

Infections by *Citrobacter*, including meningitis, brain abscess, endocarditis, urinary tract, and other sites, often have nonspecific acute or mixed acute and chronic inflammatory reactions. *Citrobacter* infections of the central nervous system may be meningitis, hemorrhagic encephalitis, and one or multiple cerebral abscesses (Figure 53–2). The spectrum of lesions in the respiratory tract includes lung abscess, pneumonia, and bronchitis. There are, however, no pathologic features that suggest *Citrobacter* infection. The gram-negative *Citrobacter* bacilli can be difficult to identify in Gram stained tissue sections and, in some specimens, there is a mixed polymicrobial flora. *Citrobacter* cannot be distinguished from other gram-negative bacilli by light or electron microscopy, and diagnosis depends on demonstrating the organism by culture.

DIAGNOSIS

The most important agents in the differential diagnosis of *Citrobacter* sp are other members of the Enterobacteriaceae, including *Escherichia, Enterobacter, Klebsiella, Salmonella,* and *Shigella*. *Citrobacter* infections are diagnosed by culture of tissues, swabs, stool, or body fluids. *Citrobacter* are motile bacilli, have a positive methyl-red reaction, a negative Voges–Proskauer test, grow on Simmons citrate medium, and most isolates slowly hydrolyze urea. Members of this genus have positive tests for β-galactosidase with O-nitrophenol-β-D-galactoside and form gas from glucose fermentation. Tests for inositol fermentation, DNase, lysine, and phenylalanine deamination are negative. The production of H_2S on triple sugar iron agar occurs only with *C freundii,* but unlike *Salmonella* sp, which also produces H_2S, *Citrobacter* usually grow in the presence of potassium cyanide (KCN). *Citrobacter freundii* is indole negative and H_2S positive, differentiating it from *C diversus*. *Citrobacter amalonaticus* differs from *C diversus* by the former's inability to ferment malonate (Figures 53–3 and 53–4).[1]

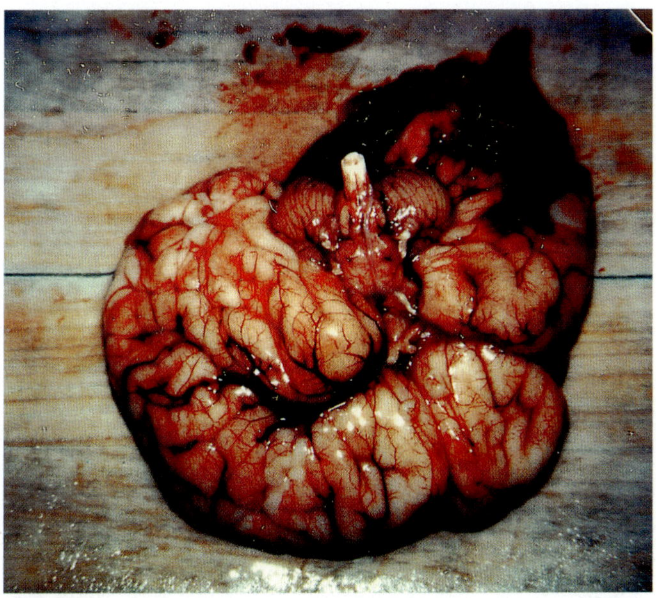

Figure 53–2. Basal view of a brain obtained from the autopsy of a 3-day-old infant with *C diversus* septicemia. Meningitis and hemorrhagic encephalitis were present. *(Photograph courtesy of Centers for Disease Control and Prevention, Atlanta, Georgia.)*

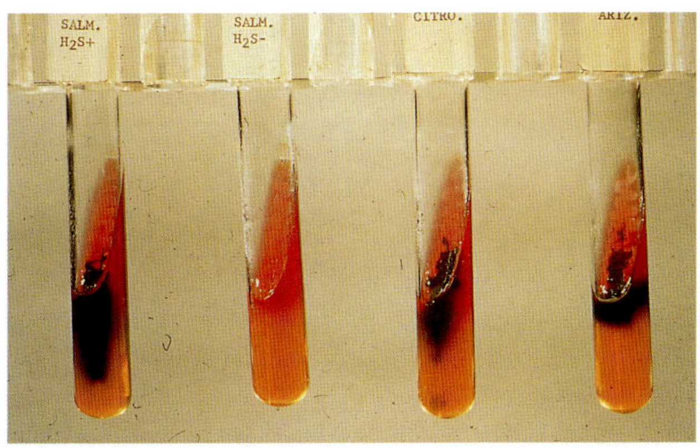

Figure 53–4. *Citrobacter* reaction on triple sugar iron (TSI) showing H_2S production.

REFERENCES

1. Eisenstein BI. Enterobacteriaceae. In: Mandell GL, Bennett JE, Dolin R, eds. *Principles and Practice of Infectious Diseases.* 4th ed. New York: Churchill Livingstone; 1995: 1964–1979.
2. Ewing WH. *Edwards and Ewing's Identification of Enterobacteriaceae.* 4th ed. New York: Elsevier Science Publishing; 1986.
3. Werkman CH, Gillen GF. Bacteria producing trimethylene glycol. *J Bacteriol.* 1932;23:167–182.
4. Barnes LA, Cherry CB. A group of paracolon organisms having apparent pathogenicity. *Am J Public Health.* 1946; 36:481–483.
5. Harris D, Cone TE Jr. *Escherichia freundii* meningitis: report of two cases. *J Pediatr.* 1960;56:774–777.
6. Graham DR, Band JD. *Citrobacter diversus* brain abscess and meningitis in neonates. *JAMA.* 1981;245:1923–1925.
7. McCracken GH Jr, Mize SG. A controlled study of intrathecal antibiotic therapy in gram-negative enteric meningitis of infancy. Report of the Neonatal Meningitis Cooperative Study Group. *J Pediatr.* 1976;89:66–72.
8. Graham DR, Anderson RL, Arier FE, et al. Epidemic nosocomial meningitis due to *Citrobacter diversus* in neonates. *J Infect Dis.* 1981;144:203–209.
9. Finn A, Talbot GH, Anday E, et al. Vertical transmission of *Citrobacter diversus* from mother to infant. *Pediatr Infect Dis J.* 1988;7:293–294.
10. Parry MF, Hutchinson JH, Brown NA, et al. Gram-negative sepsis in neonates: a nursery outbreak due to hand carriage of *Citrobacter diversus. Pediatrics.* 1980;65:1105–1109.
11. Madrazo A, Geiger J, Lauter CB. *Citrobacter diversus* at Grace Hospital, Detroit, Michigan. *Am J Med Sci.* 1975; 270:497–501.
12. Hodges GR, Degener CE, Barnes WG. Clinical significance of *Citrobacter* isolates. *Am J Clin Pathol.* 1978;70:37–40.
13. Williams RD, Simmons RL. *Citrobacter* perinephric abscess presenting as pneumoscrotum in transplant recipient. *Urology.* 1974;3:478–480.
14. MacCulloch D, Menzies R, Cornere BM. Endocarditis due to *Citrobacter diversus* developing resistance to cephalothin. *NZ Med J.* 1977;85:182.
15. Lipsky BA, Hook ER III, Smith A, et al. *Citrobacter* infections in humans: experience at the Seattle Veterans Administration Medical Center and a review of the literature. *Rev Infect Dis.* 1980;2:746–760.

CHAPTER 54

Clostridial Infections

David A. Schwartz and Stanley J. Geyer

The history of gas gangrene is the history of wars of the twentieth century.

A. T. Willis

Executive Mansion
Washington, Nov. 21, 1864
To Mrs. Bixby, Boston, Mass.
Dear Madam,
I have been shown in the files of the War Department a statement of the Adjudant General of Massachusetts that you are the mother of five sons who have died gloriously on the field of battle. I feel how weak and fruitless must be any word of mine which should attempt to beguile you from the grief of a loss so overwhelming. But I cannot refrain from tendering you the consolation that may be found in the thanks of the republic they died to save. I pray that our Heavenly Father may assuage the anguish of your bereavement and leave you only the cherished memory of the loved and lost, and the solemn pride that must be yours to have laid so costly a sacrifice upon the altar of freedom.

Yours very sincerely and respectfully,
A. Lincoln

INTRODUCTION TO THE GENUS *CLOSTRIDIUM*

The genus *Clostridium* includes almost 90 recognized species of anaerobic, spore-forming bacilli. Fewer than 20 species, however, are associated with human disease. The ultrastructural characteristics of clostridial cell walls indicate that they are gram-positive, but many strains appear gram-variable or even gram-negative. The loss of gram-positivity occurs most frequently in preparations of clinical material, in cultures following prolonged incubation, and in those species having terminal spores. The clostridia appear straight or slightly curved, vary in length and width, and have blunt, rounded, or slightly tapered ends. The bacilli may be single organisms, in pairs, or in chains (Figures 54–1 through 54–3). Some clostridia, such as *C novyi,* are motile by means of peritrichous flagella and produce swarming on the surface of blood agar plates (Figure 54–4).

Members of the genus *Clostridium* are ubiquitous in the environment, in decaying vegetation; soil; ocean sediment; and in the gastrointestinal tract of humans, other vertebrates, and insects. Many clostridial infections are endogenous, from clostridial species on the skin and mucous membranes of the host. Because clostridia are commonly isolated as a component of polymicrobial flora, it may be difficult to establish their role in pathogenesis. The most common and well-established clostridial diseases are a group of histotoxic syndromes caused by a variety of clostridial toxins. These

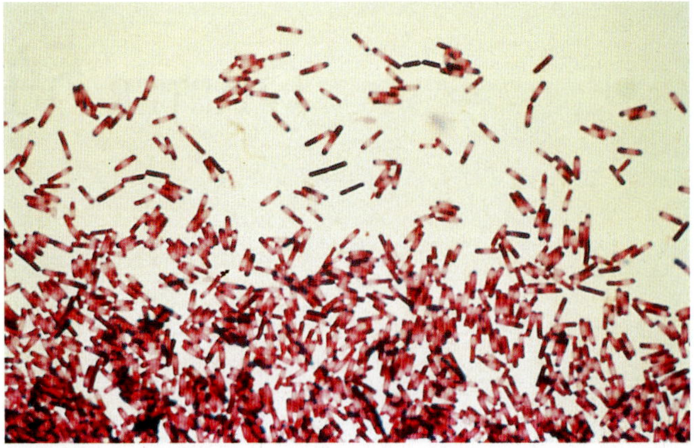

Figure 54–1. *Clostridium difficile.* Typical appearance of bacilli on impression smear following 72 hours of anaerobic growth on blood agar (Gram's stain, ×1000).

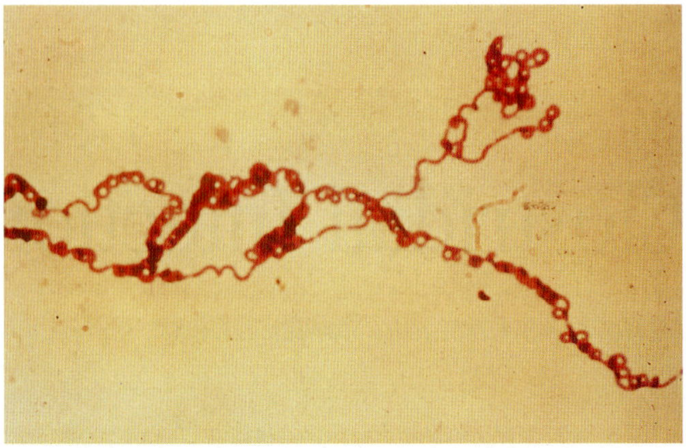

Figure 54–3. *Clostridium ramosum* from laboratory culture, showing the unusual shape of this bacillus. This species, along with *C perfringens,* does not readily sporulate (Gram's stain, ×1000).

syndromes include myonecrosis (gas gangrene), cellulitis, food poisoning, tetanus, botulism, antibiotic-associated colitis, neutropenic enterocolitis, and segmental enteritis necroticans ("pig-bel," see Chapter 77). A unique feature of some clostridial infections is the production of nitrogen or hydrogen gas at the infected site, causing gas gangrene, crepitant cellulitis, and emphysematous cystitis and cholecystitis.

The clostridia vary in their motility, nutritional requirements, temperatures for optimal growth, and tolerance of oxygen. Some species, including *C novyi* and *C haemolyticum,* are strict anaerobes and will not divide when oxygen concentration exceeds 0.05%. Other clostridia, such as *C histolyticum* and *C tertium,* are partially aerotolerant and may replicate, but not sporulate, under aerobic conditions.

Clostridial endospores are spherical or ovoid, and may be central, subterminal, or terminal within the bacillus (Figure 54–5). Most species readily sporulate at incubation temperatures below those necessary for optimal growth (usually 30°C). Some clostridial species, including *C perfringens* and *C ramosum,* do not readily form spores (Figure 54–3). Sporulation can be induced by heating starch-broth cultures to 70° to 80°C for 10 minutes or by ethanol shock following exposure to an equal volume of 95% ethanol for 45 minutes.

Clostridial toxins are biologically active proteins that demonstrate strong antigenicity and are neutralized by the specific antisera. Some of these toxins are lethal for animals. Among these toxins are α-toxin (lecithinase), β-toxin, enterotoxins, botulinal toxins A-G, and such virulence factors as neuraminidase (sialidase), non–α-δ-θ hemolysins, and the organism's metabolic activity. The production of lecithinase can be demonstrated by using agar plates containing egg yolk (Figure 54–6). When α-toxin is present, an opaque zone sur-

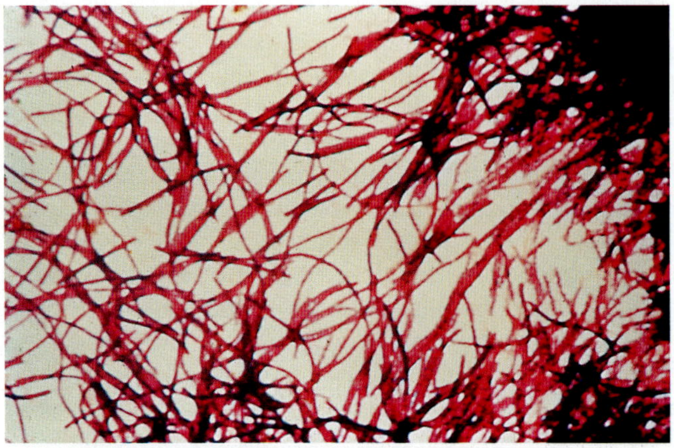

Figure 54–2. *Clostridium difficile* grown on cycloserine mannitol blood agar. This medium interrupts normal cell division, resulting in filamentation (Gram's stain, ×1000).

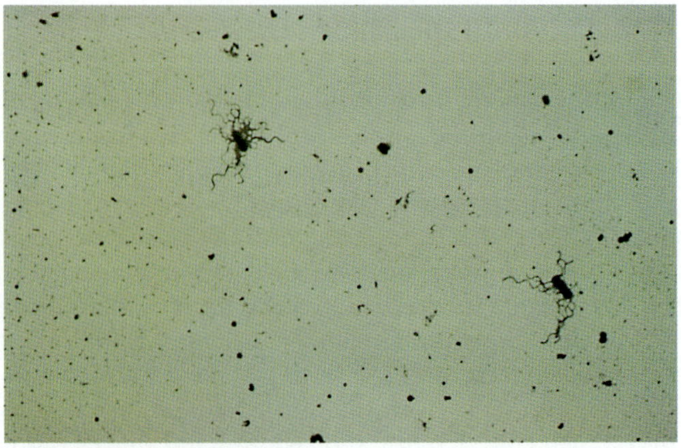

Figure 54–4. Peritrichous flagella are in this smear of *Clostridium novyi,* an important agent of clostridial myonecrosis (Leifson flagella stain, ×1000).

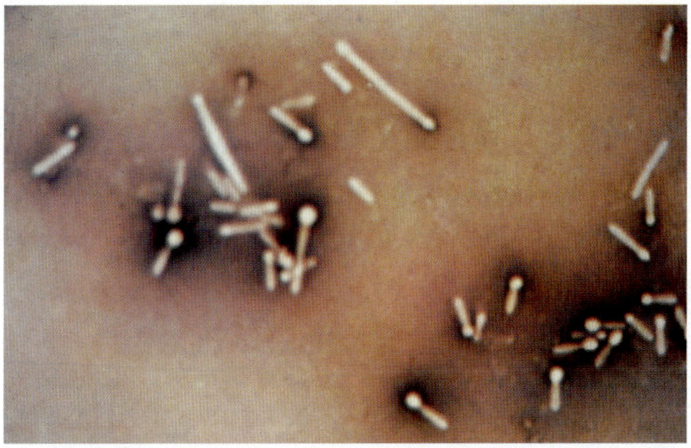

Figure 54–5. Large, spherical terminal spores of *C tetani* (Nigrosin stain, original magnification, ×2000).

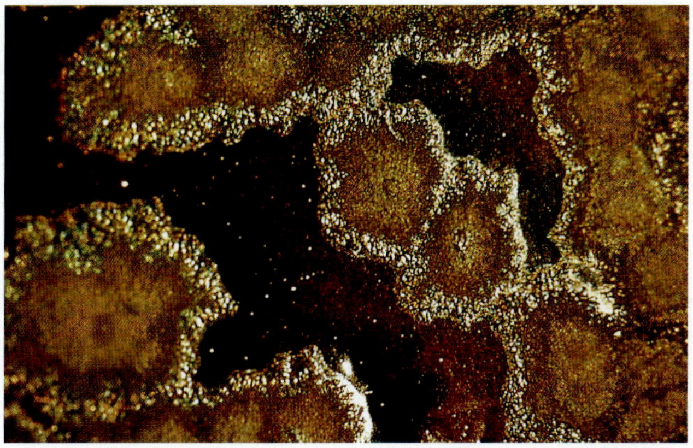

Figure 54–7. Lipase reaction of *C sporogenes* on a 48-hour egg yolk agar plate. *(Photograph courtesy of Centers for Disease Control and Prevention, Atlanta.)*

rounds the growing colonies. Egg yolk agar can also be used to test for lipase. Lipase-producing clostridia, such as *C sporogenes, C botulinum,* and *C novyi* type A, break down the fats in egg yolk to release free fatty acids, appearing as an oily, iridescent sheen (Figure 54–7). Additional features used to speciate clostridia include the ability to ferment carbohydrates, hydrolyze gelatin, and digest casein.[1–6]

Classification

Tetanus is caused by *Clostridium tetani,* an obligate anaerobic bacillus. *Clostridium tetani* is gram-positive in fresh cultures, but it may have variable staining in old cultures or in tissue.

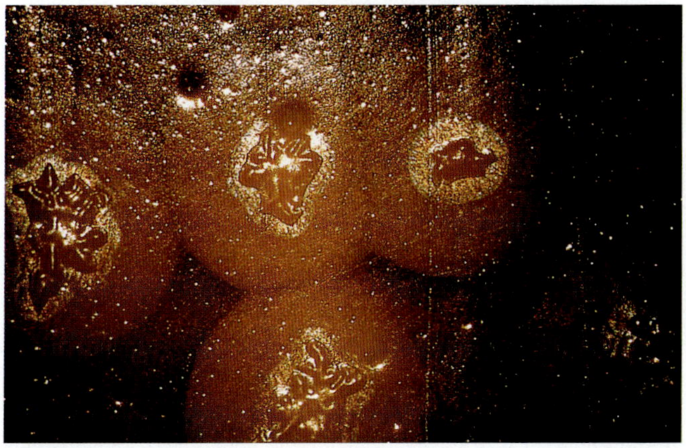

Figure 54–6. *Clostridium novyi* type A lipase and lecithinase reactions on a 48-hour egg yolk agar plate. *(Photograph courtesy of Centers for Disease Control and Prevention, Atlanta.)*

History

Tetanus has been known and described by Egyptian and Greek physicians, who described the association between injuries and lethal spasms, since ancient times. In 1884, Nicolaier isolated a toxin from the soil with "strychnine-like" properties. Recognition of the clinical and experimental associations between small local infection by this organism and the profound toxemia with neuromuscular manifestations led to the discovery of the tetanus toxin and, shortly thereafter, the specific anti-toxin. In 1890, Behring and Kitasato reported active immunization using tetanus toxoid.

Epidemiology

Although effective immunization has existed for tetanus for more than 100 years, the global incidence is approximately 1 million per year. The mortality rate in North America is only 0.1 per 100,000, but is as high as 28 per 100,000 in some developing countries. In the United States, about 70 infections are reported annually, which is probably an underestimate. In developed nations, most reported infections are in those over the age of 60, suggesting that decreasing levels of immunity are a significant risk factor. In developing countries, neonatal tetanus causes about one half of known infections, with as many as one-third of these infants born to mothers with a previously infected child.

Neonatal tetanus usually is caused by infection of the umbilical stump, most often from failure of aseptic technique and when mothers are not adequately immunized. In some regions, the application of mud or dirt to the umbilical stump to prevent bleeding contributes to the high incidence of neonatal tetanus.

In the United States, about 70% of all tetanus is caused by an acute injury, divided equally between lac-

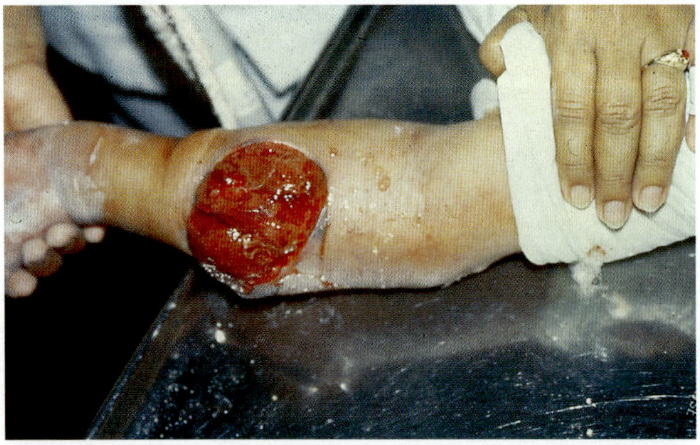

Figure 54–8. This contaminated wound on the arm provided entry of *C tetani* and caused generalized tetanus. *(Photograph courtesy of Anastacio de Queiroz Sousa, MD, Universidade Federal do Ceara, Fortaleza, Brazil, and Martin Cetron, MD, Centers for Disease Control and Prevention, Atlanta.)*

erations and punctures (Figure 54–8). Cryptogenic tetanus afflicts about 7% of patients.

Biology

The tetanus bacillus is long and thin compared to other clostridial species and ranges in size from 3 to 8 by 2 to 5 μm. *Clostridium tetani* is an obligate anaerobe and moderately fastidious in its requirement for anaerobiasis. It possesses numerous peritrichous flagella that are slowly motile during growth. Flagella are lost by mature bacilli, and the organisms develop a terminal spore and resemble a squash racket or drumstick (Figure 54–5). Spores do not take Gram's stain and appear as colorless round structures in the bacillus. The spores are stable in the environment and remain infectious indefinitely. An important factor for pathologists and laboratory workers is that spores can tolerate exposure to a variety of organic solvents and fixatives, including formalin, phenol, and ethanol, and still retain their ability to germinate.

There are two toxins produced by *C tetani*—tetanospasmin, commonly termed tetanus toxin, and tetanolysin. Tetanospasmin is encoded on a plasmid and is produced by all toxigenic strains. It is initially synthesized as a 151 kD chain that is cleaved extracellularly into a 100 kD heavy chain and a 50 kD light chain (fragment A). The heavy chain (composed of fragments B and C) mediates binding to cell surface receptors and transport proteins. The light chain causes presynaptic inhibition of release of neurotransmitter. Following entry of the tetanospasmin into the nervous system via the presynaptic terminals of lower motor neurons, it stops neuromuscular transmission. The toxin is then carried via the retrograde axonal transport system to the cell bodies of these neurons in the spinal cord and brain stem, causing the characteristic symptoms of tetanus. Tetanospasmin most likely acts by selective cleavage of synaptobrevin II, a protein component of synaptic vesicles. The functions of tetanolysin are unknown. Toxin binding is an irreversible event.[7]

Clinical Features

There are four distinct clinical types of tetanus—generalized, localized, cephalic, and neonatal. Following the implantation of spores of *C tetani* into an appropriate (aneorobic) site, there is an incubation period of 4 to 10 days.

Generalized tetanus is the most common form. Initial symptoms are usually trismus (termed "lockjaw" from the rigidity of the masseter muscle) and risus sardonicus (from increased tone of the orbicularis oris muscle) (Figures 54–9 and 54–10). The generalized spasm consists of opisthotonos, which resembles decorticate posturing, with painful flexion of arms and extension of the legs (Figure 54–11). The diaphragm can be involved in these spasms, and the upper airway can be obstructed, occasionally causing fatal asphyxiation. The spasms can be triggered by sensory stimulation such as loud noises, and the patient remains con-

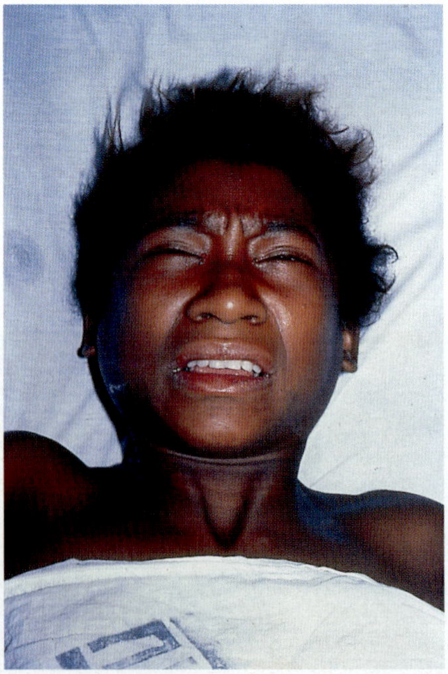

Figure 54–9. Tetanus with typical facies of trismus, which is difficulty in opening the mouth from painful masseter muscles. *(Photograph courtesy of Anastacio de Queiroz Sousa, MD, Universidade Federal do Ceara, Fortaleza, Brazil, and Martin Cetron, MD, Centers for Disease Control and Prevention, Atlanta.)*

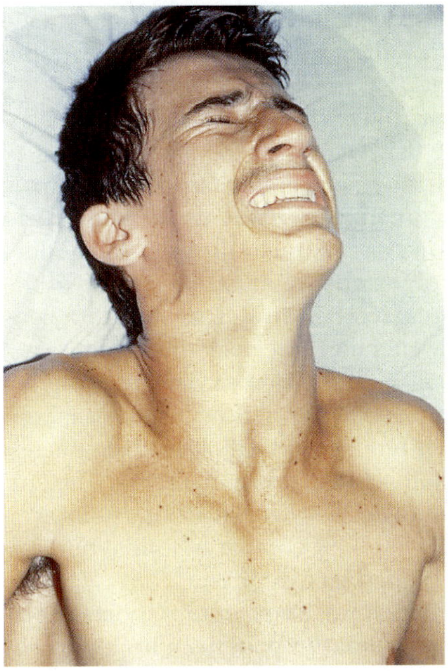

Figure 54–10. Painful spasm of generalized tetanus with risus sardonicus. *(Photograph courtesy of Anastacio de Queiroz Sousa, MD, Universidade Federal do Ceara, Fortaleza, Brazil, and Martin Cetron, MD, Centers for Disease Control and Prevention, Atlanta.)*

scious during the spastic episodes. Generalized tetanus progresses for approximately 2 weeks and is a function of the time necessary for transport of toxin. Dysfunction of lower motor neurons may not be diagnosed until the muscular spasms decrease in severity.

Localized tetanus follows traumatic inoculation of *C tetani* spores, causing rigidity of muscles at the site of inoculation. Localized tetanus is often mild and persistent, but usually resolves spontaneously. There is often damage to the lower motor neuron, which causes weakness and decreased tone in the involved muscle. Although localized tetanus may develop in patients with partial immunity to tetanus, it can be also a prodrome to generalized disease if sufficient toxin reaches the central nervous system.

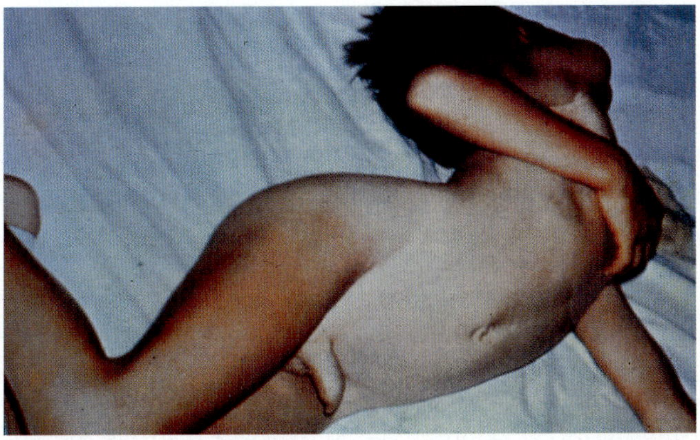

Figure 54–11. Opisthotonic posturing caused by involvement of spinal musculature in a child with generalized tetanus. *(Photograph courtesy of Anastacio de Queiroz Sousa, MD, Universidade Federal do Ceara, Fortaleza, Brazil, and Martin Cetron, MD, Centers for Disease Control and Prevention, Atlanta.)*

The initial symptoms of neonatal tetanus (tetanus neonatorum) are often generalized weakness and failure to nurse. Muscular rigidity and spasms develop later, often causing delays in the development of surviving infants. The mortality rate of neonatal tetanus is more than 90%.

Cephalic tetanus is a specialized type of localized tetanus that involves muscles supplied by the cranial nerves. Although some patients with cephalic tetanus die, in others the disease is mild. There is often a lower motor neuron lesion, which causes weakness of the facial nerve, and there may be also involvement of the extraocular muscles.[1,3]

Pathology

There are no characteristic microscopic features of *C tetani* infection in infected wounds, fractures, or umbilical stumps. Because contaminated wounds usually have polymicrobial growth, performing gram-stained smears or biopsies of these lesions is not helpful (see next sections).

Diagnosis

The diagnosis of tetanus is made by clinical history and symptoms. Laboratory testing does not help diagnose tetanus, except to exclude some intoxications (especially strychnine poisoning), which may mimic tetanus. Culturing *C tetani* from wounds of those suspected of having tetanus is not useful because *C tetani* may grow from the wound of an immunized patient even when the patient does not have tetanus. Nor does a culture of *C tetani* indicate whether the isolate contains the toxigen-producing plasmid. Biopsy does not play a role in the diagnosis of tetanus.

Treatment

Virtually all tetanus is preventable with a regimen of vaccinations and properly managing wounds. Treating tetanus requires maintaining respiratory function throughout the course. Benzodiazepines are the mainstay of medical therapy for the syndrome of tetanus. Passive immunization with human tetanus immunoglobulin (HTIG) lessens the severity and shortens the course of tetanus. The advantages of antimicrobial therapy are controversial.[1]

GAS GANGRENE (CLOSTRIDIAL MYONECROSIS)

Classification

Gas gangrene is a fulminant and potentially life-threatening infection caused by *Clostridium perfringens* and some other clostridial species. Gas gangrene is characterized by severe tissue damage associated with gas and fluid-filled bullae in necrotic tissues, particularly in skeletal muscle and overlying soft tissues, caused by potent bacterial exotoxins.

Because involvement of skeletal muscle is nearly universal in gas gangrene, synonyms include clostridial myonecrosis and clostridial myositis. The latter term is misleading because inflammation in the gangrenous muscle is usually absent or scant. *Clostridum perfringens* has been previously called *Bacillus aerogenes capsulatus, Bacillus perfringens,* and *Clostridium welchii.*

History

Clostridium perfringens was first characterized by Welch and Nuttall in 1892 from the blood vessels of autopsied patients. *Clostridium perfringens* was associated with gas gangrene and other clinical syndromes by Welch and Flexner in 1896. During World War I, the prevalence of gas gangrene, as a complication of combat wounds, was 5%. The prevalence decreased during successive conflicts—0.3% to 0.7% in World War II, 0.2% during the Korean War, and 0.0002% during the Vietnam War. These decreases were from better medical care, including prompt management of traumatic wounds and rapid transport of patients to surgical treatment facilities.

Epidemiology

Clostridium perfringens has been isolated from the soil of almost every region of the world except the Sahara desert. In addition, *C perfringens* has been identified in the feces of virtually every vertebrate, including domestic and wild herd animals, marine mammals, rodents, birds, carnivores, and pets. It is widespread in the human population, with one study showing that *C perfringens* was present in the feces of 28 out of 40 adults examined.[8] *Clostridium perfringens* is the major cause of gas gangrene, causing about 80% of infections.[9–11] *Clostridum septicum* is the second most frequent agent, with other clostridial agents including *C novyi, C histolyticum, C sordelli, C bifermentans,* and *C fallax.*[9] *Clostridium perfringens* and *Clostridium septicum* are the most common organisms to cause nontraumatic gas gangrene.[11,12] Some infections have more than one clostridial species isolated from the infected site. The species of *Clostridium* implicated in gas gangrene collectively produce at least 12 exotoxins, including 7 that are lethal to mice when inoculated in the peritoneum.

Penetrating wounds, contaminated with soil or feces containing clostridial organisms, are the most important risk factors in the pathogenesis of gas gangrene. Most gas gangrene occurs in patients with severely contaminated soft tissue and muscle injuries, usually combat wounds and farm incidents. The combination of extensive muscle damage with an inadequate circulation and gross contamination favors clostridial infection because the organisms are anaerobes and require the low oxygen tension of injured tissues with reduced blood flow. Cultures taken from traumatic open wounds reveal clostridial species in 20% to 80%. In spite of this, gas gangrene is rare. In one study from World War II, clostridial organisms were cultured from 20% to 30% of combat wounds, but only 0.32% of them developed gas gangrene.[13]

Gas gangrene also occurs spontaneously (in the absence of trauma) in patients who have reduced resistance to infections and an insult to the small or large intestine, permitting the entrance of clostridial organisms into the wall of the bowel and subsequently into the blood, producing clostridial sepsis. *Clostridium septicum* is the most common cause of spontaneous gas gangrene in patients with underlying carcinoma of the bowel, hematological malignancy, diabetes mellitus, and cyclic neutropenia.[11,14–16] Occasionally, gas gangrene complicates burns, amputations, biliary tract surgery, or vascular insufficiency of the lower limbs associated with diabetes and decubitus ulcers. Uterine gas gangrene (Figure 54–12) can follow septic abortion.

Biology

Clostridium perfringens is a short, wide rod with squarish ends and strong gram-positive staining. The bacilli are uniform and range from 2 to 4 by 1 to 1.5 μm. *Clostridium perfringens* is nonmotile, relatively aerotolerant, and does not form spores in routine cultures or in infected tissues. Spores, however, can develop in the organism's natural habitat or with the special culture media. Capsules may appear in smears from wound exudates, but are not uniformly demonstrable in culture.

Clostridium perfringens produces a number of antigenic, biologically active toxins, the most important of which is α-toxin (phospholipase C), a 43 kD lecithinase that splits lecithin into phosphoryl choline, diglyceride, and a thiol-activated hemolysin (θ-toxin or perfringolysin O) (Figure 54–13). α-toxin disrupts the cell membranes of erythrocytes, white blood cells, and muscle cells. Among the 12 toxins produced by *C perfringens,* there are 4 major lethal toxins that are used to classify the species into five serologic types—A to E.

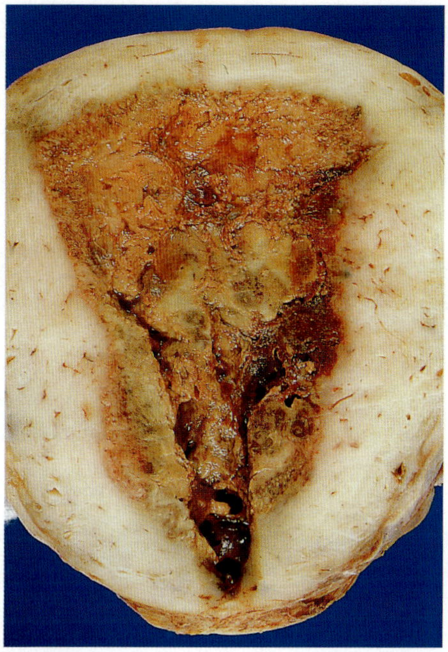

Figure 54–12. Clostridial infection of the uterus, with necrosis and hemorrhage. Shown are the placental implantation site and adjacent endometrium and myometrium. The patient was 16 years old. Mixed anaerobic organisms, including *C perfringens,* were grown in culture.

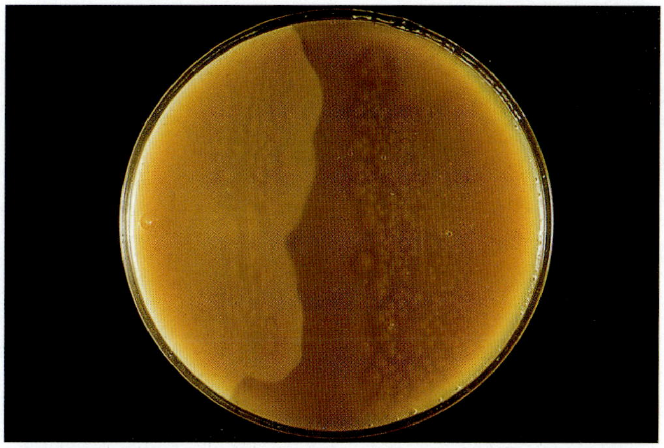

Figure 54–13. *Clostridial perfringens* growing on a half anti-toxin plate. The inhibition of opalescence on the antitoxin-treated portion of the plate is not totally specific for this species. *(Photograph courtesy of Centers for Disease Control and Prevention, Atlanta.)*

Other virulence factors produced by *C perfringens* include enterotoxin, neuraminidase (sialidase), non–α-δ-θ-hemolysins, and the organism's metabolic activity. Type A strains are the only ones found both in the soil and the intestine.

Clostridium septicum is another cause of gas gangrene. *Clostridium septicum* has a subterminal spore, is motile, and produces a number of toxins in vivo, including lecithinase, deoxyribonuclease, a hemolysin, and hyaluronidase. *Clostridium novyi,* a rare cause of gas gangrene, is also motile with a subterminal spore and produces lecithinase.[3,5,9,10]

Clinical Features

The most common predisposing factors for gas gangrene are traumatic injury or penetrating wounds, usually on a limb; surgery that usually involves the biliary tract or intestine; lesions of soft tissue associated with vascular insufficiency, including burns; septic or criminal abortion or delivery; preexisting colorectal cancer or pelvic cancer; and neutropenia associated with leukemia or cytotoxic therapy.

The incubation period of gas gangrene is relatively short—1 to 4 days, with a range of 6 hours to 3 weeks. The initial symptoms are sudden, with steady, severe pain or a feeling of pressure at the site of the wound. At this time the wound may be unremarkable. The infection progresses rapidly, and within minutes to hours of first symptoms, there is pallor, tenderness, and localized edema. The skin is pale at first, but changes to magenta or bronze. This is followed by hemorrhagic bullae and subcutaneous emphysema. With increasing severity there may be a serosanguineous discharge with a "sweet" or "mousy" odor. Gas is present in the involved tissues and can be detected by palpation, radiographs, or scans. Crepitus is late and is neither sensitive nor specific for gas gangrene (Figures 54–14 through 54–17).

Accompanying these local findings are diaphoresis, tachycardia beyond that expected for the degree of fever, and anxiety. Fever is often low or absent in the early stages. Late complications include hypotension, renal failure, hemoglobinuria, intravascular hemolysis, and metabolic acidosis. Before death the patient becomes comatose, and the entire body is crepitant with widespread discoloration of skin.[3,5]

Pathology

The lecithinase produced by *C perfringens* and other histotoxic clostridial species diffuses along muscle cells, disrupting cell membranes and killing cells, including white blood cells and muscle cells, thereby extending the zone of myonecrosis. Leukocytes are killed by the toxin, and muscle cells lose their nuclei and their cytoplasm stains unevenly (Figure 15–18, A and B). *Clostridium perfringens* ferments muscle carbohydrates,

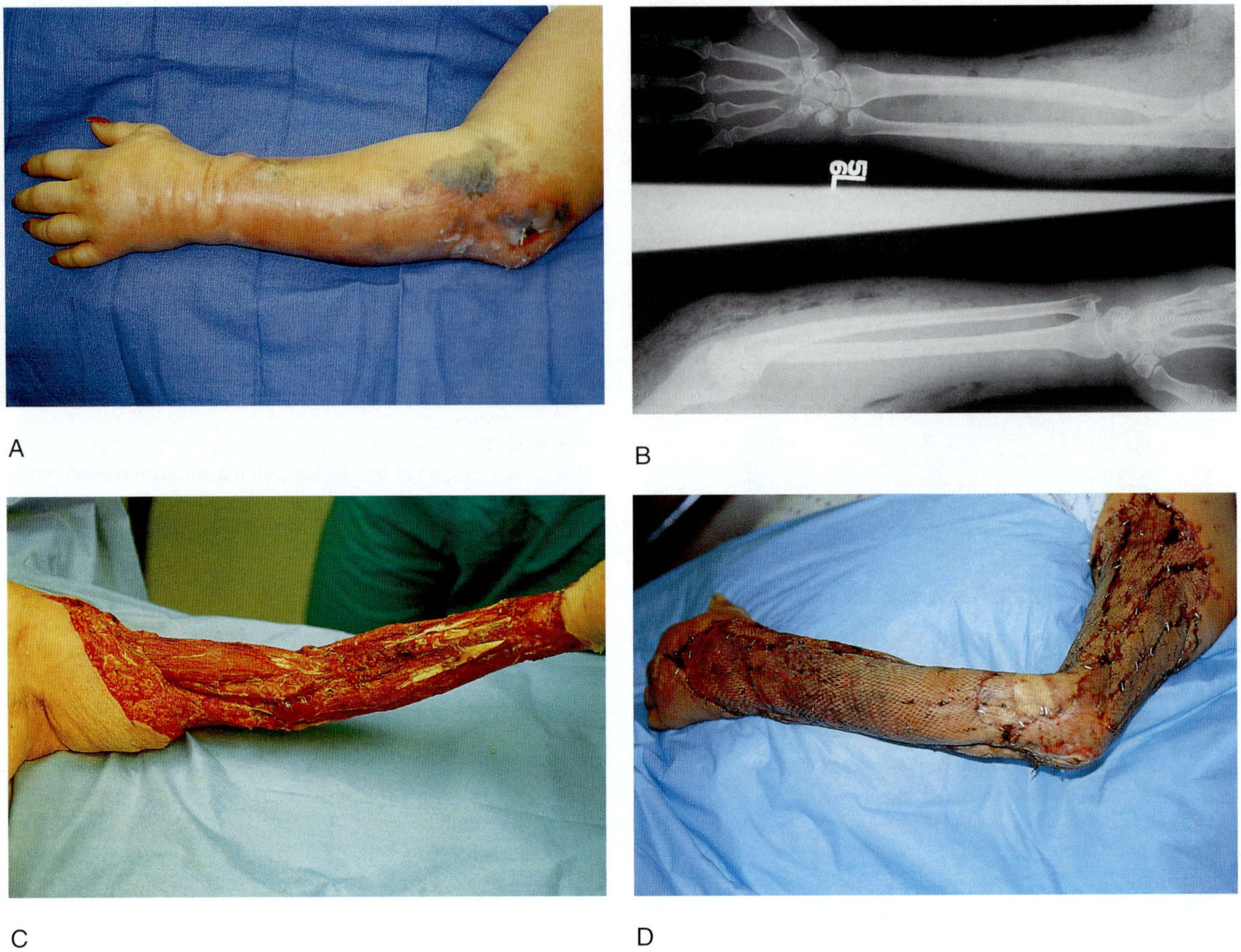

Figure 54–14. (**A**) Arm of a female drug abuser with ulcers of left wrist at site where needle entered ("skin-popper"). She has gas gangrene of left arm with an ulcer of the left medial wrist and extensive swelling. Cultures grew *Clostridium* sp. (**B**) (Same patient as in **A**). Radiographs demonstrate the typical appearance of subcutaneous emphysema. (**C**) (Same patient as in **A**). Massive surgical debulking ("skeletonization") of affected tissues, extending down to skeletal muscle. (**D**) (Same patient as in **A**). Arm after skin grafting. *(Photographs courtesy of Dr. David J. Wages, Emory University Department of Surgery.)*

yielding large amounts of hydrogen and carbon dioxide. This causes the crepitation in the gangrenous muscle and creates empty cystic spaces that are conspicuous microscopically and often macroscopically as well. The myonecrosis seen microscopically is often greater in extent than was suspected at the time of debridement. Tissue gram-staining usually reveals numerous gram-positive bacilli (Figure 54–18, B). A variety of necrotizing lesions, as well as gas gangrene, have been induced in animals experimentally infected with histotoxic clostridial species.

Diagnosis

The diagnosis of gas gangrene is made from the clinical features, myonecrosis at surgery, and appropriate microbiologic findings. The affected muscle has a pale or darkened appearance during surgery (Figure 54–16) and fails to contract when electrically stimulated. Bleeding is often absent from the cut surface. Frozen sections during surgical debridement, massive debulking ("skeletonization") (Figure 54–14, C), or amputation may help estimate the extent of clostridial myonecrosis. Radio-

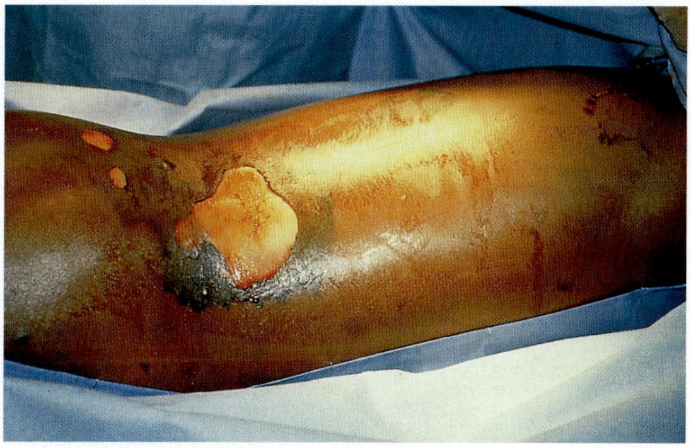

A

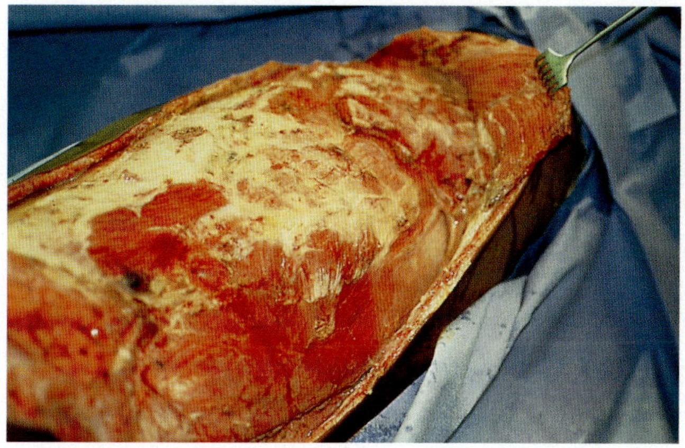

B

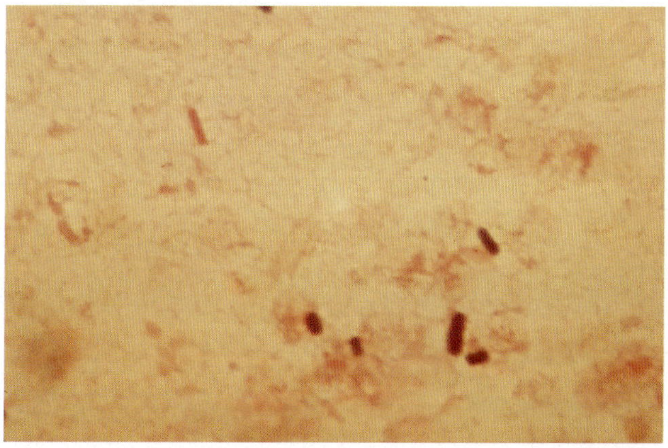

C

Figure 54–15. (**A**) Young male patient was stabbed above his left nipple and subsequently developed epidermolysis and gas gangrene caused by clostridial infection of left lower thorax, hip, and flank. (**B**) (Same patient as in **A**). Surgical debridement was performed. (**C**) (Same patient as in **A**). Gram's stain of exudate showing gram-positive clostridial organisms in the necrotic tissue. *(Photographs courtesy of Dr. David J. Wages, Emory University Department of Surgery.)*

logic studies showing gas-filled cysts or subcutaneous emphysema, and computed tomography (CT) scans demonstrating gas in a muscle compartment and in the fascial planes (Figures 54–14, 54–15, and 54–17) support the diagnosis. A Gram's stain of the discharge often shows large numbers of typical gram-positive or gram-variable rods in devitalized tissue but with few or no inflammatory cells (Figures 54–15, C). Laboratory confirmation is made by isolating a *Clostridium* sp in cultures of material obtained from the gangrenous tissue or blood. Only 10% to 15% of patients with gas gangrene, however, will have demonstrable bacteremia.[5]

Gas gangrene must be differentiated from cellulitis and other infections that cause extensive soft tissue and muscle necrosis. Cellulitis can be caused by a variety of bacterial organisms. When clostridial infection produces cellulitis, the infection originates in contaminated wounds, as with gas gangrene, but the cellulitis does not extend to muscle and is not associated with gas. If clostridial cellulitis is severe or resists treatment, gas gangrene may develop. Anaerobic streptococcal infections may cause myonecrosis similar to gas gangrene, but these conditions can be easily differentiated by microbiological testing.

Treatment

The most important component of life therapy for gas gangrene is the rapid and extensive surgical debridement of affected tissues, leaving a wide surgical margin of unaffected tissues. In patients with an involved extremity, amputation is usually required, whereas women with uterine infection require hysterectomy. Antibiotics therapy, usually with penicillin G, consistently enhance survival. Hyperbaric oxygen therapy has been used for treatment of gas gangrene for more than 30 years, but

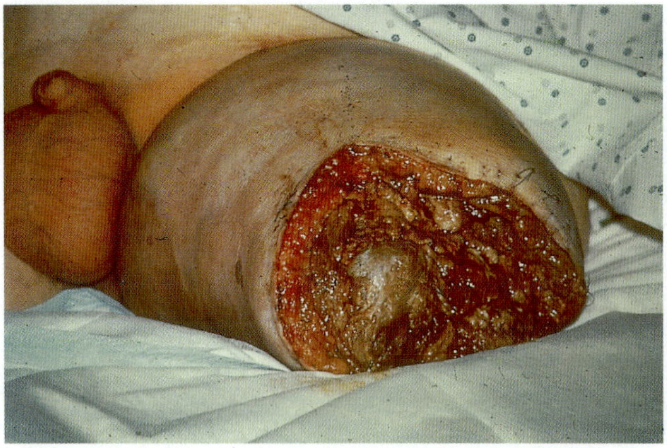

Figure 54–16. Gas gangrene of amputation stump caused by *C septicum,* requiring surgical revision of margin. Note discoloration of skeletal muscle and swelling of thigh and scrotum. *(Photograph courtesy of Dr. Robert Fass, Ohio State University and Centers for Disease Control and Prevention, Atlanta.)*

there is no agreement on its value. Antitoxin for gas gangrene, which was originally developed in 1918, is not efficacious and is no longer commercially available.[5]

PSEUDOMEMBRANOUS COLITIS

Definition

Pseudomembranous colitis is a severe, potentially lethal infection of the colon. The most common agent is *Clostridium difficile,* which overgrows other organisms in the large intestine of patients whose normal bowel flora has been altered by treatment with some antibiotics.

Other names for this condition are antibiotic-associated pseudomembranous colitis, antibiotic-associated colitis, and pseudomembranous enterocolitis.

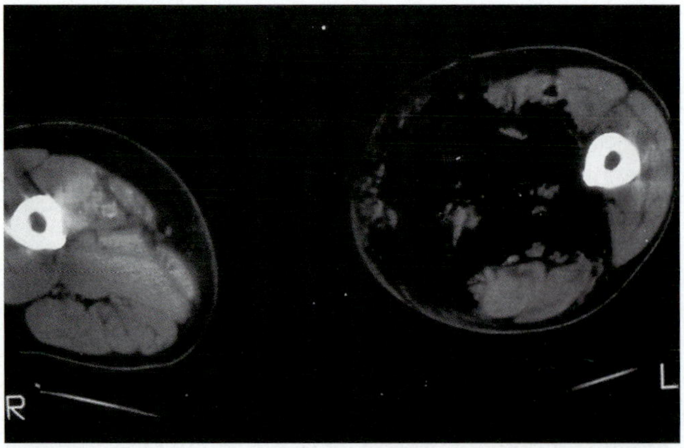

Figure 54–17. CT scan of thigh in a patient with gas gangrene. There is prominent gas production with myonecrosis in the medial compartment of the left thigh caused by *C septicum. (Photograph courtesy of Martin Cetron, MD, Centers for Disease Control and Prevention, Atlanta.)*

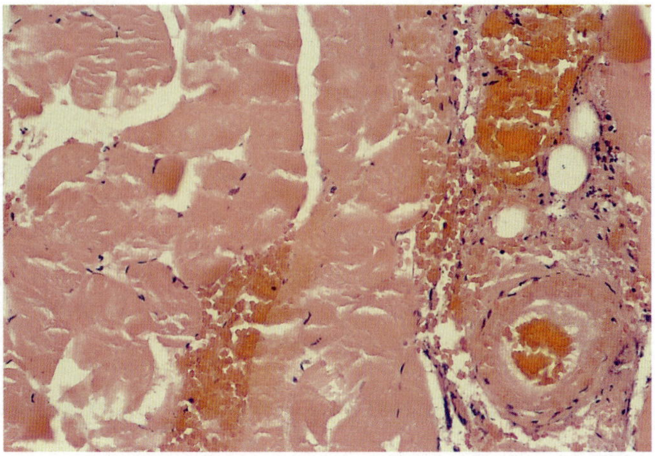

A

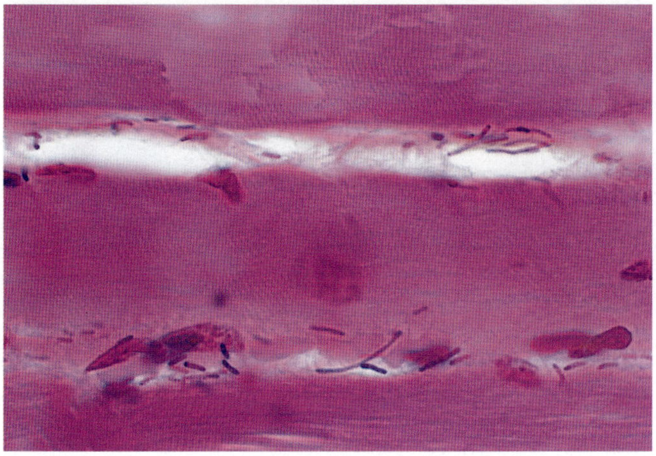

B

Figure 54–18. (**A**) Microscopic features of skeletal muscle with gas gangrene caused by *C septicum.* Low magnification shows loss of muscle nuclei and hemorrhage (hematoxylin-eosin, ×40). (**B**) (Same patient as in **A**). High magnification of clostridial organisms in and around the myofiber (Tissue Gram's stain, ×1000).

Epidemiology

Clostridium difficile colitis has been reported from patients of all ages, but is most frequent in middle-age or older adults, debilitated persons, patients with cancer or burns, and those in intensive care or who have had recent surgery. Pseudomembranous colitis can erupt even after a short course of appropriate antibiotic, which allows the spores of *C difficile* to germinate, overgrow the normal flora, produce toxins, and cause colitis. The list of inciting antibiotics is long, but includes penicillin G, rifampin, ciprofloxacin, metronidazole, lincomycin, clindamycin, ampicillin, erythromycin, tetracycline, cephalosporins, and aminoglycosides. The antibiotic therapy may inhibit growth of bacterial flora normally found in the intestine, permitting the overgrowth of *C difficile*. The colitis may start while receiving antibiotics or several weeks after discontinuing the antibiotic.[17,18]

Biology

Clostridium difficile is an obligate anaerobic, gram-positive rod (Figures 54–1 and 54–2) that produces a wide variety of acid fermentation products that are detectable by gas-liquid chromatography. The organism can be isolated from the feces of 2% to 4% of healthy adults and 10% to 20% of patients in hospital. Isolation rates as high as 64% have been reported in infants. *Clostridium difficile* only rarely invades the colonic mucosa, although it may do this in infants or patients with neutropenia.[17] Approximately 25% of strains isolated from humans lack the genes for the production of toxins, and these strains are nonpathogenic. Pathogenic strains produce at least two antigenically distinct toxins—toxin A (enterotoxin) and toxin B (cytotoxin)—both of which are important in the development of pseudomembranous colitis. Toxin A is weakly cytotoxic, causes intestinal hemorrhage, and kills some rodents. Toxin B is strongly cytotoxic to cells in standard cell culture assays (Figure 54–19). These toxins probably attack the membranes and microfilaments of host cells, causing them to leak fluid and contract. The toxins also cause hemorrhage and inflammation.[17–21]

Clinical Features

Clostridium difficile produces a spectrum of clinical findings, ranging from asymptomatic carriage to severe and life-threatening diarrhea in patients with pseudomembranous colitis. Milder forms of diarrhea may resolve when antibiotic therapy is stopped. When diarrhea persists, however, or when the patient remains severely ill after the withdrawal of the responsible antibiotic, the diagnosis of pseudomembranous colitis must still be considered.

In the past, *Staphylococcus aureus* was believed to cause a form of enterocolitis resembling pseudomembranous colitis. Staphylococcal enterocolitis, however, is rarely encountered in contemporary practice, and *Staphylococcus* is generally not believed to cause pseudomembranous colitis.[17]

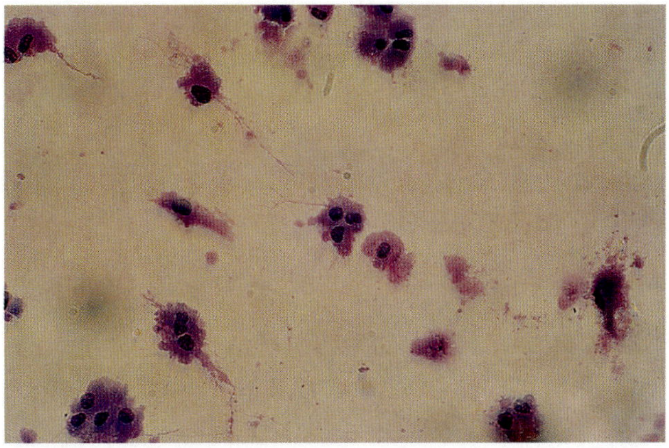

Figure 54–19. The cytotoxic effects of the toxins of *C difficile* are illustrated in this tissue culture of MRC-5 cells. These cells, normally spindle-shaped, are retracted and degenerated after exposure to the bacteria present in a stool filtrate from a patient with pseudomembranous colitis.

Pathology

Active colitis is the most important lesion of pseudomembranous colitis because in some patients pseudomembranes may be small or absent. In typical infections, there are multiple, shaggy, yellow and white exudates, varying in size from a few mm to 20 mm, scattered over the colonic mucosa. The intervening mucosa may be normal or hyperemic and edematous. These lesions are easily seen during colonoscopy, permitting a tentative diagnosis of pseudomembranous colitis (Figure 54–20). In early stages the lesions are

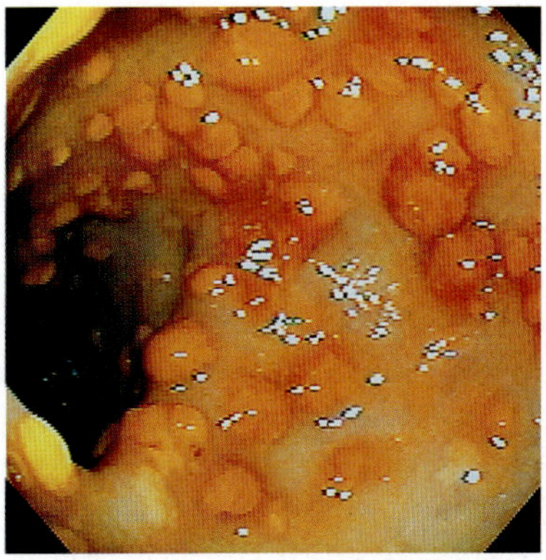

Figure 54–20. High resolution colonoscopic photograph of the typical endoscopic appearance of pseudomembranous colitis. *(Photograph courtesy of C. Mel Wilcox, MD, Department of Medicine, University of Alabama at Birmingham.)*

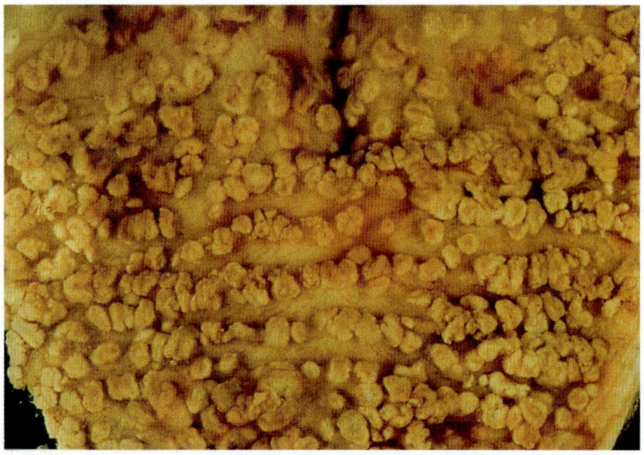

Figure 54–21. Colonic mucosa from a patient with antibiotic-induced pseudomembranous colitis caused by *C difficile.* Each focus of pseudomembrane is a discrete ulcer.

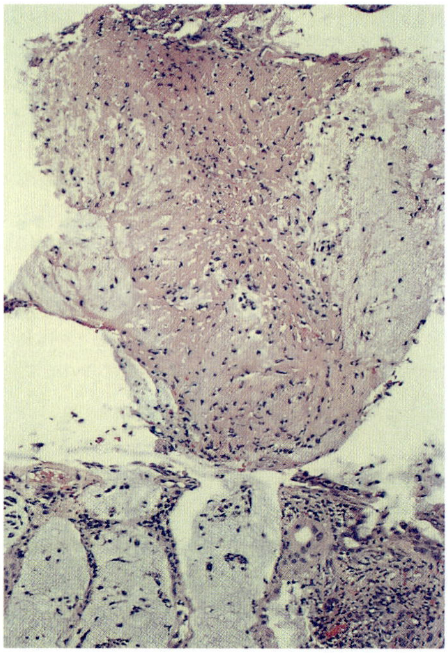

Figure 54–22. Typical "volcano-like" eruptive appearance of the active colitis associated with *C difficile.* Fibrin is mixed with inflammatory cells, mostly neutrophils (hematoxylin-eosin, ×200).

punctate, but as the disease progresses the exudates coalesce, forming a friable "membrane" that peels from the underlying ulcerated mucosa (Figure 54–21). In most patients the disease is not segmental and involves the mucosa of the entire colon. In approximately one third of patients, however, the disease may be confined to the proximal segment of the colon and spare the distal portion.[19] Pseudomembranes are usually most common in the rectosigmoid. The ileum is usually spared unless the patient has an ostomy.

Microscopically the mucosa is acutely inflamed and ulcerated, epithelial cells of the crypts are focally necrotic, and an acute inflammatory exudate covers the mucosal surface. The exudate contains neutrophils, necrotic debris, and abundant mucus, and appears to erupt from the surface, similar to a volcano spewing lava (Figure 54–22). As the exudate spreads and merges with adjacent exudative materials, an inflammatory pseudomembrane forms and covers the ulcerated mucosa.

Diagnosis

The diagnosis can be confirmed by endoscopy with biopsy specimens to confirm the characteristic histopathologic features of pseudomembranous colitis. Findings from biopsy, however, are diagnostic only when the fully developed eruptive lesions are present. In approximately 10% of patients, the pseudomembranous changes are confined to the proximal part of the colon, and these may be missed if colonoscopy is performed only on the distal portion of colon. The colonic mucosa of patients with early or mild infections may be erythematous, edematous, and only mildly inflamed, with only a scant or absent pseudomembrane. In these patients, biopsy diagnosis is difficult because the findings are nonspecific early in the disease.

Isolation of *C difficile* from the feces, immunologic identification of the toxins produced by the organism, or cell culture cytotoxicity assay identification of toxin B have varying degrees of effectiveness in supporting the diagnosis. Because the organism is in the feces of 10% to 20% of hospitalized patients, culture of *C difficile* is nonspecific and has limited predictive value in establishing a diagnosis of pseudomembranous colitis. Counterimmunoelectrophoresis, enzyme-linked immunosorbent assay (ELISA), and latex agglutination assays are available for the immunologic detection of the toxins produced by the organism. Cell culture cytotoxicity assay for the detection of toxin B, however, appears to provide greater predictive value than other laboratory tests in supporting a diagnosis of pseudomembranous colitis.

Treatment

Patients with mild to moderate pseudomembranous colitis caused by *C difficile* may require supportive treatment only. This includes discontinuing treatment with the inciting antibiotic and giving fluids and electrolytes accompanied by careful monitoring. Patients with severe colitis, or those having leukocytosis, high fever, prominent abdominal pain, or signs of peritoneal inflammation should be treated promptly with antibiotics specific for *C difficile,* including vancomycin, metronidazole, or bacitracin. Opiates and other antiperistaltic agents should be avoided, and steroids are of no proved value.[17]

BOTULISM

Classification

Botulism is not an infection, but an acute systemic toxemia caused by absorption of a preformed toxin produced by *Clostridium botulinum*—botulinum toxin. Botulinum toxin is a bacterial neurotoxin and one of the most potent toxins known. Although the disease is a predominantly sporadic or epidemic food-borne illness, wound infections can also occur.

History

The term botulism is derived from the Latin word *botulus,* meaning sausage, because poisonings were caused by eating sausage in 19th-century Europe. Sausage poisoning was first made a reportable disease in 1820 following a large epidemic in southern Germany. The initial description of *C botulinum* was made by van Ermengen in 1897, who demonstrated that the bacillus produced a toxin that caused illness in animals. Wound botulism was first described in 1943, and infant botulism was first noted in 1976.

Epidemiology

Botulism is mostly in the northern hemisphere, between 30° and 65° northern latitude. Most outbreaks have been in seven countries—United States, the former Soviet Union, Japan, Canada, Poland, France, and Germany. Food-borne botulism most commonly causes outbreaks, and the source is usually home-canned fruits, vegetables, and fish. In Alaska, local food preparation practices involving fermentation of fish cause botulism, while in parts of China, home preparation of fermented beans is the most common source of the toxin. In the United States, 124 outbreaks of food-borne botulism were reported to the Centers for Disease Control and Prevention between 1976 and 1984. Large outbreaks were associated with restaurants, whereas small outbreaks (mean 2.7 cases) were usually from home-prepared foods. In the United States, type A botulism occurs most commonly in the west and type B in the east; the geographic distribution of type F is not as well defined.[2] Infant botulism (also from Type A and B toxins) occurs predominantly in California. Botulism from raw or lightly smoked fish is caused by type E neurotoxin, common in Japan, Scandinavian countries, the former Soviet Union, and the Great Lakes regions of the United States.

Biology

Clostridium botulinum is a gram-positive bacillus that is strictly anaerobic. The bacillus is straight to slightly curved, with a size range of from 3.4 to 8.6 by 0.5 to 1.3 μm. It is motile with peritrichous flagella and produces spores that are oval, subterminal, and tend to distend the bacillus. The spores are found globally in marine sediment and soil and show the greatest heat resistance of any anaerobe. Because they withstand 100°C at one atmosphere for several hours, boiling may enhance the growth of the bacillus by making solutions more anaerobic. The spores are also resistant to irradiation and can survive cold temperatures up to −190°C.

Botulinum toxin is synthesized as a single polypeptide chain varying from 150 to 165 kD. This polypeptide is of low potency, but is subsequently nicked by bacterial protease to form two chains connected by a disulfide bond. The nicked toxin type A becomes, on the basis of molecular weight, the most potent naturally occurring toxin. Unlike the spores of *C botulinum,* the toxin is heat-labile. The botulinum neurotoxins are termed types A through G based on antigenic differences.

Clostridium botulinum is composed of four physiologic types—Groups I to IV. Group I organisms are proteolytic in vivo and product toxin types A, B, or F. Group II bacilli are nonproteolytic and synthesize toxin types B, E, or F. The organisms belonging to Group III produce toxin type C or D, and Group IV bacilli produce only toxin type G. In general, a single strain of *C botulinum* produces only one type of toxin. It is typical for each strain of *C botulinum* to contain several plasmids, but, unlike the plasmid-encoded toxins of *C tetani,* only toxin type G is encoded on a plasmid.

Botulinum neurotoxins produce most of their clinical effects by affecting the peripheral neuromuscular junctions and autonomic synapses. Once at the synapse, botulinum toxin inhibits release of acetylcholine. The result is that stimulation of the presynaptic cell fails to produce neurotransmitter release, causing motor paralysis. Autonomic dysfunction can occur when parasympathetic nerve terminals or the autonomic ganglia are affected. The damage to the synapse is permanent. Although botulinum toxin can be transported through the nerves and gain access to the central nervous system (CNS), symptoms referable to this tissue are rare.[2]

Clinical Features

The three main clinical presentations of botulism are food-borne botulism, infant botulism, and wound botulism. Fever is not a feature of any form of botulism.

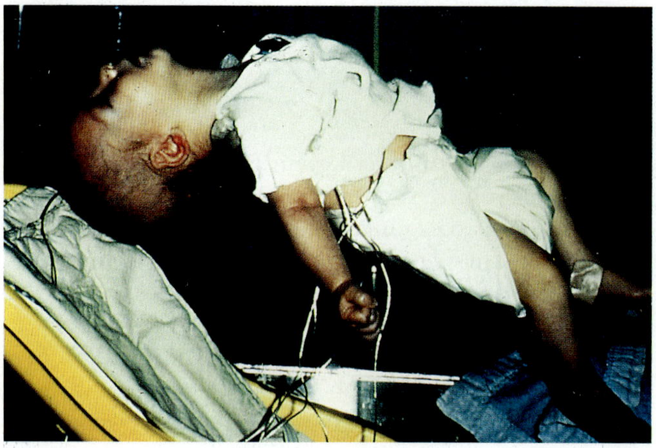

Figure 54–23. A 6-week-old infant with botulism, demonstrating the systemic effects, including marked loss of muscle tone and loss of head control.

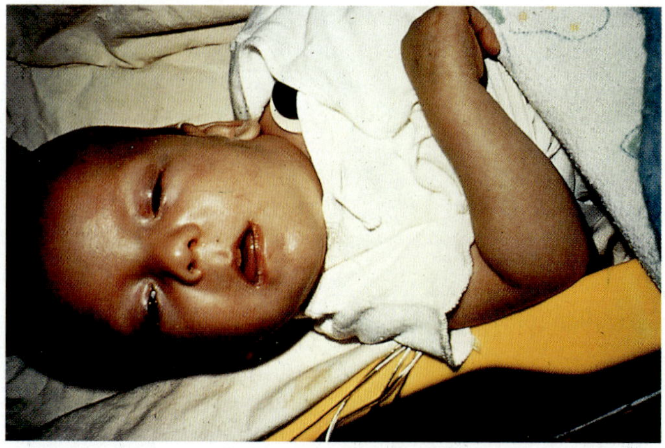

Figure 54–24. Same infant as in Figure 54–23 showing flaccid facial musculature, ptosis, and lack of expression.

The incubation period of food-borne botulism is 12 to 36 hours after ingestion of toxin. Neurotoxin leads to a symmetrical, descending pattern of weakness or paralysis of the cranial nerves (especially nerve IV), limbs, and trunk. First symptoms include nausea, dry mouth, and diarrhea. Later, there is cranial nerve involvement with blurring of vision from pupillary dilation, nystagmus (especially in type A disease), dysphagia, dysarthria, and hypoglossal weakness. Weakness can spread to the upper and lower limbs and trunk. Respiratory embarrassment may be caused by diaphragmatic weakness or upper airway obstruction, and either may require mechanical ventilation. Autonomic problems can include urinary retention, variations in resting heart rate, hypothermia, and loss of responsiveness to change in posture or hypotension.

Infant botulism can present with constipation, followed by difficulties in feeding, weak cry, hypotonia, and increased drooling (Figures 54–23 and 54–24). In infants with severe disease, there may be upper airway obstruction, respiratory weakness, and cranial neuropathies. Ventilatory failure occurs in approximately one half of patients. Infantile botulism may be one cause of sudden infant death syndrome (SIDS).

Wound botulism follows traumatic introduction of spores into a wound, where the bacilli germinate, infection becomes established, and toxin is produced. Thus, this form of the disease lacks the initial gastrointestinal complaints that occur in food-borne botulism, but is otherwise similar in the range of clinical manifestations (Figures 54–25 and 54–26). Incubation varies from 4 to 14 days after injury.[2,22–24]

Pathology

The histologic changes of botulism are nonspecific and include CNS hyperemia and microthromboses of the small vessels. Respiratory paralysis and vascular stasis can cause hypoxic damage to sensitive organs. Mechanical ventilation may cause secondary pulmonary changes.

Diagnosis

Because the differential diagnosis of botulism is limited to just a few conditions, the most important diagnostic feature of botulism is the clinical history. Both myasthenia gravis and Lambert-Eaton myasthenic syndrome share some clinical features with botulism, but they lack the autonomic features and are rarely fulminant. Other diseases in the clinical differential diagnosis include acute inflammatory polyneuropathy, tick paralysis, polio, and poisoning from organophosphates or magnesium. Biopsy does not have a role in the diagnosis of botulism.

Laboratory evaluation of suspected patients include anaerobic cultures and botulinum toxin testing on specimens of serum, stool, and suspected foods. In approximately 75% of patients, toxin typing and confirmation will be obtained. The most sensitive test for botulinum toxin is the mouse bioassay, but serum from patients with other diseases (Guillain-Barré syndrome) can also produce paralysis in mice. Excretion of toxin may persist for a month after onset of illness.

Treatment

The most important aspects of treatment for botulism include ventilatory support and other critical care measures to treat the symptoms of infection. In patients for whom contaminated food remains in the digestive tract, purgatives can be useful unless there is ileus. Antitoxin therapy is important; trivalent (types A, B, and E) equine serum is usually used. Patients with wound bot-

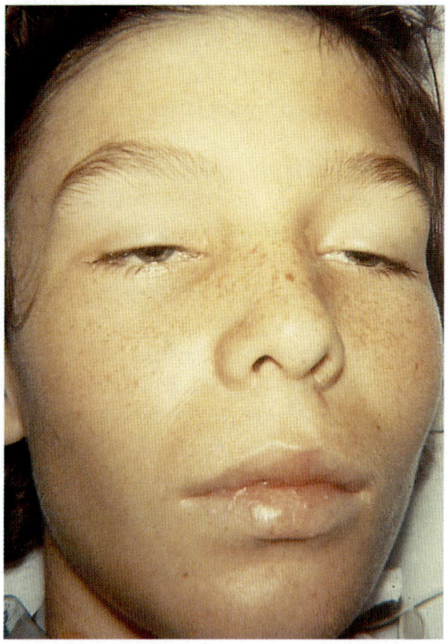

Figure 54–25. A 14-year-old boy fractured the right ulna and radius, and wound botulism followed. He has drooping eyelids and lack of expression caused by the systemic effects of botulinum toxin.

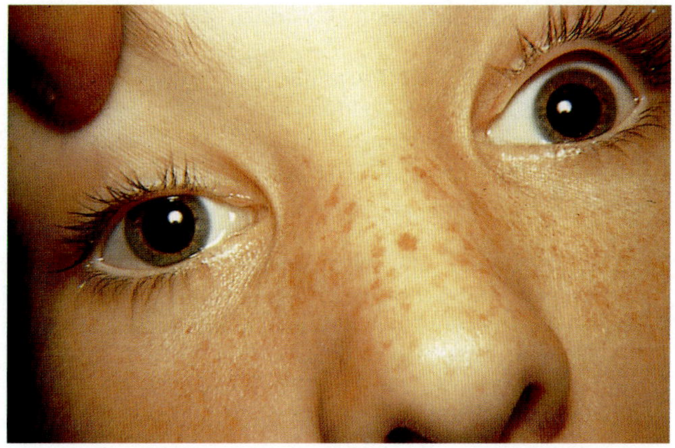

Figure 54–26. Same patient as in Figure 54–25 with pupils dilated and fixed.

ulism also need local care of the wound site, especially surgical debridement. Immunity to botulinum toxin does not develop after exposure, and repeated attacks have been reported.[2]

OTHER CLOSTRIDIAL INFECTIONS

Biliary Tract Infections

Clostridial infections, in particular *C perfringens,* are associated with more than 50% of emphysematous cholecystitis. Clostridial organisms in bile are also the presumed source of gas gangrene of the abdominal wall, a complication of biliary tract surgery. Clostridial sp have been identified in from 10% to 20% of all diseased gall bladders removed at surgery.

Female Genital Tract Infections

Clostridial species are present in 4% to 20% of women having genital tract infections not from sexually transmitted infections. Tubo-ovarian and pelvic abscesses are the most frequent gynecologic manifestation; however, clostridia are present in the vaginal flora of from 5% to 10% of normal women. Recently, *C sordelli* has been identified as an agent of gas gangrene of the uterus and a possible agent of toxic-shock syndrome.

Pulmonary Infections

The clostridia have been identified in 8% to 10% of pulmonary infections associated with anaerobic bacteria, and *C perfringens* is responsible for one half of these isolates. Clostridial infections of lung have followed a penetrating injury of the chest, thoracotomy for lung resection, thoracentesis, and pleural biopsy. Rarely, clostridial infection of lung has followed pulmonary infarction.

Neutropenic Enterocolitis

Also known as typhilitis, neutropenic enterocolitis occurs in those with congenital neutropenia, leukemia, or neutropenia from cytotoxic chemotherapy. It is caused primarily by *C septicum* and presents with watery or bloody diarrhea, abdominal pain, and fever. Pathologic findings of excised cecum or large intestine are nonspecific, including edema, hemorrhage, and necrosis. Gram's stains often show gram-positive bacilli invading the bowel wall.

Enteritis Necroticans (Pig-Bel)

This rare clinical entity is a necrotizing infection of small intestine caused by the β-toxin of *C perfringens* type C. It is described in Chapter 77.

REFERENCES

1. Bleck TB. *Clostridium tetani.* In: Mandell GL, Bennett JE, Dolin R, eds. *Principles and Practice of Infectious Diseases.* 4th ed. Churchill Livingstone; 1995:2173–2178.
2. Bleck TB. *Clostridium botulinum.* In: Mandell GL, Bennett JE, Dolin R, eds. *Principles and Practice of Infectious Diseases.* 4th ed. Churchill Livingstone; 1995:2178–2182.

3. Hatheway CL. Toxigenic clostridia. *Clin Microbiol Rev* 1990;3:66–98.
4. Willis AT. *Anaerobic Bacteriology: Clinical and Laboratory Practice.* 3rd ed. London: Butterworth; 1977:68–172.
5. Lorber B. Gas gangrene and other *Clostridium*-associated diseases. In: Mandell GL, Bennett JE, Dolin R, eds. *Principles and Practice of Infectious Diseases.* 4th ed. New York: Churchill Livingstone; 1995:2182–2195.
6. Cato EP, George WL, Finegold SM. Genus *Clostridium* Prazmowski 1880. In: Sneath PHA, Mair NS, Charpe ME, et al, eds. *Bergey's Manual of Systematic Bacteriology.* Vol. 2. Baltimore: Williams & Wilkins; 1986:1141–1200.
7. Matsuda M. The structure of tetanus toxin. In: Simpson LL, ed. *Botulinum Neurotoxin and Tetanus Toxin.* San Diego: Academic Press; 1989:69–92.
8. Finegold SM, Attebary HR, Sutter VL. Effect of diet on human fecal flora: comparison of Japanese and American diets. *Am J Clin Nutr.* 1974;27:1456–1469.
9. Hill GB, Osterhout S, Willett HP. *Clostridium.* In: Joklik WK, Willett HP, Amos DB, et al, eds. *Zinsser Microbiology.* Norwalk: Appleton & Lange; 1988:537–554.
10. Sherris JC, Plorde JJ. Clostridia, gram-negative anaerobes and anaerobic cocci. In: Sherris JC, ed. *Medical Microbiology: An Introduction to Infectious Disease.* New York: Elsevier Science Publishing; 1990:325–342.
11. Stevens DL, Musher DM, Watson DA, et al. Spontaneous, nontraumatic gangrene due to *Clostridium septicum. Rev Infect Dis.* 1990;12:286–296.
12. Jendrzejewski JW, Jones SR, Newcombe RL, Gilbert DN. Nontraumatic clostridial myonecrosis. *Am J Med.* 1978, 65:542–546.
13. MacLennan JD. The histotoxic clostridial infections of man. *Bacteriol Rev.* 1962;26:177–276.
14. Kornbluth AA, Danzig JB, Bernstein LG. *Clostridium septicum* infection and associated malignancy. *Medicine.* 1989;68:30–37.
15. Bretzke ML, Bubrick MP, Hitchcock CR. Diffuse spreading *Clostridium septicum* infection, malignant disease and immune suppression. *Surg Gynecol Obstet.* 1988;166:197–199.
16. Brown-Harrell V, Nitta AT, Goble M. Recurrent episodes of spontaneous clostridial myonecrosis related to colorectal carcinoma. *Clin Infect Dis.* 1996;22:582–583.
17. Fekety R. Antibiotic-associated colitis. In: Mandell GL, Bennett JE, Dolin R, eds. *Principles and Practice of Infectious Diseases.* 4th ed. New York: Churchill Livingstone; 1995:978–987.
18. Borrielo SP. Clostridial disease of the gut. *Clin Infect Dis.* 1995;20(supp 2):S242–S250.
19. Bartlett JG. *Clostridium difficile:* clinical consideration. *Rev Infect Dis.* 1990;12(Supp 2):s243-s251.
20. Tedesco FJ, Barton RW, Alpers HD. Clindamycin-associated colitis. *Ann Intern Med.* 1974;81:429–433.
21. Bartlett JG. Antibiotic-associated colitis. *Disease of the Month.* 1984;30:1–54.
22. Hughes JM, Blumenthal JR, Merson MH, et al. Clinical features of type A and B foodborne botulism. *Ann Intern Med.* 1981;95:442–445.
23. Hughes JM. Botulism. In: Scheld WM, Whitley RJ, Durack DT, eds. *Infections of the Central Nervous System.* New York: Raven Press; 1991:589–602.
24. Cherington M. Botulism. *Semin Neurol.* 1990;10:27–31.

CHAPTER 55

Corynebacterial Infections

David A. Schwartz, A. Bennett Jenson, and Lai Y. Lim

. . . and living long having given me frequent opportunities of seeing certain remedies cried up as curing everything, and yet soon after totally laid aside as useless, I cannot but fear that expectation of great advantage from the new method of treating diseases will prove a delusion. That delusion may however in some cases be of use while it lasts.

Ben Franklin (1706–1790)

Just think of it. A hundred years ago there were no bacilli, no ptomaine poisoning, no diphtheria, and no appendicitis. Rabies was but little known, and only imperfectly developed. All of these we owe to medical science. Even such things as psoriasis and parotitis and trypanosomiasis, which are now household names, were known only to the few, and were quite beyond the reach of the great mass of people.

Stephen B. Leacock (1869–1944)

INTRODUCTION

Corynebacteria (from the Greek words *koryne,* meaning "club," and *bacterion,* meaning "little rod") compose a diverse genus of Gram-positive, catalase-positive, aerobic or facultatively anaerobic, nonsporulating rods that are usually nonmotile. Species of *Corynebacterium* are widely distributed in nature and are commonly found in soil and water, as well as on the skin and mucous membranes of humans and animals. In some species, the bacterial cell wall is weaker at one end, resulting in a club-shaped bacillus. *Corynebacterium diphtheriae* is the only major human pathogen in this genus, which includes a number of opportunistic species as well as nonpathogenic and poorly described saprophytes frequently found on the surfaces of mucous membranes.

CLASSIFICATION

In 1896, Lehmann and Neumann suggested that the agent of diphtheria and all other bacteria resembling it be grouped into the genus *Corynebacterium.* Since then, the non-diphtheria species of this genus have been known commonly as *diphtheroids. Corynebacterium diphtheriae,* medically the most important member, causes the characteristic syndrome of necrotic pseudomembrane formation in the throat and other tissues termed *diphtheria.* Other potentially pathogenic corynebacterial species and the diseases they produce include *C minutissimum* (erythrasma), *C ulcerans* (pharyngitis), *C striatum* (bacteremia and sepsis, purulent conjunctivitis, chorioamnionitis, infectious keratitis, and pyogenic granuloma), *C xerosis* (opportunistic disease), *Corynebacterium* group D2 (urinary tract infections), *Actinomyces (Corynebacterium) pyogenes* (suppurative disease), *C bovis* (endocarditis, central nervous system [CNS] disease), *C pseudodiphthericum* (endocarditis, lower respiratory infection), *C jeikeium* (wound infection and septicemia), *C pseudotuberculosis* (lymphadenitis), and *Arcanobacterium (Corynebacterium) haemolyticum* (pharyngitis, skin ulceration). The exact family affiliation of this genus is unclear, but corynebacteria are related taxonomically to the mycobacteria and

Nocardia because of the similarity in cell-wall composition.

Corynebacterium diphtheriae

History

The history of identifying the bacterial cause of diphtheria, of unraveling of the epidemiology of this lethal disease, and subsequent development of an effective vaccine is one of the most interesting in the annals of bacteriology. Descriptions of a syndrome of sore throat, membrane production, and suffocation appear as early as the Hippocratic writings.[1] The autopsy findings of diphtheria were recorded by the French physician Guillame de Baillou during an epidemic of diphtheria in Paris in 1576, and his record is one of the earliest autopsy-based descriptions of an epidemic disease. Following the postmortem examination of a 7-year-old boy whose pharynx was slightly swollen before death, de Baillou identified the false membrane characteristic of diphtheria. His description stated that "sluggish resisting phlegm was found which covered the trachea like a membrane and the entry and exit of air to the exterior was not free."[2] Diphtheria was first established as a specific clinical entity in 1826, after publication of a classic monograph by Pierre Bretonneau. The bacterial cause of diphtheria, however, was not completely established until 1883, when Klebs described chaining cocci and bacilli in microscopic preparations of diphtheric membranes.[3] While working in Robert Koch's laboratory 1 year later, Friedreich Loeffler isolated and morphologically characterized the diphtheria bacillus in a culture medium that bears his name.[4] Loeffler demonstrated that 1) the organism could produce disease when inoculated into guinea pigs, and fulfilled Koch's postulates for proof that it caused diphtheria; 2) healthy asymptomatic people could harbor the organism in their throats, thus identifying a carrier state; and 3) the bacillus remained localized to the pseudomembrane and did not invade the tissues. Loeffler also predicted that the neurologic and cardiac manifestations were caused by a toxin that was elaborated by the diphtheria bacillus,[4] which was confirmed at the Pasteur Institute in 1888, when Roux and Yersin[5] separated the toxin from the bacillus by filtration. Two years later, von Behring demonstrated that antiserum against the toxin protected animals after they were experimentally infected. Following this, Roux reported in 1894 that antitoxin produced in horses reduced mortality from diphtheria among foundlings in Paris from 51% to 24%. Horses were ideal animals in which to produce antitoxin because they were not only large and highly reactive to diphtheria toxin, but they were also relatively insensitive to the toxin. However, horses used for long-term antibody production eventually died of amyloidosis, and approximately 10% of diphtheria patients vaccinated with horse antiserum developed acute serum sickness. In 1897, Ehrlich[6] developed a bioassay for the toxin using guinea pigs to determine the minimum lethal dose.

Theobold Smith and von Behring immunized children successfully with a toxin–antitoxin mixture in 1923. At the same time in Paris, Ramon developed an effective "toxoid" vaccine by rendering the toxin nontoxic through treatment with dilute formalin and heat.[7] Identifying and characterizing *C diphtheriae* by culture was a focus of interest to bacteriologists during the late 19th and early 20th centuries. In 1886, Babes,[8] and in 1888, Ernst[9] distinguished toxigenic *C diphtheria* from nontoxigenic diphtheroids by metachromatic granules in the former. In 1926, Cornwell, and Cowan in 1927 separated avirulent and virulent strains into three categories depending on its ability to produce disease—*gravis, intermedius,* and *mitis.*[10]

Epidemiology

Diphtheria is worldwide in distribution but is now rare in the United States and other developed nations. The dramatically changing incidence of diphtheria during the past decades in developed countries is at least partially the result of widespread childhood immunization, although a full explanation is not clear. For example, from 1921 to 1924 diphtheria was the leading cause of death in Canadian schoolchildren aged 2 to 14 years, and 147,991 infections were reported in the United States in 1920.[1,11] Since 1980, 5 or fewer diphtheria infections per year have been reported in the United States, and in 1993 no new cases were reported to the Centers for Disease Control and Prevention.[11] Tragically, diphtheria remains an endemic public health problem where less than 10% of infants are immunized, including Brazil, India, Indonesia, the Philippines, Nigeria, and the eastern Mediterranean, and it is estimated that diphtheria kills 1 million persons each year. Beginning in 1990, Russia and other former states of the Soviet Union experienced significant numbers of new cases of diphtheria, with 3897 cases reported in 1992 alone.[1]

Humans are the only identified reservoirs for *C diphtheriae,* and symptom-free carriers and persons in the incubation stage of infection are the major sources of infection. Most respiratory tract diphtheria occurs in the colder months in temperate climates, and is associated with crowded indoor living and hot, dry air. The primary mechanisms of transmission are airborne respiratory droplets and by direct contact with respiratory secretions or infected skin. Fomites also serve as a source of infection, and epidemics have been associated with infected milk. In tropical areas, *C diphtheriae* on the skin is an important source of transmission, and data indicate that person-to-person transmission of diphtheria from infected cutaneous sites is more efficient than respiratory transmission.[1]

Immunity to diphtheria depends on antitoxin in the blood as a result of clinical or subclinical infection or from active immunization with toxoid. Infants younger than 6 months of age are passively protected by transplacental passage of antitoxin from immune mothers. Immunization reduces the probability of a person becoming a carrier, and although immunized people can still develop diphtheria, prior immunization reduces the frequency and severity of the disease.

Recent epidemics have involved not only children younger than age 15 years, but also nonimmunized or poorly immunized adults, especially the rural and urban poor. There have been recent reports of pharyngeal carriage of nontoxigenic strains of *C diphtheriae* in homosexual men[12] and invasive infections in injecting drug abusers.[13]

Biology

Corynebacterium diphtheriae is a slender, Gram-positive, nonsporulating, nonencapsulated, and nonmotile pleomorphic bacillus. The species name is derived from the Greek word *diphtheria,* meaning "leather hide," and refers to the characteristic leathery membrane that forms in infected tissues. The bacillus is club-shaped at both ends, measures approximately 1.5 to 5 μm long and 0.5 to 1 μm wide. In Gram-stained smears of organisms grown on Loeffler's medium, the bacilli may contain metachromatic granules, and the bacteria are characteristically arranged in palisades or at sharp angles to one another in V and L configurations. These "Chinese character" arrangements result from the "snapping" movement of two cells during cell division. Special diagnostic reagents are required for isolating *C diphtheriae* by culture and subsequent subculture for toxigenic and biochemical testing. Selective media containing potassium tellurite inhibit many of the normal throat commensals, and *C diphtheriae* appears as gray-black colonies containing reduced tellurite. The species is divided into three types—*gravis, intermedius,* and *mitis*—based on differences in colonies on tellurite agar, fermentation reactions, and hemolytic patterns (Figure 55–1). Similar to other corynebacterial species as well as the nocardia and mycobacteria, the peptidoglycans of the cell wall of *C diphtheriae* contain meso-α, ε-diaminopimelic acid, and the major cell wall sugars are arabinose and galactose. The lipids associated with the outer envelop also contain significant amounts of mycolic acids, which are similar to the large saturated, α-branched, β-hydroxy fatty acids of the mycobacteria.

Current knowledge of the toxigenic characteristics of the diphtheria toxin is extensive.[14–16] Exotoxin production by *C diphtheriae* depends on the presence of a

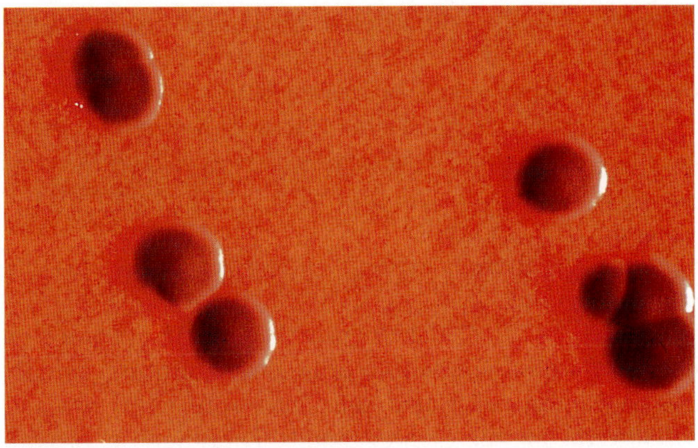

Figure 55–1. Morphologic appearance of *mitis* colonies of *Corynebacterium diphtheriae* cultivated on cystine tellurite medium. *(Courtesy of the Centers for Disease Control and Prevention, Atlanta.)*

lysogenic bacteriophage that carries the gene encoding for production of toxin (tox$^+$). During the lysogenic phase, the bacteriophage's circular DNA strand integrates with the genetic material of the host bacterium as a prophage, resulting in the ability of the bacillus to express the gene necessary for production of the toxin polypeptide. The exotoxin is a 62 kD polypeptide composed of two parts—an enzymatically active part (fragment A) at its amino terminus and a carboxy-terminus fragment (fragment B) that attaches to specific receptors on the membranes of susceptible host cells. Diphtheria toxin binds to the precursor of a heparin-binding epidermal growth factor (EGF)–like growth factor on the surface of a susceptible eukaryotic host cell. After internalization and attachment to cell membranes by the B fragment, the A fragment is translocated into the cytosol of the cell. Fragment A inactivates the transfer RNA (tRNA) translocase, termed "elongation factor 2," which is in eukaryotic but not bacterial cells. The loss of this enzyme prevents the interaction of mRNA and tRNA, halting further addition of amino acids to elongating polypeptide chains.

Significant toxin production depends not only on the presence of the lysogenic tox$^+$ bacteriophage but also on bacterial growth being slowed by exhaustion of iron in the environment. Although diphtheria toxin affects all cells in the body, it exerts its most prominent effects on the nerves, kidneys, and heart. Minuscule amounts of toxin halt protein synthesis in cultured HeLa cells within 3 hours, and only 0.1 μg/kg is necessary to kill a susceptible animal. These properties make diphtheria toxin one of the most potent known to humankind. In general, the incidence of toxin production in *C diphtheriae* correlates with the strain biotype—98.9% of *intermedius* strains are toxigenic, compared with 84% of *gravis* strains and 34.1% of *mitis* strains.[17] Usually, diphtherial infections produced by *mitis* strains tend to be less severe than infections produced by either *gravis* or *intermedius* strains.

Strains of *C diphtheriae* lacking lysogenic phage produce no toxin. These strains, however, can be converted to toxin production in vitro by infection with the lysogenic tox$^+$ phage, a process termed *lysogenization.* Significantly, there is evidence that this process also can occur in nature.[16]

Growth of *C diphtheriae* in infected tissues is restricted to the epithelium of mucosal surfaces, usually the respiratory tract and skin, and only rarely does *C diphtheriae* invade deeper tissues. Diphtheria exotoxin, however, is absorbed into the systemic circulation, and can produce pathologic effects on many deep tissues, especially the nerves, heart and kidneys.

Clinical Features

The clinical presentation of diphtheria can be divided into two major types—respiratory tract and extra-respiratory infections. Clinical manifestations of respiratory tract disease are variable and depend on the virulence of the organism, state of host resistance, and anatomic location of the lesion. The incubation period varies from 2 to 4 days, after which local signs and symptoms of infection can develop at various sites within the respiratory tract. Faucial diphtheria is the most common clinical presentation, and can involve infection of the posterior structures of the mouth, tonsils, and proximal pharynx. It usually begins abruptly with sore throat, mild pharyngeal injection, malaise, and low-grade fever. Development of the characteristic pseudomembrane usually begins on one or both tonsils and extends to one or more of the following structures: uvula, tonsillar pillars, oropharynx, hypopharynx, soft palate, and nasopharynx (Figure 55–2). The pseudomembrane at first is white and glossy but later becomes gray, with focal areas of green or black necrosis. The extent of the pseudomembrane correlates with the severity of symptoms. Thus, the disease caused by a localized tonsillar pseudomembrane is often mild, but extension of the pseudomembrane into the posterior pharynx, soft palate, and periglottal mucosa is associated with severe malaise, prostration, and weakness. Cervical lymph nodes become tender and edematous, distorting the normal contour of the submental and cervical areas and resulting in the "bull neck" appearance (Figure 55–3). The larynx may be infected primarily or by spread from the pharynx. Symptoms of laryngeal involvement include hoarseness, dyspnea, respiratory stridor, and cough. Pseudomembrane with edema involving the trachea and bronchi can further complicate respiration. These patients are anxious, cyanotic, use accessory muscles of respiration, and demonstrate inspiratory retractions. Mechanical obstruction of the airways by

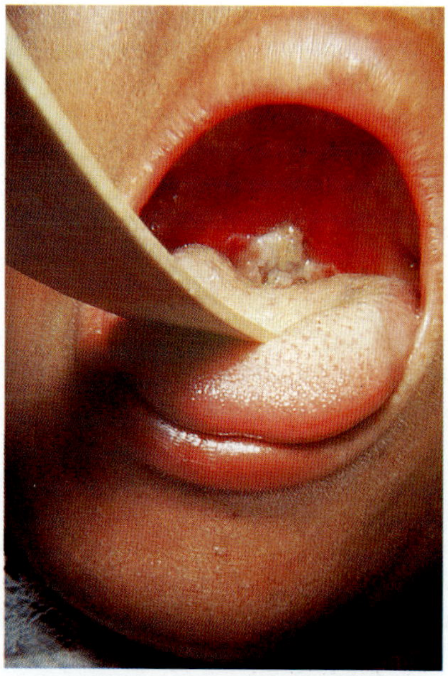

Figure 55–2. Typical appearance of the diphtheritic pseudomembrane in the oropharynx of a child with mild diphtheria.

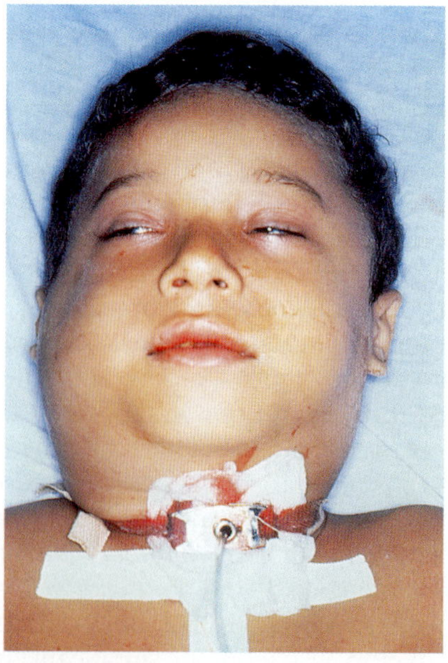

Figure 55–3. Severe laryngeal diphtheria causing respiratory distress and requiring intubation. This Brazilian boy shows dramatic swelling of the face and neck, causing "bull neck." *(Courtesy of Anastacio de Queiroz Sousa, MD, Universidade Federal do Ceara, Fortaleza, Brazil, and Martin Cetron, MD, Centers for Disease Control and Prevention, Atlanta.)*

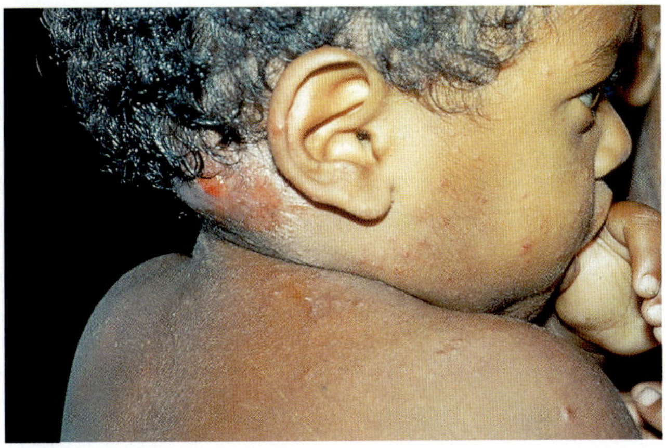

Figure 55–4. Ulcer of cutaneous diphtheria at the hairline of the base of the neck in a Brazilian infant. The gross appearance of this lesion is not distinctive for *Corynebacterium diphtheriae*. *(Courtesy of Anastacio de Queiroz Sousa, MD, Universidade Federal do Ceara, Fortaleza, Brazil, and Martin Cetron, MD, Centers for Disease Control and Prevention, Atlanta.)*

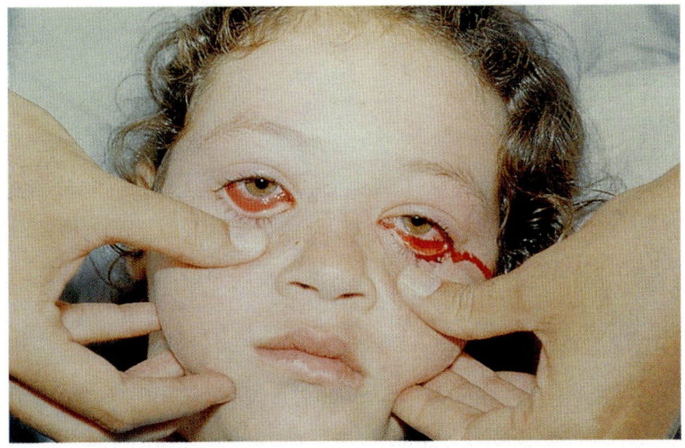

Figure 55–5. "Bloody tears" from infection of this Brazilian girl's left eye with *Corynebacterium diphtheriae*. Involvement of the eyes is an unusual manifestation of diphtherial infection. *(Courtesy of Anastacio de Queiroz Sousa, MD, Universidade Federal do Ceara, Fortaleza, Brazil, and Martin Cetron, MD, Centers for Disease Control and Prevention, Atlanta.)*

diphtherial pseudomembranes is a medical emergency, and the risk of suffocation is high without immediate medical intervention, including tracheostomy or intubation.[1]

Extra-respiratory diphtheria is most common in the tropics. Cutaneous infection is the most common extra-respiratory manifestation of diphtheria (Figure 55–4). The classic diphtheritic cutaneous ulcer is nonhealing and covered with a dirty-gray pseudomembrane. However, 85% of diphtheritic ulcers cannot be distinguished from other dermatologic conditions, including eczema and psoriasis. The clinical presentation of cutaneous diphtheria is indolent and is rarely associated with systemic signs of toxicity. Most cutaneous diphtheritic ulcers are associated with *Staphylococcus aureus* and Group A streptococci. The cornea and conjunctiva also are occasional sites of diphtheria. The diphtheritic pseudomembranes on the mucosal surfaces of the eye resemble those in other parts of the body, and may be accompanied by hemorrhage ("bloody tears") when the pseudomembrane is torn or shed (Figure 55–5). Other unusual sites of diphtheria include the vagina, nose, and ear. Infection of these sites is almost always associated with pharyngeal or cutaneous infection.

Systemic complications of diphtheria are caused by diphtheria toxin produced by the bacteria, and the effects of this toxin are most severe in the heart and in nerve tissues. In up to two thirds of patients, the first evidence of cardiac involvement usually begins after 1 to 2 weeks of illness. From 10% to 25% of patients develop clinical signs of cardiac dysfunction, which can present clinically as congestive heart failure, circulatory collapse, progressive dyspnea, or weakness. As with cardiac toxicity, neurologic toxicity is proportional to the severity of primary infection. Although mild infections only infrequently develop neurologic manifestations, as many as 75% of patients with severe disease develop neuropathy. Neurologic involvement usually begins with local paralysis of the soft palate and the posterior pharyngeal wall. Cranial neuropathies can develop, and later, peripheral neuritis. Occasionally, motor nerves of the upper limbs, neck, and trunk are involved.[1] The mortality rates of diphtheria vary from 3.5% to 12% and have not changed since the mid 1950s. The majority of deaths are in the first 3 to 4 days, and are the result of myocarditis or asphyxia.

Pathology

After invasion, *C diphtheriae* multiplies rapidly on epithelial cells at the site of infection. Exotoxin destroys the cells at the site of infection, and inflammatory cells accumulate, accompanied by a fibrin-rich exudate. At first the exudate is patchy, but later the exudative lesions coalesce to form a resilient pseudomembrane that adheres tightly to the underlying ulcerated tissue (Figure 55–6). Initially, the membrane is white and shiny, then becomes gray to black. It is composed of lymphocytes, neutrophils, erythrocytes, and necrotic epithelial cells in a matrix of fibrin (Figure 55–7). Tissue Gram's staining can reveal large numbers of Gram-positive, club-shaped bacilli within the exudate (Figures 55–8 and 55–9), especially in the early stages. With progression of disease, neutrophilic infiltration of the underlying tissues becomes more intense, and is accompanied by edema, vascular congestion, fibrin exudation, and perivascular cuffing (Figure 55–10). In laryngeal infections, the epiglottis, false cords, and true cords may be covered by a pseudomembrane that can

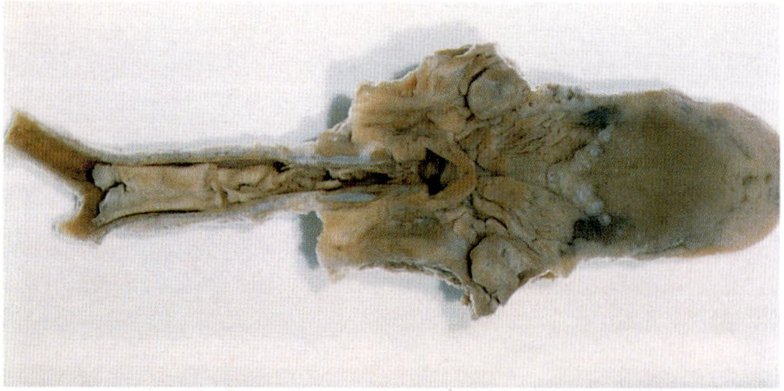

Figure 55–6. Posterior view of tongue, larynx, trachea, and bronchi removed at autopsy of a child with laryngeal diphtheria. The diphtheritic pseudomembrane extends to larynx and main bronchi. *(Courtesy of the Pathology Department, Grady Memorial Hospital, Atlanta.)*

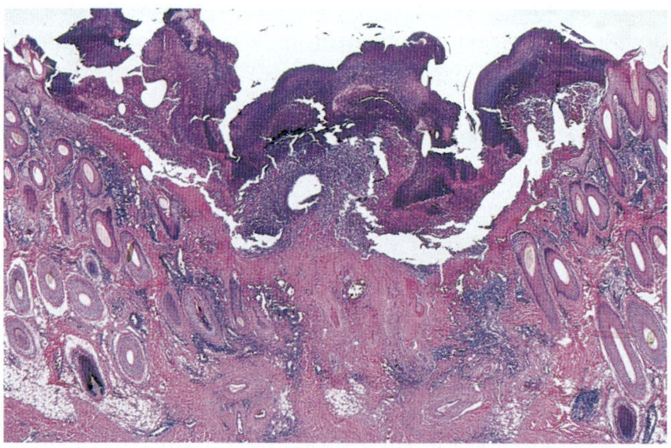

Figure 55–7. Ulcer from scalp of a 31-year-old soldier serving in the Pacific during World War II. On 30 November 1943 he was admitted to the area Army Hospital for malaise, anuria, nausea, and fever—all of approximately 12 days' duration. Ulcers on his face and scalp were treated with sulfadiazine by mouth and $KMnO_4$ soaks. Most of the ulcers healed, but one on the scalp persisted. On 23 December he complained of severe precordial pain. He had a rapid pulse, a "mitral configuration" of his heart by chest x ray, and evidence of myocardial damage by EKG. He died a few hours later on 24 December. The clinical diagnosis was mitral stenosis and coronary occlusion, but an autopsy performed 5 hours later by Captain Victor M. Thompkins MC, US Army (subsequently director of laboratories for the State of New York) revealed fatal pulmonary edema, a severely degenerated heart, and, on the scalp, an ulcer covered by a "glassy membrane," from which Dr. Thompkins cultured a toxigenic strain of *Corynebacterium diphtheriae*. This low-power photomicrograph shows the pseudomembrane and underlying hair-bearing skin (hematoxylin-eosin, ×10).

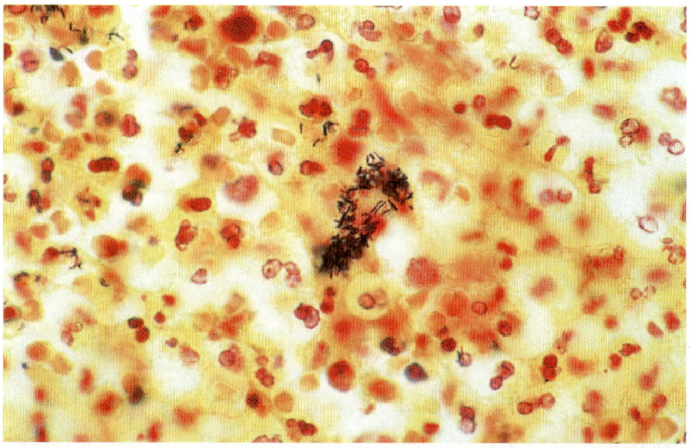

Figure 55–8. Clusters of Gram-positive bacilli in the base of the ulcer shown in Figure 55–7 (Brown–Hopps tissue Gram stain, ×240).

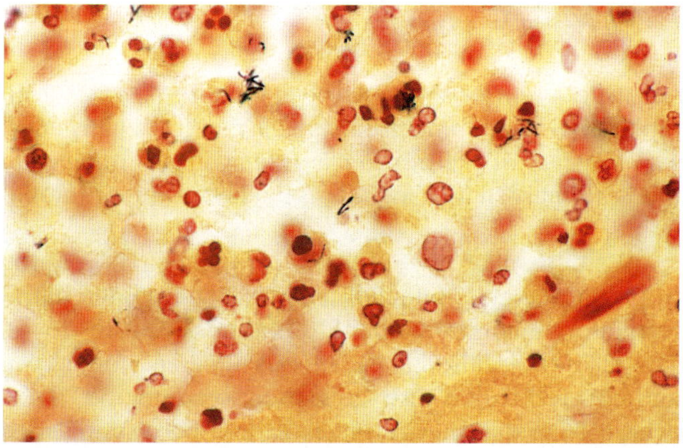

Figure 55–9. Many of the bacilli are club-shaped, as is the bacillus in the center of the picture from a tissue section of the diphtheritic pseudomembrane shown in Figure 55–7 (Brown–Hopps tissue Gram stain, ×300).

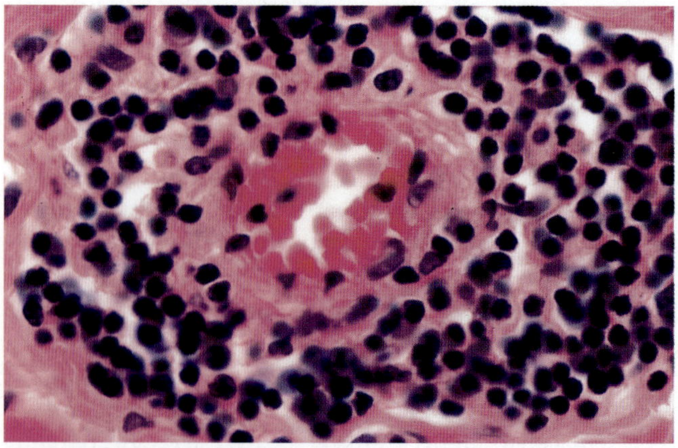

Figure 55–10. Dermis underlying the cutaneous ulcer from Figure 55–7, showing perivascular lymphocytic cuffing (hematoxylin-eosin, ×300).

extend into the trachea (Figure 55–6). On the deeper aspects, the laryngeal epithelium is included in the pseudomembrane, and the submucosal seromucinous glands beneath the pseudomembrane often are necrotic. In cases in which the epithelium is of the columnar respiratory type, the membrane peels or is coughed off easily from the basement membrane. In the squamous epithelium-lined vocal cords, however, the pseudomembrane separates with difficulty, and there may be airway obstruction. In some infections, inflammation and necrosis of subjacent tissues cause spontaneous separation of the pseudomembrane, with aspiration and respiratory embarrassment. After resolution with treatment, the pseudomembrane is either expelled or digested by enzymes, the inflammatory reaction subsides, and the ulcerated mucosa heals by regeneration.

When there is diphtheritic neurotoxicity, the changes in nerves are nonspecific and include degeneration of myelin sheaths and axon cylinders. With diphtheritic myocarditis, the heart is pale, flabby, and has yellow streaks.[18] Microscopically, myofibers have hyaline, granular, and fatty changes. Myocarditis, when present, consists of necrosis of single or of clusters of myofibers associated with infiltrates of mononuclear cells and neutrophils (Figure 55–11). As a result of the systemic effects of exotoxin, patients with diphtheria may develop generalized reticuloendothelial hyperplasia of the spleen and the lymph nodes. The nodes in the neck can enlarge dramatically in patients with respiratory tract infection, causing the "bull neck" appearance (Figure 55–3). In severe infections, there may be fatty change and focal necrosis of the liver cells, adrenal glands, and kidneys. In addition, the kidneys may show interstitial inflammation, nephrocalcinosis, and degenerative and regenerative changes of renal tubules with epithelial casts (Figures 55–12 and 55–13).

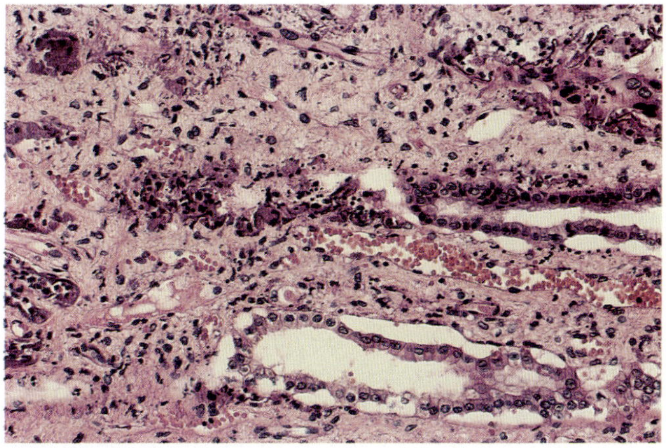

Figure 55–12. Kidney with interstitial inflammation and degenerative changes in the renal tubules from the patient in Figure 55–7. These changes are caused by circulating diphtheria exotoxin, not direct tissue invasion by the organisms (hematoxylin-eosin, ×100).

Diagnosis

When diphtheria is suspected, laboratory personnel should be warned that the specimen may contain toxigenic *C diphtheriae*. Specimens should be inoculated onto blood agar and tellurite media (Downie's media) immediately. Tellurite media is whole sheep blood in an agar base that supports the characteristic shape of *C diphtheriae* while suppressing other bacteria. After incubating overnight in tellurite media, *gravis* colonies are large, flat, and gray to black with a dull surface; *mitis* organisms (Figure 55–1) produce medium-sized

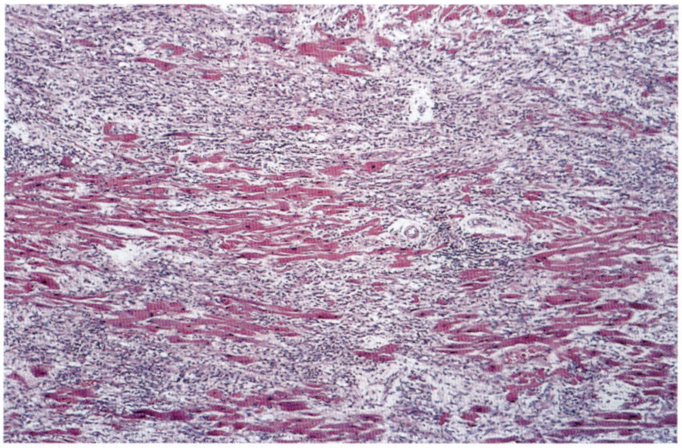

Figure 55–11. Section of myocardium from patient described in Figure 55–7. There are myocardial necrosis and prominent myocarditis (hematoxylin-eosin, ×400).

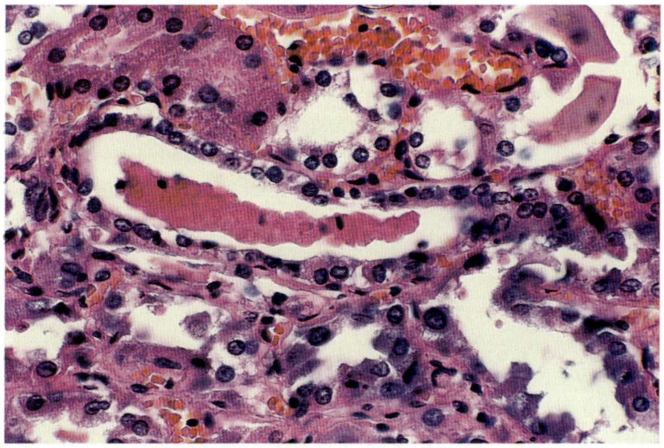

Figure 55–13. Higher magnification of degenerative changes in the renal tubules. An epithelial cast is in the lumen of one renal tubule (hematoxylin-eosin, ×250).

colonies that are blacker, glossy, and more convex; and *intermedius* colonies are very small and can be smooth or rough. Each colony type is subcultured on Columbia blood agar plate for toxigenic and biochemical testing. For microscopic morphology, the colonies are subcultured on Dorset's egg medium, then smeared on slides. The slides are stained by Loeffler's methylene blue and Albert's stain, both of which allow identification of metachromatic granules. However, immediate microscopic diagnosis by morphologic features of *C diphtheriae* from culture may be difficult. In some microbiologic media, the bacteria may stain variably or negatively, unlike the classic descriptions of organisms grown on Loeffler's serum medium or Dorset's egg medium. In fact, the organisms may have to be cultured on the more classic medium before they can be recognized by their morphologic features. *Corynebacterium diphtheriae* initially outgrows other throat flora when inoculated onto Loeffler's media, so that the culture plate should be examined within 24 hours for evidence of growth.

Although biochemical testing is irrelevant to patient management, it is an essential tool for biotyping, contact tracing, and epidemiologic studies. Biotyping is best performed on cultures that have incubated 24 to 28 hours.

Testing for toxigenicity is important and should be performed immediately. Although the test can be performed in vivo using guinea pigs, results are slow to develop. A more rapid method in vitro uses the modified Elek's immunodiffusion method, which can be done in a clinical laboratory. Results are available within 24 to 36 hours.

Vero cell bioassays, polymerase chain reaction, and ribotyping with restriction enzymes are also used to identify the tox^+ genes of *C diphtheriae.*[19] Few laboratories, however, are equipped to identify *C diphtheriae* rapidly and isolates can be sent to the Centers for Disease Control and Prevention, the central public health institution, for confirmation.

Although pathologic examination of infected tissues, including membranes, may reveal suggestive microscopic changes and bacilli that resemble *C diphtheriae,* definitive diagnosis rests on clinical and microbiologic results.[1,20]

Treatment and Prevention

The only specific treatment for diphtheria is antitoxin given when the diagnosis is first suspected. *Corynebacterium diphtheriae* is susceptible to a variety of antibiotics, and penicillin G is the drug of choice. Although antibiotics may prevent secondary infections, thereby reducing the subsequent carrier rate, they are an adjunct to therapy and given only in combination with antitoxin.

A diphtheria toxoid has been incorporated into a vaccine (DPT) that includes preparations of pertussis and tetanus toxoid. In the past, combination vaccines contained impure mixtures of formalin-inactivated diphtheria toxin that were 40% antigenically active. Newer vaccines, however, are pure and consist of cross-reacting mutants of diphtheria toxin containing toxoid more than 90% antigenically active. Revaccination every 10 years is recommended to maintain immunity.[21]

Corynebacterium minitissimum

Erythrasma is a cosmopolitan superficial skin infection that was described in 1859. Its etiology, however, remained unknown until 1961, when *C minitissimum* was identified as the cause. In addition to erythrasma, there have been scattered reports of other human infections with this agent: four patients had bacteremia, including three patients with hematologic malignancies and one patient undergoing hemodialysis with a pseudoaneurysmal fistula. Additional reports of infection by *C minitissimum* include breast abscess, a deep abscess following cervical discectomy, endocarditis, peritonitis associated with peritoneal dialysis, and a single patient with nonfluorescent erythrasma of the vulva.[22]

Corynebacterium ulcerans

Corynebacterium ulcerans is a commensal of horses that produces mastitis in cows. The organism has been isolated from cow's milk and many strains produce the diphtheria toxin and, occasionally, a dermonecrotic toxin as well. The majority of isolates of *C ulcerans* from humans have been from the respiratory tract, usually the throat in asymptomatic persons. A diphtheria-like disease, including exudative pharyngitis, pseudomembrane, and cardiac and neurologic manifestations due to *C ulcerans,* has been reported.[23]

Corynebacterium striatum

Corynebacterium striatum is a component of the normal bacterial flora of the anterior nares and skin. Although it is not highly pathogenic, it has caused a variety of human diseases. *Corynebacterium striatum* usually infects debilitated or immunodeficient patients who have underlying malignancies, neutropenia, or who are undergoing catheterization. Bacteremias and sepsis, infections of catheter sites, native valve endocarditis, purulent conjunctivitis, chorioamnionitis, infectious keratitis, and pyogenic granuloma have all been associated with *C striatum.*[22]

Corynebacterium xerosis

Corynebacterium xerosis is a commensal, nontoxigenic corynebacterium of humans, inhabiting the skin, nasopharynx, and conjunctival sac.[24] Similar to other species of nondiphtherial corynebacteria, it has been associated with a variety of infections, including septic arthritis, meningitis, endocarditis, bacteremia, pneumonia, intra-abdominal infection, keratitis, vertebral osteomyelitis, and mediastinitis.[22]

Corynebacterium Group D2

This organism was described by King in 1972 and has been isolated widely from the skin of hospitalized patients, especially women, and the organisms are highly resistant to multiple antibiotics. Group D2 organisms have been associated with alkaline-encrusted cystitis, a severe chronic urinary tract infection that is difficult to treat,[25] and also with pneumonia, peritonitis, endocarditis, osteomyelitis, wound infection, and bacteremia.

Actinomyces (Corynebacterium) pyogenes

Actinomyces pyogenes, until recently known as *Corynebacterium pyogenes,* was described in 1893 by Lucet. It is a commensal and pathogen of domestic animals and causes a variety of suppurative diseases (Figure 55–14) in cattle, sheep, swine, and goats. Rare infections of humans have been reported that were probably zoonotic. Infections have been well-documented, including bacteremia associated with colon cancer, abscesses, otitis media, cystitis, intra-abdominal infection, and bacteremic mastoiditis.[22,26] In addition, an annual outbreak of leg ulcers in Thai schoolchildren has been attributed to this agent.

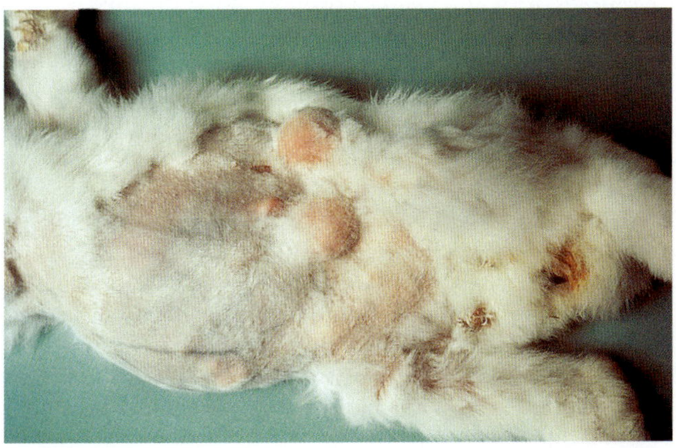

Figure 55–14. *Actinomyces* (*Corynebacterium*) *pyogenes* causing multiple subcutaneous abscesses in an experimentally infected rabbit. *(Courtesy of the Centers for Disease Control and Prevention, Atlanta.)*

Corynebacterium bovis

These bacilli are common commensals in the udders of cows, and in milk they hydrolyze butterfat, making the milk rancid. There are eight reports of human infection with *C bovis*[22]: Three patients had infections of the central nervous system, three patients had endocarditis of prosthetic valves, one patient had chronic otitis media and mastoiditis, and one patient had a chronic leg ulcer after falling on a meat bone in a butcher's shop.[27]

Corynebacterium pseudodiphtheriticum

Corynebacterium pseudodiphtheriticum was first described in 1896 as *Bacillus pseudodiphtheriticum,* and is a normal, nontoxigenic member of the pharyngeal flora in humans. It has been associated with endocarditis in 18 persons with both native and prosthetic valvular disease.[24,28] In addition, *C pseudodiphtheriticum* has been associated with malakoplakia of the urinary tract, infections of upper and lower respiratory tracts, suppurative lymphadenitis, and infection of a skin graft donor site, all in immunodeficient hosts.[22]

Corynebacterium jeikeium (Group JK)

Corynebacterium jeikeium was first described in 1976, and has been renamed JK.[29] This organism causes sepsis in patients with malignant diseases and concomitant risk factors, including prolonged hospitalization and neutropenia, treatment with multiple antibiotics, and integumentary disruption. *Corynebacterium jeikeium* appears to be a normal inhabitant of the skin of hospitalized patients, especially males, and the most common sites of colonization are the rectum, inguinal, and axillary areas. Most infections are nosocomial, and approximately one third to one half of patients admitted to cancer centers are colonized with this agent.[22] Diseases attributable to *C jeikeium* include septicemia, infections of the skin and soft tissue, endocarditis, abscesses, pneumonitis, peritonitis, and wound infections.

Corynebacterium pseudotuberculosis

This agent had been previously termed the Preisz–Nocard bacillus after the investigators who discovered it, and *Corynebacterium ovis* because of its initial isolation from the necrotic kidney of a sheep. Although *C pseudotuberculosis* is an important infectious agent, producing pneumonia, abscesses, and suppurative lymphadenitis in a variety of animals including horses, cattle, deer, and goats, human infection was not reported until 1966. Almost all strains of

C pseudotuberculosis produce a dermonecrotic toxin, and some isolates produce a diphtheria toxin. The majority of human infections with this agent produced suppurative and granulomatous lymphadenitis in persons who had contact with animals, drank raw milk, or handled animal offal and hides.[24,30]

Arcanobacterium (*Corynebacterium*) *haemolyticum*

This agent was first isolated during World War II from infected American soldiers stationed in the South Pacific. Although previously called a *Corynebacterium*, it has been reclassified into the new genus *Arcanobacterium*. It is a commensal of the skin and pharynx of asymptomatic persons and is rarely found in animals. The majority of human infections result in pharyngitis and chronic skin ulcers, but there have been occasional reports of *A haemolyticum* associated with osteomyelitis, meningitis, brain abscess, endocarditis, septicemia, and cavitary pneumonia.[22]

REFERENCES

1. MacGregor RR. *Corynebacterium diphtheriae.* In: Mandell GL, Bennett JE, Dolin R, eds. *Principles and Practice of Infectious Diseases.* 4th ed. New York: Churchill Livingstone, Inc.; 1995:1865–1872.
2. Schwartz DA, Herman CJ. The importance of the autopsy in emerging and reemerging infectious diseases. *Clin Infect Dis.* 1996;23:in press.
3. Agrifoglio L. Historical delineation of diphtheria. *Riv Ital Igiene.* 1961;21:205.
4. Loeffler F. Untersuchungen über die Bedeutung der Mikroorganismen für die Entstehung der Diphtherie. *Mitt Kaiserlichen Gesundheitsamt.* 1884;2:421–499.
5. Roux E, Yersin A. Contribution a l'etude de la diphtherie. *Ann Inst Pasteur.* 1889;iii:273–288.
6. Ehrlich P. Die Werthbemessung des Diphtherieheilserums und deren theoretische Grundlagen. *Klin Jahrb.* 1897;vi:299–326.
7. Rosenthal R. The story of diphtheria. *Minn Med.* 1960;43:627.
8. Babes. Les spores des bacilles de la diphtherie humaine; nouvelle coloration des tissus normaux et pathologiques. *Progres Med Par.* 1886;2:154.
9. Ernst P. Ueber Kern-und Sporenbildung in Bacterien. *Ztschr f Hyg.* 1988;99:428–486.
10. Cowan ML. Separation of virulent cultures of *B diphtheriae* into virulent and avirulent types. *Brit J Exper Path.* 1927;8:6–11.
11. Centers for Disease Control and Prevention. Summary of Notifiable Diseases, United States—1993.
12. Wilson APR, Efstratiou A, Weaver E, et al. Unusual non-toxigenic *Corynebacterium diphtheriae* in homosexual men. *Lancet.* 1992;339:998.
13. Millar OS, Cooper ON, Kakkar VV, et al. Invasive infection with *Corynebacterium diphtheriae* among drug users. *Lancet.* 1992;339:1359.
14. Melby EL, Jacobsen J, Olsnes S, et al. Entry of protein toxins in polarized epithelial cells. *Cancer Res.* 1993;53:1755–1759.
15. Pappenheimer AM, Gill DM. Diphtheria: recent studies have clarified the molecular mechanisms involved in its pathogenesis. *Science.* 1973;182:353–358.
16. Pappenheimer AM, Murphy JR. Studies in the molecular epidemiology of diphtheria. *Lancet.* 1983;ii:923–926.
17. Brooks GF, Bennett JV, Feldman RA. Diphtheria in the United States, 1959–1970. *J Infect Dis.* 1974;129:172–178.
18. Edington GM, Gilles HM. *Pathology in the Tropics.* 2nd ed. London: Edward Arnold; 1976:372.
19. Zoysa AD, Efstratiou A, George RC, et al. Molecular epidemiology of *Corynebacterium diphtheriae* from northwestern Russia and surrounding countries studied by using ribotyping and pulsed-field electrophoresis. *J Clin Microbiol.* 1995;33:1080–1083.
20. Brooks R, Joynson DHM. Bacteriological diagnosis of diphtheria. *J Clin Pathol.* 1990;43:576–580.
21. Popovic T, Wharton M, Wenger JD, et al. Are we ready for diphtheria? *J Inf Dis.* 1995;171:765–767.
22. Brown AE. Other corynebacteria and *Rhodococcus.* In: Mandell GL, Bennett JE, Dolin R, eds. *Principles and Practice of Infectious Diseases.* 4th ed. New York: Churchill Livingstone; 1995:1872–1878.
23. Meers PD. A case of classical diphtheria and other infections due to *Corynebacterium ulcerans. J Infect.* 1979;1:139–142.
24. Lipsky BA, Goldberger AC, Tompkins LS, et al. Infections caused by non-diphtheria corynebacteria. *Rev Infect Dis.* 1982;4:1220–1235.
25. Soriano F, Ponte C, Santamaria M, et al. *Corynebacterium* group D2 as a cause of alkaline encrusted cystitis: report of four cases and characterization of the organisms. *J Clin Microbiol.* 1985;21:788–792.
26. Gahrn-Hansen B, Federiksen W. Human infection with *Actinomyces pyogenes* (*Corynebacterium pyogenes*). *Diagn Microbiol Infect Dis.* 1992;15:349–354.
27. Vale JA, Scott GW. *Corynebacterium bovis* as a cause of human disease. *Lancet.* 1977;2:682–684.
28. Murray BA, Karchmer AW, Moellering RC. Diphtheroid prosthetic valve endocarditis. *Am J Med.* 1980;69:838–848.
29. Coyle MB, Lipsky BA. Coryneform bacteria in infectious diseases: clinical and laboratory aspects. *Clin Microbiol Rev.* 1990;3:227–246.
30. Richards M, Hurse A. *Corynebacterium pseudotuberculosis* abscesses in a young butcher. *Aust NZ J Med.* 1985;15:85–86.

CHAPTER 56

Ehrlichial Infections

J. Stephen Dumler and David H. Walker

Man sees it (infections) from his own prejudiced point of view; but clams, oysters, insects, fish, flowers, tobacco, potatoes, tomatoes, fruit, shrubs, trees, have their own varieties of small pox, measles, cancer, or tuberculosis. Incessantly, the pitiless war goes on, without quarter or armistice—a nationalism of species against species.

Hans Zinsser (1878–1940)

DEFINITION

Ehrlichioses are infections caused by obligate intracellular bacteria of the genus *Ehrlichia.* Although veterinary ehrlichial infection is well known, human infection has been identified only recently.[1] Two ehrlichial agents cause human disease: *Ehrlichia sennetsu,*[2] the agent of a mononucleosis-like illness in the Far East, and *E chaffeenis,*[3,4] the newly characterized agent of ehrlichiosis in the United States.

The agents of ehrlichiosis are grouped in the family *Rickettsiaceae.*[7] They are obligate intracellular bacteria and live part of their life in an invertebrate host. Unlike rickettsiae that infect endothelial cells, the target cell of the *Ehrlichia* are the phagocytic cells derived from the hematopoietic system. Depending on the species of *Ehrlichia,* the infected cells are macrophages/monocytes or neutrophils. The *Ehrlichia* attach by means of a surface protein to a host cell receptor, gain access to an endosome, and actively inhibit lysosome fusion.[8] Within the cytoplasmic vacuole, the ehrlichiae proliferate by binary fission to form clusters bound by a trilaminar host cell cytoplasmic membrane. In vitro infection causes cytolysis of host cells, yet in vivo the organisms may be difficult to detect, indicating that a mechanism of injury not mediated by the bacteria may exist.[9]

Human infection by an *E canis*-like agent was first documented in 1986 in a patient who had a tick bite and suffered a near-fatal illness.[1] The initial clinical impression was Rocky Mountain spotted fever, a diagnosis not confirmed by serology. Intraleukocytic inclusions resembling those in canine ehrlichiosis were noted during the acute phase of illness, and a serologic response to *E canis* antigens was demonstrated in convalescent serum. After this discovery, many additional patients thought to have Rocky Mountain spotted fever were found to have ehrlichiosis instead.[10–12] In 1991, the first human isolate of an ehrlichia in the United States was reported.[3] The new agent is serologically similar to *E canis,* but genetic typing showed significant DNA sequence differences.[4] The new species was named *E chaffeensis.*

Recently, a granulocytotropic ehrlichia has been identified in circulating neutrophils of febrile patients.[5] The bacteria were closely related to the veterinary agents, *E phagocytophila* and *E equi,* by molecular methods.[6]

Studies of Japanese patients with infectious mononucleosis in the 1950s led to the isolation of a rickettsial agent in some cases.[2] The clinical illness associated with infection by *E sennetsu* is rarely recognized and is called *sennetsu ehrlichiosis* or *sennetsu fever.*[13]

GEOGRAPHIC DISTRIBUTION

Human monocytic ehrlichiosis, as described in the United States, has been documented in 27 states,[3] and recently cases from Portugal[14] in Europe and from Mali in Africa[15] have been recognized. Human granulocytic ehrlichiosis has been documented in the upper Midwest and the northeastern states. The exact distribution of the human ehrlichioses in the United States is still being determined. Sennetsu ehrlichiosis occurs in Japan and specific areas of Malaysia.[16] No cases have been identified elsewhere.

LIFE CYCLE, NATURAL HISTORY, AND EPIDEMIOLOGY

Ehrlichioses in the United States are associated with exposure to ticks and to tick bites.[11,12] *Ehrlichia chaffeensis*-specific DNA sequences have been detected mainly in the Lone Star tick (*Amblyomma americanum*)[17] and less frequently in the American dog tick (*Dermacentor variabilis*), which have geographic distributions closely approximating human monocytic ehrlichiosis.[4] The related species, *E canis,* is maintained in nature through horizontal transmission from tick to canid to tick. Transovarial transmission of infection does not occur in ticks.[18] In fact, dogs are susceptible to prolonged asymptomatic infection by *E chaffeensis* and may be a reservoir.[19] White-tailed deer, which also are susceptible to infection and ehrlichemia of 2 weeks duration, are a likely reservoir.[20,21]

Both human monocytic and granulocytic ehrlichioses are seen during seasons with tick activity, and infection is acquired most often in rural areas. Most patients are male, and the incubation period is usually 7 to 10 days.[11,12] Infection with *E chaffeensis* is more common than previously suspected, with a prevalence rate of 27% in febrile patients after recent tick exposure in a highly endemic area of Arkansas.[22] *Ixodes scapularis* is the suspected vector of human granulocytic ehrlichiosis.

The specific vector of sennetsu ehrlichiosis is unknown. Some authors suggest ticks; others suggest ingestion of seafood infested with ehrlichia-containing helminths.[23]

MORPHOLOGIC FEATURES OF THE ORGANISM

Ehrlichiae are small (0.2 to 1.0 μm), pleomorphic coccoid bacteria (Figure 56–1). Because their obligate intracellular lifestyle is adapted to the environment of endosomes,[8] *E chaffeensis* and the human granulocytic ehrlichia grow into clusters called *morulae* located in the cytoplasm[3] of the infected host phagocytes, usually macrophages and monocytes for *E chaffeensis* and neutrophils for the *E phagocytophila*-like agent.[9] Each morula may contain many ehrlichial "elementary bodies" and thus may be as large at 10 μm in diameter. In vivo usually only one morula is present per infected cell, and even in severe infection morulae of *E chaffeensis* are extremely difficult to locate in peripheral blood, bone marrow, and tissue.[9] When stained by Giemsa, Wright, or Leishman methods, the morulae and elementary bodies are dark violet-blue and stippled (Figure 56–2, A). The majority of cases of human granulocytic ehrlichiosis diagnosed thus far have had morula-containing neutrophils in blood smears. Ultrastructural study of *E chaffeensis* reveals bacteria with a gram-negative cell wall clustered within a membrane-bound vacuole in the cytoplasm of the host cell.[3] Morphologically, *E sennetsu* is similar but tends to occur as individual membrane-bound organisms.

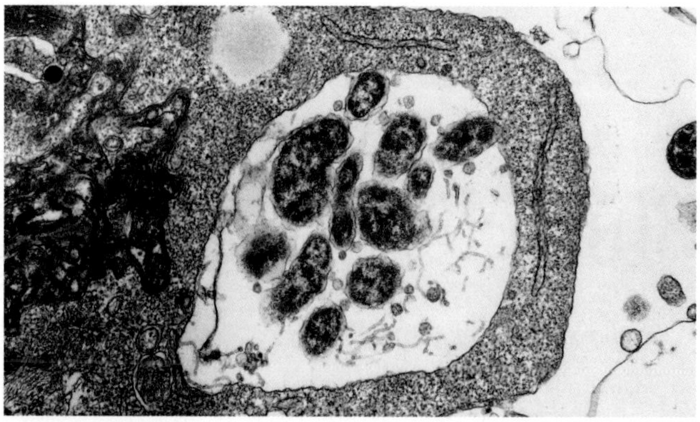

Figure 56–1. Electron photomicrograph of *E chaffeensis* cultivated in vitro in a histiocytic tissue culture cell line. Note the pleomorphic coccoid and bacillary forms sequestered within a cytoplasmic vacuole (×24,375).

CLINICAL FEATURES

The clinical presentation frequently involves headache, fever, and myalgias; gastrointestinal symptoms such as nausea and vomiting are slightly less frequent.[11,12,24] Rash occurs in less than half of adult patients, but is common in children.[11,24,25] No specific skin lesion has been consistently identified, and petechial lesions are inconstant. Occasional patients suffer from meningitis,[24,26–30] pneumonitis,[31] renal failure,[28] cholestatic jaundice,[32] or hepatitis.[11] Important laboratory features are mild to moderate leukopenia, thrombocytopenia, and elevations of serum hepatic transaminases.[11,12] The nadir of leukopenia averages from 1300 to 4000 cells/μL, and concentrations of both neutrophils and lymphocytes in the circulation may be decreased.[11,12] Thrombocytopenia is concurrent with leukopenia, usually between 50,000 and 140,000 platelets/μL, but may be severe (<20,000 platelets/μL).[9,11] Clinical severity ranges from asymptomatic[22] to fatal,[9,29,33,34] and tetracycline therapy may promote rapid recovery.[28] Most patients recover, but convalescence may be prolonged.[1,11] Reliable mortality data are not available, but approximately 2% have died.

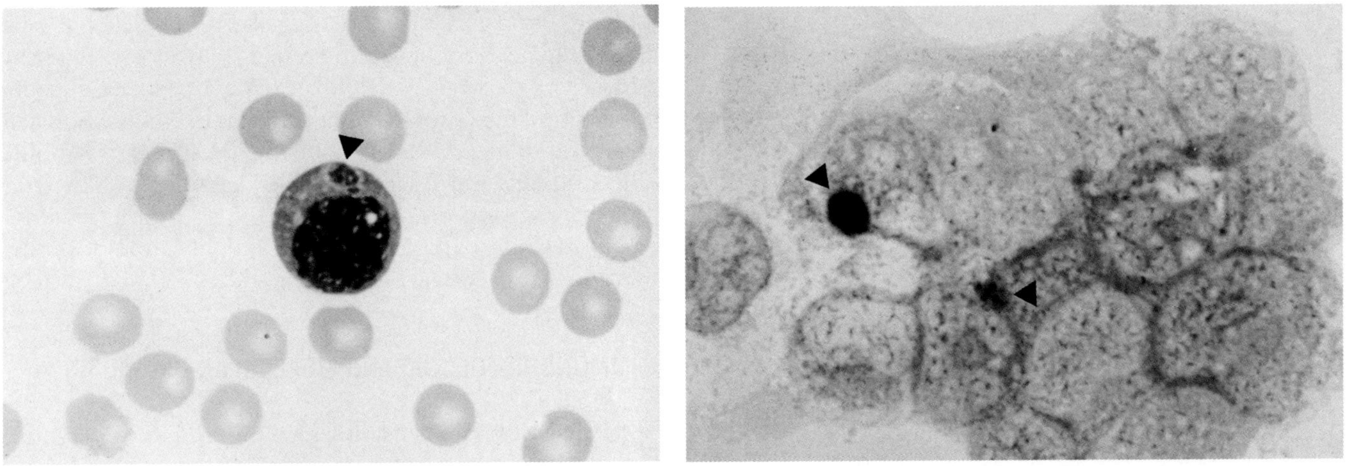

A B

Figure 56–2. *Ehrlichia chaffeensis* morula (*arrows*) in (**A**) a peripheral blood mononuclear cell (Wright's stain, ×1600) and in (**B**) a cerebrospinal fluid mononuclear cell (labeled streptavidin-biotin immunoalkaline phosphatase with hematoxylin counterstain, ×1600). Note the intracytoplasmic location, and often a stippled appearance corresponding to individual ehrlichia.

PATHOLOGY

Because of the frequent hematologic alterations in human monocytic ehrlichiosis, bone marrow changes have been examined extensively. Marrow hyperplasia, due to myeloid or pancellular proliferation and megakaryocytosis, is most common, although hypocellular and normocellular marrows occasionally are encountered.[9,35,36] Three fourths of patients have increased mononuclear phagocytic activity in the bone marrow, with granulomas, ring granulomas, or poorly formed granulomatous or foamy histiocytic infiltrations (Figure 56–3).[9] Nonspecific findings include erythrophagocytosis, plasmacytosis, and lymphoid aggregates. Necrosis is rarely encountered in nonfatal infections. Fatal cases often have poorly formed granulomas or collections of foamy histiocytes in bone marrow and other tissues.[9] Bone marrow hyperplasia associated with leuko-, thrombo-, or pancytopenia is strong evidence that these hematopoietic elements are consumed or destroyed during infection. In spite of these findings, there is no evidence of thrombosis or vasculitis with consumptive coagulopathy.

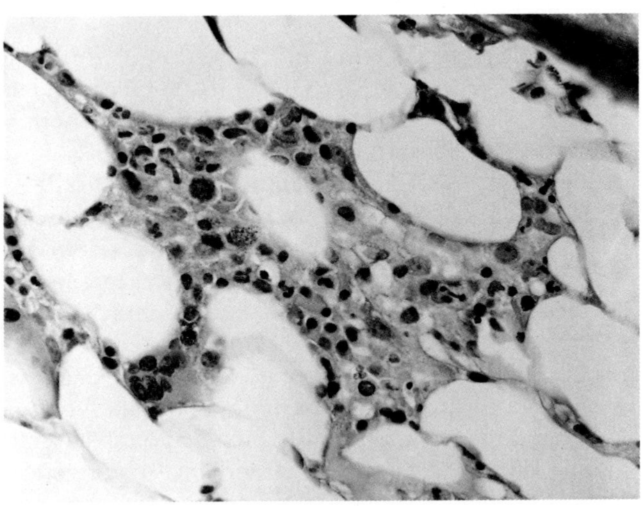

Figure 56–3. Small focus of foamy histiocytes infiltrating hypocellular bone marrow in fatal ehrlichiosis (hematoxylin-eosin; ×460).

Although mild perivascular lymphohistiocytic infiltrates are in almost every tissue, organs with active mononuclear phagocytic systems have the most pronounced changes.[31] The liver may have mild Kupffer's cell hyperplasia with occasional intrasinusoidal foamy histiocytes, periportal and perivascular lymphohistiocytic infiltrates, and focal hepatocytic necrosis (Figure 56–4). Hepatic granulomas and cholestasis also may be present.[31,32] Similarly, the liver and spleen may have focal necroses on a background of mild histiocytosis.[31] Depletion of lymphocytes, as described in veterinary ehrlichioses,[23] is infrequent. Pulmonary changes may be minimal but include interstitial mononuclear cell pneumonitis; secondary changes such as pulmonary hemorrhage and viral or bacterial superinfection may intervene to worsen and obscure the original ehrlichial pathologic pattern.[37] Diffuse alveolar damage may result in a macrophage-rich organizing pneumonia in the absence of known complicating infections. Involvement of the central nervous system is dem-

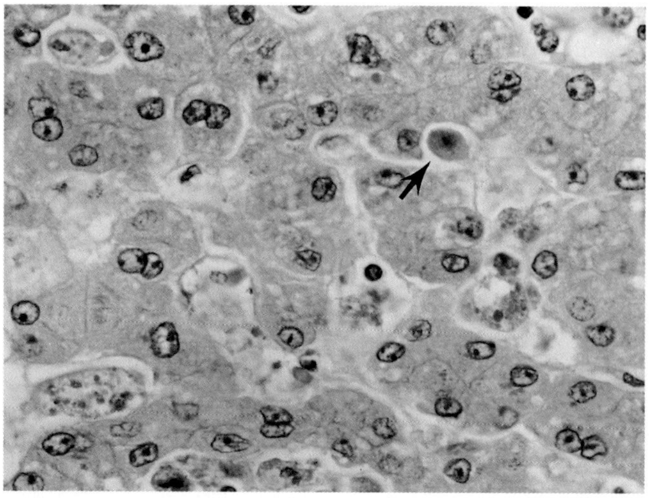

Figure 56–4. Hepatic changes in ehrlichiosis include focal and individual cell hepatic necroses (acidophil bodies; *arrow*) and Kupffer's cell hyperplasia. Note the foamy histiocytes (presumably Kupffer's cells) in the sinusoidal spaces (hematoxylin-eosin, ×580).

onstrated by cerebrospinal fluid mononuclear cell pleocytosis and mild to moderate perivascular lymphohistiocytic infiltrates in the meninges and less commonly in brain.[11,26–28] Because of the concurrent ehrlichia-induced thrombocytopenia and leukopenia, severe infection may result in hemorrhagic or secondary infectious complications.[37]

The use of special stains may suggest the cause, because morulae may be identified by Giemsa or silver impregnation methods.[38] These techniques are nonspecific and lack sensitivity. Furthermore, even if a few ehrlichiae are present, they may resemble cellular granules, and thus these nonspecific methods may be of little diagnostic value. The observation of typical morulae in appropriate cells warrants the use of more specific confirmatory methods.[30,31,39]

DIFFERENTIAL DIAGNOSIS

The clinical presentation of undifferentiated fever invokes a wide differential diagnosis.[37,40] Entities such as Rocky Mountain spotted fever, meningococcemia, bacterial sepsis or endocarditis, toxic shock syndrome, influenza, typhoid fever, Q fever, Kawasaki disease, infectious mononucleosis, other viral infections, and idiopathic or thrombotic thrombocytopenic purpura may be considered. With involvement of a specific organ system the differential diagnosis also changes, and may include viral hepatitis, viral meningoencephalitis, acute gastroenteritis, or pneumonia. In patients with severe leukopenia, hematologic or lymphoid neoplasia may be suggested.[41] A tick bite suggests Lyme borreliosis, tularemia, babesiosis, relapsing fever, or Colorado tick fever. The nonspecific pathologic findings provide evidence to exclude neoplastic and vasculitic disorders, but the presence of granulomas widens the list of possible diagnoses. Knowledge of the local occurrence of ehrlichiosis and its potential clinical and pathologic presentations should prompt further diagnostic evaluation.

IMMUNOHISTOLOGIC AND MOLECULAR DIAGNOSIS

Because nonspecific stains may be useless in diagnosis, the immunochemical demonstration of ehrlichial morulae may provide specific and timely evidence of infection.[28,31,42] Although currently available only in research institutions, the immunoperoxidase method has been used to identify *E chaffeensis* in tissues and cytologic preparations from patients with suspected infection (Figure 56–2, B). The method is equally applicable to paraffin-embedded, formalin-fixed tissues and fresh acetone-fixed frozen sections or air-dried, fixed smears. The added advantage of increased contrast and demonstration of specific antigens make this procedure potentially very useful. Unfortunately, this method also is somewhat insensitive, and the absence of demonstrable ehrlichiae does not exclude the diagnosis because so few organisms are in tissues. The polymerase chain reaction technique has been developed for blood taken in the acute phase of infection and appears to be the most sensitive and useful technique for timely and early diagnosis.[30,39]

CONFIRMATIONAL TESTING AND DIAGNOSIS

Although desirable, the in vitro cultivation of ehrlichiae is difficult.[3] Aside from specialized tissue culture methods and cell lines, isolation of ehrlichiae from peripheral blood may require longer than 1 month of cultivation and observation.[3] Because of these problems, microbiologic culture in its current state is not useful. The predominant method of diagnosis relies on the retrospective demonstration of a serologic response in convalescent serum tested with specific ehrlichial antigens by an indirect immunofluorescence method.[43] This is done in very few laboratories or at the Centers for Disease Control and Prevention, and thus serologic confirmation is not useful during the acute infection. In time, a better understanding of ehrlichial pathogenesis will foster creative methods for timely diagnosis and will result in early effective therapy for this potentially fatal zoonosis.

REFERENCES

1. Maeda K, Markowitz N, Hawley RC, Ristic M, Cox D, McDade JE. Human infection with *Ehrlichia canis*, a leukocytic rickettsia. *N Engl J Med.* 1987;316:853–856.
2. Misao T, Kobayashi Y. Studies on infectious mononucleosis (glandular fever): I. Isolation of etiologic agent from blood, bone marrow and lymph node of a patient with infectious mononucleosis by using mice. *Kyushu J Med Sci.* 1955;6:145–152.
3. Dawson JE, Anderson BE, Fishbein DB, et al. Isolation and characterization of an *Ehrlichia* sp. from a patient diagnosed with human ehrlichiosis. *J Clin Mircobiol.* 1991;29:2741–2745.
4. Anderson BE, Dawson JE, Jones DC, Wilson KH. *Ehrlichia chaffeensis*, a new species associated with human ehrlichiosis. *J Clin Microbiol.* 1991;29:2838–2842.
5. Bakken JS, Dumler JS, Chen S-M, Eckman MR, Van Etta LL, Walker DH. Human granulocytic ehrlichiosis in the upper Midwest United States: a new species emerging? *JAMA.* 1994;272:212–218.
6. Chen S-M, Dumler JS, Bakken JS, Walker DH. Identification of a granulocytotropic *Ehrlichia* species as the etiologic agent of human disease. *J Clin Microbiol.* 1994;32:589–595.
7. Ristic M, Huxsoll DL. Ehrlichiae. In: Kreig NR, Holt JG, eds. *Bergey's Manual of Systematic Bacteriology.* Baltimore, Md: Williams & Wilkins; 1984:704–709.
8. Wells M, Rikihisa Y. Lack of lysosomal fusion with phagosomes containing *Ehrlichia risticii* in P388D_1 cells: abrogation of inhibition with oxytetracycline. *Infect Immun.* 1988;56:3209–3215.
9. Dumler JS, Dawson JE, Walker DH. Human ehrlichiosis: hematopathology and immunohistologic detection of *Ehrlichia chaffeensis. Hum Pathol.* 1993;24:391–396.
10. Fishbein DB, Sawyer LA, Holland CJ, et al. Unexplained febrile illnesses after exposure to ticks: infection with an *Ehrlichia? JAMA.* 1987;257:3100–3104.
11. Eng TR, Harkess JR, Fishbein DB, et al. Epidemiologic, clinical, and laboratory findings of human ehrlichiosis in the United States, 1988. *JAMA.* 1990;264:2251–2258.
12. Rohrbach BW, Harkess JR, Ewing SA, Kudlac J, McKee GL, Istre GR. Epidemiologic and clinical characteristics of persons with serologic evidence of *Ehrlichia canis* infection. *Am J Public Health.* 1990;80:442–445.
13. Tachibana N. Sennetsu fever: the disease, diagnosis, and treatment. In: Leive L, ed. *Microbiology—1986.* Washington, DC: American Society for Microbiology; 1986:205–208.
14. Morais J, Dawson JE, Greene C, Filipe AR, Galhardas LC, Bacellar F. First European case of ehrlichiosis. *Lancet.* 1991;338:633–634.
15. Uhaa IJ, MacLean JD, Greene CR, Fishbein DB. A case of human ehrlichiosis acquired in Mali: clinical and laboratory findings. *Am J Trop Med Hyg.* 1992;46:161–164.
16. Rapmund G. Rickettsial disease in the Far East: new perspectives. *J Infect Dis.* 1984;149:330–338.
17. Anderson BE, Sims KG, Olson JG, et al. *Amblyomma americanum*: a potential vector of human ehrlichiosis. *Am J Trop Med Hyg.* 1993;49:239–244.
18. Smith RD, Sells DM, Stephenson EH, Ristic M, Huxsoll DL. Development of *Ehrlichia canis,* causative agent of canine ehrlichiosis, in the tick *Rhipicephalus sanguineus* and its differentiation from a symbiotic rickettsia. *Am J Vet Res.* 1976;37:119–126.
19. Dawson JE, Ewing SA. Susceptibility of dogs to infection with *Ehrlichia chaffeensis,* the causative agent of human ehrlichiosis. *Am J Vet Res.* 1992;53:1322–1327.
20. Dawson JE, Childs JE, Biggie KL, et al. White-tailed deer as a potential reservoir of *Ehrlichia* spp. *J Wildl Dis.* 1994;30:162–168.
21. Dawson JE, Stallknecht DE, Howerth EW, et al. Susceptibility of white-tailed deer (*Odocoileus virginianus*) to infection with *Ehrlichia chaffeensis,* the etiologic agent of human ehrlichiosis. *J Clin Microbiol.* 1994;32:2725–2728.
22. Uhaa IJ, Sanchez JL, Dawson JE, Greene CR, Kardatzke JT, Fishbein DB. Epidemiologic, clinical, and serologic investigation of patients with suspected tick-borne illnesses. In: Program and Abstracts of the Ninth Sesqui-Annual Meeting of the American Society of Rickettsiology and Rickettsial Diseases, 1991:45.
23. Rikihisa Y. The tribe *Ehrlichieae* and ehrlichial diseases. *Clin Microbiol Rev.* 1991;4:286–308.
24. Fishbein DB, Dawson JE, Robinson LE. Human ehrlichiosis in the United States, 1985 to 1990. *Ann Intern Med.* 1994;120:736–743.
25. Harkess JR, Ewing SA, Brumit T, Mettry CR. Ehrlichiosis in children. *Pediatrics.* 1991;87:199–203.
26. Dimmitt DC, Fishbein DB, Dawson JE. Human ehrlichiosis associated with cerebrospinal fluid pleocytosis: a case report. *Am J Med.* 1989;87:677–678.
27. Golden SE. Aseptic meningitis associated with *Ehrlichia canis* infection. *Pediatr Infect Dis J.* 1989;8:335–337.
28. Dunn BE, Monson TE, Dumler JS, et al. Identification of *Ehrlichia chaffeensis* morulae in cerebrospinal fluid mononuclear cells. *J Clin Microbiol.* 1992;30:2207–2210.
29. Fichtenbaum CJ, Peterson LR, Weil GJ. Ehrlichiosis presenting as a life-threatening illness with features of the toxic shock syndrome. *Am J Med.* 1993;95:351–357.
30. Everett ED, Evans KA, Henry RB, McDonald G. Human ehrlichiosis in adults after tick exposure. *Ann Intern Med.* 1994;120:730–735.
31. Dumler JS, Brouqui P, Aronson JF, Taylor JP, Walker DH. Identification of *Ehrlichia* in human tissues. *N Engl J Med.* 1991;325:1109–1110. Letter.
32. Moskovitz M, Fadden R, Min T. Human ehrlichiosis: a rickettsial disease associated with severe cholestasis and multisystemic disease. *J Clin Gastroenterol.* 1991;13:86–90.
33. Dumler JS, Sutker WL, Walker DH. Persistent infection with *Ehrlichia chaffeensis. Clin Infect Dis.* 1993;17:903–905.
34. Paddock CD, Suchard DP, Grumbach KL, et al. Brief report: fatal seronegative ehrlichiosis in a patient with HIV infection. *N Engl J Med.* 1993;329:1164–1167.
35. Pearce CJ, Conrad ME, Nolan PE, Fishbein DB, Dawson JE. Ehrlichiosis: a cause of bone marrow hypoplasia in humans. *Am J Hematol.* 1988;28:53–55.

36. Harkess JR. Ehrlichiosis: a cause of bone marrow hypoplasia in humans. *Am J Hematol.* 1989;30:265–266. Letter.
37. Dumler JS, Walker DH. Human ehrlichiosis. *Curr Op Infect Dis.* 1991;4:597–602.
38. Steele KE, Rikihisa Y, Walton AM. Ehrlichia of Potomac horse fever identified with a silver stain. *Vet Pathol.* 1986; 23:531–533.
39. Anderson BE, Sumner JW, Dawson JE, et al. Detection of the etiologic agent of human ehrlichiosis by polymerase chain reaction. *J Clin Microbiol.* 1992;30:775–780.
40. Harkess JR. Ehrlichiosis. *Infect Dis Clin North Am.* 1991; 5:37–51.
41. Caldwell CW, Poje E, Cooperstock M. Expansion of immature thymic precursor cells in peripheral blood after acute marrow suppression. *Am J Clin Pathol.* 1991;95:824–827.
42. Yu X, Brouqui P, Dumler JS, Raoult D. Detection of *Ehrlichia chaffeensis* in human tissue by using a species-specific monoclonal antibody. *J Clin Mircobiol.* 1993;31: 3284–3288.
43. Dawson JE, Rikihisa Y, Ewing SA, Fishbein DB. Serologic diagnosis of human ehrlichiosis using two *Ehrlichia canis* isolates. *J Infect Dis.* 1991:163:564–567.

CHAPTER 57

Erythrasma

Jacqueline M. Junkins-Hopkins and Thomas D. Griffin

And Asa in the thirty and ninth year of his reign was diseased in his feet, until his disease was exceeding great: yet in his disease he sought not to the Lord, but to the physicians.

II Chronicles 16:12

Mankind, it has been said, is always advancing, man is always the same. The love, hope, fear and faith that make humanity, and the elemental passions of the human heart, remain unchanged, and the secret of inspiration in any literature is the capacity to touch the cord that vibrates in a sympathy that knows nor time nor place.

Sir William Osler (1849–1919), A Way of Life

DEFINITION

Erythrasma is a superficial bacterial infection of the skin caused by *Corynebacterium minutissimum,* which typically involves the intertriginous sites. It is characterized by scaly red to brown patches or scaling between the toes that emit a red-orange fluorescence when examined with Wood's light.

ETIOLOGY AND PATHOGENESIS

Erythrasma has been recognized since 1859.[1] Initially the causative agent was called *Microsporum minutissimum,* erroneously assuming it was a fungus. Erythrasma continued to be ascribed to various filamentous organisms such as *Nocardia* until 1961,[1] when the organism was established as a gram-positive diphtheroid and thus renamed *Corynebacterium minutissimum* (from Greek, n. *coryne,* "a club," and n. *bakterion,* "a small rod"; Latin sup. adj. *minutissimus,* "very small"). These organisms are nonmotile, non-spore-forming facultative anaerobes, which are pleomorphic, straight to slightly curved rods with tapered and occasionally club-shaped ends.[2]

As with other diphtheroids, *C minutissimum* is a component of the normal skin flora.[3] It may, however, cause lesions, which are enhanced by an occlusive, humid environment. The fluorescence, emitted at 365 nm of ultraviolet light, is caused by a water-soluble porphyrin produced by the organism.[1] Fluorescent diphtheroids also have been cultured from sites without lesions,[4,5] and it has been suggested that the condition of erythrasma be limited to the classic brawny, round, scaly, truncal lesions. Moreover, some have questioned whether *C minutissimum* plays a primary or secondary causal role in erythrasma.[5] In support of a secondary role is the fact that scaling from maceration and chafing can precede colonization with fluorescent diphtheroids.[6] Nevertheless, lesions of erythrasma have been induced experimentally in healthy volunteers,[1] and it appears there is some causal role of *C minutissimum* in erythrasma, albeit not completely defined.

EPIDEMIOLOGY

Erythrasma is seen in many parts of the world. It is typically in adults—both men and women—but all ages are susceptible, afflicting patients as young as 1 year.[7]

The prevalence may be underestimated, but has been documented to range from 3% to 25%, depending on the population studied.[7] As a mild subclinical form involving the toe webs, it may be quite common,[8] occurring in more than 50% of male recruits in the Danish armed forces.[8] Genitocrural lesions are more prominent in men, although clinically apparent truncal disease, in general, is seen less frequently.[7] Widespread or generalized lesions are rare and more prevalent in tropical and subtropical climates and in middle-aged black women.[7] Diabetics[9] and people in institutions[10] are also more prone to erythrasma.

CLINICAL

Mild forms of erythrasma present as asymptomatic scaling or maceration between the toes, especially between the lateral two toe webs. Clinically apparent erythrasma typically appears as irregularly shaped, well-circumscribed patches that are initially smooth, but later develop a fine wrinkling or obvious scale (Figure 57–1). The color may vary, ranging from red or pink in earlier lesions, to orange-tan or brown in more established lesions (Figures 57–2 and 57–3). Examined with a Wood's lamp, these lesions characteristically emit a coral-red fluorescence. Washing the affected area before examination, however, may eliminate this fluorescence.[7] Culture of *C minutissimum* is possible, in spite of negative fluorescence. The lesions tend to be asymptomatic, but may be slightly pruritic. Commonly afflicted areas include the groin, scrotum, and axillae but any intertriginous site may be affected, including the periumbilical region and anogenital area, where it may present as vulvar pruritus[11] or pruritus ani.[12] A concomitant infection by a dermatophyte such as in tinea cruris[13] or tinea pedis[8,14,15] is common. Erythrasma may also coexist with other coryneform-like disorders such as trichomycosis axillaris and pitted keratolysis.[16] Generalized lesions may appear atrophic and disciform,[17,18] simulating lichen sclerosus et atrophicus or parapsoriasis. The infection usually remains localized to the superficial epidermis, but *C minutissimum* abscesses have been reported.[19,20] In addition, septicemia[20] and endocarditis[21] have been documented in immunodeficient patients.

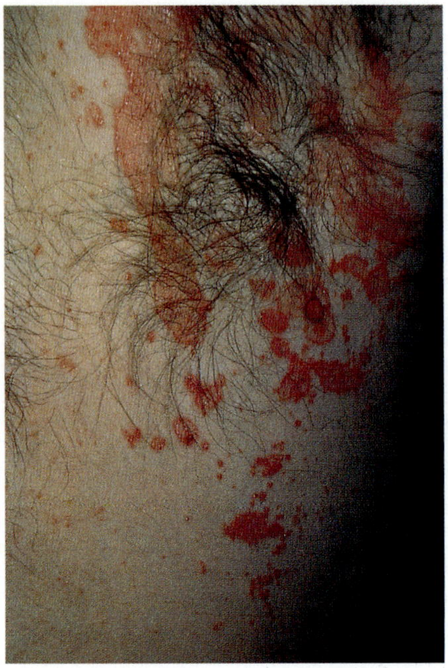

Figure 57–2. Orange-brown, well-circumscribed, scaly macules and plaques involving the axilla.

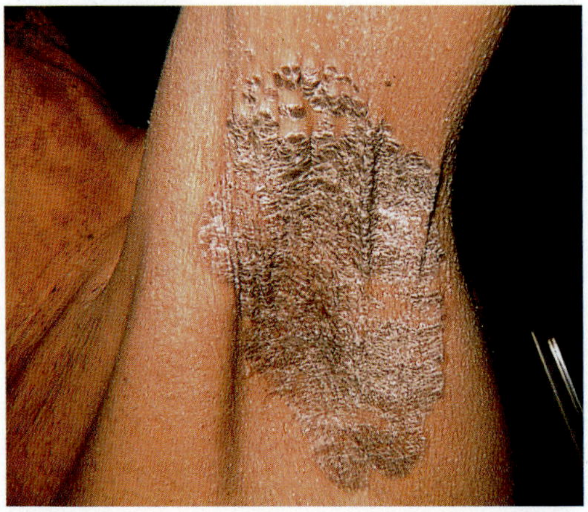

Figure 57–1. Well-circumscribed, hyperpigmented, scaly plaques involving the axilla.

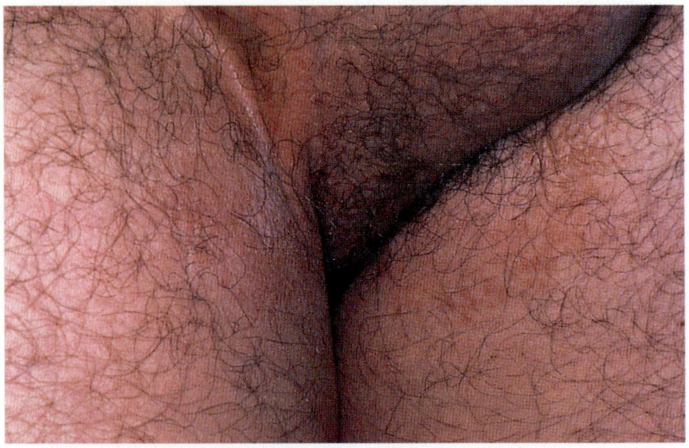

Figure 57–3. Pink to orange, minimally scaly patches involving the groin and upper thighs.

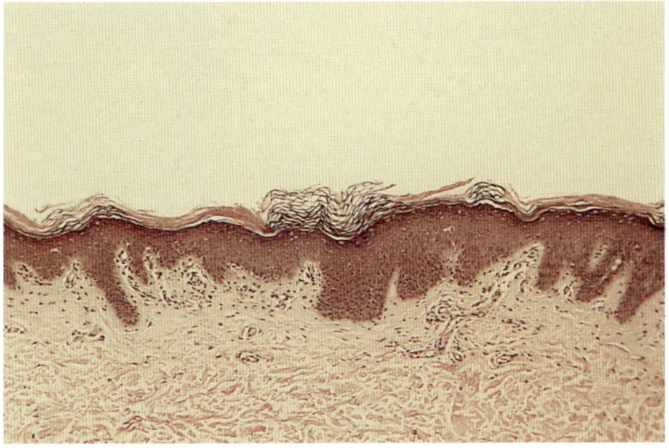

Figure 57–4. Erythrasma with alternating orthokeratosis and loose hyperkeratosis, hypergranulosis, and irregular acanthosis (hematoxylin-eosin, ×50). *(Photograph courtesy of Lisa M. Cohen, MD, Cambridge, Massachusetts.)*

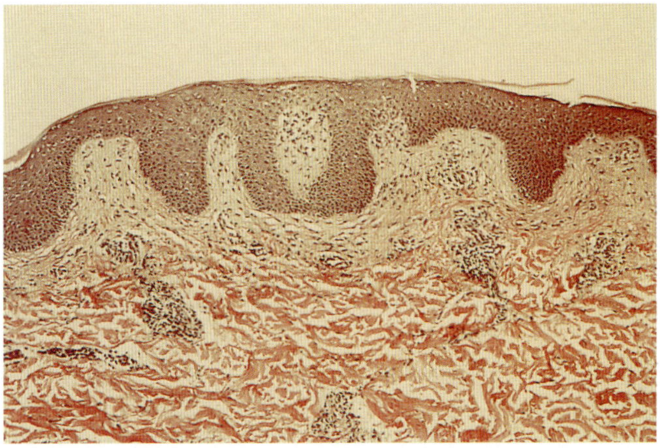

Figure 57–6. Erythrasma with acanthosis, spongiosis, and a perivascular lymphocytic infiltrate (hematoxylin-eosin, ×50).

PATHOLOGY

Because of the distinct clinical features, biopsy of erythrasma is rarely necessary. Histopathologic features of erythrasma, therefore, are only sporadically described.[11,22] In general, the histologic features are nonspecific. The epidermal changes include compact hyperkeratosis, which may alternate with loose hyperkeratosis, occasional parakeratosis, hypergranulosis, variable acanthosis and atrophy, mild spongiosis, and exocytosis of mononuclear cells (Figures 57–4 through 57–7). Vacuolated cells in the granular layer and upper layers of the stratum malpighii, epidermal hyperpigmentation, and disruption of the dermal/epidermal interface also may be seen.[22] A mild to moderate superficial lymphohistiocytic infiltrate with occasional plasma cells, interstitial edema, mild capillary proliferation, vascular ectasia, or disruption with erythrocyte extravasation are some of the dermal findings. With only hematoxylin-eosin staining, the differential diagnosis includes chronic eczematous processes, dermatophytosis, parapsoriasis, and pityriasiform dermatoses. On routine stains, organisms, when abundant, may be seen concentrated in the areas of compact hyperkeratosis[22] (Figure 57–8).

The organisms are gram-positive, although uneven staining is common, and there may be metachromatic granules.[2] The organisms are 1 to 2 × 0.3 to 0.6 μm.

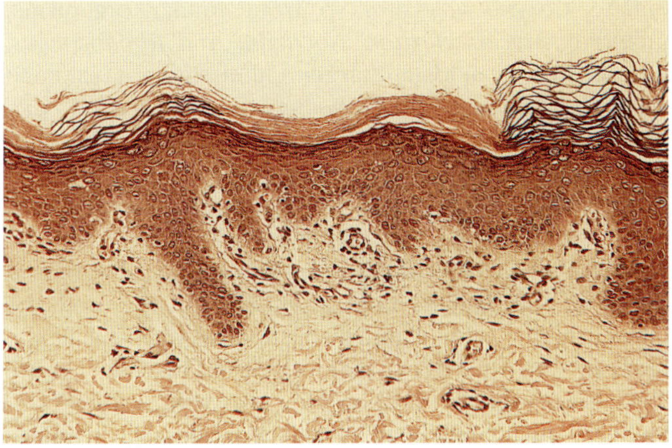

Figure 57–5. Erythrasma with alternating orthokeratosis, hypergranulosis, acanthosis, exocytosis of lymphocytes, and a superficial perivascular lymphocytic infiltrate (hematoxylin-eosin, ×100).

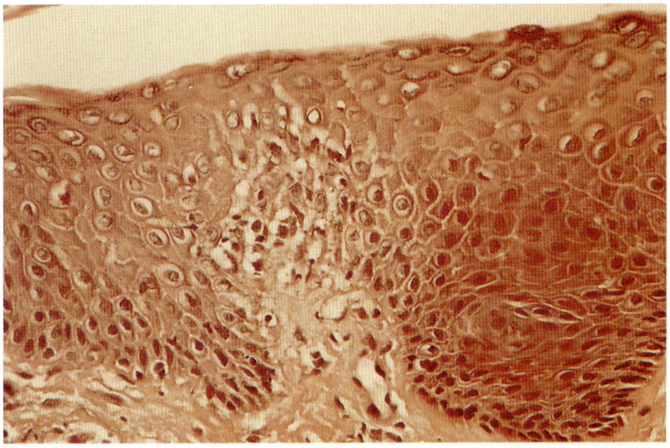

Figure 57–7. Erythrasma showing mild spongiosis and exocytosis of lymphocytes (hematoxylin-eosin, ×200).

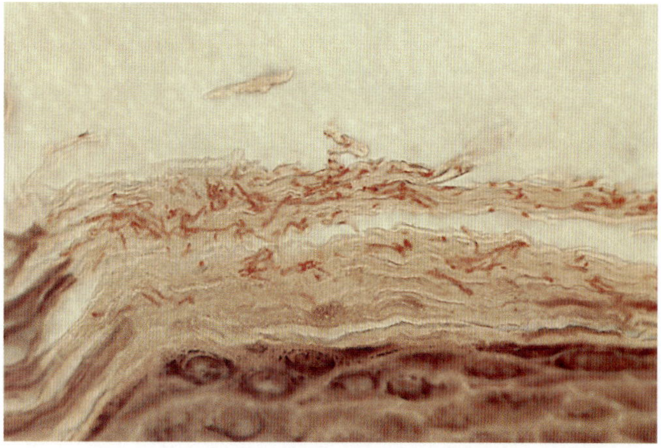

Figure 57–8. Compact orthokeratosis containing scattered *C minutissimum* organisms (hematoxylin-eosin, ×500). *(Photograph courtesy of Lisa M. Cohen, MD, Cambridge, Massachusetts.)*

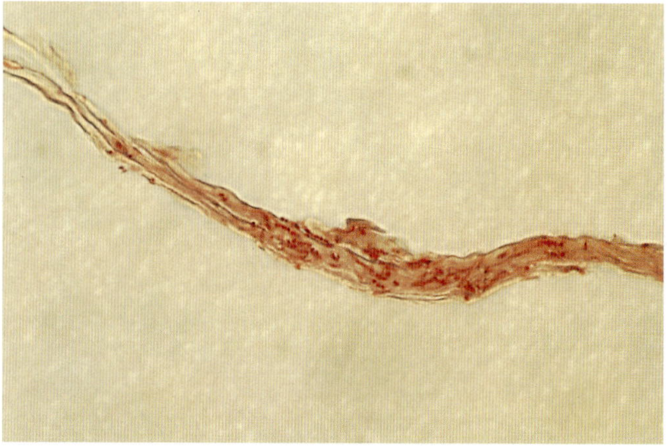

Figure 57–10. Cocco-bacillary and filamentous *C minutissimum* organisms seen within scale (PAS, ×500).

Snapping division produces V-shaped, angular, and palisaded cells. Gram or periodic acid–Schiff (PAS) staining of paraffin tissue sections may reveal a mixture of coccal, bacillary, and branching or filamentous forms (Figure 57–9). On occasion, the organisms may be sparse and fragmented. Shorter bacillary forms are more typical of toe web lesions, whereas filamentous forms are more typical of groin lesions.[7] Giemsa and methylene blue stains also may highlight the organisms.[22] Alternatively, the diagnosis may be made without a biopsy by microscopic examination of the scales stained with some of the stains mentioned (Figure 57–10).

Ultrastructurally, bacteria are at different levels of the stratum corneum—superficially, between the cornified cells, penetrating these cells, and intracellularly within the keratinized cells. Areas of decreased cytoplasmic density may be around bacteria within the cells, suggesting keratolysis. The organisms on the surface have a homogenous fine structure, whereas those within the stratum corneum may be pleomorphic.[23]

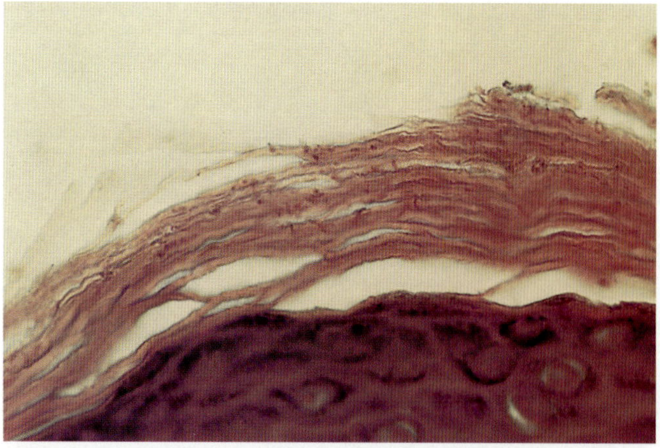

Figure 57–9. Stratum corneum containing multiple pleomorphic *C minutissimum* organisms. Multiple angulated filamentous forms are present (PAS, ×500). *(Photograph courtesy of Lisa M. Cohen, MD, Cambridge, Massachusetts.)*

BACTERIOLOGY

Biochemically, members of the *Corynebacterium* genus have 1) cell walls containing arabinose, galactose, and meso-diaminopimelic acid (meso-DAP); 2) DNA base compositions in the range of 51% to 63% guanine + cytosine (G + C) (56.4% to 58.9% for *C minutissimum*) and contain dihydrogenated menaquinones with eight and/or nine isoprene units [predominantly MK-8 (H2) and MK-9 (H2) in *C minutissimum*]; and 3) predominantly straight-chain saturated and monounsaturated fatty acids, and mycolic acids approximately 22 to 36 carbon atoms long. These short-chain lipids help differentiate *Corynebacterium* sp from similar organisms, including *Mycobacterium, Nocardia,* and *Rhodococcus,* whose mycolic acids are larger. Other similar taxa, such as *Brevibacterium, Arthrobacter, Curtobacterium, Cellulomonas,* and *Microbacterium,* lack these lipids in addition to having other differentiating characteristics. *Caseobacter* also are quite similar, but are aerobic and possess a higher G + C content.[2]

Culture of *C minutissimum* is rarely necessary and not done routinely in most laboratories. If required, the organism can be isolated from the scales of the lesion cultured on media containing 20% bovine serum, 78% tissue culture medium No. 199 without bicarbonate, 2% agar, and 0.05% tris(hydroxymethy)-aminomethane at optimal temperatures of 37°C. Growth occurs within 12 to 14 hours as 1- to 2-mm shiny, moist, white to gray, translucent, slightly convex colonies.

There is a coral-red to orange fluorescence under Wood's light (365 nm); however, it may disappear by the end of 96 hours.[1] Cell wall determination to differentiate *C minutissimum* from other similar organisms is impractical and rarely performed. The Centers for Disease Control and Prevention system for identification of gram-positive rods may be more practical and reliable.[24] Tests available to routine laboratories for preliminary diagnosis of these organisms include catalase and urease production, motility, nitrate reduction, and rapid carbohydrate fermentation reactions.[20]

Differentiating *C minutissimum* from *C jeikeium* or *C bovis* can be exceedingly difficult, if not impossible.[20,24] Characteristics that favor *C minutissimum* over the other two include nonlipid dependency, growth on triple sugar iron agar (producing an acid or alkaline slant), and growth on unsupplemented peptone water.[20,24] Fluorescence of the colonies also supports the diagnosis of *C minutissimum;* however, *C bovis, C ulcerans, C xerosis, C pseudotuberculosis,* and *C renale* emit some kind of fluorescence.[24] In addition, using a blood agar medium containing delta-aminolevulinic acid, a precursor of protoporphyrin, fluorescence may be seen with *Staphylococcus* sp, Enterobacteriaceae, *C hofmannii, X xerosis,* and *C diphtheriae.*[24]

TREATMENT

Lesions of erythrasma respond well to a 5-day course of erythromycin, 500 mg, four times a day.[1] Other antibiotics, such as ampicillin, doxycyline, rifampin, ciprofloxacin, vancomycin, and gentamycin, may also be effective, but resistance to these as well as the macrolides has been reported.[25] The use of topical erythromycin,[1] miconazole, and Whitfield's ointment[26] may offer partial clearing. Topical treatment with antibacterial soaps is also beneficial, but there may be recurrences.[27]

REFERENCES

1. Sarkany I, Taplin D, Blank H. The etiology and treatment of erythrasma. *J Invest Dermatol.* 1961;37:283–288.
2. Collins MD, Cummins CS. Irregular nonsporing gram-positive rods. In: Sneath P, Mair N, Sharpe M, Holt J, eds. *Bergey's Manual of Systematic Bacteriology.* Baltimore: Williams & Wilkins; 1986;2:1266–1272.
3. Marples RR. Diphtheroids of normal human skin. *Br J Dermatol.* 1969;81(supp 1):47–54.
4. Somerville DA. Erythrasma in normal young adults. *J Med Microbiol.* 1970;3:57–64.
5. Burns RE, Greer JE, Mikhail G, et al. The significance of coral-red fluorescence of the skin. *Arch Dermatol.* 1967; 96:436–440.
6. Somerville DA. A quantitative study of erythrasma lesions. *Br J Dermatol.* 1972;87:130–137.
7. Sarkany I, Taplin D, Blank H. Incidence and bacteriology of erythrasma. *Arch Dermatol.* 1962;85:578–582.
8. Svejgaard E, Christophersen J, Jelsdorf H-M. Tinea pedis and erythrasma in Danish recruits. *J Am Acad Dermatol.* 1986;14:993–999.
9. Montes LF, Dobson H, Dodge BG, et al. Erythrasma and diabetes mellitus. *Arch Dermatol.* 1969;99:674–680.
10. Somerville DA, Seville RH, Cunningham RC, et al. Erythrasma in a hospital for the mentally subnormal. *Br J Dermatol.* 1970;82:355–360.
11. Mattox TF, Rutgers J, Yoshimori RN, et al. Nonfluorescent erythrasma of the vulva. *Obstet Gynecol.* 1993;81:862–864.
12. Jillson OF. Pruritus ani: disputing the passage. *Cutis.* 1984; 33:537–548.
13. Schlappner OLA, Rosenblum GA, Rowden G, et al. Concomitant erythrasma and dermatophytosis of the groin. *Br J Dermatol.* 1979;100:147–151.
14. Temple DE, Boardman CR. The incidence of erythrasma of the toewebs. *Arch Dermatol.* 1962;86:518–519.
15. Maglietta T, Detwiler DE, Capogna L. Tinea pedis and erythrasma. Differential diagnosis and a case report. *J Am Podiatry Assoc.* 1983;73:315–318.
16. Shelley WB, Shelley ED. Coexistent erythrasma, trichomycosis axillaris, and pitted keratolysis: An overlooked corynebacterial triad? *J Am Acad Dermatol.* 1982;7: 752–757.
17. Engber PB, Mandel EH. Generalized disciform erythrasma. *Int J Dermatol.* 1979;18:633–635.
18. Tschen JA, Ramsdell WM. Disciform erythrasma. *Cutis.* 1983;31:541–547.
19. Berger SA, Gorea A, Stadler J, et al. Recurrent breast abscesses caused by *Corynebacterium minutissimum. J Clin Microbiol.* 1984;20:1219–1220.
20. Golledge CL, Phillips G. *Corynebacterium minutissimum* infection. *J Infect.* 1991;23:73–76.
21. Herschorn BJ, Brucker AJ. Embolic retinopathy due to *Corynebacterium minutissimum* endocarditis. *Br J Ophthalmol.* 1985;69:29–31.
22. Graham JH. Superficial fungus infection. In: Graham JH, Johnson WC, Helwig EB, eds. *Dermal Pathology.* Hagerstown: Harper & Row; 1972:249–253.
23. Montes LF, McBride ME, Johnson WP, et al: Ultrastructural study of the host-bacterium relationship in erythrasma. *J Bacteriol.* 1965;90:1489–1491.
24. Coyle MB, Lipsky BA. Coryneform bacteria in infectious diseases: clinical and laboratory aspects. *Clin Microbiol Rev.* 1990;3:227–246.
25. Soriano F, Zapardiel J, Nieto E. Antimicrobial susceptibilities of *Corynebacterium* species and other non-spore-forming gram-positive bacilli to 18 antimicrobial agents. *Antimicrob Agents Chemother.* 1995;39:208–214.
26. Pitcher DG, Noble WC, Seville RH. Treatment of erythrasma with miconazole. *Clin Exp Dermatol.* 1979;4: 453–456.
27. Dodge BG, Knowles WR, McBride ME, et al. Treatment of erythrasma with an antibacterial soap. *Arch Dermatol.* 1968:97:548–552.

CHAPTER 58

Escherichia coli Diarrhea

James K. Kelly and David A. Owen

I am poured out like water, and all my bones are out of joint: my heart is like wax; it is melted in the midst of my bowels.

Psalms 22:14

INTRODUCTION

Escherichia coli, named after the German pediatrician Theodore Escherich who described it in 1885, is the most common aerobe among the normal human colonic flora and is also the most common Gram-negative human pathogen. It causes purulent neonatal meningitis, cystitis, pyelonephritis, diarrheal disease, and dysentery.[1,2] It is the most common cause of travelers' diarrhea and a major cause of infantile and childhood diarrhea in underdeveloped countries, where diarrhea contributes significantly to malnutrition, growth retardation, and death of infants. *Escherichia coli* is transmitted by the fecal–oral route, by food, animals, and animal products. Achlorhydria increases the risk of infection.[3] *Escherichia coli* is serotyped by three antigen groups: the lipopolysaccharide O antigens, the heat-labile flagellar H antigens, and the capsular (K) antigens. Approximately 170 O antigens and 60 H antigens are recognized. The *E coli* that cause diarrhea are currently classified into five groups, each possessing distinctive virulence attributes: enteropathogenic (EPEC), enterotoxigenic (ETEC), enteroinvasive (EIEC), enterohemorrhagic (EHEC), and enteroadherent.[4]

Enterovirulent *E coli* colonize the intestine by elaborating surface proteins that bind complementary receptors on host epithelial cells. Three distinct patterns of adherence of *E coli* to monolayers of HeLa and HEp-2 cells are described: localized adherence (LA), in which microcolonies of bacteria bind to localized areas on the cell surface; diffuse adherence (DA), in which bacteria surround the cell surface uniformly[5–8]; and aggregative adherence (AggA), in which bacteria aggregate in a "stacked brick" pattern on cells or on the glass surface in between cells.[7] This last form of adherence is the basis for recognition of enteroaggregative *E. coli* (EAggEC).[4,9,10] Diffusely adherent *E coli* (DAEC), unlike LA or AggA stains, often are not diarrheagenic[5,6] but have been implicated in infantile and adult diarrhea and in travelers' diarrhea.[9,11] Some diffusely adhering strains belong to EPEC class II.[12] A fourth pattern of interaction is that some *E coli* cause detachment of HEp-2 cell monolayers from the coverslip when examined in the adherence assay. This is of uncertain significance.[13]

ENTEROPATHOGENIC *ESCHERICHIA COLI*

EPEC were defined by Neter[14] according to the following criteria: single serotypes found to be the predominating aerobic organism in the majority of affected infants in outbreaks of diarrhea; the serotype was isolated in much lower frequency from healthy individuals; antibiotics effective in vitro usually were effective in therapy; specific serum antibody response often could be shown; virus isolation was negative; and disease was reproducible experimentally in volunteers.

Epidemiology

Enteropathogenic *E coli* strains are a major cause of seasonal and sporadic diarrheas, and contribute substantially to the high mortality from diarrhea in neonates and infants in developing countries. EPEC cause diarrheal outbreaks in day nurseries and hospitals worldwide. Like other strains of diarrhea-causing *E coli,* EPEC appear to be endemic in the community and cause outbreaks of diarrhea when circumstances are favorable.

Nonhuman sources for EPEC have not been identified, and EPEC were in the stools of 2% of nondiarrheal controls, possibly an asymptomatic reservoir.[15] Breast-feeding prevents most EPEC infection. Strict isolation of diarrheal infants and rigorous asepsis are necessary to prevent nosocomial outbreaks.[3]

Pathogenesis

EPEC do not elaborate heat-labile (LT) or heat-stable (ST) enterotoxins, do not cause disseminated sepsis, and belong to certain classic strains including O serogroups 18, 26, 44, 55, 86, 111, 114, 119, 125, 126, 127, 128ab, 142, and 158.[14] EPEC are divided into two classes. Class I possesses EPEC adherence factor (EAF), bundle-forming pili (BFP), *E coli* attachment-effacement (*eae*) genes, show localized adherence to HEp-2 cells, and include O serogroups 55, 86, 111, 119, 125, 127, 128, and 142. Class II is rarely EAF-positive, displays diffuse adherence or nonadherence to HEp-2 cells, and includes members of O serogroups 44, 86, 114, 125, and 128.[16] EPEC can induce diarrhea in healthy adult volunteers.[17] Attachment–effacement is a primary pathogenic mechanism in class I EPEC. The bacteria attach to the plasma membranes of enterocytes, effacing the microvilli, and forming intimate cup-shaped adhesion complexes that often project from the cell surface on pedestals. The actin filaments, which normally form bundles beneath the microvilli, aggregate in the cytoplasm beneath the adhesion complex.[17] EPEC cured of the *eae* gene induce less severe diarrhea in human volunteers than wild-type strains.[18] LA is mediated in part by a 60-Md plasmid[19] through its product EAF.[16] Strains cured of the plasmid are less diarrheagenic in volunteer studies than the noncured strains.[20,21] EAF also confers the ability to elicit endocytosis by cells in tissue culture,[22] but the endocytosis determinant, a single gene, is not an essential component of the attachment–effacement determinant.[23] Another virulence factor, BFP, is expressed by EPEC that display LA, and is encoded by a 92-kilobase plasmid. BFP create a close-knit community of organisms by binding bacteria into a meshwork of fibers.[24,25]

Class II EPEC possess 50- to 70-Md plasmids that lack EAF genes but encode the 100-kd adhesin involved in diffuse adhesion (AIDA-I). Their pathogenic mechanism does not involve HEp-2 adhesiveness.[20]

Clinical Manifestations

Infants present with watery diarrhea without blood or mucus, accompanied by vomiting, low-grade fever, and, in severe infections, dehydration and electrolyte imbalance. The average total duration of diarrhea is about 9 days, but the duration tends to be longer in younger children[26] and may persist beyond 14 days.[27] Treatment consists of rehydration, antibiotics, and, in severe infections, total parenteral nutrition and zinc replacement.[28] EPEC often are antibiotic resistant, but may be sensitive to neomycin, gentamicin, chloramphenicol, tobramicin, trimethaprim–sulfamethoxazole, and mecillinam.[3] Oral neomycin often is given until the results of sensitivity testing are available. Three-day courses of antibiotics often are as effective as longer courses.[29]

Pathology

Biopsy is not a practical diagnostic method but in a small number of infections, attachment–effacement has been shown in endoscopic biopsies either of the duodenum or the rectum.[28,30,31] Duodenal biopsies show flat mucosa with crypt hyperplasia and a row of bacteria attached diffusely or patchily along the brush border. Biopsy specimens of the duodenum and the rectum from children with prolonged diarrhea (more than 10 days) associated with EPEC do not show adherent bacteria, but this does not exclude adherence earlier in the infection.[32] Some class I strains elicit internalization by epithelial cells,[23] but what contribution this makes to human disease is not known.

ENTEROHEMORRHAGIC *ESCHERICHIA COLI*

Enterohemorrhagic *E coli* would be better termed verotoxinogenic *E coli,* because hemorrhage is not a constant feature of these strains whereas verotoxin production is. After the first reports in 1982 of outbreaks of hemorrhagic diarrhea and colitis associated with *E coli* O157:H7, there was a flood of confirmatory reports.[33–42] Sporadic infections of hemorrhagic colitis occur throughout the world[34,41] with marked seasonality, the majority during the summer months.[43] The prototypic EHEC, serotype O157:H7, is readily identified by its sorbitol-nonfermenting phenotype, but other non–O157:H7 serotypes can be identified by direct fecal verotoxin detection using a cell culture assay.[44] DNA probes for verotoxin I and II may ultimately replace the biologic assay. Non–O157:H7 serotypes account for about 25% of EHEC infections and include some serogroups formerly regarded as EPEC, such as O26 and O128.[44–47] Antimicrobial treatment did not influence the duration of symptoms or the risk of developing complications but has not been studied systematically.[48,49] The fatality rate is up to 26% in outbreaks in nursing homes[35] but less than 1% in sporadic infections.[50] Approximately 12% of patients infected with *E coli* O157:H7 develop either hemolytic uremic syndrome (HUS) or thrombotic/thrombocytopenic purpura.[48] The mean interval from onset of diarrhea to diagnosis of HUS is 7 days (range of 2 to 12).[49] Up to 75% of patients with HUS of childhood have evidence of preceding EHEC infection,[43,49] and HUS is the leading cause of renal failure in childhood.

Epidemiology

Outbreaks occur in the general population, in nursing homes, and in day care centers. In North America the highest incidence is in the northern United States and Canada. The incidence is highest in children younger than 5 years of age, followed by children between 6 and 14 years of age, and those 65 years or older.[43] The source of infection most often implicated is ground beef.[33,35,37,51] Other sources are raw milk, apple cider, swimming in infected pools or waters, and person-to-person transmission.[52,53] Proper cooking of food is the preventive measure of choice.[50] EHEC is much more frequent in patients with bloody diarrhea than in those with watery diarrhea.[34,41,42] In Washington state, the incidence of *E coli* O157:H7 is similar to that of *Shigella* but considerably lower than *Campylobacter* or *Salmonella.*[48] The isolation rate of non–O157:H7 serotypes in Washington is higher than *Shigella* or *Yersinia* but lower than *Campylobacter, E coli* O157:H7, or *Salmonella.*[46]

Pathogenesis

The pathogenesis of mucosal colonization, diarrhea, colitis, and HUS are distinct but related areas being investigated. EHEC possess a plasmid-encoded adherence protein mediating early mucosal interaction.[54] This is followed by attachment–effacement, identical to that of EPEC, mediated in part by intiminO157, a 97-kd outer membrane protein encoded on the *eae* gene[55] (Figures 58–1 through 58–3). These adherence factors permit colonization of the gut and may contribute to diarrhea.

In addition, EHEC produce phage-encoded verotoxin I (VT-I), verotoxin II (VT-II), or both.[56–60] Also called Shiga-like toxins, these toxins were initially identified as toxic to the Vero cell line. VT-I is identical to Shiga-toxin, the toxin of *S dysenteriae*-I, whereas VT-II is 56% homologous to Shiga-toxin at the deduced amino-acid level. Both toxins consist of a single A subunit in association with a pentamer of B subunits. The B subunits bind the holotoxin to the glycolipid receptor globotriosylceramide (Gb_3), permitting endocytosis of the complex. The A subunit is a specific *N*-glycosidase that cleaves a single adenine residue from the 28SrRNA component of the 60S eukaryotic ribosome complex, inhibiting protein synthesis and killing the cell.[60] VT-I is usually the sole VT gene in non–O157:H7 EHEC.[46] Experimental infection of infant rabbits with *E coli* O157:H7 showed not only attachment–effacement to

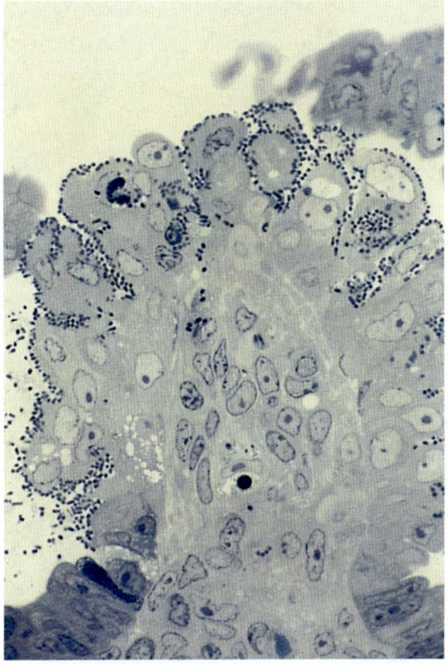

Figure 58–1. Appendix of an infant rabbit showing attaching-effacing *E coli* O157:H7.

ileum, appendix, cecum, and proximal colon, but also a severe distal colopathy characterized by extensive apoptosis of epithelial cells. Colonic mucosal apoptoses were reproducible by feeding the animals partially purified preparations of toxin by stomach tube.[61,62] Verotoxins are believed to cause in part the colitis and to be responsible for HUS.[61,63]

Recent studies find that neither verotoxins nor plasmid are essential for the production of diarrhea.[64] Furthermore, the prevalence of diarrhea, the severity of the mucosal abnormalities, and the alteration of colonic handling of electrolytes are lessened by inhibition of neutrophil migration, suggesting that factors released by

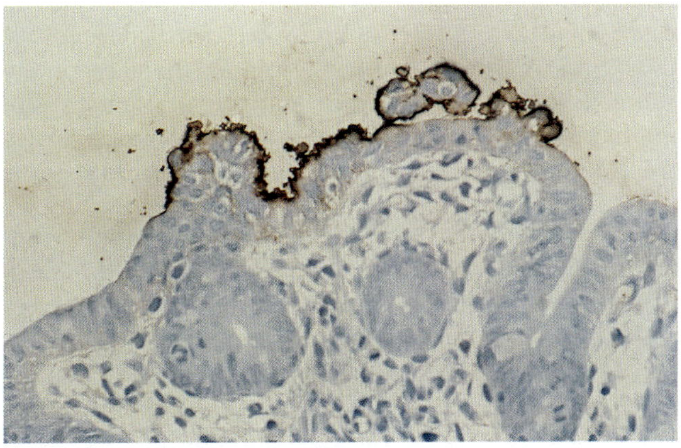

Figure 58–2. Cecum of an infant rabbit showing attaching-effacing *E coli* immunostained with anti-O157 antiserum.

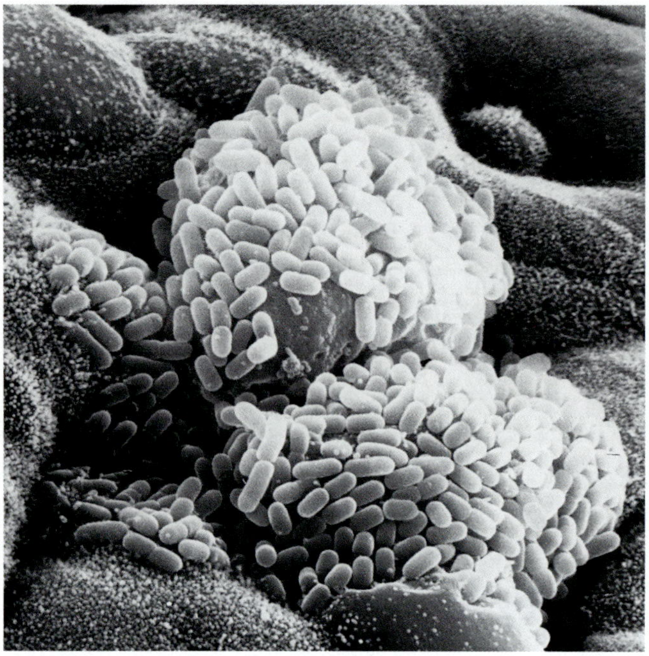

Figure 58–3. Cecum of an infant rabbit showing adherent *E coli*.

neutrophils contribute to the diarrhea.[65] At present, neural mechanisms of diarrhea have not been investigated.

The pathogenesis of the HUS or thrombotic/thrombocytopenic purpura (TTP) may involve combined effects of absorbed Shiga-toxin and endotoxin on vascular endothelial cells[66,67] with swollen glomerular endothelial cells, fibrin deposits, and infiltrates of inflammatory cells in the kidneys.[62]

Clinical Manifestations

Infection with *E coli* O157:H7 exhibits a spectrum of illness from asymptomatic infection through mild diarrhea to hemorrhagic colitis with HUS and death.[33–45] Typically, crampy abdominal pain is soon followed by watery diarrhea. Within 48 hours the diarrhea becomes bloody, lasts for 3 to 4 days, and then gradually wanes.[68] Fever is uncommon and never high. About one half of patients have nausea and vomiting.[45,67] Between one third and two thirds of patients in outbreaks have bloody diarrhea, but in sporadic infections, bloody diarrhea is reported in almost 100%, probably reflecting the fact that patients with bloody diarrhea are more likely to seek medical attention than those with nonbloody diarrhea.[69] There is a mild neutrophil leukocytosis and a small number of fecal leukocytes.[69] Endoscopically, the rectum and sigmoid usually are normal, and lesions are mainly on the right side of the colon. These include erythema, edema, hemorrhage, erosions, large ulcers, and pseudomembranes.[70] Barium enema may show an inverted "thumb-printing" pattern in the ascending and transverse colon caused by severe submucosal edema.

Histopathology

Endoscopic Biopsies

The main pathologic lesions usually are in the ascending and transverse colon. Biopsy specimens of the rectosigmoid show normal mucosa or mild acute inflammation indistinguishable from other infectious colitides.[62] Colonoscopic biopsy specimens show a spectrum of change from edema and neutrophil infiltration characteristic of infectious colitis, to superficial mucosal necrosis and exudation resembling ischemic colitis, or pseudomembranous colitis similar to that caused by *Clostridium difficile*[63,70–73] (Figures 58–4 and 58–5). These lesions may be associated with fibrin/platelet thrombi in mucosal capillaries. The pseudomembranes contain a mixture of neutrophils, mucin, and fibrin, and the underlying mucosa shows necrosis of the surface epithelium and crypts dilated with mucus and lined by flattened epithelium; however, the basal portions of the crypts remain viable, except in the most severe infections. The lamina propria has an infiltrate of neutrophils, hemorrhage, edema, and fibrinous exudation. More severe pseudomembranous lesions display confluent surface exudate overlying necrotic mucosa. The ghost outlines of dilated crypts may be filled with mucin.

Resection Specimens

The right side of the colon is predominantly affected, but the entire colon may be involved. Specimens show patchy, shallow ulcers, some covered by a layer of

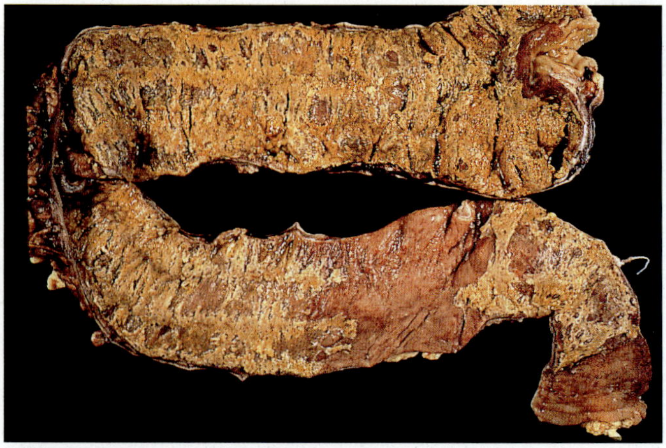

Figure 58–4. Pseudomembranous colitis pattern caused by *E coli* O157:H7.

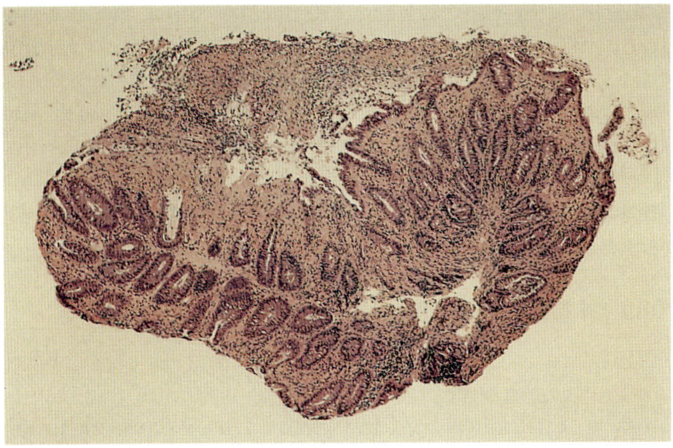

Figure 58–5. Neutrophil cryptitis and laminal edema in *E coli* 0157:H7 infection.

greenish exudate or pseudomembrane (Figure 58–6). Pseudomembranes form discrete plaques of yellow-green friable material in some areas and a confluent membrane in other areas.[70,73–75] Severe submucosal edema and hemorrhage can obliterate the lumen and the mucosa may be friable, hemorrhagic, and ulcerated.[63,73] Microscopically, in infections with HUS or TTP, there have been acute inflammation, lymphoid follicular necrosis in Peyer's patches, and colonic lymphoid tissue.[63] The mucosa may display necrosis, pseudomembranes similar to those with *C difficile*, capillary thrombi in the mucosa and submucosa, and extreme submucosal edema with hemorrhage and fibrinous exudate.[74] In the most severe infections, necrosis extends into the submucosa and muscle.[63,73] In patients with HUS or TTP, fibrin thrombi may be in all levels of the gut, including the larger arteries.[63] The widespread microangiopathy and endothelial cell damage support the hypothesis that HUS and TTP are mediated by a systemic toxemia, and that endothelial cells are the primary target cells for verotoxins,[63] but verotoxins may also injure the mucosa directly. At autopsy, the kidneys are pale, swollen, and purpuric in HUS. They display glomerular thrombotic microangiopathy and acute tubular necrosis. Glomerular capillary walls are thickened and fibrin thrombi occlude the lumens. Afferent arterioles frequently are occluded by fibrin thrombi.[63]

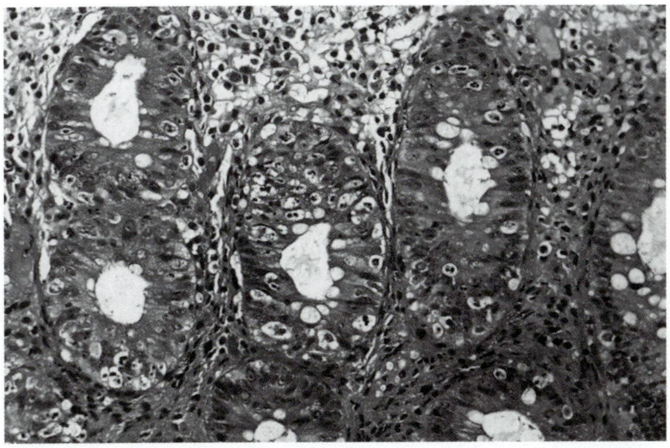

Figure 58–6. Subtotal colectomy infected with *E coli* 0157:H7. There are diffuse pseudomembranous exudates in the right side and transverse colon, and the remaining mucosa is extremely congested. *(Photograph courtesy of Dr. Steve Rasmussen.)*

Differential Diagnosis

The differential diagnosis includes other infectious colitides, *C difficile*–associated colitis, ischemic colitis, and idiopathic inflammatory bowel disease. If the biopsy shows only edema and neutrophil infiltration, it is indistinguishable from other infectious colitides. The pseudomembranous lesions are indistinguishable from those caused by *C difficile*. Both may be associated with capillary thrombi. The clinical history provides more clues than the histology; recent antibiotic treatment makes *C difficile*–associated disease more likely, whereas acute diarrhea followed by bloody diarrhea makes EHEC more likely. The distinction between ischemic colitis and EHEC colitis also may be impossible, but typical acute ischemic lesions show coagulative necrosis, ulceration, and minimal inflammation. Features of infectious colitis, in addition to mucosal necrosis, favor EHEC infection. The gold standard for diagnosis continues to be culture and toxin detection.

ENTEROTOXIGENIC *ESCHERICHIA COLI*

Enterotoxigenic *E coli* produce LT or ST enterotoxins, which promote fluid secretion by the gut and secretory diarrhea.[76] Classic LT is a cholera-like toxin, which is neutralized by antibodies to cholera toxin and activates adenyl cyclase and promotes chloride secretion, presumably through stimulation of endocrine cells and neural reflexes relayed through the myenteric plexus.[77] A second LT-like toxin is not neutralizable by antibodies to cholera toxin.[76] ST include STa, a family of heat-stable enterotoxins that activate guanylate cyclase; and STb, a toxin that causes secretion by an undefined means in piglets.[78] ETEC strains may also produce colonization factors and colonization factor antigens (CFAs). They do not invade or produce attachment–effacement.

Epidemiology

ETEC is a major cause of diarrhea in children and adults in developing countries, in travelers to developing countries, and in outbreaks in the developed world.[76,78–80] In developing countries approximately 15% to 20% of childhood diarrheas are associated with ETEC and strains that produce only STa predominate.[78] Children being weaned from breast milk are at particular risk for ETEC infection in the wet season, as contaminated food and water are the main sources of infection.[81] ETEC is the main cause of travelers' diarrhea, which affects 25% to 50% of travelers in the first week of travel from industrialized to developing tropical countries.[78]

Pathogenesis

A relatively large inoculum of 10^6 to 10^{10} organisms is required to cause disease in the normal host.[82] The two main virulence attributes of ETEC are colonization factors and enterotoxins.[83,84] Three colonization factor antigens, CFA1, 2, and 3, are recognized, and several putative colonizing factors that include six coli surface (CS) antigenic specificities located on either fimbriae (pili) or fibrillae. CFAs are plasmid encoded, with the exception of CS1 and CS2, which are chromosomally encoded. CFA expression, however, requires a regulatory gene always present on a high-molecular-weight plasmid. Several ETEC strains have no known colonizing factor. CFAs allow bacterial adherence to mucosal epithelium and proliferation to significant numbers. Studies in humans have shown that CFAs are necessary for diarrhea. Serotypes tend to be associated with specific CFAs and specific toxins, that is, CFA2 with ST, CFA1 with ST and LT, and CFA3 with ST, LT, or both.[85–87] ETEC that produce CFAs are richly fimbriate bacteria that adhere to the brush border of enterocytes or tissue culture cells in vitro but do not damage the microvilli.[88,89] They may form a fibrillar webbing that interlinks the bacteria[90] resembling BFP.[24]

Four enterotoxins are recognized.[76] Heat-labile toxin is a high-molecular-weight protein composed of five binding B subunits and one active A subunit, resembling cholera toxin. The cellular receptor is the ganglioside GM_1, on which the binding site is the terminal galactose. The A subunit is a proenzyme that must be nicked by proteolysis yielding an A1-enzyme and an A2-"linker" peptide. A1 is translocated across the membrane of epithelial cells, possibly after endocytosis, and catalyses the ADP ribosylation of the G protein $G_{s\alpha}$ of adenylate cyclase, thereby stimulating production of cyclic adenosine monophosphate (AMP). Subsequent reflex neural stimulation causes secretion of fluid and electrolytes. The second toxin is an LT-like toxin but is not neutralized by anticholera toxin and is chromosomally, not plasmid, encoded. The third, heat-stable toxin (ST), is a family of low-molecular-weight proteins that bind intestinal brush border membrane receptors, stimulate guanylate cyclase, and cause chloride and fluid secretion through poorly understood mechanisms. The fourth toxin, heat stable toxin B, is also a low-molecular-weight protein but has not yet been shown to cause human disease.[76]

Clinical Manifestations

ETEC cause small bowel diarrhea that is cholera-like and ranges in severity from mild to voluminous. The illness is self-limited and lasts from 1 to 5 days, although rarely infections may persist up to 3 weeks. About one quarter of patients also suffer from malaise, anorexia, abdominal cramps, nausea, vomiting, and low-grade fever.[80,88,91] Dehydration is the main complication and may be more common in adults than in children. Treatment consists of rehydration. Antibiotics or bismuth may diminish the frequency of stools and can be employed in prophylaxis. An intestinal calmodulin "inhibitor" also can decrease the severity and duration of diarrhea.[92] Definitive diagnosis rarely is made because of the cost and difficulty of diagnosis. Differential diagnosis includes cholera, infection by a noncholera vibrio, giardiasis, cryptosporidiosis, Norwalk or *Rotavirus* diarrhea, and preformed bacterial toxin in food.[78]

Pathology

The histopathology of human infection with ETEC has not been described, but the changes in calves are mild and consist of villous blunting, focal degeneration of enterocytes, and exfoliation of epithelial cells.[93]

ENTEROAGGREGATIVE *ESCHERICHIA COLI*

EAggEC are a cause of acute and persisting pediatric diarrhea in both underdeveloped and developed countries.[94–96] In England, EAggEC are isolated from 3% of children with diarrhea, a frequency similar to better known pathogens such as EPEC, *Campylobacter, Salmonella, Shigella, Giardia lamblia,* and *Cryptosporidium.* EAggEC cause travelers' diarrhea and are an important cause of secretory diarrhea in India.[97] In Thailand, however, EAggEC were isolated with similar frequencies from controls as from diarrheal children.

Pathogenesis

EAggEC do not invade epithelial cells, do not elaborate Shiga-like toxin or classic enterotoxins characteristic of ETEC, and do not usually have O:H serotypes associated with EPEC or other markers of EPEC, although some serogroups (O44, O55, O86, O111, O126, and O127) include both EPEC and EAggEC. A sensitive and specific DNA probe to identify EAggEC has been described.[97,98] One strain caused diarrhea in adult volunteers.[99] Other strains adhere in vitro to human enterocytes, mucus, and mucosa in an aggregative pattern, through fimbriae.[100,101] (In gnotobiotic piglets, EAggEC elicit hyperemia of the distal small intestine and cecum and swelling of small intestinal villi but no inflammatory response.)[102] In rabbit and rat intestinal loops, EAggEC induced shortening of the villi, hemorrhagic necrosis of the villous tips, and a mild inflammatory response, with edema and mononuclear infiltration of the submucosa.[7] In humans, EAggEC are believed to colonize the distal ileum and colon. EAggEC evince a mannose-resistant aggregative adherence to HEp-2 cells, which is mediated by bundle-forming fimbriae encoded on a 60-Md plasmid[7] that is highly conserved among these strains.[94,98,103] A heat-stable protein enterotoxin of low molecular weight that is associated with the 60-Md plasmid has been described in several strains of EAggEC.[102] This toxin is named EAST (enteroaggregative *E coli* heat-stable enterotoxin).[102] It is not cross-reactive immunologically with STa and is the leading candidate to cause the diarrhea.

Pathology

Histopathology of human infection has not been described.

ENTEROINVASIVE *ESCHERICHIA COLI*

EIEC cause a dysenteric illness resembling shigellosis.[104] Most EIEC share antigenic and physiologic similarities with *Shigella,* closely related genera. EIEC are usually nonmotile, lactose negative, and lysine decarboxylase negative. EIEC include members of O serogroups 28, 29, 42, 112, 124, 136, 143, 144, 152, 164, and 167.[105]

Epidemiology and Pathogenesis

A small number of outbreaks or individual infections caused by EIEC have been identified in various countries. EIEC invade epithelial cells in animal models, eliciting mucosal inflammation and epithelial necrosis and ulceration.[104] These organisms give a positive Sérény test (invade rabbit conjunctiva) and invade HeLa cell monolayers. Unlike *Shigella,* a high infective dose of EIEC is necessary to cause illness in volunteers.[104] A 140-md plasmid encodes several polypeptides essential for inducing phagocytosis by epithelial cells and replication of the bacteria in the cell. This plasmid is homologous with the plasmid encoding invasiveness in *Shigella* species.[106] As in *Shigella,* chromosomal genes are necessary for full expression of invasiveness and for survival in experimental animal hosts. A second potential virulence factor is Shiga toxin, which is produced in quantities similar to *S flexneri* 2A.[56] EIEC also elaborate a third virulence factor, the siderophore aerobactin, which chelates ferric iron.[105]

Pathology

Descriptions of the morphology of the gut in humans infected by EIEC have not yet been reported, but features similar to shigellosis would be expected.

REFERENCES

1. Robins-Browne RM. Traditional enteropathogenic *Escherichia coli* of infantile diarrhea. *Rev Infect Dis.* 1987;9: 28–53.
2. Levine MM. *Escherichia coli* infections. *N Engl J Med.* 1985;313:445–447.
3. Boedeker EC. Enteroadherent (enteropathogenic) *Escherichia coli.* In: MJG Farthing, GT Keusch, eds. *Enteric Infection: Mechanisms, Manifestations and Management.* London: Chapman and Hall; 1989.
4. Levine MM. *Escherichia coli* that cause diarrhoea: enterotoxigenic, enteropathogenic, enteroinvasive, enterohemorrhagic, and enteroadherent. *J Infect Dis.* 1987;155: 377–389.
5. Scaletsky ICA, Silva MLM, Trabulsi LR. Distinctive patterns of adherence of enteropathogenic *Escherichia coli* to HeLa cells. *Infect Immun.* 1984;45:534–536.
6. Nataro JP, Scaletsky ICA, Kaper JP, Levine MM, Trabulsi LR. Plasmid mediated factors conferring diffuse and localized adherence of enteropathogenic *Escherichia coli. Infect Immun.* 1985;48:378–383.
7. Vial PA, Robins-Browne R, Lior H, et al. Characterization of enteroadherent-aggregative *Escherichia coli,* a putative agent of diarrheal disease. *J Infect Dis.* 1988;158: 70–79.
8. Levine MM, Prado V, Robins-Browne R, et al. Use of DNA probes and HEp-2 cell adherence assay to detect diarrheagenic *Escherichia coli. J Infect Dis.* 1988;158: 224–228.
9. Brook MG, Smith HR, Bannister BA, et al. Prospective study of verocytotoxin-producing, enteroaggregative and diffusely adherent *Escherichia coli* in different diarrhoeal states. *Epidemiol Infect.* 1994;112:63–67.
10. Paul M, Tsukamoto T, Ghosh AR, et al. The significance of enteroaggregative *Escherichia coli* in the etiology of hospitalized diarrhoea in Calcutta, India and the demonstration of a new honey-combed pattern of aggregative adherence. *FEMS Microbiol Lett.* 1994;117:319–325.
11. Jallat C, Livrelli V, Darfeuille-Michaud A. *Escherichia coli* strains involved in diarrhea in France: high prevalence and heterogeneity of diffusely adhering strains. *J Clin Microbiol.* 1993;31:2031–2037.
12. Benz I, Schmidt MA. Isolation and serologic character-

ization of AIDA-1, the adhesion mediating the diffuse adherence phenotype of the diarrhea-associated *Escherichia coli* strain 2787 (O126:H27). *Infect Immun.* 1992;60:13–18.

13. Gunzburg ST, Chang BJ, Elliott SJ, Burke V, Gracey M. Diffuse and enteroaggregative patterns of adherence of enteric *Escherichia coli* isolated from aboriginal children from the Kimberley region of Western Australia. *J Infect Dis.* 1993;167:755–758.
14. Neter E. Enteritis due to enteropathogenic *Escherichia coli*. *Am J Dig Dis.* 1965;10:883–886.
15. Rademaker CM, Fluit AC, Jansze M, et al. Frequency of enterovirulent *Escherichia coli* in diarrhoeal disease in The Netherlands. *Eur J Clin Microbiol Infect Dis.* 1993; 12:93–97.
16. Nataro JP, Baldini MM, Kaper JB, Black RE, Bravo N, Levine MM. Detection of an adherence factor of enteropathogenic *Escherichia coli* with a DNA probe. *J Infect Dis.* 1985;152:560–565.
17. Levine MM, Bergquist EJ, Nalm DR, et al. *Escherichia coli* strains that cause diarrhea but do not produce heat-labile or heat-stable enterotoxins and are not invasive. *Lancet.* 1978;1:1119–1122.
18. Donnenberg MS, Tacket CO, James SP, et al. Role of the *eaeA* gene in experimental enteropathogenic *Escherichia coli* infection. *J Clin Invest.* 1993;92:1412–1417.
19. Baldini MM, Kaper JB, Levine MM, Candy DCA, Moon HW. Plasmid-mediated adhesion in enteropathogenic *Escherichia coli*. *J Pediatr Gastroenterol Nutr.* 1983;2: 534–538.
20. Levine MM, Nataro JP, Karch H, et al. The diarrhoeal response of humans to some classic serotypes of enteropathogenic *Escherichia coli* is dependent on a plasmid encoding an enteroadhesiveness factor. *J Infect Dis.* 1985;152:550–559.
21. Baldini MM, Nataro JP, Kaper JB. Localization of a determinant for HEp-2 adherence by enteropathogenic *Escherichia coli*. *Infect Immun.* 1986;52:334–336.
22. Donnenberg MS, Donohue-Rolfe A, Keusch GT. Epithelial cell invasion: an overlooked property of enteropathogenic *Escherichia coli* (EPEC) associated with the EPEC adherence factor. *J Infect Dis.* 1989;160:452–459.
23. Fletcher JN, Embaye HE, Getty B, Batt RM, Hart CA, Saunders JR. Novel invasion determinant of enteropathogenic *Escherichia coli* plasmid pLV501 encodes the ability to invade epithelial cells and HEp-2 cells. *Infect Immun.* 1992;60:2229–2236.
24. Giron JA, Ho ASY, Schoolnik GK. An inducible bundle-forming pilus of enteropathogenic *Escherichia coli*. *Science.* 1991;254:710–713.
25. Giron JA, Donnenberg MS, Martin WC, Jarvis KG, Kaper JB. Distribution of the bundle-forming pilus structural gene (bfpA) among enteropathogenic *Escherichia coli*. *J Infect Dis.* 1993;168:1037–1041.
26. Gurwith MJ, Wiseman DA, Chow P. Clinical and laboratory assessment of the pathogenicity of serotyped enteropathogenic *Escherichia coli*. *J Infect Dis.* 1977;133: 736–743.
27. Penny MT, Harendra de Silva DG, McNeish AS. Bacterial contamination of the small intestine of infants with enteropathogenic *Escherichia coli* and other enteric infections: a factor in the aetiology of persistent diarrhoea? *Brit Med J.* 1986;292:1223–1261.
28. Rothbaum R, McAdams AJ, Giannella R, Partin JC. A clinicopathologic study of enterocyte-adherent *Escherichia coli:* a cause of protracted diarrhoea in infants. *Gastroenterology.* 1982;83:441–454.
29. Nelson JD. Duration of neomycon therapy for enteropathogenic *Escherichia coli* diarrheal disease: a comparative study of 113 cases. *Pediatrics.* 1971;48:248–258.
30. Ulshen MH, Rollo JL. Pathogenesis of *Escherichia coli* gastroenteritis in man: another mechanism. *N Engl J Med.* 1980;302:99–101.
31. Clausen CR, Christie DL. Chronic diarrhoea in infants caused by adherent enteropathogenic *Escherichia coli*. *J Pediatr.* 1982;100:358–361.
32. Sherman PM, Drumm B, Karmali M, Cutz E. Adherence of bacteria to the intestina in sporadic cases of enteropathogenic *Escherichia coli*-associated diarrhea in infants and young children: a prospective study. *Gastroenterology.* 1989;96:86–94.
33. Riley LW, Remis RS, Helgerson SD, et al. Outbreaks of hemorrhagic colitis associated with a rare *E. coli* serotype. *N Engl J Med.* 1983;308:681–685.
34. Remis RS, MacDonald KL, Riley LW et al. Sporadic cases of haemorrhagic colitis associated with *Escherichia coli* O157:H7. *Ann Intern Med.* 1984;101:624–626.
35. Ryan CA, Tauxe RV, Hosek GW, et al. *Escherichia coli* O157:H7 diarrhea in a nursing home: clinical epidemiological, and pathological findings. *J Infect Dis.* 1986; 154:631–638.
36. Spika JS, Parsons JE, Nordenberg D, Wells JG, Gunn RA, Blake PA. Hemolytic uremic syndrome and diarrhea associated with *Escherichia coli* O157:H7 in a day care center. *J Pediatr.* 1986;109:287–291.
37. Stewart PJ, Desormeaux W, Chene H. Haemorrhagic colitis in a home for the aged—Ontario. *Can Dis Weekly Rep.* 1983;9-8:29–32.
38. Belsheim MR, Lewis J, Brien W. Clinical and laboratory observations on patients from a nursing home outbreak of verotoxin-producing *E. coli* (O157:H7 strain). *Clin Gastroenterol.* 1988;2:57–59.
39. Pudden D, Tuttle N, Korn D, et al. Haemorrhagic colitis in a nursing home in Ontario. *Can Med Assoc J.* 1986; 134:50.
40. Carter AO, Borczyk AA, Carlson JAK, et al. A severe outbreak of *Escherichia coli* O157:H7-associated hemorrhagic colitis in a nursing home. *N Engl J Med.* 1987; 317:1496–1500.
41. Pai CH, Gordon R, Sims HV, Bryan LE. Sporadic cases of hemorrhagic colitis associated with *Escherichia coli* O157:H7: clinical, epidemiologic, and bacteriologic features. *Ann Intern Med.* 1984;101:738–742.
42. Ratnam S, March SB. Sporadic occurrence of haemorrhagic colitis associated with *Escherichia coli* O157:H7 in Newfoundland. *Can Med Assoc J.* 1986;134:43–45.
43. Grandsen WR, Damm MAS, Anderson JD, Carter JE, Lior H. Further evidence associating hemolytic uremic syndrome with infection by verotoxin-producing *Escherichia coli* O157:H7. *J Infect Dis.* 1986;154:522–524.

44. Ritchie M, Partington S, Jessop J, Kelly MT. Comparison of a direct fecal Shiga-like toxin assay and sorbitol-MacConkey agar culture for laboratory diagnosis of enterohemorrhagic *Escherichia coli* infection. *J Clin Microbiol.* 1992;30:461–464.
45. Pai CH, Ahmed N, Lior H, Sims HV, Johnson WM, Woods DE. Epidemiology of sporadic diarrhea due to verocytotoxin-producing *Escherichia coli* (VTEC): a two-year prospective study. *J Infect Dis.* 1988;157:1054–1057.
46. Bokete TN, O'Callahan CM, Clausen CR, et al. Shiga-like toxin-producing *Escherichia coli* in Seattle children: a prospective study. *Gastroenterology.* 1993;105:1724–1731.
47. Scotland SM, Willshaw GA, Smith HR, Said B, Stokes N, Rowe B. Virulence properties of *Escherichia coli* strains belonging to serogroups O26, O55, O111 and O128 isolated in the United Kingdom in 1991 from patients with diarrhoea. *Epidemiol Infect.* 1993;111:429–438.
48. Ostroff SM, Kobayashi JM, Lewis JH. Infections with *Escherichia coli* O157:H7 in Washington State. *JAMA.* 1989;262;355–359.
49. Karmali MA, Petric M, Lim C, Fleming PC, Argus GS, Lior H. The association between idiopathic hemolytic uremic syndrome and infection by verotoxin-producing *Escherichia coli. J Infect Dis.* 1985;151:775–782.
50. Bryant HE, Athar MA, Pai CH. Risk factors for *Escherichia coli* O157:H7 infection in an urban community. *J Infect Dis.* 1989;160:858–863.
51. Update: multistate outbreak of *Escherichia coli* O157:H7 infections from hamburgers—western United States, 1992–1993. *MMWR.* 1993;42:258–263.
52. McDonald KL, O'Leary MJ, Cohen ML et al. *Escherichia coli* O157:H7, an emerging gastrointestinal pathogen: results of a one-year, prospective, population-based study. *JAMA.* 1988;259:3567–3570.
53. Rowe PC, Orrbine E, Ogborn M, et al. Epidemic *Escherichia coli* O157:H7 gastroenteritis and hemolytic-uremic syndrome in a Canadian Inuit community: intestinal illness in family members as a risk factor. *J Pediatr.* 1994;124:21–26.
54. Knutton S, Baldini MM, Kaper JB, McNeish AS. Role of plasmid-encoded adherence factors in adhesion of enteropathogenic *Escherichia coli* to HEp-2 cells. *Infect Immun.* 1987;55:78–85.
55. Louie M, de Azavedo JC, Handelsman MY, et al. Expression and characterization of the *eaeA* gene product of *Escherichia coli* serotype O157:H7. *Infect Immun.* 1993;61:4085–4092.
56. O'Brien AD, Leveck GD, Thomson MR, Formal SB. Production of *Shigella dysenteriae* 1-like cytotoxin by *Escherichia coli. J Infect Dis.* 1982;146:763–769.
57. Newland JW, Strockbine NA, Miller SF, O'Brien AD, Holmes RK. Cloning of Shiga-like structural genes from a toxin converting phage of *Escherichia coli. Science.* 1985;230:179–181.
58. Scotland SM, Smith HR, Willishaw GA, Rowe B. Vero cytotoxin production in strain of *Escherichia coli* is determined by genes carried on bacteriophage. *Lancet.* 1983;2:216.
59. Strockbine NA, Marques LM, Newland JW, Williams-Smith H, Holmes RK, O'Brien AD. Two toxin-converting phages from *Escherichia coli* O157:H7 strain 933 encode antigenically distinct toxins with similar biological activities. *Infect Immun.* 1986;53:135–140.
60. Bobak DA, Guerrant RL. New developments in enteric bacterial toxins. *Adv Pharmacol.* 1992;23:85–108.
61. Pai CH, Kelly JK, Meyers GL. Experimental infection of infant rabbits with vero-toxin producing *Escherichia coli. Infect Immun.* 1986;51:16–23.
62. Keenan KP, Sharpnack DD, Collins H, Formal SB, O'Brien AD. Morphologic evaluation of the effects of Shiga toxin and *E. coli* Shiga-like toxin on the rabbit intestine. *Am J Pathol.* 1986;125:69–80.
63. Richardson SE, Karmali MA, Becker LE, Smith CR. The histopathology of the hemolytic uremic syndrome associated with verocytotoxin-producing *Escherichia coli* infections. *Hum Pathol.* 1988;19:1102–1108.
64. Li Z, Bell C, Buret A, Robins-Browne R, Stiel D, O'Loughlin EV. The effect of enterohemorrhagic *Escherichia coli* O157:H7 on intestinal structure and solute transport in rabbits. *Gastroenterology.* 1993;104:467–474.
65. Elliott E, Li Z, Bell C, et al. Modulation of host response to *Escherichia coli* O157:H7 infection by anti-CD18 antibody in rabbits. *Gastroenterology.* 1994;106:1554–1561.
66. Louise CB, Obrig TG. Shiga toxin-associated hemolytic uremic syndrome: combined cytotoxic effects of shiga toxin and lipopolysaccharide (endotoxin) on human vascular endothelial cells in vitro. *Infect Immun.* 1992;60: 1536–1543.
67. Tesh VL, Samuel JC, Perera LP, Sharefkin JB, O'Brien AD. Evaluation of the role of shiga and shiga-like toxins in mediating direct damage to human vascular endothelial cells. *J Infect Dis.* 1992;164:344.
68. Pai CH, Kelly JK. Shiga-like toxin-producing *Escherichia coli.* In: MJG Farthing, GT Keusch, eds. *Enteric Infections, Mechanisms, Manifestations and Management.* London: Chapman and Hall; 1989:141–153.
69. Griffin PM, Ostroff SM, Tauxe RV, et al. The broad spectrum of illness associated with *Escherichia coli* O157:H7. *Ann Intern Med.* 1988;109:705–712.
70. Morrison DM, Tyrrell DLJ, Jewell LD. Colonic biopsy in verotoxin-induced hemorrhagic colitis and thrombotic thrombocytopenic purpura (TTP). *Am J Clin Pathol.* 1986;86:108–112.
71. Kelly JK, Pai CH, Jadusingh H, Macinnis ML, Shaffer EA, Hershfield NB. The histopathology of rectosigmoid biopsies from adults with bloody diarrhea due to verotoxin-producing *Escherichia coli. Am J Clin Pathol.* 1987;88: 78–82.
72. Griffin PM, Olmstead LC, Petras RE. *Escherichia coli* O157:H7–associated colitis. A clinical and histological study of 11 cases. *Gastroenterology.* 1990;99:142–149.
73. Eidus LB, Guindi M, Drouin J, Gregoire S, Barr JR. Colitis caused by *Escherichia coli* O157:H7: a study of six cases. *Can J Gastroenterol.* 1990;4:141–146.
74. Kelly JK, Oryshak A, Wenetsek M, Grabiec J, Handy S. The colonic pathology of *Escherichia coli* O157:H7 infection. *Am J Surg Pathol.* 1990;14:87–92.
75. Hunt CM, Harvey JA, Youngs ER, Irwin ST, Reid TM. Clinical and pathological variability of infection by en-

terohaemorrhagic (verocytoxin producing) *Escherichia coli*. *J Clin Pathol.* 1989;42:847–852.
76. Guerrant RL, Moore RA, Kirschenfeld PM, Sande MA. Roles of toxigenic and invasive bacteria in acute diarrhoea in childhood. *N Engl J Med.* 1975;293:567–573.
77. Jodal M, Holmgren S, Lundgren O, Sjoquist A. Involvement of the myenteric plexus in the cholera toxin-induced net fluid secretion in the rat small intestine. *Gastroenterology.* 1993;105:1286–1293.
78. Wanke CA, Guerrant RL. Enterotoxigenic *Escherichia coli*. In: MJG Farthing, GT Keusch, eds. *Enteric Infections: Mechanisms, Manifestations and Management.* London: Chapman and Hall; 1989:253–263.
79. Echeverria P, Blacklow NR, Vollet JL, et al. Reovirus like agent and ETEC in pediatric diarrhoea in the Philippines. *J Infect Dis.* 1978;138:326–331.
80. Sack DA, Kaminski DC, Sack RB, et al. Prophylactic doxycyclin for travellers diarrhoea: results of a prospective double blind study of Peace Corps volunteers in Thailand. *Johns Hopkins Med J.* 1977;141:63–70.
81. Black RE, Brown KH, Becker S, Alim ARMA, Merson MH. Contamination of weaning foods and transmission of enterotoxigenic *E. coli* diarrhea in children in rural Bangladesh. *Trans Roy Soc Trop Med Hyg.* 1982;76:259–264.
82. Levine MM, Caplan ES, Wakman D, Cans RA, Hornick R, Synair MJ. Diarrhoea caused by *E. coli* that produce only heat stable enterotoxin. *Infect Immun.* 1977;17:78–82.
83. Satterwhite TK, Evans DG, DuPont HL, Evans DJ. Role of *E. coli* colonization factor antigens in acute diarrhoea. *Lancet.* 1978;2:181–184.
84. Smith HW, Linggood MA. Observations on the pathogenic properties of the K88, Hly and Ent plasmids of *E. coli* with particular reference to porcine diarrhoea. *J Med Microbiol.* 1978;14:467.
85. Echeverria P, Seriwatana J, Taylor DN, et al. Plasmids coding for colonization factor antigens 1 and 2, heat-labile enterotoxin and heat stable enterotoxin A2 in *E. coli*. *Infect Immun.* 1986;51:626–630.
86. Thomas LV, Cravioto A, Scotland SM, Rowe B. New fimbrial antigens type (E8775) that may represent a colonization factor in ETEC in humans. *Infect Immun.* 1982;35:1119–1124.
87. Viboud GI, Binsztein N, Svennerholm AM. Characterization of monoclonal antibodies against putative colonization factors of enterotoxigenic *Escherichia coli* and their use in an epidemiological study. *J Clin Microbiol.* 1993;31:558–564.
88. Echeverria P, Blacklow NR, Sanford LB, Cakor G. Travellers diarrhoea among Peace Corp volunteers in Thailand. *J Infect Dis.* 1981;143:767–771.
89. Knutton S, Lloyd DR, McNeish AS. Adhesion of enterotoxigenic *Escherichia coli* to human intestinal enterocytes and to cultured human intestinal mucosa. *Infect Immun.* 1987;55:69–77.
90. Knutton S, Lloyd DR, Candy DCA, McNeish AS. Adhesion of enterotoxigenic *Escherichia coli* to human intestinal enterocytes. *Infect Immun.* 1985;48:824–831.
91. Guerrant RL, Rouse JD, Hughes JM, Rose B. Turista among members of the Yale Glee Club in Latin America. *Am J Trop Med Hyg.* 1980;29:895–900.
92. DuPont HL, Ericsson CD, Mathewson JJ, et al. Zaldaride maleate, an intestinal calmodulin inhibitor, in the therapy of traveller's diarrhea. *Gastroenterology.* 1993;104:709–715.
93. Bellamy JEC, Acres SD. Enterotoxigenic coli bacillosis in colostrum-fed calves: pathological changes. *Am J Vet Res.* 1979;40:1391–1397.
94. Bhan MK, Raj P, Levine MM, et al. Enteroaggregative *Escherichia coli* associated with persistent diarrhea in a cohort of rural children in India. *J Infect Dis.* 1989;159:1061–1064.
95. Chan KN, Phillips AD, Knutton S, Smith HR, Walker-Smith JA. Enteroaggregative *Escherichia coli:* another cause of acute and chronic diarrhea in England? *J Pediatr Gastroenterol Nutr.* 1994;18:87–91.
96. Baldwin TJ, Knutton S, Sellers L, et al. Enteroaggregative *Escherichia coli* produce a secreted protein immunologically related to *E. coli* hemolysin. *Infect Immun.* 1992;60:2092–2095.
97. Paul M, Tsukamoto T, Ghosh AR, et al. The significance of enteroaggregative *Escherichia coli* in the etiology of hospitalized diarrhoea in Calcutta, India and the demonstration of a new honey-combed pattern of aggregative adherence. *FEMS Microbiol Lett.* 1994;117:319–325.
98. Baudry B, Savarino SJ, Vial P, Kaper JB, Levine MM. A sensitive and specific DNA probe to identify enteroaggregative *Escherichia coli,* a recently discovered diarrheal pathogen. *J Infect Dis.* 1990;161:1249–1251.
99. Mathewson JJ, Johnson PC, DuPont HL, Satterwhite TK, Windsor DK. Pathogenicity of enteroadherent *Escherichia coli* in adult human volunteers. *J Infect Dis.* 1986;154:524–527.
100. Yamamoto T, Endo S, Yokota T, Echeverria P. Characteristics of adherence of enteroaggregative *Escherichia coli* to human and animal mucosa. *Infect Immun.* 1991;59:3722–3739.
101. Haider K, Faruque SM, Shahid NS, et al. Enteroaggregative *Escherichia coli* infections in Bangledeshi children: clinical and microbiological features. *J Diarrheal Dis Res.* 1991;9:318–322.
102. Savarino SJ, Fasano A, Robertson DC, Levine MM. Enteroaggregative *Escherichia coli* elaborate a heat-stable enterotoxin demonstrable in an in vitro rabbit intestinal model. *J Clin Invest.* 1991;87:1450–1455.
103. Nataro JP, Deng Y, Maneval DR, German AL, Martin WC, Levine MM. Aggregative adherence fimbriae of enteroaggregative *Escherichia coli* mediate adherence to HEp-2 cells and hemagglutination of human erythrocytes. *Infect Immun.* 1992;60:2297–2304.
104. Dupont HL, Formal SB, Hornick RB, et al. Pathogenesis of *Escherichia coli* diarrhoea. *N Engl J Med.* 1971;285:1–9.
105. Sansonetti PJ. Enteroinvasive *Escherichia coli.* In: MJG Farthing, GT Keusch, eds. *Enteric Infections: Mechanisms, Manifestations and Management.* London: Chapman & Hall; 1989:283–287.
106. Sansonetti PJ, d'Hauteville H, Ecobichon C, Pourcel C. Molecular comparison of virulence plasmids in *Shigella* and enteroinvasive *Escherichia coli*. *Ann Microbiol (Inst Pasteur).* 1983;134A:295–318.

CHAPTER 59

Granuloma Inguinale (Donovanosis)

Bhagirath Majmudar

Look wise, say nothing, and grunt. Speech was given to conceal thought.

Sir William Osler (1849–1919)

DEFINITION

Granuloma inguinale (donovanosis, granuloma venereum) is infection by a minute coccobacillus *Calymmatobacterium granulomatis* and is characterized by a progressive inflammatory disease primarily of the genital and anal skin and subcutaneous tissue. It may also affect other genital and nongenital tissues. Although a sexually transmitted disease, nonvenereal transmission of granuloma inguinale is well documented.

EPIDEMIOLOGY

Granuloma inguinale exists as small endemic foci in all continents, minimally in Europe,[1] and primarily in tropical and subtropical countries, most commonly India, Brazil, the West Indies, South China, and the west coast of Africa.[2–5] Large series have recently been reported from Africa.[6,7] In the United States, fewer than 100 infections are reported annually.[4] Indeed, the low incidence of reported donovanosis could be spurious because of incomplete reporting and incomplete investigation of patients with genital ulcer. Appropriate laboratory techniques are vital to diagnosis.[8]

Granuloma inguinale is considered a venereal disease because there is a preponderance of infection in the 20- to- 30-year-old group, coinciding with the peak ages for sexually transmitted diseases. Granuloma inguinale, however, also afflicts the young and old, and there may be a lack of coexistent infection in sexual partners,[7] thus indicating that transmission is not exclusively venereal. The male-to-female ratio is about 2.5:1. Spontaneous regression of well-developed lesions is uncommon, but response to therapy is usually satisfactory.

A bacterium resembling *C granulomatis* has been isolated from feces,[9] suggesting *C granulomatis* might be a member of the family Enterobacteriaceae normally residing in the intestine. It is presumed that the organisms are inoculated as a result of minor trauma, such as a break in the skin or mucosa, and produce the clinical lesions of donovanosis. This suggests transmission during coitus or close physical contact with the anogenital region. Two possible modes of transmission of this disease are therefore suggested: direct contact during rectal intercourse and indirect contact through vaginal contamination by feces or fecal organisms.

The latter mode might explain the rarity of granuloma inguinale in prostitutes, most of whom douche regularly, which would tend to reduce fecal contamination of the vagina. In addition, those who develop granuloma inguinale, particularly the disseminated form, may have some deficiency of cellular immune response. In a study of subpopulations of tissue level lymphocytes, the T4:T8 ratio in ulcerogranulomatous lesions was significantly higher than that in hypertrophic variants, indicating a greater cell-mediated immune response in the former.[10] This line of investigation should be pursued. It may also enhance our knowledge to study the biological course of granuloma inguinale in patients with acquired immunodeficiency syndrome.

ETIOLOGY

Diagnosis of granuloma inguinale is based on the demonstration of intracellular *C granulomatis,* also called "Donovan bodies," in cytologic smears or in tissue sections. The bodies generally are not seen unless special stains are employed.

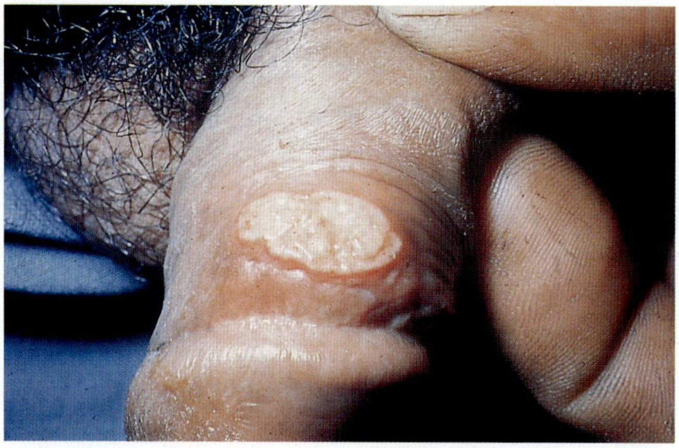

A

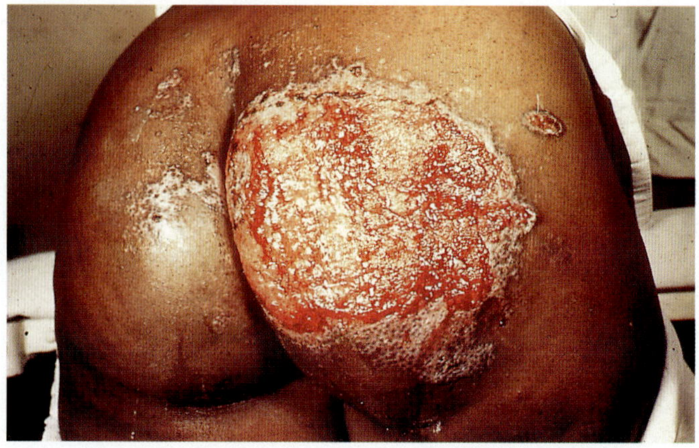

B

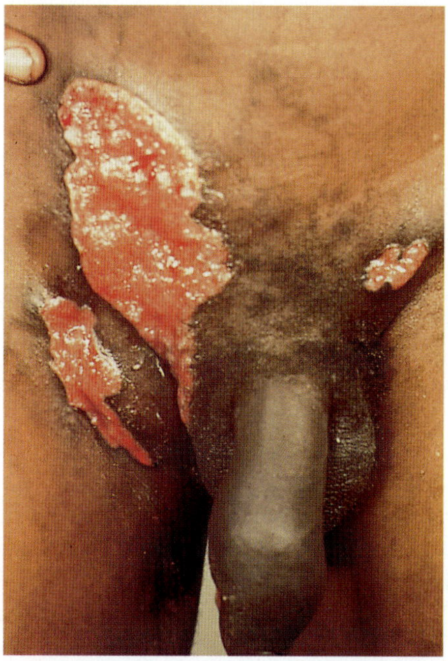

C

Figure 59–1. Donovanosis, penile lesions. (**A**) Punched-out, clean, and shallow ulcer is seen on the penile shaft. (**B**) Occasionally the ulcer can be large and simulate malignancy. (**C**) An ulcer exhibiting red granulation tissue in its base.

The cause of granuloma inguinale is *C granulomatis,* a minute, gram-negative, nonmotile, asporogenic, and encapsulated coccobacillus (0.5 to 1.5 μm by 1 to 2 μm). It is classified in its own genus associated with the family Enterobacteriaceae. Morphologically and antigenically, *C granulomatis* resembles members of the genus *Klebsiella,* in particular *K rhinoscleromatis.* It has been cultured only under microaerophilic to anaerobic conditions and will not grow on the surface of ordinary laboratory media, simple or complex. *Calymmatobacterium granulomatis* has been grown in special liquid media, egg yolk slant fluid, and yolk sacs of 5-day-old chick embryos. Optimal temperature for growth is 37°C, and it has not been grown on artificial media. Electron microscopy[11,12] confirms ultrastructural characteristics of a gram-negative bacillus and demonstrates also bacteriophage-like particles within Donovan bodies. *Calymmatobacterium granulomatis* may be part of the intestinal flora that is made pathogenic by a bacteriophage.

CLINICAL MANIFESTATIONS

Donovanosis is an acute or chronic infection manifested by ulcerating, necrotizing lesions of the skin and subcutaneous tissues in the anogenital areas.[4,13] In most patients, the period from exposure to development of lesions is from 7 to 30 days. The initial lesion is a small papule that erodes the surface of the skin, breaking down into ulcers that enlarge progressively (Figure

59–1, A–C). Lesions are the same in both male and female patients (Figures 59–2, A–C). Old lesions are hypertrophic, velvety, beefy red, indurated granulation tissue. Uncomplicated lesions are painless, but secondary infection induces pain and suppuration. Lesions most commonly are on the inner aspect of the labia or the fourchette in female patients and on the penis in male patients. The disease progresses by extension to adjacent skin, and frequently spreads by autoinoculation and lymphatic or systemic dissemination.

In women, massive swelling of the labia is common. The lymphatics are widely dilated but unobstructed because dye injected into the tissues reaches the regional lymph nodes rapidly. Even in extensive infection, the regional lymph nodes are not enlarged, painful, or tender. Absence of lymphadenopathy is a diagnostic characteristic, but secondary infection produces inguinal lymphadenopathy. Inguinal swellings do appear, however; they are indurated or fluctuant abscesses, called "pseudobuboes" because they represent subcutaneous granulation tissue and not enlarged lymph nodes (Figure 59–3), and they eventually break down to be replaced by ulcers. Large destructive lesions may be mistaken for malignancy.[5,14] A combination of biopsy and cytology is necessary to exclude malignant tumor in these patients. Proper treatment heals and completely resolves all lesions. In general, the response to treatment is very satisfactory, but in long-standing infections there may be genital deformities, such as residual depigmentation of skin, stenosis of urethral, vaginal, and anal orifices, and massive edema.

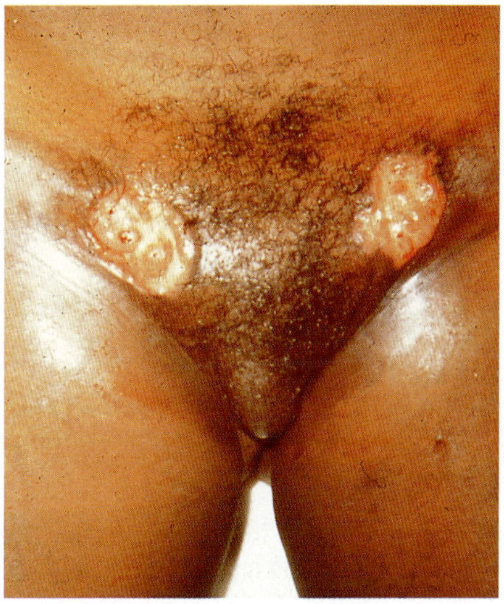

Figure 59–3. Destruction of inguinal soft tissue creating bilateral "pseudobuboes."

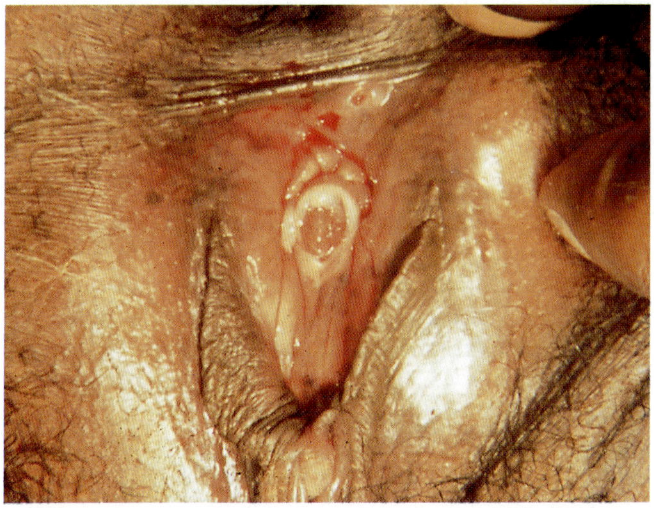

A

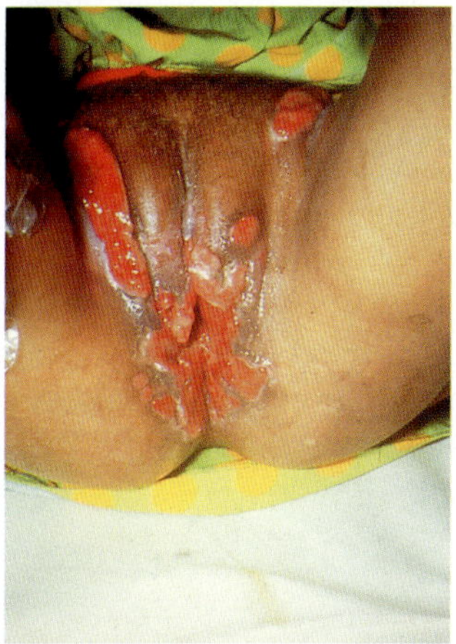

B

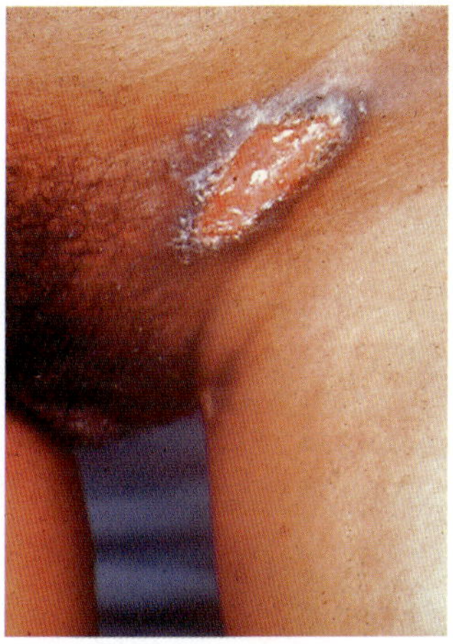

C

Figure 59–2. Donovanosis in female patients. The ulcers in male and female patients resemble each other. A–C have a striking resemblance to Figures 59–1, A–C, respectively.

Extragenital lesions have been reported on the face, neck, mouth, and throat, and metastatic lesions involving bones, joints, and viscera have been encountered.[15–17] These patients often had associated cervical or uterine lesions, and some patients had a history of a prior pregnancy or an operation. There is no record of congenital transmission. Clinical manifestations are different in pregnant and nonpregnant women. Genital tract bleeding and multiple sites of infection (vulva, vagina, cervix) are much more common in nonpregnant patients.[6]

DIAGNOSIS

Biopsy and cytologic smears (Figure 59–4) of the lesion are the most dependable methods of diagnosis. Biopsy specimens reveal a dense mixed cellular infiltrate in the

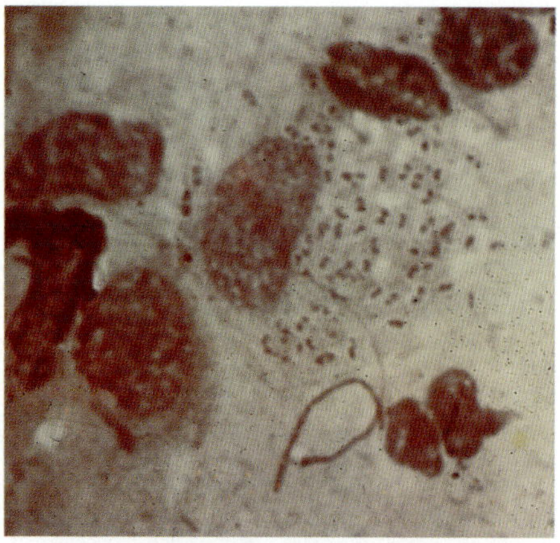

Figure 59–4. Smeared exudate from the edge of an ulcer. Donovan bodies are in the cytoplasm of a macrophage. Some are paired and some have a distinct (clear) capsule (Wright–Giemsa, ×1000).

dermis, composed predominantly of macrophages, with occasional foci of neutrophils. Granulation tissue and, later, fibrous tissue are prominent (Figure 59–5). The epithelial border is frequently acanthotic. Other features include intraepidermal abscess, elongation of rete ridges, and pseudoepitheliomatous hyperplasia. Caseation, suppuration, and Langhans' giant cells are not typical. Both biopsy specimens and cytologic smears reveal *C granulomatis* within histiocytes. These are "pathognomonic cells" and establish the diagnosis (Figure 59–6, A and B). These cells are enlarged (20 to 90 μm), have an eccentric nucleus, and contain single or clusters of bacilli in capsular or cystlike compartments of the cytoplasm. Neutrophils are rare, except near the surface of the lesion. Pathognomonic cells are scattered in variable numbers in the upper half of the granulation tissue, particularly near the margins of the ulcer. The capsules are believed to protect the organism from degradation. The only currently effective laboratory procedure for the diagnosis of donovanosis is a properly prepared and stained tissue section or smear.

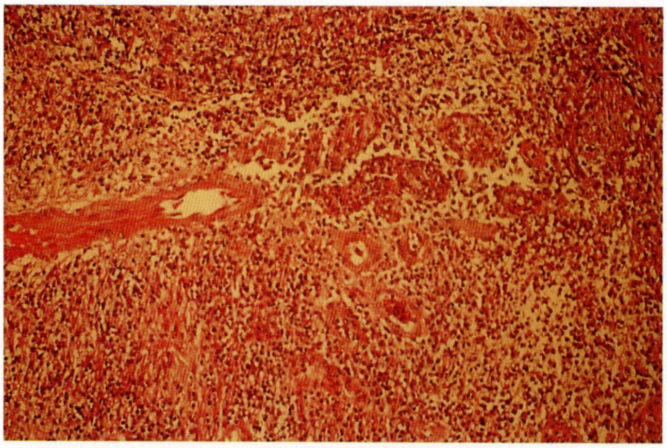

Figure 59–5. Section of the ulcer showing acute inflammation with microabscesses and granulation tissue (hematoxylin-eosin, ×50).

DIFFERENTIAL DIAGNOSIS

The diagnosis of donovanosis may be overlooked primarily because it is rare in the United States and thus not remembered as a cause of genital lesions. Furthermore, the ulcers of syphilis and chancroid resemble granuloma inguinale. Also, antibiotic therapy may alter the appearance. At present, the only conclusive method of diagnosis is to demonstrate Donovan bodies in large mononuclear cells by biopsy or cytology of the lesion. It must also be remembered that a patient may have more than one venereal disease, and infection by human immunodeficiency virus must be considered as well in a patient with any venereal disease. A clinical and laboratory search should be directed accordingly. The chancre of early syphilis may be confused with early ulcers of granuloma inguinale. Syphilis can be excluded, usually, by negative serology and lack of spirochetes by darkfield examination of the exudate. Lymphogranuloma venereum is characterized by bilateral, tender, inguinal nodes (buboes) that often suppurate and, in untreated patients, may lead to elephantiasis of the external genitalia. Exclusion is aided by serology with lymphogranuloma venereum (LGV) titers less than 1:15. Chancroid is manifested by shallow, painful, exudate-filled ulcers and tender inguinal adenopathy. The causative agent (*Haemophilus ducreyi*) can be cultured on a modified selective chocolate agar medium. Nodes heal spontaneously. Herpes simplex II causes asymptomatic initial vesicles that quickly break down to form shallow, clean-based ulcers. Local edema and enlargement of inguinal lymph nodes may be present. Exclusion is by detection of intranuclear inclusions and multinucleated giant cells in smear or cultures for the herpesvirus. Vulvar cancer and cervical cancer are excluded by biopsy. Exophytic lesions or large necrotic ulcers of granuloma inguinale may resemble carcinoma on clinical examination. Parametrial involvement may add to the confusion.

Granuloma inguinale should always be considered when genital lesions are long-standing and have slow progression of weeks to months.

LABORATORY DIAGNOSIS

Specimen Collection

For a biopsy specimen, use granulation tissue near the periphery of the lesion, cleaned with several saline-

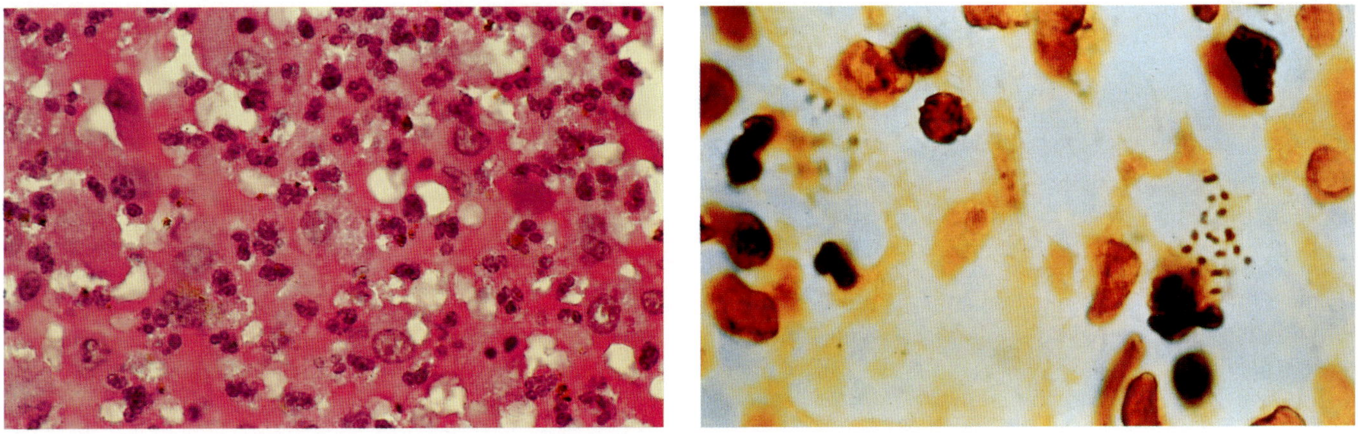

A B

Figure 59–6. (**A**) Section through the margin of an ulcer. The macrophage in the center of the field has abundant granular amphophilic cytoplasm that contains many Donovan bodies—not discernible at this magnification (hematoxylin-eosin, ×290). (**B**) The intracytoplasmic Donovan bodies are seen by the Warthin–Starry stain (×1000).

soaked gauze squares, then dried with gauze. Blood does not affect the specimen. Take the specimen with a punch, forceps, or small curette.

Take smears from the underside of the ulcer. Do not respread any area, and cease spreading when the specimen begins to dry. The dry areas will contain rubbed and broken cells of no use in diagnosis. Air dry the specimen, fix in 95% ethanol for 5 minutes, and stain. With hematoxylin-eosin stains, the bacilli may be faintly stained but are usually not seen unless present in large numbers. Wright, Giemsa, Pinacyanole, or Warthin–Starry stains show the organisms more clearly in tissue sections and on smears. With Wright's stain, however, the dye should remain on the smear for 1.5 minutes before diluting with 6.4-pH phosphate buffer. The bacilli appear as small, straight, or curved dumbbell-shaped ("closed safety pin") coccobacilli having a blue to deep purple color and surrounded by pink capsules. Broken tissue cells are not satisfactory for examination because there are many other extracellular objects of similar size and shape in the specimen. The pathognomonic cells can be detected with the high dry lens (×450) and confirmed with the oil lens (×1000).

Culture Specimen and Examination

A specimen obtained as described in the last section is placed between two sterile glass slides and crushed between them with a twisting motion. Separate the slides and add 0.2 to 0.5 mL of sterile saline to each surface. Emulsify the tissue debris with a sterile toothpick or loop.

For isolation of *C granulomatis* in chick embryos, inoculate 0.2 mL of the tissue debris into the yolk sac of a 5-day-old chick embryo and incubate at 37°C for 72 hours. Growth of *C granulomatis* occurs in the yolk sac. The organisms may be demonstrated in stained smears as described previously.

For isolation of *C granulomatis* on "Dulaney slants," inoculate 0.2 mL of the suspension of tissue debris onto the coagulated egg yolk slants, then cover three quarters of the surface of the slant with Locke's salt solution. Close the tubes and incubate upright at 37°C for 48 to 72 hours. Slants made of egg yolks from range-fed chickens (as well as ducks, geese, and turkeys) are effective, whereas those made from egg yolks obtained from diet-fed birds are ineffective; the reasons for this are unknown.

IMMUNITY AND PATHOGENICITY

There is no serologic procedure currently available either for detecting antibodies to *C granulomatis* in human sera or for identifying the organism as an isolate; however, antibodies have been detected in human sera using complement-fixing procedures. Significant serum titers were only in sera from patients in whom the duration of a lesion exceeded 3 months. The lack of protection by circulating antibodies is similar to other diseases in which the organism is found intracellularly, for example, lepromatous leprosy, tuberculosis, and chronic mucocutaneous candidiasis. It has been found that *C granulomatis* has antigenic cross-reactivity with *K pneumoniae* and *K rhinoscleromatis.* Other than the chick embryo, *C granulomatis* is pathogenic only for humans.

TREATMENT

Effective antibiotics include streptomycin, chloramphenicol, erythromycin, lincomycin, co-trimoxazole, and the tetracyclines.[1] More recently, norfloxacin and thiamphenicol have been effective.[1] Granuloma inguinale tends to relapse after successful treatment; therefore prolonged follow-up is necessary. Lincomycin combined with erythromycin has been satisfactory in treating pregnant patients. Penicillin is not effective, and ampicillin or erythromycin alone have given inconsistent results.

PROGNOSIS

As a rule, lesions resolve with proper treatment. Untreated lesions distort, mutilate, and destroy as they spread, and spread may be contiguous or systemic. Death is rare and is usually a consequence of complications, such as pneumonia, cardiac failure, and hemorrhage.

ASSOCIATION WITH CARCINOMA

Granuloma inguinale may cause vulvar ulcers and lesions on the cervix or vagina that are necrotizing and proliferating and sometimes thicken the parametrial tissues. It is not surprising therefore that granuloma inguinale and carcinomas of the genital region are confused. However, in addition, an association of granuloma inguinale and genital carcinoma has been suspected because 1) there is a higher incidence of genital carcinoma where donovanosis is endemic, 2) carcinoma has occurred within depigmented areas of healed donovanosis, and 3) there has been concurrence of carcinoma and donovanosis in the same lesion. The histologic distinction of the two is usually clear-cut, but the acanthosis and pseudoepitheliomatous hyperplasia of granuloma inguinale might raise some confusion at first glance. When a biopsy from a large necrotic lesion that is clinically suspicious for carcinoma shows only inflammatory changes, a possibility of granuloma inguinale should be considered and special stains obtained to demonstrate *C granulomatis*. However, when the lesion remains unaltered or grows in spite of treatment, multiple biopsies should be obtained to ascertain whether a malignancy coexists with granuloma inguinale. An association between donovanosis and carcinoma, although reported, is distinctly uncommon.

REFERENCES

1. Richens J. The diagnosis and treatment of donovanosis (granuloma inguinale). *Genitourin Med.* 1991;67:441–452.
2. Goldberg J. Studies on granuloma inguinale VII. Some epidemiological considerations of the disease. *Br J Vener Dis.* 1964;40:140–145.
3. Kuberski T. Granuloma inguinale (donovanosis): a review. *Sex Transm Dis.* 1980;7:29–36.
4. Kellogg D, Majmudar B. Granuloma Inguinale. In: Morse SA, Moreland AA, Thompson SE, eds. *Atlas of Sexually Transmitted Diseases.* Philadelphia: JB Lippincott Company; New York, London: Gower Medical Publishing; 1990:4.2–4.12.
5. Wysoki RS, Majmudar B, Willis D. Granuloma inguinale (donovanosis) in women. *J Reprod Med.* 1988;33:709–713.
6. Bassa AG, Hoosen AA, Moodley J, Bramdev A. Granuloma inguinale (donovanosis) in women. An analysis of 61 cases from Durban, South Africa. *Sex Transm Dis.* 1993;20:164–167.
7. O'Farrell N. Clinico-epidemiological study of donovanosis in Durban, South Africa. *Genitourin Med.* 1993;69:108–111.
8. Joseph AK, Rosen T. Laboratory techniques used in the diagnosis of chancroid, granuloma inguinale, and lymphogranuloma venereum. *Dermatol Clin.* 1994;12:1–8.
9. Goldberg J. Studies on granuloma inguinale V. Isolation of a bacterium resembling *Donovania granulomatis* from the faeces of a patient with granuloma inguinale. *Br J Vener Dis.* 1964;38:99–102.
10. Sehgal VN, Gupta MM, Jain VK. Tissue level lymphocyte sub-populations in donovanosis. *Int J Dermatol.* 1991;30:857–859.
11. Chandra M, Jain AK, Ganguly DD, Sharma AK, Bhargava NC. An ultrastructural study of donovanosis. *Indian J Med Res.* 1989;89:158–164.
12. Kuberski T, Papadimitriou JM, Phillips P. Ultrastructure of *Calymmatobacterium granulomatis* in lesions of granuloma inguinale. *J Infect Dis.* 1980;142:744–749.
13. Goens JL, Schwartz RA, DeWolf K. Mucocutaneous manifestations of chancroid, lymphogranuloma venereum and granuloma venereum. *Am Fam Phys.* 1994;49:415–418, 423–425.
14. Hoosen AA, Draper G, Moodley J, Cooper K. Granuloma inguinale of the cervix: a carcinoma look-alike. *Genitourin Med.* 1990;66:380–382.
15. Barnes R, Masood S, Lammert N, Young RH. Extragenital granuloma inguinale mimicking a soft-tissue neoplasm: a case report and review of the literature. *Hum Pathol.* 1990;21:559–561.
16. Kirkpatrick DJ. Donovanosis (granuloma inguinale): a rare cause of osteolytic bone lesions. *Clin Radiol.* 1970;21:101–105.
17. Spagnola DV, Coburn PR, Cream JJ, Azadian BS. Extragenital granuloma inguinale (donovanosis) diagnosed in the United Kingdom: a clinical, histological, and electron microscopical study. *J Clin Pathol.* 1984;37:945–949.

Chapter 60

Helicobacter pylori

Robert R. Pascal and C. Mel Wilcox

By the Incisura Angularis, lookin' northward to the head,
There's a rough mucosal pattern, an' it looks like it 'as bled.
It's a picture worth rememb'rin', tho' it's ugly an' it's gory;
It's the gastric inflammation that's produced by H. pylori.
Tho' I've pampered it an' soothed it,
I admit I've plain abused it,
An' the bile comes up like thunder every hour of the day.

I've eaten spices from the Indies, from New Guinea, an' Malaysia,
An' I always thought that they 'ad caused my colonic metaplasia.
But now the Goddamn journals tell a very different story:
It ain't the stuff I've eaten; it's the dev'lish H. pylori.
Yes, I've been a glutton,
Eatin' jook an' curried mutton,
So hot it makes ol' Satan's fires a pleasant place t'play.

Now all that is nothin' compared to a tiny spiral rod,
That makes a man put down his gin, an' wish 'e was with God.
An' there's no one to prevent that; no soldier, judge, or jury,
An there ain't no ocean big enough to escape that H. pylori.
I've used Gelusil an' Maalox,
(I've 'ad Bismuth for the Pox)
An' I've even tried some 'eathen brews, but dyspepsia's 'ere to stay.

So 'ere's to you, Fuzzy-Wuzzy bug, on my foveolar cell
I'll drown my gut with British gin, an' you can go to Hell
An' if I meet my maker, well, I won't say that I'm sorry
For you'll be there inside me, eatin' mucus, H. pylori.
God knows when first I ate you,
But you're there, and tho' I hate you,
You'll be with me, H. pylori, 'till 'eaven's judgement day.

Robert R. Pascal, 1995

INTRODUCTION

Although bacterial colonization of the stomach was described as early as the 1800s, it was not until 1983 when Warren[1] and Marshall[2] identified and cultured a bacterium—called *Campylobacter pyloridis*—from the gastric mucosa, that interest in gastric bacteriology was renewed. These investigators observed curved bacilli in association with the histologic findings of active chronic gastritis, most commonly in the antrum. Since these reports, there has been an explosion of information culminating in the characterization of the organism and the establishment of a causal role in human disease. Subsequently named *Helicobacter pylori,* it is now believed to cause antral (type B) gastritis and it fulfills Koch's postulates for gastritis.

EPIDEMIOLOGY AND NATURAL HISTORY

Helicobacter pylori has been found throughout the world in all human populations studied. Although the infection—and gastritis—appear to be worldwide, differences in prevalence have emerged not only between but within countries.[3] Regardless of the population evaluated, the frequency of infection increases with age. For example, in the United States the prevalence of *H pylori* increases from approximately 10% in those less than 30, to 60% or more in those 60 years or older.[4] Seroepidemiologic studies from developing countries demonstrate early acquisition of the bacteria such that the seropositivity rate may be as high as 80% by age 20. In the United States, there appears to be an inverse correlation with socioeconomic status, and for all levels, blacks are more commonly infected than whites.[3] There is no strong association with the use of alcohol, tobacco, or nonsteroidal anti-inflammatory drugs.

The mode of transmission is unknown; however, the differences in prevalence rates between industrialized and developing nations suggests a fecal–oral route. In addition, studies of families document a clustering of infection, suggesting spread within the family.[5] Furthermore, the infection rate in groups of people in close contact, such as in orphanages, also demonstrate a high prevalence rate.[6] Nucleic acid-based studies of *H pylori* in these infected populations reveal the organisms to be the same. Once acquired, the infection appears to be lifelong. Although *H pylori* may be successfully eradicated by antibiotics and remain undetectable for 1 to 2 years, the long-term eradication rate remains to be determined. Studies of up to 6 years' duration suggest a low rate (less than 1% per year) of reacquisition.[7]

MORPHOLOGIC FEATURES

Helicobacter pylori is a gram-negative, highly motile, microaerophilic, nonsporulating bacterium.[8] It is approximately 3.5 μm long and 0.5 to 1 μm wide, typically S-shaped and has four to seven unipolar flagella. Although previously thought to be of the *Campylobacter* species, DNA hybridization studies have more closely linked it to the other spiral bacteria. Thus, the new genus *Helicobacter* has been created, of which *H pylori* is the major organism. A unique feature of *H pylori* is the presence of the enzyme urease, which has been employed diagnostically (see later discussion).

CLINICAL FEATURES

Helicobacter pylori infection appears to be asymptomatic in most patients. Gastrointestinal symptoms have been described in experiments where an uninfected person ingests the organism, causing acute infection.[7] Within days of infection, dyspepsia (and acute gastritis histologically) develops but improves spontaneously. Acute infection is also associated with hypochlorhydria. By definition, infection by *H pylori* is associated histologically with gastritis. It does not, however, appear to be associated with other forms of gastritis such as pernicious anemia or eosinophilic gastroenteritis.[8] Studies have attempted to determine the role of *H pylori* in the genesis of nonulcer dyspepsia, given the frequent occurrence of gastritis in this syndrome.[9] Controlled trials have, however, failed to establish a causal role of *H pylori* and gastritis in this syndrome.[10]

Epidemiologic studies have suggested *H pylori* as a potential factor in gastric adenocarcinoma, presumably through chronic gastritis and intestinal metaplasia.[11–20] There is also epidemiologic and experimental evidence of a causal relationship between *H pylori* and gastric lymphoma of mucosa-associated lymphoid tissue, or MALT-oma.[21–26] Clinical trials in which patients with MALT-oma were treated with antibiotics without surgery, radiation, or cytotoxic agents have been successful.[27]

More recently, infection by *H pylori* has been indicted as a permissive factor in the genesis of peptic ulcer disease. Antral gastritis can be histologically identified almost uniformly in patients with duodenal ulcer and in 75% to 80% of patients with gastric ulcer.[10] Recent placebo-controlled studies, in which the organism has been eradicated, document a dramatic reduction in the rate of ulcer recurrence.[28,29] In the series of Graham and colleagues,[29] the duodenal ulcer relapse after *H pylori* eradication at 40 weeks was 12% but was

95% in those not receiving antibiotic treatment. Similarly, for patients with gastric ulcer the recurrence rates were 13% and 74%, respectively. These studies strongly suggest that eradication of *H pylori* alters the natural history of peptic ulcer disease. Further long-term studies are ongoing to determine the most effective and least toxic antibiotic regimen, and to assess the long-term eradication rate.

PATHOLOGY

The initial acute gastritis produced by *H pylori* is rarely seen histologically.[7,30] It consists of an inflammatory infiltrate, composed primarily of neutrophils, with edema in the lamina propria and gastric glands, and degeneration of surface epithelium, but no erosion or lymphoplasmacytic expansion of the lamina propria. Experimentally, this phase was seen 5 days after ingesting *H pylori*,[7] and was restricted to the antrum. Characteristic organisms were demonstrable histologically.

By the time most patients are examined by a physician and endoscopic biopsy specimen is evaluated, the disease has progressed to the stage of active chronic gastritis. This has been observed experimentally on the 11th day following ingestion of *H pylori*.[7] At that time, the lamina propria in the foveolar regions is expanded by a mixed inflammatory cell infiltrate, rich in plasma cells and with a variable number of neutrophils. Neutrophilic infiltration of the glands with damage to the epithelium is observed mainly in the antrum but sometimes in both the antrum and body of the stomach (Figures 60–1 and 60–2). The acute inflammation is usually most intense at the junction of the gastric gland and neck, corresponding to the zone of epithelial proliferation.[30] It is almost always possible to see the curved forms of *H pylori* in the mucus overlying or beside the affected areas using Romanowsky stains or various silver impregnation techniques.[31] (Figures 60–3 through 60–6). Infections of longer duration, if untreated, show a progression of both the intensity and extent of the acute and chronic inflammatory reaction.[32] With further chronicity, the inflammation involves deeper portions of the glands, but always remains mucosal, with progressive loss of endocrine cells and specialized glandular epithelium. Eventually, a picture of chronic atrophic gastritis with intestinal metaplasia is produced.[33] At that late stage, it may be impossible to visualize the organisms. Longstanding infection with *H pylori* also leads to the accumulation of lymphoid aggregates, and to the formation of lymphoid follicles with germinal centers.[34] The picture of follicular gastritis has an extremely high correlation with the presence of *H pylori*.[34–36]

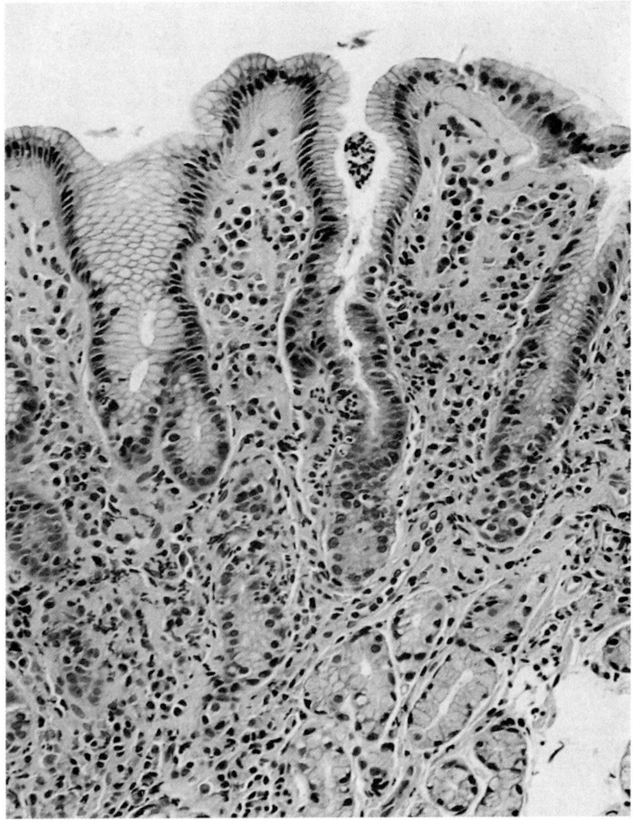

Figure 60–1. Active chronic gastritis associated with *H pylori*. The superficial lamina propria of the antrum is expanded by chronic inflammation, and the midportion of the gland is infiltrated by neutrophils [hematoxylin-eosin (H&E), ×200].

In the active phase of the gastritis, *H pylori* may be more numerous adjacent to, rather than within, the most intensely inflamed areas. That seems to be related to the requirement of the bacteria for gastric mucus, and the mucus depletion that accompanies the inflammation. The mucus depletion is also liable to increase the vulnerability of the gastric mucosa to injury by acid and a variety of ingested substances.[37,38] That gastric mucosa is the target for *H pylori* attack is supported by several studies. Among patients with gastroenteric anastomoses following antrectomy, *H pylori* infected areas of antral metaplasia in the duodenum, but not the normal duodenal mucosa.[39,40] Similarly, in patients with Barrett's esophagus, *H pylori* colonized the metaplastic gastric mucosa.[41] One patient had *H pylori* infection of gastric mucosa in a Meckel's diverticulum.[42] It has been postulated that bacterial ligands of *H pylori* bind to receptors that are exclusively present in gastric epithelial cells with resultant loss of epithelial microvilli and subsequent damage of the function and structure of the cell.[30]

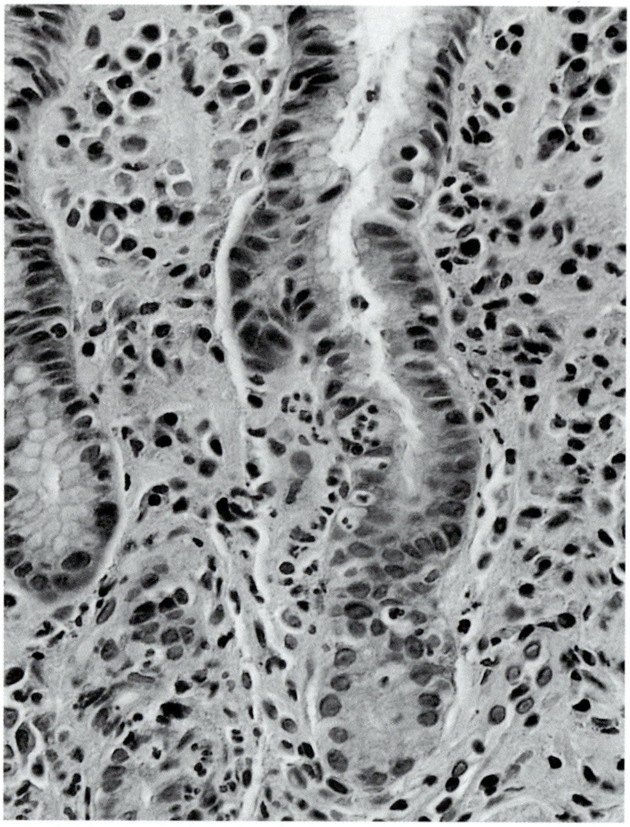

Figure 60–2. The junction of the antral gland and gland neck, where cell regeneration takes place, is infiltrated by neutrophils with accompanying destruction of epithelial cells. The lamina propria is widened by a lymphoplasmacytic infiltrate (H&E, ×400).

Ultrastructural studies have shown the organism to be in intimate contact with the host cell membrane of the surface mucus cells.[43] Some patients have had alterations in the host cell membrane.[44] The organism may occasionally be in the cytoplasm of epithelial cells.[44]

The intensity of symptoms may be related to the histologic severity of the active gastritis,[45,46] but that may not be apparent from a single biopsy specimen. Generous sampling of the gastric mucosa by the endoscopist is an important factor in correlation. At least two antral samples may be necessary to relate the histopathologic features to the clinical features.[45]

Helicobacter infection is almost uniformly in the antrum, and may proceed to involve the proximal stomach.[47] Nevertheless, the disease may be patchy and multiple biopsies throughout the stomach may be needed to document its presence. *Helicobacter pylori* is almost always present with active chronic gastritis. Occasionally the organism may be identified in areas of otherwise normal gastric mucosa. In these patients, biopsies of additional areas of gastric mucosa may demonstrate active chronic gastritis.[47,48]

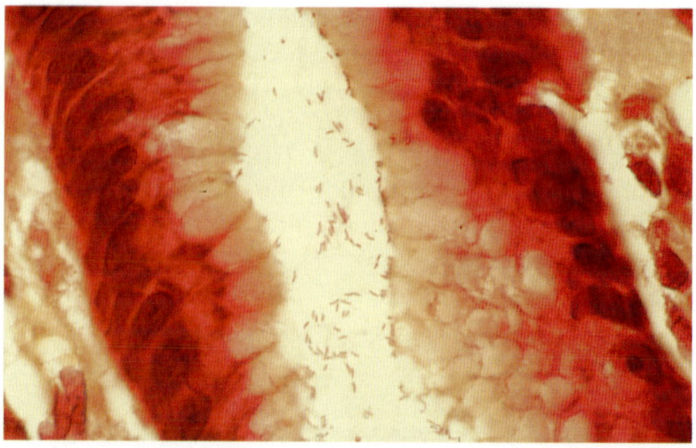

Figure 60–3. Numerous *H pylori* are in the superficial mucus of this gastric mucosal biopsy. The bacilli are easily seen with H&E staining when organisms are numerous (H&E, ×290). *(Contributed by David A. Schwartz, MD, Emory University.)*

Spiral organisms other than *H pylori* have frequently been reported in association with active chronic gastritis.[49–52] Although little is known about these bacteria, one appears to be an inhabitant of the stomachs of cats, dogs, and other mammals and has been named *Spirillum rappini.*[49]

CONFIRMATIONAL TESTING AND DIAGNOSIS

Invasive Tests

Most commonly, *H pylori* is identified on endoscopic biopsy specimens of the gastric mucosa. When multiple

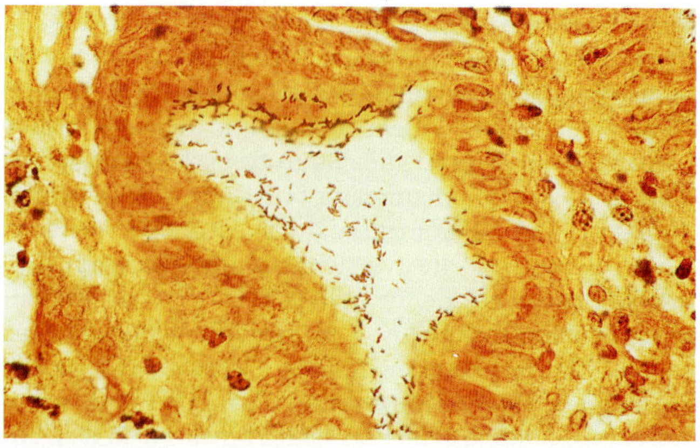

Figure 60–4. The Steiner silver staining method is optimum for demonstrating *H pylori* in biopsy specimens. This specimen of stomach reveals a heavy infection, even at this intermediate magnification (Steiner stain, ×180). *(Contributed by David A. Schwartz, MD, Emory University.)*

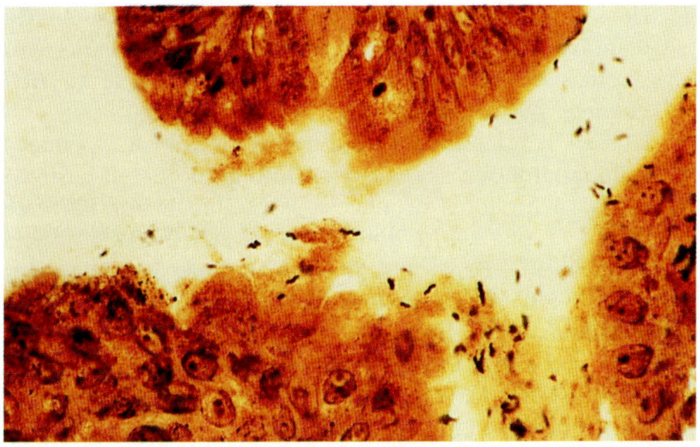

Figure 60–5. Higher magnification demonstrates characteristic gull-winged and spiral shapes of *H pylori* in gastric mucus (Steiner stain, ×290). *(Contributed by David A. Schwartz, MD, Emory University.)*

biopsies are taken, sensitivity for diagnosis is high. The "gold standard" for diagnosis is culture, although this technique appears to be less sensitive than other non-invasive tests. Commercially available tests that utilize the organisms' urease activity have been developed.[53] The biopsy specimen is placed in a solution or gel containing urea and a pH-sensitive dye. If urease is present (and therefore *H pylori*), urea will be split, producing carbon dioxide and ammonia; ammonia will increase the pH of the gel causing a color change. This test has a sensitivity of higher than 90% and is usually positive within an hour. False-negative results may be obtained if a small number of organisms are present, or if an area of *H pylori* infection is not appropriately sampled.

Noninvasive Tests

Breath tests have been developed that take advantage of the bacteria's urease activity. A ^{13}C or ^{14}C-labeled urea is ingested with a liquid meal.[54] In the presence of urease in the stomach, the labeled urea is split into ammonia and C^{14} labeled CO_2, which are absorbed, and then expired in the breath, which can be measured. This test is a highly reliable, noninvasive way to determine the presence of the organism, as well as to monitor eradication after antibiotic therapy.

Serologic Tests

Serologic antibody tests have also been developed, further implicating *H pylori* in the pathogenesis of gastritis. Using the enzyme-linked immunosorbent assay technique, *H pylori*–specific IgG, IgA, and IgM antibodies can be detected in association with *H pylori* infection.[55,56] Current evidence suggests that the presence of serologically identifiable antibody to *H pylori* predicts

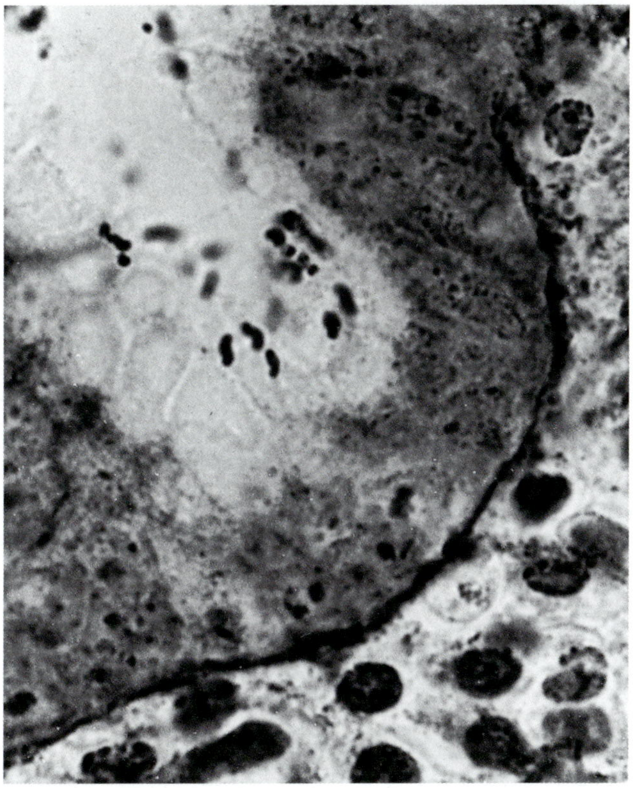

Figure 60–6. In an infected antral gland, numerous curved bacteria typical of *H pylori* are clearly demonstrated by silver impregnation. The bacilli are coated with silver and thus appear black with transmitted light and they are made to appear larger with the coat of silver (Steiner stain, ×1000).

the presence of gastritis. It appears that IgA and IgG antibody titers remain at stable high levels with persistence of the infection. Serologic testing has a high sensitivity and specificity and can obviate the need for endoscopic mucosal biopsy. Antibody titers appear to fall with successful eradication of the infection.[57]

REFERENCES

1. Warren JR. Unidentified curved bacilli on gastric epithelium in active chronic gastritis. *Lancet.* 1983;1:1273. Letter.
2. Marshall B. Unidentified curved bacilli on gastric epithelium in active chronic gastritis. *Lancet.* 1983;1:1273–1275. Letter.
3. Graham DY, Malaty HM, Evans DG, Evans DJ Jr, Klein PD, Adam E. Epidemiology of *Helicobacter pylori* in an asymptomatic population in the United States. Effect of age, race and socioeconomic status. *Gastroenterology.* 1991;100:1495–1501.
4. Dooley CP, Cohen H, Fitzgibbons PL, et al. Prevalence of *Helicobacter pylori* infection and histologic gastritis in asymptomatic persons. *N Engl J Med.* 1989;321:1562–1566.

5. Drumm B, Perez-Perez GI, Blaser MJ, Sherman PM. Intrafamilial clustering of *Helicobacter pylori* infection. *N Engl J Med.* 1990;322:359–363.
6. Perez-Perez GI, Taylor DN, Bodhidatta L, et al. Seroprevalence of *Helicobacter pylori* infections in Thailand. *J Infect Dis.* 1990;161:1237–1241.
7. Morris A, Nicholson G. Ingestion of *Campylobacter pyloridis* causes gastritis and raised fasting gastric pH. *Am J Gastroenterol.* 1987;82:192–199.
8. Ormand JE, Talley NJ. *Helicobacter pylori:* controversies and an approach to management. *Mayo Clin Proc.* 1990; 65:414–426.
9. Sobala GM, Dixon MF, Axon ATR. Symptomatology of *Helicobacter pylori*–associated dyspepsia. *J Gastroenterol Hepatol.* 1990;2:445–449.
10. Peterson WL. *Helicobacter pylori* and peptic ulcer disease. *N Engl J Med.* 1991;324:1043–1048.
11. Nomura A, Stemmermann GN, Chyou P-H, et al. *Helicobacter pylori* infection and gastric carcinoma among Japanese Americans in Hawaii. *N Engl J Med.* 1991;325: 1132–1136.
12. Parsonnet J, Friedman GD, Vandersteen DP, et al. *Helicobacter pylori* infection and the risk of gastric carcinoma. *N Engl J Med.* 1991;325:1127–1131.
13. Nogueira AMM, Ribeiro GM, Rodrigues MAG, et al. Prevalence of *Helicobacter pylori* in Brazilian patients with gastric carcinoma. *Am J Clin Pathol.* 1993;100:236–239.
14. Hansson L-E, Engstrand L, Nyren O, et al. *Helicobacter pylori* infection: independent risk indicator of gastric carcinoma. *Gastroenterology.* 1993;105:1098–1103.
15. Kato T, Saito Y, Niwa M, et al. *Helicobacter pylori* infection in gastric carcinoma. *Eur J Gastroenterol Hepatol.* 1994;6(suppl 1):S93–S96.
16. Recavarren-Arce S, Leon-Barua R, Cok J, et al. *Helicobacter pylori* and progressive gastric pathology that predisposes to gastric cancer. *Scand J Gastroenterol.* 1991; 26(suppl 181):51–57.
17. Munoz N, Crespi M, Correa P, et al. Prevalence of precancerous lesions of the stomach and *Helicobacter pylori* in China. *Ital J Gastroenterol.* 1991;23(suppl 2):5–6.
18. Munoz N, Pisani P. *Helicobacter pylori* and gastric cancer. *Eur J Gastroenterol Hepatol.* 1994;6:1097–1103.
19. Correa P. How does *Helicobacter pylori* infection increase gastric cancer risk? *Eur J Gastroenterol Hepatol.* 1994;6: 1117–1118.
20. DobAlla G, Benvenuti S, Amplatz S, Zancanella L. Chronic gastritis, intestinal metaplasia, dysplasia and *Helicobacter pylori* in gastric cancer: putting the pieces together. *Ital J Gastroenterol.* 1994;26:449–458.
21. Isaacson PG, Spencer J. Malignant lymphoma of mucosa-associated lymphoid tissue. *Histopathology.* 1987;11:445–462.
22. Wotherspoon A, Ortiz-Hidalgo C, Diss T, Falzon MR, Isaacson PG. *Helicobacter pylori*–associated gastritis and primary B-cell gastric lymphoma. *Lancet.* 1991;338:1175–1176.
23. Doglioni C, Wotherspoon AC, Moschini A, de Boni M, Isaacson PG. High incidence of primary gastric lymphoma in northeastern Italy. *Lancet.* 1992;339:834–835.
24. Hussell T, Isaacson PG, Crabtree JE, Spencer J. The response of cells from low-grade B-cell gastric lymphomas of mucosa-associated lymphoid tissue to *Helicobacter pylori*. *Lancet.* 1993;342:571–574.
25. Hussell T, Isaacson PG, Crabtree JE, Dogan A, Spencer J. Immunoglobulin specificity of low grade B-cell gastrointestinal lymphoma of mucosa-associated lymphoid tissue (MALT) type. *Am J Pathol.* 1993;142:285–292.
26. Isaacson PG, Banks PM, Best PV, McLure SP, Muller-Hermelink HK, Wyatt JI. Primary low-grade hepatic B-cell lymphoma of mucosa-associated lymphoid tissue (MALT)-type. *Am J Surg Pathol.* 1995;19:571–575.
27. Wotherspoon AC, Doglioni C, Diss TC, Pan L, Moschini A, de Boni M. Regression of primary low-grade B-cell lymphoma of mucosa-associated lymphoid tissue type after eradication of *Helicobacter pylori*. *Lancet.* 1993;342: 575–577.
28. Rauws EA, Tytgat GN. Cure of duodenal ulcer associated with eradication of *Helicobacter pylori*. *Lancet.* 1990;335: 1233–1235.
29. Graham DY, Lew GM, Klein PD, et al. Effect of treatment of *Helicobacter pylori* infection on the long-term recurrence of gastric or duodenal ulcer. *Ann Intern Med.* 1992;116:705–708.
30. Dixon MF. Morphological aspects of *H pylori* gastritis. In: Proceedings of 3rd Tokyo Int. Symposium on *Helicobacter pylori*. Tokyo: UI Publishing Co; 1990:10–17.
31. Genta RM, Robason GO, Graham DY. Simultaneous visualization of *Helicobacter pylori* and gastric morphology: a new stain. *Hum Pathol.* 1994;25:221–226.
32. Niemela S, Karttunen T, Kerola T. *Helicobacter pylori*–associated gastritis. Evolution of histologic changes over 10 years. *Scand J Gastroenterol.* 1995;30:542–549.
33. Eidt S, Stolte M. Prevalence of intestinal metaplasia in *Helicobacter pylori* gastritis. *Scand J Gastroenterol.* 1994; 29:607–610.
34. Genta RM, Hamner HW, Graham DY. Gastric lymphoid follicles in *Helicobacter pylori* infection: frequency, distribution and response to triple therapy. *Hum Pathol.* 1993;24:577–583.
35. Eidt S, Stolte M. Prevalence of lymphoid follicles and aggregates in *Helicobacter pylori* gastritis in antral and body mucosa. *J Clin Pathol.* 1993;46:832–835.
36. Genta RM, Hamner HW. The significance of lymphoid follicles in the interpretation of gastric biopsy specimens. *Arch Pathol Lab Med.* 1994;118:740–743.
37. Ormand JE, Talley NJ. *Campylobacter pylori,* mucus and peptic ulceration. A dynamic interaction. *J Clin Gastroenterol.* 1989;5:492–495.
38. Dixon MF. *Helicobacter pylori* and peptic ulceration: histopathological aspects. *J Gastroenterol Hepatol.* 1991;6: 125–130.
39. Fitzgibbons PL, Dooley CP, Cohen H, Appleman MD. Prevalence of gastric metaplasia, inflammation, and *Campylobacter pylori* in the duodenum of members of normal population. *Am J Clin Pathol.* 1988;90:711–714.
40. Offerhaus GJA, Molyvas EN, Hoedemaeker PG. *Helicobacter pylori* infection of gastric mucin cell metaplasia: the duodenum revisited. *J Pathol.* 1990;162:239–243.

41. Talley NJ, Cameron AJ, Shorter RG, Zinsmeister AR, Phillips SF. *Campylobacter pylori* and Barrett's esophagus. *Mayo Clin Proc.* 1988;63:1176–1180.*Comm Gut.* 1990;31: 243.
42. Morris A, Nicholson G, Zwi J, Vanderwee M. *Campylobacter pylori* infection in Meckel's diverticula containing gastric mucosa. *Gut.* 1989;30:1233–1235.
43. Bode G, Malfertheiner P, Ditschuneit H. Pathogenetic implications of ultra-structural findings in *Campylobacter pylori* related gastroduodenal disease. *Scand J Gastroenterol.* 1988;23(suppl 142):25–39.
44. Evans DG, Evans DJ, Graham DY. Adherence and internalization of *Helicobacter pylori* by Hep-2 cells. *Gastroenterology.* 1992;102:1557–1567.
45. Morris A, Ali MR, Brown P, Lane M, Patton K. *Campylobacter pylori* infection in biopsy specimens of gastric antrum: laboratory diagnosis and estimation of sampling error. *J Clin Pathol.* 1989;42:727–732.
46. Czinn SJ, Bertram TA, Murray PD, Yang P. Relationship between gastric inflammatory response and symptoms in patients infected with *Helicobacter pylori. Scand J Gastroenterol.* 1991;26(suppl 181):33–37.
47. Bayerdorffer E, Lehn N, Hatz R, et al. Difference in expression of *Helicobacter pylori* gastritis in antrum and body. *Gastroenterology.* 1992;102:1575–1582.
48. Peterson WL, Lee E, Feldman M. Relationship between-*Campylobacter pylori* and gastritis in healthy humans after administration of placebo or indomethacin. *Gastroenterology.* 1988;95:1185–1197.
49. Morris A, Ali MR, Thomsen L, Hollis B. Tightly spiral shaped bacteria in the human stomach: another cause of active chronic gastritis? *Gut.* 1990;31:139–143.
50. Dye KR, Marshall BJ, Frierson HF, Guerrant RL, McCallum RW. Ultrastructure of another spiral organism associated with human gastritis. *Dig Dis Sci.* 1989;34:1787–1791.
51. Oliva MM, Lazenby AJ, Permen JA. Gastritis associated with *Gastrospirillum hominis* in children: comparison with *Helicobacter pylori* and review of the literature. *Mod Pathol.* 1993;6:513–515.
52. Vanzanten SJOV, Malatjalian DA, Desormeau LM, Pereira LV. Gastritis induced by the *Helicobacter gastrospirillum hominis. Can J Gastroenterol.* 1994;8:257–260.
53. Marshall BJ, Warren JR, Francis GJ, Langton SR, Goodwin CS, Blincow ED. Rapid urease test in the management of *Campylobacter pyloridis*–associated gastritis. *Am J Gastroenterol.* 1986;82:200–210.
54. Royan EAJ, Langenberg W, Woensel JV, Urij AA, Tytgat GN. 14C-urea breath test in *C pylori* gastritis. *Gut.* 1989; 30:798–803.
55. Musgrove C, Bolton FJ, Krypczyk AM, et al. *Campylobacter pylori*: clinical, histological, and serological studies. *J Clin Pathol.* 1988;41:1316–1321.
56. Perez-Perez GI, Dworkin BM, Chodos JE, Blaser MJ. *Campylobacter pylori* antibodies in humans. *Ann Intern Med.* 1988;109:11–17.
57. Morris AJ, Ali MR, Nicholson GI, Perez-Perez GI, Blaser MJ. Long-term follow-up of voluntary ingestion of *Helicobacter pylori. Ann Intern Med.* 1991;114:662–663.

CHAPTER 61

Haemophilus influenzae Infection

Edith F. Marley and Joseph M. Campos

. . . but people in good health were all of a sudden attacked by violent heats in the head, and redness and inflammation in the eyes, the inward parts, such as the throat or tongue, becoming bloody and emitting an unnatural and fetid breath . . .

Thucydides (471?–400? BC)

DEFINITION

Members of the genus *Haemophilus* are small, nonmotile, gram-negative coccobacillary or pleomorphic bacilli.[1] They are facultative anaerobes. Most species require hemin and/or nicotinamide adenine dinucleotide (NAD) (X and V factors) for growth. These may be supplied by the lysed erythrocytes of chocolate agar, by nutritionally enriched growth media, or may be excreted by other organisms present in mixed cultures.

Robert Koch first described *Haemophilus*-like organisms in conjunctival exudates in 1882. Pfeiffer, however, is generally recognized as discovering the primary pathogen *Haemophilus influenzae* in 1892. He isolated the organism from the sputum and lung tissue of patients who died during the human influenza pandemic of that year.[1] In retrospect, the organism likely represented a secondary bacterial invader in those who died from influenza virus infection.

Alexander and others established encapsulated (typeable) *H influenzae* strains as significant agents of infection, particularly meningitis and bacteremia. Capsular serotype b *H influenzae* was recognized as the most frequent agent of invasive infection in children. Elucidation and purification of the type b capsular polysaccharide antigen led to the development of highly immunogenic vaccines, the first introduced in 1985. Although there has been a marked reduction in the incidence of infection caused by this serotype, *Haemophilus* sp remain an important cause of a varied spectrum of human infections.

EPIDEMIOLOGY

The 10 human species in the genus *Haemophilus* are primarily colonizers of the upper respiratory tract. They may be considered part of the commensal flora of the nasopharynx and oropharynx. *Haemophilus ducreyi* is the exception; it is a pathogen of the genital tract. *Haemophilus influenzae* is the species that most frequently causes human disease.

The nasopharynx is the portal of entry for *H influenzae*, and person-to-person spread is by inhalation of respiratory droplets. Respiratory tract colonization rates for all strains may be as high as 50% of the population.[2] Most species that populate the upper airway are nonencapsulated *H influenzae* and *H parainfluenzae* strains. Infections caused by the nonencapsulated strains usually occur at sites contiguous with the upper respiratory tract. However, these may cause severe respiratory tract disease in patients with any form of respiratory compromise, or invasive disease in the immunodeficient patient. Colonization by capsular type b strains of *H influenzae* is fairly uncommon in healthy infants, children, and adults.

CLINICAL MANIFESTATIONS

Haemophilus infections range from those that are frequent, mild, and uncomplicated (eg, conjunctivitis, otitis media) to those that are uncommon, severe, difficult to manage, and with significant sequelae.

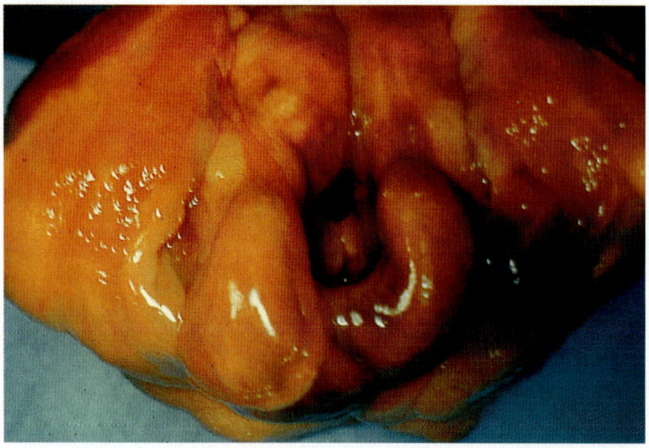

Figure 61–1. Fatal infection in a child with acute laryngeal edema and laryngeal obstruction caused by *H influenzae* (1956). The patient was a 5-year-old girl who was well until 1 week before admission, when she complained of sore throat. The morning of admission she had noisy respirations, and by the time a physician reached her home she was cyanotic and moribund. When she arrived at the hospital, a laryngoscope was passed to establish a clear airway. The epiglottis was purple-red and edematous. In spite of supportive measures, she died. At autopsy, bacteriologic cultures of specimens from heart, lung, and esophagus grew *H influenzae* type b. The epiglottis, aryepiglottic folds, and vocal cords were edematous, causing almost complete obstruction of the lumen. *(Courtesy of Harry P. W. Kozakewich, MD, and Ernest E. Lack, MD.)*

Until recently, *H influenzae* type b was the leading cause of bacterial meningitis and epiglottitis (Figure 61–1), both of which are potentially life-threatening infections. *Haemophilus influenzae* type b was also a major cause of pericarditis, pneumonia, septic arthritis, osteomyelitis, and facial cellulitis.[3] Routine culture techniques used for urine specimens do not recover this bacterium, so the true incidence of urinary tract infections caused by *H influenzae* may be higher than the few reported. A combination of vaccination, rifampin prophylaxis of contacts, and use of more efficacious therapeutic agents has sharply reduced the incidence of invasive infections. Adults now represent up to 24% of cases of invasive *H influenzae* infections, and bacteremic pneumonia accounts for 70% of these infections.[4] Other antecedent events for invasive *H influenzae* infections in adults are obstetric infections, epiglottitis, and tracheobronchitis. Underlying debilitating conditions are present in the vast majority of these patients.

Nontypeable strains frequently cause lower respiratory tract infections (febrile tracheobronchitis and community-acquired pneumonia) in both adults and children. These infections may cause exacerbations of chronic bronchitis, and occasionally invasive infections in neonates, children, adults, and immunodeficient patients.[4–6] In children, these organisms are the most common cause of purulent bacterial conjunctivitis and, after *Streptococcus pneumoniae,* the most frequent cause of otitis media.[6]

Haemophilus influenzae has been associated with acute chorioamnionitis.[7] Although recognized as a major pathogen of young children, its role as an infection that can be transferred vertically to the fetus or newborn is less well known. One study showed *H influenzae* to be a definite cause of early neonatal bacteremia.[8]

In São Paulo, Brazil, in 1984, strains of *H influenzae* (biogroup *aegyptius*) caused an outbreak of Brazilian purpuric fever, a severe childhood illness characterized by high fever, abdominal pain, vomiting, hemorrhagic skin lesions, vascular collapse, and death.[9]

PATHOLOGY

The sites and nature of *H influenzae* infections are such that few biopsy specimens need to be procured or examined. Localized infections (such as conjunctivitis) may generate clinical specimens. Although direct Gram staining techniques are not as sensitive as culture, their sensitivity may be improved by cytocentrifugation of specimens onto microscopic slides. As with other bacterial infections, the inflammatory response is acute, primarily neutrophils (Figure 61–2, A and B). There may be accompanying tissue damage and necrosis. The meningitis, like other bacterial meningitides, is suppurative and may be hemorrhagic (Figures 61–3 and 61–4). Purulent discharges or body fluids [eg, cerebrospinal fluid (CSF)] may be examined microscopically following Gram stain at the time of culturing (Figure 61–5). Intra-amnionic infection may result in the examination of the placenta. Criteria for acute chorioamnionitis are 1) evidence of a maternal and/or fetal inflammatory response, 2) neutrophils in the chorioamnion, and 3) chorionic plate and umbilical cord vasculitis. There are no histopathologic features distinctive for *H influenzae* infection.

PATHOGENESIS

The establishment of infection after intranasal inoculation of *H influenzae* depends on several steps: 1) the ability to colonize and penetrate the oro/nasopharyngeal mucosa, 2) the ability to reach, survive, and multiply in the bloodstream, and 3) the ability to infect target tissues.[10] Possession of a polysaccharide capsule is an important virulence factor for *Haemophilus* strains

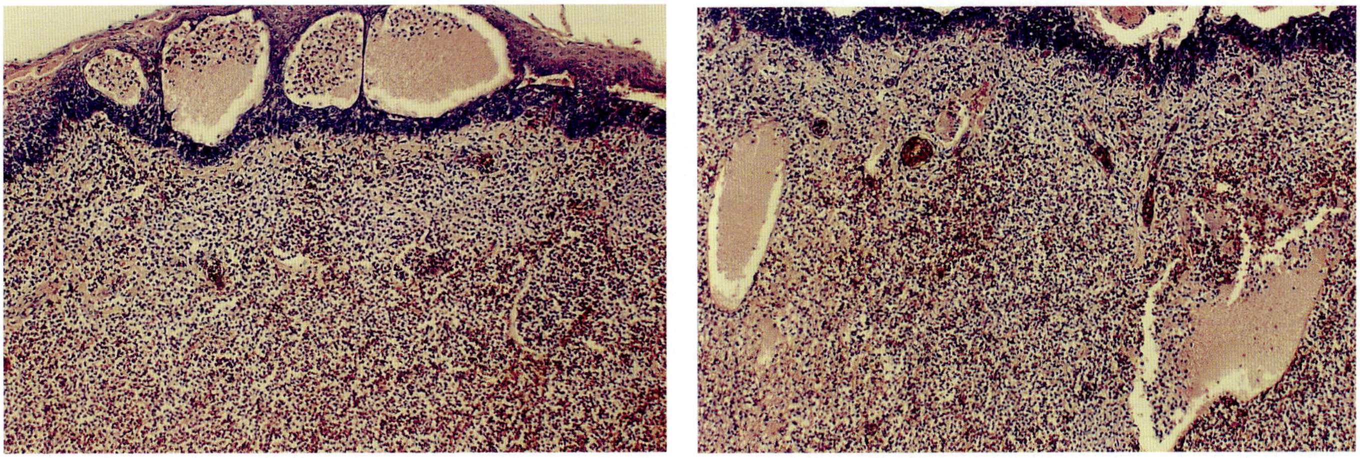

A B

Figure 61–2. (**A**) Epiglottis shown in Figure 61–1. There is mucosal ulceration with severe edema and acute inflammation throughout all layers of the epiglottis, except the cartilage. Scattered gram-negative bacilli were identified in the tissue (toluidine-blue eosin, ×100). (**B**) Same epiglottis showing marked acute ulceration and inflammation caused by *H influenzae* (toluidine-blue eosin, ×150).

that cause systemic infections. The capsule may facilitate colonization and protect against complement mediated destruction and/or phagocytosis. Production of IgA protease may also play a role. Lipopolysaccharide (LPS) composition varies among *Haemophilus* strains and differs from that of the Enterobacteriaceae, but all exhibit endotoxic activity. LPS may cause the production of local inflammation in the meninges and elsewhere.[10]

DIAGNOSIS

Recovery of *Haemophilus* sp from specimens containing commensal flora is difficult, because of the fastidious growth requirements of the organism and the ease with which the small colonies of *Haemophilus* can be obscured by those of other microorganisms.[2] Blood, body fluids, and ocular and respiratory specimens may

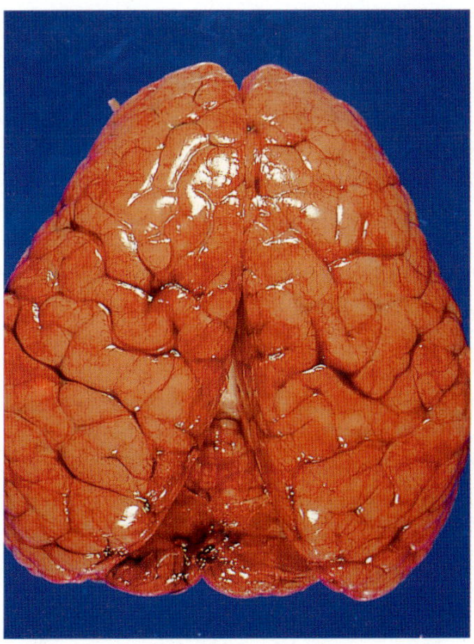

Figure 61–3. Diffuse suppurative meningitis caused by *H influenzae*. There is a diffuse milky discoloration to the surface of the brain, most prominent over the frontal lobes. Patchy hemorrhage is also a conspicuous feature. *(Courtesy of Ernest E. Lack, MD.)*

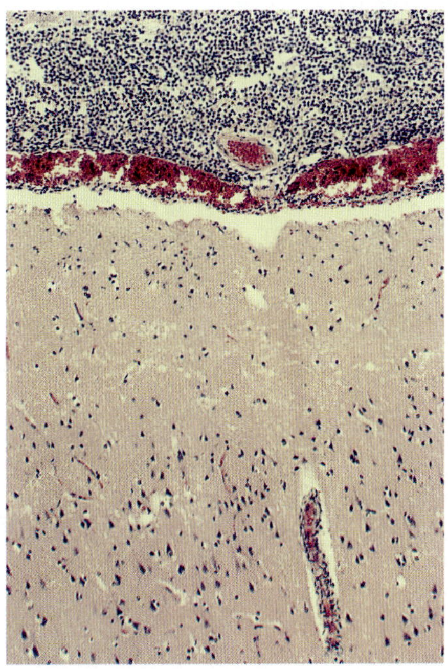

Figure 61–4. Acute suppurative meningitis shown in Figure 61–3. The subarachnoid space is expanded by a purulent exudate and the subarachnoid vessels are congested (luxol-fast-blue-eosin, ×120).

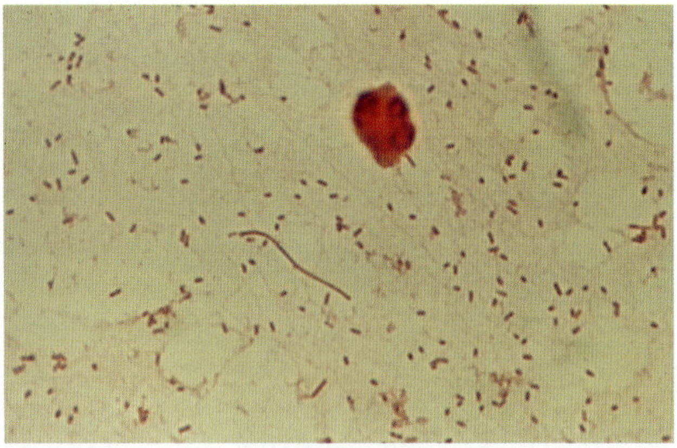

Figure 61–5. Small gram-negative pleomorphic bacilli in smear of CSF. This fluid was from a patient with *H influenzae* meningitis (Gram stain, ×1000).

be cultured. Documenting *Haemophilus* sp as the cause of lower respiratory tract infection is difficult because it is part of the colonizing flora of the upper respiratory tract. Specimens should be inoculated to chocolate agar and/or a suitable enrichment broth. In addition to determining growth requirements, key biochemical tests are performed to identify isolates to the species level.

In direct specimen smears, the Gram stain lacks sensitivity; in addition, the organisms are relatively small. The tiny, gram-negative coccobacilli of *H influenzae* can be camouflaged very effectively by the gram-negative proteinaceous strands and stained cellular debris present in inflamed body fluids. Use of the methylene blue stain highlights dark-blue bacteria against a lighter gray background. Smears stained with acridine orange from specimens in which bacteria are expected to be in low concentration may be examined under a fluorescence microscope. This DNA binding stain detects fluorescent orange-stained bacilli. Gram stain must then be used to determine the bacteria's differential staining characteristics.

Serotyping methods exist for identifying encapsulated strains of *H influenzae*. Particle agglutination methods, enzyme immunoassay, radioimmunoassay, and indirect immunofluorescence assays for *H influenzae* type b antigens have been developed. An immunoperoxidase method using a monoclonal antibody directed against an outer membrane protein of *H influenzae* has been employed in sputum specimens from patients with cystic fibrosis.[2]

TREATMENT

Until approximately the mid-1970s, ampicillin was uniformly effective for treating *Haemophilus* infections. Since that time ampicillin–penicillin resistance has become commonplace. Chloramphenicol resistance also exists, especially where this drug is still in common use. Trimethoprim–sulfamethoxazole-, tetracycline-, and rifampin-resistant strains also are being detected with increasing frequency. Resistance is primarily by a plasmid-mediated beta lactamase in the case of ampicillin, and microbial production of an inactivating enzyme (chloramphenicol acetyl transferase) for chloramphenicol. Cefotaxime or ceftriaxone are the drugs of choice for treating invasive infections. Because the sensitivity of *Haemophilus* sp to other antimicrobial agents is unpredictable, routine testing of clinically significant isolates is recommended.

REFERENCES

1. Koneman EW. *Haemophilus.* In: Koneman EW, Allen SD, Janda WM, et al, eds. *Diagnostic Microbiology.* Philadelphia: JB Lippincott; 1992:279–301.
2. Campos JM. *Haemophilus.* In: Murray PR, ed. *Manual of Clinical Microbiology.* Washington, DC: American Society for Microbiology; 1995:556–565.
3. Dajani AS, Asman BI, Thirumoorthi MC. Systemic *Haemophilus influenzae* disease: an overview. *J Pediatr.* 1979;94:355–364.
4. Farley MM, Stephens DS, Brachman PS Jr, et al. Invasive *Haemophilus influenzae* disease in adults: a prospective population-based surveillance. *Ann Intern Med.* 1992;116: 806–812.
5. Friesen CA, Cho CT. Characteristic features of neonatal sepsis due to *Haemophilus influenzae. Rev Infect Dis.* 1986;8:777–780.
6. Gilsdorf JR. *Haemophilus influenzae* non-type b infections in children. *Am J Dis Child.* 1987;141:1063–1065.
7. Benirschke K. Infectious disease. In: Benirschke K, Kaufman P, eds. *Pathology of the Human Placenta.* New York: Springer-Verlag; 1995:537–624.
8. Brazilian Purpuric Fever Study Group. Brazilian purpuric fever: epidemic purpura fulminans associated with antecedent purulent conjunctivitis. *Lancet.* 1987;ii:761–763.
9. Rusan P, Adam RD, Petersen EA, Ryan KJ, Sinclair NA, Weinstein L. *Haemophilus influenzae.* An important cause of maternal and neonatal infections. *Obstet Gynecol.* 1991;77:92–96.
10. Turk DC. The pathogenicity of *Haemophilus influenzae. J Med Microbiol.* 1984;18:1–16.

CHAPTER 62

Intestinal Spirochetosis

Heidrun Rotterdam

An ounce of illness is felt more than an hundredweight of health.

Dutch Proverb

HISTORIC ASPECTS

Intestinal spirochetes were first described by the inventor of the light microscope, Leeuwenhoek, who is said to have discovered these organisms in his own stool in 1719.[1] It was not until the late nineteenth century that Escherich in Germany made these bacteria known to the medical public when he saw spirochetes in the stool of patients with cholera.[1] In the early twentieth century, reports from France,[2] England,[3] and Africa[4] confirmed the global presence of intestinal spirochetes. They were noted in a variety of intestinal illnesses, but soon the organisms were found in the feces of healthy individuals also,[5] and the question of whether intestinal spirochetes are innocent commensals or pathogens has remained. The frequencies with which spirochetes have been isolated from human feces in the more recent past does not depend on the presence or absence of symptoms, but on nationality and lifestyle.

In West Africans, a frequency of 100% was reported in 1917,[4] but a much lower figure of 23% came from a study of Rwandans in 1986.[6] Certain Asian populations have a relatively high frequency: 27% of Gulf Arabs in Oman[7] and 4.6% of Indian nationals in Great Britain have spirochetes in their intestines.[8] By contrast, spirochetes were in only 1.2% of British soldiers in 1916,[3] and in 1.5% of 1527 subjects living in England in 1986, all of whom were either Asians or homosexuals.[8] Homosexuals in Scotland had spirochetes in their stools in 21%[8] and 36%[9] even before the acquired immunodeficiency syndrome epidemic, although none had symptoms.

Attachment of spirochetes to the colonic surface epithelium was first described by electron microscopy in 1967.[10] Interestingly, spirochetosis was recognized by light microscopy only when the specimen was reviewed after electron microscopy.

DEFINITION

The presence of spirochetes in stool specimens is not necessarily synonymous with intestinal spirochetosis. Intestinal spirochetosis has been variously defined as "overgrowth of spirochetes"[8,11] or as "infestation of intestinal epithelium by spirochetes."[12] Because "overgrowth" implies that there is a baseline normal growth that is exceeded, and no such normal baseline is established for spirochetes, the latter definition of epithelial infestation by spirochetes is more objective and used in this chapter.

Not all patients whose stool cultures are positive for intestinal spirochetes have tissue involvement. In one study of human immunodeficiency virus (HIV)-infected patients whose stool cultures were positive for spirochetes, only 50% had spirochetosis on subsequent biopsies.[13]

GEOGRAPHIC DISTRIBUTION

Intestinal spirochetosis so defined requires a biopsy for diagnosis. Its incidence should show the same geographic distribution as that of spirochete-positive stool specimens. The few studies of African and Asian populations available, however, did not employ biopsies, although most of the recent studies of Western populations did.

Incidences in Europeans vary from 2.5% to 16.5%.[12,14–16] Of 1205 Norwegians undergoing colorectal biopsies during 1990, 2.5% had intestinal spirochetosis.[14] Similarly, 5% of 200 Danish patients undergoing sigmoidoscopy,[15] 10% of 100 consecutive rectal biopsies from British patients,[16] and 16.5% of 145 consecutive colon biopsies from Greek patients[12]—groups with a variety of intestinal conditions—also had intestinal spirochetosis.

These incidences are slightly higher than those based on stool specimens, suggesting that intestinal spirochetosis may be more common in patients with underlying intestinal diseases. However, no biopsy studies of healthy subjects are available to confirm this impression. In two U.S. series, intestinal spirochetosis was found in 2%[17] and less than 1%[18] of rectal biopsies. In homosexual men, the incidence of intestinal spirochetosis diagnosed on rectal or colonoscopic biopsies was 30%, regardless of whether they were HIV positive.[13,19] This figure is similar to the frequencies of 21%[8] and 36%[9] reported for stool specimens. Therefore it is most probable that the majority of patients with spirochetes in their stool would also have intestinal spirochetosis on biopsy.

MORPHOLOGIC, BIOCHEMICAL, AND GENETIC FEATURES OF INTESTINAL SPIROCHETES

The spirochetal bacteria noted in human feces and large intestinal biopsies are probably a heterogeneous group. In 1982, Danish investigators isolated a species of nontreponemal spirochete from patients with intestinal spirochetosis, described its morphologic features and culture requirements, and named it *Brachyspira aalborgii.*[20] The organism is a regularly coiled spirochete 4 to 6 μm long and 2 to 3 μm wide. A second, irregularly coiled, larger type of spirochete, more common in Eastern and African populations than in Europeans,[7] has been identified by electronmicroscopy and varies in length from 4 to 20 μm and in width from 0.2 to 0.5 μm. This type of spirochete was named *Spirochaeta eurygyrata,*[4] a term no longer accepted taxonomically. *Spirochaeta eurygyrata* now is placed tentatively in the genus *Treponema.*[21] Recent reports refer to this at-present nameless organism simply as *fecal* or *intestinal spirochete.*[7,21] By scanning electron microscopy, a third type of intestinal spirochete, 1.9 μm long and 0.2 μm in diameter, was in a rectal biopsy of a 70-year-old woman with diarrhea. The bacteria were only slightly wavy and had only a few tight spirals.[22] These varying descriptions suggest that intestinal spirochetosis may be caused by more than one strain of spirochete.

Several different biotypes of intestinal spirochetes were discerned on microbiologic and biochemical characterization of spirochetes isolated from the feces of homosexual males.[23] Intestinal spirochetes are anaerobes and grow poorly or not at all in broth or on solid media in the absence of serum supplements. The best medium suggested is a trypticase soy agar, supplemented with spectinomycin, polymyxin B, and either citrated human blood or defribinated horse blood.[23] Two distinct morphologic types of spirochetes could be distinguished: colony-forming and haze-forming types. Furthermore, differences in biochemical, enzyme, and volatile fatty-acid profiles support the notion that intestinal spirochetes are a heterogeneous group. Biochemically, they produce esterases C4 and C8, and B-galactosidase, and by activity they metabolize a wide range of carbohydrates.[8,24]

Comparative analysis of the genomes of intestinal spirochetes of human and animal origin has yielded interesting results.[25] First, human intestinal spirochetes are genetically unrelated to nonintestinal spirochetes, such as *Treponema pallidum.* Second, human intestinal spirochetes are closely related to *Treponema hyodysentericae,* the etiologic agent of swine diarrhea. Third, there is great variation in the degree of DNA homology between the swine *T hyodysentericae* and 21 human intestinal spirochetes tested—30% to 100%—indicating again that human intestinal spirochetes comprise a genetically heterogeneous group. Thus, morphologic, biochemical, and genetic observations come to the same conclusion.

CLINICAL FEATURES

No single specific clinical feature is associated with intestinal spirochetosis. Intestinal spirochetosis has been found in patients with a variety of intestinal diseases, which prompted endoscopy and biopsy; however, most are unrelated etiologically. These include appendicitis,[26] irritable bowel syndrome, colonic diverticulosis, colonic carcinoma, colonic polyps, ulcerative colitis, megacolon, malabsorption, gastric or duodenal ulcer, dyspepsia, hemorrhoids, and diarrhea of unknown cause.[12,15] It has been suggested that chronic stasis may favor spirochetal replication and mucosal infestation.[12] This would explain some of the noted associations, such as with colonic carcinoma, diverticulosis, megacolon, and appendicitis. In routine surgical pathology specimens, intestinal spirochetosis most often afflicted patients with adenomatous polyps and diarrhea of unknown cause (personal observation). In homosexual men, gonorrhea was significantly associated with spirochetosis.[19] A perianal condyloma in a 12-year-old boy was superinfected with intestinal spirochetes.[27] In children, intestinal spirochetosis has been associated with diarrhea and rectal bleeding, ascariasis, and enterobiasis, as well as with a variety of nonspecific symptoms.[28,29] Spirochetes were in the appendix and colon. In HIV-infected patients, intestinal spirochetosis affects primarily homosexual men.[13,30,31] In some of these patients, diarrhea could not be ascribed to any other infectious agent, and both symptoms and spirochetes disappeared after treatment with metronidazole,

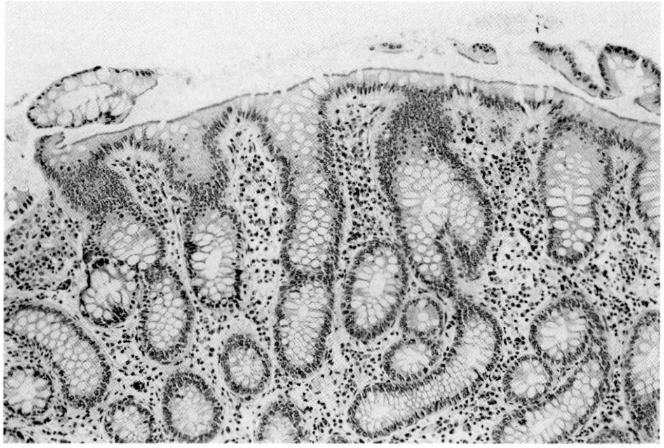

Figure 62–1. Intestinal spirochetosis, low magnification: A dark band covers the luminal surface of the colonic epithelium (hematoxylin-eosin, ×100).

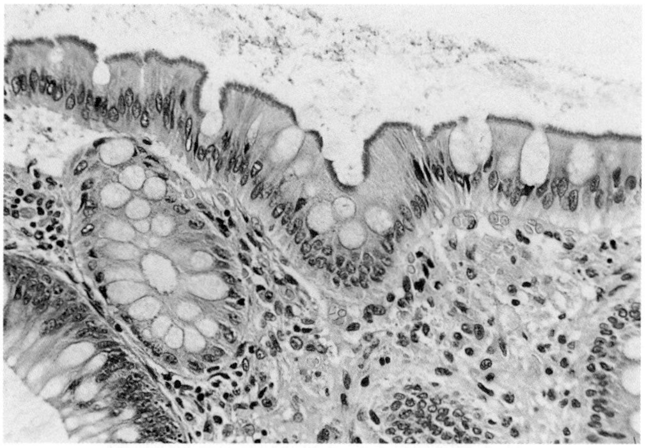

Figure 62–2. Intestinal spirochetosis, higher magnification: Spirochetes are attached to the surface of absorptive cells but not to goblet cells (hematoxylin-eosin, ×250).

suggesting that intestinal spirochetes may become pathogenic in HIV-infected patients. Spirochetosis in HIV-infected patients is exclusively in those not treated previously with antibiotics or antiparasitic medications.[13] There was no correlation between the degree of infestation and the degree of immune suppression as determined by T4 cell counts. In non–HIV-infected patients, clinical and histopathologic evidence of cure after antibiotic therapy was provided in rare patients with unexplained diarrhea,[11] and in one 16-year-old girl with amoxycillin-therapy–related diarrhea and intestinal spirochetosis.[24] In most other patients, treatment eradicated the organism but not the symptoms, suggesting that in these patients intestinal spirochetosis had no clinical significance.[11,15] Controversy over treatment and pathogenicity persists.[32] The situation in humans is thus similar to that of other mammals, in which there exists a spectrum of intestinal spirochetosis with apparently asymptomatic excretion in rodents, mucosal colonization without symptoms in primates, and epithelial attachment and damage leading to diarrhea in swine.[33]

PATHOLOGY

The appendix, sigmoid colon, and rectum are most commonly involved in humans. In healthy rhesus monkeys, used for various experiments, intestinal spirochetosis—morphologically identical to human spirochetosis—involved the entire large intestine but not the small intestine.[17] In 1930, appendiceal involvement was reported in 9.6% of patients with appendicitis-like symptoms,[33] and in 1974, in 2.1% of 388 patients, many of whom had an appendectomy incidental to other surgery.[17] As previously mentioned, rectal spirochetosis was demonstrated in up to 10% of unselected rectal biopsy specimens[10] and in 30% of homosexuals with[13] or without[19] known HIV infection. In HIV-infected patients, spirochetosis was shown to involve several segments of the colon and even to extend into the distal ileum.[13] In the majority of these latter patients, other pathogens coexisted.

There are no distinctive gross pathologic features of intestinal spirochetosis. Microscopically, however, the features are distinctive, and once encountered, they are easy to recognize. Hematoxylin-eosin–stained sections reveal a basophilic fringe, 2 to 3 μm thick, on the luminal aspect of the surface epithelium. Although visible at low magnification (Figure 62–1), this fringe is best seen at high magnification (Figure 62–2). To pathologists unfamiliar with spirochetosis, this fringe or band may be mistaken for a brush border comprised of microvilli. Microvilli, however, are shorter and eosinophilic (pink), whereas the fringe of spirochetes appears as a radially striate blue layer (Figure 62–3). If the junction of normal and abnormal surface epithelium is included, the distinction is obvious. The spirochetal band covers the lumenal surfaces of absorptive cells, spares goblet cells (Figure 62–2), and extends for a short distance into the neck of crypts. Deeper portions of the crypt epithelium are not affected. In adenomatous polyps, spirochetes do not usually colonize the neoplastic epithelium (Figures 62–4, A and B), with the possible exception of one case described but not illustrated.[12] The organism stains with periodic acid–Schiff (PAS), Giemsa, Masson–Fontana, and the Warthin–Starry and Dieterle silver stains (Figure 62–5). The strong staining with PAS and weak staining with Alcian blue indicate the presence of a large amount of neutral and a small amount of acid mucosubstances.[16] In one study,

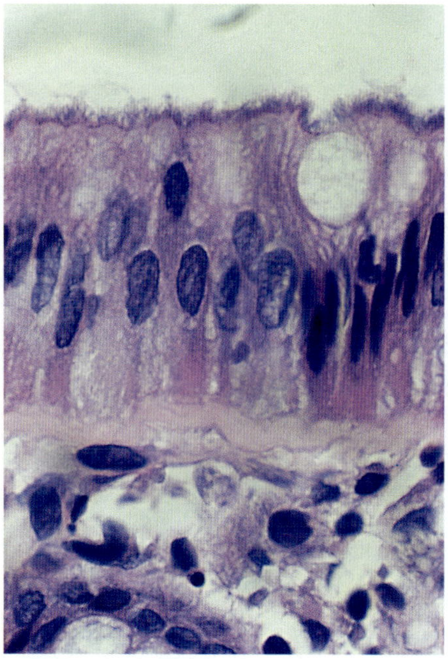

Figure 62–3. Intestinal spirochetosis. Surface epithelium and the luminal portion of crypt epithelium are colonized. Spirochetes are basophilic in contrast to the eosinophilic microvilli (hematoxylin-eosin, ×1000).

silver stains doubled the number of infections recognized visible by light microscopy.[19] Organisms can be detached from the surface within mucus (Figure 62–5). Darkfield illumination also demonstrates the organism as well (Figure 62–6). Typically, the crypt architecture is intact and the number of inflammatory cells in the lamina propria appears normal or only mildly increased,[11,29] unless there is a coexisting infection or inflammatory disorder. Immunohistochemical studies of mucosal plasma cells have yielded conflicting results.[11,34] An increase in IgE-producing plasma cells, up to 30% of the entire plasma cell population, and a decrease in IgA-producing plasma cells was found in one study.[11] This shift reversed to normal—with only single, scattered IgE cells—after eradication of the organisms, suggesting that the IgE plasmacytosis was directly related to the spirochetosis. Another study demonstrated a decrease in IgD- and IgE-positive cells and an increase in IgA cells.[34] These differences may reflect differences in patient populations. All tissues with increases in IgA cells were derived from patients who underwent resections for colon cancer.[34]

Electronmicroscopy discloses additional changes, which may reflect the pathogenic mechanisms for diarrhea associated with some cases of intestinal spirochetosis: The spirochetes are attached vertically to the surface of the epithelial cell and between the microvilli (Figure 62–7), or, less frequently, along the length of the bacterial surface.[24] The length of the spirochetes varies within the same patient. For instance, long spirochetes (4 to 6 μm long × 0.18 to 0.2 μm wide), may alternate with shorter and thicker spirochetes less than 4 μm long and 0.3 to 0.4 μm wide.[24] Microvilli may be well preserved, reduced in number in some regions, or blunted and destroyed in others.[11,24] Spirochetes also may be in the cytoplasm of the absorptive epithelial

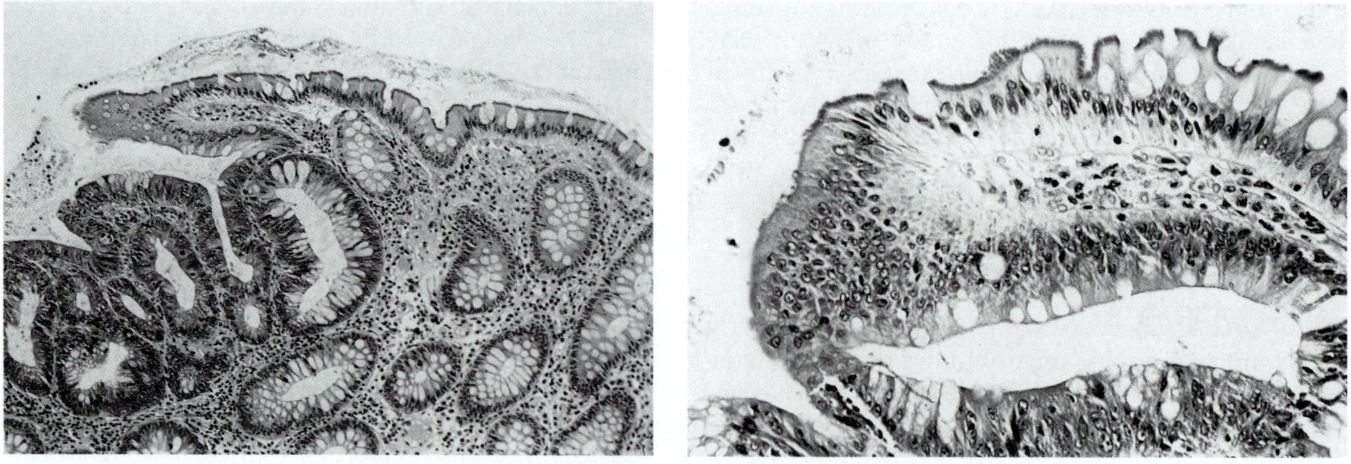

A B

Figure 62–4. (**A**) Intestinal spirochetosis associated with a tubular adenoma. The neoplastic epithelium is not affected (hematoxylin-eosin, ×100). (**B**) Same lesion showing the fringe of spirochetes involving the non-neoplastic surface epithelium adjacent to the tumor (hematoxylin-eosin, ×250).

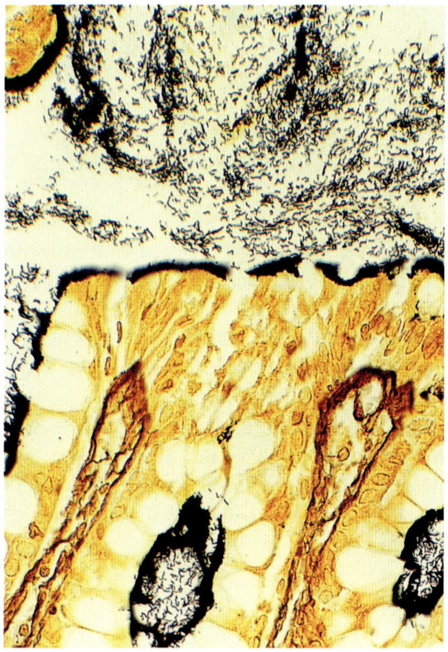

Figure 62–5. Intestinal spirochetosis. Organisms are intensely silvered and are attached to colonic surface epithelium as well as lying freely within mucus. Surface of crypt epithelium is also involved (Dieterle, ×400).

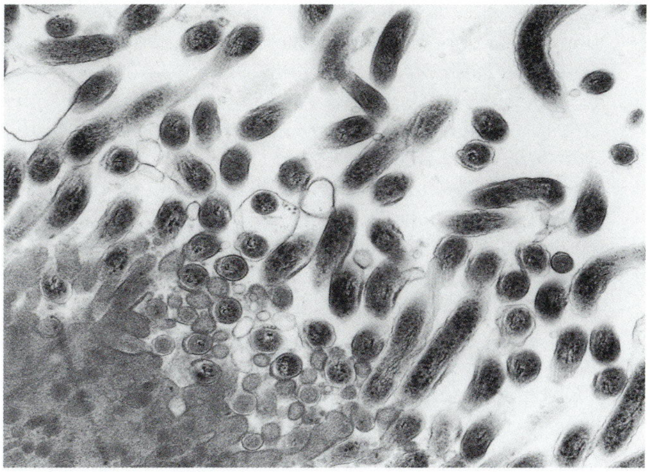

Figure 62–7. Intestinal spirochetosis. By electronmicroscopy, spirochetes (dark) are between microvilli (light). Individual spirochetes are within a membranous sheath and display spirally arranged flagella, which appear dotlike on cross-section and wavy on longitudinal section (EM, ×35,500). *(Courtesy of Dr. Gurdip S. Sidhu, Manhattan Veterans Administration Hospital, New York.)*

cells, within well-circumscribed inclusions or randomly distributed, and singly or in clusters within macrophages of the lamina propria. These findings establish a potential for invasion and cell damage. The finding of partially degranulated intraepithelial mast cells with large cytoplasmic vacuoles, is another interesting feature not previously noted in any other intestinal inflammatory condition.[11]

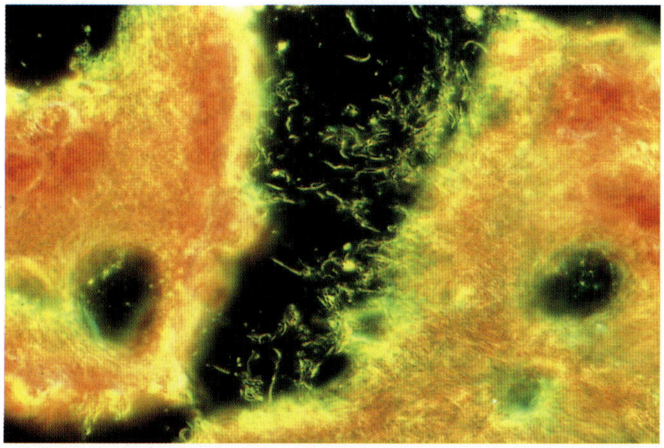

Figure 62–6. Intestinal spirochetosis. Darkfield illumination shows numerous spirochetes in the mucus layer and attached to the surface epithelium (Darkfield, ×1000).

REFERENCES

1. Escherich T. Klinisch-therapeutische Beobachtungen aus der Cholera-Epidemie in Neapel. *Arztliches Intelligenz-Blatt.* 1884;31:561–564.
2. Le Dantec M: Dysenterie spirillaire CR. *Soc Biol (Paris).* 1903;55:617–618.
3. Fantham HB. Observations on *Spirochaeta eurygyrata* as found in human feces. *Br Med J.* 1916;I:815–816.
4. Macfie JWS. The prevalence of *Spirochaeta eurygyrata* in Europeans and natives in the Gold Coast. *Lancet.* 1917: 336–340.
5. Parr LW. Intestinal spirochetes. *J Infect Dis.* 1923;33: 369–383.
6. Goossens H, Lejour M, De Mol O, et al. Isolation of *Treponema hyodysentericae* from human faecal specimens; a curiosity or a new enteropathogen? In: First European Congress of Clinical Microbiology, 1983; Bologna. Abstract 267. As cited by Tompkins DS, Foulkes SJ, Godwin PGR, West AP. Isolation and characterization of intestinal spirochaetes. *J Clin Pathol.* 1986;39:535–541.
7. Barrett SP. Intestinal spirochaetes in a Gulf Arab population. *Epidemiol Infect.* 1990;104:261–266.
8. Tompkins DS, Foulkes SJ, Godwin PGR, et al. Isolation and characterization of intestinal spirochaetes. *J Clin Pathol.* 1986;39:535–541.
9. Tompkins DS, Waugh MA, Cooke EM. Isolation of intestinal spirochaetes from homosexuals. *J Clin Pathol.* 1981; 34:1385–1387.
10. Harland WA, Lee FD. Intestinal spirochaetosis. *Br Med J.* 1967;III:718–719.

11. Gebbers IO, Ferguson DJP, Mason C, et al. Lokale Immunreaktion bei intestinaler Spirochätose des Menschen. *Schweiz Med Wschr.* 1987;117:1087–1091.
12. Delladetsima K, Markaki S. Papadimitriou. Intestinal spirochaetosis. Light and electron microscopic study. *Pathol Res Pract.* 1987;182:780–782.
13. Kasbohrer A, Gelderblom HR, Arasteh W, et al. Intestinale Spirochätose bei HIV-Infektion. *Dtsch Med Wschr.* 1990;115:1499–1506.
14. Lindboe CF, Tostrup NE, Nersund R, et al. Human intestinal spirochetosis in mid-Norway. A retrospective histopathologic study with clinical correlations. *APMIS.* 1993; 101:858–864.
15. Nielsen RH, Orholm M, Pedersen JO, et al. Colorectal spirochetosis. Clinical significance of the infestation. *Gastroenterology.* 1983;85:62–67.
16. Lee FD, Kraszewski A, Gordon J, et al. Intestinal spirochetosis. *Gut.* 1971;12:126–133.
17. Takeuchi A, Jervis HR, Nakazawa H, et al. Spiral-shaped organisms on the surface colonic epithelium of the monkey and man. *Am J Clin Nutr.* 1974;27:1287–1296.
18. Gear EV, Dobbins WO. Rectal biopsy. *Gastroenterology.* 1968;55:522–544.
19. Surawicz CM, Roberts PL, Rompalo A, et al. Intestinal spirochetosis in homosexual men. *Am J Med.* 1987; 82:587–592.
20. Hovind-Hougen K, Birch-Anderson A, Henrik-Nielsen R, et al. Intestinal spirochetosis; morphological characterization and cultivation of the spirochete *Brachyspira aalborgi;* gen. nov. sp. nov. *J Clin Microbiol.* 1982;16: 1127–1136.
21. Cooper C, Cotton DWK, Hudson MJ, et al. Rectal spirochetosis in homosexual men; characterization of the organism and pathophysiology. *Genitourin Med.* 1986; 62:47–52.
22. Lager DJ, Landas SK. Correlative light and scanning electron microscopy of intestinal giardiasis, cryptosporidiosis, and spirochetosis. *Ultrastruc Pathol.* 1991;15:585–591.
23. James MJ, Miller NJ, George L. Microbiological and biochemical characterization of spirochetes isolated from the feces of homosexual males. *Clin Microbiol.* 1986;24: 1071–1074.
24. Rodgers FG, Rodgers C, Shelton AP, et al. Proposed pathogenic mechanism for the diarrhea associated with human intestinal spirochetes. *Am J Clin Pathol.* 1986;679–682.
25. Coene M, Agliano AM, Paques AT, et al. Comparative analysis of the genomes of intestinal spirochetes of human and animal origin. *Infect Immun.* 1989;57: 138–145.
26. Henrik-Nielsen R, Lundbeck FA, Teglebjaerg PS, et al. Intestinal spirochetosis of the vermiform appendix. *Gastroenterology.* 1985;88:971–977.
27. Sagerman PM, Kadish AS, Niedt GW. Condyloma acuminatum with superficial spirochetosis simulating condyloma latum. *Am J Dermatol.* 1993;15:176–179.
28. While J, Roche D, Chan YF, et al. Intestinal spirochetosis in children: report of two cases. *Ped Pathol.* 1994;14: 191–199.
29. da Cunha RMC, Ferreira RM, Phillips AD, et al. Intestinal spirochetosis in children. *J Ped Gastroenterol Nutr.* 1993;17:333–336.
30. Lafeuillade A, Quilichini R, Benderitter T, et al. Intestinal spirochetosis in HIV-infected homosexual men. *Postgrad Med J.* 1990;66:253–254.
31. Nathwani D, McWhinney PHM, Green ST, et al. Intestinal spirochetosis in a man with the acquired immune deficiency syndrome (AIDS). *J Infect.* 1990;21:318–319. Letter.
32. Lo TC, Heading RC, Gilmour HM. Intestinal spirochetosis. *Postgrad Med J.* 1994;70:134–137.
33. Harris DL, Kinyou JM. Significance of anaerobic spirochetes in the intestines of animals. *Am J Clin Nutr.* 1974;27:1297–1304.
34. Lindboe CF, Engesvoll I, Darell M, et al. Immunoglobulin-containing cells in the colonic mucosa in patients with human intestinal spirochetosis. *APMIS.* 1994;102:849–854.

CHAPTER 63

Klebsiella and Rhinoscleroma

David A. Schwartz and Stanley J. Geyer

A faith healer may or may not start out with fraud in mind. But to his amazement, his patients actually seem to be improving. Their emotions are genuine, their gratitude heart-felt. Whenever the healer is criticized, such people rush to his defense.

Carl Sagan (1934–), The Demon Haunted World

INTRODUCTION

The *Klebsiella* are gram-negative bacteria and are an important component of the normal flora of the gastrointestinal tract. They cause a wide variety of clinical illnesses, including pneumonia, urinary tract infections, bacteremia, and a chronic granulomatous disease of the upper airways. These organisms are most frequently associated with disease in the setting of nosocomial infections and in debilitated or immunodeficient patients.

CLASSIFICATION

Members of the genus *Klebsiella* belong to the family Enterobacteriaceae, a large heterogeneous group of gram-negative bacilli that contains some of the most medically important pathogens of humans. The genus *Klebsiella* shares the tribe Klebsielleae with three other genera: *Enterobacter, Hafnia,* and *Serratia.* Collectively, members of the tribe Klebsielleae have become the third leading cause of nosocomial infections in the United States. Four species belong to the genus *Klebsiella: K pneumoniae, K ozaenae, K rhinoscleromatis,* and *K oxytoca. Klebsiella pneumoniae* was previously termed Friedländer's bacillus.[1] Rhinoscleroma has been termed scrofulous lupus and scleroma, and the causative agent, *K rhinoscleromatis,* has been previously known as the "encapsulated diplococcus of Frisch."

EPIDEMIOLOGY

Although *K pneumoniae* is well known as an important cause of community-acquired pneumonia, the population at high risk for pulmonary infection includes those with underlying illnesses, including diabetes mellitus, alcoholism, and chronic obstructive pulmonary disease. Thus, this agent behaves as an opportunistic or nosocomial pathogen more frequently than it does as a community-acquired disease. Capsular type 1, 3, 4, and 5 have been most often associated with respiratory tract illness, which usually presents as nosocomial-acquired bronchiectasis or bronchopneumonia.

Klebsiella sp have been isolated from the feces and upper respiratory tract of 5% to 10% of healthy persons. *Klebsiella* sp have been reported to cause 8% of all documented nosocomial bacterial infections, including (in order of decreasing frequency) infection of the urinary tract, lower respiratory tract, biliary tract, and surgical wound sites. Most clinical isolates of *Klebsiella* are associated with urinary tract sepsis. A recent study from the Centers for Disease Control and Prevention showed that *Klebsiella* was the cause of 9% of urinary tract infections and 14% of primary bacteremias in hospitalized patients.[2] Indwelling and invasive devices used in patient care are an important source of nosocomial *Klebsiella* infections, including intravenous and urinary catheters and endotracheal tubes. The isolates of *Klebsiella* in hospitalized patients usually demonstrate multiple antibiotic resistance. Bloodstream infections caused by *K pneumoniae* have been reported in hemodialysis patients following nosocomial contamination of dialyzers by poor glove-changing techniques and inadequate sterilization procedures.[3] Multiple drug-resistant strains of *K pneumoniae* with plasmid-borne extended-spectrum beta-lactamases are an increasingly alarming source of concern in nosocomial infections.[4]

Klebsiella pneumoniae has been reported also as an agent of nursery epidemics. During these outbreaks, colonization rates of neonates is high, but most patients are asymptomatic. The primary source of nosocomial infection in these patients is contaminated fomites.

Other species of *Klebsiella,* notably *K ozaenae* and *K rhinoscleromatis,* are associated with upper respiratory tract infections, usually outside the United States. The role of *K ozaenae* in chronic atrophic rhinitis, or ozaenia, is not well established. *Klebsiella rhinoscleromatis* is the etiologic agent of rhinoscleroma, a chronic granulomatous disease of the upper respiratory tract. Although the initial reports of this disease were from Central and Eastern Europe, rhinoscleroma is now rare or absent in those areas. Currently, rhinoscleroma is mostly among impoverished and rural inhabitants of Central and South America, Egypt and parts of Africa, the Middle East, Philippines, and India. Rhinoscleroma does not appear to be highly communicable.[1]

BIOLOGY

Klebsiella is the second most populous genus of bacteria present in the intestinal flora of humans. The *Klebsiella* are lactose-fermenting (with the exception of *K rhinoscleromatis*), nonmotile bacilli. *Klebsiella pneumoniae* is approximately 6 μm in length and 0.6 μm in width, whereas *K rhinoscleromatis* is a smaller organism measuring from 2 to 3 μm in length. They are facultative anaerobes, and are H_2S and indole negative. Greater than 95% of isolates of *K pneumoniae* give a positive Voges–Proskauer reaction, can grow in KCN, and utilize citrate as a sole carbon source. Members of this genus form large, mucoid colonies on agar (Figure 63–1), and appear microscopically as large bacilli with Gram staining, both of which are caused by a prominent polysaccharide capsule. This capsule contains the K (capsular) antigens, which are more useful for serotyping purposes than the five identified O (somatic) antigens. Immunization of rabbits stimulates antibodies that cause serotype-specific agglutination and microscopic demonstration of the capsule, termed the quellung reaction. This reaction is caused by increased visibility of the capsule because the binding of antibody renders it refractile (Figure 63–2). More than 70 types of K (capsular) antigens have been identified by precipitin, agglutination, or quellung reactions, although none has been identified as conferring a greater probability of infection. The capsule is an important virulence factor for *Klebsiella,* because it has been associated with prevention of neutrophil migration into infected tissues, and also in inhibiting phagocytosis. Some K antigens of *Klebsiella* demonstrate cross-reactivity with the capsules of *H influenzae* and the pneumococcus. The majority of *K ozaenae* strains belong to capsular type 4, while most *K rhinoscleromatis* strains are type 3.[1]

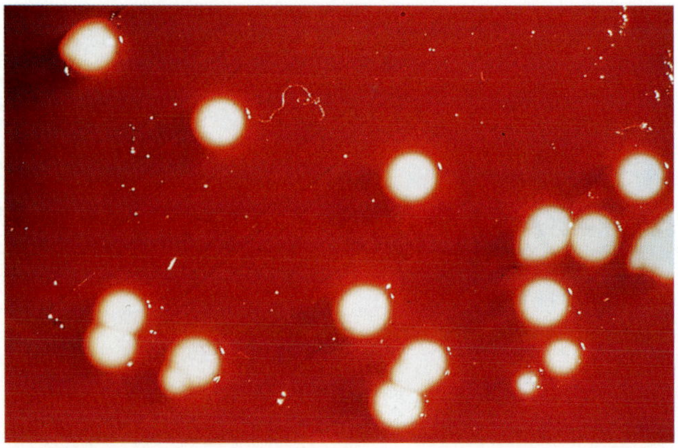

Figure 63–1. Typical appearance of *K pneumoniae* colonies on blood agar.

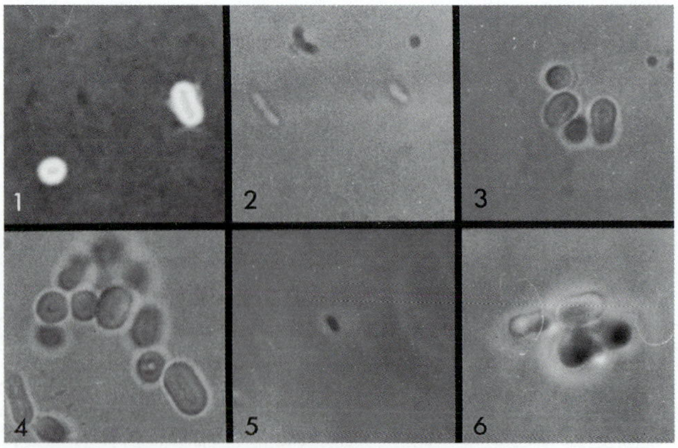

Figure 63–2. Photomicrographs of *K pneumoniae* in clinical and laboratory specimens. (*1*) India ink preparation showing capsule (×1000); (*2*) *K pneumoniae* type 60 in heterologous antiserum (×1000); (*3*) *K pneumoniae* type 60 in type 60 antiserum showing typical appearance of positive quellung reaction (×1000); (*4*) *K pneumoniae* type 60 in type 60 antiserum (×1000); (*5*) *K pneumoniae* type 60 in heterologous antiserum phase contrast (×1000); (*6*) *K pneumoniae* type 60 in type 60 antiserum, (phase contrast, ×1000). *(Photograph contributed by Dr. Eickhoff, Centers for Disease Control and Prevention, Atlanta, Georgia.)*

CLINICAL FEATURES

Pulmonary Disease

Most *Klebsiella* infections of lung are bronchopneumonia or bronchiolitis. Characteristically, patients have an abrupt onset with chills, high fever, productive cough with hemoptysis, pleuritic chest pain, and shortness of breath. Sputum from patients with *Klebsiella* pulmonary disease is often described as "currant jelly" because of the hemorrhagic, necrotic, and inflammatory changes in the lung and airways. Radiographic findings often show a swollen, infiltrated lobe, producing the "bowed fissure" radiologic sign. Pneumonia caused by *K pneumoniae* is a severe illness and can produce destructive lung lesions. Patients with *Klebsiella* pneumonia are at high risk of abscesses, cavitations, bronchiectasis, empyema, and pleural adhesions, and mortality remains high. Leukopenia is common in patients with severe infections. In a recent study of alcoholic patients with community-acquired *Klebsiella* pneumonia, the overall mortality rate was 64%. In 39% of these patients, there was a concomitant *Klebsiella* bacteremia, which was associated with a high (100%) mortality rate.[5]

In addition to debilitated and immunosuppressed adults, *Klebsiella* can also produce pneumonia and septicemia in neonates and infants,[6] but infection in these age groups is unusual. The case fatality rate in sporadic pediatric infections is approximately 50%.

Rhinoscleroma

Rhinoscleroma is an unusual granulomatous disease caused by *K rhinoscleromatis,* an organism that is not a normal inhabitant of the nasal flora. Rhinoscleroma involves the mucosa of the upper respiratory tract, and leads, in severe infections, to bony invasion and airway obstruction. The disease receives its name from the tendency of the lesions to undergo fibrosis, developing "scleromatous" nodules. The initial symptoms can resemble a common cold; but in fully developed disease there can be upper airway obstruction, dysphonia, aphonia, and anosmia. Anesthesia of the soft palate and hypertrophy of the uvula should suggest the clinical diagnosis of rhinoscleroma. In patients with completely developed rhinoscleroma, there are large, firm, intramucosal nasal masses having a coarsely granular surface. These lead to external expansion of the nose, especially involving the nasal cartilage. Nodules may also be in the subcutaneous tissues around the nose. In the proliferative stage of development, nasal involvement may be severe, causing a deformity known as "Hebra nose" (Figure 63–3). Recent reports include a patient with systemic infection[7] and two human immunodeficiency virus (HIV)-infected patients with oropharyngeal rhinoscleroma.[8]

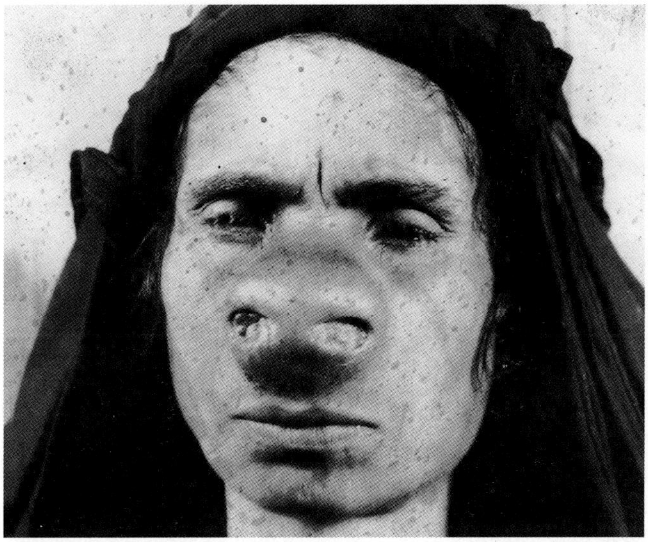

Figure 63–3. Typical "Hebra nose" in a patient with fully developed rhinoscleroma. *(Photograph contributed by the Armed Forces Institute of Pathology, Washington, DC.)*

Other Presentations

Extrapulmonary infections by *K pneumoniae* and *K oxytoca* have been reported. Enterotoxin-producing strains of *K pneumoniae* have been described from patients with a tropical spruelike illness.[9] In a 5-year review of patients with meningitis, *Klebsiella* species caused 15% of 61 cases of gram-negative bacterial meningitis.[10] Brain abscesses and wound infections also have been described.[11] One of us has seen a unique case of suppurative mastitis in a nonpuerperal woman caused by *K oxytoca* (Figures 63–4 through 63–7). Liver abscesses and septic endophthalmitis caused by *K pneumoniae* can occur, especially in patients with diabetes mellitus.[12] *Klebsiella oxytoca* has caused endocarditis following transurethral resection of the prostate,[13] and has been associated with spontaneous peritonitis in a patient with cardiac ascites.[14]

An etiologic role of *K ozaenae* has been proposed in chronic atrophic rhinitis. This is associated with necrosis of the nasal mucosa accompanied by a foul mucopurulent nasal discharge. This organism has also been isolated from patients with bacteremia and urinary tract and soft tissue infections.[1]

PATHOLOGY

Pneumonia

The acute pneumonia may be patchy, lobular, or lobar (Figures 63–8 and 63–9). There may be a consolidating infiltrate involving an entire lobe, which grossly and

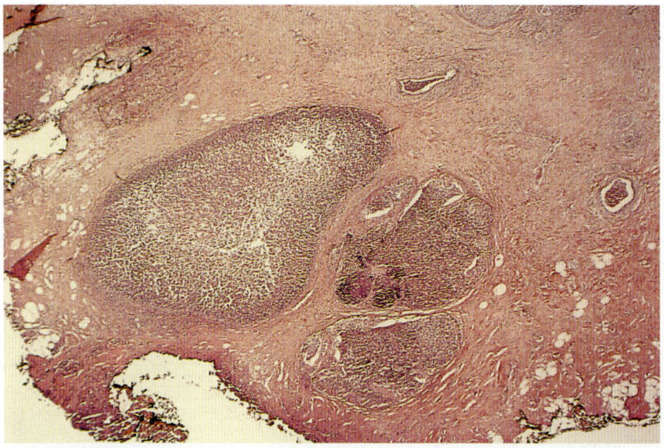

Figure 63–4. Acute suppurative mastitis in a 41-year-old nonpuerperal woman with sudden onset of breast pain, fever, and chills. Cultures were positive only for *K oxytoca*. Multiple ducts are filled with neutrophils and necrotic material [hematoxylin-eosin (H&E), ×20].

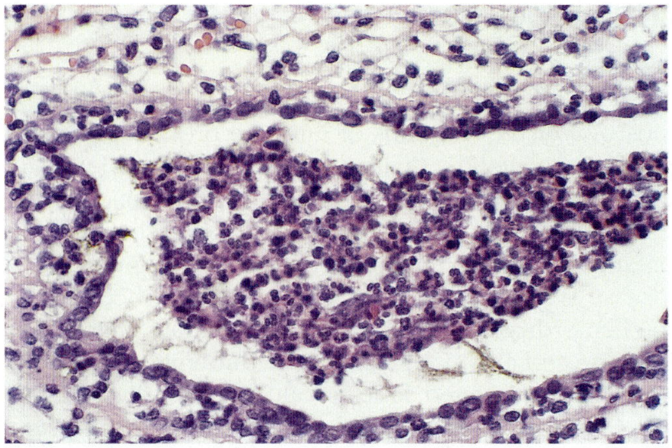

Figure 63–6. The microscopic changes in this inflamed duct are not specific for *Klebsiella* infection. Culture is essential to define the cause (H&E, ×400).

radiographically resembles the lobar pneumonia caused by the pneumococcus. Compared with pneumococcal pneumonia, however, parenchymal destruction tends to be more severe and abscess formation is more common. Empyema is a frequent complication of *Klebsiella* pneumonia.

In the acute stages of infection, *Klebsiella* pneumonia resembles other bacterial pneumonias, with parenchymal consolidation and loss of crepitation (Figures 63–10 and 63–11). Neutrophils fill the alveolar spaces, and the alveolar septal capillaries are congested. Foamy macrophages are in alveolar spaces and areas of inflammation, and gram-negative bacilli can be seen in the cytoplasm of some cells using tissue Gram staining. Because of their thick polysaccharide capsules, the bacilli are blackened with the Gomori methenamine-silver technique. In chronic pulmonary infection, there is extensive scarring, which may efface large areas of alveolar architecture. The bronchi can show acute and chronic inflammation, glandular hyperplasia, luminal dilatation, and fibrosis. In areas of bronchiolitis or bronchopneumonia, there is necrotizing bronchitis, and necrotic material fills the lumina of the airways. Abscess can be severe and multicentric (Figure 63–9).

Massive pulmonary gangrene is a rare but severe complication in which early diagnosis and surgical intervention are necessary to save the patient's life. The pulmonary parenchyma shows extensive necrosis, but

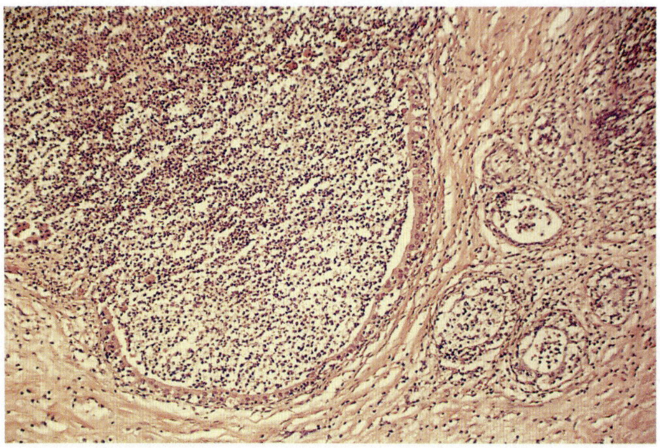

Figure 63–5. Same lesion shown in Figure 63–4. Both small-order and larger, ectatic lactiferous ducts are involved (H&E, ×100).

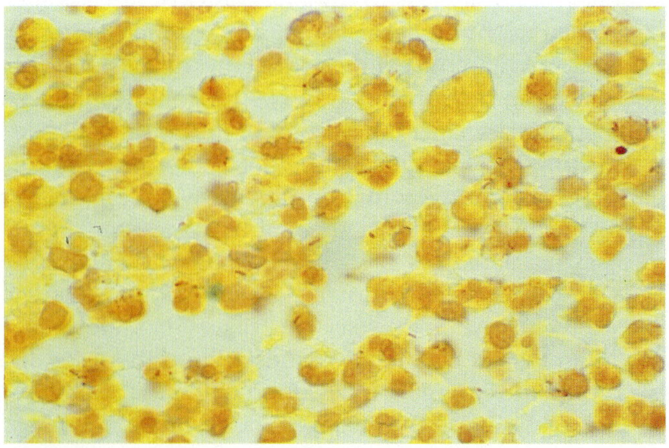

Figure 63–7. Gram-negative bacilli, consistent with culture findings of *Klebsiella,* are in the necrotic and inflamed material in a lactiferous duct (tissue Gram stain, Brown–Hopps, ×1000).

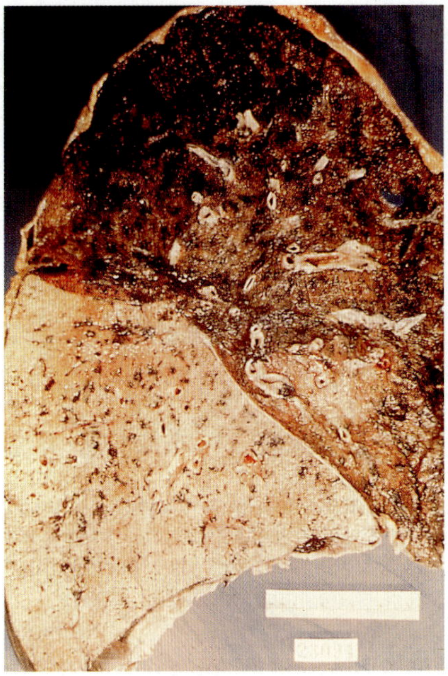

Figure 63–8. Lung from autopsied patient with fatal lobar pneumonia caused by *K pneumoniae*. Note the sharp contrast between the involved lower lobe and uninvolved upper lobe.

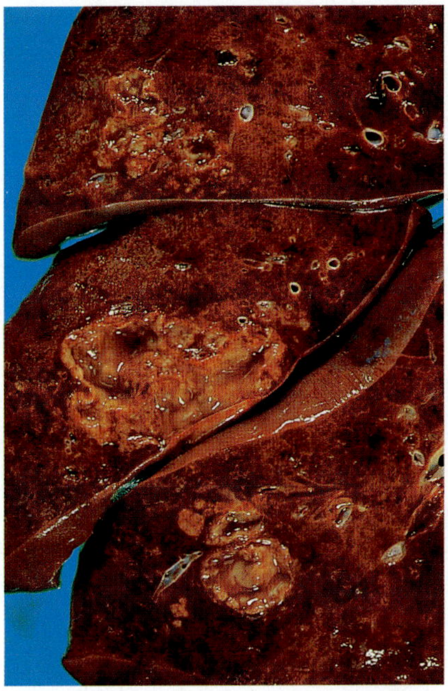

Figure 63–9. Lung from a patient with *Klebsiella* bronchopneumonia. Multiple lobes are involved, with abscesses.

the underlying architecture of the lung can still be identified. Thrombosis[15] and acute vasculitis without organisms in the inflamed vessels have been reported.[16]

Rhinoscleroma

Rhinoscleroma passes through three microscopic stages of development—the catarrhal (or rhinitis) stage, proliferative (or granulomatous) stage, and fibrotic stage. In the catarrhal or rhinitis stage, the mucosa contains nonspecific inflammatory changes with abundant neutrophils, cellular debris, and granulation tissue. In the proliferative or granulomatous stage, there is intense granulomatous inflammation that involves the nasal mucosa and, occasionally, the upper lip, paranasal sinuses, lacrimal duct, orbit, pharynx, larynx, and trachea. The characteristic lesion of rhinoscleroma shows a thickened, hyperplastic mucosa in which there may be squamous metaplasia. Under the epithelium is an intense submucosal inflammatory cell infiltrate composed of plasma cells, Russell bodies, and large foamy nonlipid containing histiocytes called "Mikulicz cells" (Figures 63–12 and 63–13). These cells are present in variable numbers, but often are in large sheets. Mikulicz cells have a single rounded and hyperchromatic nucleus, which is usually peripheral. The cells vary in size, but can attain up to 200 μm in diameter. Within the cytoplasm of Mikulicz cells the rod-shaped bacteria can be seen using Steiner or Warthin–Starry silver stains, or with Giemsa (Figure 63–14). When bacteria are plentiful, they may be seen with routine H&E staining. By electron microscopy, Mikulicz cells contain many large phagosomes filled with scanty *Klebsiella* bacilli, and a finely granular or fibrillar material.[17] Occasional neutrophils or eosinophils can also be present in the inflammatory infiltrate. In the final, or fibrotic, stage there are variable degrees of fibrosis. Mikulicz cells are characteristically absent in this stage. At least two

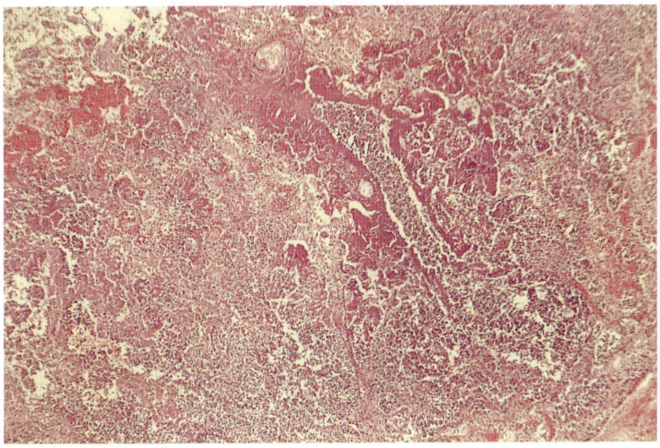

Figure 63–10. Typical appearance of *Klebsiella* pneumonia: inflammation, consolidation, hemorrhage, and necrosis (H&E, ×40).

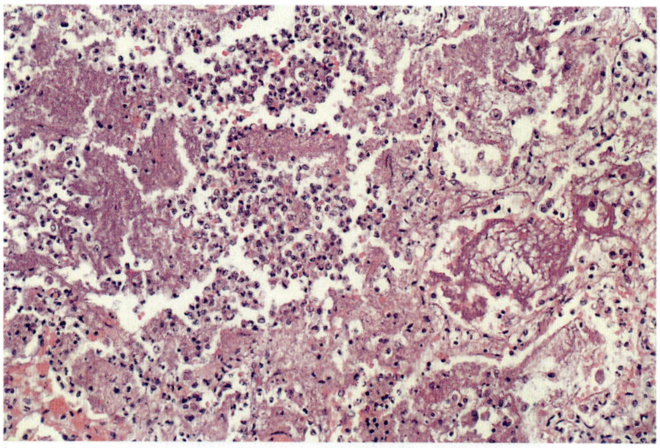

Figure 63–11. Fatal necrotizing pneumonia caused by *K pneumoniae* in a premature neonate. This section of lung shows extensive necrotizing inflammation and intra-alveolar fibrin (H&E, ×100).

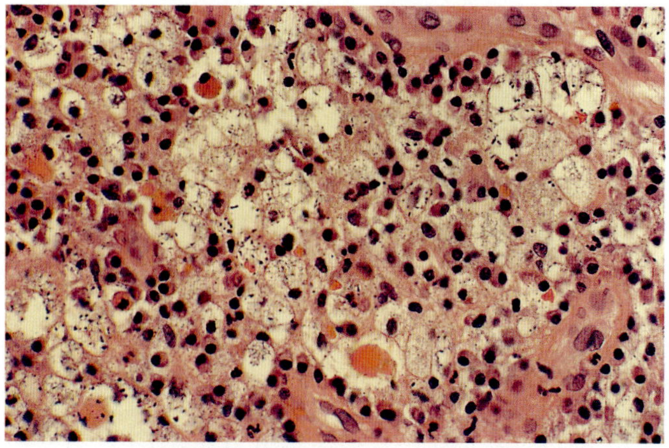

Figure 63–13. Numerous foamy histiocytes, or Mikulicz cells, are present in the nasal submucosa from this patient with rhinoscleroma. The bacilli are abundant and easily seen in this H&E stained section. Plasma cells are numerous (H&E, ×400).

patients have had squamous cell carcinoma arising at the site of rhinoscleroma infections.[18]

DIAGNOSIS

With the exception of rhinoscleroma, the pathologic features of *Klebsiella* infections are not specific, so that microbiological culture remains the mainstay of diagnosis. The diagnosis of *Klebsiella* pneumonia is often performed by isolating the organism from sputum. The use of sputum as a diagnostic specimen is complicated by the fact that *Klebsiella* may be a normal component of the oropharyngeal flora.

The differential diagnosis of rhinoscleroma is broad, and includes leprosy, sarcoidosis, lymphoma, tuberculosis, primary and metastatic tumors, mucocutaneous leishmaniasis, and such mycotic infections as paracoccidioidomycosis and rhinosporidiosis.[19] Diagnosis can be performed by biopsy and by microbiological culture.

Treatment of *Klebsiella* infections has been complicated by the development of multiple drug-resistant strains. Antibiotic treatment of nosocomial-acquired *Klebsiella* infections requires susceptibility testing of bacterial isolates, and empirical treatment should be tailored to the susceptibility pattern present at the individual hospital.[1,4,20]

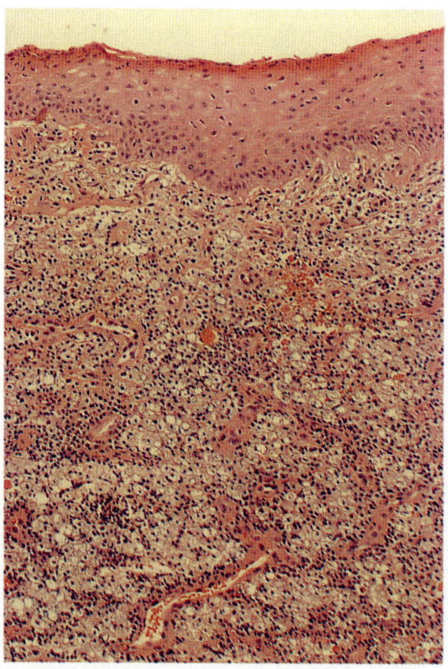

Figure 63–12. Rhinoscleroma involving nasal mucosa. There is squamous metaplasia with an underlying inflammatory infiltrate composed mostly of sheets of vacuolated histiocytes (H&E, ×100).

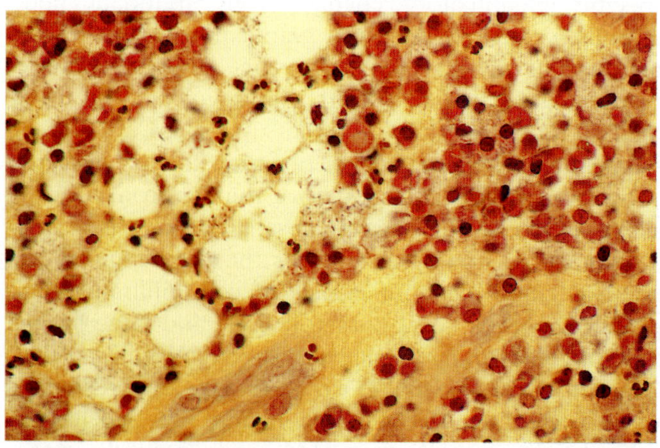

Figure 63–14. Gram-negative *K rhinoscleromatis* are in Mikulicz cells in this Gram-stained section of rhinoscleroma (AFIP Neg 79-15301; Brown–Hopps stain, ×1000).

REFERENCES

1. Eisenstein BI. Enterobacteriaceae. In: Mandell GL, Bennett JE, Dolin R, eds. *Principles and Practice of Infectious Diseases.* 4th ed. New York: Churchill Livingstone; 1995: 1964–1980.
2. Centers for Disease Control and Prevention. National nosocomial infection study report. Annual summary 1979. Atlanta, Georgia; March 1992.
3. Welbel SF, Schoendirf K, Bland LA, et al. An outbreak of Gram-negative bloodstream infections in chronic hemodialysis patients. *Am J Nephrol.* 1995;15:1–4.
4. Eisen D, Russlee EG, Tymms M, et al. Random amplified polymorphic DNA and plasmid analyses used in investigation of an outbreak of multiresistant *Klebsiella pneumoniae. J Clin Microbiol.* 1995;33:713–717.
5. Jong GM, Hsiue TR, Chen CR, Chang HY, Chen CW. Rapidly fatal outcome of bacteremic *Klebsiella pneumoniae* pneumonia in alcoholics. *Chest.* 1995;107:214–217.
6. Fryklund B, Tullus K, Burman LG. Epidemiology and attack index of Gram-negative bacteria causing invasive infection in three special-care neonatal units and risk factors for infection. *Infection.* 1995;23:76–80.
7. Porto R, Hevia O, Hensley GT, et al. Disseminated *Klebsiella rhinoscleromatis* infection. *Arch Pathol Lab Med.* 1989;113:1381–1383.
8. Paul C, Pialoux G, Dupont B, et al. Infection due to *Klebsiella rhinoscleromatis* in two patients infected with human immunodeficiency virus. *Clin Infect Dis.* 1993;16: 441–442.
9. Klipstein FA, Engert RF. Purification and properties of *Klebsiella pneumoniae* heat-stable enterotoxin. *Infect Immun.* 1976;13:1307.
10. Mangi RJ, Quintillani R, Andriole VT. Gram-negative bacillary meningitis. *Am J Med.* 1975;59:829.
11. Nagast T, Wada S, Nakamura R, et al. Magnetic resonance imaging of multiple brain abscesses of the bilateral basal ganglia. *Intern Med.* 1995;34:554–558.
12. Han SH. Review of hepatic abscess from *Klebsiella pneumoniae.* An association with diabetes mellitus and septic endophthalmitis. *West J Med.* 1995;162:220–224.
13. Pascual J, Sureda A, Garcia-Hoz F, et al. Spontaneous peritonitis due to *Klebsiella oxytoca* in a patient with cardiac ascites. *Am J Gastroenterol.* 1988;83:1313–1314.
14. Watanakunakorn C. *Klebsiella oxytoca* endocarditis after a transurethral resection of the prostate gland. *South Med J.* 1985;78:356–357.
15. Humphreys DR. Spontaneous lobectomy. *Br Med J.* 1945: II:185.
16. Knight L, Fraser RG, Robson HG. Massive pulmonary gangrene: a severe complication of *Klebsiella* pneumonia. *Can Med Assoc J.* 1975;112:196–198.
17. Michaels L. *Ear, Nose and Throat Histopathology.* Berlin: Springer-Verlag; 1987:141.
18. Attia OM. Rhinoscleroma and malignancy: two cases of rhinoschleroma associated with carcinoma. *J Laryngol Otol.* 1958;72:412–415.
19. Hyams VJ. Rhinoscleroma. In: Binford CH, Connor DH, eds. *Pathology of Tropical and Extraordinary Diseases.* Washington, DC: Armed Forces Institute of Pathology; 1976;1:187–189.
20. Jett BD, Ritchie DJ, Reichley R, Bailey TC, Sahm DF. In vitro activities of various beta-lactam antimicrobial agents against clinical isolates of *Escherichia coli* and *Klebsiella* sp resistant to oxymino cephalosporins. *Antimicrob Agents Chemo.* 1995;39:1187–1190.

Chapter 64

Legionellosis

Phyllis R. Vezza, Ernest E. Lack, and Francis W. Chandler

It is like a Roman mob,
Small, taken one by one, but my god, together!

Sylvia Plath (1932–1963)

INTRODUCTION

Legionellosis is a bacterial infection caused by species of the genus *Legionella* (particularly *Legionella pneumophila*), which are gram-negative bacilli having fastidious growth requirements in vitro. Synonyms include legionnaires' disease and Pontiac fever. The *Legionella* bacillus was first described by McDade et al in 1977, following an outbreak of pneumonia at an American Legion convention in Philadelphia during July 1976.[1] Since the initial isolation of the organism, more than 40 different species of *Legionella* and 52 serotypes have been identified in the family Legionellaceae. There are 15 serogroups of *L pneumophila,* three of which cause 85% of human infections; the second most common is *L micdadei.* Others include *L longbeachae, L dumoffii, L bozemanii,* and *L feeleii. Tatlockia* is the genus name used by some authors when referring to the *micdadei* and *maceachernii* species, and *Fluoribacter* for the species *dumoffii, gormanii,* and *bozemanii.*[2] Exposure to this organism can actually produce two very distinct illnesses, legionnaires' disease and Pontiac fever. Although caused by the same agent, these infections have different epidemiologies, symptoms, and sequelae. These factors have contributed to make *Legionella* sp unusual and important human pathogens.

GEOGRAPHIC DISTRIBUTION

The *Legionella* sp have a ubiquitous aquatic distribution. Cases of legionnaires' disease have been reported in most countries in which appropriate diagnostic studies are available. Natural reservoirs include lakes, rivers, ponds, and wet soil, and a symbiotic relationship with organisms such as amebae and other protozoa has been documented. These organisms provide the bacilli with nutrients and an intracellular environment for replication. Protozoa in which the *Legionella* sp have been isolated include *Hartmannella veriformis,*[3] *Acanthamoeba castellanii,*[4] and *Tetrahymena pyriformis.*[5] This symbiotic relationship has been likened to a "Trojan horse," in that the amebae carry the infectious bacilli into the host.

Human infection from natural water is rare, having been reported in near drownings.[6,7] Artificial reservoirs, however, play a major role in the propagation of disease. Many water-associated systems are habitats for these bacteria. These include evaporator pans and cooling towers of air conditioners, aerosolizing machines, respiratory therapy equipment, humidifiers, hot water tanks, whirlpool spas, decorative fountains, shower heads, water outlets, and household potable water supplies.[8] Infections originating from these sources have occurred in hospitals, hotels, and nursing homes. All public institutions with commercial air conditioning systems or devices that generate aerosolized water are potential sites of dissemination. In one study, 24 of 46 (52%) cooling water systems of air conditioners contained *Legionella* bacilli.[9] Very few infections have been contracted in private homes.[10] Although water temperatures of 25 to 40°C appear to favor growth, the organisms can survive at 0 to 60°C. Other factors conducive to bacterial proliferation include obstruction and stagnation, biofilms, rust-laden plumbing fixtures, minerals, and commensal microflora. *Legionella* sp appear to resist low concentrations of chlorine, such as those usually found in man-made reservoirs.

EPIDEMIOLOGY

Serologic studies of stored sera at the Centers for Disease Control and Prevention (CDC) have shown that *L pneumophila* caused outbreaks of pneumonia as early as 1947.[11] Currently, 1000 to 1300 infections are reported to the CDC annually, but because many infections are undiagnosed, the incidence may be much higher.[12] Some authors estimate that there are more than 25,000 infections annually in the United States.

Infection may be sporadic or epidemic, and approximately 65% to 80% of infections are believed to be sporadic,[13,14] typically with no identifiable source. Epidemic infections, however, are clustered in time and place, often with a proved source. There were more than 200 victims in the Philadelphia epidemic. *Legionella* sp cause approximately 10% of nosocomial pneumonias,[15] and up to 15% of community-acquired pneumonias.[16] The overall fatality rate in those treated is approximately 10%,[17] compared with 20% to 30% for untreated patients.[15] Survival depends on early diagnosis, antibiotic therapy, and lack of adverse host factors such as debilitating illness, immunodeficiency, old age, smoking, and alcohol consumption. Legionellosis occurs predominantly during periods of warm temperatures. Some studies report up to 75% of infections between June and October, a pattern related, perhaps, to water systems such as air conditioning units and exposure to lakes, ponds, and rivers. The mortality rate in untreated immunodeficient patients is 80%, and approximately 25% in treated patients with immunodeficiencies.[15] Interestingly, patients with acquired immunodeficiency syndrome (AIDS) have not had a higher incidence of legionnaires' disease. Also at increased risk are those with chronic bronchitis, emphysema, renal failure, cancer, and diabetes mellitus. Infections in men are 2.6 times more common than in women. Although infection has been documented from 16 months to 89 years, the median age is 55 years.[18] Infections in children are rare and the majority are immunosuppressed.[19]

MORPHOLOGY OF *LEGIONELLA* SPECIES

Legionella sp are aerobic, fastidious, gram-negative, and 0.3 to 1.0 μm wide by 2.5 μm long. They are facultative, intracellular organisms that proliferate in and ultimately destroy phagocytic cells. Although usually found as individual bacilli, the organisms can form chains or long filaments up to 20 μm, especially when grown in culture (Figure 64–1). Flagella or pili can be seen when the organisms are cultured. Electron microscopy has revealed numerous intracytoplasmic vacuoles and granular inclusions that are usually composed of lipid or polyhydroxybutyrate. An envelope is present as in other gram-negative bacteria. This structure is 75 Å wide and consists of an inner and outer triple-layered unit membrane separated by a periplasmic space (Figure 64–2). The bacterial cell walls have a distinctive fatty-acid and ubiquinone composition that aids in identification by gas chromatography.[20] The bacteria lack mitochondria, nuclear membranes, and endoplasmic reticulum. Replication is by binary fission (division by central pinching).

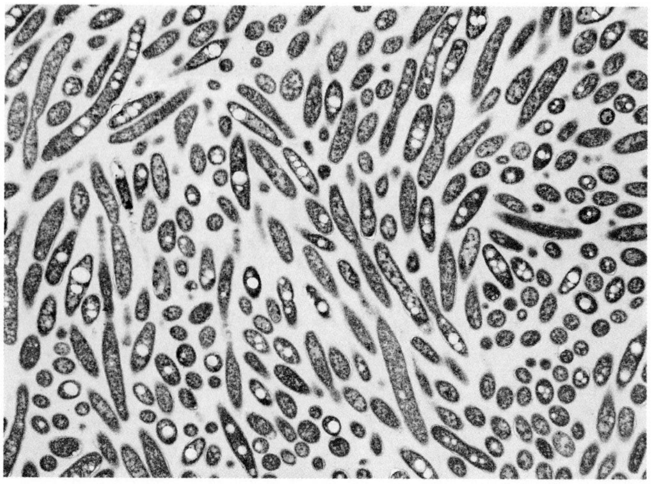

Figure 64–1. Transmission electron micrograph of *L pneumophila* grown on bacteriologic medium. Note bacilli dividing by central pinching. Many of the bacilli have vacuolated cytoplasm (uranyl acetate and lead citrate, ×9000). *(Courtesy of Francis W. Chandler, DVM, PhD.)*

PATHOGENESIS AND VIRULENCE

Most investigators believe that legionnaires' disease is caused by inhaling aerosolized water containing *Legionella* bacilli; some also believe that ingestion of the organism causes infection. Rare localized infections from inoculation of skin or wounds have been reported. There is no evidence for person-to-person or in utero transmission. Cell-mediated immunity is the primary defense mechanism. Activated macrophages destroy the organism. Specific antibodies and complement proteins help sequester bacilli in pulmonary macrophages. Although humoral activity may play a role in immunity, it is not essential for bacterial eradication. A unique coiling phagocytosis without specific antibodies has been described in legionnaires' disease.[21] Unless the host can mount an effective cell-mediated response, the humoral activity can be more detrimental than beneficial by providing the bacillus

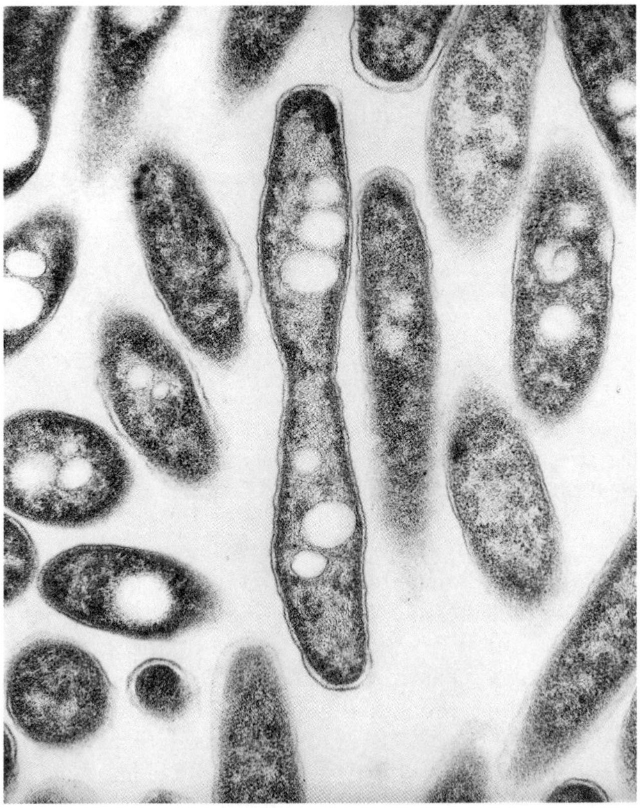

Figure 64–2. Transmission electron micrograph of *L pneumophila* grown on bacteriologic medium. Bacilli are enclosed by a double envelope, which consists of inner and outer triple-layered "unit" membranes. Most organisms contain vacuoles (uranyl acetate and lead citrate, ×72,000). *(Courtesy of Francis W. Chandler, DVM, PhD.)*

with an appropriate environment for proliferation. In patients with immunodeficiencies or in those infected with particularly virulent strains of *Legionella* sp, phagosomes do not fuse with lysosomes, resulting in an environment conducive to bacterial replication. Bacilli eventually overgrow the cell, rupture its membranes, and spill into the surrounding tissues, thus continuing the reproductive cycle. Neutrophils and circulating monocytes engulf bacilli but are less effective. Phagocytosis by neutrophils requires both complement and specific antibodies. Virulence depends on many factors, including host susceptibility, size of inoculum, and mode of transmission. One report suggests that exposure to one colony-forming unit per 50 L of air can cause infection. The concentration and size of the infecting dose, therefore, may be extremely small.[22] Virulence is also strain specific. Contributing factors include antigenicity, complement sensitivity, macrophage toxicity, plasmid content, oxidative burst sensitivity, and intracellular replication. Many of these factors are thought to be governed by toxins elaborated by the bacteria, including proteases, hemolysins, cytotoxins, phospholipases, DNAse, and RNAse.[23] Extrathoracic and systemic manifestations also may be a consequence of these products. The most abundant polypeptide produced by the bacillus, major secretory protein (MSP), plays a role in proteolytic, hemolytic, and cytotoxic activities.

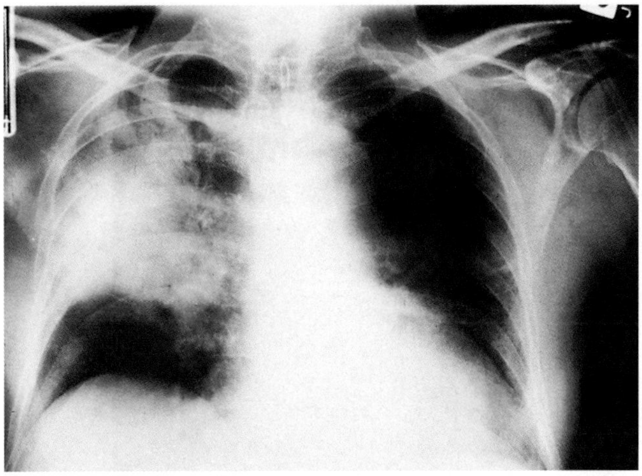

Figure 64–3. Pulmonary legionellosis. Posterior-anterior chest radiograph shows consolidation of right upper and middle lobes.

CLINICAL FEATURES

Patients with legionnaires' disease can have a broad spectrum of signs and symptoms. Although asymptomatic infections and minimal respiratory illnesses can occur, infection is typically systemic and characterized by a life-threatening pneumonia (Figure 64–3). The disease has a low attack rate and an incubation period of 2 to 10 days. Early symptoms include progressive headache, malaise, and myalgia. High fever (40°C) usually appears 24 to 48 hours after infection in 50% of patients. A relative bradycardia is common. Chills and rigors occur in 75% of patients. A nonproductive or mucoid cough is present in 50% of patients. Patients may also complain of shortness of breath and pleuritic pain. Rales often are present. There may be confusion, lethargy, delirium, and ataxia. Nausea, vomiting, and diarrhea may develop in a few days. Abnormal laboratory values include hyponatremia and hypophosphatemia. Increased lactate dehydrogenase, creatinine kinase, alkaline phosphatase, and aldolase have been documented.[15,24] The white blood count is normal or elevated. Studies of cerebrospinal fluid may be normal, even when there are neurologic symptoms.

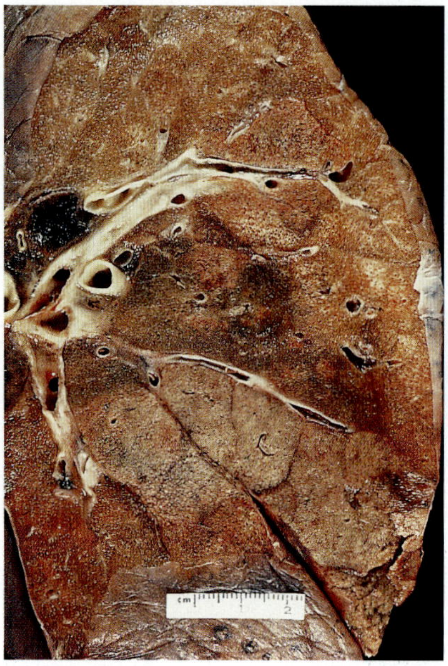

Figure 64–4. Section of lung in fatal legionnaires' disease. The lung is firm. Note irregular consolidation with hemorrhage.

PATHOLOGY

The lungs are consolidated, firm, and rubbery (Figure 64–4), and the involved portions bulge forth when the chest is opened at autopsy—a feature characteristic of expanding pneumonias. Microscopically there is an early infiltrate of macrophages and fewer neutrophils. Later there is necrosis of inflammatory cells, with hemorrhage that may proceed to cavitation (Figure 64–5). Segmental or diffuse pneumonitis is prominent and often accompanied by lysis of septa and focal hemorrhage. Intra-alveolar macrophages and neutrophils are abundant and may form near-confluent sheets separated by delicate alveolar septa (Figures 64–6 and 64–7). Bacteria can be detected in many of the pulmonary macrophages (Figure 64–8, A and B) by using any of the silver impregnation stains—Steiner, Warthin–Starry, Dieterle (Figure 64–9) or the modified Brown–Hopps tissue Gram stain with 1% basic fuchsin (Figure 64–10). *Legionella micdadei* and *L pneumophila* (rarely) are weakly acid fast in routine processed tissue sections stained with modified acid-fast procedures that use an aqueous solution of a weak acid for decolorization. *Legionella* sp also can be identified in imprint smears and in frozen sections by using the Gimenez stain (Figure 64–11) and, more specifically, immunoperoxidase (Figure 64–12) and immunofluorescence procedures (Figure 64–13). The last two immunohistologic procedures also can be applied to formalin-fixed, deparaffinized tissue sections. Necrosis and proteinaceous

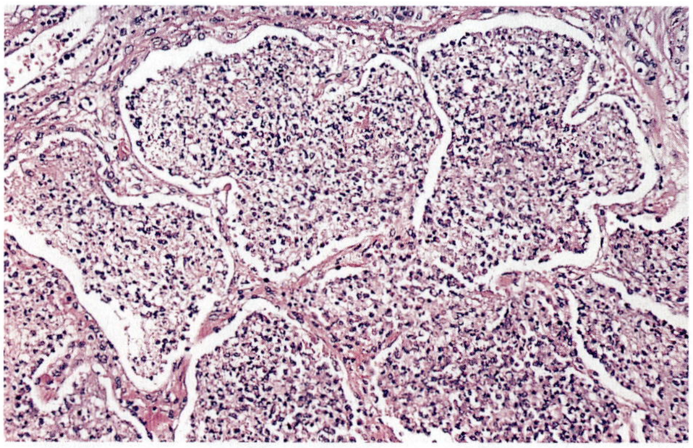

Figure 64–6. Pulmonary legionellosis. Fibrinosuppurative exudate fills alveolar spaces. Some alveolar septa are beginning to degenerate (hematoxylin-eosin, ×100).

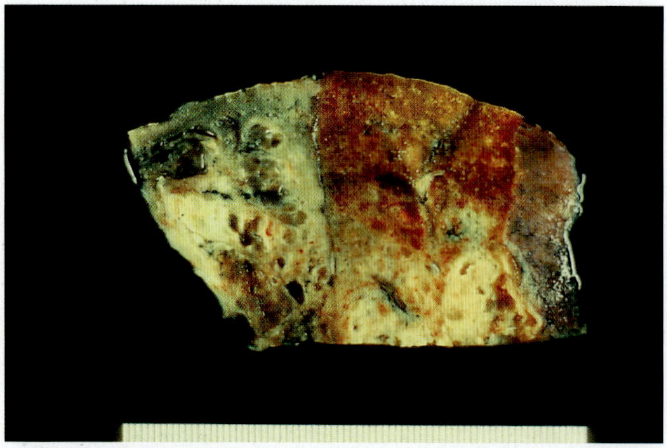

Figure 64–5. Legionnaires' pneumonia. More advanced necrosis with multiple areas of cavitation. *(Courtesy of Daniel H. Connor, MD.)*

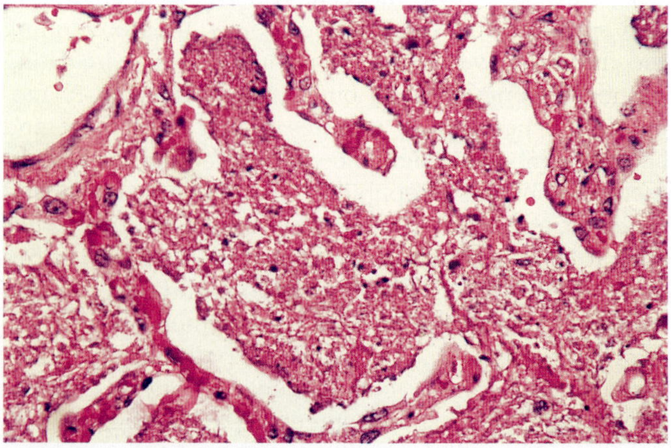

Figure 64–7. Legionnaires' pneumonia. The alveolar exudate is necrotic (hematoxylin-eosin, ×160).

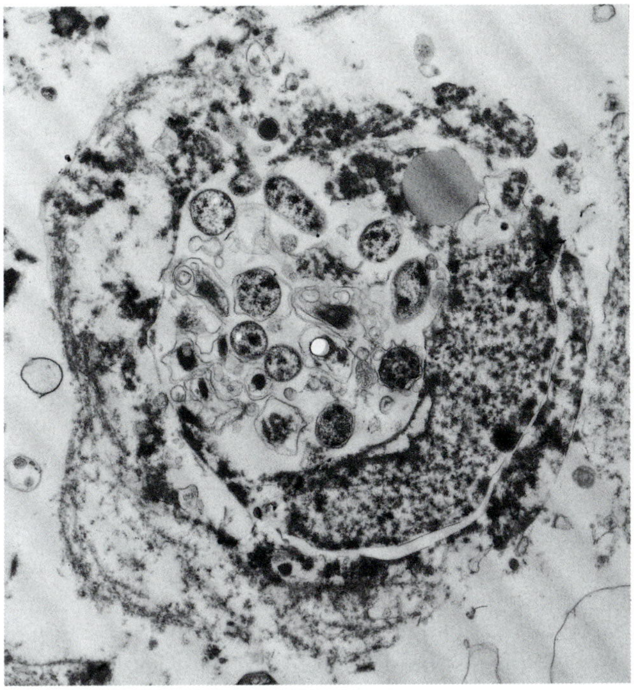

A

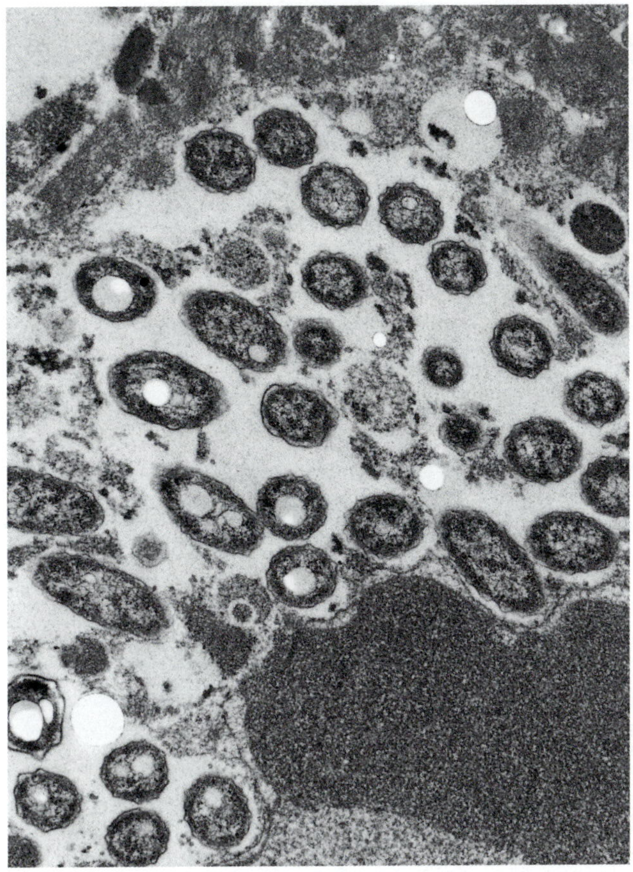

B

Figure 64–8. (**A**) Pulmonary legionellosis. Electron micrograph of alveolar macrophage that contains numerous intact and degenerating *L pneumophila*. Note enclosure of bacilli by a double envelope, characteristic of gram-negative bacteria (uranyl acetate and lead citrate, ×16,055). (**B**) Electron micrograph of *L pneumophila* in a phagocytic vacuole of an alveolar macrophage (uranyl acetate and lead citrate, ×23,000).

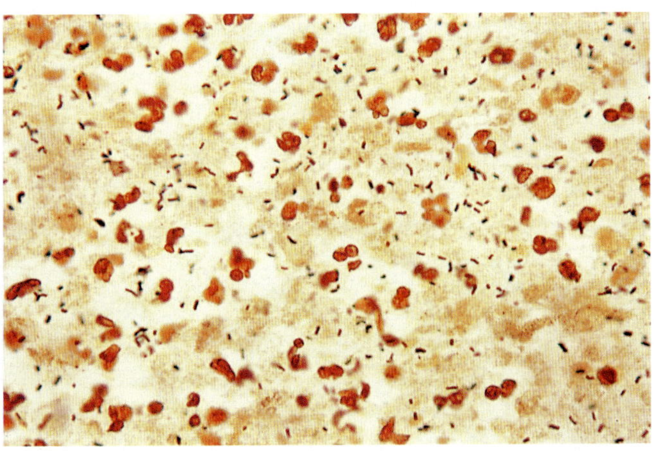

Figure 64–9. Legionnaires' pneumonia. Bacilli of *L pneumophila* have been coated with silver, making them opaque and larger. Bacilli also are in the pulmonary interstitium of this immunosuppressed patient (Dieterle silver impregnation, ×250).

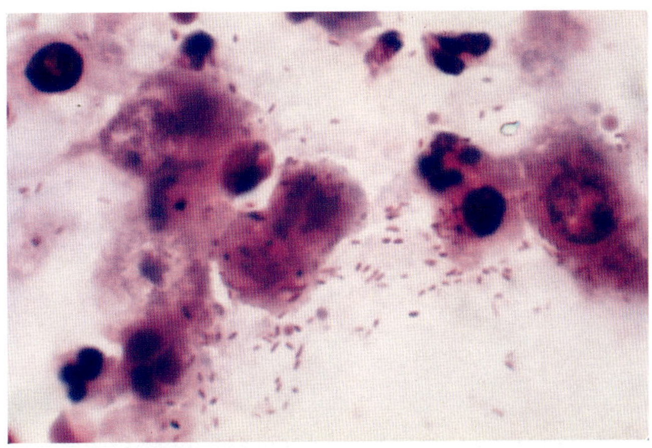

Figure 64–10. Imprint smear of lung from a patient with legionnaires' pneumonia. The bacilli are gram-negative and are intra- and extracellular (modified Brown–Hopps with 1% basic fuchsin, ×250).

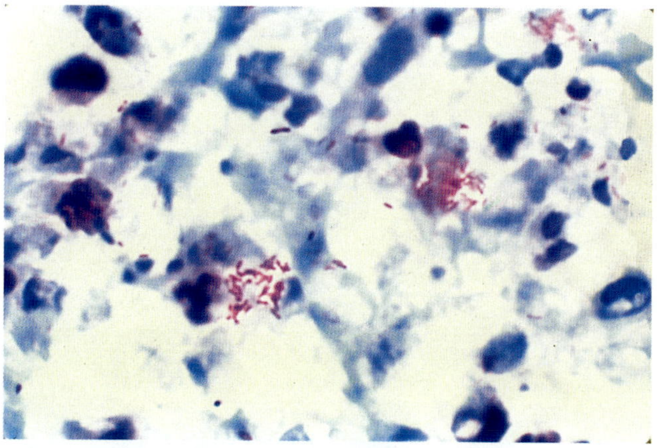

Figure 64–11. Imprint smear of lung in legionnaires' disease. The bacilli are red and clustered in alveolar macrophages (Gimenez stain, ×250).

debris develop in the areas of infection. These infiltrates progress from patchy localized involvement to confluent multilobular consolidations that may be bilateral. Thirty percent of patients have pleural effusions. Small abscesses occasionally are apparent. There may be cavitation, but empyema is rare. Healing is by fibrosis. Severe protracted infections may show bronchiolitis obliterans or fibrosing alveolitis. The major ensuing complications are respiratory distress and adult respiratory distress syndrome (ARDS), and can result in death.

Spread of infection may be contiguous, hematogenous, or lymphatic. Bacteria have been recovered from extrapulmonary sites including the kidneys, liver, brain, heart, bone marrow, spleen, lymph nodes, cutaneous lesions, and nasal sinuses. The kidneys may show mesangial proliferation, interstitial nephritis, glomerulonephritis, and acute tubular necrosis. Clinically there may be complete renal failure. Urine studies sometimes reveal hyaline or granular casts, hematuria, proteinuria, and myoglobinuria.[20] Rhabdomyolysis and disseminated intravascular coagulation also have been reported.[25]

Localized infections have rarely been documented. These have no anatomic or epidemiologic pattern. Involved sites have included prosthetic cardiac valves, the heart, kidneys, peritoneum, nasal sinuses, brain, cutaneous wounds, and arteriovenous fistulas of renal dialysis patients. Infection of these extrapulmonary sites can be caused by direct inoculation of tissues with contaminated water or by infected circulating monocytes.[15]

LABORATORY DIAGNOSIS

Tracheal aspirations, sputum, bronchoalveolar lavage samples, pleural effusions, and lung biopsies are all excellent specimens for diagnostic purposes. Culturing the organism from one or more samples has been the "gold standard" for diagnosis. The organism will not grow in vitro on conventional laboratory media. The most effective culture medium is supplemented buffered charcoal yeast extract in humidified air at 35°C. Some species of *Legionella* require an additional 2.5% CO_2 for optimum growth. Modified Mueller–Hinton agar also is useful. Growth is usually apparent within 3 to 5 days; however, it may be necessary to retain cultures longer for adequate colony formation. Colonies are characteristically gray to blue-green, glistening, and measure 3 to 4 mm in diameter. Antimicrobial agents (eg, cefamandole) may be added to the media to prevent contamination by other organisms. Pretreatment of the specimen with acid also is helpful in eradicating

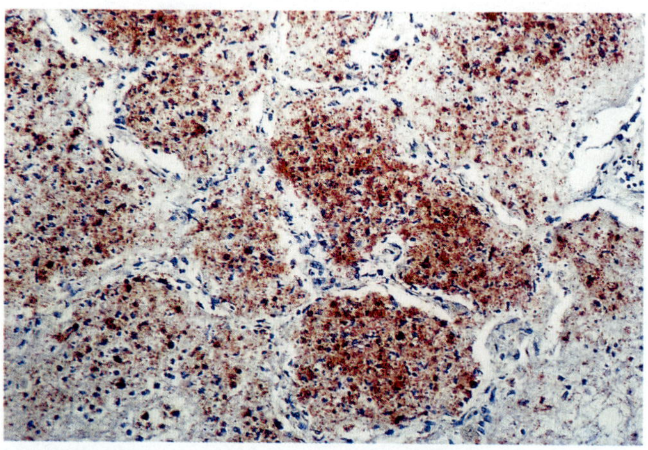

Figure 64–12. Legionnaires' pneumonia. Immunoperoxidase stain for *Legionella* sp shows strong reactivity for antigens in the alveolar exudate (×25).

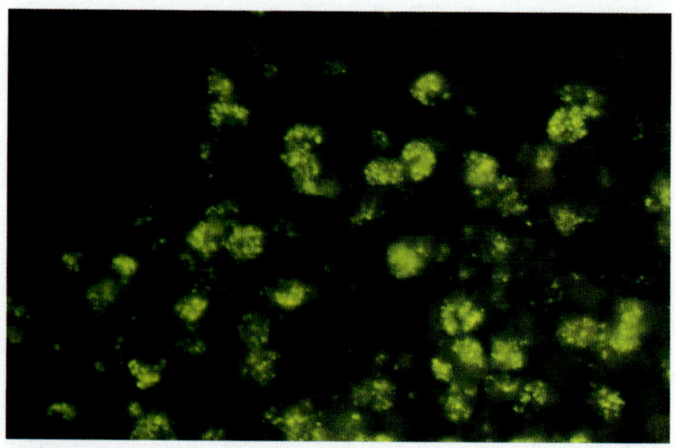

Figure 64–13. Direct immunofluorescence of *L pneumophila* in a formalin-fixed deparaffinized section of human lung. Numerous bacilli in alveolar macrophages are brightly decorated with a species-specific conjugate (×150).

contaminants. Culture specificity approaches 100%, but sensitivity is slightly lower (90% to 100%), depending on the appropriate sampling and handling of tissues or fluids.

Serologic studies with a specificity of 90% and a sensitivity of 75%, are useful in diagnosis. Indirect fluorescent antibody (IFA) detection can show evidence of infection in serum. A fourfold increase in antibody titers from acute and convalescent phase samples at 1:128 or greater can be expected, but may require several weeks for a definitive result. A single high titer of 1:256 also is considered adequate for confirmation. The direct fluorescent antibody (DFA) procedure can be used to identify *Legionella* sp in routinely processed specimens (Figure 64–13). DFA is rapid, with a sensitivity of 70% and specificity of 99%, and it can be performed on tissue that has been formalin-fixed for 24 hours or less, but interpretation of this test requires skill. Antigenic studies on urine samples can be performed by radioimmunoassay (RIA), enzyme-linked immunosorbent assay (ELISA), and latex agglutination. There is a 60% to 80% sensitivity and high specificity, approaching 100% for RIA and ELISA. These rapid tests are excellent for diagnosis.[26] Viable *Legionella* bacilli can be detected using polymerase chain reaction and gene probe techniques, which are especially useful for identifying environmental sources for bacterial dissemination. Nucleic acid probes for detecting *Legionella* sp are now commercially available.[27] Cultures within the peritoneum of guinea pigs and coculturing the bacillus with amebae and other protozoa also have been used successfully. Gas chromatography and electron microscopy also are good investigative tools. Electrophoresis has been effective in identifying different serotypes.[28]

TREATMENT

The most effective drug is erythromycin, an antimicrobial agent that should initially be given intravenously (1 g every 6 hours) and then orally if there is improvement in clinical status within a few days. Therapy should be continued for 3 weeks to prevent relapse. Immunodeficient patients likely will require a more extended course. An adjunct drug, such as rifampin (600 mg every 12 hours) often is beneficial in more resistant infections. Other antimicrobial agents that may be effective include trimethoprim–sulfamethoxazole, doxycycline, clarithromycin, and ciprofloxacin.

PREVENTION

Filtration of potable water supplies with frequent filter replacement can aid in the removal of *Legionella* sp as well as other organisms that may be present. Hyperchlorination coupled with flushing of distal outlets also is an effective method of eradication. Other techniques include ultraviolet treatment of the water system and thermal destruction at extreme temperatures. Vaccines also are being explored. High levels of antibody have been achieved by inoculating guinea pigs with proteins isolated from the *Legionella* sp. Both humoral and cell-mediated immunity were acquired using major secretory protein in experimental animals, making this a possible component for a vaccine.[29] The results of human trials have not yet been published.

PONTIAC FEVER

This is an acute, self-limited, nonpneumonic form of legionellosis that may be sporadic or epidemic. Pontiac fever has a very high attack rate with an incubation period of 24 to 48 hours. Symptoms are characteristically influenza-like and include chills, fever, dry cough, headache, and malaise. The first reported outbreak was in July 1968, in a county health department building in Pontiac, Michigan. During this initial epidemic, 144 employees and visitors were affected, with an attack rate of 95%; most affected had been in good health. No causal agent was identified at the time, but an airborne pathogen was suspected, thus implicating the cooling system. Since then there have been many other epidemics. Four species of *Legionella* have been implicated in Pontiac fever. *L pneumophila,*[30] *L micdadei,*[31] *L feeleii,*[32] and *L anisa.*[24,33] Unlike its more serious counterpart, legionnaires' disease, there is typically no progression to pneumonia in Pontiac fever, although the upper respiratory tract may be involved. There also are no fatalities or serious persistent complications. Resolution is in 2 to 5 days, although in some patients it may be prolonged and recurrent. No treatment is required for this illness because it is self-limited.

It is paradoxical that exposure to the same organisms can produce two very different illnesses, but several theories have been postulated to explain this. Host status is an important consideration; many of those with Pontiac fever are essentially healthy before infection. Other hypotheses suggest that Pontiac fever may arise from exposure to nonviable bacteria (eg, bacilli incapable of intracellular replication), inactive or attenuated toxic substances, or hypersensitivity to amebae or other protozoa coexisting with the organism.[30]

REFERENCES

1. McDade JE, Shepard CC, Fraser DW, Tsai TR, Redus MA, Dowdle WR. Legionnaires' disease: isolation of a bac-

terium and demonstration of its role in other respiratory disease. *N Engl J Med.* 1977;297:1197–1203.
2. Baron EJ, Peterson LR, Finegold SM. *Bailey and Scott's Diagnostic Microbiology.* St. Louis, Mo: Mosby-Year Book; 1994:570–575.
3. Breiman RF, Fields BS, Sanden GN, Volmer L, Meier A, Spika JS. Association of shower use with Legionnaires' disease: possible role of amoebae. *JAMA.* 1990;263: 2924–2926.
4. Moffat JF, Tompkins LS. A quantitative model of intracellular growth of *Legionella pneumophila* in *Acanthamoeba castellanii. Infect Immun.* 1992;60:296–301.
5. Fields BS, Shotts EB, Feeley JC, Gorman GW, Martin WT. Proliferation of *Legionella pneumophila* as an intracellular parasite of the ciliated protozoan *Tetrahymena pyriformis. Appl Environ Microbiol.* 1984;47:467–471.
6. Lavocat MP, Berthier JC, Rousson A, Bornstein N, Hartemann E. Légionellose pulmonaire chez un infant après noyade en eau douce. *Presse Med.* 1987;16:780.
7. Farrent JM, Drury AEC, Thompson RPH. Legionnaire's disease following immersion in a river. *Lancet.* 1988;2 (8608):460. Letter.
8. Barbaree JM, Gorman GW, Martin WT, Fields BS, Morrill WE. Protocol for sampling environmental sites for Legionellae. *Appl Environ Microbiol.* 1987;53:1454–1458.
9. The Chartered Institute of Building Services Engineers. Minimizing the risk of Legionnaires' disease. Technical memorandum no 13. London: The Chartered Institute of Building Services Engineers; 1987.
10. Stout JE, Yu VL, Muraca P. Legionnaires' disease acquired within the homes of two patients. Link to the home water supply. *JAMA.* 1987;257:1215–1217. [Published erratum appears in *JAMA.* 1987;257:2595.]
11. McDade JE, Brenner DJ, Bozeman FM. Legionnaires' disease bacterium isolation in 1947. *Ann Intern Med.* 1979; 90:659–661.
12. Legionnaires' disease associated with cooling towers—Massachusetts, Michigan, and Rhode Island, 1993. *MMWR.* 1994;43:491–493, 499.
13. Summaries of notifiable disease in the United States, 1989. *MMWR.* 1990;38:53.
14. Cases of specified notifiable disease in the United States. *MMWR.* 1990;39:93.
15. Edelstein PH, Meyer RD. *Legionella* pneumonias. In: Pennington JE, ed. *Respiratory Infection: Diagnosis and Management.* New York: Raven Press; 1994:455–484.
16. Yu VL. *Legionella pneumophila* (Legionnaires' disease). In: Mandell GL, Douglas RG, Bennett JE, eds. *Principles and Practice of Infectious Diseases.* New York: Churchill Livingstone; 1995;2087–2097.
17. Falco V, de Sevilla TF, Alegre J, Ferrer A, Vazquez JMM. *Legionella pneumophila:* a cause of severe community-acquired pneumonia. *Chest.* 1991;100:1007–1011.
18. Gilpin RW. *Legionella* and *Legionella*-like organisms. In: Levison ME, ed. *The Pneumonias.* Boston: John Wright, PSG; 1984;358–371.
19. Goldberg DJ, Emslie JA, Fallon RJ, Green ST, Wrench JG. Pontiac fever in children. *Pediatric Infect Dis J.* 1992;11: 240–241.
20. Palutke WA, Crane LR, Wentworth BB, et al. *Legionella feeleii*-associated pneumonia in humans. *Am J Clin Pathol.* 1986;86:348–351.
21. Sout JE, Yu VL. *Legionella pneumophila.* In: Chmel H, Bendinelli M, Friedman H, eds. *Pulmonary Infections and Immunity.* New York: Plenum Press; 1994:97–111.
22. Breiman RF, Cozen W. Fields BS, et al. Role of air sampling in investigation of an outbreak of Legionnaires' disease associated with exposure to aerosols of an evaporator condenser. *J Infect Dis.* 1990;161:1257–1261.
23. Skerrett SJ, Locksley RM. Legionellosis: ecology and pathogenesis. In: Sande MA, Hudson LD, Root RK, eds. *Respiratory Infections.* New York: Churchill Livingstone; 1968:161–190.
24. Fields BS, Barbaree JM, Sandan GN, Morrill WE. Virulence of a *Legionella anisa* strain associated with Pontiac fever: an evaluation using protozoan, cell culture and guinea pig models. *Infect Immun.* 1990;58:3139–3142.
25. Olderburger D, Carson JP, Gundlach WJ, Ghaly FI, Wright WH. Legionnaires' disease: association with *Mycoplasma pneumonia* and disseminated intravascular coagulation. *JAMA.* 1979;241:1269–1270.
26. Birtles RJ, Harrison TG, Samuel D, Taylor AG. Evaluation of urinary antigen ELISA for diagnosing *Legionella pneumophila* serogroup 1 infection. *J Clin Pathol.* 1990;43: 685–690.
27. Falkingham JO. Nucleic acid probes. In: Gerhardt P, Murray RGE, Wood WA, Krieg NR, eds. *Methods for General and Molecular Bacteriology.* Washington, DC: American Society for Microbiology; 1994:701–710.
28. Roig J, Domingo C, Morera J. Legionnaires' disease. *Chest.* 1994;105:1817–1825.
29. Blander SJ, Horwitz MA. Vaccination with the major secretory protein of *Legionella pneumophila* induces cell-mediated and protective immunity in a guinea pig model of Legionnaires' disease. *J Exp Med.* 1989;169:691–705.
30. Miller LA, Beebe JL, Butler JC, et al. Use of polymerase chain reaction in an epidemiologic investigation of Pontiac fever. *J Infect Dis.* 1993;168:769–772.
31. Goldberg DJ, Wrench JG, Collier PW, et al. Lochgoilhead fever: outbreak of non-pneumonic legionellosis due to *Legionella micdadei. Lancet.* 1989;1(8633):316–318.
32. Herwaldt LA, Gorman WW, McGrath T, et al. A new *Legionella* species, *Legionella feeleii* species nova, causes Pontiac fever in an automobile plant. *Ann Intern Med.* 1984;100:333–338.
33. Fenstershieb MD, Miller M, Diggins C, et al. Outbreak of Pontiac fever due to *Legionella anisa. Lancet.* 1990;336: 35–37.

CHAPTER 65

Leprosy

Clay J. Cockerell

. . . his clothes shall be rent, and the hair of his head shall go loose, and he shall cover his upper lip, and shall cry: 'Unclean, unclean'.

Leviticus 13:45

Jesus put forth his hand, and touched him, saying, . . . be thou clean. And immediately his leprosy was cleansed.

Matthew 8:3

DEFINITION

Leprosy is a systemic infection caused by *Mycobacterium leprae.* Synonyms include Hansen's disease, Hanseniasis, elephantiasis grecorum, and Lucio's disease.

GEOGRAPHIC DISTRIBUTION

The disease is most common in the tropics and subtropics including south and southeast Asia, Mexico and Central America, Africa, China, the Middle East, India, southern Europe, and the southern United States. Worldwide, 10 to 12 million people are infected. In the United States, patients may be in any state but most are in California, Hawaii, Florida, Texas, and Louisiana. About one half of American patients acquire their infections outside the United States.[1,2]

NATURAL HISTORY

The most common sites of involvement are skin and peripheral nerves but bacteria may be in respiratory mucosa, in endothelial cells, and in phagocytic cells of the reticuloendothelial (RE) system (Figures 65–1, 65–2, and 65–3). A patient's clinical features, course, and prognosis depend on the efficiency of the cell-mediated reaction to antigens of *M leprae.*[3] Leprosy has thus been divided into two principal types: lepromatous leprosy, when there is little or no cell-mediated response, and tuberculoid leprosy when there is a vigorous cell-mediated response. These are the polar forms of leprosy; polar in the sense that they are at opposite ends of an immunologic spectrum. Many patients, however, have varying degrees of cell-mediated reaction and lie between these polar forms. These patients are said to have borderline leprosy. In addition, humoral immunity in patients with leprosy may be quite strong and circulating antibodies to *M leprae* can be identified.[4]

Important contrasting features of untreated lepromatous and tuberculoid leprosy include these:

Lepromatous	Tuberculoid
Progressive and fatal	Limited and self-healing
Nodular and diffuse	Macular and one or a very few lesions
Histiocytes	Epithelioid cells and Langhans' giant cells
Massive numbers of organisms	Few organisms
Negative lepromin test	Positive lepromin test
Treatment is lifelong	Treatment stopped with healing

Subclinical infection follows contact with the bacillus, after which there may be no disease or only one or

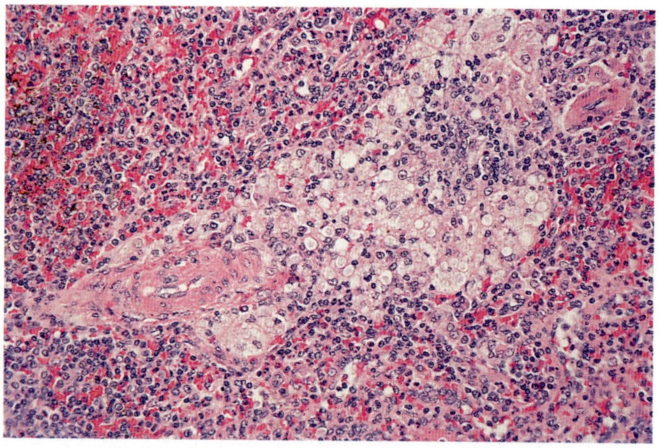

Figure 65–1. Spleen, lepromatous leprosy. Collections of foamy histiocytes are clustered around the penicilliary arterioles. The cytoplasm of the histiocytes is gray-blue, characteristics of enormous numbers of acid-fast bacilli in the histiocytes (hematoxylin-eosin, ×72).

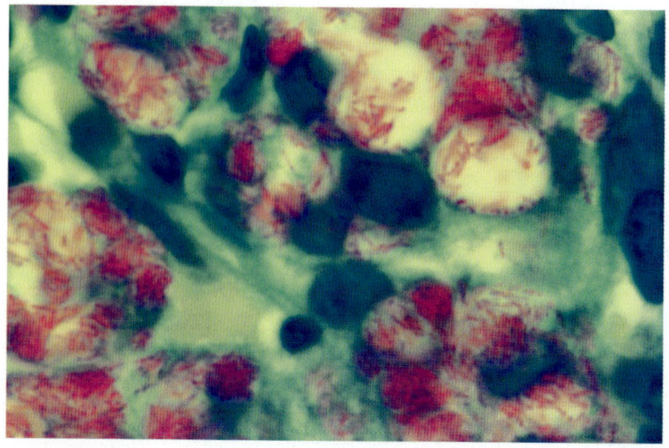

Figure 65–3. Specially stained section to show the individual bacilli. *M leprae* is partially acid-fast and stains weakly or not at all with standard acid-fast stains including the Ziehl-Neelsen. (Fite-Faraco ×490).

a few hypopigmented slightly scaly macular lesions. Biopsy specimens taken at this stage reveal few bacilli and mild "nonspecific" inflammatory changes—changes that are too early to assess the patient's cell-mediated response or allow a diagnosis of leprosy. These patients, therefore, are said to have indeterminate leprosy. Clinical and pathologic features of leprosy are consequences of host cell-mediated immunity and consequences also of the multiplication and spread of bacilli. *Mycobacterium leprae* invades and destroys nerves, and in time nerve damage may cause contraction deformities (Figure 65–4) and chronic debilitation. Anesthesia may also lead to trophic ulcers and tissue destruction.[5]

Although the exact mechanism of transmission is unclear, untreated lepromatous patients discharge large numbers of *M leprae* in their respiratory secretions and for this reason it is assumed that transmission is by aerosolized particles landing on and passing through nasal mucosa.[6] Percutaneous transmission is rare and poorly documented.

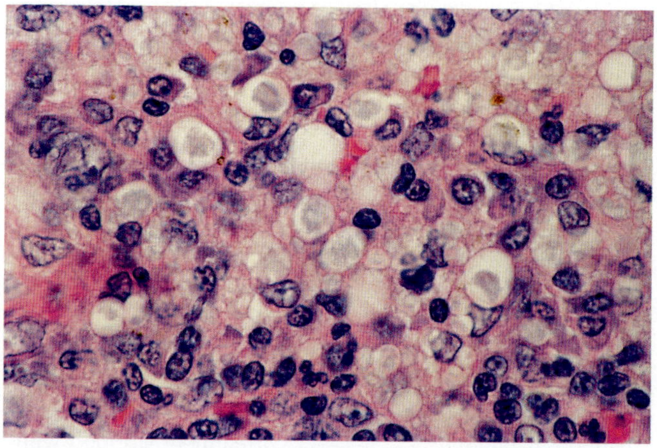

Figure 65–2. Higher magnification showing the gray-blue cytoplasm. Note the lack of necrosis. Leprosy of skin, mucous membranes, and RE organs is non-necrotizing (hematoxylin-eosin, ×290).

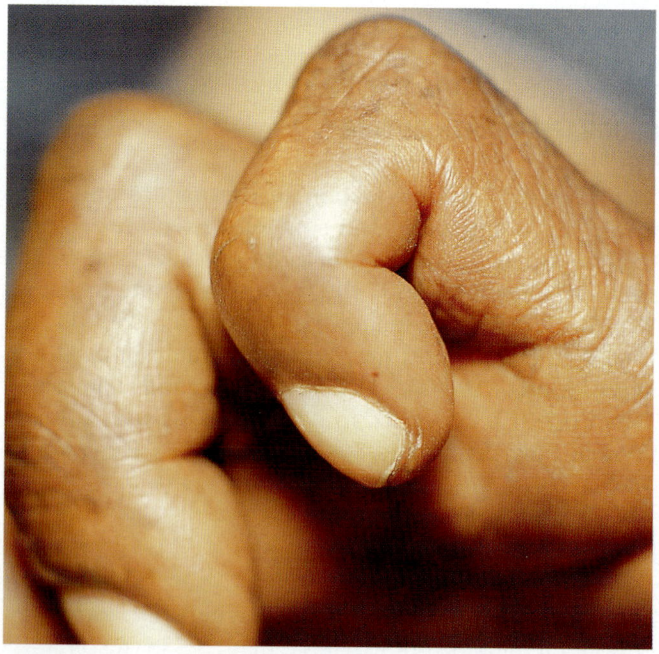

Figure 65–4. This contraction deformity has been caused by damage to the ulnar nerve. This patient has a "claw" hand. *(Patient at Nkone Leprosarium near Lotumbe, Republic of Zaire. Photograph by Daniel H. Connor, MD, 1972.)*

THE ORGANISM

Mycobacterium leprae is the first microorganism to be recognized as a cause of human disease yet it has not been cultivated in vitro. (Although more than 100 reports have been made since the turn of the century describing cultivation of *M leprae* on artificial media, the cultivation techniques in none of these reports has been repeated successfully nor has any of these reports been retracted.[7]) However, *M leprae* does replicate in the mouse footpad and it infects the nine-banded armadillo.[8] It appears to grow best at 33°C dividing every 12 to 18 days. It is, thus, the slowest replicating bacterial pathogen. The phenolic glycolipid in the capsule is, in part, related to the pathogenesis and causes foamy histiocytes to accumulate.[9] Other unusual features are 1) *M leprae* provokes a broad cell-mediated response that is non-necrotizing in skin and RE organs, 2) *M leprae* is the only bacteria that invades and destroys nerves, 3) it invades tissues that are below the body's core temperature including skin, testis, anterior segment of eye, mucous membranes of nasal passages and ear lobes (Figures 65–5 through 65–7), 4) *M leprae* has limited acid fastness and, finally, 5) it causes a disease mentioned in the bible.

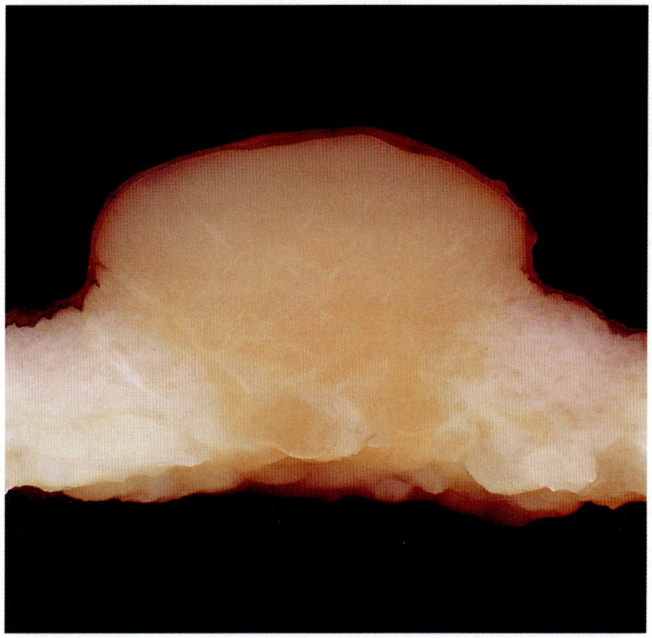

Figure 65–6. Excised nodule of lepromatous leprosy. The cut surface is pale yellow—characteristic of a collection of histiocytes either inflammatory or tumorous. The epidermis is stretched thinly over the surface and the margins of the lesion are not circumscribed nor encapsulated. In fact, the margins of lepromatous lesions tend to blend with each other. Microscopically lepromatous infiltrates are collections of histiocytes, each containing enormous numbers of acid-fast bacilli. *(Photograph by Daniel H. Connor, MD, 1975.)*

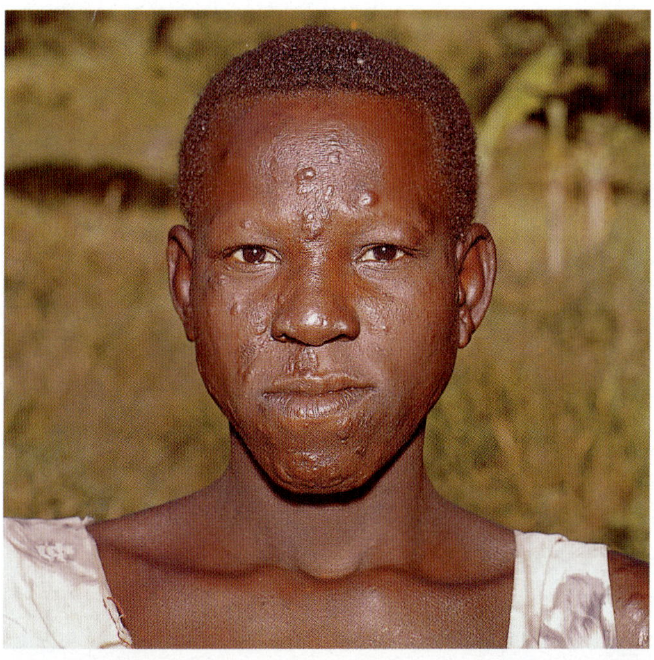

Figure 65–5. Advanced lepromatous leprosy in an African woman. Characteristic features include nodules, plaques, and poorly defined infiltrates of skin including ear lobes, and loss of eyebrows and eyelashes. Untreated lepromatous leprosy may progress to grotesque distortion of features. With dapsone (diamino-diphenyl sulfone) and other antileprosy microbials, however, the patient's nodules will regress and the lesions gradually become bacteriologically negative. *(Photograph by Daniel H. Connor, MD, 1972.)*

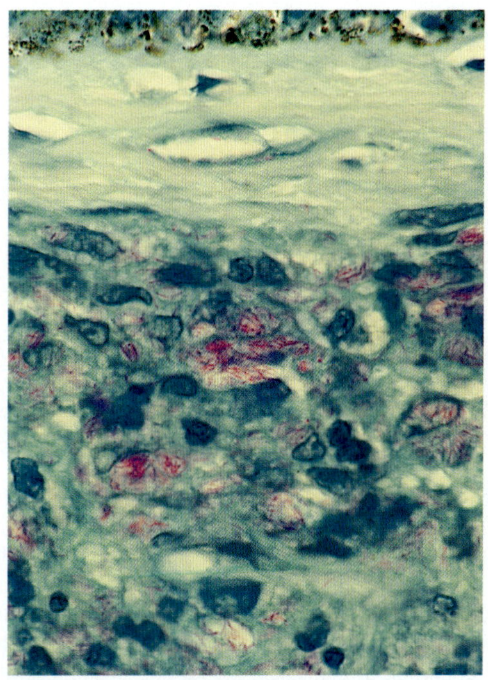

Figure 65–7. Higher magnification showing the pigmented basal layer at the top. Note the clear uninvolved zone ("grenz") immediately beneath the basal layer. The lesion is histiocytes with a few lymphocytes intermixed. The histocytes contain enormous numbers of mycobacteria (Fite-Faraco, ×290).

CLINICAL FEATURES

Indeterminate leprosy follows initial contact with the bacillus (in susceptible individuals) and is characterized by one or more slightly scaly macules often on the face but occasionally on limbs, buttocks, or trunk. Occasionally, indeterminate leprosy may present with more characteristic lesions or with weakness or anesthesia. Rarely, a reaction is the presenting sign. Polar tuberculoid leprosy is clinically manifested by localized skin lesions, which are often hypopigmented, have sharp borders, hypesthesia, or anesthesia and have an asymmetrical distribution (Figures 65–8 and 65–9). Enlargement of cutaneous nerves is common (Figure 65–10). The number of organisms in skin is few. At the other end of the spectrum is polar lepromatous leprosy in which patients have widely distributed symmetrical lesions manifest as either macules, papules, plaques, or nodules, often erythematous. In some patients, there may be diffuse thickening of the skin with loss of eyebrows and eyelashes—the "Bonita" (pretty) form (Figure 65–5). Between these two poles are three named points on this immunologic continuum—borderline tuberculoid, true borderline, and borderline lepromatous, each of which has varying features of tuberculoid and lepromatous leprosy both clinically and histopathologically (Figure 65–11).[4]

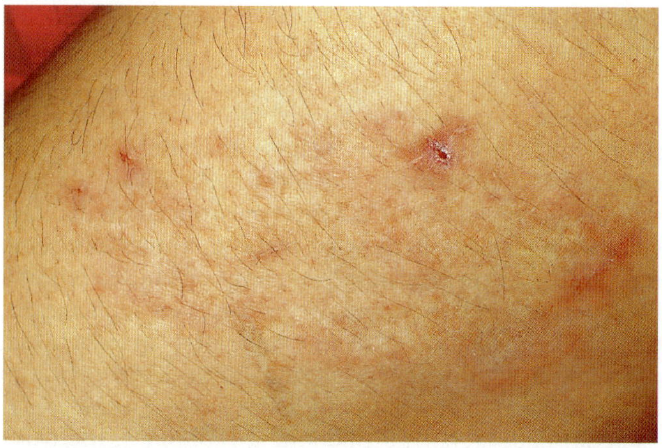

Figure 65–9. Macule of tuberculoid leprosy in white skin. The margin of the macule is raised and irregularly erythematous (AFIP Neg 80-12027).

Reactional leprosy takes two forms. Type I reactions are induced by cell-mediated immunity and consist of upgrading and downgrading reactions. Upgrading (reversal) reactions are in patients with borderline lepromatous leprosy. After treatment is begun, lesions progress toward the tuberculoid end of the spectrum.

Figure 65–8. A macule of tuberculoid leprosy in black skin. When there is more than one lesion, the lesions have an asymmetrical distribution on the body. The central portion of the macule is hypopigmented and hypesthetic, and the margin is infiltrated—ie, raised—by granulomas and other inflammatory changes. Dermal nerves and nerve twigs are inflamed in the infiltrated margin and destroyed in the central portion of the lesion. Biopsy specimens taken for diagnosis, therefore, should include the infiltrated margin (as the best hunting ground for *M leprae*) as well as skin on both sides of the margin so the presence and appearance of dermal nerves in the burnt out center, infiltrated margin, and adjacent normal skin can be compared. *(Photograph by Daniel H. Connor, MD, 1970.)*

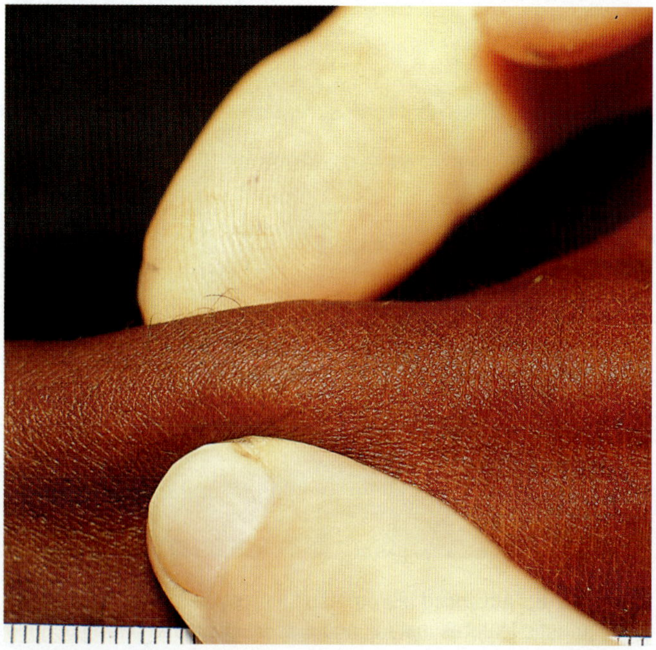

Figure 65–10. Thickened radial nerve over the wrist of an African patient with leprosy. Unlike lesions in skin and RE organs, lesions in nerves may be necrotizing and resemble the caseation necrosis of tuberculosis. *(Patient of Wayne M. Meyers, MD; photograph by Daniel H. Connor, MD, 1970.)*

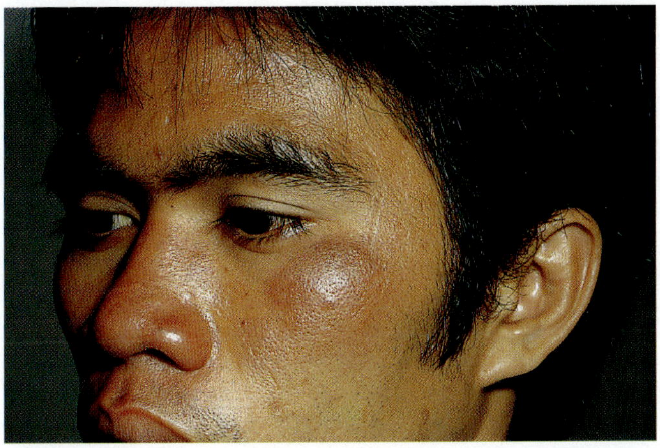

Figure 65–11. Borderline lepromatous leprosy (BL) in a young Thai patient. Features of lepromatous (nodules) and tuberculoid (macules) are present. *(Photograph by Daniel H. Connor, MD, 1980.)*

Downgrading reactions progress from tuberculoid toward the lepromatous end of the spectrum, often in the absence of treatment. In these patients there is inflammation of the existing lesions associated with painful neuropathy.[10] Type II reactions are primarily immune complex mediated and include erythema nodosum leprosum (ENL) (Figure 65–12) and Lucio's phenomenon. Both of these are manifestations of immune-complex-mediated vasculitis, which causes acute inflammation, often with ulceration and acute damage to nerves.

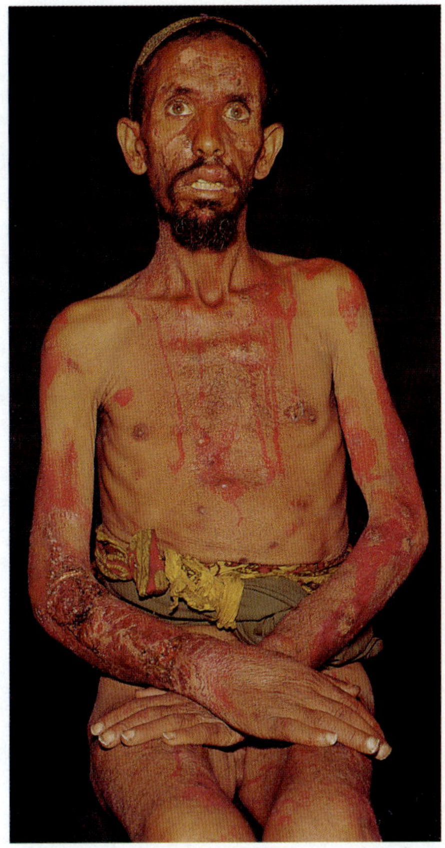

Figure 65–12. ENL in a 38-year-old Yemenite farmer. He had painful nodules on his trunk and limbs, a nodule in his left eye (conjunctiva), and was being treated for streptococcal dermatitis with a red solution. Biopsy of the nodule below his xiphoid process revealed lepromatous leprosy as well as the vascular changes of ENL. Note also the clinical features of pellagra: hyperpigmentation, scaling and ulceration of exposed skin, and perhaps a vacant stare of dementia. Chronic infections such as tuberculosis and leprosy aggravate the features of pellagra. *(Photograph by Daniel H. Connor, MD, 1972.)*

HISTOPATHOLOGY

Indeterminate Leprosy

Histologically, indeterminate leprosy is characterized by a sparse lymphohistiocytic infiltrate surrounding blood vessels of the superficial and deep vascular plexuses. There is often a perineural and sometimes intraneural infiltrate of lymphocytes and histiocytes (Figure 65–13). Sometimes small numbers of foamy histiocytes contain a few acid-fast bacilli. Patients with these are more likely to progress toward lepromatous leprosy, whereas those with epithelioid histiocytes without bacilli tend to progress toward tuberculoid leprosy.[11] When confronted with a perivascular dermatitis involving nerves, leprosy should be remembered and further studies done. Finally, lesions of indeterminate leprosy may be encountered in patients with well-established lepromatous leprosy or tuberculoid leprosy.[11]

Polar Tuberculoid Leprosy

Tuberculoid leprosy is characterized histologically by tubercles comprised of epithelioid cells and Langhans' giant cells surrounded by lymphocytes and plasma cells (Figures 65–14 and 65–15).[12] Granulomas develop in and around cutaneous nerves infected with *M leprae* and silver stains for axons demonstrate the residua of nerves within them. Because the granulomas tend to follow the course of nerve twigs, they often are elongated which aids in distinguishing tuberculoid leprosy from sarcoidosis. In addition to nerves, adnexal structures and arrector pili muscles may be involved.[12] The number of lymphocytes and plasma cells surrounding the epithelioid granulomas in tuberculoid leprosy varies with the host's immunity.[13] In some patients, furthermore, epithelioid cell granulomas invade the papillary dermis and obscure the dermo-epidermal junction.

Lepra bacilli in tuberculoid leprosy are few and may be difficult to find. Sometimes a prolonged search

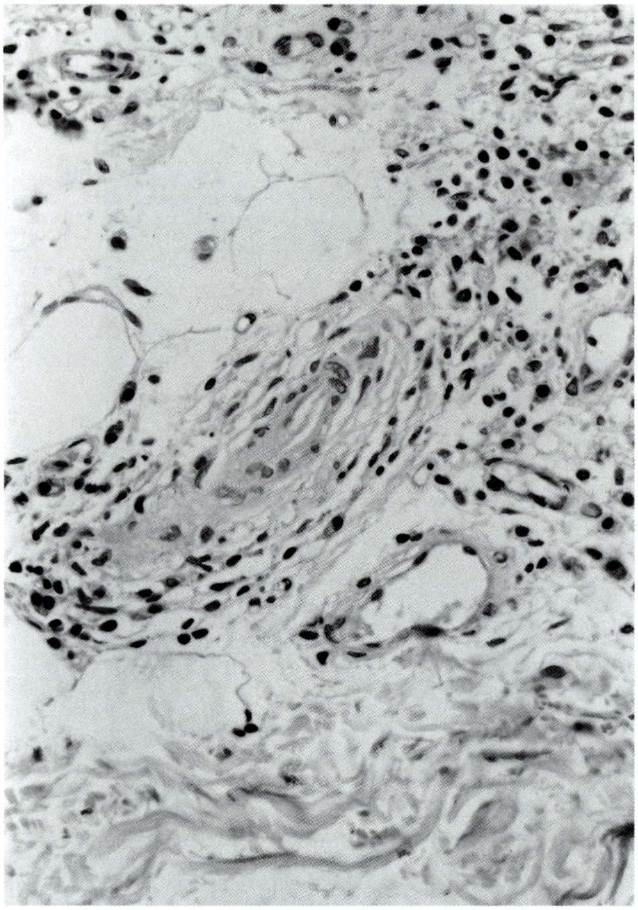

Figure 65–13. Indeterminate leprosy. An inflammatory infiltrate has the overall appearance of nonspecific dermatitis but if it is centered around nerves, it should raise the suspicion of leprosy and prompt studies for acid-fast bacilli. At this stage, however, leprosy is usually missed unless there is a clue in the history (hematoxylin-eosin, ×400).

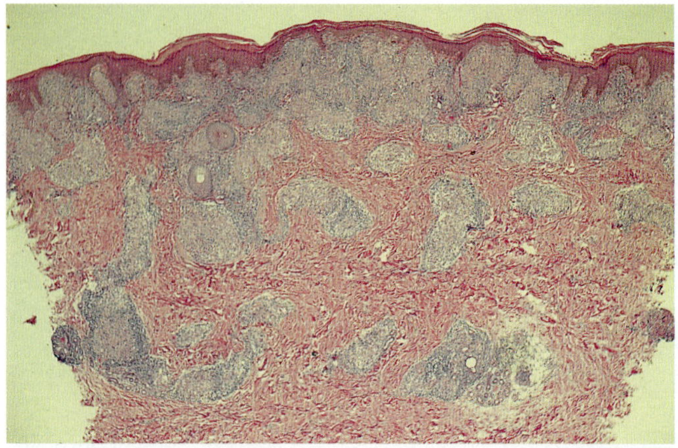

Figure 65–14. Section through the margin of a macule of tuberculoid leprosy. Discrete tubercles composed of epithelioid histiocytes, Langhans' giant cells, lymphocytes, and plasma cells are throughout the dermis. Some tubercles (perhaps most of them) surround damaged nerves and some of the tubercles touch the epidermis. Leprosy bacilli are very few (hematoxylin-eosin, ×7.2).

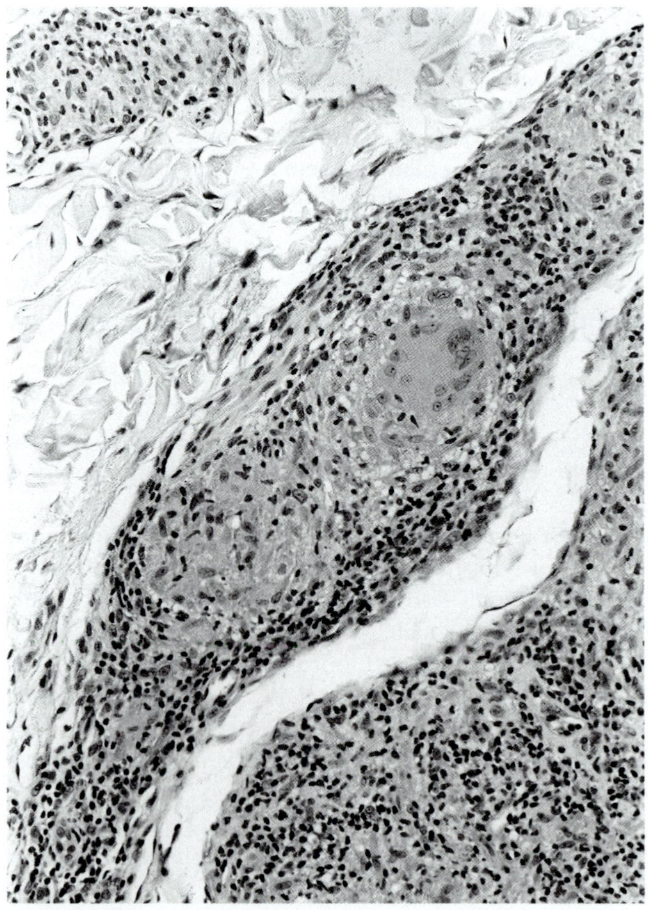

Figure 65–15. Tuberculoid leprosy. This elongated granuloma probably follows the course of a destroyed dermal nerve. The granuloma is comprised of epithelioid histiocytes, some of which are multinucleated. The granuloma is surrounded by a mantle of T helper lymphocytes (hematoxylin-eosin, ×250).

of many Fite–Faraco-stained sections is required (Figure 65–16). Nerve twigs, granulomas and arrector pili muscles are the most rewarding sites to search. If, after a prolonged search, the diagnosis remains in doubt, a second biopsy may be the best next step. It is often helpful for the pathologist and clinician to evaluate the patient together and to be sure the most rewarding site for biopsy is chosen (Figure 65–8). When persistence fails to reveal even a single acid-fast bacillus, immunoperoxidase stains using antibodies against mycobacterial antigens,[14] electron microscopy,[15] and the polymerase chain reaction[16] may all help confirm or exclude leprosy.

Borderline Tuberculoid Leprosy

In general, the features of borderline tuberculoid leprosy resemble those of polar tuberculoid leprosy but there is less involvement of the papillary dermis and lit-

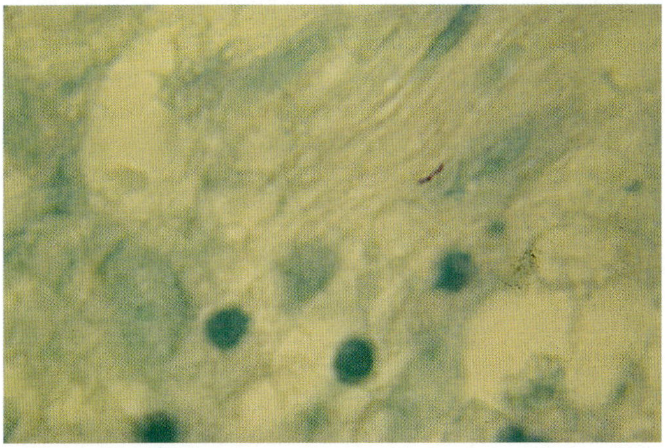

Figure 65–16. Tuberculoid leprosy. This solitary, beaded, slightly curved, faintly stained acid-fast bacillus appears to be degenerating and was found after a prolonged search of multiple sections from a macule of tuberculoid leprosy. Even when a bacillus is partially degenerated, such as this one, it confirms the diagnosis in the right clinical setting (Fite–Faraco, ×1000).

tle if any involvement of the dermo-epidermal junction. Histiocytes are less differentiated and are less spindled than those in polar tuberculoid leprosy. Dermal nerve twigs are more readily identified and although there are few organisms, there are more than there are in polar tuberculoid leprosy.

Borderline Lepromatous Leprosy

As the spectrum progresses further toward the lepromatous pole, there are greater numbers of foamy macrophages, decreased numbers of lymphocytes, and fewer epithelioid histiocytes. Nerves are inflamed and thickened. Acid-fast bacilli are in dermal macrophages and nerves. The degree of inflammation in nerves is less than that in tuberculoid forms of leprosy although there is greater perineural involvement.[17]

Subpolar Lepromatous Leprosy

In this form there is a clear separation of the epidermis from the dermal inflammatory reaction, which is characterized by a diffuse infiltrate of many histiocytes with grayish "foamy" cytoplasm. Lymphocytes are fewer than in tuberculoid leprosy. Perineural thickening with a laminated perineurium giving an "onion skin" appearance is characteristic of subpolar lepromatous leprosy. Innumerable intact bacilli, often in clusters known as globi, are in foamy histiocytes throughout the dermis and in affected nerves.[18]

Polar Lepromatous Leprosy

In polar lepromatous leprosy there is a distinct clear zone separating epidermis from the dermal infiltrate (Figure 65–7), which is comprised of an almost pure collection of "foamy" histiocytes containing many bacilli (Figures 65–6 and 65–7). Some of these foamy histiocytes become vacuolated and enlarged with age and the bacilli within them become packed in tight bundles. These were first identified by Rudolph Virchow and are often referred to as "Virchow" or "lepra" cells. Dermal granulomas may be elongated and distributed along the course of cutaneous nerves but in severe forms, there is a dense diffuse infiltrate that involves the entire dermis and subcutis with destruction of adnexal structures. The cytoplasm of these histiocytes is often gray as a consequence of the abundant mycobacterial lipid and this a helpful clue to diagnosis on routinely stained H&E sections (Figure 65–1 and 65–2). The number of lymphocytes and plasma cells is minimal.[19] A variant of lepromatous leprosy, histoid leprosy, is characterized by fibroplasia, which partly replaces the infiltrate of foam cells.[20]

Reactional Leprosy

Leprosy in reaction exhibits different histologic findings depending on the type of reaction. Reversal reactions (upgrading) are shifts from either subpolar lepromatous or borderline lepromatous to borderline tuberculoid leprosy and usually follows initiation of treatment. The downgrading reaction is a shift from borderline tuberculoid leprosy toward the lepromatous end of the spectrum. Downgrading usually is associated with progression in the absence of treatment. Both upgrading and downgrading may be inflammation of preexisting skin lesions with acute painful neuropathy that may progress to sensory loss and permanent deformities. Histologically these reactions have increased numbers of lymphocytes, fibroblasts, and histiocytes in the lesions in the dermis as well as in and around nerves. It may be difficult to distinguish these reactions from stable disease histologically, and clinical correlation or comparison with a previous biopsy specimen of a stable lesion may be necessary.[21]

The type II reaction is erythema nodosum leprosum. This is most often in patients with lepromatous leprosy, usually polar or subpolar forms, and rarely with borderline lepromatous leprosy. ENL may develop at any point during the course of lepromatous leprosy either before or after treatment. Clinically patients develop malaise, fever, and eruptive skin lesions. Many organs other than the skin may be involved including eyes, synovia, and testes.[22] ENL is thought to be generated by an immune-complex-mediated vasculitis associated with antigen excess from the heavy bacterial load.[23] Histologically there is an influx of neutrophils in granulomatous areas in the dermis and subcutis as well as leukocytoclastic vasculitis (Figure 65–17).[23] Abundant necrosis, abscesses and ulceration may develop.

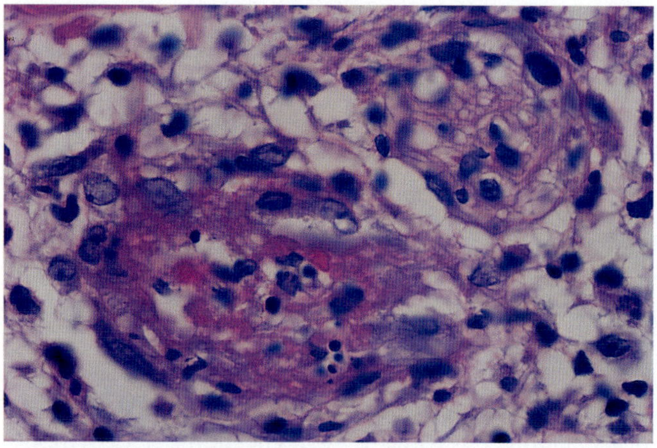

Figure 65–17. Erythema nodosum leprosum, skin from the 38-year-old Yemenite farmer shown in Figure 65–12. The wall of the vessel (*lower left*) is damaged by neutrophils and fibrin. The gray-blue masses in the histiocytes in the nerve (*upper right*) are clusters of *M leprae* (hematoxylin-eosin, ×1000).

The Lucio phenomenon is thought to be a variant of ENL in severe diffuse forms of lepromatous leprosy most commonly in patients from South and Central America. Heavy colonization of vascular endothelium by lepra bacilli damages vessels caused by a brisk immune-complex-mediated vasculitis that arises as a consequence of antigen excess in the setting of a massive bacterial load. Virtually all small and medium-sized blood vessels are affected. Clinically, this causes deep cutaneous infarcts and ulcers.[24]

LEPROSY AND AIDS

Patients with the acquired immunodeficiency syndrome are susceptible to progressive and fatal infection by other mycobacteria including in particular *M tuberculosis* and the *M avium-intracellulare* complex. The few descriptions of patients infected with both human immunodeficiency virus and *M leprae,* however, have not as yet revealed a pattern of acceleration of their leprosy or of downgrading of their leprosy.[25]

DIFFERENTIAL PATHOLOGIC DIAGNOSIS

Indeterminate leprosy may be difficult to diagnose histopathologically and may mimic other diseases associated with perivascular lymphocytic infiltrates. In general, the density of the lymphocytic infiltrate is less in indeterminate leprosy than in other cutaneous lymphocytic infiltrates. Involvement near a nerve, especially if there are foamy histiocytes, is evidence for leprosy.

Polar tuberculoid leprosy may be mimicked by other granulomatous processes associated with epithelioid histiocytes such as sarcoidosis, berylliosis, and silica-induced granulomas. Elongated granulomas that follow the course of cutaneous nerves or inflamed nerve twigs, so characteristic of leprosy, are not features of these other disorders. Other entities associated with epithelioid cell granulomas include infection by other mycobacteria, fungi, protozoa, zirconium-induced granulomas, and granuloma multiforme. If acid-fast bacilli are in skin and nerves, and stain with the Fite–Faraco technique but not with the Ziehl–Neelsen, the argument for a diagnosis of leprosy is very strong (Figure 65–18, A and B). Silica granulomas contain birefringent crystals recognized by polarized light. Granuloma multiforme, a rare tropical disorder that resembles granuloma annulare, usually contains many plasma cells and exhibits a clear zone beneath the basal layer. Adnexal structures are usually involved in tuberculoid leprosy and usually there is neither spongiosis, epithelial hyperplasia, nor caseation necrosis.[26]

Erythema nodosum leprosum may histologically mimic other forms of leukocytoclastic vasculitis. Once again, the demonstration of bacilli by the Fite–Faraco stain or their breakdown products helps establish the diagnosis.

Lepromatous leprosy may mimic other xanthogranulomatous inflammatory disorders such as adult xanthogranuloma or true xanthomata. Abundant foamy histiocytes with grayish cytoplasm should prompt one to perform a Fite–Faraco stain, which will demonstrate bacilli.

Histoid leprosy histologically resembles dermatofibroma but the foam cells, thinning of the epidermis rather than epidermal hyperplasia, and lack of epidermal hyperpigmentation usually distinguishes between these two entities. Fite–Faraco-stained sections demonstrate innumerable intact viable bacilli in many of the spindle-shaped cells as well as in the foam cells.[19]

MOLECULAR PATHOLOGIC DIAGNOSIS

Monoclonal and polyclonal antibodies directed to mycobacteria such *Mycobacterium paratuberculosis* and *Mycobacterium duvallii* also stain *M leprae* and can be used to confirm the diagnosis or detect small numbers of bacilli in formalin-fixed paraffin-imbedded tissue.[16] The polymerase chain reaction has also been used diagnostically in tuberculoid or indeterminate leprosy in which there are few microorganisms.

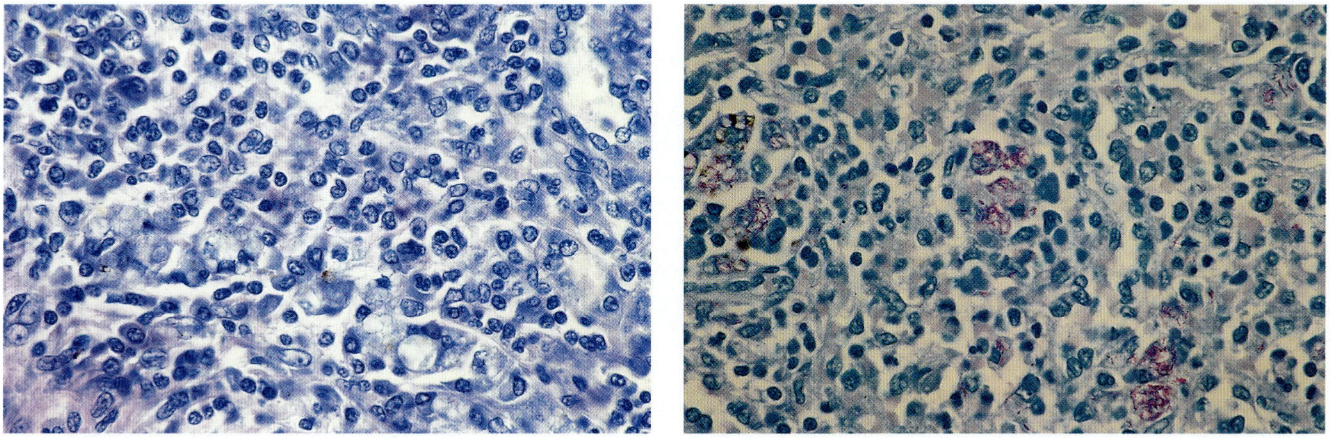

A B

Figure 65–18. (**A**) Lepromatous leprosy of spleen stained by Ziehl–Neelsen. Although there are many foamy histiocytes containing blue-gray masses (clusters of *M leprae*), they are not acid-fast (Ziehl–Neelsen, ×180). (**B**) Section of the same spleen stained with the Fite–Faraco acid-fast technique. Now the clumps of bacilli are clearly acid fast. The acid fastness of *M leprae* is limited and a modified acid-fast stain—such as the Fite–Faraco—must be used (Fite–Faraco, ×180).

CONFIRMATIONAL TESTING AND DIAGNOSIS

Injection of tissue into mouse footpads or into armadillos may be used to replicate *M leprae* although no successful in vitro culture techniques have been developed.[7] The lepromin skin test is neither specific nor diagnostic and has been used to evaluate the patient's type of leprosy.[4]

Some "Don'ts" for Surgical Pathologists and Dermatopathologists

1. Don't diagnose leprosy without being certain. Leprosy is far too serious a disease to suggest it until doubts are resolved. Many patients without leprosy have this diagnosis in their records because someone has suggested it prematurely. And it is very difficult to "undiagnose" leprosy once it gets into a patient's record. Problems in diagnosis tend to be at the tuberculoid end of the spectrum when bacilli are few and very difficult or impossible to find. If patients without demonstrable bacilli have a) dermal granulomas, b) a selective destruction of dermal nerves, and c) unequivocal hypesthesia then a presumptive diagnosis of leprosy is sometimes made. It may be better in such patients, however, to rebiopsy and continue the search for bacilli or its antigens until doubts are resolved.
2. It follows from point 1 that terms such as "compatible with leprosy" or "consistent with leprosy" should be avoided.
3. Don't use the word "leper." "Leper" has a harsh and even cruel connotation dating back to biblical days. With modern methods of diagnosis and treatment, leprosy can be controlled and, in most patients, cured. "Leper" is forbidden in the circles of medical science.

Some "Do's" for Surgical Pathologists and Dermatopathologists

1. Do remember the possibility of leprosy when you see any granulomatous dermatitis, or an infiltrate of foamy histiocytes in the skin or in the RE system.
2. Do remember to use the Fite–Faraco stain. If there is reason to suspect leprosy, search for acid-fast bacilli on Fite–Faraco-stained sections—not Ziehl–Neelsen-stained sections.
3. Consult with the physician or dermatologist before biopsy if possible and, if not, before rebiopsy.
4. Refer questions about treatment to the National Hansen's Disease Center.

REFERENCES

1. Lockwood DNJ, McAdam KPWJ. Leprosy. In: Gorbvach SL, Bartlett JG, Blacklow NR, eds. *Infectious Diseases.* Philadelphia: WB Saunders; 1992:1256–1266.
2. Binford CH, Meyers WM. Leprosy. In: Binford CH, Connor DH, eds. *Pathology of Tropical and Extraordinary Diseases.* Washington, DC: Armed Forces Institute of Pathology; 1976:205–225.
3. Myrvang B, Godal T, Ridley DS, et al. Immune responsiveness to *Mycobacterium leprae* and other mycobacterial antigens throughout the clinical and histopathological spectrum of leprosy. *Clin Exp Immunol.* 1973;14:541–553.
4. Bryceson ADM. Leprosy. In: Champion RH, Burton JL, Ebling FJG, eds. *Textbook of Dermatology.* 5th ed. London: Blackwell; 1992:1065–1083.
5. Ridley DS. *The Pathogenesis of Leprosy and Related Diseases.* London: Wright; 1988.
6. Davey TF, Rees RJW. The nasal discharge in leprosy: clinical and bacteriological aspects. *Lepr Rev.* 1974;45: 121–134.
7. The late Chapman H. Binford, MD, personal communication to Daniel H. Connor, 1982.
8. Storrs EE. The nine banded armadillo: a model for leprosy and other biomedical research. *Int J Lepr.* 1971;39: 703–714.
9. Brennan PJ. Carbohydrate containing antigens of *Mycobacterium leprae. Lepr Rev.* 1986;57(suppl 2):39–51.
10. Jolliffe DS. Leprosy reactional states and their treatment (review). *Br J Dermatol.* 1977;97:345–352.
11. Browne SG. Indeterminate leprosy. *Int J Dermatol.* 1985; 24:555–559.
12. Ridley DS. *Skin Biopsy in Leprosy.* Basel: Documenta Geigy; 1977.
13. Turk JL, Bryceson ADM. Immunological phenomena in leprosy and related diseases. *Adv Immunol.* 1971;39: 703–716.
14. Mshana RN, Humber DF, Harboe M, et al. Demonstration of mycobacterial antigens in nerve biopsies from leprosy patients using peroxidase–antiperoxidase immunoenzyme techniques. *Clin Immunol Immunopathol.* 1983;29:359–368.
15. Imaeda T. Electron microscopy of leprosy lesions. *Dermatol Int.* 1968;7:116–118.
16. Northcutt AD, Tschen JA. New ways to demonstrate pathogenic organisms. *Clin Dermatol.* 1991;9:205–215.
17. Kwittken J, Peck SM. Borderline leprosy. *Arch Dermatol.* 1967;95:50–56.
18. Fields JP, Meyers WM. Leprosy. In: Farmer ER, Hood AF, eds, *Pathology of the Skin.* Norwalk, Conn: Appleton and Lange; 1990:340–350.
19. Ackerman AB. *Histologic Diagnosis of Inflammatory Skin Diseases.* Philadelphia: Lea and Febiger; 1978:775.
20. Sehgal VN, Srivastava G. Histoid leprosy. *Int J Dermatol.* 1985;24:286–292.
21. Ridley DS. Reactions in leprosy. *Lepr Rev.* 1969;40:77–81.
22. Kramarsky B, Edmondson HA, Peters RL, et al. Lepromatous leprosy in reaction. *Arch Pathol.* 1968;85:516–531.
23. Sanchez NP, Mihm MC Jr, Soter NA. Erythema nodosum leprosum—an immune complex mediated necrotizing vasculitis. *J Invest Dermatol.* 1980;75:461. Abstract.
24. Quismorio FP, Rea T, Chandor S, et al. Lucio's phenomenon: an immune complex deposition syndrome in lepromatous leprosy. *Clin Immunol Immunopathol.* 1978;9: 184–193.
25. Moran CA, Nelson AM, Tuur SM, Luengu M, Fonseca L, Meyers WM. Leprosy in five immunodeficiency virus-infected patients. *Mod Pathol.* 1995;8:662–664.
26. Lever WF, Schaumberg-Lever G, eds. *Histopathology of the Skin.* Philadelphia: JB Lippincott; 1990:333–338.

CHAPTER 66

Leptospirosis

Phillip F. Pierce, John P. Utz, and Ernest E. Lack

And some there be, which have no memorial.

Ecclesiasticus XLIV 8

DEFINITION

Leptospirosis (from Greek *leptos,* meaning "fine," and *speira,* meaning "a coil") is a disease caused by a variety of pathogenic spirochetes of the genus *Leptospira,* and is one of the most widespread zoonoses in the world, occurring in both tropical and temperate climates.

INTRODUCTION

Leptospirosis was first recognized as a disease of sewer workers by Landouzy in 1883,[1] but the severe form of the illness was characterized as a clinical entity by Adolf Weil of Heidelberg in 1886 who reported four men with fever, jaundice, hemorrhage, and renal failure.[2] The causative organism was independently isolated in 1915 by German[3,4] and Japanese[5] investigators. Leptospirosis, one of the seven spirochetal diseases of man, may have varied clinical manifestations ranging from a mild nonicteric infection to a more severe illness, which may prove fatal (Weil's disease). The protean clinical manifestations have spawned different designations for the disease such as Fort Bragg fever[6] (or "pretibial fever"[7] with rash on anterior aspect of the legs), swamp fever, swineherd's disease, and 7-day fever.

ETIOLOGY

Spirochetes of the genus *Leptospira* are composed of seven officially recognized pathogenic genomic species: *L interrogans, L biflexa, L borgpetersenii, L weilli, L santarosai, L kirshneri,* and *L noguchi.*[8,9] These seven pathogenic genomic species along with four nonpathogenic species are divided into more than 250 serovars by serotyping using microagglutination. Precise identification and classification of species of *Leptospira* is important for epidemiologic and public health surveillance because different serovars have different host specificities and cause different clinical forms of the disease.[9]

EPIDEMIOLOGY AND PREVALENCE

Leptospirosis is primarily a disease of animals (zoonosis), which are the reservoir for organisms causing human disease. Transmission to humans is usually indirect by exposure to water or soil contaminated by animal urine, usually from dogs, rats, cattle, or pigs. Leptospires favor warm, alkaline, and moist environments. The bite of the rat flea also transmits infection. Men are more often infected, particularly those with occupational exposure such as in canals, sewers, harbors, sugar cane plantations, taro fields, and coal mines. Skin abrasions or cuts may facilitate transmission, but the organism can penetrate moist skin and mucous membranes including conjunctiva. Also at risk are military troops operating in trenches or jungle terrain. In the autopsy study by Arean of 33 fatal infections (24 male, 9 female) most patients lived in homes heavily infested with rats.[10] Human-to-human spread is rare, as is vertical transmission from mother to fetus. Neves et al[11] reported the first patient with the acquired immunodeficiency syndrome (AIDS).

Transmission is most common in tropical climates such as southeast Asia. In the United States the annual incidence has been estimated to be 0.05 per 100,000 while in Hawaii an annual incidence of 128 per 100,000 person-years has recently been reported with one of the risk factors being household use of rainwater.[12] The prevalence of infection may be underestimated in many parts of the world, particularly milder forms of the disease, which may go unrecognized. Inner city population-based surveys in the United States have studied the prevalence of leptospiral antibodies, finding 16% of patients positive in a clinic for sexually transmitted diseases in Baltimore[13] and 30% of children under 6 years old in Detroit.[14] Some patients are travelers who have returned from the tropics with fever.[15]

Leptospires can live for long periods in the kidneys of animals such as the brown Norway rat, in which they adhere to the brush border of the proximal tubular epithelium. Here they proliferate and enter the urine (leptospiruria).[16] Some animals, such as dogs, may become symptomatic and die of leptospiral nephritis.

MORPHOLOGY OF LEPTOSPIRA

The first description of pathogenic leptospires was given by Stimson in 1907 in sections of kidneys of patients who supposedly died of yellow fever.[17] The organisms appeared as ". . . irregularly curved . . . having a regular series of alternating curves . . . one or both extremities bent back in the form of a hook . . . entire length up to 14 μ; width estimated at 0.5 μ. . . ."[17] As depicted schematically in Figure 66–1, the spirals are regular and tightly coiled, and when a hook is at one end, the shape of the organism has been likened to a shepherd's crook. The outer membrane of the leptospire acts as an osmotic barrier, enabling the organism to exchange solutes with water in which it lives. The organism cannot survive dessication or a saltwater environment because the plasma membrane becomes completely disorganized. Leptospires are unable to multiply in water because they are unable to synthesize fatty acids, which have to be provided by an animal or human host.[16]

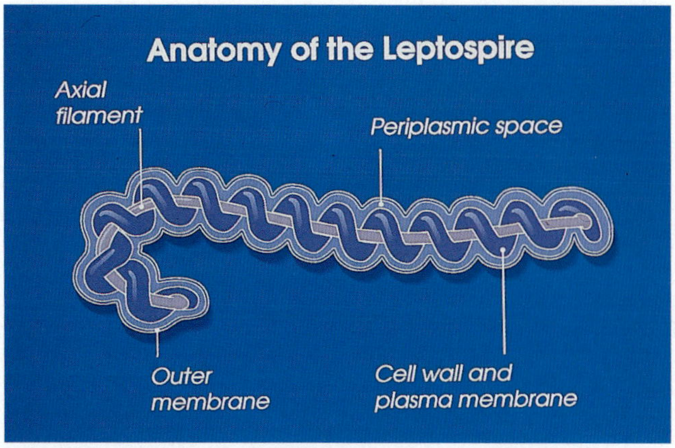

Figure 66–1. Schematic illustration of leptospire showing regular closely grouped coils or spirals with hook at one end.

CLINICAL FEATURES

From 30 to 60 infections (a reportable disease until 1995) are listed annually in *The Morbidity and Mortality Weekly Report.* The incubation period is from 2 to 30 days, usually 5 to 14 days, and the illness is biphasic. Initially, the septicemic (also termed leptospiremic) phase is marked by nonspecific symptoms of acute illness: "flulike" with abrupt onset, remittent fever, headache, myalgia, and malaise. *Leptospira* sp may be cultured from blood, cerebrospinal fluid (CSF), or from various tissues. This phase has a duration of 4 to 7 days. Subsequently, the patient enters the "immune" phase at which time kidneys, liver, meninges, eyes, skin, and other organs are involved. At this point leptospires can be recovered only from the urine.

In a study of 150 military personnel in Vietnam, the most common symptoms were headache (98%), fever (97%), myalgia (79%), chills (78%), nausea (41%), diarrhea (29%), abdominal pain (28%), and cough (20%); in the same study the most common signs were conjunctival suffusion (42%), splenomegaly (22%), lymphadenopathy (21%), pharyngeal erythema (17%), hepatomegaly (15%), nuchal rigidity (12%), rash (7%), and jaundice (2%).[18] Pancreatitis may cause abdominal pain and in a recent report pancreatitis was associated with acute acalculous cholecystitis.[19] Despite these findings and percentages, Weil's disease, an historically important manifestation of infection, is recognized by jaundice and hematuria. It is the more severe form and may be fatal.

PATHOLOGY

In fatal leptospirosis, death is usually from renal failure and uremia, but with the availability of hemodialysis some of these patients may be saved. Other fatal complications include hemorrhage and occasionally myocarditis. The gross appearance of organs depends on the severity of jaundice and azotemia. Hemorrhages can be in many tissues usually as petechiae, but extensive hemorrhage in the abdomen and diffuse subarachnoid hemorrhage have been described. The liver is often a distinct yellow-green (Figure 66–2) and may be enlarged. Microscopically the architecture overall is preserved, but there may be a conspicuous or subtle dissociation or disorganization of liver cell plates, which is

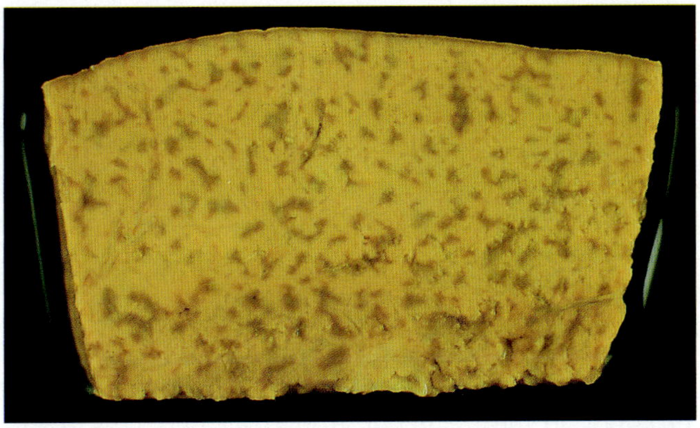

Figure 66–2. Fatal human leptospirosis. Liver is grossly bile stained on section and mildly enlarged.

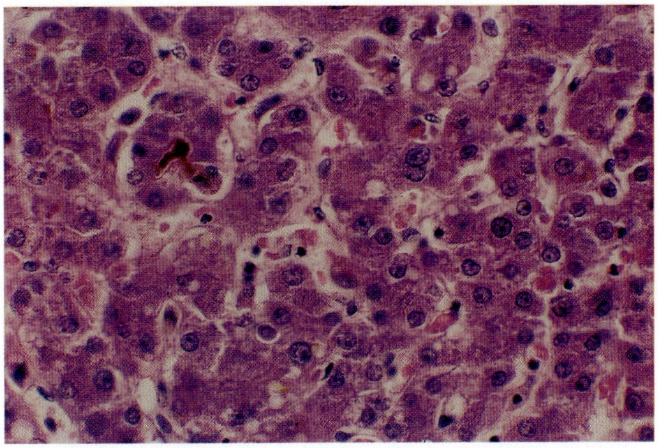

Figure 66–4. Liver in fatal leptospirosis. There is slight dissociation of liver cell plates and area of canalicular bile stasis in left upper quadrant of field (hematoxylin-eosin, ×375).

an agonal change (Figure 66–3). These changes may be associated with regeneration such as binucleated and trinucleated hepatocytes, anisonucleosis, and occasional mitotic figures. Necrotic hepatocytes ("acidophilic" bodies) may be in sinusoids usually in central and midzones but also may be periportal (Figure 66–3). Ballooning degeneration is a feature also. Plugs of bile may be in ductules or canaliculi (Figure 66–4). Leptospires are found in about 25% of patients, but without any special localization.[20]

The kidneys are enlarged and may be icteric. Microscopically there is an interstitial chronic inflammatory cell infiltrate composed of lymphocytes and plasma cells. The lumens of the tubules may be distended by hyaline or granular casts (Figure 66–5). Epithelium of proximal convoluted tubules may be necrotic. In general, the alterations vary depending on the duration of illness. Leptospires have been identified in 65% of patients[10] and may be in the lumen (Figure 66–6) or epithelial cells of the tubules.

Lesions are not confined to liver and kidney, but involve a variety of other organs and tissues causing myocarditis, encephalitis, pancreatitis, and necrosis and inflammation of skeletal muscle.[10]

DIAGNOSIS

Definitive diagnosis can be made by culture of body fluids. In the first week of illness, blood and CSF are most likely to be productive; thereafter, cultures from these sources are unusual. During the second week, leptospires are excreted in the urine, which becomes the highest yielding body fluid for culture. Leptospires

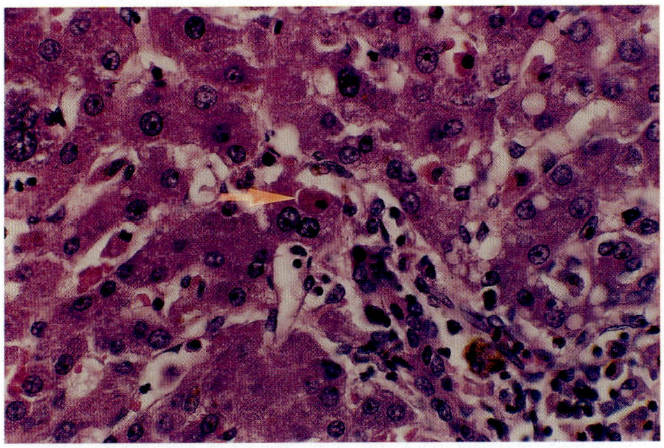

Figure 66–3. Mild degree of dissociation or disorganization of liver plates in fatal human leptospirosis. Note also "acidophilic body" or necrotic hepatocyte in periportal region (*arrow*) and mild portal chronic inflammation (hematoxylin-eosin, ×375).

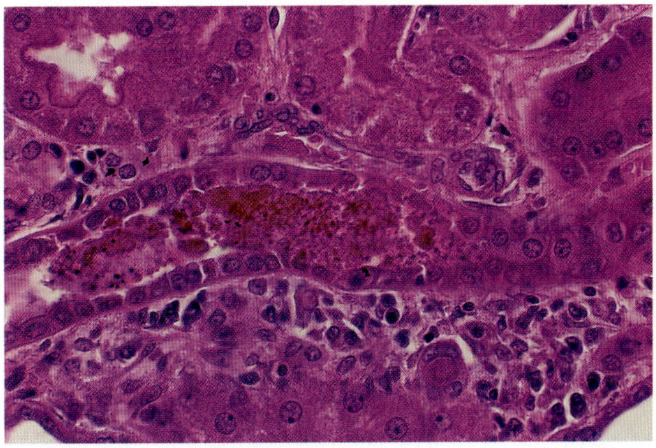

Figure 66–5. Kidney in fatal human leptospirosis. Note interstitial chronic inflammation and granular cast with focal necrosis of tubular epithelium (hematoxylin-eosin, ×375).

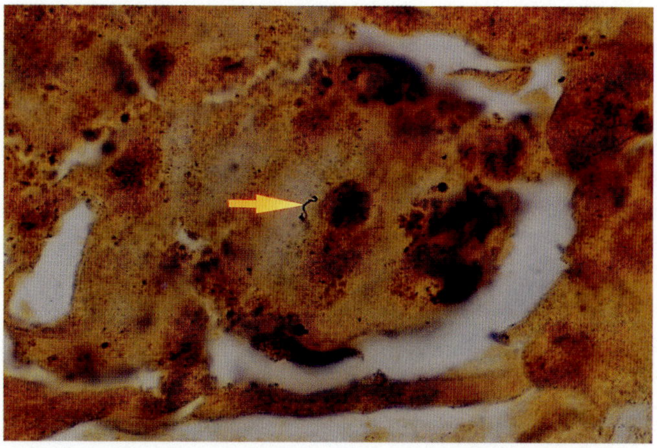

Figure 66–6. Leptospire in lumen of renal tubule in fatal leptospirosis in human (Warthin–Starry stain, ×1000).

can be propagated by inoculating the body fluid on Fletcher's media, incubating for an extended period (ie, up to 8 weeks at 25°C), with growth visualized using darkfield microscopy. Serologic diagnosis is standard, as often leptospirosis has not been suspected early when cultures of body fluids are likely to yield leptospires. The most commonly employed test is the agglutination test, eg, microscopic agglutination test (MAT), which measures IgG and IgM antibodies directed against surface antigens. Cross agglutinating antibodies prevent speciation of the strain by this test. Antibodies appear late in the first week and peak during the third to fourth week. The persistence of antibodies for years after an infection limits the diagnosis by a single serum specimen. Enzyme immunoassay detects other antigens, but has not allowed earlier or more specific diagnosis.[21] Ten percent of culture-proven infections have a negative serology. This may be related to treatment with antimicrobics, infection by an unrecognized serovar, or delayed host response. A recent study showed that DNA extraction and subsequent polymerase chain reaction on freshly voided urine samples was twice as sensitive as culturing the organism, and that leptospiruria may be detected during the first 7 days of illness. Some urine samples were still positive for leptospires years after the infection, indicating that shedding of the organism may last much longer than generally assumed.[22]

TREATMENT

The earliest useful antimicrobial agent was penicillin G, given intravenously in a daily dosage of 2,400,000 to 3,600,000 units. Later tetracycline (in daily dosage of 2 g) provided an oral route of administration. To be effective, treatment should begin before the fourth day of recognized illness. Currently doxycycline, 100 mg twice daily or amoxicillin, 500 mg three times daily (either drug orally for 7 days), is recommended.

The evaluation of the effectiveness of antimicrobial therapy has been limited by inadequate trial designs and the sporadic infections. Two randomized controlled trials both have demonstrated the efficacy of tetracycline in moderate infection. McClain et al[23] reported a series of 29 patients, 14 receiving doxycycline and 15 placebo. Doxycycline significantly reduced duration of illness as manifested by diminished fever, headache, myalgias, and malaise. Leptospiruria was eliminated promptly in the treatment group, but persisted in 95% of the placebo group. There were no differences in clearance rates of leptospires. Chemoprophylaxis with weekly doxycycline reduced the attack rate from 4.3% to 0.2% among 940 U.S. soldiers deployed in Panama for 3 weeks. Thus doxycycline may be used as an intense but short-term preventive.[24] Jarisch–Herxheimer reactions after penicillin treatment have been described in varying frequencies. As in other spirochetal diseases, a flare of symptoms and hypotension may follow penicillin.

Techniques to reduce risk of infection have been recommended. Precautions include 1) eliminating rodents, 2) wearing protective clothing, 3) avoiding immersion in natural waters, 4) covering abrasions, 5) showering after exposure to natural water, and 6) using footwear. These techniques may be impractical for those with occupational exposure. Vaccination of domestic livestock and pets is available, but leptospirosis has been transmitted experimentally to dogs despite vaccination.[25] A human vaccine for those at risk has been produced, but is not available in Britain nor in the United States.

REFERENCES

1. Landouzy. Fièvre bilieuse ou hépatique. *Gaz hôp.* 1883;56:809–810.
2. Weil A. Über eine eigenthümliche, mit milztumor, icterus und nephritis einhergehende, acute infektionskrankheit. *Dtsch Arch Klin Med.* 1886;39:209–232.
3. Hübener, Reiter: Beiträge zur aetiologie der weilschen krankheit. *Deuts Med.* 1915;41:1275–1277.
4. Uhlenhuth P, Fromme W. Zur aetiologie der sog weil'schen krankheit (austeckende gelbsucht). *Berl Klin Wchnschr.* 1916;53:269–273.
5. Inada R, Ido Y, Hoki R, Kaneko R, Ito H. The etiology, mode of infection and specific therapy in Weil's disease (spirochaetosis icterohemorrhagica). *J Exp Med.* 1916;23:377–402.
6. Gochenouer WS Jr, Smadel JE, Jackson EB, Evans LB, Yager RH. Leptospiral etiology of Fort Bragg fever. *Publ Health Rep.* 1952;67:811–813.

7. Daniels WB, Grennan HA. Pretibial fever. *JAMA.* 1943; 122:361–365.
8. Gravekamp C, Van de Kemp H, Franzen M, et al. Detection of seven species of pathogenic leptospires by PCR using two sets of primers. *J Gen Microbiol.* 1993;139: 1691–1700.
9. De Caballero OLSD, Neto ED, Koury MC, Romanha AJ, Simpson AJG. Low-stringency PCR with diagnostically useful primers for identification of leptospira serovars. *J Clin Microbiol.* 1994;32:1369–1372.
10. Arean VM. The pathologic anatomy and pathogenesis of fatal human leptospirosis (Weil's disease). *Am J Pathol.* 1962;40:393–423.
11. Neves E de S, Pereira MM, Galhardo MCG, et al. Leptospirosis patient with AIDS the first case recorded. *Rev Soc Bras Med Trop.* 1994;27:39–42.
12. Sasaki DM, Pang L, Minette HP, et al. Active surveillance and risk factors for leptospirosis in Hawaii. *Am J Trop Med Hyg.* 1993;48:35–43.
13. Childs JE, Schwartz BS, Ksiazek TG, Graham RR, LeDuc JW, Glass GE. Risk associated with antibodies to leptospires in inner-city residents of Baltimore: a protective role for cats. *Am J Public Health.* 1992;82:597–599.
14. Detmers RY, Frank RR, Thierman AB, Demers PA. Exposure to *Leptospira icterohemorrhagia* in inner-city and suburban children: a serologic comparison. *J Fam Pract.* 1983;17:1007–1011.
15. van Crevel R, Speelman P, Gravekamp C, Terpstra WJ. Leptospirosis in travelers. *Clin Inf Dis.* 1994;19:132–134.
16. Clinical conferences at the Johns Hopkins Hospital. Leptospirosis. *Johns Hop Med J.* 1980;147:65–69.
17. Stimson AM. Note on an organism found in yellow fever tissue. *Publ Health Rep.* 1907;22:541.
18. Berman SJ, Tsai C, Holmes K, Fresh JW, Watten RH. Sporadic anicteric leptospirosis in South Vietnam. *Ann Intern Med.* 1973;79:167–170.
19. Monno S, Mizushima Y. Leptospirosis with acute acalculous cholecystitis and pancreatitis. *J Clin Gastroenterol.* 1993;16:52–54.
20. Dooley JR, Ishad KG. Leptospirosis. In: Binford CC, Connor DH, eds. *Pathology of Tropical and Extraordinary Diseases.* Washington, DC: Armed Forces Institute of Pathology, 1976:101–106.
21. Lupidi R, Sinco M, Balanzin D, Delprete E, Varaldo PE. Serological follow-up of patients involved in a localized outbreak of leptospirosis. *J Clin Microbiol.* 1991;29:805–809.
22. Bal AE, Gravekamp C, Hartskeerl RA. Meza-Brewster J de, Korver H, Terpstra WJ. Detection of leptospires in urine by PCR for early diagnosis of leptospirosis. *J Clin Microbiol.* 1994;32:1894–1898.
23. McClain JBL, Ballou WR, Harrison SM, Steinweg DL. Doxycycline therapy for leptospirosis. *Ann Intern Med.* 1984;100;696–698.
24. Takafuji ET, Kirkpatrick JW, Miller RN, et al. An efficacy trial of doxycycline chemoprophylaxis against leptospirosis. *N Engl J Med.* 1984;310:497–500.
25. Schmidt DR, Winn RE, Keefe TJ, Leptospirosis. Epidemiological features of a sporadic case. *Arch Intern Med.* 1989;149:1878–1880.

CHAPTER 67

Listeriosis

Martin E. A. Mielke, Thomas K. Held, and Matthias Unger

. . . slay both man and woman, infant and suckling, ox and sheep, camel and ass.

First Samuel 15:3

DEFINITION

Listeriosis is a bacterial infection caused by the facultative intracellular, gram-positive bacillus *Listeria monocytogenes*. *Listeria monocytogenes* is distributed throughout the world—in mankind, in numerous animals, and in soil and contaminated foods. The illness occurs sporadically or in clusters and usually presents as bacteremia with or without septicemia, meningitis, meningoencephalitis, or, less commonly, as a characteristic encephalitis of the brainstem. Immunodeficient patients, the elderly, and pregnant women are at increased risk of infection. During pregnancy, infection may cause abortion, stillbirth, or neonatal infection. The disseminated *Listeria*-induced lesions in various organs show a broad histologic pattern, ranging from focal necroses and microabscesses to mononuclear granulomas, usually without giant cells. Diagnosis is presumed when intracellular gram-positive bacilli are in the lesions and confirmed by culture. Effective antibiotic therapy is available, but encephalitis, especially of the brainstem, is often fatal, particularly if diagnosis is delayed. Any infection with disseminated microabscesses and granulomas, especially in liver or brain, containing gram-positive bacilli, suggests listeriosis. Antibodies are not protective, and immunity to listeriosis depends on an interaction of specific T cells with infected parenchymal cells and phagocytes.

INTRODUCTION

Listeria monocytogenes was first described by Murray et al,[1,2] who reported a septic illness in laboratory rabbits caused by a hitherto undescribed gram-positive bacillus. Because the organism caused a marked peripheral monocytosis in these animals, it was initially named *Bacterium monocytogenes*. In 1927, Pirie[3] detected a similar bacillus in mice with characteristic liver lesions and named the organism *Listerella hepatolytica* after Lord Lister. When it was discovered that both diseases were caused by the same bacillus, the bacillus was named *Listerella monocytogenes* and, finally, according to the current taxonomy, *Listeria monocytogenes*.

Human listeriosis and even the bacillus had been seen before 1926, however. One of the first descriptions of listeriosis was probably by Henle[4] in 1893 as "pseudotuberculosis in newborn twins." Outbreaks of meningoencephalitis in animals, most likely caused by *L monocytogenes,* were described in sheep and pigs in the United States, Germany, and the Soviet Union in the late 1920s. Infected animals had a characteristic pathologic gait so their illness was called "circling disease."[5]

It was not until 1933 that *L monocytogenes* was recognized as a cause of encephalitis in humans.[6] In the following years, Burn[7] described several neonatal infections with meningitis and ventriculitis with ventricular hemorrhages, as well as listerial meningitis in an adult.

Reports of listeriosis remained rare between 1933 and 1950. Since then, the number of reported infections has increased, and severe outbreaks with central nervous system (CNS) manifestations have been reported.[8–10]

GEOGRAPHIC DISTRIBUTION, PREVALENCE, PREDISPOSING FACTORS, AND TRANSMISSION

Listeriosis has been described on all continents except Antarctica with some concentration in certain regions such as France.[10] Symptomatic infection is diagnosed in 2 to 7 per million persons per year in Europe and the United States.

Those at highest risk are patients with immunodeficiencies from leukemia, malignant lymphomas, rheumatoid arthritis, organ transplants with corticosteroid or cyclosporin A therapy, hepatic cirrhosis, pregnancy, and fetuses and newborns of infected mothers.[9,11]

Among the various manifestations of listeriosis, CNS infection is the most common form of postnatal infection. Of 467 reported infections, 77% presented with meningitis or encephalitis.[12] CNS involvement, however, may be overrepresented in the literature since infections without CNS involvement have nonspecific clinical features of septicemia. *Listeria monocytogenes* accounts for 0.8% to 4.7% of all bacterial infections of the CNS.[13–15] Among immunodeficient patients, however, this figure rises to 22%.[11] Only about 3% of reported infections present as other than bacteremia or meningoencephalitis.

The age distribution of patients has shifted over the years. Almost all infections during the 1960s and 1970s were in newborns, whereas now, most infections are in those over 45.[16] Prolonged survival of patients suffering from malignant diseases may explain this shift.

Listeriosis usually presents sporadically, probably through endogenous infection from the gastrointestinal tract, which harbors *Listeria* in 1% to 5% of the healthy population. From time to time, however, there are outbreaks caused mostly by contaminated food. Vegetables, meat and sausage, and even pasteurized milk have been sources of infection. In this context, it is of interest that *Listeria* multiply even while refrigerated. Contaminated soft cheese caused several epidemics during the 1980s[8,17] and there have been outbreaks in hospitals. The fetus becomes infected transplacentally during maternal bacteremia or by a primary ascending infection of amniotic fluid followed by tracheobronchial and oral ingestion of bacteria.

DESCRIPTION OF *LISTERIA MONOCYTOGENES*

Listeria monocytogenes is a gram-positive, non-spore-forming, nonencapsulated, facultatively anaerobic, nonbranching rod (Figure 67–1).[18] It is motile at room temperature and has a narrow zone of β-hemolysis when grown on blood agar. The bacilli resemble Corynebacteria, although in Gram stains of clinical specimens, they may look like streptococci, especially pneumococci or enterococci. Sometimes they stain poorly and may be mistaken for *Haemophilus influenzae* or other gram-negative bacilli. *Listeria monocytogenes* has a close genetic relationship with other gram-positive bacilli, including *Clostridia* sp, staphylococci, and streptococci.[19,20] Among the seven known species of the genus *Listeria,* only *L monocytogenes* is an important human pathogen. The common clinical isolates are serotypes 1/2a, 1/2b, and 4b.

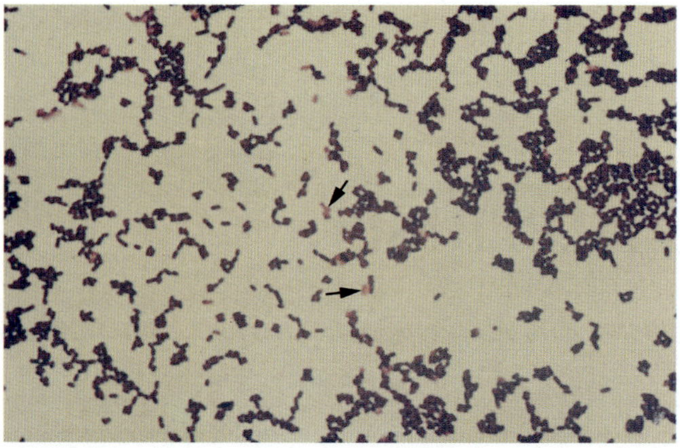

Figure 67–1. Gram stain of *L monocytogenes* demonstrating imperfect gram-positivity (*arrows*) (×1000).

The virulence of *L monocytogenes* depends on the ability to invade, reproduce in, and spread from cell to cell.[21] It therefore belongs to the group of facultative intracellular bacteria,[22] sharing this feature with other genera afflicting the CNS, like *Mycobacteria, Nocardia, Treponema, Borrelia, Francisella,* and *Rickettsia.* Among these, *Listeria* causes the most fulminating infection with the highest mortality, probably because of its potent toxin production, short replication time, and the ability to spread rapidly.

CLINICAL FEATURES

Although many people carry *L monocytogenes* in their gastrointestinal tract or vagina, there are very few infections. These are best divided into three groups: 1) infection during pregnancy, 2) transplacental or ascending infection of the fetus, and 3) perinatal or postnatal infections in newborns or infection in adults other than pregnant women.

Infection during pregnancy may cause nothing more than a brief, flulike illness; indeed, 40% may be asymptomatic and positive blood cultures are the only sign of infection. As a consequence of maternal bacteremia and transplacental transmission, listeriosis in pregnant women may cause abortion, premature birth, or infected liveborn babies. *Listeria monocytogenes* has been isolated from the cervix. Accordingly, septicemia may follow delivery or abortion. In some patients, persistent vaginal colonization manifests itself in subsequent pregnancies, so that mothers of infants with congenital listeriosis may already have had abortions or stillborn infants.

Neonatal listeriosis may appear as early onset or late onset disease similar to group B streptococcal infection. Transplacental transmission is most common in the third trimester and appears during the first week of the infant's life in a form that resembles neonatal sepsis (early onset disease). Often the amniotic fluid is meconium stained, and the newborn has leukocytosis with a shift to the left as well as immature red cells from severe anemia. General signs and symptoms may be nonspecific, and include respiratory distress or circulatory failure. There may be vomiting, refusal of food, or diarrhea. Hypotonia, altered deep reflexes, or convulsions indicate involvement of the CNS. Hepatomegaly and splenomegaly are common but not constant. Signs more specific for listeriosis are papular cutaneous lesions (Figure 67–2) and mucosal nodules—on a congested posterior pharyngeal mucosa, for example. These signs are thought to be pathognomonic of severe early onset neonatal listeriosis, the so-called "granulomatosis infantiseptica." Mortality of untreated, early onset, neonatal listeriosis is virtually 100%; the few survivors have sequelae including hydrocephalus and mental retardation.

Late onset listeriosis appears between the second and the eighth week of life. These infants probably become infected at delivery from the colonized genital tract or from the gastrointestinal tract of the mother who is almost always asymptomatic. Late onset listeriosis more closely resembles infection in adults, in that CNS infection dominates the clinical setting.

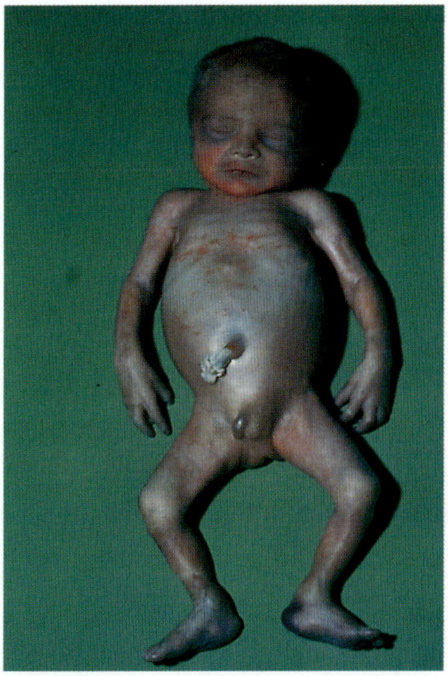

Figure 67–2. Stillborn with "granulomatosis infantiseptica." Typical cutaneous lesions are papules surrounded by red margins. They are most pronounced on the right arm and trunk. *(Contributed by Dr H.P.R. Seeliger, Würzburg, Germany.)*

Symptoms and signs of listerial meningitis and/or meningoencephalitis cannot be distinguished from other bacterial infections. Listerial meningoencephalitis may even resemble a viral infection. Differentiation requires culture of blood and cerebrospinal fluid. Although onset is usually acute, some patients have prodromal symptoms, including fatigue, headache, low-grade fever, nausea, vomiting, or diarrhea.

In contract to listerial meningitis, listerial rhombencephalitis is unique for a bacterial infection. It is the human equivalent of "circling disease" in ruminants. Eck[23] was first to describe listerial meningoencephalitis of the brainstem. Occurring in 5% to 10% of listerial CNS infections, rhombencephalitis affects mainly the middle aged and elderly, although occasionally it may develop in neonates. It typically has two phases; first the prodromal phase lasting up to 10 days is characterized by increasing fever, headaches, nausea, and vomiting or change in personality. The bulbar phase follows with ptosis, diplopia, dysarthria, dysphagia, hemiparesis, or tetraparesis, or an insidious disturbance of consciousness. Ataxia is particularly common. Approximately 90% of these patients have cranial nerve palsies with involvement of facial, glossopharyngeal, trigeminal, vagus, abducens, and accessory nerves—in decreasing frequency.[24] Patients die of respiratory and circulatory failure.

RARE MANIFESTATIONS OF LISTERIOSIS

Oculoglandular listeriosis is more localized and characterized by fever, purulent conjunctivitis, and enlargement of parotid and submandibular lymph nodes. Patients with this form of listeriosis have been infected by animals.

Similarly, cervicoglandular listeriosis is a localized form of infection afflicting cervical lymph nodes after entry of the bacillus through the nasopharynx. It may cause an abscess or a fistula resembling tuberculosis.

Postnatal cutaneous listeriosis is a rare primary infection of skin. It is usually on the forearms and arms of veterinarians or farmers who have handled infected animals or handled contaminated animal material. The cutaneous eruptions, mainly papular or pustular, develop in 48 to 72 hours after exposure and are sometimes preceded by fever, chills, and leukocytosis.

Listerial endocarditis, although rare, usually complicates underlying rheumatic heart disease. All endocardial infections have been in adults. In most patients, vegetations involved the mitral, or mitral and aortic valves and there has been septic embolization to brain.[25] The whole spectrum of clinical manifestations of listeriosis is presented in Table 67–1.

TABLE 67–1. CLINICAL MANIFESTATIONS OF INFECTION BY *LISTERIA MONOCYTOGENES*

I. Asymptomatic carrier
    Intestinal or vaginal
II. Infection during pregnancy
    Transient bacteremia
    Panmetritis
    Placentitis
    Chorioamnionitis
III. Fetal or early onset neonatal listeriosis
    Spontaneous abortion or stillbirth
    Premature birth
    Granulomatosis infantiseptica
IV. Perinatal and postnatal infection (late onset listeriosis) or listeriosis in the adult
    1. Sepsis
        Infection of the small and large intestine, appendicitis, mesenteric lymphadenitis
        Infection of liver, spleen, and adrenals
        Infection of lung and pleura
        Nephritis
        Peritonitis, intra-abdominal abscesses
        Endocarditis
        Osteomyelitis, arthritis
    2. CNS manifestations
        Meningitis
        Meningoencephalitis
        Rhombencephalitis
        Brain and spinal cord abscess
        Endophthalmitis
    3. Local infections
        Skin infection
        Conjunctivitis
        Infection of the middle ear and paranasal sinuses
        Cervical lymphadenitis
        Cholecystitis

PATHOGENESIS

The essential knowledge about the pathogenesis of listeriosis derives from epidemiologic studies[26] and from experimental infections in rabbits, sheep, and mice.[5,21,27–30] All clinical isolates of *L monocytogenes* are virulent for mice. Also, the course of infection, the histologic pattern, and the factors predisposing to infection are strikingly similar in humans and mice[31–33]—so that data obtained from mice have been directly applicable to the current view of pathogenesis in man. In fact, the broad spectrum of lesions seen at autopsy can best be understood from experimental infections.

Entry and Dissemination

As mentioned, listerial infection is usually acquired by invasion from the gastrointestinal tract or by hematogenous transmission through the placenta. In gastrointestinal infections, the M cells of Peyer's patches are usually the first to be infected,[34] although enterocytes or cells of the oral mucosa may also be invaded.[35–38] *Listeria monocytogenes* has no fimbriae or pili to help it adhere to the mucosal surface.[39] Virulent organisms, however, possess superficial α-D-galactose residues, which enable them to bind to specific receptors on the surface of human cells.[40] In addition, lipoteichoic acid of the cell wall may play a role in initial adhesion. Subsequent cellular invasion is being promoted by two proteins called invasin and internalin, which induce active endocytosis of *L monocytogenes.*[41–43] Uptake by professional phagocytes is facilitated by opsonization with complement C3b and especially C3bi.

After ingestion, virulent strains survive, multiply, and spread within the cell.[21,44] The most important bacterial factor toward this is listeriolysin O,[45,46] a secreted, pore-forming cytotoxin, which can easily be detected by its ability to lyse erythrocytes, eg, when the bacteria are cultured on blood agar. All clinical isolates show this trait. Virulent strains producing listeriolysin O are able to evade the phagocytotic vacuole and thereby escape destruction in the phagolysosome. The capability to produce listeriolysin O, however, is necessary but not sufficient by itself for virulence.[47] The toxin enables the bacteria to multiply intracytoplasmically but not to spread to other cells. The latter process is induced by an actin-binding protein on the posterior surface of the bacteria, which mediates a polar effect on the cytoskeleton of the infected cell.[48] In this way the bacteria are able to infect adjacent cells without leaving the intracellular milieu, thereby avoiding any contact with humoral mechanisms of defense.

After the mucosal phase of infection, *L monocytogenes* is transported in phagocytes or free in lymphatics to mesenteric lymph nodes and finally, via the thoracic duct, into the circulation.[49,50] In transplacental transmission, infection of the fetus starts immediately with bacteremia. It is this type of infection that experimental intravenous infection resembles most.

Listeria circulating in the blood are rapidly taken up by resident macrophages and hepatocytes, the former being mainly in spleen and liver, but also in lungs and adrenals.[27,51] Most of the bacteria are killed within hours. About 20%, however, survive in macrophages and parenchymal cells (eg, hepatocytes), in which they grow exponentially.[52] The generation time of *L monocytogenes* in epithelial cells is 1 hour, ie, not substantially longer than growth under optimal conditions of bacterial culture.[41,46]

Early Tissue Reaction

During the early phase of infection, before a specific immune response begins, *Listeria*-infected cells, mainly macrophages and epithelial cells, provoke an intense

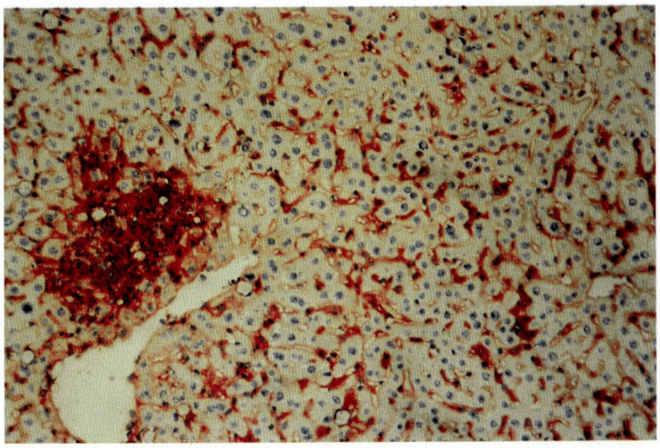

Figure 67–3. Experimental infection of mouse liver. Expression of Ia antigen demonstrated by immunohistochemistry. Ia antigen is concentrated in an abscess beside a sublobular vein and in Kupffer's cells (counterstaining with Meyer's hematoxylin, ×640).

infiltration by neutrophils. The invasion of phagocytes is induced by chemotactic factors [bacterial components and complement, essentially C5a, as well as proinflammatory cytokines such as tumor necrosis factor alpha (TNF-α), interleukin (IL)-1, IL-6, and IL-8] and is mediated by the activation of adhesion molecules like CD18/CD11b.[53] The invading phagocytes are able to selectively lyse infected hepatocytes and can thereby prevent unrestricted growth in permissive cells.[52] If invasion of phagocytes is inhibited, eg, by specific antibodies against CD18/CD11b or against neutrophils, *L monocytogenes* grows unhindered in parenchymal cells and causes acute progression of infection with focal necrosis but without reaction of surrounding tissue.

Even in this early, preimmune phase, interferon gamma (IFN-γ) is usually present. It is produced by natural killer cells stimulated by macrophage-derived TNF-α and IL-12.[54] The cytokine leads to T-cell–independent activation of monocytes and macrophages as well as endothelial cells—evident by an early increase in MHC class II expression (Figure 67–3).

If these early proinflammatory events are blocked as has been done experimentally by gene knockout procedures or by specific antibodies against IL-1, IL-6, TNF-α, IL-12, or IFN-γ or by the application of IL-10, mechanisms of resistance become impaired and susceptibility to infection rises dramatically.[30] This explains why corticosteroid treatment predisposes to listeriosis.

Specific Immunity

Patients with severe or fatal infections may not mount a specific immune response. The histologic picture at necropsy, therefore, is likely to be dominated by microabscesses rather than by granulomas. In patients who survive this critical phase, the ensuing activation of specific T lymphocytes promotes the formation of granulomas that characterize the subsequent stages of disease.[27,55–57] *Listeria*-induced granulomas contain mononuclear phagocytes and lymphocytes but no giant cells.

Listeria monocytogenes activates CD4+, CD8+ and double-negative, γ/δ-receptor-positive T cells. The role of different T-cell subpopulations during infection and their interaction with phagocytes has been investigated immunohistochemically, as well as experimentally by adoptive transfer of T cells, T-cell depletion in vivo, and, most recently, by the use of gene knockout mice.[30,58] The results can be summarized as follows:

1. While the number of CD8+ T cells remains almost constant while granulomas are forming, CD4+ T cells accumulate substantially within 72 hours after their activation. Consequently, they form the main component of mature granulomas besides bloodborne monocytes. Moreover, in contrast to CD8+ lymphocytes, CD4+ T cells are necessary for granuloma formation, delayed type hypersensitivity, and splenomegaly. Their presence is closely associated with the production of IL-2, IL-3, and IL-4, as well as with an increased amount of TNF-α, IFN-γ, and GM-CSF in infected tissues, a finding that suggests a role for these cytokines in *Listeria*-induced antigen-specific inflammatory phenomena. Studies using neutralizing antibodies as well as the effects of administered recombinant cytokines point to a critical role for TNF-α and IFN-γ in granuloma formation as well as in central coagulative necrosis. Although most potent in mediating inflammation, the protective efficacy of CD4+ T cells is minor compared to CD8+ T cells.
2. The activation of *Listeria*-specific CD8+ T cells depends on the presence of viable bacteria. These cells do not cause granulomas but have marked protective potency, which is thought to be caused by the lysis of permissive infected host cells. Bacteria liberated by this mechanism are most probably killed by invading neutrophils.
3. CD4−/CD8− γ/δ and T cells appear before CD8+ and CD4+ T cells but little is known about the mechanisms by which they are induced nor about their function or antigen specificity. Studies using CD4+/CD8+ T-cell–depleted mice or α/β-T-cell receptor gene knockout mice suggest that these cells may regulate the degree of *Listeria*-induced tissue necrosis in granulomas. The different phases of experimental murine listeriosis and their outcomes are summarized in Figure 67–4.

The minor protective role of CD4+ T cells may account for the rarity of listeriosis in patients with

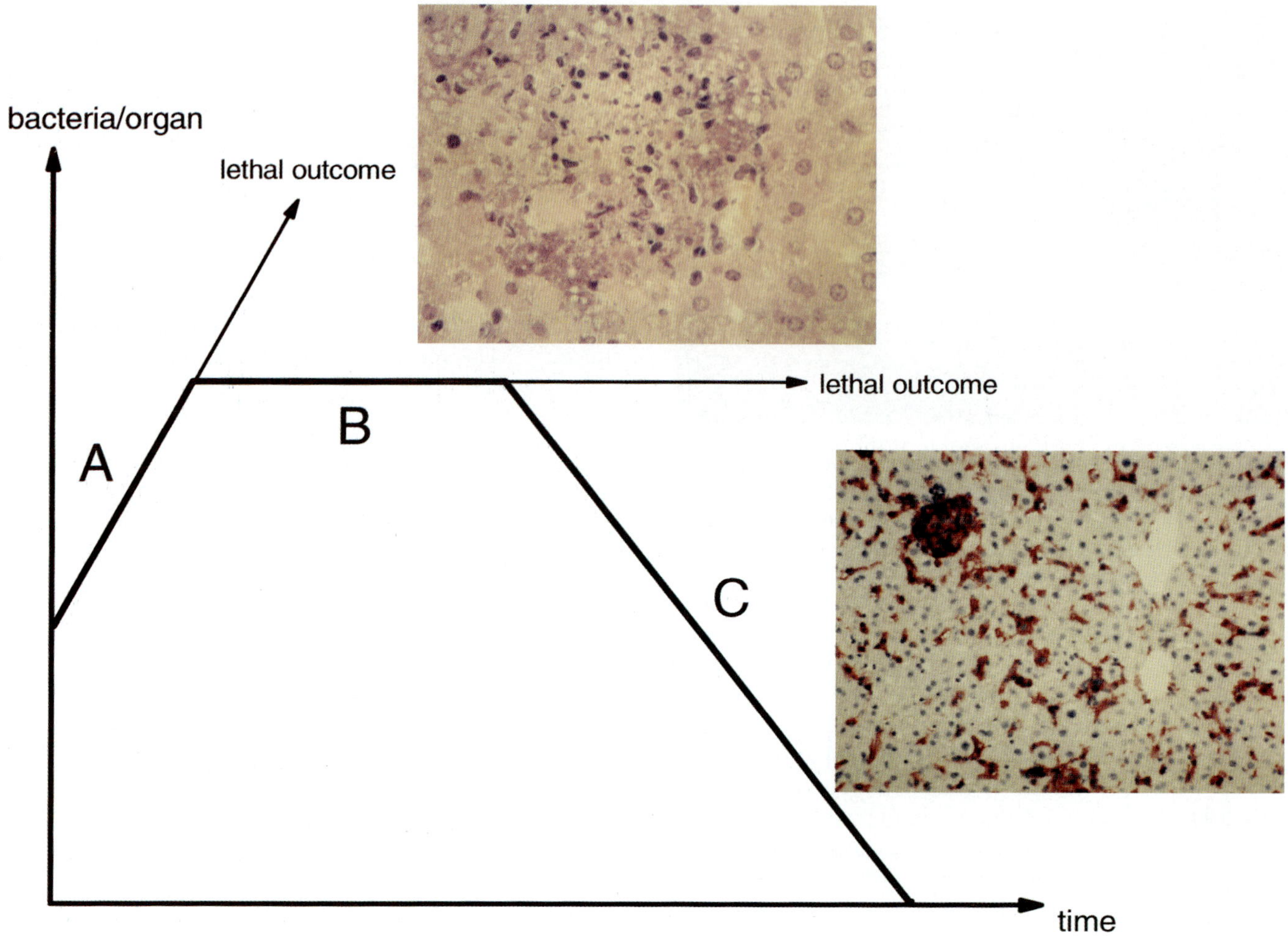

Figure 67–4. Course of experimental murine listeriosis demonstrating the relationship between histopathology and immune response. (**A**) Phase 1: Invasion and unrestrained multiplication of *L monocytogenes* in permissive host cells (eg, hepatocytes). (**B**) Phase 2: Preimmune phase of host response (T-cell–independent resistance). Microabscess in severe infection with parenchymal necrosis (H&E, ×640). (**C**) Phase 3: Immune phase of host response. Granuloma-like focal mononuclear cell aggregates and diffuse infiltrates dominated by CD4+ T cells and bloodborne monocytes with few CD8+ T cells at the periphery (immunohistochemical stain demonstrating CD4+ T cells and counterstained with Meyer's hematoxylin, ×640).

acquired immunodeficiency syndrome.[59,60] Most of these patients had an additional risk factor, such as treatment with corticosteroids. They resemble other patients both clinically and in their response to therapy.[61]

PATHOLOGY

Comprehensive reviews of *Listeria*-induced lesions in humans were published mainly in the 1950s and early 1960s.[9,23,62,63] Findings depend on the patient's age, predisposing conditions, mode and dose of infection, and site of lesions.

Fetal or early onset neonatal listeriosis is caused by transplacental or ascending infection. In some patients, placental abscesses may be seen macroscopically (Figure 67–5). More often, however, there are irregularly distributed small yellow nodules in the placenta (Figure 67–6) or on the surface of the chorionic plate, placental membranes, or umbilical cord.[64,65] With transplacental transmission, typical findings include intervillous and/or intravillous microabscesses (Figure 67–7) as well as villus necrosis and necrotizing villitis. From this location, bacteria seed into the fetus through the umbilical vein. Circulating bacteria infect various organs and may be excreted by the kidneys, thus contaminating the amniotic fluid. Aspiration, in turn, leads to infection of the gastrointestinal and pulmonary tracts of the fetus. In ascending infection, there is acute chorioamnionitis and funiculitis with tiny foci of necrosis or abscesses. The infection may extend to the amnion and the subsequent

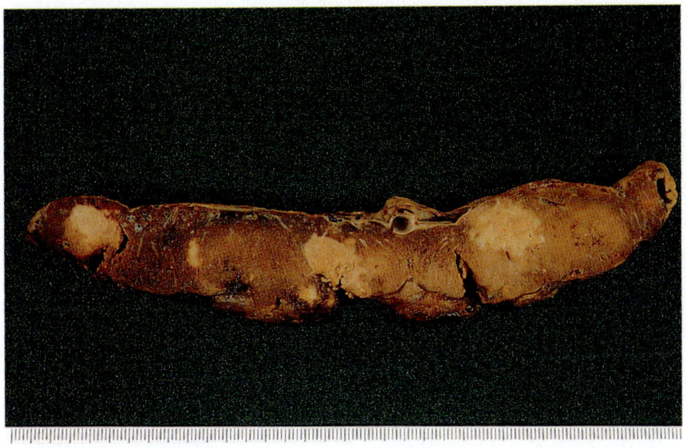

Figure 67–5. Thirty-third week of gestation. Placental macroabscesses with perifocal circulatory disturbances caused by listerial infection.

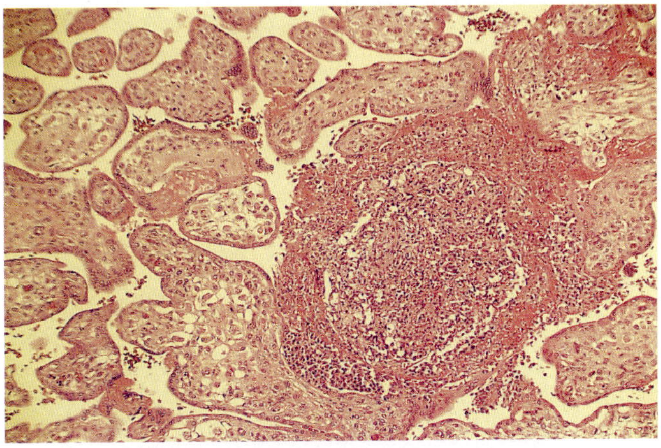

Figure 67–7. Placenta, fetal listeriosis with an intravillous microabscess and intervillous suppuration. The villus is partially destroyed and a coagulum of fibrin and neutrophils surrounds it (hematoxylin-eosin, ×4). *(Contributed by David A. Schwartz, MD.)*

tracheobronchial and bowel infection results in secondary septicemia of the fetus. This may lead to retrograde infection of the placenta, featuring listerial embolism in the villous vessels, acute villitis, and *intra*villous abscesses without alterations of the *inter*villous space. With extended placental infection, however, it may be impossible to distinguish between a primarily infected placenta from maternal bacteremia and a secondarily infected organ from fetal sepsis.

Listerial septicemia causes widespread focal necroses, microabscesses, and granulomas in potentially all organs of the fetus and newborn. Although the extreme form of infection is termed "granulomatosis infantiseptica" many focal lesions are indeed microabscesses. There may be fetal hydrops. In addition, meconium staining of placental membranes and fetal surfaces is common. Characteristic are elevated gray-white papules, surrounded by a red margin on the skin of the back and limbs (Figure 67–2).

Multiple organs and tissues, including liver, spleen, adrenal, lung, pleura, posterior pharyngeal wall, esophagus, stomach, intestine, lymph nodes, and tonsils are studded with grayish white or gray-yellow nodules varying from less than a millimeter to a few millimeters in diameter (Figure 67–8). In the intestine, lymphatic structures of small intestine and appendix are preferentially affected.

Microscopically, most of the lesions are foci of necrosis or microabscesses dominated by neutrophils that often show karyorrhexis. Larger lesions contain amorphous basophilic necrotic debris and have centers of coagulation necrosis and/or a rim of eosinophilic parenchymal cells (Figure 67–9). Tissue Gram stains reveal gram-positive pleomorphic rods, 0.4 to 0.5 μm by 0.5 to 2.0 μm (Figure 67–10). Silver methods such

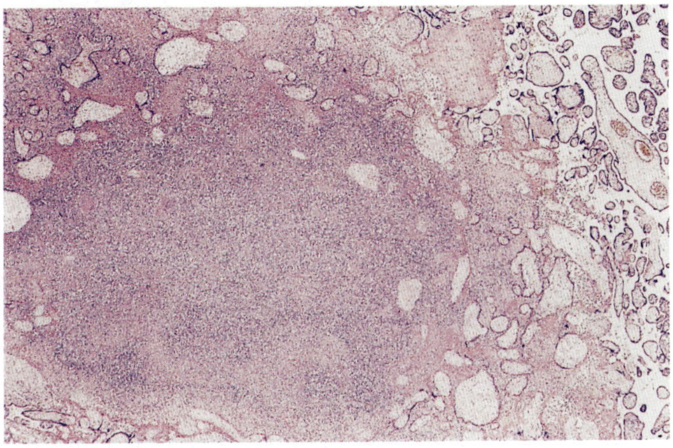

Figure 67–6. Placenta, 22nd week of gestation. Intervillous listerial abscess 4 mm in diameter (hematoxylin-eosin, ×8). *(Contributed by Dr H. Kühn, Fürth, Germany.)*

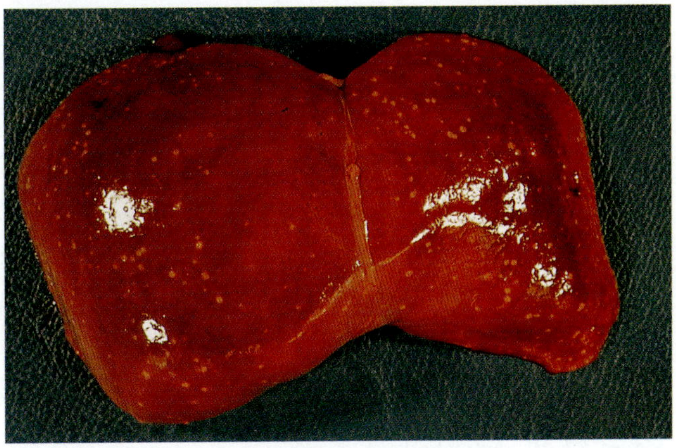

Figure 67–8. Early onset listeriosis in a preterm neonate (31st week of gestation). There are miliary nodules throughout the liver.

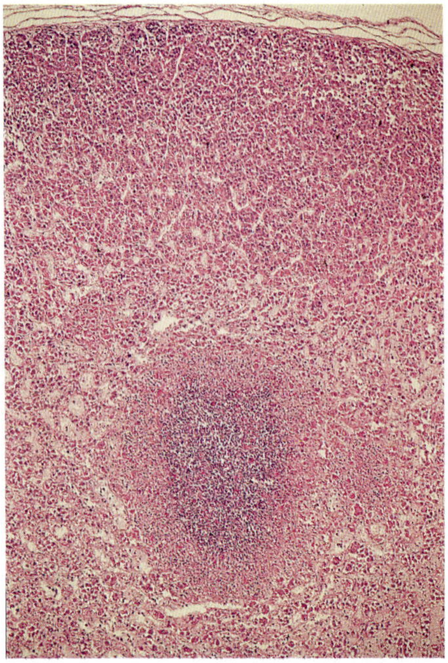

Figure 67–9. Congenital listeriosis. This lesion in adrenal cortex is necrotic, contains neutrophils, and is surrounded by degenerating cortical cells (hematoxylin-eosin, ×20).

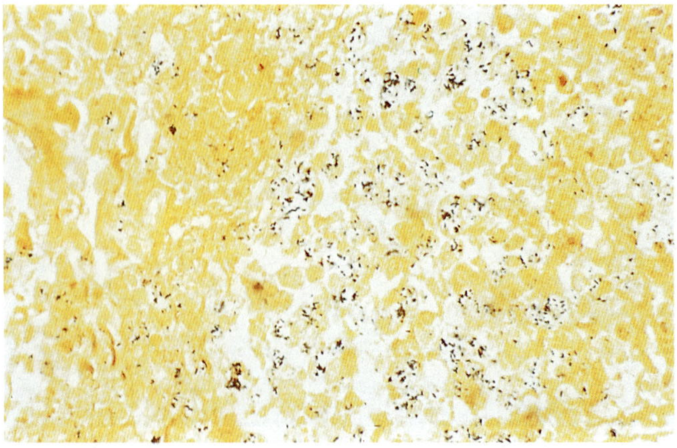

Figure 67–11. Liver, fatal fetal listeriosis. *Listeria monocytogenes* demonstrated by Dieterle stain (×400).

Kidneys often show nephritis at the corticomedullary junction from bloodborne infection and therefore may shed bacteria. Lungs have foci of bronchopneumonia from aspirated amniotic fluid in addition to miliary nodules on pleura and in the lung seeded from the bloodstream. Sometimes the walls of bronchi and/or

as Gomori's methenamine-silver stain, Warthin–Starry, Levaditi, or Dieterle stains (Figure 67–11) also demonstrate *L monocytogenes.*

As described earlier, numerous monocytes/macrophages and T cells may appear at the perimeter of the necroses or microabscesses and migrate inward until the lesion is transformed into a granuloma. Granulomas may contain epithelioid cells but giant cells are not a feature (Figure 67–12). In still older lesions, fibrous tissue may surround the granulomas.

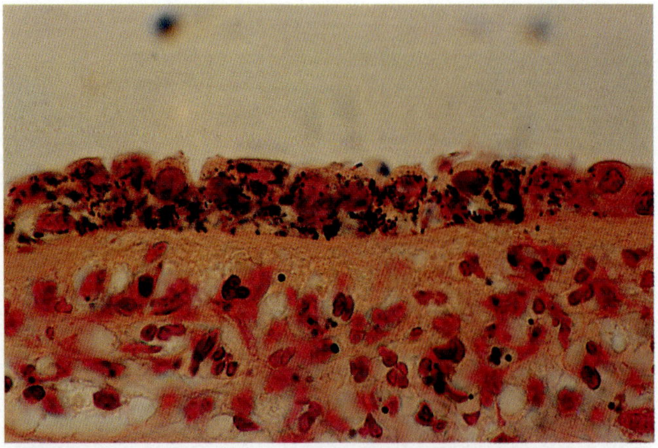

Figure 67–10. Amniotic layer of placenta in a neonate born with disseminated listeriosis. Clusters of gram-positive bacilli are in the cells of the amnion (Brown–Hopps, ×290).

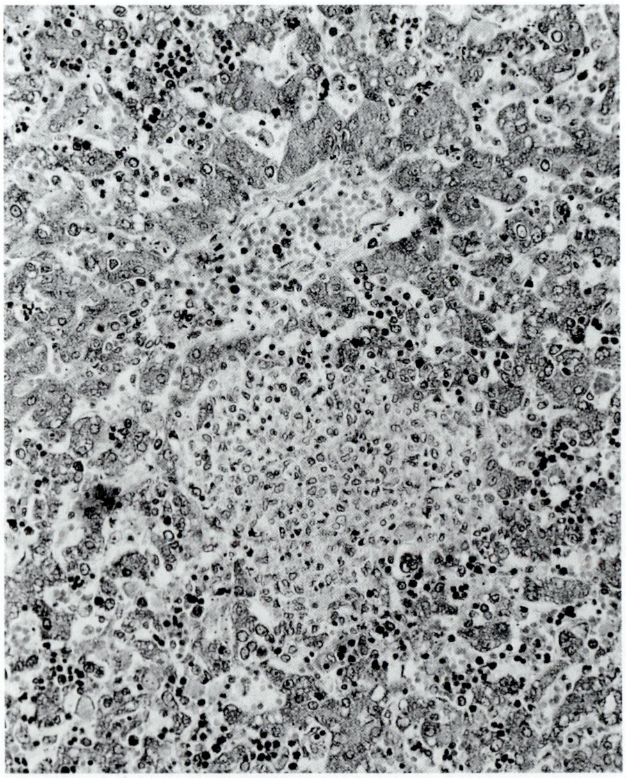

Figure 67–12. Liver, neonatal listeriosis. The parenchymal cells have vanished and are replaced by macrophages, some of which have elongated nuclei that are progressing toward epithelioid cells (AFIP Neg 65-12926; hematoxylin-eosin, ×195).

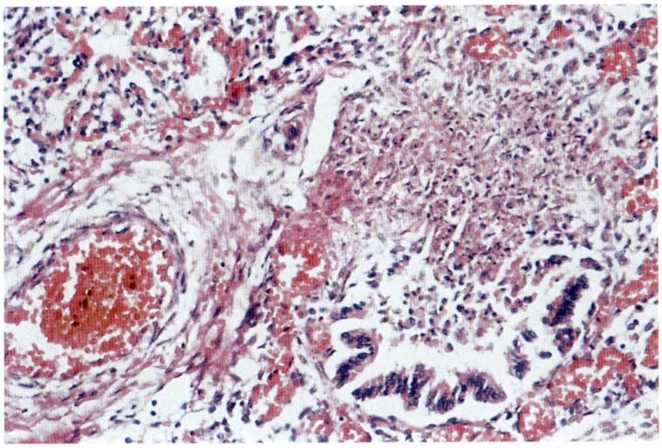

Figure 67–13. Lung, neonatal listeriosis. A purulent exudate has extended into and destroyed the wall of this bronchiole (hematoxylin-eosin, ×30).

bronchioles are necrotic (Figure 67–13). Even the heart may contain scattered foci of necrosis.

Late onset neonatal listeriosis, like listeriosis in adults, is dominated by infection of the CNS, which may present as meningitis, meningoencephalitis, or, on rare occasions, isolated rhombencephalitis. The meninges contain small yellow-gray areas or diffuse suppuration. Histologically, there are miliary foci in leptomeninges or suppuration of the subarachnoid space (Figure 67–14). The underlying glia may react to a minor degree. Sometimes, there are diffusely distributed areas of nonreactive liquefactive necrosis. These are mostly in white matter. Infiltrates of neutrophils are less common in these lesions. The most affected areas in newborn CNS listeriosis are the periventricular region and the ventricular wall, which contain lymphocytic infiltrates in the form of an ependymitis and subependymitis, respectively. Neonatal CNS listeriosis may cause occlusive hydrocephalus. Sinus thrombosis and thrombotic lesions of the internal venous system of the CNS have been reported as well as subependymal hemorrhages. Gram stains may reveal bacilli in the leptomeninges, the choroid plexus, the periventricular space, and cortex. Any necrotic focus may contain free bacilli or bacilli in phagocytes or parenchymal cells. Immunohistochemistry may allow specific identification of *L monocytogenes.*[66,67]

Compared to listeriosis in neonates, infection in adults less frequently involves organs other than CNS. More than 60% of adult patients with listeriosis have infection of the CNS only.[11] The remaining patients have at least lesions in the liver. Sometimes a local infection of nasal cavity, paranasal sinuses, middle ear, pharynx, or conjunctiva precedes infection of the CNS.

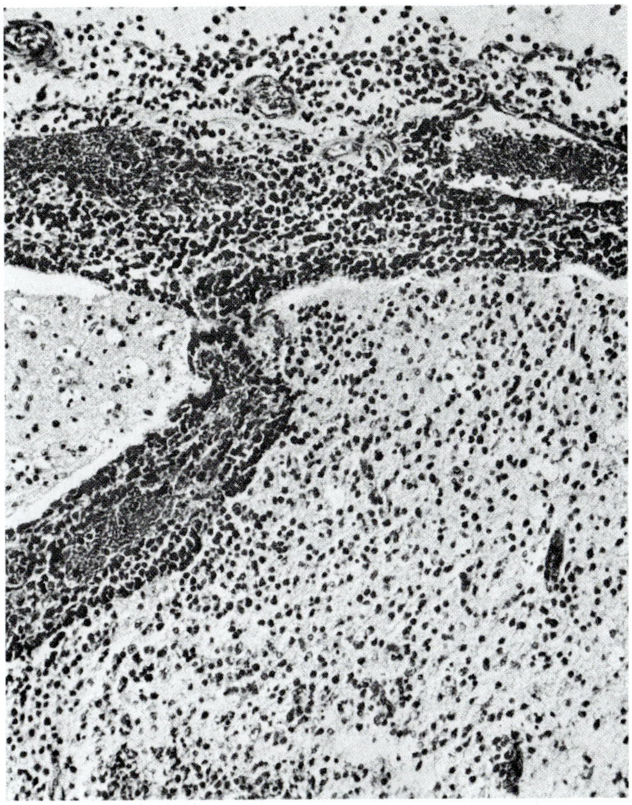

Figure 67–14. Brain, neonatal listeriosis. The inflammatory exudate, mainly neutrophils, has expanded the subarachnoid space and extends into the Virchow–Robin spaces. There are inflammatory cells also in adjacent cortex (AFIP Neg 13263; hematoxylin-eosin, ×130).

This might point to a local transport of the bacilli via axons of cranial nerves, in which the bacteria have been demonstrated.[35]

Macroscopically, listerial meningitis in adults does not differ from other forms of bacterial meningitis. Pus is often at the base of the brain, but may also be above the cerebellum, brainstem, and over the cerebral hemispheres. There may be hemorrhagic lesions throughout the brain. Sometimes, miliary nodules in the leptomeninges appear as small white spots on the surface of the brain. Poorly defined gray-red lesions, occasionally cavitating, may be in pons or medulla oblongata. The brain may be edematous, hyperemic, and contain petechiae.

Histologically, the leptomeninges contain lymphocytes, macrophages, and a variable number of neutrophils. The inflammation extends along the adventitial spaces from the leptomeninges into the brain, with lymphocytic cuffing. The ependymal lining of ventricles and the choroid plexuses may be extensively involved.

Cerebrum or brainstem may contain foci of necrosis or abscesses with central cavitation; these often are surrounded by macrophages containing phagocytosed debris. As a rule, there is some proliferation of capillaries around the abscesses, and adjacent vessels may show fibrinoid necrosis or perivascular lymphocytic and plasmacytic cuffing. Small hemorrhages may be near the abscesses, which contain bacilli demonstrable by special stains (see earlier discussion).

Rhombencephalitis and Brain Abscess

Rhombencephalitis caused by *L monocytogenes*[23,24,68–70] causes edematous swelling of brain or brainstem. Cross-sections reveal disseminated, partly hemorrhagic, necrotic foci in the mesencephalon, pons, medulla oblongata, and upper cervical cord. Sometimes, although not often, those foci are in cerebellum and parathalamic regions. Gross lesions may be absent in listerial encephalitis. The CNS may contain lesions in different phases of infection. In the early phase, there are circumscribed necroses with adjacent edema. Neutrophils, proliferation of microglia, and foamy macrophages follow. Later there are perivascular infiltrates of mononuclear cells and/or collections of mononuclear cells, irregularly distributed. Seldom is there necrosis at the centers of these granulomas. If located in the upper cervical cord, those infiltrates may spread into the anterior and posterior nerve roots and cause a radiculomyelitis. Gram-positive bacilli are in these infiltrates. Another typical feature is fibrinoid necrosis of vessel walls with or without inflammatory cells.

Brain abscesses account for less than 5% of listerial lesions of the CNS.[71–73] They cannot be distinguished from abscesses caused by other bacteria. Usually, they are in the hemispheres, but have been in thalamus, basal ganglia (Figures 67–15 and 67–16), brainstem, and spinal cord.

CLINICAL AND LABORATORY DIAGNOSIS

Signs and symptoms of listeriosis as well as laboratory data and hematologic alterations are nonspecific. Features that suggest infection in pregnant women are fever during pregnancy accompanied by flulike symptoms and followed by abortion or stillbirth; in neonates they are meconium-stained amniotic fluid, asphyxia, suppurating conjunctivitis, and/or miliary changes of skin and mucous membranes, or signs of meningoencephalitis in the first 7 days of life; there may be also neonatal sepsis or meningitis.

Clinical features of immunodeficient or elderly patients pointing to listerial infection include sepsis of unknown origin, fever and headache with or without a stiff neck, changes in behavior or mental status, focal neurologic deficits, hemiplegia or seizures, signs and symptoms of brainstem or cerebellar involvement such as cranial nerve palsies, difficulties in swallowing or speaking, ataxia, nausea, and vomiting.

In all forms of CNS listeriosis, the cerebrospinal fluid (CSF) may be clear or slightly cloudy. Suppuration is rare. Accordingly, in most patients the CSF cell count is modestly elevated, ranging between 8 to 26,500 cells/mm^3.[11] Sometimes, the CSF may be hemorrhagic caused by increased vascular permeability.

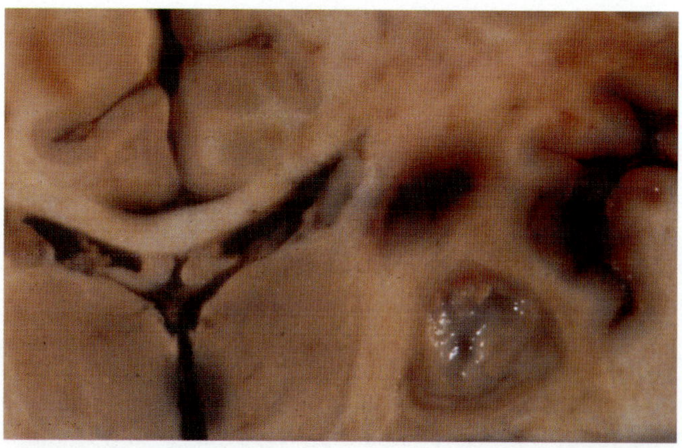

Figure 67–15. This patient had a renal transplant followed by neurologic deterioration. Radiographic studies revealed an abscess in the left putamen. Attempted aspiration missed the lesion and caused hemorrhage in the internal capsule and insula above and to the right of the abscess. The patient died shortly thereafter and autopsy revealed these lesions. Postmortem culture of material from this abscess grew *L monocytogenes. (Contributed by Dr H. J. Manz.)*

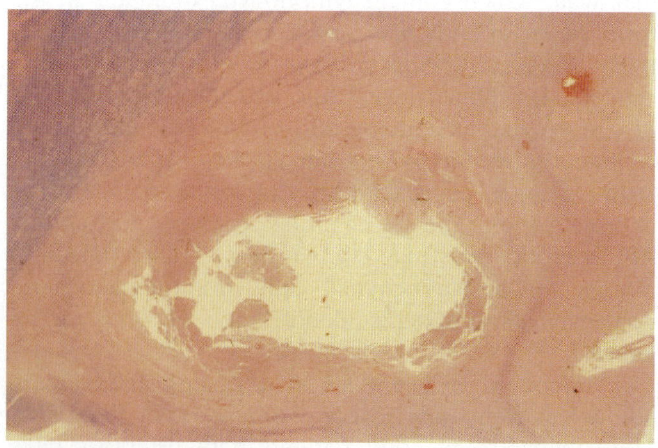

Figure 67–16. Abscess shown in Figure 67–15. It has a purulent liquefied core. The internal capsule (blue) is in the left upper corner. The insular cortex is on the right. (Luxol fast blue–H&E, ×3). *(Contributed by Dr H. J. Manz.)*

TABLE 67–2. SPECIMENS SUITED FOR CULTURE OF *LISTERIA MONOCYTOGENES*

I. General
- Blood
- Cerebrospinal fluid
- Liver biopsy

II. In neonatal listeriosis
- Vaginal secretion of the mother
- Lochial secretion
- Meconium
- Amniotic fluid
- Placental tissue
- Gastric aspirate
- Swabs from ear or conjunctiva
- Skin biopsy

Patients with brainstem encephalitis usually have low cell counts between 10 to 980/mm^3.[74] Indeed, there are reports in which the CSF cell count was normal.[75] CSF protein varies substantially, ranging from 250 to 10,000 mg/L. It tends to be initially high (>30,000 mg/L) in patients with a poor prognosis.[11] Gram stain of CSF sediment almost never reveals bacteria, even when *L monocytogenes* is grown from CSF. Aside from clinical signs, brainstem involvement in most patients can be demonstrated, if at all, only by magnetic resonance imaging.[76]

The definitive diagnosis is made by culturing *L monocytogenes.* The most important specimen for culture in all patients with listeriosis is blood. Blood cultures, for instance, are positive in 75% of patients with listerial meningitis. CSF should, of course, be cultured in all patients having a spinal tap. Other specimens that may yield a positive culture are summarized in Table 67–2. Usually, *L monocytogenes* grows on simple media in 18 to 24 hours, but the microbiologic laboratory should be notified so selective media are used. Reports of isolations of "diphtheroids" or "nonpathogens" must always be challenged. Instead, a statement that *L monocytogenes* has been excluded is required. Other available methods of confirming the diagnosis are DNA hybridization[77] and immunohistochemistry.[49,66] Serologic assays are of no avail.

PROGNOSIS AND TREATMENT

Despite available antibiotic therapy, mortality is estimated at 10% to 60%, depending on age, nature of underlying disease, and delay between clinical onset and initiation of effective therapy.[11,24,78,79] Ampicillin in combination with an aminoglycoside (eg, gentamicin) is the most widely used regimen. An alternative for patients with allergy to beta-lactam antibiotics is trimethoprim–sulfamethoxazole.[80] Controlled studies to establish the best regimen, however, are still lacking. Depending on the clinical syndromes and the response to treatment, duration of therapy varies from 2 to 6 weeks or more in patients with brain abscess.

REFERENCES

1. Murray EGD, Webb RE, Swann MBR. A disease of rabbits characterized by a large mononuclear leucocytosis, caused by a hitherto undescribed bacillus *Bacterium monocytogenes. J Pathol Bacteriol.* 1926;29:407–439.
2. Murray EGD. The story of *Listeria. Trans Roy Soc Can.* 1953;47:15–21.
3. Pirie JHH. A new disease of veld rodents. "Tiger river disease." *South African Inst Med Res.* 1927;3:163–186.
4. Henle A. Pseudotuberkulose bei neugeborenen Zwillingen. *Arb a d Pathol Inst Göttingen.* 1893;143–146.
5. Gill D. A circling disease. A meningoencephalitis of sheep in New Zealand. *Vet J.* 1934;89:258–270.
6. Burn CG. Unidentified gram positive bacillus associated with meningo-encephalitis. *Proc Soc Exp Biol Med.* 1934; 31:1095–1097.
7. Burn CG. Clinical and pathological features of an infection caused by a new pathogen of the genus *Listerella. Am J Pathol.* 1936;12:341.
8. Schlech WF III, Lavigne PM, Bortolussi RA, et al. Epidemic listeriosis—evidence for transmission by food. *N Engl J Med.* 1983;308:203–206.
9. Seeliger HPR. *Listeriosis.* Basel: Karger; 1961.
10. Seeliger HPR. Listeriosis. History and actual developments. *Infection.* 1988;16:80–84.
11. Nieman RE, Lorber B. Listeriosis in adults: a changing pattern. Report of eight cases and review of the literature. *Rev Infect Dis.* 1980;2:207–227.
12. Gray ML. Listeric infection in man in the United States. In: Gray ML, ed. *Second Symposium of Listeric Infection.* Montana: Artcraft Printers; 1963.
13. Bouvet EF, Stuter F, Gibert C, Witchitz C, Bazin C, Vachon F. Severe meningitis due to *Listeria monocytogenes. Scand J Infect Dis.* 1982;14:267–270.
14. Spanjaard L, Bol J, Zanen C. Non-neonatal meningitis due to less common bacterial pathogens. *J Hyg.* 1986;97: 219–228.
15. Windorfer A, Fischer P, Gobel F. Epidemiologie bakterieller Meningitiden bei Kindern und Erwachsenen. *Sozialpädiatrie in Praxis und Klinik.* 1986;8:419–425.
16. Albritton, WL, Cocahi SH, Feeley JC. Overview of neonatal listeriosis. *Clin Invest Med.* 1984;7:311–314.
17. Schlech WF III. New perspectives on the gastrointestinal mode of transmission in invasive *Listeria monocytogenes* infection. *Clin Invest Med.* 1984;7:321–324.
18. Bille J, Doyle MP. Listeria and erysipelothrix. In: Balows A, Hausler W, Herrmann KL, Isenberg HD, Shadony HJ, eds. *Manual of Clinical Microbiology.* 5th ed. Washington, DC: American Society for Microbiology; 1995:287–295.
19. Jones D. The place of Listeria among gram-positive bacteria. *Infection.* 1988;16(suppl 2):S85–S88.

20. Rocourt J. Taxonomy of the genus *Listeria*. *Infection.* 1988;16:89–91.
21. Cossart P, Mengaud J. *Listeria monocytogenes*: a model system for the molecular study of intracellular parasitism. *Mol Biol Med.* 1989;6:463–474.
22. Moulder JW. Comparative biology of intracellular parasitism. *Microbiol Rev.* 1985;49:298–337.
23. Eck H. Encephalomyelitis listeriaca apostematosa. *Schweiz Med Wochenschr.* 1957;9:210–214.
24. Trautmann M, Wagner M. Stoltenburg-Didinger G, Brückner O, Bringmann A. Rhombenzephalitis durch *Listeria monocytogenes:* Klinische und pathologisch-anatomische Befunde bei einer seltenen Enzephalitisform. *Nervenarzt.* 1982;53:705–709.
25. Buchner LH, Schneierson S. Clinical and laboratory aspects of *Listeria monocytogenes* infections. With a report of ten cases. *Am J Med.* 1968;45:904–921.
26. Farber JM, Peterkin PI. *Listeria monocytogenes,* a foodborne pathogen. *Microbiol Rev.* 1991;55:476–511.
27. Mackaness GB. Cellular resistance to infection. *J Exp Med.* 1962;118:381–406.
28. Osebold JW, Inouye T. Pathogenesis of *Listeria monocytogenes* infections on natural hosts. I. Rabbit studies. *J Infect Dis.* 1954;95:52–66.
29. Osebold JW, Inouye T. Pathogenesis of *Listeria monocytogenes.* II. Sheep studies. *J Infect Dis.* 1954;95:67–78.
30. Mielke MEA, Ehlers S, Hahn H. The role of cytokines in experimental listeriosis. *Immunobiol.* 1993;189:285–315.
31. Klatt EC, Pavlova Z, Teberg AJ, Yonekura ML. Epidemic perinatal listeriosis at autopsy. *Hum Pathol.* 1986;17: 1278–1281.
32. North RJ. The action of cortisone acetate on cell-mediated immunity to infection; suppression of host cell proliferation and alteration of cellular composition of infective foci. *J Exp Med.* 1971;134:1485–1500.
33. Schaffner A, Douglas H, Davis CE. Models of T cell deficiency in listeriosis: the effects of cortisone and cyclosporin A on normal and nude BALB/c mice. *J Immunol.* 1983;131:450–453.
34. MacDonald TT, Carter PB. Cell-mediated immunity to intestinal infection. *Infect Immun.* 1980;28:516–523.
35. Asahi O, Hosoda T, Akiyama Y. Studies on the mechanism of infection of the brain with *Listeria monocytogenes*. *Am J Vet Res.* 1957;18:147–157.
36. Racz P, Tenner K, Mero E. Experimental *Listeria* enteritis: I. An electron microscopic study of the epithelial phase in experimental *Listeria* infection. *Lab Invest.* 1972;26: 694–700.
37. Berche P, Gaillard JL, Richard S. Invasiveness and intracellular growth of *Listeria monocytogenes*. *Infection.* 1988;16(suppl 2):S145–S148.
38. Okamota M, Nakane A, Minagawa T. Host resistance to an intragastric infection with *Listeria monocytogenes* in mice depends on cellular immunity and intestinal bacterial flora. *Infect Immun.* 1994;62:3080–3085.
39. Fiedler F. Biochemistry of the cell surface of *Listeria* strains: a locating general view. *Infection.* 1988;16(suppl 2):S92–S97.
40. Cowart RE, Lashmet J, McIntosh ME, Adams TJ. Adherence of a virulent strain of *Listeria monocytogenes* to the surface of a hepatocarcinoma cell line via lectin-substrate interaction. *Arch Microbiol.* 1990;153:282–286.
41. Gaillard JL, Berche P, Mounier J, Richard S, Sansonetti P. In vitro model of penetration and intracellular growth of *Listeria monocytogenes* in the human enterocyte-like cell line Caco-2. *Infect Immun.* 1987;55:2822–2829.
42. Kuhn M. Goebel W. Identification of an extracellular protein of *Listeria monocytogenes* possibly involved in intracellular uptake by mammalian cells. *Infect Immun.* 1989;57:55–61.
43. Gaillard JL, Berche P, Frehel C, Gouin E, Cossart P. Entry of *Listeria monocytogenes* into cells is mediated by internalin, a repeat protein reminiscent of surface antigens from gram-positive cocci. *Cell.* 1991;65:1127–1141.
44. Chakraborty T, Goebel W. Recent developments in the study of virulence of *Listeria monocytogenes*. *Curr Topics Microbiol Immunol.* 1988;138:41–58.
45. Bielecki JP, Youngman P, Connelly P, Portnoy DA. *Bacillus subtilis* expressing a haemolysin gene from *Listeria monocytogenes* can grow in mammalian cells. *Nature.* 1990;345:175–176.
46. Portnoy DA, Jacks PS, Hinrichs DJ. Role of hemolysin on the intracellular growth of *Listeria monocytogenes*. *J Exp Med.* 1988;167:1459–1471.
47. Kuhn M, Prevost M-C, Mounier J, Sansonetti PJ. A nonvirulent mutant of *Listeria monocytogenes* does not move intracellularly but still induces polymerization of actin. *Infect Immun.* 1990;58:3477–3486.
48. Pistor S, Chakraborty T, Walter U, Wehlund J. The bacterial actin nucleator protein ActA of *Listeria monocytogenes* contains multiple binding sites for host microfilament proteins. *Curr Biol.* 1995;5:517–525.
49. Marco AJ, Domingo M, Prab M, Briones V, Pumarola M, Dominguez L. Pathogenesis of lymphoid lesions in murine experimental listeriosis. *J Comp Pathol.* 1991;105: 1–15.
50. Roll JT, Czuprynski CJ. Hemolysin is required for extraintestinal dissemination of *Listeria monocytogenes* in intragastrically inoculated mice. *Infect Immun.* 1990;58: 3147–3150.
51. North RJ. The relative importance of blood monocytes and fixed macrophages to the expression of cell-mediated immunity to infection. *J Exp Med.* 1970;132:521–534.
52. Conlan JW, North RJ. Neutrophil-mediated dissolution of infected host cells as a defense strategy against a facultative intracellular bacterium. *J Exp Med.* 1991;174:741–744.
53. Rosen H, Law SKA. The leukocyte cell surface receptor(s) for the iC3b product of complement. *Curr Topics Microbiol Immunol.* 1990;153:99–122.
54. Bancroft GJ, Schreiber RD, Unanue ER. Natural immunity: a T cell-independent pathway of macrophage activation, defined in SCID mouse. *Immunol Rev.* 1991;124:5–24.
55. Deschryver-Kecskemeti K, Bancroft GJ, Bosma GC, Bosma MJ, Unanue ER. Pathology of *Listeria* infection in murine severe combined immunodeficiency. A study by immunohistochemistry and electron microscopy. *Lab Invest.* 1988;58:698–705.
56. Heyme B, Hof H, Emmerling P, Finger H. Morphology and time course of experimental listeriosis in nude mice. *Infect Immun.* 1976;14:832–835.

57. Mielke MEA. Niedobitek G, Stein H, Hahn H. Acquired resistance to *Listeria monocytogenes* is mediated by Lyt-2+ T cells independently of the influx of monocytes into granulomatous lesions. *J Exp Med.* 1989;170:589–594.
58. Kaufmann SHE. Immunity against intracellular bacteria. Biological effector functions and antigen specificity of T lymphocytes. *Curr Top Microbiol Immunol.* 1988;138: 141–176.
59. Jacobs JL, Murray HW. Why is *Listeria monocytogenes* not a pathogen in the acquired immunodeficiency syndrome? *Arch Intern Med.* 1986;146:1299–1300.
60. Mullin GE, Sheppell AL. *Listeria monocytogenes* and the acquired immunodeficiency syndrome. *Arch Intern Med.* 1987;147:176.
61. Decker CF, Simon GL, DiGioia RA, Tuazon CU. *Listeria monocytogenes* infections in patients with AIDS: report of five cases and review. *Rev Infect Dis.* 1991;13:413–417.
62. Colmant HJ. Neuropathologie der Listeriose. *Dtsch Z Nervenheilkunde.* 1961;182:492–515.
63. Hirasawa H. Morphologischer Beitrag zur Kenntnis der Listeria-Meningoenzephalitis beim Erwachsenen und beim Säugling. *Arch Psych Nervenkrkh.* 1958;197:449–462.
64. Kloos KH, Vogel M. *Pathologie der Perinatalperiode.* Stuttgart: Georg Thieme; 1995:213–214.
65. Benirschke K, Kaufmann P. *Pathology of the Human Placenta.* New York: Springer-Verlag; 1995:560–564.
66. Domingo M, Ramos JA, Dominguez L, Ferrer L, Marco A. Demonstration of *Listeria monocytogenes* with the PAP technique in formalin fixed and paraffin embedded tissues of experimentally infected mice. *Zentralblatt für Veterinarmedizen Reihe B.* 1986;33:537–542.
67. McLauchlin J, Black A, Green HT, Nash JQ, Taylor AG. Monoclonal antibodies show *Listeria monocytogenes* in necropsy tissue samples. *J Clin Pathol.* 1988;41:983–988.
68. Duffy PE, Sassin JF, Summers DS, Lourie H. Rhombencephalitis due to *Listeria monocytogenes. Neurology.* 1964;14:1067–1072.
69. Kennard C, Howard AJ, Scholtz C, Swash M. Infection of the brainstem by *Listeria monocytogenes. J Neurol Neurosurg Psychiatr.* 1979;42:931–933.
70. Weinstein A, Schiavone WA, Furlan AJ. Listeria rhombencephalitis. *Arch Neurol.* 1982;39:514–516.
71. Lechtenberg MD, Sierra MF, Prugle GF, Shucar WA, Butt KMH. *Listeria monocytogenes:* brain abscess or meningoencephalitis? *Neurology.* 1979;29:86–90.
72. Viscoli C, Garaventa A, Ferrea G, Manno G, Taccone A, Terragna A. *Listeria monocytogenes* brain abscess in a girl with acute lymphoblastic leukaemia after late central nervous system relapse. *Eur J Cancer.* 1991;27:435–437.
73. Dee RR, Lorber B: Brain abscess due to *Listeria monocytogenes:* case report and review. *Rev Infect Dis.* 1986;8: 968–977.
74. Kohler J, Winkler T, Wakhloo AK. *Listeria* brainstem encephalitis: two own cases and literature review. *Infection.* 1991;19:36–40.
75. Delacour JL, Floriot C, Ritz A, Wagschal G, Ory JP. Rhombencephalitis listeriennes sans atteinte meningee. *Presse Med.* 1987;16:735.
76. Just M, Kramer G, Higer HP, Thomke F, Pfannenstiel P. MRI of *Listeria* rhombencephalitis. *Neuroradiology.* 1987; 29:401–402.
77. Notermans S, Chakraborty T, Leimeister-Wächter M, et al. A specific gene probe for the detection of bio- and serotyped Listeria strains. *Appl Environ Microbiol.* 1989;55: 902–906.
78. John JF Jr. *Listeria* monocytogenes. In: Vinken PJ, Bruyn GW, Klawans HL, eds. *Handbook of Clinical Neurology.* Vol 8, *Microbial Disease.* New York: Elsevier; 1988: 89–101.
79. Brun-Buisson CJ, de Gialluly E, Gharardi R, Otterbein G, Gray F, Rapin M. Fatal nonmeningitic *Listeria* rhombencephalitis. Report of two cases. *Arch Intern Med.* 1985; 145:1982–1985.
80. Marget W, Seeliger HPR. *Listeria monocytogenes* infections. *Infection.* 1988;16(suppl 2):S175–S177.

CHAPTER 68

Lyme Disease

Paul H. Duray and Francis W. Chandler

Oh give me a home where the buffalo roam,
Where the deer and the antelope play.

American Cowboy Song

DEFINITION

Lyme disease (LD), also called Lyme borreliosis, is infection by *Borrelia burgdorferi,* an elongated spirochete (Figure 68–1) closely related to spirochetes of the relapsing fever group.[1] The natural reservoirs for *B burgdorferi* vary depending on geographic location and environmental conditions (usually mice), and *B burgdorferi* is passed to humans by several species of ticks of the genus *Ixodes.* In recent years LD has become more common because urban areas continue to encroach on the natural habitat of the vector tick that harbors *B burgdorferi.*[2,3] Some of the increase, furthermore, is blamed on the increasing population of deer and rodents in the suburbs[3] and finally, awareness of LD by physicians contributes to the increasing number of patients diagnosed with the disease.[4] LD has protean manifestations and in the past, for instance, has been confused with Guillain–Barré syndrome, presenile dementia, Still's disease, lupus erythematosus, idiopathic myocardiopathy, localized scleroderma, and chronic fatigue (Table 68–1).[4–7]

GEOGRAPHIC DISTRIBUTION AND HISTORICAL PERSPECTIVE

LD was first described in Europe in 1909 when a Swedish dermatologist reported an unusual cutaneous rash on the forehead of a young woman. Her rash followed a tick bite. As more patients were recognized in Europe, a variety of names were used, including erythema migrans,[8–11] Bannwarth's syndrome, and Boujadoux–Garin syndrome.[12–14] Many, however, tended to be associated with an attached and engorged tick complicated by a variety of conditions including cutaneous lymphocytomas,[15,16] encephalomyelitis,[17] meningoradiculitis,[18,19] and chronic infections of the skin.[20–24] These syndromes (each a pattern of chronic involvement) tended to be clustered in selected geographic areas of western Europe. Chronic skin conditions (acrodermatitis chronica atrophicans) were in certain parts of Sweden and Scandinavia,[11,22,25] while meningoradiculitis was clustered in parts of Germany and Austria.[17,18,26]

In the United States, LD was recognized by Steere in 1975 following an epidemic of oligoarthritis in Lyme, Connecticut.[27] The small orange-brown tick of the *Ixodes ricinus* species complex was identified as vector. In 1982, Burgdorfer isolated the causal spirochete, subsequently named *Borrelia burgdorferi,* from *Ixodes* ticks originating in Shelter Island, New York.[28] Thereafter, it was shown that *B burgdorferi* could be cultivated in vitro,[29] but it is, however, difficult to culture from tissues and body fluids.[4,23,30–32]

MOLECULAR PATHOGENESIS

Borrelia burgdorferi invades many tissues and body fluids,[4] and the inflammatory responses are probably caused by the direct presence of spirochetes. Most of the clinical features are a consequence of the interplay among interleukin-1 (IL-1), IL-2, tumor necrosis factor, and other cytokines.[33–35] During chronic large joint disease, collagenase is elaborated by synovial cells in response to IL-1. Collagenase and other proteases produced in a sustained manner erode articular hyaline cartilage. IL-6 also may be involved in the pathogenesis

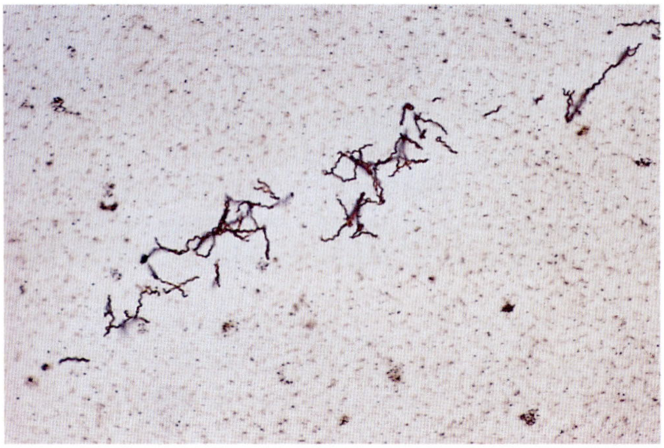

Figure 68–1. *Borrelia burgdorferi* cultivated in vitro and embedded in agar block. Note variable lengths and undulations of the spirochetes (Steiner silver impregnation, ×250).

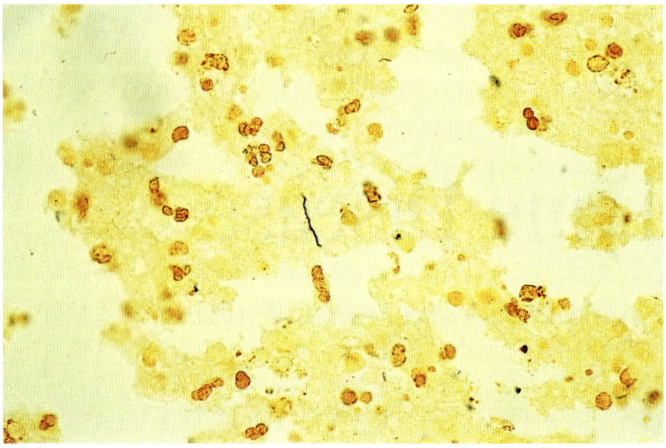

Figure 68–2. Site of tick bite showing single borrelia-like spirochete in the center. Inflammatory cells also are visible (Steiner silver impregnation, ×250).

of Lyme arthritis.[35] Circulating immune complexes have been identified in serum and joint fluid of patients with LD, but it is not known if these are important in pathogenesis.[36,37]

DIAGNOSTIC TESTS

Serologic tests to detect infection are based on immunoglobulin response to the spirochetal membranes.[37–41] Serum IgM peaks about 6 weeks after infection.[37] IgG rises in response to spirochetal protein and persists longer than IgM. Serum immunoglobulin levels do not appear to correlate with clinical severity or tissue damage.

TABLE 68–1. PATHOLOGIC FEATURES OF LYME DISEASE SUMMARIZED BY SYSTEMS AND ORGANS OTHER THAN SKIN

Lymphoreticular system	Follicular hyperplasia, necrotic foci, and atypical immunoblasts in lymph nodes and spleen
Liver	Portal triaditis; sinusoidal mononuclear infiltrates; hepatocellular injury
Heart	Endocarditis; transmyocarditis; fibrinous pericarditis
Central nervous system	Pleocytosis; cortical microgliosis; oligodendrogliosis; perivascular infiltrates; spongiform changes
Peripheral nervous system	Chronic lymphoplasmacytic infiltrates in autonomic ganglia and longitudinal nerves
Musculoskeletal system	Myositis; tendinitis; carpal tunnel syndrome; periosteitis; arthritis and synovitis

B burgdorferi are sparse and difficult to detect in tissue (Figure 68–2) and this is true also for experimentally infected animals[42] (Figure 68–3). This limits the routine silver impregnation and immunohistologic techniques for diagnosis.[5–7,43]

CLINICAL FEATURES

LD has an acute phase and a disseminated phase,[4] but the possibility of persistent infection in humans is controversial and awaits further study.

The acute phase starts with a characteristic rash called erythema migrans (EM), a macular, circular to ovoid area of erythema, that expands centrifugally from

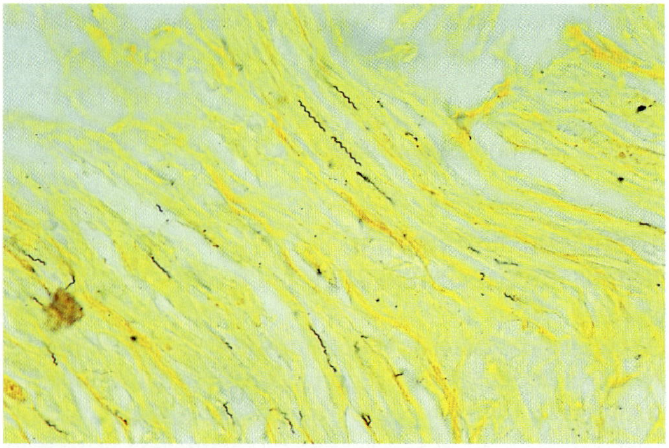

Figure 68–3. Extracellular location of *B burgdorferi* in myocardium of experimentally infected mouse (Steiner silver impregnation, ×250).

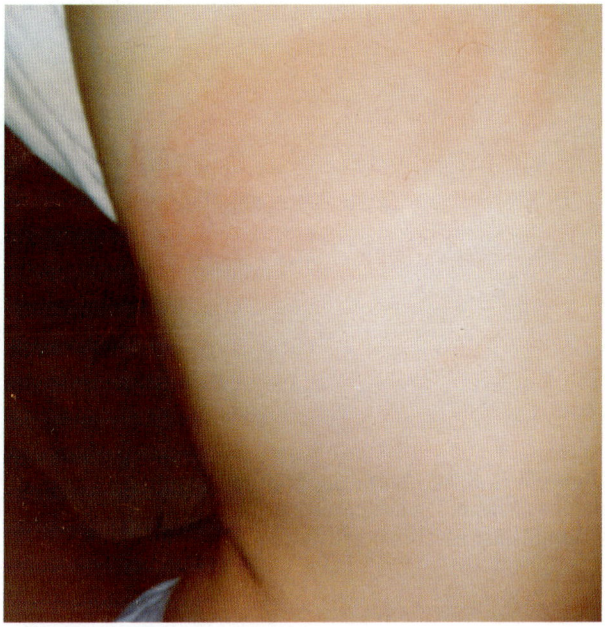

Figure 68–4. Expanding macular rash of erythema migrans, the best clinical marker for early Lyme disease.

the site of the tick bite (Figure 68–4).[44–48] The center often clears rapidly as the red border expands. This pattern is characteristic and is a clinical marker for LD in endemic areas. The rash begins 3 to 30 days after infection and may persist for weeks before resolution. About 60% of patients have erythema migrans. There may be fever, headache, photophobia, nausea, vomiting, myalgia, chills, and generalized lymphadenopathy during the acute phase. Patients are often febrile at the end of the day. Fatigue may be the most incapacitating clinical feature and is described as "dragging." It makes difficult even menial tasks such as driving and bathing. Children may be anorexic, listless, and inactive but have no localizing signs.

Unilateral or bilateral Bell's palsy, cranial nerve radiculopathy, meningoradiculitis, meningitis, and encephalitis are all features of involvement of the central nervous system (CNS). Cardiac involvement may cause first, second, and third degree AV heart block.[49–54] In disseminated LD some patients have myalgia of one or more muscle groups in the limbs. The pain may be incapacitating or mild, and associated with swollen muscles. Meningoradiculitis, encephalitis, and cranial neuropathy, when present, comprise a triad that suggests LD.[50,51] Patients also may complain of pain of the temporomandibular joint while eating and there may be transient pain in other joints without signs of arthritis.

Disseminated LD is best characterized by oligoarthritis of large joints, typically the knee.[27,55–57] There is discomfort while walking and there may be swelling around the joint and effusion. Proteins in the joint fluid are elevated and the third component of complement is usually less than serum levels. The arthritis is remitting with periods of quiescence followed by recurrent bouts, a pattern sometimes persisting for several years, or the arthritis may disappear or become persistent. When persistent, there may be erosive osteoarthritis and loss of cortical bone.

A few patients have peripheral neuropathy, often in western and central Europe.[26,53,54] This is largely a sensorimotor neuropathy that is prone to strike the purely sensory sural nerve. Clinical signs of transverse myelitis have been reported.[58] Some patients with late-phase LD have acrodermatitis chronica atrophicans (ACA), a bilaterally symmetrical purplish-red discoloration of skin of hands, wrists, ankles, and feet and over the proximal tibia.[22] When long standing, there is cutaneous atrophy and yellowish discoloration of venules. Soft tissue swellings may accompany ACA, especially over ulnar regions of the forearms.[11,45] ACA occurs mostly in Europeans. Focal sclerodermoid reactions are rare.[59]

THE ORGANISM

Borrelia burgdorferi varies from 10 μm after division to 42 μm for senescent forms. In tissue it may be elbow shaped, bacillus-like, or more typical with undulations and spirals (Figures 68–1 and 68–2). One or both ends may taper, but this is variable. In tissue sections, *B burgdorferi* can be distinguished from protocollagen, elastin, and other tissue fibers because *B burgdorferi* are never as wide as connective tissue fibers and, as previously mentioned, they are difficult to find because they are so few—in contrast to connective tissue fibers.

PATHOLOGY

Erythema Migrans (EM)

The initial skin lesion is the site of tick attachment and is a papule containing a mixed inflammatory cell infiltrate and rare spirochetes. We have encountered a characteristic focal hemorrhage in these tick-associated papules.[6] Microscopically, in EM, there are lymphocytes, plasma cells, histiocytes, and occasional mast cells around small blood vessels in the papillary and reticular dermis (Figure 68–5).[60] In the papule where the tick was attached, there is a dense inflammatory cell infiltrate around a focus of hemorrhage.[47] This is often the best site to demonstrate *B burgdorferi* (Figure 68–2). *Borrelia burgdorferi* can be demonstrated in selected

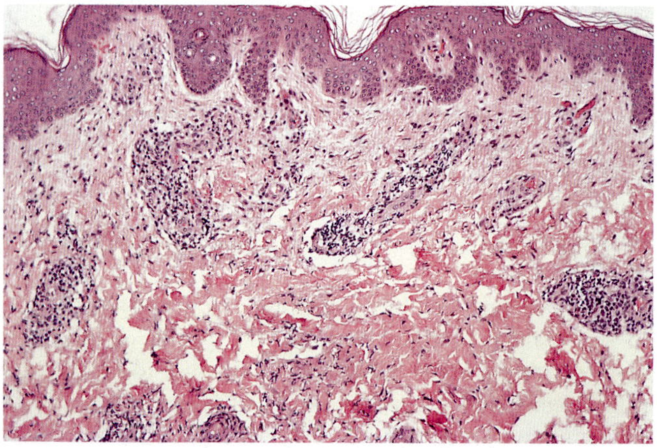

Figure 68–5. Histopathologic features of erythema migrans. Plasma cells, lymphocytes and histiocytes are clustered around dermal blood vessels. H&E, ×50.

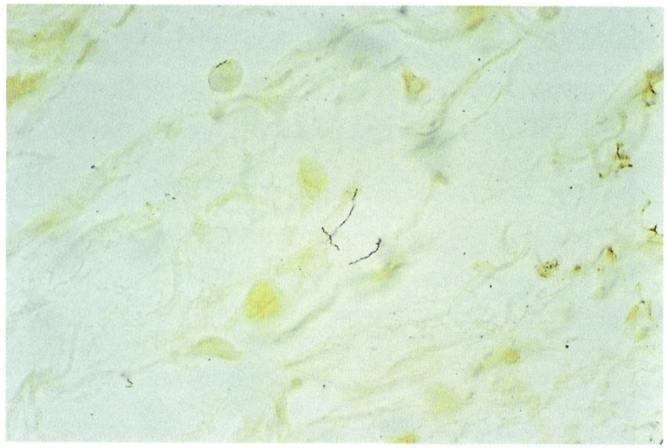

Figure 68–7. Biopsy specimen from an erythema migrans lesion. Note the shape of the slender, relatively straight spirochetes in this patient (Steiner silver impregnation, ×250).

biopsy specimens by any of the silver impregnation stains (Dieterle, Steiner, Warthin–Starry). Of these, we prefer the modified Dieterle or the Steiner methods.[61,62] In EM, spirochetes are haphazardly distributed in the dermis and mostly extracellular (Figures 68–6 and 68–7). They are often around dermal blood vessels but are not confined to these areas. Hemorrhagic nodules at the site of the tick bite may contain more borreliae than surrounding collagen. The mild to moderately severe lymphohistiocytic perivascular infiltrate of EM can be distinguished from other lymphoid perivascular disorders of the skin by the presence of plasma cells. Plasma cells in the perivascular areas should always alert pathologists to the possibility of EM. The vasculitis of secondary syphilis characterized by lymphoplasmacellular infiltrates in and around small vessels is not a feature of LD.

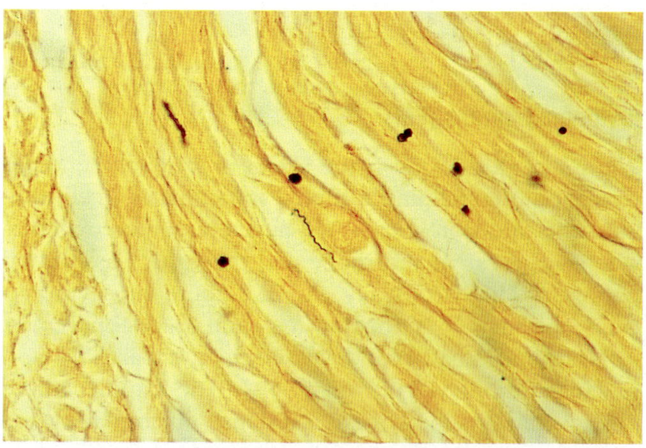

Figure 68–6. *Borrelia burgdorferi* in the dermis of a patient with erythema migrans (Steiner silver impregnation, ×250).

Urticaria, Angioedema

Urticarial lesions in the acute stage of LD have been on the face and upper trunk.[48] The lesions are plaquelike with erythema. Histologically, there is dermal and perivascular edema associated with lymphocytes and plasma cells. Red cell extravasation is usually absent.

Borrelia Lymphocytoma (Cutaneous Lymphoid Hyperplasia, Lymphadenosis Benigna Cutis)

Most patients with borrelial lymphocytoma have been Europeans. Typically, borrelial lymphocytoma involves the inferior earlobes, nipples and areolae, and axillary folds.[47,63,64] Clinically the lesions are bulbous, erythematous swellings. Histologically, the epidermis may be attenuated but otherwise intact, and there is a clear zone (a "grenz") between the base of the epidermis and the upper borders of the lymphoid hyperplasia in the dermis.[7,47] The lymphoid hyperplasia ranges from dense, highly cellular, nodular and follicular infiltrates that fill the dermis and suggest cutaneous lymphoma, to asymmetric, irregular lymphoid follicles with a mild, intervening dermal infiltrate. The lymphoid infiltrate consists of sheets of polymorphic lymphocytes and well-delineated lymphoid follicles with germinal centers. Germinal centers resemble those of normal tonsil and of reactive lymph nodes. The number of lymphoid follicles varies, but cutaneous lesions of borrelial lymphoid hyperplasia have at least a few follicles. The follicular hyperplasia in Europeans mimics follicular lymphoma at low magnification. *Borrelia burgdorferi* can be cultured from these lesions and demonstrated with relative ease by silver impregnation stains. Borreliae are more numerous in these lesions than in other cutaneous forms of LD.

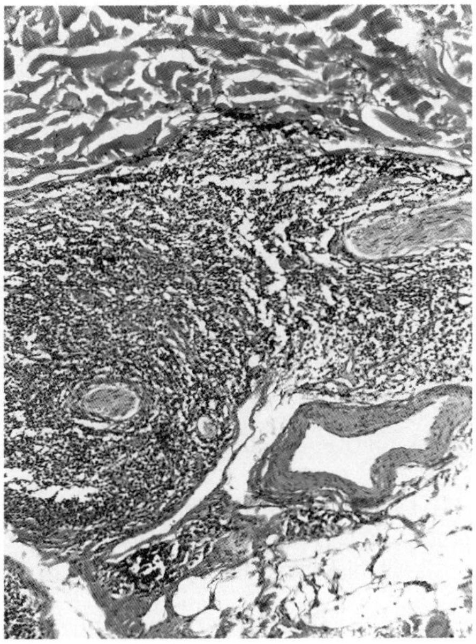

Figure 68–8. Deep, subcutaneous lymphocytic panniculitis in a patient with a plaquelike induration caused by cutaneous borreliosis following acute erythema migrans. The differential diagnosis included lupus profundus as well as other causes of nodular panniculitis [hematoxylin-eosin (H&E), ×150].

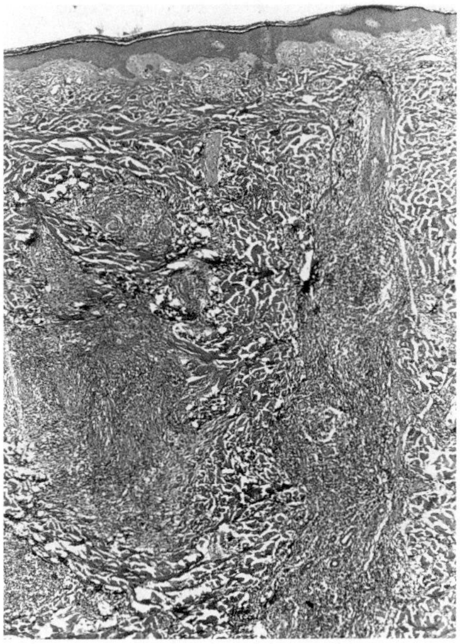

Figure 68–9. Acrodermatitis chronica atrophicans. This is not the long-standing lesion where atrophy and effacement of rete ridges are hallmarks; illustrated is the rarely seen early hypertrophic phase (H&E, ×50).

Borrelial Plaque (Lupus Profundus–Like)

This rare lesion is a raised purplish plaque on the limbs and commonly the shoulders. Microscopically there are dense infiltrates of lymphocytes and plasma cells around dermal vessels. Lumens of some vessels are obliterated by the inflammatory cells. Infiltrates are in the deeper vessels, including those in the subcutaneous fat (Figure 68–8). This pattern resembles lupus erythematosus profundus, from which it must be distinguished. Immunofluorescence may be required to adequately exclude lupus profundus. *Borrelia burgdorferi* can be demonstrated in borrelial plaque, especially between collagen fibers in areas near dermal blood vessels.

Acrodermatitis Chronica Atrophicans (ACA)

This is the classic lesion of chronic cutaneous involvement in LD, and is more prevalent in Europe than in the United States.[21–23] ACA takes several clinical forms but typically is a bilaterally symmetrical, variably erythematous (may have variegated discoloration) area of the acral skin of hands, wrists, elbows, feet, ankles, and lower tibia. It also can involve other sites. Clinically, ACA does not resemble the scaling papulosquamous disorders of psoriasis, parapsoriasis enplaque, seborrheic dermatitis, and pityriasis rosea. ACA is caused by *B burgdorferi* or possibly other *Borrelia* sp, and the spirochetes can be cultured from the lesion and demonstrated by silver impregnation stains in histologic sections. If untreated, ACA can persist for many years and cause cutaneous atrophy.

Long-standing ACA of feet and ankles also can be associated with periosteal involvement and underlying joint disease with subluxation. Microscopically, ACA of recent onset causes dermal thickening and elongation of rete ridges with hyperkeratosis (Figure 68–9), in addition to a severe transdermal polymorphic inflammatory cell infiltrate. Unlike psoriasis, there is little evidence of subcorneal neutrophilic microabscesses.

In early lesions of ACA, there are plasma cells, histiocytes, mast cells, lymphocytes, and a few neutrophils in the dermis. The infiltrate is angiocentric at first, and then spreads to contiguous dermal zones. The initial inflammatory response is hypertrophic. In time, this progresses to hyperkeratosis and thinning of the epidermis with loss of rete ridges. The dermal changes of chronic, well-developed ACA are nonspecific: dermal blood vessels are dilated and have attenuated endothelium, and there is diffuse infiltration of lymphocytes, plasma cells, and histiocytes (Figure 68–10). Eventually, the dermis is thinned and the microvasculature may become occluded.

Lichen Sclerosis et Atrophicans

It is unclear if lichen sclerosis et atrophicans (LSEA) is caused by cutaneous spirochetosis, is an immunologic

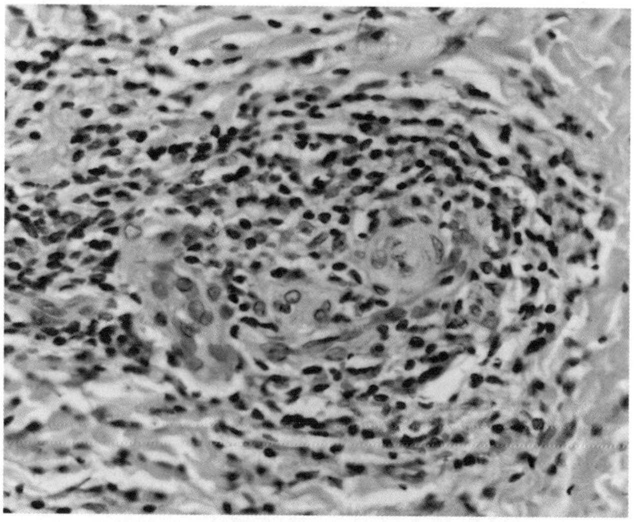

Figure 68–10. Later stage of acrodermatitis chronica atrophicans showing dermal plasmacytic and lymphohistiocytic perivascular infiltration (H&E, ×500).

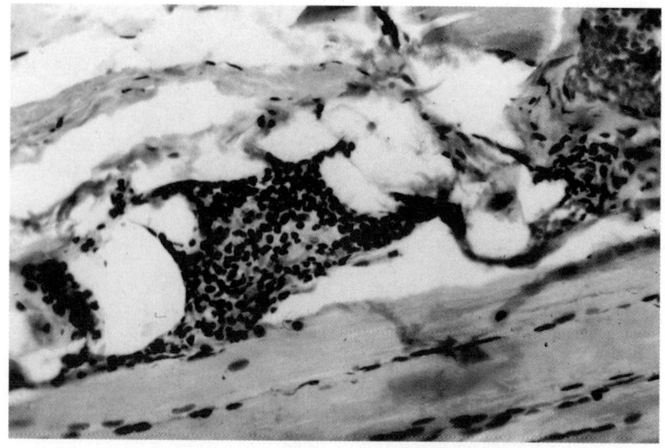

Figure 68–11. Lyme-associated diffuse fasciitis. Although infrequent, the process is characterized by lymphoid aggregates in the deep dermis, fascial thickening, edema, and myositis (H&E, ×450).

complication, or is simply coincidental. LSEA, however, has developed close to lesions of ACA so is probably spirochete associated in some patients. Microscopically it is typical LSEA, with orthohyperkeratosis, thinning of the epidermis, basal epidermal vacuolar degeneration, edematous and amorphic papillary dermal collagen, and a deeper zone of mononuclear inflammatory cells in the subjacent reticular dermis.

Morphea (Localized Scleroderma)

This cutaneous lesion has been proven to be spirochete associated by culture and by silver stains. Morphea is synonymous with localized scleroderma, neither of which should be confused with the scleroderma of progressive systemic sclerosis of lungs, gastrointestinal tract, myocardium, and skin. Inflammatory infiltrates in morphea vary from relatively few lymphoid cells to moderately heavy perivascular infiltrates. In *B burgdorferi*–induced morphea, collagen expands into subcuticular adipose tissue, as it does in typical scleroderma.

Diffuse Fasciitis with Eosinophilia

Diffuse fasciitis is rare.[65] It is a subcutaneous induration, follows EM by 1 to 2 months, and is usually at the same site. There are plasma cells and lymphocytes around dermal vessels, more than in EM, and there is a patchy plasmacytic panniculitis with edema, lymphoid cells, histiocytes, mast cells, plasma cells, and scattered eosinophils (Figure 68–11). This resembles the sclerodermoid-diffuse fasciitis with eosinophilia of Shulman's syndrome. There are sparse spirochetes between collagen fibers in the lower reticular dermis. The lesion is rare but has been seen in Americans and Europeans.[65] Peripheral eosinophilia as seen in classic Shulman's syndrome may be present in Lyme fasciitis.

Myositis

The painful swelling of muscles 6 to 8 weeks after infection is characterized histologically by aggregates of plasma cells, lymphocytes, histiocytes, and mast cells around intramuscular blood vessels.[66,67] Even the extraocular muscles have been involved.[68–70] Individual muscle fibers may be swollen, but striations are usually preserved. Inflammation is confined to intramuscular vessels. Rare extracellular spirochetes are in the interstitium.

Lymph Nodes

Generalized or regional lymphadenopathy can develop with EM, but is more common after the rash resolves. Lymphadenopathy is most common within the first 6 weeks of infection and subsides in one to several weeks. Cervical lymphadenopathy of LD may resemble lymphadenopathy of infectious mononucleosis in some patients. The histologic pattern ranges from follicular hyperplasia to interfollicular expansion without prominent germinal centers. The paracortical T-cell zones are expanded and contain plasma cells and sometimes large transformed B immunoblasts (Figure 68–12). These blastlike lymphocytes sometimes can be labeled with anti-IgM. Lymphoplasmacytic vasculitis, characteristic of syphilitic lymphadenitis, is not a feature of LD lymphadenitis. Spirochetes usually can be demonstrated after a careful search in Lyme lymphadenitis.

Tonsillitis and hyperplastic adenoidal tissue develop in young patients with LD. This may be from

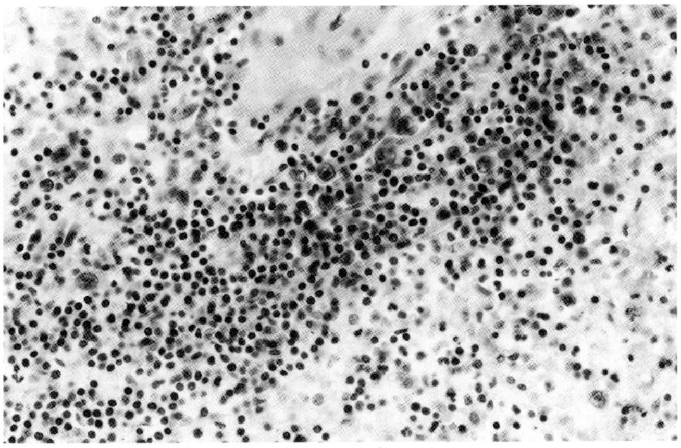

Figure 68–12. Immunoblasts in a lymph node from the groin of a patient with clinical lymphadenitis and recent-onset Lyme disease. The lymph node was enlarged and removed because lymphoma was suspected. Similar atypical immunoblasts may appear in the cerebrospinal fluid in meningoencephalitis. These cells should not be considered malignant until Lyme disease is excluded (H&E, ×450).

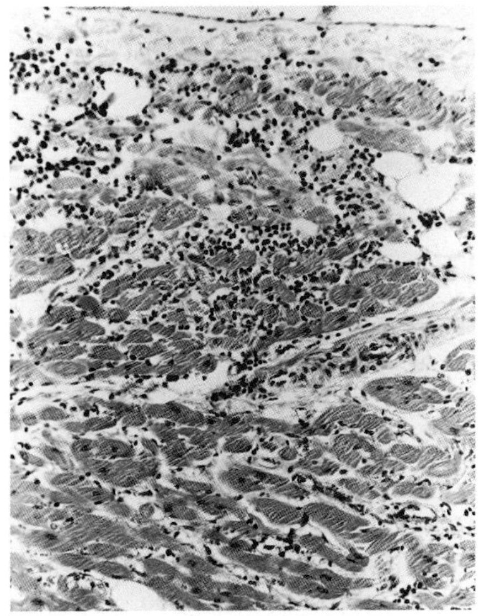

Figure 68–13. Lyme-associated myocarditis. The interstitial lymphocytes and plasma cells resemble viral myocarditis (H&E, ×200).

direct spirochetal invasion or an immune response to infection in other sites, or possibly from a coincidental viral infection.

Spleen

The spleen may be tender and enlarged, resembling the spleen of infectious mononucleosis. There are two histologic patterns. The first is follicular hyperplasia, with congested red pulp. Large, atypical B immunoblasts may be in the white pulp. These have atypical, hyperchromatic nuclei with mitotic figures and increased nuclear:cytoplasmic ratios. The second is in patients who present with acute abdominal pain. This pattern is typified by scattered necrotic foci in the spleen. A few neutrophils and macrophages surround discrete areas of necrosis, and numerous plasma cells are between necrotic foci. *Borrelia burgdorferi* were numerous in one spleen.[71]

Liver

The extent of hepatic involvement in LD is unknown. There is the suspicion that other tick-borne pathogens cause mild elevations in hepatic enzymes. Intrahepatic jaundice is not a feature. Hepatocytes may be swollen and vacuolated[72] and there are hepatocellular mitoses—more numerous than in other inflammatory conditions of the liver. The sinusoids and portal tracts contain mononuclear inflammatory cells, and Kupffer's cells are prominent.

Cardiovascular System

Fifteen percent of patients have carditis during the first 2 to 3 months of infection.[4,73] Lymphocytes, plasma cells, and macrophages are in the myocardial interstitium[74] (Figure 68–13). All layers of the myocardium are usually involved, but especially endocardium in which there is a bandlike collection of lymphoid cells. This band is characteristic of Lyme myocarditis, and its presence (in the right ventricle in specimens taken by transvenous catheter) should alert pathologists to LD.[43] Transvenous biopsies usually do not include intramyocardial vessels, but they may show adventitial and periadventitial inflammatory cells. In one patient who died of Lyme carditis, there was a myocardial vessel with sloughed endothelial cells and thrombosis.[74] Focal lymphoplasmacytic infiltrates often extend into the visceral pericardium and into the pericardial fat. Rarely, there may be fibrinous pericarditis, in which the pericardium is thickened by fibrin and leukocytes. *Borrelia burgdorferi* often can be demonstrated in the myocardium in Lyme carditis. The organism has been isolated from the heart,[75] and *B burgdorferi* may persist despite antibiotic therapy.[76,77] In histologic sections, spirochetes are extracellular in the interstitium or over individual muscle fibers (Figure 68–14).

Cerebrospinal Fluid

Several weeks after infection, 25% of patients develop clinical meningism with or without cranial nerve palsies, and these patients have mononuclear cells in the cerebrospinal fluid (CSF) (pleocytosis).[14,78,79] The pleocytosis can resemble lymphoid neoplasia because of the increased numbers of lymphocytes and because some of the precursor lymphocytes are atypical. Binucleate plasmacytoid blasts and precursor T cells are in the centrifuged and stained preparations of the CSF.

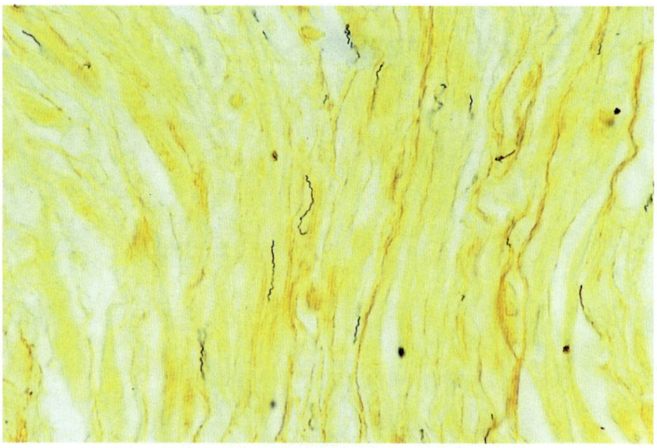

Figure 68–14. *Borrelia burgdorferi* in myocardium. Spirochetes are extracellular and in the interstitium or superimposed over individual muscle fibers (Steiner silver impregnation, ×250).

Brain

Pathologic changes in the cerebral cortex were first identified in autopsies done on rare fatal infections in Europe, but recently, biopsy specimens have been studied from patients with serious CNS deterioration. In these patients, herpes encephalitis had to be excluded by biopsy and these are the basis of our current knowledge. Magnetic resonance imaging (MRI) scans have suggested a cerebrocortical pseudotumor, and a diffuse pattern of small and scattered lucent areas has suggested capillaritis. The range of histologic patterns and clinical correlations is still evolving. To date, the few cortical biopsy specimens have revealed:

1. Minimal or no change[80,81]
2. Mild to moderate perivascular collections of lymphoid cells[7]
3. Edema; perivascular edema[5]
4. Moderate spongiform encephalopathy without inflammation
5. Microfoci or aggregated microglial cells, with or without spongiform changes[82]
6. Increase in oligodendrocytes.

We have demonstrated spirochetes in the CNS of five patients, using silver impregnation techniques, but spirochetes have been difficult to identify.[81] Experience is required to distinguish candidate spirochetes from neuronal dendritic processes, but it can be done with proper staining, patience, and experience. Immunohistochemical methods are recommended on fresh tissue imprints. These methods are more efficient and specific for detecting *B burgdorferi* than is prolonged searching of silver-stained tissue sections.

To our knowledge, stereotactically directed biopsy specimens have not been obtained from the multiple, lucent areas in the white matter by MRI. We postulate that either capillaritis or microglial foci are present; however, this must await further study.

Eye

One patient had necrotizing retinitis after parenteral penicillin culminating in what may have been a Jarisch–Herxheimer reaction; spirochetes were in the vitreous contents.[83] Uveitis and keratitis are being increasingly recognized in ocular LD,[84,85] but conjunctivitis is more common.

Autonomic Ganglia

The dorsal roots, autonomic ganglia, and cranial nerves are intermittently and unpredictably involved in intermediate-phase LD. Microscopically there are lymphocytes and fewer plasma cells in tight clusters around autonomic ganglion cells, and also in the ganglion capsules where they are perivascular. It is not known whether *B burgdorferi* is in these tissues, or whether the inflammation is caused by another mechanism such as autoimmunity based on molecular mimicry.

Peripheral Nerves

Biopsies of peripheral nerves in LD patients with peripheral neuropathy have two major patterns of inflammation.[5,7,18,54] One is an infiltrate of lymphocytes and plasma cells in the perivascular spaces of the perineurium, while the other is of lymphocytes and plasma cells in the axon cylinders. Even in the latter, inflammatory cells involve the microvasculature in most patients.[12] There is often axonal degeneration and mild to moderate demyelination. Sections 1 μm thick reveal that vascular endothelial cells are targeted by inflammatory cells and that these endothelial cells have proliferative features sometimes referred to as histiocytoid or epithelioid. Spirochetes have not been identified in longitudinal sections of nerve.

Periarticular Soft Tissues

Intramuscular lesions have been described in the section on skin involvement. Similarly involved are the periarticular tendons, periosteum, perichondrium, and bursae of involved joints, where swelling of soft tissues is probably caused by lymphocytes and plasma cells in the vicinity of tendon sheaths. Periarticular swelling can mask Lyme disease.

Joints and Synovia

Lyme arthritis (synovitis) is clinically expressed as either 1) intermittent recurring oligoarthritis or, less commonly, 2) persistent arthritis without intervening resolution. Each recurrence is heralded by an effusion of synovial fluid that contains neutrophils and increased proteins. The synovial membrane becomes hyperplastic, and the villi have accentuated folds and proliferations that may resemble the macroscopic appearance of small intestine. This villous change is accompanied by hyperplasia of synovial cells on the surface in multilayers and in subjacent stroma. In chronic arthritis, synovial cells are often more numerous than macrophages. In about 50% of patients, fibrin on synovial surfaces is mixed with fragments of synovial villi.[86] Fibrin in the villous stroma is more characteristic of Lyme synovitis than of Reiter's disease or rheumatoid arthritis where fibrin, characteristically, is on the villous surfaces. Fibrin and fibrinogen can be confirmed histochemically. Thus, abundant fibrin in the villous stroma suggests Lyme arthritis–synovitis.

Another pattern in Lyme synovitis is lymphoid hyperplasia in which there are collections of lymphocytes and histiocytes resembling those in small lymph nodes. The inflammatory cells form multiple nodules that often display a "starry sky" pattern. This pattern may be associated with more spirochetes rather than other types of Lyme synovitis.

In the usual Lyme synovitis, there are focal microscopic aggregates of lymphoid cells that usually do not form well-delineated germinal centers. The aggregates contain T cells, B cells, IgD-bearing cells, and follicular dendritic cells.[87] T cells are usually clustered around vessels of the synovium, while plasma cells are dispersed within patchy areas of the synovial stroma and within some of the lymphoid aggregates.[88] Plasma cells also cluster near the base of synovial cells. Mast cells are abundant and may form isolated infiltrates, especially where plasma cells are sparse.

In a subset of Lyme synovitis patients, the synovium has obliterative vascular changes (Figure 68–15). These changes are caused by proliferating endothelial cells and hyperplastic adventitia mixed with lymphocytes and other mononuclear inflammatory cells. Lumens of blood vessels become obliterated, and these changes probably are a form of vasculopathy seen in about 25% of patients with Lyme synovitis. Obliterative vascular changes are more closely associated with those with fibrin in the synovial stroma. This change may be in patients with recurring attacks of Lyme synovitis. The combination of prominent stromal fibrin and hypercellular vascular obliteration suggests Lyme synovitis. With the trichrome stain, fibrin–fibrinogen deposits stain deep red from reaction with basic fuchsin. Stains for amyloid are nonreactive. Two patients with Lyme arthritis had non-necrotic, epithelioid cell granulomas—one an 8-year-old and the other a 35-year-old man. Both had positive serologic titers.

Lyme arthritis usually presents in one of three clinical forms. The first is a clear-cut attack on one of the

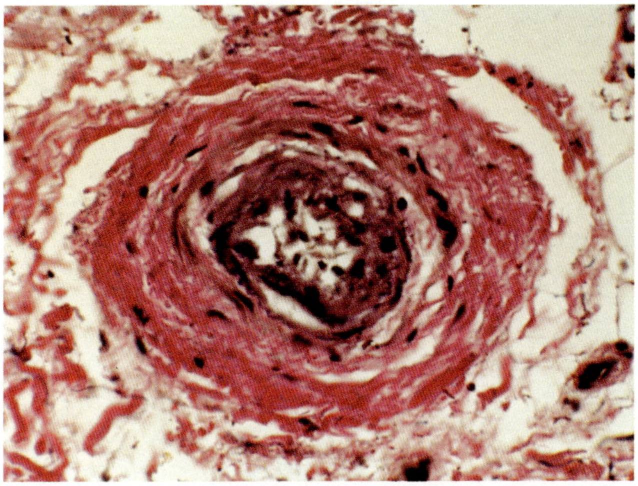

Figure 68–15. Vascular obliteration in chronic Lyme synovitis (arthritis) (VVG elastic stain, ×750).

larger joints such as the knee. There is spontaneous resolution without sequelae, with or without antibiotic therapy. The second is characterized by recurring attacks of arthritis in one or more joints over several years. The attacks last for a few weeks to several months. The third form is a chronic persistent arthritis that can lead to erosion of cortical bone around the joints. Because these clinical forms of Lyme arthritis are time dependent, histologic changes vary. Spirochetes have been repeatedly demonstrated in the synovial membranes,[86,89] but they are sparse and difficult to detect. Spirochetes can be found near the synovial membrane, near vessels, or deep in the collagenous stroma (Figure 68–16). We have found them in areas of edema as well, but searching for spirochetes is laborious and often fruitless. There is evidence that some borreliae colonize specific sites. Molecular differences in the 16S ribosomal RNA and other genes may contribute to this and to the differences in clinical presentations between U.S. and European patients.[90] Localized autoimmunity also may prove to be a major contributing factor in persistent tissue damage.[91]

Transplacental Infections

Neonatal death caused by maternal infection with *B burgdorferi* is very rare. Spirochetes have been identified in brain, spleen, myocardium, and bone marrow of neonatal and fetal tissues, but inflammatory changes are much less than in adult patients and sometimes absent. There are no histopathologic clues in these tissues to suggest the diagnosis of LD.

Because inflammation is minimal or absent, however, spirochetes may be more numerous than in adult tissues.[92,93] Neonates infected during pregnancy have

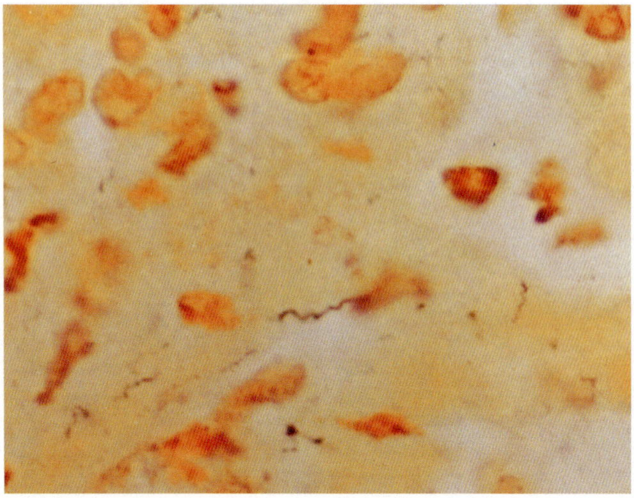

Figure 68–16. Synovium from a patient with Lyme arthritis. The sparse spirochetes resemble those in erythema migrans (modified Dieterle silver impregnation, ×750).

had atrial or ventricular septal defects and anomalous pulmonary venous drainage, but these are rare. Placental changes have ranged from unremarkable to chorionic villitis with increased Hofbauer cells, plasma cells, and macrophages. Spirochetes are in the intervillous areas and in villi and chorionic membranes. They can be demonstrated by immunofluorescence using polyclonal and monoclonal antibodies on fixed, paraffin-embedded, or frozen tissue sections.

TREATMENT

The best antimicrobial therapy remains controversial. All agree, however, that the sooner antibiotics are given, the better the chance for eradication of the organism. Delay increases the risk for prolonged infection. Most clinicians agree that the tetracyclines, particularly doxycycline (100 mg BID for 3 weeks), are the best choices in early infection; amoxicillin (1 g TID, with 500 mg Benemid TID, for 3 weeks) is recommended for pregnant patients and children (dosage is varied for body weight). For early disseminated infection or multiple EM, the same therapy is extended to 30 days.[94] Potentially life-threatening myocarditis with third-degree heart block, and symptomatic meningoencephalitis are managed by either aqueous penicillin G (10 to 20 million units IV for 14 days) or ceftriaxone (2 g IV for 14 days). Advanced, longer term infections such as chronic arthritis and symptomatic encephalopathy also are treated with ceftriaxone or penicillin in the same dosages.[95]

REFERENCES

1. Barbour AG. Antigenic variation of surface proteins of *Borrelia* species. *Rev Infect Dis.* 1988;10(suppl 2): S399–S402.
2. Anderson JF, Magnarelli LA, McAninch JB. New *Borrelia burgdorferi* antigenic variant isolated from *Ixodes dammini* from upstate New York. *J Clin Microbiol.* 1988; 26:2209–2212.
3. Anderson JF, Magnarelli LA, Stafford KC. Bird-feeding ticks transtadially transmit *Borrelia burgdorferi* that infect Syrian hamsters. *J Wildl Dis.* 1990;26:1–10.
4. Steere AC. Lyme disease (review). *N Engl J Med.* 1989; 321:586–596.
5. Duray PH, Steere AC. Clinical pathologic correlations of Lyme disease by stage. *Ann NY Acad Sci.* 1988;539:65–79.
6. Duray PH, Steere AC. The spectrum of organ and systems pathology in human Lyme disease. *Zbl Bakt Hyg A.* 1986;263:169–178.
7. Duray PH. The surgical pathology of human Lyme disease. An enlarging picture. *Am J Surg Pathol.* 1987; 11(suppl 1):47–60.
8. Weber K, Puznik A, Becker T. Erythema-migrans-Krankheit. Beitrag zur Klinik und Beziehung zur Lyme-Krankheit. *Dtsch Med Wochenschr.* 1983;108:1182–1190.
9. Weber K, Neubert U. Clinical features of early erythema migrans disease and related disorders. *Zbl Bakt Hyg A.* 1986;263:209–228.
10. Asbrink E, Olsson I. Clinical manifestations of erythema chronicum migrans Afzelius in 161 patients; a comparison with Lyme disease. *Acta Derm Venereol.* 1985;65:43–52.
11. Asbrink E. Erythema chronicum migrans Afzelius and acrodermatitis chronica atrophicans. Early and late manifestations of *Ixodes ricinus*-borne borrelia spirochetes. *Acta Derm Venereol (Stockh).* 1985;(suppl 118):1–63.
12. Camponovo F, Meier C. Neuropathy of vasculitic origin in a case of Garin–Boujadoux–Bannwarth syndrome with positive borrelia antibody response. *J Neurol.* 1986; 233:69–72.
13. Pfister HW, Einhaupl KM, Preac-Mursic V, Wilske B. The spirochetal etiology of lymphocytic meningoradiculitis of Bannwarth (Bannwarth's syndrome). *J Neurol.* 1984;231: 141–144.
14. Preac-Mursic V, Wilske B, Schierz G, Pfister HW, Einhaupl KM. Repeated isolation of spirochetes from the cerebrospinal fluid of patients with meningoradiculitis Bannwarth. *Eur J Clin Microbiol.* 1984;3:564–565.
15. Paschoud JM. Lymphocytom nach Zeckenbiss. *Dermatologica.* 1954;108:434–437.
16. Paschoud JM. Die Lymphadenosis benigna cutis als übertragbare Infektionskrankheit. *Hautarzt.* 1957;8:197–211.
17. Ackermann R, Rehse-Kupper B, Gollmer E. Progressive borrelia encephalomyelitis. *Zbl Bakt Hyg A.* 1986;263: 201–205.
18. Kristoferitsch W, Sluga E, Graf M. et al. Neuropathy associated with acrodermatitis chronica atrophicans. *Ann NY Acad Sci.* 1988;539:35–45.
19. Vallet JM, Hugon J, Lubeau M, Leboutet MJ, Dumas M,

Desproges-Gutteron R. Tick-bite meningoradiculoneuritis: clinical, electrophysiologic, and histologic findings in 10 cases. *Neurology.* 1987;37:749–753.
20. Ehrmann S, Falkenstein S. Uber Dermatitis atrophicans und ihre Pseudo-sklero-dermatischen Formen. *Arch Dermtol Syph (Berl).* 1925;149:142–175.
21. Hauser W. Zur Kenntenis der Acrodermatitis chronica atrophicans. *Arch Dermatol Syph.* 1955;199:350–393.
22. Buechner SA, Rufli T, Erb P. Acrodermatititis chronica atrophicans. A chronic T cell–mediated immune reaction against *Borrelia bergdorferi. J Am Acad Dermatol.* 1993; 28:399–405.
23. Asbrink E, Brehmer-Andersson E, Hovmark A. Acrodermatitis chronica atrophicans—a spirochetosis: clinical and histopathological picture based on 32 patients; course and relationship to erythema migrans Afzelius. *Am J Dermatopathol.* 1986;8:209–219.
24. Bafverstedt B. Uber Lymphadenosis benigna cutis. *Acta Derm Venereol (Stockh).* 1943;11(suppl):1–202.
25. Asbrink E, Hovmark A. Cuteneous manifestations in Ixodes-borne borrelia spirochetosis. *Int J Dermatol.* 1987;26:215–223.
26. Ackerman R, Rehse-Kupper B, Gollmer E, Schmidt R. Chronic neurologic manifestations of erythema migrans borreliosis. *Ann NY Acad Sci.* 1988;539:16–23.
27. Steere AC, Malawista SE, Snydman DR, et al. Lyme arthritis: an epidemic of oligoarticular arthritis in children and adults in three Connecticut communities. *Arthr Rheum.* 1977;20:7–17.
28. Burgdorfer W, Barbour AG, Hayes SF, Benach JL, Grunwaldt E, Davis JP. Lyme disease—a tick-borne spirochetosis? *Science.* 1982;216:1317–1319.
29. Barbour AG. Cultivation of borrelia: a historical overview. *Zbl Bakt Hyg A.* 1986;263:11–14.
30. Karlsson M, Hovindho K, Svenungs, Stiernst G. Cultivation and characterization of spirochetes from cerebrospinal fluid of patients with Lyme borreliosis. *J Clin Microbiol.* 1990;28:473–479.
31. Nadelman RB, Pavia CS, Magnarelli LA, Wormser GP. Isolation of *Borrelia burgdorferi* from the blood of 7 patients with Lyme disease. *Am J Med.* 1990;88:21–26.
32. Wilske B, Preac-Murisc V, Schierz G. Antigenic heterogeneity of European *Borrelia burgdorferi* strains isolated from patients and ticks. *Lancet.* 1985;1:1099.
33. Beck G, Habicht GS, Benach JL, Coleman JL, Lysik RM, O'Brien RF. A role for interleukin-1 in the pathogenesis of Lyme disease. *Zbl Bakt Hyg A.* 1986;263:133–136.
34. Habicht GS, Beck G, Benach JL. The role of interleukin-1 in the pathogenesis of Lyme disease. *Ann NY Acad Sci.* 1988;539:80–86.
35. Garciamo JC, Benach JL. The pathogenesis of Lyme disease. *Rheum Dis.* 1989;15:711–726.
36. Hardin JA, Steere AC, Malawista SE. Immune complexes and the evolution of Lyme arthritis. Dissemination and localization of abnormal C1q binding activity. *N Engl J Med.* 1979;301:1358–1363.
37. Craft JE, Fischer DK, Shimamoto GT, Steere AC. Antigens of *Borrelia burgdorferi* recognized during Lyme disease—appearance of a new immunoglobulin M response and expansion of the immunoglobulin G response late in the illness. *J Clin Invest.* 1986;78:934–939.
38. Benach JL, Gruber BL, Coleman JL, Habicht GS, Golightly MG. An IgE response to spirochete antigen in patients with Lyme disease. *Zbl Bakt Hyg A.* 1986;263:127–132.
39. Coleman JL, Benach JL. Isolation of antigenic components from the Lyme disease spirochete: the role in early diagnosis. *J Infect Dis.* 1987;155:756–765.
40. Benach JL, Coleman JL, Carcia-Monco JC, Deponte PC. Biological activity of *Borrelia burgdorferi* antigens. *Ann NY Acad Sci.* 1988;539:115–125.
41. Dattwyler RJ, Luft BJ. Immunodiagnosis of Lyme borreliosis. *Rheum Dis C.* 1989;15:727–734.
42. Duray PH, Johnson RC. The histopathology of experimentally infected hamsters with the Lyme disease spirochete, *Borrelia burgdorferi* (42251). *Proc Soc Exp Biol Med.* 1986;181:263–269.
43. Duray PH. Histopathology of clinical phases of human Lyme disease. *Rheum Dis C.* 1989;15:691–710.
44. Steere AC, Bartenhagen NH, Craft JE, et al. The early clinical manifestations of Lyme disease. *Ann Intern Med.* 1983;99:76–82.
45. Weber K, Schierz G, Wilske B, Preac-Mursic V. European erythema migrans disease and related disorders. In: Steere AC, Malawista SE, Craft JE, Fischer DK, Garcia-Blanco M, eds. *Lyme Disease: First International Symposium. Yale J Biol Med.* 1984;57:463–471.
46. Weber K, Schierz G, Wilske B, et al. Reinfection in erythema migrans disease. *Infection.* 1986;19:32–35.
47. Duray PH, Asbrink E, Weber K. The cutaneous manifestations of human Lyme disease: a widening spectrum. *Adv Dermatol.* 1989;4:255–276.
48. Berger BW. Cutaneous manifestations of Lyme borreliosis. *Rheum Dis C.* 1989;15:627–634.
49. Pachner AR, Steere AC. Neurologic findings of Lyme disease. In: Steere AC, Malawista SE, Craft JE, Fischer DK, Garcia-Blanco M, eds. *Lyme Disease: First International Symposium. Yale J Biol Med.* 1984;57:313–314.
50. Pachner AR. *Borrelia burgdorferi* in the nervous system: the new "great imitator." *Ann NY Acad Sci.* 1988; 539:56–64.
51. Reik L, Steere AC, Bartenhagen NH, Shope RE, Malawista SE. Neurologic abnormalities of Lyme disease. Medicine. 1979;58:281–294.
52. Baumwackl U, Kristoferitsch W, Sluga E, Stanek G. Neurological manifestations of *Borrelia burgdorferi* infections: the enlarging clinical spectrum. *Zbl Bakt Hyg A.* 1986;263:334–336.
53. Halperin JJ. Nervous system manifestations of Lyme disease. *Rheum Dis C.* 1989;15:635–645.
54. Kristoferitsch W. Lyme borreliosis in Europe—neurologic disorders (review). *Rheum Dis C.* 1989;15:767–774.
55. Steere AC, Malawista SE, Hardin JA, Ruddy S, Askenase PW, Andiman WA. Erythema chronicum migrans and Lyme arthritis: the enlarging clinical spectrum. *Ann Intern Med.* 1977;86:685–698.
56. Herzer P, Wilske B. Lyme arthritis in Germany. *Zbl Bakt Hyg A.* 1986;263:268–274.
57. Steere AC, Gibofsky A, Patarroyo ME, Winchester RJ,

Hardin JA, Malawista SE. Chronic Lyme arthritis: clinical and immunogenetic differentiation from rheumatoid arthritis. *Ann Intern Med.* 1979;90:286–291.
58. Kohler J. Lyme borreliosis—a case of transverse myelitis with syrinx cavity. *Neurology.* 1989;39:1553–1554. Technical note.
59. Aberer E, Stanek G. Histological evidence for spirochetal origin of morphea and lichen sclerosus et atrophicans. *Am J Dermatopathol.* 1987;9:374–379.
60. Berger B. Erythema chronicum migrans of Lyme disease. *Arch Dermatol.* 1984;120;1017–1021.
61. Duray PH, Kusnitz A, Ryan J. Demonstration of the Lyme disease spirochete *Borrelia burgdorferi* by a modification of the Dieterle stain. *Lab Med.* 1985;16:685–687.
62. de Koning J, Hoogkamp-Korstanje JAA. Demonstration of spirochetes in biopsies. *Zbl Bact Hyg A.* 1986;263:179–188.
63. Hovmark A, Asbrink E, Olsson I. The spirochetal etiology of lymphadenosis benigna cutis. *Acta Derm Venereol (Stockh).* 1986;66:479–484.
64. Weber K, Schierz G, Wilske B, Preac-Mursic V. Das lymphozytom—eine Borreliose? *Z Hautkr.* 1985;60: 1585–1598.
65. Granter SR, Barnhill RL, Hewins ME, Duray PH. Identification of *Borrelia burgdorferi* in diffuse fasciitis with peripheral eosinophilia: borrelial fasciitis. *JAMA.* 1994; 272:1283–1285.
66. Reimers CD, Pongratz DE, Neubert U, et al. Myositis caused by *Borrelia burgdorferi:* report of four cases. *J Neurol Sci.* 1989;91:215–226.
67. Atlas E, Novack SN, Steere AC, Duray PH. Lyme myositis. *Ann Intern Med.* 1988;109:245–246.
68. Seidernberg KB, Leib ML. Orbital myositis with Lyme disease. *Am J Ophthalmol* 1990;109:13–16.
69. Reimers CD, deKoning J, Neubert A, Preac-Mursic W, et al. *Borrelia burgdorferi* myositis: report of eight patients. *J Neurol.* 1993;240:278–283.
70. Horowitz HW, Sanghera K, Goldberg N, Pechmon D, et al. Dermatomyositis associated with Lyme disease: case report and review of Lyme myositis. *Clin Infect Dis.* 1994;18:166–171.
71. Rank EL, Dias S, Hasson J, Duray PH, et al. Human necrotizing splenitis caused by *Borrelia burgdorferi*. *Am J Clin Pathol.* 1989;91:493–498.
72. Goellner M, Agger WA, Duray PH. Hepatitis due to recurrent Lyme disease. *Ann Intern Med.* 1988;108:707–708.
73. Steere AC, Batsford WP, Weinberg M, et al. Lyme carditis: cardiac abnormalities of Lyme disease. *Ann Intern Med.* 1980;93:8–16.
74. Marcus LC, Steere AC, Duray PH, Anderson AE, Mahoney EB. Fatal pancarditis in a patient with coexisting Lyme disease and babesiosis. *Ann Intern Med.* 1985;103:374–376.
75. Stanek G, Klein J, Bittner R, Glogar D. Isolation of *Borrelia burgdorferi* from the myocardium of a patient with longstanding cardiomyopathy. *N Engl J Med.* 1990; 322:249–252.
76. Preacmur V, Weber K, Pfister HW, Wilske G, Gross B, Baumann A, Prokop J. Survival of *Borrelia burgdorferi* in antibiotically treated patients with Lyme borreliosis. *Infection.* 1989;17:355–359.
77. Cary NRB, Fox B, Wright DJM, Cutler SJ, Shapiro LM, Grace AA. Fatal Lyme carditis and endodermal heterotopia of the atrioventricular node. *Postg Med J.* 1990; 66:134–136.
78. Pfister HW, Preac-Mursic V, Wilske B, Einhaupl KM, Weinberger K. Latent Lyme neuroborreliosis: presence of *Borrelia burgdorferi* in the cerebrospinal fluid without concurrent inflammatory signs. *Neurology.* 1989;39:1118–1120.
79. Kruger H, Reuss K, Pulz M, et al. Meningoradiculitis and encephalomyelitis due to *Borrelia burgdorferi*—a follow-up study of 72 patients over 27 years. *J Neurol.* 1989; 236:322–328.
80. Weber K, Bratzke HJ, Neubert U, Wilske B, Duray PH. *Borrelia burgdorferi* in a newborn despite oral penicillin for Lyme borreliosis during pregnancy. *Pediatr Infect Dis J.* 1988;7:286–289.
81. Shadick NA, Phillips CB, Logigian EL, et al. The long-term clinical outcomes of Lyme disease. A population-based retrospective cohort study. *Ann Intern Med.* 1994; 121:560–567.
82. Pachner AR, Duray PH, Steere AC. Central nervous system manifestations of Lyme disease. *Arch Neurol.* 1989;46: 790–795.
83. Steere AC, Duray PH, Kaufmann DJH, Wormser GP. Unilateral blindness caused by infection with the Lyme disease spirochete, *Borrelia burgdorferi*. *Ann Intern Med* 1985;103:382–384.
84. Winward KE, Smith JL, Culberts WW, Parisham A. Ocular Lyme borreliosis. *Am J Ophthalmol.* 1989;108:651–657.
85. Smith JL. Lyme disease appears to have many ocular manifestations. *Arch Ophthalmol.* 1990;108:337. Letter.
86. Johnston YE, Duray PH, Steere AC, et al. Lyme arthritis: spirochetes found in synovial microangiopathic lesions. *Am J Pathol.* 1985;118:26–34.
87. Steere AC, Duray PH, Butcher EC. Spirochetal antigens in lymphoid cell surface markers in Lyme synovitis: comparison with rheumatoid synovium and tonsillar lymphoid tissue. *Arth Rheum.* 1988;31:487–495.
88. Neumann A, Schlesie M, Schneide H, Vogt A, Peter HH. Frequencies of *Borrelia burgdorferi* reactive lymphocytes-T in Lyme arthritis. *Rheum Int.* 1989;9:237–241.
89. Valesova M, Trnavsky K, Hulinska D, Alusik S, Janousek J, Jirous J. Detection of borrelia in the synovial tissue from a patient with Lyme borreliosis by electron microscopy. *J Rheumatol.* 1989;16:1502–1505.
90. Duray PH, Zhang L. Current concepts in the biology of Lyme disease: pathologic effects from molecular strains of spirochetes. *Adv Pathol Lab Med.* 1994;7:161–178.
91. Aberer E, Brunner C, Suchanek G, et al. Molecular mimicry and Lyme borreliosis—a shared antigenic determinant between *Borrelia burgdorferi* and human tissue. *Ann Neurol.* 1989;26:732–737.
92. MacDonald AB. Gestational Lyme borreliosis—implications for the fetus. *Rheum Dis C.* 1989;15:657–677.
93. Schlesinger PA, Duray PH, Burke BA, Steere AC, Stillman MT. Maternal–fetal transmission of the Lyme disease spirochete, *Borrelia burgdorferi*. *Ann Intern Med.* 1985;103:67–68.
94. Steere AC. Lyme disease. *N Engl J Med.* 1989;321:586–596.
95. Rahn DW, Malawista SE. Lyme disease: recommendations for diagnosis and treatment. *Ann Intern Med.* 1991; 114:472–481.

CHAPTER 69

Melioidosis

Frederick A. Meier

All our science, measured against reality, is primitive and childlike—and yet it is the most precious thing we have.

Albert Einstein (1879–1955)

DEFINITION

Melioidosis is a bacterial infection with manifold, sometimes deceptive, manifestations.[1,2,3] It has a limited geographic range[4] as a human pathogen[5] and tends to prey on patients with impaired host defenses.[6] Endemicity is limited to Southeast Asia,[4] where more people show evidence of exposure to the infectious agent than develop clinical disease[6]; however, among émigrés, sojourners, or travelers who leave the endemic region, melioidosis has developed years later, usually in the context of impaired defenses.[7]

The bacterial agent of these infections is *Burkholderia pseudomallei.*[8] *Burkholderia* is the genus that makes up ribosomal RNA group II among the family *Pseudomonadaceae.*[9] *Burkholderia pseudomallei* was called *Pseudomonas pseudomallei* before group II was distinguished as its own genus. The clinical manifestations of *B pseudomallei* infections range from skin abscesses through necrotizing pneumonia to septicemia with metastatic abscesses in solid viscera; however, the agent has sometimes been overlooked in purulent material from all of these sites.[5]

Other members of the genus *Burkholderia* share clinically relevant characteristics with *B pseudomallei.* Another species of the genus, *Burkholderia mallei,* causes the predominantly equine zoonoses glanders and farcy.[3] Melioidosis, in its pulmonary presentation, is the human equivalent of glanders; in its cutaneous–lymphatic presentation it is the human equivalent of farcy. Therefore, the agent of melioidosis has received the species cognomen *pseudomallei* ("false glanders"), whereas the name of the disease that this agent causes is conversely *melioidosis* ("glanders-like"). From the viewpoint of human medicine, the big difference between these two agents is that, whereas human glanders can usually be traced to an animal source, animal to human spread of melioidosis has been difficult to document,[1] even though *B pseudomallei* is also a veterinary pathogen both within and outside its endemic Southeast Asian range for causing human disease.[4] The type species of the genus *Burkholderia, B cepacia,* shares with *B pseudomallei* a tropism for the lung (Figure 69–1) and predilection for patients with altered host defenses.[10–12] *Burkholderia cepacia* has been recognized as a cause of progressive lung disease among patients with cystic fibrosis.[13] *Burkholderia cepacia* and other constituents of the genus *Burkholderia* have a tropism for specific plants, a characteristic that has led to some species having names such as *B gladioli* and being major plant pathogens.[8] *Burkholderia pseudomallei* shares with these relatives an ecological association with vegetable material, water (especially still surface water), and soil (especially moist soil) in a warm ambient atmosphere (most isolations of *B pseudomallei* have been in the tropics between latitudes 20°N and 20°S.[5] Given these peferences, the typical association of melioidosis with exposure to the landscape of rice paddies, replete with vegetable, aqueous, and soil components, seems natural.[6]

Although *B pseudomallei* is a powerful stimulus to purulence in its local, pulmonary, and systemic presentations, the paucity of the characteristic gram-negative bipolar bacillus morphotype in smears of purulent exu-

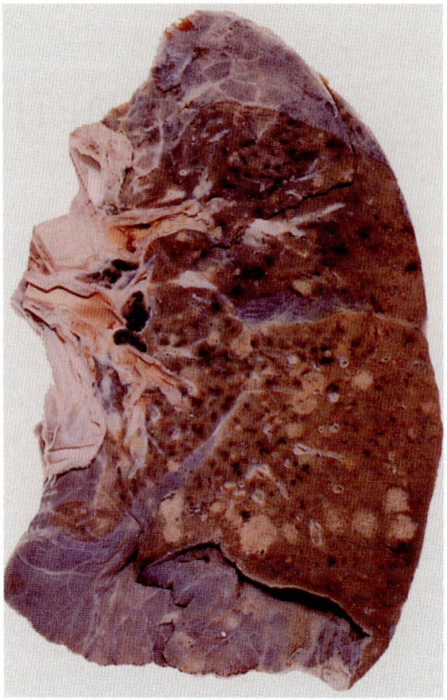

Figure 69–1. Fixed lung including a cut surface showing multiple abscesses of *B pseudomallei* acute necrotizing pneumonia, appearing as round tan lesions of various sizes concentrated in the posterior segment of the lower lobe. *(Photograph courtesy of David A. Schwartz, MD.)*

dates or aspirates has led to *B pseudomallei* acquiring a reputation as a deceptive "great mimicker" among pathogens in its characteristic milieu.[14]

GEOGRAPHIC DISTRIBUTION

Melioidosis is a true tropical disease.[7] In the tropics, human infection is almost completely limited to residents, sojourners, or travelers in Southeast Asia, its contiguous archipelagos, and adjacent regions of Oceania. *Burkholderia pseudomallei* was first detected as a cause of necrotizing pneumonia and subcutaneous abscesses in Burma (Myanmar) in 1911[15]; it is also endemic in adjacent Thailand[16] and Indochina,[17] as well as in subjacent Malaysia[14] and Singapore.[18] The endemic zone continues through Indonesia[19] to Papua New Guinea[20] (at least as a zoonosis), then on to northern Australia.[21] In addition, there is a focus at Hong Kong[22] and, probably, on mainland China[23] and in the Philippines.[24] The most systematic studies of the bacterium's geographic distribution have been in Malaya[25] and Thailand.[26]

Animal disease caused by *B pseudomallei* is less geographically confined than is human infection.[4,5] Infections have been initially misinterpreted as distemper among laboratory animals within the endemic zone in Malaya[27] and as glanders outside the zone during an outbreak in a zoological garden in Paris (in which the index case may have been a panda presented to the zoo by Chairman Mao).[28] *Burkholderia pseudomallei* also has been recognized as the cause of lethal epizootics within the zone of human infection; among marine animals at an oceanarium in Hong Kong[29,30]; and among sheep, calves, and other animals in Australia.[31–33] The agent, however, also has been potentially incriminated in veterinary disease in the Amazon basin[34] and in the Caribbean.[35] It has definitely caused animal disease in Niger and Upper Volta (Burkina Faso), in West Africa,[36] and on the islands of Madagascar and Le Reunion off the coast of East Africa.[34]

Outside of Southeast Asia, nevertheless, indigenous human infection is very rare, limited to case reports from Central America,[37,38] east[39] and west[40] Africa, and, most persuasively, from Iran, where both animal disease[41] and human infection[42,43] among rice growers were documented in the early 1970s. This hint of a presence in Persia makes the paucity of reports of the disease from apparently similar geographic areas in Pakistan,[44] India,[45–47] and Bangladesh[48] all the more remarkable. Until recently, all human infections in North America and Europe could be traced to Southeast Asia, either directly, through patient history, or indirectly by laboratory-acquired infections,[49] or by sexual transmission.[50]

ECOLOGICAL DISTRIBUTION

In endemic areas, *B pseudomallei* flourishes as a free-living bacterium in the soil and surface water of not only rice paddies,[6] but also newly planted oil palm gardens and monsoon drains.[5] Consistent with this pattern of environmental growth, its presence is greater in rural versus urban soil samples, in the rainy versus the dry season, and in still rather than running water.[5]

In such ecological circumstances, human subclinical infection, measured by serologic positivity, exceeds human disease by many fold.[5] In Thailand, there is about 15% population-wide seropositivity, with a range of 8% to 29% within various subpopulations.[5] In Malaya, this range is from 2% to 16%, with the highest prevalence among rice growers.[5] In northern Australia, 6% overall were positive, as were 8% to 11% of aborigines and 29% of Vietnamese refugees.[5] Pertinent to North America, 1% to 2% of US soldiers who sojourned in Vietnam between 6 and 12 months were seropositive.[2]

In general, the geographical distribution of *B pseudomallei* is tropical, Southeast Asian, and rural, whereas its ecological distribution is in warm, damp, muddy growth zones. In these areas, human exposure (subclinical infection) is much more frequent than human disease.

BIOLOGICAL BEHAVIOR

As the discrepancy between subclinical infection and illness suggests, *B pseudomallei* behaves as an opportunistic pathogen. From this characterization, it follows that subclinical and mild or local infections can easily be overlooked or not characterized, and that clinical manifestations of infection can be delayed years or even decades after exposure, at least up to a quarter of a century.[51] The opportunistic pattern also is reflected in the high frequency of comorbidities that diminish host defenses in patients with clinical disease.[5] These conditions include diabetes mellitus, cancers and their treatment, chronic renal or hepatic failure, immunosuppressive therapy, and conditions otherwise known to decrease immunity or splenic function.[5]

Similar to other pseudomonads, *B pseudomallei* has the potential to flourish in a variety of aqueous hospital environments, posing a risk of nosocomial infection.[52] Similarly, as an airborne pathogen, it also presents a risk to laboratorians tempted to smell its distinctive odor when the organism has been isolated on agar plates.[50] The most striking clinical consequence of *B pseudomallei's* indolent biological behavior is the tendency for clinical disease, in some cases, to declare itself slowly.[1,2] In particular, there is often a localized mild infection days before systemic infection.[5] The missed diagnostic opportunity can, in retrospect, be mortifying.

NATURAL HISTORY/VIRULENCE PROFILE

Natural History

As with many infections that are usually recognized only late in their courses, the natural history of melioidosis is controversial. There is relative agreement, however, in accord with *B pseudomallei's* known ecology, that it is usually acquired either through the skin, which may be frequently abraded, cut, or ulcerated in the rural tropics, via contaminated water, mud, soil, or vegetable matter, or through the respiratory tract by inhalation of infectious water droplets or particles of dirt. Whether squamous or other epithelia are colonized to any significant degree remains disputed; however, the very long incubation periods mentioned previously suggest that there is a reservoir in human tissue, perhaps the colonic epithelium.[53] Also, some local or systemic defect in host defenses seems almost always necessary for clinically apparent infection, although some investigators have argued that this element in the natural history is caused by only contemplating "the tip of the iceberg" of endemic melioidosis.[4] Certainly, many infections afflicting rural people in Southeast Asia without immune defects could very easily be overlooked.[6]

At the other end of the spectrum of host defenses, observers have also studied the impact of the introduction, over the past decade, of human immunodeficiency virus (HIV) into the melioidosis endemic area.[54]

Virulence Profile

The virulence characteristics of *Burkholderia* sp in general, and *B pseudomallei* in particular, are much less understood than they are for the fluorescent *Pseudomonas* in general and *P aeruginosa* in particular (see Chapter 80). *Burkholderia pseudomallei* appears to have at least one proteolytic enzyme[55] (defined 30 years ago) and a (heat sensitive) exotoxin,[56] whereas *P aeruginosa* has several well-characterized entities in each of these categories. Similar to other *Pseudomonadaceae, B pseudomallei's* cell wall also contains endotoxin.[57] The bacterium also has its own siderophore.[58] An important focus of investigation is *B pseudomallei's* putative ability to survive intracellularly for long periods.[59] This capacity may contribute to the striking delays between infection and disease. Another area of research into the virulence of *B pseudomallei,* pursued by a group of Anglo-American and Thai investigators, is the impact of melioidosis on cytokine expression.[60,61]

EPIDEMIOLOGY

In summary, *B pseudomallei* is a free-living, hardy bacterium from warm, wet, vegetative, rural, tropical environments. In these environments there is evidence of a low to moderate rate of infection among both travelers and sojourners, as well as in indigenous populations (especially agricultural people). Such infection appears to be by transcutaneous inoculation or respiratory inhalation. The bacterium's subsequent mechanisms of colonization are either epithelial or intracellular. The bacterium's long-term survival in the host remains a subject of investigation, as does the mechanism(s) that triggers clinical disease. A third point requiring further investigation is the prevalence of clinical disease. It is clear, however, that patients with vascular conditions, organ dysfunctions, (auto)immune defects and diseases, and splenic malfunction are at greatest risk for clinical disease. Clinical infection usually presents as a local suppurative lesion before systemic manifestations or with metastatic foci. After dissemination, antimicrobial treatment may be ineffective, even with agents to which the organism shows in vitro susceptibility.[5]

MORPHOLOGY

Burkolderia pseudomallei is a typical pseudomonad. A small gram-negative bacillus takes up stain with increased intensity at the ends of its long axis and grows as variable smooth to rough colonies on sheep blood or MacConkey agar culture media.[62] The tendency of these colonies to become wrinkled on prolonged incubation and the "pungent odor of putrefaction,"[5] described by others as a "sweet earthy smell,"[4] that the colonies emit are potentially helpful characteristics of growth. When tested by routine bacteriologic methods, *B pseudomallei* is motile; has polar flagella; is oxidase positive, as is typical of pseudomonads; and reduces nitrate to nitrite. In clinical microbiologic jargon, it is an "oxidase positive gram-negative nonfermenter."[5] It has a typical behavior in the standard triple sugar iron agar tube test: it produces, initially, an acid slant with neutral butt (at 16 to 24 hours) that becomes wholly acid (at 48 to 72 hours)[62] but does not produce gas. Unlike fluorescent *Pseudomonas* sp, *B pseudomallei* does not produce pigment.

Some commercial test batteries have demonstrated excellent identification of *B pseudomallei.*[62] For endemic areas, Dance and colleagues[62] also have validated a "screening profile" for identifying *B pseudomallei* presumptively: 1) oxidase positivity, 2) bipolar Gram's staining, 3) growth on Columbia agar adjacent to gentamicin and colistin 10 microgram disks, and 4) confluent growth at 48 to 72 hours on a modified version of Ashdown's selective (gentamicin containing) agar. The latter growth has a metallic sheen, the distinctive odor, and consists of opaque, purple, rugose colonies with no discoloration of surrounding medium (which contains crystal violet and neutral red, the latter producing the purple colonies).[62] Ashdown's medium has been used also to screen both contaminated clinical specimens (from throat, sputum, wound, or stool) and environmental samples for *B pseudomallei.*[53,63] It appears to have greatest clinical utility in sorting through respiratory specimens in which the relatively slow growing *B pseudomallei* may be obscured by faster growing colonies of normal flora.[5,62] Ashdown's medium also is the means by which colonic carriage of the organism, one of the potential mechanisms of long-term asymptomatic infection, has been documented.[53] *Burkholderia pseudomallei* cannot always be detected in tissue sections stained with any of the Gram procedures, even when basic fuchsin is increased from 0.1% to 1.0%. The bacilli are blackened and readily detected, however, when silver impregnation techniques are used (Steiner, Dieterle, or Warthin–Starry).

HISTOPATHOLOGY

Two patterns of histopathologic reaction to *B pseudomallei* have been described, both of which can be confusing.[64–66] The more common pattern is acute necrotizing inflammation dominated by neutrophils[64,66] but also containing macrophages (some of which qualify as giant cells) and lymphocytes.[64] This infiltrate may be focal or diffuse but the gram-negative intra- and extracellular bacilli can be disproportionately few given the intensity of suppuration.[5,64,66] This is the usual pattern in acute subcutaneous abscesses (Figures 69–2 and 69–3), metastatic acute abscesses in patients with septicemia, and septic arthritis and prostatitis caused by *B pseudomallei.*[64] Even when the Gram's stain is negative, cultures of such exudates often reveal the bacillus; however, growth may be delayed until after 48 hours incubation,[5] especially when a patient is being treated with partially effective antimicrobials.

The less common pattern is loose granulomas (aggregates of macrophages), usually with but sometimes without (particularly in metastatic infections) necrosis.[64,65] Wong and colleagues[64] also stressed the diagnostic utility of demonstrating giant cells and macrophages that contain "globi" (tangled clumps of bacilli) of *B pseudomallei* in this second pattern of inflammation.[64] This chronic pattern was seen more often, in Wong's series,[64] in zones of myositis (representing the clinical presentation of deep soft tissue infection) and in the spleen (Figure 69–4) and other viscera in patients with more subacute courses, or among whom systemic melioidosis was first appreciated at autopsy, than it was in patients presenting abruptly with acute disease. Wong and colleagues[64,65] further stressed that bacilli were difficult to demonstrate in biopsy specimens with the acute suppurative pattern (in the majority of their patients); however, they were easier to demonstrate in the intracellular "globi," in mixed acute and chronic granulomatous lesions, and in those that

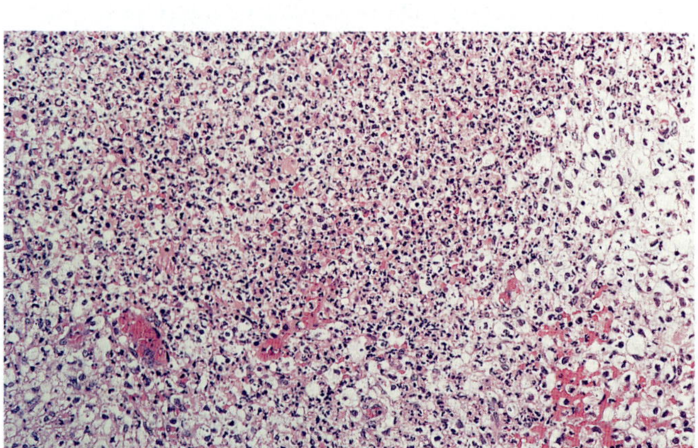

Figure 69–2. Sinus tract leading from a subcutaneous abscess. The central area of necrosis is surrounded by an inflammatory cell exudate composed of neutrophils and macrophages (hematoxylin-eosin ×100). *(Photograph courtesy of Francis W. Chandler, DVM, PhD.)*

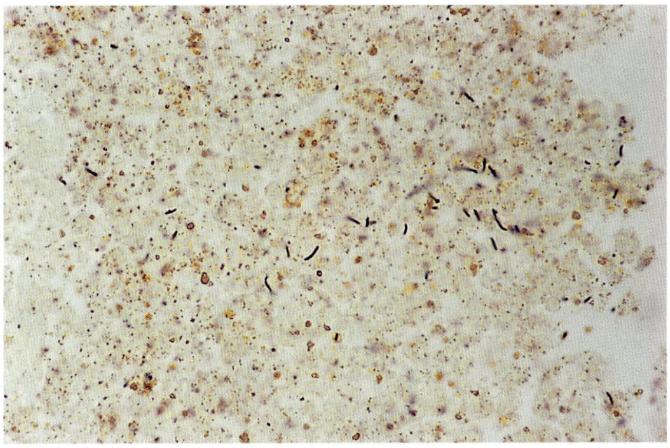

Figure 69–3. Same lesion showing blackened curved bacilli in the exudate (Steiner silver impregnation technique, ×250). *(Photograph courtesy of Francis W. Chandler, DVM, PhD.)*

were purely granulomatous. Intracellular bacilli in these lesions are evidence of the intracellular survival of *B pseudomallei.*[64]

CLINICOPATHOLOGIC FEATURES

Leelarasamee and Bovornkitti[5] make six excellent clinical pathologic points in introducing their 1989 review

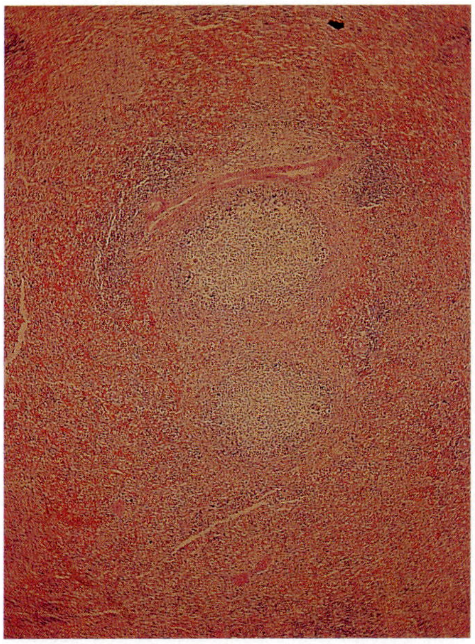

Figure 69–4. Low power photomicrograph of a spleen showing two necrotizing granulomas, a typical finding at postmortem in patients with a subacute or chronic course of systemic melioidosis (AFIP Neg 69-5770).

of melioidosis: 1) localized active melioidosis usually becomes evident several days before septicemic symptoms herald disseminated disease; 2) as already stressed, examination of aspirates of these local suppurative lesions usually reveals many neutrophils but few bacilli; 3) aspirates usually grow gram-negative bacilli, but they may be identified as "norfermentative (oxidase positive) gram-negative bacilli" or "*Pseudomonas* sp" rather than specifically as *B pseudomallei;* 4) in patients with a history of exposure to the endemic ecosystem, especially in patients with immunodeficiencies, "septicemic melioidosis should be included in the differential diagnosis when there is a primary site of infection and subsequent dissemination to joint and lung"; 5) overwhelming septicemia may ensue within 2 to 3 days of presentation with local infections, particularly if the abscesses are visceral; and 6) in vitro antimicrobial activity does not always predicate clinical success in patients with septicemic melioidosis.[5,67,68]

Syndromes of melioidosis can be divided into three groups: 1) respiratory, 2) skin, lymphatic, soft tissue, and musculoskeletal; and 3) bacteremic–visceral.[1,2,5] Respiratory infection usually presents as acute suppurative (necrotizing) pneumonia with its expected complications—abscess and empyema. It more rarely presents as miliary pneumonia with a granulomatous pattern of inflammation described previously. Cutaneous, soft tissue, lymphatic, and musculoskeletal infection usually present as subcutaneous abscess or an infected superficial wound, a deeper cellulitis, or septic arthritis, with or without suppurative or mixed suppurative granulomatous lymphadenitis. It more rarely presents as osteomyelitis with or without subperiosteal abscess. Visceral disease frequently follows or accompanies septicemia. The latter is usually abrupt and obvious, especially in patients with demonstrable respiratory, skin, soft tissue, or musculoskeletal infections. More rarely, however, the septicemia is insidious and subtle, presenting as prolonged fever of obscure cause. In the more common and more dramatic presentation, focal findings may include ecthyma gangrenosum, pyomyositis, or visceral abscesses (hepatic, splenic, and pancreatic in the deep viscera; prostatic, testicular, and parotid superficially). In the less common and more subtle constellation, endocarditis and widely dispersed metastatic abscesses may eventually declare themselves (eg, ophthalmitis, meningoencephalitis, intracerebral abscess, or pericarditis); otherwise, in more subtle disease, one sees only granulomas in liver, elsewhere in the biliary tree, or in spleen. Superficially, such inflammation may involve muscle.

Septicemia without demonstrable sites of metastatic infection has a much better prognosis than does septicemia with evidence of disseminated disease.[5] In the latter, the prognosis can be grim, even with appropriate antimicrobial therapy. The prognosis of skin, soft tissue, lymphatic, and musculoskeletal disease is more variable depending on the site. Infections of the lung that remain localized are often slowly responsive (Figure 69–1). In all types of *B pseudomallei* infection, relapse is relatively common. The tardiness of response in respiratory infection and the tendency to relapse in the skin, soft tissue, bone, joint, prostate, and lung has lead to the prolongation of antimicrobial regimens for localized *B pseudomallei* infections at those sites.[69]

TREATMENT

In the recent past, two approaches to antimicrobial therapy have found advocates.[1,2] One features oral trimethoprim–sulfamethoxazole, chloramphenicol, and doxycycline. The other is intravenous "antipseudomonal" drugs: third-generation, cephalosporins, such as ceftazidime, or antipseudomonal penicillins, such as piperacillin or amoxicillin–clavulanic acid. The latter appears to have been successful in the hands of Anglo–Thai experts,[1,5] in spite of in vitro data suggesting that ceftazidime is not bactericidal for "selected strains."[68] A US publication suggests trimethoprim–sulfamethoxazole for subacute or chronic infection with the oral multidrug regimen for acute infection, but intravenous ceftazidime or amoxicillin–clavulanic acid for "severe" acute sepsis.[70] "Coverage" by one or the other regimen seems especially important in the context of surgical drainage of abscesses that, in the Thai experience, were associated with subsequent bacteremia and metastatic infection in an alarmingly high proportion of patients.[5]

A final disputed clinical feature of melioidosis is the propensity toward person-to-person infection, particularly from patients with lung or prostatic infection, by droplet[71] or sexual[49] transmission. Currently, well-documented instances of this sort of transmission appear limited to case reports.

DIFFERENTIAL DIAGNOSIS

The diagnosis of *B pseudomallei* infection in a subcutaneous site or wound, bone, joint, or inflamed muscle can be difficult. In a patient exposed in an endemic area, melioidosis joins the differential diagnosis, particularly when gram-positive cocci cannot be demonstrated. The similarity of *B pseudomallei* to *Pseudomonas* sp, more frequently encountered in immunodeficient patients outside of endemic areas, can also confuse the diagnosis, unless *B pseudomallei* is considered.

As a necrotizing pneumonia, pulmonary melioidosis joins a differential diagnosis that is commonly headed by *Staphylococcus aureus* and *Streptococcus pyogenes* among gram-positive pathogens, and *Klebsiella pneumoniae* and *Pseudomonas aeruginosa* among gram-negative pathogens. As with *P aeruginosa* pneumonia, *B pseudomallei* pneumonia strikes patients with local and/or systemic immunodeficiencies. The combination of 1) exposure to an endemic zone, 2) immunodeficiency, 3) a pattern of "hematogenous" spread of small necrotic zones on chest x ray in a patient without evidence of one of the other pathogens listed earlier (to which in some areas *L pneumophilia* would need to be added), and 4) growth of a "nonfermenter" or a "pseudomonad" should prompt a suspicion of *B pseudomallei* pneumonia. Less commonly, *B pseudomallei* pneumonia should also be considered in patients with a miliary pattern in which intracellular bacilli are seen but are not acid-fast.

Burkholderia pseudomallei should stand highest on a differential diagnosis of septicemia following discovery of local superficial or visceral abscess(es) in a immunodeficient patient with endemic exposure. Then, *B pseudomallei* joins its relative *P aeruginosa* in the differential diagnosis of ecthyma gangrenosum. In these patients, the combination of prostatitis[72] and necrotizing pneumonia or septic arthritis[73] and necrotizing pneumonia are striking presentations of *B pseudomallei.* In patients with diabetes, *B pseudomallei* causes invasive necrotizing soft tissue infections.[74]

Ophthalmic pathologists should be aware that *B pseudomallei* causes corneal ulcers in Southeast Asia.[75] In Singapore, *B pseudomallei* septicemia may cause sudden death,[76] and in northern Australia, Woods and colleagues[77] describe systemic *B pseudomallei* infection as causing a distinctive brainstem encephalitis, "aseptic" meningitis, and pneumonia, presenting initially with acute paresis or paralysis. In addition, Wong and colleagues[64] describe pyogranulomatous lymphadenitis resembling cat scratch disease. Finally, in patients with previous melioidosis, all pathologists should remember the potential for relapse in any of these presentations,[69] especially if the primary site has been one noted for resisting treatment, such as bone or prostate.[78]

DIAGNOSTIC TECHNIQUES FOR ANATOMIC PATHOLOGISTS

The key diagnostic techniques are Gram's stain and culture. Typical bacilli may be rare in the acute suppurative lesions, where they can be both extra- and intracellular. Bacilli are more likely to appear within cells in the subacute chronic granulomatous pattern (Figures 69–5 and 69–6). In the latter, they appear in

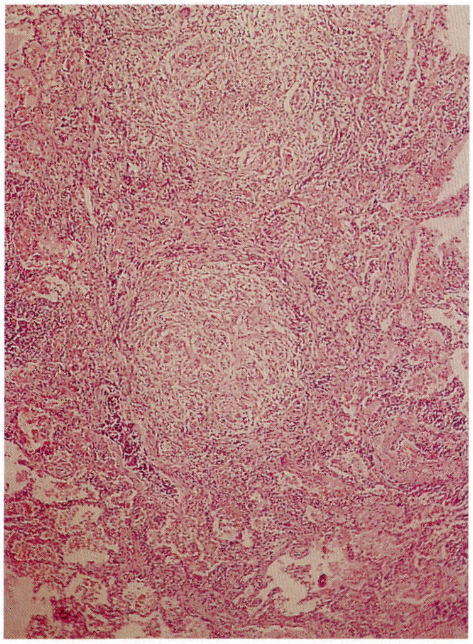

Figure 69–5. Low magnification photomicrograph of two microabscesses on a background of organizing pneumonia, a typical appearance at postmortem examination of fatal acute pneumonic melioidosis (AFIP Neg 68-1214).

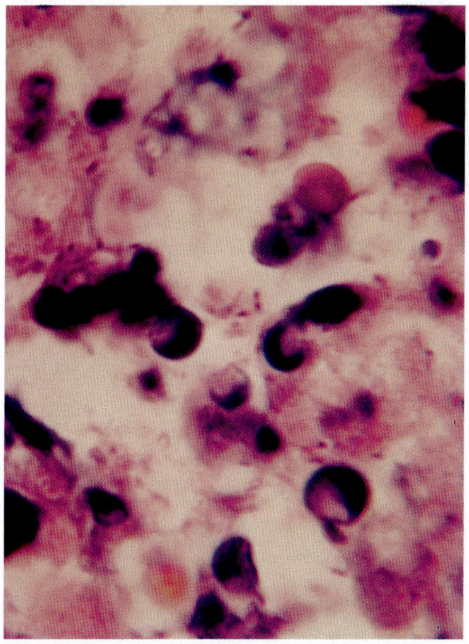

Figure 69–6. High magnification photomicrograph of *B pseudomallei* bacilli against a typical background of neutrophils, lymphocytes, macrophages, and necrotic debris. Note the three extracellular bacilli in the center of the photomicrograph and the multiple intracellular bacilli in the apparently multinucleated cell at the top of the field. Fields containing so many bacilli are relatively rare in smears of purulent material collected antemortem from patients with melioidosis (AFIP Neg 68-905).

macrophages and giant cells as "globi" of crisscrossed bacilli. In culture, *B pseudomallei* is not fastidious, but indolent. *Burkholderia pseudomallei* grows in routine media under routine aerobic conditions, but growth may take longer than the conventional 48 hours. For the same reason, *B pseudomallei* may be obscured in cultures of sputum by faster growing contaminants. Ashdown's selective medium[63] is a proven strategy for dealing with this difficulty, especially in regions where melioidosis is endemic.

Blood culture is an important adjunct to diagnosis whenever melioidosis is possible. To detect *B pseudomallei,* the volume of blood is the most important variable in the technique's sensitivity. Studies by Wuthiekanun and colleagues[79] suggest that more dilute (1:10) cultures, those subcultured earlier and more often, and those incubated in a resin-containing medium improve the likelihood of isolating *B pseudomallei* in patients already receiving antibiotics. However, isolation rates were high (86%) among patients not being treated with antibiotics at the time of culture, even when a small volume (5 mL) of blood was incubated at a high blood-to-broth ratio (1:4) in an unsupplemented broth bottle.

Because seropositivity is evidence of infection rather than evidence of disease, it is difficult to see what role serology could play in diagnosis beyond confirming what has already been learned from the patient.[80] However, a rapid antigen detection assay using a monoclonal antibody has been described with a 75% sensitivity and 98% specificity that may have practical utility.[81] For monitoring therapeutic effect and surveillance for relapse, Ashdown[82] has presented evidence that serial assays for C-reactive protein are valuable.

Any discussion of diagnostic techniques for *B pseudomallei* should conclude by stressing the importance of eliciting the clinical history of venturing through or living in the endemic area of the organism, almost always essential for diagnosis.

REFERENCES

1. Dance DAB. Melioidosis and glanders. In: Weatherall DJ, Ledingham JGG, Warrell DA, eds. *Oxford Textbook of Medicine.* 3rd ed. Oxford: Oxford Medical Publications; 1996:590–595.
2. Sanford JP. *Pseudomonas* species (including melioidosis and glanders). In: Mandell GL, Bennett JE, Dolin R, eds. *Principles and Practice of Infectious Diseases.* 4th ed. New York: Churchill Livingstone; 1995:2003–2008.
3. Mayr A (ed). *Rolle/Mayr medizinische Mikrobiologie, Infektions-und Seuchenlehre für Tierärzte, Biologen, und Agrarwissenschaftler.* 5th ed. Stuttgart: Ferdinand Enke Verlag; 1984:718.
4. Dance DAB. Melioidosis: the tip of the iceberg? *Clinical Microbiology Reviews.* 1991;4:52–60.

5. Leelarasamee A, Bovornkitti S. Melioidosis: review and update. *Rev Infect Dis.* 1989;11:413–425.
6. Dance DAB. *Pseudomonas pseudomallei:* danger in the paddy fields. *Trans Roy Soc Trop Med Hyg.* 1991;85:1–3.
7. Koponen MA, Zlock D, Palmer DL, Merlin TL. Melioidosis: forgotten but not gone! *Arch Int Med.* 1991;151: 605–608.
8. Gilligan PH. *Pseudomonas* and *Burkholderia.* In: Murray PR, ed. *Manual of Clinical Microbiology.* 6th ed. Washington, DC: ASM Press; 1995:509–519.
9. Yabuuchi E, Kosako Y, Oyaizu H, et al. Proposal of *Burkholderia* gen. nov. and transfer of seven species of the genus *Pseudomonas* homology group II to the new genus, with the type species *Burkholderia cepacia* (Palleroni and Holmes 1981) comb. nov. *Microbiol Immunol.* 1992;36:1251–1275.
10. O'Neil KM, Herman JH, Modlin JF, Moxon ER, Winkelstein JA. *Pseudomonas cepacia:* an emerging pathogen in chronic granulomatous disease. *J Ped.* 1986;108:940–942.
11. Snell GI, deHoyos A, Krajden M, Winton T, Maurer JR. *Pseudomonas cepacia* in lung transplant recipients with cystic fibrosis. *Chest.* 1993;103:466–471.
12. Pegues DA, Carson LA, Anderson RL, et al. Outbreak of *Pseudomonas cepacia* bacteremia in oncology patients. *Clin Inf Dis.* 1993;16:407–411.
13. Gilligan PH. Microbiology of airway disease in patients with cystic fibrosis. *Clin Microbiol Reviews.* 1991;4:35–51.
14. Yee KC, Lee MK, Chua CT, Puthucheary SD. Melioidosis, the great mimicker: a report of 10 cases from Malaysia. *J Trop Med Hyg.* 1988;91:249–254.
15. Whitmore A, Krishnaswami CS. A account of the discovery of a hitherto undescribed infectious disease occurring among the population of Rangoon. *Indian Med Gaz.* 1912;47:262–267.
16. Chaowagul W, White NJ, Dance DAB, et al. Melioidosis: a major cause of community-acquired septicemia in northeastern Thailand. *J Infect Dis.* 1989;159:890–899.
17. Howe C, Sampath A, Spotnitz M. The pseudomallei group: a review. *J Infect Dis.* 1971;124:598–606.
18. Tan AL, Ang BSP, Ong YY. Melioidosis: epidemiology and antibiogram of cases in Singapore. *Singapore Med J.* 1990; 31:335–337.
19. Bezemer F. Melioidosis op Celebes. *Geneeskunde Tijdschrift de Nederlandse Indie.* 1935;75:1577–1579.
20. Egerton JR. Melioidosis in a tree climbing kangaroo. *Austral Vet J.* 1963;39:243–244.
21. Guard RW. Melioidosis in Australia: a review. *Austral Fam Phys.* 1987;16:119–123.
22. So SY, Chau PY, Leung YK, Lam WK. First report of septicemic melioidosis in Hong Kong. *Transactions of the Roy Soc Trop Med Hyg.* 1984;78:456–459.
23. Galimand M, Dodin A. Répartition de *Pseudomonas pseudomallei* en France et dans le monde: la mélio dose. *Bull du Soc Vet Practique Francaise.* 1982;66:651–667.
24. Prevatt AL, Hunt JS. Chronic systemic melioidosis: review of literature and report of a case, with a note on visual disturbance due to chloramphenicol. *Amer J Med.* 1957; 23:810–823.
25. Strauss JM, Groves MG. Mariappan M, Ellison DW. Melioidosis in Malaysia: II. Distribution of *Pseudomonas pseudomallei* in soil and surface water. *Amer J Trop Med Hyg.* 1969;18:698–702.
26. Punyagupta S, Sirisanthana T, Stapatayovong B, ed. *Melioidosis.* Bangkok: Bangkok Medical Publisher; 1989.
27. Stanton AT, Fletcher W. Melioidosis: A new disease of the tropics. *Transactions of the Fourth Congress for the Far Eastern Association for Tropical Medicine.* 1921;2: 196–198.
28. Mollaret HH. "L'affaire du jardin des plantes" ou comment la méliodose fit son apparition en France. *Med Mal Infect.* 1988;18:643–654.
29. Huang CT. What is *Pseudomonas pseudomallei? Elixir.* 1976;70:2.
30. Vedros NA, Chow D, Liong E. Experimental vaccine against *Pseudomonas pseudomallei* infections in captive cetaceans. *Dis Aquat Organisms.* 1988;5:157–161.
31. Ketterer PJ, Bamford VW. A case of melioidosis in lambs in south western Australia. *Austral Vet J.* 1967;43:79–80.
32. Ketterer PJ, Donald B, Rogers RJ. Bovine melioidosis in south eastern Queensland. *Austral Vet J.* 1975;51:395–398.
33. Laws L, Hall WTK. Melioidosis in animals in North Queensland: IV. Epidemiology. *Austral Vet J.* 1964;40: 309–314.
34. Galimand M, Dodin A. Le point sur la mélioidose dans le monde. *Bull Soc Pathol Exot.* 1982;75:375–383.
35. Sutmoller P, Kraneveld FC, van der Schaaf A. Melioidosis (pseudomalleus) in sheep, goats, and pigs on Aruba (Netherlands Antilles). *J Amer Vet Med Ass.* 1957;130: 415–417.
36. Dodin A, Ferry D. Découverte du bacille de Whitmore en Afrique. *Med Mal Infect.* 1975;5:97–101.
37. McDowell F, Varney PL. Melioidosis: report of first case from the Western Hemisphere. *J Amer Med Ass.* 1947;134: 361–362.
38. Larionov GM. The transfer of melioidosis and an epidemiological review of its dissemination. *Zh Mikrobiol Epidemiol Immunobiol.* 1987;36:93–97.
39. Bremmelgaard A, Bygbjerg IB, Hoiby N. Microbiological and immunological studies in a case of human melioidosis diagnosed in Denmark. *Scand J Infect Dis.* 1982;14: 271–275.
40. Wall RA, Mabey DCW, Corrah PT, Peters L. A case of melioidosis in West Africa. *J Infect Dis.* 1985;152:424–425.
41. Baharsefat M, Amjadi AR. Equine melioidosis in Iran. *Arch Inst Razi.* 1970;22:209–213.
42. Pourtaghva M, Machoun A, Dodin A. Mise en évidence de *Pseudomonas pseudomallei* (bacille de Whitmore) dans la boue des rizières iraniennes. *Bull Soc Pathol Exot.* 1975; 68:367–370.
43. Pourtaghva M, Dodin A, Portovi M, Teherani M, Galimand M. Premier cas de mélioidose pulmonaire humaine en Iran. *Bull Soc Pathol Exot.* 1977;70:107–109.
44. Thurnheer U, Novak A, Michel M, Ruchti C, Jutzi H, Weiss M. Septische Melioidose nach Aufenthalt im indischen Subkontinent. *Schweiz Med Wochenschr.* 1988;118: 558–564.
45. Sheppard MJ, Marriot RM, Brown TJ. *J Infect.* 1990; 20:83–84. (Letter).

46. Ives JCJ, Thomson TJ. Chronic melioidosis: the first report of a case infected in Central India. *Glasgow Med J.* 1953; 34:61–67.
47. Raghavan KR, Shenoi RP, Zaer F, Aiyer R, Ramamoorthy P, Mehta MN. Melioidosis in India. *Indian Pediatrics.* 1991;28:184–188.
48. Kibbler CC, Roberts CM. Ridgway GL, Spiro SG. Melioidosis in a patient from Bangladesh. *Postgrad Med J.* 1991;67:764–766.
49. McCormick JB, Sexton DJ, McMurray JG, Carey E, Hayes P, Feldman RA. Human-to-human transmission of *Pseudomonas pseudomallei. Ann Intern Med.* 1975;83: 512–513.
50. Schlech WF III, Turchik JB, Westlake RE Jr, Klein GC, Band JC, Weaver RE. Laboratory-acquired infection with *Pseudomonas pseudomallei* (melioidosis). *N Engl J Med.* 1981;305:1133–1135.
51. Mays EE, Ricketts EA. Melioidosis: recrudescence associated with bronchogenic carcinoma twenty-six years following initial geographic exposure. *Chest.* 1975;68: 261–263.
52. Ashdown LR. Nosocomial infection due to *Pseudomonas pseudomallei:* two cases and an epidemiologic study. *Rev Infect Dis.* 1979;1:891–894.
53. Wuthiekanun V, Dance DAB, Wattanagoon Y, Supputtamongkol Y, Chaowagul W, White NJ. The use of selective media for the isolation of *Pseudomonas pseudomallei* in clinical practice. *J Med Microbiol.* 1990;33:121–126.
54. Tanphaichitra D, Sahaphong S, Srimuang S, Wangroongsarb Y. A case comparison of acquired immune deficiency syndrome (AIDS) in homosexual males with spindle-endothelial cell abnormalities and with recrudescent melioidosis. *Asian Pacific J Allergy Immunol.* 1985;3: 200–204.
55. Heckly RJ. Differentiation of exotoxin and other biologically active substances in *Pseudomonas pseudomallei* filtrates. *J Bacteriol.* 1964;88:1730–1736.
56. Ismail G, Embi MN, Omar O, Allen JC, Smith CJ. A competitive immunosorbent assay for detection of *Pseudomonas pseudomallei* exotoxin. *J Med Microbiol.* 1987;23: 353–357.
57. Rapaport FT, Millar WJ, Ruch J. Endotoxic properties of *Pseudomonas pseudomallei. Arch Pathol.* 1961;71: 429–436.
58. Yang H, Chaowagul W, Sokol PA. Siderophore production by *Pseudomonas pseudomallei. Infect Immun.* 1991; 59:776–780.
59. Pruksachartvuthi S, Aswapokee N, Thankerngpol K. Survival of *Pseudomonas pseudomallei* in human phagocytes. *J Med Microbiol.* 1990;31:109–114.
60. Suputtamongkol Y, Kwiatkowski D, Dance DAB, Chaowagul W, White NJ. Tumor necrosis factor in septicemic melioidosis. *J Infect Dis.* 1992;165:561–564.
61. Brown AE, Dance DAB, Suputtamongkol Y, et al. Immune cell activation in melioidosis: increased serum levels of interferon-gamma and soluble interlukin-2 receptors without change in soluble CD8 protein. *J Infect Dis.* 1991; 163:1145–1148.
62. Dance DAB, Wuthiekanun V, Naigowit P, White NJ. Identification of *Pseudomonas pseudomallei* in clinical practice: use of simple screening tests and API 20 NE. *J Clin Pathol.* 1989;42:645–648.
63. Ashdown LR. An improved screening technique for isolation of *Pseudomonas pseudomallei* from clinical specimens. *Pathology.* 1979;11:293–297.
64. Wong KT, Puthucheary DS, Vadivelu J. The histopathology of human melioidosis. *Histopathology.* 1995;26:51–55.
65. Piggott JA, Hochholzer L. Human melioidosis: a histopathologic study of acute and chronic melioidosis. *Arch Pathol.* 1970;90:101–111.
66. Greenawald KA, Nash G, Foley FD. Acute systemic melioidosis. *Am J Clin Pathol.* 1969;52:188–198.
67. Yamamato T, Naigowit P, Dejsirilert S, et al. In vitro susceptibilities of *Pseudomonas pseudomallei* to 27 antimicrobial agents. *Antimicrob Agents Chemother.* 1990;34: 2027–2029.
68. Sookpranee T, Sookpranee M, Mellencamp MA, Preheim LC. *Pseudomonas pseudomallei:* a common pathogen in Thailand that is resistant to the bactericidal effects of many antibiotics. *Antimicrob Agents Chemother.* 1991;35: 484–489.
69. Chaowagul W, Suputtamongkol Y, Dance DAB, Rajchanuvong L, Pattara-arechachai J, White NJ. Relapse in melioidosis: incidence and risk factors. *J Infect Dis.* 1993;168: 1181–1885.
70. Sanford JP. Melioidosis (Whitmore Disease). In: Benenson AS, ed. *Control of Communicable Diseases Manual.* 16th ed. Washington, DC: American Public Health Association; 1995:299–300.
71. Kunakorn M, Jayanetra P, Tanphaichitra D. Man-to-man transmission of melioidosis. *Lancet.* 1991;337:1290–1291. Letter.
72. Bouvy JJ, Degener JE, Stijnen C, Gallee MPW, van der Berg B. Septic melioidosis after a visit to Southeast Asia. *Eur J Clin Microbiol.* 1986;5:655–656.
73. Saengnipanthkul S, Laupattarakasem W, Kowsuwon W, Mahaisavariya B. Isolated articular melioidosis. *Clin Orthopaed Related Res.* 1991;267:182–185.
74. Elango S, Sivakumaran S. Parapharyngeal space melioidosis in a diabetic. *J Laryngol Otol.* 1991;105:582–583.
75. Siripanthong S, Teerapantuwat S, Prugsanusak W, et al. Corneal ulcer caused by *Pseudomonas pseudomallei:* report of three cases. *Rev Infect Dis.* 1991;13:335–337.
76. Yap EH, Chan YC, Goh KT, et al. Sudden unexplained death syndrome: a new manifestation in melioidosis? *Epidemiol Infect.* 1991;107:577–584.
77. Woods ML II, Currie BJ, Howard DM, et al. Neurological melioidosis: seven cases from the Northern Territory of Australia. *Clin Infect Dis.* 1992;5:163–169.
78. Desmarchelier PM, Dance DAB, Chaowogul W, Suputtamongkol Y, White NJ, Pitt TL. Relationships among *Pseudomonas pseudomallei* isolates from patients with recurrent melioidosis. *J Clin Microbiol.* 1993;31:1592–1595.
79. Wuthiekanun V, Dance D, Chaowagul W, Suputtamongkol Y, Wattanagoon Y, White N. Blood culture techniques for the diagnosis of melioidosis. *Eur J Clin Microbiol Infect Dis.* 1990;9:654–658.
80. Kanaphun P, Therawattanasuk N, Supputtamongkol Y, et

al. Serology and carriage of *Pseudomonas pseudomallei:* a prospective study in 1000 hospitalized children in northeast Thailand. *J Infect Dis.* 1993;167:230–233.
81. Anuntagood A, Intachote P, Naigowit P, Sirisinha S. Rapid antigen detection assay for identification of *Burkholderia (Pseudomonas) pseudomallei*. *J Clin Microbiol.* 1996;34: 975–976.
82. Ashdown LR. Serial serum C-reactive protein levels as an aid to the management of melioidosis. *Am J Trop Med Hyg.* 1992;46:151–157.

CHAPTER 70

Mycobacterium avium Complex (MAC) Infection

Heidrun Rotterdam

Public health is more than a local responsibility. Disease knows nothing about town lines, nor do bacilli undertake to inquire about local jurisdictions.

Franklin D. Roosevelt (1882–1945)

DEFINITION AND SYNONYMS

Mycobacterium avium complex (MAC) is a group of nontuberculous mycobacteria that includes *M avium, M intracellulare,* and rare other nontuberculous strains.[1] A survey in 1980 of mycobacterial isolates from all state laboratories in the United States identified one third as nontuberculous. Among these, the single largest group was MAC (61%).[2] The taxonomy of these mycobacteria has changed remarkably in recent years. The increasing frequency of acquired immunodeficiency syndrome (AIDS)-related MAC infections and the development of new molecular techniques have revealed new divisions and new distinct subtypes of MAC.

The avian tubercle bacillus, now known as *M avium,* was first described in 1890 as the causal agent of an economically important disease in chickens.[1] The mycobacterium now known as *M intracellulare* was first cultured in 1969 from the sputum of tuberculosis patients in the Battey State Hospital of Rome, Georgia, and was therefore originally referred to as "Battey bacillus."[1] Runyon, in 1971, divided nontuberculous mycobacteria into three groups: 1) the photochromogens, such as *M kansasii,* 2) the scotochromogens, such as *M scrofulaceum* and *M xenopi,* and 3) the nonphotochromogens, such as MAC.[3]

On the basis of glycolipid typing, MAC has been divided into 28 serotypes, also referred to as serovars.[4] Serotypes 1 to 6 and 8 belong to *M avium* and serotypes 7, 12, 14, 16, and 18 to *M intracellulare.* The other serotypes remain unclassified. MAC infections in AIDS patients are almost exclusively caused by serotypes of *M avium.* Among AIDS patients in the United States, serotypes 4, 8, 1, and 6 are more common (in decreasing order of frequency), whereas in Sweden, serotype 6 is more common.[4,5] Among immunocompetent patients, infections by *M intracellulare* and *M avium* are almost of equal frequency.[6]

On the basis of restriction fragment length polymorphism (RFLP), *M avium* has been divided into two types: type A, isolated from tissues of most infections by MAC, and type A1, isolated from the wood pigeon and also from intestinal tissues of patients with inflammatory bowel disease, especially those with Crohn's disease.[7]

Conventional studies of RFLP employ endonucleases that result in large numbers of small chromosomal DNA fragments. These are used to assess genetic relatedness but do not allow strain-specific identification.[8] Large DNA restriction fragments (LRF) can be produced by digesting DNA with infrequently cutting endonucleases. Such LRF patterns have shown differences within identical serotypes of isolates from different patients but remained the same within different isolates from the same patient.[8]

Nucleotide sequence analysis allows the degree of difference between bacterial strains to be quantified.[9] The use of the variable 16S-23S and rDNA internal transcriber spacer (ITS) in the sequence analysis of MAC has defined four sequevars, Mav-A to D. All isolates from AIDS patients belonged to Mav-A or B and showed a high degree of relatedness when compared to sequevars from pulmonary sources of non-AIDS patients, which were genetically more diverse.[9]

GEOGRAPHIC DISTRIBUTION AND EPIDEMIOLOGY

Mycobacteria of the *M avium* complex are ubiquitous and have been isolated, worldwide, from soil, dust, freshwater, ocean water, animal feed, chickens and other birds, swine, sheep, and cattle.[9,10] The organism has been cultured also from the sputum, saliva, and urine of healthy persons in rural areas, or patients with nonmycobacterial lung disease. Certain serotypes seem to be nonpathogenic saprophytes, common in house dust.

Human infection with MAC is also worldwide and particularly frequent in Western Australia and Japan.[11] Before the AIDS pandemic, MAC in the United States was primarily known as a cause of pulmonary infections in the southeast, especially Georgia and Florida, where clinical and subclinical infections are common. More than 65% of healthy naval recruits from the southeastern and Gulf-bordering states reacted to tuberculin derived from *M intracellulare*.[12] Pulmonary infections were typically in elderly white men with underlying chronic lung disease such as chronic obstructive pulmonary disease, inactive or active tuberculosis, bronchiectasis, pneumoconiosis, chronic aspiration pneumonia, or bronchogenic carcinoma, and in patients who had undergone gastrectomy.[9] One fifth of patients had had thoracic operations and one third were under 60 years of age and without predisposing conditions.[11] More recently, pulmonary infections by MAC have been increasingly frequent in immunocompetent patients without predisposing conditions.[13] Between 24% and 46% have been among so-called "normal" persons, especially elderly women.[14] Among these "normal" persons, there is a high prevalence of pectus excavatum, causing a narrowed distance from sternum to vertebral column, of thoracic scoliosis, and of mitral-valve prolapse, suggesting that multisystem connective-tissue disorders may predispose to infection by MAC. The rising incidence in this population may reflect the increasing longevity of the general population, which enlarges the pool of vulnerable subjects, as well as the increasing virulence of the microorganism. Plasmid-associated enhancement of virulence among certain strains isolated from patients with AIDS has been documented,[15] a development that parallels the evolution of more virulent strains of *M tuberculosis* in the same clinical setting.

AIDS-related MAC infection is now a well-known complication that occurs relatively late in the course of AIDS and is usually disseminated by the time it is diagnosed. Disseminated MAC infection affected 5.7% of patients with AIDS between 1985 and 1988, and 15% to 24% in 1989–1990.[16] These figures underestimate the true incidence, since disseminated MAC is found at autopsy in more than 50% of those dying in the United States with AIDS.[17] In the United States, as of December 1990, an estimated 24,000 to 39,000 with AIDS were infected with MAC.[16] Initially only recognized at autopsy, MAC infection in AIDS was variously misinterpreted as either a colonizer of moribund patients not responsible for illness or, because of the histologic resemblance of the MAC-infested macrophage with the Whipple macrophage, as Whipple's disease.[18] In contrast to MAC infection in immunocompetent hosts, which tends to be mild and limited to lungs, MAC in AIDS is usually disseminated and contributes substantially to morbidity and mortality. Disseminated infection before the onset of the AIDS pandemic was so rare that only 24 cases were in the medical literature by 1980.[13] There is no difference in the frequency of disseminated MAC infection in AIDS according to gender or risk group in adults. In children, however, the overall incidence of disseminated MAC infection is much lower than in adults (11.4% versus 25%), and the incidence is significantly higher in hemophilia and transfusion-associated AIDS than in perinatally acquired AIDS (12.9% and 13.8% versus 4.6%).[19] Hispanic patients are less likely to be infected than non-Hispanic whites or blacks and the frequency declines with age.[13]

Regional differences in frequency are small in the United States, Europe, and Australia, indicating ubiquitous environmental exposure. It may be different in Africa, where rare infections have been reported,[16] but none was found in a survey of 50 patients with AIDS from Uganda.[20] Since MAC is in the African environment and human exposure proven by means of positive skin tests,[21] the reasons for the rarity of MAC infection in African patients with AIDS cannot be easily explained. Perhaps the high prevalence of tuberculosis and of BCG vaccination in Africa causes broad antimycobacterial immunity, which protects the patient from disseminated MAC. Furthermore, African AIDS patients may not live long enough to reach the stage of profound immune depression necessary for disseminated MAC.

MAC infection also occurs in patients with immunodeficiency states other than AIDS, such as malignant neoplasms[22] or prolonged steroid therapy,[23] but much less frequently so, suggesting that the immunologic defect in AIDS selectively favors MAC infection. Rarely, infection by MAC has been described in patients with bone marrow transplants, severe combined immunodeficiency,[24] renal transplant,[25] and eosinophilic granuloma of the femur treated with radiotherapy, chemotherapy, and steroids.[26] Patients with cystic fibrosis have a high yield of MAC from cultured sputum, especially in the southeastern United States,[27] but whether this reflects colonization or infection is not clear.

NATURAL HISTORY

Data derived from epidemiologic surveys indicate that MAC infection results from primary acquisition of the pathogen rather than reactivation of old disease.[10,20] The infection is acquired through ingestion or inhalation. In addition to dust, soil, water, and food, hot water systems contain MAC as do airborne particles generated and concentrated in showers, which have been implicated as the source of infection.[10] Pet birds were implicated as the source of infection in a child.[28]

Analyses of MAC strains using commercially available gene probes have shown that the vast majority of AIDS-related MAC infections (more than 90%) are due to *M avium* and of non-AIDS MAC infections to *M intracellulare.* Restriction fragment profiles have demonstrated multiple strains supporting the hypothesis that infection is acquired from environmental sources and not from other patients.[29] Bacteremic patients may be infected with more than one strain.

In immunocompetent hosts, asymptomatic colonization of the respiratory or gastrointestinal tracts may progress to an indolent infection, usually pulmonary.[2,4,6] In the southeastern part of the United States, pulmonary disease caused by MAC is now as common as pulmonary tuberculosis.[2] The disease tends to follow a slow, indolent, yet progressive course. Dissemination in non-AIDS patients is rare but may occur in patients treated with high doses of corticosteroids.[15]

In AIDS patients, symptomatic infection develops after an unknown duration of colonization late in the course. Colonization of the gastrointestinal tract is increasingly frequent as human immunodeficiency virus (HIV) infection progresses. MAC was isolated from feces of 1.3% of patients with symptomatic HIV infection and 14.8% of patients with full-blown AIDS.[30] No asymptomatic HIV seropositive or seronegative person was shown to harbor MAC in their gastrointestinal tract. MAC is isolated from the gastrointestinal tract twice as frequently as from the respiratory tract,[31] a finding in accordance with the experience in surgical pathology that gastrointestinal biopsies are much more likely to show the infection than lung biopsies.[32]

Retrospective studies have demonstrated that 30% to 60% of HIV-infected persons with respiratory MAC colonization and 80% of those with gastrointestinal MAC colonization progress to disseminated infection.[33] The major risk factor that determines progression is the mean number of CD4 cells. Infection is rare in patients with CD4 cell counts above 100/mm^3.[31] Most AIDS patients with disseminated MAC infection have CD4 cell counts of less than 60/mm^3.[16]

In a prospective study of AIDS patients with CD4 cell counts below 200/mm^3, one fifth developed bacteremia (23% per year). Only 21% of patients with MAC bacteremia, however, had evidence of previous colonization (such as positive sputum or stool cultures or positive acid-fast smears) within 3 or more months before bacteremia was demonstrated.[34] These studies suggest that the period of colonization before dissemination is variable and may be short, perhaps less than 3 months. The risk of developing disseminated MAC infections depends on the presence of colonization and the degree of immune suppression. For patients with no evidence of colonization and CD4 cell counts below 50 mm^3, the risk is 45%; for patients with evidence of colonization and the same CD4 cell counts, the risk rises to 60%.[35]

Symptomatic infection is rarely localized, although focal pneumonia[36] and localized gastrointestinal infections[37] have been reported in a small percent of patients prior to the development of disseminated disease. MAC is the most common systemic bacterial infection in AIDS[38] and was documented in virtually all initial AIDS patients who were autopsied.[39–41] Once disseminated, MAC can be in virtually every organ, typically within histiocytes, which phagocytose the mycobacteria, but are unable to kill them. Disseminated MAC infection in AIDS is associated with shortened survival, reducing average life expectancy to 4.1 months. AIDS patients without MAC infection have a median survival of 11.1 months.[42] The cause of death is rarely attributed directly to MAC infection, rather, it is malnutrition and severe immune suppression that hasten death from other infections.[16] Prolonged therapy with four or five agents is recommended and has provided symptomatic relief, clearing of bacteremia, and, rarely, has extended life for more than a year.[38]

MORPHOLOGIC AND MICROBIOLOGIC FEATURES

The mycobacteria of MAC are beaded rods, 4 to 6 μm long and less than 1 μm in diameter. They are acid fast and on smears stained with Ziehl–Neelson cannot be distinguished by virtue of their shape or size from other mycobacteria including *M tuberculosis.* Their intracellular location and their tendency to align themselves into stacks are distinctive features.

As do some other mycobacteria, MAC stain positively with the periodic acid–Schiff (PAS) technique. Carbohydrate residues of bacterial peptidoglycolipids, unique to MAC, are thought to be responsible for this reaction.[43] Mycobacteria, including MAC, also stain positively with Gomori's methenamine-silver (GMS) stain, which may give rise to confusion with fungi. The small size and lack of branching and budding, however, clearly distinguish MAC from fungi. The intensity of GMS staining of MAC is comparable to that of acid-fast staining in most tissues and may be even greater, except for bone marrow specimens in which decalcification procedures seem to diminish GMS staining intensity.[44]

With the immunoperoxidase technique, MAC stains strongly for cytoskeletal filaments (such as desmin, actin, and tubulin) and moderately for keratin.[45]

CLINICAL FEATURES

Since MAC can infect any organ and can infect immunocompetent as well as immunosuppressed patients, the clinical presentations are varied. Clinical features fall into three main categories: 1) patients without predisposing conditions, 2) patients with predisposing conditions other than AIDS, and 3) patients with AIDS. In groups 2 and 3, clinical features of the predisposing conditions may dominate and make it difficult to define clearly the symptoms of MAC infection.

Most immunocompetent patients without predisposing conditions develop pulmonary disease and present with persistent cough and purulent sputum, usually without fever or weight loss. Fever, when present, is low grade. Constitutional symptoms and features of chronic disease, such as anemia or leukocytosis, are usually absent. Chest x rays reveal slowly progressive nodular opacities (71%) and rarely cavitary disease, usually in more than one lobe, but occasionally restricted to the upper lobes.[1,11,13] In elderly women, isolated involvement of the lingula or middle lobe has been attributed to habitual voluntary suppression of cough and subsequent nonspecific inflammation in these poorly draining regions, predisposing them to MAC infection. The term "Lady Windermere's syndrome" has been suggested for this unique presentation.[46] In children, primary infection may produce lesions of lung and hilar lymph node, similar to the Ghon complex of tuberculosis.[28]

Several otherwise healthy patients have had tenosynovitis.[47] All involved wrist, hand, or digits and none had pulmonary disease or other evidence of dissemination. Isolated MAC infection of a chronic gastric ulcer was identified in one immunocompetent patient.[48]

Spinal osteomyelitis has been described, in the absence of lung disease, in an elderly patient with collagen vascular disease and steroid-induced osteoporosis.[49] Clinically indistinguishable from tuberculosis, the diagnosis was delayed for weeks until mycobacterial cultures grew MAC.

Arthritis is a rare presenting symptom of MAC infection in immunocompetent as well as immunosuppressed patients.[50] MAC peritonitis may complicate peritoneal dialysis,[51] alcoholic cirrhosis,[52] or AIDS.[53]

In AIDS patients, MAC infection is usually disseminated when first discovered and the symptoms reflect bacteremia and preferential involvement of the gastrointestinal tract. Symptoms include, in decreasing order of frequency, weight loss, fever accompanied by sweats and chills, diarrhea, and abdominal pain.[54] The mean duration of AIDS before the diagnosis of MAC is 7.7 months. The gastrointestinal tract is more often infected than the lungs, and endoscopy and biopsy usually yield a diagnosis. Other infections of GI tract coexist in more than 50% of patients and include infections with *Candida* sp, cytomegalovirus, *Cryptosporidia,* Herpes simplex, *Giardia lamblia, Campylobacter,* and *Salmonella* sp.[54] Malabsorption, as shown by an abnormal D-xylose absorption test, can be demonstrated in about one half of the patients.[54,55]

By endoscopy, fine white nodules may be in the duodenal mucosa but the majority of patients have no endoscopic abnormalities. Infection of the lower gastrointestinal tract is less frequent. Rarely, intestinal ulceration and hemorrhage[56] and isolated terminal ileitis[57] have been attributed to MAC. Mesenteric lymph nodes may be massively enlarged and present as a palpable mass and can cause intestinal obstruction secondary to compression, intussusception, or volvulus.[58] Enlarged cervical and axillary lymph nodes may present as pseudotumors.[45,59] Infection of spleen may cause splenomegaly and necessitate splenectomy.[60] Rarely described disseminated cutaneous infection reflects the bacteremic state and may be caused by dual mycobacterioses such as MAC and *M tuberculosis* or MAC and *M simiae.*[61]

Involvement of bone marrow is common and bone marrow biopsy and culture provide the diagnosis of MAC infection in the majority (72%) of patients.[62] Anemia, common in AIDS patients with or without MAC infections, is more profound in MAC-infected AIDS patients than in those not infected. MAC-infected macrophages secrete a soluble factor that is thought to suppress erythroid progenitor cells and thus impair erythropoiesis.[63]

Liver dysfunction is common in patients with AIDS and may be caused by MAC hepatitis. Mycobacterial infection is the most frequent diagnostic finding in liver biopsies of patients with AIDS (42%).[64] Depending on risk group, either *M tuberculosis* (IV drug abusers)[65] or MAC (homosexual men)[66] is the most commonly reported hepatic pathogen.

PATHOLOGY OF MAC INFECTION

Gross Features

There is no special gross feature of MAC infection that is uniformly present in all organs affected. Since the infection is focal, affected organs are often grossly normal. MAC pneumonia produces consolidation and nodules and rarely cavities.[1,11] Gastrointestinal involvement is characterized by yellow mucosal nodules and flattening of small intestinal villi.[54,55] Enlarged lymph nodes grossly resemble neoplasms, since they are solid and firm. Necrosis may be present but is focal.[45,59]

Microscopic Features

The light microscopic appearance of MAC infection differs according to the immune status of the patient. In immunocompetent patients, granulomas are typically present and may be non-necrotizing[47] or necrotizing.[1,13] Acid-fast bacilli are difficult to find. In patients with AIDS, well-formed granulomas are usually absent.

Regardless of severity or organ involved, MAC infection in patients with AIDS is characterized by aggregates of foamy or striated histiocytes containing mycobacteria. The severity of infection determines the number of mycobacteria and histiocytes. Massive infiltrates are commonly seen in the small bowel and lymph nodes (Figure 70–1). Singly scattered infected histiocytes are common in bone marrow, Kupffer's cells, and intestinal mucosa (Figure 70–2), but may be in any organ, often perivascular, reflecting hematogenous dissemination. Poorly formed granulomas composed of

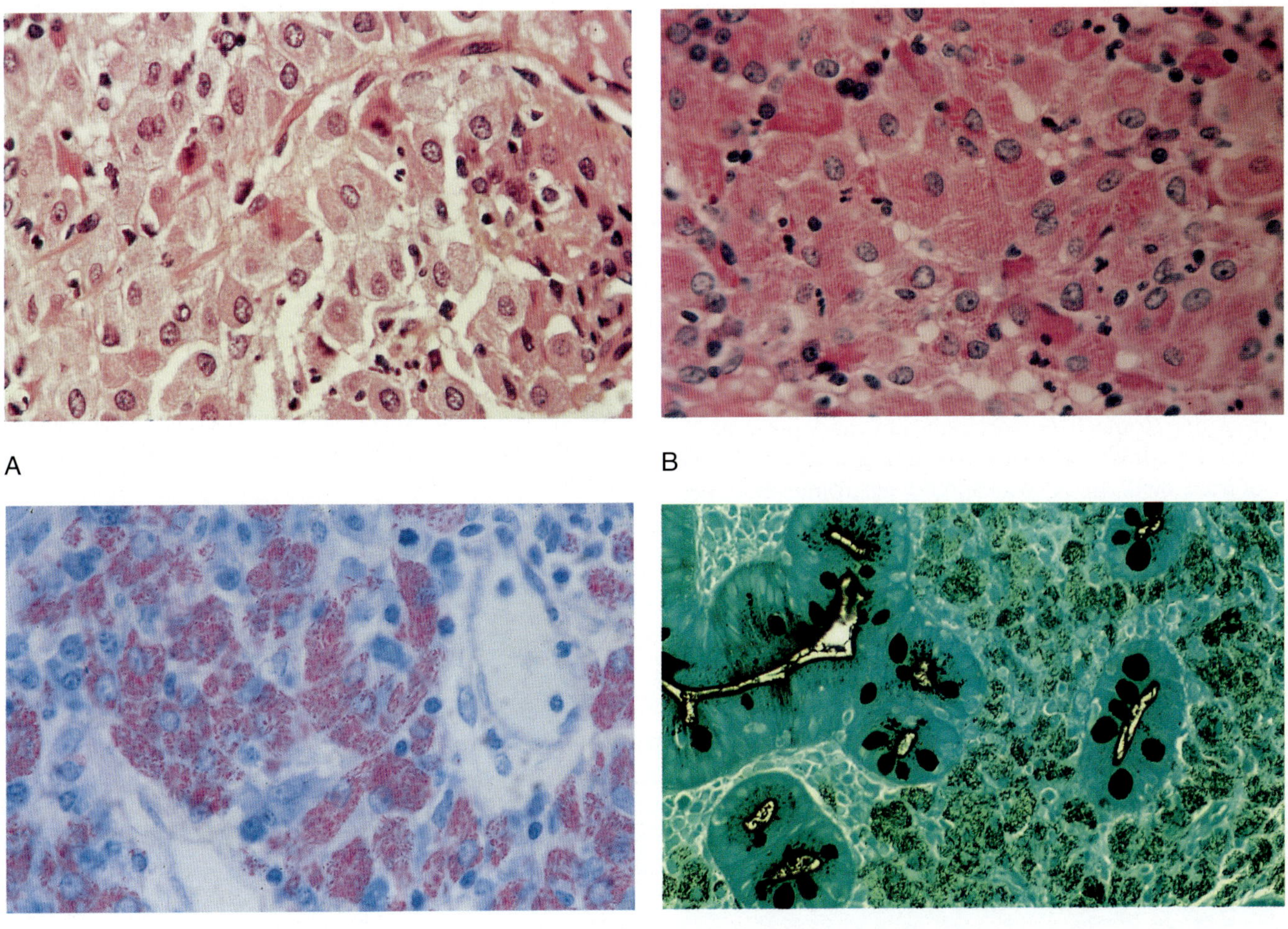

A B C D

Figure 70–1. MAC infection, histologic appearance. Diffuse histiocytic infiltrates are seen typically in the small bowel and lymph nodes. (**A**) On hematoxylin-eosin, the histiocytes are pale and have foamy or striated cytoplasm (hematoxylin-eosin, ×250). (**B**) With PAS, the striated cytoplasm is more evident and reflects the intracellular stacks of bacilli (PAS, ×250). (**C**) Acid-fast staining demonstrates numerous intracytoplasmic bacilli (Ziehl–Neelsen, ×250). (**D**) Bacilli are silvered with Gomori's methenamine-silver technique. Intestinal goblet cells stain black (GMS, ×250).

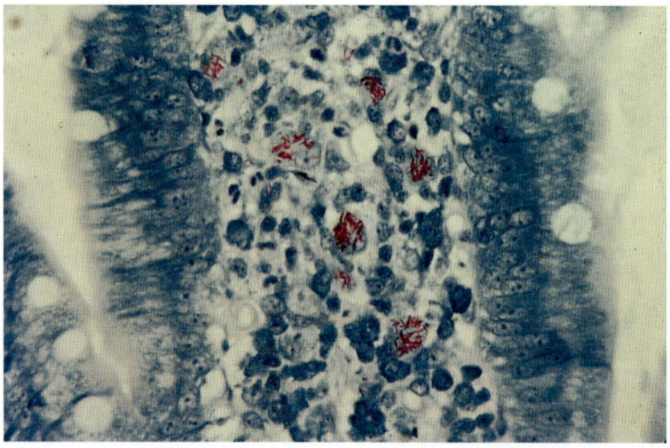

Figure 70–2. MAC infection of jejunum. Single infected histiocytes can be recognized only with the acid-fast stain (Ziehl–Neelsen, ×250).

epithelioid histiocytes and occasionally giant cells may be in bone marrow and liver (Figure 70–3). Intestinal involvement, in our experience, produces no granulomatous reaction but always a focal or diffuse histiocytic infiltrate.[67] In the proximal small bowel, the site most commonly and most severely infected, the histiocytic infiltrate may be so marked as to produce villous blunting and flattening of the mucosa, resembling Whipple's disease (Figure 70–4).[18] In the colon, histiocytic infiltrates are usually less marked. In one patient with massive involvement of the small and large intestines, however, a colostomy was done to manage diarrhea. The colon contained infected macrophages in all layers including the mesentery (personal observation). Infection of the stomach is extremely rare and presents as scattered foamy histiocytes containing acid-fast bacilli associated with more widespread gastrointestinal disease. Esophageal involvement is the least common type of gastrointestinal infection,[68] but may result in fistula formation.[69]

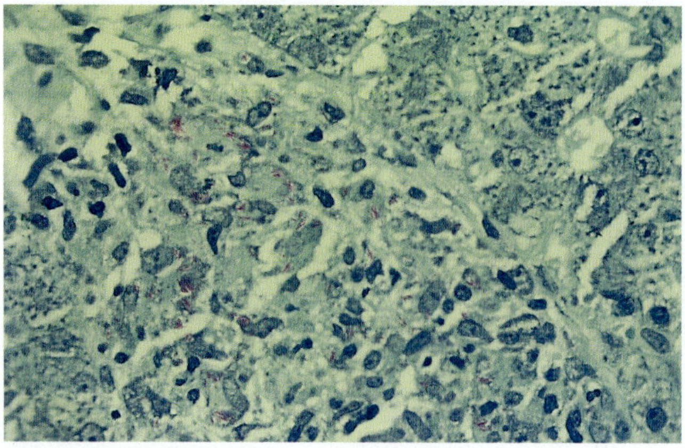

Figure 70–3. MAC infection of liver. Ill-defined granulomas containing MAC are typical for involvement of liver and bone marrow (Ziehl–Neelsen, ×200).

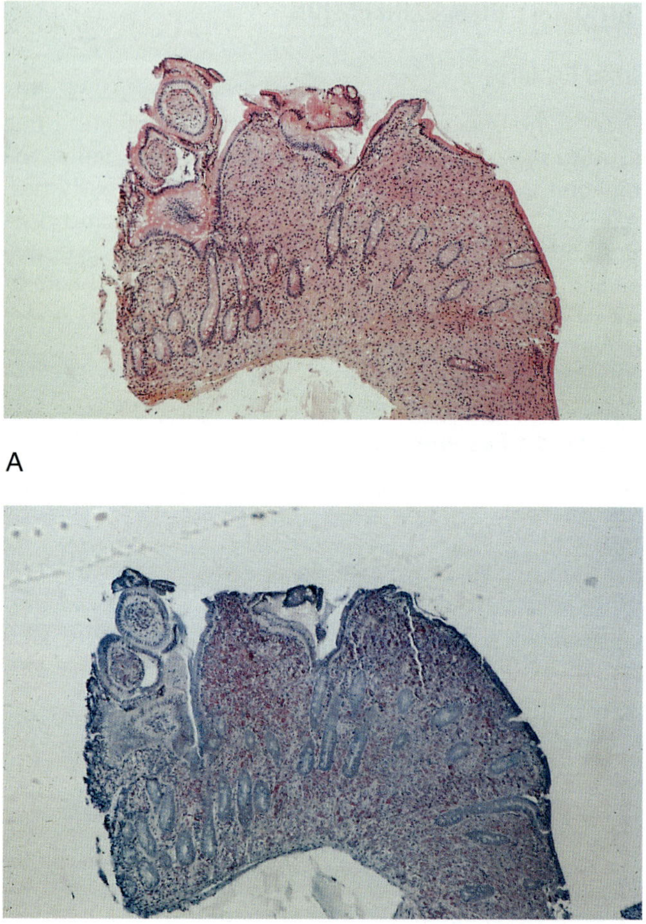

A

B

Figure 70–4. MAC infection of duodenum. (**A**) Massive histiocytic infiltrate expands the entire mucosa and flattens the villi, mimicking Whipple's disease (hematoxylin-eosin, ×40). (**B**) (Ziehl–Neelsen, ×40).

In lymph nodes, and occasionally in bone marrow, infected macrophages may appear spindly and mimic a spindle cell tumor, such as leiomyoma, fibrous histiocytoma, or epithelioid hemangioma (Figures 70–5 and 70–6).[59] Necrosis is usually absent but may be present in massively involved lymph nodes and in bone and soft tissue lesions.

Intrahistiocytic bacilli are conspicuous, acid-fast, PAS positive (Figure 70–1, B),[43] silvered with the GMS stain (Figure 70–1, D)[44] and are decorated by immunoperoxidase for desmin, actin, tubulin, and keratin.[45] In Romanowsky-stained bone marrow smears, extra- and intracellular bacilli are clear or red refractile bacilli or nonrefractile negative images.[70] Smears of bone mar-

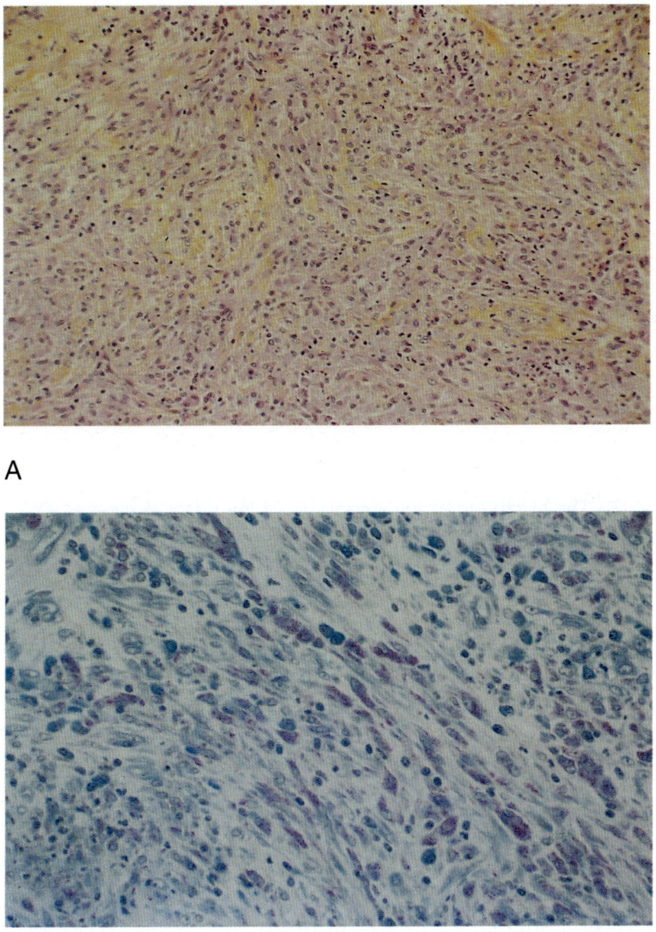

A

B

Figure 70–5. MAC infection of lymph node. (**A**) Compressed infected histiocytes appear spindly and may be mistaken for a spindle cell tumor (hematoxylin-eosin, ×100). (**B**) Acid-fast staining demonstrates numerous acid-fast bacilli in these spindle cells (Ziehl–Neelson, ×100).

row tend to be positive more often for MAC than are biopsy specimens. In Wright-stained peripheral blood smears, negatively stained linear bacilli are in monocytes and in neutrophils.[71]

CYTOPATHOLOGY OF MAC INFECTION

Enlarged lymph nodes are commonly sent for intraoperative consultation. Because frozen sections on tissue from HIV-infected patients carry the risk of contamination and the need of decontamination of the cryostat, most pathologists are reluctant to perform them. Cytologic preparations may enable an early specific diagnosis and allow for the subsequent correct handling of the specimen. Touch preparations of MAC-infected lymph nodes, stained with Diff-Quik show negatively stained bacilli as empty rod-shaped spaces or linear striations in histiocytes as well as extracellularly (Figure 70–7).[72] Fine-needle aspiration of mediastinal lymph nodes has also proven successful.[73]

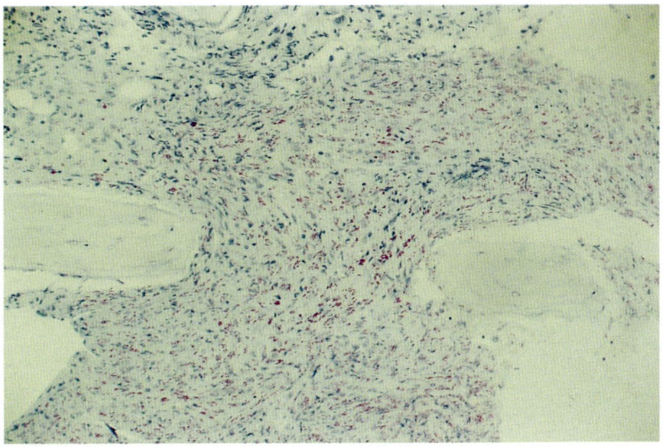

Figure 70–6. MAC infection of bone marrow. A geographic infiltrate of spindly histiocytes mimics a spindle cell tumor (Ziehl–Neelsen, ×100).

DIFFERENTIAL DIAGNOSIS OF MAC INFECTION

Biopsy specimens of small bowel stained with H&E and PAS resemble Whipple's disease. The similarity, both clinically and histopathologically, of these two conditions has been pointed out repeatedly.[18,74] Acid-fast stains, mandatory on all intestinal biopsy specimens from patients with AIDS, resolve any diagnostic confusion.

In biopsy specimens of lymph nodes, spindle-shaped histiocytes may be mistaken for fibroblasts, endothelial cells, or smooth muscle cells. Again, the acid-fast stain identifies the lesion as a mycobacterial infection rather than a spindle cell tumor.[45,59]

Alveolar macrophages in sputum or specimens taken by bronchoalveolar lavage may contain crystalline inclusions sometimes mistaken for intracellular mycobacteria. These are clofazimine crystals and have been described in alveolar macrophages of AIDS patients with MAC infection treated with a multidrug regimen, which includes clofazimine.[75] The crystals are red-orange and of variable shape and dissolve with oil immersion oil.

The main problem in the differential diagnosis of MAC infection involves the distinction of MAC from other mycobacteria. Distinguishing MAC from *M tuberculosis* is important, because treatment regimens differ markedly. Histopathologic features highly suggestive of

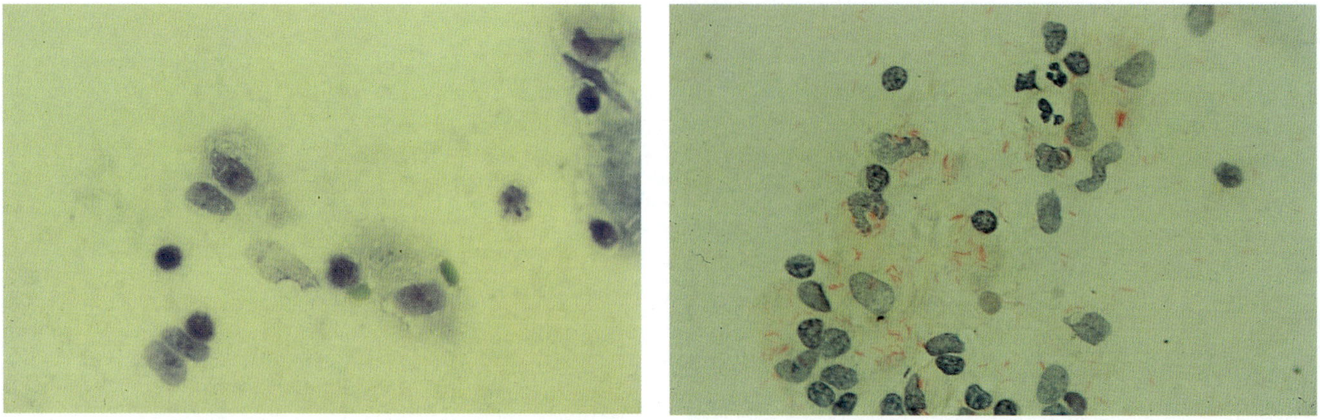

A B

Figure 70–7. Touch preparations of a MAC infected lymph node. (**A**) The striations of the cytoplasm of the infected histiocytes represent the negative image of the intracytoplasmic bacilli (Diff-Quik, ×400). (**B**) An acid-fast stain provides the positive image (Ziehl–Neelsen, ×400).

MAC infection include diffuse infiltrates of histiocytes, poorly formed granulomas, an abundance of intracellular bacilli, and, in a majority of patients, the absence of necrosis. Using these criteria, MAC infection could be distinguished from tuberculosis in 100% of intestinal biopsies and 83% of lymph nodes. In the bone marrow, the distinction is more difficult, because both *M tuberculosis* and MAC cause small non-necrotizing granulomas.[67]

Mycobacterium kansasii infection differs from MAC infection by producing well-formed necrotizing and non-necrotizing granulomas, sometimes associated with acute inflammation and necrosis.[72] In Diff-Quik-stained cytologic preparations, MAC and *M kansasii* have similar appearances but were distinguished on the basis of the greater length and more marked beading of *M kansasii* and its tendency to form long cords and coils from intertwining of bacilli.[72]

DIAGNOSIS BY CULTURE

Since MAC is a frequent contaminant of microbiologic cultures and may colonize the respiratory and gastrointestinal tracts without invasion, diagnostic criteria include both positive cultures and evidence of disease. For the immunocompetent host with pulmonary disease, the American Thoracic Society recommended the following diagnostic criteria in 1982: roentgenographic changes such as infiltrates, particularly asymmetric shadows or cavitation, isolation of multiple colonies of the same species, and absence of other potential pathogens.[76] More recently, it has been suggested that two or more isolations of MAC in the sputum in the first few days after onset of clinical disease are sufficient to make a diagnosis of MAC infection of lung.[77]

In AIDS patients, the diagnosis of MAC infection is based on either positive blood cultures or a tissue diagnosis of mycobacterial infection suggestive of MAC and confirmed by culture. Cultures of blood detect disseminated MAC infections in most patients. Blood cultures were positive in 45 of 46 and 24 of 25 patients with disseminated infection.[78,79] However, the minimum or optimum number of blood cultures required to detect MAC septicemia reliably has not been established. Using a special culture system for the recovery of MAC, called the Isolator (EI Du Pont de Nemours, Wilmington, Delaware) mycobacteremia could be demonstrated by two consecutive blood cultures in 98.2% of patients.[80] Recovery of MAC from blood cultures can be expedited by methods that involve radiometry and lysis centrifugation. The nonradiometric BACTEC NR 660 aerobic 6A blood culture medium uses infrared spectroscopy for detection of carbon dioxide released by metabolically active microorganisms and is especially useful in identifying MAC in blood cultures.[81] Differential susceptibilities of *M avium* and *M intracellulare* to sodium nitrite (*M intracellulare* grows in media containing sodium nitrite, *M avium* does not) can be used to subclassify strains.[82]

TISSUE DIAGNOSIS

The disadvantage of mycobacterial cultures is the 1 to 2 weeks required for growth. The more rapid identification of acid-fast bacilli in tissue sections or cytologic preparations (see earlier discussion), therefore, enables immediate diagnosis and treatment. As mentioned, MAC can be distinguished from *M tuberculosis* by virtue of its unique tissue reaction.[67,72] Biopsy specimens of the gastrointestinal tract, lymph nodes, and soft tissue are most likely to show changes characteristic of MAC infection.

DNA PROBES

The identification of MAC by microbiologic culture involves two steps: the primary culture and subsequent subcultures for biochemical testing. DNA probes applied to the primary culture eliminate the need for subcultures and biochemical testing and therefore allow for a more rapid diagnosis. The Gen-Probe culture confirmation test (Gen-Probe Corporation, San Diego, California) employs nucleic acid hybridization probes complementary to ribosomal mycobacterial RNA.[83] These I-labeled DNA probes are commercially available for the identification of *M avium, M intracellulare* (MAC), and *M tuberculosis.* When tested against a large number of other mycobacteria they proved highly specific. Cross-reactivity with *M paratuberculosis,* however, has been described.[84]

The alkaline-phosphatase-labeled DNA probe (SNAP) developed by Syngene, San Diego, California, includes three separate probes: A (*M avium*), I (*M intracellulare*), and X. The X probe hybridized with mycobacterial strains, which were identified as MAC by biochemical tests and mycolic acid analysis but not by either SNAP assays A nor I nor with the Gen-Probe assay.[85] Furthermore, a fourth group of mycobacteria, biochemically identified as MAC, failed to hybridize with either SNAP assays A, I, or X.[85] Thus, the use of DNA probes not only leads to more rapid isolation of MAC but also to the discovery of previously unrecognized strains. X-positive MAC strains were isolated exclusively from sputa of recent immigrants to the United States who presented with hemoptysis.[86] Although more than 90% of MAC isolates from HIV-infected patients are *M avium, M intracellulare* serotypes have recently been identified with increasing frequency.[86]

The chemiluminescent Accu Probe system employs acridinium ester as the probe label. Applied to BACTEC broth cultures containing MAC, sensitivity was 96% and specificity 100%.[87] Misdiagnosis of MAC by conventional culture and as *M tuberculosis* by Accu Probe, however, has been described.[88]

Cloning and sequencing of DNA fragments (DT1 and DT6) from *M avium* serotype 2 were successfully used to create DNA probes that hybridized with specific serovars (DT1 with serovars 2, 3, 7, 12 to 20, and 23 to 25; DT6 with serovars 1 to 6, 8 to 11, and 21).[89] Whether DT1- and DT6-derived oligonucleotides can be used as primers of a reliable diagnostic polymerase chain reaction (PCR) remains to be seen.

POLYMERASE CHAIN REACTION

Amplification of mycobacterial DNA fragments with the use of *M avium*-specific PCR primers and subsequent detection by hybridization with a radiolabeled probe has been successfully employed on MAC-infected blood specimens.[90] Sensitivity was 80%, with PCR inhibition accounting for culture-positive/PCR-negative cases. Specificity was 86%. The majority of patients that were positive by PCR but negative by culture tested positive with primers specific for the genus *Mycobacterium.* Thus, PCR appears to be more sensitive than culture. PCR has been successfully applied also to sputum specimens.[91] All culture-positive sputa were PCR positive. PCR proved superior to fluorescent antibody staining, which detected only 91% of culture-positive cases. PCR can detect as few as 10 copies of the mycobacterial genome and is completed in 48 hours.

CONFIRMATORY TESTING

Skin test antigens prepared from nontuberculous mycobacteria have been employed in epidemiologic studies but, as yet, have not proven useful for diagnosis. Although the sensitivity of a skin test antigen prepared from *M intracellulare* (PPD-B) made bioequivalent to PPD-T, derived from *M tuberculosis,* was high, the specificity was too low for clinical usefulness.[92]

Mycobacterial lipoproteins are important targets for host immune responses. The diagnostic usefulness of specific immunodiagnostic reagents reactive to a variety of cell-wall-related lipoproteins and the possibility of vaccine development are being explored.[93] Seroagglutination and monoclonal antibodies to glycolipid antigens have been used for the differentiation of serovars of MAC[94] and multilocus enzyme electrophoresis in association with serotyping for locating specific infection sources.[95]

Recently, nucleotide sequence data of the variable 16S-23S rDNA ITS defined six ITS sequences, each defining a MAC sequevar.[96] Disseminated disease-associated MAC strains belonged to two sequevars that differed in ITS sequence by only one nucleotide, whereas localized disease (mainly pulmonary) associated MAC strains belonged to a greater number of sequevars and showed greater variability in nucleotide sequence, among each other as well as in comparison to the disseminated disease-associated sequevars. Thus, ITS sequence analysis may become a useful diagnostic tool to differentiate virulent from less virulent strains of MAC.

Similarly, nucleotide sequence analysis isolated mycobacterial insertion sequences IS900 and IS901, which distinguish two distinct subtypes of MAC, differing in host range, virulence, plasmid possession, and serotyping antigens.[97]

TREATMENT AND PROGNOSIS

MAC organisms are generally resistant to available antituberculous drugs. All MAC strains are resistant to isoniazid, 81% are resistant to rifampin, and 64% to streptomycin. The mechanisms of drug resistance are currently under investigation. Preliminary data suggest that drug resistance is conferred by mutations in the ribosomal S12 protein.[98] Whereas early studies showed no convincing improvement in either microbiologic indicators of infection or survival, more recent trials with multiple agents including ethambutol, rifabutin, and amikacin administered over longer periods have demonstrated relief of symptoms, decrease in bacteremia and prolonged survival.[99,100] Patients with untreated disseminated MAC infection have a median survival of 4 months, compared to 11 months for treated patients.[99] Treatment with zidovudine has no influence on the frequency of MAC infection. Prophylactic treatment with rifabutin is recommended for the prevention of disseminated MAC infection in AIDS patients who have CD4 cell counts of less than $200/mm^3$.[101]

REFERENCES

1. Wolinsky E. Mycobacterial diseases other than tuberculosis. *Clin Infect Dis.* 1992;15:1–12.
2. Good RC. Isolation of nontuberculous mycobacteria in the United States, 1980. *J Infect Dis.* 1982;146:829–833.
3. Runyon EH. Whence mycobacteria and mycobacterioses. *Ann Intern Med.* 1971;75:467–468.
4. Tsang AY, Denner JC, Brenman PJ, et al. Clinical and epidemiological importance of typing of *Mycobacterium avium* complex isolates. *J Clin Microbiol.* 1992;30: 479–484.
5. Mc Fadden, Junze ZM, Portaels F, et al. Epidemiological and genetic markers, virulence factors and intracellular growth of *Mycobacterium avium* in AIDS. *Res Microbiol.* 1992;143:423–430.
6. Yamori S, Tsukamura M. Comparison of prognosis of pulmonary diseases caused by *Mycobacterium avium* and by *Mycobacterium intracellulare. Chest.* 1992;102: 89–90.
7. Mc Fadden J, Collins J, Beaman B, et al. Mycobacteria in Crohn's disease: DNA probes identify the wood pigeon strain of *Mycobacterium avium* and *Mycobacterium paratuberculosis* from human tissue. *J Clin Microbiol.* 1992;30:3070–3073.
8. Mazurek GH, Hartman S, Zhang Y, et al. Large DNA restriction fragment polymorphism in the *Mycobacterium avium–M. intracellulare* complex: a potential epidemiologic tool. *J Clin Microbiol.* 1993;31:390–394.
9. Von Reyn CF, Waddell RD, Eaton T, et al. Isolation of *Mycobacterium avium* complex from water in the United States, Finland, Zaire, and Kenya. *J Clin Microbiol.* 1993; 31:3227–3230.
10. Horsburgh Jr, CR. Epidemiology of mycobacterial diseases in AIDS. *Res Microbiol.* 1992;143:372–377.
11. Rosenzweig DY, Schlueter DP. Spectrum of clinical disease in pulmonary infection with *Mycobacterium avium-intracellulare. Rev Infect Dis.* 1981;3:1046–1051.
12. O'Brien RJ, Geiter LJ, Snider Jr, DE. The epidemiology of nontuberculous mycobacterial diseases in the United States: results from a national survey. *Am Rev Respir Dis.* 1987;135:1007–1014.
13. Prince DS, Petersen DD, Steiner RM, et al. Infection with *Mycobacterium avium* complex in patients without predisposing conditions. *N Engl J Med.* 1989;321:863–868.
14. Iseman MD. *Mycobacterium avium* complex and the normal host. *N Engl J Med.* 1989;321:896–898.
15. Gangadharam PR, Perumal VK, Crawford JT, et al. Association of plasmids and virulence of *Mycobacterium avium* complex. *Am Rev Respir Dis.* 1988;137:212–214.
16. Horsburgh CR Jr. *Mycobacterium avium* complex infection in the acquired immunodeficiency syndrome. *N Engl J Med.* 1991;324:1332–1338.
17. Whimbey E, Kiehn TE, Armstrong D. Disseminated *Mycobacterium avium-intracellulare* disease: diagnosis and therapy. *Curr Clin Top Infect Dis.* 1986;7:112–133.
18. Roth RI, Owen RL, Keren DF, et al. Intestinal infection with *Mycobacterium avium* in acquired immune deficiency syndrome (AIDS). Histological and clinical comparison with Whipple's disease. *Dig Dis Sci.* 1985;5: 497–504.
19. Horsburgh Jr. CR, Caldwell MB, Simonds RJ. Epidemiology of disseminated nontuberculous mycobacterial disease in children with acquired immunodeficiency syndrome. *Pedr Infect Dis J.* 1993;12:219–222.
20. Morrissey AB, Aisu TO, Falkinham JO, et al. Absence of *Mycobacterium avium* complex disease in patients with AIDS in Uganda. *J Acquir Immune Defic Syndr.* 1992;5: 477–478.
21. Von Reyn CF, Barber TW, Arbeit RD, et al. Evidence of previous infection with *Mycobacterium avium–Mycobacterium intracellulare* complex among healthy subjects: an international study of dominant mycobacterial skin test reactions. *J Infect Dis.* 1993;168:1553–1558.
22. Feld R, Bodey G, Groschel D. Mycobacteriosis in patients with malignant disease. *Arch Intern Med.* 1976;136: 67–70.
23. Horsburgh Jr. CR, Masson III UG, Farhi DC, et al. Disseminated infection with *Mycobacterium avium-intracellulare. Medicine (Baltimore).* 1985;64:36–48.
24. Ozkaynak MF, Lenarsky C, Kohn D, et al. *Mycobacterium avium-intracellulare* infections after allogeneic bone marrow transplantation in children. *Am J Ped Hematol Oncol.* 1990;12:220–224.
25. Sumrani N, Hong JH, Sommer BG. *Mycobacterial avium-intracellulare* infection of a renal allograft. *Clin Nephrol.* 1991;35:45–46.
26. DeBerker D, Paterson IC. Pulmonary *Mycobacterium avium-intracellulare* infection in eosinophilic granuloma. *Respir Med.* 1992;86:61–62.

27. Kilby JM, Gilligan PH, Yankaskas JR, et al. Nontuberculous mycobacteria in adult patients with cystic fibrosis. *Chest.* 1992;102:70–75.
28. Reich J. Primary pulmonary disease due to *Mycobacterium avium-intracellulare. Chest.* 1992;101:1447–1448.
29. Arbeit RD, Slutsky A, Barbara TW, et al. Genetic diversity among strains of *Mycobacterium avium* causing monoclonal and polyclonal bacteremia in patients with AIDS. *J Infect Dis.* 1993;167:1384–1390.
30. Hellyer TJ, Brown IN, Taylor MB, et al. Gastrointestinal involvement in *Mycobacterium avium-intracellulare* infection of patients with HIV. *J Infect.* 1993;26:55–66.
31. Wallace JM, Hannah JB. *Mycobacterium avium* complex infection in patients with the acquired immunodeficiency syndrome. *Chest.* 1988;93:926–932.
32. Vasquez M, Rotterdam H, Vamvakas E. Diagnostic yields of surgical specimens from patients with AIDS or at risk for AIDS. *Progr AIDS Pathol.* 1990;2:187–194.
33. Horsburgh Jr. CR, Metchock BG, Mc Gowan JE, et al. Clinical implications of recovery of *Mycobacterium avium* complex from the stool or respiratory tract of HIV-infected individuals. *AIDS.* 1992;6:512–514.
34. Havlik JA, Metchock BG, Thompson III SE, et al. A perspective evaluation of *Mycobacterium avium* complex colonization of the respiratory tracts of persons with human immunodeficiency virus infection. *J Infect Dis.* 1993;168:1045–1048.
35. Chin DP, Hopewell PC, Yajko DM, et al. *Mycobacterium avium* complex in the respiratory or gastrointestinal tract and the risk of *M avium* complex bacteremia in patients with human immunodeficiency virus infection. *J Infect Dis.* 1994;169:289–295.
36. Ruf B, Schuermann D, Berhmer W, et al. Pulmonary manifestations due to *Mycobacterium avium–Mycobacterium intracellulare* in AIDS patients. *Am Rev Resp Dis.* 1990;141(suppl);A611. Abstract.
37. Gray JR, Rabeneck L. Atypical mycobacterial infection of the gastrointestinal tract in AIDS patients. *Am J Gastroenterol.* 1989;84:1521–1524.
38. Young LS. *Mycobacterium avium. J Infect Dis.* 1988; 157:863–867.
39. Green JB, Sidhu GS, Lewin S, et al. *Mycobacterium avium-intracellulare*: a cause of disseminated life-threatening infection in homosexuals and drug abusers. *Ann Intern Med.* 1982;97:539–546.
40. Zakowsky P, Fligid S, Berlin GW, et al. Disseminated *Mycobacterium avium-intracellulare* infection in homosexual men dying of acquired immunodeficiency. *JAMA.* 1982;248:2980–2983.
41. Sohn CC, Schnoff RW, Kliewer KE, et al. Disseminated *Mycobacterium avium-intracellulare* infection in homosexual men with acquired cell-mediated immunodeficiency: a histologic and immunologic study of two cases. *Am J Clin Pathol.* 1983;79:247–252.
42. Horsburgh Jr. CR, Harlik JA, Thompson SE. Survival of AIDS patients with disseminated *Mycobacterium avium* complex infection (DMAC): a case control study. In: Final Program and Abstracts of the Sixth International Conference on AIDS; June 20–21, 1990; San Francisco; Vol I.
43. Pappolla MA, Mehta VT. PAS reaction stains phagocytosed atypical mycobacteria in paraffin sections. *Arch Pathol Lab Med.* 1984;108:372–373.
44. Beckman EN, Broussard Jr. WA, Genre CF. Methenamine silver positivity of the *Mycobacterium avium-intracellulare* complex. *J Infect Dis.* 1993;168:1338–1339.
45. Umlas J, Federman M, Crawford C, et al. Spindle cell pseudotumor due to *Mycobacterium avium-intracellulare* in patients with acquired immunodeficiency syndrome (AIDS). Positive staining of mycobacteria for cytoskeleton filaments. *Am J Surg Pathol.* 1991;15: 1181–1187.
46. Reich J, Johnson RE. *Mycobacterium avium* complex pulmonary disease presenting as an isolated lingular or middle lobe pattern. The Lady Windermere syndrome. *Chest.* 1992;101:1605–1609.
47. Meijer FE, Kroon FP, Dijkmans BAC, et al. Tenosynovitis due to *Mycobacterium avium-intracellulare:* a case report and a review of the literature. *Clin Exp Rheumatol.* 1992;10:169–171.
48. Cappell MS, Taunk JL. A chronic gastric ulcer refractory to conventional antiulcer therapy associated with localized gastric *Mycobacterium avium-intracellulare* infection. *Am J Gastroenterol.* 1991;86:654.
49. Pirofsky JG, Huang C-T, Waites KB. Spinal osteomyelitis due to *Mycobacterium avium-intracellulare* in an elderly man with steroid-induced osteoporosis. *Spine.* 1993;18:1926–1929.
50. Vinetz JM, Rickman LS. Chronic arthritis due to *Mycobacterium avium* complex infection in a patient with the acquired immunodeficiency syndrome. *Arthritis Rheum.* 1991;1339–1340.
51. Pulliam JP, Vernon DD, Alexander SR, et al. Nontuberculous mycobacterial peritonitis associated with continuous ambulatory peritoneal dialysis. *Am J Kidney Dis.* 1983; 2:610–614.
52. Fernandez-Miranda C, Medina J, Palenque E, et al. Peritonitis with *Mycobacterium avium* in a patient with hepatic cirrhosis. *Am J Gastroenterol.* 1993;88:615. (Letter).
53. Perazella M, Eisen T, Brown E. Peritonitis associated with disseminated *Mycobacterium avium* complex in an acquired immunodeficiency syndrome patient on chronic ambulatory peritoneal dialysis. *Am J Kidney Dis.* 1993;21:319–321.
54. Gray JR, Rabeneck L. Atypical mycobacterial infection of the gastrointestinal tract in AIDS patients. *Am J Gastroenterol.* 1989;84:1521–1524.
55. Gillin JS, Shike M, Alcock N, et al. Malabsorption and mucosal abnormalities of the small intestine in the acquired immunodeficiency syndrome. *Ann Intern Med.* 1985;102:619–622.
56. Cappell MS, Gupta A. Gastrointestinal hemorrhage due to gastrointestinal *Mycobacterium avium-intracellulare* or esophageal candidiasis in patients with the acquired immunodeficiency syndrome. *Am J Gastroenterol.* 1992; 87:224–229.
57. Schneebaum CW, Novick DM, Chabon AB, et al. Terminal ileitis associated with *Mycobacterium avium-intracellulare* infection in a homosexual man with acquired immunodeficiency syndrome. *Gastroenterology.* 1987;92: 1127–1132.

58. Cappell MS, Hassan T, Rosenthal S, et al. Gastrointestinal obstruction due to *Mycobacterium avium-intracellulare* associated with the acquired immunodeficiency syndrome. *Am J Gastroenterol.* 1992;87:1823–1827.
59. Chen KTK. Mycobacterial spindle cell pseudotumor of lymph nodes. *Am J Surg Pathol.* 1982;16:276–281.
60. Mathew A, Raviglione MC, Niranjan U, et al. Splenectomy in patients with AIDS. *Am J Hematol.* 1989;32: 184–189.
61. Lombardo P, Weitzman I. Isolation of *Mycobacterium tuberculosis* and *M avium* complex from the same skin lesions in AIDS. *N Engl J Med.* 1990;323:916–917.
62. Nicholas L, Florentine B, Lewis W, et al. Bone marrow examination for the diagnosis of mycobacterial and fungal infections in the acquired immunodeficiency syndrome. *Arch Pathol Lab Med.* 1991;115:1125–1132.
63. Gascon P, Sathe SS, Rameshwar P. Impaired erythropoiesis in the acquired immunodeficiency syndrome with disseminated *Mycobacterium avium* complex. *Am J Med.* 1993;94:41–48.
64. Cappell MS, Schwartz MS, Bempica L. Clinical utility of liver biopsy in patients with serum antibodies to the human immunodeficiency virus. *Am J Med.* 1990;88: 123–130.
65. Comer GM, Mukherjee S, Scholes JV, et al. Liver biopsies in the acquired immune deficiency syndrome. Influence of endemic disease and drug abuse. *Am J Gastroenterol.* 1989;84:1525–1531.
66. Schneiderman DJ, Arenson DM, Cello JP, et al. Hepatic disease in patients with the acquired immune deficiency syndrome (AIDS). *Hepatology.* 1987;7:925–930.
67. Yee HT, Doniguian AE, Della-Latta P, et al. Mycobacterial infections: a correlative study of culture and tissue diagnoses. In: Platform Presentation, US and Canadian Academy of Pathology; March 10, 1994; San Francisco.
68. Bonacini M, Young T, Laine L. The causes of esophageal symptoms in human immunodeficiency virus infection. *Arch Intern Med.* 1991;151:1567–1572.
69. DeSilva R, Stoopack PM, Raufman JP. Esophageal fistulas associated with mycobacterial infection in patients at risk for AIDS. *Radiology.* 1990;175:449–453.
70. Torlakovic E, Clayton F, Ames E. Refractile mycobacteria in Ramanowsky-stained bone marrow smears. *Am J Clin Pathol.* 1992;97:318–321.
71. Godwin JH, Stopeck A, Chang VT, et al. Mycobacteremia in acquired immunodeficiency syndrome. *Am J Clin Pathol.* 1991;95:369–375.
72. Jannotta FS, Sidaway MK. The recognition of mycobacterial infections by intraoperative cytology in patients with acquired immunodeficiency syndrome. *Arch Pathol Lab Med.* 1989;113:1120–1123.
73. Baron KM, Aranda CP. Diagnosis of mediastinal mycobacterial lymphadenopathy by transbronchial needle aspiration. *Chest.* 1991;100:1723–1724.
74. Gillin JA, Urmacher C, West R, et al. Disseminated *Mycobacterium avium-intracellulare* infection in acquired immunodeficiency syndrome mimicking Whipple's disease. *Gastroenterology.* 1983;85:1187–1191.
75. Sandler ED, Ng VL, Hadley K. Clofazimine crystals in alveolar macrophages from a patient with the acquired immunodeficiency syndrome. *Arch Pathol Lab Med.* 1992;116:541–543.
76. Ahn CH, McLarty JW, Ahn SS, et al. Diagnostic criteria for pulmonary disease caused by *Mycobacterium kansasii* and *Mycobacterium intracellulare. Am Rev Resp Dis.* 1982;125:388–391.
77. Tsukamura M. Diagnosis of disease caused by *Mycobacterium avium* complex. *Chest.* 1991:99:667–669.
78. Kiehm TE, Edwards FF, Brannon P, et al. Infections caused by *Mycobacterium avium* complex in immunocompromised patients: diagnosis by blood culture and fecal examination, antimicrobial susceptibility tests and morphological and seroagglutination characteristics. *J Clin Microbiol.* 1985;21:168–173.
79. Hawkins CC, Gold JWM, Whimbey E, et al. *Mycobacterium avium* complex infections in patients with the acquired immunodeficiency syndrome. *Ann Intern Med.* 1986;105:184–188.
80. Yagupsky P, Menegus MA. Cumulative positive rates of multiple blood cultures for *Mycobacterium avium-intracellulare* and *Cryptococcus neoformans* in patients with the acquired immunodeficiency syndrome. *Arch Pathol Lab Med.* 1990;114:923–925.
81. Motyl MR, Saltzman B, Levi MH, et al. The recovery of *Mycobacterium avium* complex and *Mycobacterium tuberculosis* from blood specimens of AIDS patients using the nonradiometric BACTEC NR 660 medium. *Am J Clin Pathol.* 1990;94:84–86.
82. Katsumasa S, Tomioka H, Saito H. Differential susceptibilities of *Mycobacterium avium* and *Mycobacterium intracellulare* to sodium nitrite. *J Clin Microbiol.* 1992;30:2994–2995.
83. Body BA, Warren NG, Spicer A, et al. Use of Gen-Probe and BACTEC for rapid isolation and identification of mycobacteria. *Am J Clin Pathol.* 1990;93:415–420.
84. Thoresen OF, Saxegaard F. Gen-Probe rapid diagnostic system for the *Mycobacterium avium* complex does not distinguish between *Mycobacterium avium* and *Mycobacterium paratuberculosis. J Clin Microbiol.* 1991;29: 625–626.
85. Woodley CL, Floyd MM, Silcox VA. Evaluation of Syngene DNA-DNA probe assays for the identification of the *Mycobacterium tuberculosis* complex and the *Mycobacterium avium* complex. *Diagn Microbiol Infect Dis.* 1992;15:657–662.
86. Cregan P, Yajko DM, Ng VL, et al. Use of DNA probes to detect *Mycobacterium intracellulare* and "X" mycobacteria among clinical isolates of *Mycobacterium avium* complex. *J Infect Dis.* 1992;66:191–194.
87. Evans KD, Nakasone AS, Sutherland PA, et al. Identification of *Mycobacterium tuberculosis* and *Mycobacterium avium-intracellulare* directly from primary BACTEC cultures by using acridinium ester-labeled DNA probes. *J Clin Microbiol.* 1992;30:2427–2431.
88. Bull TJ, Shanson DC. Rapid misdiagnosis by *Mycobacterium avium-intracellulare* masquerading as tuberculosis in PCR/DNA probe tests. *Lancet.* 1992;340:1360.
89. Thierry D, Vincent V, Clement F, et al. Isolation of specific DNA fragments of *Mycobacterium avium* and their

possible use in diagnosis. *J Clin Microbiol.* 1993;31: 1048–1054.

90. Iralu JV, Srithavan VK, Pieciak WS, et al. Diagnosis of *Mycobacterium avium* bacteremia by polymerase chain reaction. *J Clin Microbiol.* 1993;31:1811–1814.
91. Snyder S, Viscot B, Miller C, et al. PCR increases the sensitivity of mycobacterial culture and staining in sputum. In: 93rd General Meeting of the American Society for Microbiology; Atlanta, Georgia; 1993. Abstract 159774.
92. Huebmer RE, Schein MF, Cauthen GM, et al. Evaluation of the clinical usefulness of mycobacterial skin test antigens in adults with pulmonary mycobacteriosis. *Am Rev Resp Dis.* 1992;145:1160–1166.
93. Nair J, Rouse DA, Morris SL. Nucleotide sequence analysis and serologic characterization of a 27-kilodalton *Mycobacterium intracellulare* lipoprotein. *Infect Immun.* 1993;61:1074–1081.
94. Denner JC, Tsang AY, Chatterjee D, et al. Comprehensive approach to identification of serovars of *Mycobacterium avium* complex. *J Clin Microbiol.* 1992;30:473–478.
95. Yakrus MA, Reeves MW, Hunter S. Characterization of isolates of *Mycobacterium avium* serotypes 4 and 8 from patients with AIDS by multilocus enzyme electrophoresis. *J Clin Microbiol.* 1992;30:1472–1478.
96. Frothingham R, Wilson KH. Molecular phylogeny of the *Mycobacterium avium* complex demonstrates clinically meaningful divisions. *J Infect Dis.* 1994;169:305–312.
97. Kunze ZM, Portaels F, McFadden JJ. Biologically distinct subtypes of *Mycobacterium avium* differ in possession of insertion sequence IS 901. *J Clin Microbiol.* 1992;30: 2366–2372.
98. Nair J, Rouse D, Morris S. Nucleotide sequence analysis of the ribosomal S12 gene of *Mycobacterium intracellulare. Nucl Acid Res.* 1993;21:1039.
99. Horsburgh CR, Havlik JA, Ellis DA, et al. Survival of patients with acquired immune deficiency syndrome and disseminated *Mycobacterium avium* complex infection with and without antimycobacterial chemotherapy. *Am Rev Resp Dis.* 1991;144:557–559.
100. Jorup-Ronstrom C, Julander I, Petrini B. Efficacy of triple drug regimen of amikacin, ethambutol and rifabutin in AIDS patients with symptomatic *Mycobacterium avium* complex infection. *J Infect.* 1993;26:67–70.
101. Nightingdale SD, Cameron DW, Gordin FM, et al. Two controlled trials of rifabutin prophylaxis against *Mycobacterium avium* complex infection in AIDS. *N Engl J Med.* 1993;329:828–833.

CHAPTER 71

Mycobacterium marinum Infections

Shukdeo Sankar and Princy N. Kumar

Make haste and use all new remedies before they lose their effectiveness.

Sir William Withey Gull (1816–1890)

INTRODUCTION

Mycobacterial infections other than those caused by *Mycobacterium tuberculosis* have been increasingly recognized during the last 15 years.[1] This is in part attributable to the growing population of patients who are immunodeficient. *Mycobacterium marinum* causes disseminated infection in immunodeficient hosts.[2,3] In those with competent immunity, it usually causes localized infections of the limbs and is often referred to as "swimming pool granuloma" and "fish tank granuloma."

HISTORY

Mycobacterium marinum was first isolated in 1926 by Aronson[4] from tubercles of dead fish at the Philadelphia aquarium. Infected fish may develop a disseminated granulomatous disease (fish tuberculosis) that causes wasting and ultimately death. Norden and Linell,[5] in 1951 isolated a new mycobacterium from swimming pools that was named *Mycobacterium balnei.* They subsequently isolated the same organism from skin lesions of swimmers in Sweden.[6] *Mycobacterium marinum* and *M balnei* were later found to be identical and are now called *M marinum.*

EPIDEMIOLOGY

Mycobacterium marinum is a Runyon Group I photochromogen. It lives in marine life of both saltwater and freshwater. Patients with localized infections frequently have had puncture wounds while in or around open bodies of water. Others have had traumatic contact with marine life[7] and some have had minor traumas while cleaning aquariums.[8] Shrimp, snails, and water fleas, however, have been reported to be vectors of *M marinum* and to have caused human infection.[9]

MICROBIOLOGY

As a photochromogen, *M marinum* prefers cooler temperatures and grows optimally at 30 to 32°C. It may grow poorly or not at all at 37°C, temperatures often used for incubating mycobacteria. At optimum temperatures, it usually grows in 7 to 14 days. It shares a variety of antigens with other mycobacteria including *M tuberculosis.* Most strains are resistant to isoniazid (INH) in vitro.

CLINICAL FEATURES

Mycobacterium marinum infects all age groups. Men are more commonly infected than women. Most patients, as noted earlier, have been exposed to marine life while fishing, diving, swimming, boating, or cleaning fish tanks. The clinical presentations of infection by *M marinum* tend to be similar. Infection involves skin and sometimes underlying structures and is usually confined to one limb. The hand is the most common site, but the elbows, knees, and foot are other recognized sites of involvement.[10] Superficial infections are more common than deep infections, probably because *M marinum* grows optimally at temperatures below the body's normal core temperature. In spite of this *M marinum* is a relatively common cause of tenosynovitis.[7] Patients with tenosynovitis may be mistreated for ex-

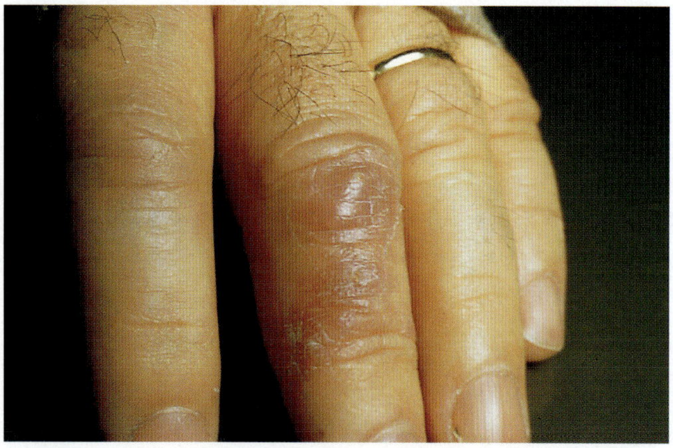

Figure 71–1. Adult male patient whose middle phalanx is infected with *M marinum*. The patient had cleaned and scraped the inside of a fish tank. The lesion is papular, erythematous, has ill-defined borders, and was associated with lymphangitis. *(Photograph contributed by Jeffrey D. Hubbard, MD, and Ernest E. Lack, MD.)*

tended periods before the correct diagnosis is made.[11] Osteomyelitis,[12] infection of larynx,[13] sclerokeratitis,[14] and disseminated infections[2,3] have all been described.

The incubation period is usually 2 to 4 weeks. The typical presentation is a single papulonodular lesion (Figure 71–1) with pain, swelling, and warmth. One patient had numbness and tingling.[15] With time, the lesion may become verrucous or ulcerated. Some patients have presented with multiple nodules along lymphatics. This nodular lymphangitis[16] is often referred to as the sporotrichoid form of *M marinum* infection. There are some claims that surgical exploration may precipitate rapid lymphatic spread.[8] Patients with superficial infections tend to have minimal symptoms. They may complain only of a cosmetic deformity or may have mild, persistent pain or itching in the affected area of infection. Patients with tenosynovitis may have pain and limited movement of fingers and hands. Tenderness and swelling may be present early in the course. Chronic infection may cause significant deformity[16] and there may be a draining sinus. Paresthesias and other symptoms of carpal tunnel syndrome may be a feature of tenosynovitis caused by *M marinum*. Patients are usually afebrile and regional nodes are not enlarged or tender.

PATHOLOGY

A broad range of inflammatory changes is seen in lesions produced by *M marinum*[15] and this range is seen in infections of skin and synovial tissues. In spite of this a characteristic synovitis has been described in one series.[17] Rice bodies in a synovial specimen taken at surgical exploration should alert the pathologist to the possibility of *M marinum*.[16]

Granulomas are in most specimens but sometimes these are poorly formed. Varying degrees of acute or subacute inflammation and subtle granulomatous changes may be present[15] (Figure 71–2, A). Well-formed granuloma when present are usually non-necrotizing and noncaseating. Foreign body reactions or even suppuration may be present. Langhans' giant cells are occasionally present (Figure 71–2, B) and to some extent the reaction depends on the age of the lesion.

With synovitis, there is synovial proliferation with hypertrophy of the lining cells. Fibrin may cover synovial surfaces. The synovium is thickened by a lymphohistiocytic infiltrate with a relative paucity of plasma cells. Giant cells of both Langhans' and foreign body

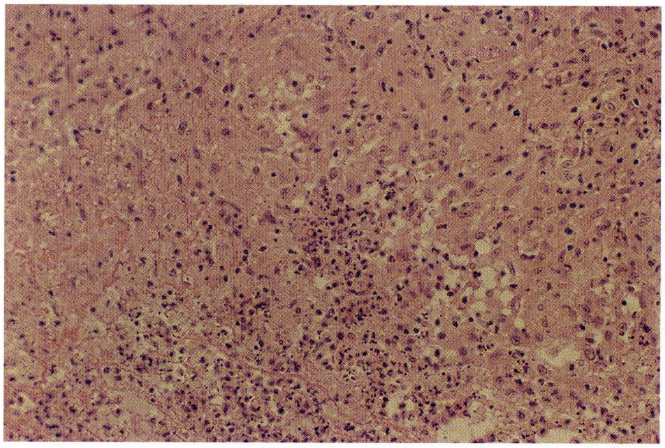

A

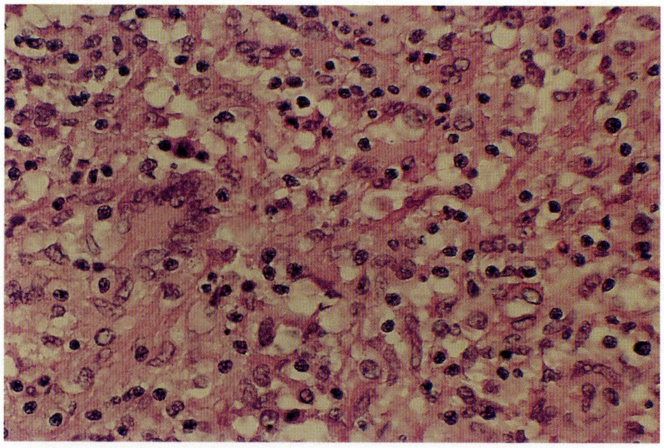

B

Figure 71–2. *Mycobacterium marinum* infection. **(A)** The reaction is granulomatous mixed with a few neutrophils seen in the lower portion of the field (hematoxylin-eosin, ×120). **(B)** Chronic inflammatory cells are scattered among epithelioid histiocytes. Note the Langhans' giant cell on the left (hematoxylin-eosin, ×350).

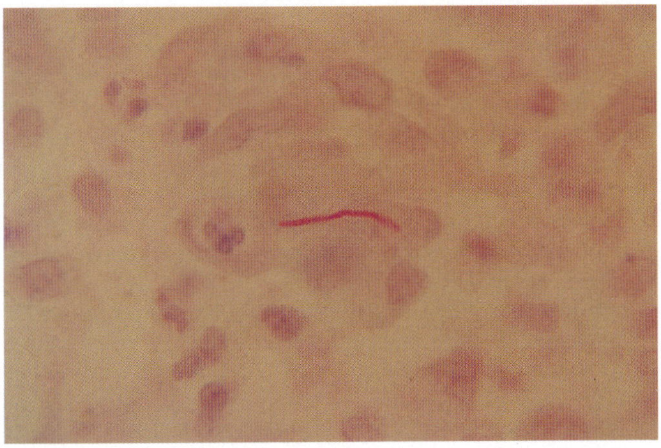

Figure 71–3. Infection with *M marinum*. Rare acid-fast bacilli are in epithelioid histiocytes (Ziehl–Neelsen, ×1000).

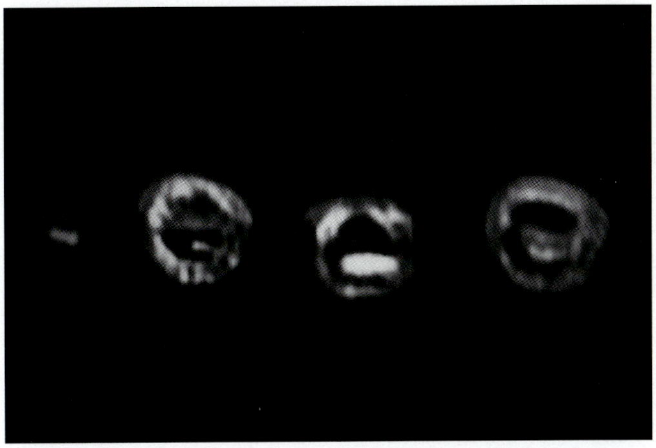

Figure 71–4. MRI of middle phalanx infected with *M marinum*. On the T_2-weighted axial image, there is soft tissue swelling of the second, fourth, and to a lesser extent the fifth digit. Similar changes are around the flexor digitorum superficialis tendons.

types may be present. Granulomas vary in quality, number, and distribution but are usually well defined and without caseation.[17] This combination of microscopic features resembles those of sporotrichosis and other deep fungal infections.

Acid-fast bacilli are few and thus usually difficult to find even with well-stained preparations (Figure 71–3). In one series of soft tissue infections only 2 of 24 biopsy specimens contained demonstrable acid-fast bacilli.[18] In another series of *M marinum* synovitis, only 1 of 8 specimens contained demonstrable acid-fast bacilli.[17] This yield may be greatly increased if multiple sections are studied and searched by a pathologist experienced in finding acid-fast bacilli.

DIAGNOSIS

The diagnosis is suspected when the patient gives an appropriate history and has characteristic clinicopathologic features and the diagnosis is confirmed by culture and/or by identifying acid-fast bacilli in the lesions. A high index of suspicion should be maintained because infection by *M marinum* tends to be unfamiliar to those outside the specialties of dermatology, infectious disease, and hand surgery.

A specific history of antecedent trauma, contact with fish, or keeping an aquarium should be sought. In one series of deep infections of the hand, 16 of 24 patients had a puncture wound from contact with a fish, crabs, or shrimp, and only three had no contact with fish.[7] In another series of skin infections,[18] 16 of 31 patients had been exposed to fish tanks (52%). There may be a history of ill or dead fish in the aquarium or of cleaning the fish tank ungloved and/or with broken skin.[8]

Laboratory studies are not helpful. White blood cell counts are normal as are sedimentation rates. Biopsy and culture are essential in making the diagnosis. Routine bacterial, fungal, and mycobacterial smears and cultures should be done. Cultures should be incubated at 30 to 32°C as well as the usual temperature of 37°C. If cultures are incubated at 37°C, the organism may grow slowly or not at all. (This is a common cause of failure of *M marinum* to grow.) Imaging procedures such as magnetic resonance imaging (MRI) are helpful in the diagnosis (Figure 71–4).[19]

The pathologist should be forewarned about possible *M marinum* infection so multiple sections can be searched for acid-fast bacilli (AFB). Due to the paucity of AFB in this infection, mycobacterial stains are usually negative underlying the utmost importance of appropriate cultures.

Skin testing is not helpful in diagnosis. The PPD for *M tuberculosis* is often positive. Specific testing with *M marinum* antigens is also unhelpful since patients with *M marinum* infection involving deep tissues appear to have an antigen-specific T-cell anergy.[20]

DIFFERENTIAL DIAGNOSIS

The most common diagnostic pitfall is mistaking multinodular *M marinum* for sporotrichosis. Other causes of nodular lymphangitis includes nocardiosis, leishmaniasis, and tularemia.[16] Rare causes include *M chelonei, M kansasii,* and fungal infections including blastomycosis, coccidiomycosis, and cryptococcosis.

The differential diagnosis of granulomatous synovitis also includes sarcoidosis, foreign body granulomas, brucellosis, fungal diseases, Crohn's disease, tuberculosis, and other "atypical" mycobacterial infections.[17]

TREATMENT

There are no controlled studies to determine the best treatment for *M marinum* infections and this may persist because of the low frequency of infection. Treatment is based on clinical experience. The most commonly used agents are TMP–SMX, the tetracyclines including minocycline, amikacin, and the antituberculosis agents. In reviewing the literature the best regimen seems to be rifampin 600 mg/day and ethambutol at approximately 15 mg/kg/day.[21] *Mycobacterium marinum* infections usually resist INH and pyrazinamide. There appears to be a higher failure rate with minocycline than with the combination of rifampin and ethambutol.[18]

There is even less agreement about the optimum duration of therapy. This has ranged from a few weeks to 18 months. Treatment with rifampin and ethambutol for 6 to 9 months appears to be sufficient. With deep seated infections, eg, tenosynovitis, it seems wise to err on the side of a longer course of treatment. Some authors advocate treating skin and soft tissue infections for 3 to 6 months or for 4 to 6 weeks after the lesion has disappeared. Clinical response is variable and there may be no improvement for 3 weeks.[21]

In addition to medical therapy, surgery may have a role in deep-seated infections, eg, tenosynovitis for debridement, synovectomy, and obtaining adequate specimens for pathologic examination and for culture.

PREVENTION

Fish fanciers should know this infection can be acquired from their hobby. Sick and dead fish should be handled carefully. Gloves should be worn before cleaning fish tanks especially if breaks on the skin are present.

REFERENCES

1. Wolinsky E. Mycobacterial diseases other than tuberculosis. *Clin Infect Dis.* 1992;15:1–12.
2. Enzenauer RJ, McKoy J, Vincent D, Gates R. Disseminated cutaneous and synovial *Mycobacterium marinum* infection in a patient with SLE. *South Med J.* 1990;83(4): 471–474.
3. Gombert MD, Goldstein EJC, Corrado ML, et al. Disseminated *Mycobacterium marinum* infection after renal transplantation. *Ann Intern Med.* 1981;94:486–487.
4. Aronson JD. Spontaneous tuberculosis in saltwater fish. *J Infect Dis.* 1926;39:315–320.
5. Norden A. Linell F. A new type to pathogenic mycobacteria. *Nature.* 1951;168:826.
6. Linell F, Norden A. *Mycobacterium balnei:* a new acid-fast bacillus occurring in swimming pools and capable of producing skin lesions in humans. *Acta Tuberc Scand.* 1954;33(suppl):1–84.
7. Chow SP, Ip FK, Lau JH, et al. *Mycobacterium marinum* infection of the hand and wrist. Results of conservative treatment in twenty-four cases. *J Bone Joint Surg (Am).* 1987;69:1161–1168.
8. Gray SF, Stanwell Smith R, Reynolds NJ, Williams EW. Fish tank granuloma. *Br Med J.* 1990;300:1069–1070.
9. Huminer D, Pitlik SD, Block C, et al. Aquarium-borne *Mycobacterium marinum* skin infection. Report of a case and review of the literature. *Arch Dermatol.* 1986;122: 698–703.
10. Woods GL, Washington JA II. Mycobacteria other than *Mycobacterium tuberculosis*: Review of microbiologic and clinical aspects. *Rev Infect Dis.* 1987;9:275–294.
11. Gunther SF. Non tuberculous mycobacterial infections of the hand. In: Flynn JE, ed. *Hand Surgery.* 3rd ed. Baltimore, Md: Williams and Wilkins; 1982:730–739.
12. Jolly HW, Seabury JH. Infections with *Mycobacterium marinum. Arch Dermatol.* 1972;106:32–36.
13. Gould WM, McMeekin DR, Bright RD. *Mycobacterium marinum (balnei)* infection. Report of a case with cutaneous and laryngeal lesions. *Arch Dermatol.* 1968;97: 159–162.
14. Schonherr U, Naumann GO, Lang GK, Bialasiwicz AA. Sclerokeratitis caused by *Mycobacterium marinum. Am J Opthalmol.* 1989;108:607–608.
15. Travis WD, Travis LB, Roberts GD, Weiland LW. Histopathologic spectrum in *Mycobacterium marinum* infection. *Arch Pathol Lab Med.* 1985;109(112):1109–1113.
16. Kostman JR, DiNubile MJ, Nodular lymphangitis: a distinctive but often unrecognized syndrome. *Ann Intern Med.* 1993;118:833–838.
17. Beckman EN, Pankey, McFarland GB. The histopathology of *Mycobacterium marinum* synovitis. *Am J Clin Pathol.* 1985;83(4):457–462.
18. Edelstein H. *Mycobacterium marinum* skin infections. Report of 31 cases and review of the literature. *Arch Intern Med.* 1994;154(12):1359–1364.
19. Brody GH, Stoller DW. The wrist and hand. In: Stoller DW, ed. *Magnetic Resonance Imaging in Orthopaedics & Sports Medicine.* Philadelphia: JB Lippincott; 1993:683–806.
20. Dattwyler RJ, Thomas J, Hurst LC. Antigen-specific T-cell anergy in progressive *Mycobacterium marinum* infection in humans. *Ann Intern Med.* 1987;107:675–677.
21. Wallace RJ Jr. American Thoracic Society. Diagnosis and treatment of disease caused by non tuberculous mycobacteria. *Am Rev Respir Dis.* 1990;142:940–953.

CHAPTER 72

Mycoplasma pneumoniae Infections

Anthony A. Gal

How art thou out of breath, when thou hast breath
To say to me that thou art out of breath?

William Shakespeare (1564–1616), Romeo and Juliet, II

INTRODUCTION

Mycoplasma are the smallest free-living organisms capable of causing disease in humans. Currently 10 species have been identified in humans: *M pneumoniae* is a major respiratory pathogen and is discussed in this chapter. *Mycoplasma hominis, M genitalium,* and related *Ureaplasma urealyticum* are implicated in respiratory and urogenital infections.[1]

Mycoplasma are filamentous, pleomorphic organisms that measure 200 × 10 nanometers and divide by binary fission.[2] They can grow aerobically or anaerobically and require proteins, sterols, and peptides for growth. Unlike bacteria, *Mycoplasma* lack a bacterial cell wall, but show a triple-layered unit membrane, 75 to 100 Å, with outer and inner electron-dense layers.[2] Because of the absence of a cell wall, *Mycoplasma* do not stain with Gram stain and show insensitivity for β-lactam cell-wall-type antibiotics.[3,4] Like viruses, however, *Mycoplasma* can readily pass through filters.

While *Mycoplasma* have only recently been recognized as a distinct genera, they were isolated before the turn of the century.[1,2] Advancements during the 1930s and 1940s led to the ultimate characterization of this distinctive class of organisms.[5] In 1943, Peterson et al[6] described cold isohemagglutinin in atypical pneumonia. The following year, Eaton et al[7] reproduced pneumonia in rodents. This filterable infectious pathogen isolated from sputa and lungs of patients with primary atypical pneumonia later became known as the Eaton agent. In 1962 Channock[8] grew Eaton's agent on agar and it was subsequently named *Mycoplasma pneumoniae*.[5,9]

PATHOGENESIS

Mycoplasma pneumoniae is a respiratory pathogen that is principally acquired by close contact. The organism is believed to be transmitted by large droplet secretions.[2,4] *Mycoplasma* penetrate the mucociliary blanket and attach to ciliated respiratory epithelium via a specialized terminal filament (0.1 × 2 nm) that is mediated by P1 protein (168-kd) attachment factor.[10] Subsequent extracellular replication of the organism inhibits ciliary motility. The local production of hydrogen peroxide, superoxides, and cytotoxins causes ciliary stasis, epithelial necrosis, and mucosal sloughing.[2]

CLINICAL

Mycoplasma pneumoniae accounts for 30% to 50% of community-acquired pneumonia.[11] Infections occur in all seasons, but there is an increased incidence in fall and winter. Most *Mycoplasma* pneumonia occurs in otherwise healthy children and young adults. Infection is uncommon in young children and patients older than 40 years of age.[2] Severe *Mycoplasma* pneumonia has been described in children with sickle cell disease[12] and in immunodeficient patients.[13,14] Because of the close contact associated with mycoplasmal infection, outbreaks have occurred in schools, universities, and military camps.[2,15,16]

The clinical presentation typically evolves from an upper to a lower respiratory tract infection.[3] After a 12- to 14-day incubation period, the onset of infection is

TABLE 72–1. EXTRAPULMONARY MANIFESTATIONS OF *MYCOPLASMA PNEUMONIAE* INFECTION

Hematopoietic
Autoimmune hemolytic anemia
Myelosuppression
Thrombocytopenia
Disseminated intravascular coagulation
Central Nervous System
Meningoencephalitis
Aseptic meningitis
Transverse myelitis
Neuropathies
Mononeuritis multiplex
Guillain-Barré
Sensorineural hearing loss
Cerebrovascular thromboses
Cerebellar ataxia
Cranial nerve palsies
Skin
Transient erythematous maculopapular or vesicular rash
Urticaria
Erythema nodosum
Erythema multiforme
Stevens–Johnson syndrome
Gastrointestinal tract
Hepatitis
Hepatosplenomegaly
Pancreatitis
Renal
Glomerulonephritis
Tubulointerstitial nephritis
Cardiac
EKG changes: ST segment and T wave alterations
Pericarditis
Myocarditis
Congestive heart failure
Hemopericardium
Complete heart block
Musculoskeletal
Myalgia and arthralgia
Polymyositis
Arthritis

From Refs. 2, 3, and 15–17.

characterized by a prodrome of malaise, headache, anorexia, fever up to 101°F, and other constitutional symptoms.[11,15] While the symptoms resemble influenza virus infection, the onset in *Mycoplasma* infection is more insidious.[4]

Upper respiratory tract involvement leads to pharyngitis, sinusitis, conjunctivitis, laryngotracheobronchitis, or cervical lymphadenopathy.[2,17] Otalgia or hearing disturbances may indicate bullous or hemorrhagic myringitis.[3] Of those infected with *M pneumoniae,* pneumonia develops in 3% to 10%.[2] In the lower respiratory tract, *Mycoplasma* pulmonary infection leads to an "atypical pneumonia" that is characterized by pulmonary infiltrates, normal white blood cell counts, and the absence of a bacterial pathogen.[7] Pulmonary involvement is associated with a persistent, intractable nonproductive cough. On occasion, however, sputa may be purulent, but no bacteria are identified with Gram staining.[11] Patients typically complain of mild respiratory discomfort and chest tightness, and chest auscultation reveals rales and rhonchi. Involvement of the pleura leads to pleuritis and pleural effusion in 20% of patients.[2] The chest radiograph can show a variety of patterns: unilateral segmental lower infiltrate, bilateral patchy infiltrate, nodular densities, pleural effusion, or hilar adenopathy.[18]

Most uncomplicated infections of *Mycoplasma* pneumonia are self-limiting with complete recovery in 3 to 4 weeks. Sometimes, however, there may be clinical relapse 7 to 10 days following initial resolution of pneumonia. Other pulmonary complications that may follow *Mycoplasma* infection include bronchiolitis obliterans,[19–21] bronchiectasis,[22,23] Swyer–James (Macleod) syndrome,[24] Stevens–Johnson syndrome,[20,22] interstitial fibrosis,[25,26] abscess,[27,28] septicemia,[29,30] persistent infection,[31] and adult respiratory distress syndrome.[32,33] There are rare reports of fatal *Mycoplasma* pneumonia.[19,20,23,25,28–30, 33–36]

Mycoplasma pneumoniae infections may be associated with diverse extrapulmonary manifestations.[2,3,15–17] Involvement of the central nervous system, skin, gastrointestinal, hematologic, and musculoskeletal systems result in the clinical complications listed in Table 72–1. The pathogenesis of extrapulmonary infection is uncertain, but has been attributed to the production of autoantibodies, toxins, hypercoagulability, or altered host response.[2,16]

PATHOLOGY

The histopathologic features of *Mycoplasma* pneumonia are nonspecific and overlap with other infectious pulmonary processes.[37] There are only a few reports describing the antemortem pathologic findings.[14,21,26,32,37] Tissue biopsies are seldom performed since the diagnosis of *Mycoplasma* pneumonia is primarily based on clinical grounds. Nevertheless, in open lung biopsy specimens, *Mycoplasma* pneumonia is characterized by a cellular bronchiolocentric inflammatory process primarily affecting the small airways (Figure 72–1).[14,37] As previously mentioned, the loss of mucosal integrity leads to tissue damage, necrosis, and mucosal sloughing. The corresponding biopsy specimens show degenerated, ulcerated epithelium, and neutrophils and fibrin in the bronchiolar lumen (Figure 72–2).[14] These features indicate a cellular bronchioli-

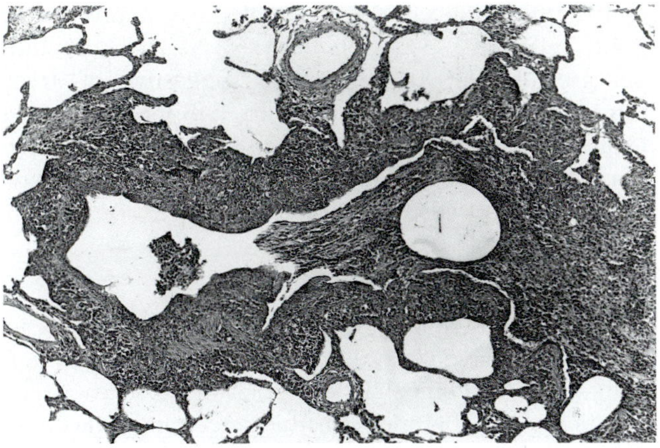

Figure 72–1. *Mycoplasma pneumoniae* bronchiolitis. This low-power magnification demonstrates the bronchiolocentric pattern of injury common in *M pneumoniae* infection (hematoxylin-eosin, ×25).

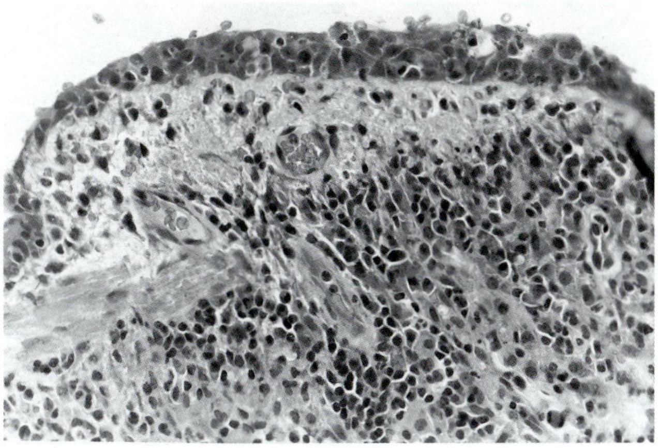

Figure 72–3. Cellular bronchiolitis. The thickened, edematous bronchiolar wall is heavily infiltrated by plasma cells and lymphocytes (hematoxylin-eosin, ×100).

tis.[37] The thickened, edematous bronchiolar wall is heavily infiltrated by a dense chronic inflammatory cell infiltrate composed of lymphocytes and plasma cells (Figure 72–3). In some patients, a plug of loose granulation tissue in small bronchioles causes bronchiolitis obliterans (Figure 72–4).[21] There is an interstitial pneumonitis when the lymphoplasmacytic infiltrate extends beyond the bronchiolar wall into adjacent alveolar septa (Figure 72–5). Vascular congestion is frequent in open lung biopsy specimens.

Autopsy studies have shown a similar bronchiolocentric pattern of injury exemplified by necrotizing bronchiolitis and bronchitis.[23,34,35] The lungs may additionally show features of diffuse alveolar damage (DAD) (ie, hyaline membranes, type II pneumocyte hyperplasia, interstitial organization, and squamous metaplasia).[19,23,30,34,36] Some autopsy studies have shown a pattern of an acute bronchopneumonia with microabscesses.[28,33] Pulmonary fibrosis may develop in some patients, probably resulting from resolving diffuse alveolar damage.[25] Occasionally, intraalveolar hemorrhage,[19] vascular thrombosis,[19,28,33–36] bronchiectasis,[23] and bronchiolitis obliterans[19,20] have been identified at autopsy.

CULTURE

The most reliable method of diagnosis is by microbial culture. Moreover, since *M pneumoniae* is not part of

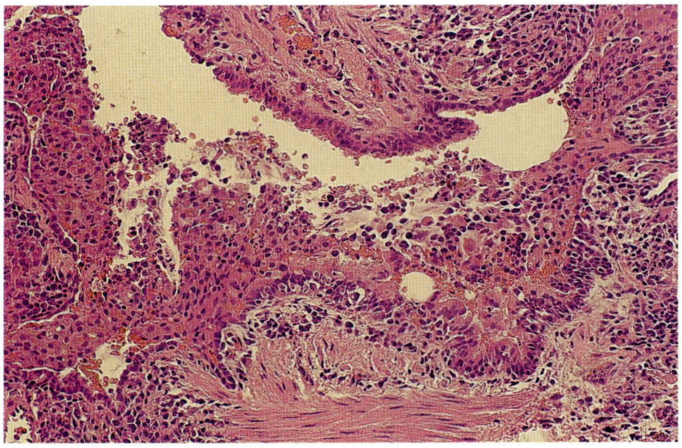

Figure 72–2. Destruction of bronchiolar wall. Ensuing mycoplasmal infection causes epithelial necrosis and mucosal ulceration (hematoxylin-eosin, ×50).

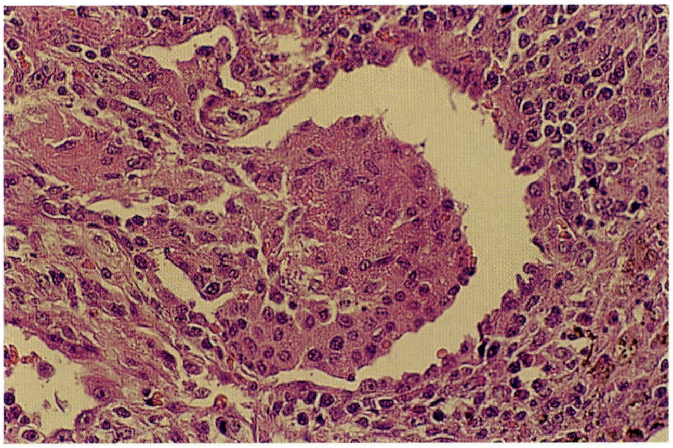

Figure 72–4. Bronchiolitis obliterans. Mucosal damage in a small bronchiole causes a plug of granulation tissue to form in the lumen (hematoxylin-eosin, ×100).

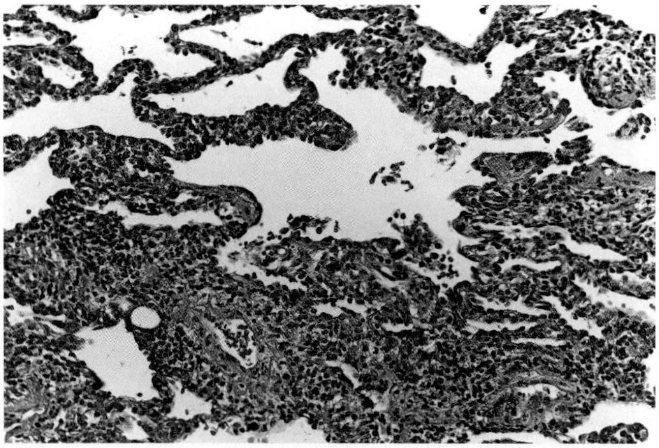

Figure 72–5. Interstitial pneumonitis. The lymphoplasmacytic infiltrate extends beyond the bronchiolar wall into adjacent alveolar septa (hematoxylin-eosin, ×50).

the normal microbial flora, its isolation from respiratory tract specimens (ie, throat or nasopharyngeal swabs) is clinically significant.[3] *Mycoplasma pneumoniae* organisms require an enriched broth or agar base for growth.[1,2] Hayflicks medium or SP-4 enriched medium improves recovery of the organism. In clinical isolates, *Mycoplasma* produces spherical, dense, granular rough-surfaced colonies 10 to 300 μm in diameter.[1] The "fried egg" appearance is not seen, as it is with other *Mycoplasma* species.[1] The organism ferments glucose, xylose, mannose, maltose, and dextrin.[2] There is beta hemolysis with sheep red blood cells and this is a confirmatory test. *Mycoplasma* are slow growing and cultures take 2 to 3 weeks.

SEROLOGIC TESTS

Complement Fixation Test

The complement fixation test utilizes an antigen prepared from lipid extract of organisms and is the most frequently utilized test to identify *Mycoplasma.* The IgM titer appears 7 to 9 days postinfection, peaks at 4 to 6 weeks, and declines in 4 to 6 months.[16] A presumptive diagnosis of *Mycoplasma* infection is made on a fourfold rise in paired titer. A single titer greater than 1:64 suggests recent infection.[15,38] The serologic response may be minimal or absent in immunodeficient patients.

Cold Hemagglutinins

Cold hemagglutinins may occur in 33% to 76% of patients with *Mycoplasma* infection.[2] They are characterized by an IgM immunoglobulin with anti-I specificity. At 4°C, the antibody fixes complement, binds to red blood cells, and causes hemolysis. A cold agglutinin titer greater than 1:64 is highly suggestive of *Mycoplasma* infection.[15] Patients with lymphoproliferative disorders, infectious mononucleosis, syphilis, influenza virus, adenovirus, and *Legionella* infections may have lower titers and false positive reactions.[4,15]

Other Related Tests

Several enzyme-linked immunosorbent assay tests for *Mycoplasma* have been described but they are not generally used in clinical laboratories because they lack specificity.[3] By this method, the detection of IgG does not necessarily indicate acute infection caused by the persistence of antibodies. Advances in molecular biology have led to the development of DNA probes to identify infectious pathogens. A commercially available kit has been reported to be highly sensitive and specific when compared to conventional methods.[30,39–42] Recently the polymerase chain reaction has been developed to identify *Mycoplasma.*[43]

OTHER LABORATORY FINDINGS

In most patients, the white blood count (WBC) is normal but in 25% it may be elevated over 10,000 cells/mm.[15,16] Differential WBC counts may show a mild to moderate relative increase in the proportion of neutrophils with shifts to right or left.[15] Other laboratory findings include elevated ALT and AST, C-reactive protein, and erythrocyte sedimentation rate. A positive direct Coombs' test may be caused by cold hemaagglutinins. False-positive VDRL, antinuclear antibodies, and tuberculin skin tests have been reported.

DIAGNOSIS

In patients with the presentation of an atypical pneumonia, the diagnosis of *Mycoplasma* pneumonia is largely made on clinical grounds by demonstrating an appropriate antibody response or by culture. The differential diagnosis encompasses other important pathogens including *Legionella pneumophila, Coxiella burnetii, Chlamydia pneumoniae,* and influenza virus.[3] Lung biopsy specimens are seldom obtained in this clinical setting, but a cellular bronchiolitis, luminal neutrophils, and lymphoplasmacytic mural infiltrates should alert the pathologist to *Mycoplasma* infection.[37]

Acknowledgments. Thomas V. Colby, MD, provided illustrative material and Faye Sanders provided secretarial assistance.

REFERENCES

1. Couch RB. Introduction to *Mycoplasma* diseases. In: Mandell GL, Douglas RG, Bennett JE, eds. *Principles and Practice of Infectious Diseases.* 3rd ed. New York: Churchill Livingstone; 1990:1445–1446.
2. Broughton RA. Infections due to *Mycoplasma pneumoniae* in childhood. *Ped Infect Dis.* 1986;5:71–85.
3. Luby JP. Pneumonia caused by *Mycoplasma pneumoniae* infection. *Clin Chest Med.* 1991;12:237–244.
4. Leigh MW, Clyde WA. Chlamydial and mycoplasmal pneumonias. *Sem Respir Infect.* 1987;2:152–158.
5. Marmion BP. Eaton agent-science and scientific acceptance: a historical commentary. *Rev Infect Dis.* 1990;12: 338–353.
6. Peterson OL, Han TH, Finland M. Cold agglutins (autohemagglutins) in primary atypical pneumonia. *Science.* 1943;97:167.
7. Eaton MD, Meiklejohn G, van Herick W. Studies on the etiology of primary atypical pneumonia. *J Exp Med.* 1944; 79:649–668.
8. Channock RM, Hayflick L, Barlie MF. Growth on artificial medium of an agent associated with atypical pneumonia and its identification as a PPLO. *Proc Natl Acad Sci USA.* 1962;48:41–49.
9. Channock RM, Dientes H, Eaton MD, et al. *Mycoplasma pneumonaie:* proposed nomenclature for atypical pneumonia organism (Eaton agent). *Science.* 1963;140:662.
10. Hu PC, Cole RM, Huang YS, et al. *Mycoplasma pneumoniae* infection: role of a surface protein in the attachment organelle. *Science.* 1982;216:313–315.
11. Mansel JK, Rosenow EC, Smith TF, Martin JW. *Mycoplasma pneumoniae* pneumonia. *Chest.* 1989;95:639–646.
12. Shulman ST, Bartlett J, Clyde WA, Ayoub EM. The unusual severity of *Mycoplasma* pneumonia in children with sickle-cell disease. *N Engl J Med.* 1972;287:164–167.
13. Foy HM, Ochs H, Davis SD, Kenny GE, Luce RR. *Mycoplasma pneumoniae* infections in patients with immunodeficiency syndromes. *J Infect Dis.* 1973;127:388–393.
14. Ganick DJ, Wolfson J, Gilbert EF, Joo P. *Mycoplasma* infection in the immunosuppressed leukemic patient. *Arch Pathol Lab Med.* 1980;104:535–536.
15. Levine DP, Lerner AM. The clinical spectrum of *Mycoplasma pneumoniae* infections. *Med Clin North Am.* 1978; 62:961–978.
16. Tuazon CU, Murray HW. Atypical pneumonias. In: Pennington JE, ed. *Respiratory Infections: Diagnosis and Management.* 2nd ed. New York: Raven Press; 1988: 341–363.
17. Murray HW, Masur H, Senterfit LB, Roberts RB. The protean manifestations of *Mycoplasma pneumoniae* infection in adults. *Am J Med.* 1975;58:229–242.
18. Brolin I, Wernstedt L. Radiologic appearance of *Mycoplasma* pneumonia. *Scand J Respir Dis.* 1978;59(suppl): 179–189.
19. Meyers BR, Hirschman SZ. Fatal infections associated with *Mycoplasma pneumoniae. Mt Sinai J Med.* 1972;39: 258–264.
20. Edwards C, Penny M, Newman J. *Mycoplasma* pneumonia, Stevens–Johnson syndrome, and chronic obliterative bronchitis. *Thorax.* 1983;38:867–869.
21. Coultas DB, Samet JM, Butler C. Bronchiolitis obliterans due to *Mycoplasma pneumoniae. West J Med.* 1986;144: 471–474.
22. Whyte KF, Williams GR. Bronchiectasis after *Mycoplasma* pneumonia. *Thorax.* 1984;39:390–391.
23. Halal F, Brochu P, Delage G, Lamarre A, Rivard G. Severe disseminated lung disease and bronchiectasis probably due to *Mycoplasma pneumoniae. CMAJ.* 1977;117: 1055–1056.
24. Stokes D, Siegler A, Khouri NF, Talamo RC. Unilateral hyperlucent lung (Swyer–James syndrome) after severe *Mycoplasma pneumoniae* infection. *Am Rev Respir Dis.* 1978;117:145–152.
25. Kaufman JM, Cuvelier CA, Van Der Straeten M. *Mycoplasma* pneumonia with fulminant evolution into diffuse interstitial fibrosis. *Thorax.* 1980;35:140–144.
26. Tablan OC, Reyes MP. Chronic interstitial pulmonary fibrosis following *Mycoplasma pneumoniae* pneumonia. *Am J Med.* 1985;79:268–270.
27. Siegler DIM. Lung abscess associated with *Mycoplasma pneumoniae* infection. *Br J Dis Chest.* 1973;67:123–127.
28. Koletsky RJ, Weinstein AJ. Fulminant *Mycoplasma pneumoniae* infection. *Am Rev Respir Dis.* 1980;122:491–496.
29. Naftalin JM, Wellisch G, Kahana Z, Diengott D. *Mycoplasma pneumoniae* sepiticemia. *JAMA.* 1974;228: 565.
30. Donat WE, Mark E, Kalmas S, et al. Case records of the Massachusetts General Hospital case 5-1992. *N Engl J Med.* 1992;326:324–336.
31. Holt S, Ryan WF, Epstein EJ. Severe *Mycoplasma* pneumonia. *Thorax.* 1977;32:112–115.
32. Fishman RA, Marschall KE, Kislak JW, Greenbaum DM. Adult respiratory distress syndrome caused by *Mycoplasma pneumoniae. Chest.* 1978;74:471–473.
33. Fraley DS, Ruben FL, Donnelly EJ. Respiratory failure secondary to *Mycoplasma pneumoniae* infection. *South Med J.* 1979;72:437–440.
34. Parker F, Jolliffe LS, Finland M. Primary atypical pneumonia. *Arch Pathol.* 1947;44:581–608.
35. Maisel JC, Babbitt LH, John TJ. Fatal *Mycoplasma pneumoniae* infection with isolation of organisms from lung. *JAMA.* 1967;202:139–142.
36. Benisch BM, Fayemi A, Gerber MA, Axelrod J. Mycoplasmal pneumonia in a patient with rheumatic heart disease. *Am J Clin Pathol.* 1972;58:343–348.
37. Rollins S, Colby T, Clayton F. Open lung biopsy in *Mycoplasma pneumoniae* pneumonia. *Arch Pathol Lab Med.* 1986;110:34–41.
38. Lee SH, Charoenying S, Brennan T, Markowski M, Mayo DR. Comparative studies of three serologic methods for the measurement of *Mycoplasma pneumoniae* antibodies. *Am J Clin Pathol.* 1989;92:342–347.
39. Edelstein PH. Use of DNA probes for the diagnosis of infectious caused by *Mycoplasma pneumoniae* and *Legionella*—a review. In: Kleger B, ed. *Rapid Methods in Clinical Microbiology.* New York: Plenum Press; 1988: 58–69.

40. Dular R, Kajioka R, Kasatiya S. Comparison of Gen-Probe commercial kit and culture technique for the diagnosis of *Mycoplasma pneumoniae* infection. *J Clin Microbiol.* 1988;26:1068–1069.
41. Kleemola SRM, Karjalainen JE, Raty RKH. Rapid diagnosis of *Mycoplasma pneumoniae* infection. *J Infect Dis.* 1990; 162:70–75.
42. Hata D, Kuze F, Mochizuki Y, et al. Evaluation of DNA probe test for rapid diagnosis of *Mycoplasma pneumoniae* infections. *J Pediatr.* 1990;116:273–276.
43. Bernet C, Garret M, de Barbeyrac B, Bebear C, Bonnet J. Detection of *Mycoplasma pneumoniae* by using the polymerase chain reaction. *J Clin Microbiol.* 1989;27:2492–2496.

CHAPTER 73

Neisserial Infections

Gonorrhea

David A. Schwartz and Ernest E. Lack

. . . when any man has a discharge . . . , his discharge is unclean. . . . Every bed on which he who has the discharge lies shall be unclean; and everything on which he sits shall be unclean.

Leviticus 15, 2–4

Gonococci exert their effect
On the genital tract more direct
Urethra and tube
Inflame and occlude
Obstruction most hard to correct.

Leslie H. Sobin (1934–), A Pathology Primer in Verse, 2nd ed, Nomad Press, Washington, DC, 1991

CLASSIFICATION

Neisseria gonorrhoeae is the causative agent of gonorrhea, one of the most common of the sexually transmitted diseases (STDs). The organism is a member of the family Neisseriaceae. Morphologically, it resembles closely the related *Neisseria meningitidis,* and several nonpathogenic *Neisseria* species. *Neisseria gonorrhoeae* is differentiated from other members of this genus by its ability to grow on selective media, reduce nitrites, utilize glucose but not maltose, lactose nor sucrose, and by its inability to grow well at reduced temperatures or on simple nutrient agar. Gonorrhea has been referred to colloquially as the "clap" (Middle French *clapoir,* "bubo").

INTRODUCTION AND HISTORY

Gonorrhea is one of the most ancient of recognized medical illnesses. There are numerous references to gonococcal urethritis in Chinese writings dating back 2500 years. Sarah, the wife of Abraham (Genesis, Chapter 12) could have had an STD, perhaps gonorrhea, and the book of Leviticus describes a similar infection (*Vide supra*). The term gonorrhea, meaning "flow of seed" (*gonos,* seed; *rhoia,* flow), was introduced by Galen in about 130 A.D., who confused the purulent urethral exudate from infected men with semen. Additional descriptions of gonorrhea can be found in the Papyrus of Ebers and the writings of Hippocrates. The causative agent was first described by Neisser in 1879, and it was first cultivated by Leistikow and Loeffler in 1882. Koch's postulates for the gonococcus were fulfilled in 1885 by Bumm. Because of the fastidious growth requirements of the gonococcus, laboratory cultivation was difficult until the development of chocolatized blood agar supplemented with growth factors. Isolation of *N gonorrhoeae* was made even simpler following the development of selective media containing antimicrobial and antifungal agents, such as Thayer–Martin medium, in the 1960s. Now, biochemical and serologic tests permit identification of the gonococcus within a few hours of isolation.

EPIDEMIOLOGY

Gonorrhea is a public health problem of global importance. In the United States, it remains the most frequently reported STD.[1] There has been a dramatic increase in gonorrhea during the past 25 years in many nations. In the United States, the number of reported cases tripled between 1965 and 1975. Fortunately, this trend has leveled off or decreased slightly in the United States and other Western countries since 1975. In 1993, there were 439,673 cases of gonorrhea reported in the United States, which represents a total rate of 172.40 cases per 100,000 population.[2] This number is probably low from underreporting of new infections. In fact, it has been estimated that only one half of new infections are reported.[3] The incidence for gonorrhea can be adjusted upward considerably if the denominator includes only sexually active men who are in nonmonogamous relations.[4] Many more male infections are reported than female infections—partly because more infections are diagnosed in men. The male : female case ratio fell steadily from 1.5 : 1 in the 1970s to 1.3 : 1 in 1987, largely because the number of infected homosexual men decreased during this period. An increased risk of gonorrhea was noted among adolescents from 1981 through 1991, consistent with the findings of an increased proportion of women who reported having premarital sex during the 1980s.[1]

Transmission of the gonococcus is almost exclusively by sexual contact. Nonsexual transmission (skin to skin, skin to mucous membrane, or autoinoculation) or fomite transmission (excluding laboratory accident) of *N gonorrhoeae* has not been documented.[2] Those persons who are at highest risk for infection are those under 25 years with multiple sexual contacts. The rates of gonorrhea are highest among males and in minority and inner city populations. The transmission efficiency (probability of acquiring infection following a single episode of sexual contact) of *N gonorrhoeae* is believed to be 50% to 60% from an infected man to an uninfected woman, and 22% from an infected woman to an uninfected man. After two contacts the transmission efficiency (woman to man) is 35%.[5] More than 90% of men with urethral infection develop symptoms within 5 days of exposure; infections in women, however, are far less likely to produce early symptoms. The prevalence of positive cultures for the gonococcus varies between different populations: less than 1% of military prenatal patients, 25% of women attending STD clinics, 5% of women at nonprivate clinics, and 1% to 2% of women attending private gynecology clinics.[6] The presence and survival of *N gonorrhoeae* in fresh and frozen semen have been well documented. Women artificially inseminated with semen from asymptomatic donors have been infected and had the complication of pelvic inflammatory disease too.[7]

Although gonococci were exquisitely sensitive to penicillin for many years, the spread throughout the world of strains resistant to penicillin and other antibiotics has developed into a major impediment for controlling gonorrhea. Strains of penicillinase-producing *N gonorrhoeae* (PPNG) were described almost simultaneously in 1976 in the United States, western Europe, the Philippines, and western Africa. Both chromosomal and plasmid-mediated types of gonococcal resistance occur. The gonococcus has a variety of plasmids (termed the Pc^r determinant) of differing sizes that produce beta lactamase. PPNG strains currently cause one half of all gonococcal infections in some regions of Africa and Asia, and were first reported in the United States in 1981. During 1993, PPNG strains were 9.6% of all gonococcal isolates, and an additional 6.1% were resistant to penicillin because of apparent chromosomal mutations. Currently, strains of *N gonorrhoeae* with chromosomal resistance to penicillin, tetracycline, erythromycin, and cefoxitin, as well as decreased sensitivity to ceftriaxone, have been reported throughout the world and especially Southeast Asia. Recent reports from North America, Asia, Australia, and the United Kingdom have described gonococcal strains with greatly decreased susceptibility to fluoroquinolones, which is most likely caused by one or more mutations in genes encoding for DNA gyrase and/or changes in membrane permeability.[8]

BIOLOGY AND PATHOGENESIS

Neisseria gonorrhoeae are gram-negative, spherical, or ovoid cocci that are usually in pairs with flattened adjacent sides. They are non-spore-forming, are generally nonmotile, and are 0.6 to 2.0 μm in diameter. In the laboratory, culture depends on high humidity, a carbon dioxide atmosphere, specific nutrients, an optimal pH of 7.2 to 7.4, and a temperature of 35 to 36°C. In the human, gonococci grow preferentially in columnar and transitional epithelium. Similar to other gram-negative bacteria, the gonococcus has a cell envelope composed of three layers: an inner cytoplasmic membrane, middle peptidoglycan cell wall, and outer membrane. The outer membrane contains lipooligosaccharide (LOS), phospholipid, and several types of proteins. Porin, previously called Protein I, has a molecular weight of 32 to 36 kd and is closely associated in the membrane with LOS. It provides channels through which aqueous solutes pass the outer membrane, and is thought to serve an important role in pathogenesis. Because porin demonstrates stable antigenic variation between gonococcal strains, it is the major protein involved in serologic typing systems based on outer membrane antigens. Opacity proteins, formerly termed Protein II, include several related proteins with molecular weights of 20 to 28 kd, and these proteins vary in quantity or may be absent from a strain of *N gonorrhoeae.* Opacity proteins increase adhesion of gonococci to one another, and also to a variety of eukaryotic cells, including phagocytic cells. Loss of these proteins is associated with resistance to phagocytic killing by neutrophils. Reduction-modifiable protein, formerly known as Protein III, is present in all gonococcal strains as a complex with porin and LOS, and has a molecular weight of 30 to 31 kd. It can stimulate blocking antibodies that reduce serum bactericidal activity against the gonococcus.

Gonococcal LOS is composed of lipid A and a core oligosaccharide that lacks O-antigenic side chains. It has endotoxic properties, is lethal to experimental animals, and mediates ciliary destruction and death of adjacent uninfected cells in the fallopian tube explant model. Antigenic variations in the components of the LOS form the basis for an alternative gonococcal serotyping system, but these types have not yet been associated with clinical disease or epidemiologic factors.

The peptidoglycan layer may promote the host inflammatory response in gonorrheal infections. Fragments of gonococcal peptidoglycan are toxic in the fallopian tube explant model, and they have been isolated from otherwise sterile synovial fluid in patients with gonococcal arthritis–dermatitis syndrome.

Distinctive colony types of *N gonorrhoeae* occur when the organism is grown on translucent agar. Recently isolated strains produce types P^+ and P^{++} colonies, and the organisms have numerous pili extending from their surfaces. Following 20 to 24 hours of cultivation, nonpiliated organisms predominate, forming P^- colonies. This transition is mediated by chromosomal rearrangements. Nonpiliated gonococci are avirulent in human inoculation experiments. Piliated organisms are better able to attach to human mucosal surfaces and show greater virulence in animal models than do nonpiliated organisms. The pili of *N gonorrhoeae* are composed of repetitive protein subunits (pilin) and show areas of both antigenic homology and diversity between strains. The pili play an important role in attachment of the gonococcus to host cells. Piliated organisms are mostly extracellular and usually in clumps. Short pili are seen in nonpathogenic organisms, whereas long pili are present in both pathogenic and nonpathogenic strains. More than 50 serotypes of pili have been identified.[8–11] Because the gonococcus is a strictly human pathogen without a good experimental model of infection, experimental urethritis has been induced in male human volunteers by inoculation of various strains of *N gonorrhoeae* to study molecular features in pathogenesis[12] and possibly facilitate development of an effective vaccine.[13]

CLINICAL FEATURES AND PATHOLOGY

Genital Tract Infection in Men

The most frequent manifestation of gonorrhea in men is acute urethritis, presenting as urethral discharge and dysuria. The initial discharge usually appears 2 to 5 days after exposure, and consists initially of scant mucoid material, which rapidly becomes abundant and purulent (Figure 73–1) and contains gonococci (Figure 73–2). A small number of men with gonococcal urethritis are asymptomatic (1% to 5%).[2] If untreated, most infections resolve spontaneously after several weeks. The most common complication of gonococcal urethritis is acute epididymitis, but this is uncommon in Western nations. Some rare complications of gonorrheal infection in men include penile edema (Figure 73–3), penile lymphangitis, gangrenous balanitis, periurethral

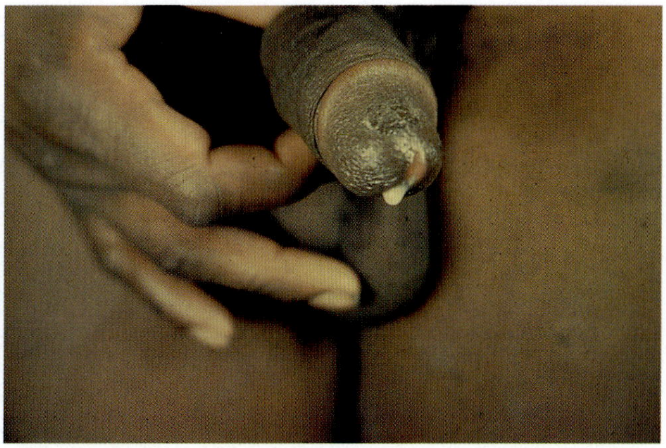

Figure 73–1. Gonorrheal urethritis. The urethral exudate has the color and consistency of coffee cream.

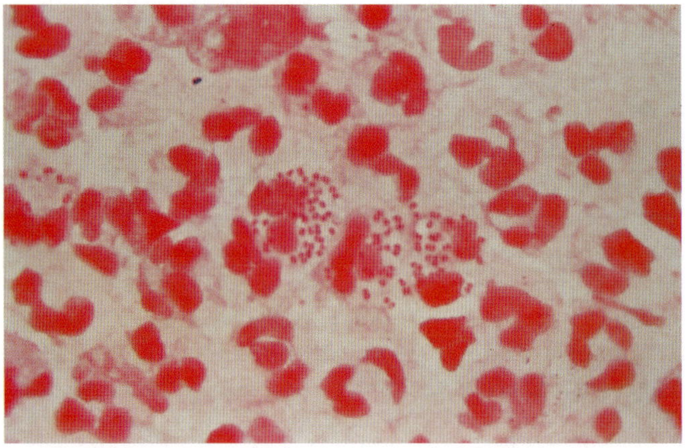

Figure 73–2. Swab of urethral discharge, showing numerous inflammatory cells, some containing intracytoplasmic gram-negative diplococci of *N gonorrhoeae* (Gram stain, ×500).

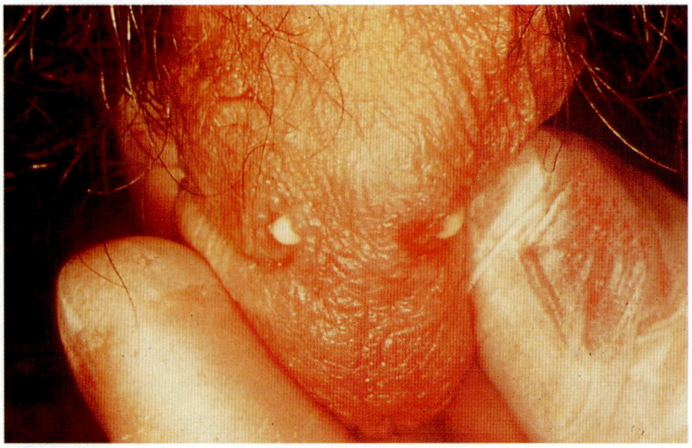

Figure 73–4. An unusual infection of Tyson's glands by *N gonorrhoeae*.

abscess, acute prostatitis, seminal vesiculitis, and infections of Cowper's and Tyson's glands (Figure 73–4).[8,9]

Genital Tract Infection in Women

The endocervix is the primary site of genital tract gonococcal infection in women. The organisms are rarely isolated from the paraurethral (Skene's) glands and the ducts of Bartholin's glands. Most women who develop symptoms of gonorrhea do so 10 days after infection, but a substantial number of infected women are asymptomatic or do not seek medical attention. The most common symptoms include any combination of cervicitis, urethritis, vaginal discharge, intermenstrual bleeding, and menorrhagia.[14,15] Physical examination reveals a mucopurulent cervical exudate, erosions, and other signs of cervicitis (Figures 73–5 and 73–6). Occasionally, mucopurulent discharge can be expressed from the ducts of Bartholin's glands (Figure 73–7) or the urethra. Prepubertal females may develop vulvovaginitis.[2]

Pelvic Inflammatory Disease

Pelvic inflammatory disease (PID) is an important chronic complication of gonorrhea that results from an ascending infection in approximately 10% to 20% of infected women.[16] PID is a major reproductive health problem in young women because of its association with infertility and ectopic pregnancy. Although the gonococcus is a major cause of PID, other organisms, notably *Chlamydia trachomatis,* are also implicated and mixed infections with these two agents are not uncommon.[16] Fifteen percent to 20% of women having a single episode of PID are infertile, and 50% to 80% of women with three or more episodes of PID are infertile.[17,18] Infertility may be more common with PID

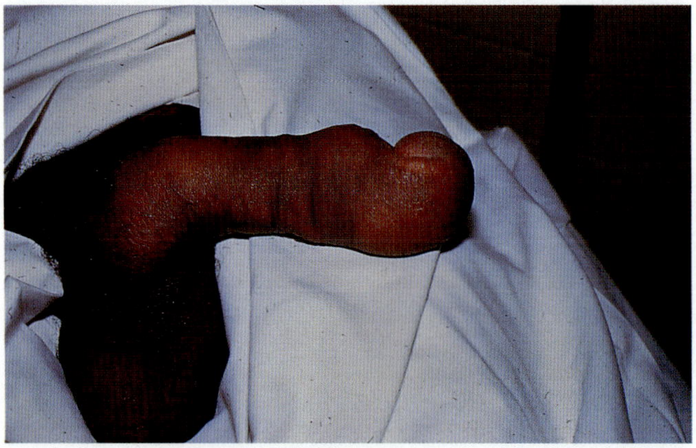

Figure 73–3. Gonococcal penile edema, termed "bullheaded clap," is an unusual manifestation of gonorrhea in men.

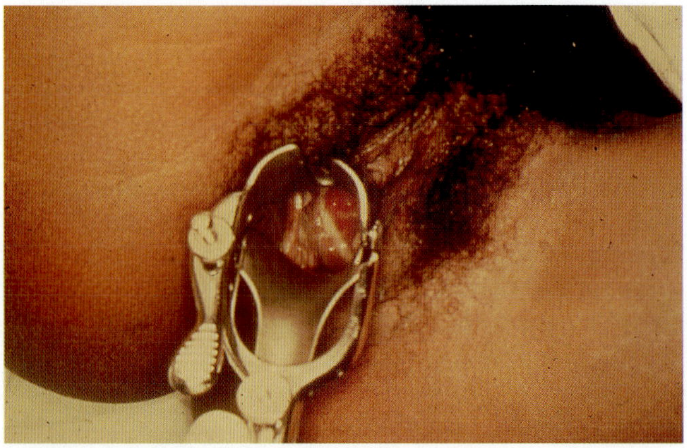

Figure 73–5. Uncomplicated gonorrhea of the female genital tract, showing cervicitis with mucopurulent discharge.

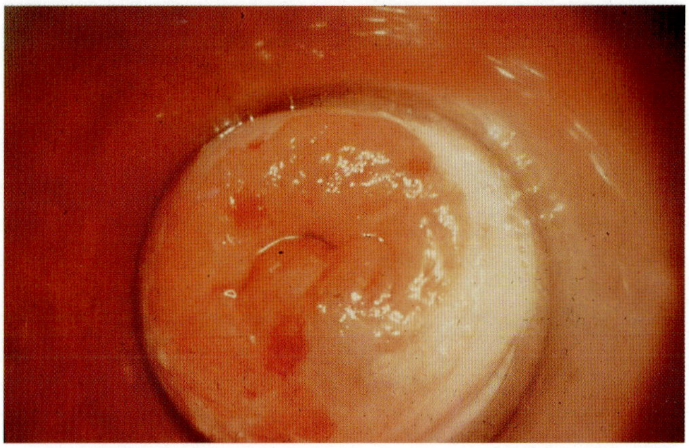

Figure 73–6. Cervical erosion caused by *N gonorrhoeae.*

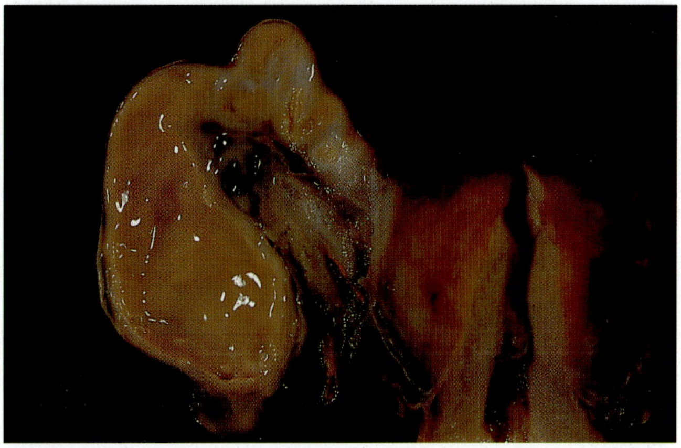

Figure 73–8. Fallopian tube with purulent salpingitis and pyosalpinx caused by *N gonorrhoeae.*

caused by *C trachomatis,* because *N gonorrhoeae* causes more severe clinical manifestations of gonococcal salpingitis and thus results in more rapid treatment. Fifty percent to 80% of fallopian tubes from women with ectopic pregnancies have histologic evidence of previous salpingitis.[18]

The most common clinical finding with PID is lower abdominal pain, which is usually bilateral. Most women have symptoms of infection of the lower genital tract as well. Examination usually demonstrates pelvic adnexal tenderness, pain with movement of the cervix, and tender adnexal masses. Some patients have fever, nausea, vomiting, leukocytosis, and elevation of the erythrocyte sedimentation rate or of C-reactive protein. These symptoms are caused by one or more of the following manifestations of PID: endometritis, salpingitis, pyosalpinx (Figure 73–8), tubal, ovarian, or tubo-ovarian abscess (Figures 73–9 and 73–10), and peritonitis. Other complications of PID include pelvic thrombophlebitis, ruptured abscess, chronic pelvic pain, and menstrual abnormalities.[16]

Anorectal Infection

Approximately 40% of women and homosexually active men with uncomplicated gonorrhea have positive rectal cultures for the gonococcus. In 40% of homosexual men and 5% of women with gonorrhea, the rectum is the only site found to be infected (Figure 73–11). Although most persons with positive rectal cultures are asymptomatic, those with symptoms have tenesmus, anal pruritus, and purulent rectal discharge or bleeding. The findings of a mucopurulent exudate in the anorectal area suggest gonorrhea, but other sexually transmit-

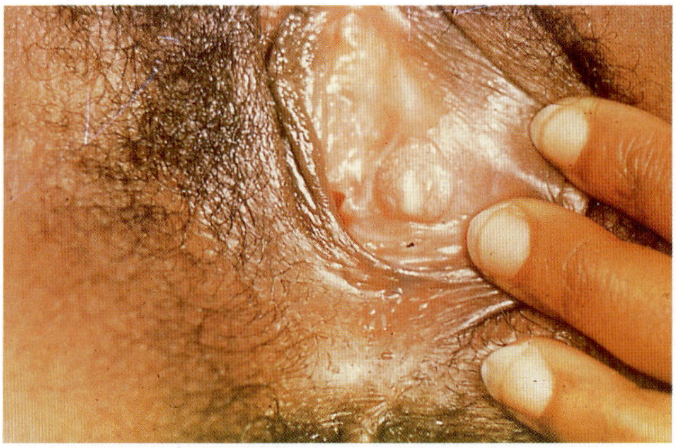

Figure 73–7. Bartholin's abscess of vagina associated with gonorrhea.

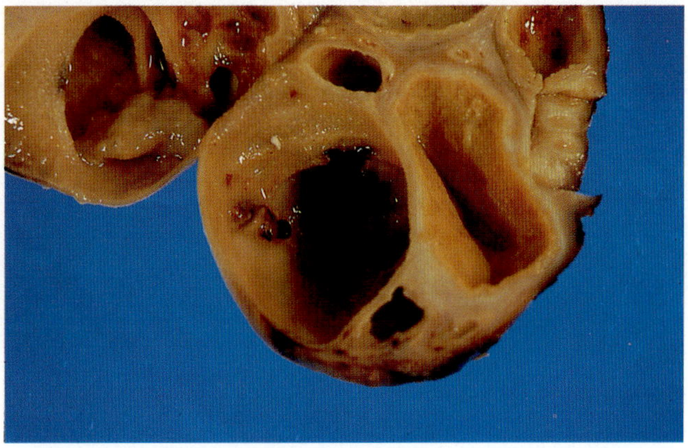

Figure 73–9. Ovarian abscess associated with gonococcal PID.

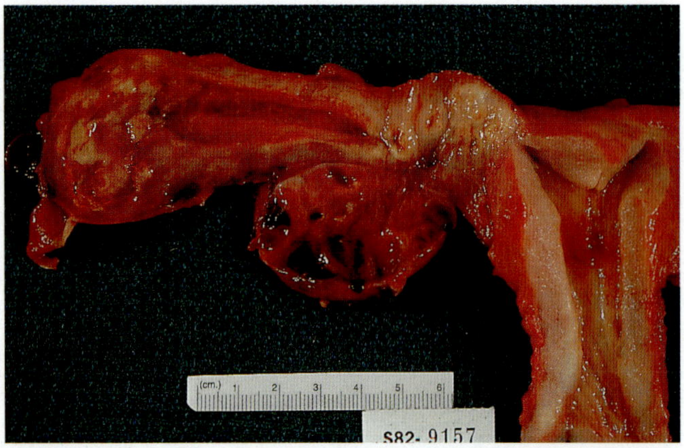

Figure 73–10. Tubo-ovarian abscess is an important complication of upper genital tract infection with gonorrhea.

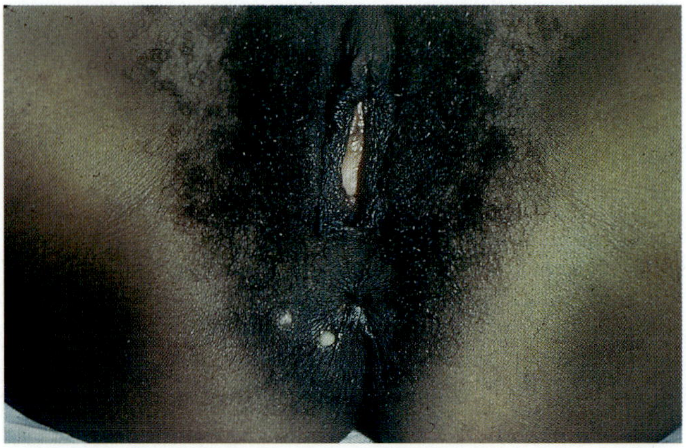

Figure 73–12. *Fistula-in-ano* is an unusual complication of anorectal gonorrhea.

ted infections can produce these findings.[19] Complications of anorectal infection include fistulas (Figure 73–12).

Pharyngeal Infection

The majority of patients with pharyngeal gonococcal infection are asymptomatic, but some have purulent pharyngitis and cervical lymphadenitis. The major risk factor for developing pharyngeal gonococcal infection is oral–genital sexual exposure with an infected partner. Ten percent to 20% of heterosexual women and 10% to 25% of homosexual men with gonorrhea have gonococcal pharyngitis, but only 3% to 7% of heterosexual men with gonorrhea have gonococcal pharyngitis.

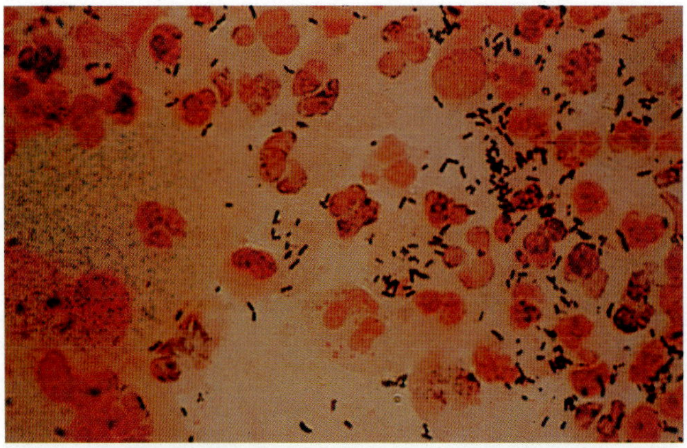

Figure 73–11. Gram-stained rectal smear from a patient with anorectal gonorrhea. The predominant bacteria are gram-positive rods, but a neutrophil containing gram-negative diplococci is in the center (Gram stain, ×500).

Perihepatitis

Approximately 15% to 30% of women with gonococcal PID develop gonococcal perihepatitis, also termed the Fitz–Hugh–Curtis syndrome (FHCS). For many years, this syndrome was thought to be in women only. Current literature, however, indicates that *C trachomatis* can also cause this syndrome in men.[20,21] FHCS is caused by the spread of the organisms from the fallopian tube through the peritoneum and onto the liver capsule. Lymphangitic or hematogenous transmission may also cause the FHCS, explaining gonococcal perihepatitis in men. The FHCS can mimic a variety of abdominal emergencies, such as perforated peptic ulcer.[22] In the early phase of perihepatitis, there is a fibrinopurulent exudate on the capsule of the liver and hemorrhagic areas on the adjacent parietal peritoneum. The very fine adhesions that are characteristic of healed FHCS have been called "violin-string" adhesions. They form between the liver capsule and parietal peritoneum.

Disseminated Gonococcemia

About 0.5% to 3% of patients have bacteremia and dissemination. Patients deficient in late complement components may not clear gram-negative bacteria because of an inability to kill or lyse bacteria.[23] The most common manifestations are septic arthritis and polyarthritis. Rare complications of dissemination include endocarditis, meningitis, osteoarthritis, severe sepsis accompanied by Waterhouse–Friderichsen syndrome, and the adult respiratory distress syndrome.

Arthritis and dermatitis are the most frequent clinical presentation of disseminated gonococcemia. Patients complain at first of polyarthralgias involving

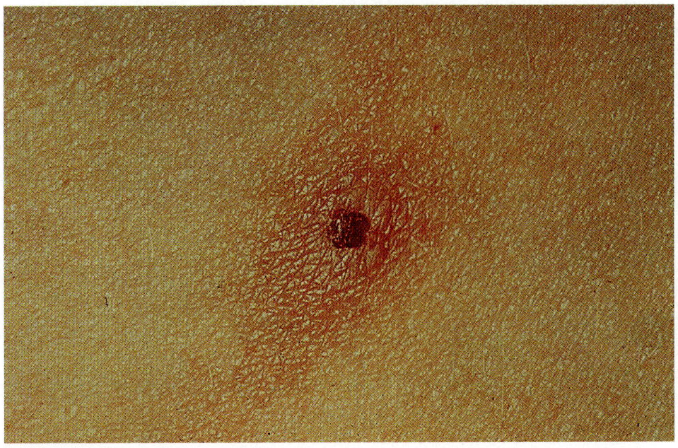

A

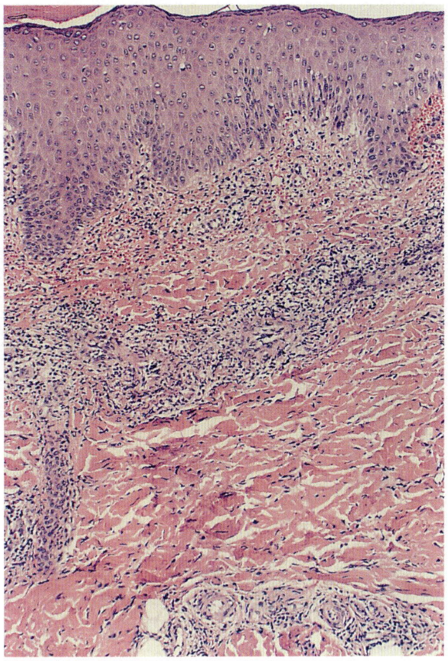

B

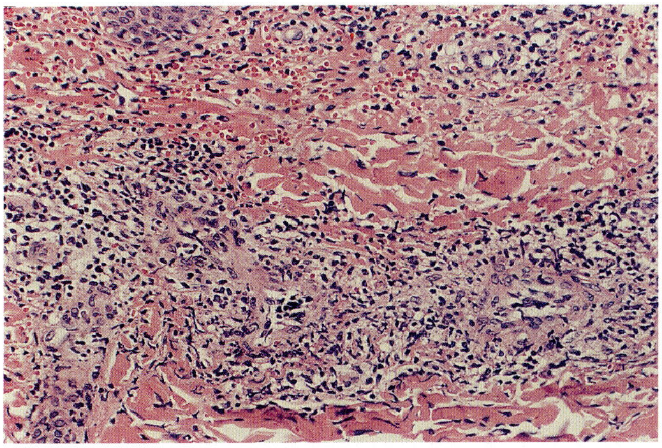

C

Figure 73–13. (**A**) Typical appearance of the papular skin lesion of gonococcemia. (**B**) Purpuric skin lesion in patient with disseminated gonococcemia. Inflammatory infiltrates involve small vessels in dermis (hematoxylin-eosin, ×150). (**C**) Inflammatory infiltrate consists of lymphocytes and neutrophils with some evidence of karyorrhexis. Lesion resembles small vessel leukocytoclastic vasculitis. Note extravasation of red blood cells; cocci could not be identified on special stains (hematoxylin-eosin, ×200).

knees, elbows, and more distal joints.[24] These patients typically have clinical arthritis or tenosynovitis in two or more joints. The polymerase chain reaction (PCR) may confirm the clinical diagnosis of gonococcal arthritis in patients whose synovial fluid is sterile by culture.[25] About 75% of patients have a characteristic dermatitis, consisting of papules and pustules with a hemorrhagic component (Figure 73–13, A–C). Other types of skin lesions may be present, including hemorrhagic bullae and necrotic lesions, which mimic ecthyma gangrenosum or the lesions of neutrophilic dermatitis (Figures 73–14 and 73–15).[8,9]

Gonorrhea and Pregnancy

Gonococcal infection during pregnancy is associated with a variety of poor obstetric outcomes, including spontaneous abortion, premature labor, chorioamnionitis (Figure 73–16) with early rupture of membranes, and perinatal infant mortality (discussion follows).[26] It is unclear whether the gonococcus is directly responsible for these untoward outcomes, or is simply a marker for high risk caused by other factors.

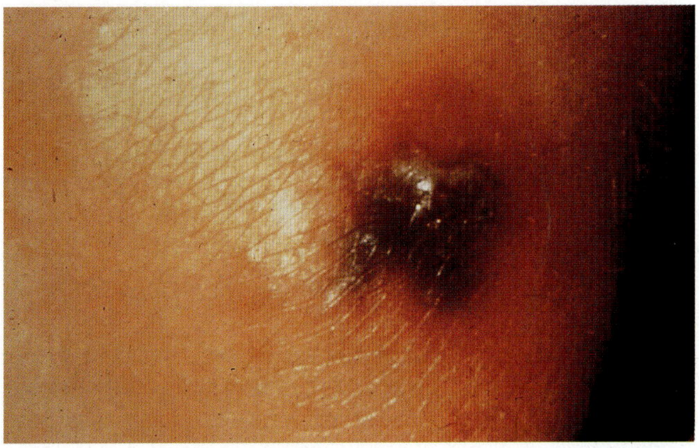

Figure 73–14. Hemorrhagic skin lesion associated with gonococcemia.

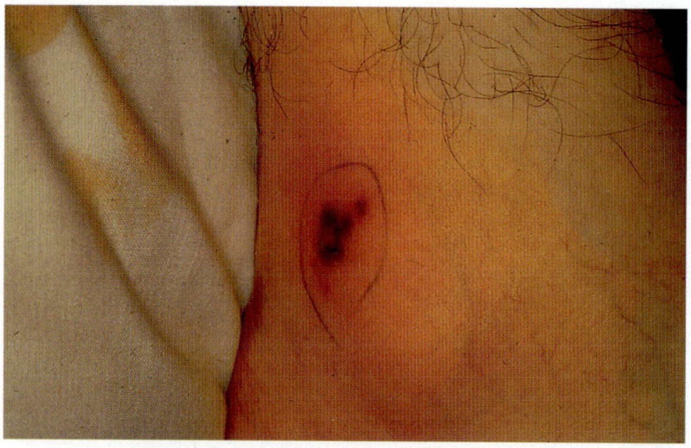

Figure 73–15. Patient with gonococcemia and a necrotic skin lesion resembling ecthyma gangrenosum.

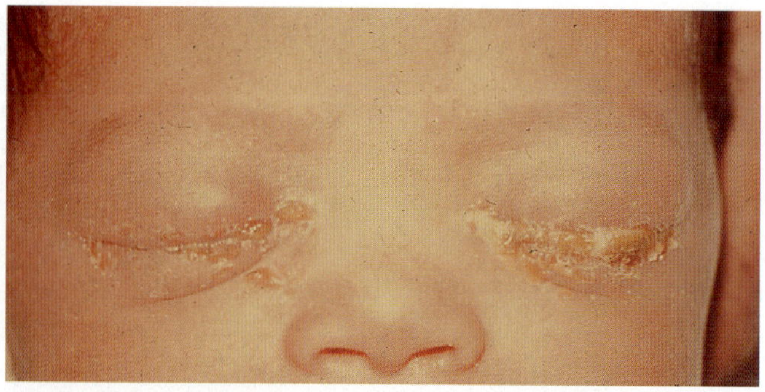

Figure 73–17. Ophthalmia neonatorum in an infant delivered to a mother with gonorrhea.

Neonatal and Pediatric Infections

Mothers infected with *N gonorrhoeae* can transmit the organism to infants in utero, during delivery, or postpartum. Gonococcal conjunctivitis of the newborn (ophthalmia neonatorum) is the most frequent clinical manifestation of neonatal infection. At one time in the United States it was the most common cause of blindness, and it remains a pediatric public health problem in many developing nations. Ophthalmia neonatorum usually develops from 3 to 7 days after delivery as a bilateral, profuse, purulent conjunctivitis (Figures 73–17 and 73–18). Extension to the cornea causes keratitis or panophthalmitis. Fibrosis during the healing phase of ophthalmia neonatorum can cause partial or complete blindness. Fortunately, the incidence of ophthalmia neonatorum has declined dramatically with the routine instillation of a solution of 1% silver nitrate or erythromycin ophthalmic ointment into the eyes of newborns.[20]

Newborns exposed to the gonococcus can also develop septicemia and arthritis, but these are uncommon. Pediatric gonococcal infections before the first year of life are probably congenital infections; those after the first year are almost always from sexual abuse by an infected individual.

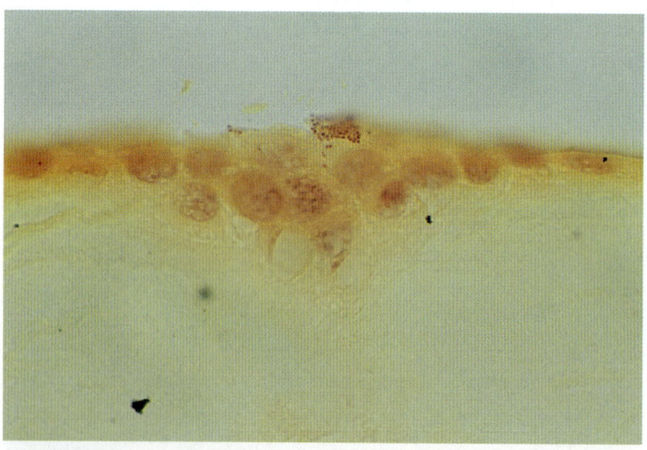

Figure 73–16. Tissue Gram stain of extraplacental membrane with severe chorioamnionitis. The placenta is from a stillborn infant delivered to a mother with cocaine use and a positive vaginal culture for *N gonorrhoeae*. A cluster of gram-negative gonococci is in the center of the figure, adherent to the outer surface of the amnionic epithelium (modified Brown–Hopps stain, ×1000).

DIAGNOSIS AND TREATMENT

Conventional diagnosis of gonorrhea relies on culture and demonstration of intracellular gram-negative diplococci in Gram-stained smears of genital discharge or swabs. Gram-stained smears from genital sites must be interpreted with caution, since they can be colonized by other gram-negative bacteria (eg, *N meningitidis*); also

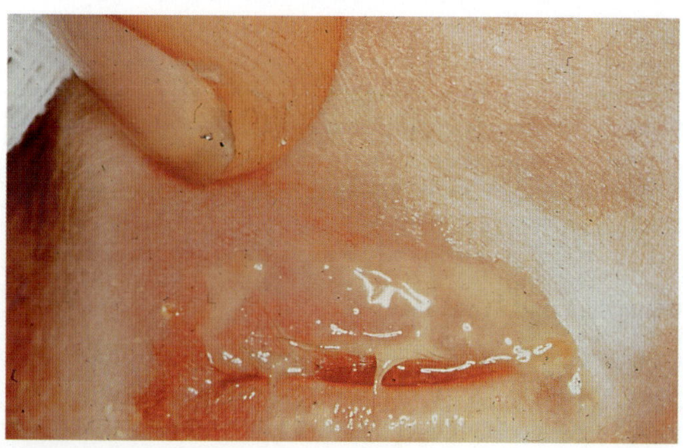

Figure 73–18. Close-up of suppurative exudate from the eye of the infant in Figure 73–17.

one cannot automatically assume that an organism with diplococcal morphology that grows on a selective medium is a pathogenic species of *Neisseria.*[27] Rapid identification of *N gonorrhoeae* has been improved by direct fluorescent antibody testing of presumptive isolates.[28] The Accu Probe culture confirmation test is also a rapid and accurate means of identifying cultured isolates of *N gonorrhoeae.*[29] A nonisotopic DNA probe assay (PACE 2) has been used to detect the gonococcus in urethral and endocervical specimens with sensitivity and specificity of 100% and 99.3%[30] and overall concordance with culture of 98.4%.[30] This DNA probe has also been used as a test for cure; a positive result more than 6 days after treatment with intramuscular ceftriaxone was considered evidence of reinfection.[31] A ligase chain reaction has been applied to urine samples as a practical alternative to culture for detection of the gonococcus in women.[32] Recently a duplex PCR assay was developed for simultaneous detection of *N gonorrhoeae* and *C trachomatis* in clinical specimens.[33]

The changing resistance patterns of *N gonorrhoeae* necessitate periodic modification in treatment. In the Gonococcal Isolate Surveillance Project (GISP) study group, 32.4% of isolates were resistant to penicillin or tetracycline, and the proportions of isolates with high-level plasmid-mediated resistance to one or both drugs had increased significantly in the United States during 1988–1991.[34] Other data also support the recommendation that penicillin and tetracycline should not be used for the primary treatment of uncomplicated gonorrhea in PID and salpingitis; it has also been recommended that gonococci isolated from women with PID be tested routinely to confirm susceptibility to therapeutic agents.[35] Therapeutic efficacy of single-dose treatment of uncomplicated gonorrhea has been shown for the following: 1) cefotaxime 500 mg IM (together with 7-day course of doxycycline to cover possible coinfection with *Chlamydia*),[36] 2) ceftriaxone 250 mg IM, 3) ciprofloxacin 500 mg pO, or 4) cefixime 400 mg pO.[37,38] Changes in patterns of antimicrobial susceptibility may be related not only to antimicrobial selection pressures, but also shifts among gonococcal strains in a community.[39]

REFERENCES

1. Webster LA, Berman SM, Greenspan JR. Surveillance for gonorrhea and primary and secondary syphilis among adolescents, United States—1981–1991. *MMWR.* 1993;42 (SS-3):1–11.
2. Centers for Disease Control and Prevention. Summary of notifiable diseases, United States, 1993. *MMWR.* 1993; 42:1–73.
3. Knapp JS, Rice RJ. *Neisseria* and *Branhamella.* In: Murray PR, Baron EJ, Pfaller MA, Tenover FC, Yolken RH, eds. *Manual of Clinical Microbiology.* 6th ed. Washington, DC: ASM press; 1995.
4. Kassler WJ, Tanfer K, Aral SO. Gonorrhea rates among US men adjusted for sexual activity. *Am J Pub Health.* 1994; 84:1524–1525.
5. Holmes KK, Johnson DW, Trostle HJ. An estimate of the risk of acquiring gonorrhea by sexual contact with infected women. *Am J Epidemiol.* 1970;91:170–174.
6. Mascola L, Guinan ME. Screening to reduce transmission of sexually transmitted diseases in semen used for artificial insemination. *N Engl J Med.* 1986;314:1354–1359.
7. Spence M. Gonorrhea. *Clinic Obstet Gynecol.* 1983;25: 111–124.
8. Whittington W, Ison C, Thompson S. Gonorrhea. In: Morse SA, Moreland AA, Holmes KK, eds. *Atlas of Sexually Transmitted Diseases and AIDS.* 2nd ed. London: Mosby-Wolfe; 1996:99–117.
9. Handsfield HH, Sparling PF. *Neisseria gonorrhoeae.* In: Mandell GL, Bennett JE, Dolin R, eds. *Principles and Practice of Infectious Diseases.* 4th ed. New York: Churchill Livingstone; 1995:1909–1926.
10. Britigan BE, Cohen MS, Sparling PF. Gonococcal infections: a model of molecular pathogenesis. *N Engl J Med.* 1985;312:1683–1694.
11. Morello JM, Janda WM, Doern GV. *Neisseria* and *Branhamella.* In: Balows A, Hausler WJ, Herrmann KL, et al, eds. *Manual of Clinical Microbiology.* 5th ed. Washington, DC: American Society for Clinical Microbiology; 1991: 258–276.
12. Schneider H, Cross AS, Kuschner RA, et al. Experimental human gonoccocal urethritis: 250 *Neisseria gonorrhoeae* M51mkC are infective. *J Infect Dis.* 1995;172:180–185.
13. Cohen MS, Cannon JG, Jerse AE, Charniga LM, Isbey SF, Whicker LG. Human experimentation with *Neisseria gonorrhoeae:* rationale, methods, and implications for the biology of infection and vaccine development. *J Infect Dis.* 1994;169:532–537.
14. McCormack WM, Stumacher RJ, Johnson K, Donner A. Clinical spectrum of gonococcal infections in women. *Lancet.* 1977;1:1182–1185.
15. Barlow D, Phillips I. Gonorrhoea in women: diagnostic, clinical and laboratory aspects. *Lancet.* 1978;1:761–764.
16. Rice R, Schwartz DA, Knapp J, Paavonen J. Pelvic inflammatory disease. In: SA Morse, AA Moreland, KK Holmes, eds. *Atlas of Sexually Transmitted Diseases and AIDS.* 2nd ed. London: Mosby-Wolfe; 1996:133–147.
17. Sweet RL. Pelvic inflammatory disease and infertility in women. *Infect Dis Clin N Am.* 1987;1:199–215.
18. Weström L. Incidence, prevalence and trends of acute pelvic inflammatory disease and its consequences in industrialized countries. *Am J Obstet Gynecol.* 1980;138: 880–892.
19. Klein EJ, Fisher CS, Chow AW, Guze LB. Anorectal gonococcal infection. *Ann Intern Med.* 1977;86:340–346.
20. Biswas MK, Summers PR. Gonorrhea. In: Pastorek JG II, ed. *Obstetric and Gynecologic Infectious Disease.* New York: Raven Press; 1994:467–478.
21. Lopez-Zano JA, Keith LG, Berger GS. The Fitz–Hugh–Curtis syndrome revisited: changing perspectives after half a century. *J Reprod Med.* 1985;30:567–582.

22. Counselman FL. An unusual presentation of Fitz–Hugh–Curtis syndrome. *J Emerg Med.* 1994;12:167–170.
23. Case records of the Massachusetts General Hospital. Case 44-1993. *N Engl J Med.* 1993;329:1411–1416.
24. Lewis DA, Pollock LM, Randell J, Wilson P, Kopelman PG. Acute gonococcal arthritis: an unusual host and pathogen combination. *J Clin Pathol.* 1995;48:86–88.
25. Liebling MR, Arkfeld DG, Michelini GA, et al. Identification of *Neisseria gonorrhoeae* in synovial fluid using the polymerase chain reaction. *Arthrit Rheum.* 1994;37:702–709.
26. Edwards LE, Barrada MMI, Harmann AA, et al. Gonorrhea in pregnancy. *Am J Obstet Gynecol.* 1978;132:637–641.
27. Baron EJ, Peterson LR, Finegold SM, eds. *Baily and Scott's Diagnostic Microbiology.* 9th ed. St. Louis, Mo.: Mosby; 1994.
28. Beebe JL, Rau MP, Flageolie S, Calhoon B, Knapp JS. Evidence of *Neisseria gonorrhoeae* isolates negative by Syva direct fluorescent antibody test but positive by Gen-Probe AccuProbe test in a sexually transmitted disease clinic population. *J Clin Microbiol.* 1993;13:2535–2537.
29. Young H, Moyes A. Comparative evaluation of AccuProbe culture identification test for *Neisseria gonorrhoeae* and other rapid methods. *J Clin Microbiol.* 1993;31:1996–1999.
30. Stary A, Kopp W, Zahel B, Nerad S, Teodorowicz L, Hörting-Müller I. Comparison of DNA-probe test and culture for the detection of *Neisseria gonorrhoeae* in genital samples. *Sex Transm Dis.* 1993;20:243–247.
31. Hanks JW, Scott CT, Butler CE, Wells DW. Evaluation of a DNA probe assay (Gen-Probe PACE2) as the test of cure for *Neisseria gonorrhoeae* genital infections. *J Pediatr.* 1994;125:161–162.
32. Smith KR, Cling S, Lee H, et al. Evaluation of ligase chain reaction for use with urine for identification of *Neisseria gonorrhoeae* in females attending a sexually transmitted disease clinic. *J Clin Microbiol.* 1995;33:455–457.
33. Wong KC, Ho BSW, Egglestone SI, Lewis WHP. Duplex PCR system for simultaneous detection of *Neisseria gonorrhoeae* and *Chlamydia trachomatis* in clinical specimens. *J Clin Pathol.* 1995;48:101–104.
34. Gorwitz RJ, Nakashima AK, Moran JS, Knapp JS. Sentinel surveillance for antimicrobial resistance to *Neisseria gonorrhoeae*—United States, 1988–1991. The Gonococcal Isolate Surveillance Project Study Group. *MMWR CDC Surveill Summ.* 1993;42:29–39.
35. Rice RJ, Knapp JS. Susceptibility of *Neisseria gonorrhoeae* associated with pelvic inflammatory disease to cefoxitin, ceftriaxone, clindamycin, gentamycin, doxycycline, azithromycin, and other antimicrobial agents. *Antimicrob Agents Chemother.* 1994;38:1688–1691.
36. McCormack WM, Mogabgab WJ, Jones RB, Hook EW III, Wendel GD Jr, Handsfield HH. Multicenter comparative study of cefotaxime and ceftriaxone for treatment of uncomplicated gonorrhea. *Sex Transm Dis.* 1993;20:269–273.
37. Haizlip J, Isbey SF, Hamilton HA, et al. Time required for evaluation of *Neisseria gonorrhoeae* from urogenital tract in men with symptomatic urethritis: comparison of oral and intramuscular single-dose therapy. *Sex Transm Dis.* 1995;22:145–148.
38. Mogabgab WJ, Lutz FB. Randomized study of cefotaxime versus ceftriaxone for uncomplicated gonorrhea. *South Med J.* 1994;87:461–464.
39. Schwebke JR, Whittington W, Rice RJ, Handsfield HH, Hale J, Holmes KK. Trends in susceptibility of *Neisseria gonorrhoeae* to ceftriaxone from 1985 through 1991 *Antimicrob Agents Chemother.* 1995;39:917–920.

Meningococcal Infections

Elena R. Ladich and Ernest E. Lack

Acute pain of the ear with continual and strong fever is to be dreaded; for there is danger that the man may become delirious and die.

Hippocrates, Book of Prognostics, 22

INTRODUCTION

Neisseria meningitidis causes a wide range of infections in humans including meningitis, arthritis, endocarditis, and primary pneumonia. *Neisseria meningitidis* can have a fulminating course killing a previously healthy person within a few hours of onset of symptoms. Among species of *Neisseria* only *N meningitidis* and *N gonorrhoeae* are pathogens for humans,[1] although rare exceptions of infections by "nonpathogenic" *Neisseria* are reported, eg, endocarditis, meningitis, and pneumonia caused by *N sicca* and *N mucosa.*[2]

CLASSIFICATION

Neisseria sp and *Branhamella catarrhalis* are classified, along with the genera *Moraxella, Kingella,* and *Acinetobacter,* in the family Neisseriaceae. The genera *Eikenella, Simonsiella,* and *Alysiella* have also been assigned to the same family.[1] *Neisseria* sp are gram-negative diplococci with adjacent sides flattened, which gives the appearance of a kidney or "coffee bean" in stained smears. Sometimes there are tetrads when the bacteria divide at right angles to each other.[1] *Neisseria meningitidis* is oxidative, producing acid from glucose and maltose.[3]

EPIDEMIOLOGY

Neisseria meningitidis can colonize the oropharynx or nasopharynx of asymptomatic carriers. Colonization may occur in 2% to 15% of healthy individuals,[1,4] or in an even greater proportion in crowded or confluent populations, such as military recruits.[1] Colonization is so common that *N meningitidis* could arguably be considered part of the normal human oral flora.[4] Thirteen serogroups are currently recognized based on acidic capsular polysaccharides: A, B, C, D, 29E, H, I, K, L, W135, X, Y, and Z,[1,4] and can be further classified according to type, subtype, and immunotype.[5] Strains belonging to groups A, B, C, Y, and W135 most frequently cause systemic disease; classically group A and C strains cause epidemic meningococcal disease. In England and Wales, most infections (69%) are caused by group B followed by group C (28%).[4] During the last 15 years, Norway has had the highest incidence of meningococcal disease in Northern Europe with 80% of infections caused by serogroup B meningococci.[6] The incidence of meningococcemia is highest in school-age children, adolescents, and young adults.[1]

In Africa, epidemic meningitis is in a wide band of countries lying south of the Sahara in the so-called "meningitis belt." The region consists of broad, grassy savanna plains extending from Gambia in West Africa across the continent to Ethiopia.[4] In the African meningitis belt epidemics of meningococcal meningitis occur at intervals of 8 to 12 years, and are usually caused by serogroup A strains. Typically epidemics start well after the beginning of the dry season and spread in the population with dramatic speed until ending abruptly with the onset of the rainy season.[7] Perhaps mass migration of pilgrims plays an important role in the spread of meningococcal infections in these parts of the world.[7] Epidemics reaching prevalence rates of up to 500 to 1600 per 100,000 inhabitants have caused major public health problems.[7] The annual incidence in other parts of the world is much lower, eg, 2 per 100,000 population in Sweden.[8] Recent studies suggest that "antigenic shifts" in group A meningococcal clones may trigger an outbreak of disease by suddenly decreasing immunity within a population.[9]

Because meningococci do not survive well outside the human host and have no alternative host, transmission is usually by direct contact with contaminated respiratory secretions or airborne droplets. Sexual transmission of meningococci has been reported, causing lower genital tract infections in both women and homosexual men, representing anogenital carriage in addition to oropharyngeal and nasopharyngeal carrier states.[1] In a recent study only 5% of patients had a history of contact with another patient with meningococcal infection.[8] Prevention of spread is based on mass vaccination and chemoprophylaxis of close contacts of patients with infections. Recently polymerase chain reaction (PCR) amplicon restriction endonuclease analysis (AREA) has been useful in identifying the strain, and has potential for studying the spread of a pathogenic strain in a population.[10]

PATHOGENESIS

Structurally the meningococcus has two cell membranes and about 50% of the outer leaflet of the outer membrane consists of amphophilic lipooligosaccharide (LOS) molecules. Outside the outer membrane is a capsule consisting of acidic polysaccharide, which is highly antigenic (except in group B strains) and is the basis for the major epidemiologic subdivision of meningococci.[5] The major toxic factors of *N meningitidis* are LOS, which is toxic for human endothelial and epithelial cells in vitro.[11] Pili are filamentous protein appendages that facilitate adherence to cells. They extend considerable distances from the bacterial surface, and probably cause interaction with host epithelial cells first and then with endothelial cells.[5] Pili may have a synergistic effect in toxicity.[11] Piliation appears to be required for colonization of host mucosal surfaces, and for at least some stages of invasive disease.[5]

Studies suggest that LOS is an important activator of complement in systemic meningococcal disease. Activation of the complement system is essential in protecting humans from invading *N meningitidis*. Formation and deposition of C3b on the bacterial surface enhances phagocytosis and intracellular killing of the bacteria. At the same time proper assemblage and insertion of the membrane attack complex (MC5b-9) on the bacterial surface are the basis for serum bactericidal activity.[12] A defect in one or more of the higher complement factors, C5 through C9, is associated with recurrent meningococcal infections, and defects in properdin may cause fulminating meningococcal septicemia and death.[12] In the process of complement activation, anaphylotoxins (C3a, C4a, C5a) are formed that are potent mediators of inflammatory effects and promote activation of coagulation; these split products may have a profound effect on the vascular bed and contribute to pathophysiology. The complement system, therefore, may have potentially beneficial and detrimental effects on the host, depending on the degree of activation.[12] During the process of disseminated intravascular coagulation (DIC) there may be depletion of naturally occurring anticoagulants, eg, protein C and protein S, and the magnitude of decline, degree of thrombocytopenia, and presence of fibrin split products are directly related to clinical severity.[13]

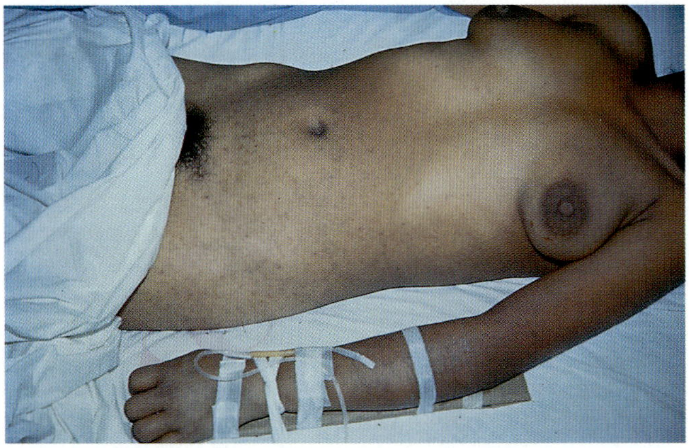

Figure 73–19. Woman in terminal meningococcal septicemia. She had DIC and there are scattered petechiae over abdomen and trunk.

CLINICAL MANIFESTATIONS

Clinical manifestations may be dominated by a fulminating, rapidly progressive septicemia with fever, vascular collapse, and DIC as manifested by petechial (Figure 73–19) or purpuric skin lesions (Figure 73–20). The combination of skin rash and fever led to the descriptive term "spotted fever," which has also been applied to other infections such as typhoid fever. The course of the infection may be brief with death in a few hours of onset. Meningitis may not be clinically apparent in fulminating infections and at autopsy the brain may be only slightly hyperemic. Other manifestations of meningococcal septicemia include acute polyarthritis and endocarditis. There may be primary meningococcal pneumonia without preceding bloodstream invasion.[14]

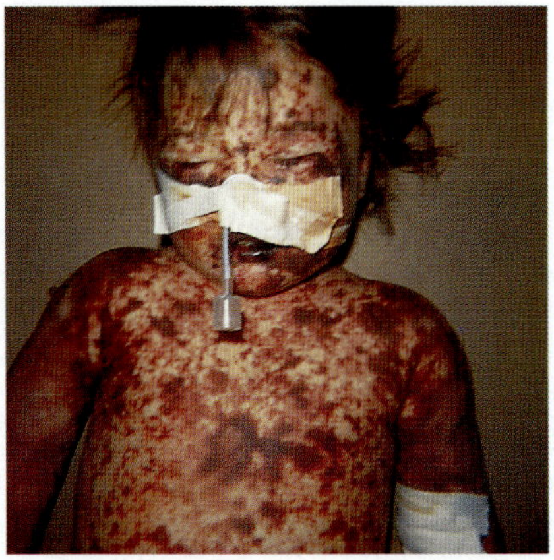

Figure 73–20. Fatal meningococcal septicemia in an infant with Waterhouse–Friderichsen syndrome. Hemorrhages in skin are confluent.

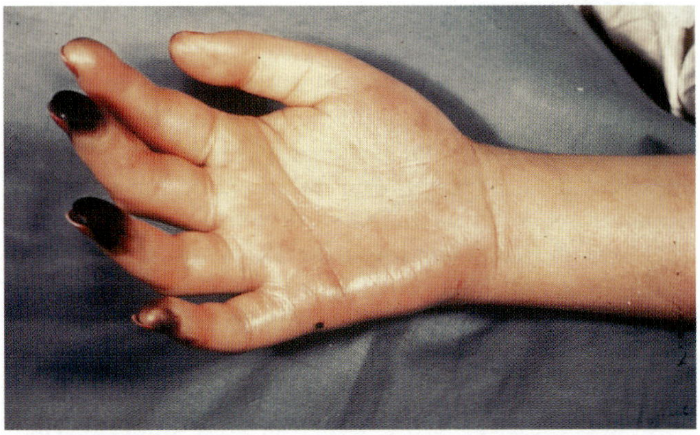

A

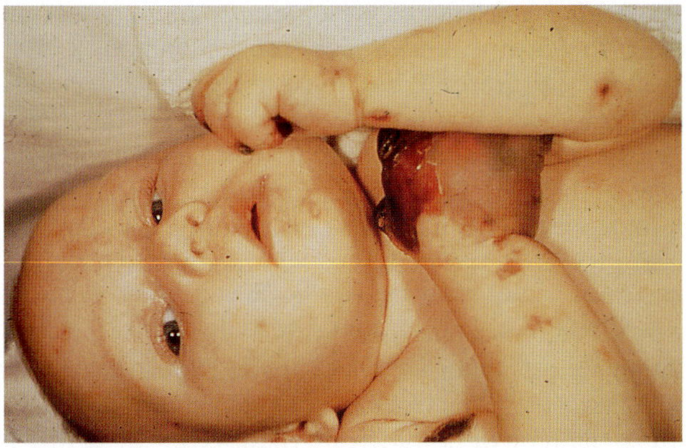

B

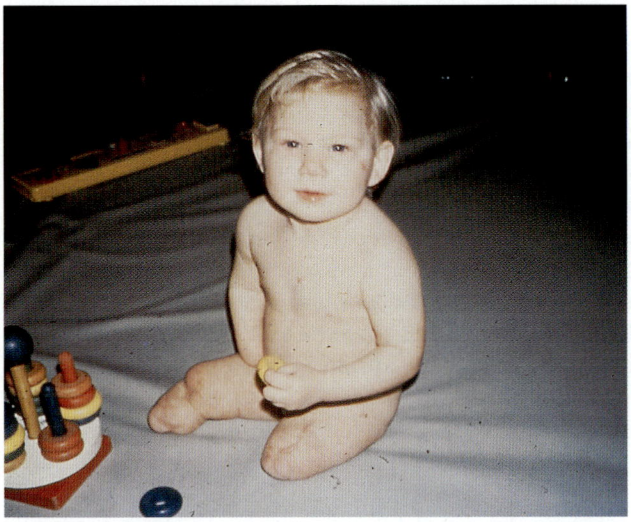

C

Figure 73–21. (**A**) Purpura fulminans in a child with fatal meningococcal septicemia. Note gangrene of terminal digits of right hand. (**B**) Purpura fulminans with asymmetrical acral gangrene of right hand. *(Contributed by David A. Schwartz, MD.)* (**C**) Partial loss of limbs in an infant who survived purpura fulminans caused by meningococcal septicemia. This 20-month-old child had both feet and the right wrist amputated. *(Contributed by David A. Schwartz, MD.)*

Purpura fulminans is a catastrophic febrile illness with initial hemorrhagic skin lesions that progress to gangrene.[15] The confluent purpura and gangrene are usually in the distal portion of the limbs in a symmetrical or asymmetrical distribution (Figure 73–21, A and B). If the patient survives the initial crisis, amputation of a gangrenous limb may be required (Figure 73–21, C) and sometimes revision to a higher level is necessary.[16] Purpura fulminans has been reported also with hematogenous infections by other bacteria such as *Escherichia coli, Streptococcus pneumoniae, Proteus mirabilis,*[15] and viruses, including varicella[15] and rubella.[16] The fatality rate in several recent series was 6.6%[8] to 10%.[6,17]

Several studies have identified prognostic factors of meningococcal infections.[17] Grave prognostic signs include circulatory insufficiency, less than 10,000 circulating white cells per cubic millimeter, or coagulopathology. The likelihood of death increases dramatically when multiple organ systems fail.[18] Overall mortality rate was accurately predicted by the pediatric risk of mortality (PRISM) score.[18–21] Other poor prognostic indicators include hypothermia, seizures or shock, platelet count below 100,000/mm^3 and purpura fulminans.[17]

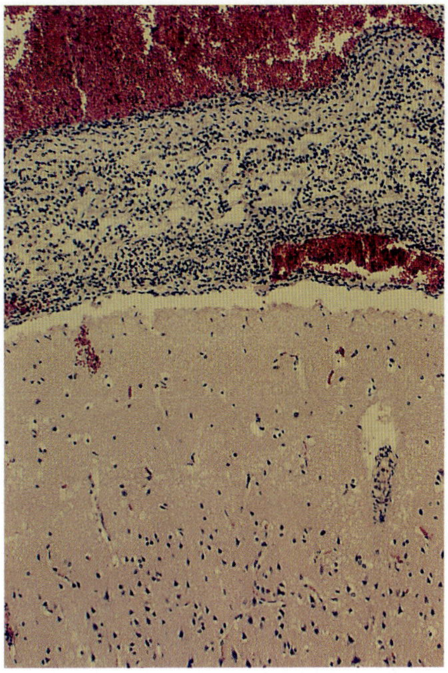

Figure 73–23. Acute suppurative leptomeningitis caused by *N meningitidis.* The exudate is comprised of neutrophils, fibrin, and interspersed foci of hemorrhage (hematoxylin-eosin, ×175).

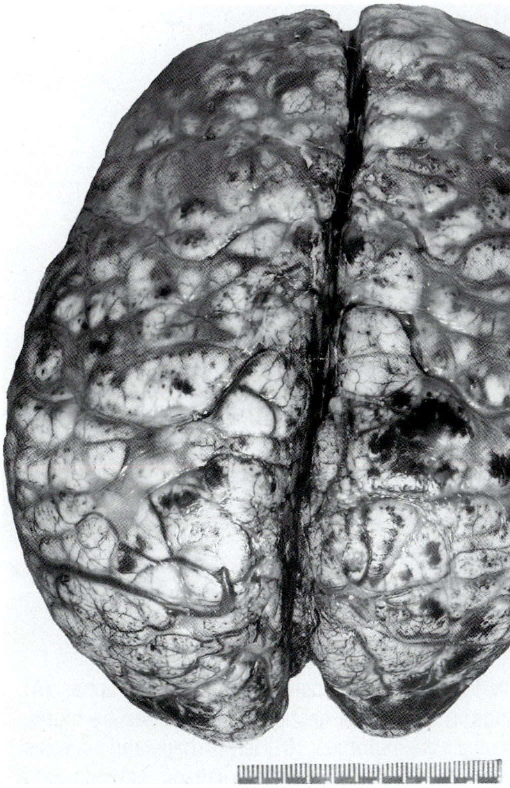

Figure 73–22. Acute suppurative leptomeningitis caused by *N meningitidis.* Leptomeninges are cloudy to opaque from a purulent exudate in the subarachnoid space. The dark patches are hemorrhage. Note background of congestion with swollen gyri and flattened sulci.

Postmeningitic adhesions may also obstruct cerebrospinal fluid (CSF). The acute inflammatory exudate distends the leptomeninges and there may be foci of hemorrhage (Figures 73–22 and 73–23). The brain may swell and compromise function of the brain stem. A "post-basic" form of meningococcal meningitis has been described in young children which affects meninges over the base of the brain, particularly in the posterior fossa, which may be confused clinically with tuberculous meningitis.

WATERHOUSE–FRIDERICHSEN SYNDROME

Waterhouse–Friderichsen syndrome (W-FS) is a well-defined clinicopathologic syndrome described by Waterhouse in 1911 and Friderichsen in 1918, although it may have been recognized in 1901.[22] Although W-FS is classically associated with meningococcal septicemia it is caused also by *Haemophilus influenzae, Streptococcus pneumoniae,* and varicella infections. W-FS typically has an abrupt onset, usually in a previous healthy patient, and has a rapid course characterized by septicemia, shock, and cutaneous petechiae. At autopsy there is hemorrhage into both adrenal glands. In most patients the adrenals are dark red and retain their shape

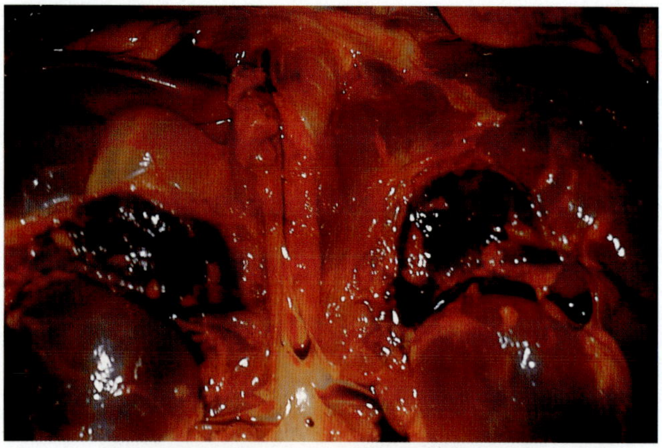

Figure 73–24. W-FS caused by meningococcal septicemia in a young child. Both adrenal glands are hemorrhagic but retain relatively normal shape.

(Figure 73–24), but sometimes hemorrhage into the cortex is extensive and disrupts the normal anatomy. The adrenals may look like hematomas with distention of the capsules (Figure 23–25, A); hemorrhage may extend into periadrenal adipose tissue (Figure 73–25, B and C). Histologically there may be cortical necrosis and deposits of fibrin in sinusoids (Figure 73–26). The adrenal hemorrhage in the W-FS is probably caused by direct action of bacterial endotoxins on a gland that is already "stressed" from septicemia. The generalized Shwartzman phenomenon has been proposed as an experimental model for the W-FS. The generalized Shwartzman reaction follows a second injection of endotoxin (24 hours after the first injection).

PURPURIC SKIN LESIONS

Biopsy of purpuric skin lesions in patients with meningococcal septicemia reveals extravasated red blood cells around small vessels in the dermis associated with fibrin thrombi and sparse to moderate accu-

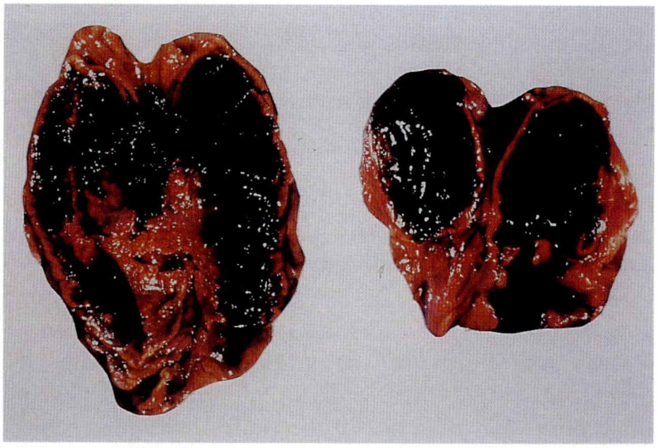

A

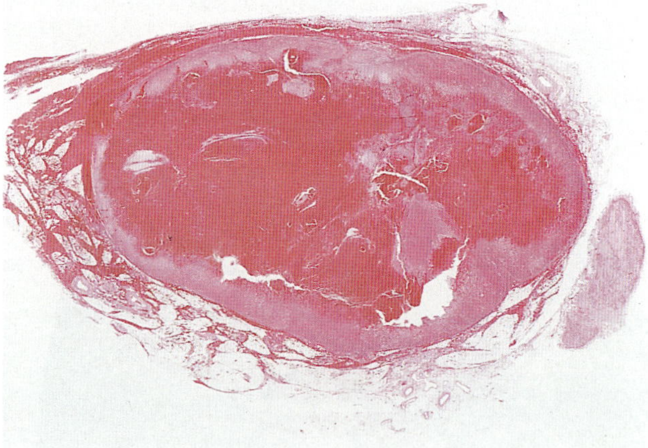

B

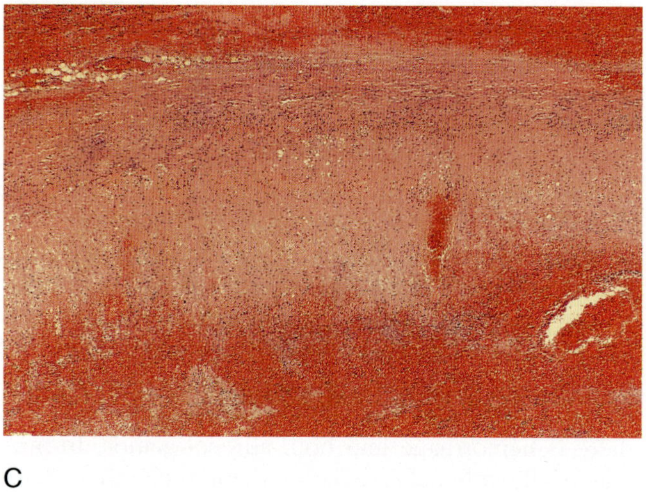

C

Figure 73–25. W-FS caused by meningococcal septicemia. (**A**) Both adrenal glands in transverse section are distended by blood, giving the appearance of hematomas. (**B**) Hemorrhage and necrosis obliterate cortical architecture. Some hemorrhage extends into periadrenal adipose tissue (hematoxylin-eosin, ×4). (**C**) Higher magnification showing pericapsular hemorrhage and a hematoma of the medulla encroaching on the cortex (hematoxylin-eosin, ×40).

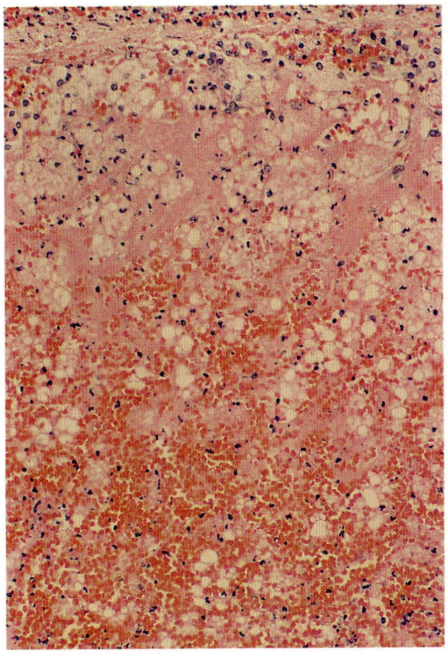

Figure 73–26. W-FS caused by meningococcal septicemia. Fibrin thrombi are in sinusoids of adrenal cortex and there is a background of necrosis and hemorrhage. Adrenal capsule is at top of field (hematoxylin-eosin, ×120).

mulation of neutrophils (Figure 73–27, A and B). Special stains such as Brown–Hopps (Figure 73–27, C) or Giemsa (Figure 73–28) may reveal cocci free within the lumen of the vessel and/or the perivascular space or within cytoplasm of neutrophils. This is not the most expeditious way to make the diagnosis of meningococcal septicemia, and in a significant number of patients identification of cocci is equivocal or absent.

DIAGNOSIS AND TREATMENT

The hallmark of meningococcal disease is its rapid, fulminating course. Thus, early specific diagnosis and treatment are essential. A diagnosis of meningococcal disease is normally first suspected on clinical grounds and confirmed by isolation of *N meningitidis* from blood or CSF, or by microscopic detection of Gram-negative diplococci in CSF (Figure 73–29). Cultures of blood are positive in about one third of the patients with meningococcal meningitis and in 50% to 75% of those with clinical meningococcemia or meningococcemia-meningitis. In about 90% of patients with meningococcal meningitis, *N meningitidis* can be cultured from the CSF (Figure 73–30) or identified on Gram-stained smears of CSF. Cultures of blood or CSF take 12 to 24 hours and may not grow *N meningitidis* if the patient has been treated with an antibiotic.[23]

Several rapid diagnostic techniques, including counterimmunoelectrophoresis, coagglutination, and latex agglutination are used to detect antigen in biologic fluids. Although counterimmunoelectrophoresis has been used by many laboratories for several years, latex agglutination is more effective.[24] Latex agglutination offers serogroup identification, an essential aspect of diagnosis both for initial therapy and prophylaxis.[25] In addition, accurate serotyping provides important epidemiologic information critical in application of specific meningococcal vaccines and is useful in following epidemic trends worldwide.

In recent years, molecular diagnostic techniques such as PCR have been developed, allowing rapid and early detection of *N meningitidis*. PCR detects the organism even when cultures are negative, and may be especially useful when diagnosis is difficult because the patient has already been treated with antibiotics. Kristiansen et al[26] used PCR for diagnosis with primers homologous to the *N meningitidis* gene encoding dihydropteroate synthetase. Others have described PCR primers utilizing an insertion sequence IS1106 with a sensitivity and specificity of 91%.[27] Specificity and sensitivity of 95% have been reported with the use of 16sRNA nested primers.[28]

TREATMENT

Up until the dawn of the twentieth century, standard medical treatment of meningococcal disease was primitive. Therapies included cold water baths, medicinal extracts of bark and wine, and copious bloodletting.[29] In 1906, the first effective treatment of meningococcal meningitis was introduced by Branham[30] with her discovery of meningococcal antiserum. Flexner, by targeting specific serotypes, improved the efficacy of meningococcal antiserum during an epidemic in New York City in 1915. The use of therapeutic serum reached its zenith in World War I, when meningococcal infections afflicted military recruits and civilians of all involved nations. Treatment with intrathecal injections of polyvalent antimeningococcal serum lowered the mortality rate from approximately 75% to 39%.[31]

Antibiotics

A second milestone in the treatment of infectious diseases occurred in 1934 when the antimicrobial activity of the red dye prontosil (the generic precursor of the sulfonamides) was discovered by Domagk. In 1937, the first patient with meningococcal meningitis was successfully treated with sulfanilamide, and by 1941, sulfonamides had become standard therapy for meningococcal infections.[32] In 1942, with the discovery of penicillin, and its clinical efficacy in the treatment of

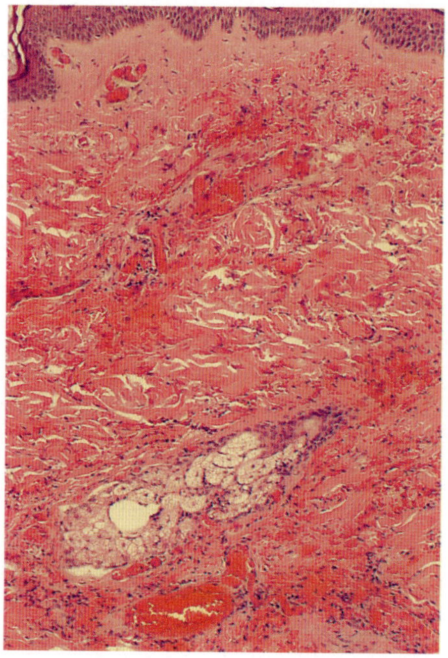

A

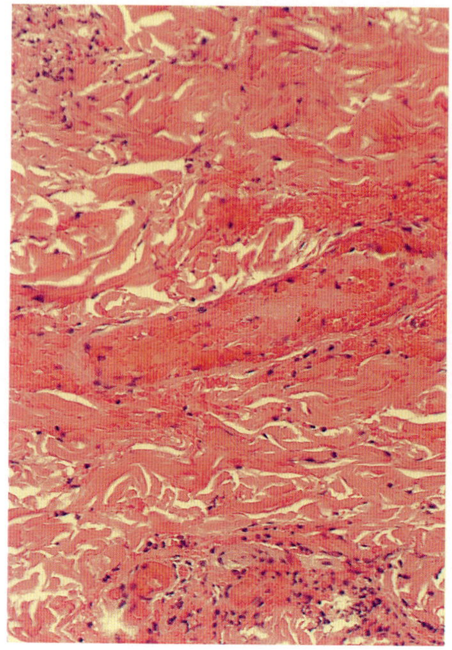

B

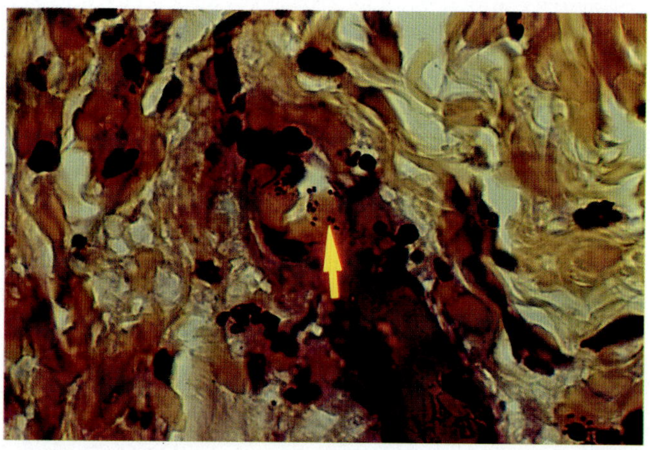

C

Figure 73–27. Meningococcal septicemia in a 19-year-old woman. Patient had sore throat, stiff neck, and a purpuric rash. (**A**) Biopsy of skin was done to rule out sepsis. *Neisseria meningitidis* was cultured from the CSF. Note fibrin thrombi in small dermal vessels and extravasated red blood cells (hematoxylin-eosin, ×100). (**B**) Fibrin thrombi are associated with scattered neutrophils and extravasated blood. Patient had clinical and laboratory evidence of DIC (hematoxylin-eosin, ×208). (**C**) A few diplococci are in the fibrin thrombus in vessel (*arrow*). (Brown–Hopps, ×1000).

meningococcal infections, new possibilities of treatment were offered.

The prophylactic value of sulfadiazine was tested during World War II during an epidemic of meningococcal meningitis among U.S. recruits, and following the prophylactic therapy with sulfadiazine the fatality rate dropped to 3.7%.[33] These results have not been improved. Today bacterial meningitis has a mortality rate of 3% to 6%. The use of sulfa drugs came to a halt in the United States after an outbreak of sulfadiazine-resistant group B meningococci at the U.S. Naval training center in San Diego, California, in 1963.[29] Since then, epidemics of sulfa-resistant groups A, B, and C meningococcal infections have been reported throughout most of the world.

Current Treatment

Intravenous penicillin G remains the drug of choice for treatment of meningococcal meningitis as well as acute meningococcemia. In the last several years, however, penicillin-resistant isolates of *N meningitidis* have been reported worldwide. Resistant meningococci appear to produce altered forms of penicillin-binding proteins, thus decreasing the organism's affinity for antibiotic. Given the fulminating nature of *N meningitidis* infections, simple and reliable antimicrobial susceptibility testing is becoming important in identifying penicillin-resistant isolates. The E-test is a relatively new approach to test such antimicrobial susceptibility. The method is based on the diffusion of a continuous concentration

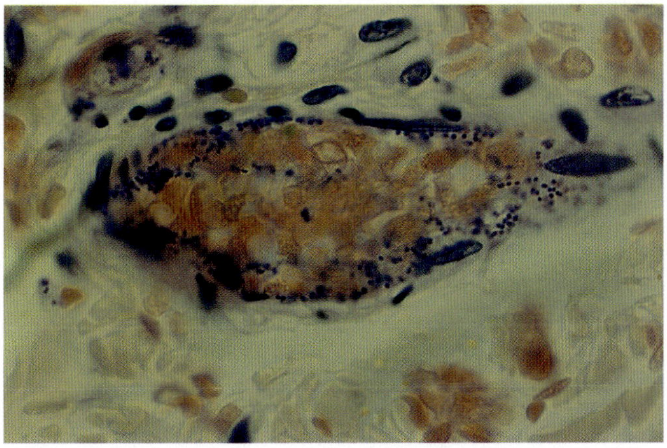

Figure 73–28. Fatal meningococcal septicemia. There were purpuric lesions at autopsy. There are numerous diplococci in and along the wall of the vessel (Giemsa stain, ×1000).

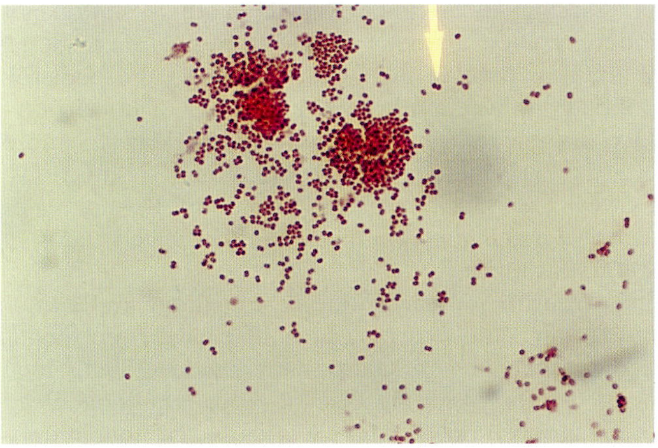

Figure 73–30. Meningococcal meningitis. *Neisseria meningitidis* was cultured from CSF of patient in Figure 73–27 and shown here are numerous gram-negative diplococci in smear of culture plate. Note occasional tetrad (Gram stain, ×1000).

gradient of an antimicrobial agent from a carrier strip into an agar medium. Current dilution tests are expensive, cumbersome, and have not been standardized. The E-test is a simple and accurate method for the emerging need to test meningococci and other pathogenic species of *Neisseria*.[34]

Chloramphenicol, introduced in 1947, is a recommended alternative in patients allergic to penicillin. Also, *N meningitidis* has remarkable sensitivity to the third-generation cephalosporins such as ceftriaxone and cefotaxin showing an average potency 8- to 64-fold greater than that of penicillin.[34] Ceftriaxone was effective even when given as a single injection in an epidemic in Africa. This promises good results for mass treatment in the African meningitis belt.[35]

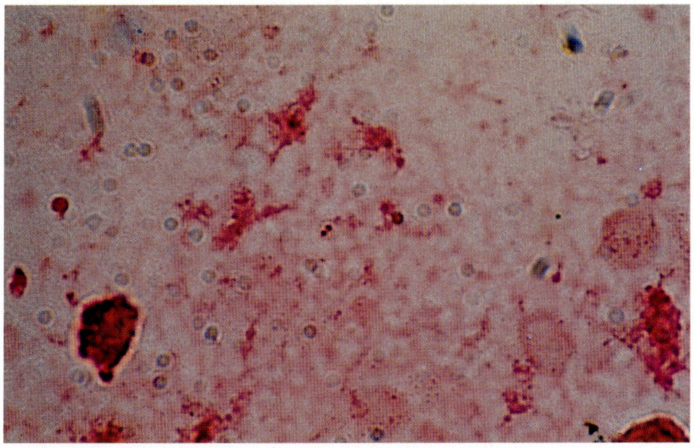

Figure 73–29. Meningococcal meningitis. Gram stain of CSF shows few gram-negative cocci (Gram stain, ×1000). *(Contributed by Grace M. Thorne, PhD.)*

Other Aspects of Treatment

Severe meningococcemia requires supportive measures for shock and other complications such as DIC and purpura fulminans. Despite advances in critical care, mortality rates associated with meningococcal sepsis have improved little during the last 30 years and range between 10% and 28%. Sepsis-associated purpura fulminans is more frequent in children than adults, and may have a 50% to 60% mortality. The pathogenesis of purpura fulminans appears to be related, at least in part, to a deficiency of proteins C and S. Studies have indicated that early replacement of protein C arrests the development of clinical signs of purpura fulminans in children and has been shown to reverse the associated organ dysfunction.[36]

Other therapies such as heparin, frozen plasma, and antithrombin III have had varying degrees of success in treating DIC. Heparin has been controversial, but ultimately has not improved the outcome of patients with fulminating meningococcemia and DIC. Antithrombin III has prevented endotoxin-induced DIC, and has been used in clinical trials.[37] Fresh frozen plasma is recommended instead of coagulation factors for DIC.

PROPHYLAXIS

Goldschneider et al[38] have shown that much of the bactericidal effect of antisera was from antibodies directed against capsular polysaccharide, demonstrating the potential of these antigens in developing vaccines. Currently, a quadrivalent vaccine is commercially available (groups A, C, W, W135). Vaccines based on capsular polysaccharides are immunogenic in adults, but do not induce a good antibody response in children under 2 years, thus limiting their effectiveness in the pediatric population. Recent advances in the use of novel polysaccharide conjugate vaccines should lead to more effective vaccines against group A and C infections. However, a vaccine against serogroup B, the major cause of meningococcal disease in the United States, is still not available.[39]

Group B polysaccharide is structurally and immunologically similar to molecules that have been identified on human cells, particularly in developing fetal brain tissue, suggesting that the poor immunogenicity of the group B polysaccharide is caused by an immunologic tolerance. Recent trials with vaccines derived from outer membrane protein are encouraging because they show it is possible to induce protection against group B meningococci.[39] Routine immunization is not recommended because of the low risk of disease in the absence of outbreaks. In some epidemiologic situations, however, such as in sub-Saharan Africa, routine vaccination is an important preventive measure.

Chemoprophylaxis

Chemoprophylaxis reduces nasopharyngeal carriage of the meningococcus and thereby interrupts transmission. Several antimicrobial agents have been successful prophylactically. Sulfonilamides have been used extensively since World War II, and historically were safe and effective. Unfortunately, sulfonamide-resistant meningococci are now prevalent, thus decreasing the utility of this class of drugs. Rifampin is now the drug of choice for prophylaxis. A 2-day course of rifampin eradicates meningococcal throat carriage in 95% to 98% of cases.[39] Minocycline also is an effective prophylactic for meningococcal meningitis, although it causes side effects. Recent reports suggest that ciprofloxacin eradicates nasopharyngeal carriage in 89% to 97% of those treated.[40] Also, ceftriaxone eradicates the carrier state when given as a single intramuscular injection.

Who should receive chemoprophylaxis? It is recommended that close household contacts of the patient receive prophylactic therapy. These individuals are usually defined as those sleeping in the same household, and as those likely to have exchanged saliva through kissing or coughing. There is no evidence that hospital personnel are at greater risk unless they have given mouth-to-mouth resuscitation. Prophylaxis should begin when the infection is identified. Since penicillin does not eradicate nasopharyngeal carriage, rifampin should be given to the index patient prior to discharge.

REFERENCES

1. Knapp JS, Rice RJ. *Neisseria* and *Branhamella*. In: Murray PR, Baron EJ, Pfaller MA, Tenover FC, Yolken RH, eds. *Manual of Clinical Microbiology*. 6th ed. Washington, DC: ASM Press; 1995.
2. Herbert DA, Ruskin J. Are the "nonpathogenic" *Neisseriae* pathogenic? *Am J Clin Pathol.* 1981;75:739–743.
3. Baron EJ, Peterson LR, Finegold SM, eds. *Bailey and Scott's Diagnostic Microbiology*. 9th ed. St. Louis, Mo.: Mosby; 1994.
4. Moore PS, Broome CV. Cerebrospinal meningitis epidemics. *Sci Am.* 1994;271:38–45.
5. Hart CA, Rogers TRF, eds. Meningococcal disease. *J Med Microbiol.* 1993;39:3–25.
6. Bjune G, Hoiby EA, Gronnesby JK, Arnesen O, Fredriksen JH, Haltensen A, Holten E, Linbak A-K, Nokleby H, Rosenqvist E, et al. Effect of outer membrane vesicle vaccine against group B meningococcal disease in Norway. *Lancet.* 1991;338:1093–1096.
7. Bjorvatn B, Hassan-King M, Greenwood B, Haimanot RT, Fekade D, Sperber G. DNA finger printing in the epidemiology of African serogroup A *Neisseria meningitidis*. *Scand J Infect Dis.* 1992;24:323–332.
8. Berg S, Trollfors B, Alestig K, Jodal U. Incidence, serogroups and case fatality rate of invasive meningococcal infections in a Swedish region 1975–1989. *Scand J Infect Dis.* 1992;24:333–338.
9. Moore PS, Meningococcal meningitis in sub-Saharan Africa: a model for the epidemic process. *Clin Infect Dis.* 1992;14:515–525.
10. Kristiansen B-E, Fermér C, Jenkins A, Ask E, Swedberg G, Sköld O. PCR amplicon restriction endonuclease analysis of chromosome *dhps* gene of *Neisseria meningitidis:* a method for studying spread of the disease-causing strain in contacts of patients with meningococcal disease. *J Clin Microbiol.* 1995;33:1174–1179.
11. Dunn KLR, Virji M, Moxon ER. Investigations into the molecular basis of meningococcal toxicity for human endothelial and epithelial cells: the synergistic effect of LPS and pili. *Microbiol Pathogenesis.* 1995;18:81–96.
12. Brandtzaeg P, Mollnes TE, Kierulf P. Complement activation and endotoxin levels in systemic meningococcal disease. *J Infect Dis.* 1989;160:58–65.
13. Powars D, Larsen R, Johnson J, et al. Epidemic meningococcemia and purpura fulminans with induced protein C deficiency. *Clin Infect Dis.* 1993;17:254–261.
14. Irwin RS, Woelk WK, Coudon WL III. Primary meningococcal pneumonia. *Ann Intern Med.* 1975;82:493–498.
15. Chu DZJ, Blaisdell FW. Purpura fulminans. *Am J Surg.* 1982;143:356–362.
16. Genoff MC, Hoffer MM, Achauer B, Formosa P. Extremity amputations in meningococcemia-induced purpura fulminans. *Plastic Reconstr Surg.* 1992;89:878–881.
17. Wong VK, Hitchcock W, Mason WH. Meningococcal infections in children: a review of 100 cases. *Pediatr Infect Dis J.* 1989;8:224–227.
18. Stiehm ER, Damrosch DS. Factors in the prognosis of meningococcal infection. *J Pediatr.* 1966;68:457–467.

19. Pollack MM, Ruttimann VE, Getson PR. Pediatric risk of mortality (PRISM) score. *Crit Care Med.* 1988;16:1110–1116.
20. Algren JT, Lah S, Cutliff SA, Richman BJ. Predictors of outcome in acute meningococcal infection in children. *Crit Care Med.* 1993;21:447–452.
21. Tesoro LJ, Selbst SM. Factors affecting outcome in meningococcal infections. *Am J Dis Child.* 1994;145:218–220.
22. Sloper JC. The adrenal glands and extra-adrenal chromaffin tissue (revised by B. Fox). In: Symmers W, ed. *Systemic Pathology.* 2nd ed. Edinburgh: Churchill Livingstone; 1978:1914–1974.
23. Schwartz MN, Dodge PR. Bacterial meningitis: a review and selected aspects I. General clinical features, special problems and unusual reactions mimicking bacterial meningitis. *N Engl J Med.* 1965;272:779–787.
24. Kaldon JR, Asznowicz Buist DG. Latex agglutination in diagnosis of bacterial infections with special reference to meningitis and septicemia. *Am J Clin Pathol.* 1977;68:284–287.
25. Nato F, Mazie JC, Fournier JM, et al. Production of polyclonal and monoclonal antibodies against group A, B, and C capsular polysaccharides of *Neisseria meningitidis* and preparation of latex reagents. *J Clin Microbiol.* 1991;29:1447–1452.
26. Kristiansen BE, Ask E, Jenkins A, Fermér C, Rädström P, Sköld O. Rapid diagnosis of meningococcal meningitis by polymerase chain reaction. *Lancet.* 1991;337:1568–1569.
27. Ni H, Knight AI, Cartwright K, Palmer WH, McFadden J. Polymerase chain reaction for diagnosis of meningococcal meningitis. *Lancet.* 1992;340:1432–1434.
28. Rädström P, Bäckman A, Qian N, Kragsbjerg P, Påhlson C, Olcén P. Detection of bacterial DNA in cerebrospinal fluid by an assay for simultaneous detection of *Neisseria meningitidis, Haemophilus influenzae,* and streptococci using a seminested PCR strategy. *J Clin Microbiol.* 1994;32:2738–2744.
29. Vedros NA, Gold R. Clinical aspects of meningococcal disease. In: *Evolution of Meningococcal Disease.* Boca Raton, Fla.: CRC Press; 1987;2:69–97.
30. Branham S. Milestones in the history of the meningococcus. *Can J Microbiol.* 1956;2:175–188.
31. Brundage JF, Zollinger W. Evolution of meningococcal disease epidemiology in the U.S. Army. In: *Evolution of Meningococcal Disease.* Boca Raton, Fla.: CRC Press; 1987;1:paper 5-25.
32. Etienne J. Development of antibiotic sensitivity of the meningococci. In: *Evolution of Meningococcal Disease.* Boca Raton, Fla.: CRC Press; 1987;2:57–68.
33. Kuhns DM, Nelson CT, Feldman HA, Kuhn LR. The prophylactic value of sulfadiazine in the control of meningococcic meningitis. *J Am Med Assoc.* 1943;123:335–339.
34. Hughes JH, Biedenbach DJ, Erwin ME, Jones RN. E test as susceptibility test and epidemiologic tool for evaluation of *Neisseria meningitidis* isolates. *J Clin Microbiol.* 1993;31:3255–3259.
35. Schwartz B, Al-Tobaiqi A, Al-Ruwais A, et al. Comparative efficacy of ceftriaxone and rifampicin in eradicating pharyngeal carriage of group A *N. meningitidis. Lancet.* 1988;1:1239–1242.
36. Rivard GE, Michile D, Farrell C, Schwartz HP. Treatment of purpura fulminans in meningococcemia with protein C concentrate. *J Pediatr.* 1995;126:646–652.
37. Fourrier F, Chopin C, Huart JJ, Runge I, Caron C, Goudemand J. Double-blind, placebo-controlled trial of antithrombin III concentrates in septic shock with disseminated intravascular coagulation. *Chest.* 1993;104:882–888.
38. Goldschneider I, Gotschlich EC, Artenstein MS. Human immunity to the meningococcus II. Development of natural immunity. *J Exp Med.* 1969;129:1327–1348.
39. Hart CA, Rogers TRF. Meningococcal disease review. *J Med Microbiol.* 1993;39:17–20.
40. Cuevas LE, Kazembe P, Mughogho GK, Tillotson GS, Hart CA. Eradication of nasopharyngeal carriage of *Neisseria meningitidis* in children and adults in rural Africa: a comparison of ciprofloxacin and rifampicin. *J Infect Dis.* 1995;171:728–731.

CHAPTER 74

Nocardiosis

Francis W. Chandler

Humanity has but three great enemies; fever, famine and war; of these by far the greatest, by far the most terrible, is fever.

Sir William Osler (1849–1919), Journal of the American Medical Association 1896; 26:999

DEFINITION

Nocardiosis is a systemic or localized infection caused by aerobic, filamentous bacteria in the genus *Nocardia* and the order Actinomycetales.[1–5] Unlike actinomycosis (Chapter 40), nocardiosis is an exogenous disease that is usually opportunistic. It most often afflicts those who are immunodeficient[6–12] or who have diseases such as lymphoma (especially Hodgkin's disease),[13,14] leukemia, granulocytopenia, chronic granulomatous disease,[15,16] collagen–vascular diseases,[17] and chronic pulmonary disorders (especially alveolar proteinosis).[18–20] Patients with dysfunction of cellular immunity are most susceptible, but those with functional abnormalities of neutrophils and defects in humoral immunity are also at increased risk for nocardiosis.[4,5,21] Most infections begin in the lung and result from inhaled nocardiae that live as saprophytes in soil and decaying vegetable matter. Pulmonary infection may be asymptomatic and self-limited or progressive. Hematogenous or lymphatic dissemination from a primary pulmonary focus can involve virtually any organ, but the central nervous system (CNS) and skin are most often affected.[22–24] Primary cutaneous and subcutaneous infections are rare and result from the accidental percutaneous inoculation of nocardiae in the environment.[25–29] Primary nocardial infection of the brain following direct inoculation by penetrating foreign objects has been described in an adult[30] and in a child.[31]

The term nocardiosis, as used here, refers to infection in which bacterial filaments are randomly scattered within the invaded tissue.[32] *Nocardia* sp, on rare occasions, form grains or granules in tissue. This kind of nocardiosis remains localized, is usually seen in otherwise healthy patients, and is classified as actinomycotic mycetoma (see Chapter 113).

EPIDEMIOLOGY

Infections caused by the *Nocardia* sp are worldwide. Approximately 500 to 1000 new cases of nocardiosis are diagnosed annually in the United States,[33] and the incidence of nocardial infections, especially in patients with acquired immunodeficiency syndrome (AIDS), is increasing.[4,5,34] More than 50% of patients with systemic nocardiosis are immunocompromised.[4] Systemic infections occur three times as often in males as in females, and most patients are between the ages of 21 and 50 years.[4,5,33] Nocardiosis is uncommon in children, and the usual clinical presentation is pneumonia with rapid dissemination and death.[3,35] Human-to-human or animal-to-human transmission has not been documented, and nocardiosis is not a contagious disease.

Fewer than 0.5% of patients with AIDS have nocardiosis as a complicating infection, and nocardiosis is not considered to be an AIDS-defining infection according to criteria established by the Centers for Disease Control and Prevention (CDC). About 60 cases of nocardiosis in AIDS patients from the United States have been reported.[4,5]

ETIOLOGIC AGENTS

The three medically most important species that cause nocardiosis are *Nocardia asteroides, N brasiliensis,* and *N otitidiscaviarum* (formerly *N caviae*). Rarely, other species such as *N transvalensis, N farcinica,* and *N nova* can cause similar infections.[4,5,36–39] Approximately 85% of nocardial infections in humans are caused by *N asteroides,* and this species is most often implicated in pulmonary infections. The remaining species can also cause pneumonia but are more often implicated in localized cutaneous and subcutaneous infections[21,28,29,40–44] or as agents of actinomycotic mycetoma (Chapter 113).

CLINICAL FEATURES

Nocardiosis usually presents either as chronic pneumonia in immunocompetent individuals or as an acute and progressive pneumonia in those patients with profound immunodeficiencies or with underlying diseases.[3–5] Pulmonary infection is characterized by consolidation, abscesses, pleural involvement, and empyema (Figure 74–1). Symptoms mimic those of tuberculosis and include fever, chills, dyspnea, cough, hemoptysis, chest pain, night sweats, and weight loss. Chest radiographs, which are nonspecific, often reveal bilateral infiltrates and thin-walled cavities.

Pulmonary infection can remain localized or spread to other organs via hematogenous and lymphatic pathways. Occasionally, primary pulmonary lesions may heal spontaneously and not be apparent when signs and symptoms of metastatic disease appear. Dissemination occurs in about one third of patients, and secondary lesions are most frequently found in the CNS and skin.[4,5] Patients with nocardiosis of the CNS may be asymptomatic, or they may present with headache, nausea, vomiting, stiff neck, mental confusion, convulsions, and paralysis. Brain abscesses are often multiloculated, and meningitis is rare. Other common sites of secondary infection include the bones and joints, heart, kidneys, eyes (especially the retinas), and the peritoneum.[4,5,32,45]

Cutaneous and subcutaneous infections result from hematogenous dissemination or, rarely, traumatic percutaneous implantation.[25–27] Patients with secondary lesions usually present with solitary or multiple subcutaneous abscesses and draining sinus tracts, whereas those with primary lesions often present with the lymphocutaneous (sporotrichoid) form of nocardiosis. The latter mimics classic lymphocutaneous sporotrichosis and consists of a chain of subcutaneous nodules along lymphatics leading from a primary cutaneous ulcer.[46] In either primary or secondary (disseminated) lesions of the skin and soft tissues, swelling, induration, and fistulous tracts are not as common as in actinomycosis (Chapter 40).

PATHOLOGIC FEATURES

The usual host reaction in nocardiosis is suppurative necrosis with ill-defined abscesses (Figure 74–2). In chronic infections, there are solitary or multiple encapsulated abscesses and sinus tracts filled with thick, greenish-yellow, odorless pus and separated by areas of fibrosis.[32] The abscesses are 1 mm to 2 cm or more in diameter, and contain neutrophils, macrophages, necrotic debris, and varying numbers of nocardial fila-

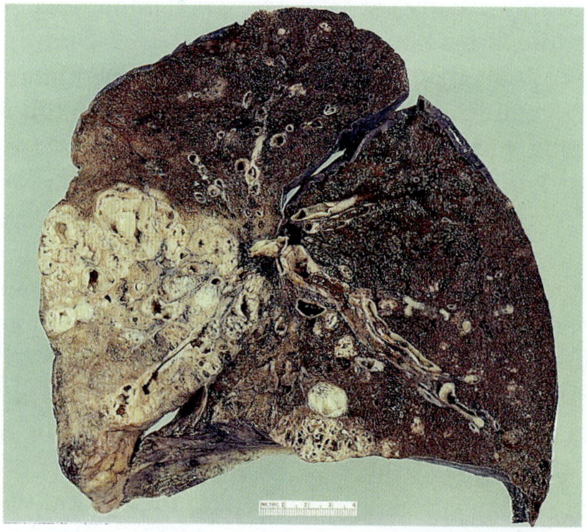

A

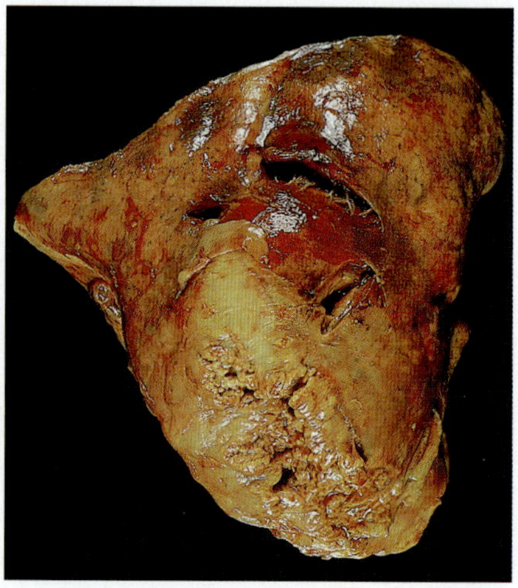

B

Figure 74–1. Chronic pulmonary nocardiosis. (**A**) Cut surface of lung reveals multiple confluent abscesses with fibrotic walls. *(Courtesy of John C. Watts, MD.)* (**B**) Large necrotizing nocardial abscess in the right lower lobe of a patient with Hodgkin's disease. Empyema resulted from direct extension of infection through the pleura.

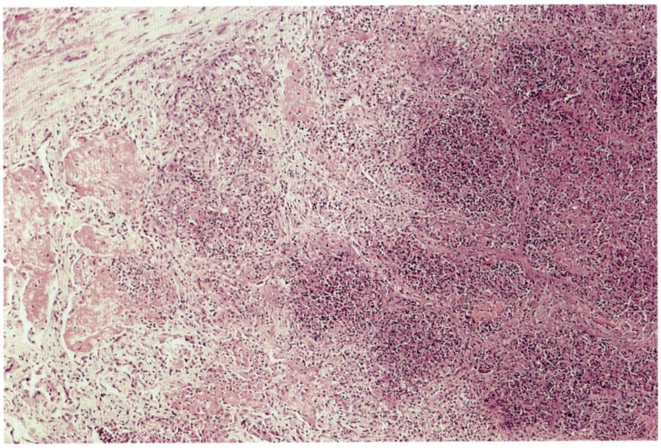

Figure 74–2. Acute pulmonary nocardiosis. The usual host reaction is suppurative necrosis with the formation of ill-defined abscesses (*right*) (hematoxylin-eosin, ×25).

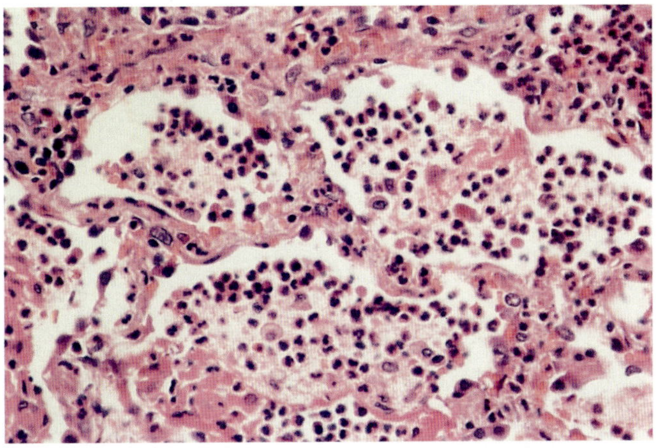

Figure 74–4. Acute pulmonary nocardiosis. The fibrinosuppurative bronchopneumonia is similar to that caused by nonfilamentous bacterial pathogens. Individual filaments of *Nocardia asteroides* (culture proved) are not delineated with hematoxylin-eosin (hematoxylin-eosin, ×160).

ments (Figure 74–3). Large abscesses are often cavitating. Epithelioid histiocytes and giant cells are sometimes at the periphery of encapsulated abscesses and blend imperceptibly with the suppurative center. As nocardial filaments age, they fragment into pleomorphic coccobacillary forms that are more readily phagocytosed by macrophages and giant cells. In the lungs, lesions vary from focal necrotizing and often multiloculated abscesses to diffuse fibrinosuppurative pneumonia with consolidation (Figure 74–4). The lower lobes are most frequently involved. Fibrinosuppurative pleuritis with empyema is a frequent complication (Figure 74–5). Rarely, the *Nocardia* sp colonize preexisting pulmonary cavities and produce "fungus balls."[4,5]

Immunodeficient patients with pulmonary nocardiosis usually present with progressive infection that appears as lobar, lobular, or fulminant necrotizing pneumonia.[32,47] Histologically, fibrosis is minimal and the pneumonia is similar to that caused by more commonly encountered nonfilamentous bacteria (Figure 74–6). In this fulminant form of nocardiosis, myriad nocardiae are often present and appear as faintly basophilic filaments in hematoxylin-eosin (H&E)-stained sections of lung.[32] Large numbers of entangled nocar-

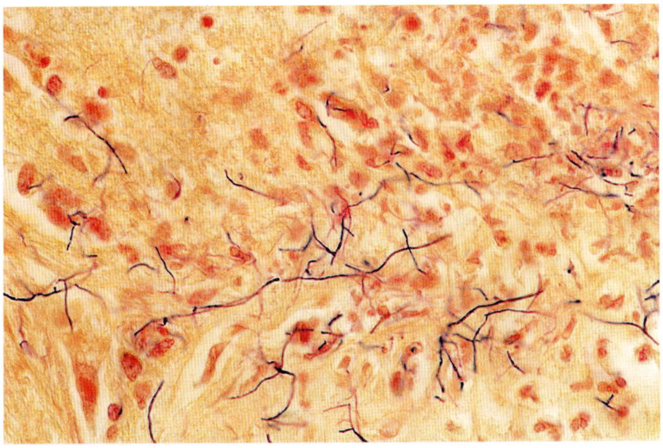

Figure 74–3. Pulmonary nocardiosis caused by *Nocardia asteroides*. An abscess contains delicate, gram-positive, randomly oriented, bacterial filaments that are approximately 1 μm wide and branch predominantly at right angles (Brown–Brenn, ×160).

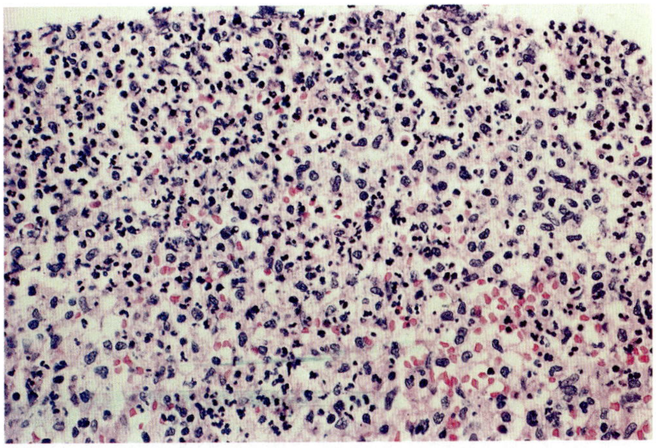

Figure 74–5. Chronic pleuritis caused by *Nocardia asteroides*. Pleural involvement and empyema are common complications of pulmonary nocardiosis and result from direct extension of the infection. Nocardial filaments within the thickened pleura do not stain with hematoxylin-eosin (hematoxylin-eosin, ×100).

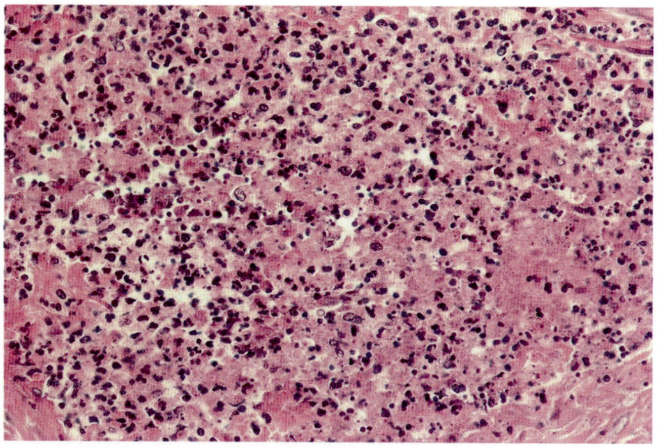

Figure 74–6. Pulmonary nocardiosis in an immunocompromised patient. Myriad nocardiae provoke a fulminant suppurative and necrotizing bronchopneumonia similar to that caused by certain nonfilamentous bacteria (hematoxylin-eosin, ×100).

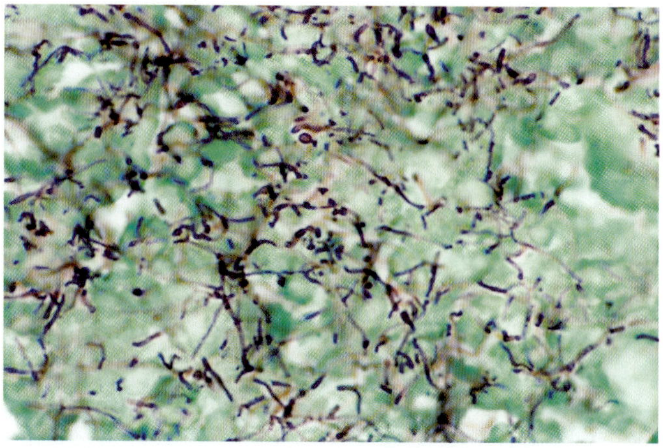

Figure 74–8. Nocardiosis caused by *Nocardia otitidiscaviarum.* A tangled mass of delicate, randomly oriented filaments and fragmented coccobacillary forms are embedded in an abscess. A terminal, spherical conidium (usually produced in culture) is at top center (GMS, ×400).

dial filaments can form loose aggregates within abscesses and alveolar spaces (Figures 74–7 and 74–8), but these aggregates do not resemble the compact "sulfur granules" of actinomycosis. The nocardial filaments are not ensheathed by clublike, intensely eosinophilic Splendore-Hoeppli material, a common feature of the granules in actinomycosis.[32]

In lesions of nocardiosis, the *Nocardia* sp appear as slender bacterial filaments, about 1 μm wide, that branch at predominantly right angles (Figure 74–3). Nocardial filaments are characteristically beaded because of irregular staining with Gram, GMS, and acid-fast procedures. Frequently, organisms are so numerous and so highly branched that they have been described as resembling "Chinese characters." In tissue sections, the filaments are randomly distributed in the inflammatory exudate, predominantly extracellular, and readily demonstrated with GMS (Figure 74–8) and modified Gram stains, such as Brown–Brenn and Brown–Hopps (Figure 74–3). However, the *Nocardia* sp are not reliably stained with H&E, the periodic acid-Schiff reaction, and Gridley fungus procedure. *Nocardia* sp are partially acid-fast and nonalcohol-fast in tissues and primary cultures when stained with modified acid-fast procedures (eg, Kinyoun, Coates–Fite, and Fite–Faraco) that use an aqueous solution of a weak acid for decolorization (Figure 74–9). Partial acid-fastness is lost, however, in older cultures or when nocardiae are subcultured.[4,5] All

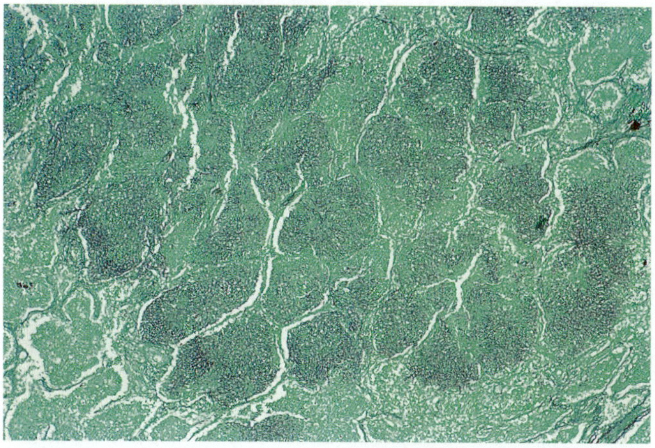

Figure 74–7. Pulmonary nocardiosis caused by *Nocardia otitidiscaviarum* in a child with leukemia. Tangled masses of argyrophilic bacterial filaments fill and distend alveolar spaces (GMS, ×16).

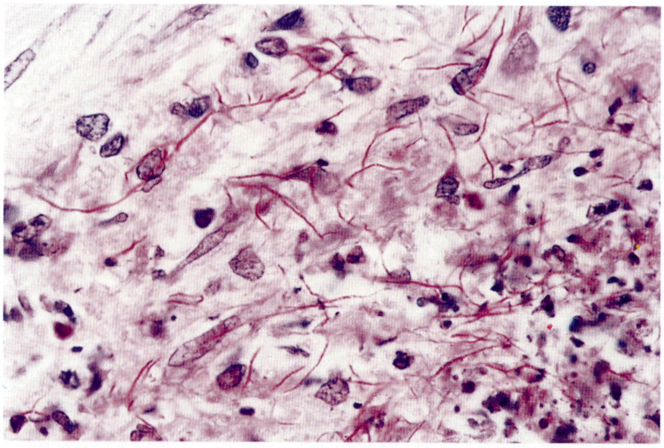

Figure 74–9. Disseminated nocardiosis. The wall of this cerebral abscess contains partially acid-fast filaments of *Nocardia asteroides,* about 1 μm in width, that branch at right angles (Modified Ziehl-Neelsen, ×250).

pathogenic species of *Nocardia* are morphologically and tinctorially similar in tissue.[32,48,49]

CONFIRMATIONAL TESTING AND DIAGNOSIS

Nocardial infections are difficult to diagnose, and lung biopsy or bronchoalveolar lavage is often required for isolation and identification in culture. Recovery of nocardiae in blood cultures is most successful in patients who are severely immunodeficient.[5] Even when appropriate cultures are instituted, 1 to 2 weeks are often required to obtain definitive results.[2–4] *Nocardia* sp may not be isolated from clinical specimens if plates are routinely discarded after 48 hours. Diagnosis can be made more quickly and easily by direct microscopic examination of stained smears of lesional exudate or sputum (Figure 74–10) and of routinely processed tissue specimens stained with Gram and modified acid-fast procedures.[32] Because smears and cultures are reported to be simultaneously positive in only one third of cases, multiple clinical specimens should be submitted to increase the diagnostic yield.[5] Reliable immunofluorescence reagents are not yet available for identifying the *Nocardia* sp. Serologic tests lack sensitivity and specificity, and are not recommended for diagnosis.[4,5]

All of the *Nocardia* sp are aerobic and grow readily on Lowenstein–Jensen medium at 30° to 37°C (Figure 74–11). They also grow on blood agar and Sabouraud's agar that are antibiotic-free. Charcoal-yeast extract agar and modified Thayer–Martin medium have also been reported to enhance recovery of *Nocardia* sp.[3] Colonies usually develop within 3 to 7 days, are heaped and folded, cream to yellowish-orange, and have a surface that is either moist and glabrous or covered with a powdery white aerial mycelium. The nocardiae are morphologically and tinctorially similar in cultures and clinical materials, appearing as delicate, branched, nonmotile, nonencapsulated, gram-positive, bacterial filaments about 1 μm in width and 10 to 50 μm or more in length.[32] The filaments in culture are often irregularly stained or beaded because of alternating segments of gram-positive and non–gram reactivities, and fragmented bacillary and coccoid forms are sometimes seen. Isolates can be identified in culture by studying their physiologic and biochemical properties.[3]

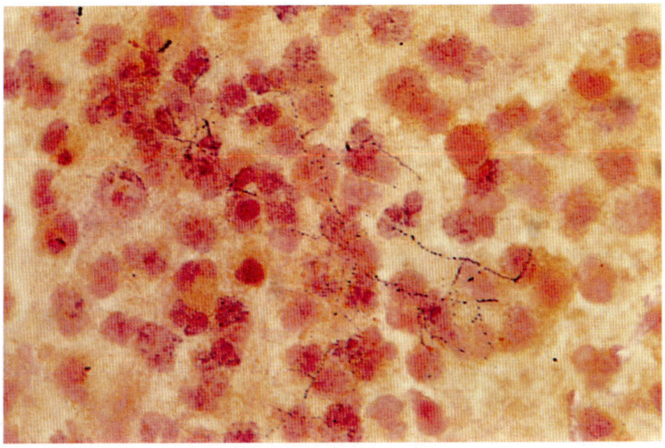

Figure 74–10. Cytospin preparation of sputum from a patient with pulmonary nocardiosis. Delicate, gram-positive filaments of *Nocardia asteroides* branch at right angles. Irregular gram reactivity gives the filaments a beaded or granular appearance (Gram stain, ×250). (*Courtesy of John C. H. Steele, Jr, MD.*)

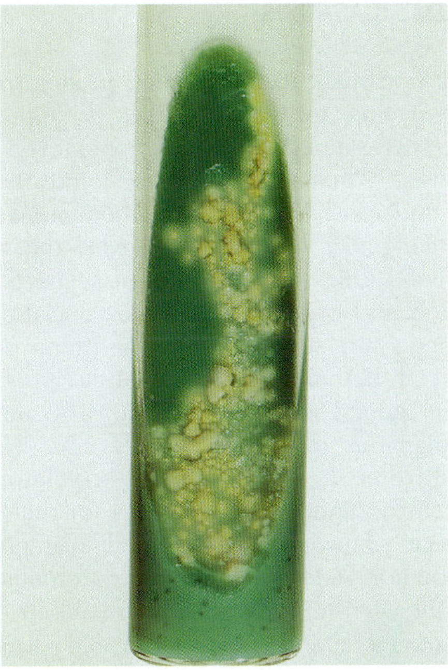

Figure 74–11. Colonies of *Nocardia asteroides* on Lowenstein–Jensen medium after 7 days' growth. The bacterium was isolated from sputum of an immunocompromised patient with bilateral pulmonary infiltrates. (*Courtesy of John C. H. Steele, Jr, MD.*)

MOLECULAR DIAGNOSIS

DNA amplification and restriction endonuclease analysis have been used to rapidly differentiate clinically significant taxa and recognized pathogenic species within the genus *Nocardia* in culture.[50] Polymerase chain reaction (PCR) also has been used in combination with restriction endonuclease analysis of amplified products to separate mycobacteria from nocardiae[51] and to identify species of *Nocardia*.[52,53] At present, however, molecular methods to not contribute to the pathologic diagnosis of nocardiosis.

DIFFERENTIAL DIAGNOSIS

Individual nocardial filaments and pleomorphic coccobacillary forms are very difficult or impossible to detect in H&E-stained tissue sections, even at high magnification. When seen, they are faintly hematoxylinophilic and most conspicuous when numerous and loosely entangled.[32] Usually, however, the diagnosis will be missed unless the pathologist suspects a bacterial infection and orders appropriate special stains. Of the modified Gram stains, the Brown–Brenn procedure has produced the most consistent results in our laboratory. When stained with GMS or one of its more rapid variants, filaments may stain weakly and unevenly if the staining time in the silver nitrate solution is not increased. If modified acid-fast stains for the *Nocardia* sp are done improperly, individual filaments interpreted to be non–acid-fast cannot be differentiated from those of the *Actinomyces* sp and members of other actinomycete genera in Gram- and GMS-stained sections. Even when modified acid-fast stains are done properly, merely observing unbranched, partially acid-fast bacilli in lesions is an insufficient basis for making a diagnosis of nocardiosis. Certain other bacteria such as *Legionella micdadei* and *Rhodococcus equi* also are partially acid-fast.

When stained with modified acid-fast procedures, the novice may mistake elongated and beaded *Mycobacterium* sp for the *Nocardia* sp.[32,54] This is especially true when nontuberculous mycobacteria are numerous and overlie one another to give the false impression of branching (Figure 74–12). When in doubt, one should remember that mycobacteria remain acid-fast when an acid–alcohol decolorizer is used in conventional acid-fast staining procedures, whereas the nocardiae do not. Mycobacteria also are shorter bacilli, do not branch, and often do not appear beaded or irregularly acid-fast.

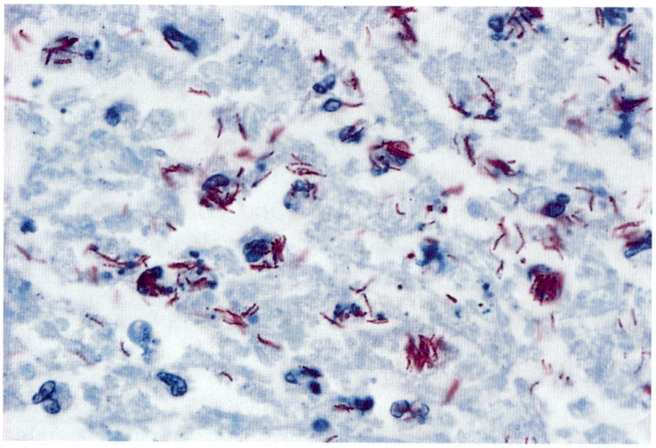

Figure 74–12. Disseminated *Mycobacterium avium* complex infection in an AIDS patient. When stained with modified acid-fast procedures, elongated and beaded mycobacteria can be mistaken for the *Nocardia* sp. This is especially true when mycobacteria are numerous and overlie one another to give the false impression of branching, as illustrated here. The mycobacteria do not branch, and in conventional acid-fast staining procedures they remain acid fast when an acid-alcohol decolorizer is used; the nocardiae do not (Modified Ziehl-Neelsen, ×250).

TREATMENT

Sulfonamides or trimethoprim–sulfamethoxazole given alone or in combination with antibacterial antibiotics are the drugs of choice for treating nocardiosis.[4,5,55,56] Minocycline also has been used with success, especially in less severe infections. Because of the tendency of nocardial infections to recur and disseminate, treatment must be prolonged (6 to 12 months). When indicated, surgical excision or drainage of abscesses is a valuable adjunct to antimicrobial therapy.

REFERENCES

1. Causey WA, Lee R. Nocardiosis. In: Vinken PJ, Bruyn GW, eds. *Handbook of Clinical Neurology*. Vol. 35. *Infections of the Nervous System*. Part III. Amsterdam: North Holland Publishing Company; 1978.
2. Beaman BL, Boiron P, Beaman L, et al. Nocardia and nocardiosis. *J Med Vet Mycol.* 1992;30(suppl 1):317–331.
3. McNeil MM, Brown JM. The medically important aerobic actinomycetes: epidemiology and microbiology. *Clin Microbiol Rev.* 1994;7:357–417.
4. Beaman BL, Beaman L. *Nocardia* species: host–parasite relationships. *Clin Microbiol Rev.* 1994;7:213–264.
5. Lerner PI. Nocardiosis. *Clin Infect Dis.* 1996;22:891–905.
6. Krick JA, Stinson EB, Remington JS. Nocardia infection in heart transplant patients. *Ann Intern Med.* 1975;82:18–26.
7. Simpson GL, Stinson EB, Egger MJ, et al. Nocardial infections in the immunocompromised host: a detailed study in a defined population. *Rev Infect Dis.* 1981;3:492–507.
8. Stevens DA, Pier AC, Beaman BL, et al. Laboratory evaluation of an outbreak of nocardiosis in immunocompromised hosts. *Am J Med.* 1981;71:928–934.
9. Smego RAJ, Gallis HA. The clinical spectrum of *Nocardia brasiliensis* infection in the United States. *Rev Infect Dis.* 1984;6:164–180.
10. Kim J, Minamoto GY, Grieco MH. Nocardial infection as a complication of AIDS: report of six cases and review. *Rev Infect Dis.* 1991;13:624–629.
11. Javaly K, Horowitz HW, Wormser GP. Nocardiosis in patients with human immunodeficiency virus infection: report of 2 cases and review of the literature. *Medicine.* 1992;71:128–138.
12. Wilson JP, Turner HR, Kirchner KA, Chapman SW. Nocar-

dial infections in renal transplant recipients. *Medicine.* 1989;68:38–53.
13. Young LS, Armstrong D, Blevins A, Lieberman P. *Nocardia asteroides* infection complicating neoplastic disease. *Am J Med.* 1971;50:356–367.
14. Pinkhas J, Oliver I, deVries A, Spitzer SA, Henig E. Pulmonary nocardiosis complicating malignant lymphoma successfully treated with chemotherapy. *Chest.* 1973;63: 367–370.
15. Casale TB, Macher AM, Fauci AS. Concomitant pulmonary aspergillosis and nocardiosis in a patient with chronic granulomatous disease of childhood. *South Med J.* 1984; 77:274–275.
16. Jonsson S, Wallace RJ Jr, Hull SI. Recurrent *Nocardia* pneumonia in an adult with chronic granulomatous disease. *Am Rev Respir Dis.* 1986;133:932–934.
17. Garty BZ, Stark H, Yaniv I. Pulmonary nocardiosis in a child with systemic lupus erythematosus. *Pediatr Infect Dis.* 1985;4:66–68.
18. Burbank B, Morrione TG, Cutler SS. Pulmonary alveolar proteinosis and nocardiosis. *Am J Med.* 1960;28: 1002–1007.
19. Carlsen ET, Hill RB, Rowlands DT. Nocardiosis and pulmonary alveolar proteinosis. *Ann Intern Med.* 1964;60: 275–281.
20. Clague HW, Harth M, Hellyer D, et al. Septic arthritis due to *Nocardia asteroides* in association with pulmonary alveolar proteinosis. *J Rheumatol.* 1982;9:469–472.
21. Bradsher RW, Monson TP, Steele RW. Brain abscess due to *Nocardia caviae:* report of a fatal outcome associated with abnormal phagocyte function. *Am J Clin Pathol.* 1982;78:124–127.
22. Frazier AR, Rosenow EC, Roberts GD. Nocardiosis: a review of 25 cases occurring during 24 months. *Mayo Clin Proc.* 1975;50:657–663.
23. Curry WA. Human nocardiosis: a clinical review with selected case reports. *Arch Intern Med.* 1980;140:818–826.
24. Stevens DA. Clinical and clinical laboratory aspects of nocardial infection. *J Hyg* (London). 1983;91:377–384.
25. Kahn FW, Gornick CC, Tofte RW. Primary cutaneous *Nocardia asteroides* infection with dissemination. *Am J Med.* 1981;70:859–863.
26. Kalb RE, Kaplan MH, Grossman ME. Cutaneous nocardiosis: case reports and review. *J Am Acad Dermatol.* 1985; 13:125–133.
27. Tsuboi R, Takamori K, Ogawa H. Lymphocutaneous nocardiosis caused by *Nocardia asteroides. Arch Dermatol.* 1986;122:1183–1185.
28. Moeller CA, Burton CS. Primary lymphocutaneous *Nocardia brasiliensis* infection. *Arch Dermatol.* 1986;122: 1180–1182.
29. Schwartz JG, McGough DA, Thorner RE, et al. Primary lymphocutaneous *Nocardia brasiliensis* infection: three case reports and a review of literature. *Diagn Microbiol Infect Dis.* 1988;10:113–120.
30. Poretz DM, Smith MN, Park CH. Intracranial suppuration secondary to trauma: infection with *Nocardia asteroides. JAMA.* 1975;232:730–731.
31. Stallworth JR, Perina D, Boykin D, Young FH Jr, Porter RC. Central nervous system nocardiosis associated with a traumatic polymicrobial brain abscess. *Pediatr Infect Dis.* 1985;4:412–413.
32. Chandler FW, Watts JC. *Pathologic Diagnosis of Fungal Infections.* Chicago: ASCP Press; 1987:279–286.
33. Beaman BL, Burnside J, Edward B, et al. *Nocardia* infections in the United States, 1972–1974. *J Infect Dis.* 1976; 134:286–289.
34. Coker RJ, Bignardi G, Horner P, et al. *Nocardia* infection in AIDS: a clinical and microbiological challenge. *J Clin Pathol.* 1992;45:821–822.
35. Baghdadlian H, Sorger S, Knowles K, McNeil M, Brown J. *Nocardia transvalensis* pneumonia in a child. *Pediatr Infect Dis J.* 1989;8:470–471.
36. McNeil MM, Brown JM, Georghiou PR, Allworth AM, Blacklock ZM. Infections due to *Nocardia transvalensis:* clinical spectrum and antimicrobial therapy. *Clin Infect Dis.* 1992;15:453–463.
37. McNeil MM, Brown JM, Magruder CH, et al. Disseminated *Nocardia transvalensis* infection: an unusual opportunistic pathogen in severely immunocompromised patients. *J Infect Dis.* 1992;165:175–178.
38. Parmentier L, Salmon-Ceron D, Boiron P, et al. Pneumopathy and kidney abscess due to *Nocardia farcinica* in an HIV-infected patient. *AIDS.* 1992;6:891–893.
39. Schiff TA, McNeil MM, Brown JM. Cutaneous *Nocardia farcinica* infection in a nonimmunocompromised patient: case report and review. *Clin Infect Dis.* 1993;16:756–760.
40. Berd D. *Nocardia brasiliensis* infection in the United States: a report of nine cases and a review of the literature. *Am J Clin Pathol.* 1973;60:254–258.
41. Karassik SL, Subramanyan L, Green RE, et al. Disseminated *Nocardia brasiliensis* infection. *Arch Dermatol.* 1976;112:370–372.
42. Salh B, Fegan C, Hussain A, et al. Pulmonary infection with *Nocardia caviae* in a patient with diabetes mellitus and liver cirrhosis. *Thorax.* 1988;43:933–934.
43. Torre NP, Kim BK. Septic arthritis due to *Nocardia caviae. Ann Rheum Dis.* 1991;50:968–969.
44. Sieratzki HJ. *Nocardia brasiliensis* infection in patients with AIDS. *Clin Infect Dis.* 1992;14:977–978.
45. Boudoulas O, Camisa C. *Nocardia asteroides* infection with dissemination to skin and joints. *Arch Dermatol.* 1985;121:898–900.
46. Wlodaver CG, Tolomeo T, Benear JB. Primary cutaneous nocardiosis mimicking sporotrichosis. *Arch Dermatol.* 1988;124:659–660.
47. Neu HC, Silva M, Hazen E. Necrotizing nocardial pneumonitis. *Ann Intern Med.* 1967;66:274–284.
48. Robboy SJ, Vickery AL. Tinctorial and morphologic properties distinguishing actinomycosis and nocardiosis. *N Engl J Med.* 1970;282:593–596.
49. Oddo D, Gonzalez S. Actinomycosis and nocardiosis: a morphologic study of 17 cases. *Pathol Res Pract.* 1986; 181:320–326.
50. Steingrube VA, Brown BA, Gibson JL, et al. DNA amplification and restriction endonuclease analysis for differentiation of 12 species and taxa of *Nocardia,* including recognition of four new taxa within the *Nocardia asteroides* complex. *J Clin Microbiol.* 1995;33:3096–3101.
51. Lungu O, Latta PD, Weitzman I, Silverstein S. Differentia-

tion of *Nocardia* from rapidly growing *Mycobacterium* species by PCR–RFLP analysis. *Diagn Microbiol Infect Dis.* 1994;18:13–18.
52. Cook SM, Bartos RE, Pierson CL, Frank TS. Detection and characterization of atypical mycobacteria by the polymerase chain reaction. *Diagn Mol Pathol.* 1994;3:53–58.
53. Wallace RJ Jr, Brown BA, Blacklock Z, et al. New *Nocardia* taxon among isolates of *Nocardia brasiliensis* associated with invasive disease. *J Clin Microbiol.* 1995;33: 1528–1533.
54. Kamat BR, Dvorak AM. The electron microscopic appearance of *Nocardia asteroides* in human lung tissue. *Arch Pathol Lab Med.* 1984;108:862–864.
55. Palmer DL, Harvey RL, Wheeler JK. Diagnostic and therapeutic considerations in *Nocardia asteroides* infection. *Medicine.* 1974;53:391–401.
56. Adams HG, Beeler BA, Wann LS, et al. Synergistic action of trimethoprim and sulfamethoxazole for *Nocardia asteroides:* efficacious therapy in five patients. *Am J Med Sci.* 1984;287:8–12.

CHAPTER 75

Noma

Jerome T. O'Connell II and Daniel H. Connor

We are threatened with suffering . . . from the external world, which may rage against us with overwhelming and merciless forces of destruction; . . .

Sigmund Freud (1856–1939)

DEFINITION

Noma is a severe tissue-destroying, infectious disease of the orofacial tissues characterized by a constellation of clinical signs: an apthous lesion initially, soft tissue necrosis, alveolar and mandibular bone destruction, and a septic-appearing patient with or without positive blood cultures (Figure 75–1). The disease can be divided into three age groups: neonates, children (classical noma), and adults. The results are often facial deformities with subsequent psychological consequences (Figure 75–2). Noma is readily diagnosed by any clinician who is familiar with the disease.[1]

SYNONYMS

Cancrum oris, gangrenous stomatitis, and necrotizing ulcerogingivostomatitis are synonyms.

GEOGRAPHIC DISTRIBUTION

Today noma is rare in North America and Western Europe but is still frequent in Africa, Asia, and South America. Neonatal noma is more common in the Western world than are the childhood and adult types. As the number of immunosuppressed adult patients increases in the United States, so probably will patients with noma.[2]

NATURAL HISTORY AND EPIDEMIOLOGY

The clinical picture of noma is similar across all age groups and rarely will a clinician with prior exposure to noma overlook the diagnosis. The classical predisposing factors include malnutrition (especially protein/energy deficiencies and vitamin A deficiency), immunodeficiencies, poor oral hygiene, trauma to the orofacial soft tissues, and recent debilitating infection, especially measles.[3] In neonates additional risk factors include intrauterine growth retardation, prematurity, and infants small for their gestational age. These neonatal risk factors are likely analogous to in utero malnutrition and exacerbate the immaturity of their immune status.

MORPHOLOGY OF ORGANISM

Cultures of infected/necrotic tissues usually reveal a mixed flora including bacilli, cocci, and filamentous organisms, and occasionally diplococci and spirochetes.[4] In neonates *Pseudomonas aeruginosa* is almost always cultured from the lesion and 86% of neonates will have positive blood cultures for *Pseudomonas*. This is not the case with adults. Often, *P aeruginosa* is cultured in the orofacial region of children and adults but positive blood cultures are much less frequent.[5]

Within the lesions of both children and adults the organisms can be divided into the mixed flora and a group of homogeneous filamentous organisms along the leading edge of bone destruction (Figure 75–3). These filamentous organisms are multicellular with septa and have a gram-positive envelope surrounding the entire filamentous structure. They average 0.6 μm in

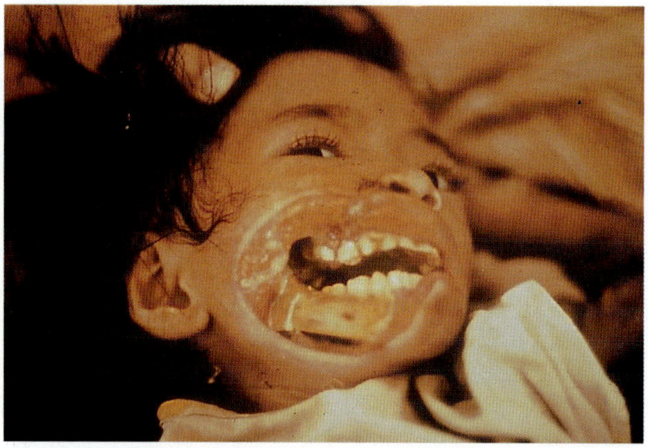

Figure 75–1. Noma. Extensive erosion of lips and cheek, exposing the mandible (AFIP Neg 74-19325).

diameter and have variable lengths up to several microns.[5]

The most commonly cultured organisms other than *P aeruginosa* include alpha hemolytic streptococci, *Staphylococcus aureus,* anaerobic corynebacterium, *Klebsiella pneumoniae,* and *Candida albicans.*[4]

CLINICAL FEATURES

Noma is an insidious gangrenous process that usually follows a febrile illness and often begins with an aphthous ulcer or trauma to the oral mucosa. The disease process erodes and destroys, most commonly, cheeks, lips, gingival mucosa, gums, and, in severe untreated patients, the alveolar and mandibular bone (Figure 75–1). The earliest signs are excessive salivation, bad breath, and facial swelling.[3] There may be systemic manifestations including fluctuating fever, tachycardia, malaise, and prostration.[1] Systemic features vary from profound to nonexistent but the severity of orofacial involvement does not correlate with the severity of systemic manifestations. The older the patient, the less common are systemic features. The end result is facial deformity and social stigmatism (Figure 75–2).

GROSS PATHOLOGY

The orofacial tissues undergo a wet gangrenous destructive course resulting in grotesque distortion of form and function. In neonates an aphthous lesion usually appears on the gingival mucosa and this is followed by a gangrenous slough and, if untreated, invasion of alveolar and mandibular bone by microorganisms.[5] Lesions of the cervicofacial tissues consist of a frank red mass, which eventually extends into a large fistula in the buccal mucosa. This fistulous track provides access to the deeper tissues of the region. The result is destruction of maxillary and mandibular tissue with concomitant loss of teeth.[4]

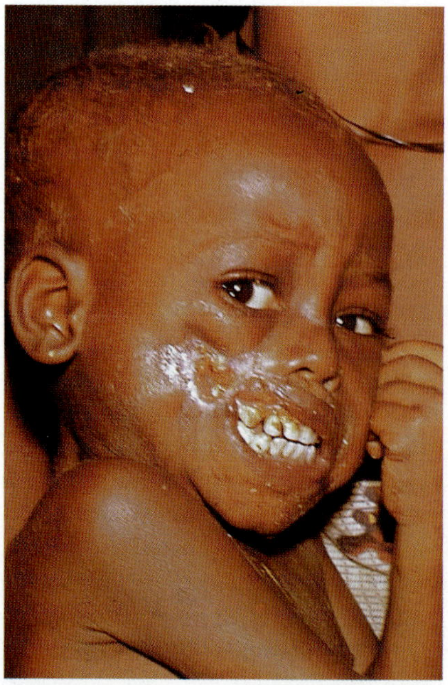

Figure 75–2. Noma. Healing ulcer in a Zairian child. *(Photograph by Daniel H. Connor, MD, 1968.)*

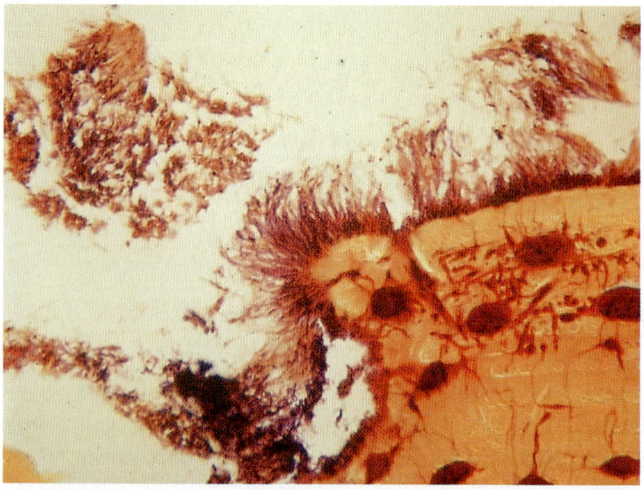

Figure 75–3. Noma. Fragment of maxilla with masses of filamentous bacteria attached to the surface of bone. (AFIP Neg 75-3947; Brown–Hopps, ×675).

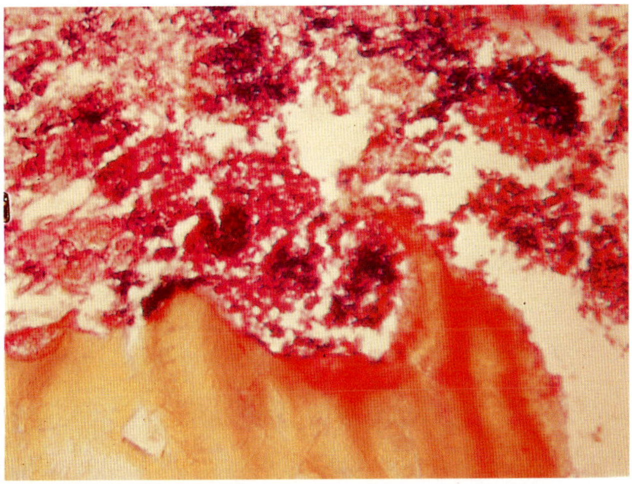

Figure 75–4. Noma. Biopsy specimen of facial bone showing masses of bacteria in eroded bone (AFIP Neg 75-2641, ×970).

LIGHT MICROSCOPY

A mixed flora of bacteria invade soft tissue and bone without significant inflammatory cell response.[4] Late lesions show necrosis with a ghost outline of previously viable tissue.[1] Cells at the margin of the necrotic tissue lack both nuclei and a capillary circulation. Bacteria appear as blue granular masses on routine hematoxylin-eosin-stained sections. Special stains reveal a variety of gram-positive and gram-negative bacteria including spirochetes and yeasts (Figures 75–3 and 75–4). Healing, as noted, leaves a disfiguring scar (Figure 75–2).

ELECTRON MICROSCOPY

Electron microscopy reveals a regular arrangement of filamentous organisms along the resorbing bone mass. These organisms are uniform, aligned perpendicularly to the tissue, and adherent to the resorbing bone. They are long, and perpendicular to the leading edge of bone resorption. They are also in lacunae of intact matrix.

TREATMENT

Patients are given intravenous antibiotics, necrotic tissue is debrided, and their nutritional deficiencies corrected.[1,6–9] The advent and availability of intravenous antibiotics has reduced the mortality of children and adults to less than 10%.[3] Mortality rates for neonatal noma, however, remain high.[5]

REFERENCES

1. Joseph SW, Duncan JF. Noma. In: Binford CH, Connor DH, eds. *Pathology of Tropical and Extraordinary Diseases.* Washington, DC: Armed Forces Institute of Pathology; 1976:202–204.
2. Muzyka BC. Glick M. HIV and necrotizing stomatitis. *General Dentistry.* 1992;42:66–68.
3. Enwonwu CO. Noma—a neglected Third World disease. *World Health.* 1994;47:23.
4. Merrel BW, Joseph SW, Casazza LJ, Duncan JF. Bacterial bone resorption in noma (gangrenous stomatitis). *J Oral Pathol.* 1981;10:173–185.
5. Juster-Reicher A, Moligner BM, Levi G, Flidel O, Amitai M. Neonatal noma. *Am J Perinatol.* 1993;10:409–411.
6. Biswal N, Mahadevan S, Srinivasan S. Gangrenous stomatitis following measles. *Indian Pediatr (India).* 1992;29: 509–511.
7. Dutasta B. Eight cases of African noma. The therapeutic importance of nutrition. *Rev Stomatol Chir Maxillofac.* 1987;88:139–142.
8. Enwonwu CO. Infectious oral necrosis (cancrum oris) in Nigerian children: a review. *Community Dent Oral Epidemiol (Denmark).* 1985;13:190–194.
9. Sawyer DR, Nwoku AL. Malnutrition and the oral health of children in Ogbomosho, Nigeria. *ASDC J Dnt Child (United States).* 1987;52:141–145.

CHAPTER 76

Ornithosis (Psittacosis)

Alfonso J. Strano

A dry cough is the trumpeter of death.

English Proverb

DEFINITION

Human ornithosis (psittacosis, parrot fever) is a zoonosis contracted most commonly from exposure to infected avian species as well as by human-to-human spread (aerosol). It is characterized by pneumonitis, fever, myalgia, and malaise.

ETIOLOGIC AGENT

Ornithosis is caused by a group B chlamydia serovar of *Chlamydia psittaci.* These bacteria are obligate intracellular parasites that cannot be cultured on artificial media. They require living host cells for replication. The life cycle consists of the intracellular reticulate body, the replicative stage, dividing by binary fission (see also Chapter 51). After a defined number of divisions, each reticulate body condenses into an elementary body, which is shed extracellularly and is an infectious particle. The elementary body is approximately 350 nm in diameter and the intracellular reticulate body is 850 nm. Both stages contain RNA and DNA. *Chlamydia psittaci* are heat labile and killed at 56°C for 30 minutes and by common disinfectants. They withstand desiccation for months.

EPIDEMIOLOGY

Chlamydia psittaci infection was first described in Switzerland in the 1870s and subsequently in outbreaks throughout the world including a large outbreak in the bayou region of Louisiana in 1943.[1–3] A majority of the early outbreaks were associated with psittacine birds but in the 1950s it was discovered in poultry and noted to be an important occupational hazard to employees in poultry processing plants.[4] Infection in birds is usually intestinal with the infectious particles and elementary bodies in the feces and transmitted by aerosol to humans. Human-to-human transmission, although rare, is also by aerosol.

CLINICAL MANIFESTATIONS

The incubation period is usually 7 to 21 days. The prodrome is nonspecific, with the onset abrupt or insidious. Earliest features can resemble the common cold or an influenza–like syndrome. It can also present as a severe pneumonitis with fever (37.8 to 40.5°C), severe headache, nonproductive cough, and oxygen hunger. Other features can include x-ray evidence of a pneumonic process and hepatosplenomegaly.[5] It has also presented as a generalized toxic state.[1] Before the introduction of tetracycline therapy, the mortality rate was as high as 40% but now death is uncommon with recovery varying from 1 to several weeks.[6]

PATHOLOGY

Since the advent of antibiotic therapy, death as a result of ornithosis is rare and anatomic studies even more so. The pathologic manifestations were described by autopsy studies performed before the advent of antibiotic therapy.[2,3]

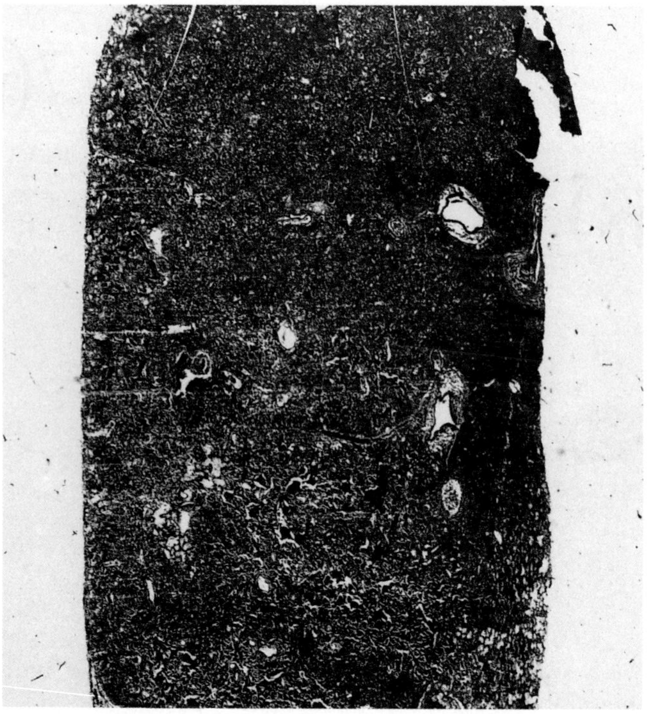

Figure 76–1. Lung. Van Gieson stain showing consolidation sharply demarcated from nonconsolidated area (AFIP Neg 75-6865-10; ×3.5).

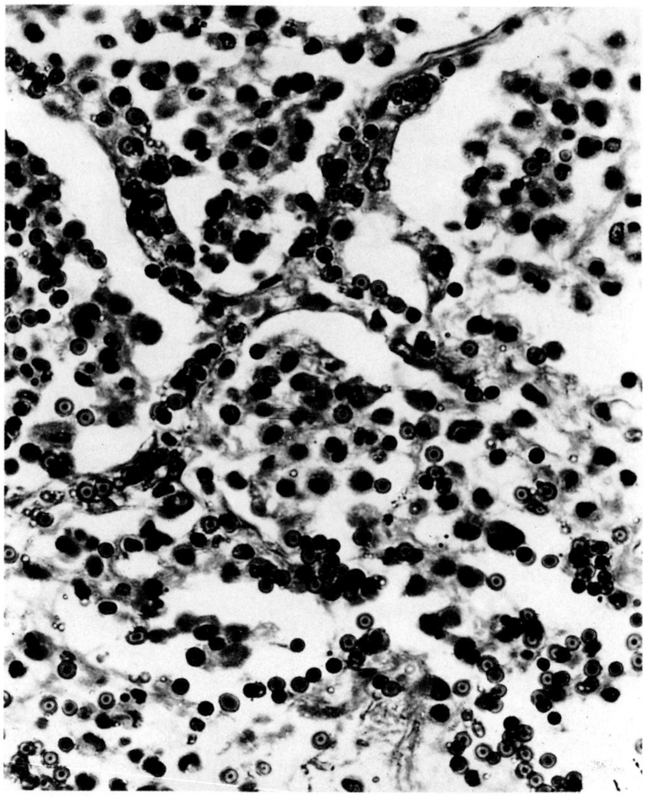

Figure 76–2. Lung. Romanovsky stain showing widened septa and intra-alveolar exudate comprised of mononuclear cells and alveolar lining cells (AFIP Neg 75-6865-5; ×560).

Gross

Lillie[2] in reporting 9 autopsies of his own and 43 others stated "psittacosis in man is anatomically characterized by a pulmonary inflammatory process which goes on to consolidation." The consolidation was primarily lobular but often became lobar. The sequence was congestion, edema, and inflammatory infiltrates progressing through red and gray hepatization. This was confirmed by Binford and others (Figure 76–1).[3]

Microscopic

Histopathologically fibrin, red cells, neutrophils, and epithelial cells of alveolar lining origin appear early in the alveolar exudate. Later neutrophils break up into debris and disappear and alveoli become filled with large mononuclear cells and alveolar epithelial lining cells (Figure 76–2). In the early stages the interstitial infiltrate was lacking, but with progressive infiltration by lymphocytes and monocytes, becomes prominent (Figure 76–3). Bronchioles were severely affected while larger bronchioles and bronchi maintained luminal patency but were cuffed with lymphocytes and macrophages. Binford, as did Lillie, identified intracytoplasmic minute basophilic coccobacillary inclusions in the epithelial lining cells (Figure 76–4). In the liver, swelling, vacuolization, and phagocytic activity of Kupffer's cells were often found along with focal hepatocellular necrosis.

DIAGNOSIS

Anatomically, ornithosis cannot be separated from other interstitial pneumonitides. In the laboratory, *C psittaci* is potentially dangerous and should be handled only in laboratories with proper containment equipment and experienced personnel. There is considerable variability in the identification of the various *Chlamydia* in tissues and tissue cultures by special stains for inclusion bodies and organisms by fluorescent antibodies. *Chlamydia psittaci* are the least specific by these methods.[7] Isolation is readily accomplished by tissue culture, animal inoculation, and inoculation of yolk sac but these are highly complex and time-consuming techniques and not readily available in most clinical laboratories. The most widely used diagnostic procedure for *C psittaci* is the complement fixation test (CFT). This requires paired

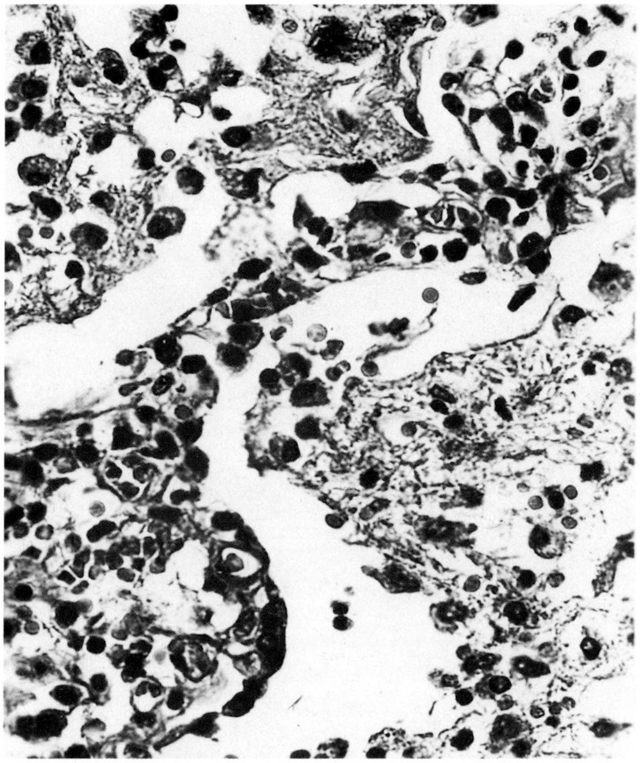

Figure 76–3. Lung. Van Gieson stain showing fibrinomononuclear cell alveolar exudate, thickened septum and swollen alveolar lining cells (AFIP Neg 75-6865-7; ×400).

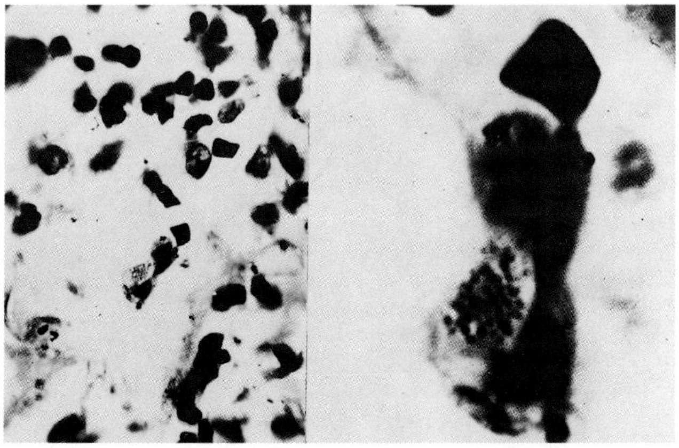

Figure 76–4. Lung. Romanovsky stain showing alveolar lining cells with basophilic cytoplasmic coccobacillary bodies—probably elementary bodies (AFIP Neg 75-6865-9; left×1000; right×4500; right is an enlargement of left).

sera and must show a fourfold rise in titer. After the acute stage of infection, any titer above 1:16 should be considered not specific but positive evidence of exposure to chlamydia. Microimmunofluorescence is a more complex and demanding procedure but is more sensitive than the CFT, and may be used in the diagnosis of *C psittaci*. Paired sera will show rising titers of immunoglobulin G.[7]

Electron Microscopy

Except for the occasional identification of developmental forms of chlamydia within the cytoplasm of epithelial cells, electron microscopy does not define significant anatomic features on which a definitive diagnosis can be made.

REFERENCES

1. Schacter J, Davison CF. Human chlamydial infections. New York: Littleton, PSG Publishing; 1978.
2. Lillie RD. Pathology of psittacosis in man. *NIH Bull.* May 1933;161:1.
3. Binford CH, Hauser GH. An epidemic of a severe pneumonitis in the bayou region of Louisiana. III. Report of autopsy on two cases. *Pub. Health Rep.* 1944;59(42): 1363–1374.
4. Meyer KF. Ornithosis. In: Biester HE, Schwarte LH, eds. *Diseases of Poultry.* Ames: Iowa State University Press; 1965:675.
5. Treuting WL, Olson BJ. An epidemic of a severe pneumonitis in the bayou region of Louisiana, II. Clinical features of the disease. *Pub. Health Rep.* 1944;59(41): 1331–1350.
6. Schacter J. Chlamydiaceae: the chlamydia. In: Lennette EH, Halonen P, Murphy F, eds. *Laboratory Diagnosis of Infectious Diseases, Principles and Practice.* New York: Springer-Verlag; 1988;II:847–863.
7. Schachter J, Stamm WE. Chlamydia. In: Murry PR, Baron EF, Pfaller MA, Tenover FC, Yolken RH, eds. *Manual of Clinical Microbiology.* 6th ed. Washington, DC: ASM Press; 1995:669–677.

CHAPTER 77

Pig-Bel and Other Necrotizing Disorders of the Gut Involving *Clostridium perfringens*

Stephen D. Allen

A cat looks down at you, a dog looks up to you, but a pig looks you straight in the eye.

Attributed to Winston S. Churchill (1874–1965)

DEFINITION AND HISTORIC CONSIDERATIONS

Pig-bel is a necrotizing infection of the small intestine caused by β-toxin-producing strains of *Clostridium perfringens* type C.[1] First recognized in the highlands of Papua New Guinea (PNG), where it was the most common cause of mortality in children,[2,3] pig-bel occurs both in sporadic and epidemic form and has commonly been associated with pig feasts. The appellation "pig-bel" was proposed by Murrell and colleagues "because this is the pidgin English name used by medical orderlies [in the highland hospitals of PNG] to describe the abdominal discomfort which follows [eating] a large pork meal."[3]

Pig-bel is probably the same disease as "Darmbrand" ("fire bowels" or "burnt bowels"), which was reported from post-war Germany in the mid- to late-1940s.[4,5] Several hundred people were affected with the disease, and about 20% to 60% of them died. Fortunately, by about 1950, Darmbrand mysteriously disappeared.

There has been considerable dispute about the cause and pathogenesis, as well as confusion regarding the nomenclature and definition of this disease.[6] Thus, as reviewed by Murrell[4] and by Walker,[5] in addition to the names pig-bel and Darmbrand, it has been called enteritis gravis, necrotizing jejunitis, jejunitis actua phlegmonosa, and necrotic enteritis. In 1949, Zeissler and Rassfeld-Sternberg[7] called the condition "enteritis necroticans" (EN) and thought it was caused by *C perfringens* type "F," but it was later determined that the strains that caused the outbreaks in Germany were variants of type C.[4]

Murrell[4] has argued convincingly that the history of enteritis necroticans dates back to the time of Hippocrates. Could the prevention of pig-bel have been part of the reason for the Old Testament prohibition against eating pork, where it was written that swine "is unclean" and "of its flesh you shall not eat" *(Leviticus 11:7–8)?* The human ecology during medieval times was probably similar to that which currently exists in Third World countries.[1] Thus, in those times, people undoubtedly were subject to some of the same dietary and unhygienic conditions that occur today in PNG or in other Third World populations.[1]

In 1900, William H. Welch[8] of Johns Hopkins University reported on a variety of morbid conditions that had been recognized in the United States to be caused by the organism now known as *C perfringens.* Thus, by the turn of the 20th century, several cases had been described in which so-called "gas-bacilli" (*C perfringens)* were observed in large numbers within superficial necrotizing lesions of intestinal mucous membranes. Also, at the same time, many cases had been observed in which clostridia invaded from the intestine and spread to extraintestinal sites (with or without intestinal lesions). The gastrointestinal lesions, which were noted to occur with or without gas cysts, were commonly found beneath the folds of the valvulae conniventes and were characterized by "absence of nuclear staining and disintegration of the cells and tissue." In the early observations of what probably was intestinal necrosis produced by *C perfringens,* a marked inflammatory reaction was not usually seen, a finding that is known to be consistent with clostridial toxin–mediated disease. Peritonitis involving *C perfringens,* with and without perforation of the intestine, was also well known in the early days of anaerobic bacteriology.[8]

GEOGRAPHIC DISTRIBUTION AND EPIDEMIOLOGY

Smith[9] and Murrell[1,10] have emphasized that EN is an international disease that is widespread in tropical regions of the world. It occurs in several countries of Southeast Asia, including Thailand,[11] Vietnam,[12] southern parts of China,[13] Nepal,[14] Malaysia,[15] and others. Intestinal illness with similar features has been reported also in Uganda,[16] Bangladesh, and the British Solomon Islands.[5] Since the late 1940s, sporadic cases of necrotizing enteropathies with similar clinical and pathologic features to those of EN also have been reported in the United States,[17,18,19] Great Britain,[20,21] and the Netherlands.[22,23]

Geographically, pig-bel has occurred mostly in the middle of PNG in the highlands, but not in the coastal areas. There, the role of *C perfringens* in pig-bel has been studied most extensively in children from 1 to 10 years old and in young adults. It has been rare in those younger than 1 year. Interestingly, most patients with Darmbrand in Germany ranged from 40 to 60 years.[5] In PNG, the incidence of the disease and the mortality in children have been very high, and the disease has been more common in males.[5,24]

The earliest reports of pig-bel emphasized the association of pork consumption at pig feasts.[2,24] As a result of case-controlled epidemiologic studies, Millar et al[25] reported that the episodic consumption of pork is a powerful risk factor for pig-bel in PNG. Not all patients, however, have provided a history of meat consumption prior to the disease.[26] Pig-bel has also been associated epidemiologically with the ingestion of other foods, especially sweet potatoes and raw peanuts.

In PNG, the evidence that *C perfringens* type C causes pig-bel is strong. Although type C strains were isolated from several resected specimens of bowel and feces of patients who had the disease, it was isolated only rarely from healthy people or from pigs.[27] Subsequently, based on the use of a fluorescent antibody technique, Lawrence et al[28] reported that *C perfringens* type C was present in about 50% to 80% of the human fecal samples tested from different areas, about 80% to 100% of pig fecal samples, and was widespread in the soil. Serologic studies for serum antibodies to the beta toxin of *C perfringens* type C revealed detectable levels of antitoxin in 23 of 24 patients with pig-bel and significant levels of antitoxin in >70% of the healthy population in PNG. In contrast, about 10% of sera from a European control population had beta antitoxin titers.[3]

THE ORGANISM AND PATHOGENESIS

The morphology of *C perfringens* is illustrated in Figure 77–1. The organisms are relatively large gram-positive rods with blunt ends, usually about 2 to 4 μm by about 0.6 to 1 μm. In tissue, they often appear "boxcar-shaped."[29] In broth cultures that have incubated only a few hours, the rods are usually short or even coccoid, whereas in older broth cultures, some of the cells may be elongated to 10 to 20 μm and filamentous. In culture, as well as in tissue, they occur as single cells, pairs, or short chains, and they are nonmotile. Although sporulation of *C perfringens,* correlated with enterotoxin production, takes place within the upper small bowel in patients with type A food-borne illness, it is usually possible to demonstrate the subterminal spores of *C perfringens* only under special growth conditions. Spores are uncommon in routinely used media.[30] Likewise, it is rare to observe the spores of *C perfringens* in tissue (eg, in *C perfringens* myonecrosis).[29] In contrast, *C difficile* and *C septicum,* two other species of *Clostrid-*

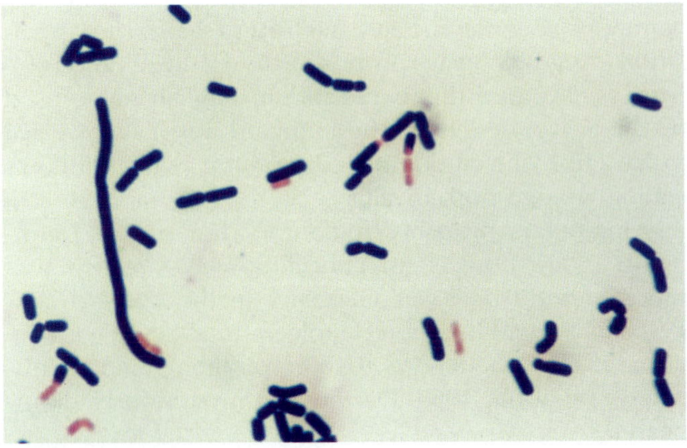

Figure 77–1. Gram-stained smear of *Clostridium perfringens* in fluid aspirated from an infected site in which there are relatively broad, gram-positive rods, varying from short forms ~2 μm long to a "snake-like" form >15 μm long. The presence of gram-negative forms, indicating gram-variability, and the absence of spores in direct smears of body fluids, tissue, and in cultures is typical of the appearance of *C perfringens* (×500).

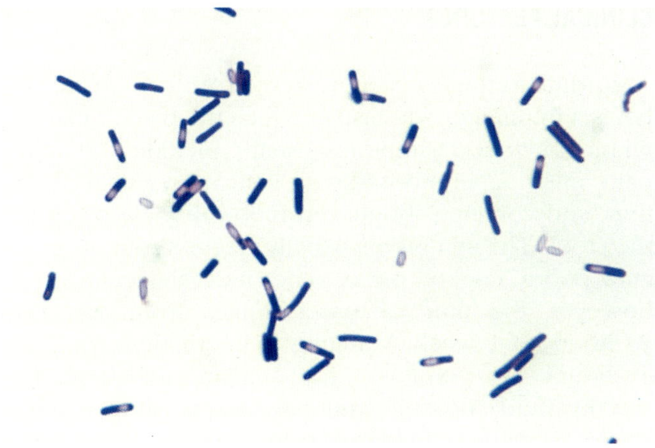

Figure 77–2. Gram-stained smear of *Clostridium difficile* prepared from a broth culture to compare with Figure 77–1. The rod-shaped vegetative cells are shorter and narrower than those of *C perfringens;* abundant subterminal and "free" spores are present (×500).

ium that cause intestinal illness in humans, are smaller in diameter and produce spores readily in culture media. For comparison, the microscopic features of *C difficile* and of *C septicum* are shown in Figures 77–2 and 77–3.

Although *C perfringens* is an obligate anaerobe, some strains may be aerotolerant. Nonetheless, proper anaerobic media and anaerobic systems for cultivation should be used for its isolation and cultivation.[29] Colonies of *C perfringens* on rabbit or sheep blood agar are usually surrounded by a double zone of hemolysis—an inner, narrow zone of complete hemolysis caused by theta toxin and an outer, wider zone of incomplete hemolysis caused by the alpha toxin. On egg yolk agar, an opaque zone is produced within the agar by the action of lecithinase produced by alpha toxin. The optimal temperature for growth of most strains of *C perfringens* is 45°C, but their temperature range for good growth is broad (eg, 20°C to 50°C). When attempting to isolate *C perfringens* from specimens containing a mixture of organisms, it is useful to incubate cultures at 45°C. With its extremely fast growth rate (ie, generation time of only 8 minutes) at this temperature, it can outgrow other microorganisms that may be present.[31] Described in detail elsewhere,[30] a spore selection technique (eg, heat-shock or alcohol) can aid in isolating the organisms from specimens containing mixtures of bacteria. In peptone-yeast extract-glucose broth, the organisms produce major amounts of acetic and butyric acids with a minor amount of proprionate. They produce "stormy fermentation" in milk; reduce nitrate; ferment glucose, lactose, maltose, and sucrose; and liquefy gelatin. Further details about the isolation and identification of *C perfringens* are available elsewhere.[29,30]

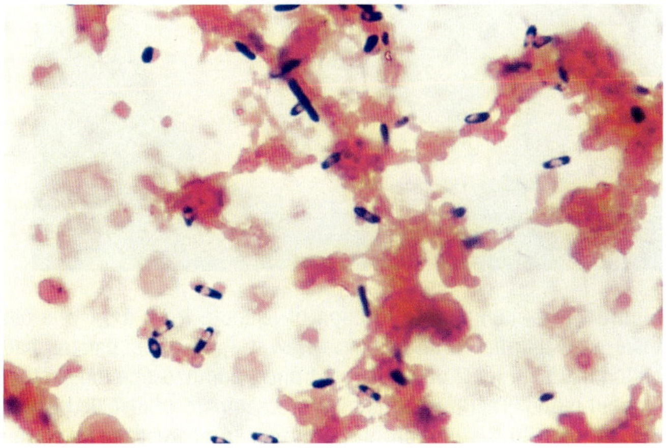

Figure 77–3. Gram-stained smear of *Clostridium septicum* prepared from a blood culture. Numerous ovoid subterminal spores, some of which are "citron-shaped," are present (×500).

Clostridium perfringens has been divided into five types (A, B, C, D, and E), originally based on the elaboration of at least 12 different toxins by members of the species.[30,32] The typing scheme currently used in reference laboratories, however, is based on the demonstration of its four major lethal toxins—alpha, beta, epsilon, and iota. The alpha toxin, produced by all toxin types of *C perfringens,* is a phospholipase C; it is a zinc metalloprotease that cleaves lecithin into phosphorylcholine and a diglyceride. Type A strains produce alpha toxin as the only major lethal toxin; type C strains produce both alpha and beta major lethal toxins. Types A and C are both found in human diseases. Types B, D, and E *C perfringens* are intestinal pathogens encountered in veterinary medicine but not in humans. Type A strains of *C perfringens* have caused almost all the outbreaks of *C perfringens* food-borne gastroenteritis in the United States. As mentioned previously, type C strains have been incriminated in PNG and in most parts of Southeast Asia where the toxin types have been studied.[28,33]

Although *C perfringens* is probably best known for its role in gas gangrene,[31] it has come to be recognized as an intestinal pathogen of humans associated with an array of diseases. The organism is not only capable of causing life-threatening necrotizing enteritis, but it is also reported to cause colitis, or a combination of the two (ie, necrotizing enterocolitis in adults).[34] In addition to the necrotizing lesions, *C perfringens* is also a major cause of a much less severe and usually self-limited food-borne illness caused by type A strains.[30] Although not widely regarded as a cause of antibiotic-associated diarrhea in the United States, *C perfringens* ranks second to *C difficile* as a cause of this condition in England.[35] Also, there have been some tantalizing leads that suggest *C perfringens* plays a role in neonatal necrotizing enterocolitis, but the evidence for this is lacking.[36] In addition, *C perfringens* type C causes outbreaks of necrotic enteritis in pigs, sheep, goats, cattle, and chickens.[31] It is particularly a problem in young animals.

In the highlands of PNG, Lawrence and Walker[37] observed that the diet of the highlanders "was very low in protein," that these people ate meat rarely (mostly they ate pig contaminated with *C perfringens* type C), and that they "depend on sweet potato" as their dietary staple. They hypothesized that EN occurs in these people because they have low levels of pancreatic trypsin in the intestinal lumen. The low pancreatic trypsin levels were postulated to be caused by a low protein diet and the presence of heat-stable trypsin inhibitors in the sweet potatoes. The beta toxin of *C perfringens* type C is very susceptible to the proteolytic action of trypsin; absence of pancreatic trypsin in the upper small intestine thus would allow the beta toxin to cause the disease. During pig feasts, the meat is cooked in the ground in crude "ovens" containing hot stones wrapped in palm leaves. The meat, which is prepared unhygienically and contaminated with intestinal bacteria of the pig, only reaches 70°C during the two or so hours it is "cooked." Subsequently, viable *C perfringens* type C is eaten along with the meat.

In their guinea pig model of pig-bel, Lawrence and Walker[37] and Lawrence and Cooke[38] produced EN in the animals by injecting *C perfringens* type C into the small intestine at laparotomy, but not by oral or intragastric dosing of the organism by itself. If they fed the guinea pigs *C perfringens* type C culture plus crushed soy beans, which contain trypsin inhibitors, or dried raw sweet potato, the animals died. The intestinal lesions, both macroscopically and microscopically, were typical of those in humans.[37,38] Protein-deprived monkeys produce trypsin only at reduced levels and cease producing chymotrypsin. In addition to the cases of pig-bel associated with eating sweet potato, others have been associated with meals containing raw peanuts and poorly cooked beans. Peanuts and beans contain trypsin inhibitors. Thus, the elegant studies of Lawrence and colleagues have firmly established the important role of a low protein diet, dietary trypsin inhibitors, and the presence of β toxin producing *C perfringens* type C in the pathogenesis of pig-bel in PNG. An additional factor in the pathogenesis of pig-bel can be the production of another trypsin inhibitor by the parasite *Ascaris lumbricoides,* which also may be found in a number of these individuals.[1] Factors that appear to have predisposed patients to EN in the sporadic cases reported from Western countries include alcoholism,[39] malabsorption,[18] overeating with gastric dilatation,[39] and gastric or pancreatic surgery.[21]

CLINICAL FEATURES

According to the excellent review of Walker,[5] acute pig-bel is a fulminating disease in which the patient may die within 24 hours. Symptoms usually include abdominal pain, often superimposed with colic, abdominal distention, and vomiting. Bright red blood may be passed in the stool. The symptoms usually begin about 48 hours after poorly cooked pig or other meat has been eaten; however, the time of onset ranges from less than 24 hours to 1 week. Vomiting is intermittent for 24 to 48 hours. The vomitus is foul-smelling and looks like "murky fluid" flecked with particles of shed mucosa. There is marked tenderness in the upper abdomen. Severe shock may develop, probably related more to septicemia and fluid and electrolyte loss than to the effects of the clostridial toxins per se.[5]

PATHOLOGY

The pathology of pig-bel has been investigated rather extensively by Cooke,[40] reviewed by Walker,[5] and more recently by Murrell,[1] and is illustrated in Figures 77–4 through 77–10. Just as there is a spectrum of clinical findings ranging from mild illness (resembling gastroenteritis) to acute fulminant, life-threatening pig-bel, and even a subset of patients with so-called "chronic

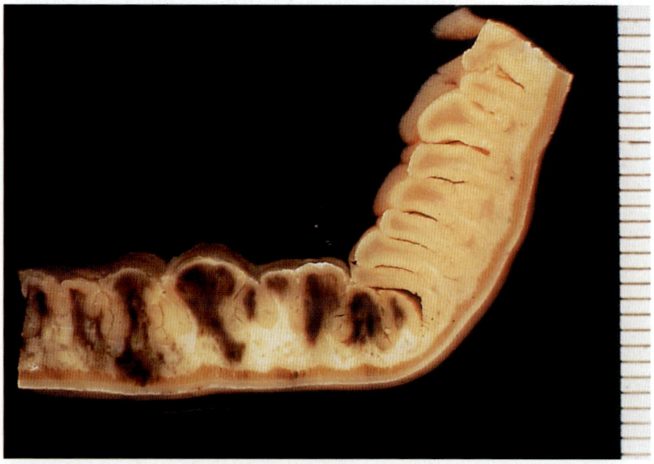

Figure 77–4. Longitudinal section of jejunum from a 14-year-old male with pig-bel from Goroka, New Guinea. The patient had abdominal pain for 2 days, vomited once, and had one loose stool without blood. There was one localized segment of involved bowel 16 cm long. In the portion of the specimen nearest the ruler, the mucosa is thickened, but intact, and there is prominent submucosal edema. The darker portions of the specimen contain foci of hemorrhagic necrosis that extends from the mucosa to involve nearly the full thickness of bowel. *(Specimen courtesy of Robin A. Cooke, MD; photograph courtesy of Daniel H. Connor, MD.)*

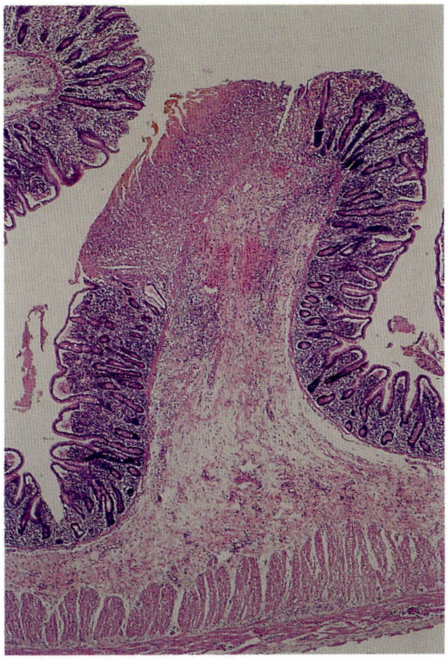

Figure 77–5. Pig-bel. Section from a relatively superficial, sharply demarcated ulcer, surrounded by thickened but intact mucosa, with underlying submucosal edema (hematoxylin-eosin, ×50).

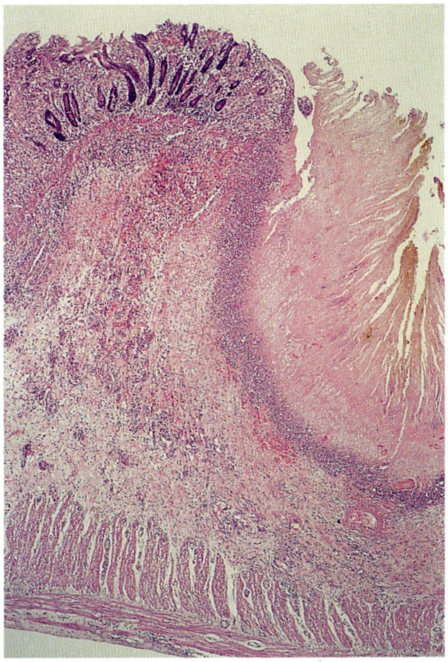

Figure 77–7. Pig-bel. Deep ulcer with a sharp line of demarcation between nonviable tissue on right and viable tissue on left. The dark line of demarcation was produced by an infiltrate of neutrophils that penetrate deeply in the submucosa. Numerous small vessels are in the edematous submucosa on the left (hematoxylin-eosin, ×25).

pig-bel" who present with malnutrition and/or obstruction caused by strictures or constricting bands, there is a similar spectrum of pathologic findings in this disease.[3,5] In many cases of pig-bel, the jejunum is the primary site of involvement, although the entire small intestine may be involved. Pathologically, this is an acute, patchy, hemorrhagic, necrotizing, ulcerative, and inflammatory disease of the small bowel. There may be pseudomembranes. Some patients have gas cysts but most do not. In some areas, the necrosis may involve

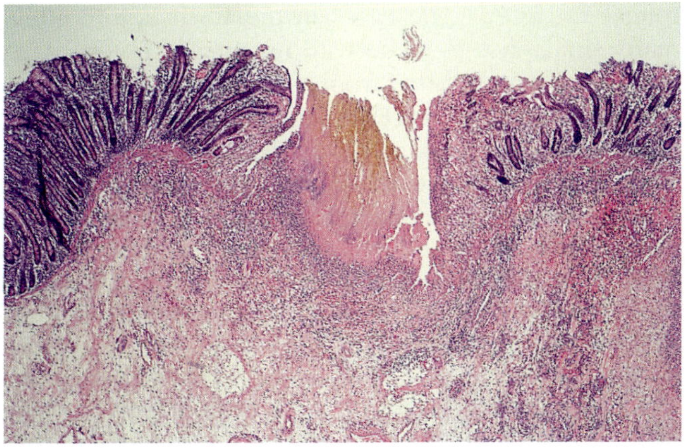

Figure 77–6. Pig-bel. A larger and deeper area of ulceration than that in Figure 77–5 is shown (hematoxylin-eosin, ×25).

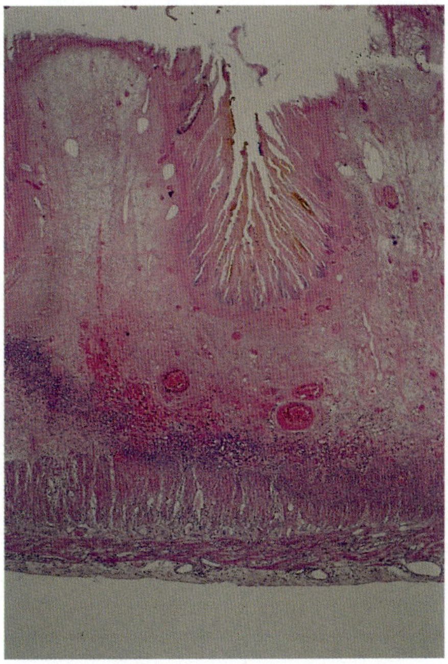

Figure 77–8. Pig-bel. Infarcted area with full thickness necrosis; neutrophils have infiltrated through the external muscle layer to the serosa (hematoxylin-eosin, ×10).

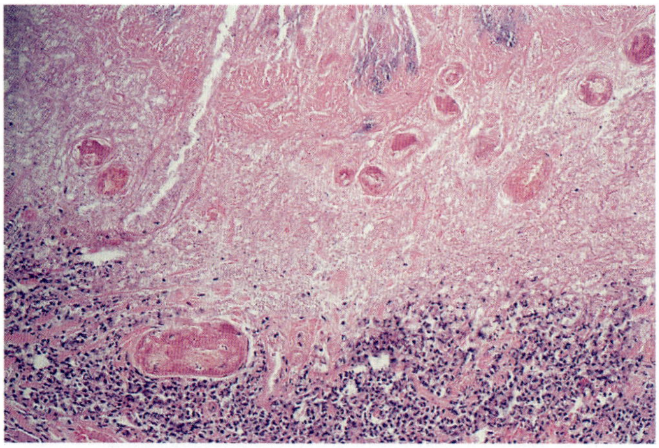

Figure 77–9. Higher magnification of Figure 77–8 showing thrombi in numerous small vessels with extravasated erythrocytes at the junction of the infarcted mucosa and the submucosa (hematoxylin-eosin, ×50).

only mucosa or extend only superficially beneath it (Figure 77–5). The submucosa may show edema and inflammatory cells in some areas, but in others, inflammatory cell infiltration may not be prominent (Figures 77–5 through 77–7). In still other areas, particularly in advanced disease, there is full thickness necrosis through the wall (Figure 77–8), and there may be perforation.

The pathology of pig-bel appears to be identical to that of Darmbrand. In the 1980s a rapidly fatal case of necrotizing enterocolitis in a 24-year-old diabetic man was reported from the Netherlands.[22] He had *C perfringens* type C in his feces and was inoperable because of the rapid and extensive necrosis of his intestine. The

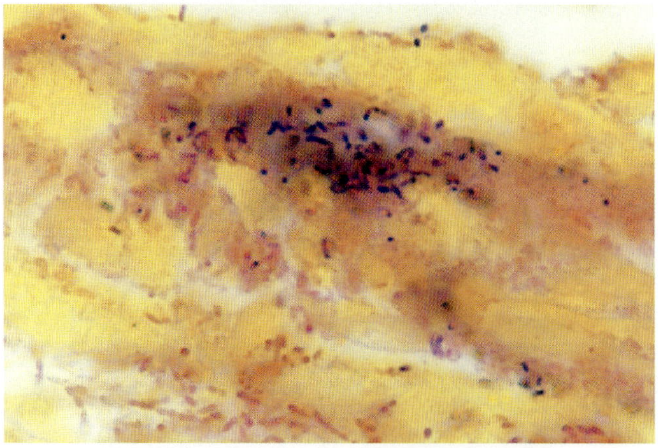

Figure 77–10. Brown-Hopps tissue Gram's stain revealing a typical mixture of gram-positive rods, gram-positive cocci, and gram-negative rods within necrotic mucosa. The gram-stained section of necrotic bowel wall does not permit differentiation between organisms of the gut flora and potentially pathogenic clostridia (×500).

entire small intestine, beginning at about 15 cm from the Treitz ligament, and large parts of the colon were involved. This case offers important evidence that necrotizing enterocolitis caused by *C perfringens* type C occurs outside the endemic area of New Guinea, Southeast Asia, and post-war Germany. More recently, a second report from the Netherlands by Van Kessel et al[23] implicated *C perfringens* type A in a 17-year-old woman who had necrotizing enteritis. Although small numbers of *C perfringens* type C may have been missed as Lawrence suggested,[41] the authors suggested that type A strains might be underestimated as causal agents in this kind of intestinal illness.

Sporadic cases of necrotizing bowel disease caused by *C perfringens* that have either not been typed or were caused by *C perfringens* type A have been reported from various other countries in the world, including England, Canada, and the United States. In the United States in 1952, Patterson and Rosenbaum[18] described a patient with primary *C perfringens* infection of the small intestine. The intestinal ulceration and necrosis resembled previously reported cases of Darmbrand that had been described in the previously cited German and British publications. Another form of intestinal illness called acute hemorrhagic enterocolitis was reported in patients in Cincinnati[42]; however, the role of *Clostridium* sp in these patients (if any) was not certain. In 1962, another case with hemorrhagic necrosis of the ileum and cecum was reported in the United States by Jarkowski and Wolf.[43] The patient was 21 years old, had acute lymphocytic leukemia (not involving the intestine), and had been treated with corticosteroids and 6-MP. He died with disseminated *C perfringens,* probably originating endogenously from the bowel wall, and there were gas cysts in many viscera. In yet another patient from the United States, a 24-year-old with underlying Crohn's disease developed necrotizing jejunitis and ileitis complicated by multiple perforations of the ileum. *Clostridium perfringens* (plus *Escherichia coli*) was isolated from the purulent peritoneal exudate.[44] The cases in the US literature show many similarities to those with necrotizing enterocolitis that have been reported from New Guinea, many countries in Southeast Asia, Europe, Britain, and Canada. In many of the US cases, however, definitive microbiologic studies, combined with the clinical and pathologic descriptions, were lacking, thus making it difficult to interpret the reports.

DIFFERENTIAL DIAGNOSIS

The differential diagnoses include ischemic bowel disease (eg, caused by an atheroma, a thrombus, an embolus, or vasculitis), as well as lesions of nonocclusive ischemia. In situations that cause low blood flow to the gut, the splanchnic blood vessels may constrict, resulting in a reduced blood supply to the small or large bowel. Left ventricular failure, aortic insufficiency, and shock are among the most common causes of bowel ischemia. Obstruction from adhesions, volvulus, intussusception, tumor, or other mechanical or nonmechanical causes, and other inflammatory disorders such as appendicitis, as well as disorders including infections caused by identifiable or cultivable microorganisms should be considered. Murrell[1] pointed out that typhoid fever, intestinal tuberculosis, and ascariasis are among the infections that can be confused with EN. Disease produced by other clostridia (eg, *C septicum* or *C difficile*) also should be considered.[30]

In addition to this discussion, it seems likely that diseases of the bowel that cause stasis or obstruction, trauma (including surgery), transient ischemia, shock, or decreased splanchnic blood flow could predispose the gut to overgrowth of the indigenous anaerobes (including *Clostridium* sp) in an involved segment. Then clostridia could invade the mucosa and produce toxins. Thus, clostridia can be the primary or secondary cause of necrotizing bowel disease. To further complicate the situation of autopsy examination of the intestines, there can be postmortem invasion of the gut and other areas of the body by clostridia, although it is not likely to occur before a postmortem interval of about 4 hours in a refrigerated body. Also, clostridia may cause disease by producing toxin without significant inflammatory response. This kind of toxin-mediated intestinal disease may be difficult to distinguish between postmortem autolysis when the postmortem interval goes beyond 4 hours. In addition to producing toxin, clostridia may produce infection (ie, mediated by invasiveness and other virulence factors) and may produce a toxico-infectious disease (or a combination of toxins and other virulence factors may be involved).

DIAGNOSIS

At this writing, there are no commercially available molecular diagnostic methods (eg, hybridization, PCR) to aid in the diagnosis of EN. A few research laboratories are working with PCR methods to detect the beta toxin gene, and these techniques are promising. Lawrence, Walker, and colleagues[28] have described immunofluorescent antibody reagents to demonstrate *C perfringens* type C in PNG. Unfortunately, such reagents are not available in the United States.

If EN is suspected, feces, blood, bowel wall (if available), and peritoneal fluid should be collected for culturing, isolating, identifying, and typing *C perfringens*. If a delay in processing is anticipated, specimens should not be refrigerated because *C perfringens* does not survive well at refrigeration temperatures.[31] No direct assay for the beta toxin of type C strains is currently available.

In the United States, in spite of reservations about the extent of microbiology reported in some earlier studies, necrotizing enterocolitis caused by *C perfringens* has been documented since the turn of the 20th century. Necrotizing intestinal diseases caused by other clostridia, particularly *C difficile* and *C septicum,* have emerged more recently. Perhaps life-threatening intestinal disease caused by *Clostridium* sp is overlooked by clinicians and pathologists in the United States and thus is underdiagnosed. Details of the procedures that are used to provide microbiologic confirmation of the clostridial intestinal diseases are given elsewhere.[30,31]

TREATMENT

The conservative management of acute pig-bel includes the rapid replacement of fluid and electrolytes (large amounts of fluid and potassium are lost), intestinal decompression, and intravenous administration of antibiotics. Benzyl (crystalline) penicillin has been given in the treatment of patients with mild illness; chloramphenicol and metronidazole have been recommended for patients with severe pig-bel.[1] Surgical measures in pig-bel are controversial. Surgery is "contraindicated in mild cases where diagnosis is uncertain and conservative measures are likely to succeed." In addition, surgery is contraindicated "in very severe cases where resuscitative measures cannot reverse the trend to shock." Surgery has been undertaken in patients who remained toxic in spite of appropriate medical management or because of intestinal obstruction and continued pain, suspected perforation, and/or recurrent severe bleeding.[5]

VACCINATION TO PREVENT PIG-BEL IN PAPUA NEW GUINEA

In 1980, following a controlled trial in which a *C perfringens* type C beta-toxoid vaccine protected against pig-bel for more than 2 years, a program to immunize children using two injections of the toxoid was begun in PNG.[12] By 1987, when a high proportion of the children had been vaccinated, a marked decrease in cases of pig-bel was reported, which coincided with an increase in immunity. Because immunity was relatively short lived in some children (eg, 2.5 years in a few after a third dose of toxoid), booster injections of toxoid might be needed. Nonetheless, Lawrence and colleagues[12] found a "striking benefit from immunization against pig-bel in Papua New Guinea," a success story that theoretically could be repeated in other countries where the incidence of the disease remains high, such as Vietnam.[12]

REFERENCES

1. Murrell TGC. Enteritis necroticans. In: Finegold SM, George WL, eds. *Anaerobic Infections in Humans.* San Diego: Academic Press; 1989:639–659.
2. Murrell TGC, Roth L. Necrotizing jejunitis: a newly discovered disease in the highlands of New Guinea. *Med J Austral.* 1963;1:61–69.
3. Murrell TG, Roth L, Egerton J, Samels J, Walker PD. Pig-bel: enteritis necroticans. A study in diagnosis and management. *Lancet.* 1966;1:217–222.
4. Murrell TG. A history of enteritis necroticans. *P N G Med J.* 1979;22:5–17.
5. Walker PD. Pig-Bel. In: Borriello SP, ed. *Clostridia in Gastrointestinal Disease.* Boca Raton: CRC Press; 1985:94–115.
6. Finegold SM. Intoxications due to anaerobic bacteria. In: Finegold SM, ed. *Anaerobic Bacteria in Human Disease.* New York: Academic Press; 1977:472–512.
7. Zeissler J, Rassfeld-Sternberg L. Enteritis necroticans due to *Clostridium welchii* type F. *Brit Med J.* 1949;1:267–269.
8. Welch WH. Morbid conditions caused by *Bacillus aerogenes capsulatus. Bull Johns Hopkins Hosp.* 1900;11: 185–204.
9. Smith F. Enteritis necroticans—an international disease of tropical communities? Personal observation of an itinerant surgeon. *P N G Med J.* 1979;22:60–61.
10. Murrell TG. Pigbel in Papua New Guinea: an ancient disease rediscovered. *Int J Epidemiol.* 1983;12:211–214.
11. Johnson S, Echeverria P, Taylor DN, et al. Enteritis necroticans among Khmer children at an evacuation site in Thailand. *Lancet.* 1987;2:496–500.
12. Lawrence GW, Lehmann D, Anian G, et al. Impact of active immunization against enteritis necroticans in Papua New Guinea. *Lancet.* 1990;336:1165–1167.
13. Shann F, Lawrence G, Jun-Di P. Enteritis necroticans in China. *Lancet.* 1979;1:1083–1084. Letter.
14. Murrell TG. Enteritis necroticans in Nepal. *Lancet.* 1979; 1:279. Letter.
15. Mukherjee AP, Foong WC, Ferguson BR. Necrotizing enteritis. *The Medical Journal of Malaya.* 1971;25:285–287.
16. Wright DH, Stanfield JP. Enteritis necroticans in Uganda. *J Pediatr.* 1967;71:264–268.
17. Clarke LE, Diekmann-Guiroy B, McNamee W, Java DJ Jr, Weiss SM. Enteritis necroticans with midgut necrosis caused by *Clostridium perfringens. Arch Surg.* 129:557–560.
18. Patterson M, Rosenbaum HD. Enteritis necroticans. *Gastroenterol.* 1994;21:110–118.
19. Hitchcock CR, Bubrick MP. Gas gangrene infections of the small intestine, colon and rectum. *Dis Colon Rectum.* 1976;19:112–119.
20. Blenkinsopp WK, Dupont PA. Bacteria in necrotising enterocolitis. *Lancet.* 1977;2:617. Letter.
21. Williams MR, Pullan JM. Necrotising enteritis following gastric surgery. *Lancet.* 1953;2:1013–1018.
22. Severin WP, de la Fuente AA, Stringer MF. *Clostridium perfringens* type C causing necrotising enteritis. *J Clin Pathol.* 1984;37:942–944.
23. Van Kessel LJP, Verbrugh HA, Stringer MF, Hoekstra JBL. Necrotizing enteritis associated with toxigenic type A *Clostridium perfringens. J Infect Dis.* 1985;151:974–975.
24. Murrell TGC. Some epidemiological features of pig-bel. *Papua New Guinea Med J.* 1967;9:39–50.
25. Millar JS, Smellie S, Coldman AJ. Meat consumption as a risk factor in enteritis necroticans. *Int J Epidemiol.* 1985; 14:318–321.
26. Watson DA, Andrew JH, Banting S, Mackay JR, Stillwell RG, Merrett M. Pig-bel but no pig: enteritis necroticans acquired in Australia. *Med J Aust.* 1991;155:47–50.
27. Lawrence G, Brown R, Bates J, et al. An affinity technique for the isolation of *Clostridium perfringens* type C from man and pigs in Papua New Guinea. *J Appl Bacteriol.* 1984;57:333–338.
28. Lawrence G, Walker PD, Garap J, Avusi M. The occurrence of *Clostridium welchii* type C in Papua New Guinea. *Papua New Guinea Med J.* 1979;22:69–73.
29. Koneman EW, Allen SD, Janda WM, Schreckenberger PC, Winn WC Jr. *Color Atlas and Textbook of Diagnostic Microbiology.* Philadelphia: JB Lippincott Co; 1992.
30. Onderdonk AB, Allen SD. *Clostridium.* In: Murray PR, Baron EJ, Pfaller MA, Tenover FC, Yolken RH, eds. *Manual of Clinical Microbiology.* Washington, DC: ASM Press; 1995:574–586.
31. Smith LDS, Williams BL. *The Pathogenic Anaerobic Bacteria.* Springfield: Charles C. Thomas. 1984.
32. Hatheway CL. Toxigenic clostridia. *Clinical Microbiology Reviews.* 1984;3:66–98.
33. Murrell TG, Walker PD. The pigbel story of Papua New Guinea. *Trans R Soc Trop Med Hyg.* 1991;85:119–122.
34. Schwartz JN, Hamilton JP, Fekety CR, et al. Ampicillin-induced enterocolitis: implication of toxigenic *Clostridium perfringens* type C. *Brief Clinical and Laboratory Observations.* 1980;97:661–663.
35. Borriello SP, Barclay FE, Welch AR, et al. Epidemiology of diarrhoea caused by enterotoxigenic *Clostridium perfringens. J Med Microbiol.* 1985;20:363–372.
36. Kosloske AM, Ulrich JA. A bacteriologic basis for the clinical presentations of necrotising enterocolitis. *J Pediatr Surg.* 1980;15:558–564.
37. Lawrence G, Walker PD. Pathogenesis of enteritis necroticans in Papua New Guinea. *Lancet.* 1976;1:125–126.
38. Lawrence G, Cooke R. Experimental Pigbel: the production and pathology of necrotizing enteritis due to *Clostridium welchii* type C in the guinea-pig. *Brit J Experimental Pathol.* 1980;61:261–271.
39. Devitt PG, Stamp GW. Acute clostridial enteritis—or pigbel? *Gut.* 1983;24:678–679.
40. Cooke R. The pathology of Pig Bel. *Papua New Guinea Med J.* 1979;22:35–49.
41. Lawrence G. Necrotizing enteritis and *Clostridium perfringens. J Inf Dis.* 1986;153:803–804.
42. Wilson R, Qualheim RE. A form of acute hemorrhagic enterocolitis afflicting chronically ill individuals: a description of twenty cases. *Gastroenterol.* 1954;27:431–444.
43. Jarkowski TL, Wolf PL. Unusual gas bacillus infections including necrotic enteritis. *J Amer Med Assoc.* 1962;181: 845–850.
44. Mogadam M, Priest RJ. Necrotizing enteritis in Crohn's disease of the small bowel. *Gastroenterol.* 1969;56:337–341.

CHAPTER 78

Pitted Keratolysis

Ernest E. Lack and Monica V. E. Gallivan

The cow eats the plant. Man eats both of them; and bacteria eat the man.

Hans Zinsser (1878–1940), Rats, Lice and History

DEFINITION

Pitted keratolysis, also referred to in the earlier literature as keratoma (or keratoderma) plantare sulcatum, is a multifocal superficial bacterial infection of stratum corneum with predilection for soles. Characteristically there are sharply defined, punched-out pits in the epidermis.

GEOGRAPHIC DISTRIBUTION AND EPIDEMIOLOGY

Pitted keratolysis has a worldwide distribution,[1–6] and a particular predilection for those in the tropics where higher humidity and moist conditions may be factors. Men are more commonly infected than women. People in temperate climates may also be affected, particularly those with hidrosis or body parts exposed to increased moisture.[7] Combat troops in training or at war in the tropics may be affected. *Dermatophilus congolensis,* the bacterium usually believed to be the cause of pitted keratolysis, causes also a dermatitis of animals, mainly cattle, sheep ("mycotic dermatitis," "lumpy wool," "strawberry foot rot"), and horses.[8,9]

CLINICAL FEATURES

Pitted keratolysis derives its name from the pits in the keratin layer, which often have vertical walls giving a punched-out appearance (Figure 78–1, A–C). The pits usually cause no pain or other symptoms,[7] but when severe can cause soreness and disability.[10] In the tropics, particularly during rainy seasons, the pits may coalesce to form more extensive excavated or crateriform lesions (Figure 78–2).[11] Rarely, bullae have been described.[7] Infection of oral mucosa by *D congolensis* has simulated "hairy" leukoplakia in a male homosexual.[12]

ETIOLOGY

Pitted keratolysis is an infection caused by the gram-positive bacterium *D congolensis,* which is aerobic (facultatively anaerobic). It can be isolated only on complex media; the minimal nutritional requirements are unknown.[9,13] Typical lesions of pitted keratolysis have also been attributed to species of *Corynebacterium, Actinomyces,* and *Micrococcus sedentarius.*[14–17] There may be some overlap in clinical manifestations of pitted keratolysis and erythrasma, which may cause confusion in pinpointing the precise causal agent. A patient with pitted keratolysis had coexistent erythrasma and trichomycosis axillaris.[18] Extracellular proteolytic activity of *D congolensis* is an important factor in keratinolysis and may explain why keratinized surfaces are the main sites of infection.[19]

PATHOLOGY

In pitted keratolysis the pits are usually 1 to 3 mm in diameter, sharply defined, and in biopsy specimens may have a near-vertical wall giving a punched-out appearance (Figure 78–3). Biopsy specimens at the Armed Forces Institute of Pathology had gram-positive organisms in the base and walls of the pits (Figure 78–4), which were not acid fast and formed branching, septate, filamentous structures. The filaments were 0.5 to 1 μm wide and divided and separated longitudinally

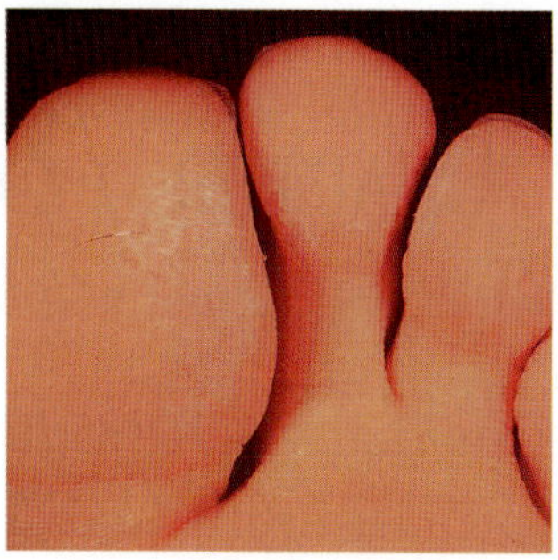

A

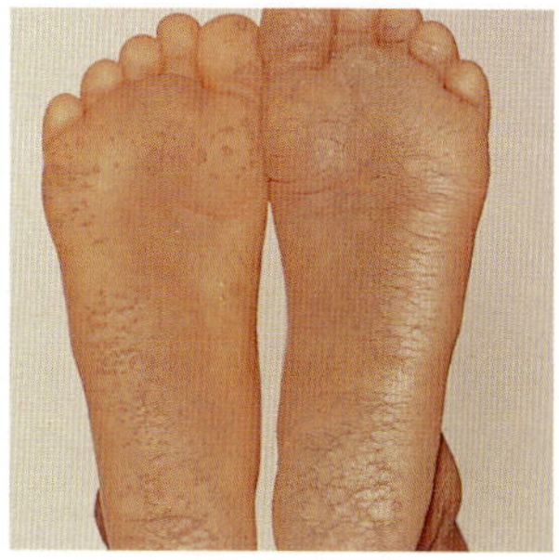

B

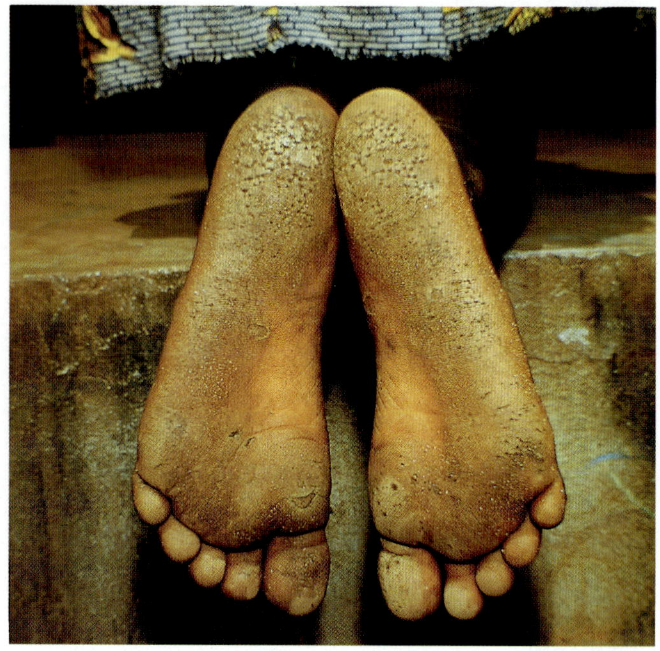

C

Figure 78–1. Pitted keratolysis. (**A**) Note small pitted to confluent areas in keratin layer on plantar aspect of first two toes. Here the pits are shallow. (**B**) Pitted keratolysis with deeper pits on feet in a patient living in the tropics. Pits are discrete and concentrated on the weight-bearing areas of the soles. (**C**) There are numerous distinct pitted lesions on the heels and on the balls of the feet. Instep is spared. *(Photographs by Daniel H. Connor, MD, 1968, 1970.)*

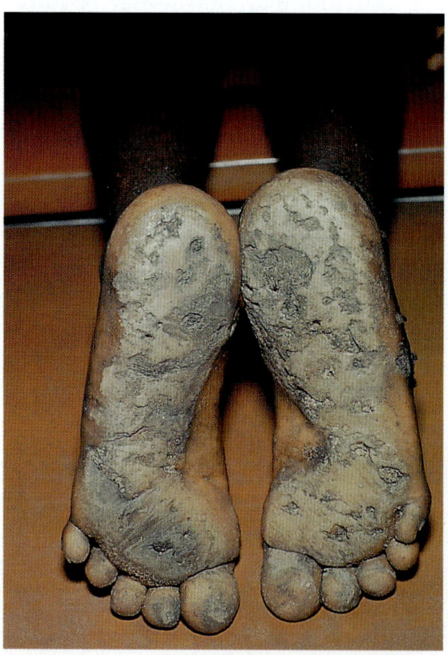

Figure 78–2. An extreme example of pitted keratolysis with concentration of lesions on weight-bearing areas of soles. Many pitted areas are confluent with geographic configuration. *(Photograph by Daniel H. Connor, MD, 1968.)*

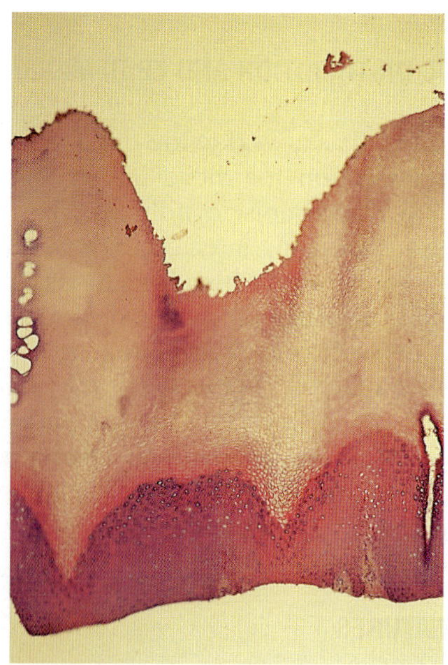

Figure 78–3. Pitted keratolysis. Pit in keratin layer in center of field has almost vertical borders. Note opaque material on surface, which may be seen on sole of barefooted people. Coils of intraepidermal sweat duct (acrosyringium) are on either side of field. The cause—*D congolensis*—is in keratin lining the pit, but cannot be seen with this stain and at this magnification (AFIP Neg 69-5003; hematoxylin-eosin, ×50).

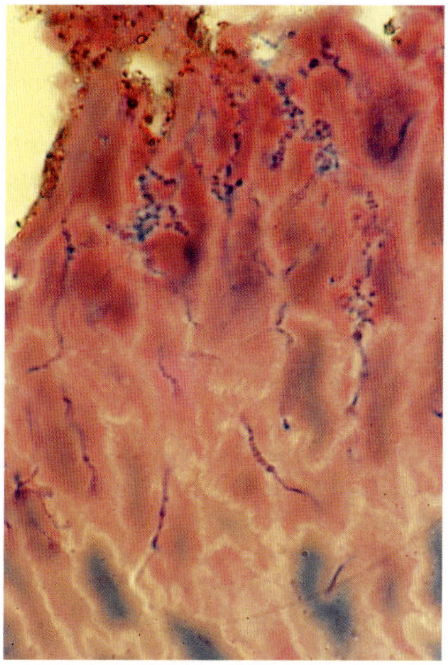

Figure 78–4. Pitted keratolysis. Section through wall of pit or crater reveals branching filaments. A characteristic feature is separation of the organism both transversely and longitudinally into small coccoid bodies (Giemsa stain, ×1000).

as well as transversely, giving the organism a distinctive beaded appearance that could be mistaken for micrococci (Figure 78–5). The branching filaments are highlighted in sections stained with Gomori's methenamine silver (Figure 78–6, A and B). The morphology of *D congolensis* is unique among known microorganisms, and permits accurate diagnosis.

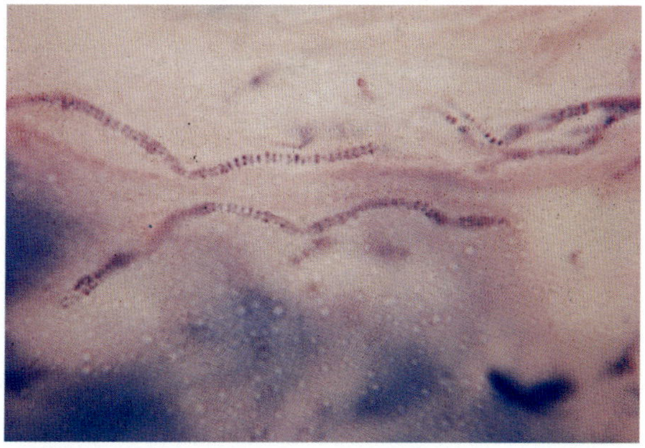

Figure 78–5. Pitted keratolysis. Characteristic filaments of *D congolensis* are broken up into chains of small coccoid bodies (Giemsa stain, ×1000).

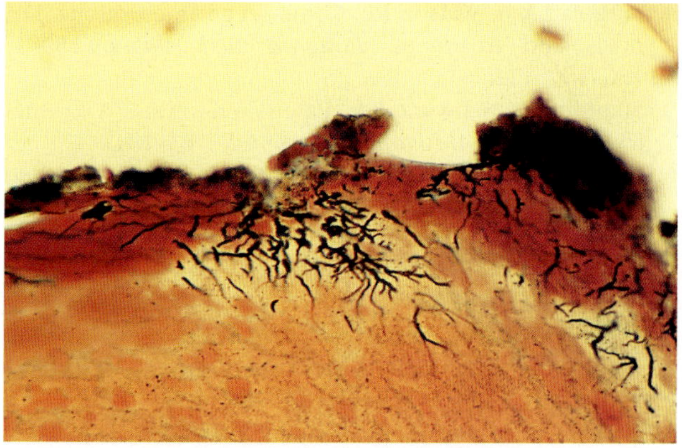

A

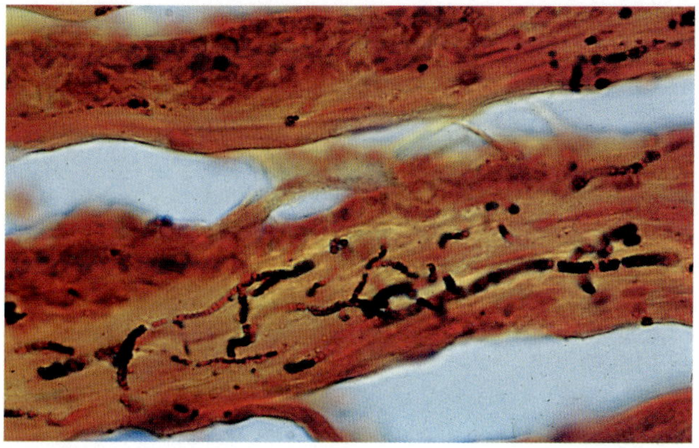

B

Figure 78–6. Pitted keratolysis. (**A**) Numerous branching filamentous forms of *D congolensis* are in the superficial epidermis (mainly stratum corneum) (Gomori's methenamine-silver stain, ×100). (**B**) Filaments of *D congolensis* are separated into smaller rectangular or coccoid bodies (Gomori's methenamine-silver stain, ×1000).

TREATMENT

Treatment of pitted keratolysis may involve thorough and persistent drying of affected areas (ie, soles), but the etiologic agent is susceptible to a variety of antimicrobial agents such as penicillin, streptomycin,[8] and topical ointment of 40% formalin.[7]

REFERENCES

1. Gill KA Jr, Buckels LJ. Pitted keratolysis. *Arch Dermatol.* 1968;98:7–11.
2. Rubel LR. Pitted keratolysis and *Dermatophilus congolensis. Arch Dermatol.* 1972;105:584–586.
3. Tilgen W. Pitted keratolysis (keratolysis plantare sulcatum). *J Cutan Pathol (Denmark).* 1979;6:18–30.

4. Fragola LA Jr, Watson PE. Common groin eruptions. Diagnosis and treatment. *Postgrad Med.* 1981;69:159–163, 166–169, 172.
5. Stanton RL, Schwarz RA. Pitted keratolysis: A common foot problem. *Am Fam Phys.* 1983;27:183–184.
6. Gillum RL, Qadri SM, Al-Ahdal MN, Connor DH, Strano AJ. Pitted keratolysis: a manifestation of human dermatophilosis. *Dermatologica (Switzerland).* 1988;177: 305–308.
7. Connor DH, Neafie RC. Pitted keratolysis. In: Binford CH, Connor DH, eds. *Pathology of Tropical and Extraordinary Diseases.* Washington, DC: Armed Forces Institute of Pathology; 1976.
8. Gordon MA. Aerobic pathogenic *Actinomycetaceae.* In: Lennette EH, ed. *Manual of Clinical Microbiology.* 3rd ed. Washington, DC: American Society for Microbiology; 1980.
9. Beaman BL, Sanbolle MA, Wallace RJ. *Nocardia, Rhodococcus, Streptomyces, Oerskovia,* and other aerobic actinomycetes of medical importance. In: Murray PR, ed. *Manual of Clinical Microbiology.* 6th ed. Washington, DC: American Society for Microbiology; 1995.
10. Lamberg SI. Symptomatic pitted keratolysis. *Arch Dermatol.* 1969;100:10–11.
11. Sehgal VU, Ramesh V. Crateriform depression—an unusual clinical expression of pitted keratolysis. *Dermatologica (Switzerland).* 1983;166:202–211.
12. Bunker ML, Chewning L, Wang SE, Gordon MA. *Dermatophilus congolensis* and "hairy" cell leukoplakia. *Am J Clin Pathol.* 1988;89:683–686.
13. *Bergey's Manual of Determinative Bacteriology.* 9th ed. Baltimore, Md: Williams and Wilkins; 1994.
14. Valente NY, Ribeiro Costa A, Pessoa Mendes J. Pitted keratolysis. Presentation of 2 cases with culture of lesions positive for bacteria of the genus *Corynebacterium. Med Cutaneo Ibero Lat Am (Portugal).* 1983;11:61–64.
15. Conti Diaz IA, Cestau de Peluffo I, Civila E, Calegari L, Sanabria D, Viegas MC. Pitted keratolysis of hyperkeratotic form and isolation of the etiologic agent: *Corynebacterium* sp. *Med Cutaneo Ibero Lat Am (Portugal).* 1987; 15:157–160.
16. Nordstrom KM, McGinley KJ, Cappiello L, Zechman JM, Leyden JJ. Pitted keratolysis. The role of *Micrococcus sedentarius. Arch Dermatol.* 1987;123:1320–1325.
17. Holland KT, Marshall J, Taylor D. The effect of dilution rate and pH on biomass and proteinase production by *Micrococcus sedentarius* growth on continuous culture. *J Appl Bacteriol (England).* 1992;72:429–434.
18. Shelley WB, Shelley ED. Coexistent erythrasma, trichomycosis axillaris and pitted keratolysis: an overlooked corynebacterial triad? *J Am Acad Dermatol.* 1982;7: 752–757.
19. Hanel H, Kalisch J, Keil M, Marsch WC, Buslau M. Quantitation of keratinolytic activity from *Dermatophilus congolensis. Med Microbiol Immunol (Berlin).* 1991;180: 45–51.

CHAPTER 79

Plague

Jerome H. Smith and Barbara S. Reisner

Lord! how sad it is to see the streets empty of people, and very few upon the 'Change. Jealous of every door that one sees shut up, lest it should be the plague; and about us two shops in three, if not more, generally shut up.

Samuel Pepys Diary, August 16, 1665

DEFINITION

Plague is an acute, febrile, contagious infectious disease, caused by *Yersinia pestis* (formerly *Pasteurella pestis*), a bipolar gram-negative bacillus of the family Enterobacteriaceae. Plague has three clinicopathologic forms—bubonic, primary pneumonic, and primary septicemic—and two epidemiologic forms—arthropod-borne and aerosol spread.[1–3]

SYNONYMS

Plague has also been called the black plague, the black death, the pest, pestis, bubonic plague, septicemic plague, and pneumonic plague.

GEOGRAPHIC DISTRIBUTION

Plague has had a worldwide distribution in historic times in four great pandemics. The first great pandemic started in Egypt in the sixth century AD (probably originating in Central Africa and spreading down the Nile) and extended through Turkey into Europe, killing 100 million people. The second pandemic started in Asia Minor and/or Africa in the fourteenth century spreading into Europe, killing approximately a quarter of the population. The third pandemic was in Europe during the fifteenth to eighteenth centuries. The fourth pandemic started in China in the province of Yunnan in 1860 killing tens of millions of people, spread to Hong Kong, and then throughout the world by ships. In the early part of the nineteenth century, India bore the heaviest burden of plague, but this was exhausted by 1950. In the 1960s, Vietnam had 10,000 deaths per year.[2,4]

In recent times, plague has existed principally as sylvatic foci (see Epidemiology section) in the southwestern United States of America, Africa (South Africa, Zimbabwe, Angola, Zaire, Kenya, Uganda, Tanzania, and Madagascar), South America (Peru, Ecuador, Bolivia, and Brazil), and the Far East (China and Southeast Asia); sporadic accidental human infections occur within these sylvatic foci. Plague becomes epidemic on entering lower economic urban areas where environmental barriers separating rats, fleas, and human habitations are not strict.[2] A recent epidemic emerged in Calcutta in late 1994.[5]

NATURAL HISTORY AND EPIDEMIOLOGY

Epidemics of the black death are recorded in the earliest writings. Plague pandemics in the Middle Ages destabilized European society sufficiently to bring about and end the Dark Ages. Epidemics have traditionally descended the Nile from Central Africa spreading around the Mediterranean and to Europe.

Plague is an anthropozoonosis. Small mammals, principally rodents, are the natural hosts. Transmission from mammal to mammal is by the bites of fleas; the most important vector species is *Xenopsylla cheopis,* the rat flea. On ingesting blood from an infected mammal, *Y pestis* replicates unchecked in the flea's foregut, obstructing its proventriculus and preventing the flea from digesting and absorbing the blood meal. These bacilli produce a coagulase active at 20 and 28°C (but inactive at 35 to 37°C),[6] which clots the blood meal; this may provoke the proventricular obstruction. Eventually the flea dies of starvation, but before death, it attempts repeatedly to feed, each time inoculating its host with *Y pestis.*

The susceptibility of the domestic rat *(Rattus rattus)* is so great that during an epizootic, most of the rats die. The true reservoir of plague is wild rodents (sylvatic plague), which are relatively resistant to infection. Domestic rats, after straying into the enviroment of wild rodents, bring the disease back to the urban rat population. Carnivores, both wild (coyotes, wolves, bobcats, other species of wild cats) and domestic (dogs and cats), become infected when they eat infected prey or when they are bitten by fleas from their infected prey. Humans are an accidental host and are infected when they handle infected mammals or when bitten by an infected flea. Since fleas "prefer" their natural hosts, human infection from flea bites usually develops only when most of the natural hosts die of infection or other causes. In the southwestern United States, ground squirrels are the principal reservoir, but jack rabbits and prairie dogs are reservoirs also. Different rodents in different parts of the world serve as reservoir hosts for sylvatic plague.

Epizootics and epidemics are strikingly focal and seasonal. Focal limitations of plague are probably a consequence of the parochial behavior of rats and other rodents. Plague strikes in warm, moist seasons, but disappears in hot seasons when ambient temperatures are too high for the coagulase of *Y pestis* to "plug" the flea's proventriculus, thus rendering the flea an inefficient vector.

Once plague enters a human population, human fleas, principally *Pulex irritans,* and body lice *(Pediculus humanus)* may transmit the infection from man to man. Exhaled droplets and sputum from a patient with terminal plague (secondary pneumonic plague, *vide infra*) are highly infectious and may cause primary pneumonic plague in contacts.

CHARACTERISTICS OF THE ORGANISM

Yersinia pestis, an aerobic, facultatively anaerobic, nonmotile, gram-negative, plump coccobacillus, is bipolar with Wayson's stain. Its cell wall contains gram-negative lipopolysaccharides capable of inducing macrophage production of interleukin-1 (IL-1) and tumor necrosis factor alpha (TNF-α), as well as several specific endotoxins and exotoxins (see Pathogenesis section). Temperature-dependent regulation of production of adaptive proteins lends a bimodal adaptability of the organism to life in homeothermic mammals at 35 to 37°C and in insects at ambient temperatures. While the precise mechanism remains uncertain, *Y pestis* incites increased capillary permeability and elicits a "fluid wave" of edema and increased lymph flow in infected tissues, which spreads the organism to regional lymph nodes or throughout the airways. There is also clinical evidence of a cardiotoxin in the human disease. The lesions of plague are relatively devoid of neutrophils, considering the numbers of bacilli and extent of necrosis; this suggests that plague bacilli do not elicit a neutrophilic response in tissue. In peripheral blood, however, there is a leukocytosis that approaches a leukemoid reaction. The paucity of neutrophils in tissue therefore is probably caused by local destruction possibly from Yop E, a cytotoxin, and/or Yop H, a phosphotyrosine phosphatase (see discussion later) and possibly by other as yet undetermined factors.

CLINICAL FEATURES

There are three clinical forms: bubonic, primary septicemic, and primary pneumonic. *Bubonic plague,* the most common type, is contracted by the bite of an infected flea on a limb; there is a minute lesion at the site of the bite in up to a quarter of patients. The lesion may be vesicular, pustular, macular, papular, or gangrenous.

After incubation of 2 to 4 days, there is sudden onset of chills, high fever, tachycardia, tachypnea, oliguria, and anxiety accompanied by the appearance of the bubo with its sharp, "stabbing" pain and swollen, nonfluctuant lymphadenitis. There is neutrophilic leukocytosis with the white blood count commonly reaching 40,000/μL and, occasionally in children, 100,000/μL. Blood cultures are positive in approximately 50% of patients. Disseminated intravascular coagulation caused by lipopolysaccharides in the wall of the bacilli is a common complication. Liver enzymes and bilirubin may be elevated.

The "bubo," an acute hemorrhagic lymphadenitis involving single or multiple lymph nodes that drains the site of the flea bite, appears on the second to fifth day (Figures 79–1 and 79–2). It is exquisitely painful and tender, commonly 4 or 5 cm in diameter, but may reach 10 cm in diameter. In adult patients the inguinal nodes are most commonly involved, but in children axillary and cervical nodes are more frequently involved. Skin over the bubo is erythematous and may be taut. Buboes may suppurate, become fluctuant, ulcerate, and drain spontaneously. If fluctuant, they should be incised and drained.

Lymphangitis and lymphadenitis progress proximally along the lymphatic drainage (with distal nodes

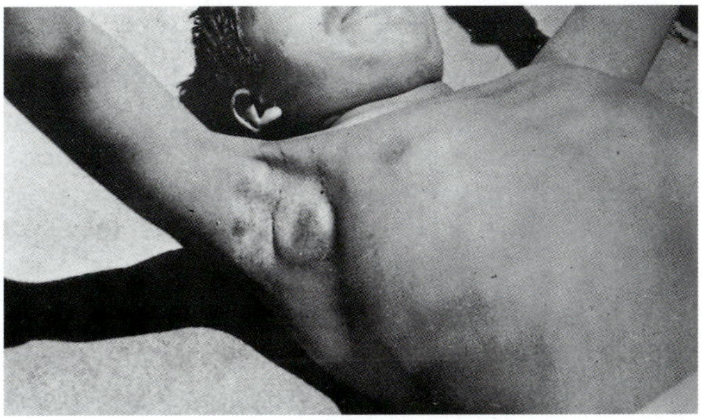

Figure 79–1. Axillary bubo. Ulceration appears imminent (AFIP Neg 219900).

having "older" stages of lymphadenitis than proximal nodes), leading to lymphohematogenous spread. Septicemia and secondary pneumonic plague follow. Terminally, petechiae and hemorrhagic cutaneous infarcts caused by disseminated thromboses (DIC) in the microvasculature and massive ecchymoses prompted the name "black death." Untreated, mortality is 60% to 90% and death may be rapid, sometimes within 24 hours, but usually within 5 days of onset. If treatment is delayed, the endotoxemia may kill the patient even though all bacilli are dead.

Plague minor is a variant of bubonic plague in which endotoxemia is minimal, buboes are small, and patients ambulatory. Although the plague bacillus may be in blood, sputum, or bubo, establishing the diagnosis, patients almost always recover. Also, transient pharyngeal carrier states have been noted in people with no apparent illness.

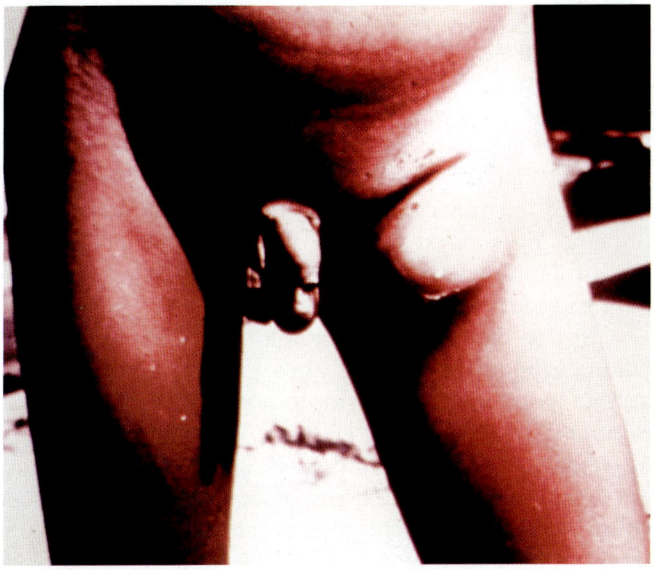

Figure 79–2. Inguinal bubo, origin unknown.

Primary septicemic plague accounts for only about 1% of infections. The clinical onset is sudden, with fever, chills, anxiety, and prostration. Meningitis is common and a rare patient, especially one with undertreated bubonic plague, may present as "meningitic plague" without other localizing symptoms or signs. The course of primary septicemic plague is rapid and 90% fatal within in 24 to 48 hours. Pneumonia and hemorrhage are common. The pathogenesis is not clear, but some postulate that the flea may introduce bacilli directly into the blood. Or primary septicemic plague may result when the infected flea bites the skin of the head or neck or bacilli enter the nose or pharynx; consequently, an early lymphohematogenous spread results from the short length of the lymphatic chain into the thoracic duct, which drains into the left subclavian vein.

Primary pneumonic plague develops when airborne bacilli are inhaled, usually from cadavers or carcasses of animals or more commonly from the cough of a patient with pneumonic plague. After 24 to 60 hours of incubation, sudden chills, high fever, severe cough, and dyspnea mark the onset. Sputum is watery, frothy, occasionally bloody, and teeming with bacilli. Auscultation reveals few signs of pneumonia. In untreated patients, there is 90% mortality in 8 to 24 hours from onset. Death is from acute respiratory insufficiency or endotoxic shock.

PATHOLOGY

Pathogenesis

Entry of the plague bacillus into a mammalian host with its 37°C temperature induces expression of several virulence factors (helping it to evade host defenses) and rapid replication (which produces enormous burdens of bacilli—as high as 10^{10} bacilli/gram of tissue.)[7] Bacteria induce an inflammatory response at the site of inoculation and this effusion carries bacilli into lymphangioles and then regional nodes. Experimental infections have identified several virulence factors necessary for *Y pestis* to survive in mammals.

Low Calcium Response

Low Calcium Response (LCR) genes are on a 75-kb plasmid, one of three plasmids in *Y pestis*. The LCR is characterized by the regulated expression of 12 surface and released proteins specifically at 37°C in the presence of low amounts of Ca^{++} (< 1 mM).[8–12] These proteins include a secreted protein called V antigen and 11 surface and secreted proteins called Yops (for *Y*ersinial outer membrane proteins). Many of the Yops have been shown, through mutational analysis, to be essential for full virulence in mice. In vitro studies with the purified Yop proteins have identified activities that appear important in survival of *Y pestis* in mammals:

- *Yop H* has antiphagocytic activity against mouse peritoneal macrophages[13] and phosphotyrosine phosphatase activity.[14] Bacteria rarely phosphorylate tyrosine; this activity probably targets host phosphoproteins, possibly disrupting intracellular signaling.
- *Yop E* is cytotoxic[15] and acts by disrupting host cell microfilaments.[16] Yop E was associated with microtubules, potentially using them for transport within the cell.
- *Yop M* binds human thrombin[17] and competes with platelets for thrombin, potentially sequestering thrombin in lesions and causing an anti-inflammatory effect.[18]

Bacterial Capsule Fraction 1

Bacterial capsule fraction 1, encoded by a gene on a 110-kb plasmid, is maximally expressed at 37°C and is antiphagocytic for neutrophils and monocytes.[19,20] Although *Y pestis* survives in macrophages, it is killed by neutrophils,[21,22] so inhibition of phagocytosis by these cells has important survival value for the bacteria.

pH 6 Antigen

The *pH 6 antigen* is expressed specifically at 37°C and at an acidic pH; it probably plays a role in survival within acidic phagolysosomes and necrotic lesions.[23–25] Recent studies indicate that it is also probably involved in adhernce.[26]

Pigmentation

Pigmentation phenotype is observed as pigmented colonies on hemin[27] or Congo red[28] agar at 26°C and is involved in the temperature-dependent storage of hemin. Avirulent strains do not express pigment.[29] Such attenuated strains are used for laboratory study of plague and have a large chromosomal deletion encoding the gene *hms* (involved in hemin storage) and at least one gene involved in high-affinity iron acquisition at 37°C.[30]

Coagulase/Fibrinolysin

The 9.5-kb plasmid pPCP1 encodes three proteins,[31] including a bifunctional protein called coagulase/fibrinolysin. This protein acts as a coagulase at ambient temperatures in a flea,[6] whereas it acts as a fibrinolysin (which precludes bacterial entrapment and, thus, promotes dissemination in mammals) and cleaves complement C3 at 37°C.[32]

The local lesions of plague are accompanied by such remarkable proliferation of *Y pestis* that it resembles postmortem bacterial growth. The earliest response to these myriad bacteria is a profuse protein- and mucopolysaccharide-rich effusion, presumably the initial vascular phase of acute inflammation combined with direct endothelial toxicity of yersinial toxins. At this stage, there are no inflammatory cells, and vascular lesions are minimal. Later, toxin-induced necrosis without actual bacterial invasion destroys vessels causing hemorrhage. In the final phase, which may coincide with or follow shortly after the necrosis, there is a paltry neutrophilic infiltrate. Even though macrophages actively phagocytose bacilli, they are unable to kill them and, instead, bacillary toxin destroys the phagocytes.

The lesions of plague result from the local and systemic effects of endotoxins, some of which invoke peripheral vascular collapse and disseminated intravascular coagulation. DIC more frequently complicates plague in children than in adults.

Pathology

Crowell, Strong, and Teague,[33–35] working in both the Manila and Manchurian epidemics of plague, defined the portals of entry and macropathogenesis of the several forms of plague which comprise the usual clinicopathologic presentations. Their careful and scholarly studies at autopsy and in experimental animals, published in now obscure journals (available from the National Library of Medicine), are classics that more recent pathologic studies have improved and modified only slightly. Most infections fall into three clinicopathologic categories: bubonic, primary septicemic, and primary pneumonic.

Bubonic Plague

A cutaneous lesion at the site of the flea's bite develops in less than a quarter of patients with bubonic plague.[2] Grossly, it is usually inapparent, but it may be macular, papular, vesicular, pustular, or a small eschar. It is rarely sampled, so microscopy is not well described in humans. Effusion at the site of inoculation swiftly carries proliferating bacilli into lymphangioles to regional lymph nodes.

At first, lymph nodes exhibit slight congestion and edema (Figure 79–3); then, aggregates of bacilli appear at the junction of the lymph nodal sinuses and the periphery of the follicles (Figure 79–4). These bacillary aggregates have a ground-glass amphophilic appearance typical of plague; special stains, such as tissue Gram stains or metachromatic stains (methylene blue or Giemsa stain) (Figures 79–5 and 79–6), and electron microscopy demonstrate that these exudates are com-

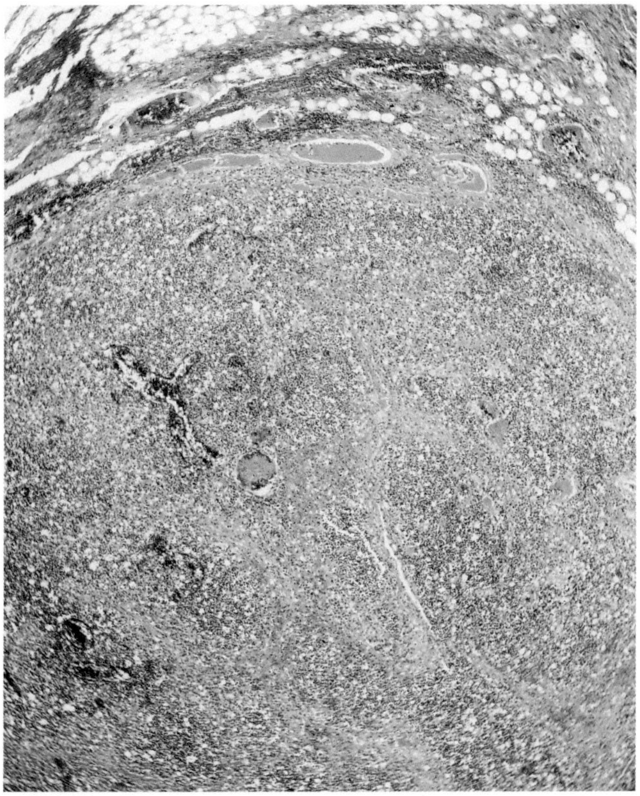

Figure 79–3. Early stage of plague lymphadenitis with congestion and edema (AFIP Neg 73-5760; hematoxylin-eosin, ×50).

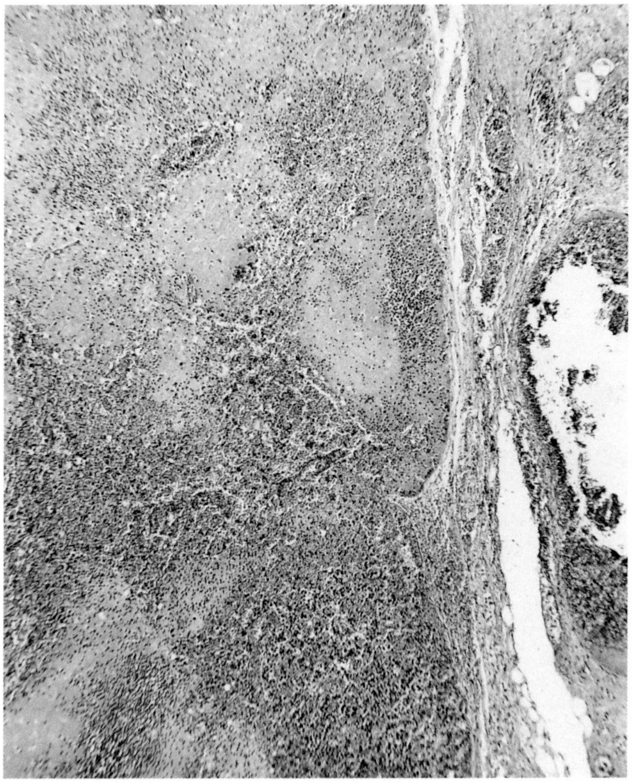

Figure 79–4. Later stage of plague lymphadenitis; gray homogeneous areas with finely granular or ground-glass amphophilic appearance (AFIP Neg 73-5757; hematoxylin-eosin, ×80).

prised almost entirely of plague bacilli, ie, a pure culture in vivo. Ground-glass exudates may occur in other diseases, but when they are identified in sections from sick or dead patients, plague must be suspected. Subsequently, lympholysis spreads from these loci as bacteria proliferate. The exact mechanism of lympholysis is not certain, but some lymphocytes appear unaffected and are, for a time, isolated in a sea of ground-glass bacillary colonial growth. This suggests that some subsets of B and T lymphocytes may resist some of the bacterial cytotoxins. Eventually, there is lysis of all cells in the area, including vascular walls, and hemorrhage ensues, both within and outside of the affected lymph nodes (Figure 79–7). Hemorrhage appears to be low pressure; that is, extravasated erythrocytes do not displace and compress surrounding soft tissue, but infiltrate it. This pattern suggests lysis of small low-pressure venules, rather than of high-pressure arterioles. Adjacent nodes undergoing these changes become edematous, boggy, and hemorrhagic, that is, the bubo.

Lymphadenitis in nodes along the course of the lymphatic drainage evolves into buboes. In swollen lymph nodes, the architecture is obliterated by massive serosanguinous effusion, hemorrhage, and necrosis. The hemorrhagic effusion spreads into perinodal tissues and makes the necrosis in adjacent nodes confluent. Necrosis may lead to ulceration and cutaneous fistulae. Suppuration is late. Lymphohematogenous spread from the foot takes longer to cause systemic sepsis because of the greater length of the lymphatic chain. Thus, patients bitten on the leg or foot are slower to develop a bubo and sepsis than are patients bitten on the arm or head.

Lymphatic spread continues until lymphohematogenous bacteremia and septcemia seeded through the thoracic duct follow. Gram-negative sepsis with septic shock and disseminated intravascular coagulation follow. Disseminated lesions and secondary pneumonic plague also develop. Disseminated intravascular coagulation is often prominent with ecchymoses and may result in microvascular thrombotic lesions with multiple small cutaneous infarcts, especially along the distal parts of the limbs.[2] Microvascular thromboses in renal glomeruli (Figure 79–8) may cause changes in urine.

Secondary Pneumonic Plague

This lesion occurs in nearly all patients with severe untreated bubonic plague. It starts as a peribronchial,

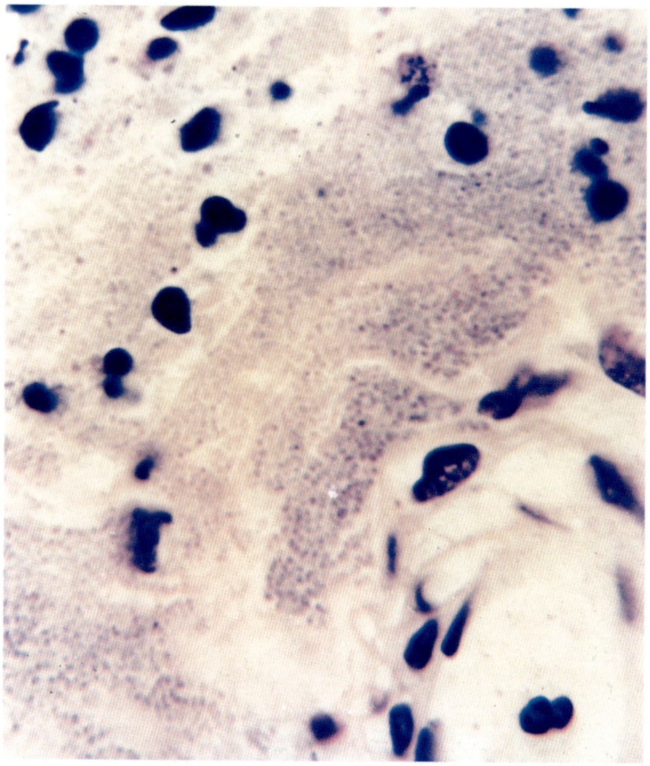

Figure 79–5. Higher magnification showing the ground-glass amphophilic material to be masses of plague bacilli. (AFIP Neg 74-6327; Giemsa, ×1500).

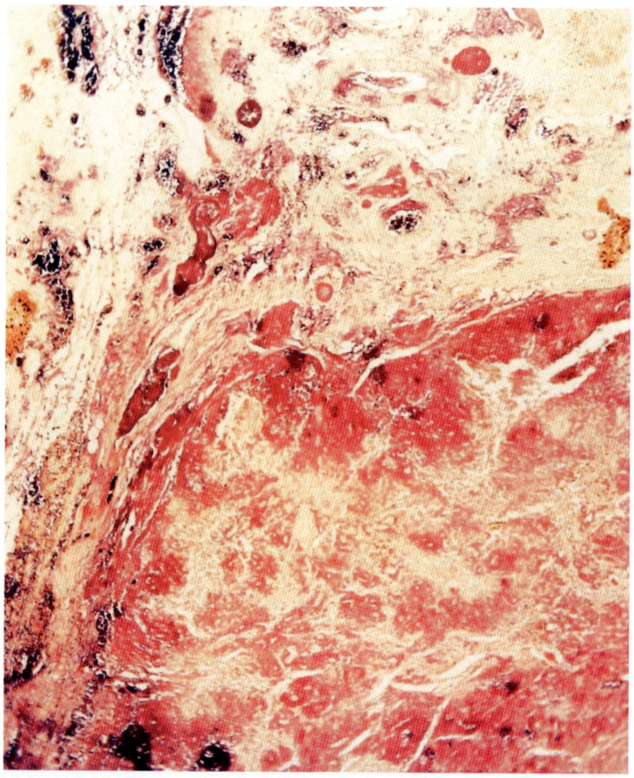

Figure 79–6. Tissue Gram stain of plague lymphadenitis. Red granular areas are masses of closely packed plague bacilli filling peripheral sinuses of node and extending into efferent lymphangioles. Confusion with postmortem bacterial growth is compounded by paucity of neutrophils (AFIP Neg 73-5758; Humberstone stain, ×250).

perivascular interstitial process, but soon breaks into the air spaces to produce hemorrhagic necrotizing bronchopneumonia. It may be a significant factor in the patient's death (among the other serious complications of plague sepsis), but its real significance is that it causes coughing with aerosol spread that may lead to a calamitous epidemic starting with the exposed family and health care workers.

Handling unfixed postmortem and surgical specimens requires extreme caution because pneumonic plague is contagious and progresses with alarming speed. Inhaled bacilli may cause a rapidly fatal infection, so in areas of high risk, pathologists should maintain immunization.

Autopsies of dead rodents are vitally important in defining epidemic foci, but lesions may be insignificant for diagnosis in animals infected naturally. Typically, their spleens are enlarged, severely congested, friable, and hemorrhagic. Serosal hemorrhages and blood-stained serosal fluids may be present. There may be congestion and focal necrosis in adrenals and liver. Buboes usually involve cervical lymph nodes. *Yersinia pestis* usually can be cultured from spleen.

Primary Pneumonic Plague

This type of plague is caused by aerosol spread (inhalation) of droplets laden with plague bacilli either from improper handling of tissues or bodies of plague victims or more commonly from patients with bubonic plague and terminal secondary plague pneumonia. It begins as a lobular pneumonia, with myriads of bacilli in alveoli and a proteinaceous effusion. Subsequently, alveolar walls become necrotic and hemorrhage ensues. Infiltration of neutrophils, while present, is disproportionately sparse with respect to the number of bacteria or the amount of necrosis. The relative neutropenia results from dilution by superimposed pulmonary edema (congestive heart failure) and lysis of neutrophils by bacillary toxins. This process usually spreads by confluence, becomes lobar, then multilobar, and is accompanied by fibrinopurulent pleuritis. Spread is accelerated by pulmonary edema—a consequence of left-sided heart failure from plague cardiotoxin. The spread is rapid and produces pulmonary insufficiency, toxemic shock, and septicemia with complications of gram-negative sepsis. The lungs are purple or black and have large necrotic areas (Figure 79–9). Microscopic examination reveals hemorrhage, large foci of necrosis,

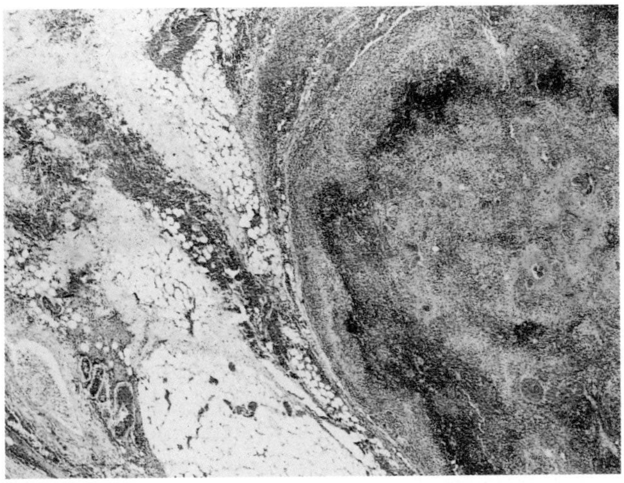

Figure 79–7. Fully developed plague lymphadenitis (bubo). There is edema and hemorrhage of perinodal fat and areolar tissue; the lymph node embedded in this boggy mass is necrotic and hemorrhagic. Myriad plague bacilli are clearly seen under higher magnification (AFIP Neg 76067; hematoxylin-eosin, ×30).

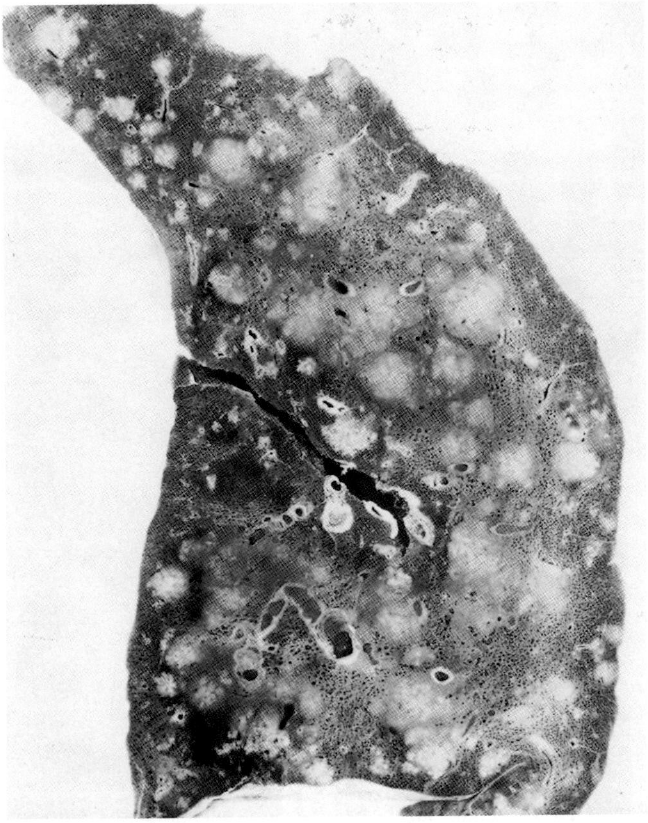

Figure 79–9. Lung in primary pneumonic plague. Necrotic nodules with intense hyperemia and hemorrhage are in the lower lobe, but the upper lobe contains only necrotic nodules. Intervening "normal" pulmonary parenchyma has foci of compensatory emphysema (AFIP Neg 40657).

scant suppuration, and large numbers of bacilli in most of the alveoli (Figure 79–10). The exudate in the alveoli usually has the same ground-glass amphophilic appearance (Figures 79–11 and 79–12) seen in lymph nodes with bubonic plague. This exudate is relatively devoid of fibrin, presumably a consequence of bacterial fibrinolysin (plasminogen activator).

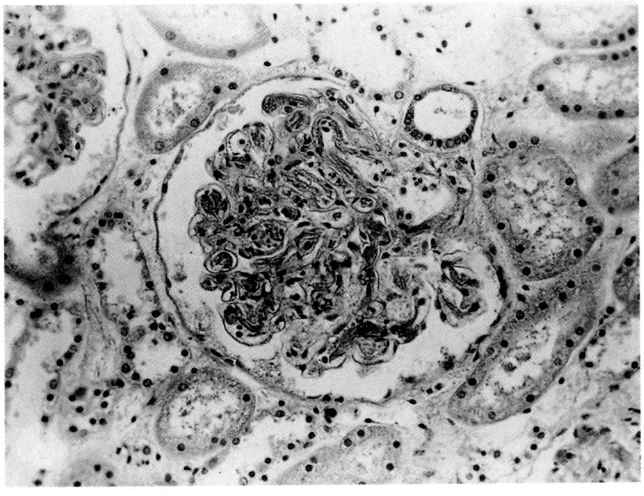

Figure 79–8. Glomerulus with capillaries distended with fibrin thrombi. This is the initial phase of disseminated intravascular coagulation—a complication of septicemic plague (AFIP Neg 80167; hematoxylin-eosin, ×250).

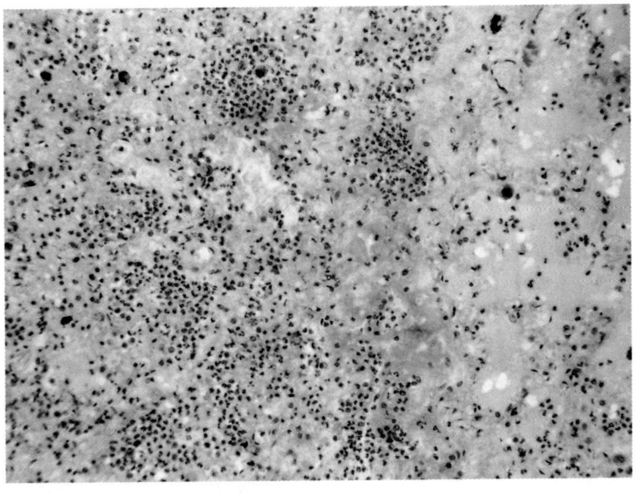

Figure 79–10. Masses of plague bacilli *(Y pestis)* form the gray background of this pneumonic focus in which there is no intact parenchyma. Fibrin is conspicuously absent. (AFIP Neg 77335; hematoxylin-eosin, ×230).

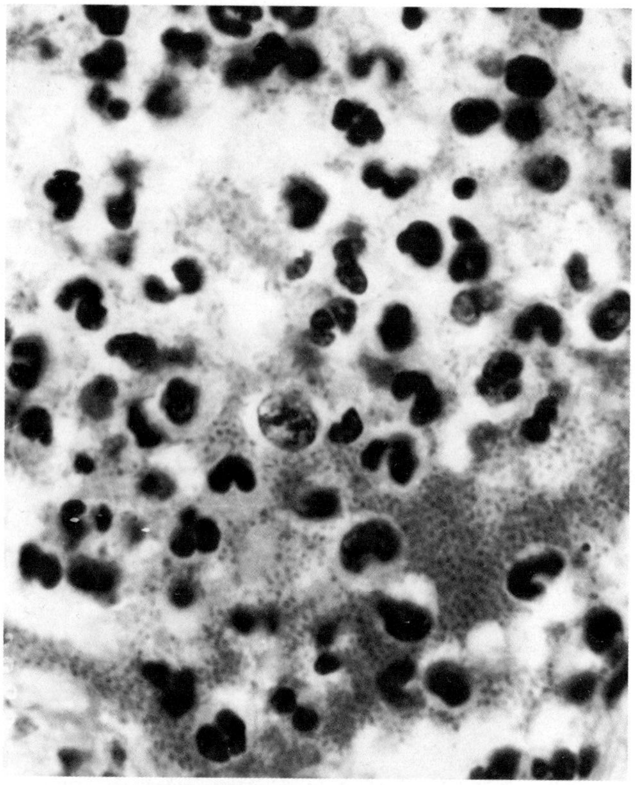

Figure 79–11. Lung. Masses of bacilli in edema-diluted purulent exudate (AFIP Neg 74-6326; Giemsa, ×1400).

Primary Septicemic Plague

Primary septicemic plague is uncommon. In Manila, it was associated with oral, tonsillar, or pharyngeal portals of entry and occasional flea bites on the head.[33] Oropharyngeal and tonsillar portals of entry were caused by crushing fleas between the teeth during reciprocal grooming. The short length of the lymphatic system (mouth to thoracic duct) permitted lymphohematogenous spread before a bubo developed in the regional nodes. Cervical lymph nodes are enlarged, erythematous, and boggy and exhibit microscopic congestion and edema; small ground-glass aggregates begin at the junction of the lymph nodal sinusoid and the periphery of the follicles. Tissue Gram stains show these ground-glass exudates to be colonies of gram-negative bacilli.

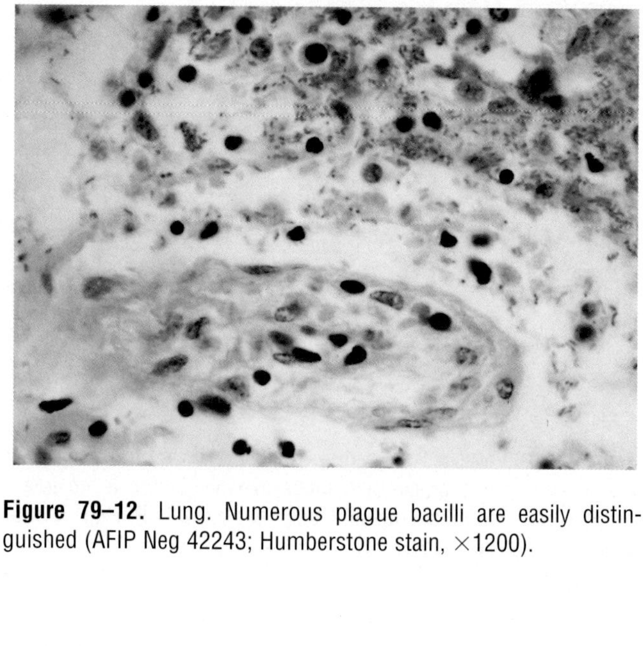

Figure 79–12. Lung. Numerous plague bacilli are easily distinguished (AFIP Neg 42243; Humberstone stain, ×1200).

In septicemic plague, whether primary or secondary, there are bacilli in all vessels. Fibrin casts of renal glomerular capillaries are often present and petechiae or ecchymoses in skin, mucosa, and serosal surfaces are caused by toxemic vascular necrosis and/or disseminated intravascular coagulation. The heart is dilated, may be flabby (probably an effect of the cardiotoxin), and, if the patient lives long enough, may develop a diffuse interstitial myocarditis. The liver has multifocal necrosis, and there is diffuse hemorrhagic necrosis of an enlarged spleen.

DIFFERENTIAL DIAGNOSIS (PATHOLOGY)

Bubonic plague is distinctive grossly and clinically as a severe *acute febrile* illness with buboes. Buboes or pseudobuboes may also appear in some patients with tularemia, sporotrichosis, chancroid, lymphogranuloma venereum, and cat scratch disease, but these maladies rarely present with a sudden onset; also they present different histologic patterns and clinical microbiologic findings. Similarly, syphilis, granuloma inguinale, brucellosis, tuberculosis, *Pasteurella multocida* infection of a bite, and pyogenic coccal infections may present with regional lymphadenopathy, especially inguinal, but primary foci of these diseases at the portal of entry are usually quite apparent.

Definitive diagnosis is accomplished by making smears and cultures of aspirates of the bubo or enlarged lymph nodes. Aspirates of plague buboes contain bipolar bacilli on Wayson's stain; these are gram-negative. Lesions and exudates of chancroid contain streaming "schools of fish" of gram-negative bacilli. Streptococcal and staphylococcal lymphadenitis contains gram-positive cocci in chains or clusters, respectively, and lesions of tuberculosis contain acid-fast bacilli. Syphilis may show spirochetes on darkfield examination of aspirates. Macrophages containing Donovan bodies (encapsulated gram-negative bacilli) may be seen on Gram stain or Giemsa stains and are silvered by Warthin–Starry and other silver impregnation techniques. Tularemia, *P multocida* infections, brucellosis, sporotrichosis, lymphogranuloma venereum, and cat scratch disease rarely demonstrate pathognomonic organisms on smears of aspirates. Culture for some of these requires specialized techniques and is not routine. The clinician or pathologist submitting the specimen therefore must tell the microbiologist of any suspicions.

Histologically, plague buboes may be differentiated from other lymphadenitis on the basis of the pattern of cellular response as well as the teeming gram-negative bacilli in the inflammatory, cell-poor, hemorrhagic, necrotic lesions described. Chancroid, *P multocida* infections and pyogenic coccal infections have prominent neutrophilic infiltrates, even abscesses. Tularemia, lymphogranuloma venereum and cat scratch disease (and sometimes lesions of *P multocida*) usually show stellate microabscesses, which are irregularly "geographic" and enclosed by palisaded macrophages. The reactions in granuloma inguinale, brucellosis, and tuberculosis are dominated by macrophages, mostly activated with soft or otherwise typical granulomas. Syphilis exhibits prominent perinodal fibrosis, plasmacytosis, and endarteritis; spirochetes may be demonstrated with silver impregnation stains (Warthin–Starry or Dieterle).

CONFIRMATION OF DIAGNOSIS BY MICROBIOLOGIC CULTURE, SEROLOGY, AND IMMUNOLOGY

Yersinia pestis may be isolated from exudates of buboes, sputum, or blood on a variety of broth and agar media, including blood agar. At 24 hours on blood agar media, colonies are pinpoint in size but by 48 hours are 1 to 1.5 mm in diameter, gray to grayish-white, and may appear mucoid. *Yersinia pestis* is nonmotile at either room or body temperature and is relatively unreactive with routine biochemical tests (urea hydrolysis, sugar fermentation such as adonitol, L-rhamnose or melibiose), but it shows nonuniform turbidity ("stalactites") in liquid media, exhibits *Yersinia* phage susceptibility at 20 and 37°C, produces coagulase (at 20°C, but not at 37°C) and fibrinolysin (at 37°C, but not at 20°C), and reacts with specific antisera. It is pathogenic for mice, white rats, Guinea pigs, and gerbils, but not hamsters.[1] Prompt presumptive identification is essential because untreated, 60% of patients die. Furthermore, the rapid course dictates that appropriate antibiotic therapy be started early. Pus (aspirated from buboes or swabbed from fistulous buboes) or sputum in the pneumonic phase characteristically teems with organisms, and blood culture is usually positive (especially in primary septicemic plague).

TREATMENT

Antibiotics (streptomycin, tetracycline, and chloramphenicol), when given early, are very effective. After chemotherapy, fluctuant buboes should be incised and drained. Supportive therapy (rehydration and support of blood pressure) is critical. Heparin therapy for DIC has been of no benefit.[2]

REFERENCES

1. Farmer JJ, Kelly MT. Enterobacteriaceae. In: Balows A, Hausler WJ, Herrmann KL, Isenberg HD, Shadomy JH, eds. *Manual of Clinical Microbiology*. 5th ed. Washington, DC: American Society of Microbiology; 1991:380–381.
2. Butler T. Plague. In: Strickland GT, ed. *Hunter's Tropical Medicine*. 7th ed. Philadelphia: WB Saunders, 1991:408–416.
3. Butler T. *Yersinia* species. In: Mandell GL, Bennett JE, Dolin R, eds. *Principles and Practice of Infectious Disease*. 4th ed. New York: Churchill Livingstone; 1995:2070–2076.
4. Cravens G, Marr JS. *The Black Death*. New York: Ballantine Books; 1977.
5. Sternberg S. Plague epidemic. Bottleneck keeps existing vaccine off the market. *Science*. 1994;266:22–23.
6. McDonough KA, Falkow S. A *Yersinia pestis* specific DNA fragment encodes temperature-dependent coagulase and fibrinolysin associated phenotypes. *Molecul Microbiol*. 1989;3:767–775.
7. Butler T. *Plague and Other Yersinia Infections*. New York: Plenum Medical Book Company; 1983.
8. Bolin I, Portnoy DA, Wolf-Watz H. Expression of the temperature-inducible outer membrane proteins of yersinieae. *Infect Immun*. 1985;48:234–240.
9. Perry RD, Haddix P, Atkins EB, Soughers TK, Straley SC. Regulation of expression of V antigen and outer membrane proteins of *Yersinia pestis*. *Contrib Microb Immun*. 1987;9:173–178.
10. Portnoy DA, Wolf-Watz H, Bolin I, Beeder AB, Falkow S. Characterization of common virulence plasmids in *Yersinia* species and their role in the expression of outer membrane proteins. *Infect Immun*. 1984;43:108–114.
11. Straley SC, Bowmer WS. Virulence genes regulated at the transcriptional level by Ca^{2+} in *Yersinia pestis* include structural genes for outer membrane proteins. *Infect Immun*. 1986;51:445–454.
12. Straley SC, Brubaker RR. Cytoplasmic and membrane proteins of yersinieae cultivated under conditions simulating mammalian intracellular environment. *Proc Natl Acad Sci USA*. 1981;78:1224–1228.
13. Rosqvist R, Skurnik M, Wolf-Watz H. Increased virulence of *Yersinia pseudotuberculosis* by two independent mutations. *Nature*. 1988;334:522–525.
14. Guan K, Dixon JE. Protein tyrosine phosphatase activity of an essential virulence determinant in *Yersinia*. *Science*. 1990;249:553–556.
15. Rosqvist R, Forsberg A, Rimpilainen M, Bergmen T, Wolf-Watz H. The cytotoxic protein Yop E of *Yersinia* obstructs the primary host defense. *Molecul Microbiol*. 1990;4:657–667.
16. Rosqvist R, Fosberg A, Wolf-Watz H. Intracellular targeting of the *Yersinia* Yop E cytotoxin in mammalian cells

induces actin microfilament disruption. *Infect Immun.* 1991;59:4562–4569.
17. Leung KY, Reisner BS, Straley SC. Yop M inhibits platelet aggregation and is necessary for virulence of *Yersinia pestis* in mice. *Infect Immun.* 1990;58:3262–3271.
18. Reisner BS, Straley SC. Function and regulation of *Yersinia pestis* Yop M: thrombin binding and overexpression. *Infect Immun.* 1992;60:5242–5252.
19. Smith H, Keppie J, Cocking EC, Witt K. The chemical basis of the virulence of *Pasteurella pestis.* I. The isolation and the aggressive properties of *Pasteurella pestis* and its products from infected guinea pigs. *Br J Exp Pathol.* 1960;41:452.
20. Brubaker RR. Expression of virulence in yersinieae. In Schlessinger D, ed. *Microbiology.* Washington, DC: American Society for Microbiology; 1979.
21. Cavanaugh DC, Randal R. The role of multiplication of *Pasteurella pestis* in mononuclear phagocytes in the pathogenesis of flea-borne plague. *J Bacteriol.* 1959;83: 348–363.
22. Burrows TW, Bacon GA. The basis of virulence in *Pasteurella pestis:* the development of resistance to phagocytosis in vitro. *Br J Exp Pathol.* 1956;37:286–299.
23. Ben-Efraim S, Aronson M, Bichowsky-Slomnicki L. New antigenic component of *Pasteurella pestis* formed under specific conditions of pH and temperature. *J Bacteriol.* 1961;81:704–714.
24. Bichowsky-Slomnicki L, Ben-Efraim S. Biological activities in extracts of *Pasteurella pestis* and their relation to the "pH 6 antigen." *J Bacteriol.* 1963;86:101–111.
25. Lindler LE, Klempner MS, Straley SC. *Yersinia pestis* pH 6 antigen, genetic, biochemical and virulence characterization of a protein involved in the pathogenesis of bubonic plague. *Infect Immun.* 1990;58:2569–2577.
26. Lindler LE, Tall BD. Yersinia pH 6 antigen forms fimbriae and is induced by intracellular association with macrophages. *Molecul Microbiol.* 1993;8:311–324.
27. Jackson S, Wurrow, TW. The pigmentation of *Pasturella pestis* on a defined medium containing haemin. *Br J Exp Pathol.* 1956;37:570–576.
28. Surgall MJ, Beesley ED. Congo red-agar plating medium for detecting pigmentation in *Pasteurella pestis. Appl Microbiol.* 1969;18:834–837.
29. Une T, Brubaker RR. In vivo comparison of avirulent Vwa^- and Pgm^- or Pst^r phenotypes of yersinieae. *Infect Immun.* 1984;43:895–900.
30. Pendrak JL, Perry RD. Characterization of a hemin-storage locus of *Yersinia pestis. Biol Metals.* 1991;4:41–47.
31. Sodiende OA, Goguen JD. Genetic analysis of the 9.5-kilobase virulence plasmid of *Yersinia pestis. Infect Immun.* 1988;56:2743–2748.
32. Sodiende OA, Subrahmanyam YVBK, Stark K, Quan T, Bao Y, Goguen JD. A surface protease and the invasive character of plague. *Science.* 1992;258:1004–1007.
33. Strong RP, Teague O. Studies on pneumonic plague and plague immunization. IV. Portal of entry of infection and method of development of the lesions in pneumonic and primary septicemic plague: experimental pathology. *Philippine J Sci B Philippine J Trop Med.* 1912;7:173–180.
34. Strong RP, Crowell BC, Teague O. Studies on pneumonic plague and plague immunization. VII. Pathology. *Philippine J Sci B Philippine J Trop Med.* 1912;7:203–221.
35. Crowell BC. Pathologic anatomy of bubonic plague. *Philippine J Sci B Trop Med.* 1915;10:249–306.

CHAPTER 80

Pseudomonas aeruginosa

Frederick A. Meier

Infectious disease is one of the great tragedies of living things—the struggle for existence between different forms of life.

Hans Zinsser (1878–1940)

Sur les Colorations bleue et verte des linges à pansements.

C. Gessard[1]

DEFINITION AND SYNONYMS

In 1994, the generic designation *Pseudomonas* achieved its centenary; however, the genus for which *Pseudomonas aeruginosa* is the type species has recently experienced a striking contraction.[2]

The contraction has been due to the application of the taxonomic technique of ribosomal RNA (rRNA) grouping to the phylogenic tree of the purple bacteria in general and the family Pseudomonadaceae in particular.[3] The distinctions made by the differences in rRNA types have been integrated successfully with phenotypic diagnostic properties that yield reproducible results from seven simple tests: 1) colony structure (helpful when it is characteristic), 2) odor (an important sign to generations of clinical microbiologists at the bench), 3) production of phenazine pigments (the most salient of these phenotypic markers), 4) capacity for growth at 42°C (most helpful in sorting among pigment producers), 5) gelatin liquefaction (of second-line utility among pigment producers), 6) denitrification, and 7) growth utilizing specified carbon compounds that are assimilated differentially among similar bacteria (the last two phenotypes are particularly helpful in classifying nonpigmented isolates). The rRNA-based taxonomy yields five related groups within the family Pseudomonadaceae.[4] Only members of a single group, Palleroni's rRNA group I, still bear the genus name *Pseudomonas*.

Within the new genus, there are only three phenotype clusters.[5] The first cluster of organisms manifests the fluorescent *Pseudomonas* phenotype; it includes the type species *P aeruginosa* [also known, earlier in the 100-year history of this colorful nomenclature, as *Pseudomonas pyocyanea* (pyocyanea = blue pus) (Migula, 1900) and, earlier still, as *Bacterium aeruginosa* (aeruginosa = verdigris, the green color of oxidized copper) (Schroeter, 1872)], as well as two other species, *Pseudomonas fluorescens* and *Pseudomonas putida* (putida = fetid, stinking); these three related species produce characteristic water-soluble pigments that fluoresce white to blue-green under long-wavelength (400-nm) ultraviolet light. Among the fluorescent *Pseudomonas,* only *P aeruginosa* grows at 42°C, distinguishing it from its companions in the pigment-producing phenotype. The other two organisms are, in turn, separated from one another by the ability to liquefy gelatin, an ability that *P fluorescens* possesses but *P putida* does not.

A second cluster of members of the current genus *Pseudomonas* is ubiquitous soil and water bacteria that play an important ecological role by performing denitrification, when growing anaerobically; these organisms rarely cause human infection. The species of this cluster are *P stutzeri* and the relatively rare *P mendocina.*

The final phenotype within the current genus consists of bacteria that are only weakly saccharolytic in the low peptone oxidative-fermentative bacteriologic medium: *P alcaligenes* and its slight variants, *P pseudoalcaligenes* and *P denitrificans.* They are also only rare causes of human infection. From this list one can see that, except for the type species, all clinically significant prior members of the genus *Pseudomonas* have been banished to other taxa.

The other genera[6] corresponding to Pseudomonadaceae rRNA groups II–IV are group II: *Burkholderia;* group III: *Comamonas* and *Acedovorax;* group IV: *Brevundemonas;* and group V: *Stenotrophomonas. Burkholderia* includes, besides some economically important plant pathogens, three important infectious agents of mammals: *B mallei,* the cause of the equine disease glanders; *B pseudomallei,* the cause of melioidosis, a glanders-like disease in humans, and *B cepacia,* an occasional respiratory pathogen in humans associated with progressive lung disease in patients with cystic fibrosis. *Stenotrophomonas* consists solely of the species *Stenotrophomonas maltophilia,* which, as *Xanthomonas maltophilia,* attracted clinical interest during the 1980s for two, probably related, reasons: 1) its increased incidence as an opportunistic infectious agent among immunodeficient patients treated with broad-spectrum antibiotics and 2) its own broad spectrum of antimicrobial resistance achieved through an impressive variety of resistance mechanisms.[7] Two other causes of opportunistic infection that once bore the genus designation *Pseudomonas* have been expelled even from the family Pseudomonadaceae.[8] These exiles are *Shewanella putrefaciens* and *Sphingomonas paucimobilis.* This chapter focuses on the pathologic patterns, appearances, and mechanisms of *P aeruginosa* and how these bacteria are distinguished from the fluorescent *Pseudomonas* sp whose phenotypes may be confused with the type species.

GEOGRAPHIC AND ECOLOGIC DISTRIBUTION

Geographically, *P aeruginosa* is an ubiquitous bacterium with a cosmopolitan distribution. Ecologically, it occupies three related niches[9]: First, it is a remarkably hardy inhabitant of watery environments, including some aqueous media naively considered inhospitable to bacteria. Examples of such media are whirlpool bath and hot-tub water or disinfectant solutions. Infected bath and tub water has caused skin infection. Contaminated disinfectants have produced outbreaks of pseudo- (rather than *Pseudomonas*) bacteremia. Second, *P aeruginosa* is also a soil bacterium throughout a wide variety of terrestrial milieu. Third, it maintains remarkably stable relationships with other denizens of rhizospheres, the wet soil environments that form complex ecosystems surrounding plant roots.

From this ecological distribution, the potential reservoirs for human contact with *Pseudomonas* follow[10]: 1) water-related reservoirs outside hospitals—swimming pools, whirlpools, and hot tubs, as well as contact lens solutions; 2) water-related reservoirs in hospital respirator equipment, dialysis fluid and equipment, other equipment washed by aqueous solutions, aqueous medicines and disinfectants, and wet surfaces such as sinks, damp mops, and food mixers; 3) soil-related reservoirs outside hospital, like nails, splinters, and dirt itself introduced into wounds; and 4) plant-related reservoirs both outside and in hospital, like salads, vegetables, and flowers.

Pseudomonas aeruginosa econiches also predict the usual sites of epithelial colonization in healthy humans[11]: dark, moist, warm surface zones resembling rhizospheres. These zones are the external ear canal, axilla, perineum, and colon. Human colonization rates are, however, low in subjects outside hospital: 0% to 2% on squamous, 0% to 6% on respiratory, and 2.6% to 24% on colonic epithelia. In hospital, these colonization rates increase, especially on altered epithelia exposed, during treatment, to environmental solutions and broad-spectrum antimicrobials (eg, in burn patients and patients supported by mechanical ventilation). In cancer patients colonization appears to precede infection.[12] In a neonatal intensive care unit, colonization was associated with the presence of ecological reservoirs.[13]

BIOLOGIC BEHAVIOR

Growth Conditions[14]

Pseudomonas aeruginosa has three growth characteristics that contribute to its ecological adaptability and its success as an agent of opportunistic infection: ability to flourish across a broad spectrum of physical conditions, especially of temperature; minimum nutritional requirements, due to remarkable biochemical versatility; and relative resistance to widely used antimicrobials, thanks to a variety of both cell wall and cytosolic resistance mechanisms.

Bacteriologically, *P aeruginosa* is, among aerobic, non-spore-forming gram-negative rods, the most frequent clinically significant isolate that is not a member of the family Enterobactereaceae.[15] The organism's status as a nonenteric was recognized early in its history; this recognition is reflected in the modifying first syllable of its generic name (pseudo = false, in this case, not an enteric, motile bacterium). This 1- to 5-μm-long and 0.5- to 1.0-μm-wide bacillus does, however, possess the polar flagella characteristic of many enteric bacteria. The flagella are responsible not only for the motility of *Pseudomonas* but also for the stem of its Latin generic name (monas = unit; the flagella appear to be the "unit" that Migula was using to group motile bacteria when, a century ago, he introduced the generic designation). *Pseudomonas* distinguishes itself from the enteric bacteria biochemically by its nonfermenter (colorless) colony morphotype on MacConkey or EMB agar and by being oxidase positive (producing a color change with a standard oxidase reagent).[16]

In most clinical isolates, the agar plate morphotype is a spreading flat colony with a serrated edge and metallic sheen, however, there is a variant colony morphotype of raised domed colonies with entire edges and a mucoid surface[17]; this variant is seen most frequently in isolates from cystic fibrosis patients with chronic infection. *Pseudomonas aeruginosa* also produces a distinctive smell that is usually described as both grape-like and musty or fetid. The even more characteristic phenazine pigment phenotype is complex[18]: the visible bright green, which is usually observed, combines the blue of pyocyanin (unique to *P aeruginosa*) with the yellow of pyoverdin (produced by all fluorescent *Pseudomonas*). *Pseudomonas aeruginosa* may also produce pyorubin (red) or pyomelanin (black) pigment variants. The species' nutritional versatility is reflected in its ability to utilize as carbon sources a variety of simple and complex carbohydrates, their derivative alcohols, and amino acids. In the clinical microbiology laboratory, *P aeruginosa* is usually identified by four findings[5]: 1) a positive oxidase test, 2) a triple sugar ion (TSI) agar reaction of alkaline slant over unchanged butt, 3) production of blue, blue-green, red, or brown diffusible pigments on Mueller–Henton (non-dye-containing) agar, and 4) 42°C growth. The last characteristic can also separate yellow (pyoverdin) pigment-producing *P aeruginosa* from the other two members of the genus; *P fluorescens* and *P putida* produce this yellow pigment, but do not grow at 42°C.

Some *P aeruginosa* strains, especially of the mucoid colony phenotype, fail to form any pigment. For these, a second line of biochemical tests needs to be deployed[16]: nitrate reduction and production of nitrogen gas, oxidation of glucose but not disaccharides (eg, glucose and xylose but not maltose, among standard carbohydrate substrates), and arginine dihydrolase activity but not lysine or ornithine decarboxylase activity (among amino acid substrates) is the usual second-line profile. In the "classic" bacteriologic battery of biochemical tests, *P aeruginosa* is also typically citrate and indophenol positive. Although commercial bacterial identification test kits and automated identification systems identify most *P aeruginosa* reliably, many commercial methods have difficulty differentiating the other members of the genus from the type species. Thus, identification by kit and automated methods of other *Pseudomonas* species or of atypical *P aeruginosa* isolates should be handled with gentle skepticism until confirmed by reference techniques.

Antimicrobial susceptibility phenotypes of *P aeruginosa* distribute themselves along a spectrum that correlates, roughly, with the duration and intensity of exposure to antibacterial agents.[19] Community-acquired *Pseudomonas* isolates are usually susceptible to the antipseudomonal penicillins (ticarcillin, piperacillin, mezlocillin, and combinations containing these agents). As their descriptive name suggests, these penicillins were introduced to deal with *P aeruginosa*'s uniform resistance to the previously developed antistaphylococcal penicillins. Community-acquired isolates are also usually susceptible to aminoglycoside, third-generation cephalosporin, monobactam, carbapenim, and quinolone agents. The latter statement is not true for hospital-acquired agents. The latter are now (1995) often resistant to, at least, some of the broad-spectrum cephalosporins and, increasingly, to quinolones. Among heavily treated patients, primarily chronically infected cystic fibrosis patients, resistance to the mainstays of antipseudomonal therapy (the penicillins listed earlier, and the two most effective cephalosporins—cefoperazone and ceftazidime) has sometimes emerged in ominous, multidrug-resistant phenotypes.[20]

By all measures of growth conditions, adaptability to various physical environments, versatile metabolism, and broad-spectrum antimicrobial resistance, *P aeruginosa* is a strikingly tough organism. This realistic adaptation to a wide variety of growth conditions fits the natural history of *P aeruginosa* as the quintessential opportunist.[21]

NATURAL HISTORY AND VIRULENCE PROFILE

The natural history of *P aeruginosa* is indeed that of an opportunistic infectious agent. Unlike most opportunists, however, its virulence profile is complex.

Natural History

As an opportunist, *P aeruginosa* must exploit one or more defects in host defenses. Typically these defects are 1) disruption of cutaneous or mucosal epithelial surfaces (eg, by maceration, burns, or wounds) or contiguous spread through defective or penetrated epithelial surfaces (eg, causing contiguous soft tissue infections and osteomyelitis); 2) circumvention of anatomic barriers (eg, by therapeutic devices like intravascular and urinary catheters or endotracheal tubes); and 3) immune dysfunction (eg, caused by neutropenia in patients being treated with immunosuppressive therapy).

The first sort of defect disruption, of epithelial surfaces, underpins most community-acquired cases of *P aeruginosa* infection. Macerated skin in a moist environment usually accounts for primary infection of the cutaneous epithelium and its appendages. Examples of this mechanism of infection, listed in order of increasing severity, are *Pseudomonas* dermatitis, folliculitis, pyoderma, and "malignant" otitis externa ("swimmer's ear"). Especially severe cases of this mechanism of integumentary defect are *Pseudomonas* burn wound infection,[22] unmanageable exacerbations of acne vulgaris in which ecosuccession by *Pseudomonas* is implicated,[23] and noma neonatorum.[24] The last is a fortunately rare necrotizing *Pseudomonas* infection of the oral, nasal, or perianal regions in newborn infants. Subepithelial wound infections, and other soft tissue, bone, and joint *Pseudomonas* infections, if they are not due to bacteremia, are manifestations of deep inoculation through a surface defect. Soft tissue infections present, again in order of increasing severity, as deep abscess, cellulitis, and necrotizing fasciitis. These occur in areas below sometimes trivial penetrating trauma or in structures subjacent to an ulcerated epithelium. The same is true of contiguous, as distinct from post septicemic, *Pseudomonas* osteochondritis and osteomyelitis. In particular, *P aeruginosa* is the most common cause of osteochondritis following puncture wounds of the foot.[25] Interestingly, this lesion appears due to inoculation, by the penetrating object, of *P aeruginosa* that colonized the rubber sole of the tennis shoe of the victim rather than by bacteria from the penetrating object itself or the surrounding soil.[26] *Pseudomonas aeruginosa* is also one of the most commonly isolated gram-negative causes of contiguous osteomyelitis in other anatomic sites.[27] When *P aeruginosa* is the cause of bone infection, contiguity is often to an overlying or adjacent puncture wound or irrigated skin ulcer.[28] The isolation of *P aeruginosa* from debrided tissue or a sampled lesion signals an uncertain prognosis for success in systemic antimicrobial therapy; in one study, failure in the treatment of *P aeruginosa* osteomyelitis was more likely when the infection's focus was in a long bone than when the focus was in a flat bone.[27]

The second sort of defect, circumvention of anatomic barriers, accounts for most nosocomial infection in patients without immune defects. It is also a contributing factor in most infections among immunodeficient patients. In contact lens wearers *P aeruginosa* eye infections cause bacterial keratitis to the anterior segment of the eye as well as bacterial endophthalmitis involving the posterior parts of the eye, which are examples of this kind of mechanism in which the presence of a prosthetic device gives the bacterium an opportunity to adhere to an epithelial surface, to proliferate, and then to invade adjacent structures.[29] *Pseudomonas* urinary tract infections usually occur in catheterized patients, especially patients who also undergo urologic instrumentation.[30] It seems that only relatively minor epithelial trauma from the catheter or instrument is required to initiate the infectious process; however, once begun, the process develops rapidly into a destructive and deep infectious focus. A third instance of this mechanism is central nervous system (CNS) infection (meningitis and brain abscess) due to extension from contiguous soft tissue or bone infection foci.[31] Another, potentially lethal, example is the complex of consequences following *Pseudomonas* bacteremia in drug addicts: endocarditis, hematogenous pneumonia, and hematogenous (especially vertebral and pelvic) osteomyelitis.[32] These metastatic infections are typically traced to standing water in the injection paraphernalia or "works" of intravenous drug abusers. The latter introduce waterborne *Pseudomonas* into the intravascular compartment by nonsterile intravenous injection.[33] From the bloodstream the bacteria seed heart valves, lung tissue, and the bones of the axial skeleton. The fifth and last of these instances of the circumvention of anatomic barriers is found in cystic fibrosis (CF) patients: The defect here is the inability of the ciliary escalator to move secretions up the lower respiratory tract's epithelial surface.[17] The lower respiratory tract's anatomy is subsequently distorted by inspissated mucus. This loss of a natural barrier to bacterial inoculation and growth contributes to the intractable nature of the bronchocentric lung lesions in cystic fibrosis patients. Through indolent, but relentless, infection by highly resistant mucoid strains,[34] *P aeruginosa* renders progressive the initial physiologic, then anatomic, distortion of the airway in CF.

The third genre of host defect that contributes to the variety of natural histories of *P aeruginosa* infection is immune suppression. Many types of immune compromise have been associated with increased frequencies of *Pseudomonas* infection: diabetes, hematologic malignancies, congenital hypogammaglobulinemia congenital hypocomplementemia, therapeutic immune suppression following organ transplantation, and acquired immunodeficiency syndrome.[10] However, the defect most often associated with systemic *Pseudomonas* infection has been neutropenia induced by antineoplastic chemotherapy. In patients undergoing chemotherapeutic regimens, mucosal sloughing and ulceration, particularly of the lower gastrointestinal tract, provides access via an injured epithelium (*vide* the first mechanism mentioned), as do intravascular prostheses (*vide* the second mechanism). Nevertheless, two other, overriding factors seem to dominate the development of increased risk for patients receiving intense antitumor treatment: neutropenia cripples the immediate host defense response to *Pseudomonas* bacteremia by decreasing the population of active phagocytes; broad-spectrum, long-term, multidrug antimicrobial prophylaxis, or similar episodic treatment during febrile episodes, also selects for resistant bacterial invaders of the bloodstream.[35]

The increase in populations of immunosuppressed patients and variations in their treatment together appear to have had a major impact on the historical epidemiology of *Pseudomonas* infection.[9] From the late 1880s to the late 1940s, identifiable *P aeruginosa* infections depended almost entirely on the disruption of epithelial surfaces in immune competent hosts and were rare. From the late 1940s until the late 1970s, the frequency, morbidity, and mortality of nosocomial *P aeruginosa* infection all climbed in the expanding populations of immunodeficient, hospitalized patients (including burn patients and premature infants as well as cancer chemotherapy and CF patients). Since 1980, the proportion of nosocomial infections due to *P aeruginosa* has declined. Two plausible causes for this fall in relative incidence are changes in cancer therapy, including, on the positive side, the advent of antipseudomonal penicillins and, on the negative side, the increased association of gram-positive bacteria with septicemia in patients with indwelling catheters.[36]

Pseudomonas aeruginosa, however, continues to precipitate lethal septicemia among the immunodeficient. *Pseudomonas* bacteremia also remains a cause of major metastatic infectious complications of immunosuppressive therapy. These complications appear in every organ or system discussed earlier: endocarditis, hematogenous pneumonia, and postbacteremic osteomyelitis (as with IV drug abusers), as well as brain abscess and meningitis (seeded by a similar mechanism), and, most typically, ecthyma gangrenosum of epithelial surfaces. This last lesion is particularly characteristic and instructive to pathologists.[37] It usually presents as small, round, indurated nodules, that begin as vesicles then undergo hemorrhagic necrosis and ulceration.[38] Its presence raises the likelihood that a patient is suffering from *Pseudomonas* bacteremia. The ecthyma gangrenosum lesion is described later in detail because it is one of the two common histopathologic patterns that recur throughout the tripartite natural history of human *Pseudomonas* infections.

Virulence Profile

The three patterns of *P aeruginosa* natural history depend to the greatest extent on host status. The patterns of bacterial behavior are, however, mediated by a complex profile of *Pseudomonas* virulence factors.[21]

Students of bacterial pathogenesis divide these factors into three functional groups: *adhesins, invasins,* and *defensins*.[39] *Adhesins* mediate bacteria's attachment to epithelial surfaces. *Invasins* facilitate their penetration of tissues deep to the epithelia and into the bloodstream. *Defensins* parry the efforts of host mechanisms to neutralize or destroy the bacterial invaders.

The primary *adhesins* of *P aeruginosa* are pili or fimbriae. In the case of *Pseudomonas,* these threadlike structures that project from the bacterial cells preferentially attach to injured epithelial surfaces.[40] Among mucoid *P aeruginosa* phenotypes surface exopolysaccharide or capsule also plays the role of an attachment device. Both the fimbrial and capsular adhesins appear to bind to cell surface structures composed of glycolipids bearing sialic acid residues (especially asialo-GM-1). The latter may need to be exposed by loss of the physiologic surface protection from fibronectin or by the enzymatic effect of the *Pseudomonas*'s own neuramidase[21] before such binding can take place. Within the pilus or fimbria, galactosemannose lectins have been demonstrated to be the molecular ligands that attach specifically to the host cell surface binding sites.[41] Alginate, a recurring series of residues in the surface exopolysaccharide, has been shown to play the same ligand role in the mucoid phenotype. The *Pseudomonas* exopolysaccharide is often, in fact, referred to as alginate in discussions of pathogenesis.[42]

Redundancy is a key strategy for *P aeruginosa.* This is true not only in its metabolic pathways and defense mechanisms against antimicrobial agents, but also in its virulence profile. Besides pili and exopolysaccharide, evidence suggests that *P aeruginosa* has at least two other adhesive mechanisms available.[43] One of these adhesins may be exoenzyme S, whose more studied invasive function is discussed later.[44]

Whatever its repertoire of adhesive devices, the overall strategy of *P aeruginosa* is one of opportunistic adherence. This strategy is applied not only to epithelia themselves, but also, at least in some instances, to the overlying layer of mucus. For the mucoid *P aeruginosa* phenotype, the inspissated mucus of cystic fibrosis patients contains receptor sites binding the *P aeruginosa* exopolysaccharide alginate.[45] This melding of bacterial and host mucoid layers creates a biofilm that surrounds *P aeruginosa* colonies.[46] The biofilm combines the features of an adherence opportunity with those of a bacterial countermeasure, in this instance against both host humoral and phagocytic defense mechanisms. Histopathologic appearances at postmortem in CF patients demonstrated the encapsulated colonies of gram-negative bacilli deep in the distorted, mucus-clogged branches of the distal bronchial tree; this feature has been cited as evidence for this phenomenon.[47]

The invasins of *P aeruginosa* are extracellular toxins, other extracellular products primarily toxic to neutrophils, proteases, membranolysins, and phenazine pigments. Various experimental models have defined at least two diphtheria-like toxins that are produced by *P aeruginosa,* (exo)toxin A and exoenzyme S.[44] Two other toxic molecules produced by *P aeruginosa,* leukocidin[48] (a cytotoxin with a tropism for neutrophils), and lipopolysaccharide (endotoxin) are extracellular products that combine invasive with bacterial defensive functions. The proteases fall into at least two classes of histolytic enzymes: an alkaline protease and a pair of elastases.[49] The membranolysins include at least two enzymes that attack lipid bilayers: phospholipase C, which is a heat-labile hemolysin, and rhamnolipid, which is heat stable and nonhemolytic.[21] Pyocyanin, one of the phenazine pigments discussed earlier as a taxonomic marker among the fluorescent *Pseudomonas* (pyocyanin is the pigment that identifies *P aeruginosa*), has been shown to have a variety of effects toxic to mammalian hosts.[18] The toxic effects are inhibition of mitochondrial respiration by binding to cytochrome B (these pigments are siderophores), interference with neutrophil production of superoxide (a bacterial countermeasure), inhibition of lymphocyte proliferation (also a countermeasure), interference with the function (rhythmic beating) of respiratory epithelial cilia, and triggering of the contraction of vascular smooth muscle.[50] The pigments have also been shown to be directly cytotoxic to human epithelial and endothelial cells. This variety of toxic devices, mechanisms, and effects facilitates bacterial invasion. They sound again the leitmotif of redundancy: multiple means to a particular end and multiple functions for a particular means.

(Exo)toxin A and exoenzyme S are both adenosine diphosphate (ADP) ribosyl transferases. They thus share a toxic mechanism, but not a chemical structure, with diphtheria toxin. In this mechanism, one domain (A) contains the surface binding site by which attachment to the host cell and internalization are achieved; the other domain (B) incorporates the enzymatic active site which ADP ribosylates and inactivates ribosomal protein elongation factor 2 (EF-2).[51] This inactivation interferes with mammalian protein synthesis. (Exo)toxin A is expressed by most clinical isolates and has different substrate profiles from exoenzyme S, which is less uniformly expressed.[52] Indeed, exoenzyme S expression is, according to some investigators, a differential marker of *P aeruginosa* strain virulence in animal models.[53]

As already mentioned, in some experimental models, exoenzyme S appears to have only domain A (ligand) and not domain B (enzymatic) activity. This may be because a host factor activating (exo)S (FAS) is necessary to the toxic function.[54] This observation may be explained by *P aeruginosa*'s opportunistic *modus operandi,* in which a trigger, perhaps associated with host injury, is required before the toxic effect can be exerted.

Along with redundancy of mechanisms, regulation by environmental stimuli is a hallmark of *Pseudomonas* virulence. *Pseudomonas* virulence factors are subject to a high degree of genetic regulation.[55] The genes regulating toxin production are, in turn, stimulated or repressed by environmental stimuli. For example, for both the *Pseudomonas* diphtheria-like toxins, gene expression is inhibited by increased environmental iron but stimulated by the stationary phase of growth in the milieu.[56] While iron has a similar inhibitory effect on diphtheria toxin,[57] in *Pseudomonas,* the stimulation during the stationary growth phase is mediated through a fascinating recently described feedback mechanism called *quorum sensing.*[58]

There are other examples of genetic regulation by environmental stimuli in *P aeruginosa:* Both pilus and capsule adhesins are regulated by an ambient nitrogen level.[59] Similarly, the *Pseudomonas* neuraminidase, which enhances pilus-mediated adherence by clipping off host sialic acid residues, thus revealing binding sites, is regulated by osmolarity[21] and so is alginate synthesis.[60] Exoenzyme S's variability may, in fact, be due to differences in the physical environment, temperature, and oxygen tension that control its gene expression.

The complexity of the *Pseudomonas* regulatory mechanisms is most completely anatomized for alginate production, in which eight regulatory proteins are characterized.[61] The redundancy of these mechanisms is most aptly illustrated by the control of (exo)toxin A transcription, which involves not only a repressor, like the gene product regulating other iron-repressed diphtheria-like toxin genes, but also a transcription activator, controlled by a repressor.[62]

Pseudomonas lipopolysaccharide's effect on the mammalian host is similar to that of endotoxin produced by other gram-negative bacilli; however, the control of its expression is of special interest because it illustrates a third characteristic of *Pseudomonas* virulence factors: coregulation.[63] The switch from the usual to the mucoid *Pseudomonas* phenotype involves not only the environmentally stimulated and complex promotion of alginate production, but also a variation in the backbone structure and side-chain composition of *Pseudomonas* lipopolysaccharide (LPS), from a negatively charged to an electrically neutral LPS.[21] The latter structural alteration is associated with a decrease in membrane permeability. This decrease in membrane permeability, in turn, mediates resistance to aminoglycoside and quinalone antimicrobials.[64] Such covariation suggests a survival strategy of complex integrated packages of bacterial virulence factors whose expression is modulated by environmental stimuli via complex genetic control mechanisms.

The next package of phenotypic factors in *P aeru-*

ginosa's virulence profile can be thought of as a tool kit for tissue necrosis. Leukocidin is a cytotoxin with an appetite, which suggested its name, for polymorphonuclear phagocytes.[65] The alkaline protease(s) attack(s) sites of vulnerability in host cellular proteins,[66] while the two elastases work in coordinated fashion: one, Las A, a serine protease, nicks elastin molecules permitting the other, Las B, to degrade them. This elastase enzyme system is also both responsive to environmental stimuli, including zinc and iron levels, and redundantly regulated.[67] Two phospholipases[68] play the same role among lipids that the protease and elastases play among proteins, increasing the versatility of *P aeruginosa* as an agent of necrosis.

The virulent action of the pigments other than pyocyanin is uncertain. Pyocyanin, however, appears to act as an oxygen sink, not only depriving host cells of the substrate of respiration but also catalyzing superoxide and hydrogen peroxide mediated tissue damage.[69] (Other pigments and bacterial siderophores may play this latter role as well.)

The histolytic activities just outlined, in general, and several of the virulence factors listed, in particular, are powerful stimuli of the host inflammatory and immune responses. This stimulation creates a challenge for *Pseudomonas* defensins to parry the blows that phagocytes, complement, antibodies, and lymphocytes then shower on the bacterial invaders. Neutrophils and complement are the main components of the initial host response: They are countered primarily by proteases[70]: 1) denaturing chemotactic messenger compounds, slowing neutrophil chemotaxis, and 2) inhibiting complement mediated opsonic phagocytosis, by denaturing both complement components and specific antibodies. Leukocidin then attacks the neutrophils directly, while another extracellular product of *P aeruginosa,* neutrophil inhibitor,[71] interferes with their bacterial killing function. The antiphagocytic effect of the exopolysaccharide capsule in the mucoid phenotype has already been cited, as has phenazine pigment's ability to interfere with phagocytes' respiratory burst, should *Pseudomonas* cells be ingested and a killing mechanism driven by the burst be necessary to their demise.

The mediators of a final pair of bacterial countermeasures are less apparent. The effects of these countermeasures are suppression of cell-mediated immunity (decreased T-cell function) and the disordering of humoral immunity (by polyclonal B-cell activation).[72] In general, however, one would imagine that the themes of redundancy, environmental stimulation, complexity of genetic control, and coregulation will appear again as the defensins causing these effects are delineated, particularly in the phenotypic packages induced when *Pseudomonas* adapts to chronic infection.

EPIDEMIOLOGY

A survey of *P aeruginosa*'s ecological distribution and natural history predicts correctly that the epidemiology of the agent should be mostly that of a nosocomial pathogen. In the hospital milieu, *P aeruginosa* remained, at the beginning of the 1990s, the fourth most frequently isolated nosocomial agent, accounting for 10.1% of all hospital-acquired infections.[10] During the late 1980s, however, the overall incidence of nosocomial *Pseudomonas* infections fell, as noted earlier, from 4.8/1000 hospital discharges in 1985 to 3.4/1000 discharges in 1991.[10]

Within the hospital, *P aeruginosa* has a primary focus: It is the most frequent cause of infections in intensive care units (ICUs) where it caused 12.4% of all such infections in 1991.[15]

Consideration of the three patterns of *Pseudomonas* infection already described—in light of the focus of *Pseudomonas* infections in ICUs, where respiratory, urinary, and intravascular devices that circumvent anatomic barriers are the rule rather than the exception—leads one to a second set of accurate predictions: *P aeruginosa* is 1) the most frequent cause of nosocomial pneumonia (causing 16.8% of these lower respiratory infections overall and 17.5% of those occurring in ICU patients in the 1991 survey); 2) the third most common cause of hospital-acquired urinary tract infection (UTI) (accounting for 12% of nosocomial UTIs overall and 12.1% of those from ICUs); and 3) the eighth most frequent cause of nosocomial septicemia overall (accounting for 13.6% of bacteremic episodes), but the sixth most common cause of septicemia in ICU patients.

A second hospital focus of *Pseudomonas* infection is in surgical wounds. Among wound infections, *P aeruginosa* is the fifth most frequent pathogen overall (incriminated as the cause in 8.2% of wound infections), but, again, more common in ICUs where it is the third most frequent agent of wound infections (accounting for 10.9% of isolates from infected ICU surgical wounds).

Two other epidemiologic foci occur in patients frequently in hospital and in special care units: 1) children and young adults with CF (in this population the incidence of *P aeruginosa* in respiratory secretions increases with patient age from 21% at 1 year old to greater than 80% at 26 years or older,[73] and 2) burn patients (among whom *P aeruginosa* is, luckily, not a frequent pathogen; it is, however, despite therapeutic advances, still the bacterial pathogen associated with highest mortality[74]).

Non-nosocomial epidemiologic foci of *P aeruginosa* infection have already been mentioned as examples of the agent's natural history. 1) While the association of *P aeruginosa* with involuntary water emersion continues (it is the most common cause of tropical immersion foot[10]), skin infections associated with voluntary immersion have been increasing—these include point-source outbreaks associated with immersive therapeutic and leisure activities from physical therapy and whirlpool baths through spas and hot tubs[75] (with loofah sponges[76]) to swimming pools.[77] 2) *Pseudomonas aeruginosa* is the most common pathogen isolated from patients with acute ("malignant") otitis externa[78] or chronic otitis media.[79] 3) *Pseudomonas aeruginosa* competes for first place among the bacterial pathogens that cause bacterial keratitis in contact lens wearers, particularly in humid environments[80]; among the usual bacterial agents of this infection, *P aeruginosa* is also the most destructive. 4) *Pseudomonas aeruginosa* does maintain most frequent pathogen status for bone infections in two very different epidemiologic settings: osteochondritis following puncture wounds of the foot among sneaker wearers,[81] and disseminated hematogenous osteomyelitis of the axial skeleton (vertebrae[82] and pelvis[83]) among intravenous drug abusers. 5) *Pseudomonas aeruginosa* is also the most common gram-negative cause of acute and chronic contiguous (nonbacteremic) osteomyelitis,[84] and the cause most frequently associated with therapeutic failure.[27] Indeed, whenever a patient presents with one of the clinical conditions listed in this paragraph, adequate treatment of potential *P aeruginosa* infection is the main therapeutic issue.

PATHOLOGY

Two histologic lesions are characteristic of *P aeruginosa* infection. The appearance of either pattern should bring the agent to mind, particularly if the epidemiologic and clinical features of the case fit one of *P aeruginosa*'s natural histories; however, neither pattern is specific for *Pseudomonas.* The differential diagnosis of these lesions almost always includes infections caused by other gram-negative bacilli morphologically indistinguishable from *P aeruginosa.* For this reason, culture evidence is usually necessary to make the specific diagnosis; however, such evidence is usually forthcoming, either from culture of the examined tissue itself or from companion cultures of blood or other anatomically appropriate body fluids.

The first and more characteristic histopathologic lesion is that seen associated with the bacteremic pattern of spread in immunosuppressed patients. The second and more variable lesion is found more in local or contiguous spread patterns of infection and in patients with intact host defenses.

The first lesion, in all tissues where it occurs, has four components: 1) necrosis, 2) easily demonstrable gram-negative bacilli, particularly in vessel walls, especially the medial layer, and—most strikingly—3) hemorrhage, with these three elements arranged in a 4) vasocentric pattern. This tetrad is called "*Pseudomonas* vasculitis."[85] It appears most typically and vividly in skin and mucosae as ecthyma gangrenosum[86] and in the lung as hemorrhagic pneumonia (Figures 80–1 through 80–3).[87] In both locations, it involves small arteries and veins invaded by many gram-negative bacilli but few neutrophils, with surrounding coagulation necrosis. Hemorrhage spreads from the center of the lesion and defines its edge. In the skin this edge is a narrow rim of erythema; in the lung it is usually a wide border of hemorrhage. One can often demonstrate a few neutrophils in the zone of necrosis and a sparse mixed inflammatory infiltrate around it; however, in both epithelial and parenchymal lesions, the hemorrhagic component is usually more striking than in other inflammatory vasculitides, especially when compared to other vasculitides due to infection.

The same histologic tetrad also appears in other sites: in soft tissues as cellulitis and necrotizing fasciitis; in bones as vertebral osteomyelitis; and in the brain as hemorrhagic cerebritis. *Pseudomonas* endocarditis and mycotic aneurysm, with their striking perivalvular necrosis and perivascular hemorrhage, can be considered variations of this theme in larger blood vessels.

The second lesion, in its many manifestations, demonstrates three common elements: 1) necrosis; and 2) gram-negative bacilli are prominent once again, but in contrast to "*Pseudomonas* vasculitis," 3) a dense infiltrate of neutrophils or abscess formation is prominent, without a vasocentric arrangement. This pattern can be contrasted to the first pattern in the skin and lung. In epithelia, it presents itself as a pustular infiltrate of neutrophils, forming microabscesses and causing ulcers; eg, in the skin, it usually presents as a pustular folliculitis.[88] On the epithelial surface, this inflammatory infiltrate produces superficial bulla and ulcers (or a sloughed mucosa); in deeper tissues there is subjacent spread of neutrophils toward soft tissue structures below the zone of most intense involvement. If this lesion becomes chronic, it elicits mixed lymphoplasmacytic infiltrates, usually coexisting with ongoing neutrophil infiltration and scarring fibrosis.[89] In the lung, this lesion appears as a necrotizing brochocentric (rather than vasculocentric) pneumonia with microabscesses and alveolar septal necrosis. In severe cases this process leads to confluent zones of liquefactive necrosis.[90] There can, of course, be secondary hemorrhage into these areas, but this lesion is not predominantly a hemorrhagic pneumonia. The often umbilicated nodules of necrosis are,

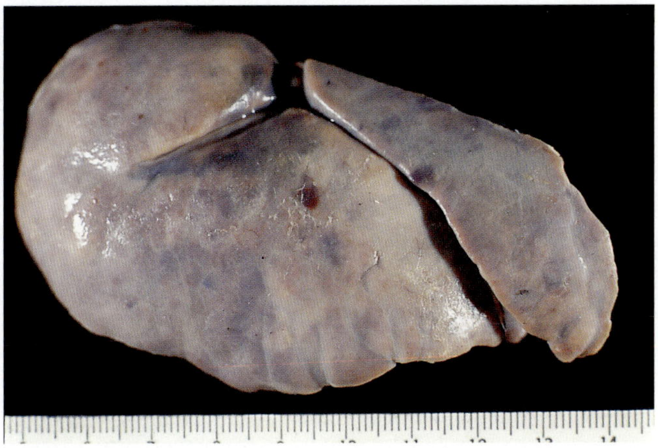

A

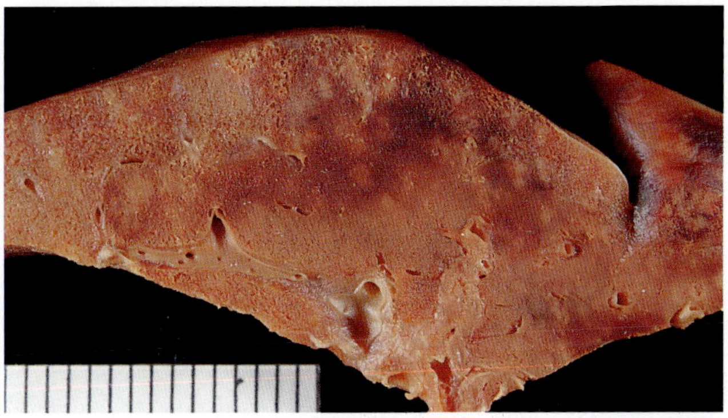

B

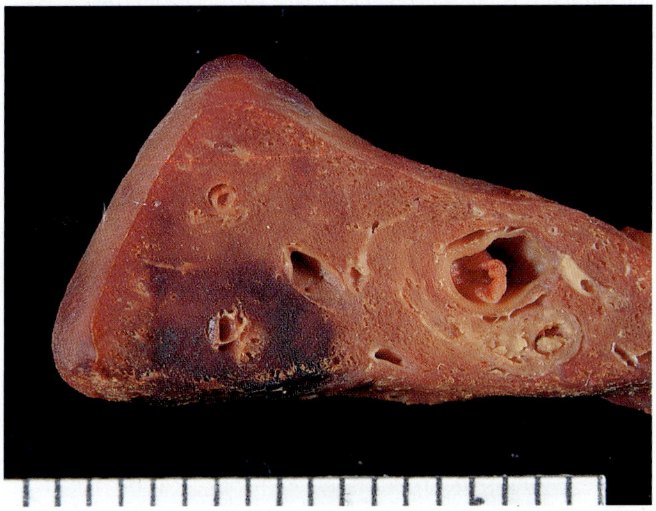

C

Figure 80–1. (**A**) Fatal *P aeruginosa* pneumonia in a child who died at age 3 months after surgical repair of an omphalocele. The lungs were firm and all lobes retained their contour during dissection. Note the subpleural hemorrhage (gross ×.75). (**B**) Same lung. Note areas of necrosis and hemorrhage (gross, ×2.5). (**C**) Same lung showing orientation of hemorrhage around a thrombosed vessel. Invasion of a vessel wall by *P aeruginosa* is followed by septic thrombosis, hemorrhage, and septic infarction. (gross, ×3.5). *(Photographs by Daniel H. Connor, MD, 1995.)*

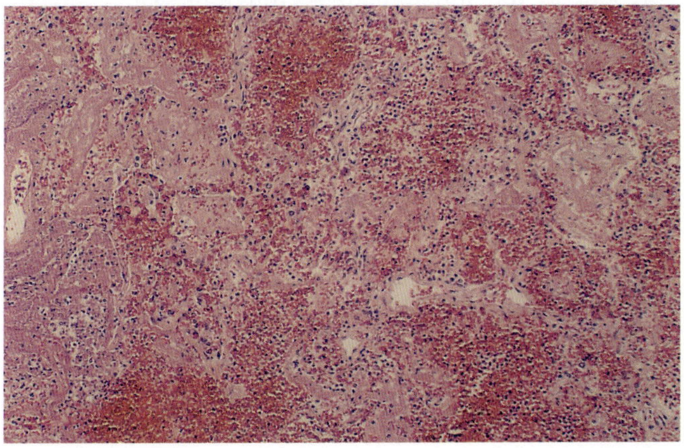

A

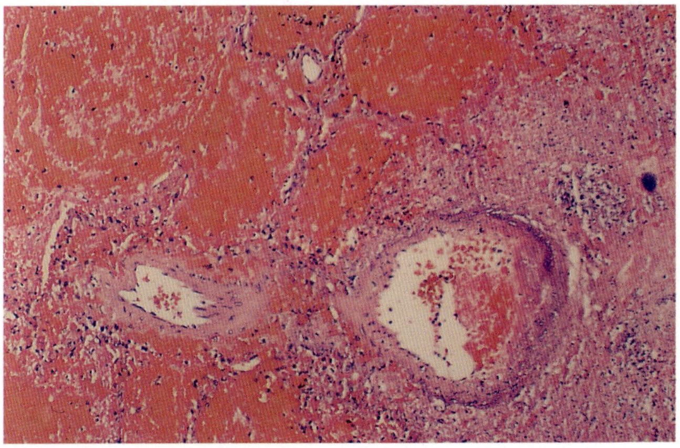

B

Figure 80–2. Fatal *P aeruginosa* pneumonia in an adult with granulocytopenia complicating treatment for a malignancy. (**A**) Consolidated lung with hemorrhage, fibrin-rich exudate, and a few neutrophils (hematoxylin-eosin, ×100). (**B**) The dark blue band in the vessel wall is tightly packed *P aeruginosa*. A septic thrombus is forming over the infected wall (hematoxylin-eosin, ×200).

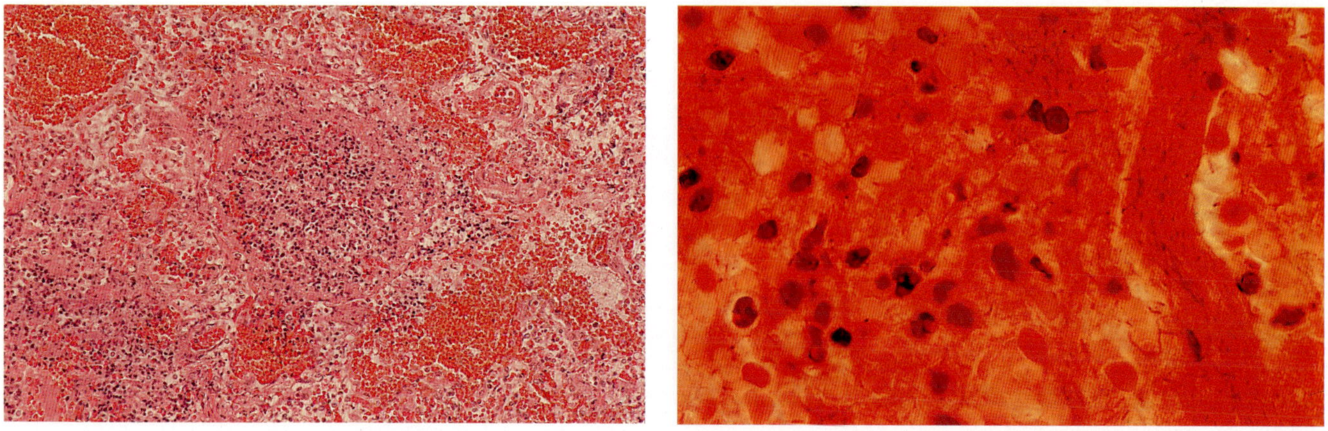

A B

Figure 80–3. Sections of lung shown in Figure 80–1. (**A**) A septic thrombus is in the center of the field surrounded by pulmonary hemorrhage. Note the large number of neutrophils, compared to Figure 80–2, A and B (hematoxylin-eosin, ×200). (**B**) There are many gram-negative bacilli in the wall of this vessel and in the adjacent hemorrhagic lung. (Brown–Hopps tissue, Gram stain, ×450).

however, usually surrounded by a demarcating zone of congested and hemorrhagic lung.

This triad morphologic pattern also presents in other sites: in soft tissues as deep abscesses; in bones as acute osteochondritis and acute and chronic contiguous osteomyelitis; and in the brain as meningitis or brain abscess. Most ear infections caused by *Pseudomonas,* including malignant otitis externa, are examples of this pattern. The corneal ulcerations associated with contact lens contamination and primary burn wound infections are other specific examples of this pattern that occur in epithelia. In the lung, *Pseudomonas* chronic bronchopulmonary infection in cystic fibrosis patients is a particular variant of this lesion.

In summary, for both morphologic presentations, the hallmarks of *P aeruginosa* infection are striking necrosis and almost as striking evidence of bacterial proliferation. In the first instance, they combine with hemorrhage in the absence of an appropriate inflammatory response in a vasocentric pattern. In the second instance, they do evoke such an appropriate inflammatory response, but tend to be epithelially based rather than vasocentric.

CLINICOPATHOLOGIC FEATURES

These features of *P aeruginosa* infection are organized below by organ and syndrome: first, those associated with superficial infection of the skin, external and middle ear, cornea and eye, and urinary and enterocolonic epithelia; second, those associated with deep infections of the lung, soft tissues, cartilage, bone, and brain; and third, the vascular lesions associated with bacteremia.

Skin

Primary *P aeruginosa* skin infections usually present in patients with a history of aquatic exposure, with lesions appearing in the areas of the cutaneous surface that were damp the longest: feet, the bathing suit area, or external ear canal. Infected skin is red, itchy, and weeps an exudate containing neutrophils and necrotic debris. These findings are associated with local pain and swelling, but not signs of systemic illness (fever, leukocytosis, etc). The inflammation may be diffuse and produce bullae, as in immersion foot,[91] or be focal and progress to ulceration, as in folliculitis.[92] The characteristic blue-green pigment and fetid, fruity odor may be present in the inflammatory effluvium, especially that from ulcers or burn eschar.[93]

Secondary *P aeruginosa* skin infections usually occur in patients with an obvious immune defect, circumvention of usual anatomic barriers to deep sites of *Pseudomonas* infection, or an apparent wound or other primary focus of infection at a cutaneous site distant from the new skin lesion. The ecthyma gangrenosum lesion is the pivotal finding[94]: singular or scattered, small, round, firm nodules that are usually found on the trunk. Most often they present initially as vesicles containing cloudy, but not purulent, bacteria-laden fluid, then progress through a sequence of hemorrhage, necrosis, and ulceration, within a rim of erythema, but with strikingly little suppuration in either the vesicle fluid, exudate, or involved tissues. Since the secondary skin lesions are most often due to septicemia, fever and the other signs of systemic sepsis are usually present. A primary cutaneous focus of infection can also be the incendiary nidus from which secondary infection seeds distant skin sites: This was the mechanism detected in the first report that linked *P aeruginosa* to ecthyma gangrenosum, nearly a hundred years ago.[95]

Ear

In otitis externa due to *P aeruginosa*, pain and swelling of the pinna, along with green exudate from the canal, are the salient clinical findings. In malignant external otitis, the necrotizing infection usually spreads down soft tissue planes rather than along the canal.[96]

Besides being the most common cause of malignant otitis externa, *P aeruginosa* is also the most common cause of chronic suppurative otitis media.[97] The latter presents with deep ear pain and persistent purulent discharge from the ear canal through a ruptured tympanic membrane. Important complications are mastoiditis and bacteremia. The former is difficult to treat and the latter can be immediately life threatening.

Eye

History of trauma to the corneal epithelium can be elicited in most cases of *P aeruginosa* keratitis. The most common occasion for such trauma is contact lens use.[98] Mucopurulent discharge heralds the rapid development of one or more expanding corneal ulcers that soon cloud the vision. Eyelids may also be infected (Figure 80–4). As with the other primary epithelial syndromes of *Pseudomonas* infection, signs and symptoms of systemic disease are absent.

Posterior penetration of the corneal ulcers or penetrating trauma, either accidental or surgical, can lead to *Pseudomonas* endophthalmitis, which often follows a fulminant course. The rapidity with which eye pain, orbital erythema and edema, and loss of ocular motion and acuity all occur distinguish this catastrophe from endophthalmitis caused by less virulent but more frequent bacterial agents, like coagulase negative staphylococci and alpha hemolytic streptococci.[99] Both superficial and deep *Pseudomonas* eye infections are regarded as ophthalmologic emergencies.

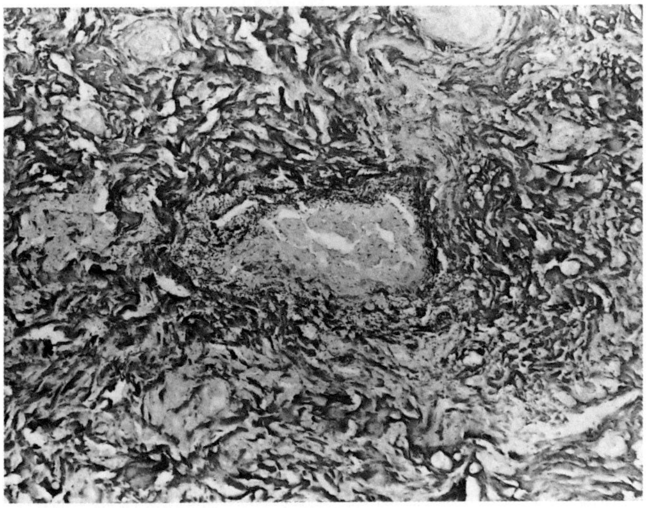

Figure 80–4. Infection of eyelid by *P aeruginosa.* The bacilli are "swarming" in and around the wall of a vessel in necrotic fascia of the eyelid (hematoxylin-eosin, ×250).

Urinary Tract

Whereas skin, ear, and eye *P aeruginosa* infections occur relatively frequently in non-nosocomial situations, *Pseudomonas* urinary tract infection is usually hospital acquired.[100] A history of catheterization and/or instrumentation and surgery of the lower urinary tract is usually forthcoming. Where these historical predisposing factors are absent, findings of obstruction (particularly by stones), chronic infection (particularly of the prostate), and chronic antimicrobial treatment are usually present, sometimes in combination.

Beyond the usual signs of pain and pyuria, which fail to distinguish *Pseudomonas* urinary tract infections from those caused by other bacterial agents, *Pseudomonas* infection is particularly likely to produce two other findings: hematuria, associated with much necrotic debris in the urinary sediment, and bacteremia. These are consequences, respectively, of the ulcerative and invasive aspects of *Pseudomonas* urothelial infection.

Three quarters of a century ago, Fraenkel observed and described how, when *Pseudomonas* infections of the lower urinary tract ascend to the kidney, they may also provoke the lesion of *Pseudomonas* vasculitis in that organ: The bacteria cluster in the walls of medium-sized blood vessels and produce the typical vasocentric hemorrhagic necrosis emphasized earlier.[101]

Gastrointestinal Tract

Pseudomonas aeruginosa infections of the gastrointestinal tract are also mostly nosocomial. Among hospital populations, these infections are focused in immunodeficient patients, especially those who are neutropenic. In such patients, the pattern of presentation is, once again, one that combines superficial ulceration and deep invasion, with the latter sometimes demonstrating the vasocentric, hemorrhagic, necrotizing lesion of *Pseudomonas* vasculitis. In one immunodeficient population, premature infants, this lesion presents as the syndrome of necrotizing enterocolitis (NEC); with NEC an infant rapidly develops vomiting, bloody diarrhea, abdominal distention, and dehydration.[102] This ominous presentation is then quickly followed by signs of peritonitis and systemic sepsis. In another immunodeficient population, neutropenic patients receiving cancer chemotherapy, particularly therapy for leukemia, the clinical course is often similar to that of NEC; however, the characteristic lesion is often localized to the ileocecal segment of gut. This localization of the ulcerated, penetrating, necrotizing lesion has given the associated acute abdominal syndrome in immunodeficient adults the name typhlitis, from the Greek designation for the secum.[103] Finally, also in neutropenic cancer chemotherapy patients, anorectal ulceration may be the epithelial defect that permits the entry of *P aeruginosa* into subjacent soft tissue planes.[104] Such defects can be the occasions for horrifying examples of the syndromes of necrotizing soft tissue infection described later.

Lung

Pseudomonas aeruginosa lower respiratory infections usually occur against the background of an altered host. The alteration can either be local, of lung structure or function, or systemic, of host defenses. The clinical features are different, depending on whether the infection is bronchocentric or vasocentric. These patterns correlate roughly with whether the infection is primary (arising in the airways) or secondary (seeded from the bloodstream).

Bronchocentric *P aeruginosa* pneumonia fits on the spectrum of gram-negative bacillary pneumonia.[105] Among the gram-negative bacilli, *Pseudomonas* is one of the most frequent causes of fulminant bronchopneumonia. Such infection presents with sudden onset of severe dyspnea; the patient coughs up copious purulent sputum, develops cyanosis, and progresses rapidly to respiratory failure. Chest x ray shows diffuse bronchopneumonia, with the nodular infiltrates often showing central clearing. The nodular infiltrates correlate with the bronchocentric areas of coagulation necrosis and the central lucencies with the bronchial abscesses found postmortem.[106]

Vasocentric *Pseudomonas* pneumonia fits into a different spectrum of fulminant disease. The syndrome is usually announced by an episode of gram-negative sepsis, followed by rapidly progressive respiratory failure. Chest x ray shows pulmonary congestion and infiltrates in an interstitial-alveolar distribution that, over 2 to 3 days, gives rise to irregular lucent zones that can be correlated later with the zones of hemorrhagic necrosis found at postmortem examination.[107]

Not all clinical presentations of *Pseudomonas* lower respiratory infection are as dramatically disastrous as these two genres of catastrophe. Indeed, *P aeruginosa* has been isolated from infections associated with the full range of airway inflammation.

The range of presentations of *Pseudomonas* lung infection is particularly apparent among CF patients,[108] where clinical presentations can range from persistent cough, through discrete episodes of dyspnea and fever, followed by progressively worsening productive cough, then wheezing, to terminate with the secondary features of combined chronic obstructive and restrictive lung disease. This clinical deterioration, usually played out over years, finds its x-ray correlates in peribronchial thickening, waxing and waning patchy infiltrates, bronchiectasis and patchy atelectasis, then progressive overaeration and increased interstitial markings. Pathologically, these findings correlate, in turn, with the severe bronchitis and peribronchitis, patchy parenchymal scarring, from multiple episodes of bronchopneumonia, mucus plugging of bronchi, associated with widespread bronchiectasis and cyst formation, and finally interstitial fibrosis, all findings documented at autopsy (Figures 80–5 and 80–6).

Soft Tissue

Primary soft tissue infections tend to occur deep to zones of epithelial infection or disruption. They present as deep abscesses, (sometimes nodular) cellulitis, or necrotizing fasciitis. These presentations represent a necrotizing process of varying degrees of aggressiveness—from well-localized necrosis in the abscesses to rapidly spreading tissue destruction in necrotizing fasciitis. Such processes tend to invade along tissue planes. For example, as mentioned earlier regarding malignant external otitis, the necrotizing infection usually spreads through the retromandibular and parotid spaces, rather than along the ear canal. In those soft tissue spaces, it leads to palsies of the facial and other cranial nerves.[109]

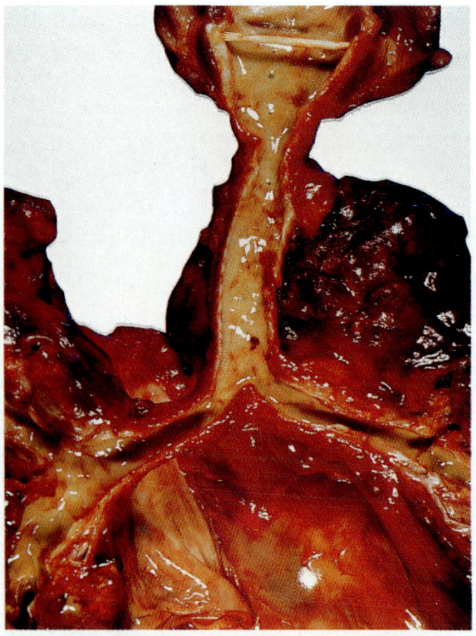

Figure 80–5. Lungs of young adult who died of cystic fibrosis. There is extensive suppuration of trachea, bronchi, and bronchioles. *Pseudomonas aeruginosa* was grown from the exudate. The patient had many endobronchial abscesses with bronchiectasis. *(Contributed by Ernest E. Lack, MD.)*

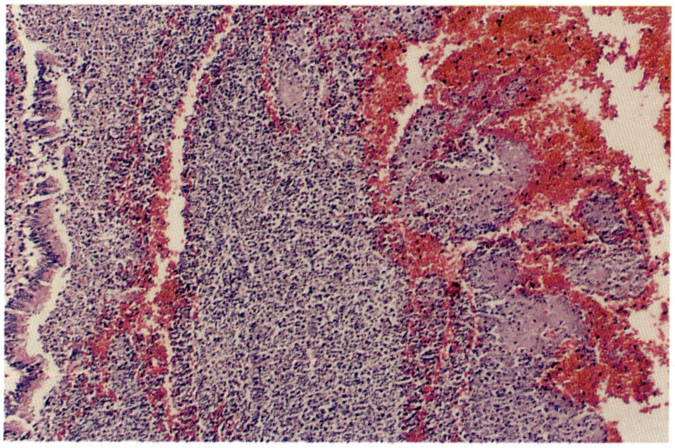

Figure 80–6. Section of lung from patient who died of CF showing endobronchial abscess with abundant mucopurulent exudate. Desquamated bronchial epithelium is on the left (hematoxylin-eosin, ×200).

The latter findings are sometimes the initial clinical evidence of deep tissue invasion from a superficial, chronically infected site.

Secondary *P aeruginosa* soft tissue infections demonstrate striking hemorrhage, rather than inflammation. As in other tissues, this hemorrhagic necrosis tends to follow the course of blood vessels in the pattern stressed earlier as *Pseudomonas* vasculitis.

Cartilage and Bone

Pseudomonas aeruginosa manifests a peculiar tropism for cartilage.[110] This attraction is most strikingly illustrated in primary osteochondritis of the foot. Clinically, it leads to a delay in the presentation of this deep infection, often a week or more after the initial puncture wound. This delay may prompt the patient to report a biphasic pattern of pain and swelling, the immediate phase separated by a relatively asymptomatic period from the subsequent phase. The tropism for cartilage is also associated with relatively indolent behavior in bone and joint sites, especially in comparison to some of the pulmonary and soft tissue syndromes just described. It is further associated with a lack of systemic signs of infection; however, for example, the tarsal osteochondritis can eventually spread locally to involve several bones and joints of the foot.

Chronic contiguous *Pseudomonas* osteomyelitis shares with osteochondritis these indolent, but persistent, and finally destructive characteristics. Clinically, besides puncture wounds, contiguous osteomyelitis is precipitated not only by obviously "dirty" wounds, such as compound fractures and skin ulcers, but also by apparently "clean" wounds, even including closed fractures and median sternotomy in coronary artery bypass patients.[111]

The clinical features of hematogenous infections by *Pseudomonas* of cartilage and bone make a study in contrast to those of contiguous infection. Hematogenous infections tend to involve flat bones in the axial skeleton rather than the tubular bones of the extremities.[111] The hematogenous infections also differ in tending to occur in well-defined, high-risk populations, intravenous drug abusers, immunodeficient patients, and those with *Pseudomonas* urinary tract infections complicated by bacteremia. Bacteremic infections are, of course, also more closely associated with intravascular rather than contiguous initial foci of infection.

Contiguous and hematogenous infections of bone and cartilage, nevertheless, also have characteristics in common: 1) their mutual attraction to cartilage, which leads to a facility for invading joint spaces, and 2) their relatively indolent infectious behavior. The latter feature makes them appear less aggressive, but more stubborn, than *Staphylococcus aureus* infection in the same bony sites: vertebrae, pelvic rami, and the symphysis pubis (where it can cause a pyarthrosis).[112]

Central Nervous System

The distinction between, on one hand, infection due to penetrating trauma and contiguous spread and, on the other, bacteremic spread, which we have just used to sort among *Pseudomonas* cartilage and bone infection, applies equally well to infectious lesions in CNS. For example, the clinical onset of penetrating or contiguous *Pseudomonas* meningitis or brain abscess may be subtle, obscured by the antecedent or adjacent injury, and appear gradual.[113] In contrast, bacteremic infection in the same sites tends to produce an abrupt onset of fulminant disease, associated with hemorrhagic necrosis in the affected layers of tissue.

Bacteremia

Much of the clinical profile of *Pseudomonas* bacteremia has already been presented: 1) the high-risk populations of intravenous drug addicts and immunodeficient patients; 2) the signal lesion of ecthyma gangrenosum; 3) the catastrophic rapidity of hematogenous lung, soft tissue, and CNS infections; 4) the more indolent post-bacteremic bone and cartilage infections of the axial skeleton; 5) the association with hemorrhagic necrotizing rather than inflammatory necrotizing lesions; and 6) the vasocentric pattern of those hemorrhagic lesions.

Four additional points can be added to this list: 7) clinically, *Pseudomonas* sepsis is indistinguishable at presentation from gram-negative sepsis caused by other species; 8) along with its affinity for cartilage adjacent to tarsal bones and between vertebrae, *P aeruginosa* shows an equally striking affinity for connective tissue of heart valves (Figure 80–7)[114]; although the presenta-

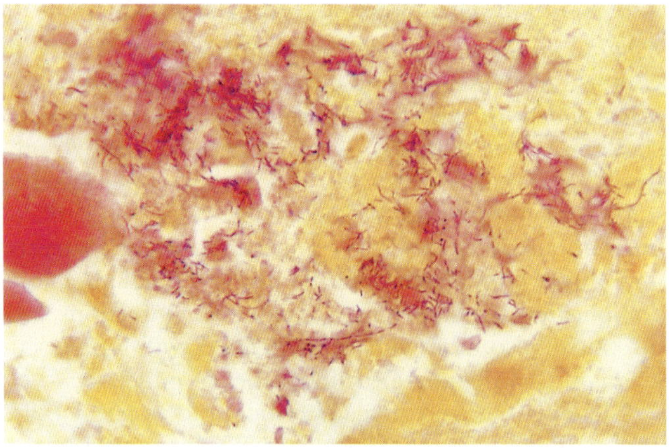

Figure 80–7. A cluster of *P aeruginosa* in a vegetation and in the connective tissue of aortic valve (Brown–Hopps, ×400).

tion of *Pseudomonas* acute endocarditis is no different from that caused by other aggressive bacteria, well armed with extracellular toxins and enzymes, it has singular abilities to deform heart valves, induce necrosis of the surrounding valve ring, and seed septic emboli; 9) because of the intravenous injection of contaminated water by drug addicts and the presence of indwelling catheters adjacent to the right heart in many immunosuppressed cancer patients, most *Pseudomonas* endocarditis is right sided, producing septic pulmonary rather than systemic emboli[115]; and 10) finally, although the necrotizing tropism of *P aeruginosa* bacilli for vessel walls primarily affects medium-sized vessels in the skin or lung, the same bacterial agent can also cause necrosis of larger vessel walls and, consequently, induce mycotic aneurysms in larger blood vessels.[10]

DIFFERENTIAL DIAGNOSIS FOR ANATOMIC PATHOLOGISTS

The potential diagnosis of *P aeruginosa* infection is raised by the presence of gram-negative bacilli in a necrotizing lesion. It is also raised by the pattern of vasocentric necrosis, particularly if the necrosis is associated with a paucity of acute inflammatory cells.

Three overlapping groups of infectious agents enter into the differential diagnosis of the *Pseudomonas* infections described: 1) bacteria, mostly other gram-negative rods, especially other nonfermenters, that cause aquatic or other water-associated infections; 2) bacterial agents causing the clinicopathologic syndromes of a) rapidly progressive bronchopneumonia, particularly with cavitation, b) hemorrhagic pneumonia, particularly in immunodeficient patients, c) probable contiguous osteomyelitis especially of long bones, d) probable hematogenous osteoarthritis especially of flat bones, e) necrotizing fasciitis, f) brain abscess, necrotizing cerebritis, and meningitis, and g) progressive airway disease in patients with cystic fibrosis, again, particularly, if the apparent agent is a gram-negative bacillus; and 3) any potential infectious cause of vasocentric necrosis, not limited to gram-negative rods.

Among the many bacterial infectious agents associated with aquatic and other damp environments, several gram-negative rods share with *P aeruginosa* the characteristics of precipitating necrotizing inflammation, being highly resistant to antimicrobial treatment, and having the epidemiology of an opportunistic infectious agent: most frequently *Acinetobacter* sp; next, the other highly resistant pseudomonads: *Burkholderia* sp, *Stenotrophomonas maltophilia,* and *Alcaligenes* sp; and the former pseudomonad *Sphingomonas paucimobilis;* but also, *Legionella* sp. *Acinetobacter* of the *calcoaceticus-baumanii* complex (mostly *A baumanii*) is, after *P aeruginosa,* the second most common nonfermenter isolated from clinically significant infections[8]; *Stenotrophomonas* (*Xanthomonas,* nee *Pseudomonas*) *maltophilia* is the third most common pathogenic nonfermenter isolate.[5] *Burkholderia pseudomallei* shares *P aeruginosa*'s propensities for skin infection, soft tissue and bone abscesses, pneumonia, and fulminant sepsis, but exposure is limited almost entirely to swampy environments in Southeast Asia and Oceania. However, it has occurred in former sojourners in those environments long after they had left the region for drier and more temperate climes.[116] *Burkholderia cepacia* mimics *P aeruginosa*'s role as a waterborne (and even disinfectant-borne) pathogen (and pseudopathogen).[117] *Burkholderia cepacia* has also proven equally, if not more, virulent than *P aeruginosa* in patients with cystic fibrosis.[17] *Alcaligenes* sp and *Sphingomonas* (nee *Pseudomonas*) *paucimobilis* are less frequent, waterborne opportunists whose proven ability to cause clinical disease is almost completely restricted to the immunodeficient, frequently intravenously catheterized populations,[8] the same populations that are victimized primarily by *P aeruginosa. Legionella* sp also reside in water, are often water aerosol-borne, and have been associated with, especially, necrotizing pneumonia.[118]

Rapidly progressive bronchopneumonia of the clinicopathologic sort caused by *P aeruginosa* can be produced by both gram-positive and gram-negative bacteria. Among gram-positives, the most frequent causes of necrotizing bronchopneumonia are virulent, usually community-acquired pathogens: *S aureus* and *Streptococcus pyogenes* (group A streptococcus). Among the gram-negatives, there is one enteric rod, *Klebsiella pneumoniae* (Friedlander's bacillus), that has a reasonable rate of community acquisition. The rest are opportunists; the syndrome that they create—of rapidly progressive bronchopneumonia, sometimes with cavitation—is gram-negative pneumonia.[119] Agents of this syndrome, besides *P aeruginosa,* include *E coli* and *Proteus* sp (both often colonize the upper respiratory tract in hospitalized patients), *Enterobacter* sp (which, like *P aeruginosa,* can display multidrug antimicrobial resistance), and *Serratia marcescens* (although some clinical authorities doubt the latter's ability to cause tissue necrosis).[120]

Two of the agents just cited also shared *P aeruginosa*'s role in causing hematogenous pneumonia, mostly among hospitalized neutropenic patients. These agents are *K pneumoniae* and *E coli.* In both lung and skin, the latter can produce a vasocentric lesion identical to that characteristic of *P aeruginosa,*[121] and so can, with allowance for the strikingly different morphologies of the agents themselves, three types of fungi: *Candida* sp,[122] *Aspergillus* sp, and the agents of zygomycosis.[37]

Bacterial osteomyelitis remains primarily caused by *S aureus,*[123] but, like *P aeruginosa,* the other aerobic gram-negative opportunists mentioned earlier, as well as anaerobic gram-negative bacilli, can produce osteomyelitides that are, on average, more indolent than those caused by *S aureus.* The infections they cause are clinically identical to the bone infections caused by *P aeruginosa,* but are usually more easily treated by antimicrobial regimens.

In hematogenous osteoarthritis, *S aureus* takes first place among pathogens, however, especially in patients with a urinary tract source seeding the septicemia. *E coli* and *Proteus* sp can instigate a *Pseudomonas*-like vertebral osteomyelitis.

Recently, the gram-positive coccus, *S pyogenes,* returned to prominence as the most important cause of necrotizing fasciitis. Some students of this condition have separated that infection (in which group A streptococci predominates, designated as hemolytic streptococcal gangrene) from the infections, like those in which *P aeruginosa* can play a role, where a combination of bacterial morphotypes is often seen.[124] In the latter infections, both gram-negative aerobes and at least one anaerobic species (which may be gram-positive or gram-negative) are typically isolated. *Escherichia coli, Proteus* sp, *Enterobacter* sp, and *Klebsiella* sp are all more frequent components of such a mix than is *P aeruginosa.*

As a cause of necrotizing infection in the CNS, *P aeruginosa* tends to be second in various lists of opportunists that cause these infections in immunodeficient patients[10]: second to *Listeria monocytogenes* as a cause of meningitis among the neutropenic and second to *E coli* as a cause of brain abscess in the same group. Interestingly, both of these agents can demonstrate vasocentric tropism in CNS.

The ability of *B cepacia* to mimic and tragically outdo *P aeruginosa* as a bacterial cause of progressive airway disease in patients with CF has already been mentioned. In patients with CF, there is often a microbiologic succession of prominent pathogens. As one specific dominant organism succeeds the next, from *S aureus* to *P aeruginosa* to *B cepacia,*[17] antimicrobial therapy is less and less successful. The other present and former pseudomonads listed at the beginning of this section can intrude on this sequence as well as can the relatively resistant respiratory pathogen *Moraxella (Branhamella) catarrhalis.*[17]

DIAGNOSTIC TECHNIQUES FOR ANATOMIC PATHOLOGISTS

From biopsy material, bacterial culture and adequate species identification remain the basic diagnostic techniques in the specific diagnosis of *P aeruginosa* infection. For bacteriologic purposes, as in most other situations, sterile fresh tissue, aspirated fluid, or aspirated exudate are superior to swabs for culture and isolation. Routine culture media and conditions usually suffice to isolate *P aeruginosa,* although species identification may sometimes be a maneuver beyond the capacity of routine kit or automated methods and require multitest batteries of biochemical tests. Antimicrobial susceptibility testing results are usually reproducible. Blood cultures may, of course, be useful in the differentiation of invasive versus (post)bacteremic patterns of infection. Regarding morphologic tissue examination itself, in the author's experience, Brown–Hopps stain sometimes will clearly demonstrate culture-confirmed *P aeruginosa* in areas of tissue necrosis where the bacilli are not visible by the Brown–Brenn tissue Gram stain.

REFERENCES

1. Gessard C. Sur les Colorations bleue et verte des linges à pansements. *Comptes Rendus Hebdomadaires des Séances de l'Académie des Sciences.* 1882;94:536–538.
2. Palleroni NJ. Present situation of the taxonomy of aerobic pseudomonads. In: Galli E, Silver S, Witholt B, eds. *Pseudomonas: Molecular Biology and Biotechnology.* Washington, DC: American Society for Microbiology; 1992:105–115.
3. Palleroni NJ, Kunisawa R, Contopoulou R, Doudoroff M. Nucleic acid homologies in the genus *Pseudomonas. Int J Syst Bacteriol.* 1973;23:333–339.
4. Schreckenberger PC. Update on taxonomy of nonfastidious, glucose-nonfermenting gram-negative bacilli. *Clin Microbiol Newsl.* 1995;17(6):41–48.
5. Gilligan PH. *Pseudomonas* and Burkholderia. In: Murray PR, Baron EJ, Pfaller MA, Tenover FC, Yolken RH, eds.

Manual of Clinical Microbiology. 6th ed. Washington, DC: American Society for Microbiology; 1995:509–519.
6. DeVos P, van Landschoot A, Segers P, et al. Genotypic relationships and taxonomic localization of unclassified *Pseudomonas* and *Pseudomonas*-like strains by deoxyribonucleic acid: ribonucleic acid hybridizations. *Int J Syst Bacteriol*. 1989;39:35–49.
7. Nagai T. Association of *Pseudomonas maltophilia* with malignant lesions. *J Clin Microbiol*. 1984;20:1003–1005.
8. von Graevenitz A. *Acinetobacter, Alcaligenes, Moraxella,* and other nonfermentative gram-negative bacteria. In: Murray PR, Baron EJ, Pfaller MA, Tenover FC, Yolken RH, eds. *Manual of Clinical Microbiology*. 6th ed. Washington, DC: American Society for Microbiology; 1995: 520–532.
9. Botzenhart K, Doring G. Ecology and epidemiology of *Pseudomonas aeruginosa*. In: Campa M, Bendinelli M, Friedman H, eds. *Pseudomonas aeruginosa as an Opportunistic Pathogen*. New York: Plenum Press; 1993:1–18.
10. Pollack M. *Pseudomonas aeruginosa*. In: Mandell GL, Bennett JE, Dolin R, eds. *Principles and Practice of Infectious Diseases*. 4th ed. New York: Churchill Livingstone; 1995:1980–2003.
11. Morrison AJ, Wenzel RP. Epidemiology of infections due to *Pseudomonas aeruginosa*. *Rev Infect Dis*. 1984; 6(suppl):S627–S647.
12. Schimpff SC, Moody M, Young VM. Relationship of colonization with *Pseudomonas aeruginosa* to development of *Pseudomonas* bacteremia in cancer patients. In: Hobby GL, ed. *Antimicrobial Agents and Chemotherapy—1970*. Washington, DC: American Society for Microbiology; 1971:240–244.
13. Brown DG, Baublis J. Reservoirs of *Pseudomonas* in an intensive care unit for newborn infants: mechanisms of control. *J Pediatr*. 1977;90:453–489.
14. Sewell DL. *Pseudomonas* infections. In: Wentworth BB, ed. *Diagnostic Procedures for Bacterial Infections*. 7th ed. Washington, DC: American Public Health Association; 1987:455–469.
15. Jarvis WR, Martone WJ. Predominant pathogens in hospital infections. *J Antimicrob Chemother*. 1992;29(suppl A):19–24.
16. Baron EJ, Peterson LR, Finegold SM. Nonfermentative gram-negative bacilli and coccobacilli. In: Baron EJ, Peterson LR, Finegold SM, eds. *Diagnostic Microbiology* 9th ed. St. Louis, MO: Mosby; 1994:386–405.
17. Gilligan PH. Microbiology of airway disease in patients with cystic fibrosis. *Clin Microbiol Rev*. 1991;4:35–51.
18. Sorenson RU, Joseph F Jr. Phenazine pigments in *Pseudomonas aeruginosa* infection. In: Campa M, Bendinelli M, Friedman H, eds. *Pseudomonas aeruginosa as an Opportunistic Pathogen*. New York: Plenum Press; 1993:43–57.
19. Bellido F, Hancock REW. Susceptibility and resistance of *Pseudomonas aeruginosa* to antimicrobial agents. In: Campa M, Bendinelli M, Friedman H, eds. *Pseudomonas aeruginosa as an Opportunistic Pathogen*. New York: Plenum Press; 1993:321–348.
20. Pederson SS, Pressler T, Jenson T, et al. Combined imipenem/cilastatin and tobramycin therapy of multiresistant *Pseudomonas aeruginosa* in cystic fibrosis. *J Antimicrob Chemother*. 1987;19:101–107.
21. Salyers AA, Whitt DD. *Pseudomonas aeruginosa*. In: Salyers AA, Whitt DD, eds. *Bacterial Pathogenesis: A Molecular Approach*. Washington, DC: American Society for Microbiology; 1994:260–269.
22. Holder IA. *Pseudomonas aeruginosa* burn infections: pathogenesis and treatment. In: Campa M, Bendinelli M, Friedman H, eds. *Pseudomonas aeruginosa as an Opportunistic Pathogen*. New York: Plenum Press; 1993: 275–295.
23. Leyden JJ, McGinley KJ, Mills OH. *Pseudomonas aeruginosa* gram-negative folliculitis. *Arch Dermatol*. 1979; 115:1203–1204.
24. Lin J-Y, Wang D-W, Peng C-T, et al. Noma neonatorum: an unusual case of noma involving a full-term neonate. *Acta Paediatr*. 1992;81:720–722.
25. Faden H, Grossi M. Acute osteomyelitis in children: reassessment of etiologic agents and their clinical characteristics. *Am J Dis Child*. 1991;145:64–69.
26. Fisher MC, Goldsmith JF, Gilligan PH. Sneakers as a source of *Pseudomonas aeruginosa* in children with osteomyelitis following puncture wounds. *J Pediatr*. 1985;106:607–609.
27. Gilbert DN, Tice AD, Marsh PK, et al. Oral ciprofloxacin therapy for chronic contiguous osteomyelitis caused by gram-negative bacilli. *Am J Med*. 1987;82(suppl 4A): 254–258.
28. Bodey GP, Bolivar R, Fainstein V, Jadeja L. Infections caused by *Pseudomonas aeruginosa*. *Rev Infect Dis*. 1983;5:279–313.
29. Liesegang TJ. Bacterial keratitis. *Infect Dis Clin North Am*. 1992;6:815–829.
30. Moore B, Forman A. An outbreak of urinary *Pseudomonas aeruginosa* infection acquired during urological operations. *Lancet*. 1966;2:929–931.
31. Bray DA, Calcaterra TC. *Pseudomonas* meningitis complicating head and neck surgery. *Laryngoscope*. 1976; 86:1386–1390.
32. Sapico FL, Montgomerie JZ. Vertebral osteomyelitis in intravenous drug abusers: report of three cases and review of the literature. *Rev Infect Dis*. 1980;2:196–200.
33. Rajashehekaraiah KR, Rice TW, Kallick CA. Recovery of *Pseudomonas aeruginosa* from syringes of drug addicts with endocarditis. *J Infect Dis*. 1981;144:482.
34. Fick RB Jr. Pathogenesis of *Pseudomonas aeruginosa* lung lesion in cystic fibrosis. *Chest*. 1989;96:158–164.
35. Pizzo P. *Pseudomonas* [Use of third-generation cephalosporins] *Hosp Pract*. 26(suppl 4):18–21;48–50.
36. Ehni WF, Reller LB, Ellison RT III. Bacteremia in granulocytopenic patients in a tertiary-care general hospital. *Rev Infect Dis*. 1991;13:613–619.
37. Bodey GP. Dermatologic manifestations in infections in neutropenic patients. *Infect Dis Clin North Am*. 1994;8: 655–675.
38. van den Brock PJ, van der Meer JWM, Kunst MW. The pathogenesis of ecthyma gangrenosum. *J Infect*. 1979;1: 263–267.

39. Mims CA, Dimmock N, Nash A, Stephen J. *The Pathogenesis of Infectious Disease.* 4th ed. London: Academic Press; 1995.
40. Irvin RT. Attachment and colonization of *Pseudomonas aeruginosa:* role of the surface structures. In: Campa M, Bendinelli M, Friedman H, eds. *Pseudomonas aeruginosa as an Opportunisitic Pathogen.* New York: Plenum Press; 1993:19–42.
41. Gilboa-Garber N, Mizrahi L. Interaction of the Mannose-philic lectins of *Pseudomonas aeruginosa* with luminous species of marine enterobacteria. *Microbios.* 1979;26: 31–36.
42. Doig P, Smith NR, Todd T, Irvin RT. Characterization of the binding of *Pseudomonas aeruginosa* alginate to human epithelial cells. *Infect Immun.* 1987;55:1517–1522.
43. Simpson DA, Ramphal R, Lory S. Genetic analysis of *Pseudomonas aeruginosa* adherence: distinct genetic loci control attachment to epithelial cells and mucins. *Infect Immun.* 1992;60:3771–3779.
44. Galloway DR. Role of exotoxins in the pathogenesis of *Pseudomonas aeruginosa* infections. In: Campa M, Bendinelli M, Friedman H, eds. *Pseudomonas aeruginosa as an Opportunistic Pathogen.* New York: Plenum Press; 1993:107–127.
45. Ramphal R, Guay C, Pier GB. *Pseudomonas aeruginosa* adhesins for tracheobronchial mucin. *Infect Immun.* 1987;55:600–603.
46. Schwartzmann S, Boring JR III. Antiphagocytic effect of slime from a mucoid strain of *Pseudomonas aeruginosa. Infect Immun.* 1971;3:762–767.
47. Lam J, Chan R, Lam K, et al. Production of mucoid microcolonies by *Pseudomonas aeruginosa* within infected lungs in cystic fibrosis. *Infect Immun.* 1980;28: 546–556.
48. Scharmann W. Cytotoxic effects of leukocidin from *Pseudomonas aeruginosa* on polymorphonuclear lymphocytes from cattle. *Infect Immun.* 1976;13:836–843.
49. Galloway DR. *Pseudomonas aeruginosa* elastase and elastolysis revisited: recent developments. *Mol Microbiol.* 1992;6:1155–1162.
50. Arena F, Baiqiang C, Sorensen RU, Hyman A, Lippton H. Pyocyanin: a bacterial product with novel vascular properties. *Circulation.* 1990;82:111–121
51. Li J. Bacterial toxins. *Curr Opin Struct Biol.* 1991;2: 545–556.
52. Coburn J. *Pseudomonas aeruginosa* exoenzyme S. *Curr Top Microbiol Immunol.* 1992;175:133–143.
53. Woods DE, Sokol PA. Use of transposon mutants to assess the role of exoenzyme S in chronic pulmonary disease due to *Pseudomonas aeruginosa. Eur J Clin Microbiol.* 1985;4:163–169.
54. Fu H, Coburn J, Collier R. The eukaryotic host factor that activates exoenzyme S of *Pseudomonas aeruginosa* is a member of the 14-3-3 protein family. *Proc Natl Acad Sci USA.* 1993;90:2320–2324.
55. Lory S, Tai PC. Biochemical and genetic aspects of *Pseudomonas aeruginosa* virulence. *Curr Top Microbiol Immunol.* 1985;118:53–69.
56. Shumard CM, Wozniak DJ, Galloway DR. Regulation of toxin A synthesis in *Pseudomonas aeruginosa.* In: Campa M, Bendinelli M, Friedman H, eds. *Pseudomonas aeruginosa as an Opportunistic Pathogen.* New York: Plenum Press; 1993:59–77.
57. Schmidt M, Holmes RK. Analysis of diphtheria toxin repressor-operator interactions and characterization of a mutant repressor with decreased binding activity of divalent metals. *Mol Microbiol.* 1993;9:173–181.
58. Passador L, Iglewski BH. Quorum sensing and virulence gene regulation in *Pseudomonas aeruginosa.* In: Roth JA, Bolin CA, Brogden KA, Mineon FC, Wannemuehler MJ, eds. *Virulence Mechanisms of Bacterial Pathogens.* 2nd ed. Washington, DC: American Society for Microbiology; 1995:65–78.
59. Strom MS, Lory S. Structure—function and biogenesis of the type IV pili. *Annu Rev Microbiol.* 1993;47:565–596.
60. Kimbara K, Chakrabarty AM. Control of alginate synthesis in *Pseudomonas aeruginosa:* regulation of the *alg R1* gene. *Biochem Biophys Res Commun.* 1989;164:601–608.
61. Maharaj R, Zielinski NA, Chakrabarty AM. Environmental regulation of alginate gene expression by *Pseudomonas aeruginosa.* In: Galli E, Silver S, Witholt B, eds. *Pseudomonas: Molecular Biology and Biotechnology.* Washington, DC: American Society for Microbiology; 1992:65–74.
62. Gambello MJ, Kaye S, Iglewski BH. LasR of *Pseudomonas aeruginosa* is a transcriptional activator of the alkaline protease gene *(apr)* and an enhancer of exotoxin A expression. *Infect Immun.* 1993;61:1180–1184.
63. Deretic V, Schurr MJ, Boucher JC, Martin DW. Conversion of *Pseudomonas aeruginosa* to mucoidy in cystic fibrosis: environmental stress and regulation of bacterial virulence by alternative sigma factors. *J Bacteriol.* 1994; 176:2773–2780.
64. Kaduruganueva J, Lam J, Beveridge T. Interaction of gentamicin with the A band and B band lipopolysaccharides of *Pseudomonas aeruginosa* and its possible lethal effect. *Antimicrob Agents Chemother.* 1993;37:715–721.
65. Baltch AL, Hammer MC, Smith RP, et al. Effects of *Pseudomonas aeruginosa* cytotoxin on human serum and granulocytes and their microbicidal, phagocytic, and chemotactic functions. *Infect Immun.* 1985;48:498–506.
66. Steadman R, Heck LW, Abrahamson DR. The role of proteases in the pathogenesis of *Pseudomonas aeruginosa* infections. In: Campa M, Bendinelli M, Friedman H, eds. *Pseudomonas aeruginosa as an Opportunistic Pathogen.* New York: Plenum Press; 1993:129–143.
67. Hector J, Azghrani A, Johnson A. Genetic regulation and expression of elastase in *Pseudomonas aeruginosa.* In: Campa M, Bendinelli M, Friedman H, eds. *Pseudomonas aeruginosa as an Opportunistic Pathogen.* New York: Plenum Press; 1993:145–162.
68. Ostroff RM, Vasil AI, Vasil M. Molecular comparison of a nonhemolytic and a hemolytic phospholipase C from *Pseudomonas aeruginosa. J Bacteriol.* 1990;172:5915–5923.
69. Sorensen RU, Klinger JD. Biological effects of *Pseudomonas aeruginosa* phenazine pigments. *Antibiot Chemother.* 1987;39:113–124.

70. Speert DP. *Pseudomonas aeruginosa*—phagocytic cell interaction. In: Campa M, Bendinelli M, Friedman H, eds. *Pseudomonas aeruginosa as an Opportunistic Pathogen.* New York: Plenum Press; 1993:163–181.
71. Nonyama S, Kojo H, Mine Y, Nishida M, Geto S, Kuwahara S. Inhibitory effect of *Pseudomonas aeruginosa* on the phagocytic and killing activity of rabbit polymorphonuclear leukocytes: purification and characterization of an inhibitor of polymorphonuclear leukocyte function. *Infect Immun.* 1979;24:394–398.
72. Campa M, Marelli P, Lupetti A. Effects of *Pseudomonas aeruginosa* on immune function. In: Campa M, Bendinelli M, Friedman H, eds. *Pseudomonas aeruginosa as an Opportunistic Pathogen.* New York: Plenum Press; 1993:207–222.
73. Fitzsimmons SC. The changing epidemiology of cystic fibrosis. *J Pediatr.* 1993;122:1–9.
74. McManus AT, Mason, AD Jr, McManus WF, et al. Twenty-five year review of *Pseudomonas aeruginosa* bacteremia in a burn center. *Eur J Clin Microbiol.* 1985;4:219–223.
75. Centers for Disease Control and Prevention. Otitis due to *Pseudomonas aeruginosa* 0:10 associated with a mobile redwood tub system—North Carolina. *MMWR.* 1982;31: 541–542.
76. Bottone EJ, Perez II AA. *Pseudomonas aeruginosa* folliculitis acquired through the use of a contaminated loofah sponge: an unrecognized public health problem. *J Clin Microbiol.* 1993;31:480–483.
77. Thomas P, Moore M, Bell E, et al. *Pseudomonas aeruginosa* dermatitis associated with a swimming pool. *JAMA.* 1985;253:1156–1159.
78. Chandler JR. Malignant external otitis. *Laryngoscope.* 1968;1257–1294.
79. Kenna MA, Bluestone CD. Microbiology of chronic suppurative otitis media in children. *Pediatr Infect Dis.* 1986;5:223–225.
80. Liesegang TJ, Forester RK. Spectrum of microbial keratitis in South Florida. *Am J Ophthalmol.* 1980;90:38–47.
81. Jacobs RF, McCarthy RE, Elser JM. *Pseudomonas* osteochondritis complicating puncture wounds of the foot in children. a 10-year evaluation. *J Infect Dis.* 1989;160: 657–661.
82. Wiessman GJ, Wood VE, Kroll LL. *Pseudomonas* vertebral osteomyelitis in heroin addicts: report of five cases. *J Bone Joint Surg.* 1973;55:1416–1424.
83. delBusto R, Quinn EL, Fisher EJ, et al. Osteomyelitis of the pubis: report of seven cases. *JAMA.* 1982;241: 498–500.
84. Waldvogel FA, Vasey H. Osteomyelitis: the past decade. *N Engl J Med.* 1980;303:360–370.
85. Teplitz C. Pathogenesis of *Pseudomonas* vasculitis and septic lesions. *Arch Pathol.* 1965;80:297–307.
86. Greene SL, Su WPD, Muller SA. Ecthyma gangrenosum: report of clinical, histopathologic, and bacteriologic aspects of eight cases. *J Am Acad Dermatol.* 1984;11: 781–787.
87. Soave R, Murray HW, Litrenta MM. Bacterial invasion of pulmonary vessels: *Pseudomonas* bacteremia mimicking pulmonary thromboembolism with infarction. *Am J Med.* 1978;65:864–867.
88. Fox AB, Hambrick GW Jr. Recreationally associated *Pseudomonas aeruginosa* folliculitis. *Arch Dermatol.* 1984;120:1304–1307.
89. Murphy GF. Pustular folliculitis. In Murphy GF, ed. *Dermatopathology.* Philadelphia: WB Saunders; 1995:142–145.
90. Tillotson JR, Lerner AM. Characteristics of nonbacteremic *Pseudomonas* pneumonia. *Ann Intern Med.* 1968;69: 287–294.
91. Hall JH, Callaway JL, Tindall JP, et al. *Psudomonas aeruginosa* in dermatology. *Arch Dermatol.* 1968:97: 312–324.
92. Silverman AR, Nieland ML. Hot tub dermatitis. A familial outbreak of *Pseudomonas* folliculitis. *J Am Acad Dermatol.* 1983;8:153–156.
93. Pruitt BA Jr. Infections of burns and other wounds caused by *Pseudomonas aeruginosa.* In: Sabath LD, ed. *Pseudomonas aeruginosa: The Organism, Diseases It Causes, and Their Treatment.* Bern: Hans Huber; 1980: 55–70.
94. El Baze P, Thyss A, Vinte H, Deville A, Dellamonica P, Ortonne J-P. A study of nineteen immunocompromised patients with extensive skin lesions caused by *Pseudomonas aeruginosa* with and without bacteremia. *Acta Derm Venereal (Stockh).* 1991;71:411–415.
95. Hitschman F, Kreibich K. Zur Pathogenese des Bacillus pyocyaneus und zur Aetiologie des Ekthyma Gangrenosum. *Wien Klin Wochenschr.* 1897;10:1093–1101.
96. Damiani JM, Damiani KK, Kinney SE. Malignant external otitis with multiple cranial nerve involvement. *Am J Otol.* 1979;1:115–120.
97. Brook I, Finegold SM. Bacteriology of chronic otitis media. *JAMA.* 1979;241:487–488.
98. Alfonso E, Mandelbaum S, Fox MJ, et al. Ulcerative keratitis associated with contact lens wear. *Am J Ophthalmol.* 1986;101:429–433.
99. Irvine WD, Flynn HW Jr, Miller D, et al. Endophthalmitis caused by gram-negative organisms. *Arch Ophthalmol.* 1992;110:1450–1454.
100. Marrie TJ, Majot H, Gurwith M, et al. Prolonged outbreak of nosocomial urinary tract infection with a single strain of *Pseudomonas aeruginosa. Can Med Assoc J.* 1978;119: 593–598.
101. Fraenkel E. Weitere Untersuchungen uber die Menschenpathogenitat des Bacillus pyocyaneus Z. *Hyg Infekt.* 1917;84:369–423.
102. Motil KJ. Necrotizing enterocolitis. In: Oski FA, ed. *Principles and Practice of Pediatrics.* 2nd ed. Philadelphia: JB Lippincott; 1994:436–443.
103. Stone HH, Kolb LD, Geheber CE. Bacteriologic consideration in perforated necrotizing enterocolitis. *South Med J.* 1979;72:1540–1544.
104. Angel C, Patrick CC, Lobe T, et al. Management of anorectal-perineal infection caused by *Pseudomonas aeruginosa* in children with malignant diseases. *J Pediatr Surg.* 1991;26:487–493.
105. Crane LR, Komshian S. Gram-negative bacillary pneumonia. In: Pennington JE, ed. *Respiratory Infections: Diagnosis and Management.* New York: Raven Press; 1988:314–340.

106. Lerner AM. The gram-negative bacillary pneumonias. *Dis Month*. 1980;27:1–56.
107. Iannini PB, Claffey T, Quintiliani R. Bacteremic *Pseudomonas* pneumonia. *JAMA*. 1974;230:558–561.
108. Nagaki M, Shimura S, Tanno Y, et al. Role of chronic *Pseudomonas aeruginosa* infection in the development of bronchiectasis. *Chest*. 1992;102:1464–1469.
109. Maqbool M, Ahmad R, Qazi S. Necrotizing fasciitis in the head and neck region. *Br J Plast Surg*. 1992;45:481–483.
110. Cumberworth VL, Hogarth TB. Hazards of ear-piercing procedures which traverse cartilage: a report of *Pseudomonas* perichondritis and review of other complications. *Br J Clin Pract*. 1990;44:512–513.
111. Salahuddin NI, Madhavan T, Fisher EJ, et al. *Pseudomonas* osteomyelitis: radiographic features. *Radiology*. 1973;109:41–47.
112. Sequeira W, Jones E, Seigel ME, et al. Pyogenic infections of the pubic symphysis. *Ann Intern Med*. 1982;96: 604–606.
113. Wise BL, Mathis JL, Jawetz E. Infections of the central nervous system due to *Pseudomonas aeruginosa*. *J Neurosurg*. 1969;31:432–434.
114. Gould K, Ramerez-Ronda CH, Holmes RK, et al. Adherence of bacteria to heart valves in vitro. *J Clin Invest*. 1975;56:1364–1370.
115. Reyes MP, Lerner AM. Current problems in the treatment of infective endocarditis due to *Pseudomonas aeruginosa*. *Rev Infect Dis*. 1983;5:314–321.
116. Koponen MA, Zlock D, Palmer DL, Merlin TL. Melioidosis: forgotten, but not gone! *Arch Int Med*. 1991;151: 605–608.
117. Pallent LJ, Hugo WB, Grant DJW, Davies A. *Pseudomonas* cepacia as contaminant and infective agent. *J Hosp Infect*. 1983;4:9–13.
118. Edelstein PH, Meyer RD. Legionella pneumonias. In: Pennington JE, ed. *Respiratory Infections: Diagnosis and Management*. 2nd ed. New York: Raven Press; 1988: 381–402.
119. Torres A, Serra-Batiles J, Ferrer A, et al. Severe community acquired pneumonia: epidemiology and prognostic factors. *Am Rev Respir Dis*. 1991;144:312–318.
120. Cunha BA. Historical, physical, and laboratory clues to the diagnosis of pneumonia. In: Karetzky M, Cunha BA, Brandstetter RD, ed. *The Pneumonias*. New York: Springer Verlag; 1993:106–144.
121. Rajan RK. Spontaneous bacterial peritonitis with ecthyma gangrenosum due to *Escherichia coli*. *J Clin Gastroenterol*. 1982;4:145–148.
122. Fine JD, Miller JA, Harrist TJ, Haynes HA. Cutaneous lesions in disseminated candidiasis mimicking ecthyma gangrenosum. *Am J Med*. 1981;70:1133–1135.
123. Mader JT, Colhoun J. Osteomyelitis. In: Mandel GL, Bennett JE, Dolin R, eds. *Principles and Practice of Infectious Diseases*. 4th ed. New York: Churchill Livingstone; 1995: 1039–1051.
124. Swartz MN. Cellulitis and subcutaneous tissue infection. In: Mandell GL, Bennett JE, Dolin R, eds. *Principles and Practice of Infectious Diseases*. 4th ed. New York: Churchill Livingstone; 1995:909–936.

Chapter 81

Pyomyositis

Philip E. S. Palmer

But swoln . . .
Rot inwardly and foul contagion spread.

John Milton (1608–1674), Lycidas, 1 123

INTRODUCTION

Pyomyositis, a suppurative disease of skeletal muscle, occurs with varying frequency worldwide, but is most common in the tropics (Figure 81–1). Pyomyositis is now separated into two forms, *tropical* and *temperate* or nontropical. The distinction is imperfect because the only difference is whether the patient has some obvious precipitating factor (temperate) or is otherwise seemingly healthy (tropical). So there are patients with tropical pyomyositis who have never been to the tropics and there are patients with temperate pyomyositis who live in the tropics but have recognized sources of infection. This is not a new disease, although it had become much less common with the availability of chemotherapy for bacteria, and even less frequent when antibiotics were developed. Now frequency is rising again, mainly because of immunosuppression, together with penicillin-resistant *Staphylococcus aureus*. Both factors are influencing the increasing number of infections in the tropics as well as in temperate climates.

In tropical pyomyositis the origin of the infection is not clear, but "spontaneous" infections are a significant problem. It has accounted for more than 2% of surgical admissions in eastern Ecuador, and even more, about 4%, of surgical patients in Uganda. The temperate forms were first described by Scriba[1] in 1885 and the tropical variety by Zieman[2] in 1904 followed in 1912 by a similar series from Jamaica.[3] Since then there have been many patients in Malaysia, Indonesia, Africa, Brazil, and other South American countries.[4–8]

Tropical pyomyositis is a single or multiple intramuscular abscess, not caused by, or related to trauma, human immunodeficiency virus (HIV), or other infections: There is no clear explanation to account for these often life-threatening abscesses, nor is there any obvious reason why the incidence is rising in some countries, while decreasing in others. It is surprisingly variable in age-incidence, being more common in men over 30 to 40 years in some areas, but elsewhere being more common under 20, even in children. It is generally more common in men than women. No predisposing climatic or other geographic factors have been identified except that in countries such as Ecuador it is 20 times more common in those who live in tropical forests than in the mountains. Altitude, however, does not provide full protection.[8] In Uganda it is much more common in the rainy season and in rural populations, but occurs throughout the year and regardless of living conditions. It cannot be related to parasites (eg, guinea worm).[9,10] In truth, the origin of tropical pyomyositis remains an enigma. Some authors have (without convincing proof) blamed a preceding viral infection, probably the Coxsackie B virus and subsequent staphylococcal infection.[11] The Coxsackie B virus is common in the tropics and can produce muscle necrosis. Another theory suggested a deficit of vitamin C, causing latent scurvy. In 1990 Idoko et al[12] studied this possibility in Nigerian patients with tropical pyomyositis. Their patients had, if anything, higher plasma vitamin C levels than the control series. Similarly, patients in New Guinea, Swaziland, and elsewhere in Southern Africa

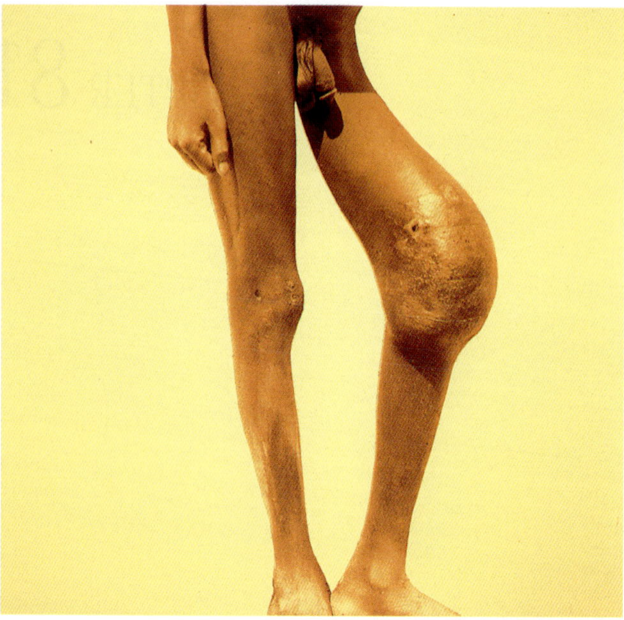

Figure 81–1. Tropical pyomyositis in the thigh of a West African. The patient had visited local health practitioners and their treatments account for some of the damage to the skin. The abscess was huge by the time he came to hospital *(From Palmer PES, Reeder MM.* The Imaging of Tropical Diseases. *2nd ed. Heidelberg: Springer Verlag;1996.)*

have not shown any vitamin deficiency.[13,14] Nowhere is there a convincing history of local, previous injury related to the abscess or abscesses.

Nontropical pyomyositis is a complication of immunosuppression, intravenous drug abuse, trauma, diabetes, or intravenous catheterization. With these possible precipitating factors, this pyomyositis can occur at any age and in either sex. Unlike the tropical variety, patients are often clinically ill before the onset of the myositis.

CLINICAL FINDINGS

Patients with temperate pyomyositis complain of pain and local swelling: because they are often ill already, the recognition of the usually deep-seated infection can be difficult unless ultrasound, computed tomography (CT), or magnetic resonance imaging (MRI) is available. They can be a challenging diagnostic problem, whereas patients with tropical pyomyositis usually delay seeking treatment, so that when the abscess or abscesses are first seen, the majority are large and tense. In the few early lesions described, the muscle has been pale and edematous, without pus. Patients first have local pain restricting movement and sometimes joint pain also. Almost all will have swelling in the infected area, with local warmth, and in about one third, fluctuation. In others, the pain and swelling are the major complaint: Some patients are afebrile, others have a low-grade fever.[15–17]

About two thirds of the patients have a solitary abscess, most commonly in the thigh muscles (Figure 81–2). Others have either multiple abscesses or no clinically detected suppuration. Only in one third or less is there regional lymphadenopathy. In some patients, the whole process is acute and leads to septic shock, sufficient in one instance to kill a 10-year-old. The abscesses may be large: In one elderly patient the brachial artery was compressed and, as a result, the forearm became gangrenous and the patient died. Metastatic abscess may be in multiple organs, including brain, lung, liver, kidney, spine, and abdomen; rupture of these abscesses in some situations can be fatal. Pyogenic pericarditis and bacterial endocarditis can cause cardiac failure and death.[18–20]

DIAGNOSIS

The pain, fever, local swelling, localized tenderness, and, in some patients, fluctuation make the clinical diagnosis fairly straightforward, except when the patient is afebrile. Ultrasound (Figure 81–3), CT, or MRI may show the extent of any abscess and surrounding edema.[21–26] When the patient is immunodeficient, focal fluid within the muscles develops more rapidly. The mass formed by the edema can be quite large and deep pelvic infections can involve many muscle groups, and more than one muscle may be involved. Some progress to gangrenous myositis and necrotizing fasciitis may occur. Gadolinium-enhanced MRI may show rim enhancement; the focal fluid collections usually have a high signal intensity and are hypointense on T2-weighted images. Rim enhancement can also be seen when contrast is used with CT. The bones near the abscess may show local resorption, sometimes with a lamellar reaction; this may resemble a tumor. Chronic abscesses may cause adjacent bone sclerosis, eg, in the pelvis. Only rarely is there osteomyelitis.[5,7,10,15,16,27,28]

The differential diagnosis in the tropics includes an abscess caused by guinea worm, although this is more likely to be extramuscular. Mycotic and tuberculous abscesses often develop sinuses. In the abdominal muscles, the abscess may be mistaken for an intra-abdominal event, such as appendicitis or, in toxic patients, even typhoid fever or hepatitis.[27] Liver or cerebral metastatic abscesses will only be misdiagnosed if the primary pyomyositis has not been recognized.

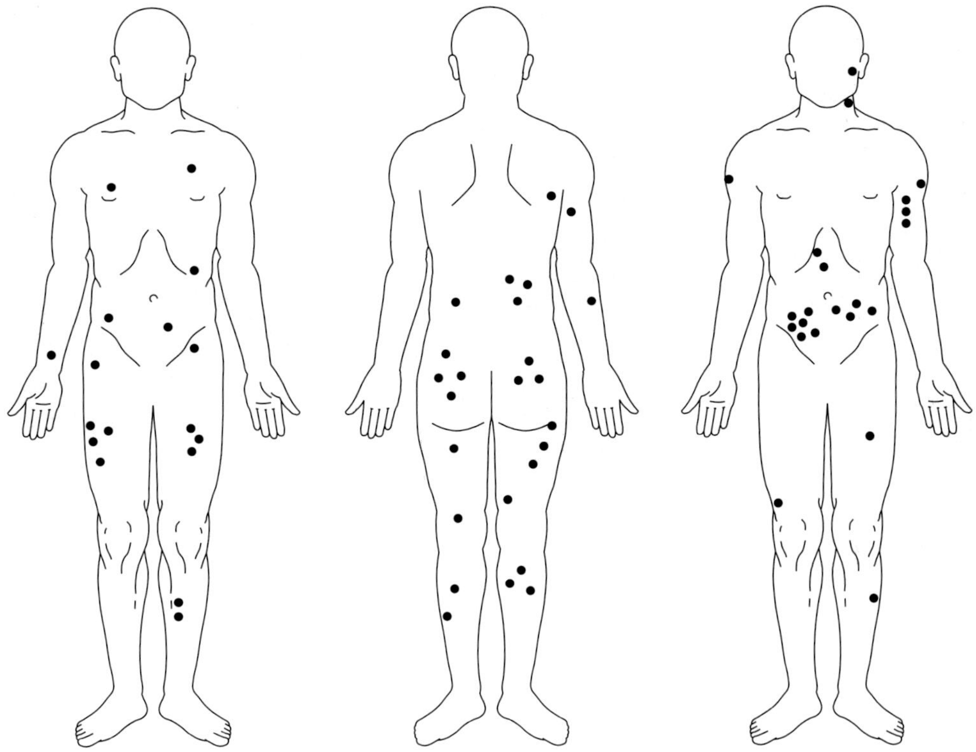

Figure 81–2. (*Left*) Anatomic location of abscesses of pyomyositis in 12 patients in Malaysia and (*middle and right*) of 46 abscesses in 26 patients in New Guinea *(Left, redrawn from Robin*[4]*; middle and right, redrawn from Sayers.*[9]*)*

PATHOLOGY

The abscesses of tropical pyomyositis arise most commonly in the thigh and gluteal muscles, but involve also muscles around the shoulder, in the upper limb, abdomen, pelvis, and around the spine. There is, again, no significant link with geography, tribe, or climate to account for the variation in sites.

About 90% of abscesses contain *S aureus;* other organisms, eg, *Escherichia coli,* hemolytic streptococci, and *S albus,* have been grown but may be contaminants. The *S aureus* in Uganda was type 11, single phase 3a, 3b, 3c, 55/71, but no other tropical series has been accurately typed and it is not certain that Ugandan cultures are applicable everywhere.[21,27–31]

Patients with nontropical pyomyositis have predominantly staphylococcal infections. In the Solomon Islands all the bacteria were identified as group 2. (Most of these infections were preceded by trauma or by preexisting pyoderma.) Beta-hemolytic streptococci have caused severe infections and *S pyogenes* have been identified in two cases. In other patients, bacterial culture has been negative. It has been suggested that *Neisseria gonorrhoeae* should also be a consideration, but no strains of *N gonorrhoeae* have yet been cultured.[1,22,23,30,32–34]

Histologic studies have shown edema between the myofibrils, coagulation necrosis, cytolysis, and glandular infiltration. Even when there is little or no frank pus, there is loss of muscle striations (Figures 81–4 through 81–9). In the 19 autopsies reported by Taylor et al[10] the earliest changes (identified in premortem biopsies) were separation of myofibers, presumably from edema fluid. Other changes identified before the appearance of an inflammatory exudate were a patchy myocytolysis, foci of coagulation necrosis, and, more rarely, granular degeneration of myofibers. With disintegration of muscle there were lymphocytes, plasma cells, and eosinophils around the dead muscle fibers and sometimes around adjacent vessels. In 4 autopsies there were inflammatory infiltrates beneath the pericardium and within the myocardium and in three of these hearts there were cocci in myocardium surrounded by neutrophils. In lungs and pleura 50% had bronchpneumonia and 30% had staphylococcal abscesses. One patient had empyema. Other organs with metastatic abscesses were kidney, liver (two patients), and brain (three patients).

TREATMENT

Surgery is nearly always necessary; antibiotics are not usually successful. Pus may form rapidly. Ultrasound-guided needle aspiration/biopsy can be used to reduce tension and type the causal organism. The pus can be

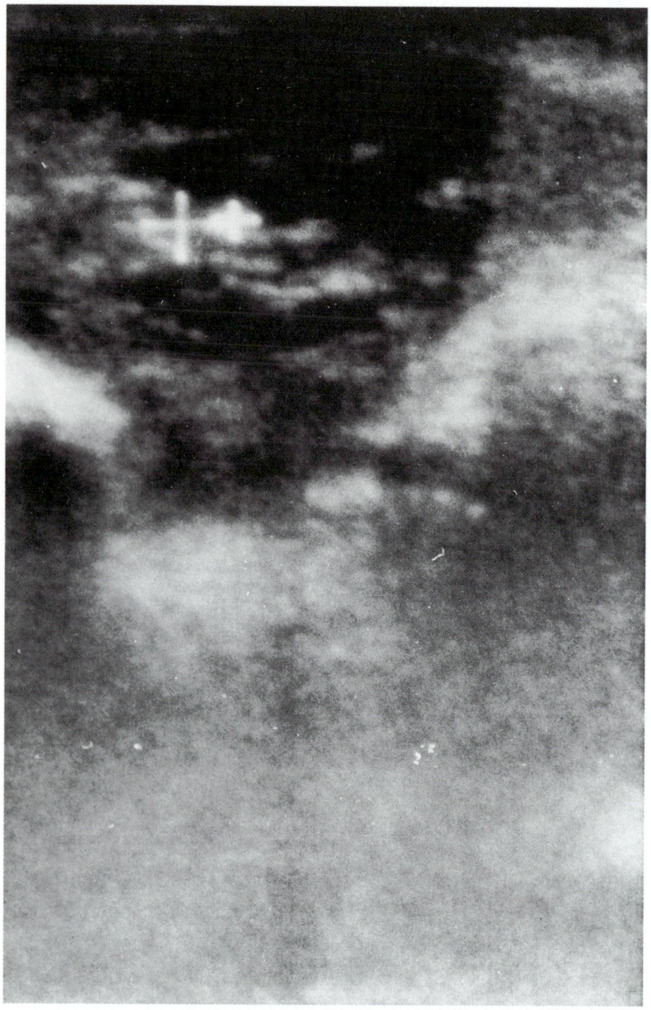

Figure 81–3. Ultrasonography of an African patient in Uganda with pyomyositis. There is infiltrating edema and a developing abscess (++). *(Contributed by Professor L. Belli, Veronese, and with permission of* Skeletal Radiology.*)*

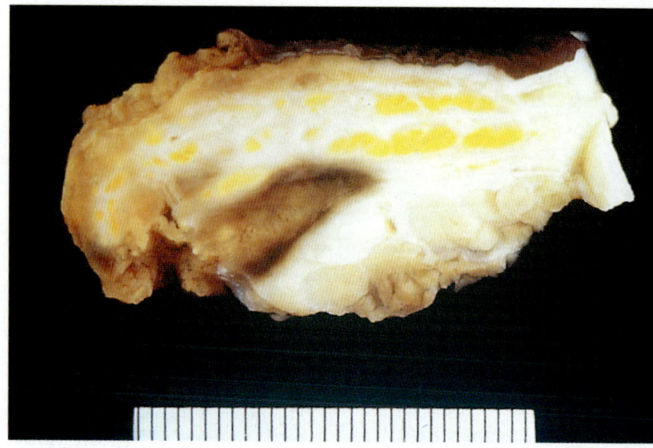

Figure 81–4. Excised skin including a draining sinus, subcutaneous tissue and deep fascia from a Zairian patient with pyomyositis. The draining sinus is on the left and the dagger-shaped area near the center is an extension of the abscess into the subcutaneous tissue. *(Contributed by Daniel H. Connor, MD, 1977.)*

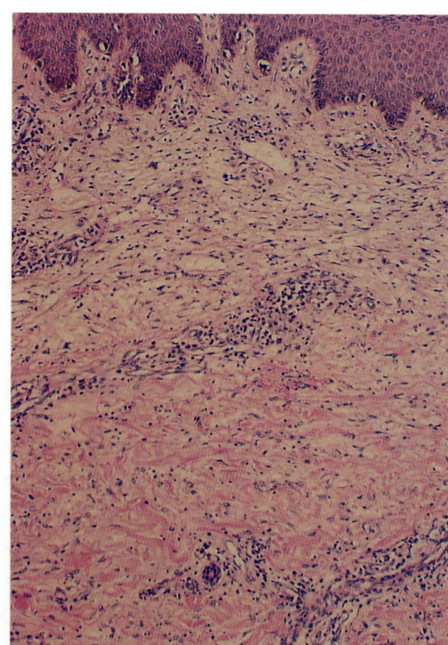

Figure 81–5. Inflammatory change in skin over the abscess. Edema of the dermis and dilated dermal lymphatics and lymphocytes are all present, as well as plasma cells and neutrophils around vessels and appendages (hematoxylin-eosin, ×80).

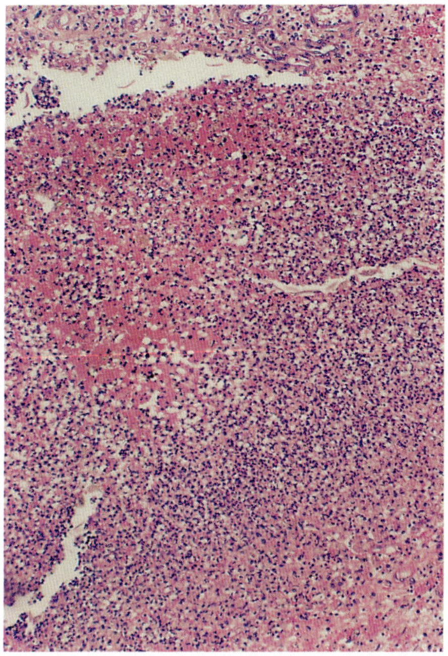

Figure 81–6. The exudate in the abscess contains fibrin and degenerating macrophages and neutrophils (hematoxylin-eosin, ×80).

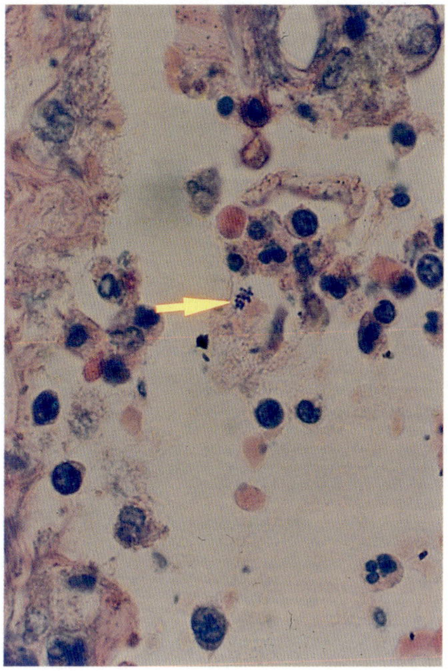

Figure 81–8. Necrotic tissue near the lining of the lesion. There are clumps of cocci in a degenerating phagocytic cell (tip of arrow) (Giemsa, ×1000).

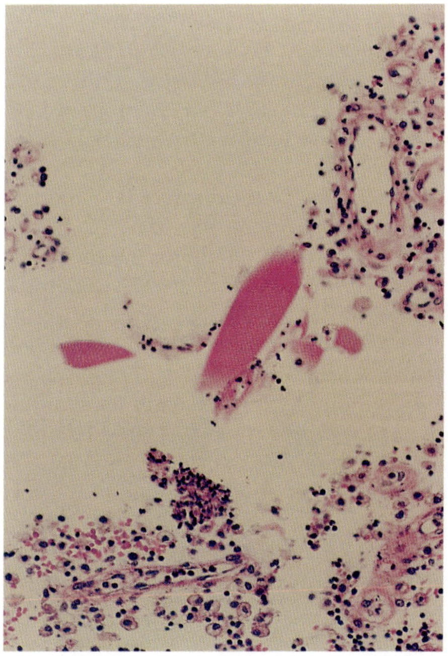

Figure 81–7. The cavity of the abscess contains fragments of degenerating skeletal muscle (hematoxylin-eosin, ×250).

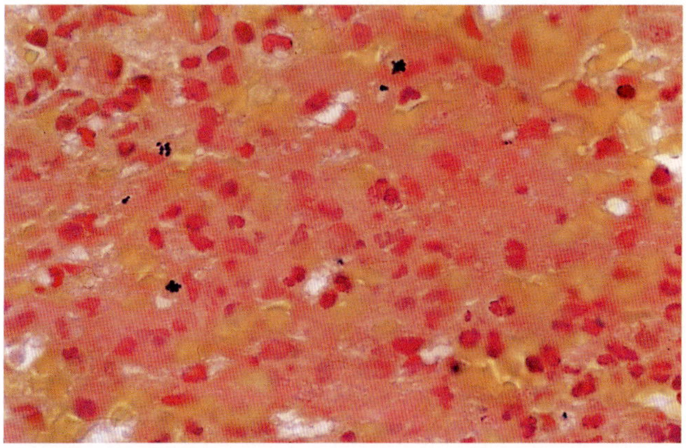

Figure 81–9. From the wall of an abscess in the calf of a 24-year-old American Peace Corps volunteer. There are clusters of gram-positive cocci in macrophages. While serving in West Africa he developed leukopenia and intermittent fevers and returned to the United States for treatment. CT scans revealed abscesses in his left calf and right biceps. These were drained and *S aureus* was cultured from the pus. The abscesses resolved with antibiotic therapy but then leukemia was discovered. The patient had a bone marrow transplant and subsequently died (tissue gram stain, ×1000). *(Specimen contributed by Drs Herbert J. Manz and Princy Kumar, Georgetown University Hospital.)*

difficult to aspirate when thick, and difficult to locate without ultrasonography. Premature incision does not cause harm and there is seldom any postincisional hemorrhage. Healing is quite rapid, usually in about 2 weeks.[6,8,10,35,36]

It is recommended that a chest radiograph precede surgery, to exclude a metastatic lung abscess. Similarly, sonology of the liver and kidneys is useful, particularly when the clinical condition of the patient fails to improve as expected.

The outcome can vary. When the abscess or abscesses are well drained, there may be little deformity, but the necrotic muscle does not regenerate, so there may be a persistent wasting defect and disability. In children, skeletal growth near the abscess may be retarded. But in many patients the healing process leaves little evidence of what may have been a significant abscess.

REFERENCES

1. Scriba J. Beitrag zur Aetiologie der Myositis acuta. *Deutsch Ztschr f Chir.* 1885;22:497–502.
2. Zieman H. Cited in an article by Ransford ON. *East Afric Med J.* 1946;23:278–281.
3. Scott HH. Deep suppuration of the thigh associated with a peculiar bacillus. *Am J Trop Med Hyg.* 1912;15:97–99.
4. Robin GC. Tropical myositis in Malaysia. *Am J Trop Med Hyg.* 1961;64:288–291.
5. Ryan BP. Pyomyositis in Papuan children. *Trans R Soc Trop Med Hyg.* 1962;56:312–318.
6. Chiedozi LC. Pyomyositis. Review of 205 cases in 112 patients. *Am J Surg.* 1979;137:255–259.
7. Chaudry NFAM. Pyomyositis. *East Afr Med J.* 1972;49: 466–469.
8. Kerrigan UR, Nelson ST. Tropical myositis in eastern Ecuador. *Trans R Soc Trop Med Hyg.* 1992;86:90–91.
9. Sayers EG. Tropical myositis and muscle abscess. *Trans R Soc Trop Med Hyg.* 1930;23:385–400.
10. Taylor JF, Templeton AC, Henderson B. Pyomyositis, a clinico-pathological study based on 19 autopsy cases at Mulago Hospital 1964–1968. *East Afr Med J.* 1970;47: 493–501.
11. Horn D, Masters CV. Pyomyositis Tropicans in Uganda. *East Afric Med J.* 1968;45:463–471.
12. Idoko JA, Jimoh O, Onyewoth II. Has lack of vitamin C any role in the etiology of tropical pyomyositis? *J Infect.* 1990;21:7–9.
13. Tilma A. Pyomyositis in Swaziland. *S Afr Med J.* 1979; 51:39–41.
14. vanNiekerk JP de V. Pyomyositis in African mine workers. Unpublished series, personal communication, 1977.
15. Lapido GOA, Fakunie YF. Tropical pyomyositis in the Nigerian savanna. *Trop Geogr Med.* 1979;29:223–228.
16. Marcus RT, Foster WD. Observations on the clinical features, etiology and geographical distribution of pyomyositis in East Africa. *East Afr Med J.* 1968;45:167–170.
17. Gambhir IS, Singh DS, Gupta SS, Gupta PR, Kumar M. Tropical pyomyositis in India: a clinico-histopathological study. *Am J Trop Med Hyg.* 1992;95:42–46.
18. Andy JJ, Ekpo EB. Cardiovascular complications of pyomyositis. *Trop Geogr Med.* 1987;39:260–264.
19. Dasgupta DJ, Prachar BS, Bhardnaj PK, et al. Tropical myositis complicated by arrhythmias and pleuritis. *J Assoc Physicians India.* 1991;39:300–301. Letter.
20. Thomas GE, Francis TI, Smith JA. Cardiac complications of tropical pyomyositis. *Nig Med J.* 1974;4:29–31.
21. Gordon BA, Martinez S, Collins AJ. Pyomyositis: characteristics and CT and MR imaging. *Radiology.* 1995;197: 279–286.
22. Vicens JL, Aubspin D, Buchon R, et al. Pyomyositis in AIDS: appropos of a case. *Ann Radiol (Paris).* 1990;33: 200–203.
23. Jimenez-Megias ME, de Leon LF, Alfaro-Garcia MJ, et al. Pyomyositis caused by *Staphylococcus aureus. Med Clin (Barc).* 1992;99:201–205.
24. Radvany NG, Chandnani VP. Tropical pyomyositis. *Australas Radiol.* 1995;39:78–79.
25. Yuh WT, Schreiber AE, Montgomery WJ, et al. Magnetic resonance imaging of pyomyositis. *Skeletal Radiol.* 1988; 17:190–193.
26. Belli L, Aeggivori R, Cocozza E, et al. Ultrasound in tropical radiology. *Skeletal Radiol.* 1992;21:107–109.
27. Hansen LB, Baekgaard N, Reske-Nielsen E. Focal myositis of the rectus abdominal muscles. *Acta Chir Scand.* 1985;151:77–80.
28. Foster WD. The bacteriology of tropical pyomyositis in Uganda. *East Afr Med J.* 1968;45:463–471.
29. Christin L, Sarosi GA. Pyomyositis in North America: case reports and review. *Clin Infect Dis.* 1992;15:668–677.
30. Farrag N, Kavanagh TG, Chin T. Pyomyositis; an underreported disease in temperate climates. *J Infect.* 1988;17: 256–263.
31. Taylor JF, Fluck D. Tropical myositis: ultrastructural studies. *J Clin Pathol.* 1976;29:1081–1084.
32. Birkbeck D, Watson JT. Obturator internus pyomyositis. A case report. *Clin Orthop (US).* 1995;316:221–226.
33. Eason R, Osbourne J, Ashford T, et al. Tropical pyomyositis in the Solomon Islands: clinical and aetiological features. *Trans R Soc Trop Med Hyg.* 1989;83:275–278.
34. Muscat I, Anthony PP, Cruickshank JG. Non-tropical pyomyositis. *J Clin Pathol.* 1986;39:1116–1118.
35. Davey WW. Pyomyositis (tropical myositis). In: *A Companion to Surgery in Africa.* Edinburgh: E & S Livingstone; 1968.
36. Pinto DJ. The treatment of pyomyositis. *East Afr Med J.* 1972;49:9:644–651.

CHAPTER 82

Q Fever

Joseph T. Newsome

It is better to have a lion at the head of an army of sheep than to have a sheep at the head of an army of lions.

Daniel Defoe (1660–1731)

This fever, that hath troubled me so long,
Lies heavy on me; O, my heart is sick!

William Shakespeare (1564–1616), King John, V, III

DEFINITION

Q fever is infection by *Coxiella burnetii* and has worldwide distribution. Although commonly considered nonpathogenic in most species of domestic animals, it is an occupational hazard for those exposed to infected animals, their tissues, or the causative agent. This disease is an acute febrile illness with headache, malaise, and interstitial pneumonitis. Pathologically it leads to fibrin ring granulomas in affected tissues.

SYNONYMS AND HISTORY

The causal agent is a rickettsial organism named *Coxiella burnetii,*[1] (*Rickettsia burnetii*[2] or *R diaporica*[3]). Animal infection with *C burnetii* is known as coxiellosis.[4,5] Abattoir fever[4] and Balkan grippe[4,6] were early synonyms cited for this disease. In 1937 Derrick described a febrile illness in Australian meat workers and isolated a small gram-negative bacillus from their blood and urine.[2,5] He queried the relationship between the bacillus and the fever and the name "Q" (for "query") fever stuck. Burnet and Freeman[7] first characterized this agent as a rickettsial-like filterable bacterium obtained from guinea pigs infected by Derrick. An epidemiologic report in 1940 showed that *R burnetii* could be isolated from the tick *Haemaphysalis humerosa.*[8] As the epidemiology of Q fever was being investigated in Australia, two reports by Cox[9,10] described a filterable rickettsia-like bacterial agent isolated from the tick *D andersoni* in North America that was similar to an agent described by Noguchi in 1926. After accidental infection by a staff scientist in Cox's lab while attempting to isolate the organism on fertile chicken eggs, the isolates from humans and vectors in both Australia and North America were postulated to be the same microorganism.[4] From 1938 to 1953 the epidemiology of *C burnetii* was limited until the phase variations were discovered.[4,11] Since 1956 and the development of sensitive serologic assays that account for the variations of specific serodiagnostic antigens, the distribution of Q fever has been well defined.[4,12,13] Several recent books give excellent historical accounts of the discovery of Q fever and the elucidation of its cause.[1,4,14,15]

DESCRIPTION OF *COXIELLA BURNETII*

Coxiella burnetii is the only member of the genus *Coxiella* of the family Rickettsiaceae.[4,16,17] It is a mildly acidophilic obligate intracellular bacterium that grows exclusively in the phagolysosome of eukaryotic cells.[18] Three distinct cell types grow in the phagolysosome. They are the large cell variant, small cell variant, and spore form. Ultrastructural evidence supports the view that these variants are a consequence of the unique developmental biology of *C burnetii.* Replication consists of both transverse binary fission and sporogenic cellular differentiation. Both are necessary and vital events in the life cycle of the organism.[19]

A new genus was designated because of the unique differences between the Q fever agent and other Rickettsiaea.[20] These include large guanine plus cytosine ratios, transmission by inhalation rather than cutaneous inoculation, exclusive growth in cytoplasmic vacuoles, and increased resistance to environmental conditions. No other bacterium has this unique combination—phagolysosome tropism, synthesis of a weakly endotoxic lipopolysaccharide (LPS), and sporulation.[1,4]

Immunologically *C burnetii* has a distinct variation that is important in diagnosis, disease state, and characterization of the organism.[21] This variation relates to changes in the surface LPS of *C burnetii* that is environmentally influenced. The virulent strain is known as phase I. The avirulent phase II strain is seen only after serial passage in the laboratory. Differences in amino acid content, sugar moieties, immunogenic protein presentation, cell size, cell density, and resistance to phagocytosis are recognized between phases.[20,22] LPS subtypes (smooth, S-LPS, and rough, R-LPS) are described for both phase I and phase II. Mutational shifts from smooth to rough correlate with decreasing virulence. *Coxiella burnetii* also contains an endogenous plasmid that can integrate with the genome. Plasmid type and LPS subtypes appear to be associated with different clinical syndromes.[4,23]

A recent classification is based on review of more than 34 banked isolates using recombinant DNA techniques. Genomic restriction fragment length polymorphisms (RFLP) after BamH1 restriction endonuclease digest and polyacrylamide gel electrophoresis (PAGE) revealed approximately six distinct groups. These groups allow characterization based on genomic hybridization, plasmid type, LPS variants, genome mapping, disease entity, and animal virulence.[4]

Although difficult to grow and isolate routinely, *C burnetii* has historically been cultivated using chicken embryo or inoculation into whole animals. *Coxiella burnetii* grows in cell cultures of chick embryo, mouse embryo fibroblasts (L929), kidneys of African green monkeys, tick tissue, and macrophage-like tumor cell lines.[20]

GEOGRAPHIC DISTRIBUTION

Worldwide in its distribution, Q fever is considered globally enzootic. Marrie[24] and others[1,11,25] have documented that Q fever is on every continent. *Coxiella burnetii* has an extremely diverse host range with disparate cycles of transmission, leading to a plethora of infected species in varied habitats.[1,11,13,24,25] Aerosols are the primary mode of transmission and arthropod vectors, including *Acarina, Anoplura,* mites, *Diptera, Hemiptera,* and *Siphonaptera* families of arthropods are a secondary mode of transmission,[4] although annelid, poikilotherm, and other homiotherm reservoirs have been described.[4,22,24,26,27] The host–microorganism interaction enhances a complicated cycle of transmission in nature.

LIFE CYCLE, NATURAL HISTORY, AND EPIDEMIOLOGY

Coxiella burnetii is maintained in nature through an animal–tick cycle. The primary reservoirs are ixodid and argasid ticks in which *C burnetii* is in all stages of the tick life cycle—adult, egg, larva, and nymph. This ensures life cycles in rodents, larger animals, and birds. Water contaminated by feces of infected large animals can also support growth of this organism, primarily through replication of *C burnetii* in, and continued excretion by, the common leach *Hirudo medicinalis* in the United States.[15,27]

Dermacenter andersoni, the Rocky Mountain wood tick, was first identified as a carrier of *C burnetii.*[3] Other arthropods, rodents, wild mammals, and birds act as the permanent hosts and are naturally infected and may play a role in the domestic animal and human infection.[4]

Humans are a dead-end host for *C burnetii.* Transmission is by direct contact, airborne, or vectorborne routes from its diverse range of reservoir hosts. *Coxiella burnetii* infects a wide range of animals and insects, yet causes little if any disease among them. The low pathogenicity of *C burnetii* for these animal reservoirs allows it to prevail.[1,4] Because these animals secrete *C burnetii* and because the spores of *C burnetii* are stable in the environment, outbreaks of Q fever predominate where domestic animals are abundant.[1,11,25,28] This may be caused by the concentration and persistence of *C burnetii* in feces, urine, milk, and tissues (especially the placenta) of domestic animals (Figures 82–1 and 82–2), allowing fomites and infective aerosols to form easily. This route—domestic animals to man—is the cause of urban outbreaks.[11,29–34] Pet owners exposed to newborn or stillborn animals are at high risk. This is an occupational hazard for those in contact with domestic animals or their products.[1,4,20,35] Transmission by inhalation of infected aerosols and by ingestion of raw milk has been documented. Sheep, cattle, and goats are the principal mammalian reservoirs of human infection[36]; otherwise humans rarely acquire Q fever from arthropod bites. It is more likely that airborne inhalation of feces rich in *C burnetii* from infected arthropods is a route of infection.

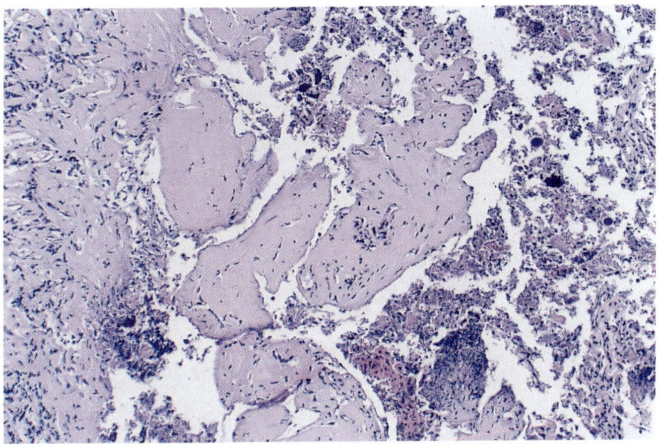

Figure 82–1. Placenta illustrating a necrotizing subacute, diffuse, severe placentitis from a spontaneous abortion in a pygmy goat (hematoxylin-eosin, ×100). *(Contributed by Dr Bruce Williams, AFIP Registry of Veterinary Pathology, Washington, DC.)*

Transmission is facilitated by the stability of this agent in the environment. Its extremely long biologic half-life and resistance to temperature, desiccation, osmotic shock, ultraviolet light, and chemical disinfectants is a function of its spore-forming ability.[1,27,37,38] The environmental stability and the variable antigenic forms expressed while *C burnetii* grows in phagolysosomes of cells of the host prevent immune responses and account for airborne transmission as the primary mode of dissemination. Inhalation of particulate microorganisms causes systemic spread, eventually localizing to the placenta and mammary glands. Animals shed *C burnetii* in all bodily fluids and harbor organisms in almost all tissue types. At time of parturition, placental tissue may contain as many as 10^9 bacilli per gram of tissue (Figures 82–1 and 82–2). Contaminated wool, feces, and other animal by-products also can carry this *Rickettsia.*

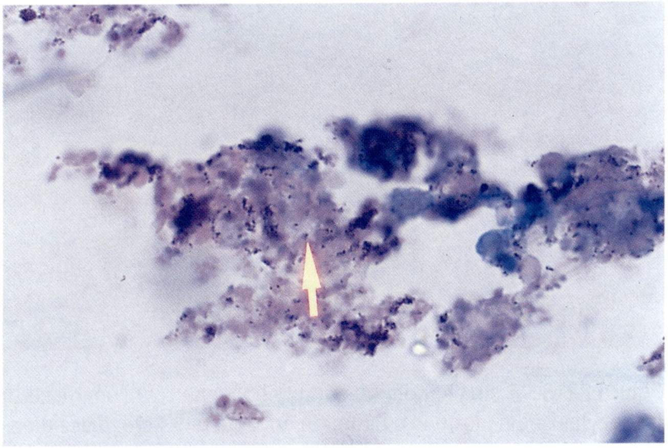

Figure 82–2. Giemsa stain of goat abortive placenta. Note the numerous intracytoplasmic organisms of *C burnetii* (Giemsa stain, ×1000). *(Contributed by Dr Bruce Williams, AFIP Registry of Veterinary Pathology, Washington, DC.)*

CLINICAL DISEASE

Exposure to *C burnetii* frequently leads to asymptomatic or mild illness. In a population that seroconverted, only 50% had clinical disease.[20,39] Clinically apparent infections by *C burnetii* are described as acute or chronic Q fever.[6]

Symptoms and signs in acute Q fever are variable and are related to dose, strain of *C burnetii,* route of infection, host immune status, and age.[40] The incubation period varies from 9 to 28 days (average 18 to 30 days). An abrupt onset of fever may reach 40°C in 2 to 4 days and persist to 3 to 6 weeks in an undulating biphasic pattern. A bifrontal headache with severe retrobulbar pain, malaise, anorexia, myalgia, chills, sweats, and occasional chest pains accompany the acute febrile stage. Rarely there is a rash. Pulmonary Q fever is bronchitis with "atypical pneumonitis" often associated with a nonproductive cough and sore throat. Also present are acute hepatitis with hepatomegaly, splenomegaly, and elevated liver enzymes and gastrointestinal disturbances.[41]

Less commonly, acute Q fever is associated with encephalitis, encephalomyelitis, optic neuritis, thyroiditis, myocarditis, pericarditis, lesions of bone marrow, hemolytic anemia, polyarthritis, pancreatitis, and disorders of the genitals.[20]

The most serious, although uncommon, complication of chronic Q fever is subacute endocarditis. Symptoms are slow in onset, sometimes 1 to 20 years after exposure. Typical signs are consistent with aortic and mitral valve dysfunction. They include fever, cardiac failure, splenomegaly, elevated liver enzymes, hematuria, hypergammaglobulinemia, petechiae, digital clubbing, and/or arterial embolisms. The aortic valve alone is most commonly infected. Second is the mitral valve alone and third is infection of both aortic and mitral valves. Unique to Q fever endocarditis is repeated negative blood cultures. Approximately one third of the patients with chronic Q fever may also have chronic hepatitis. In addition, chronic Q fever polyarthritis, valvular graft disease, osteomyelitis, and uterine infections are described.[20,39]

Perinatal Q fever is rare but *C burnetii* has been demonstrated in human placenta and breast milk with antibodies in breast milk and fetal cord blood. No abortifacient or teratogenic alterations have been attributed to this organism.[4,20]

PATHOLOGY

Mortality is low and there are few autopsy studies of *C burnetii* infection in man. In fatal Q fever there is lobar consolidation that resembles bacterial pneumonia. Histologic changes, however, are more consistent with a histiocytic infiltrate as seen with psittacosis and certain viral pneumonias. There is an intense interstitial infiltrate about bronchioles and vasculature that extends into adjacent alveolar walls. Plasma cells are numerous. The lumens of bronchioles may contain neutrophils. Alveolar lining cells are swollen and the alveoli contain desquamated lining cells and large mononuclear cells. This lobar pneumonia may be particularly severe in aged, debilitated, or immunodeficient patients.[20,42]

Biopsy specimens of liver and bone marrow from patients with hepatitis or osteomyelitis have diffuse granulomatous changes. Granulomas may be nonspecific and unorganized (Figure 82–3) or may exhibit classic "doughnut" granulomas of Q fever. The term "doughnut-type" granuloma has been used to describe these lesions.[41] They have a central empty space, rimmed by neutrophils and epithelioid cells and are surrounded by eosinophilic fibrinoid material (Figures 82–4 and 82–5). These central spaces may be accumulations of immunoglobin proteins in response to *C burnetii.* These granulomas have no elastic or basement membrane components. *Coxiella burnetii* may be identified in these granulomas by immunofluorescence or immunohistochemistry. Other changes include decreases in myeloid series, necrosis, and hemophagocytosis by histiocytes.[43]

Chronic valvular endocarditis is primarily associated with preexisting valvular disease or prosthetic valves and only rarely with normal valves. Native valves may have perforations, small pale yellow and brown vegetations and small nodular calcifications. Prosthetics have vegetative inflammatory responses associated with the valve material and surfaces.[20]

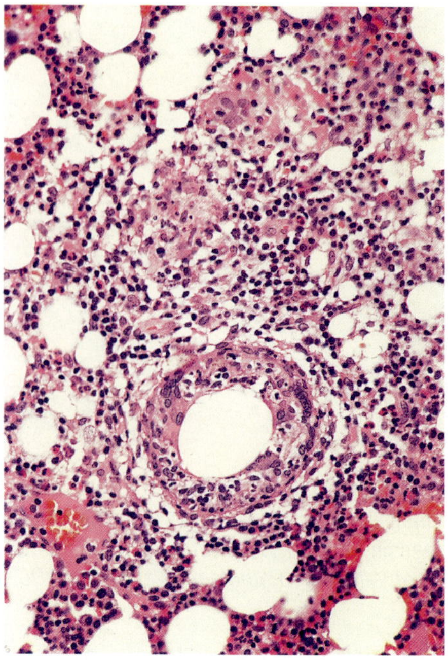

Figure 82–4. Bone marrow with lipid and trilinear cellular elements. There is a background of granulomatous inflammation containing a characteristic "doughnut-like" structure that is sharply circumscribed and composed of epithelioid cells, giant cells, and neutrophils (hematoxylin-eosin, ×400). *(Contributed by Dr William Travis, AFIP Washington, DC.)*

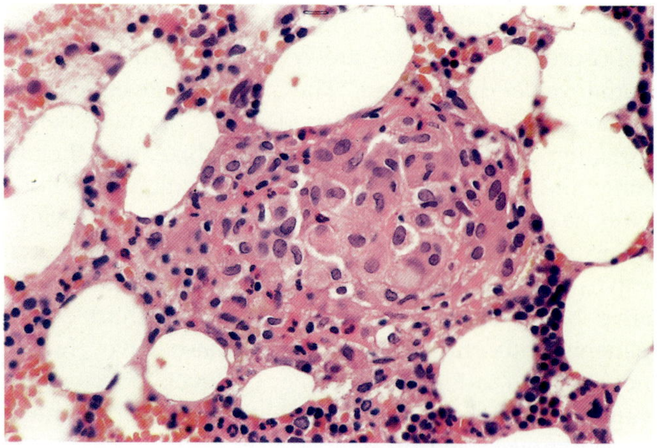

Figure 82–3. Large focal unorganized granuloma in bone marrow. Note clusters of macrophages with some evidence of conversion to epithelioid cells and giant cells (hematoxylin-eosin, ×400). *(Contributed by Dr William Travis, AFIP, Washington, DC.)*

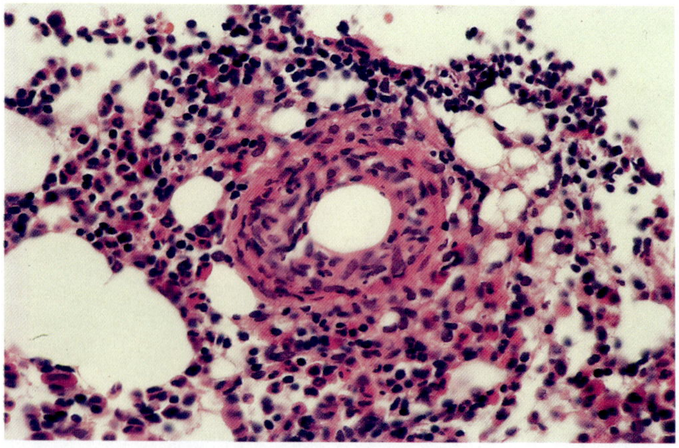

Figure 82–5. A small granuloma in the bone marrow comprised of histiocytes and neutrophils. Although not apparent here, these granulomas form around a lipid droplet, suggesting that the response is to *C burnetii* antigens expressed on the cell surface (hematoxylin-eosin, ×400). *(Contributed by Dr William Travis, AFIP Washington, DC.)*

The necrosis is presumed to be caused by *C burnetii* entering the phagolysosomes of cells, replicating and rupturing the cell, leading to lysosomal release and adjacent destruction.[44]

DIFFERENTIAL DIAGNOSIS

Acute Q fever imitates many infections (eg, influenza, other viral infections, salmonellosis, malaria, hepatitis, brucellosis, and so forth). Later stages mimic bacterial, viral, and mycoplasmal pneumonias. Differential diagnosis of chronic Q fever hepatitis should include other infections of liver that cause granulomas, including tuberculosis, sarcoidosis, histoplasmosis, brucellosis, tularemia, and syphilis.[42] Other diseases that may be confused with the fibrin-ring ("doughnut") granulomas are visceral leishmaniasis, boutonneuse fever, toxoplasmosis, Hodgkin's disease, allopurinol hypersensitivity, and hepatitis A.[43,44]

DIAGNOSIS

Diagnosis is made by clinical suspicion and demonstration of phase I antibodies in the patient's serum. History of exposure to animals, animal products, and/or ticks is an important clue. Unlike other rickettsial diseases, Q fever is not associated with cutaneous exanthems nor does it agglutinate *Proteus* strains (negative Weil–Felix reaction). The organism is identifiable in tracheal washes using modified Ziehl–Neelsen or Macchiavello stains.[17] Antibodies in human sera have been detected against both phase I and II antigens using indirect immunofluorescence.[45] Differentiation between immune responses to either phase I or phase II antigens has been demonstrated with Western immunoblotting[46] and culture using the L929 immortalized fibroblast cell line.[47] *Coxiella burnetii* can be isolated from the blood. Specific complement fixating and agglutinating antibodies appear during convalescence. Immunofluorescence techniques, including enzyme-linked immunosorbent assay (ELISA), are the current choice for detecting specific antibodies. Antibodies against phase II antigens reflect exposure to acute Q fever strains. Phase I organisms rarely produce detectable antibodies in human sera but when present, they reflect chronic Q fever. Recently, restriction fragment length polymorphisms and polymerase chain reaction techniques have been used to detect infection. Specifically, oligonucleotide primers derived from the *Qp*HI plasmid gene sequence identified *C burnetii* in human heart valve and liver (frozen and paraffin-embedded), sheep placenta, and in sheep amniotic fluid and blood.[26,47–51] Both high-voltage and transmission electronmicroscopy have been used to demonstrate *C burnetii* in cell culture[47] and fixed heart valves, respectively.[50]

PREVENTION

Q fever is a proven occupational hazard for personnel working in the livestock and meat processing industry, in small and large animal clinics, and in medical research laboratories. In addition, both pet owners and hunters are at risk.[4,49] Prevention is by blocking animal-to-man transmission: Milk should be pasteurized; dust controlled in affected industries; education of those at risk; and animal placentas, animal feces, and urine should be incinerated. Hospitalized patients with Q fever should be isolated and their sputum and urine autoclaved. Serologic surveillance and vaccination of animals and man in endemic areas reduce the frequency of shedding. Immunization of humans with high occupational risk is recommended.[49] A vaccine against phase 1 Henzerling strain rickettsiae is effective and should be used to protect those at risk in slaughterhouses, dairies, vivaria, rendering plants, and sheep herders, woolsorters, and farmers.[30] Recent studies have focused on safety and vaccines with more specific subunit immunogenic fractions of phase I *C burnetii*.[17,46] These include a chloroform-methanol extraction residue vaccine for Q fever. Expanded clinical research on these preparations should help elucidate their future applicability. Because prior exposure may lead to severe localized reactions with formalin-inactivated whole-cell vaccine preparations, prior immunologic screening is recommended. These vaccines, although not commercially available in the United States, may be obtained from specialty laboratories, eg, U.S. Army Medical Research Institute of Infectious Diseases in Frederick, Maryland, or from Australia, to be used under an investigational new drug (IND) protocol.[16,35]

TREATMENT

Treatment is consistent with other rickettsial infections. Tetracyclines and doxycycline are effective. In acute disease, treat until the patient has been afebrile for at least 5 days. Recent literature indicates that a 2-week therapeutic regimen of doxycycline is sufficient.[42] Patients with chronic Q fever warrant long-term chemotherapy usually with rifampin and doxycycline. Preferred therapy for patients with endocarditis is long-term tetracyclines. If antibiotic therapy is only partially effective, damaged valves may be surgically replaced although there are reports of cures without surgical intervention. Clear-cut regimens for chronic hepatitis or polyarthritis have not been determined.

REFERENCES

1. Weiss E, Williams JC, Thompson HA, eds. The place of *Coxiella burnetii* in the microbiological world. In: *Q Fever: The Biology of Coxiella burnetii.* Boca Raton, Fla: CRC Press; 1991:1–10.
2. Derrick EH. "Q" fever, a new fever entity: clinical features, diagnosis, and laboratory investigation. *Med J Aust.* 1937; 2:281–289.
3. Cox HR. Studies of a filter passing infectious agent isolated from ticks. V. Further attempts to cultivate in cell-free media suggested classification. *Public Health Rep.* 1939;54:1822–1827.
4. Williams JC, Sanchez V. Q fever and coxiellosis. In: Beran GW, ed. *Handbook of Zoonoses.* Boca Raton, Fla: CRC Press; 1994:429–446.
5. Lang GH. Coxiellosis. (Q Fever) in animals. In: Marrie TJ, ed. *Q Fever, Vol. 1, The Disease.* Boca Raton, Fla: CRC Press; 1990:23–27.
6. Derrick EH. *Rickettsia burnetii:* the cause of "Q" fever. *Med J Aust.* 1939;1:14–19.
7. Burnet FM, Freeman M. Experimental studies of the virus of "Q" fever. *Med J Aust.* 1937;2:299–305.
8. Smith DJW, Derrick EH. Studies in the epidemiology of Q fever. I. The isolation of six strains of *Rickettsia burnetii* form the tick *Haemaphysalis humerosa. Aust J Exp Biol Med Sci.* 1940;18:1–19.
9. Cox HR. A filter passing infectious agent isolated from ticks. III. Descriptions of organism and cultivation experiments. *Public Health Rep.* 1983;53:2270.
10. Davis GE, Cox AR. A filter passing infectious agent isolated from ticks I. Isolation from *Dermacentor andersoni:* reactions in animals and filtration experiments. *Public Health Rep.* 1938;53:2270–2278.
11. Berge TO, Lennette EH. World distribution of Q fever: human, animal and anthropod infection. *Am J Hyg.* 1953;57:125–139.
12. Stoker MGP, Fiset P. Phase variation of the Nine Mile and other strain of *Rickettsia burnetii. Can J Microbiol.* 1956; 2:310–321.
13. Fiset P. Phase variation of *Rickettsia (Coxiella) burnetii;* a study of antibody response in guinea pigs and rabbits. *Can J Microbiol.* 1957;3:435.
14. McDade JE. Historical aspects of Q fever. In: Marrie TJ, ed. *Q Fever, Vol 1, The Disease.* Boca Raton, Fla: CRC Press; 1990:5–25.
15. Rehacek J, Tarasevich IV. Q fever: *Coxiella burnetii.* In Rehacek J, Tarasevich IV, eds. *Acari-borne Rickettsiae and Rickettsiosis in Eurasia.* Bratslavia: VDEA Publishing; 1988:204–215.
16. Behymer D, Riemann HP. *Coxiella burnetii* infection (Q fever), zoonosis update. *JAVMA.* 1989;194:764–766.
17. Jubb KVF, Kennedy PC, Palmer N, eds. The female genital system: diseases of the pregnant uterus. In: *Pathology of Domestic Animals.* 3rd ed. San Diego: Academic Press; 1985;3:355–357.
18. Hackstadt T, Williams JC. Biochemical strategem for obligate parasitism of Eukaryotic cells by *Coxiella burnetii. Proc Natl Acad Sci USA.* 1981;78:3240–3244.
19. McCaul TF, Williams JC, eds. Localization of DNA in *Coxiella burnetii* by post-embedding immunoelectron microscopy. *Ann NY Acad Sci.* 1990;590:136–147.
20. Reimer LG. Q fever. *Clin Microbiol Rev.* 1993;6:193–198.
21. Amano KI, Williams JC, Missler R, Reinhold VR. Structure and biological relationship of *Coxiella burnetii* lipopolysaccharides. *J Biol Chem.* 1980;262:4740–4746.
22. Shurong Y. *Coxiella burnetii* in China. In: Williams JC, Thompson HA, eds. *Q Fever: The Biology of Coxiella burnetii.* Boca Raton, Fla: CRC Press; 1991:327–338.
23. Sammuel JE, Frazier ME, Mallavia LP. Correlation of plasmid type and disease caused by *Coxiella burnetii. Infect Immun.* 1985;49:775–779.
24. Marrie TJ. Epidemiology of Q fever. In: Marrie TJ, ed. *Q Fever Vol 1. The Disease.* Boca Raton, Fla: CRC Press; 1990: 49–61.
25. Stoker MGP, Fiset P. The spread of Q fever from animal to man: the natural history of *Rickettsia burnetii. Can. J Microbiol.* 1956;2:310–321.
26. Waag DM, Williams JC, Peacock MG, Raoult HD. Methods of isolation, amplification, and purification of *Coxiella burnetii* in Q fever etc. In: Williams JC, Thompson HA, eds. *Q Fever: The Biology of Coxiella burnetii.* Boca Raton, Fla: CRC Press; 1991:73–95.
27. Williams JC. Infectivity, virulence and pathogenicity of *C burnetii* for various hosts in Q fever. In: Williams JC, Thompson HA, eds. *The Biology of Coxiella burnetii.* Boca Raton, Fla: CRC Press; 1991:21–45.
28. Kaplar MM, Bertagna P. The geographical distribution of Q fever. *Bull WHO.* 1955;13:829–834.
29. Embil J, Williams JC, Marrie TJ. The immune response in a cat-related outbreak of Q fever measured by indirect immunofluorescence and ELISA. *Can J Microbiol.* 1990; 36:292.
30. Dupont HT, Raoult D, Brouqui P, et al. Epidemiologic features of clinical presentation of acute Q fever. *Am J Med.* 1992;93:427–434.
31. Langly JM, Marrie TJ, Covert A, Waas DM, Williams JC. Poker player's pneumonia. An urban outbreak of Q fever following exposure to a parturient cat. *N Engl J Med.* 1988;319:354–361.
32. Marrie TJ, Durant H, Williams JC, Mintz E, Waas DM. Exposure to parturient cats: a risk factor for acquisition of Q fever in maritime Canada. *J Infect Dis.* 1988;158: 101–106.
33. Marrie TJ, Langille D, Papkuna V, Yates L. Tracking pneumonia, an outbreak of Q fever in a truck repair plant due to aerosols from clothing contaminated by contact with newborn kittens. *Epidemiol Infect.* 1989;102:119–123.
34. Pinsky RL, Fishbein DB, Greene CR, Gensheimer KF. An outbreak of cat associated Q fever in the United States. *J Infect Dis.* 1991;162:202–208.
35. Q fever. In: Fraser CM, ed. *The Merck Veterinary Manual.* 7th ed. Rahway, NJ: Merck & Co; 1993:386–388.

36. Babaderi B. Q fever a zoonosis. *Adv Vet Sci.* 1959;5: 81–154.
37. Scott GH, Williams JC. Susceptibility of *Coxiella burnetii* to chemical disinfectants. *Ann NY Acad Sci.* 1990;590: 291–296.
38. Thompson HA, Williams JC. Ph and membrane physiology in *Coxiella burnetii.* In: *Q Fever: The Biology of Coxiella burnetii.* Boca Raton, Fla: CRC Press; 1991:117–127.
39. Baca OG, Paretsky D. Q fever and *Coxiella burnetii:* a model for host parasite interactions. *Microbiol Rev.* 1983; 47:127–149.
40. Raoult D. Host factors in the severity of Q fever. *Ann NY Acad Sci.* 1990;33–37.
41. Travis LB, Travis WA, Li LY, Pierre RV. Q fever: a clinicopathologic study of five cases. *Arch Pathol Lab Med.* 1986;110:1017–1020.
42. Q-fever. In: Berkow R, ed. *The Merck Manual of Diagnosis and Therapy,* 16th ed. Rahway, NJ: Merck & Co. 1992: 177–178.
43. Marazuela M, Moreno A, Yebra M, Cerezo E, Gomez-Gesto C, Vargas JA. Hepatic fibrin-ring granulomas: a clinicopathologic study of 23 patients. *Hum Pathol.* 1991;22: 607–613.
44. Ruel M, Sevestre H, Henny-Biaband E, Couroace AM, Capron JP, Erlinger S. Fibrin-ring granulomas in hepatitis A. *Digestive Dis Sci.* 1992;37:1915–1917.
45. Htwe KK, Yoshida T, Hayashi S, et al. Prevalence of antibodies to *Coxiella burnetii* in Japan. *J Clin Microbiol.* 1993;31:722–723.
46. Blondeu JM, Williams JC, Marrie TJ. The immune response to phase I and phase II coxiella antigens as measured by Western immunoblotting. *Ann NY Acad Sci.* 1990;590:187–202.
47. Hechemy KE, McKee M, Marko M, Sampsonoff WA, Roman M, Baca O. Three dimensional reconstruction of *Coxiella burnetii* infected L929 cells by high voltage electron microscopy. *Infect Immun.* 1993;61:4485–4488.
48. Stein A, Raoult D. Detection of *Coxiella burnetii* by DNA amplification using polymerase chain reaction. *Clin Microbiol.* 1992;30:2462–2466.
49. Williams JC, Peacock MG, Wang DM, et al. Vaccines against coxiellosis and Q fever. *Ann NY Acad Sci.* 1990; 590:88–108.
50. McCaul TF, Dare AJ, Gannon JP, Galbreth AJ. In vivo endogenous spore formation by *Coxiella burnetii* in Q fever endocarditis. *J Clin Pathol.* 1994;47:978–981.
51. Ernel R, Rindell L, Wallace C, Griffey S, Chomel B, Brooks D. Detection of *Coxiella burnetii* by DNA amplification using polymerase chain reaction. Applications for control of Q fever in sheep research. *Cont Topics-AALAS.* 1995; 35:26.

Chapter 83

Relapsing Fever

Isam A. Eltoum and Michael Lewin-Smith

Either socialism will defeat the louse or the louse will defeat socialism.

Vladimir Ilyich Lenin (1870–1924)

It is not the function of our government to keep the citizen from falling into error; it is the function of the citizens to keep the government from falling into error.

Robert H. Jackson (1892–1954)

DEFINITION

The relapsing fevers (louse-borne relapsing fever, tick-borne relapsing fever, recurrent fever, sweating sickness, famine fever) are a complex of acute infections caused by spirochetes of the genus *Borrelia* and characterized by episodes of fever separated by apyrexial intervals. The disease is transmitted to vertebrates by lice or ticks.

HISTORY

Relapsing fever was known to the ancient civilizations of Greece and Egypt. It was recorded by Hippocrates in Thasos as "ardent fever."[1] In the period from 1843 to 1848, Criagie and Henderson used the term *relapsing fever* to differentiate this febrile illness from typhus.[1] David Livingstone in 1857 described "tick disease," which was thought by Africans to be transmitted by ticks.[2] In 1868, Otto Obermeier discovered spirochetes in the blood of a patient with relapsing fever.[3] Munch who inoculated himself with infected blood and developed the disease in 1874, investigated bedbugs and fleas as possible vectors.[4] In 1904, Dutton and Todd described infection of the tick *Ornithodoros moubata* by spirochetes.[1] In 1907, Mackie suggested lice as the possible vectors.[2] In the first half of this century, more than 50 million people were affected worldwide. There were epidemics in Europe, Asia, and Africa during World War II. During the Russian revolution, Lenin said in reference to relapsing fever "either socialism will defeat the louse or the louse will defeat socialism."[5]

While socialism was perhaps successful in defeating lice in Russia, it failed in Sudan and Ethiopia where the last known epidemics of louse-borne fever occurred, respectively, in 1974 and 1988–1991 during socialist regimes.[6–8] Today, small foci of endemic tick-borne relapsing fever exist throughout the world, with the exception of Australia, New Zealand, and parts of the Pacific (Figure 83–1). Like the disease itself, interest in relapsing fever has relapsed and remitted. The discovery of *Borrelia burgdorferi* as the cause of Lyme disease has recently revived interest in *Borrelia,* including the agents of relapsing fever.

CAUSATIVE ORGANISM

Members of the genus *Borrelia* are gram-negative, and from 0.2 to 0.5 μm by 3 to 30 μm.[9] The organism belongs to the genus *Borrelia,* which belong to the family Spirochaetaceae in the bacterial order Spirochaetales. Spirochetes, unlike eubacteria, are helically shaped and have flagella that originate in the tip of the protoplasm and lie between an outer and inner membrane. Within the spirochetes, *Borrelia* was classified as a genus because they are transmitted by hematophagous arthropods. They are further classified into species by the susceptibility of arthropod vectors. Lice

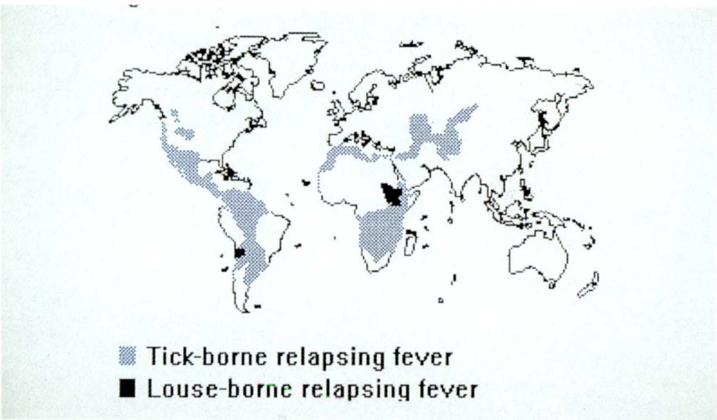

Figure 83–1. Global distribution of relapsing fever.

transmit *B recurrentis,* which causes louse-borne relapsing fever (LBRF), whereas argasid ticks transmit *B hermsii, B turcatae, B parkeri,* and *B duttoni,* which cause tick-borne relapsing fever (TBRF). Hard-shell ticks transmit *B burgdorferi,* which causes Lyme disease.

GEOGRAPHIC DISTRIBUTION

The relapsing fevers have been historically ubiquitous. Presently, tick-borne relapsing fever is seen in rural environments of less than 2000 m in elevation, corresponding to the habitats of the argasid vectors (soft ticks) of the genus *Ornithodoros.* Louse-borne relapsing fever is geographically unrestricted but most infections are now in the mountains of East Africa, especially Ethiopia (Figure 83–1 and Table 83–1).

EPIDEMIOLOGY

Epidemiologic differences divide relapsing fever into louse- and tick-borne varieties (Table 83–1). Transmission of louse-borne fever is epidemic. Outbreaks follow disastrous events such as wars, famine, and floods when overcrowding, malnutrition, and poor personal hygiene are widespread.[10,11] The body louse, *Pediculus humanus corporis* (Figure 83–2), and, rarely, the head louse, *Pediculus humanus capitis,* become infected by feeding on patients with relapsing fever. There is no known reservoir except humans. The organism crosses the gut of the arthropod to reach the hemocele where it multiplies. Because the microorganism does not remain in the insect's gut or infect its salivary glands, uncomplicated louse bites do not transmit relapsing fever. The disease occurs when an infected louse is crushed over breaks in the epidermis causing contamination with the louse hemolymph. After an incubation period of approximately 1 week, the disease starts with fever that relapses and remits, and if untreated, progresses to death in up to 70% of patients.[12,13] Because *Borrelia* are not transmitted transovarially in the louse, epidemics of LBRF are self-limited.

In tick-borne relapsing fever the *Borrelia* are acquired by the argasid vectors more commonly from small mammals (the natural reservoir) than from humans. TBRF is endemic in certain areas depending on the habitat of the vector. In Africa for example, ticks are present in dwellings year-round and therefore, transmission of infection is continuous. On the other hand, in mountainous areas of the United States such as Colorado, relapsing fever is seen during the summer when rodents infested with ticks come out of hibernation and contact large numbers of human visitors.[14–16] Because of the limited mobility of the argasid vectors, TBRF is usually endemic and is often a "place disease."

Ticks become infected by feeding on infected rodents. *Borrelia* survive in the tick because the tick's gut has no extracellular digestive mechanisms.[17] *Borrelia* are taken up with a blood meal, enter the enterocytes, and then penetrate to reach the hemocele where they multiply and spread to invade the salivary glands, ganglia, and ovaries or testes.[9] Ticks remain infected for life. They transmit *Borrelia* to mammals during feeding,

TABLE 83–1. SPECIES, VECTORS, HOSTS, AND GEOGRAPHIC DISTRIBUTION OF ARTHROPOD-BORNE FEVER

***Borrelia* sp**	**Vector**	**Reservoir**	**Distribution**	**Disease**
B recurrentis	*P humanus*	Humans	Worldwide	LBRF, epidemic
B duttoni	*O moubata*	Humans	Africa	TBRF, East African
B hispanica	*O erraticus*	Rodents	North Africa	TBRF, Hispano-African
B crocidurae	*O erraticus*	Rodents	North Africa	TBRF, North African
B persica	*O tholozani*	Rodents	Asia	TBRF, Asiatic-African
B caucasica	*O verrucosus*	Rodents	Asia	TBRF, Caucasian
B hermsii	*O hermsii*	Rodents	Western United States	TBRF, American
B turcatae	*O turcatae*	Rodents	Southwestern United States	TBRF, American
B parkeri	*O parkeri*	Rodents	Western United States	TBRF, American
B venzuelensis	*O rudis*	Rodents	South America	TBRF, American

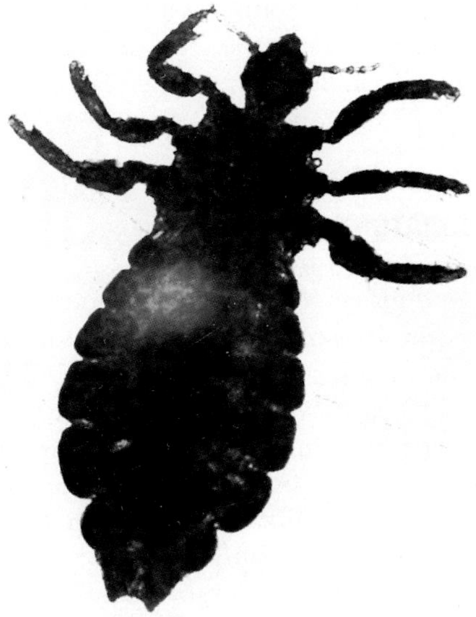

Figure 83–2. *Pediculus humanus corporis,* the vector of louse-borne relapsing fever.

to tick offspring transovarially, and, rarely, from male to female tick venereally. Unlike LBRF, trauma to the tick is not required for infection. Infection is mediated by contamination of the tick bite with its saliva or the fluid of the coxal gland (a special organ that excretes excess fluid and solute). Humans are infected inadvertently and play no role in the maintenance of the life cycle of tick-borne *Borrelia.*

CLINICAL FEATURES

The two varieties of relapsing fever are clinically and histopathologically indistinguishable. LBRF tends to be a more severe disease. The illness begins abruptly and affects multiple organs.[8,14,16,18] The cardinal signs are high fever (94% to 100% of patients), chills (76%), and headache (69%). Other nonspecific symptoms include prostration, myalgia, arthralgia (69%), nausea (60%), vomiting (40%), and abdominal pain (60%). Nonproductive cough (40%) and epitaxis are also common (25%). Bleeding in sites such as brain, gastrointestinal tract, and urinary tract may be profound and fatal when there is intracranial hemorrhage.

On examination, patients usually look ill with alteration in the sensorium. They have high fever (39 to 40°C) and 66% have tachycardia. About 50% have meningism or icterus. Ten to 60% of patients have a fleeting pleomorphic skin rash. Splenomegaly and hepatomegaly, often with tenderness, are common. After several relapses of TBRF, some patients have iritis and iridocyclitis.[16] Ten percent have pneumonia. Abortion and/or premature labor is reported in up to 49% of women with relapsing fever; some live-born infants have congenital relapsing fever.[19] Neurologic complications resembling the neurologic complications of Lyme disease have been reported. Some have suggested that *Borrelia* are a causal factor in multiple sclerosis.[20,21]

The initial episode lasts 6 to 9 days, with an apyrexial interval of 4 to 7 days before the next bout of illness (Table 83–2). Subsequent relapses tend to be less severe.[16] Spontaneous and therapeutically induced remissions are attended by a febrile crisis that is identical to the Jarisch–Herxheimer reaction. Transient chills, fever, profuse sweating, tachycardia, and hypertension are followed by severe prolonged hypothermia, hypotension, and bradycardia. Murmurs and gallop rhythm corroborate the clinical impression of myocarditis.

The diagnosis of relapsing fever depends on the epidemiologic setting, clinical picture, and laboratory findings. The differential diagnosis in areas of LBRF include any acute febrile illness, especially malaria, kala-azar, typhoid fever, and typhus. In areas of TBRF, the differential diagnosis includes Colorado tick fever, juvenile rheumatoid arthritis, tularemia, Lyme disease, and brucellosis.[15]

LABORATORY DIAGNOSIS

Borrelia are demonstrable in thick or thin blood films taken during the febrile stage. They stain blue by Romanowsky stains (Wright–Giemsa, Diff-Quik, and Field's stain) (Figure 83–3).[22] They stain negatively with Gram's stain, and black with Dieterle's silver stain.[23] Acridine orange stain is rapid and more sensitive than Romanowsky methods for detecting low-level spiro-

TABLE 83–2. CLINICAL FEATURES OF RELAPSING FEVER

Clinical Feature	TBRF	LBRF
Sex = male	60%	40%
Age <20	Majority	Minority
Incubation period	7 days	Not available
Duration of febrile attack	3.1 days	5.5
Duration of afebrile period	6.8 days	9.3
Duration of relapse	2.5 days	1.9
Number of relapses	3.0	1.0
Temperature		99%
Chill		83%
Body pain and aches		50%
Splenomegaly	41%	77%
Hepatomegaly	17–18%	66%
Jaundice	7%	36%
Rash	28%	8%
Respiratory symptoms	16%	Not available
CNS involvement	9%	30%

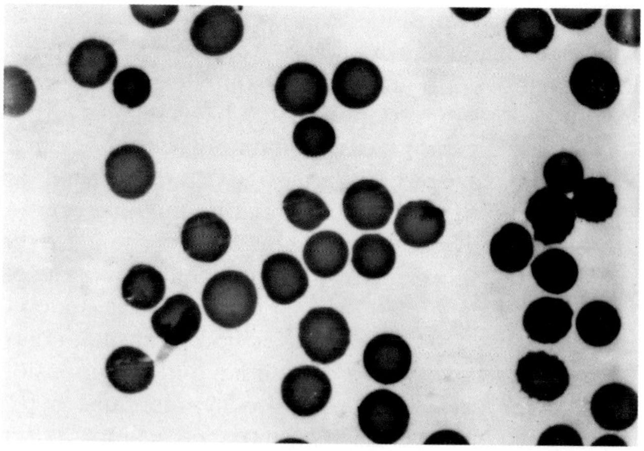

Figure 83–3. *Borrelia recurrentis* spirochetes are in the blood during febrile stages (AFIP Neg 75-6873; thin blood film stained with Giemsa, ×2000).

chetemia.[24] A wet preparation, one drop of blood and sodium citrate, examined under phase contrast microscopy is a simple way of demonstrating the organism. In tissue sections, the organisms are easily seen when blackened with silver impregnation stains.

In the past, animal inoculation was used for the isolation and propagation of the organism. Kelly's medium, however, or its modification, the Barbour–Stoenner–Kelly (BSK) II, are now used for isolating even one organism.[25,26] Cryopreservation is used routinely for storing and maintaining *Borrelia* in specialized laboratories.

The cumbersome xenodiagnosis, which exploits the *Borrelia*–vector specificity to classify the organisms, is now superseded by molecular techniques that are specific, sensitive, and easy to perform compared to xenodiagnosis.

Pulse field electrophoresis of DNA shows a profile of plasmid and chromosome patterns that distinguishes the different species of *Borrelia.*[27] Plasmid profiles for different isolates, however, may change over prolonged culture.[28] Amplification of an internal sequence in the flagellin gene using polymerase chain reaction and detection of the product with a specific probe are specific and sensitive in detection of *B hermsii.*[29] DNA–DNA hybridization and analysis of 16 rRNA sequences were used for the taxonomic classification of *Borrelia* in general.[30,31] The results of these methods show that some *Borrelia,* such as *B turcatae, B hermsii,* and *B parkeri* may not be separate species.

The fatty acid methyl ester (FAME) profile of *B hermsii* is different than *B turcatae* and *B parkeri.*[32] Detection of antibodies raised against the organism using immunofluorescence and enzyme immunoassay is neither specific nor sensitive. Sera from patients with relapsing fever react strongly with antigens of *B burgdorferi.*[27] On the other hand, the detection of flagellar antigen, with monoclonal antibody (H9826), is specific for *B hermsii.*[33]

OTHER LABORATORY FINDINGS

Moderate anemia is common. The peripheral blood leukocyte count is usually normal except for a leukopenia during febrile episodes. The erythrocyte sedimentation rate (ESR) is elevated. Thrombocytopenia and a prolonged bleeding time and partial prothrombin time are common.[6,16,18] There may be reduced levels of factor V and elevated fibrin degradation products. Derangement of renal function is seen especially in LBRF. Serum glutamic-oxalacetic transaminase (SGOT) and lactic dehydrogenase (LDH) are elevated. Serum albumin is reduced while globulins and bilirubin are raised. Urinary urobilinogen is increased in the majority of patients. Marked elevations in creatine phosphokinase (CPK) usually signify parenchymal hemorrhage in the central nervous system.

PATHOGENESIS

Relapsing fever is an acute bacteremia; spirochetemia may reach 10,000 to 100,000/mm^3. No borrelial endotoxin has been found, but fever, the cardinal sign of the disease, is directly related to spirochetes in the blood and subsides when the organisms disappear.[34] Clearance of the organism is complement- or antibody-mediated and is continuous.[34] Brisk phagocytosis is induced during crisis after an antibody surge and following specific treatment. A cascade of cytokines, tumor necrosis factor alpha (TNF-α), interleukin-6 (IL-6), and IL-8, follows and possibly causes the various pathophysiologic features of relapsing fever and the Jarisch–Herxheimer reaction.[35]

When antigenic variants of *Borrelia* fail to induce an immune response during the first attack (either because there are few *Borrelia* or because they are in a privileged site such as brain), they proliferate and cause spirochetemia/clinical relapse.[36] Antigenic variation is a spontaneous phenomenon that is not related to host reaction and can occur in culture or in mice that are unable to mount an immune response. An estimated 40 different serotypes may arise from a single organism at a rate of 1×10^{-3} to 10^{-4} per generation.[36] The diversity is caused by variation of the surface major protein (Vmp), which is accomplished through somatic mutation and recombination in a manner similar to and synchronous with antibody production by the host.[37] Relapse and remission continue until the host is treated or dies. Some animals, however, clear the infection without treatment.

JARISCH–HERXHEIMER REACTION

The Jarisch–Herxheimer reaction is a constellation of signs and symptoms following treatment of spirochetal and some bacterial and protozoal infections.[34] The most severe form of Jarisch–Herxheimer reaction follows treatment of relapsing fever, where it affects 20% of patients and has a 20% mortality.[38] The Jarisch–Herxheimer reaction develops about 60 minutes after treatment with antibiotics, especially tetracycline. The Jarisch–Herxheimer reaction is characterized by 1) a rise in body temperature and rigors followed by a fall in temperature and sweating; 2) a worsening of existing lesions, especially myocarditis; and 3) hyperventilation and increased blood pressure early, and decreased blood pressure later. The reaction is mediated by TNF-α, IL-6, and IL-8. The kinetics of these cytokines are closely associated with the pathophysiological changes of Jarisch–Herxheimer reaction.[35]

PATHOLOGY

The fatality rate of untreated patients may reach 40%, but of those treated only 5% die. Myocarditis is a common cause of death in relapsing fever (Figure 83–4), but patients die also of hepatic insufficiency, hyperpyrexial convulsions, or hemorrhage.[18,39,40] Every patient who dies has jaundice. Hemorrhagic areas are in pleura, peritoneum, lungs, and gastrointestinal mucosa. Large amounts of blood may be in the gastrointestinal tract. The liver is enlarged, congested, and has accentuated markings. The spleen is enlarged and contains numerous small areas of necrosis scattered haphazardly throughout the pulp. These are miliary, yellow, and usually have geographic outlines. The kidneys are enlarged and pale. The brain is often edematous with hemorrhagic foci in the cortex.

Although *Borrelia* may be in any or all organs at the time of death, the most characteristic features of the disease are in the spleen where the organisms are most numerous. *Borrelia* collect around miliary "abscesses." These lesions may be seen grossly and are randomly scattered or are sometimes around or near a lymphoid follicle (Figure 83–5). The "abscess" is an accumulation of histiocytes, scattered plasma cells, and relatively few, if any, neutrophils. In sections stained with H&E, a zone of bluish amorphous material surrounds the lesion. As demonstrated by silver impregnation stains, this zone is a tightly tangled solid mass of *Borrelia*. The organisms at the perimeter are relatively intact, whereas in the center, small fragments of argyrophilic material are assumed to be fragments of dead organisms. There is often hemorrhage in the pulp around the lesion. The sinuses are packed with blood and histiocytes that contain hemosiderin, cells, and other debris. There may be chronic myocarditis, which is predominantly lymphocytic. The liver has hypertrophic Kupffer's cells and focal necrosis of hepatocytes in the mid and central zones. The lungs are congested, edematous, and have occasional patches of bronchopneumonia. The renal tubules may be dilated and contain proteinaceous casts. Focal to massive hemorrhage without significant cellular reaction is often found in the central nervous system.

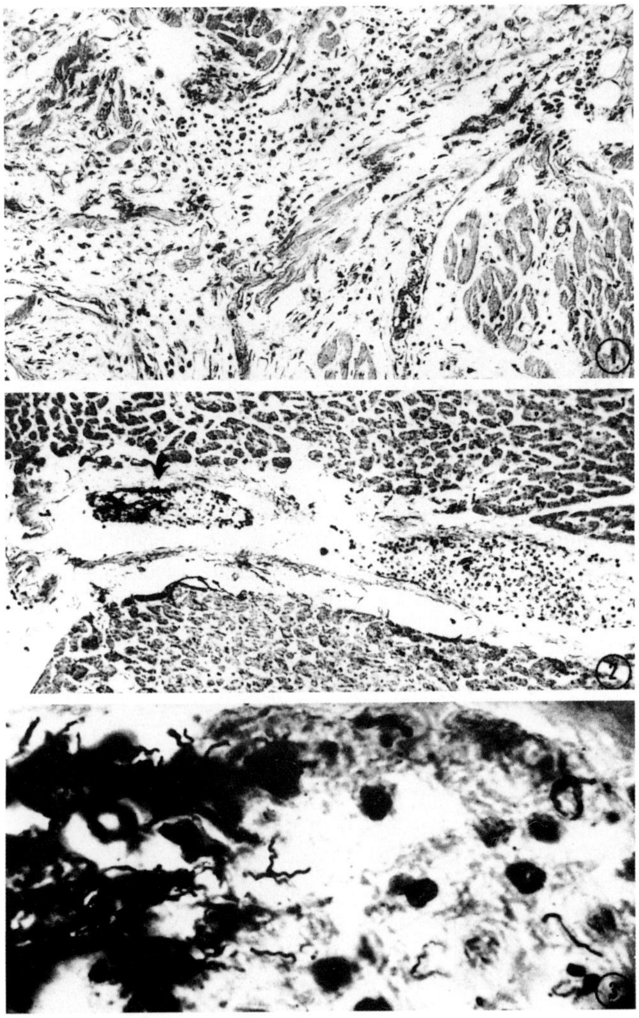

Figure 83–4. Myocarditis. In Panel 1 there are interstitial myocardial edema and an inflammatory cell infiltrate [hematoxylin-eosin (H&E), ×100]. In Panel 2 there is an inflamed and infected intramyocardial vessel (H&E, ×100). Panel 3 is a higher magnification of Panel 2 showing silvered *Borrelia*. *Borrelia* are most often in the lumens of vessels, as in this coronary artery (AFIP Neg 75-9240; Warthin–Starry, ×1780).

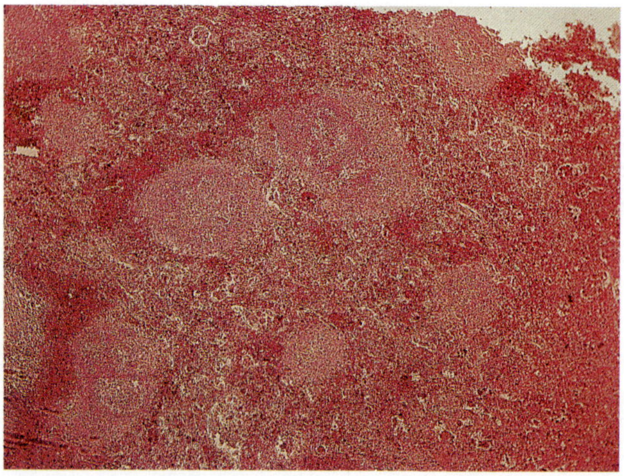

Figure 83–5. Microabscesses in spleen are the most characteristic postmortem finding. The microabscesses involve both follicles and extrafollicular tissues. The pale area of extrafollicular necrosis is clearly demarcated from the surrounding pulp (AFIP Neg 75-8838; H&E, ×71).

Occasionally, there is hemorrhagic meningitis with *Borrelia* in the cerebral cortex. Postmortem the organisms are most often identified in splenic microabscesses. They may be seen in the parenchyma as well as in the walls of blood vessel.

THERAPY, PROGNOSIS, AND CONTROL

The treatment of choice in LBRF is tetracycline, chloramphenicol, or erythromycin. For TBRF, the treatment is tetracycline or erythromycin. Jarisch–Herxheimer reaction is treated symptomatically with fluid, vitamin K, and antipyretics. Meptazinol (an opiate antagonist) diminishes this reaction.[41] Most patients with LBRF are debilitated and often have intercurrent illnesses such as salmonellosis, shigellosis, and typhus. Attention to these illnesses helps reduce mortality.

Epidemics are controlled by treating those infected with antibiotics and by controlling or eliminating the vector by delousing the population.[42] Epidemics of relapsing fever are as frequent as famines and wars, which, in east Africa, have become endemic.[12,13,42] Dealing with these issues as well as social and economic development, is important not only for controlling relapsing fever, but for diarrheal diseases, malaria, and leishmaniasis as well.

Tick-borne fever on the other hand is a place disease. Control depends on avoiding areas infested with ticks. Vector control may be tried in huts or in frequently visited caves, though this is a difficult task. Immunization against relapsing fever is not available.

REFERENCES

1. Scott HH. *A History of Tropical Medicine.* Baltimore: Williams & Wilkins; 1942:781.
2. Carlisle RJ. Two cases of relapsing fever with notes of occurrence of this disease throughout the world at the present day. *J Infect Dis.* 1906;3:233.
3. Obermeier O. Die ersten Fälle und der Character der Berliner Flecktyphusepidemie von 1873. *Berlin Klin Wschr.* 1873;10:349, 364.
4. Morsund W. Historical introduction to the symposium on relapsing fever. Symposium on relapsing fever in the Americas. *AAAS Monograph.* 1942;18:1.
5. Sigerist HE. *Civilization and Disease.* Ithaca, NY: Cornell University Press; 1943:121.
6. Salih SY, Mustafa D, Abdel Wahab SM, Ahmed AM, Omer A. Louse-borne relapsing fever: I. A clinical and laboratory study of 363 cases in the Sudan. *Trans R Soc Trop Med Hyg.* 1977;71:43–51.
7. Borgnolo G, Hailu B, Chiabrera F. Louse-borne relapsing fever in Ethiopia. *Lancet.* 1991;338:827.
8. Borgnolo G, Denku B, Chiabrera F, Hailu B. Louse-borne relapsing fever in Ethiopian children: a clinical study. *Ann Trop Paediatr.* 1993;13:165–171.
9. Barbour AG, Hayes SF. Biology of *Borrelia* species. *Microbiol Rev.* 1986;50:381–400.
10. Daniel E, Beyene H, Tessema T. Relapsing fever in children. Demographic social and clinical features. *Ethiop Med J.* 1992;30:207–214.
11. Borgnolo G, Hailu B, Ciancarelli A, Almaviva M, Woldemariam T. Louse-borne relapsing fever. A clinical and an epidemiological study of 389 patients in Asella Hospital, Ethiopia. *Trop Geogr Med.* 1993;45:66–69.
12. Beveridge CEG. The louse-borne type of relapsing fever as prevalent in the Anglo-Egyptian Sudan, 1926 and 1927. *Med J Aust.* 1928;1:110–112.
13. Maurice GK. The epidemiology of relapsing fever in the Anglo-Egyptian Sudan. *Ann Trop Med Parasitol.* 1939;33: 125–140.
14. Rawlings JA. An overview of tick-borne relapsing fever with emphasis on outbreaks in Texas. *Tex Med.* 1995; 91:56–59.
15. Horton JM, Blaser MJ. The spectrum of relapsing fever in the Rocky Mountains. *Arch Intern Med.* 1985;145:871–875.
16. Southern PM, Sanford JP. Relapsing fever: a clinical and microbiological review. *Medicine.* 1969;48:129–149.
17. Akov S. Blood digestion in ticks. In: Obenchain FD, Galun R, eds. *Physiology of Ticks.* Oxford: Pergamon. 1982: 197–212.
18. Ahmed MA, Abdel Wahab SM, Abdel Malik MO, et al. Louse-borne relapsing fever in the Sudan. A historical review and a clinico-pathological study. *Trop Geogr Med.* 1980;32:106–111.
19. Barclay AJ, Coulter JB. Tick-borne relapsing fever in central Tanzania. *Trans R Soc Trop Med Hyg.* 1990;84:852–856.
20. Kurtz SK. Relapsing fever/Lyme disease. Multiple sclerosis. *Med Hypotheses.* 1986;21:335–343.
21. Lange WR, Schwan TG, Frame JD. Can protracted relapsing fever resemble Lyme disease? *Med Hypotheses.* 1991;35:77–79.

22. Weiss E. A simple method for staining spirochetes. *J Lab Clin Med.* 1929;14:1191.
23. Dieterle RR. Method for the demonstration of *Spirochaeta pallida* in single microscopic sections. *Arch Neurol Psychol.* 1927;18:73–80.
24. Sciotto CG, Lauer BA, White WL, Istre GR. Detection of Borrelia in acridine orange-stained blood smears by fluorescence microscopy. *Arch Pathol Lab Med.* 1983;107:384–386.
25. Kelley RT. Cultivation and physiology of relapsing fever borreliae. In: Johnson RC, ed. *The Biology of Parasitic Spirochaetes.* New York: Academic Press; 1976:87–94.
26. Barbour AG. Isolation and cultivation of Lyme disease spirochetes. *Yale J Biol Med.* 1984;54:421–425.
27. Cutler SJ, Fekade D, Hussein K, Knox KA, et al. Successful in-vitro cultivation of *Borrelia recurrentis. Lancet.* 1994;22:343(8891):242. Letter.
28. Barbour AG. Antigenic variation of a relapsing fever *Borrelia* species. *Annu Rev Microbiol.* 1990;44:155–171.
29. Picken RN. Polymerase chain reaction primers and probes derived from flagellin gene sequences for specific detection of the agents of Lyme disease and North American relapsing fever. *J Clin Microbiol.* 1992;30:99–114.
30. Hyde FW, Johnson RC. Genetic relationship of Lyme disease spirochetes to *Borrelia, Treponema,* and *Leptospira* spp. *J Clin Microbiol.* 1984;20:151–154.
31. Marconi RT, Garon CF. Phylogenetic analysis of the genus *Borrelia:* a comparison of North and European isolates of *Borrelia burgdorferi. J Bacteriol.* 1992;174:241–244.
32. Livesley MA, Thompson IP, Gern L, Nuttal PA. Analysis of intra-specific variation in the fatty acid profiles of *Borrelia burgdorferi. J Gen Microbiol.* 1993;139:2197–2201.
33. Schwan TG, Gage KL, Karstens RH, Schrumpf ME, Hayes SF, Barbour AG. Identification of the tick-borne relapsing fever sprirochete *Borrelia hermsii* by using a species-specific monoclonal antibody. *J Clin Microbiol.* 1992;30:790–795.
34. Bryceson AD. Clinical pathology of the Jarisch–Herxheimer reaction. *J Infect Dis.* 1976;133:696–704.
35. Negussie Y, Remick DG, DeForge LE, Kunkel SL, Eynon A, Griffin GE. Detection of plasma tumor necrosis factors, interleukins 6, and 8 during the Jarisch–Herxheimer reaction of relapsing fever. *J Exp Med.* 1992;175:1207–1212.
36. Stoenner HG, Dodd T, Larsen C. Antigenic variation of *Borrelia hermsii. J Exp Med.* 1982;156:1297–1311.
37. Restrepo BI, Barbour AG. Antigen diversity in the bacterium *B hermsii* through somatic mutations in rearranged vmp genes. *Cell.* 1994;78:867–876.
38. Zein ZA. Louse borne relapsing fever (LBRF): mortality and frequency of Jarisch–Herxheimer reaction. *J R Soc Health.* 1987;107:146–147.
39. Judge DM, Samuel I, Perine PL, Vukotic D. Louse-borne relapsing fever. *Arch Pathol.* 1974;97:136–140.
40. Anderson RT, Zimmerman IE. Relapsing fever in Korea. *Am J Pathol.* 1955;31:1083.
41. Teklu B, Habte-Michael A, Warrell DA, White NJ, Wright DJ. Meptazinol diminishes the Jarisch–Herxheimer reaction of relapsing fever. *Lancet.* 1983;16:835–839.
42. Sundness KO, Hiamanot AT. Epidemic of louse-borne relapsing fever in Ethiopia. *Lancet.* 1993;13:1213–1215.

CHAPTER 84

Rhodococcus equi Infections

Stephen D. Allen

There is a common saying . . . , 'He hath as many diseases as a horse', but 'is false, for man *hath many more.*

James Howell (1594?–1666), The Parley of the Beasts, Sec. 5

DEFINITION AND HISTORICAL AND TAXONOMIC CONSIDERATIONS

Rhodococcus equi (formerly called *Corynebacterium equi*) is an aerobic, gram-positive, nonmotile, pleomorphic coccobacillus, which varies from coccoid to bacillary, depending on the growth medium or conditions within the specimen. Although it is described as partially acid fast, its "acid fastness" is not constant in tissue, in touch preparations, or in smears of fresh clinical materials; its acid fastness depends on staining technique, composition of the medium, and age of culture. Since 1923, when it was first isolated from lungs of foals with pneumonia, *R equi* has been recognized in veterinary medicine as an important pathogen of horses, cattle, swine, and other animals.[1,2] The first infection involving *R equi* in a human was not reported until 1967,[3] and the excellent review by Van Etta et al in 1983 cited only 11 additional human infections.[4] Since then *R equi* has been receiving increasing attention as an opportunistic pathogen in immunodeficient patients, particularly in those infected with human immunodeficiency virus (HIV).[5–7]

Rhodococci share several morphologic and biochemical characteristics with the genera *Corynebacterium, Gordona, Mycobacterium, Nocardia,* and *Tsukamurella.*[8] The taxonomic classification of bacteria now included in this group has had a long and confusing history. Formerly known as *Mycobacterium rhodochrous,* or the "rhodochrous complex," the genus "*Rhodococcus* Zopf" was reinstated by Goodfellow and Alderson in 1977 as the home for the type species *Rhodococcus rhodochrous,* plus nine additional species of the former "rhodochrous complex."[9] This change in classification was based on the results of a numerical taxonomic study, together with data from chemical, serologic, and nucleic acid studies and previous reports in the literature. Accordingly, Goodfellow and Alderson described the rhodococci as aerobic actinomycetes that grow on the surface of agar media and form rudimentary to extensively branched hyphae. The hyphae typically fragment into rod-shaped to coccoid bacterial elements, which can give rise to a primary mycelium. The peptidoglycan of their cell walls characteristically contains mesodiaminopimelic acid, arabinose, and galactose. The formation of pigmented pink, orange or red, smooth, rough or mycobacteria-like colonies is common but some strains form only colorless colonies.[8,9] In 1988, Strackebrandt et al[10] revived the names *Gordona bronchialis* and *G terrae* and created the names *G rubropertinctus* and *G sputi* for these species that had been formerly placed in the genus *Rhodococcus.* The species previously called *Rhodococcus aichciensis* was recently transferred to the genus *Gordona* as *Gordona aichciensis.*[11] The former *R chubuensis* was found to be a later subjective synonym of *G sputi* and *R chubuensis* no longer has standing in the nomenclature.[12] *Rhodococcus luteus,* likewise, no longer has standing in nomenclature, because it was found to be a later subjective synonym of *Rhodococcus fascians.*[13] The species formerly called *R aurantiacus* is now *Tsukamurella paurometabolum.*[14] Thus, reports of infections involving "*Rhodococcus bronchialis,*"[15] and of "*Rhodococcus aurantiacus*"[16] should now be regarded as infections involving *G bronchialis* and *T paurometabolum,* instead of *Rhodococcus* sp. Except for *R equi,* little is known about the pathogenic potential of the 12 species remaining in the genus *Rhodococcus.*

DISTRIBUTION OF THE ORGANISM AND EPIDEMIOLOGY

Rhodococcus equi is widely distributed in soils around the world, and in the feces of several warm-blooded animals. There have been reports of human infections from five continents: North America, Europe, Africa, Australia, and Asia and from 11 countries. Infections have been reported from 15 states in the United States.[5] As reviewed recently by Prescott,[2] *R equi* has been isolated from the intestines and/or manure of herbivores or omnivores including horses, pigs, cattle, sheep, goats, and deer. Its widespread presence in herbivore feces probably results from ingestion of feed contaminated with the organism.[2] *Rhodococcus equi* is an important cause of pneumonia in horses, particularly foals. High numbers of organisms have been found in surface soils of certain farms where *R equi* infections of horses have been endemic, particularly in the summertime in temperate climates. Nutrients in herbivore manure appear to meet the nutritional requirements of the organism, allowing for *R equi* to multiply, provided that the temperature is within 10 to 40°C and that the pH stays in a favorable range.[2,8] *Rhodococcus equi* has been isolated from the feces of a number of wild birds, but has not been found commonly in the excreta of chickens. It has been isolated only rarely from the feces of dogs, but not from cats. Using a selective medium described by Woolcock et al,[17] Mutimer et al[18] found only two strains of *R equi* in 521 specimens of human feces. As pointed out by Prescott, it seems unlikely that *R equi* could multiply in the anaerobic regions of the adult intestinal tract because it is an obligate aerobe.[2] However, during the first 8 weeks of life before an adult-type flora is established, it multiplies in the intestinal tract of foals.[2,19]

In spite of recent attention in the literature, reports of human infections involving *R equi* are rare.[20] Collectively, about 29% to 32% of these patients have had a history of some kind of exposure to animals, especially horses (eg, contact with farm animals or manure). It is assumed that both animals and humans usually acquire the infection by the respiratory route. Inhalation of the organism in dust is likely to be the major way that foals acquire the infection.[2] As reviewed recently, however, localized infections with *R equi* have followed direct inoculation of soil or contaminated materials from animals.[20] Soil, including dust, is probably the source of infection in a number of patients who recalled no contact with animals.

CLINICAL FEATURES

Although at least half of the over 100 infections have been in HIV-positive patients, about 40% have involved patients who were immunodeficient from other conditions, while the remaining 10% were immunocompetent.[5,21–35] Ages of the 72 patients in the review of Verville et al[5] ranged from 9 months to 77 years (median of 34 years), and the male:female ratio was 3.5:1. Possible explanations for the higher occurrence of *R equi* infections in males than in females could include the higher prevalence of HIV-infected men than HIV-infected women, and possible differences in soil/farm animal environmental exposures in men compared with women. Pneumonia was diagnosed in about three fourths of the patients; 18% of these patients who had pneumonia also had infection with the organism in an extrapulmonary site. Nearly one fourth of all the 72 patients reviewed had infection in extrapulmonary sites without documentation of pulmonary infection.[5]

Predisposing Factors

As indicated, the majority of patients studied also had acquired immunodeficiency syndrome (AIDS). This association has become so strong that the diagnosis of *R equi* lung infection in a patient with pulmonary illness should be considered a presumptive diagnosis of AIDS until proven otherwise.[36] In addition to AIDS, other predisposing factors include leukemia,[34] lymphoma,[35,37] small cell lung cancer,[35] renal transplantation, IV drug abuse, treatment with corticosteroids, rheumatoid arthritis, toxic epidermal necrolysis, diabetes mellitus,[35] alcoholism, sarcoidosis, burns, penetrating eye injuries, surgical procedures on the eye, open heart surgery, IV catheters, and contact with soil/manure (eg, gardening) or animals (eg, horses/swine).[36–39]

Clinical Manifestations

In either HIV-positive or HIV-negative patients who have pulmonary infections involving *R equi*, the most common presenting complaints are fever, cough (either productive or nonproductive), pleuritic chest pain, and dyspnea.[4,7,34–37] Evidence of pneumonia is usually detected on chest radiography, and pulmonary cavitation is frequently present—in up to one half of patients with pneumonia.[35–37] High on the list of differential diagnoses of the pulmonary infiltrates would be tuberculosis, fungal infections such as histoplasmosis, nocardiosis, or neoplasm (eg, involvement with malignant lymphoma or primary lung tumor).

Chest radiographs have commonly revealed an opaque pulmonary infiltrate, often involving only a single upper lobe. The pulmonary infiltrates were bilateral, however, in 6 of 8 patients described by Scott et al.[35] When first visualized, the lesions may vary from a 2-cm nodular infiltrate to an infiltrate involving most of a lobe. During the next 2 to 4 weeks, especially if not treated effectively, the infiltrate may enlarge slowly, may develop cavitation with an air-fluid level within the lesion, or may develop multiloculated cavities. Air-fluid levels in chest films are not a characteristic of tuberculosis.[2,7] Pleural effusions[40] or thoracic empyema[41] are also included among the clinical manifestations encountered most commonly in these patients.

Although an invasive procedure such as bronchoscopy, thoracentesis, or thoracotomy may be done to establish a diagnosis, cultures of blood and sputum may aid in diagnosing *R equi* pneumonia.[7,37]

Extrapulmonary infections by *R equi* include brain abscess,[42] endophthalmitis following penetrating eye injury,[39] prostatic abscess in a patient with AIDS,[43] skin lesion of the foot of an IV drug abuser with AIDS and dissemination to lymph nodes, lungs, and brain,[21] bacteremia, psoas abscess and pelvic mass in a patient with AIDS,[44] bacteremia in an adult with leukemia,[34] osteomyelitis in a renal transplant patient,[45] a paraspinal, soft tissue abscess in a renal transplant patient,[41] a disseminated infection in an IV drug abuser with AIDS involving the lungs, kidneys, brain, and bloodstream,[46] peritonitis in a patient receiving chronic ambulatory peritoneal dialysis,[47] and cervical lymphadenitis in a child.[48]

PATHOLOGY

Gross examination of lung tissue removed as lobectomy specimens has revealed cavitary lesions surrounded by consolidated lung. The lung abscesses have been of varying sizes, often ranging up to 6 or 8 cm in diameter. Pulmonary malakoplakia with cavitation, or necrotizing pneumonia with abscess have been the pathologic findings reported most frequently.[26]

Extrapulmonary lesions that are nodular and firm may also be removed surgically. At the operating table, abscesses may be aspirated and drained, and a few drops to several milliliters of pinkish-tan exudate may be collected for microbiologic examination. Samples of soft tissue from the walls of wounds or abscesses have consisted of flat, irregular pieces of yellow and pink tissue measuring up to a few centimeters in greatest dimension (SD Allen, personal observations).

Light microscopic examination of hematoxylin-eosin-stained sections of lesions surrounding abscess cavities typically reveals an unusual type of suppurative and granulomatous inflammatory reaction characterized by sheets or aggregates of macrophages with eosinophilic cytoplasm (Figure 84–1). In early lesions or in areas near an abscess cavity, there may be numerous neutrophils, but there may be few neutrophils in other, more peripheral areas. Plasma cells and lymphocytes may also be present, but not usually in large numbers.

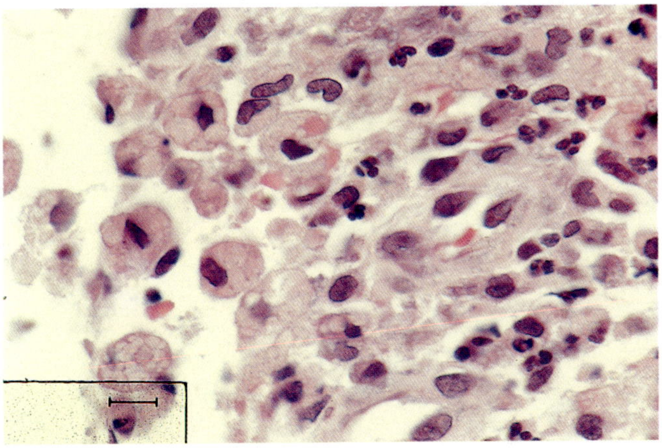

Figure 84–1. The section was taken from the wall of a soft tissue mass that had cavitated. Sheets of macrophages with eosinophilic material in the cytoplasm are a prominent feature (hematoxylin-eosin, ×63 oil immersion objective).

Granulation tissue may be a prominent feature in some areas (Figure 84–2). In sections stained with periodic acid–Schiff (PAS) (Figure 84–3), the granular material in the cytoplasm of macrophages is pinkish to red PAS-positive inclusions, ranging up to 10 μm in diameter, some of which may be "target shaped."

Malakoplakia

Recently, it has been recognized that the PAS-positive materials in macrophages are accumulations of giant phagolysosomes containing degenerated bacteria and debris, which can be visualized by electron microscopy;

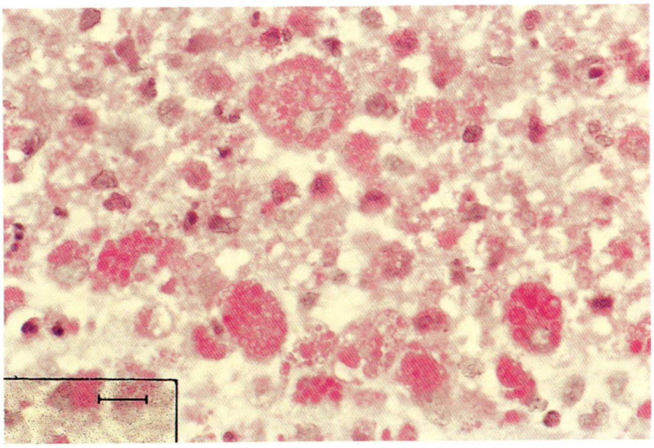

Figure 84–2. Numerous macrophages filled with aggregates of PAS-positive granular material, often having the appearance of membrane-bound spherical inclusions. In addition, extracellular aggregates of PAS-positive granular material are present. Diastase digestion had no effect on the PAS-positive material (PAS with diastase, ×40 objective).

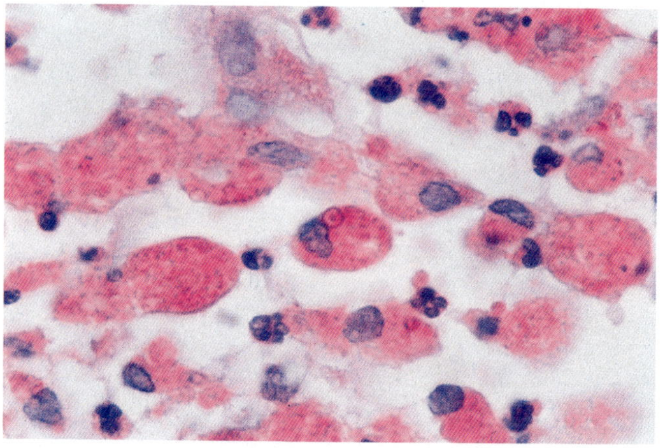

Figure 84–3. The PAS-positive, target-like inclusion in the macrophage located in the center of the photograph is characteristic of a Michaelis–Gutmann body. Details are given in the text (PAS with diastase, ×100 objective).

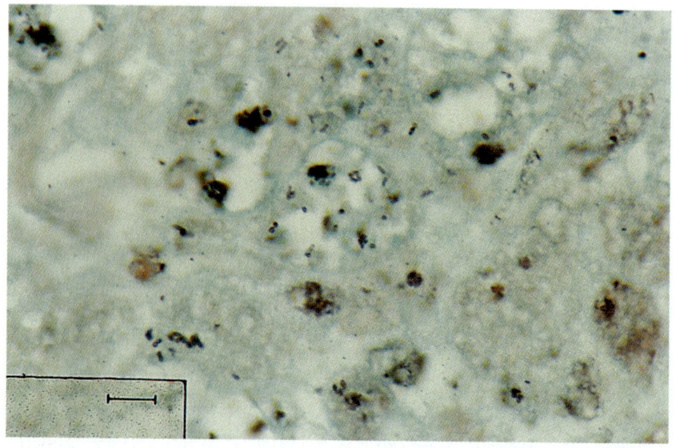

Figure 84–5. There are laıge numbers of small, pleomorphic, "diphtheroid" coccobacilli within macrophages and some that are extracellular. *Rhodococcus equi* was the only organism isolated (same case as in Figures 84–1 through 84–4) (GMS, ×100 objective).

when they become calcified, they are referred to as Michaelis–Gutmann (MG) bodies.[22,26,33,49] Defective and incomplete digestion of engulfed intracellular bacteria within phagolysosomes by macrophages, which have been called von Hansemann's cells, is believed to be important in the pathogenesis of MG bodies.[2,49,50]

MG bodies have a rounded, target-shaped appearance, are up to 10 μm in diameter, and are in macrophages and extracellularly, mainly within macrophages (Figure 84–3). The special stain findings of MG bodies in *R equi* pneumonia were summarized recently by Kwon and Colby[26] and included the following: PAS (stained pink-red), Gomori's methanamine silver (dark brown), Grocott (green), Giemsa (dark blue), von Kossa (brown-red), Alizarin red (orange), Prussian blue (dark blue), and S100 (not stained).

Malakoplakia has most often been described in the setting of bacterial infections in nonpulmonary sites involving other microorganisms, especially *Escherichia coli.* Other gram-negative bacteria, and gram-positive bacteria including mycobacteria, as well as fungi, have also been identified in malakoplakia. Currently, as reviewed by Kwon and Colby[26] and De Peralta-Venturina et al,[22] there are at least 13 cases of pulmonary

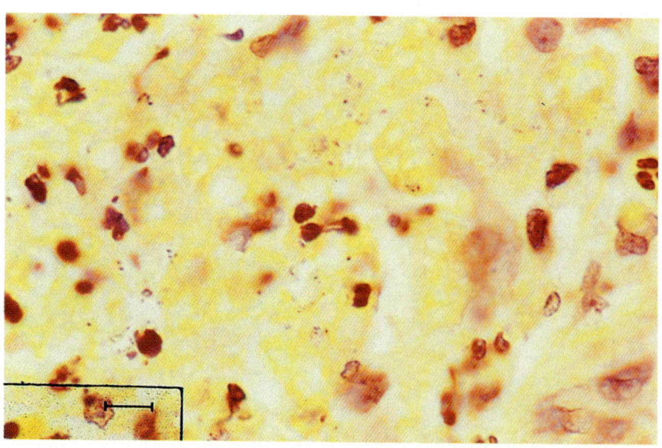

Figure 84–4. Small, pleomorphic, gram-variable, "diphtheroid," coccobacilli from the same tissue specimen as in Figures 84–1 through 84–3. *Rhodococcus equi* was isolated and identified in the clinical microbiology laboratory of the Indiana University Medical Center. It was the only organism that grew from the specimen (Brown–Hopps tissue gram stain, ×100 objective).

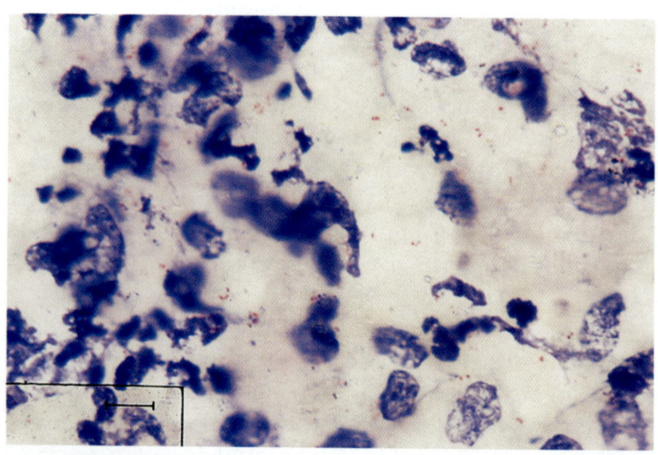

Figure 84–6. There are numerous tiny partially acid-fast coccobacilli, morphologically suggestive of *Rhodococcus equi,* in this sediment of a bronchoalveolar lavage specimen from an HIV-positive man. *Rhodococcus equi* was isolated and identified from the specimen (modified Kinyoun acid-fast stain, ×100 objective).

malakoplakia in the literature; the most commonly isolated microorganism was *R equi*—in 9/13 or 69%. Other organisms isolated from patients with pulmonary malakoplakia were *E coli* (in 3/13 or 23%) and *Acinetobacter* sp in one.

Malakoplakia may appear grossly as tumorlike nodules, thus leading the surgeon or pathologist to suspect neoplasm. In addition to malakoplakia involving lungs, this benign inflammatory reaction historically has been described most frequently in the setting of chronic infections involving the urinary bladder. It has also been described in several other sites and organs including the kidneys, urethra, prostate, testis, epididymis, endometrium, vagina, broad ligament, adrenal, stomach, appendix, intestine, anus, retroperitoneum, lymph nodes, tonsil, conjunctiva, bone, skin, and subcutaneous tissue.[49,51]

Rhodococcus equi is a facultatively intracellular bacterial pathogen that can be easily detected in lesions using modified Gram stains including the Brown–Hopps or Brown–Brenn stains (Figure 84–4). These stains may demonstrate large numbers of small, pleomorphic, gram-positive or gram-variable bacilli, tiny coccoid forms (< 1 μm in diameter) or coccobacilli within cytoplasm of macrophages. Likewise, Gomori's methanamine-silver (GMS) stain reveals large numbers of intracellular bacteria within macrophages (Figure 84–5). *Rhodococcus equi* may stain partially acid fast in tissue with either the Fite stain or Fite–Farraco stain, or with the modified Kinyoun acid-fast stain in touch preparations or imprint smears of fresh specimens (ie, some, but not all, of the bacteria will be acid fast, see Figure 84–6). Regardless of the modified acid-fast stain, the organisms are usually harder to find in tissue sections than in fresh imprints or smears. *Rhodococcus equi* will not be acid fast with the routine Ziehl–Neelsen stain. The presence of PAS-positive inclusions in macrophages (with or without diastase), presence of gram-positive coccobacilli that also can be seen in the GMS stain, and the presence of small coccoid to ovoid, partially acid-fast bacteria in abscesses suggest infection by *R equi.*

DIFFERENTIAL DIAGNOSIS

The differential diagnosis of pulmonary and extrapulmonary conditions involving the immunosuppressed patient in which there are large numbers of foamy or eosinophilic macrophages can be problematic. It is important clinically to be able to differentiate between *R equi* infection, infections involving other microorganisms, and other conditions, especially in HIV-positive patients. The recognition of MG bodies, diagnostic of malakoplakia, especially in an HIV-infected or other immunodeficient patient is a valuable clue to the presumptive diagnosis of *R equi* infection, although it is not definitively diagnostic by itself. As mentioned earlier, and at the risk of redundancy, the organisms can be easily demonstrated in tissue using a modified tissue Gram stain, such as the Brown–Brenn, GMS stain, and a modified acid-fast stain such as the Fite stain or modified Kinyoun. They are not acid fast with the routine Ziehl–Neelsen stain. HIV-positive patients with mycobacterial infections of lung caused by a variety of organisms including *Mycobacterium tuberculosis, M avium-intracellulare* complex, *Histoplasma capsulatum, Cryptococcus neoformans,* and *Pneumocystis carinii,* may contain foamy macrophages frequently filled with the causal organism. In hematoxylin-eosin-stained sections, the macrophages are most likely to be eosinophilic in *R equi* infections,[35] but not in the other infections mentioned. Likewise in the other conditions, PAS-positive phagolysosomes and the calcified MG bodies are not likely to be seen. The other microorganisms listed can be differentiated with special stains and by microbiologic isolation and identification procedures, Pulmonary Whipple's disease, caused by *Tropheryma whippelii,* is rare but may need to be considered because of its morphologic similarity to *R equi* infection.[35,52] In Whipple's disease, the macrophages are more likely to be foamy and not eosinophilic, more likely to be found in the pulmonary interstitium, and they may infiltrate peribronchiolar smooth muscle.[22,26,49] Noninfectious processes that could be considered in the differential diagnosis include obstructive pneumonia with foam cells, suppurative bronchiolitis, exogenous lipoid pneumonia, lipid-storage disorders including Niemann–Pick disease and Gaucher's disease, and pulmonary alveolar proteinosis.[22,26,35,49]

Microbiologic Confirmation of the Diagnosis

On microscopic examination of *R equi* in smears of clinical specimens or in smears prepared from primary isolation media, the organism is gram-positive or gram-variable, and the cells vary from short rods arranged singly, or with a pleomorphic "diphtheroid" appearance, or they may be in the form of tiny coccoid cells to short coccobacilli.[54] They may form "Chinese letters" or picket fence arrangements or simply sheets and masses of tiny ovoid to nearly spherical bacterial forms. One may see traces of branching in early stages of growth on culture media. The rod-shaped forms of *R equi,* like those of other species of *Rhodococcus* and *Nocardia,* fragment into coccoid cells.[9,53] Thus, their size may be extremely variable. Like other *Rhodococcus* and *Nocardia* species, *R equi* may be partially acid fast using the modified Kinyoun stain, but not acid fast in either the Ziehl–Neelsen or auramine-rhodamine acid-fast stains that are commonly used in microbiology laboratories.[54] Details for preparation and application of these stains are available elsewhere.[54]

The organism grows aerobically at 35°C on blood agar, chocolate agar, phenylethylalcohol blood agar, and on colistin nalidixic acid agar, but does not grow on MacConkey or other agar media used selectively for the isolation of gram-negative bacilli. Aerial hyphae are not formed on these media. Colonies are usually smooth and usually not pigmented at first, but may become salmon-pink to coral with prolonged incubation, especially if the plates are held at room temperature (eg, 22 to 25°C). *Rhodococcus equi* is nonmotile, catalase positive, arylsulfatase negative, sensitive to lysozyme, variable for urease production, variable for nitrate reduction, negative for production of acid from glucose, and negative for production of β-galactosidase. Additionally, more detailed differential characteristics are given by Goodfellow in *Bergey's Manual of Systematic Bacteriology*[53] and by Koneman et al.[54]

TREATMENT

Because *R equi* is a facultative intracellular pathogen that persists and multiplies inside macrophages, antimicrobial agents that concentrate within macrophages should be selected for treatment.[36] These include erythromycin, azithromycin, clarithromycin, roxithromycin, quinolones, and rifampin. Erythromycin and rifampin act synergistically and are probably the most potent combination.[55,56] Although successful therapy may require many weeks (eg, 4 to 8 weeks) of parenteral antimicrobial treatment, the treatment probably should be continued until the patient is no longer culture positive and his or her condition is stable.[36] Surgical measures (eg, segmental resection or lobectomy; incision and drainage of an abscess in soft tissue) may be required for a successful outcome.

REFERENCES

1. Magnusson H. Spezifische infektiöse pneumonie beim fohlen. Ein neuer eitererreger beim pferd. *Arch Wiss Prakt Tierheilkd.* 1923;50:22–38.
2. Prescott JF. *Rhodococcus equi:* an animal and human pathogen. *Clin Microbiol Rev.* 1991;4:20–34.
3. Golub B, Falk G, Spink WW. Lung abscess due to *Corynebacterium equi*. Report of first human infection. *Ann Intern Med.* 1967;66:1174–1177.
4. Van Etta LL, Filice GA, Ferguson RM, Gerding DN. *Corynebacterium equi:* a review of 12 cases of human infection. *Rev Infect Dis.* 1983;5:1012–1018.
5. Verville TD, Huycke MM, Greenfield RA, Fine DP, Kuhls TL, Slater LN. *Rhodococcus equi* infections of humans. *Medicine.* 1994;73:119–132.
6. Drancourt M, Bonnet E, Gallais H, Peloux Y, Raoult D. *Rhodococcus equi* infection in patients with AIDS. *J Infect.* 1992;24:123–131.
7. Emmons W, Reichwein B, Winslow DL. *Rhodococcus equi* infection in the patient with AIDS: literature review and report of an unusual case. *Rev Infect Dis.* 1991;13:91–96.
8. Holt JG, Krieg NR, Sneath PH, Staley JT, Williams ST, eds. *Bergey's Manual of Determinative Bacteriology.* 9th ed. Baltimore, Md: Williams & Wilkins; 1994:625–650.
9. Goodfellow M, Alderson G. The actinomycete-genus *Rhodococcus:* a home for the '*rhodochrous*' complex. *J Gen Microbiol.* 1977;100:99–122.
10. Stackebrandt E, Smida J, Collins MD. Evidence of phylogenetic heterogeneity within the genus *Rhodococcus:* revival of the genus *Gordona (Tsukamura)*. *J Gen Appl Microbiol.* 1988;34:341–348.
11. Klatte S, Rainey FA, Kroppenstedt RM. Transfer of *Rhodococcus aichiensis Tsukamura* 1982 and *Nocardia amarae* Lechevalier and Lechevalier 1974 to the genus *Gordona* as *Gordona aichiensis* comb. nov. and *Gordona amarae* comb. nov. *Int J Syst Bacteriol.* 1994;44:769–773.
12. Riegel P, Kamne-Fotso MV, De Briel D, et al. *Rhodococcus chubuensis* Tsukamura 1982 is a later subjective synonym of *Gordona sputi* (Tsukamura 1978) Stackebrandt 1989 comb. nov. *Int J Syst Bacteriol.* 1994;44:764–768.
13. Klatte S, Jahnke KD, Kroppenstedt RM, Rainey F, Stackebrandt E. *Rhodococcus luteus* is a later subjective synonym of *Rhodococcus fascians*. *Int J Syst Bacteriol.* 1994;44:627–630.
14. Collins MD, Smida J, Dorsch M, Stackebrandt E. *Tsukamurella* gen. nov. harboring *Corynebacterium paurometabolum* and *Rhodococcus aurantiacus*. *Int J Syst Bacteriol.* 1988;38:385–391.
15. Richet HM, Craven PC, Brown JM, et al. A cluster of *Rhodococcus (Gordona) bronchialis* sternal-wound infections after coronary-artery bypass surgery. *N Engl J Med.* 1991;324:104–109.
16. Tsukamura M, Hikosaka K, Nishimura K, Hara S. Severe progressive subcutaneous abscesses and necrotizing tenosynovitis caused by *Rhodococcus aurantiacus*. *J Clin Microbiol.* 1988;26:201–205.
17. Woolcock JB, Farmer A-MT, Mutimer MD. Selective medium for *Corynebacterium* isolation. *J Clin Microbiol.* 1979;9:640–642.
18. Mutimer WD, Woolcock JB, Sturgess BR. *Corynebacterium equi* in human faeces. *Med J Aust.* 1979;2:422.
19. Takai S, Ohkura H, Watanabe Y, Tsubaki S. Quantitative aspects of fecal *Rhodococcus (Corynebacterium) equi* in foals. 1986;23:794–796.
20. McNeil MM, Brown JM. The medically important aerobic Actinomycetes: epicoccus equi in a drug abuser seropositive for human immunodeficiency virus. *Rev Infect Dis.* 1991;13:509–510.
21. Antinori S, Esposito R, Cernuschi M, et al. Disseminated *Rhodococcus equi* infection initially presenting as foot mycetoma in an HIV-positive patient. *AIDS.* 1992;6:740–742.

22. De Peralta-Venturina MN, Clubb FJ, Kielhofner MA. Pulmonary malakoplakia associated with *Rhodococcus equi* infection in a patient with acquired immunodeficiency syndrome. *Am J Clin Pathol.* 1994;102:459–463.
23. Frame BC, Petkus AF. *Rhodococcus equi* pneumonia: case report and literature review. *Ann Pharmacother.* 1993; 27:1340–1342.
24. Gray BM. Case report: *Rhodococcus equi* pneumonia in a patient infected by the human immunodeficiency virus. *Am J Med Sci.* 1992;303:180–183.
25. Gillet-Juvin K, Stern M, Israël-biet D, Penaud D, Carnot F. A highly unusual combination of pulmonary pathogens in an HIV infected patient. *Scand J Infect Dis.* 1994;26: 215–217.
26. Kwon KY, Colby TV. *Rhodococcus equi* pneumonia and pulmonary malakoplakia in acquired immunodeficiency syndrome. *Arch Pathol Lab Med.* 1994;118:744–748.
27. Legras A, Lemmens B, Dequin P, Cattier B, Besnier J. Tamponade due to *Rhodococcus equi* in acquired immunodeficiency syndrome. *Chest.* 1994;106:1278–1279.
28. Libanore M, Rossi MR, Bicocchi R, Ghinelli F. *Rhodococcus equi* pneumonia and occult HIV infection. *Lancet.* 1993;342:496–497.
29. Magnani G, Elia GF, McNeil MM, et al. *Rhodococcus equi* cavitary pneumonia in HIV-infected patients: an unsuspected opportunistic pathogen. *J AIDS.* 1992;5:1059–1064.
30. Mastrianni CM, Lichtner M, Vullo V, Salvatore D. Humoral immune response to *Rhodococcus equi* in AIDS patients with *R equi* pneumonia. *J Infect Dis.* 1994;169:1179–1180.
31. Moyer DV, Bayer AS. Progressive pulmonary infiltrates and positive blood cultures for weakly acid-fast, gram-positive rods in a 76-year-old woman. *Chest.* 1993; 104:259–261.
32. Nordmann P, Rouveix E, Guenounou M, Nicolas MH. Pulmonary abscess due to a rifampin and fluoroquinolone resistant *Rhodococcus equi* strain in a HIV infected patient. *Eur J Clin Microbiol Infect Dis.* 1992;11:557–558.
33. Russell GM, Mills AE. Pulmonary malakoplakia related to *Rhodococcus equi* occurring in the acquired immunodeficiency syndrome. *Med J Austral* 1994;160:308–309.
34. Sladek GG, Frame JN. *Rhodococcus equi* causing bacteremia in an adult with acute leukemia. *South Med J.* 1993;86:244–246.
35. Scott MA, Graham BS, Verrall R, Dixon R, Schaffner W, Tham KT. *Rhodococcus equi*—an increasingly recognized opportunistic pathogen. Report of 12 cases and review of 65 cases in the literature. *Am J Clin Pathol.* 1995;103: 649–655.
36. Walsh RD, Schoch PE, Cunha BA. *Rhodococcus* infections. *Infect Dis Newsletter.* 1993;12:36–37.
37. Harvey RL, Sunstrum JC. *Rhodococcus equi* infection in patients with and without human immunodeficiency virus infection. *Rev Infect Dis.* 1991;13:139–145.
38. Hillerdal G, Riesenfeldt-Orn I, Pederson A, Ivanicova E. Infection with *Rhodococcus equi* in a patient with sarcoidosis treated with corticosteroids. *Scand J Infect Dis.* 1988;20:673–677.
39. Hillman D, Garretson B, Fiscella R. *Rhodococcus equi* endophthalmitis. *Arch Ophthalmol.* 1989;107:20. Letter.
40. LeBar WD, Pensler MI. Pleural effusion due to *Rhodococcus equi. J Infect Dis.* 1986;154:919–920.
41. Jones MR, Neale TJ, Say PJ, Horne JG. *Rhodococcus equi:* an emerging opportunistic pathogen? *Aust NZ J Med.* 1989;19:103–107.
42. Obana WG, Scannell KA, Jacobs R, et al. A case of *Rhodococcus equi* brain abscess. *Surg Neurol.* 1991;35: 321–324.
43. Mandarino E, Rachlis A, Towers M, Simor AE. Prostatic abscess due to *Rhodococcus equi* in a patient with acquired immunodeficiency syndrome. *Clin Microbiol. Newsletter.* 1994;16:14–16.
44. Fierer J, Wolf P, Seed L, Gay T, Noonan K, Haghighi P. Non-pulmonary *Rhodococcus equi* infections in patient with acquired immune deficiency syndrome (AIDS). *J Clin Pathol.* 1987;40:556–558.
45. Novak RM, Polisky EL, Janda WM, Libertin CR. Osteomyelitis caused by *Rhodococcus equi* in a renal transplant recipient. *Infection.* 1988;16:186–188.
46. Sirera G, Romeu J, Clotet B, et al. Relapsing systemic infection due to *Rhodococcus equi* in a drug abuser seropositive for human immunodeficiency virus. *Rev Infect Dis.* 1991;13:509–510.
47. Franklin DB, Yium JJ, Hawkins SS. *Corynebacterium equi* peritonitis in a patient receiving peritoneal dialysis. *South Med J.* 1989;82:1046–1047.
48. Thomsen VF, Henriques U, Magnusson M. *Corynebacterium equi* Magnusson isolated from a tuberculoid lesion in a child with adenitis colli. *Dan Med Bull.* 1968;15: 135–138.
49. Schwartz DA, Ogden PO, Blumberg HM, Honig E. Pulmonary malakoplakia in a patient with the acquired immunodeficiency syndrome: differential diagnostic considerations. *Arch Pathol Lab Med.* 1990;114:1267–1272.
50. Shapiro JM, Romney BM, Weiden MD, White CS, O'Toole KM. *Rhodococcus equi* endobronchial mass with lung abscess in a patient with AIDS. *Thorax.* 1992;47:62–63.
51. McClure J. Malakoplakia. *Pathology.* 1983;140:275–330.
52. Relman DA, Schmidt TM, MacDermott RP, Falkow S. Identification of the uncultured bacillus of Whipple's disease. *N Engl J Med.* 1992;327:293–301.
53. Goodfellow M. Genus *Rhodococcus* Zopf 1891, 28[AL]. In: Williams ST, Sharpe ME, eds. *Bergey's Manual of Systematic Bacteriology,* Baltimore, Md: Williams & Wilkins; 1989;4:2362–2371.
54. Koneman EW, Allen SD, Janda WM, Schreckenberger PC, Winn WC Jr. *Color Atlas and Textbook of Diagnostic Microbiology.* 4th ed. Philadelphia: JB Lippincott; 1992: 467–518.
55. Nordmann P, Ronco E. In-vitro antimicrobial susceptibility of *Rhodococcus equi. J Antimicrob Chemother.* 1992;29: 383–393.
56. Nordmann P, Kerestedjian J, Ronco E. Therapy of *Rhodococcus equi* disseminated infections in nude mice. *Antimicrob Ag Chemother.* 1992;36:1244–1248.

CHAPTER 85

Rickettsial Infections

David H. Walker and J. Stephen Dumler

The microbe is so very small
You cannot make him out at all,
But many sanguine people hope
To see him through a microscope

Hilaire Belloc (1870–1953)

DEFINITION

Rickettsiae are obligately intracellular bacteria that are ecologically associated with an arthropod host. The genus *Rickettsia* includes three antigenically defined groups: spotted fever group (SFG), typhus group, and scrub typhus group.[1] The spotted fever and typhus groups are closely related genetically, but the scrub typhus rickettsia, *Orientia* (formerly *Rickettsia*) *tsutsugamushi*, has no established evolutionary relationship with them. Phenotypically, *O tsutsugamushi* differs from SFG and typhus group organisms in its lack of lipopolysaccharide and peptidoglycan in the cell wall.[2] Nevertheless, all the diseases caused by the rickettsiae have similar target tissues (blood vessels) and organs with the result that the histopathology has many common themes. These microbiologically distinct pathogens cause diseases with many similar features (Table 85–1).

SYNONYMS

- Rocky Mountain spotted fever (exanthematic typhus of São Paulo, Tobia fever)
- Boutonneuse fever (Mediterranean spotted fever, Marseille fever, South African tick-bite fever, Kenya tick typhus, Israel tick typhus, Indian tick typhus)
- North Asian tick typhus (Siberian tick typhus)
- Oriental spotted fever (Japanese spotted fever)
- Rickettsialpox (Kew Gardens spotted fever)
- Epidemic typhus (louse-borne typhus, jail fever, ship fever, tabardillo)
- Murine typhus (endemic typhus, shop typhus)
- Scrub typhus (chigger-borne typhus, akamushi fever, flood fever, tsutsugamushi disease, Japanese river fever, Shishito fever, kedani fever, mite typhus, rural typhus)

GEOGRAPHIC DISTRIBUTION, NATURAL HISTORY, AND EPIDEMIOLOGY

The geographic distribution and epidemiology of rickettsial diseases are determined by the ecologic conditions that maintain the arthropod host and its vertebrate host (Table 85–1).[3–5] Humans are infected when bitten by infected ticks and mites, or by contacting feces of infected lice and fleas. *Orientia tsutsugamushi* and SFG rickettsiae are maintained in nature by transovarial transmission, although pathogenic SFG rickettsiae also are maintained by a minor component of horizontal transmission.[4,5] Louse-borne typhus fever occurs as explosive deadly epidemics in contrast with the endemic, widespread occurrence of Rocky Mountain spotted fever, other SFG rickettsioses, murine typhus, sylvatic typhus, and scrub typhus. Knowledge of the seasonality of the vector assists in the epidemiologic diagnosis (eg, spring–summer season of *Dermacentor variabilis* activity and Rocky Mountain spotted fever in

TABLE 85–1. ETIOLOGY, EPIDEMIOLOGY, AND ECOLOGY OF RICKETTSIAL DISEASES

Disease	Agent	Geographic Distribution	Natural History	Transmission to Humans
Rocky Mountain spotted fever	*R rickettsii*	North, Central, and South America	Transovarial maintenance in *Dermacentor, Rhipicephalus,* and *Amblyomma* ticks; less extensive horizontal transmission from tick to mammal to tick	Tick bite
Boutonneuse fever	*R conorii*	Mediterranean basin, Africa, Asia	Transovarial maintenance in *Rhipicephalus, Hyalomma,* and *Amblyomma* ticks; role of horizontal transmission is not clear	Tick bite
North Asian tick typhus	*R sibirica*	Russia, China, Mongolia Pakistan, Kazakhstan, Girgizistan, Tadzhikistan	Transovarial maintenance in *Dermacentor, Haemaphysalis,* and *Hyalomma* ticks; horizontal transmission from tick to mammal to tick	Tick bite
Oriental spotted fever	*R japonica*	Japan	Presumably a transovarial tick host; the role of horizontal transmission is not clear	Tick bite
Queensland tick typhus	*R australis*	Eastern Australia	Transovarial transmission in *Ixodes* ticks; the role of horizontal transmission is not clear	Tick bite
Rickettsialpox	*R akari*	United States, Ukraine, Croatia, possibly worldwide	Transovarial transmission in *Liporyssoides sanguine* mites; horizontal transmission from mite to *Mus musculus* to mite	Mite bite
Murine typhus-like illness	*R felis*	California, Texas	Transovarial transmission in cat fleas; role of horizontal transmission is not clear	Presumably flea feces
Murine typhus	*R typhi*	Worldwide, predominantly tropical and subtropical especially coastal California and Texas in the United States	*Rattus* to rat flea to *Rattus;* opossum to cat flea to opossum	Flea feces scratched into skin, rubbed into conjunctiva, or inhaled
Epidemic typhus	*R prowazekii*	South America, Africa, Asia, Central America, Mexico	Human to *Pediculus corporis humanus* louse to human	Louse feces scratched into skin
Sylvatic typhus	*R prowazekii*	United States	Flying squirrel to louse and flea ectoparasites to flying squirrels	Ectoparasite of flying squirrels to humans
Recrudescent typhus	*R prowazekii*	Worldwide	Reactivation of latent human infection years after acute illness	None
Scrub typhus	*O tsutsugamushi*	Japan, southern and eastern Asia, northern Australia, islands of the western and southwestern Pacific	Transovarial transmission in *Leptothrombidium* chiggers	Chigger bite

the eastern United States), and a travel history can suggest the diagnosis (eg, boutonneuse fever in travelers returning from tick-infested areas of South Africa, Kenya, or the Mediterranean coast).

MORPHOLOGIC FEATURES OF THE ORGANISMS

Rickettsiae are small (0.3 × 1.0 μm) bacilli and have a cell wall with the ultrastructural characteristics of a gram-negative bacterium (Figure 85–1). The outer envelope of the SFG and typhus group rickettsiae has a thin outer electron-dense layer of 2.5 nm and a thick inner layer of 6.2 to 7.7 nm and differs from *O tsutsugamushi*, which has a thick outer layer of 8.5 nm and a thin inner layer of 2.5 nm.[6] Presumably, the protein composition and presence of lipopolysaccharide and peptidoglycan in the cell wall of SFG and typhus group rickettsiae explain these ultrastructural differences from *O tsutsugamushi*. Scrub typhus rickettsiae also lack the prominent electron-lucent zone that surrounds the cell wall of SFG and typhus rickettsiae and is thought to be a capsule-like slime layer.

CLINICAL FEATURES

Rickettsial diseases are initiated by the inoculation of rickettsiae into the skin by the bite of a tick or mite or by scratching infected feces deposited by a louse or flea.[7] Some species of *Rickettsia* such as *R conorii, R sibirica, R akari, R japonica,* and *O tsutsugamushi* frequently cause local epidermal and dermal necrosis known as an eschar or *tache noire* (black spot) at the inoculation site.[8,9] Other rickettsiae seldom (*R rickettsii* and Israel SFG rickettsia)[10] or never (*R prowazekii* and *R typhi*) naturally produce an eschar. During the incubation period, which averages 7 days for Rocky Mountain spotted fever, rickettsiae spread via the bloodstream, attach to the cell membrane of endothelial cells throughout the body, and induce the endothelial cells to engulf them.[11] The organisms then escape from the phagosome into the cytosol where they divide by binary fission. The major pathophysiologic effects of rickettsial diseases ensue because of injury to infected endothelium, and the major targets are the blood vessels in the skin, lungs, brain, and gastrointestinal tract.[12–23]

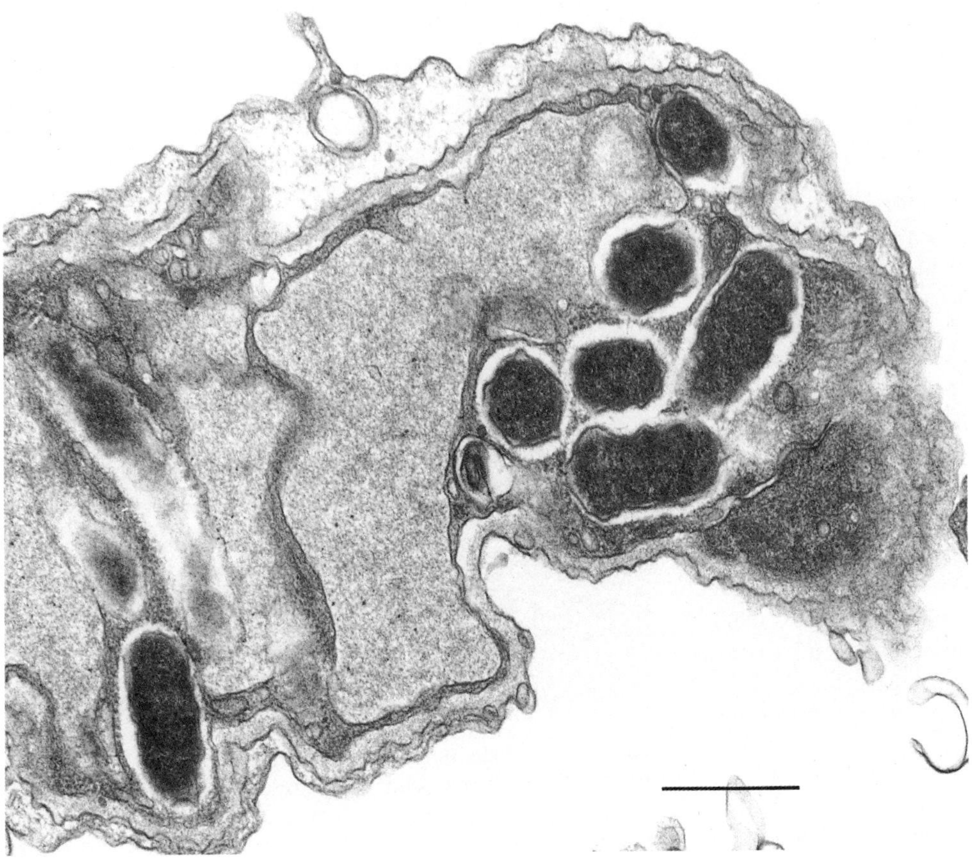

Figure 85–1. SFG rickettsiae in an endothelial cell of a pulmonary alveolar capillary of an experimentally infected mouse (bar, 0.5 μm; ×55,000).

During the first 3 days after the onset of illness, the symptoms (fever, severe headache, myalgia, nausea, and vomiting) do not point to a specific diagnosis.[24,25] Some of the stereotyped clinical manifestations of the acute phase response are likely mediated by cytokines such as interleukin-1 and tumor necrosis factor alpha. The principal direct effect of rickettsial injury to the endothelium of the microcirculation is increased vascular permeability with consequent edema and hypovolemia.[13,26,27] Edema may accumulate not only in the soft tissues of the skin but may manifest as life-threatening noncardiogenic pulmonary edema.[7,28] Decreased perfusion of the organs accounts for some pathophysiologic effects (eg, prerenal azotemia or, in more severe infections, acute tubular necrosis).[29] The focal vascular lesions in the skin, brain, and gastrointestinal tract are the basis of the rash, encephalitis, nausea, vomiting, and abdominal pain. Severe injury to the blood vessel wall results in extravasation of erythrocytes into the center of the petechial cutaneous maculopapule. Many of these patients manifest thrombocytopenia because of consumption of platelets in hemostatic plugs in the numerous foci of denuded endothelium. Mortality rates of 20% and higher were reported for Rocky Mountain spotted fever, epidemic typhus, and scrub typhus in the preantibiotic era. Mortality rates are substantially lower for these rickettsioses after early treatment with tetracyclines or chloramphenicol and even without specific treatment for the other rickettsioses.

PATHOLOGY

The pathologic lesions of rickettsial diseases are the result of vascular infection and injury by intracellular rickettsiae in the endothelium and additionally for Rocky Mountain spotted fever in vascular smooth muscle cells. Early lesions are subtle, and cause only functional alterations in vascular permeability (Figure 85–2). Later in the course, the histopathologist recognizes the host response to the focal intracellular infection, namely, perivascular accumulations of lymphocytes and macrophages (Figures 85–3 and 85–4). The occurrence of thrombi has been overemphasized, for they are in only a small fraction of foci of vascular damage and they are usually nonocclusive (Figures 85–5 and 85–6). Consequently, there are few microinfarcts in rickettsial infections. The most impressive clinical form of a rickettsial disease, fulminant Rocky Mountain spotted fever, is characterized by a rapidly fatal course within 5 days after the onset of illness. The microscopic lesions reflect the short, severe course; there are many thrombi and microinfarcts, but essentially no perivascular lymphohistiocytic host response (Figure 85–7).[30]

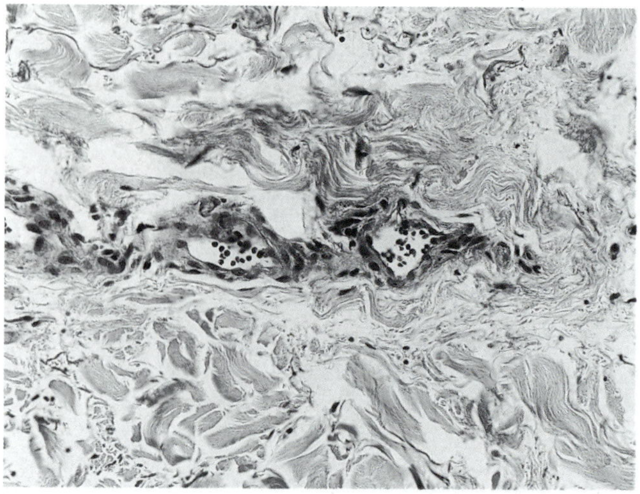

Figure 85–2. Early vascular changes in Rocky Mountain spotted fever are predominantly functional; note the prominence of the endothelial cells, the perivascular edema, and the lack of a significant inflammatory cell infiltrate (hematoxylin-eosin, ×250).

The vascular lesions affect mainly the microcirculation and may be observed in any organ. The most characteristic lesions are the petechial maculopapular rash, eschar, cerebral glial nodules, interstitial pneumonia, interstitial mononuclear myocarditis, and lymphohistiocytic vasculitis in the wall of the gastrointestinal tract.

Skin Lesions

The diagnosis of a rickettsial disease can be established by the surgical pathologist in the acute stage of the illness only after the onset of a rash. A biopsy of a maculopapular lesion, preferably an advanced lesion with a central petechia, can be examined by immunohistology

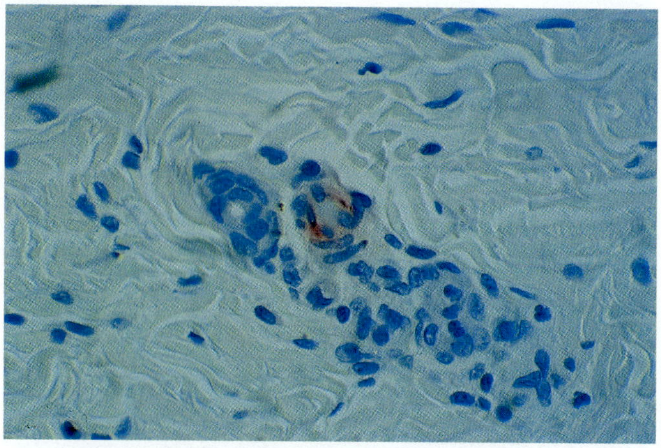

Figure 85–3. Skin from a patient with a later stage of Rocky Mountain spotted fever shows immunoperoxidase-stained *R rickettsii* and a mild perivascular lymphohistocytic infiltrate (anti-spotted fever rickettsia immunoperoxidase, ×100).

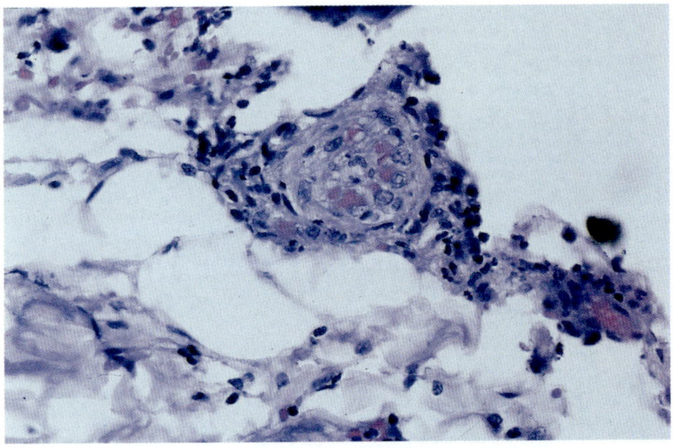

Figure 85–4. The host response to endothelial cell infection by *R typhi* is most frequently perivascular infiltrates of lymphocytes and histiocytes; also note swollen, injured endothelial cells in this small vessel in the skin (hematoxylin-eosin, ×160).

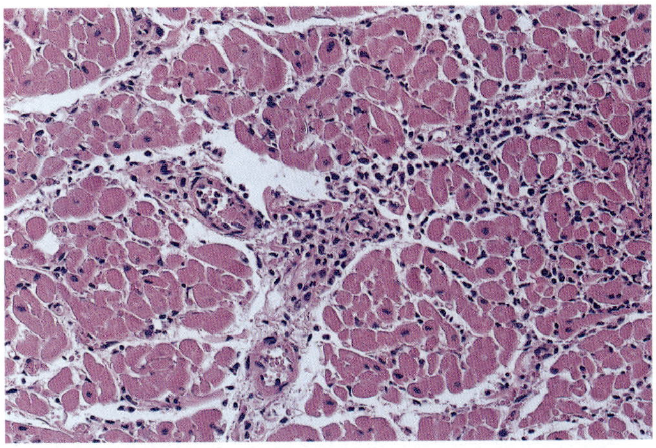

Figure 85–6. Interstitial myocarditis, generally a pathophysiologically unimportant lesion, reflects vascular infection and the host immune response. There is a nonocclusive thrombus in an injured blood vessel and adjacent perivascular and interstitial infiltration by lymphocytes and macrophages (hematoxylin-eosin, ×50).

for rickettsial organisms (Figure 85–8).[31–34] Wolbach used a Giemsa stain, a superb research tool in his laboratory, to demonstrate *R prowazekii* in endothelial cells in the rash of Polish patients with epidemic typhus in the aftermath of World War I.[23] Subsequently frozen sections of cutaneous biopsy specimens cut at levels to include particularly the center of the maculopapule, where the intensity of rickettsial infection is greatest, have been used to diagnose Rocky Mountain spotted fever at the time when critical therapeutic decisions are being made.[32,34,35] Recently the immunoperoxidase method has been applied successfully to the demonstration of SFG rickettsiae in formalin-fixed, paraffin-embedded tissues (Figure 85–6).[31]

Microscopic examination of the eschar at the site of the tick bite reveals a more vigorous host immune and phagocytic response than is observed in the rash with numerous perivascular T-helper and T-cytotoxic/suppressor lymphocytes and macrophages and usually relatively few rickettsiae.[9,36] Thrombi are seldom extensive despite the apparent ischemic necrosis of the epidermis and dermis.

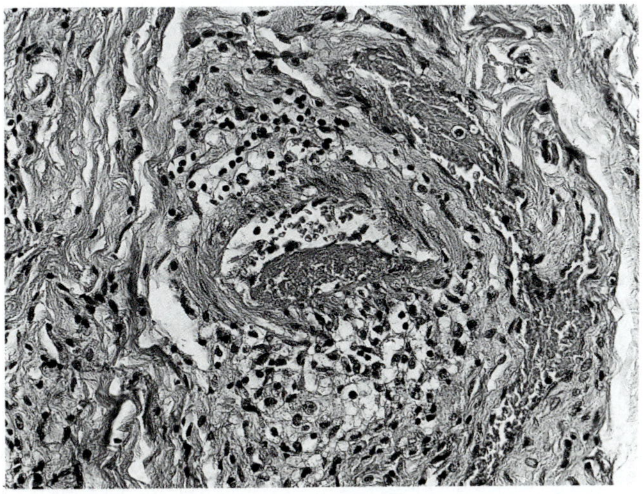

Figure 85–5. Eccentric, nonocclusive thrombi are infrequent in Rocky Mountain spotted fever. The eccentric localization of the thrombus corresponds to focal, heavily infected endothelial cells (hematoxylin-eosin, ×250).

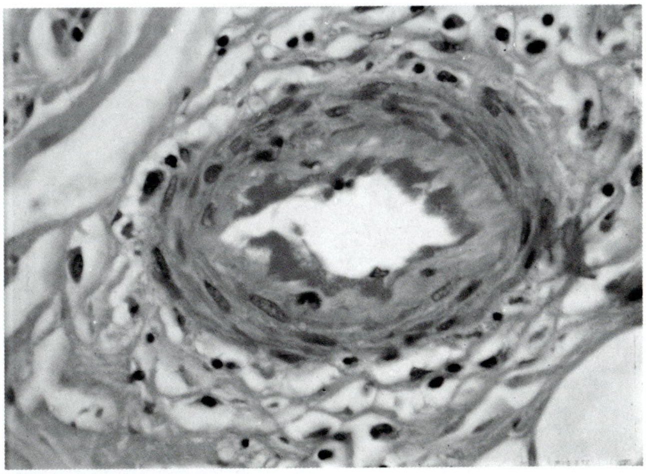

Figure 85–7. Fulminant Rocky Mountain spotted fever is characterized by rapid course and death within 5 days after onset. There is severely damaged vasculature at foci of infection and an absence of a significant inflammatory cell response to the infection. Here the endothelium is denuded and replaced by a fibrin thrombus (hematoxylin-eosin, ×780).

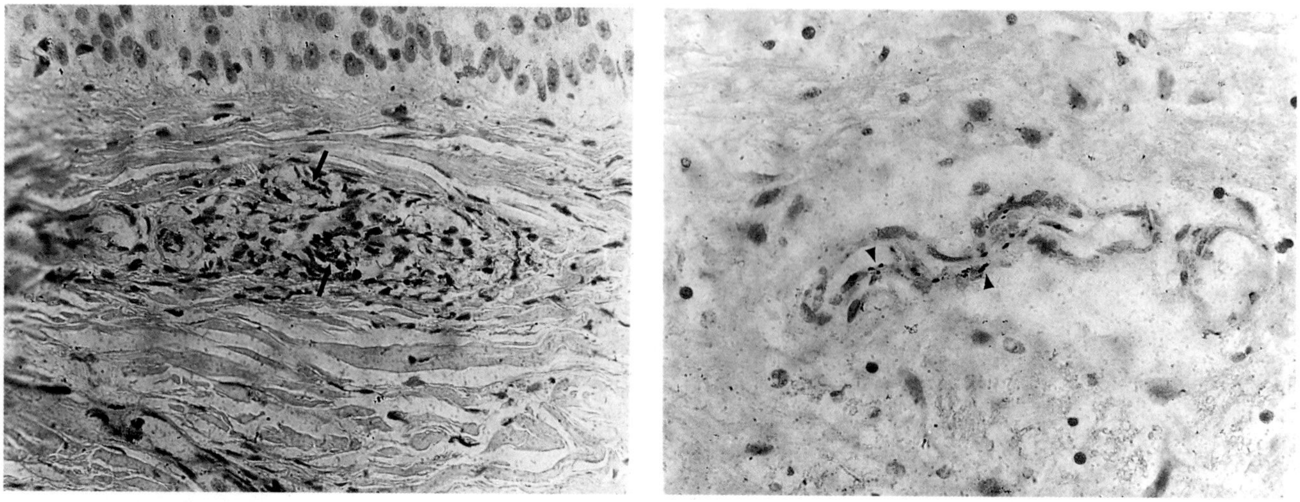

A B

Figure 85–8. Immunohistologic demonstration of *R rickettsii* (*arrows*) in (**A**) a superficial dermal vessel with necrotizing lymphohistiocytic vasculitis, and (**B**) a cerebral vessel with little or no inflammatory cell infiltrate. This method or an immunofluorescent detection method may be used to make a timely diagnosis of spotted fever rickettsiosis, or may establish the diagnosis where serologic studies have failed (labeled-streptavidin-biotin immunoperoxidase with rabbit anti-*R rickettsii,* hematoxylin counterstain; ×630 and ×500, respectively).

Central Nervous System Lesions

The so-called glial nodule is highly characteristic of rickettsial encephalitis.[7,14,15,18,20,22,23,37–39] It comprises focal perivascular infiltration of the neurophil by predominantly macrophages (Figures 85–9 through 85–11). Sometimes lymphocytes are also in the affected perivascular space. In some patients, vascular damage causes microinfarcts or perivascular ring hemorrhages. The leptomeninges may manifest a mild lymphohistiocytic, frequently perivascular, infiltrate.

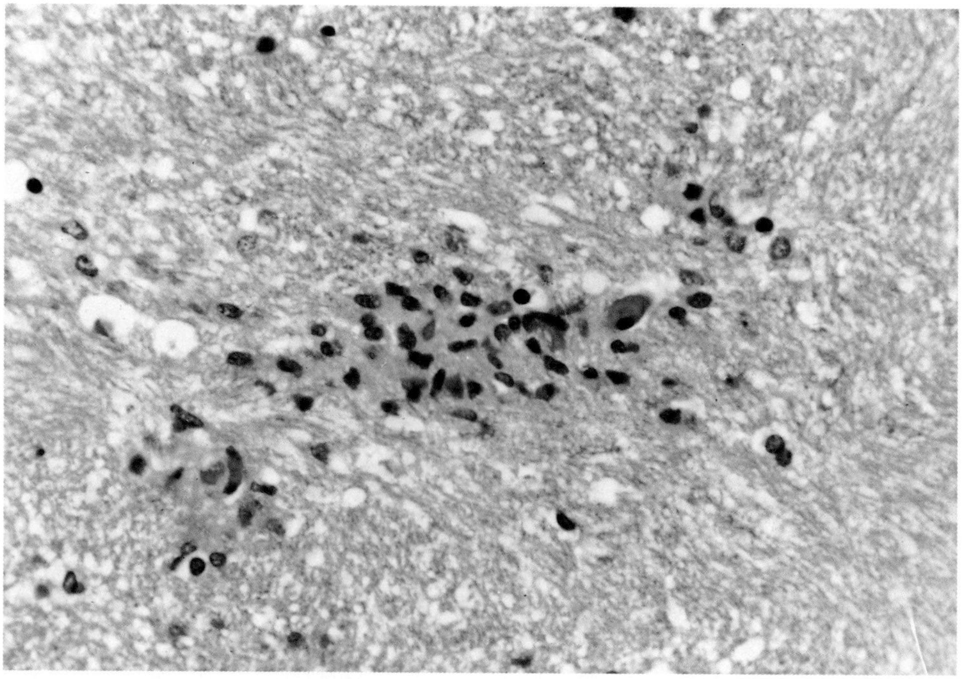

Figure 85–9. Small glial nodule in the pons from a patient with Rocky Mountain spotted fever (hematoxylin-eosin, ×600).

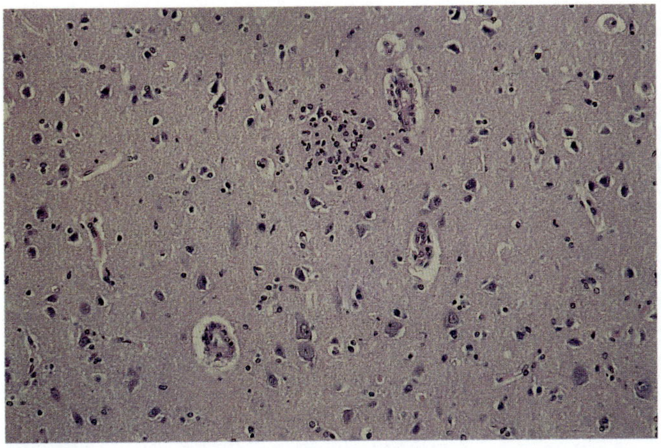

Figure 85–10. A similar lesion in scrub typhus (hematoxylin-eosin, ×50).

Pulmonary Lesions

The microcirculation of the lungs is a major target of rickettsial infection, and the result in severe infections is often noncardiogenic pulmonary edema or adult respiratory distress syndrome.[28] Microscopic lesions vary from primarily alveolar edema at times with hyaline membranes to lymphohistiocytic infiltration of the alveolar sepia (interstitial pneumonia) and perivascular space (pulmonary vasculitis) (Figures 85–12 and 85–13).[16,17,39] Additional observations include alveolar septal congestion, interstitial edema, increased quantities of alveolar macrophages, alveolar and interlobular septal hemorrhages, and focal alveolar fibrinous exudates.

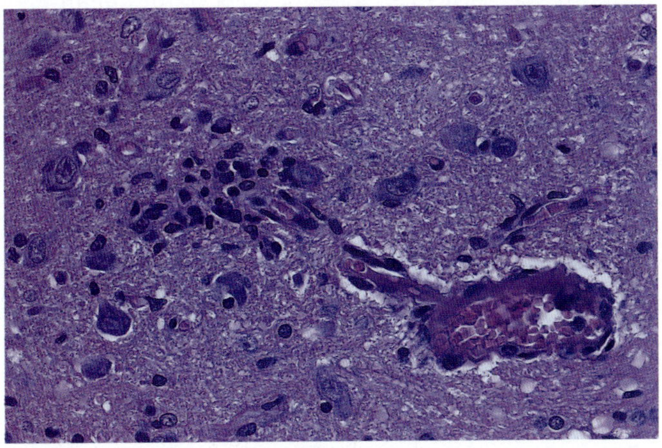

Figure 85–11. The perivascular mononuclear cell infiltrates of the neuropil are apparent in this lesion in the brain of a patient with epidemic louse-borne typhus fever (hematoxylin-eosin, ×100).

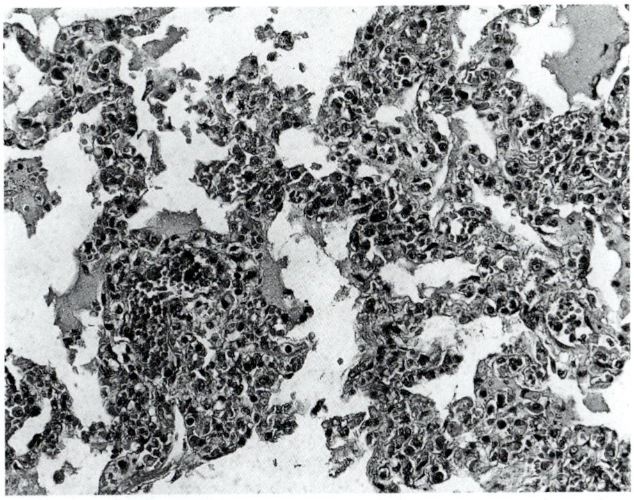

Figure 85–12. Interstitial pneumonitis and hyaline membranes in Rocky Mountain spotted fever. Note the thickening of the alveolar septa secondary to infiltration with lymphocytes, histiocytes, and edema fluid. The alveolar wall is focally necrotic where hyaline membranes are noted (hematoxylin-eosin, ×250).

Myocardial Pathology

The histologic appearance of the myocardium is occasionally the first abnormal finding to be detected by the pathologist. Interstitial and perivascular accumulations of macrophages and lymphocytes trigger the diagnostic designation of myocarditis (Figure 85–6).[40] Note that the heart does not manifest myocardial necrosis, flabby dilated ventricles, nor the echocardiographic and cardiopulmonary dynamics of overt cardiac failure in rickettsial diseases. Thus, the pathologic diagnosis of myocarditis can be confusing or misleading to the clinicians who cared for the patient. The pathologist who pursues the cause to identification of a particular *Rickettsia* species will have achieved a more useful diagnosis.

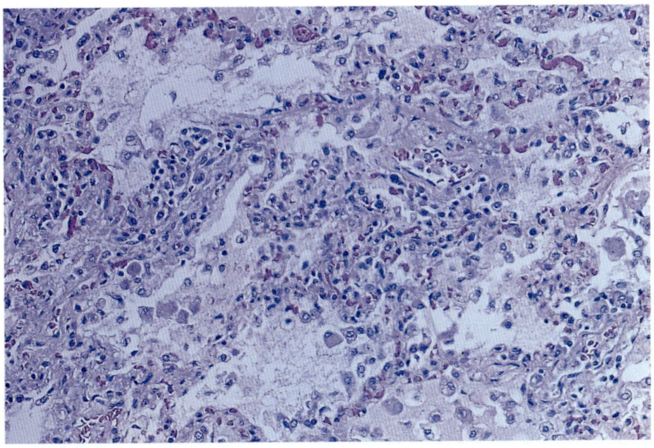

Figure 85–13. Interstitial pneumonia and consequent alveolar edema are important pulmonary lesions in scrub typhus (hematoxylin-eosin, ×50).

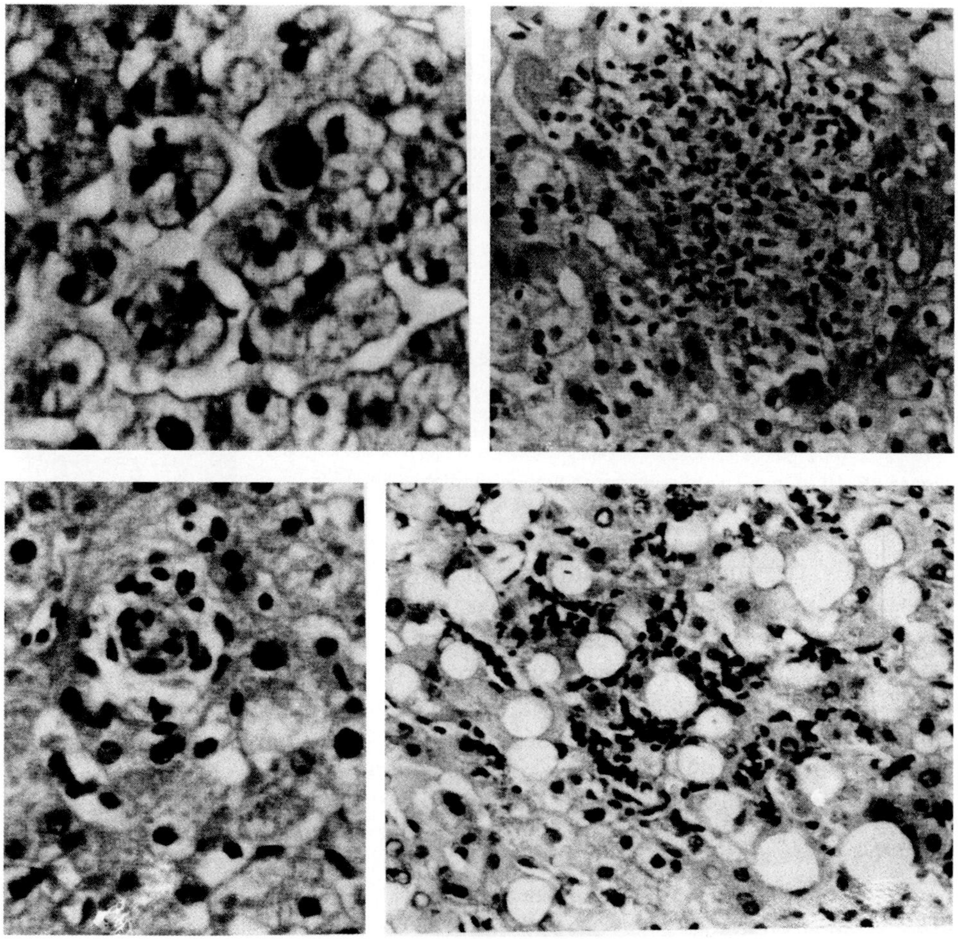

Figure 85–14. Hepatic biopsy specimens in boutonneuse fever. Note the aggregates containing predominantly lymphocytes and histiocytes associated with a focus of hepatocellular necrosis (hematoxylin-eosin, ×240). *Upper left:* acidophilic hepatocellular necrosis, ×375; *upper right:* lobular focus of hepatocellular necrosis and leukocytic infiltration, ×240; *lower left:* lobular granuloma-like focus of necrosis and lymphohistiocytic infiltration, ×375; *lower right:* multifocal mononuclear cell infiltrates and moderate steatosis, ×240 (hematoxylin-eosin). *(Photomicrograph from Walker et al.[44])*

Other Lesions

Search for lesions reveals lymphohistiocytic vasculitis in the gastrointestinal tract, pancreas, hepatic portal triads, and renal parenchyma, particularly near the corticomedullary junction.[15,19,20,29,41–43] In addition, the liver in boutonneuse fever frequently contains foci of hepatocellular necrosis and host cellular response that results in hepatic granuloma-like lesions (Figure 85–14).[44]

IDENTIFICATION OF ORGANISMS IN TISSUE

Giemsa and Brown–Hopps stains have been used to demonstrate rickettsiae in tissue sections.[21–23] However, most histology laboratories are not able to stain rickettsiae in formalin-fixed tissue by the routine Giemsa method, and only a small fraction of the organisms present are demonstrated by the modified Brown–Hopps technique. In contrast, numerous intracellular thin bacilli are demonstrated by immunohistologic methods including immunofluorescence on frozen sections[32,34,35,46,47] and immunofluorescence[33] and immunoperoxidase[31] on protease-digested, formalin-fixed, paraffin-embedded sections. Ultrastructural search for rickettsiae is usually difficult because their distribution is multifocal with large volumes of intervening uninfected tissue. However, identification of thin gram-negative bacilli in the cytosol of endothelial cells may be considered as indicative of a rickettsial disease.[46,47]

DIFFERENTIAL DIAGNOSIS

The clinical differential diagnosis in the early days of the illness prior to the appearance of the rash is vast and includes influenza, enteroviral infection, typhoid fever, and many entities suggested by the specific geographic exposure (eg, malaria, Lassa fever). If nausea, vomiting, and abdominal pain are prominent, viral, bacterial, and protozoal agents of enterocolitis are considered. Cough and clinical and radiologic chest abnormalities may suggest pneumonia. Fever, coma, seizures, and neurologic signs suggest meningitis and herpes simplex or arboviral encephalitis. Even after the recognition of local cutaneous necrosis, the possibilities include cutaneous anthrax, tularemia, syphilis, and chancroid. After the onset of rash, the diagnostic considerations include meningococcemia, gram-negative sepsis, toxic shock syndrome, leptospirosis, disseminated gonococcal infection, secondary syphilis, measles, rubella, enteroviral exanthem, immune thrombocytopenic purpura, thrombotic thrombocytopenic purpura, and immune complex vasculitis (eg, systemic lupus erythematosus).

The pathologic differential diagnosis depends on which stage of the vascular lesion is encountered histologically. Whether perivascular edema, thrombi, or a perivascular lymphohistiocytic response is prominent, there are too many viral, bacterial, fungal, and protozoal diseases with a vasculocentric host immune and inflammatory response to recount. What is most important is to include rickettsioses in the differential diagnosis and to apply the appropriate, specific, sensitive assays to establish a rickettsial diagnosis.

CONTEMPORARY DIAGNOSTIC APPROACHES

In addition to the immunohistologic diagnosis of SFG or typhus group rickettsiosis by immunofluorescence or immunoperoxidase staining as already discussed, Rocky Mountain spotted fever has been diagnosed by polymerase chain reaction amplification of DNA of the gene for the 17-kD surface protein from patients' blood and tissue specimens.[45,48,49] A clever approach to the diagnosis of boutonneuse fever relies on separation of circulating *R conorii* infected endothelial cells that have become dislodged from their moorings.[51] Immunomagnetic beads coated with a monoclonal antibody to a surface epitope on human endothelial cells capture these cells. After washing away the other blood components, rickettsiae are detected by specific immunofluorescent staining. The principles of these approaches are likely to be applicable to any of the vasculopathic rickettsioses.

CONFIRMATIONAL TESTING AND DIAGNOSIS

The gold standard of diagnosis for infectious diseases is isolation and identification of the etiologic agent from the patient's blood or tissues. Cultivation of rickettsiae is seldom undertaken. Rickettsiae, although classically recovered by inoculation of guinea pigs, other susceptible animals, or yolk sac of embryonated hen's eggs, can be isolated in antibiotic-free cell culture. Recently numerous cases of boutonneuse fever have been confirmed by isolation of *R conorii* in shell vial centrifugation-enhanced cell culture.[52] With biohazard containment facilities equipped with laminar flow hoods, rickettsiae should be no more daunting to cultivate in the small quantities required for diagnostic identification than are viruses.

Most often rickettsial diagnoses are confirmed by demonstration of a fourfold or greater rise in antibody titer by a specific assay utilizing rickettsial antigens. Reagents are available commercially for the diagnosis of Rocky Mountain spotted fever, boutonneuse fever, and murine typhus by immunofluorescent antibody (IFA) assay,[53] latex agglutination test,[54] and enzyme immunoassay. Among these assays, the one that currently is considered the most sensitive, specific, and reliable is the IFA test.[55,56] It should be emphasized that one does not expect to detect diagnostic antibodies in the acute stage of illness, and patients often die before producing antibodies to the offending rickettsia. Thus, serologic diagnosis is retrospective and requires collection of serum during convalescence. Although demonstration of seroconversion is preferred, a single convalescent titer of 64 by IFA, 128 by latex agglutination, or 16 by complement fixation strongly supports the diagnosis of Rocky Mountain spotted fever.

Indirect immunoperoxidase assay is similar in its usefulness to IFA[57] and has been utilized extensively for the diagnosis of scrub typhus and Israel spotted fever. It is important to recognize that many state public health laboratories offer highly reliable serologic tests for rickettsial diseases.

REFERENCES

1. Weiss E, Moulder JW. The rickettsias and chlamydias. In: Kreig MR, Holt JG, eds. *Bergey's Manual of Systematic Bacteriology*. Baltimore: Williams & Wilkins; 1984: 687–739.
2. Amano K-I, Tamura A, Ohashi N, Urakami H, Kaya S, Fukushi K. Deficiency of peptidoglycan and lipopolysaccharide components in *Rickettsia tsutsugamushi*. *Infect Immun.* 1987;55:2290–2292.
3. Azad AF. Epidemiology of murine typhus. *Annu Rev Entomol.* 1990;35:553–569.
4. Burgdorfer W. Ecological and epidemiological considerations of Rocky Mountain spotted fever and scrub typhus. In: Walker DH, ed. *Biology of Rickettsial Diseases.* Boca Raton, Fla: CRC Press; 1988:33–50.
5. McDade JE, Newhouse VF. Natural history of *Rickettsia rickettsii*. *Am Rev Microbiol.* 1986;40:287–309.
6. Silverman D, Wisseman CL, Jr. Comparative ultrastructural study on the cell envelopes of *Rickettsia prowazekii, Rickettsia rickettsii,* and *Rickettsia tsutsugamushi*. *Infect Immun.* 1978;21:1020–1023.
7. Walker DH. Pathology and pathogenesis of the vasculotropic rickettsioses. In: Walker DH, ed. *Biology of Rickettsial Diseases.* Boca Raton, Fla: CRC Press; 1988:115–137.
8. Brettman LR, Lewin S, Holzman RS, et al. Rickettsialpox:

report of an outbreak and a contemporary review. *Medicine.* 1981;60:363–382.
9. Walker DH, Occhino C, Tringali GR, Di Rosa S, Mansueto S. Pathogenesis of rickettsial eschars: the tache noire of boutonneuse fever. *Hum Pathol.* 1988;19:1449–1454.
10. Walker DH, Gay RM, Valdes-Dapena M. The occurrence of eschars in Rocky Mountain spotted fever. *J Am Acad Dermatol.* 1981;4:571–576.
11. Walker TS. Rickettsial interactions with human endothelial cells in vitro: adherence and entry. *Infect Immun.* 1984; 44:205–210.
12. Davidson MG, Breitschwerdt EB, Walker DH, et al. Vascular permeability and coagulation during *Rickettsia rickettsii* infection in dogs. *Am J Vet Res.* 1990;51:165–170.
13. Harrell GT, Aikawa JK. Pathogenesis of circulatory failure in Rocky Mountain spotted fever. Alterations in the blood volume and the thiocyanate space at various stages of the disease. *Arch Intern Med.* 1949;83:331–347.
14. Horney LF, Walker DH. Meningoencephalitis as a major manifestation of Rocky Mountain spotted fever. *South Med J.* 1988;81:915–918.
15. Lillie RD. I. The pathology of Rocky Mountain spotted fever. *NIH Bull.* 1941;177:1–46.
16. Roggli VL, Keener S, Bradford WD, Pratt PC, Walker DH. Pulmonary pathology of Rocky Mountain spotted fever (RMSF) in children. *Pediatr Pathol.* 1985;4:47–57.
17. Walker DH, Crawford CG, Cain BG. Rickettsial infection of the pulmonary microcirculation: the basis for interstitial pneumonitis in Rocky Mountain spotted fever. *Hum Pathol.* 1980;11:263–272.
18. Walker DH, Gear JHS. Correlation of the distribution of *Rickettsia conorii,* microscopic lesions, and clinical features in South African tick bite fever. *Am J Trop Med Hyg.* 1985;34:361–371.
19. Walker DH, Herrero-Herrero JI, Ruiz-Beltran R, Bullon-Sopelana A, Ramos-Hidalgo A. The pathology of fatal Mediterranean spotted fever. *Am J Clin Pathol.* 1987; 87:669–672.
20. Walker DH, Parks FM, Betz TG, Taylor JP, Muehlberger JW. Histopathology and immunohistologic demonstration of the distribution of *Rickettsia typhi* in fatal murine typhus. *Am J Clin Pathol.* 1989;91:720–724.
21. Wolbach SB. The etiology of Rocky Mountain spotted fever. (A preliminary report). *J Med Res.* 1916;34:121–128.
22. Wolbach SB. Studies on Rocky Mountain spotted fever. *J Med Res.* 1919;41:1–218.
23. Wolbach SB, Todd JL, Palfrey FW. Pathology of typhus in man. In: *The Etiology and Pathology of Typhus.* Cambridge: League Red Cross Soc Harvard Univ; 1922; 152–221.
24. Helmick CG, Bernard KW, D'Angelo LJ. Rocky Mountain spotted fever: clinical, laboratory, and epidemiological features of 262 cases. *J Infect Dis.* 1984;150:480–488.
25. Kaplowitz LG, Fischer JJ, Sparling PF. Rocky Mountain spotted fever: a clinical dilemma. *Curr Clin Top Infect Dis.* 1981;2:89–108.
26. Ruiz R, Herrero JI, Martin AM, et al. Vascular permeability in boutonneuse fever. *J Infect Dis.* 1984;149:1036.
27. Vicente V, Alberca I, Ruiz R, Herrero I, Gonzalez R, Portugal J. Coagulation abnormalities in patients with Mediterranean spotted fever. *J Infect Dis.* 1986;153: 128–131.
28. Lankford HV, Glauser FL. Cardiopulmonary dynamics in a severe case of Rocky Mountain spotted fever. *Arch Intern Med.* 1980;140:1357–1360.
29. Walker DH, Mattern WD. Acute renal failure in Rocky Mountain spotted fever. *Arch Intern Med.* 1979;139: 443–448.
30. Walker DH, Hawkins HK, Hudson P. Fulminant Rocky Mountain spotted fever. Its pathologic characteristics associated with glucose-6-phosphate dehydrogenase deficiency. *Arch Pathol Lab Med.* 1983;107:121–125.
31. Dumler JS, Gage WR, Pettis GL, Azad AF, Kuhadja FP. Rapid immunoperoxidase demonstration of *Rickettsia rickettsii* in fixed cutaneous specimens from patients with Rocky Mountain spotted fever. *Am J Clin Pathol.* 1990; 93:410–414.
32. Walker DH, Burday MS, Folds JD. Laboratory diagnosis of Rocky Mountain spotted fever. *South Med J.* 1980; 73:1443–1447.
33. Walker DH, Cain BG. A method for specific diagnosis of Rocky Mountain spotted fever on fixed, paraffin-embedded tissue by immunofluorescence. *J Infect Dis.* 1978;137:206–209.
34. Walker DH, Cain BG, Olmstead PM. Laboratory diagnosis of Rocky Mountain spotted fever by immunofluorescent demonstration of *Rickettsia rickettsii* in cutaneous lesions. *Am J Clin Pathol.* 1978;69:619–623.
35. Kaplowitz LG, Lange JV, Fischer JJ, Walker DH. Correlation of rickettsial titers, circulating endotoxin, and clinical features in Rocky Mountain spotted fever. *Arch Intern Med.* 1983;143:1149–1151.
36. Herrero-Herrero JI, Walker DH, Ruiz-Beltran R. Immunohistochemical evaluation of the cellular immune response to *Rickettsia conorii* in *Taches noires. J Infect Dis.* 1987;155:802–805.
37. Binford CH, Ecker HD. Endemic (murine) typhus. Report of autopsy findings in three cases. *Am J Clin Pathol.* 1947;17:797–806.
38. Settle EB, Pinkerton H, Corbett AJ. A pathologic study of tsutsugamushi disease (scrub typhus) with notes on clinicopathologic correlation. *J Lab Clin Med.* 1945;30:639–661.
39. Levine HD. Pathologic study of thirty-one cases of scrub typhus fever with especial reference to the cardiovascular system. *Am Heart J.* 1946;31:314–328.
40. Walker DH, Paletta CE, Cain BG. Pathogenesis of myocarditis in Rocky Mountain spotted fever. *Arch Pathol Lab Med.* 1980;104:171–174.
41. Adams JS, Walker DH. The liver in Rocky Mountain spotted fever. *Am J Clin Pathol.* 1981;75:156–161.
42. Bradford WE, Croker BP, Tisher CC. Kidney lesions in Rocky Mountain spotted fever. *Am J Pathol.* 1979;97: 381–392.
43. Randall MB. Rocky Mountain spotted fever. Gastrointestinal and pancreatic lesions and rickettsial infection. *Arch Pathol Lab Med.* 1984;108:963–967.
44. Walker DH, Staiti A, Mansueto S, Tringali G. Frequent occurrence of hepatic lesions in boutonneuse fever. *Acta Trop.* 1986;43:175–181.
45. Sexton DJ, Kanj SS, Wilson K, et al. The use of polymerase

chain reaction as a diagnostic test for Rocky Mountain spotted fever. *Am J Trop Med Hyg.* 1994;50:59–63.

46. Moe JB, Mosher DF, Kenyon RH, et al. Functional and morphologic changes during experimental Rocky Mountain spotted fever in guinea pigs. *Lab Invest.* 1976; 35:235–245.
47. Walker DH, Harrison A, Henderson F, Murphy FA. Identification of *Rickettsia rickettsii* in a guinea pig model by immunofluorescent and electron microscopic techniques. *Am J Pathol.* 1977;86:343–358.
48. Carl M, Tibbs CW, Dobson ME, Paparello S, Dasch GA. Diagnosis of acute typhus infection using the polymerase chain reaction. *J Infect Dis.* 1990;161:791–793.
49. Tzianabos T, Anderson BE, McDade JE. Detection of *Rickettsia rickettsii* DNA in clinical specimens by using polymerase chain reaction technology. *J Clin Microbiol.* 1989;27:2866–2868.
50. Kass EM, Szaniawski WK, Levy H, Leach J, Srinivasan K, Rives C. Rickettsialpox in a New York City hospital, 1980 to 1989. *N Engl J Med.* 1994;331:1612–1617.
51. Drancourt M, George F, Brouqui P, Sampol J, Raoult D. Diagnosis of Mediterranean spotted fever by indirect immunofluorescence of *Rickettsia conorii* in circulating endothelial cells isolated with monoclonal antibody-coated immunomagnetic beads. *J Infect Dis.* 1992; 166:660–663.
52. Marrero M, Raoult D. Centrifugation-shell vial technique for rapid detection of Mediterranean spotted fever rickettsia in blood culture. *Am J Trop Med Hyg.* 1989;40: 197–199.
53. Philip RN, Casper EA, Ormsbee RA, Peacock MG, Burgdorfer W. Microimmunofluorescence test for the serological study of Rocky Mountain spotted fever and typhus. *J Clin Microbiol.* 1976;3:51–61.
54. Hechemy KE, Michaelson E, Anacker RL, et al. Evaluation of Latex-*Rickettsia rickettsii* test for Rocky Mountain spotted fever in 11 laboratories. *J Clin Microbiol.* 1983; 18:938–946.
55. Kaplan JE, Schonberger LB. The sensitivity of various serologic tests in the diagnosis of Rocky Mountain spotted fever. *Am J Trop Med Hyg.* 1986;35:840–844.
56. Walker DH, Peacock MG. Laboratory diagnosis of rickettsial diseases. In: Walker DH, ed. *Biology of Rickettsial Diseases.* Boca Raton, Fla: CRC Press; 1988:135–155.
57. Raoult D, De Micco C, Chaudet H, Tamalet J. Serological diagnosis of Mediterranean spotted fever by the immunoperoxidase reaction. *Eur J Clin Microbiol.* 1985;4:441–442.

CHAPTER 86

Sago Palm Disease

Alfonso J. Strano

This disease is beyond my practice.

William Shakespeare (1564–1616), Macbeth, V, i, 57

DEFINITION AND EPIDEMIOLOGY

Sago palm disease (SPD) is a chronic cutaneous infection caused by an as-yet uncultured and unclassified gram-positive bacillus. Limbs, trunk, and face may be involved. SPD is characterized by contiguous spreading hyperkeratotic dermal nodules (Figures 86–1 and 86–2). The disease has been reported only in the East Sepic district of Papua New Guinea. There have been a dozen known infections; 11 in Melanesians and 1 in a Scot living in the area.[1–3] The geographic area has extensive swamp woodlands containing groves of sago palms (Metrozylon). Most of the patients were pricked or traumatized at the sight of primary lesion, while handling sago palms. Attempts to culture the organism and to infect animals have been unsuccessful.[3]

CLINICAL MANIFESTATION

The incubation period is unknown but primary lesions usually appear several months after the episode of trauma. Lesions are intradermal, first at the sight of trauma and then followed by contiguous intradermal spread over a period of months to years. The lesions do not ulcerate, bleed, or become necrotic. The lesions have shown no tendency to systemic dissemination and the patients have no constitutional symptoms. Treatment with antibiotic and antifungal drugs has been unsuccessful.[3] The only therapeutic success has been early wide excision of the primary lesion.

PATHOLOGY

The nodules are of variable size with sharply demarcated edges and covered by scaly hyperkeratotic epidermis. There is no ulceration, erosion, or necrosis. On cross-section the nodules are sharply defined, firm, and have a variegated white and yellowish color. There is no necrosis or hemorrhage (Figure 86–3). The nodules are composed of masses of large foamy histiocytes intermixed with fibroblasts, bundles of collagen, amorphous ground substance, organisms, and inflammatory infiltrates of lymphocytes and plasma cells (Figures 86–4 and 86–5). The organisms stain poorly with hematoxylin-eosin but are silvered by Gomori's methenamine-silver (GMS) technique (Figures 86–6 and 86–7). The bacilli vary in shape, sometimes appearing beaded and branching. They are thin and filamentous forming a mass resembling a syncytium. They are gram-positive, not acid fast, and are about 0.5 μm by 1.8 μm.

ELECTRON MICROSCOPY

All specimens studied to date have been fixed in formalin. For electron microscopy the formalin-fixed tissues were prepared by standard electron microscopy (EM) methods. The results were adequate but less than optimal. The organism is readily defined as a prokaryote with a cell wall averaging 175 nm in thickness and easily defined internal features of a bacterium (Figure 86–8). They divide by inward growth of the cell wall at

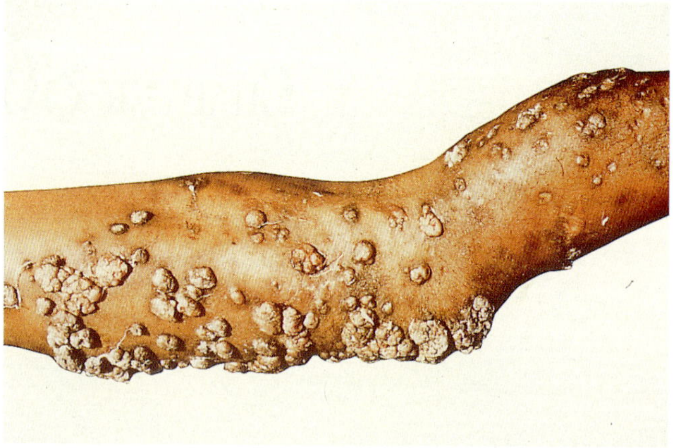

Figure 86–1. Thigh, knee, and upper leg of a young Melanesian woman. These lesions spread from a single nodule over a period of 6 years. There is no ulceration or other evidence of necrosis or hemorrhage (AFIP Neg 74-9542).

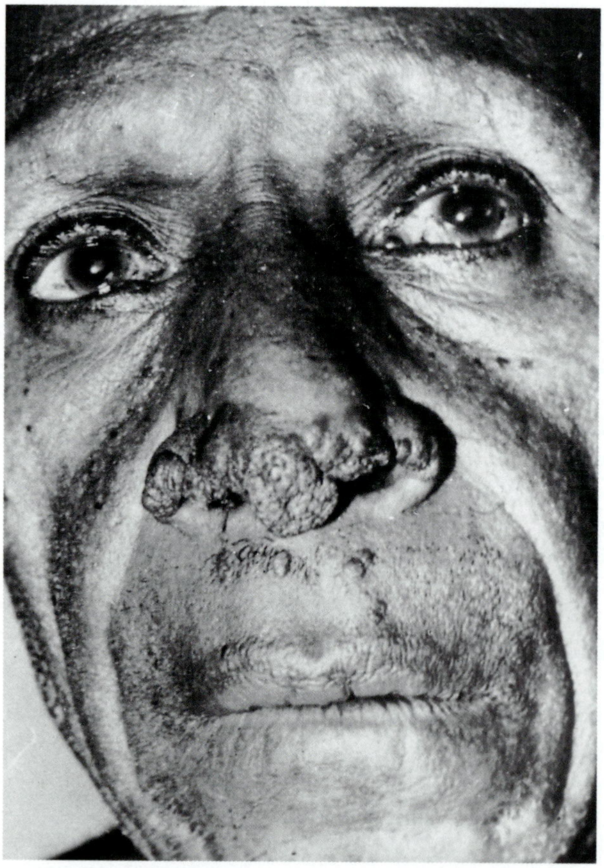

Figure 86–2. An elderly Melanesian male with lesions of the nose and upper lip (AFIP Neg 72-1005-13).

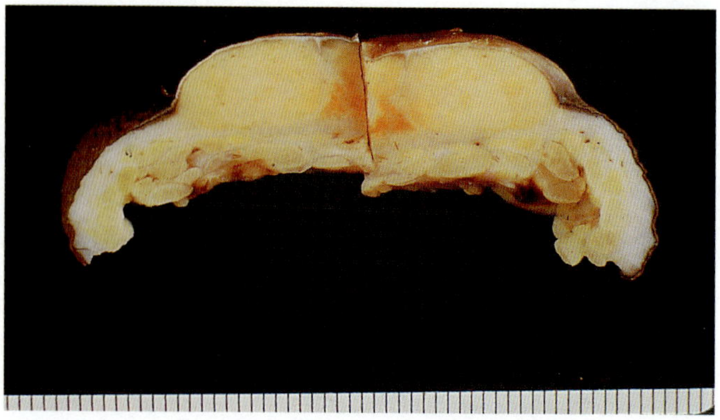

Figure 86–3. Section of a sharply demarcated nodule demonstrating the intradermal localization (gross; AFIP Neg 72-11626).

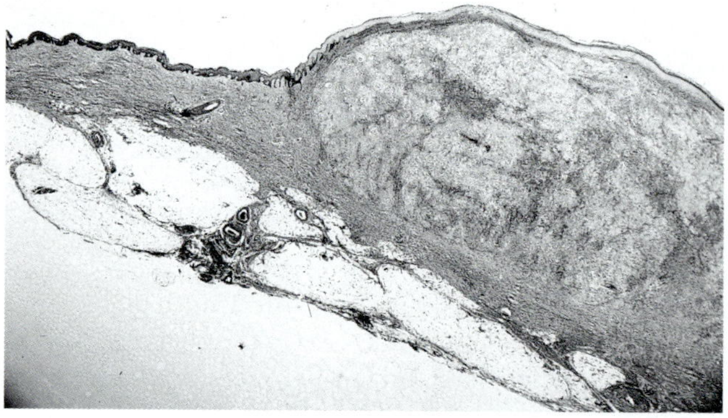

Figure 86–4. Section of the nodule shown in Figure 86–3, composed of foamy histiocytes. Note contour of the nodule and its intradermal location (AFIP Neg 72-1444; hematoxylin-eosin, ×6.5)

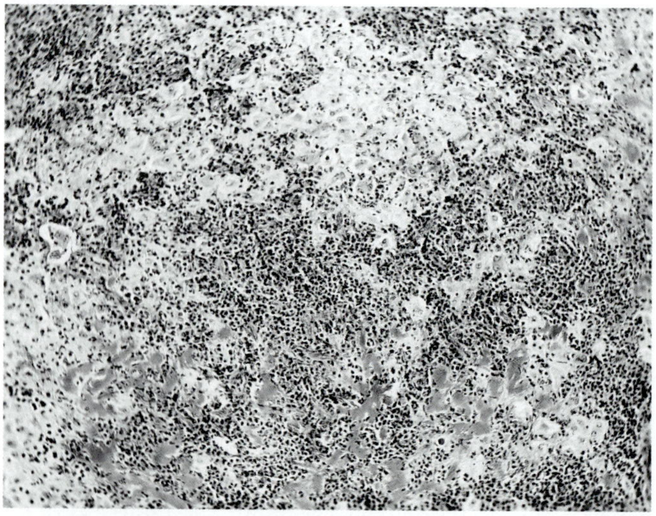

Figure 86–5. Higher magnification to show the foamy histiocytes and in addition fibroblasts, collagen bundles, and an inflammatory cell infiltrate of lymphocytes and plasma cells (AFIP Neg 72-1442; hematoxylin-eosin, ×115).

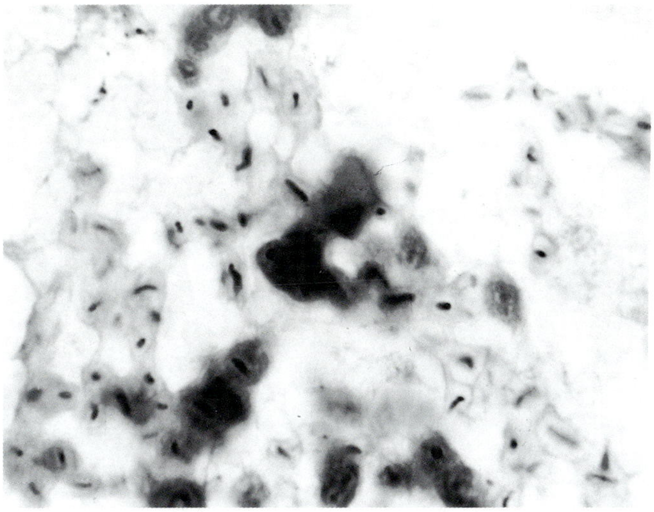

Figure 86–6. Here are shown many cross-sections and tangential sections of branching and dividing bacilli that resembles a syncytium (AFIP Neg 72-1437; GMS, ×2040).

various angles; thus before separating they give the appearance of branching. Also clearly demonstrated is that the structures, which on light microscopy appeared as a syncytium, are actually individual bacilli embedded in an amorphous proteinaceous ground substance surrounded and infiltrated with collagen (Figure 86–8).

DIAGNOSIS

The clinical, gross, light microscopic, and electron microscopic features are distinctive, so distinctive in fact that the diagnosis is readily made.

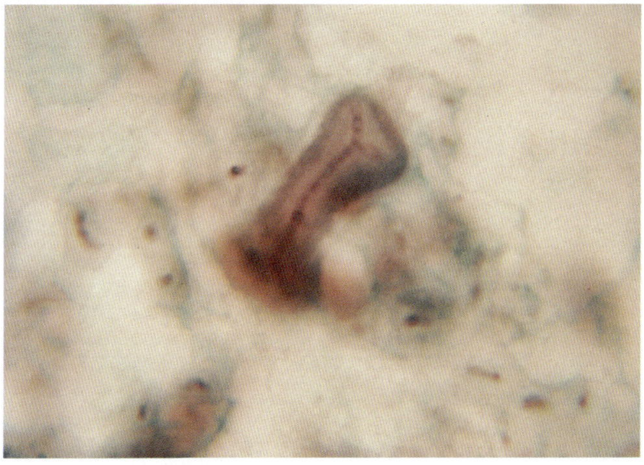

Figure 86–7. A branching filament surrounded by material that resembles ground substance (GMS, ×865).

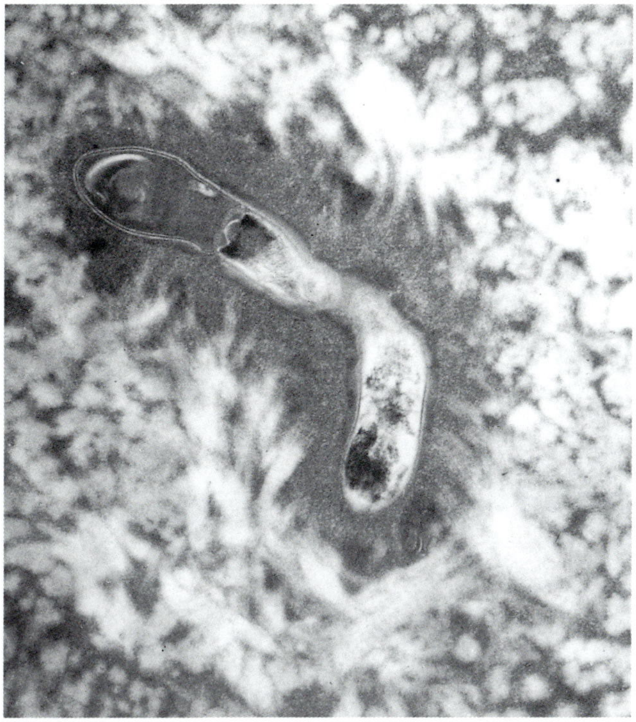

Figure 86–8. Electron micrograph of the gram-positive bacterium surrounded by ground substance and interwoven collagen fibers (AFIP Neg 75-4194; EM, ×15,000).

REFERENCES

1. Wilkey IS, Strano AJ. An unusual cutaneous infection from Papua, New Guinea. *Pathology.* 1973;5:335.
2. Strano AJ. Sago palm disease. In: Binford CH, Connor DE, eds. *Pathology of Tropical and Extraordinary Diseases, Atlas.* Washington, DC: Armed Forces Institute of Pathology, 1976.
3. Wilkey IS, 1976, personal communication.

CHAPTER 87

Staphylococcal Infections

John M. Kissane

Thou art a boil,
A plague sore, an embossed carbuncle
In my corrupted blood.

William Shakespeare (1564–1616), King Lear, II, iv, 226

GENERAL CONCEPTS

Staphylococci are members of the family Micrococcaceae.[1] *Staphylococcus aureus* is the usual pathogen; *S epidermidis* and *S saprophyticus* produce lesions in special circumstances. Staphylococci are gram-positive 0.7 to 1.2 μm in diameter with a tendency to grow in clusters.[2] Cluster formation is most prominent in solid media and can be inapparent in liquid media.[3] Organisms phagocytosed by neutrophils may be only weakly gram-positive or even gram-negative in smears or sections. Several laboratory tests are important in differentiating *S aureus* from *S epidermidis* and *S saprophyticus:* 1) catalase production, 2) coagulase production, 3) mannitol fermentation, and 4) deoxyribonuclease production.[4] Staphylococci can survive many unfavorable environmental conditions. They can be cultured from dried surfaces after several months, are relatively heat resistant, and can survive high salt concentrations.

Staphylococcus aureus produces and secretes a large array of enzymes and toxins.[5] It has become popular to ascribe to such agents one or another aspect in the pathogenicity of the parent organism. Such interpretations should be made cautiously. Purification of these agents is difficult because of their instability. Demonstration of a particular activity in vitro does not establish that the agent has an analogous activity in vivo, and the attribution of one or another aspect in the pathogenesis of lesions associated with *S aureus* is often an *a priori* analogy not established by experimental or clinical evidence.

Enzymes

- *Catalase:* All staphylococcal strains produce hydrogen peroxide that is converted to oxygen and water by catalase. It has been suggested that catalase contributes to the pathogenicity of staphylococci by splitting toxic oxygen radicals important in killing phagocytosed bacteria.[6]
- *Coagulase:* Both cell-bound and soluble coagulase mediate coagulation by steps that differ from those that participate in normal thrombosis.
- *Hyaluronidase:* This enzyme hydrolyses hyaluronic acids, acid mucopolysaccharides in the extracellular matrix of connective tissue.
- *Beta-lactamase:* These enzymes hydrolyze β-lactams. Their role in bacterial homeostasis in the absence of β-lactam antibiotics is unknown.

Other Enzymes

Staphylococcus aureus produces a phosphodiesterase whose hydrolytic action on DNA is used for taxonomic studies. It also produces several lipases.

Toxins

- *Alpha toxin:* Among five toxins that damage cell membranes this electrophoretically heterogeneous protein acts on erythrocytes, leukocytes, platelets, fibroblasts, and HeLa cells but not bacterial cell membranes. Alpha toxin is dermonecrotic when injected subcutaneously.

- *Beta-toxin:* This enzyme degrades sphingomyelin, an important component of cell membranes.
- *Gamma-toxin:* This toxin lyses erythrocytes of many species including human beings. This electrophoretically heterogeneous toxin disrupts surface membranes by a detergent-like action and also stimulates production of cyclic AMP in rabbit and guinea pig ileum, an action that may play a role in the pathogenesis of diarrhea associated with staphylococcal infections.
- *Leukocidin:* This toxin produces a prominent reversible granulocytopenia when injected into rabbits and human beings probably by forming pores in the membranes of granulocytes, allowing entry of cations.
- *Exfoliatins:* This group of proteins causes dermatologic features of several staphylococcal diseases, including staphylococcal scalded skin syndrome and toxic shock syndrome.[7]
- *Enterotoxins:* About half of all strains of *S aureus* produce one or more enterotoxins of which six (A through F) have been demonstrated.

EPIDEMIOLOGY

Shortly after birth, staphylococci from the contiguous human environment colonize the infant's umbilical stump, skin, perineum, and sometimes the gastrointestinal tract.[8] Older children and adults become carriers of staphylococci either transiently or more persistently.[9] The most common site of such carriage is the anterior nasal vestibule. The nasal carrier rate in randomly cultured adults is 20% to 40% depending on the season and other factors. Over time, about 30% of adults are prolonged carriers and about 50% are intermittent carriers, while about 20% are never colonized. Of importance in the pathogenesis of the toxic shock syndrome (TSS), about 10% of premenopausal women have staphylococci in vaginal secretions, more during menstrual periods.[10] Some groups have staphylococcal carrier rates higher than the general population. Physicians, nurses, and hospital ward attendants are particularly prone to staphylococcal colonization.[11] Diabetic patients receiving insulin injections,[12] patients on hemodialysis,[13–15] and intravenous drug abusers[16,17] more frequently harbor staphylococci than do members of the general population. There is no significant nonhuman reservoir.

PATHOLOGY

From its primary focus in the anterior nasal cavity or on the skin, *S aureus* gains access to subcutaneous tissues either of the carrier or of another person when the protective barrier of the skin is breached, inadvertently or deliberately. In the subcutaneous tissue or another site that it is has reached by direct implantation or by blood or lymphatics, the staphylococcus evokes a typical acute inflammatory reaction of which the major cellular component is the neutrophil. More than this, the staphylococcus is the quintessential pyogen (pus former) that early and characteristically produces a localized area of acute inflammation surrounding a focus of necrosis, that is, an abscess.

Abscesses vary from the limit of naked-eye visibility to confluent roughly spherical lesions many centimeters in diameter that contain semiliquid white or grayish-yellow material, pus, surrounded by a dusky mantle of viable tissue and, peripheral to that, a circumferential halo of hyperemic tissue recognizable as a fine dark red line. Microscopically the contents of an abscess include dead and dying neutrophils, fibrin, the products of necrosis of parent tissue, and dead, dying, and viable cocci, often recognizable in routine tissue stains as clouds of amphophilic granular material. The staphylococcus produces a variety of cutaneous and subcutaneous lesions[18] conveniently divided between localized infectious lesions, collectively referred to as staphylococcal pyodermas, and generalized lesions associated with a diffuse skin rash.[19]

LOCALIZED INFECTIONS

The clinical diagnosis of a staphylococcal pyoderma is usually readily made and confirmed by Gram stain and culture of extruded purulent material that usually produces a pure culture of *S aureus.* These infections are favored by poor personal hygiene, minor trauma, insect bites, or maceration, and underlying cutaneous disorders such as eczema and acne. Most infections are centered about a hair follicle. Systemic features are usually absent.

Folliculitis

The simplest staphylococcal infection is an acute inflammation involving hair follicles that presents as a series of varied, usually tender pink to red papules that rapidly undergo central suppuration and extrude pus from the orifice of the involved follicle. Resolution may be spontaneous or by local antiseptic measures. If the infection spreads to perifollicular subcutaneous tissue, a furuncle (boil) may result.[20] These are raised lesions, up to a centimeter in diameter, and usually painful. They tend to be on hairy portions of the body such as the scalp, face, axilla, shoulders, or buttocks. If not drained by incision, furuncles promptly break down centrally and discharge pus after which they usually resolve, although satellite lesions may be produced by autoinoculation. A still larger lesion, a carbuncle, results from spread of infection more deeply along fascial planes (Figure 87–1) from which it may drain to the surface through multiple sinuses. Surgical treatment is usually necessary. Carbuncles are dangerous. They may cause staphylococcal septicopyemia or spread locally to vital structures as, for instance, a lesion on the upper lip or around the eye (Figure 87–2) may spread centrally to involve the cavernous sinus and subarachnoid space.

Three special forms of furunculosis are referred to as the follicular obstruction triad because they share obstruction of the pilosebaceous apparatus by epithelial proliferation and the infectious complications of this obstruction.[21–27] Hidradenitis suppurativa involves the axilla or anoinguinal region[21,22]; acne conglobata involves the chest and shoulders, less commonly the face; *perifolliculitis capitis abscedens et suffodiens* involves the scalp.[23–26] Each of these disorders is featured by recurrent folliculitis, abscesses, draining sinuses, and distortion by fibrosis. Infection of cystically dilated follicles, often by *S aureus,* is not the primary disease but a complication of the underlying obstructive disorder that is incompletely understood.[22,27] Early, the obstructed pilosebaceous apparatuses are tender nodules, the contents of which soon become infected and communicate with each other and with the overlying surface by a series of sinus tracts accompanied by fibrosis. Early involved follicles are infiltrated by neutrophils, eosinophils, lymphocytes, plasma cells, and histiocytes. Later foreign body giant cells become prominent as a reaction to extravasated sebum and keratin. The discontinuous lining of the sinus tracts often undergoes focal squamous metaplasia that may be mistaken for epidermoid carcinoma.[27] Epidermoid carcinoma has complicated hydradenitis suppurativa and *perifolliculitis capitis abscedens et suffodiens.* The differential diagnosis, when axillae, inguinal, or perianal regions are infected, includes mycoses, lymphogranuloma venereum, and cat scratch disease.

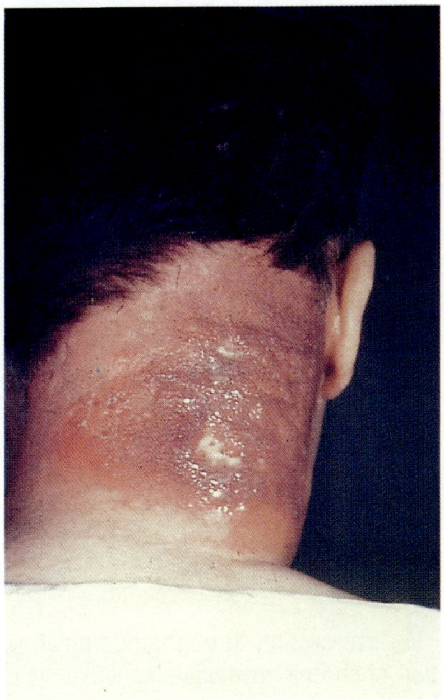

Figure 87–1. Deeply invading staphylococcal cellultis/carbuncle in nape of neck.

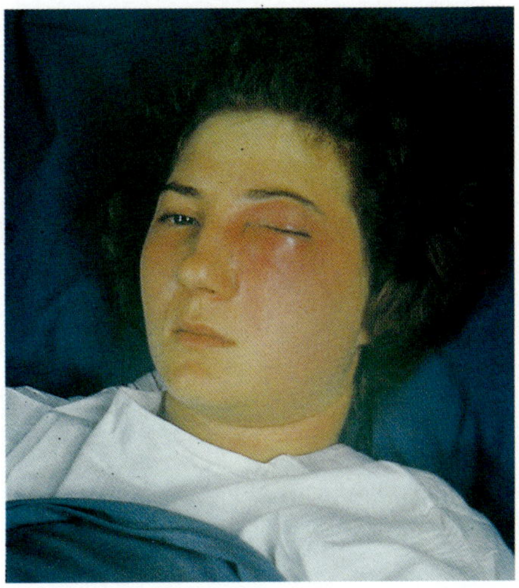

Figure 87–2. Massive periorbital cellulitis caused by *S aureus* with thrombosis of the cavernous sinus. *(Contributed by Ernest E. Lack, MD.)*

Impetigo

Impetigo[28–30] is an infection of the epidermis usually of exposed skin of children, most commonly on face and legs. Lesions begin as minute red macules that rapidly become vesicular and contain cloudy fluid or frank pus on an erythematous base (Figure 87–3).

About 80% of impetigo is staphylococcal. About 10% is streptococcal (clinically and pathologically indistinguishable) and about 10% is mixed staphylococcal and streptococcal.[29,30] The differential diagnosis early includes herpes (simplex or zoster) and varicella. Heal-

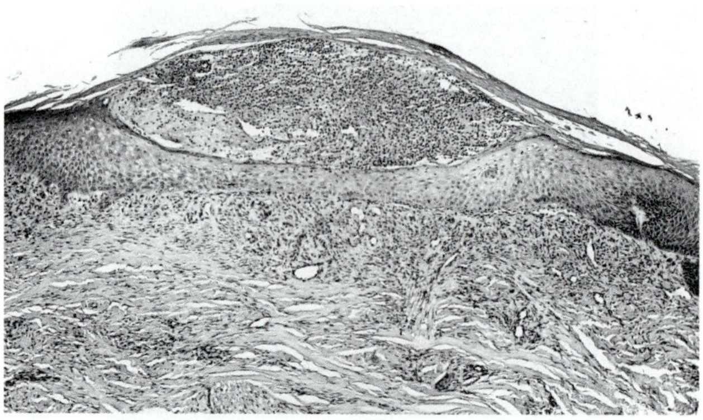

Figure 87–3. Impetigo. A focus of intraepidermal purulent exudate (hematoxylin-eosin, ×100).

ing usually proceeds without scarring. Impetigo is highly contagious, among children in a family, and among contacts in circumstances of crowding and close interpersonal contact such as orphanages and day care centers. Antiseptic measures are important to prevent spread from autoinoculation and contagion.

Staphylococcal Scalded Skin Syndrome

Staphylococcal scalded skin syndrome (SSSS or Ritter's disease)[31] is most typically in newborns[32,33] and less commonly in older children or adults—the latter often with lymphoma (Figures 87–4 and 87–5),[34] or otherwise with impaired immunity.[35–37] The disease begins with a zone of perioral erythema, which rapidly becomes generalized and is followed within hours by large flaccid bullae. These promptly rupture and extrude clear fluid that is initially sterile. Clinically uninvolved skin can be made to exfoliate by friction (Nikolsky's sign). Fluid loss and sepsis are complications. Mortality in infants is 3% to 5%. The disease is a toxic response of epidermis to exfoliatin, a soluble product of some strains of staphylococci.[38–42] The responsible staphylococci are usually in the patient's nose. The Nikolsky's sign and exfoliation can be produced in newborn mice by subcutaneous or intraperitoneal injection of supernatant from staphylococci cultured from the patient.[33] Relevant staphylococci are usually of phage group II in the United States; group I, III, or mixed I and III are more common in Japan.[39]

Exfoliatins are soluble exotoxins of which two distinct serotypes have been identified.[40] Staphylococcal exfoliatin has been shown to bind to filaggrins, a group of proteins associated with keratohyaline granules in squamous epithelium that elaborates keratin intermediate filaments that radiate to the cell surface, notable to desmosomes.[41] Labeled exfoliatin is less rapidly excreted in the urine by newborn than adult mice. This and a hypothetical immaturity of the intraepidermal cellular attachment mechanism are thought to explain the preponderance of SSSS in newborn infants. Microscopically, the bullae form by coalescence of intraepidermal clefts that form between the stratum corneum and stratum granulosum of the epidermis (Figure 87–6).[43,44] Electron microscopically, the clefts are occupied by microvilli, and contiguous epithelial cells show "half desmosomes"[35] and later no desmosomes.[44] Fluid aspirated from bullae contains few or no inflammatory cells and no keratolytic cells and is sterile—at least in early lesions. The most important differential diagnosis is toxic epidermal necrolysis (TEN) or Lyell's disease.[45] TEN is a toxic exfoliation of epithelium of skin and internal squamous epithelia, in response to a variety of drugs, usually in adults. The separation in TEN is at the dermal–epidermal junction[46] and fluid from bullae contains keratolytic cells.[46,47] Some regard TEN as a very severe form of bullous erythema multiforme. The situation is made more complicated by the fact that some authors call SSSS "staphylococcal TEN." In bullous impetigo, the aspirated fluid contains microorganisms, and the dermis is moderately inflamed.[48] A localized, limited form of SSSS is sometimes called "pemphigus neonatorum." "Scarlatiniform eruption" is better regarded as a *forme fruste* of TSS (see next section).[48–52]

Toxic Shock Syndrome[53–70]

In 1978, Todd and associates described, in seven children and adolescents, a syndrome characterized by fever, shock, diarrhea, renal failure, mental confusion,

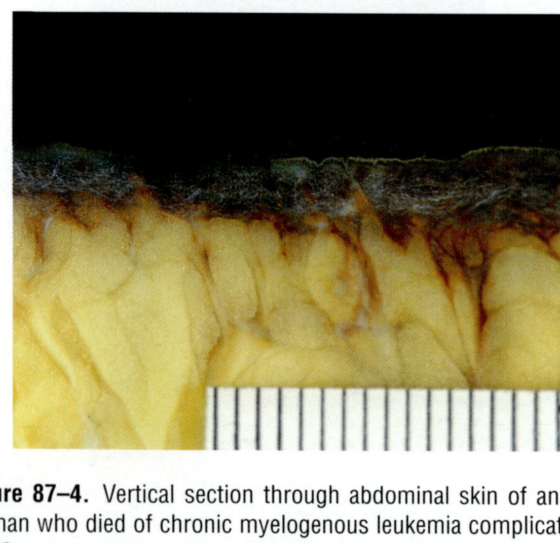

Figure 87–4. Vertical section through abdominal skin of an adult woman who died of chronic myelogenous leukemia complicated by SSSS and staphylococcal septicemia. The upper dermis and epidermis are hemorrhagic and necrotic. The epidermal slough contained clusters of staphylococci. *(Photograph by Daniel H. Connor, MD, 1992.)*

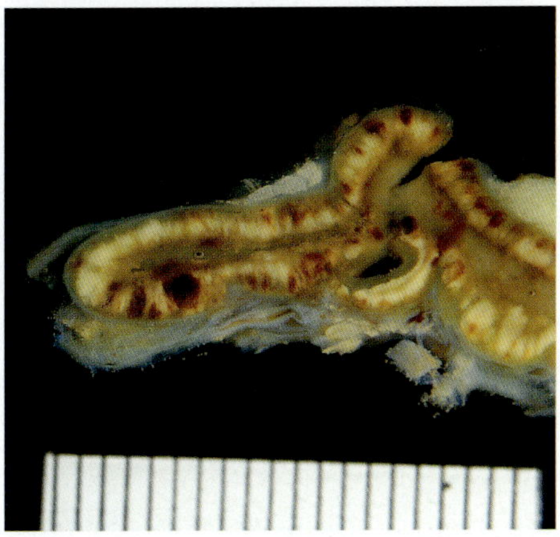

Figure 87–5. Adrenal of same patient as Figure 87–4 with hemorrhagic abscesses containing staphylococci. *(Photograph by Daniel H. Connor, MD, 1992.)*

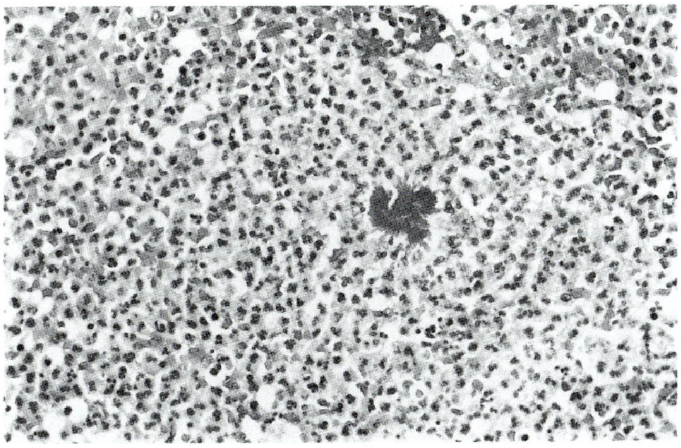

Figure 87–7. Botryomycosis. A cluster of staphylococci embedded in an eosinophilic matrix (Splendore–Hoeppli) in an abscess (hematoxylin-eosin, ×200).

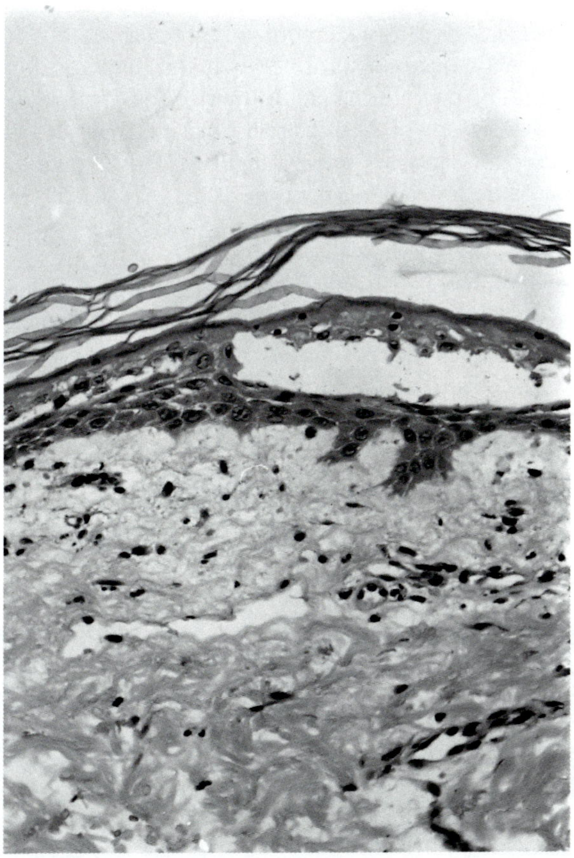

Figure 87–6. SSSS. An intraepidermal cleft (hematoxylin-eosin, ×100).

and erythroderma.[53] One of the patients died. Five were colonized with phage group 1 *S aureus*. In 1980 the disease emerged as a multisystem disorder mainly of menstruating women, the frequency of which was probably caused by recently developed hyperabsorptive vaginal tampons. Langmuir and associates[57] suggested that the mysterious "Plague of Athens" that killed Pericles in the fifth century BC may have been a toxic-shock-like syndrome associated with staphylococcal post influenzal pneumonia.*

TSS is rare in men and nonmenstruating women. Mortality is currently about 3%. *Staphylococcus aureus* is cultured from vaginal secretions of 98% of menstruating women with TSS and from other sites in all nonmenstruating patients.[56] Rarely, an identical syndrome may be associated with streptococcal infection.[58,59] The disease has been attributed to enterotoxin F or exotoxin type C (probably the same) produced by phage group I staphylococci, usually of type 29 or 52.[64–67] Early, in the skin, there is perivasculitis. Later there is sloughing at the dermal–epidermal junction.[69] Cervicovaginal mucosa may be focally inflamed and ulcerated. Changes in kidneys, liver, lungs, lymphoid tissue, and central nervous tissues are nonspecific.[70]

Botryomycosis

Botryomycosis[71–83] is a disorder in which solitary or multiple abscesses contain basophilic granules set in an acellular eosinophilic matrix rich in immunoglobulins (Figure 87–7). Rarely granules can be seen grossly.

* Whether this suggestion is true or not, it is good to have a translation of Thucydides, who himself contracted the disease but survived.

Botryomycotic abscesses are most common in deep subcutaneous tissue but also may be in liver, kidneys, lung, prostate, and lymph nodes. Trauma or foreign bodies are occasionally inciting factors. The clusters of staphylococci usually are surrounded by an eosinophilic coagulum (Splendore–Hoeppli substance) and lie in an abscess that is surrounded by a granulomatous reaction. Pulmonary botryomycosis has been identified in patients with cystic fibrosis.[77] *Staphylococcus aureus* is most commonly isolated from botryomycotic abscesses, but botryomycosis may be caused by other organisms[75,79] including *Pseudomonas aeruginosa.* No immunologic defect has been identified in these patients.[81–83] The major differential diagnosis is a variety of deep mycotic infections, which can be distinguished from botryomycosis by culture or by demonstrating the organism in histopathologic sections.

COAGULASE-NEGATIVE STAPHYLOCOCCI

Previously often regarded as contaminants of cultures, coagulase-negative staphylococci are assuming importance as agents of human infections.[84] These are often related to implanted foreign devices. The taxonomy of coagulase-negative staphylococci is complex[1,85] and not relevant to this discussion.

Coagulase-negative staphylococci are natural inhabitants of human skin. *Staphylococcus epidermidis* is the most prevalent, and *S saprophyticus* is occasionally in the genitourinary tract or on skin. Except for occasional patients with native or prosthetic valvular endocarditis, all infections by *S epidermidis* are hospital acquired, while *S saprophyticus* causes urinary tract infections in sexually active women outside the hospital setting.[86,87] Some strains of *S epidermidis* elaborate an extracellular eosinophilic material known as "slime" that enmeshes organisms in contact with plastic or vitreous materials (Figure 87–8). These "slimes" may contribute to the pathogenicity of these organisms related to implanted foreign materials.[87–95]

ORGAN INFECTIONS

Besides causing cutaneous infections, purulent infections of wounds, and as an agent in septicemia without an identified focus of infection,[96,97] staphylococci are important agents in a variety of deep organ infections.

Endocarditis

Staphylococci cause 20% to 30% of bacterial endocarditis,[97–111] and 80% to 90% of these are caused by coagulase-positive *S aureus.* In about one third of patients, staphylococci attack normal valves. Staphylococcal endocarditis characteristically produces bulky vegetations very destructive of valve tissue. Hemodynamic "jet lesions" are important in pathogenesis.[98,99] Infective endocarditis most frequently involves valves on the left side of the heart,[10] but occasionally, especially in intravenous drug abusers, may involve right-sided valves[102–104] (Figure 87–9).

Bacterial endocarditis is an important complication of cardiac valve replacement.[107] Infection of prosthetic valves may occur intraoperatively or may result from subsequent bacteremia. A distinctive lesion that results from infection of the fibroelastic annulus of native valves or by spread from infection of the sewing ring of prosthetic valves is the "ring abscess" (Figure 87–10).[105,106] This is a destructive purulent concentric lesion in the valve annulus. About one third are staphylococcal and two thirds streptococcal. Besides being a source of bacteremia and septic emboli, ring abscesses may cause valve dysfunction (more common of mitral valves) or cardiac conduction defects (more common with aortic valve lesions). Emboli, often septic, giving rise to abscesses may be in myocardium, kidneys, or brain in about 40% of patients with staphylo-

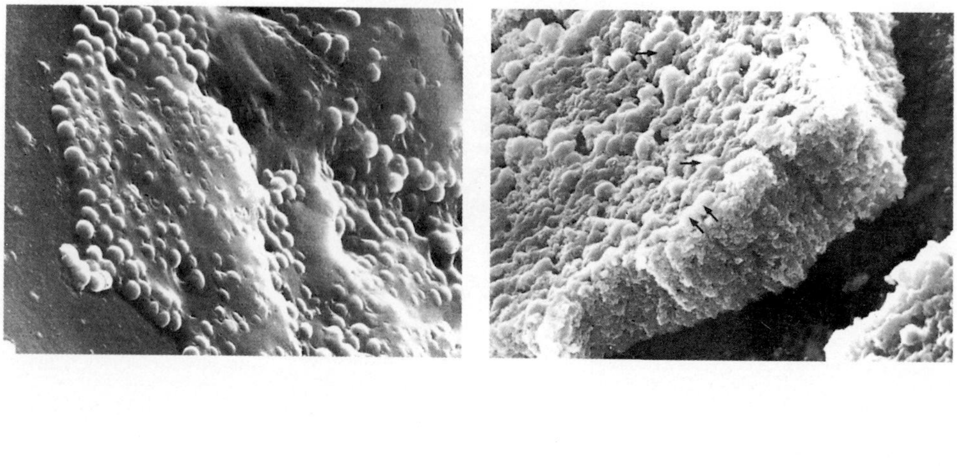

Figure 87–8. Scanning electron micrograph showing slimy material produced by coagulase-negative staphylococci on the surface of a polyethylene catheter after 48 hours (*left*) and (*right*) embedding staphylococci (*arrows*) after incubation for 96 hours. *(From Peters et al.[90])*

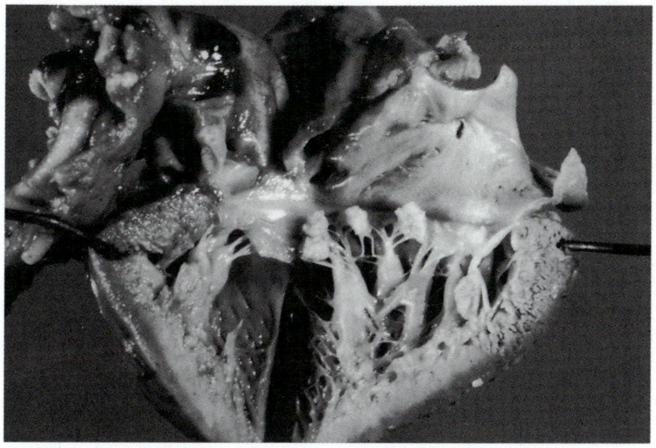

Figure 87–9. Vegetations of acute staphylococcal endocarditis of tricuspid valve in an intravenous drug abuser.

coccal endocarditis. Immune-complex-mediated glomerulonephritis is an uncommon complication.[109] Purulent pericarditis often complicates myocardial abscesses.[110,111]

Lungs

Staphylococcal pneumonia may complicate aspiration, bronchial foreign bodies or antecedent pulmonic infections often viral such as influenza.[104] Staphylococcal pneumonia is now a less common complication of cystic fibrosis than is pseudomonas pneumonia. In newborn infants, staphylococcal pneumonia may complicate maternal mastitis or endobronchial instrumentation of infants.[112–116] Staphylococcal pneumonia, whatever its pathogenesis, undergoes necrosis early, forming multiple abscesses, which may invade pleura, causing staphylococcal pleuritis and empyema (Figure 87–11).

Bone

Staphylococci are the commonest cause of osteomyelitis, accounting for about half of all infections.[117–132] Osteomyelitis is characteristically a purulent inflammation of metaphyseal cancellous bone, a site that is a consequence of the shape and course of epiphysial venules.[109] Subperiostial dissection of pus may produce a lytic lesion of cortical bone (Brodie's abscess) often associated with subperiosteal bone formation. Garre's osteomyelitis is a chronic lesion, more fibroblastic than purulent, typically of the mandible in association with dental infections.[128]

Implanted Devices

Staphylococci are the commonest cause of infected prosthetic cardiac valves, prosthetic joints, ocular implants, vascular grafts, arteriovenous anastamoses, ventriculovenous shunts, breast implants, pacemakers, power packs, and endovascular catheters.[133–138] A distinctive glomerulonephritis, "shunt nephritis," may complicate infection of ventriculovenous shunts.[139]

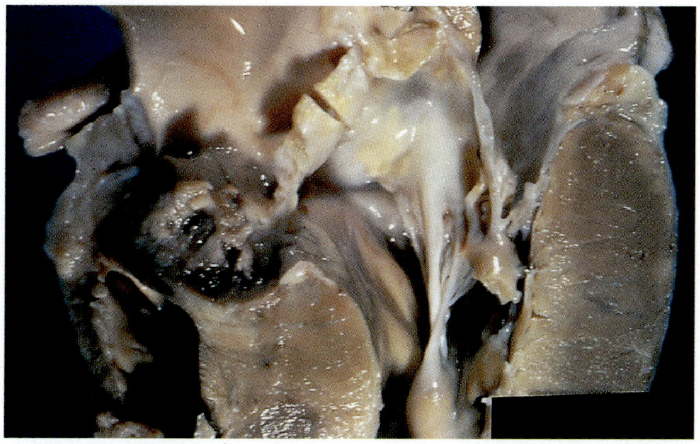

Figure 87–10. Staphylococcal ring abscess involving the annulus of the mitral valve.

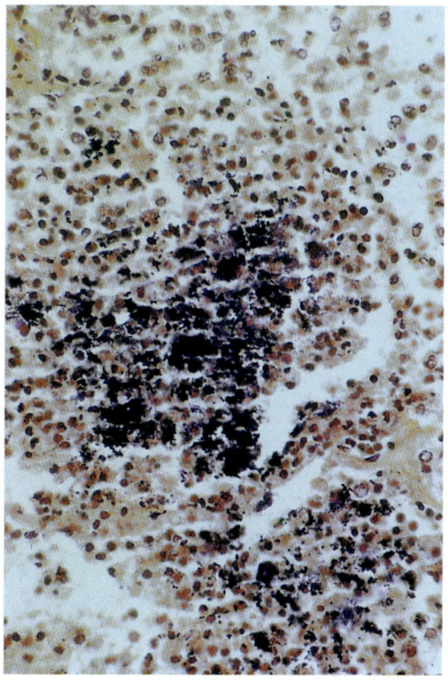

Figure 87–11. Staphylococcal pneumonia. An abscess containing clusters of staphylococci (tissue Gram stain, ×400).

STAPHYLOCOCCAL FOOD POISONING

Staphylococcal food poisoning[140–145] is not an infection but a toxemia caused by one of several heat-stable staphylococcal enterotoxins (A to F). About half of all isolates of *S aureus* produce one of these enterotoxins. Staphylococcal food poisoning is caused by ingestion of food containing enterotoxin-producing staphylococci, often originating in cutaneous lesions on the hands of those preparing the food. Staphylococci proliferate and elaborate toxin under conditions of inadequate refrigeration. Creamed foods or salads with the preformed toxin that are ingested are often the source in the United States, and meats, fish, or poultry are more common in Great Britain.[140] Vomiting begins within a few hours. There is occasionally diarrhea without blood or pus. The disorder is almost always self-limited, and recovery ensues within 24 to 48 hours. The mechanism of action of staphylococcal enterotoxin is unknown but appears to be central on the vomiting center in response to impulses carried in the vagi or abdominal sympathetic chain.[144,145]

REFERENCES

1. Smith PH, Mair NS, Sharpe ME, Holt JG, eds. *Bergey's Manual of Systematic Bacteriology*. Baltimore: Williams Wilkins; 1989:1013–1035.
2. Kasper DL: Introduction. In: Mandel GL, Douglas RG Jr, Bennett JE, eds. *Principles and Practice of Infectious Diseases*. 3rd ed. New York: Churchill Livingstone; 1990: 1484–1489.
3. Waldvogel FA. *Staphylococcus aureus* (including toxic-shock syndrome). In Mandel GL, Douglas RG Jr, Bennett JE, eds. *Principles and Practice of Infectious Diseases*. 3rd ed. New York: Churchill Livingstone; 1990:1484–1489.
4. Kloos WE, Schleifer KH. Simplified scheme for routine identification of human *Staphylococcus* species. *J Clin Microbiol.* 1975;1:82–88.
5. Kaplan MH, Tenenbaum MJ. *Staphylococcus aureus:* cellular biology and clinical application. *Am J Med.* 1982;72:248–258.
6. Mandell GS. Catalase, superoxide dismutase, and virulence of *Staphylococcus aureus.* In vitro and in vivo studies with emphasis on staphylococcal–leukocyte interaction. *J Clin Invest.* 1975;55:561–566.
7. Rogolsky M. Nonenteric toxins of *Staphylococcus aureus*. *Microbiol Rev.* 1970;43:320–360.
8. Fekety FR Jr. The epidemiology and prevention of staphylococcal infection. *Medicine.* 1964;42:593–613.
9. Rogers DE, ed. Staphylococcal infections. *Ann NY Acad Sci.* 1956;65:57–246.
10. Martin RR, Buttram V, Besch P, Kirkland JJ, Petty GP. Nasal and vaginal *Staphylococcus aureus* in young women: quantitative studies. *Ann Intern Med.* 1982;96 (part2):951–953.
11. Godfrey MI, Smith IM. Hospital hazards of staphylococcal sepsis. *JAMA.* 1958;166:1197–1201.
12. Tuazon CU, Perez A, Kishato T, Sheagren JN. *Staphylococcus aureus* among insulin-injecting diabetic patients. An increased carriage rate. *JAMA.* 1975;231:1272.
13. Kirmani N, Tuazon CU, Murray HW, Parish AE, Sheagren JN. *Staphylococcus aureus* carriage rate of patients receiving long-term hemodialysis. *Arch Intern Med.* 1978;138:1657–1659.
14. Vas SI. Infections associated with peritoneal and hemodialysis. In: Bisno AL, Waldvogel FA, eds. *Infections Associated with Indwelling Medical Devices.* Washington, DC: American Society for Microbiology; 1989:215–248.
15. Archer GL. Antimicrobial susceptibility and selection of resistance among *Staphylococcus epidermidis* isolates recovered from patients with infections if in-dwelling foreign devices. *Antimicrob Agents Chemother.* 1978; 14:353–359.
16. Tuazon CU, Sheagren JN. Increased rate of carriage of *Staphylococcus aureus* among narcotic addicts. *J Infect Dis.* 1974;129:725–727.
17. Saravolatz LD, Pohlod DJ, Arking LM. Community-acquired methecillin-resistant *Staphylococcus aureus* infections: a new source for nosocomial outbreaks. *Ann Int Med.* 1982;97:325–329.
18. Musher DM, McKenzie SO. Infections due to *Staphylococcus aureus*. *Medicine.* 1977;56:383–409.
19. Zeisler EP. Pyogenic infections of the skin. *Med Clin North Am.* 1942;6:83–96.
20. Pinkus M. Furuncle. *J Cutan Pathol.* 1979;6:517–518.
21. Brunsting HA. Hidradenitis suppurativa: abscess of the apocrine sweat glands. A study of the disease and pathologic features with a report of twenty-two cases and a review of the literature. *Arch Dermatol Syphilol.* 1939;39: 108–120.
22. Dvorak VC, Root RK, MacGregor RR. Host-defensive mechanisms in hidradenitis suppurativa. *Arch Dermatol.* 1977;113:450–453.
23. McMullan FM, Zeliman I. *Perifolliculitis capitis abscedens et suffodiens.* Its successful treatment with x-ray epilation. *Arch Dermatol.* 1956;73:256–263.
24. Moyer DG, Williams RM. *Perifolliculitis capitis abscedens et suffodiens.* A report of six cases. *Arch Dermatol.* 1962;85:378–384.
25. Moschella SL, Klein MH, Miller RJ. *Perifolliculitis capitis abscedens et suffodiens. Arch Dermatol.* 1967;96: 195–197.
26. Curry SS, Gaither DM, King LE Jr. Squamous cell carcinoma arising in dissecting perifolliculitis of the scalp. A case report and review of secondary squamous cell carcinomas. *J Am Acad Dermatol.* 1981;4:673–678.
27. Hyland CM, Kheir SM. Follicular occlusion disease with elimination of abnormal elastic tissue. *Arch Dermatol.* 1980;116:925–928.
28. Coskey RJ, Coskey LA. Diagnosis and treatment of impetigo. *J Am Acad Dermatol.* 1987;17:62–63.
29. Noble WC, Presbury D, Connor BL. Prevalence of streptococci and staphylococci in lesions of impetigo. *Br J Dermatol.* 1974;91:115–116.
30. Parker MT, Tomlinson AJH, Williams RED. Impetigo con-

tagiosa. The association of certain types of *Staphylococcus aureus* and *Staphylococcus pyogenes* in superficial skin infections. *J Hyg Cambridge.* 1955;53:458–473.
31. Ritter von Rittershain C. Die exfoliative Dermatitis jüngerer Säuglinge. *Zentralzeitschrift für Kinderheilkunde.* 1878;2:3–23.
32. Melish ME, Glasgow LA, Turner MD. The staphylococcal scalded-skin syndrome: isolation and partial characterization of the exfoliative toxin. *J Infect Dis.* 1972;125: 129–140.
33. Melish ME, Glasgow LA. The staphylococcal scalded skin syndrome: development of an experimental model. *N Engl J Med.* 1970;282:1114–1119.
34. Ridgeway MB, Lowe NJ. Staphylococcal scalded skin syndrome in an adult with Hodgkins' disease. *Arch Dermatol.* 1979;115:589–590.
35. Diem E, Konrad K, Graninger W. Staphylococcal scalded-skin syndrome in an adult with fatal disseminated staphylococcal sepsis. *Acta Derm Venereol (Stockh).* 1982;62:295–299.
36. Reid LM, Weston WL, Humbert JR. Staphylococcal scalded-skin syndrome. *Arch Dermatol.* 1974;109:239–241.
37. Borchers SL, Gomez EC, Isseroff RR. Generalized staphylococcal scalded skin syndrome in an anephric boy undergoing hemodialysis. *Arch Dermatol.* 1989;120: 912–918.
38. Wuepper KD, Dimond RL, Knutson DD. Studies of the mechanism of epidermal injury by a staphylococcal epidermolytic toxin. *J Invest Dermatol.* 1975;65:191–200.
39. Sarai Y, Nakahara H, Ishikawa T, Konda I, Futaki S, Hirakama K. A bacteriologic study on children with staphylococcal toxic epidermal necrolysis in Japan. *Dermatologica.* 1977;134:161–167.
40. Kondo I, Sakurai S, Sarai Y, Futaki S. Two stereotypes of exfoliatin and their distribution in staphylococcal strains isolated from patients with scalded skin syndrome. *J Clin Microbiol.* 1975;1:397–400.
41. Smith TP, Baily CJ. Epidermolytic toxin from *Staphylococcus aureus* binds to filaggrins. *FEBS.* 1986;194: 309–312.
42. Fritsch P, Elias P, Varga J. The fate of Staphylococcus exfoliatin in newborn and adult mice. *Brit J Dermatol.* 1976;95:275–284.
43. Dimond RL, Wuepper KD. Das staphylogene Lyell–Syndrom. *Hautarzt.* 1977;28:447–455.
44. Dimond RL, Wolff HH, Braun-Falco O. The staphylococcal scalded-skin syndrome. *Br J Dermatol.* 1977;96: 483–492.
45. Lyell A. Toxic epidermal necrolysis: an eruption resembling scalding of the skin. *Br J Dermatol.* 1936;68: 355–361.
46. Amon RB, Dimond RL. Toxic epidermal necrolysis. Rapid differentiation between staphylococcal- and drug-induced disease. *Arch Dermatol.* 1975;111:1433–1437.
47. Manzella JP, Hall CB, Green JL, McMeechin TO. Toxic epidermal necrolysis in childhood: differentiation from staphylococcal scalded skin syndrome. *Pediatrics.* 1980; 66:291–294.
48. Elias PM, Levy SW. Bullous impetigo. Occurrence of localized scalded-skin syndrome in an adult. *Arch Dermatol.* 1976;112:856–858.
49. Goldstein SM, Wintroub BW, Elias PM, Wuepper KD. Toxic epidermal necrolysis. Unmuddying the waters. *Arch Dermatol.* 1987;123:1153–1155.
50. Levine J, Norden CW. Staphylococcal scalded-skin syndrome in an adult. *N Engl J Med.* 1972;287:1339–1340.
51. Konskoukis CE, Ackerman AB. What histologic finding distinguishes superficial pemphigus and bullous impetigo? *Am J Dermatopathol.* 1984;6:179–181.
52. Dancer SJ, Poston SM, East J, Simmons NA, Noble WC. An outbreak of pemphigus neonatorum. *J Infect Dis.* 1990;20:73–82.
53. Todd J, Fishaut M. Toxic-shock syndrome associated with phage-group-I staphylococci. *Lancet.* 1978;2:1116–1121.
54. Davis JP, Chesney PJ, Wand PJ, LaVenture M, and the Investigative and Laboratory team. Toxic-shock syndrome. *N Engl J Med.* 1980;303:1429–1435.
55. Findley RF, Odom RB. Toxic shock syndrome (review). *Int J Dermatol.* 1982;21:117–121.
56. Huntley AC, Tanabe JL. Toxic shock syndrome as a complication of dermatologic surgery. *J Am Genet Dermatol.* 1987;16:227–229.
57. Langmuir AD, Worthen TD, Solomon J, Ray CG, Petersen E. The Thucydides syndrome. A new hypothesis for the cause of the plague of Athens. *N Engl J Med.* 1985; 313:1027–1030.
58. Bartter T, Dascal A, Carrol K, Curle FJ. "Toxic strep syndrome." A manifestation of group A streptococcal infection. *Arch Intern Med.* 1988;148:1421–1424.
59. Cone LA, Woodward DR, Schlievert PM, Tomory GS. Clinical and bacteriologic observations of a toxic-shock like syndrome due to *Streptococcus pyogenes. N Engl J Med.* 1987;317:146–149.
60. Chesney PJ, Davis JP, Purdy WK, Ward PJ, Chesney RW. Clinical manifestations of toxic shock syndrome. *JAMA.* 1981;246:741–748.
61. Larkin SM, Williams DN, Osterholm MT, Tofte RW, Posalsky ZA. Toxic shock syndrome; clinical, laboratory and pathologic findings in non fatal cases. *Ann Intern Med.* 1982;96:858–864.
62. Osterholm MT, David JP, Gibson RW, et al, and the Investigative Team. Tri-state toxic-shock syndrome study. I. Epidemiologic findings. *J Infect Dis.* 1982;145:431–440.
63. Davis JP, Osterholm MT, Helms CM, et al, and the Investigative Team: Tri-state toxic-shock syndrome study. II. Chemical and laboratory findings. *J Infect Dis.* 1982;145: 441–448.
64. Bergdoll MS, Crass B, Reiser RF, Robbins RN, Davis JP. A new staphylococcal enterotoxin, enterotoxin F, associated with toxic-shock syndrome *Staphylococcus aureus* isolates. *Lancet.* 1981;1:1017–1021.
65. Schlievert PM, Shands KN, Dan BB, Schmid GP, Nishimura RD. Identification and characterization of an exotoxin from *Staphylococcus aureus* associated with toxic-shock syndrome. *J Infect Dis.* 1981;143:509–516.
66. Schlievert PM. Alteration of immune function by staphylococcal pyrogenic exotoxin type C: possible role in toxic-shock syndrome. *J Infect Dis.* 1983;147:391–398.

67. Kass EH, Parsonnet J. On the pathogenesis of toxic shock syndrome. *Rev Infect Dis.* 1987;9:482–489.
68. Abdul-Karim FW, Lederman MM, Carter JR, Hewlett EL, Newman AJ, Greene BM. Toxic shock syndrome: clinicopathologic findings in a fatal case. *Hum Pathol.* 1981; 12:16–22.
69. Elbaum DJ, Wood C, Albuabara F, Morhenn VB. Bullae in a patient with toxic shock syndrome. *J Am Acad Dermatol.* 1984;10:267–272.
70. Paris AL, Herwaldt LA, Blum D, Schmid GP, Shands KN, Broome CV. Pathologic findings in twelve fatal cases of toxic shock syndrome. *Ann Intern Med.* 1982;96: 852–857.
71. Wilson DJ. Botryomycosis. *Am J Pathol.* 1959;35:153–167.
72. Hacker P. Botryomycosis. *Int J Dermatol.* 1983;22:455–458.
73. Patterson JW, Kitces EN, Neafie RC. Cutaneous botryomycosis in a patient with acquired immunodeficiency syndrome. *J Am Acad Dermatol.* 1987;16:238–242.
74. Toth IR, Kazal ML. Botryomycosis in acquired immunodeficiency syndrome. *Arch Pathol.* 1987;111:246–249.
75. Leibowitz MR, Asvat MS, Kalla AA. Extensive botryomycosis in a patient with diabetes and chronic active hepatitis. *Arch Dermatol.* 1981;117:739–742.
76. Kansky A. Botryomycosis. *Acta Derm Venereol (Stockh).* 1964;44:369–376.
77. Katznelsen D, Vawter GF, Foley GE, Schwachman M. Botryomycosis, a complication in cystic fibrosis. Report of 17 cases. *J Pediatr.* 1964;65:525–539.
78. Williams HM Jr, Stone OJ. Blastomycosis-like pyoderma. Case report of unusual entity with response to curettage. *Arch Dermatol.* 1966;93:226–228.
79. Su WPD, Duncan SC, Perry HO. Blastomycosis-like pyoderma. *Arch Dermatol.* 1979;115:170–173.
80. Picou K, Batres E, Jarratt M. Botryomycosis. A bacterial cause for mycetoma. *Arch Dermatol.* 1979;115: 609–610.
81. Bishop GF, Greer KE, Horwitz DA. *Pseudomonas* botryomycosis. *Arch Dermatol.* 1976;112:1568–1570.
82. Waisman M. Staphylococcal actinophytosis (botryomycosis). Granular bacteriosis of the skin. *Arch Dermatol.* 1962;86:525–529.
83. Harman RRN, English MP, Halford M, Sachen EM, Greenham LW. Botryomycosis. *Br J Dermatol.* 1980;102: 215–222.
84. Klein JO. From harmless commensal to invasive pathogen: coagulase-negative staphylococci. *N Engl J Med.* 1990;323:339–340. Editorial.
85. Archer GL. *Staphylococcus epidermidis* and other coagulase-negative staphylococci. In: Mandell GL, Douglas RG Jr, Bennett JE, eds. *Principles and Practice of Infectious Diseases.* 3rd ed. New York: Churchill Livingstone; 1990:1511–1518.
86. Jordan PA, Iravani A, Richard GA, Baer H. Urinary tract infection caused by *Staphylococcus saprophyticus. J Infect Dis.* 1980;142:510–515.
87. Tojo M, Yamashita N, Goldmann DA, Pier GB. Isolation and characterization of a capsular polysaccharide adhesion from *Staphylococcus epidermidis. J Infect Dis.* 1988; 157:713–722.
88. Nicolle LE, Hoban SA, Harding GKM. Characterization of coagulase-negative staphylococci from urinary tract infections. *J Clin Microbiol.* 1983;17:267–271.
89. Geesey GG. Microbial exopolymers: ecological and economic considerations. *Am Soc Microbiol. News.* 1982; 48:9.
90. Peters G, Locci R, Pulverer G. Adherence and growth of coagulase-negative staphylococci on surfaces of intravenous catheters. *J Infect Dis.* 1982;146:479–482.
91. Christensen GD, Simpson WA, Bisno AL, Beachey EH. Experimental foreign body infections in mice challenged with slime-producing *Staphylococcus epidermidis. Infect Immun.* 1983;38:407–416.
92. Christensen GD, Simpson WA, Bisno AL, Beachey EH. Adherence of slime producing strains of *Staphylococcus epidermidis* to smooth surfaces. *Infect Immun.* 1982;37: 318–326.
93. Marrie TJ, Costerton JW. Scanning and transmission electron microscopy of in vitro bacterial colonization of intravenous and intraperitoneal catheters. *J Clin Microbiol.* 1984;19:687–693.
94. Franson TR, Sheth NK, Rose HD, Sohnle PG. Scanning electron microscopy of bacteria adherent to intravascular catheters. *J Clin Microbiol.* 1984;20:500–505.
95. Christensen GD, Baddour LM, Simpson A. Phenotypic variation of *Staphylococcus epidermidis. Infect Immun.* 1987;55:2870–2877.
96. Mendell TH. Staphylococcal septicemia. A review of thirty-five cases with six recoveries, twenty nine deaths and sixteen autopsies. *Arch Intern Med.* 1939;63: 1068–1083.
97. Eykyn SJ. Staphylococcal sepsis. The changing pattern of disease and therapy. *Lancet.* 1988;1:100–104.
98. Weinstein L, Schlesinger JJ. Pathoanatomic, pathophysiologic and clinical correlations in endocarditis. *N Engl J Med.* 1974;291:832–837.
99. Gonzalez-Levin L, Lise M, Ross D. The importance of the "jet lesions" in bacterial endocarditis involving the left heart. Surgical considerations. *J Thorac Cardiovasc Surg.* 1970;59:185–192.
100. Wilson LM. Etiology of bacterial endocarditis. Before and since the introduction of antibiotics. *Ann Intern Med.* 1963;58:946–952.
101. Buchbinder NA, Roberts WC. Left-sided valvular active infective endocarditis. A study of forty-six necropsy patients. *Am J Med.* 1972;53:20–35.
102. Roberts WC, Buchbinder NA. Right-sided valvular infective endocarditis. A clinicopathologic study of twelve necropsy patients. *Am J Med.* 1972;53:7–19.
103. Levine DP, Cushing RD, Jui J, Brown WJ. Community-acquired methicillin-resistant *Staphylococcus aureus* endocarditis in the Detroit Medical Center. *Ann Intern Med.* 1982;97:330–338.
104. Reisberg BE. Infective endocarditis in the narcotic addict. *Prog Cardiovasc.* 1979;22:193–204.
105. Sheldon WH, Golden A. Abscesses of the valve rings of the heart: a frequent but not well recognized complica-

tion of acute bacterial endocarditis. *Circulation.* 1951;4: 1–12.

106. Arnett MM, Roberts WC. Valve ring abscess in active infective endocarditis. Frequency, location and clues to clinical diagnosis from the study of 95 necropsy patients. *Circulation.* 1976;54:140–145.
107. Anderson DJ, Buckley BH, Hutchins GM. A clinicopathologic study of prosthetic valve endocarditis in 22 patients: morphologic basis for diagnosis and therapy. *Am Heart J.* 1977;94:325–332.
108. Arnett EN, Roberts WC. Prosthetic valve endocarditis. Clinicopathologic analysis of 22 patients with active infective endocarditis involving natural left-side cardiac valves. *Am J Cardiol.* 1976;38:281–292.
109. Perez GO, Rothfield N, Williams RC. Immune complex nephritis in bacterial endocarditis. *Arch Intern Med.* 1976;136:334–336.
110. Klacsman PG, Bulkey BH, Hutchins GM. The changed spectrum of purulent pericarditis. An 86 year autopsy experience in 200 patients. *Am J Med.* 1977;63:666–673.
111. Rubin RH, Moellering RC Jr. Clinical microbiologic and therapeutic aspects of purulent pericarditis. *Am J Med.* 1975;59:68–78.
112. Willenman OJ Jr, Finland M. Pathology of staphylococcal pneumonia complicating clinical influenza. *Am J Pathol.* 1943;19:23–41.
113. Eischenwald ME, Shinefield MR. The problem of staphylococcal infection in newborn infants. *J Pediatr.* 1960;56:665–674.
114. Slim MS, Firzli SS, Melhem RE. Staphylococcal pneumonia in infants under the age of six months. *Dis Chest.* 1965;48:6–13.
115. Huxtable KA, Tucker AS, Wedgewood RJ. Staphylococcal pneumonia in childhood. Long-term follow-up. *Am J Dis Child.* 1964;108:262–269.
116. Pryles CV. Staphylococcus pneumonia in infancy and childhood; an analysis of 24 cases. *Pediatrics.* 1958;21: 609–623.
117. Waldvogel JA, Medoff G, Swartz MN. Osteomyelitis: a review of clinical features, therapeutic considerations and unusual aspects; I: Hematogenous osteomyelitis; II: Osteomyelitis secondary to a contiguous infection and secondary to vascular insufficiency; III: Unusual organisms and unusual locations. *N Engl J Med.* 1970; 282:198–206.
118. Beekman F. Acute hematogenous osteomyelitis. Its pathology, with special reference to involvement of joints, its diagnosis and the present day concepts of treatment. *Bull NY Acad Med.* 1930;6:792–807.
119. Norden CW, ed. Osteomyelitis. *Inf Dis Clin North Am.* 1990;4:361–554.
120. Nade S. Acute hematogenous osteomyelitis in infancy and childhood. *J Bone Joint Surg.* 1983;65(B):109–119.
121. Wiley AM, Trueta J. The vascular anatomy of the spine and its relationship to pyogenic vertebral osteomyelitis. *J Bone Joint Surg.* 1959;41:796–809.
122. Dich VG, Nelson JD, Haltalin DC. Osteomyelitis in infants and children: a review of 163 cases. *Am J Dis Child.* 1975;129:1273–1278.
123. Waldvogel FA, Vasey H. Osteomyelitis: the past decade. *N Engl J Med.* 1983;303:360–370.
124. LaMont RL, Anderson PA, Dajami AS, Thirumoorthi MC. Acute hematogenous osteomyelitis in children. *J Ped Orthopaedics.* 1987;7:579–583.
125. Vaughan PA, Newman NM, Rosman MA. Acute hematogenous osteomyelitis in children. *J Ped Orthopaedics.* 1987;7:652–655.
126. Scott RJ, Christofersen MR, Robertson WW Jr, Davidson RS, Rankin L, Drummond DS. Acute osteomyelitis in children: a review of 116 cases. *J Ped Orthopaedics.* 1990;10: 649–652.
127. Faden M, Grossi M. Acute osteomyelitis in children. Reassessment of etiologic agents and their clinical characteristics. *Am J Dis Child.* 1991;145:65–69.
128. Jensen DR. Chronic sclerosing osteomyelitis: Garre. *Am J Surg.* 1941;54:377–383.
129. Reich RS. Purulent arthritis. *J Bone Joint Surg.* 1928;10: 554–578.
130. Ogden JA. Pediatric osteomyelitis and septic arthritis: the pathology of neonatal disease. *Yale J Biol Med.* 1979;52: 423–448.
131. Barton LL, Dunkle LM, Habib FH. Septic arthritis in childhood. A 13-year review. *Am J Dis Child.* 1987;141: 898–900.
132. Flynn JE. Acute suppurative tenosynovitis of the hand. *SGO.* 1943;6:227–235.
133. Younger JJ, Christensen GD, Bartley DL, Simmons JCH, Bennett FF. Coagulase-negative staphylococci isolated from cerebrospinal fluid shunts; importance of slime production, species identification, and shunt removal to clinical outcome. *J Infect Dis.* 1987;156:548–554.
134. Christensen GD, Boddour LM, Hasty DL, Lawrence JH, Simpson A. Microbiologic and foreign body factors in the pathogenesis of medical device infections. In: Bisno AL, Waldvogel FA, eds. *Infections Associated with Indwelling Medical Devices.* Washington, DC: American Society for Microbiology; 1989:27–60.
135. Brause BD. Infected orthopedic prostheses. In: Bisno AL, Waldvogel FA, eds, *Infections Associated with Indwelling Medical Devices.* Washington, DC: American Society for Microbiology; 1989:111–128.
136. Bisno AL. Infections of central nervous system shunts. In: Bisno AL, Waldvogel FA, eds. *Infections Associated with Indwelling Medical Devices.* Washington, DC: American Society for Microbiology; 1989:93–110.
137. Karchmer DW, Bisno AL. Infections of prosthetic heart valves and vascular grafts. In: Bisno AL, Waldvogel FA, eds. *Infections Associated with Indwelling Medical Devices.* Washington, DC: American Society for Microbiology; 1989:129–160.
138. Baker AS, Schein OD. Ocular infections. In: Bisno AL, Waldvogel FA, eds. *Infections Associated with Indwelling Medical Devices.* Washington, DC: American Society for Microbiology; 1989:75–92.
139. Dobrin RS, Day NK, Quie PG. The role of complement, immunoglobulin, and bacterial antigen in coagulase-negative staphylococcal shunt nephritis. *Am J Med.* 1975; 59:660–673.

140. Gilbert RJ. Staphylococcal food poisoning and botulism. *Postgrad Med J.* 1974;50:603–611.
141. Effersol P, Kjerulf K. Clinical aspects of outbreak of staphylococcal food poisoning during air travel. *Lancet.* 1975;2:599–600.
142. Breckenridge JC, Bergdoll MS. Outbreak of foodborne gastroenteritis due to a coagulase-negative enterotoxin-producing staphylococcus. *N Engl J Med.* 1971;284:541–543.
143. Elias J, Shields R. Influence of staphylococcal enterotoxin on water and electrolyte transportation in the small intestine. *Gut.* 1976;17:527–535.
144. Clark WG, Vanderhooft GF, Borison HL. Emetic effect of purified staphylococcal enterotoxin in cats. *PSEM.* 1962;111:205–207.
145. Sugiyama H, Hayama T. Abdominal viscera as site of emetic action for staphylococcal enterotoxin in the monkey. *J Infect Dis.* 1965;115:330–336.

CHAPTER 88

Streptococcal Infections and Infections by "Streptococcus-like" Organisms

John M. Kissane

He prayeth best who loveth best
All things both great and small.
The Streptococcus is the test—
I love it least of all.

Wallace Wilson (fl. 20th Cent.)

INTRODUCTION

The family Streptococcaceae consists of gram-positive, nonsporulating, catalase-negative cocci. Except for pneumococci, now classified as *Streptococcus pneumoniae* that grow as lancet-shaped diplococci and members of the genus *Aerococcus* that grow as tetrads or clumps, members of the family characteristically grow as chains in liquid media.

Streptococci are gram-positive catalase-negative bacteria that tend to grow in pairs or chains of spherical or ovoid cells 0.6 to 1.0 μm in diameter. Streptococci are facultative anaerobes. Some strains grow better than others, particularly in primary isolation, under anaerobic conditions, and many are stimulated by an atmosphere that is enriched with 5% to 7% carbon dioxide. Medically important *Streptococci, Enterococci,* and *Aerococci* are homofermentative, that is, the sole product of their fermentation of glucose is lactic acid. Some viridans streptococci require for their growth thiol compounds, cysteine, or active forms of vitamin B6.

Classification of gram-positive cocci is elaborate.[1–4] Clinically defined "pneumococci" are now placed in the genus *Streptococcus* as *S pneumoniae.* Other species including *S hemolyticus, S scarletinae,* and *S erysipelatis* have no formal status. Certain important organisms are now classified in the separate genus *Enterococcus.* Streptococcus-like gram-positive cocci of genera *Leuconostoc, Lactococcus, Aerococcus, Pediococcus,* and *Gemella,* primarily environmental and plant saprophytes, are occasional opportunistic human pathogens. Some anaerobic gram-positive cocci that cause human infections under special circumstances are found in the genera *Peptostreptococcus* and *Peptococcus.*

The description of hemolysis produced by streptococci growing on blood agar is very old (1919 or perhaps 1903). Beta hemolysis (complete hemolysis), alpha hemolysis (hemolysis with greening), and the oxymoron "gamma hemolysis" (better nonhemolytic) are widely understood although those attributes interdigitate with other systems of classification.[5] The cell wall of streptococci, like that of other gram-positive organisms, consists primarily of peptidoglycans with which various carbohydrates, teichoic acids, lipoproteins, and surface proteins are associated (Figure 88–1, A).[6] The Lancefield system of grouping beta-hemolytic streptococci is based on cell wall polysaccharide antigens or lipoteichoic acids. Groups A to H and K to U are identified. Groups A, B, C, D, F, and G are most commonly isolated from human beings; groups E, L, M, P, and U are rarely if ever isolated from human beings, but a facial abscess caused by group L streptococcus has been reported in a previously healthy 35-year-old man.[7] Group A streptococci are further divided into serotypes

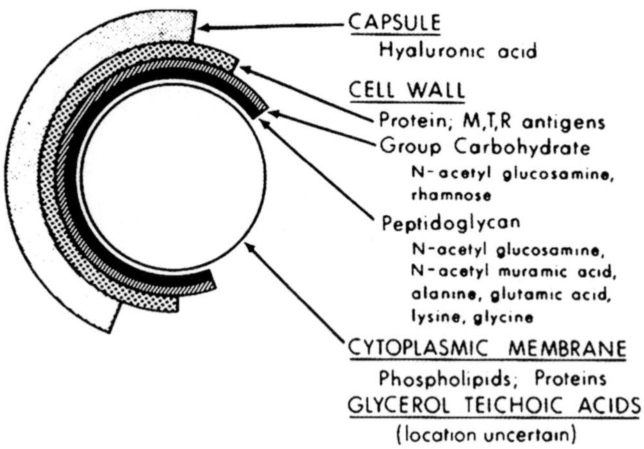

A

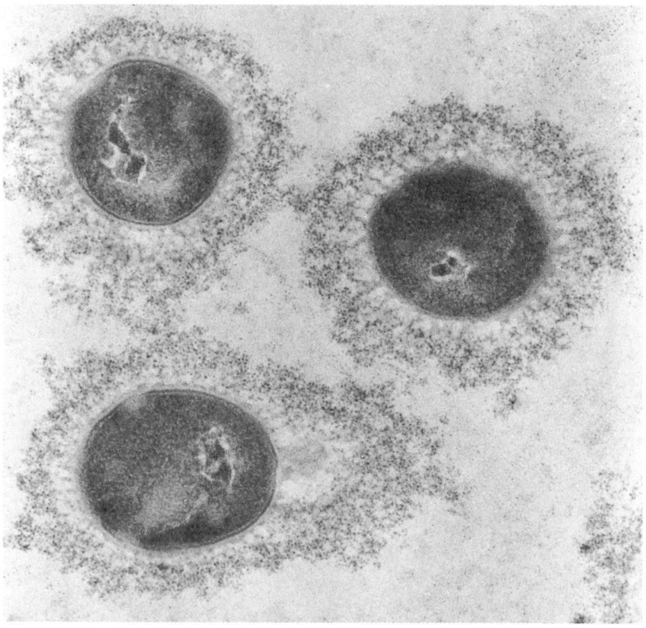

B

Figure 88–1. (**A**) Diagram showing components of the cell wall of group A streptococci. *(From Krause RM, Bact Rev. 1963;27:369.)* (**B**) Electron micrograph of *Streptococci* in culture.

of which at least 70 have been identified, based on immunologic differences in the M protein of their cell walls[8] (Figure 88–1, B). The M protein coating of streptococcal fimbriae seems less important in binding of group A streptococci to epithelial surfaces than the lipoteichoic acid moiety of the cell wall.[9] Huskins and Kaplan[10] could not support earlier observations of others that an inhibitory substance elaborated by indigenous viridans streptococci affected colonization of the upper respiratory tract by group A streptococci.

STREPTOCOCCUS PYOGENES (GROUP A BETA HEMOLYTIC STREPTOCOCCI)

Virulence Factors

Group A beta-hemolytic streptococci elaborate a variety of extracellular products during growth in vitro or in vivo. Not all of these have been well characterized.[11]

Hemolysins: Group A streptococci elaborate two hemolysins. Streptolysin O (for oxygen sensitivity) hemolyzes erythrocytes of several species and is also toxic to neutrophils, platelets, tissue culture cells, and isolated mammalian and amphibian hearts. Streptolysin S (produced in presence of serum) damages membranes of neutrophils, platelets, and subcellular organelles. Most streptococci produce both hemolysins.

Enzymes: Several enzymes, at least theoretically, facilitate spreading of alpha streptococcal infection by liquefying pus or tissue fluid. Among these are 1) four antigenically distinct deoxyribonucleic acid hydrolases (DNAses A, B, C, and D); 2) a hyaluronidase; 3) streptokinase that liquefies fibrin; and 4) other enzymes including nicotinamide adenine deoxynucleotidase (NADase), proteinase, amylase, and esterase.[1] Many of these are also produced by streptococci that are other than beta hemolytic.

Pathology

Although *S pyogenes,* as the name implies, is regarded as a pus former, streptococci less commonly evoke the formation of frank pus than do staphylococci. The inflammatory response to streptococcal infections is undeniably acute, that is, characterized by neutrophils, but it is characteristically a spreading reaction, and the formation of abscesses ordinarily depends on local factors such as impaired bronchial drainage of a pneumonic focus. Of great theoretical interest as well as clinical importance is the association of streptococcal infections, usually by group A organisms, with "nonsuppurative" sequelae, acute rheumatic fever, and acute glomerulonephritis.

Tonsillopharyngitis caused by group A streptococcus is the commonest cause of bacterial tonsillopharyngitis, one of the commonest bacterial infections of man.[12,13] Although it can occur at any age, the disease is most frequent in children from 4 to 6 years. The infection involves epithelial crypts embedded in lymphoid tissue, either solitary aggregates or confluent masses of lymphoid tissue such as the faucial tonsils. Exudation of serofibrinopurulent exudate from the crypts produces the familiar "crypt abscesses" that stud the tonsillar surfaces. Related lymph nodes undergo acute hyperplasia and, if bacteria reach them via afferent lymphatic channels, may suppurate (Figures 88–2

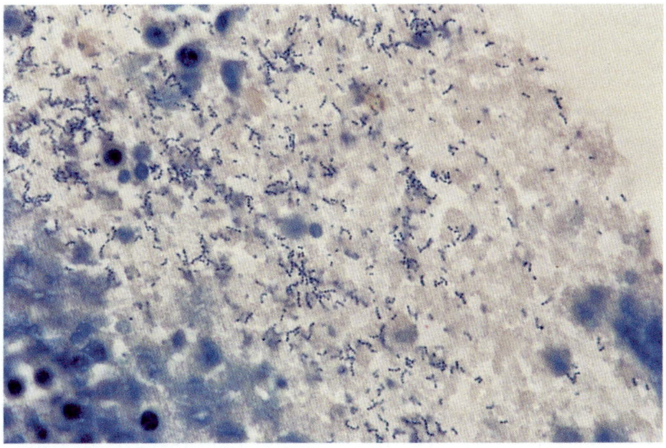

Figure 88–2. Focus of necrosis and suppuration in cervical lymph node following streptococcal pharyngitis (Ziehl–Neelsen, ×400).

and 88–3). Spread of infection to peritonsillar tissues accounts for peritonsillar abscess (quinsy).[14,15] These are pathologically undistinguished acute purulent inflammations. Spread of infection from the throat may involve paranasal sinuses or the middle ear. If the cribriform plate is traversed, purulent meningitis, dural sinus thrombosis, or brain abscess may result.

Scarletina (scarlet fever) is produced by scarletinal toxin elaborated by some strains of group A streptococci infected by a temperate bacteriophage. Experimentally, erythrogenic toxin is pyrogenic, cytotoxic, and enhances the action of endotoxin. Four serologically distinct forms (toxins A to D), each capable of inhibition by specific antibody, are recognized. Scarletina usually accompanies tonsillopharyngitis although it may result from pyoderma or endometritis produced by toxigenic streptococci. The cutaneous lesion of scarletina is rarely examined microscopically.[16] The dermis is edematous and hyperemic. There is a scanty perivascular dermal infiltrate of lymphocytes and other mononuclear cells. In the epidermis, keratinization is accelerated in the middle layer (pseudokeratosis), and there is desquamation through this plane. The differential diagnosis includes viral exanthemata, drug or other allergies, toxic shock syndrome, and Kawasaki disease.

Erysipelas is an acute infection of skin caused by group A streptococci (rarely group C).[17–19] The disease occurs predominantly in infants and in adults over 30. The disease most often involves the face (Figure 88–4), in which case there is often a history of antecedent streptococcal tonsillopharyngitis. Erysipelas of the trunk or limbs most often results from infection of a wound, either surgical or accidental. The cutaneous lesion begins as a patch of erythema and swelling that expands rapidly with elevated red margins and often central clearing. Microscopically the dermis is expanded by edema that soon becomes fibrinopurulent although, particularly early, there may be surprisingly few neutrophils (Figure 88–5). As the lesion progresses there may be a loosely palisaded perivascular accumulation

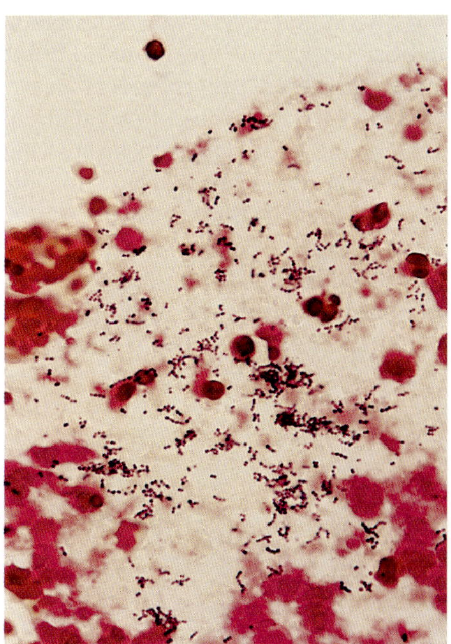

Figure 88–3. Same lesion showing clusters and chains of streptococci (tissue gram stain, ×1000).

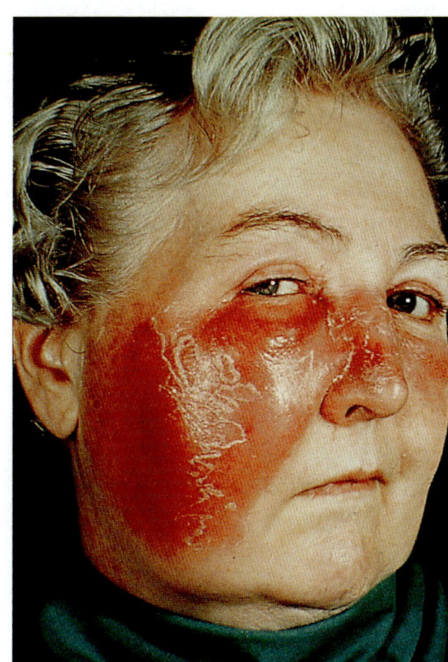

Figure 88–4. Erysipelas of face in an adult woman.

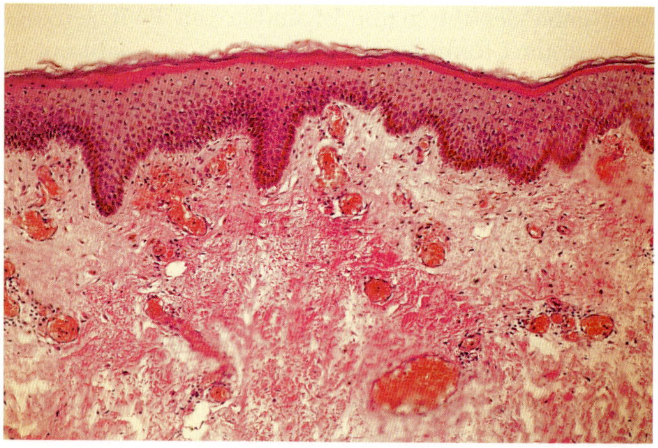

Figure 88–5. Erysipelas. Photomicrograph showing characteristic acute congestion and scanty inflammatory cell reaction. The dermal blood vessels and lymphatics are dilated and congested. There is dermal edema and some tinctorial change of collagen fibers, probably a consequence of toxic damage (hematoxylin-eosin, ×40).

of histiocytes, lymphocytes and neutrophils. The dermal expansion may be sufficiently marked to form a dermal–epidermal cleavage plane with the development of vesicles or even small bullae. The epidermis shows nonspecific spongiosis. Streptococci are ordinarily easily seen in Gram-stained sections.

Other infections of skin and connective tissue include a variety of pyodermas: impetigo,[20,21] a more deeply ulcerating pyoderma known as ecthyma,[22] and clinically nondescript infections of wounds[23] or burns. Streptococcal cellulitis (spreading infection of cellular connective tissue) may complicate postmastectomy lymphedema or filariasis. Cellulitis, presumed to be streptococcal because of its response to penicillin, may occur in lower limbs that have been donor sites of saphenous vein coronary arterial bypass grafts.

Rare cases of toxic shock syndrome have been associated with streptococcal (as "toxic strep syndrome") rather than staphylococcal infection.[24–26] This clinical presentation correlates strongly with elaboration of streptococcal pyrogen (scarletinal) exotoxin, especially type A.[25]

A severe infectious lesion in deep subcutaneous tissues has been termed "hospital gangrene," "necrotizing erysipelas," and, most recently, "necrotizing fasciitis."[27–30] This disorder was recognized during the American Civil War, World War I,[31] and importantly by Meleney in China.[32] The infection practically always follows trauma, but this may be trivial or even overlooked. In young patients, necrotizing fasciitis usually follows street trauma or appendicitis; in older patients congestive heart failure or diabetes may be underlying conditions or the disorder may begin as infection of a surgical wound. Clusters of cases have occurred.[33] Early the skin may be uninvolved but soon becomes bluish-purple and sloughs, revealing undermining inflammation of fascial planes (Figure 88–6). Thrombosis may be present. Sometimes the necrosis is crepitant. Myositis, necrosis of muscle, is uncommon, unlike (tropical) pyomyositis, a different disease, almost always staphylococcal.[34] Systemic toxicity and impaired consciousness are often conspicuous, sometimes resembling the toxic shock syndrome. The commonest bacterial agent is the beta-hemolytic streptococcus Lancefield group A, less commonly group C. The molecular pathogenesis of the process has not been established. Often the responsible streptococcus has been toxigenic.[25,35] Streptococcal protease has been suggested as having a role.[36] Other bacteria such as staphylococci, clostridial species, or anaerobic cocci can cause a similar lesion.

Streptococcal pneumonia, usually caused by group A organisms, is not common. Usually it complicates preexisting infectious diseases, influenza, measles, or pertussis. It is an undistinguished neutrophilic bronchopneumonia. Streptococcal bacteremia is rarely nosocomial. In California, the commonest associated condition is drug abuse.[37]

Streptococci collectively are the commonest causes of bacterial endocarditis.[38–48] Groups A or B are typically associated with acute bacterial endocarditis, alphahemolytic ("viridans") streptococci with subacute bacterial endocarditis. Although prolonged antibiotic therapy currently blurs the morphologic differences between the two forms of bacterial endocarditis, the distinction remains useful clinically. Streptococcal endocarditis is more common on left-sided valves[41] than right-sided ones.[42] Right-sided lesions are more common in intravenous drug abusers.[43] Streptococci are important agents in infective endocarditis of prosthetic valves.[41,49] Vegetations in acute bacterial endocarditis (Figure 88–7) are classically more luxuriant than in subacute bacterial endocarditis (Figures 88–8 and 88–9). Bacterial vegetations consist of three zones: 1) a luminal mantle of sparsely cellular fibrin, 2) an intermediate zone of leukocytes, predominantly neutrophils, and bacteria, and 3) a basal layer, more sparsely inflamed consisting

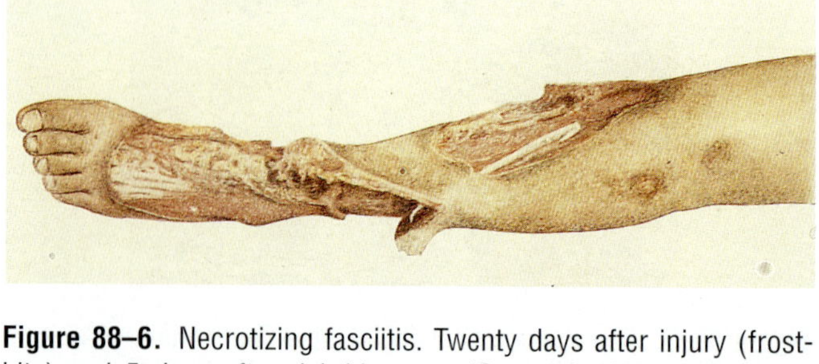

Figure 88–6. Necrotizing fasciitis. Twenty days after injury (frostbite) and 5 days after debridement. *(Copyright AMA 1924; from Meleney.[32])*

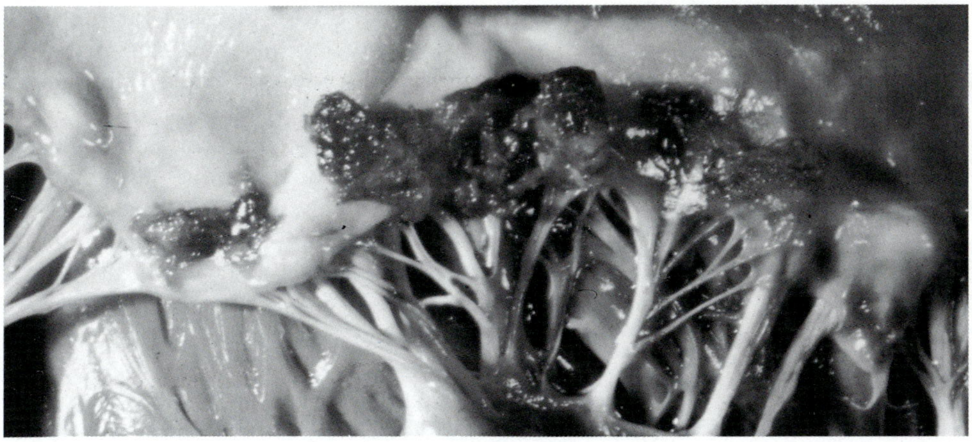

Figure 88–7. Acute streptococcal endocarditis of mitral valve. The vegetations have destroyed some of the anterior leaflet and most of the posterior leaflet.

of a partially vascularized zone of damaged valvular or endocardial tissue (Figure 88–10). The localization of bacterial vegetations is in areas of endocardium damaged by jet lesions of which the location can be understood by hydrodynamic principles. Either focal or diffuse glomerulonephritis are occasional complications.[48] Purulent pericarditis may occur[49,50] less commonly than as a complication of lobar pneumonia.

Nonsuppurative Complications

Rheumatic fever is an acute inflammatory process that involves heart, joints, skin, and central nervous system (CNS).[51] The disease follows infections by Lancefield group A beta-hemolytic streptococci in susceptible individuals and is prone to recur following subsequent streptococcal infections, ultimately resulting in cardiac valvular deformity and chronic valvular heart disease. Classically a disease of fall and winter months in temperate climates, rheumatic fever has become less common in medically advanced countries.[52] It remains an important medical problem in developing countries in Africa, Asia, and Latin America where, in spite of emphasis on other forms of cardiovascular disease such as endomyocardial fibrosis and Kawasaki disease, rheumatic heart disease remains by far the commonest form of heart disease in the young. In the United States there have been recent outbreaks of acute rheumatic fever in many localities including New York City, Pittsburgh, Salt Lake City, and Fort Leonard Wood, Missouri.[53] Several factors may contribute to the recrudescence of rheumatic fever, among them changes in the streptococcus not only in its "rheumatogenicity" but in its clinical manifestations so that its clinical diagnosis, particularly differences from viral pharyngitis, becomes more difficult and, importantly, diminishing frequency of throat cultures and lack of compliance by patients in completing their antibiotic regimens.

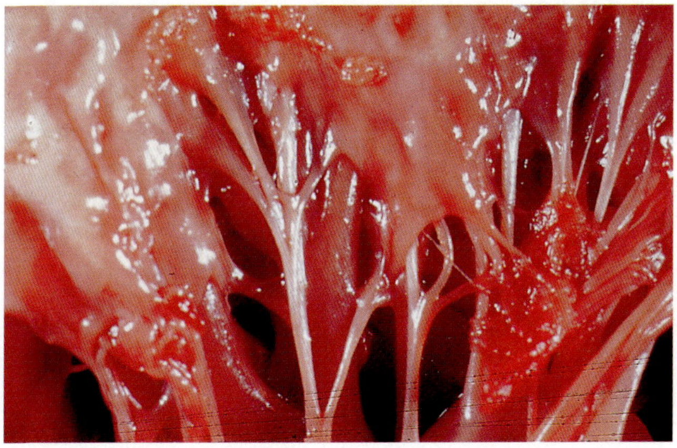

Figure 88–8. Subacute streptococcal (viridans) endocarditis of posterior leaflet and chordae tendineae of mitral valve, probably damaged by chronic rheumatic endocarditis.

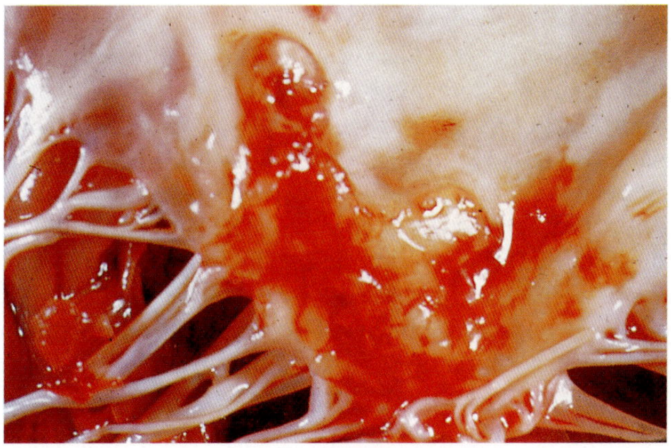

Figure 88–9. Subacute bacterial endocarditis of mitral valve. Characteristically, as seen here, the vegetations are on the closing surface.

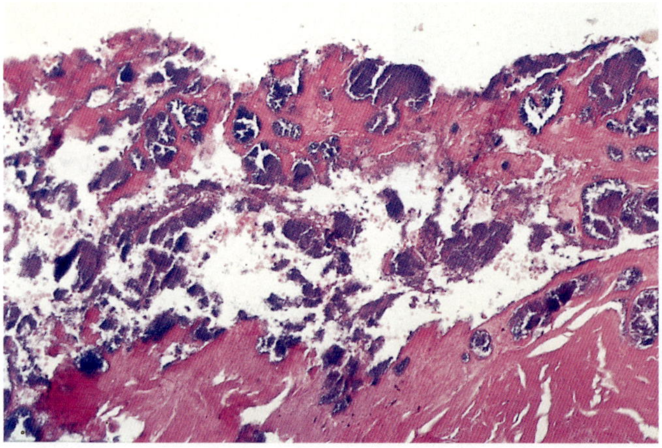

Figure 88–10. Subacute bacterial endocarditis of mitral valve. The masses of organisms are hematoxylinphilic (hematoxylin-eosin, ×20).

As stated in the definition, rheumatic fever follows streptococcal infections in susceptible individuals. The relevant streptococcal infection is practically always an acute tonsillopharyngitis caused by beta-hemolytic organisms of Lancefield group A. The attack rate of acute rheumatic fever is about 3% of those infected by appropriate streptococci. The degree of "rheumatogenicity" by various capsular serotypes of group A streptococci has recently received attention. Serotype 18 is more prone than other serotypes to produce rheumatic fever. Tissues involved in acute rheumatic fever are not infected by streptococci. Inflammation in these tissues is thought to be immunologically mediated,[54,55] and an enormous literature, beyond the scope of this discussion, has accumulated. Participation of involved tissue in a reaction to nonspecific immune complexes and autoimmunity triggered by antigens common to the streptococcus and human tissues have both been investigated.[56]

Rheumatic carditis is a specific granulomatous inflammation that involves all layers of the heart.[57] Grossly this process produces rows of opalescent warty excrescences, rheumatic veruccae, at lines of closure of cardiac valves and less conspicuously on chordae tendineae or mural endocardium. The process begins in microscopic foci of edema, swelling, and increased eosinophilia of connective tissue in the cardiac interstitium. These foci of what is termed "fibrinoid necrosis" become inflamed, initially by lymphocytes and plasma cells and soon by cardiac histocytes, Anitchkoff "myocytes," large ameboid cells with bean-shaped nuclei and prominent nucleoli that, depending on the plane of section, present either an "owl's eye" or "caterpiller" configuration. The Anitchkoff cell is not specific and occurs in foci of myocardial injury of varying pathogenic mechanisms, not all of them inflammatory. Although early termed "myocytes,"[58] these cells are currently thought to be modified tissue macrophages. Ultimately Anitchkoff cells coalesce to form multinucleated cells in the granulomatous foci that, at this stage, are termed Aschoff bodies (Figure 88–11). This process ultimately undergoes fibrosis and persists as roughly rhomboidal foci of interstitial fibrosis characteristically related to small blood vessels. It is this fibrosing process that distorts the heart valves, producing chronic valvular dysfunction.

Periarticular tissues from patients with acute rheumatic fever are rarely examined. These are the site of chronic perivascular inflammation of lymphocytes, plasma cells, and histiocytes, the latter often arrayed in perivascular pallisades similar to or indistinguishable from lesions of rheumatoid arthritis. Unlike periarticular lesions of rheumatoid arthritis, those of rheumatic fever resolve completely. In subcutaneous (rarely other) tissues, acute rheumatic fever may give rise to rheumatoid nodules. These are split pea to bean-sized slightly tender nodules that microscopically consist of flame-shaped foci of fibrinoid necrosis surrounded by radially arranged palisades of histocytes and mixed round cells set in a fibrovascular connective tissue reaction. Distinction from nodules of rheumatoid arthritis may be impossible. The differential diagnosis also includes other dermal necrobioses including erythema nodosum and necrobiosis lipoidica diabeticorum.

Lesions in the CNS that account for the bizarre motor disturbances of Sydenham's chorea are rarely documented. Nonspecific scanty perivascular accumulations of lymphocytes have been described.

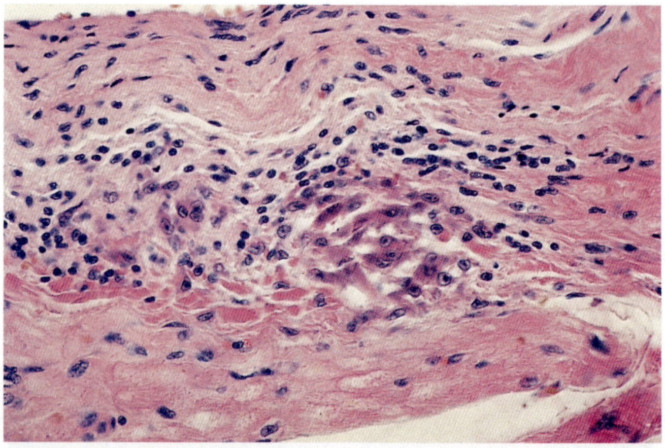

Figure 88–11. Aschoff body. The reacting cells and immune complexes damage the connective tissue and lead to scarring (hematoxylin-eosin, ×200).

Acute glomerulonephritis is an important renal disease that occurs throughout the world.[51,59,60] The disease usually follows an extrarenal infection, typically by streptococci of Lancefield group A. Not only may other streptococci, eg, Lancefield group C, D, or G, rarely be followed by glomerulonephritis, but infections by other bacteria or even viruses may be followed by acute glomerulonephritis. The group A streptococcus is the commonest agent of antecedent infection, however, and is the agent that precipitates perhaps 85% of cases of acute glomerulonephritis. Acute glomerulonephritis may occur at any age, but like the associated infection, is most common between 4 and 6 years. The antecedent infection is usually a tonsillopharyngitis but, unlike acute rheumatic fever, acute glomerulonephritis is rather frequently associated, particularly in economically depressed populations, with streptococcal pyodermas, usually impetigo.

The tendency for acute glomerulonephritis to follow group A streptococcal infections is greater with some capsular serotypes than others. Serotype 12 is most strikingly "nephritogenic" but types 4, 25, and 49 are also prone to be followed by glomerulonephritis. Glomerulonephritis has followed infection by serotypes 1, 2, 18, 57, and 60. Unlike rheumatic fever, acute glomerulonephritis is not prone to recur after subsequent streptococcal infections. Oddly, rheumatic fever and acute glomerulonephritis rarely coexist. Like acute rheumatic fever, acute glomerulonephritis is thought to be immunologically mediated, and a prodigious clinical and experimental literature relates to the disease. Renal injury by immune complexes trapped in renal glomeruli has received much attention. There has been variable success in identifying nephritogenic antigenic products of streptococcal infection.

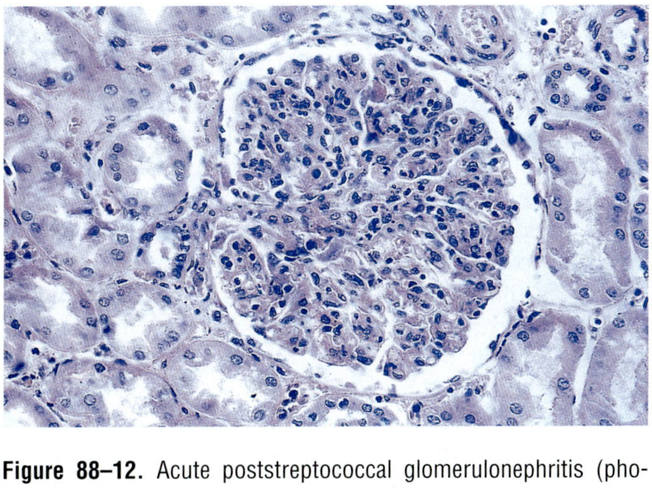

Figure 88–12. Acute poststreptococcal glomerulonephritis (photomicrograph).

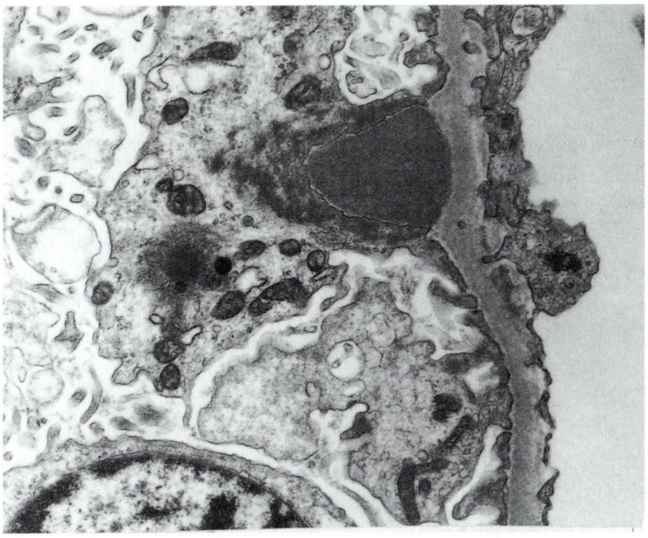

Figure 88–13. Electron micrograph of glomerular capillary wall in acute poststreptococcal glomerulonephritis showing hemispherical electron-dense deposit ("humps") in subepithelial space.

Glomeruli in acute glomerulonephritis are diffusely swollen and hypercellular (Figure 88–12). The hypercellularity is contributed to by each of the resident cells of the renal glomerulus: epithelial cells (both parietal and visceral), endothelial cells, and mesangial cells and also by cells from the circulating blood, neutrophils, and macrophages derived from circulating monocytes.

Electron microscopy characteristically demonstrates large but variable-sized aggregates of granular electron-dense material ("humps") thought to be immune complexes irregularly arrayed in the glomerular subepithelial space among foot processes of glomerular epithelial cells (Figure 88–13). These aggregates ordinarily bind fluorescein-labelled antibodies to IgG and various components of the complement cascade plus IgA and IgM.

The differential diagnosis includes the very large number of glomerular inflammatory lesions.

STREPTOCOCCUS AGALACTIAE (GROUP B BETA-HEMOLYTIC STREPTOCOCCI)

Perinatal infections by the group B streptococcus are an important cause of pneumonia, meningitis, and sepsis without organ localization in newborn infants.[61] In 20% to 40% of adult women the lower reproductive tract is colonized by group B streptococci.[62,63] Pregnancy does not itself affect the incidence of colonization. Streptococci reach the infant either during labor or during passage through the birth canal. Nosocomial transmission by nursery personnel, for instance, during times of overcrowding, is less common. Both asymptomatic colonization and clinical infection are increased in preterm infants and infants born after premature rupture of fetal membranes, prolonged labor, or by instrumental delivery.

Congenital pneumonia results from contamination of amniotic fluid after premature rupture of membranes or during prolonged labor. Any microbial resident of the birth canal can cause congenital pneumonia. Congenital pneumonia is often of lobar distribution because the lungs of the fetus are partially expanded with fluid that disseminates organisms throughout both lungs. Microscopically, congenital pneumonia is an acute neutrophilic inflammation that lacks fibrin because of the fibrinolytic properties of amniotic fluid. Squamous debris and other elements of meconium are increased. Interstitial participation in the inflammation is important in distinguishing true congenital pneumonia from the lungs of a newborn infant who "drowns in pus" (because of purulent chorioamnionitis).

In neonatal streptococcal pneumonia, intra-alveolar fibrin hyaline membranes are often conspicuous (Figure 88–14).[64] Distinction from noninfectious neonatal hyaline membrane disease is important and can usually be made by more pronounced neutrophilic exudate in neonatal pneumonia and by the presence of gram-positive cocci, usually in large numbers in the hyaline membranes (Figure 88–15).

Purulent meningitis is often present in cases of perinatal streptococcal infection because the group B streptococcus vies with *Escherichia coli* for first place among bacterial causes of neonatal meningitis.[65]

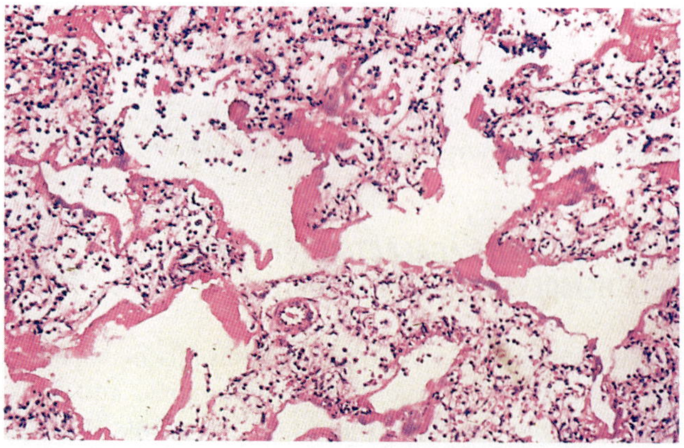

Figure 88–14. Pneumonia caused by group B streptococcus in a newborn infant. Hyaline membranes line the air spaces. *(Contributed by Dr Anna L. Katzenstein, Syracuse, New York.)*

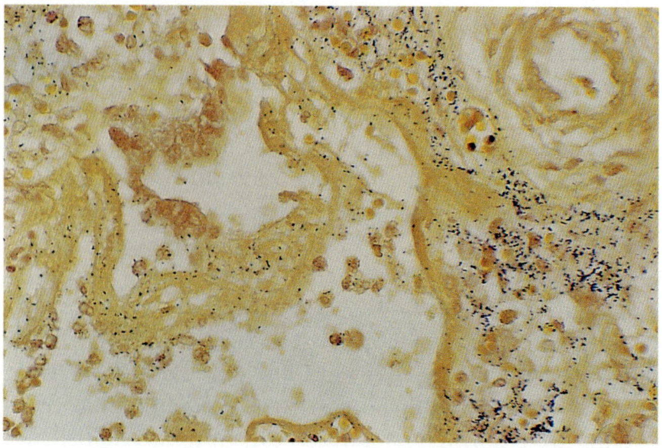

Figure 88–15. Gram stain of a group B streptococcal pneumonia. There are many cocci, some in hyalin membranes (Brown–Brenn, ×400).

Beyond the newborn period, group B infections are rare in infancy and childhood.[66]

Endometritis caused by the group B streptococcus is one of the commonest causes of postpartum endometritis.[67,68] Prolonged rupture of membranes, prolonged or instrumental delivery, and septic abortion are factors. It is an undistinguished acute purulent inflammation. The frequency of infected parametrial thrombophlebitis contributes to infected pulmonary infarcts. Postpartum meningitis is rare.[69] Other than in postpartum women, group B streptococcal infections are rare in adults. Myositis has been described.[70]

Beta-hemolytic streptococci of Lancefield group C fall into three species: *S equisimilis, S zooepidemicus,* and *S equi.* A fourth species, *S dysgalactiae,* has been described, but it is alpha hemolytic or nonhemolytic although it has a group C capsular antigen. Some "small colony" streptococci of the *S milleri* group also carry the group C or group F antigen and are beta hemolytic. These organisms are called *S anginosus.* Other members of the *S milleri* group are alpha hemolytic.

The most common human pathogen of group C,[71] *S equisimilis,* has been isolated from asymptomatic carriers and from patients with pharyngitis.[72,73] It has also caused cellulitis, necrotizing fasciitis, epiglottitis, pneumonia, empyema, meningitis, brain abscess, osteomyelitis, arthritis,[74–77] and endocarditis as well as bacteremia and postpartum sepsis.[78–80] Many of the patients have had underlying diseases such as diabetes, immunosuppression, cardiopulmonary disease, malignancy, or alcoholism.[79]

Streptococcus zooepidemicus causes a variety of infections in domestic animals and outbreaks of pharyngitis in human beings.[80,81] Often these have been attributed to unpasteurized milk or homemade cheese.

Postinfectious glomerulonephritis has occurred.[81,82] *Streptococcus equi* causes "strangles" in horses but rarely causes human infections. Meningitis caused by *S dysgalactiae* has occurred in an infant.[83]

Group D streptococci include *S bovis* and *S equi*. Some former members of group D are now classified in the genus *Enterococcus*. Human infections by *S bovis* are importantly associated with gastrointestinal lesions, most conspicuously carcinoma of the colon but also including other neoplasms both benign and malignant[84–88] and non-neoplastic diseases such as Crohn's disease and ulcerative colitis.[89,90] *Streptococcus bovis* has been implicated also in meningitis,[91–95] brain abscess,[96] bacteremia,[97] endocarditis,[98,99] and splenic abscess.[100]

Streptoccus suis sometimes placed in group D (or in groups R, S, RS, or T)[101] causes bacteremia or meningitis almost confined to pork handlers[102] including a poacher who ate the meat of a wild boar.[103]

Streptococcus anginosus (*S milleri* in the British taxonomic scheme) is a beta-hemolytic organism that possesses the group F (or group C) capsular polysaccharide and grows as "minute colonies." These organisms cause severe deep suppurative infections,[104] osteomyelitis, and endocarditis.[105,106] Other "small colony" beta-hemolytic streptococci carry capsular antigens of group A, C, or G.

Group G streptococci are part of the normal oropharyngeal, gastrointestinal, vaginal, and cutaneous flora.[107] They can cause infections related to these sites that include pharyngitis, otitis media, cellulitis, pleuropulmonary infection, septic arthritis, endocarditis, and meningitis. Bacteremia has occurred in drug abusers.[108,109] Others of these patients often have had malignancies, congestive heart failure, or chronic pulmonary disease.[110,111] Group G streptococcal meningitis has occurred in acquired immunodeficiency syndrome patients.[112] Acute glomerulonephritis has followed pharyngitis[113,114] and purulent arthritis,[115] and other infections caused by group G streptococci.[116] Secretion of neuraminidase has been associated with nephritogenicity.[117]

ALPHA-HEMOLYTIC STREPTOCOCCI (*STREPTOCOCCUS* VIRIDANS)

Streptococci other than pneumococcus that produce partial (alpha) hemolysis of erythrocytes in solid media are often designated streptococcus viridans or green streptococci.[118–120] "Viridans" is not a systematic taxonomic designation and should not be italicized.

Alpha-hemolytic streptococci are commensals on many human body surfaces such as the oral cavity, urogenital system, alimentary tract, and skin. Clinically significant infections may originate from these sites or be topographically related to them.[118–120] The most important diseases caused by viridans streptococci include

1. dental plaque and caries,
2. infective endocarditis, and
3. organ abscesses.

Oral species such as *S mutans* and *S sanguis* participate in the formation of dental plaque and initiate the formation of dental caries because they elaborate complex glycans from fructose. From the mouth, the streptococci may enter the bloodstream after oral trauma, surgery, or manipulations as benign as brushing the teeth.

Alpha-hemolytic species are the commonest agents in streptococcal endocarditis usually clinicopathologically characterized as "subacute bacterial endocarditis" and often related to previously damaged valves as by rheumatic fever or congenital cardiovascular lesions. The ability to produce solitary or multiple abscesses is a lesser known attribute of some alpha-hemolytic streptococci. In the British taxonomy, these organisms are often designated as *S milleri* (mainly *S constellatus* and *S intermedius* in the American nomenclature).[121–144] The abscesses may occur in soft tissues or in any viscus. The liver is frequently involved (Figure 88–16)[137–140]; brain and lung may be sites.[141] Abscesses occur in the myocardium both with and without bacterial endocarditis.[142] Pyometra has occurred after myomectomy.[142] Meningitis is uncommon.[144]

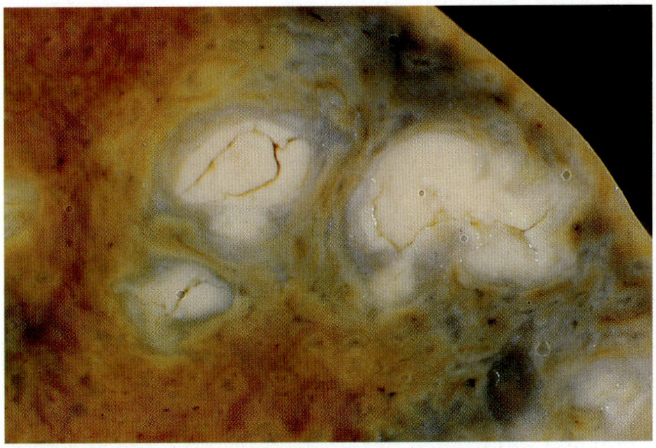

Figure 88–16. Streptococcal abscesses of liver complicating subacute bacterial endocarditis. *(Photograph by Daniel H. Connor, MD, 1982.)*

Enterococcus Species

These organisms previously included with members of group D streptococci are normal inhabitants of the gastrointestinal tract of human beings and many animal species.[145,146] They are the commonest streptococci found in blood cultures,[147–151] are important agents in nosocomial infections, and cause about 15% of cases of bacterial endocarditis.[152–154] Adherence to valve tissue is a factor.[155,156] They also can cause abdominal and pelvic infections,[157] urinary tract infections,[158,159] wound infections, meningitis,[160] perinatal sepsis, and pneumonia.[161,162] There are currently 14 species among which *E faecalis* causes 80% to 90% of human infections. *Enterococcus faecium* causes another 10% to 15%.[163] Antibiotic resistance is a continuing problem.[164,165]

STREPTOCOCCUS PNEUMONIAE (THE PNEUMOCOCCUS)

Streptococcus pneumoniae, the "pneumococcus," is an important human pathogen. The organism is the most common cause of community-acquired pneumonia,[166] the second commonest cause of purulent meningitis[167] and the commonest cause of otitis media, purulent sinusitis, and mastoiditis.[168] Pneumococci are gram-positive, nonmotile, non-spore-forming cocci that occur in pairs in clinical material, and in pairs or short chains in liquid culture. They are alpha hemolytic.

The major factor in *S pneumoniae* that is associated with pathogenicity is the presence of capsular polysaccharides, complex hydrophilic polymers that form on the cell surface.[169,170] Chemical structures of several are known. Organisms that produce capsular polysaccharide (formerly SSS, soluble specific substance) form smooth colonies on solid media and are pathogenic for man or experimental animals while those that do not form such a substance grow in rough colonies and are nonpathogenic. Capsular polysaccharides are antigenically specific and constitute the basis for primary typing of *S pneumoniae.* Some 84 antigenically distinct types are currently recognizable. Pathogenicity differs among the various capsular types, types 1, 2, 3, 4, 7, 8, 12, and 14 being more pathogenic than others.[171] The demonstration of conversion of capsular type by heat-killed organisms was the beginning of microbial genetics when the component responsible for capsular conversion was shown to be deoxyribonucleic acid.

Pneumococci also produce as components of their cell wall C substance or C polysaccharide, precipitation of which by a serum β globulin in the presence of calcium is an indicator of acute inflammatory disease. Type specific M protein and an R protein from rough pneumococci have been demonstrated. They appear not to contribute to pathogenesis.

Pathogenecity of *S pneumoniae* appears to reside in its ability to invade tissue because of the antiphagocytic properties of C polysaccharide. These organisms produce a variety of other factors that may have toxic or toxin-like properties. These include pneumolysin, a purpura-producing factor, and a neuraminidase.

Streptococcus pneumoniae are frequently found in the respiratory tracts of normal individuals.[172] The frequency varies from 5% to 70% and the distribution of capsular types depends on many factors that include age (more frequent in the young), season of the year, presence of children in the household, and presence of respiratory disease in the community.[173,174]

Like other gram-positive cocci, S pneumoniae is a classic extracellular pathogen that evokes an acute neutrophilic inflammatory response in the host. The distribution of capsular types shows that six types (8, 4, 1, 14, 3, and 7) contribute 50% of infections of pneumococcal diseases. More than 90% of pneumococcal infections are caused by types against which currently available antipneumococcus vaccine offers protection. Important among these are pneumococcal pneumonia[166] and its complications: empyema,[174] lung abscess, and purulent pericarditis.[175] The pneumococcus is the commonest cause of purulent otitis and acute inflammation of the paranasal sinuses and mastoid.[176]

Streptococcus pneumoniae distantly follows *Haemophilus influenzae* as a cause of acute epiglottitis.[177] The pneumococcus is the second commonest cause of bacterial meningitis.[167] About half of all cases have pneumonia. Others have pneumococcal sinusitis, mastoiditis, or otitis media. Pneumococci are a recognized cause of primary purulent peritonitis (peritonitis without perforation of a viscus) especially in patients with ascites due to cirrhosis of the liver[178] or the nephrotic syndrome. An uncommon but important cause of bacterial endocarditis, the pneumococcus may form luxurient mural vegetations as well as the more typical valvular lesions. Pneumococci occasionally colonize the female reproductive tract and have caused endometritis, salpingitis, pelvic abscess, and postpartum sepsis.[145,179,180] Pelvic infections caused by pneumococcus have occurred in prepubertal, even newborn girls.[145] Other circumstances in which pneumococcal infections are particularly common are postsplenectomy and other conditions with impaired host response such as hemoglobinopathy, certain hematologic diseases, alcoholism, hypogammaglobulinemia, neutropenic states, and diabetes mellitus.[146] Typing of pneumococci isolated in disease states had become relatively neglected but has resumed importance with the availability of polyvalent pneumococcal vaccines. Pathologic features of organ-specific pneumococcal infections are considered in discussions of the various organ systems.

MISCELLANEOUS GRAM-POSITIVE ("STREPTOCOCCUS-LIKE") COCCI

Many genera of gram-positive cocci occur in the environment, often as plant saprophytes or associated with water. The taxonomy of these organisms is complicated by variable definitions of *anaerobic,*[2] and by the lack of inclusion of modern genetic information in their classification. Several of these genera are of economic importance in brewing and wine making, as additives to processed foods, and as sileage additives. A few genera are occasional human pathogens almost entirely as opportunists. These include members of genera *Aerococcus,*[181] *Leuconostoc,*[182–189] *Lactococcus, Pediococcus,* and *Gemella.*[190,191] There are no distinctive pathologic features of lesions caused by these organisms.

Anaerobic Gram-Positive Cocci

A group of gram-positive anaerobic cocci is second to *Bacteroides* species in clinical importance among anaerobic organisms. Chief among these are *Peptostreptococci,* notably *P magnus* and *P anaerobius.* Recent reclassification has left *Peptococcus magnus,* a rare human pathogen, as the only species of the genus *Peptococcus.*[191,192]

Peptostreptococci usually infect surgical wounds that follow gastrointestinal procedures or hysterectomies. Approximately 10% of infections are mixed.

REFERENCES

1. Bridge PD, Sneath PH. Numerical taxonomy of *Streptococcus. J Gen Microbiol.* 1983;129;565–597.
2. Facklam RR, Smith PB. The gram positive cocci. *Hum Pathol.* 1976;7:187–194.
3. Schleifer KH, Kilpper-Bälz R. Molecular and chemotaxonomic approaches to the classification of streptococci, enterococci and lactococci: a review. *Syst Appl Microbiol.* 1980;10:1–19.
4. Smith PH, Mair NS, Sharpe ME, Holt JG, eds. *Bergey's Manual of Systematic Bacteriology.* Baltimore: Williams Wilkins; 1989:1043–1071.
5. Bisno AL. Classification of streptococci. In: Mandell GL, Douglas RG Jr, Bennett JE, eds. *Principles and Practice of Infectious Diseases.* 3rd ed. New York: Churchill Livingstone; 1990:1518–1519.
6. McCarty M. The streptococcal cell wall. *Harvey Lect.* 1971;65:73–96.
7. Smalley DL, Doyle VR, Hollis CH, Duckworth JK. Facial abscess due to group L streptococcal infection. *South Med J.* 1981;74:511–512.
8. Fischetti VA. Streptococcal M protein: molecular design and biological behavior. *Clin Microbiol Rev.* 1989;2: 285–314.
9. Beachey EH, Ofek I. Epithelial cell bindings of group A streptococci by lipoteichoic acid on fimbriae denuded of M protein. *J Exp Med.* 1976;143:759–771.
10. Huskins WC, Kaplan EL. Inhibitory substances produced by *Streptococcus salivarius* and colonization of the upper respiratory tract with group A streptococci. *Epidem Inf.* 1989;102:401–412.
11. Bisno AL. Streptococcus pyogenes. In: Mandell GL, Douglas RG Jr, Bennett JE, eds. *Principles and Practice of Infectious Diseases.* 3rd ed. New York: Churchill Livingstone; 1990:1519–1528.
12. Rammelkamp CH Jr. Natural history of streptococcal infections. *Bull NY Acad Med.* 1955;31:103–112.
13. Peter G, Smith AL. Group A streptococcal infections of the skin and pharynx. *N Engl J Med.* 1977;297:311–317.
14. deMarie S, Richenel TO, Tham TA, et al. Clinical infections and nonsurgical treatment of parapharyngeal space infections complicating throat infection. *Rev Infect Dis.* 1989;11:975–982.
15. Grodinsky M. Retropharyngeal and lateral pharyngeal abscesses. An anatomic and clinical study. *Ann Surg.* 1939;110:177–199.
16. Brody H, Smith LW. The visceral pathology in scarlet fever and related streptococcus infections. *Am J Pathol.* 1936;12:373–394.
17. Culatta CS. Erysipelas in children under two years of age. *J Pediatr.* 1935;7:16–20.
18. Francis T Jr. Studies on pathogenesis and recovery in erysipelas. *J Clin Invest.* 1928;6:221–230.
19. Tappeiner J, Pfleger L. Zur Histopathologie cutaner Lymphgefasse beim chronisch-rezidivierenden Erysipel der unteren Extremitaten. *Hautarzt.* 1964;15:218–223.
20. Noble WC, Presbury D, Connor BL. Prevalence of streptococci and staphylococci in lesions of impetigo. *Br J Dermatol.* 1974;91:115–116.
21. Parker MT, Tomlinson AJH, Williams REO. Impetigo contagiosa. The association of certain types of *Staphylococcus aureus* and *Streptococcus pyogenes* in superficial skin infections. *J Hyg Cambridge.* 1955;53:458–473.
22. Kelly C, Toplin D, Allen AM. Streptococcal ecthyma. *Arch Dermatol.* 1971;103:306–310.
23. Mastro TD, Farley TA, Elliott JA, et al. An outbreak of surgical-wound infections due to group A streptococcus carried on the scalp. *N Engl J Med.* 1990;323:968–972.
24. Bartter T, Dascal A, Carrol K. Curley FJ. "Toxic strep syndrome." A manifestation of group A streptoccal infection. *Arch Intern Med.* 1988;148:1421–1424.
25. Cone LA, Woodward DR, Schlievert PM, Tomory GS. Clinical and bacteriologic observations of a toxic-shock like syndrome due to streptococcus pyogenes. *N Engl J Med.* 1987;317:146–149.
26. Hoge CW, Schwartz B, Talkington DF, Breiman RF, MacNeill EM, Englender SJ. The changing epidemiology of invasive group A streptococcal infections and the emer-

gence of streptococal toxic-shock like syndrome. A retrospective population based study. *JAMA.* 1993;269: 384–389.

27. Working group on severe streptococcal infections. Defining the group A streptococcal toxic shock syndrome: rationale and concensus definition. *JAMA.* 1993;269: 390–391.
28. Rea WJ, Wyrick WJ. Necrotizing fasciitis. *Ann Surg* 1970; 172:957–964.
29. Stevens DL. Invasive group A streptococcal infections. *Clin Infect Dis.* 1992;14:2–11.
30. Stevens DL, Tanner MH, Winship J, et al. Severe group A streptococcal infections associated with a toxic shock-like syndrome and scarlet fever toxin A. *N Engl J Med.* 1989;321:1–7.
31. Pfanner W. Zur Kenntnis und Behandlung des nekrotisierenden Erysipels. *Dtschr Ztschrf Chir.* 1918;14: 108–119.
32. Meleney FL. Hemolytic streptococcal gangrene. *Arch Surg.* 1924;9;317–364.
33. Schwartz B, Elliot JA, Buller JC, et al. Clusters of invasive group A streptococcal infections in family, hospital, and nursing-home settings. *Clin Infect Dis.* 1992;15:277–284.
34. Gibson RK, Rosenthal SJ, Lukert BP. Pyomyositis: increasing recognition in temperate climates. *Am J Med.* 1984;77:768–772.
35. Invasive group A streptococcal infections—United Kingdom, 1994. *JAMA.* 1994;272:16.
36. Talkington DF, Schwartz B, Black CM, et al. Association of phenotypic and genotypic characteristics of invasive *Streptococcus pyogenes* isolates with clinical components of streptococcal toxic shock syndrome. *Infect Immun.* 1993;61:3369–3374.
37. Braunstein H. Characteristics of group A streptococcal bacteremia in patients at the San Bernardino County Medical Center. *Rev Infect Dis.* 1991;1:8–11.
38. Wilson LM. Etiology of bacterial endocarditis. Before and since the introduction of antibiotics. *Ann Intern Med.* 1963;58:946–952.
39. Weinstein L, Schlesinger JJ, Pathoanatomic, pathophysiologic and clinical correlations in endocarditis. *N Engl J Med.* 1974;291:832–837,1122–1126.
40. Gonzalez-Lavin L, Lise M, Ross D. The importance of the "jet lesions" in bacterial endocarditis involving the left heart. Surgical considerations. *J Thorac Cardiovasc Surg.* 1970;59:185–192.
41. Buchbinder NA, Roberts WC. Left-sided valvular acute infective endocarditis. A study of forty-five necropsy patients. *Am J Med.* 1972;53:20–35.
42. Roberts WC, Buchbinder NA. Right-sided valvular infective endocarditis. A clinocopathologic study of twelve necropsy patients. *Am J Med.* 1972;53:7–19.
43. Reisberg BE. Infective endocarditis in the narcotic addict. *Prog Cardiovasc Dis.* 1979;22:193–204.
44. Anderson DJ, Buckley BH, Hutchins GM. A clinicopathologic study of prosthetic valve endocarditis in 22 patients: morphologic basis for diagnosis and therapy. *Am Heart J.* 1977;94:325–332.
45. Arnett EN, Roberts WC. Prosthetic valve endocarditis. Clinicopathologic analysis of 22 necropsy patients with active infective endocarditis involving natural left-sided cardiac valves. *Am J Cardiol.* 1976;38:281–292.
46. Arnett MM, Roberts WC. Valve ring abscesses in active infective endocarditis. Frequency, location and clues to clinical diagnosis from the study of 95 necropsy patients. *Circulation.* 1976;54:140–145.
47. Sheldon WM, Golden A. Abscesses of the valve rings of the heart: a frequent but not well recognized complication of acute bacterial endocarditis. *Circulation.* 1951;4: 1–12.
48. Perez GO, Rothfield W, Williams RC. Immune complex nephritis in bacterial endocarditis. *Arch Intern Med.* 1976;136:334–336.
49. Rubin RH, Moellering RC Jr. Clinical microbiologic and therapeutic aspects of purulent pericarditis. *Am J Med.* 1975;59:68–78.
50. Klacsman PG, Bulkley BH, Hutchins GM. The changed spectrum of purulent pericarditis. An 86 year autopsy experience in 200 patients. *Am J Med* 1977;63:666–673.
51. Bisno AL. Nonsuppurative poststreptococcal sequelae: rheumatic fever and glomerulonephritis. In: Mandell GL, Douglas RG Jr, Bennett JE, eds. *Principles and Practice of Infectious Diseases.* 3rd ed. New York: Churchill Livingstone; 1990:1528–1539.
52. Stollerman GH. Rheumatogenic group A streptococci and the return of rheumatic fever. *Adv Intern Med.* 1990;35:1–25.
53. Quinn RW. Comprehensive review of morbidity and mortality trends for rheumatic fever, streptococcal disease, and scarlet fever: the decline of rheumatic fever. *Rev Infect Dis.* 1989;11:928–953.
54. Bisno AL. Group A streptococcal infections and acute rheumatic fever. *N Engl J Med.* 1991;325:783–793.
55. Dale JB, Beachey EH. Protective antigenic determinant of streptococcal M protein shared with sarcolemmal membrane protein of human heart. *J Exp Med.* 1982; 156:1165–1176.
56. Kaplan MH. Rheumatic fever, rheumatic heart disease, and the streptococcal connection: the role of streptococcal antigens cross-reactive with heart tissue. *Rev Infect Dis.* 1979;1:988–995.
57. Saphir O. The Aschoff nodule. *Am J Clin Pathol.* 1959;31: 534–539.
58. Murphy GE. The characteristic rheumatic lesions of striated and non-striated or smooth muscle cells of the heart. Genesis of the lesions known as Aschoff bodies and those myogenic components known as Aschoff cells or as Anitchkow cells or myocytes. *Medicine.* 1963;42: 73–117.
59. Silva FG. Acute postinfectious glomerulonephritis complicating persistent bacterial infections. In Heptinstall RH, ed. *Pathology of the Kidney.* 4th ed. Boston: Little Brown; 1992:297–388.
60. Kaplan EL, Anthony BF, Chapmann SS. Epidemic acute glomerulonephritis associated with type 49 streptococcal pyoderma. *Am J Med.* 1970;48:9–27.
61. Eickhoff TC, Klein JO, Daly AK, Ingall D, Finland M. Neonatal sepsis and other infections due to group B beta-hemolytic streptococci. *N Engl J Med.* 1964;271: 1221–1228.

62. Baker CJ, Group B streptococcal infections. *Adv Intern Med.* 1980;25:475–501.
63. Jones DE, Friedl EM, Kanarek KS, Williams JK, Lim DV. Rapid identification of pregnant women heavily colonized with group B streptococci. *J Clin Microbiol.* 1983;18:558–560.
64. Katzenstein AL, Davis C, Braude A. Pulmonary changes in neonatal sepsis due to Group B β-hemolytic *Streptococcus.* Relation to hyaline membrane disease. *J Infect Dis.* 1976;133:430–435.
65. Sáez-Llorens X, McCracken GH Jr. Bacterial meningitis in neonates and children. *Infect Dis Clin North Am.* 1990; 4:623–644.
66. Arditi M, Shulman ST, Davis AT, Yogev R. Group C β-hemolytic streptococcal infections in children: nine pediatric cases and review. *Rev Infect Dis.* 1989;11:34–45.
67. Colebrook L, Hare B. Anaerobic streptococci associated with puerpural fever. *J Obstet Gynecol Br Emp.* 1933;40: 609–629.
68. Novy MJ. Post partum infections. In: Pernall, Benson RC, eds. *Current Obstetric and Gynecologic Diagnosis and Treatment.* 6th ed. Los Altos: Lange Medical Publications; 1989:226–227.
69. Aharoni A, Potasman I, Levitan Z, Golan D, Sharf M. Postpartum maternal group B streptococcal meningitis. *Rev Infect Dis.* 1990;12:273–276.
70. Back SA, O'Neill T, Fishbein G, Gwinn PG. A case of group B streptococcal pyomyositis. *Rev Infect Dis.* 1990;12:784–787.
71. Stamm AM, Cobbs CG. Group C streptococcal pneumonia: report of a fatal case and review of the literature. *Rev Infect Dis.* 1980;2:889–898.
72. Cimolai N, Elford RW, Bryan L, Anand C, Berger P. Do the β-hemolytic non-group A streptococci cause pharyngitis? *Rev Infect Dis.* 1988;10:587–601.
73. Rudensky B, Isacosohn M. β-hemolytic group C streptococci and pharyngitis. *Rev Infect Dis.* 1989;11:668.
74. Rose HD, Allen JR, Witte G. *Streptococcus zooepidemicus* group C pneumonia in a human. *J Clin Pathol.* 1980;11: 76–78.
75. Gorman PW, Collins DN. Group C streptococcal arthritis: a case report of equine transmission. *Orthopedics.* 1987; 10:615–616.
76. Mitnick H, Mitnick JS, Rafii M, Wetherbee R. Septic arthritis secondary to group C streptococcus. *J Rheumatol.* 1982;9:974–976.
77. Ortel TL, Kallianos J, Gallis HA. Group C streptococcal arthritis: case report and review. *Rev Infect Dis.* 1990; 12:829–837.
78. Salata RA, Lerner PI, Shlaes DM. Infections due to Lancefield group C streptococci. *Medicine.* 1989;68:225–239.
79. Bradley SF, Gordon JJ, Baumgartner DD, Marasco WA, Kauffman CA. Group C streptococcal bacteremia: analysis of 88 cases. *Rev Infect Dis.* 1991;13:270–280.
80. Barnham M, Ljunggren A, McIntyre M. Human infection with *Streptococcus zooepidemicus* (Lancefield group C): three case reports. *Epidem Inf.* 1987;98:183–190.
81. Barnham M, Thornton TJ, Lange K. Nephritis caused by *Streptococcus zooepidemicus* (Lancefield group C). *Lancet.* 1983;1:945–948.
82. Duca E, Teodorovici G, Radu C, et al. A new nephritogenic streptococcus. *J Hyg Cambridge.* 1969;67:691–698.
83. Kuskie MR. Group C streptococcal infections. *Pediatr Infect Dis J.* 1987;6:856–859.
84. Burns CA, McCaughey R, Lauter CB. The association of *Streptococcus bovis* fecal carriage and colon neoplasia: possible relationship with polyps and their malignant potential. *Ann J Gastroenterol.* 1985;80:42–46.
85. Emilani VJ, Chodos JE, Comer GM, Holness LG, Schwartz AJ. *Streptococcus bovis* brain abscess associated with an occult colonic villous adenoma. *Am J Gastroenterol.* 1990;85:78–80.
86. Jadeja L, Kantarjian H, Boliver R. *Streptococcus bovis* septicemia and meningitis associated with chronic radiation enterocolitis. *South Med J.* 1983;76:158–159.
87. Kewal N, Seneviratne BIB, Wilkinson RR, Seneviratne EME. Asymptomatic colonic carcinoma revealed by investigation of *Streptococcus bovis* bacteremia. *Aust N Z J Med.* 1983;13:173–174.
88. Klein RS, Catalano MT, Edberg SC, Casey JL. Steigbigel MH. *Streptococcus bovis* septicemia and carcinoma of the colon. *Ann Intern Med.* 1990;91:560–562.
89. Moshkowitz M, Arber N, Wajsman R, Baratz M, Gilat T. *Streptococcus bovis* endocarditis as a presenting manifestation of idiopathic ulcerative colitis. *Postgrad Med J.* 1992;68:930–931.
90. Reynolds JB, Silva E, McCormack WM. Association of *Streptococcus bovis* bacteremia with bowel disease. *J Clin Microbiol.* 1983;17:696–697.
91. Robbins W, Wisoff HS, Klein RS. Vertebral osteomyelitis caused by *Streptococcus bovis. Am J Med Sci.* 1986;291: 128–129.
92. Trajber I, Solomon A, Michowitz M, Yust I. *Streptococcus bovis* subacute bacterial endocarditis as a presenting symptom of occult double carcinoma of the colon. *J Surg Oncol.* 1984;27:186–188.
93. Gavryck WA, Sattler FR. Meningitis caused by *Streptococcus bovis. Arch Neurol.* 1982;39:307–308.
94. Purdy RA, Cassidy B, Marrie JJ. *Streptococcus bovis* meningitis. Report of 2 cases. *Neurology.* 1990;40: 1782–1784.
95. Fikar CR. *Streptococus bovis* meningitis in a neonate. *Am J Dis Child.* 1979;133:1149–1150.
96. Leibovitch G, Maaravi Y, Sholev O. Multiple brain abscess caused by *Streptococcus bovis. J Infect.* 1991;23: 195–196.
97. Ruoff KL, Miller SJ, Gavner CV, Ferraro JM, Calderwood SB. Bacteremia with *Streptococcus bovis* and *Streptococcus salivarius:* clinical correlates of more accurate identification of isolates. *J Clin Microbiol.* 1989;27:305–308.
98. Fung JC, Gadbow JJ Jr, Donta ST, Tilton RC. Infective endocarditis due to penicillin-tolerant *Streptococcus bovis. Diagn Microbiol Infect Dis.* 1986;5:171–176.
99. Savitch CB, Barry AL, Hoeprich PD. Infective endocarditis caused by *Streptococcus bovis* resistant to the lethal effect of penicillin G. *Arch Intern Med.* 1978;138: 931–939.
100. Belinkie SA, Narayanan NC, Russell JC, Becker DR. Splenic abscess associated with *Streptococcus bovis* sep-

ticemia and neoplastic lesions of the colon. *Dis Colon Rectum.* 1983;26:823–824.

101. Perch B, Pedersen KB, Henrichsen J. Serology of capsulated streptococci pathogenic for pigs: six new serotypes of *Streptococcus suis. J Clin Microbiol.* 1983;17:993–996.
102. Arends JP, Zanen HC. Meningitis caused by *Streptococcus suis* in humans. *Rev Infect Dis.* 1988;10:131–137.
103. Bonmarchand G, Massani P, Humbert G, et al. Group R streptococci: wild boars as a second reservoir. *Scand J Infect Dis.* 1985;17:121–122.
104. Libertin CR, Hermans PE, Washington JA II. Beta-hemolytic group F streptococcal bacteremia: a study and review of the literature. *Rev Infect Dis.* 1985;7:498–503.
105. Gopalakrishna KV, Kwon DH, Shah A. Metastatic myocardial abscess due to group F streptococci. *Am J Med Sci.* 1977;274:329–332.
106. Shlaes DM, Lerner PI, Wolinsky E, Gopalakrishna KV. Infections due to Lancefield group F and related streptococci (*S milleri, S anginosus*). *Medicine.* 1981;60:197–207.
107. Vartian C, Lerner PI, Shlaes DM, Gopalakrishna KV. Infections due to Lancefield group G streptococci. *Medicine.* 1985;64:75–88.
108. Goldshlack P, Blackburn G. Lancefield group G streptococcus septic arthritis in a heroin user: report of a case. *J Am Osteopath Assn.* 1984;84:60–61.
109. Craven DE, Rixinger AI, Bisno AL, Goularte TA, Mccabe WR. Bacteremia caused by group G streptococci in parenteral drug abusers: epidemiological and clinical aspects. *J Infect Dis.* 1986;153:988–992.
110. Auckenthaler R, Hermans PE, Washington JA II. Group G streptococcal bacteremia: Clinical study and review of the literature. *Rev Infect Dis.* 1983;5:196–204.
111. Watsky KL, Kollisch N, Denson P. Group G streptococcal bacteremia. The clinical experience at Boston University Medical Center and a critical review of the literature. *Arch Intern Med.* 1985;145:58–61.
112. Raviglione MC, Tierno PM, Orruso P, Klemes AB, Davidson M. Group G streptococcal meningitis and sepsis in a patient with AIDS. A method to biotype group G streptococcus. *Diagn Microbiol Infect Dis.* 1990;13:261–264.
113. Reid HF, Basset DCJ, Poon-King T, Zabriskie JB, Read SE. Group G streptococci in healthy school children and in patients with glomerulonephritis in Trinidad. *J Hyg London.* 1985;94:61–68.
114. Hill HR, Wilson E, Caldwell GG, Hager D, Zimmerman RA. Epidemic of pharyngitis due to streptococci of Lancefield group G. *Lancet.* 1969;2:371–374.
115. Clinicopathologic Conference. Septic polyarthritis and acute renal failure in a 57-year-old man. *Am J Med.* 1991; 91:293–299.
116. Gnann JW Jr, Gray BM, Griffin FM Jr, Dismukes WE. Acute glomerulonephritis following group G streptococcal infections. *J Infect Dis.* 1987;156:411–412.
117. Mosquera JA, Katiyar VN, Coello J, Rodriguez-Iturbe B. Neuraminidase production by streptococci from two patients with glomerulonephritis. *J Infect Dis.* 1985;151: 259–263.
118. Coykendall AL. Classification and identification of the viridans streptococci. *Clin Microbiol Rev.* 1989;2: 315–328.
119. Facklam RR. Physiological differentiation of viridans streptococci. *J Clin Microbiol.* 1977;5:184–201.
120. French GL, Talsania H, Charlton JRH, Phillips I. A physiological classification of the viridans streptococci by use of the APL-20 STREP system. *J Med Microbiol.* 1989;28: 275–286.
121. Ruoff KL. Nutritionally variant streptococci. *Clin Microbiol Rev.* 1991;4:184–190.
122. Shlaes DM, Marino J, Jacobs MR: Infection caused by vancomycin-resistant *Streptococcus sanguis:* II. *Antimicrob Agents Chemother.* 1984;25:527–528.
123. Coto H, Berk SL. Endocarditis caused by *Streptococcus morbillorum. Am J Med Sci.* 1984;287(3):54–58.
124. McCarthy LR, Bottone EJ. Bacteremia and endocarditis caused by satelliting streptococci. *Am J Clin Pathol.* 1974;61:585–591.
125. Barrios H, Bump CM. Conjuctivitis caused by a nutritionally variant. *Streptococcus. J Clin Microbiol.* 1986;23: 379–380.
126. Carey RB, Gross KC, Roberts RB. Vitamin B_6-dependent *Streptococcus mitior (mitis)* isolated from patients with systemic infections. *J Infect Dis.* 1975;131:722–726.
127. Bignardi GE, Isaacs D. Neonatal meningitis due to *Streptococcus mitis. Rev Infect Dis.* 1989;11:86–88.
128. Catto BA, Jacobs MR, Shlaes DM. *Streptococcus mitis.* A cause of serious infection in adults. *Arch Int Med.* 1987;147:885–888.
129. Roberts RB, Krieger AG, Schiller NL, Gross KC. Viridans streptococcal endocarditis: the role of various species, including pyoridoxal-dependent streptococci. *Rev Infect Dis.* 1979;1:955–965.
130. Ezaki T, Facklam R, Takeuchi N, Yabuuchi E. Genetic relatedness between the type strain of *Streptococcus anginosus* and minute-colony-forming beta-hemolytic streptococci carrying different Lancefield grouping antigens. *J Syst Bacteriol.* 1986;36:345–347.
131. Gossling J. Occurrence and pathogenecity of the *Streptococcus milleri* group. *Rev Infect Dis.* 1988;10:257–275.
132. Lawrence J, Yajko DM, Hadley WK. Incidence and characterization of beta-hemolytic *Streptococcus milleri* and differentiation from *S pyogenes* (group A), *S equisimilis* (group C), and large-colony group G streptococci. *J Clin Microbiol.* 1985;22:772–777.
133. Molina J.-M, Leport C, Bur A, Wolff M, Michon C, Vilde JL. Clinical and bacterial features of infections caused by *Streptococcus milleri. Scand J Infect Dis.* 1991;23:659–666.
134. Ruoff KL. *Streptococcus anginosus* ("*Streptoccus milleri*"): the unrecognized pathogen. *Clin Microbiol Rev.* 1988;1: 102–108.
135. Ruoff KL, Kunzl J, Ferraro MJ. Occurrence of *Streptococcus milleri* among beat-hemolytic streptococci isolated from clinical specimens. *J Clin Microbiol.* 1985;22:149–151.
136. Singh KP, Morris A, Lang SDR, MacCulloch DM, Bremner DA. Clinically significant *Streptococcus anginosus* (*Streptococcus milleri*) infections: a review of 186 cases. *NZ J Med.* 1988;101:813–816.

137. Allison HF, Immelman EJ, Forder AA. Pyogenic liver abscess caused by *Streptococcus milleri*. Case reports. *South Afr Med J.* 1984;65:432–435.
138. Bateman NT, Eykyn SJ, Phillips I. Pyogenic liver abscess caused by *Streptococcus milleri. Lancet.* 1975;1:657–659.
139. Chua D, Reinhart HH, Sobel JD. Liver abscess caused by *Streptococcus milleri. Rev Infect Dis.* 1989;11:197–202.
140. Gelfand MS, Hodgkiss T, Simmons BR. Multiple hepatic abscesses caused by *Streptococcus milleri* in association with an intrauterine device. *Rev Infect Dis.* 1989;11: 983–987.
141. Murray HW, Gross KC, Masur M, Roberts RB. Serious infections caused by *Streptococcus milleri. Am J Med.* 1978;64:759–764.
142. Levandowski RA. *Streptococcus milleri* endocarditis complicated by myocardial abscess. *South Med J.* 1985;78: 892–893.
143. Prichard JG, Lowenstein MH, Silverman IJ, Brennan JC. *Streptococcus milleri* pyometra simulating infective endocarditis. *Obet Gynic.* 1986;68:465–495.
144. Gelfand MS, Bachtian BJ, Simmons BP. Spinal sepsis due to *Streptococcus milleri:* Two cases and review. *Rev Infect Dis.* 1991;13:559–563.
145. Berntesson E, Cullberg G, Trollfors B. Intraabdominal pneumococcal abscess. *Scand J Infect Dis.* 1978;10: 249–250.
146. Bisno AL. Hyposplenism and overwhelming pneumococcal infection: a reappraisal. *Am J Med Sci.* 1971;262: 101.
147. Murray BE. The life and times of the enterococcus. *Clin Microbiol Rev.* 1990;3:46–65.
148. Ruoff KL. Recent taxonomic changes in the genus *Enterococcus. Eur J Clin Microbiol Infect Dis.* 1990;9:75–79.
149. Boulanger JM, Ford-Jones EL, Matlow AG. Enterococcal bacteremias in a pediatric institution: a four year review. *Rev Infect Dis.* 1991;13:847–856.
150. Gullberg RM, Homann SR, Phair JP. Enterococcal bacteremia: an analysis of 75 episodes. *Rev Infect Dis.* 1989;11:74–85.
151. Maki D, Agger WA. Enterococcal bacteremia. Clinical features, the risk of endocarditis, and management. *Medicine.* 1988;67:248–269.
152. Dealler SF, Grace RJ, Norfolk DR. *Enterococcus avium* septicemia in an immunocompromised patient. *Eur J Clin Microbiol Infect Dis.* 1990;9:367–368.
153. Lipman ML, Silva J Jr. Endocarditis due to *Streptococcus faecalis* with high-level resistance to gentamicin. *Rev Infect Dis.* 1989;11:325–328.
154. Rice LB. Calderwood SB, Eliopoulos GM, Farber BF, Karchmer AW. Enterococcal endocarditis: a comparison of prosthetic and native valve disease. *Rev Infect Dis.* 1991;13:1–7.
155. Drake TA, Rodgers GM, Sande MA. Tissue factor is a major stimulus for vegetation formation in enterococcal endocarditis in rabbits. *J Clin Invest.* 1984;73:1750–1753.
156. Gould K, Ramirez-Ronda CH, Holmes RK, Sanford JP. Adherence of bacteria to heart valves in vitro. *J Clin Invest.* 1975;56:1364–1370.
157. Gibbs RS, Listwa HM, Dreskin RB. A pure enterococcal abscess after caesarian section. *J Reprod Med.* 1977;19: 17–20.
158. Morrison AJ, Wenzel RP. Nosocomial urinary tract infections due to enterococcus. Ten years' experience at a university hospital. *Arch Intern Med.* 1986;146:1549–1551.
159. Felmingham D, Wilson APR, Quintana AI, Gruneberg RN. *Enterococcus* species in urinary tract infections. *Clin Infect Dis.* 1992;15:295–301.
160. Ryan JL, Pochner A, Andriole VT, Root RK. Enterococcal meningitis: combined vancomycin and rifampin therapy. *Am J Med.* 1980;68:449–451.
161. Berk SL, Verghese A, Holtsclaw SA, Smith JK. Enterococcal pneumonia. Occurrence in patients receiving broad-spectrum antibiotic regimens and enteral feeding. *Am J Med.* 1983;74:153–154.
162. Thomas CT, Berk SL, Thomas E. Enterococcal liver abscess associated with moxalactam therapy. *Arch Intern Med.* 1983;143:1780–1781.
163. Schliefer KM, Kilpper-Bälz R: Transfer of *Streptococcus faecalis* and *Streptococcus faecaium* to the genus *Enterococcus* nom. rev. as *Enterococcus faecalis* comb. nov. and *Enterococcus faecium* comb. nov. *Int J Syst Bacteriol.* 1984;34:31–34.
164. Eliopoulos GM, Eliopoulos CT. Therapy of enterococcal infections. *Eur J Clin Microbiol Infect Dis.* 1990;9: 118–126.
165. Lewis CM, Zervos MJ. Clinical manifestations of enterococcal infection. *Eur J Clin Microbiol Infect Dis.* 1990;9: 111–117.
166. Johnston RB Jr. Pathogenesis of pneumococcal pneumonia. *Rev Infect Dis.* 1991;13(suppl 6):509–517.
167. Wispelwey B, Tunkel AR, Scheld WM. Bacterial meningitis in adults. *Infect Dis Clin North Am.* 1990;4:645–659.
168. Austrian R, Howie VM, Ploussard J. The bacteriology of pneumococcal otitis media. *Johns Hopkins Med J.* 1977; 141:104–111.
169. Johnston RB. The host response to invasion by *Streptococcus pneumoniae:* Protection and the pathogenesis of tissue drainage. *Rev Infect Dis.* 1981;3:282–288.
170. Tomasz A. Surface components of *Streptococcus pneumoniae.* Rev Infect Dis. 1981;3:190–211.
171. Klugman KP, Koornhof HJ. Drug resistance patterns and serogroups or serotypes of pneumococcal isolates from cerbrospinal fluid or blood, 1979–1986. *J Infect Dis.* 1988;5:956–964.
172. Broome CV, Facklam RR. Epidemiology of clinically significant isolates of *Streptococcus pneumoniae* in the United States. *Rev Infect Dis.* 1981;3:277–280.
173. Klein JO. The epidemiology of pneumococcal disease in infants and children. *Rev Infect Dis.* 1981;3:246–253.
174. Varkey B, Rose HD, Kesavan K, Politis J. Empyema thoracis during a ten-year period. Analysis of 72 cases and comparison to a previous study (1952–1967). *Arch Intern Med.* 1981;141:1771–1776.
175. Hendley JO, Sande MA, Stewart PM, Gwaltney JM, Jr. Spread of *Streptococcus pneumoniae* in families. I. Carriage rates and distribution of types. *J Infect Dis.* 1975;132:55–61.

176. Musher DM. Infections caused by *Streptococcus pneumoniae:* clinical spectrum, pathogenesis, immunity, and treatment. *Clin Infect Dis.* 1992;14:801–807.
177. Khilanani U, Khabib R. Acute epiglotitis in adults. *Am J Med Sci.* 1984;287(1):65–70.
178. Conn HO, Fessel JM. Spontaneous bacterial peritonitis in cirrhosis: variations on a theme. *Medicine.* 1971;50:161.
179. Robinson EN Jr. Pneumonococal endometritis and neonatal sepsis. *Rev Infect Dis.* 1990;12:799–801.
180. Raha VG, Ben-David L, Persitz E. Post menopausal pneumococcal tubo-ovarian abscess. *Rev Infect Dis.* 1991;13: 896–897.
181. Bosley GS, Wallace PL, Moss CW, et al. Phenotypic characterization, cellular fatty acid composition and DNA relatedness of Aerococci and comparison to related genera. *J Clin Microbiol.* 1990:28:416–422.
182. Buu-Hoi A, Branger C, Acar JF. Vancomycin-resistance streptococci or *Leuconostoc* sp. *Antimicrob Agents Chemother.* 1985;28:458–460.
183. Coovadia YM, Solwa Z, van den Ende J. Meningitis caused by vancomycin-resistant *Leuconostoc* sp. *J Clin Microbiol.* 1987;25:1784–1785.
184. Friedland IR, Snipelisky M, Khoosa IM. Meningitis in a neonate caused by *Leuconostoc* sp. *J Clin Microbiol.* 1990;28:2125–2126.
185. Handwerger S, Horowitz H, Coburn K. Kolokathis A, Wormser GP. Infection due to *Leuconostoc* species: six cases and review. *Rev Infect Dis.* 1990;12:602–610.
186. Hardie S, Ruoff KL, Catlin EA. Santos JI. Catheter-associated infection with a vancomycin-resistant gram-positive coccus of the *Leuconostoc* sp. *Pediatr Infect Dis.* 1988;7:519–520.
187. Horowitz HW, Handwerger S, Van Horn KG, Wormser GP. *Leuconostoc,* an emerging vancomycin-resistant pathogen. *Lancet.* 1987;2:1329–1330.
188. Rubin LG, Vellozzi E, Shapiro J, Isenberg HD. Infection with vancomycin-resistant "streptococci" due to *Leuconostoc* species. *J Infect Dis.* 1988;157:216.
189. Wenocur HS, Smith MA, Vellozzi EM, Shapiro J, Isenberg HD. Odontogenic infection secondary to *Leuconostoc* species. *J Clin Microbiol.* 1988;26:1893–1894.
190. Golledge CL, Stringemore N, Aravena M, Joske D. Septicemia caused by vancomycin-resistant *Pedicoccus acidilactici. J Clin Microbiol.* 1990;28:1678–1679.
191. Mastro TD, Spike JS, Lozano P, Appel J, Facklam RR. Vancomycin-resistant *Pediococcus acidilactici:* nine cases of bacteremia. *J Infect Dis.* 1990;161:956–960.
192. Pien FD, Thompson RL, Martin WJ. Clinical and bacteriologic studies of anaerobic gram-positive cocci. *Mayo Clin Proc.* 1972;47:251–257.

CHAPTER 89

Syphilis

Steven E. Kolker, Herbert J. Manz, and David A. Schwartz

He first wore buboes dreadful to the sight
Felt strange pains, and sleepless passed the night.
From him the malady received its name
The neighbouring shepherds catch'd the spreading flame.

Fracastorius, 1530

Syphilitic lesions widespread
From the skin to aorta and head
With endarteritis
Leutic orchitis
Then paresis tabes to dread.

Leslie H. Sobin (1934–) A Pathology Primer in Verse, 2nd ed., Nomad Press, Washington, DC, 1991.

CLASSIFICATION

Syphilis is caused by the spirochete, *Treponema pallidum* sp *pallidum* and is one of four pathogenic treponemes in the order Spirochetales. Other pathogenic treponemes include *T pallidum* sp *pertenue* (yaws), *T pallidum* sp *endemicum* (endemic syphilis or bejel), and *T carateum* (pinta) (see chapter 97). These pathogenic treponemes are morphologically, genomically, and antigenically similar, but they produce distinct diseases. Within the same group are the nonpathogenic commensal treponemes, which live in the mouth and gastrointestinal tract. These latter spirochetes are morphologically similar to the pathogenic types, but lack the genomic and antigenic homology.

A sexually transmitted disease of chronic and indolent nature, syphilis's rich history spans the last five centuries, occupying many volumes, and challenging the minds of some of the world's greatest scientific thinkers. Syphilis can affect almost any organ, and produce a variety of cutaneous and systemic manifestations. Syphilis progresses through three clinical stages, interrupted by a latent period lasting many years. Syphilis may mimic many other diseases, giving it the distinction as the "great imitator." Sir William Osler expanded on this motif by his declaration, "Know syphilis in all its manifestations and relations, and all great things clinical will be added unto you."

EPIDEMIOLOGY

Syphilis, also known as venereal lues, is a worldwide disease that before the 1940s was a major cause of morbidity and mortality. The advent of penicillin reduced the number of infections in the United States and Europe, but, despite the predictions of syphilologists, failed to eradicate the disease. During the 1980s the number of new infections rose dramatically in the United States, but in the 1990s, the rate has so far remained stable. Approximately 130,000 new infections are reported each year to the Centers for Disease Control and Prevention, but the actual incidence is believed to be much higher. The most common group affected in the United States is the young, urban, black, heterosexual.[1]

HISTORY

The origin of syphilis has spawned a centuries-old, unresolved debate about whether the illness is a New World disease taken to Europe by Christopher Columbus's crew or an isolated Old World disease that simply flourished in the face of war.[2] Variably known as *morbus gallicus* (the French disease), the buboes, and the "great pox," the first European pandemic of syphilis was a severe, subacute illness that killed an estimated 25% of those infected.[3] Over the centuries, the virulence of *T pallidum* diminished; death during the early stages of infection is now exceedingly rare. The name of the disease is derived from Fracastorius's 1530 poem about the afflicted shepherd, Syphilis.

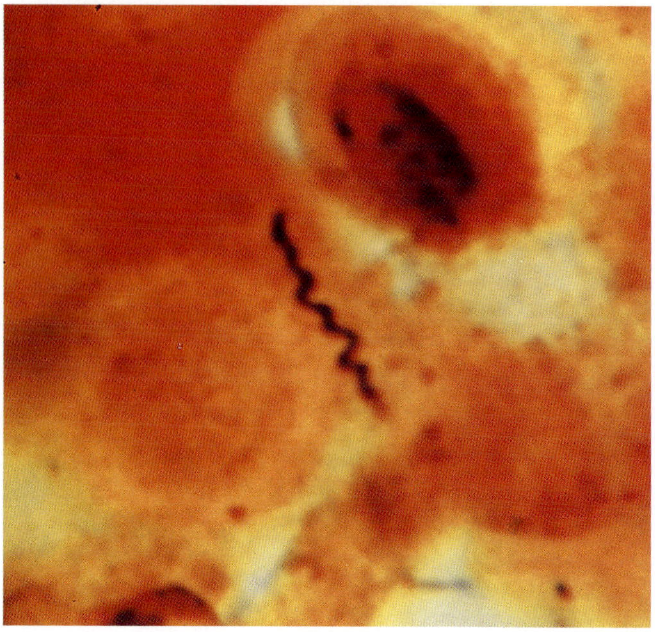

Figure 89–1. *Treponema pallidum* in skin showing the tight regular coils (Warthin–Starry, ×1500).

LIFE CYCLE

Humans are the only natural reservoir of *T pallidum*. Outside the body, the organism is extremely labile and quickly killed by disinfectants, soaps, heating, and drying. Transmission is most common by direct sexual contact when an infected partner has active primary or secondary syphilis. Transplacental infection causes congenital syphilis. Rarer modes of transmission include transfusion of contaminated blood and nonsexual contact with an infectious lesion.

MORPHOLOGY OF THE SPIROCHETE AND PATHOGENESIS OF LESIONS

Treponema pallidum is a thinly coiled, double-membraned, 6- to 15-μm-long, 0.1- to 0.2-μm-wide, motile bacterium (Figure 89–1), which penetrates mucous membranes and abraded skin. Once inside the host, and long before the primary lesion appears, the spirochetes spread rapidly through lymph and blood, and invade regional lymph nodes. Humoral and cellular immunologic and inflammatory responses ensue, causing what is thought to be the principal pathogenetic mechanism of disease.[4,5]

During the primary stage, or shortly after, the host develops resistance to new infection. Although this establishes protective immunity, it is ineffective against progression of the current infection. Titers of antibody to *T pallidum* rise during the early stages of syphilis. Instead of indicating control of infection, however, these rising titers are associated with increasing clinical manifestations. *Treponema pallidum* is initially resistant to the immune response of the host and this may be caused by a paucity of antigenic integral membrane proteins located on the organism's outer membrane.[6,7] Other authors have ascribed the resistance and persistence of virulent *T pallidum* to surface-associated host proteins, such as fibronectin.[8] While both the humoral and cellular immune systems are activated in syphilis, studies in animal models suggest that T-cell-mediated delayed hypersensitivity and subsequent macrophage clearance of organisms play the more significant role in transiently confining the infection.[9] After several weeks or months, most of the spirochetes are cleared by the immune system. Following effective treatment, protective immunity established during infection is lost, and the host is again susceptible to infection.

While most of the treponemes are cleared late in the secondary stage of disease, a few organisms survive. It is thought that these surviving treponemes represent a subpopulation of *T pallidum* that resists phagocytosis.[10] This surviving group continues to divide during the latent period, gradually provoking the inflammatory changes and scarring that characterize tertiary syphilis.

Treponema pallidum invades small arteries and arterioles via its ability to bind to endothelial cells. This propensity to adhere to endothelial cells is thought to be mediated by the glycoprotein, fibronectin.[11,12] Throughout the course of disease, *T pallidum*'s inherent tendency to invade blood vessel walls is responsible for initiating what is known as a luetic vasculitis. As plasma

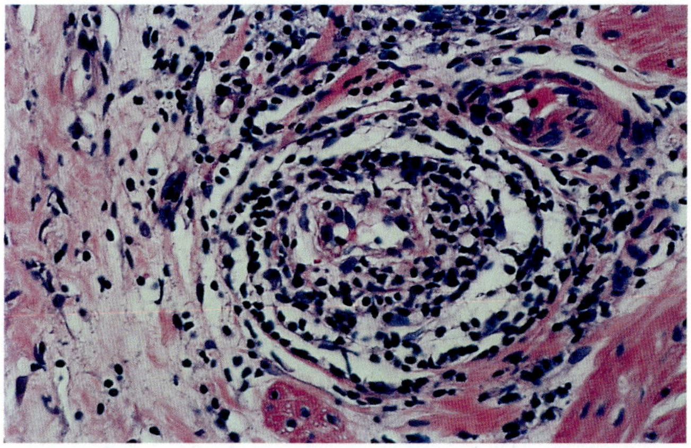

Figure 89–2. Scrotal skin. Dense perivascular mononuclear cellular cuff in and around vessel wall. The lumen is narrowed (hematoxylin-eosin, ×400).

cells and lymphocytes infiltrate the vessel wall, they form an angiocentric pattern of inflammation, often referred to as perivascular cuffing or coat sleeving. Proliferation of fibroblasts causes fibrosis and thickening of the vessel walls (Figure 89–2), while endothelial cells within the lumen hypertrophy and proliferate. This endothelial proliferation causes the lumen of the vessel to become concentrically narrowed in an onion skin pattern. The progressive stenosis causes an obliterative endarteritis, producing ischemic lesions in various organs and tissues.

CLINICAL FEATURES

The primary stage is heralded by the chancre. This usually develops 10 to 90 days (average, 21 days) after the inoculation of *T pallidum* and appears as a solitary, painless ulcer. The chancre is most common on the external genitalia, cervix, anus, or mouth. Following the chancre's appearance, unilateral or bilateral painless regional lymphadenopathy often develops 1 to 2 weeks later (Figure 89–3). The primary lesion heals in 3 to 6 weeks, but the lymphadenopathy may persist for months.

Secondary syphilis usually becomes apparent 2 to 6 weeks after the chancre heals, but may develop while the chancre is still present, or up to 6 months later. Secondary syphilis is the stage of the hematogenous dissemination of *T pallidum* and is characterized by mucocutaneous lesions and constitutional symptoms, including low-grade fever, malaise, anorexia, headache, sore throat, and a generalized, nontender lymphadenopathy. Immune complexes, cytokines, and chemical mediators responding to the spirochetemia are thought to account for these systemic manifestations.[13]

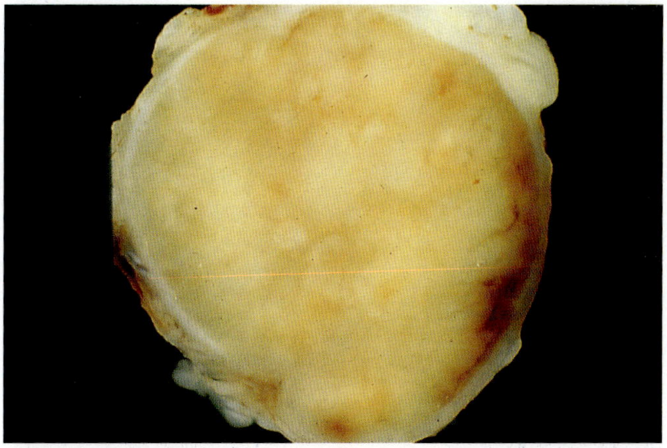

Figure 89–3. Inguinal lymph node excised for diagnosis. In this section, the pale areas are hyperplastic lymphoid tissue. The capsule is thickened (gross photograph, ×2). *(Photograph courtesy of D. H. Connor, MD.)*

Secondary syphilis usually lasts for several weeks, then resolves. Relapses of secondary syphilis may develop, however, in approximately 25% of patients.

Secondary syphilis is followed by a period of latency. This latent stage is characterized by positive syphilis serology in the absence of clinical symptoms. Patients with latent syphilis may remain asymptomatic for life, or their disease may resolve spontaneously (become seronegative), or they may progress to tertiary syphilis.

Following a latent period of 2 to 20 years, 30% of untreated patients will develop clinical features of tertiary syphilis. This stage is characterized by lesions in the central nervous system and cardiovascular system, as well as by the formation of gummas. Gummas are granulomatous lesions that can affect any organ or tissue. As opposed to the earlier self-limited stages of syphilis, tertiary syphilis is progressively destructive and may kill the patient. The advent of penicillin virtually eliminated the tertiary stage, but with the arrival of the acquired immunodeficiency syndrome (AIDS) pandemic and the concomitant increase in syphilis, there has been an upsurge in neurosyphilis.[14]

PATHOLOGY

Primary Syphilis

Primary syphilis begins the moment *T pallidum* enters the body but does not become clinically apparent until the chancre appears at the site of inoculation in 3 to 6 weeks. The classical primary chancre begins as a solitary, circular, reddened papule (Figure 89–4), from a few millimeters to several centimeters, which quickly erodes, forming a shallow ulcer. It is slightly raised,

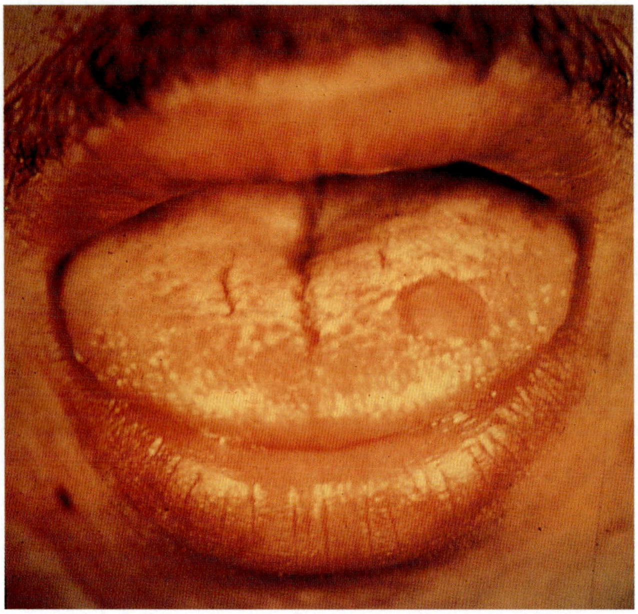

Figure 89–4. Chancre of the tongue at the preulcerative papular stage.

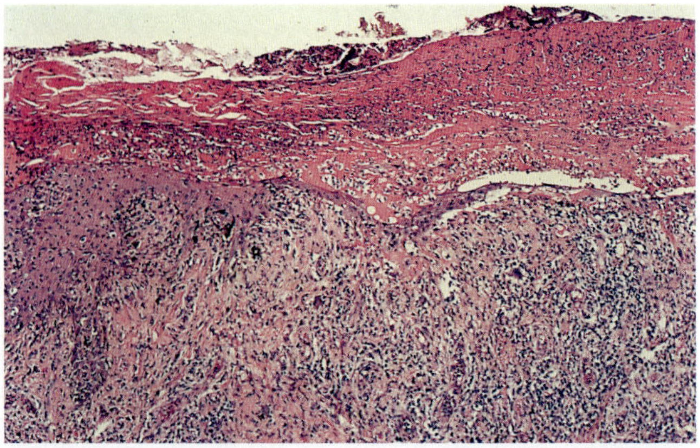

Figure 89–5. Biopsy specimen taken through the margin of a chancre, with intact epithelium on the left, ulceration on the right. There is an intense inflammatory infiltrate in the ulcer bed (hematoxylin-eosin, ×100).

with sharp, firm, cartilaginous-like edges, and a smooth, red, indurated base. A gray-yellow slough or a hemorrhagic crust often covers the surface of the lesion. Squeezing the chancre produces a thin serous discharge that teems with spirochetes, as seen by darkfield microscopy.

Although this is the description of the classical chancre, there are many variations. Multiple lesions and "atypical morphology" are common.[4,15] Chancres in women and those in extragenital sites lack the cartilaginous firmness, but instead are characterized by an edematous induration.[16]

In a typical biopsy specimen, the surface of the ulcer is covered with fibrin and necrotic debris. The bordering epidermis is acanthotic, and except for the center of the lesion, which is completely eroded, is hyperplastic. Jagged projections of squamous epithelium protrude into the dermis. Within the dermis there is an inflammatory infiltrate composed mostly of lymphocytes and plasma cells; a few histiocytes and macrophages are also present. The inflammation is dense and extensive in the center, while near the periphery it is reduced and confined to the perivascular zones (Figure 89–5). Edema is significant. The endothelium lining the arterioles is swollen and proliferative, and there is marked neovascularization. Spirochetes cannot be seen in the chancre by standard hematoxylin-eosin staining, but are seen clearly by electron microscopy, silver impregnation, immunohistochemistry, and immunofluorescence. Spirochetes are mostly concentrated in the exudative fluid around the blood vessels, but are also in and around endothelial cells, leukocytes, and epidermal cells.[1]

Traumatic ulcers, chancroid ulcers, and herpes simplex lesions are the most common genital ulcers that must be distinguished from the primary lesion.[15]

Secondary Syphilis

The disseminated lesions of secondary syphilis vary in severity, number, and appearance. They may present as a skin rash, as erosions of mucous membranes (mucous patches), or as flat wart-like growths known as condylomata lata. These lesions, especially the moist ones, are extremely contagious.

Although a wide variety of cutaneous lesions have been described, the most common types are the macular, maculopapular, papular, and annulopapular eruptions.[17] The first cutaneous lesion to appear is the macular rash. This is comprised of circular, 1- to 2-cm rose-colored lesions that are located at first on the torso and proximal surfaces of upper limbs. The rash then spreads to other regions, including palms and soles, but avoids the face. The macular eruptions may then evolve into maculopapules or papules. These are reddish-brown circular lesions that are often on the face and the genitalia. They may be also on palms and soles, where they are frequently surrounded by a thin collar of white scale (the "collarette of Biette")[17] (Figure 89–6). Sometimes the papules form oval or ringlike patterns called annular syphilids. These predominate in black people and have a predilection for the face. Their shape and size resemble coins, and are often referred to as "nickel and dime" lesions (Figure 89–7).

Histologically, the cutaneous lesions are variable, but most commonly there is a vasculitic process. Characteristics of these lesions include a vascular and peri-

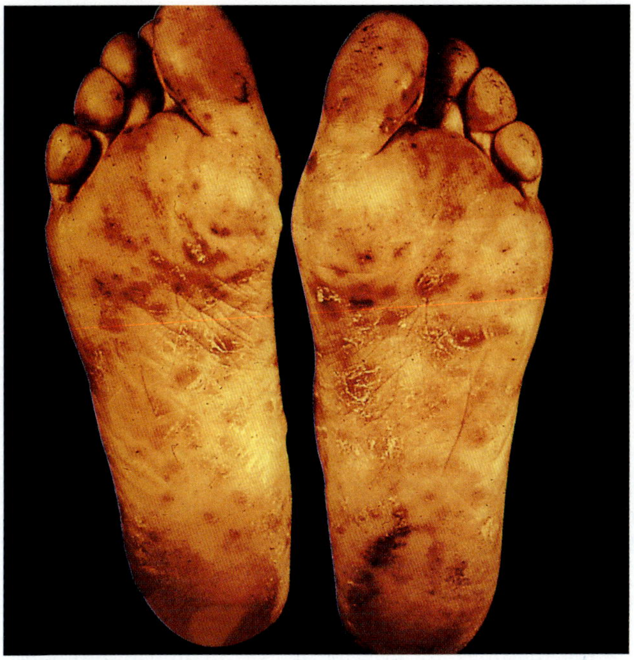

Figure 89–6. Secondary syphilis. Multiple red papules with surrounding white scale on soles.

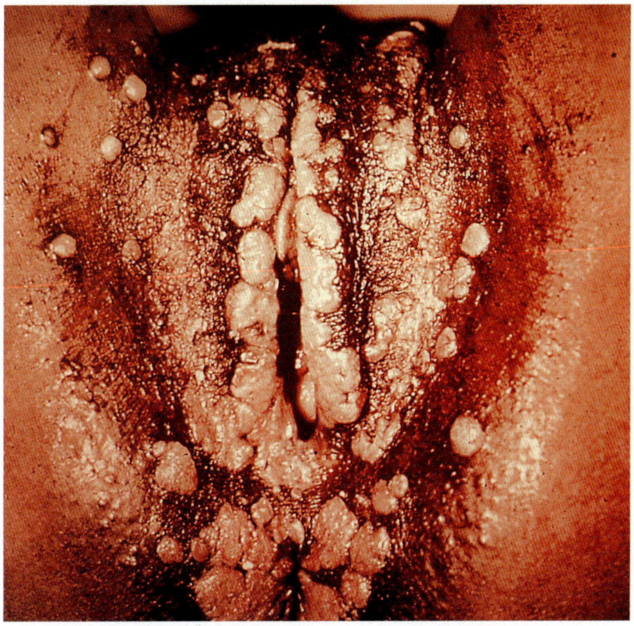

Figure 89–8. Condylomata lata on vulva, perineum, and anus demonstrating smooth and papillary features.

vascular lymphoplasmacytic infiltrate, thickened and fibrosed blood vessels, swollen and proliferating endothelial cells, and epidermal hyperplasia.[18]

Mucosal ulcers ("mucous patches") may affect mucous membranes of the mouth, esophagus, anorectal region (Figure 89–8), pharynx, larynx, and genitals.

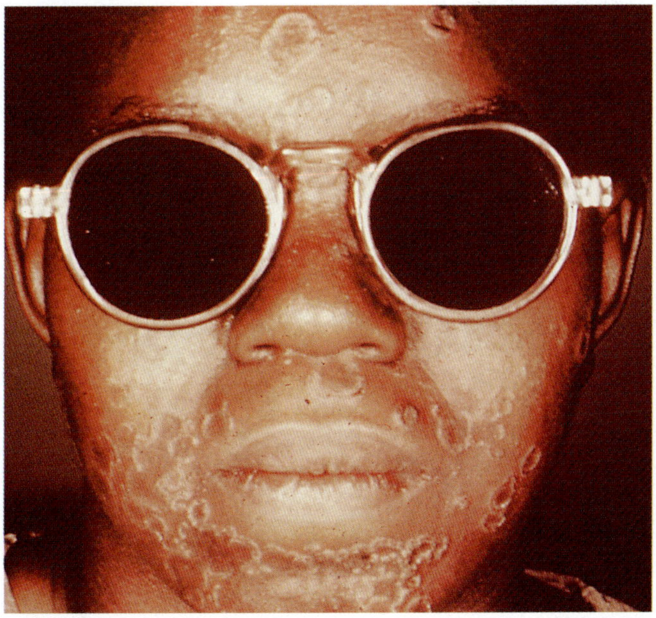

Figure 89–7. Annular, "nickel and dime" lesions of secondary syphilis.

These lesions are typically round and either flat or slightly raised. They are covered by a grayish white slough, and bordered by a dull, red ring. The mucous ulcers also may appear as thin, serpiginous lesions, known as "snail tracks." These are silvery, with an erythematous border. Histologically, the mucosal ulcers resemble the other cutaneous lesions.

Within the intertriginous zones of the body, flesh-colored or hypopigmented oozing papules may become confluent, forming broad-based, 2- to 3-cm-long, flattened lesions. These lesions, known as condylomata lata, are usually multiple and are most common on the perineum. Their surfaces are smooth, papillary, or cauliflower-like.[16] The epidermis is acanthotic and hyperplastic, with elongation and broadening of rete ridges (Figure 89–9). Vascular and perivascular inflammation is present, as are numerous spirochetes. In contrast to the cutaneous and mucous lesions, which heal in weeks, condylomata lata often persist for months.

The variety of lesions in secondary syphilis creates a large differential diagnosis. Cutaneous lesions may be confused with measles, pityriasis rosea, lichen planus, psoriasis, and erythema multiforme; mucous patches may resemble aphthous ulcers; condylomata lata may be confused with hemorrhoids or virally induced condylomata accuminata.[19]

In addition, the lymph nodes of early syphilis are enlarged, discrete, firm, and movable. Histologically, there are a variety of changes, including fibrous thickening of the capsule, follicular hyperplasia,

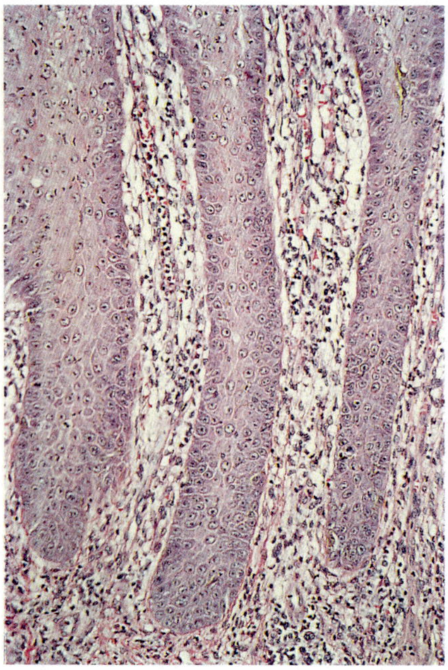

Figure 89–9. Secondary syphilis. Elongated, rounded rete ridges of condyloma latum (hematoxylin-eosin, ×45).

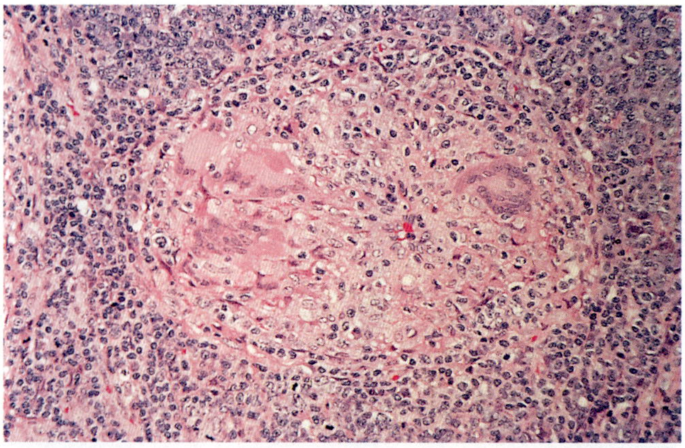

Figure 89–10. Lymph node in the late secondary stage of syphilis, with a discrete granuloma containing Langhans' giant cells, macrophages, lymphocytes, and plasma cells. Spirochetes were few (hematoxylin-eosin, ×125).

reticuloendothelial proliferation, and numerous invading spirochetes, most commonly in the walls of the vessels. A plasmacytosis is present and this contributes to the characteristic syphilitic vasculopathy. Later, the lymph nodes may also contain small noncaseating granulomatous foci (Figure 89–10).[20]

The gastrointestinal tract, particularly stomach, may also be involved in secondary syphilis. *Treponema pallidum* may infect any region of the stomach, but the antrum is almost universally affected. The organism initiates a syphilitic gastritis, characterized during the early stages by superficial erosions or ulcers, and a preponderant plasma cell infiltrate. Necrosis is also evident. Grossly, syphilitic gastritis may appear as a mass, as nodules, or simply as rugal hypertrophy. In later phases of gastric infection, a linitis plastica appearance is produced, which may radiographically and endoscopically mimic malignancy.[21,22] There is an intense mucosal and submucosal infiltrate of plasma cells, as well as a proliferative endarteriolitis (Figure 89–11). Plasma cells are occasionally arranged in a vasocentric pattern. Silver staining with Steiner or Dieterle methods usually reveals numerous spirochetes.

The liver may be involved in all stages of syphilis. During the secondary stage, syphilitic hepatitis occurs in 10% of patients, often accompanied by jaundice, tender hepatomegaly, and an elevated alkaline phosphatase. The histologic findings of syphilitic hepatitis are variable and nonspecific. They include focal hepatocellular necrosis, Kupffer's cell hyperplasia, and a granulomatous, mononuclear, or acute inflammatory cell infiltrate. This inflammation is concentrated in the portal and parenchymal areas (Figure 89–12). Syphilis seldom causes cholestasis, but in some patients there is pericholangitis with edema surrounding the bile ductules. Identifying the spirochetes in the liver may be difficult or impossible.[23]

Tertiary Syphilis

Cardiovascular syphilis, neurosyphilis, and benign tertiary syphilis (gumma) are the three categories of tertiary syphilis.

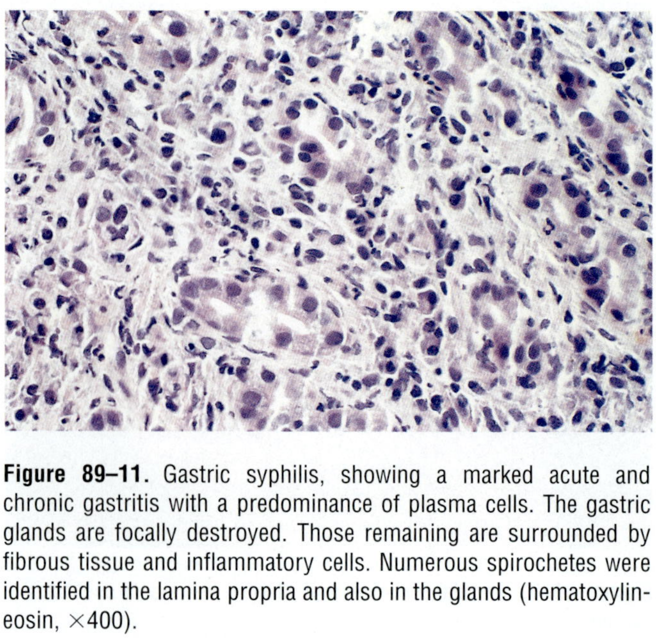

Figure 89–11. Gastric syphilis, showing a marked acute and chronic gastritis with a predominance of plasma cells. The gastric glands are focally destroyed. Those remaining are surrounded by fibrous tissue and inflammatory cells. Numerous spirochetes were identified in the lamina propria and also in the glands (hematoxylin-eosin, ×400).

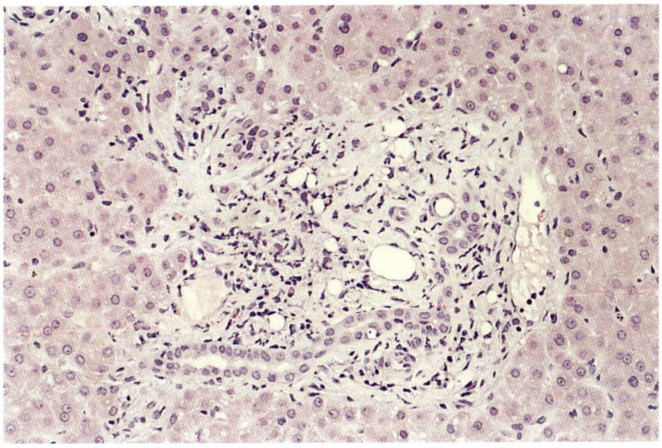

Figure 89–12. Hepatitis from a patient with secondary syphilis. There is an inflammatory cell infiltrate in the portal tract (hematoxylin-eosin, ×200).

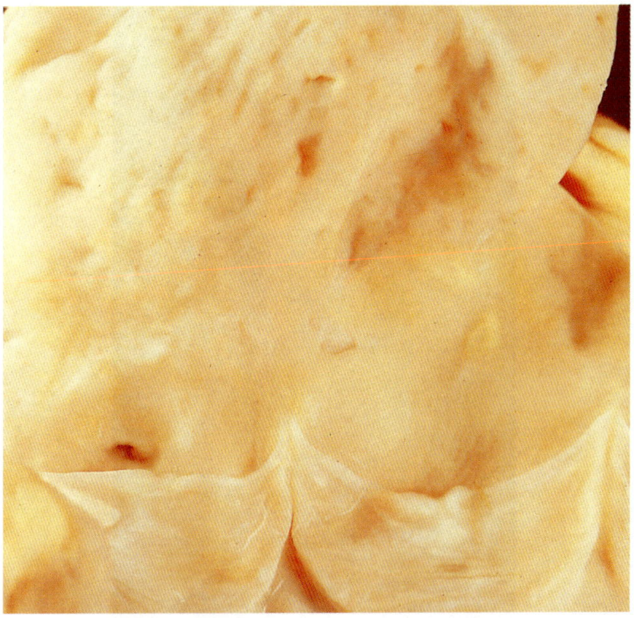

Figure 89–13. Cardiovascular syphilis. Tree bark appearance of ascending aorta with pitting. The roughened intima is a consequence of ischemic necrosis and fibrous scarring of the media.

Cardiovascular Syphilis

Cardiovascular syphilis is an inflammation of the aortic wall that becomes clinically recognizable 20 to 40 years after infection. *Treponema pallidum* is rarely isolated from these lesions, but the obliterative endarteritic changes may cause aortic aneurysm, aortic valvular incompetence, and stenosis of the ostia of the coronary arteries.

The changes in the wall of the aorta begin shortly after resolution of the secondary stage when *T pallidum* invades the vasa vasorum of the aortic wall and provokes an inflammatory response. This reaction occurs most commonly in the ascending and transverse arch of the aortic wall, a tendency that is probably related to the rich supply of blood vessels and lymphatics in this area (Figure 89–13). Within the adventitia of the aortic wall, an infiltrate composed mostly of lymphocytes and plasma cells induces a periarteritis and endarteritis of the vasa vasorum. The intimal cells within the vasa vasorum proliferate, progressively narrow and eventually obliterate the lumen. The resulting ischemia produces patchy necrosis of the media, as well as thickening and fibrosis of the adventitia. The delicate weave of collagen, elastica, and smooth muscle that gives the aorta its strength and elasticity is gradually replaced by inelastic, weak scar. Furthermore, scarring of the media induces reactive proliferation of the myointimal and endothelial cells; the intima appears stretched and longitudinally wrinkled, a pattern characteristically known as "tree barking" of the aorta. The intima is also lined with pits and radial scars. Overall, these intimal changes are often obscured by an accelerated deposition of atherosclerotic plaque.

Continued weakening and stretching of the aortic wall lead to a variety of clinical complications. The most common is aneurysm, mostly of the saccular type, which may eventually rupture, causing exsanguination. Furthermore, stretching of the ascending aorta may cause dilatation of the aortic valve ring, widening of the commissures, and aortic valvular incompetence. The valve cusps are thickened, fibrotic, shortened, and often have rolled edges. Lastly, intimal proliferation and overlying atherosclerosis may obstruct one or both coronary ostia, producing angina-like symptoms.

Cardiovascular syphilis may be treated surgically; for instance, a syphilitic aortic aneurysm may be replaced with a synthetic graft (Figure 89–14).

Benign Tertiary Syphilis (The Gumma)

Granulomas, known as gummas, characterize the benign tertiary stage of syphilis. These lesions are rare today, but were once common in patients with untreated syphilis. The gumma is not as benign as its name implies and may cause significant tissue and organ damage. Involvement of heart and brain have even caused death. The formation of the gumma is based on a delayed type of hypersensitivity to a scant number of treponemes. This reaction is slowly progressive, usually becoming evident 3 to 7 years after the secondary stage resolves. The lesions may affect almost any organ or tissue of the body, but the skin, bones, and subcutaneous tissues are the most common sites.[4] The gummas appear as nodules, which vary from microscopic to several centimeters in diameter. Histologically, they are solitary foci of necrotic tissue surrounded by epithelioid cells and occasional giant cells.

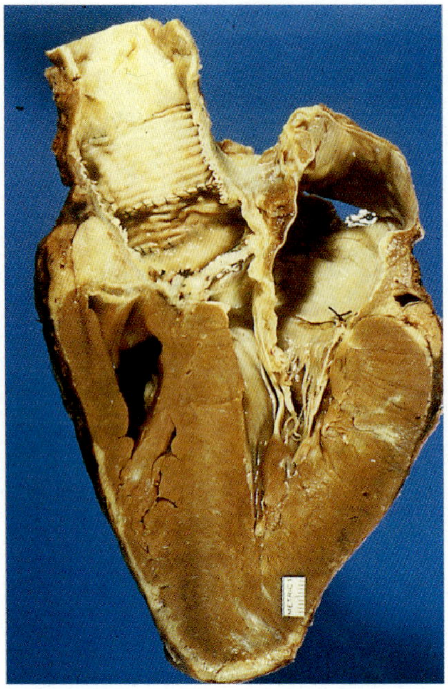

Figure 89–14. Axially sectioned heart. Dacron graft in aortic root was the surgical treatment for a syphilitic aneurysm.

The lesions are further surrounded by a lymphoplasmacytic infiltrate, and encased by a dense layer of fibrous scar. Although *T pallidum* initiates the gumma, a prolonged search is required to find spirochetes in the lesion.

Gummas form different patterns in different tissues. In skin, they resemble a punched-out ulcer, with sharp, hyperpigmented borders and a caseating center. In the liver, gummas may be single or multiple, healing by a distinctive, multilobulated form of scarring, called hepar lobatum.

Neurosyphilis

The first evidence of central nervous system (CNS) syphilis is pleocytosis and elevated protein in the cerebrospinal fluid (CFS). The diagnosis is confirmed by positive serology of the CSF. CNS syphilis occurs early, and is initially asymptomatic. These changes are demonstrable in approximately 12% of patients in the primary stage and 30% during the secondary stage.[24] When the CNS changes persist beyond early syphilis, late manifestations may develop. These late lesions have been classified as meningovascular and parenchymatous; the latter includes general paralysis of the insane (GPI) and tabes dorsalis.

Meningovascular Syphilis

The meningeal and vascular changes of meningovascular syphilis usually begin during the secondary stage, but progression is so slow that symptoms do not appear until 5 to 12 years later. The reaction that ensues involves a plasma cell and lymphocytic vasculitis of the arterioles and arteries of the brain. Within the larger vessels, the vasa vasorum also are involved. This vasculitis causes an obliterative endarteritis (Heubner's endarteritis) of the cerebral vasculature, which becomes narrowed and eventually occluded. The ischemia of the media causes necrosis, fibrosis, and eventually scarring. This scarring induces fibrous proliferation of the intima, which concentrically narrows the lumen of the artery. At the same time endothelial cells proliferate, eventually narrowing the lumen, sometimes to the point of causing thrombosis. This subsequently leads to infarction, gliosis, and cavitation of brain tissue. In addition, the meninges, particularly the dura and pia-arachnoid at the base of the brain, are affected by the inflammatory reaction. They are thickened and fibrosed, often with a cloudy exudate, and are infiltrated with lymphocytes and plasma cells (Figure 89–15). The thickened meninges at the base of the brain may obstruct the flow of CSF and cause hydrocephalus, or may irritate or compromise nerves, producing cranial nerve palsies.

Parenchymatous Syphilis

Parenchymatous syphilis is the last of the neurosyphilitic syndromes. As opposed to meningovascular syphilis, which largely causes its damage by an ischemic vasculitis and fibrosing meningitis, general paralysis of the insane and tabes dorsalis are unique in that the pathogenesis of the disease is based on progressive neuronal and axonal destruction.[25,26] Furthermore, GPI is distinguished from other forms of tertiary syphilis by the fact that spirochetes are abundant within the lesions.

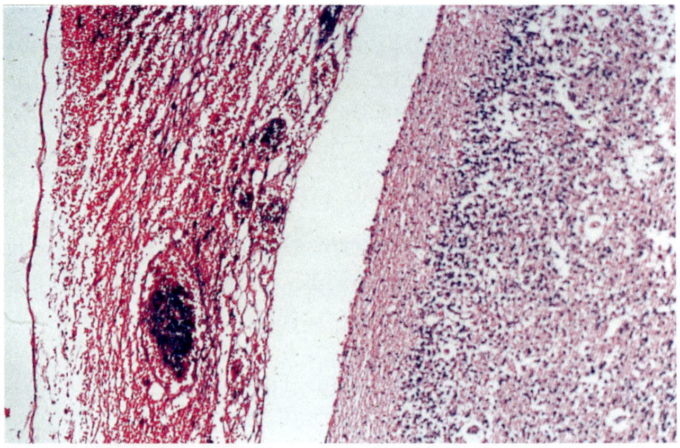

Figure 89–15. Cerebellum and subarachnoid space of infant with congenital syphilis. There is severe fibrosis of the subarachnoid space (luxol-fast blue–nematoxylin-eosin, ×100).

General Paralysis of the Insane

General paralysis of the insane (paretic dementia, general paresis) is a chronic, progressive, syphilitic meningoencephalitis that commonly appears 10 to 20 years after infection. Once a common cause of psychiatric admissions, it is now rare. Grossly, the brains of patients with GPI are atrophied, with dilated ventricles, a granular ependymitis, and a thickened, opaque, meningeal layer. The cortical atrophy is diffuse, but is most pronounced in the frontal and temporal lobes. Microscopically, the meninges and cortex are inflamed, with the infiltrate composed mostly of lymphocytes and plasma cells. The infiltrate is diffuse in the meninges, but limited to perivascular cuffs within the cortex. Within the cortex, there is severe neuronal degeneration, with loss of neurons and gliosis. There are abundant microglial cells, which are elongated and hypertrophied (rod cells). Astrocytes are also increased in number, and appear as transependymal tufts giving the ependyma a fine granular surface (granular ependymitis). *Treponema pallidum* may be located in the subcortical gray matter in about 50% of brains of patients with GPI.[27]

Tabes Dorsalis

Tabes dorsalis ("wasting") is caused by progressive inflammation and destruction of the lumbosacral posterior nerve roots, which produce secondary degeneration and atrophy (ascending Wallerian degeneration) of the posterior columns. This usually affects patients 15 to 20 years after infection. Grossly, the degenerated posterior columns appear flat or even sunken and the leptomeninges around the spinal cord are fibrotic. Microscopically, the axons and myelin of the posterior columns are replaced by astrocytes and their fibers (Figure 89–16). Patients lose proprioception, which becomes evident as a wide-based (tabetic) gait and a positive Romberg sign. They also lose their sense of joint position, manifested as foot slap, leading to the neuropathic destruction of large joints (Charcot's joints).

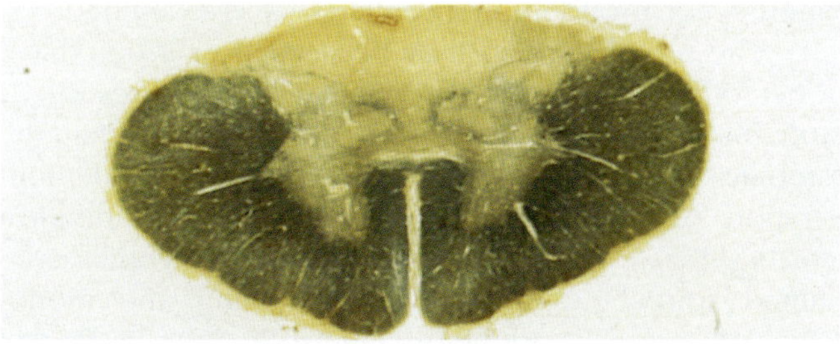

Figure 89–16. Tabes dorsalis. Loss of axons and myelin is evident in the posterior columns of the spinal cord (Woelke stain). *(Courtesy of the late Dr O. Solnitzky, former professor and chairman, Department of Anatomy, Georgetown University.)*

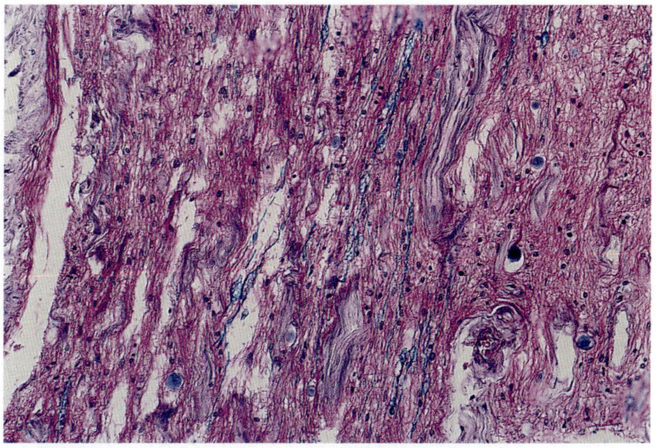

Figure 89–17. Substantial loss of myelinated axons in optic nerve caused by constricting fibrosis of the meningeal sheaths of the optic nerve (LFB–hematoxylin-eosin, ×400).

Other common symptoms include the Argyll Robertson pupil and optic atrophy (Figure 89–17). Rarely, tabes dorsalis and GPI may occur together (taboparesis).

Congenital Syphilis

Treponema pallidum can cross the placental barrier and infect the developing fetus. The incidence of congenital syphilis has been increasing, caused by the rising incidence of syphilis in young women. Although hematogenous transmission of *T pallidum* across the placenta was originally thought to occur only in the second and third trimesters, there are reports of first trimester infection of the fetus, which in one patient was associated with syphilitic endometritis. The likelihood of infection in the fetus is greatest during the early stages of maternal infection, but fetal infection during the latent stages of maternal disease has also occurred. Complications of congenital syphilis include spontaneous abortion, stillbirth, early congenital syphilis, and late congenital syphilis.

In the perinatal period and in infancy, the early manifestations of congenital syphilis often resemble those found in secondary syphilis, but in addition may present with extensive, vesiculobullous, desquamating, cutaneous lesions. Found on the palms, soles, perineum (Figures 89–18 and 89–19), and around the mouth, these lesions weep and teem with spirochetes. Other manifestations of congenital syphilis include osteochondritis and periostitis. These lesions affect the joints, long bones, palate, and the bones and cartilage of the nose. Furthermore, lung involvement may produce a fulminant interstitial fibrosis. The lungs appear pale, heavy, and airless (pneumonia alba). Usually the liver is affected too with diffuse inflammation and isolated nests of hepatocytes that are separated by fibrosis.

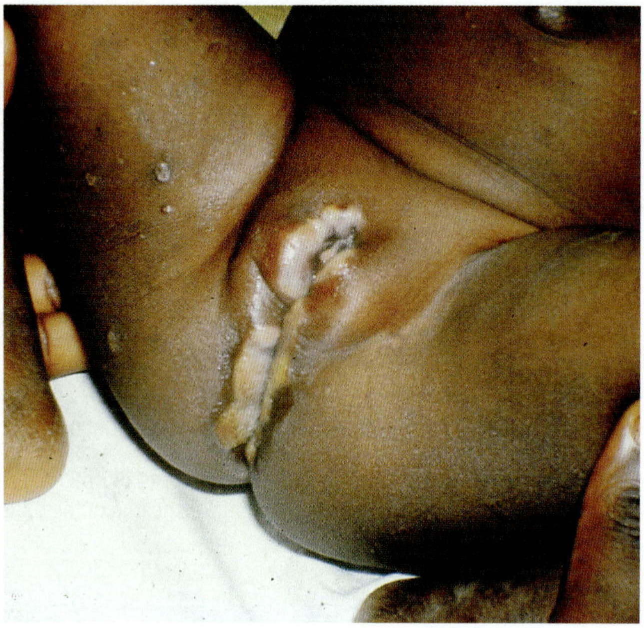

Figure 89–18. Congenital syphilis. Vesiculobullous lesions on vulva and perineum in an 18-month-old Zairian. *(Contributed by Dr Leo O. Lanoie.)*

Ultimately, any organ may be affected by the spirochetemia of congenital syphilis, as the spirochetes infiltrate the tissues and induce a diffuse interstitial inflammatory response.

The late complications of congenital syphilis include an interstitial keratitis, which may cause vascularization and opacification of the cornea; gummas, which may perforate the palate or cause collapse of the bridge of the nose (saddle nose); and a meningovasculitis, which can lead to eighth nerve deafness and optic atrophy. The incisors of children with congenital syphilis may appear short and screwdriver-shaped, a condition called Hutchinson's teeth. Also, periostitis and new bone formation of the tibias result in the characteristic anterior bowing known as "saber shins."

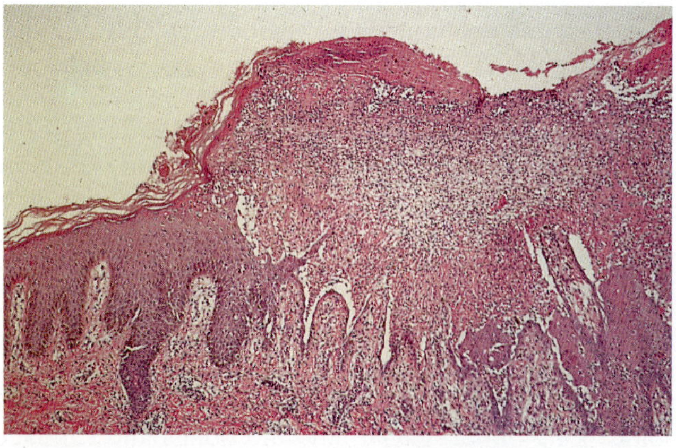

Figure 89–19. Biopsy specimen of vulvar lesion of Figure 89–18. Destruction of epidermis, elongation of rete ridges, and lymphocytes and plasma cells in the dermis are seen. Deeper in the dermis the infiltrate is concentrated around vessels and in vessel walls (hematoxylin-eosin, ×18).

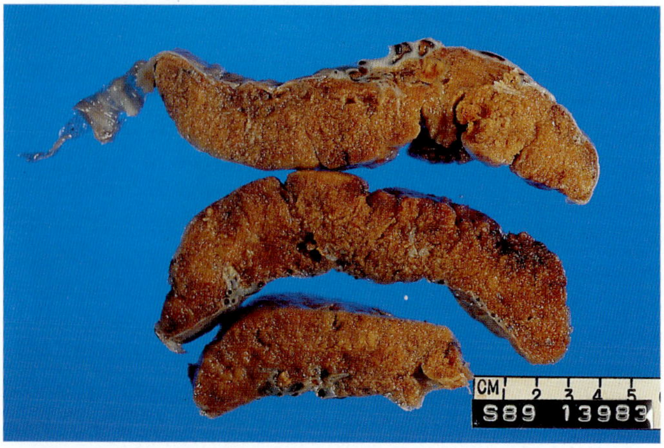

Figure 89–20. Cut surfaces of a syphilitic placenta. Syphilitic placentas are firm and heavy for their gestational ages, but usually are not hydropic.

Examining the placenta of an infant with suspected congenital syphilis may be critical for obtaining an early diagnosis. Grossly, the placenta of the infant born with congenital syphilis is often large, heavy, and bulky for gestational age (Figure 89–20). Microscopically, there is dysmaturity of the chorionic villi, hyperplasia of villous stromal macrophages (termed Hofbauer cells), and, in some placentas, acute or chronic villitis. The vasculature is characterized by perivascular and adventitial fibrosis, and endarteritis, which sometimes obliterates the lumen of the chorionic vessels. Within the fetal vasculature, an increased number of nucleated red blood cells can often be found (Figure 89–21).[28,29] The decidual tissue may be infiltrated by plasma cells, and the placental membranes may either be normal, or they may exhibit a chorioamnionitis, with or without necrosis.[28] Spirochetes can be difficult to demonstrate in chorionic villi, and false-negative diagnostic results will often occur if only the placental body is examined.

The umbilical cord may be normal or it may have a necrotizing, acute, or chronic funisitis (Figures 89–22 and 89–23).[30] Schwartz et al[30] demonstrated that the umbilical cord may be the optimal tissue for demonstration of *T pallidum.* Twenty-two of 25 umbilical cords (88%) from infants with congenital syphilis contained spirochetes—using silver staining and monoclonal fluorescent antibody (Figure 89–24). Twelve of these cords were histologically normal, in spite of the fact that 11 contained spirochetes. Subamnionic collections of spirochetes were in some cords, providing histologic evidence of infection of amniotic fluid.[30,31]

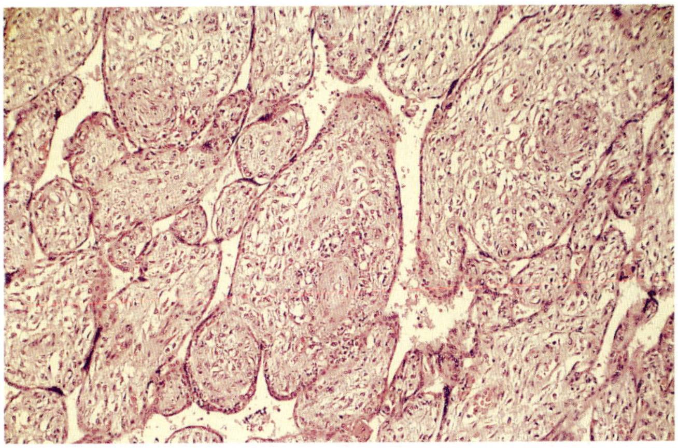

Figure 89–21. Placenta from an infant with congenital syphilis. The chorionic villi are dysmature, hypercellular, and there is erythroblastosis (hematoxylin-eosin, ×100).

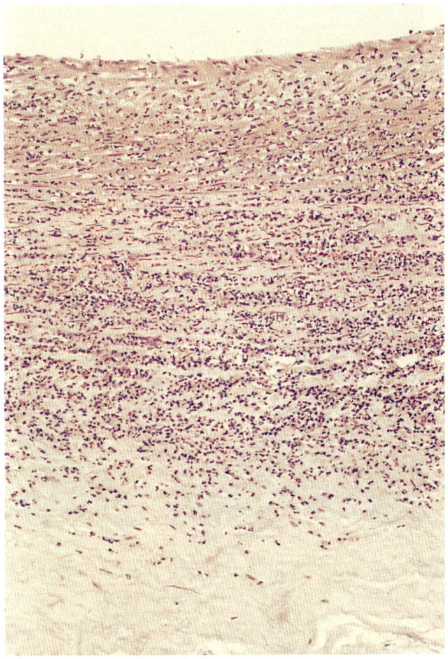

Figure 89–23. Necrotizing funisitis. This lesion is characterized by zones of inflammatory cells, predominantly mononuclear, that infiltrate the umbilical vessels and extend into Wharton's jelly. This lesion is the most common abnormality of the umbilical cord in congenital syphilis and is associated with active destruction of the wall of the umbilical vein. Spirochetes were in this vessel (hematoxylin-eosin, ×100).

The pathologist is often requested to evaluate a stillborn or macerated fetus (Figure 89–25) for the possibility of congenital syphilitic infection. In most specimens, the internal organs have undergone extensive autolytic degeneration, and the characteristic histopathologic features of congenital syphilis (ie, pancreatitis, endocarditis, hepatic fibrosis) are difficult to recognize. The spirochetes, however, usually remain intact within the necrotic tissues, and are most likely to be detected in sections of liver, brain, kidneys, pancreas, and heart.

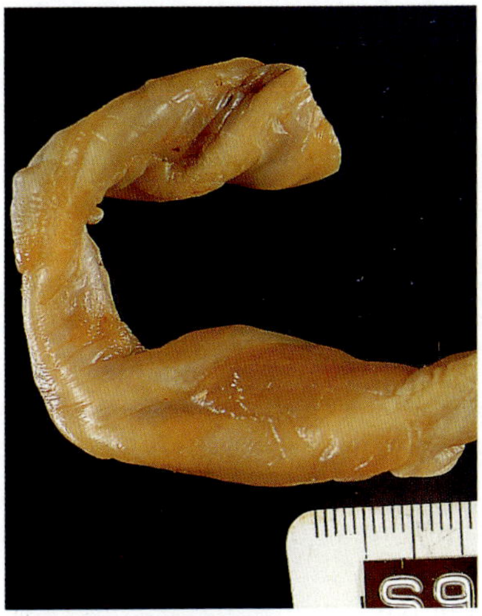

Figure 89–22. The gross features of necrotizing funisitis are recognizable in the delivery room. The cord has a "barber pole" appearance, and the vessels are white or brown, which is caused by sclerosis, necrosis, or calcification.

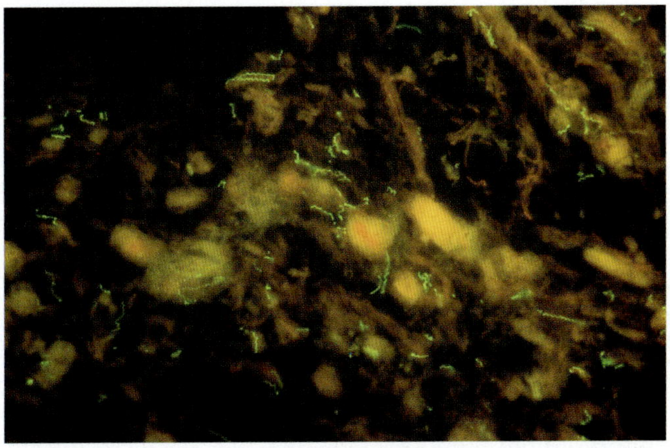

Figure 89–24. Formalin-fixed section of umbilical cord stained with fluorescent antibody to *T pallidum*. The spirochetes are easily visualized (×1000).

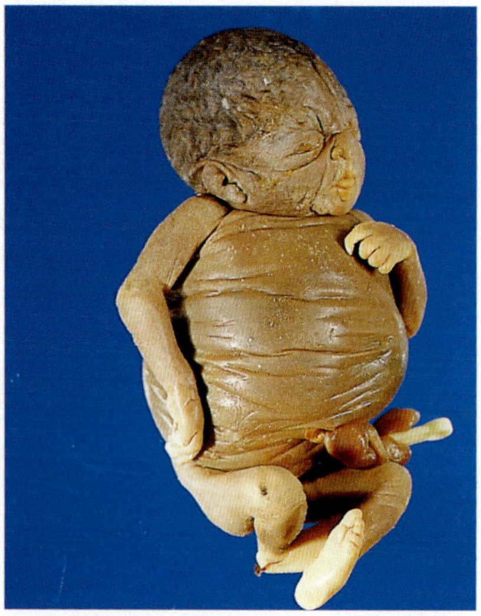

Figure 89–25. Macerated stillborn fetus with congenital syphilis. The fetus is hydropic, and the umbilical stump is swollen and dark red-brown. Spontaneous abortion is frequent in women with untreated active syphilis.

DIAGNOSIS AND SEROLOGY

Treponema pallidum is a microaerophilic organism that cannot be continuously cultured in vitro. It is not visible by Gram stain, but can be visualized by immunofluorescence, immunohistochemistry, silver stains, or darkfield microscopy.

The quickest and most specific method of identifying *T pallidum* is by direct microscopic evaluation using darkfield microscopy or the direct fluorescent antibody test for *T pallidum* (DFA-TP).[32] Serum obtained from primary lesions, secondary lesions, or aspirated lymph nodes may be used to visualize the organism. The DFA-TP uses polyclonal antibodies specific for *T pallidum*. This test is especially advantageous in oral and anal lesions, since it is capable of distinguishing *T pallidum* from commensal spirochetes that reside in these areas.

Serologically, syphilis may be diagnosed by two basic methods. One involves the detection of antibody directed against *T pallidum* (treponemal tests), while the other involves detection of antibodies formed against products of tissue destruction (nontreponemal tests; reagin).[17]

The two most common nontreponemal tests in use today are the RPR (rapid plasma reagin) and VDRL (Venereal Disease Research Laboratory); both are sensitive, but they lack specificity. These tests screen for anticardiolipin antibodies, which are formed during treponemal disease. Antibody titers become positive after the third or fourth weeks of infection, peak during the secondary stage of disease, and decrease afterward. These tests are most sensitive during the secondary stage, but less so during the primary and late stages. The nontreponemal tests may be positive in a variety of other conditions, resulting in biologic false-positives (BFPs). As opposed to the treponemal tests, titers of antibody in nontreponemal tests may be used as a reflection of disease activity or as a screen for cure. The VDRL test may also be used on CSF to diagnose neurosyphilis (provided the lumbar puncture is atraumatic).

The fluorescent treponemal antibody absorption test (FTA-Ab) is currently the most commonly used treponemal test. This test uses fixed *T pallidum* antigen, which is reacted against tested sera and incubated with a fluorescein-labeled human gamma globulin antibody. The FTA-Ab is more sensitive and specific than the RPR or VDRL and becomes positive before any other test. Following a reactive nontreponemal test, the FTA-Ab is typically used for diagnostic confirmation. Even following effective treatment, the FTA-Ab usually remains positive for life. Another treponemal test is the microhemagglutination test for *T pallidum* (MHA-TP or TPHA). This test measures antibodies which agglutinate erythrocytes that are coated with *T pallidum*. The sensitivity and specificity of the TPHA test are comparable to the FTA-Ab during the secondary and late stages of syphilis, but appear to be slightly less sensitive during the primary stage. The 19S IgM FTA-ABS test for syphilis is a recently approved test for the diagnosis of congenital syphilis. During the neonatal period, this test is able to distinguish the antitreponemal IgM produced by the infant from the antitreponemal IgG that has been passively transferred from the mother to the fetus during pregnancy.

Monoclonal antibodies, antigen detection kits using cloned antigens, and PCR (polymerase chain reaction) are other methods that can be used to diagnose syphilis, but these tests are not yet readily available.[4,30]

SYPHILIS AND HUMAN IMMUNODEFICIENCY VIRUS

Studies have shown that syphilis is a risk factor for the contraction of human immunodeficiency virus (HIV).[33,34] These studies suggest that the chancre, with its predominance of lymphocytes, may serve as a portal of entry for HIV and, vice versa, may serve as a source for transmission.[4] In addition, since syphilis depends on cellular immunity to control infection, the defect in cellular immunity caused by HIV infection predisposes patients to a more severe infection and also more frequent late complications.[35]

Patients concomitantly infected with syphilis and HIV are more likely to progress to neurosyphilis.[14,36,37] Several reports suggest that this progression is more rapid, more destructive, and often follows failed penicillin treatment.[14,36–39] The most common manifestations after failed penicillin treatment include meningeal, meningovascular, and ocular syphilis.[40] Ocular syphilis is a unique manifestation of neurosyphilis in HIV patients, and commonly presents as uveitis, papillitis, vitreitis, retinitis, or an optic neuritis.[35] In addition, a particularly florid and aggressive form of neurosyphilis, known as "quaternary" syphilis has been documented. In one patient, this was characterized by a progressive meningitis, with infarction, moya-moya* disease, and a necrotizing encephalitis. Massive numbers of treponemes had infiltrated the brain.[41]

Although a few reports have suggested delayed or absent seroreactivity in patients with syphilis, serologic testing is still a reliable diagnostic indicator of syphilis in patients with HIV.[14,42] In fact, compared with HIV-negative patients, those with HIV infection produce significantly higher nontreponemal antibody titers. In undiluted blood samples, this antibody excess has caused false-negative serologic tests for syphilis, or the so-called prozone phenomenon.[43]

A more difficult problem arises when diagnosing neurosyphilis. First, because the CSF VDRL is not a very sensitive test (only 22% to 69% sensitive)[42,44] and, second, while the presence of pleocytosis and elevated protein in CSF is suggestive of neurosyphilis in non-HIV patients, approximately 40% of HIV-infected patients may have similar CSF profiles even without nervous system infection by *T pallidum*.[45,46]

*Moya-moya disease (Japanese for "puff of smoke," as depicted by cerebral angiography) is caused by a number of different processes. It refers to the compensatory enlargement and proliferation of the lenticulostriate arterioles as a result of stenosis or occlusion of the distal segment of the internal carotid arteries.

REFERENCES

1. Lukehart SA, Holmes KK. Syphilis. In: Isselbacher KJ et al, eds. *Harrison's Principles of Internal Medicine.* 13th ed. New York: McGraw-Hill; 1994;chap 133:726–737.
2. Felman YM. Syphils: from 1495 Naples to 1989 AIDS. *Arch Dermatol.* 1989;125:1698–1699.
3. Sell S, Norris SJ. The biology, pathology and immunology of syphilis. *Int Rev Exp Pathol.* 1983;24:203–276.
4. Hutchinson CM, Hook EW III. Syphilis in adults. *Med Clin North Am.* 1990;74:1389–1416.
5. Lukehart SA. Prospects for development of a treponemal vaccine. *Rev Infect Dis.* 1985;7(suppl 2):S305–S313.
6. Norris SJ and the *Treponema pallidum* Polypeptide Research Group. Polypeptides of *Treponema pallidum:* progress toward understanding their structural, functional, and immunologic roles. *Microbiol Rev.* 1993;57:750–779.
7. Radolf JD, Norgard MV, Schulz WW. Outer membrane ultrastructure explains the limited antigenicity of virulent *Treponema pallidum. Proc Natl Acad Sci USA.* 1989; 86:2051–2055.
8. Alderete JF, Baseman JB. Surface-associated host proteins on virulent *Treponema pallidum. Infect Immun.* 1979; 26:1048–1056.
9. Fitzgerald TJ. The Th1/Th2-like switch in syphilitic infection: is it detrimental? *Infect Immun.* 1992;60:3475–3479.
10. Lukehart SA, Shaffer JM, Baker-Zander SA. A population of *Treponema pallidum* is resistant to phagocytosis: possible mechanism of persistence. *J Infect Dis.* 1992;166: 1449–1453.
11. Thomas DD, Baseman JB, Alderete JF. Enhanced levels of attachment of fibronectin-primed *Treponema pallidum* to extracellular matrix. *Infect Immun.* 1986;52:736–741.
12. Peterson KM, Baseman JB, Alderete JF. *Treponema pallidum* receptor binding proteins interact with fibronectin. *J Exp Med.* 1983;157:1958–1970.
13. Jorizzo JL, McNeely MC, Baughn RE, et al. Role of circulating immune complexes in human secondary syphilis. *J Infect Dis.* 1986;153:1014–1022.
14. Musher DM, Hamill RJ, Baughn RE. Effect of human immunodeficiency virus (HIV) infection on the course of syphilis and on the response to treatment. *Ann Intern Med.* 1990;113:872–881.
15. Chapel TA. The variability of syphilitic chancres. *Sex Trans Dis.* 1978;5:68–70.
16. Sanchez M, Luger FA. Syphilis. In: Fitzpatrick TB et al, eds. *Dermatology in General Medicine.* 4th ed. New York: McGraw-Hill; 1993;chap 218:2703–2743.
17. Crissey JT. Syphilis. In: Parish LC, Gschnait F, eds. *Sexually Transmitted Diseases: A Guide for Clinicians.* New York: Springer. 1988;chap 3:11–31.
18. Jeerapaet P, Ackerman AB. Histologic patterns of secondary syphilis. *Arch Dermatol.* 1973;107:373–377.
19. Mroczkowski TF. Syphilis. In: Mroczkowski TF, ed. *Sexually Transmitted Diseases,* New York: Igaku-Shoin Medical Publishers; 1990;chap 8:164–227.
20. Hartsock RJ, Halling LW, King FM. Luetic lymphadenitis: a clinical and histologic study of 20 cases. *Am J Clin Pathol.* 1970;53:304–314.
21. Greenstein DS, Wilcox CM, Schwartz DA. Gastric syphilis: report of seven cases and review of the literature. *J Clin Gastro.* 1994;18:4–9.
22. Fenoglio-Preiser CM, Lantz PE, Listrom MB, et al. *Gastrointestinal Pathology. An Atlas and Text.* New York: Raven Press; 1989:144.
23. Grases PJ. Bacterial, protozoal, helminthic, and spirochaetal inflammatory diseases. In: Peters RL, Craig JR, eds. *Liver Pathology.* New York: Churchill Livingstone; 1986: 139.
24. Hahn RD, Clark ES. Asymptomatic neurosyphilis: a review of the literature. *Am J Syph Gonor Ven Dis.* 1946;30: 305–316.
25. Hook EW III. Central nervous system syphilis. In: Scheld WM, et al, eds. *Infections of the Central Nervous System.* New York: Raven Press; 1991;chap 27:639–656.
26. Merritt HH, Adams RD, Solomon HC. *Neurosyphilis.* New York: Oxford University Press; 1946.

27. Walton J, ed. *Syphilis of the nervous system.* In: *Brain's Diseases of the Nervous System.* 9th ed. New York: Oxford University Press; 1985;chap 9:263–273.
28. Schwartz DA, Zhang W, Larsen S, et al. Placental pathology of congenital syphilis—immunohistochemical aspects. *Troph Res.* 1994;8:223–229.
29. Benirschke K, Kaufmann P. *Pathology of the Human Placenta.* 2nd ed. Berlin: Springer-Verlag; 1990:575–578.
30. Schwartz DA, Larsen S, Beck-Sague C, et al. Pathology of the umbilical cord in congenital syphilis: analysis of 25 specimens using histochemistry and immunofluorescent antibody to *Treponema pallidum*. *Hum Pathol.* 1995;26: 784–791.
31. Wendel GD, Maberry MC, Christmas JT, et al. Examination of amniotic fluid in diagnosing congenital syphilis with fetal death. *Obstet Gynecol.* 1989;74:967–970.
32. Larsen SA. Syphilis. *Sex Trans Dis.* 1989;9:545–557.
33. Quinn TC, Glasser D, Cannon RO, et al. Human immunodeficiency virus infection among men with sexually transmitted diseases. *N Engl J Med.* 1988;318:197–203.
34. Greenblatt RM, Lukehart SA, Plummer FA, et al. Genital ulceration as a risk factor for human immunodeficiency virus infection. *AIDS.* 1988;2:47–50.
35. Tramont EC. Syphilis in HIV-infected persons. In: Volberding P, Jacobson MA, eds. *AIDS Clinical Review 1993/1994.* New York: Marcel Dekker; 1994;chap 4: 61–72.
36. Johns DR, Tierney M, Felsenstein D. Alteration in the natural history of neurosyphilis by concurrent infection with the human immunodeficiency virus. *N Engl J Med.* 1987;316:1569–1572.
37. Berry CD, Hooton TM, Collier AC, Lukehart SA. Neurologic relapse after benzathine penicillin therapy for secondary syphilis in a patient with HIV infection. *N Engl J Med.* 1987;316:1587–1589.
38. Katz DA, Berger JR. Neurosyphilis in acquired immunodeficiency syndrome. *Arch Neurol.* 1989;46:895–898.
39. Engelkens HJH, van der Sluis JJ, Stolz E. Syphilis in the AIDS era. *Int J Dermatol.* 1991;30:254–256.
40. Hook EW III, Marra CM. Acquired syphilis in adults. *N Engl J Med.* 1992;326:1060–1067.
41. Morgello S, Laufer H. Quaternary neurosyphilis in a Haitian man with human immunodeficiency virus infection. *Hum Pathol.* 1989;20:808–811.
42. Matlow AG, Rachlis AR. Syphilis serology in human immunodeficiency virus-infected patients with symptomatic neurosyphilis: case report and review. *Rev Infect Dis.* 1990;12:703–707.
43. Jurado RL, Campbell J, Martin PD. Prozone phenomenon in secondary syphilis: has its time arrived? *Arch Intern Med.* 1993;153:1496–1498.
44. Hart G. Syphilis tests in diagnostic and therapeutic decision making. *Ann Intern Med.* 1986;104:368–376.
45. Hollander H. Cerebrospinal fluid normalities and abnormalities in individuals infected with human immunodeficiency virus. *J Infect Dis.* 1988;158:855–858.
46. Appleman ME, Marshall DW, Brey RL, et al. Cerebrospinal fluid abnormalities in patients without AIDS who are seropositive for the human immunodeficiency virus. *J Infect Dis.* 1988;158:193–198.

CHAPTER 90

Tropical Phagedenic Ulcer

Kurt F. Heim

One of our Zanzibaris named Mrima, impatient at the slow progress towards recovery from a large and painful ulcer, shot himself with a Remington rifle today. Poor fellow, I remember him as a cheery, willing, and quick boy.[1]

SYNONYMS

Tropical phagedenic ulcer has been referred to as Aden ulcer, Annamite sore, cochin sore, Delagoa sore, Guadeloupe ulcer, Guiana ulcer, *kidonda ndugu* (Swahili), Madi sore, Malabar ulcer, Malagache ulcer, malarial ulcer, mango sore, Mozambique sore, Naga sore, Natal sore, Rhodesian sore, *sarmes du Congo,* tropical septic ulcer, tropical sloughing phagedena, tropical ulcer, *ulcus tropicum,* Yemen ulcer, and Zambesi ulcer.[2–7]

DEFINITION

Tropical phagedenic ulcer (TPU) is a painful, malodorous, and disabling infection of the lower leg and foot (Figures 90–1 and 90–2) affecting mainly young adults and older children in the tropics.[8,9] There is necrosis of the skin and subcutaneous tissues. A characteristic foul-smelling slough overlies a soft, tender, easily bleeding, granulomatous base with surrounding edema.[6] It has been described as "once seen, once smelled, never forgotten."[10] Although usually solitary, multiple ulcers on a single patient do occur.[11]

GEOGRAPHIC DISTRIBUTION

Tropical phagedenic ulcer is limited to the tropics and subtropics. Tropical Africa (including Gambia, Zambia, Nigeria, Zimbabwe, Malawi, Ethiopia, Uganda, Zaire, and South Africa), tropical Asia, tropical South America, the Pacific Islands (including Papua New Guinea, Fiji, and Kiribati), Central America, the West Indies, and southern India are endemic regions.[6,8,9,12–21]

HISTORY

The first documentation of TPU appears to have come from proceedings surrounding a Dutch medical hearing in 1775.[22] In December 1774, a ship named the *Ouwerkerk,* which belonged to the Dutch East India Company, sailed from Batavia along Java's north coast and landed in Castle Nieuw Victoria, on the Isle of Ambon, on March 9, 1775. The ship's first surgeon, Adriaan van Brakel, was accused of inappropriately treating an outbreak of ulcers on the lower limbs of the crew. The disease struck so many on board that it was considered at one point to be "a punishment from heaven." The descriptions of the wounds and the surrounding circumstances leave little doubt that the lesions were TPUs.

CLINICAL FEATURES

Often beginning after a scratch, thorn prick, or other penetrating trauma, TPU is limited to the leg below the knee.[8] Trauma, however, may not be necessary.[23] The skin becomes red, swollen, and acutely painful, following which a pustule 1 to 1.5 cm in diameter develops. In about a week the lesion discharges blood-stained pus and may remain very painful. The base has a gray fibrin cover and emits a putrid odor that may draw flies (Figure 90–3). Several days later, the slough disintegrates, revealing an orange-brown base.[3] The diameter of a TPU rarely exceeds 10 cm, usually measuring from 2 to 4 cm. If neglected, however, it will spread quickly to involve deeper tissues, including tendons, muscles, and bone (Figure 90–4).[10] The ulcer margin is raised and firm, and the edges are slightly everted but not

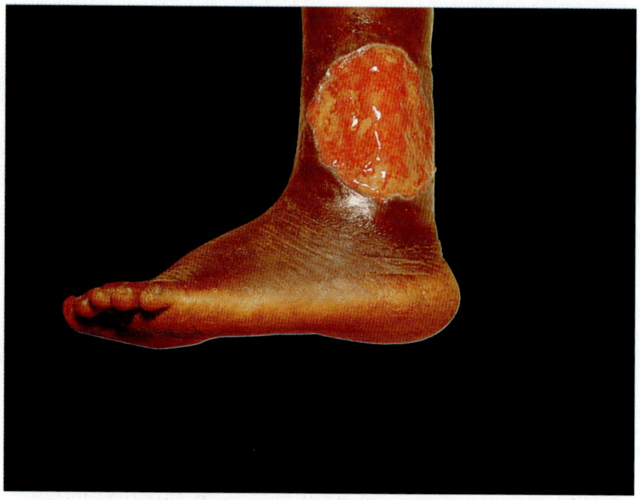

Figure 90–1. Typical tropical phagedenic ulcer. It involves skin of lower leg and upper ankle, its margins are slightly raised but not undermined, and it had a putrid odor. *(By Daniel H. Connor, MD, 1968.)*

undermined (Figure 90–5). Malaise, fever, and tender regional lymphadenopathy may develop but subside as the acute stage passes. With time, the ulcer margin becomes harder and thicker, further deepening the crater. Secondary bacterial infections (Figure 90–6) cause acute exacerbations and asymmetrical expansion. New epithelium that grows over the fibrotic base may be destroyed by secondary infections. The ulcer may continue for years, partially healing and breaking down over old scar.[8] In fact, the old Swahili name for the

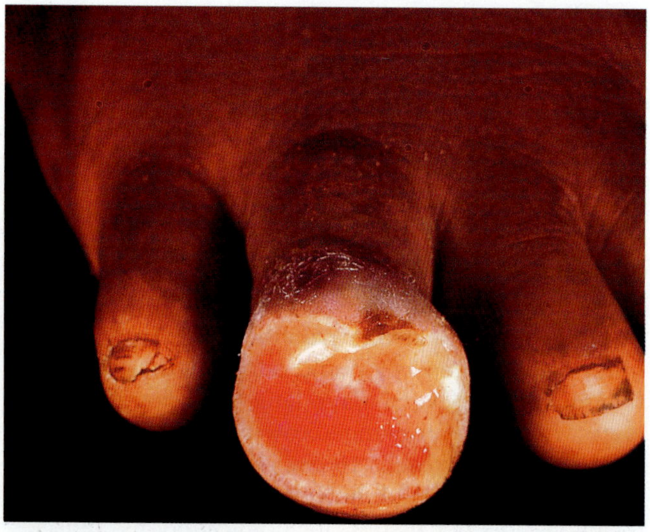

Figure 90–2. A tropical phagedenic ulcer on the toe of a Zairian patient. The ulcer has eroded much of the soft tissue of the distal phalanx. *(By Daniel H. Connor, MD, 1968.)*

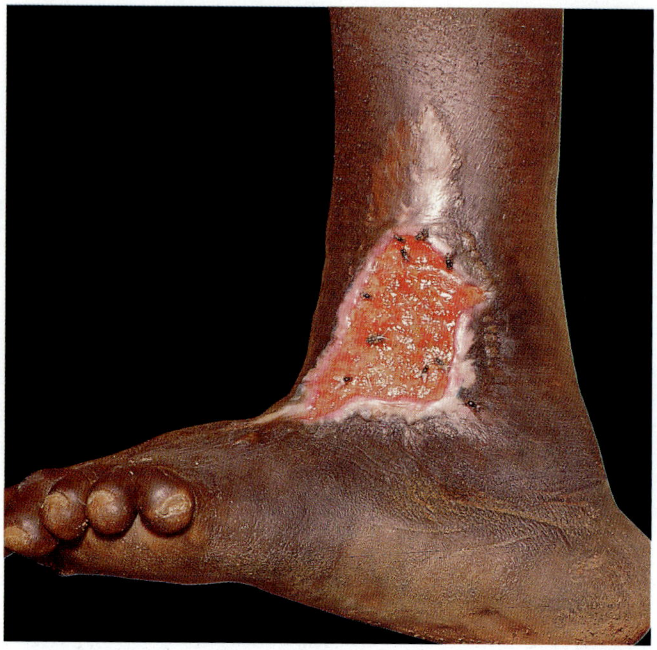

Figure 90–3. Many flies are feeding on the exudate in the crater of this tropical phagedenic ulcer. Flies, which have been implicated in the development and progression of these lesions, are drawn to the ulcers by their putrid odor. There is a thin rim of nonpigmented epithelium at the margin. *(By Daniel H. Connor, MD, 1968.)*

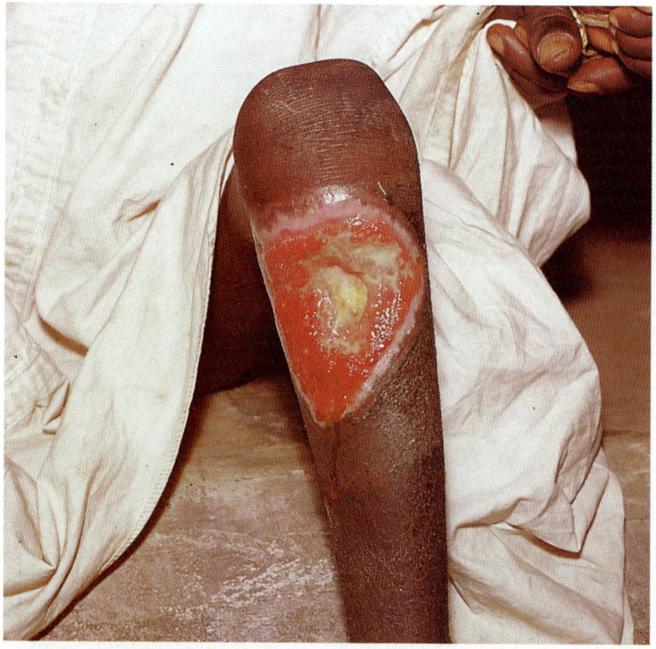

Figure 90–4. This was an acutely painful, progressive tropical phagedenic ulcer. Bloody fluid from the crater runs down the leg. A margin of nonpigmented epithelium surrounds the ulcer, but the destruction in the center of the crater has exposed the tibia. *(By Daniel H. Connor, MD, 1968.)*

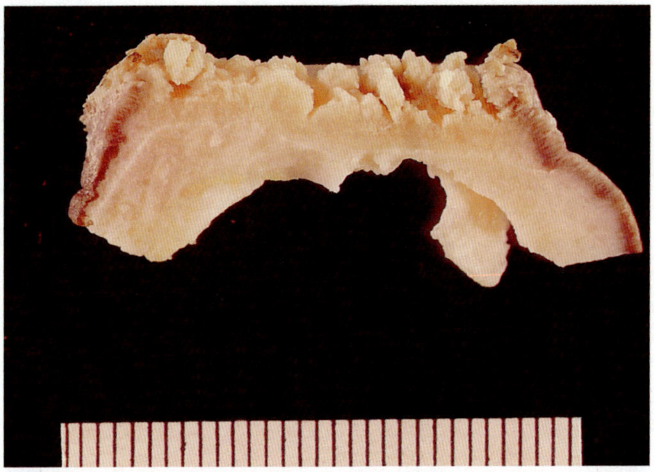

Figure 90–5. This ulcer, shown in cross-section, was excised from the pretibial skin of a young Ethiopian male patient on the suspicion that it was cancer. The ulcer's contour is shown in profile. Note the raised margins and the gray exudate covering the crater. The ulcer is 23 mm across (AFIP Neg 68-1539-2).

ulcer, *kidonda ndugu,* means "my brother sore," signifying a sore that lives with the patient and does not go away.[24] Its persistence may be caused by inappropriate treatment, undernutrition, unhygienic living conditions, contamination of the ulcer, poor blood supply to the pretibial area, venous stasis, and excessive scarring.[8] The end result is a broad crusting scar covered by thin nonpigmented epithelium.[3]

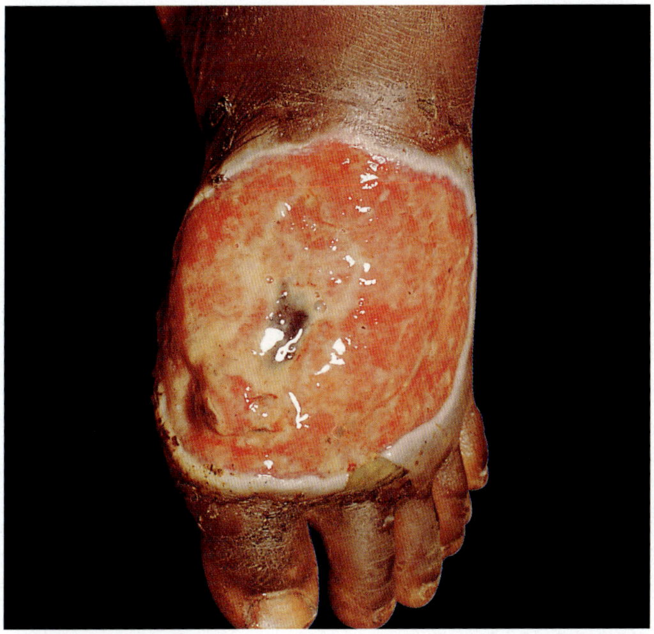

Figure 90–6. Secondary bacterial infections, like the one in the center of this ulcer, complicate the course of tropical phagedenic ulcers. This organism is producing black pigment and has invaded to bone. *(By Daniel H. Connor, MD, 1977.)*

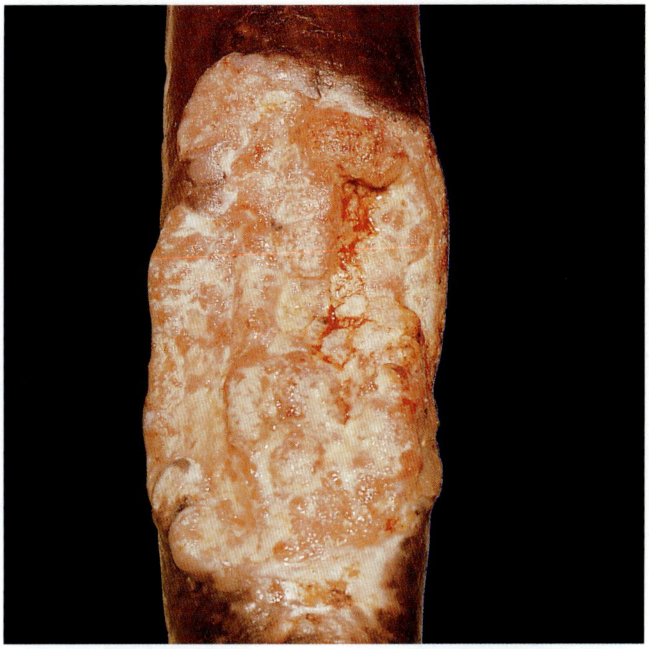

Figure 90–7. This patient, in a rural hospital in Uganda, has a squamous cell carcinoma (sometimes called invasive acanthosis) at the site of a tropical phagedenic ulcer. These lesions invade locally but do not metastasize. The cause of the malignant change may be actinic damage to the nonpigmented epithelium at the margin of the ulcer (see Figures 90–3 and 90–4). *(By Daniel H. Connor, MD, 1963.)*

Complications of chronic, inappropriately treated TPUs include tibial osteomyelitis and squamous cell carcinoma (Figure 90–7).[3,13,24] The latter may be caused by actinic rays reaching nonpigmented skin at the margin of the ulcer.[3] Although invading squamous projections may destroy adjacent tissues (Figures 90–8 through 90–12), metastases to regional lymph nodes and to distant organs have not been documented.[8] Sarcomas have been seen in a small proportion of cases.[21] Finally, hepatitis B surface antigen and e antigen have been found in exudates from these ulcers.[20]

ETIOLOGY AND EPIDEMIOLOGY

Some reports of the disease as early as 1924 describe this lesion in cachectic individuals whose health was impaired by unsanitary surroundings.[2] It appeared to be common among those who walked barefoot through wet and muddy areas and was more prevalent during damp months. At the time, the disease was thought to be contagious, being found among school children who were in constant contact with one another,[2] but later studies indicated little person-to-person infectivity.[9,13] It has been suggested that malnutrition is an important causal factor, but objective studies have not confirmed this.[13]

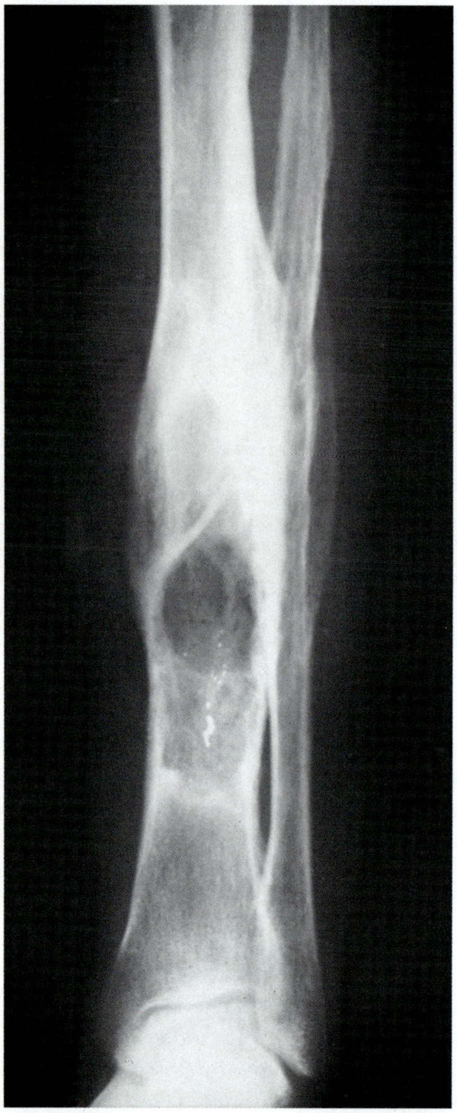

Figure 90–8. A radiograph of the lower leg of a patient with a chronic tropical phagedenic ulcer. A low-grade squamous cell carcinoma has invaded the tibia and caused this circumscribed lytic lesion.

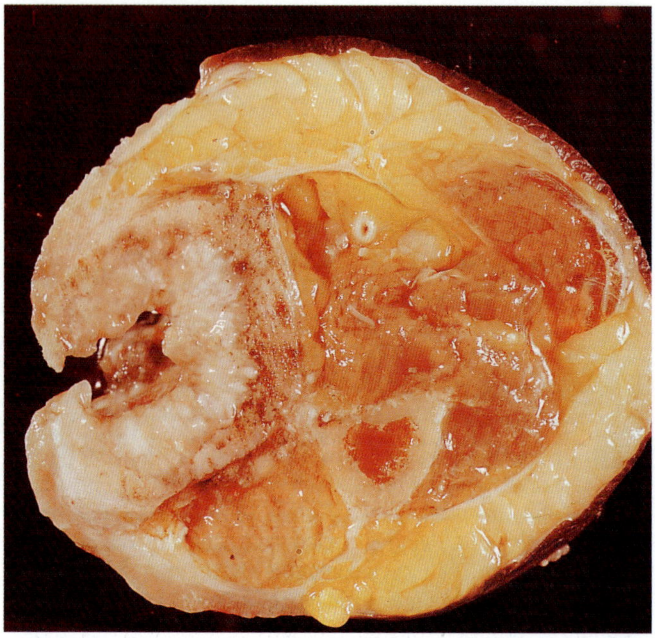

Figure 90–9. The leg shown in the radiograph in Figure 90–8 was amputated and this is a cross-section through the defect in the tibia. The squamous cell carcinoma has almost completely destroyed the tibia at this level.

The definitive cause of TPU remains unclear, but it is presumed that the lesion results from a synergistic bacterial infection involving a spirochete, *Borrelia vincentii* or *Treponema vincentii,* and a gram-positive or gram-negative anaerobic bacillus, *Fusobacterium fusiforme, Bacillus fusiforme, B fusiformis,* or *Fusiformis fusiformis.*[8,10,15,25–30] Fusiforms were first observed in the exudate of ulcers in Guiana in 1884.[31] One study has suggested that the species found in these ulcers is different from previously identified fusobacteria.[32] Further characterization of the fusiform component in one report has identified the organism *Fusobacterium nucleatum.*[6] *Fusobacterium ulcerans* (named for its source, the ulcer itself) has been mentioned as well.[33]

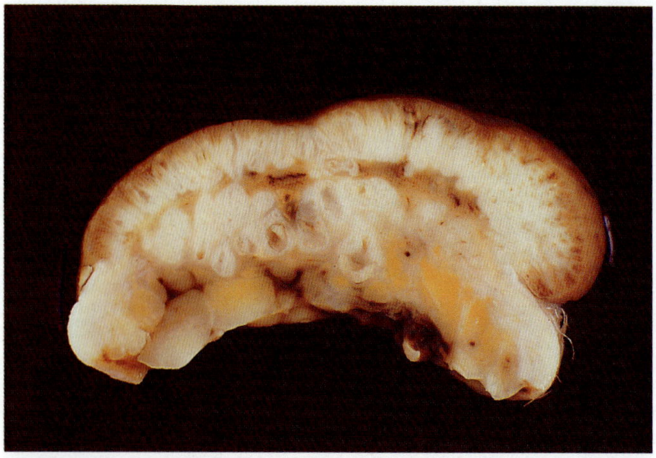

Figure 90–10. This squamous cell carcinoma, arising in a tropical phagedenic ulcer, has overgrown the surface of the ulcer, giving it a cauliflower-like appearance, and has invaded the dermis and the subcutaneous fatty tissue. *(By Daniel H. Connor, MD, 1970.)*

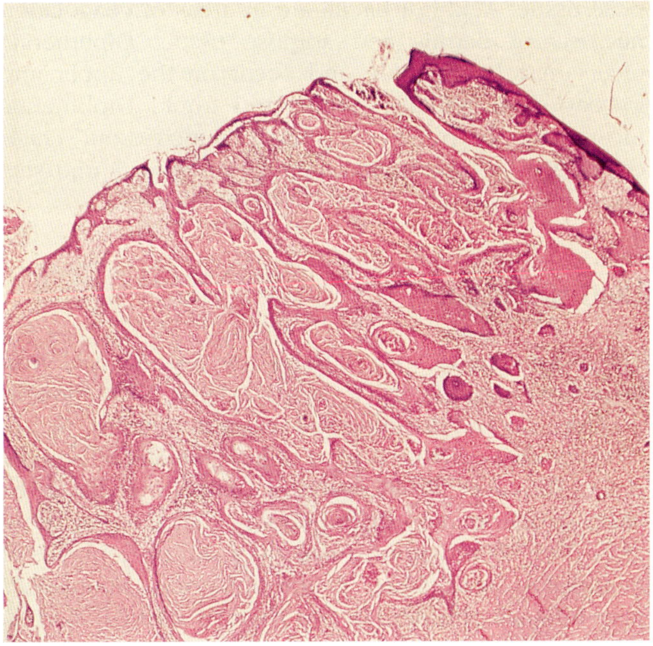

Figure 90–11. A section through the margin of a squamous cell carcinoma that has developed in a chronic tropical phagedenic ulcer. There is an abrupt transition from neoplastic to non-neoplastic epithelium. The tumor is undermining adjacent epidermis (AFIP Neg 68-1312; hematoxylin-eosin, ×8).

Rapid destruction of tissue may be caused by the cytotoxicity of butyrate, which is the major metabolic end product of *Fusobacterium*.[30,33] Other anaerobes recovered from TPUs include *Bacteroides,* anaerobic cocci, *Veillonella,* and propionibacteria.[34] Aerobes recovered include coliforms, *Staphylococcus aureus,* coagulase negative staphylococci, and streptococci.

Although these organisms are in established ulcers, it is not known if they are primary infecting agents. Once the ulcer becomes chronic or the patient is treated with antibiotics, there is nonspecific bacterial overgrowth.[10] One report has suggested that saliva may be a source of wound contamination since organisms in the ulcers are also in the mouth.[6] Sweating during humid seasons, followed by skin maceration and scratching, which may introduce organisms, have been suggested as causal factors as well.[10,16] Also, it is unclear whether fecal contamination of mud or slow-moving freshwater in endemic regions may be a factor,[13] but flies drawn to wounds of people using public latrines may carry contaminating organisms from fecal material to skin. The role of flies as a potential vector has been postulated.[5]

A recent survey showed that 96% of TPUs involve the foot or lower leg, with about 6% lasting more than 6 months.[13] Most TPUs are in children and teenagers of rural populations (Figures 90–13 and 90–14). Another large study showed that these ulcers are more common

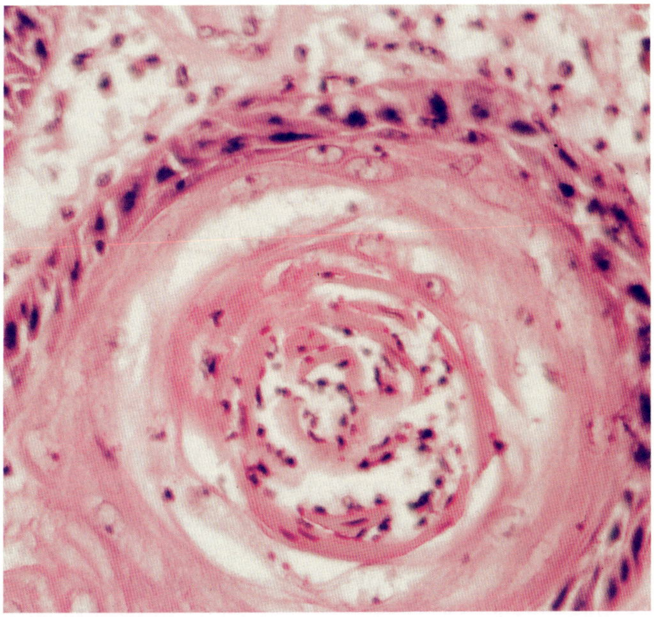

Figure 90–12. This nest of squamous cell carcinoma has retained regular maturation and exhibits three distinct layers: 1) an outer layer of hyperchromatic pleomorphic basal cells, 2) an inner layer of prickle cells, and 3) a central parakeratotic mass (AFIP Neg 68-1310; hematoxylin-eosin, ×180).

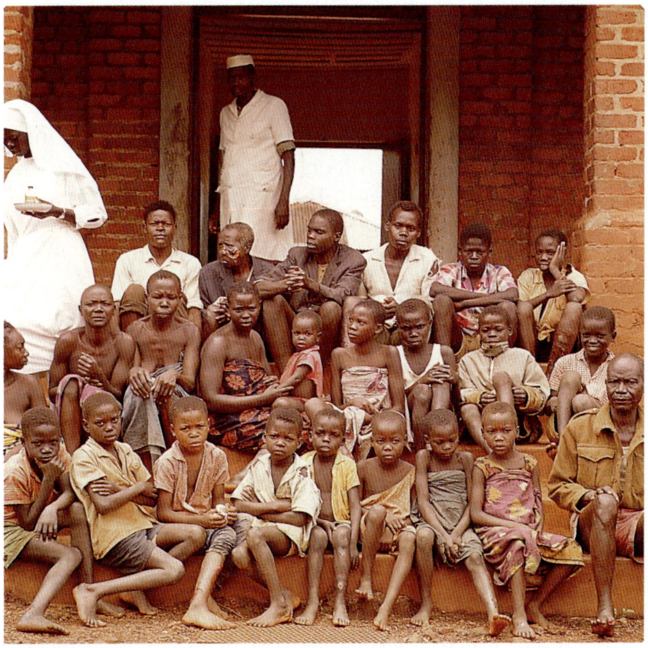

Figure 90–13. Patients attending the ulcer clinic at Watsa, Eastern Zaire, on August 29, 1968. Most of these patients have a tropical phagedenic ulcer and the children in the front rows are displaying the ulcers on their lower legs. *(By Daniel H. Connor, MD, 1968.)*

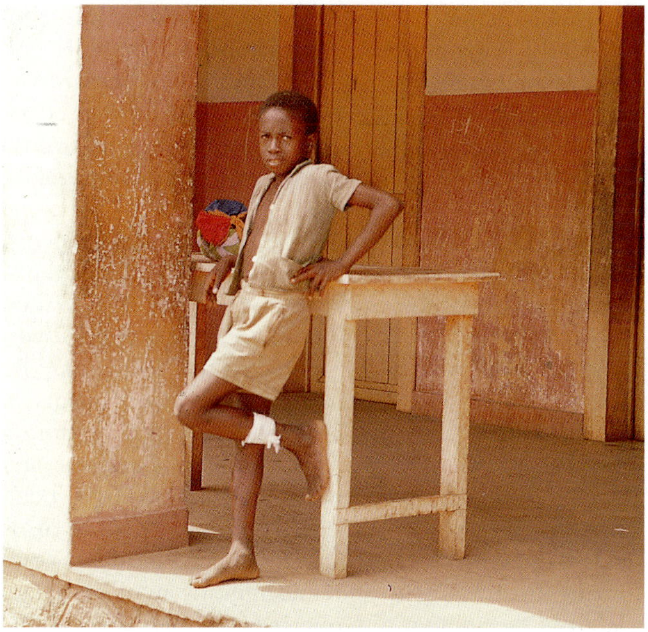

Figure 90–14. A common sight throughout the tropics. The ulcer on the leg of this boy in Businga, Zaire, has just been treated and dressed at a rural dispensary. *(By Daniel H. Connor, MD, 1968.)*

in the wet and humid months, with 63% in the 5- to 14-year-old age group.[16] Male:female ratio is 1.4:1, according to that report. In a province of New Guinea, an estimated 5000 TPUs are seen annually in a rural population of 260,000.[35]

IMMUNOLOGY

Although some authors have denied evidence of immunity following the first ulcer,[10] others have noted that development of a second ulcer is rare.[3]

DIFFERENTIAL DIAGNOSIS

Although the appearance is usually very characteristic, TPU must be differentiated from primary yaws, Buruli ulcer *(Myocobacterium ulcerans),* diphtheritic ulcers, and deep fungal infections.[36] The cutaneous lesions of yaws are usually multiple and occur on the thighs, calves, buttocks, and upper limbs. When ulcerated, yaws lesions are more irregular and they do not have raised or hard edges. Biopsy reveals hyperplasia of the epithelium and large numbers of plasma cells and lymphocytes in the exudate. Lesions caused by *M ulcerans* are usually larger than TPUs and are mostly in patients inhabiting swampy lowlands and river valleys. They are painless, have undermined edges, and are associated with swelling and induration of the subcutaneous adipose tissue. Acid-fast bacilli are in areas of coagulation necrosis of dermis and adipose tissue. Diphtheritic ulcers may be multiple and occur on the upper and lower limbs, genitalia, scalp, and trunk. Diphtheritic ulcers have sharp flat edges and a "punched-out" crater covered by a diphtheritic membrane. Smears and sections from the crater reveal diphtheroids.

LIGHT MICROSCOPY

The main microscopic findings are loss of epidermis associated with extensive dermal edema, infiltration by neutrophils, and disruption of collagen bundles.[7] Acanthosis, with a variable degree of hyperkeratosis, is at the rim of the ulcer. Proliferation of vessels may be at the base. In lesions less than 1 month old, there is spongiosis, which is accompanied by a diffuse infiltrate of neutrophils in all layers of the epidermis. Neutrophils may infiltrate the dermis and there is dermal vascular dilatation. In older lesions, a coagulum composed of fibrin, degenerating cellular debris, and masses of intermixed bacteria lies over the surface of the ulcer.[8] Granulation tissue infiltrated by leukocytes supports the coagulum. There is elongation of the rete ridges and pronounced epidermal thickening.[7] Thickening of the vessel walls with endothelial proliferation is also in the dermis of chronic ulcers. The base of the ulcer contains a variety of inflammatory cells, including histiocytes, eosinophils, neutrophils, plasma cells, and lymphocytes.[8] Clusters of lymphocytes, plasma cells, and histiocytes are prominent around vessels in adjacent scar tissue and occasional giant cells may also be in the deeper layers of the scar.

The most commonly identified bacteria are gram-negative pleomorphic bacilli (Figure 90–15), but spiral bacteria (Figure 90–16) may be in the slough or at the ulcer rim in untreated lesions.[7] Gram-positive cocci may also be in the epidermis.

ELECTRON MICROSCOPY

In general, light microscopic findings are confirmed by electron microscopy. Predominating bacteria are rod-shaped, round, or elongated with a thin, irregular cell wall, an appearance most resembling fusobacteria from culture.[7] Spirochetes may be in deeper layers of the dermis. Disrupted bundles of collagen have been seen in the vicinity of clusters of bacteria, suggesting that toxins induce necrosis.[7]

One study found the spirochetes to have three flagellae and morphologically identified them as treponemes,[7] but examination of negatively stained spirochetes by transmission electron microscopy revealed

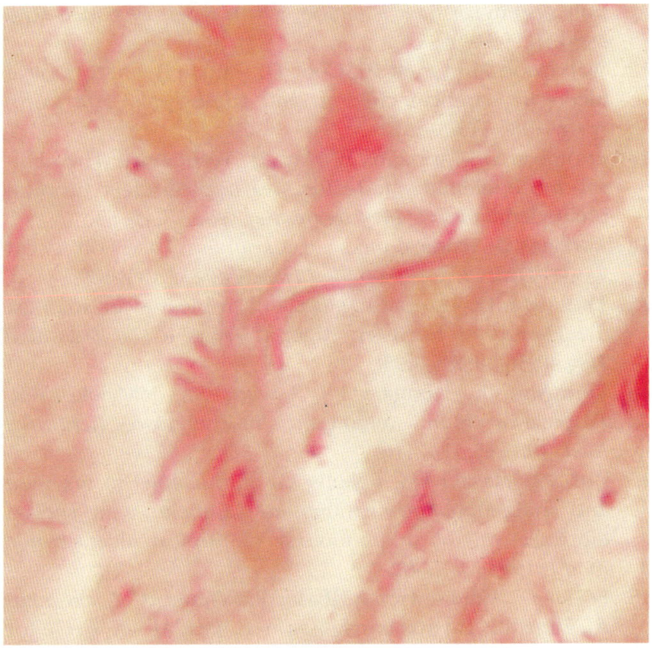

Figure 90–15. Large numbers of bacilli are in the superficial exudates of tropical phagedenic ulcers. They are gram-negative, pleomorphic, and have pointed ends, characteristic features of fusiform bacilli (AFIP Neg 68-1876; Brown–Hopps, ×1200).

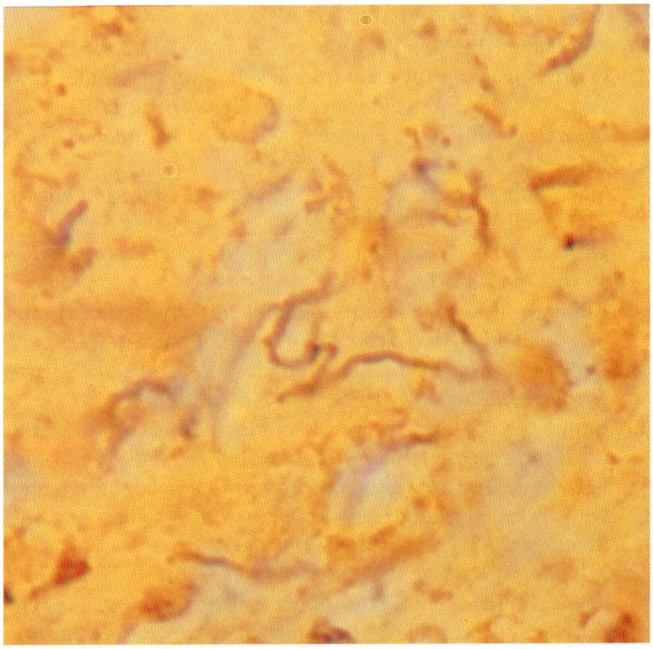

Figure 90–16. Silver impregnation stains reveal spirochetes mixed with the fusiform bacilli. Unlike *Treponema pallidum,* these spirochetes have loose irregular spirals (AFIP Neg 74-11309; Warthin–Starry, ×1440).

spirochetal cells with the characteristic spiral shape and eight periplasmic flagellae originating from one end of the cell.[6] This suggests the probability of a typical 8-16-8 periplasmic flagellar arrangement.

CULTURE

Although transport media are available and putative organisms can be seen in biopsies or smears, the techniques and facilities required make laboratory confirmation impractical in remote areas.[35] One group suggests transporting samples in Hungate tubes with prereduced peptone yeast broth and agar.[11] Using this method, viable anaerobes were still present 6 weeks after procurement of specimens. Samples were taken from beneath the established edge of an advancing ulcer and from the center of early papules after deroofing. Following transport, samples were plated on blood agar and cysteine lactose electrolyte-deficient plates for aerobes; supplemented brain heart infusion agar (BHIA) with 10% horse blood, supplemented BHIA with kanamycin and vancomycin, supplemented BHIA with netilmycin, supplemented BHIA with nalidixic acid, and Veillonella agar for anaerobes.[32,34] Several other selective media have been suggested for isolation of fusobacteria.[30,37,38] Identification of fusobacteria is aided by their production of large amounts of butyrate.[30,33] *Fusobacterium ulcerans* does not produce extracellular DNAase, does not digest casein, and is nonhemolytic.[33]

MOLECULAR ASPECTS

Several methods beyond culture and biochemical characterization have been used to speciate and subspeciate the fusobacteria. They include DNA probes,[39] polyacrylamide gel electrophoresis,[40] and pyrolysis mass spectrometry.[41] The most powerful methods have been comparative analysis of small-subunit rRNA sequences[42] and the use of rRNA gene restriction patterns.[43]

TREATMENT

Older treatments short of surgery included daily saline injections beneath the ulcer following initial curetting, intramuscular injections of arsphenamin with potassium iodide by mouth, moist dressings covered by a banana leaf, and, when the ulcer was clean and granulating, dusting with Vincent's powder, which consisted of one part sodium hypochlorite and nine parts boric acid.[2] A more recent study advocated the topical application of framycetin to speed healing.[44]

The course of the disease can be interrupted in the early stages by the administration of antibiotics, but later administration has little effect.[14] Primary therapy usually includes intramuscular penicillin and regular dressings with an antiseptic like Eusol.[35] Infection in the ulcer crater has been controlled with penicillin, 500,000 units, and streptomycin, 1 g, twice weekly.[8] However, β-lactamase activity has been reported.[45] Metronidazole has been effective also.[46]

Healing is promoted by improving general health, eliminating infection in the ulcer crater, thorough cleansing, and skin grafting when necessary.[8] Immersing the affected area for 1 hour in 1% to 2% hydrogen peroxide helps loosen inspissated material. Potassium permanganate solution (1:5000) has been used effectively and occlusive dressings may also help.[8] Ulcers less than 5 cm will heal within 2 weeks with proper treatment.[3] Larger ulcers may require grafting. Access to grafting facilities reduces the need for long-term dressings and the risk of chronic ulcerations. Hospitalized patients require a minimum of 15 days of therapy compared to 10 days if lesions are grafted early.[35] Although skin grafting produces excellent responses, there is a high drop-out rate.

REFERENCES

1. Stanley HM. *In Darkest Africa.* New York: Charles Scribner's Sons; 1890;II:158.
2. Corpus T. A survey of ulcus tropicum. *JAMA.* 1924; 82:1192–1194.
3. Connor DH. Tropical phagedenic ulcer. In: *The Skin.* Baltimore: Williams and Wilkins; 1971:448–454.
4. Apostolides G. Note on the recent epidemic septic ulcer in Palestine (tropical sloughing phagedaena). *J Trop Med Hyg.* 1922;25:81–88.
5. Fox ECR. Naga sore. *Indian J Med Res.* 1920;8:694–698.
6. Falkler WA, Montgomery J, Nauman RK, Alpers M. Isolation of *Fusobacterium nucleatum* and electron microscopic observations of spirochetes from tropical skin ulcers in Papua New Guinea. *Am J Trop Med Hyg.* 1989;40:390–398.
7. Adriaans B, Hay R, Lucas S, Robinson DC. Light and electron microscopic features of tropical ulcer. *J Clin Pathol.* 1987;40:1231–1234.
8. Connor DH, Neafie RC. Tropical phagedenic ulcer. In: Binford CH, Connor DH, eds. *Pathology of Tropical and Extraordinary Diseases.* Washington: Armed Forces Institute of Pathology; 1976;1:199–200.
9. Robinson DC, Hay RJ. Tropical ulcer in Zambia. *Trans R Soc Trop Med Hyg.* 1986;80:132–137.
10. Kariks J. Tropical ulcer amongst the natives of New Guinea. *Med J Aust.* 1957;2:346–350.
11. Adriaans B, Hay RJ, Drasar BS, Robinson DCA. Anaerobic bacteria in tropical ulcer—the application of a new transport system for their isolation. *Trans R Soc Trop Med Hyg.* 1986;80:793–794.
12. Watkinson M, Aggett PJ, Cole TJ. Zinc and acute tropical ulcers in Gambian children and adolescents. *Am J Clin Nutr.* 1985;41:43–51.
13. Robinson DC, Adriaans B, Hay RJ, Yesudian P. The clinical and epidemiologic features of tropical ulcer (tropical phagedenic ulcer). *Int J Dermatol.* 1988;27:49–53.
14. Adriaans B. Tropical ulcer—a reappraisal based on recent work. *Trans R Soc Trop Med Hyg.* 1988;82:185–189.
15. Thomson IG. The pathogenesis of tropical ulcer amongst the Hausas of Northern Nigeria. *Trans R Soc Trop Med Hyg.* 1956;50:485–495.
16. Tumwine JK, Dungare PS, Tswana SA, Maoneke WR. Tropical ulcers in a remote area in Zimbabwe. *Cent Afr J Med.* 1989;35:413–416.
17. Bulto T, Maskel FH, Fisseha G. Skin lesions in resettled and indigenous populations in Gambela, with special emphasis on the epidemiology of tropical ulcer. *Ethiop Med J.* 1993;31:75–82.
18. Foster O, Ajdukiewicz A, Ryder R, Whittle H, Zuckerman AJ. Hepatitis B virus transmission in West Africa: a role for tropical ulcer? *Lancet.* 1984;1:576–577.
19. Gear JH. Aetiology of tropical ulcer. *Trans R Soc Trop Med Hyg.* 1990;84:753.
20. Tibbs CJ. Hepatitis B, tropical ulcers, and immunisation strategy in Kiribati. *Br Med J.* 1987;294:537–540.
21. Fletcher CDM. Soft tissue sarcomas apparently arising in chronic tropical ulcers. *Histopathology.* 1987;11:501–510.
22. Bruijn IDR, Bruijn GW. An eighteenth-century medical hearing and the first observation of tropical phagedaena. *Med Hist.* 1991;35:295–307.
23. McAdam I. Tropical phagedenic ulcers in Uganda. *J R Coll Surg Edinb.* 1966;11:196–205.
24. Goodacre TEE. Tropical ulcers. *Lancet.* 1987;2:1152.
25. O'Brien JP. Tropical ulcer and desert sore. In: Hunter GW, Frye WW, Swartzwelder JC, eds. *A Manual of Tropical Medicine.* 4th ed. Philadelphia: WB Saunders; 1967: 628–631.
26. Maegraith B, ed. *Clinical Tropical Diseases.* Oxford: Blackwell; 1984:467–473.
27. Obrien HD. Treatment of tropical ulcers. *Br Med J.* 1951;2:1544–1551.
28. Kuberski T, Koteka G. An epidemic of tropical ulcer in the Cook Islands. *Am J Trop Med Hyg.* 1980;29:291–297.
29. James CS. Tropical phagedenic ulcer in the Pacific. *Trans R Soc Trop Med Hyg.* 1938;31:647–666.
30. Bennett KW, Eley A. Fusobacteria: new taxonomy and related diseases. *J Med Microbiol.* 1993;39:246–254.
31. LeDanteg. The phagedaena of warm climates; its identity with hospital gangrene, its pathology, symptoms and treatment. *J Trop Med.* 1899;1:308–312.
32. Adriaans B, Drasar BS. The isolation of fusobacteria from tropical ulcers. *Epidemiol Infect.* 1987;99:361–372.
33. Adriaans B, Garelick H. Cytotoxicity of *Fusobacterium ulcerans*. *J Med Microbiol.* 1989;29:177–180.
34. Adriaans B, Hay R, Drasar B, Robinson D. The infectious aetiology of tropical ulcer—a study of the role of anaerobic bacteria. *Br J Dermatol.* 1987;116:31–37.

35. Morris GE, Hay RJ, Srinivasa A, Bunat A. The diagnosis and management of tropical ulcer in East Sepik Province of Papua New Guinea. *J Trop Med Hyg.* 1989;92:215–220.
36. Barnetson RS. Skin diseases in the tropics. *Med J Aust.* 1993;159:321–325.
37. Morgenstein AA, Citron DM, Finegold SM. New medium selective for *Fusobacterium* species, and differential for *Fusobacterium necrophorum*. *J Clin Microbiol.* 1981;13: 666–669.
38. Brazier JS, Citron DM, Goldstein EJC. A selective medium for *Fusobacterium* spp. *J Appl Bacteriol.* 1991;71:343–346.
39. Bolstad AI, Skang N, Jensen HB. Use of synthetic oligonucleotide DNA probes for the identification of different strains of *Fusobacterium nucleatum*. *J Period Res.* 1991;26: 519–526.
40. Calhoon DA, Mayberry WR, Slots J. Cellular fatty acid and soluble protein profiles of oral fusobacteria. *J Dent Res.* 1983;62:1181–1185.
41. Magee JT, Hindmarch JM, Bennett KW, Duerden BI, Aries RE. A pyrolysis-mass spectrometry study of fusobacteria. *J Med Microbiol.* 1989;28:227–236.
42. Lawson PA, Gharbia SE, Shah HN, Clarke DR, Collins MD. Intrageneric relationships of members of the genus *Fusobacterium* as determined by reverse transcriptase sequencing of small-subunit rRNA. *Int J Syst Bacteriol.* 1991; 41:347–354.
43. Lawson PA, Gharbia SE, Shah H, Clarke DR. Recognition of *Fusobacterium nucleatum* subgroup Fn-1, Fn-2 and Fn-3 by ribosomal RNA gene restriction patterns. *FEMS Microbiol Lett.* 1989;65:41–45.
44. Gupta SN, Jha B, Jha SN. Role of topical dressings in tropical ulcer leg. *J Indian Med Assoc.* 1984;82:161–164.
45. Tuner K, Lindqvist L, Nord CE. Characterization of a new β-lactamase from *Fusobacterium nucleatum* by substrate profiles and chromatofocusing patterns. *J Antimicrob Chemother.* 1985;16:23–30.
46. Yesudrian P, Thambiah AR. Metronidazole in the treatment of tropical phagedenic ulcer. *Int J Dermatol.* 1979;18:755–757.

CHAPTER 91

Tuberculosis

Ernest E. Lack and Daniel H. Connor

> *. . . Where youth grows pale, and spectre-thin, and dies; . . .*
> *You must not look at me in my dying gasp, nor breathe my passing breath . . .*
> *That drop of blood is my death warrant. I must die.*
>
> *John Keats (1795–1821)*

DEFINITION

Tuberculosis is infection by *Mycobacterium tuberculosis* and is the historical and classical example of granulomatous inflammation. Any organ or tissue may be involved. *Mycobacterium tuberculosis* is also known as the "tubercle bacillus" and "Koch's bacillus." Strains of *M tuberculosis* virulent for mankind are referred to as H37RV ("H" for human, "37" for optimal growth at 37°C, "R" for rough colony, and "V" for virulent).

INTRODUCTION

Tuberculosis has had a tremendous impact on human societies throughout the ages.[1] More than a century ago tuberculosis was the most common killer in the western world claiming those of all rank. John Keats died of tuberculosis in 1821 in his 26th year.[2,3] Chopin, Paganini, Simonetta Vespucci (the model for Botticelli's venus), Jean Jacques Rousseau, Goethe, Chekhov, Schiller (the dramatist who wrote "Ode to Joy" in the chorale of Beethoven's ninth symphony), Cardinal Richelieu, Laurence Sterne, Shelley, Poe, Eugene O'Neill, and Sir Walter Scott are a few of the many artists, writers, composers, and statesmen who suffered with or died of tuberculosis.[4] Tuberculosis, in fact, tended to be associated with genius, youth, and great art and these associations lent an ambiance of romance and glamour to its victims. Mimi in *La Boheme* and Violetta in *La Traviata* are two touching examples of the romantic aura that attended fatal tuberculosis. Some even thought tuberculosis inspired genius, and many patients, even those with terminal tuberculosis, were energetic, hopeful, and optimistic to the end—the so-called *spes phthisica.* Throughout most of the nineteenth century the cause of tuberculosis was unknown and contagion, although suspected in southern Europe,[5] was dismissed as unlikely in northern Europe and in Britain. All romanticism vanished abruptly on the evening of March 24, 1882, however, when Robert Koch described the cause of tuberculosis to the Berlin Physiological Society. Ryan tells us that at the end of his presentation Koch was baffled by the reaction of the audience.[4] There were no questions, applause, or congratulatory remarks. Rudolph Virchow donned his hat and left without a word. Perhaps the audience was stunned by the significance of the findings, for they must have realized they had just witnessed a great moment in history. For on that night Koch established that tuberculosis was caused not by a "tubercular diathesis," not by "humors," nor by the other popular speculations of the day, but by an infectious and contagious agent. Koch had described a new kind of bacterium–one with a tough waxy wall that gave it unusual staining properties. Doubts about its causal role were swept away by the presentation of his careful studies, for he demonstrated that the bacterium could 1) be isolated from tuberculous lesions, 2) be grown in pure culture, 3) produce tubercles when inoculated into animals, and 4) be reisolated from the lesions of animals.[1] These four steps, now known as Koch's postulates, had been established earlier during his work on anthrax and he now applied them elegantly to the tubercle bacillus. From that moment tuberculosis was recognized as a contagious disease. The illusion of beauty and genius

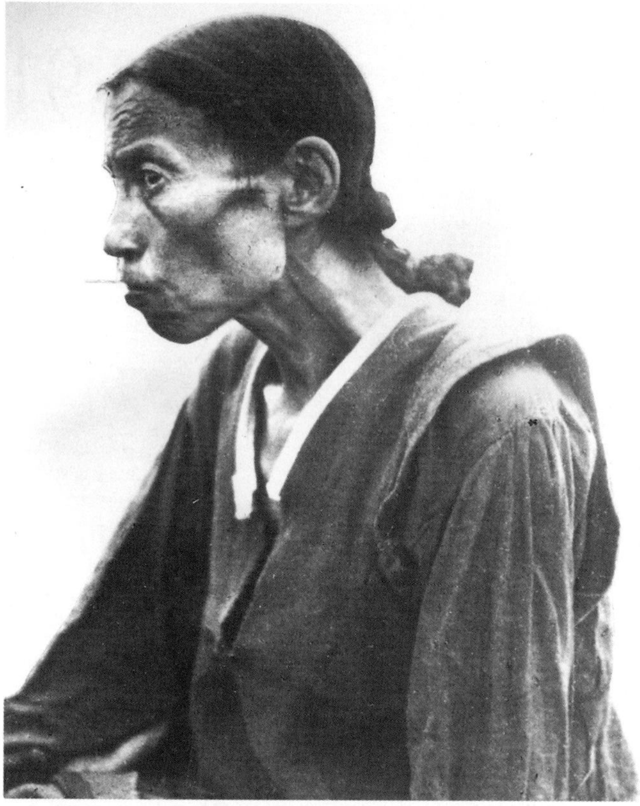

Figure 91–1. This Esquimaux woman has a thermometer in her mouth. She is 38 years old, came out of the Arctic hinterland with her family in June 1951, after the long Arctic night, and encamped just above the tide flats in the Esquimaux village at Frobisher Bay, Baffin Island. She was cachectic, febrile, had signs of vitamin C and B complex deficiencies, and had a cough that produced sputum containing enormous numbers of acid-fast bacilli. She spat on the dirt floor of her small hut until given a container for collection. She died 3 months later. *(Photograph by Daniel H. Connor, MD, 1951.)*

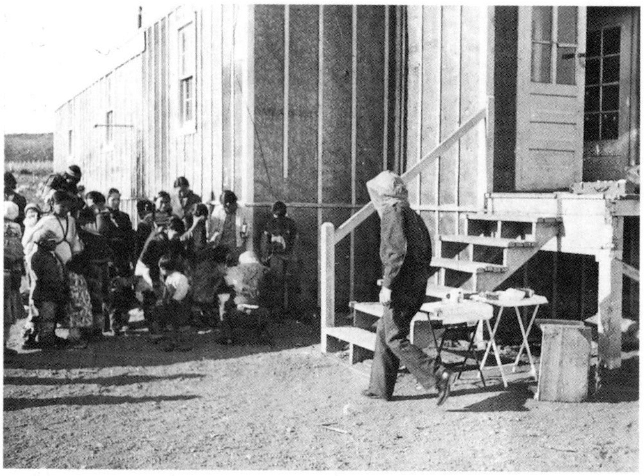

Figure 91–2. Two hundred Esquimaux at the Frobisher Bay village were tuberculin-tested one day in July 1951 by three then-medical students: the late Dr. Emmett T. Cleary, Dr. Ronald Ziegler, and one of us (DHC). Of the 200 tested, 199 were positive—the sole nonreactor being an infant in arms. Head nets protected duty personnel from mosquitoes. *(Photograph by Daniel H. Connor, MD, 1951.)*

attending its victims was gone. Patients with consumption were shunned and tubercular youths, once thought tragically beautiful and artistic, were abandoned by friends and society.[6] But Koch's identification of the tubercle bacillus failed to stem the tide and tuberculosis has continued its worldwide slaughter of the ordinary and great, killing, for example, two of the most accomplished women of our own century, Vivien Leigh and Eleanor Roosevelt.

PREDISPOSING FACTORS

The elderly urban poor are predisposed, as are the homeless, prisoners, and all who suffer from malnutrition and crowding. Some occupations increase one's likelihood of tuberculosis. Patients with pneumoconiosis have increased risk of tuberculosis too and these occupations include stonecutters, masons, and miners. Dairy workers exposed to infected cows are at increased risk as are those who care for tuberculous patients. In the United States 20% of those with tuberculosis have been foreign born. It has been said that some racial groups—including blacks, Amerindians, and Esquimaux—are more susceptible to tuberculosis, but this may have been too convenient an explanation. In decades past, for instance, when it was claimed that Esquimaux had a racial predisposition, their dwellings were crowded, their sputa accumulated on the floors of their huts and dried there, and they suffered episodes of exposure and malnutrition during the long Arctic nights (Figures 91–1 and 91–2).

PREVALENCE AND EPIDEMIOLOGY

Tuberculosis has declined in the United States from 84,304 reported in 1953 to 22,255 in 1984, but increased by 5% to 23,495 in 1989 and by 6% in 1990.[7] This upward blip in the downward trend has been attributed to three phenomena—the acquired immunodeficiency syndrome (AIDS) epidemic, the influx of immigrants from Southeast Asia and Haiti, and the increasing numbers of homeless people.[8] Overall about 6% of the U.S. population is tuberculin positive but the distribution of tuberculosis is uneven and influenced by a variety of factors including age, race, occupation, and socioeconomic status. In 1982, throughout the world, there were an estimated 8 to 10 million new human infections. About 3 million die of tuberculosis each year.[8] The highest per capita incidence is in Africa, where an estimated 165 per 100,000 are infected each year. In Asia the total number infected is about 3.5 times that of Africa—based on its larger population.[8] Tuberculosis continues to be an ominous public health problem throughout the world and complicating the problem is the rising prevalence of strains of *M tuberculosis* resistant to combinations of antituberculous drugs, so-called triple-resistant strains.[9–12]

MODE OF TRANSMISSION

Transmission from person to person is by aerosolized droplets or dust containing *M tuberculosis.* To establish infection, the droplets must pass the respiratory bronchioles and alveolar ducts to reach alveoli. Larger droplets are stopped in the proximal airways, phagocytosed, and carried up by the mucociliary escalator. Tuberculosis may be acquired also by ingesting contaminated milk from infected cows. *Mycobacterium tuberculosis* and *M bovis* are both passed to humans in contaminated milk. Rarely, tuberculosis is acquired by inoculation of skin. One hundred years ago, for instance, pathologists acquired cutaneous tuberculous nodules at autopsy, but the nodules tended to remain localized and heal slowly so were regarded as a nuisance rather than a threat. They were called "postmortem wart," "pathologist's nodule," "verruca necrogenica," and "tuberculosis cutis verrucosa." Not only those doing autopsies but health care workers involved in cough-inducing procedures are also at high risk, even in institutions with few tuberculous patients.[13] Infection in congenital tuberculosis is from the mother's tuberculous bacillemia during pregnancy, with infection of the maternal genital tract and placenta followed by hematogenous spread to the fetus through the umbilical vein. The fetus may be infected also by inhaling or ingesting amniotic fluid containing *M tuberculosis* from placenta or genitalia.[14]

PATHOLOGY

Stimulate the phagocytes. Drugs are a delusion.

George Bernard Shaw, The Doctor's Dilemma, Act I (1913)

General Considerations

When tubercle bacilli enter an alveolus and establish infection, neutrophils phagocytose the bacilli but fail to kill them and are soon destroyed by the bacilli. This brief acute inflammatory response is soon overshadowed by an influx of monocytes. They leave the circulation, migrate into the area of infected lung, and "take up the battle," so to speak. This is the beginning of the granulomatous reaction and the pathogenesis of tuberculosis is, in large part, the reaction of monocytes, macrophages, and their derivatives to *M tuberculosis.* Derivatives include activated macrophages, epithelioid cells, and Langhans' giant cells. As monocytes/macrophages accumulate in and around the focus of infection they form a tumorlike swelling—the granuloma (Figure 91–3). Macrophages phagocytose tubercle bacilli and "process" the mycobacterial antigens. Macrophages then "present" the antigen on their surfaces, allowing T lymphocytes with corresponding surface receptors to bind to the antigen. This "sensitizes" the lymphocytes and they proliferate to form a clone of sensitized progeny. The macrophages induce the clone of T lymphocytes to liberate cytokines, which attract more macrophages to the site of infection, "activate" them, and immobilize them holding them at the site of infection. Activation of macrophages is the key to the granuloma's ability to destroy microorganisms. There are five reasons for this: 1) Some activated macrophages have increased phagocytic activity, 2) some secrete cytokines that organize and promote the development of the granuloma, 3) other activated macrophages produce oxidative and digestive enzymes that kill tubercle bacilli, 4) some activated macrophages become epithelioid cells that function in two ways—by killing bacilli and by surrounding and containing the infection. In making the transformation to epithelioid cells, macrophages become flattened—and broad too, like pancakes. Finally, 5) some epithelioid cells fuse to form Langhans' giant cells, which also have direct killing effects. The nuclei of these fused epithelioid cells persist and frequently form a "horseshoe" arrangement

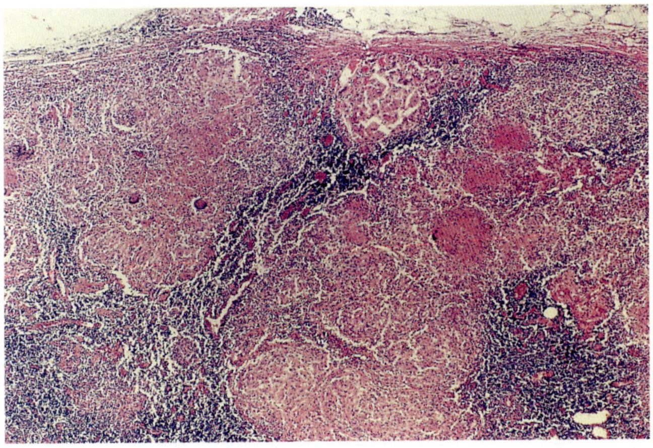

Figure 91–3. Adrenal cortex almost completely replaced by discrete and confluent tuberculous granulomas. Foci of caseation necrosis are apparent in some of the granulomas. The tissue between the granulomas contains lymphocytes and plasma cells (hematoxylin-eosin, ×40).

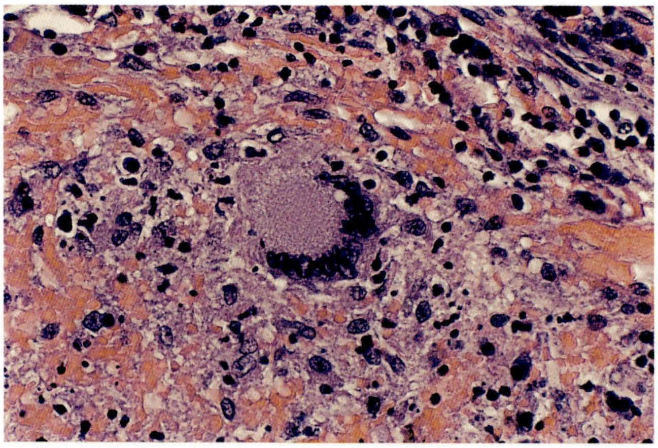

Figure 91–4. Langhans' giant cell in tuberculosis has multiple nuclei having a "horseshoe-like" configuration. Giant cells are a fusion of epithelioid cells. Although not specific for tuberculosis, foci of caseation necrosis with adjacent or surrounding Langhans' giant cells are characteristic (hematoxylin-eosin, ×400).

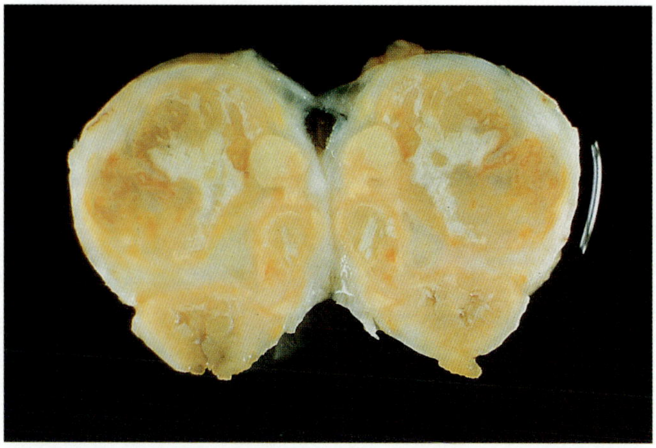

Figure 91–5. Bisected lymph node containing multiple areas of caseation necrosis; the largest is stellate and near the center of the node. The white semisolid caseous material reminded earlier pathologists of cottage cheese, hence "caseation" necrosis. *(Photograph by Daniel H. Connor, MD, 1970.)*

around the perimeter of the cell giving the Langhans' giant cell its distinctive appearance (Figure 91–4). Some cytokines promote the formation of the granuloma. Interleukin-2 (IL-2), produced by sensitized T lymphocytes, stimulates a variety of cytokines, which contribute to activation of macrophages. Some cytokines attract macrophages to the site and immobilize them, thus holding them at the site. Finally γ (gamma) interferon and IL-4 contribute to activation of macrophages, and both accelerate the development of epithelioid cells and their fusion to form Langhans' giant cells.

Caseation Necrosis

Tuberculous granulomas tend to have a concentric arrangement—necrotic tissue in the center surrounded by a mixture of macrophages/histiocytes, epithelioid cells, and giant cells. This is surrounded by a cuff of lymphocytes and plasma cells and these in turn are surrounded by a perimeter of granulation tissue. As healing proceeds, the granulation tissue matures to a layer of scar that surrounds the lesion. Necrosis is a constant feature of active tuberculosis and the necrotic tissue has a characteristic appearance. Grossly, foci of caseation necrosis are creamy-white, semisolid, and resemble cottage cheese, hence "caseation" (Figure 91–5). Microscopically, foci of caseation necrosis are eosinophilic, bland, usually structureless, and have some blue stippling ("salt and pepper") from mineral deposits (Figure 91–6). Areas of caseation necrosis are, by themselves, mycobacteriostatic because, being avascular, they have low oxygen tension and their pH is low too, from released fatty acids. The consequences of this are seen in tissue sections; the numbers of mycobacteria in the centers of the caseating areas decrease abruptly and eventually vanish, whereas surviving bacilli tend to be at the perimeter of the caseating area where oxygen tension and pH are both higher. The necrosis in tuberculosis is unusual for infections characterized by granulomatous reactions because it develops before macrophages are activated. In other infectious granulomas (histoplasmosis for example) necrosis develops only after macrophages are activated and able to produce toxic oxygen species and proteolytic enzymes. But this is not so in tuberculosis. Necrosis begins early and persists throughout active infection. Thus the necrosis in early tuberculosis must be caused by a direct action of tubercle bacilli rather than by the toxic substances

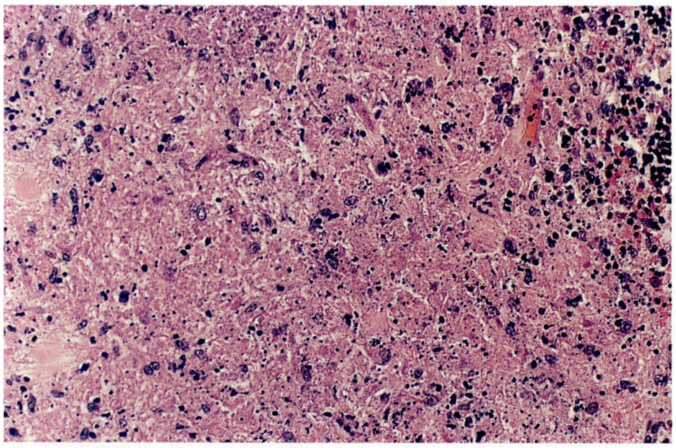

Figure 91–6. Section of lymph node showing caseation necrosis. The "salt and pepper" appearance is a feature of early mineralization (hematoxylin-eosin, ×200).

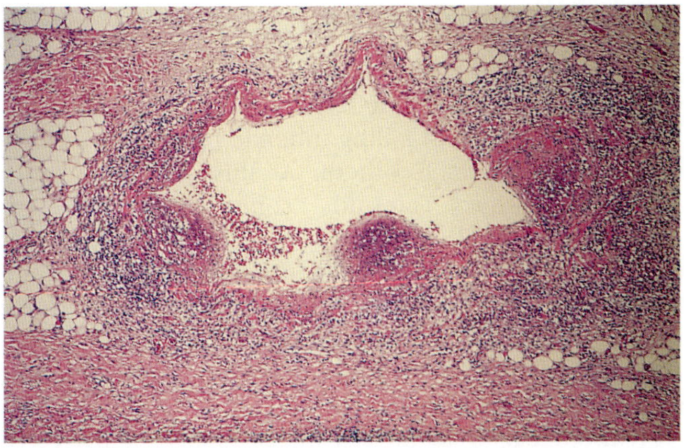

Figure 91–7. Tuberculous lesions invading a pulmonary vein near the hilum of the lung. These nodules are comprised of degenerating macrophages and fibrin, ie, "tuberculous thrombi" (hematoxylin-eosin, ×4).

produced by activated macrophages. Cord factor, a toxic glycolipid of the mycobacterial wall, may cause this early necrosis. Other factors in pathogenesis include the sulfatides of virulent strains of *M tuberculosis* that prevent fusion of phagosomes with lysosomes of macrophages. Leukocyte adhesion molecules (LAM) heteropolysaccharide, akin to gram-negative endotoxins, inhibits activation of macrophages and also induces IL-10, which suppresses T-cell proliferation. If infection continues, progressive necrosis causes malaise, fever, sweating, and cough. The mechanism may be by means of LAM inducing macrophages to secrete tumor necrosis factor.

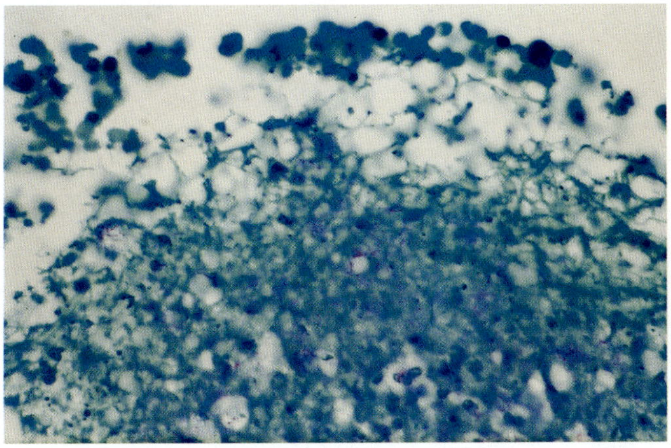

Figure 91–8. Higher magnification of one of the "tuberculous thrombi" shown in Figure 91–7. There are enormous numbers of bacilli being shed into the blood (Ziehl–Neelsen, ×400).

Miliary Tuberculosis

Tuberculous lesions may invade vessels and shower the bloodstream with bacilli (Figures 91–7 and 91–8). The result is widespread seeding. Disseminated "miliary lesions" are the consequence. Grossly they are small, creamy-white, discrete, spherical, and up to several millimeters across (Figures 91–9 and 91–10), reminding older pathologists of millet seeds—hence "miliary" tuberculosis (Figure 91–11). Miliary lesions may be in

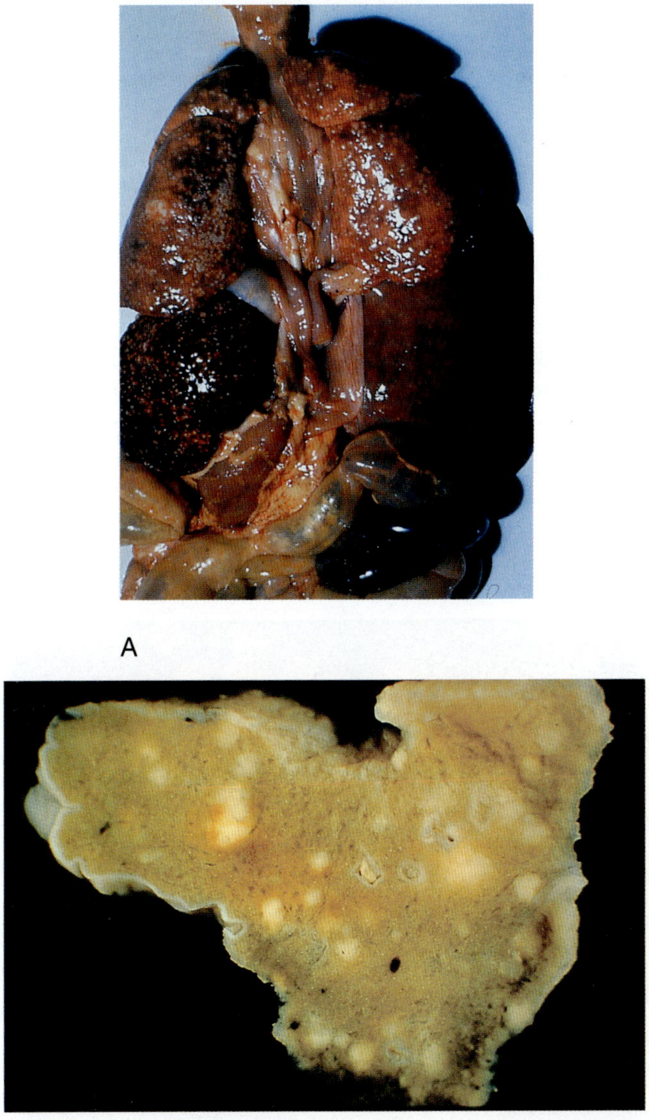

A

B

Figure 91–9. (**A**) Disseminated miliary tuberculosis in a young child. Note small miliary tubercles on surfaces of kidney and lung. The patient was anergic. (**B**) Miliary tuberculosis of lung. Most of the lesions are 1 to 2 mm across, discrete, and creamy-white. The patient also had miliary lesions in spleen, liver, lymph nodes, bone marrow, and kidney. *(Photograph by Daniel H. Connor, MD, 1978.)*

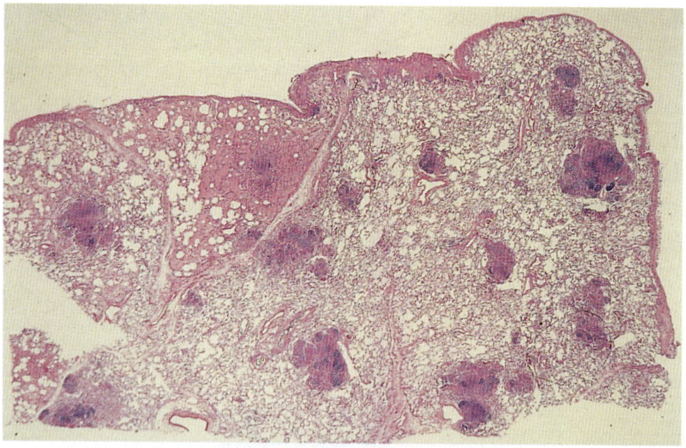

Figure 91–10. Same lung shown in Figure 91–9, B. Microscopically the lesions are foci of caseation necrosis. There is no fibrous tissue surrounding the lesions and very little cellular reaction (AFIP Neg 78-3355; hematoxylin-eosin, ×4).

almost any organ, but lung, kidney, spleen, liver, lymph nodes, and bone marrow are most heavily involved. Patients with miliary lesions may have anergic reactions or hypersensitivity reactions, but when miliary tuberculosis develops in those with immunodeficiencies, including those with AIDS, the reaction is anergic.

Anergy Versus Hypersensitivity

Before macrophages are activated, tubercle bacilli are unchecked and infection advances quickly. The macrophages, rather than killing tubercle bacilli, act instead as microincubators for them. At this stage the granuloma is anergic. Tragically, some patients do not develop activated macrophages and their reaction, therefore, remains anergic. In these patients infection progresses quickly to death. Sometimes the reason for persistent anergy is obvious. Patients receiving immunosuppressive therapy or who have AIDS, for instance, remain anergic (Figure 91–12).

In other patients the reason for persistent anergy is unclear. Perhaps they have an immunologic "blind spot." For instance, their macrophages may lack the ability to process or present antigens of the tubercle bacillus, or perhaps the patient lacks lymphocytes with sufficiently congruent receptors. Fortunately, however, most patients develop activated macrophages and when they do the reaction becomes hypersensitive. Then they have a cell-mediated immune response. Activated macrophages have the ability to kill tubercle bacilli, and the number of bacilli in tissue drops precipitously. Activation of macrophages does not guarantee healing but it gives the patient a "fighting chance."

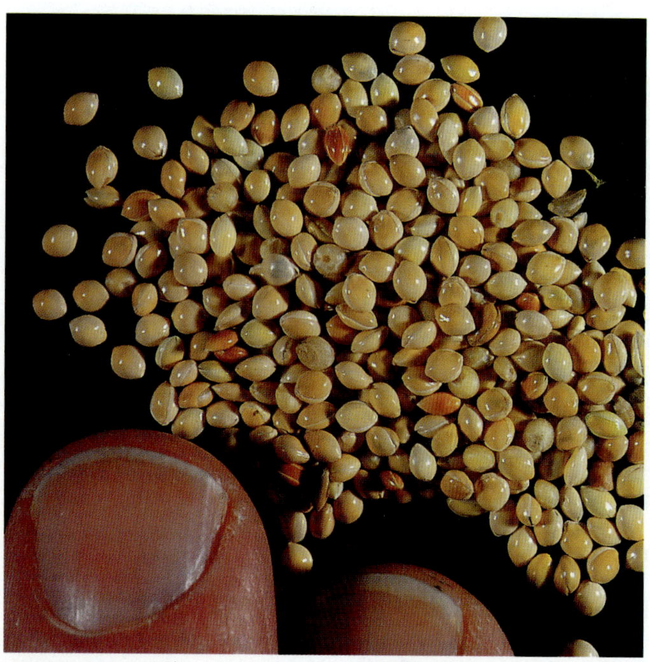

Figure 91–11. Millet. The seeds are about the size, shape, and color of the miliary lesions of tuberculosis. *(Photograph by Daniel H. Connor, MD, 1991.)*

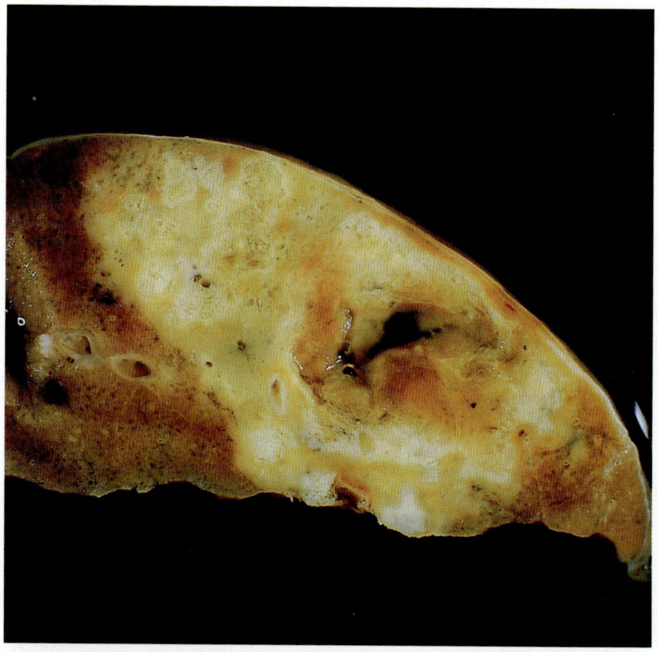

Figure 91–12. Pulmonary tuberculosis in a patient with AIDS. Note the diffuse consolidation around a central cavity. Microscopically, tubercle bacilli were abundant and there was a poorly developed granulomatous reaction. *(Photograph by Daniel H. Connor, MD, 1984.)*

PRIMARY TUBERCULOSIS

Primary tuberculosis begins when tubercle bacilli first proliferate in the body. Lung is the most common site but skin and bowel also may be primary sites. When lung is involved a focus of bronchopneumonia develops, usually in the lower lung fields.[15] In those with good nutrition and competent immunity, primary infection progresses through necrosis, granulomatous inflammation, granulation tissue, fibrosis, and finally healing with mineralization of the lesion. Macrophages sometimes carry bacilli through lymphatics to hilar nodes where a second focus of infection develops. The two lesions, parenchymal and hilar, are called the "Ghon complex" (Figure 91–13). When both become mineralized they are recognized on chest x-ray films as healed tuberculosis.[16] An early feature of hypersensitivity and healing is "palisading" of epithelioid cells. They are closely packed to form a layer around the necrotic center. They wedge themselves around the caseous areas like stacked pancakes. They are not layered, as one might suspect, with their flat surfaces against the caseous focus but are arranged radially with their long axes pointing through the granuloma. Another characteristic of hypersensitivity is the giant cell with long ("antigenic") points (Figure 91–14). These points are the ends of recently joined epithelioid cells and are a feature of antigenic stimulation and hypersensitivity. Most people heal their primary infection without clinical evidence of disease. In 5% to 15%, however, primary infection progresses to cause clinical illness with malaise, fever, night sweats, and weight loss.[7,17,18] With early diagnosis and good management, most of these patients recover. The remainder die of progressive infection.

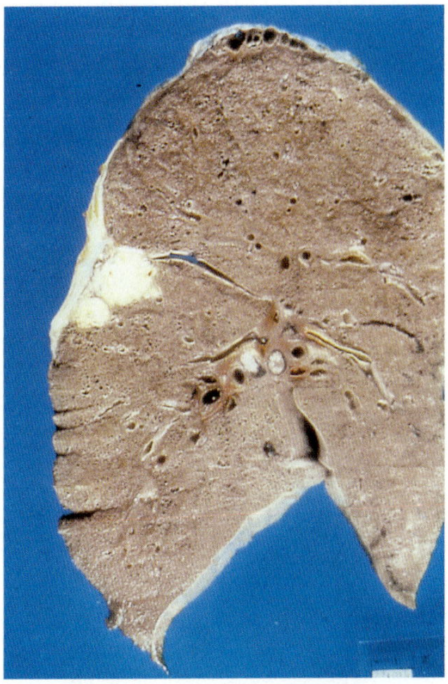

Figure 91–13. Primary tuberculosis of lung. There are two dominant lesions, both subpleural and in the upper portion of the right middle lobe. They appear to be separate but are probably confluent in a different plane. The lesions are yellow-white, indistinctly circumscribed, stony hard from advanced mineralization, and the overlying pleura is thickened and scarred. In addition, two hilar lymph nodes are also involved. They have advanced to the same stage of healing as the primary lesion, that is, they are yellow-white and stony hard from mineralization. Hilar nodes become infected when macrophages carry organisms to them from the primary focus. The mineralized primary focus in the lung and the mineralized hilar lymph nodes have a characteristic picture on chest x ray. These combined lesions are called the Ghon complex.

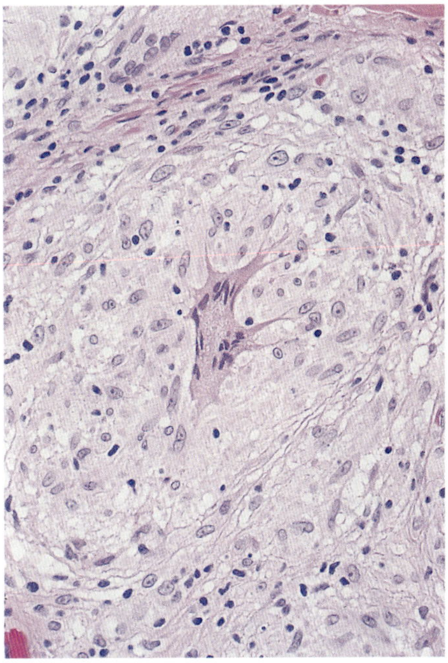

Figure 91–14. Langhans' giant cell with "antigenic points." The long tapering points on this Langhans' giant cell are residues of epithelioid cells that have recently fused to form the giant cell. They indicate active infection and a hypersensitive reaction (hematoxylin-eosin, ×400).

"Healing" in primary tuberculosis is conditional—conditional because tubercle bacilli in healed lesions continue to divide at a slow rate and antigens continue to leak out of the granuloma. Thus the patient's cellular immunity continues to be stimulated, the granuloma remains hypersensitive, and the bacilli remain incarcerated. The healed tuberculoma of primary tuberculosis therefore is a dynamic balance between contained bacilli and a perimeter of host defenses comprised of activated macrophages, epithelioid cells, Langhans' giant cells, and fibrous tissue.

REACTIVATION TUBERCULOSIS

If the patient's immune mechanisms wane, the wall of the healed primary lesion loses its integrity; tubercle bacilli proliferate more rapidly and escape through the barrier of epithelioid cells and scar tissue. The granulomas of reactivation tuberculosis may be anergic or hypersensitive, but for reasons not always clear, the balance now favors the invading bacilli. Corticosteroid therapy and infection with the human immunodeficiency virus, for instance, are two factors that promote reactivation of healed primary lesions. The infection is now destructive and continues to be so until the patient dies or until cell-mediated immunity is restored and the infection is once again contained. The various paths infection takes are summarized in Figure 91–15.

The lesions of reactivation tuberculosis vary greatly in size and distribution. Most are confined to the lung, and are characteristically in the apices of the upper lobes. They are usually hypersensitive and extensively caseating. Cavities are a characteristic feature. When caseation necrosis erodes a bronchus or bronchiole, necrotic tissue is coughed up, leaving a cavity. Bacilli proliferate in the warm, dark, moist, nutritious, aerated lining of the cavity and when these are coughed up and spit out they become a source of epidemic contagion. The outcome may be chronic cavitary tuberculosis or bacilli may spread by blood to seed meninges, causing tuberculous meningitis, and to other organs especially spleen, liver, bone marrow, adrenal, kidney, and lymph nodes. A caseating hilar or bronchial lymph node may rupture into a bronchus, another source of bacilli in sputum. Reactivation tuberculosis may involve vertebrae (Pott's disease), other bones, and sometimes the tendon sheath.[10] Tuberculomas of brain may develop. These are usually large, solitary, caseating, and in the cerebellum. Tuberculosis of fallopian tube can cause architectural distortion with fusion of tubal plicae, an appearance that has been mistaken for well-differentiated adenocarcinoma (Figure 91–16). Extensive necrocaseous tuberculosis of the adrenals can cause Addison's disease (Figures 91–17 and 91–18).[19] In one study (between 1900 and 1929) of 566 patients with Addison's disease, 70% were caused by tuberculosis.[20] Tuberculosis of bone marrow can cause a variety of hematologic abnormalities including anemia, leukopenia, monocytosis, and leukocytosis.[21] Occasionally there are leukemoid reactions and other changes resembling leukemia.

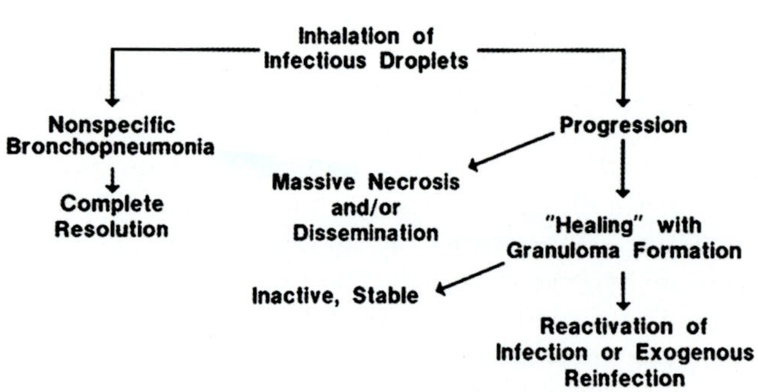

Figure 91–15. Possible consequences of tuberculosis range from early healing to miliary dissemination and death.

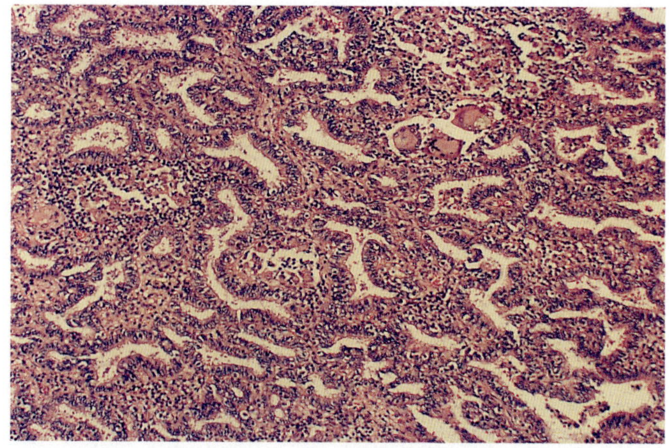

Figure 91–16. Tuberculous salpingitis with complex architectural distortion of plicae caused by inflammation and fusion. Note small granulomas and Langhans' giant cells (hematoxylin-eosin, ×100).

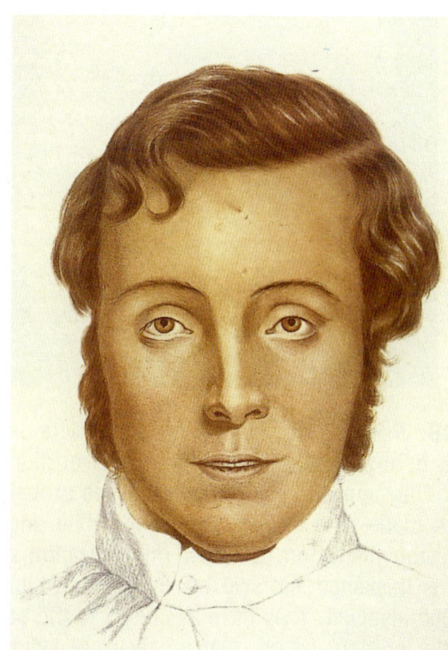

Figure 91–17. Addison's disease. Young man with pulmonary tuberculosis had diseased vertebrae with a psoas abscess on right side, which contained about a pint of "flaky" pus. Note olive hue of skin.[17]

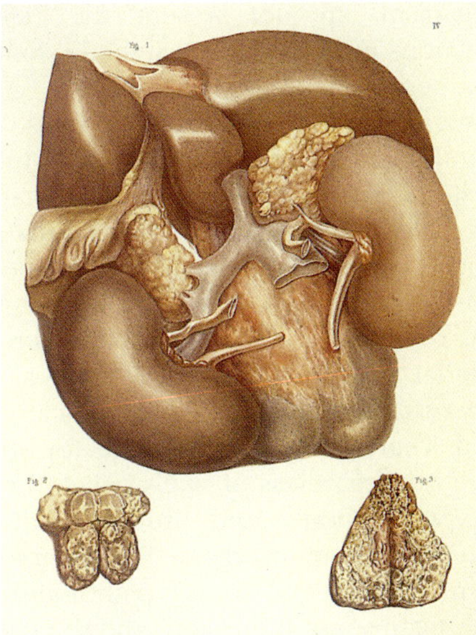

Figure 91–18. At autopsy of patient shown in Figure 91–17, both adrenal glands were enlarged and "converted into a mass of strumous disease."[19] Adrenal glands are present in situ with organ block and are bisected below.

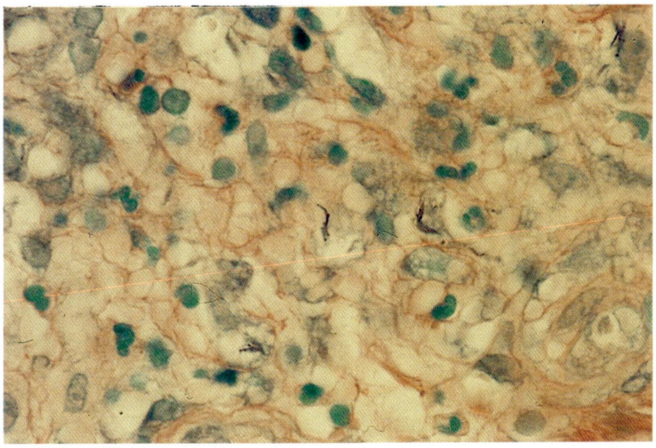

Figure 91–19. This specimen teems with acid-fast bacilli but only a few are seen with routine stains (Giemsa, ×400).

Although bovine tuberculosis, caused by *M bovis,* is now rare in the United States it was so common in the early 1900s that the cream on top of milk was called popularly "tuberculous pus."[22]

IDENTIFICATION OF TUBERCLE BACILLI

The key to diagnosis is finding mycobacteria in tissue sections. Although occasional acid-fast bacilli may stain with simple aniline dyes (Figure 91–19), the Ziehl–Neelsen stain is preferred, and in searching for acid-fast bacilli most pathologists prefer the oil immersion lens especially if organisms are scarce. In early infections and in all patients with anergic tuberculosis, organisms are numerous—sometimes massive—and are easily identified. In necrotizing granulomas, when bacilli are few, the best "hunting ground" for tubercle bacilli is the caseous center of the granuloma[23] (Figure 91–20). Later, however, when the reaction becomes hypersensitive, tubercle bacilli in the caseating centers become scarce. Their numbers are reduced for a variety of reasons—hypersensitivity, hypoxia, and a lowered pH. Then the best hunting ground shifts to the perimeter, especially in epithelioid cells and Langhans' giant cells, around the caseous center. Acid-fast bacilli, stained with carbol fuchsin, are intensely red, slender, curved, sometimes beaded, and usually 0.5×4 to 5 μm. The tubercle bacillus is also periodic acid–Schiff (PAS)-positive along with a number of other mycobacterial species,[24] and may be gram-positive although Gram staining is variable. "Acid fastness" is a consequence of the lipid-rich, hydrophobic outer membrane, which retains carbol fuchsin even when flushed with strong acid/alcohol solutions. When tubercle bacilli cannot be seen with the Ziehl–Neelsen stain, the Gomori's methenamine-silver (GMS) technique may help identify organisms because carcasses and fragments of acid-fast bacilli are silvered after they have lost their acid fastness (Figure 91–21).

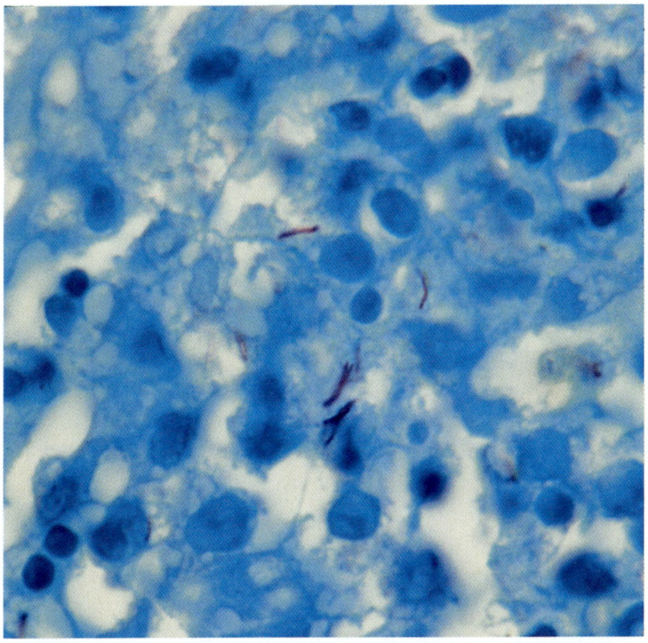

Figure 91–20. Numerous linear to curvilinear acid-fast bacilli in the caseous center of a lesion from a patient with disseminated tuberculosis (Ziehl–Neelsen stain, ×1000).

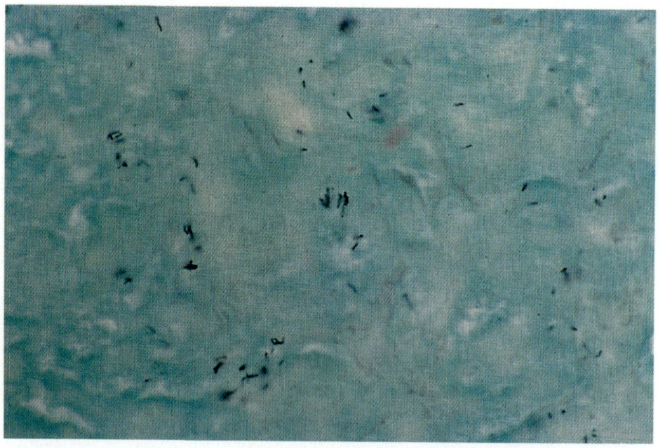

Figure 91–21. Pulmonary tuberculosis. Carcasses and fragments of tubercle bacilli are silvered by GMS. No acid-fast bacilli were identified with the Ziehl–Neelsen stain. Silvering with the GMS persists long after the bacilli lose their acid fastness (GMS, ×290).

Having identified an acid-fast bacillus, the question may arise, "Is it the cause?" Mycobacteria from extraneous sources show up regularly on slides. These spurious mycobacteria may come from tap water, or be in the water bath as holdovers from previous specimens that contained mycobacteria, or mycobacteria may contaminate solutions used to process and stain specimens. These spurious mycobacteria are called "floaters" and three guidelines help distinguish floaters from pathogens. First, microorganisms causing infections are *in,* not *on* or *under* the tissue. Thus, by focusing up and down through the tissue, floaters can usually be distinguished from pathogens. Second, the orientation of infectious organisms in tissue varies from flat to vertical, whereas floaters are typically flat. If a mycobacterium is flat it may be a floater and if there are many bacilli and they are all flat they are certain to be floaters. Third, pathogens are "in context." That is, infectious bacilli are *in* the lesions and usually concentrated in the centers of the lesions. Another practical point is that tubercle bacilli are not in the mix of lymphocytes, plasma cells, granulation tissue, and scar tissue that surrounds the caseous center. A final tip: If the lesion is caseating and granulomatous and without evidence of suppuration, then the infection—in the American context at least—is almost certain to be tuberculosis or histoplasmosis. The presence of neutrophils does not exclude tuberculosis because neutrophils are in early tuberculous lesions and also in lesions when the patient is immunodeficient,[25] but their presence broadens the differential diagnosis to include other infectious granulomas. Histoplasmosis can be excluded because the yeasts and carcasses of *Histoplasma capsulatum* are centered in the areas of caseation and readily silvered with GMS. They are thus quickly identified, when present. If *H capsulatum* organisms are not present, the Ziehl–Neelsen stained sections must then be searched—sometimes for prolonged periods.

Having identified a mycobacterial cause for a caseating granuloma, can one then diagnose tuberculosis? This question begs for debate and perhaps endless definition. One argument claims "yes"—that any mycobacterial infection with caseation *is* tuberculosis. This is the "inclusive" definition. The opposite or "exclusive" definition reserves a diagnosis of tuberculosis for mycobacterial infections caused by "typical" strains of *M tuberculosis.* This presumes that "typical" strains can be defined. There are good arguments for both sides of this debate but regardless of one's belief, the important problems of taxonomy and drug-resistant strains of *M tuberculosis* belong to others. The pathologist's role, however, remains unique, for the pathologist alone sees the causal organism in the lesion, and the pathologist is thus alone among specialists in seeing and being certain of the cause.

The fluorescent Auramine–Rhodamine stain is a rapid and sensitive technique for demonstrating mycobacteria (Figure 91–22). Mycobacteria can be seen at low magnifications and frequently even with the scanning objective.[26] This is so because the Auramine–Rhodamine stain shows bacilli "glowing in the dark," but the dark background obscures the relationship of the mycobacteria and host tissue. A positive identification, therefore, requires that a slide be stained by the Ziehl–Neelsen method to be certain a bacillus is not a floater. Most pathologists, therefore, prefer to use the Ziehl–Neelsen stain as the first and only stain. DNA "fingerprinting" using the polymerase chain reaction (PCR) has detected mycobacterial DNA in formalin-fixed paraffin-embedded tissue.[27–29] PCR may even permit specific identification.[30] Of special interest are speci-

Figure 91–22. Fluorescence microscopy shows bacilli reactive with the Auramine–Rhodamine stain (×120).

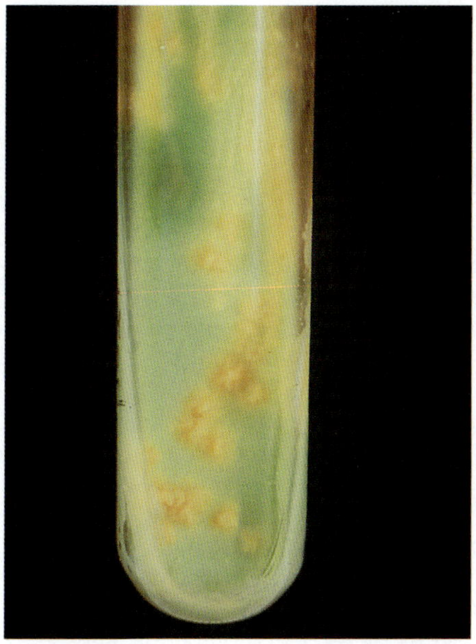

Figure 91–23. Growth of *M tuberculosis* on a slant of Lowenstein–Jensen medium. Colonies have a buff hue and rough surface. Biochemical testing confirmed the isolate.

mens from patients with sarcoid containing mycobacterial DNA.[27]

Isolation of *M tuberculosis* in pure culture permits specific identification and sensitivity studies to screen for drug susceptibility.[31,32] Colonies of *M tuberculosis* can be identified as early as 3 weeks, although some isolates require 6 weeks or longer to grow. Colonies are typically eugonic with a buff tint and rough contour caused by serpentine cording on the surface (Figure 91–23). Rapid identification of *M tuberculosis* and other mycobacteria is possible by automated DNA sequencing, which is PCR based and therefore may be used with primary specimens or early cultures with the BACTEC radiorespiratory detection system. Preliminary data demonstrate the feasibility of specific identification of mycobacteria and the potential to identify mutations associated with antimicrobial resistance in less than 48 hours.[33]

TUBERCULIN SKIN TEST

A skin test for tuberculosis utilizes a purified protein derivative (PPD) of the tubercle bacillus. When the response is positive, the skin becomes slightly raised, indurated, and red in 1 to 3 days. Microscopically the reaction is an epithelioid cell granuloma. On rare occasions skin test antigens provoke extensive necrosis and sloughing (Figure 91–24). Patients who fail to react to PPD are those who 1) have never been infected by *M tuberculosis,* or 2) have been infected but are anergic, or 3) have an infection so recent that hypersensitivity has not had time to develop. A small number of patients fail to react even though they have normal immune mechanisms. These are the so-called nonreactors. Why they fail to react is uncertain. If they form healing granulomas to antigens released by their infecting mycobacteria but fail to form granulomas at the test site, the antigens from the infecting bacillus and the test antigens must not be congruent. A patient can be converted iatrogenically from negative to positive by vaccination with bacille Calmette–Guérin and sometimes by repeated injections of PPD.

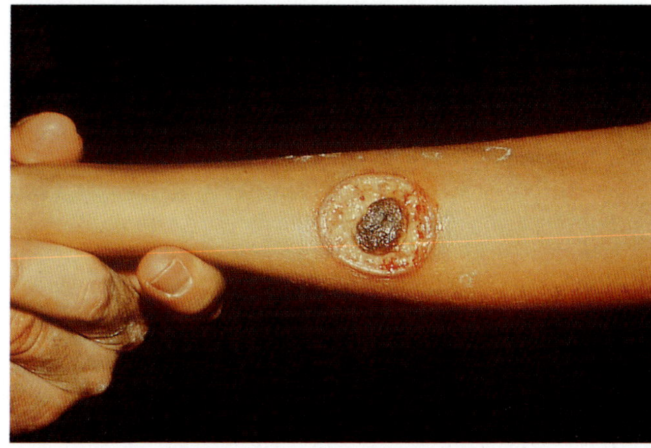

Figure 91–24. Sloughing of skin and subcutis at the site of injection of tuberculin. Patient had a hyperimmune response with dermal and subcutaneous necrosis.

REFERENCES

1. Lin JI. Centennial discovery of tubercle bacillus. *Lab Med.* 1982;13:699–702.
2. Dubos R, Dubos J. *The White Plague: Tuberculosis, Man and Society.* Boston: Little, Brown; 1952.
3. Smith H. John Keats: poet, patient, physician. *Rev Infect Dis.* 1984;6:390–404.
4. Ryan F. *The Forgotten Plague.* New York: Little, Brown; 1993.
5. Abbott CE. Composers and tuberculosis: the effects on creativity. *Can Med Assoc J.* 1982;126:534, 536–538, 543–544.
6. Krause RM. After AIDS: the risk of other plagues. *Cosmos.* 1991;1:15–21.
7. Barnes PF, Bloch AB, Davidson PT, Snider DE Jr. Tuberculosis in patients with human immunodeficiency virus infection. *N Engl J Med.* 1991;324:1644–1650.
8. Gracey DR. Commentary: tuberculosis in the world today. *Mayo Clin Proc.* 1988;63:1251–1255.
9. Iseman MD. Treatment of multidrug-resistant tuberculosis. *N Engl J Med.* 1993;329:784–791.
10. Small PM, Shafer RW, Hopewell PC, et al. Exogenous reinfection with multidrug-resistant *Mycobacterium tuberculo-*

sis in patients with advanced HIV infection. *N Engl J Med.* 1993;328:1137–1144.

11. Goble M, Iseman MD, Madsen LA, Waite D, Ackerson L, Horsburgh CR Jr. Treatment of 171 patients with pulmonary tuberculosis resistant to isoniazid and rifampin. *N Engl J Med.* 1993;328:527–532.
12. Frieden TR, Sterling T, Pablos-Mendez A, Kilburn JO, Cauthen GM, Dooley SW. The emergence of drug-resistant tuberculosis in New York City. *N Engl J Med.* 1993;328:521–526.
13. Menzies D, Fanning A, Yuan L, Fitzgerald M. Tuberculosis among health care workers. *N Engl J Med.* 1995;332:92–98.
14. Cantwell MF, Shehab ZM, Costello AM, et al. Brief report: congenital tuberculosis. *N Engl J Med.* 1994;330:1051–1054.
15. Boom WH, Patel RJ. Tuberculosis: diagnostic methods for a resurgent disease. *Lab Management.* January 1987: 37–42.
16. Midthun DE, Swensen SJ, Jett JR. Approach to the solitary pulmonary nodule. *Mayo Clin Proc.* 1993;68:378–385.
17. Youmans GP. *Tuberculosis.* Philadelphia: WB Saunders; 1979.
18. Glassroth J, Robins AG, Snider DE Jr. Tuberculosis in the 1980's. *N Engl J Med.* 1980;302:1441–1450.
19. Addison T. *On the Constitutional and Local Effects of Disease of the Suprarenal Capsules.* London: Samuel Highley; 1855. Reproduced by Classics of Medicine Library, 1980.
20. Guttman PH. Addison's disease. A statistical analysis of five hundred and sixty-six cases and study of the pathology. *Arch Pathol.* 1930;10:742–785, 895–935.
21. Glasser RM, Walker RI, Herion JC. The significance of hematologic abnormalities in patients with tuberculosis. *Ann Intern Med.* 1970;125:691–695.
22. Dunlop D. Eighty-six cases of Addison's disease. *Br Med J.* 1963;2:887–891.
23. Ulbright TM, Katzenstein A-LA. Solitary necrotizing granulomas of the lung. Differentiating features and etiology. *Am J Surg Pathol.* 1980;4:13–28.
24. Wear DJ, Hadfield TL, Connor DH, et al. Periodic acid–Schiff reaction stains *Mycobacterium tuberculosis, Mycobacterium leprae, Mycobacterium ulcerans, Mycobacterium chelonei (abscessus)* and *Mycobacterium kansasii. Arch Pathol Lab Med.* 1985;109:701–702.
25. Lucas S, Nelson AM. Pathogenesis of tuberculosis in human immunodeficiency virus infected people. In: Bloom BR, ed. *Tuberculosis: Pathogenesis, Protection and Control.* Washington, DC: American Society for Microbiology: 1994:503–513.
26. Kommareddi S, Abramowsky CR, Swinehart GL, Hrabak L. Nontuberculous mycobacterial infections: comparison of the fluorescent auramine-O and Ziehl–Neelsen techniques in tissue diagnosis. *Hum Pathol.* 1984;15:1085–1089.
27. Popper HH, Winter E, Höfler G. DNA of *Mycobacterium tuberculosis* in formalin-fixed, paraffin-embedded tissue in tuberculosis and sarcoidosis detected by polymerase chain reaction. *Am J Clin Pathol.* 1994;101:738–741.
28. Small PM, Hopewell PC, Singh SP, et al. The epidemiology of tuberculosis in San Francisco; a population-based study using conventional and molecular methods. *N Engl J Med.* 1994;330:1703–1709.
29. Ghossein RA, Ross DG, Salomon RN, Rabson AR. A search for mycobacterial DNA in sarcoidosis using the polymerase chain reaction. *Am J Clin Pathol.* 1994;101:733–737.
30. Ghossein RA, Ross DG, Salomon RN, Rabson AR. Rapid detection and species identification of mycobacteria in paraffin-embedded tissues by polymerase chain reaction. *Diagn Mol Pathol.* 1992;1:185–191.
31. Runyon EH, Karlson AG, Kubica GP, Wayne LG. Mycobacterium. In: Lennette EH, Spaulding EH, Truant JP, eds. *Manual of Clinical Microbiology.* 2nd ed. Washington, DC: American Society for Microbiology; 1974.
32. Sommers HM. The identification of Mycobacteria. *Lab Med.* 1978;9:34–43.
33. Kapur V, Li L-L, Hamrich MR, et al. Rapid *Mycobacterium* species assignment and unambiguous identification of mutations associated with antimicrobial resistance in *Mycobacterium tuberculosis* by automated DNA sequencing. *Arch Pathol Lab Med.* 1995;119:131–138.

CHAPTER 92

Tularemia

Stanley J. Geyer, Adam Burkey, and Francis W. Chandler

Medicine is a science of uncertainty and an art of probability.

Sir William Osler (1849–1919)

DEFINITION

Tularemia, a zoonotic bacterial infection caused by the small gram-negative pleomorphic coccobacillus *Francisella tularensis,* is typically characterized by a mucocutaneous ulcer at the site of entry, high fever, severe constitutional symptoms, and enlargement of regional lymph nodes. Tularemia was discovered in 1910 by George W. McCoy during his investigation of a plague-like epizootic among ground squirrels in Tulare County, California. In 1912, Drs. McCoy and Charles W. Chapin isolated *F tularensis* (formerly *Pasteurella tularensis*) and demonstrated that it could cause infection of humans. In 1919, Dr. Edward Francis demonstrated that deerfly fever, described 8 years earlier, was tularemia, and he began investigations on its epidemiology and immunology.

Tularemia is sometimes referred to as rabbit fever or deerfly fever because the causative organism infects wild animals such as rabbits, rodents, squirrels, deer, and raccoons, and insect vectors such as deerflies and ticks.

EPIDEMIOLOGY

Tularemia occurs throughout the Northern Hemisphere. In the United States, most infections are in the south central region. Infections occur throughout the year but peak in summer from tick transmission and in winter from infected animal carcasses. Water contaminated by infected beavers, muskrats, and voles has caused outbreaks, and laboratory workers have been infected by breathing aerosolized organisms.[1] Infections have been caused also by consumption of contaminated water. More than 100 species of animals have been infected and each of these animals has been reported to be a source of human infection. Most are lagomorphs (rabbits and hares), rodents, raccoons, squirrels, and cats. In addition to wild animals, domestic animals can become infected and be a source of infection for humans. At least six patients have acquired infections from cats.[2]

ETIOLOGIC AGENT

Francisella tularensis is a weakly gram-negative, nonmotile coccobacillus, that is 0.2 by 0.2 to 0.7 μm in size. It has a bipolar staining pattern with Giemsa and other polychrome stains. A thick capsule surrounds virulent organisms, and loss of the capsule is associated with a loss of virulence.[3] The organism is an obligate aerobe and grows in culture over a temperature range of 24 to 39°C. Optimal growth is at 37°C. Exposure to 56°C for 10 minutes kills *F tularensis,* but freezing does not. Although all strains of *F tularensis* are serologically identical, there are two types: Jellison type A, which is more virulent, and Jellison type B, which causes milder infections. Culture in modified Mueller–Hinton broth is a reliable in vitro indicator for the efficacy of antimicrobial therapy.[4]

CLINICAL FEATURES

Infection by *F tularensis* usually causes inflammation and necrosis in some combination of lymph node, skin, eye, oropharynx, and lung.[5] Incubation varies from 1 day to 3 weeks, and onset is usually abrupt with malaise, fever, chills, and headache dominating. The six

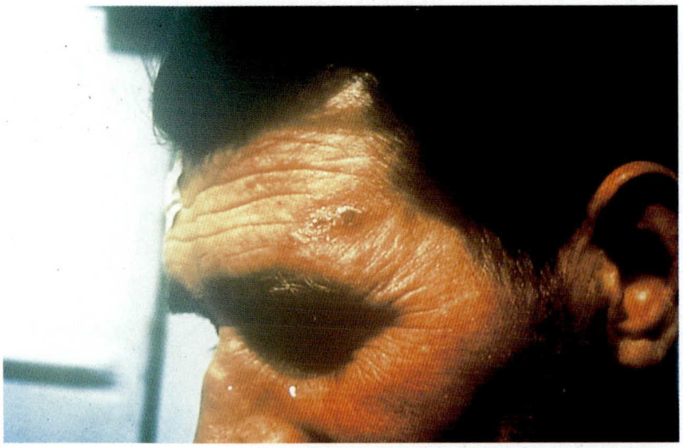

Figure 92–1. Ulcerative facial lesion of tularemia in a muskrat trapper. *(Contributed by the Centers for Disease Control and Prevention, Atlanta.)*

clinical types of tularemia are ulceroglandular, glandular, typhoidal, oculoglandular, oropharyngeal, and pneumonic. *Ulceroglandular tularemia* is most common, accounting for 70% to 80% of all infections. Lymph nodes draining a site of cutaneous inoculation become enlarged, firm, and painful. Skin at the site of inoculation develops small, red papules that become ulcers with sharp borders (Figures 92–1 and 92–2). Eventually a dark crust covers the ulcers, which finally heal and leave residual scars. *Glandular tularemia* is less common, accounting for 10% to 15% of infections, and is characterized by painful enlargement of lymph nodes. This clinical type is the same as ulceroglandular tularemia except that the site of inoculation is not apparent. *Typhoidal tularemia* also accounts for 10% to 15% of infections. It has features of sepsis, but there is no lymphadenopathy or other localizing features. Diagnosis is established by blood culture. About half the patients with typhoidal tularemia have pulmonary infiltrates that may be misdiagnosed as legionellosis. *Oculoglandular tularemia* is rare, accounting for 1% to 5% of infections. Conjunctiva is the portal of entry. Ulcers appear on the palpebral conjunctiva, and draining lymph nodes in the preauricular, submandibular, and cervical regions become enlarged and painful. *Oropharyngeal tularemia* is a variant of the ulceroglandular form and occurs when the pharynx is the portal of entry, usually from eating contaminated and inadequately cooked meat. Also, oropharyngeal tularemia may be associated with the typhoidal form. In the series reviewed by Dienst,[5] one third of those with typhoidal tularemia had oropharyngeal lesions. Ulcerative pharyngitis, tonsillitis, and cervical lymphadenopathy are characteristic. Patients may present with a gray necrotic pseudomembrane that resembles a diphtheritic membrane and covers the posterior pharyngeal wall and tonsils. It is removed with difficulty but does not normally bleed. Infection may spread to soft palate, uvula, and buccal mucosa.[5] There is primary or secondary involvement of lung in most fatal infections. *Primary pulmonary tularemia* is caused by inhaled aerosolized droplets containing *F tularensis*.[6,7] It is rare when compared with the fairly high prevalence of secondary pleuropulmonary tularemia.[8] Organisms spread to lungs through blood and lymph. Patients have a dry cough, dyspnea, pleuritic pain, cyanosis, rales, dullness on percussion, bronchophony, and pleural friction rubs. About two thirds of patients have bilateral involvement, and chest radiographs reveal any combination of bronchopneumonia, hilar adenopathy, pleural effusion, consolidation, apical infiltrates, and focal densities. Residual lesions of pulmonary tularemia may include areas of calcification and fibrosis.[8]

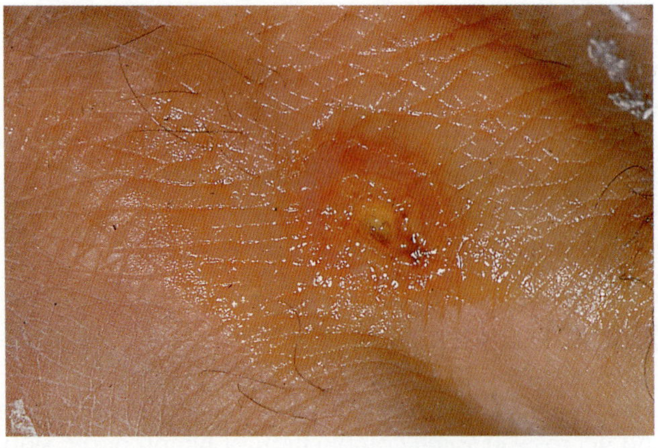

Figure 92–2. Cutaneous ulcer, caused by *F tularensis* on the hand of a trapper with tularemia. *(Contributed by the Centers for Disease Control and Prevention, Atlanta.)*

Regardless of portal of entry, onset and general features of tularemia tend to be the same. The usual incubation period is 3 to 5 days, with a range of 1 to 21 days. There is abrupt onset with fever, chills, headache, cough, generalized myalgia, and vomiting.[9] The initial symptoms usually disappear in 1 to 4 days, followed by remission for 1 to 3 days, and then recurrence for an additional 2 to 3 weeks. The cause of death in untreated patients appears to be septicemia or a lower nephron syndrome manifested by uremia, oliguria, acidosis, and sometimes hypoglycemia. Pneumonic symptoms also can be severe and usually portend a poor prognosis; a 55% mortality rate has been reported.[5] Rhabdomyolysis with myoglobinuria and extremely high CPK levels have been documented and can lead to renal failure. Renal involvement, however, may occur without rhabdomyolysis.[10] Finally, bacteremia has been associated with more severe infections.[11]

PATHOLOGY

The acute inflammatory response to the invading bacteria is intense and consists of fibrin, neutrophils, macrophages, and T lymphocytes (Figure 92–3). In early lesions, neutrophils and macrophages surround clusters of degenerating and necrotic inflammatory cells. Later there are lymphocytes, epithelioid cells, and a few giant cells. There may be extensive necrosis and cavitation of lung (Figure 92–4) and extensive necrosis of lymph nodes that begins beneath the capsule (Figures 92–5 through 92–7). Necrotic areas may resemble infarcts. Thrombosis and necrosis of small and medium-sized veins and arteries are common. The organisms, although concentrated in areas of necrosis and inflammation, are difficult to demonstrate in tissue sections. In our experience, *F tularensis* cannot be satisfactorily demonstrated in tissue sections stained by any of the modified Gram techniques (Figure 92–8). The silver impregnation techniques (Steiner, Dieterle, Warthin–Starry), however, coat the organisms with metallic silver, enlarge their silhouettes, and make them black and opaque (Figure 92–9). Organisms are usually in macrophages and epithelioid cells. Gallivan et al[2] reported that organisms were seen in Dieterle-stained sections of necrotic lung, after which bacilli were specifically identified in sections of lung by immunofluorescence. In kidney, acute tubular necrosis, glomerulonephritis, and acute interstitial nephritis have been described.[12] Organizing abscesses in the rectus abdominis muscles of some patients suggest that the acute rhabdomyolysis associated with tularemia can be caused by direct involvement of skeletal muscle.[10] Residual lesions of pulmonary tularemia include areas of caseation, calcification, and fibrosis.[8]

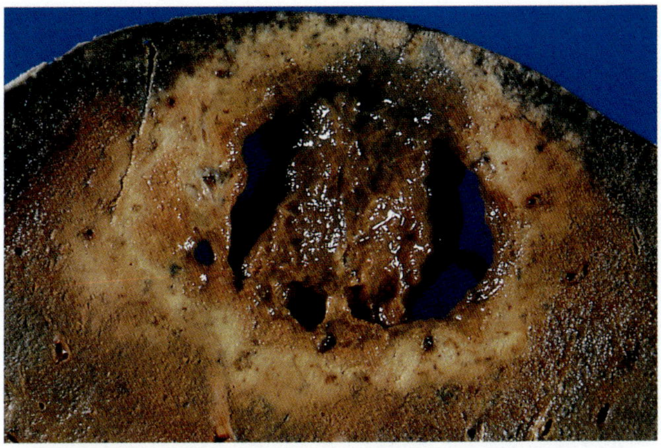

Figure 92–4. Fatal case of cat-transmitted tularemia. A 65-year-old man was accidentally bitten by his pet cat and developed an ulcer at the site on the back of his left hand. Five days later he had sudden onset of spiking fever and shaking chills. On examination he had a nonhealing ulcer at the site of the bite and tender lymphadenopathy in the left axilla. He died after 3 weeks in hospital of tularemia involving lungs, lymph nodes, spleen, liver, and peritoneum. The combined weight of the lungs was 4000 g and they were diffusely consolidated. In addition, there were areas of necrosis and cavitation. This picture shows a pulmonary cavity with a liquid, necrotic center surrounded by a yellow zone of consolidated lung. *(Contributed by Monica Gallivan, MD.)*

IMMUNITY

Protective antibodies diminish with time, and by 25 years, serum agglutination titers are low (usually below 40). T-cell memory for infection by *F tularensis,* however, is long—perhaps lasting for the life of the patient.[13]

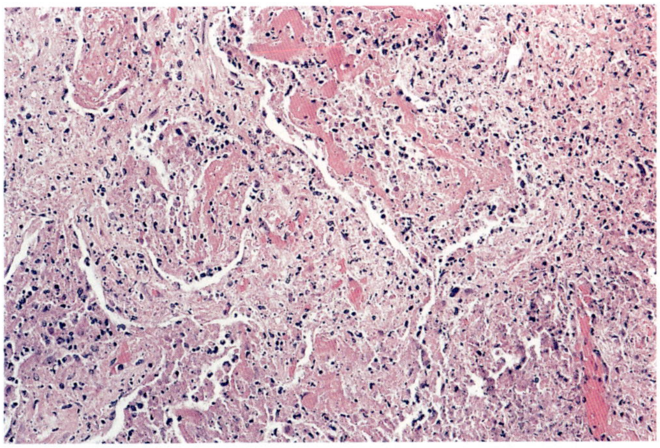

Figure 92–3. Acute tularemic pneumonia. Alveolar spaces and terminal bronchioles contain abundant fibrin and necrotic macrophages. There is extensive necrosis of alveolar septa (hematoxylin-eosin, ×25).

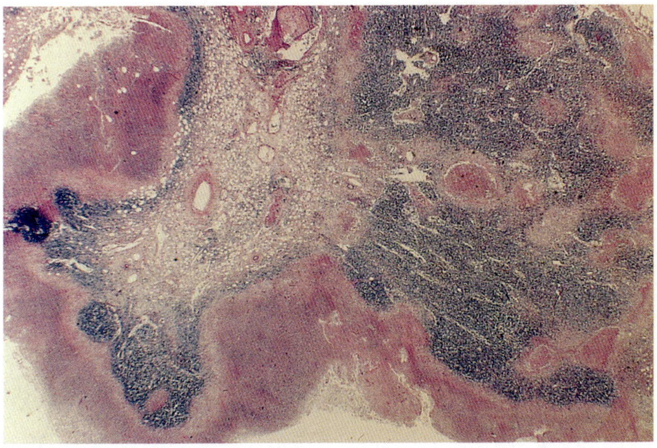

Figure 92–5. An axillary lymph node contains geographic areas of confluent liquefactive necrosis. The necrosis involves the outer cortex (hematoxylin-eosin, ×10).

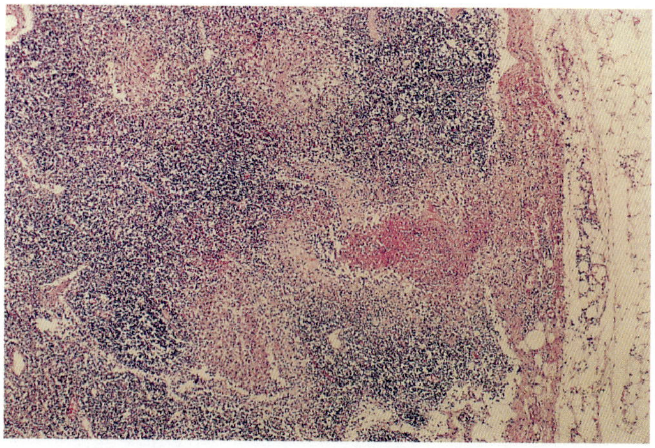

Figure 92–6. Early necrosis of the same lymph node shown in Figure 92–5. The necrosis is subcapsular, centered in an abscess, and intensely eosinophilic. Localization of the necrotic areas to the subcapsular region suggests that *F tularensis* entered the node through the afferent lymphatics (hematoxylin-eosin, ×100). *(Contributed by Ernest E. Lack, MD.)*

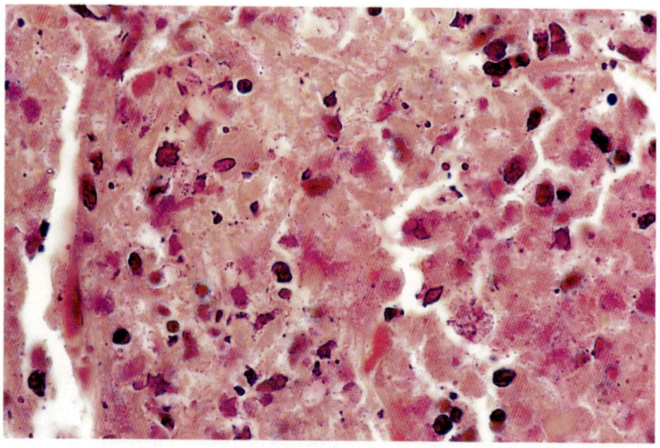

Figure 92–8. Tularemic pneumonia. Alveolar macrophages contain weakly gram-negative coccobacilli that are *F tularensis* (modified Brown–Hopps stain using 1% basic fuchsin, ×100).

LABORATORY CONFIRMATION

Because *F tularensis* is not a laboratory contaminant, its identification by culture establishes a diagnosis of tularemia. *Francisella tularensis* can be isolated from primary ulcers, lymph nodes, bone marrow, and other tissues. In culture, *F tularensis* is an obligate aerobe, requires the amino acids cystine and cysteine for growth, and is stimulated by increased CO_2. Colonies may not be visible for 3 to 5 days on agar. *Francisella tularensis* is oxidase negative, grows poorly on MacConkey agar, is biochemically inert, and can be isolated on buffered charcoal yeast extract agar. Agglutination tests with antisera enable specific identification of *F tularensis*. Handling organisms and cultures poses a risk to laboratory personnel because the organism can penetrate small breaks in the skin. Specimens from patients with suspected tularemia, therefore, must be handled with great care under a safety hood. The antigen skin test and the agglutination test are equally sensitive in detecting tularemia between 4 weeks and 2 years after infection.[14,15] Outside this interval, however, the skin test is more sensitive, becoming positive in the first or second week of illness. It can be read after 48 hours and may remain positive for up to 40 years.[14] Serologic testing is helpful, especially when culture is

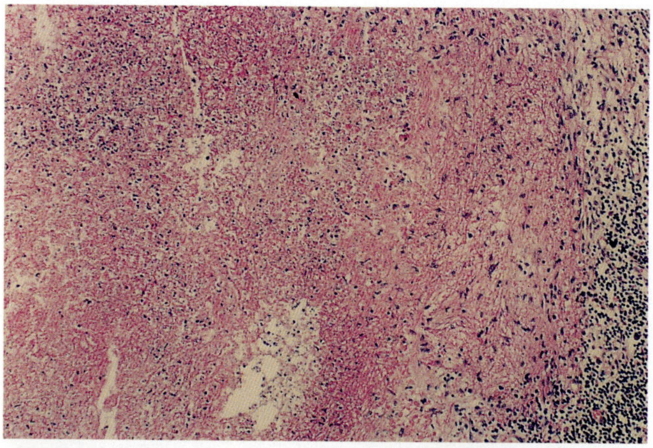

Figure 92–7. Higher magnification of the lymph node shown in Figures 92–5 and 92–6. There is a sharply defined area of coagulation necrosis (hematoxylin-eosin, ×10). *(Contributed by Ernest E. Lack, MD.)*

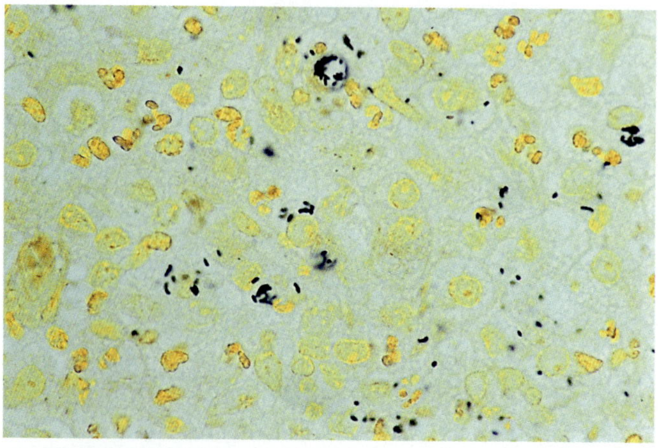

Figure 92–9. Tularemic pneumonia. Small coccobacilli—*F tularensis*—are mostly in macrophages and are silvered and blackened by the Steiner silver impregnation technique (×100).

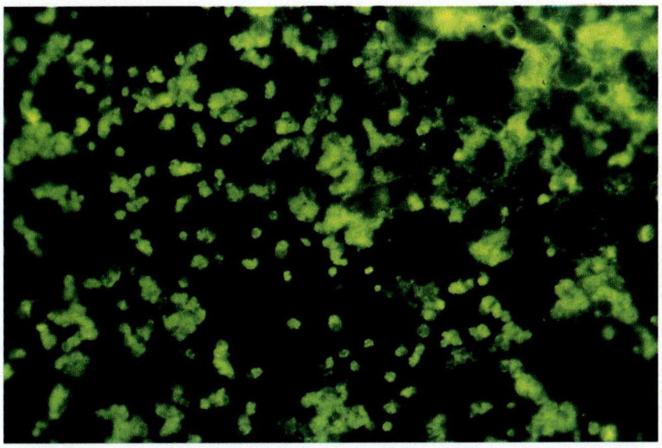

Figure 92–10. Liver of a mouse infected with *F tularensis* and stained with a specific fluorescent antibody. Numerous short plump bacilli are present (×1000). *(Contributed by the Centers for Disease Control and Prevention, Atlanta.)*

not available or negative. A microagglutination assay detects IgM anti–*F tularensis* antibodies.[15] *Francisella tularensis* can be identified also by direct immunofluorescence (Figure 92–10) in smears of exudates from lesions and in formalin-fixed, deparaffinized tissue sections.[2]

TREATMENT

Streptomycin is the drug of choice, and when begun promptly at the appropriate dose, cures the patient. Delayed or inappropriate therapy is the most common cause of persistent infection and death.[16] About 5% of untreated patients die. Rapid therapy with aminoglycosides has been recommended for anyone with suspected tularemia, and especially for those with an underlying debilitating disease such as chronic lung disease, ischemic heart disease, diabetes, or chronic glomerulonephritis.[16] Dramatic improvement is usual within 3 days when 7.5 mg/kg body weight is given intramuscularly every 12 hours. This is continued for 10 days. Erythromycin, tetracycline, gentamycin, and chloramphenicol also are effective, but patients are likely to relapse when not treated with streptomycin.[17] Doxycycline, a tetracycline metabolized mostly by the liver, has been used successfully in patients with renal impairment. Intravenous administration once per day avoids inactivation by the antacids used in treating renal failure.[12]

REFERENCES

1. Taylor JP, Istre GR, McChesney TC, Satalowich FT, Parker RL, McFarland LM. Epidemiologic characteristics of human tularemia in the southwest-central states, 1981–1987. *Am J Epidemiol.* 1991;133:1032–1038.
2. Gallivan MVE, Davis WA II, Garagusi VF, Paris AL, Lack EE. Fatal cat-transmitted tularemia: demonstration of the organism in tissue. *South Med J.* 1980;73:240–242.
3. Gutman LT. *Francisella.* In: Joklik WK, Willet HP, Amos DB, Wilfert CM, eds. *Zinsser Microbiology.* 20th ed. Norwalk, Conn: Appleton & Lange; 1992:595–599.
4. Baker CN, Hollis DG, Thornsberry C. Antimicrobial susceptibility testing of *Francisella tularensis* with a modified Mueller–Hinton broth. *J Clin Microbiol.* 1985;22:212–215.
5. Dienst FT. Tularemia: a perusal of three hundred thirty-nine cases. *J Louisiana State Med Soc.* 1963;115:114–127.
6. Stuart BM, Pulley RL. Tularemic pneumonia. Review of American literature and report of 15 additional cases. *Am J Med Sci.* 1945;210:223–236.
7. Avery FW, Barnett TB. Pulmonary tularemia. A report of five cases and a consideration of pathogenesis and terminology. *Am Rev Resp Dis.* 1967;95:584–591.
8. Miller RP, Bates JH. Pleuropulmonary tularemia: a review of 29 patients. *Am Rev Resp Dis.* 1969;99:31–41.
9. Evans ME, Gregory DW, Schaffner W, McGee ZA. Tularemia: a 30 year experience with 88 cases. *Medicine.* 1985;64:251–269.
10. Kaiser AB, Rieves D, Price AH, et al. Tularemia and rhabdomyolysis. *JAMA.* 1985;253:241–243.
11. Provenza JM, Klotz SA, RL Penn. Isolation of *Francisella tularensis* from blood. *J Clin Microbiol.* 1986;24:453–455.
12. Tilley WS, Garman RW, WJ Stone. Tularemia complicated by acute renal failure. *South Med J.* 1983;76:273–274.
13. Ericsson M, Sandström G, Sjöstedt, Tärnvik A. Persistence of cell-mediated immunity and decline of humoral immunity to intracellular bacterium *Francisella tularensis* 25 years after natural infection. *J Infect Dis.* 1994;170: 110–114.
14. Buchanan TM, Brooks GF, Brachman PS. The tularemia skin test: 325 skin tests in 210 persons: serologic correlation and review of the literature. *Ann Intern Med.* 1971; 74:336–343.
15. Sato T, Fujita H, Ohara Y, Homma M. Microagglutination test for early specific serodiagnosis of tularemia. *J Clin Microbiol.* 1990;28:2372–2374.
16. Penn RL, GT Kinasewitz. Factors associated with a poor outcome in tularemia. *Arch Intern Med.* 1987;147:265–268.
17. Westerman EL, McDonald J. Tularemic pneumonia mimicking Legionnaires' disease: isolation of organism on CYE agar and successful treatment with erythromycin. *South Med J.* 1983;76:1169–1170.

CHAPTER 93

Typhoid Fever

Jerome H. Smith

She died of a fever, and no one could save her,
And that was the end of sweet Molly Malone;
Her ghost wheels her barrow through streets broad and narrow,
Crying, Cockles and Mussels! A-live, A-live oh!

Irish Folk Song

In typhoid gut changes are found
Great patches of Peyer profound
Have cell infiltration
And then ulceration
From which Salmonella abound.

Leslie H. Sobin (1934–), A Pathology Primer in Verse, 2nd ed., Nomad Press, Washington, DC, 1991.

DEFINITION

Typhoid fever is an acute febrile systemic illness caused by motile gram-negative bacilli of the genus *Salmonella,* usually by *Salmonella typhi* and *S paratyphi A,* occasionally by *S paratyphi B (S schottmuelleri)* and *S paratyphi C (S hirschfeldii)* and rarely by other *Salmonellae* and *Citrobacter freundii.*[1,2] Other species of *Salmonella* produce assorted gastroenterocolitides causing diarrhea with transient bacteremia, but these are differentiated from typhoid or enteric fever, which is a systemic infection. Typhoid fever is also known as enteric fever and paratyphoid fever.

GEOGRAPHIC DISTRIBUTION

Typhoid fever is cosmopolitan, striking where sanitary controls break down or are not yet established. Strains of *S typhi* resistant to traditionally effective antibiotics have emerged in Southeast Asia, the Indian subcontinent, subsaharan Africa, and western South America.[3–18]

EPIDEMIOLOGY

Although worldwide, typhoid fever is endemic where sanitary controls are inadequate. Water and dairy products contaminated with human excreta cause major outbreaks; minor outbreaks and isolated infections result from ingesting shellfish harvested from contaminated waters. The 5 F's of typhoid transmission are food, fingers, flies, fomites, and feces. Throughout history, typhoid fever has been a scourge of armies and refugees. Today, in countries with modern sanitary control of water and milk, typhoid fever is sharply reduced. Although vaccination provides some protection, it cannot replace sanitary control. Routine vaccination is no longer recommended in the United States. It is restricted to travelers to endemic areas and to those in a community or institution where outbreaks have occurred. Recent progress in vaccines has increased their efficacy and may simultaneously include immunization to cholera.[19–24]

MORPHOLOGY OF ORGANISM

All species causing typhoid fever are facultative anaerobic gram-negative bacilli of the family Enterobacteriaceae. All have in common the Vi antigen.

CLINICAL FEATURES

Typhoid fever may present in various ways, such as sustained fever, headache, diarrhea or constipation, anorexia, vomiting, abdominal distention, cough, or apathy. Classically, untreated typhoid fever progresses through five stages: incubation, active invasion, fastigium, lysis, and convalescence (Figure 93–1). Incubation is usually 10 to 14 days, but varies from 5 to 30 days, depending on the size of the infecting dose. Each of the other stages lasts approximately 1 week. Typically, symptoms progress gradually. There are daily, stepwise elevations in temperature during active invasion. In some patients, rose spots resembling petechial hemorrhages develop on the trunk. Leukopenia and bradycardia may be prominent, even when temperature is elevated. At the fastigium, symptoms are maximal and there is continuous fever with only slight daily fluctuations. During lysis, symptoms wane and fever slowly falls, but daily fluctuations in temperature are extreme. In convalescence, weakness and fatigue occur, but no other symptoms, and temperatures may be slightly subnormal.

While the classical presentation and course still occur in untreated nonimmune adults, many patients in the antibiotic era present with a more ambiguous syndrome characterized by fever, headache, diarrhea, abdominal pain, and some respiratory symptoms (cough and sore throat) with prominent hepatosplenomegaly.[25–31] Signs and symptoms are even more obscure among children and infants.[32–35] A good prognosis depends mainly on early specific treatment. Clinical differential diagnoses include malaria, typhus, bacterial endocarditis, appendicitis, relapsing fever, miliary tuberculosis, trichinosis, undulant fever, and meningitis.

LABORATORY FINDINGS

Leukopenia with relative lymphocytosis is usual in classical presentations, but leukocytosis has often been noted in nonclassical infections. During incubation, salmonellae may be cultured from blood. In stages of active invasion and fastigium, cultures of blood are usually positive, but salmonellae are less frequently grown from urine and stool. Cultures of urine and stool become positive toward the end of the fastigium. Blood cultures are usually negative during lysis and convalescence, but stool cultures may remain positive until late convalescence (Figure 93–1).

The Widal (agglutination) test, using O or H antigens, may be positive from 10 days after onset and continues to rise into convalescence (Figure 93–1).[36] The agglutination test, using H (flagellar) antigens, does not help with diagnosis if the patient has had previous immunization, previous typhoid or paratyphoid fever, or subclinical exposure. Antibody levels against the O (somatic) antigen above 1 : 50 are significant.

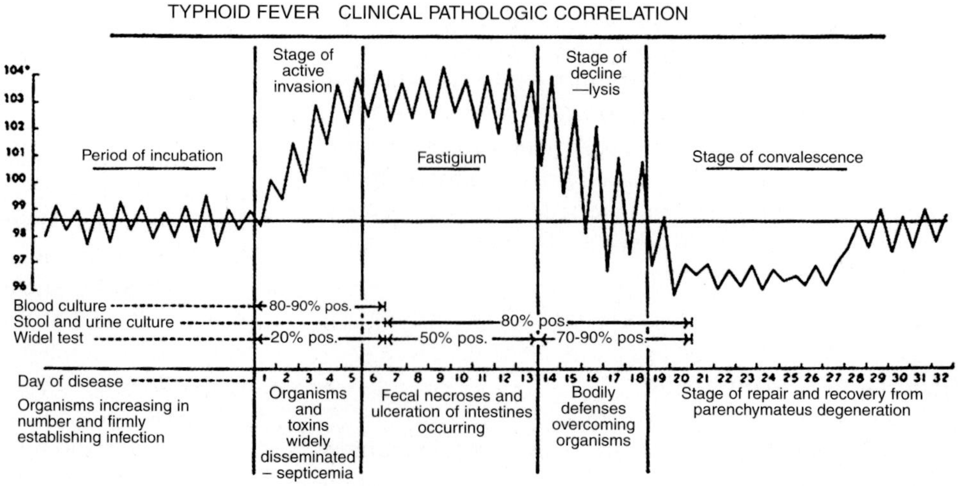

Figure 93–1. Typhoid fever, clinicopathologic correlation (AFIP Neg 75-3946). *(Contributed by Dr Howard C. Hopps, University of Missouri, Columbia, Missouri. Published in Pathology, 6th ed. Edited by W.A.D. Anderson. C.V. Mosby Co., St. Louis, 1971.)*

PATHOGENESIS

Infection is by the oral route, and in normal adults the critical infective dose is 10^5 bacilli with lower critical infective doses in patients with gastric atrophy or previous gastrectomy. The duration of incubation, and perhaps the severity of the disease, is related to the size of the infecting dose, but is not associated with a phage type.[37–39]

Following adhesion-dependent attachment of bacilli to the apex of the enterocyte (luminal surface), bacilli enter the enterocyte by a receptor-mediated endocytotic process. Cytoplasmic translocation of the endosome delivers the *Salmonella* bacterium to the basal surface of the enterocyte, which culminates in its release into the lamina propria. During this process, the bacillus secretes a heat-labile enterotoxin, which causes a net efflux of water and electrolytes into the intestinal lumen.[40–43] While typhoid bacilli exhibit adhesion and endocytosis in cultured enterocytes (and a variety of other cultured cells), some studies suggest that the M cells of the epithelium overlying the Peyer's patches of the ileum are most actively phagocytic and are a major route for invasive organisms into the lamina propria.

Once in the lamina propria, typhoid bacilli enter the lacteals (lymphangioles) and small blood vessels. Lymphatic invasion allows dissemination to regional mesenteric lymph nodes and then lymphohematogenous spread via the cisterna chyli and thoracic duct. Invasion of blood vessels—primarily capillary and venular—carries bacilli to the liver where Kupffer's cells phagocytose them, after which they enter the biliary tract. Since growth of *Salmonella* is not inhibited by bile (which is used by the clinical microbiologist to enhance bacteriologic isolation), they proliferate in bile and this amplification is emptied back into the small intestine to repeat the cycle, a bacterial enterohepatic circulation with increasing numbers of bacilli.[40–44]

With effective humoral and cellular response, *Salmonellae* are lysed, endotoxin is released causing endotoxemia, activation of the kallikrein–kinin system, secretion of tumor necrosis factor alpha (TNF-α) and interferon γ, induction of a serum TNF-α inhibitor (in mice), consumptive coagulopathy, and probably numerous lymphokines, which activate macrophages.[45–51]

Typhoid fever is characterized by diffuse enterocolitis associated with hypertrophy, then necrosis of intestinal and mesenteric lymphoid tissues. At first, the hypertrophy of intestinal lymphoid tissues is caused by edema (stage of incubation and active invasion) and then by influx of mononuclear cells (both lymphocytes and macrophages with the latter predominant). There are focal "soft" granulomas throughout the macrophage–phagocyte system (reticuloendothelial organs) wherever bacilli spread. Inflammatory lesions are dispersed throughout the body. The host cellular reaction is exclusively mononuclear, rather than neutrophilic, and bacteria are mostly in macrophages throughout the body but concentrated in the reticuloendothelial system. The bacilli are demonstrated in tissue sections by Gram staining (Brown–Hopps, Brown–Brenn, Humberstone stains) or by any metachromatic stain (eg, Giemsa stain).

PATHOLOGY

Even though clinicopathologic correlation may be inexact, in most untreated infections, "classic" clinical stages correlate with the "classic" gross and light microscopic pathologic findings. For simplicity, therefore, pathology is discussed by stage. During incubation, there is a mild "catarrhal" enteritis and mesenteric lymphadenitis in which macrophages predominate and hyperplasia of intestinal lymphoid tissue begins. Catarrhal enteritis (Figure 93–2) is manifest grossly by diffuse hyperemia and mucosal edema associated with secretion of excessive mucin by enteric epithelia. Microscopically there is hyperemia of the lamina propria, and edema of both lamina propria and submucosa; this is most striking in Peyer's patches of ileum. Later, in the stage of incubation, especially when prolonged, mononuclear cells begin to infiltrate the lamina propria, especially in the Peyer's patches.

During active invasion, the bacteremia, which is intermittent during incubation, becomes continuous (Figure 93–1). Focal inflammatory lesions caused by disseminated bacilli predominate, but widespread lesions caused by endotoxins may also appear. The small intestine is dilated, has a light red mildly injected serosa and, rarely, a fibrinous exudate on the serosa. The mucosa is red and edematous. Peyer's patches and small lymphoid aggregates throughout the intestine and

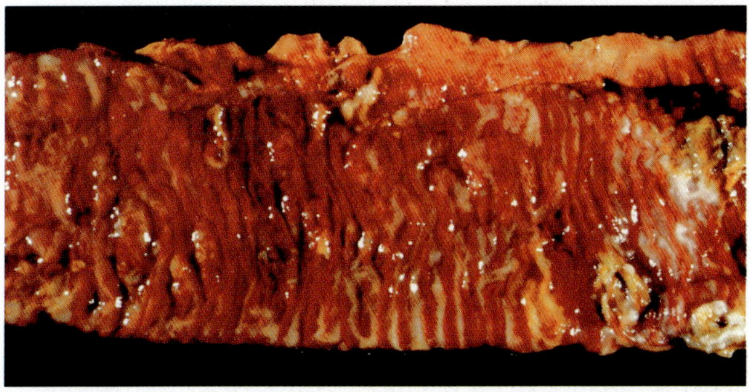

Figure 93–2. Unfixed small intestine with catarrhal enteritis. The mucosa and submucosa are congested and edematous; surfaces weep fluid. Tenacious mucus adheres to the surface.

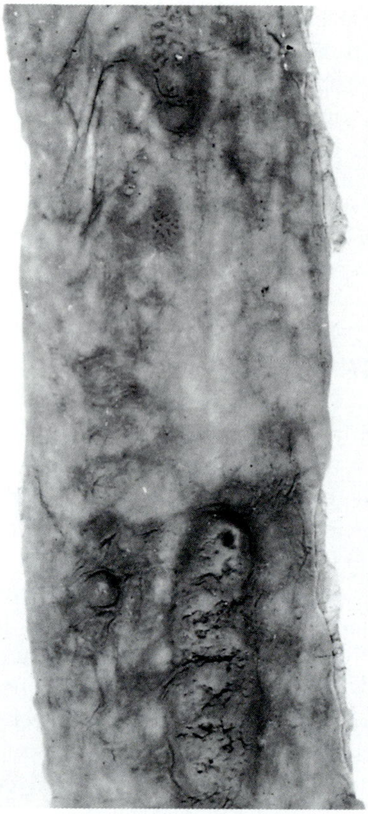

Figure 93–3. Formalin-fixed small intestine and Peyer's patch in stage of active invasion. The Peyer's patch is elongated (on the longitudinal axis of the bowel), and has a convoluted surface covered with intact mucosa (AFIP Neg 30457).

colon enlarge progressively and are raised from 0.1 to 0.4 cm. Peyer's patches are soft, erythematous, and covered by convoluted mucosa (Figure 93–3). The cut surface is reddish and adjacent mucosa and submucosa are edematous. Peyer's patches are on the antimesenteric border, round to oval, and concentrated in the terminal ileum. They are aggregates of lymphoid tissue. During the hypertrophy induced by typhoid fever, they elongate and smaller intestinal lymphoid aggregates throughout the small intestine and colon enlarge to become visible. In typhoid fever Peyer's patches may be in the proximal jejunum and even in the duodenum. *Salmonella paratyphi B* produces similar lesions in stomach and rectum.

Microscopically, intestinal lymphoid tissues are hyperplastic, hyperemic, edematous, and infiltrated with macrophages (typhoid or Mallory's cells), plasma cells, and lymphocytes; neutrophils are rare (Figures 93–4 through 93–6). "Typhoid" cells predominate and actively phagocytose bacilli, erythrocytes, and degenerating lymphocytes. The vermiform appendix is frequently involved and its lymphoid tissue undergoes the same changes.

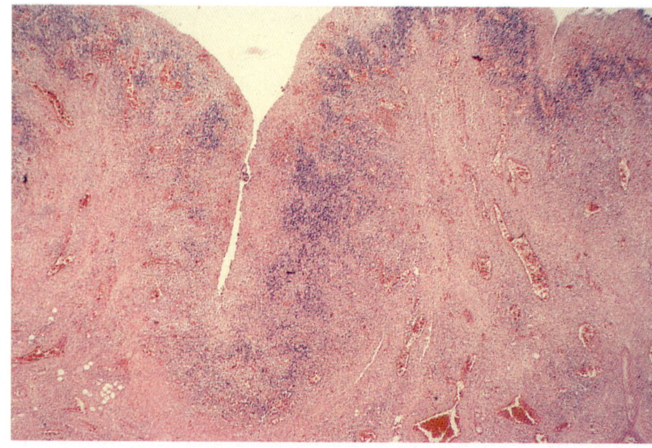

Figure 93–4. Low magnification of ileum in early stage of active invasion. The surface is ulcerated. Lymphoid tissue is hyperemic and edematous and contains a mononuclear cell infiltrate (hematoxylin-eosin, ×25).

Mesenteric lymph nodes are enlarged, soft, and red (Figure 93–7). Microscopically, the changes resemble those of the intestinal lymphoid tissues. Spleen is enlarged, red, soft, and congested; its serosa may have a fibrinous exudate (Figure 93–8). Microscopically, the red pulp is congested and contains aggregates of macrophages (typhoid nodules). The white pulp may be hyperplastic. The liver is slightly enlarged. Typhoid nodules may be in liver, usually in the outer third of the lobule (Figure 93–9), as well as in bone marrow, kidney, testis, and parotid gland.

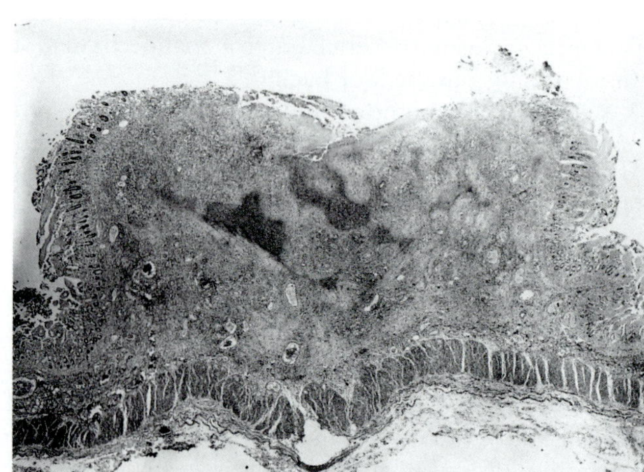

Figure 93–5. Low magnification of ileum in late stage of active invasion showing the contour of a Peyer's patch. There is hyperemia and a prominent mononuclear cell infiltrate. The overlying mucosa is necrotic (AFIP Neg 78460; hematoxylin-eosin, ×13).

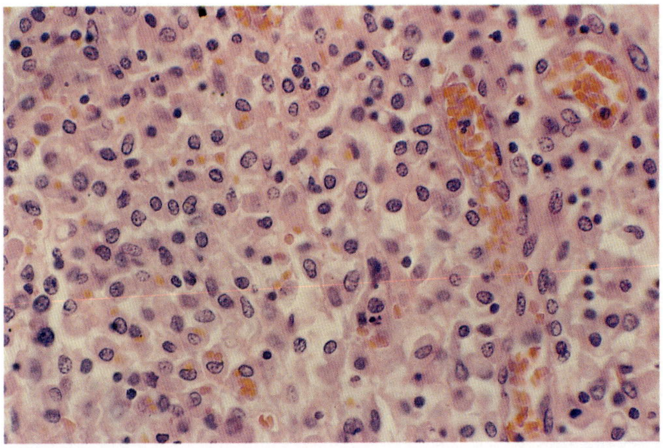

A

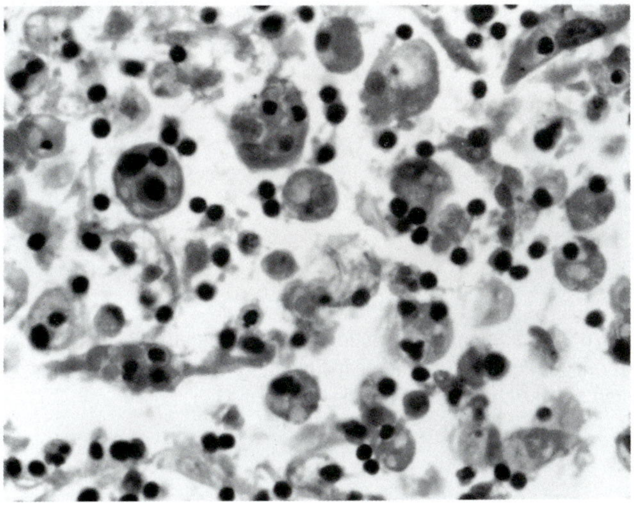

B

Figure 93–6. (**A**) Sheets of histiocytes in a Peyer's patch. Some contain erythrocytes. A single neutrophil is in the upper part of the field (hematoxylin-eosin, ×400). (**B**) Higher magnification of the Peyer's patch in Figure 93–5, showing the characteristic mononuclear cell infiltrate of typhoid fever. The cells are macrophages mixed with lymphocytes and plasma cells. Neutrophils are few (AFIP Neg 72-4598; hematoxylin-eosin, ×750).

Salmonellae persist during fastigium, but since this stage lasts for 10 days to 2 weeks, effective humoral and cellular immunity has been mounted by the host. Many bacteria are being killed by the immune response, and dying bacilli release endotoxins causing systemic toxemia. Necrosis of typhoid mononuclear infiltrates and nodules is prominent, and intestinal lymphoid tissues begin to ulcerate during fastigium. Macroscopically, the intestine resembles that of active invasion, but erythema and injection are more severe. Catarrhal enteritis continues. Peyer's patches remain elevated with discrete hyperemic margins, but their surfaces are shaggy, gray-tan and friable (Figure 93–10). The surfaces of the Peyer's patches are devoid of mucosa and often green from bile staining of necrotic lymphoid tissue. Necrosis of intestinal lymphoid tissue extends to the muscularis propria but rarely through it. Intestinal lymphoid tissues of colon, vermiform appendix, and ileal Peyer's patches all become necrotic (Figure 93–11).

Mesenteric lymph nodes remain large but are firmer than during active invasion. Their cut surfaces are gray-tan friable and necrotic (Figure 93–12) and may resemble caseation necrosis. Microscopically, the necrosis of macrophages begins multifocally, becomes confluent, and, finally, may destroy the entire node.

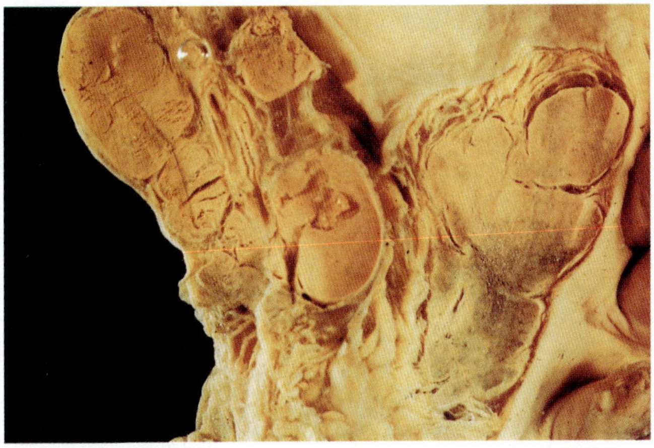

Figure 93–7. Formalin-fixed mesenteric lymph nodes late in the stage of active invasion. They are enlarged, focally hemorrhagic, and necrotic (AFIP Neg 64-3208-1).

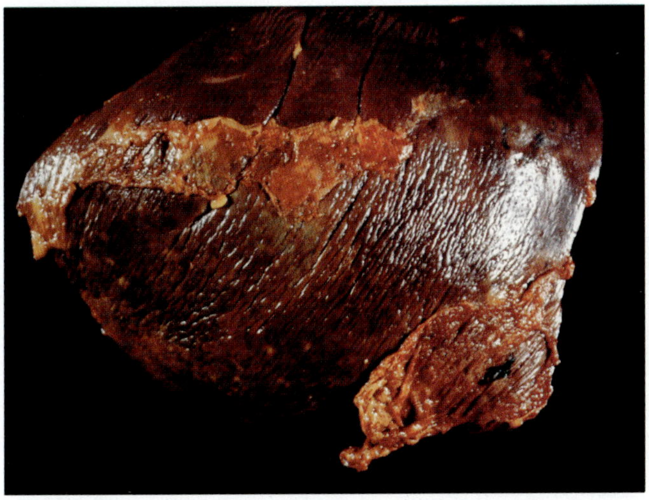

Figure 93–8. Unfixed spleen. A fibrinous exudate is on the capsule. The pulp is congested soft and flabby. The pale spots on the surface are "typhoid nodules."

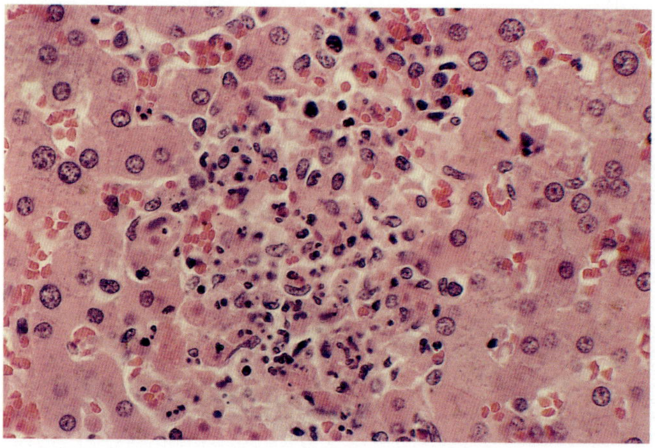

Figure 93–9. Photomicrograph of liver in stage of active invasion, with "classic" typhoid nodule. This lesion is comprised of macrophages *(center)* with lymphocytes and plasma cells at the periphery. Hepatocytes are obliterated in the granuloma but the reticulin framework is intact (hematoxylin-eosin, ×250).

The spleen enlarges three to four times and is more congested than during active invasion. Microscopically, the typhoid nodules are larger, may become confluent, and may be centrally necrotic. Typhoid nodules in liver and other organs may become confluent and necrotic (Figure 93–13). Typhoid nodules in other organs expand as do the areas of central necrosis they contain.

Toxemic lesions appear late during active invasion but are most prominent in fastigium. There is swelling and fatty metamorphosis of myocytes, hepatic parenchymal cells, and renal tubular cells. The heart is flabby and ventricles dilated. Interstitial pneumonitis (diffuse alveolar damage probably caused by endotoxin on pulmonary endothelia), "ring" hemorrhages in brain, and multiple capillary microthrombi are present. Zenker's

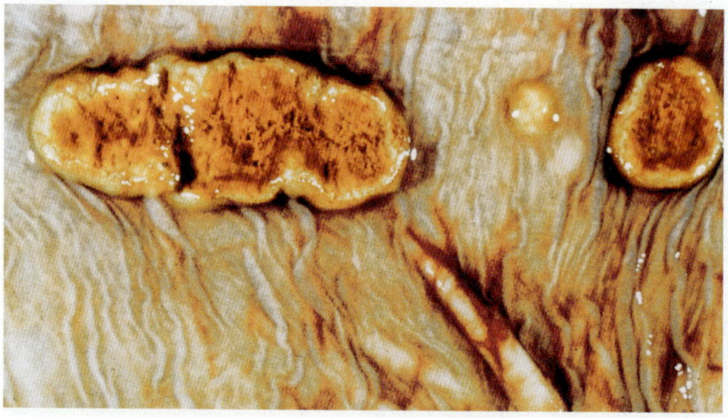

Figure 93–10. Formalin-fixed Peyer's patches of ileum in early fastigium. The Peyer's patches are raised, convoluted, and have a shaggy necrotic base (AFIP Neg 62-4724-3).

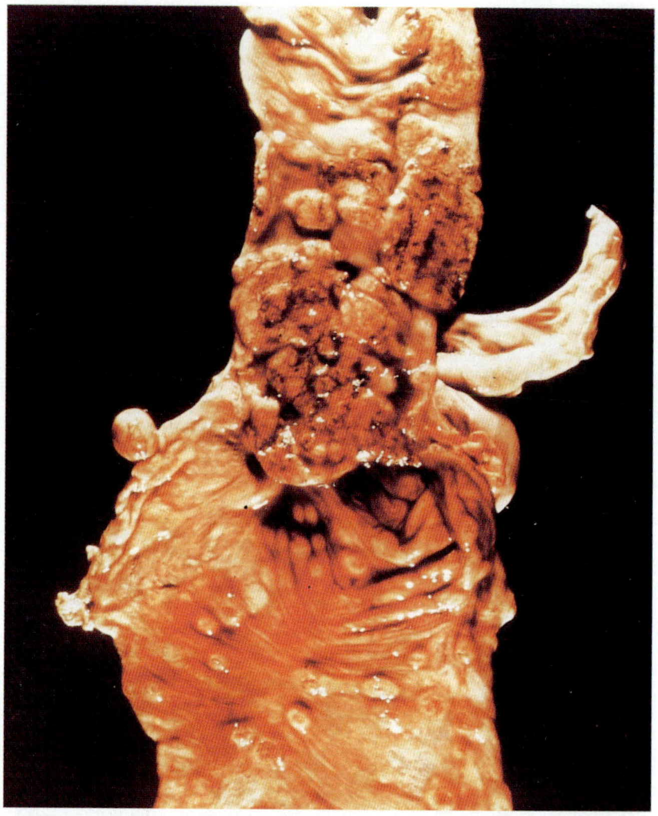

Figure 93–11. Ileocecal junction during fastigium. Peyer's patches are raised, necrotic, and appear fungating. Cecal lymphoid masses show similar changes (AFIP Neg 62-4724-1).

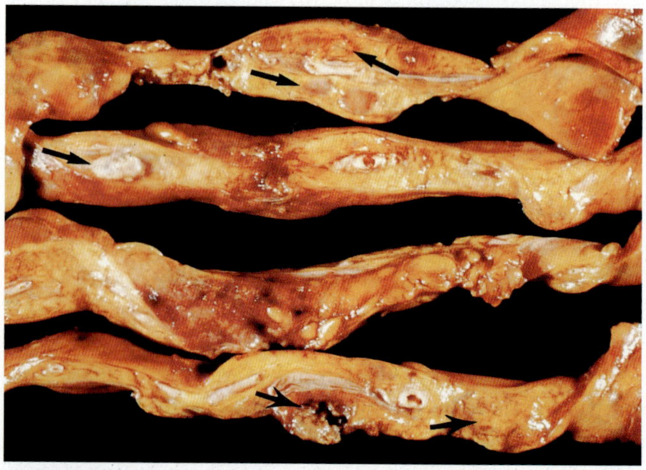

Figure 93–12. Gross appearance of transected mesentery showing necrotic lymph nodes *(arrows)* in patient who died during the stage of fastigium.

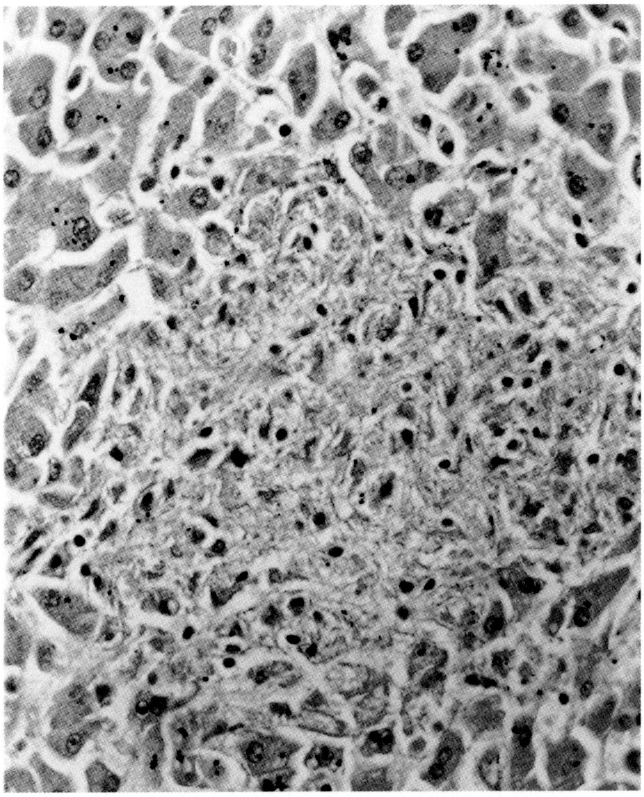

Figure 93–13. Typhoid nodule in liver during fastigium. The macrophages have become necrotic (AFIP Neg 72-4599; hematoxylin-eosin, ×395).

degeneration of skeletal muscle (Figure 93–14) may be severe in untreated patients and is most frequent in those muscles that continue to be active in the bedridden patient (chest, diaphragm, abdomen, and thigh); rupture of and hemorrhage into the *rectus abdominis* muscle may simulate a surgically "acute abdomen."

During lysis, necrotic intestinal lymphoid tissues slough (Figure 93–15), producing characteristic oval ulcers with raised erythematous margins orientated with the long axis of the bowel. At first the ulcer has a gray-green shaggy base, but later it becomes clean, and the underlying exposed pink muscle is often stained green with bile. By the end of this stage, granulation tissue changes the color of the base to red, and the catarrhal enteritis shows resolution. Necrotic material in lymph nodes and in typhoid nodules is slowly absorbed.

The mucosa regenerates during convalescence, converting the necrotic oval ulcer into a stellate ulcer with a base of granulation tissue. Then the intestine returns to normal, with minimal scarring of mucosa and only rare adhesions. Typhoid nodules in the liver and spleen are reabsorbed without distortion, unless there has been extensive coalescent necrosis. The fibrinous exudate on the splenic capsule may become organized

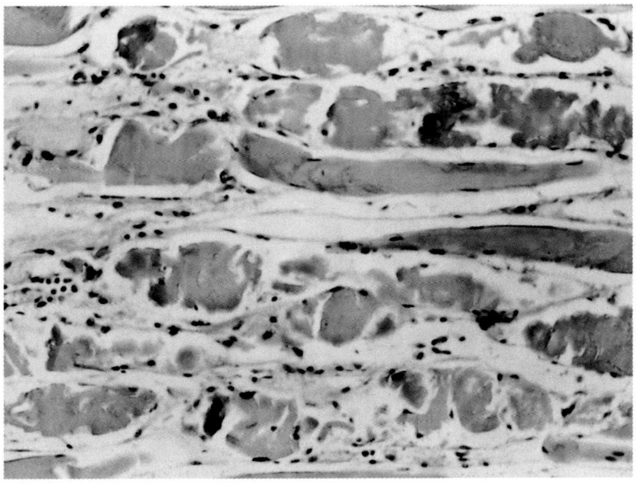

Figure 93–14. Zenker's hyaline degeneration of skeletal muscle, a manifestation of the toxemia of typhoid fever. Zenker's is most prominent during fastigium (AFIP Neg 80985; hematoxylin-eosin, ×160).

and fibrotic, producing the classic "zuckergleiss" (sugar-coated) spleen. Toxic changes in the heart disappear and skeletal muscle regenerates.

CARRIERS

A small portion (<1% to 5%) of patients with acute typhoid fever do not clear their infections and have persistent chronic low-grade infection of the biliary tract.

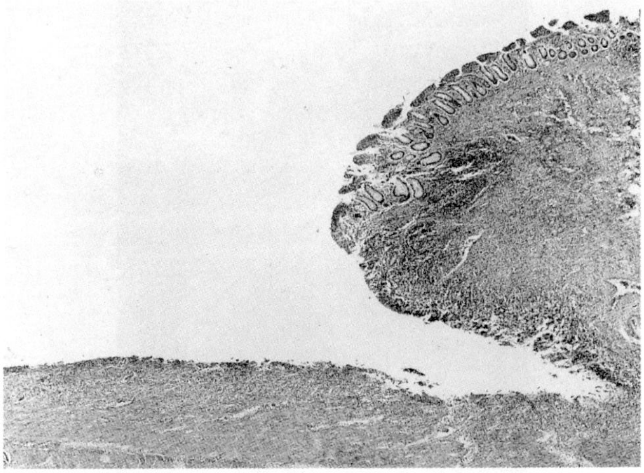

Figure 93–15. Low magnification of ileum at the margin of a Peyer's patch during the stage of lysis; the mucosa and submucosa have sloughed, leaving a base that is nearly bare muscularis propria (AFIP Neg 72-4602; hematoxylin-eosin, ×22).

Chronic biliary infections are important epidemiologically and clinically too because they cause acalculous cholecystitis (along with other *Salmonellae*) and have also been implicated in increased incidences of cholangiocellular carcinoma.[52,53]

COMPLICATIONS

Complications are numerous and account for most deaths, but complications are not related to dose or phage type.[39] Most complications are during the second or third week (fastigium and early stage of lysis). Early in the disease enterotoxins may cause ileus, acute renal tubular necrosis, and sudden death from cardiac arrhythmia. The most frequent and most feared complication is massive intestinal hemorrhage from Peyer's patches (Figure 93–16) and it develops in 5% to 10% of untreated patients. While this complication is usually in the fastigium or the early stage of lysis (the second or third week of illness), it is apparently not related to size of ulcerated Peyer's patches nor to the size of the infecting dose. Consumptive coagulopathy during fastigial toxemia (resulting from gram-negative sepsis) may contribute to the hemorrhage, but some patients have consumptive coagulopathy without demonstrable disseminated intravascular coagulation (DIC). Hemorrhage from ulcerated necrotic hypertrophic lymphoid tissues in the large intestine may be massive.[54–56]

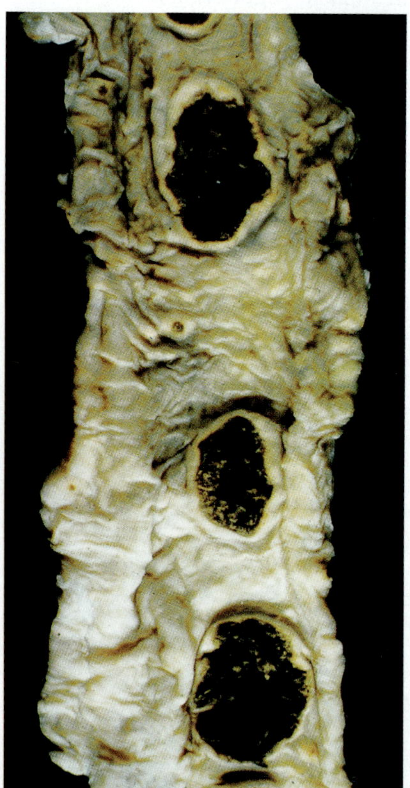

Figure 93–16. Formalin-fixed ileum during fastigium. The mucosa is bile-stained and the Peyer's patches are hemorrhagic. Massive gastrointestinal hemorrhage is the most feared complication. Compare these Peyer's patches with those in Figure 93–10.

Perforation of intestinal ulcers may cause peritonitis. This may be a subtle clinical event because there is usually paralytic ileus, and lesions of skeletal muscle (Zenker's degeneration) inhibit the reflex that causes the rigid boardlike abdomen of peritonitis. Thus the abdomen is soft, even with multiple perforations and peritonitis. The suspicion of peritonitis can be confirmed on x rays by demonstrating "free air" under the diaphragm. This complication must be diagnosed quickly and corrected surgically if the patient's life is to be saved. Untreated, the mortality is 40% to 60%.[57–63]

Typhoid nodules may coalesce into abscesses of liver, spleen, or kidney and typhoid nodules lead to multifocal hepatocytic necrosis that may raise liver enzymes. Endotoxic hepatocellular lesions also alter liver function tests. Indeed, typhoid hepatitis may result in massive hepatic necrosis in children.[64–67] Spontaneous splenic rupture may be associated with typhoid fever. Kidneys may manifest typhoid glomerulonephritis, especially associated with schistosomiasis mansoni and tubular dysfunction.[68,69] Pancreatic dysfunction has been described during the course of typhoid fever.[70]

Atypical localizations and manifestations of typhoid fever include pneumonitis,[71] pericarditis, osteomyelitis, arthritis, sacroiliitis,[72] meningitis, and cerebellar ataxia.[73,74] Osteomyelitis is common in patients with sickle cell hemoglobinopathies and *Salmonella* is the commonest cause of osteomyelitis in these patients. Thrombophlebitis of femoral or saphenous veins develops in approximately 5% to 10% of patients.

Hematologic abnormalities are common in typhoid fever. Typhoid nodules of bone marrow may coalesce causing massive myelonecrosis with leukopenia.[75–77] Intestinal hemorrhages may cause anemia. Other causes of anemia include DIC or a generalized hemophagocytic syndrome involving macrophages in liver, bone marrow, lymph node, and spleen.[78–81]

DIFFERENTIAL DIAGNOSIS (PATHOLOGY)

Typhoid "ulcers" begin in Peyer's patches located on the antimesenteric aspect of intestine; as the hypertrophic typhoid-infected Peyer's patch enlarges it elongates, becoming an ovoid longitudinal ulcer. This longitudinal ulcer differentiates typhoid from tuberculous enteritis, which also begins in Peyer's patches but enlarges circumferentially as granulomas involve the lymphatics, which are mainly circumferential. Both tuberculosis and typhoid fever may involve regional lymph nodes, but the necrosis in typhoid fever is tan and soft while the caseation necrosis of tuberculous lymphadenitis is white and dry. Tuberculous granulomas contain activated macrophages, epithelioid macrophages, Langhans' giant cells and in older lesions fibrosis and calcification; typhoid "granulomas" are aggregates of "bland" macrophages without epithelioid cells nor giant cells and rarely have fibrosis; they are "soft" granulomas, resembling the granulomas of brucellosis and Q fever.

A variety of infectious enteritides may cause Peyer's patches to enlarge. These include enteric tularemia, enteric infection by *Yersinia pseudotuberculosis* and *Y enterocolitica;* these all produce "stellate abscesses" in the hypertrophic Peyer's patches and mesenteric lymph nodes. "Stellate abscesses" present microscopic profiles that are geographic and comprised of an outer epithelioid macrophage boundary surrounding a central collection of neutrophils or liquefaction necrosis. The lesions of typhoid fever rarely contain significant numbers of neutrophils.

"Soft granulomas" in liver, spleen, and other reticuloendothelial organs in typhoid fever (typhoid nodules) cannot be reliably differentiated from the loose aggregates of macrophages in brucellosis, Q fever, melioidosis, *Mycobacterium avium-intracellulare* infections and *M tuberculosis* (in AIDS patients or other immunosuppressed states) on a histologic basis alone.

CONFIRMATION OF DIAGNOSIS BY MICROBIOLOGIC CULTURE, SEROLOGY, AND IMMUNOLOGY

Establishing a diagnosis of typhoid fever quickly is paramount for the patient's survival. The "gold standard" of microbiologic diagnosis is culture, so culture material should be collected before antibiotic therapy is begun, otherwise the typhoid bacillus may never be grown from the patient. In many endemic areas laboratory support is not sufficient and clinical algorithms for diagnosis and treatment have been devised.[82,83]

Although the methods of cultivation are well established, the positive yield is disappointingly low, either because of previous therapy or because the organisms vary greatly in their concentrations among sources and stages of disease. To counter these variables, a variety of ingenious methods and culture sources are used, including blood, streptokinase-lysed blood clots, the mononuclear cell-platelet fraction (or buffy coat) of blood, bone marrow, stool, urine, and duodenal contents[84–90]; in general, cultures of bone marrow and buffy coat are most often positive.

A positive Widal test is an effective criterion for cogently initiating lifesaving specific therapy[91–95] despite the theoretical objections that it may not become positive until later in the disease and that previous exposure to other *Salmonellae* may give a false-positive test. Recent refinements include more specific antigens and/or antibodies,[96–99] more sensitive detection systems,[100,101] including passive hemagglutination[102,103] and various permutations of the enzyme-linked immunosorbent assay.[98,99,104–110] Although each of these has increased sensitivity and specificity over the simple Widal test, each has also increased the complexity, cost, and distance from the critical bedside decision.

To increase sensitivity of diagnosis in the earliest stage, tests using DNA probes have been developed to detect bacilli or their derivatives in the blood,[111–114] and urine.[115] Polymerase chain reaction has been used to detect bacilli in blood.[116] Finally, sonography has been used to diagnose both typhoid and its complications.[117,118]

TREATMENT

In the past, treatment of typhoid fever with chloramphenicol has been effective in lessening severity, shortening the course, and reducing complications. The mortality, formerly 10% to 20%, had been greatly reduced. Tetracycline, used by some clinicians, also appeared to be effective, as did ampicillin and SMX–TMP. Multiple drug-resistant strains of typhoid bacilli arose in the Orient and have spread throughout Asia, especially India, Africa, and South America.[3–18] At present, quinolone antibiotics, such as ciprofloxacin and ofloxacin, appear effective in vitro and in vivo against typhoid and paratyphoid bacilli. Supportive care, such as adequate hydration and maintaining electrolyte balance and blood pressure are important, but steroids and anticoagulants (to counteract DIC) have not proven beneficial. The single most important factor in survival is early diagnosis and treatment.

REFERENCES

1. Edington GM, Gilles HM. *Pathology in the Tropics.* London: Edward Arnold; 1969.
2. Flegg PJ, Mandal BK. *Citrobacter freundii* bacteraemia presenting as typhoid fever. *J Infect.* 1989;18:171–173.
3. Pape JW, Gerdes H, Oriol L, Johnson WD Jr. Typhoid fever: successful therapy with cefoperazone. *J Infect Dis.* 1986;153:272–276.
4. Soe GB, Overturf GD. Treatment of typhoid fever and other systemic salmonelloses with cefotaxime, ceftriaxone, cefoperazone, and other newer cephalosporins. *Rev Infect Dis.* 1987;9:719–736.
5. Keusch GT. Antimicrobial therapy for enteric infections

and typhoid fever: state of the art. *Rev Infect Dis.* 1988;10(suppl 1):S199–S205.
6. Wang F, Gu XJ, Zhang MF, Tai TY. Treatment of typhoid fever with ofloxacin. *J Antimicrob Chemother.* 1989;23: 785–788.
7. Pithie AD, Wood MJ. Treatment of typhoid fever and various infectious diarrhea with ciprofloxacin. *J Antimicrob Chemother.* 1990;26(suppl F):47–53.
8. Mandal BK. Modern treatment of typhoid fever. *J Infect.* 1991;22:1–4.
9. Verghese SL, Manonmani R, Balasubramanian S, Chandrasekharan S. Multi-drug resistance in salmonellae isolated from enteric fever cases at Porur—a semi urban area near Madras City. *J Commun Dis.* 1992;24:12–15.
10. Threlfall EJ, Ward LR, Rowe B, et al. Widespread occurrence of multiple drug-resistant *Salmonella typhi* in India. *Eur J Clin Microbiol Infect Dis.* 1992;11:990–993.
11. Girgis NI, Kilpatrick ME, Farid Z, Sultan Y, Podgore JK. Cefixime in the treatment of enteric fever in children. *Drugs Exp Clin Res.* 1993;19:47–49.
12. de Silva HJ, Wijewickrema R, Thevanesam V. Chloramphenicol resistant typhoid fever. *Ceylon Med J.* 1993;38: 33–34.
13. Rao PS, Rajashekar V, Varghese GK, Shivananda PG. Emergence of multidrug-resistant *Salmonella typhi* in rural southern India. *Am J Trop Med Hyg.* 1993;48: 108–111.
14. Mirza SH, Hart CA. Plasmid encoded multi-drug resistance in *Salmonella typhi* from Pakistan. *Ann Trop Med Parasitol.* 1993;87:373–377.
15. Dutta P, Rasaily R, Saha MR, et al. Ciprofloxacin for treatment of severe typhoid fever in children. *Antimicrob Agents Chemother.* 1993;37:1197–1199.
16. Du Pont HL. Quinolones in *Salmonella typhi* infection. *Drugs.* 1993;45(suppl 3):119–124.
17. Rasaily R, Dutta P, Saha MR, Mitra U, Lahiri M, Pal SC. Multi-drug resistant typhoid fever in hospitalized children. Clinical, bacteriological and epidemiological profiles. *Eur J Epidemiol.* 1994;10:41–46.
18. Gotuzzo E, Echevarria J, Carrillo C, et al. Randomized comparison of aztreonam and chloramphenicol in treatment of typhoid fever. *Antimicrob Agents Chemother.* 1994;38:558–562.
19. Forrest BD. The development of a bivalent vaccine against diarrheal disease. *Southeast Asian J Trop Med Public Health.* 1988;19:449–457.
20. Levine MM, Ferreccio C, Black RE, Tacket CO, Germanier R. Progress in vaccines against typhoid fever. *Rev Infect Dis.* 1989;11(suppl 3):S552–S567.
21. Izhar M, DeSilva L, Joysey HS, Hormaeche CE. Moderate immunodeficiency does not increase susceptibility to *Salmonella typhimurium* aroA live vaccines in mice. *Infect Immun.* 1990;58:2258–2261.
22. Woodruff BA, Pavia AT, Blake PA. A new look at typhoid vaccination. Information for the practicing physician. *JAMA.* 1991;265:756–759.
23. Simanjuntak CH, Paleologo FP, Punjabi NH, et al. Oral immunization against typhoid fever in Indonesia with Ty21a vaccine. *Lancet.* 1991;338(8774):1055–1059.
24. Holmgren J, Svennerholm AM. Bacterial enteric infections and vaccine development. *Gastroenterol Clin North Am.* 1992;21:283–302.
25. Roy SK, Speelman P, Butler T, Nath S, Rahman H, Stoll BJ. Diarrhea associated with typhoid fever. *J Infect Dis.* 1985;151:1138–1143.
26. Gupta SP, Gupta MS, Bhardwaj S, Chugh TD. Current clinical patterns of typhoid fever: a prospective study. *J Trop Med Hyg.* 1985;88:377–381.
27. Mishra S, Patwari AK, Anand VK, et al. A clinical profile of multidrug resistant typhoid fever. *Indian Pediatr.* 1991;28:1171–1174.
28. Ndububa DA, Erhabor GE, Akinola DO. Typhoid and paratyphoid fever: a retrospective study. *Trop Gastroenterol.* 1992;13:56–63.
29. Gupta S, Meena HS. Changing profile of enteric fever—in summer–91. *J Assoc Physicians India.* 1992;40:726–729.
30. Carmeli Y, Raz R, Schapiro JM, Alkan M. Typhoid fever in Ethiopian immigrants to Israel and native-born Israelis: a comparative study. *Clin Infect Dis.* 1993; 16:213–215.
31. Mandal BK. *Salmonella typhi* and other salmonellas. *Gut.* 1994;35:726–728.
32. de Juan Martin F, Perez-Gascon M, Martin Espildora N. Typhoid and paratyphoid fevers in childhood: apropos of 210 cases. *An Esp Pediatr.* 1986;25:170–176.
33. Thisyakorn U, Mansuwan P, Taylor DN. Typhoid and paratyphoid fever in 192 hospitalized children in Thailand. *Am J Dis Child.* 1987;141:862–865.
34. Choo KE, Razif A, Ariffin WA, Sepiah M, Gururaj A. Typhoid fever in hospitalized children in Kelantan, Malaysia. *Ann Trop Paediatr.* 1988;8:207–212.
35. Green SD, Cheesbrough JS. *Salmonella* bacteraemia among young children at a rural hospital in western Zaire. *Ann Trop Paediatr.* 1993;13:45–53.
36. Hoffman SL, Flanigan TP, Klaucke D, et al. The Widal slide agglutination test, a valuable rapid diagnostic test in typhoid fever patients at the Infectious Diseases Hospital of Jakarta. *Am J Epidemiol.* 1986;123:869–875.
37. Olubuyide IO. Factors that may contribute to death from typhoid infection among Nigerians. *West Afr J Med.* 1992; 11:112–115.
38. Sharma A, Gathwala G. Clinical profile and outcome in enteric fever. *Indian Pediatr.* 1993;30:47–50.
39. Finch MJ, Franco A, Gotuzzo E, et al. Plasmids in *Salmonella typhi* in Lima, Peru, 1987–1988: epidemiology and lack of association with severity of illness or clinical complications. *Am J Trop Med Hyg.* 1992;47:390–396.
40. Goodpasture EW. Concerning the pathogenesis of typhoid fever. *Am J Pathol.* 1937;13:175–185.
41. Edsall G, Gaines S, Landy M, et al. Studies on infection and immunity in experimental typhoid fever. I. Typhoid fever in chimpanzees orally infected with *Salmonella typhosa*. *J Exp Med.* 1960;112:143–157.
42. Gaines S, Sprinz H, Tully JG, et al. Studies on infection and immunity in experimental typhoid fever. VII. The distribution of *Salmonella typhi* in chimpanzee tissue following oral challenge, and the relationship between the

numbers of bacilli and morphologic lesion. *J Infect Dis.* 1968;118:293–306.
43. Hornick RB, Greisman SE, Woodward TE, et al. Typhoid fever; pathogenesis and immunologic control. *N Engl J Med.* 1970;283:686–691, 739–746.
44. Sprinz H, Gangarosa EJ, Williams M, et al. Histopathology of the upper small intestines in typhoid fever, Biopsy study of experimental disease in man. *Am J Dig Dis.* 1966;11:615–624.
45. Yabuuchi E, Ikedo M, Ezaki T. Invasiveness of *Salmonella typhi* strains in HeLa S3 monolayer cells. *Microbiol Immunol.* 1986;30:1213–1224.
46. Elsinghorst EA, Baron LS, Kopecko DJ. Penetration of human intestinal epithelial cells by *Salmonella:* molecular cloning and expression of *Salmonella typhi* invasion determinants in *Escherichia coli. Proc Nat Acad Sci USA.* 1989;86:5173–5177.
47. D'Aoust JY. Pathogenicity of foodborne *Salmonella. Int J Food Microbiol.* 1991;12:17–40.
48. Adinolfi LE, Utili R, Gaeta GB, Perna P, Ruggiero G. Presence of endotoxemia and its relationship to liver dysfunction in patients with typhoid fever. *Infection.* 1987; 15:359–362.
49. DeLa Cadena RA, Laskin KJ, Pixley RA, et al. Role of kallikrein–kinin system in pathogenesis of bacterial cell wall-induced inflammation. *Am J Physiol.* 1991;260: 213–219.
50. Mastroeni P, Villareal-Ramos B, Hormaeche CE. Role of T cells, TNF-α and interferon γ in recall of immunity to oral challenge with virulent salmonellae in mice vaccinated with live attenuated aro-*Salmonella* vaccines. *Microb Pathog.* 1992;13:477–491.
51. Mastroeni P, Villareal B, Demarco de Hormaeche R, Hormaeche CE. Serum TNF-α inhibitor in mouse typhoid. *Microb Pathog.* 1992;13:343–349.
52. Callea F, Sergi C, Fabretti G, Brisgotti M, Cozzutto C, Medicina D. Precancerous lesions of the biliary tree. *J Surg Oncol.* 1993;3(suppl):131–133.
53. Caygill CP, Hill MJ, Braddick M, Sharp JC. Cancer mortality in chronic typhoid and paratyphoid carriers. *Lancet.* 1994;343(8889):83–84.
54. Reyes E, Hernandez J, Gonzales A. Typhoid colitis with massive lower gastrointestinal bleeding, an unexpected behavior of *Salmonella typhi. Dis Colon Rectum.* 1986; 29:511–514.
55. Himal HS. Benign cecal ulcer. *Surg Endosc.* 1989;3: 170–172.
56. Dob'on Rasc'on MA, Fat'as Cabeza JA, Navarro Vega ML, et al. Massive lower digestive hemorrhage caused by typhoid fever. *Rev Esp Enferm Apar Dig.* 1989;76: 491–493.
57. Butler T, Knight J, Nath SK, Speelman P, Roy SK, Azad MA. Typhoid fever complicated by intestinal perforation: a persisting fatal disease requiring surgical management. *Rev Infect Dis.* 1985;7:244–256.
58. Bitar R, Tarpley J. Intestinal perforation in typhoid fever: a historical and state-of-the-art review. *Rev Infect Dis.* 1985;7:257–271.
59. Meier DE, Imediegwu OO, Tarpley JL. Perforated typhoid enteritis: operative experience with 108 cases. *Am J Surg.* 1989;157:423–427.
60. Gibney EJ. Typhoid perforation. *Br J Surg.* 1989;76: 887–889.
61. Kayabali I, Gokcora IH, Kayabali M. A contemporary evaluation of enteric perforations in typhoid fever: analysis of 257 cases. *Int Surg.* 1990;75:96–100.
62. Richens J. Management of bowel perforation in typhoid fever. *Trop Doct.* 1991;21:149–152.
63. Akoh, JA. Prognostic factors in typhoid perforation. *East Afr Med J.* 1993;70:18–21.
64. Khosla SN, Singh R, Singh GP, Trehan VK. The spectrum of hepatic injury in enteric fever. *Am J Gastroenterol.* 1988;83:413–416.
65. Bhutta ZA. Fulminant hepatic failure with typhoid fever in childhood. *JPMA J Pak Med Assoc.* 1991;41:123–126.
66. Morgenstern R, Hayes PC. The liver in typhoid fever: always affected, not just a complication. *Am J Gastroenterol.* 1991;86:1235–1239.
67. Dutta P, Lahiri M, Bhattacharya SK, et al. Hepatitis-like presentation in typhoid fever. *Trans R Soc Trop Med Hyg.* 1992;86:92.
68. Khosla SN, Lochan R. Renal dysfunction in enteric fever. *J Assoc Physicians India.* 1991;39:382–384.
69. Martinelli R, Pereira LJ, Brito E, Rocha H. Renal involvement in prolonged *Salmonella* bacteremia: the role of schistosomal glomerulopathy. *Rev Inst Med Trop Sao Paulo.* 1992;34:193–198.
70. Hermans P, Gerard M, van Laethem Y, de Wit S, Clumeck N. Pancreatic disturbances and typhoid fever. *Scand J Infect Dis.* 1991;23:201–205.
71. Sharma AM, Sharma OP. Pulmonary manifestations of typhoid fever. Two case reports and a review of the literature. *Chest.* 1992;101:1144–1146.
72. Menon KP, Gupta A. Atypical salmonellosis: two cases of sacroiliitis. *Indian J Pathol Microbiol.* 1993;36:84–86.
73. Wadia RS, Ichaporia NR, Kiwalkar RS, Amin RB, Sardesai HV. Cerebellar ataxia in enteric fever. *J Neurol Neurosurg Psychiatry.* 1985;48:695–697.
74. Sawhney IM, Prabhakar S, Dhand UK, Chopra JS. Acute cerebellar ataxia in enteric fever. *Trans R Soc Trop Med Hyg.* 1986;80:85–86.
75. Mallouh AA, Sadi AR. White blood cells and bone marrow in typhoid fever. *Pediatr Infect Dis J.* 1987;6: 527–529.
76. Gupta RK. Extensive fatal bone marrow necrosis in typhoid fever. *Indian J Pathol Microbiol.* 1992;35:66–68.
77. Shin BM, Paik IK, Cho HI. Bone marrow pathology of culture proven typhoid fever. *J Korean Med Sci.* 1994;9:57–63.
78. Fame TM, Engelhard D, Riley HD Jr. Hemophagocytosis accompanying typhoid fever. *Pediatr Infect Dis.* 1986; 5:367–369.
79. Udden MM, Banez E, Sears DA. Bone marrow histiocytic hyperplasia and hemophagocytosis with pancytopenia in typhoid fever. *Am J Med Sci.* 1986;291:396–400.
80. Tsui WM, Wong KF, Tse CC. Liver changes in reactive hemophagocytic syndrome. *Liver.* 1992;12:363–367.

81. Ramanathan M, Karim N. Hemophagocytosis in typhoid fever. *Med J Malaysia.* 1993;48:240–243.
82. Ross IN, Abraham T. Predicting enteric fever without bacteriological culture results. *Trans R Soc Trop Med Hyg.* 1987;81:374–377.
83. Richens J, Smith T, Mylius T, Spooner V. An algorithm for the clinical differentiation of malaria and typhoid: a preliminary communication. *PNG Med J.* 1992;35:298–302.
84. Vallenas C, Hernandez H, Kay B, Black R, Gotuzzo E. Efficacy of bone marrow, blood, stool and duodenal contents cultures for bacteriologic confirmation of typhoid fever in children. *Pediatr Infect Dis.* 1985;4: 496–498.
85. Hoffman SL, Edman DC, Punjabi NH, et al. Bone marrow aspirate culture superior to streptokinase clot culture and 8 ml 1:10 blood-to-broth ratio blood culture for diagnosis of typhoid fever. *Am J Trop Med Hyg.* 1986;35: 836–839.
86. Escamilla J, Florez-Ugarte H, Kilpatrick ME: Evaluation of blood clot cultures for isolation of *Salmonella typhi, Salmonella paratyphi-A,* and *Brucella melitensis. J Clin Microbiol.* 1986;24:388–390.
87. Simanjuntak CH, Hoffman SL, Darmowigoto R, Lesmana M, Soeprawoto, Edman DC. Streptokinase clot culture compared with whole blood culture for isolation of *Salmonella typhi* and *S. paratyphi A* from patients with enteric fever. *Trans R Soc Trop Med Hyg.* 1988;82: 340–341.
88. Duthie R, French GL. Comparison of methods for the diagnosis of typhoid fever. *J Clin Pathol.* 1990;43: 863–865.
89. Rubin FA, McWhirter PD, Burr D, et al. Rapid diagnosis of typhoid fever through identification of *Salmonella typhi* within 18 hours of specimen acquisition by culture of the mononuclear cell-platelet fraction of blood. *J Clin Microbiol.* 1990;28:825 –827.
90. Farooqui BJ, Khurshid M, Ashfaq MK, Khan MA. Comparative yield of *Salmonella typhi* from blood and bone marrow cultures in patients with fever of unknown origin. *J Clin Pathol.* 1991;44:258–259.
91. Chow CB, Wang PS, Cheung MW, Yan WW, Leung NK. Diagnostic value of the Widal test in childhood typhoid fever. *Pediatr Infect Dis J.* 1987;6:914–917.
92. Buck RL, Escamilla J, Sangalang RP, et al. Diagnostic value of a single, pre-treatment Widal test in suspected enteric fever cases in the Philippines. *Trans R Soc Trop Med Hyg.* 1987;81:871–873.
93. West B, Richens JE, Howard PF. Evaluation in Papua New Guinea of a urine coagglutination test and a Widal slide agglutination test for rapid diagnosis of typhoid fever. *Trans R Soc Trop Med Hyg.* 1989;83:715–717.
94. Chew SK, Cruz MS, Lim YS, Monteiro EH. Diagnostic value of the Widal test for typhoid fever in Singapore. *J Trop Med Hyg.* 1992;95:288–291.
95. Choo KE, Razif AR, Oppenheimer SJ, Ariffin WA, Lau J, Abraham T. Usefulness of the Widal test in diagnosing childhood typhoid fever in endemic areas. *J Paediatr Child Health.* 1993;29:36–39.
96. Chaicumpa W, Thin-Inta W, Khusmith S, et al. Detection with monoclonal antibody of *Salmonella typhi* antigen 9 in specimens from patients. *J Clin Microbiol.* 1988;26: 1824–1830.
97. Sadallah F, Brighouse G, Del Giudice G, Drager-Dayal R, Hocine M, Lambert PH. Production of specific monoclonal antibodies to *Salmonella typhi* flagellin and possible application to immunodiagnosis of typhoid fever. *J Infect Dis.* 1990;161:59–64.
98. Verdugo-Rodriguez A, Lopez-Vidal Y, Puente JL, Ruiz-Placios GM, Calva E. Early diagnosis of typhoid fever by an enzyme immunoassay using *Salmonella typhi* outer membrane protein preparations. *Eur J Clin Microbiol Infect Dis.* 1993;12:248–254.
99. Sippel JE, Hanafy HM, Diab AS, Prato C, Arroyo R. Serodiagnosis of typhoid fever in pediatric patients by anti-LPS ELISA. *Trans R Soc Trop Med Hyg.* 1987;81: 1022–1026.
100. Rai GP, Zachariah K, Shrivastava S. Detection of typhoid fever by Widal and indirect fluorescent antibody (IFA) tests. A comparative study. *J Hyg Epidemiol Microbiol Immunol.* 1989;33:331–336.
101. Jesudason MV, Sridharan G, Mukundan S, John TJ. Vi-specific latex agglutination for early and rapid detection of *Salmonella* serotype *typhi* in blood cultures. *Diagn Microbiol Infect Dis.* 1994;18:75–78.
102. Coovadia YM, Singh V, Bhana RH, Moodley N. Comparison of passive hemagglutination test with Widal agglutination test for serological diagnosis of typhoid fever in an endemic area. *J Clin Pathol.* 1986;39:680–683.
103. Petchclai B, Ausavarungnirun R, Manatsathit S. Passive hemagglutination test for enteric fever. *J Clin Microbiol.* 1987;25:138–141.
104. Losonsky GA, Ferreccio C, Kotloff KL. Development and evaluation of an enzyme-linked immunosorbent assay for serum Vi antibodies for detection of chronic *Salmonella typhi* carriers. *J Clin Microbiol.* 1987;25:2266–2269.
105. Heiba I, Girgis NI, Farid Z. Enzyme-linked immunosorbent assays (ELISA) for the diagnosis of enteric fever. *Trop Geogr Med.* 1989;41:213–217.
106. Brown A, Hormaeche CE. The antibody response to salmonellae in mice and humans studied by immunoblots and ELISA. *Microb Pathog.* 1989;6:445–454.
107. Quiroga T, Goycoolea M, Tagle R, Gonzalez F, Rodriguez L, Villarroel L. Diagnosis of typhoid fever by two serologic methods. Enzyme-linked immunosorbent assay of antilipopolysaccharide of *Salmonella typhi* antibodies and Widal test. *Diagn Microbiol Infect Dis.* 1992;15: 651–656.
108. Nandakumar KS, Palanivel V, Muthukkaruppan V. Diagnosis of typhoid fever: detection of *Salmonella typhi* porins-specific antibodies by inhibition ELISA. *Clin Exp Immunol.* 1993;94:317–321.
109. Qadri A, Ghosh S, Prakash K, Kumar R, Moudgil KD, Talwar GP. Sandwich enzyme immunoassays for detection of *Salmonella typhi. J Immunoassay.* 1990;11:251–269.
110. Choo KE, Oppenheimer SJ, Ismail AB, Ong KH. Rapid serodiagnosis of typhoid fever by dot enzyme immu-

noassay in an endemic area. *Clin Infect Dis.* 1994;19: 172–176.

111. Rubin FA, Kopecko DJ, Noon KF, Baron LS. Development of a DNA probe to detect typhoid fever. *J Clin Microbiol.* 1985;22:600–605.
112. Rubin FA, Kopecko DJ, Sack RB, et al. Evaluation of a DNA probe for identifying *Salmonella typhi* in Peruvian and Indonesian bacterial isolates. *J Infect Dis.* 1988; 157:1051–1053.
113. Rubin FA, McWhirter PD, Punjabi NH, et al. Use of a DNA probe to detect *Salmonella typhi* in the blood of patients with typhoid fever. *J Clin Microbiol.* 1989;27: 1112–1114.
114. Casanueva V, Cid X, Cavicchioli G, Oelker M, Cofre J, Chiang MT. Serum adenosine deaminase in the early diagnosis of typhoid fever. *Pediatr Infect Dis J.* 1992; 11:828–830.
115. Chaicumpa W, Ruangkunaporn Y, Burr D, Chongsa-Nguan M, Echeverria P. Diagnosis of typhoid fever by detection of *Salmonella typhi* antigen in urine. *J Clin Microbiol.* 1992;30:2513–2515.
116. Song JH, Cho H, Park MY, Na DS, Moon HB, Pai CH. Detection of *Salmonella typhi* in the blood of patients with typhoid fever by polymerase chain reaction. *J Clin Microbiol.* 1993;31:1439–1443.
117. Cohen EK, Stringer DA, Smith CR, Daneman A. Hydrops of the gallbladder in typhoid fever as demonstrated by sonography. *JCU J Clin Ultrasound.* 1986;14:633–635.
118. Puylaert JB, Kristjandottir S, Golterman KL, de Jong GM, Knecht NM. Typhoid fever: diagnosis by using sonography. *Am J Roentgenol.* 1989;153:745–746.

CHAPTER 94

Vibrio vulnificus

Yanina Bednov and Edwin Beckman

The oyster's a confusing suitor:
It's masc., and fem., and even neuter.
At times it wonders, may what come,
Am I husband, wife, or chum?

Ogden Nash (1902–1971), Verses From 1929 On

Science is an attempt, largely successful, to understand the world, to get a grip on things, to get hold of ourselves, to steer a safe course. Microbiology and meteorology now explain what only a few centuries ago was considered sufficient cause to burn women to death.

Carl Sagan (1934–   ), The Demon Haunted World

INTRODUCTION

Vibrio vulnificus is one of the free-living species of marine vibrios. It is halophilic (salt-loving), asporogenous, gram-negative, actively motile, rod-shaped, and curved. This bacterium originally was thought to be a lactose-positive variant of *Vibrio parahaemolyticus,*[1] but *V vulnificus* infection has a distinct clinical course. Because of its lactose positivity and pathogenicity, *V vulnificus* now has a separate taxonomic identity.[1,2] *Vulnificus* is Latin for "wound inflicting," which reflects its ability to cause severe soft tissue damage as well as life-threatening septicemia.

HISTORY

Hippocrates likely made the first recorded description of *V vulnificus* infection.[3] A fisherman named Criton from the island of Thasos, presumably after exposure to the organism in seawater, presented with "violent pain in foot," fever, delirium, and black skin blisters. He died on the second day after the onset of symptoms.

EPIDEMIOLOGY

Vibrio vulnificus is part of the normal marine flora, rather than being a pollutant from waste.[4,5] *Vibrio vulnificus* grows along with *V parahaemolyticus* and *V alginolyticus* in coastal water and in brackish inland waters along the Gulf of Mexico,[6] the Atlantic[7] and Pacific coasts, and off the Hawaiian Islands. It has been identified in lakes in New Mexico and Oklahoma and in the Great Salt Lake in Utah. Human infections have been reported from widely scattered countries, including Japan, Belgium, Australia, China,[8] Taiwan,[9] and Korea.[10] *Vibrio vulnificus* grows best when the water temperature approaches 20°C and salinity is 0.7% to 1.6%.[11] Growth in the Northern Hemisphere is maximal from March through December, with the peak in July and August. Infection follows eating contaminated raw or undercooked shellfish (primarily oysters, which are "sea filters") resulting in septicemia, or by exposure of broken skin to vibrio-bearing seawater, leading to a rapidly progressing wound infection.[4] The male-to-female ratio of patients is 4 : 1. Primary septicemia occurs disproportionately more frequently in older patients, with half or more patients 60 years or older.[5,12,13] This may be a consequence of older persons with chronic diseases concentrating in coastal areas such as Florida and along the Gulf Coast. Because saltwater-related trauma is more common in young people, young patients are more frequently among those with wound infection, but many patients acquiring significant wound infections are older. More than 90% of patients with primary septicemia have eaten raw or undercooked oysters within 24 to 48 hours of clinical onset (range: 7 hours to 4 days). The number of consumed oysters has ranged from 3 to 48. The United States Food and Drug Administration (FDA) reports that more than 50% of oysters and 10% of crabs contain *V vulnificus*. The potential for infection seems to exist regardless of the source of the oysters, and eating raw oysters is now recognized as the primary mode of acquiring *V vulnificus* infection in the United States. Primary septicemia follows colonization of the gastrointestinal tract and invasion of the bloodstream.[14] *Vibrio vulnificus* has emerged as the leading cause of death from food-borne illness in some areas of the United States.[15]

RISK FACTORS

Risk factors for developing septicemia after eating oysters include chronic liver disease, low gastric acidity,[12] immunodeficiency (cancer, diabetes, chronic intestinal disease, corticosteroid therapy), and iron overload states (hemochromatosis, thalassemia). Proliferation of *V vulnificus* continues at 5°C, and thus infectious oysters are transported to the inland United States. Proliferation stops at 4°C and below; *V vulnificus* is killed by boiling or freezing.

PATHOPHYSIOLOGY

Vibrio vulnificus is the most invasive of the vibrios and one of the most invasive of any genus. It produces pili, cytotoxic hemolysins, a mucinase, chondroitinsulfase, hyaluronidase, elastase, phospholipase A2, collagenase, lipase, siderophores, and antiphagocytic surface antigen.[10] *Vibrio vulnificus* has an acidic mucopolysaccharide capsule that, along with antiphagocytic antigen, resists phagocytosis and bactericidal activity by human serum. The presence of this capsule correlates directly with the virulence of the organism,[16] and spontaneous mutants that lack this capsule are nonpathogenic in mice. Production of collagenase and lipase can contribute to invasion of healthy tissue. Proteases permit invasion of tissues containing elastin and collagen and elicit rapidly extending dermal necrosis. Protease causes edema by enhancing vascular permeability through histamine release activation of the plasma kallikrein–kinin system, which generates bradykinin. Extracellular cytolysin possesses four toxic activities, including cytolytic, cytotoxic, vascular permeability increasing, and lethal activities; hemolysin is probably identical to lethal toxin. Intradermal infection with *V vulnificus* and intradermal injection of the cytolysin produces acute cellulitis in mice, characterized by edema and necrosis of cells. The production of cytolysin, protease, and hemolysin is significant in the pathogenesis of *V vulnificus* septicemia, causing edema, tissue necrosis, bullae, and death. After being ingested, *V vulnificus* attaches to the gastrointestinal mucosa, colonizes, disseminates as a gram-negative septicemia, and produces several toxins, causing severe hypotension and shock. Vascular invasion may cause thromboses and tissue necrosis.

Vibrio vulnificus is an unusual organism that requires elevated serum iron to predominate. Iron in vitro and in vivo increases the pathogenicity of *V vulnificus* and decreases bactericidal properties of the serum.[17] The bacteria's enzymes can break down hemoglobin to obtain iron. The released hemoglobin can be chelated by haptoglobin, but *V vulnificus* can overcome the haptoglobin binding and still utilize iron.[18] For this reason, *V vulnificus* is especially pathogenic for patients with hemochromatosis,[19] thalassemia, alcoholic cirrhosis, and chronic aggressive hepatitis. After the organisms invade muscle, infection is often accompanied by severe myositis with rapid progression to myonecrosis and gangrene, which suggests that *V vulnificus* obtains iron from myoglobin.

The association of cirrhosis and infection by *V vulnificus* may be related to decreased blood flow through the liver, shunting *V vulnificus* into the major circulation without the bacteria being phagocytosed or possibly detoxified by Kupffer cells. The defense mechanisms of the cirrhotic liver are not effective in killing bacteria. Other deficiencies of the immune system, such as decreased opsonization, defective white blood cell function, and decreased serum bactericidal activity, contribute to the increased susceptibility of cirrhotic patients to develop septicemia.[20] Chronic alcohol consumption is believed to affect iron availability in one of two ways: 1) alcohol may cause increased absorption by stimulating gastric acid secretion, resulting in more ferric ions that are more readily absorbed by the small intestine; and 2) alcohol consumption can also result in decreased production of carrier proteins, such as transferrin, either through resultant malnutrition or decreased synthetic capabilities from the alcohol-induced liver disease. Low levels of transferrin and elevated transferrin saturation are more important than total iron stores in the pathogenesis of *V vulnificus*.[21]

CLINICAL FEATURES

Vibrio vulnificus causes two major clinical pictures: 1) primary septicemia, and 2) wound infection.[4] Gastroenteritis and a spectrum of assorted other illnesses have also been described. From 1981 to 1992, 125 infections were reported to the Florida Department of Health and Rehabilitation Services.[13] Overall, 44 patients (35%) died. Seventy-two patients (58%) had primary septicemia, 35 (28%) had wound infections, and 18 (14%) had gastroenteritis (78% were oyster associated). Fifty-eight patients (81%) with primary septicemia had eaten raw oysters in the week before the onset. The mean age of these patients was 60 years (range 33 to 90 years); 51 (88%) were male. Forty patients (69%) with primary septicemia died; of these, 35 (88%) had eaten raw oysters. The case fatality rate from raw oyster associated *V vulnificus* septicemia among patients with preexisting liver disease was 67% (30 of 45), but only 38% (5 of 13) among those without liver disease.

Patients with liver disease are more likely to contract septicemia from oysters than those in the general population. In one study, 75% with primary septicemia had liver disease.[4] The annual rate of death from *V vulnificus* for adults with liver disease who eat raw oysters is 45 per million—more than 200 times greater than the death rate for persons without known liver disease who eat raw oysters (0.2 per 1 million).

Primary septicemia begins with abrupt chills, fever, and malaise. At initial presentation, a third of patients are in shock. More than 90% of patients who develop hypotension within 12 hours of admission will die.[11] In a majority of patients (up to 90%) characteristic secondary skin lesions arise,[4] including ecchymoses, bullae, vesicles, and necrotic ulcers on the limbs, usually within 24 hours of onset of generalized symptoms. *Vibrio vulnificus* is often (56%) isolated from the skin lesions, pointing to hematogenous seeding as the basis.[22] Cultures of blood are usually positive. The intense pain of the lower limbs from swelling, cellulitis, myositis, and gangrene may necessitate fasciotomy. Thrombocytopenia, leukopenia, and disseminated intravascular coagulation may also complicate the infection.

Wound infection by *V vulnificus* is most often seen in otherwise healthy people following exposure of open wounds or after injury in seawater during fishing, crabbing, swimming, or oyster shucking. Symptoms include swelling, erythema, and intense pain with rapidly progressive cellulitis, fasciitis, and myositis, which may be complicated by gangrene, thus necessitating amputation. Blood cultures are positive in only 30% of these patients, and there is a correspondingly lower mortality than for primary septicemia. The prognosis is much worse for those with wound infections who also have an underlying disease such as cirrhosis,[5,14] which raises the mortality from wound infection to 24%.

Approximately 11% of patients present with gastroenteritis. Clinical features include vomiting, diarrhea, abdominal pain, and a positive stool culture for *V vulnificus*. These patients do not die of infection. *Vibrio vulnificus* can cause a wide spectrum of additional illnesses, including pneumonia and septicemia after near drowning and aspiration of seawater,[23] meningitis, spontaneous bacterial peritonitis, endometritis after sexual intercourse in seawater, corneal ulcers, otitis after diving into seawater with a perforated ear drum, acute osteomyelitis, and endocarditis.

PATHOLOGY

Gross

Skin lesions, whether in primary septicemia or from local injury, proceed from ecchymoses to vesicles and bullae (Figures 94–1 and 94–2) to necrotic ulcers (Figure 94–3)[4,24]; areas may become denuded.[5] The skin lesions in primary septicemia are on the limbs but may extend onto the trunk. Fasciitis and myositis can progress to gangrene of muscles and soft tissues. If disseminated intravascular coagulation has developed, there may be widespread purpura.[25] Internal organs are grossly congested.[24,26]

Histopathology

The picture in the skin is similar whether it follows primary septicemia or a saltwater-related local injury.[25] The salient alteration is an intense cellulitis.[5,27] An intense neutrophilic infiltrate traverses the subcutaneum

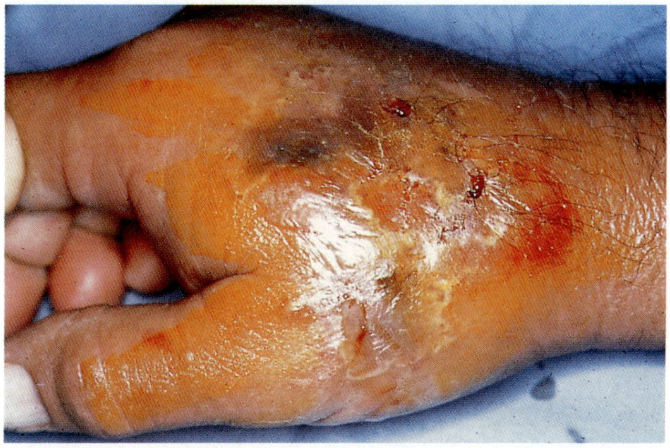

Figure 94–1. Swollen hand with bullae in a man in septic shock with *Vibrio vulnificus* following shrimp wound. The patient was taking prednisone for hepatitis with cirrhosis.

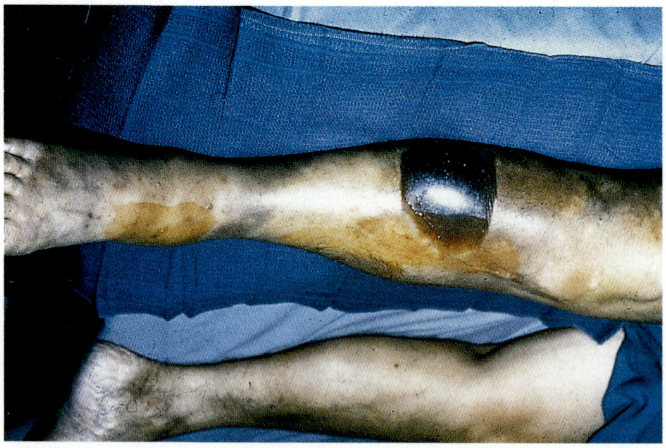

Figure 94–2. Marked edema and hemorrhagic and nonhemorrhagic bullae of the leg of a man acquiring *V vulnificus* from fire ant bites after wading in the sea. In spite of amputation and vigorous therapy, the patient died 6 days after the initial incident. Hepatic cirrhosis was established at autopsy. *(By permission: Fernandez CR, Pankey GA. Tissue invasion by unnamed marine vibrios. JAMA. 1976;233: 1173–1176.)*

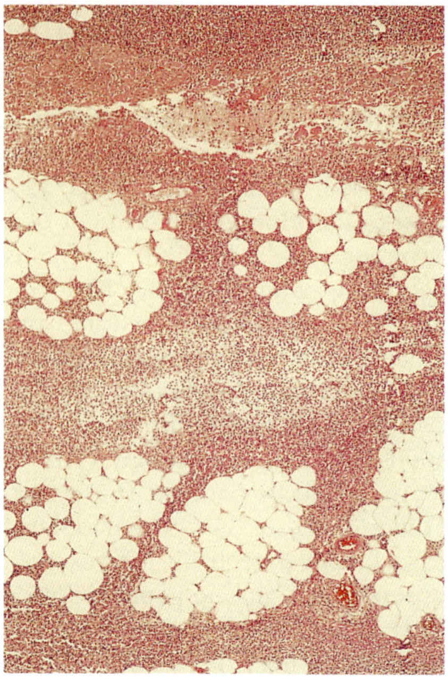

Figure 94–4. Bands of intense acute inflammation traverse the subcutaneous tissue in the cellulitis of *V vulnificus* wound infection. The inflammation may extend into skeletal muscle and/or dermis [hematoxylin-eosin (H&E), ×40].

in a septal pattern (Figures 94–4 and 94–5). Typically, there are numerous bacteria amidst the inflammatory infiltrate (Figure 94–6). Neutrophils traverse the walls of vessels of the subcutaneum (Figure 94–7), but there is not the fibrinoid necrosis characteristic of a primary collagen vascular disease.[27] The vessels may be thrombosed,[5,27] and the endothelium of the vessels is typically hyperplastic and swollen (Figure 94–8). Often, many bacteria are centered around the vessels.[24,26] The inflammation may extend into adjacent skeletal muscle (Figures 94–9 and 94–10). Such involvement of the muscle may be profound, and there may be areas of advanced necrotizing vasculitis, myositis, and fasciitis. Intense acute inflammation extends into the adjacent dermis. The more superficial portions of the dermis may be devoid of an inflammatory infiltrate or may have acute inflammation.[24] In any case, there is relatively less inflammation of the superficial dermis than of the deep dermis and subcutaneum (Figure 94–11). The dermis and epidermis may be devitalized.[24] Bullae form at the

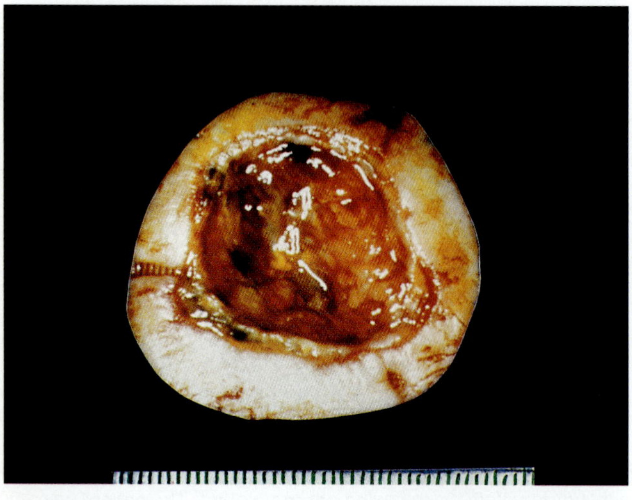

Figure 94–3. Deep necrotic ulcer caused by halophilic marine *Vibrio.*

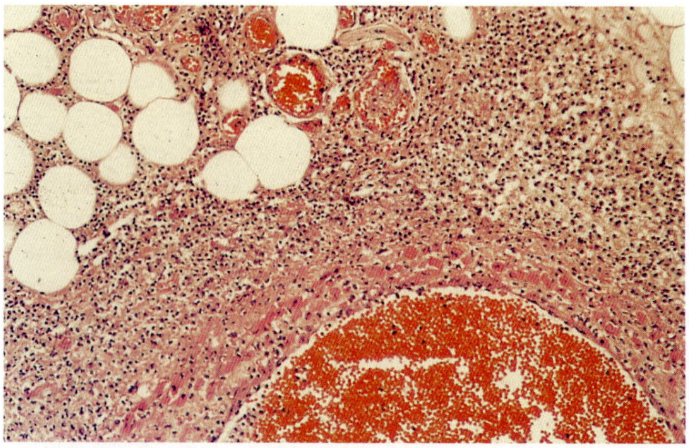

Figure 94–5. Intense cellulitis and vascular inflammation in *V vulnificus* wound infection (H&E, ×100).

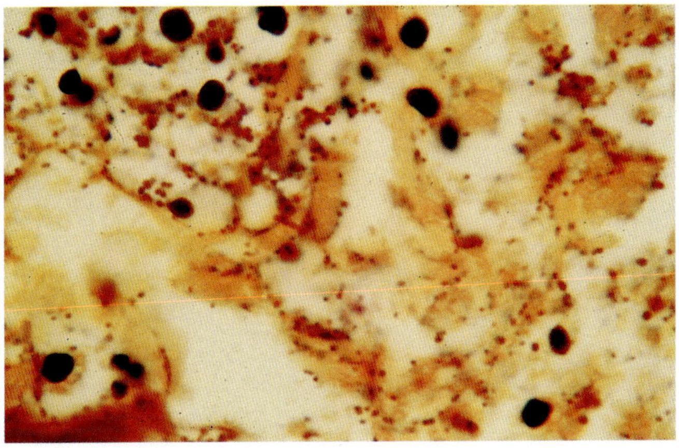

Figure 94–6. Numerous gram-negative organisms of *V vulnificus* in cellulitis (tissue gram stain, ×1000).

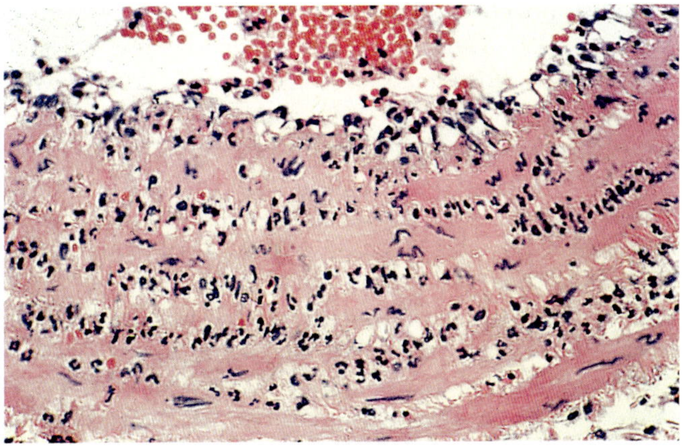

Figure 94–7. Intense neutrophilic infiltrate of wall of a vessel of the subcutaneum in *V vulnificus* wound infection (H&E, ×220).

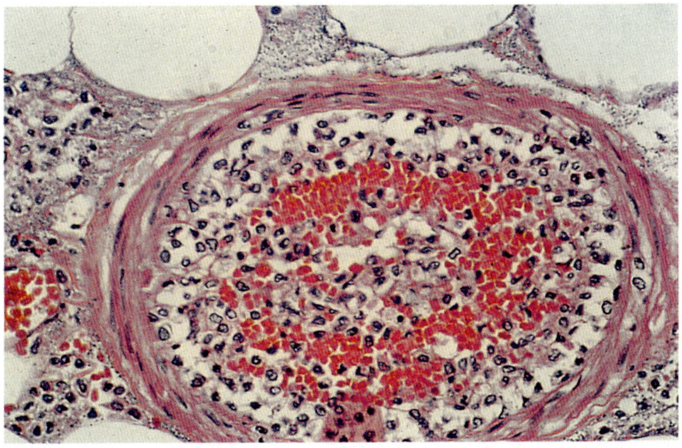

Figure 94–8. Endothelial hyperplasia in cellulitis of *V vulnificus* wound infection. Many bacteria surround the vessel (H&E, ×220).

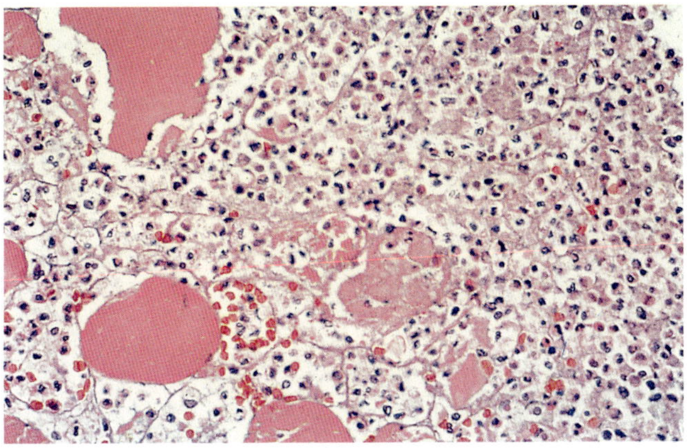

Figure 94–9. Muscle necrosis and intense neutrophilic infiltrate in *V vulnificus* wound infection (H&E, ×220).

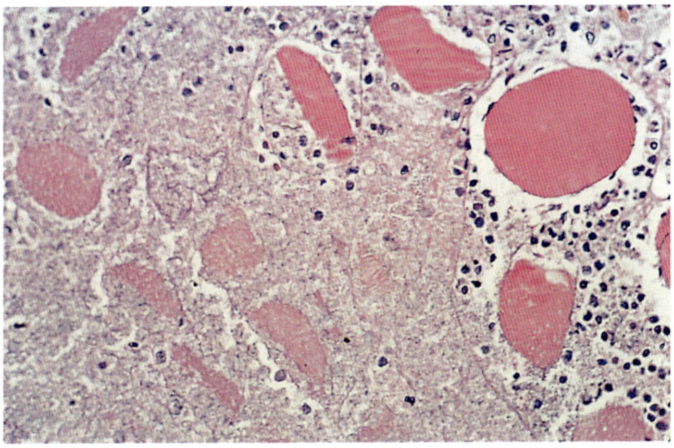

Figure 94–10. Muscle necrosis and intense neutrophilic infiltrate in *V vulnificus* wound infection (H&E, ×220).

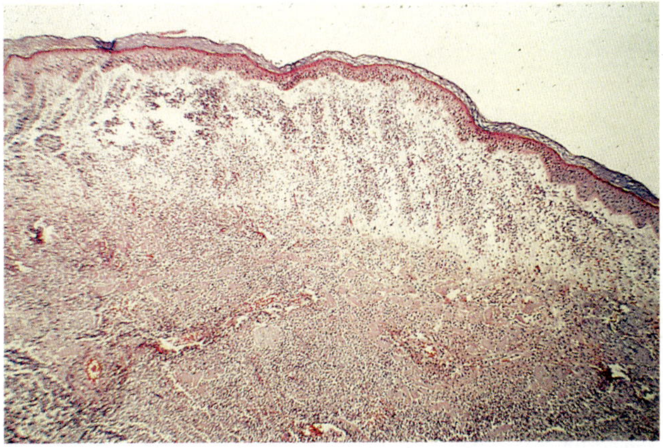

Figure 94–11. Intense inflammation of the dermis in *V vulnificus* wound infection, but with edema and relatively less inflammation of the superficial dermis (H&E, ×20).

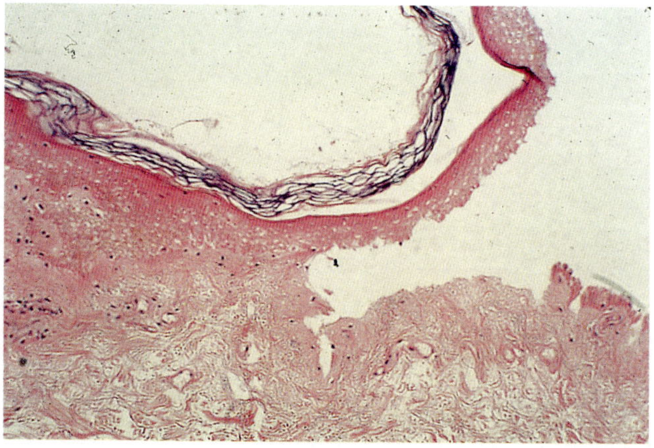

Figure 94–12. Noninflammatory bulla of necrotic skin in *V vulnificus* wound infection. Intense inflammation may involve the dermis as well as the subcutaneum. Typically there are numerous bacteria in the base of the bullae (H&E, ×100).

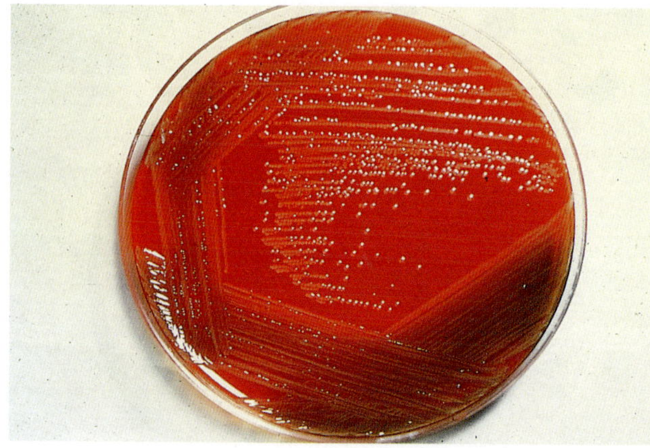

Figure 94–14. Culture of *V vulnificus* on rabbit blood plate.

dermal–epidermal interface. The bullae are of the noninflammatory type, as neutrophils are not typically in the fluid of the bulla (Figure 94–12). There may be numerous bacteria at the base of the bullae (Figure 94–13) and throughout the dermis.

Vessels of internal organs may have an intense neutrophilic infiltrate.[24,26] Abscesses in such organs as the spleen and testis can occur in septicemia.[24]

IDENTIFICATION

Vibrio vulnificus is a gram-negative, motile, slightly curved rod, morphologically identical to other vibrios. It can be misidentified as an enteric organism. In fact, when grown on enteric media, it looks very much like a lactose-positive member of the family *Enterobacteriaceae*. Unlike those, however, it is oxidase positive. Although *V vulnificus* is a halophile, it can grow in media with as little as 0.5% sodium chloride. It can, therefore, be recovered from most blood culture media (Figure 94–14), as well as from trypticase soy agar with 5% sheep blood, MacConkey, xylose-lysine deoxycholate (XLD), and Hectoen-enteric agar plates.[18] The Centers for Disease Control and Prevention (CDC) recommends, after 24 hours of incubation, subculturing from blood culture bottles to a high salt content medium such as marine agar. If *V vulnificus* is suspected, TCBS (thiosulfate citrate bile salts sucrose agar) is the medium of choice (Figure 94–15). TCBS can differentiate the sucrose fermenters that produce yellow colonies (*V cholera* and *V alginolyticus*) from *V vulnifi-*

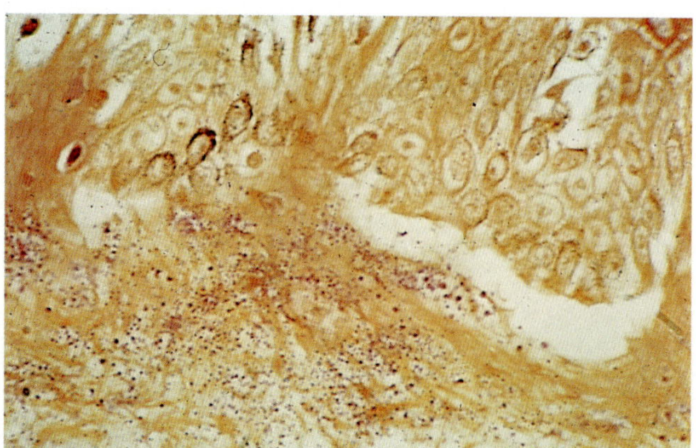

Figure 94–13. Large numbers of gram-negative organisms of *V vulnificus* at the base of developing bulla (tissue gram stain, ×600).

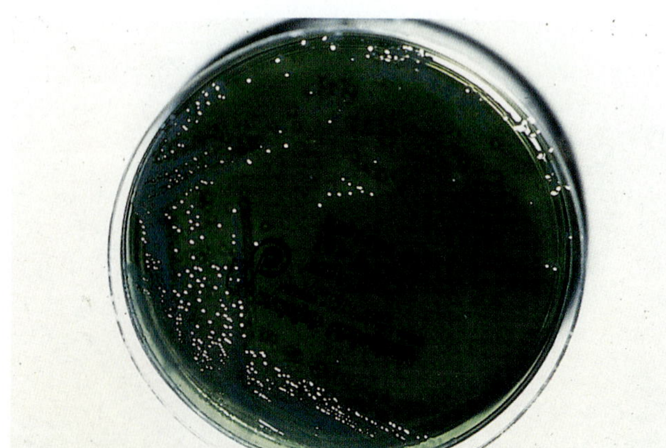

Figure 94–15. Culture of *V vulnificus* on TCBS (thiosulfate citrate bile salts sucrose agar) plate.

cus and *V parahaemolyticus,* which yield olive-green colonies and usually do not ferment sucrose. After 48 hours of incubation on ENDO agar, *V vulnificus* produces red colonies that achieve the diameter of 2 to 4 mm, a feature enabling differentiation from *V alginolyticus, V parahaemolyticus,* and *V fluvialis.*[28] Key biochemical characteristics that suggest *V vulnificus* include lactose fermentation, a positive ortho-nitrophenyl-galactoside (ONPG) test for delayed fermentation, and a positive oxidase test, as well as other differentiating reactions. Monoclonal antibodies for rapid identification of members of the genus *Vibrio* have been developed. Genus-specific monoclonal antibodies (MAb) may be useful for identifying vibrios rapidly in the screening of acute infection, whereas the species-specific MAb may be useful for completing the diagnosis. For example, the genus specific MAb F11P411F recognizes the isolates as *Vibrio* species, whereas the species-specific MAb F31P46F identifies the isolates as *V vulnificus.*[29]

TREATMENT AND PROPHYLAXIS

Because *V vulnificus* infection is life threatening and can progress rapidly, antibiotic therapy must be initiated as soon as this disease is suspected, even before the organism is identified.[10] Septicemia and/or wound infection accompanied by characteristic skin lesions in a patient in the appropriate epidemiological setting should spur the clinician to obtain a history of eating raw shellfish or exposure to the marine environment. *Vibrio vulnificus* is sensitive to many broad spectrum antibiotics, especially to the third generation cephalosporins,[9] but tetracycline[30] and chloramphenicol are still the treatment of choice. Rapid identification of the organism and aggressive management of the patients, including surgical debridement of wounds or amputation of the limb, can reduce the high morbidity and mortality caused by infection by *V vulnificus.* Patients in high-risk groups (those with chronic liver disease, immunodeficiencies, hemochromatosis, thalassemia, organ transplants, hematologic disorders, and corticosteroid therapy) should not eat raw or undercooked shellfish, especially oysters. Nutrition education remains the most important preventive measure.[31] Furthermore, trauma in the marine environment and exposure of preexisting skin wounds should be avoided, especially if a patient is in one of the high-risk groups.

REFERENCES

1. Hollis DG, Weaver RE, Baker CN, Thornsberry C. Halophilic vibrio species isolated from blood cultures. *J Clin Microb.* 1976;3:425–431.
2. Farmer JJ. *Vibrio* ("Beneckea") *vulnificus,* the bacterium associated with sepsis, septicemia, and the sea. *Lancet.* 1979;2:903.
3. Baethge BA, West BC. *Vibrio vulnificus:* did Hippocrates describe a fatal case? *Rev Inf Dis.* 1988;10:614–615.
4. Blake PA, Merson MH, Weaver RE, Hollis DG, Heublein PC. Disease caused by a marine vibrio—clinical characteristics and epidemiology. *NEJM.* 1979;300:1–5.
5. Case records of the Massachusetts General Hospital (case 41-1989). *NEJM.* 1989;321:1029–1038.
6. Johnston JM, Becker SF, McFarland LM. *Vibrio vulnificus. JAMA.* 1985;253:2850–2853.
7. Levine WC, Griffin PM, Gulf Coast Vibrio Working Group. *Vibrio vulnificus* infections on the Gulf Coast: results of first year regional surveillance. *J Inf Dis.* 1993;167:479–483.
8. Chuang YC, Young C, Chen CW. *Vibrio vulnificus* infection. *Scand J Infect Dis.* 1989;21:721–726.
9. Chuang YC, Yuan CY, Liu CY, Lan CK, Huang AH. *Vibrio vulnificus* infection in Taiwan: report of 28 cases and review of clinical manifestations and treatment. *Clin Infect Dis.* 1992;15:271–276.
10. Park SD, Shon HS, Joh NJ. *Vibrio vulnificus* septicemia in Korea: clinical and epidemiologic findings in seventy patients. *J Amer Acad Dermat.* 1991;24:397–403.
11. Koenig KL, Muller J, Rose T. *Vibrio vulnificus*—hazard on the half shell. *West J Med.* 1991;155:400–403.
12. Barrett E. *Vibrio vulnificus* infections, Virginia, 1974–1992. *Epidemiol Bull* (Virginia). 1993;93:1–3.
13. *Vibrio vulnificus* infections associated with raw oyster consumption–Florida, 1981–1992. *Morbidity and mortality weekly report.* 1993;42:405–407.
14. Janda JM. A lethal leviathan: *Vibrio vulnificus. West J Med.* 1991;155:421–422.
15. Kizer KW. *Vibrio vulnificus* hazard in patients with liver disease. *West J Med.* 1994;161:64–65.
16. Reddy GP, Hayat U, Bush A, Morris JG Jr. Capsular polysaccharide structure of a clinical isolate of *Vibrio vulnificus* strain B062316 determined by heteronuclear NMR spectroscopy and high performance anion-exchange chromatography. *Analyt Biochem.* 1993;214:106–115.
17. Bullen JJ, Spalding PB, Ward CG, Gutteridge JM. Hemochromatosis, iron, and septicemia caused by *Vibrio vulnificus. Arch Int Med.* 1991;151:1606–1609.
18. Karnaugh L. *Vibrio vulnificus*: Neptune's revenge? *Diag Med.* 1984;7:21–25.
19. Muench KH. Hemochromatosis and infection: alcohol and iron, oyster and sepsis. *Am J Med.* 1989;87:3-40N–3-43N.
20. Warnock EW III, MacMath TL. Primary *Vibrio vulnificus* septicemia. *J Emerg Med.* 1993;11:153–156.
21. Brennt CE, Wright AC, Dutta SK, Morris JG Jr. Growth of *Vibrio vulnificus* in serum from alcoholics: association with high transferrin iron saturation. *J Infect Dis.* 1991;164:1030–1032.
22. Blake PA, Weaver RE, Hollis DG. Diseases of humans (other than cholera) caused by vibrios. *Ann Rev Microbiol.* 1980;34:341–367.
23. Hoge CW, Watsky D, Peeler RN, Libonati JP, Israel E, Morris JG Jr. Epidemiology and spectrum of *Vibrio* infections in a Chesapeake Bay community. *J Infect Dis.* 1989; 160:985–992.

24. Matusuo T, Kohno S, Ikeda T, Saruwatari K, Ninomiya H. Fulminating lactose-positive vibrio septicemia. *Acta Path Jap.* 1978;28:937–948.
25. Tyring SK, Lee PC. Hemorrhagic bullae associated with *Vibrio vulnificus* septicemia: report of two cases. *Arch Dermatol.* 1986;122:818–820.
26. Shirouzu K, Miyamoto Y, Yasaka T, Matsubayashi Y, Morimatsu M. *Vibrio vulnificus* septicemia. *Acta Path Jap.* 1985;35:731–739.
27. Beckman EN, Leonard GL, Castillo LE, Genre CF, Pankey GA. Histopathology of marine vibrio wound infection. *Am J Clin Path.* 1981;76:765–772.
28. Desmond EP, Janda JM, Adams FI, Bottone EJ. Comparative studies and laboratory diagnosis of *Vibrio vulnificus,* an invasive *Vibrio* sp. *J Clin Microb.* 1984;19:122–125.
29. Chen D, Hanna PJ, Altmann K, Smith A, Moon P, Hammond LS. Development of monoclonal antibodies that identify *Vibrio* species commonly isolated from infections of humans, fish, and shellfish. *Appl Environ Microbiol.* 1992;58:3694–3700.
30. Fang FC. Use of tetracycline for treatment of *Vibrio vulnificus* infections. *Clin Infect Dis.* 1992;15:1071.
31. Ross EE, Guyer I, Varnes J, Rodrick G. *Vibrio vulnificus* and molluscan shellfish: the necessity of education for high-risk individuals. *J Amer Diet Assoc.* 1994;94:312–313.

CHAPTER 95

Whipple's Disease

William O. Dobbins III

Of the three prize-winners it was Whipple who first occupied himself with the investigations for which the prize has now been awarded.

Professor I. Holmgren, official presentation of the Nobel Prize, 1934

As a matter of fact, men go into this branch of work . . . (research on infectious diseases) . . . from a number of motives, the last of which is a self-conscious desire to do good. The point is that it remains one of the few sporting propositions left for individuals who feel the need of a certain amount of excitement. Infectious disease is one of the few genuine adventures left in the world. The dragons are all dead, and the lance grows rusty in the chimney corner.

Hans Zinsser (1878–1940)

The jejunum is more exempt from morbid conditions than any other portion of the alimentary canal.

Sir William Withey Gull (1816–1890), St. Bartholomew's Hospital Reports 52:45,1916

ETIOLOGY

Whipple's disease is a bacterial infection, even though the causative agent has not been cultured nor has the infection been reproduced in animals.[1] Whipple described great numbers of a "rod-shaped organism" in silver-stained sections of a small mesenteric lymph node,[2] but his observation was not confirmed until 1960–1961, when three reports describing the electron microscopy of Whipple's disease showed bacilli in involved tissues. The bacilli were stained by the periodic acid–Schiff (PAS), Gram, and Giemsa methods, and had the fine structural features of bacteria. The organism provoked an infiltrate of macrophages, reacted with tissue stains for bacteria (Brown–Brenn), was silvered by Gomori's methenamine-silver (GMS) method but was not acid fast. The organism was 0.25 μm by 1.0 to 2.0 μm and it is now accepted that Whipple's disease is caused by a specific and unique bacillus.

CLASSIFICATION OF THE ORGANISM

Wilson et al,[3] by nucleotide sequencing and amplification by polymerase chain reaction (PCR) on the bacterial 165 ribosomal DNA, concluded that the Whipple's bacillus belonged to a hitherto undefined genus most closely related to *Rhodococcus, Arthrobacter,* and *Streptomyces* genera. Relman et al,[4] however, using PCR, amplified the bacterial 16S ribosomal RNA sequence and identified a unique 1321 base pair 16S RNA sequence. On the basis of this they believe the Whipple's bacillus is a gram-positive actinomycete and not closely related to any known genus of bacteria. They thus proposed a new genus and species, naming the bacterium *Tropheryma whippelii* (from the Greek *trophe*, "nourishment," and *eryma*, "barrier," because it causes malabsorption and for Dr. George Whipple).

Whipple bacilli share antigens with streptococcal groups B and G, and with *Shigella flexneri*. This is explained by the fact that similar polysaccharides are in different bacteria. These immunologic reactions do not necessarily give a clue to the identity of the organism involved. Rather, the importance of these observations is that there is a distinctive bacterial antigen profile, as defined with a battery of bacterial antisera, which further supports the concept that a single (antigenically definable) bacterial species is the cause of Whipple's disease. This "fingerprint" of reactivity with bacterial antisera may be utilized to establish or confirm the diagnosis of Whipple's disease.

PATHOGENESIS

The bacillus, though largely extracellular, invades (or is taken up by) a large number of cells including macrophages, neutrophils, mast cells, intestinal epithelial cells, capillary and lymphatic endothelia, smooth muscle, lymphocytes, and plasma cells. It has been found in the intestine, colon, lymph nodes, central nervous system (CNS), eye, heart, liver, lung, synovium, kidney, bone marrow, and skin. The organism clearly has low virulence in man. Although there may be large numbers of organisms, tissue injury is minimal. In the intestinal mucosa Whipple's disease is characterized by two remarkable histologic features: 1) histiocytes containing many bacilli in varying stages of digestion are packed into the lamina propria and 2) there are many extracellular bacilli just below the basal lamina of the epithelial cells and with a progressive decrease in numbers of bacilli towards the submucosa.[5]

In some ways, Whipple's disease resembles lepromatous leprosy. Both are characterized by local accumulations of macrophages containing large numbers of bacilli, in both there is a lack of tissue necrosis, and both have macrophages containing indigestible remnants of phagocytosed bacteria. Finally, neither the bacillus causing leprosy nor the bacillus causing Whipple's disease has been cultured.

There may be an unusual host susceptibility to the Whipple bacillus. Indeed, there is considerable evidence of immunodeficiency in the untreated patient, but this may be a consequence of malnutrition, obstruction to lymphatic drainage from the intestine, and the transient anergy of infection. Following successful treatment, most immune functions return to normal. There is, however, virtually no antibody response to *T whippelii,* suggesting immune tolerance to the bacillus, and there may be defective ability of macrophages to degrade ingested antigen. There is clear evidence that the clinically well patient has a subtle defect in cellular immunity. There is a persistent lymphocytopenia (with normal ratios of helper to suppressor cells), there is diminished responsiveness of T cells to nonspecific mitogens, and the cutaneous response to antigens (delayed hypersensitivity) is depressed. Immune complexes may play a role in the pathogenesis of arthralgias in Whipple's disease. There is a clear association of Whipple's disease with HLA-B27. Nineteen of 82 (23%) patients tested were B27 positive.

PATHOLOGY

General Remarks

Whipple's disease is characterized by a striking infiltrate of involved tissues with histiocytes containing myriads of ingested bacilli in varying stages of degradation. Occasionally there is also a prominent infiltrate of granulocytes. The inflammatory response may be granulomatous; indeed, 9% of patients have granulomatous changes, mainly in the liver and lymph nodes,[6] and less frequently in intestine, brain, and lung. Some of the early reports emphasized this aspect and called the disease "lipophagia granulomatosis." The similarity of Whipple's disease to sarcoidosis is often emphasized and a number of patients have been misdiagnosed at first as having sarcoidosis. The distinction of the two diseases is sometimes difficult because in Whipple's disease the noncaseating granulomas may be PAS negative. Detection of *T whippelii* within the granulomas, however, indicates that the granulomas represent a response to the Whipple bacillus, and are not a response to an unknown antigen.

Gastrointestinal Tract

The gut and its mesentery are almost always involved. The mesentery tends to be thickened with enlarged lymph nodes (Figure 95–1, A). When the mucosa is severely involved it may be grossly thickened and granular (Figure 95–1, B). Retroperitoneal and mesenteric lymph nodes may be so large that the patient presents with an abdominal mass. Duodenojejunal biopsy is the diagnostic procedure of choice (Figure 95–2). The duodenum, jejunum, and ileum are almost always infiltrated by characteristic macrophages (Figure 95–3), which are intensely positive with the PAS stain (Figure 95–4). The infiltrate is usually mucosal and rarely submucosal. Intestinal mucosa may be extensively involved with blunting and widening of villi (Figure 95–5), but may

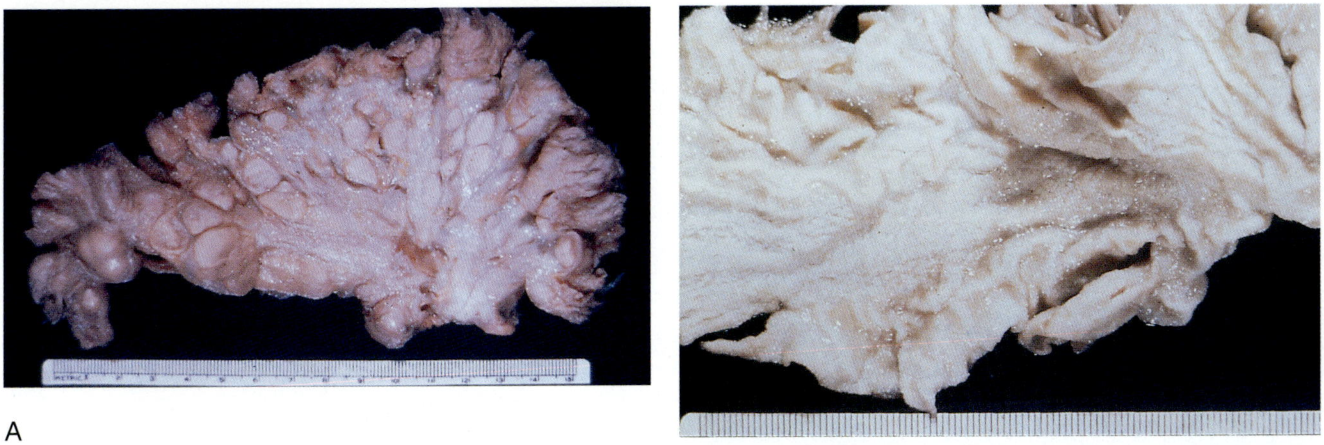

A

B

Figure 95–1. (**A**) Mesentery from an autopsy of an adult man who died of Whipple's disease. The mesenteric lymph nodes are involved and greatly enlarged. (**B**) Small bowel with extensive Whipple's disease. The mucosa is pale and finely granular. *(Photographs contributed by Ernest E. Lack, MD.)*

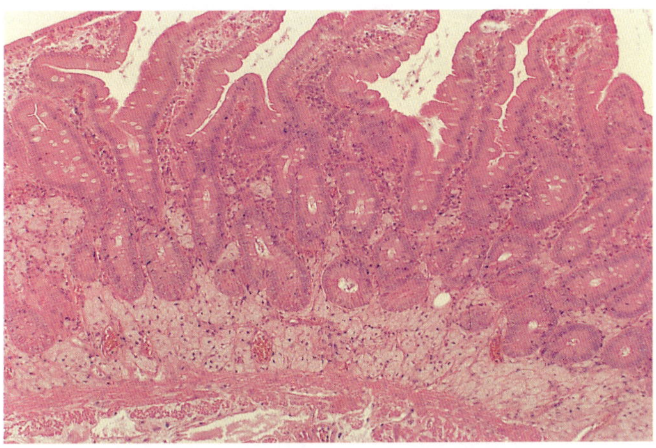

Figure 95–2. Whipple's disease of small intestine with characteristic macrophages along the base of the lamina propria and between crypts. A more superficial biopsy would have missed these characteristic cells (hematoxylin-eosin, ×75).

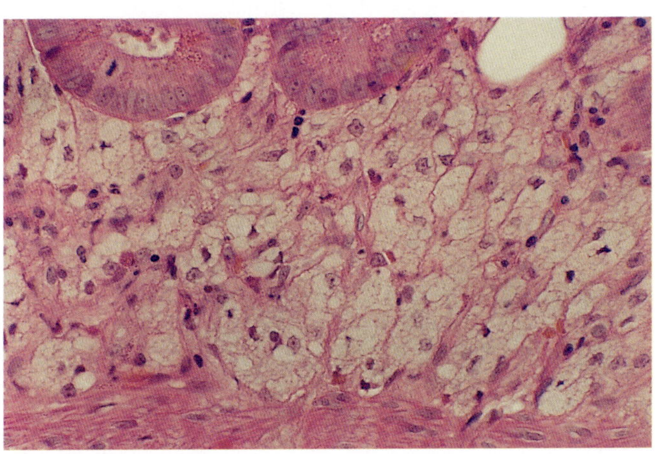

Figure 95–3. Whipple's disease of small intestine. Note confluent clusters of macrophages with pale staining cytoplasm characteristic of Whipple's disease (hematoxylin-eosin, ×400).

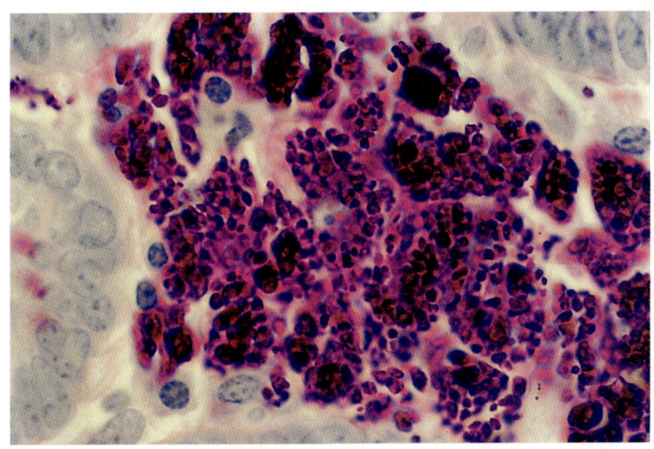

Figure 95–4. Macrophages in Whipple's disease contain abundant coarsely granular, punctate to elongate structures, which stain intensely with PAS (×1000).

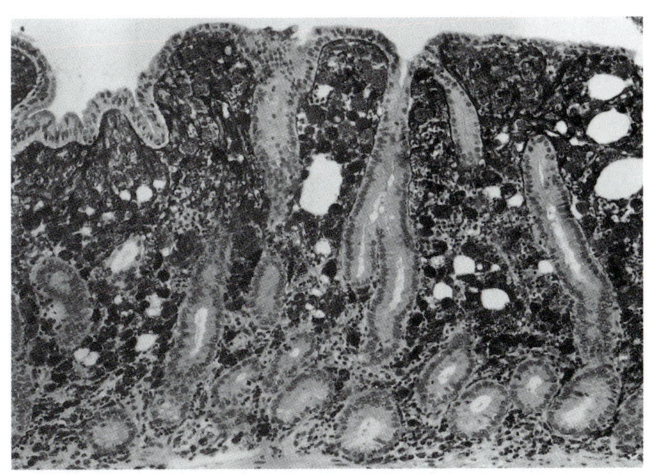

Figure 95–5. Small bowel mucosa with severe involvement by Whipple's disease. Villi are clubbed and flattened and the lamina propria is packed with histiocytes containing abundant PAS-positive material (PAS, ×250).

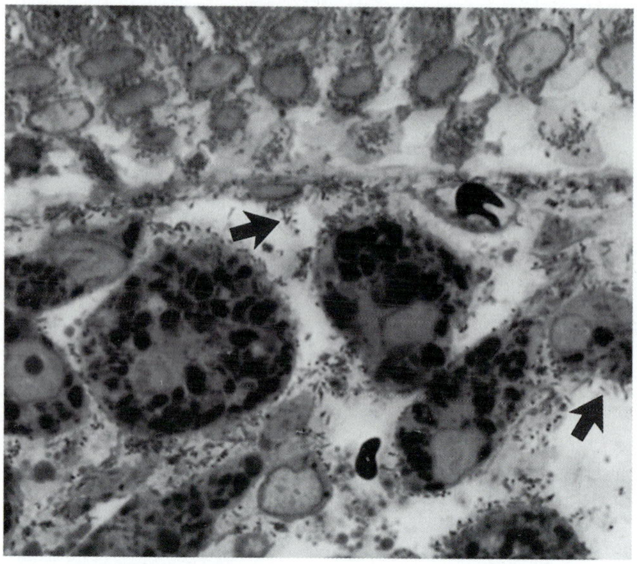

Figure 95–6. Whipple's disease; light microscopic appearance of macrophages in the small intestinal lamina propria. Note that most of the inclusions are either rounded or sickle shaped. This appearance is virtually diagnostic, especially when present in the intestinal mucosa. Note numerous rod-shaped bacilli throughout the lamina propria. Tangentially sectioned epithelial cells are at the top of the illustration (toluidine-blue stain of thick section, ×1500).

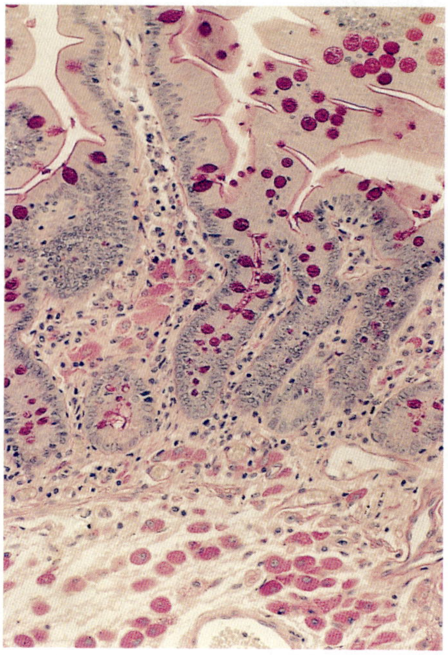

Figure 95–7. Post-treatment small bowel biopsy specimen from patient with Whipple's disease. The density of PAS-positive macrophages in the lamina propria is diminished when compared with the pretreatment biopsy specimen (PAS, ×120).

have normal contours as seen in Figure 95–2. Occasionally, there may be a severe intestinal mucosal lesion comparable to that seen in untreated celiac sprue.

The lamina propria is packed with macrophages, numerous bacilli, and frequent, large, free, lipid inclusions. The macrophages and bacilli are most frequent at the apex of the villi, but are occasionally in the submucosa. Lacteals are dilated but rarely contain lipid inclusions. Many bacilli are extracellular but may invade epithelial cells. The macrophages often appear to be actively "ingesting" bacilli. They contain numerous sickle-shaped inclusions, which are unique to Whipple's disease (Figure 95–6). Ultrastructural study shows that these membrane-bound inclusions contain a myriad of bacilli in various stages of digestion. It is the polysaccharide content of these inclusions that permits intense PAS staining. Following treatment, bacilli clear rapidly while the marophages clear slowly (Figure 95–7). They may still be prominent at the end of a year's course of antibiotic treatment and are still present in small numbers for as long as 11 years after completing treatment. The stomach and colon are rarely involved in Whipple's disease. It is important to note that PAS-positive macrophages may be seen in gastric and in intestinal mucosa in conditions other than Whipple's disease, eg, "lipophages" in stomach and "muciphages" in rectum (Figure 95–8). Patients with acquired immunodeficiency syndrome (AIDS) and infection of intestinal mucosa with *Mycobacterium avium-intracel-*

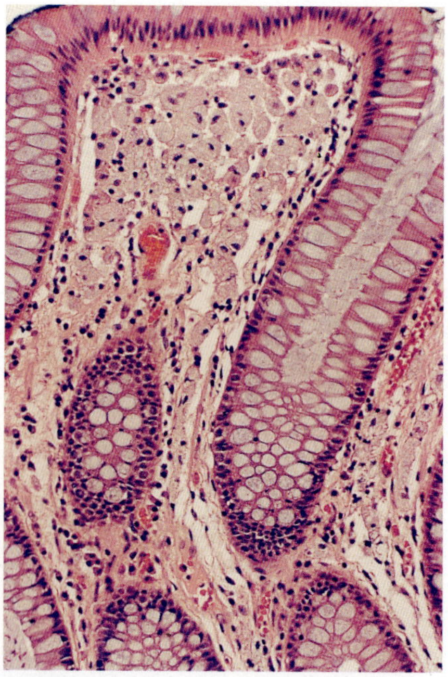

Figure 95–8. "Muciphages" in lamina propria of rectal mucosa should not be mistaken for macrophages of Whipple's disease nor for a systemic storage disease. These macrophages contain extravasated mucus from the crypt mucosal cells (hematoxylin-eosin, ×100).

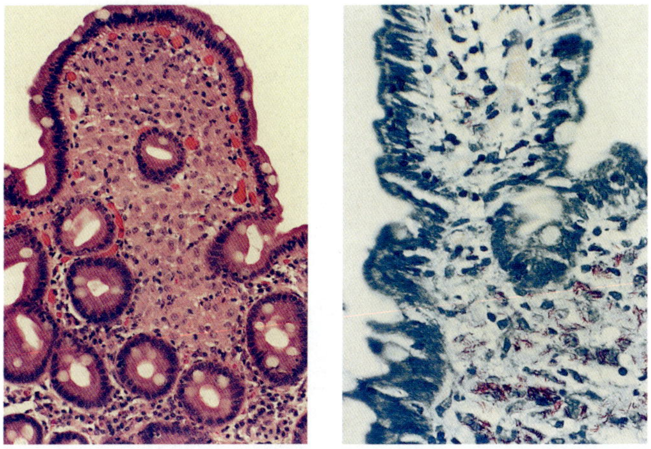

A B

Figure 95–9. (**A**) MAC infection in a patient with AIDS. The lamina propria is distended by macropahges swollen by enormous numbers of acid-fast bacilli (hematoxylin-eosin, ×100). (**B**) Same biopsy specimen shown in part (A). There are clusters of acid-fast bacilli in macrophages (Ziehl–Neelsen, ×400).

lulare complex (MAC) have many macrophages in the lamina propria (Figure 95–9, A). These can be distinguished from the macrophages of Whipple's disease with the Ziehl–Neelsen stain, which reveals intracellular acid-fast bacilli (Figure 95–9, B).

Capsular thickening of the spleen and liver are frequent, whereas hepatosplenomegaly is infrequent. Liver biopsy specimens are usually not helpful because the infiltrates in liver tend to be PAS negative. Pancreas and gallbladder are rarely involved. With lymph node involvement there may be vacuolar spaces suggesting lipid accumulation (Figure 95–10), and in early stages there may be a granulomatous reaction resembling lymphangiogram effect.

Cardiovascular System

At autopsy pericarditis and endocarditis are prominent findings in untreated patients, while clinically important cardiac manifestations are infrequent. Adhesive pericarditis is present in 75%, fibrosis and/or deformity of cardiac valves with marantic lesions in about 50%, myocardial fibrosis in 10%, and lymphocytic myocarditis in 1%. Replacement of aortic and mitral valves has sometimes been required. Vasculitis is uncommon.

Central Nervous System and Eye

The clinical manifestations of involvement of the CNS are protean, and reflect the widespread distribution of lesions usually consisting of 1- to 2-mm infiltrates of histiocytes. Hemispheric involvement results in personality changes, dementia, and rarely hemiparesis and seizures.

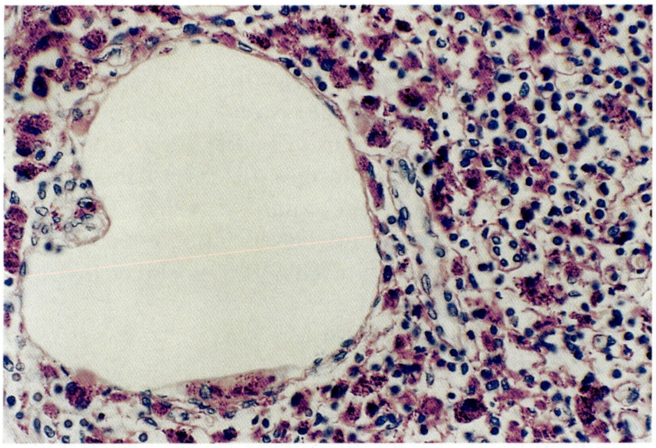

Figure 95–10. Whipple's disease involving a regional mesenteric lymph node. Lymphatic channels are dilated and numerous PAS-positive macrophages characteristic of Whipple's disease are present.

Involvement of hypothalamus results in insomnia, hypersomnia, hyperphagia, or polydipsia. Cerebellar ataxia, mesencephalic lesions causing ophthalmoplegia or nystagmus, and Wernicke's encephalopathy are all complications. Dementia, ophthalmoplegia, and myoclonus are the most frequent manifestations and when present simultaneously constitute a virtually diagnostic triad. Hypothalamic changes are the fourth most frequent CNS manifestation. Rhythmic convergence of the eyes associated with synchronous contractions of masticatory muscles—oculomasticatory myorhythmia—though rare, is unique to Whipple's disease.

A number of patients with CNS disease have had minimal features of gastrointestinal involvement even though characteristic histologic changes were in intestinal biopsy specimens. More importantly, a few patients have had CNS disease without involvement of the gut. Finally, many patients have developed, years after initially successful treatment, relapse manifested by irreversible and progressive dementia leading to death. Peripheral neuropathy and polyradiculoneuropathy (Guillain-Barré) are rare.

Manifestations of eye involvement include uveitis, vitritis, retinitis, retrobulbar neuritis, and papilledema. The usual clinical manifestation is that of change or loss of vision usually caused by involvement of the CNS. Some patients present with eye involvement in the absence of intestinal or CNS symptoms, and Whipple's disease should be considered in patients with "chronic idiopathic bilateral retinitis and vitritis."

Musculoskeletal System

The disease often presents as a seronegative enteropathic arthritis, 65% of patients having arthralgias and/or arthritis affecting the large joints during the course of their disease. The clinical combination of polyarthralgias and fever prior to intestinal symptoms may lead to early diagnosis. Destructive joint changes are unusual and synovial fluid reveals only nonspecific changes of inflammatory arthropathy. Axial arthritis is also associated with Whipple's disease. Clinical and radiologic sacroiliitis are common (20% to 30%), whereas ankylosing spondylitis is rare, even though 23% (19/82) of patients are HLA B27 positive. Involvement of skeletal muscle is rare.

Lungs and Pleura

Chronic nonproductive cough, dyspnea on exertion, and pleuritic chest pain are common. The disease may mimic sarcoidosis, both clinically and radiologically. Pleural effusions, and diffuse and focal infiltrates may be in the chest x ray.

Skin and Peripheral Lymph Nodes

Increased skin pigmentation, not involving the buccal mucosa, and of undefined mechanism, is present in 50% to 60% and is a hallmark of the disease. Rarely, PAS-positive macrophages have been in the skin, or in subcutaneous nodules. Several patients have had scurvy. Peripheral lymphadenopathy, localized in 25% and generalized in 15%, may be prominent.

Genitourinary System

The kidney is rarely involved and the genitourinary tract is even less likely to be involved. Renal biopsy specimens may show a variety of nonspecific changes but did show granulomas and Whipple bacilli in one patient.

Endocrine System

Involvement of endocrine organs is virtually nonexistent. Whipple's disease often presents clinically like Addison's disease, but Addison's disease has not been established in such patients.

ELECTRON MICROSCOPY

Electron microscopy shows that the core of the bacillus is enclosed within a plasma membrane (Figure 95–11). External to the plasma membrane is a 20-nm-thick cell wall consisting of distinct areas. The inner dense layer contains polysaccharides, possibly teichoic acid, and accounts for the PAS staining reaction, and is the final remnant of digested bacilli within macrophages. The outer dense layer has a trilaminar appearance similar to that of plasma membranes, is conceivably of host origin, and may account for the apparent antigenic tolerance to the bacillus and for its indolent growth.

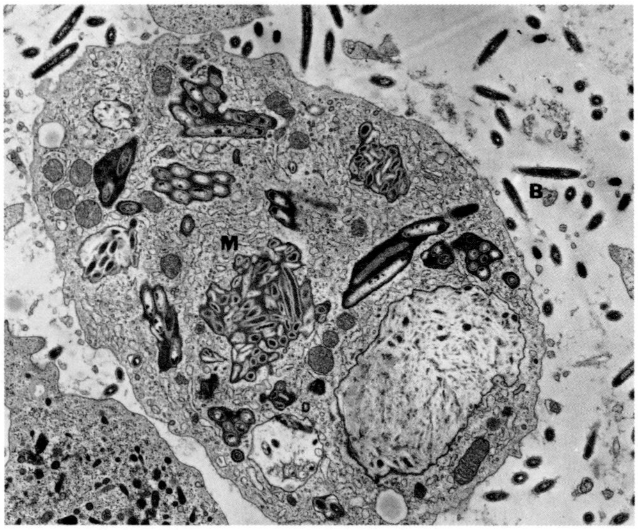

Figure 95–11. Electron micrograph of intestinal lamina propria showing numerous bacilli (B) in the extracellular spaces and ingested bacilli in varying stages of digestion within a macrophage (M) (×11,000).

DIAGNOSIS

The diagnostic procedure of choice is peroral intestinal biopsy. The disease process is usually diffuse but may be focal and thus the biopsy specimen should be obtained endoscopically. The duodenoscopic appearance is characteristic: thickened mucosal folds are coated with yellow granular material, or with 1- to 2-mm yellow-white plaques. These may be diffuse or have a patchy distribution.

The appearance alone of the PAS-stained section is sufficient to establish the diagnosis in most patients, and electron microscopic demonstration of bacilli is not essential. Occasional macrophages or histiocytes are in the normal intestinal lamina propria; they may stain faintly or even strongly with the PAS reaction, but the inclusions are not sickle shaped. There are three infrequent occasions when numerous PAS positive macrophages in the intestinal lamina propria may be misleading: 1) AIDS with MAC infection,[7] 2) systemic histoplasmosis, and 3) macroglobulinemia. The pathologist should distinguish the faintly staining, homogeneously PAS-positive macrophages of macroglobulinemia, and the PAS-positive, rounded, encapsulated histoplasma organisms in large macrophages, from those of Whipple's disease. More care must be taken to distinguish Whipple's disease from the intestinal mucosa in patients with AIDS and with a lamina propria filled with macrophages containing MAC (Figure 95–9, A and B). In the latter, the lamina propria is packed with histiocytes, which, with the hematoxylin-eosin stain and with the PAS stain, resemble those of Whipple's disease. However, MAC bacilli are acid fast, easily cultured, and have an electron microscopic appearance quite different from that of Whipple bacilli.

Rarely (10/760 patients) the diagnosis has been established in the *absence* of intestinal involvement. In these patients the diagnosis was established by the electron microscopic demonstration of bacilli in cerebrospinal fluid, in computer tomography guided or surgical brain biopsy specimens, or in peripheral lymph nodes. More recently a patient with chronic bilateral uveitis, caused by Whipple's disease, had no clinical or pathologic evidence of gastrointestinal Whipple's disease but the diagnosis was confirmed by polymerase chain reaction assay on specimens taken from the vitreous and the duodenal mucosa.[8]

Caution is required in the interpretation of gastric and rectal biopsy specimens. PAS-positive macrophages are frequent in normal gastric and rectal mucosa, as well as in many diseases of the stomach and rectum. The stomach often contains faintly PAS-positive, lipid-containing macrophages (lipophages), whereas the rectal mucosa usually contains strongly PAS-positive muciphages and pigment-containing macrophages. Generally, electron microscopic demonstration of Whipple bacilli in these tissues is necessary to establish the diagnosis.

REFERENCES

1. Dobbins WO III. *Whipple's Disease.* Springfield, Ill: CC Thomas; 1987.
2. Whipple GH. A hitherto undescribed disease characterized anatomically by deposits of fat and fatty acids in the intestinal and mesenteric lymphatic tissues. *Johns Hopkins Hosp Bull.* 1907;18:382–391.
3. Wilson KH, Blitchington R, Frothingham R, Wilson JA. Phylogeny of the Whipple's disease—associated bacterium. *Lancet.* 1991;338:474–475.
4. Relman DA, Schmidt TM, MacDermot RP, Falkow S. Identification of the uncultured bacillus of Whipple's disease. *N Engl J Med.* 1992;327:293–301.
5. Enzinger FM, Helwig EB. Whipple's disease—a review of the literature and report of fifteen patients. *Virchows Arch Path Anat.* 1963;336:238–268.
6. Southern JF, Moscicki RA, Magro C, Dickersin GR, Fallon JT, Bloch HJ. Lymphedema, lymphocytic myocarditis, and sarcoid-like granulomatosis. Manifestations of Whipple's disease. *JAMA.* 1989;261:1467–1470.
7. Maliha GM, Hepps KS, Mala DM, Gentry KR, Fraire AE, Goodgame RW. Whipple's disease can mimic chronic AIDS enteropathy. *Am J Gastroenterol.* 1991;86:79–81.
8. Rickman LS, Freeman WR, Green WR, et al. Brief report: uveitis caused by *Tropheryma whippelii* (Whipple's bacillus). *N Engl J Med.* 1995;332:363–366.

CHAPTER 96

Whooping Cough (Pertussis)

Ernest E. Lack and Harry P. W. Kozakewich

The needs of children should not be made to wait.

John F. Kennedy (1917–1963), Message to Congress on the Nation's Youth, February 14, 1963

DEFINITION

Pertussis [Latin, *per*, "very (intensive)," and *tussis*, "cough"], also known as whooping cough, is an acute bacterial infection of the respiratory tract caused by the gram-negative coccobacillus (short rod) *Bordetella pertussis* (Bordet–Gengou bacillus). A mild form of pertussis may be caused by *B parapertussis*. The "whoop" refers to the sonorous labored inspiration at the termination of a paroxysm of coughing, but it is important to note that not all patients with pertussis whoop,[1] and in some patients a whoop may be caused by an entirely different infectious agent,[2,3] or rarely a mixed infection.[4] Because whooping cough may be a clinical syndrome, the more specific term *pertussis* will be used throughout this chapter.

EPIDEMIOLOGY

Pertussis is a highly communicable disease particularly when it is introduced into a susceptible population. Transmission usually requires contact with an infected patient; infants between 1 and 2 months of age are at highest risk for pertussis.[5] Infants and children who are not immunized and children who are incompletely immunized are particularly prone to infection. Adolescents and adults with decreased immunity and mild atypical infection have an important role in transmitting *B pertussis* to susceptible patients.[6] From the 1920s, when pertussis became a nationally reportable disease, until the early 1940s, when pertussis vaccines first became available, the average annual incidence for reported cases was 150 per 100,000 population with an average death rate of 6 per 100,000 in the United States.[5] Following the introduction and widespread use of whole-cell pertussis vaccines combined with diphtheria and tetanus toxoids (DTP vaccine) the incidence of reported cases of pertussis declined dramatically (about 99% reduction by 1970) (Table 96–1), and since 1981 pertussis has been listed as an underlying cause of death on less than eight death certificates per year.[5] Throughout the world, however, pertussis remains a major cause of morbidity and mortality among infants, causing an estimated 600,000 deaths yearly.[7]

In 1993 there was a resurgence of pertussis in the United States with 6335 infections reported, the most in 26 years.[8,9] The figures reported, however, may underestimate the true incidence of pertussis because of incomplete reporting. In a recent microbiologic surveillance of a pertussis epidemic in Cincinnati in 1993, infections were primarily among children who had been appropriately immunized, indicating that the whole-cell pertussis vaccine failed to give full protection.[6] There was a shift in incidence from young infants to older children, and 11% of patients were more than 12 years old.[6] Other studies also report that protection provided by conventional pertussis vaccine is evidently short lived,[10,11] and as immunity wanes in adulthood, there may develop a new epidemiologic status quo with an enlarging reservoir of potential infection for the hosts at greatest risk, young infants. There is no known prolonged carrier state in this disease. Despite the availability of an effective (80% to 90% protective) whole-cell vaccine as well as new acellular vaccines, pertussis remains a disease of worldwide distribution, because some developing countries lack resources for effective mass vaccination.[12]

TABLE 96–1. FEATURES OF 16 CASES OF FATAL PERTUSSIS FROM THE AUTOPSY FILES OF THE CHILDREN'S HOSPITAL, BOSTON, 1929–1971

Year	Age/Sex	Duration of Illness	Presentation	Course	WBC (per microliter)	Autopsy Findings
1. 1929	4 wk/F	—	Cough paroxysm	Persistent cough, hypoxia	—	Bronchitis
2. 1933	1 mo/F	2 wk	Cough, convulsions	Cough paroxysm, respiratory arrest	97,000; 34% lymphocytes	Laryngotracheobronchitis, superimposed sepsis
3. 1934	19 mo/F	1 wk	Cough paroxysm	Increasing fever	128,000; 78% lymphocytes	Tracheobronchitis, acute bronchopneumonia, superimposed sepsis
4. 1934	15 mo/F	3 wk	Cough paroxysm, respiratory distress	Cardiorespiratory failure	—	Acute bronchopneumonia and superimposed sepsis
5. 1936	5 yr/F	4 wk	Delirium	Sepsis	68,000; 75% neutrophils	Otitis media, superimposed sepsis
6. 1936	5 mo/F	several wk	Cough paroxysm	Apnea	170,000; 43% lymphocytes	Acute tracheobronchitis, bronchopneumonia
7. 1937	4 mo/F	6 wk	Cough, fever	Seizures, respiratory failure	118,000; 78% lymphocytes	Bronchopneumonia, otitis media, sepsis
8. 1937	2 yr/F	—	Respiratory distress	Progressive dyspnea, shock	—	Interstitial pneumonitis, bronchiolitis obliterans organizing pneumonia (BOOP)
9. 1938	4 mo/F	—	Respiratory distress	Progressive pneumonia	10,300; 68% lymphocytes	Acute bronchopneumonia, otitis media, sepsis
10. 1939	6 mo/M	1 mo	Progressive cough, fever	Cardiorespiratory failure	—	Acute tracheobronchitis
11. 1945	8 mo/F	—	Cough paroxysm	Progressive cough, seizures	92,000; 95% lymphocytes	Bronchitis, interstitial pneumonia, pneumococcal meningitis
12. 1945	11 mo/M	—	Spasmodic cough, fever, seizures	Shock	—	Bronchitis, otitis media, respiratory syncytial virus pneumonia
13.1947	5 mo/F	3 wk	Cough paroxysm, fever	Respiratory failure	—	Acute tracheobronchitis, bronchopneumonia
14. 1950	2 yr/M	—	Cough, seizure, fever	Convulsions, encephalopathy	53,000; 47% lymphocytes	Bronchitis
15. 1960	18 mo/F	4 wk	Cough, fever, apnea	Pneumonia, cardiac arrest	74,000: 65% lymphocytes	Pneumonia, sepsis
16. 1971	8 wk/F	—	Cough paroxysm	Pneumonia, seizures, apnea	49,000; 68% lymphocytes	Tracheobronchitis, adenovirus pneumonia

CLINICAL FEATURES

The incubation period of pertussis varies from 6 to 20 days (average of about 7 days), and symptomatic illness is divided into three stages: catarrhal, paroxysmal, and convalescent.[1,12] In the catarrhal stage (1 to 2 weeks) there are nonspecific signs or symptoms that can mimic a cold or other viral upper respiratory tract infection. During this stage the disease is highly communicable, organisms may be isolated from cultures of the posterior nasopharynx, and appropriate antibiotic treatment may significantly modify the course of disease.[12] In the paroxysmal phase (2 to 4 weeks or longer[1]), cough increases in frequency and severity often with a whoop due to sudden marked inspiratory effort as air is inhaled forcefully against a narrowed glottis. This may be associated with vomiting, cyanosis, bulging eyes, salivation, lacrimation, or distention of neck veins. Paroxysms of coughing may be exhausting. In infants under 6 months there may be apneic episodes and the whoop may be absent.[12] Patients often appear normal between paroxysms. There is usually a marked lymphocytosis (Table 96–1). At this stage it is increasingly difficult to isolate *B pertussis* from the respiratory tract, and treatment with antibiotics has little or no effect on course of the disease.[12]

Important complications may occur during the paroxysmal stage, including secondary bacterial infections (eg, pneumonia and otitis media), toxic central nervous system manifestations (eg, convulsions and encephalopathy), and conditions directly related to severe coughing, such as hernia, pneumothorax, and rectal prolapse. In the convalescent stage (1 to 2 weeks) there is a decrease in frequency and severity of coughing episodes, and complete recovery may require weeks or months. Immunity from naturally acquired infection is characteristically lifelong, while immunity from vaccination may be short lived.[11] *Bordetella parapertussis* may cause a mild form of pertussis, and in the United States and Europe has caused 5% or less of documented *Bordetella* infections.[13]

PATHOLOGY

All members of the genus *Bordetella* are respiratory pathogens of warm-blooded animals, and share a tropism for ciliated respiratory epithelial cells. *Bordetella pertussis* and *B parapertussis* are uniquely human pathogens and multiply among and remain localized to ciliated cells of the respiratory tract.[12] Infection therefore is largely noninvasive. The histopathology in the lung is bronchitis and bronchiolitis with only slight extension of the interstitial inflammatory cell infiltrate into the neighboring alveoli (Figure 96–1). Neutrophils characteristically infiltrate in the area of the junction between epithelium and lamina propria (Figure 96–2) and cluster about degenerating epithelial cells.[14] Severe sloughing of respiratory epithelium can leave segments of bronchial wall denuded. An acute inflammatory exudate may accompany the sloughed, degenerated epithelial cells in the lumen of conducting airways. The tropism of *B pertussis* for ciliated respiratory epithelial cells has been studied in vitro using scanning electron microscopy of hamster tracheal organ cultures with selective attachment to specialized cell types.[15] Filamentous hemagglutin (FHA), a toxin of *B pertussis*, facilitates the attachment of bacteria to ciliated epithelium.[14] *Bordetella pertussis* remains localized on the epithelial surface, and can be demonstrated in sections stained for bacteria, particularly in early stages of the

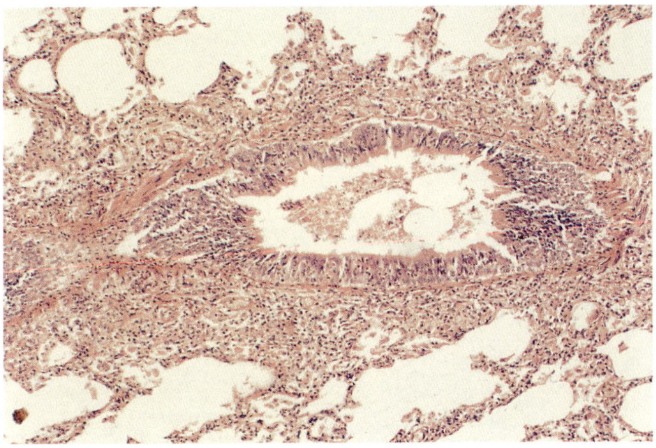

Figure 96–1. Fatal pertussis in infant who succumbed to the disease in the preantibiotic era. Bronchiole is involved by moderate degree of inflammation, which extends into adjacent alveolar septa (hematoxylin-eosin, ×100).

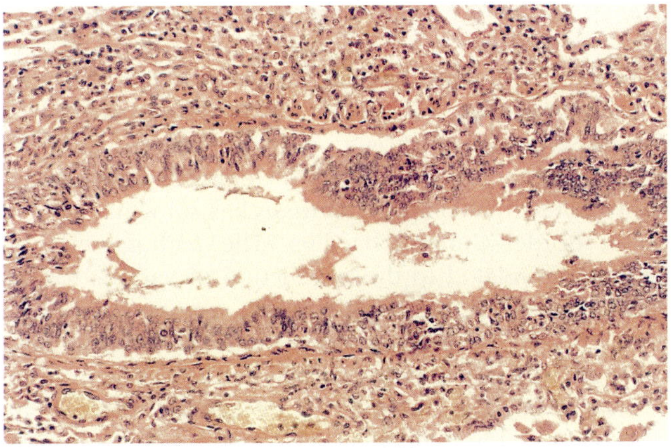

Figure 96–2. Fatal pertussis, same case as Figure 96–1, but at higher magnification in a different area. Note neutrophils permeating respiratory epithelium of terminal bronchiole with extension into adjacent lung (hematoxylin-eosin, ×200).

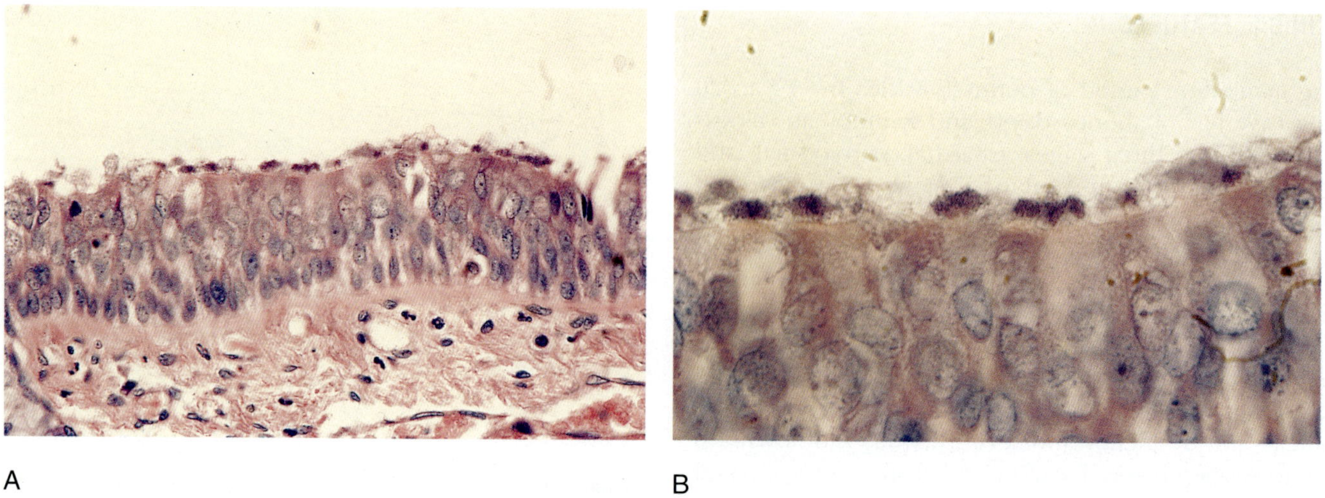

Figure 96–3. Fatal case of pertussis in 1934 (Table 96–1, case 3). Nineteen-month-old infant had "cold-like" symptoms and signs for 2 weeks, and 1 week before admission had paroxysmal attacks of coughing, some associated with vomiting. The white blood count was 128,000 per microliter with 78% lymphocytes. Sections of trachea show intact pseudostratified respiratory-type epithelium with immense numbers of small bacilli arranged along ciliated border. There was no viral cytopathic effect. Similar findings were noted also in respiratory epithelium of bronchioles. (**A**) Giemsa, ×400 and (**B**) Giemsa, ×1000.

disease (Figure 96–3, A and B).[16] Several earlier studies identified intranuclear inclusions, suggesting a possible role for a filterable virus in this disease,[17,18] but *B pertussis* remains the true causative agent of pertussis. Some of these infections may have been caused by adenovirus.

MICROBIOLOGY AND PATHOGENESIS

The genus *Bordetella* includes two additional species, *B bronchiseptica* and *B avium*, which are commensal and opportunistic pathogens of the respiratory tracts of various animals; eg, *B bronchiseptica* causes infectious tracheobronchitis in dogs ("kennel cough").[12] *Bordetella* sp are minute gram-negative coccobacilli arranged singly or in pairs, rarely in chains, and may be mobile from the peritrichous flagella.[19] *Bordetella pertussis* and *B parapertussis* are nonmotile.[12] *Bordetella pertussis* has the most fastidious growth requirements for primary isolation in culture.[12] Bordet and Gengou[20] first isolated the bacillus in 1906 and *B pertussis* has sometimes been called Bordet–Gengou bacillus. The pathogenesis of pertussis is related to the production of various toxins and virulence factors by *B pertussis*, among them pertussis toxin (PT), adenyl cyclase toxin (ACT), and FHA. PT is an exotoxin thought to play an important role in pathogenesis, and antibody to PT can be effective in protecting children against severe pertussis.[12] Secretion of PT, not simply production, is required for maximum virulence, and the toxin subunits must traverse both the inner and outer membranes of *B pertussis*. The *ptl* locus of *B pertussis* encodes proteins necessary for the secretion of PT into the extracellular medium, and localization of the promoter for *ptl* genes may be useful in the design of strains capable of secreting large quantities of PT into the culture supernatant.[21] Since inactivated PT is a component of all acellular pertussis vaccines developed to date, increased availability might reduce production costs.

The ACT produced by *B pertussis* can bind to calmodulin and calcium when taken up by macrophages or neutrophils, and become activated to generate cAMP, which suppresses chemotactic, phagocytic, and bactericidal activity; this may help explain the long persistence of organisms in airways of patients with infection and contribute to development of secondary infections.[22]

LABORATORY DIAGNOSIS

Collection, transport, and culture of *Bordetella* sp from clinical specimens has improved from the time of the "cough plate" technique, but isolation of the organism is probably at best 50% sensitive for laboratory diagnosis of pertussis compared with comprehensive serologic testing to establish seroconversion.[12] Direct and rapid examination of clinical specimens (eg, nasopharyngeal material obtained by suction or paranasal swab) can be done using a fluorescent antibody test in conjunction with culture to enhance sensitivity and specificity. Sensitivity in detection may be low, late in the disease process. Detection of *B pertussis*–specific nucleic acids with DNA amplification methods based on the polymerase chain reaction shows great potential in the diagnosis of pertussis. An isolate is not required for antimicrobial susceptibility testing because the organism is predictably susceptible to erythromycin, which is the drug of choice for both treatment and prophylaxis.

PREVENTION

Prophylaxis against pertussis, introduced in the 1940s, initially utilized conventional whole-cell vaccines composed of killed inactivated *B pertussis* organisms that contained a multitude of antigens[23]; although being efficacious overall, this has been associated with some untoward effects, such as anaphylaxis or unexplained encephalopathy after a previous dose.[24] A recent large population-based control study showed no significantly increased risk of serious neurologic illness in the 7 days after DTP vaccine exposure for young children.[25] Because severity of illness and mortality are highest in infancy, preventive measures such as vaccination should be done early in life; for instance, infants born to apparently immune mothers are highly susceptible to infection, particularly if maternal immunity was vaccine induced.[26] Recent studies indicate that acellular pertussis vaccine containing detoxified PT, FHA, and pertactin (also involved in adhesion of the bacterium to epithelium of the respiratory tract) produces fewer adverse reactions and provides a high antibody response against the antigens of *B pertussis* involved in bacterial adhesion and systemic toxic effects.[27] Controversy surrounds the various aspects of vaccination for prophylaxis against pertussis in the United States as well as in developing countries.

REFERENCES

1. Feigin RD. Pertussis. In: Feigin RD and Cherry JD, eds. *Textbook of Pediatric Infectious Diseases.* Philadelphia: WB Saunders; 1981.
2. Pereira MS, Candeias JA. Association of viruses with clinical pertussis. *J Hyg (Camb).* 1971;69:399–403.
3. Keller MA, Aftandelians R, Connor JD. Etiology of pertussis syndrome. *Pediatrics.* 1980;66:50–55.
4. Klenk EL, Gaultney JF, Bass JW. Bacteriologically proved pertussis and adenovirus infection. *Am J Dis Child.* 1972; 124:203–207.
5. Farizo KM, Cochi SL, Zell ER, Brink EW, Wassilak SG, Patriarca PA. Epidemiological features of pertussis in the United States, 1980–1989. *Clin Infect Dis.* 1992;14: 708–719.
6. Christie CDC, Marx ML, Marchant CD, Reising SF. The 1993 epidemic of pertussis in Cincinnati. Resurgence of disease in a highly immunized population of children. *N Engl J Med.* 1994;331:16–21.
7. Six killers of children. *World Health.* January/February 1987:7.
8. Resurgence of pertussis—United States, 1993. *MMWR.* 1993;42:952–953, 959–960.
9. Reported vaccine-preventable diseases—United States, 1993, and the childhood immunization initiative. *MMWR.* 1994;43:57–60.
10. He Q, Viljanen MK, Nikkari S, Lyytikäinen R, Mertsola, J. Outcomes of *Bordetella pertussis* infection in different age groups of an immunized population. *J Infect Dis.* 1994; 170:873–877.
11. Mulholland K. Measles and pertussis in developing countries with good vaccine coverage. *Lancet.* 1995;345: 305–307.
12. Marcon MJ. *Bordetella.* In: Murray RR, Baron EJ, Pfaller MA, Tenover FC, Yolken RH, eds. *Manual of Clinical Microbiology.* 6th ed. Washington, DC: ASM Press; 1995.
13. Linnemann CC Jr, Perry EB. *Bordetella parapertussis.* Recent experience and a review of the literature. *Am J Dis Child.* 1977;131:560–563.
14. Kuhn C III. Bacterial infections. In: Thurlbeck WM, Churg AM, eds. *Pathology of the Lung.* 2nd ed. New York: Thieme Medical Publishers; 1995.
15. Muse KE, Collier AM, Baseman JB. Scanning electron microscopic study of hamster tracheal organ cultures infected with *Bordetella pertussis.* *J Infect Dis.* 1977;136: 768–777.
16. Mallory FB. The bacillus of whooping cough and the lesion it produces. *Am J Publ Health.* 1913;3:589–592.
17. McCordock HA, Muckenfuss RS. The similarity of virus pneumonia in animals to epidemic influenza and interstitial bronchopneumonia in man. *Am J Pathol.* 1933;9: 221–251.
18. Goodpasture EW, Auerbach SH, Swanson HS, Cotter EF. Virus pneumonia of infants secondary to epidemic infections. *Am J Dis Child.* 1939;57:997–1011.
19. Holt JG, Krieg NR, Sneath PHA, Staley JT, Williams ST. *Bergey's Manual of Determinative Bacteriology.* 9th ed. Baltimore: Williams and Wilkins; 1994.
20. Bordet J, Gengou O. Le microbe de la coqueluche. *Ann de l'Inst Pasteur Paris.* 1906;20:731–741.
21. Kotob SI, Hausman SZ, Burns DL. Localization of the promotor for the *ptl* genes of *Bordetella pertussis,* which encode proteins essential for secretion of pertussis toxin. *Infect Immun.* 1995;63:3227–3230.
22. Confer DL, Eaton JW. Phagocyte impotence caused by an invasive bacterial adenylate cyclase. *Science.* 1982;217: 948–950.
23. Rabinovich R, Robbins A. Pertussis vaccines. A progress report. *JAMA.* 1994;271:68–69.
24. Burgess M. Pertussis vaccine—time to stop the confusion. *Med J Aust.* 1994;161:293–294.
25. Gale JL, Thapa PB, Wassilak SGF, Bobo JK, Mendelman PM, Foy HM. Risk of serious acute neurological illness after immunization with diphtheria-tetanus-pertussis vaccine. A population-based case-control study. *JAMA.* 1994; 271:37–41.
26. Statement on pertussis immunization. *Can Med Assoc J.* 1993;149:1132–1134.
27. Podda A, De Luca EC, Contu B, et al. Comparative study of a whole-cell pertussis vaccine and a recombinant acellular pertussis vaccine. *J Pediatr.* 1994;124:921–926.

CHAPTER 97

Yaws, Bejel, and Pinta

Herbert J. Manz and Alfred A. Buck

A physician is obligated to consider more than a diseased organ, more even than the whole man—he must view the man in his world.

Harvey Cushing (1869–1939)

INTRODUCTION

Three well-defined, clinically distinct, nonvenereal treponematoses are recognized.[1] Belonging to the same genus as the spirochete causing syphilis, these organisms are genomically, antigenically, and morphologically virtually indistinguishable, but appear to have different virulence and, specifically, a nonvenereal route of transmission. They also have different specificities for experimental transmission to laboratory animals.[2] *Treponema pallidum* sp *pertenue* causes yaws, *T pallidum* sp *endemicum* causes bejel (or "endemic" syphilis), and *T carateum* causes pinta. The difference in a single nucleotide is apparently not a definitive distinguishing trait between *T pallidum* sp *pallidum* and *T pallidum* sp *pertenue*.[3] In almost all patients serologic tests for syphilis are positive in these clinical syndromes[4]; transplacental transmission is not recognized.

In addition to bejel, yaws, and pinta, there are still other treponemal infections, whether singly or in conjunction with other microorganisms. For example, *T denticola* is implicated in periodontal disease; *T vincentii* and *Bacillus fusiformis* combine to contribute to the chronicity of tropical phagedenic ulcer; in trench mouth (Vincent's stomatitis) and Vincent's angina, anaerobic fusobacteria and *T vincentii* cooperate in causing necrotizing ulceration of mouth and pharynx and even lung abscesses and bronchiectasis; *T vincentii, B fusiformis, Corynebacterium,* and *Bacteroides* have most frequently been identified as causal agents in noma (cancrum oris). In these latter diseases, the variety of bacteria appear to act synergistically. Only yaws, bejel, and pinta are discussed further.

EPIDEMIOLOGY AND PATHOGENESIS

The nonvenereal treponematoses tend to be restricted to tropical and subtropical climates and to affect children and young adults. Even though transmission is nonvenereal, all three diseases are most likely acquired by direct personal contact, though bejel may also be transmitted by fomites; there is tentative evidence that arthropod vectors might transmit pinta and yaws. Pinta ("painted" in Spanish) is largely restricted to Central and South America; the disease manifestations are generally confined to the skin, thus making pinta the least virulent. Yaws is a disease of humid, tropical environments, and is transmitted during childhood by direct contact. Bejel (nonvenereal or endemic syphilis) exists in generally arid regions of the Balkans, Near East and Middle East, and Africa. In all three treponematoses, spirochetes multiply at the site of primary infection and disseminate to regional lymph nodes, causing lymphadenitis. In both bejel and yaws, a systemic spirochetemia may ultimately cause tertiary lesions in bones and about joints; however, aortitis and central nervous system (CNS) involvement are very rare and transplacental transmission apparently does not occur. Similarly, the obliterative endarteritis so characteristic of venereal syphilis is not a feature of the nonvenereal treponematoses. In all three diseases, the regional lymphadenopathy mimics syphilis.

Like syphilis, the clinical course of the nonvenereal treponematoses can be divided into early and late lesions, separated by periods of latency. In communities with endemic treponematoses, the prevalence of infection, based on positive reactions (treponemal antibody testing), is much higher than is the frequency of those with lesions. The estimated ratio for these diagnostic criteria varies between 1 : 2 to 1 : 5. In other words, in endemic areas the seropositives outnumber those with clinical disease by two to five times.

The World Health Organization and the United Nations Children's Fund launched massive campaigns in the 1950s and 1960s to eradicate the nonvenereal treponematoses and there were dramatic reductions.[5,6] Nevertheless, in the 1970s and 1980s, there was a dramatic resurgence of yaws[7–9] and several international symposia were convened to define the problem, to plan strategies, to assess research needs, and to implement protocols for worldwide control and eradication.[10–12] Recent comprehensive reviews have been published.[13–15]

YAWS

Yaws (frambesia, derived from "raspberry" in French) is a systemic treponematosis of children in humid, tropical areas. The primary lesion, or mother yaw, occurs at the site of inoculation, perhaps at an abrasion, by contact with a contagious lesion or perhaps an insect vector. This primary yaw appears 2 or more weeks after inoculation, is an elevated, papillomatous, crusted lesion resembling a raspberry (Figure 97–1), and may enlarge to many centimeters, forming an ulcerated mass. Serum expressed from it teems with spirochetes morphologically identical to *T pallidum*. Histologically, there are florid epidermal hyperplasia (Figure 97–2), a dense lymphocytic and plasmacellular infiltrate in the dermis (Figures 97–3 through 97–5), and even neutrophilic leukocytes, if the lesion is ulcerated. Spirochetes are readily demonstrable in the lesion (Figure 97–6) and regional lymph node by silver impregnation or indirect immunofluorescence.[16] The mother yaw may heal in several weeks, but may persist for months.

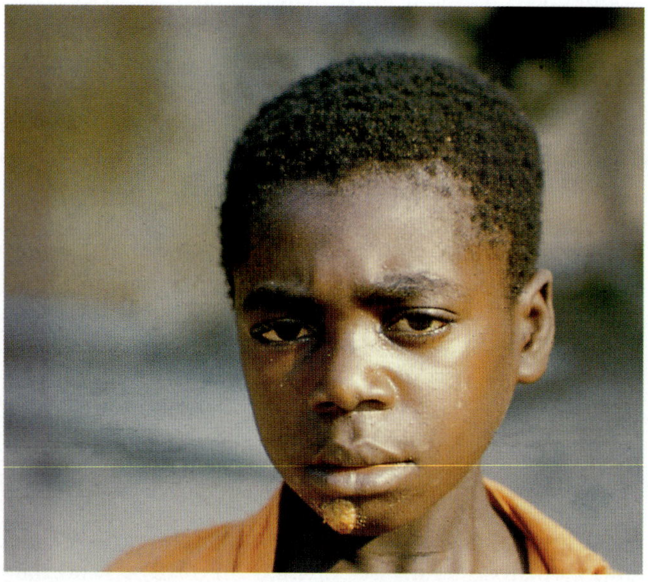

Figure 97–1. Primary "mother yaw" on the chin of a teenage African. The lesion is an elevated, papillomatous structure resembling a yellow raspberry.

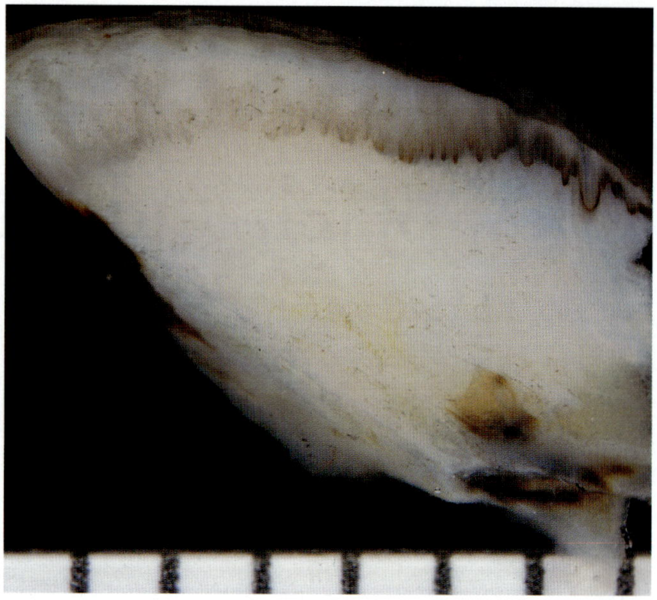

Figure 97–2. Cross-section of biopsied early yaws lesions, depicting hyperplastic epidermis whose basal layer is hypopigmented when compared to the normally pigmented epidermis on the right (×5). *(Photograph contributed by Dr Daniel H. Connor.)*

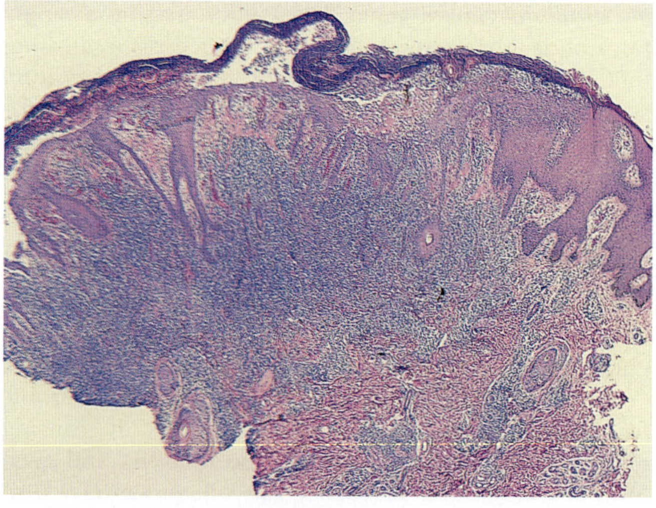

Figure 97–3. On histologic section, the lesion is hyperkeratotic, acanthotic, and acantholytic, with sawtooth-like elongated rete ridges and a dense, chronic, inflammatory cell infiltrate in the reticular dermis (hematoxylin-eosin, ×3.5). *(Photograph contributed by Dr Daniel H. Connor.)*

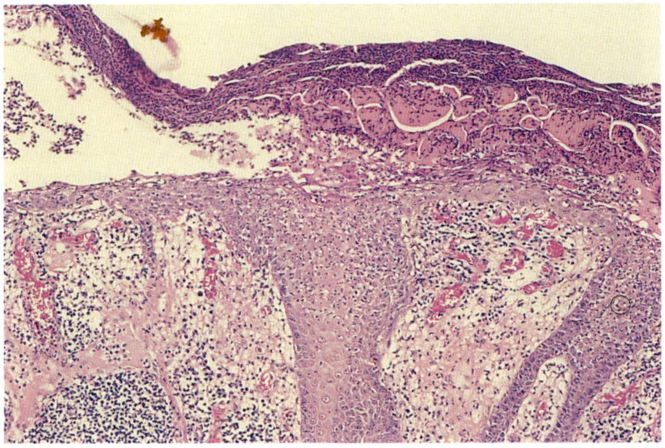

Figure 97–4. Higher magnification discloses the intraepidermal vesicle with epidermal necrosis and crusting, marked acanthosis, prominent microvasculature in the papillary dermis, and chronic inflammation (hematoxylin-eosin, ×50). *(Photograph contributed by Dr Daniel H. Connor.)*

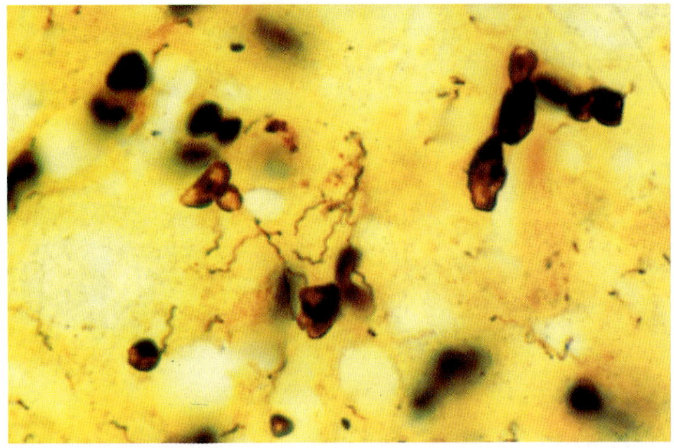

Figure 97–6. Tightly coiled spirochetes and chronic inflammatory cells in the papillary dermis (Warthin–Starry, ×1000). *(Photograph contributed by Dr Daniel H. Connor.)*

At this time, secondary yaws develop at multiple sites in the skin; these may be scaly, macular, verrucose, or oozing raspberry-like lesions that may resolve over weeks to months; however, new crops of similar yaws or maculopapules akin to those of secondary syphilis may appear recurrently for years, particularly at mucocutaneous junctions. Early lesions tend to be pruritic, so that scratching may result in autoinoculation as well as facilitate transmission within the household and community by contaminated fingers. The oozing lesions attract flies. A generalized or local lymphadenopathy is a prominent feature, but constitutional symptoms of fever and malaise are minor complaints. Palms, and particularly soles, develop hyperkeratoses with painful fissures; these lesions cause the patient to walk with soles inverted, producing the distinctive "crab yaws" gait.

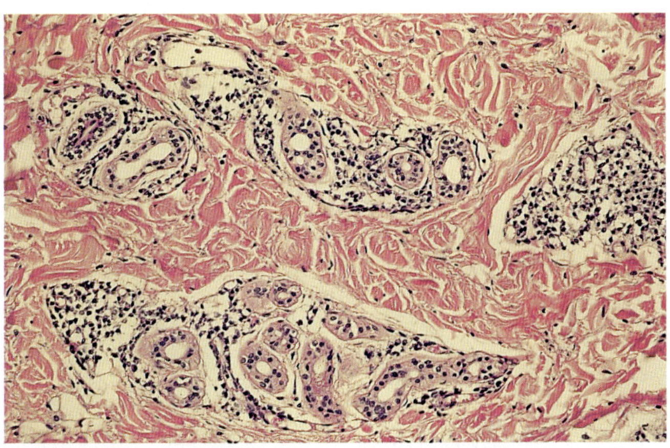

Figure 97–5. In the deep dermis, the sweat glands and ducts are surrounded by a chronic inflammatory cell infiltrate (hematoxylin-eosin, ×160). *(Photograph contributed by Dr Daniel H. Connor.)*

There may also be tender and painful periostitis. The disease may arrest or progress; a latent phase may intervene to be followed by late lesions several years later (not decades, as in syphilis); these are typical gummas in skin, subcutaneous, and periarticular areas and gummatous ulceration of the central face; the florid periosteal inflammation and reaction deform maxillae and tibiae (goundou and saber shins, respectively). Cardiovascular and CNS lesions are distinctly rare.[17]

BEJEL

Treponema pallidum sp *endemicum* is transmitted by direct, but nonvenereal contact, usually in childhood, and children serve as the reservoir of infection. Since the disease is commonly familial, and since oral lesions prevail, the spirochetes may be transmitted by kissing, by shared drinking or eating utensils, and by fingers contaminated with saliva. The primary lesion is only occasionally identified, and is most strikingly apparent on the breast of a nursing mother (Figure 97–7) whose infant acquired the disease by an unknown route but not across the placenta. Grossly and histologically, the primary site of inoculation resembles the syphilitic ulcer or chancre, including epidermal acanthosis, spongiosis, perivascular lymphoplasmacytic infiltrate, and numerous spirochetes. Mucocutaneous lesions are the most prevalent and involve not only the mouth (Figure 97–8), but also the nasopharynx and upper airway; these are identical to those of syphilis. There are also secondary cutaneous rashes, often in the moister body regions, such as axilla (Figure 97–9) and groin. Rarely, typical condylomata lata occur in the perineum.[5] Late lesions

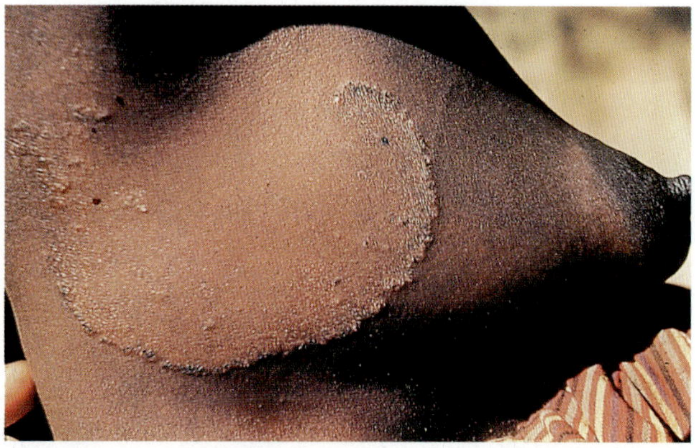

Figure 97–7. Endemic syphilis on breast of an African woman, with small, secondary lesions in axilla.

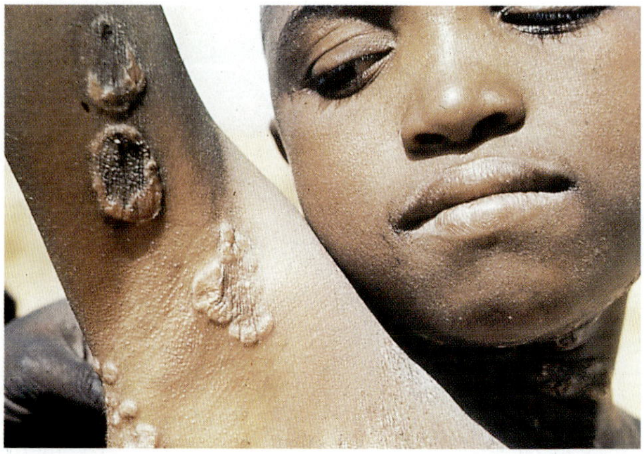

Figure 97–9. Large, secondary lesions of endemic syphilis in the axilla of an African person.

of the nose and bones are gummatous; periosteal inflammation and proliferation cause disfigurement of face (gangosa) (Figure 97–10) and limbs, particularly the lower legs.

PINTA

Pinta, a treponemal dermatosis, derives its name from the discolored lesions of skin and is caused by *T pallidum* sp *carateum*. The spirochetes are most likely transmitted by direct skin contact, since the lesions tend to be first evident on the uncovered limbs and frequently not until adulthood. This epidemiologic fact suggests that *T carateum* is not particularly virulent; further support for this suggestion derives from the confinement of the disease to skin and regional lymph nodes.

Several weeks after inoculation, usually by direct skin contact with a contagious lesion or possibly from the bite of reduviid bugs, a papule appears generally on the leg, the dorsum of the foot or hand, or the forearm. This lesion enlarges over weeks to months as a scaly, dyschromic, serpiginous plaque (Figure 97–11); the draining lymph nodes enlarge. In dark-skinned indigenous populations, the lesion initially is pink, erythematous, or violaceous, generally turns slate-blue later, and becomes hypopigmented over the years. Secondary pintids appear as pale, pink macules on exposed surfaces after several months. These lesions, too, become dyschromic, depigmented, and scaly. The multitude of shades and hues of skin coloration and haphazard distribution of the lesions account for the name, pinta. Histologically, both the primary lesion and subsequent pintids are characterized by epidermal hyperplasia (Figure 97–12), papillomatosis, acanthosis, hyperkeratosis, in-

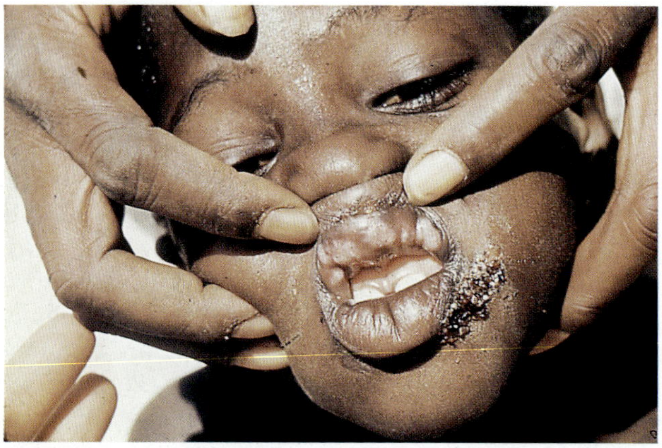

Figure 97–8. African child with labial and perioral lesions of endemic syphilis; the mucocutaneous lesions teem with spirochetes and are contagious.

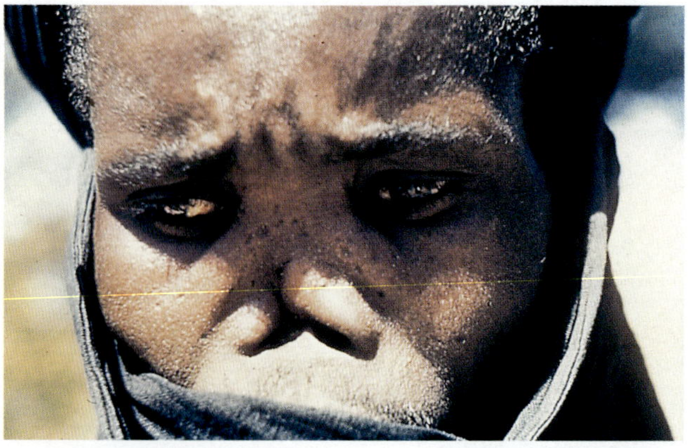

Figure 97–10. Destructive late lesions, "rhinopharyngitis mutilans," or gangosa in an African as a late sequel to endemic syphilis.

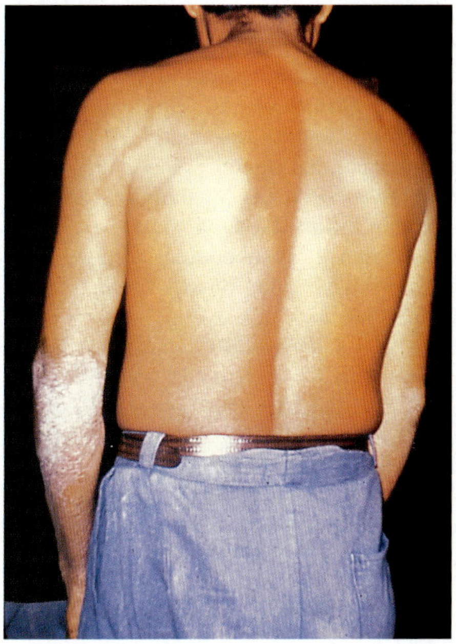

Figure 97–11. Irregular, whitish, elevated, squamopapular lesion of pinta involving the left elbow in a Mexican man. *(Photograph contributed by Dr Francis W. Chandler.)*

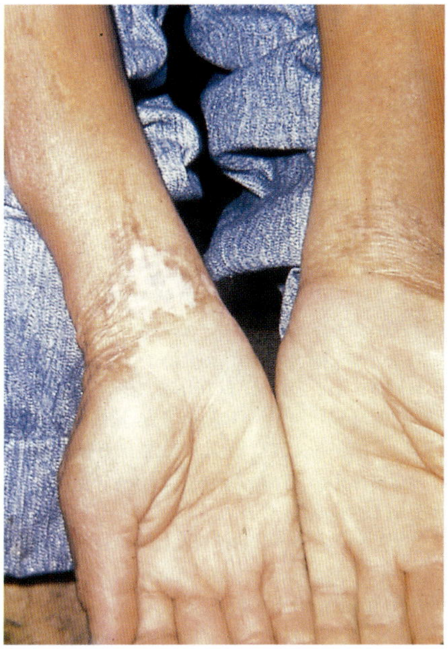

Figure 97–13. Healed lesion of pinta on right wrist and forearm. The hypopigmentation mimics vitiligo. *(Photograph contributed by Dr Francis W. Chandler.)*

traepidermal microabscesses, and loss of melanocytes in the basal layer, and numerous melanophages in the upper dermis. Dense lymphoplasmacytic inflammatory cell cuffs surround dermal vessels; the degree of vascularity and state of congestion of vessels also account for the clinical presentation. Spirochetes are readily demonstrable by silver impregnation stains. The primary and secondary cutaneous lesions are contagious. In the late tertiary stage, the degree of inflammation is markedly abated; the epidermis may be atrophic or hyperkeratotic with loss of melanocytes and a corresponding increase in numbers of Langerhans' cells[18]; these depigmented areas mimic vitiligo (Figure 97–13). The dermis is fibrotic; spirochetes are rare. The lesions tend to occur over bony prominences (Figure 97–14) and joints.[19]

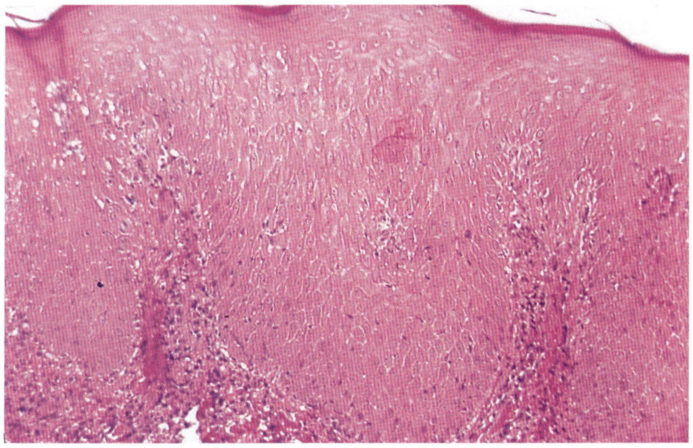

Figure 97–12. Histologic section of early pinta illustrating epidermal hyperplasia and chronic inflammation in papillary dermis (hematoxylin-eosin, ×125). *(Photograph contributed by Dr Francis W. Chandler.)*

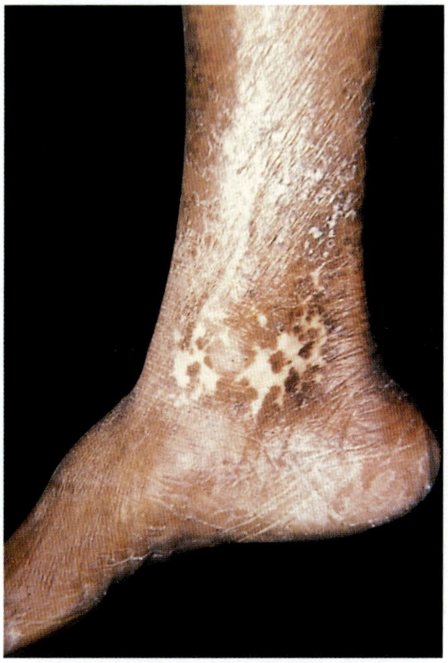

Figure 97–14. Chronic, residual effect of pinta over lower leg, particularly the medial malleolus. *(Photograph contributed by Dr Francis W. Chandler.)*

REFERENCES

1. Dooley JR, Binford CH. Treponematoses. In: Binford CH, Connor DH, eds. *Pathology of Tropical and Extraordinary Diseases.* Washington, DC: Armed Forces Institute of Pathology; 1976;1:110–117.
2. Gutman LT. The Spirochetes. In: Joklik et al, eds. *Zinsser Microbiology.* 20th ed. Norwalk, Conn: Appleton and Lange; 1992:657–666.
3. Noordhoek GT, Wieles B, van der Sluis JJ, van Embden JDA. Polymerase chain reaction and synthetic DNA probes: a means of distinguishing the causative agents of syphilis and yaws? *Infect Immun.* 1990;58:2011–2013.
4. Fohn MJ, Wignall FS, Baker-Zander SA, Lukehart SA. Specificity of antibodies from patients with pinta for antigens of *Treponema pallidum* subspecies *pallidum*. *J Infect Dis.* 1988;157:32–37.
5. Grin EI. Epidemiology and control of endemic syphilis. Report on a mass-treatment campaign in Bosnia. *WHO Monograph Series.* 1953;11:1–84.
6. Arslanagic N, Bokonjic M, Macanovic K. Eradication of endemic syphilis in Bosnia. *Genitourin Med.* 1989;65:4–7.
7. Hopkins DR. After smallpox eradication: yaws? *Am J Trop Med Hyg.* 1976;25:860–865.
8. Sehgal VN, Jain S, Bhattacharya SN, Thappa DM. Yaws control/eradication. *Int J Dermatol.* 1994;33:16–20.
9. Engelkens HJH, Niemel PLA, van der Sluis JJ, Stolz E. The resurgence of yaws. Worldwide consequences. *Int J Dermatol.* 1991;30:99–101.
10. Burke JP, Hopkins DR, Hume JC, Perine PL, St. John R, eds. International symposium on yaws and other endemic treponematoses. *Rev Infect Dis.* 1985;7(suppl 2):S217–S351.
11. Perine PL, Hopkins DR, Niemal PLA, St John RK, Causse G, Antal GM. *Handbook of Endemic Treponematoses.* Geneva: World Health Organization; 1984.
12. Fogarty International Center Symposium. *Yaws and Other Endemic Treponematoses.* Washington, DC: Pan American Health Organization; 1984.
13. Koff AB, Rosen T. Nonvenereal treponematoses: yaws, endemic syphilis, and pinta. *J Am Acad Dermatol.* 1993;29:519–535.
14. Engelkens HJH, Judanarso J, Oranje AP, et al. Endemic treponematoses. Part I. Yaws. *Int J Dermatol.* 1991;30:77–83.
15. Engelkens HJH, Niemel PCA, van der Sluis JJ, Meheus A, Stolz E. Endemic treponematoses. Part II. Pinta and endemic syphilis. *Int J Dermatol.* 1991;30:231–238.
16. Engelkens HJH, ten Kate JW, Judanarso J, et al. The localization of treponemes and characterization of the inflammatory infiltrate in skin biopsies from patients with primary or secondary syphilis, or early yaws. *Genitourin Med.* 1993;69:102–107.
17. Román GC, Román LN. Occurrence of congenital, cardiovascular, visceral, neurologic and neuro-ophthalmologic complications in late yaws: a theme for future research. *Rev Infect Dis.* 1986;8:760–770.
18. Rodriguez HA, Albores-Saavedra J, Lozano MM, Smith M, Feder W. Langerhans' cells in late pinta. *Arch Pathol.* 1971;91:302–306.
19. Fuchs J, Milbradt R, Pecher SA. Tertiary pinta: case report and overview. *Cutis.* 1993;51:425–430.

CHAPTER 98

Yersiniosis

A. Brian West

Disease generally begins that equality which death completes.

Samuel Johnson (1709–1784)

DEFINITION AND GENERAL DESCRIPTION

Yersinia enterocolitica and *Y pseudotuberculosis* cause yersiniosis. *Yersinia pestis*, the organism that causes plague, is closely related genetically to *Y pseudotuberculosis*, but is described in Chapter 79. The Yersiniae are facultatively anaerobic, non–lactose-fermenting, gram-negative coccobacilli that belong to the Enterobacteriaceae.[1] *Yersinia enterocolitica* and *Y pseudotuberculosis* share the important characteristics of being motile at 25°C (but not at 37°C) and of growing well at 4°C. The ability of these organisms to grow at low temperatures may account for the fact that milk, vegetables, refrigerated foods and drinking water act as common sources of infection. Whereas iron is an essential growth factor for Yersiniae, they are unusual among bacteria in lacking siderophores to capture iron. For iron uptake, therefore, Yersiniae depend on siderophores synthesized by other microorganisms or administered therapeutically (desferrioxamine), or on an exceptionally iron-rich environment such as blood stored for transfusions. *Yersinia pseudotuberculosis*, first isolated in 1884, was formerly assigned to the genus *Pasteurella*. It was given its specific name because of the resemblance of the gross appearance of the lesions it causes in the guinea pig to lesions of *Mycobacterium tuberculosis*. *Yersinia pseudotuberculosis* is a common pathogen of birds and domestic mammals, and is well known to veterinary pathologists. Infection in nonhuman species, however, is often strikingly different from that seen in human infections. *Yersinia enterocolitica* was first described in 1939, and was known under a variety of names until the current nomenclature was introduced in 1964.[2] Strains pathogenic to humans are carried harmlessly by several species of mammal and bird, which act as reservoirs for human infection.

YERSINIA ENTEROCOLITICA

Epidemiology

More than 50 serotypes of *Y enterocolitica* are known, but the majority are nonpathogenic, and 3 account for more than 90% of human infections: serotypes O:3, O:8, and O:9. Serotypes O:3 and O:8 cause most of the infections in North America (O:3 is more common in Canada, O:8 in the United States), O:3 and O:9 in Europe. For reasons that are not fully understood, there is marked geographic variation in the frequency of infection. *Yersinia enterocolitica* infections occur worldwide, but are more common in colder climates, and in winter than in summer. In Scandinavia and other parts of northern Europe, *Y enterocolitica* is second only to *Salmonella* sp as a cause of gastroenteritis. However, while *Y enterocolitica* is a common gastrointestinal pathogen in Belgium, it is much less often encountered in nearby France. Several studies suggest that in both Europe and North America infections with *Y enterocolitica* are being recognized with increasing frequency. Whether this is from a greater number of infections or more effective diagnosis is not clear.[3,4]

Most infections arise by the oral route. Sporadic infections and occasional epidemics result from consumption of contaminated food or drinking water. Food products are sometimes contaminated by being washed in water containing pathogens. Strains of *Y enterocolitica* pathogenic to humans occur as commensals in the upper respiratory and alimentary tracts of pigs, and undercooked pig meat has been recognized as a source of infection both in Europe[5] and North America.[6,7] Parental transmission of *Y enterocolitica* also occurs occasionally, usually as a result of growth of the organism in blood products stored at 4°C prior to transfusion.

Pathology

Acute Self-Limited Enterocolitis

Acute self-limited enterocolitis is the commonest presentation of *Y enterocolitica* in both adults and children, and in various parts of the world including Northern Europe and Canada. *Yersinia enterocolitica* rivals *Salmonella* and *Campylobacter* as a cause of acute diarrhea.[8] The symptoms of crampy abdominal pain and diarrhea, sometimes with nausea and vomiting, are usually short lived, though infants in particular may require hospitalization and a proportion of them develop septicemia.[9] Patients are rarely subjected to endoscopic examination or mucosal biopsy and, consequently, there are few descriptions of the pathologic features.

At endoscopy diseased mucosa is boggy, erythematous, and friable, or there may be aphthoid ulcers covered with a fibrinopurulent exudate that rarely forms a pseudomembrane.[10,11] On histologic examination the mucosal architecture shows no chronic changes. Early in the course there are mucin depletion and occasional crypt abscesses, and the lamina propria is expanded by neutrophils with few lymphocytes and histiocytes (Figure 98–1). Foci of superficial mucosal ulceration correspond to the aphthoid ulcers seen endoscopically, and often overlie lymphoid follicles (lymphoglandular complexes). If the process is biopsied late in its evolution the neutrophil-predominant infiltrate in the lamina propria is replaced by one rich in plasma cells and lymphocytes, and areas that were ulcerated will show mucosal regeneration.

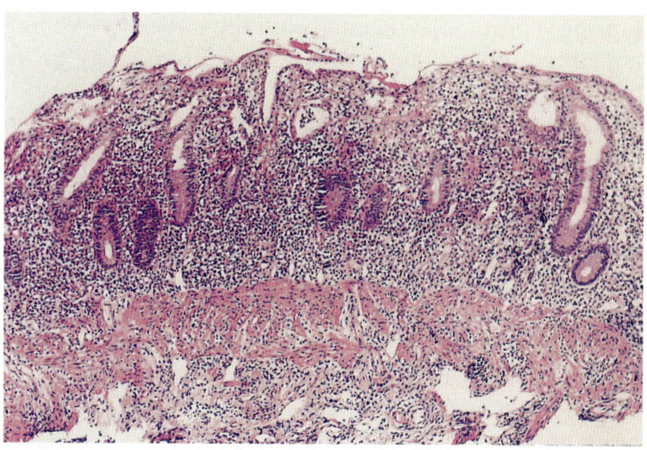

Figure 98–1. Acute colitis in a 19-year-old woman caused by *Y enterocolitica* O:9. The histologic features are those of acute self-limited colitis; mucosa of normal architecture with mucin depletion, increased inflammatory cells in the lamina propria including neutrophils, focal cryptitis, and surface epithelial injury. Injury is most severe in the superficial half of the mucosa (hematoxylin-eosin, ×10).

The histologic differential diagnosis of the diffuse lesions includes enterocolitides caused by other enteroinvasive pathogens such as *Salmonella, Campylobacter,* enteroinvasive *Escherichia coli,* and *Shigella.* The aphthoid lesions raise the possibility of *Salmonella typhi* infection and Crohn's disease, and if the pseudomembrane becomes confluent the process may be confused endoscopically (though not histologically) with pseudomembranous colitis. On resolution, regenerative changes in the previously ulcerated areas may lead to marked architectural distortion in mucosal biopsies, which is easily confused with ulcerative colitis.

Mesenteric Adenitis and Acute Appendicitis

Mesenteric adenitis is a common consequence of *Y enterocolitica* infection in teenagers.[12] Typically, these patients present with abdominal pain, nausea, and mild pyrexia. In time the pain may localize to the right lower quadrant of the abdomen, and it is often difficult to distinguish the signs and symptoms from those of acute appendicitis. If the patient proceeds to laparotomy or laparoscopy, the appendix, which appears grossly normal, is excised, but the enlarged mesenteric lymph nodes are not usually removed.

The lymph nodes are generally less than 1.5 cm in diameter and soft, without macroscopically visible necrosis.[13,14] On histologic examination the architecture is preserved. The capsule is thickened by edema and an infiltrate composed mainly of lymphocytes with a few eosinophils, plasma cells, and other inflammatory cells. This process also involves the trabeculae running inward from the capsule. Germinal centers are commonly small and inactive, though reactive follicles may be found. The cortical and paracortical pulp is expanded by large numbers of immunoblasts, plasmablasts, and plasma cells. The sinusoids are dilated and contain a mixture of lympyhoid cells including small lymphocytes, conspicuous immunoblasts, plasmablasts and immature plasma cells, and groups of transformed lymphocytes ("immature sinus histiocytosis") and cells in mitosis. Small clusters of histiocytes may be in the cortical pulp, and may contain central accumulations of neutrophils with or without necrosis (central microabscesses). Epithelioid granulomas are usually not present.

The histologic differential diagnosis of the lesions in the lymph nodes includes infections by *Y pseudotuberculosis, Salmonella typhi, Toxoplasma gondii,* the cat-scratch bacillus, and Epstein–Barr virus (infectious mononucleosis). The features of *Y pseudotuberculosis* lymphadenitis are described later. Nodes infected by *S typhi* typically contain prominent accumulations of activated phagocytes ("typhoid nodules") and few if any neutrophils. Cat-scratch disease is unlikely to affect the mesenteric nodes, and infectious mononucleosis is usually diagnosed clinically or by biopsy of a more superficial lymph node. Clusters of epithelioid histiocytes, typical of toxoplasmosis, are not seen in *Y enterocolitica* lymphadenitis. In uncomplicated mesenteric adenitis the appendix is grossly normal. In most cases no acute inflammation is observed histologically, but there is usually reactive hyperplasia of the lymphoid follicles. In some cases thorough sampling will reveal small foci of ulceration of the mucosa overlying lymphoid follicles (Figure 98–2), and occasionally the germinal centers contain microabscesses that erupt into the lumen.[12,13]

Yersinia enterocolitica has been implicated as the cause in some 4% to 10% of cases of acute appendicitis.[15,16] The histologic findings in the appendix, however, are not specific, and are indistinguishable from those seen in *Yersinia*-negative patients with acute appendicitis (Figure 98–2).

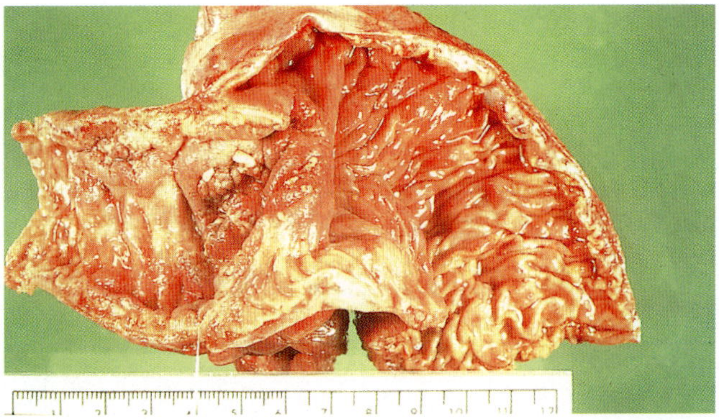

Figure 98–3. Terminal ileitis caused by *Y enterocolitica*. The terminal ileum is thickened by edema and enlargement of the Peyer's patches, which appear erythematous and focally ulcerated with a creamy surface exudate. In the cecum, nodules of erythematous mucosa represent inflamed lymphoglandular complexes. *(Photograph by Dr David Owen, Department of Pathology, Vancouver General Hospital, Vancouver, BC, Canada.)*

Terminal Ileitis

Among anatomic pathologists, acute terminal ileitis is probably the best recognized manifestation of infection by *Y enterocolitica*. Its striking characteristics have been well described.[8,17–19] It can occur at any age. Infants and small children tend to present with diarrhea and pyrexia, older patients with abdominal pain, nausea, vomiting, and fever suggestive of acute appendicitis. Rarely it presents as intestinal perforation. In almost all severe infections the terminal ileum and right colon are resected.

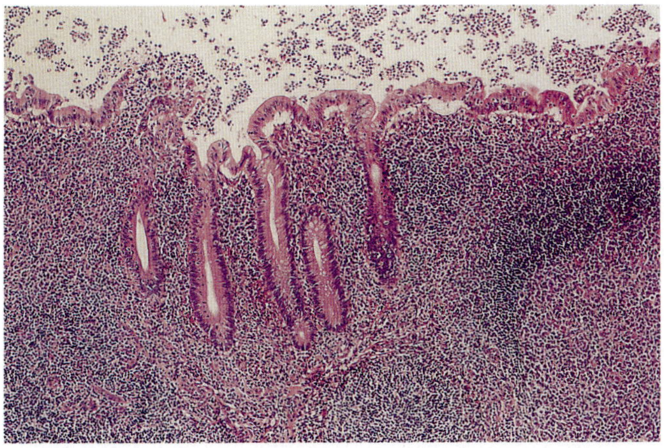

Figure 98–2. Acute appendicitis in a 14-year-old boy caused by *Y enterocolitica* O:3. There is reactive follicular lymphoid hyperplasia, with increased lymphocytes and plasma cells throughout the lamina propria and acute inflammation that has erupted through the surface epithelium at multiple points. Ulceration and features of more developed acute appendicitis were evident elsewhere in the specimen (hematoxylin-eosin, ×10).

The terminal ileum is the main focus, though the cecum and ascending colon are usually involved to some degree. The terminal ileum appears thickened, there is often fibrinous serositis, and the mesenteric lymph nodes are enlarged. The ileal mucosa contains numerous erythematous areas with shallow central ulcers varying in size from a few millimeters to 5 cm, mostly overlying the Peyer's patches (Figure 98–3). A fibrinopurulent exudate covers the floor of these ulcers, which are often sharply defined with a punched-out appearance or a surrounding rim of slightly exuberant mucosa. The intervening mucosa appears congested and edematous. The ileocecal valve, cecum, and ascending colon have numerous small erythematous elevations or punctate ulcers scattered over the mucosa; when close together, the surface exudates may become confluent, forming a pseudomembrane. The ileal wall is thickened, boggy, and edematous.

The ulcers involve the Peyer's patches (Figure 98–4), the colonic lymphoglandular complexes, and the superficial lymphoid tissue of the appendix. In early lesions neutrophil microabscesses are present in the germinal centers of the lymphoid follicles. These necrotizing processes erupt through the overlying surface epithelium, covering the area with a fibrinomucopurulent exudate. Immediately beneath this, in the inflamed and disrupted germinal center, the bacteria proliferate and form colonies of gram-negative coccobacilli that may readily be seen in sections stained with hema-

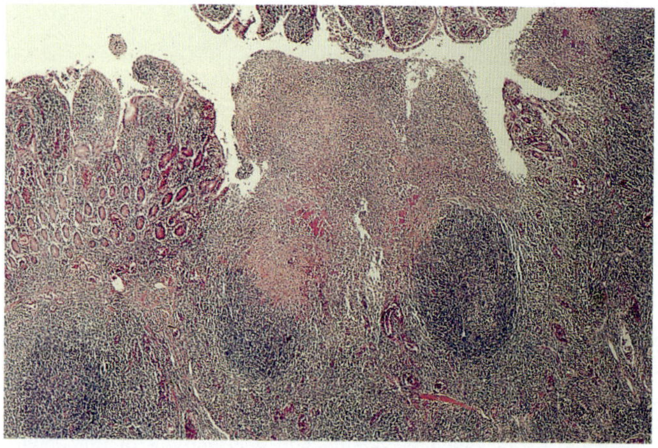

Figure 98–4. Peyer's patch from the specimen illustrated in Figure 98–3. The mucosa overlying the hyperplastic lymphoid follicles is ulcerated, and histologically viable lymphocytes in the luminal pole of affected follicles give way to a zone of coagulative necrosis and then a layer of acute inflammatory exudate, which erupts into the lumen (hematoxylin-eosin, ×4).

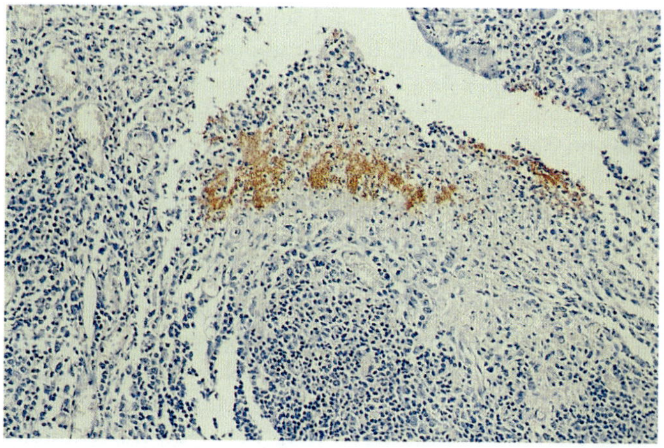

Figure 98–6. Section of terminal ileum from the same block illustrated in Figure 98–5, immunostained with an antibody specific to *Y enterocolitica*. The bacteria in the colonies forming the corona are immunoreactive with this antibody. The majority of the bacteria in the intestinal lumen in this section were not immunoreactive *(×20; immuonocytochemistry by Dr Richard Cartun, Department of Pathology, Hartford Hospital, Hartford, Connecticut.)*

toxylin-eosin (H&E) (Figures 98–5 and 98–6). Deep to the bacterial colonies is a loose layer of histiocytes, and this in turn is surrounded by lymphocytes. There are no granulomas. Entire Peyer's patches become ulcerated. The edges of the ulcers are sharply defined at the microscopic level. The surrounding mucosa is edematous and mildly inflamed, but ulceration and severe inflammation generally are confined to the mucosa overlying lymphoid tissue. In the ileum an infiltrate of eosinophils, lymphocytes, and neutrophils often accompanies transmural edema, which distends the submucosa and thickens the intestinal wall.

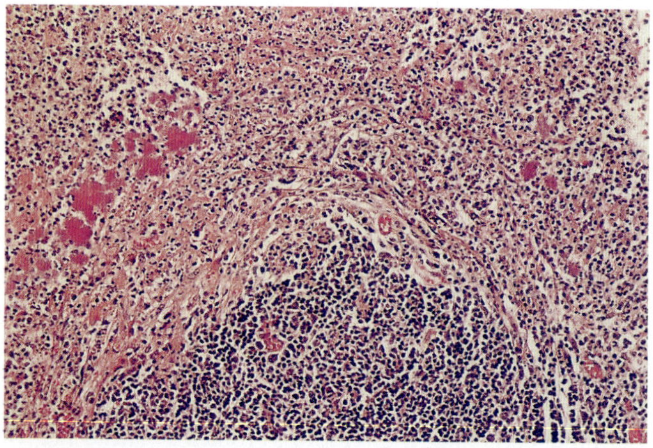

Figure 98–5. Higher magnification of the upper portion of a lymphoid follicle illustrated in Figure 98–4. At the border between the inflammatory exudate and the necrotic tissue overlying the follicle is an incomplete corona of colonies of bacteria that stain magenta on this H&E preparation. This feature is characteristic of *Y enterocolitica* ileitis and colitis (hematoxylin-eosin, ×20).

The mesenteric nodes are enlarged with features similar to those seen in mesenteric adenitis, as described earlier, but in addition with foci of necrosis that often contain colonies of *Y enterocolitica.*

The differential diagnosis includes typhoid, intestinal tularemia, brucellosis, tuberculosis, pseudotuberculosis, lymphogranuloma venereum, and Crohn's disease. In typhoid, neutrophil microabscesses are typically absent from the lesions of the Peyer's patches and "typhoid nodules" of activated phagocytes may be present. Granulomas may be in all the other entities in the differential. In Crohn's disease, there are usually features of chronicity and transmural fibrosis, and the ulcers tend to be deeper and more fissure-like than the shallow ulcers of *Y enterocolitica.*

Chronic Intestinal Yersiniosis and Extraintestinal Manifestations

Enteric *Y enterocolitica* infections may have three phases: primary, comprising acute enterocolitis, appendicitis, or mesenteric adenitis; secondary, occurring 1 to 2 weeks after the primary phase, and exemplified by sterile lesions at remote sites (polyarthritis, erythema nodosum, erythema multiforme, uveitis, iridocyclitis, glomerulonephritis, Reiter's syndrome); and tertiary, involving chronic diseases such as rheumatoid arthritis and ankylosing spondylitis.[20]

Most primary infections are self-limited and do not progress further. Occasionally, however, a primary infection becomes chronic and may persist for months or years, simulating Crohn's disease.[10–21] *Yersinia en-*

terocolitica has been demonstrated by immunofluorescence in sections of ileum and lymph nodes in patients with chronic ileitis and lymphadenitis and with persistent elevations of *Y enterocolitica*–specific IgA (see later discussion).[21] The morphologic features of these persistent primary infections have not yet been described in detail, however.

The pathology of the extraintestinal lesions seen in the secondary and tertiary phases of *Y enterocolitica* infection is typical for the lesions, and is not peculiar to this pathogen. Although cultures of the remote lesions are consistently negative for *Y enterocolitica*, evidence for persistence of infection is accumulating. In serum of patients with tertiary phase disease who are seronegative by the routine assays, de Koning and colleagues have documented persistent *Y enterocolitica*–specific IgA by Western blotting, which is more sensitive than the tests used routinely.[22] They argued that because IgA has a half-life of only a few days, persistent *Y enterocolitica* antigen must be present to stimulate production of this antibody continuously; and that because the predominant antibody was IgA, the most likely location of the pathogen was in the mucosa. By immunofluorescence they were able to demonstrate small numbers of persistent virulent organisms in intestinal mucosa, apparently in macrophages, including in patients with extraintestinal but no gastrointestinal symptoms.[22] Consistent with these findings, *Y enterocolitica* antigen, but not intact organisms, was demonstrated in inflammatory cells in synovial fluid from patients with post-*Yersinia* arthritis, in one of whom the disease had been present for 11 years.[23]

Bacteremia and Its Complications

Bacteremia occurs mainly in two settings: in patients with iron overload, especially those on the iron chelator, desferrioxamine; and in patients receiving contaminated blood transfusions.

In patients with iron overload, it seems that iron is more readily available to these siderophore-deficient bacteria, and may also inhibit host defense mechanisms. In patients treated with desferrioxamine, a siderophore produced by *Streptomyces pilosus* and for which *Y enterocolitica* has a receptor, the availability of iron to the pathogen is enormously increased. Thus, in these circumstances *Y enterocolitica* has a significant growth advantage.[24] Contamination of blood products with *Y enterocolitica* would seem unlikely because there are many more common pathogens for which this rarely occurs. If present in a blood pack, however (either from contamination or from undetected bacteremia at the time of donation), *Yersinia* will continue to grow in this iron-rich environment during storage at 4°C.

Bacteremia may lead to the development of active infection at virtually any location in the body, including septicemia, endocarditis, mycotic aneurysm, meningitis, suppurative arthritis, pyomyositis, osteomyelitis, renal abscess, lung abscess, and pneumonia.[2] The possibility of unsuspected hemochromatosis should be considered in any patient with *Y enterocolitica* bacteremia or its complications, since in one series of patients with liver abscesses caused by *Y enterocolitica* at least 63%, and possibly as many as 92%, had hemochromatosis.[25]

YERSINIA PSEUDOTUBERCULOSIS

Epidemiology

There are six major serotypes of *Y pseudotuberculosis*, types I through VI. Because it is much less commonly diagnosed than *Y enterocolitica*, this species has been less thoroughly studied in the clinical setting, and information on the pathogenicity of the serotypes is incomplete. In contrast, much is now known about aspects of its pathogenicity at a molecular level.[26] *Yersinia pseudotuberculosis* type I is a frequent cause of mesenteric adenitis, and type IV a cause of acute terminal ileitis and acute appendicitis.[3] *Yersinia pseudotuberculosis* is found in a wide variety of domestic and wild mammals and birds. Infection of humans is thought to be zoonotic, resulting either from direct contact with carrier animals, or from consumption of contaminated food or water. In Japan, *Y pseudotuberculosis* infection in children has been reported to cause a syndrome of fever, desquamative rash, crusted lips, strawberry tongue, conjunctivitis, and lymphadenopathy termed Izumi fever, and elevated serum antibody titers to *Y pseudotuberculosis* have been found in a proportion of patients with Kawasaki disease, suggesting that it may play a role in the etiology of this condition.[27]

Pathology

Mesenteric Adenitis and Associated Lesions

Mesenteric adenitis is generally considered to be the commonest presentation of infection by *Y pseudotuberculosis*. Patients, predominantly males from 2 to 25 years, typically complain of abdominal pain that may localize to the right lower quadrant, with nausea, fever, and vomiting. The clinical features may be indistinguishable from acute appendicitis. At laparotomy the appendix usually appears normal, the terminal ileum may be slightly swollen, and the mesenteric lymph nodes in the ileocolic region are enlarged, hyperemic, and sometimes matted. In severe cases the terminal ileum, cecum, appendix, and associated nodes form an inflammatory mass and there is a serosanguinous fluid in the peritoneal cavity. The majority of infections, however, are mild. Usually, if laparotomy or laparoscopy is performed in these circumstances, a histologically normal appendix is removed, the nodes are not biopsied, and the self-limited infection resolves.

El-Maraghi and Mair,[28] in a histologic analysis of tissues from 70 patients with *Y pseudotuberculosis* infection including 69 mesenteric nodes, 18 appendices, and 5 terminal ileums, interpreted their observations on the mesenteric nodes as showing four stages of progression. The first is characterized by lymphoid hyperplasia with enlarged reactive germinal centers in the follicles; the second by diffuse "histiocytic cell" hyperplasia; the third stage by multiple epithelioid granulomas, which are commonly related to the paracortical sinuses, and which may occasionally contain giant cells; and the fourth by centrally located neutrophil microabscesses and necrosis within the granulomas. The series included 35 patients with *Y pseudotuberculosis* type I, 18 with type II, 2 with type III, 3 with type IV, and 1 with type V. On histologic grounds, these authors could not distinguish between infections with types I through IV. The patient with type V infection had large necrotizing granulomas with extensive caseous necrosis surrounded by palisaded histiocytes and occasional giant cells of Langhans' type, indistinguishable from tuberculosis.

In contrast to the previous findings, Bohm and Wybitul[29] observed no granulomas in mesenteric nodes from six patients with type I infection; rather there was paracortical expansion and immunoblastic ("reticulum cell") proliferation with loose aggregates of neutrophils or sharply defined microabscesses in the paracortical areas, and germinal centers were not enlarged, as illustrated in Figures 98–7 and 98–8. In a node from one of their patients with type II *Y pseudotuberculosis*, epithelioid granulomas were present and some contained microabscesses and giant cells.

These differences in morphology may reflect different stages of progression, as El-Maraghi and Mair suggested, or differences in strain pathogenicity or in host response. These studies were performed before immunohistochemical methods for characterizing inflammatory cell populations were widely available, and their interpretation will depend on a better understanding of the nature of the infiltrates in these conditions.

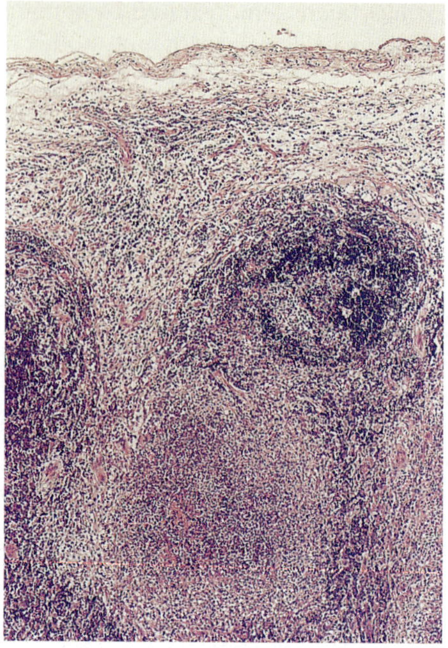

Figure 98–7. Lymph node from a 13-year-old boy with mesenteric adenitis caused by *Y pseudotuberculosis* type I. The follicle near the surface *(right)* has a reactive germinal center with lysis of some follicle center cells that give it a moth-eaten appearance. Deep to this is a cortical microabscess in which a central region populated by neutrophils is surrounded by a paler staining area that contains lymphocytes and histiocytes. Inflammation and edema are in the capsule and extend along a trabecula toward the hilum (hematoxylin-eosin, ×10).

Acute Appendicitis, Enterocolitis, and Extraintestinal Manifestations

Relatively little has been written about the pathology of *Y pseudotuberculosis* infections other than those causing mesenteric adenitis. This organism may cause acute mucosal infections, including simple acute appendicitis (Figure 98–9), granulomatous appendicitis (Figures 98–10 and 98–11), and terminal ileitis as mentioned earlier. Acute enterocolitis may also occur, and may be severe (Figure 98–12) or self-limited. In one series *Y pseudotuberculosis* infection was reported in as many as 27% of patients with acute appendicitis, though this may have represented an epidemic.[15] Extraintestinal complications are similar to those described for *Y enterocolitica*. Septicemia, related to iron overload and administration of siderophores, and its complications are documented.[3,4]

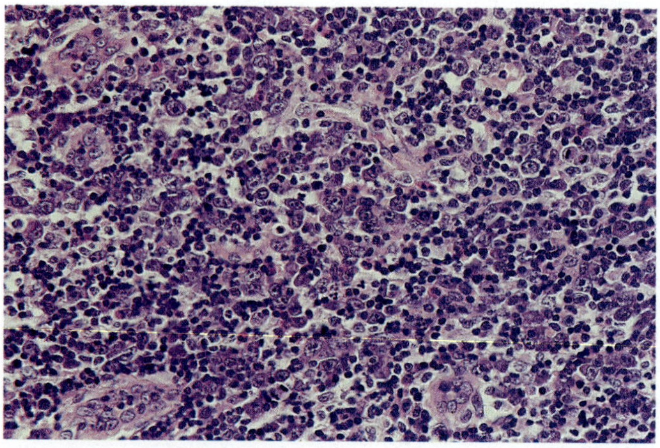

Figure 98–8. Reactive immunoblasts are prominent in the paracortical area of the lymph node illustrated in Figure 98–7 (hematoxylin-eosin, ×40).

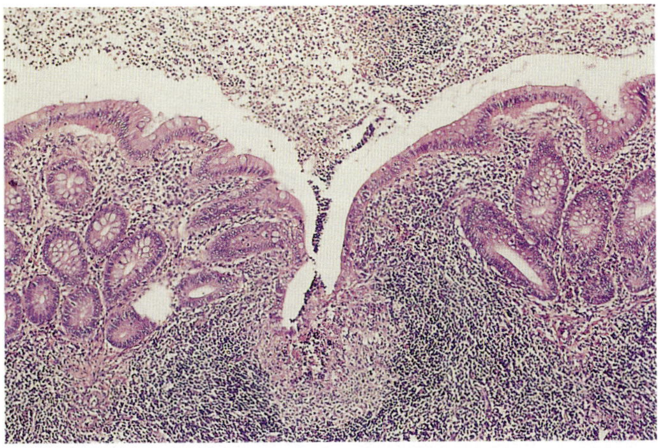

Figure 98–9. Acute appendicitis in a 9-year-old boy with *Y pseudotuberculosis* type IV infection. In most appendicitides caused by *Y pseudotuberculosis* the histologic features are indistinguishable from those of appendicitis of nonspecific cause. Breakdown of reactive germinal centers with eruption of the contents into the lumen, as illustrated here, is common in the early lesions (hematoxylin-eosin, ×10).

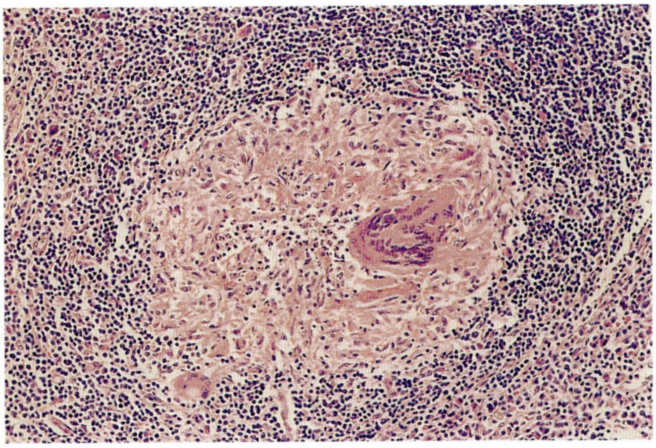

Figure 98–11. High-power view of a granuloma from the specimen illustrated in Figure 98–10. This granuloma contains a central region of necrosis with small numbers of neutrophils, surrounded by epithelioid histiocytes and a giant cell. Many other granulomas, however, did not show central necrosis (hematoxylin-eosin, ×20).

DIAGNOSIS

The most satisfactory way to diagnose yersiniosis is by culture of the organism and determination of its species and serotype. While this is relatively easy in patients with septicemia or a *Yersinia* abscess, it may be difficult to obtain *Yersinia* by culture of stool, because first the organisms may have left the intestinal lumen by the time cultures are taken and, second, because they are slow growing they are readily overgrown by other enteric flora and may escape detection unless selective media and cold enrichment procedures are used.[30] If intestinal yersiniosis is suspected, culture of pharyngeal swabs should be undertaken because the organisms may cause a mild pharyngitis also and be readily isolated from this site.

Many cases of yersiniosis can be diagnosed by serology. Markedly elevated antibody titers or a fourfold increase in titer in sequential samples is commonly taken as indicative of infection. However, the test is

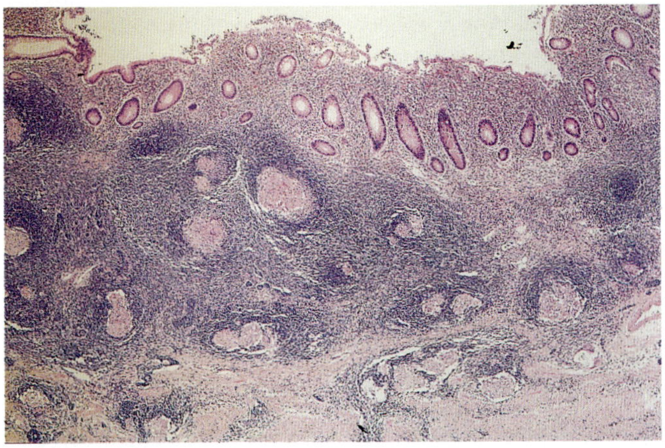

Figure 98–10. Acute appendicitis with numerous epithelioid granulomas in a 15-year-old boy with *Y pseudotuberculosis* type IV infection. The granulomas in this infection were transmural. Appendicitis was more severe in other sections, and in addition to ulceration and transmural inflammation, microabscesses were present focally outside the muscularis propria (hematoxylin-eosin, ×4).

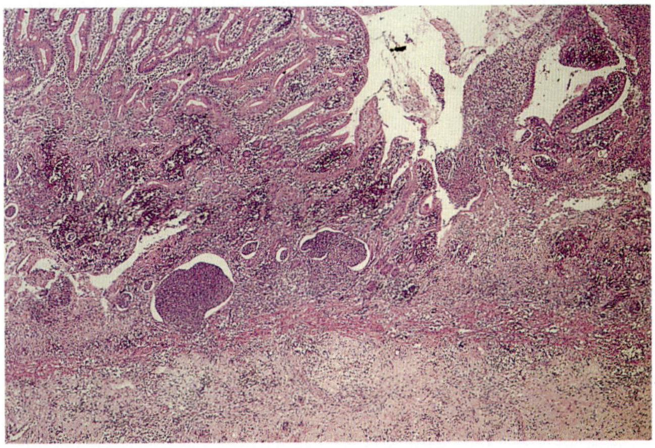

Figure 98–12. Acute enteritis in an 18-year-old man caused by *Y pseudotuberculosis* type IV. In this specimen there is severe acute inflammation of the mucosa with destructive crypt abscesses that, in adjacent parts of the specimen, had become confluent, undermining the overlying mucosa and causing it to slough. Necrotic mucosa is in the right side of the field. The submucosa is edematous and inflamed (hematoxylin-eosin, ×4).

cumbersome because it has to be repeated for each serotype. Moreover, there is cross-reactivity between *Y enterocolitica* O:9 and *Brucella* sp and between *Y pseudotuberculosis* types II and IV and *Salmonella* of groups B and D, respectively, necessitating absorption of serum samples against these antigens if screening tests are positive. Agglutination tests, enzyme-linked immunosorbent assays, and fluorescent antibody tests have all been used, and are satisfactory for diagnosing acute infections, though samples of convalescent serum should be assayed if serum collected in the acute phase is negative, since antibodies to *Y pseudotuberculosis* often rise very late.[31] Serologic diagnosis of chronic yersiniosis appears to be more difficult since agglutinating IgM and IgG antibodies are commonly negative, and an immunoblot for assay for IgA may be necessary.[21]

Yersinia infections have also been diagnosed by immunostaining, using serotype-specific antibodies, as illustrated in Figure 98–6, though this procedure is not widely available in diagnostic laboratories. Detection by polymerase chain reaction and by in situ hybridization will undoubtedly supplement these other techniques in the future.

REFERENCES

1. Cover TL. *Yersinia enterocolitica* and *Yersinia pseudotuberculosis*. In: Blaser MJ, Smith PD, Ravdin JI, Greenberg HB, Guerrant RL, eds. *Infections of the Gastrointestinal Tract.* New York: Raven Press; 1995:811–823.
2. Cover TL, Aber RC. *Yersinia enterocolitica*. *N Engl J Med.* 1989;321:16–24.
3. Attwood SEA, Cafferkey MT, Keane FBV. *Yersinia* infections in surgical practice. *Br J Surg.* 1989;76:499–504.
4. Butler T. *Yersinia* species (including plague). In: Mandell GL, Bennett JE, Dolin R, eds. *Principles and Practice of Infectious Diseases.* 4th ed. New York: Churchill Livingstone; 1994:2070–2078.
5. Tauxe RV, Vandepitte J, Wauters G, et al. *Yersinia enterocolitica* infections and pork: the missing link. *Lancet.* 1987;1:1129–1132.
6. Lee LA, Gerber AR, Lonsway DR, et al. *Yersinia enterocolitica* O:3 infections in infants and children, associated with the household preparation of chitterlings. *N Engl J Med.* 1990;322:984–987.
7. Lee LA, Taylor J, Carter GP, Quinn B, Farmer III JJ, Tauxe RV. *Yersinia enterocolitica* O:3: an emerging cause of pediatric gastroenteritis in the United States. *J Infect Dis.* 1991;163:660–663.
8. Anon. Case 28-1990. *N Engl J Med.* 1990;323:113–123.
9. Naqvi SH, Swierkosz EM, Gerard J, Mills JR. Presentation of *Yersinia enterocolitica* enteritis in children. *Pediatr Infect Dis J.* 1993;12:386–389.
10. Vantrappen G, Agg HO, Ponette E, Geboes K, Bertrand P. *Yersinia* enteritis and enterocolitis: gastroenterological aspects. *Gastroenterology.* 1977;72:220–227.
11. Brown R, Tedesco FJ, Assad RT, Rao R. *Yersinia* colitis masquerading as pseudomembranous colitis. *Dig Dis Sci.* 1986;31:548–551.
12. Sternby NH. Morphologic findings in appendix in human *Yersinia enterocolitica* infection. *Contrib Microbiol Immunol.* 1973;2:141–143.
13. Ahlqvist J, Ahvonen P, Rasanen JA, Wallgren GR. Enteric infection with *Yersinia enterocolitica*. *Acta Pathol Microbiol Scand A.* 1971;79:109–122.
14. Schapers RFM, Reif R, Lennert K, Knapp W. Mesenteric lymphadenitis due to *Yersinia enterocolitica*. *Virchows Arch Pathol Anat.* 1981;390:127–138.
15. Attwood SEA, Mealy D, Cafferkey MT, et al. *Yersinia* infection and acute abdominal pain. *Lancet.* 1987;1:529–533.
16. Bennion RS, Thompson JE, Gil J, Schmit PJ. The role of *Yersinia enterocolitica* in appendicitis in the southwestern United States. *Am Surgeon.* 1991;57:766–768.
17. Bradford WD, Noce PS, Gutman LT. Pathologic features of enteric infection with *Yersinia enterocolitica*. *Arch Pathol.* 1974;98:17–22.
18. Gleason TH, Patterson SD. The pathology of *Yersinia enterocolitica* ileocolitis. *Am J Surg Pathol.* 1982;6:347–355.
19. Mazzoleni G, deSa D, Gately J, Riddell RH. *Yersinia enterocolitica* infection with ileal perforation associated with iron overload and deferoxamine therapy. *Dig Dis Sci.* 1991;36:1154–1160.
20. Larsen JH. Significance of specific IgA antibodies in infections due to *Yersinia enterocolitica* and their complications. *Contr Microbiol Immunol.* 1987;9:136–140.
21. Hoogkamp-Korstanje JAA, de Koning J, Heesemann J. Persistence of *Yersinia enterocolitica* in man. *Infection.* 1988;16:81–85.
22. de Koning J, Heesemann J, Hoogkamp-Korstanje JAA, Festen JJM, Houtman PM, van Oijen PLM. *Yersinia* in intestinal biopsy specimens from patients with seronegative spondyloarthropathy: correlation with specific serum IgA antibodies. *J Infect Dis.* 1989;159:109–112.
23. Merilahti-Palo R, Pelliniemi LJ, Granfors K, et al. Electron microscopy and immunolabelling of *Yersinia* antigens in human synovial fluid cells. *Clin Exper Rheumatol.* 1994;12:255–259.
24. Robins-Browne RM, Prpic JK. Effects of iron and desferrioxamine on infections with *Yersinia enterocolitica*. *Infect Immun.* 1985;47:774–779.
25. Vadillo M, Corbella X, Pac V, Fernandez-Viladrich P, Pujol R. Multiple liver abscesses due to *Yersinia enterocolitica* discloses primary hemochromatosis: three case reports and review. *Clin Infect Dis.* 1994;18:938–941.
26. Cornelis GR. *Yersinia* pathogenicity factors. *Curr Top Microbiol Immunol.* 1994;192:243–263.
27. Sato K, Ouchi K, Taki M. *Yersinia pseudotuberculosis* infection in children, resembling Izumi fever and Kawasaki syndrome. *Pediatr Infect Dis.* 1983;2:123–126.

28. El-Maraghi NRH, Mair NS. The histopathology of enteric infection with *Yersinia pseudotuberculosis. Am J Clin Pathol.* 1979;71:631–639.
29. Bohm N, Wybitul K. Different histologic types of mesenteric lymphadenitis in *Yersinia pseudotuberculosis* type I and type II infection. *Pathol Res Pract.* 1978;162:301–315.
30. Kontiainen S, Sivonen A, Renkonen O-V. Increased yields of pathogenic *Yersinia enterocolitica* strains by cold enrichment. *Scand J Infect Dis.* 1994;26:685–691.
31. Cafferkey MT, Buckley TF. Comparison of saline agglutination, antibody to human gammaglobulin, and immunofluorescence tests in the routine serological diagnosis of yersiniosis. *J Infect Dis.* 1987;156:845–848.

Pathology of Infectious Diseases

Volume II

Editors

Daniel H. Connor, MD
Visiting Professor
Department of Pathology
Georgetown University School of Medicine
Washington, DC

Francis W. Chandler, DVM, PhD
Professor of Pathology
Department of Pathology
Medical College of Georgia
Augusta, Georgia

David A. Schwartz, MD, MS Hyg
Associate Professor of Pathology
Assistant Professor of Medicine (Infectious Diseases)
Emory University School of Medicine
Atlanta, Georgia

Herbert J. Manz, MD
Professor of Pathology
Department of Pathology
Georgetown University School of Medicine
Washington, DC

Ernest E. Lack, MD
Professor of Pathology
Department of Pathology
Georgetown University School of Medicine
Washington, DC

Assistant Editors

J. Kevin Baird, PhD
Lieutenant Commander
Medical Service Corps, United States Navy
and
Naval Medical Research Institute
Malaria Program
Rockville, Maryland

John P. Utz, MD
Professor Emeritus
Department of Medicine
Georgetown University School of Medicine
Washington, DC

APPLETON & LANGE
Stamford, Connecticut

97 98 99 00 01 / 10 9 8 7 6 5 4 3 2 1

Prentice Hall International (UK) Limited, *London*
Prentice Hall of Australia Pty. Limited, *Sydney*
Prentice Hall Canada, Inc., *Toronto*
Prentice Hall Hispanoamericana, S.A., *Mexico*
Prentice Hall of India Private Limited, *New Delhi*
Prentice Hall of Japan, Inc., *Tokyo*
Simon & Schuster Asia Pte. Ltd., *Singapore*
Editora Prentice Hall do Brasil Ltda., *Rio de Janeiro*
Prentice Hall, *Upper Saddle River, New Jersey*

Library of Congress Cataloging-in-Publication Data

Pathology of infectious diseases / [edited by] Daniel H. Connor . . . [et al.].
p. cm.
ISBN 0-8385-1601-7 (case : alk. paper)
1. Communicable diseases—Diagnosis. 2. Diagnosis. Laboratory.
I. Connor, Daniel H. 1928– .
[DNLM: 1. Communicable Diseases—pathology WC 100P297 1997]
RC113.3.P36 1997
616.9′047—dc20
DNLM/DLC
for Library of Contgress 96-31452
CIP

Managing Editor, Development: Kathleen McCullough
Production Service: Spectrum Publisher Services, Mercedes Jackson
Designer: Mary Skudlarek

PRINTED IN HONG KONG

Note: Most of the magnifications stated in the figure legends are the original magnifications of the 35-mm transparencies or photographs.

ISBN 0-8385-1601-7
90000
9 780838 516010

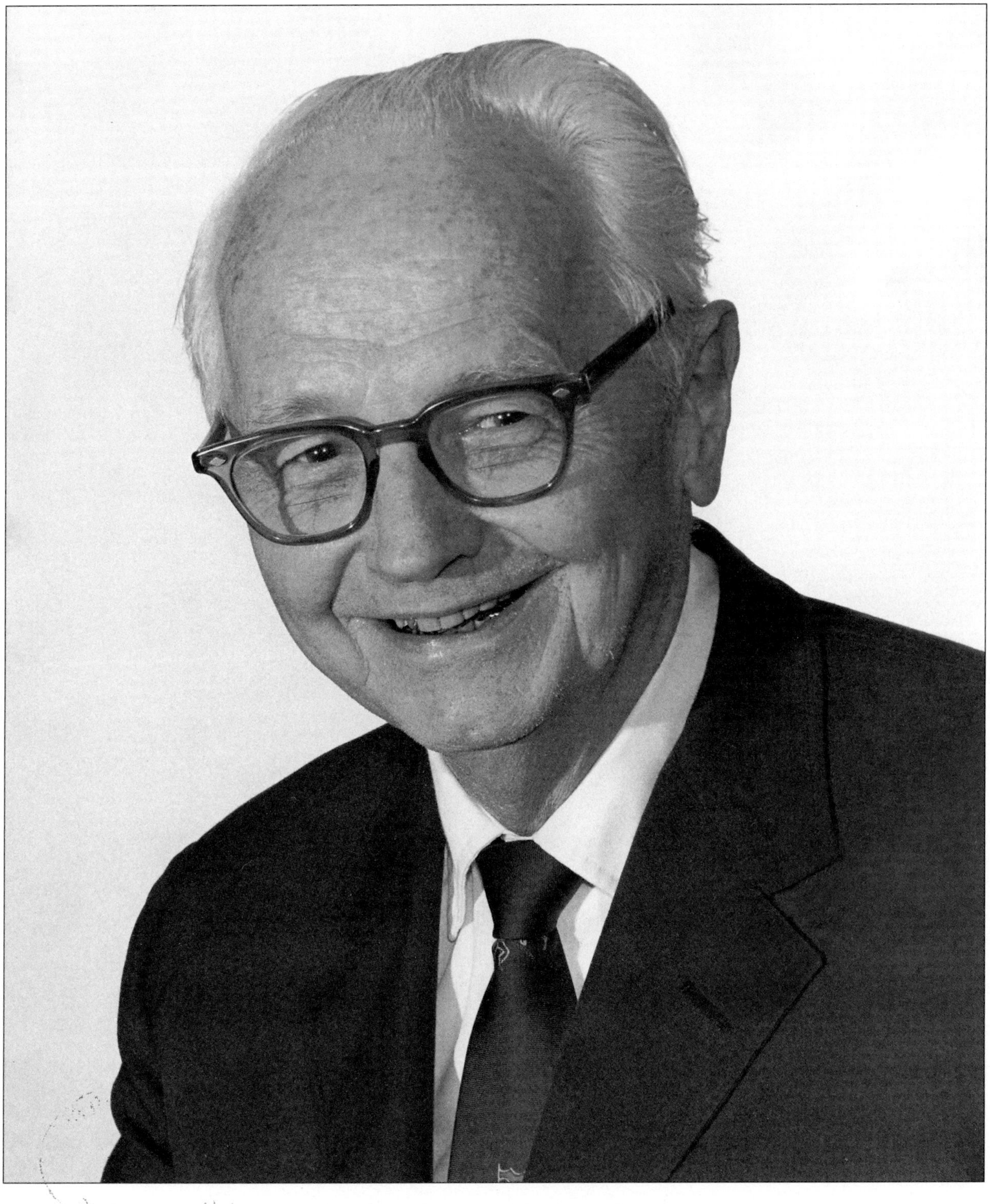

Dedicated to the memory of
Chapman H. Binford, AB, MD, DSc (Hon), DSc (Hon)
1900–1990

by those who worked with him and for him, to whom he was a trusted, selfless, and loyal friend; gifted teacher; dedicated medical scientist and leprologist; writer; editor; and, above all, devoted humanitarian.

Contents

Contributors

Carlos R. Abramowsky, MD
Director of Pediatric Pathology
and
Professor of Pathology
Emory University School of Medicine
Atlanta, Georgia

Masazumi Adachi, MD, ScD
Director of Laboratories
Kingsbrook Jewish Medical Center
Professor of Pathology
State University of New York, Health Science Center at Brooklyn
Brooklyn, New York

Ann M. Adams, PhD
Research Parasitologist
Seafood Products Research Center
United States Food and Drug Administration
Seattle District
Bothell, Washington

Masamichi Aikawa, MD
Professor
Institute of Medical Sciences
Tokai University
Kanagawa, Japan

Libero Ajello, PhD
Adjunct Professor
Ophthalmic Research Section
Emory Eye Center
Emory University School of Medicine
Atlanta, Georgia

Stephen D. Allen, MD
Professor of Pathology and Laboratory Medicine
and
Director
Division of Clinical Microbiology
Indiana University School of Medicine
Indianapolis, Indiana

Geoffrey Altschuler, MB, BS
Clinical Professor of Pathology
University of Oklahoma Health Sciences Center
and
Children's Hospital of Oklahoma
Oklahoma City, Oklahoma

Norio Azumi, MD, PhD
Medical Director
Molecular Diagnostic Laboratory
Georgetown University Medical Center
Professor of Pathology
Georgetown University School of Medicine
Washington, DC

J. Kevin Baird, PhD
Lieutenant Commander
Medical Service Corps, United States Navy
and
Naval Medical Research Institute
Malaria Program
Rockville, Maryland

John G. Banwell, MD
Attending Physician
Togus VA and Regional Medical Center
Adjunct Professor of Medicine
Case Western Reserve University School of Medicine
Cleveland, Ohio

Edwin Beckman, MD
Clinical Associate Professor of Pathology
Ochsner Medical Institutions
Tulane Medical School
New Orleans, Louisiana

Yanina Bednov, MD
Department of Pathology
Georgetown University School of Medicine
Washington, DC

William J. Bellini, MD
Chief
Measles Virus Section
Centers for Disease Control and Prevention
Atlanta, Georgia

Charles E. Binkley, BA
Medical Student
Georgetown University School of Medicine
Washington, DC

H. Braunstein, MD
Honorary Medical Staff
and
Retired Chairman
Department of Laboratories
San Bernardino County Medical Center
San Bernardino, California
Former Professor in Residence
Biomedical Sciences
University of California
Riverside, California

John Bryan, MD
Fellow in Pathology
George Washington University School of Medicine
Washington, DC

Alfred A. Buck, MD, DRPH
Professor of International Health, Molecular Biology, and Immunology
Johns Hopkins University
Baltimore, Maryland

James M. Burke, MD
Georgetown University School of Medicine
Washington, DC

Adam R. Burkey, MD
Research Fellow
Department of Neurosurgery
Georgetown University School of Medicine
Washington, DC

Joseph M. Campos, MD, PhD
Director
Microbiology Laboratory and Laboratory Informatics
Children's National Medical Center
Professor
Department of Pediatrics, Pathology and Microbiology/Immunology
George Washington University Medical Center
Washington, DC

Michael J. Carey, MD
Staff Pathologist (Resident)
University of Utah
Salt Lake City, Utah

Christopher L. Carroll, MD
Georgetown University School of Medicine
Washington, DC

Francis W. Chandler, DVM, PhD
Professor of Pathology
Department of Pathology
Medical College of Georgia
Augusta, Georgia

Clay J. Cockerell, MD
Director
Freeman–Cockerell Laboratories
and
Aston Dermatology Clinic
Associate Professor of Dermatopathology
and
Director
HIV Associated Skin Disease Clinic
University of Texas Southwestern Medical Center
Dallas, Texas

Daniel H. Connor, MD
Visiting Professor
Department of Pathology
Georgetown University School of Medicine
Washington, DC

Richard M. Conran, MD, PhD
Associate Professor of Pathology
Uniformed Services University of the Health Sciences
Bethesda, Maryland

James D. Cotelingam, MD
Captain
Medical Service Corps, United States Navy
Adjunct Professor of Pathology
Uniformed Services University of the Health Sciences
Bethesda, Maryland

John H. Cross, PhD
Professor of Tropical Public Health
Department of Preventive Medicine and Biometrics
Uniformed Services University of the Health Sciences
Bethesda, Maryland

Deborah Dean, MD, MPH
Assistant Professor
University of California at San Francisco School of Medicine
Francis I. Proctor Foundation
San Francisco, California

Ellen C. DeNigris, MD
Commander
Medical Service Corps, United States Navy
Assistant Professor of Pathology
Uniformed Services University of the Health Sciences
Bethesda, Maryland

William O. Dobbins III, MD
Professor Emeritus
Department of Medicine
University of Michigan Medical Center
Ann Arbor, Michigan

J. Stephen Dumler, MD
Director
Medical Microbiology Division
Johns Hopkins Hospital
Associate Professor of Pathology
Johns Hopkins School of Medicine
Baltimore, Maryland

Paul H. Duray, MD
Attending Surgical Pathologist
Warren G. Magnuson Clinical Center
Special Expert in Pathology
National Cancer Institute
National Institutes of Health
Bethesda, Maryland

Mark L. Eberhard, PhD
Division of Parasitic Diseases
National Center for Infectious Diseases
Centers for Disease Control and Prevention
Atlanta, Georgia

Isam A. Eltoum, MD, MRCPath
Fellow in Anatomic Pathology
University of Alabama at Birmingham
Birmingham, Alabama

Armando Filie, MD
Fellow in Cytology
George Washington University School of Medicine
Washington, DC

Sydney D. Finkelstein, MD
Associate Professor of Pathology
University of Pittsburgh Medical Center
Pittsburgh, Pennsylvania

James L. Fishback, MD
Associate Professor of Pathology
University of Kansas School of Medicine
Kansas City, Kansas

Nancy Fishback, MD, CDr, MC, USNR
Associate Professor of Pathology
Uniformed Services University of the Health Sciences
Bethesda, Maryland

Heather E. Fork, MD
Private Practice
Austin, Texas

Elie K. Fraiji, Jr., MD
Georgetown University School of Medicine
Washington, DC

J. K. Frenkel, MD, PhD
Professor Emeritus
University of Kansas
Lawrence, Kansas
Adjunct Professor
University of New Mexico
Santa Fe, New Mexico

David L. Fritz, DVM
Supervisor
Ultrastructural Pathology Group
US Army Medical Research Institute
of Infectious Diseases
Fort Detrick
Frederick, Maryland

Anthony A. Gal, MD
Staff Surgical Pathologist
Emory University Hospital
Associate Professor of Pathology
Emory University School of Medicine
Atlanta, Georgia

Monica V. E. Gallivan, MD
Associate Pathologist
Mount Vernon Hospital
Alexandria, Virginia

David L. Gang, MD
Chief
Anatomic Pathology
Baystate Medical Center
Springfield, Massachusetts
Professor of Pathology
Tufts University School of Medicine
Medford, Massachusetts

Fernando U. Garcia, MD
Director of Surgical Pathology
Allegheny University Hospital
Associate Professor of Pathology
Allegheny University School of Medicine—Center City
Philadelphia, Pennsylvania

David F. Garvin, MD
Director of Diagnostic Services
and
Professor of Pathology
Georgetown University School of Medicine
Washington, DC

Robert M. Genta, MD
Chief
Pathology and Laboratory Medicine
Veterans Affairs Medical Center
Professor of Medicine and Professor of Microbiology and Immunology
Baylor College of Medicine
Houston, Texas

Stanley J. Geyer, MD
Chairman
Department of Pathology and Laboratory Medicine
Western Pennsylvania Hospital
Clinical Professor of Pathology
University of Pittsburgh School of Medicine
Pittsburgh, Pennsylvania

Zachary D. Goodman, MD, PhD
Chief
Hepatic Pathology Division
Armed Forces Institute of Pathology
Washington, DC

M. Alba Greco, MD
Director of Pediatric Pathology
New York University–Bellevue Hospital
Associate Professor of Pathology
New York University Medical Center
New York, New York

H. G. Greenberg, MD
Professor of Medicine and Medical Investigation
Palo Alto Veterans Administration
Palo Alto, California
Stanford University Medical Center
Stanford, California

Thomas D. Griffin, MD
Johnson Griffin Dermatopathology Associates
Glenside, Pennsylvania

Max Grogl, PhD
United States Army Medical Research Unit
Brazil

Hans E. Grossniklaus, MD
F. Phinizy Calhoun Jr. Professor of Ophthalmic Pathology
and
Director
L. F. Montgomery Ophthalmic Laboratory
Emory University School of Medicine
Atlanta, Georgia

Robin Hampton, MD, PhD
Department of Pathology and Laboratory Medicine
Emory University School of Medicine
Atlanta, Georgia

Mark G. Hanly, MBChB, MRCPath, FCAP
Attending Pathologist
Medical College of Georgia Hospital and Clinics
Assistant Professor
Medical College of Georgia
Augusta, Georgia

Christian H. Hansen, MD
Resident Physician
Department of Pathology
Georgetown University Medical Center
Washington, DC

Abida K. Haque, MD
Professor and Director of Anatomic Pathology
University of Texas Medical Branch
Galveston, Texas

Phillip J. Harrity, MD
Staff Pathologist
Sinai Samaritan Medical Center
Clinical Assistant Professor of Pathology
Medical College of Wisconsin
Milwaukee, Wisconsin

Rod J. Hay, DM, FRCP, FRCPath
Professor of Cutaneous Medicine
and
Dean of the Institute of Dermatology
UMDS
Department of Dermatology
Guy's Hospital
London, England

Kurt F. Heim, MD, PhD
Senior Staff Fellow
Department of Transfusion Medicine
Clinical Center
National Institutes of Health
Bethesda, Maryland

Thomas K. Held, MD
Fellow in Hematology and Oncology
Humbolt University
Virchow Clinic
Berlin, Germany

Jeffrey F. Hines, MD
Staff Physician
Division of Gynecologic Oncology
Department of Obstetrics and Gynecology
Brooke Army Medical Center
San Antonio, Texas

Scott R. Hyde, PhD
Assistant Professor of Pathology
University of Oklahoma College of Medicine—Tulsa
Scientific Director of Perinatal Pathology and Diagnostic Molecular Biology
South Tulsa Pathology at Saint Francis Hospital
Tulsa, Oklahoma

Nancy K. Jaax, DVM
Colonel
United States Army
Chief
Pathology Division
United States Army Medical Research Institute of Infectious Diseases
Fort Detrick
Frederick, Maryland

Elaine S. Jaffe, MD
Chief
Hematopathology Section
Laboratory of Pathology
National Cancer Institute
National Institutes of Health
Bethesda, Maryland

A. Bennett Jenson, MD
Professor of Pathology
Georgetown University School of Medicine
Washington, DC

Jacqueline M. Junkins-Hopkins, MD
Johnson Griffin Dermatopathology Associates
Glenside, Pennsylvania

Juntra Karbwang, MD
Faculty of Tropical Medicine
Mahidol University
Bangkok, Thailand

David Katz, MD
Laboratory of Neuropathology
National Institute of Neurological Disorders and Stroke
Bethesda, Maryland

Kevin R. Kazacos, DVM, PhD
Director
Clinical Parasitology Laboratory
and
Professor of Parasitology
School of Veterinary Medicine
Purdue University
West Lafayette, Indiana

James W. Kazura, MD
Chief
Division of Georgraphic Medicine
and
Professor of Medicine and International Health
Case Western Reserve University School of Medicine
Cleveland, Ohio

James K. Kelly, MD
Chief
Anatomical Pathology
Greater Victoria Hospital Society
Victoria, British Columbia, Canada

Francisco A. Kerdel, MD
Professor of Clinical Dermatology
University of Miami
School of Medicine
Department of Dermatology
Cedars Medical Center
Miami, Florida

Mahmoud A. Khalifa, MD, PhD, FRCP(C)
Department of Pathology
General Hospital
Memorial University of Newfoundland
Saint John's, Newfoundland

Jung H. Kim, MD
Attending Physician
Yale–New Haven Hospital
Associate Professor
Section of Neuropathology
Yale University School of Medicine
New Haven, Connecticut

John M. Kissane, MD
Pathologist
Barnes–Jewish Hospital and Saint Louis Children's Hospital
Professor of Pathology and Pediatrics
Washington University School of Medicine
St. Louis, Missouri

Steven E. Kolker, MD
Resident in Pathology
University of California at San Francisco
San Francisco, California

Harry P. W. Kozakewich, MD
Associate Professor of Pathology
Children's Hospital
and
Harvard Medical School
Boston, Massachusetts

Princy N. Kumar, MD
Assistant Professor of Medicine
Division of Infectious Diseases
Georgetown University School of Medicine
Washington, DC

Ernest E. Lack, MD
Professor of Pathology
Department of Pathology
Georgetown University School of Medicine
Washington, DC

Elena R. Ladich, MD
Department of Pathology
Georgetown University School of Medicine
Washington, DC

Philip E. LeBoit, MD
Co-Director
Dermatopathology Service
and
Associate Professor of Clinical Pathology and Dermatology
University of California at San Francisco
San Francisco, California

Michael R. Lewin-Smith, MD
Department of Pathology
George Washington University Medical Center
Washington, DC

Lai Y. Lim, MT, ASCP
Department of Pathology
Georgetown University School of Medicine
Washington, DC

Alberto Thomaz Londero, MD
Emeritus Professor
Department of Microbiology
School of Medicine
Federal University of Santa Maria
Santa Maria, Brazil

Mario A. Luna, MD
Director
Autopsy Service
and
Professor of Pathology
University of Texas
M.D. Anderson Cancer Center
Houston, Texas

Bhagirath Majmudar, MD
Professor of Pathology
and
Associate Professor of Obstetrics and Gynecology
Emory University School of Medicine
Atlanta, Georgia

Elias E. Manuelidis, MD (Deceased)
Professor of Pathology
Yale University School of Medicine
New Haven, Connecticut

Laura Manuelidis, MD
Section of Neuropathology
Yale University School of Medicine
New Haven, Connecticut

Herbert J. Manz, MD
Professor of Pathology
Department of Pathology
Georgetown University School of Medicine
Washington, DC

Edith F. Marley, MD
Pathologist
Sunrise Hospital and Medical Center
and
Sunrise Children's Hospital Laboratory Consultants
Las Vegas, Nevada

Augusto Julio Martinez, MD
Professor of Pathology
Department of Gastrointestinal Sciences
University of Pittsburgh School of Medicine
Pittsburgh, Pennsylvania

M. Mathan, MD
Professor of Pathology
and
Head
Department of Gastrointestinal Sciences
Christian Medical College and Hospital
Tamil Nadu, India

Michael R. McGinnis, PhD
Professor of Pathology
University of Texas Medical Branch
Associate Director
WHO Collaborating Center for Tropical Diseases
Director
Medical Mycology Research Center
Galveston, Texas

Richard A. McPherson, MD
Chairman
Division of Clinical Pathology
Medical College of Virginia Hospitals
Professor of Pathology
Virginia Commonwealth University
Richmond, Virginia

Frederick A. Meier, MD
Chairman
Clinical and Anatomic Pathology
Alfred I. DuPont Institute
Wilmington, Delaware

Martin E. A. Mielke, MD
Associate Medical Director
Medical Microbiology and Infectious Diseases/Immunology
and
Associate Professor
Institute for Medical Microbiology
Free University (Berlin)
Berlin, Germany

James Patrick Mixon, MD
Department of Pathology
Emory University School of Medicine
Atlanta, Georgia

Elizabeth A. Montgomery, MD
Associate Professor of Pathology
Georgetown University School of Medicine
Washington, DC

Zuher M. Naib, MD
Professor Emeritus of Pathology
Emory University School of Medicine
Atlanta, Georgia

Kei-Ichiro Nakamura, MD
Department of Anatomy
Faculty of Medicine
Kyushu University
Fukuoka, Japan

Lydia Navarro-Román, MD
Humana Health Care Plans
San Antonio, Texas

Joseph T. Newsome, DVM
Staff Veterinarian
Research Resources Facility
Georgetown University School of Medicine
Washington, DC

Gregory Nikolaidis, MD
Resident in Pediatrics
Texas Children's Hospital
Baylor College of Medicine
Houston, Texas

Jerome T. O'Connell II, MD
Resident Physician
Department of Pathology
University of California at Los Angeles Medical Center
Los Angeles, California

Daniel P. O'Neill, MD
Resident Physician
California Pacific Medical Center
San Francisco, California

Jan Marc Orenstein, MD
Professor of Pathology
George Washington University Medical Center
Washington, DC

David A. Owen, MB, BCh, FRCPath, FRCP(C)
Head
Division of Anatomical Pathology
Vancouver Hospital and Health Sciences Centre
Professor of Pathology
University of British Columbia
Vancouver, British Columbia, Canada

Robert L. Owen, MD
Environmental Health Physician
Cell Biology and Aging Section
VA Medical Center
Professor of Medicine, Epidemiology, and Biostatistics
University of California at San Francisco
San Francisco, California

Philip E. S. Palmer, MD
Department of Radiology
University of California School of Medicine
Davis, California

Demosthenes Pappagianis, MD, PhD
Professor
Department of Medical Microbiology and Immunology
University of California School of Medicine
Davis, California

Robert R. Pascal, MD
Director
Division of Anatomic Pathology
Emory University Hospital
Profesor and Vice-Chairman
Department of Pathology and Laboratory Medicine
Emory University School of Medicine
Atlanta, Georgia

Claire M. Payne, PhD
Research Professor
Arizona Research Laboratories
Division of Biotechnology and Department of Microbiology and Immunology
University of Arizona College of Medicine
Tucson, Arizona

Gary R. Pearson, PhD
Professor
Department of Microbiology and Immunology
Georgetown University School of Medicine
Washington, DC

Philip E. Pellet, MD
Chief
Herpes Virus Section
Centers for Disease Control and Prevention
Atlanta, Georgia

Daniel P. Perl, MD
Director
Neuropathology Division
Mount Sinai Medical Center
Professor of Pathology
Mount Sinai School of Medicine
New York, New York

David H. Persing, MD
Director
Molecular Microbiology Laboratory
Mayo Clinic
Rochester, Minnesota

C. J. Peters, MD
Centers for Disease Control and Prevention
Atlanta, Georgia

Catherine P. Picken, MD
Assistant Professor
Department of Otolaryngology, Head and Neck Surgery
Georgetown University Medical Center
Washington, DC

Phillip F. Pierce, MD
Associate Professor of Medicine and Microbiology
Georgetown University Medical Center
Washington, DC

Duane Pinto, MD
Medical Resident
Beth Israel Hospital/Harvard Medical School
Boston, Massachusetts

Lisa G. Portnoy, DVM
Staff Veterinarian
Research Resources Facility
Georgetown University Medical Center
Instructor of Pathology
Georgetown University School of Medicine
Washington, DC

Ewald Pretner, MD
Staff Physician
Georgetown University Hospital
Washington, DC

David T. Purtilo, MD (Deceased)
Department of Pathology and Microbiology
University of Nebraska Medical Center
Omaha, Nebraska

John R. Rabbege, BS
Assistant Professor
Case Western Reserve University
Cleveland, Ohio

Evette Ramsay, MD
Resident Physician
Georgetown University School of Medicine
Washington, DC

Robert L. Rausch, DVM, PhD
Professor Emeritus
Department of Pathology
School of Public Health and Medicine
and
Department of Comparative Medicine
University of Washington School of Medicine
Seattle, Washington

Barbara S. Reisner, PhD
Associate Director
Clinical Microbiology Laboratory
and
Assistant Professor
Department of Pathology
University of Texas Medical Branch
Galveston, Texas

Gustavo C. Román, MD
Humana Health Care Plans
San Antonio, Texas

Theodore Rosen, MD
Chief of Dermatology
Houston VA Medical Center
Professor of Dermatology
Baylor College of Medicine
Houston, Texas

Marc K. Rosenblum, MD
Chief
Neuropathology and Autopsy Service
Memorial–Sloan Kettering Cancer Center
Associate Professor of Pathology
Cornell University Medical College
New York, New York

Leonard J. Rosenthal, PhD
Professor of Microbiology and Immunology
Georgetown University School of Medicine
Washington, DC

Heidrun Rotterdam, MD
Attending Pathologist
Columbia Presbyterian Medical Center
Professor of Clinical Pathology
College of Physicians and Surgeons of Columbia University
New York, New York

L. J. Saif, PhD
Professor of Virology and Immunology
Food Animal Health Research Program
Department of Veterinary Preventive Medicine
Ohio Agricultural Research and Development Center
Ohio State University
Wooster, Ohio

Nirmal K. Saini, MD
Acting Chief
Department of Anatomic Pathology
Pathologic Medicine Laboratory Service
Assistant Pathologist
George Washington University Medical Center
Washington, DC

Judy A. Sakanari, PhD
Assistant Adjunct Professor
University of California at San Francisco
San Francisco, California

Shukdeo Sankar, MD
Staff Physician
Whitman Walker Clinic and Max Robinson Center
Silver Spring, Maryland

Gerhard A. Schad, PhD
Department of Pathobiology
University of Pennsylvania School of Veterinary Medicine
Philadelphia, Pennsylvania

Stephen P. Schiffer, DVM, MS
Director
Research Resources Facility
and
Associate Professor of Cell Biology
Georgetown University School of Medicine
Washington, DC

David A. Schwartz, MD, MS Hyg
Associate Professor of Pathology
and
Assistant Professor of Medicine (Infectious Diseases)
Emory University School of Medicine
Research Scientist
National Center for Infectious Diseases
Centers for Disease Control and Prevention
Atlanta, Georgia

Christopher M. Seniw, MD
Resident Physician
Georgetown University Hospital
Washington, DC

John A. Shadduck, DVM
Texas A&M College of Veterinary Medicine
College Station, Texas

Robert J. Siegel, MD
Director
Pathology Laboratories
Crawford Long Hospital
Associate Professor
Department of Pathology and Laboratory Medicine
Emory University School of Medicine
Atlanta, Georgia

Bharatha Sinniah, MD
Professor and Chairman
Department of Parasitology
University of Malaya
Kuala Lumpur
Malaysia

Jerome H. Smith, MD
Pathologist
Autopsy Service
and
Professor of Pathology
University of Texas Medical Branch
Galveston, Texas

J. Thomas Stocker, MD
Professor of Pathology
Uniformed Services University of the Health Sciences
Bethesda, Maryland
Clinical Professor of Pathology
Georgetown University School of Medicine
Washington, DC

Melissa Conrad Stöppler, MD
Assistant Professor of Pathology
Georgetown University School of Medicine
Washington, DC

Alfonso J. Strano, MD, PhD
Director (Retired)
Microbiology Laboratory
Saint John's Hospital
Clinical Professor of Pathology
Southern Illinois University School of Medicine
Springfield, Illinois

Kimberly Studeman, MD
Resident Physician
Jackson Memorial Hospital
Miami, Florida

Ramiah Subramanian, MD
Medical Officer
United States Food and Drug Administration
Adjunct Associate Professor of Pathology
Georgetown University School of Medicine
Washington, DC

Tsieh Sun, MD
Director
Flow Cytometry Laboratory
VA Medical Center
Professor of Pathology
University of Colorado School of Medicine
Denver, Colorado

Donald E. Sweet, MD
Chairman
Department of Orthopedic Pathology
Armed Forces Institute of Pathology
Bethesda, Maryland

Bernard Tandler, PhD
Department of Geographical Medicine
Case Western Reserve University
Cleveland, Ohio

Van Q. Telford, DVM, MD
Medical Director
Department of Pathology
RHD Memorial Hospital
Dallas, Texas

Elizabeth R. Unger, MD, PhD
Associate Professor of Pathology
Emory University School of Medicine
Atlanta, Georgia

Matthias Unger, MD
Pathologist
Department of Pediatric Pathology and Placentology
Humbolt University
Virchow Clinic
Berlin, Germany

John P. Utz, MD
Professor Emeritus
Department of Medicine
Georgetown University School of Medicine
Washington, DC

Patrick J. Vaughan, MD
Department of Orthopedic Surgery
Medical College of Virginia
Richmond, Virginia

Phyllis R. Vezza, MD
Department of Pathology
Georgetown University School of Medicine
Washington, DC

Tuyethoa N. Vinh, MD
Department of Bone and Joint Pathology
Armed Forces Institute of Pathology
Washington, DC

Govinda S. Visvesvara, PhD
Parasitic Disease Branch
Centers for Disease Control and Prevention
Atlanta, Georgia

Franz von Lichtenberg, MD
Senior Pathologist
Brigham and Women's Hospital
Professor of Pathology Emeritus
Harvard Medical School
Boston, Massachusetts

David H. Walker, MD
Professor and Chairman
Department of Pathology
University of Texas Medical Branch
Director
WHO Collaborating Center for Tropical Diseases
Galveston, Texas

John C. Watts, MD
Chief
Surgical Pathology
William Beaumont Hospital
Associate Clinical Professor of Pathology
Wayne State University School of Medicine
Royal Oak, Michigan

A. Brian West, MB, FRCPath
Director of Surgical Pathology
and
Professor of Pathology
University of Texas Medical Branch
Galveston, Texas

Jacqueline A. Wieneke, MD
Resident in Pathology
Georgetown University Medical Center
Washington, DC

C. Mel Wilcox, MD
Director of Clinical Research
and
Associate Professor of Medicine
Division of Gastroenterology and Hepatology
University of Alabama at Birmingham
Birmingham, Alabama

Washington C. Winn, Jr., MD, MBA
Director
Clinical Microbiology Laboratory
Fletcher Allen Health Care
Professor of Pathology
University of Vermont College of Medicine
Burlington, Vermont

Edward J. Young, MD
Chief of Staff
VA Medical Center
Professor of Medicine
Baylor College of Medicine
Houston, Texas

Neal S. Young, MD
Chief
Clinical Service
Hematology Branch
National Institutes of Health
Bethesda, Maryland

David Zagzag, MD, PhD
Assistant Professor of Pathology
New York University Medical School
New York, New York

Sherif R. Zaki, MD
Chief
Molecular Pathology and Ultrastructural Activity
Centers for Disease Control and Prevention
Atlanta, Georgia

Introduction

Infectious diseases are the leading cause of death worldwide. In the United States, infectious diseases are the third leading cause of death. The World Health Organization estimates that approximately 17 million of the 52 million deaths (33%) worldwide in 1995 were caused by microbial agents. Infection with human immunodeficiency virus (HIV) is now the leading cause of death in the United States in persons between 25 and 44 years of age. In view of these facts, it is ironic that we are, in some ways, less prepared to address infectious diseases in the United States than we were in the mid-1960s.

As a result of improvements in sanitation and overall living conditions during the early part of the 20th century and the subsequent introduction of many vaccines and antibiotics, considerable complacency has developed regarding infectious diseases that many regarded as either preventable by immunization or treatable by antibiotics. The 1970s produced the beginning of a series of what, in retrospect, should have been loud wake-up calls regarding the challenges infectious diseases continue to pose domestically and globally. Rotaviral gastroenteritis, Lyme disease, legionnaires' disease, and toxic shock syndrome are a few of the infectious diseases first recognized during the 1970s. The most dramatic example of an emerging infectious disease, the acquired immunodeficiency syndrome (AIDS), was recognized in 1981, and hemorrhagic colitis caused by *Escherichia coli* O157:H7 was identified in 1982. The end of the 1980s saw the reemergence of measles and tuberculosis in the United States and the emergence of multiple drug resistance in *Mycobacterium tuberculosis* strains causing disease predominantly in persons infected with HIV.

Experiences with these and other emerging and reemerging diseases should have alerted physicians, microbiologists, researchers, public health officials, policy makers, and the public to the critical importance of ensuring the capacity to detect, respond to, and control these infections. In the fall of 1992, the Institute of Medicine (IOM) published a report entitled "Emerging Infections: Microbial Threats to Health in the United States." This report, developed under the leadership of Drs. Joshua Lederberg and Robert Shope, highlighted the complacency regarding emerging infections and identified the important factors in disease emergence and reemergence (changes in human demographics and behaviors, advances in technology and industry, economic development and changes in land use, increases in travel and commerce, microbial adaptation and change, and deterioration in the public health system at the local, state, national, and global levels). The IOM committee made 15 recommendations that stressed the need to improve surveillance and response capacity and also identified research issues and training priorities.

Since publication of this report, physicians, microbiologists, and public health officials have faced numerous challenges from microorganisms in the United States and abroad. Domestic challenges have included an interstate outbreak of hemorrhagic colitis caused by *E coli* O157:H7 associated with contaminated hamburger, a large waterborne disease outbreak of cryptosporidiosis associated with contaminated drinking water in Milwaukee, the outbreak of hantavirus pulmonary syndrome caused by a previously unrecognized hantavirus, the continued emergence of vancomycin-resistant enterococci and penicillin-resistant *Streptococcus pneumoniae*, and nationwide outbreaks of *Salmonella* serotype Enteritidis infection associated with contaminated ice cream and *Cyclospora* gastroenteritis associated with raspberries.

Internationally, a number of outbreaks have served as reminders that the world is a global village. Examples include plague in India and equine morbillivirus infection in Australia in 1994, Ebola hemorrhagic fever in Zaire and leptospirosis in Nicaragua in 1995, and a new variant of Creutzfeldt–Jakob disease (CJD) in the United Kingdom and a large outbreak of *E coli* O157:H7 hemorrhagic colitis in Japan in 1996. Each of these outbreaks illustrates the critical importance of adequate surveillance and response capacity, the critical role of the laboratory and the discipline of pathology in addressing emerging infections, and the global implications of a local problem.

The ability to address these emerging and reemerging microbial threats requires adequate surveillance and response capacity, ongoing research programs, strengthened prevention and control programs, and repair of the public health system at the local, state, national, and international levels. The discipline of pathology has played an important role in the recognition and characterization of the hantavirus pulmonary syndrome outbreak, diagnosis and subsequent prospective surveillance of Ebola hemorrhagic fever in Central Africa, identification of the etiologic agent in the leptospirosis outbreak in Nicaragua, and characterization of the variant form of CJD in the United Kingdom. Pathologists have also made vital contributions to recognition of opportunistic infections in HIV-infected and other immunodeficient patients. The chapters in this book clearly document the role of classic and modern molecular methods in assessing disease etiology and pathology of infectious diseases. The challenges that these diseases continue to pose demand a multidisciplinary approach and a supply of trained clinicians, microbiologists, pathologists, rodent and vector biologists, ecologists, behavioral scientists, and public health officials.

Future challenges are difficult to predict but certainly include more problems with antimicrobial-resistant infections, the threat of another influenza pandemic, the likelihood of increasing problems of dengue hemorrhagic fever, and the risk of urban yellow fever in the Western Hemisphere. The global HIV epidemic will put large numbers of people at risk for currently recognized and new opportunistic infections. The roles of hepatitis B virus in chronic liver disease and hepatocellular carcinoma, human papillomavirus in cervical cancer, and *Helicobacter pylori* infection in peptic ulcer disease and gastric cancer are now well established. It is likely that more chronic diseases will be found to have an infectious etiology. Pathologists clearly have an important role in the future in surveillance, diagnosis, and response to emerging and reemerging infections. This book should serve as a valuable source of information for them and for their colleagues in related disciplines.

James M. Hughes, MD
Assistant Surgeon General
Director, National Center for Infectious Diseases
Centers for Disease Control and Prevention
Atlanta, Georgia
September 1996

Foreword

We were all aware of the deaths of 34 people of legionnaires' disease in Philadelphia in 1976, of the 32 deaths by hantavirus infection in the southwestern United States in 1993, of the sudden outbreaks of Ebola virus in Africa in 1995, and, of course, of the worldwide spread of human immunodeficiency virus (HIV) and acquired immunodeficiency syndrome (AIDS). The intense drama of lethal infectious diseases has been highlighted in the mass media to focus public attention on microorganisms that threaten human health. A striking feature of the diseases mentioned is that every one of them was discovered only since the early 1970s and they were unknown when I studied microbiology in medical school. Moreover, during this relatively short time frame many other pathogenic human microbes have been discovered that cause diarrhea, hepatitis, arthritis, and leukemia. As if this were not enough, scourges of the past have begun to reemerge, and resistant strains of malaria, tuberculosis, *Escherichia coli,* and pneumococcus are taking hold.

Why are these epidemics happening now? The conquest and prevention of infectious diseases are arguably the greatest victories of medicine. The era of antibiotics and vaccines has brought under control such dread diseases as influenza, which killed more than half a million Americans in one season early in the 20th century, and smallpox, which has been eliminated altogether. Infectious diseases, however, remain a great threat to public health. Emerging and reemerging infections are being encountered for many reasons. Antibiotics themselves select for genetic changes and impart resistant phenotypes. Changes in society have a profound impact: population explosions, declining public health, and the efficient transmission of disease across geographic boundaries brought by modern day travel. The days have long past when the dying Duke of Gaunt could claim:

This fortress built by Nature herself
Against infection and the hand of war,
This blessed plot, this earth, this realm, this
England . . .

William Shakespeare (1564–1616), Richard II, II, i

Even then, infectious diseases still managed to spread through populations. Such plagues helped shape our species by inflicting severe selective pressures. Indeed, our genome carries the archeologic vestiges of past epidemics. These relics have left their imprint in the variable antibody genes of our immune system, in our blood types, and in our histocompatibility antigens. Humans and their microorganisms have been parallel evolutionary partners, and the human genome has molded a formidable immune system and tissue reaction in response to its microorganisms. This pattern of infection, disease, and the reshaping of the host response will inevitably continue.

For medicine to combat infectious disease requires great familiarity with it. This text, *Pathology of Infectious Diseases,* is a milestone toward that objective. Here we are taken into the diagnosis of human infectious disease as manifested by invasion of the organism, by its propagation, and by the ensuing host response. Detailed observations made by pathologists have been brought together in a single reference work that substantially encompasses the known infectious diseases that affect humankind. This comprehensive work underscores the principle that the microscope is still essential in revealing subtle clues linking a microorganism to a clinical disease process. Under the experienced leadership of Dr. Daniel H. Connor, together with Drs. Chandler, Schwartz, Manz, and Lack, the current body of knowledge of diagnostic pathology of human infectious disease has been assembled. Few could tackle the daunting task and credit is due to Dr. Connor and his colleagues for bringing this text to fruition. It is hoped that this special volume serves those who embark on the discovery, prevention, and treatment of the diseases described herein and the diseases that await discovery.

Jeffrey Cossman, MD
Chairman, Department of Pathology
Georgetown University School of Medicine
Washington, DC
August 1996

Preface

Winston Churchill said, "Writing a book is an adventure. At first it's a toy; then it becomes a mistress, then a master, and just when you become resigned to your servitude, you kill the monster and fling it about at the public."

This book, conceived in the fall of 1990, is the culmination of the efforts of many people, among whom we are most grateful to the contributing authors. As the saying goes, to accomplish a task, ask a busy person; this we did—repeatedly and persistently in our attempt to make the book comprehensive and timely. But 6 years is a long incubation period, and as a consequence, some authors updated their manuscripts once, twice, and even three times while awaiting publication—a reflection of the rapidly changing world of infectious diseases.

The idea of using quotations at the beginning of certain chapters started capriciously, almost as an afterthought, and at first were used only when they were pertinent to the subject—for instance, rabies (Chapter 30). But the quotations gained popularity with authors and editors, so our goal escalated to find one for each chapter. Dr. Sarah Frankel and Dr. Ann Marie Nelson, both at the US Armed Forces Institute of Pathology, furnished reference books that fueled our interest in pursuing quotations. And we took liberties. The chapter on clostridial infections (Chapter 54), for instance, was the vehicle for our favorite prose—President Lincoln's letter to Mrs. Lydia Bixby. How noble is such eloquence and humility! As Viscount Bryce has said of these four sentences, "I do not know where the nobility of self-sacrifice for a great cause, and the consolation which the thought of a sacrifice so made should bring, is set forth with such simple and pathetic beauty. Deep must be the fountains from which there issues so pure a stream." (Maybe one, or perhaps two, of Mrs. Bixby's sons died of a gas infection complicating a battlefield wound.) As our resources broadened, at least one quotation was selected for each chapter. This broader approach is best exemplified perhaps by Maxwell's equations used for Chapter 132 (Free-Living Amebic Infections). We hope the association of these equations and the subject need no explanation or justification. Finally, it seemed appropriate that Chapter 36 (Viral Infections by Human Herpesviruses 6, 7, and 8), which was completed on July 4, should have a quotation by Thomas Jefferson.

If there were stages of "toy" or "mistress" in the preparation of this book, they were fleeting. Now our "servitude" is over. We hope that this book will not be "flung about" but used regularly and with benefit by pathologists, clinicians, epidemiologists, veterinarians, and other medical scientists. We welcome helpful comments for any future editions. Our final prayer is that this century's great advances in medical science, including prevention, therapy, and technology, will become available soon to all people everywhere.

Daniel H. Connor, MD
Long Lake, Ontario, Canada
August 1996

Acknowledgments

Lorenz E. Zimmerman, MD, helped in many ways, reading some chapters and making his collection of pictures available. Evelma Jones at the Armed Forces Institute of Pathology located many of the illustrations. Cathy Cataldo typed, scanned, and mailed many manuscripts. We are especially grateful to the entire staff of the Georgetown University Dahlgren Memorial Medical Library, who were enormously helpful and always cheerful. Jeanne Larsen was never defeated by a remote or very old reference. Lilia Frilles, Alexandra Gomes, Terry Tobias, Tony Pasieka, Martha Cohn, and Brian Dobbs helped continuously with library work that sometimes seemed unending. Amanda Hall and Joni Douglass in Educational Media at Georgetown University School of Medicine helped produce many of the illustrations expertly and on time. We are grateful also to Carolyn James, Gloria Baptist, Patricia Jones, and Joan Edmondson of the Division of Media and Training Services, Public Health Practice Office, Centers for Disease Control and Prevention, Atlanta, Georgia, for assistance in obtaining some of the illustrative materials.

Pathology of Infectious Diseases

Volume II

Part IV

Fungal and Algal Infections

Chapter 99

Adiaspiromycosis

John C. Watts and Francis W. Chandler

For there is in man the bitter and the salt, the sweet and the acid, the sour and the insipid, and a multitude of other things having all sorts of powers both as regards power and strength. These, when all mixed and mingled up with one another, are not apparent, neither do they hurt a man; but when any of them is separate, and stands by itself, then it becomes perceptible, and hurts a man.

Hippocrates (460–377 B.C.)

DEFINITION

Human adiaspiromycosis is an extremely rare, self-limited pulmonary infection caused by the soil saprophyte *Chrysosporium parvum* var *crescens* (formerly *Emmonsia crescens*). The other variety of this species, *C parvum* var *parvum*, is primarily a pathogen of rodents and other small mammals and is not known to infect humans. Synonyms include haplomycosis and adiasporosis. The name of the disease, adiaspiromycosis, derives from the unusual asexual conidia of this fungus, the adiaconidia (formerly adiaspores), which are fungal conidia that enlarge progressively at body temperature (and in vitro at 40°C) but do not propagate or disseminate in host tissues.[1,2]

GEOGRAPHIC DISTRIBUTION

Human adiaspiromycosis has been reported from France, Czechoslovakia, the Soviet Union (Commonwealth of Independent States), Honduras, Guatemala, Venezuela, and Brazil.[3–5] The fungus itself, however, is widely distributed throughout the world, predominantly in temperate zones. Autochthonous human cases have not been reported from the United States.

LIFE CYCLE AND MORPHOLOGIC FEATURES

Chrysosporium parvum var *crescens*, a dimorphic fungus, grows as a septate, branched mycelium in culture at room temperature. Small aleurioconidia, 2 to 4 μm in diameter, are borne on conidiophores at right angles to the vegetative hyphae of the mycelium. When these conidia are incubated at 40°C in vitro or are introduced into the lungs, they transform into spherical adiaconidia, which manifest the unusual property of progressive, massive enlargement under these conditions of growth.

Mature adiaconidia are thick-walled spherules that measure 200 to 400 μm or more in diameter. With the hematoxylin-eosin (H&E) stain, the refractile walls of these conidia, 20 to 70 μm thick, are comprised of two layers: a narrow, outer, eosinophilic layer that contains periodic fenestrations; and a broad, inner, hyaline layer composed predominantly of chitin[6] (Figure 99–1). The conidial walls stain uniformly and completely with the Gomori's methenamine-silver (GMS) stain, which accentuates the fenestrated layer (Figure 99–2). The Gridley fungus stain, however, delineates three layers in the conidial wall (Figure 99–3) that correspond to those demonstrated by electron microscopy.[7] The adiaconidia in human lung tissue are usually empty, but they may contain small, refractile, eosinophilic hyaline globules

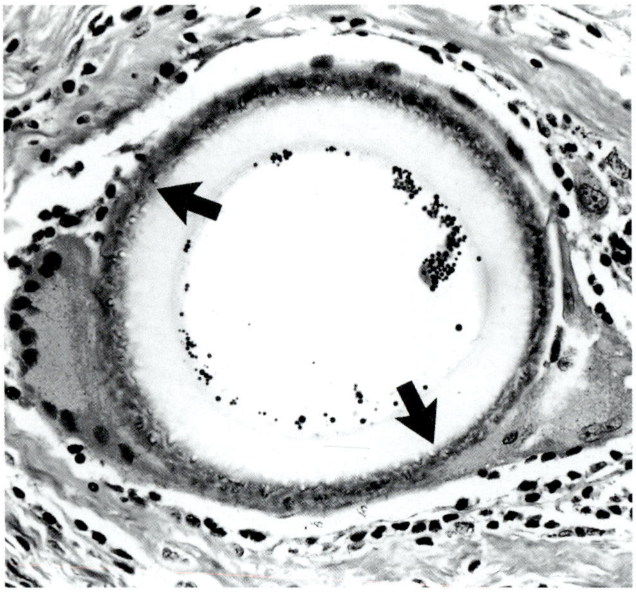

Figure 99–1. Adiaconidium of *C parvum* var *crescens*. The conidial wall is composed of an outer, eosinophilic and an inner, hyaline layer. Fenestrations are barely visible at the junction of these two layers *(lower left, between arrows)*. The interior of the conidium contains eosinophilic, hyaline globules but is otherwise empty (hematoxylin-eosin, ×300).

along the inner surfaces of their walls (Figure 99–1). Adiaconidia, however, do not contain nuclei or other cellular organelles, and they show no evidence of replication (eg, budding or endosporulation).[4] Tangentially cut adiaconidia may appear solid rather than ring-shaped (Figure 99–4).

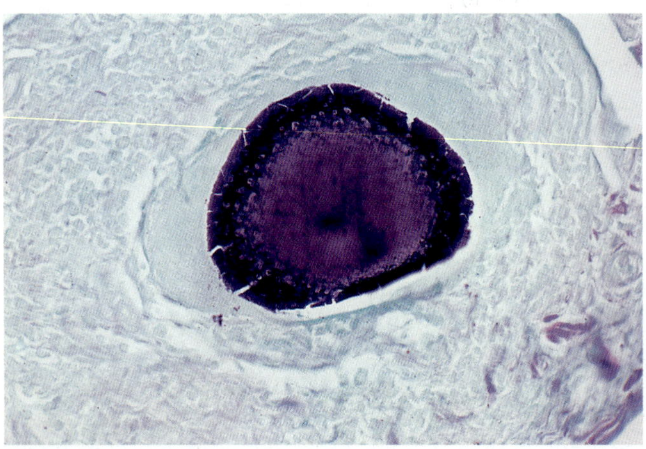

Figure 99–2. Fenestrations in the wall of this tangentially cut adiaconidium are seen more clearly with a methenamine-silver stain (GMS, ×100).

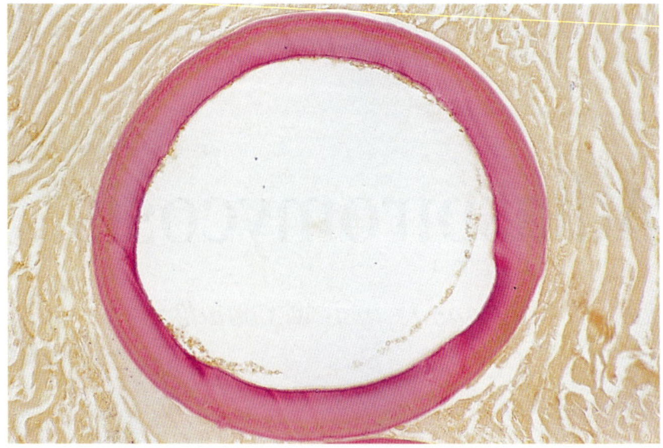

Figure 99–3. The Gridley fungus stain defines three layers in the wall of the adiaconidium (Gridley, ×100).

CLINICAL FEATURES

Most reported patients with documented adiaspiromycosis have been asymptomatic. A clinicopathologic classification of human infections based on the density and distribution of lesions in the lungs, developed by Czechoslovakian workers, includes the following: solitary granuloma, localized granulomatous disease, and diffuse, disseminated granulomatous disease.[3,4] Patients in the last category may experience symptoms such as fever, cough, and dyspnea.[5,8] Adiaspiromycosis, however, is an incidental finding in most patients, including

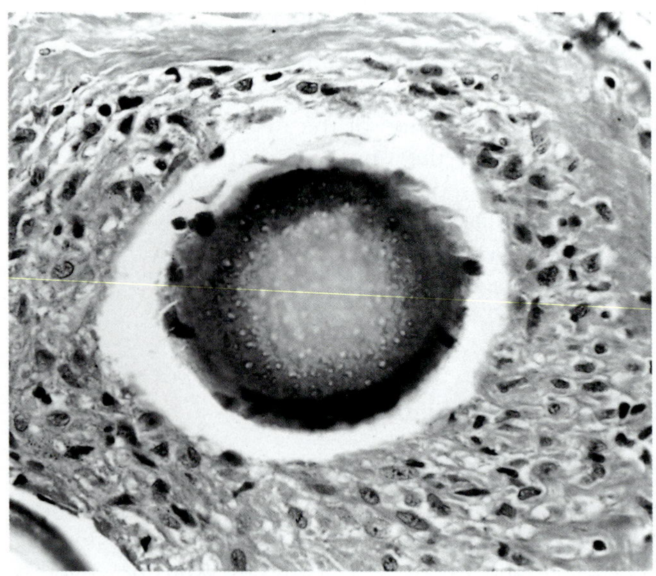

Figure 99–4. Tangential section through the wall of an adiaconidium. The conidium is enveloped by an epithelioid granulomatous response (hematoxylin-eosin, ×300).

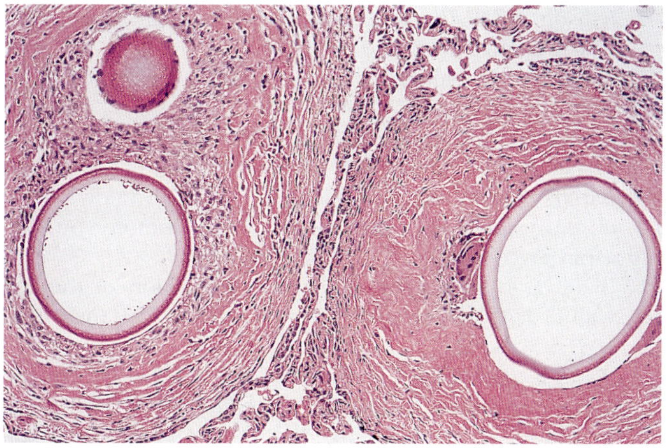

Figure 99–5. Diffuse, densely nodular pulmonary adiaspiromycosis. Each adiaconidium has evoked a fibrogranulomatous response. The intervening lung is normal (hematoxylin-eosin, ×40).

some of those with disseminated pulmonary nodules discovered either radiographically or pathologically.[9] Dissemination to extrapulmonary sites has not been reported in natural human infection. Because the pulmonary infection is self-limited, specific antifungal therapy is not necessary.

PATHOLOGY

The inflammatory response in adiaspiromycosis is fibrogranulomatous. Each adiaconidium is surrounded by an epithelioid and giant cell granulomatous response, which in turn is encompassed by a dense capsule of fibrous connective tissue (Figure 99–5). In the densely nodular form of the disease, the miliary granulomas are often confluent. Individual granulomas vary in size from 0.5 to 3 mm, and the adiaconidia contained within them are sometimes large enough to be just visible with the naked eye. All granulomas are at a similar stage of development, indicating evolution from a one-time exposure without subsequent replication of the conidia in the lungs. Clinical symptoms, when they occur, are apparently caused by compression and displacement of distal airways and alveolar parenchyma by the expanding granulomas (Figure 99–6).

DIFFERENTIAL DIAGNOSIS

Other fungi that produce large spherules or sporangia in host tissues are occasionally mistaken for the adiaconidia of *C parvum* var *crescens*. The sporangia of *Rhinosporidium seeberi* are distinguished by the distinctive appearance and zonation of their sporangiospores. The spherules of *Coccidioides immitis* are smaller than the adiaconidia of *C parvum* var *crescens*, and when mature they contain abundant endospores, which are not found within adiaconidia. No other human fungal pathogens have walls as thick as those of the adiaconidia of *C parvum* var *crescens*. The large size and thick, chitinous walls of the adiaconidia may suggest a pulmonary helminthic infection.[5] Adiaconidia, however, lack the somatic musculature and internal

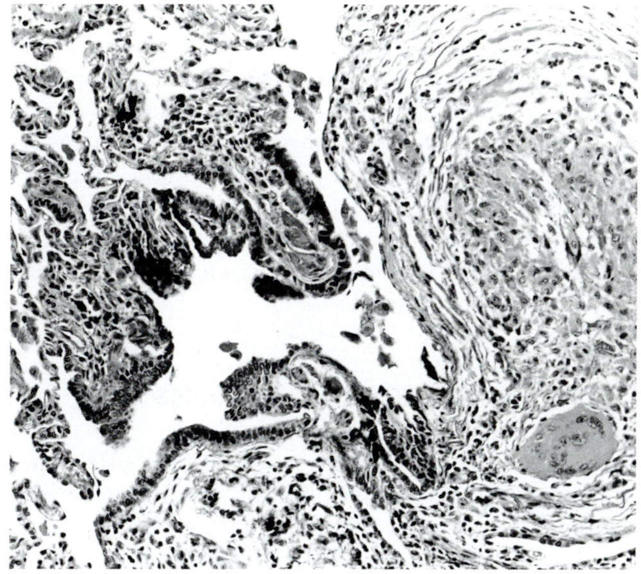

Figure 99–6. Adiaspiromycotic granuloma compresses the lumen of a respiratory bronchiole (hematoxylin-eosin, ×120).

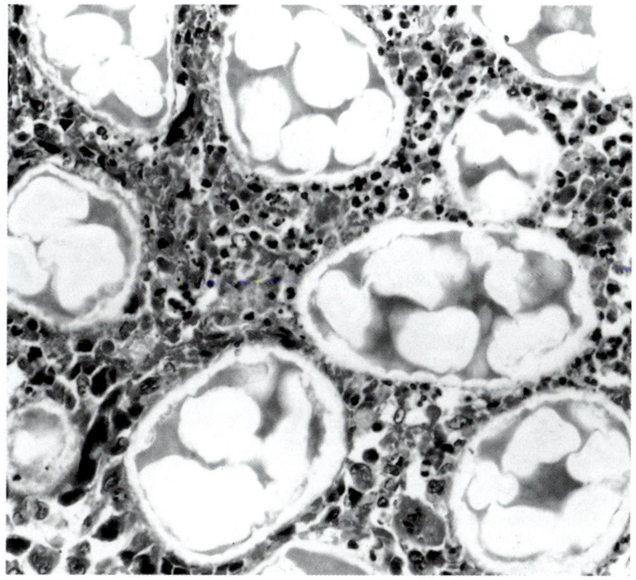

Figure 99–7. Lentil pneumonia. Aspirated starch granules can be mistaken for adiaconidia but are distinguished by their loculated starch content (hematoxylin-eosin, ×300).

organs that characterize the parasitic metazoa, and they are spherical rather than tubular, which can be shown by step sectioning the tissue specimen. Finally, the starch granules of lentils and other leguminous vegetables stimulate a suppurative, necrotizing, and granulomatous pneumonitis (lentil pneumonia) following their aspiration into the lungs[10] (Figure 99–7). The individual starch granules can be distinguished easily from adiaconidia by their loculated starch content with the periodic acid–Schiff reaction.

CONFIRMATIONAL TESTING AND DIAGNOSIS

The diagnosis of adiaspiromycosis is usually established by histopathologic identification of the distinctive adiaconidia in lung tissue. A skin test antigen, haplosporangin, is available,[5] but its reliability is unknown. Because the adiaconidia in human lung are presumed to be sterile cells, confirmation of the histopathologic diagnosis by culture of respiratory secretions or lung tissue is unlikely to be helpful.

REFERENCES

1. Emmons CW, Jellison WL. *Emmonsia crescens* sp n and adiaspiromycosis (haplomycosis) in mammals. *Ann NY Acad Sci.* 1960;89:91–101.
2. Jellison WL. *Adiaspiromycosis (= Haplomycosis).* Missoula, Mont: Mountain Press; 1969.
3. Kodousek R. Adiaspiromycosis. *Acta Univ Palacki Olomuc Fac Med.* 1974;70:5–68.
4. Schwarz J. Adiaspiromycosis. *Pathol Annu.* 1978;13(part 1):41–53.
5. Barbas Filho JV, Amato MBP, Deheinzelin D, Saldiva RHN, de Carvalho CRR. Respiratory failure caused by adiaspiromycosis. *Chest.* 1990;97:1171–1175.
6. Blank F. Note on the chemical composition of the cell wall of *Haplosporangium parvum. J Histochem Cytochem.* 1957;5:500–502.
7. Watts JC, Callaway CS, Chandler FW, Kaplan W. Human pulmonary adiaspiromycosis. *Arch Pathol.* 1975;99:11–15.
8. Kodousek R, Vortel V, Fingerland A, et al. Pulmonary adiaspiromycosis in man caused by *Emmonsia crescens*: report of a unique case. *Am J Clin Pathol.* 1971; 56:394–399.
9. Bambirra EA, Nogueira AMMF. Human pulmonary granulomas caused by *Chrysosporium parvum* var *crescens (Emmonsia crescens). Am J Trop Med Hyg.* 1983; 32:1184–1185.
10. Knoblich R. Pulmonary granulomatosis caused by vegetable particles. So-called lentil pulse pneumonia. *Am Rev Respir Dis.* 1969;99:380–389.

CHAPTER 100

Aspergillosis

John C. Watts and Francis W. Chandler

> ***aspergillum*** *n. pl. -la or -lums (1649): a brush or small perforated container with a handle that is used for sprinkling holy water in a liturgical service.*
>
> *Webster's Ninth New Collegiate Dictionary, 1988*

DEFINITION

Aspergillosis encompasses a disparate group of diseases of varying pathogeneses, having in common their association with mycelial pathogens of the genus *Aspergillus.* The pathogenetic spectrum of aspergillosis includes 1) allergic reactions involving the nasal cavity, paranasal sinuses, and lower respiratory tract in hypersensitized hosts; 2) colonization of obstructed paranasal sinuses, bronchi, and preformed pulmonary cavities, with formation of fungus balls in persons with normal immunity; 3) superficial cutaneous infections; 4) limited invasive infection of bronchi and pulmonary parenchyma in mildly immunodeficient patients; and 5) frankly invasive pulmonary infection in severely immunodeficient patients, often complicated by systemic dissemination and death.[1]

GEOGRAPHIC DISTRIBUTION

Aspergillus sp are common throughout the world. Their conidia are ubiquitous in the environment. Favored habitats include soil and decaying organic material. These fungi are frequent contaminants in the clinical laboratory.

EPIDEMIOLOGY

Because conidia of the *Aspergillus* sp are ubiquitous, they are constantly being inhaled. Those who are allergic or have underlying pulmonary disease, respiratory obstruction, or immunologic deficiencies are susceptible to one or more forms of aspergillosis. The type of host reaction, the associated pathologic findings, and the ultimate outcome depend more on host factors than on virulence or pathogenesis of the invading aspergilli. The respiratory tract is the most frequent and most important portal of entry for human infection.

LIFE CYCLE AND MORPHOLOGIC FEATURES

Although hundreds of species of *Aspergillus* are known, only about 10 species cause human disease. Species classified in the *A fumigatus, A flavus,* and *A niger* groups are the most frequent pathogens.[2,3] These fungi are widespread in the environment, so a cultured species of *Aspergillus* should not be accepted as a pathogen unless it fits with the clinical, radiologic, and pathologic findings.

Aspergilli are asexual mycelial fungi that, with rare exception, cannot be distinguished histologically from each other (or from certain other hyalohyphomycetes). In the environment, in culture, and in infected tissues, the aspergilli grow as branched, septate hyphae that produce conidial heads when exposed to air. A conidial head consists of a conidiophore with a terminal vesicle, on which are borne one or two layers of phialides, or sterigmata (Figure 100–1). These elongated cells in turn produce columns of spherical conidia, which are the infectious propagules from which the mycelial phase of the fungus develops. Identification of individual species depends, in part, on differences of their conidial heads.[4]

In sections, well-preserved hyphae of *Aspergillus* sp are homogeneous and uniform, measuring 3 to 6 μm in width. They have parallel contours, are regularly sep-

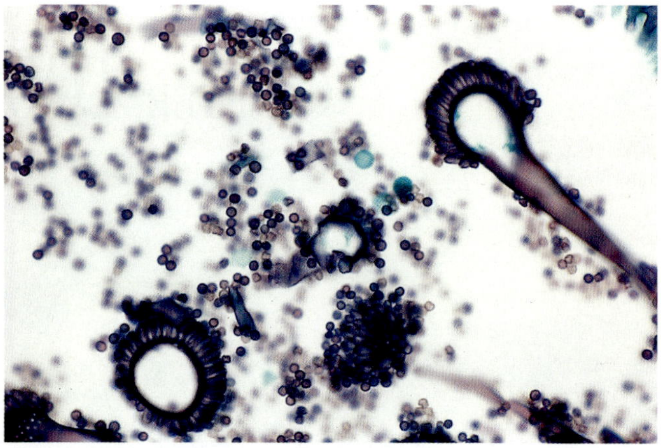

Figure 100–1. Conidial heads of *A fumigatus* in a pulmonary cavity. Uniseriate phialides cover the upper two thirds of the vesicles. The small spherical conidia, most of which have fallen off the heads, are normally attached in columns to the tips of the phialides [Gomori's methenamine-silver (GMS) stain, ×250].

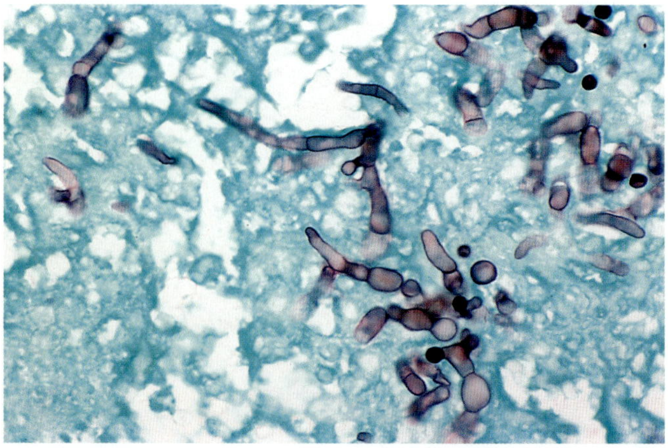

Figure 100–3. Aleurioconidium of *A terreus*. The small, spherical conidium is borne laterally from the hyphal fragment on a short conidiophore (GMS, ×250).

tate, and have a progressive, arboreal pattern of branching (Figure 100–2). Branches are dichotomous (of a size similar to the hyphae of origin) and usually arise at acute angles. The viable mycelium has basophilic walls, but a necrotic mycelium is either eosinophilic or colorless in routine sections. Although usually visible with hematoxylin-eosin staining, hyphal morphology is demonstrated much better with a special stain for fungi, such as GMS. The same is true of the conidial heads. *Aspergillus terreus* can be identified by its spherical or oval aleurioconidia, 6 or 7 μm in maximum size, that develop from the lateral walls of the mycelium[5,6] (Figure 100–3). Otherwise, the hyphae of the pathogenic

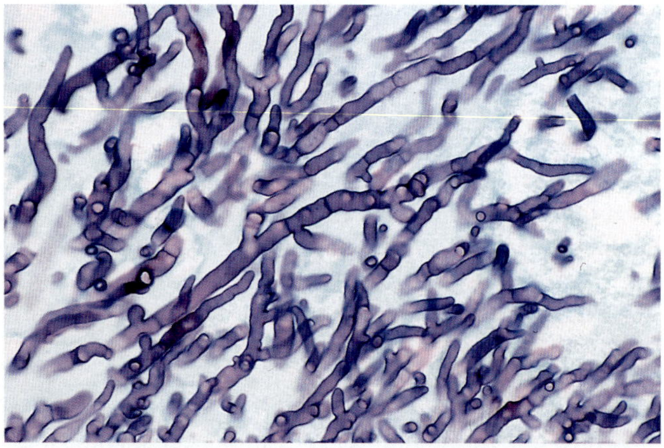

Figure 100–2. Typical hyphae of an *Aspergillus* sp. These hyphae, which are uniform and regularly septate, have a progressive, arboreal, and dichotomous pattern of branching (GMS, ×250).

aspergilli are morphologically indistinguishable from each other. Conidial heads are only rarely produced in the lesions of human aspergillosis, being most frequent when the aspergilli are exposed to air such as with fungus balls in pulmonary cavities and sinonasal aspergillomas, tracheobronchial aspergillosis, cutaneous aspergillosis, and otomycosis. Typical conidial heads in these lesions justify a histopathologic diagnosis of aspergillosis, even in the absence of culture and studies using immunofluorescent techniques.

CLINICAL FEATURES

Allergic aspergillosis is a clinicopathologic spectrum, a consequence of hypersensitivity to aspergillus antigens. Clinical features of allergic bronchopulmonary aspergillosis include asthma, pulmonary infiltrates, peripheral eosinophilia, elevated levels of serum IgE, and serologic evidence of hypersensitivity to *Aspergillus* antigens.[7,8] A similar spectrum of allergic reactions, termed *allergic aspergillus sinusitis*, involves the upper respiratory tract. The clinical features include nasal obstruction and discharge, headache, and facial pain together with laboratory evidence of allergy as described earlier.[9]

Colonizing forms of aspergillosis include obstructive bronchial aspergillosis and true aspergilloma. Obstructive bronchial colonization may complicate cystic fibrosis, asthma, chronic bronchitis, bronchiectasis, and bronchogenic neoplasm. The symptoms are those of the underlying disease, no tissue injury results, and no treatment is needed. An aspergilloma, or fungus ball, can form either in the paranasal sinuses or, more often, in a preformed pulmonary cavity, the latter usually a

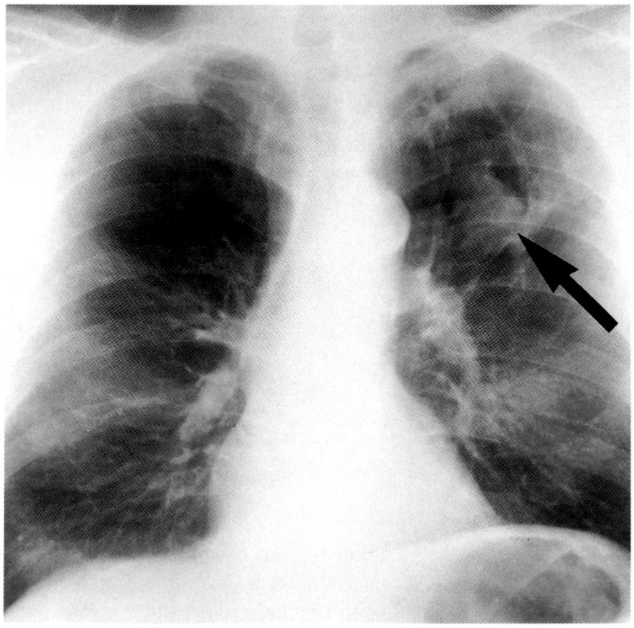

Figure 100–4. An intracavitary aspergilloma is in the left upper lobe *(arrow)*. The radiodense fungus ball is partially surrounded superiorly by air crescents, a characteristic radiographic feature.

consequence of tuberculosis or other chronic cavitary lung disease.[10] Fungus balls often remain clinically silent until hemorrhage supervenes. Radiographic studies demonstrate an intracavitary mass (Figure 100–4) that can be identified as an aspergilloma by culture or serologic studies.[10] Life-threatening hemorrhage is the major indication for surgical excision of these pulmonary cavities or radical debridement of the paranasal sinuses.

Invasive aspergillosis includes all forms of aspergillosis in which host tissues are invaded or destroyed. Almost always these patients have some underlying immunodeficiency. Mild immunodeficiency, such as that associated with mild leukopenia, low-dose corticosteroid therapy, collagen-vascular diseases, alcoholism, or diabetes mellitus, may result in only limited or superficial invasion. Clinicopathologic syndromes of this type include necrotizing pseudomembranous bronchial aspergillosis[11,12] and chronic necrotizing ("semi-invasive") pulmonary aspergillosis (CNPA),[13,14] both of which are infrequent. Bronchial aspergillosis may cause dyspnea, wheezing, cough, or hemoptysis. Most patients with CNPA have underlying noncavitary structural pulmonary disease, and some have received low-dose corticosteroids.[15] The appearance of new cavities in radiographic areas of infiltration should suggest the diagnosis, particularly if fungus balls develop in the cavities. CNPA is a chronic infection that is not associated with vascular invasion or dissemination. Most patients respond to surgical resection or drainage and antifungal chemotherapy, and about 80% of patients so treated survive. Other examples of limited or superficial infection include otomycosis and infection of burns.

Invasive pulmonary aspergillosis (IPA) and disseminated aspergillosis are devastating infections of severely immunodeficient patients.[16] Factors that predispose to these severe forms of invasive infection include granulocytopenia (leukocyte count less than 500/mm^3), cytotoxic chemotherapy, and corticosteroid therapy.[17] Patients usually present with fever and pulmonary infiltrates,[2] or with symptoms of hemorrhagic pulmonary infarction such as pleuritic chest pain and hemoptysis. Because the symptoms are nonspecific, and sputum and blood cultures are negative in most patients, diagnosis and subsequent systemic antifungal chemotherapy are often delayed, and more than 70% of patients die.[18,19] Hematogenous dissemination, a frequent complication of IPA, results from the propensity of the *Aspergillus* sp to invade medium-sized and large blood vessels. Disseminated lesions frequently involve the central nervous system, heart, kidneys, gastrointestinal tract, liver, and spleen.[20]

PATHOLOGY

Allergic bronchopulmonary aspergillosis (ABPA) is characterized by a variety of pathologic lesions that involve conducting airways and more distal air spaces. There are similar changes in the upper respiratory tract in allergic *Aspergillus* sinusitis.[21] The major pulmonary findings include mucoid impaction of bronchi, bronchocentric granulomatosis, exudative bronchiolitis, chronic eosinophilic pneumonia, and microgranulomatous hypersensitivity pneumonitis.[7,22] Although these changes may be in pure form, they often coexist. In mucoid impaction, casts of viscid, rubbery mucus obstruct and distend the lumens of proximal bronchi.[7] The "allergic mucin" that composes these casts consists of serpiginous layers of eosinophils, epithelial cells, necrotic cellular debris, and Charcot–Leyden crystals embedded in dense, eosinophilic mucus[23] (Figure 100–5). The distinctive microscopic appearance of these casts should immediately suggest the diagnosis of allergic fungal disease, which can be confirmed by demonstrating hyphae with an appropriate special stain. As a rule, however, the hyphae in these casts are sparse, fragmented, and distorted. Because the aspergilli are only one of several genera of mycelial pathogens that have been implicated in the cause of mucoid impaction and allergic bronchopulmonary fungal disease, their specific identification as an *Aspergillus* sp may require immunohistology or culture.

Bronchocentric granulomatosis is characterized by extensive destruction of the walls of small bronchi and

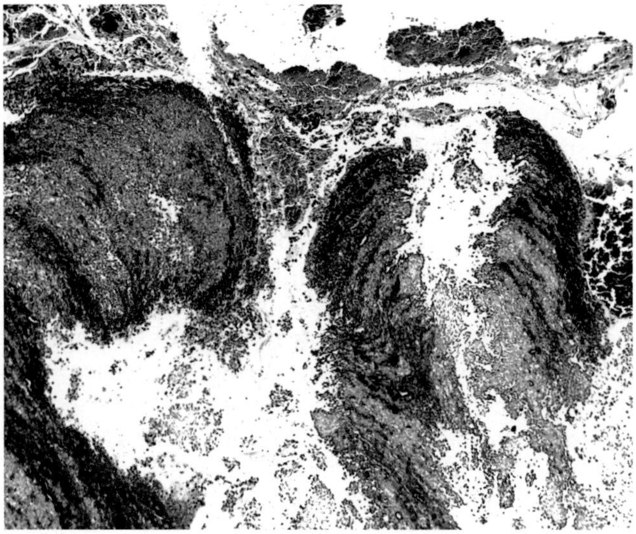

Figure 100–5. Fragments of bronchial plug from a patient with mucoid impaction caused by allergic bronchopulmonary aspergillosis. Note prominent parallel lamination caused by interposing layers of mucus with layers of degenerated eosinophils. This histopathologic pattern is characteristic of allergic bronchopulmonary fungal disease (hematoxylin-eosin, ×50).

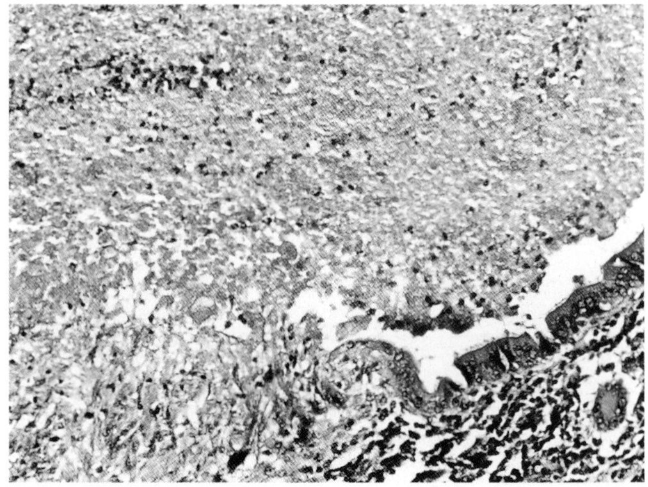

Figure 100–6. Bronchocentric granulomatosis caused by hypersensitivity to aspergillus antigens. The normal bronchial epithelial lining *(right)* is abruptly replaced by a granulomatous inflammatory response. The bronchial lumen *(above)* is filled with necrotic debris that contains degenerated eosinophils (hematoxylin-eosin, ×120).

bronchioles, with replacement by granulomatous inflammation[24] (Figure 100–6). The lumens of affected airways contain necrotic debris with scattered eosinophils and distorted hyphal fragments. Similar changes can be caused by endobronchial tuberculosis or histoplasmosis, so the diagnosis requires specific identification of the etiologic agent. *Exudative bronchiolitis*[22] is characterized by an exudate in the lumen composed of necrotic neutrophils and eosinophils and cellular debris, often with segmental destruction of the bronchiolar wall (Figure 100–7). The nongranulomatous exudate usually contains strands of mucus, but it does not have the distinctive appearance of the "allergic mucin" of mucoid impaction of bronchi.

Chronic eosinophilic pneumonia as a manifestation of ABPA is indistinguishable from eosinophilic pneumonia of other causes.[25] Cellular infiltrates composed of eosinophils, macrophages, and Charcot–Leyden crystals fill alveolar spaces (Figure 100–8). Interstitial cellular infiltrates involve the alveolar septa, and organizing eosinophilic endobronchiolitis is also seen. *Microgranulomatous hypersensitivity pneumonitis* is an allergic reaction to the antigens of *A clavatus* ("malt-workers lung"). Although rarely biopsied, the changes are indistinguishable from those of other forms of extrinsic allergic alveolitis.

Colonizing aspergillosis, whether in the upper or lower respiratory tract, is characterized by a fungus ball in a cavity[26] (Figure 100–9). Fungus balls are macrocolonies that are formed of concentric layers of mycelium. Hyphae in the outer layers of the fungus ball are viable, whereas those nearer the center may be degenerated and quite bizarre, with prominent vesicles and inconspicuous septa (Figure 100–10). Conidial heads may be on the surface of the fungus balls, and

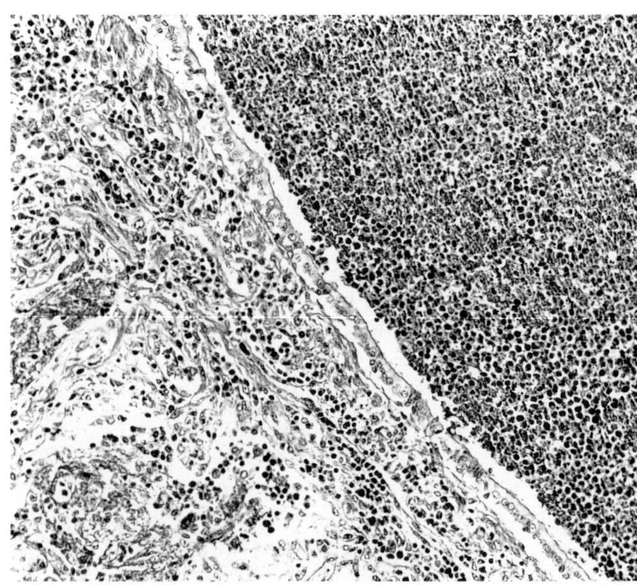

Figure 100–7. Exudative bronchiolitis in allergic bronchopulmonary aspergillosis. The lumen of this bronchiole *(upper right)* is occluded by an inflammatory exudate composed of degenerated eosinophils and neutrophils, mucus, fibrin, and Charcot–Leyden crystals (hematoxylin-eosin, ×120).

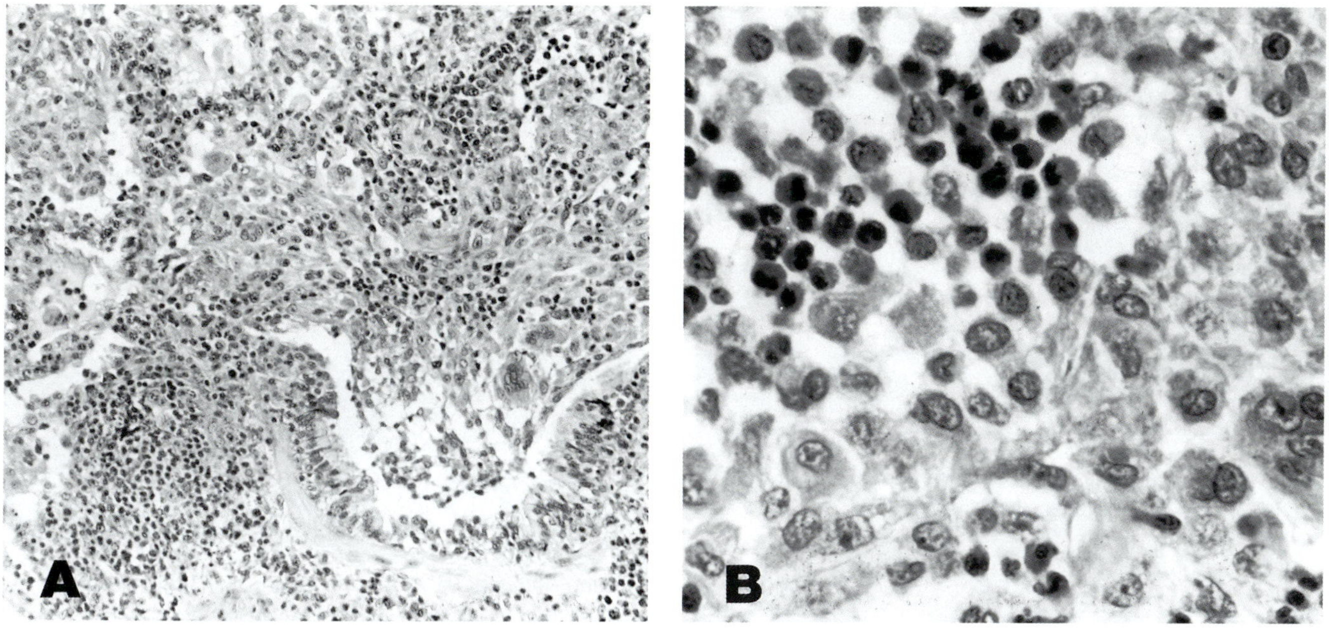

Figure 100–8. Chronic eosinophilic pneumonia. (**A**) Cellular exudate occupies the lumen of a respiratory bronchiole and extends into an adjacent alveolar duct and alveolar spaces (hematoxylin-eosin, ×120). (**B**) The cellular exudate is composed of macrophages, eosinophils, and occasional giant cells (hematoxylin-eosin, ×480).

calcium oxalate crystals may deposit in and between the mycelial layers[27,28] (Figure 100–11). The fungus balls move freely in the cavities, eroding the epithelial lining and causing hemorrhage (Figure 100–12). Ordinarily, hyphae do not invade the wall of the cavity, unless host defenses are deficient.

Necrotizing bronchial aspergillosis is characterized by a pseudomembrane that undermines and replaces the bronchial epithelium.[29] Pseudomembranes are an acute inflammatory exudate mixed with mucus, necrotic

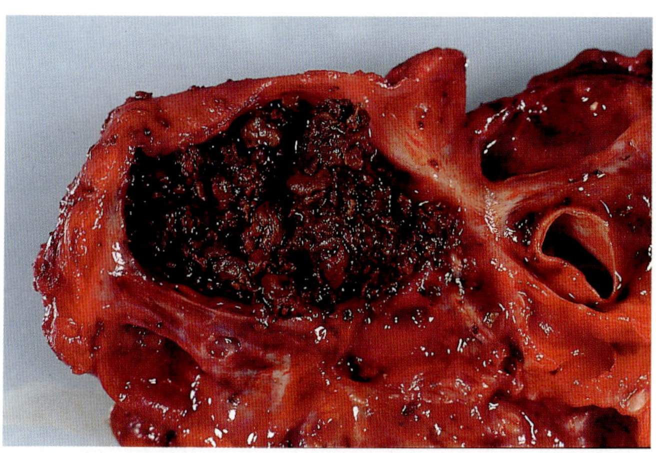

Figure 100–9. Intracavitary aspergilloma. The friable mycelium that composes the fungus ball is attached loosely to the thin, fibrous wall of the cavity.

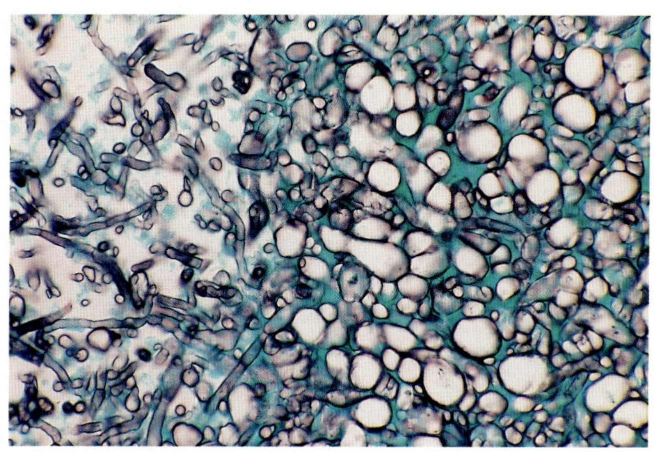

Figure 100–10. Zonation of mycelium in an intracavitary aspergilloma. The more superficial layer *(left)* is composed of hyphae with normal morphology. Degenerated hyphae in the deeper layer *(right)* are swollen and have developed prominent vesicles (GMS, ×160).

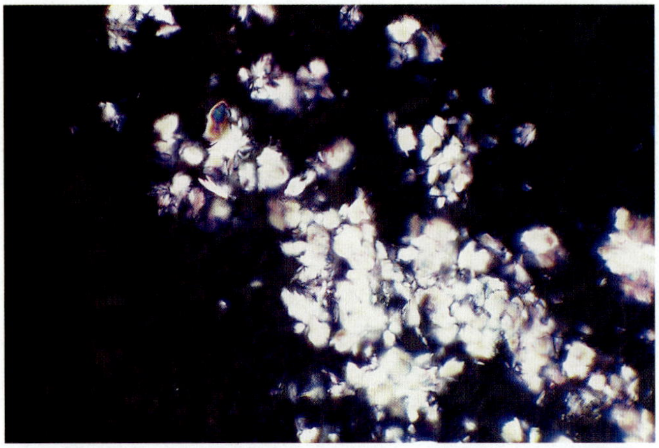

Figure 100–11. Birefringent deposits of calcium oxalate crystals in an intracavitary aspergilloma (hematoxylin-eosin, ×160, plane polarized light).

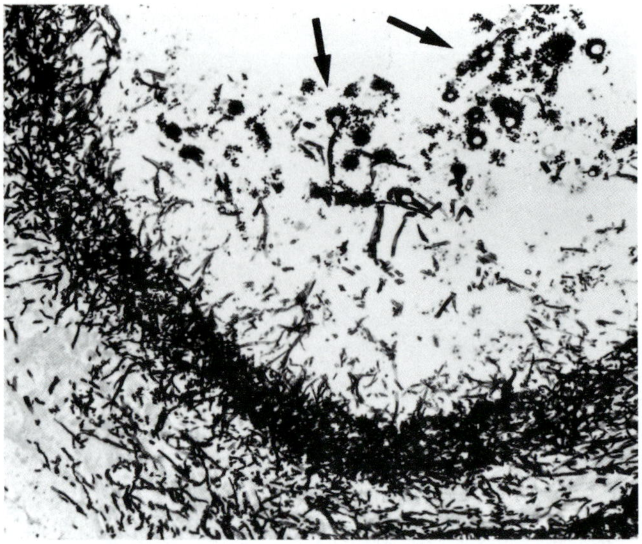

Figure 100–13. Necrotizing pseudomembranous bronchial aspergillosis. The bronchial mucosa is replaced by matted hyphae that invade the bronchial wall. Note conidial heads in the bronchial lumen *(arrows)* (GMS, ×120).

inflammatory cells, and abundant hyphae, occasionally with conidial heads[12] (Figure 100–13). Hyphae typically invade and destroy segments of the bronchial wall, and they may ultimately extend into peribronchial parenchyma. There is no hematogenous spread unless the patient has granulocytopenia or other severe immunodeficiency.

The pathologic findings in *CNPA* have not been thoroughly described, but this entity has features of both aspergilloma and invasive aspergillosis. The lungs contain cavities that are surrounded by fibrotic pulmonary parenchyma. Aggregates of mycelium or well-formed fungus balls are in these cavities.[30] It is the dynamic development of these cavities and fungus balls in previously normal lung that distinguishes CNPA from colonizing aspergilloma, a noninvasive form of aspergillosis that develops in a preexisting pulmonary cavity. In CNPA, apparently, there is parenchymal infection with limited invasion of surrounding lung. Cavities form by sequestration of necrotic lung, and overgrowth of mycelium in these sequestra leads to an intracavitary fungus ball.[31,32]

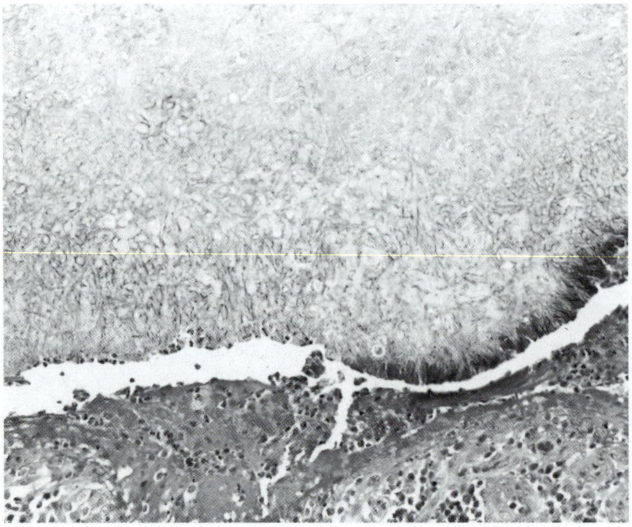

Figure 100–12. The fungus ball *(above),* composed of hyaline mycelium, has eroded the wall of the cavity *(below),* which is covered by a fibrin-rich exudate. Hemorrhage from eroded vessels in the lining of the cavity may require lobectomy (hematoxylin-eosin, ×120).

The pathologic hallmark of *IPA* is vascular invasion and occlusion with secondary nodular pulmonary infarction.[33] The respiratory tract is the portal of entry. Local overgrowth of mycelia in the bronchial tree gives rise, in the granulocytopenic host, to transmural hyphal invasion. Hyphae can then invade adjacent pulmonary arteries in the bronchovascular bundles (Figure 100–14), which undergo thrombotic occlusion. The resulting nodular infarcts, several millimeters to 3 cm or more in diameter, are composed of a central sphere of pulmonary parenchyma that has undergone ischemic necrosis, surrounded by a peripheral rim of parenchymal hemorrhage[33] (Figure 100–15). An occluded blood vessel is often in or at the margin of a nodular infarct, and aspergillus hyphae extend radially through the vascular wall and proliferate in the infarcted tissue, occasionally extending into adjacent viable lung. Other pathologic changes described in IPA include suppurative bronchopneumonia (in the nongranulocytopenic

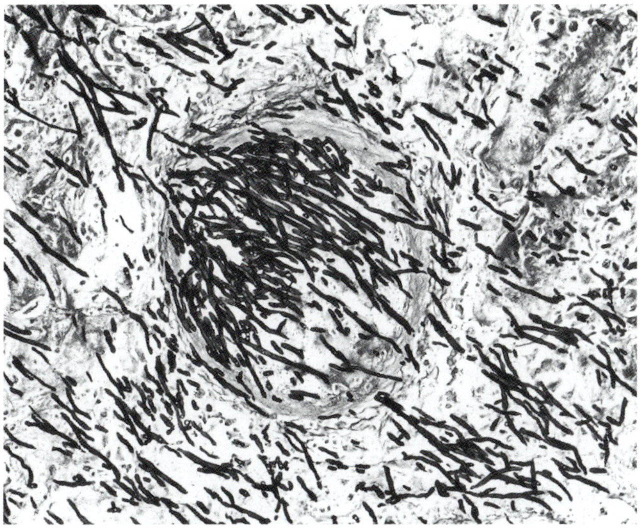

Figure 100–14. Invasion of a blood vessel by hyphae of *Aspergillus* sp. This is a pathologic hallmark of invasive and disseminated forms of aspergillosis. Angioinvasion is characteristic also of some zygomycetes and less commonly of other fungi as well, so this pattern of vascular invasion is not a specific feature of aspergillosis (Gridley fungus stain, ×100).

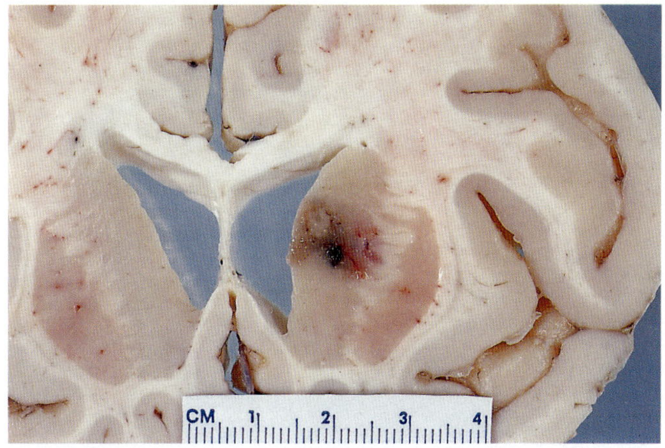

Figure 100–16. Disseminated aspergillosis. A granular infarct with surrounding hemorrhage is in the caudate nucleus in the left cerebral hemisphere.

host) and wedge-shaped, pleural based pulmonary infarcts, the latter a consequence of large vessel occlusion.

Hematogenous dissemination of aspergillosis, a serious complication of IPA, occurs in 25% to 33% of profoundly immunodeficient patients. Disseminated visceral lesions, caused by septic thromboembolism, are hemorrhagic or ischemic infarcts (Figure 100–16) that contain abundant aspergillus hyphae.

Chronic, smoldering infections of immunocompetent patients, and those treated with antifungal chemotherapy, may develop a prominent granulomatous response. This reaction occurs most often in patients with chronic *Aspergillus* sinusitis.

The diagnosis of invasive aspergillosis can be made by fine-needle aspiration, although the same qualifications regarding the nonspecificity of hyphal morphology in sections also pertain to cytology specimens. Electron microscopy has no role in the diagnosis of aspergillosis.

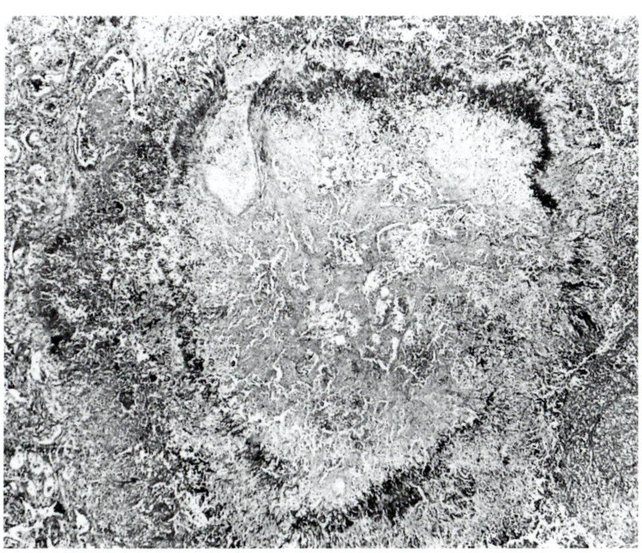

Figure 100–15. Nodular infarct in invasive pulmonary aspergillosis. The central, pale zone of ischemic pulmonary parenchyma is demarcated by a hemorrhagic rim. This lesion is a consequence of vascular occlusion caused by hyphal angioinvasion (hematoxylin-eosin, ×40).

DIFFERENTIAL DIAGNOSIS

Aspergillus hyphae in human tissues may undergo degenerative changes that distort the hyphae and may complicate identification. For example, degenerated hyphae in the core of an aspergilloma are often bizarre, with varicose or globose segments up to 15 μm in diameter, inconspicuous septa, and sparse branching. These degenerated hyphae can resemble those of the Zygomycetes. The correct diagnosis of aspergillosis is often suggested by the morphologically typical hyphae or conidial heads elsewhere in the lesion.

The hyphae of other opportunistic, angioinvasive hyalohyphomycetes, notably the *Fusarium* sp and *Pseudallescheria boydii*, are both branched and septate, and can be mistaken for hyphae of the *Aspergillus* sp.[34] The hyphae of *Fusarium* sp are 3 to 8 μm in width, slightly wider than those of the aspergilli. Their hyphal branches, however, tend to arise at right angles rather than acute angles, and the branches are typically constricted at their sites of origin from parent hyphae,

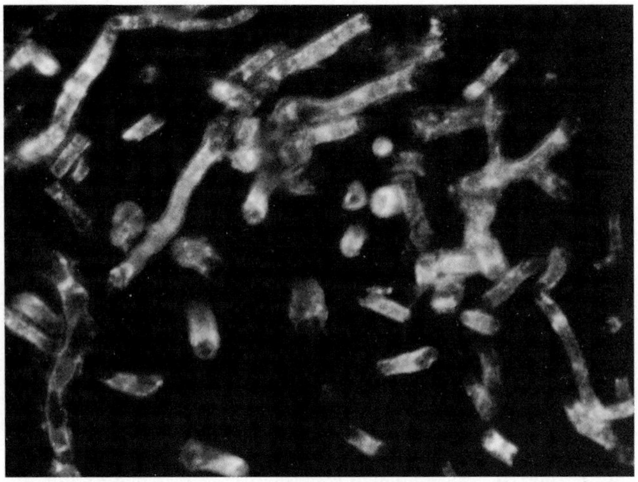

Figure 100–17. The hyphae of the *Aspergillus* sp can be identified generically by direct immunofluorescence in sections of routinely processed tissue (direct immunofluorescence, ×750).

unlike the hyphal branches of the aspergilli.[34] *Pseudallescheria boydii* is an agent of colonizing and invasive pulmonary infections in immunodeficient hosts, and these infections can be indistinguishable from corresponding forms of pulmonary aspergillosis. The hyphae of *P boydii*, 2 to 5 μm wide, are slightly narrower than those of the aspergilli, and their pattern of branching is haphazard rather than progressive.[34] Furthermore, the hyphae of *P boydii* frequently contain prominent vesicles, and they may produce ovoid conidia, 5 by 10 μm in size, on short conidiophores. Nevertheless, despite the morphologic differences, it may be difficult or impossible to distinguish the hyphae of these pathogens from each other by routine methods alone. Therefore, unless distinctive conidial heads are recognized, a histopathologic diagnosis of aspergillosis is best confirmed by culture or immunohistology.

MOLECULAR PATHOLOGIC DIAGNOSIS

Although molecular methods may have limited diagnostic application in the clinical laboratory,[35] they currently contribute little to the pathologic diagnosis of aspergillosis.

CONFIRMATIONAL TESTING AND DIAGNOSIS

Isolation of an *Aspergillus* sp from a normally sterile site is the best way to confirm the pathologic diagnosis of aspergillosis. As already noted, however, the ubiquity of aspergillus conidia warrants caution in the interpretation of the clinical significance of a culture. Unequivocal evidence of invasion usually requires a biopsy specimen. When cultures are negative or cannot be done (eg, because of prior fixation), immunohistochemistry can confirm a presumptive histopathologic diagnosis of aspergillosis.[34,36,37] Immunoreagents can be applied to deparaffinized sections of formalin-fixed tissue (Figure 100–17) but are specific for genus only and are not widely available.

Serologic studies help establish the clinical diagnosis of ABPA and can confirm the diagnosis of intracavitary aspergilloma. The value of antigen detection in the diagnosis of invasive aspergillosis has yet to be determined.[38]

REFERENCES

1. Chandler FW, Watts JC. Fungal infections. In: Dail DH, Hammar SP, eds. *Pulmonary Pathology.* 2nd ed. New York: Springer-Verlag; 1994:351–427.
2. Young RC, Bennett JE, Vogel CL, Carbone PP, DeVita VT. Aspergillosis: the spectrum of the disease in 98 patients. *Medicine (Baltimore).* 1970;49:147–173.
3. Young RC, Jennings A, Bennett JE. Species identification of invasive aspergillosis in man. *Am J Clin Pathol.* 1972; 58:554–557.
4. Rippon JW, ed. *Medical Mycology: The Pathogenic Fungi and the Pathogenic Actinomycetes.* Philadelphia: WB Saunders; 1988:618–650.
5. Pore RS, Larsh HW. Aleuriospore formation in four related *Aspergillus* species. *Mycologia.* 1967;59:318–325.
6. Tracy SL, McGinnis MR, Peacock JE, et al. Disseminated infection by *Aspergillus terreus. Am J Clin Pathol.* 1983;80:728–733.
7. Katzenstein AL, Liebow AA, Friedman PJ. Bronchocentric granulomatosis, mucoid impaction, and hypersensitivity reactions to fungi. *Am Rev Respir Dis.* 1975;111:497–537.
8. Ricketti AJ, Greenberger PA, Mintzer RA, et al. Allergic bronchopulmonary aspergillosis. *Arch Intern Med.* 1983; 143:1553–1557.
9. Waxman JE, Spector JG, Sale SR, Katzenstein AA. Allergic aspergillus sinusitis: concepts in diagnosis and treatment of a new clinical entity. *Laryngoscope.* 1987;97:261–266.
10. Glimp RA, Bayer AS. Pulmonary aspergilloma: diagnostic and therapeutic considerations. *Arch Intern Med.* 1983; 143:303–308.
11. Niimi T, Kajita M, Saito H. Necrotizing bronchial aspergillosis in a patient receiving neoadjuvant chemotherapy for non-small cell lung cancer. *Chest.* 1991;100:277–279.
12. Pervez NK, Kleinerman J, Kattan M, et al. Pseudomembranous necrotizing bronchial aspergillosis: a variant of invasive aspergillosis in a patient with hemophilia and acquired immune deficiency syndrome. *Am Rev Respir Dis.* 1985;131:961–963.
13. Binder RE, Faling LJ, Pugatch RD, Mahasaen C, Snider GL. Chronic necrotizing pulmonary aspergillosis: a discrete clinical entity. *Medicine (Baltimore).* 1982;61:109–124.

14. Gefter WB, Weingrad TR, Epstein DM, Ochs RH, Miller WT. "Semi-invasive" pulmonary aspergillosis: a new look at the spectrum of *Aspergillus* infections of the lung. *Radiology.* 1981;140:313–321.
15. Palmer LB, Greenberg HE, Schiff MJ. Corticosteroid treatment as a risk factor for invasive aspergillosis in patients with lung disease. *Thorax.* 1991;46:15–20.
16. Rinaldi MG. Invasive aspergillosis. *Rev Infect Dis.* 1983;5: 1061–1077.
17. Gerson SL, Talbot GH, Hurwitz S, Strom BL, Lusk EJ, Cassileth PA. Prolonged granulocytopenia: the major risk factor for invasive pulmonary aspergillosis in patients with acute leukemia. *Ann Intern Med.* 1984;100:345–351.
18. Herbert PA, Bayer AS. Fungal pneumonia (part 4): invasive pulmonary aspergillosis. *Chest.* 1981;80:220–225.
19. Fisher BD, Armstrong D, Yu B, Gold JWM. Invasive aspergillosis: progress in early diagnosis and treatment. *Am J Med.* 1981;71:571–577.
20. Lemos LB, Jensen AB. Pathology of aspergillosis. In: Al-Doory Y, Wagner GE, eds. *Aspergillosis.* Springfield, Ill: Charles C Thomas; 1985:156–195.
21. Katzenstein ALA, Sale SR, Greenberger PA. Pathologic findings in allergic aspergillus sinusitis. *Am J Surg Pathol.* 1983;7:439–443.
22. Bosken CH, Myers JL, Greenberger PA, Katzenstein ALA. Pathologic features of allergic bronchopulmonary aspergillosis. *Am J Surg Pathol.* 1988;12:216–222.
23. Jelihovsky T. The structure of bronchial plugs in mucoid impaction, bronchocentric granulomatosis and asthma. *Histopathology.* 1983;7:153–167.
24. Koss MN, Robinson RG, Hochholzer L. Bronchocentric granulomatosis. *Hum Pathol.* 1981;12:632–638.
25. Warnock ML, Fennessy J, Rippon J. Chronic eosinophilic pneumonia, a manifestation of allergic aspergillosis. *Am J Clin Pathol.* 1974;62:73–81.
26. Schwarz J. Aspergillosis. *Pathol Annu.* 1973;8:81–107.
27. Kurrein F, Green GH, Rowles SL. Localized deposition of calcium oxalate around a pulmonary *Aspergillus niger* fungus ball. *Am J Clin Pathol.* 1975;64:556–563.
28. Lee SH, Barnes WG, Schaetzel WP. Pulmonary aspergillosis and the importance of oxalate crystal recognition in cytology specimens. *Arch Pathol Lab Med.* 1986;110: 1176–1179.
29. Clarke A, Skelton J, Fraser RS. Fungal tracheobronchitis. Report of 9 cases and review of the literature. *Medicine (Baltimore).* 1991;70:1–14.
30. Wiggins J, Clark TJH, Corrin B. Chronic necrotizing pneumonia caused by *Aspergillus niger. Thorax.* 1989;44: 440–441.
31. Przyjemski C, Mattii R. The formation of pulmonary mycetomata. *Cancer.* 1980;46:1701–1704.
32. Kibbler CC, Milkins SR, Bhamra A, Spiteri MA, Noone P, Prentice HG. Apparent pulmonary mycetoma following invasive aspergillosis in neutropenic patients. *Thorax.* 1988;43:108–112.
33. Orr DP, Myerowitz RL, Dubois PJ. Patho-radiologic correlation of invasive pulmonary aspergillosis in the compromised host. *Cancer.* 1978;41:2028–2039.
34. Chandler FW, Watts JC. *Pathologic Diagnosis of Fungal Infections.* Chicago: ASCP Press; 1987:55–74.
35. Burnie JP, Coke A, Matthews RC. Restriction endonuclease analysis of *Aspergillus fumigatus* DNA. *J Clin Pathol.* 1992;45:324–327.
36. El Nageeb S, Hay RJ. Immunoperoxidase staining in the recognition of *Aspergillus* infections. *Histopathology.* 1981; 5:437–444.
37. Phillips P, Weiner MH. Invasive aspergillosis diagnosed by immunohistochemistry with monoclonal and polyclonal reagents. *Hum Pathol.* 1987;18:1015–1024.
38. Rogers TR, Haynes KA, Barnes PA. Value of antigen detection in predicting invasive pulmonary aspergillosis. *Lancet.* 1990;2:1210–1213.

CHAPTER 101

Blastomycosis

Francis W. Chandler

Sciences may be learned by rote, but Wisdom not.

Laurence Sterne (1713–1768), Tristram Shandy, Bk. V, Ch. 32

There is nothing which can better serve our patronage than the promotion of science and literature. Knowledge is in every country the surest basis of public happiness.

George Washington, address to Congress, January 8, 1790

Adapted from Carl Sagan (1934–), The Demon Haunted World

DEFINITION

Blastomycosis is a systemic infection caused by the thermally dimorphic fungus *Blastomyces dermatitidis*.[1–3] Previously this mycosis was thought to be restricted to North America, but in recent years autochthonous cases have been diagnosed in Africa, the Middle East, Asia, and Europe.[4–7] The vast majority of cases, however, originate in North America. In the United States, blastomycosis is endemic in the Mississippi River basin, around the Great Lakes, and in the Southeast.[3–8] Synonyms include North American blastomycosis, Chicago disease, and Gilchrist's disease.

EPIDEMIOLOGY

Clinical and epidemiologic studies indicate that humans and animals usually contract blastomycosis after inhaling aerosolized infectious conidia of the mycelial form of the fungus growing as a saprophyte in soil, and that the primary focus of infection is in the lungs.[9,10] Most primary pulmonary infections are asymptomatic or mildly symptomatic but self-limited in immunocompetent hosts.[11] Primary cutaneous infection is rare and usually caused by accidental inoculation of the fungus into the skin and subcutaneous tissues.[3,11] This form of blastomycosis is an occupational hazard for clinical microbiologists and pathologists, and it has occurred following dog bites.[12,13] Laboratory-acquired pulmonary blastomycosis also has been reported.[14] Blastomycosis, however, is not contagious.

Because a reliable skin test is not available, it is impossible to determine if there is a benign subclinical form of blastomycosis as there is for histoplasmosis capsulati (Chapter 109). In endemic regions of North America, epidemiologists estimate that as many as 4 cases of symptomatic blastomycosis requiring antifungal therapy occur per 100,000 each year.[5,15] The disease is usually sporadic, and is more frequent in persons 30 to 50 years old who are often outdoors. There is no racial predilection. The male-to-female ratio is as high as 15 to 1. Epidemics of blastomycosis are rare, affect all ages and both sexes, and are usually related to a point-source exposure.[3,4] Of the domestic animals, dogs are most susceptible; the infection rate is estimated to be 10 times that for humans.[5]

CLINICAL FEATURES

The two major clinical forms of blastomycosis are cutaneous and systemic. Both forms have a pulmonary inception, but their clinical presentation, course, pathologic features, and prognosis differ.[8–10] Patients with the cutaneous form of blastomycosis present with papular,

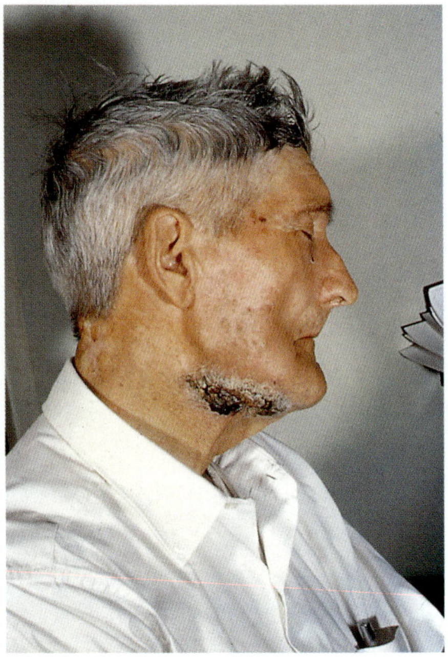

Figure 101–1. Cutaneous blastomycosis. A typical dry, crusted, sharply circumscribed, blastomycotic lesion involves the chin. *(Contributed by Centers for Disease Control and Prevention, Atlanta, Georgia.)*

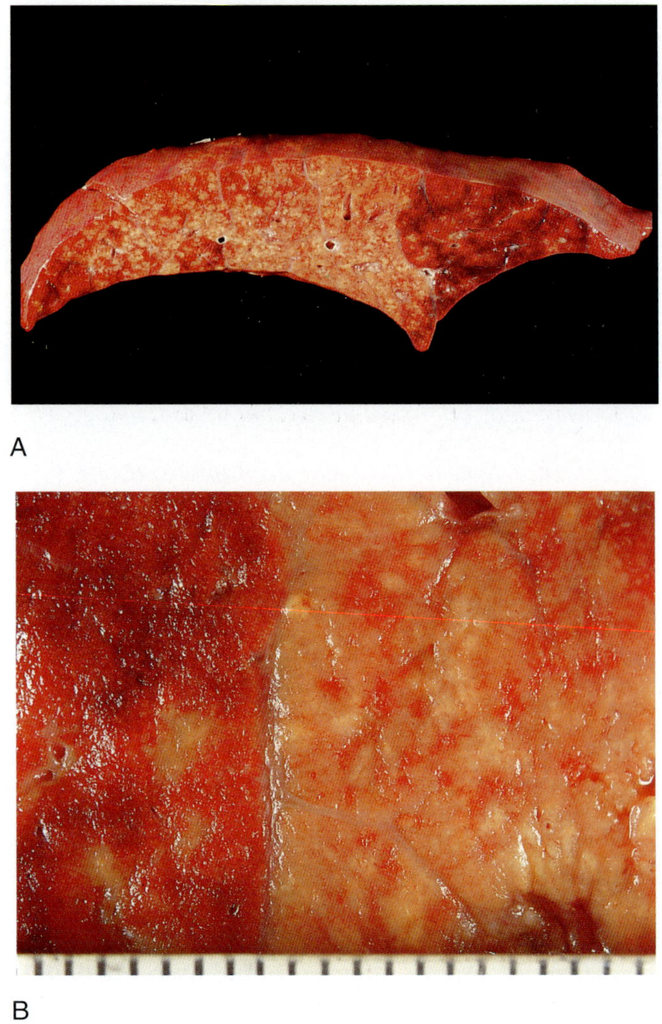

Figure 101–2. (**A**) Fatal chronic progressive pulmonary blastomycosis involving all lobes of both lungs of a 15-year-old youth from Richmond, Virginia. The white areas throughout most of the lung, shown here on the cut surface, are multifocal, discrete, and confluent pyogranulomatous lesions. Some areas are hyperemic and hemorrhagic. In this lung, the pleura is not thickened. (**B**) A closer view of the lung in Part (A) showing discrete and confluent white pyogranulomatous lesions. *(Both by Daniel H. Connor, MD, 1995.)*

pustular, or indolent, ulcerative-nodular and verrucous skin lesions with crusted surfaces and raised, serpiginous, sharply slanted borders (Figure 101–1). Lesions are usually painless, do not itch, and are often on exposed parts of the body, particularly the face, neck, and hands. Clinically, they are sometimes mistaken for squamous cell carcinoma and widely excised. There is minimal or no erythema of adjacent skin, and lymphangitis and lymphadenopathy are uncommon. In cutaneous blastomycosis, primary pulmonary lesions are usually inapparent, systemic symptoms are absent or mild, and the general health of the patient is not impaired.[9–11] If left untreated, the clinical course of cutaneous blastomycosis can range from months to years, with remissions and exacerbations and progressive increase in the size of lesions. As lesions enlarge, they heal centrally and leave thin, atrophic, depigmented scars. The rare primary cutaneous lesions of blastomycosis are localized, self-limited infections that are accompanied by regional lymphadenopathy and almost never disseminate.[12]

Systemic blastomycosis begins in lung and remains confined to lung or disseminates hematogenously to other organs, particularly skin, larynx, bones and joints, male genitourinary tract (especially the prostate), central nervous system, lymph nodes, heart, and adrenal glands[16–20] (Figure 101–2, A and B). Overwhelming primary infection with *B dermatitidis* can cause severe diffuse pneumonitis and adult respiratory distress syndrome, even in immunocompetent hosts.[15] Untreated systemic infections are often severe, progressive, and fatal; the mortality rate is greater than 90%.[8] Patients usually present with chronic respiratory symptoms, including productive cough, dyspnea, pleuritic chest pain, low-grade fever, night sweats, and weight loss. Concomitantly, about two thirds of patients have skin lesions, one third have bone lesions, and one fifth of male patients have lesions of the genitourinary tract.[2,3,11] Residual pulmonary nodules or "coin lesions," frequent in histoplasmosis capsulati and coccidioidomycosis, seldom develop in blastomycosis, and calcification of such lesions is even rarer.[21–23]

Like most other fungal infections, severely immunodeficient patients are at increased risk for blastomycosis.[24,25] The clinical presentation of primary pulmonary blastomycosis in immunodeficient patients is similar to that in immunocompetent patients. However, infection tends to disseminate more often (especially to the central nervous system) and is more rapidly progressive in patients who are immunodeficient, including those with acquired immunodeficiency syndrome (AIDS).[26,27] Endogenous reactivation of residual pulmonary lesions also has been described.[28] However, unlike cryptococcosis and histoplasmosis capsulati, blastomycosis is seldom encountered as an opportunistic mycosis in patients with AIDS or other profound cell-mediated immunodeficiencies. It is not one of the AIDS-defining infections according to criteria established by the Centers for Disease Control and Prevention.[27] There is also a low incidence of blastomycosis among bone marrow and solid organ transplant recipients.[29] Progressive dissemination of primary cutaneous blastomycosis, the rare localized and self-limited form in otherwise healthy hosts, has been reported in immunodeficient patients.[30]

MORPHOLOGIC FEATURES OF THE ORGANISM

Because *B dermatitidis* is dimorphic, it produces nonencapsulated yeastlike cells in host tissues and in vitro at 37°C on enriched media, and white-to-tan, downy-to-fluffy moulds at room temperature on standard mycologic media. In tissue sections stained with hematoxylin-eosin (H&E), typical yeastlike cells are morphologically distinctive.[21,22] They are spherical, hyaline, 8 to 15 μm in diameter, multinucleated, and have vacuolated cytoplasm and thick "double-contoured" walls with sharply defined inner and outer tables (Figure 101–3). Because of shrinkage during fixation and processing, the amphophilic cytoplasm is sometimes

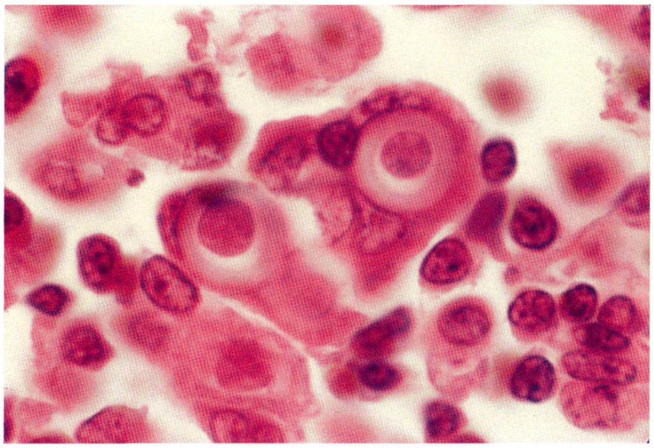

Figure 101–4. Cutaneous blastomycosis. Two spherical yeast forms of *B dermatitidis* with thick, "double-contoured" walls are located within a dermal granuloma. Retraction of cytoplasmic contents from the rigid fungal cell walls creates optically clear spaces or "halos" (H&E, ×400).

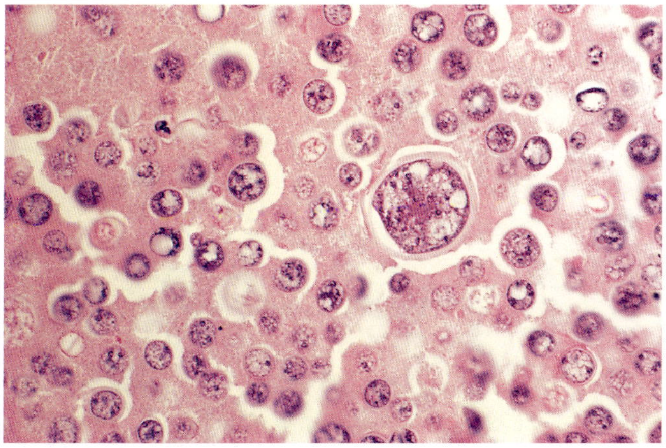

Figure 101–3. Blastomycotic pneumonia. Numerous hyaline, spherical to oval yeast forms of *B dermatitidis* have multiple, hematoxylinophilic nuclei and thick, "double contoured" walls (H&E, ×160).

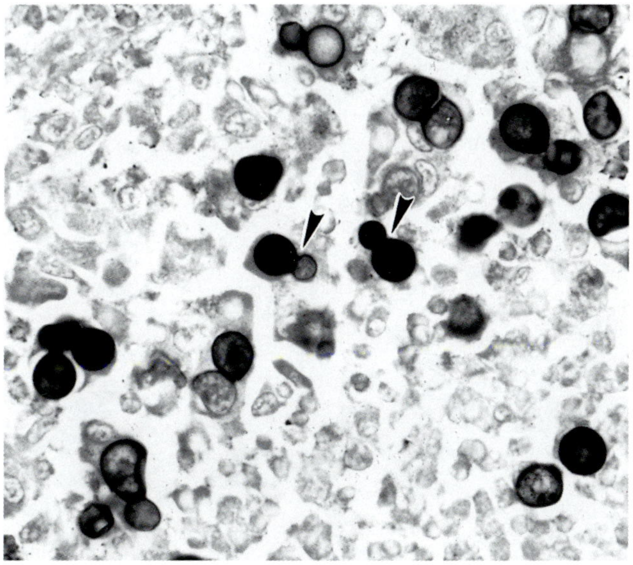

Figure 101–5. Pulmonary blastomycosis. The suppurative center of a granuloma contains numerous single and budding yeast forms of *B dermatitidis*. The "double-contoured" walls of fungal cells are not readily apparent when stained with Gomori's methenamine silver (GMS). Persistent broad-based budding *(arrowheads)* is diagnostic for this fungus (GMS, ×480).

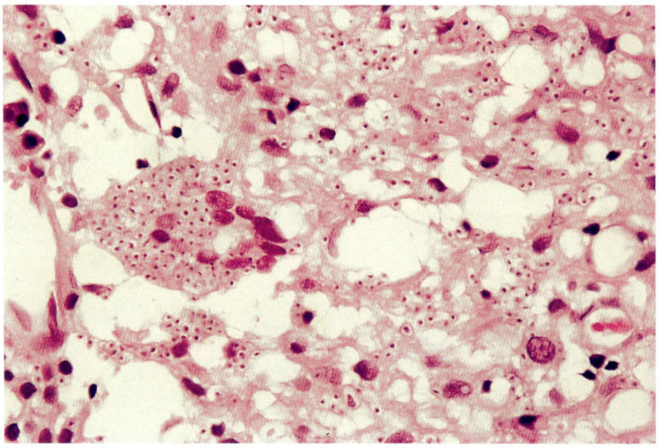

Figure 101–6. Small forms (microforms) of *B dermatitidis* in a cerebellar granuloma. Epithelioid histiocytes and giant cells contain myriad, compact yeast forms, 2 to 4 μm in diameter, that have centrally retracted, hematoxylinophilic cytoplasm and resemble the small, uniform, yeastlike cells of *Histoplasma capsulatum* var *capsulatum* (H&E, ×160).

retracted from the rigid fungal cell wall, leaving an optically clear space that surrounds all or part of the internal contents (Figure 101–4). The yeastlike cells reproduce by budding, and buds (blastoconidia) are attached to their parent cells by broad bases (Figure 101–5). Generally, only one bud is produced, and the broad-based buds are often connected to parent cells by large (4- to 5-μm-diameter) bud pores. Very small (2- to 4-μm) but morphologically typical forms of *B dermatitidis* (so-called "microforms") are occasionally in blastomycotic lesions[21,22,31] (Figure 101–6). When

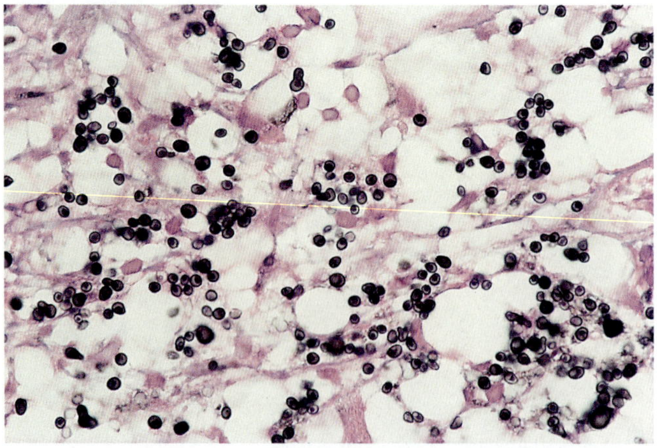

Figure 101–7. Microforms of *B dermatitidis*. Although unusually small, the yeastlike cells bud by a diagnostic broad base, have thick walls, and are morphologically similar to the larger yeast forms typical of this fungus. The presence of unusually small and typical forms of *B dermatitidis* in a lesion should not be mistaken for coexisting mycoses (GMS–H&E, ×160).

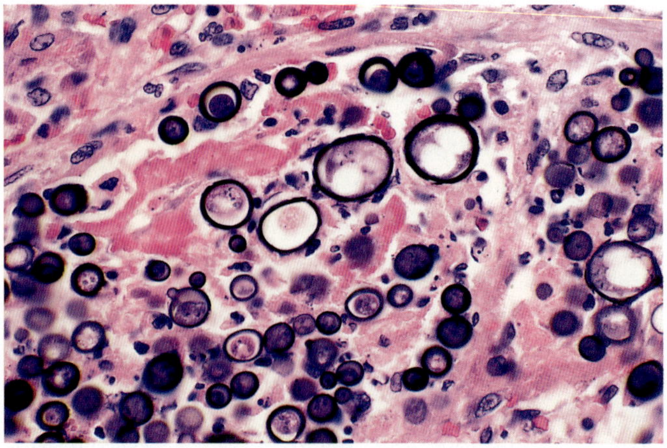

Figure 101–8. Blastomycotic pneumonia. Typical yeast forms of *B dermatitidis,* 8 to 15 μm in diameter, are mixed with unusually large forms, 20 to 40 μm in diameter, with vacuolated cytoplasm. A blastomyces cell with two buds is seen at lower left (GMS–H&E, ×160).

encountered, these microforms are usually numerous and may be the majority of the fungal cell population (Figure 101–7). However, they are always present as part of a continuous series of sizes ranging from the unusually small (2 to 4 μm) to the larger yeast forms (8 to 15 μm) typical of this fungus. Rarely, giant forms (macroforms) of *B dermatitidis* also are encountered in the lesions of blastomycosis.[22,32] These abnormally large yeast forms are 20 to 30 μm in diameter and occasionally reach 40 μm (Figure 101–8). Otherwise they resemble the adjacent, typical blastomyces cells. The giant forms, which are sometimes empty and often lack blastoconidia, form a minor part of a continuous series of sizes ranging from the usual to the gigantic. Germinating yeast forms (Figure 101–9), cells with multiple buds, septate hyphae, and thin-walled yeast forms of

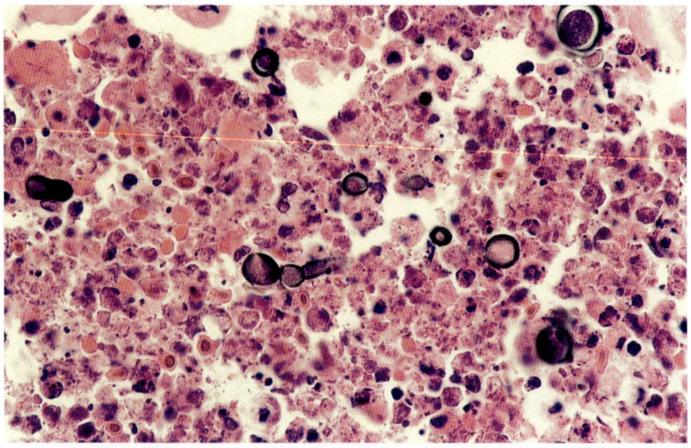

Figure 101–9. Acute pulmonary blastomycosis. A germinating yeast form of *B dermatitidis (center)* is mixed with typical forms in the necrotic center of an abscess (GMS–H&E, ×160).

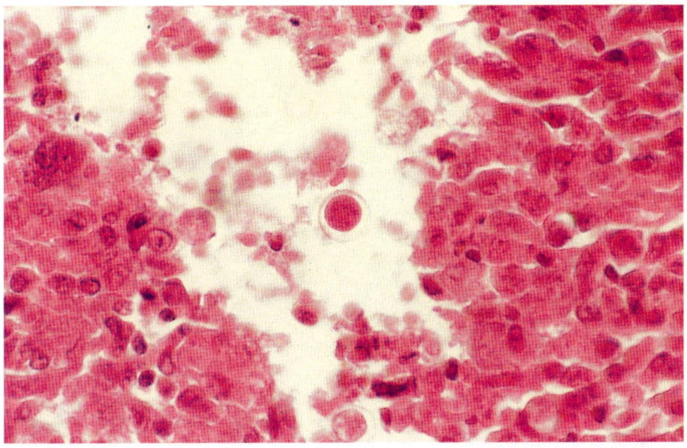

Figure 101–10. Cutaneous blastomycosis. An atypical, thin-walled yeast form of *B dermatitidis,* considered to be a cell-wall-deficient spheroplast, is located in a dermal granuloma (H&E, ×160).

B dermatitidis that are thought to represent cell-wall-deficient spheroplasts (Figure 101–10) are rarely produced in blastomycotic lesions.[21,22,33] When these aberrant forms are encountered, typical budding blastomyces cells also are usually present. A definitive diagnosis can be based on the presence of typical forms.

GMS and other special stains for fungi help locate organisms, especially when fungal cells are sparse, and the special stains also help delineate their morphology. The cell walls of *B dermatitidis* are sometimes lightly colored with mucin stains such as mucicarmine, Alcian blue, and colloidal iron[21,22] (Figure 101–11). Because *B dermatitidis* cells are not encapsulated, the staining reaction is confined to the thick cell wall rather than to true capsular material. Modified Gram's stains do not reliably demonstrate the yeast forms of *B dermatitidis* in tissue.

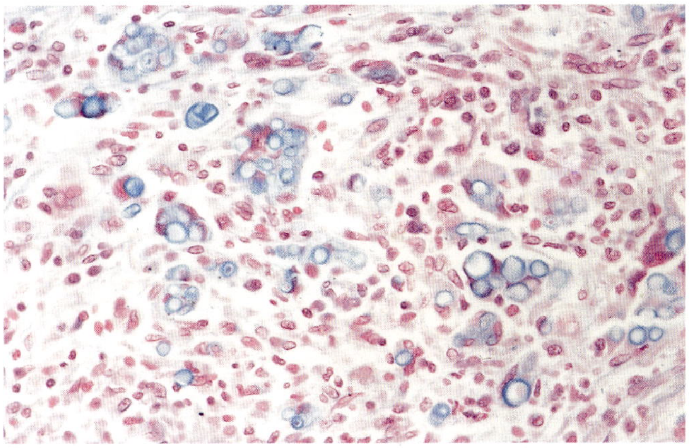

Figure 101–11. Pulmonary blastomycosis in an African. The thick walls of *B dermatitidis* cells react weakly with mucin stains. Note clustering of yeast forms within epithelioid and giant cells, and persistent broad-based budding (Alcian blue, ×100).

PATHOLOGY

The predominant inflammatory reaction in the lesions of acute blastomycosis is suppurative, with infiltration of neutrophils and abscesses.[10,22,23] Fungal cells are usually extracellular, numerous, and scattered throughout the lesions or localized to well-defined abscesses (Figure 101–12). In chronic lesions, there is a mixed suppurative and granulomatous inflammatory reaction; either component may dominate, depending on the age of the lesion and the immunologic status of the host[22,23] (Figure 101–13). Fungal cells in chronic lesions are usually sparse and sometimes distorted; examination of several GMS-stained serial sections may be necessary to detect typical organisms with diagnostic single, broad-based buds. In the lungs, classical tuberculoid granulomas composed of compact epithelioid histiocytes, giant cells, lymphocytes, and fibroblasts can be seen in interstitial or intra-alveolar locations, but caseation and calcification are uncommon.[23] Multifocal or confluent granulomas with suppurative and necrotic centers also can be in the lungs as well as in other organs. These lesions closely resemble those in chronic active tuberculosis. Fibrosis and hyalinization of granulomas occur frequently in long-standing infections, and in the lungs, may be accompanied by cavitation.[21,23] Chronic fibrosing mediastinitis is most often a complication of histoplasmosis capsulati (Chapter 109), but blastomycosis may cause superior vena caval obstruction from fibrosing mediastinitis.[34]

In rapidly progressive lesions and in profoundly immunodeficient patients, fungal cells sometimes pro-

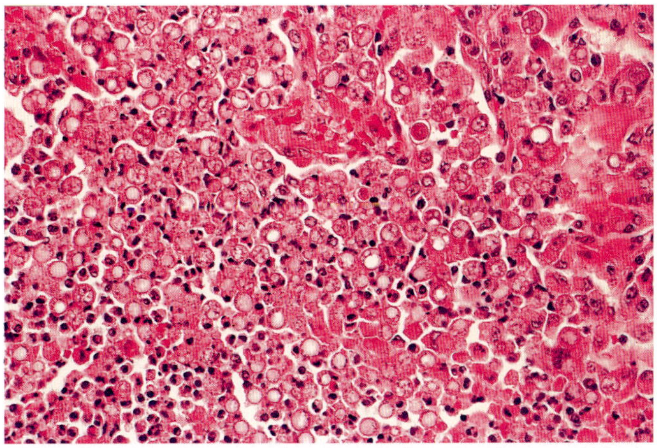

Figure 101–12. Acute pulmonary blastomycosis. Alveolar spaces contain neutrophils, macrophages, cellular debris, and numerous intra- and extracellular, spherical to oval yeast forms of *B dermatitidis* with thick walls. Many of the fungal cells have vacuolated cytoplasms (H&E, ×100).

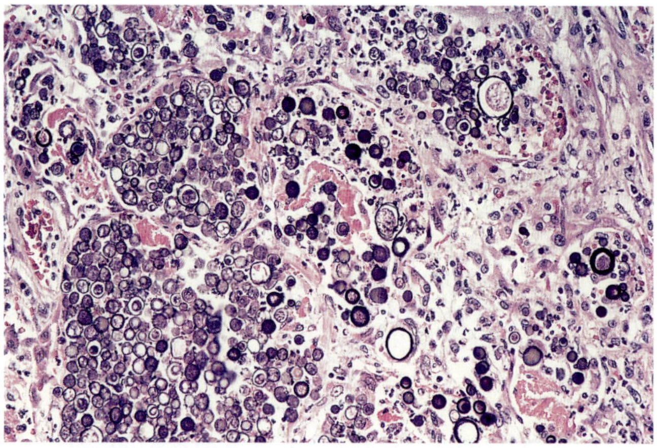

Figure 101–13. Progressive pulmonary blastomycosis. A mixed suppurative and granulomatous inflammatory reaction is accompanied by interstitial fibrosis. Numerous, pleomorphic, rapidly dividing, intra- and extracellular yeast forms are seen. Note the marked variation in size of fungal cells (GMS–H&E, ×100).

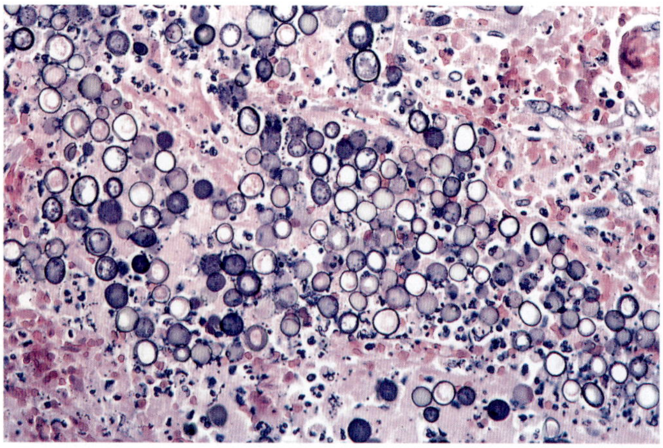

Figure 101–15. Systemic blastomycosis in an AIDS patient. Compact aggregates of *B dermatitidis* cells ("yeast lakes") efface the normal pulmonary architecture. Suppurative inflammation is minimal (GMS–H&E, ×160).

liferate in great numbers, and solid sheets or compact clusters of organisms ("yeast lakes") with minimal inflammation may be in many organs; epithelioid cell granulomas are rarely formed.[22] In the lungs, alveolar spaces are sometimes filled with and distended by myriad rapidly proliferating yeast forms of *B dermatitidis* that elicit little or no inflammatory response (Figures 101–14 and 101–15), resembling the paucireactive pattern of opportunistic cryptococcosis (Chapter 106).

In cutaneous blastomycosis, the *B dermatitidis* cells incite florid pseudoepitheliomatous hyperplasia that is usually more extensive than is seen in chromoblastomycosis, sporotrichosis, and coccidioidomycosis[21] (Figure 101–16). Intraepidermal microabscesses

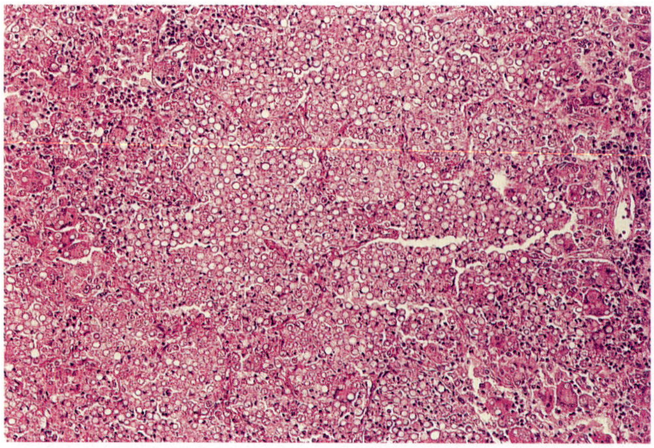

Figure 101–14. Rapidly progressive pulmonary blastomycosis in an immunocompromised patient. Myriad, rapidly dividing fungal cells that are predominantly extracellular fill and distend alveolar spaces (H&E, ×40).

result from transepidermal elimination characterized by extensive downgrowth of rete ridges and incorporation of dermal microabscesses or their draining sinuses. Fungal cells can be in microabscesses in the dermis and epidermis, within giant and epithelioid cells at the periphery of dermal microabscesses, in transepidermal elimination channels, and in the hyperkeratotic layer of the epidermis (Figure 101–17). There may be similar hyperplastic lesions in the larynx or on other mucous membranes lined by stratified squamous epithelium.[22] Although not pathognomonic, this histologic pattern suggests blastomycosis.

CONFIRMATIONAL TESTING AND DIAGNOSIS

Whenever fresh tissues are available, microbiologic culture should complement histopathologic studies. The mycelial form of *B dermatitidis* can be readily isolated from blastomycotic lesions on synthetic media at 25°C, but growth is slow and often requires 4 weeks or more. Microscopically, the mycelium consists of spherical to oval conidia, 3 to 5 μm in diameter, borne on the sides of hyphae and on the ends of simple conidiophores.[2,13] Once isolated, subculture on blood agar at 37°C converts the dimorphic fungus to the yeast phase.[13] More rapid diagnosis is possible by direct microscopic demonstration in sputum (Figure 101–18), or in autopsy and biopsy specimens, of classical yeast forms with persistent broad-based budding, multiple nuclei, and thick "double-contoured" walls. When typical yeast forms are present, a definitive histopathologic diagnosis can be made.[21,22] Diagnosis by direct examination of lesional exudates digested with 10% KOH, and of Papanicolaou

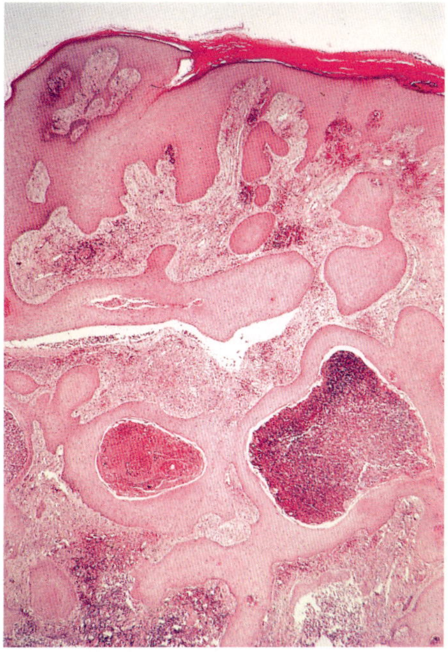

Figure 101–16. Cutaneous blastomycosis. Florid pseudoepitheliomatous hyperplasia of the epidermis is accompanied by mixed suppurative and granulomatous inflammation in the dermis (H&E, ×20).

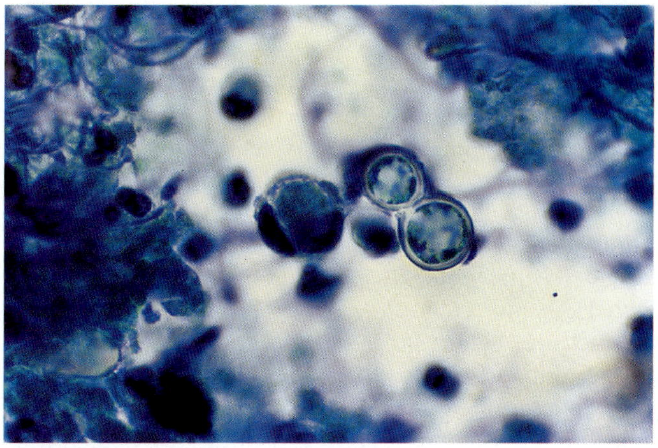

Figure 101–18. Antemortem sputum from a patient with chronic progressive pulmonary blastomycosis (same case as in Figure 101–2). The specimen contained numerous classical yeast forms with broad-based buds, multiple nuclei, and thick "double-contoured" walls (Diff-Quik stain, ×1000). *(Contributed by Ernest E. Lack, MD.)*

and GMS stained smears of respiratory secretions is also possible.[35] When there are sparse or atypical fungal cells, direct immunofluorescence using a specific conjugate directed against the cell wall polysaccharide antigens of *B dermatitidis* is useful for rapid, definitive identification of the fungus in smears and formalin-fixed, deparaffinized tissue sections[36] (Figure 101–19). Serologic tests (enzyme-linked immunosorbent assay, immunodiffusion, Western blot) that use a purified *B dermatitidis* "A" antigen are rapid, sensitive, and provide presumptive evidence of infection.[37] They are especially useful for early diagnosis and monitoring of the course of blastomycosis.

MOLECULAR DIAGNOSIS

Rapid diagnosis of blastomycosis during early culture is possible using DNA-based assays for *B dermatitidis*.[35] At present, however, molecular methods do not contribute to the pathologic diagnosis of blastomycosis.

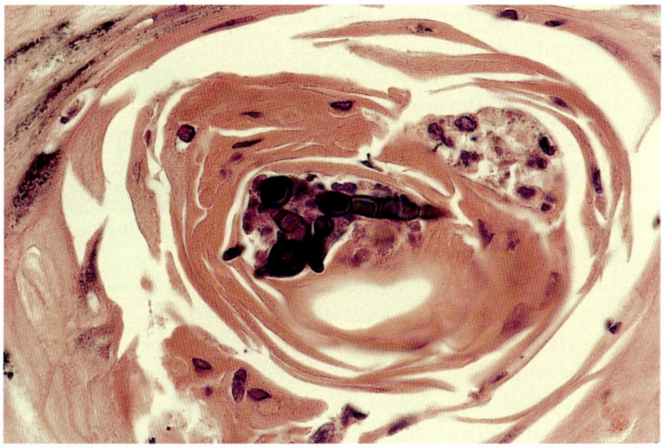

Figure 101–17. Cutaneous blastomycosis. Typical yeast forms and a short, frequently septate hypha of *B dermatitidis* are located within a transepithelial elimination channel (GMS–H&E, ×160).

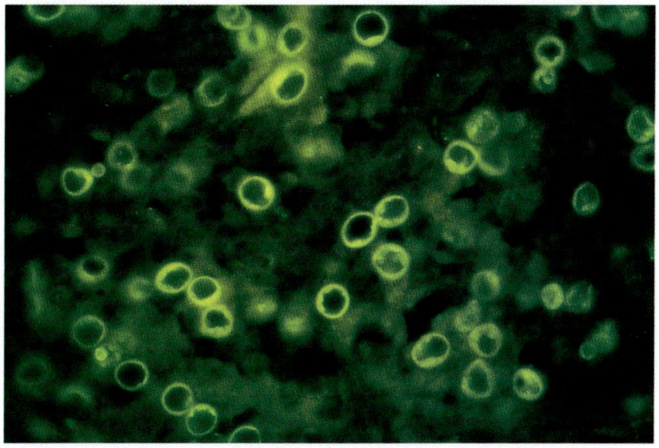

Figure 101–19. Direct immunofluorescence of *B dermatitidis* cells in formalin-fixed, deparaffinized lung section. The walls of single and budding yeast forms are brightly decorated with a conjugate specific for this fungus (×160).

DIFFERENTIAL DIAGNOSIS

Because the yeast forms of *B dermatitidis* and *H capsulatum* var *duboisii* (Chapter 110) both have thick walls and are similar in size and shape, they can be mistaken for each other in tissue sections.[21] The latter, however, usually bud by a narrower base with typical "double-cell" forms, whereas the diagnostic budding form of *B dermatitidis* is broad based. When stained with H&E, the cells of *H capsulatum* var *duboisii* are uninucleate, whereas *B dermatitidis* cells each contain multiple hematoxylinophilic nuclei. When these differentiating features are equivocal, a presumptive morphologic diagnosis can be confirmed by microbiologic culture or immunofluorescence of fungal elements in formalin-fixed, paraffin-embedded tissue sections[36] (Figure 101–19).

TREATMENT

Amphotericin B is the drug of choice for severe, life-threatening blastomycosis; 2-hydroxystilbamidine, either alone or in combination with amphotericin B, also has been successfully used.[38,39] The azole antifungal agents ketoconazole and itraconazole may be effective in patients who are not seriously ill, and these antifungals can be used when toxicity precludes the use of amphotericin B.[40,41] Fluconazole given for at least 6 months is a moderately effective treatment for nonmeningeal, non-life-threatening blastomycosis.[42] Surgical excision of localized lesions may be a valuable adjunct to antifungal therapy.

REFERENCES

1. Vanek J, Schwarz J, Haken S. North American blastomycosis. *Am J Clin Pathol.* 1970;54:384–400.
2. Tenenbaum MJ, Greenspan J, Kerkering TM. Blastomycosis. *Crit Rev Microbiol.* 1982;9:139–163.
3. Bradsher RW. Blastomycosis. *Clin Infect Dis.* 1992;14 (suppl 1):S82–S90.
4. Schwarz J. Epidemiology and epidemics of blastomycosis. *Mykosen.* 1983;16:7–14.
5. Al-Doory Y. Introduction. In: Al-Doory Y, DiSalvo AF, eds. *Blastomycosis.* New York: Plenum; 1992:1–7.
6. Emerson PA, Higgins E, Branfoot A. North American blastomycosis in Africans. *Br J Dis Chest.* 1984;78:286–291.
7. Baily GG, Robertson VJ, Neill P, Garrido P, Levy LF. Blastomycosis in Africa: clinical features, diagnosis, and treatment. *Rev Infect Dis.* 1991;13:1005–1008.
8. Sarosi GA, Davies SF. Blastomycosis. *Am Rev Respir Dis.* 1979;120:911–938.
9. Busey JF, ed. Blastomycosis: I. A review of 198 collected cases in Veterans Administration hospitals. *Am Rev Respir Dis.* 1964;89:659–672.
10. Schwarz J, Salfelder K. Blastomycosis: a review of 152 cases. In: Grundmann E, Kirsten WH, eds. *Current Topics in Pathology.* Berlin: Springer-Verlag; 1977;65:165–200.
11. Bradsher RW. A clinician's view of blastomycosis. *Curr Top Med Mycol.* 1993;5:181–200.
12. Larson DM, Eckman MR, Alber RL, et al. Primary cutaneous (inoculation) blastomycosis: an occupational hazard to pathologists. *Am J Clin Pathol.* 1983;79:253–255.
13. Rippon JW. *Medical Mycology. The Pathogenic Fungi and the Pathogenic Actinomycetes.* 3rd ed. Philadelphia: WB Saunders; 1988:474.
14. Baum GL, Lerner PI. Primary pulmonary blastomycosis: a laboratory acquired infection. *Ann Intern Med.* 1970; 73:263–265.
15. Meyer KC, McManus EJ, Maki DG. Overwhelming pulmonary blastomycosis associated with the adult respiratory distress syndrome. *N Engl J Med.* 1993;329:1231–1236.
16. Rippon JW, Zvetina JR, Reyes C. Case report: miliary blastomycosis with cerebral involvement. *Mycopathologia.* 1977;60:121–125.
17. Inoshita T, Youngberg GA, Boelen LJ, Langston J. Blastomycosis presenting with prostatic involvement: report of 2 cases and review of the literature. *J Urol.* 1983;130: 160–162.
18. Steel RW, Abernathy RS. Systemic blastomycosis in children. *Pediatr Infect Dis.* 1983;2:304–307.
19. Payne J, Koopmann CF Jr. Laryngeal carcinoma—or is it laryngeal blastomycosis? *Laryngoscope.* 1984;94:608–611.
20. Rader PA, Neel HB III. Blastomycosis in otolaryngology: review of a large series. *Laryngoscope.* 1993;103:53–58.
21. Chandler FW, Watts JC. *Pathologic Diagnosis of Fungal Infections.* Chicago: ASCP Press; 1987:149–160.
22. Chandler FW, Watts JC. Pathologic features of blastomycosis. In: Al-Doory Y, DiSalvo AF, eds. *Blastomycosis.* New York: Plenum; 1992:189–220.
23. Chandler FW, Watts JC. Fungal infections. In: Dail DH, Hammar SP, eds. *Pulmonary Pathology.* 2nd ed. New York: Springer-Verlag; 1994:364–368.
24. Recht LD, Davies SF, Eckman MR, et al. Blastomycosis in immunosuppressed patients. *Am Rev Respir Dis.* 1982; 125:359–362.
25. Pappas PG, Threlkeld MG, Bedsole GD, et al. Blastomycosis in immunocompromised patients. *Medicine (Baltimore).* 1993;72:311–325.
26. Harding CV. Blastomycosis and opportunistic infections in patients with acquired immunodeficiency syndrome. An autopsy study. *Arch Pathol Lab Med.* 1991;115:1133–1136.
27. Pappas PG, Pottage JC, Powderly WG, et al. Blastomycosis in patients with the acquired immunodeficiency syndrome. *Ann Intern Med.* 1992;116:847–853.
28. Laskey WL, Sarosi GA. Endogenous reactivation in blastomycosis. *Ann Intern Med.* 1978;88:50–52.
29. Serody JS, Mill MR, Detterbeck FC, Harris DT, Cohen MS. Blastomycosis in transplant recipients: report of a case and review. *Clin Infect Dis.* 1993;16:54–58.
30. Butka BJ, Bennett SR, Johnson AC. Disseminated inoculation blastomycosis in a renal transplant recipient. *Am Rev Respir Dis.* 1984;130;1180–1183.
31. Tuttle JG, Lichtwardt HE, Altshuler CH. Systemic North American blastomycosis. Report of a case with small

forms of blastomycetes. *Am J Clin Pathol.* 1953;23: 890–897.

32. Watts JC, Chandler FW, Mihalov ML, Kammeyer PL, Armin AR. Giant forms of *Blastomyces dermatitidis* in the pulmonary lesions of blastomycosis. Potential confusion with *Coccidioides immitis*. *Am J Clin Pathol.* 1990;93:119–122.
33. Atkinson JB, McCurley TL. Pulmonary blastomycosis: filamentous forms in an immunocompromised patient with fulminating respiratory failure. *Hum Pathol.* 1983;14: 186–188.
34. Lagerstrom CF, Mitchell HG, Graham BS, Hammon JW Jr. Chronic fibrosing mediastinitis and superior vena caval obstruction from blastomycosis. *Ann Thorac Surg.* 1992; 54:764–765.
35. Goodman NL. Diagnosis of blastomycosis. In: Al-Doory Y, DiSalvo AF, eds. *Blastomycosis.* New York: Plenum; 1992:105–121.
36. Chandler FW, Kaplan W, Ajello L. *Color Atlas and Text of the Histopathology of Mycotic Diseases.* Chicago: Year Book Medical Publishers; 1980:23–25.
37. Kaufman L. Immunodiagnosis of blastomycosis. In: Al-Doory Y, DiSalvo AF, eds. *Blastomycosis.* New York: Plenum; 1992:123–132.
38. Lockwood WR, Allison F, Blair BE, et al. The treatment of North American blastomycosis: ten years' experience. *Am Rev Respir Dis.* 1969;100:314–320.
39. Bradsher RW. Prognosis and therapy of blastomycosis. In: Al-Doory Y, DiSalvo AF, eds. *Blastomycosis.* New York: Plenum; 1992:237–247.
40. National Institute of Allergy and Infectious Diseases Mycoses Study Group. Treatment of blastomycosis and histoplasmosis with ketoconazole: Results of prospective randomized clinical trials. *Ann Intern Med.* 1985;103: 861–872.
41. Dismukes WE, Bradsher RW, Cloud GC, et al. Itraconazole therapy for blastomycosis and histoplasmosis. NIAID Mycoses Study Group. *Am J Med.* 1992;93:489–497.
42. Pappas PG, Bradsher RW, Chapman SW, et al. Treatment of blastomycosis with fluconazole: a pilot study. The National Institute of Allergy and Infectious Diseases Mycoses Study Group. *Clin Infect Dis.* 1995:20:267–271.

Chapter 102

Candidiasis

Mario A. Luna

And thou shalt have great sickness by disease of thy bowels, until thy bowels fall out by reason of the sickness day by day.

2 Chronicles 21:15

DEFINITION

Candidiasis is an infection caused by species of fungi of the genus *Candida*. Many *Candida* sp are common inhabitants of the human respiratory, gastrointestinal, and genitourinary tracts. In normal hosts, these organisms usually do not invade. In immunodeficient patients, however, they are capable of invading and causing severe disease. Although different forms of candidiasis vary in severity, most are localized, superficial diseases, limited to a particular mucocutaneous site. During the last three decades, however, these organisms have assumed increasing prominence as major pathogens. According to data from the National Nosocomial Infections Surveillance System, *Candida* sp are the fifth most common primary bloodstream organisms and the seventh most common cause of nosocomial infections.[1]

GEOGRAPHIC DISTRIBUTION

Candida organisms are readily detectable as harmless commensals in the flora of the mouth, pharynx, vagina, and skin. Patients with candidiasis have been reported from all parts of the world, but because *Candida* sp are ubiquitous and so frequent in healthy people in such a variety of clinical forms, it is impossible to obtain accurate data on the geographic distribution of the disease.

EPIDEMIOLOGY AND PATHOGENESIS

Candida sp are confined to human and animal reservoirs, although they are frequently recovered from soil, food, hospital personnel, and occasionally from the air.[2] The gastrointestinal tract is believed to be the major colonizing habitat of *Candida* sp. The true prevalence of yeasts in the gastrointestinal tract of humans is unclear because of problems involved in obtaining reliable samples. Cohen et al,[3] using a special double lumen tube placed under fluoroscopic guidance, cultured *Candida* sp from the jejunum of 55% of adults. Furthermore, *Candida* sp were cultured with increased frequency as samples were obtained from more distal sites in the gastrointestinal tract.

The female genital tract and the urine of patients with indwelling catheters also are colonized frequently with *Candida* sp, but they rarely colonize normal skin unless there are breaks or damage that promote colonization. Consequently, the potential for endogenous infection clearly exists if *Candida* sp are present in adequate numbers and host factors are conducive.

Systems for typing *C albicans* and other *Candida* sp[4–7] include the DNA restriction-fragment analysis of Stevens et al,[5] the biotyping system of Odds and Abbott,[6] and the killer system of Polonelli et al.[7] Epidemiologic studies have been performed using these techniques in a wide range of situations to further delineate the epidemiology[8,9] and the nosocomial transmission of *Candida* sp.[10,11]

Mechanical barriers, inflammatory cells, humoral immunity, and cell-mediated immunity restrict *Candida* sp to superficial, nonsterile sites.[12] In turn, the resident bacterial flora normally limit the number of fungal organisms. Bacteria block candidal attachment to epithelial cells, compete with the fungi for nutrients, and prevent conversion of the fungus to its tissue-invasive forms. When any one of these defenses is deficient, candidal infections can occur. Antibiotic therapy most commonly precipitates candidiasis, because antibiotics suppress competing bacterial flora. Under conditions of unopposed growth, the yeast converts to its invasive form (hyphae or pseudohyphae), invades superficially, and incites an inflammatory or immunologic response.

Severe candidal infections have increased in recent years, partly because there are now more patients with neutropenia and other immunodeficiencies. Other aspects of contemporary medical care also predispose to candidiasis, including the more frequent use of intravascular catheters and monitoring devices, endotracheal tubes, and urinary catheters.[13] Each of these provides a route to a normally sterile site. Contamination of infusion fluid may lead to intravascular candidiasis.[14] Candidemia may follow peritoneal dialysis or may develop after surgery for a ruptured viscus. Intravenous drug users also develop deep candidal infections when they inoculate fungi into their bloodstreams.

TAXONOMY OF *CANDIDA* SP

Candida sp are anamorphic (asexual/imperfect) yeasts classified in the Form-Division Fungi Imperfecti, Form-Class Blastomycetes. Some *Candida* species mate, producing a teleomorphic (sexual/perfect) form. All species of *Candida* are identified primarily by their ability to assimilate and/or ferment various substrates, most notably carbohydrates.[15]

More than 81 species of *Candida* are known. Only a small number are pathogenic for mankind. *Candida albicans* is the most frequently isolated species and accounts for up to 75% of species from sites of infection.[16,17] *Candida tropicalis, C pseudotropicalis, C parapsilosis, C krusei, C lusitaniae, C stellatoidea*, and *C guilliermondii* are other pathogenic species. *Candida tropicalis* is the most frequently isolated fungal pathogen from patients with hematologic malignancies.[16,18]

Candida krusei is an emerging agent of opportunistic disease, inciting serious infections in neutropenic patients, as well as diarrhea in infants. When invasive, the organism is most often isolated from cases of septicemia and endophthalmitis.[19] Recently, awareness of candidiasis caused by *C krusei* has been amplified as a result of its apparent innate resistance to fluconazole.[20]

CLINICAL FEATURES

The clinical features of candidiasis are so varied, depending on the location of the infection, that they are discussed separately under the anatomic sites involved.[21–27]

MORPHOLOGIC FEATURES OF *CANDIDA* ORGANISMS

By light microscopy, in sections stained with hematoxylin and eosin (H&E), the organisms are pale blue or lilac colored yeast cells intermingled with pseudohyphae and, occasionally, true hyphae. The yeastlike forms or blastoconidia are oval and measure 3 to 5 μm in diameter (Figure 102–1). The pseudohyphae are 3 to 5 μm wide and have periodic constrictions at points where budding yeast cells are joined end to end. With appropriate special stains such as periodic acid–Schiff (PAS) and Gomori's methenamine-silver (GMS) stain, oval blastoconidia with thin walls are clearly visible (Figure 102–1). *Candida* sp stain bright magenta with the PAS technique. The GMS stain has been the most consistent of the silver stains for fungi and should be used as the single screening stain for fungal pathogens. The GMS procedure deposits silver along the thin walls of *Candida* cells.

By electron microscopy the appearance of the candidal cell wall depends on the fixative.[28] The cell walls and cytoplasmic contents of both blastoconidia and pseudohyphae are similar in appearance. Most investigators have described at least three layers in the *Candida* cell wall: 1) an outer floccular electron-dense coat of variable thickness (50 to 150 nm), 2) a middle, thin, electron-dense band (13 to 16 nm), and 3) an inner electron-lucent zone (60 to 70 nm) (Figure 102–2). Internal to these structures is a plasma membrane formed by a trilaminar unit membrane of about 12 nm in total thickness. This membrane has frequent folds forming structures called lomasomes.[29] The cytoplasmic

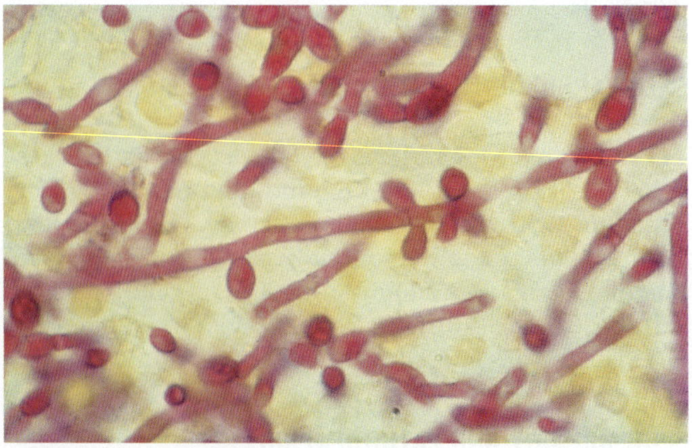

Figure 102–1. Hyphae, pseudohyphae, and yeastlike forms in disseminated candidiasis (Gridley fungus stain, ×400).

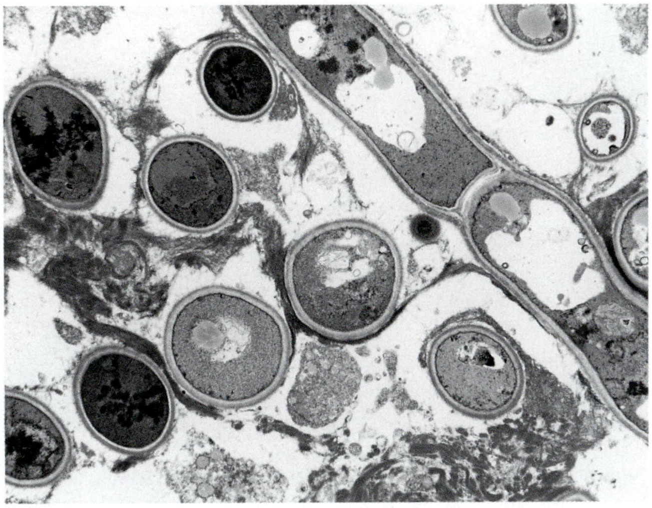

Figure 102–2. Candidal organisms, electron microscopic appearance. Note septation in a pseudohypha (×8500).

contents consist primarily of numerous electron-dense dots. Some cells exhibit numerous cristate mitochondria. A single round-to-oval nucleus is present. Only slight differences in morphologic characteristics have been noted between the different *Candida* sp.[28]

PATHOLOGY

Pathologic studies have demonstrated three varieties of human candidiasis: 1) superficial, 2) locally invasive, and 3) deeply invasive or disseminated. Each of these clinicopathologic forms of candidiasis has a characteristic gross appearance.

Superficial candidiasis, the most common form, is characterized by infections limited to lining surfaces such as the skin, oropharynx (Figure 102–3), gastrointestinal tract (Figure 102–4), and upper and lower respiratory tracts. In this form, there is no vascular invasion or deep organ involvement. In superficial candidiasis, the surface of the lesion has a velvety appearance, and the adjacent mucous membrane is dark red and swollen. Ulcerative or necrotic lesions indicate deeper tissue invasion.

Locally invasive candidiasis afflicts patients with immunodeficiencies and causes a variety of severe localized forms of candidiasis including pneumonia, cystitis, esophagitis, and pyelonephritis. The most frequently invasive localized lesions are ulcerations of the intestinal (Figure 102–5), respiratory, and genitourinary tracts. Typically, the ulcers have sharp margins, shaggy or granular bases, with an ochre exudate that may cover the entire ulcer base or be limited to its periphery (Figure 102–6).

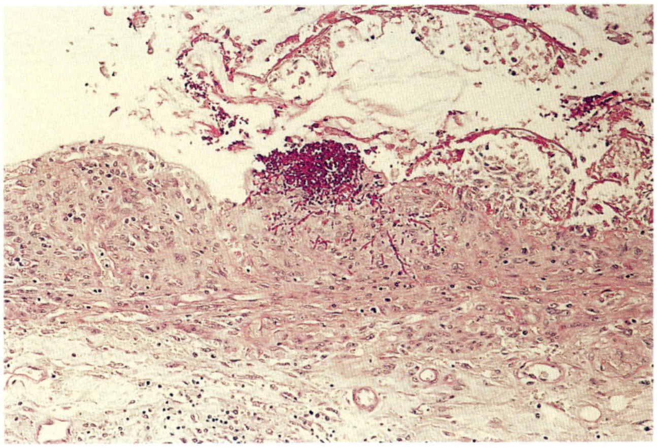

Figure 102–3. Candidal organisms are readily identified in oral mucosa with routine H&E staining, but their appearance is more striking when special stains are used (PAS, ×100).

Disseminated candidiasis, in its most severe form, is deep or disseminated and characterized by intraparenchymal lesions usually in heart, kidney (Figures 102–7 through 102–9), liver, spleen, lungs, and brain, but any organ may be involved. Disseminated candidiasis is an invasive infection involving the parenchyma of two or more organs, excluding the mucosa of the gastrointestinal, respiratory, or genitourinary tracts.[30,31]

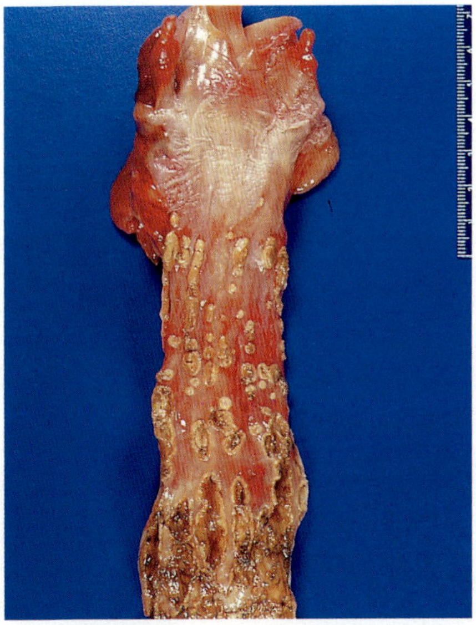

Figure 102–4. Lower pharynx and esophagus of a patient with candidal esophagitis. There are multiple candidal ulcers, which are punctate to linear and in the lower esophagus are confluent. Borders of the ulcers are raised, tan-yellow and friable. *(Contributed by Ernest E. Lack, MD.)*

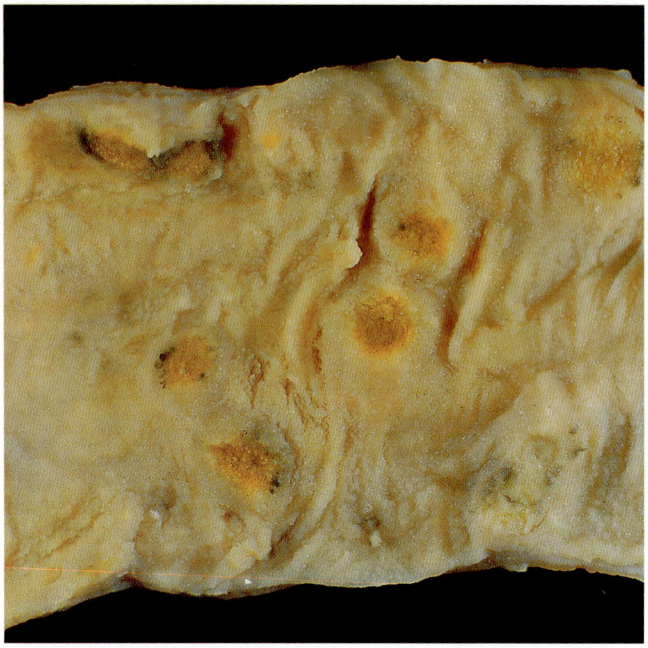

Figure 102–5. Multiple candidal ulcers of colon. The margins of the ulcers are raised and the base contains a necrotic slough with candidal organisms. *(Contributed by Daniel H. Connor, MD.)*

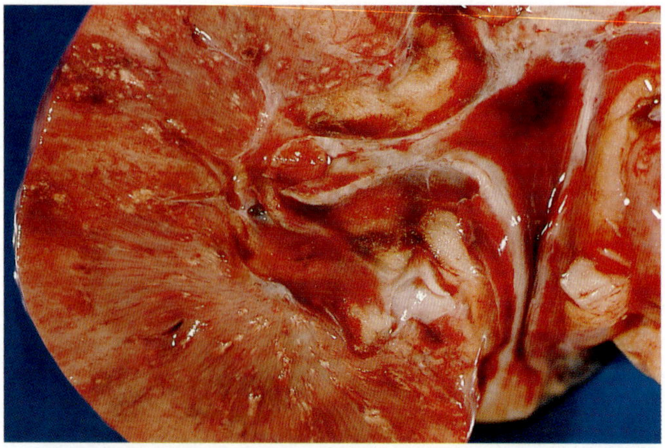

Figure 102–7. Kidney with lesions of disseminated candidiasis. The lesions are white and have a red margin. A few of the lesions are small and punctate but most are linear with pointed ends, which are shaped as the *Candida* organisms proliferate along the tissue planes of the tubules. *(Contributed by G. Frederick Worsham, MD.)*

Disseminated candidiasis is characterized by the formation of multiple parenchymal abscesses. On gross inspection, they resemble lesions of miliary tuberculosis (Figure 102–10) or of diffuse metastatic carcinoma. The most common sites at autopsy are gastrointestinal tract, followed by lung and kidney. The median number of organs involved is four, the most common combination being the gastrointestinal tract, liver, kidney, and lung.[30,32]

The pathology of disseminated candidiasis in neutropenic patients who have acute leukemia or in those receiving organ transplants is characteristic. Involvement of gastrointestinal tract is invariably present in leukemic patients and is probably the source of infection in most of them.[33] The primary source of infection in patients with adequate neutrophils who develop disseminated candidiasis may be an infected intravenous catheter or candidal contamination of an infusion fluid, especially hyperalimentation fluid.[14] Another potential route of bloodstream infection in these patients is peritoneal cavity following prolonged abdominal surgery.

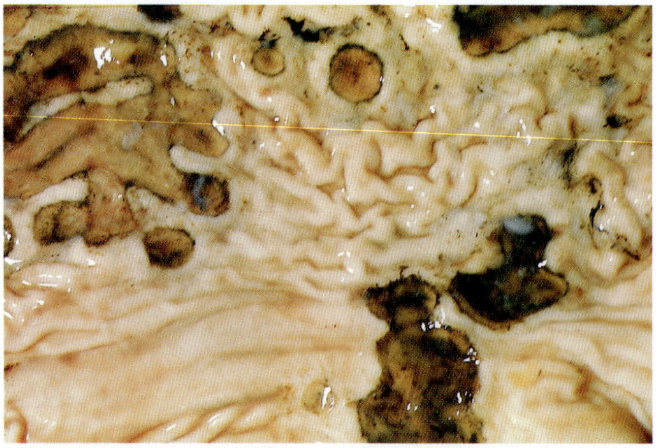

Figure 102–6. Gastric candidiasis. There are circumscribed to confluent ulcers with slightly raised borders involving the mucosa of the stomach. *(Contributed by G. Frederick Worsham, MD.)*

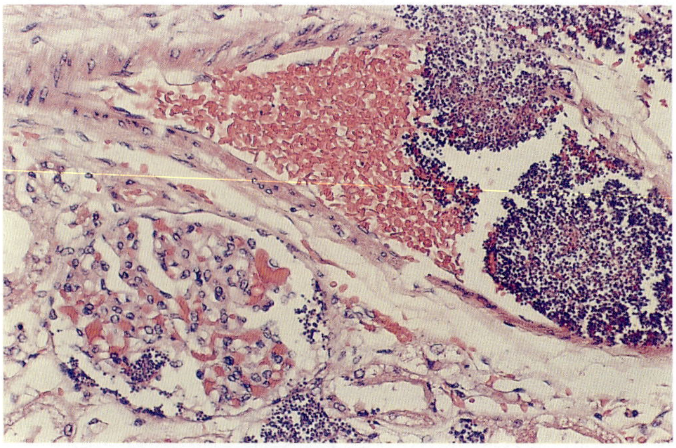

Figure 102–8. Disseminated candidiasis of kidney. Candidal blastoconidia have colonized a renal vein. The blastoconidia are migrating freely through the vessel wall and renal tissues. Some have penetrated the capsule of the glomerulus (hematoxylin-eosin, ×150).

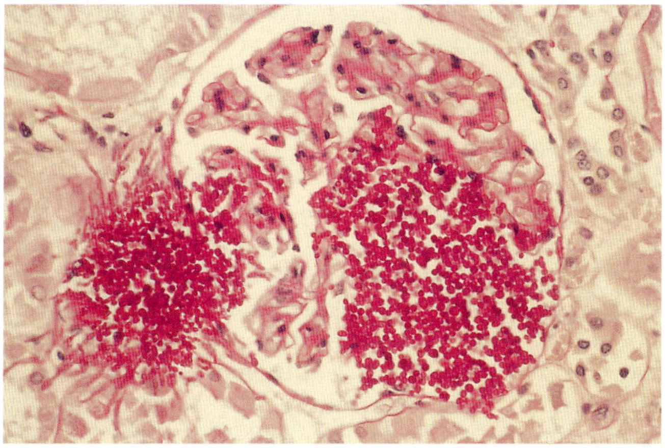

Figure 102–9. Disseminated candidiasis. Many candidal blastoconidia have invaded Bowman's space (PAS, ×300).

Patients with adequate neutrophil counts who develop disseminated candidiasis after abdominal surgery, or from intravenous catheter-induced phlebitis, tend to have myocardial, pulmonary, renal, ocular, and cerebral involvement. Lesions of liver, spleen, and skin are unusual in these patients. The gastrointestinal tract is the most common source of systemic candidiasis in patients with hematologic malignancies and neutropenia; as a result, they have a high incidence of hepatic and splenic involvement. Ocular candidiasis is extremely unusual.[30,32] The kidneys are involved with the same frequency in patients with and without neutropenia.[30]

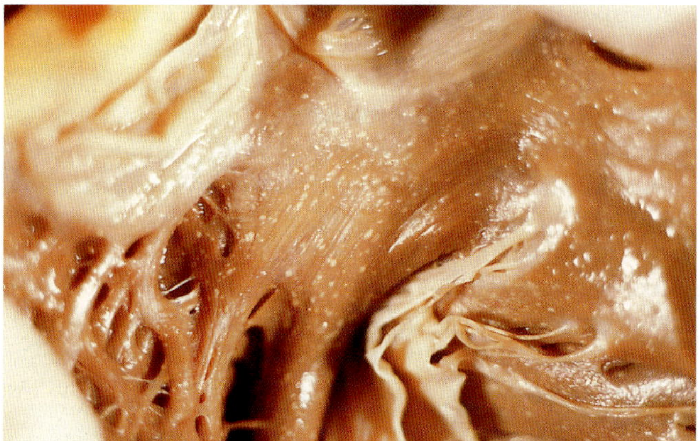

Figure 102–10. Heart from a 66-year-old man who had lymphoma and secondary acute myelogenous leukemia with severe neutropenia and disseminated candidiasis. Terminally he had sepsis, shock, and cardiac arrest. At autopsy small white nodules were throughout the heart. Microscopically these were foci of *Candida* sp, in the heart as well as in all organs studied microscopically including lung, kidney, spleen, brain, liver, lymph node, marrow, gall bladder, thyroid, adrenal, pancreas, and large and small intestine. *(Contributed by Mary A. Furlong, MD.)*

Microscopic Pathology

The usual response to *Candida* sp is an acute inflammatory reaction, with neutrophils predominating and causing microabscesses. In sections stained with H&E, pale blue yeastlike bodies with pseudohyphae are between pus cells. With appropriate special stains such as PAS and GMS, oval blastoconidia with thin walls are clearly visible and measure 3 to 6 μm (Figure 102–1). Pseudohyphae are usually present. On a surface, the organisms are abundant as true hyphae; usually interposed between them are clusters of oval blastoconidia.

Microscopic examination of the white patches of superficial candidiasis of mucous membranes reveals that they consist of a mass of yeastlike cells, pseudohyphae, necrotic debris, and inflammatory cells. The latter are composed largely of neutrophils. The surface epithelium is totally or partially destroyed, and hyphae may extend into the underlying tissue. The histologic changes are entirely nonspecific, except for the identification of the fungus.

In the localized form of invasive candidiasis, there is mural invasion beneath the superficial membranes, leading to submucosal growth of fungi and necrosis of overlying mucosa. Microscopically, a pseudomembrane consisting of a mat of pseudohyphae embedded in fibrin and necrotic debris covers the base of the ulcer. Infection may extend into the deeper layers with subsequent angioinvasion. Neutropenic patients mount no cellular response, but there is coagulative necrosis usually associated with hemorrhage.

Histologically, the lesions in disseminated candidiasis are small abscesses composed of neutrophils and mononuclear cells such as lymphocytes, plasma cells, and macrophages. In neutropenic patients, the inflammatory reaction is replaced by coagulative necrosis. Because dissemination is hematogenous, localized vascular lesions and vasculitis may be in any organ, although they are most often inconspicuous. Rarely, the tissue response is granulomatous with giant cells (Figure 102–11). Blastoconidia and sometimes fragments of hyphae are within the giant cells. A granulomatous reaction to *Candida* sp is commonly found in patients with chronic systemic candidiasis and in those with treated "*Candida* granuloma," the most severe form of chronic mucocutaneous candidiasis.[34,35]

Pathologic Features by Organ Systems

Oropharynx and Esophagus

Oropharyngeal and esophageal candidiasis are common in patients with cell-mediated dysfunction, such as primary immune deficiency diseases of infants, chronic

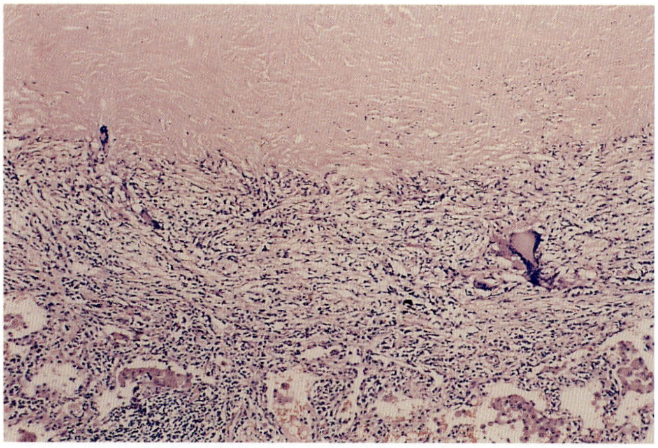

Figure 102–11. Necrotizing granuloma caused by *Candida* sp in a patient with treated chronic hepatosplenic candidiasis. Note the typical caseating granuloma with Langhans' giant cells (hematoxylin-eosin, ×60).

mucocutaneous candidiasis, diabetes, and acquired immunodeficiency syndrome.[36,37] Symptoms most frequently associated with esophageal candidiasis include dysphagia, retrosternal pain, and odynophagia.[38] Histologically, the esophageal lesions are superficial erosions and focal ulcerations with sharp margins. The ulcers have granulation tissue and a lymphocytic–plasmacytic infiltrate at the base. *Candida* organisms also can secondarily involve ulcerations caused by Herpes simplex virus and other microorganisms.

Lower Gastrointestinal Tract

Certain conditions promote candidiasis of the gastrointestinal tract. These include neoplasms; diabetes; localized lesions of the gastrointestinal tract; and therapy with antibiotics, steroids, cancer chemotherapeutic agents, and antacids. These conditions cause anatomic, functional, or microbial changes. Infection of the lower gastrointestinal tract commonly complicates malignant disease. In one autopsy study of 2517 cancer patients, 109 had gastrointestinal candidiasis.[33] Esophagus was the most common site followed by stomach (23%), bowel (7%), and multiple sites in 28%. The overall frequency of lower gastrointestinal infections was 0.6% in patients with solid tumors, but it was 30% in patients with leukemia and lymphoma.

The most common gross lesion of candidiasis is mucosal ulceration, with or without a pseudomembrane (Figure 102–4). There may be exophytic granulation tissue, but this is unusual. Microscopically, the pseudomembrane is composed of a mixture of yeasts and pseudohyphae embedded in necrotic debris and fibrin. In deeply invasive lesions, pseudohyphae extend into the deepest portion of the muscle layer, but pseudohyphae seldom, if ever, extend beyond the serosa. Peritonitis from perforation of bowel rarely complicates candidal ulceration.[33]

Liver and Spleen

Hepatic and splenic candidiases are more common in leukemic patients with gastrointestinal candidal lesions than in patients with solid tumors.[32] Hepatic and splenic lesions frequently occur together and are identical. Grossly, they resemble metastatic carcinoma. The nodules are large and round with necrotic centers, and they are scattered throughout the parenchyma in a miliary fashion. Characteristically, the largest candidal lesions are more often in liver and spleen than in other organs. They are best imaged with computed tomography or sonography, allowing computed tomography-guided fine-needle aspiration biopsy to be performed for diagnosis.[34]

Depending on the status of host defenses and/or the rate of recovery of immune competence, hepatic candidiasis may have two histologic patterns: microabscesses and granulomas. The latter are common in patients with treated chronic hepatosplenic candidiasis (Figure 102–11), whereas microabscesses complicate the acute phase of infection.[34]

Chronic disseminated candidiasis, also known as hepatosplenic candidiasis, is a form of candidal infection that has been recognized for less than two decades. It occurs predominantly in patients with leukemia, although a few patients have had other hematologic malignancies and aplastic anemia. The common denominator in all of these patients is prolonged severe neutropenia. The frequency of this infection has increased substantially during the past decade.[39]

Candidal Abscess and Hypersplenism

Candidal abscesses of the spleen are a manifestation of disseminated infection and are almost always associated with liver involvement. Only a few cases have been reported in which splenic involvement represented the major manifestation of candidal infection.[40] Hypersplenism secondary to disseminated candidiasis was first recognized in a patient who achieved a complete remission of acute leukemia after chemotherapy but remained pancytopenic.[25]

Lung

The lung is commonly involved in disseminated candidiasis. In an autopsy study, Myerowitz et al[32] reported that the lung was involved in 81% of patients with acute leukemia and in 48% of other patients. In another study of disseminated candidiasis, Maksymiuk et al[30] found lung infection in 50% of patients with fungemia, and in 95% of patients without fungemia. Among 16 patients with confirmed pulmonary mycoses after renal allografts, 2 had candidiasis.[41]

Pulmonary invasion by *Candida* sp may result from seeding of the lung during hematogenous spread, or it may follow aspiration from the upper respiratory tract. Endobronchial dissemination of pulmonary candidiasis is characterized by very small, asymmetric, patchy lesions of predominantly the lower lobes. Microscopically, the fungi are endobronchial; vascular invasion is absent, and an upper respiratory tract candidal lesion (ie, laryngeal ulceration) is present.

In hematogenous candidiasis there are round, nodular, well-circumscribed lesions with a necrotic center and a hemorrhagic rim. The lesions are bilateral and miliary and involve parenchyma and pleura. Microscopically, the most specific finding is the intravascular distribution of pseudohyphae and yeast forms. Evidence of intravascular invasion, however, may not be present in all cases of hematogenous candidiasis.[31]

Primary candidal pneumonia is an uncommon infection. Unequivocal evidence of primary candidal pneumonia has been reported in only 55 cases.[24] At two large cancer centers, the frequency of this infection at autopsy was 0.2% and 0.4%.[24,42]

Heart

Candidal abscesses are seldom seen grossly. The lesions are miliary, and may involve myocardium of both ventricles and septum, as well as the subendocardium and subepicardium (Figure 102–10). Myocardial microabscesses with yeasts and pseudohyphae are the most common manifestations of cardiac infection in disseminated candidiasis.[43] Endocarditis and pericarditis are much less common. Because of the small size of the lesions, the heart compromised by candidiasis may manifest subtle alterations in function, and most cases of *Candida* myocarditis are clinically undetectable.[43–45]

Candidal endocarditis is a threat to patients following cardiac surgery, particularly when prosthetic valves have been inserted, and is also encountered in drug addicts and in patients with long-term venous catheters.[44,45] The valvular vegetations tend to be bulkier than those caused by bacteria (Figure 102–12). In any of these circumstances, the fungus may evoke little or no inflammatory reaction or may induce a suppurative response. Hyphal and yeast forms of *Candida* sp are in the vegetations. The organisms are usually located in the superficial portion of the vegetations; in other vegetations, the fungi are in the interior as well as on the surface. Arterial emboli from candidal endocarditis are generally larger than those from bacterial infections and, consequently, larger vessels are involved with subsequent infarctions often in spleen, kidneys, brain, and lower limbs.[45]

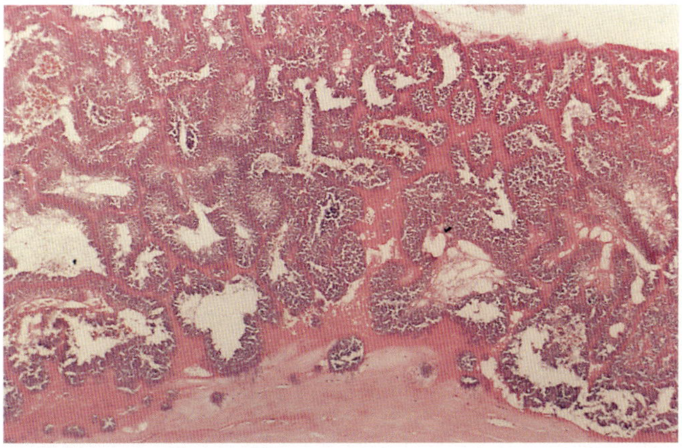

Figure 102–12. Candidal endocarditis. There are masses of *Candida* organisms on the endocardium of a heart valve (hematoxylin-eosin, ×120).

Central Nervous System

Cerebral involvement by *Candida* sp usually is not recognized until autopsy[46,47] because the patient's severe underlying primary disease masks the cerebral candidiasis. Furthermore the lesions tend to be small and focal. Grossly, the lesions are scattered randomly throughout the cerebral hemispheres, the basal ganglia, and the cerebellum, and typically are most numerous near the middle cerebral artery. The lesions include intraparenchymal abscesses and small vessel thromboses formed by pseudohyphae. Microinfarcts surrounding areas of vasculitis are the rule. The inflammatory reaction depends on the immunologic status of the patient.

Urinary Tract

Candidiasis often involves the lower urinary tract, especially in catheterized patients treated with antibiotics. In the noninvasive form of mucosal candidiasis, the urinary bladder, ureters, or renal pelves may be reddened, edematous, and covered with a velvety pseudomembrane. This is conspicuous in urinary tract obstruction or in ascending infection.

Candidal pyelonephritis, caused by obstruction or ascending infection, grossly is indistinguishable from acute bacterial pyelonephritis. The renal medullae are more frequently involved than cortex. Lesions are small, white, multiple, and asymmetric. Pyelitis, hydronephrosis, hydroureter, and cystitis are often present. Microscopically, pseudohyphae and yeasts are usually in the lumens of tubules, invading the tubular wall and extending into the interstitium. There is no vascular invasion.

Most candidiasis of the renal pelvis follows hematogenous seeding. The rich vascularity of the kidney and the large volume of blood circulating through the kidney make this route probable.[48] Grossly there are small, round, white foci with necrotic centers and hyperemic rims. The lesions are bilateral and miliary, involving cortex and medulla. When seeding is hematogenous, the lower urinary tract is spared. Microscopically, yeast forms and pseudohyphae in glomeruli (Figures 102–8 and 102–9) distinguish hematogenous spread. The absence of lower urinary tract lesions is one of the most reliable features of hematogenous renal infection.

Eye

Candidiasis of the eye is uncommon.[26] Candidal keratitis may follow minor corneal trauma but more frequently complicates other prolonged treatment with topical antibiotics and steroids.[49] Hematogenous candidal endophthalmitis is often in patients with disseminated candidiasis,[26] but it also has been reported weeks after spontaneous clearing of transient candidemia and after treatment of candidal septicemia.[50] Eyes taken at autopsy have an inflammatory infiltrate with neutrophils predominating, and granulomatous inflammation with giant cells.[26] The characteristic yeasts and hyphal elements are demonstrated with PAS and GMS stains.

Skin

Bodey and Luna[27] described a characteristic macronodular skin lesion in patients with systemic candidiasis. The lesions usually involve the entire body but can be localized. The lesions vary in size and number and appear as raised, firm nodules with well-circumscribed borders. Microscopically, the epidermis is intact, but there is a fibrinous exudate and focal hemorrhage in the middle and lower dermis. Some blood vessels have edematous walls with edema of surrounding tissue. There is minimal mononuclear inflammation around the blood vessels and skin appendages. Pale-blue yeast-like organisms and pseudohyphae are in the dermis and blood vessels. The organisms are best demonstrated with PAS and GMS stains.

Biopsy of the lesion will establish the diagnosis if the pathologist is alerted to the possibility of candidiasis. Several different levels of the specimen must be examined because the organisms may not be in a single section.

Biopsy specimens of lesions of skin or mucous membranes in patients with chronic mucocutaneous candidiasis have hyphae in the superficial tissues. There is only limited invasion of the dermis or deeper tissues.[35,51] The underlying tissues have an intense inflammatory infiltrate with neutrophils and mononuclear cells.

Genital Tract

Vulvovaginal candidiasis (VVC) is the most common candidal infection in women, and balanitis is the most common in men.[52] VVC is worldwide and is the most common cause of acute vaginitis in tropical climates. In the United States, candidiasis is the second most common cause of vaginal infection, with bacterial vaginosis almost twice as common as VVC.[53] Based on the numbers of prescriptions written to treat yeast infections between 1980 and 1990, the incidence of candidal vaginitis has almost doubled,[54] with about 13 million prescription users in 1990.

Recurrent and chronic genital candidiasis is usually transmitted sexually. As in oral candidiasis, chronic intractable vaginal infection also may reflect increasing immunodeficiency and may herald the onset of other opportunistic infections in women with acquired immunodeficiency syndrome.[55,56]

HISTOPATHOLOGIC DIFFERENTIAL DIAGNOSIS

Most pathogenic fungi can be identified, at least by genus, by biopsy or fine-needle aspiration. Tissues stained with H&E, used in combination with special techniques such as PAS (Figure 102–9), GMS (Figure 102–13), or Gridley staining (Figure 102–1), can help distinguish between different fungi, but there is a need for more specific differentiation.[57] This is especially true when examining tissues of immunosuppressed patients. Immunosuppression appears to create conditions in tissue that are conducive to complete or partial transformation of fungi into developmental forms usually observed only in cultures. Kenney[58] has illustrated examples of such abnormal development of fungi and parasites in histopathologic sections of tissues from immunosuppressed patients.

The histopathologic diagnosis of fungal infections in immunodeficient patients is based on the recognition of characteristic features of the fungi. The patient's response, although sometimes giving clues to an invading fungus, cannot be used as a basis for diagnosis. Furthermore, the host response depends on immunologic status, which may change with therapy and state of underlying disease. Pathologists who deal with these infections must be familiar with the many therapeutic and supportive measures that alter the host's reaction. Pathologists must know also the specific procedures for handling various types of specimens in order to provide a rapid and accurate diagnosis.

The *Candida* sp must be distinguished from *Aspergillus*, *Histoplasma*, and *Trichosporon beigelii*. Identification of *Aspergillus* in tissue generally rests on four points: 1) uniform-sized hyphae of 4 to 6 μm width, 2) characteristic dichotomy, with branching at

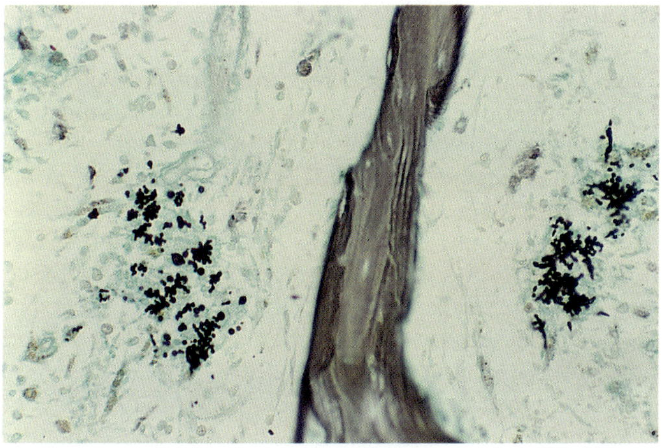

Figure 102–13. Disseminated candidiasis in patient with acute leukemia and severe neutropenia. Special stains demonstrate candidal organisms in vascular spaces of hypocellular bone marrow (GMS, ×150).

about 45 degrees, 3) better staining of hyphae with special stains than with H&E, and 4) septation of hyphae. These four characteristics can be used to distinguish an *Aspergillus* sp from a *Candida* sp. In tissue, a *Candida* sp shows 1) a mixture of yeasts and pseudohyphae, 2) thin pseudohyphae with no true branching, and 3) poor staining with H&E but a strong magenta stain with PAS (Figures 102–3 and 102–9). Thus, the major features distinguishing *Candida* from *Aspergillus* are 1) the difference in hyphal width, 2) the presence of true dichotomous branching in *Aspergillus*, and 3) most importantly, the blastoconidia in *Candida* sp.[59] In addition, the *Aspergillus* sp can be identified by immunohistochemical techniques.[60]

The major differential point between *Histoplasma* and *Candida* sp is the absence of pseudohyphae in the former. When there are only yeast cells and no pseudohyphae, rare elements of *Candida* sp are impossible to differentiate from *H capsulatum* on morphologic grounds alone because measurements of the *Candida* yeast cell and *H capsulatum* overlap. In these rare instances, additional histologic sections usually help in finding the diagnostic features of *Candida* sp. The intracellular location of fungi and the presence of granulomas favor the diagnosis of histoplasmosis rather than candidiasis.

Trichosporon beigelii is the other opportunistic fungus that produces yeasts and pseudohyphae in tissue; therefore, the histologic distinction from *Candida* sp is extremely difficult. The larger average diameter (5 versus 2.5 μm) and the pleomorphism of *Trichosporon* yeast forms are helpful differential features. *Trichosporon* pseudohyphae are poorly formed and narrow, whereas *Candida* pseudohyphae can be recognized by the regular areas of constriction. Another important distinction is radially arranged fungal growth and arthroconidia in the former. In addition, *Candida* sp show a bright, strong, magenta stain with the PAS technique. Application of immunohistochemistry has consistently identified *T beigelii* in formalin-fixed, paraffin-embedded tissue.[61]

SPECIAL TISSUE TECHNIQUES

Several techniques aid in the histopathologic detection of fungi. These include fungal autofluorescence,[62] whitening agents such as Calcofluor white,[63] 2-hydroxystilbamidine isethionate,[64] Blakophor BA 267,[65] and diaethanol.[66] In general, these methods are more rapid but somewhat less sensitive or specific than conventional fungal stains.

Direct immunofluorescence (IF) staining of fungi in formalin-fixed, paraffin-embedded tissue sections is a rapid, relatively inexpensive and extremely helpful procedure for confirming a presumptive histologic diagnosis of a mycosis, especially with atypical forms of a fungus.[58,67,68] Because of the unavailability of commercial reagents, only a few specialty laboratories perform IF staining for fungi in tissue sections and smears.

Fungal immunohistochemistry utilizing polyclonal and/or monoclonal antibodies offer potential advantages. Application of the immunoperoxidase technique has been successful in identifying several fungi including *Candida* sp.[68] Antibodies against fungi, however, have not been widely available for clinical diagnosis. As a result, fungal immunohistochemical testing has remained a service provided by a few reference laboratories. Furthermore, improved reagents are needed to increase specificity.

The two principal molecular techniques used in the detection of microorganisms are 1) nucleic acid hybridization, the binding of the probe to its target with a specific DNA or RNA probe, and 2) DNA amplification by the polymerase chain reaction.[69,70] These techniques are useful for the direct detection of organisms in clinical samples or for confirming results of microbial cultures. In tissues obtained for mycologic diagnosis, however, these techniques have remained as research and epidemiologic tools because conventional stains (PAS and GMS) are sensitive and reliable.

DIAGNOSIS AND CONFIRMATIONAL TESTING

The diagnosis of candidiasis can be made conclusively only by direct demonstration of candidal organisms in tissue. A section with invading candidal organisms confirms the diagnosis. Biopsy may not be feasible, however, and small candidal lesions may be missed. Then the following laboratory findings are helpful: 1) repeated isolation of candidal organisms from blood in the absence of an intravenous catheter, 2) isolation of candidal organisms from normally self-sterile sites or body fluids (pleural, peritoneal, cerebrospinal, subarachnoid and joint spaces, or peritoneal cavity), and 3) presence of 10,000 or more *Candida* organisms per milliliter of fresh urine obtained by catheterization in the absence of a Foley catheter or other indwelling catheter.[71]

Laboratory identification of *Candida* to the species level has been found to carry prognostic and therapeutic significance, and this can be accomplished only by culturing. The conventional microbiologic methods of diagnosis include 1) direct examination of specimens and 2) cultures of blood and other normally sterile body fluids, tissues, and surfaces. Direct examination of a specimen may provide rapid diagnosis. In addition, it provides a semiquantitative estimate of the number of *Candida* sp and reveals the morphologic features of the organisms. Direct examination further provides information about the cellular composition of an inflammatory exudate, and the presence of any other organisms, such as bacteria and noncandidal fungi.[71]

Detection of *Candida* sp in blood is one of the most substantial advances in diagnosing invasive candidiasis during the past two decades. In the past, cultures of blood often did not recover *Candida* sp and led to a disparity between postmortem findings of invasive candidiasis and the paucity of premortem positive blood cultures. Various methods, especially the lysis-centrifugation technique, have improved the detection of *Candida* sp in blood and thus the rate and quickness of recovery of *Candida* sp.[72] The lysis-centrifugation technique for processing blood cultures has improved the yield of positive cultures in fungal infections, especially in candidiasis. In several studies, fungi were recovered from about 60% of specimens by using conventional culture methods, whereas the yield was increased to 90% with the lysis-centrifugation technique.[73–75]

Numerous investigators have invested considerable effort toward developing an immunologic test to assist in the diagnosis of candidiasis. These approaches include 1) immunologic detection of anti-*Candida* antibodies[76] and candidal antigens such as cell–wall mannan,[77] *Candida* enolase-antigen,[78] anti-*Candida* enolase antibody,[79] and HSP 90–related *Candida* antigen[80]; 2) analytic detection of *Candida* metabolites,[81] and cell–wall components[82]; and 3) detection of *Candida* DNA by polymerase chain reaction.[83] These new approaches are promising diagnostic and epidemiologic tools.

TREATMENT

Superficial candidal infections can be treated with topical preparations, whereas major organ or disseminated infections require systemic therapy. Topical preparations have been effective against superficial infections of skin and, to a lesser extent, the nails. They are also useful for treating gastrointestinal and vaginal infections, but recent studies indicate that orally absorbable agents are superior to topical preparations for these latter infections, especially in patients with compromised host defenses or recurrent infections.[84]

For many years, amphotericin B was the only agent available for disseminated candidiasis.[85] Subsequently, flucytosine was developed and, more recently, the azole compounds (miconazole, ketoconazole, fluconazole, and itraconazole).[84] Amphotericin B given in lipid vehicles reduces toxicity, permitting higher doses that may be more effective.[86] In addition to the commercially available azole compounds, others have been synthesized that have promising characteristics such as improved pharmacokinetic properties or expanded activity against fungi.[87]

REFERENCES

1. Banerjee SN, Emori TG, Culver DH, et al. Secular trends in nosocomial primary bloodstream infections in the United States, 1980–1989. *Am J Med.* 1991;91:86S–89S.
2. Bauer TM, Ofner E, Just HM, Just H, Faschner FD. An epidemiological study assessing the relative importance of airborne and direct contact transmission of microorganisms in a medical intensive care unit. *J Hosp Inf.* 1990; 15:301–309.
3. Cohen R, Roth JF, Delgado E, Ahearn DG, Kalser MH. Fungal flora of the normal human small and large intestine. *N Engl J Med.* 1968;279:340–344.
4. Denning DW. Epidemiology and pathogenesis of systemic fungal infections in the immunocompromised host. *J Antimicrob Chemother.* 1991;28:1–16.
5. Stevens DA, Odds FC, Scherer S. Application of DNA typing methods to *Candida albicans* epidemiology and correlations with phenotype. *Rev Infect Dis.* 1990;12:258–266.
6. Odds FC, Abbott AB. Modification and extension of tests for differentiation of *Candida* species and strains. *Sabouraudia.* 1983;21:79–81.
7. Polonelli L, Archibusacci C, Sestito M, Morace G. Killer system: a simple method for differentiating *Candida albicans* strains. *J Clin Microbiol.* 1983;17:774–780.
8. Clemons KV, Shankland GS, Richardson MD, Stevens DA. Epidemiologic study by DNA typing of a *Candida albicans* outbreak in heroin addicts. *J Clin Microbiol.* 1991;29:205–207.
9. Powderly WG, Robinson K, Keath EJ. Molecular typing of *Candida albicans* isolated from oral lesions of HIV-infected individuals. *AIDS.* 1992;6:81–84.

10. Reagan DR, Pfaller MA, Hollis RJ, Wenzel RP. Characterization of the sequence of colonization and nosocomial candidemia using DNA fingerprinting and a DNA probe. *J Clin Microbiol.* 1990;28:2733–2738.
11. Pfaller MA. Strain variation among *Candida* species: application of various typing methods to study the epidemiology and pathogenesis of candidiasis in hospitalized patients. *Inf Control.* 1987;8:273–276.
12. Vartivaran S, Smith CB. Pathogenesis, host resistance, and predisposing factors. In: Bodey GP, ed. *Candidiasis: Pathogenesis, Diagnosis and Treatment.* 2nd ed. New York: Raven Press; 1993:59–84.
13. Karabinis A, Hill C, Leclerco B, Tancrede C, Baume D, Andremont A. Risk factors for candidemia in cancer patients: a case-controlled study. *J Clin Microbiol.* 1988; 26:429–432.
14. Pockros PJ, Silberman H. Parenteral nutrition complicated by candidiasis. *J Infect Dis.* 1982;145:592–593.
15. Barnett JA, Payne RW, Yarrow D. *Yeasts—Characteristics and Identification.* 2nd ed. New York: Cambridge University Press; 1991.
16. Goodrich JM, Reed EC, Mori M, et al. Clinical features and analysis of risk factors for invasive candidal infection after marrow transplantation. *J Infect Dis.* 1991;164:731–740.
17. Leen CLS, Brettle RP. Fungal infections in drug users. *J Antimicrob Chemother.* 1991;28:83–96.
18. Marina NM, Flynn PM, Rivera GK, Hughes WT. *Candida tropicalis* and *Candida albicans* fungemia in children with leukemia. *Cancer.* 1991;68:594–599.
19. McQuillen DP, Zingman BS, Meunier F, Levitz SM. Invasive infections due to *Candida krusei:* report of ten cases of fungemia that include three cases of endophthalmitis. *Clin Infect Dis.* 1992;14:272–278.
20. Wingard JR, Merz WG, Rinaldi MG, Johnson TR, Karp JE, Saral R. Increase in *Candida krusei* infection among patients with bone marrow transplantation and neutropenia treated prophylactically with fluconazole. *N Engl J Med.* 1991;325:1274–1277.
21. Roth JS, Grossman ME. Images in clinical medicine. Cutaneous lesions of disseminated candidiasis. *N Engl J Med.* 1994;330:1650.
22. Lewis MA, Samaranyake LP, Lamey PJ. Diagnosis and treatment of oral candidosis. *J Oral Maxillofac Surg.* 1991;49:996–1002.
23. Jorizzo JL. The spectrum of mucosal and cutaneous candidosis. *Dermatol Clin North Am.* 1984;2:19–27.
24. Haron E, Vartivarian S, Annissie E, Dekmezian R, Bodey G. Primary *Candida* pneumonia: experience at a large cancer center and review of the literature. *Medicine.* 1993; 72:137–142.
25. Bodey GP, DeJongh D, Isassi A, Freireich EJ. Hypersplenism due to disseminated candidiasis in a patient with acute leukemia. *Cancer.* 1969;26:417–420.
26. Edwards JE, Foos RY, Montgomerie JZ, Guze LP. Ocular manifestations of *Candida* septicemia: review of seventy-six cases of hematogenous *Candida* endophthalmitis. *Medicine.* 1974;53:47–75.
27. Bodey GP, Luna M. Skin lesions associated with disseminated candidiasis. *JAMA.* 1974;229:1466–1468.
28. Nagai Y, Takeshita N, Saku T. Histopathologic and ultrastructural studies of oral mucosa with *Candida* infection. *J Oral Pathol Med.* 1992;21:171–175.
29. Myerowitz RL. Ultrastructural observations in disseminated candidiasis. *Arch Pathol Lab Med.* 1978;102:512–514.
30. Maksymiuk AW, Thongprasert S, Hopfer R, Luna MA, Fainstein V, Bodey GP. Systemic candidiasis in cancer patients. *Am J Med.* 1984;77:20–27.
31. Myerowitz RL. Localized and disseminated candidiasis. In: Myerowitz RL, ed. *The Pathology of Opportunistic Infections.* New York: Raven Press; 1983:95–114.
32. Myerowitz RL, Pazin GJ, Allen CM. Disseminated candidiasis. Changes in incidence, underlying disease, and pathology. *Am J Clin Pathol.* 1977;68:29–38.
33. Eras P, Goldstein MJ, Sherlock P. *Candida* infection of the gastrointestinal tract. *Medicine.* 1972;51:367–379.
34. Shirkhoda A, Lopez-Berestein G, Holbert JM, Luna MA. Hepatosplenic fungal infection: CT and pathologic evaluation after treatment with liposomal Amphotericin B. *Radiology.* 1986;159:349–353.
35. Shama SK, Kirkpatrick CH. Dermatophytosis in patients with chronic mucocutaneous candidiasis. *J Am Acad Dermatol.* 1980;2:285–294.
36. Odden K, Schenck K, Koppang H, Hurlen B. Candidal infection of the gingiva in HIV-infected persons. *J Oral Pathol Med.* 1994;23:178–183.
37. Macher AM, DeVinatea M, Tuur SM, Amgrit P. AIDS and the mycoses. *Infect Dis Clin North Am.* 1988;2:827–838.
38. Wheeler RR, Peacock JE, Cruz JM, Richter JE. Esophagitis in the immunocompromised host: role of esophagoscopy in diagnosis. *Rev Infect Dis.* 1987;9:88–96.
39. Thaler M, Pastakia B, Shawker TH, O'Leary T, Pizzo PA. Hepatic candidiasis in cancer patients: the evolving picture of the syndrome. *Ann Intern Med.* 1988;108:88–100.
40. Johnson JD, Raff MJ. Fungal splenic abscess. *Arch Intern Med.* 1984;144:1987–1993.
41. Mills SA, Seigler HF, Wolfe WF. The incidence and management of pulmonary mycosis in renal allograft patients. *Ann Surg.* 1975;182:617–626.
42. Masur H, Rosen PP, Armstrong D. Pulmonary disease caused by *Candida* species. *Am J Med.* 1977;63:914–925.
43. Parker JC. The potentially lethal problem of cardiac candidiasis. *Am J Clin Pathol.* 1980;73:356–361.
44. Walsh TJ, Hutchins GM, Bulkley BH, Mondolsohn G. Fungal infections of the heart. Analysis of 51 autopsy cases. *Am J Cardiol.* 1980;45:357–366.
45. Hallum JL and Williams TW. *Candida* endocarditis. In: Bodey GP, ed. *Candidiasis: Pathogenesis, Diagnosis and Treatment.* 2nd ed. New York: Raven Press; 1993:357–369.
46. Parker JC. Human cerebral candidiasis. A postmortem evaluation of 19 patients. *Hum Pathol.* 1981;12:23–28.
47. Moyer DV, Edwards JE. *Candida* endophthalmitis and central nervous system infection. In: Bodey GP, ed. *Candidiasis: Pathogenesis, Diagnosis and Treatment.* 2nd ed. New York: Raven Press; 1993:346–355.
48. Clark RE, Minagi H, Palubinskas AJ. Renal candidiasis. *Radiology.* 1971;101:567–572.
49. Cameron JA, Antonios SR, Cotter JB, Habash NR. Endoph-

thalmitis from contaminated donor corneas following penetrating keratoplasty. *Arch Ophthalmol.* 1991;109: 54–59.
50. Brooks R. Prospective study of *Candida* endophthalmitis. *Infect Immun.* 1980;27:628–634.
51. Kirkpatrick CH. Chronic mucocutaneous candidiasis. In: Bodey GP, ed. *Candidiasis: Pathogenesis, Diagnosis and Treatment.* 2nd ed. New York: Raven Press; 1993:167–184.
52. Odds FC. Genital candidosis. *Clin Exp Dermatol.* 1982; 7:345–354.
53. Centers for Disease Control. Non-reported sexually transmitted diseases. *MMWR.* 1979;28:61.
54. Kent HL. Epidemiology of vaginitis. *Am J Obstet Gynecol.* 1991;165:1168–1176.
55. Rhoads JL, Wright C, Redfield RR. Chronic vaginal candidiasis in women with human immunodeficiency virus infection. *JAMA.* 1987;257:3105–3107.
56. Bykov VL. Histopathology of human vaginal candidosis. *Mycoses.* 1992;35:77–82.
57. Rolph L, Austwick PKC. Differential staining of fungi in tissues. *J Sci Technol.* 1987;17:22–26.
58. Kenney M. Misleading morphology of parasites and fungi in tissue sections. *Pathol Annu.* 1981;16:313–335.
59. Chandler FW, Watts JC. *Pathologic Diagnosis of Fungal Infections.* Chicago: ASCP Press; 1987.
60. Phillips P, Weiner MH. Invasive aspergillosis diagnosed by immunohistochemistry with monoclonal and polyclonal reagents. *Hum Pathol.* 1987;18:1015–1024.
61. Kobayashi M, Kotani S, Fujishita M, et al. Immunohistochemical identification of *Trichosporon beigelii* in histologic sections by immunoperoxidase method. *Am J Clin Pathol.* 1988;89:100–105.
62. Mann JL. Autofluorescence of fungi: an aid to detection in tissue sections. *Am J Clin Pathol.* 1983;79:587–590.
63. Monheit JE, Cowan DF, Moore DG. Rapid detection of fungi in tissue using calcofluor white and fluorescence microscopy. *Arch Pathol Lab Med.* 1984;108:616–618.
64. Murgatroyd LB. 2-Hydroxystilbamidine isethionate: a new fluorochrome for use in general pathology II. *Diag Histopathol.* 1982;5:219–222.
65. Hollander H, Keiling W. A reliable fluorescent stain of fungi in tissue sections and clinical specimens. *Mycopathology.* 1984;88:131–134.
66. Koch HA, Pimsler M, Walsh GP. Nonspecific fluorescent stains for detecting and identifying fungal elements in tissue. In: Program of the Annual Meeting of the American Society of Microbiology; 1986; Washington, DC. Abstract F-62.
67. Jackson JA, Kaplan W, Kaufman L. Development of fluorescent-antibody reagents for demonstration of *Pseudallescheria boydii* in tissue. *J Clin Microbiol.* 1983;18: 668–673.
68. Reiss E, de-Repentgny L, Kuykendall J, et al. Monoclonal antibodies against *Candida tropicalis* mannans antigen detection by enzyme immunoassay and immunofluorescence. *J Clin Microbiol.* 1986;24:796–802.
69. Naber PS. Molecular pathology—diagnosis of infectious disease. *New Engl J Med.* 1994;331:1212–1215.
70. Symposium: molecular techniques in diagnostic pathology. *Hum Pathol.* 1994;25:555–614.
71. Walsh TJ, Pizzo PA. Laboratory diagnosis of candidiasis. In: Bodey GP, ed. *Candidiasis: Pathogenesis, Diagnosis and Treatment.* 2nd ed. New York: Raven Press; 1993: 109–135.
72. Telenti A, Roberts GD. Fungal blood cultures. *Eur J Clin Microbiol Infect Dis.* 1989;8:825–831.
73. Kiehn TE, Wong B, Edwards FF, Armstrong D. Comparative recovery of bacteria and yeasts from lysis-centrifugation and a conventional blood culture system. *J Clin Microbiol.* 1983;18:300–304.
74. Bodey GP. Hematogenous and major organ candidiasis. In: Bodey GP, ed. *Candidiasis: Pathogenesis, Diagnosis and Treatment.* 2nd ed. New York: Raven Press; 1993: 279–329.
75. Telenti A, Guerra L, Roberts GD, Wilson WR. Usefulness of the lysis-centrifugation blood culture system for the clinical management of patients having fungemia. In: *Interscience Conference on Antimicrobial Agents and Chemotherapy*; September 28–October 1, 1986; New Orleans, La; 1986:119. Abstract 129.
76. Taschdjian CL, Kozinn PJ, Cuesta MV, Toni EF. Serodiagnosis of candidal infections. *Am J Clin Pathol.* 1971;57: 195–205.
77. Jones JM. Laboratory diagnosis of invasive candidiasis. *Clin Microbiol Rev.* 1990;3:32–45.
78. Franklyn KM, Warmington JR, Ott AK, Ashman RB. An immunodominant antigen of *Candida albicans* shows homology to the enzyme enolase. *Immunol Cell Biol.* 1990;68:173–178.
79. Walsh TJ, Maret SM, Cates DA, Schaufele RS, Pizzo PA. Complementary role of anti-*Candida* enolase antibody and *Candida* enolase antigen in detection of invasive candidiasis. ICAAC, Chicago; 1991.
80. Matthews RC, Burnie JP. Diagnosis of systemic candidiasis by an enzyme-linked dot immunobinding assay for a circulating immunodominant 47 kD antigen. *J Clin Microbiol.* 1988;26:459–463.
81. Roboz J, Suzuki R, Holland JF. Quantification of arabinitol in serum by selected ion monitoring as a diagnostic technique in invasive candidiasis. *J Clin Microbiol.* 1980;12: 594–602.
82. Obayashi T, Tamura H, Tanaka S, et al. A new chromogenic endotoxin-specific assay using recombined *Limulus* coagulation enzyme and its clinical applications. *Clin Chem Acta.* 1985;149:55–65.
83. Kan VL. Polymerase chain reaction for the diagnosis of candidemia. *J Infect Dis.* 1993;168:780–783.
84. Bodey GP. Antifungal agents. In: Bodey GP, ed. *Candidiasis: Pathogenesis, Diagnosis and Treatment.* 2nd ed. New York: Raven Press; 1993:371–406.
85. Perfect JR, Pickard WW, Hunt DL, Palmer B, Schell WA. The use of amphotericin B in nosocomial fungal infection. *Rev Infect Dis.* 1991;13:474–479.
86. Lopez-Berestein G, Bodey GP, Fainstein V, et al. Treatment of systemic fungal infections with liposomal amphotericin B. *Arch Intern Med.* 1989;149:2533–2536.
87. Bodey GP. What's new in fungal infection in leukemic patients. *Leukemia Lymphoma.* 1993;11:127–135.

CHAPTER 103

Chlorellosis

Christopher M. Seniw, Francis W. Chandler, and Daniel H. Connor

A green wound is soon healed.

English proverb

DEFINITION

Chlorellosis is infection of man and animals by unicellular green algae, belonging to the genus *Chlorella*.[1] A single human infection has been documented (vide infra), and at least 16 infections in animals have been reported, most being in cattle and sheep.[1–4] *Prototheca* sp are related organisms but lack chloroplasts and are thought to be achloric mutants of green algae.[5–7] Chloroplasts give the fresh lesions of chlorellosis a distinct green color, but lesions of protothecosis are not green. Microscopically, chloroplasts of *Chlorella* sp have a characteristic appearance and allow them to be easily distinguished from the *Prototheca* sp.[2]

CHLORELLOSIS IN A HUMAN

The tongue of a trailer fell on the right foot of a 30-year-old woman in Nebraska.[1] The injury was blunt, nonpenetrating, but caused persistent pain, swelling, and numbness. Four months after the injury, scar tissue and a traumatic neuroma were excised from the injured site. Healing of the wound was uneventful until a short time later, when she went canoeing on a river. There, the dressing became contaminated with river water. The lesion became inflamed and continued to drain in spite of two subsequent debridements. Ten months after the initial injury, and following a third and final debridement, the lesion healed completely.

Routine and special stains prepared from sections of debrided tissue revealed chronic inflammation surrounding a sinus tract lined by fibrin and neutrophils (Figure 103–1). Adjacent granulation tissue and scar tissue contained numerous lymphocytes, with fewer mast cells, neutrophils, and scattered clusters of Langhans' giant cells. Gomori's methenamine-silver (GMS) stain and the periodic acid–Schiff (PAS) reaction revealed clusters of microorganisms in the wall of the sinus tract (Figure 103–2). In hematoxylin-eosin (H&E) stained sections, the organisms were poorly delineated and appeared as clear vacuoles with traces of stainable contents (Figure 103–3). The cell walls of the organisms and their cytoplasmic contents were strongly silvered with GMS and reacted intensely with PAS (Figures 103–4 and 103–5). Although most of the organisms were in the lining of the sinus tract, a few were in adjacent connective tissue and in the cytoplasm of Langhans' giant cells, which were surrounded by neutrophils (Figure 103–6). The algae were ovoid or spherical or polygonal and varied from 3 to 10 μm in diameter. Some were elongated, while others were collapsed and crescentic. All had a thin, limiting membrane and many contained numerous distinct cytoplasmic granules that, by electron microscopy, proved to be chloroplasts. The chloroplasts were 1 to 3 μm in diameter and stained with GMS and PAS (Figure 103–7). In summary, the reaction was pyogranulomatous, specifically—microabscesses surrounded by macrophages and epithelioid cells. Immunofluorescence conjugates specific for *P zopfii* and *P wickerhamii*, the two known pathogenic *Prototheca* sp,[3,8] did not stain the algal cells.[9] All tissue was processed for histopathologic examination, so cultures could not be done. Studies of the patient's serum were normal. By transmission electron microscopy, stacked cytoplasmic membranes surrounded electron-dense granules (1 to 4 μm) in a few of the cells. These membranous profiles and cytoplasmic granules are characteristic of chloroplasts.

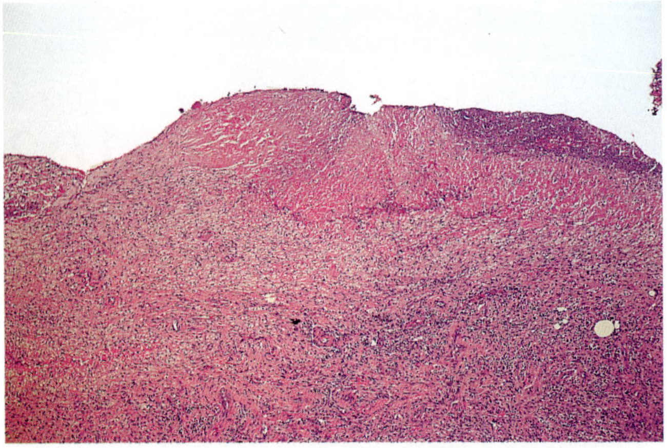

Figure 103–1. Sinus tract at top surrounded by neutrophils and fibrin supported by chronically inflamed granulation tissue in the only known human infection by a *Chlorella* sp (hematoxylin-eosin, ×18).

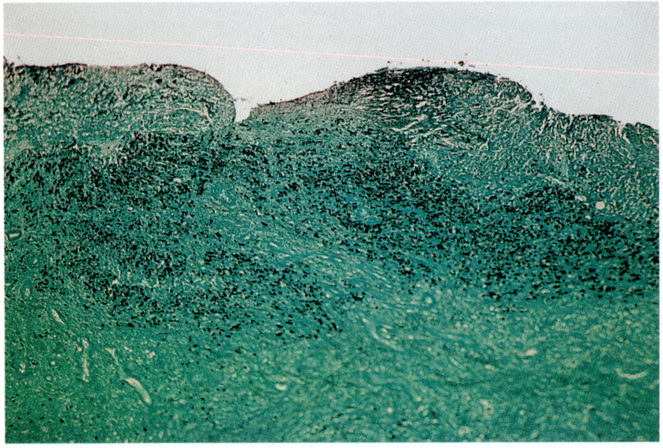

Figure 103–2. A parallel adjacent section of the lesion in Figure 103–1 reveals a band of algal cells concentrated beneath the lining of the sinus tract. The algae are black because they are silvered by the GMS technique (×18).

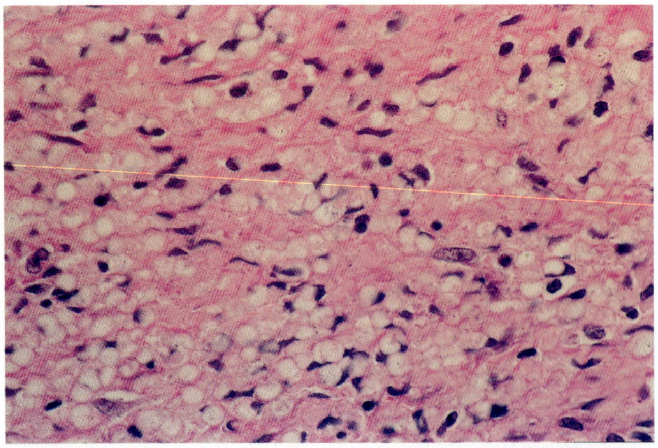

Figure 103–3. Although silvered by the GMS stain, *Chlorella* sp appear as clear round spaces in sections stained with hematoxylin-eosin. Under higher magnification, some of the algal cells have traces of stainable (eosinophilic) contents, including structures that may be chloroplasts (×180).

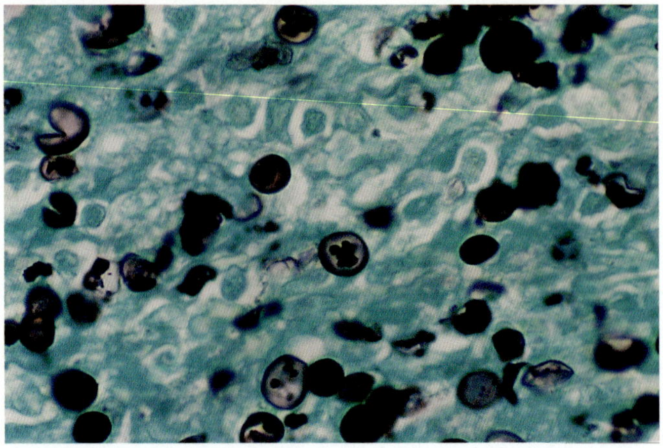

Figure 103–4. Higher magnification of Figure 103–3 reveals walls of the chlorellae. The chloroplasts in the cytoplasm are also silvered (GMS, ×400).

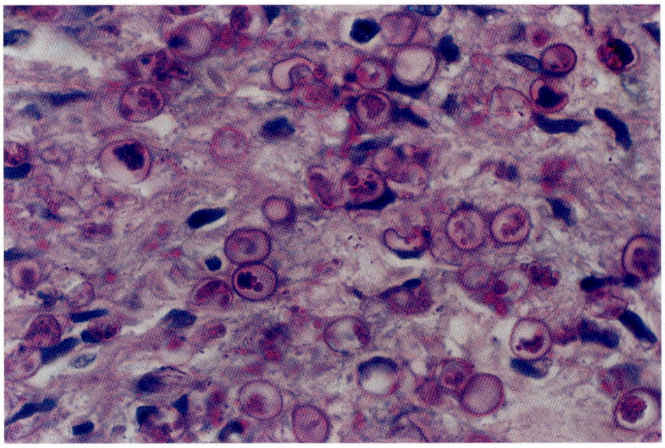

Figure 103–5. The walls and chloroplasts of the algae react with PAS (×400).

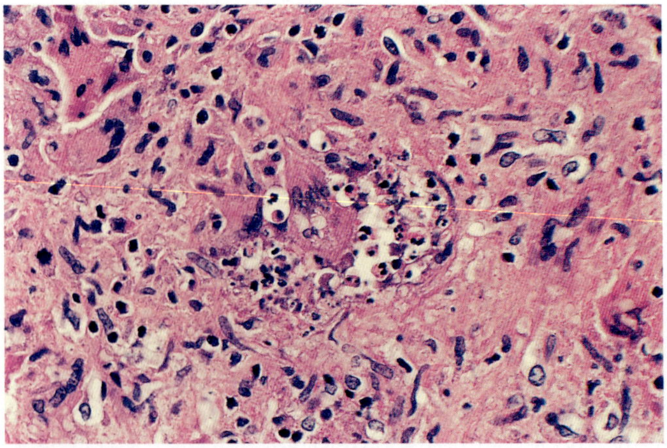

Figure 103–6. A pyogranulomatous focus comprised of a Langhans' giant cell containing at least two algae. Neutrophils surround the giant cell, and two neutrophils are in its cytoplasm (hematoxylin-eosin, ×400).

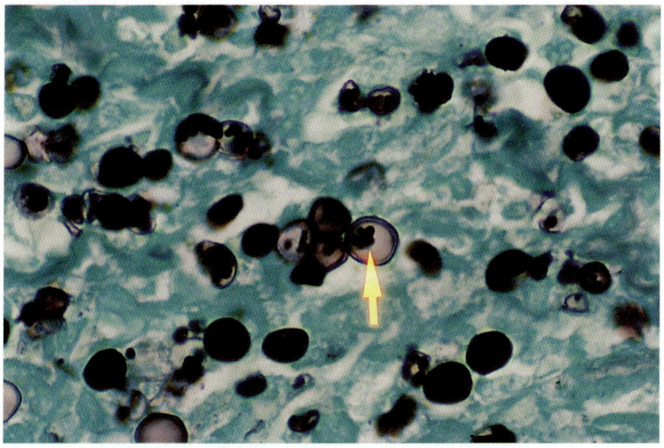

Figure 103–7. Cell walls of *Chlorella* sp sometimes appear doubly contoured. The arrow points to a cluster of chloroplasts within the organism (GMS, ×400).

CHLORELLOSIS IN ANIMALS

Chlorellosis in animals has involved mainly lymph nodes and deep organs (Figure 103–8). Cutaneous and subcutaneous nodules have been seen also in the pelt of a beaver from Canada.[3] Clinically and on gross examination, the fresh lesions were green, and smears revealed organisms that contained green, refractile granules (chloroplasts). The green color of the lesions was lost when specimens were fixed and embedded in paraffin.[1] In our experience, however, paraffin blocks may retain a green hue (Figure 103–9). As in the human infection, organisms did not stain uniformly with H&E, but reacted intensely with PAS, were silvered with GMS (Figure 103–10), and stained clearly with the Gridley fungus (GF) procedure. Immunologic and cultural studies suggest that these organisms belonged to the genus *Chlorella*.[1] In lesions of animals the *Chlorella* cells have been ovoid or spherical, and single or endosporulating, ranging from 4 to 15 μm in diameter.[2–4] Microscopically, most of the cells contained multiple cytoplasmic granules that varied from 0.5 to 4 μm in diameter. These granules are components of chloroplasts, and they are morphologically and tinctorially distinctive. The gran-

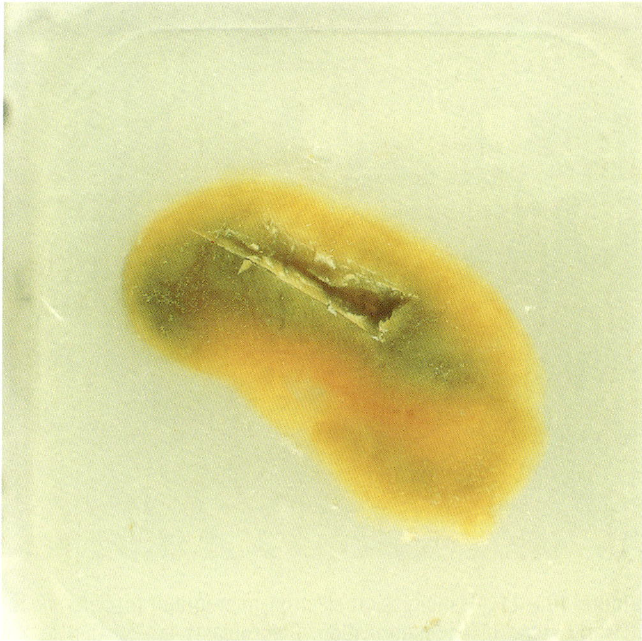

Figure 103–9. Paraffin block containing formalin-fixed lymph node from a lamb with disseminated chlorellosis. Note partial retention of green color even though the specimen has been fixed and embedded. *(By Daniel H. Connor, MD 1978.)*

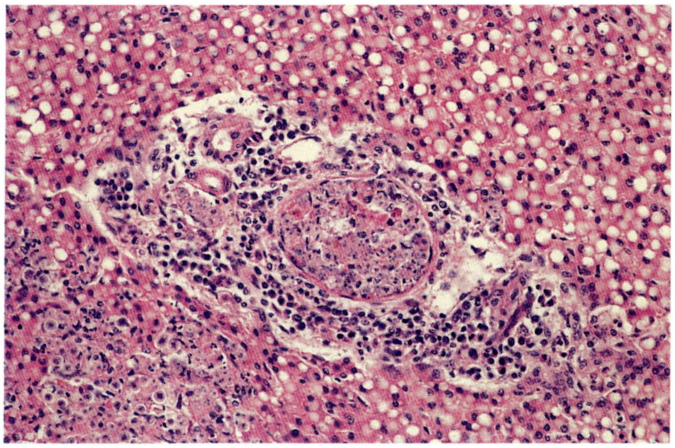

Figure 103–8. Disseminated chlorellosis involving the liver in a sheep. There is fatty change of parenchymal cells and clusters of poorly stained algae in sinusoids and portal tracts, causing septic thrombosis of portal veins (hematoxylin-eosin, ×70).

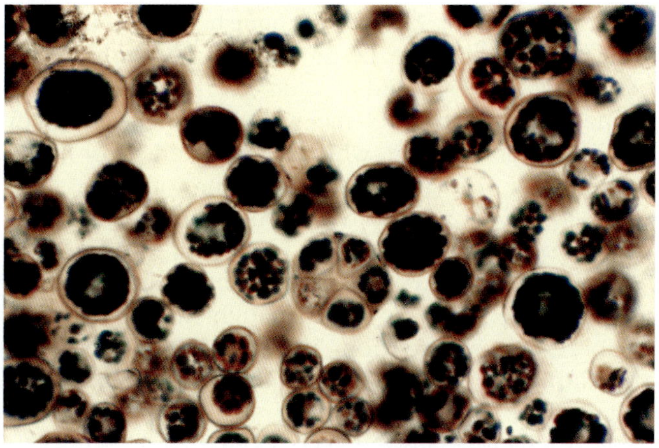

Figure 103–10. Microscopic view of the lymph node in Figure 103–9 shows intensely silvered chloroplasts within the algal cells. The walls of the algae are not as argyrophilic as are those in the human case. (GMS, ×400).

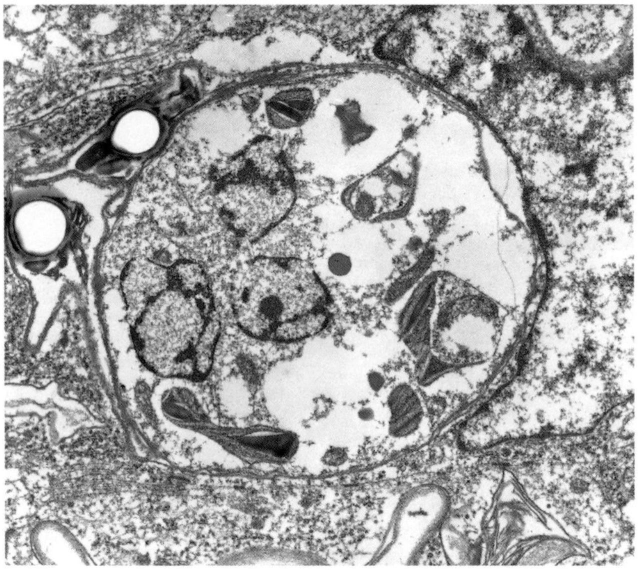

Figure 103–11. Transmission electron micrograph of *Chlorella* sp in early stage of endosporulation. Chloroplasts are located in the cytoplasm and consist of central, electron-dense, and elongated starch granules intimately surrounded by highly organized, stacked and twisted lamellae (uranyl acetate and lead citrate, ×6000).

ules, which are starch, stain uniformly and intensely with PAS, GMS, and GF procedures, and are often birefringent in plane-polarized light.[10] By transmission electron microscopy, the starch granules are the central components of chloroplasts in the cytoplasm of green algal cells, and are intimately surrounded by membranes composed of alternating bands of narrow lamellae (Figure 103–11).[2]

DIFFERENTIAL DIAGNOSIS

Fungi and bacteria can be distinguished from algae by size, shape, and type of reproduction.[1] Furthermore, both *Chlorella* sp and *Prototheca* sp lack glucosamine—a component of the walls of fungi—and they lack also muramic acid, which is characteristic of bacteria.[11–13] The causative agents of protothecosis and chlorellosis are spherical or ovoid, unicellular, have hyaline sporangia, and range from 3 to 30 μm. They reproduce asexually by internal septation and cytoplasmic cleavage, with up to 20 daughter cells (sporangiospores) produced from the parent cell (the sporangium). When mature, the outer wall (theca) of the parent cell ruptures, releasing the sporangiospores, each of which begins the cycle anew.[1,2,7,14,15]

Histopathologically, *Chlorella* sp must be distinguished from *Prototheca* sp. The morphologic and tinctorial features of the green algae resemble those of *P zopfii* and *P wickerhamii*. *Chlorella* sp, for instance, range from 6 to 14 μm and form endosporulating sporangia in tissue. In H&E stained tissue sections, cell walls of the sporangia are hyaline, and the cytoplasm, like that of *P zopfii*, is finely vacuolated. These two algae, however, can be distinguished in tissue by the following criteria: 1) lesions caused by *Chlorella* sp are distinctly green before fixation and processing; 2) *Chlorella* sp contain chloroplasts, which are numerous, large, diastase-sensitive, intracytoplasmic, birefringent granules that stain intensely with PAS, GF, and GMS procedures. All developmental forms of *Chlorella* sp, including sporangiospores, contain these granules, whereas cells of the *Prototheca* sp lack them; 3) chloroplasts have a distinctive appearance by transmission electron microscopy and consist of smoothly contoured, electron-dense starch granules, 0.5 to 4 μm or more in diameter. The granules are surrounded by or contiguous to tightly appressed, alternating membranes or multidisk bands. Some of the alternating membranes may be spirally twisted and associated with several starch granules in a single plane. When starch granules (plastids) are in *Prototheca* sp, they are either membrane free or surrounded by a single membrane, and lack the stacked lamellar component of true chloroplasts; 4) in formalin-fixed, paraffin-embedded sections, the two pathogenic species of *Prototheca* can be distinguished from *Chlorella* sp (and from each other) by direct immunofluorescence using species-specific conjugates.

TREATMENT

Infection in the only human documented to have chlorellosis resolved after several debridements, whirlpool treatments with dilute chlorine solution, irrigation of the wound with Dakin's solution, and gauze packing and gradual removal for drainage and granulation.[1] If such conservative treatment is not effective, an alternate and successful treatment reported for protothecosis might be tried: intravenous amphotericin B in combination with tetracycline. In vitro studies have revealed that the *Prototheca* sp are sensitive to these drugs.[16,17]

REFERENCES

1. Jones J, McFadden H, Chandler F, et al. Green algal infection in a human. *Am J Clin Pathol.* 1983;80:102–107.
2. Chandler FW, Kaplan W, Callaway CS. Differentiation between *Prototheca* and morphologically similar green algae in tissue. *Arch Pathol Lab Med.* 1978;102:353–356.
3. Kaplan W. Protothecosis and infections caused by morphologically similar green algae. In: *Proceedings of the Fourth International Conference on the Mycoses,* June 1977; Sci Pub 356, PAHO, Washington, DC; 1978:218–232.

4. Rogers RJ, Connole MD, Norton J, Thomas A, Ladds PW, Dickson J. Lymphadenitis of cattle due to infection with green algae. *J Comp Pathol.* 1980;90:1–9.
5. Cooke WB. Studies in the genus *Prototheca*: I. Literature review. *J Elisha Mitchell Sci Soc.* 1968;84:213–216.
6. Cooke WB. Studies in the genus *Prototheca*: II. Taxonomy. *J Elisha Mitchell Sci Soc.* 1968;84:217–220.
7. Sudman MS. Protothecosis. A critical review. *Am J Clin Pathol.* 1974;61:10–19.
8. Connor DH, Gibson DW, Ziefer A. Diagnostic features of three unusual infections: Micronemiasis, phaeomycotic cyst, and protothecosis. In: Majno G, Cotran RS, eds. *Inflammatory Disease.* International Academy of Pathology Monograph. Baltimore: Williams and Wilkins; 1982: 205–239.
9. Sudman MS, Kaplan W. Identification of the *Prototheca* species by immunofluorescence. *Appl Microbiol.* 1973;25: 981–990.
10. Chandler FW, Watts JC. *Pathologic Diagnosis of Fungal Infections.* Chicago: ASCP Press; 1987:43–53.
11. Connor DH, Neafie RC. Protothecosis. In: Binford CH, Connor DH, eds. *Pathology of Tropical and Extraordinary Diseases.* Washington, DC: Armed Forces Institute of Pathology; 1976:684–689.
12. Emmons CW, Binford CH, Utz JP, et al. Protothecosis. In: *Medical Mycology.* 3rd ed. Philadelphia: Lea & Febiger; 1977:511–517.
13. Garcia de Lomas J, Penalver Martinez J, Altuna Cuesta A, et al. Infecciones por algas: protothecosis (Algal infections: protothecosis). *Rev San Hig Pub.* 1979;53:437–470.
14. El-Ani AS. Life cycle and variation of *Prototheca wickerhamii. Science.* 1967;156:1501–1503.
15. Klintworth GK, Fetter BF, Nielsen HS Jr. Protothecosis, an algal infection: report of a case in man. *J Med Microbiol.* 1968;1:211–216.
16. Nelson AM, Neafie RC. Protothecosis. In: Strickland GT, ed. *Hunter's Tropical Medicine.* 7th ed. Philadelphia: WB Saunders; 1991:522–523.
17. Nelson AM, Neafie RC, Connor DH. Cutaneous protothecosis and chlorellosis, extraordinary "aquatic borne" algal infections. In: Mandojana RM, ed. *Clinics in Dermatology.* Philadelphia: JB Lippincott, 1987:76–87.

CHAPTER 104

Chromoblastomycosis

Michael R. McGinnis and Francis W. Chandler

Things medical and gruesome have a singular attraction for people.

Sir William Osler (1849–1919)

DEFINITION

Chromoblastomycosis is a chronic fungal infection of the skin and subcutaneous tissues that develops following traumatic implantation of one of several dematiaceous (naturally pigmented) fungi. The causal agents of chromoblastomycosis divide by internal septation, frequently appearing as cells with vertical and horizontal lines (muriform cells) and hyphae that are chestnut brown from melanin pigment in their cell walls.[1] The currently recognized agents include *Cladophialophora carrionii* (syn. *Cladosporium carrionii*), *Exophiala jeanselmei, E spinifera, Fonsecaea compacta, F pedrosoi, Phialophora verrucosa*, and *Rhinocladiella aquaspersa*.

GENERAL COMMENTS

Synonyms include chromomycosis, as well as numerous other names contained in the older literature.[2,3] The distribution of chromoblastomycosis is worldwide but it is most common in tropical and subtropical regions among bare-footed agricultural workers. The causal fungi grow on woody plants and in the soil. Infection probably develops after an agent is introduced into the patient's skin and subcutaneous tissues by traumatic implantation such as by a sliver or splinter. Although rarely detected in lesions of chromoblastomycosis, slivers and splinters are commonly detected in lesions of a closely related infection—phaeohyphomycosis (Chapter 116). Chromoblastomycosis remains localized to skin, but there have been rare disseminations to other organs. Most infections have been in men, probably a consequence of exposure at their occupations. Most infections involve legs and arms, sites often injured during agricultural work. Other body sites include buttocks, face, ears, shoulders, and trunk. There are no indications that infection is contagious, nor are there any reports of person-to-person spread.

Most infections are caused by *F pedrosoi*. In the Americas, this is the principal cause, and infections most often involve lower limbs. In Australia, the most common cause is *C carrionii*, and the lesions are most frequently on the upper limbs, especially the hands.[2,4]

MORPHOLOGIC FEATURES OF THE ORGANISMS

The fungi that cause chromoblastomycosis are dematiaceous and many are probably asexual forms of loculoascomycetes. With the exception of *P verrucosa*, these fungi are pleomorphic, ie, they may produce several different asexual forms known as anamorphs when grown in culture. Conidia-bearing cells called annellides characterize *E jeanselmei* and *E spinifera*, as well as a yeast form that is typically present in recently isolated colonies. *Phialophora verrucosa* forms flask-shaped collarettes with cup-shaped collarettes and conidia that accumulate in balls at the apices of the phialides. *Cladophialophora carrionii* forms branching chains of blastoconidia upon hypha-like to distinct conidiophores. *Fonsecaea compacta* and *F pedrosoi* develop complex conidial heads consisting of series of sympodial cells that ultimately give rise to a single series of apically located blastoconidia. These two species may also form phialides with collarettes, branching chains of blastoconidia arising from distinct conidiophores, and sympodial conidiogenous cells that have acropleurogenously arranged conidia.

In infected tissues, the fungi that cause chromoblastomycosis characteristically form muriform cells (sclerotic bodies, Medlar bodies) that are chestnut brown from melanin pigmentation of their cell walls, thick-walled, 5 to 12 μm in diameter, and divide by septation in two planes. Fungal elements may be free in the tissue but more commonly are in macrophages and giant cells.[1,2,5,6] Hyphae, when present, are usually in the hyperkeratotic epidermis, and are only rarely formed in the dermis.[7]

CLINICAL FEATURES

Chromoblastomycosis tends to be chronic, pruritic, progressive, indolent, and resistant to treatment (Figures 104–1 through 104–4). Infections spread contiguously or, if the patient scratches, satellite lesions can develop from autoinoculation. Spread by cutaneous lymphatics, although sometimes suggested by the linear distribution of lesions, is unlikely because the fungi do not invade lymphatics nor do they involve regional lymph nodes (Figure 104–1). Carrion described five types of lesions, which can occur in various combinations.[8] At first there is a small scaly papule, which develops into a superficial nodule. The nodule grows to form raised, purplish, superficial, irregular plaques that may have scaly, cracked, or verrucous centers. The infection can progress to form a large, papillomatous growth involving a large portion of a limb (Figure 104–2). Secondary bacterial infections cause regional lymphadenitis, lymph stasis, and elephantiasis. Nodular lesions are either smooth, verrucous, or scaly, and moderately elevated, soft, dull, and pink to violet. They gradually become tumorous, papillomatous, and occasionally lobulated (Figure 104–3). In time, tumorous lesions grow and have roughened surfaces resembling a cauliflower. Verrucous lesions are hyperkeratotic and frequently on the borders of the foot. The plaque is the least common lesion, and frequently has clusters of fungi in parakera-

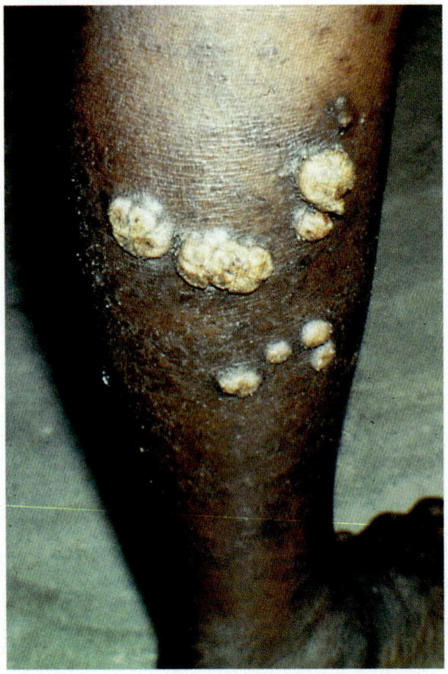

Figure 104–1. Chromoblastomycosis limited to the leg of a Zairian male agricultural worker. These multiple lesions could be contiguous with a satellite pattern of spread or they could be from autoinoculation—a consequence of itching and scratching. Lymphocutaneous spread, although suggested by the pattern of lesions at upper and lower right, seems unlikely because microscopically the fungi are not in lymphatics and regional lymph nodes do not become involved. *(Contributed by Leo O. Lanoie, MD, Karawa Mission Hospital, Republic of Zaire.)*

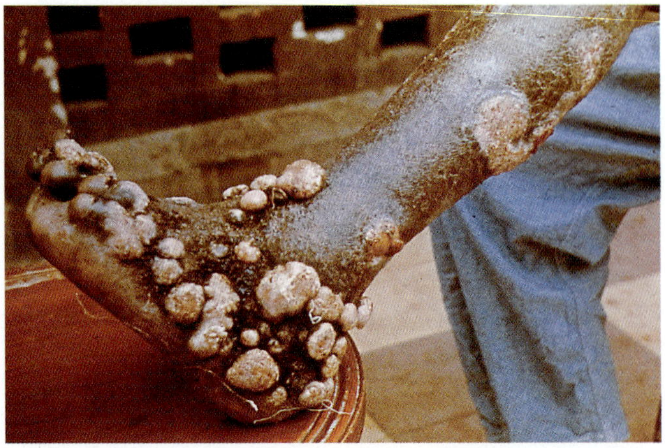

Figure 104–2. Chromoblastomycosis. Multiple verrucous nodules involve the skin of leg and foot.

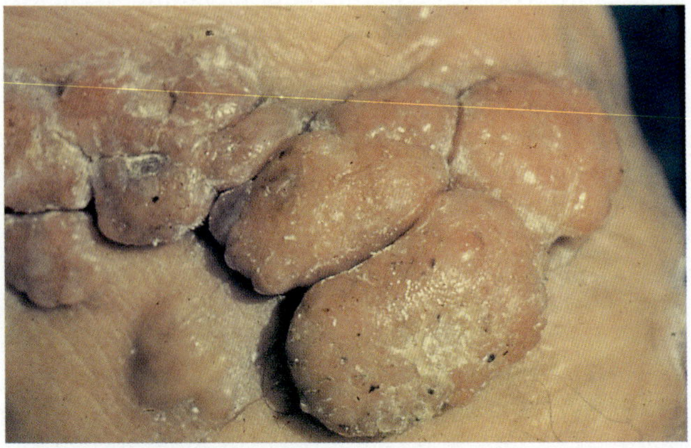

Figure 104–3. Chromoblastomycosis of the lower leg characterized by lobulated, confluent, cutaneous nodules with focal ulcerations.

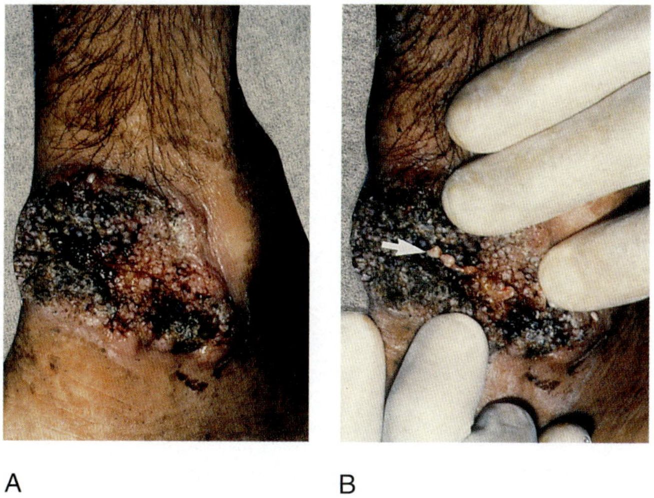

Figure 104–4. (**A**) Panamanian agricultural worker with chromoblastomycosis on the ankle. The lesion is verrucous and papillary with areas of depigmentation and hyperpigmentation. (**B**) The white structures at the arrow tip have been squeezed from the surface of the lesion. They are collections of neutrophils mixed with parakeratotic debris and fungi. *(By Ernest E. Lack, MD.)*

totic material that can be expressed from the surface of the lesion. Parakeratotic masses squeezed from the surface contain the typical fungi and confirm the diagnosis (Figures 104–4, B, and 104–5). The elimination of microorganisms and other structures from the surface of a lesion has been called transepithelial elimination (TEE).[5,9,10] In some lesions, fibrous tissue dominates and these lesions are annular or arciform or serpiginous, and develop by expanding centrifugally. These lesions have depressed centers from atrophic scarring.[1,8]

PATHOLOGY

The inflammatory reaction is characteristically suppurative and granulomatous (Figure 104–6) with dermal fibrosis and pseudoepitheliomatous hyperplasia (Figure 104–7). Dermal microabscesses contain the fungi (Figure 104–6) and may be surrounded by granulation tissue. Uribe et al[10] found suppurative inflammation and granulomas with macrophages, lymphocytes, giant cells, and epithelioid histiocytes in 96% of lesions. They also saw muriform brown fungi, most often in microabscesses in the interpapillary areas at the dermoepidermal junction. They identified pseudoepitheliomatous hyperplasia in 89% of lesions. Banks et al,[5] however, found a prominent infiltrate of eosinophils in the lesions of 15 of 17 (88%) Zairian patients (Figure 104–6).

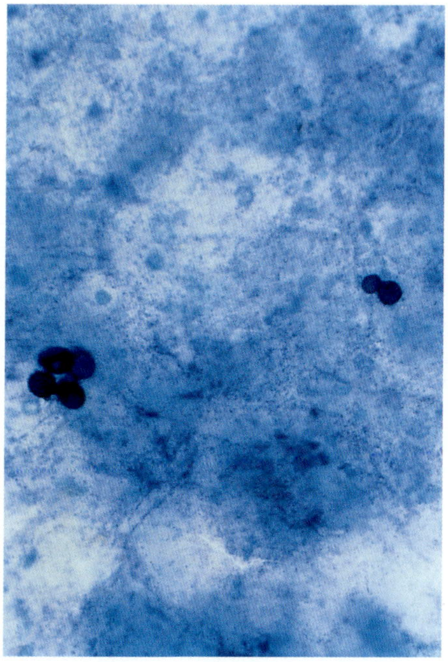

Figure 104–5. The parakeratotic material expressed from the lesion shown in Figure 104–4 was smeared and stained. A cluster of four and a cluster of two fungi are in this field and diagnostic of chromoblastomycosis (modified Giemsa stain, ×400). *(By Ernest E. Lack, MD.)*

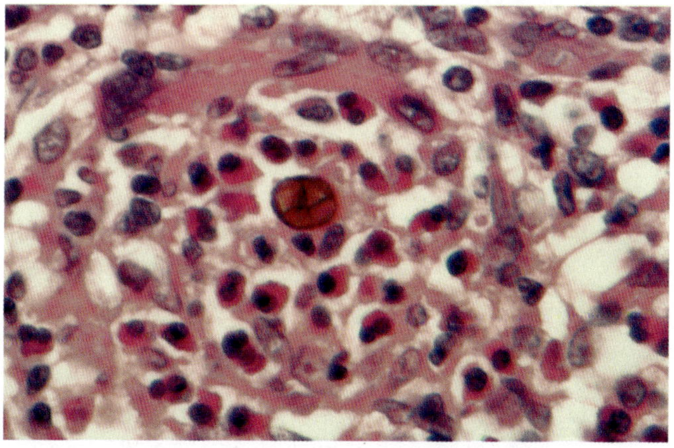

Figure 104–6. Typical dermal abscess in chromoblastomycosis. There is a quadrate cluster of organisms in the center surrounded by a mixture of neutrophils, macrophages, and numerous eosinophils. There is a giant cell at the perimeter *(top center).* The organisms, which have been called "copper pennies," "sclerotic bodies," and "Medlar bodies," are brown from melanin in their cell walls. They divide by internal septation frequently forming "back-to-back D's" and sometimes, as seen here, a quadrate cluster with opposed flattened surfaces (hematoxylin-eosin, ×250).

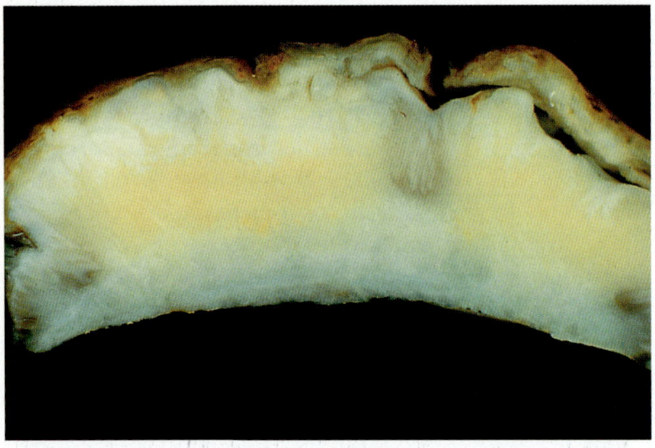

Figure 104–7. Cutaneous chromoblastomycosis showing the cut surface of a single nodule with a roughened cauliflower-like surface. The lesion is raised and has pinched-in margins and elongated rete ridges projecting into the dermis (gross, ×2). *(By Daniel H. Connor, MD, 1979.)*

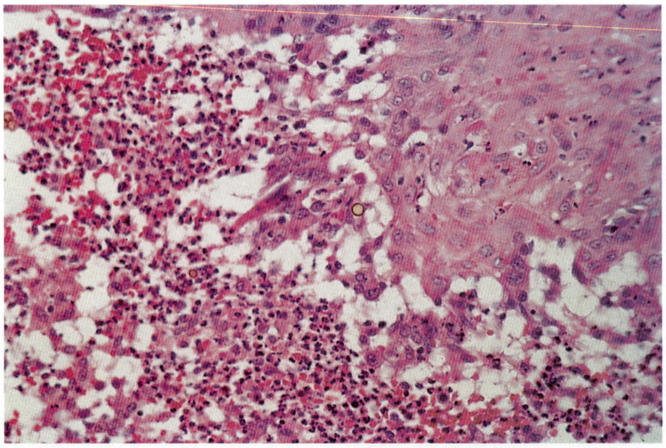

Figure 104–9. Epithelial hyperplasia begins when the fungi contact and provoke the basal layer. Here a single organism in the dermis, in contact with the epidermis, has stimulated the basal layer to form microscopic projections. These have begun to surround and enclose the fungus (AFIP Neg 83-9595; hematoxylin-eosin, ×120).

Although not a constant feature, plasma cells and Russell bodies are prominent in some lesions (Figure 104–8). Batres et al.[9] first identified TEE in chromoblastomycosis and noted that pseudoepitheliomatous hyperplasia was probably an expression of TEE. They showed also that elongated rete ridges first surround and trap clusters of fungi in the dermis (Figures 104–9 and 104–10), then incorporate the fungi in the epidermis (Figure 104–11). Their findings were confirmed in the larger series by Banks et al[5] who noted that fungi trapped in the epidermis continue to divide and, at the same time, migrate to the surface of the epidermis through tortuous columns that could be dilated ducts of sweat glands (Figure 104–11). When clusters of fungi

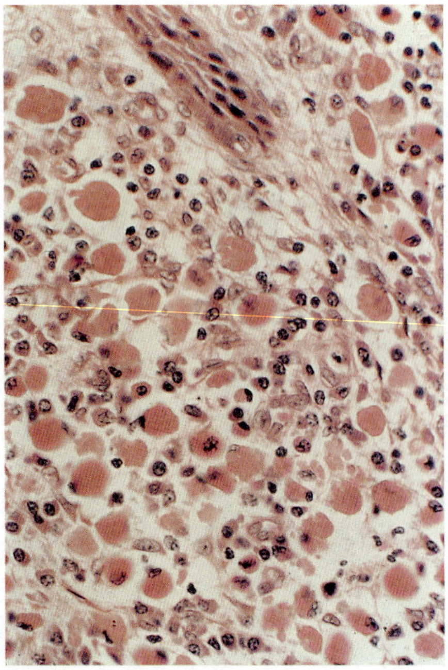

Figure 104–8. Although not always conspicuous, some lesions of chromoblastomycosis contain, as shown here, many plasma cells and Russell bodies in the exudate hematoxylin-eosin, ×250).

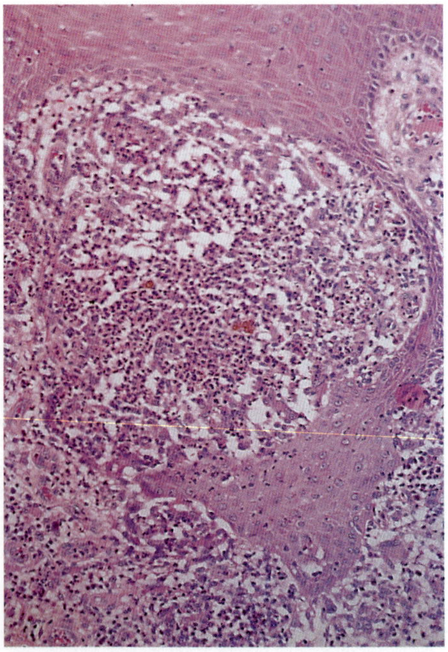

Figure 104–10. Cutaneous chromoblastomycosis. A greatly elongated rete ridge has formed a sweeping "pincers" movement around a cluster of fungi. Fungi that are enclosed by epithelial projections are incorporated into the epidermis and eventually shed from the surface by transepidermal elimination (AFIP Neg 83-9600; hematoxylin-eosin, ×150).

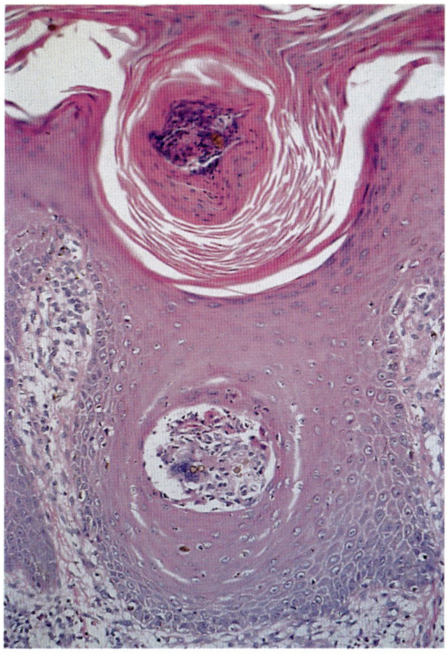

Figure 104–11. Chromoblastomycosis. Two cross-sections of an intraepidermal channel through which the organisms move to reach the surface. The location and tortuosity of these channels suggest that they may be expanded ducts of sweat glands. (AFIP Neg 83-9596; hematoxylin-eosin, ×150).

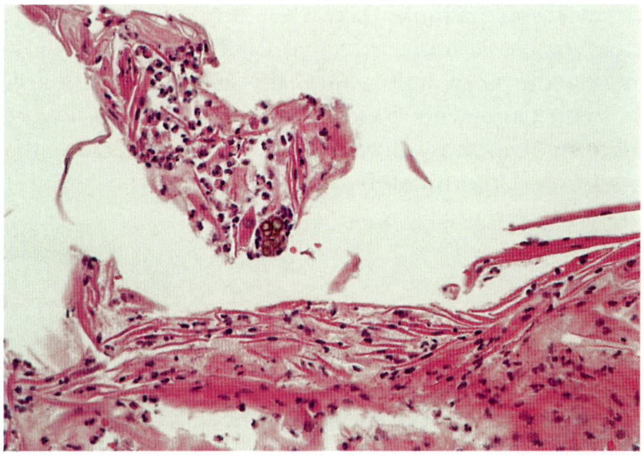

Figure 104–12. Chromoblastomycosis. A cluster of fungi is being sloughed from the surface of the skin in a parakeratotic scale. Microscopic identification of typical brown fungi in the scrapings from the surface of a lesion confirms a diagnosis of chromoblastomycosis (hematoxylin-eosin, ×70).

are sufficiently large and are shed in the keratin scales, they appear as black dots on the surface (Figure 104–12). These suggest a diagnosis of chromoblastomycosis, which can be confirmed when the muriform fungi are identified microscopically (Figure 104–5). Another cause of dark spots on the surface of the lesions of chromoblastomycosis is focal hemorrhage into the epidermis from dilated capillaries in the dermal papillae—hemorrhages that are shed with the parakeratotic scales.[5] Finally, while in the surface keratin, the organisms sometimes form short hyphae (Figure 104–13).

DIAGNOSIS

Clinically, a variety of lesions has been mistaken for chromoblastomycosis. Phaeohyphomycosis (phaeomycotic cyst) is occasionally mistaken for chromoblastomycosis.[11] Other lesions include keratoacanthoma, leishmaniasis, lepromatous leprosy, Kaposi's sarcoma, lobomycosis, paracoccidioidomycosis, sarcoidosis, squamous cell carcinoma, mossy foot, and cutaneous tuberculosis. Other dermatoses that can resemble chromoblastomycosis are blastomycosis, cutaneous leishmaniasis, and tropical lymphangitis.[8] The clinical presentation, histopathologic findings of chestnut brown muriform cells, and recovery, by culture, of one of the causal fungi, confirm the diagnosis. The fungi that cause this disease are readily grown on routine mycologic media. Monoclonal antibodies specific for surface antigens of *F pedrosoi* have been developed.[12]

TREATMENT

In early stages of chromoblastomycosis, surgical excision of the entire lesion may be curative. Cryosurgery and localized heat also have been effective in some patients with small lesions. The causal fungi tend to resist amphotericin B, and because these fungi are often sensitive to 5-fluorocytosine, these two drugs are used together to achieve synergism, which has proven effec-

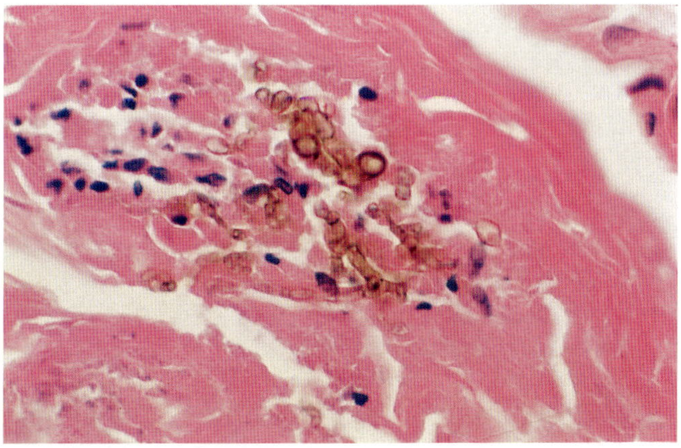

Figure 104–13. Chromoblastomycosis caused by *P verrucosa*. Dematiaceous hyphae and muriform cells are in the hyperkeratotic layer of the epidermis (hematoxylin-eosin, × 160).

tive in some patients. Likewise, amphotericin B plus ketoconazole is more effective than either drug alone. Fluconazole is of little value. In contrast, itraconazole has been used with good response. *Cladophialophora carrionii* responds more rapidly to itraconazole than *F pedrosoi.* Unfortunately, relapse is common.[13,14]

COMMENT

One can wonder at the variety of reactions mounted by the body against the organisms that cause chromoblastomycosis. Suppuration, cell-mediated immunity as expressed by the granulomatous reaction, humoral immunity as expressed by the many lymphocytes, plasma cells and Russell bodies, the vigorous reaction of eosinophils, and the phenomenon of TEE are all conspicuous, yet all ineffective. Why should this be? Any one or a combination of these reactions would be expected to eliminate an infection. But unlike so many successful parasites of mankind, the causes of chromoblastomycosis do not keep a low antigenic profile. In fact, they appear to engage vigorously every element of the body's defenses. Yet in spite of this, the infection smolders on, month after month, and year after year—no one of the reactions, nor combination of reactions, able to overcome the infection.

REFERENCES

1. Fader RC, McGinnis MR. Infections caused by dematiaceous fungi: chromoblastomycosis and phaeohyphomycosis. *Infect Dis Clin N Am.* 1988;2:925–938.
2. McGinnis MR. Chromoblastomycosis and phaeohyphomycosis: new concepts, diagnosis, and mycology. *J Am Acad Dermatol.* 1983;8:1–16.
3. McGinnis MR, Ajello L, Schell WA. Mycotic diseases: a proposed nomenclature. *Int J Dermatol.* 1985;24:9–15.
4. Milam CP, Fenske NA. Chromoblastomycosis. *Dermatol Clin.* 1989;7:219–225.
5. Banks IS, Palmieri JR, Lanoie LO, Connor DH, Meyers WM. Chromomycosis in Zaire. *Int J Dermatol* 1985;24:302–307.
6. Rosen T, Gyorkey F, Joseph LM, Batres E. Ultrastructural features of chromoblastomycosis. *Int J Dermatol.* 1980;19:461–468.
7. Okuda C, Ito M, Oka K. Relationship between tissue reactions and morphological changes of the fungi in chromoblastomycosis: morphometry and electron microscopy. *Arch Dermatol Res.* 1992;284:95–99.
8. Carrion AL. Chromoblastomycosis. *Ann NY Acad Sci.* 1950;50:1255–1282.
9. Batres E, Wolf JE, Rudolph AH, Knox JM. Transepithelial elimination of cutaneous chromomycosis. *Arch Dermatol.* 1978;114:1231–1232.
10. Uribe JF, Zuluaga AI, Leon W, Restrepo A. Histopathology of chromoblastomycosis. *Mycopathologia.* 1989;105:1–6.
11. Connor DH, Gibson DW. Association of splinters with chromomycosis and phaeomycotic cysts. *Lett Arch Dermatol.* 1985;121:168.
12. Esterre P, Ravisse P, Peyrol S, et al. Immunopathologie de la lésion cutanée de chromomycose. *J Mycol Méd* 1991;1:201–207.
13. Restrepo A. Treatment of tropical mycoses. *J Am Acad Dermatol* 1994;31:S91–S102.
14. Queiroz-Telles F, Purim KS, Fillus JN, et al. Itraconazole in the treatment of chromoblastomycosis due to *Fonsecaea pedrosoi. Int J Dermatol.* 1992;31:805–812.

CHAPTER 105

Coccidioidomycosis

Demosthenes Pappagianis and Francis W. Chandler

I tell thee that those viewless beings,
Whose mansion is the smallest particle
Of the impassive atmosphere,
Think, feel and live like man.

Percy Bysshe Shelley (1792–1822) (Queen Mab, Sect. II)

Always note and record the unusual. Keep and compare your observations. Communicate or publish short notes on anything that is striking or new.

Sir William Osler (1849–1919), Bulletin of the Johns Hopkins Hospital 1919;30:198

DEFINITION

Coccidioidomycosis is an infectious disease caused by *Coccidioides immitis,* a terricolous fungus. The disease usually is acquired by inhaling fungal conidia and may range from silent infection (in most people) to progressive infection and death. Coccidioidomycosis causes a wide variety of lesions and, like syphilis, is called a "great imitator."[1,2] Synonyms for coccidioidomycosis include coccidioidal granuloma, San Joaquin Valley fever, desert rheumatism, the bumps, cox, coccy, or cocci (this term should be avoided as its use, appropriate for certain bacteria, has caused confusion).

GEOGRAPHIC DISTRIBUTION

Coccidioides immitis exists in soil in limited areas of the New World from 40°N latitude in northern California to 40°S latitude in Argentina. The fungus favors arid climates with low rainfall, hot summers, and mild winters. The soil is often sandy and alkaline, and abundant ash is in soil where archaeologists have acquired coccidioidomycosis while digging for artefacts. In North America, many soils containing *C immitis* are coterminous with a geologic zone termed the Lower Sonoran Life Zone.[3]

LIFE CYCLE, NATURAL HISTORY, AND EPIDEMIOLOGY

Coccidioides immitis is diphasic and multimorphic with a hyphal/arthroconidial "saprobic" phase in nature and in routine culture, and a spherule/endospore "parasitic" phase in human tissues (and under special culture conditions). Arthroconidia, borne in chains on aerial hyphae, disarticulate and disperse in air currents. When inhaled, arthroconidia reach small airways where they replicate by endosporulation and provoke a pyogranulomatous response, cell-mediated immunity, hypersensitivity to coccidioidal antigens, and resolution with lasting immunity. In a few patients, however, organisms disseminate beyond the primary pulmonary focus. Dissemination is reported to be more common in African-Americans, Filipinos, and other Asians than among Caucasians. Mexicans and Native Americans also have a slightly higher rate of pulmonary dissemination than do Caucasians.[3] Other factors that adversely affect infection are blood group B, certain hematopoietic neoplasms,[4] acquired immunodeficiency syndrome

(AIDS),[5] immunosuppression for an organ transplant,[6,7] a "locus minoris resistentiae," and onset during the second and third trimesters of pregnancy. The nonpregnant adult Caucasian female, however, is less likely to have disseminated infection than the adult Caucasian male.

Transmission of *C immitis* from one human to another has not been documented, nor has transmission from one mammal to another except for a veterinarian who may have acquired infection while performing necropsy on a horse.[8] Dogs, horses, and other animals also become infected by inhaling arthroconidia.

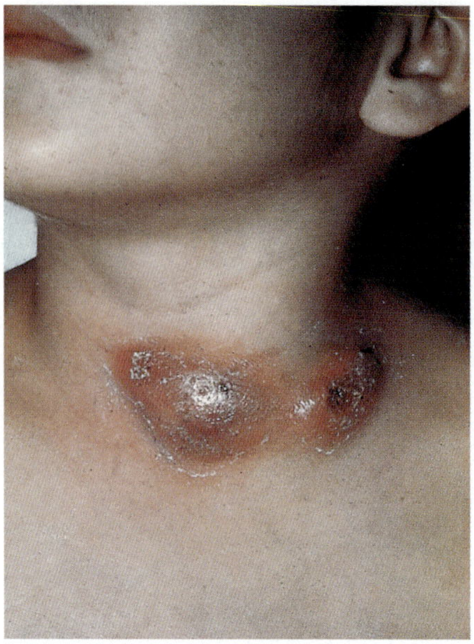

Figure 105–1. Disseminated coccidioidomycosis. Cutaneous lesions are large, sharply circumscribed, erythematous nodules. Microscopically, the lesions contained abundant fungal cells. *(Photograph courtesy of Centers for Disease Control and Prevention, Atlanta.)*

CLINICAL FEATURES

There are four basic clinical forms of coccidioidomycosis: pulmonary (asymptomatic or symptomatic), disseminated, residual pulmonary, and primary cutaneous. Approximately 60% of primary pulmonary infections are silent and detected by coccidioidin or spherulin skin tests. Of the 40% of patients with clinically apparent infections, manifestations are varied. In acute primary pulmonary coccidioidomycosis, there is chest pain (71%), cough (65%), fever (64%), and malaise (41%). Primary pulmonary infection is usually detected on chest radiographs (see the Differential Diagnosis section), and approximately 20% of patients have a rash that manifests in various forms. An estimated 5% of patients with clinically apparent primary pulmonary coccidioidomycosis have disseminated infections. These patients may continue to have pulmonary manifestations, but may also develop lesions in cutaneous and subcutaneous tissues (Figures 105–1 and 105–2), bones and joints, viscera, and the meninges. About 10% of patients with symptomatic primary pulmonary infection develop residual pulmonary coccidioidomycosis presenting as single cavities, fibrocaseous nodules (coccidioidomas) and fibrocavitary lesions that resemble those of chronic tuberculosis (Figure 105–3). The primary cutaneous form of coccidioidomycosis is rare and is caused by direct percutaneous inoculation of the fungus. An ulcer or chancre usually develops at the site of inoculation and is often accompanied by regional lymphadenopathy.

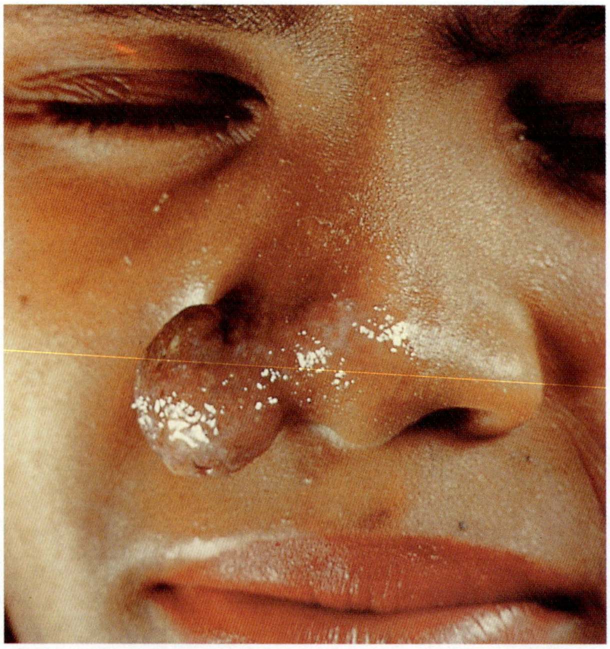

Figure 105–2. Cutaneous lesion in disseminated coccidioidomycosis. An enlarging, erythematous nodule involves the nose. *(Photograph courtesy of Centers for Disease Control and Prevention, Atlanta.)*

MORPHOLOGIC FEATURES OF THE ORGANISM

The saprophytic ("saprobic") or in vitro phase of *C immitis,* in nature and the usual culture medium, is represented by hyphae 2 to 4 μm wide that may produce shorter hyphae 1 to 2 μm wide on which are borne infectious arthroconidia. Arthroconidia are typically barrel-shaped and 2 to 4 μm by 5 to 6 μm, but they also may be cylindrical or oval. They are usually separated

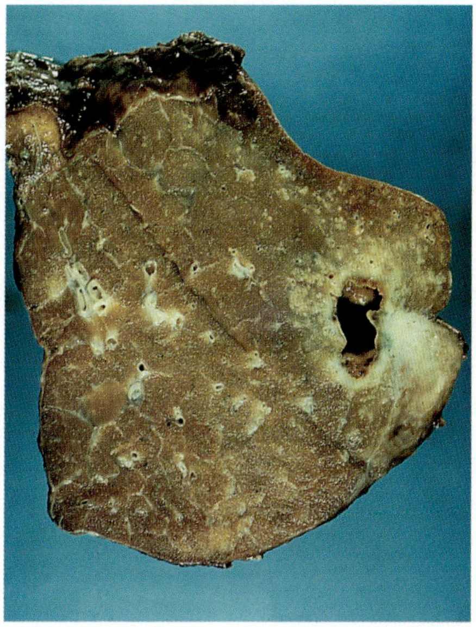

Figure 105–3. Residual pulmonary coccidioidomycosis. The lung contains a solitary, thin-walled, fibrocavitary lesion *(right)* that resembles those of chronic tuberculosis. *(Photograph courtesy of David H. Dail, MD.)*

from each other in the chain by empty degenerate cells that can fracture, permitting disarticulation ("rhexolytic dehiscence") and dispersion.

In a suitable medium, arthroconidia are formed in 5 to 7 days at 34°C to 37°C. This interval is significant because opening a culture at less than 5 days is less risky. After arthroconidia are inhaled or inoculated, they become spherical, increase in size, and, in approximately 48 hours (in the experimental host), become thick-walled endosporulating spherules 20 to 100 μm in diameter (Figure 105–4). In succeeding hours, the spherules rupture and release uninucleate endospores 2 to 5 μm in diameter (Figure 105–5). Each endospore then enlarges to become a mature spherule and repeats the reproductive cycle (Figure 105–6). Branched, septate hyphae and barrel-shaped arthroconidia sometimes are produced in pulmonary cavities, especially those that communicate with the bronchial tree (Figure 105–7). However, these have not led to infections in other individuals. Hyphal fragments of *C immitis* are in 10% to 30% of coccidioidal cavities. The endosporulating spherule is diagnostic in tissue, but in vitro, colonies of *C immitis* may be indistinguishable from several nonpathogenic fungi.

PATHOLOGY

Pulmonary lesions may be miliary and from 1 to 3 mm up to several centimeters across. The "thin-walled" cavity noted on chest radiographs often has a wall several millimeters thick. Coccidioidal fungus ball (mislabeled

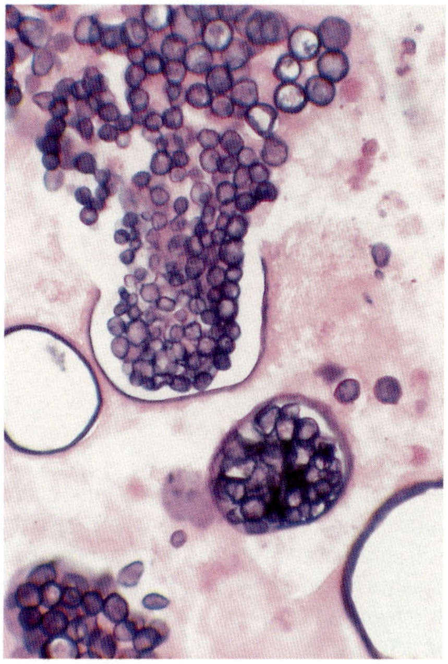

Figure 105–4. Immature (empty) and endosporulating spherules of *Coccidioides immitis*. The walls of immature spherules and endospores are uniformly blackened with the GMS stain, but walls of endosporulating spherules vary in their staining intensity. One of the endosporulating spherules has ruptured *(top)*, and many endospores are being released (Gomori's methenamine silver–hematoxylin-eosin, ×250).

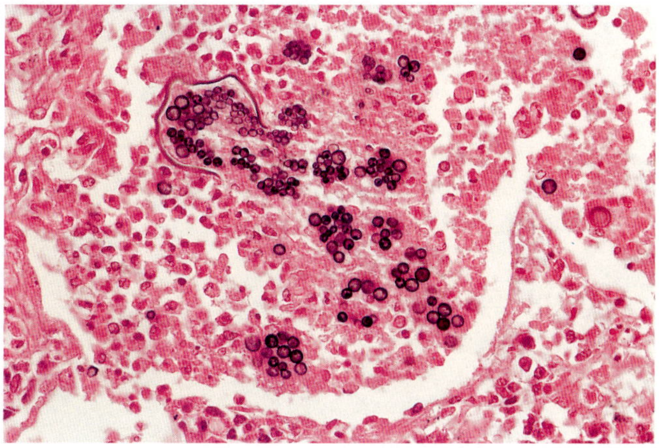

Figure 105–5. Ruptured endosporulating spherule of *Coccidioides immitis*. The recently released endospores, 2 to 5 μm in diameter, elicit a suppurative inflammatory reaction. Note that released endospores tend to cluster in small packets (Gomori's methenamine silver–hematoxylin-eosin, ×100).

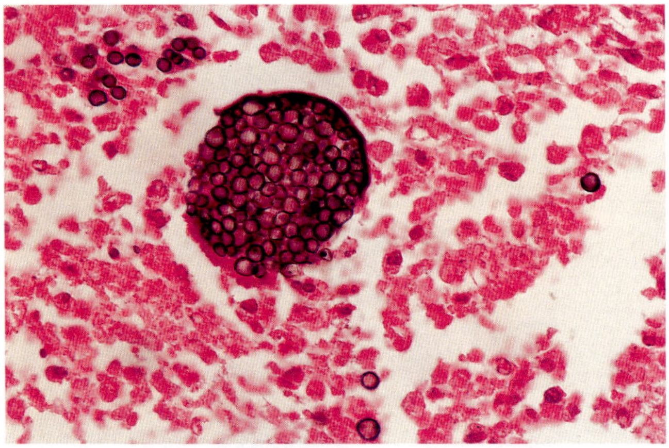

Figure 105–6. *Coccidioides immitis.* A large endosporulating spherule (approximately 100 μm in diameter) has ruptured, and many spherical, compact endospores are being released. Endospore walls are intensely silvered with the GMS stain. Only a portion of the spherule wall remains intact *(top)* (Gomori's methenamine silver–hematoxylin-eosin, ×160).

"pulmonary mycetoma") has been reported by several authors.[9] Osseous lesions may be lytic or proliferative, and villous synovitis often complicates coccidioidal arthritis. Cutaneous lesions, which include erythema nodosum and erythema multiforme and may be urticarial, papular, morbilliform, or vesicular, are probably hypersensitivity reactions to coccidioidal antigens. Cutaneous lesions from dissemination of *C immitis* from a primary pulmonary infection may be pustular, crusted, verrucous, plaque-like, or granulomatous, and contain intact fungal cells.[10] Direct inoculation of the skin has caused "chancriform complex"—a pustular or ulcerated lesion with regional lymphadenopathy.[11] Coccidioidal chorioretinitis varies from large exudative or oval, edematous lesions to sharply punched-out chorioretinal scars with varying degrees of hyper-pigmentation or depigmentation.[12]

Many animals with coccidioidomycosis have similar lesions, but there are exceptions. Osseous lesions in humans tend to be lytic,[13] but in dogs they are destructive and productive (periosteal and endosteal).[14]

Microscopically, *C immitis* can be identified in synovial, pleural, pericardial, or peritoneal fluids, but the diagnosis is more successful when tissue specimens are examined.[15] Active lesions usually contain numerous organisms, and diagnostic endosporulating spherules are easily seen in hematoxylin-eosin stained tissue sections (Figure 105–8). Resolving and residual lesions contain fewer organisms, which are best seen with the Gomori's methenamine silver (GMS) stain. Endospores and immature spherules also are periodic acid–Schiff (PAS)-positive, but the walls of mature spherules stain weakly or not at all with the PAS reaction and other special stains for fungi because of their high phospholipid content (Figure 105–9). Other GMS-positive organisms, eg, *Pneumocystis carinii,* may be coincidentally present.

Histopathologically, there is a predominantly suppurative reaction to recently released endospores and a granulomatous reaction to maturing spherules (Figure 105–10).[16] The typical active lesion, therefore, tends to have central suppuration and a surrounding granulomatous reaction (Figure 105–11). Detection of *C immitis* distinguishes these granulomas from other pyogran-

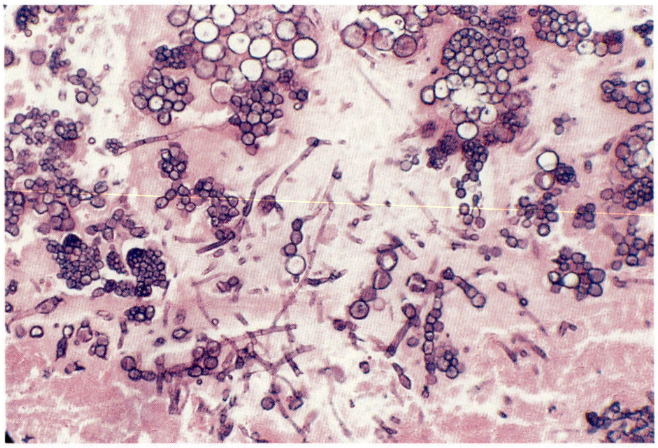

Figure 105–7. Miliary pulmonary coccidioidomycosis in an immunosuppressed patient. The center of a necrotic nodule contains numerous immature and endosporulating spherules, septate hyphae, and typical arthroconidia of *Coccidioides immitis.* Arthroconidia are produced by septal disarticulation of hyphae *(bottom center)* (Gomori's methenamine silver–hematoxylin-eosin, ×40).

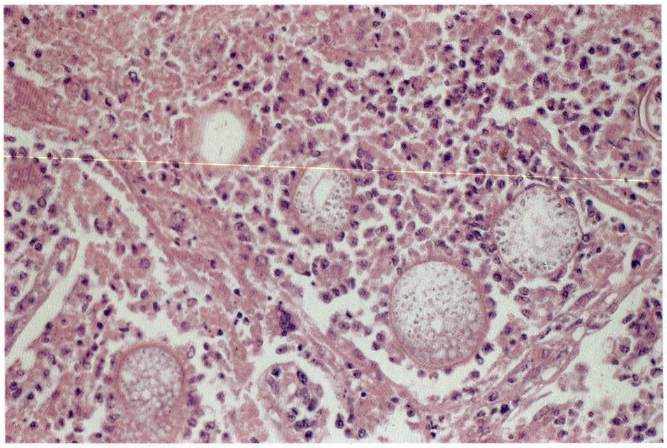

Figure 105–8. Acute pulmonary coccidioidomycosis. Mature endosporulating spherules and recently released endospores are lightly hematoxylinophilic and elicit a mixed suppurative and granulomatous inflammatory reaction (hematoxylin-eosin, ×40).

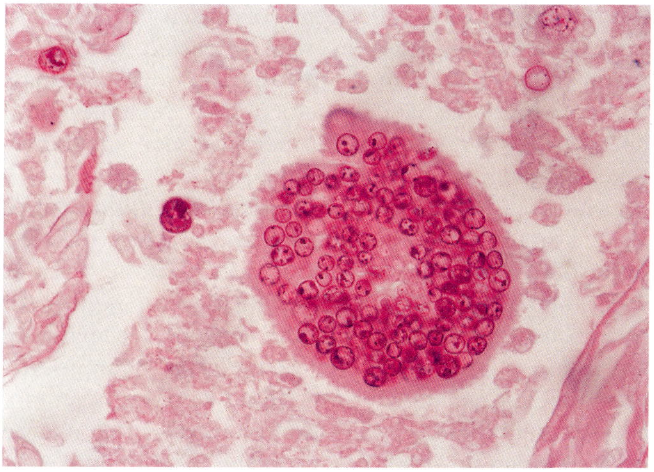

Figure 105–9. Mature spherule of *Coccidioides immitis*. When treated with the PAS reaction, the walls and cytoplasmic inclusions of endospores are intensely reactive, but the walls of spherules are nonreactive because of their high phospholipid content (periodic acid–Schiff, ×250).

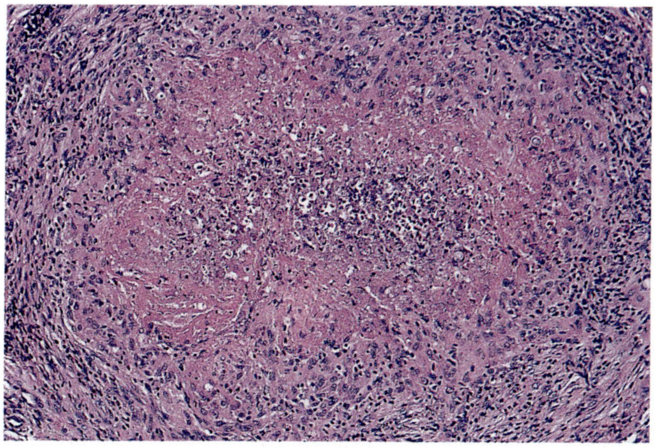

Figure 105–11. Miliary pulmonary coccidioidomycosis. The typical active lesion consists of an epithelioid and giant cell granuloma with central suppuration and necrosis (hematoxylin-eosin, ×40). *(Photograph courtesy of John C. Watts, MD.)*

ulomatous lesions, especially those of blastomycosis (see Chapter 101), paracoccidioidomycosis (see Chapter 114), and certain other granulomatous diseases. Often, there is a mixed inflammatory reaction with a microabscess and granuloma side by side. In other lesions, there is a preponderance of dispersed epithelioid macrophages. Spherules and aggregates of endospores are sometimes surrounded by radiating, intensely eosinophilic Splendore-Hoeppli material (Figure 105–12). Eosinophilia may cause eosinophilic pneumonia.[17–19]

Caseous necrosis with or without calcification, fibrosis, and peripheral collections of lymphocytes are features of residual coccidioidal granulomas (coccidioidomas) (Figure 105–13). Residual granulomas often do not contain detectable or morphologically distinctive organisms (Figure 105–14); culture and/or serology are then needed to confirm the diagnosis.

The inflammatory response and rate of replication of *C immitis* are influenced by the patient's immune status and by underlying disease. For example, lungs of

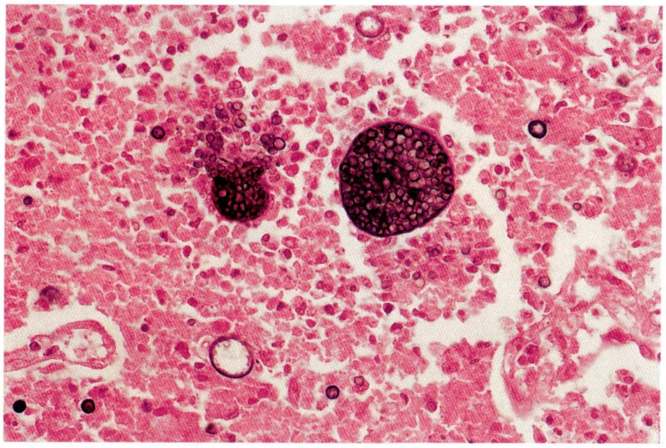

Figure 105–10. Primary pulmonary coccidioidomycosis. There is a predominantly suppurative reaction to recently released endospores of *Coccidioides immitis (left center)* and a granulomatous reaction to maturing spherules of this fungus (Gomori's methenamine silver–hematoxylin-eosin, ×100).

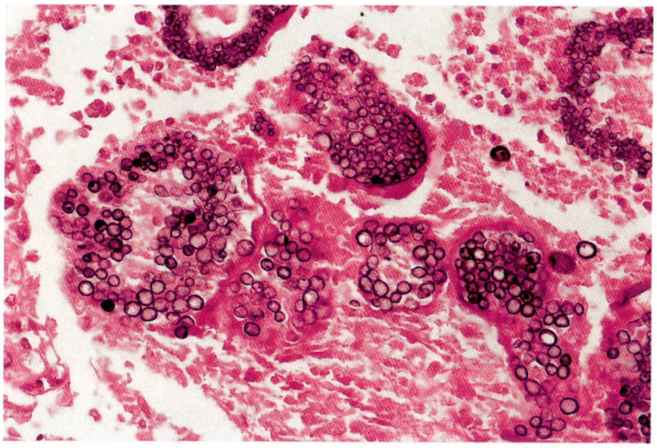

Figure 105–12. Intact and ruptured endosporulating spherules of *Coccidioides immitis* within a pulmonary granuloma. Intensely eosinophilic Splendore-Hoeppli material coats the spherules. Walls of spherules are variably stained with GMS. Endospores are strongly GMS-positive (Gomori's methenamine silver–hematoxylin-eosin, ×100).

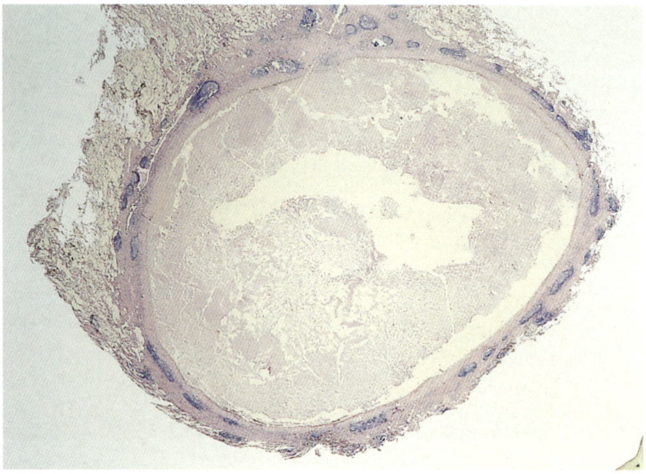

Figure 105–13. Residual pulmonary coccidioidomycosis (coccidioidoma). A large central zone of caseous necrosis is surrounded by a fibrous capsule that contains prominent lymphoid aggregates and scattered epithelioid cells and giant cells. Spherules of *Coccidioides immitis* within the central caseous residuum are not readily visible at this magnification (hematoxylin-eosin, ×8).

experimentally infected monkeys previously immunized by subcutaneous inoculation of *C immitis* or of formaldehyde-killed spherules had less necrosis, more mature granulomas, and fewer *C immitis* cells than those of nonimmunized monkeys.[20,21] In patients with coccidioidomycosis and AIDS, pulmonary lesions have an "abortive or poorly developed granulomatous response."[22] Also, there are fewer lymphocytes, only loosely organized collections of macrophages, and fewer giant cells than in well-organized epithelioid granulomas of immunocompetent controls. Vasculitis with perivascular inflammatory cell infiltrates and endarteritis obliterans are sometimes seen in coccidioidal meningitis and encephalitis.[23]

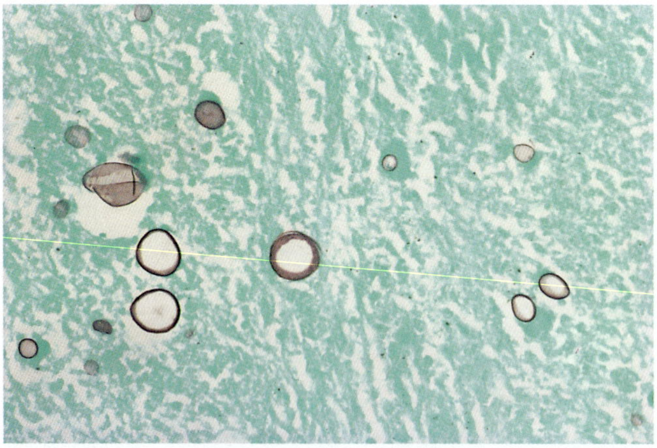

Figure 105–14. Necrotic center of residual pulmonary nodule (coccidioidoma). Empty and distorted immature spherules of *Coccidioides immitis* resemble yeast-form fungi, especially *Cryptococcus neoformans*. Other fields should be searched for typical endosporulating spherules of *C immitis* or collapsed spherule walls contiguous to packets of recently released endospores. The combination of any of these morphologic forms is diagnostic for coccidioidomycosis (Gomori's methenamine silver, ×160).

As noted previously, spherules of *C immitis* provoke a granulomatous reaction, and recently released endospores provoke a suppurative reaction (Figures 105–5 and 105–10).[24,25] Progressive development of an outer phospholipid layer in the wall of the maturing spherule is associated with a change from granulocytic to monocytic inflammation.[26] Thus, there are microabscesses within the centers of granulomas (ie, mature endosporulating spherules inducing a granulomatous response, and recently released endospores eliciting suppurative inflammation and microabscesses) (Figure 105–11). When released, endospores are held together in a matrix thought to be glycoprotein (although it is not stained by PAS or GMS).[27] This matrix impedes phagocytosis of endospores.[28] Huntington[29] described "Schiff-positive dust" within giant cells in pulmonary coccidioidomycosis.

The host reaction in coccidioidomycosis also is influenced by soluble coccidioidal substances that, in the presence of heat-labile serum components (possibly complement), are chemotactic for human neutrophils.[30] Chemotaxis is facilitated by cytokines from host leukocytes[31] and perhaps by complement activated by antigen–antibody complexes that precipitate in fibrin as well as in agar used for gel diffusion.[32] Suppression of the cellular response in mice is achieved by administering soluble coccidioidal antigen.[33,34] Cox[35] demonstrated that extracts of *C immitis* cell walls suppressed T lymphocytes by activating splenic suppressor cells. Patients with AIDS and coccidioidomycosis tend to deteriorate when CD_4 lymphocyte counts drop below $200/mm^3$.[35]

ELECTRON MICROSCOPIC FEATURES

The arthroconidia, uninucleate or multinucleate, are borne on a short hyphal strand (conidiophore?) that is narrower than the usual nonfertile (vegetative) hypha. Arthroconidia often alternate with disjunctor cells and have a bilaminar wall composed of an outer electron dense layer and an inner less dense layer. The disjunctor cells retain only the thin electron dense outer layer and lose intracellular components. The disjunctors fracture, permitting release and dispersion of adjacent arthroconidia.

Germination of arthroconidia produces hyphae with bilaminar septa that have pores and nearby granules (Woronin bodies) as found in the Ascomycotina.[36–38] The wall of the spherule also is bilaminar,[36,37,39,40] and in vivo there is a peripheral (possibly phospholipid) layer.[26] Invagination of the plasma membrane of young multinucleate spherules also includes the inner less dense layer that produces cytoplasmic compartments.[38] The cleavage planes, consisting of chitin and beta-glucan and later alpha-glucan and mannoprotein,[41] ultimately partition the cytoplasm into uninucleate endospores arrayed in clusters in a fibrillar matrix that may be antiphagocytic.[39–43] Clusters of endospores are released through a rupture or ostiole of the wall of the spherule.[38] Neutrophils damage the outer wall of the spherule,[43] but there is limited killing of *C immitis*. In the presence of sensitized human lymphocytes, monocytes undergo phagosome–lysosome fusion and kill phagocytosed *C immitis* cells.[44]

DIFFERENTIAL DIAGNOSIS

Because coccidioidomycosis affects almost any organ system, it mimics many diseases and thus provokes a broad differential diagnosis. Only rarely, however, does coccidioidomycosis involve the endocardium and gastrointestinal mucosa.[45] Presence in an endemic area is helpful in suspecting coccidioidomycosis.

Acute primary pulmonary coccidioidomycosis may cause a mild influenza-like illness in which the complaints do not suggest a pulmonary lesion, or there may be pneumonitis. Pneumonitis does not usually impair respiratory function, but in some patients there may be rapid progression to respiratory insufficiency and death. There may be lobar, segmental, patchy, discrete unifocal or multifocal pulmonary infiltrates that are usually homogeneous but may vary from "a veil-like haze or vague mottling" to dense consolidations.[16] Peribronchial and miliary or diffuse reticulonodular infiltrates frequently result from hematogenous dissemination and often complicate coccidioidomycosis in patients with AIDS.[5] These varied patterns resemble other pneumonitides, including those caused by bacteria and other fungi, and rarely may be interpreted as "eosinophilic pneumonia."[18,19] There is often hilar adenopathy, usually associated with parenchymal disease. Lesions may resemble sarcoidosis, and when accompanied by peripheral eosinophilia may prompt premature mediastinoscopy in anticipation of Hodgkin's disease. The adenopathy may extend to the mediastinal, paratracheal, and even supraclavicular lymph nodes. Pleural and pericardial effusions and transient pulmonary cavities add to the spectrum of acute primary coccidioidomycosis.

Equally varied are the chronic pulmonary changes: a solitary pulmonary nodule (coccidioidoma) must be distinguished from a neoplasm or a tuberculoma; bilateral apical fibrocavitary disease may resemble tuberculosis and histoplasmosis capsulati and have a dismal and gradually progressive course in spite of antifungal therapy. The pulmonary cavity in coccidioidomycosis may resemble other fungal diseases or mycobacterial infections, and when a fluid level is present it can resemble a bacterial abscess. Rupture through the pleura can cause hydropneumothorax or empyema. A coccidioidal fungus ball ("pulmonary mycetoma") has been described and must be differentiated from fungus balls caused by other fungi.[9] Less frequently, bronchiectasis is a residuum of chronic pulmonary coccidioidomycosis.

Because disseminated coccidioidomycosis can involve almost any organ, many diseases, including those that are infectious and neoplastic, also must be considered. Coccidioidomycosis has caused dysuria and the suspicion of benign prostatic hyperplasia,[46] and even recurrent carcinoma of the prostate was suspected in a patient with coccidioidal prostatitis.[47] Both extraocular and intraocular coccidioidomycosis can resemble inflammatory ophthalmic diseases of other causes.

Coccidioidomycosis has kept company with neoplastic conditions.[4,48] In general, malignancies of the hematopoietic system adversely affect concomitant coccidioidomycosis, whereas other malignancies do not.[48] Lymphocytopenia was correlated with risk of dissemination of coccidioidomycosis.[4] Coexistent coccidioidomycosis and tuberculosis also have been reported,[49] as have coccidioidomycosis and histoplasmosis capsulati or blastomycosis.[50,51] Progressive and lethal coccidioidomycosis has been reported in many patients with AIDS,[5,52] and often there has been concomitant infection with other agents (eg, *Pneumocystis carinii*).[52] The inflammatory response elicited by *C immitis* has been mistaken for malignancy (in lung and pulmonary lymph nodes). Sometimes, a needle biopsy has led to a diagnosis of carcinoma, followed by pneumonectomy and lymphadenectomy; postoperatively, the tissues had only coccidioidal disease. In an unusual proximity, *Cryptococcus neoformans* and *C immitis* were in the same lesion in the lung of a cheetah in the San Diego Zoo.[53] Both organisms were recovered by culture.

Histologically, myospherulosis, a pseudomycosis characterized by pigmented bodies (parent bodies) and internal spherules (endobodies) within cystic stromal spaces of the soft tissues and upper respiratory tract, is an entity that may be confused with coccidioidomycosis.[54] The pigmented (brown) bodies of myospherulosis are erythrocytes altered by lipid, and they may superficially resemble endosporulating spherules of *C immitis* (Figure 105–15). Tissue forms of *C immitis,* however, are never pigmented. In addition, the pigmented bodies of myospherulosis do not stain with GMS and other special stains for fungi.

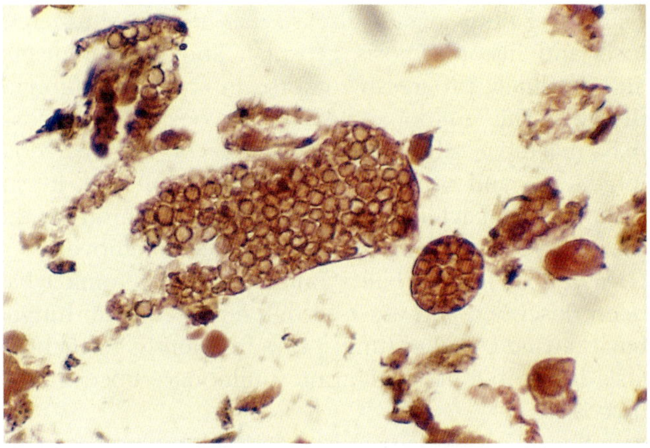

Figure 105–15. Myospherulosis. A cystic stromal space within the nasal mucosa contains pigmented bodies that superficially resemble endosporulating spherules of *Coccidioides immitis*. (Spherical endobodies within the parent bodies are not blackened with the GMS stain, a feature that readily distinguishes them from the GMS-positive endospores of *C immitis*) (hematoxylin-eosin, ×160).

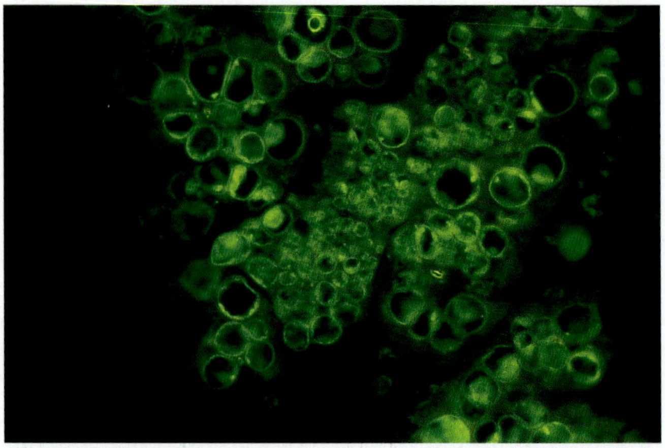

Figure 105–16. Immunofluorescence of *Coccidioides immitis* within a necrotizing pulmonary granuloma. Walls of endospores and immature spherules are brightly decorated with a species-specific conjugate, but walls of mature spherules are not decorated. The pattern of fluorescence resembles the PAS reaction (see Figure 105–9) (Direct immunofluorescence, ×160).

MOLECULAR DIAGNOSIS

A nucleic acid "hybrid protection assay" has been developed for the rapid (45 minutes) identification of *C immitis* (Gen-Probe, Inc., San Diego).[55] Ribosomal RNA is extracted from the suspect colony and allowed to hybridize with a reference DNA probe to which is attached an acridinium ester. If hybridization takes place (ie, coccidioidal rRNA is present), the hybrid containing the attached acridinium will withstand hydrolysis and be luminescent. If noncoccidioidal RNA is present, there will be no hybridization and unhybridized DNA-acridinium ester will be hydrolyzed and therefore nonluminescent.

Monoclonal antibodies can be used to identify certain components of *C immitis* in clinical specimens, but they are not yet more useful than polyclonal antibodies. Direct immunofluorescence using a polyclonal antibody has been applied for the detection of *C immitis* in fixed, deparaffinized tissue sections (Figure 105–16).[54,56]

CONFIRMATIONAL TESTING AND DIAGNOSIS

Direct Microscopy

The presence of typical endosporulating spherules is diagnostic. Spherules can be demonstrated in tissues or body fluids with conventional stains (eg, hematoxylin-eosin and GMS for tissues[29,54]; Papanicolaou for respiratory secretions[57]). Calcofluor, a nonspecific whitening agent, also can be used to detect *C immitis* (eg, in bronchoalveolar lavage fluid).

Culture

If tissues or body fluids are unavailable or unrevealing for confirming coccidioidomycosis, cultures should be prepared. Sputum, lesional exudates, effusions, cerebrospinal fluid (CSF), peripheral blood, urine, biopsy specimens (tissue or bone marrow), and gastric, bronchial, or transtracheal washings or stools may yield *C immitis*. Usually, it is not difficult to recover *C immitis* because the fungus is not exacting in its nutritional requirements (summarized in ref. 58); however, specimens must be cultured prior to digestion or other treatment of sputum used for the recovery of *Mycobacterium tuberculosis*[59] because pretreatment can damage *C immitis*. To reduce the chance of overgrowth by other organisms, the specimen can be pretreated with penicillin G and streptomycin or another aminoglycoside. A cycloheximide- and chloramphenicol-containing agar medium can be used, as can a medium with elevated pH (eg, by the addition of NH_4OH or K_3PO_4 with or without $CuSO_4$[0.04%]) to select for *C immitis*. Ordinary bacteriologic agar media (sheep blood, brain-heart infusion, trypticase soy, Sabouraud's glucose) yield colonies 1 to 4 mm across by 48 hours and 2 to 9 mm across by 72 hours, but the cultures should not be discarded as "no growth" until at least 14 days have elapsed.

Growth of *C immitis* is at first grayish-white, cottony, and web-like. Later, colonies become granular and faintly cream colored on the obverse, whereas the reverse is tan to brownish. However, because there is sufficient variation in colonial morphology of different isolates, a definitive diagnosis cannot be made from the

TABLE 105–1. DIAGNOSTIC TESTS FOR COCCIDIOIDOMYCOSIS

Biopsy, necropsy, sputum, effusion,[a] exudate
- Direct: endosporulating spherule
- Animal inoculation: endosporulating spherule

Culture
- Exoantigen test
- Hybrid protection assay of ribosomal RNA
- Animal inoculation for endosporulating spherule

Serologic
- Serum, CSF, synovial and pleural fluid
- Latex particle, immunodiffusion, complement fixation, enzyme-linked immunosorbent assay

Skin test
- Coccidioidin or spherulin; diagnostic only if recent conversion (−) to (+); helpful for asymptomatic pulmonary disease

[a] Infected tissue of site is positive more often than fluid.

gross and microscopic features alone. Members of the nonpathogenic genera *Arachniotus, Auxarthron, Malbranchea, Pseudoarachniotus,* and *Uncinocarpus* may contaminate clinical specimens and produce catenulate arthroconidia resembling those of *C immitis.*[60] Specific identification requires one of the following (see also Table 105–1):

1. Identification of the endosporulating spherule after inoculation of laboratory animals or of special culture media
2. Exoantigen identification of suspect culture
3. Nucleic acid hybridization (hybrid protection assay) as described previously

Serologic and Immunologic Procedures

Specimens may not be readily available for biopsy or culture. If cultures are obtained, it may take up to 2 weeks to identify *C immitis.* (This could be reduced to 1 week or less with the DNA-hybrid protection assay.) Serologic tests are sensitive and specific. Smith[61] established that the usual patient with symptomatic, acute, primary, coccidioidal infection will develop a positive delayed hypersensitivity cutaneous response to coccidioidin and an early "precipitin" antibody (now known to be IgM) and later complement fixing antibody (now known to be IgG).[32] (It is evident that a patient may be, for various reasons, unreactive to coccidioidin or spherulin. Serologic studies should be done regardless of whether the skin test is reactive.) The antigen reactive with IgG in fixing complement is a chitinase.[62] Available evidence indicates that antigen(s) that react(s) with IgM contain(s) abundant polysaccharide[63] and may be a β-glucosidase (or glucanase),[64] but a protease also has been proposed to react with IgM.[65] IgM may be the only antibody in early infection. It can be detected by tube precipitin (TP), latex particle agglutination (LA), immunodiffusion corresponding to TP (IDTP), and enzyme-linked immunosorbent assay (ELISA) (Table 105–2).

Later-appearing IgG can be detected by complement fixation (CF) or by immunodiffusion that detects the same antibody (IDCF). The titer by CF (or by quantitative IDCF) corresponds to the extent of coccidioidal disease. Thus, a rising titer of IgG indicates extension (worsening), whereas a declining titer indicates improvement. Depending on the technique, a CF titer exceeding 1 : 16 should alert clinicians to the possibility of metapulmonary dissemination. Potentially lethal infections (acute pulmonary, meningeal), however, may occur in spite of a low CF titer (eg, 1 : 2 to 1 : 8). The detection and measurement of antibody can be done on other body fluids. For example, CF titers on CSF usually indicate coccidioidal meningitis, but may also indicate a juxtadural lesion. Coccidioidal IgM in the CSF (barring gross contamination with blood) indicates coccidioidal meningitis. Caution is needed in the interpretation of more sensitive tests (eg, immunodiffusion after concentrating the CSF or ELISA) as they may detect coccidioidal IgG in the CSF even in the absence of coccidioidal meningitis.[66,67]

TABLE 105–2. SEROLOGIC CATEGORIES OF COCCIDIOIDOMYCOSIS

	Type of Disease				
	Very Early and Most Asymptomatic Primary; Some Immunodeficient	*Primary*		*Continuing Disseminated; Old Pulmonary Cavity*	*Past*
		Early	*Later*		
Precipitin (IgM) = IDTP[a]	(−)	(+)	(+)	(+) or (−)	(−)
CF[a] (IgG) = IDCF[a]	(−)	(−)	(+)	(+)	(+) or (−)

[a] CF, complement fixation; IDCF, immunodiffusion corresponding to CF; IDTP, immunodiffusion corresponding to tube precipitin and latex particle agglutination.

TREATMENT

Depending on the form of coccidioidomycosis, surgical or medical therapy may be required.[68] The chronic pulmonary cavity rarely responds to antifungal therapy. Parenteral amphotericin B may be used for rapidly progressive acute pulmonary or widespread disseminated coccidioidomycosis. Additional chemotherapy is now available in the form of ketoconazole or the triazoles—fluconazole or itraconazole—which can be administered orally, have fewer side effects than amphotericin B, and can be used for more indolent forms, including disseminated coccidioidomycosis. Meningitis, which had long been treated by intrathecal or intraventricular injection of amphotericin B, can be treated with oral fluconazole or itraconazole, although these azoles may have to be continued for the lifetime of the patient.[69] Even in patients without meningitis, prolonged (and expensive) treatment may be required because the azoles are fungistatic, and relapses have occurred even after treatment for longer than 1 year.

REFERENCES

1. Ampel NM, Wieden MA, Galgiani JN. Coccidioidomycosis: clinical update. *Rev Infect Dis.* 1989;11:897–911.
2. Huntington RW Jr. Coccidioidomycosis: a great imitator disease. *Arch Pathol Lab Med.* 1986;110:182. Editorial.
3. Pappagianis D. Epidemiology of coccidioidomycosis. *Current Topics Med Mycol.* 1988;2:199–238.
4. Deresinski SC, Stevens DA. Coccidioidomycosis in compromised hosts. Experience at Stanford University Hospital. *Medicine.* 1974;54:377–395.
5. Fish DG, Ampel NM, Galgiani JN, et al. Coccidioidomycosis during human immunodeficiency virus infection. A review of 77 patients. *Medicine.* 1990;69:384–391.
6. Cohen IM, Galgiani JN, Potter D, Ogden DA. Coccidioidomycosis in renal replacement therapy. *Arch Intern Med.* 1982;142:489–494.
7. Brewer JH, Parrott CL, Rimland D. Disseminated coccidioidomycosis in a heart transplant recipient. *Sabouraudia.* 1982;20:261–265.
8. Kohn GJ, Linné SR, Smith CM, et al. Acquisition of coccidioidomycosis at necropsy by inhalation of coccidioidal endospores. *Diagn Microbiol Infect Dis.* 1992;15:527–530.
9. Rohatgi PK, Schmitt RG. Pulmonary coccidioidal mycetoma. *Am J Med Sci.* 1984;287:27–30.
10. Hobbs ER. Coccidioidomycosis. *Dermatol Clin.* 1989;7: 227–239.
11. Wilson JW. The importance of the portal of entry in certain microbial infections. The primary cutaneous "chancriform" syndrome. *Dis Chest.* 1968;54(suppl 1):S299–S304.
12. Rodenbiker HT, Ganley JP, Galgiani JN, Axline SG. Prevalence of chorioretinal scars associated with coccidioidomycosis. *Arch Ophthalmol.* 1981;99:71–75.
13. Dalinka MK, Dinnenberg S, Greendyke WH, Hopkins R. Roentgenographic features of osseous coccidioidomycosis and differential diagnoses. *J Bone Joint Surg.* 1971;53: 1157–1164.
14. Millman TM, O'Brien TR, Suter PF, Wolf AM. Coccidioidomycosis in the dog: its radiographic diagnosis. *J Am Vet Radiol Soc.* 1979;20:50–65.
15. Lonky SA, Catanzaro A, Moser KM, Einstein H. Acute coccidioidal pleural effusion. *Am Rev Resp Dis.* 1976;114: 681–688.
16. Fiese M. *Coccidioidomycosis.* Springfield, IL: Charles C. Thomas; 1958.
17. Echols RM, Palmer DL, Loney GW. Tissue eosinophilia in human coccidioidomycosis. *Rev Infect Dis.* 1982;4:656–664.
18. Huntington RW. Acute fatal coccidioidal pneumonia. In: Ajello L, ed. *Coccidioidomycosis: Current Clinical and Diagnostic Status.* Miami: Symposia Specialists; 1977:127–137.
19. Lombard CM, Tazelear HD, Frasne DL. Pulmonary eosinophilia in coccidioidal infections. *Chest.* 1987;91:734–736.
20. Pappagianis D, Miller RL, Smith CE, Kobayashi GS. Response of monkeys to respiratory challenge following subcutaneous inoculation with *Coccidioides immitis*. *J Immunol.* 1961;86:28–34.
21. Levine HB, Miller RL, Smith CE. Influence of vaccination on respiratory coccidioidal disease in cynomolgous monkeys. *J Immunol.* 1962;89:242–251.
22. Graham AR, Sobonya R, Bronniman DA, Galgiani JN. Quantitative pathology of coccidioidomycosis in acquired immunodeficiency syndrome. *Hum Pathol.* 1988;19:800–806.
23. Williams PL, Johnson R, Pappagianis D, et al. Vasculitic and encephalitic complications associated with *Coccidioides immitis* infections of the central nervous system in humans: report of 10 cases. *Clin Infect Dis.* 1992;14: 673–682.
24. Ophuls W. Coccidioidal granuloma. *JAMA.* 1905;45:1291–1296.
25. Forbus WD, Bestebreurtje AM. Coccidioidomycosis: a study of 95 cases of the disseminated type with special reference to the pathogenesis of the disease. *Milit Surgeon.* 1946;99:653–719.
26. Tarbet JE, Breslau AM. Histochemical investigation of the spherule of *Coccidioides immitis* in relation to host reaction. *J Infect Dis.* 1953;92:183–190.
27. Collins MS, Pappagianis D. Effects of lysozyme and chitinase on the spherules of *Coccidioides immitis* in vitro. *Infect Immun.* 1973;7:817–822.
28. Frey CL, Drutz DJ. Influence of fungal surface components on the interaction of *Coccidioides immitis* with polymorphonuclear neutrophils. *J Infect Dis.* 1986;153: 933–943.
29. Huntington RW Jr. Diagnostic and biologic complications of the histopathology of coccidioidomycosis. *Proc Sympos Coccidioidomycosis,* US Public Health Service Publ No. 575, 1957;36–46.
30. Galgiani JN, Isenberg RA, Stevens DA. Chemotaxigenic activity of extracts from the mycelial and spherule phases of *Coccidioides immitis* for human polymorphonuclear leukocytes. *Infect Immun.* 1978;21:862–865.
31. Slagle DC, Cox RA, Kuranganti U. Induction of tumor

necrosis factor alpha by spherules of *Coccidioides immitis*. *Infect Immun.* 1989;57:1916–1921.

32. Pappagianis D, Zimmer BL. Serology of coccidioidomycosis. *Clin Microbiol Rev.* 1990;3:247–268.
33. Ibrahim AB, Pappagianis D. Experimental induction of anergy to coccidioidin by antigens of *Coccidioides immitis*. *Infect Immun.* 1973;7:786–794.
34. Cox RA. Immunosuppression by cell wall antigens of *Coccidioides immitis*. *Rev Infect Dis.* 1988;10(suppl 2):S415–S418.
35. Cox RA, Kennell W. Suppression of T-lymphocyte response by *Coccidioides immitis* antigen. *Infect Immun.* 1988;56:1424–1429.
36. Cutler JE, Erke KH. Ultrastructural characteristics of *Coccidioides immitis,* a morphological variant of *Cryptococcus neoformans* and *Podosypha ravenelii*. *J Bacteriol.* 1971;105:438–444.
37. O'Hern EM, Henry BS. A cytological study of *Coccidioides immitis* by electron microscopy. *J Bacteriol.* 1956;72: 632–645.
38. Huppert M, Sun SH. Overview of mycology, and the mycology of *Coccidioides immitis.* In: Stevens DA, ed. *Coccidioidomycosis: A Text.* New York: Plenum Press; 1980:21–46.
39. Cole GT, Sun SH. Arthroconidium-spherule-endospore transformation in *Coccidioides immitis.* In: Szaniszlo PJ, ed. *Fungal Dimorphism.* New York: Plenum Press; 1985: 281–333.
40. Donnelly WH, Yunis EJ. The ultrastructure of *Coccidioides immitis*. *Arch Pathol.* 1974;98:227–232.
41. Hector RF, Pappagianis D. Enzymatic degradation of the walls of spherules of *Coccidioides immitis*. *Experimental Mycology.* 1982;6:136–152.
42. Sun SH, Huppert M. A cytological study of morphogenesis in *Coccidioides immitis*. *Sabouraudia.* 1976;14:185–198.
43. Drutz DJ, Huppert M. Coccidioidomycosis: factors affecting the host-parasite interaction. *J Infect Dis.* 1983;147: 372–390.
44. Beaman L, Pappagianis D. Fate of *Coccidioides immitis* arthroconidia in human peripheral blood monocyte cultures in vitro. Coccidioidomycosis. Proceedings of the 4th International Conference on Coccidioidomycosis; Washington, DC, National Foundation for Infectious Diseases; 1985:170–180.
45. Weisman IM, Moreno AJ, Parker AL, Sippo WC, Liles WJ. Gastrointestinal dissemination of coccidioidomycosis. *Am J Gastroenterol.* 1986;81:589–593.
46. Price MJ, Lewis EL, Carmalt JE. Coccidioidomycosis of the prostate gland. *Urology.* 1982;19:653–655.
47. Bellin HJ, Bhagavan BS. Coccidioidomycosis of the prostate gland. *Arch Pathol.* 1973;96:114–117.
48. Pappagianis D. Opportunism in coccidioidomycosis. In: Chick EW, Ballows A, Furcolow ML, eds. *Opportunistic Fungal Infections.* Springfield, IL: Charles C. Thomas; 1975:221–234.
49. Cotton BH, Penido JRF, Birsner JW, Babcock CE. Coexisting pulmonary coccidioidomycosis and tuberculosis: a review of twenty-four cases. *Am Rev Tuberc.* 1954;70: 109–120.
50. Perry LV, Jenkins DE, Whitcomb FC. Simultaneously occurring pulmonary coccidioidomycosis and histoplasmosis. *Am Rev Resp Dis.* 1965;92:952–957.
51. Davidson W, Sarosi GA. Disseminated blastomycosis and coccidioidomycosis in the same patient. *Am Rev Resp Dis.* 1981;124:179.
52. Wolf JE, Little JR, Pappagianis D, Kobayashi GS. Disseminated coccidioidomycosis in a patient with acquired immune deficiency syndrome. *Diagn Microbiol Infect Dis.* 1986;5:331–336.
53. Griner L. *Pathology of Zoo Animals.* Zoological Society of San Diego; 1983:440.
54. Chandler FW, Watts JC. *Pathologic Diagnosis of Fungal Infections.* Chicago: ASCP Press; 1987:13–25.
55. Clark KAM, Talbot LAM, Bee G, Gordon PC, Pusateri KD. Development of rapid non-isotopic DNA probe assays for fungi: *Coccidioides immitis*. *Amer Soc Microbiol,* Washington, DC; 1991;420. Abstract.
56. Kaplan W, Kraft D. Demonstration of pathogenic fungi in formalin-fixed tissues by immunofluorescence. *Am J Clin Pathol.* 1969;52:420–432.
57. Warlick MA, Quan SF, Sobonya RE. Rapid diagnosis of pulmonary coccidioidomycosis. Cytologic v potassium hydroxide preparations. *Arch Intern Med.* 1983;143: 723–725.
58. Pappagianis D. Coccidioidomycosis. In: Balows A, Hausler WJ Jr, Lennette EH, eds. *Laboratory Diagnosis of Infectious Diseases.* New York: Springer-Verlag; 1988; 599–622.
59. Reep BR, Kaplan W. The use of *N*-acetyl-L-cysteine and dithiothreitol to process sputa for mycological and fluorescent antibody examinations. *Health Lab Sci.* 1972;9: 118–124.
60. Sigler L, Carmichael JW. Taxonomy of *Malbranchea* and some other hyphomycetes with arthroconidia. *Mycotaxon.* 1976;4:349–488.
61. Smith CE, Saito MT, Simons SA. Pattern of 39,500 serologic tests in coccidioidomycosis. *JAMA.* 1956;160:546–552.
62. Johnson SM, Pappagianis D. The coccidioidal complement fixation and immunodiffusion-complement fixation antigen is a chitinase. *Infect Immun.* 1992;60:2588–2592.
63. Pappagianis D, Putman EW, Kobayashi GS. Polysaccharide of *Coccidioides immitis*. *J Bacteriol.* 1973;82:714–723.
64. Cole GT, Kruse D, Seshan KR. Antigen complex of *Coccidioides immitis* which elicits a precipitin antibody response in patients. *Infect Immun.* 1991;59:2434–2446.
65. Resnick S, Zimmer B, Pappagianis D, Eakin A, McKerrow J. Purification and amino-terminal sequence analysis of the complement-fixing and precipitin antigens from *Coccidioides immitis*. *J Clin Microbiol.* 1991;28:385–388.
66. Pappagianis D, Saito MT, Van Hoosear K. Antibody in cerebrospinal fluid in non-meningitic coccidioidomycosis. *Sabouraudia.* 1972;10:173–179.
67. Talbot RC, Johnson RC, Leonard J. Enzyme-linked immunosorbent assay of coccidioidal antibody in CSF specimens. *Proc Annual Coccidioidomycosis Study Group.* 1986;1.
68. Stevens DA. Coccidioidomycosis. *N Engl J Med.* 1995; 332:1077–1082.
69. Tucker RM, Denning DW, Dupont B, Stevens DA. Itraconazole therapy for chronic coccidioidal meningitis. *Ann Intern Med.* 1990;112:108–112.

CHAPTER 106

Cryptococcosis

Francis W. Chandler and John C. Watts

A long disease does not always tell a lie; it will kill at last.

Irish Proverb

Enter his chamber, view his breathless corpse,
And comment then upon his sudden death.

William Shakespeare (1564–1616), 2 Henry VI, III, ii

DEFINITION

Cryptococcosis is a systemic mycosis caused by the encapsulated basidiomycetous, yeast-like fungus *Cryptococcus neoformans*.[1,2] The fungus is widespread in nature and worldwide in distribution. It is a ubiquitous saprophyte of soil and most abundant in avian habitats, particularly those heavily contaminated with pigeon excreta.[3] There are two varieties of *C neoformans: C neoformans* var *neoformans* and *C neoformans* var *gatti*.[2] The prevalence of cryptococcosis caused by var *neoformans* is far greater than that caused by var *gatti*. Synonyms for cryptococcosis include torulosis, European blastomycosis, and Busse-Buschke disease.

EPIDEMIOLOGY

Cryptococcosis is not a contagious disease. It is usually acquired by inhaling aerosolized cells of *C neoformans* that are produced in the environment.[4,5] Primary cutaneous cryptococcosis is very rare and usually results from accidental inoculation of skin. Although the fungus is pathogenic for those with competent immunity, it is more often encountered as an opportunistic infectious agent and is the most common cause of fungal meningitis.[6] Surveys indicate that the majority of patients with cryptococcosis have defective cellular immunity or severe underlying disease.[6,7] Factors that predispose to opportunistic cryptococcosis include acquired immunodeficiency syndrome (AIDS), hematologic malignancies (especially Hodgkin's disease), long-term corticosteroid therapy, sarcoidosis, diabetes mellitus, and other conditions that are known to impair cell-mediated immunity.[8–12] In patients with AIDS, cryptococcosis is one of the more common life-threatening infections and it varies in frequency from 6% to 10% in different geographic areas of the United States, western Europe, and Australia, and from 15% to 30% in sub-Saharan Africa.[6] Worldwide, patients with AIDS and cryptococcosis are infected almost exclusively with *C neoformans* var *neoformans* serotype A.[6]

CLINICAL FEATURES

Clinically, cryptococcosis occurs in two basic forms: pulmonary cryptococcosis and, by hematogenous or lymphatic dissemination from a primary pulmonary focus, cerebromeningeal cryptococcosis.[13–15] Cutaneous, mucocutaneous, osseous, and visceral forms of the disease develop less often through dissemination from a primary pulmonary infection. Cutaneous lesions occur in 10% to 20% of patients and vary from papules and pustules to large ulcerated nodules (Figure 106–1).[16–18] Osteolytic lesions, particularly of long bones, pelvis, vertebrae, and ribs, occur in about 10% of patients with disseminated cryptococcosis. A benign, asymptomatic,

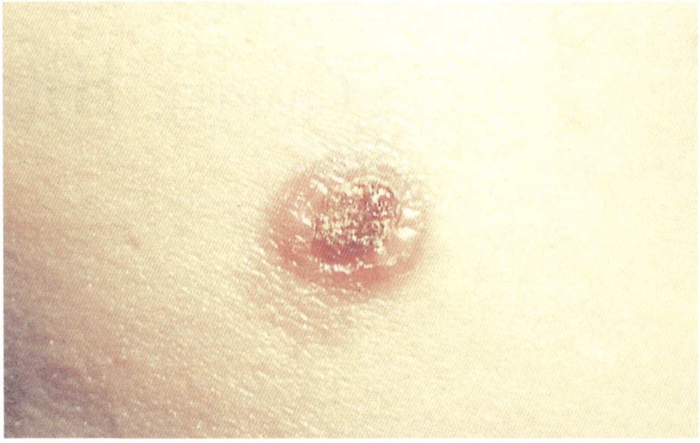

Figure 106–1. Cutaneous lesion in disseminated cryptococcosis. A solitary, sharply circumscribed, ulcerative nodule is on the trunk. *(Courtesy of Centers for Disease Control and Prevention, Atlanta.)*

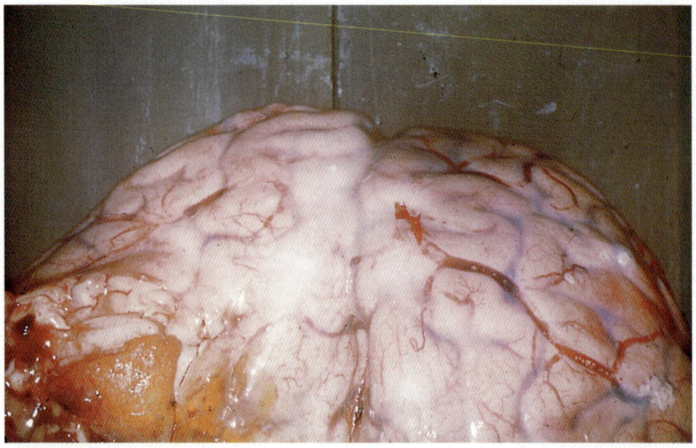

Figure 106–2. Cerebromeningeal cryptococcosis. The meninges are thickened, milky white, glistening, and slimy on gross examination. Microscopically, the leptomeninges were distended with myriad, closely packed cryptococci with wide, mucoid capsules. *(Courtesy of Centers for Disease Control and Prevention, Atlanta.)*

or mildly symptomatic but self-limited pulmonary form of cryptococcosis no doubt exists, but the absence of a sensitive and specific skin test antigen has prevented its verification.

The clinical manifestations of symptomatic pulmonary cryptococcosis are not pathognomonic.[14,15] Pulmonary cryptococcosis evolves over 1 to 4 weeks and may involve one or both lungs. Chest radiographs often reveal multiple nodular densities, but in severe infections the areas of infiltration are more diffuse or there may be marked peribronchial infiltrates. Cavitation, caseation, and calcification are rare.[15,19] Pulmonary infections with capsule-deficient cryptococci are almost always in those without underlying immunodeficiencies or other predisposing illness, and extrapulmonary dissemination is exceedingly rare.[19,20] A diagnosis of pulmonary cryptococcosis is based on the yeast-like cells of *C neoformans* in respiratory fluids or lung biopsy specimens and on microbiologic culture.

The predominant clinical form of cryptococcosis is cerebromeningeal and is the most common form of cryptococcosis in patients with AIDS (Figure 106–2).[6,9,10] For reasons that are not understood, *C neoformans* is extremely neurotropic and frequently disseminates to the central nervous system (CNS) from apparent or inapparent primary pulmonary infections. Duration of the disease varies from a few days to 20 years or more. The clinical course, however, is usually fulminant and if untreated is almost always fatal. Definitive diagnosis of cerebromeningeal infection is made by demonstrating *C neoformans* in tissue specimens or India ink preparations of cerebrospinal fluid (CSF) (Figure 106–3) and, whenever possible, by culture. A diagnosis also can be made by detecting cryptococcal polysaccharide antigen in the CSF by latex agglutination.[21,22] This test is more sensitive than direct examination of India ink preparations, and it detects cryptococcal polysaccharide antigen in the CSF in about 90% of patients with cerebromeningeal cryptococcosis.

MORPHOLOGIC FEATURES OF THE ORGANISM

Isolation of *C neoformans* from clinical materials generally is not difficult.[1,2] Unlike most yeast-like pathogens, *C neoformans* is not dimorphic. On Sabouraud's agar without cycloheximide, typical isolates grow rapidly at either 25°C or 37°C and develop moist, smooth, mucoid, white to pale yellow colonies. Microscopically, the colonies are composed of spherical to oval, encap-

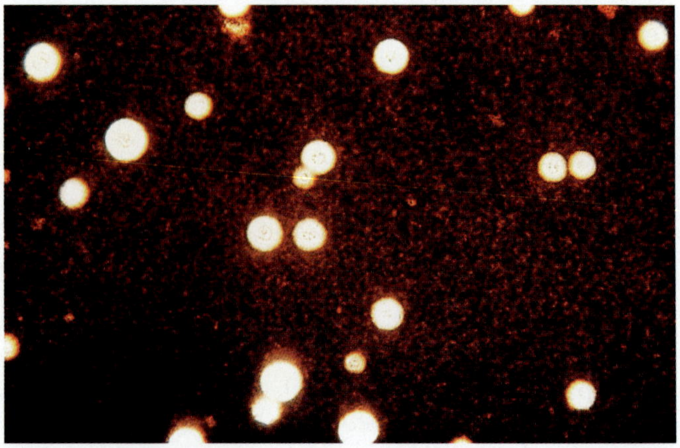

Figure 106–3. Cerebromeningeal cryptococcosis. An India ink preparation of cerebrospinal fluid reveals numerous cryptococci surrounded by wide, optically clear capsules (India ink, ×160).

sulated, yeast-like cells, 2 to 20 μm in diameter, that replicate by budding from a relatively narrow base. Single buds are usually produced, but multiple buds and chains of budding cells are sometimes present. The colonies of capsule-deficient cryptococci are smaller, more convex, drier, and more wrinkled than the larger, mucoid colonies of typically encapsulated yeast forms.[2] *Guizotia abyssinica* seed extract (birdseed) agar as the primary culture medium increases sensitivity and facilitates the isolation of *C neoformans*.[23] *Cryptococcus neoformans* produces brown colonies when grown on this selective medium, and is the species that usually causes cryptococcosis; however, two other species—*C albidus* and *C laurentii*—have rarely caused similar disease.[24–26]

In hematoxylin-eosin-stained tissue sections, the pleomorphic yeast-like cells of *C neoformans* are eosinophilic or lightly basophilic, uninucleate, have thin walls, and vary in size from 2 to 20 μm but usually measure 4 to 10 μm in diameter (Figure 106–4). The fungal cell bodies are occasionally refractile. Typical fungal cells are spherical, oval, or elliptical, and surrounded by optically clear, smoothly contoured spherical zones or "halos" that are unstained or weakly stained mucinous capsules and impart a "soap bubble" appearance at low magnification (Figure 106–5). The capsules are distinctive diagnostic markers, may have a diameter up to five times that of the fungal cells they surround, and are readily detected with mucin stains such as Mayer's mucicarmine, colloidal iron, and Alcian blue (Figure 106–6). With mucin stains, the capsular material often has a spinous or crenated appearance caused by uneven shrinkage during tissue processing (Figure 106–7). With Gomori's methenamine silver (GMS) and other special stains for fungi, the cell walls of cryptococci are deeply colored and readily demonstrated (Figure 106–8). In active lesions that contain abundant fungal cells, budding is frequent. Single budding by a narrow base is common, but multiple budding and short chains of yeast-form cells may also be present (Figure 106–9). Germ tubes, pseudohyphae, and true hyphae are rare in tissues (Figure 106–10).[27]

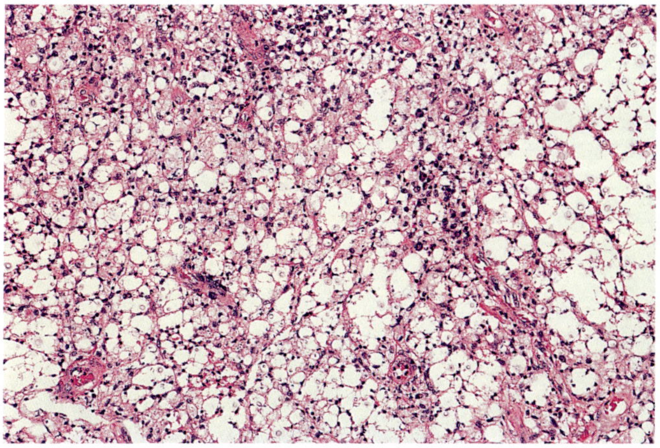

Figure 106–5. Primary cutaneous cryptococcosis. Myriad cryptococci in the dermis and subcutaneous tissue are surrounded by unstained, smoothly contoured, mucinous capsules that impart a "soap bubble" appearance at low magnification (hematoxylin-eosin, ×40).

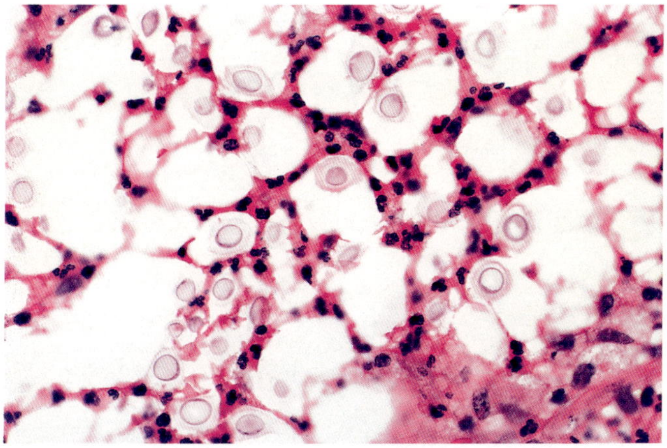

Figure 106–4. Primary cutaneous cryptococcosis. Numerous pleomorphic yeast forms in the dermis are surrounded by optically clear or faintly eosinophilic spherical zones ("halos") that are the wide mucopolysaccharide capsules. The fungal cells are embedded in a suppurative inflammatory cell infiltrate (hematoxylin-eosin, ×160).

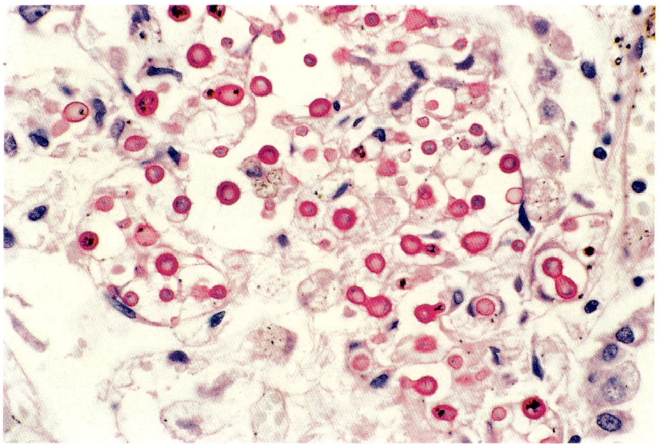

Figure 106–6. Cryptococcal pneumonitis. Single and budding cryptococci distend the interstitium and are surrounded by brilliant carminophilic capsules. The capsules are distinctive diagnostic markers and readily detected with mucin stains (Mayer's mucicarmine, ×100).

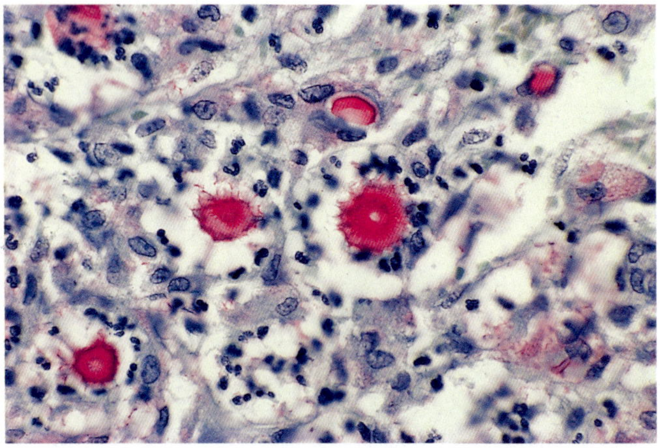

Figure 106–7. Primary cutaneous cryptococcosis. Pleomorphic cryptococci in the dermis are surrounded by wide, intensely carminophilic capsules that have a spinous or crenated appearance caused by uneven shrinkage during tissue processing (Mayer's mucicarmine, ×160).

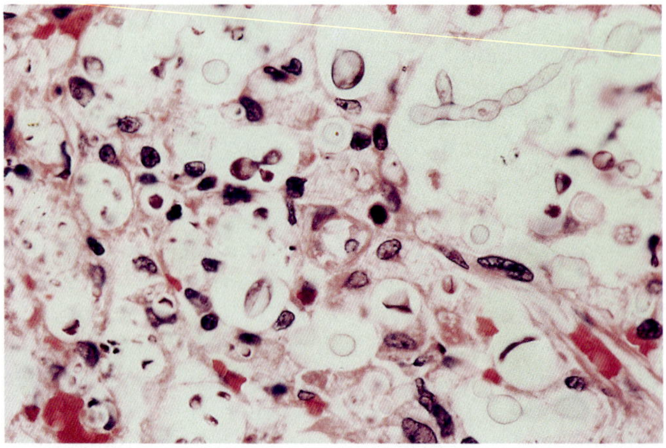

Figure 106–9. Disseminated cryptococcosis in an AIDS patient. Pleomorphic cryptococci with wide capsules occupy a "cystic" lesion of the thyroid gland. A multiple budding cell *(upper left)* and a germinating cell *(upper right)* are mixed with typical cryptococci (hematoxylin-eosin, ×250).

PATHOLOGY

The host reaction to *C neoformans* is variable and usually depends on the immunologic status of the patient, the presence of underlying disease, and the extent of encapsulation of the cryptococcal cells.[19,27] In anergic patients, it may be difficult to detect any host reaction at all. In this paucireactive pattern, the cryptococci multiply profusely, displace normal tissues, and form a "cystic" lesion filled with myriad closely packed fungal cells in which wide mucoid capsules give the lesion a glistening appearance and slimy consistency on gross examination. This appearance is particularly striking in some patients with cryptococcal meningitis in which compact masses of fungi in the leptomeninges displace the underlying brain parenchyma. In patients with AIDS and other profound cell-mediated immunodeficiencies, proliferating cryptococci may produce large extracellular aggregates or "yeast lakes" that efface the normal architecture of an organ (Figure 106–11). In AIDS

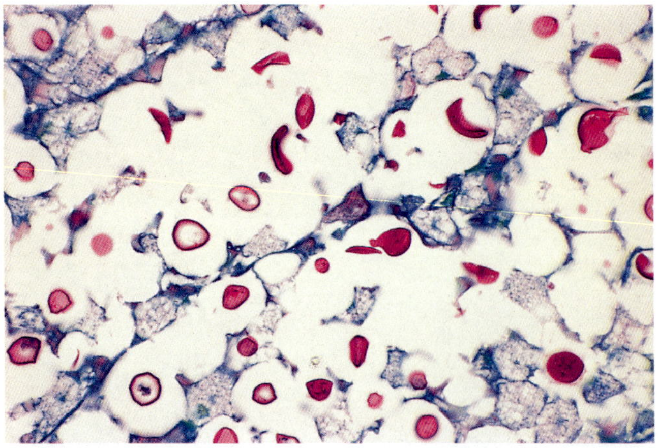

Figure 106–8. Cryptococcal meningitis. Compact yeast-like cells of *Cryptococcus neoformans* distend the leptomeninges and evoke minimal inflammation. Fungal cell walls are deeply colored with the PAS reaction and other special stains for fungi. The clear zones around fungal cells represent the wide, unstained capsules. Note the variability in size and shape of the cryptococci (PAS, ×160).

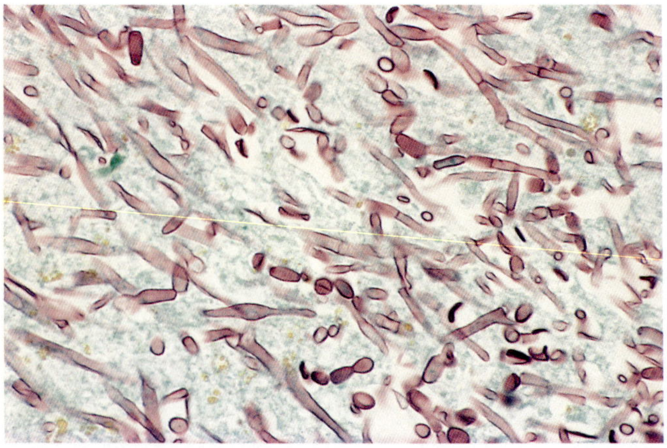

Figure 106–10. Disseminated cryptococcosis in an immunodeficient patient. Pseudohyphae and septate, branched hyphae of *Cryptococcus neoformans* are mixed with typical yeast forms. Mycelial elements of this fungus are only rarely produced in tissue (GMS, ×250).

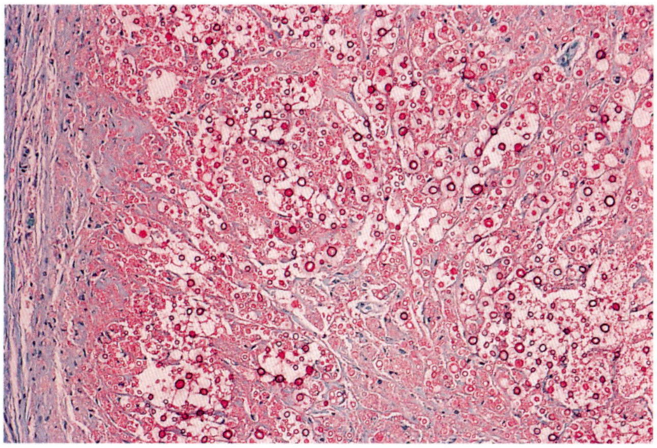

Figure 106–11. Cryptococcal lymphadenitis in an AIDS patient. There is total effacement of the nodal architecture by compact masses of encapsulated cryptococci. The capsules of fungal cells are intensely carminophilic in this section stained with Mayer's mucicarmine procedure. Inflammation is minimal (Mayer's mucicarmine, ×40).

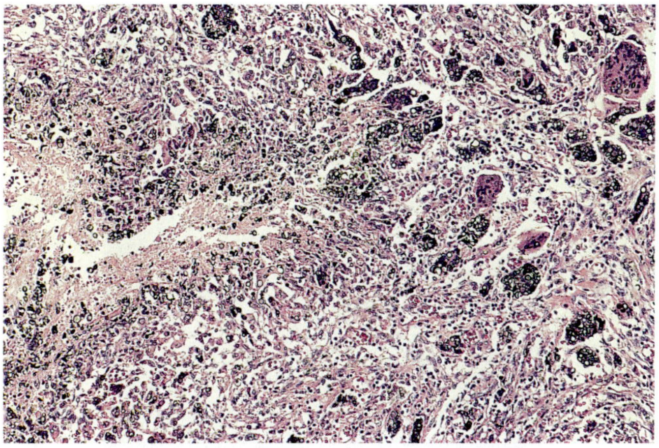

Figure 106–13. Pneumonitis caused by capsule-deficient cryptococci. There is a dispersed granulomatous inflammatory reaction with areas of necrosis and minimal suppuration. The dark masses are compact fungal cells within phagocytes (GMS–hematoxylin-eosin, ×40).

patients with pulmonary cryptococcosis, there are often numerous cryptococci in the interstitium with little or no inflammation (Figure 106–12).[19,28]

In otherwise healthy, immunocompetent patients, *C neoformans* usually elicits a mixed suppurative and granulomatous inflammatory cellular reaction or a purely granulomatous reaction with varying degrees of necrosis. If the cryptococci are capsule-deficient, they almost always elicit a focal or dispersed granulomatous inflammatory reaction with areas of necrosis and minimal suppuration (Figure 106–13).[29,30] Confluent fibrosis may be prominent in chronic infections and, at low magnification, often has a storiform pattern. Pleomorphic yeast forms without conspicuous capsules are present in varying numbers, many of which are located within epithelioid histiocytes and giant cells (Figure 106–14).

Long-standing infections by *C neoformans* can cause residual pulmonary granulomas (cryptococcomas) that usually appear as "coin lesions" on chest radiographs (Figure 106–15).[19,31] However, unlike residual fibrocaseous granulomas caused by *Histoplasma*

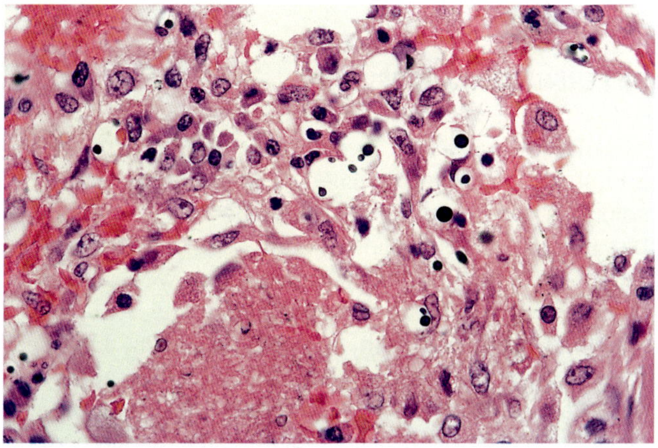

Figure 106–12. Hematogenous cryptococcal pneumonitis in an AIDS patient. Several encapsulated, GMS-positive cryptococci in the pulmonary interstitium are associated with minimal inflammation. A contiguous alveolar space contains aggregated cysts and trophozoites of *Pneumocystis carinii* (GMS–hematoxylin-eosin, ×100).

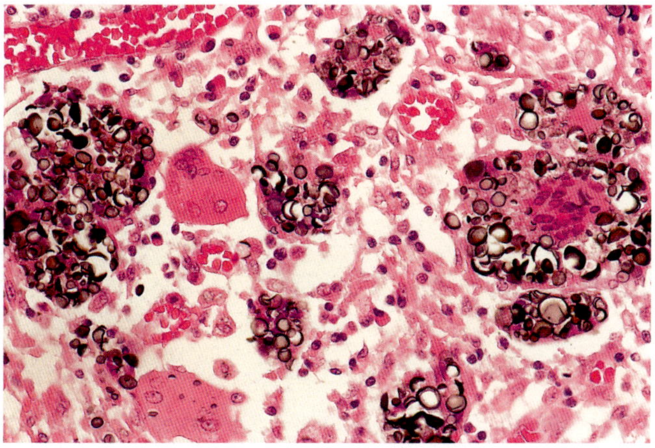

Figure 106–14. Granulomatous pneumonitis caused by capsule-deficient *Cryptococcus neoformans*. Numerous pleomorphic yeast forms without conspicuous capsules are in epithelioid histiocytes and giant cells (GMS–hematoxylin-eosin, ×160).

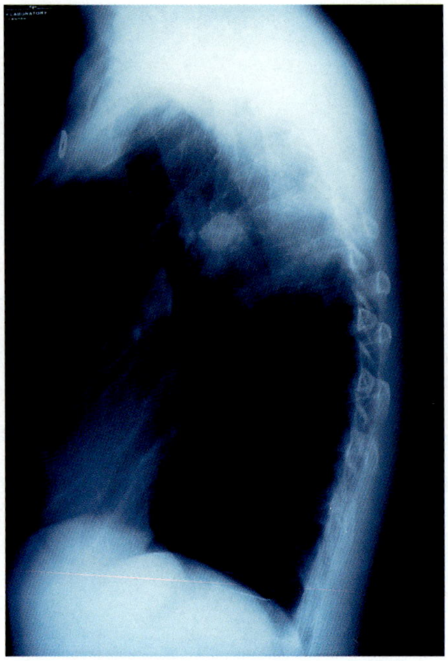

Figure 106–15. Residual pulmonary cryptococcosis (cryptococcoma). This chest radiograph reveals a solitary "coin lesion" in the left upper lobe.

capsulatum var *capsulatum* (histoplasmomas) and *Coccidioides immitis* (coccidioidomas), cryptococcomas rarely calcify.[19,32,33] They are often found incidentally at autopsy or are suspected of being neoplasms in chest radiographs and resected (Figure 106–16). In these lesions, the cells of *C neoformans* are difficult to detect with hematoxylin-eosin because they are often atypical,

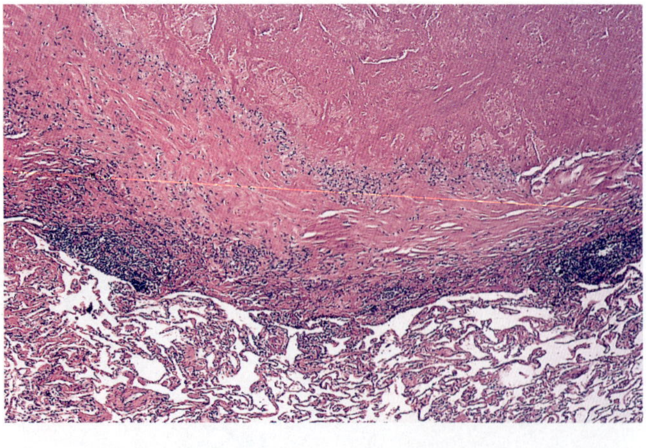

Figure 106–16. Residual pulmonary cryptococcosis (cryptococcoma). A solitary fibrocaseous nodule is partially surrounded by prominent lymphoid aggregates. In cryptococcomas, intact and fragmented fungal cells are in the central caseous material. They are difficult to detect with hematoxylin-eosin, but usually can be demonstrated with the GMS procedure (hematoxylin-eosin, ×16).

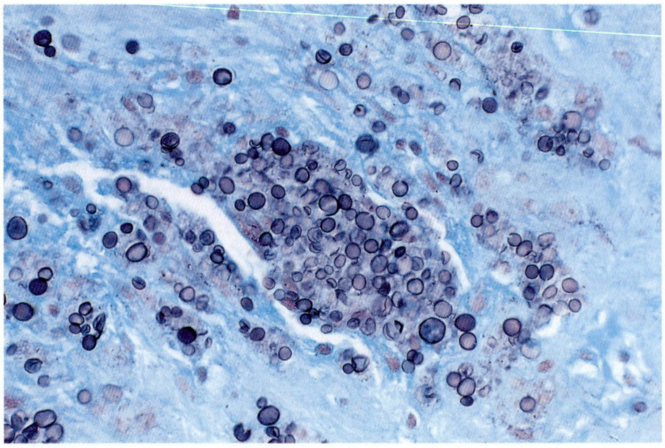

Figure 106–17. Residual pulmonary cryptococcosis. Small, pleomorphic yeast forms within the central caseous material of the cryptococcoma are distorted, fragmented, unevenly stained, and capsule deficient (GMS, ×160).

distorted, and fragmented.[19,27] They can, however, be demonstrated readily with the GMS stain within the central caseous material and at the periphery of the granuloma within epithelioid histiocytes and giant cells (Figure 106–17). Usually, the cryptococci are small (2 to 5 μm in diameter), unevenly stained, and capsule deficient, and it is difficult to culture the fungus from these residual lesions. When sparse and atypical, the fungal cells can be mistaken for those of *H capsulatum* var *capsulatum* and other yeast-like fungi in GMS-stained tissue sections.[19,30] In these instances, examination by direct immunofluorescence of cryptococcomas in replicate, deparaffinized tissue sections is a valuable diagnostic aid.[27,34]

DIFFERENTIAL DIAGNOSIS

Because the cells of *C neoformans* vary greatly in size and shape, and encapsulated cells are not always conspicuous, cryptococcosis should be considered in the histopathologic differential diagnosis of virtually any yeast-form infection.[27] Cryptococci with well-developed capsules are readily visible and can usually be identified in sections stained with hematoxylin-eosin. However, their morphology can be studied to better advantage with the special stains for fungi. When the capsule of a yeast stains intensely with mucin stains, a diagnosis of cryptococcosis can be made with confidence because the *Cryptococcus* sp are the only pathogenic fungi that produce mucinous capsules. A histologic diagnosis of cryptococcosis is more difficult to establish when most or all of the cryptococci in a lesion are capsule deficient

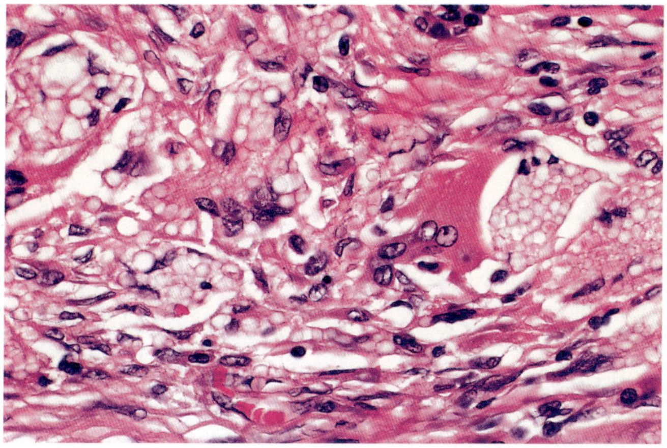

Figure 106–18. Granulomatous pneumonitis caused by capsule-deficient *Cryptococcus neoformans*. The pleomorphic yeast forms are small (2 to 5 μm in diameter), spherical, weakly stained, predominantly intracellular, and do not have conspicuous capsules (hematoxylin-eosin, ×160).

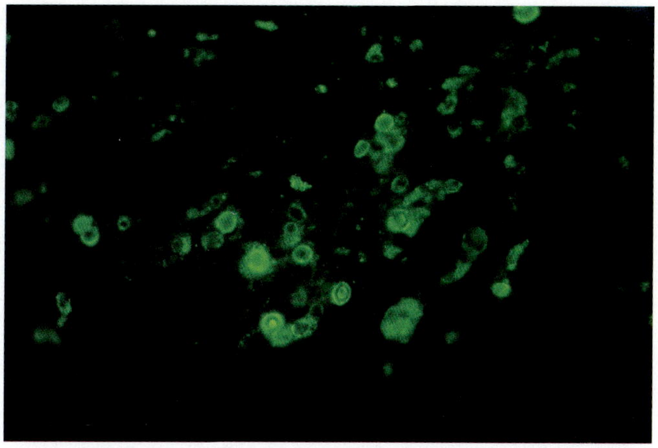

Figure 106–20. Direct immunofluorescence of capsule-deficient cryptococci within the central necrotic residuum of a cryptococcoma. Intact and fragmented fungal cells are in this deparaffinized section of formalin-fixed tissue. The immunofluorescence conjugate is species-specific and directed against capsular polysaccharide antigens (Direct immunofluorescence, ×160).

(Figure 106–18).[27,35] In our experience, however, at least some weakly encapsulated cells can almost always be detected in such lesions when mucin-stained sections are examined carefully at high magnification (Figure 106–19). Capsule-deficient *C neoformans* can simulate *H capsulatum* var *capsulatum* and *Blastomyces dermatitidis* with small tissue forms (so-called microforms), and the potential for confusion with *Sporothrix schenckii, Torulopsis glabrata,* blastoconidia of the *Candida* sp, and immature spherules of *C immitis* also exists.[27] If a mycosis is not suspected clinically, fresh tissue may not be available for culture. Given this situation, several adjunctive methods can be used to identify cryptococci in fixed tissues.

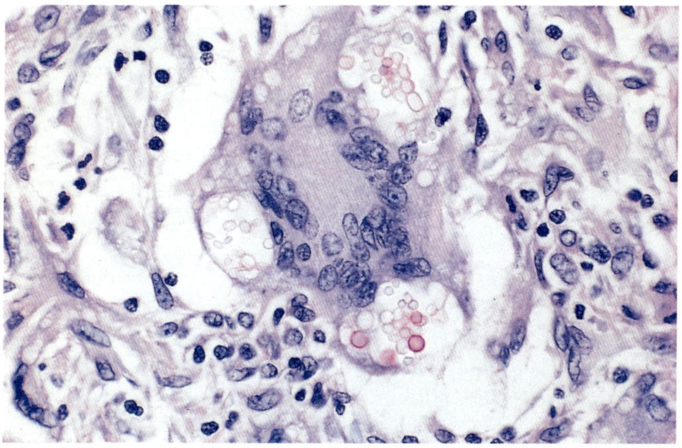

Figure 106–19. Capsule-deficient *Cryptococcus neoformans* within a pulmonary granuloma. The attenuated capsules of the cryptococci are either weakly reactive or nonreactive in this section stained with Mayer's mucicarmine procedure (Mayer's mucicarmine, ×160).

Direct Immunofluorescence

Cryptococcus neoformans can be identified in formalin-fixed, paraffin-embedded tissue sections by direct immunofluorescence.[27,34] Unfortunately, specific fluorescent antibody conjugates are not widely available. The conjugate used at the Centers for Disease Control and Prevention, considered specific for *C neoformans* when used to test clinical specimens, is directed against capsular polysaccharide antigens. Therefore, capsule-deficient cells are only weakly stained, but at least some immunoreactive cells are present (Figure 106–20).

Electron Microscopy

The capsule of *C neoformans* has a distinct and characteristic ultrastructural appearance.[27] It is separated from the underlying electron-dense cell wall by an electron-lucent zone and is composed of a finely granular matrix that contains radiating filaments and tubules. Most capsule-deficient *C neoformans* cells that are mucicarmine negative by light microscopy have attenuated capsules that can be detected easily by electron microscopy (Figure 106–21).

Fontana-Masson Stain for Silver-Reducing Substances

The Fontana-Masson stain, as modified by Kwon-Chung et al,[36] stains the cell walls of the *Cryptococcus* sp brown or black in tissue sections (Figure 106–22). A positive reaction highlights silver-reducing substances

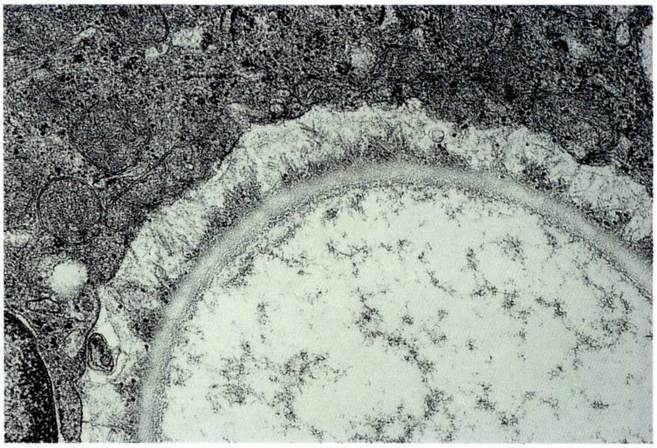

Figure 106–21. Transmission electron micrograph of a capsule-deficient *Cryptococcus neoformans* cell. The attenuated capsule is composed of a finely granular matrix that contains radiating filaments and tubules. Most capsule-deficient cryptococci that are mucicarmine negative by light microscopy have thin capsules that can be detected easily by electron microscopy (Uranyl acetate and lead citrate, ×49,200).

(melanin-like substances derived from dihydroxyphenylalanine) in the cell walls and does not depend on the presence of capsular mucopolysaccharide.[37] Unfortunately, the reaction is not specific for the cryptococci; the cells of *S schenckii* and the immature spherules of *C immitis* may also react with this stain. Occasionally, the cell walls of *Rhinosporidium seeberi* and *B dermatitidis* also show varying degrees of carminophilia when stained with Mayer's and other mucicarmine procedures.[27,35] These two fungi, however, are unencapsulated, morphologically distinct, and unlikely to be confused with *C neoformans;* mucin stains are not required for their identification in tissue sections.

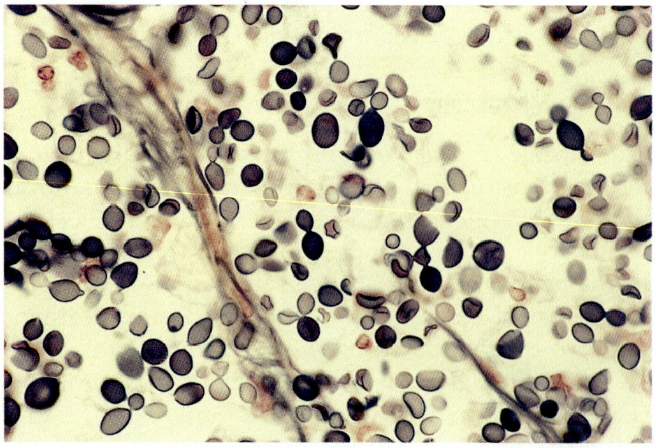

Figure 106–22. Disseminated cryptococcosis. Because cryptococcal cell walls contain silver-reducing substances, they react positively with a modified Fontana-Masson stain for melanin. A positive reaction does not depend on capsular mucopolysaccharide. Note the characteristic budding of cryptococci by a narrow base (Modified Fontana-Masson, ×250).

MOLECULAR DIAGNOSIS

Several DNA-based techniques have been used in epidemiologic studies to identify the variety, serotype, or individual strain of *C neoformans.*[38] Specific primers and probes for polymerase chain reaction (PCR) amplification and detection of defined DNA sequences of *C neoformans* in clinical materials also have been developed.[39–41] Currently, however, molecular methods have had limited application for diagnosis in the clinical laboratory, and they contribute little to the pathologic diagnosis of cryptococcosis.

TREATMENT

The combination of intravenous amphotericin B and oral 5-fluorocytosine is synergistic against *C neoformans* and the treatment of choice for the progressive pulmonary and cerebromeningeal forms of cryptococcosis.[42,43] Oral fluconazole, a new triazole antifungal drug, has been effective as suppressive therapy for disseminated cryptococcosis in patients with AIDS.[44] This antifungal alone, however, is not effective for the primary treatment of cryptococcal meningitis. Surgical resection of localized pulmonary lesions may be a valuable adjunct to antifungal therapy.[45]

REFERENCES

1. Rippon JW. Cryptococcosis. In: Rippon JW, ed. *Medical Mycology.* 3rd ed. Philadelphia: WB Saunders; 1988: 582–609.
2. Kwon-Chung KJ, Bennet JE. Cryptococcosis. In: *Medical Mycology.* Philadelphia: Lea and Febiger; 1992:397–446.
3. Powell KE, Dahl BA, Weeks RJ, Tosh FE. Airborne *Cryptococcus neoformans:* particles from pigeon excreta compatible with alveolar deposition. *J Infect Dis.* 1972;125: 412–415.
4. Neilson JB, Fromtling RA, Bulmer GS. *Cryptococcus neoformans:* size range of infectious particles from aerosolized soil. *Infect Immun.* 1977;17:634–638.
5. Ellis DH, Pfeiffer TJ. The ecology of *Cryptococcus neoformans. Eur J Epidemiol.* 1992;8:321–325.
6. Mitchell TG, Perfect JR. Cryptococcosis in the era of AIDS—100 years after the discovery of *Cryptococcus neoformans. Clin Microbiol Rev.* 1995;8:515–548.
7. Schimpff SC, Bennett JE. Abnormalities in cell-mediated immunity in patients with *Cryptococcus neoformans* infections. *J Allergy Clin Immunol.* 1975;55:430–441.

8. Kaplan MH, Rosen PP, Armstrong D. Cryptococcosis in a cancer hospital. Clinical and pathological correlates in forty-six patients. *Cancer.* 1977;39:2265–2274.
9. Zuger A, Louie E, Holzman RS, et al. Cryptococcal disease in patients with the acquired immunodeficiency syndrome. *Ann Intern Med.* 1986;104:234–240.
10. Dismukes WE. Cryptococcal meningitis in patients with AIDS. *J Infect Dis.* 1988;157:624–628.
11. Clark RA, Greer D, Atkinson W, Valainis GT, Hyslop N. Spectrum of *Cryptococcus neoformans* infection in 68 patients infected with human immunodeficiency virus. *Rev Infect Dis.* 1990;12:768–777.
12. Chechani V, Kamholz SL. Pulmonary manifestations of disseminated cryptococcosis in patients with AIDS. *Chest.* 1990;98:1060–1066.
13. Lewis RL, Rabinovich S. The wide spectrum of cryptococcal infections. *Am J Med.* 1972;53:315–322.
14. Kerkering TM, Duma RJ, Shadomy S. The evolution of pulmonary cryptococcosis: clinical implications from a study of 41 patients with and without compromising host factors. *Ann Intern Med.* 1981;94:611–616.
15. Diamond RD. *Cryptococcus neoformans* pneumonia. In: Pennington JE, ed. *Respiratory Infections: Diagnosis and Management.* New York: Raven; 1983:341–351.
16. Schupbach CW, Wheeler CE, Briggaman RA, Warner NA, Kanof EP. Cutaneous manifestations of disseminated cryptococcosis. *Arch Dermatol.* 1976;112:1734–1740.
17. Borton LK, Wintroub BU. Disseminated cryptococcosis presenting as herpetiform lesions in a homosexual man with acquired immunodeficiency syndrome. *J Am Acad Dermatol.* 1984;10:387–390.
18. Rico MJ, Penneys NS. Cutaneous cryptococcosis resembling molluscum contagiosum in a patient with AIDS. *Arch Dermatol.* 1985;121:901–902.
19. Chandler FW, Watts JC. Fungal Infections. In: Dail DH, Hammar SP, eds. *Pulmonary Pathology.* 2nd ed. New York: Springer-Verlag; 1993:351–428.
20. Harding SA, Scheld WM, Feldman PS, Sande MA. Pulmonary infection with capsule-deficient *Cryptococcus neoformans. Virchows Arch* [A]. 1979;382:113–118.
21. Bloomfield N, Gordon MA, Elmendorf DF Jr. Detection of *Cryptococcus neoformans* antigen in body fluids by latex particle agglutination. *Proc Soc Exp Biol Med.* 1963;114: 64–67.
22. Tanner DC, Weinstein MP, Fedorciw B, et al. Comparison of commercial kits for detection of cryptococcal antigen. *J Clin Microbiol.* 1994;32:1680–1684.
23. Denning DW, Stevens DA, Hamilton JR. Comparison of *Guizotia abyssinica* seed extract (birdseed) agar with conventional media for selective identification of *Cryptococcus neoformans* in patients with acquired immunodeficiency syndrome. *J Clin Microbiol.* 1990;28:2565–2567.
24. Krumholz RA. Pulmonary cryptococcosis: a case due to *Cryptococcus albidus. Am Rev Respir Dis.* 1972;105: 421–424.
25. Lynch JP III, Schaberg DR, Kissner DG, Kauffman CA. *Cryptococcus laurentii* lung abscess. *Am Rev Respir Dis.* 1981;123:135–138.
26. Horowitz ID, Blumberg EA, Krevolin L. *Cryptococcus albidus* and mucormycosis empyema in a patient receiving hemodialysis. *Southern Med J.* 1993;86:1070–1072.
27. Chandler FW, Watts JC. *Pathologic Diagnosis of Fungal Infections.* Chicago: ASCP Press; 1987:161–175.
28. Khardori N, Butt F, Rolston KVI. Pulmonary cryptococcosis in AIDS. *Chest.* 1988;93:1319–1320.
29. Farmer SG, Komorowski RA. Histologic response to capsule-deficient *Cryptococcus neoformans. Arch Pathol.* 1973;96:383–387.
30. Gutierrez F, Fu YS, Lurie HI. Cryptococcosis histologically resembling histoplasmosis. A light and electron microscopical study. *Arch Pathol.* 1975;99:347–352.
31. Menon A, Rajamani R. Giant "cryptococcoma" of the lung. *Br J Dis Chest.* 1976;70:269–272.
32. Cohen AA, Davis W, Finegold SM. Chronic pulmonary cryptococcosis. *Am Rev Respir Dis.* 1965;91:414–423.
33. Baker RD. The primary pulmonary lymph node complex of cryptococcosis. *Am J Clin Pathol.* 1976;65:83–92.
34. Kaplan W, Kraft DE. Demonstration of pathogenic fungi in formalin-fixed tissues by immunofluorescence. *Am J Clin Pathol.* 1969;52:420–432.
35. Lazcano O, Speights VO Jr, Strickler JG, et al. Combined histochemical stains in the differential diagnosis of *Cryptococcus neoformans. Modern Pathol.* 1993;6:80–84.
36. Kwon-Chung KJ, Hill WB, Bennett JE. New, special stain for histopathological diagnosis of cryptococcosis. *J Clin Microbiol.* 1981;13:383–387.
37. Wheeler MH, Bell AA. Melanins and their importance in pathogenic fungi. *Curr Topics Med Mycol.* 1987;2:338–387.
38. Mitchell TG, Sandin RL, Bowman BH, Meyer W, Merz WG. Molecular mycology: DNA probes and applications of PCR technology. *J Med Vet Mycol.* 1994;32(supp 1): 351–366.
39. Huffnagle KE, Gander RM. Evaluation of Gen-Probe's *Histoplasma capsulatum* and *Cryptococcus neoformans* AccuProbes. *J Clin Microbiol.* 1993;31:419–421.
40. Mitchell TG, Freedman EZ, White TJ, Taylor JW. Unique oligonucleotide primers in PCR for identification of *Cryptococcus neoformans. J Clin Microbiol.* 1994;32:253–255.
41. Sandhu GS, Kline BC, Stockman L, Roberts GD. Molecular probes for diagnosis of fungal infections. *J Clin Microbiol.* 1995;33:2913–2919.
42. Larsen RA, Leal MAE, Chan LS. Fluconazole compared with amphotericin B plus flucytosine for cryptococcal meningitis in AIDS. A randomized trial. *Ann Intern Med.* 1990;113:183–187.
43. Dismukes WE. Management of cryptococcosis. *Clin Infect Dis.* 1993;17(supp 2):S507–S512.
44. Sugar AM, Saunders C. Oral fluconazole as suppressive therapy of disseminated cryptococcosis in patients with acquired immunodeficiency syndrome. *Am J Med.* 1988; 85:481–489.
45. Smith FS, Gibson P, Nicholls TT, Simpson JA. Pulmonary resection for localized lesions of cryptococcosis (torulosis): a review of eight cases. *Thorax.* 1976;31:121–126.

Chapter 107

Fusariosis

John C. Watts and Francis W. Chandler

All things are hidden, obscure and debatable if the cause of the phenomena be unknown, but everything is clear if this cause be known.

Louis Pasteur (1822–1895), The Germ Theory and Its Application to Medicine and Surgery, Ch. 2 (tr. by H. C. Ernst)

DEFINITION

The *Fusarium* sp cause a variety of superficial and invasive infections in humans, the latter occurring almost exclusively in immunodeficient hosts. These opportunistic fungi of low virulence are grouped among the hyalohyphomycetes. The three medically most important species are *F moniliforme*,[1,2] *F oxysporum*,[3] and *F solani*.[4,5] More recently described occasional pathogens in this genus include *F chlamydosporum*[6] and *F proliferatum*.[7]

GEOGRAPHIC DISTRIBUTION

The *Fusarium* sp are soil saprophytes and plant pathogens of worldwide distribution.

LIFE CYCLE AND EPIDEMIOLOGY

The *Fusarium* sp grow rapidly in culture at room temperature or at 37°C. The mycelium is composed of hyaline, septate hyphae that branch frequently and may produce intercalated or terminal chlamydoconidia. The genus is characterized by the production in vitro of fusoid, multiseptate hyaline macroconidia, and most species also produce chains of microconidia.[1]

These soil-inhabiting fungi are apparently ubiquitous in the environment, and they are isolated occasionally as contaminants in the clinical laboratory. Of relatively low pathogenicity, the *Fusarium* sp usually require deficient host defenses to initiate invasive infection.

MORPHOLOGIC FEATURES

In tissue, the *Fusarium* sp produce hyaline, branched, septate hyphae 3 to 8 μm wide. Although there may be regular, acute-angle branching of hyphae similar to those of the aspergilli, more often the pattern of branching is irregular and haphazard, and branches often arise at right angles to their hyphae of origin (Figure 107–1). The hyphal branches, furthermore, may be prominently constricted at their sites of origin. Varicosities and terminal or intercalated chlamydoconidia are in some of the hyphae in tissue sections (Figure 107–2). We studied one wound infected with *F solani*, in which microconidia were produced by the mycelium on the surface of the wound. These ovoid conidia superficially resembled yeastlike cells but could be distinguished from the latter because some were septate (Figure 107–3), and none showed evidence of budding. The characteristic macroconidia are not produced in tissue. It may be difficult or impossible to distinguish hyphae of the *Fusarium* sp from those of the aspergilli and other hyalohyphomycetes in tissue sections. A specific histopathologic diagnosis of fusariosis, therefore, is not justified unless confirmed by culture or immunohistology.

CLINICAL FEATURES

The *Fusarium* sp are well-recognized agents of mycotic keratitis, onychomycosis, superficial cutaneous infections, osteomyelitis, and mycetoma. Their major importance, however, is as invasive pathogens in immunodeficient hosts. Thus, invasive and disseminated fusariosis has been reported in burned patients,[8,9] in patients

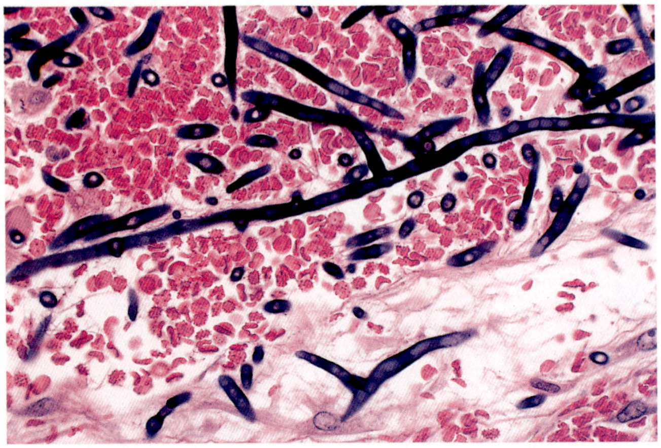

Figure 107–1. Septate hyphae of a *Fusarium* sp. Unlike hyphae of *Aspergillus* sp, those of fusarium branch haphazardly, and branches often arise perpendicularly to their hyphae of origin [Gomori's methenamine silver (GMS)/hematoxylin-eosin, ×480].

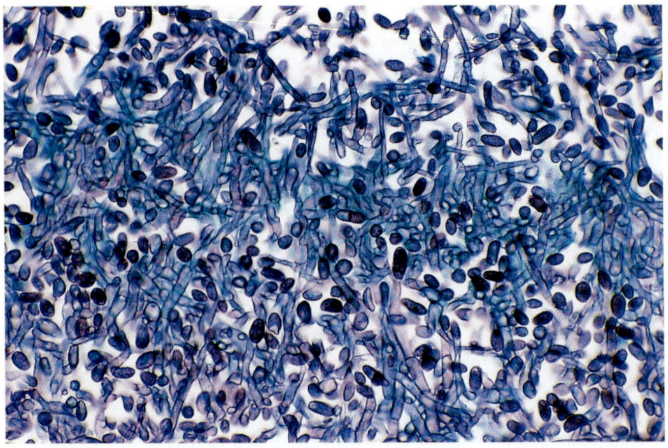

Figure 107–3. Microconidia of *F solani* produced by the mycelium at the surface of an invasive wound infection. These oval conidia, which resemble yeastlike cells, can be mistaken for a *Candida* sp. Detection of septa in the microconidia is an important clue to the diagnosis (GMS, ×480).

treated for acute leukemia[5,10,11] and malignant lymphoma,[1] and in renal[3] and bone marrow[12] transplant recipients. Granulocytopenia and treatment with immunosuppressive cytotoxic drugs and corticosteroids all predispose to invasive fusariosis. Patients may present with fever, respiratory symptoms, and chest radiographic infiltrates. Painful, erythematous, ulcerated, or necrotic cutaneous nodules resembling ecthyma gangrenosum are a frequent clinical manifestation, and the diagnosis can often be conveniently confirmed by culture of a *Fusarium* sp from one of these nodules.[2–5,7,10] Because these fungi are angioinvasive, dissemination of the infection to multiple organs (especially lungs, kidneys, and myocardium) is a significant and often fatal complication if the diagnosis is not made quickly and appropriate antifungal chemotherapy begun. Many isolates are resistant to amphotericin B, and most are resistant to flucytosine. Invasive cutaneous infections may require debridement as well as antifungal chemotherapy. Most invasive infections in immunodeficient hosts have been fatal.

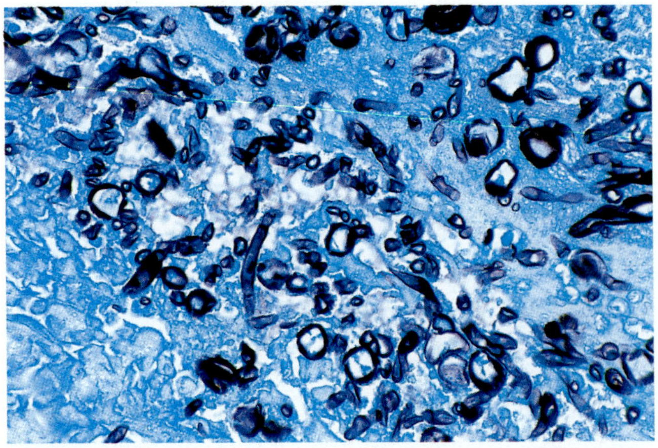

Figure 107–2. Thick-walled chlamydoconidia produced by the mycelium of a *Fusarium* sp in an invasive wound infection (GMS, ×480).

PATHOLOGY

The gross lesions of invasive fusariosis may resemble abscesses (in the nongranulocytopenic host), infarcts, or granulomas. Microscopically, the lesions are abscesses or nodular infarcts (Figure 107–4), the latter a consequence of septic thrombosis. Hyphae, typically abundant in these lesions, can be seen quite well with the hematoxylin-eosin stain. However, a special stain for fungi is usually needed to demonstrate the details of hyphal morphology.

DIFFERENTIAL DIAGNOSIS AND CONFIRMATIONAL TESTING

Distinguishing features of the hyphae of the *Fusarium* sp include constriction of hyphal branches at their sites of origin, terminal and intercalated chlamydoconidia, and intrahyphal vesicles. The hyphae are narrower, and their septations more frequent and prominent, than the hyphae of the zygomycetes. Nevertheless, none of these morphologic features is entirely reliable in distin-

separates *G candidum* from species of the other two genera. Jensen et al[11] have developed an indirect immunofluorescence technique that is used to identify *G candidum* in tissue sections.

CONFIRMATIONAL TESTING AND DIAGNOSIS

The clinical presentation, hyphae that form only arthroconidia in tissue, and the isolation of *Geotrichum* sp in culture confirm the diagnosis of geotrichosis.

TREATMENT

Cutaneous geotrichosis has been successfully treated with isoconazole.[12] Ketoconazole was successfully used in conjunction with surgical drainage of a joint infection.[1] For disseminated geotrichosis in immunodeficient patients, amphotericin B should be considered.

REFERENCES

1. Chang WWL, Buerger L. Disseminated geotrichosis. *Arch Intern Med.* 1964;113:356–360.
2. Ghamande AR, Landis FB, Snider GL. Bronchial geotrichosis with fungemia complicating bronchial carcinoma. *Chest.* 1971;59:98–101.
3. Fishbach RS, White ML, Finegold SM. Bronchopulmonary geotrichosis. *Am Rev Respir Dis.* 1973;108:1388–1392.
4. Sheehy TW, Honeycutt BK, Spency JT. *Geotrichum* septicemia. *JAMA.* 1976;235:1035–1037.
5. Hardy DB, Nassar NN, Rinaldi MG. Traumatic joint infection due to *Geotrichum candidum. Clin Infect Dis.* 1995; 20:468–469.
6. Kassamali H, Anaissie E, Ro J, et al. Disseminated *Geotrichum candidum. J Clin Microbiol.* 1987;25:1782–1783.
7. Heinic GS, MacPhail LA, Greenspan JS. Oral *Geotrichum candidum* infection associated with HIV infection. A case report. *Oral Surg Oral Med Oral Pathol.* 1992;73:726–728.
8. Anaissie E, Bodey GP, Kantarjian H, et al. New spectrum of fungal infections in patients with cancer. *Rev Infect Dis.* 1989;11:369–378.
9. Jagirdar J, Geller SA, Bottone EJ. *Geotrichum candidum* as a tissue invasive human pathogen. *Hum Pathol.* 1981; 12:668–671.
10. Chandler FW, Watts JC. *Pathologic Diagnosis of Fungal Infections.* Chicago: ASCP Press; 1987:117–121.
11. Jensen HE, Hau J, Aalbaek B, Schonheyder H. Indirect immunofluorescence staining and crossed immunoelectrophoresis for differentiation of *Candida albicans* and *Geotrichum candidum. Mycoses.* 1990;33:519–526.
12. Gugnani HC, Akpata LE, Gugnani MK, Srivastava R. Isoconazole nitrate in the treatment of tropical dermatomycosis. *Mycoses.* 1994;37:39–41.

CHAPTER 109

Histoplasmosis Capsulati

Francis W. Chandler and John C. Watts

One must assume that the infective material is alive or, at least, can survive on the outside. A healthy body is not a proper soil for it, and pre-existing tissue changes might be required to permit its growth and proliferation.

Jacob Henle (1805–1885), Pathologische Untersuchungen

DEFINITION

Histoplasmosis capsulati is a systemic fungal infection contracted by inhaling airborne infectious conidia of the classic, small-celled, or *capsulatum* variety of *Histoplasma capsulatum* originating in soil.[1–4] The primary sources of most infections are avian and chiropteran habitats that favor growth and multiplication of this thermally dimorphic fungus in soil, enriched with feces. Synonyms include classical histoplasmosis, small-form histoplasmosis, small-cell histoplasmosis, Darling's disease, and Tingo Maria fever. In the interest of clarity and uniformity, Chandler, Kaplan, and Ajello[2] coined the term histoplasmosis capsulati in 1980 for infections caused by *H capsulatum* var *capsulatum*. The precedent for this was set by Cockshott and Lucas[5] in 1964 when they first used the name histoplasmosis duboisii for infections caused by *H capsulatum* var *duboisii*.

GEOGRAPHIC DISTRIBUTION

Histoplasmosis capsulati has a global distribution, and there is no evidence that it is contagious. In the United States, highly endemic areas include the broad regions of the Ohio and Mississippi River valleys. In the Western Hemisphere, other endemic countries include Guatemala, Mexico, Peru, and Venezuela.

African histoplasmosis caused by the large form or *duboisii* variety of *H capsulatum* is confined to the African continent.[5] Infections caused by the *capsulatum* variety of this fungus also occur in Africa, but African histoplasmosis is discussed separately (Chapter 110) because it is a distinct clinical and pathologic entity in which skin and bone lesions dominate.

CLINICAL FEATURES

Epidemiologists estimate that 500,000 new infections occur each year in the United States, and that 90% to 95% of these are asymptomatic.[6–8] Primary pulmonary lesions in histoplasmosis capsulati are usually subclinical and heal without antifungal therapy, but they may calcify and be discovered in chest radiographs or at autopsy.[8,9] The remaining 5% to 10% of new infections are symptomatic and fall into three broad clinical forms: 1) acute pulmonary, 2) disseminated, and 3) chronic pulmonary.[3,10,11] Patients with the acute pulmonary form have influenza-like symptoms that usually last for a few days to 2 weeks before recovery. Most patients have a history of exposure to conidial aerosols of *H capsulatum* var *capsulatum* from disturbed chicken coops, bird roosts, or other avian habitats, or from areas such as caves and attics where bat guano has accumulated. The incubation period ranges from 3 to 14 days, and the severity and duration of disease depend on host resistance and the number of conidia inhaled. Most acute pulmonary infections resolve with bed rest and other supportive therapy; antifungal therapy is seldom required. Rare sequelae of acute pulmonary infection include persistent lymphadenopathy with bronchial obstruction, granulomatous and sclerosing mediastinitis caused by direct extension of infection from hilar lymph nodes, and pericarditis.[6,12,13]

Disseminated histoplasmosis capsulati, the most severe and life-threatening form, usually occurs in infants, the elderly, and in profoundly immunodeficient patients.[14] It frequently complicates hematologic malignancies, cytotoxic chemotherapy, immunosuppressive therapy in patients with transplanted organs, and the acquired immunodeficiency syndrome (AIDS), all of which have deficient cell-mediated immunity.[15–21] Hematogenous dissemination results in slow but progressive spread of infection to various organs via the mononuclear phagocyte system, or in fulminating infection with rapid clinical deterioration and death. Patients often have fever, chills, productive cough, dyspnea, hemoptysis, purpura, weight loss, malaise, headache, drowsiness, diarrhea, generalized lymphadenopathy, hepatosplenomegaly, ulcerations of the oropharynx and intestines, and bone marrow suppression with one or more cytopenias.[22–24] Involvement of mediastinal and cervical lymph nodes can mimic rapidly progressive lymphoma.[12,13] Patients also may have symptoms of Addison's disease from massive involvement of adrenals. Papular and nodular–ulcerative lesions of skin and oral mucosa are frequent in patients with AIDS (Figure 109–1). The mortality rate in the disseminated form is as high as 80% without antifungal therapy.

The chronic pulmonary form of histoplasmosis capsulati is most commonly a disease of middle-aged men.[25] Symptoms are indistinguishable from those of other chronic pulmonary infections. Chronic pulmonary histoplasmosis may immediately follow the acute pulmonary form or become clinically apparent after a long dormancy. Cavitary lesions are usually endogenous reinfections similar to those seen in tuberculosis. The solitary residual nodule or histoplasmoma is usually subpleural, sharply circumscribed, discretely rounded, from 0.5 to several centimeters across (most are between 1 and 2 cm), and often contains granular deposits of mineral usually concentrated in the necrotic center (Figure 109–2, A and C). What fungal cells remain are mostly collapsed carcasses and concentrated in the necrotic center (Figure 109–2, D). Histoplasmomas also may be accompanied by enlarged, caseous, and calcified hilar lymph nodes. In chest radiographs, histoplasmomas appear as "coin" lesions and resemble carcinoma when they are noncalcified and enlarge progressively on sequential examinations.[9,26] Residual nodules are less frequent in spleen, liver, extrathoracic lymph nodes, and other organs.

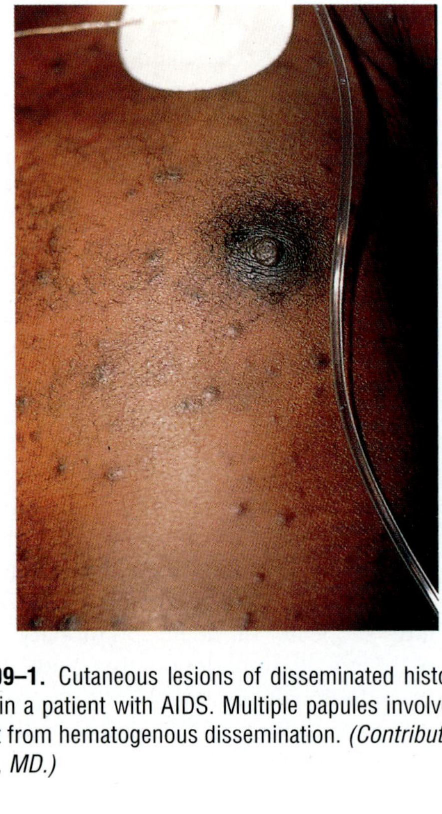

Figure 109–1. Cutaneous lesions of disseminated histoplasmosis capsulati in a patient with AIDS. Multiple papules involve the trunk and result from hematogenous dissemination. *(Contributed by Jack L. Lesher, MD.)*

MORPHOLOGIC FEATURES OF THE ORGANISM

Histoplasma capsulatum var *capsulatum* is thermally dimorphic. The yeast form, produced in culture at 37°C on enriched media, is morphologically similar to that found in infected tissues. The mycelial form, produced in soil and on Sabouraud's medium at 25°C, produces downy, white to golden brown colonies and has two types of asexual conidia: small (2- to 4-μm), smooth-surfaced microconidia (the infectious particles), and large (8- to 14-μm), thick-walled, tuberculate macroconidia with digitate protuberances.[1,27] Once inhaled, the microconidia are rapidly transformed at body temperature into proliferating yeastlike cells.

PATHOLOGY

In tissue sections, cells of *H capsulatum* var *capsulatum* are yeastlike, hyaline, spherical to oval, uniform, 2 to 4 μm in diameter, uninucleate, have single buds attached by a relatively narrow base, and are often clustered because of their initial confinement within macrophages. The fungal cells are more easily detected with H&E when they are numerous and intracellular. In H&E stained tissue sections, the basophilic cytoplasm of the fungal cells is retracted from the thin, weakly stained cell wall, creating a clear zone or "halo" that gives the false impression of an unstained capsule (Figure 109–3). This capsular effect is eliminated when sections are stained with GMS or other special stains for fungi that color the walls (Figure 109–4). Germinating cells and pseudohyphae are occasionally seen in

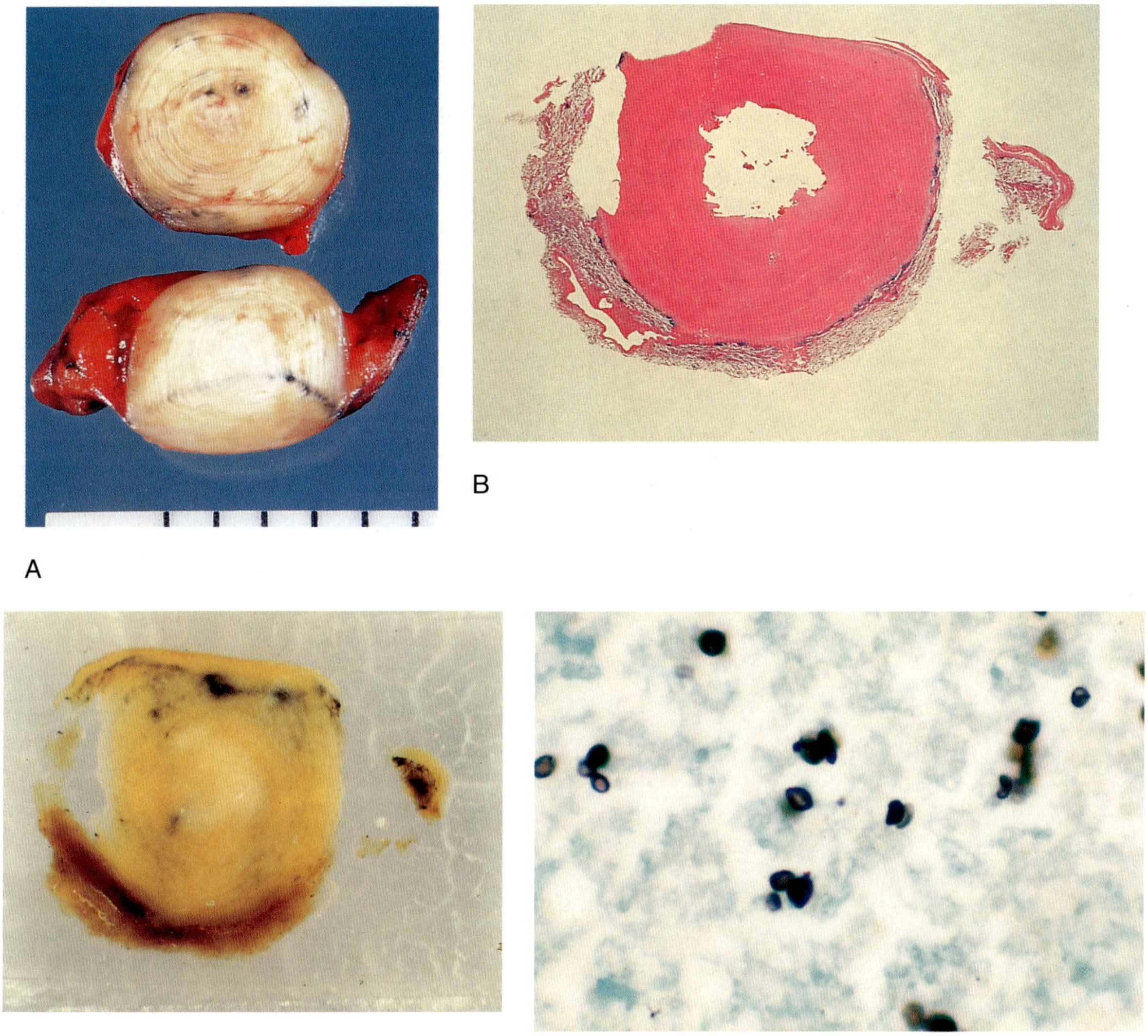

A B C D

Figure 109–2. Residual pulmonary histoplasmosis capsulati. (**A**) Two surgically excised, discretely rounded, subpleural nodules (histoplasmomas) are composed of concentric layers of calcification and caseation, all characteristic features. In radiographs of the chest, histoplasmomas appear as "coin" lesions and resemble carcinoma when the mineralization does not yet show and when they enlarge progressively on sequential examinations. *(Contributed by David H. Dail, MD.)* (**B**) When cutting and staining sections of histoplasmomas, the central necrotic material frequently "falls out." This lost material, unfortunately, is the site of what remains of the yeast forms. Faced with a "hole in the middle," the pathologist should locate the paraffin block and discuss the problem with the technician [whole mount, hematoxylin-eosin (H&E), ×2.5]. *(Contributed by Daniel H. Connor, MD.)* (**C**) Paraffin block of the lesion in part (B). The central necrotic area is, in fact, present and must be retained. *(Contributed by Daniel H. Connor, MD.)* (**D**) Histoplasmoma. The chromic acid in the Gomori's methenamine-silver (GMS) procedure removes mineral salts from the necrotic center of the granuloma while the fungal carcasses are silvered (blackened). The carcasses are misshapen and collapsed but can almost always be identified (GMS, ×630).

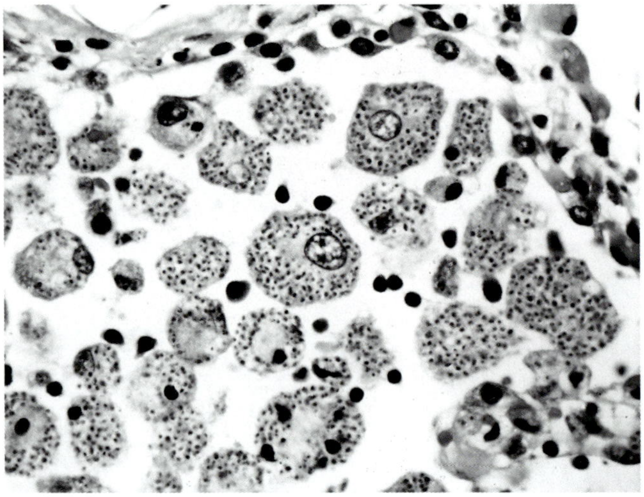

Figure 109–3. Acute pulmonary histoplasmosis capsulati. Alveolar macrophages contain myriad fungal cells 2 to 4 μm in diameter. In H&E stained tissue sections, the hematoxylinophilic cytoplasm of each fungal cell is retracted from the thin, weakly stained but rigid cell wall, creating an optically clear zone or "halo" that gives the false impression of an unstained capsule (H&E, ×500).

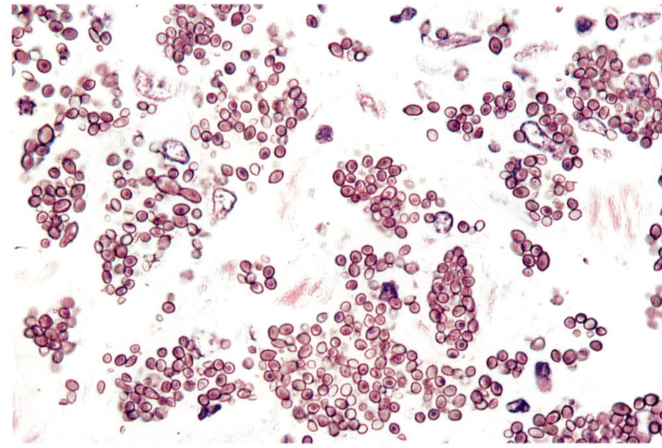

Figure 109–5. Disseminated histoplasmosis capsulati in a mesenteric lymph node of a patient with a transplanted kidney. Intra- and extracellular aggregates of proliferating fungal cells efface the normal histologic architecture of the node. A germinating yeast form is at left center (GMS–H&E, ×250).

rapidly progressive lesions that contain myriad yeast forms[9] (Figure 109–5); both hyphae and huge, thick-walled yeast forms up to 25 μm in diameter may form on or near the surface of valvular vegetations in histoplasma endocarditis[28–31] (Figure 109–6).

The host response to *H capsulatum* var *capsulatum* varies with the number of conidia inhaled and the age and immunologic status of the host.[2,32,33] When many conidia are inhaled, pulmonary lesions are often rapidly progressive and contain myriad proliferating intra-alveolar and interstitial yeast forms accompanied by necrosis and mononuclear cell infiltrates (Figures 109–7 and 109–8). In the very young and in the immunodeficient or anergic, the host response is usually histiocytic, characterized by intracellular multiplication of abundant fungal cells. Dispersed infiltrates of yeast-laden histiocytes often efface the normal architecture of an organ, and there may be bland necrosis and widespread involvement of the mononuclear phagocyte system. In patients with AIDS or other profound cell-mediated immunodeficiencies, rapidly dividing yeast forms

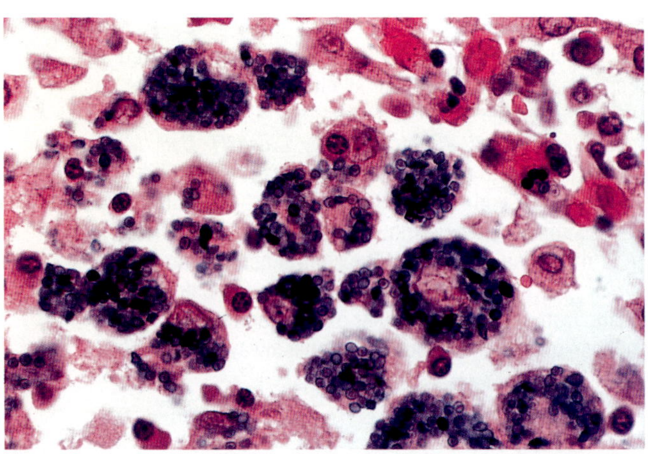

Figure 109–4. Acute pulmonary histoplasmosis capsulati. Many yeast forms are crowded into the alveolar macrophages. When tissue sections are stained with GMS or other special stains for fungi, the walls of the fungal cells are intensely colored, indicating the true size of organisms. There is no capsular or "halo" effect (GMS–H&E, ×250).

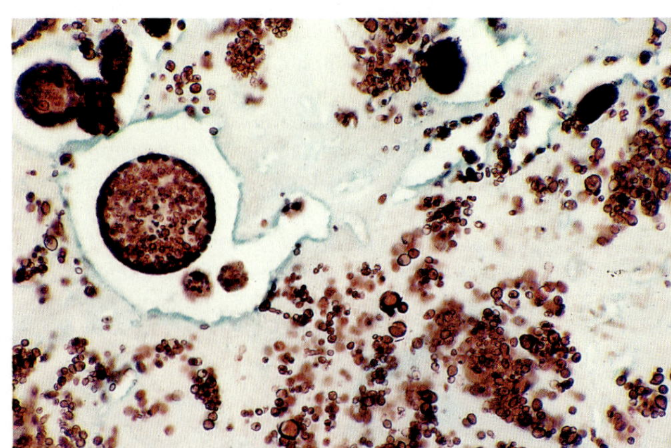

Figure 109–6. Endocarditis caused by *H capsulatum* var *capsulatum*. Large, bizarre yeast forms with thick walls are among compact aggregates of typical organisms near the surface of a valvular vegetation. This lesion also contained short hyphae and germinating yeast forms (GMS, ×160).

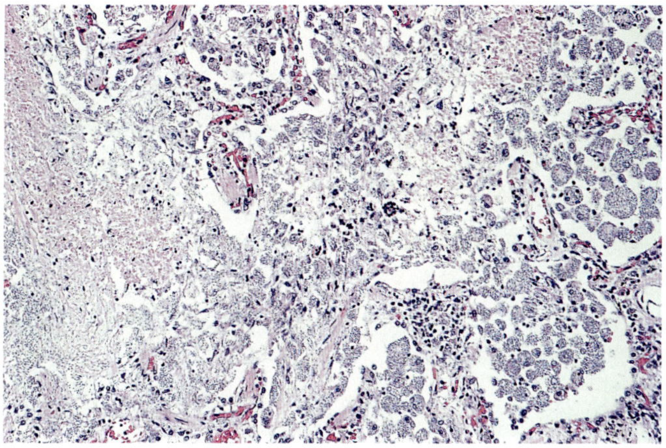

Figure 109–7. Acute pulmonary histoplasmosis capsulati. Alveolar spaces contain macrophages that have phagocytosed yeast forms of *H capsulatum* var *capsulatum*. The pulmonary parenchyma is focally necrotic *(left center)* (H&E, ×40).

may produce large extracellular aggregates or "yeast lakes"[9] (Figure 109–9). In immunocompetent persons, *H capsulatum* var *capsulatum* usually elicits an epithelioid and giant cell granulomatous response with or without caseation (Figure 109–10); fungal cells are relatively sparse in these lesions[7,9] (Figures 109–11 and 109–12).

The residual nodule, or histoplasmoma, consists of a large and often irregularly mineralized central zone of caseous necrosis surrounded by a thick fibrous capsule that contains epithelioid histiocytes, giant cells, and peripheral lymphoid aggregates[9,26] (Figure 109–13). All

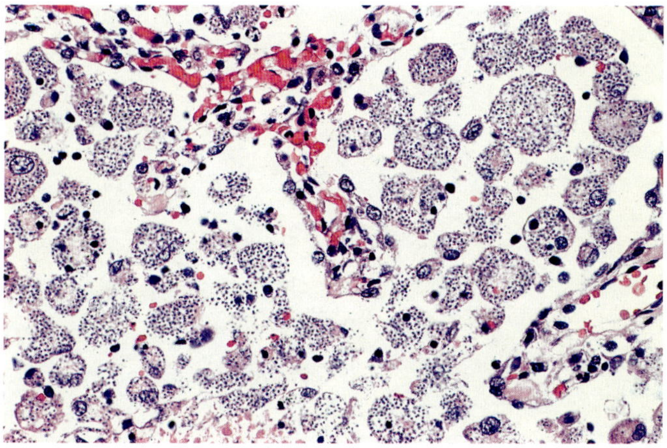

Figure 109–8. Acute pulmonary histoplasmosis capsulati. Alveolar macrophages contain myriad, compact fungal cells. The hematoxylinophilic cytoplasm of individual histoplasma cells is retracted from the thin cell wall, giving the false impression of an unstained capsule. Interstitial inflammation is minimal (H&E, ×100).

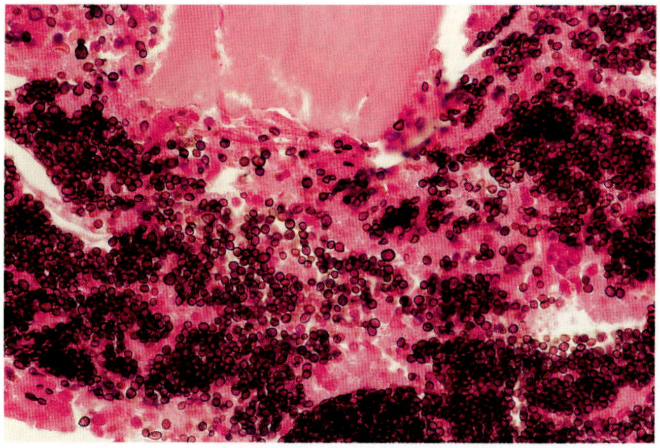

Figure 109–9. Disseminated histoplasmosis capsulati involving the bone marrow in an AIDS patient. The dark masses are large extracellular aggregates or "yeast lakes" of rapidly dividing histoplasma cells. Smaller numbers of fungal cells are within macrophages (GMS–H&E, ×160).

too often, however, the necrotic, calcified center is so loose that it floats away and is "lost" in the water bath (Figure 109–2, B). Unfortunately this is where the organisms are concentrated. When this happens, it is helpful to identify the necrotic center with the histotechnologist before the block is recut (Figure 109–2, C). When the center is retained and stained with GMS, the fungal carcasses ("ghost forms") can usually be identified (Figure 109–2, D) in spite of the fact that they may be collapsed, distorted, fragmented, and weakly or unevenly stained. Here the GMS does double duty, for it not only silvers (blackens) the walls of the yeast forms

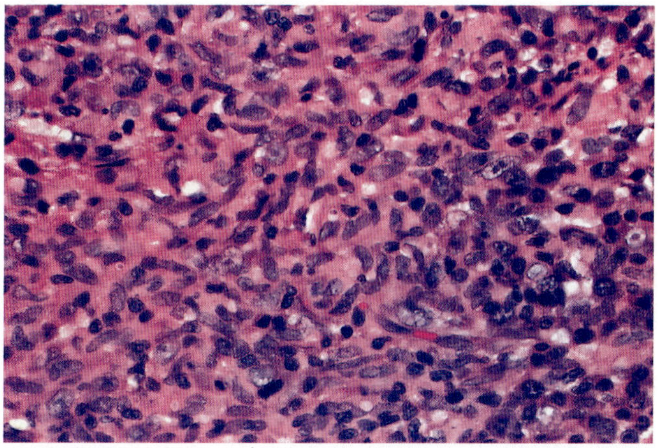

Figure 109–10. Disseminated histoplasmosis capsulati involving the tongue. A dispersed granulomatous reaction is present in the submucosa. Scattered, weakly stained histoplasma cells are located in epithelioid histiocytes (H&E, ×160).

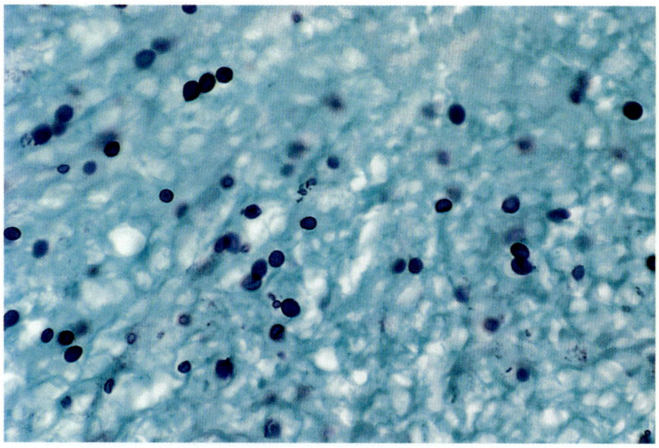

Figure 109–11. Disseminated histoplasmosis capsulati. A replicate, GMS stained section of the lingual granuloma shown in Figure 109–10 reveals isolated, single and budding yeast forms of *H capsulatum* var *capsulatum.* The fungal cells bud by a relatively narrow base *(lower center)* (GMS, ×250).

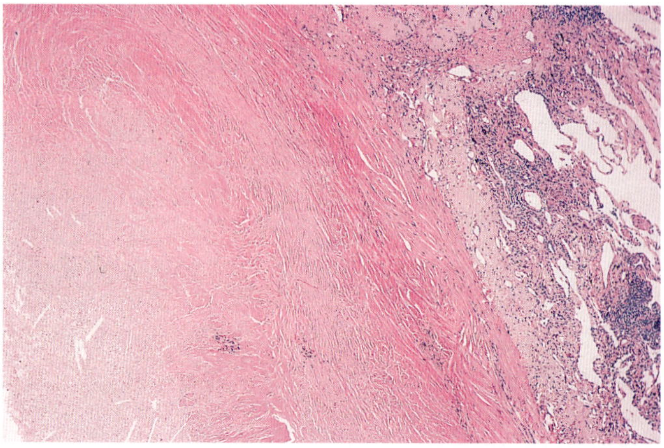

Figure 109–13. Outer wall of a residual pulmonary nodule (histoplasmoma). The nodule consists of a central area of caseous necrosis surrounded by a fibrous capsule that contains varying numbers of epithelioid histiocytes and giant cells. Histoplasma cells are limited to the caseous center of the lesion and usually appear as collapsed carcasses. The GMS stain is required to identify them as they are not visible in H&E stained sections (H&E, ×16).

but also removes the mineral deposits from the necrotic tissue, thus preventing confusion between organisms and small spherules of calcium. The organisms may be in clusters because of their previous intracellular confinement, and budding cells are few (Figure 109–14). Attempts to culture *H capsulatum* var *capsulatum* from these lesions are usually unsuccessful, but a definitive histopathologic diagnosis can be made by direct immunofluorescence of formalin-fixed, deparaffinized tissue sections that contain either intact or fragmented fungal cells[2,27] (Figure 109–15).

DIFFERENTIAL DIAGNOSIS

The yeast-like pathogens most often confused with *H capsulatum* var *capsulatum* in tissue sections are *Torulopsis glabrata,* the cause of torulopsosis (Chapter 123), and *Penicillium marneffei,* the cause of penicilliosis marneffei (Chapter 115). In GMS stained tissue sections, cells of *T glabrata* are spherical to oval, 2 to 5 μm in diameter, have single buds, and resemble those of histoplasma, especially when clustered within histiocytes.[34–36] Unlike histoplasma, however, *T glabrata*

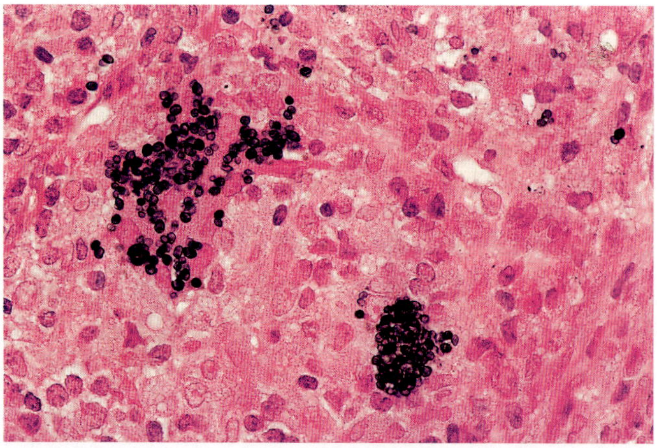

Figure 109–12. Histoplasma lymphadenitis presenting as pseudolymphoma in an immunocompetent patient. Epithelioid histiocytes and giant cells efface the normal architecture of the node. The histoplasma cells, 2 to 4 μm in diameter, are in giant cells (GMS–H&E, ×160).

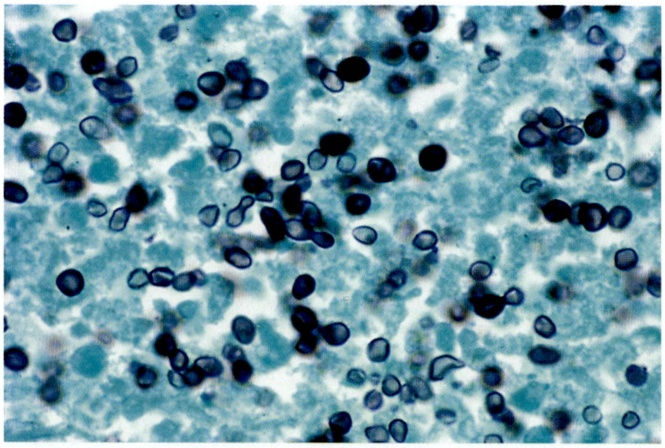

Figure 109–14. Residual pulmonary histoplasmosis capsulati. A replicate, GMS stained section of the histoplasmoma shown in Figure 109–13 reveals distorted and unevenly stained yeast forms of *H capsulatum* var *capsulatum* in the central necrotic residuum (GMS, ×400).

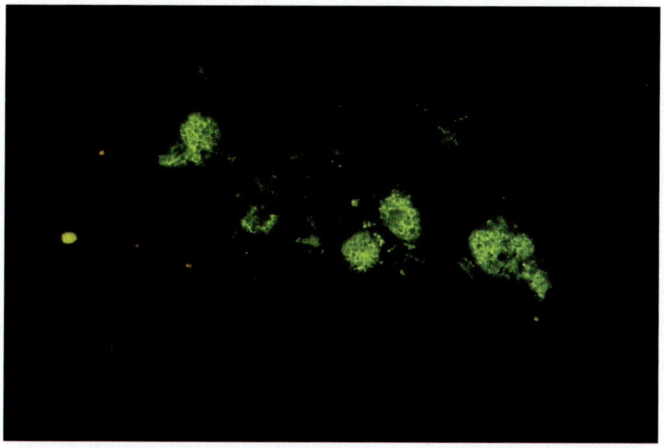

Figure 109–15. Immunofluorescence of *H capsulatum* var *capsulatum* in a deparaffinized section of formalin-fixed lymph node. The walls of fungal cells in epithelioid histiocytes are brightly decorated using a species-specific conjugate (direct immunofluorescence, ×160).

cells are amphophilic, more variable in size, and stain entirely with H&E; a pseudocapsular effect is not observed. The spherical to oval yeastlike cells of *P marneffei* measure 2.5 to 5.0 μm or more, are often sequestered within mononuclear phagocytes, and also resemble those of histoplasma. However, *P marneffei* does not bud. Instead, this fungus reproduces by schizogony (fission) with the formation of a prominent transverse septum.[37,38] In addition to classic septate cells, short hyphal forms and elongated, oval, and curved "sausage" forms up to 20 μm long with rounded ends and one or more septa are occasionally produced in tissue.

Capsule-deficient cryptococci (Chapter 106) and microforms of *B dermatitidis* (Chapter 101) also can resemble the yeastlike cells of *H capsulatum* var *capsulatum*.[9] Most capsule-deficient cryptococci, however, are at least weakly carminophilic when stained with Mayer's or other mucicarmine procedures. Cryptococci also are more pleomorphic, ranging in size from 2 to 20 μm. Microforms of *B dermatitidis* are multinucleated, have thick "double-contoured" cell walls, bud by a broad base, and are usually mixed with yeast forms of typical size (8 to 15 μm). When these differentiating features are equivocal, immunofluorescence using species-specific conjugates is invaluable for confirming a presumptive histopathologic diagnosis.[2,27]

In H&E stained tissue sections, amastigotes of the *Leishmania* sp (Chapter 135) and *Trypanosoma cruzi* (Chapter 143) mimic histoplasma. Under oil immersion, however, the distinguishing bar-shaped kinetoplasts (paranuclear bodies) of these protozoans can be seen with H&E and are even better demonstrated with Wolbach's Giemsa or Wilder's reticulum stains. The histoplasma cells have no such structure and reproduce by budding. Cells of *Toxoplasma gondii* (Chapter 140) also can be confused with histoplasma, but they are smaller, stain entirely with H&E, lack a clear zone or "halo" around each organism, do not bud, and usually parasitize somatic cells. Special histologic stains for fungi do not reliably stain any of these protozoans.

CONFIRMATIONAL TESTING AND DIAGNOSIS

Definitive diagnosis is based on culturing the fungus from clinical materials, or by demonstrating characteristic yeast forms in smears and tissue sections.[2,27] A chemiluminescence-labeled DNA probe or the exoantigen test can be used for rapid confirmation in culture.[39,40] Screening of Wright's stained smears of peripheral blood and bone marrow for histoplasma cells in monocytes and neutrophils is also useful (Figure 109–16); blood smears are positive in up to 50% of patients with AIDS and severe disseminated histoplasmosis capsulati.[41] Serologic tests, such as complement fixation and agar gel double diffusion techniques on acute and convalescent sera, may provide presumptive evidence of infection.[27] Measurement of antigen levels of *H capsulatum* var *capsulatum* in blood and urine by radioimmunoassay helps diagnose some forms of histoplasmosis, and is useful for detecting relapse in AIDS patients and for managing maintenance therapy.[42] Williams et al[43] reported that tests for histoplasma antigen in blood were most useful in patients with disseminated infection or in those with severe pulmonary

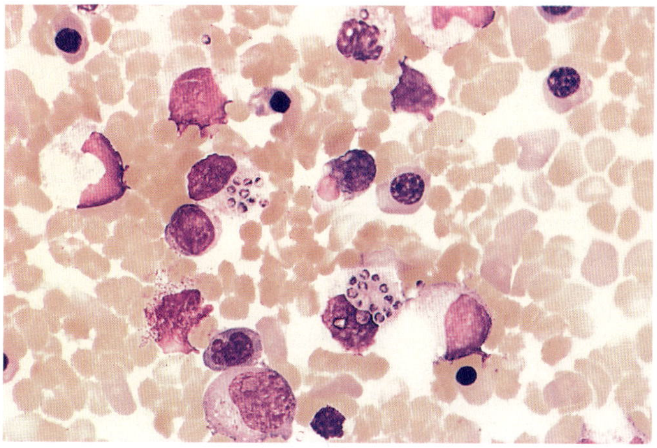

Figure 109–16. Peripheral blood smear from a patient with severe, disseminated histoplasmosis capsulati. Monocytes contain compact histoplasma cells. With Wright's stain the chromatin of individual yeast forms is a dark violet, eccentric, oval or crescentic mass in the weakly stained cytoplasm (Wright's, ×250).

infections, especially during the first few weeks of illness when serologic tests are usually negative. To confirm a presumptive histologic diagnosis in formalin-fixed, deparaffinized tissue sections, direct immunofluorescence using a screening conjugate directed against polysaccharide antigens of all known serotypes of *H capsulatum* is a valuable adjunctive procedure.[2,9]

Models using polymerase chain reaction and specific oligonucleotide probes for detecting and identifying *H capsulatum* var *capsulatum* and other fungal pathogens in clinical specimens have been developed.[44,45] To date, however, these systems have had limited use in the clinical laboratory, and contribute little to the pathologic diagnosis of histoplasmosis capsulati. When refined to optimize sensitivity, a definitive diagnosis using these systems should be possible within hours after receiving a clinical sample.[46]

TREATMENT

Antifungal therapy with amphotericin B is not usually needed in the acute pulmonary form of histoplasmosis capsulati, but is indicated in progressive pulmonary and disseminated infections, and in chronic cavitary pulmonary histoplasmosis.[1,4] Indolent, chronic infections also have been successfully treated with fluconazole and ketoconazole,[47–49] and disseminated infections in AIDS patients have been effectively treated with itraconazole.[50] Amphotericin B, however, remains the treatment of choice for disseminated histoplasmosis. Surgery may be beneficial for patients with chronic cavitary pulmonary lesions and those with fibrosing mediastinitis and pericarditis.[25]

REFERENCES

1. Goodwin RA Jr, Des Prez RM. Histoplasmosis: state of the art. *Am Rev Resp Dis.* 1978;117:929–956.
2. Chandler FW, Kaplan W, Ajello L. *Color Atlas and Text of the Histopathology of Mycotic Diseases.* Chicago: Year Book Medical Publishers; 1980:63–66.
3. Domer JE, Moser SA. Histoplasmosis: a review. *Rev Med Vet Mycol.* 1980;15:159–182.
4. Schwarz J. *Histoplasmosis.* New York: Praeger Publishers; 1981.
5. Cockshott WP, Lucas AO. Histoplasmosis duboisii. *Quart J Med.* 1964;33:223–238.
6. Vanek J, Schwarz J. The gamut of histoplasmosis. *Am J Med.* 1971;50:89–104.
7. Goodwin RA Jr, Loyd JE, Des Prez RM. Histoplasmosis in normal hosts. *Medicine (Baltimore).* 1981;60:231–266.
8. Sarosi GA, Davies SF. *Histoplasma capsulatum* pneumonia. In: Pennington JE, ed. *Respiratory Infections: Diagnosis and Management.* New York: Raven Press; 1983:375–379.
9. Chandler FW, Watts JC. Fungal infections. In: Dail DH, Hammar SP, eds. *Pulmonary Pathology.* 2nd ed. New York: Springer-Verlag; 1993:355–362.
10. Straus SE, Jacobson ES. The spectrum of histoplasmosis in a general hospital: a review of 55 cases diagnosed at Barnes Hospital between 1966 and 1977. *Am J Med Sci.* 1980;279:147–158.
11. Sutliff WD. Histoplasmosis in Veterans Administration hospitals in middle America. *Mycopathologia.* 1983;83:57–62.
12. Zeanah CH, Zusman J. Mediastinal and cervical histoplasmosis simulating malignancy. *Am J Dis Child.* 1979;133:47–49.
13. Gaebler JW, Kleiman MB, Cohen M, et al. Differentiation of lymphoma from histoplasmosis in children with mediastinal masses. *J Pediatr.* 1984;104:706–709.
14. Goodwin RA Jr, Shapiro JL, Thurman GH, et al. Disseminated histoplasmosis: clinical and pathologic correlations. *Medicine (Baltimore).* 1980;59:1–33.
15. Kauffman CA, Israel KS, Smith JW, et al. Histoplasmosis in immunosuppressed patients. *Am J Med.* 1978;64:923–932.
16. Walsh TJ, Catchatourian R, Cohen H. Disseminated histoplasmosis complicating bone marrow transplantation. *Am J Clin Pathol.* 1983;79:509–511.
17. Bonner JR, Alexander WJ, Dismukes WE, et al. Disseminated histoplasmosis in patients with the acquired immune deficiency syndrome. *Arch Intern Med.* 1984;144:2178–2181.
18. Wheat LJ, Slama TG, Zeckel ML. Histoplasmosis in the acquired immune deficiency syndrome. *Am J Med.* 1985;78:203–210.
19. Mandell W, Goldberg DM, Neu HC. Histoplasmosis in patients with the acquired immune deficiency syndrome. *Am J Med.* 1986;81:974–978.
20. Wheat J. Histoplasmosis and coccidioidomycosis in individuals with AIDS. A clinical review. *Infect Dis Clin North Am.* 1994;8:467–482.
21. Wheat J. Endemic mycoses in AIDS: a clinical review. *Clin Microbiol Rev.* 1995;8:146–159.
22. Miller RL, Gould AR, Skolnick JL, et al. Localized oral histoplasmosis: a regional manifestation of mild chronic disseminated histoplasmosis. *Oral Surg.* 1982;53:367–374.
23. Sathapatayavongs B, Batteiger BE, Wheat J, et al. Clinical and laboratory features of disseminated histoplasmosis during two large urban outbreaks. *Medicine (Baltimore).* 1983;62:263–270.
24. Cappell MS, Mandell W, Grimes MM, et al. Gastrointestinal histoplasmosis. *Dig Dis Sci.* 1988;33:353–360.
25. Goodwin RA Jr, Owens FT, Snell JD, et al. Chronic pulmonary histoplasmosis. *Medicine (Baltimore).* 1976;55:413–452.
26. Ulbright TM, Katzenstein ALA. Solitary necrotizing granulomas of the lung. *Am J Surg Pathol.* 1980;4:13–28.
27. Kaufman L. Laboratory methods for the diagnosis and confirmation of systemic mycoses. *Clin Infect Dis.* 1992;14(suppl 1):S23–S29.
28. Canlas MS, Dillon ML Jr. *Histoplasma capsulatum* endocarditis: report of a case following heart surgery. *Angiology.* 1977;28:454–463.
29. Gaynes RP, Gardner P, Causey W. Prosthetic valve endo-

carditis caused by *Histoplasma capsulatum*. *Arch Intern Med.* 1981;141:1533–1537.

30. Hutton JP, Durham JB, Miller DP, et al. Hyphal forms of *Histoplasma capsulatum:* a common manifestation of intravascular infections. *Arch Pathol Lab Med.* 1985; 109:330–332.
31. Svirbely JR, Ayers LW, Buesching WJ. Filamentous *Histoplasma capsulatum* endocarditis involving mitral and aortic valve porcine bioprostheses. *Arch Pathol Lab Med.* 1985;109:273–276.
32. Binford CH. Histoplasmosis: tissue reactions and morphologic variations of the fungus. *Am J Clin Pathol.* 1955;25: 25–36.
33. Baker RD. Histoplasmosis in routine autopsies. *Am J Clin Pathol.* 1964;41:457–470.
34. Grimley PM, Wright LD, Jennings AE. *Torulopsis glabrata* infection in man. *Am J Clin Pathol.* 1965;43:216–223.
35. Aisner J, Sickles EA, Schimpff SC, et al. *Torulopsis glabrata* pneumonitis in patients with cancer. Report of three cases. *JAMA.* 1974;230:584–585.
36. Hickey WF, Sommerville LH, Schoen FJ. Disseminated *Candida glabrata:* report of a uniquely severe infection and a literature review. *Am J Clin Pathol.* 1983;80: 724–727.
37. Deng Z, Connor DH. Progressive disseminated penicilliosis caused by *Penicillium marneffei:* report of eight cases and differentiation of the causative organism from *Histoplasma capsulatum*. *Am J Clin Pathol.* 1985;84: 323–327.
38. Deng Z, Ribas JL, Gibson DW, et al. Infections caused by *Penicillium marneffei* in China and Southeast Asia: review of eighteen published cases and report of four Chinese cases. *Rev Infect Dis.* 1988;10:640–652.
39. Hall GS, Pratt-Rippin K, Washington JA. Evaluation of a chemiluminescent probe assay for identification of *Histoplasma capsulatum* isolates. *J Clin Microbiol.* 1992;30: 3003–3004.
40. Padhye AA, Smith G, McLaughlin D, et al. Comparative evaluation of a chemiluminescent DNA probe and an exoantigen test for rapid identification of *Histoplasma capsulatum*. *J Clin Microbiol.* 1992;30:3108–3111.
41. Hemochowicz S, Sahovic E, Pistole M, et al. Histoplasmosis diagnosed on peripheral blood smear from a patient with AIDS. *JAMA.* 1985;253:3148.
42. Wheat LJ, Kohler RB, Tewari RP. Diagnosis of disseminated histoplasmosis by detection of *Histoplasma capsulatum* antigen in serum and urine specimens. *N Engl J Med.* 1986;314:83–88.
43. Williams B, Fojtasek M, Connolly-Stringfield P, Wheat J. Diagnosis of histoplasmosis by antigen detection during an outbreak in Indianapolis, Ind. *Arch Pathol Lab Med.* 1994;118:1205–1208.
44. Bowman BH. A model PCR/probe system for the identification of fungal pathogens. In: Persing DH, Smith TF, Tenover FC, White TJ, eds. *Diagnostic Molecular Microbiology: Principles and Applications.* Washington, DC: American Society for Microbiology; 1993:423–430.
45. Sandhu GS, Kline BC, Stockman L, Roberts GD. Molecular probes for diagnosis of fungal infections. *J Clin Microbiol.* 1995;33:2913–2919.
46. Mitchell TG, Sandin RL, Bowman BH, Meyer W, Merz WG. Molecular mycology: DNA probes and applications of PCR technology. *J Med Vet Mycol.* 1994;32(suppl 1): 351–366.
47. Slama TG. Treatment of disseminated and progressive cavitary histoplasmosis with ketoconazole: proceedings of a symposium on new developments in therapy for the mycoses. *Am J Med.* 1983;74:70–73.
48. Dismukes WE, Cloud G, Bowles C, et al. Treatment of blastomycosis and histoplasmosis with ketoconazole. *Ann Intern Med.* 1985;103:861–872.
49. Maholtz MS, Dauber JH, Yousem SA. Case report: fluconazole therapy in histoplasma mediastinal granuloma. *Am J Med Sci.* 1994;307:274–277.
50. Wheat J, Hafner R, Korzun AH, et al. Itraconazole treatment of disseminated histoplasmosis in patients with the acquired immunodeficiency syndrome. *Am J Med.* 1995; 98:336–342.

CHAPTER 110

Histoplasmosis Duboisii

Francis W. Chandler and Libero Ajello

A disease also is farther on the road to being cured when it breaks forth from the concealment and manifests its power.

Seneca (4? B.C.–A.D. 65), Moral Epistles to Lucilius, LVI, tr. by Richard M. Gummere

The Lord shall smite thee with the botch of Egypt, and with the emerods, and with the scab, and with the itch, whereof thou canst not be healed.

Deuteronomy 28:35

DEFINITION

Histoplasmosis duboisii is a progressive mycosis with a pulmonary inception and a marked tendency to disseminate to skin, lymph nodes, and bones.[1–3] It is caused by the thermally dimorphic, large-celled, *duboisii* variety of *Histoplasma capsulatum.* Like histoplasmosis capsulati, caused by the small-celled, *capsulatum* variety of this fungus, many infections are thought to be asymptomatic and to resolve spontaneously. Histoplasmosis duboisii occurs in immunocompetent hosts, but rapidly progressive disseminated infection is most common in profoundly immunodeficient patients, especially those with acquired immunodeficiency syndrome.[4,5] Diseases caused by the *duboisii* and *capsulatum* varieties of *H capsulatum* are clinically and histopathologically distinct.[2,6]

The *duboisii* variety of *H capsulatum* was so named formally by Ciferri in 1960.[7] Four years later, Cockshott and Lucas coined the disease term histoplasmosis duboisii.[8] The varietal status of the *duboisii* variety was confirmed by Kwon-Chung[9] in 1975 when she mated isolates of this variety with the tester strains of *Ajellomyces capsulatus* (as *Emmonsiella capsulata*), the teleomorphic or perfect state of *H capsulatum.* Synonyms include African histoplasmosis, large-form histoplasmosis, and large-cell histoplasmosis.

GEOGRAPHIC DISTRIBUTION

With the exception of two reported cases—one from Japan[10] and the other from Madagascar[11]—natural infection by *H capsulatum* var *duboisii* is only in Africa where it infects humans, bats, and nonhuman primates, from the Tropic of Cancer south to the Cape of Good Hope[6,12] (Figure 110–1). The disease is occasionally seen in the United States and other nonendemic areas in those who have lived or traveled in Africa.[13–15] Soil is thought to be the natural reservoir for *H capsulatum* var *duboisii,* and infection follows inhalation of aerosolized microconidia produced by the saprophytic mycelial form of the fungus. The first authentic isolation from soil and bats was documented by Gugnani et al[16] in 1994.

CLINICAL FEATURES

The two clinical forms of histoplasmosis duboisii are localized and disseminated.[8,17] Both forms are thought to have a pulmonary inception but, unlike classic histoplasmosis, pulmonary lesions are uncommon and often subtle when detected.[1] The localized form has a chronic course and is characterized by regional lymphadenopathy with lesions of skin and bone (Figures 110–2 and

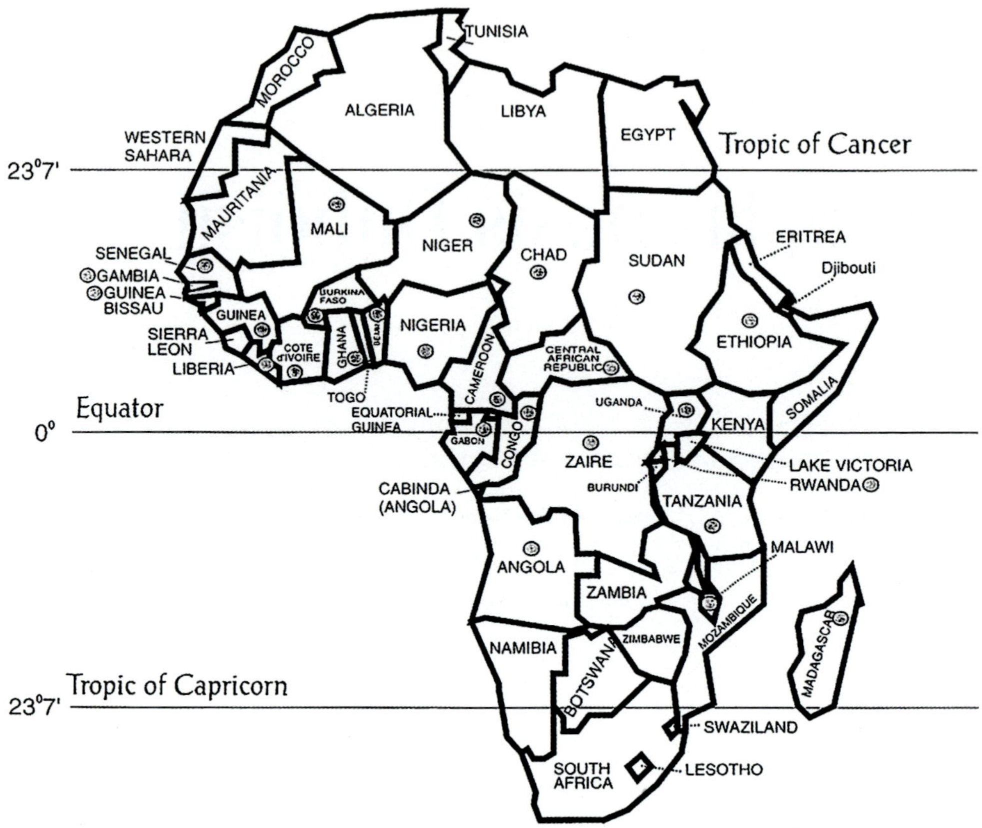

Figure 110–1. Endemic distribution of the *duboisii* variety of *H capsulatum* in Africa and on the island of Madagascar. The shaded circles identify the countries in which infection by *H capsulatum* var *duboisii* has been identified.

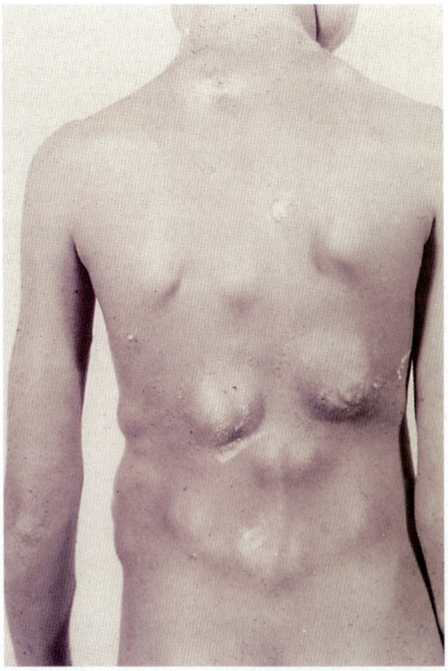

Figure 110–2. Disseminated histoplasmosis duboisii in a Nigerian patient. Multiple, large, subcutaneous nodules involve the neck, shoulders, and trunk. Note ulceration of skin overlying some of the nodules. *(From Centers for Disease Control and Prevention, Atlanta, Georgia.)*

110–3). Skin lesions are most common, and they are papules or nodules that eventually form abscesses and ulcerate[18] (Figure 110–4). Bone lesions occur in one third of patients and are characterized by osteolysis and involvement of contiguous joints.[19,20] Almost any bone can be affected, but the cranium, ribs, sternum, scapula, vertebrae, and long bones are most frequently involved. Osteomyelitis often involves multiple sites, and there may be overlying subcutaneous abscesses and draining sinus tracts. Chronic, localized infections have persisted for several decades.

Although histoplasmosis duboisii is usually localized and chronic, a more rapidly progressive and disseminated form with fever, anemia, weight loss, hepatosplenomegaly, and prominent lymphadenopathy has been reported, especially in patients who are profoundly immunodeficient.[4,5] Hematogenous or lymphatic dissemination from a primary pulmonary or other localized focus to the liver, spleen, intestine, and other organs can be rapidly progressive and fatal unless promptly diagnosed and treated.[21–24]

MORPHOLOGIC FEATURES OF THE ORGANISM

In cultures grown at 25°C on standard mycologic media, the mycelial forms of the *capsulatum* and

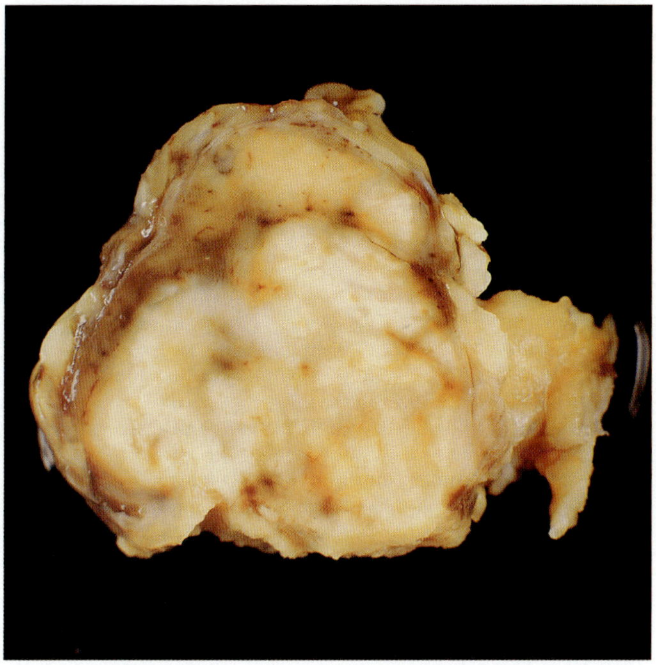

Figure 110–3. Chronic, localized histoplasmosis duboisii in a patient from Zaire. An enlarged inguinal lymph node is effaced by multifocal and confluent granulomas. *(Contributed by Daniel H. Connor, MD, 1976.)*

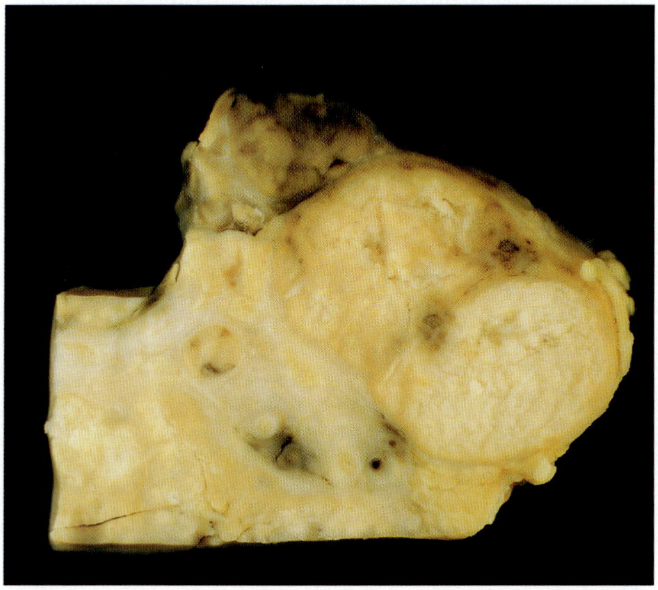

Figure 110–4. Chronic, localized histoplasmosis duboisii. The skin and soft tissues contain large, circumscribed granulomas. Some of the granulomas are encapsulated by fibrous connective tissue. *(Contributed by Daniel H. Connor, MD, 1978.)*

duboisii varieties of *H capsulatum* develop within 1 to 3 weeks and cannot be distinguished from each other either macroscopically or microscopically.[6] The yeast forms of the two varieties, grown at 37°C on enriched culture media, are also morphologically identical. Cultures can be identified with certainty only by infecting laboratory animals and seeing the difference in size of their yeast forms in tissue.[6,25]

In tissue sections, cells of *H capsulatum* var *duboisii* are yeastlike, spherical to oval, uninucleate, 8 to 15 μm in diameter, have thick "doubly contoured" walls, and bud from a relatively narrow base[2] (Figure 110–5). The budding daughter cells commonly enlarge until they are about the size of the parent cells, to which they remain attached by a narrow isthmus, thus creating classical "double-cell" or "figure-eight" forms (Figure 110–6). When "double-cell" forms share a centrally constricted cytoplasm, they are referred to as "hourglass" cells. Germinating yeast forms and short chains of three to five budding cells are common, especially in lesions that contain abundant, rapidly proliferating fungal cells (Figure 110–7). When stained with H&E, the walls of the fungal cells are hyaline, and their cytoplasm is lightly hematoxylinophilic and often vacuolated (Figure 110–5). Special histologic stains for fungi readily color the cell walls of *H capsulatum* var *duboisii*, but staining of the cytoplasmic contents varies.

PATHOLOGY

In both natural and experimental infections, *H capsulatum* var *duboisii* characteristically elicits a dispersed

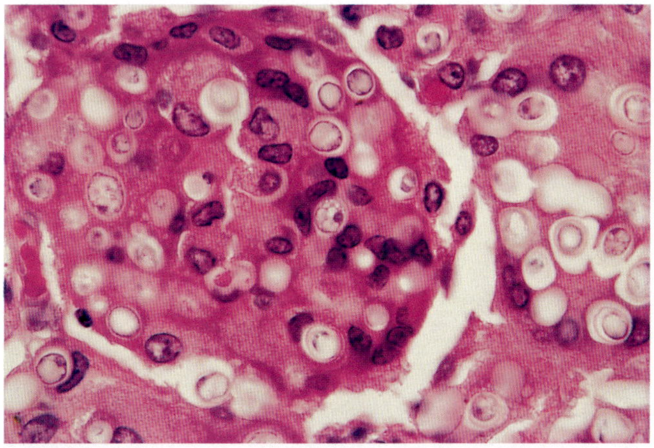

Figure 110–5. Disseminated histoplasmosis duboisii. In tissue, cells of *H capsulatum* var *duboisii* are yeastlike, spherical to oval, uninucleate, 8 to 15 μm in diameter, have thick "doubly contoured" walls, and they bud from a relatively narrow base *(left center)*. Fungal cells are usually in macrophages and giant cells (hematoxylin-eosin, ×250).

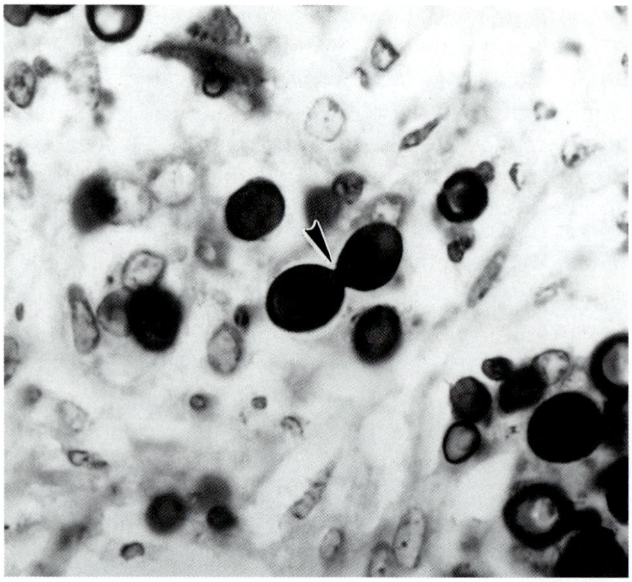

Figure 110–6. Histoplasmosis duboisii. A classical "double-cell" form of *H capsulatum* var *duboisii (arrowhead)* is produced when the budding daughter cell enlarges until it is equal in size to the parent cell, to which it remains attached by a narrow isthmus [Gomori's methenamine silver (GMS)–H&E, ×760].

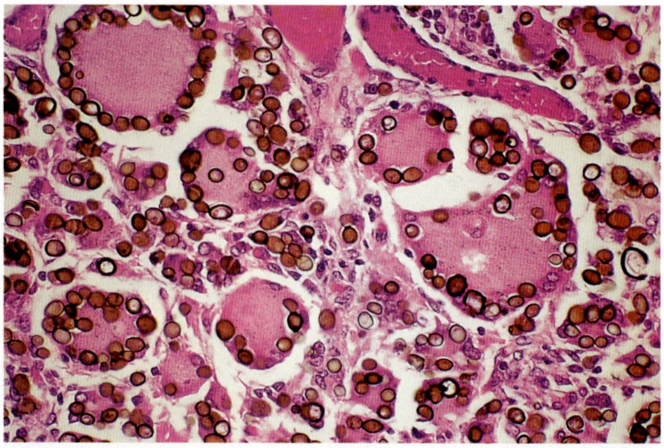

Figure 110–8. Chronic, localized histoplasmosis duboisii. Dispersed macrophages and giant cells within a subcutaneous granuloma contain myriad single and budding yeast forms of *H capsulatum* var *duboisii* (GMS–H&E, ×100).

granulomatous inflammatory reaction in which numerous yeastlike cells are in the cytoplasm of epithelioid histiocytes and giant cells of both the foreign-body and Langhans' types[2,17] (Figures 110–8 and 110–9). Lesions are microscopically similar in all organs. In chronic infections, there is almost total effacement of some organs, and the granulomatous response is sometimes accompanied by focal necrosis and fibrosis (Figure 110–10). Almost every phagocyte contains fungal cells, and it is not unusual to see enormous giant cells up to 150 μm in diameter that contain 20 or more yeast forms in a single plane of section (Figure 110–11). Although most fungal elements are intracellular, small numbers also may be extracellular, either singly or in clusters. Extracellular collections of degenerated, weakly stained fungal cells are especially observed in foci of caseous necrosis. Occasionally, lymphocytes, plasma cells, and neutrophils are scattered among the epithelioid cells and giant cells. Neutrophils do not contain organisms and are only a minor component of the inflammatory cell infiltrate.

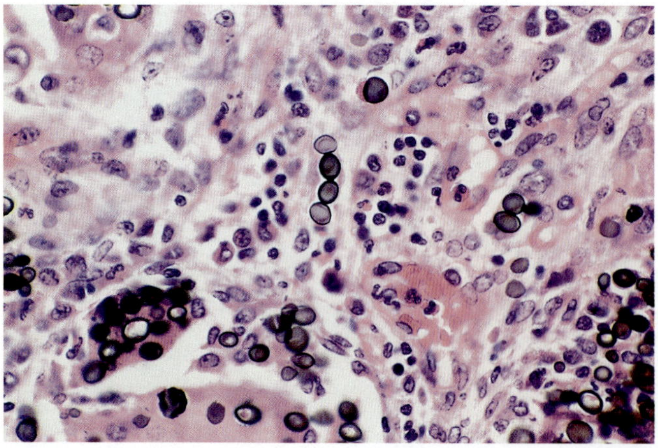

Figure 110–7. Disseminated histoplasmosis duboisii. A splenic granuloma contains a chain of four budding yeast forms *(center)*, each connected by a narrow isthmus. Typical nonbudding and single budding cells of *H capsulatum* var *duboisii* are also present (GMS–H&E, ×160).

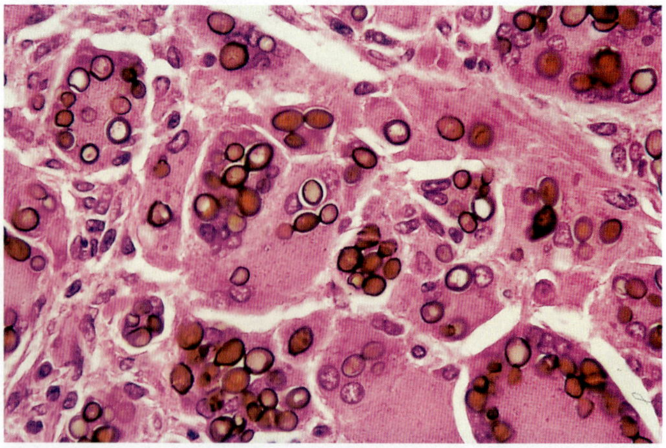

Figure 110–9. Histoplasmosis duboisii. Numerous spherical to oval yeastlike cells, 8 to 15 μm in diameter, have thick cell walls and are located within giant cells. Note classical "double-cell" yeast form *(top center)* and short chains of budding cells *(center)* (GMS–H&E, ×260).

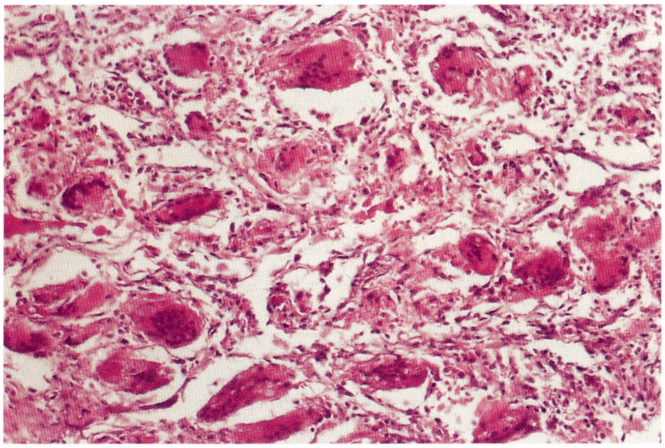

Figure 110–10. Primary pulmonary histoplasmosis duboisii. Note dispersed granulomatous inflammation and interstitial fibrosis. Yeastlike cells of *H capsulatum* var *duboisii* within the huge foreign body-type giant cells are not readily visible at this magnification (H&E, ×40).

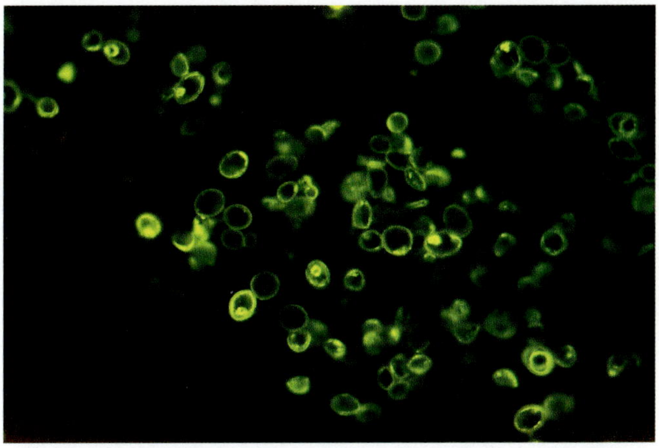

Figure 110–12. Direct immunofluorescence of *H capsulatum* var *duboisii* in a deparaffinized section of formalin-fixed tissue. The walls of histoplasma cells are brightly decorated using a species-specific conjugate (direct immunofluorescence, ×160).

DIFFERENTIAL DIAGNOSIS

Because of their similarity in size and shape and their thick, "doubly contoured" walls, cells of *H capsulatum* var *duboisii* and *Blastomyces dermatitidis* can be easily mistaken for each other in tissue sections.[2,3] The former, however, usually bud from a narrower base with typical "double-cell" forms, whereas the diagnostic budding form of *B dermatitidis* is always broad based. When stained with H&E, yeastlike cells of the *duboisii* variety of *H capsulatum* are uninucleate (Figure 110–11), whereas *B dermatitidis* cells each contain multiple, hematoxylinophilic nuclei. When these differentiating features are equivocal, a presumptive morphologic diagnosis can be confirmed by culture and immunofluorescence staining of fungi in formalin-fixed, deparaffinized tissue sections[2,6,26] (Figure 110–12).

In tissue, yeast forms of *H capsulatum* var *duboisii* are easily distinguished from those of the *capsulatum* variety of *H capsulatum*. The former are much larger, bud more frequently with classical "double-cell" forms, and are predominately within huge giant cells instead of histiocytes.

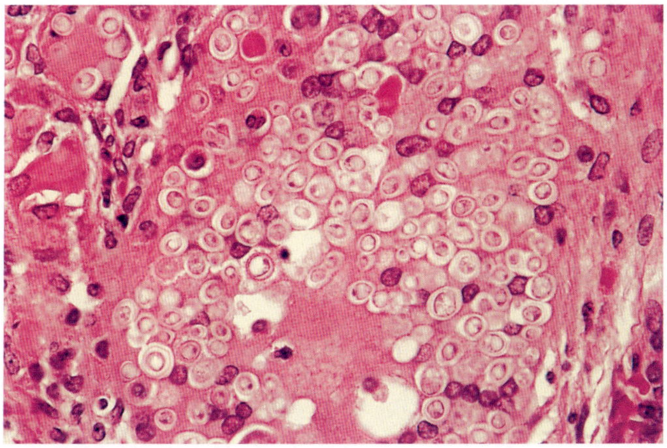

Figure 110–11. Disseminated histoplasmosis duboisii. An enormous giant cell contains many spherical to oval yeast forms, 8 to 15 μm in diameter. Note that the yeastlike cells are uninucleate, a feature that helps distinguish them from cells of *B dermatitidis* in H&E stained tissue sections (H&E, ×160).

TREATMENT

Intravenously administered amphotericin B is the treatment of choice for both the localized and disseminated forms of histoplasmosis duboisii, but relapse is common in the latter. Oral ketoconazole has been used successfully as an alternative to amphotericin B, and favorable responses also have been reported when a combination of trimethoprim and sulfamethoxazole is used.[27] Localized, readily accessible lesions have been successfully treated by excision alone, or by excision combined with antifungal therapy.

REFERENCES

1. Clark BM, Greenwood BM. Pulmonary lesions in African histoplasmosis. *J Trop Med Hyg*. 1968;71:4–10.
2. Chandler FW, Watts JC. *Pathologic Diagnosis of Fungal Infections*. Chicago: ASCP Press; 1987:141–147.

3. Chandler FW, Watts JC. Fungal infections. In: Dail DH, Hammar SP, eds. *Pulmonary Pathology.* 2nd ed. New York: Springer-Verlag; 1994:362–364.
4. Arendt V, Coremans-Pelseneer J, Gottlob R, et al. African histoplasmosis in a Belgian AIDS patient. *Mycoses.* 1991; 34:59–61.
5. Carme B, Ngaporo AI, Ngolet A, et al. Disseminated African histoplasmosis in a Congolese patient with AIDS. *J Med Vet Mycol.* 1992;30:245–248.
6. Ajello L. Histoplasmosis. A dual entity: histoplasmosis capsulati and histoplasmosis duboisii. *Igiene Moderna.* 1983;79:3–30.
7. Ciferri R. *Manuale di Micologia Medica.* 3rd ed. Parte speciale. Casa Editrice Renzo Cortina; 1960;2:796.
8. Cockshott WP, Lucas AO. Histoplasmosis duboisii. *Q J Med.* 1964;33:223–238.
9. Kwon-Chung KJ. Perfect state *(Emmonsiella capsulata)* of the fungus causing large-form African histoplasmosis. *Mycologia.* 1975;67:980–990.
10. Yamato H, Hitomi H, Maekawa S, Mimura K. A case of histoplasmosis. *Acta Med Okayama.* 1957;11:347–364.
11. Coulanges P, Raveloarison G, Ravisse P. Existence of histoplasmosis with *Histoplasma duboisii* outside continental Africa (on the first Malagash case). *Bull Soc Pathol Exot Filliales.* 1982;75:400–403.
12. Walter J, Spooner ETC. Natural infection of the African baboon *(Papio papio)* with the large cell form of histoplasmosis. *J Pathol Bacteriol.* 1960;8:436–439.
13. Nethercott JR, Schachter RK, Givan KF, et al. Histoplasmosis due to *Histoplasma capsulatum* var *duboisii* in a Canadian immigrant. *Arch Dermatol.* 1978;114:595–598.
14. Shore RN, Waltersdorff RL, Edelstein MV, et al. African histoplasmosis in the United States. *JAMA.* 1981;245:734.
15. Lobdell DH, Cappiello MA, Riccio FJ. African histoplasmosis in Connecticut. *Conn Med.* 1982;46:187.
16. Gugnani HC, Muotoe-Okafor FA, Kaufman L, Dupont B. A natural focus of *Histoplasma capsulatum* var *duboisii* in a bat cave. *Mycopathologia.* 1994;127:151–157.
17. Williams AO, Lawson EA, Lucas AO. African histoplasmosis due to *Histoplasma duboisii. Arch Pathol.* 1971;92: 306–318.
18. Lucas AO. Cutaneous manifestations of African histoplasmosis. *Br J Dermatol.* 1970;82:435–447.
19. Lunn HF. A case of histoplasmosis of bone in East Africa. *J Trop Med Hyg.* 1960;63:175–180.
20. Cockshott WP, Lucas AO. Radiological findings in *Histoplasma duboisii* infections. *Br J Radiol.* 1964;37:653–660.
21. Lanceley JL, Lunn NF, Wilson AMM: Histoplasmosis in an African child. *J Pediatr.* 1961;59:756–764.
22. Cole ACE, Ridley DS, Wolfe HRI. Bowel infections with *Histoplasma duboisii. J Trop Med Hyg.* 1965;68:92–96.
23. Olurin O, Lucas AO, Oyediran ABO. Orbital histoplasmosis due to *Histoplasma duboisii. Am J Ophthalmol.* 1969; 68:14–18.
24. Adekunle OO, Sudhakaran P, Timeyin ED. African histoplasmosis of the jejunum: report of a case. *J Trop Med Hyg.* 1978;81:88–90.
25. Duncan JT. A unique form of *Histoplasma. Trans Roy Soc Trop Med Hyg.* 1946;40:364–365.
26. Standard PG, Kaufman L. Specific immunological tests for the rapid identification of members of the genus *Histoplasma. J Clin Microbiol.* 1976;3:191–199.
27. Brown KGE, Molesworth BD, Boerrigter FGG, et al. Disseminated histoplasmosis duboisii in Malawi: partial response to sulphonamide/trimethoprim combination. *East Afr Med J.* 1974;51:584–590.

CHAPTER 111

Lobomycosis

Gregory Nikolaidis and Theodore Rosen

A wound, 'tho cured, yet leaves behind a scar.

John Oldham, Satires upon the Jesuits, 1680

DEFINITION

First described by Jorge Lobo in 1931, lobomycosis is a chronic fungal infection of the skin caused by *Loboa loboi.*[1] The condition is characterized by nodules, which may coalesce into plaques, and resembles keloid in its clinical appearance. It does not involve the internal organs, and except for occasional involvement of the regional lymph nodes, is limited to the skin.[2,3] The disease is sporadic, and arises primarily in the South and Central American tropics. Natural infections have been reported only in humans and dolphins.

SYNONYMS

Lobomycosis is known also as Amazonian blastomycosis, South American blastomycosis, keloidal blastomycosis, blastomycoid granuloma, pseudoleprosy, and Jorge Lobo's disease.[2,4]

ETIOLOGY

The fungus that causes lobomycosis has been isolated but not been cultured on synthetic media, and confusion surrounds its taxonomy. Mycologists have classified it as possibly belonging to one of three different genera: *Paracoccidioides, Glenosporella,* or *Blastomyces.*[5,6] The name *Loboa loboi* is preferred because no consensus has been reached, and because it does not imply any relationship to other organisms.[7,8]

EPIDEMIOLOGY

More than 300 confirmed cases of lobomycosis have been reported in humans since the disease was first described in 1931.[2] More than two thirds of these infections have been in the Brazilian and Colombian Amazon regions.[9,10] In addition, lobomycosis has been described in Surinam, French Guinea, Venezuela, Panama, Costa Rica, Peru, Ecuador, Bolivia, Guyana, Mexico, and France.[9–16]

Lobomycosis predominates in areas with thick vegetation and tropical climate, such as the Amazon rain forests. The fungus is believed to be a saprophyte of soil or vegetation, and cutaneous trauma is presumed to be the means of acquiring the disease. A plant reservoir, however, has not been reported. Since the disease is in dolphins, it may have an aquatic habitat.[17] Although dolphin-to-human transmission has been reported,[16] there is no evidence of human-to-human transmission.

Lobomycosis affects all races and no racial prevalence has been described. Men are more commonly affected than women, apparently because men work in close contact with the environment that harbors the fungus. The incidence of lobomycosis is higher in women in those tribes where women have a more active role in farming and jungle clearing.[18] In addition to farmers, hunters and rubber plant workers have an increased incidence of this disease. Lobomycosis affects all age groups, and the usual age of onset is between 20 and 40 years.[9]

LIFE CYCLE

The natural habitat of *L loboi* is unknown. It is believed to live in water, soil, or on vegetation, and to enter the skin through trauma. The organism is phagocytosed by macrophages in the dermis and begins a slow cycle of growth.[9] The incubation period usually lasts a few years.

MORPHOLOGY OF *LOBOA LOBOI*

The organism is spherical to oval, yeastlike, 6 to 12 μm in diameter, and has a thick, hyaline doubly refractile wall.[19] It reproduces by budding, and forms chains of up to 20 fungal cells, each connected by a narrow, tubelike isthmus.[5] Although it may be extracellular, *L loboi* is primarily an intracellular organism.[19,20]

CLINICAL FEATURES

The lesions of lobomycosis are polymorphic. Even in the same patient one may find macules, papules, keloidal nodules, plaques, and verrucous and ulcerated lesions (Figure 111–1, A–C).[21] The nodular keloid lesion is most common.[19] The disease spares mucous membranes and does not involve internal organs. Lesions tend to arise on traumatized areas of exposed skin, such as the face, ears, arms, legs, and feet. Initially, patients may have an inflammatory or pruritic reaction at the site of inoculation.[22] Otherwise, patients are asymptomatic and have no systemic manifestations of the disease. The affected area may be hypesthetic or anesthetic, resembling leprosy.[2,19] Cutaneous lesions of lobomycosis are usually isolated, but may become disseminated, and are believed to be spread by autoinoculation.[23] The course of the disease is slow, yet progressive. Although macular lesions may regress, they do not heal spontaneously.[24] They are amenable to surgical treatment, but only in the early circumscribed stage of disease.[25]

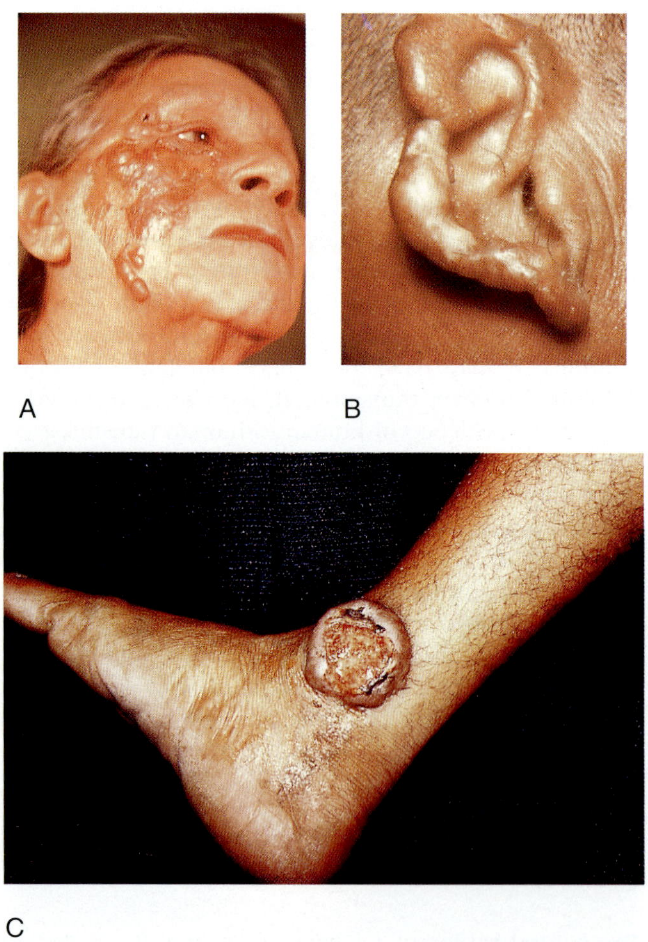

Figure 111–1. Clinical presentation of lobomycosis showing the polymorphous character of the lesions. Macules, papules, keloidal nodules, plaques, and a raised lesion on the ankle with central ulceration are displayed in these three patients. *(From the Centers for Disease Control and Prevention, Atlanta.)*

PATHOLOGY

The histologic picture of lobomycosis is characteristic and distinctive.[26] Biopsy reveals a dispersed granulomatous infiltrate along with numerous fungi in the lower dermis and subcutaneous tissue (Figures 111–2 and 111–3).[2,27] The epidermis is often atrophic, and may show a loss of rete ridges. A narrow clear zone (Grenz) separates the epidermis from the granuloma.[28] The granuloma is comprised primarily of giant cells, macrophages, and epithelioid cells. Occasional lymphocytes and plasma cells are also noted.[2,28] Both the giant cells and macrophages contain phagocytosed fungi. The macrophages are loaded with phagolysosomes that contain incompletely digested fungal elements, and thus resemble the foamy macrophages of Gaucher's disease.[27] Fibrosis is minimal even in long-

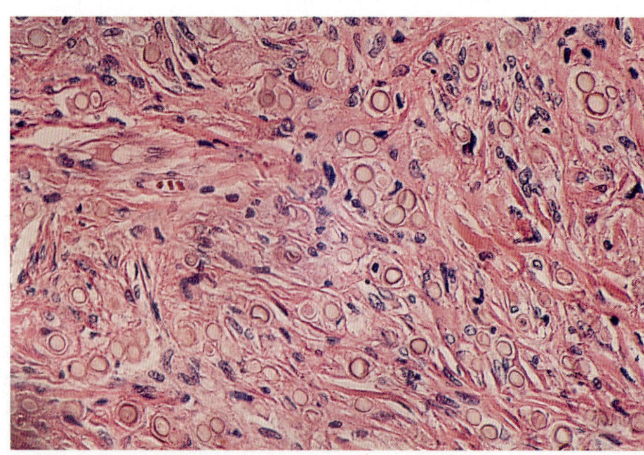

Figure 111–2. Dermis of a patient with lobomycosis. There is minimal fibrosis and an infiltrate of macrophages. Yeastlike cells of *L loboi* are numerous. Characteristically, as shown here, there are pairs, short chains, and clusters of yeast forms in macrophages and giant cells (hematoxylin-eosin, ×400).

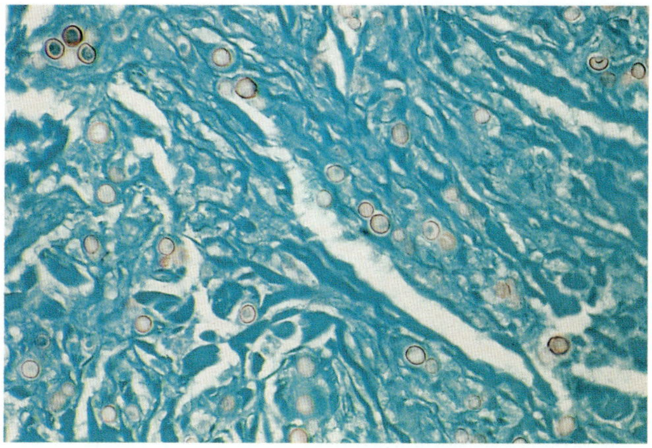

Figure 111–3. *Loboa loboi.* The walls of fungal cells are lightly silvered and easily recognized. Yeast forms occur singly, in pairs, and in clusters in this field. Most of the fungi are in macrophages [Gomori's methenamine silver (GMS), ×400].

standing infections. Immunohistochemistry shows that most of these macrophages are quiescent; only a few are activated.[20] The fungi have a thick, doubly contoured wall, and usually form single chains of budding cells joined by narrow tubelike bridges (Figure 111–4). Occasionally, there may be multiple (secondary) buds.[28] Although the organism ranges from 5 to 12 μm in diameter, most are uniform in size. The granulomatous infiltrate may spread to underlying muscle, and may be exuberant enough to damage cutaneous adnexa and nerves.[27]

The cell wall and cytoplasm of *L loboi* are strongly GMS- and periodic acid–Schiff (PAS)-positive. Hematoxylin-eosin stain reveals the double silhouette of the cell wall and one or more small, hematoxylinophilic nuclei. GMS and other stains for fungi readily demonstrate the characteristic budding of the organism.[27,28]

Electron microscopy reveals marked variation of the internal structure of the fungal cells.[28] Some have a homogeneous cytoplasm without organelles, while others have multiple nuclei, along with mitochondria, endoplasmic reticulum, ribosomes, and vesicles. The cell wall has internal and external layers with small pores through which the filopodial processes of macrophages may penetrate.[29]

DIFFERENTIAL DIAGNOSIS

Microscopically, keloids and other scars have marked fibrosis, which is rare in lobomycosis.[2] In addition, keloids lack granulomatous inflammation and fungi. *Paracoccidioides brasiliensis* reproduces by multiple budding ("steering wheel" forms) and has much more variability in its size (1 to 40 μm). *Loba loboi,* however, produces multiple buds that can be mistaken for those of *P brasiliensis* (Figures 111–5 and 111–6). *Blastomyces dermatitidis* and *Histoplasma capsulatum* var *duboisii* usually do not form chains of cells when budding. *Sporothrix schenckii* (2 to 8 μm) and *Histoplasma capsulatum* var *capsulatum* (3 to 4 μm) are both smaller than *L loboi.*[24]

DIAGNOSIS

Although the clinical features of lobomycosis may be confusing, biopsy shows a characteristic picture that confirms the diagnosis. The morphology and pattern of

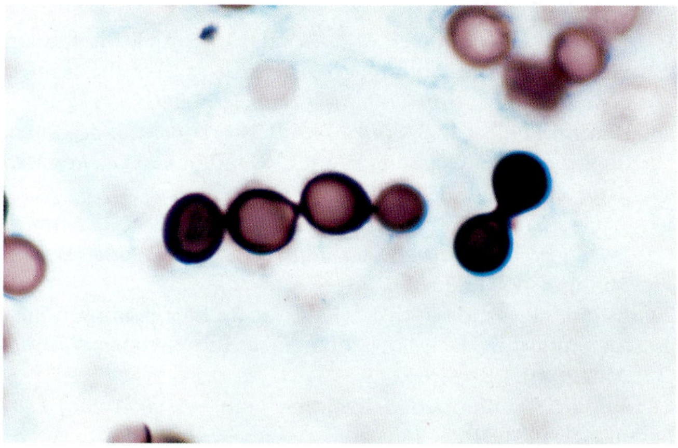

Figure 111–4. *Loboa loboi.* The fungi have a thick, doubly contoured wall, and form a single chain with individual cells joined by narrow tubelike bridges (GMS, ×500). *(Contributed by Francis W. Chandler, DVM, PhD.)*

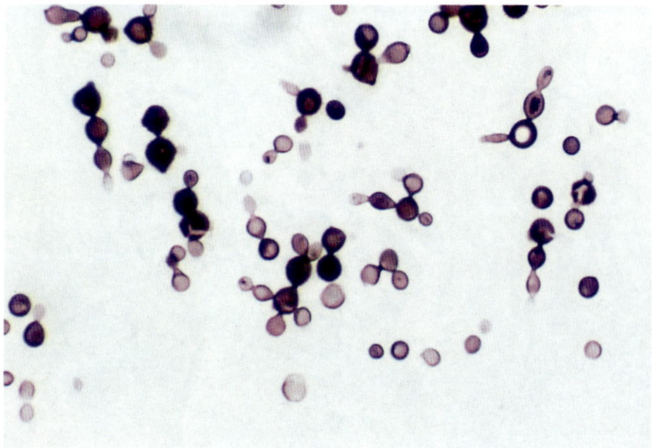

Figure 111–5. Human lobomycosis. Some of the *L loboi* cells have secondary buds, a pattern that resembles somewhat the "steering wheel" buds of *P brasiliensis* (GMS, ×200). *(Contributed by Francis W. Chandler, DVM, PhD.)*

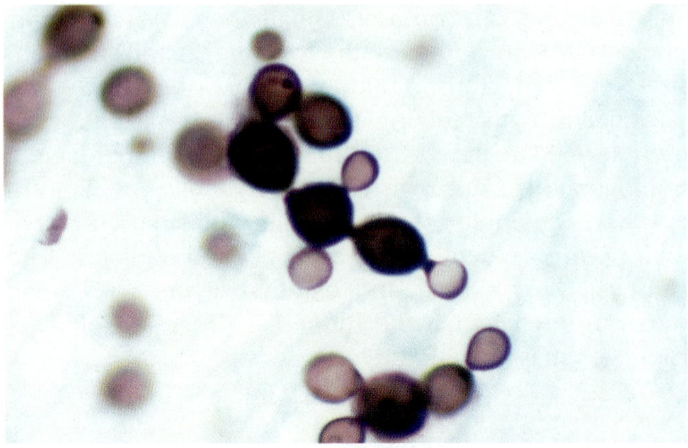

Figure 111–6. Lobomycosis in a dolphin. Short chains and secondary buds are seen in a cutaneous granuloma. (GMS, ×500). *(Contributed by Francis W. Chandler, DVM, PhD.)*

budding of *L loboi* are morphologically distinctive. Although serologic tests are not available, increased titers of IgG and IgM to the polysaccharide antigens of the fungus have been shown.[28] Lobomycosis in dolphins resembles lobomycosis in humans both microscopically and clinically (Figures 111–6 and 111–7).

TREATMENT

Isolated lesions are amenable to surgical excision. The disseminated form of lobomycosis, however, recurs when treated surgically and usually does not respond to antifungal therapy.[24–26]

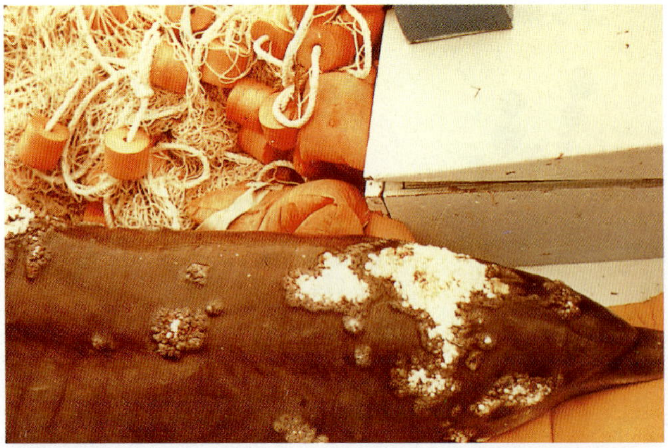

Figure 111–7. Cutaneous lobomycosis in a captured Florida dolphin. The lesions are verrucous, depigmented, probably a consequence of epithelial hyperplasia, but not ulcerated. *(Contributed by David A. Schwarz, MD.)*

REFERENCES

1. Lobo J. Um caso de Blastomicose, produzido per uma especia nova, encontrada em Recife. *Rev Med Pernambuco.* 1931;1:763–775.
2. Rodriguez-Toro G. Lobomycosis. *Int J Dermatol.* 1993;32: 324–332.
3. Azulay RD, Carneiro JA, Da Graca M, Cunha S, Reis LT. Keloidal blastomycosis with lymphatic involvement: a case study. *Int J Dermatol.* 1976;15:40–42.
4. Boreli D. Lobomycosis: nomenclatura de su agente. *Med Cutan.* 1968;3:152–156.
5. Azulay RD. Die Blastomycose vom Typ Jorge Lobo. In: Marchioni A, ed. *Handbuch der Haut und Geschlechtskrankheiten.* Berlin: Springer; 1963:175.
6. Emmons CW, Binford CM, Utz J. Paracoccidioides and lobomycosis. In: *Diseases in Medical Mycology.* Philadelphia: Lea and Febiger; 1970:342–346.
7. Rippon JW. Lobomycosis. In: *Medical Mycology.* Philadelphia: WB Saunders; 1982:315–324.
8. Ciferri R, Carniero LS, Campos S, et al. Advances in the knowledge of fungus of Jorge Lobo's disease. *J Trop Med Hyg.* 1956;59:214–215.
9. Lacaz CS, Baruzzi RG, Rosa MCB. *Doneca de Jorge Lobo.* Sao Paolo: Editoria da USP-IPSIS Grafica e Editoria; 1986.
10. Rodriguez-Toro G, Tellez N. Lobomycosis in Colombian Amerindian patients. *Mycopathologia.* 1982;80:65–72.
11. Pardinard R. Entre le Yucatan, la Floride et al Guyane Francaise, la lobomycose existe telle aux Antilles? *Bull Soc Path Exot.* 1984;77:392–394.
12. Tapia A, Torres-Calcindo A, Aromena R. Keloidal blastomycosis in Panama. *Int J Dermatol.* 1978;17:572–578.
13. Arrese EJ, Rurangirwa A, Pierrando GE. Lobomycosis. *Ann Pathol.* 1988;8:325–327.
14. Rose P, Hay RJ. Lobo's disease. Report of a case from Guyana. *Am J Trop Med Hyg.* 1975;24:105–114.
15. Zavala-Velasquez J, Perez AR. Enfermedad de Lobo. Primer caso Mexicano. *Dermatologia.* 1978;22:5–12.
16. Symmers W. A possible case of Lobo's disease acquired in Europe from a bottle-nosed dolphin. *Bull Soc Path Exot.* 1983;76:777–784.
17. Caldwell DK, Caldwell MC, Woodard JC, Ajello L, Kaplan W, McClure HM. Lobomycosis as a disease of the bottled nose dolphin. *Am J Trop Med Hyg.* 1975;24:105–114.
18. Baruzzi RG, Lacaz S, Souza PAA. Historia natural de donca de Jorge Lobo. Occurencia entre os indios Caibai. *Rev Med Trop Sao Paulo.* 1979;21:302–308.
19. Wiersema JD. Lobo's disease. In: Baker RD, ed. *Human Infection with Fungi, Actinomycetes and Algae.* Berlin: Springer; 1971:577.
20. Esterre P, Pradinaud R, Ravisse P. Etude immunohistochimque de la lesion cutanee de lobomycose. *J Mycol Med.* 1991;1:276–283.
21. Talhari S. Enfermedad de Jorge Lobo. *Arch Argent Dermatol.* 1981;31:23–26.
22. Borelli D. Lobomycosis experimental. *Dermatol Venez.* 1961;3:72–82.
23. Roscoe J, Farmer ER. Diseases caused by fungi. In: Farmer ER, Hood AF, eds. *Pathology of the Skin.* Norwalk, Conn: Appleton & Lange; 1990:381–382.

24. Dias LB, Sampaio MM, Silva D. Jorge Lobo's disease. *Rev Inst Med Trop Sao Paulo.* 1970;12:8–15.
25. Baruzzi RG, Marcopito LF, Michalany NS, et al. Early diagnosis and prompt treatment by surgery in Jorge Lobo's disease. *Mycopathologia.* 1981;174:51–54.
26. Pecher SA. Cosideracoes sobre cinco casos de Lobomycosis. *Ann Braz Dermatol.* 1976;51:40–42.
27. Fuchs J, Milbradt R, Pecher S. Lobomycosis. *Cutis.* 1990; 46:227–234.
28. Bawan J, Bain RW, Purtilo DT, et al. Lobomycosis. *J Cutan Pathol.* 1976;3:5–16.

CHAPTER 112

Malasseziasis

Melissa Conrad Stöppler

A disease which is new and obscure to you, Doctor, will be known only after death; and even then not without an autopsy will you examine it with exacting pains.

Hermann Boerhaave (1668–1738)

DEFINITION AND HISTORY

Malassezia furfur, also known historically as *Pityrosporum orbicularis* and *P ovale*, is the traditional cause of pityriasis (tinea) versicolor, a common and usually innocuous patchy and scaling dermatophytosis. Much less common, more recently discovered, and much more serious, are the deep infections caused by *M furfur*. Tied to these very different infections of skin and deep organs, however, is an unusual growth requirement of *M furfur*. Lacking the ability to synthesize long-chain fatty acids, *M furfur* requires an exogenous supply of these lipids. In the skin these are supplied by the sebaceous glands. In the deep organs they are supplied by deeply placed venous catheters delivering nutrients to the patient. In the keratin layer of skin, *M furfur* is dimorphic, forming hyphae of 2.5 to 4 μm in diameter as well as round and oval yeasts 3 to 8 μm across. In deep organs *M furfur* grows as a yeast, causing septic thrombosis and septic infarction. Fortunately for the diagnostic pathologist, yeasts of *M furfur* have a characteristic type of reproduction—budding is unipolar with the daughter being extruded from the parent through a distinctive collarette. After separation of the daughter yeast, another bud is produced by the parent yeast at the same site.[1]

CLINICAL MANIFESTATIONS

As noted, *M furfur* causes two distinct types of infection: superficial infection of the skin and more aggressive deep infections.[2] Excessive proliferation of *M furfur* in skin causes tinea versicolor, usually an asymptomatic benign infection of the stratum corneum layer of skin characterized by flat or slightly raised macules. The macules are oval, may be hypo- or hyperpigmented, are usually scaling, and are most commonly on the upper trunk, shoulders, arms, and neck. Tinea versicolor tends to be chronic, with the macules enlarging and coalescing, then regressing and recurring for many years. Tinea versicolor is most common in warm climates but is found throughout the world, and, apart from cosmetic change, is innocuous. Other superficial skin infections in which *M furfur* has been implicated include folliculitis[3] and seborrheic dermatitis in patients with acquired immunodeficiency syndrome (AIDS). In 10 patients with AIDS and seborrheic dermatitis, a correlation was established between the severity of the dermatitis and the number of *M furfur* organisms on Giemsa-stained smears of skin scrapings.[4]

In addition to skin infections, *M furfur* has been associated with dacryoliths,[5] maxillary sinusitis,[6] mastitis,[7] peritonitis in patients undergoing peritoneal dialysis,[8,9] and septic arthritis.[10] The role of *M furfur* as a pathogen in these infections has been difficult to define since there has been no histologic demonstration of tissue invasion or reaction to *M furfur*. Nearly all other *M furfur*–associated illnesses are sepsis in patients receiving total parental nutrition including lipid infusions through central venous catheters. In 1981 Redline and Dahms[11] described an aggressive infection by *M furfur* in a premature infant who had received intravenous lipid infusions. At 6 weeks of age the infant developed respiratory distress and had bilateral pulmonary infiltrates. An open-lung biopsy revealed vasculitis and bronchopneumonia—both caused by *M furfur*. The infant ultimately died and autopsy confirmed the presence of *M furfur* and showed the organism within the walls of pulmonary vessels. No extension of the organism beyond lungs was described in this report. Since then, other reports have documented the presence of *M furfur* sepsis in neonates in intensive care settings receiving intravenous lipids,[12–18] but *M furfur* sepsis has also been reported in children[12,19] and adults.[12,20]

Common to the vast majority of cases of *M furfur* sepsis is the presence of 1) an indwelling central venous catheter used for the administration of hyperalimentation including lipid infusions, and 2) colonization and occlusion of central venous catheters by *M furfur*[21,22] with attachment of the organisms to the luminal surface of central venous catheters.[23] How the catheters become colonized by *M furfur* is not clear, but colonization may result from contamination at the time of placement, infusion of contaminated lipids, hematogenous spread from a distant source, migration of *M furfur* from skin along the catheter tract, or migration of *M furfur* from a contaminated catheter bulb through the lumen.[2] While skin of healthy, full-term newborns is not colonized with *M furfur*,[24] it is known that colonization of neonatal skin in intensive care units by *M furfur* correlates with low gestational age, with increasing time in the intensive care unit, and with handling of the infants by multiple adults.[15] It is likely that catheter contamination results from migration of organisms from colonized infant skin.

Although several of the infants reported with *M furfur* sepsis expired, recovery from *M furfur* sepsis has been documented,[10,12,15,17,20] by removing the central venous catheter, or by antifungal chemotherapy, or by a combination of the two. Recovery from *M furfur* sepsis has also been documented in a neonate on discontinuation of intravenous lipid therapy without removal of the central venous catheter.[18]

PATHOLOGIC FINDINGS

A few reports describe lesions caused by *M furfur* and they reveal a recurring pattern of cardiopulmonary lesions. These include mycotic thrombi around the tips of central venous catheters, vegetations of endocardium, and lesions of the lung including mycotic thromboemboli, alveolitis (Figure 112–1), infarcts, and vasculitis with vessels containing *M furfur* mixed with droplets of lipid (Figure 112–2).[11–13] "Target thrombi" (Figure 112–3), with alternating concentric layers of organisms and thrombus material, have been in vessels, and the mechanism of their formation is uncertain. It is possible that lipid is first deposited in walls of pulmonary vessels predisposing to growth of *M furfur* on the intima, followed by layers of fibrin and proliferating organisms. Also possible is that an embolus containing

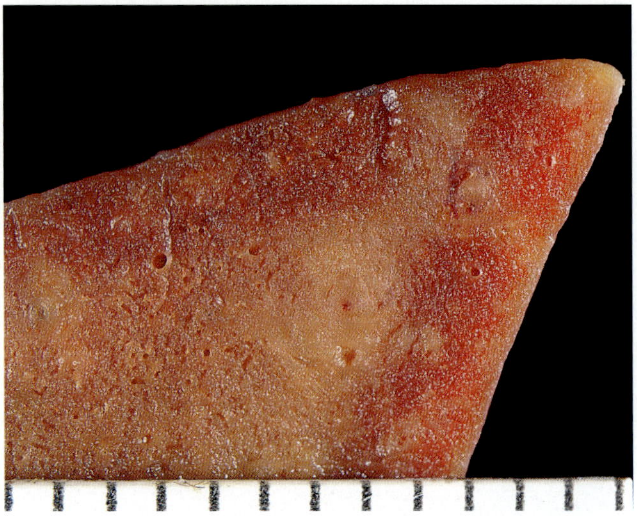

Figure 112–1. Gross photograph of lung from a male infant twin who had necrotizing entercolitis on day 2. After segmental resection of the ileum he was given total parenteral nutrition by Broviac catheter and did well for about 2 weeks, when he developed increasing respiratory distress. He was treated for viral pneumonia but at autopsy had disseminated *M furfur* infection. The vessel near the center of the picture contains a septic thrombus and is surrounded by white (consolidated) lung. *Malassezia furfur*, fibrin, and macrophages have consolidated the alveoli around this vessel. Small areas of consolidation around pulmonary arterioles are characteristic of pulmonary infection by *M furfur* (gross, ×5.5). *(Autopsy by Dr. Mary A. Furlong; photograph by Daniel H. Connor, MD, 1995.)*

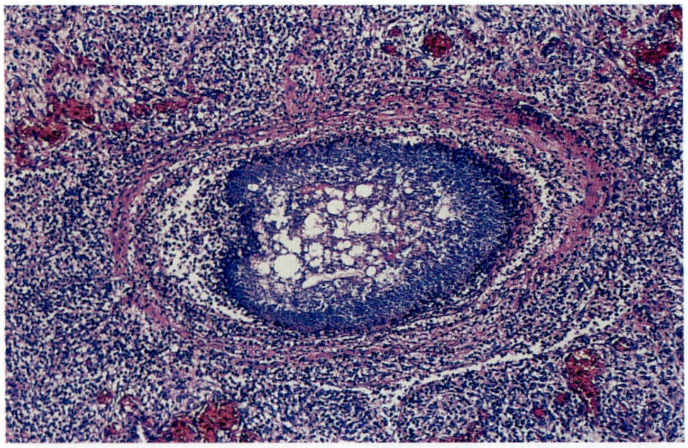

Figure 112–2. Pulmonary artery occluded by a septic thrombus containing a mixture of *M furfur* and lipid droplets, which appear as open spaces in the lumen of the vessel. Many yeasts are in the lumen, and the surrounding alveoli are consolidated with neutrophils and macrophages (hematoxylin-eosin, ×100).

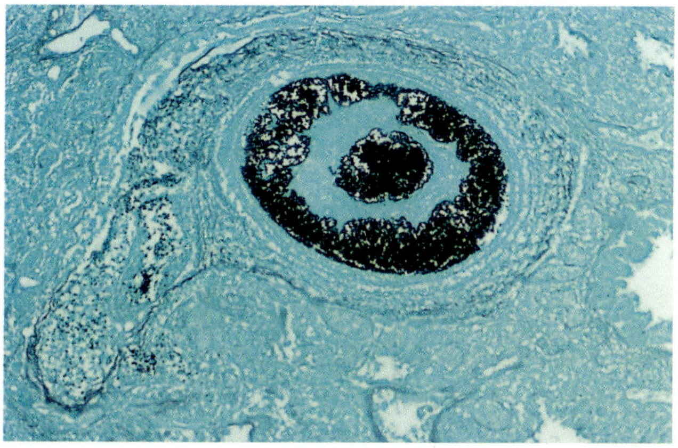

Figure 112–3. A "target thrombus" in a pulmonary artery. The central area ("bull's eye") is comprised of organisms and lipid, and is surrounded by a layer of leukocytes and fibrin, which is surrounded by a further layer of organisms against the intima of the vessel [Gomori's methenamine silver (GMS), ×100].

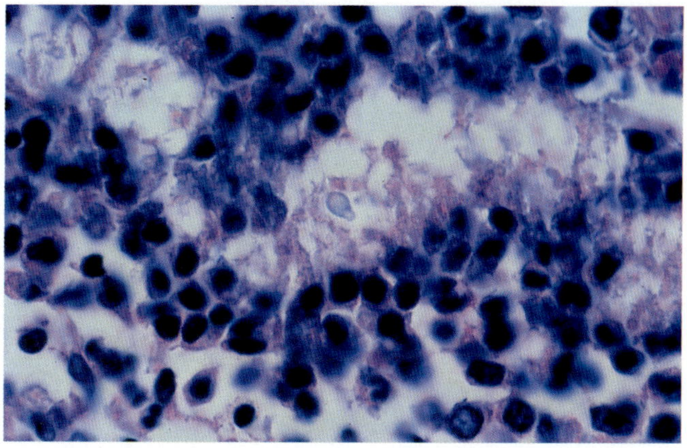

Figure 112–5. Higher magnification of a budding yeast of *M furfur* associated with lipid droplets within a septic embolus in the lung. Note the daughter cell emerging through the collarette (hematoxylin-eosin, ×400).

M furfur arrests in an artery or arteriole and acts as a nidus for growth by accretion—with deposits of successive layers of fibrin and organisms. In addition to the cardiopulmonary lesions described, *M furfur* may cause disseminated disease. Disseminated infections by *M furfur* reported in 1989 by Shek et al[13] described three infants, each of whom died after prolonged courses of neonatal intensive care. All three had disseminated lesions including acute meningitis, necrotizing encephalitis (Figure 112–4), and interstitial nephritis. These infants also had *M furfur* lesions in other organs including heart, adrenal, colon, and pancreas.

While *M furfur* is dimorphic in the stratum corneum layer of skin, only yeast forms are in the deep and disseminated lesions. *Malassezia furfur* appears in tissue sections as monomorphous yeasts that are round to oval, up to 5 μm across, with many unipolar budding forms characterized by the daughter cells sprouting from one pole of the parent through a collarette (Figure 112–5). With routine hematoxylin and eosin staining, masses of *M furfur* are lightly hematoxylinophilic but characteristic morphologic features are not distinct (Figures 112–2 and 112–6). The periodic acid–Schiff (PAS), GMS, Gridley fungus stain, and tissue Gram stains all stain yeast forms of *M furfur.* Although the GMS stain appears to stain the greatest number of organisms (Figure 112–7), the distinctive features of the organism are particularly well demonstrated with the Brown–Hopps

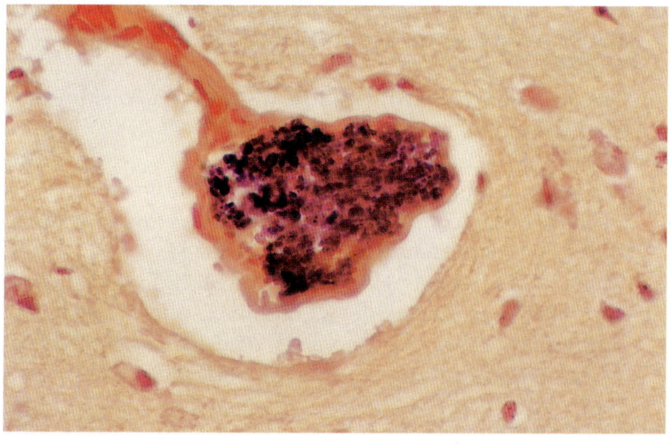

Figure 112–4. Focus of organisms *(M furfur)* in vessel in cerebral cortex of an infant with necrotizing encephalitis caused by malasseziasis (Brown–Hopps tissue Gram stain, ×400).

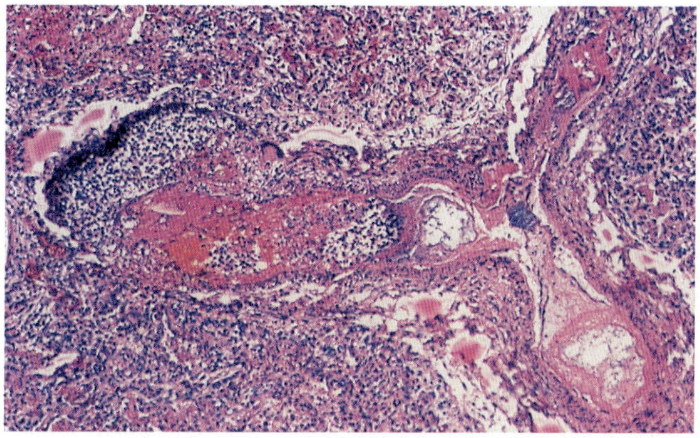

Figure 112–6. A septic thrombus with multiple organisms of *M furfur* within lipid droplets occluding a branch of a pulmonary artery. The adjoining alveolar spaces are consolidated (hematoxylin-eosin, ×100).

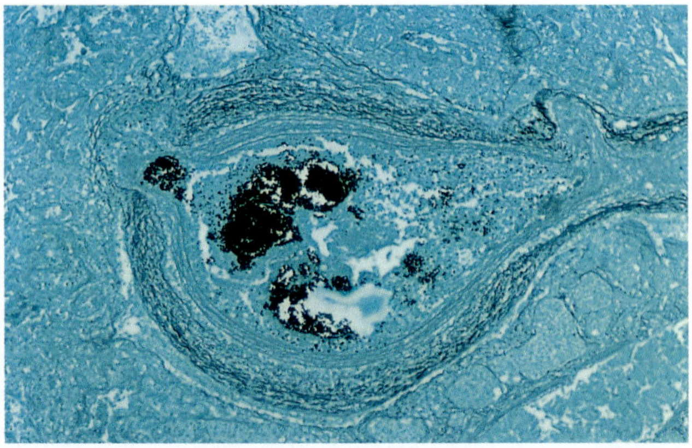

Figure 112–7. The GMS technique appears to silver most of the *M furfur* yeasts, which appear here as solid black masses. The yeasts are the nidus of a septic thrombus, which occludes a branch of a pulmonary artery. The organisms also are invading through the vessel wall into surrounding lung (GMS, ×100).

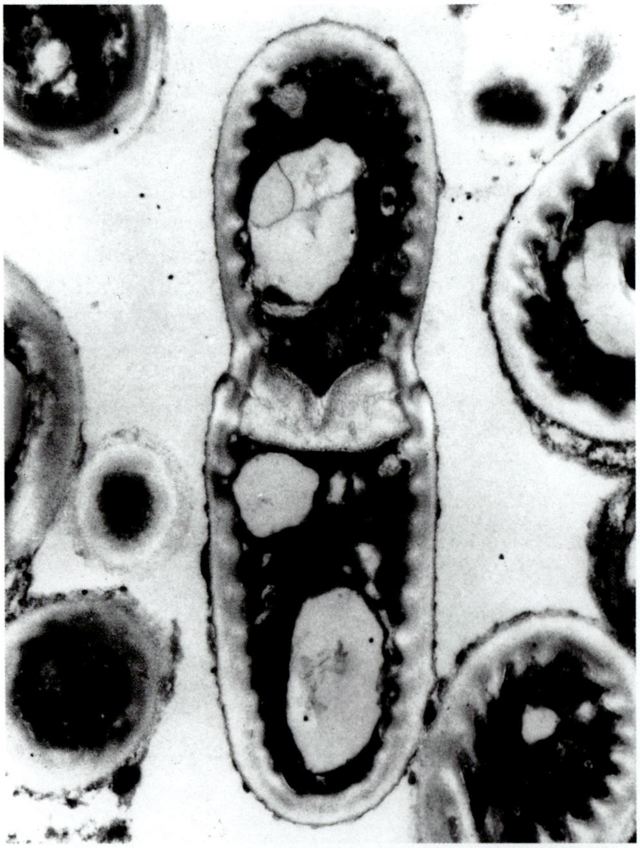

Figure 112–8. Electron micrograph of *M furfur*. The daughter cell *(upper)* is growing out of the parent cell. After separating, another daughter cell is produced at the same site. The thick cross-wall separating the two, the phialitic ring, the thick capsule and the internal corrugations of the capsule are all apparent in this picture and characteristic of *M furfur* (×27,000).

tissue Gram stain. *Malassezia furfur* also has a characteristic appearance when examined by electron microscopy. Electron micrographs reveal a thick wall with corrugations on the inner surface and a circumferential thickening of the wall forming the distinct collarette (Figure 112–8).

The distinctive features of *M furfur* enable the pathologist to readily distinguish *M furfur* from the other common pathogenic yeasts. Although *H capsulatum* is approximately the same size as *M furfur*, *H capsulatum* has narrower neck buds. *Cryptococcus neoformans* also possesses narrow neck buds and additionally has a much greater range in size (2 to 10 μm) than *M furfur*. Unlike *M furfur*, *Candida* species are usually polymorphous in tissue sections, with hyphae, pseudohyphae, and yeasts all present, and they do not show unipolar buds. Although anatomic location and tissue reaction cannot be used to identify a specific fungus, the location of yeasts in septic thrombi or in intravascular collections of lipid should signal the possibility of *M furfur*, particularly in patients receiving long-term intravenous lipid infusions.

REFERENCES

1. Chandler FW, Kaplan W, Ajello L. *Color Atlas and Text of the Histopathology of Mycotic Diseases.* Chicago: Year Book Medical Publishers; 1980:120, 293.
2. Marcon MJ, Powell DA. Human infections due to *Malassezia* spp. *Clin Microbiol Rev.* 1992;5:100–119.
3. Potter B, Burgoon CF, Johnson SC. *Pityrosporum* folliculitis. Report of seven cases and review of the *Pityrosporum* organism relative to cutaneous disease. *Arch Dermatol.* 1973;107:388–391.
4. Groisser D, Bottone EJ, Lebwohl M. Association of *Pityrosporum orbiculare (Malassezia furfur)* with seborrheic dermatitis in patients with acquired immunodeficiency syndrome (AIDS). *J Am Acad Dermatol.* 1989;20:770–773.
5. Wolter J. *Pityrosporum* species associated with dacroliths in obstructive dacryocystitis. *Am J Ophthalmol.* 1977;84: 806–809.
6. Oberle AD, Fowler M, Grafton WD. *Pityrosporum* isolate from the upper respiratory tract. *Am J Clin Pathol.* 1981; 76:112–116.
7. Bertini B, Kuttin E, Beemer A. Cytopathology of nipple discharge due to *Pityrosporum orbiculare* and cocci in an elderly woman. *Acta Cytol.* 1975;19:38–42.
8. Wallace M, Bagnall H, Glen D, Averill S. Isolation of lipophilic yeast in "sterile" peritonitis. *Lancet.* 1979;2:956.
9. Gidding H, Hawes L, Dwyer B. The isolation of *Malassezia furfur* from an episode of peritonitis. *Med J Aust.* 1989;151:603.
10. Wurtz RM, Knospe WN. *Malassezia furfur* fungemia in a patient without the usual risk factors. *Ann Intern Med.* 1989;109:432–433.
11. Redline R, Dahms B. *Malassezia* pulmonary vasculitis in

an infant on long-term intralipid therapy. *N Engl J Med.* 1981;305:1395–1398.

12. Redline R, Redline S, Boxerbaum B, Dahms B. Systemic *M furfur* infections in patients receiving intralipid therapy. *Hum Pathol.* 1985;16:815–822.
13. Shek YH, Tucker MC, Viciana AL, Manz HJ, Connor DH. *Malassezia furfur*–disseminated infection in premature infants. *Am J Clin Pathol.* 1989;92:595–603.
14. Dankner W, Spector S. *M furfur* sepsis in neonates. *J Pediatr.* 1985;107:643–644. Letter.
15. Powell D, Aungst J, Snedden S, Hansen N, Brady M. Broviac catheter-related *M furfur* sepsis in five infants receiving intravenous fat emulsions. *J Pediatr.* 1984;105: 987–990.
16. Long J, Keyserling H. Catheter-related infection in infants due to an unusual lipophilic yeast. *Pediatrics.* 1985;76: 896–900.
17. Alpert G, Bell L, Campos J. *M furfur* fungemia in infancy. *Clin Pediatr.* 1987;26:528–531.
18. Weiss SJ, Schoch PE, Cunha BA. *Malassezia furfur* fungemia associated with central venous catheter lipid emulsion infusion. *Heart Lung.* 1991;20:87–90.
19. Hassall E, Ulich T, Ament M. Pulmonary embolus and *Malassezia* pulmonary infection related to urokinase therapy. *J Pediatr.* 1983;102:722–725.
20. Middleton C, Lowenthal RM. *Malassezia furfur* fungemia as a treatable cause of obscure fever in a leukemia patient receiving parenteral nutrition. *Aust NZ J Med.* 1987;17: 603–604.
21. Aschner JL, Punsalang A, Maniscalco WM, Menegus MA. Percutaneous central venous catheter colonization with *Malassezia furfur:* incidence and clinical significance. *Pediatrics.* 1987;80:535–539.
22. Azimi PH, Levernier K, Lefrak LM, et al. *Malassezia furfur:* a cause of occlusion of percutaneous central venous catheters in infants in the intensive care nursery. *Pediatr Infect Dis J.* 1988;7:100–103.
23. Powell DA, Marcon MJ, Durrell DE, Pfister RM. Scanning electron microscopy of *Malassezia furfur* attachment to Broviac catheters. Hum Pathol. 1987;18:740–745.
24. Bell LM, Alpert G, Slight PH, Campos JM. *Malassezia furfur* skin colonization in infancy. *Infect Control Hosp Epidemiol.* 1988;9:151–153.

CHAPTER 113

Mycetoma

Francis W. Chandler and Libero Ajello

All the causes of things cannot be seen, because they appear to depend on circumstances which are unknown, or appear to be accidental.

John Hunter (1728–1793)

DEFINITION

Mycetomas are chronic, localized, progressive infections of skin, subcutaneous tissues, muscle, fascia, and bone caused by a wide variety of free-living or exogenous, geophilic, aerobic actinomycetes and fungi.[1,2] These microorganisms form, in tissue, grains or granules that are organized mycelial aggregates, which are the diagnostic hallmarks of mycetomas. The recognized causal agents of actinomycotic mycetomas caused by actinomycetes (filamentous bacteria) are listed in Table 113–1. Mycetomas caused by true fungi are termed *eumycotic* and the causal agents form either hyaline (white) or dematiaceous (black) granules in tissue. The currently known agents of eumycotic mycetomas are listed in Table 113–2. The causal agents of actinomycosis (Chapter 40) also form granules in tissue. Actinomycosis, however, is an endogenous disease and therefore not included in this chapter on mycetomas. Synonyms of mycetoma include madura foot and maduromycosis.

EPIDEMIOLOGY AND GEOGRAPHIC DISTRIBUTION

Mycetomas are not contagious. All patients are infected from sources in nature by traumatic percutaneous implantation of the causal agent into those parts of the body that are usually exposed, eg, a foot or hand, and less often the head, neck, chest wall, shoulders, and back. Although mycetomas can develop at any age, the highest incidence coincides with the most active years of adulthood. Men are more often affected than women. Although mycetomas occur worldwide, they are most prevalent in tropical and subtropical regions between latitudes 15°S and 30°N, especially in Asia, northern Africa, South America, and Mexico. The actinomycetes and fungi that cause mycetomas differ from country to country, and the agents that are common in one region are infrequently reported from others.[3–7]

MORPHOLOGIC FEATURES OF THE ORGANISMS

Once an offending actinomycete or fungus begins to develop at the site of implantation, its mycelium proliferates and becomes organized into aggregates known as granules or grains. These granules are of various sizes, shapes, colors, and degrees of hardness, depending on the causal agent.[2,8] To determine if a granule is actinomycotic (caused by actinomycetes) or eumycotic (caused by true fungi), special stains for bacteria (eg, Brown–Brenn modified Gram procedure) and fungi [eg, Gomori's methenamine-silver (GMS) procedure] are usually needed. The granules of actinomycotic mycetomas are either white, yellow, or red on gross examination. Histologically, they are identified by the presence of delicate, branched, gram-positive and sometimes beaded or fragmented bacterial filaments 1 μm or less in width. Generally, the bacterial filaments are radially oriented and more numerous at the periphery of the granules. In contrast, the granules of eumycotic mycetomas are composed of septate, fungal hyphae that are 2 to 6 μm or more in width and are either dematiaceous (black grained) or hyaline (white grained), depending on the causal agent. The hyphae that form eumycotic granules are frequently distorted

TABLE 113–1. CAUSAL AGENTS OF ACTINOMYCOTIC MYCETOMAS

Actinomadura madurae	*N otitidiscaviarum*
A pelletieri	*N transvalensis*
Nocardia asteroides	*Nocardiopsis dassonvillei*
N brasiliensis	*Streptomyces somaliensis*

TABLE 113–2. CAUSAL AGENTS OF EUMYCOTIC MYCETOMAS

White Grain	Black Grain
Acremonium falciforme	*Chaetosphaeronema larense*
A kiliense	*Curvularia geniculata*
A recifei	*C lunata*
Aspergillus nidulans	*Exophiala jeanselmei*
Corynespora cassiicola	*Leptosphaeria senegalensis*
Cylindrocarpon cyanescens	*L tompkinsii*
C destructans	*Madurella grisea*
Fusarium moniliforme	*M mycetomatis*
F solani [a]	*Plenodomus arramii*
Neotestudina rosatii	*Pyrenochaeta mackinnonii*
Polycytella hominis	*P romeroi*
Pseudallescheria boydii	
Pseudochaetosphaeronema larense	

[a] var *coeruleum* has been reported to produce black grains in tissue.

and bizarre in form and size. In addition, they often form large, spherical to oval, thick-walled, terminal chlamydoconidia, especially at the periphery of the granules. Chlamydoconidia are not formed in actinomycotic mycetomas. In both actinomycotic and eumycotic mycetomas, the mycelium within the granules may be embedded in an amorphous cement-like substance depending on the species involved. On low-power examination, discrete zones of mycelial growth may be apparent in some granules. Frequently, the granules are bordered by refractile, intensely eosinophilic, finely to coarsely dentate Splendore–Hoeppli material that represents a localized antigen–antibody reaction in the hypersensitized host. The Splendore–Hoeppli material often interdigitates with proliferating mycelial elements at the periphery of the granules.

The diagnostic characteristics of the granules in actinomycotic and eumycotic mycetomas are summarized in Tables 113–3 and 113–4, respectively. Experienced pathologists and mycologists often can correlate the color, shape, size, texture, and microscopic architecture of a granule with a specific causal agent or with a particular group to which it belongs. However, culture is usually needed for definitive identification of the actinomycete or fungus involved.

CLINICAL FEATURES

Mycetomas are usually insidious because, in their early stages, discomfort is minimal. As a mycetoma progressively develops, the affected area gradually enlarges and becomes disfigured as a result of chronic inflammation and fibrosis (Figures 113–1 through 113–5).[9–12] Abscesses develop and multiple draining sinus tracts emerge to give the classical clinical picture. These tracts discharge serosanguinous fluid that often contains the grossly visible, telltale granules that range from 0.2 to 5 mm in diameter and may be white, black, gray, yellow, pink, or red. The infection destroys muscle, eventually reaches bone, and frequently causes severe, destructive osteomyelitis. Although mycetomas are usually localized infections, they commonly breach tissue planes and spread to adjacent tissues by local invasion

TABLE 113–3. DIAGNOSTIC CHARACTERISTICS OF GRANULES IN ACTINOMYCOTIC MYCETOMAS

Causal Agent	Color	Size Range	Texture	Cement	Staining Properties
Actinomadura madurae	White	0.5–5 mm	Soft	No	Non–acid-fast filaments; periphery of granules intensely hematoxylinophilic
A pelletieri	Red	0.3–0.5 mm	Soft to hard	No	Non–acid-fast filaments; granules uniformly hematoxylinophilic
Nocardia asteroides[a]	White	25–200 μm	Soft	No	Variably acid-fast filaments; granules amphophilic with H&E
N brasiliensis[a]	White	25–200 μm	Soft	No	Variably acid-fast filaments; granules amphophilic with H&E
N otitidiscaviarum[a]	White	<1 mm	Soft	No	Variably acid-fast filaments; granules amphophilic with H&E
N transvalensis	White	<1 mm	Hard	No	Variably acid-fast filaments; granules amphophilic with H&E
Nocardiopsis dassonvillei	White	<0.5 mm	Soft	No	Non–acid-fast filaments
Streptomyces somaliensis	Yellow	0.5–2 mm	Hard	Yes	Non–acid-fast filaments; granules are homogeneous and weakly eosinophilic

[a] Granules formed by these three species are morphologically and tinctorially indistinguishable.

TABLE 113–4. DIAGNOSTIC CHARACTERISTICS OF GRANULES IN EUMYCOTIC MYCETOMAS

Causal Agent	Color	Size Range	Texture	Cement	Histologic Features[a]
Acremonium falciforme	White	0.5–1 mm	Soft	No	Eosinophilic border darker than interior; intricate network of hyaline mycelium and chlamydoconidia
A kiliense	White	0.5–1 mm	Soft	No	Eosinophilic border darker than interior; intricate network of hyaline mycelium and chlamydoconidia
A recifei	White	0.5–1 mm	Soft	No	Eosinophilic border darker than interior; intricate network of hyaline mycelium and chlamydoconidia
Aspergillus nidulans	White	0.5–4 mm	Soft	No	Eosinophilic with light and dark zones; dense network of mycelium with extremely large chlamydoconidia, 10–40 μm in diameter
Corynespora cassiicola	Black	<0.5 mm	Hard	No	Eosinophilic
Curvularia geniculata	Black	0.5–>1 mm	Hard	Yes	Lobulated; dark periphery with loose network of mycelium and large chlamydoconidia in cemented periphery (similar to granules of *L senegalensis* and *L tompkinsii*)
C lunata	Black	1–2 mm	Hard	Yes	Lobulated; dark periphery with loose network of mycelium and large chlamydoconidia in cemented periphery (similar to granules of *L senegalensis* and *L tompkinsii*)
Cylindrocarpon cyanescens	White	0.3–3.0 mm	NA[b]	No	NA
C destructans	White	0.5 mm	Soft	No	Eosinophilic periphery
Exophiala jeanselmei	Black	0.2–0.3 mm	Soft	No	Irregularly shaped (spherical, oval, and crescentic); dark periphery composed of mycelium and chlamydoconidia
Fusarium moniliforme	White	0.5–1.0 mm	Soft	No	Eosinophilic, entire or lobulated granules composed of a tangled mass of mycelium; hyphae in peripheral zone swollen and distorted
Leptosphaeria senegalensis	Black	0.5–2 mm	Hard	Yes, in periphery	See description of *C geniculata* and *C lunata* granules
L tompkinsii	Black	0.5–2 mm	Hard	Yes, in periphery	See description of *C geniculata* and *C lunata* granules
Madurella grisea	Black	0.3–0.6 mm	Hard	Variable	Dark peripheral zone, variably shaped; dense internal network of mycelium with chlamydoconidia
Madurella mycetomatis	Black	0.5–4 mm	Hard	Yes	Two basic types of granules: 1. Compact, filamentous type of variable size and form; may be lobulated; cement throughout granule stained uniformly brown 2. Vesicular type more irregular in size and form than compact type; cement, only in periphery, stained dark brown; mycelium in periphery with chlamydoconidia; central zone lightly stained. Both types of development may be found in a single granule.
Neotestudina rosatii	White	0.5–1 mm	Hard	Yes, in periphery	Irregular in form; eosinophilic border; central zone with disintegrated mycelium and chlamydoconidia
Plenodomus arramii	Black	0.5–0.8 mm	Soft	No	NA
Polycytella hominis	White	0.5–1.0 mm	Soft	No	Eosinophilic fringe
Pseudallescheria boydii	White	0.5–1 mm	Soft	No	Eosinophilic border darker than interior; composed of dense network of hyaline interwoven mycelium with prominent chlamydoconidia
Pseudochaetosphaeronema larense	Black	0.3–0.6 mm	Soft	Variable	Dark peripheral zone; interior with interwoven mycelium
Pyrenochaeta mackinnonii	Black	1.0 mm	NA	Yes	NA
P romeroi	Black	0.3–0.6 mm	Soft	Variable	Dark peripheral zone; variably shaped; internal dense network of mycelium without chlamydoconidia

[a] H&E stain.
[b] Not available.

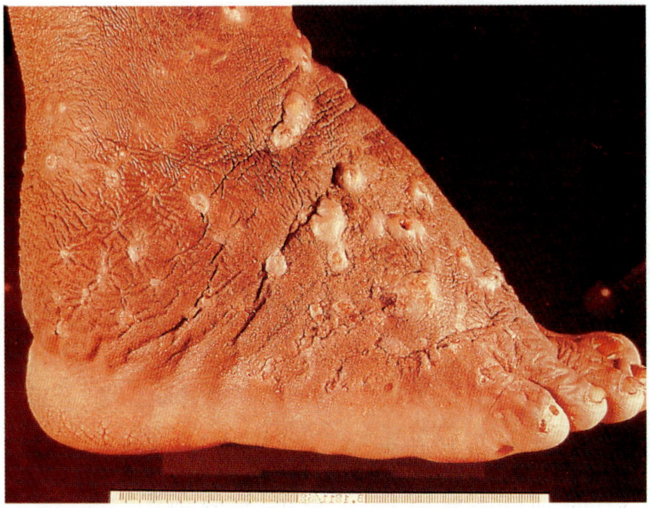

Figure 113–1. Eumycotic mycetoma of the foot. Note swelling and openings of draining sinuses. *(By Daniel H. Connor, MD, 1963.)*

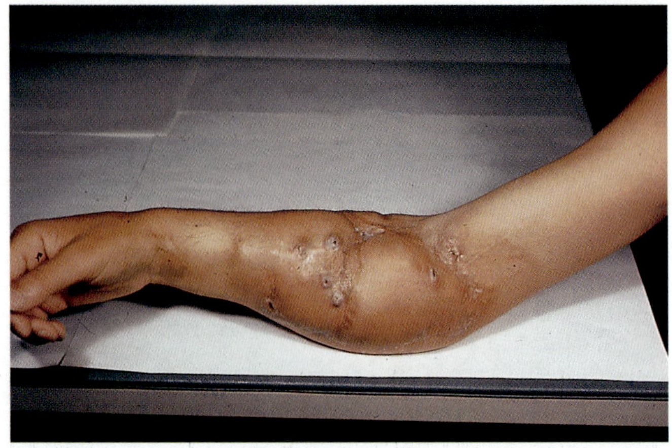

Figure 113–3. Eumycotic mycetoma of the arm caused by *M mycetomatis.*

of their mycelial elements or granules and their fragments. Hematogenous dissemination or lymphatic spread from a primary cutaneous or subcutaneous infection is extremely rare.[2,13]

TREATMENT

Treatment of eumycotic mycetomas is limited primarily to surgical excision or amputation; debridement and antifungal therapy are usually ineffective.[14–16] In contrast, if patients with actinomycotic mycetomas are treated early and aggressively for an extended period, they usually respond to dapsone and streptomycin or to trimethoprim–sulfamethoxazole and streptomycin.[14,15,17] Since actinomycotic mycetomas usually respond to treatment with antibiotics and eumycotic mycetomas do not, the histopathologic distinction between granules formed by actinomycetes and fungi is of fundamental importance. When cultures are not available, accurate histopathologic differentiation is crucial in determining the form of treatment and the prognosis.[18]

PATHOLOGY

Both actinomycotic and eumycotic mycetomas elicit a similar host reaction regardless of the causative organisms.[2,8] The dermis and subcutaneous tissues contain

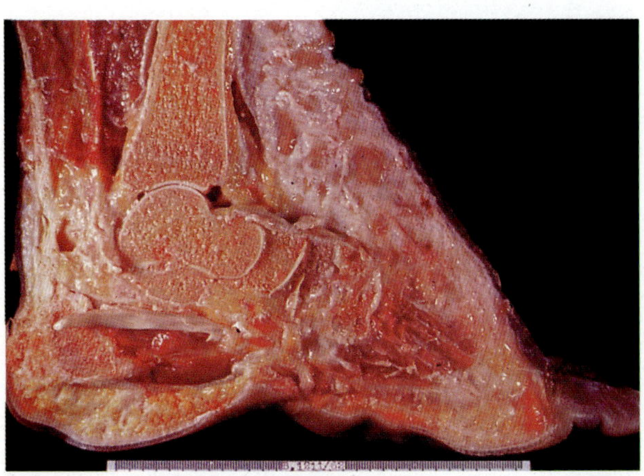

Figure 113–2. Cut surface of foot shown in Figure 113–1 reveals deformity, marked fibrosis, and destructive osteomyelitis. *(By Daniel H. Connor, MD, 1963.)*

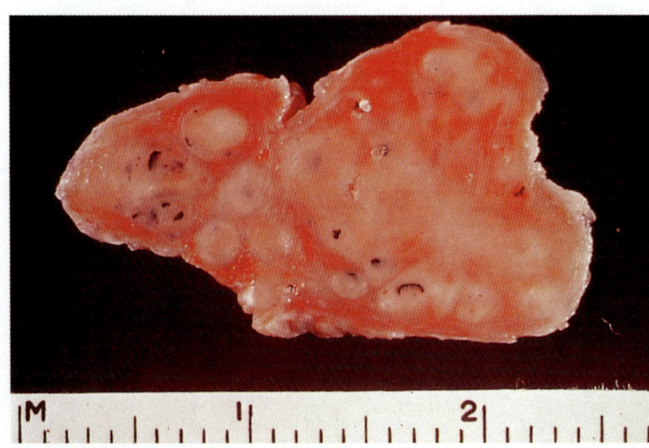

Figure 113–4. Eumycotic black grain mycetoma. The cut surface of this subcutaneous nodule reveals multiple pigmented granules embedded in a fibrotic stroma. *(Contributed by Daniel H. Connor, MD.)*

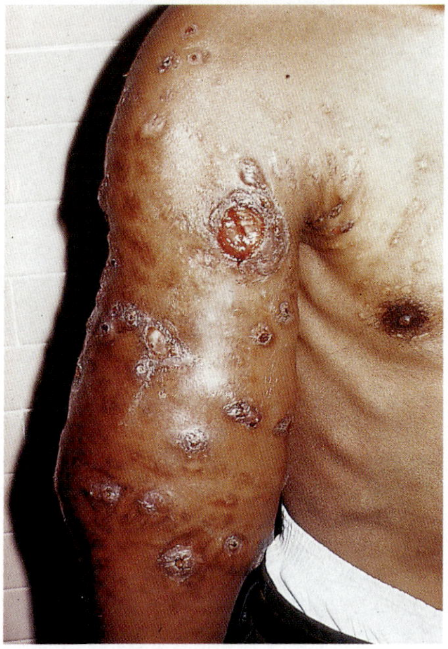

Figure 113–5. Actinomycotic mycetoma of upper arm and shoulder. There are swelling and multiple openings of draining sinuses. The causal agent was *N brasiliensis*.

sinus tracts and localized abscesses of varying sizes, each of which usually contains abundant neutrophils, necrotic debris, and one or more spherical, subspherical, or lobular granules that range from 0.25 mm to several millimeters in diameter, depending on the causal agent. The granules are either pigmented or nonpigmented in hematoxylin-eosin (H&E) stained tissue sections, contain either true fungi or actinomycetes, and are usually bordered by finely serrate or broad, clublike projections of intensely eosinophilic Splendore–Hoeppli material. In addition, organic foreign materials such as thorns or splinters are sometimes contiguous to the granules and are presumed to have been the vehicles of infection.[19,20] Surrounding each abscess or sinus tract is a chronic inflammatory reaction that usually consists of palisaded epithelioid histiocytes and giant cells of both the foreign body and Langhans' types mixed with fibroblasts, macrophages, plasma cells, and lymphocytes. In the stroma, there is dense granulation tissue that may be highly vascular and infiltrated with mononuclear inflammatory cells. Occasional giant cells also may be in the reactive stroma. Fibrosis, particularly in long-standing infections, is severe and results in tumefaction and deformity that may be mistaken clinically for neoplasia. Because the host response in mycetomas is not pathognomonic, one must demonstrate the characteristic granules before a diagnosis can be made.

DIAGNOSIS

Frequently, the granules that occur in clinical materials can be detected with the unaided eye, primarily when the material (pus, serosanguinous fluid) is distributed in a thin layer over the bottom plate of a sterile Petri dish. Single granules should be picked out and repeatedly washed by shaking them in several changes of sterile physiologic saline. This procedure will often remove adherent contaminating bacterial and fungal propagules. Some of the cleansed granules should be examined directly on a glass slide after crushing under a coverslip, or if hard, with another slide. Other granules should be inoculated onto agar slants or plates of isolation media, eg, Sabouraud dextrose agar with and without cycloheximide and chloramphenicol. Because specific identification of the causal agents usually requires careful correlation of cultural and histologic findings, the reader should consult Refs. 1, 2, 8, and 21.

Excised tissue should be examined grossly before fixation for granules (Figure 113–4). The granules occur in solid lesions and abscesses, and in draining sinus or fistulous tracts that exude pus or serosanguinous fluid. Other materials, such as curettings or exudates from sinus tracts, as well as protective gauze bandages, also should be carefully examined. If granules are present, they should be gently removed with tweezers, cleansed by serial washings in physiologic saline, and placed on a glass slide in a drop of 10% potassium hydroxide. The granules should then be flattened by applying pressure with a coverslip or with another slide, if hard, and examined under a microscope. The nature of the mycelial filaments should be noted: whether they are narrow and aseptate (actinomycotic) or broad and septate (eumycotic). Other granules and tissue specimens should be fixed and processed by standard histologic procedures to better observe their constituent elements and, if desired, to prepare a photographic record of the granules' microscopic architecture (see Tables 113–3 and 113–4).

Each species or group of species of the causal agents of mycetomas is characterized by a specific type of granule. With experience and a battery of appropriate histologic stains, one can correlate the color, shape, size, and internal configuration (microscopic architecture) of a granule with a specific causal agent or with a group of agents. Definitive identification basically depends on isolation and characterization of the organism in culture. Specific fluorescent antibody conjugates are available for the immunohistologic identification of *P boydii,* the most common agent of eumycotic mycetomas in the United States.[8] The histopathologic features of the more common actinomycotic and eumycotic mycetomas are illustrated in Figures 113–6 through 113–25. For detailed information on the

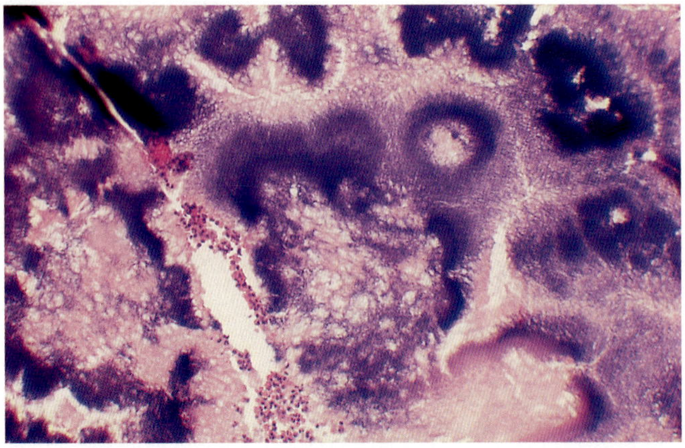

Figure 113–6. Actinomycotic mycetoma caused by *A pelletieri*. Multiple lobulated granules contain compact bacterial filaments that are intensely hematoxylinophilic and radiate from the periphery of the granules into surrounding tissue (hematoxylin-eosin, ×25).

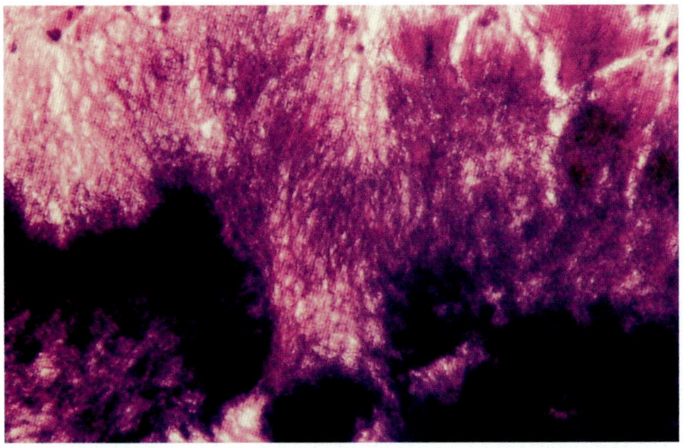

Figure 113–7. *Actinomadura pelletieri* granule. Wavy, tangled, hematoxylinophilic filaments project from the periphery of the granule. The delicate, advancing filaments, about 1 μm wide, are embedded in Splendore–Hoeppli material that borders the granule (H&E, ×250).

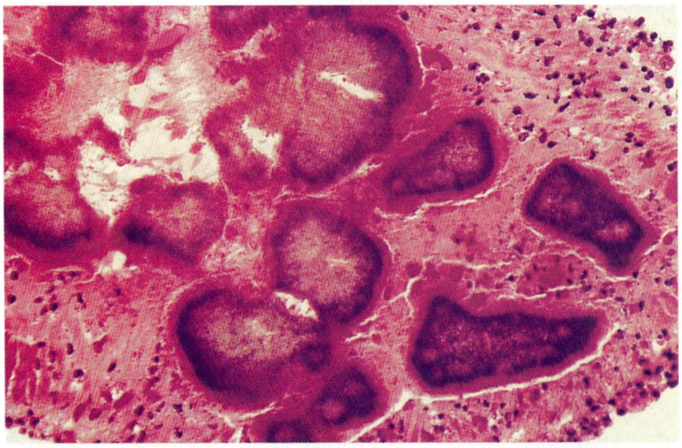

Figure 113–8. Actinomycotic mycetoma caused by *A madurae*. Individual granules in a subcutaneous abscess are intensely hematoxylinophilic and have eosinophilic centers. Brightly eosinophilic Splendore–Hoeppli material borders the granules. *Actinomadura madurae* granules are the largest produced by actinomycetes; granules produced by the *Nocardia* sp are the smallest (H&E, ×25).

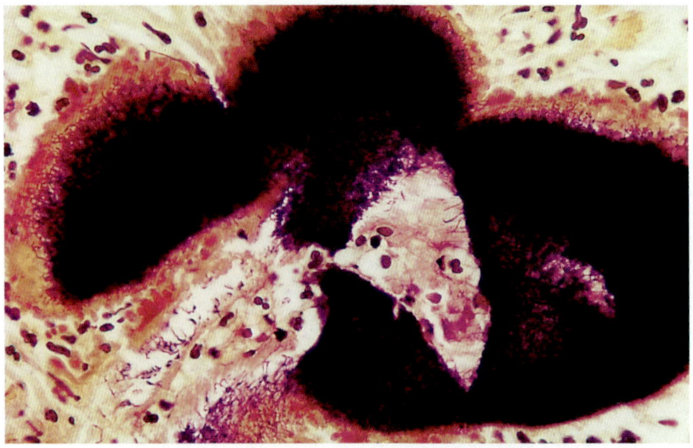

Figure 113–9. *Actinomadura madurae* granule. The entire granule is scalloped and intensely gram-positive. Numerous, gram-positive actinomycetes, about 1 μm wide, are more easily seen at the periphery of the granule. Some of the bacterial filaments radiate within gram-negative Splendore–Hoeppli material that envelopes the granule (Brown–Brenn, ×160).

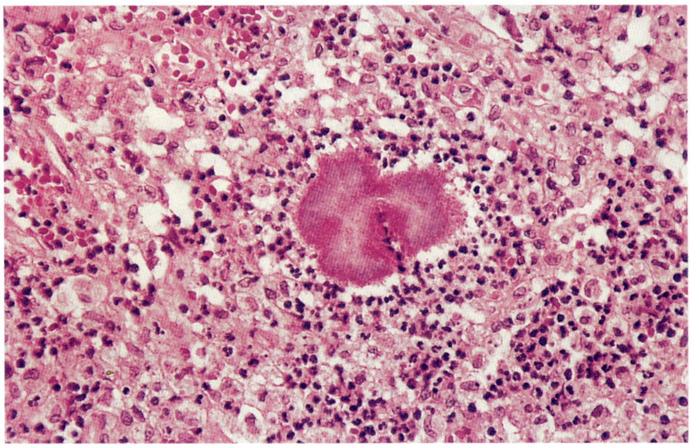

Figure 113–10. *Nocardia brasiliensis* granule in actinomycotic mycetoma. The interior of the granule is finely granular, lightly hematoxylinophilic, and surrounded by dentate, intensely eosinophilic, Splendore–Hoeppli material. Individual filaments of the actinomycete are not visible in H&E stained sections (×25).

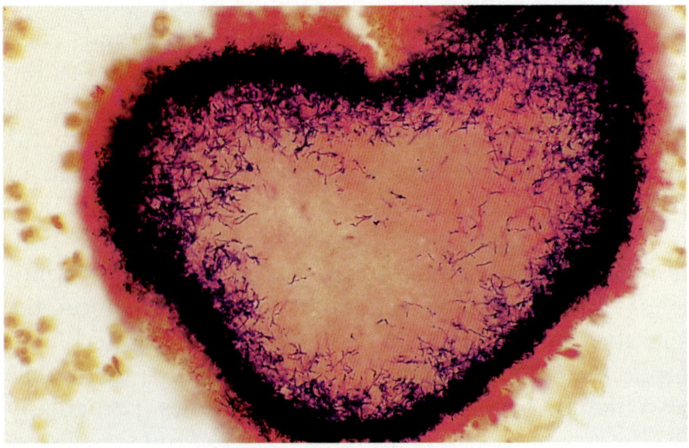

Figure 113–11. *Nocardia brasiliensis* granule. Delicate, branched, gram-positive filaments are randomly embedded in the matrix of the granule. The filaments are compact and most numerous at the periphery, and project into gram-negative Splendore–Hoeppli material that surrounds the granule (Brown–Brenn, ×160).

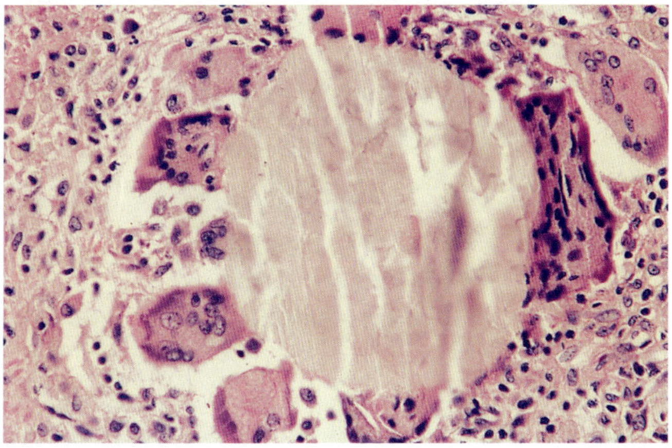

Figure 113–12. Actinomycotic mycetoma caused by *S somaliensis.* A subcutaneous granuloma contains a single, eosinophilic, smoothly contoured granule. Note absence of Splendore–Hoeppli material at periphery, and undulating fracture lines through the hard, cement-like matrix of the granule caused by the microtome knife. Although the entire granule is stained with H&E, individual filaments within its matrix are not visible (×50).

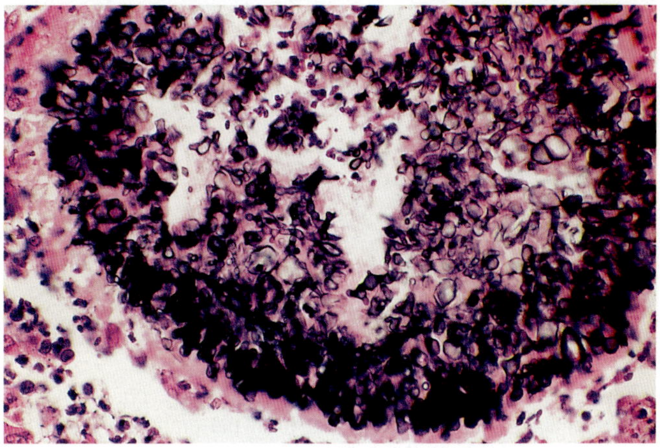

Figure 113–14. Granule caused by *N rosatii.* The silvered fungal elements that form the granule consist of degenerated hyphae and occasional chlamydoconidia. The surrounding suppurative reaction is clearly demonstrated with the H&E counterstain (GMS-H&E, ×160).

histomorphologic features of mycetoma granules, several texts and atlases are recommended.[2,8,21]

DIFFERENTIAL DIAGNOSIS

The most difficult differential diagnostic problem is encountered with mycetoma-like infections termed deep dermatophytic granulomas or pseudomycetomas.[21–24] Dermatophytes comprise 28 taxonomically related fungi in the genera *Epidermophyton, Microsporum,* and *Trichophyton,* and they commonly infect the nonviable keratinous portions of the skin, ie, stratum corneum, hair, and nails. The superficial infections that dermatophytes produce are contagious and known as tineas or ringworm. Rarely, these fungi invade the deeper nonkeratinized skin and subcutaneous tissues where they produce nodular or dispersed lesions and evoke a mixed suppurative and granulomatous inflammatory reaction (Figure 113–26). Occasionally,

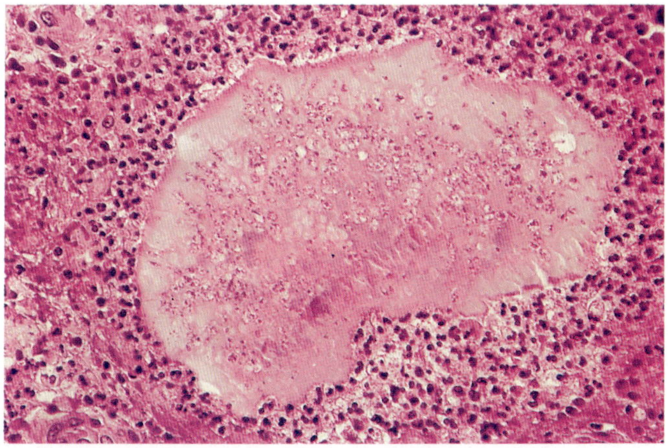

Figure 113–13. White grain mycetoma caused by *N rosatii.* The irregularly shaped granule is embedded in an abscess and consists of hematoxylinophilic hyphae that are more abundant in the interior of the granule. The hyphae are embedded in a homogeneous, eosinophilic, cement-like matrix. A narrow, incomplete layer of Splendore–Hoeppli material borders the granule (H&E, ×50).

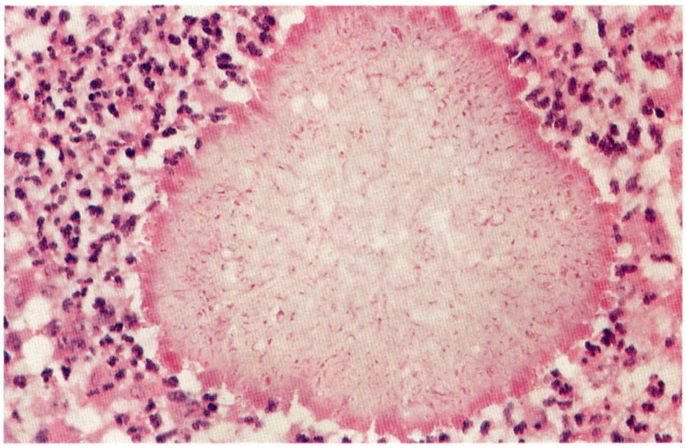

Figure 113–15. White grain mycetoma caused by *P boydii.* The hyaline granule is composed of a dense network of interwoven hyphae and prominent chlamydoconidia with optically clear centers. The granule lacks cement substance and resembles those produced by *Acremonium* sp and *A nidulans,* but it differs from them because its chlamydoconidia are more numerous and larger (H&E, ×100).

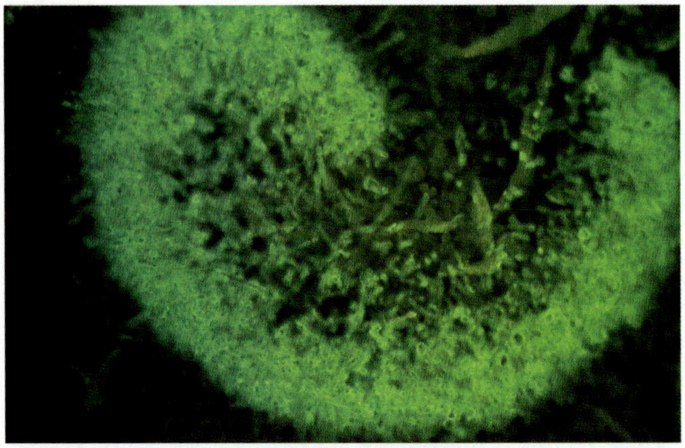

Figure 113–16. Eumycotic mycetoma caused by *P boydii*. Hyphae and vesicular chlamydoconidia that form the granule are brightly decorated in a formalin-fixed, deparaffinized tissue section stained with a species-specific immunofluorescence conjugate (direct immunofluorescence, ×100).

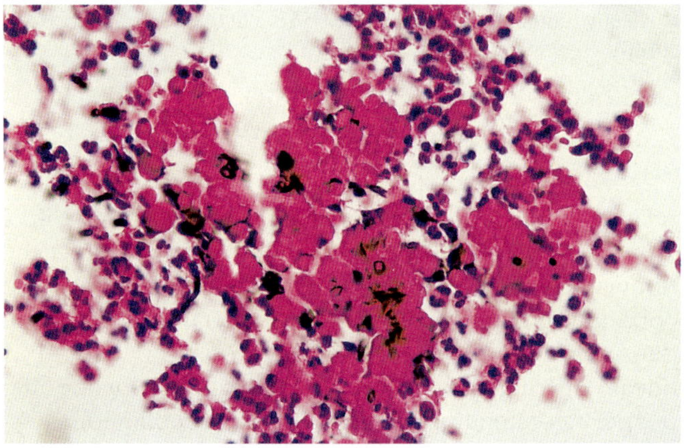

Figure 113–17. *Acremonium falciforme* granule in early stage of development. The small granule within a draining sinus tract consists of a loose network of hyphae and small chlamydoconidia ensheathed by abundant, intensely eosinophilic, Splendore–Hoeppli material (GMS-H&E, ×160).

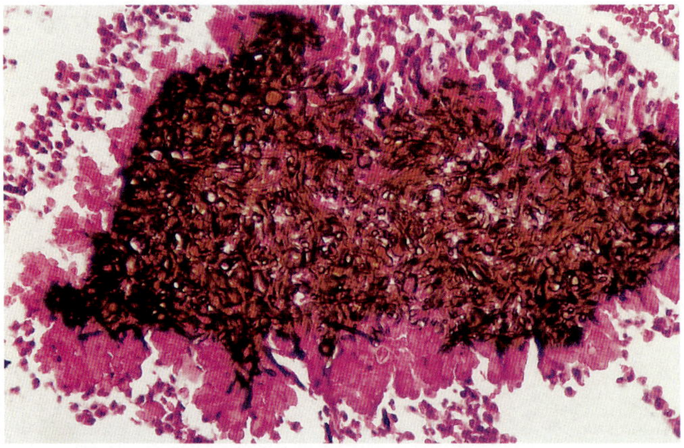

Figure 113–18. White grain mycetoma caused by *A falciforme*. This mature granule is composed of an intricate network of compact, randomly oriented hyphae and small chlamydoconidia. The granule is bordered by broad, irregular projections of Splendore–Hoeppli material, and it closely resembles those formed by *A recifei* and *P boydii* (GMS-H&E, ×100).

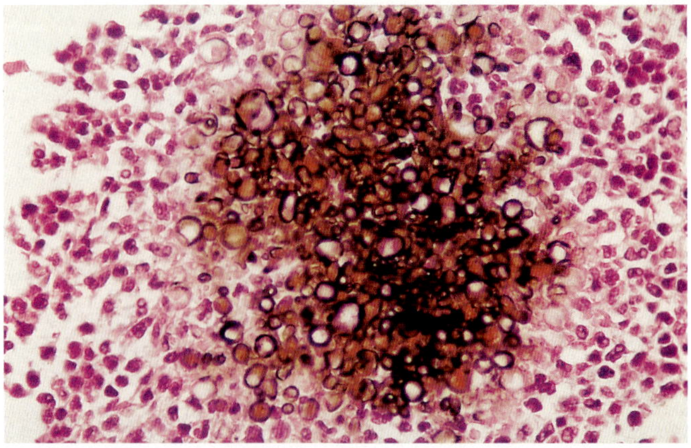

Figure 113–19. *Aspergillus nidulans* granule in early stage of development. The granule is small and consists of an intricate network of compact hyphae and small, thick-walled chlamydoconidia. Because the granule resembles those caused by certain other hyaline hyphomycetes, specific identification of the causative agent requires cultural studies (GMS-H&E, ×160).

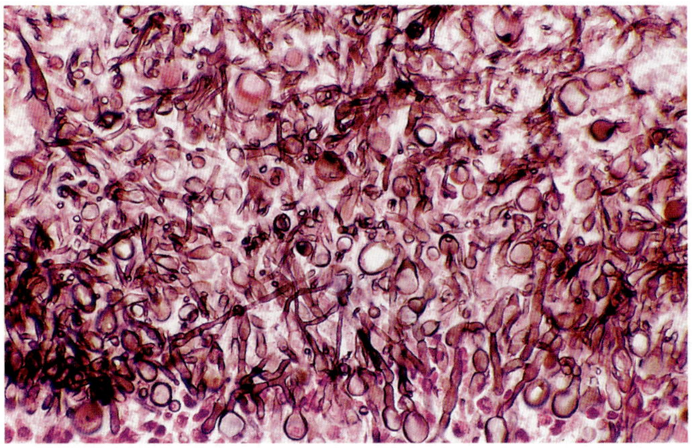

Figure 113–20. White grain mycetoma caused by *A nidulans*. The periphery of this mature granule consists of compact hyphae and small, spherical chlamydoconidia. The interior of the granule is composed of a loose network of randomly oriented fungal elements (GMS-H&E, ×160).

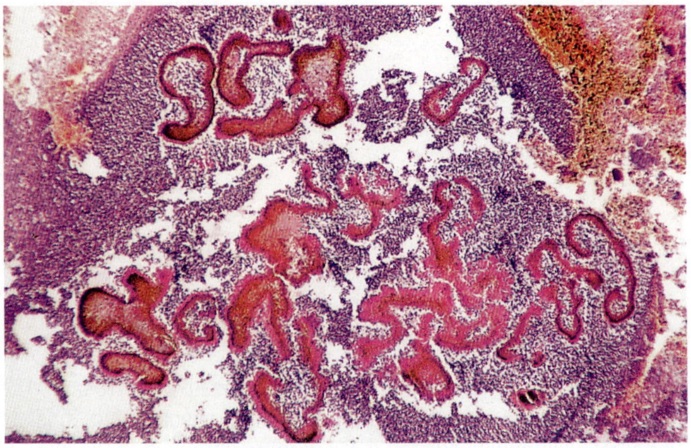

Figure 113–21. Black grain mycetoma caused by *E jeanselmei*. Dematiaceous (naturally brown) granules and abundant neutrophils occupy a draining sinus tract (H&E, ×10).

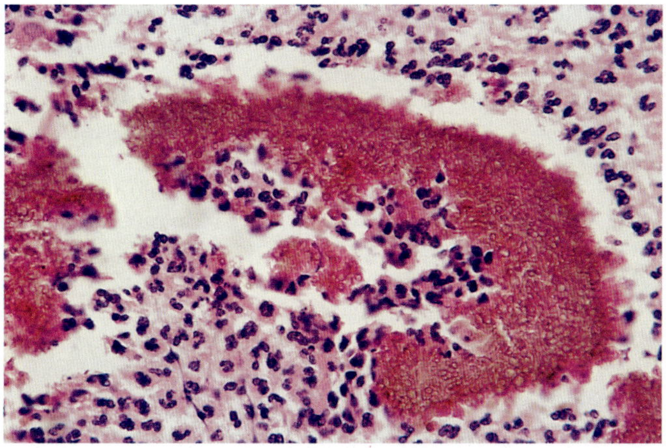

Figure 113–22. *Exophiala jeanselmei* granule. Note that the granule is crescent shaped and composed of compact, brown chlamydoconidia and fewer hyphae. Neutrophils surround the granule (H&E, ×160).

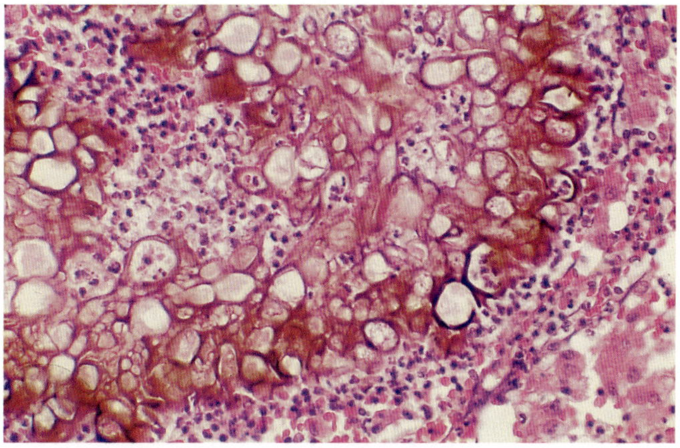

Figure 113–24. *Curvularia geniculata* granule. The periphery of the granule is composed of compact, brown hyphae and prominent, thick-walled chlamydoconidia embedded in cement-like material. The interior of the granule consists of a loose network of weakly pigmented mycelium. *Curvularia geniculata* granules resemble those produced by *L senegalensis* (H&E, ×100).

intrafollicular dermatophytic elements can be seen invading the contiguous dermis through defects in the follicular wall. In some of these deep-seated infections, extrafollicular fungal elements within the dermis occur as individual hyphae and arthroconidia, and the lesion is referred to as Majocchi's dermatophytic granuloma. In other infections, the organized clustering of individual fungal elements forms loose or compact aggregates of varying sizes that resemble the granules of eumycotic, white grain mycetomas. The aggregated fungal elements are frequently embedded in and surrounded by abundant, PAS-positive Splendore–Hoeppli–like material (Figure 113–26). These endogenous mycelial aggregates are erroneously considered by some to be granules or grains and the lesion to be a mycetoma. The mycelial aggregates, however, are almost always associated with and contiguous to individual fungal elements and are more properly termed pseudogranules. The microscopic appearance of dermatophytic pseudomycetomas is strikingly similar irrespective of the causal agent, and the histopathologic pattern resembles that seen in mycetomas. In addition, typical dermatophytic elements can often be demonstrated in overlying, intact hair follicles. Such pseudomycetomas have been caused

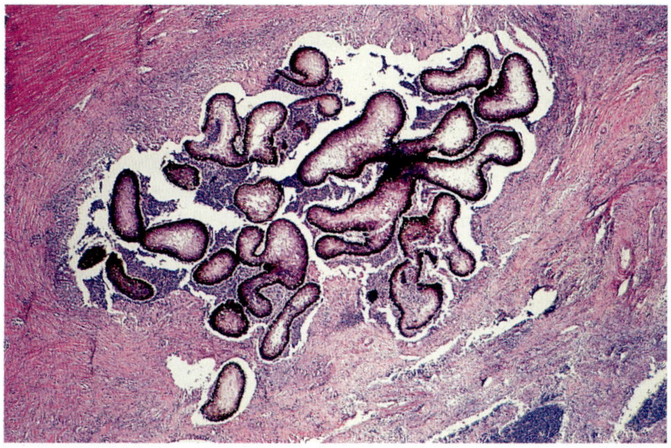

Figure 113–23. Black grain mycetoma of soft tissue and bone caused by *C geniculata*. The irregular dark masses are clusters of pigmented granules. Note extensive fibrosis and destructive osteomyelitis (H&E, ×5).

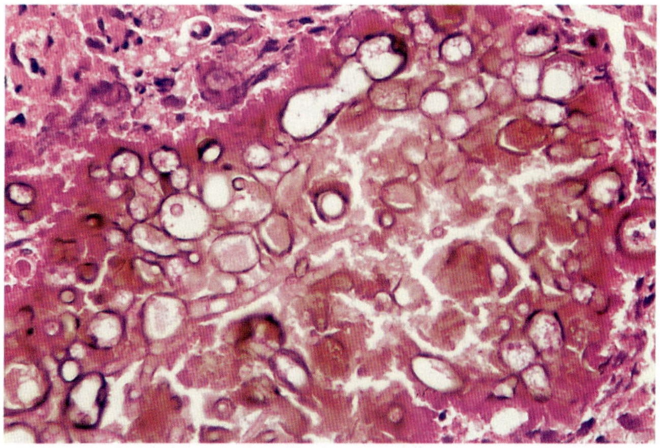

Figure 113–25. *Leptosphaeria senegalensis* granule in black grain mycetoma. The granule has a dark perimeter of pigmented chlamydoconidia and hyphae embedded in a brownish cement-like material. Granules produced by this fungus are morphologically and tinctorially similar to those of *C geniculata* (see Figure 113–24) (H&E, ×160).

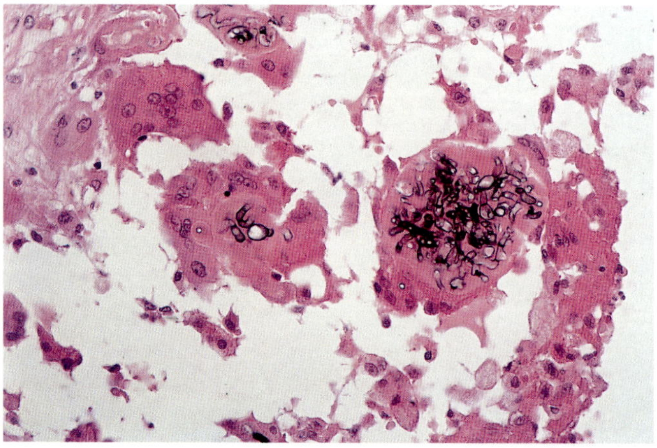

Figure 113–26. Dermatophytic pseudomycetoma caused by *Microsporum canis.* Individual hyphae and hyphal aggregates within a dermal granuloma are ensheathed by abundant Splendore–Hoeppli–like material. Typical dermatophytic fungi were in overlying, intact hair follicles (GMS-H&E, ×100).

by the following species of dermatophytes: *Microsporum audouinii, M canis, M ferrugineum, Trichophyton mentagrophytes, T rubrum, T tonsurans,* and *T violaceum.*[25]

Another major problem in the histopathologic differential diagnosis of mycetomas is botryomycosis, a chronic, localized bacterial pseudomycosis usually of the skin and subcutaneous tissues caused by nonfilamentous gram-positive and gram-negative bacteria that form compact aggregates or granules.[26,27] These granules are almost always bordered by Splendore–Hoeppli material, and like those of the mycetomas, are in encapsulated abscesses. In H&E stained tissue sections, entire botryomycotic granules are usually hematoxylinophilic or amphophilic and resemble those in mycetomas, especially actinomycotic mycetomas, because the bacteria that form these granules are poorly delineated. Histopathologic differentiation is achieved with tissue Gram stains, such as the Brown–Hopps and Brown–Brenn procedures, which demonstrate bacterial cocci and bacilli in botryomycosis and delicate, branched, gram-positive filaments in actinomycotic mycetomas.

REFERENCES

1. Mahgoub ES, Murray IG. *Mycetoma.* London: William Heinemann Medical Books; 1973.
2. Winslow DJ. Mycetoma. In: Baker RD et al, eds. *The Pathologic Anatomy of Mycoses. Human Infection with Fungi, Actinomycetes and Algae.* New York: Springer-Verlag; 1971:589–613.
3. Green WO, Adams TE. Mycetoma in the United States: a review and report of seven additional cases. *Am J Clin Pathol.* 1964;42:75–91.
4. Klokke AH, Swamidasan G, Anguli R, Verghese A. The causal agents of mycetoma in South India. *Trans R Soc Trop Med Hyg.* 1968;62:509–516.
5. Cameron HM, Gatei D, Bremner AD. The deep mycoses in Kenya: a histopathological study. 1. Mycetoma. *East Afr Med J.* 1973;50:382–395.
6. Hay RJ, Mackenzie DWR. Mycetoma (Madura foot) in the United Kingdom: a survey of forty-four cases. *Clin Exp Dermatol.* 1983;8:553–563.
7. Bendl BJ, Mackey D, Al-Saati F, et al. Mycetoma in Saudi Arabia. *J Trop Med Hyg.* 1987;90:51–59.
8. Chandler FW, Kaplan W, Ajello L. *A Colour Atlas and Textbook of the Histopathology of Mycotic Diseases.* London: Wolfe Medical Publications; 1980:76–82, 222–239.
9. Oyston JK. Madura foot: a study of twenty cases. *J Bone Joint Surg.* 1961;43B:259–267.
10. Zaias N. Mycetoma. *Arch Dermatol.* 1969;99:215–225.
11. Palestine RF, Rogers RS. Diagnosis and treatment of mycetoma. *J Am Acad Dermatol.* 1982;6:107–111.
12. Magana M. Mycetoma. *Int J Dermatol.* 1984;23:221–236.
13. El Hassan AM, Mahgoub ES. Lymph node involvement in mycetoma. *Trans R Soc Trop Med Hyg.* 1972;66:165–169.
14. Vanbreuseghem R. Early diagnosis, treatment and epidemiology of mycetoma. *Rev Med Vet Mycol.* 1967;6:49–60.
15. Mahgoub ES. Medical management of mycetoma. *Bull WHO.* 1976;54:303–310.
16. Mahgoub ES, Gumaa SA. Ketoconazole in the treatment of eumycetoma due to *Madurella mycetomi. Trans R Soc Trop Med Hyg.* 1984;78:376–379.
17. Tight RR, Bartlett MS. Actinomycetoma in the United States. *Rev Infect Dis.* 1981;3:1139–1150.
18. Winslow DJ, Steen FJ. Considerations in the histologic diagnosis of mycetoma. *Am J Clin Pathol.* 1964;42:164–169.
19. MacKinnon JE. Mycetomas as opportunistic wound infections. *Lab Invest.* 1962;11:1124–1131.
20. Burkus JK. Primary mycetoma infection of the distal tibia secondary to an occult foreign body. *Foot Ankle.* 1985;6:47–52.
21. Chandler FW, Watts JC. *Pathologic Diagnosis of Fungal Infections.* Chicago: ASCP Press; 1987:251–263.
22. Ajello L, Kaplan W, Chandler FW. Dermatophyte mycetomas: fact of fiction? In: *Proceedings of the Fifth International Conference on the Mycoses: Superficial, Cutaneous, and Subcutaneous Infections.* Sci Pub 396; Washington, DC: Pan American Health Organization; 1980:135–140.
23. West BC, Kwon-Chung KJ. Mycetoma caused by *Microsporum audouinii:* first reported case. *Am J Clin Pathol.* 1980;73:447–454.
24. West BC. Five year follow-up of a man with subcutaneous mycetomas caused by *Microsporum audouinii. Am J Clin Pathol.* 1982;77:767–769.
25. Rinaldi MG, Lamazor EA, Roeser EH, Wegner CJ. Mycetoma or pseudomycetoma? A distinctive mycosis caused by dermatophytes. *Mycopathologia.* 1983;81:41–48.
26. Winslow DJ. Botryomycosis. *Am J Pathol.* 1959;35:153–167.
27. Greenblatt M, Heredia R, Rubenstein L, Alpert S. Bacterial pseudomycosis ("botryomycosis"). *Am J Clin Pathol.* 1964;41:188–193.

CHAPTER 114

Paracoccidioidomycosis

Alberto Thomaz Londero and Francis W. Chandler

A discovery is rarely, if ever, a sudden achievement, nor is it the work of one man; a long series of observations, each in turn received in doubt and discussed in hostility, are familiarized by time, and lead at last to the gradual disclosure of truth.

Sir Berkeley Moynihan (1865–1936), Surg Gynecol Obstet. 1920;31:549.

DEFINITION

Paracoccidioidomycosis (PCM) is a systemic infection caused by the thermally dimorphic fungus *Paracoccidioides brasiliensis*. Primary lesions of paracoccidioidomycosis are usually seen in young people as a self-limited pulmonary infection, rarely displaying a progressive acute or subacute course. Years later, reactivation of a primary quiescent lesion may become progressive chronic PCM of the lungs, with or without involvement of other organs. Synonyms include South American blastomycosis, Lutz–Splendore–Almeida's disease, and paracoccidioidal granuloma.

GEOGRAPHIC DISTRIBUTION

PCM is endemic or acquired in continental Latin American countries, with the exception of Belize, Nicaragua, Guiana, Surinam, and Chile.[1,2] Two cases of PCM were reported and another one diagnosed in the Caribbean islands of Trinidad, Grenada, and Guadeloupe.[1]

MORPHOLOGIC FEATURES OF THE ORGANISM

Paracoccidioides brasiliensis grows in culture in its mycelial phase at 25°C and in its yeastlike phase in tissue and in culture at 35 to 37°C. At 25°C the fungus grows slowly. White colonies with short aerial hyphae appear in 3 to 4 weeks. Later on, they become velvety. Glabrous, cerebriform, brownish colonies also are sometimes formed. The colonies are composed of interlaced, septate, branched, delicate hyphae with intercalated chlamydoconidia 15 μm in diameter. On natural media (soil agar, yeast agar), single-celled conidia (3 to 4 μm) and plain or bulging arthroconidia (3 × 6 μm) are produced.[3,4]

At 35 to 37°C, yeastlike, opaque, cream-colored, cerebriform colonies appear in 5 to 10 days. In tissue and in culture at 35 to 37°C, the fungus appears as spherical or oval yeastlike cells, 3 to 30 μm or more in diameter, with double, refractile walls. These cells reproduce by single or multiple buds—the blastoconidia—which are connected to the parent cell by a narrow isthmus (Figure 114–1, A–C). Six or more blastoconidia of various sizes may be produced, some of which also bud. The variability in size and number of blastoconidia, and their connection to parent cells, are characteristic (Figure 114–2, A–C). These features are clearly seen in clinical specimens mounted in 10% KOH. Multiple budding cells can be recognized in hematoxylin-eosin (H&E) stained tissue sections, but the peculiar features of the fungus are best disclosed by Gomori's methenamine-silver (GMS) stain. In tissue sections, large cells completely covered with small buds, 1 to 3 μm in diameter, are also seen. These structures ("steering-wheel" forms) are pathognomonic (Figures 114–1 and 114–2). The thick walls of larger fungal cells sometimes fracture to produce "mosaic" or "soccer-ball" forms.

LIFE CYCLE

Although *P brasiliensis* has been recovered from soil, its natural habitat and ecology remain unknown.[3,5] In

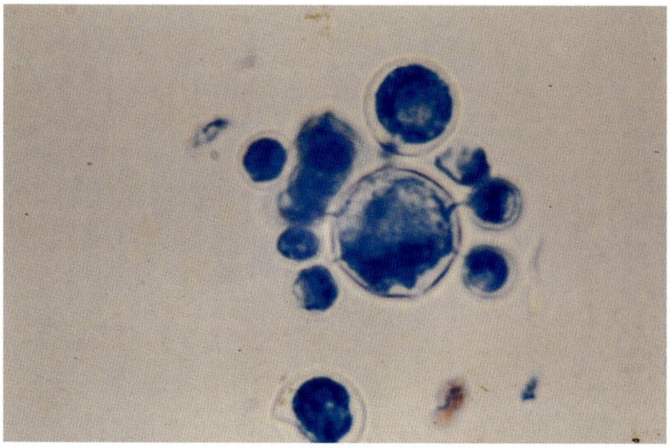

A

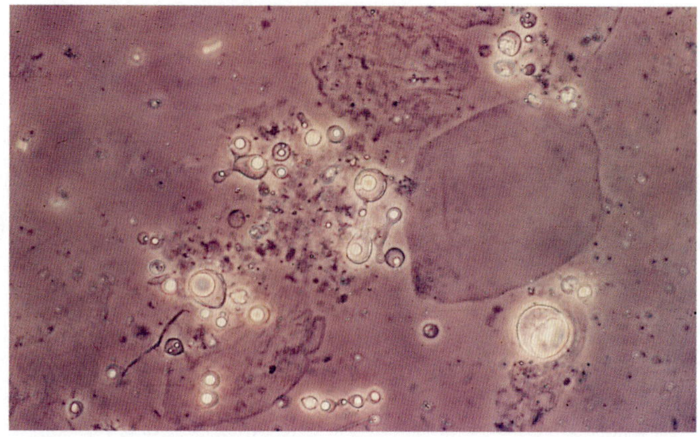

B

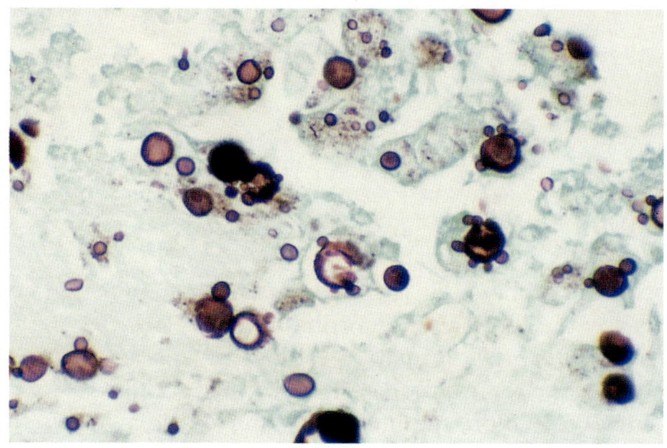

C

Figure 114–1. *Paracoccidioides brasiliensis.* (**A**) Lactophenol cotton blue mount of multiple budding yeast forms grown in culture at 35°C (×400). (**B**) A 10% KOH preparation revealing numerous thick-walled yeast forms in sputum (×160). (**C**) Pathognomonic (multiple budding) yeast forms in lung section stained with GMS (×160).

nature, the fungus may exist in the mycelial phase because it grows and regularly produces infective propagules on very simple natural substrates.[3,4] Humans and possibly nine-banded armadillos are the hosts for *P brasiliensis,* but overt disease has not been demonstrated in the latter.[1,3]

EPIDEMIOLOGY

PCM is not a notifiable disease, so its epidemiology is based on case reporting and on surveys using paracoccidioidin skin tests. These data, however, are not available from vast regions. Consequently, the real incidence and prevalence of PCM cannot be estimated.[1] Endemic areas have high humidity, rich vegetation, moderate temperatures, and acid soil.[3] These areas are distributed along rivers from the Amazonian jungle[6] to small indigenous forests in Uruguay.[5]

In children, infection has been reported in early infancy, with a peak incidence in the 10- to 19-year-old age group.[1,7] Overt disease, however, is uncommon in children (no sex difference) and adolescents (slight male predominance).[7,8] Clinical disease is more frequent in adults (30 to 50 years), and there is a striking male predominance.[2] The greatest number of patients with PCM has been recorded in Brazil, Colombia, and Venezuela. The majority of children and adolescents with disease has been reported in the Brazilian states between 15°S and 25°S.[8] Rural people who maintain close contact with soil are usually affected. All races are susceptible. There is no report of epidemics or of human-to-human transmission.

NATURAL HISTORY

Paracoccidioides brasiliensis enters the body by the respiratory passages, eliciting a primary pulmonary–lymph node complex.[9,10] Simultaneously, fungal cells may bypass regional lymph nodes and disseminate to any organ hematogenously. Primary infection evolves in two ways, depending on the immunologic status of the host: spontaneous regression or progressive dis-

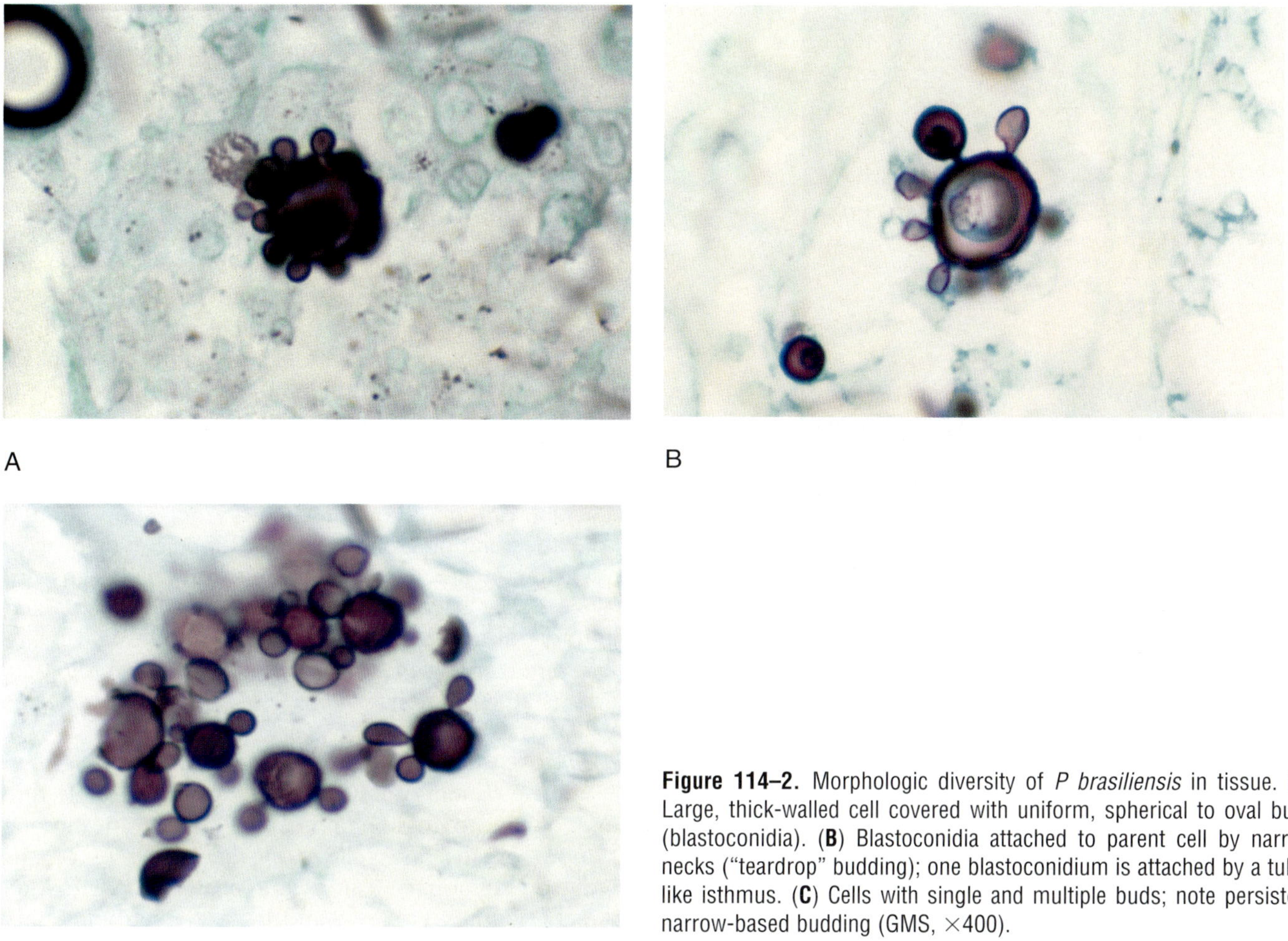

A

B

C

Figure 114–2. Morphologic diversity of *P brasiliensis* in tissue. (**A**) Large, thick-walled cell covered with uniform, spherical to oval buds (blastoconidia). (**B**) Blastoconidia attached to parent cell by narrow necks ("teardrop" budding); one blastoconidium is attached by a tube-like isthmus. (**C**) Cells with single and multiple buds; note persistent narrow-based budding (GMS, ×400).

ease. In normal hosts, primary lesions evolve subclinically or as spontaneously regressing, nonspecific respiratory infections. Within healed lesions, the fungus is destroyed or remains viable.[9] Nevertheless, there is host sensitization—revealed by a reactive paracoccidioidin skin test. In the abnormal host, primary lesions may progress with an acute or subacute course. Fungemia is commonly detected, consequently any organ may be involved.[2,7]

In adults over 30 years of age, overt disease usually results from endogenous reactivation of quiescent lesions.[9–11] Reactivation can occur in infections acquired many years before. The disease is protracted, and is either confined to the lungs or may involve other organs.[2,9]

CLINICAL FEATURES

PCM presents with a regressive course (subclinical and primary pulmonary forms) or as a progressive disease (acute pulmonary, acute or subacute disseminated, chronic pulmonary, and chronic disseminated forms).[2,9]

Subclinical Infection. Skin test surveys in Brazil and Colombia indicate that 10% of the population of both countries is, or has been, infected by *P brasiliensis.*[2] One patient with spontaneously resolving asymptomatic pulmonary lesions and a few patients with fibrotic or calcified residual pulmonary lesions also have been reported.[1,9,10]

Primary Pulmonary Paracoccidioidomycosis. Symptoms of respiratory infection associated with infiltrative lung lesions and hilar adenopathy on chest radiographs were reported in a girl and followed for 10 years after resolution.[12]

Acute Pulmonary Paracoccidioidomycosis. Symptoms of acute respiratory infection, radiologic evidence of progressive consolidation in both lung bases, and bilateral pleural effusion (empyema) were reported in a boy with PCM.[9]

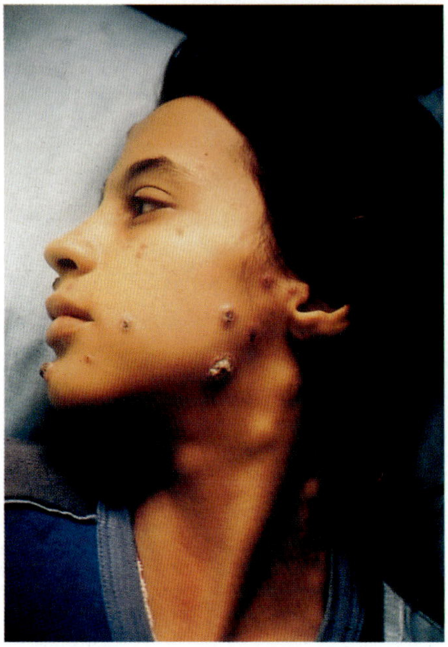

Figure 114–3. Subacute disseminated paracoccidioidomycosis (juvenile type) in a 15-year-old girl. Note ulcerative–nodular lesions of the face and accompanying cervical lymphadenopathy.

Acute or Subacute Disseminated Paracoccidioidomycosis. This form occurs in children, adolescents, and young adults. All organ systems may be involved, but the mononuclear phagocyte system is the most severely affected.[10] Signs and symptoms are more prominent in groups of organs, resulting in a variety of clinical pictures (Figure 114–3). The first and most evident manifestations may be 1) generalized lymphadenopathy, 2) gastrointestinal symptoms (diarrhea, abdominal pain, or masses), 3) signs of osteoarticular involvement simulating osteomyelitis, or 4) acute abdominal syndrome.[7] Presentation as a cutaneous or respiratory infection is exceptional.[7,8] Hepatosplenomegaly, weight loss, and fever are usually present. Bouts of fungemia explain the frequency of multiple skin lesions, acuteness of the clinical picture, and relapses. Although the fungus can be demonstrated in sputum or bronchial washings, lesions are infrequently seen on chest radiographs.[2] Lesions of mucous membranes are uncommon.

Chronic Pulmonary Paracoccidioidomycosis. This form occurs in adults and evolves for months or years as a recurrent or continuous respiratory infection. Cough and expectoration, followed by dyspnea, weight loss, and asthenia are usual symptoms. Physical signs are few, and vary according to the extent of lesions. Mixed infiltrates distributed throughout the middle and lower lobes are very suggestive, but nonspecific radiologic findings are common.[2,11]

Chronic Disseminated Paracoccidioidomycosis. More than 90% of the patients are adult males. The clinical picture depends on progression and extension of lesions in one or more organs, as well as the sequence of organs involved. Pulmonary lesions are present in almost all patients (Figures 114–4, A and B).[2,9,12] Extrapulmonary lesions are more frequently localized to mucous mem-

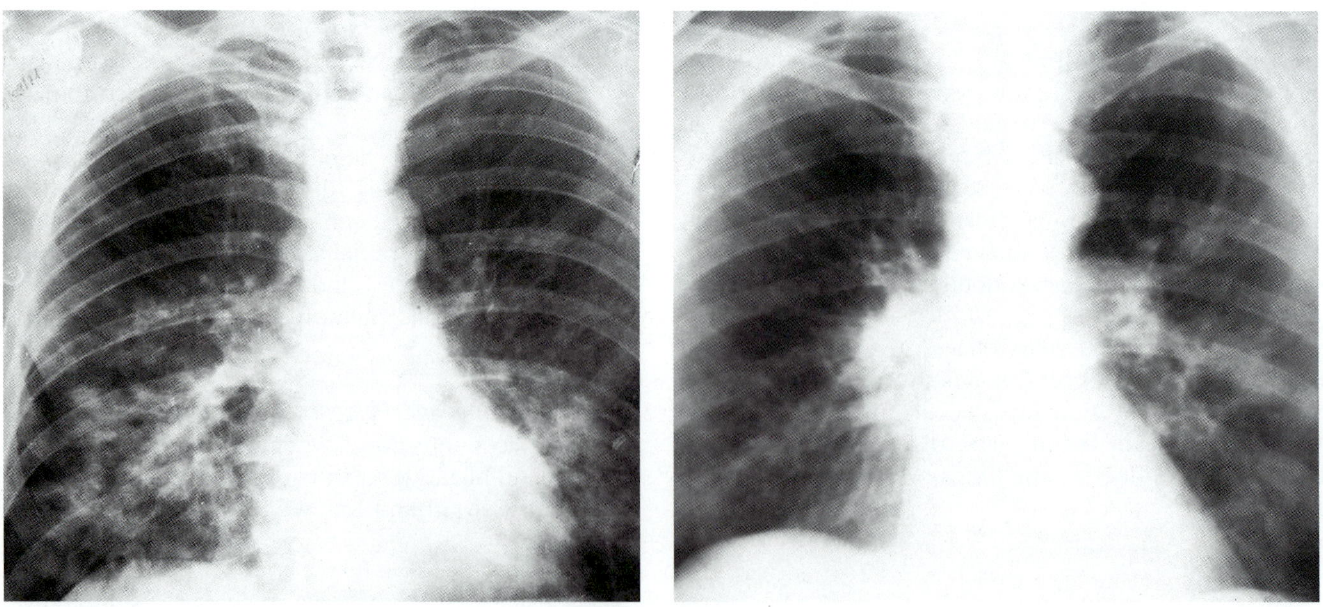

A B

Figure 114–4. Chronic disseminated paracoccidioidomycosis. Chest radiographs reveal (**A**) nodular and interstitial lesions in the lower portions of both lungs and (**B**) pulmonary lesions suggesting metastatic malignancy.

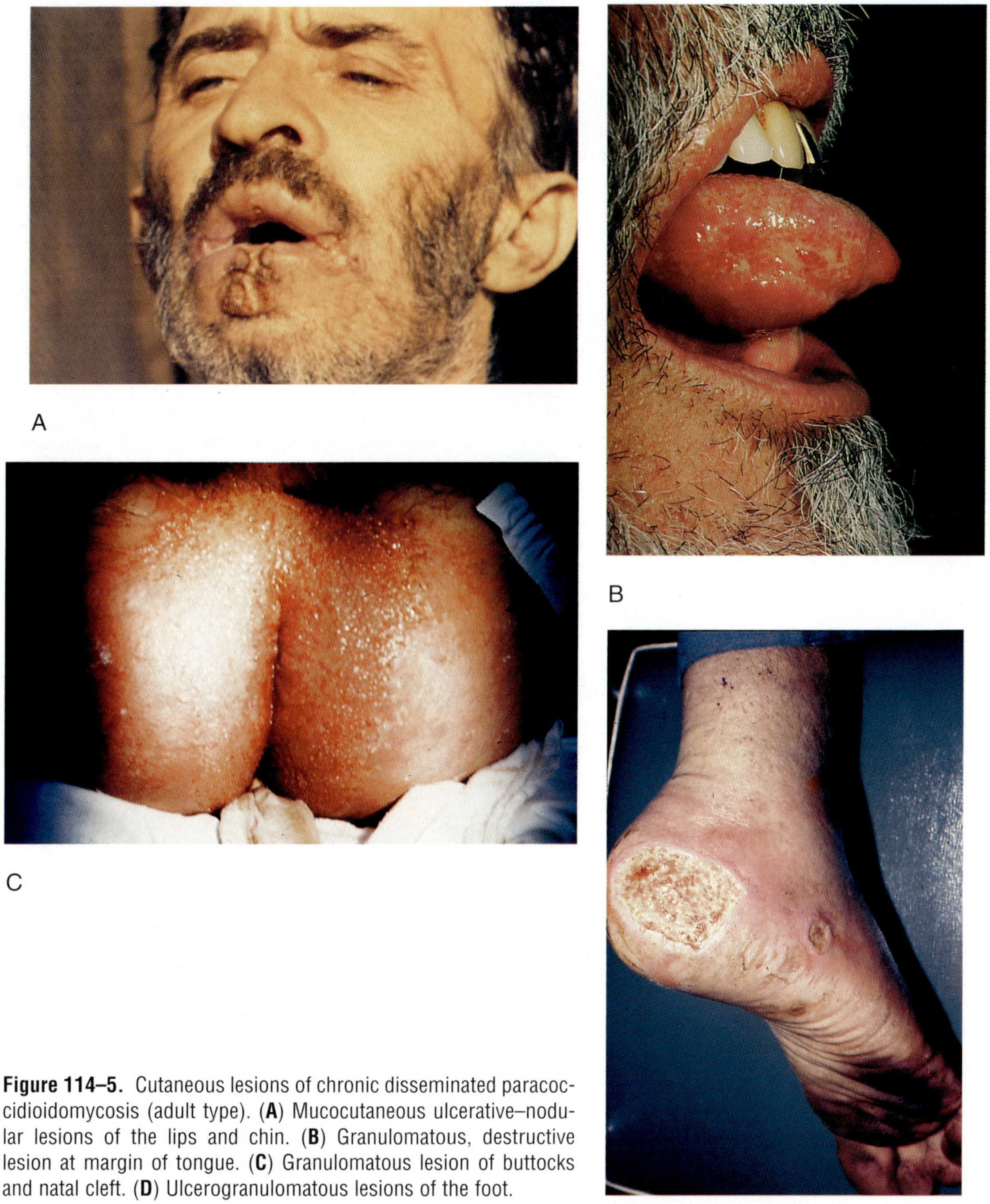

Figure 114–5. Cutaneous lesions of chronic disseminated paracoccidioidomycosis (adult type). (**A**) Mucocutaneous ulcerative–nodular lesions of the lips and chin. (**B**) Granulomatous, destructive lesion at margin of tongue. (**C**) Granulomatous lesion of buttocks and natal cleft. (**D**) Ulcerogranulomatous lesions of the foot.

branes, lymph nodes, and skin (Figure 114–5, A–D), and less frequently to genitals, central nervous system, intestines, liver, and spleen. However, magnetic resonance imaging, photoscanning with gallium-67, ultrasonography, and computed tomography reveal lesions that are unsuspected clinically or are not disclosed radiographically.[13,14] Weight loss, adynamia, and asthenia are common complaints. Although lung lesions are very extensive, signs and symptoms are scarce and nonspecific. Ulceration of the mouth occurs in 30% to 50% of patients. Less frequently, granulomatous or ulcerative lesions of the pharynx, larynx, nasal mucosa, and skin are seen. Mandibular and cervical lymphadenopathies are associated with buccal lesions. Asymptomatic involvement of endocrine glands may be detected. Addison's disease may be the presenting feature or may occur later in the course of infection.[14] Involvement of the gastrointestinal tract is uncommon. Liver, spleen, and pancreas may be mildly affected. Lesions of brain, epididymitis, and tumefaction of the testes have been observed.[2,12] Involvement of the heart, aorta, bones, kidneys, and eyes is rare.

Opportunistic Paracoccidioidomycosis. Acute, disseminated PCM has been induced by immunosuppressive drugs.[15] PCM in AIDS patients has been reported rarely.[16]

PATHOLOGY

A primary pulmonary–lymph node complex has been documented in PCM. Spontaneously regressing lesions have been described as small fibrotic or calcified nodules in the lungs and adrenal glands.[1] Solitary residual nodules or "coin" lesions also have been reported.[10] The pathologic anatomy of PCM, however, has been mainly described from autopsies of patients at an advanced or terminal stage of disease.[17] In the acute or subacute disseminated form of PCM, there are extensive involvement of lymphoid tissues, widespread lesions of the intestines, and multiple bone lesions. Lymphadenopathy is commonly multifocal and sometimes confluent. Suppurative nodes contain a greenish-yellow pus. Isolated or confluent ulcerations are distributed throughout the ileum, colon, and rectum. Single or multiple bone lesions consist of osteolytic foci or diffuse osteomyelitis.[17]

In the chronic disseminated form of PCM, pulmonary and adrenal lesions are present in almost all patients. Ulcerations of the mucous membranes are common. The lungs have a bosselated appearance caused by areas of fibrotic retraction and emphysema, and there is focal thickening of the pleura. On cut surface, the most common findings are thickening of the centrilobular septa, a netlike appearance from dilated alveoli, or numerous, grayish, isolated or confluent nodules 1 to 4 mm in diameter.[17] Cavitation is not uncommon. Miliary, pneumonic, or bronchopneumonic lesions are rare. Enlarged adrenal glands have multiple necrotic or granulomatous foci, or diffuse necrosis. Lesions of the spleen, liver, and genitals are similar to those of tuberculosis. In the central nervous system, granulomas or abscesses are observed.

The histopathologic features of PCM resemble those of other mycoses, and lesions are recognized only when the distinctive tissue forms of *P brasiliensis* are disclosed (Figures 114–1 and 114–2). The most common host response is granulomatous or mixed granulomatous and suppurative (Figure 114–6). In the same specimen, there may be multifocal and confluent microabscesses in one field and epithelioid granulomas in another. Granulomas may be either well formed or poorly defined, isolated or confluent, and consist of epithelioid cells, foreign-body and Langhans' giant cells, macrophages, lymphocytes, plasma cells, and fibroblasts. They may be centrally necrotic, similar to those of tuberculosis, or solid, mimicking those of sarcoidosis.[17] Destructive lesions with massive caseous necrosis surrounded by a granulomatous reaction also may be observed, particularly in lymph nodes and adrenals. In immunodeficient patients, there may be bland necrosis associated with abundant, rapidly proliferating fungal cells (Figure 114–7). Pseudoepitheliomatous hyperplasia is seen in the epidermis and mucosa, while mixed granulomatous and suppurative inflammation with microabscesses is found in the dermis and submucosa (Figure 114–8). Fibrogranulomatous, fibrocaseous, and

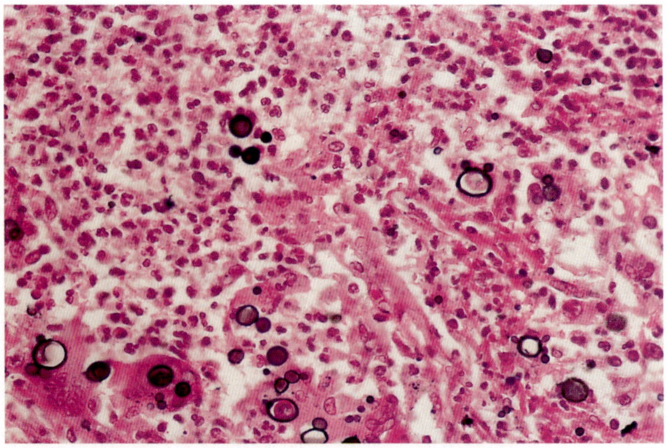

Figure 114–6. Acute paracoccidioidal pneumonia. Alveolar spaces are filled with neutrophils, macrophages, giant cells, and sparse yeast forms of *P brasiliensis* (GMS–H&E, ×100).

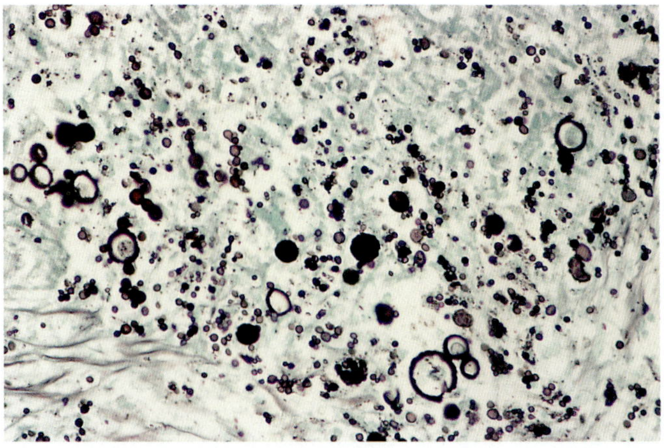

Figure 114–7. Acute paracoccidioidal pneumonia in an immunodeficient patient. Note marked pleomorphism of abundant fungal cells, including several thick-walled macroforms. Multiple budding is evident, even at low magnification (GMS, ×100).

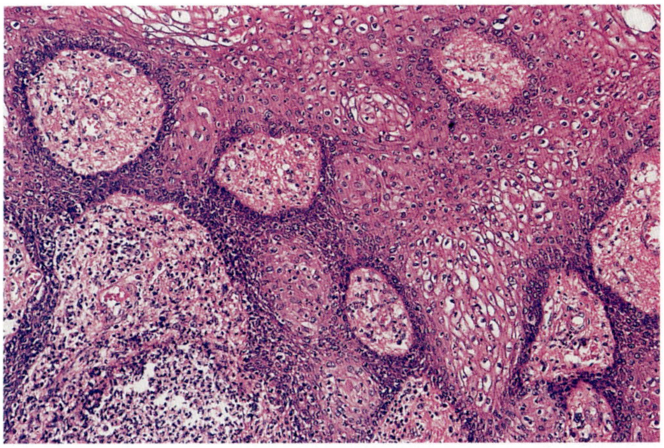

Figure 114–8. Tongue showing disseminated paracoccidioidomycosis characterized by florid pseudoepitheliomatous hyperplasia of the lingual mucosa and mixed suppurative and granulomatous inflammation in the submucosa (H&E, ×10).

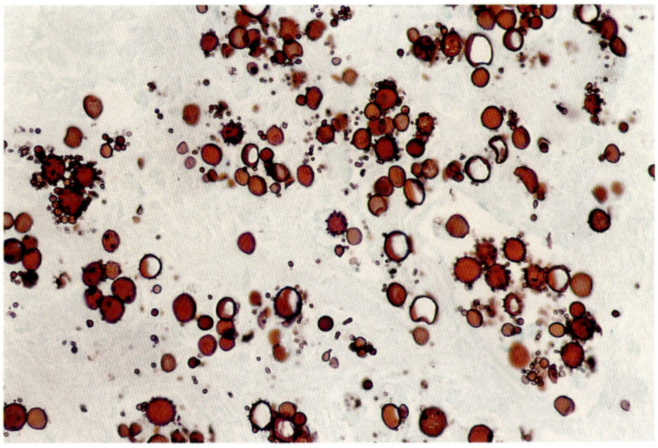

Figure 114–10. Chronic disseminated paracoccidioidomycosis. A replicate section of the granulomatous lesion in Figure 114–9 reveals numerous yeastlike cells of *P brasiliensis* that vary in size and shape. Many fungal cells contain multiple buds that are diagnostic (GMS, ×100).

calcified pulmonary lesions are encountered incidentally.[9,17]

Paracoccidioides brasiliensis can be recognized in H&E stained tissue sections that contain active lesions, but the characteristic features of pathognomonic tissue forms are best defined by GMS. When stained with H&E, the fungus appears as globose cells with relatively thin, refractive walls. The multinucleated cytoplasm is lightly hematoxylinophilic and commonly is separated from the cell wall by an optically clear space or "halo" (Figure 114–9). Fungal cells of various sizes, distributed within giant cells or extracellularly, are seen in the same section (Figure 114–10). Connections of buds to parent cells are undefined, and buds appear to surround parent cells. Nevertheless, fungal elements are not readily visible with H&E when they are small to medium-sized and distributed in sarcoid-like foci, or when they are present as predominantly small forms in any lesion.[17] On the other hand, small intracellular forms may be confused with *Histoplasma capsulatum* var *capsulatum* (Figure 114–11); medium-sized forms may be mistaken for *Blastomyces dermatitidis* or with capsule-deficient *Cryptococcus neoformans*. Occasionally, large empty forms mimic immature spherules of *Coccidioides immitis* (Figure 114–12). Replicate, GMS stained sections readily reveal the characteristic multiple budding forms

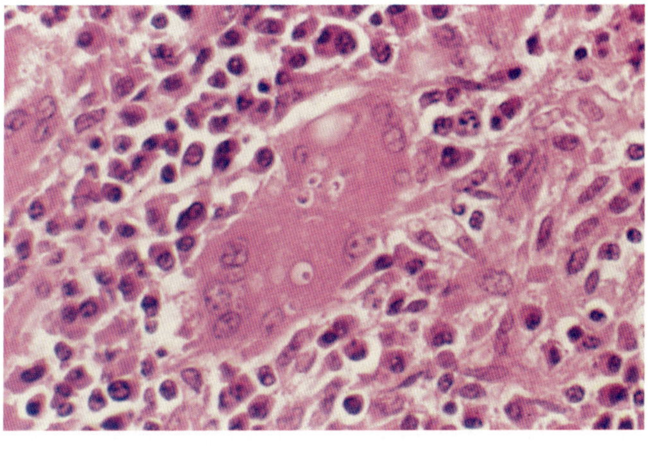

Figure 114–9. Granulomatous orchitis in a patient with chronic disseminated paracoccidioidomycosis. A giant cell contains several weakly stained yeast forms of *P brasiliensis* (H&E, ×160).

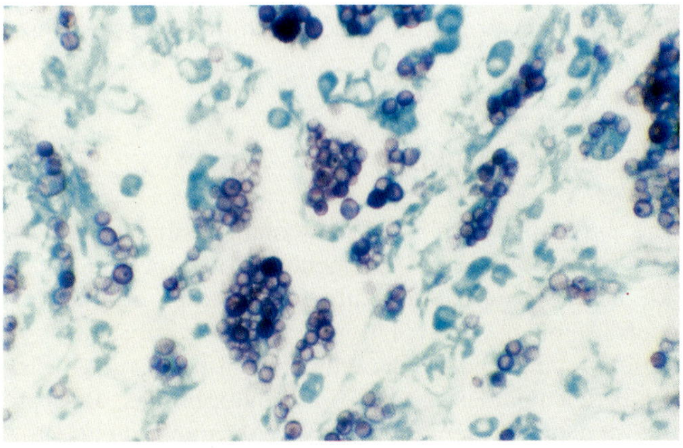

Figure 114–11. Chronic disseminated paracoccidioidomycosis. The normal architecture of a hilar lymph node is effaced by dispersed collections of epithelioid and giant cells that contain small (2 to 5 μm), spherical, nonbudding forms of *P brasiliensis*. Small, compact, intracellular forms of this fungus can be mistaken for yeast forms of *H capsulatum* var *capsulatum* (GMS, ×160).

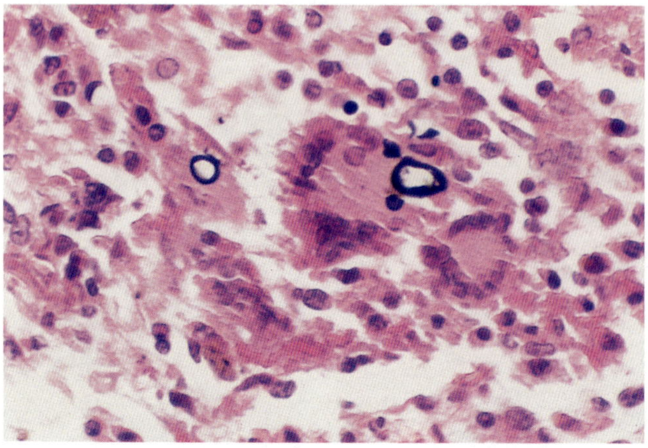

Figure 114–12. Paracoccidioidal pneumonia. Note the large, thick-walled, and empty forms of *P brasiliensis* within epithelioid cells and giant cells. When devoid of buds, these forms mimic empty, immature spherules of *C immitis* (GMS–H&E, ×160).

of *P brasiliensis.*[17] Mayer's mucicarmine stains capsular material of *C neoformans* and differentiates *C neoformans* from *P brasiliensis.* Germinating yeastlike cells and hyphae of *P brasiliensis* are rarely produced in tissue.[18]

Mycelial and yeastlike cultures of *P brasiliensis* have been studied by transmission and scanning electron microscopy.[4] The ultrastructure of the fungus in human tissue also has been documented.[18] Characteristic cells of *P brasiliensis* can be detected by cytologic examination of sputum and bronchial secretions. The fungus is recognizable in Schorr or Papanicolaou stained preparations, but it is more readily delineated with the GMS stain.[19] Specimens obtained by fine-needle aspiration of lymph node and lung have been useful for diagnosis.[20]

DIFFERENTIAL DIAGNOSIS

The two types of clinical presentations in which PCM can be suspected are mucocutaneous ulcerations in adults, and lymphadenopathies in children and adolescents. Similar presentations also are observed in patients with chronic disseminated histoplasmosis capsulati, leishmaniasis, and certain lymphomas. Because the clinical presentations of PCM are protean, this mycosis should be suspected in any patients with a respiratory tract infection living in an endemic area.[2,9] In highly endemic areas, PCM also should be suspected in infections of bones, lymph nodes, and gastrointestinal tracts of children and adolescents.[7,10]

MOLECULAR DIAGNOSIS

A purified 43-kd glycoprotein (gp43) has been obtained from *P brasiliensis* grown in tomato juice–enriched complex medium. This gp43 component corresponds to previously described antigens: immunoelectrophoretic arc E and immunodiffusion band 1.[21] It has been identified as a concanavalin A–binding glycoprotein. The gp43 is the predominant IgG reactive antigen recognized in sera from all patients with overt disease. Patient's sera and murine monoclonal antibodies recognize conformational peptide epitopes of the purified gp43 antigen. Other antigens, eg, 70 kd, also are being studied.[21]

CONFIRMATIONAL TESTING AND DIAGNOSIS

Diagnosis of PCM is based on direct demonstration of the classical tissue forms of the fungus, but this should be complemented by microbiologic culture. For direct microscopic examination, lesional exudates, pus, sputum, bronchial washings or brushings, body fluids, feces, and teased tissues should be examined in a drop of 10% KOH. Before examination, body fluids and *N*-acetyl-cysteine-treated sputum should be centrifuged. Tissue samples collected in fixatives should be processed and stained with H&E and GMS. For culture studies, specimens should be planted on Mycosel (BBL), Sabouraud's or SABHI (Difco) media, and incubated at 25 and 35°C. Isolation from sputum is best achieved on Mycosel medium at 36°C.[2,9]

Various techniques have been used to detect antibodies to *P brasiliensis.* They are very useful for obtaining a presumptive diagnosis, for screening, and for monitoring therapy. Complement fixation has been used for monitoring treatment but not for diagnosis because of cross-reactions with antibodies to other fungal pathogens. Immunodiffusion (ID) is the preferred and most commonly used test; it is simple, 90% sensitive, and 100% specific.[21,22] Immunodiffusion, however, is time consuming and cannot be a criterion for diagnosis in patients with a history of treated PCM. Counterimmunoelectrophoresis is more sensitive than ID and less time consuming, making it an attractive screening procedure. ELISA and MELISA are very sensitive and versatile tests that detect different classes of immunoglobulins. ELISA is useful for serodiagnosis and prognosis, but cross-reactions can occur in patients with other mycoses.[22] Direct immunofluorescence is useful for the direct identification of *P brasiliensis* when only deparaffinized sections of formalin-fixed tissues are available.[23]

TREATMENT

The antifungal agent of choice for most patients with active infection is ketoconazole.[24,25] Amphotericin B and itraconazole are also effective.[26] Surgical excision of localized lesions may be a valuable adjunct to antifungal therapy.

REFERENCES

1. Wake B, Londero AT. Epidemiology and paracoccidioidomycosis infection. In: Franco M, Lacaz CS, Restrepo A, Del Negro G, eds. *Paracoccidioidomycosis.* Boca Raton, Fla: CRC Press; 1994:109–120.
2. Bethlem NM, Lemle A, Bethlem E, et al. Paracoccidioidomycosis. *Semin Respir Med.* 1991;12:81–97.
3. Restrepo A. Ecology of *Paracoccidioides brasiliensis.* In: Franco M, Lacaz CS, Restrepo A, Del Negro G, eds. *Paracoccidioidomycosis.* Boca Raton, Fla: CRC Press; 1994: 121–130.
4. Edwards MR, Salazar ME, Samsonof WA, et al. Electron microscopic study of conidia produced by the mycelium of *Paracoccidioides brasiliensis. Mycopathologia.* 1991; 114:169–177.
5. Conti-Diaz IA, Rila FD. Hipotesis sobre el nicho ecologico de *Paracoccidioides brasiliensis.* Rev Med Uruguay. 1989;5:97–103.
6. Naif RD, Barret TV, Arias JR, et al. Encuesta epidemiologica de histoplasmosis, paracoccidioidomicosis y leishmaniasis mediante pruebas cutaneas. *Bol Sanit Panam.* 1988; 104:35–50.
7. Londero AT, Rios-Goncalves AJ, Cruz MES, et al. Paracoccidioidomicose disseminada "infanto-juvenil" em adolecentes. Arq Bras Med. 1987;61:5–12.
8. Terra GMF, Rios-Goncalves AJ, Londero AT, et al. Paracoccidioidomicose em criancas. Apresentacão de casos. *Arq Bras Med.* 1991;65:8–15.
9. Londero AT. Paracoccidioidomicose. Patogenia, formas clinicas, manifestacões pulmonares de diagnostico. *J Pneumonol.* 1986;12:41–57.
10. Restrepo A, Robledo M, Giraldo R, et al. The gamut of paracoccidioidomycosis. *Am J Med.* 1976;61:33–42.
11. Londero AT, Severo LC. The gamut of progressive pulmonary paracoccidioidomycosis. *Mycopathologia.* 1981; 75:65–74.
12. Londero AT, Ramos CD. Paracoccidioidomicose. Estudo clinico e micologico de 260 casos observados no interior do Estado do Rio Grande do Sul. *J Pneumonol.* 1990; 16:129–132.
13. Calegaro JUM, Gomes EF, Carvalho ACM, et al. 67-Ga na blastomicose: nossa experiencia. *Radiol Bras.* 1990;25: 59–63.
14. Tendrich M, Wanke B, Del Negro G, et al. Adrenocortical involvement. In: Franco M, Lacaz CS, Restrep M, Del Negro G, eds. *Paracoccidioidomycosis.* Boca Raton, Fla: CRC Press; 1994:303–312.
15. Londero AT, Santos JW, Silva LA, et al. Paracoccidioidomicose associada por droga immunosupressora em paciente com lupus eritematoso sistêmico. *J Pneumonol.* 1987;13:224–226.
16. Marques SA, Shikanai-Yasuda MA. Paracoccidioidomycosis associated with immunosuppression, AIDS and cancer. In: Franco M, Lacaz CS, Restrepo A, Del Negro G, eds. *Paracoccidioidomycosis.* Boca Raton, Fla: CRC Press; 1994:393–405.
17. Angulo-Ortega A, Pollak L. Paracoccidioidomycosis. In: Baker RD, ed. *The Pathologic Anatomy of Mycoses. Human Infection with Fungi, Actinomycetes and Algae.* Berlin: Springer-Verlag; 1971:507–576.
18. Furtado JS, Brito T, Freymuller E. The structure and reproduction of *Paracoccidioides brasiliensis* in human tissue. *Sabouraudia.* 1967;5:226–229.
19. Tani EM, Franco M. Pulmonary cytology in paracoccidioidomycosis. *Acta Cytologica.* 1984;28:571–575.
20. Matos MCFI, Schmitt FCL, Marques MEA, et al. Puncão aspirativa de gânglio, linfatico: revisão de 283 casos puncionados no Hospital de Clinicas da faculdade de Medicina de Botucatu. *LAES.* 1991;73:32–40.
21. Puccia R, Travassos LR. 43-Kilodalton glycoprotein from *Paracoccidioides brasiliensis.* Immunochemical reactions with sera from patients with paracoccidioidomycosis, histoplasmosis and Jorge Lobo's disease. *J Clin Microbiol.* 1991;29:1610–1615.
22. Brumer E, Castaneda E, Restrepo A. Paracoccidioidomycosis: an update. *Clin Microbiol Rev.* 1993;6:89–117.
23. Chandler FW, Kaplan W, Ajello L. *Color Atlas and Text of the Histopathology of Mycotic Diseases.* Chicago: Year Book Medical Publishers; 1980:23–25.
24. Cohen J. Antifungal chemotherapy. *Lancet.* 1982;ii:532–537.
25. Hermans PE, Key TF. Antifungal agents used for deep-seated mycotic infections. *Mayo Clin Proc.* 1983;58: 223–231.
26. Restrepo A, Gomez I, Robledo J, Patino MM, Cano LE. Itraconazole in the treatment of paracoccidioidomycosis. A preliminary report. *Rev Infect Dis.* 1987;9(suppl 1): S51–S56.

CHAPTER 115

Penicilliosis Marneffei

Michael R. McGinnis and Francis W. Chandler

What we call experience is often a dreadful list of ghastly mistakes.

J. Chalmers Da Costa (1863–1933)

DEFINITION

Penicilliosis marneffei is a disseminated fungal infection that involves the mononuclear phagocyte system and occurs primarily in human immunodeficiency virus (HIV)-infected patients living in Thailand and southern China.[1,2] The etiologic agent is the thermally dimorphic fungus *Penicillium marneffei,* which grows as an intracellular yeast in tissue and as a typical species of *Penicillium* on standard mycologic media at 25°C. At one time, "Chinese histoplasmosis" was used as a synonym—before the specific features of *P marneffei* were recognized.

GEOGRAPHIC DISTRIBUTION

Penicillium marneffei is endemic in Thailand, the Guangxi Province of China, Hong Kong, Vietnam, and Indonesia. Infections also have been reported in patients from France, the United Kingdom, the United States, Italy, The Netherlands, and Australia. These patients were immunodeficient and had traveled to one or more of the endemic areas. Supparatpinyo et al[2] speculate that *P marneffei* probably exists in Cambodia, Laos, Malaysia, and Burma. The fungus has been isolated from rodents (*Rhizomys sinensis, R pruinosus, R pruinosus senex,* and *Cannomys badius*)[1,3,4] and from soil in the burrows of bamboo rats.[4]

EPIDEMIOLOGY

Penicillium marneffei was isolated in 1956[5] and subsequently described as a new species of *Penicillium* in 1959 by Segretain.[6] It is believed that the conidia are inhaled, which establishes primary pulmonary infection. Before 1987, most infections were in non–acquired immunodeficiency syndrome (non-AIDS) patients, especially those in southern China. Between 1987 and 1992, 92 patients with penicilliosis marneffei were seen at Chiang Mai University Hospital, Thailand.[2] Eighty-six of these patients were infected with HIV or had AIDS. During the same period, 438 patients were diagnosed as having AIDS. In 1993, 35% of 400 AIDS patients at the same hospital had penicilliosis marneffei.[7] This fungal infection has become an early indicator of HIV infection in that region of the world.[8]

LIFE CYCLE AND MORPHOLOGIC FEATURES OF THE ORGANISM

Among the known species of *Penicillium,* only *P marneffei* is a pathogenic dimorphic fungus. The fungus appears to be restricted to endemic areas in Southeast Asia.

Penicillium marneffei is a biverticillate species that is closely related to the ascomycetous genus *Talaromyces.*[9] *Penicillium marneffei* forms colonies on Sabouraud glucose agar that vary from gray to white and have yellowish-green to olive drab to brown to yellowish-brown areas. Colonies are flat, thin, velvety, and have radial folds. A red pigment diffuses into the agar. The conidia are globose, becoming elliptical to limoniform, occur in tangled chains, and are 3 to 4 × 6 to 7 μm.[1,10,11] Growth of *P marneffei* is inhibited by cycloheximide. At 37°C, *P marneffei* grows as a yeast. The yeast cells divide in their centers by fission. They are approximately the same size as *Histoplasma capsula-*

tum var *capsulatum,* but do not reproduce by budding. The ontogeny of the yeast form of *P marneffei* has been studied using electron microscopy.[12]

CLINICAL FEATURES

In patients without AIDS who have had disseminated penicilliosis marneffei, predisposing conditions included tuberculosis, Hodgkin's disease, lymphoproliferative disorders, systemic lupus erythematosus, herpes zoster, active cytomegalovirus infection, osteomyelitis, and poor nutrition.[1,4] In these patients, the most common clinical signs were, in order of decreasing frequency, fever with or without chills; respiratory signs such as pneumonitis, persistent cough, dyspnea, and thoracic pain; cutaneous and subcutaneous lesions; lymphadenopathy; hepatomegaly and splenomegaly; and osteoarticular lesions. In contrast, AIDS patients exhibited fever with or without chills; respiratory signs such as persistent cough and pulmonary infiltrates; cutaneous and subcutaneous lesions; septicemia; and gastrointestinal lesions. Cutaneous lesions consisted of papules, rashes, necrotic pustules, acne-like pustules, and nodules. Weight loss, anorexia, asthenia, and profound cachexia also occurred in disseminated infections.[1]

PATHOLOGY

Histopathologic examination is the most rapid and reliable means of diagnosis. The most frequently examined specimens are lymph node, liver and skin biopsies, and pus from subcutaneous abscesses. In non-AIDS patients, lymph nodes, liver, lung, and kidney are most commonly involved, whereas in AIDS patients, lymph nodes, skin, bone, and bone marrow are the most frequent organs involved.[1] Deng et al[4] have described three inflammatory patterns in penicilliosis marneffei: granulomatous, suppurative, and anergic or necrotizing. The first two reactions are seen in those who have intact immunity (Figure 115–1), and the third occurs in patients with deficient immunity.

In tissue sections, *P marneffei* is yeastlike and multiplies within histiocytes that enlarge to accommodate the fungus (Figure 115–2). The intracellular yeast forms are oval to slightly elongated and 2.5 to 5 μm (Figure 115–3). When extracellular, the yeast cells are sometimes much longer, approaching 8 μm in length, and have rounded ends (Figure 115–4). The cells divide at a central septum by fission (schizogony); they do not bud (Figure 115–5). The central transverse septum usually stains more intensely with Gomori's methenamine silver (GMS) and is wider than the external fungal cell wall. This division process clearly distinguishes yeast forms of *P marneffei* from those of *H capsulatum* var *capsulatum,* which only reproduce by budding.[13]

Suppurative lesions tend to be more common in pulmonary, cutaneous, and subcutaneous sites. The anergic and necrotizing reactions in immunodeficient patients also involve lung, skin, and liver. In addition to the histopathology described by Deng et al,[4] the ultrastructural aspects of penicilliosis marneffei have been described.[1,14,15] In an AIDS patient, a fine-needle aspirate of an enlarged cervical lymph node was used to make the diagnosis.[16]

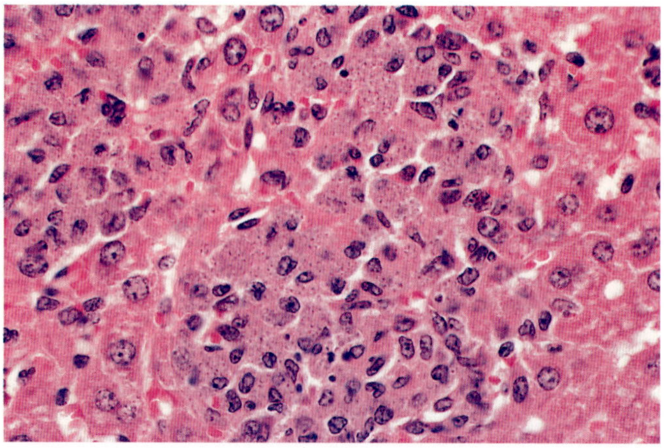

Figure 115–1. Disseminated penicilliosis marneffei in an immunocompetent patient. This hepatic granuloma contains numerous intracellular yeast forms of *P marneffei,* 2.5 to 5 μm in diameter [hematoxylin-eosin (H&E), ×160].

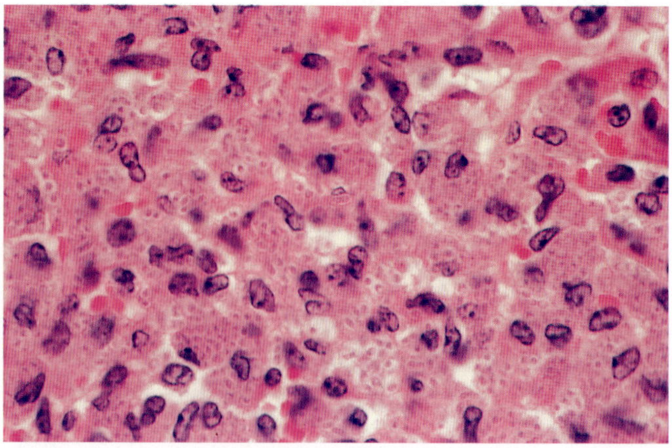

Figure 115–2. Yeast forms of *P marneffei* in a hepatic granuloma. The cytoplasm of individual fungal cells is retracted from their unstained walls, giving the false impression of an unstained capsule. In H&E stained sections, cells of *P marneffei* resemble yeast forms of *H capsulatum* var *capsulatum*, especially when intracellular (H&E, ×250).

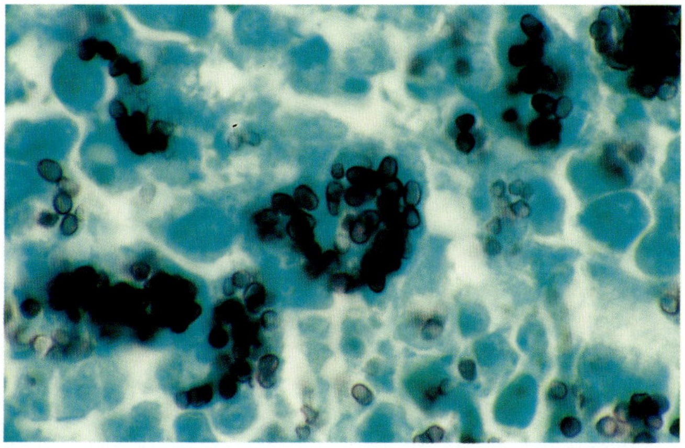

Figure 115–3. Disseminated penicilliosis marneffei. Septate and nonseptate yeast forms of *P marneffei* within histiocytes. Fungal cell walls stain intensely and there is no halo (pseudocapsular) effect as seen in H&E stained sections (GMS, ×400).

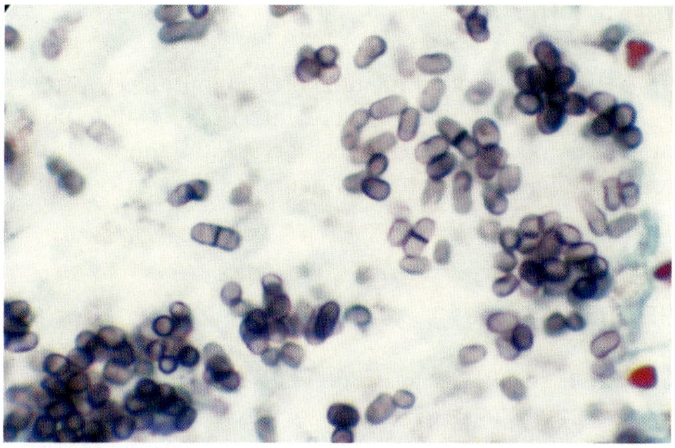

Figure 115–5. Penicilliosis marneffei. Individual and clustered yeast forms of *P marneffei* in a splenic abscess. Three yeast forms at center contain single, wide, transverse septa that stain more intensely than the external walls. Unlike *H capsulatum* var *capsulatum* and other yeast-form pathogens, the cells of *P marneffei* do not bud (GMS, ×500).

DIFFERENTIAL DIAGNOSIS

Because of their similarity in size and shape, the intracellular yeast forms of *H capsulatum* var *capsulatum* and *P marneffei* can be confused. However, differences in the division process (budding for *H capsulatum* and septation for *P marneffei*) readily separates these two fungal pathogens.[1] Special stains for fungi are needed to demonstrate these differences.

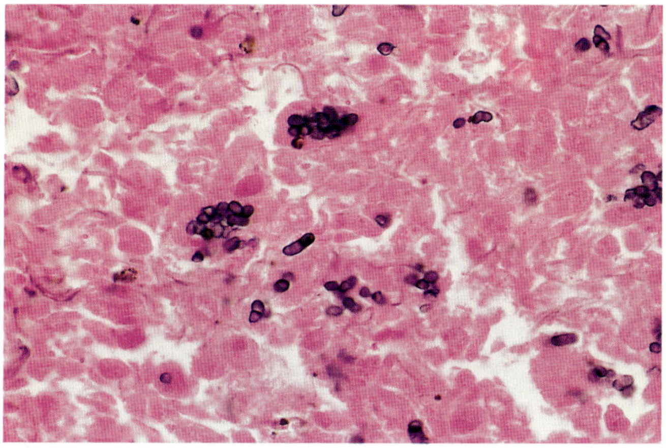

Figure 115–4. Disseminated penicilliosis marneffei in an immunodeficient patient. This splenic infarct contains individual and clustered cells of *P marneffei*. An elongated cell with a single transverse septum and rounded ends is at center (GMS-H&E, ×250).

MOLECULAR DIAGNOSIS

LoBuglio and Taylor[9] developed a specific probe for *P marneffei* by using unique oligonucleotide primers from the nuclear ribosomal DNA internal transcribed spacer region that might be incorporated in a polymerase chain reaction assay for use with clinical specimens. Using their own reagents, Yuen et al[17] developed an indirect immunofluorescent antibody test that needs further evaluation in patients with a variety of mycotic infections. For the tissue recognition of the fungus, a monoclonal antibody that detects a specific galactomannan has been developed. Unfortunately, it cross-reacts with *Aspergillus* sp.[18]

CONFIRMATIONAL TESTING AND DIAGNOSIS

Penicillium marneffei is readily recovered from clinical specimens. In AIDS patients, the fungus is most frequently isolated from bone marrow aspirates, blood, skin lesions, and bronchoalveolar lavage specimens.[1]

Identification of isolates is confirmed by converting them to their corresponding tissue form. Sekhon et al[19] developed an exoantigen test that can be used to identify *P marneffei*. The Pastorex *Aspergillus* latex agglutination test for the detection of circulating *Aspergillus* galactomannan may have some diagnostic value in penicilliosis marneffei because it cross-reacts with *P marneffei*.[20]

TREATMENT

Itraconazole or ketoconazole is recommended for treating mild to moderately severe infections. Maintenance oral therapy may be necessary with these drugs. Amphotericin B is recommended for seriously ill patients.[21]

REFERENCES

1. Drouhet E. Penicilliosis due to *Penicillium marneffei:* A new emerging systemic mycosis in AIDS patients travelling or living in southeast Asia. Review of 44 cases reported in HIV infected patients during the last 5 years compared to 44 cases of non AIDS patients reported over 20 years. *J Mycol Med.* 1993;4:195–224.
2. Supparatpinyo K, Khamwan C, Baosoung V, Nelson KE, Sirisanthana T. Disseminated *Penicillium marneffei* infection in Southeast Asia. *Lancet.* 1994;344:110–113.
3. Ju-chang L, Le-quan P, Shao-xi W. Mycologic investigation on *Rhizomys pruinosus senex* in Guangxi as natural carrier with *Penicillium marneffei. Chinese Med J.* 1989;102: 477–485.
4. Deng Z, Ribas JL, Gibson DW, Connor DH. Infections caused by *Penicillium marneffei* in China and Southeast Asia: review of eighteen published cases and report of four more Chinese cases. *Rev Infect Dis.* 1988;10;640–652.
5. Capponi M, Sureau P, Segretain G. Pénicilliose de *Rhizomys sinensis. Bull Soc Pathol Exot.* 1956;49:418–421.
6. Segretain G. Description d'une nouvelle espèce de *Penicillium: Penicillium marneffei,* n sp. *Bull Soc Mycol Fr.* 1959;75:412–416.
7. Sirisanthana T. Mycotic infections in patients infected with HIV. Paper presented at IX International Congress on AIDS; June 6–11, 1993; Berlin. Abstract PS-07-2.
8. Li PCK, Tsui MS, Ma KF. *Penicillium marneffei:* indicator disease for AIDS in South East Asia. *AIDS.* 1992;6:240–241.
9. LoBuglio KF, Taylor JW. Phylogeny and PCR identification of the human pathogenic fungus *Penicillium marneffei. J Clin Microbiol.* 1995;33:85–89.
10. Pracharktam R, Srivrairatna S, Jayanetra P. Morphological variation in pathogenic strains of *Penicillium marneffei. J Med Assoc Thai.* 1992;75(suppl 1):172–179.
11. Ramiréz C. *Manual and Atlas of the Penicillia.* Amsterdam: Elsevier Biomedical Press; 1982:503–506.
12. Garrison RG, Boyd KS. Dimorphism of *Penicillium marneffei* as observed by electron microscopy. *Can J Microbiol.* 1973;19:1305–1309.
13. McGinnis MR. *Penicillium marneffei,* dimorphic fungus of increasing importance. *Clin Microbiol Newsl.* 1994;4: 29–31.
14. Drouhet E, Ravisse P, Ave P, deBievre C, Dupont B, Pielfroid A. Etude mycologique, ultrastructurale et experimentale sur *Penicillium marneffei* isole d'une penicilliose disseminee chez un sida. *Bull Soc Fr Mycol Med.* 1988; 17:77–82.
15. Chan Y, Chow TC. Ultrastructural observations on *Penicillium marneffei* in natural human infection. *Ultrastruct Pathol.* 1990;14:439–452.
16. Ma K, Tsui M, Tsang DNC. Fine needle aspiration diagnosis of *Penicillium marneffei* infection. *Acta Cytol.* 1991;35: 557–559.
17. Yuen K, Wong SS, Tsang DNC, Chau P. Serodiagnosis of *Penicillium marneffei* infection. *Lancet.* 1994;344:444–445.
18. Estrada JA, Stynen D, van Cutsem J, Piérard-Franchimont C, Piérard GE. Immunohistochemical identification of *Penicillium marneffei* by monoclonal antibody. *Int J Dermatol* 1992;31:410–412.
19. Sekhon AS, Li JSK, Garg AK. *Penicillium marneffei:* serological and exoantigen studies. *Mycopathologia.* 1982;77: 51–57.
20. van Cutsem J, Meulemans L, van Gerven F, Stynen D. Detection of circulating galactomannan by Pastorex *Aspergillus* in experimental invasive aspergillosis. *Mycoses.* 1990;33:61–69.
21. Supparatpinyo K, Nelson KE, Merz WG, et al. Response to antifungal therapy by human immunodeficiency virus-infected patients with disseminated *Penicillium marneffei* infections and *in vitro* susceptibilities of isolates from clinical specimens. *Antimicrob Agents Chemother.* 1993;37: 2407–2411.

CHAPTER 116

Phaeohyphomycosis

Francis W. Chandler and John C. Watts

The physician without physiology and chemistry flounders along in an aimless fashion, never able to gain any accurate conception of disease, practicing a sort of popgun pharmacy, hitting now the malady and again the patient, he himself not knowing which.

Sir William Osler (1849–1919), Aequanimitas, with Other Addresses, "Teaching and Thinking"

DEFINITION

Phaeohyphomycosis comprises a heterogeneous group of fungal infections caused by a wide variety of dematiaceous (phaeoid or naturally pigmented) fungi that develop as black moulds in culture (Figure 116–1) and as dark-walled (brown), moniliform fungal elements in tissue.[1–4] The etiologic agents of this mycosis include more than 80 recognized genera and species of opportunistic, phaeoid fungi that are common saprophytes of soil, wood, and decaying vegetable matter (Table 116–1). Because these fungi are ubiquitous in the environment, proof of their etiologic role in disease requires direct microscopic detection of morphologically and tinctorially typical fungal elements in tissue; isolation of a black mould in culture in the absence of compatible histopathologic findings is insufficient for diagnosis.[5] Synonyms include chromomycosis (in the past), phaeosporotrichosis, phaeomycotic cyst, cerebral chromomycosis, and cerebral dematiomycosis.

GEOGRAPHIC DISTRIBUTION AND EPIDEMIOLOGY

Phaeohyphomycosis occurs worldwide in both humans and animals, and there is no apparent geographic prevalence. Infection is more common in immunodeficient or debilitated hosts but also may occur in healthy subjects. Because the agents of phaeohyphomycosis are saprophytes of soil and plant materials, this mycosis is more common in those who spend much of their time outdoors. There is no age or gender predilection, nor any racial difference in the incidence of infection. Recent experimental studies using animal models suggest that immunosuppression may be the most important predisposing factor in systemic phaeohyphomycosis.[6]

CLINICAL FEATURES AND TREATMENT

The two major clinical forms of phaeohyphomycosis are subcutaneous (phaeomycotic cyst) and systemic (cerebral phaeohyphomycosis). The subcutaneous form is more common, and the most frequently encountered agents include *Exophiala (Phialophora) jeanselmei, Phialophora parasitica, P richardsiae, Wangiella dermatitidis, Bipolaris (Drechslera) spicifera,* and *Alternaria alternata.*[7–10] Patients present with solitary or multiple, firm to fluctuant, painless, subcutaneous abscesses on an exposed part, usually the hand, arm, face, or neck (Figure 116–2). The abscess follows traumatic implantation of fungi by a wooden splinter or other foreign object that serves as a vehicle of infection, or when fungi enter the body through a skin wound.[11,12] Lesions develop at the site of inoculation, enlarge slowly, range from 0.4 to 7.0 cm or more in diameter, and are occasionally mistaken clinically for a synovial cyst, foreign body granuloma, or giant cell tumor of tendon sheath.[13] Lymphangitis and regional lymphadenopathy are unusual, and excision of local-

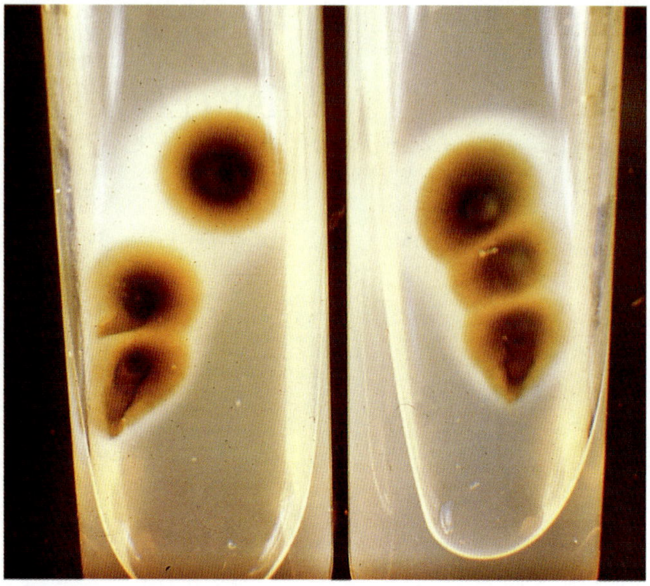

Figure 116–1. Culture of *Exophiala (Phialophora) jeanselmei,* from the content of the cyst in Figure 116–2. Note the black colonies. *(By Daniel H. Connor, MD, 1968.)*

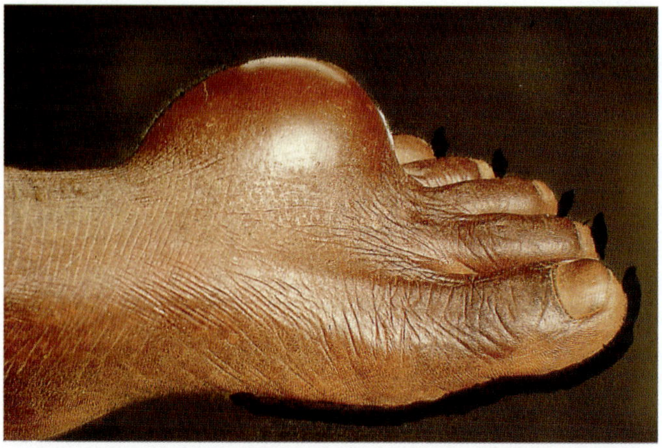

Figure 116–2. Phaeomycotic cyst on the foot of a Zairian man living in Mbwasenge, a small village in the Ubangi Territory. The cyst is solitary, painless, tensely fluctuant, and 7.0 cm across—perhaps a world record for size. The overlying skin is smooth but a sliver was lodged in the dermis over the cyst. Phaeomycotic cysts may be mistaken for synovial cysts, foreign body granulomas, or giant cell tumors of tendon sheath. *(By Daniel H. Connor, MD, 1986.)*

TABLE 116–1. SELECTED ETIOLOGIC AGENTS OF PHAEOHYPHOMYCOSIS IN HUMANS AND LOWER ANIMALS

Alternaria alternata	*E spinifera*
A chartarum	*Exserohilum longirostratum*
A dianthicola	*E mcginnisii*
A infectoria	*E rostratum*
A stemphyloides	*Lasiodiplodia theobromae*
A tenuis	*Lecythophora hoffmannii*
A tenuissima	*Mycocentrospora acerina*
Anthopsis deltoidea	*Mycolettodiscus indicus*
Aureobasidium pullulans	*Nattrassia mangiferae*
Bipolaris australiensis	*Ochroconis constricta*
B hawaiiensis	*Oidiodendron cerealis*
B spicifera	*Onychocola canadensis*
Chaetomium funicolum	*Phialophora parasitica*
C globosum	*P repens*
C perpulchrum	*P richardsiae*
Cladophialophora bantiana	*Phoma cava*
C debriesii	*P cruris-hominis*
Cladosporium cladosporoides	*P hibernica*
Curvularia clavata	*P oculo-hominis*
C geniculata	*Phyllosticta citricarpa*
C lunata	*Pseudomicrodochium suttonii*
C pallescens	*Pyrenochaeta unguis-hominis*
C senegalensis	*Scedosporium prolificans*
Cylindrocarpon tonkinensis	*Scytalidium lignicola*
Exophiala jeanselmei	*Thermomyces lanuginosus*
E moniliae	*Wangiella dermatitidis*

ized lesions is usually curative. Progressive disseminated infection following percutaneous inoculation is extremely rare (Figure 116–3).[14–17]

In the systemic or cerebral form of phaeohyphomycosis, the route of infection is usually the respiratory tract following inhalation of fungal elements growing as a mycelium in the environment.[18–20] The most frequently encountered agent is *Cladophialophora bantiana* (formerly *Xylohypha bantiana* and *Cladosporium bantianum*), a pigmented fungus that is particularly neurotropic.[21–25] Following hematogenous dissemination from a primary pulmonary focus, most infections are confined to the brain and meninges (Figure 116–4), with only occasional involvement of other organs. Moreover, the primary pulmonary focus is often inapparent. Other authenticated agents of cerebral phaeohyphomycosis in humans include *Bipolaris hawaiiensis, B spicifera, Curvularia pallescens, Dactylaria constricta* var *gallopava,* and *W dermatitidis.*[2–4,10,19,26,27] Symptoms may include headache, nausea, vomiting, fever, confusion, hemiparesis, and nuchal pain and rigidity. Cerebral lesions, either solitary or multiple and up to 5 cm in diameter, are either encapsulated abscesses similar to those encountered in phaeomycotic cyst (Figure 116–4), or more dispersed inflammatory infiltrates with necrosis. Surgical extirpation of encapsulated lesions and aggressive antifungal therapy with itraconazole or amphotericin B are the treatments of choice for systemic infections.[3,4,10,28]

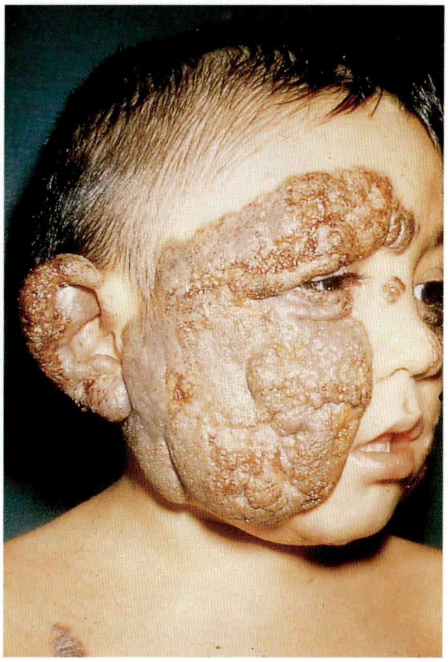

Figure 116–3. Progressive disseminated phaeohyphomycosis in a child following percutaneous inoculation of the right cheek 2 years previously. This infection was caused by *E spinifera*.

In addition to subcutaneous and cerebral infections, unusual clinical presentations of phaeohyphomycosis include severe disseminated infection, osteomyelitis, sinusitis, intrasinus and pulmonary fungus balls, granulomatous pulmonary disease, keratitis, endocarditis, peritonitis associated with continuous ambulatory peritoneal dialysis, saprophytic wound colonization, and allergic bronchopulmonary disease.[4,10,14–17,29–31]

PATHOLOGY

The host reaction in phaeohyphomycosis is similar regardless of the etiologic agent and the anatomic site of involvement.[5] It is characterized by cystic or, rarely, dispersed granulomas that are usually solitary and encapsulated by dense collagenous connective tissue, with central geographic or stellate foci of suppurative necrosis (Figures 116–5 and 116–6). The walls of the granulomas contain compact aggregates of epithelioid histiocytes and numerous giant cells of both the Langhans' and foreign body types (Figure 116–7). In subcutaneous phaeohyphomycosis (phaeomycotic cyst), the lesions are located in the deep dermis and subcutaneous tissue, and the overlying epidermis is usually unaffected and of normal thickness (Figures 116–8 and 116–9).[5,8,9] Wooden splinters or thorns, presumed to be the vehicles of infection, can sometimes be demonstrated within or near the cyst (Figures 116–10).[11,12]

A histopathologic diagnosis of phaeohyphomycosis is made by detecting pigmented (brown), moniliform fungal elements within giant cells in the cyst walls and extracellularly within the central necrotic debris (Figure 116–11). The fungi may vary in their degree of pigmentation, and appear as infrequently branched hyphae, 2 to 6 μm wide, that are often closely septate and constricted at their prominent septations. The hyphae occur singly or in small, loose aggregates, and

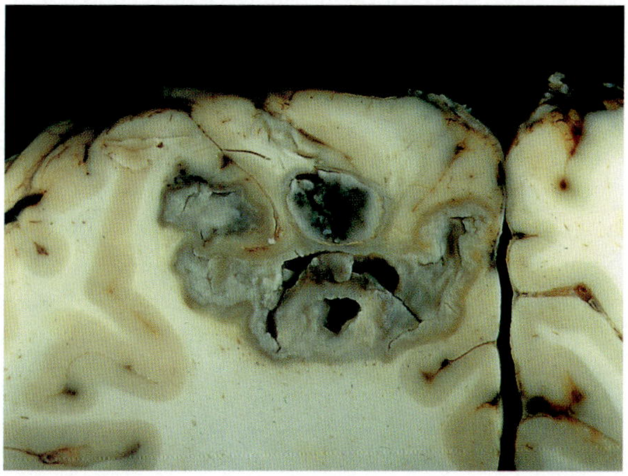

Figure 116–4. Cerebral phaeohyphomycosis caused by *Cladophialophora* sp. A coronal section of the brain reveals multiple circumscribed abscesses similar to those encountered in subcutaneous phaeohyphomycosis (phaeomycotic cyst). The patient was a 39-year-old diabetic man from Durban, South Africa. *(By Daniel H. Connor, MD, 1985.)*

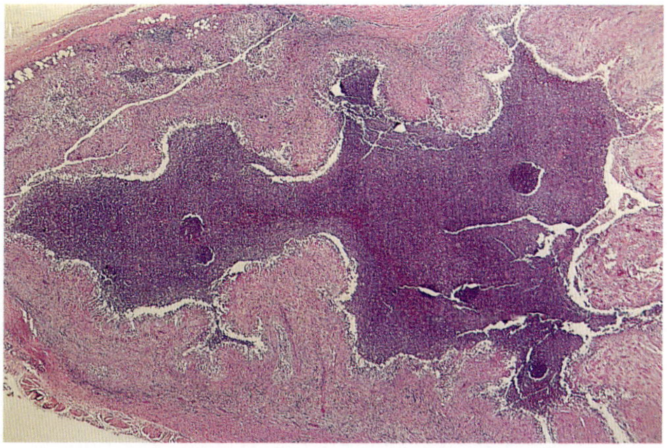

Figure 116–5. Phaeomycotic cyst with a prominent stellate outline. The central area of suppuration is formed by coalescence of multiple smaller abscesses [hematoxylin-eosin (H&E), ×4.5].

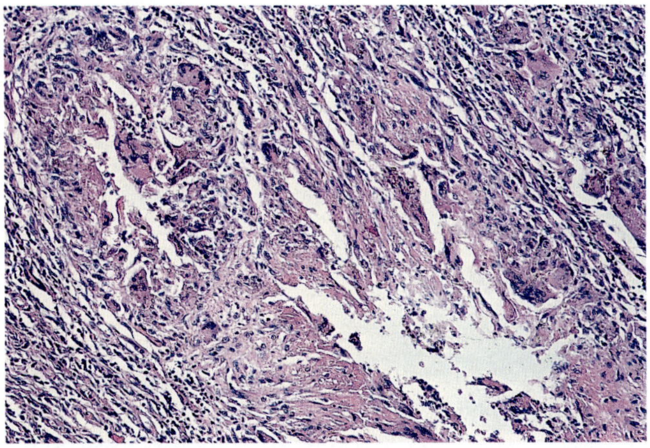

Figure 116–6. Phaeomycotic cyst caused by *E jeanselmei.* The internal cyst wall consists of compact aggregates of epithelioid histiocytes and giant cells of both the Langhans' and foreign body types. Phaeoid (naturally pigmented) fungi are not visible at this magnification (H&E, ×40).

sometimes contain bizarre, thick-walled, terminal, or intercalated vesicular swellings, 25 μm or more in diameter, that resemble chlamydoconidia (Figure 116–12). Yeastlike cells that produce buds singly or in chains, and spherical to oval cells that reproduce by septation in only one plane, also may be present (Figure 116–13).

Occasionally, the natural brown pigmentation of the agents of phaeohyphomycosis may not be readily apparent (Figure 116–14). A detailed search under high magnification with the oil objective will almost always reveal at least some fungal elements with lightly pigmented walls in either H&E stained or unstained

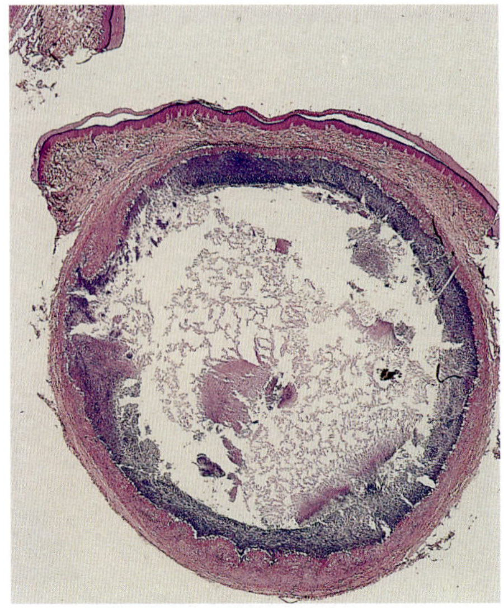

Figure 116–8. More advanced phaeomycotic cyst on the finger of a 60-year-old woman with lymphoma. She punctured her finger while tending roses. The cyst is now spherical, but stellate indentations are preserved at the perimeter of the abscess. A fragment of sliver is in the exudate on the right near the equator. The central area of suppuration has been formed by coalescence of smaller abscesses (H&E, ×2.5).

(cleared and mounted) tissue sections, or in potassium hydroxide mounts of lesional exudates. When pigmentation is not detectable or is equivocal, stains for melanin can sometimes accentuate and confirm the presence of melanoid pigments in the fungal cell walls (Figure 116–15).[5,32] The agents of phaeohyphomycosis are well demonstrated with the special stains for fungi such as GMS and periodic acid–Schiff (PAS) reaction;

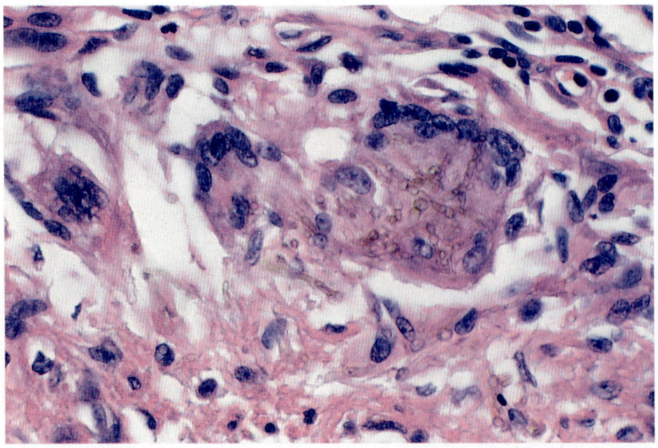

Figure 116–7. Phaeomycotic cyst caused by *E jeanselmei.* Giant cells in the cyst wall contain numerous pigmented (brown) yeastlike cells that occur singly and in chains (H&E, ×160).

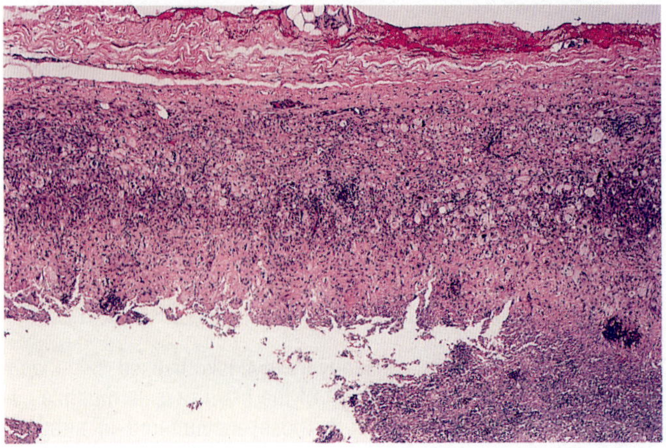

Figure 116–9. Phaeomycotic cyst. A cystic granuloma is located in the deep dermis and subcutaneous tissue. The overlying epidermis is unaffected and of normal thickness (H&E, ×16).

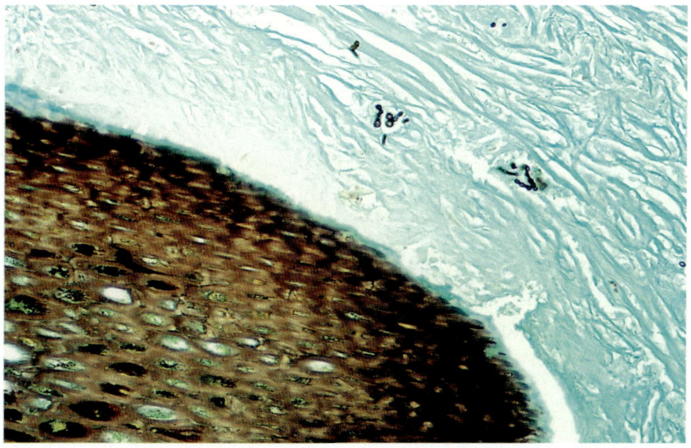

Figure 116–10. Phaeomycotic cyst. A retained wooden splinter *(lower left),* presumed to be the vehicle of percutaneous implantation, is in the wall of the cyst. Note scattered, polymorphous fungal elements near the splinter [Gomori's methenamine silver (GMS), ×25].

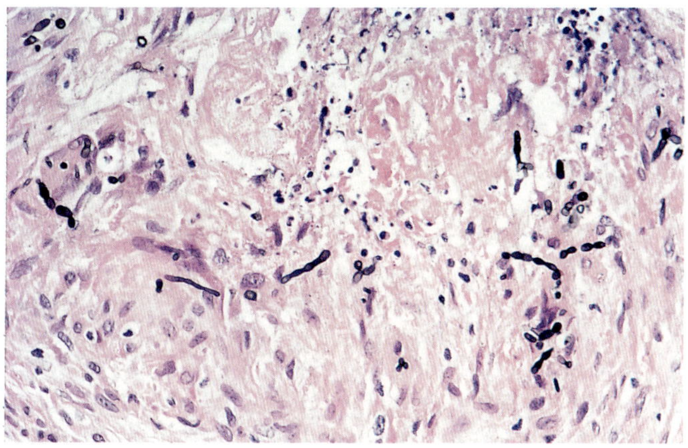

Figure 116–11. Phaeomycotic cyst caused by *P richardsiae*. Scattered moniliform fungal elements are in giant cells in the cyst wall and extracellularly in the central necrotic debris *(top center)* (GMS-H&E, ×50).

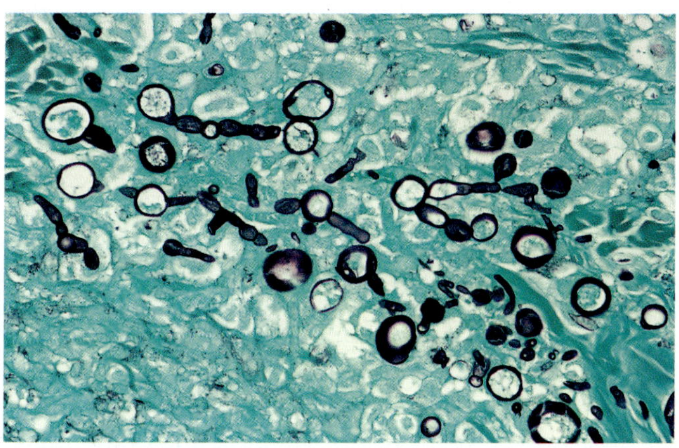

Figure 116–12. Subcutaneous phaeohyphomycosis. Polymorphous hyphae within a subcutaneous granuloma contain bizarre, thick-walled, terminal and intercalated vesicular swellings, up to 25 μm in diameter, that resemble chlamydoconidia (GMS, ×160).

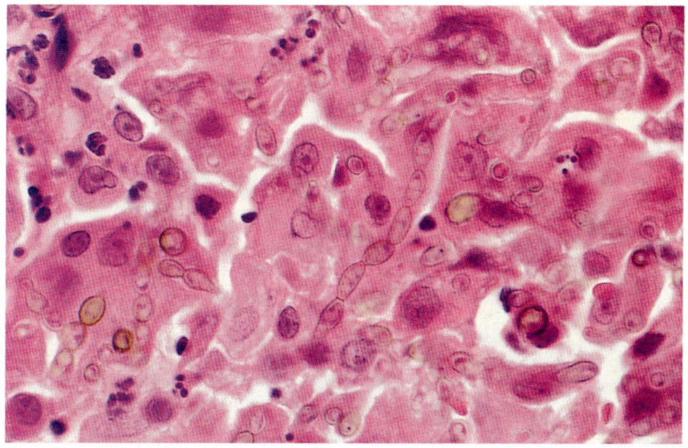

Figure 116–13. Subcutaneous phaeohyphomycosis caused by *E spinifera*. Phaeoid (naturally pigmented) yeastlike cells and chains of budding cells are readily apparent in a dispersed granulomatous infiltrate (H&E, ×250).

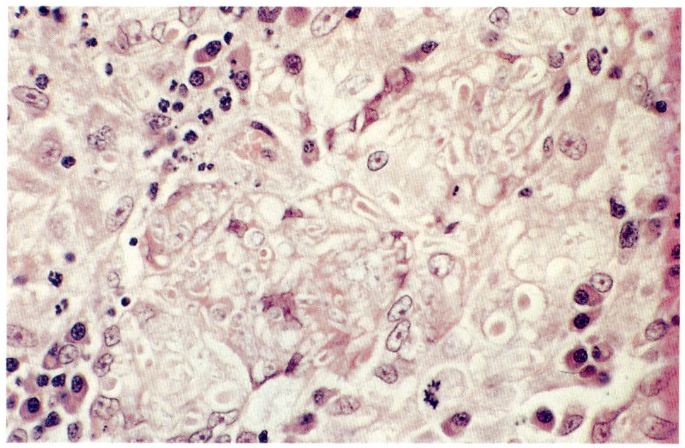

Figure 116–14. Subcutaneous phaeohyphomycosis caused by a lightly pigmented strain of *A alternata*. Even at high magnification, the usual brown pigmentation of fungal cells is difficult to demonstrate within this subcutaneous granuloma (H&E, ×160).

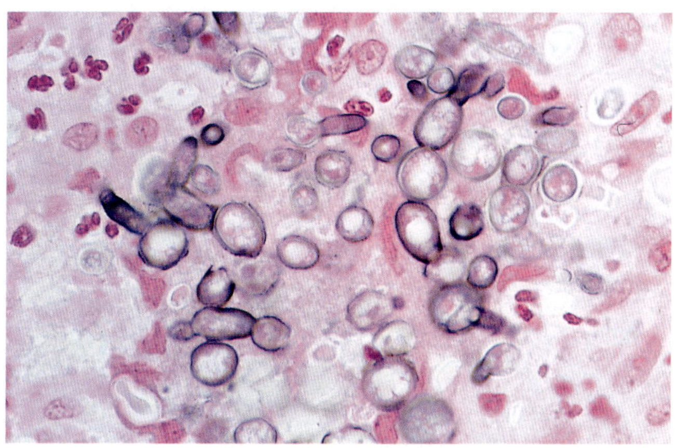

Figure 116–15. Subcutaneous phaeohyphomycosis caused by *A alternata*. When the natural brown pigmentation of phaeoid fungi is not detected or equivocal in H&E stained sections, a modified stain for melanin can sometimes accentuate and confirm the presence of melanoid pigments in fungal cell walls, as seen here (modified Fontana–Masson, ×250).

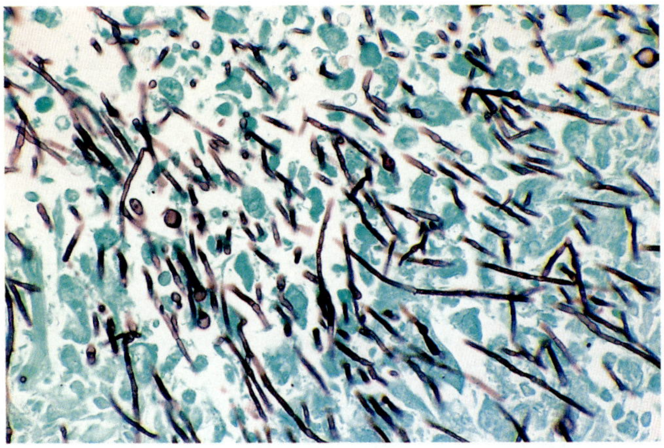

Figure 116–16. *Cladophialophora bantiana* within cerebral granuloma of a patient with systemic phaeohyphomycosis. Elongated, septate hyphae and budding yeastlike cells are intensely silvered and readily demonstrated. The distribution, morphology, and actual number of phaeoid fungi are much more evident when special histologic stains are used (GMS, ×160).

moreover, the distribution, detailed morphology, and actual number of fungal elements are much more evident when these stains are used (Figures 116–16 and 116–17). However, in most cases, special stains are unnecessary because the dark pigmentation of the cell walls highlights the fungal elements, making them easily detectable in H&E stained sections or cytologic preparations. Special stains also mask the natural brown color of the fungi, recognition of which is important for diagnosis.

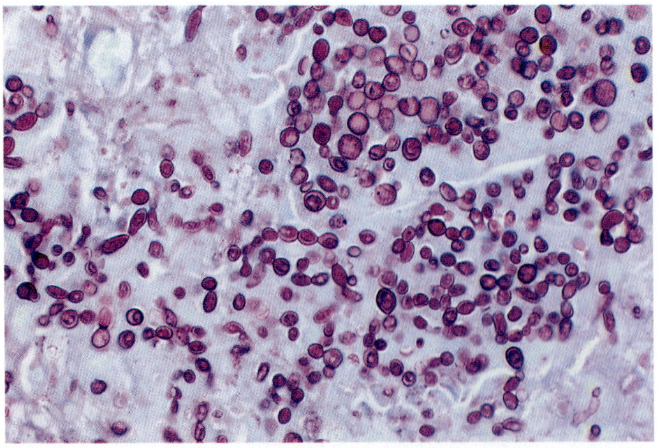

Figure 116–17. Subcutaneous phaeohyphomycosis. A dispersed granulomatous infiltrate contains numerous yeastlike cells, chains of budding cells, and short hyphae of *E spinifera*. Special stains for fungi mask the natural brown pigmentation of fungal elements. Compare with Figure 116–13 (PAS, ×160).

DIFFERENTIAL DIAGNOSIS

In tissue sections, phaeohyphomycosis can be confused with black grain eumycotic mycetomas caused by pigmented fungi (see Chapter 113).[5] However, the causative agents of mycetoma form distinct grains or granules up to 3 mm in diameter that are composed of organized, interwoven mycelial aggregates. The agents of phaeohyphomycosis never form true granules but rather appear as scattered, individual, polymorphous fungal elements or small, unorganized aggregates of hyphae. Furthermore, fungal elements in phaeohyphomycosis are often intracellular, whereas the granules in mycetomas are nearly always extracellular.

The major problem in the histopathologic differential diagnosis of phaeohyphomycosis is chromoblastomycosis (see Chapter 104), a chronic cutaneous and subcutaneous mycosis of humans caused by any one of several dematiaceous fungi—*Fonsecaea pedrosoi, Phialophora verrucosa, Cladophialophora carrionii, F compacta,* and *Rhinocladiella aquaspersa,* listed in descending order of frequency.[33–37] All of these pigmented fungi exist as saprophytes in soil and organic matter. Although the disease is cosmopolitan, most infections are encountered in the tropical regions of South America and Africa. Infection results from the accidental percutaneous inoculation of exposed body parts with matter containing the etiologic agent, and a locally spreading verrucous plaque or nodule develops at the site of implantation. Satellite lesions often develop because of regional lymphatic spread or autoinoculation, but widespread dissemination is rare. The agents of chromoblastomycosis are easily distinguished from one another in culture, but their tissue forms are morphologically and tinctorially similar.[5,33,34] In tissue sections, they appear as brown, spherical to polyhedral, thick-walled muriform cells or "sclerotic bodies" 5 to 12 μm in diameter. The muriform cells reproduce by septation in one or two planes, and the latter process produces a tetrad of daughter cells. In addition to septate cells, nonseptate cells are also present; and branched, septate, dematiaceous hyphae are occasionally observed in the hyperkeratotic surface layer of cutaneous lesions.[5,38] Fungal cells occur singly or in compact clusters within the dermis, where they elicit a mixed suppurative and granulomatous inflammatory reaction. In chromoblastomycosis, unlike subcutaneous phaeohyphomycosis, hyperkeratosis and florid pseudoepitheliomatous hyperplasia of the overlying epidermis are common, and transepidermal elimination of fungal elements is frequent.[38] Special stains for fungi are not usually needed for diagnosis unless the fungal cells are sparse.

A histopathologic diagnosis of chromoblastomycosis can be based on the presence of dark brown muriform cells that characteristically have thick walls, divide by septation in two planes, and do not form chains of cells. Because the septate muriform cells are morphologically distinctive, they should not be mistaken for the pigmented, moniliform fungal elements of phaeohyphomycosis.

CONFIRMATIONAL TESTING AND DIAGNOSIS

Because all of the various agents of phaeohyphomycosis appear similar to each other in tissue sections, they cannot be differentiated solely on the basis of morphology. Nevertheless, a disease diagnosis can be based on the natural brown color of morphologically typical, polymorphous fungal elements in clinical specimens. Immunoreagents for the identification of these fungi in tissue sections are not presently available. Therefore, culture is needed for their specific identification.

REFERENCES

1. Ajello L. Phaeohyphomycosis: definition and etiology. In: *Mycoses.* Sci Pub 304. Washington, DC: Pan American Health Organization; 1975:126–133.
2. McGinnis MR. Human pathogenic species of *Exophiala, Phialophora,* and *Wangiella.* In: *The Black and White Yeasts.* Sci Pub 356. Washington, DC: Pan American Health Organization; 1978:37–59.
3. McGinnis MR. Chromoblastomycosis and phaeohyphomycosis: new concepts, diagnosis, and mycology. *J Am Acad Dermatol.* 1983;8:1–16.
4. Fader RC, McGinnis MR. Infections caused by dematiaceous fungi: chromoblastomycosis and phaeohyphomycosis. *Infect Dis Clin North Am.* 1988;2:925–938.
5. Chandler FW, Watts JC. *Pathologic Diagnosis of Fungal Infections.* Chicago: ASCP Press; 1987:233–263.
6. Dixon DM, Merz WG, Elliot HL, Macleay S. Experimental central nervous system phaeohyphomycosis following intranasal inoculation of *Xylohypha bantiana* in cortisone-treated mice. *Mycopathologia.* 1987;100:145–153.
7. Estes SA, Merz WG, Maxwell LG. Primary cutaneous phaeohyphomycosis caused by *Drechslera spicifera. Arch Dermatol.* 1977;113:813–815.
8. Ziefer A, Connor DH. Phaeomycotic cyst: a clinicopathologic study of twenty-five patients. *Am J Trop Med Hyg.* 1980;29:901–911.
9. Bambirra EA, Miranda D, Nogueira AMF, Barbosa CSP. Phaeohyphomycotic cyst: a clinicopathologic study of the first four cases described from Brazil. *Am J Trop Med Hyg.* 1983;32:794–798.
10. Adam RD, Paquin ML, Petersen EA, et al. Phaeohyphomycosis caused by the fungal genera *Bipolaris* and *Exserohilum:* a report of 9 cases and review of the literature. *Medicine (Baltimore).* 1986;65:203–217.
11. Iwatsu T, Miyaji M. Phaeomycotic cyst: a case with a lesion containing a wooden splinter. *Arch Dermatol.* 1984;120:1209–1211.
12. Tschen JA, Knox JM, McGavran MH, Duncan WC. Chromomycosis: the association of fungal elements and wood splinters. *Arch Dermatol.* 1984;120:107–108.
13. Moskowitz LB, Clearly TJ, McGinnis MR, Thomson CB. *Phialophora richardsiae* in a lesion appearing as a giant cell tumor of the tendon sheath. *Arch Pathol Lab Med.* 1983;107:374–376.
14. Rohwedder JJ, Simmons JL, Colfer H, Gatmaitan B. Disseminated *Curvularia lunata* infection in a football player. *Arch Intern Med.* 1979;139:940–941.
15. Padhye AA, Ajello L, Chandler FW, et al. Phaeohyphomycosis in El Salvador caused by *Exophiala spinifera. Am J Trop Med Hyg.* 1983;32:799–803.
16. de la Monte SM, Hutchins GM. Disseminated *Curvularia* infection. *Arch Pathol Lab Med.* 1985;109:872–874.
17. Ferraro FA, Morgan MA. A case of disseminated *Phialophora parasitica* infection. *Arch Pathol Lab Med.* 1989; 113:1379–1381.
18. Chandramukhi A, Ramadevi MG, Shankar SK. Cerebral cladosporiosis: a neuropathological and microbiological study. *Clin Neurol Neurosurg.* 1983;85:245–253.
19. Masini T, Riviera L, Cappricci E, et al. Cerebral pheohyphomycosis. *Clin Neuropathol.* 1985;4:246–249.
20. Borges MC Jr, Warren S, White W, Pellettiere EV. Pulmonary phaeohyphomycosis due to *Xylohypha bantiana. Arch Pathol Lab Med.* 1991;115:627–629.
21. Riley O Jr, Mann SH. Brain abscess caused by *Cladosporium trichoides:* review of 3 cases and report of a fourth case. *Am J Clin Pathol.* 1960;33:525–531.
22. Crichlow DK, Enrile FT, Memon MY. Cerebellar abscess due to *Cladosporium trichoides (bantianum):* case report. *Am J Clin Pathol.* 1973;60:416–421.
23. Seaworth BJ, Kwon-Chung KJ, Hamilton JD, Perfect JR. Brain abscess caused by a variety of *Cladosporium trichoides. Am J Clin Pathol.* 1983;79:747–752.
24. McGinnis MR, Borelli D, Padhye AA, Ajello L. Reclassification of *Cladosporium bantianum* in the genus *Xylohypha. J Clin Microbiol.* 1985;23:1148–1151.
25. Dixon DM, Walsh TJ, Merz WG, McGinnis MR. Infections due to *Xylohypha bantiana (Cladosporium trichoides). Rev Infect Dis.* 1989;11:515–525.
26. Fuste FJ, Ajello L, Threlkeld R, Henry JE Jr. *Drechslera hawaiiensis:* causative agent of a fatal fungal meningoencephalitis. *Sabouraudia.* 1973;11:59–63.
27. Morton SJ, Midthun K, Merz WG. Granulomatous encephalitis caused by *Bipolaris hawaiiensis. Arch Pathol Lab Med.* 1986;110:1183–1185.
28. Hay RJ, Dupont B, Graybill JR, eds. First international symposium on itraconazole. *Rev Infect Dis.* 1987;9(suppl): S1–S152.
29. Lampert RP, Hutto JH, Donnelly WH, Shulman ST. Pulmonary and cerebral mycetoma caused by *Curvularia pallescens. J Pediatr.* 1977;91:603–605.
30. Lobritz RW, Roberts TH, Marraro RV, et al. Granulomatous pulmonary disease secondary to *Alternaria. JAMA.* 1979; 241:596–597.
31. McAleer R, Kroenert DB, Elder JL, Froudist JH. Allergic

bronchopulmonary disease caused by *Curvularia lunata* and *Drechslera hawaiiensis*. *Thorax*. 1981;36:338–344.
32. Wood C, Russel-Bell B. Characterization of pigmented fungi by melanin staining. *Am J Dermatopathol.* 1983; 5:77–81.
33. Carrion AL. Chromoblastomycosis and related infections: new concepts, differential diagnosis, and nomenclatorial implications. *Int J Dermatol.* 1975;14:27–32.
34. Londero AT, Ramos CD. Chromomycosis: A clinical and mycologic study of thirty-five cases observed in the hinterland of Rio Grande do Sul, Brazil. *Am J Trop Med Hyg.* 1976;25:132–135.
35. Montero-Gei F. Chromoblastomycosis: host-parasite interactions. In: *Proceedings of the Fifth International Conference on the Mycoses: Superficial, Cutaneous, and Subcutaneous Infections.* Sci Pub 396. Washington, DC: Pan American Health Organization; 1980:248–251.
36. Walter P, Garin Y, Richard-Lenoble D. Chromoblastomycosis: a morphological investigation of the host–parasite interaction. *Virchows Arch (Pathol Anat).* 1982;397:203–214.
37. Banks IS, Palmieri JR, Lanoie L, et al. Chromomycosis in Zaire. *Int J Dermatol.* 1985;24:302–307.
38. Batres E, Wolf JE, Rudolph AH, et al. Transepithelial elimination of cutaneous chromomycosis. *Arch Dermatol.* 1978;114:1231–1232.

CHAPTER 117

Protothecosis

Evette Ramsay, Francis W. Chandler, and Daniel H. Connor

Hippocrates in his aphorisme, as Galen writeth sure,
Saith, foure things are needfull to every kinde of cure,
The first, saith he, to God belongeth the chiefest part,
The second to the Surgeon, who doth apply the art.
The third unto the medicine, that is dame nature's friend,
The fourth unto the patient, with whom I heere will end.
How then may a Surgeon appoint a time, a day or houre,
When three parts of the cure are quite without his power.

William Clowes (1544–1604)

DEFINITION

Protothecosis is a relatively rare infection of man and animals by *Prototheca* sp. The protothecae are unicellular, achlorophyllous organisms belonging to the same phylogenic family as green algae of the genus *Chlorella*. *Prototheca* sp reproduce asexually and produce hyaline cells termed sporangia, which, when mature, divide by endosporulation to form 2 to 20 or more sporangiospores. Two species, *P wickerhamii* and *P zopfii,* cause infection. Human protothecosis has been reported clinically in three forms: 1) cutaneous, 2) olecranon bursitis, and 3) disseminated. Because the clinical features of protothecosis are not pathognomonic, some infections may not be recognized nor reported.

GEOGRAPHIC DISTRIBUTION

Prototheca sp are ubiquitous and occur in the environment as saprophytes. The source of infection is not usually apparent, but *Prototheca* sp have been isolated from the mucous flux of trees, grass, frass, soil, potato skins, fresh and marine waters, sludges of waste stabilization ponds, collections of stagnant water, and dogs, cats, cattle, deer, sheep, wild animals, and cow's milk.[1] The first reported human infection was in a rice farmer from Sierra Leone.[2] Human protothecosis has since been reported worldwide—on all continents except Antarctica. In the United States, the majority of patients have been in the Southeast, notably North Carolina and Virginia.

HISTORY

The protothecae were originally isolated and described by Kruger in 1894. At that time, these organisms were believed to be fungi. Chadot recognized them as algae in 1913. In 1930, Ashford et al[3] isolated *Prototheca ciferrii* (now synonymous with *P zopfii*) from the stools of two Puerto Ricans with tropical sprue. This association is believed to be incidental because other patients with sprue have not had protothecae in their stools.

LIFE CYCLE

Prototheca sp reproduce asexually by internal septation and irregular cleavage. The division of the organism forms a sporangium that may contain as few as 2 and as many as 20 or more daughter cells or sporangiospores in a "morula" configuration. As the division of the parent cell continues, multiple sporangiospores form and the increasing pressure of the enlarging spores ruptures the theca of the parent cell. Once the theca ruptures, the life cycle continues as the newly released spores begin to enlarge, divide, and develop into mature endosporulating forms.[4]

MORPHOLOGIC FEATURES OF PROTOTHECAE

Protothecae are unicellular, spheroidal or ovoid organisms that measure 3 to 30 μm in diameter. They have hyaline sporangia and reproduce asexually. Seven species have been identified, but to date only two, *P zopfii* and *P wickerhamii,* have infected humans.[5] Although *P zopfii* was cultured from the first infected human, most subsequent infections have been caused by *P wickerhamii.* The protothecae can be distinguished from fungi and bacteria by size, structure, and mode of reproduction. Unlike fungi, *Prototheca* sp lack glucosamine in their cell walls and they also lack the muramic acid found in bacteria. Protothecae are believed to be mutant strains of *Chlorella* species, the chlorophyllic algae. Perhaps the most obvious distinction between protothecae and chlorellae is the lack of chloroplasts in the former.[6] Protothecae do, however, have cytoplasmic granules or plastids that are believed to be nonfunctioning chloroplasts. Protothecae also have a two-layered cell wall lined with nodules on the inner surface. The two species of *Prototheca* pathogenic for humans differ in size, but otherwise resemble each other by light microscopy. The smaller form, *P wickerhamii,* measures 3 to 15 μm in diameter, and the larger form, *P zopfii,* measures 7 to 30 μm in diameter. The walls of both the sporangia and sporangiospores are readily stained with periodic acid–Schiff (PAS), Gomori's methenamine-silver (GMS), and Gridley procedures, and they are gram-positive; heat fixing destroys their features.

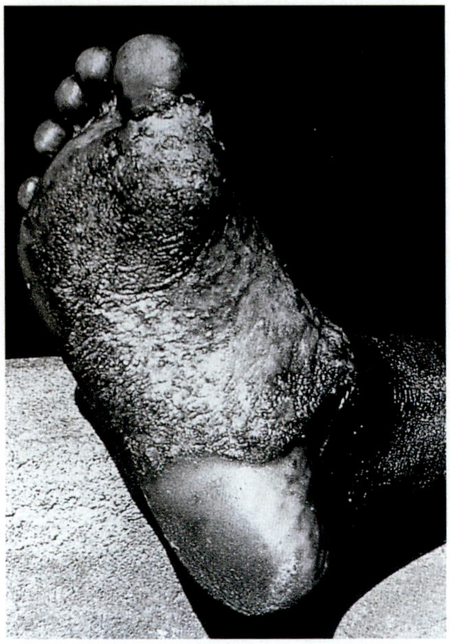

Figure 117–1. Cutaneous protothecosis caused by *P zopfii*—the first reported infection in a human. The patient was a rice farmer in Sierra Leone. There are spreading confluent keratotic papules on the skin of the right foot. *(Photograph by Dr. P. O. Wakelin.)*

CLINICAL FEATURES

Cutaneous infections account for more than half of all protothecal infections. Most patients with cutaneous protothecosis are immunodeficient. Underlying causes of immunodeficiency include immunosuppressive therapy, malnutrition, alcoholism, hepatitis, cancer, renal failure, systemic lupus erythematosus, and acquired immunodeficiency syndrome (AIDS).[7–9] Clinically, patients present with a papulonodular or eczematoid eruption and, less frequently, with herpetiform dermatitis, cellulitis, verrucous nodules, or wound infection usually limited to a limb or the face (Figures 117–1 through 117–4).[10–12] Lesions arise in areas exposed to protothecae usually by traumatic implantation, and they are indolent, developing slowly in a centrifugal manner. The regional lymph nodes are rarely involved.

The second most common clinical form of protothecosis is olecranon bursitis, which presents as a

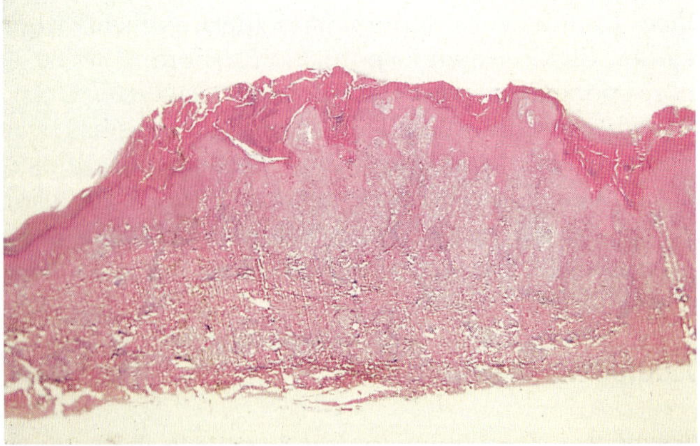

Figure 117–2. Cutaneous protothecosis. Specimen of skin from the index case shown in Figure 117–1 reveals enormous numbers of *Prototheca* organisms in the epidermis and dermis, acanthosis and hyperkeratosis, and a granulomatous reaction in the dermis [hematoxylin-eosin (H&E), ×5].

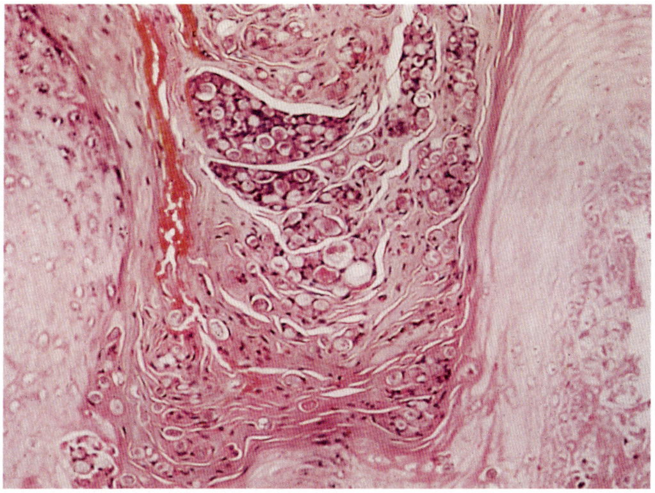

Figure 117–3. Biopsy specimen from the index human infection shown in Figures 117–1 and 117–2. The hyperkeratotic layer of epidermis contains numerous weakly stained and optically clear sporangia of *P zopfii.* Other fields revealed organisms in transepidermal elimination channels (H&E, ×100).

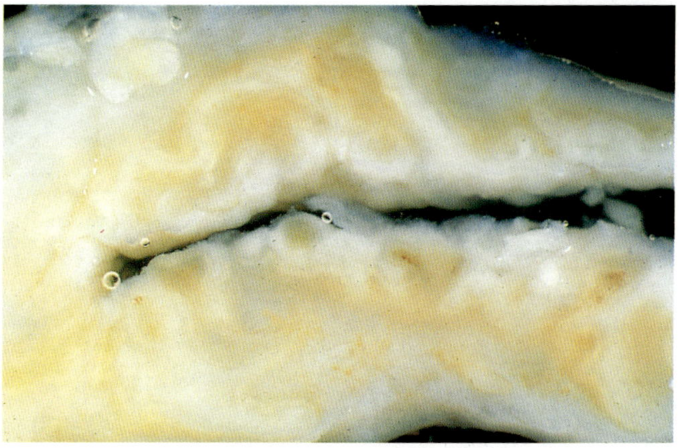

Figure 117–5. Olecranon bursitis caused by *P wickerhamii.* A 48-year-old man had a painful, swollen elbow for 2 months. Two milliliters of bloody fluid was aspirated from the olecranon bursa, with relief for several weeks, but the pain and swelling returned. The olecranon bursa was swollen and tender but attempts to further aspirate failed, after which the bursa was excised. The wall of the bursal sac is thickened and the cavity is a slitlike space. The tortuous white areas are caseation necrosis. The site healed completely after excision.

mild, slightly tender erythematous induration of the bursa (Figures 117–5 through 117–7) with production of a variable amount of serosanguineous fluid.[13] Patients are not immunodeficient but usually have had penetrating or nonpenetrating trauma to the affected elbow. Although the incubation period is unknown, symptoms typically occur several weeks after the trauma.[14]

Disseminated protothecosis is rare in humans. Some reports have described patients with competent immunity who presented with abdominal complaints. Laboratory evaluation often revealed abnormal liver function tests, elevated erythrocyte sedimentation rates, elevated immunoglobulin levels, and eosinophilia. One patient had multiple intraperitoneal nodules that resembled metastatic cancer.[15] Another patient had lesions on the forehead and nose.[16]

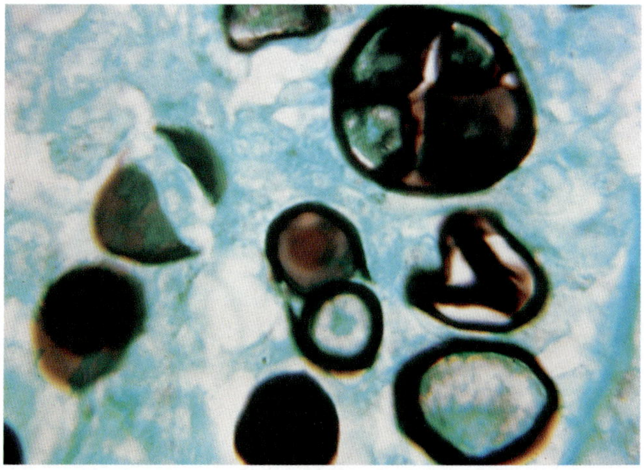

Figure 117–4. Sporangia of *P zopfii* in a dermal granuloma of the index case. One sporangium *(top right)* contains at least four sporangiospores. The wall of the sporangia and the sporangiospores are intensely silvered with the GMS stain (×400). *(By Daniel H. Connor, MD.)*

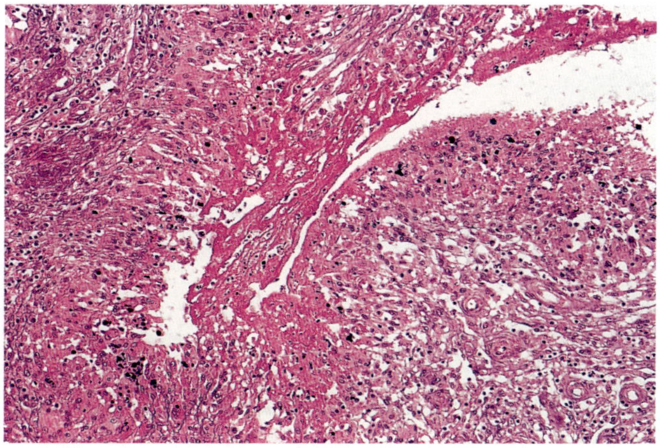

Figure 117–6. Protothecosis of the olecranon bursa. Numerous GMS-positive algal cells of *P wickerhamii* are in the wall of this necrotizing granuloma (GMS-H&E, ×10).

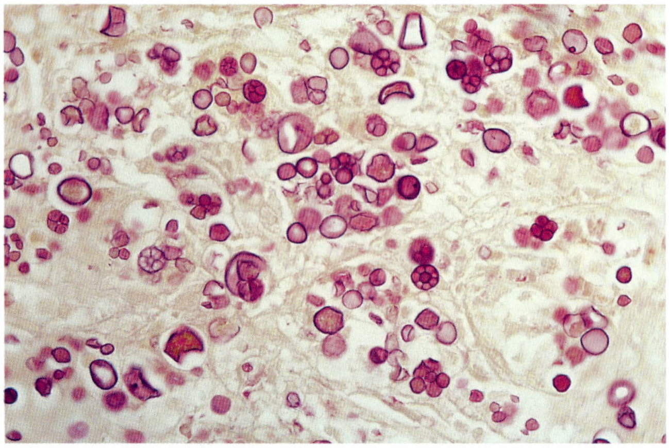

Figure 117–7. *Prototheca wickerhamii.* A necrotizing granuloma of the olecranon bursa contains single and endosporulating algal cells that are readily demonstrated with the Gridley fungus stain. A classic "morula" form is at right center (×160).

MICROBIOLOGY

Prototheca sp are easily identified by culture. Protothecae grow readily on Sabouraud's dextrose agar if incubated at 30 to 37°C, but grow poorly at room temperature. Creamy, white, yeastlike colonies form on Sabouraud's dextrose agar and these colonies are easily mistaken for yeasts (Figure 117–8). Blood agar also may be used to culture protothecae, as well as brain heart infusion agar containing 5% sheep red blood cells, eosin-methylene blue agar, MacConkey agar, and cornmeal polysorbate (Tween) 80 agar. Colonies usually are visible on the third day. A wet preparation of the culture can be stained with lactophenol cotton blue, which reveals the characteristic sporangiospores within sporangia. Growth of protothecae is inhibited by cycloheximide (50 mg/L), tetracycline hydrochloride (200 mg/L), amphotericin B (3.125 mg/L), and ketoconazole (0.02 mg/L), but not inhibited by chloramphenicol (50 mg/L), gentamycin sulfate (50 mg/L), colistin sulfate (10 mg/L), or nalidixic acid (15 mg/L).[17] Specific identification is done by sugar assimilation, comparing the pattern of assimilation of glucose, galactose, fructose, mannose, trehalose, and sucrose to the known patterns of *Prototheca* sp.

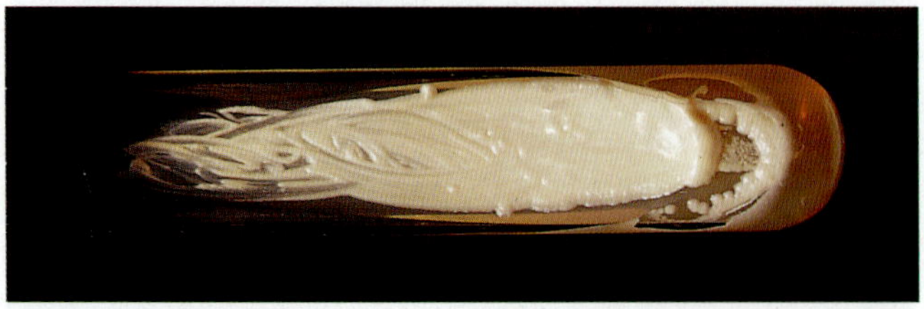

Figure 117–8. Culture of *P zopfii* on Sabouraud's dextrose agar. The *Prototheca* sp lack chloroplasts and produce cream-colored, yeastlike colonies on synthetic media. The *Chlorella* sp contain chlorophyll in their chloroplasts and produce bright green colonies.

PATHOLOGY

A histopathologic diagnosis of protothecosis is confirmed by identifying morphologically typical sporangiospores that are wedge shaped and radially arranged within a sporangium (Figure 117–9).[18] Once seen, with their characteristic internal septation and "morula" configuration, the algal cells are not forgotten. Protothecae are gram-positive, but Gram staining obscures their characteristic internal divisions. In tissue sections stained with H&E, the algal cells are either unstained or hematoxylinophilic (Figure 117–10). The protothecae are best visualized by the stains usually used to demonstrate fungi in tissue sections. These are GMS (Figure 117–4), PAS reaction, and Gridley fungus procedures (Figure 117–7). In addition to the size of individual sporangia, identification of the species of prototheca is suggested by the symmetric morula forms for *P wickerhamii* (Figures 117–7 and 117–9), and by the more random internal divisions for *P zopfii* (Figure 117–4). Typical, symmetric morula forms are rare in infections caused by *P zopfii.* Specific identification of the *Prototheca* sp can be confirmed by treating deparaffinized sections with fluorescein-conjugated antibodies (Figure 117–11).[5] The walls and contours of *Prototheca* sp have a plastic or flowing appearance by scanning electron

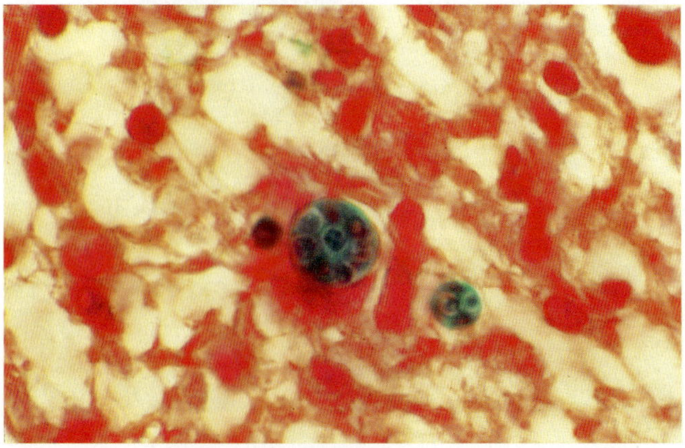

Figure 117–9. Endosporulating sporangia of *P wickerhamii.* The sporangium ("morula" form) at center contains 9 sporangiospores in a single plane of section. Note molding of the adjacent sporangiospores (Movat, ×640).

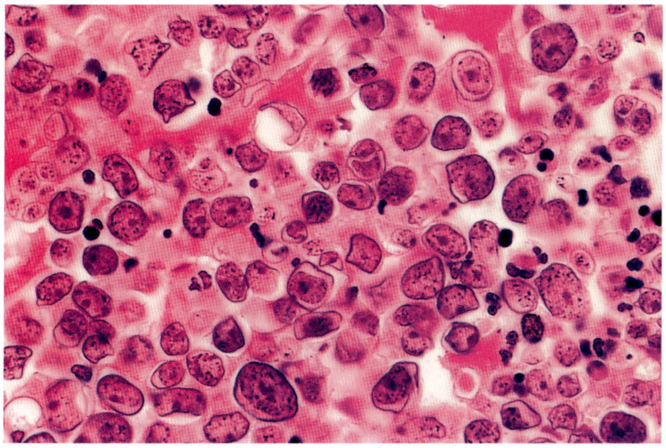

Figure 117–10. Disseminated protothecosis caused by *P zopfii.* Numerous oval and polygonal sporangia are present. Individual sporangia are hematoxylinophilic and contain single discrete nuclei (H&E, ×250).

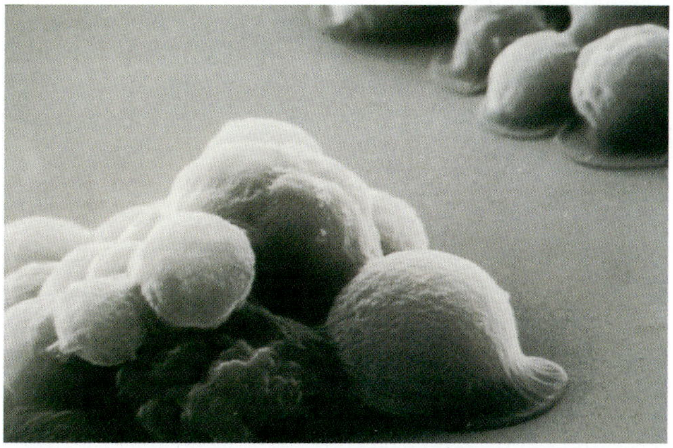

Figure 117–12. Scanning electron micrograph of *P wickerhamii* cells in culture. The walls of the protothecae spread over the surface of the culture medium and against each other, giving the individual algal cells a fluid or plastic appearance (scanning electron micrograph, ×3500).

microscopy (Figure 117–12). Transmission electron microscopy of *Prototheca* sp reveals double membrane-bound starch granules without internal organization (Figure 117–13). These prominent cytoplasmic granules are starch plastids.[19] True chloroplasts are not in the *Prototheca* sp.

Cutaneous Protothecosis

Cutaneous protothecosis usually involves both dermis and epidermis, and the inflammatory response is predominantly granulomatous (Figure 117–2).[18] The dermis contains a mixed inflammatory cell infiltrate consisting of lymphocytes, plasma cells, eosinophils, neutrophils, macrophages, epithelioid cells, and giant cells. Cutaneous lesions may be ulcerated, or there may be intraepidermal microabscesses with hyperkeratosis, parakeratosis, and acanthosis (Figure 117–3). Algal cells may be single or clustered, and are usually numerous and concentrated in areas of inflammation. Many are in macrophages and in giant cells of both foreign body and Langhans' types.[20]

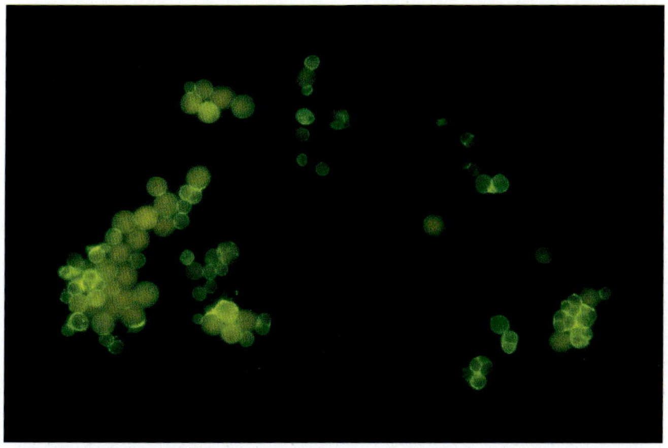

Figure 117–11. *Prototheca wickerhamii.* The walls of single and endosporulating sporangia in this deparaffinized section of formalin-fixed tissue are brightly decorated with a species-specific immunofluorescence conjugate (direct immunofluorescence, ×160).

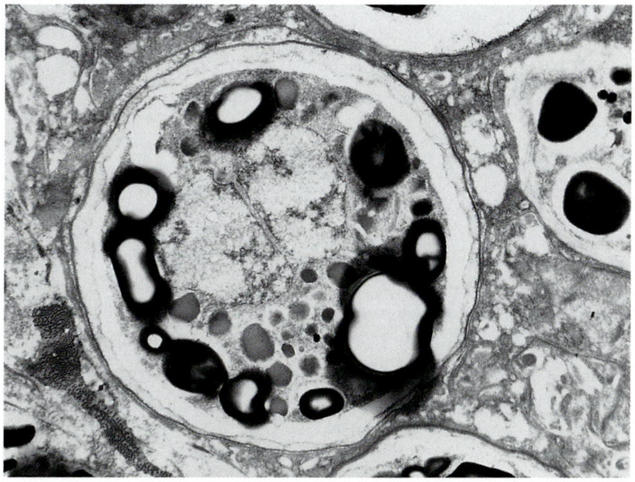

Figure 117–13. Transmission electron micrograph of *P wickerhamii* in a dermal granuloma. A sporangium in the early stage of endosporulation contains large, electron-dense plastids in its cytoplasm. The plastids contain starch and they are not surrounded by a stacked lamellar component found in chloroplasts of *Chlorella* sp (uranyl acetate and lead citrate, ×25,000).

Olecranon Bursitis

In olecranon bursitis, the inflammatory reaction is limited to the wall of the bursa without involvement of overlying skin. The wall of the bursa contains a necrotizing granuloma that resembles a rheumatic or rheumatoid nodule (Figure 117–6).[18] The granulomatous reaction usually surrounds an area of central caseation necrosis, which is in turn surrounded by palisaded epithelioid cells and Langhans' giant cells. *Prototheca* cells are usually numerous and concentrated at the margins of the caseous material[20] (Figures 117–6 and 117–7).

Disseminated Protothecosis

The intraperitoneal lesions described in this form of protothecosis were granulomatous and contained many protothecae.[15,16]

TREATMENT

Treatment of olecranon bursitis is excision of the bursa and this is curative. Repeated incision and drainage have failed. Amphotericin B injected into the bursa cured one patient (cited in Ref. 7). Treatment of cutaneous protothecosis has proven to be more difficult. Various regimens, including oral tetracycline followed by topical peroxide, systemic penicillin, flucytosine, griseofulvin, emetine, potassium permanganate, copper sulfate, Castellani's paint, and potassium iodide, have been used with little or no success. Success has been reported, however, with excision, topical amphotericin B with systemic tetracycline, and systemic ketoconazole.[10,20,21] Disseminated protothecosis appears to be best treated with systemic amphotericin B; success with ketoconazole also has been reported.[14]

REFERENCES

1. Nelson AM, Neafie RC, Connor DH. Cutaneous protothecosis and chlorellosis, extraordinary "aquatic-borne" algal infections. *Clin Dermatol.* 1987;5:76–87.
2. Davies RB, Spencer H, Wakelin PV. A case of human protothecosis. *Trans Roy Soc Trop Med Hyg.* 1964;58:448–451.
3. Ashford BK et al. A new species of *Prototheca* and a variety of same isolated from human intestine. *Arch Protistenk.* 1930;70:619–638.
4. Sudman MS. Protothecosis: a critical review. *Am J Clin Pathol.* 1974;61:10–19.
5. Sudman MS, Kaplan W. Identification of the *Prototheca* species by immunofluorescence. *Appl Microbiol.* 1973;25: 981–990.
6. Modly CE, Burnett JW. Cutaneous algal infections: protothecosis and chlorellosis. *Cutis* 1989;44:23–24.
7. Iacoviello VR, DeGirolami PC, Lucarini J, Sutker K, Williams ME, Wanke CA. Protothecosis complicating prolonged endotracheal intubation: case report and literature review. *Clin Infect Dis.* 1992;15:959–967.
8. Laeng RH, Egger C, Schaffner T, Borisch B, Pedrinis E. Protothecosis in an HIV-positive patient. *Am J Surg Pathol.* 1994;18:1261–1264.
9. Kaminski ZC, Kapila R, Sharer LR, Kloser P, Kaufman L. Meningitis due to *Prototheca wickerhamii* in a patient with AIDS. *Clin Infect Dis.* 1992;15:704–706.
10. Tyring SK, Lee PC, Walsh P, Garner JF, Little WP. Papular protothecosis of the chest. *Arch Dermatol.* 1989;125: 1249–1252.
11. Venezio FR, Lavoo E, Williams JE, Zeiss RC, et al. Progressive cutaneous protothecosis. *Am J Clin Pathol.* 1982;77: 485–493.
12. McAnally T, Parry EL. Cutaneous protothecosis presenting as recurrent chromomycosis. *Arch Dermatol.* 1985;121: 1066–1069.
13. Grocott RG, Huffaker AK, White CB. Protothecal bursitis: a case from Panama. *Lab Med.* 1979;10:89–96.
14. Nosanchuck JS, Greenberg RD. Protothecosis of the olecranon bursa caused by achloric algae. *Am J Clin Pathol.* 1973;59:567–573.
15. Chan JC, Jeffers LJ, Gould EW, et al. Visceral protothecosis mimicking sclerosing cholangitis in an immunocompetent host: successful antifungal therapy. *Rev Infect Dis.* 1990;12:802–807.
16. Cox EG, Wilson JD, Brown P. Protothecosis: a case of disseminated algal infection. *Lancet.* 1974;1:379–382.
17. Kuo T, Hsueh S, Wu JL, Wang AM. Cutaneous protothecosis: a clinicopathological study. *Arch Pathol Lab Med.* 1987;111:737–740.
18. Chandler FW, Watts JC. *Pathologic Diagnosis of Fungal Infections.* Chicago: ASCP Press; 1987:43–53.
19. Nadakavukaren MJ, McCracken DA. An ultrastructural survey of the genus *Prototheca* with special reference to plastids. *Mycopathologia.* 1977;2:117–119.
20. Chandler FW, Kaplan W, Ajello L. *A Colour Atlas and Textbook of the Histopathology of Mycotic Diseases.* London: Wolfe Medical Publications; 1980:96–100.
21. Pegram Jr PS, Kerns FT, Wasilauskas BL, Hampton KD, Scharyj M, Burke G. Successful ketoconazole treatment of protothecosis with ketoconazole associated hepatotoxicity. *Arch Intern Med.* 1983;143:1802–1805.

CHAPTER 118

Pseudallescheriasis and Scedosporiasis

David A. Schwartz

In the nineteenth century men lost their fear of God and acquired a fear of microbes.

Anonymous

CLASSIFICATION

Pseudallescheriasis is caused by the opportunistic fungus *Pseudallescheria boydii* (family Microascacae, order Microascales of the Ascomycota). It had previously been known as *Allescheria boydii* Shear, 1921; *Pseudallescheria sheari* Negroni et Fischer, 1944; and *Petriellidium boydii* (Shear) Malloch, 1970. The anamorph of *P boydii* is *Scedosporium apiospermum (Monosporium apiospermum).*

INTRODUCTION AND HISTORY

Pseudallescheria boydii was initially recognized as a human pathogen in 1911 when Saccardo described a new fungus, which he termed *Monosporium apiospermum,* which was isolated from a patient in Italy with mycetoma.[1] In 1922, Shear described the life cycle of a new ascomycetous fungus termed *Allescheria boydii,* which was isolated from a patient in Texas with mycetoma.[2] These two organisms were thought to be different causes of mycetoma until 1944 when Emmons[3] demonstrated that *M apiospermum* was the sexual state, or anamorph, of *A boydii.* Following several name changes of both teleomorphic and anamorphic states, the name *Pseudallescheria boydii* is now accepted as the correct name for the teleomorphic state. Although *P boydii* has long been recognized as an important cause of mycetoma, the importance of this agent as an opportunistic pathogen was not known until 1948, when Benham and George[4] described a patient with meningitis caused by *P boydii.* Since then, there have been numerous reports of pseudallescheriasis involving a wide variety of organs, often in immunosuppressed persons.

EPIDEMIOLOGY

Pseudallescheria boydii is a cosmopolitan saprophytic ascomycete. It has been isolated from a wide variety of natural substances, including polluted water, sewage, soil, swamps, waterlogged pastures, coastal tidelands, and poultry and cattle manure.[5] *Pseudallescheria boydii* is the most frequent cause of eumycotic (white grain) mycetoma in the United States, and is reported sporadically in rural areas of Asia, Europe, Canada, and South America.[6] It shares some epidemiologic similarities with *Aspergillus* sp as a major fungal cause of sinusitis, pulmonary colonization, and endocarditis in previously healthy hosts. An interesting epidemiologic facet of *P boydii* is its propensity to cause pneumonia in, disseminate, and kill those who have aspirated polluted freshwater. *Pseudallescheria boydii* is an important cause of disseminated infections in immunodeficient patients, either from corticosteroids or other immunosuppressive agents, or who have hematopoietic or solid malignancies, diabetes mellitus, or organ transplants.[5–12]

CLINICAL FEATURES

The clinical spectrum of *Pseudallescheria* infection is broad. In addition to its role as a cause of mycetoma in previously normal persons, *P boydii* has been implanted into bone, soft tissue, knee joints, skull, and cornea.[13,14] These patients have all presented with chronic, purulent infections without detectable grains. *Pseudallescheria* infection has been reported following surgical procedures, including craniotomy and cataract extraction. *Pseudallescheria boydii* has colonized paranasal sinuses, the external auditory canal, bronchi, and preexisting lung cavities in otherwise healthy persons.[15,16] In addition, a syndrome of allergic bronchopulmonary mycosis associated with *P boydii* has been reported.[17] There have been rare reports of invasive pulmonary pseudallescheriasis in persons with no identifiable immunologic deficits.[18]

Immunosuppressed persons and patients with underlying diseases are at high risk for localized or invasive *Pseudallescheria* infections.[19] Almost any organ can be involved after the hematogenous dissemination of *P boydii.* These infections often progress rapidly, and patients may have pneumonia, lung abscess,[20] sinusitis, brain abscess, osteomyelitis,[21] or chronic skin and subcutaneous involvement.[22,23] *Pseudallescheria boydii* is a significant ocular pathogen, causing endophthalmitis, orbital cellulitis, and corneal ulcerations.[24] *Pseudallescheria* infections have been reported in patients with acquired immunodeficiency syndrome, including sinusitis,[25] endocarditis of native valves,[26] and invasive renal and pulmonary disease.[27]

Involvement of the central nervous system by *P boydii* has been reported from at least 28 patients, of whom 11 were immunosuppressed. Although most had brain abscesses, some had meningitis and ventriculitis.[5]

MORPHOLOGY

Hyphae of *Pseudallescheria boydii* are similar to those of *Aspergillus* sp, *Fusarium,* and nonpigmented hyphae of *Alternaria alternata* and *Bipolaris* sp. These fungi cannot be reliably differentiated on morphologic grounds in tissue unless characteristic anneloconidia or "fruiting bodies" are present. *Pseudallescheria boydii* hyphae are septate, nonpigmented, hyaline, and vary from 2 to 5 μm wide (Figure 118–1). *Pseudallescheria boydii* may produce dilated swollen areas, termed chlamydoconidia, which may be terminal or intercalary and measure up to 20 μm in diameter (Figure 118–2). In some areas of densely matted hyphae, these thick-walled globose swellings may be prominent and misinterpreted as yeastlike structures. Sometimes *P boydii* can produce ovoid to pyriform, brown conidia, 5 by 10 μm, borne terminally or laterally on slender, nonpigmented, short conidiophores (Figure 118–3). The characteristic conidia are often produced in pulmonary fungomas (fungus balls), usually within densely matted hyphae at the periphery of the fungus ball. Because

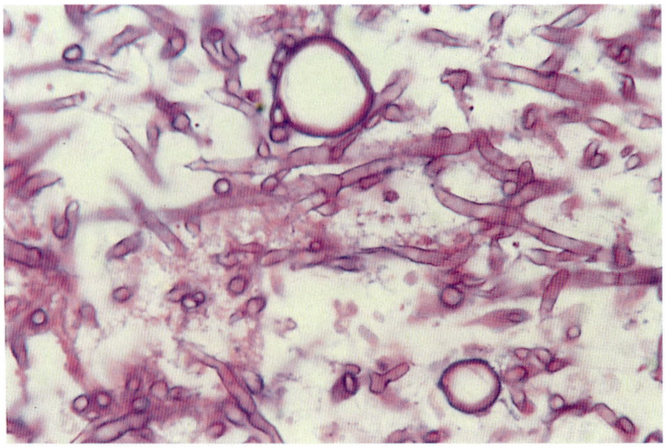

Figure 118–2. Typical appearance of the intercalary chlamydoconidia of *P boydii* (PAS, ×400).

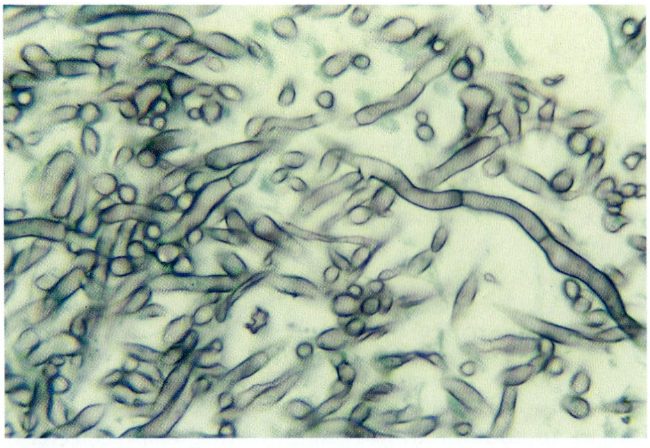

Figure 118–1. These septate hyphae of *P boydii* from infected lung are morphologically indistinguishable from those of *Aspergillus* sp (GMS, ×400).

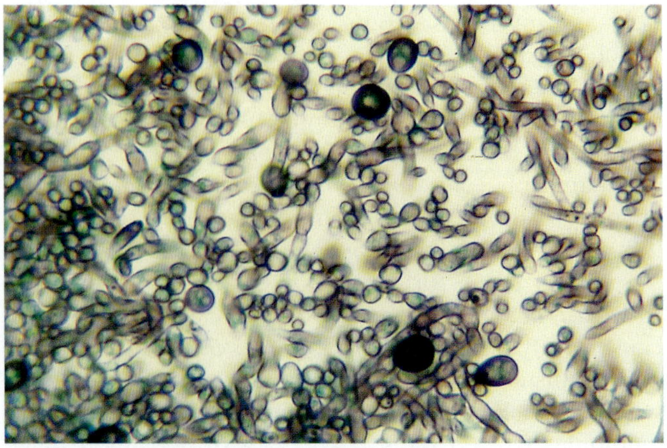

Figure 118–3. The conidia of *P boydii* confirm the diagnosis of this agent in tissue (GMS, ×400).

these structures are brown in slides stained with hematoxylin-eosin (H&E), their identification helps distinguish *P boydii* from similar fungi.

As in other fungal infections, special stains [Gomori's methenamine silver (GMS), periodic acid–Schiff (PAS) reaction] are usually necessary to study the morphologic details of the fungus and its distribution in tissues. Mycetomas caused by *P boydii* are described in Chapter 113.

PATHOLOGY

Pulmonary Infection

The most commonly encountered site of infection by *P boydii,* after pedal mycetoma, is the respiratory tract. *Pseudallescheria* infections of the lower respiratory tract can present as allergic bronchopulmonary mycosis, bronchial colonization, localized fungus balls termed "fungomas," pulmonary colonization, or invasive pulmonary disease. *Pseudallescheria boydii* can grow in poorly draining paranasal sinuses or bronchi without invading. Patients with endobronchial colonization often have bronchiectasis, and also chronic interstitial infiltrates from preexisting pulmonary disease such as tuberculosis or sarcoidosis.[28] *Pseudallescheria boydii* resembles *Aspergillus* sp by invading vessels. This explains the frequent association of pseudallescheriasis with nodular pulmonary infarcts and necrotizing pneumonitis. Although fungus balls of *P boydii* can colonize preexisting lung cavities (Figure 118–4), they originate also from necrotic host tissue by nodular infarction following mycotic thrombosis of blood vessels.[29] The fungus balls are large, spherical to ovoid, spongy, and resemble surrounding lung (Figure 118–5). They are usually loose in cavities. Microscopically, the center of the fungus ball is necrotic lung (Figures 118–6 and 118–7) infiltrated by a loose, randomly branching network of hyphae (Figure 118–8). The periphery of the fungus ball, however, is well organized and consists of alternating zones of mycelial hypercellularity and hypocellularity (Figures 118–9 and 118–10). Diagnostic conidia may be in the superficial and less cellular layers of the fungoma (Figure 118–11). The conidia are brown in H&E stained sections, and easily identified.[12,29]

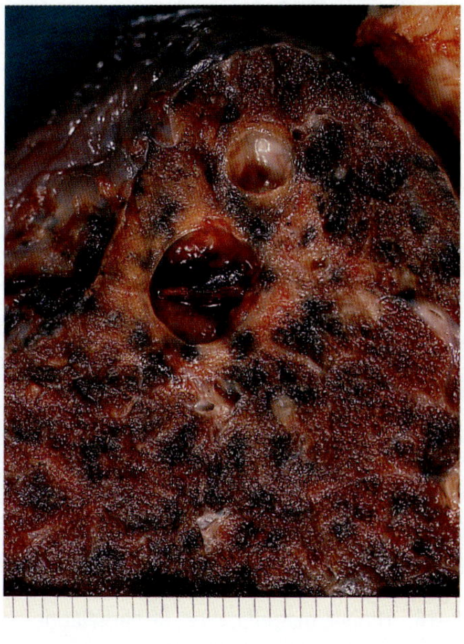

Figure 118–4. These two cavities in the lung contained fungus balls of *Pseudallescheria.*

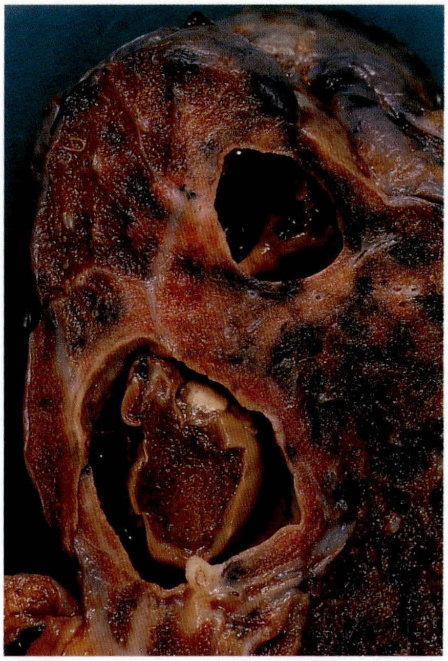

Figure 118–5. Upper lobe of lung showing a large fungus ball caused by *P boydii.* It is present in the lower cavity and is composed of necrotic lung and infiltrating fungal hyphae (see Figures 118–6 through 118–11). The patient had leukemia.

Invasive pulmonary pseudallescheriasis is pathologically similar to aspergillosis, and may produce necrotizing pneumonitis, pulmonary abscesses, and nodular infarcts. Infection can extend from lung through pleura (Figure 118–12), and invade contiguous thoracic structures including soft tissues and ribs (Figure 118–13). Many of the microscopic findings in invasive pseudallescheriasis are caused by mycotic thrombosis, resulting in parenchymal lysis and a fibrinocellular exudate in alveolar spaces. In areas of necrosis, hyphae are often fragmented and basophilic. The hyphae have a random, haphazard pattern of branching rather than the progressive, arborizing, pattern of branching characteristic of *Aspergillus* infections (Figure 118–8). Also hyphae of *P boydii* do not have the fragile, "crumpled" or "twisted ribbon" appearance of zygomycetes.[29]

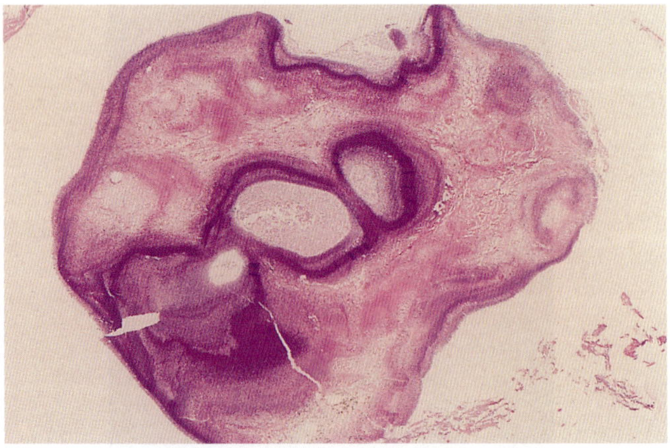

Figure 118–6. Low magnification of a *P boydii* fungus ball. The density of fungal growth corresponds to the intensity of PAS positivity (PAS, ×2).

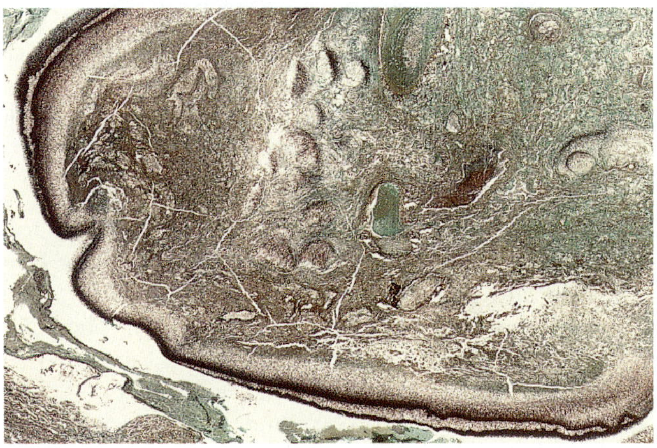

Figure 118–7. Section of the fungus ball in Figure 118–6. Superficial zones of mycelial hypercellularity can be seen at this magnification (GMS, ×4).

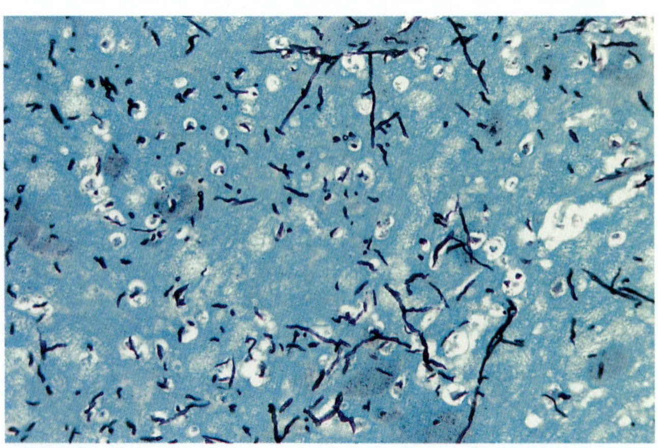

Figure 118–8. A random pattern of mycelial infiltration, in the center of this fungus ball, is typical of *P boydii* (GMS, ×100).

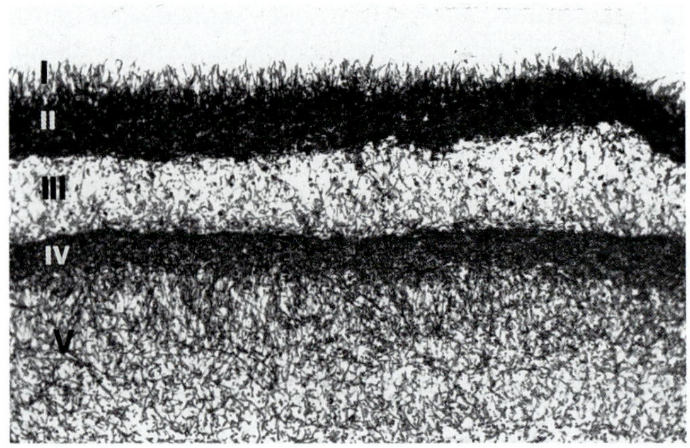

Figure 118–9. Five zones of mycelial cellularity (I–V) are easily distinguished at the periphery of this fungus ball (seen also in Figure 118–8) (GMS, ×100).

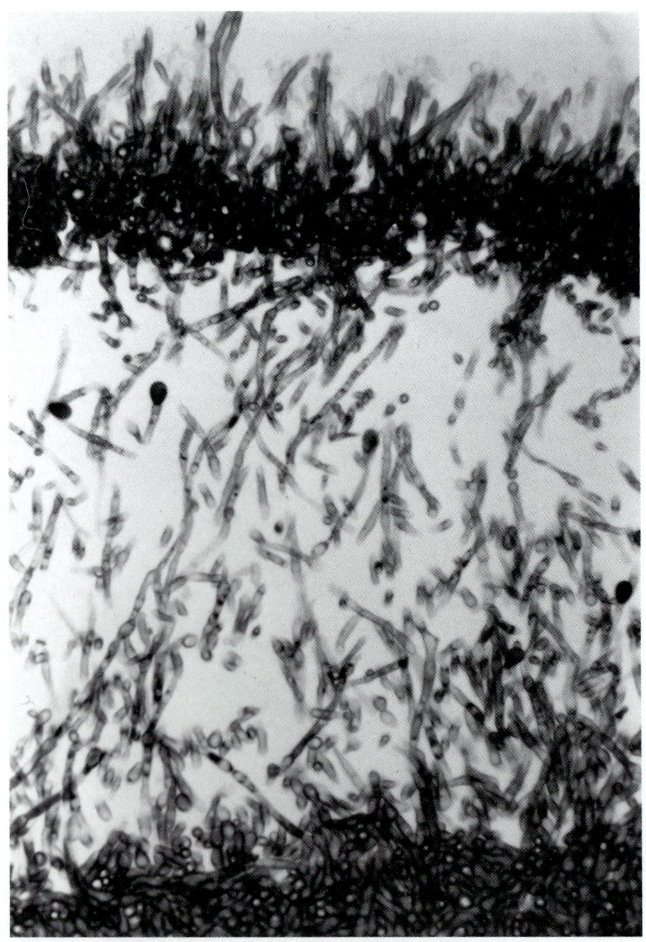

Figure 118–10. Higher magnification of conidiation zones I to IV, showing anneloconidia bearing pyriform conidia concentrated in hypocellular zone III (GMS, ×250).

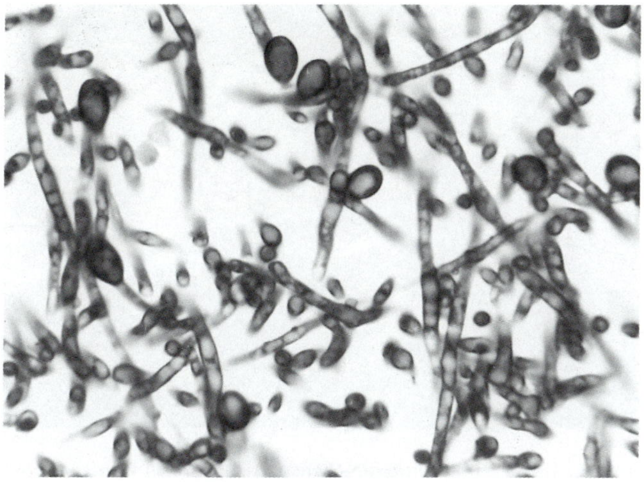

Figure 118–11. Anneloconidia and conidia in zone III of a pulmonary fungoma (GMS, ×400).

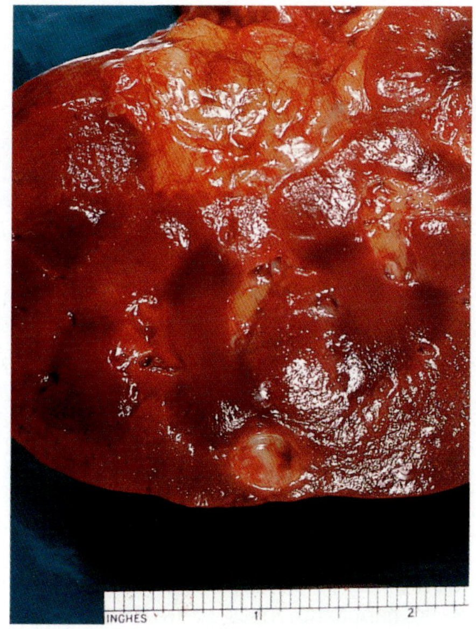

Figure 118–14. Small abscess of renal cortex caused by *P boydii.*

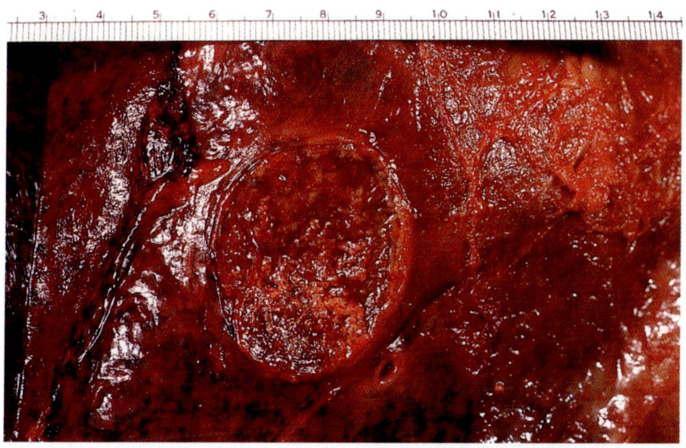

Figure 118–12. Pleural lesion of *P boydii* contiguous to the lesion of the rib cage seen in Figure 118–13.

Infections in Other Organs

The histologic appearance of pseudallescheriasis in nonpulmonary sites, including bones and joints, central nervous system, eyes, ears, thyroid, and kidneys, consists of variable amounts of fungal hyphae associated with abscesses, vascular thrombosis and infarction, and suppuration. Fungus balls have been described in extrapulmonary sites, including kidneys (Figure 118–14) and brain (Figure 118–15).[12] Because the fungus may be hematogenously disseminated in patients with systemic infection, virtually any organ can be infected. The diagnostic conidia and peripheral zones of mycelial hypercellularity, however, are usually absent in nonpulmonary tissues (Figure 118–16).[5,12,29]

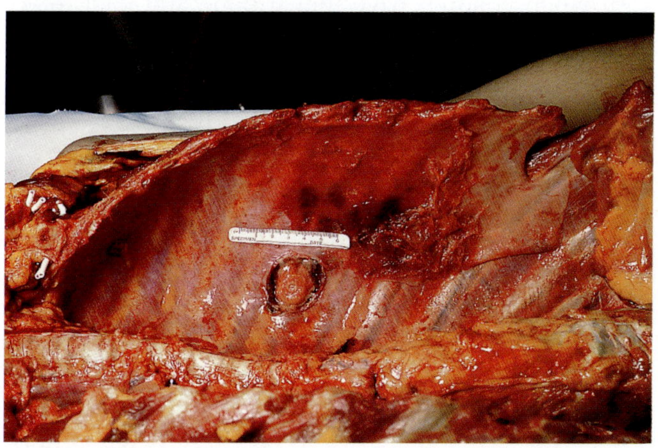

Figure 118–13. Pulmonary infection caused by *P boydii* has invaded pleura to produce this erosive lesion of the rib cage.

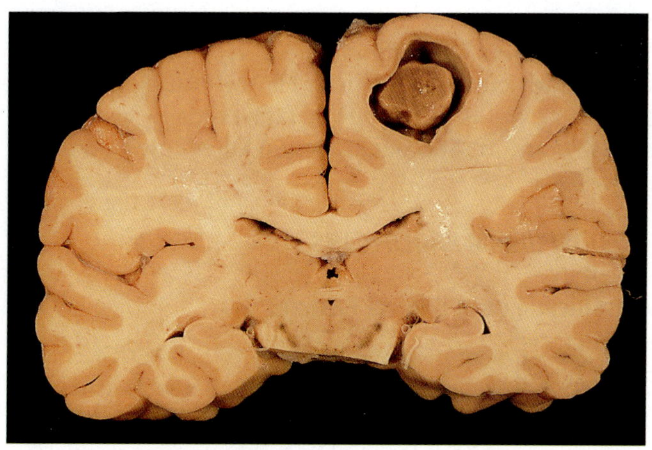

Figure 118–15. Fungus ball of *P boydii* in white matter from a patient with disseminated pseudallescheriasis.

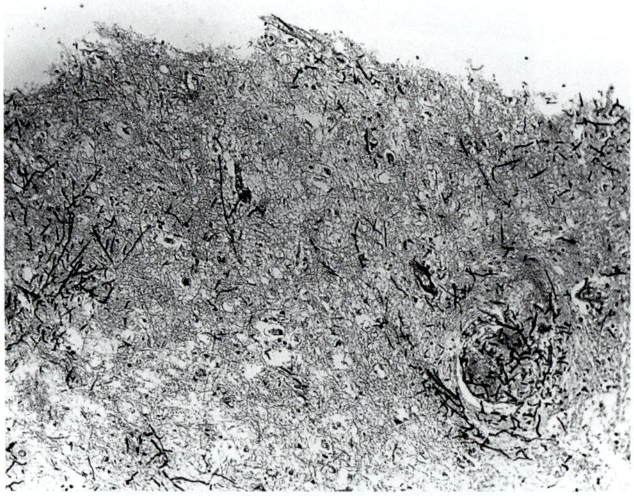

Figure 118–16. Unlike pulmonary fungus balls, this cerebral fungoma shows no peripheral zones of mycelial hypercellularity or conidiation. Note the typical haphazard branching pattern and vascular invasion of *P boydii* (GMS, ×100).

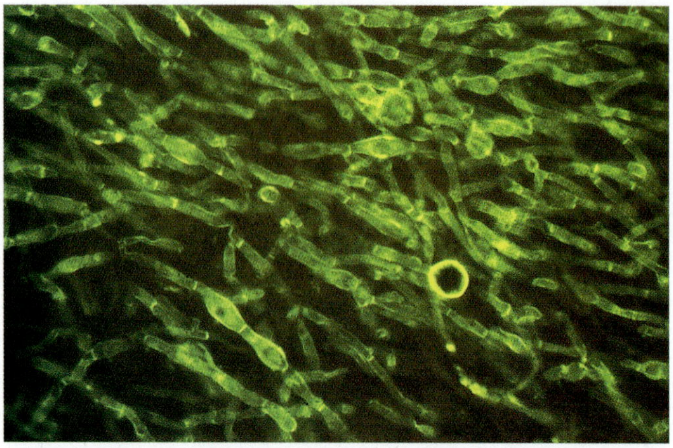

Figure 118–17. Immunofluorescence of *P boydii* in formalin-fixed, deparaffinized tissue sections is highly specific. An intercalary chlamydoconidium is present (×400).

DIAGNOSIS

Because *P boydii* has a different antifungal susceptibility pattern than both *Aspergillus* sp and *Fusarium*,[30] it is important to differentiate infections produced by these organisms. For instance, *P boydii* appears to be sensitive to imidazole derivatives, is moderately unresponsive to amphotericin B, and completely resistant to flucytosine.[5] Serologic diagnosis currently does not distinguish pseudallescheriasis from other fungal infections, and blood cultures are only rarely positive. Tissue diagnosis of pseudallescheriasis cannot be made on histologic grounds alone unless diagnostic pigmented conidia are present, although immunofluorescent methods are available for formalin-fixed and paraffin-embedded tissue (Figure 118–17). Differentiation of *P boydii* from *Aspergillus* sp from infected cavities in lung has been reported using fine-needle aspiration to obtain material for culture.[16] In most clinical situations, a portion of all fluids, scrapings, aspirates, or biopsy specimens should be submitted for fungal culture.

SCEDOSPORIUM PROLIFICANS

Classification and Clinical Features

Scedosporium prolificans (Malloch et Salkin) Guèho et de Hoog, 1991, is a recently described species that can be morphologically and physiologically distinguished from the anamorph stage of *P boydii*, termed *Scedosporium apiospermum*.[31] The designation *Scedosporium prolificans* includes the species *S inflatum*, which was first described in 1984. Several infections by *Scedosporium* have been reported, usually from young boys without any evidence of immunosuppression. Patients usually present with invasive disease, but colonization has been reported. Patients with invasive scedosporiosis have bone infections that present as arthritis or osteomyelitis. In many patients, the fungus appears to have been introduced into the affected bone or joint by contamination associated with trauma. *Scedosporium* infection producing arthritis of the hip has been reported from two intravenous drug abusers.[32]

Morphology and Pathology

The hyphae produced by *S prolificans* are indistinguishable from those of *P boydii* in tissue sections, and microbiologic culture is required to differentiate these two agents. Suspicion for *S prolificans* infection should arise when children have fungal bone and joint infections following traumatic injury.[5]

REFERENCES

1. Saccardo PA. In: *Notae Mycologicae*, Series XIII. *Ann Mycol.* 1911;9:254–255.
2. Shear CL. Life history of an undescribed ascomycete isolated from granular mycetoma of man. *Mycologia.* 1922; 14:239–243.
3. Emmons CW. *Allescheria boydii* and *Monosporium apiospermum*. *Mycologia.* 1944;36:188–193.
4. Benham RW, George LK. *Allescheria boydii,* causative agent in a case of meningitis. *J Invest Dermatol.* 1948;10: 99–110.

5. Kwon-Chung K, Bennett JE. Pseudallescheriasis and *Scedosporium* infection. In: Kwon-Chung K, Bennett JE, eds. *Medical Mycology*. Philadelphia: Lea & Febiger; 1992: 678–694.
6. Chandler FW, Watts JC. *Pathologic Diagnosis of Fungal Infections*. Chicago: ASCP Press; 1987:251–263.
7. Travis LB, Roberts GD, Wilson WR. Clinical significance of *Pseudallescheria boydii:* a review of 10 years' experience. *Mayo Clin Proc*. 1985;60:531–537.
8. Winston DJ, Jordan MC, Rhodes J. *Allescheria boydii* infections in the immunosuppressed host. *Am J Med*. 1977;63:830–835.
9. Alsip SG, Cobbs CG. *Pseudallescheria boydii* infection of the central nervous system in a cardiac transplant recipient. *South Med J*. 1986;79:383–384.
10. Gluckman SJ, Ries K, Abrutyn E. *Allescheria (Petriellidium) boydii* sinusitis in a compromised host. *J Clin Microbiol*. 1977;5:481–484.
11. Yoo D, Lee WHS, Kwon-Chung KJ. Brain abscess due to *Pseudallescheria boydii* associated with primary non-Hodgkin's lymphoma of the central nervous system: a case report and literature review. *Rev Infect Dis*. 1985;7: 272–277.
12. Schwartz DA, Amenta PS, Finkelstein SD. Cerebral *Pseudallescheria boydii* infection: unique occurrence of fungus ball formation in the brain. *Clin Neurol Neurosurg*. 1989;91:83–88.
13. Dirschl DR, Henderson RC. Patellar overgrowth after infection of the knee. *J Bone Joint Surg*. 1991;73A: 940–941.
14. Dellestable F, Kures L, Mainard D, Pere P, Gaucher A. Fungal arthritis due to *Pseudallescheria boydii (Scedosporium apiospermum)*. *J Rheumatol*. 1994;21:766–768.
15. Watters GW, Milford CA. Isolated sphenoid sinusitis due to *Pseudallescheria boydii*. *J Laryngol Otol*. 1993;107: 344–346.
16. Stanley MW, Deike M, Knoedler J, Iber C. Pulmonary mycetomas in immunocompetent patients: diagnosis by fine-needle aspiration. *Diagn Cytopathol*. 1992;8:577–579.
17. Miller MA, Greenberger PA, Amerian R, et al. Allergic bronchopulmonary mycosis caused by *Pseudallescheria boydii*. *Am Rev Resp Dis*. 1993;148:810–812.
18. Hung CC, Chang SC, Yang PC, Hsieh WC. Invasive pulmonary pseudallescheriasis with direct invasion of the thoracic spine in an immunocompetent patient. *Eur J Clin Microbiol Infect Dis*. 1994;13:749–751.
19. Vartivarian SE, Anaissie EJ, Bodey GP. Emerging fungal pathogens in immunocompromised patients: classification, diagnosis, and management. *Clin Infect Dis* 1993;17 (suppl 2):S487–491.
20. Winer-Muram HT, Vargas S, Slobod K. Cavitary lung lesions in an immunosuppressed child. *Chest*. 1994;106: 937–938.
21. Foster MR, Friedenberg ZB, Passero F. Lumbar *Petriellidium boydii* osteomyelitis with a systemic presentation. *J Spinal Dis*. 1994;7:356–360.
22. Lopes JO, Alves SH, Benevenga JP, Salla A, Khmohan C, Silva CB. Subcutaneous pseudallescheriasis in a renal transplant recipient. *Mycopathol*. 1994;125:153–156.
23. Bernstein EF, Schuster MG, Stieritz DD, Uitto J. Disseminated cutaneous *Pseudallescheria boydii*. *Br J Dermatol*. 1995;132:456–460.
24. McGuire TW, Bullock JD, Bullock JD, Elder BL, Funkhouser JW. Fungal endophthalmitis. An experimental study with a review of 17 human ocular cases. *Archiv Ophthalmol*. 1991;109:1289–1296.
25. Meyer RD, Gaultier CR, Yamashita JT, Babapour R, Pitchon HE, Wolfe PR. Fungal sinusitis in patients with AIDS: report of 4 cases and review of the literature. *Medicine*. 1994;73:69–78.
26. Raffanti SP, Fyfe B, Carreiro S, Sharp SE, Hyman BA, Ratzan KR. Native valve endocarditis due to *Pseudallescheria boydii* in a patient with AIDS: case report and review. *Rev Infect Dis*. 1990;12:993–996.
27. Scherr GR, Evans SG, Kiyabu MT, Klatt EC. *Pseudallescheria boydii* infection in the acquired immunodeficiency syndrome. *Arch Pathol Lab Med*. 1992;116:535–536.
28. Rosen P, Adelson HT, Burleigh E. Bronchiectasis complicated by the presence of *Monosporium apiospermum* and *Aspergillus fumigatus*. *Am J Clin Pathol*. 1969;93: 1125–1127.
29. Schwartz DA. Organ specific variation in the morphology of the fungomas (fungus balls) of *Pseudallescheria boydii:* development within necrotic host tissue. *Arch Pathol Lab Med*. 1980;113:476–480.
30. Walsh M, White L, Atkinson K, Eno A. Fungal *Pseudallescheria boydii* lung infiltrates unresponsive to amphotericin B in leukemic patients. *Austral NZ J Med*. 1992; 22:265–268.
31. de Hoog GS, Marvin-Sikkema FD, Lahpoor GA, Gottschall JC, Prins RA, Gueho E. Ecology and physiology of the emerging opportunistic fungi *Psedallescheria boydii* and *Scedosporium prolificans*. *Mycoses*. 1994;37:71–78.
32. Wilson CM, O'Rourke EJ, McGinnis MR, Salkin IF. *Scedosporium inflatum:* clinical spectrum of a newly recognized pathogen. *J Infect Dis*. 1990;161:102–107.

CHAPTER 119

Pythiosis Insidiosi

Michael R. McGinnis and Francis W. Chandler

The truth will always be found in some curious and interesting way, to differ from assumption and opinion.

Alan Gregg (1890–1957)

DEFINITION

In humans, pythiosis insidiosi is a cutaneous and subcutaneous vascular infection caused by *Pythium insidiosum* and characterized by rapidly developing granulomatous lesions. Progressive arterial insufficiency develops that is followed by gangrene, aneurysms, and possible death.[1] In cats, cattle, dogs, and horses, pythiosis insidiosi is a subcutaneous, osseous, or pulmonary infection. Intestinal infections also occur in dogs and horses.[2] Synonyms include bursattee, cutaneous habronemiasis (in part), equine granuloma, equine phycomycosis, Florida horse leeches, leeches, granular dermatitis, hyphomycosis destruens, hyphomycosis destruens equi, phycomycosis, phycomycotic granuloma, pythiosis, and swamp cancer.

GEOGRAPHIC DISTRIBUTION

Pythium insidiosum lives in tropical to semitropical regions. Reports of diseases caused by this microorganism have been recorded from Australia, Costa Rica, India, Japan, New Guinea, Thailand, and the United States.[3–5]

LIFE CYCLE, NATURAL HISTORY, AND EPIDEMIOLOGY

Smith[6] and Drouin[7] described the first cases of pythiosis insidiosi at the end of the 19th century. Ninety years later, Austwick and Copland[8] were the first to stimulate cultural isolates to produce biflagellate zoospores. Based on this observation, they thought that the microorganism was probably a species of *Pythium*. de Cock et al[4] proposed the name *P insidiosum,* classifying it in the order Peronosporales, phylum Oomycota. The Oomycota is best treated in the kingdom Chromista rather than the Protoctista as proposed by de Cock et al.[4]

Pythium insidiosum grows in aquatic to wet environments. Its zoospores attach and penetrate water lily and grass leaves, after which zoosporangia form from the hyphae growing in and on the plant tissue. The zoospores produced within the zoosporangia are released, and the reproductive cycle is repeated. It is speculated that oospores are produced in nature. If zoospores contact injured tissue, they encyst, form germ tubes that produce hyphae, and cause invasive disease. The zoospores have a strong tropism for skin, hair, and water lily and grass leaves.[3]

MORPHOLOGIC FEATURES OF THE ORGANISM

The oomycete *P insidiosum* can be grown on Sabouraud glucose agar where it forms sterile colonies that are white to white-yellow, with submerged vegetative and short aerial hyphae. The colonies have undulating, radiate patterns. Zoosporangia are produced in water cultures that contain the appropriate leaves. Most isolates do not form oospores.[4]

In tissue sections, *P insidiosum* occurs as hyphae and short hyphal fragments that are hyaline, thin walled, infrequently septate, irregularly branched, 5 to 7 μm wide, and have nonparallel contours (Figure 119–1). Hyphal elements are most abundant within areas of necrotizing and suppurative inflammation. Like

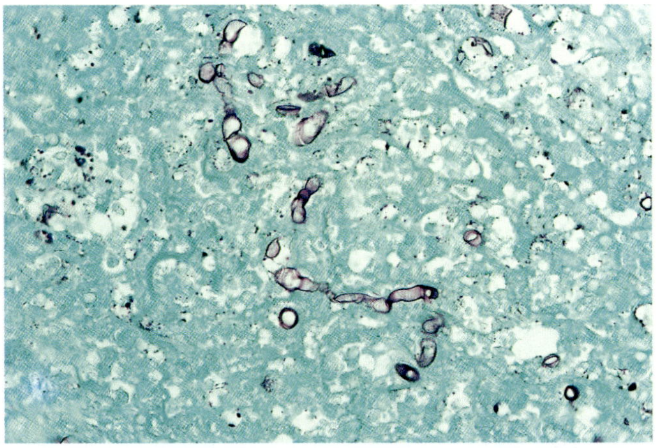

Figure 119–1. Pythiosis insidiosi of the lower limb of a patient with thalassemia hemoglobinopathy syndrome. The subcutaneous tissue contains hyphae and hyphal fragments of *P insidiosum* that are thin walled, twisted, sparsely septate, irregularly branched, 5 to 7 μm wide, and have nonparallel contours (GMS, ×160).

the zygomycetes, hyphae of *P insidiosum* are weakly and unevenly stained with Gomori's methenamine silver (GMS) and other special stains for fungi (Figure 119–2).

CLINICAL FEATURES

Several patients from Thailand who had thalassemia hemoglobinopathy syndrome developed pythiosis insidiosi of the lower limbs.[9,10] Progressive ischemia of the lower limbs, necrosis and thrombosis of the main arteries, and progressive gangrene, aneurysm formation, and ultimately fatal hemorrhage occurred when medium- to large-sized arteries were involved. *Pythium insidiosum* also has caused keratitis and localized cutaneous infections following injuries.

In horses, the legs and lower surface of the abdomen are most frequently involved. Ulcerating lesions, intense pruritus, necrotic cores (kunkers) within inflamed tissue, septic arthritis, osteitis, and tenosynovitis are typical.

PATHOLOGY

In patients who have thalassemia hemoglobinopathy syndrome, *P insidiosum* causes necrotizing arteritis and thrombosis. Infection ascends along involved arteries, and there is an acute fulminant inflammatory reaction with vascular invasion by sparsely septate, branched hyphae (Figure 119–2). Granulomas that contain sparse hyphae and hyphal fragments eventually replace perivascular tissue contiguous to infected arteries.[10] In horses, infection by *P insidiosum* produces ulcerative granulomas that contain coral-like kunkers and numerous eosinophils (Figure 119–3).[5]

DIFFERENTIAL DIAGNOSIS

Clinically, pythiosis insidiosi in humans must be differentiated from cutaneous and subcutaneous zygomycosis, sporotrichosis, mycetoma, and neoplasms. In horses, other diseases in the differential diagnosis

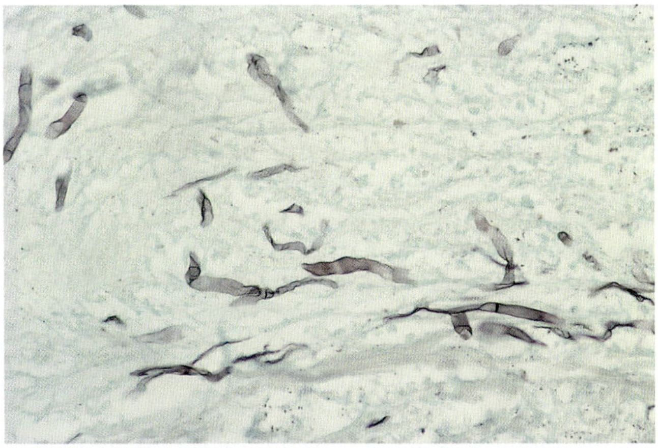

Figure 119–2. *Pythium insidiosum* causing necrotizing arteritis and thrombosis in a patient with thalassemia hemoglobinopathy syndrome. Infrequently septate, weakly stained hyphae and hyphal fragments that superficially resemble zygomycetes invade the arterial wall (GMS, ×160).

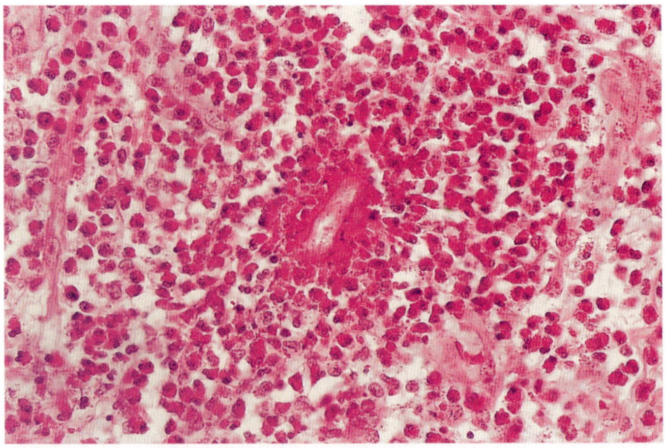

Figure 119–3. Culture-proven pythiosis insidiosi of the distal extremity in a horse. A weakly stained hyphal fragment is embedded in the center of an eosinophilic granuloma (hematoxylin-eosin, ×160).

include histoplasmosis farciminosi, cutaneous habronemiasis, and glanders.

CONFIRMATIONAL TESTING AND DIAGNOSIS

Fresh clinical specimens can be inoculated onto a mycologic medium such as Sabouraud glucose agar. Zoospores can be obtained after a 1-hour incubation at 37°C using grass or lily bait.[3] A soil-extract medium can also be used.[10] Serologic[1,2] and fluorescent antibody tests[4] also are available.

TREATMENT

In humans, there is no effective treatment. Potassium iodide has been used for cutaneous infections,[11] and surgical management has been used for other forms of pythiosis insidiosi.[10] Immunotherapy has been successfully used in horses with pythiosis insidiosi, which become anergic after the disease reaches the chronic stage.[12,13] Fluconazole, ketoconazole, and miconazole have been useful in some patients.[14]

REFERENCES

1. Pracharktam R, Changtrakool P, Sathapatayavongs B, Jayaneta P, Ajello L. Immunodiffusion test for diagnosis and monitoring of human pythiosis insidiosi. *J Clin Microbiol.* 1991;29:2661–2662.
2. Mendoza L, Nicholson V, Prescott JF. Immunoblot analysis of the humoral immune response to *Pythium insidiosum* in horses with pythiosis. *J Clin Microbiol.* 1992;30:2980–2983.
3. Mendoza L, Hernandez F, Ajello L. Life cycle of the human and animal Oomycete pathogen *Pythium insidiosum. J Clin Microbiol.* 1993;31:2967–2973.
4. de Cock AWAM, Mendoza L, Padhye AA, Ajello L, Kaufman L. *Pythium insidiosum* sp nov, the etiologic agent of pythiosis. *J Clin Microbiol.* 1987;25:344–349.
5. Connole MD. Review of animal mycoses in Australia. *Mycopathologia.* 1990;111:133–164.
6. Smith F. The pathology of bursattee. *Vet J.* 1884;19:16–17.
7. Drouin V. Sur une nouvelle mycose du cheval. *Recl Med Vet.* 1896;3:337–344.
8. Austwick PKC, Copland JW. Swamp cancer. *Nature (London).* 1974;250:84.
9. Sathapatuayavongs B, Leelachaikul P, Prachaktam R, et al. Human pythiosis associated with thalassemia hemoglobinopathy syndrome. *J Infect Dis.* 1989;159:274–280.
10. Wanachiwanawin W, Thianprasit M, Fucharoen S, et al. Fatal arteritis due to *Pythium insidiosum* infection in patients with thalassaemia. *Trans Roy Soc Trop Med Hyg.* 1993;87:296–298.
11. Thianprasit M. Human pythiosis. *Trop Dermatol.* 1990;4:1–4.
12. Mendoza L, Kaufman L, Standard PG. Immunodiffusion test for diagnosing and monitoring pythiosis in horses. *J Clin Microbiol.* 1986;23:813–816.
13. Mendoza L, Villalobos J, Calleja CE, Solis A. Evaluation of two vaccines for the treatment of pythiosis insidiosi in horses. *Mycopathologia.* 1992;119:89–95.
14. Sekhon AS, Padhye AA, Garg AK. *In vitro* sensitivity of *Penicillium marneffei* and *Pythium insidiosum* to various antifungal agents. *Eur J Epidemiol.* 1992;8:427–432.

CHAPTER 120

Rhinosporidiosis

John C. Watts and Francis W. Chandler

It is certainly a one sided opinion—even though generally adopted at the moment—that all infectious agents which are still unknown must be bacteria. Why should not other microorganisms just as well be able to exist as parasites in the body of animals?

Robert Koch (1843–1910)

DEFINITION

Rhinosporidiosis is a chronic, superficial mucocutaneous infection that primarily involves the upper respiratory tract.[1] The disease is caused by *Rhinosporidium seeberi,* a sporangial pathogen that will not grow on synthetic media. Because the morphology of *R seeberi* is so distinctive, however, a specific diagnosis can be established by direct microscopic examination of exudates from the lesions or by histopathologic examination of excised mucosal polyps.

GEOGRAPHIC DISTRIBUTION

The disease is endemic in India and Sri Lanka, where about 90% of all infections occur.[2] Autochthonous infections, however, have been reported also from Latin America, Africa, and other parts of the world, including the United States.[3]

EPIDEMIOLOGY

The natural habitat of *R seeberi* and the extent of its distribution in nature are not known. The disease seems to be associated with both rural and aquatic environments, and it primarily affects young men, 20 to 40 years old, who account for about 70% to 90% of all cases.[1,2] There is no evidence that rhinosporidiosis is contagious. Certain animals, particularly dogs and horses, are also susceptible to natural infection.[4]

LIFE CYCLE AND MORPHOLOGIC FEATURES OF THE ORGANISM

The taxonomy and life cycle of *R seeberi* are poorly understood, mainly because of the lack of a simple and effective method to cultivate it in the laboratory. *Rhinosporidium seeberi* will grow and propagate in cell culture,[5] but its identification is usually accomplished by histopathologic or cytologic methods.

Two developmental forms of *R seeberi,* termed sporangia and trophocytes, can be recognized in tissue sections.[6–8] The spherical mature form, or sporangium, measures 100 to 200 μm in diameter, although occasional sporangia achieve a size of 350 μm. The sporangial wall, about 5 μm thick, is composed of a broad, inner hyaline layer and a very thin (<1 μm), outer eosinophilic layer. The sporangium contains numerous sporangiospores (endospores), produced by nuclear fission and progressive cytoplasmic cleavage, that have a characteristic zonal arrangement. The small, flattened, uninucleated immature or germinative sporangiospores, 1 to 2 μm in maximum size, form a crescentic mass at one pole or peripherally along the wall of the sporangium. As they mature, the sporangiospores enlarge (up to 5 to 10 μm in diameter), migrate centrally, and acquire multiple refractile, eosinophilic cytoplasmic globules (Figure 120–1). The transition from immature

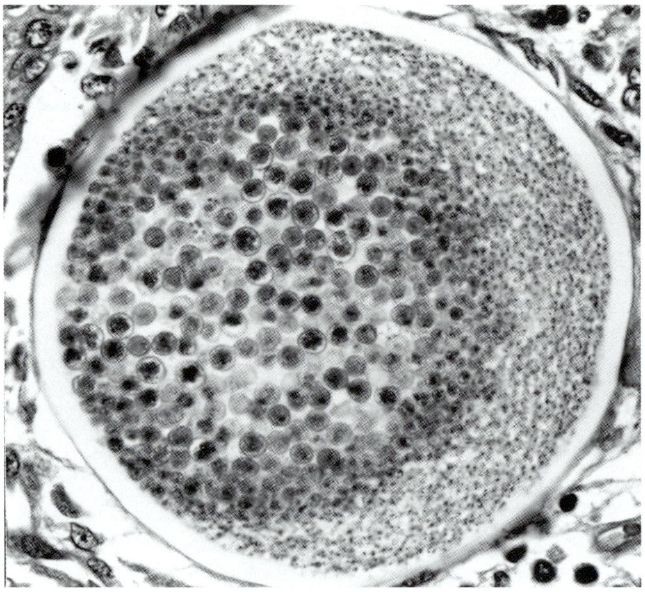

Figure 120–1. Mature sporangium of *R seeberi*. The zonal arrangement of immature, maturing, and fully mature sporangiospores is diagnostic of this pathogen. The mature sporangiospores contain characteristic eosinophilic, globular inclusions [hematoxylin-eosin (H&E), ×480].

to mature sporangiospores is usually abrupt and well delineated. The distinctive mulberry-like shape of the mature sporangiospores and the prominent polar zonation of sporangiospores within the sporangium distinguish *R seeberi* from other spherical, endosporulating pathogens in tissue sections, eg, *Coccidioides immitis* and the *Prototheca* sp.

Trophocytes are thought to develop directly from sporangiospores that are released into tissue following rupture of the sporangium. The trophocytes, 10 to 100 μm in diameter, have refractile eosinophilic walls about 2 to 3 μm thick. The cytoplasm of the trophocytes is granular or flocculent, and each trophocyte has a round, pale nucleus with a prominent nucleolus or karyosome (Figure 120–2). The trophocytes enlarge and transform ultimately into mature sporangia through a process of endosporulation.

The walls of both the mature sporangia and the sporangiospores are periodic acid–Schiff (PAS) and Gomori's methenamine silver (GMS) positive. The trophocytes, however, stain poorly or not at all with GMS (Figure 120–3). In addition, the sporangiospore walls and the inner surface of the sporangial wall stain positively with mucin stains, such as mucicarmine (Figure 120–4). None of these special stains, however, is needed for diagnosis; the distinctive appearance of the trophocytes and sporangia in routine, H&E stained sections is diagnostic.

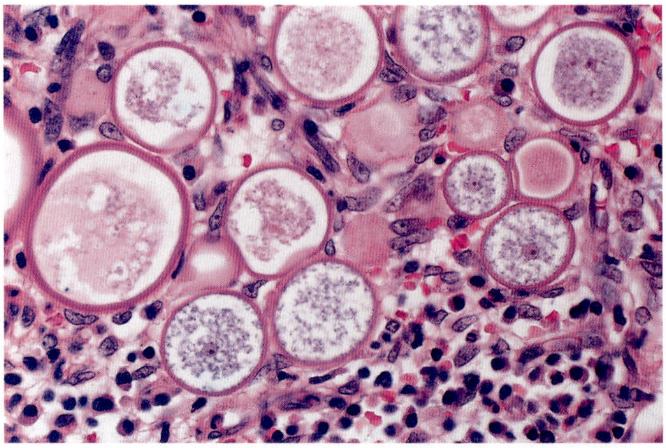

Figure 120–2. The trophocytes of *R seeberi* are characterized by densely eosinophilic walls, flocculent cytoplasm, and a single nucleus with a prominent karyosome (H&E, ×480).

CLINICAL FEATURES AND TREATMENT

Mucosal infection leads to the formation of friable, red, warty polyps or papillomas involving primarily the nasal cavity, nasopharynx, and oral cavity.[1] Less frequently, lesions arise on the conjunctivae,[3,9] paranasal sinuses, larynx, and external genitalia. The infection may spread to adjacent skin, and secondary skin lesions result from autoinoculation by scratching. Rare examples of limited systemic dissemination of rhinosporidiosis have been reported,[10] but in most patients the disease remains localized and superficial. The only effective form of treatment is surgical excision of the lesions, which tend to recur locally in mucosal sites

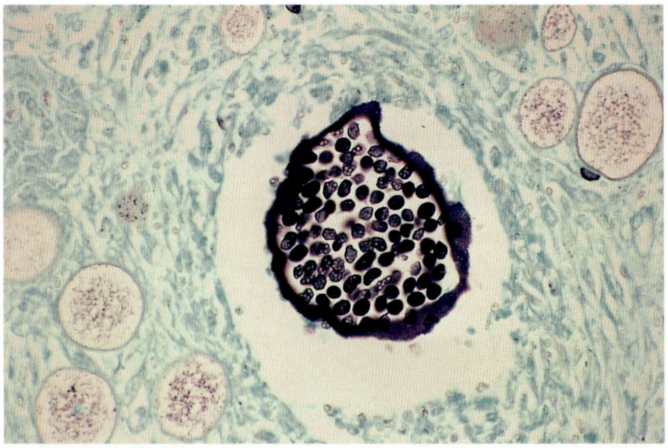

Figure 120–3. The walls of both the sporangium and the mature sporangiospores are argyrophilic with the GMS stain. Note that the trophocytes do not stain (×100).

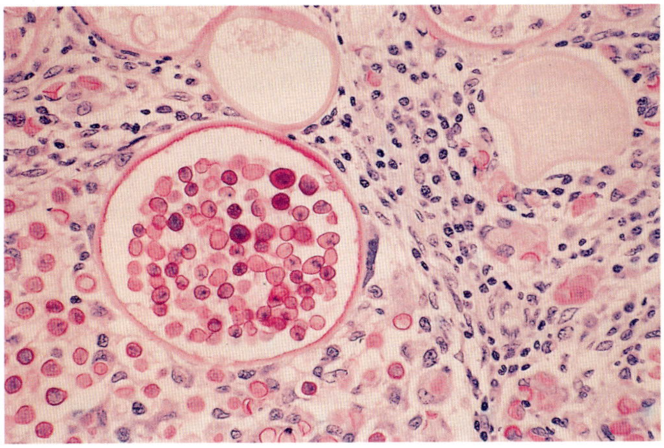

Figure 120–4. Mature sporangium of *R seeberi.* The walls of the mature sporangiospores are carminophilic. There is faint staining along the inner surface of the sporangial wall (Mayer's mucicarmine, ×100).

such as the paranasal sinuses and nasopharynx, where complete excision is difficult to achieve.

PATHOLOGY

The glistening, pink mucosal polyps may appear warty or polypoid. Microscopically, polyps arising in the upper respiratory tract are covered by respiratory or metaplastic mucosa, whereas those arising elsewhere are covered by stratified squamous mucosa (Figure 120–5). The abundant sporangia and trophocytes or *R seeberi* occupy the stromal cores of the polyps, where they elicit a chronic inflammatory response with formation of granulation tissue. There is often a granulomatous response where sporangia have ruptured into the stroma (Figure 120–6).

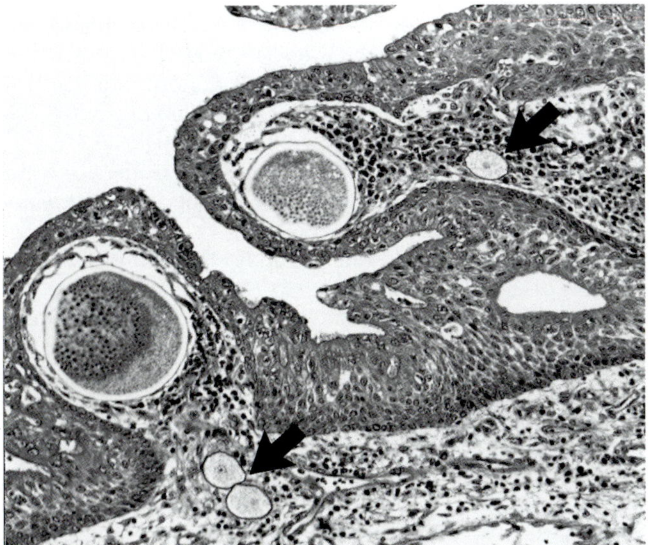

Figure 120–5. Surface of a rhinosporidial nasal polyp. The respiratory mucosa has undergone squamous metaplasia. Sporangia and trophocytes *(arrows)* of *R seeberi* are located in the stroma of the polyp, which consists of granulation tissue with a chronic inflammatory cell infiltrate (H&E, ×120).

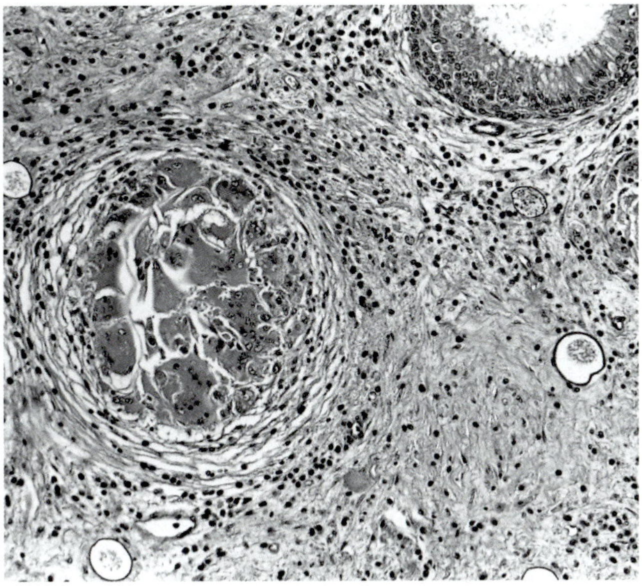

Figure 120–6. Granulomatous inflammatory response *(left)* to residual fragments of a ruptured sporangium in the stroma of a rhinosporidial nasal polyp. Several trophocytes are present in the adjacent stroma. A crypt lined by respiratory mucosa *(upper right)* extends from the surface of the polyp (H&E, ×120).

Electron microscopy has contributed to our understanding of the replicative cycle of *R seeberi,* particularly the details of its phase of endosporulation, but electron microscopy is not necessary for diagnosis. The disease can be diagnosed by cytologic examination of fluid obtained by irrigation of the paranasal sinuses.[11]

DIFFERENTIAL DIAGNOSIS

Other fungi that occur in tissue sections in the form of large spherules or sporangia can be mistaken, on occasion, for *R seeberi.* These pathogenic fungi include *C immitis* and *Chrysosporium parvum* var *crescens,* the agent of adiaspiromycosis. Recognition of the characteristic pathologic lesions—mucosal polyps—and of the distinctive morphology of rhinosporidial sporangia,

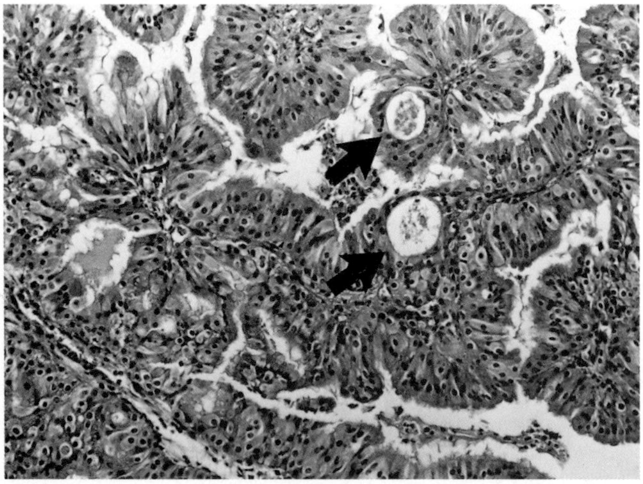

Figure 120–7. Cylindrical cell papilloma of the lateral nasal wall. The papillae are covered by stratified, columnar, oxyphilic epithelium. Mucous cysts *(arrows),* which superficially resemble rhinosporidial sporangia, are located exclusively within the epithelium rather than in the fibrovascular stromal core of the papilloma (H&E, ×120).

with zonation of sporangiospores and the presence of eosinophilic globules in the mature sporangiospores, should prevent confusion. More often, cylindrical cell (oncocytic Schneiderian) papillomas of the nasal cavity and paranasal sinuses are mistaken for rhinosporidial polyps, because the intraepithelial mucous cysts of these papillomas are confused with the sporangia of *R seeberi*[12] (Figure 120–7). Unlike the developmental forms of *R seeberi,* the mucous cysts often have a ciliated border and are located exclusively within the surface epithelium of the cylindrical cell papilloma, and they do not contain sporangiospores[13] (Figure 120–8).

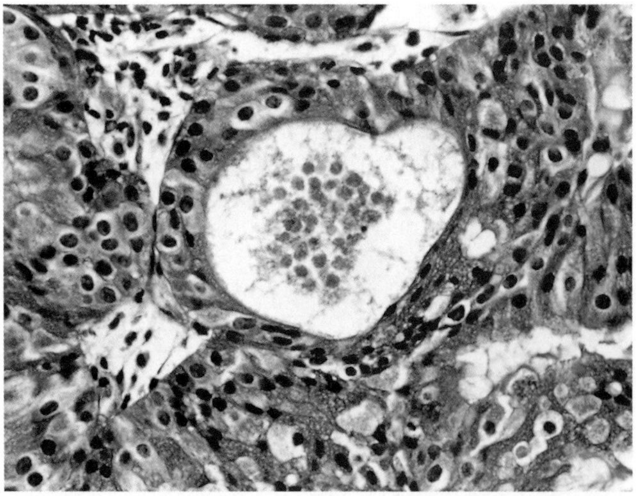

Figure 120–8. Intraepithelial mucous cyst in a cylindrical cell papilloma. Cilia are barely visible along the left border of this cyst. Mucous globules in the lumen resemble sporangiospores, but they lack nuclei and eosinophilic inclusions (H&E, ×300).

REFERENCES

1. Al-Hilli F. Infections caused by *Rhinosporidium seeberi.* In: Mukerji KG, Srivastava AK, Singh KP, Garg KL, eds. *Advances in Medical Mycology.* New Delhi, India: Aditya Books; 1992:25–38.
2. Karunaratne WAE. *Rhinosporidiosis in Man.* London: Athlone Press; 1964.
3. Jimenez JF, Young DE, Hough AJ Jr. Rhinosporidiosis: a report of two cases from Arkansas. *Am J Clin Pathol.* 1984; 82:611–615.
4. Easley JR, Meuten DJ, Levy MG, et al. Nasal rhinosporidiosis in the dog. *Vet Pathol.* 1986;23:50–56.
5. Levy MG, Meuten DJ, Breitschwerdt EB. Cultivation of *Rhinosporidium seeberi* in vitro: interaction with epithelial cells. *Science.* 1986;234:474–476.
6. Bader G, Grueber HLE. Histochemical studies of *Rhinosporidium seeberi. Virchows Arch (Pathol Anat).* 1970; 350:76–86.
7. Kannan-Kutty M, Teh EC. *Rhinosporidium seeberi:* an electron microscopic study of its life cycle. *Pathology.* 1974;6:63–70.
8. Kannan-Kutty M, Teh EC. *Rhinosporidium seeberi:* an ultrastructural study of its endosporulation phase and trophocyte phase. *Arch Pathol.* 1975;99:51–54.
9. Savino DF, Margo CE. Conjunctival rhinosporidiosis: light and electron microscopic study. *Ophthalmology.* 1983;90: 1482–1489.
10. Agrawal S, Sharma KD, Shrivastava JB. Generalized rhinosporidiosis with visceral involvement. *Arch Dermatol.* 1959;80:22–26.
11. Fortin R, Meisels A. Rhinosporidiosis. *Acta Cytol.* 1974; 18:170–173.
12. Lasser A, Smith HW. Rhinosporidiosis. *Arch Otolaryngol.* 1976;102:308–310.
13. Barnes L, Bedetti C. Oncocytic Schneiderian papilloma: a reappraisal of cylindrical cell papilloma of the sinonasal tract. *Hum Pathol.* 1984;15:344–351.

CHAPTER 121

Sporotrichosis

Francis W. Chandler and John C. Watts

Because the newer methods of treatment are good, it does not follow that the old ones were bad: for if our honorable and worshipful ancestors had not recovered from their ailments, you and I would not be here today.

Confucius (551–478 BC)

DEFINITION

Sporotrichosis is a chronic cutaneous or systemic mycosis caused by the thermally dimorphic fungus *Sporothrix schenckii.*[1,2] Infection is frequently confined to the skin, subcutaneous tissues, and contiguous lymphatics, and is caused by the accidental percutaneous inoculation of conidia of *S schenckii* growing in soil and on plant materials such as thorns, barbs, straws, and splinters.[3] Rarely, localized cutaneous and subcutaneous infections disseminate to bones, joints, lungs, meninges, genitourinary tract, and other internal organs.[4–6] Even more rarely, inhaled aerosolized fungal conidia cause a primary pulmonary infection, which also may disseminate to skin, bones, joints, and viscera.[7,8] Although sporotrichosis is not contagious, persons can become infected by accidental inoculation or contamination of skin wounds with lesional exudates or other infectious materials.

GEOGRAPHIC DISTRIBUTION

Sporotrichosis is worldwide—in temperate as well as tropical climates—where the fungus exists in nature as a saprophyte of soil, wild and domesticated plants, trees, sphagnum moss, and decaying vegetation.[3] Most documented infections have been in the United States, South Africa, Japan, Mexico, and South America.

EPIDEMIOLOGY

Sporotrichosis is usually sporadic and frequently an occupational disease. It occurs more often in gardeners, farmers, forestry workers, hay-mulching workers, miners, florists, and others who spend much of their time outdoors and are frequently exposed to plants and soil.[1,3] The largest epidemics have been in South African miners.[9,10] Those with profound immunodeficiencies, or who have serious underlying diseases, or are chronic alcoholics are at greatest risk of disseminated infection.[8,11] Disseminated sporotrichosis with extensive cutaneous or osteoarticular involvement has been reported in patients infected with the human immunodeficiency virus and with acquired immunodeficiency syndrome (AIDS).[12–15] There are no significant gender or racial predispositions and the disease may occur at any age.

MORPHOLOGIC FEATURES OF THE ORGANISM

Sporothrix schenckii is thermally dimorphic; it develops as a mycelial form when grown in vitro at room temperature, and as a yeast form when grown at 37°C in vitro or in host tissues.[16] Mycelial-form cultures grow rapidly and have a wrinkled or folded membranous surface that is white at first but later becomes brown or, occasionally, black. A fine, grayish, velvety aerial mycelium forms at the borders of some colonies. Microscopically, the cultures consist of relatively narrow, branched, septate, hyaline hyphae and abundant conidia. The oval conidia, which measure 2 × 3 μm to 3 × 6 μm, are produced on delicate sterigmata along the hyphae and terminally on conidiophores. Yeast-form colonies of *S schenckii* are moist, creamy, and white. Microscopically, they consist of single and budding yeastlike cells that are spherical, oval, or elongated, ranging from 2 to 10 μm in greatest diameter. Yeast forms identical in appearance to those in culture also occur in infected host tissues and lesional exudates.[2,17]

CLINICAL FEATURES

The two major clinical forms of sporotrichosis are cutaneous (lymphocutaneous) and systemic.[1,2,17] The classic and more familiar clinical form in humans is lymphocutaneous. Lesions consist of a linear chain of painless subcutaneous nodules that extend indolently along the course of lymphatic drainage from a primary nodular-ulcerative skin lesion, which develops at the site of traumatic percutaneous inoculation of the fungus (Figures 121–1, A and B, and 121–2). The primary lesion appears 1 week to several months after inoculation and usually occurs on an exposed part, most often the hand, arm, face, or neck, and occasionally upper chest, foot, or leg. The secondary lymphatic nodules begin to develop about 2 weeks after the appearance of the primary skin lesion and, in time, may ulcerate and discharge pus; regional lymphadenopathy is uncommon, and there are no constitutional symptoms. Primary cutaneous lesions without lymphatic involvement or with minimal lymphangitis occur more frequently than the classic lymphocutaneous form of sporotrichosis (Figure 121–3). Clinically, these solitary nodular, verrucous, or ulcerative lesions are often misdiagnosed as a neoplasm, especially squamous cell carcinoma, and excised more widely than necessary.

Systemic sporotrichosis is often localized to a single organ system, such as bone and joint or the lower respiratory tract, but, as noted, infection may occasionally disseminate to multiple organs. Dissemination is by the bloodstream and from a primary cutaneous or, rarely, a pulmonary focus. The organs most frequently involved are bones, joints, skin, brain, and lungs.

Pulmonary lesions in sporotrichosis usually develop after hematogenous dissemination from a primary cutaneous infection, where articular, osseous, and widespread cutaneous lesions predominate.[18] In disseminated sporotrichosis, the lungs are involved secondarily in fewer than 20% of cases. In both primary and secondary pulmonary sporotrichosis, clinical and radiographic features are indistinguishable from those of other chronic, progressive pulmonary infections that cause granulomatous and cavitary lesions, eg, tuberculosis and histoplasmosis capsulati.[8] Furthermore, it can be difficult to distinguish sporotrichosis from sarcoidosis, because the two diseases share a variety of pathologic and radiologic features.[19] Radiographic findings in pulmonary sporotrichosis include patchy fibronodular infiltrates, linear streaks, cavitary lesions, and, rarely, pleural effusions.

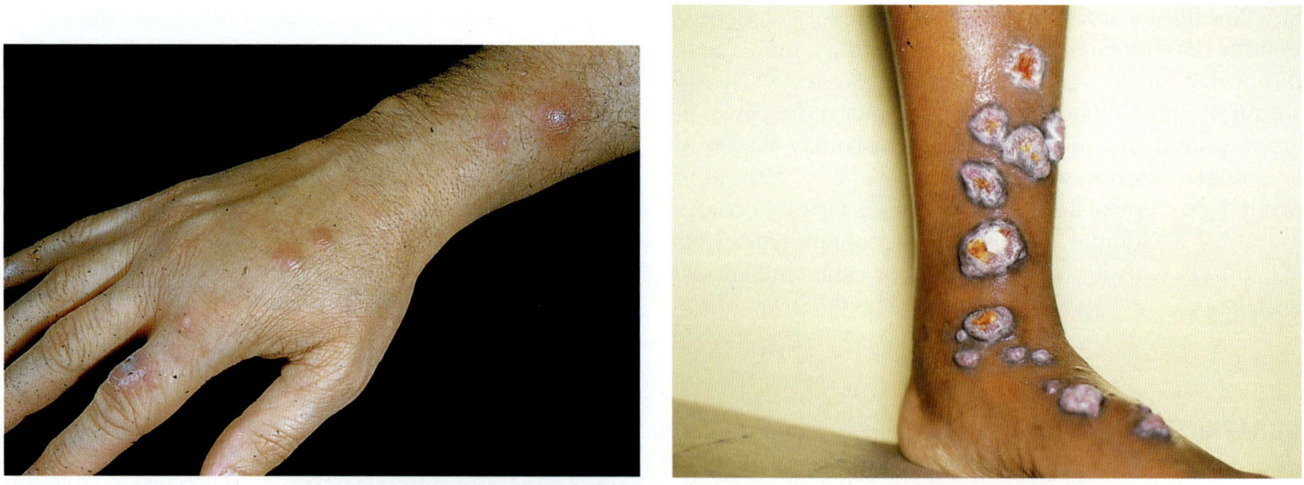

A B

Figure 121–1. (**A**) Lymphocutaneous form of sporotrichosis. A linear chain of small subcutaneous nodules extends along the course of lymphatic drainage from a primary nodular-ulcerative lesion on the forefinger. (**B**) A more striking example of lymphocutaneous sporotrichosis in a youth living in the Natal Province, Republic of South Africa. *(By Daniel H. Connor, MD, 1985.)*

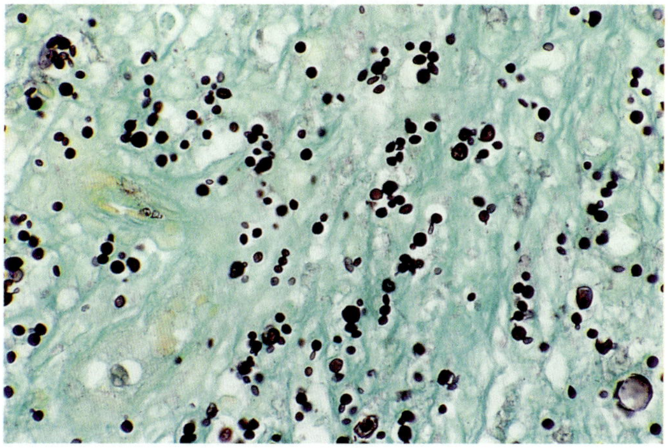

Figure 121–7. Cutaneous sporotrichosis. Proliferating yeast forms of *S schenckii* are spherical, oval, and elongated, and range from 2 to 10 μm or more in diameter. Here, unlike most primary cutaneous lesions of sporotrichosis, there are an unusually large number of fungal cells (GMS, ×160).

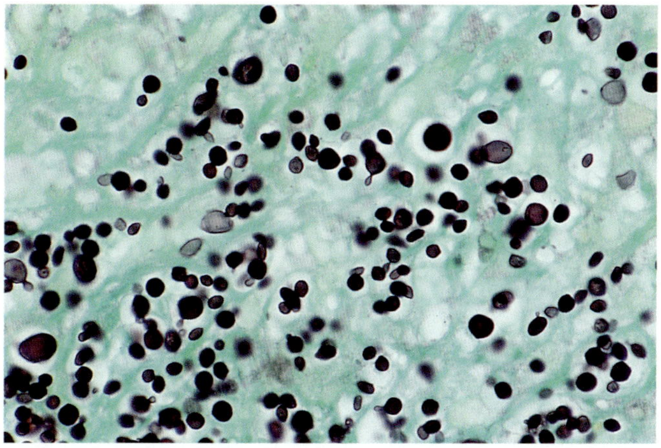

Figure 121–9. Yeastlike cells in disseminated sporotrichosis. Note variation in size and shape of unusually numerous fungal cells. Budding is by a narrow base *(top center)* (GMS, ×250).

divide by either budding or partitioning (septation).[2,27] In partitioning, daughter cells separate by dissolution of the parent cell wall, giving the appearance of a pair of eyeglasses. In spontaneous human lesions and in experimentally induced lesions in animals, both large septate and small budding forms of the *luriei* variety of *S schenckii* are usually present (Figure 121–12).

The demonstration of small numbers of morphologically typical yeast forms, either free or enveloped by Splendore–Hoeppli material (the asteroid body), justifies a presumptive histopathologic diagnosis of sporotrichosis, especially in the context of the histopathologic findings described earlier.[2,17] A definitive diagnosis, however, usually requires direct immunofluorescence of *S schenckii* cells in formalin-fixed deparaffinized tissue sections (Figure 121–13), or isolation and identification of the fungus in culture.[28–30] The asteroid body in sporotrichosis is almost always in a microabscess or in the suppurative center of a granuloma. It consists of one or more yeastlike cells intimately surrounded by a stellate, radiating corona of Splendore–Hoeppli material, 20 to 40 μm in diameter, that is refractile and intensely eosinophilic (Figure 121–14). This material is

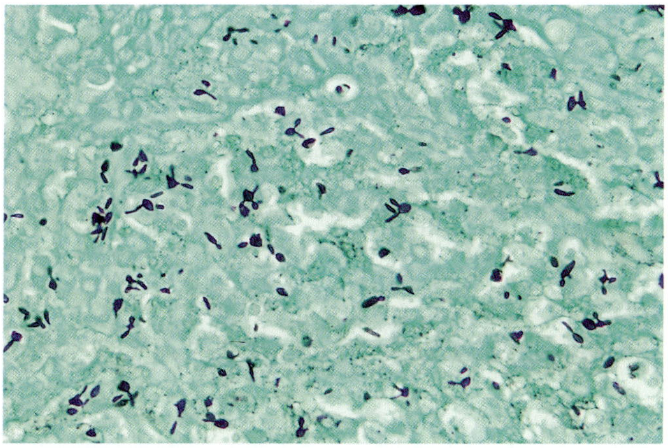

Figure 121–8. Sporotrichotic lymphadenitis. Numerous pleomorphic yeastlike cells of *S schenckii* have elongated "teardrop" and "pipestem" buds. Some of the fungal cells also have multiple buds (GMS, ×100).

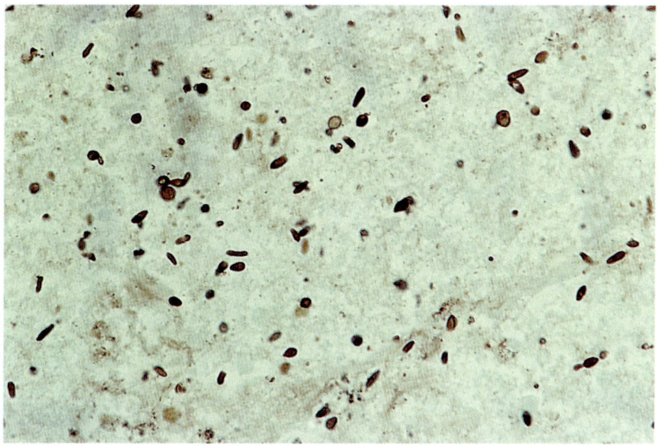

Figure 121–10. Primary pulmonary sporotrichosis. This fibrocaseous granuloma contains spherical, oval, and elongated (cigar-shaped) yeast forms of *S schenckii.* Note that buds are attached to parent cells by a narrow base *(lower right)* (GMS, ×160).

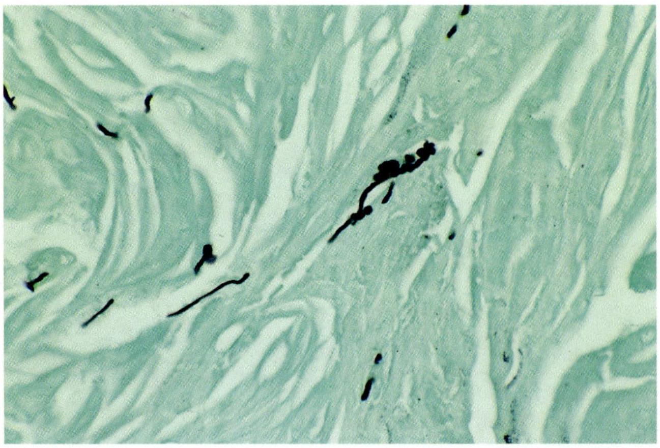

Figure 121–11. Primary cutaneous sporotrichosis. This is the superficial hyperkeratotic layer of the lesion and it contains narrow, septate, infrequently branched hyphae and hyphal fragments of *S schenckii* that bear spherical conidia. Hyphae of *S schenckii* are occasionally produced in hyperkeratotic lesions, and should not be mistaken for other fungi that typically produce hyphae in tissues (GMS, ×160).

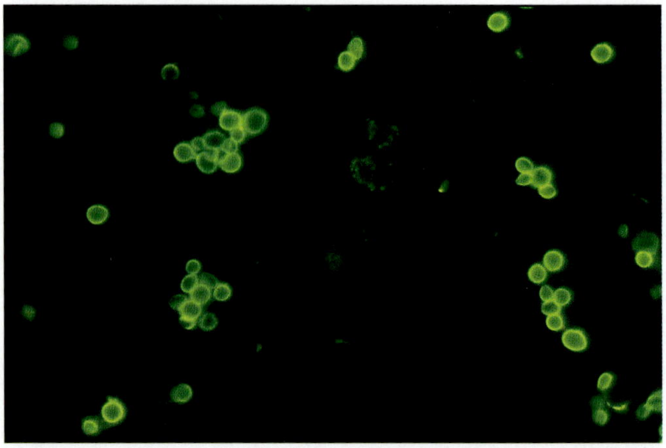

Figure 121–13. Cutaneous sporotrichosis. Brightly decorated yeastlike cells of *S schenckii* are in a deparaffinized section of formalin-fixed tissue. The section was stained with fluorescein-labeled antiglobulins specific for this fungus. Note multiple budding cells *(right center)* (direct immunofluorescence, ×250).

primarily glycoprotein of host origin that is caused by a localized antigen–antibody reaction on the surface of the *S schenckii* cells in the hypersensitized host.[2,31] There is a common misconception that the asteroid body is pathognomonic for sporotrichosis. However, Splendore–Hoeppli material also can form around compact aggregates of bacteria in the lesions of actinomycosis and botryomycosis, and around mycetoma granules, parasite ova, and foreign objects such as silk sutures, and may occur in invasive infections caused by other species of fungi, particularly *Coccidioides immitis, Aspergillus* sp, *Candida* sp and the agents of entomophthoromycosis.[2,32,33] Conversely, asteroid formation does not occur in most cases of sporotrichosis. Therefore, the absence of asteroid bodies does not rule out the possibility of sporotrichosis, and their presence does not justify a definitive diagnosis of sporotrichosis.

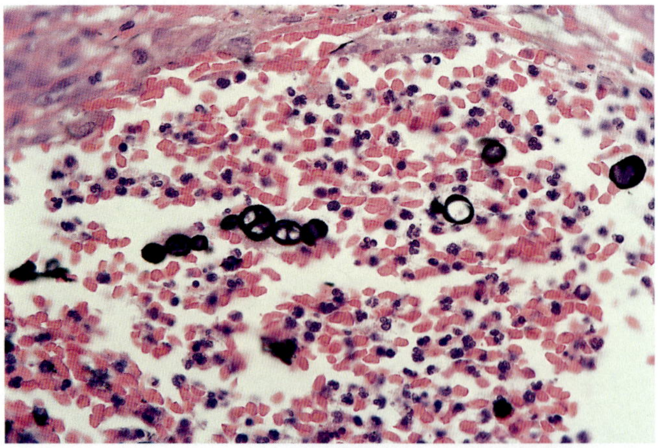

Figure 121–12. Cutaneous sporotrichosis caused by *S schenckii* var *luriei.* This rare variety produces small, budding yeast forms (morphologically similar to those of the classic variety) and large, thick-walled cells, up to 20 μm in diameter, that form transverse septa *(left center)* and divide by either budding or partitioning (septation) (GMS-H&E, ×160).

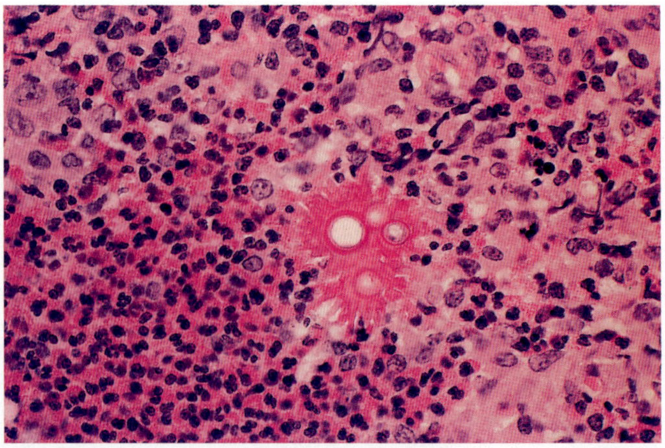

Figure 121–14. Asteroid body in sporotrichosis. Three spherical, weakly stained yeastlike cells of *S schenckii* are ensheathed by intensely eosinophilic, elongated spicules of Splendore–Hoeppli material. One fungal cell is budding *(top center)*. The asteroid body is embedded in the suppurative center of a granuloma (H&E, ×160).

DIFFERENTIAL DIAGNOSIS

Hamazaki-Wesenberg bodies (yellow-brown bodies, chromogenic bodies, elliptical bodies, Hamazaki corpuscles), commonly in the lymphoid tissues of lymph nodes with sarcoidosis and other sarcoid-like granulomas,[34–37] are occasionally mistaken for the yeastlike cells of *S schenckii* (Figure 121–15).[2] Because these bodies are GMS positive and often elliptical, they have been misidentified as the elongated "cigar bodies" of *S schenckii*. In H&E stained sections, however, Hamazaki–Wesenberg bodies have a golden-brown color, are refractile, do not bud, often have a more deeply pigmented core, and are usually much smaller and more pleomorphic than the hyaline, budding yeast forms in sporotrichosis (Figure 121–15).[2,17]

Giant cells in sarcoidosis and other granulomatous lesions may contain deeply eosinophilic, asteroid-like inclusions that can be mistaken for the asteroid bodies of sporotrichosis.[2,19] These inclusions, however, are intracellular, nonrefractile, and do not contain fungal cells, unlike the asteroid bodies of sporotrichosis.

Large, spherical, nonbudding yeastlike cells of *S schenckii* sometimes show only peripheral staining and appear empty. When these ringlike forms with optically clear centers are not accompanied by typical *S schenckii* cells, they can be mistaken for small, empty spherules of *C immitis* or large, empty, nonbudding yeastlike cells of *Blastomyces dermatitidis*.[2] Uniformly small, spherical to oval *S schenckii* cells within epithelioid histiocytes and giant cells of disseminated lesions can sometimes resemble the yeastlike cells of *Histoplasma capsulatum* var *capsulatum* and capsule-deficient *Cryptococcus neoformans*. In all of these, the diagnosis can be confirmed immunohistologically by direct immunofluorescence.[2,29]

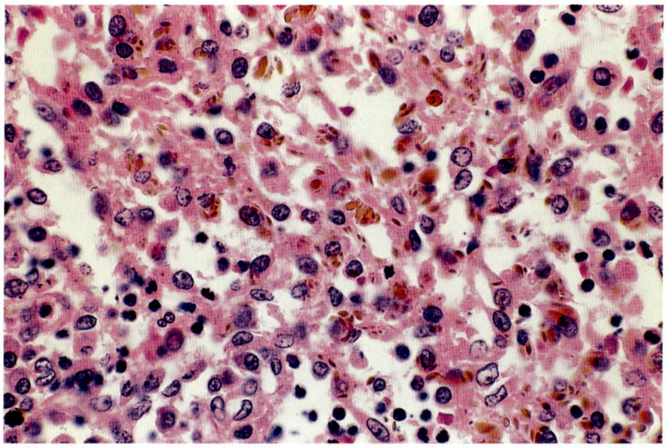

Figure 121–15. Hamazaki–Wesenberg (H–W) bodies contiguous to sarcoid granulomas in a lymph node. These bodies are sometimes mistaken for yeast forms of *S schenckii*. When stained with H&E, however, H–W bodies are brown, refractile, lack buds, and often have a deeply pigmented core. They are usually smaller and more pleomorphic than the hyaline, budding yeast forms of *S schenckii* (H&E, ×160).

CONFIRMATIONAL TESTING AND DIAGNOSIS

A definitive diagnosis of sporotrichosis is based on isolation and identification of the fungus in culture, or on direct immunofluorescence of *S schenckii* cells in tissue sections or cytologic preparations (Figure 121–13).[16,28] The fungus is readily cultured from exudates or biopsy specimens placed on Sabouraud's medium, but is sparse and sometimes difficult to demonstrate by direct examination of smears or tissue sections. A wide variety of serologic tests also are useful for diagnosis.[38] Of these, the tube agglutination, latex agglutination, and indirect enzyme immunoassay procedures have demonstrated excellent sensitivity and specificity, and are considered to be the most reliable. All of these serologic assays can be performed on either serum or cerebrospinal fluid, and they are of particular value for the diagnosis of extracutaneous infections.

REFERENCES

1. Bullpitt P, Weedon D. Sporotrichosis: a review of 39 cases. *Pathology*. 1978;10:249–256.
2. Chandler FW, Watts JC. *Pathologic Diagnosis of Fungal Infections*. Chicago: ASCP Press; 1987:193–202.
3. Powell KE, Taylor A, Phillips BJ, et al. Cutaneous sporotrichosis in forestry workers: epidemic due to contaminated moss. *JAMA*. 1978;240:232–235.
4. Marrocco GR, Tihen WS, Goodnough CP, Johnson RJ. Granulomatous synovitis and osteitis caused by *Sporothrix schenckii*. *Am J Clin Pathol*. 1975;64:345–350.
5. Brook CJ, Ravikrishnan KP, Weg JG. Pulmonary and articular sporotrichosis. *Am Rev Respir Dis*. 1977;116:141–143.
6. Smith PW, Loomis GW, Luckasen JL, et al. Disseminated cutaneous sporotrichosis: three illustrative cases. *Arch Dermatol*. 1981;117:143–144.
7. Michelson E. Primary pulmonary sporotrichosis. *Ann Thorac Surg*. 1977;24:83–86.
8. Watts JC, Chandler FW. Primary pulmonary sporotrichosis. *Arch Pathol Lab Med*. 1987;111:215–217. Editorial.
9. Sporotrichosis infection in mines of the Witwatersrand. In: *Proceedings of Transvaal Medical Officer's Association*. Johannesburg, South Africa: Transvaal Chamber of Mines; 1947.
10. Lurie HI. Five unusual cases of sporotrichosis from South Africa, showing lesions of muscles, bones, and viscera. *Br J Surg*. 1963;50:585–591.

11. Friedman SJ, Doyle JA. Extracutaneous sporotrichosis. *Int J Dermatol.* 1983;22:171–176.
12. Lipstein-Kresch E, Isenberg HD, Singer C, et al. Disseminated *Sporothrix schenckii* infection with arthritis in a patient with acquired immunodeficiency syndrome. *J Rheumatol.* 1985;12:805–808.
13. Bibler MR, Luber HJ, Glueck HI, et al. Disseminated sporotrichosis in a patient with HIV infection after treatment for acquired factor VIII inhibitor. *JAMA.* 1986;256: 3125–3126.
14. Fitzpatrick JE, Eubanks S. Acquired immunodeficiency syndrome presenting as disseminated cutaneous sporotrichosis. *Int J Dermatol.* 1988;27:406–407.
15. Viviani MA, Tortorano AM. Unusual mycoses in AIDS patients. In: Bossche HV, Mackenzie DWR, Cauwenbergh G, et al, eds. *Mycoses in AIDS Patients.* New York: Plenum Press; 1990:147–153.
16. Ajello L, Kaplan W. A new variant of *Sporothrix schenckii. Mykosen.* 1969;12:633–644.
17. Lurie HI. Histopathology of sporotrichosis. *Arch Pathol.* 1963;75:92–109.
18. Pluss JL, Opal SM. Pulmonary sporotrichosis: review of treatment and outcome. *Medicine (Baltimore).* 1986;65: 143–153.
19. Boehm D, Lynch JM, Hodges GR, et al. Case report. Disseminated sporotrichosis presenting as sarcoidosis: electron microscopic and immunologic studies. *Am J Med Sci.* 1982;283:71–78.
20. England DM, Hochholzer L. Primary pulmonary sporotrichosis: report of eight cases with clinicopathologic review. *Am J Surg Pathol.* 1985;9:193–204.
21. England DM, Hochholzer L. *Sporothrix* infection of the lung without cutaneous disease: primary pulmonary sporotrichosis. *Arch Pathol Lab Med.* 1987;111:298–300.
22. Parker JD, Sarosi GA, Tosh FE. Treatment of extracutaneous sporotrichosis. *Arch Intern Med.* 1970:125:858–863.
23. Restrepo A, Robledo J, Gomez I, et al. Itraconazole therapy in lymphangitic and cutaneous sporotrichosis. *Arch Dermatol.* 1986;122:413–417.
24. Winn WC, Jr, Chandler FW. Bacterial infections. In: Dail DH, Hammar SP, eds. *Pulmonary Pathology.* 2nd ed. New York: Springer-Verlag; 1994:255–330.
25. Maberry JD, Mullins JF, Stone OJ. Sporotrichosis with demonstration of hyphae in human tissue. *Arch Dermatol.* 1966;93:65–67.
26. Berson SD, Brandt FA. Primary pulmonary sporotrichosis with unusual fungal morphology. *Thorax.* 1977;32:505–508.
27. Alberici F, Paties CT, Lombardi G, et al. *Sporothrix schenckii* var *luriei* as the cause of sporotrichosis in Italy. *Eur J Epidemiol.* 1989;5:173–177.
28. Kaplan W, Gonzalez-Ochoa A. Application of the fluorescent antibody technique to the rapid diagnosis of sporotrichosis. *J Lab Clin Med.* 1963;62:835–841.
29. Kaplan W, Kraft DE. Demonstration of pathogenic fungi in formalin-fixed tissues by immunofluorescence. *Am J Clin Pathol.* 1969;52:420–432.
30. Font RL, Jakobiec FA. Granulomatous necrotizing retinochoroiditis caused by *Sporotrichum schenckii:* report of a case including immunofluorescence and electron microscopical studies. *Arch Ophthalmol.* 1976;94:1513–1519.
31. Lurie HI, Still WJS. The "capsule" of *Sporotrichum schenckii* and the evolution of the asteroid body: a light and electron microscopic study. *Sabouraudia.* 1969;7: 64–70.
32. Von Lichtenberg F, Smith JH, Cheever AW. The Hoeppli phenomenon in schistosomiasis: comparative pathology and immunopathology. *Am J Trop Med Hyg.* 1966;15: 886–895.
33. Liber AF, Choi HH. Splendore–Hoeppli phenomenon about silk sutures in tissue. *Arch Pathol.* 1973;95:217–220.
34. Doyle WF, Brahman HD, Burgess JH. The nature of yellow-brown bodies in peritoneal lymph nodes: histochemical and electron microscopic evaluation of these bodies in a case of suspected sarcoidosis. *Arch Pathol.* 1973;96: 320–326.
35. Moscovic EA. Sarcoidosis and mycobacterial L-forms. A critical reappraisal of pleomorphic chromogenic bodies (Hamazaki corpuscles) in lymph nodes. *Pathol Annu.* 1978;13(2):69–164.
36. Tudway AJC. Yellow bodies in superficial and deep lymph nodes. *J Clin Pathol.* 1979;32:52–55.
37. Ro JY, Luna MA, Mackay B, et al. Yellow-brown (Hamazaki–Wesenberg) bodies mimicking fungal yeasts. *Arch Pathol Lab Med.* 1987;111:555–559.
38. Scott EN, Kaufman L, Brown AC, et al. Serologic studies in the diagnosis and management of meningitis due to *Sporothrix schenckii. N Engl J Med.* 1987;317:935–940.

CHAPTER 122

Superficial Fungal Infections

Rod J. Hay and Francis W. Chandler

When excessive perspiration makes it needful to wipe the face, it ought to be done with a handkerchief, and not with the hand, except in the case of extreme necessity; by attending to this, serious inconvenience may be avoided, for the rubbing of the hand on the face may give rise to ringworm, pimples, etc.

St. Jean Baptiste de la Salle (1651–1719), The Rule of Christian Manners and Civility, I

DERMATOPHYTOSIS

Definition and Epidemiology

Dermatophytosis is a common superficial infection caused by fungi that are able to invade keratinized tissues—stratum corneum, hair, and nails.[1] Dermatophytes are worldwide in distribution, although the prevalence of different organisms varies among different parts of the world. The source of human infections may be another human (anthropophilic), an animal (zoophilic), or soil (geophilic). Infections by dermatophytes are generally endemic but sometimes they may assume epidemic proportions, for instance, in service personnel and coal miners. Infections of the scalp (tinea capitis), particularly those caused by anthropophilic dermatophytes such as *Trichophyton tonsurans,* may be epidemic in children.[2] Synonyms of dermatophytosis include ringworm and tinea.

Etiologic Agents

The dermatophytes comprise 28 taxonomically related species of the genera *Microsporum, Trichophyton,* and *Epidermophyton.* The most common dermatophyte, *T rubrum,* is isolated most commonly from tinea pedis and onychomycosis in temperate climates, and tinea cruris and tinea corporis in the tropics. In common with other anthropophilic infections, lesions caused by *T rubrum* are typically noninflamed and chronic (Figure 122–1). Invasion of the hair shafts by anthropophilic fungi also causes relatively noninflamed lesions. By contrast, infections caused by zoophilic dermatophytes such as *T verrucosum* and *M canis* are generally very inflammatory and may present with itchy, erythematous patches as well as pustules. Favus is a specific type of scalp ringworm caused by a single anthropophilic organism, *T schoenleinii,* which causes a crusted scalp infection with subsequent hair loss.[3] Tinea imbricata, or Tokelau, is infection by *T concentricum,* which causes an extensive form of tinea corporis in parts of the humid tropics such as Papua New Guinea and Malaysia. Lesions are composed of concentric rings of scales and cover large areas of the body[4] (Figure 122–2). Infections of nail (onychomycosis) caused by dermatophytes affect about 3% of the population and cause progressive destruction of the nail plate (Figure 122–3).

Clinical Features

The common varieties of clinical disease caused by the dermatophytes are well described. The archetypical pattern is a ring of inflammatory scaling with diminution of inflammation toward the center. This pattern is modified depending on the dermatophyte and the site of infection.[5] Invasion of the hair shaft generally produces scaling and eventually loss of hairs. Hairs are invaded by the fungal hyphae and break either at scalp level or a few millimeters above. In most invasions of hair shaft, the fungi form chains of vegetative spores called arthroconidia either outside the hair shaft (ectothrix) or within the hair itself (endothrix). In favus, the hair shafts are

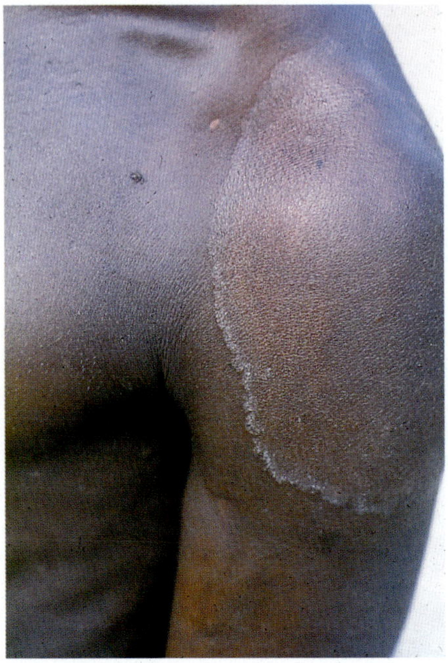

Figure 122–1. Dermatophytosis (tinea corporis) caused by *T rubrum.* A ring of scaling with minimal inflammation and central clearing involves the upper arm and shoulder.

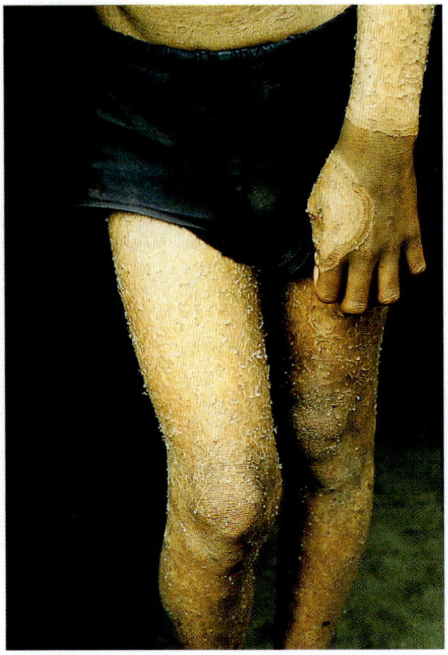

Figure 122–2. Tinea imbricata caused by *T concentricum.* Note the concentric rings of scales.

invaded by hyphae, and eventually degenerate leaving air spaces within the hair medulla.

Pathology

Infections by dermatophytes are generally diagnosed by microscopic examination of skin scrapings in 10% potassium hydroxide, or by culture. When biopsy specimens are submitted, the host reaction in dermatophytosis is variable. The epidermis often appears to be unaffected in hematoxylin-eosin (H&E) stained sections, or it may be mildly hyperkeratotic with patchy parakeratosis. In the dermis, there is a mild to intense perivascular infiltrate with lymphocytes and plasma cells. The epidermis may be spongiotic in acute lesions, and in very inflamed lesions, neutrophils accumulate in microabscesses. Hyperkeratosis may sometimes be marked. Dermatophytosis can mimic other inflammatory conditions such as eczema, erythema multiforme, or folliculitis.[6]

In tissue sections, the dermatophytes are hyaline and not readily demonstrated with H&E. Gomori's methenamine silver (GMS) and periodic acid–Schiff (PAS) procedures reveal that fungal elements are confined, in most cases, to the stratum corneum. There are hyphae and arthroconidia, which may be particularly prominent in hair follicles.

In infections of scalp, the inflammatory infiltrate is similar to that in other parts of the body, although the hair follicle becomes a focus of neutrophilic aggregation.[7] In later stages of infection, the cellular composition alters with a predominance of lymphocytes, plasma cells, and some giant cells. When special stains for fungi

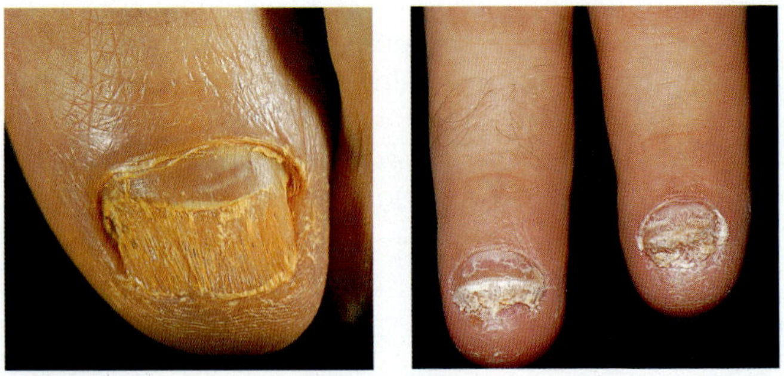

A B

Figure 122–3. (**A**) Left great toe of an old man with onychomycosis caused by *T rubrum.* Note destruction and discoloration of the nail. *(Contributed by Daniel H. Connor, MD, 1994.)* (**B**) Onychomycosis of fingernails of a young man. There is disfiguring destruction of the nails of several fingers on both hands and also of the nails of the feet.

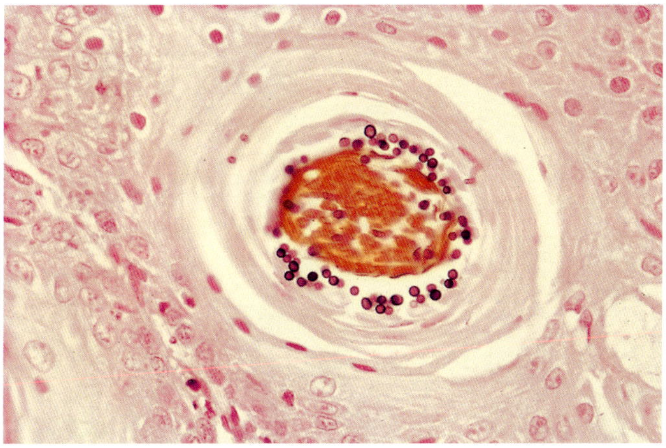

Figure 122–4. Dermatophytosis. Arthroconidia surround a hair shaft in this ectothrix scalp infection caused by *M canis* (GMS-H&E, ×160).

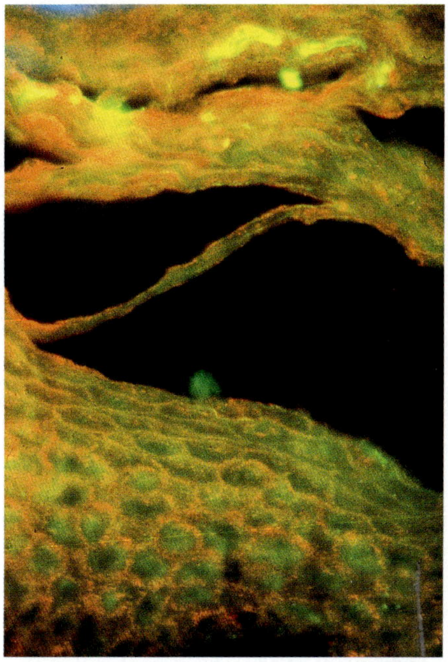

Figure 122–5. Tinea pedis caused by *T rubrum*. Fungal elements within a routinely processed skin section are brightly decorated when stained with a fluorescein-conjugated antibody to the fungus (direct immunofluorescence, ×100).

are used, hyphae can be seen within the stratum corneum of the hair shaft and the hair itself. Invasion of the hair shaft probably originates from the stratum corneum of perifollicular epidermis. Germinating hyphae penetrate the hair follicle and enter the hair cortex using expanded specialized hyphal structures called penetrating organs. Fungal growth does not occur within the hair shaft below the keratinizing zone. The typical forms of sporulation (endothrix and ectothrix, discussed earlier) can be seen in tissue sections (Figure 122–4). Arthroconidia appear as uniformly stained spherical bodies. They may be confused with yeast forms, although the absence of budding and their clustering within or around hair shafts are typical. Other stains used to demonstrate dermatophytes in smears and tissue sections include fluorescein-conjugated antibodies (Figure 122–5)[8] and fluorescein-conjugated lectins.[9] They have no specific advantage, however, over conventional methods of diagnosis.

A kerion is a severely inflamed dermatophyte infection that involves the hair shafts.[10] Spongiosis and dermal abscesses are marked. The pyogenic response has given rise to the view that kerions are secondarily infected by bacteria, but in practice this is seldom so; the host response is directed toward fungi alone. Fungal hyphae are seldom demonstrated in the inflammatory infiltrate, although small hyphal fragments may be free or in giant cells. With resolution, the inflammatory infiltrate becomes more lymphocytic (Figure 122–6). In certain chronic infections, an inflammatory or Majocchi's dermatophytic granuloma remains in the dermis and is characterized by organized granulomas with giant cells.

Favus is characterized clinically by grayish crusts called scutula that surround hairs. A scutulum consists of focal hyperkeratosis and collections of neutrophils. With well-established lesions, this may depress the stratum corneum, causing a widening of the follicular aperture, and adjacent scutula subsequently amalgamate. The undersurface of the crust is lined by neutrophils. The characteristic type of hair invasion can be seen using PAS or GMS stains.

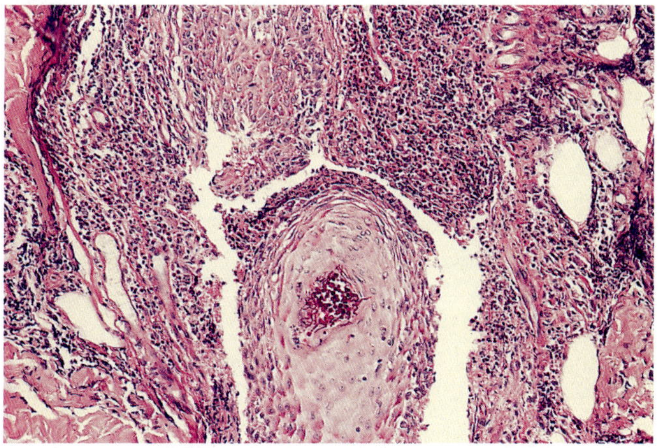

Figure 122–6. Majocchi's granuloma. Extrafollicular fungal elements of *M canis* stimulate a mixed suppurative and granulomatous inflammatory reaction in the dermis (PAS, ×40).

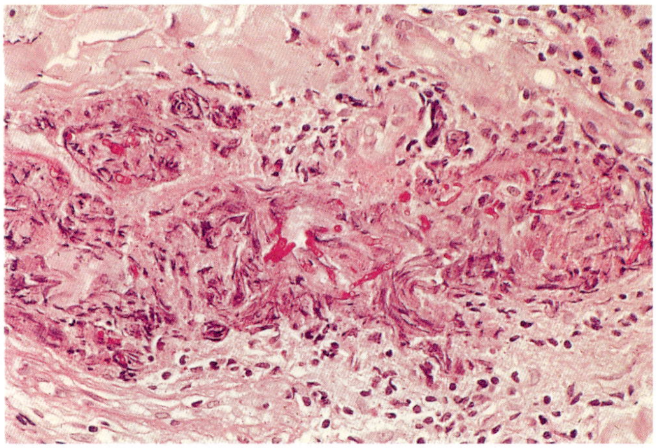

Figure 122–7. Deep dermatophyte infection caused by *T rubrum*. Individual hyphae and hyphal fragments within the dermis are surrounded by mixed inflammatory cells (PAS, ×40).

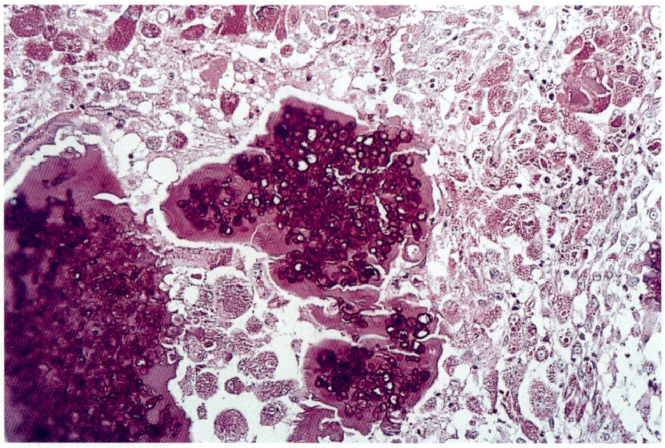

Figure 122–9. Dermatophytic pseudomycetoma. Aggregated and distorted fungal elements are embedded in and surrounded by abundant, intensely PAS-positive, Splendore–Hoeppli–like material (PAS, ×100).

Rarely, dermatophytes invade the deeper nonkeratinized skin and subcutaneous tissues where they produce nodular or dispersed lesions and evoke a mixed suppurative and granulomatous reaction (Figure 122–7). Occasionally, intrafollicular dermatophytes invade the contiguous dermis through defects in the follicular walls. In some of these deep-seated infections, extrafollicular fungal elements within the dermis occur as individual hyphae and arthroconidia, and the lesion is referred to as Majocchi's granuloma (Figure 122–6). In other lesions, the organized clustering of individual fungal elements forms loose or compact aggregates of varying sizes that resemble the granules of eumycotic, white grain mycetomas (Figure 122–8). The aggregated fungal elements are frequently embedded in and surrounded by abundant, PAS-positive Splendore–Hoeppli–like material (Figure 122–9). These endogenous mycelial aggregates are erroneously considered by some to be granules or grains and the lesion to be a mycetoma. The mycelial aggregates, however, are almost always associated with and contiguous to individual fungal elements (Figure 122–10) and are more properly termed pseudogranules. The microscopic appearance of dermatophytic pseudomycetomas is strikingly similar irrespective of the causal agent, and the histopathologic pattern resembles that seen in mycetomas.[11] In addition, typical

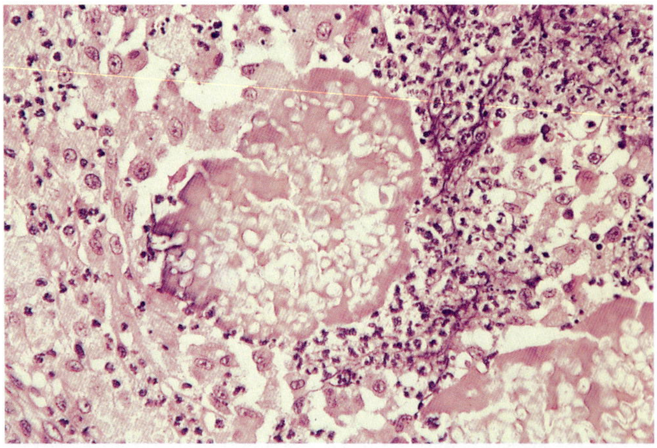

Figure 122–8. Dermatophytic pseudomycetoma caused by *M canis*. A compact aggregate of hyaline fungi (pseudogranule) is embedded in eosinophilic Splendore–Hoeppli–like material and surrounded by mixed suppurative and granulomatous inflammation (H&E, ×100).

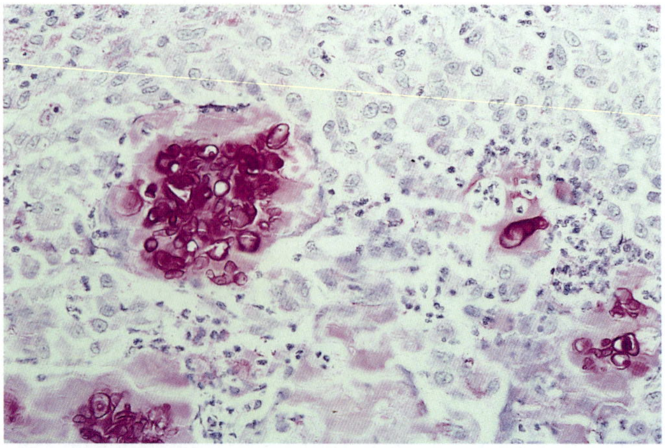

Figure 122–10. Deep dermatophytic granuloma caused by *M canis*. The dermis contains mycelial aggregates (pseudogranules) that are contiguous to individual fungal elements (PAS, ×160).

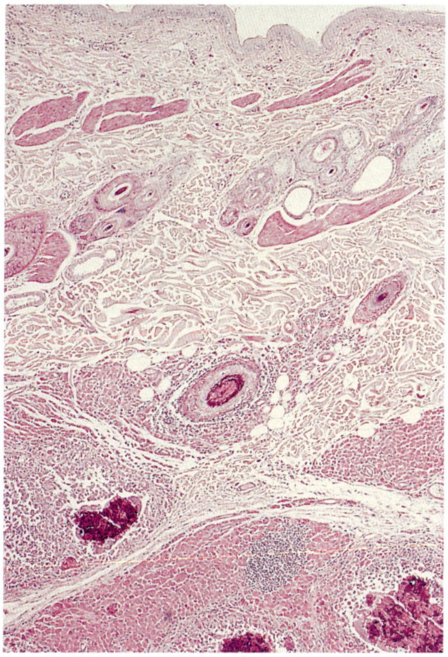

Figure 122–11. Dermatophytic pseudomycetoma caused by *M canis.* The deep dermis and subcutaneous tissue contain compact aggregates of dermatophytic hyphae. Numerous arthroconidia are seen in an adjacent, intact hair follicle (PAS, ×16).

dermatophytic elements can often be demonstrated in overlying intact hair follicles (Figure 122–11). Such pseudomycetomas have been caused by the following dermatophytes: *M audouinii, M canis, M ferrugineum, T mentagrophytes, T rubrum, T tonsurans,* and *T violaceum.* Systemic dermatophytosis is extremely rare[12–14] and its appearance resembles other deep fungal infections caused by organisms such as the *Aspergillus* sp. In addition, the dermis is often a focus of inflammation with granuloma formation, and there may be extensive hyperkeratosis. Metastatic abscesses can be in organs such as liver and brain.

Differential Diagnosis

Conventional stains for fungi (GMS and PAS) are generally sufficient to demonstrate dermatophytes in tissue. Few other organisms will cause a similar pattern of invasive disease in the stratum corneum apart from *Scytalidium dimidiatum (Hendersonula toruloidea)* and *S hyalinum;* both of these fungi cause infections of foot, hand, and nail that can clinically mimic dermatophytosis. The hyphae of these fungi in biopsy specimens resemble the dermatophytes, but they can be distinguished by culture. These infections are mainly seen in the tropics, although they may be diagnosed occasionally in the southern United States and Europe.

Confirmational Testing and Diagnosis

The diagnosis of dermatophytosis is confirmed by direct microscopy of skin scrapings, nail clippings, or hair samples mounted in 10% potassium hydroxide. The chains of arthroconidia are typical. The shapes of the colonies and microscopic appearances of dermatophytes isolated from these materials on Sabouraud's dextrose agar are diagnostic, although other confirmatory tests such as hair penetration may be used.

Treatment

Dermatophytosis of limited extent can usually be treated with one of several different topical antifungal agents ranging from benzoic acid compound (Whitfield's ointment) to azole antifungals (miconazole, clotrimazole). For widespread infections, however, or for infections involving hair or nails, oral therapy with griseofulvin, itraconazole, or terbinafine is most effective.

INFECTIONS BY *MALASSEZIA* SPECIES

Pityriasis versicolor, tinea versicolor, tinea flava, dermatomycosis furfuracea, malassezia folliculitis, seborrheic dermatitis (seborrheic eczema or dermatitis seborrheica) are synonyms for malassezia infections.

The lipophilic yeastlike fungus, *Malassezia furfur,* and other *Malassezia* sp have been implicated in a number of conditions including pityriasis versicolor (tinea versicolor), a form of folliculitis (malassezia folliculitis), and in the pathogenesis of seborrheic dermatitis.[15] Lesions of pityriasis versicolor are rarely biopsied because the organisms can be readily seen on skin scrapings (Figure 122–12). The epidermal changes are minimal with mild hyperkeratosis, follicular plugging, and acanthosis[16] (Figure 122–13). The organisms are well demonstrated with the PAS stain and appear as multiple spherical to oval yeasts that are often mixed with short, stubby, infrequently branched and curved hyphae 2.5 to 4 μm wide (Figure 122–12). Hyphal elements are sometimes difficult to demonstrate in biopsy specimens. In skin scrapings, the hyphae are often end to end. *Malassezia* yeasts, considered to be phialoconidia, are small (2 to 8 μm) and show polar bud formation. There is often a "lip" or unipolar, phialidic collarette around the point of bud initiation on the parent cell.

In malassezia folliculitis, yeast forms occupy plugged hair follicles.[17] There is often a dense perifollicular infiltrate of neutrophils and, in later stages, lymphocytes. It is not clear whether the presence of the

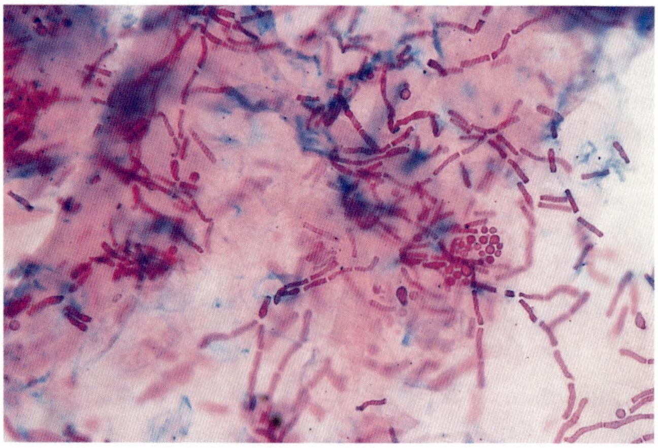

Figure 122–12. Pityriasis versicolor. Direct microscopy of a PAS-stained skin scraping reveals spherical to oval yeastlike cells, 2 to 8 μm in diameter, and short, stubby, infrequently branched and curved hyphae, 2.5 to 4 μm wide, that are often oriented end to end (×100).

fungus is cause or effect, although antifungal drugs help this condition.

Seborrheic dermatitis cannot be regarded as a true infection, although *Malassezia* yeasts are thought to be one main precipitating cause. Seborrheic dermatitis is common in both healthy subjects and AIDS patients,[18] but invasive fungal elements are not generally seen on histologic examination of lesions; surface colonization is usual.

Although *M furfur* commonly causes tinea versicolor, this lipid-dependent fungus can rarely cause fungemia and systemic infection (see Chapter 112). The latter is especially seen in patients receiving prolonged intralipid infusion through central venous catheters colonized with the fungus.[19–21] In systemic infections, the lungs are most frequently involved, probably because of increased lipid deposits in the walls of pulmonary blood vessels. Most of these infections occur in infants and in older patients with severe, chronic gastrointestinal disease. Patients often present with fever, sepsis, and thrombocytopenia. Severe systemic infections have been successfully treated with amphotericin B and other antifungals. Removal of colonized venous catheters, however, may be the only treatment necessary for *M furfur* fungemia.[19,21]

TINEA NIGRA

Pityriasis nigra, keratomycosis nigricans palmaris, microsporosis nigra, and ladosporiosis epidermica are synonyms for tinea nigra.

Tinea nigra is a superficial mycosis caused by *Exophiala werneckii (Phaeoanellomyces werneckii)*, a pigmented mycelial fungus. Seen mainly in tropical and subtropical areas, it usually presents as an asymptomatic, minimally scaly, pigmented macule on the palms or soles. Although tinea nigra is easily diagnosed by direct microscopic examination of skin scrapings, lesions may be excised in order to exclude the diagnosis of acral melanoma. The histopathologic features of tinea nigra are nonspecific and consist of hyperkeratosis and a mild mononuclear perivascular infiltrate in the dermis.[22] Pigmented hyphae in the stratum corneum, however, are easily detected with the H&E stain (Figure 122–14).

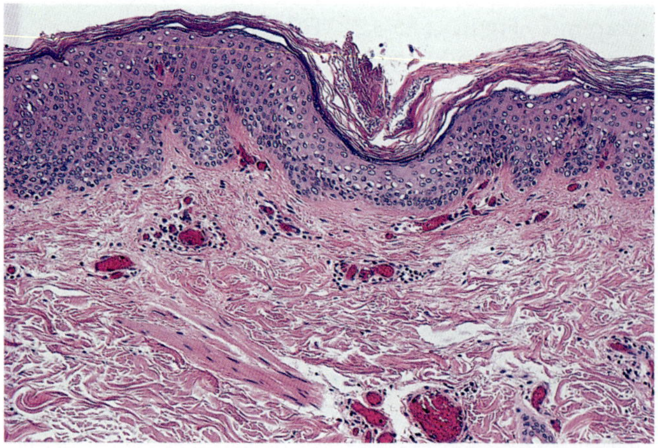

Figure 122–13. Pityriasis versicolor. A skin biopsy reveals clusters of hematoxylinophilic yeastlike cells and hyphal fragments of *M furfur* within the hyperkeratotic layer (H&E, ×40).

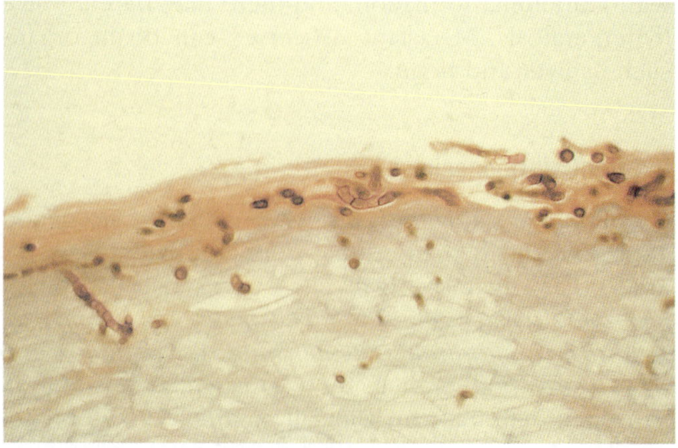

Figure 122–14. Tinea nigra. The stratum corneum contains narrow, dematiaceous (naturally pigmented) hyphae of *E werneckii* (H&E, ×100).

ONYCHOMYCOSIS

Although the appearances of fungi infecting nail plate material are nonspecific, nail biopsy is sometimes used to confirm the presence of fungi in nails that are grossly irregular, discolored, and distorted. Generally, the nail plate contains scattered mycelial elements that are best seen with PAS or GMS stains. In some infections, eg, those caused by *Scopulariopsis brevicaulis,* conidia also may be in the nail plate.[23] In *Candida* infections, a mixture of yeasts (blastoconidia), pseudohyphae, and hyphae is seen.

Other fungi may infect the skin. The lesions of many patients, however, are rarely biopsied, eg, in *Trichosporon* infections or white piedra.[24] Superficial *Candida* infections affecting the skin are common; the histopathology of candidiasis is described elsewhere (Chapter 102).

REFERENCES

1. Weitzman I, Summerbell RC. The dermatophytes. *Clin Microbiol Rev.* 1995;8:240–259.
2. Rippon JW. Epidemiology and emerging patterns of dermatophyte species. In: *Current Topics in Medical Mycology.* New York: Springer-Verlag; 1985;1:208–234.
3. Blank F. Human favus in Quebec. *Dermatologica.* 1962; 125:369–381.
4. Hay RJ, Reid S, Talwat E, MacNamara K. Endemic tinea imbricata—a study on Goodenough Island, PNG. *Trans Roy Soc Trop Med.* 1984;78:246–251.
5. Jones HE, Reinhardt JH, Rinaldi MG. A clinical, mycological and immunological survey of dermatophytosis. *Arch Dermatol.* 1973;107:61–68.
6. Strauss JS, Kligman AM. An experimental study of tinea pedis and onychomycosis of the foot. *Arch Dermatol.* 1957;76:70–79.
7. Kligman AM. The pathogenesis of tinea capitis due to *Microsporum audouinii* and *Microsporum canis. J Invest Dermatol.* 1952;18:231–246.
8. Hay RJ, Saeed EN. The immunofluorescent staining of fungi in chronic dermatophyte infections. *Clin Exp Dermatol.* 1981;18:231–246.
9. Roblez-Martinez W, Bhogal B, Morrell CA, Moore MK, Hay RJ. The use of fluorescent lectins to identify fungi in clinical material from skin. *Br J Dermatol.* 1990;123 (suppl 37):64.
10. Birt AR, Wilt JC. Mycology, bacteriology and histopathology of suppurative ringworm. *Arch Dermatol.* 1957;69: 441–448.
11. West BC, Kwon-Chung KJ. Mycetoma caused by *Microsporum audouinii. Am J Clin Pathol.* 1980;73:447–454.
12. Blank H, Smith JG. Widespread *Trichophyton rubrum* granulomas treated with griseofulvin. *Arch Dermatol.* 1960;81:779–785.
13. Liautaud B, Marill FG. La maladie dermatophytique. Observations Algeriennes recentes. *Bull Soc Fr Pathol Exotique.* 1984;77:637–648.
14. Mayou S, Calderon RA, Hay RJ, Goodfellow A. Deep dermatophyte infection. *Clin Exp Dermatol.* 1987;12:385–388.
15. Faergemann J. Lipophilic yeasts in skin disease. *Sem Dermatol.* 1985;4:173–184.
16. Roberts SOB. Pityriasis versicolor; a clinical and mycological investigation. *Br J Dermatol.* 1969;81:315–326.
17. Back O, Faergemann J, Hornquist R. Pityrosporum folliculitis: a common disease of the young and middle aged. *J Am Acad Dermatol.* 1985;12:56–61.
18. Mathes BM, Douglas MC. Seborrheic dermatitis in patients with acquired immunodeficiency syndrome. *J Am Acad Dermatol.* 1985;13:947–951.
19. Redline RW, Redline SS, Boxerbaum B, Dahms BB. Systemic *Malassezia furfur* infections in patients receiving intralipid therapy. *Hum Pathol.* 1985;16:815–822.
20. Marcon MJ, Powell DA. Epidemiology, diagnosis, and management of *Malassezia furfur* systemic infection. *Diagn Microbiol Infect Dis.* 1987;7:161–175.
21. Dankner WM, Spector SA, Fierer J, Davis CE. Malassezia fungemia in neonates and adults: complication of hyperalimentation. *Rev Infect Dis.* 1987;9:743–753.
22. Carr JF, Lewes CW. Tinea nigra palmaris. *Arch Dermatol.* 1975;111:904–905.
23. Onsberg P. *Scopulariopsis brevicaulis* in nails. *Dermatologica.* 1980;161:259–264.
24. Kalter DCA, Tschen JA, Cernoch PL, et al. Genital white piedra: epidemiology, microbiology and therapy. *J Am Acad Dermatol.* 1986;14:982–993.

CHAPTER 123

Torulopsosis

Francis W. Chandler and Libero Ajello

Variability is the law of life, and as no two faces are the same, so no two bodies are alike, and no two individuals react alike and behave alike under the abnormal conditions which we know as disease.

Sir William Osler (1849–1919), On the Educational Value of the Medical Society

DEFINITION

Torulopsosis is a rare opportunistic fungal infection caused by *Torulopsis glabrata.*[1,2] Controversy surrounds the taxonomic classification of this fungus. In 1978, David Yarrow and Sally Meyer proposed that this unicellular, asporogenous yeast be incorporated into the genus *Candida* as *C glabrata.*[3] This transfer was based on the contention that the genus *Torulopsis,* first described by Augusto Napoleone Berlese in 1894,[4] was a *nomen nudum.* To accommodate this change, Yarrow and Meyer further proposed, but did not validate, a change in the description of the genus *Candida* to incorporate yeasts, such as *T glabrata,* that do not produce pseudohyphae in vitro and in vivo.[3] The advocates of the genus *Torulopsis*[5] asserted that the genera *Candida* and *Torulopsis* are two taxonomically distinct entities distinguished by the presence or absence of pseudohyphae, respectively, in culture and in infected hosts.[4] In addition, they held that Berlese's genus was validly published. This controversy has led to confusion, and in the current literature, the two binomials (*T glabrata* and *C glabrata*) are both used. Until this controversy is resolved by definitive genetic and molecular mycologic studies, we have chosen to use the valid and well-established binomial *T glabrata,* and the name torulopsosis for infections caused by this unicellular yeast.

EPIDEMIOLOGY

Torulopsis glabrata is a ubiquitous fungus. It is part of the normal microbiota of the skin, oropharynx, gastrointestinal tract, urethra, and vagina of humans and animals, and is widely distributed as a saprophyte.[1,2] Although of low virulence, the spectrum of disease caused by *T glabrata* ranges from clinically silent fungemia and funguria to severe, life-threatening, disseminated infections.[6,7] Most fungemias and fungurias are nosocomial, and underlying diseases such as cancer and bacterial sepsis are the usual causes of death. Predisposing factors include contaminated intravenous lines, intravenous drug abuse, indwelling urethral catheters, abdominal or urologic surgery, obstructive uropathy, appendiceal abscesses, prolonged antibiotic therapy, uncontrolled diabetes mellitus, severe myelosuppression, malnutrition, and systemic therapy with corticosteroids and cytostatic agents.[8–13] Foci for hematogenous seeding of *T glabrata* include contaminated catheter tips and intravenous lines, open wounds, and sites of endogenous colonization along the gastrointestinal, urinary, and respiratory tracts.[12,13] Sometimes, however, the sources of fungemia are unexplained. The various clinical presentations of torulopsosis are worldwide, and there is no apparent geographic prevalence. Synonyms include candidiasis glabrata and candidiasis.

MORPHOLOGIC FEATURES OF THE ORGANISM

Torulopsis glabrata is a small (2 to 5 μm), spherical to oval, nonencapsulated, unicellular, haploid, yeastlike fungus that produces single buds attached to parent cells by a relatively narrow base[14] (Figure 123–1). The fungus is easily and rapidly cultured on standard mycologic media, where it produces smooth, soft, shiny, and

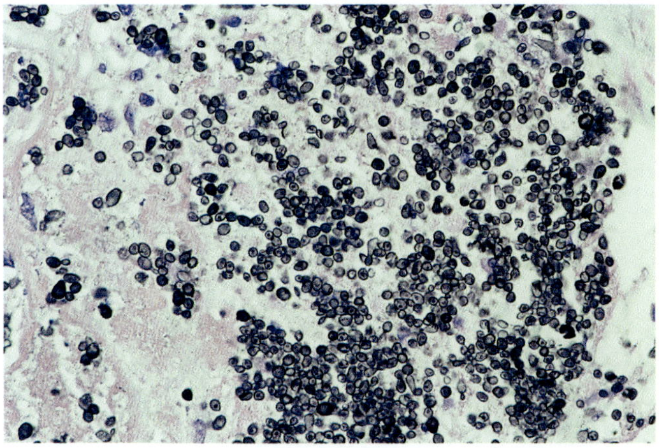

Figure 123–1. Disseminated torulopsosis. Compact aggregates of spherical to oval, single and budding yeast forms of *T glabrata,* 2 to 5 μm in diameter, are embedded in an arterial thrombus. Hyphae and pseudohyphae are not produced in tissue [Gomori's methenamine silver–hematoxylin-eosin (GMS–H&E), ×160].

creamy white yeastlike colonies that may become grayish brown with age. Colonies are composed entirely of small yeastlike cells that are quite uniform in size and shape, and morphologically similar to those seen in infected tissues; hyphae and pseudohyphae are not produced on any mycologic medium. *Torulopsis glabrata* is readily differentiated from the *Candida* sp on the basis of fermentation and assimilation reactions against a battery of sugars, and by its failure to utilize KNO_3.[5]

CLINICAL FEATURES

Approximately half of all infections by *T glabrata* are transient, self-limited, clinically inapparent fungemias and fungurias.[12] Fungemias are often superimposed on bacterial sepsis, and a positive blood culture is usually the only clue to coexisting infection.[12,15] Torulopsosis of the urinary tract with funguria can be primary (ascending) or, more commonly, secondary to disseminated infection.[13,16,17] Other patients infected with *T glabrata* have had a broad spectrum of diseases, including pyelonephritis,[18] pneumonitis,[19–21] endocarditis,[22,23] osteomyelitis,[24–26] meningoencephalitis,[27] endophthalmitis,[28] retinitis,[29] enterocolitis,[28] cholecystitis,[30] wound infection,[14,15] ulcerative esophagitis,[31] and ulcerative vaginitis.[32,33] Clinical findings in severe disseminated infections are often nonspecific and include low-grade or spiking fever with rigors and hypotension, and a rapidly deteriorating clinical course.

PATHOLOGY

Because *T glabrata* is of very low virulence, its invasive potential is minimal except in severely debilitated patients.[1] The host response to invasion by *T glabrata* varies from minimal or no inflammation to suppuration and necrosis with abscesses resembling disseminated candidiasis.[14] Single and clustered yeastlike cells are in macrophages and neutrophils, or extracellular among necrotic debris (Figure 123–1). Although amphophilic when stained with H&E (Figure 123–2), *T glabrata* cells are best demonstrated with the GMS stain and appear as uniformly blackened, spherical to oval yeast forms, 2 to 5 μm in diameter, that have single buds attached to parent cells by narrow bases (Figure 123–1). Because *T glabrata* does not produce hyphae and pseudohyphae in tissue, the formation of "fungus balls" in pulmonary and renal infections is rare.

In disseminated torulopsosis, lesions are most frequent in the kidneys, gastrointestinal tract, heart, lungs, central nervous system, and peritoneum.[1,14] About half the patients with disseminated infection have minimal to severe lesions in the kidneys.[16,17] Severe lesions usually consist of acute pyelonephritis with miliary abscesses and necrotizing papillitis. *Torulopsis glabrata* pneumonitis occurs more frequently in patients with severe myelosuppression and hematologic neoplasia,[20] or in persons who are malnourished.[21] The pneumonitis is usually primary, or, rarely, secondary to *T glabrata* fungemia. Most biopsy and autopsy specimens reveal a suppurative and necrotizing bronchopneumonia with

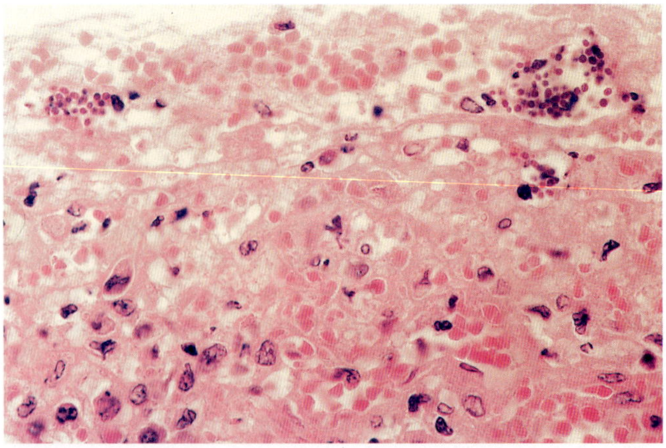

Figure 123–2. Torulopsosis. A subcutaneous necrotic nodule contains extracellular clusters of fungal cells *(top left and right),* some of which are budding. Note that the *T glabrata* cells are amphophilic and stain entirely; there is no "halo" or pseudocapsular effect as with *Histoplasma capsulatum* var *capsulatum* (H&E, ×100).

scattered intra- and extracellular yeast forms in alveolar and bronchiolar exudates.[14,19] Paucireactive inflammation often characterizes preterminal infections, where numerous yeast forms occupy alveolar spaces.

DIFFERENTIAL DIAGNOSIS

In smears and sections of infected tissue, the yeastlike cells of *T glabrata* closely resemble those of *Histoplasma capsulatum* var *capsulatum* (Figure 123–3). This is especially true when most of the *T glabrata* cells are clustered within macrophages. Careful examination, however, reveals that entire fungal cells of *T glabrata* are amphophilic when stained with H&E (Figure 123–2); there is no pseudocapsular or "halo" effect as consistently observed with the tissue forms of *H capsulatum* var *capsulatum* (see Chapter 109). The GMS stain reveals that *T glabrata* cells are slightly larger, more pleomorphic, and usually bud more frequently than histoplasma cells (Figure 123–1). Also, *T glabrata* cells are more often extracellular and do not cluster as often as the yeast forms of histoplasmosis capsulati (Figure 123–1). Although the yeast forms of *T glabrata* are usually gram-positive (Figure 123–4), this staining reaction cannot be relied on for diagnosis. Definitive identification requires direct immunofluorescence of *T glabrata* in smears and tissue sections, and isolation and identification in culture.[5,14] Unlike the *Candida* sp, *T glabrata* reproduces only by budding and occurs exclusively as a yeast form in tissue and in culture.

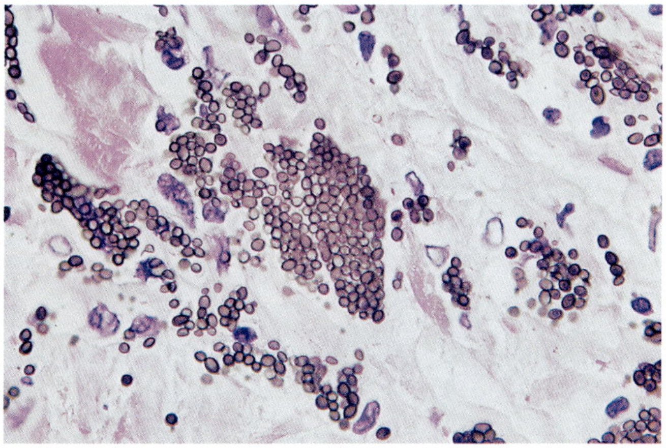

Figure 123–3. Disseminated histoplasmosis capsulati involving the adrenal gland in a patient with acquired immunodeficiency syndrome. Large intra- and extracellular aggregates of yeastlike cells efface the normal histologic architecture. Note close resemblance of the histoplasma cells to those of *T glabrata* when stained with GMS (GMS–H&E, ×160).

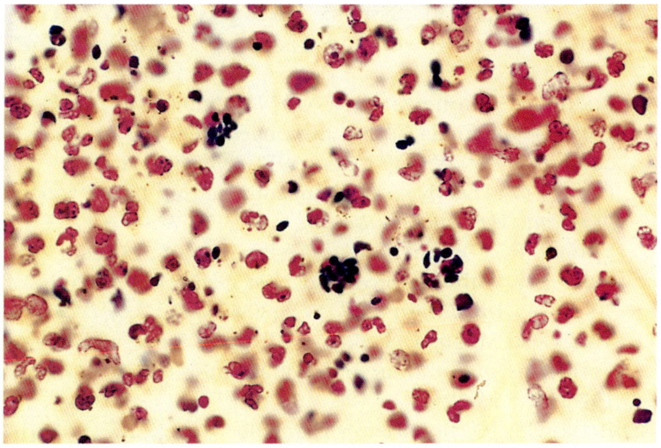

Figure 123–4. Suppurative peritonitis caused by *T glabrata.* Many of the yeast forms are uniformly gram-positive. Note clustering of fungal cells within macrophages and neutrophils (Brown–Brenn, ×250).

TREATMENT

The treatment of choice in severe, disseminated infections and persistent fungemias is amphotericin B.[2,34] Good results also have been achieved with the oral antifungals ketoconazole, miconazole, and fluconazole, especially in patients with renal failure.[29,35] Elimination of predisposing factors often results in rapid improvement without antifungal treatment, but progressive localized and disseminated infections usually require aggressive therapy.

REFERENCES

1. Grimley PM, Wright LD, Jennings AE. *Torulopsis glabrata* infection in man. *Am J Clin Pathol.* 1965;43:216–223.
2. Marks MI, Langston C, Eickhoff TC. *Torulopsis glabrata*—an opportunistic pathogen of man. *N Engl J Med.* 1970; 283:1131–1135.
3. Yarrow D, Meyer SA. Proposal for amendment of the diagnosis of the genus *Candida* Berkhout *nom cons. Int J Syst Bacteriol.* 1978;28:611–615.
4. Berlese AN. I fungi diversi dai saccaromiceti e capaci de determinare la fermentazione alcoolica. *Gior Viticolt Enol.* 1894;3:52–55.
5. McGinnis MR, Ajello L, Beneke ES, et al. Taxonomic and nomenclatural evaluation of the genera *Candida* and *Torulopsis. J Clin Microbiol.* 1984;20:813–814.
6. Louria DB, Belvins A, Armstrong D, et al. Fungemia caused by "nonpathogenic" yeasts. *Arch Intern Med.* 1967; 119:247–252.

7. Katz D, Pickard RE. Systemic *Torulopsis glabrata* infection causing shock, fever and coma. *Am J Med.* 1967;42: 151–152.
8. Rodrigues RJ, Shinya H, Wolff WI, Puttlitz D. *Torulopsis glabrata* fungemia during prolonged intravenous alimentation therapy. *N Engl J Med.* 1971;284:540–541.
9. Pankey GA, Daloviso JR. Fungemia caused by *Torulopsis glabrata. Medicine (Baltimore).* 1973;52:395–403.
10. Young RC, Bennett JE, Geelhoed GW, Levine AS. Fungemia with compromised host resistance. A study of 70 cases. *Ann Intern Med.* 1974;80:605–612.
11. Valdivieso M, Luna M, Bodey GP, et al. Fungemia due to *Torulopsis glabrata* in the compromised host. *Cancer.* 1976;38:1750–1756.
12. Berkowitz ID, Robboy SJ, Karchmer AW, Kunz LJ. *Torulopsis glabrata* fungemia—a clinical pathological study. *Medicine (Baltimore).* 1979;58:430–440.
13. Wainstein MA, Graham RD, Resnick ML. Predisposing factors of systemic fungal infections of the genitourinary tract. *J Urol.* 1995;152:160–163.
14. Chandler FW, Watts JC. *Pathologic Diagnosis of Fungal Infections.* Chicago: ASCP Press; 1987:203–208.
15. Hahn H, Condie F. Bulger RF. Diagnosis of *Torulopsis glabrata* infection. *JAMA.* 1968;203:835–837.
16. Kauffman CA, Tan JS. *Torulopsis glabrata* renal infection. *Am J Med.* 1974;57:217–224.
17. Takeuchi H, Tomoyoshi T. *Torulopsis* infection extensively involving urinary tract. *Urology.* 1983;22:173–175.
18. Vordermark JS, II, Modarelli RO, Buck AS. *Torulopsis* pyelonephritis associated with papillary necrosis. A case report. *J Urol.* 1980;123:96–97.
19. Oldfield FS, Kapica L, Pirozynski WJ. Pulmonary infection due to *Torulopsis glabrata. Can Med Assoc J.* 1968;98: 165–168.
20. Aisner J, Sickles EA, Schimpff SC, et al. *Torulopsis glabrata* pneumonitis in patients with cancer: Report of three cases. *JAMA.* 1974;230:584–585.
21. Sander LA, Young EJ, Musher DM, Clarridge JE. *Torulopsis glabrata* pneumonia in a malnourished woman. *South Med J.* 1979;72:1477–1479.
22. Heffner DK, Franklin WA. Endocarditis caused by *Torulopsis glabrata. Am J Clin Pathol.* 1978;70:420–423.
23. Holliday HD, Keipper V, Kaiser AB. *Torulopsis glabrata* endocarditis. *JAMA.* 1980;244:2088–2089.
24. Gustke KA, Wu KK. *Torulopsis glabrata* osteomyelitis: report of a case. *Clin Orthop.* 1981;154:197–200.
25. Thurston AJ, Gillespie WJ. *Torulopsis glabrata* osteomyelitis of the spine: a case report and review of the literature. *Aust NZ J Surg.* 1981;51:374–376.
26. Rubin MM, Sanfilippo RJ. Osteomyelitis of the hyoid caused by *Torulopsis glabrata* in a patient with acquired immunodeficiency syndrome. *J Oral Maxillofac Surg.* 1990;48:1217–1219.
27. Wurzel B, Goldberg P, Caroline L, et al. *Torulopsis glabrata* meningoencephalitis treated with 5-flucytosine. *Ann Intern Med.* 1972;77:814–815.
28. Baley JE, Dliegman RM, Annable WL, et al. *Torulopsis glabrata* sepsis appearing as necrotizing enterocolitis and endophthalmitis. *Am J Dis Child.* 1984;138:965–966.
29. Fitzsimons RB, Nicholls MD, Billson FA, et al. Fungal retinitis: a case of *Torulopsis glabrata* infection treated with miconazole. *Br J Ophthalmol.* 1980;64:672–675.
30. Miller DD. Postoperative acalculous cholecystitis due to *Torulopsis glabrata. Arch Surg.* 1976;111:1404–1405.
31. Tom W, Aaron JS. Esophageal ulcers caused by *Torulopsis glabrata* in a patient with acquired immune deficiency syndrome. *Am J Gastroenterol.* 1987;82:766–768.
32. Clark JFJ, Faggett T, Peters B, et al. Ulcerative vaginitis due to *Torulopsis glabrata:* a case report. *J Natl Med Assoc.* 1978;70:913–914.
33. Spinello A, Caprezzo E, Egbe TO, et al. *Torulopsis glabrata* vaginitis. *Obstet Gynec.* 1995;85:992–998.
34. Rose HD, Heckman MG. Persistent fungemia caused by *Torulopsis glabrata:* treatment with amphotericin B. *Am J Clin Pathol.* 1970;54:205–208.
35. Corbella X, Carratala J, Castells M, Berlanga B. Fluconazole treatment in *Torulopsis glabrata* upper urinary tract infection causing ureteral obstruction. *J Urol.* 1992;147: 1112–1114.

CHAPTER 124

Trichosporonosis

Michael R. McGinnis and Francis W. Chandler

This body in which we journey across the isthmus between two oceans is not a private carriage, but an omnibus.

Oliver Wendell Holmes (1809–1894)

DEFINITION

Fungal infections caused by species of *Trichosporon* can be either superficial, cutaneous, or deep. Superficial infection of the hair shaft is known as white piedra, whereas cutaneous and deep infections are called trichosporonosis. Trichosporonosis is an emerging opportunistic mycosis that is potentially life threatening because it frequently occurs in immunodeficient or postoperative patients.[1] *Trichosporon beigelii* (syn. *T cutaneum*) causes trichosporonosis and white piedra. Some mycologists believe that a number of *Trichosporon* sp are capable of causing these diseases.[2,3]

LIFE CYCLE, NATURAL HISTORY, AND EPIDEMIOLOGY

Trichosporonosis has no synonyms and its distribution is worldwide. *Trichosporon* sp are found in soil throughout the world. Isolates have been recovered from water, human feces, cabbage, rat droppings, frozen chickens, tofu cakes, shrimp, and numerous clinical specimens originating from humans and animals.[2] The fungus may colonize the throat, lower gastrointestinal tract, and skin.[4] Herbrecht et al[5] believe *T ovoides* to be the most common agent of white piedra of the scalp hair, and *Sarcinosporon inkin* (as *T inkin*) of the genital hair. Summer-type hypersensitivity pneumonitis described in patients living in Japan is caused by *T asahii* and *T mucoides*. Disseminated infections are caused by *T asahii, T mucoides,* and *S inkin*. All of these species, except *S inkin,* are treated as synonyms of *T beigelii* in this chapter because a practical method to distinguish these species is not available to diagnostic laboratories at this time.

MORPHOLOGIC FEATURES OF THE ORGANISM

Trichosporon beigelii is a yeast that forms hyaline hyphae that are branched, septate, and fragment into arthroconidia. The conidia may form blastoconidia, which frequently remain attached to each other to produce pseudohyphae. Members of the genus *Trichosporon* are distinguished from each other by differences in using various carbon and nitrogen sources for growth.

CLINICAL FEATURES

Trichosporon beigelii can cause infections in either normal or immunodeficient patients. Skin colonization of the perigenital areas has been observed in normal individuals. White piedra is characterized by soft, white to cream-colored nodules along the hair shafts that consist of hyphae and arthroconidia. Deep infections can be localized or disseminated. Localized infections have been associated with peritonitis in patients undergoing peritoneal dialysis, infection following surgery, endocarditis in an intravenous drug user, and localized pneumonia. Disseminated infections occur in immunodeficient patients, especially those who have neoplastic disease, organ transplants, or non-neoplastic cytopenia.[4,5] The most common neoplastic diseases are acute leukemia, chronic leukemia, multiple myeloma, solid tumors, non-Hodgkin's lymphoma, and Hodgkin's lymphoma. Fever, pulmonary infiltrates, cutaneous lesions, hematuria, azotemia, and fungemia are common, especially if cytotoxic chemotherapy-induced granulocytopenia has occurred.[1] There appears to be a predominance of trichosporonosis in male subjects. Host factors include cytotoxic chemotherapy-induced granulocytopenia, corticosteroids, prosthetic valve surgery, and hemochromatosis.[1]

PATHOLOGY

The host reaction in trichosporonosis is similar to that in disseminated aspergillosis. Parenchymal lesions of disseminated trichosporonosis often occur as nodular infarcts caused by mycotic angioinvasion and occlusion of blood vessels (Figure 124–1). Within infarcted tissue, proliferating fungal elements sometimes produce a radial or sunburst pattern of growth (Figure 124–2). Abscesses and granulomas also may be present. Disseminated infection involves the lungs, kidneys, heart, brain, liver, spleen, bone marrow, and other organs, and is often associated with fungemia.

In tissue, *T beigelii* forms pleomorphic yeast cells 3 to 8 μm in diameter, septate hyphae, pseudohyphae, and arthroconidia (Figure 124–3). The arthroconidia, produced by hyperseptation and disarticulation of hyphal segments, are frequently difficult to find in histopathologic material (Figure 124–4). If arthroconidia are not evident, *T beigelii* and *Candida* sp can be mistaken for each other. These two groups of yeasts can be distinguished by using immunoperoxidase and direct immunofluorescence of fungal elements in fixed, paraffin-embedded tissue sections.[6–8] Ultrastructural studies of white piedra and of *T beigelii* in culture have been reported.[2,9]

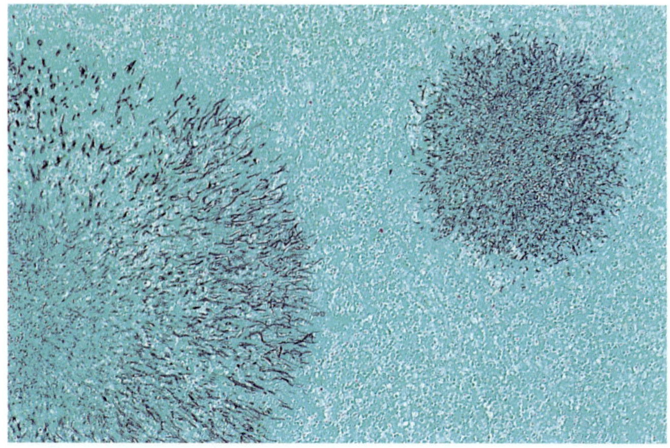

Figure 124–2. Disseminated trichosporonosis. Two radiating microcolonies of *T beigelii* occupy a nodular splenic infarct caused by mycotic invasion and occlusion of a trabecular artery branch [Gomori's methenamine silver (GMS), ×40].

DIFFERENTIAL DIAGNOSIS

Black piedra caused by *Piedraia hortae,* candidiasis, aspergillosis, pseudallescheriasis, and other opportunistic mycoses must be considered. Trichosporonosis

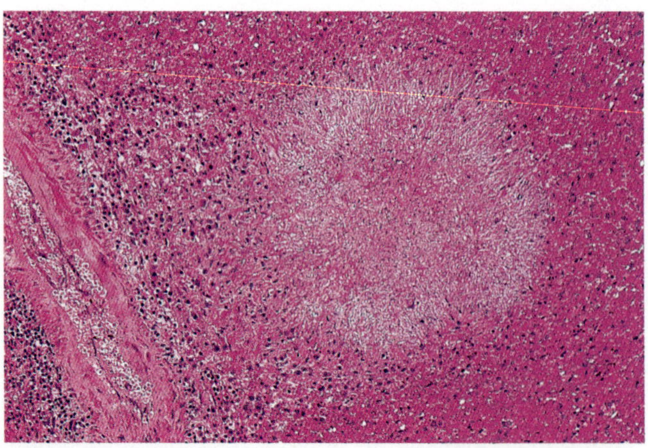

Figure 124–1. Disseminated trichosporonosis involving the spleen. Hyaline, weakly stained fungal elements proliferate from a central nidus and produce a radial or sunburst pattern within a nodular infarct [hematoxylin-eosin (H&E), ×40].

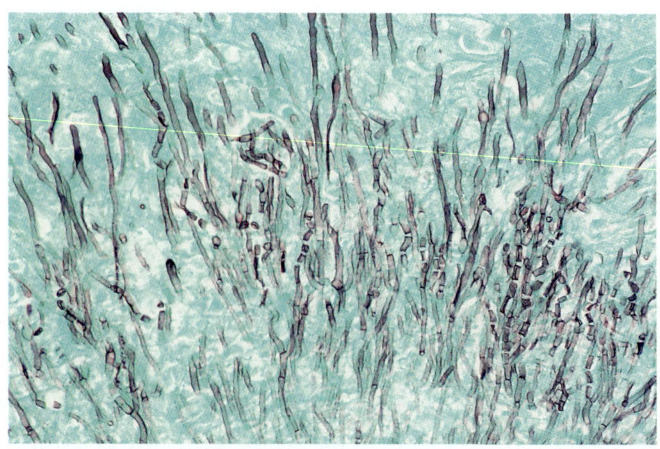

Figure 124–3. Disseminated trichosporonosis. A nodular infarct contains hyphae, yeasts, and arthroconidia of *T beigelii.* Arthroconidia *(center)* are produced by hyperseptation and disarticulation of hyphal segments (GMS, ×160).

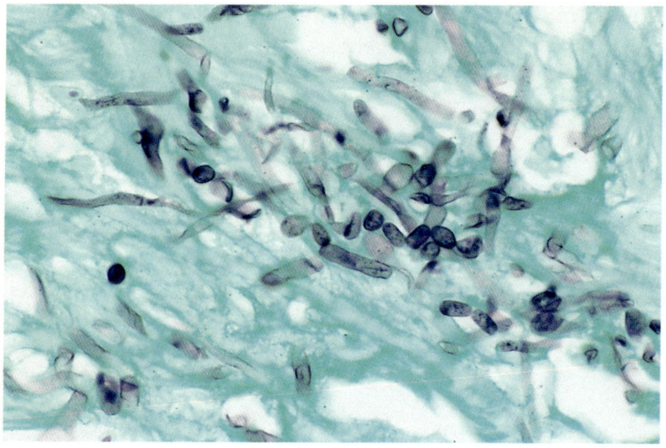

Figure 124–4. Cutaneous trichosporonosis. Intrafollicular hyphae and yeast forms extend into the contiguous dermis. Because arthroconidia are often sparse or absent in tissue specimens, the combination of pleomorphic blastoconidia (budding cells) and hyphae or pseudohyphae can be mistaken for a *Candida* sp (GMS, ×250).

may occur concurrently with pneumonia caused by *Aspergillus* sp, *Candida* sp, gram-negative bacteria, cytomegalovirus, and adenovirus.[1]

MOLECULAR DIAGNOSIS

Isoenzymes, restriction fragment length polymorphisms of rDNA, ubiquinone systems, and DNA relatedness have been used to characterize isolates of *T beigelii.*[2,10,11]

CONFIRMATIONAL TESTING AND DIAGNOSIS

Diagnosis rests on repeated isolations of the fungus from clinical specimens, and demonstration of fungal elements in biopsy specimens. *Trichosporon beigelii* is readily cultured and produces yeast-like colonies on routine mycologic media. The Vitek Yeast Biochemical Card in comparison to the API 20C Yeast Identification System does not accurately identify species of *Trichosporon.*[12] These results parallel the conclusion that *T beigelii* is a complex of several different yeasts. Serologic procedures are available for the diagnosis of summer-type hypersensitivity pneumonitis,[13] and there is some cross-reactivity with anticryptococcal antibodies detected in the latex agglutination test.[14]

TREATMENT

Isolates of *Trichosporon* sp are typically resistant to 5-fluorocytosine. Azoles and amphotericin B have been used with varying degrees of success. Recovery from granulocytopenia has a major impact on the outcome for the patient.[3,15,16]

REFERENCES

1. Walsh TJ. Trichosporonosis. *Infect Dis Clin North Am.* 1989;3:43–52.
2. Guého E, Smith MTh, de Hoog GS, Billon-Grand G, Christen R, Batenburg-van der Vegte WH. Contributions to a revision of the genus *Trichosporon*. *Antonie van Leeuwenhoek.* 1992;61:289–316.
3. Guého E, Improvisi L, de Hoog GS, Dupont B. *Trichosporon* on humans: a practical account. *Mycoses.* 1994; 37:3–10.
4. Ellner K, McGride ME, Rosen T, Berman D. Prevalence of *Trichosporon beigelii.* Colonization of normal perigenital skin. *J Med Vet Mycol.* 1991;29:99–103.
5. Herbrecht R, Koenig H, Waller J, Liu KL, Guého E. *Trichosporon* infections: clinical manifestations and treatment. *J Mycol Méd.* 1993;3:129–136.
6. Kimura M, Takahashi H, Satou T, Hashimoto S. An autopsy case of disseminated trichosporonosis with candidiasis of the urinary tract. *Virchows Archiv Pathol Anat.* 1989;416:159–162.
7. Chandler FW, Watts JC. *Pathologic Diagnosis of Fungal Infections.* Chicago: ASCP Press; 1987:113–116.
8. Kobayashi M, Kotani S, Fujishita M, et al. Immunohistochemical identification of *Trichosporon beigelii* in histologic sections by immunoperoxidase method. *Am J Clin Pathol.* 1988;89:100–105.
9. de Almeida HL, Rivitti EA, Jaeger RG. White piedra: ultrastructure and a new microecological aspect. *Mycoses.* 1990;33:491–497.
10. Sugita T, Nishikawa A, Shinoda T, Kume H. Taxonomic position of deep-seated, mucosa-associated, and superficial isolates of *Trichosporon cutaneum* from trichosporonosis patients. *J Clin Microbiol.* 1995;33:1368–1370.
11. Kemer BJ, Lehmann PF, Lee W, Walsh TJ. Distinction of deep versus superficial clinical and nonclinical isolates of *Trichosporon beigelii* by isoenzymes and restriction fragment length polymorphisms of rDNA generated by polymerase chain reaction. *J Clin Microbiol.* 1991;29:1677–1683.
12. Dooley DP, Beckius ML, Jeffrey BS. Misidentification of clinical yeast isolates by using the updated Vitek Yeast Biochemical Card. *J Clin Microbiol.* 1994;32:2889–2892.
13. Mizobe T, Yamasaki H, Doi K, Ando M, Onoue K. Analysis of serotype-specific antibodies to *Trichosporon cutaneum* types I and II in patients with summer-type hypersensitivity pneumonitis with monoclonal antibodies to serotype-related polysaccharide antigens. *J Clin Microbiol.* 1993;31:1949–1951.
14. Lyman CA, Devi SJN, Nathanson J, Frosch CE, Pizzo PA, Walsh TJ. Detection and quantitation of the glucuronoxylomannan-like polysaccharide antigen from clinical and non-clinical isolates of *Trichosporon beigelii* and implications for pathogenicity. *J Clin Microbiol.* 1995;33:126–130.

15. Anaissie E, Gokaslan A, Hachem R, et al. Azole therapy for trichosporonosis: clinical evaluation of eight patients, experimental therapy for murine infection, and review. *Clin Infect Dis.* 1992;15:781–787.
16. Walsh TJ, Lee JW, Melcher GP, et al. Experimental *Trichosporon* infection in persistently granulocytopenic rabbits: implications for pathogenesis, diagnosis, and treatment of an emerging opportunistic mycosis. *J Infect Dis.* 1992; 166:121–133.

CHAPTER 125

Zygomycosis

Francis W. Chandler and John C. Watts

Disease is very old, and nothing about it has changed. It is we who change, as we learn to recognize what was formerly imperceptible.

Jean Martin Charcot (1825–1893), De l'expectation en médecine

DEFINITION

Zygomycosis is a unifying term that encompasses various diseases caused by fungi of the class Zygomycetes (formerly Phycomycetes).[1,2] The human pathogens in this class belong to the orders Mucorales and Entomophthorales, and the corresponding diseases are mucormycosis and entomophthoromycosis, respectively. There are distinct clinical and pathologic differences between these two forms of zygomycosis.[3–6] Pathogenic genera in the order Mucorales include *Absidia, Apophysomyces, Cunninghamella, Mortierella, Mucor, Rhizomucor, Rhizopus, Saksenaea,* and *Syncephalastrum;* genera in the order Entomophthorales include *Basidiobolus* and *Conidiobolus.* The most frequent agent of mucormycosis in humans is *Rhizopus arrhizus* (formerly *R oryzae*).

EPIDEMIOLOGY

Mucormycosis (infection caused by fungi of the order Mucorales) is a sporadic disease that is worldwide.[7,8] There is no predilection based on gender, race, or occupation. Mucormycosis occurs predominantly in patients with acidosis and in those with leukemia or lymphoma or who are otherwise immunodeficient.[9–13] The opportunistic pathogens (zygomycetes) of mucormycosis are saprophytes widely distributed in nature. Infection is acquired by exposure to sporangiospores and is not contagious. The sporangiospores may be inhaled, ingested, or deposited onto sites of mucocutaneous injury, especially burns. Mucormycosis in patients infected with human immunodeficiency virus or who have acquired immunodeficiency syndrome is rare; most of these patients have had a history of active intravenous drug use.[14–19]

Entomophthoromycosis (infection caused by fungi of the order Entomophthorales) is predominantly in tropical Africa, Southeast Asia, and South America and is not an opportunistic infection.[20–22] Infection usually results from percutaneous implantation of the fungus. Sporadic cases of entomophthoromycosis are rarely encountered in the United States.

Synonyms of zygomycosis include phycomycosis, mucormycosis, entomophthoromycosis, hyphomycosis, subcutaneous phycomycosis, rhinophycomycosis, phycomycosis entomophthorae, basidiobolomycosis, oomycosis, and rhinoentomophthoromycosis.

CLINICAL FEATURES

Several clinical forms of mucormycosis are recognized. Rhinoorbitocerebral mucormycosis is a fulminating, invasive infection of the nasal cavity, paranasal sinuses, and orbit that extends to the meninges and brain[4,23,24] (Figure 125–1). The overlying facial skin becomes blackened, edematous, and necrotic. *Rhizopus* sp have been implicated in most of these infections, which usually are in acidotic patients, particularly those with uncontrolled diabetes mellitus, and in profoundly immunodeficient patients, particularly those treated for hematologic malignancies.[10,12,24] The mortality rate is high. Pulmonary mucormycosis occurs as a primary infection in immunodeficient or neutropenic patients. Pulmonary lesions are infarctive as a consequence of hyphal invasion and subsequent thrombosis of large

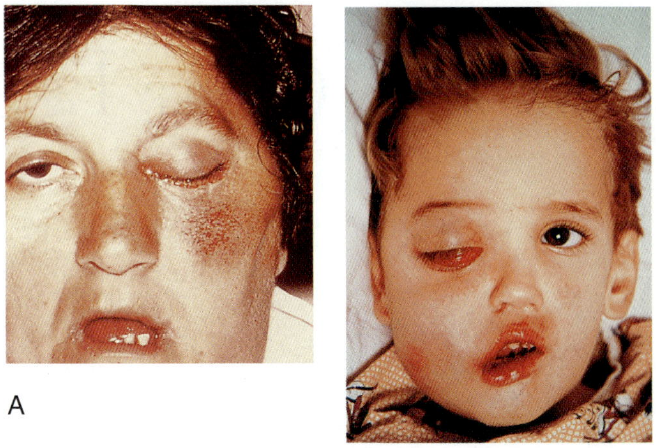

A B

Figure 125–1. (**A**) Rhinocerebral mucormycosis caused by *R arrhizus*. There is ptosis of the left eyelid and orbital and facial cellulitis. *(Contributed by Centers for Disease Control and Prevention, Atlanta, Georgia.)* (**B**) This 3-year-old boy was in good health until he developed fever, malaise, anorexia, and a foul green discharge from his right nostril. Under general anesthesia, a gelatinous mass filling the right nostril was partially removed. Five days later he had edema of the conjunctiva and reduced movements of the eye. The next day there was partial paralysis of the right side of his face and this was followed by irritability, swelling of the face, blindness, and immobility of the right eye and a dilated fixed pupil. A Caldwell–Luc procedure revealed polypoid necrotic material in the antrum. Microscopically it was inflamed granulation tissue with granulomas around nonseptate hyphae, characteristic of a zygomycete. Repeated attempts at culture grew no fungi. The left eye remained normal and there was no other systemic disease (urinalyses, blood glucose determinations, skin tests, blood cultures, and bone marrow studies revealed no abnormalities). The infection progressed slowly in spite of intravenous amphotericin B and he died suddenly of respiratory arrest 3 months and 10 days after onset.[41] *(Contributed by Frederick C. Blodi, MD, Iowa City, Iowa.)*

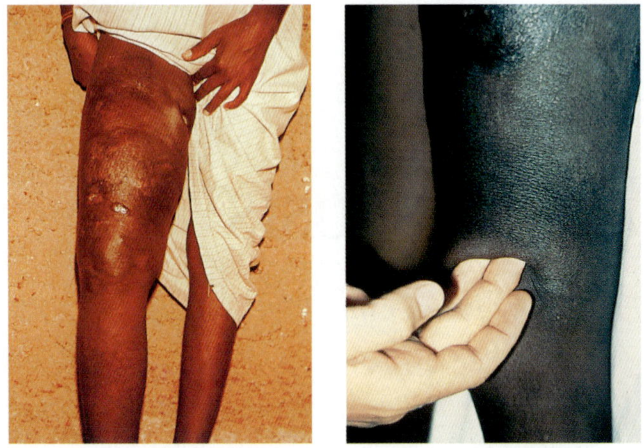

A B

Figure 125–2. (**A**) Subcutaneous entomophthoromycosis caused by *B ranarum*. *(By Daniel H. Connor, MD, 1962.)* (**B**) Clinically the hard mass has a sharp edge. By placing fingers beneath the edge, the mass can be lifted away from the deep fascia. *(Contributed by Dr. Mark H. Monson, Curran Lutheran Hospital, ZorZor, Liberia.)*

pulmonary blood vessels.[25–28] The proclivity of the mucoraceous zygomycetes to invade blood vessels often produces disseminated infection. Gastrointestinal mucormycosis is a primary ulcerative infection that affects malnourished patients and those with preexisting ulcers.[29] The stomach and colon are most often involved, and lesions consist of necrotic ulcers and segmental infarcts. Cutaneous mucormycosis usually occurs in burned patients and has been associated with the use of contaminated elastic bandages.[21,30,31] Surgical bandages have most often been contaminated with *R rhizopodiformis*.[32] Disseminated mucormycosis affects patients treated for leukemia and lymphoma, and other patients treated with immunosuppressive drugs.[33–36] Sites of predilection in disseminated infections include the lungs, brain, heart, liver, kidneys, gastrointestinal tract, and skin, but almost any organ can be involved. Often, the primary focus of infection is in the lungs. Active intravenous drug abuse is a well-documented risk factor for cerebral mucormycosis.[37,38]

There are two clinical forms of human entomophthoromycosis: subcutaneous and rhinofacial.[5,20–22] Subcutaneous entomophthoromycosis caused by *Basidiobolus ranarum* (formerly *Basidiobolus haptosporus*) produces indurated, lentiform subcutaneous masses that usually involve the limbs, trunk, or buttocks (Figure 125–2, A). A striking clinical feature is the sharply defined indurated edge that lifts freely away from the deep fascia (Figure 125–2, B). Infection is locally progressive and may ulcerate overlying skin, but dissemination is rare. Infection is probably acquired from implantation of the fungus following local penetrating injury. Rhinofacial entomophthoromycosis caused by *Conidiobolus coronatus* is a locally progressive infection of the nasal cavity, paranasal sinuses, and soft tissues of the face that rarely extends to the mediastinum and lungs. Unlike rhinoorbitocerebral mucormycosis, infection does not involve the cerebral hemispheres. Neither form of entomophthoromycosis is associated with acidosis or immunodeficiency.

MORPHOLOGY OF THE ETIOLOGIC AGENTS

Typical hyphae of the mucoraceous zygomycetes have a characteristic appearance in tissue sections.[1,2] The hyphae are broad (5 to 20 μm or more in width), irregularly contoured, and pleomorphic (Figure 125–3). Although often described as nonseptate (coenocytic), the hyphae are actually pauciseptate; septa, however, are only rarely observed in tissue sections and can be

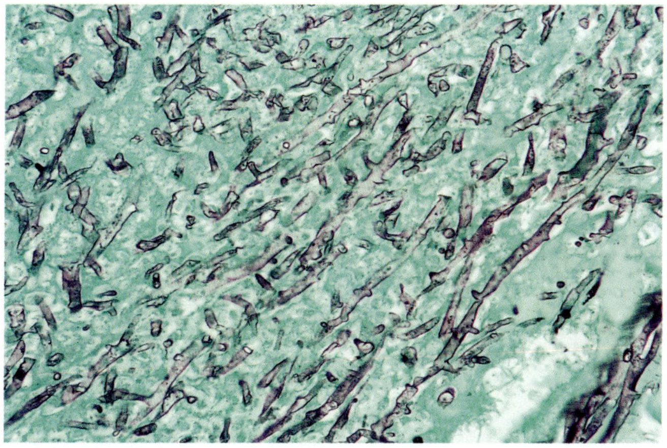

Figure 125–3. Disseminated mucormycosis. Broad, pleomorphic hyphae that vary in caliber (5 to 20 μm) and branch predominantly at right angles invade the myocardium. Note that branches are often narrower than parent hyphae (GMS, ×100).

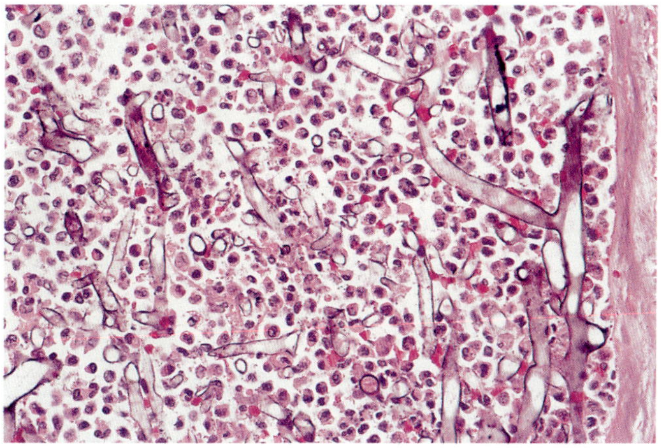

Figure 125–5. Disseminated mucormycosis. Pleomorphic, mucoraceous hyphae within an arterial thrombus are infrequently septate, irregularly contoured, and branch predominantly at right angles *(right center)* (GMS–H&E, ×160).

simulated by transverse folds and compressions of hyphal walls (Figure 125–4). The pattern of hyphal branching is haphazard and nonprogressive, and branches typically arise from parent hyphae at right angles (Figure 125–5). The walls of the hyphae are thin and appear basophilic or amphophilic in hematoxylin-eosin (H&E) stained sections; hyphae stain weakly with Gomori's methenamine silver (GMS) and other special stains for fungi, and are often more easily detected with H&E (Figure 125–6). Because the thin walls provide little structural stability, the hyphae are often twisted, folded, collapsed, and ribbon-like (Figure 125–7). The cytoplasmic contents are often absent, and hyphae appear empty with optically clear centers (Figure 125–6). Thick-walled chlamydoconidia may form within or at the ends of mucoraceous hyphae in lesions exposed to air (Figure 125–8). These chlamydoconidia, formed by hyperseptation and disarticulation, cluster in small groups after detachment from the hyphae, are intensely hematoxylinophilic or amphophilic, stain more deeply than contiguous hyphae with special stains for fungi, and can be mistaken for large, nonbudding yeastlike cells or sporangia[39] (Figure 125–9). Formation of sporangia and sporangiospores by zygomycetes is exceedingly rare in infected human tissues exposed to ambient air (Figure 125–10).

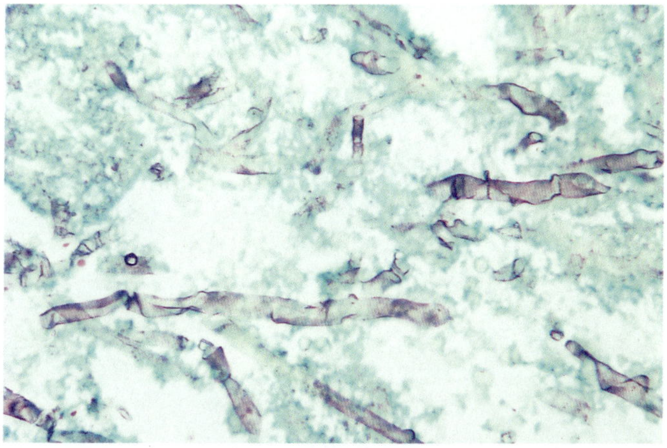

Figure 125–4. Pulmonary mucormycosis caused by a *Rhizopus* sp. This septic hemorrhagic infarct contains broad, randomly oriented, ribbon-like hyphae that have thin walls and irregular contours. Although often described as nonseptate, mucoraceous hyphae are actually pauciseptate *(right center)*. Septa, however, are rare in infected tissues and can be simulated by transverse folds and compressions of the thin delicate hyphal walls *(bottom left)* (GMS ×160).

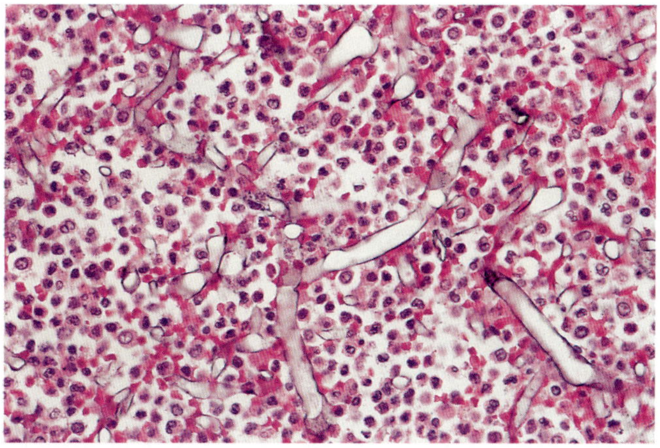

Figure 125–6. Pulmonary mucormycosis. Numerous randomly oriented hyphae within an arterial thrombus have thin walls that are weakly hematoxylinophilic. The cytoplasmic contents are absent in most of the hyphae, and they appear empty with optically clear centers (H&E, ×160).

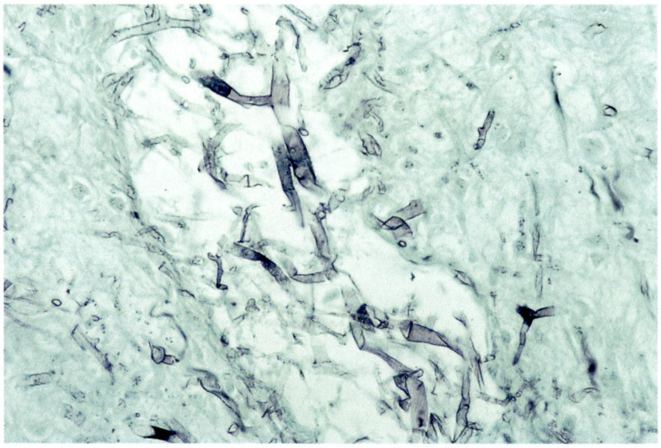

Figure 125–7. Gastrointestinal mucormycosis caused by *Cunninghamella bertholletiae*. Mucoraceous hyphae invade a submucosal blood vessel. Because the thin hyphal walls provide little structural stability, hyphae are often twisted, collapsed, and ribbon-like. The hyphae stain weakly with GMS and other special stains for fungi (GMS, ×100).

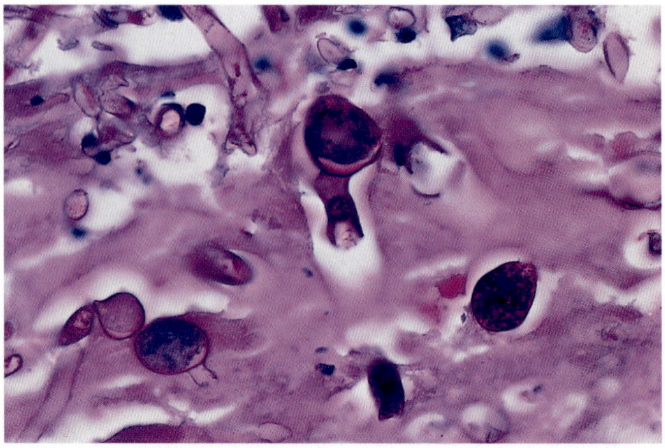

Figure 125–9. Pulmonary mucormycosis. Proliferating hyphae contain terminal chlamydoconidia that are spherical and have thick walls. Detached chlamydoconidia *(bottom)* can be easily mistaken for large yeastlike cells [periodic acid–Schiff (PAS), ×250].

PATHOLOGY

Like many other hyphal pathogens, hyphae of the mucoraceous zygomycetes are aggressively angioinvasive.[1,2] Invasion of arteries and veins, quite conspicuous in the lesions of mucormycosis, cause septic thrombosis, septic infarction, and systemic dissemination (Figure 125–11). The lesions of disseminated mucormycosis are predominantly infarctive (Figure 125–12), but also may be suppurative in nongranulocytopenic patients. The lesions in localized, indolent infections or in patients treated with amphotericin B may be granulomatous.

Entomophthoromycosis presents an altogether different histologic appearance.[1,2,5] The hyphal elements are sparse, frequently occur as short fragments, and show more conspicuous septation (Figure 125–13). Hyphal fragments are ensheathed by amorphous, intensely eosinophilic Splendore–Hoeppli material (Figure 125–14). The inflammatory response immediately surrounding hyphal fragments is eosinophilic or granulomatous, and the adjacent stroma consists of granulation tissue that is rich in eosinophils (Figure 125–14). The hyphae are not angioinvasive, which accounts for the more indolent clinical course of entomophthoromycosis when compared with mucormycosis.

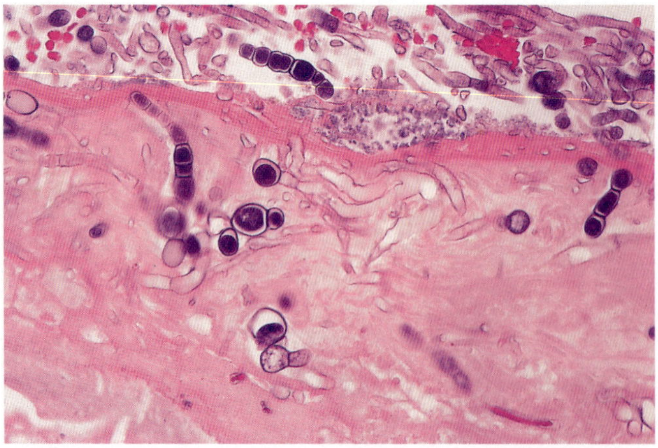

Figure 125–8. Cutaneous mucormycosis in a burned patient. Thick-walled, deeply hematoxylinophilic chlamydoconidia are produced by hyperseptation and disarticulation of mucoraceous hyphae in lesions exposed to air (H&E, ×100).

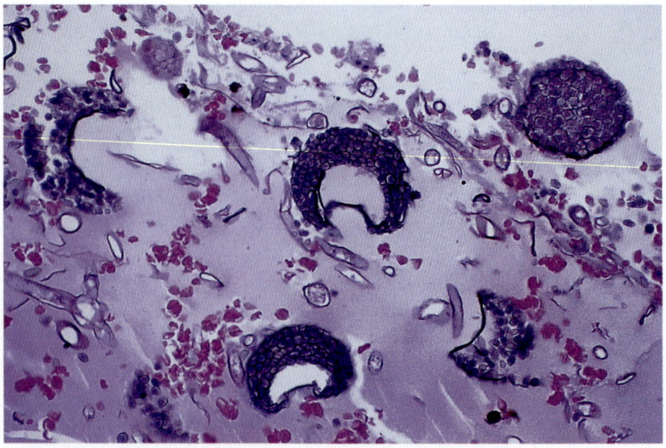

Figure 125–10. Rhinocerebral mucormycosis caused by a *Rhizopus* sp. Sporangia containing pigmented sporangiospores are located near the surface of the nasal lesion. In zygomycosis, sporangia and sporangiospores are rarely produced in tissues exposed to ambient air (H&E, ×100).

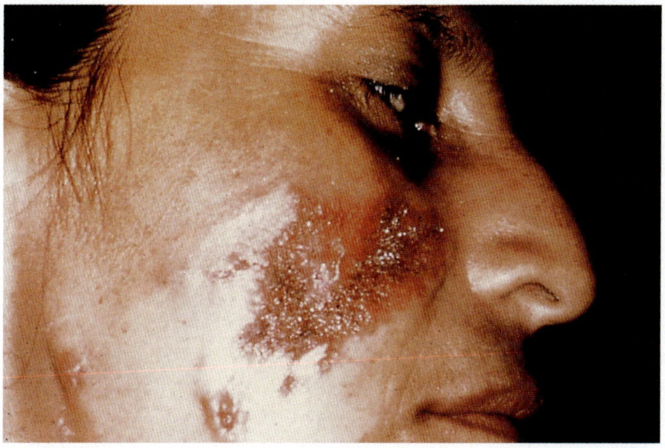

Figure 121–2. Chronic cutaneous sporotrichosis. A large, verrucous plaque on the right cheek. Note peripheral lymphangitis. *(Contributed by Centers for Disease Control and Prevention, Atlanta.)*

Primary pulmonary sporotrichosis is a progressive, bilateral, apical, cavitary, and destructive infection predominantly in middle-aged men who are alcoholics or have chronic obstructive pulmonary disease.[8,20,21] Patients often have nonspecific signs and symptoms, including fever, chills, chest pain, dyspnea, hemoptysis, cough, malaise, and weight loss; the clinical and radiographic findings closely resemble tuberculosis and histoplasmosis capsulati. Pulmonary lesions usually are large granulomas, sometimes necrotizing, that are multifocal, often confluent, and contain scattered or clustered yeast forms of *S schenckii.* Solitary, peripheral, fibrocaseous pulmonary nodules (sporotrichomas), similar to the histoplasmomas seen in residual pulmonary histoplasmosis capsulati, also have been described in a few patients with chronic pulmonary sporotrichosis.[2,8] Unlike histoplasmomas, however, calcification is rare.

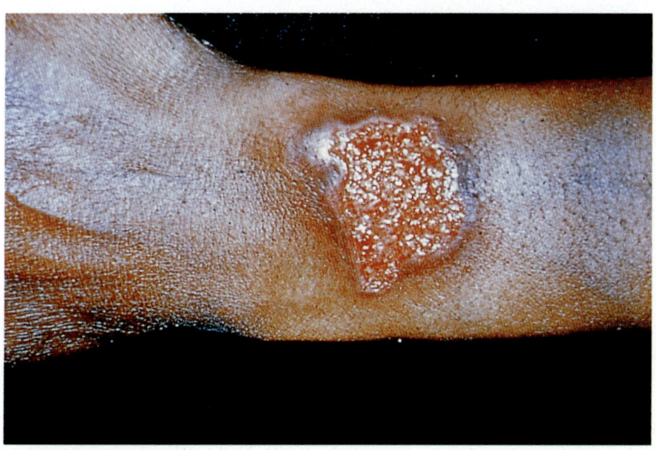

Figure 121–3. Cutaneous sporotrichosis. A large, solitary, sharply circumscribed ulcer with a prominent, raised margin on the forearm.

Occasionally, a primary cutaneous or pulmonary lesion may not be clinically apparent in patients who have disseminated sporotrichosis, and the predominant clinical findings may then be suppurative arthritis, osteomyelitis, periostitis, or tenosynovitis that frequently involves elbows and knees.[4,5,11] Without a preexisting cutaneous lesion, osteoarticular sporotrichosis may represent hematogenous spread from an inapparent pulmonary infection. In addition, many asymptomatic, otherwise healthy people who have significant antibody titers to *S schenckii* may have had previous pulmonary infection that spreads no further than hilar lymph nodes.

TREATMENT

The treatment of choice for the cutaneous and lymphocutaneous forms of sporotrichosis is an aqueous solution of saturated potassium iodide (1 g/mL) by mouth (1 to 2 mL every 8 hours until lesions disappear).[1,3] Systemic infections have been treated successfully with intravenous amphotericin B, and favorable responses have also been achieved with itraconazole and ketoconazole.[22,23] Relapse is uncommon.

PATHOLOGY

Florid pseudoepitheliomatous hyperplasia characterizes cutaneous sporotrichosis, and ulceration of the epidermis and intraepidermal microabscesses also may be present (Figure 121–4, A and B). *Sporothrix schenckii* usually elicits a mixed suppurative and granulomatous reaction that is often accompanied by fibrosis and microabscesses (Figure 121–5). This mixed pyogranulomatous reaction is typical of both localized and disseminated sporotrichosis, but it is not specific. Similar reactions can be seen in other mycoses, especially blastomycosis and chromoblastomycosis, and in bacterial diseases, eg, tuberculosis, syphilis, melioidosis, cat-scratch disease, and tularemia.[2,24]

In tissue sections, fungal elements of *S schenckii* are often sparse and difficult to visualize when stained with hematoxylin-eosin (H&E), but they usually can be demonstrated in replicate sections stained with Gomori's methenamine silver (GMS) (Figure 121–6).[2] They appear as spherical, oval, or elongated (cigar-shaped) single or budding yeastlike cells, 2 to 6 μm or more in maximum diameter (Figure 121–7). Some of the cells produce elongated buds that have a "teardrop" or "pipestem" configuration and, rarely, there are multiple buds (Figure 121–8). Cigar-shaped cells ("cigar bodies") are not regularly found except in disseminated lesions, in which they are usually mixed with a predominant

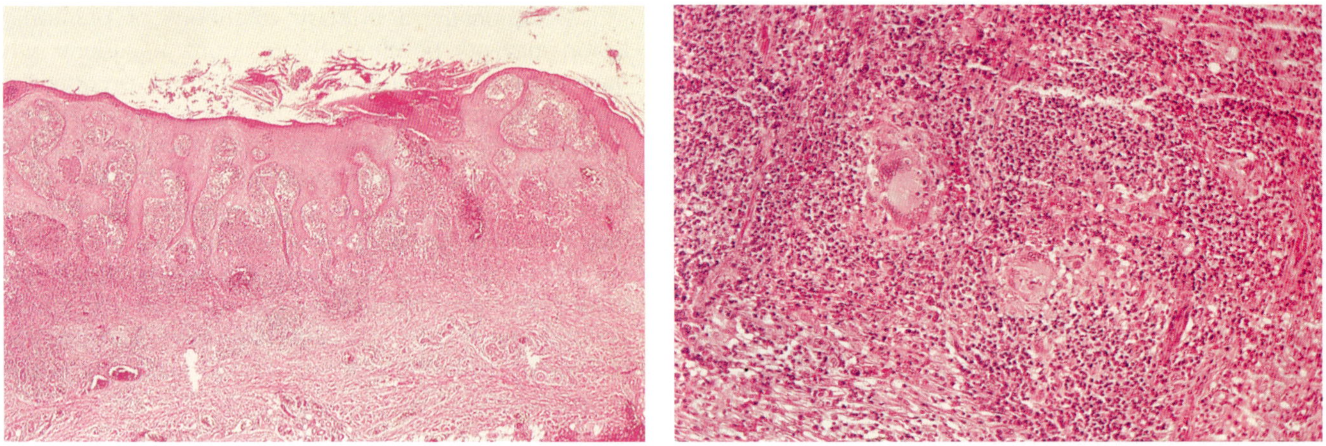

A B

Figure 121–4. (**A**) Cutaneous sporotrichosis. There is pseudoepitheliomatous hyperplasia and a mixed suppurative and granulomatous reaction in the dermis. Cutaneous ulcerative and verrucous lesions of sporotrichosis can be mistaken clinically for squamous cell carcinoma, especially when they are solitary (AFIP Neg 71-3916; H&E, ×16). (**B**) Same lesion shown in part (A). The mixed suppurative and granulomatous reaction is shown with higher magnification (AFIP Neg 71-3915; H&E, ×130).

population of spherical to oval yeast forms (Figures 121–9 and 121–10). Large, spherical yeast forms, which often appear empty and measure as much as 10 μm or more in diameter, also are occasionally encountered, particularly in disseminated lesions. These unusually large cells, with weakly stained or optically clear centers, however, are almost always mixed with typical forms of *S schenckii* (Figure 121–7). Germinating yeast forms and narrow, branched, septate hyphae of *S schenckii* that bear spherical conidia are sometimes observed in transepidermal elimination channels and in the hyperkeratotic surface layer of cutaneous lesions (Figure 121–11), but they are almost never in the dermis or in deep-seated lesions.[2,25,26]

In 1969, a new variety of *S schenckii* was described and named *S schenckii* var *luriei* by Ajello and Kaplan.[16] This unique variety was isolated from a cutaneous nodule of a South African. Since then, there have been several reported infections caused by the *luriei* variety, mostly in South Africa and Europe.[27] In culture, the *luriei* variety of *S schenckii* is indistinguishable from the classical form, but in tissue, the *luriei* variety forms not only typical budding yeastlike cells, but also distinctive, large (15 to 20 μm), spherical, thick-walled cells that

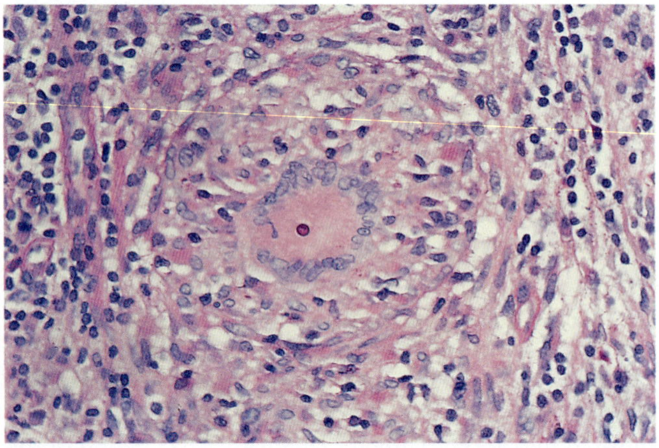

Figure 121–5. Granulomatous dermatitis caused by *S schenckii.* A Langhans' giant cell contains a single, spherical, yeastlike cell about 4 μm in diameter. Fungal elements are typically sparse in primary cutaneous lesions of sporotrichosis [periodic acid–Schiff (PAS) reaction, ×100).

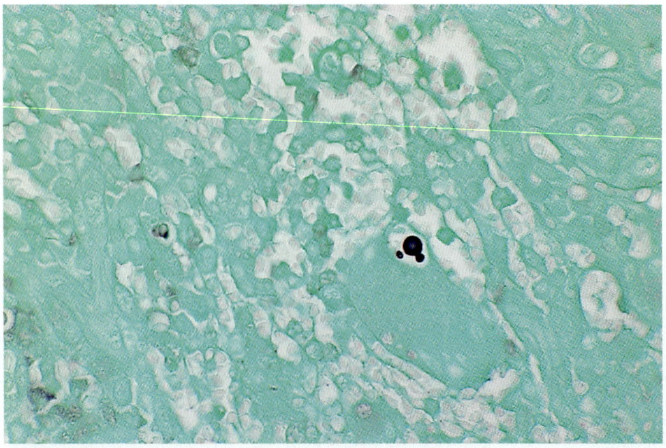

Figure 121–6. Cutaneous sporotrichosis. A dermal granuloma contains one budding cell and another small, spherical cell of *S schenckii.* Buds are attached to parent cells by relatively narrow bases (GMS, ×160).

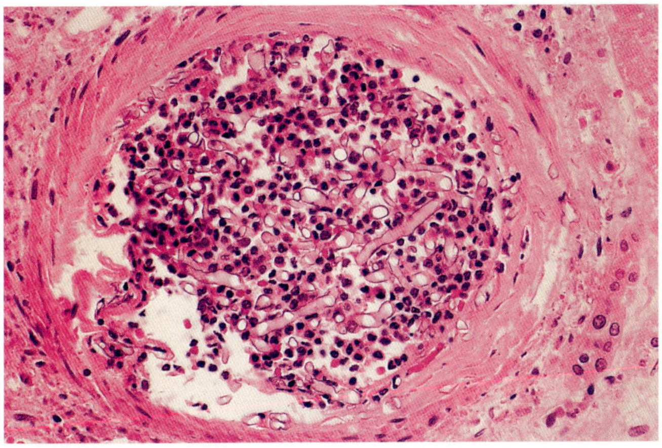

Figure 125–11. Disseminated mucormycosis. Broad, infrequently septate hyphae with thin walls penetrate the wall of a large blood vessel, causing thrombosis and infarction. Hyphae of the mucoraceous zygomycetes have a propensity for angioinvasion (H&E, ×100).

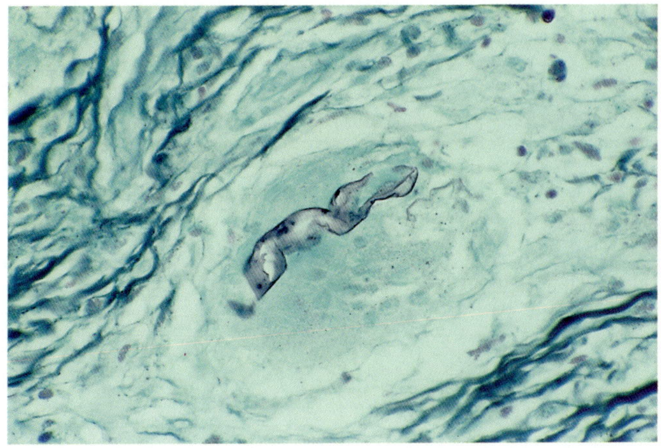

Figure 125–13. Subcutaneous entomophthoromycosis caused by *B ranarum*. A twisted, thin-walled hyphal fragment is in the center of an eosinophilic granuloma. Splendore–Hoeppli material that coats the hyphal fragment is GMS-negative (GMS, ×160).

DIFFERENTIAL DIAGNOSIS

Aspergillosis is the major infection confused with mucormycosis (Table 125–1). Usually these two mycoses are easily distinguished by hyphal morphology (width and uniformity of hyphae, frequency of septation, angle of branching, orientation of branches, and depth of staining with H&E and special stains for fungi).[2] Occasionally, however, the distinction is difficult, particularly when aspergillus hyphae are swollen and macerated or if the lesions contain only rare hyphal fragments (see Chapter 100). We have seen cases of zygomycosis, confirmed by microbiologic culture, in which the hyphae were relatively uniform with parallel contours and occasional septa. If microbiologic culture has not been performed, the diagnosis can often be resolved by direct immunofluorescence, which can generically identify the *Aspergillus* sp and the *Rhizopus* and *Absidia* sp in deparaffinized sections of formalin-fixed tissue.[1]

Hyphae of the *Fusarium* sp, 4 to 8 μm wide, resemble those of the aspergilli and also can be confused with zygomycetes in tissue sections.[2] Hyphal branches of the *Fusarium* sp characteristically arise at right angles from parent hyphae but, unlike those of the zygomycetes, are constricted at their sites of origin (see Chapter 107). The hyphae may produce terminal

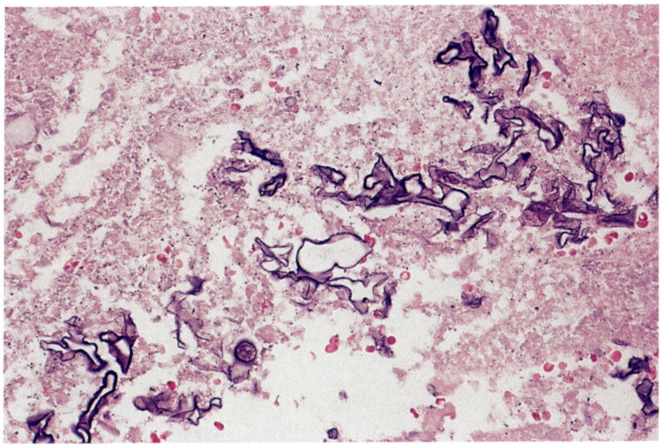

Figure 125–12. Pulmonary mucormycosis. A nodular infarct contains distorted, collapsed, and twisted hyphae that are randomly oriented and deeply hematoxylinophilic (H&E, ×100).

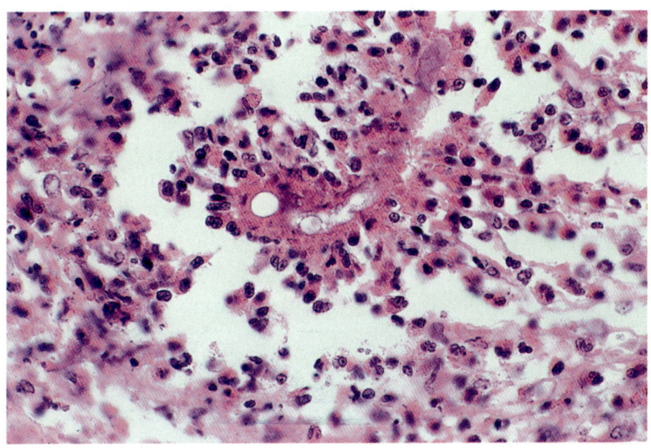

Figure 125–14. Subcutaneous entomophthoromycosis. A hyphal fragment of *B ranarum* is in an eosinophilic granuloma and ensheathed by intensely eosinophilic Splendore–Hoeppli material. The hyphal fragment has thin, weakly stained walls and an empty, optically clear center. Because hyphae are not angioinvasive, infarction and hematogenous dissemination are absent in this form of zygomycosis (H&E, ×160).

TABLE 125–1. HISTOMORPHOLOGIC FEATURES OF THE ASPERGILLI AND ZYGOMYCETES

Features	*Aspergillus* sp	*Rhizopus* sp and Other Zygomycetes
Width	Narrow (3–6 μm)	Broad (5–20 μm)
Caliber	Uniform	Variable
Branching	Regular, acute angle (dichotomous)	Haphazard, right angle
Orientation of branches	Parallel or radial	Random
Septations	Frequent	Infrequent

or intercalated chlamydoconidia; characteristic sickle-shaped macroconidia produced in culture are rarely encountered in host tissues. Definitive separation of the *Fusarium* sp from the zygomycetes requires microbiologic culture.

Transected zygomycete hyphae can resemble collapsed and empty spherules of *Coccidioides immitis,*[2] but typical mucoraceous hyphae elsewhere in the lesion and lack of endosporulating spherules serve to exclude zygomycosis. Dilated and branched capillaries, particularly in cerebral infarcts or granulation tissue, also can be mistaken for zygomycete hyphae. The basement membranes of these capillaries stain with PAS and GMS.

CONFIRMATIONAL TESTING AND DIAGNOSIS

The different genera and species of the mucoraceous zygomycetes cannot be distinguished from each other morphologically in tissue sections, although hyphae of the *Rhizopus* and *Absidia* sp can be identified generically and distinguished from the rest of the zygomycetes by direct immunofluorescence using a bivalent screening conjugate.[1] Definitive identification requires microbiologic culture on standard mycologic media.[4,8] This requires great care, since the causative agents of zygomycosis are ubiquitous in the environment and can easily contaminate cultures. The zygomycetes produce tall, cottony colonies within 3 to 5 days.

TREATMENT

Mucormycosis is a fulminating and highly aggressive opportunistic infection that is usually fatal unless promptly controlled. Successful therapy of mucormycosis depends on early recognition of the mycosis and is directed at control of the underlying disease, wide surgical debridement of accessible devitalized tissue, and antifungal chemotherapy with amphotericin B.[8,24,40]

REFERENCES

1. Chandler FW, Kaplan W, Ajello L. *Color Atlas and Textbook of the Histopathology of Mycotic Diseases.* Chicago: Year Book Medical Publishers; 1980:122–132, 294–301.
2. Chandler FW, Watts JC. *Pathologic Diagnosis of Fungal Infections.* Chicago: ASCP Press; 1987:85–95.
3. Baker RD. Mucormycosis (opportunistic phycomycosis). In: Baker RD, ed. *The Pathologic Anatomy of Mycoses: Human Infection with Fungi, Actinomycetes and Algae.* Berlin: Springer-Verlag; 1971:832–918.
4. Lehrer RI (moderator). Mucormycosis. *Ann Intern Med.* 1980;93(part 1):93–108.
5. Williams AO. Pathology of phycomycosis due to *Entomophthora* and *Basidiobolus* species. *Arch Pathol.* 1969; 87:13–20.
6. Sugar AM. Mucormycosis. *Clin Infect Dis.* 1992;14:S126–S129.
7. Meyer RD, Armstrong D. Mucormycosis: changing status. *CRC Crit Rev Clin Lab Sci.* 1973;4:421–451.
8. Marchevsky AM, Bottone EJ, Geller SA, et al. The changing spectrum of disease, etiology, and diagnosis of mucormycosis. *Hum Pathol.* 1980;11:457–464.
9. Hutter RVP. Phycomycetous infection (mucormycosis) in cancer patients: a complication of therapy. *Cancer.* 1959; 12:330–350.
10. Meyer RD, Rosen P, Armstrong D. Phycomycosis complicating leukemia and lymphoma. *Ann Intern Med.* 1972; 77:871–879.
11. Carbone KM, Pennington LR, Gimenz LF, et al. Mucormycosis in renal transplant patients: a report of two cases and review of the literature. *Q J Med.* 1985;57:825–831.
12. Parfrey NA. Improved diagnosis and prognosis of mucormycosis: a clinicopathologic study of 33 cases. *Medicine (Baltimore).* 1986;65:113–123.
13. Windus DW, Stokes TJ, Julian BA, Fenves AZ. Fatal *Rhizopus* infections in hemodialysis patients receiving desferrioxamine. *Ann Intern Med.* 1987;107:678–680.
14. Cuadrado LM, Guerrero A, Garcia-Asenjo JA, et al. Cerebral mucormycosis in two cases of acquired immunodeficiency syndrome. *Arch Neurol.* 1988;45:109–111.
15. Smith AG, Bustamante CI, Gilmor GD. Zygomycosis (absidiomycosis) in an AIDS patient. *Mycopathologia.* 1989;105:7–10.
16. Stave GM, Heimberger T, Kerkering TM. Zygomycosis of the basal ganglia in intravenous drug users. *Am J Med.* 1989;86:115–117.
17. Hopwood V, Hicks DA, Thomas S, et al. Primary cutaneous zygomycosis due to *Absidia corymbifera* in a patient with AIDS. *J Med Vet Mycol.* 1992;30:399–402.
18. Mostaza JM, Barbado RJ, Fernandez-Martin J, et al. Cutaneoarticular mucormycosis due to *Cunninghamella bertholletiae* in a patient with AIDS. *Rev Infect Dis.* 1989;11: 316–318.
19. Sanchez MR, Ponge-Wilson I, Moy JA, Rosenthal S. Zygomycosis and HIV infection. *J Am Acad Dermatol.* 1994;30:904–908.
20. Joe LK, Eng NIT. Subcutaneous phycomycosis: a new disease found in Indonesia. *Ann NY Acad Sci.* 1960;89:4–16.
21. Baker RD, Seabury JH, Schneidau JD. Subcutaneous and

cutaneous mucormycosis and subcutaneous phycomycosis. *Lab Invest.* 1962;11:1091–1102.

22. Gilbert EF, Khory GH, Pore RS. Histopathological identification of *Entomophthora* phycomycosis: deep mycotic infection in an infant. *Arch Pathol.* 1970;90:583–587.
23. Straatsma BR, Zimmerman LE, Gass JDM. Phycomycosis: a clinicopathologic study of fifty-one cases. *Lab Invest.* 1962;11:963–985.
24. Ferry AP, Abedi S. Diagnosis and management of rhino-orbitocerebral mucormycosis (phycomycosis): a report of 16 personally observed cases. *Ophthalmology.* 1983;90: 1096–1104.
25. Murray HW. Pulmonary mucormycosis with massive fatal hemoptysis. *Chest.* 1975;68:65–68.
26. Murray HW. Pulmonary mucormycosis: one hundred years later. *Chest.* 1977;72:1–2.
27. De Souza R, MacKinnon S, Spagnolo SV, Fossieck BE. Treatment of localized pulmonary phycomycosis. *South Med J.* 1979;72:609–612.
28. Donohue JF. Endobronchial mucormycosis. *Chest.* 1983; 83:585.
29. Lyon DT, Schubert TT, Mantia AG, et al. Phycomycosis of the gastrointestinal tract. *Am J Gastroenterol.* 1979;72: 379–394.
30. Ryan ME, Ochs J. Primary cutaneous mucormycosis: superficial and gangrenous infections. *Pediatr Infect Dis.* 1982;1:110–114.
31. Khardori N, Hayat S, Rolston K, et al. Cutaneous *Rhizopus* and *Aspergillus* infections in five patients with cancer. *Arch Dermatol.* 1989;125:952–956.
32. Gartenberg G, Bottone EJ, Keusch TG, et al. Hospital-acquired mucormycosis *(Rhizopus rhizopodiformis)* of skin and subcutaneous tissue: epidemiology, mycology, and treatment. *N Engl J Med.* 1978;299:1115–1118.
33. Neame P, Rayner D. Mucormycosis: a report on twenty-two cases. *Arch Pathol.* 1960;70:261–268.
34. McGinnis MR, Walker DH, Dominy IE, et al. Zygomycosis caused by *Cunninghamella bertholletiae:* clinical and pathologic aspects. *Arch Pathol Lab Med.* 1982;106: 282–291.
35. Virmani R, Connor DH, McAllister HA. Cardiac mucormycosis: a report of five patients and review of 14 previously reported cases. *Am J Clin Pathol.* 1982;78:42–47.
36. Ingram CW, Sennesh J, Cooper JN, Perfect JR. Disseminated zygomycosis: report of four cases and review. *Rev Infect Dis.* 1989;11:741–754.
37. Micozzi MS, Wetli CV. Intravenous amphetamine abuse, primary cerebral mucormycosis and acquired immunodeficiency. *J Forensic Sci.* 1985;30:504–510.
38. Gaing AA, Corbalan F, Weinberger J. Phycomycosis (mucormycosis) in differential diagnosis of cerebral mass lesions in intravenous drug users. *Mt Sinai J Med.* 1992; 59:69–71.
39. Chandler FW, Watts JC, Kaplan W, et al. Zygomycosis: report of four cases with formation of chlamydoconidia in tissue. *Am J Clin Pathol.* 1985;84:99–103.
40. Brown JF, Gottlieb LS, McCormick RA. Pulmonary and rhinocerebral mucormycosis: successful outcome with amphotericin B and griseofulvin therapy. *Arch Intern Med.* 1977;137:936–938.
41. Blodi FC, Hannah FT, Wadsworth JAC. Lethal orbito-cerebral phycomycosis. *Am J Ophthalmol.* 1969;67:698–705.

PART V

Protozoal Infections

CHAPTER 126

Cutaneous Acanthamoebiasis

Ernest E. Lack, Catherine P. Picken, and Princy N. Kumar

And then from hour to hour we rot and rot.
And thereby hangs a tale.

Shakespeare, As You Like It, II, 7

DEFINITION

Cutaneous acanthamoebiasis is an opportunistic infection of skin by free-living amebae of the genus *Acanthamoeba* and may be primary in the skin or a manifestation of disseminated infection.

CLINICAL FEATURES

Species of the genus *Naegleria* and *Acanthamoeba* are small free-living mobile amebae that only rarely cause human infection. Infection by *Acanthamoeba,* with the exception of corneal infection (keratitis), is opportunistic, and typically occurs in an immunodeficient host.[1,2] Patients at risk include those with malnutrition, cancer, or other debilitating illness and those receiving immunosuppressive therapy.[3] An increasing incidence of *Acanthamoeba* keratitis has been reported in those using contact lenses. Acanthamoebae live in soil, freshwater, pools, sewage, and in the feces of a variety of animals; some acanthamoebae have been isolated from human throat, nasal mucosa, and stool and even from dust in the air.[2] Cutaneous acanthamoebiasis is a rare opportunistic infection.[3–5] Some infections are clearly primary but in other patients hematogenous dissemination cannot be excluded.[4] Nasal mucosa is the portal of entry for the *Naegleria* that cause meningoencephalitis, but acanthamoebic meningoencephalitis is caused probably by acanthamoebae entering the lower respiratory tract with dust or aerosols.[1,2] In some patients cutaneous lesions antedate invasion of the central nervous system or they may be the sole manifestation of the infection especially in patients with human immunodeficiency virus (HIV) infection. In fact, some patients with the acquired immunodeficiency syndrome (AIDS) have had acanthamoebiasis beneath intact epidermis. These have been foci of dermal inflammation containing cysts and trophozoites.[4] Other patients have had cutaneous ulcers with undermined edges and abundant purulent exudate.[3] In one patient a disfiguring mucocutaneous ulcer involving nasal septum, the alae, and adjacent lip and face destroyed underlying soft tissue and cartilage (Figure 126–1, A and B). The pathologist must look carefully for acanthamoebae in biopsy specimens of all cutaneous inflammatory lesions from patients with AIDS and especially in those that have persisted after the usual treatments for bacterial and mycotic pathogens.

DIAGNOSIS

Biopsy of a cutaneous lesion can lead quickly to a diagnosis of acanthamoebiasis but there are caveats. First the specimen should include the advancing margin of the lesion, especially if it is raised. The raised margin (Figure 126–2) is almost certain to contain more acanthamoebae than the crater. Second, the pathologist must remember the possibility of cutaneous acanthamoebiasis and remember too what the trophozoites look like, for even when present in fair numbers they may be overlooked or mistaken for histiocytes and macrophages. In some specimens acanthamoebic trophozoites have been mistaken for *Blastomyces dermatitidis.*[4] Acanthamoebae have two stages, the trophozoite (Figures 126–2 through 126–4) and the cyst described in Chapter 132. Most species of *Acanthamoeba* resemble

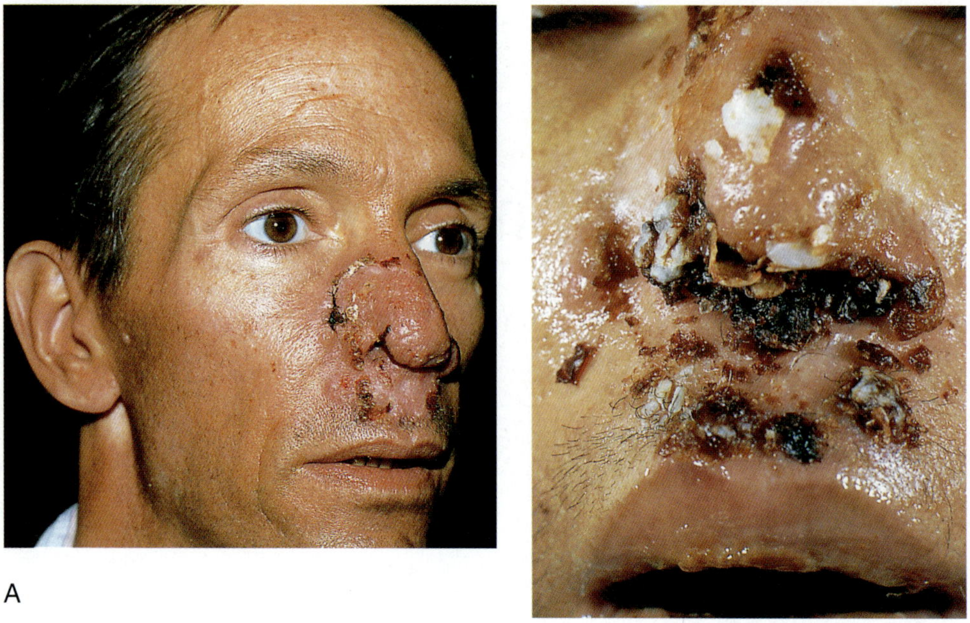

A

B

Figure 126–1. (**A**) A 44-year-old man with mucocutaneous acanthamoebiasis of nose, lip, and face. Although HIV infection was diagnosed in 1987 he remained well until August 1993, when, 2 weeks after swimming in freshwater on Cape Cod, a small "pustule" appeared on the right nostril just above the ala. The pustule ulcerated and gradually spread. Localized pain in the margin heralded expansion of the ulcer. The ulcer spread up over the nose, down to the lip, over the face, and inward to nasal septum. Beginning in September 1993 he was seen repeatedly by different physicians and given multiple cycles of antibiotics. In June and July 1994 two different biopsy specimens of the ulcer crater revealed "chronic inflammation" but in August 1994 a specimen taken at the raised expanding margin revealed acanthamoebic trophozoites. Treatment with intravenous pentamidine was begun and the lesion regressed in 2 weeks. He then developed renal failure and pentamidine had to be stopped. After a hiatus of 2 weeks pentamidine was restarted but now the lesion continued to advance. He died a month later of line-related enterococcal complications and microsporidial enteritis. Autopsy revealed acanthamoebic trophozoites in the inflamed base of the ulcer over the eroded nasal septum but there was no evidence of acanthamoebiasis in any other organ or tissue. After fluorescent antibody studies, Dr. Visvesvara thought the infectious agent probably belonged to the *Acanthamoeba castellani* group. (**B**) At postmortem there is extensive destruction of the tip of nose, alae, and septum. The lesion encroaches on cheeks and upper lip. A hemorrhagic crust covers the ulcers. The white cream is antifungal ointment. *(Photographs by Daniel H. Connor, MD, August and October 1994, respectively.)*

each other in tissue sections but antibody tagged immunofluorescent stains may allow a specific diagnosis.[6] The amebae feed on enteric gram-negative bacteria such as *Escherichia coli,* and using non-nutrient agar plates overgrown with these bacteria one may see the tracks of migrating amebae (Figure 126–5).[7]

TREATMENT

Effective treatment for disseminated acanthamoebiasis has not been established; some studies have documented sensitivity of *Acanthamoeba* species to a variety of antifungal, antibacterial, and other agents. Most recently intravenous pentamidine has been used.[3]

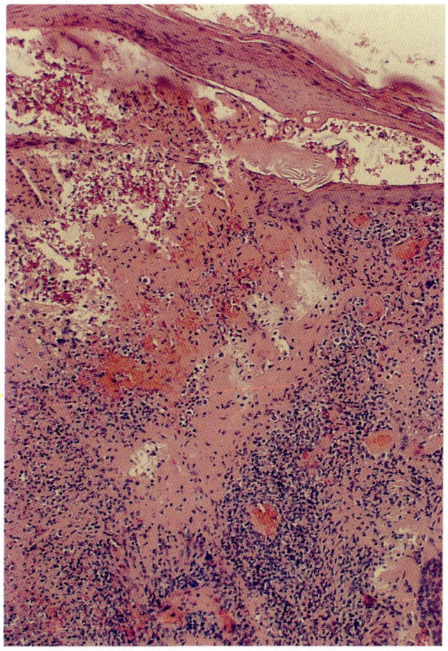

Figure 126–2. Biopsy specimen taken at the advancing margin of the ulcer. The epidermis is lifted up and there is fibrinopurulent exudate in the crater. The viable margin is hyperemic and contains many lymphocytes and plasma cells. There are trophozoites in the undermined edge [Hematoxylin-eosin (H&E), ×40].

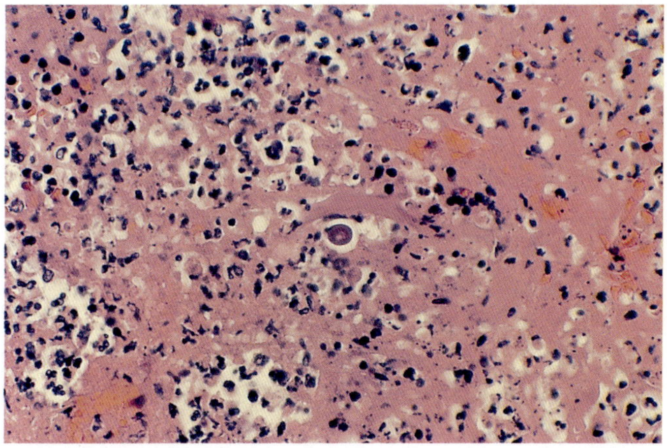

Figure 126–3. Higher magnification in the margin of the ulcer reveals a fibrin-rich exudate containing neutrophils, many of which are degenerating. In some areas there is a granulomatous component with epithelioid cells and occasional giant cells. A single trophozoite is in the center (H&E, ×200).

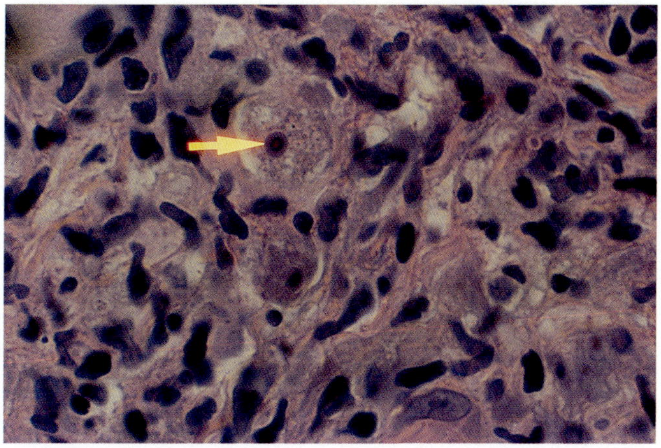

Figure 126–4. This trophozoite has distinct cell borders, and a nucleus *(arrow)* with a nucleolus surrounded by a halo. Most of the trophozoites have ameboid shapes, are 20 μm across, and have amphophilic cytoplasm sometimes containing many vacuoles, as seen here. Trophozoites are concentrated at the margin of the lesion (H&E, ×1000).

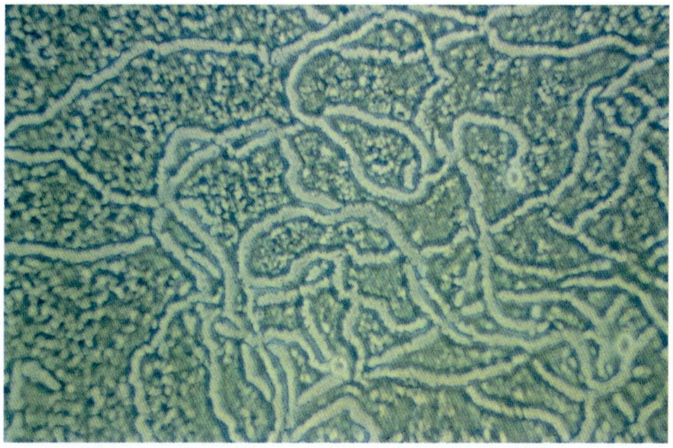

Figure 126–5. Curvilinear tracks left by mobile acanthamoebae on agar plate are highlighted with phase contrast microscopy. *(Picture courtesy of Dr. J.P. McCulley.)*

REFERENCES

1. Visvesvara GS, Stehr-Green JK. Epidemiology of free-living ameba infections. *J Protozool.* 1990;37:25S–33S.
2. Ma P, Visvesvara GS, Martinez AJ, Theodore FH, Daggett P-M, Sawyer TK. *Naegleria* and *Acanthamoeba* infections: review. *Rev Infect Dis.* 1990;12:490–513.
3. Slater CA, Sickel JZ, Visvesvara GS, Pabico RC, Gaspari AA. Brief report: successful treatment of disseminated *Acanthamoeba* infection in an immunocompromised patient. *N Engl J Med.* 1994;331:85–87.
4. Tan B, Weldon-Linne CM, Rhone DP, Penning CL, Visvesvara GS. *Acanthamoeba* infection presenting as skin lesions in patients with the acquired immunodeficiency syndrome. *Arch Pathol Lab Med.* 1993;117:1043–1046.
5. Park CH, Iyengar V, Hefter L, Pestaner JP, Vandel NM. Cutaneous *Acanthamoeba* infection associated with acquired immunodeficiency syndrome. *Lab Med.* 1994;25:386–388.
6. Visvesvara GS. Classification of *Acanthamoeba*. *Rev Infect Dis.* 1991;13:S369–S372.
7. Moore MB, McCulley JP, Luckenbach M, et al. *Acanthamoeba* keratitis associated with soft contact lenses. *Am J Ophthalmol.* 1985;100:396–403.

CHAPTER 127

Amebiasis—Infection by *Entamoeba histolytica*

H. Braunstein and Daniel H. Connor

> *Water . . . doth very greatly deject their appetite, destroy the natural heat, and overthrow the strength of the stomacke, and consequently, confounding the concoction, is the cause of crudities, fluctuations, and windinesse in the bodie.*
>
> *Tobias Venner (1577–1660)*

INTRODUCTION

Amebiasis, a term that includes all infections caused by *Entamoeba histolytica,* is cosmopolitan, enterically transmitted, and most prevalent in the Third World. In the United States most of those infected are travelers who have returned from endemic areas. Focal outbreaks in the Western world are almost always waterborne. Amebiasis has been recognized for more than 100 years; the name of the organism, *Entamoeba histolytica,* was proposed by Schaudinn, who differentiated it from the nonpathogenic *Entamoeba coli* in 1903.

THE ORGANISM

Entamoeba histolytica has a simple life cycle. Stages include cyst, precyst, and trophozoite. The cyst is both the resting stage and the infective stage. Cysts are spherical, 10 to 15 μm across and contain one to four spherical nuclei. When ingested with contaminated food or drink, the cyst excysts and becomes a trophozoite, which invades the colonic mucosa establishing infection. Here trophozoites grow and multiply. Trophozoites therefore are the tissue stage of the parasite and when identified in tissue sections confirm a diagnosis of amebiasis.

Trophozoites that do not invade colonic mucosa pass to the lower colon, encyst as uninucleated precysts, and pass in the stool becoming a source of contamination and infection. Cysts are resistant to both desiccation and temperature variation. They may remain viable for up to a month in water at 4° and for 48 hours in foods at room temperature. They are destroyed by boiling but are resistant to the chlorine concentrations usually used to treat drinking water.

PATHOGENESIS

Although *E histolytica* has a simple life cycle, the pathogenesis of human infection is complex and not completely understood. Amebic cysts resist gastric acidity.[1] After ingestion, they enter the small intestine where cyst walls are digested and metacystic trophozoites emerge. These migrate to the colon, especially the cecal region where, under favorable conditions, they multiply by binary fission. What determines pathogenicity is not clear. Strain specificity was formerly thought to be important: The "Laredo" strain was deemed less pathogenic; this has more recently been questioned.[3] "Small race" *E histolytica* is now recognized as a smaller but morphologically identical organism.

When the infecting dose is high, infection is more likely and those infections that do develop tend to be more severe. Pregnant women, the malnourished, patients with faulty immune mechanisms including those being treated with corticosteroids and victims of acquired immunodeficiency syndrome, as well as infants are all at increased risk. In fact, all of these have

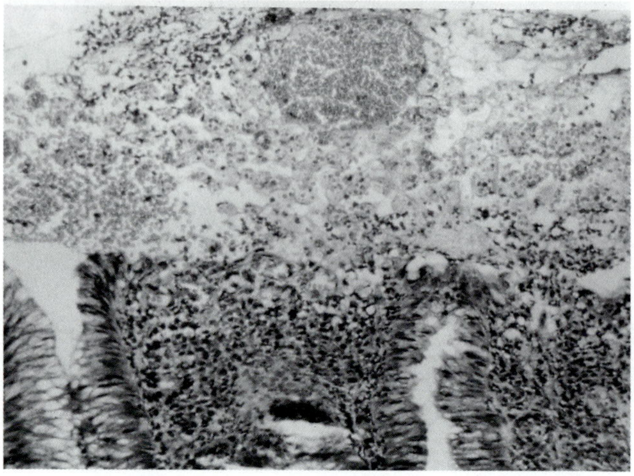

A

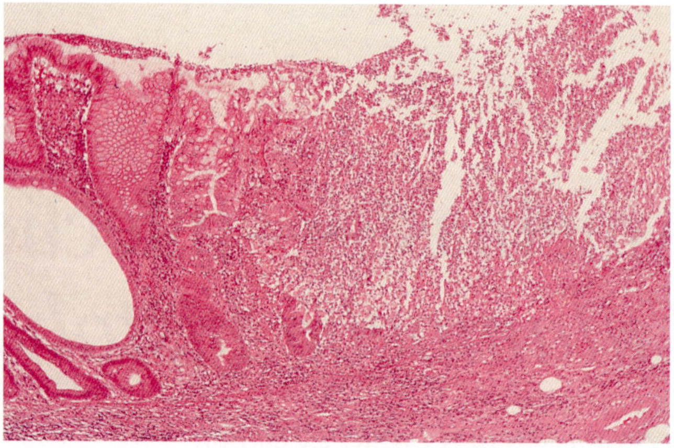

B

Figure 127–1. Sections of colon showing lytic process in amebiasis. (**A**) A cluster of trophozoites (*upper half of a picture*) has destroyed the epithelium and the supporting lamina propria. A sharp line delimits the viable margin. "Ghosts" of trophozoites are in the necrotic material on the surface [AFIP Neg 69-7842; hematoxylin-eosin (H&E), ×110]. (**B**) Same phenomenon but here the entire thickness of the mucosa is destroyed—down to and including the muscularis mucosae (AFIP Neg 68-5943; H&E, ×50).

an increased frequency of invasive amebiasis and their infections tend to be more severe. Sexual transmission may occur, especially among homosexuals.[3] Survival of pathogenic trophozoites is enhanced by microaerophilic conditions and by the presence of abundant bacterial flora.[3] Pathogenic trophozoites, under appropriate conditions, become attached to epithelial cells by lectins and produce a variety of toxic substances including proteolytic enzymes (Figure 127–1), glycosidases, and pore-forming proteins.[4–7] Trophozoites may also demonstrate enterotoxigenic activity.[3] Neutrophils are attracted to the infection, become damaged, and release enzymes that promote tissue destruction.[8–10]

Some patients are asymptomatic but continue to pass cysts. It has been suggested that these patients may have small colonic ulcers, or they may be noninfected carriers[11] complicated by other enteric problems. It is claimed that between 5% and 10% of the world's population has amebiasis or at least passes cysts.

DIAGNOSIS

Stools must be searched carefully for trophozoites and the stools must be fresh because trophozoites are fragile and disintegrate quickly. But searching stools for trophozoites may have a low yield even in patients with active colonic amebiasis, so multiple stool specimens must be searched[1,12] and, if doubt persists, a biopsy done through the margin of a colonic ulcer.

Biopsy specimens revealing trophozoites are more satisfactory than smears for diagnosis because the trophozoites are in the context of inflammation, necrosis, and ulceration. In early lesions trophozoites are concentrated on the surface of the colon (Figure 127–1) and later in the crater of the ulcer. Specimens taken through or at the margins of active lesions yield high rates of diagnosis. Trophozoites in tissue sections resemble those in fixed smears, although in tissue their nuclei may stain weakly or may be out of the plane of section. Trophozoites have characteristic features and their identification in tissue sections is diagnostic. Being an entire organism, the trophozoite has a sharply outlined cell membrane (more sharply outlined than mammalian cells for instance), amphophilic cytoplasm when the tissue has been well fixed, and the cytoplasm contains a variety of structures including vacuoles, sometimes ingested erythrocytes, fragments of nuclei, and other cellular debris. The cytoplasm of most trophozoites contains abundant glycogen, which stains intensely with periodic acid–Schiff (PAS) stain. Nuclei of *E histolytica* are 2 to 3 μm across, are distinctly smaller than mammalian nuclei, and have less chromatin—a consequence no doubt of their considerably decreased genetic information. The nucleus has a central karyosome and a concentration of chromatin around the nuclear membrane. These features serve to distinguish trophozoites of *E histolytica* from mammalian cells (Figures 127–2 and 127–3). In spite of these distinct features, however, trophozoites are regularly confused

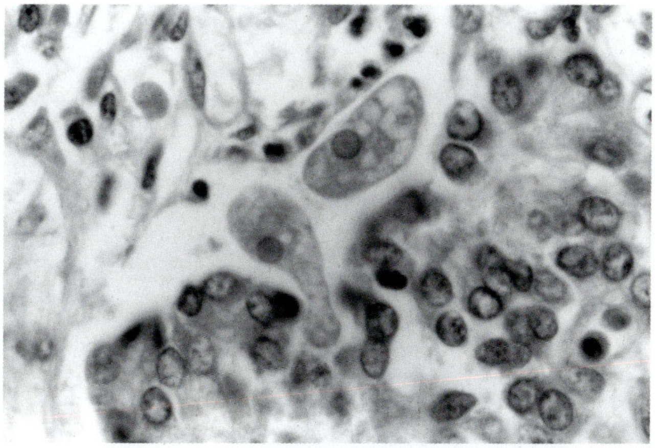

Figure 127–2. Section of lung from a 37-year-old Zairian man who had cough, hemoptysis, and emaciation and was treated for tuberculosis. The hemoptysis continued; 1 week before death he developed severe diarrhea, hectic fevers, and anemia (4.0 g of Hgb per 100 mL). At autopsy a large amebic liver abscess had eroded through the peritoneum, diaphragm, and pleura to form a large area of consolidation and cavitation in the right lower lobe. Here two trophozoites of *E histolytica* are in the viable margin of the lung abscess. Note the characteristic features: 1) a sharp cellular outline—a more distinct outline than the surrounding host cells, 2) ameboid shapes, 3) granular and vacuolated cytoplasm, 4) a single small round nucleus in each trophozoite, and 5) a karyosome in the center of each nucleus. Sometimes the karyosome is not visible in tissue sections, especially with routine H&E staining (H&E, ×2000). *(Specimen contributed by Leo O. Lanoie, MD, Karawa Mission Hospital, Zaire; photograph by Daniel H. Connor, MD, 1977.)*

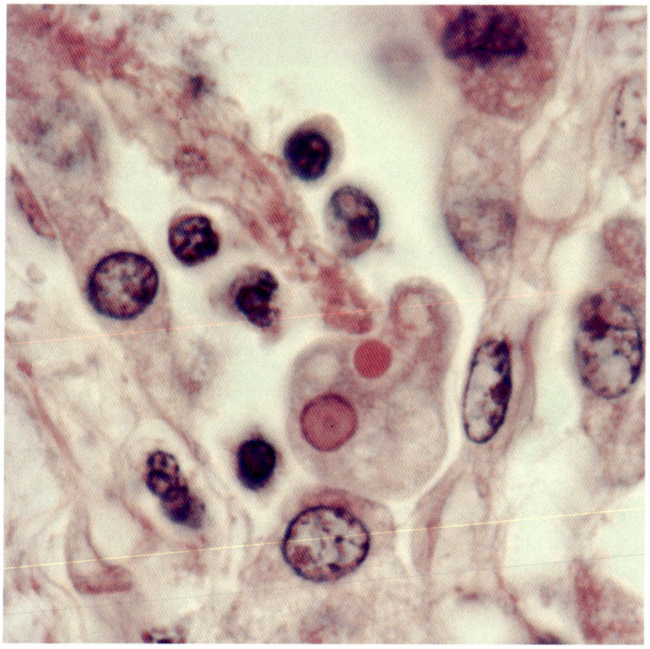

Figure 127–3. A single trophozoite of *E histolytica* is in the center of the photograph. Note the features listed for trophozoites of *E histolytica* in Figure 127–2. In addition there is an erythrocyte in the cytoplasm (H&E, ×2000). *(Photograph by Daniel H. Connor, MD, 1979.)*

with histiocytes/macrophages and sometimes with ganglion cells.

Histiocytes/macrophages tend to be smaller than trophozoites; the latter frequently measure up to 20 μm or more in diameter.[13] So too the nuclei of histiocytes/macrophages are larger than the nuclei of trophozoites and they have coarser chromatin, which is characteristic of mammalian cells in general. As noted earlier, ganglion cells may be confused with trophozoites too but they tend to be larger than trophozoites and they often have a triangular outline and are more intensely stained. Their nuclei usually contain large nucleoli and their cytoplasm often contains basophilic granules but not PAS-positive material. *Balantidium coli* may cause identical colonic lesions, but *B coli* is several times larger than *E histolytica* and has a distinctive shape. Electron microscopy is of little practical value in detecting or confirming amebae in diagnostic material. While of theoretical value, immunostaining and nucleic acid probes for detecting amebae in the routine diagnostic surgical pathology laboratory await the commercial development of specific preparations.

Immunologic detection is now of primary value in the diagnosis of extraintestinal amebiasis. Detection of antibody by indirect hemagglutination (or other techniques) is sensitive and specific.[14,15] An enzyme-linked immunosorbent assay that can detect antigen in stools has been described.[16] Although culture is readily achieved using special media, morphology and serology are almost universally used for identification.

COMPLICATIONS OF COLONIC AMEBIASIS

In severe infections the ulcers become more deeply penetrating and more broadly undermined (Figure 127–4). As the necrosis advances some ulcers become confluent (Figures 127–5 through 127–7). Other complications include amebic appendicitis, perforation of colonic ulcers into the peritoneal cavity with peritonitis, perforation of skin of trunk or abdomen, and hemorrhage from a colonic ulcer. If specific antiamebic therapy is delayed, there may be scarring with stricture or cicatricial shrinkage. When the lower colon is heavily infected there may be perianal and perineal extension (Figures 127–8 and 127–9). Not all lesions of amebiasis

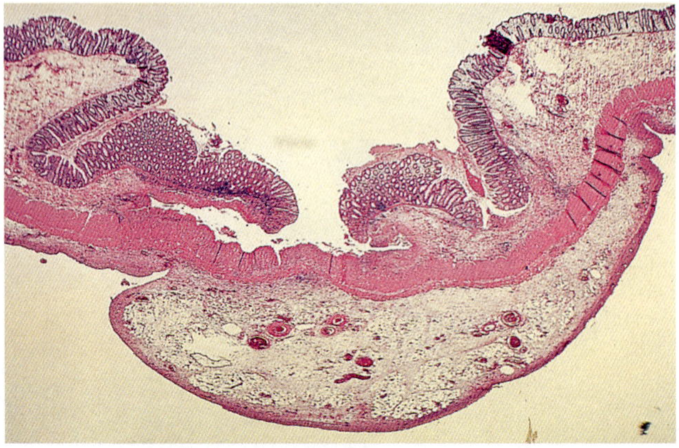

Figure 127–4. This amebic ulcer of the colon has destroyed a narrow circle of mucosa and a broader area of submucosa down to the muscularis. The serosa is edematous and hyperemic. Mucosa over the ulcer is undermined and this, with the edema of the mucosa, has produced the characteristic flask shape of the amebic ulcer (AFIP Neg 74-2981; H&E, ×6.5).

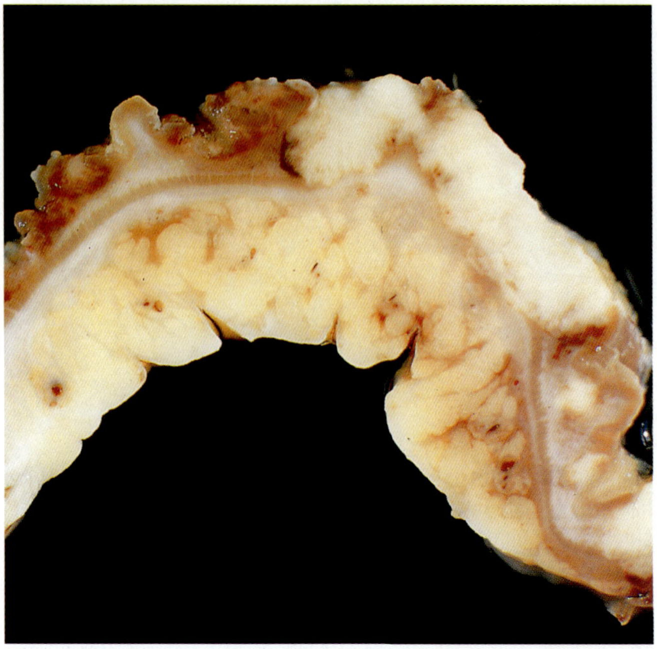

Figure 127–6. Vertical section of same colon in Figure 127–5 showing confluent amebic ulcers. The ulcers are deep, crowded together, and their craters are expanded with a fibrin-rich necrotic exudate. The entire colon was involved and the necrosis in this area has extended through the bowel wall and into periocolic fat. (gross, ×2). *(Photograph by Daniel H. Connor, MD, 1981.)*

are typical clinically or grossly and some lesions may resemble those of other enteric infections. One complication of amebic colitis is the "ameboma." This is a fibroinflammatory reaction to trophozoites in the wall of the colon. By imaging techniques and endoscopy the "ameboma" resembles a constricting or "napkin ring" adenocarcinoma. The tumefaction in amebomas is exuberant granulation tissue and scar tissue.[17] Unsuspected amebic colitis may be encountered at necropsy or in specimens resected surgically.

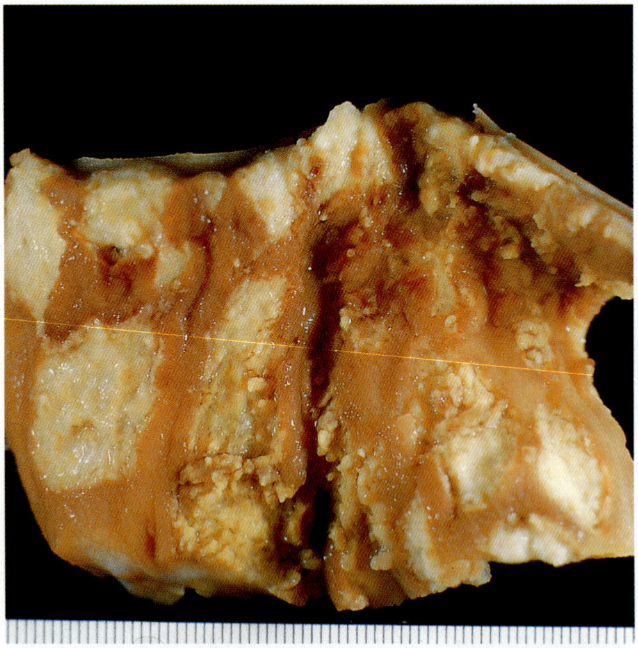

Figure 127–5. Confluent colonic ulcers in a 38-year-old woman with severe colonic amebiasis. A fibrin-rich exudate fills the craters of the ulcers. The patient had chronic diarrhea misdiagnosed as ulcerative colitis and was treated with corticosteroids. After several weeks her colitis became life threatening and a colectomy was done (gross, ×2.5). *(Photograph by Daniel H. Connor, MD, 1981.)*

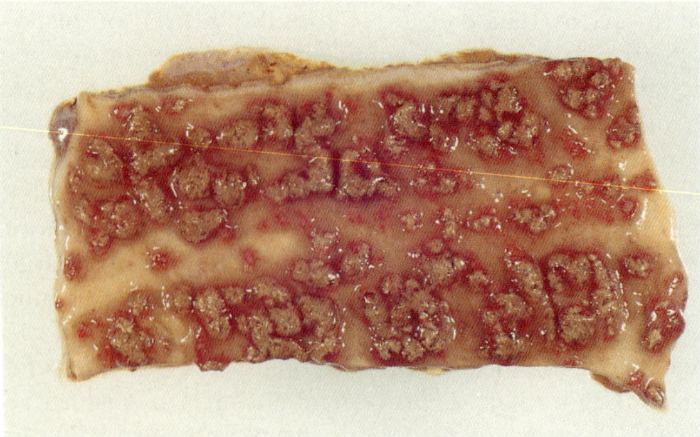

Figure 127–7. Colon taken at autopsy of an adult male Ugandan with diffuse confluent amebic ulcers of the colon. The patient's disease was misdiagnosed as plasmacytoma and treated with chemotherapeutic agents and corticosteroids (gross, ×0.9). *(Photograph by Daniel H. Connor, MD, 1962.)*

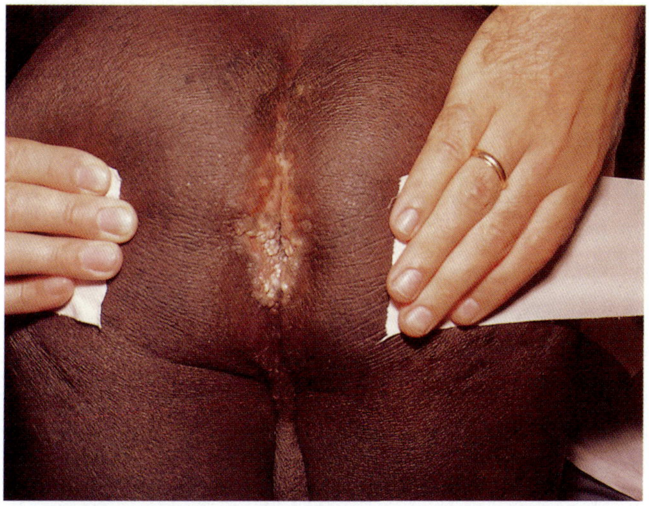

Figure 127–8. Extension of colonic and rectal amebiasis to anal skin in a 39-year-old Zairian male judge. When trophozoites invade squamous epithelium, they cause, as shown here, epithelial hyperplasia. This appearance is easily mistaken for squamous cell carcinoma. When trophozoites of *E histolytica* were identified in the biopsy specimen, the patient was treated with emetine hydrochloride and the lesion healed quickly (clinical, ×0.3). *(Patient of Dr. Roger Thorpe; photograph by Daniel H. Connor, MD, 1968.)*

SPECTRUM OF CLINICAL AMEBIASIS

Invasion of tissue by trophozoites is associated with variable clinical manifestations most of which cannot be distinguished from other infectious and noninfectious diarrheal diseases. Manifestations may be acute or chronic and the clinical manifestations of chronic amebiasis may be confused with ulcerative colitis. Patients with amebiasis, misdiagnosed and treated with corticosteroids develop overwhelming colonic amebiasis (Figures 127–5 through 127–8).

In mild infections endoscopic or gross examination reveals scattered ulcerations, characteristically having small orifices in the center and raised margins caused by inflammation of undermined mucosa. If amebic trophozoites cannot be identified in stool, exudate obtained by colonoscopy may be readily diagnostic.

Amebic Liver Abscess

The most frequent complication of invasive amebiasis of the colon is amebic liver abscess. Trophozoites enter the radicals of the portal vein and from there are carried with the portal blood to the liver. Some believe "amebic hepatitis" precedes the formation of an amebic abscess, but there is no morphologic evidence for an "amebic hepatitis." When trophozoites lodge in the liver, they cause an initial lytic lesion followed by an exudate of neutrophils. As neutrophils die and release proteolytic enzymes, there is further destruction of tissue resulting in an abscess. About two thirds of patients

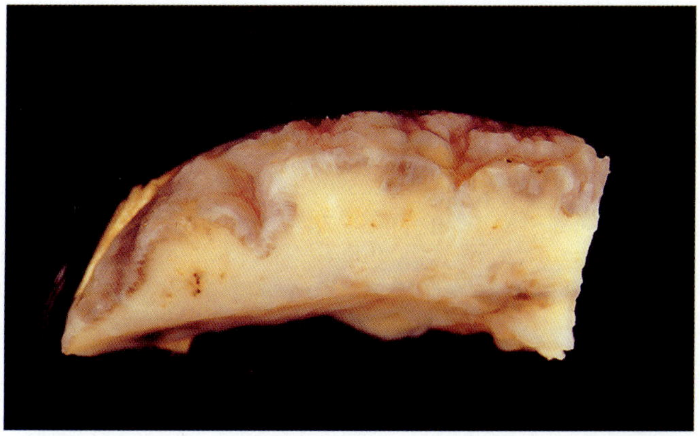

A

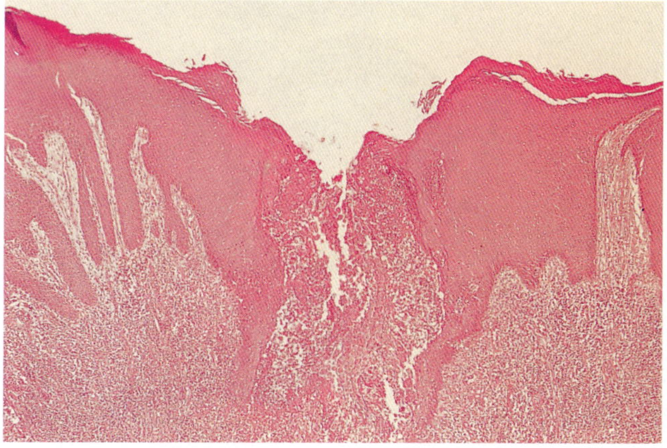

B

Figure 127–9. (**A**) Amebiasis of skin of vulva mistaken for carcinoma and widely excised. The patient was a 60-year-old Zairian woman from Kasai province. Microscopically there were epithelial hyperplasia and multiple penetrating ulcers beneath colonies of trophozoites. (**B**) Section showing the epithelial hyperplasia and a characteristic penetrating ulcer. The crater of the ulcer is filled with trophozoites enmeshed in delicate strands of fibrin (gross, ×3.5). *(Specimen contributed by Dr. Hilma Michalek; photographs by Daniel H. Connor, MD, 1976.)*

with hepatic amebiasis have a single abscess[18] and about one third have multiple abscesses. Bacterial abscesses of the liver, on the other hand, are usually multiple. Necropsy studies, however, show a higher frequency of multiple amebic abscesses than do clinical studies, indicating the progressive nature of hepatic amebiasis.[17] Grossly, amebic abscesses have a necrotic semisolid center, usually brown-orange, resembling anchovy paste (Figure 127–10). Microscopically there is an acellular necrotic center surrounded by a ring of stroma. The outermost zone of the abscess, the one adjacent to viable liver tissue, contains fibrin in which are enmeshed trophozoites often in small numbers. Material aspirated from the center of amebic abscesses contains no recognizable trophozoites. Viable trophozoites are concentrated at the perimeter of the abscess.[12] Inability to culture bacteria is helpful diagnostically. In the Western world, specimens from amebic liver abscesses are rarely encountered today because modern imaging techniques enable accurate diagnosis (Figure 127–11) and immunologic testing is about 98% sensitive.[14,15] For unknown reasons, fewer than 20% of patients with liver abscess have demonstrable amebae in their stools.[3,12]

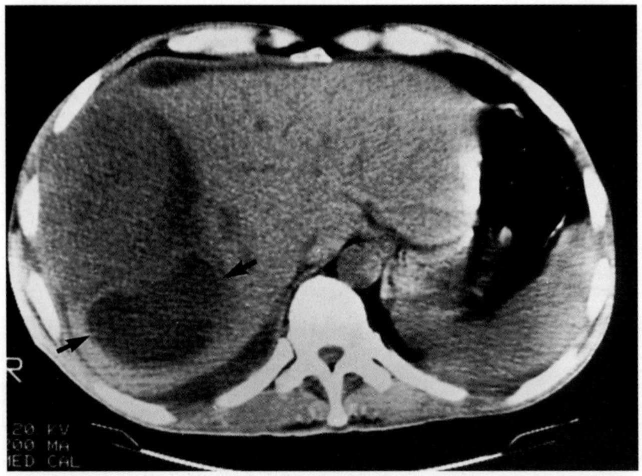

Figure 127–11. Computerized axial tomographic scan of the liver in a patient with an amebic liver abscess. The diagnosis was established by serologic testing and the good response to antiamebic therapy. The amebic abscess is the defect in the right lobe *(arrows)*.

Pleuropulmonary Amebiasis

Amebic abscesses of liver may perforate through the diaphragm and cause empyema and lung abscess. Rarely, lung abscess may result from hematogenous spread. After liver, lung is the most common site of extraintestinal amebiasis.

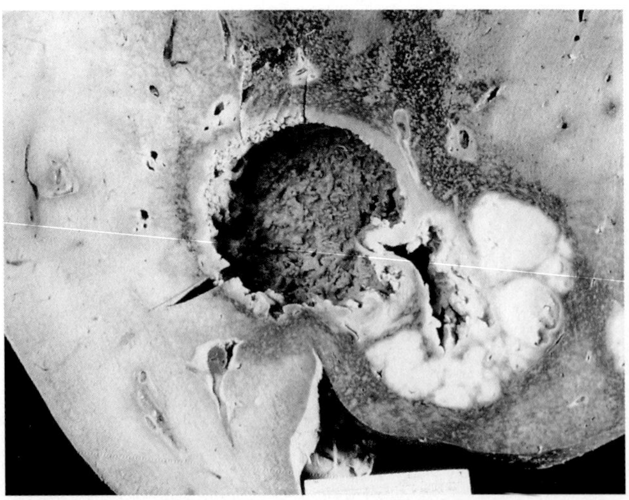

Figure 127–10. Cut of liver taken through adjoining amebic abscesses. The one to the lower right is still a coagulum—white and homogeneous—but the other contained semisolid liquid, which escaped when the liver was cut postmortem. The semisolid liquid was viscid, brown, and resembled anchovy paste (gross, ×3.5). *(Specimen contributed by Professor S. Kalichurum, Durban; photograph by Daniel H. Connor, MD, 1985.)*

Pericarditis

This is a severe complication and usually a consequence of extension from an amebic abscess in the left lobe of the liver or less often by direct extension from pleuropulmonary amebiasis. Suppurative amebic pericarditis may be preceded by a serositis at the time of initial extension. Restrictive pericarditis and tamponade are fatal complications.

Amebiasis of the Central Nervous System

The central nervous system (CNS) is rarely invaded by trophozoites of *E histolytica.* Spread to the CNS is usually hematogenous from hepatic or pleuropulmonary amebiasis. Amebic abscesses of brain vary in size and number and contain yellow green necrotic tissue which is sometimes bloodstained. The left cerebral hemisphere is most frequently involved.[17] Extension to the leptomeninges may cause purulent meningitis. Apart from the presence of trophozoites, the microscopic changes are neither characteristic nor specific.

Cutaneous Amebiasis

Sites most often involved are perianal skin, penis, vulva, and cervix. Perianal, vulvar, and cervical amebiasis is a consequence of direct extension from rectal amebiasis. Lesions of anal, penile, and vulvar amebiasis are characterized by a striking epithelial hyperplasia.[18] The hyperplasia causes a cauliflower-like surface that is mistaken clinically for squamous carcinoma (Figures 127–8 and 127–9). Also to be remembered is that carcinoma and amebiasis may coexist.[19] Microscopically trophozoites cluster on the surface of the squamous epithelium over small erosions and ulcers. Other mechanisms by which cutaneous amebiasis develops are by extension and perforation of amebic liver abscess, sexual transmission, usually involving genitalia, and rarely by direct inoculation.

Other Lesions

Virtually any part of the body may be affected—spleen, bone, respiratory tract, aorta, etc—have been sites of amebiasis.[17]

REFERENCES

1. Walsh JA. Transmission of *Entamoeba histolytica* infection. In: Ravdin JI, ed. *Amebiasis: Human Infection by Entamoeba histolytica.* New York: Churchill Livingstone; 1988:10–119.
2. Goldman M. *Entamoeba histolytica* like amoebas occurring in man. *Bull WHO.* 1969;40:355–364.
3. Ravdin JI, Petri WA Jr. *Entamoeba histolytica* (amebiasis). In: Mandell GL, Douglas RG, Bennett JE, eds. *Principles and Practice of Infectious Diseases.* 3rd ed. New York: Churchill Livingstone; 1990:2035–2049.
4. Keene WE, Pettit MG, Allen S, et al. The major neural proteins of *Entamoeba histolytica*. *J Exp Med.* 1986;163: 536–549.
5. Werries E, Nebinger P, Franz A. Degradation of biogenic oligosaccharides by beta-N-acetylglucosaminidase secreted by *Entamoeba histolytica*. *Mol Biochem Parasitol.* 1983;7:127–140.
6. Odezulo IA, Leitch GL. A membrane associated neuraminidase in *Entamoeba histolytica* trophozoites. *Infect Immun.* 1981;36:795–801.
7. Young JD-E, Cohn ZA. Molecular mechanisms of cytotoxicity mediated by *Entamoeba histolytica;* characterization of a pore forming protein. *J Cell Biochem.* 1985;29: 299–305.
8. Guerrant RL, Brush J, Ravdin JI, Sullivan JA, Mandell GL. Interaction between *Entamoeba histolytica* and human polymorphonuclear neutrophils. *J Infect Dis.* 1981;143: 83–93.
9. Ravdin JI, Guerrant RL. A review of parasite cellular mechanisms involved in the pathogenesis of amebiasis. *Rev Infect Dis.* 1982;4:1185–1207.
10. Salata RA, Ravdin JI. The interaction of human neutrophils and *Entamoeba histolytica* increases cytopathogenicity in liver cell monolayers. *J Infect Dis.* 1986;154:19–26.
11. Nanda R, Baveja U, Anard BS. *Entamoeba histolytica* cyst passers: clinical features and outcome in untreated subjects. *Lancet.* 1984;2:301–303.
12. Wolf MS. Amebiasis. In: Strickland GT, ed. *Hunter's Tropical Medicine.* 6th ed. Philadelphia: WB Saunders; 1984: 477–494.
13. Brooke MM, Melvin DM. *Morphology of Diagnostic Stages of Intestinal Parasites of Humans.* 2nd ed. US Dept of Health and Human Services Pub 84-8116. Atlanta: Centers for Disease Control and Prevention; 1984.
14. Healy GR. Serology. In: Ravdin JI, ed. *Amebiasis: Human Infection by Entamoeba histolytica.* New York: Churchill Livingstone; 1988:650–633.
15. Kessel JF, Lewis WP, Molina P, Turner JA. Indirect hemagglutination and complement fixation tests in amebiasis. *Am J Trop Med Hyg.* 1965;14:540–550.
16. Ungar BLP, Yolken RH, Quin TC. Use of a monoclonal antibody in an enzyme immunoassay for the detection of *Entamoeba histolytica* in fecal specimens. *Am J Trop Med Hyg.* 1985;34:465–472.
17. Perez-Tamayo R, Brant H. Amebiasis. In: Marcial-Rojas RA, ed. *Pathology of Protozoal and Helminthic Diseases.* Huntington, NY: Robert E. Krieger Publishing Co; 1975: 145–148.
18. Connor DH, Neafie RC, and Meyers WM. Amebiasis. In: Chapman H, Binford MD, and Connor DH, eds. *Pathology of Tropical and Extraordinary Diseases.* Washington, DC: Armed Forces Institute of Pathology; 1976:308–316.
19. Mhlanga BR, Lanoie LO, Norris HJ, Lack EE, Connor DH. Amebiasis complicating carcinomas: a diagnostic dilemma. *Am J Trop Med Hyg.* 1992;46:759–764.

Chapter 128

Babesiosis

David H. Persing

. . . or any taint of vice whose strong coruption
Inhabits our frail blood.

William Shakespeare (1564–1616), Twelfth Night, III, IV

INTRODUCTION

Protozoan parasites of the genus *Babesia,* along with their relatives the Theileridae, comprise a genetically and antigenically diverse group of intraerythrocytic pathogens of considerable veterinary, medical, and economic importance.[1–5] Collectively, *Babesia* and *Theileria* sp are called *piroplasms* because of the pear-shaped intraerythrocytic appearance of their dividing forms. All of the piroplasms described to date are tick-transmitted zoonotic agents that replicate within blood cells. In the United States, human babesiosis is an emerging tick-transmitted zoonosis, along with Lyme disease and ehrlichiosis. In some parts of the United States, all three agents (*B microti, Borrelia burgdorferi,* and the agent of human granulocytic ehrlichiosis) may be transmitted by the same tick vector, *Ixodes dammini* (also called *I scapularis*).

EPIDEMIOLOGY AND CASE DISTRIBUTION

The first recognized human case of babesiosis was documented in 1957 in a splenectomized cattle farmer from Yugoslavia; this infection was attributed to the bovine pathogen *B divergens.* Many severe and/or fatal infections with this organism have been reported in splenectomized persons in Europe. In contrast to the European cases, human infections in endemic areas in the northeastern and Great Lakes regions of the United States commonly occur in normosplenic patients and have been attributed to a small babesial parasite of rodents, *B microti.* In 1989, several infections by *B microti* were reported for the first time on the mainland of the eastern United States in Connecticut. Many subsequent infections have been observed in the northeastern and Great Lakes regions of the United States, as well as in areas that were not previously recognized as endemic. Fatal infections have been apparently contracted in geographically distinct areas of Rhode Island, Wisconsin,[6] California,[7] and Missouri. In addition to the fatal infections, several relatively severe nonfatal infections have occurred in persons from Minnesota, Washington, and California.[6–8]

Evidence for human infection with a newly recognized *Babesia*-like piroplasm is now emerging in the western United States.[8–10] These infections are produced by an as yet unnamed group of piroplasms related to the so-called WA1 piroplasm, which was recovered originally from a man from Washington state in 1991. The WA1-like piroplasms are antigenically and genetically related to *B gibsoni,* a cause of severe hemolytic anemia in dogs (Figures 128–1 and 128–2) that is often confused with autoimmune hemolytic anemia, and are antigenically and genetically distinct from *B microti.* Interestingly, this group of related organisms appears also to be phylogenetically related to members of the genus *Theileria,* even to the exclusion of some members of the genus *Babesia* itself.[7] The vector for this infection is presumed to be a tick but is currently unknown.

Babesia microti shares the same reservoir host *(Peromyscus leucopus)* and tick vector *(I dammini)* as does *B burgdorferi,* the cause of Lyme disease.[11] Concurrent infection in ticks and humans with *B burgdorferi* and *B microti* has been reported; the latter being relatively severe. The increased identification of human babesiosis in the northeastern coastal areas of the

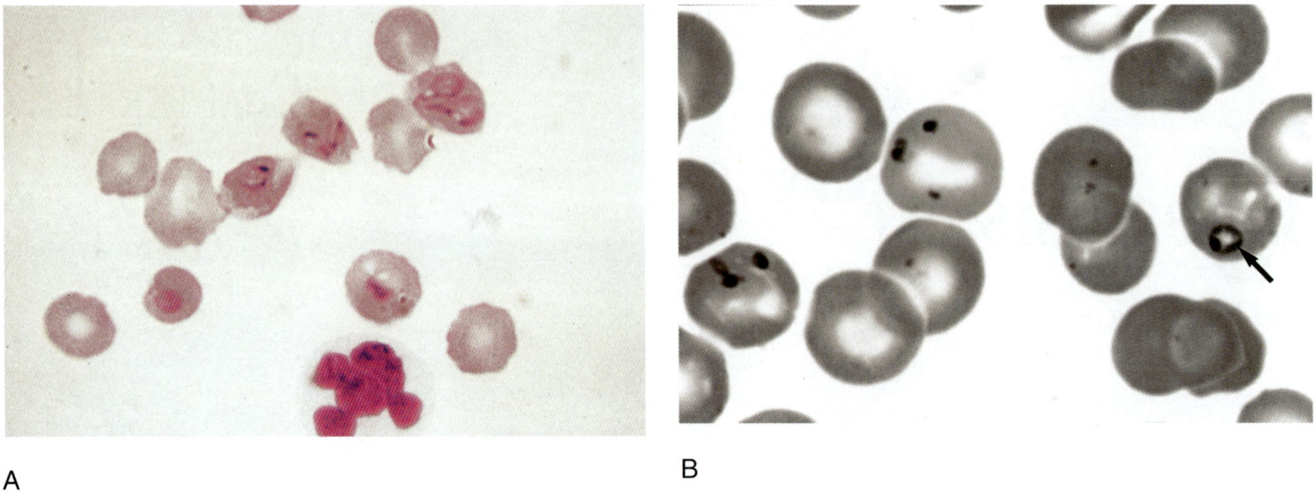

Figure 128–1. (A) Blood film of a 6-month-old male boxer in Kampala with tick fever. More than 50% of the dog's erythrocytes are parasitized. He almost died of hemolysis (Giemsa, ×1266). (B) *Babesia microti* in the blood of a 62-year-old man from Minnesota. *(From Pruthi et al.[2])*

United States parallels the increased exposure of humans to infected ticks in areas that are endemic for Lyme disease. On the northeastern terminal morraine islands of Nantucket, Martha's Vineyard, Block Island, and eastern Long Island, patients with Lyme disease are frequently seropositive for *B microti* infection.[12,13]

Studies performed in the 1970s and 1980s suggested that the majority of infections with babesial parasites are asymptomatic.[13,14] Recent prospective studies confirm this and serve to expand the clinical spectrum of babesial infection.[15] Identification of patients with apparently asymptomatic or chronic babesial infections is more difficult than the diagnosis of acute disease, since the association between seroreactivity and active infection is uncertain. Approximately 10% of 1000 sera from Lyme disease patients in Connecticut reacted positively to *B microti* antigens.[16] Such serosurveys have suggested that as many as 17 clinically inapparent infections accompany every clinically apparent case. Although the specificity of the serologic test for determining exposure to the WA1 piroplasm is less well established than for *B microti,* wide geographic variations in rates of seroreactivity have been observed for this organism. A seroepidemiologic study performed on serum samples from volunteers in Monterey County, California, revealed a 16% prevalence rate against WA1 antigen; none of the samples reacted with antigen of *B microti.*[7]

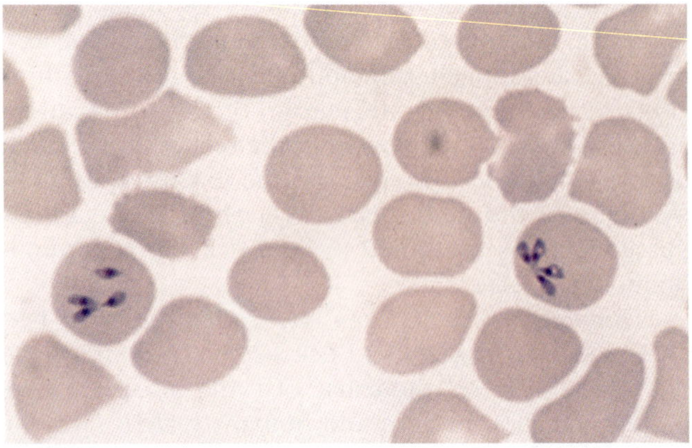

Figure 128–2. WA1 piroplasm in peripheral blood of an asplenic man from California. *(From Persing et al.[7])*

CLINICAL FEATURES

Given that the clinical spectrum of babesial infection varies from asymptomatic to severe, babesiosis might be viewed as several distinct diseases whose clinical manifestations depend on host susceptibility.[2] Clearly, at the extremes of the clinical spectrum are 1) a potentially life-threatening hemolytic disease in those predisposed to severe infection by old age, asplenia, or immunosuppression, and 2) an occult disease with few known sequelae that occurs in younger, normosplenic, immunocompetent persons. Virtually all patients described to date have presented with severe, acute hemolysis or have prolonged infections refractory to therapy. In all of these, characteristic organisms on peripheral blood smears were documented. Thus, little is known about the course of subclinical infection, during which the numbers of circulating parasites is likely to be much lower than in clinically apparent cases.

Among those with clinically apparent babesiosis reported to date, the ages of patients varied from a 3-week-old neonate to 86 years; the majority of patients were in their fifth or sixth decade. The incubation period varies from 1 to 6 weeks, although it may be as long as 3 months. The presenting complaints are usually nonspecific, with malaise, fatigue, low-grade fever or shaking chills, headache, generalized musculoskeletal complaints, emotional lability, nausea, emesis, and weight loss (Table 128–1). Icterus may be present, depending on the extent of the hemolysis. Palpable lymphadenopathy is usually absent, but there may be hepatomegaly and splenomegaly. Fever may be as high as 40°C. No consistent dermatologic manifestation of babesiosis has been documented, but concurrent infection with *B burgdorferi* may cause erythema migrans. A history of tick bite is not consistently obtained, but most patients have traveled to an endemic area. In addition, since patients with serologically confirmed Lyme disease are by definition at increased risk for concurrent babesiosis, patients failing to respond to antimicrobial agents directed at *B burgdorferi* may have underlying babesiosis.

Clinical babesiosis in New England has been markedly different from that in Europe.[17] Most of the European patients have been asplenic, and their clinical courses have been fatal in all except two patients, both from France. The organisms identified in all patients were of bovine origin; *B divergens* was implicated in all but one. In contrast, the more numerous North American infections have been mostly in normosplenic persons, except for those in the Western United States.

TABLE 128–1. SYMPTOMS ASSOCIATED WITH LYME DISEASE, BABESIOSIS, OR BOTH (IN %)

Disease Manifestations	Lyme Disease (*n* = 224)	Babesiosis (*n* = 10)	Both (*n* = 26)
Fatigue	49	60	81
Headache	42	60	77
Erythema migrans	85	0	62
Fever	42	80	58
Sweats	11	20	46
Chills	23	50	42
Myalgia	31	20	38
Anorexia	14	10	31
Arthralgia	36	50	27
Emotional lability	7	0	23
Nausea	5	10	23
Neck stiffness	21	30	23
Multiple erythema migrans	14	0	19
Cough	10	20	15
Sore throat	9	20	15
Conjunctivitis	3	0	12
Splenomegaly	0	10	8
Vomiting	4	0	8
Joint swelling	3	0	4

Adapted from Krause et al.[15]

LABORATORY DIAGNOSIS

Morphologic Features

A Wright stained or Giemsa stained smear of peripheral blood is most commonly used to demonstrate the intraerythrocytic parasites; however, a high index of suspicion is required in many patients since the level of parasitemia may be low. Factors influencing the sensitivity of this procedure include the experience of the observer and the time spent examining the smear. Although ring forms may be confused with *Plasmodium falciparum,* the absence of hemozoin should alert the observer to the possibility of babesiosis. In early falciparum infections, however, pigment may not be present. Rarely, tetrads of babesial merozoites may be visible. The typical picture in conjunction with the epidemiologic history will assist in arriving at a diagnosis. Babesiosis may be missed if the hematologic analysis is performed solely on autoanalyzers.

Serodiagnosis

Serologic evaluation with an indirect immunofluorescent antibody test (IFAT) using hamster-derived *B microti* antigen is available in a few laboratories. The cutoff titer for a positive test varies with the protocol, but in most laboratories titers >1:256 are believed to be consistent with active or recent *B microti* infection. Ten- to twenty-fold higher titers may be in those with acute babesiosis, followed by a gradual decline in titer over the ensuing weeks to months. A persistent low antibody titer or even an increase in titer has been described, but it is not known whether parasitemia recurs, associated with the increase in antibody. The serologic test is fairly specific; cross-reactivity with organisms has been described at low dilutions. Inoculations into golden hamsters can isolate the parasite and confirm the diagnosis. In cases that are difficult to diagnose based on direct examination of smears, the parasitemia is usually apparent 2 to 4 weeks later. Recent interlaboratory comparisons suggest that the sensitivity and specificity of the IFAT, similar to the one used in the studies cited, are high (>90% for both), but no study to date has challenged the IFAT with collections of sera from patients with conditions that are likely to produce serologic false positivity. Theoretically, serologic cross-reactivity might result from infection by other protozoal pathogens, and false-positive serologic results may occur in some patients, especially those with connective tissue disorders such as systemic lupus erythematosus or rheumatoid arthritis. False-negative serologic tests could occur early in the course of infection or in patients who are immunosuppressed.

Molecular Diagnosis

With the evolution of more sensitive polymerase chain reaction (PCR)-based techniques, the molecular diagnosis and monitoring of babesial infections are now possible. Detection of *B microti* by PCR was first described in 1992.[9] More recent studies, in which PCR has been used prospectively for diagnosis of suspected infections in the northeastern United States have shown that in comparison to direct examination of smears and hamster inoculation, PCR is more sensitive and equally specific for the diagnosis of acute infections.[18] PCR-based methods also may be useful for monitoring infections. In the above-mentioned study, 4 of 18 persons harbored detectable *B microti* DNA in their blood for 1 to 6 months. These studies suggest that more active recognition and treatment of babesiosis may be important not only for preventing long-term sequelae but also for protecting the blood supply from asymptomatic carriers who may later become blood donors.

TREATMENT

The fortuitous discovery of an effective therapeutic regimen for human babesiosis was made during the management of a patient with presumed transfusion-acquired malaria.[19] The patient was treated with chloroquine, but lack of response prompted a switch to quinine and clindamycin, following which the infection resolved rapidly. The diagnosis was made early in the course of treatment and was confirmed with serologic studies. Studies in animals have confirmed the value of this therapeutic combination, and this is now recommended for human babesiosis, though there have been occasional failures with this regimen. More recently, success with a combination of pentamidine and cotrimoxazole has been reported, but because of the previously mentioned side effects with pentamidine, this regimen is not recommended. Because of the phylogenetic relatedness of small babesias with members of the genus *Theileria,* treatment regimens including hydroxynaphthoquinone derivatives (similar to drugs used to treat theilerial infections in cattle) may eventually prove to be useful for managing refractory infections by *B microti.* Azithromycin also has been effective alone and in combination with quinine in a hamster model.[20] Erythrocyte exchange transfusion has been used in seriously ill patients who do not otherwise respond.

Various other pharmacologic interventions have been tried, including chloroquine, tetracycline, primaquine, sulfadiazine, and pyrimethamine, with variable results (Table 128–2). Pentamidine also has been moderately effective in improving symptoms and reducing parasitemia. Animal studies with pentamidine, however, have failed to show any clear benefit.

TABLE 128–2. THERAPEUTIC REGIMENS FOR BABESIOSIS

Proven Effective	Possibly Effective	Probably Ineffective
Clindamycin plus quinine	Azithromycin	Chloroquine
	Atovaquone	Tetracycline
	Bactrim	Primaquine
	Pentamidine	Sulfadiazine
	Cotrimoxazole	Pyrimethamine
	Clindamycin alone	Spirogermanium
		Ciprofloxacin

REFERENCES

1. Persing DH, Conrad PA. Babesiosis: new insights from phylogenetic analysis. *Infect Agents Dis.* 1995;4:182–195.
2. Pruthi RK, Marshall WF, Wiltsie JC, Persing DH. Human babesiosis. *Mayo Clin Proc.* 1995;70:853–862.
3. Taboada J, Merchant SR. Babesiosis of companion animals and man. *Vet Clin North Am Small Anim Pract.* 1991;21: 103–123.
4. Mehlhorn H, Shein E. The piroplasms: life cycle and sexual stages. *Adv Parasitol.* 1984;23:37–103.
5. Telford SR, III, Gorenflot A, Brasseur P, Spielman A. Babesial infections in man and wildlife. In: Krier JP, ed. *Parasitic Protozoa,* 2nd ed. San Diego: Academic Press; 1993:1–47.
6. Herwaldt BL, Springs FE, Roberts PP, et al. Babesiosis in Wisconsin: a potentially fatal disease. *Am J Trop Med Hyg.* 1995;53:146–151.
7. Persing DH, Herwaldt BL, Glaser C, et al. Infection with a *Babesia*-like organism in northern California. *N Engl J Med.* 1995;332:298–303.
8. Thomford JW, Conrad PA, Telford SR, III, et al. Cultivation and phylogenetic characterization of a newly recognized human pathogenic protozoan. *J Infect Dis.* 1994;169: 1050–1056.
9. Persing DH, Mathiesen D, Marshall WF, et al. Detection of *Babesia microti* by polymerase chain reaction. *J Clin Microbiol.* 1992;30:2097–2103.
10. Quick RE, Herwaldt BL, Thomford JW, et al. Babesiosis in Washington State—a new species of *Babesia. Ann Intern Med.* 1993;119:284–290.
11. Piesman J, Mather TN, Dammin GJ, Telford SD, Lastavica CC, Spielman A. Seasonal variation of transmission risk of Lyme disease and human babesiosis. *Am J Epidemiol.* 1987;126:1187–1189.
12. Benach JL, Coleman JL, Habicht GS, MacDonald A, Grunwaldt E, Giron JA. Serological evidence for simultaneous occurrences of Lyme disease and babesiosis. *J Infect Dis.* 1985;152:473–477.

13. Filstein MR, Benach JL, White DJ, et al. Serosurvey for human babesiosis in New York. *J Infect Dis.* 1980;141: 518–521.
14. Ruebush TD, Juranek DD, Chisholm ES, Snow PC, Healy GR, Sulzer AJ. Human babesiosis on Nantucket Island. Evidence for self-limited and subclinical infections. *N Engl J Med.* 1977;297:825–827.
15. Krause PJ, Telford SR III, Sikand VJ, et al. Concurrent Lyme disease and babesiosis: evidence for increased severity and duration of illness. *JAMA.* 1996;275:1657–1660.
16. Krause PJ, Telford SD, Ryan R, et al. Geographical and temporal distribution of babesial infection in Connecticut. *J Clin Microbiol.* 1991;29:1–4.
17. Brasseur P, Gorenflot A. Human babesiosis in Europe. *Memorias do Instituto Oswaldo Cruz.* 1992;87:131–132.
18. Krause PJ, Sikand VJ, Bow L, et al. PCR diagnosis of *Babesia microti* in humans. Paper presented at 33rd Interscience conference on antimicrobial agents and chemotherapy; October 17–20, 1993; New Orleans, La. Abstract 1112.
19. Wittner M, Rowin KS, Tanowitz HB, et al. Successful chemotherapy of transfusion babesiosis. *Ann Intern Med.* 1982;96:601–604.
20. Weiss LM, Wittner M, Wasserman S, Oz HS, Retsema J, Tanowitz HB. Efficacy of azithromycin for treating *Babesia microti* infection in the hamster model. *J Infect Dis.* 1993;168:1289–1292.

CHAPTER 129

Balantidiasis

David A. Schwartz and James Patrick Mixon

Our doctors . . . eat the melon and drink the new wine while they keep their patient tied down to syrups and slops.

Michel de Montaigne (1533–1592)

CLASSIFICATION

Balantidiasis is a zoonotic parasitic infection caused by the large, ciliated protozoan *Balantidium coli* (Malmsten, 1857; Stein, 1862) phylum Ciliophora, order Trichostomatida. Members of the genus *Balantidium* are parasitic in the digestive tract of a broad range of invertebrate and vertebrate hosts. Trophozoites of *B coli* are facultative anaerobes and require a normal intestinal bacterial flora for their growth. As in other ciliates, reproduction is by binary fission along the transverse axis. Characteristic cysts typify all members of the genus *Balantidium*.[1]

INTRODUCTION AND HISTORY

Balantidium coli is the largest protozoan, and the only ciliate, to cause disease in humans.[2] *Balantidium coli* was first described in 1857 by Malmsten, who identified the organisms in the feces of two patients with diarrhea and termed the parasite *Paramoecium coli*. Shortly after this report, Leuckart (1861) and Stein (1862) studied the organism in hogs, and transferred the species to the genus *Balantidium* created by Claparéde and Lachmann following the observation of the parasite in the intestines of a frog. Barret and Yarbrough first cultivated *B coli* in 1922. In 1950, Swartzwelder defined the three principal categories of clinical manifestations: 1) the asymptomatic carrier, 2) the chronic symptomatic state characterized by diarrhea alternating with constipation, and 3) dysenteric or acute disease.[3]

EPIDEMIOLOGY AND LIFE CYCLE

The geographic distribution of *B coli* is worldwide, and it commonly inhabits the intestines of a wide variety of insects (including cockroaches), fish, amphibians, fowl, and mammals in tropical and subtropical regions. Among mammals, *B coli* has been found in pigs, wild boars, horses, sheep, bovines, guinea pigs, rats, and higher primates. The pig is the most frequently and heavily naturally infected mammal, and is the most important reservoir for human infection. Approximately 25% of infected humans have had some contact with swine. *Balantidium coli* is transmitted to humans in food and water contaminated by fecal material of pigs, but infection is also associated with the handling and slaughtering of pigs and the use of pig excrement for fertilizing vegetables.[4,5] There have been sporadic outbreaks of balantidiasis throughout the world. On Truk in 1971, *B coli* infected 110 persons after a typhoon contaminated drinking water with pig feces.[6] In temperate regions, high rates of infection develop among people living in penitentiaries and in other environments where there is crowding and poor personal hygiene.[7] Person-to-person transmission has been documented, and probably caused a 4.9% rate of infection in 142 patients in a mental hospital in South Carolina in 1939. Currently, balantidiasis of humans is rare in Western countries, and in Moslem countries, where pigs are uncommon, balantidiasis is almost nonexistent. In New Guinea, where pigs are the principal domestic animal, infection rates among swineherds and slaughterhouse workers is as high as 28%.

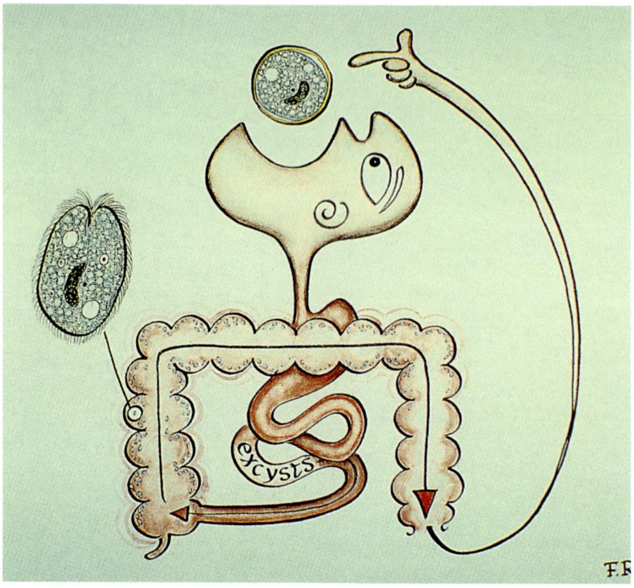

Figure 129–1. Life cycle of *B coli* (AFIP Neg 70-7334). *(By the late Frank O. Raasch, Captain, MC, USN.)*

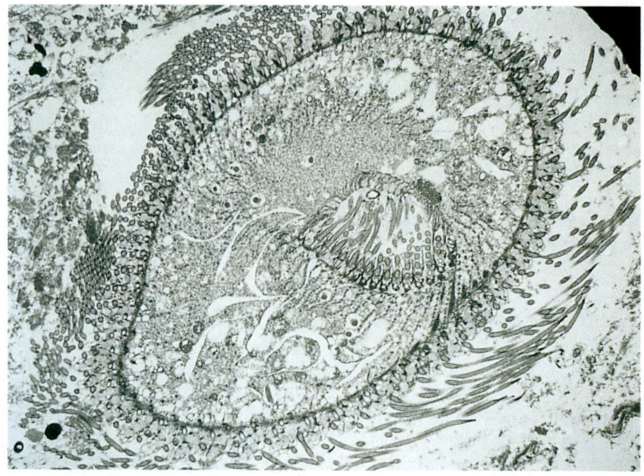

Figure 129–2. Electron micrograph of *B coli* trophozoite in colon demonstrating ciliated membrane and cytostome (AFIP Neg 75-9816; ×2000).

The life cycle of *B coli* consists of two stages: a ciliated trophozoite and an environmentally resistant cyst (Figure 129–1).[1,5,7] Trophozoites encyst while moving through the colon, or after defecation of a semiformed stool. Cysts are the infective stage and may remain viable for weeks in moist feces.[5] Infective cysts ingested with contaminated water, food, or poor hygienic practice excyst in the small intestine, and trophozoites become established in the mucosa of the terminal ileum and colon.

MORPHOLOGY

The large size of the trophozoite of *B coli* is distinctive in dysenteric feces and tissues, and should not be confused with other organisms. The length is from 50 to 200 μm, and the breadth varies from 40 to 70 μm. The organism is slipper shaped, with a partially pointed anterior end and broadly rounded posterior end. On one side of the longitudinal axis is a deep, slightly curved and inverted conical depression, called the cytostome. The trophozoite is surrounded by hundreds of short cilia, which originate from a basal granule immediately beneath the cell membrane (Figure 129–2). The cilia beat in a coordinated rhythm, and the protozoan moves either forward or backward in a partially spiral path. The cytoplasm appears granular, and contains a variety of food and storage vacuoles, and one or two contractile vacuoles. At the posterior end there is a small opening, the cytopyge, through which the residual contents of food vacuoles are periodically discharged. Microscopically, the most distinctive features of the cytoplasm of *B coli* trophozoites are the two nuclei: a large, kidney bean–shaped macronucleus (Figure 129–3), termed the "mack" by biologists, and smaller rounded micronucleus, the "mike." The micronucleus lies in the center of the inner curvature of the macronucleus, and is believed to function as a kinetic organelle. Macro- and micronuclei are characteristic of the ciliates.

The cysts of *B coli* vary from 45 to 75 μm, are round, and contain a single macro- and micronucleus. The trophozoite initially rounds up, and secretes a tough cell membrane without completely retracting its cilia. This precyst is recognizable in freshly passed stools (Figure 129–4). Eventually the cilia are lost from the surface of the precyst and the distinctive cyst is formed, containing a characteristic kidney bean–shaped macronucleus (Figure 129–5).

CLINICAL FEATURES

Infections of humans with *B coli* can be divided into intestinal and extraintestinal disease. The most common sites of *Balantidium* infection (>95%) are the terminal ileum and colon, and especially the rectosigmoid area. *Balantidium* infections are often asymptomatic, and are similar to amebiasis in that a silent carrier state may be present. Mild or chronic infections are characterized by intermittent diarrhea and constipation, weight loss, and abdominal pain. With progression of disease, patients may experience a dysenteric syndrome consisting of blood, mucus, and purulent material in the stool. Associated findings in severe infections include anorexia, nausea, tenderness over the colon, weight loss, ca-

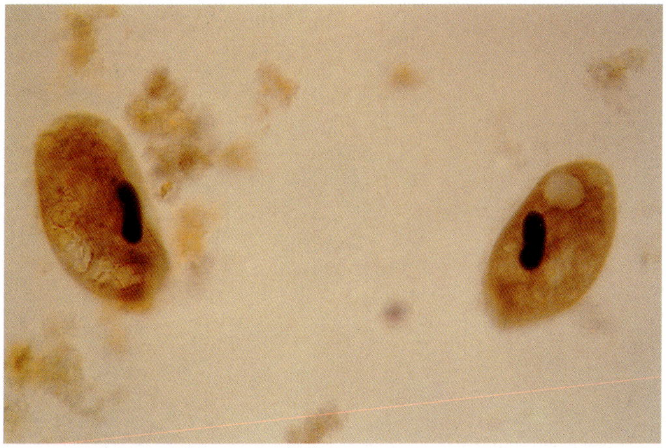

Figure 129–3. Two trophozoites of *Balantidium* in specimen of stool from a symptomatic patient. The kidney bean–shaped macronucleus is easily identified (unstained AFIP Neg 72-13051; ×325).

chexia, pallor, headache, insomnia, nausea, vomiting, anemia, dehydration, and malaise. Eosinophilia is not associated with balantidiasis.[7] In severe infections intestinal perforation and peritonitis may kill the patient.[2] Rectal examination of patients with *Balantidium* infection reveals friable, edematous, or granular mucosa, with a diffuse erythema and covered with a mucopurulent exudate.[8] Unusual intestinal manifestations of *Balantidium* infection include appendicitis,[9,10] and balantidiasis complicating ulcerative colitis.[8]

Rare extraintestinal infections with *Balantidium* have been reported, including involvement of lung, vagina, ureter, and urinary bladder.[2,3,6,8] *Balantidium* infection of liver, pleura, and mesenteric lymph nodes has been associated with peritonitis after intestinal perforation.

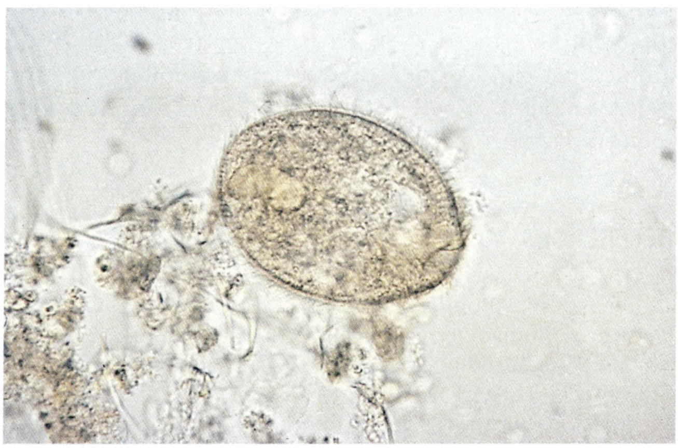

Figure 129–4. Precyst of *B coli* in unfixed stool. Features of the trophozoite stage are still present including cilia (×1000).

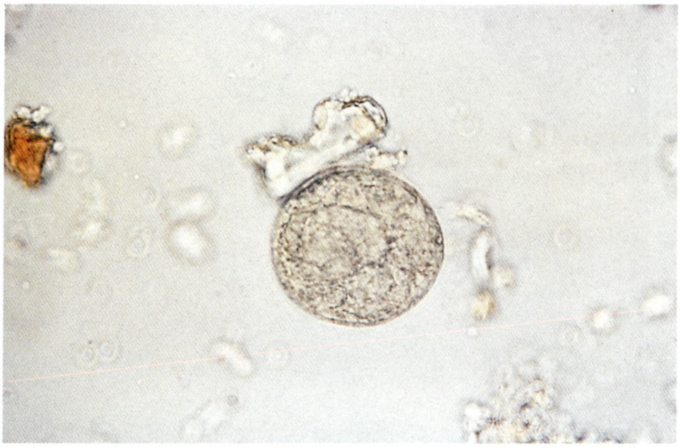

Figure 129–5. Cyst of *B coli* from unfixed stool of a patient with diarrhea (×1000).

PATHOLOGIC FEATURES

Although *B coli* is a pathogen, the organisms may reside in the lumen of the bowel without producing symptoms. Invasion of the intestinal mucosa is assisted by the production of a hyaluronidase by the trophozoite, and produces extensive necrosis, hemorrhage, and ulceration. The early lesion of *Balantidium* infection of the colon resembles that of *Entamoeba histolytica* in that both ulcers are flask shaped and have undermined edges. The ulcer crater is covered by purulent and necrotic material. Adjacent tissue is edematous and contains chronic inflammatory cells, mostly lymphocytes and plasma cells. The entire thickness of the bowel wall may become involved (Figures 129–6 and 129–7). Ulcers may communicate by interconnected passages beneath the mucosa. Trophozoites of *Balantidium* are usually single or in groups in the inflamed mucosa or

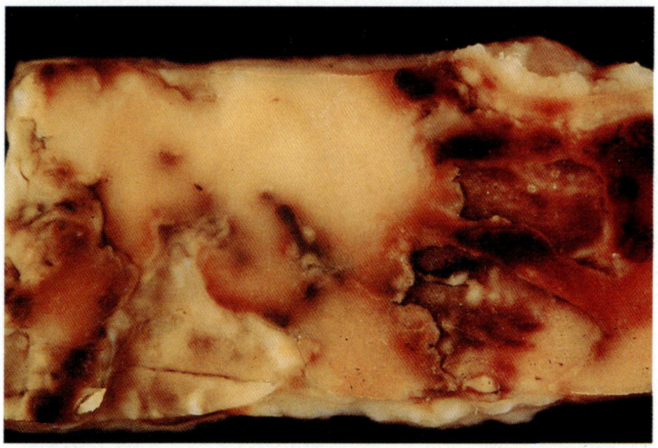

Figure 129–6. Colon with confluent ulceration and necrosis caused by *Balantidium* infection. *(By Daniel H. Connor M.D. 1972.)*

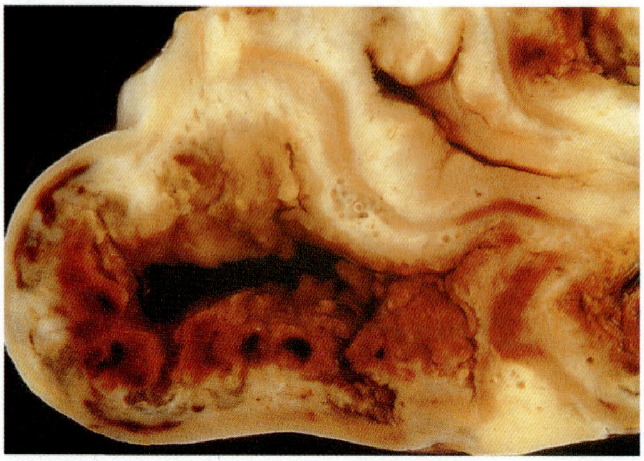

Figure 129–7. Transmural necrosis of large intestine associated with severe balantidial colitis. *(By Daniel H. Connor M.D. 1972.)*

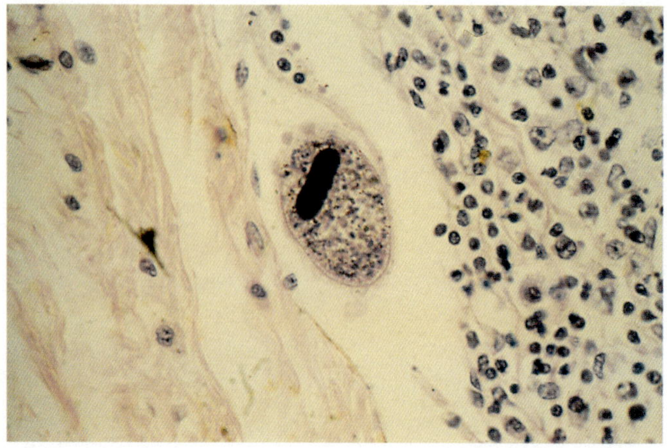

Figure 129–9. Solitary *Balantidium* trophozoite in a colonic ulcer in a chimpanzee (H&E ×400). *(By Dr. Mark Eberhard, Division of Parasitic Diseases, Centers for Disease Control and Prevention, Atlanta, GA.)*

submucosa or in the necrotic material overlying the ulcer crater (Figures 129–8 and 129–9). The characteristic ovoid trophozoites, with numerous cilia and darkly stained kidney bean–shaped macronucleus, are easily visualized in tissue sections stained with hematoxylin-eosin (H&E) (Figure 129–8), and special stains are unnecessary for identification. The trophozoites of *B coli* are so large that not all diagnostic organelles may be present in a single histologic section, and multiple levels should be examined to identify the characteristic features. After mucosal invasion, there is often secondary bacterial infection with abundant neutrophils.

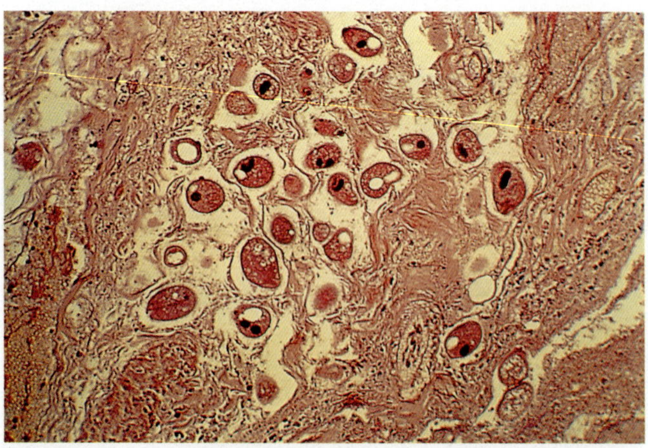

Figure 129–8. Group of *Balantidium* trophozoites in the colonic wall (H&E × 125). *(By Dr. Robert Owen, Veterans Affairs Medical Center, San Francisco, CA.)*

DIAGNOSIS

The diagnosis of balantidiasis is made by identifying characteristic cysts, precysts, or trophozoites in feces, or trophozoites in mucosal biopsy specimens obtained from the colon or other suspected sites of infection. Scrapings of ulcer exudate obtained by colonoscopy are also useful for demonstrating the organisms. *Balantidium* infection has been diagnosed cytologically in ascitic fluid from a patient with peritonitis.[11] The trophozoites of *Balantidium* are easily distinguished from those of amebae by their larger size, prominent kidney bean–shaped macronucleus, and cilia.[1,7]

TREATMENT

The treatment of choice is either tetracycline, 500 mgm four times a day for 10 days, or iodoquinol, 650 mgm three times a day for 20 days. Other useful drugs are ampicillin, carbarsone, diodoquin, nitrimidazine, and paromomycin. Mixed results have been reported with metronidazole.

REFERENCES

1. Beaver PC, Jung RC, Cupp EW, eds. *Clinical Parasitology.* 9th ed. Philadelphia: Lea & Febiger; 1984:213–217.
2. Soave R, Weikel CS. Cryptosporidium and other protozoa including *Isospora, Sarcocystis, Balantidium coli,* and *Blastocystis*. In: GL Mandell, RG Douglas, JE Bennett, eds. *Principles and Practice of Infectious Diseases.* 3rd ed. New York: Churchill Livingstone; 1990:2127–2128.

3. Ladas SD, Savva S, Frydas A, Kaloviduris A, Hatzioannou J, Raptis S. Invasive balantidiasis presented as chronic colitis and lung involvement. *Dig Dis Sci.* 1989;34:1621–1623.
4. Ravdin JI. Protozoal diseases. In: GL Mandell, RG Douglas, JE Bennett, eds. *Principles and Practice of Infectious Disease.* 3rd ed. New York: Churchill Livingstone; 1990: 2035–2036.
5. Wolfe MS. Miscellaneous intestinal protozoa. In: GT Strickland, ed. *Hunter's Tropical Medicine.* 6th ed. Philadelphia: WB Saunders Company; 1984:508–509.
6. Walzer PD, Judson FN, Murphy KB, Healy GR, English DK, Schultz MG. Balantidiasis outbreak in Truk. *Am J Trop Med Hyg.* 1973;22:33–41.
7. Neafie RC. Balantidiasis. In: Binford CH, Connor DH, eds. *Pathology of Tropical and Extraordinary Diseases.* Washington, DC: Armed Forces Institute of Pathology; 1976; 1:325–327.
8. Kamberoglou D, Savva S, Adraskelas N, Yannitsiotis A, Cocca E. Balantidiasis complicating a case of ulcerative colitis. *Am J Gastro.* 1990;85:765–766.
9. Dodd LG. *Balantidium coli* infestation as a cause of acute appendicitis. *J Infect Dis.* 1991;163:1392.
10. Dorfman S, Rangel O, Bravo LG. Balantidiasis: report of a fatal case with appendicular and pulmonary involvement. *Trans Roy Soc Trop Med Hyg.* 1984;78:833–834.
11. Lahiri VL, Elhence BR, Agarwal BM. *Balantidium* peritonitis diagnosed on cytologic material. *Acta Cytol.* 1977;21:123–124.

CHAPTER 130

Cryptosporidiosis

Jan Marc Orenstein

Time discovers truth.

Lucius Annaeus Seneca (circa 4 BC–AD 65)

DEFINITION

Infection by coccidian protozoal parasites, genus *Cryptosporidium* (phylum Apicomplexa; suborder Eimeriorina) is referred to as cryptosporidiosis.[1–4] *Cryptosporidium,* which is Greek for "hidden spore," is an ubiquitous obligate intracellular parasite primarily inhabiting the intestinal tract of vertebrates, including humans, and causing diarrhea. Taxonomically, it is closely related to three other important coccidian parasites that infect humans: *Isospora belli, Toxoplasma gondii,* and *Cyclospora cayetanensis.*

GEOGRAPHICAL DISTRIBUTION

Since the first documented human infection in 1976, cases have been reported on six continents.[4–7] The best estimates of prevalence of cryptosporidial diarrheal disease, based on stool studies, are at least 3% for the industrialized countries, 5% for Asia, and 10% for Africa. Whereas in developing countries the highest prevalence is in the crowded urban environments, as opposed to less crowded rural areas, the reverse is true for developed countries. A study of duodenal aspirates found a 12.7% asymptomatic carrier rate in immunocompetent individuals.[8] In the human immunodeficiency virus (HIV)-infected population, the prevalence of intestinal cryptosporidiosis is at least 20% in the developed world and 30% in the developing world.[9–18]

"*C. parvum* may now be one of the three most commonly found enteropathogens causing diarrheal illness in humans worldwide, especially in developing countries," and may be responsible for approximately a third of all previously undiagnosed diarrheal cases.[19] Perhaps 250 to 500 million cases of intestinal cryptosporidiosis occur in developing nations annually.[4]

Outside HIV disease, *Cryptosporidium* mostly infects the young (under 2 years of age) and malnourished, especially when the weather is warm and humid (late summer and early fall) in North America,[20] and the rainy season in South America.

EPIDEMIOLOGY

The first descriptions of cryptosporidial infection (reportedly starting in 1907) were of the gastric and intestinal epithelium of laboratory mice (*C muris* and *C parvum*).[1,4] Species were subsequently named on the basis of hosts, eg, guinea pigs, rabbits, lambs, horses, calves, pigs, poultry, and rhesus monkeys. Initially, in chickens it was found to infect cecal epithelium (1929). Many years later it was named *C baileyi* and recognized as an important cause of intestinal infection (1955) and respiratory illness (1980s) in fowl. Early in the 1970s, *Cryptosporidium* was recognized as a significant diarrheal pathogen of large animals. Cattle parasitism with *C muris* appears to be chronic and high in some dairies (to 31%) and feedlots (to 11.8%).[21]

Cryptosporidium displays little host specificity. As recently as 1980 it was suggested that there may be only a single genus with *C muris* as the type species.[1] It is now believed that the species *C parvum* accounts for the vast majority of human infections, and that there are other species infecting a wide range of hosts.[22] Only the first of the eight human cryptosporidiosis infections (reported from 1976 to 1982) was in an immunodeficient patient.

In the early 1980s, *C parvum* began to be reported as the cause of diarrhea in children in day care centers, in patients of mental institutions, and in travelers and immigrants from developing countries.[2,20] Cryptosporidiosis spreads among family members, from animals to handlers, and from patients to health care workers.[2,23,24] Transmission may be from hand to mouth (fecal–oral), by contaminated food or water, and possibly even from pets.[23,24] Cryptosporidial infection of the lung, intestine, and kidneys is relatively common in zoo birds and in pet birds.[25]

The incidence of outbreaks in day care centers has reached 63%, indicating spread among children.[5] Waterborne outbreaks have been associated with contamination of reservoirs (surface runoff from cow pastures and dairies as a result of heavy rain), inadequate filtration of swimming pool water, and contaminated drinking water and cider.[26–29] Oocysts are in 65% to 87% of samples of surface water in the United States. The largest outbreaks have been from contaminated water, eg, 13,000 patients with gastroenteritis in one county in Georgia, representing an attack rate of 40% for the county.[27] Over 400,000 people were estimated to have had diarrhea as a consequence of a *Cryptosporidium*-contaminated water treatment plant in southern Milwaukee.[29] The symptoms averaged 9 days and included watery diarrhea (93%) with a median number of daily stools of 12, abdominal cramps (84%), fever (57%), and vomiting (48%).

Unlike *I belli,* the highly resistant oocyst of *Cryptosporidium* is both fully sporulated and infectious on passage from the host.[30] The oocyst is approximately 30 times more resistant to ozone, and over 600 times more resistant to chlorine than are *Giardia lamblia* cysts.

SEROLOGY

Seropositivity [as determined by enzyme-linked immunosorbent assay (ELISA)] is common, even in preschoolers.[31–33] A study of over 800 children in Oklahoma (overall seroprevalence of 31%) found a prevalence of 13% in those less than 5 years, 38% in those 5 to 13 years old, and 58% in those 14 to 21 years old; it was higher in those at day care centers; higher if there had been a recent diarrheal episode; higher in blacks and Native Americans than in white non-Hispanics; but not different in males versus females or rural versus city dwellers. Similar IgG-positive rates were in Peace Corps volunteers before traveling (32%) and in a Wisconsin farming community (36%). Seropositivity in the developing world has exceeded 90%, eg, in a Thai orphanage. A household transmission study carried out in Brazil revealed a rate of 19%, making it comparable to the transmission rate of other highly infectious enteric pathogens.[33]

LIFE CYCLE

The ingested thick-walled, sporulated oocysts excyst during transit through the stomach, and the four freed motile sporozoites (1.5 × 0.75 μm) infect small intestinal epithelial cells of small intestine[1,3,34–36] (Figure 130–1). They then differentiate (schizogony or asexual cycle) within an intracellular but extracytoplasmic parasitophorous vacuole into schizonts or trophozoites (uninuclear meronts), which are 2 to 2.5 μm in diameter. Starting with the schizont, the parasite has a highly specialized attachment site, or feeder organelle, characterized by an electron-dense network of microfilaments. Two further divisions (total of three nuclear divisions) of the schizont yield 6 to 8 merozoites (2 to 5 × 0.4 μm). The merozoites released from these type I schizonts either reinfect the host cells (recycle) to perpetuate and amplify the infection, or develop into type II schizonts, which produce four merozoites (two nuclear divisions) that transform into gametes (gametogony, sexual cycle). It is unclear whether type II schizonts also recycle asexually.

Free merozoites, from the second-generation type II schizonts, either develop into microgamonts (microgametocytes), which contain up to 16 peripherally arranged, bullet-shaped microgametes (2 × 0.7 μm), or macrogametes (contain prominent polysaccharide and phospholipid amylopectin granule precursors of the thick oocyst wall). The macrogametes are fertilized (fuse) by freed microgametes (lack flagella, a feature of other coccidians) to form zygotes (4.5 to 6 μm), which, in turn, develop into oocysts (sporogony). Development of the oocyst's four sporozoites apparently occurs while it is still attached to the enterocytes.

Approximately 80% of zygotes develop into thick-walled (highly resistant bilayer) oocysts, which sporulate and pass in the stool. The remaining 20% are surrounded by only a single unit membrane, which allows them to release four infectious sporozoites (autoinfection) in the lumen of the bowel, to perpetuate the infection. The ability to recycle, at all levels of development, is critical to the perpetuation and amplification of infection in humans.

The merozoites and sporozoites contain the characteristic apical complex of the phylum Apicomplexa: rhoptries with their openings, micronemes, and annular ridges. These structures apparently serve as the entry apparatus.

CLINICAL FEATURES

Though the patient's immune status may not totally predict susceptibility to infection or reactivity, it does impact significantly on the degree of disease.[1,2,4,9,37,38] Regardless of the cause of the patient's immunocompromised state, the key is the ability of the patient to respond adequately and to eliminate the parasites.

Following an incubation period of from 2 to 14 days (average 5) after oocyst ingestion, most immunocompetent patients experience self-limited, flulike diarrhea, lasting from 5 to 14 days and varying in severity.[1,20,29] Infectious oocysts continue to be shed in the stool for approximately 2 more weeks. Roughly 80% of patients experience watery diarrhea (2 to 10 stools per day) that is characteristically foul smelling, mucoid, nonbloody, and essentially devoid of leukocytes. Infection is frequently associated with abdominal discomfort (often right upper quadrant), nausea, vomiting, and low-grade fever. Anorexia, weight loss (10% of body weight), malaise, weakness, myalgia, and headache are also features. The symptoms often fluctuate, apparently in parallel with oocyst shedding. Virtually all immunocompetent individuals recover, although some may require supportive care, predominantly fluid replacement. Some are symptomatic for over a month, especially the previously malnourished, and may rarely succumb to infection. A few preliminary reports suggest the occurrence of respiratory cryptosporidiosis even in immunocompetent individuals.[39]

Immunodeficient patients, especially those with acquired immunodeficiency syndrome (AIDS), experience identical symptoms, which are usually more severe and prolonged.[10,14,38,40] In the vast majority of patients, infection pursues an unrelenting course and may be the immediate cause of death. The symptoms, persistence of infection, and remissions rate usually parallel the CD4 count.[41] There are spontaneous remissions, some are coincident with commencing antiviral therapy.[42]

The diarrhea appears to be a consequence of excessive proximal small bowel fluid secretion (3 to 6 L, and more, per day), which leads to dehydration, the most striking clinical sign, often necessitating parenteral fluid therapy. In addition to carbohydrate malabsorption, there is decreased uptake of fat and vitamins, especially B_{12}, which contributes to the wasting.

By what means *Cryptosporidium* induces diarrhea and malabsorption is unclear. Suggested mechanisms include an unidentified toxin, direct decrease in absorption by loss of microvillous surface area, reduced lactase activity leading to malabsorption and intolerance, and products of enteric bacterial overgrowth.[36]

Peripheral blood leukocytosis and eosinophilia are infrequent. Nonspecific mucosal thickening and disordered small intestinal motility are the characteristic radiographic findings. The endoscopist mostly appreciates focal nonspecific atrophy, but sometimes can observe small erosions.[43]

Respiratory cryptosporidiosis has been reported in a severely immunodeficient lymphoma patient with duodenal and gall bladder infections[44] and an infant with SCID.[45] Upper respiratory, tracheobronchial, and nasal cryptosporidiosis appear to be relatively common in AIDS patients with severe small bowel disease (as seen at autopsy).[46,47]

Symptomatic infections of the biliary tract disease have been seen only in AIDS patients.[48–53] Acalculous cholecystitis and sclerosing cholangitis, with obstruction (stenosis of ampulla of Vater), have been reported in up to 7.5% of infected AIDS patients.[9] There is right upper quadrant pain, fever, nausea, and vomiting that exceeds cryptosporidial enteritis. Liver biopsy may reveal involvement of intrahepatic bile ducts.[50] Serum alkaline phosphatase is usually disproportionally elevated, hepatic transaminases (for example, gamma glutamyl transpeptidase) are moderately elevated, while bilirubin is within normal range. Radiographic studies (ultrasound) may reveal dilated and irregular intra- and extrahepatic bile ducts (characteristic of sclerosing cholangitis), a dilated thick-walled (edematous) gall bladder, and a thickened common bile duct.[52,54] Endoscopic retrograde cholangiography provides the clearest evidence of intra- and extrahepatic duct dilation and strictures. Diagnosis is made on biopsy or resected gallbladder, or by analysis of bile. Prompt relief usually follows cholecystectomy and endoscopic papillotomy or sphincterotomy.

An immunocompetent teenage girl had self-limited acute pancreatitis. Clinical features were recurrent epigastric pain, tender abdomen, dehydration, anorexia, nausea, vomiting, diarrhea, low-grade fever, white blood cell count of 29,000, elevated serum amylase (14,000 U/L), and *Cryptosporidium* oocysts in her stool.[55] The likely source of infection was the cattle that she worked with and whose untreated milk she drank. An infant with SCID had involvement of pancreatic ducts at autopsy.[45] Autopsies of AIDS patients with small bowel cryptosporidiosis often reveal involvement of pancreatic ducts.

Evidently immunity develops naturally in the maturing rodent, but not in man. Resistance apparently requires both specific intestinal secretory immunoglobulin A and adequate numbers of CD4 cells, explaining the persistence of infection in AIDS patients[56] who have diarrhea despite high levels of both serum and secretory *C parvum*–specific antibodies.[57] A recent study failed to demonstrate protection from *Cryptosporidium* infection for nursing children by antibody-positive breast milk.[58] It has been proposed that the free intraluminal forms of *C parvum* (sporozoites and merozoites) are the targets for protective secretory antibodies.[59] Apparently, the need is to block infection before the organisms are protected within parasitophorous

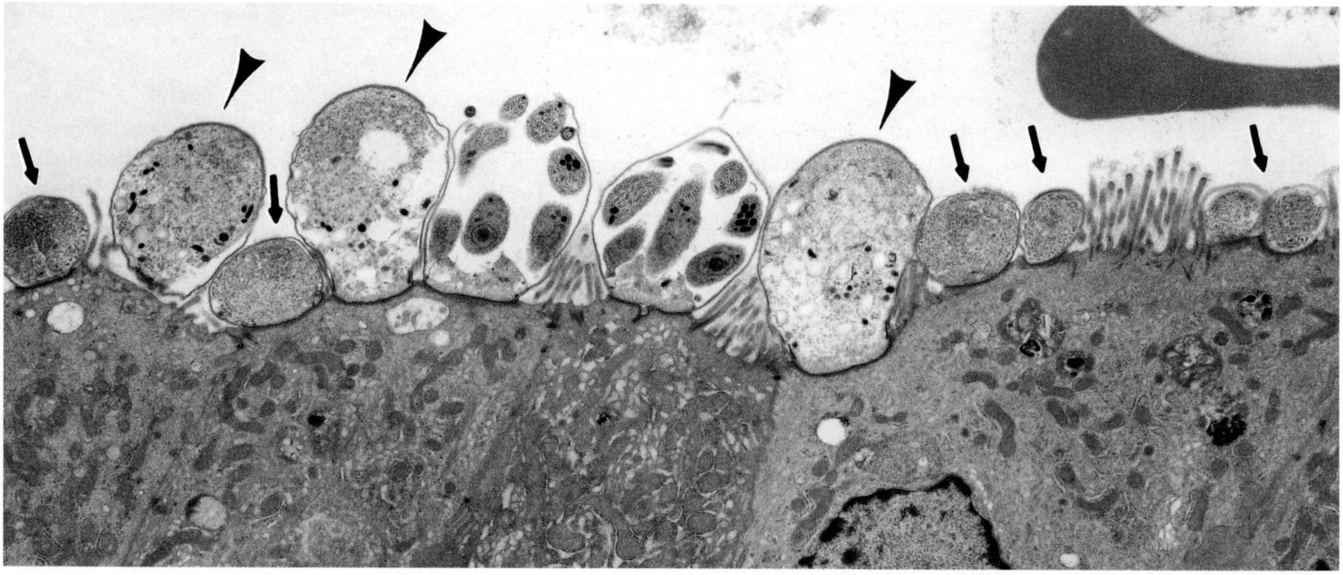

A

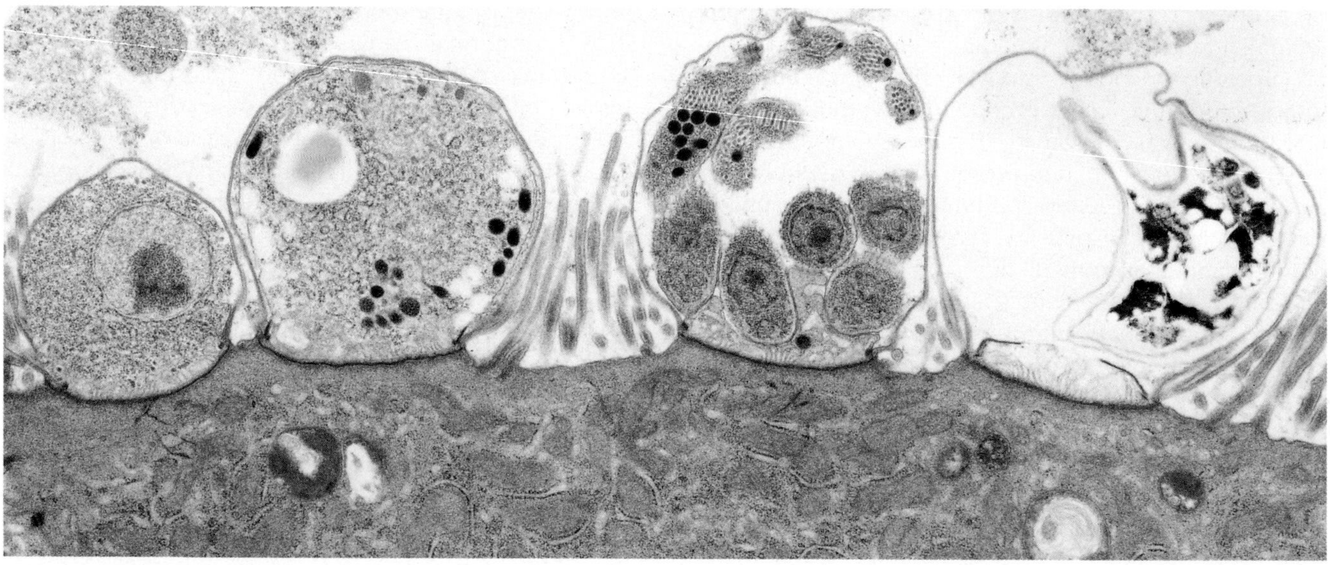

B

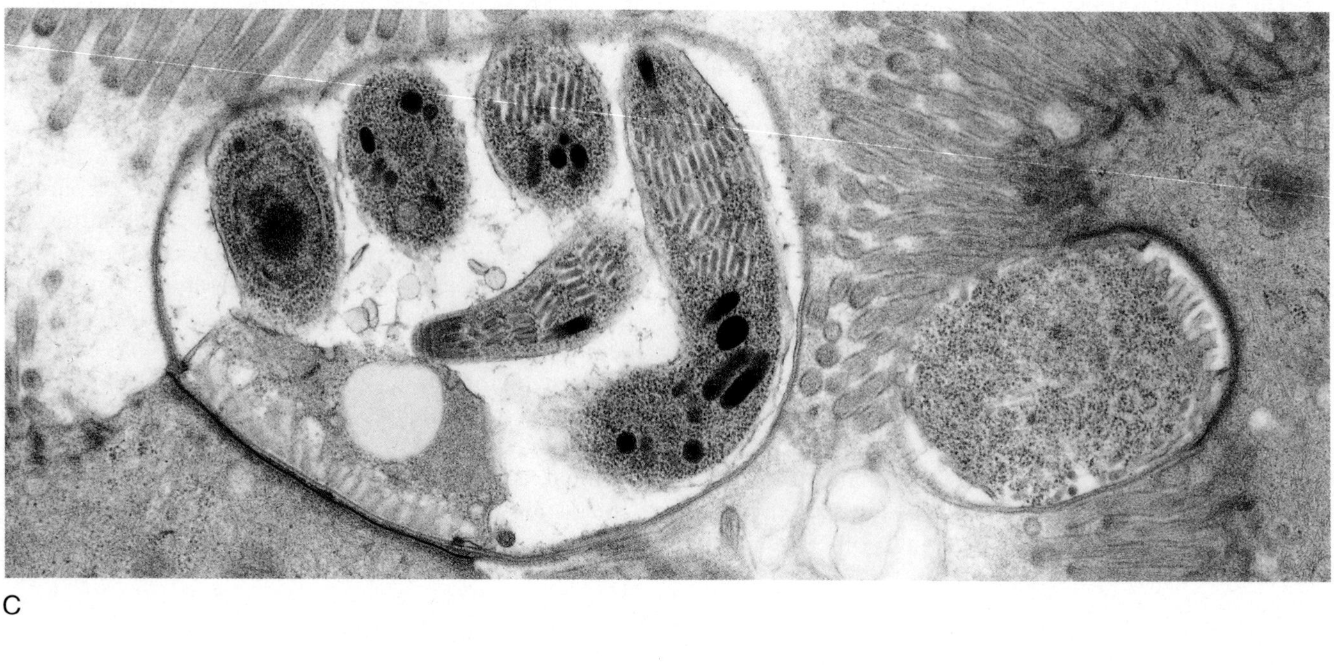

C

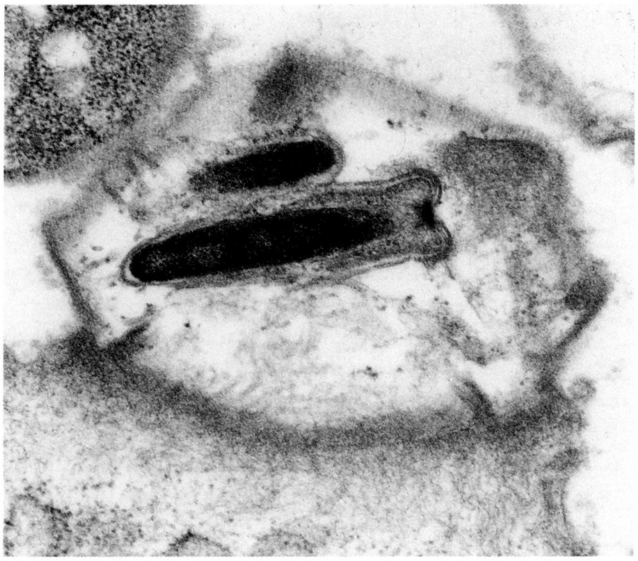

D

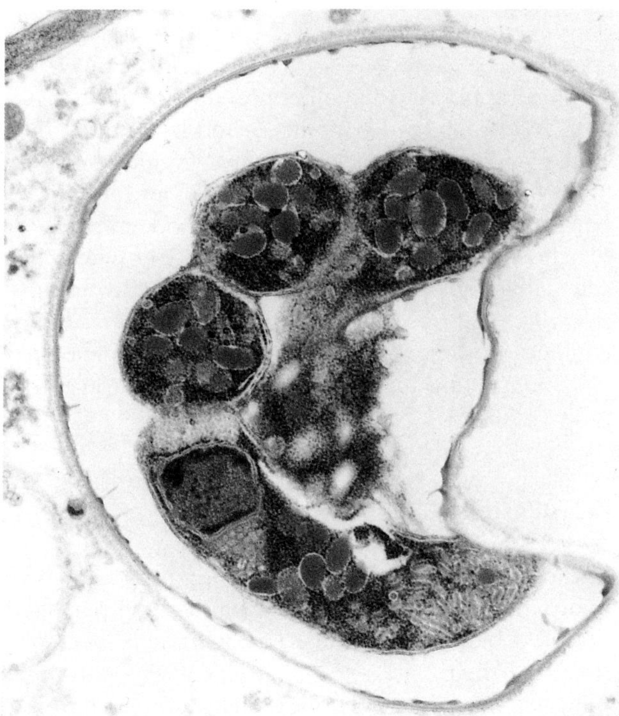

E

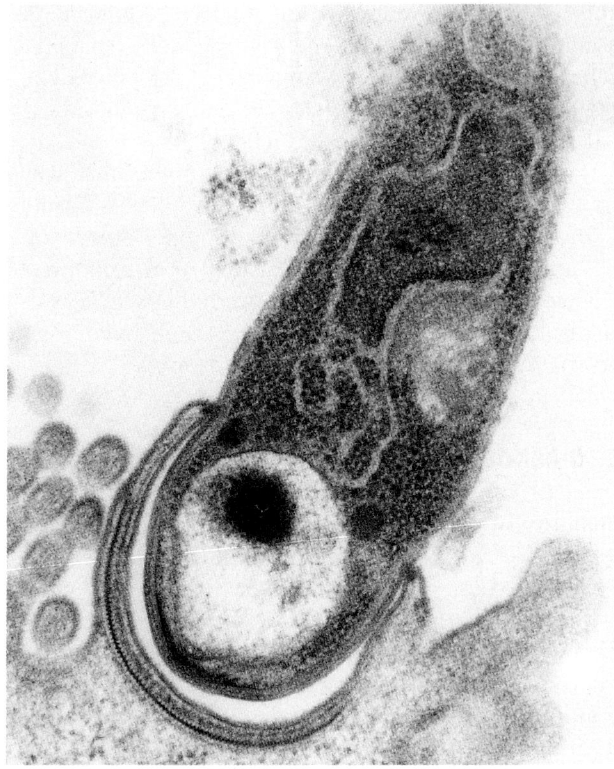

F

Figure 130–1. Transmission electron microscopy. (**A**) Virtually all the cells are infected and denuded of their microvilli. Note several smaller developing schizonts, meronts, or trophozoites (*arrows*), two type I meronts (one apparently rupturing) with multiple merozoites, and three macrogametes with light and dark bodies (*arrowheads*) (×5400). (**B**) Higher magnification of, from left to right, mononuclear meront, macrogamete, type I meront with eight merozoites, and thick-walled oocyst. Note complicated folds of the feeding plates (×11,500). (**C**) Electron-dense micronemes and granules in developing merozoites (one has prominent nucleus and nucleolus) of type I meront. Note larger feeding apparatus and schizont (*right field*) (×21,000). (**D**) Two microgametocytes of a microgamont (×33,000). (**E**) Thick-walled oocyst with four sporozoites in the stool (×25,000). (**F**) Merozoite apparently in the process of penetrating an enterocyte (×45,000).

vacuoles. It has also been suggested that the antibody-dependent, cell-mediated, cytotoxic immune response is important.

THERAPY

Over 75 agents have been tested, yet there remains no truly effective therapy for cryptosporidiosis.[2,4,9,60–69] Perhaps there is suboptimal drug absorption. As of fall 1994, paromomycin was the most promising anticryptosporidial agent.[70–73] Although relapse is common, even during maintenance therapy, resolution can be reinstituted in 80% of patients, and thus continuous therapy is required. The drug is well tolerated.

Hyperimmune bovine colostrum has had some effect in reducing diarrheal symptoms (stool remains positive for oocysts) in the small numbers of treated AIDS patients.[9,61] The active ingredient in colostrum is unknown, but is apparently not the globulin component. A cell-free supernatant (active component unknown) made from single-cell lymph node suspensions from immunized cows (transfer factor or dialyzable leukocyte extract) has had favorably preliminary clinical success with parasite reduction.[60]

Prevention of infection can be difficult, because the oocyst withstands exposure to solutions of 3% chlorine and 5% formaldehyde solutions. Temperatures of −20°C and above 65°C for at least 30 min and prolonged bleach (over 5 min) or 5% ammonia are necessary to reduce infection significantly.[4] Some have suggested that all water be boiled at least 1 min.

STOOL DIAGNOSIS

The majority of diagnoses are based on identification of oocysts in the stool, although, in some patients, endoscopic bowel biopsies are necessary.[2,4,37,43,74,75] Stool oocyst content varies with the site of bowel involvement, eg, small versus large bowel. In AIDS patients with chronic infection, oocyst excretion appears to occur continually, with relatively little stool-to-stool variation (within one order of magnitude); however, there is impressive patient-to-patient variation in mean oocyst concentration and 24-hour total oocyst numbers.[76]

Stool specimens can be submitted either fresh (least preferred) or fixed in 10% formalin or sodium acetate–acetic acid–formalin (SAF), but not in polyvinyl alcohol fixative. The oocyst burden is usually of a level (especially in AIDS patients) that a simple modified, acid-fast (Kinyoun) stain smear is adequate for diagnosis (oocysts stain red, fungi stain green). Since shedding of oocysts fluctuates widely, three stool samples should be studied before rendering a negative diagnosis.

The spores can be first concentrated from stool by sugar flotation methods, eg, Sheather's method, zinc sulfate, or saturated sodium chloride[4] or by centrifugation or sedimentation concentration methods, such as formalin–ether or formalin–ethyl acetate. All such methods may be associated with spore loss.[75] Auramine phenol, rhodamine, and safranin are also useful.[56] Phase contrast microscopy has also been used successfully on concentrated specimens.[23] The spherical oocysts (4 to 5 μm in diameter) are refractile, have up to six black granules, and often adhere to mucus. The oocysts are light pink on bright field, and bright by phase contrast microscopy. Rapid negative staining methods, using 1% and 2% aqueous solutions of merbromin (bright-field) and longer staining at high temperatures, have recently been introduced and apparently show similar sensitivity and specificity to acid-fast stains.[77,78]

More sensitive approaches to diagnosis of stool specimens are becoming available: ELISA, indirect fluorescent antibody (IFA) tests, and a direct immunofluorescence test that uses a specific murine IgM monoclonal antibody (100% specificity in stool) directed against oocyst wall antigen.[76,79] The sensitivity (compared to microscopy) of the ELISA assay has been reported to be 82.3%, and the specificity 92.4%.[74] These methods are particularly useful for rapid screening of specimens containing few oocysts. Studies have found fluorescein-labeled, monoclonal antibody (IFA) to be more sensitive than acid-fast staining in detecting oocysts in stool.[75]

The same monoclonal antibody (Merifluour™ Cryptosporidium, Meridan Diagnostics, Cincinnati, OH) used to detect oocysts in the stool, has been used, both by indirect immunofluorescence and avidin–biotin–peroxidase techniques, to stain oocysts in paraffin sections.[80] Staining is of oocyst wall, with no staining of intracellular trophozoites or macrogamonts. A second monoclonal antibody has been developed with similar staining results.[81]

Small intestinal brushing cytology has also been demonstrated as a sensitive way to diagnose cryptosporidiosis.[82]

IgG antibodies have been detected in the serum of virtually all infected patients, tested by immunofluorescence and ELISA assays, within 2 weeks of presentation. Immunocompetent individuals and HIV-infected patients, with or without documented cryptosporidial diarrhea, can generate IgG, IgM, and IgA, which indicates that the antibodies are not protective against *C parvum*.[83] Seropositivity has been found in a high percentage (approximately 50%) of asymptomatic individuals, suggesting that cryptosporidial infection is a common occurrence.

HISTOPATHOLOGIC DIAGNOSIS

The degree of malabsorption, histopathologic changes, and parasite shedding may not parallel the parasite burden in a biopsy specimen. This suggests a secretory or toxic diarrhea[1,2,43,48,84,85] (Figure 130–2). Although the parasite may have a preference for jejunum, large bowel may be heavily infected without infection of small bowel. Alternatively, small bowel can be infected while coincident biopsy specimens of large bowel contain no cryptosporidia. In time, it is more likely to find involvement of all levels of the intestine. The rectum is often involved, while the esophagus and stomach are only occasionally infected.

The effect of *Cryptosporidium* on the small bowel, as appreciated at relatively low magnification (4 to 10×), is the nonspecific pattern of injury caused by a number of other intestinal parasites, eg, *I belli, G lamblia,* and microsporidia. The degree of histopathologic change, however, often reaches a severity rarely seen with these other pathogens. The level of villus atrophy and blunting and crypt elongation (hyperplasia/hypertrophy) can leave the small bowel resembling the colon.[85] On the other hand, the changes can be surprisingly mild considering the large number of parasites.[43,85] The diagnosis of intestinal cryptosporidiosis is generally easy, even at medium magnification 16 to 25×). The diagnosis is then confirmed at higher (40×) magnification, not requiring oil-immersion lens. The unique intracellular, but extracytoplasmic, position of the parasite bulging from the apical surface of the epithelium is characteristic. Heavy burdens are usually correlated with severe mucosal damage and even infiltrates of neutrophils.[85]

Cryptosporidium stains basophilic to amphophilic by H&E, dark blue by Giemsa, and red to purple by Gram stain, respectively. A good Giemsa stain, with a light blue background, is perhaps the most reliable. Too many other structures stain with silver-based and mucin stains. Trichrome and iron-hematoxylin stains are not helpful. Acid-fast stain is much less effective on tissue section than with stool or sputum.

Infection is confined to the luminal surfaces of enterocytes, from the base of the crypts to the tips of the atrophied villi. The numbers of parasites and the degree of inflammatory change can vary from area to area, even within the same biopsy specimen. The crypts can be dilated and lined by many parasites, while the surface (colon) or villi (small bowel) may be minimal, if it is involved at all, in the same specimen. There can be cryptitis and destruction of crypts by neutrophils. There is usually relatively minimal involvement of Brunner's glands. Intraepithelial lymphocytes are relatively uncommon, while neutrophils and occasional eosinophils are often between epithelial cells and in the nearby lamina propria. Mitotic figures and cellular atypia are increased, especially in the distorted crypts.

In place of tall columnar enterocytes are distorted, disorganized cells undergoing degeneration and necrosis. The cells are often vesiculated with inconspicuous brush borders. The epithelium can appear fragile, with strips of sloughing cells.

In colorectal biopsies, parasites may be limited to the surface or the crypts, or be in both locations. There may be only focal involvement. As in the small bowel, the infected colonic crypts are often dilated, have a decreased proportion of goblets cells and increased mitotic figures.

Infection of the ducts and gall bladder is typically more spotty than uniform.[48–51] Edema and inflammation are often more pronounced than in the bowel. The ducts are usually dilated and their walls thickened. The mucosal surfaces appear granular. Parasites are in the small intrahepatic and larger biliary radicals, as well as in the glands of the wall of the common duct. The infected periductal glands are dilated and may have microabscesses. The lumen is filled with parasites, debris, and neutrophils, and there is a mixed acute and chronic inflammatory infiltrate (minimal eosinophils) in the surrounding edematous tissue. The damaged epithelial cells vary from cuboidal to flattened to irregular and there may be surface erosions.

Autopsies of patients with severe infections have revealed involvement of the main pancreatic ducts, which, unlike the bowel epithelium, undergoes squamous metaplasia.[84]

Infections of bowel can spread to respiratory tract, probably from aspiration. Infection from the pharynx to the respiratory bronchioles (not alveolar spaces), including submucosal glands, has been reported in a small number of AIDS and non-AIDS patients and is associated with squamous metaplasia.[44,45] Symptoms include cough (even croup), dyspnea, wheezing, and hoarseness. Premortem diagnosis has been made by identifying acid-fast (modified cold Kinyoun method) cryptosporidia in sputum, bronchoalveolar lavage, bronchial brushings, lung biopsies, and tracheal aspirates. Chest x ray reveals a pattern of interstitial pneumonia. The significance of respiratory cryptosporidiosis in man is unclear; however, it is an important economic problem in the poultry industry, where inhalation has been documented as a mode of spread.

EXPERIMENTAL MODELS

There is neither a good in vitro cell culture model nor a reproducible small animal model. Several cell lines appear to support asexual reproduction.[5,78,86,87] Recent breakthroughs include adult mouse and intestinal xenograft models.[88–90] The infected adult athymic mouse and T-cell subset-depleted mouse display intermittent diarrhea, weight loss, jaundice, dehydration, and have oocysts in their stools. Parasites and inflammatory changes are in the intestine, hepatobiliary tree, and pancreas.[88] Lymphoid cells from histocompatible immune mice cure infected nude mice. Manipulations that lead to a reversible increase in oocyst shedding in neonatally infected adult BALB/c mice include treatment with anti-CD4 monoclonal antibodies or anti-interferon-gamma monoclonal antibodies (even more so when combined). On the other hand, anti-CD8 and anti-interleukin-2 monoclonal antibodies apparently have no effect. This model has been used to confirm the importance of cell-mediated, and not humoral, immunity.[91] Mice infected with murine leukemia retrovirus provide another model for cryptosporidiosis in AIDS, since this virus affects T-cell immunity and susceptibility to the parasite.

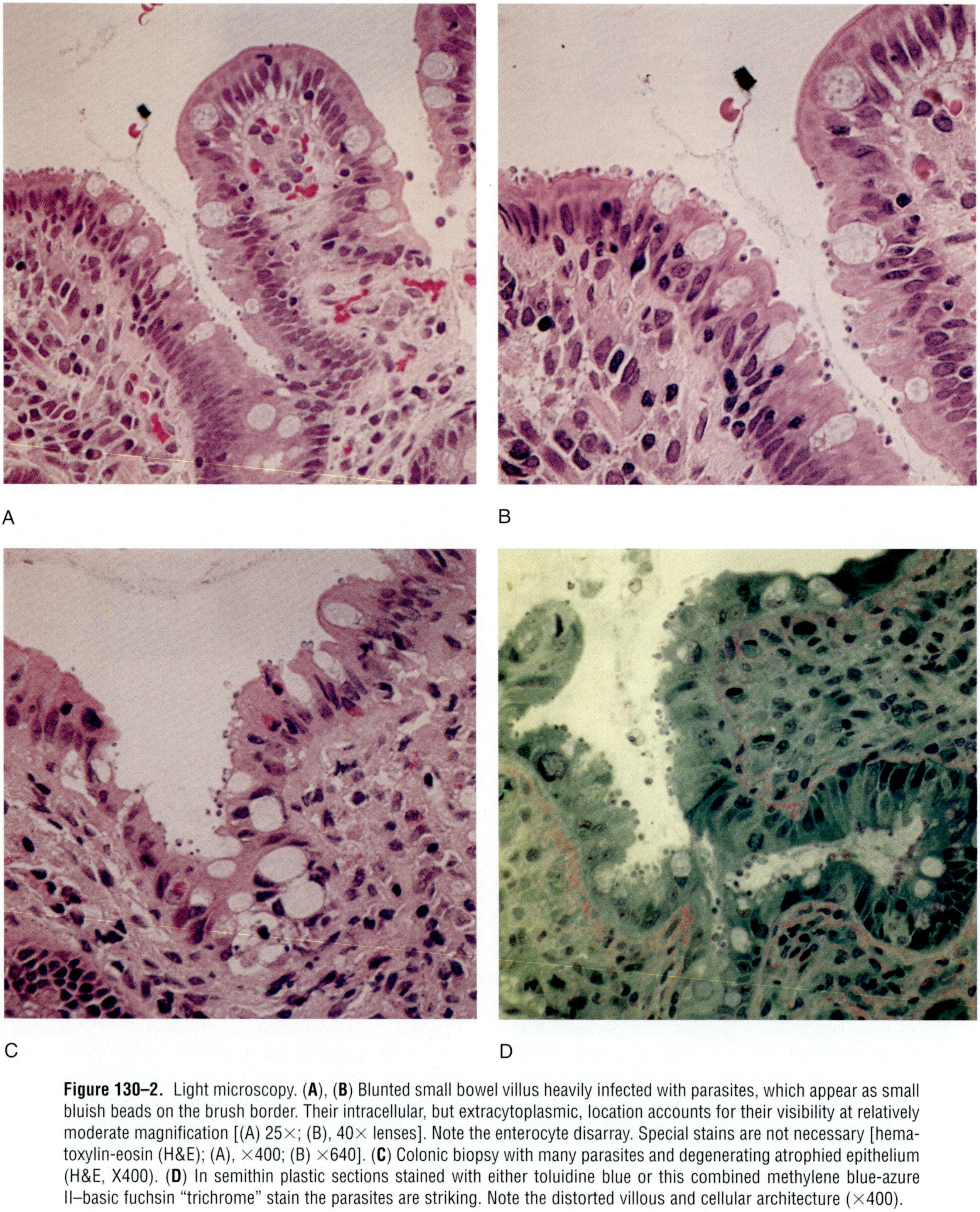

Figure 130–2. Light microscopy. (**A**), (**B**) Blunted small bowel villus heavily infected with parasites, which appear as small bluish beads on the brush border. Their intracellular, but extracytoplasmic, location accounts for their visibility at relatively moderate magnification [(A) 25×; (B), 40× lenses]. Note the enterocyte disarray. Special stains are not necessary [hematoxylin-eosin (H&E); (A), ×400; (B) ×640]. (**C**) Colonic biopsy with many parasites and degenerating atrophied epithelium (H&E, X400). (**D**) In semithin plastic sections stained with either toluidine blue or this combined methylene blue-azure II–basic fuchsin "trichrome" stain the parasites are striking. Note the distorted villous and cellular architecture (×400).

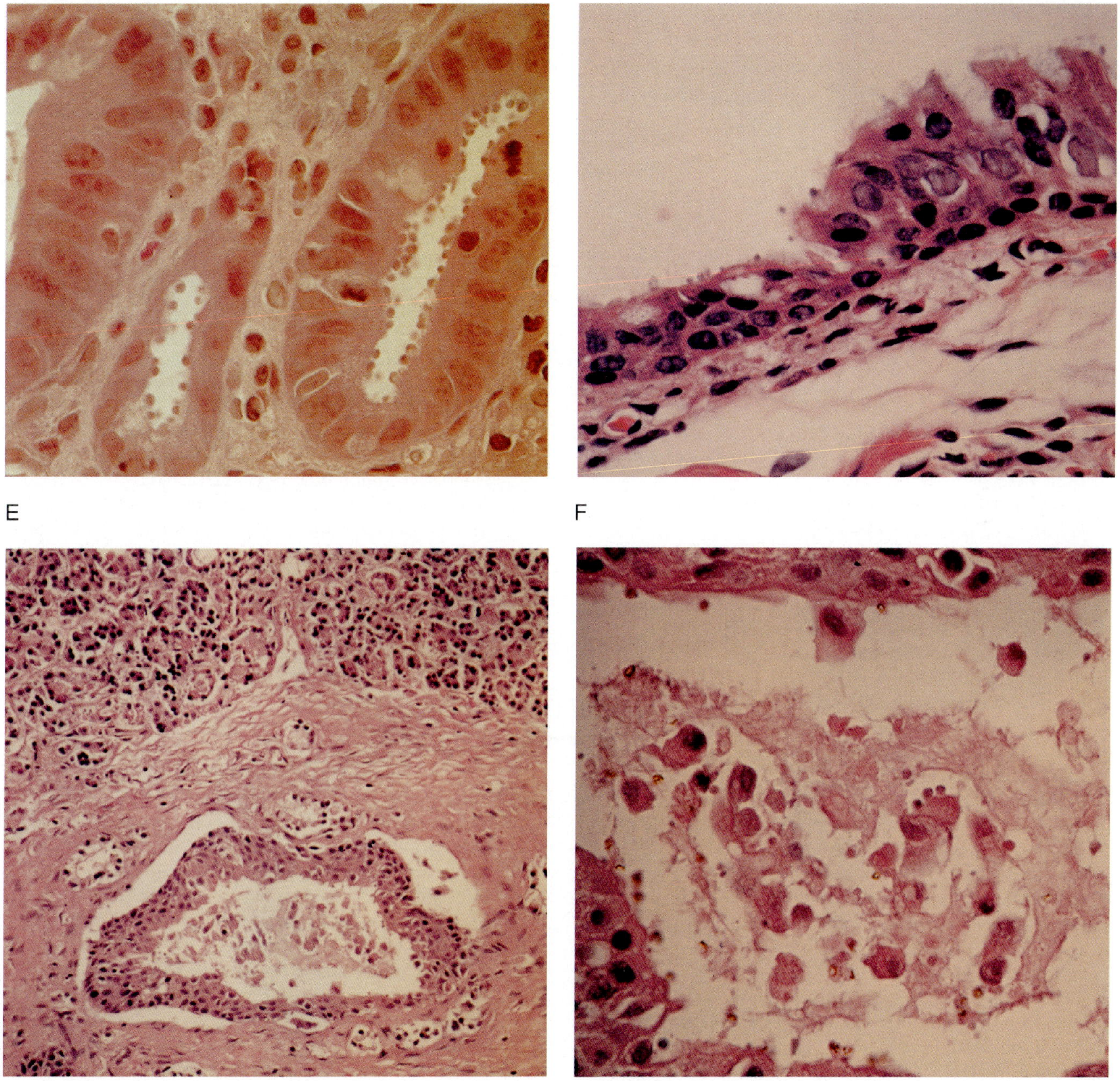

E F G H

Figure 130–2. (*Continued*) (**E**) Crypts in wall of common bile duct show heavy infection. Note the mitotic figures, disorganization and atrophy (×640). Typically, the infected tracheobronchial tree (**F**) and pancreatic ducts (**G**), (**H**) show squamous metaplasia. Note the pseudostratified columnar ciliated epithelium (F, *right*) and flattened area (*left*). Note parasites infecting attached and sloughed duct cells (**H**) [H&E; (F), ×640; (G), ×160; (H), ×640].

Hyperimmune cow colostrum inhibited *C parvum* in the HT-29.74 cell line.[92] Madin–Darby canine kidney cells apparently allow development of large numbers of *C parvum* through asexual and sexual intracellular stages (fully sporulated oocysts not identified).[93] Athymic and SCID mice, as well as SCID foals, have been used for immune reconstitution and immunotherapy studies.[94,95] An immunosuppressed rat model has recently been described for studying respiratory cryptosporidiosis.[96] The parasites induced exfoliative necrosis of epithelium and patchy alveolitis adjacent to bronchioles.

REFERENCES

1. Casemore DP, Sands RL, Curry A. Cryptosporidium species a "new" human pathogen. *J Clin Pathol.* 1985;38: 1321–1336.
2. Crawford F, Vermund SH. Human cryptosporidiosis. *Crit Rev Microbiol.* 1988;16:113–159.
3. Current WL, Owen RL. Cryptosporidiosis and microsporidiosis. In: Farthing MJG, Keusch GT, eds. *Enteric Infection: Mechanisms, Manifestations and Management.* New York: Raven Press; 1989:223–248.
4. Current WL, Garcia LS. Cryptosporidiosis. *Clin Microbiol Rev.* 1991;4:325–358.
5. Fayer R, Ungar BLP. *Cryptosporidium* spp and cryptosporidiosis. *Microbiol Rev.* 1986;50:458–483.
6. Soave R, Armstrong D. *Cryptosporidium* and cryptosporidiosis. *Rev Infect Dis.* 1986;8:1012–1023.
7. Laughon BE, Allaudeen HS, Becker JM, et al. Summary of the workshop on future directions in discovery and development of therapeutic agents for opportunistic infections associated with AIDS. *J Infect Dis.* 1991;164:244–251.
8. Roberts WG, Green PHR, Ma J, Carr M, Ginsberg AM. Prevalence of cryptosporidiosis in patients undergoing endoscopy: evidence for an asymptomatic carrier state. *Am J Med.* 1989;87:537–539.
9. Gellin BG, Soave R. Coccidian infections in AIDS: toxoplasmosis, cryptosporidiosis, and isosporiasis. *Med Clin North Am.* 1992;76:205–234.
10. Smith PD, Quinn TC, Strober W, Janoff EN, Masur H. Gastrointestinal infections in AIDS. *Ann Intern Med.* 1992;116: 63–77.
11. Colebunders R, Francis H, Mann JM, et al. Persistent diarrhea, strongly associated with HIV infection in Kinshasa, Zaire. *Am J Gastroenterol.* 1987;82:859–864.
12. Dryden MS, Shanson DC. The microbial causes of diarrhoea in patients infected with the human immunodeficiency virus. *J Infect.* 1988;17:107–114.
13. Rene E, Marche C, Regnier B, et al. Intestinal infections in patients with acquired immunodeficiency syndrome: a prospective study in 132 patients. *Dig Dis Sci.* 1989;34: 773–780.
14. Conlon CP, Pinching AJ, Perera CU, Moody A, Luo NP, Lucas SB. HIV-related enteropathy in Zambia: a clinical, microbiological, and histological study. *Am J Trop Med.* 1990;42:83–88.
15. Dallabetta GA, Miotti PG. Chronic diarrhoea in AIDS patients in the tropics: a review. *Trop Doctor.* 1992;22:3–9.
16. Cotte L, Rabododonirina M, Piens MA, Perreard M, Mojon M, Trepo C. Prevalence of intestinal protozoans in French patients infected with HIV. *J Acq Immune Def Synd.* 1993; 6:1024–1029.
17. Sauda FC, Zamarioli LA, Filho WE, Mello L de B. Prevalence of *Cryptosporidium* and *Isospora belli* among AIDS patients attending Santos Reference Center for AIDS, Sao Paulo, Brazil. *J Parasitol.* 1993;79:454–456.
18. Brandonisio O, Maggi P, Panaro MA, Bramante LA, Di Coste A, Angarano G. Prevalence of cryptosporidiosis in HIV-infected patients with diarrheal disease. *Eur J Epidemiol.* 1993;9:190–194.
19. Current WL, Blagburn BL. *Cryptosporidium* and Microsporidia: some closing comments. *J Protozool.* 1991;38: 244S–245S.
20. Wolfson JS, Richter JM, Waldron MA, Weber DJ, McCarthy DM, Hopkins CC. Cryptosporidiosis in immunocompetent patients. *N Engl J Med.* 1985;312:1278–1282.
21. Anderson BC. Prevalence of cryptosporidium muris-like oocysts among cattle populations of the United States: preliminary report. *J Protozool.* 1991;38:14S–15S.
22. Nichols GL, McLauchlin J, Samuel D. A technique for typing cryptosporidium isolates. *J Protozool.* 1991;38:237S–240S.
23. Current WL, Reese NC, Ernst JV, Bailey WS, Heyman MB, Weinstein WM. Human cryptosporidiosis in immunocompetent and immunodeficient persons. *N Engl J Med.* 1983; 308:1252–1257.
24. Casemore DP. Foodborne protozoal infection. *Lancet.* 1990;336:1427–1432.
25. Lindsay DS, Blagburn BL, Hoerr RJ, Smith PC. Cryptosporidiosis in zoo and pet birds. *J Protozool.* 1991;38: 180S–181S.
26. McAnuity JM, Fleming DW, Gonzalez AH. A community-wide outbreak of cryptosporidiosis associated with swimming at a wave pool. *JAMA.* 1994;272:1597–1600.
27. Hayes EB, Matte TD, O'Brien TR, et al. Large community outbreak of cryptosporidiosis due to contamination of a filtered public water supply. *N Engl J Med.* 1989;320: 1372–1376.
28. Millard PS, Gensheimer KF, Addiss DG, et al. An outbreak of cryptosporidiosis from fresh-pressed apple cider. *JAMA.* 1994;272:1592–1596.
29. MacKenzie WR, Hoxie NJ, Proctor ME, et al. A massive outbreak in Milwaukee of *Cryptosporidium* infection transmitted through the public water supply. *N Engl J Med.* 1994;331:161–167.
30. Current WL. The biology of *Cryptosporidium*. *ASM News.* 1988;54:605–611.
31. Kuhls TL, Mosier DA, Crawford DL, Griffis J. Seroprevalence of cryptosporidial antibodies during infancy, childhood, and adolescence. *Clin Infect Dis.* 1994;18:731–735.
32. Cordell RL, Addiss DG. Cryptosporidiosis in child care settings: a review of the literature and recommendations for prevention and control. *Pediatr Infect Dis.* 1994;13: 310–317.
33. Newman RD, Zu S-X, Wuhib T, Lima AAM, Guerrant RL, Sears CL. Household epidemiology of *Cryptosporidium*

parvum infection in an urban community in Northeast Brazil. *Ann Intern Med.* 1994;120:500–505.

34. Bird RG, Smith MD. Cryptosporidiosis in man: parasite life cycle and fine structural pathology. *J Pathol.* 1980;132: 217–233.
35. Marcial MA, Madara JL. Cryptosporidium: cellular localization, structural analysis of absorptive cell-parasite membrane-membrane interactions in guinea pigs, and suggestion of protozoan transport by M cells. *Gastroenterol.* 1986;90:583–594.
36. Ribeiro HC, Teichberg S, Sun T, Fagundes U, Lifshitz F. Ultrastructure of human cryptosporidial infection: a review. In: T. Sun, ed. *Prog Clin Parasitol.* New York; Field and Wood; 1989;1:143–158.
37. Navin TR, Juranek DD. Cryptosporidiosis: clinical, epidemiologic and parasitologic review. *Rev Infect Dis.* 1984; 6:313–327.
38. Ravn P, Lundgren JD, Kjaeldgaard P, et al. Nosocomial outbreak of cryptosporidiosis in AIDS patients. *Br Med J.* 1991;302:277–280.
39. Egger M, Mausezahl D, Odermatt P, Marti HP, Tanner M. Symptoms and transmission of intestinal cryptosporidiosis. *Arch Dis Child.* 1990;65:445–447.
40. Peterson C. Cryptosporidiosis in patients infected with the human immunodeficiency virus. *Clin Infect Dis.* 1992;15: 903–909.
41. McGowan I, Hawkins AS, Weller IVD. The natural history of cryptosporidial diarrhoea in HIV-infected patients. *AIDS.* 1993;7:349–354.
42. Greenberg RE, Mir R, Bank S, Siegal FP. Resolution of intestinal cryptosporidiosis after treatment of AIDS with AZT. *Gastroenterology.* 1989;97:1327–1330.
43. Lefkowitch JH, Krumholz S, Fengchen K, Grifin P, Despommier D, Brasitus TA. Cryptosporidiosis of the human small intestine: a light and electron microscope study. *Hum Pathol.* 1984;15:746–752.
44. Travis WD, Schmidt K, MacLowry JD, Masur H, Condron KS, Fojo AT. Respiratory cryptosporidiosis in a patient with malignant lymphoma. *Arch Pathol Lab Med.* 1990; 114:519–522.
45. Kocoshis SA, Cibull ML, Davis TE, Hinton JT, Seip M, Banwell JG. Intestinal and pulmonary cryptosporidiosis in an infant with severe combined immune deficiency. *J Ped Gastroenterol Nutr.* 1984;3:149–157.
46. Giang TT, Pollack G, Kotler DP. Cryptosporidiosis of the nasal mucosa in a patient with AIDS. *AIDS.* 1994;8: 555–556.
47. Moore JA, Frenkel JK. Respiratory and enteric cryptosporidiosis in humans. *Arch Pathol Lab Med.* 1991;115: 1160–1162.
48. Guarda LA, Stein SA, Cleary KA, Ordonez NG. Human cryptosporidiosis in the acquired immune deficiency syndrome. *Arch Pathol Lab Med.* 1983;107:562–566.
49. Margulis SJ, Honig CL, Soave R, Govoni AF, Mouradian JA, Jacobson IM. Biliary tract obstruction in the acquired immunodeficiency syndrome. *Am Intern Med.* 1986;105: 207–210.
50. Kahn DG, Garfinkle JM, Klonoff DC, Pembrook LJ, Morrow DJ. Cryptosporidial and cytomegaloviral hepatitis and cholecystitis. *Arch Pathol Lab Med.* 1987;111:879–881.
51. Schneiderman DJ, Cello JP, Laing FC. Papillary stenosis and sclerosing cholangitis in the acquired immunodeficiency syndrome. *Ann Intern Med.* 1987;106:546–549.
52. McCarty M, Choudhri AH, Helbert M, Crofton ME. Radiological features of AIDS related cholangitis. *Clin Radiol.* 1989;40:582–585.
53. Bonacini M. Hepatobiliary complications in patients with human immunodeficiency virus infection. *Am J Med.* 1992;92:404–411.
54. Hinnant K, Schwartz A, Rotterdam H, Rudzki C. Cytomegaloviral and cryptosporidial cholecystitis in two patients with AIDS. *Am J Surg Pathol.* 1989;13:57–61.
55. Hawkins SP, Thomas RP, Teasdale C. Acute pancreatitis: a new finding in cryptosporidium enteritis. *Br Med J.* 1987;294:483–484.
56. Canning EU. Protozoan infections. *Trans Roy Soc Trop Med Hyg.* 1990;84:19–24.
57. Cozon G, Biron F, Jeannin M, Cannella D, Revillard J-P. Secretory IgA antibodies to *Cryptosporidium parvum* in AIDS patients with chronic cryptosporidiosis. *J Infect Dis.* 1994;169:696–699.
58. Sterling CR, Gilman RH, Sinclair NA, Cama V, Castillo R, Diaz F. The role of breast milk in protecting urban Peruvian children against cryptosporidiosis. *J Protozool.* 1991; 38:23S–25S.
59. Heyworth MF. Immunology of *Giardia* and *Cryptosporidium* infections. *J Infect Dis.* 1992;166:465–472.
60. McMeeking A, Borkowsky W, Klesius PH, Bonk S, Holzman, Lawrence HS. A controlled trial of bovine dialyzable leukocyte extract for cryptosporidiosis in patients with AIDS. *J Infect Dis.* 1990;161:108–112.
61. Nord J, Ma P, DiJohn D, Tzipori S, Tacket CO. Treatment with bovine hyperimmune colostrum of cryptosporidial diarrhea in AIDS patients. *AIDS.* 1990;4:581–584.
62. Simon D, Weiss L, Tanowitz HB. Wittner M. Resolution of cryptosporidium infection in an AIDS patient after improvement of nutritional and immune status with octreotide. *Am J Gastroenterol.* 1991;86:615–618.
63. Kreinik G, Burstein O, Landor M, Bernstein L, Weiss LM, Wittner M. Successful management of intractable cryptosporidial diarrhea with intravenous octreotide, a somatostatin analogue. *AIDS.* 1991;5:765–767.
64. Simon DM, Cello JP, Valenzuela J, et al. Multicenter placebo-controlled trial of the effectiveness of octreotide in patients with refractory AIDS-associated diarrhea. (submitted for publication).
65. Murdoch DA, Bloss DE, Glover SC. Successful treatment of cryptosporidiosis in an AIDS patient with letrazuril. *AIDS.* 1993;7:1279–1280.
66. Cello JP, Grendell JH, Basuk P, et al. Effect of octreotide on refractory AIDS-associated diarrhea: a prospective, multicenter clinical trial. *Ann Intern Med.* 1991;115: 705–710.
67. Marshall RJ, Flanigan TP. Paromomycin inhibits *Cryptosporidium* infection of a human enterocyte cell line. *J Infect Dis.* 1992;165:772–774.
68. Rehg JE. Anticryptosporidial activity of lasalocid and other inophorous antibiotics in immunosuppressed rats. *J Infect Dis.* 1993;168:1566–1569.
69. Weikel C, Lazenby A, Belitsos P, McDewitt M, Fleming HE,

Barbacci M. Intestinal injury associated with spiramycin therapy of cryptosporidium infection in AIDS. *J Protozool.* 1991;38:147S.

70. Bissuel F, Cotte L, Rabodonirina M, Rougier P, Piens M-A, Trepo C. Paromomycin: an effective treatment for cryptosporidial diarrhea in patients with AIDS. *Clin Infect Dis.* 1994;18:447–449.
71. Fichterbaum CJ, Ritchie DJ, Powderly WG. Use of paromomycin for treatment of cryptosporidiosis in patients with AIDS. *Clin Infect Dis.* 1993;16:298–300.
72. Armitage K, Flanigan T, Carey J et al. Treatment of cryptosporidiosis with paromomycin: a report of five cases. *Arch Intern Med.* 1992;152:2497–2499.
73. Wallace MR, Nguyen M-T, Newton Jr JA. Use of paromomycin for the treatment of cryptosporidiosis in patients with AIDS. *Clin Infect Dis.* 1993;17:1070–1071.
74. Ungar BLP. Enzyme-linked immunoassay for detection of cryptosporidium antigens in fecal specimens. *J Clin Microbiol.* 1990;28:2491–2495.
75. Weber R, Bryan RT, Bishop HS, Wahlquist SP, Sullivan JJ, Juranek DD. Threshold of detection of cryptosporidium oocysts in human stool specimens: evidence for low sensitivity of current diagnostic methods. *J Clin Microbiol.* 1991;29:1323–1327.
76. Goodgame RW, Genta RM, White AC, Chappell CL. Intensity of infection in AIDS-associated cryptosporidiosis. *J Infect Dis.* 1993;167:704–709.
77. Chichino G, Bruno A, Cevini C, Atzori C, Gatti S, Scaglia M. New rapid staining methods of cryptosporidium oocysts in stools. *J Protozool.* 1991;38:212S–214S.
78. Anand A. Cryptosporidiosis in patients with AIDS. *Clin Infect Dis.* 1993;17:297–298.
79. Tsaihong JC, Ma P. Comparison of an indirect fluorescent antibody test and stool examination of cryptosporidiosis. *Eur J Clin Microbiol Infect Dis.* 1990;9:770–773.
80. Loose JH, Sedergran DJ, Cooper HS. Identification of cryptosporidium in paraffin-embedded tissue sections with the use of a monoclonal antibody. *Am J Clin Pathol.* 1989; 91:206–209.
81. Bonnin A, Petrella T, Dubremetz JF, Michiels JF, Puygauthier-Toubas D, Camerlynck P. Histopathological method for diagnosis of cryptosporidiosis using monoclonal antibodies. *Eur J Clin Microbiol Infect Dis.* 1990;9:664–666.
82. Silverman JF, Levine J, Finley J, Larkin EW, Norris T. Small-intestinal brushing cytology in the diagnosis of cryptosporidiosis in AIDS. *Diagn Cytopathol.* 1990;6:193–196.
83. Kassa M, Comby E, Lemeteil D, Brasseur P, Ballet JJ. Characterization of anti-cryptosporidium IgA antibodies in sera from immunocompetent individuals and HIV-infected patients. *J Protozool.* 1991;38:179S–180S.
84. Godwin TA. Cryptosporidiosis in the acquired immunodeficiency syndrome: a study of 15 autopsy cases. *Hum Pathol.* 1991;22:1215–1224.
85. Genta RM, Chappell CL, White Jr AC, Kimball KT, Goodgame RW. Duodenal morphology and intensity of infection in AIDS-related intestinal cryptosporidiosis. *Gastroenterology.* 1993;105:1769–1775.
86. Aji T, Flanigan T, Marshall R, Kaetzel C, Aikawa M. Ultrastructural study of asexual development of *Cryptosporidium parvum* in a human intestinal cell line. *J Protozool.* 1991;38:82S–84S.
87. Adams RB, Guerrant RL, Zu S, Fang G, Roche JK. *Cryptosporidium parvum* infection of intestinal epithelium: morphologic and functional studies in an in vitro model. *J Infect Dis.* 1994;169:170–177.
88. Ungar BP, Burris JA, Quinn CA, Finkelman FD. New mouse models for chronic cryptosporidium infection in immunodeficient hosts. *Infect Immun.* 1990;58:961–969.
89. Ungar BLP Kao TC, Burris JA, Finkelman FD. *Cryptosporidium* infection in an adult mouse model: independent roles for gamma-interferon and $CD4^+$ T lymphocytes in protective immunity. *J Immunol.* 1991;147:1014–1022.
90. Thulin JD, Kuhlenschmidt MK, Rolsma MD, Current WL, Gelberg HB. An intestinal xenograft model for *Cryptosporidium parvum* infection. *Infect Immun.* 1994;62: 329–331.
91. Fayer R, Guidry A, Blagburn BL. Immunotherapeutic efficacy of bovine colostral immunoglobulins from a hyperimmunized cow against cryptosporidiosis in neonatal mice. *Infect Immun.* 1990;58:2962–2965.
92. Flanigan T, Marshall R, Redman D, Kaetzel C, Ungar B. In vitro screening of therapeutic agents against cryptosporidium: hyperimmune cow colostrum is highly inhibitory. *J Protozool.* 1991;38:225S–227S.
93. Gut J, Peterson C, Nelson R, Leech J. *Cryptosporidium parvum:* in vitro cultivation in Madin–Darby canine kidney cells. *J Protozool.* 1991;38:72S–73S.
94. Mead JR, Arrowood MJ, Healy MC, Sidwell RW. Cryptosporidial infections in SCID mice reconstituted with human or murine lymphocytes. *J Protozool.* 1991;38:59S–61S.
95. Perryman LE, Bjorneby JM. Immunotherapy of cryptosporidiosis in immunodeficient animal models. *J Protozool.* 1991;38:98S–100S.
96. Meulbroek JA, Novilla MN, Current WL. An immunosuppressed rat model of respiratory cryptosporidiosis. *J Protozool.* 1991;38:113S–115S.

CHAPTER 131

Cyclospora Infection

Tsieh Sun

As it takes two to make a quarrel, so it takes two to make a disease, the microbe and its host.

Charles V. Chapin (1856–1941), Papers, The Principles of Epidemiology

DEFINITION

Cyclospora species is a newly discovered intestinal coccidian. Its generic name was established in 1993.[1] It belongs to the phylum Apicomplexa, class Sporozoasida, subclass Coccidiasina. The organism parasitizes enterocytes and causes diarrhea in both immunocompetent and immunodeficient patients.

HISTORICAL NOTES

Early publications credited Soave et al[2] for describing (in 1986) the first four American patients with *Cyclospora* infection. The patients had visited Haiti or Mexico. Recent articles, however, have verified that two patients from Papua New Guinea described by Ashford in 1979[3] are the first reported.[4–6]

SYNONYMS

Cyclospora has been called variably unsporulated coccidian, coccidian-like body, blue-green alga, cyanobacterium-like body, large *Cryptosporidium,* and *Cryptosporidium muris*–like oocyst.

GEOGRAPHIC DISTRIBUTION

Infection by *Cyclospora* has been reported from the United States, Nepal, Peru, the United Kingdom, Spain, and Australia.[1–3,6–18] Most patients have traveled to tropical regions, including Haiti, Mexico, Dominican Republic, Puerto Rico, Carribean Islands, India, Pakistan, Indonesia, Malaysia, Papua New Guinea, Solomon Islands, Australia, Morocco, or other unspecified areas of South and Central America, Eastern Europe, and Southeast Asia.

EPIDEMIOLOGY AND LIFE CYCLE

Although the first patients were described in 1979,[3] the report of Soave et al[2] first drew the attention of medical professionals. Since then several hundred cases have been reported. The largest outbreaks have been in Kathmandu, Nepal.[10,11,14] In the outbreak there in 1989, 55 expatriates with diarrhea passed *Cyclospora* during a 5-month period.[10] In the 1990 epidemic, 85 patients were identified[11] and in a 1993 study, 108 positive stools were recovered from 964 foreigners living in Kathmandu.[14] An outbreak of *Cyclospora* infection in Chicago during 1990, however, was traced to a water tank.[11] A pump had failed and *Cyclospora* were found later in sediment of the tank.

These outbreaks suggest that transmission is waterborne, but the organism has been in the heads of lettuce,[11] so contaminated food may be a source also. In 1996, a few hundred persons were infected with cyclospora in the United States involving several states (California, Florida, Texas, and others). The source of infection was originally considered to be contaminated strawberries, but the organism was not recovered from these fruits. In Nepal, epidemics occur between May and August—the monsoon season[10]. In Peru, the seasonal peak is between April and June.[1]

The organism was originally thought to be a coccidian[1,2] or fungal spore.[2] When examined by electron microscopy, however, thylakoid-like bodies, similar to chloroplasts of photosynthesizing organisms, were in the cytoplasm. The organism was thus designated a cyanobacterium-like body or blue-green alga.[8,9,12] *Cyclospora,* however, stain with a modified acid-fast technique and float in Sheather's solution, so are more frequently mistaken for *Cryptosporidium*[7,8,10] The study of Ortega et al[1] was, in fact, done to define the epidemiology of cryptosporidiosis in Peru but their *Cryptosporidium*-like organism did not react to the monoclonal antibody specific for *C parvum.* By inducing sporulation and excystation they concluded that their organism was a coccidian of the genus *Cyclospora.*

When purified organisms are maintained in potassium dichromate at 25 or 32°C, there is complete sporulation in 5 to 13 days.[1] Complete excystation liberates four sporozoites from the two sporocysts in the oocyst. By contrast, cryptosporidia have four naked sporozoites in each oocyst (no sporocyst stage) and in *Isospora* the oocyst contains two sporocysts but each sporocyst has four sporozoites (Table 131–1).[1] The oocysts of *Cyclospora* are 8 to 10 μm, larger than those of *Cryptosporidium* (4 to 5 μm) and smaller than those of *Isospora* (20 to 33 μm).

The oocyst of *Cyclospora* has a double cyst wall and contains of a morula about 6 to 7 μm in diameter. The morula is membrane bound and contains a cluster of refractile, also membrane-bound globules (Figures 131–1 and 131–2).[9,12] Electron microscopy shows an outer fibrillar coat on the double-layered cell wall.[1,5,8,13,16] The internal cytoplasmic mass (morula) has a cell membrane and contains light and dark granules. The unsporulated oocyst contains no nucleus, endoplasmic reticulum, or mitochondria. The sporozoite has a membrane-bound nucleus and micronemes, characteristic of coccidians of the phylum Apicomplexa.[1] The complete life cycle and host range are unknown.

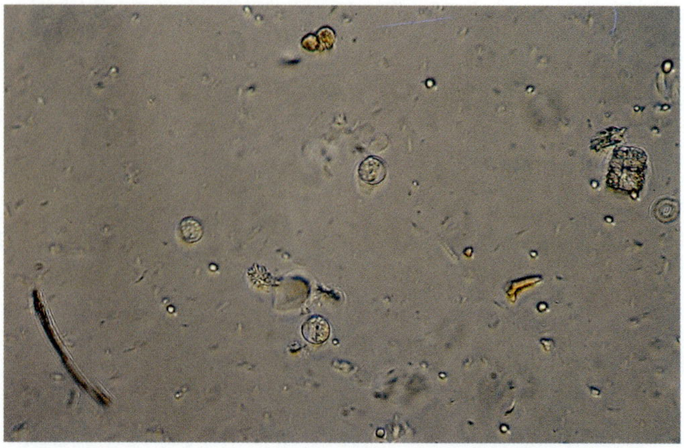

Figure 131–1. Unstained smear of stool with three oocysts of *Cyclospora*. The oocyst contains a membrane-bound morula that includes many refractile globules (×128).

CLINICAL FEATURES

The major clinical symptom is watery diarrhea or loose stools. Patients may have bowel movements 1 to 10 times per day. In one study of 55 patients in Nepal, 20% had 1 to 3 loose stools per day; 40% had 4 to 7 stools/day; and 40% had 8 or more stools/day[10]. Characteristically, the diarrhea is intermittent; patients may have diarrhea for 3 to 4 days followed by relapses that last for 1 to 15 weeks. Another study in Nepal compared patients with diarrhea and *Cyclospora* to those with diarrhea without *Cyclospora.* All patients were foreigners who visited a Canadian–American clinic in Kathmandu.[14] The study revealed that the median duration of diarrhea in the former group was 7 weeks,

TABLE 131–1. COMPARISON OF ORGANISMS

	Cyclospora	*Cryptosporidium*	*Isospora*
No. of sporocysts in each oocyst	2	0	2
No. of sporozoites in each sporocyst	2	4 naked sporozoites	4
Size in tissue (μm)	4–16	2–5	3–15
Intracellular location	Deep-seated	Intramembranous extracytoplasmic	Deep-seated
Intracellular stages	Trophozoite, schizont, merozoite	Trophozoite, schizont, merozoite, gametocyte	Trophozoite, schizont, merozoite, gametocyte
Stage in stool	Oocyst	Oocyst	Oocyst
Size of oocyst (μm)	8–10	4–5	20–23
Special stain in stool	Modified Kinyoun	Modified Kinyoun	Modified Kinyoun

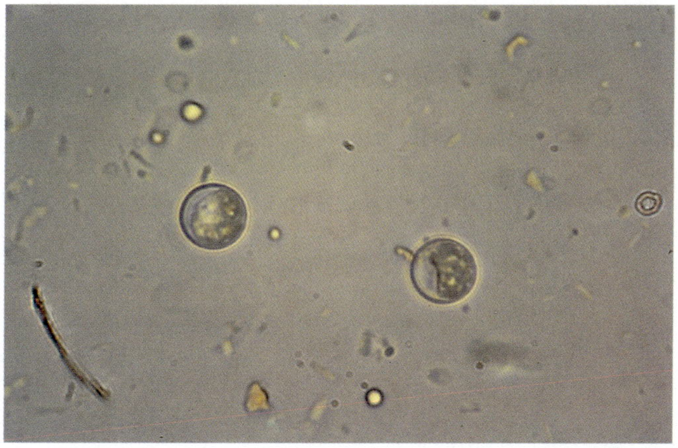

Figure 131–2. Higher magnification of two oocysts showing the detailed structure of the morula, which is separated by a space from the cell wall (×320).

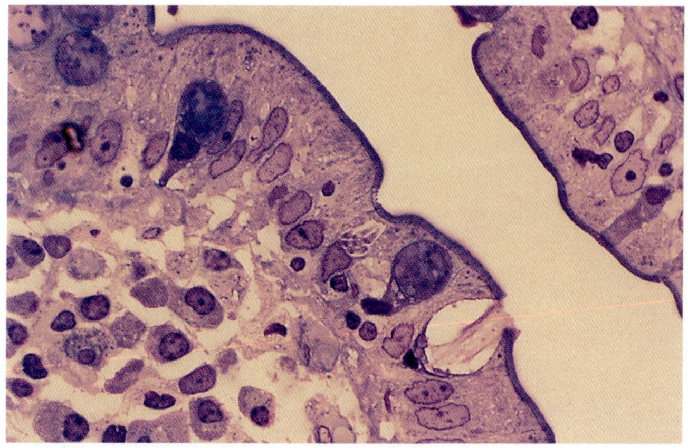

Figure 131–3. Intestinal biopsy specimen of a patient with AIDS, showing a schizont with eight merozoites inside a parasitophorous vacuole at the supranuclear location of an enterocyte (indented area). The lamina propria is infiltrated by plasma cells (toluidine blue stain on plastic section).

whereas in the latter group it was 9 days. For immunocompetent patients the diarrhea is self-limited; but patients with acquired immunodeficiency syndrome (AIDS) usually have prolonged diarrhea.[7,8,15] So far, *Cyclospora* infection has been recognized in only eight patients with AIDS.

Besides diarrhea, the most common symptoms are fatigue and anorexia.[10] Weight loss (average 3.2 to 3.6 kg) is also common in chronic infections.[10,14] Other symptoms include abdominal cramps, nausea, vomiting, flatus, belching, bloating, fever, myalgia, joint pain, and night sweats. D-xylose absorption is abnormal.[10,19]

PATHOLOGY

Histologic examination has been done in three studies.[13,19,20] In the first, jejunal biopsies were performed in two patients.[13] Both showed jejunitis with increased intraepithelial leukocytes and villous blunting. One of the biopsy specimens had villous fusion. Ultrastructural study revealed single or multiple parasites inside a parasitophorous vacuole in the cytoplasm of enterocytes. The organisms were 6 to 8 μm long, 1 to 4 μm wide, and crescent shaped in longitudinal section. *Cyclospora* has one to two nuclei with prominent nucleoli. Its cytoplasm contains rhoptries and micronemes characteristic of the phylum Apicomplexa. The second study was of nine duodenal biopsies. There were acute and chronic inflammation, surface epithelial disarray, and varying degrees of villous atrophy and crypt hyperplasia.[19] No parasites were detected in the second study.

Sun et al[20] identified *Cyclospora* in an intestinal biopsy specimen from a patient with AIDS by light microscopy (Figure 131–3). Electron microscopy further demonstrated the organism in stages of trophozoite, schizont, and merozoite.

DIAGNOSIS

The organism can be identified under light microscopy with unstained or iodine stained stool or duodenal aspirates.[18,19] It is, however, more characteristic to demonstrate the strong blue autofluorescence of the parasite with ultraviolet light.[9] Note that *Isospora* are also autofluorescent.[17] *Cyclospora* are acid fast with a modified staining technique (Figure 131–4). They stain with safranin,[8] but do not stain with iron-hematoxylin, Gomori's methenamine silver, periodic acid–Schiff, Giemsa, Gram, methylene blue, or trichrome stains.[7,8,15] The organism is visible in hematoxylin-eosin stained tissue sections.[20]

As mentioned, the differential diagnosis includes mainly cryptosporidiosis and isosporiasis (Table 131–1). Other intestinal protozoa to be excluded are microsporidiosis and sarcocystosis.[21] Microsporidians are in stool specimens as spores, much smaller (1.1 to 1.6 μm) than *Cyclospora*, and are not acid fast. A modified trichrome stain demonstrates them in stools. *Sarcocystis* is rarely detected in stools. Its oocysts are acid fast, but they are larger (25 to 33 μm) and the structural differences make them easily distinguishable from *Cyclospora*.

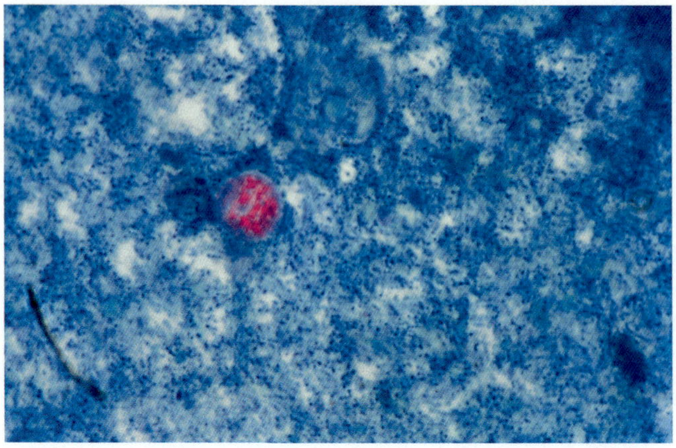

Figure 131–4. Smear of stool with a single oocyst. The globules are acid fast, whereas the membrane of the morula is not stained (modified Kinyoun stain, ×320).

TREATMENT

Varying drugs, such as metronidazole, tinidazole, ciprofloxacin, and co-trimoxazole, have stopped the excretion of oocysts.[6,15,17,22] These studies have not been controlled, however, so the patients may have recovered spontaneously. One placebo-controlled trial of co-trimoxazole in 40 patients proved that a 7-day regimen was effective in curing cyclospora infections.[23]

REFERENCES

1. Ortega YR, Sterling CR, Gilman RH, Cama VA, Diaz F. *Cyclospora* species. A new protozoan pathogen of humans. *N Engl J Med.* 1993;328:1308–1312.
2. Soave R, Dubey JP, Tummings M. A new intestinal pathogen? *Clin Res.* 1986;34:533A.
3. Ashford RW. An undescribed coccidian in man in Papua New Guinea. *Ann Trop Med Parasitol.* 1979;73:497–500.
4. Ashford RW, Warhurst DC, Reid GDF. Human infection with cyanobacterium-like bodies. *Lancet.* 1993;341:1034.
5. Sterling CR, Ortega YR. Cyanobacterium-like *Cyclospora* species. *N Engl J Med.* 1993;329:1505.
6. McDougall RJ, Tandy MW. Coccidian/cyanobacterium-like bodies as a cause of diarrhea in Australia. *Pathology.* 1993;25:375–378.
7. Hart AS, Ridinger MT, Soundarajan R, Peters CS, Swiatol AL, Kocka FE. Novel organism associated with chronic diarrhea in AIDS. *Lancet.* 1990;335:169–170.
8. Long EG, Ebrahimzadeh A, White EH, Swisher B, Callaway CS. Alga associated with diarrhea in patients with acquired immunodeficiency syndrome and in travellers. *J Clin Microbiol.* 1990;28:1101–1104.
9. Long EG, White EH, Carmichael WW, et al. Morphologic and staining characteristics of a cyanobacterium-like organism associated with diarrhea. *J Infect Dis.* 1991;164: 199–202.
10. Shlim DR, Cohen MT, Eaton M, Rajah R, Long EG, Ungar BLP. An alga-like organism associated with an outbreak of prolonged diarrhea among foreigners in Nepal. *Am J Trop Med Hyg.* 1991;45:383–389.
11. Kocka F, Peters C, Dacumos E, et al. Outbreaks of diarrheal illness associated with cyanobacteria (blue-green algae)-like bodies—Chicago and Nepal, 1989–1990. *MMWR.* 1991;40:325–327.
12. Pollok RCG, Bendall RP, Moody A, Chiodini PL, Churchill DR. Traveller's diarrhea associated with cyanobacterium-like bodies. *Lancet.* 1991;340:556–557.
13. Bendall RP, Lucas S, Moody A, Tovey G, Chiodini PL. Diarrhea associated with cyanobacterium-like bodies: a new coccidian enteritis of man. *Lancet.* 1993;341:590–592.
14. Hoge CW, Chlim DR, Rajah R, et al. Epidemiology of diarrhea illness associated with coccidian-like organism among travellers and foreign residents in Nepal. *Lancet.* 1993;341:1175–1179.
15. Wurtz RM, Kocka FE, Peters CS, Weldon-Linne CM, Kuritza A, Yungbluth P. Clinical characteristics of seven cases of diarrhea associated with a novel acid-fast organism in the stool. *Clin Infect Dis.* 1993;16:136–138.
16. Gascon J, Corachan M, Valls ME, Gene A, Bombi JA. Cyanobacteria-like body (CLB) in travellers with diarrhea. *Scand J Infect Dis.* 1993;25:253–257.
17. Butcher AR, Lumb R, Coulter E, Nielsen DJ. Coccidian/cyanobacterium-like body associated diarrhea in an Australian traveller returning from overseas. *Pathology.* 1994; 26:59–61.
18. Hale E, Aldeen W, Carroll K. Diarrhea associated with cyanobacteria-like bodies in an immunocompetent host: an unusual epidemiological source. *JAMA.* 1994;271: 144–145.
19. Connor BA, Shlim DR, Scholes JV, Rayburn JL, Reidy J, Rajah R. Pathologic changes in the small bowel in nine patients with diarrhea associated with a coccidia-like body. *Ann Intern Med.* 1993;119:377–382.
20. Sun T, Ilardi CF, Asnis D, Bresciani AR, Roberts B, Teichberg S. Light and electron microscopic identification of *Cyclospora* species in small intestine: evidence of the presence of asexual life cycle in the human host. *Am J Clin Pathol.* 1996;105:216–220.
21. Sun T. Current topics in protozoal diseases. *Am J Clin Pathol.* 1994;102:16–29.
22. Madico G, Gillman RH, Miranda E, Cabrera L, Sterling CR. Treatment of cyclospora infections with co-trimoxazole. *Lancet.* 1993;342:122–123.
23. Hoge CW, Shlim DR, Ghimire M, et al. Placebo-controlled trial of co-trimoxazole for cyclospora infections among travellers and foreign residents in Nepal. *Lancet.* 1995; 345:691–693.

CHAPTER 132

Free-Living Amebic Infections

Augusto Julio Martinez, Govinda S. Visvesvara, and Francis W. Chandler

And God said:

$$\text{“}\nabla \cdot E = 0$$
$$\nabla \cdot B = 0$$
$$\nabla \times E = -\dot{B}$$
$$\nabla \times B = \mu_0 \epsilon_0 \dot{E}\text{”}$$

And there was light.

James Clerk Maxwell (1831–1879) and the Year Book, Massachusetts Institute of Technology, 1970

DEFINITION

Since 1961 it has become apparent that several species of free-living (amphizoic) amebae can infect mammals and cause fatal disease.[1–4] Until then, *Entamoeba histolytica* was the only ameba recognized as pathogenic for humans and animals.[5]

At least three genera of pathogenic free-living amebae, *Naegleria, Acanthamoeba,* and *Balamuthia mandrillaris* (formerly leptomyxid ameba), cause disease in humans and animals[6,7] (Figure 132–1). Only one species of *Naegleria, N fowleri,* causes a fatal infection of the central nervous system (CNS). It is known as primary amebic meningoencephalitis (PAM).[8,9] *Naegleria fowleri* has been called *N aerobia* and *N invadens. Naegleria australiensis,* another species of *Naegleria,* infects experimental animals such as mice, but does not infect humans.[10]

Several species of *Acanthamoeba* and *B mandrillaris* can cause a subacute or chronic infection of the CNS known as granulomatous amebic encephalitis (GAE).[11] In addition, *Acanthamoeba* sp cause infections of the eye known as acanthamoeba keratitis.[12] In addition, different species of *Acanthamoeba* and *B mandrillaris* cause pneumonitis, subacute granulomatous dermatitis with ulcerations, granulomatous sinusitis, and osteomyelitis.[2,13,14] Infections by these free-living amebae are distinctive, with different epidemiologic patterns, clinical features, pathologic pictures, and treatments.[3,4]

NAEGLERIA FOWLERI

The morphology and life cycle of *N fowleri* are presented in Figure 132–2. Its life cycle includes a vegetative form or trophozoite, a flagellate stage, and a cyst. When placed in distilled water, some trophozoites transform in a few minutes to several hours into flagellates. A flagellate usually has two flagella, but sometimes as many as 10. The trophozoite is 15 to 25 μm in diameter and has an abundant, vacuolated, granular cytoplasm and a clear nucleus with a prominent spherical nucleolus (Figure 132–3). The rounded lobopodia or pseudopods are used for locomotion. Cysts, 10 to 20 μm in diameter, are smooth and spherical, with a dense refractile wall that has one or two plugged pores. *Naegleria fowleri* is smaller than *Acanthamoeba* sp and does not produce cysts in tissue.[1]

Geographic Distribution and Epidemiology

Naegleria amebae are ubiquitous and worldwide. They are in thermal freshwater, soil, polluted streams, sewage, cooling containers, dust, heated swimming pools, coastal waters and the thermal effluents of power

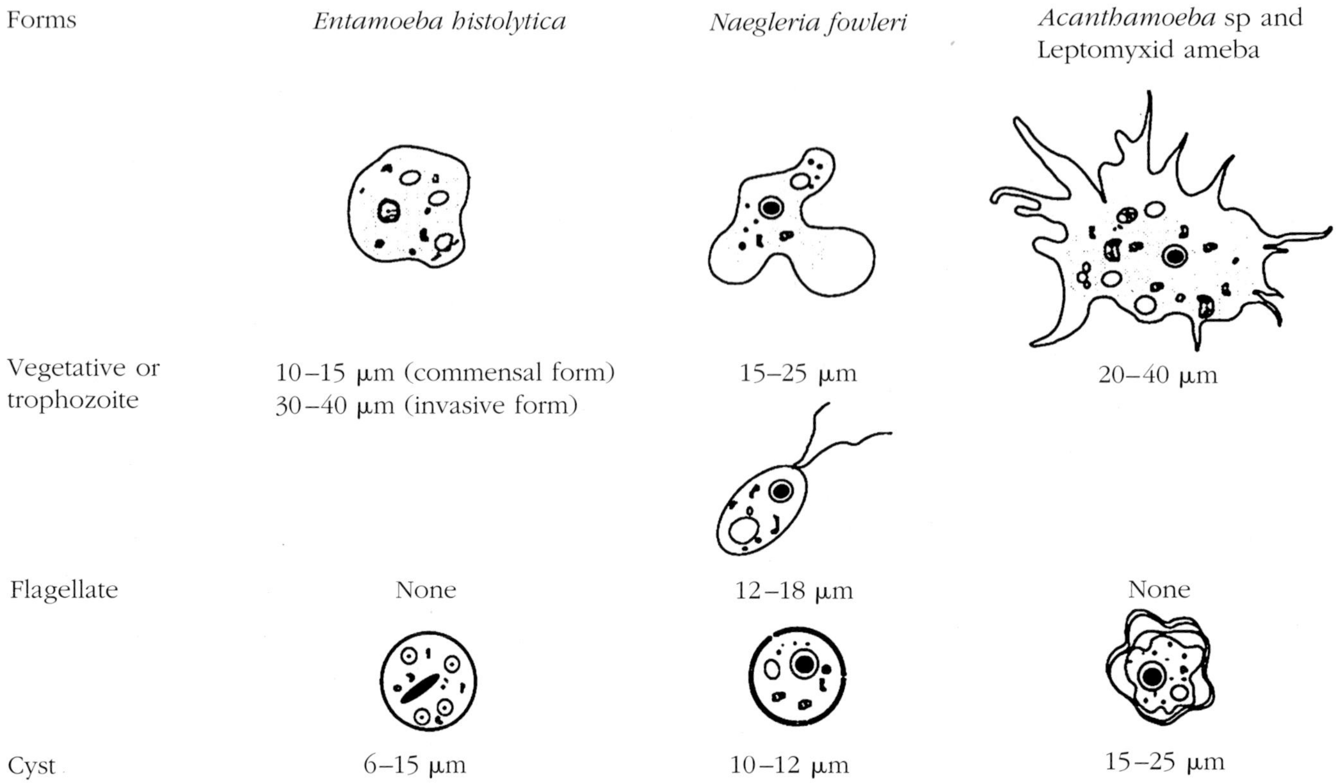

Figure 132–1. Comparative sizes, structures, and shapes of free-living and parasitic amebae.

plants (Figure 132–4). Amebic cysts can be transported and grow well in tropical climates and at high temperatures (40 to 45°C).

PRIMARY AMEBIC MENINGOENCEPHALITIS

The disease produced by *N fowleri,* called primary amebic meningoencephalitis or naegleria amebiasis,[8,9,15,16] is a rapidly fatal infection of the CNS first recognized in 1961 in Australia by Fowler and Carter.[17] By January 1996, more than 170 infections had been reported and at least 76 have been in the United States (Table 132–1).

Naegleria fowleri affects mainly healthy young persons who practice water-related sports such as swimming and diving in freshwater lakes, ponds, and heated swimming pools. Some patients, however, have had no contact with water; these are apparently caused by inhalation of aerosols, dust, or water containing trophozoites or cysts.[3,18] The epidemiologic, clinical, and pathologic features of PAM are summarized in Table 132–2.

Clinical Features

PAM is an acute, fulminant, rapidly fatal illness characterized by sudden onset of bifrontal or bitemporal headaches, fever, nausea, vomiting, and stiff neck. Infection progresses rapidly, with lethargy, confusion, coma, and death in 5 to 7 days. Generalized seizures occur, and in some patients, abnormalities of taste or smell and cerebellar ataxia. Nuchal rigidity usually occurs with positive Kernig's and Brudzinski's signs. Photophobia may be present, usually late in the clinical course. Cranial nerve palsies (third, fourth, and sixth) may indicate edema of the brain and herniations. Raised intracranial pressure has been reported in most patients.[11,19–22]

Some patients have had cardiac abnormalities and myocarditis.[23] The peripheral white blood cell count is generally elevated, with a marked increase in neutrophils. Almost all patients die within a week of onset. Cardiorespiratory arrest and pulmonary edema are the usual causes of death.

Pathologic Findings

The amebae enter the CNS through the olfactory neuroepithelium in the upper portion of the nasal mucosa and this is the site of the primary lesion in PAM. Sustentacular cells of the olfactory neuroepithelium are capable of actively phagocytosing the amebae. The route of invasion into the brain is through the fila olfac-

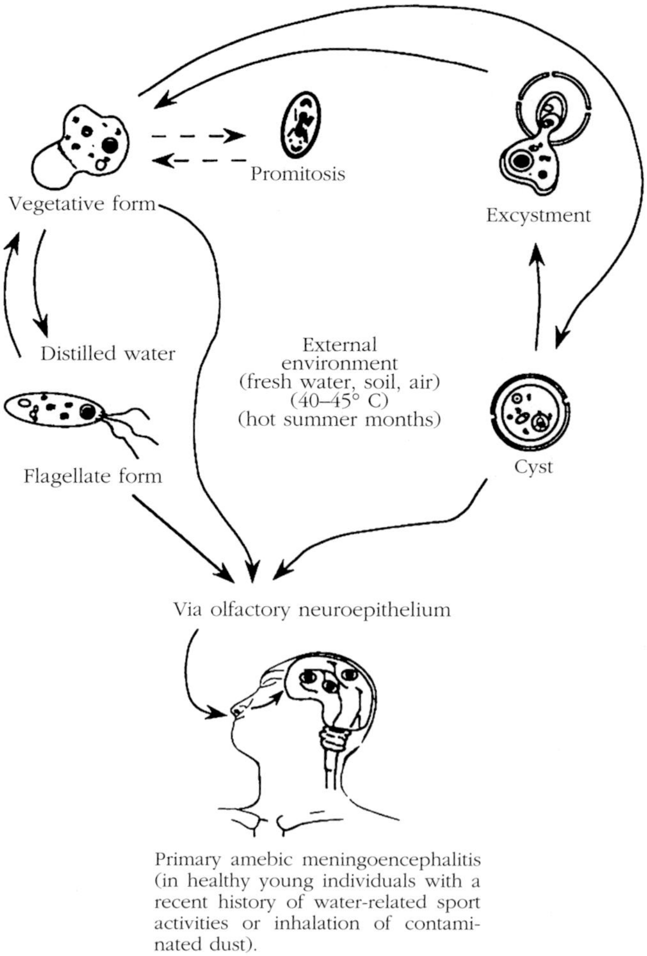

Figure 132–2. Life cycle of *N fowleri.*

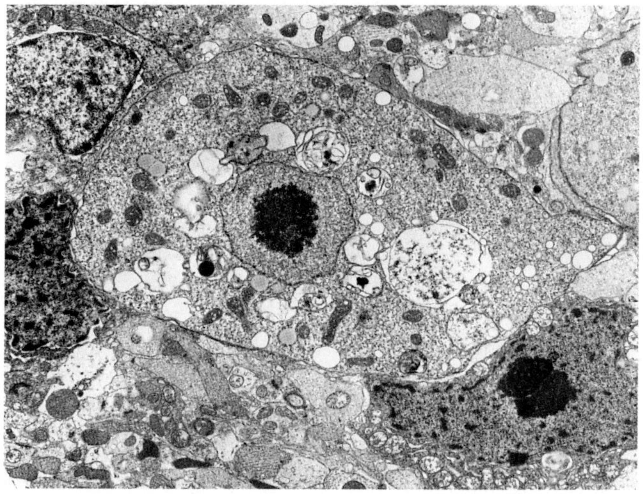

Figure 132–3. Trophozoite of *N fowleri* within infected CNS tissue (transmission electron micrograph, ×6000).

toria of the olfactory nerves. Amebic trophozoites pierce the cribriform plate of the sphenoid bone and penetrate into the subarachnoid space and the CNS.[24,25]

Modified neurons of the olfactory neuroepithelium, which are in close contact with sustentacular cells, contain sensory cilia or kinocilia, but do not phagocytose amebae. During their invasion and migration into the CNS, free-living amebae use the mesaxonal spaces of the unmyelinated olfactory nerves as a pathway. The olfactory nerve terminates in the olfactory bulb, which is located in the subarachnoid space and bathed by cerebrospinal fluid (CSF). This space is richly vascularized and constitutes the ideal medium for amebae to grow and disseminate to other areas of the brain.[24]

The incubation period of PAM varies from 2 to 15 days depending on the size of the inocula and the virulence of the amebae. Less virulent strains have a longer incubation. In experimental infections by *N australiensis,* or by a mildly virulent *N fowleri,* the incubation period has been as long as 3 to 4 weeks.[10,22]

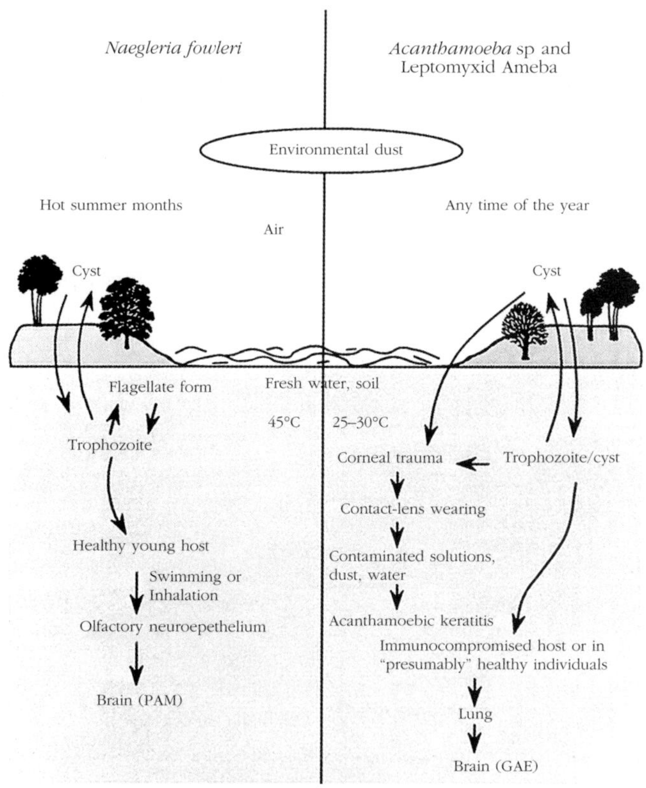

Figure 132–4. Epidemiology of free-living amebae.

TABLE 132–1. PRIMARY AMEBIC MENINGOENCEPHALITIS, GRANULOMATOUS AMEBIC ENCEPHALITIS, AND ACANTHAMOEBA KERATITIS—JANUARY 1, 1996

Location	PAM (NF)	GAE (AC)	GAE (BA)	AK
United States	76	62 (46 with AIDS)	26 (7 with AIDS)	>500[a]
Worldwide (excluding U.S.)	95	30	34	>250[a]
Total	171	92	60	>750[a]

Key: NF, *Naegleria fowleri;* AC, *Acanthamoeba* sp; BA, *Balamuthia mandrillaris.*
[a] Estimated.

Gross CNS Findings

The cerebral hemispheres are markedly swollen and edematous, with severe congestion and increased intracranial pressure. Uncal and cerebellar tonsillar herniations may be present. The arachnoid is severely congested, and there may be scant purulent exudate along the sulci. The olfactory bulbs and orbitofrontal cortices are usually necrotic and hemorrhagic.[8,9] There is hemorrhagic necrosis of the cerebral cortex, mainly in the orbitofrontal areas (Figure 132–5).

Microscopic Findings

PAM is characterized by an acute meningoencephalitis, with necrosis and foci of recent hemorrhage and edema of the CNS parenchyma. Amebic trophozoites are usually within perivascular spaces but associated with little or no inflammation (Figure 132–6). Cysts are not produced in the CNS.[10] Necrotizing vasculitis is occasionally seen, but it is not a significant feature. The leptomeninges contain fibrinopurulent exudate composed of neutrophils, eosinophils, and fewer macrophages and lymphocytes. These changes are usually at the base of the cerebral hemispheres, the brainstem, the cerebellum, and the upper portions of the spinal cord. Scant numbers of amebae can be in the purulent exudate, some phagocytosed by neutrophils and macrophages.

Laboratory Diagnosis

No distinctive clinical features exist to differentiate PAM from acute pyogenic or bacterial meningoencephalitis. Serologic tests usually are of no value in the diagnosis

TABLE 132–2. EPIDEMIOLOGIC, CLINICAL, AND PATHOLOGIC FEATURES OF GRANULOMATOUS AMEBIC ENCEPHALITIS AND PRIMARY AMEBIC MENINGOENCEPHALITIS[a]

Features	GAE	PAM
Etiologic agents	*Acanthamoeba* sp *B mandrillaris*	*N fowleri*
Predisposing factors	Immunodeficiency; debilitating diseases	None, other than exposure to contaminated freshwater
Geographic distribution	Worldwide	Worldwide
Usual portals of entry	Lungs, skin (rarely)	Nasal passages
Incubation period	Probably weeks to months	1–15 days
Clinical course	Subacute or chronic (several weeks to months)	Fulminant (5–7 days after onset of symptoms)
Cerebrospinal fluid findings	Amebae rarely observed; moderate mononuclear pleocytosis; elevated protein; low glucose	Trophozoites usually present; polymorphonuclear pleocytosis and erythrocytosis; elevated protein; low glucose
Gross pathology	Multiple, discrete, necrotic foci in brain; focal leptomeningitis; space-occupying lesions sometimes present	Hemorrhagic and necrotizing lesions of olfactory bulbs, frontal lobes, and base of brain; purulent leptomeningitis
Histopathology	Cysts and trophozoites, often perivascular; mononuclear cells with or without multinucleated giant cells; vasculitis and thrombosis	Trophozoites only (does not encyst in human host), often perivascular; polymorphonuclear leukocytes and hemorrhagic necrosis
Morphology of amebae in tissue specimens	Trophozoites, 15–35 μm in diameter, with granular or vacuolated cytoplasm and single nucleus with prominent "targetoid" karyosome; cysts, 12–30 μm in diameter, with wrinkled, GMS- and PAS-positive exocyst wall, and nucleus with karyosome; nuclear membrane lacks peripheral chromatin	Trophozoites, 10–20 μm in diameter, with granular or vacuolated cytoplasm and single, indistinct nucleus with prominent "targetoid" karyosome; nuclear membrane lacks peripheral chromatin; cysts are not produced
Extracranial involvement	Lungs, skin, eyes, kidneys, adrenal glands, and other organs	Rarely lungs

[a] Modified and expanded from Anzil et al.[44]

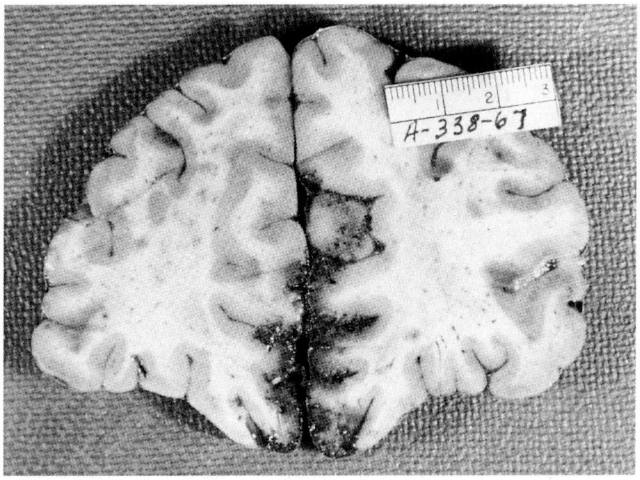

Figure 132–5. Primary amebic meningoencephalitis. Coronal section of cerebral hemispheres shows distribution of lesions, mainly in cerebral cortex. *(Contributed by Medical College of Virginia, Department of Pathology.)*

of *N fowleri* infections since most patients die within 5–7 days—before there is a detectable immune response.[20,26]

Brain Biopsy

Brain biopsy may detect amebic trophozoites and the characteristic histopathologic features within the CNS (Figure 132–6). PAM, however, has not yet been diagnosed by brain biopsy.[19]

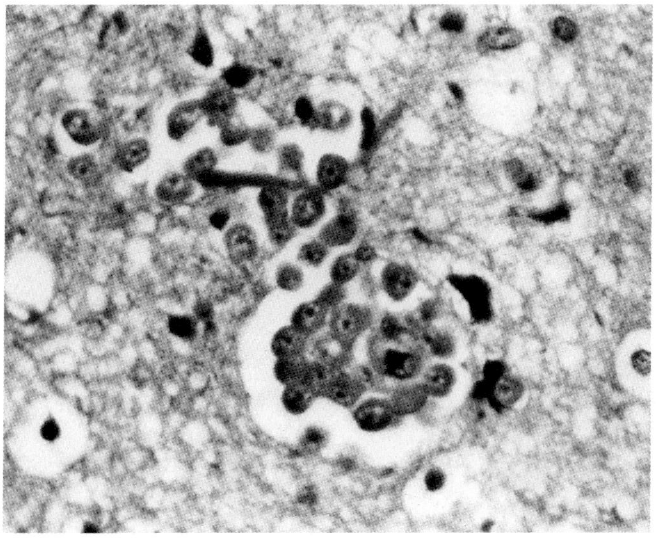

Figure 132–6. *Naegleria fowleri* trophozoites in perivascular space of brain without significant inflammatory reaction [hematoxylin-eosin (H&E), ×250].

Cerebrospinal Fluid

The CSF in PAM is characterized by pleocytosis, with a predominance of neutrophils without bacteria. The CSF pressure is elevated (300 to 600 mm H_2O). The protein content is also elevated, ranging from 100 mg/100 mL to 1000 mg/100 mL. The glucose concentration may be slightly reduced or normal. Amebic trophozoites may be detected moving in a drop of CSF, or they may be stained with Wright or Giemsa in smears. Gram's stain is not useful.[19]

Neuroimaging

Computed tomography (CT) scans show obliteration of the cisterns around the midbrain and the subarachnoid space over the cerebral hemispheres. There may be marked diffuse enhancement in these regions after administration of intravenous contrast medium.[21]

Treatment

If PAM is diagnosed early, the patient has a chance of survival. A few patients have survived and all were treated with amphotericin B (1.0 mg/kg daily). Amphotericin B, rifampin, and miconazole appear to be the drugs of choice.[22] Amphotericin B and miconazole can be administered intrathecally or intravenously, alone or in combination, and rifampin is given orally. Amphotericin B and rifampin work synergistically.

ACANTHAMOEBA SP AND *BALAMUTHIA MANDRILLARIS*

The life cycles of different species of *Acanthamoeba* and *B mandrillaris* involve a vegetative form or trophozoite, and a cyst (Figure 132–7). The *Acanthamoeba* sp that have been implicated in GAE include *A culbertsoni, A castellanii, A polyphaga, A astronyxis,* and *A healyi.* One of us (GSV) has found that *B mandrillaris* amebae probably caused some GAE previously thought to be caused by *Acanthamoeba* sp.[27,28]

The trophozoites of *Acanthamoeba* sp in tissue vary from 15 to 35 μm in diameter.[14,17,29–35] They have an irregular appearance, with filiform, spinelike projections or acanthopodia. Cytoplasm is abundant, with numerous vacuoles, granular material, and mitochondria. The nucleus is clear and contains a dense spherical nucleolus or karyosome (Figure 132–8). The cysts have double walls: The outer (ectocyst) is usually rippled and irregularly spherical, and the inner wall (endocyst) is stellate, polygonal, oval, or irregularly spherical (Figure 132–9). Based on cyst morphology and size, *Acanthamoeba* sp have been placed in three groups. Group 1 produces cysts from 18 to 28 μm in diameter, whereas the cysts of groups 2 and 3 are less

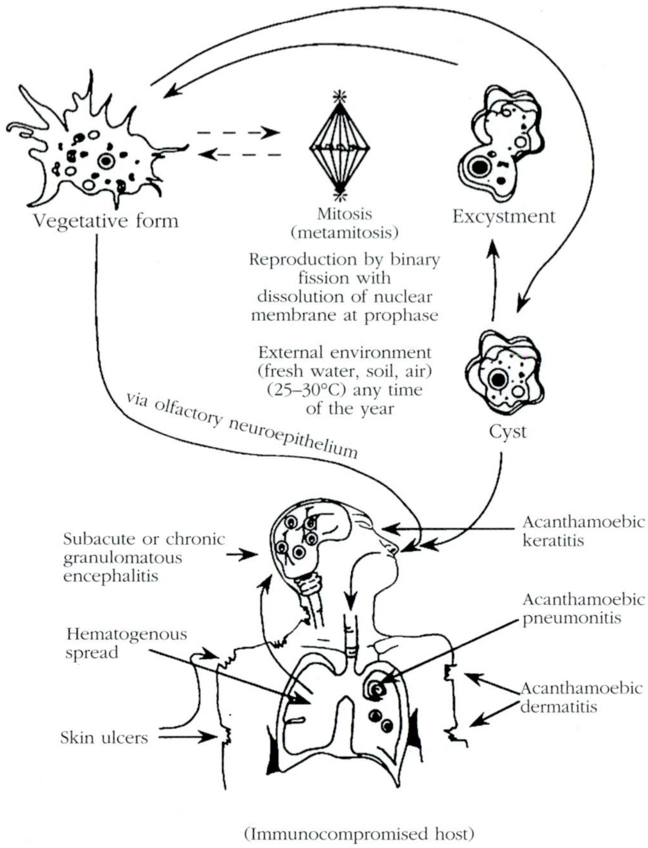

Figure 132–7. Life cycle of *Acanthamoeba* sp and probably of *B mandrillaris* (leptomyxid ameba).

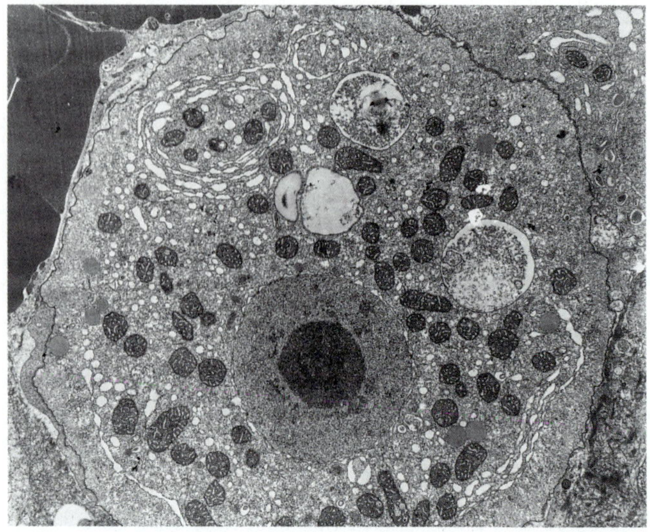

Figure 132–8. Trophozoite of *Acanthamoeba* sp. Numerous mitochondria, "digestive vacuoles," and prominent Golgi complex are in the cytoplasm. Note the conspicuous nucleolus (karyosome) enveloped by evenly granular nuclear chromatin (transmission electron micrograph, ×6500).

than 18 μm. The ectocysts of groups 1 and 2 are well developed and wrinkled, whereas the ectocysts of group 3 are not as pronounced as those of group 2. *Balamuthia mandrillaris* cysts resemble those of *Acanthamoeba* sp by light microscopy. By transmission electron microscopy, however, cysts of *B mandrillaris* are tripartite, consisting of an outer wall (the ectocyst), an inner thin wall (the endocyst), and a middle thick layer (the mesocyst). Identifying the genus of *Acanthamoeba* sp is relatively easy and is based on the characteristics of the trophozoites and cysts.[36,37] Speciating *Acanthamoeba*, however, especially those belonging to groups 2 and 3, is difficult; hence other criteria such as isoenzyme electrophoresis and restricted DNA patterns must be used.[38] In tissue sections, the characteristic features of trophozoites and cysts also may be altered because of fixation and processing. Therefore, the distinctive histopathologic features, the ultrastructural characteristics of the trophozoites and cysts, and the clinical history and immunofluorescence tests are helpful in establishing species.[38] In addition, staining the amebae by immunofluorescence or immunoperoxidase in tissue sections after reactivity with a battery of rabbit anti–*Acanthamoeba* sp antisera is useful in identifying the species.

Geographic Distribution and Epidemiology

Acanthamoeba sp and *B mandrillaris* are free-living amebae. *Acanthamoeba* sp are widely distributed in water and soil throughout the world (Figure 132–7).

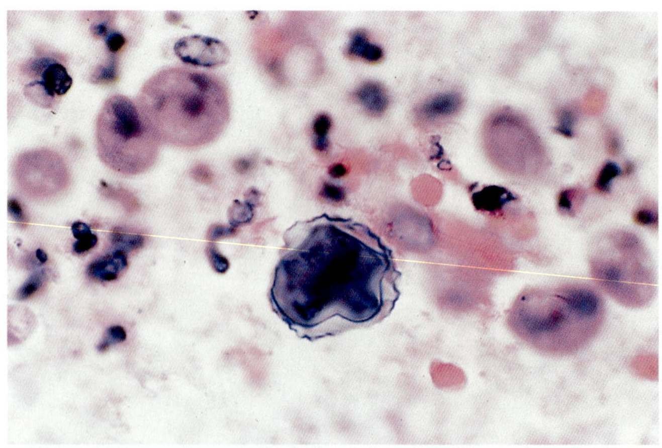

Figure 132–9. Cyst of *A culbertsoni* within necrotic lesion of cerebral cortex. Cysts of the *Acanthamoeba* sp have thick walls, are intensely hematoxylinophilic, and range from 12 to 30 μm in diameter. Some cysts, as illustrated here, have a distinctive undulating or wrinkled external wall and a polygonal or spherical internal wall. The characteristic karyosome is obscured by the deeply stained cytoplasm (H&E, ×400).

These amebae are also in brackish water; ocean sediments; heating, ventilating, and air conditioning units; bacterial, fungal, and mammalian cell cultures; contact lens paraphernalia; and cornea, lung, brain, and skin biopsy or autopsy specimens. They grow in association with *Legionella pneumophila,*[39,40] as contaminants in cell cultures of monkey kidney,[20] and in the throats of healthy people.[41] Free-living *Acanthamoeba* sp are in samples of soil and water from Antarctica, from the fjords of Norway, from high altitudes such as Lake Titicaca (elevation 5000 m), and at sea level. *Balamuthia mandrillaris,* however, has not been isolated from the environment.

Acanthamoeba sp were first described by Aldo Castellani in 1930 as saprophytic microorganisms growing in cultures of yeasts[42]; in 1958, Clyde Culbertson demonstrated their pathogenic potential.[43] It is now established that *A castellanii, A culbertsoni, A polyphaga,* and probably other species are virulent free-living opportunistic amebae capable of infecting humans and animals.[11,44] Human infection involving brain, skin, lungs, and eyes has been reported from all continents.[27,28,30–33,44–58]

GRANULOMATOUS AMEBIC ENCEPHALITIS

Acanthamoeba sp and *B mandrillaris* produce a multifocal, subacute or chronic granulomatous encephalitis with trophozoites and cysts in lesions of the CNS.[14,34,35,52,53] Granulomatous amebic encephalitis (GAE) runs a long, protracted and insidious clinical course.[14,29–31,34,35,59–66] As of January 1, 1996, at least 152 patients with GAE had been described, 88 in the United States (Table 132–1). Table 132–2 summarizes the clinical, epidemiologic, and pathologic features of GAE.

Patients with GAE tend to be chronically ill and debilitated. Many are immunosuppressed, have the acquired immunodeficiency syndrome (AIDS), or have been treated with broad-spectrum antibiotics.[44,52,54,58,59,67,68]

Clinical Features

Clinically GAE, or acanthamoebiasis, usually resembles a single or multiple space-occupying lesion(s). Localizing neurologic signs such as hemiparesis and seizures appear early. Altered mental status, headache, and stiff neck are prominent. Some patients have cranial nerve palsies (mainly third and sixth). Nausea, vomiting, and lethargy also are features. Cerebellar ataxia, diplopia, and coma signal imminent death.[11,19] Fever is sporadic and generally low grade. The direct cause of death is usually acute bronchopneumonia, hepatic or renal failure, and septicemia.

There may be ulcerations of skin with acute and chronic inflammation, and amebic trophozoites and cysts.[60] In some patients with cutaneous nodules and ulcerations, a biopsy specimen containing amebic trophozoites and cysts is diagnostic. The ulcers arise where amebae enter, or they may be "terminal"—at points of dissemination.[58] There may be pneumonitis with amebic trophozoites and cysts in alveoli, and chest radiographs often reveal consolidation.

Pathologic Features

Acanthamoebas probably spread to the CNS from lung or skin through the bloodstream. The CNS is the principal focus of clinical illness, but lesions may develop in other organs, including lung, kidney, uterus, prostate, and testis.[14,32,58]

There may be focal edema, localized cortical softening, hemorrhages, and abscesses in the cerebral hemispheres (Figures 132–10 and 132–11). Uncal notching and cerebellar tonsillar herniations may be features.[19] Areas of hemorrhagic necrosis may be in the basal ganglia, midbrain, brainstem, and cerebellum (Figure 132–10).

Microscopically there is necrotizing and granulomatous encephalitis with epithelioid cells and giant

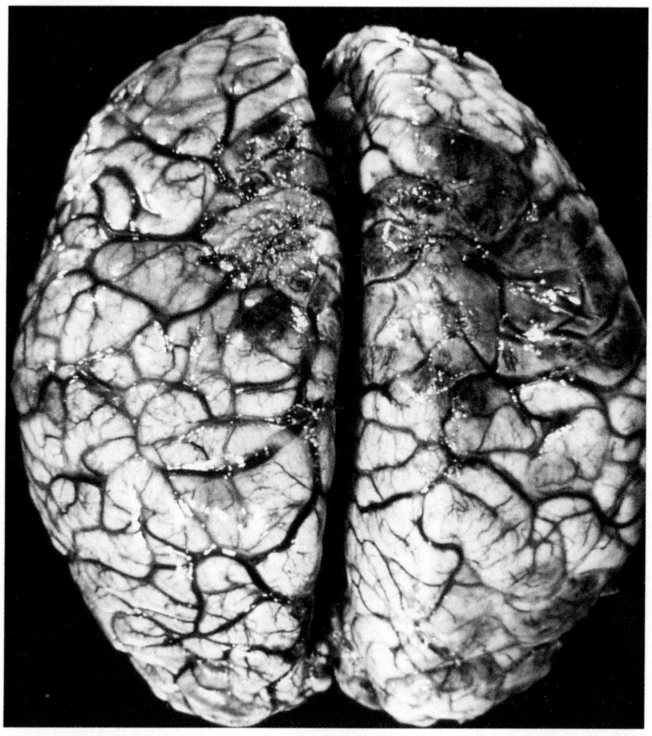

Figure 132–10. Granulomatous amebic encephalitis caused by *B mandrillaris* in a 14-year-old boy from Venezuela. Areas of hemorrhagic necrosis are in the cerebral hemispheres. *(Contributed by Jesus E. Gonzalez, MD.)*

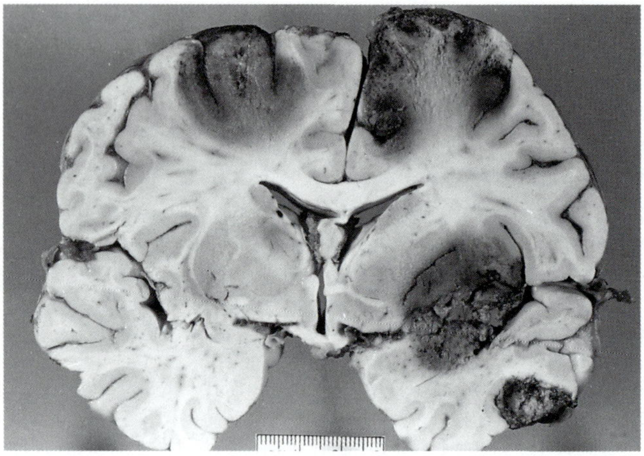

Figure 132–11. Granulomatous amebic encephalitis. Coronal section of cerebral hemispheres reveals multifocal hemorrhagic infarcts of cerebral cortex, subcortical white matter, and basal ganglia. *(Contributed by Presbyterian University Hospital of Pittsburgh.)*

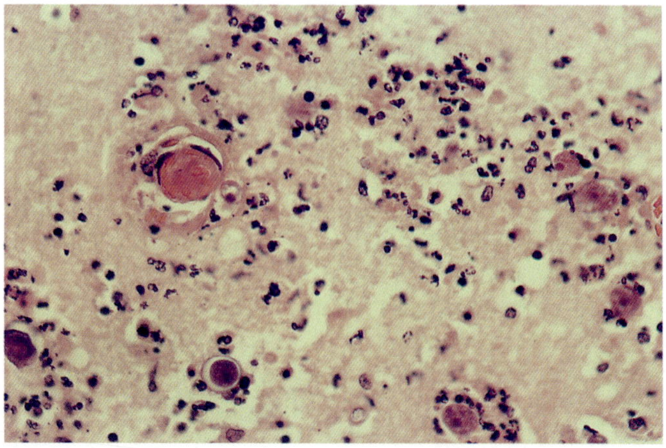

Figure 132–13. Early lesion of granulomatous amebic encephalitis. Invading trophozoites and hematoxylinophilic cysts (*lower left*) of an *Acanthamoeba* sp are intimately surrounded by neutrophils in an area of necrotizing encephalitis (H&E, ×160).

cells in the cerebral hemispheres, midbrain, basal ganglia, and cerebellum (Figure 132–12). Varying numbers of intra- and extracellular amebic trophozoites and cysts are in the lesions (Figures 132–13 and 132–14), in perivascular spaces (Figure 132–15), and in the walls of small to medium-sized blood vessels associated with perivascular hemorrhage and thrombosis (Figure 132–16). Inflammatory changes vary, depending on the immunologic status of the host. There may be chronic focal leptomeningitis. The lesions in patients with AIDS tend to be necrotic with minimal inflammation (Figure 132–17). Arteritis with trophozoites and cysts may be prominent.[69]

Laboratory Diagnosis: Brain Biopsy and Skin Biopsy

An accurate diagnosis of GAE is made when amebic trophozoites and cysts are identified in tissue or when cultured. Brain biopsy is valuable; amebic trophozoites and cysts may be present within subacute or chronic lesions. Because *N fowleri* does not encyst in tissue, amebic cysts in biopsy specimens exclude this ameba and allow a presumptive diagnosis of infection by either an *Acanthamoeba* sp or *B mandrillaris*. The cyst walls of these amebae stain with periodic acid–Schiff and Gomori's methenamine silver (GMS) (Figure 132–18). The final diagnosis in most cases of GAE has been made after biopsy or autopsy specimens have

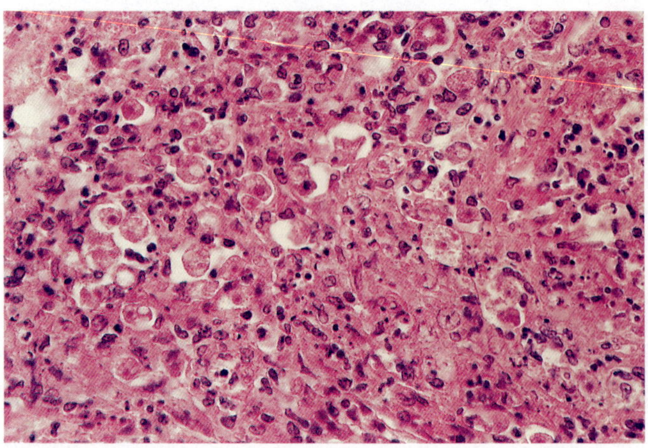

Figure 132–12. Granulomatous amebic encephalitis. Numerous thin-walled trophozoites of an *Acanthamoeba* sp elicit necrotizing and granulomatous inflammation (H&E, ×160).

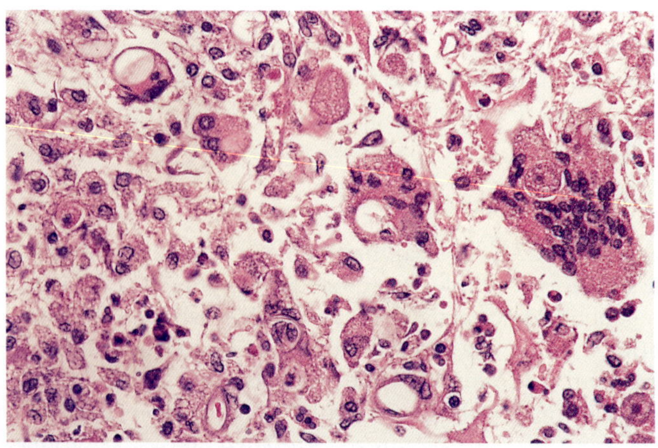

Figure 132–14. Granulomatous amebic encephalitis. Acanthamoebic cysts and trophozoites are in epithelioid cells and giant cells. Some cysts are collapsed, empty, and mimic yeast-form fungi with thick walls (H&E, ×100).

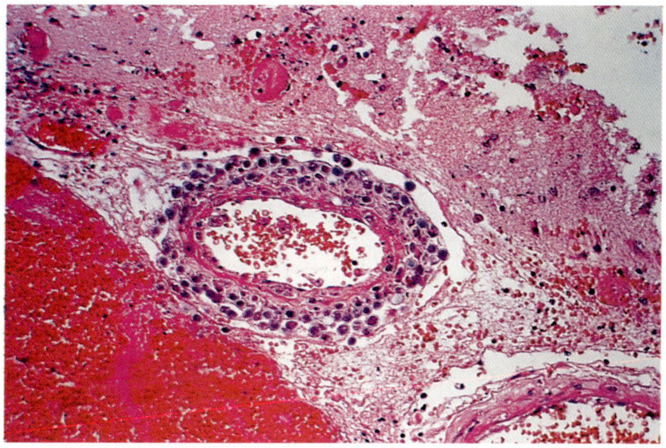

Figure 132–15. Trophozoites and cysts of *A castellanii* surround a medium-sized blood vessel in brain tissue (H&E, ×50).

been studied by light microscopy. Skin biopsy is also a valuable diagnostic procedure. Immunoperoxidase and immunofluorescence (Figure 132–19), and immunoelectrophoresis, also may be useful in identifying the causal amebae.[20,70] Specimens for culture should be processed quickly. Biopsy or autopsy tissues fixed in formalin or in Karnovsky's fixative can be embedded in plastic for electron microscopy (EM) to demonstrate features of trophozoites and cysts. Tissues embedded in paraffin can be deparaffinized, rehydrated, and embedded in plastic for EM.

Cerebrospinal Fluid

Examination of the CSF reveals lymphocytic pleocytosis, mild elevation of proteins, and normal glucose but no specific diagnostic features. Unlike *N fowleri*, *Acanthamoeba* sp and *B mandrillaris* are not readily demonstrated in the CSF. *Acanthamoeba* sp have been isolated from the CSF in only two patients, but they have been identified in brain biopsies from several patients.

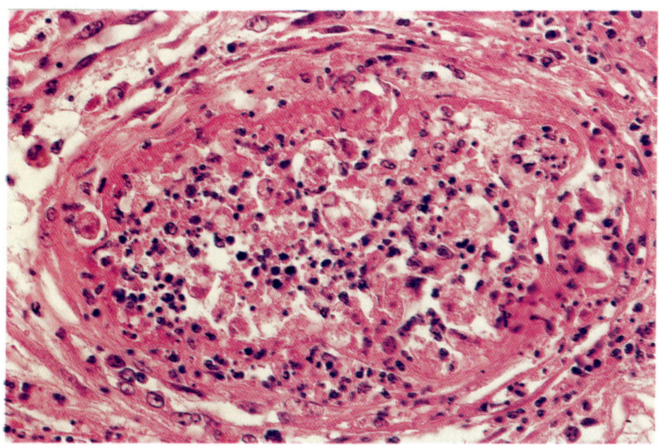

Figure 132–16. Granulomatous amebic encephalitis. Numerous trophozoites of an *Acanthamoeba* sp are in the wall and lumen of a blood vessel, associated with perivascular hemorrhage and thrombosis (H&E, ×160).

Neuroimaging

Computed tomography and magnetic resonance imaging of the head are important radiologic tests. Ring-enhancing masses after intravenous contrast fluid injection may be confused with a brain abscess or a brain tumor.

Treatment

There is no effective treatment for infections of CNS, lung, and skin. According to published reports, however, at least two patients have recovered. A Nigerian with a disorder of the CNS, from whose CSF an *Acanthamoeba* sp was isolated, was treated with sulfamethazine and recovered sufficiently to leave hospital. He was, however, lost to follow-up.[71] An Indian patient, also with an impaired CNS and a history of an isolated *Acanthamoeba* sp from the CSF, was treated with chloramphenicol and apparently recovered.[63] In vitro experiments suggest that diamidine derivatives such as pentamidine and propandine, and miconazole, ketoconazole, and 5-fluorocytosine may be effective in treating GAE. Sulfadiazine is probably ineffective, possibly because of the inadequacy of the host's impaired immune system.

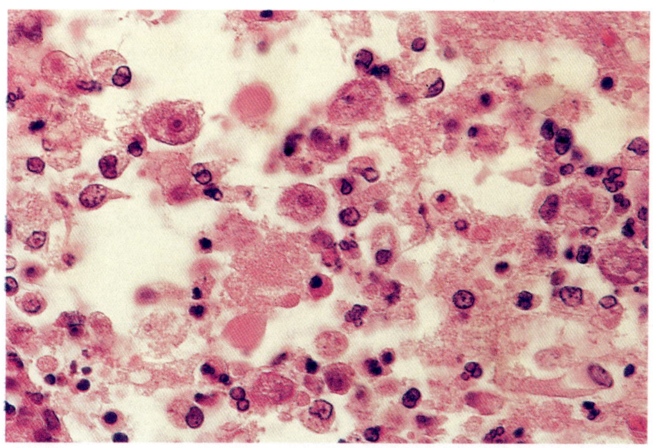

Figure 132–17. Granulomatous amebic encephalitis in a patient with AIDS. Trophozoites of an *Acanthamoeba* sp are in a necrotic lesion and elicit minimal inflammation. The trophozoites are thin walled, 15 to 35 μm in diameter, have granular and vacuolated cytoplasm, and a single, spherical amphophilic nucleus with a prominent, central, deeply hematoxylinophilic nucleolus (karyosome). The inner surface of the nuclear membrane lacks peripheral chromatin, a feature that differentiates the trophozoites from those of *E histolytica* (H&E, ×160).

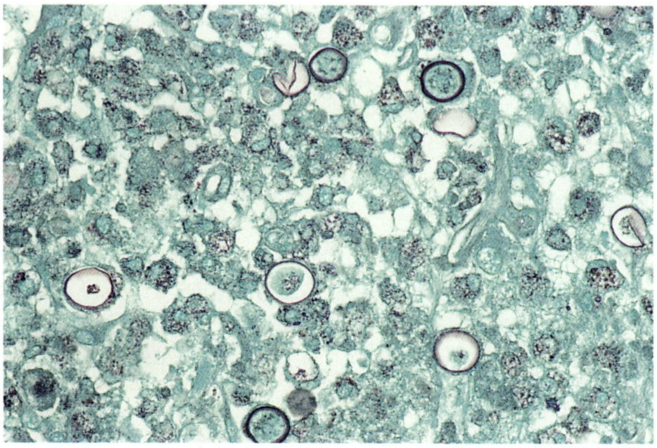

Figure 132–18. *Acanthamoeba* sp. The walls of amebic cysts are silvered (blackened) by the GMS procedure, but the thin walls of trophozoites are unstained. Cysts of *Acanthamoeba* sp and *B mandrillaris* with thick, argyrophilic, "double-contoured" walls should not be mistaken for the thick-walled yeast forms of *Blastomyces dermatitidis* (GMS, ×160).

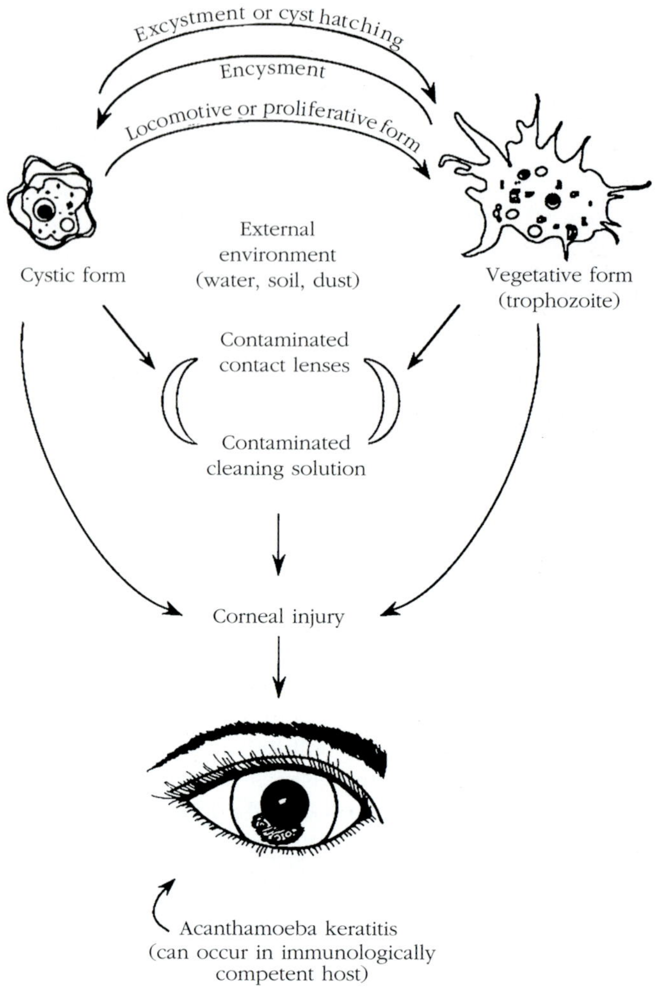

Figure 132–20. Life cycle of *Acanthamoeba* sp in acanthamoeba keratitis.

ACANTHAMOEBA KERATITIS

Definition

Acanthamoeba keratitis (AK) is chronic inflammation of the cornea from infection by *Acanthamoeba* sp, and is associated with corneal trauma and exposure to contaminated water (Figure 132–20). Contact lenses and cleansing with homemade saline solutions are risk factors.[72,73] As of January 1996, more than 750 (estimated) patients with AK had been reported worldwide.[74,75]

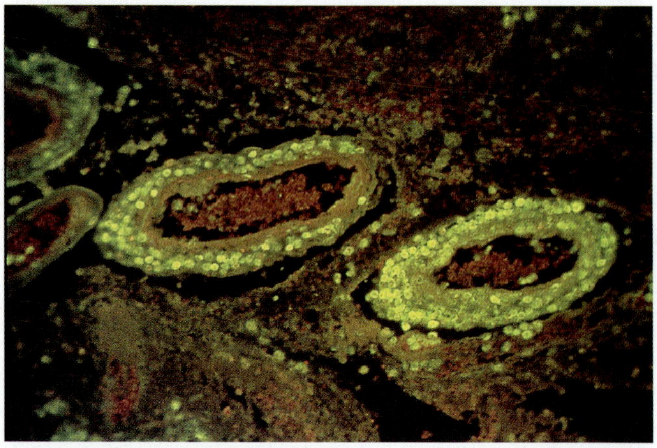

Figure 132–19. Immunofluorescence identification of *A castellanii* in formalin-fixed, deparaffinized section of brain. Trophozoites and cysts within the walls of cerebral blood vessels are brightly decorated (indirect immunofluorescence, ×50).

AK usually afflicts healthy people who damage their corneas, for instance, by wearing contact lenses, by washing their eyes with contaminated water, or by "disinfecting" their contact lenses with contaminated water.[76,77]

Gross Findings

The cornea is usually chronically inflamed with severe ocular pain and a 360° stromal ring infiltrate. Recurrent ulceration, refractory to the usual medications for bacterial, viral, or fungal infections, is the characteristic finding.[12,78–80]

Microscopic Findings

Acanthamoeba sp (*A culbertsoni, A polyphaga, A castellanii, A rhyzodes, A hatchetti*) proliferate within the cornea, usually after trauma. The trophozoite or cyst may reach the damaged cornea in contaminated water,

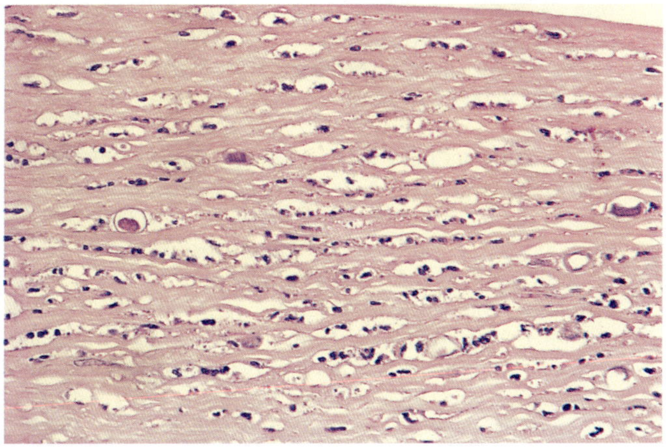

Figure 132–21. Acanthamoeba keratitis in a wearer of contact lenses. Amebic cysts and trophozoites invade the corneal stroma and elicit minimal inflammation (H&E, ×100).

cleaning solutions for contact lenses, dust, or damaged contact lenses. Amebic trophozoites and cysts are usually located deep in the corneal stroma where they produce a minimal or moderate acute inflammatory response (Figure 132–21).

Painful corneal ulcerations that do not respond to the usual antibacterial, antiviral, and antifungal therapies may be AK, which causes nonsuppurative keratitis with a waxing and waning clinical course. The damaged cornea may have a characteristic annular infiltrate and congested conjunctivae, or a "dendritiform epitheliopathy and patchy stromal infiltrate with lacunar areas."[80]

Clinical and Laboratory Diagnosis

Acanthamoeba trophozoites and especially cysts can be recovered from corneal scrapings or biopsy specimens and identified by genus in a variety of ways. The etiologic agent, however, should be isolated so that speciation by isoenzyme electrophoresis and in vitro sensitivity to various chemotherapeutic agents can both be done.[12,81]

For corneal scraping or biopsy, deep scraping is recommended. One portion of the scraped material is processed and stained and the other is cultured. Thin smears of the corneal scraping are made on at least two slides; one slide is fixed with methanol and the other with Schaudinn's fixative or a spray-on fixative. The methanol-fixed slide is stained with Wright–Giemsa or Hemacolor, and the other with Wheatly's trichrome. Hemacolor staining can be done in about a minute and is useful in identifying *Acanthamoeba* sp, especially cysts because of their distinctive shapes. Both trophozoites and cysts are stained purple. The trichrome stain is especially useful in differentiating trophozoites of *Acanthamoeba* sp from host cells, because it displays the characteristic amebic nuclei. The large nucleolus (karyosome) is reddish-pink, while the cytoplasm is greenish-purple. This stain also colors the cyst wall green or greenish purple, and the nucleus red. Other procedures used to identify *Acanthamoeba* sp are calcofluor white and immunofluorescence; both require a fluorescence microscope.[82,83]

Culture

Every effort should be made to isolate amebae. The best media are nutrient agar freshly covered with a thin suspension of *Escherichia coli* or with *Enterobacter aerogenes*. Tissue specimens should be triturated before being inoculated. The agar plate should be incubated at either 30°C, if the specimens originate from cornea or skin, or 37°C if the specimens are from brain, lung, or other internal organs, and examined under a microscope daily for at least 2 weeks. Amebae will appear as blotches on the surface of the agar plate, and a contractile vacuole can be seen as a hole inside the blotches. Often, distinctive tracts, with an ameba at the end of each tract, are on the surface. The amebae feed on the bacteria, multiply, and form cysts. The cysts are highly refractile, round, and have two walls seen under a 40× objective. *Balamuthia mandrillaris* cannot be isolated using this method, because *B mandrillaris* does not grow on bacterialized agar plates. It can, however, be isolated by inoculating macerated biopsy material into mammalian cell culture.[44,66] Generic identification of the amebae is based on the characteristic forms of trophozoites and cysts. Speciation, however, requires nonmorphologic methods such as isoenzyme analysis or DNA profiles.

The natural history of AK is corneal perforation and loss of the eye, or a vascularized scar within a thin cornea and impaired vision. The cystic forms of *Acanthamoeba* sp resist antibacterial, antifungal, and antiviral agents, probably because they are deep in the corneal stroma and because they have thick double walls.[12,81,83]

Treatment

AK has been successfully treated in some patients, but the optimal treatment is still lacking. Brolene (propamidine isethionate) and dibromopropamidine are ophthalmic medications reported to be effective. Polymyxin B, miconazole nitrate, neomycin, and neosporin also appear to be effective when combined with Brolene. Ketoconazole (Nizoral) appears to be effective both in vitro and in vivo. Clotrimazole is an antifungal agent recently reported to be effective. Other studies indicate that patients with AK who are treated topically with a combination of 1% clotrimazole (or miconazole), 0.1%

propamidine isethionate (Brolene), and neomycin or neosporin–polymyxin B–gramicidin recover with good vision. Recent studies indicate that polyhexamethylene biguanide (PHMB) has great potential.[78] PHMB has been used effectively at Moorfields Eye Hospital NHS Trust, London (Dr. Trevor Gray, personal communication).

Magainins, a group of peptide compounds originally isolated from the skin of the African clawed frog, have amebastatic and amebicidal activities that are enhanced when used with silver nitrate and other antimicrobial agents. Magainins are potentially effective in vitro.[81] Topical steroids should be used with caution in AK, even though they may reduce inflammation and tissue damage.

Penetrating keratoplasty and corneal grafting have been performed in chronic AK in which medical treatment was ineffective. Recurrence of AK has been reported following corneal transplants, probably from amebic cysts in the corneal stroma. For this reason, infection should be controlled before surgery.

Contact lenses and contact lens care solutions should be kept meticulously clean. Those who wear contact lenses should follow the directions of the manufacturers and their ophthalmologists to prevent AK.[36]

REFERENCES

1. John DT. Primary amebic meningoencephalitis and the biology of *Naegleria fowleri*. *Ann Rev Microbiol.* 1986; 36:101–123.
2. Visvesvara GS, Martinez AJ, Schuster FL, et al. Leptomyxid ameba, a new agent of amebic meningoencephalitis in humans and animals. *J Clin Microbiol.* 1990;28:2750–2756.
3. Visvesvara GS, Stehr-Green JK. Epidemiology of free-living ameba infection. *J Protozool.* 1990;37:25S–33S.
4. Visvesvara GS, Schuster FL, Martinez AJ. *Balamuthia mandrillaris,* NG, N sp, agent of amebic meningoencephalitis in humans and other animals. *J Eukaryotic Microbiol.* 1993;40:504–514.
5. Perez-Tamayo R. Pathology of amebiasis. In: Martinez-Palomo A, ed. *Amebiasis.* Amsterdam: Elsevier Biomedical Press; 1986;2:45–94.
6. Anderson MP, Oosterhuis JE, Kennedy S, Benirschke K. Pneumonia and meningoencephalitis due to amoeba in a low-land gorilla. *J Zoo Anim Med.* 1986;17:87–91.
7. Fuentealba IC, Wikse SE, Read WK, et al. Amebic meningoencephalitis in a sheep. *JAVMA.* 1992;200:363–365.
8. Butt CG. Primary amebic meningoencephalitis. *N Engl J Med.* 1966;274:1473–1476.
9. Carter RF. Primary amebic meningoencephalitis: an appraisal of present knowledge. *Trans R Soc Trop Med Hyg.* 1972;66:193–213.
10. Martinez AJ. *Free-Living Amebas: Natural History, Prevention, Diagnosis, Pathology and Treatment of Disease.* Boca Raton, Fla: CRC Press; 1985.
11. Ma P, Visvesvara GS, Martinez AJ, et al. *Naegleria* and *Acanthamoeba* infections: review. *Rev Infect Dis.* 1990;12: 490–513.
12. Moore MB, McCulley JP. Acanthamoeba keratitis associated with contact lenses. Six consecutive cases of successful management. *Br J Ophthalmol.* 1989;73:271–275.
13. Borochovitz D, Martinez AF, Patterson GT. Osteomyelitis of a bone graft of the mandible with *Acanthamoeba castellanii* infection. *Hum Pathol.* 1981;12:573–576.
14. Gullett J, Mills J, Hadley K, et al. Disseminated granulomatous *Acanthamoeba* infection presenting as an unusual skin lesion. *Am J Med.* 1979;67:891–895.
15. Callicott JH. Amebic meningoencephalitis due to free-living amebas of the *Hartmannella* (*Acanthamoeba*)-*Naegleria* group. *Am J Clin Pathol.* 1968;49:84–91.
16. dos Santos JG. Fatal primary amebic meningoencephalitis: a retrospective study in Richmond, Virginia. *Am J Clin Pathol.* 1970;54:737–742.
17. Fowler M, Carter RF. Acute pyogenic meningitis probably due to *Acanthamoeba* sp. A preliminary report. *Br Med J.* 1965;2:240–242.
18. Symmers WStC. Primary amoebic meningoencephalitis in Britain. *Br Med J.* 1969;4:449–454.
19. Martinez AJ, dos Santos Net JG, Nelson EC, et al. Primary amebic meningoencephalitis. In: Sommers SC, Rosen PP, eds. *Pathology Annual.* Part 2. Norwalk, Conn: Appleton-Century Crofts; 1977;12:225–250.
20. Martinez AJ, Visvesvara GS. Laboratory diagnosis of pathogenic free-living amoebas: *Naegleria, Acanthamoeba,* and *Leptomyxid*. *Clin Lab Med.* 1991;11:861–872.
21. Schumacher DJ, Tien RD, Lane K. Neuroimaging findings in rare amebic infection of the central nervous system. *Am J Neuroradiol.* 1995;16:930–935.
22. Seidel JS, Harmatz P, Visvesvara GS, et al. Successful treatment of primary amebic meningoencephalitis. *N Engl J Med.* 1982;306:346–348.
23. Markowitz SM, Martinez AJ, Duma RJ, Shiel FOM. Myocarditis associated with primary amebic (*Naegleria*) meningoencephalitis. *Am J Clin Pathol.* 1974;62:619–628.
24. Martinez AJ, Nelson EC, Jones MM, et al. Experimental *Naegleria* meningoencephalitis in mice. An electron microscope study. *Lab Invest.* 1971;25:465–475.
25. Martinez AJ, Duma RJ, Nelson EC, Moretta FL. Experimental *Naegleria* meningoencephalitis in mice. Penetration of the olfactory mucosal epithelium by *Naegleria* and pathologic changes produced: a light and electron microscope study. *Lab Invest.* 1973;29:121–133.
26. Visvesvara GS, Peralta MJ, Brandt FH, et al. Production of monoclonal antibodies to *Naegleria fowleri,* agent of primary amebic meningoencephalitis. *J Clin Microbiol.* 1987; 25:1629–1634.
27. Carter RF, Cullity GJ, Ojeda VJ, et al. A fatal case of meningoencephalitis due to a free-living amoeba of uncertain identity—probably *Acanthamoeba* species. *Pathology.* 1981;13:38–51.
28. Willaert E, Stevens AR, Healy GR. Retrospective identification of *Acanthamoeba culbertsoni* in a case of amoebic meningoencephalitis. *J Clin Pathol.* 1978;31:717–720.

29. Friedland LR, Raphael SA, Deutsch ES, et al. Disseminated *Acanthamoeba* infection in a child with symptomatic human immunodeficiency virus infection. *Pediatr Infect Dis J.* 1992;11:404–407.
30. Gardner HAR, Martinez AJ, Visvesvara GS, Sotrel A. Granulomatous amebic encephalitis in an AIDS patient. *Neurology.* 1991;41:1993–1995.
31. Gordon SM, Steinberg JP, DuPuis M, et al. Culture isolation of *Acanthamoeba* sp and leptomyxid amebas from patients with amebic meningoencephalitis including two patients with AIDS. *Clin Infect Dis.* 1992;15:1024–1030.
32. Gonzalez MM, Gould E, Dickinson G, et al. Acquired immunodeficiency syndrome associated with *Acanthamoeba* infection and other opportunistic organisms. *Arch Pathol Lab Med.* 1986;110:749–751.
33. Gonzales-Alfonzo JE, Martinez AJ, Garcia V, et al. Granulomatous encephalitis due to a Leptomyxid amoeba. *Trans R Soc Trop Med Hyg.* 1991;85:480.
34. Griesemer DA, Barton LL, Reese CM, et al. Amebic meningoencephalitis caused by *Balamuthia mandrillaris. Pediatr Neurol.* 1994;10:249–254.
35. Grunnet ML, Cannon GH, Kushner JP. Fulminant amebic meningoencephalitis due to *Acanthamoeba. Neurology.* 1981;31:174–178.
36. Pussard M. Comparison morphologique de 4 douches *d'Acanthamoeba* du groupe astronysix-comandoni. *J Protozool.* 1972;19:557–563.
37. Visvesvara GS, Balamuth W. Comparative studies on related free-living and pathogenic amebae with special reference to *Acanthamoeba. J Protozool.* 1975;22:245–256.
38. Visvesvara GS, Mirra SS, Brandt FH, et al. Isolation of two strains of *Acanthamoeba castellanii* from human tissue and their pathogenicity and isoenzyme profiles. *J Clin Microbiol.* 1983;18:1405–1412.
39. Newsome AL, Baker RL, Miller RD, Arnold RR. Interactions between *Naegleria fowleri* and *Legionella pneumophila. Infect Immun.* 1985;50:449–452.
40. Rowbotham T. Preliminary report on the pathogenicity of *Legionella pneumophila* from freshwater and soil amoebae. *J Clin Pathol.* 1980;33:1179–1183.
41. Wang SS, Feldman HA. Isolation of *Hartmannella* species from human throats. *N Engl J Med.* 1967;277:1174–1179.
42. Castellani A. An amoeba found in culture of a yeast: preliminary note. *J Trop Med Hyg.* June 2, 1930, p 160; second note: July 1, 1930, p 188; third note: August 1, 1930, p 221.
43. Culbertson CG, Smith JW, Minner JR. *Acanthamoeba:* observation on animal pathogenicity. *Science.* 1958;127: 1506.
44. Anzil AP, Rao C, Wrzolek MA, et al. Amebic meningoencephalitis in a patient with AIDS caused by a newly recognized opportunistic pathogen. *Arch Pathol Lab Med.* 1991;115:21–25.
45. Jaramillo-Rodriguez Y, Chavez-Macias LG, Olvera-Rabiela JE, Martinez AJ. Encefalitis por una nueva Amiba de Vida Libre, probablemente Leptomyxid. *Patologia (Mexico).* 1989;27:137–141.
46. Cox EC. Amebic meningoencephalitis caused by *Acanthamoeba* species in a four month old child. *J South Carolina Med Assoc.* 1980;76:459–462.
47. DeGregorio C, Rivasi F, Monigardo M, et al. *Acanthamoeba* meningoencephalitis in a patient with acquired immunodeficiency syndrome: First report from Europe. *Arch Pathol Lab Med.* 1992;116:1363–1365.
48. Duma RJ, Helwig WB, Martinez AJ. Meningoencephalitis and brain abscess due to a free-living amoeba. *Ann Intern Med.* 1978;88:468–473.
49. Kernohan J, Magath TB, Schloss GT. Granuloma of brain probably due to *Endolimax williamsi (Iodamoeba butschlii). Arch Pathol.* 1960;70:576–580.
50. Khalifl GE, Pambuccian SE, Visvesvara GS, Harten B. Disseminated *Acanthamoeba* infection masquerading as bacillary angiomatosis in a patient with AIDS. *Int J Surg Pathol.* 1994;2:11–16.
51. Lowichik A, Rollins N, Delgado R, et al. Leptomyxid amebic meningoencephalitis mimicking brain stem glioma. *Am J Neuroradiol.* 1995;16:926–929.
52. Martinez AJ. Is *Acanthamoeba* encephalitis an opportunistic infection? *Neurology.* 1980;30:567–574.
53. Martinez AJ, Garcia CA, Halks-Miller M, Arce-Vela R. Granulomatous amebic encephalitis presenting as a cerebral mass lesion. *Acta Neuropathol (Berlin).* 1980;51: 85–91.
54. Park CH, Lyengan V, Hefter L, et al. Cutaneous *Acanthamoeba* infection associated with acquired immunodeficiency syndrome. *Lab Med.* 1994;25:386–388.
55. Robert VB, Rorke LB. Primary amebic encephalitis probably from *Acanthamoeba. Ann Intern Med.* 1973;79: 174–179.
56. Rutherfoord GS. Amebic meningoencephalitis due to free-living amoeba. *S Afr Med J.* 1986;69:52–55.
57. Wessel HB, Hubbard J, Martinez AJ, Willaert E. Granulomatous amebic encephalitis (GAE) with prolonged clinical course: CT scan findings, diagnosis by brain biopsy and effect of treatment. *Neurology.* 1980;30:442. [Abstract.]
58. Tan B, Weldon-Linne CM, Rhone DP, et al. *Acanthamoeba* infection presenting as skin lesions in patients with acquired immunodeficiency syndrome. *Arch Pathol Lab Med.* 1993;117:1043–1046.
59. Rowen JL, Doerr CA, Vogel H, Baker CJ. *Balamuthia mandrillaris:* a newly recognized agent for amebic meningoencephalitis. *Pediatr Infect Dis J.* 1995;14: 705–710.
60. Helton J, Loveless M, White CR. Cutaneous *Acanthamoeba* infection associated with leukocytoclastic vasculitis in an AIDS patient. *Am J Dermatopathol.* 1993; 15:146–149.
61. Hoffmann EO, Garcia C, Lunseth J, et al. A case of primary amebic meningoencephalitis. *Am J Trop Med Hyg.* 1978; 27:29–38.
62. Kwame Ofori-Kwakye S, Sidebottom DG, Herbert J, et al. Granulomatous brain tumor caused by *Acanthamoeba. J Neurosurg.* 1986;64:505–509.
63. Lalitha MK, Andadi V, Srivastava A, et al. Isolation of *Acanthamoeba culbertsoni* from a patient with meningitis. *J Clin Microbiol.* 1985;21:666–667.
64. Matson DO, Rouah E, Lee RT, et al. *Acanthamoeba* meningoencephalitis masquerading as neurocysticercosis. *Pediatr Infect Dis J.* 1988;7:121–124.
65. Popek EJ, Neafie RC. Granulomatous meningoencephali-

tis due to *Leptomyxid* ameba. *Pediatr Pathol.* 1992;12: 871–881.

66. Simon MW, Wilson HD. The amebic meningoencephalitides. *Pediatr Infect Dis J.* 1986;5:562–569.
67. Anderlini P, Przepiorka D, Luna M, et al. *Acanthamoeba* meningoencephalitis after bone marrow transplantation. *Bone Marrow Transpl.* 1994;14:459–461.
68. Slater CA, Sickel JZ, Visvesvara GS, et al. Brief report: successful treatment of disseminated *Acanthamoeba* infection in an immunocompromised patient. *N Engl J Med.* 1994;331:85–87.
69. Martinez AJ. Acanthamoebiasis and immunosuppression. Case report. *J Neuropathol Exp Neuro.* 1982;41:548–557.
70. Flores BM, Garcia CA, Stamm WE, Torian BE. Differentiation of *Naegleria fowleri* from *Acanthamoeba* species by using monoclonal antibodies and flow cytometry. *J Clin Microbiol.* 1990;28:1999–2005.
71. Cleland PG, Lawande RV, Onyamelukwe G, Whittle HC. Chronic amebic meningoencephalitis. *Arch Neurol.* 1982; 39:56–57.
72. Berger ST, Mondino BJ, Hoft RH, et al. Successful medical management of *Acanthamoeba* keratitis. *Am J Ophthalmol.* 1990;110:395–403.
73. Jones DB. *Acanthamoeba*—the ultimate opportunist? *Am J Ophthalmol.* 1986;102:527–530.
74. Stehr-Green JK, Bailey TM, Visvesvara GS. The epidemiology of *Acanthamoeba* keratitis in the United States. *Am J Ophthalmol.* 1989;107:331–336.
75. Illingworth CD, Cook SD, Karabatsos CH, Easty DL. *Acanthamoeba* keratitis: risk factor and outcome. *Br J Ophthalmol* 1995;79:1078–1082.
76. Cohen EJ, Buchanan HW, Laughrea PA, et al. Diagnosis and management of *Acanthamoeba* keratitis. *Am J Ophthalmol.* 1985;100:389–395.
77. Kilvington S, Larkin DFP, White DG, Beeching JR. Laboratory investigation of *Acanthamoeba* keratitis. *J Clin Microbiol.* 1990;28:2722–2725.
78. Larkin DFP, Kilvington S, Dart JKG. Treatment of *Acanthamoeba* keratitis with polyhexan methylene biguanide. *Ophthalmology.* 1992;99:185–191.
79. Lindquist TD, Sher NA, Doughman DJ. Clinical signs and medical therapy of early *Acanthamoeba* keratitis. *Arch Ophthalmol.* 1988;106:73–77.
80. Theodore FH, Jakobiec FA, Juechter KB, et al. The diagnostic value of a ring infiltrate in acanthamoebic keratitis. *Ophthalmology.* 1985;92:1471–1479.
81. Schuster FL, Jacob LS. Effects of magainins on ameba and cyst stages of *Acanthamoeba polyphaga. Antimicrob Agents Chemother.* 1992;36:1263–1271.
82. Martinez AJ, Janitschke K. *Acanthamoeba,* an opportunistic microorganism: a review. *Infection.* 1985;13:251–256.
83. Rabinovitch J, Fook TC, Hunter WS, Ghosh M. *Acanthamoeba* keratitis in a soft-contact-lens wearer. *Can J Ophthalmol.* 1990;25:25–28.

CHAPTER 133

Giardiasis

David A. Schwartz, James Patrick Mixon, and Robert L. Owen

Falstaff. . . . what says the doctor to my water?
Page: He said, sir, the water itself was a good healthy water; but for the party that owed it, he might have moe diseases than he knew for.

William Shakespeare (1564–1616), Henry IV, I, ii, 1

CLASSIFICATION

Giardiasis is a protozoan disease caused by the flagellate *Giardia lamblia,* a member of the family Hexamitidae. The three classic morphologic types of *Giardia* organisms include *G agilis, G muris,* and *G duodenalis (lamblia).* Traditional classification schemes of the *Giardia* sp have been based on morphologic findings and host species restrictions. More recent means of classification, however, have used antigenic, isoenzyme, chromosome, and DNA analysis in addition to the more classic methods. Although *G lamblia* has been found in a variety of mammals as well as humans, it has not been classified as a true zoonosis because of the inability to definitively trace a human outbreak to an animal source.

INTRODUCTION AND HISTORY

In 1681, *G lamblia* was first observed by Antonie van Leeuwenhoek in a specimen of his own stools. He had diarrhea at the time and thought that this organism was the cause.[1,2] *Giardia lamblia* therefore, enjoys the distinction of being the first microscopic organism to be seen and recognized as an infectious agent. In 1859, Vilem Lambl, a Czechoslovakian physician, rediscovered and described the parasite, which had been recovered from the upper intestinal tract of a child with diarrhea. Nearly two centuries after the original discovery of *Giardia,* Grassi discovered the cyst form in 1859. In 1989 the in vitro completion of the entire life cycle was accomplished by Gillian and colleagues.[3,4]

Studies of giardiasis on human prisoners—to fulfill Koch's postulates—were begun in 1954. It was not until the early 1970s, however, that there was consensus on the clinical importance of this parasite as a human pathogen. Most of the disagreement revolved around the confusion arising from the wide clinical spectrum of giardial infections, which varies from asymptomatic infection to severe acute or chronic diarrhea and malabsorption. Infection by *Giardia* has been ranked as the seventh major cause of death from parasitic disease in the developing world, and giardiasis is now recognized as a frequent disease of travelers worldwide, particularly in the developing world.[3,4]

EPIDEMIOLOGY AND LIFE CYCLE

Giardia lamblia is responsible for diarrhea throughout the world, and is a common cause of diarrhea in patients with acquired immunodeficiency syndrome (AIDS).[5,6] Although *G lamblia* has a worldwide geographic distribution, the highest prevalence of giardiasis is in the tropics and subtropics, and where sanitation is poor. Specific regions of recognized increased risk for travelers include parts of the former Soviet Union, Southeast and South Asia, tropical Africa, Mexico, and western South America.[4] Persons of all ages are affected, although in endemic areas infection is more frequent in infants. In the developing world it is one of the first enteric pathogens to infect infants, with peak prevalence rates reaching 15% to 20% in children less than 10 years old.

Humans are the main reservoir of *G lamblia*.[5] *Giardia* sp, which resemble the species isolated from humans, have been identified from a broad range of mammals, including beavers, cattle, cats, coyotes, dogs, gerbils, and sheep. Among domestic companion animals, the prevalence of *Giardia* infections is 5% to 40% in dogs, and 14% to 51% in cats. The transmission of *G lamblia* can occur directly from person to person by fecal–oral contamination with cysts, or indirectly by ingestion of contaminated water and, occasionally, food. Campers and hikers are frequently infected after drinking contaminated water, including water from untreated streams, unfiltered surface waters, and shallow wells. Also at risk for giardiasis are persons who obtain their drinking and recreational water from untreated sources. In addition, outbreaks can occur within day care centers and other institutional settings, and among family members of infected children.[4]

Most infections with *Giardia* are sporadic, but many infections occur in clusters. Currently, *G lamblia* is the most frequently identified pathogen in all waterborne outbreaks in the United States.[4] In 11 outbreaks of gastroenteritis reported in the United States during 1991–1992, 45% of the infected persons were exposed to swimming/wading pools and 36% acquired *G lamblia*. During three nonconsecutive months during 1991–1992, four outbreaks of giardiasis, affecting an estimated 123 persons, were reported from California, Idaho, Nevada, and Pennsylvania; three outbreaks were associated with groundwater supplies and one was associated with unfiltered surface water containing low levels of *Giardia* cysts.[7] In 1977, epidemic giardiasis in day care centers was first reported with infection rates varying up to 25%.[8] Another mode of infection involves oral–anal sexual practices, especially among homosexual men. In 60 human immunodeficiency virus (HIV)-infected patients with past or current gastrointestinal symptoms, 18 patients were homo/bisexual men and 18 patients (30%) were positive for *G lamblia;* 17 patients (94.4%) with *G lamblia* were symptomatic.[9] Ingestion of 100 or more cysts is required to ensure infection in humans, but ingestion of as few as 10 cysts has infected volunteers. Approximately 4% of stool specimens submitted to laboratories in the United States contain *Giardia*.[8]

The life cycle of *G lamblia* consists of two stages: the trophozoite, which exists freely within the lumen and crypts of the small bowel, and the environmentally resistant cyst, which is passed with the stool. When cysts are ingested, the low pH of stomach contents stimulates excystation, resulting in release of two daughter trophozoites that remain joined to each other for a short time by a stringlike artifact between their caudal ends. The trophozoites then multiply in the small bowel. As trophozoites move to the lower intestine, they encyst within a protective wall, and cysts are passed into the environment, with feces, from which they can contaminate food and water and infect the next host.

MORPHOLOGY

The trophozoite of *G lamblia* is pear-shaped, dorsally convex, and has a distinctive shallow, ventral concave adhesion disk. The disk consists of a rigid cytoskeleton of evenly spaced microtubules 50 to 60 nm apart, linked by microribbons. Important antigenic and structural components of the disk include tubulin within the microtubules and low-molecular-weight (29 to 38 kd) giardins within the microribbons. Giardins, a prominent double band in the electrophoretic separation of the cytoskeleton protein, are significant antigenically because specific genetic probes attach to them and assist in the detection of cysts in drinking water. The dorsal surface apparently provides an area for absorption of nutrients. Attachment of the adhesion disk to the mucosal surface is thought to be from negative pressure, which develops in the concavity, in association with the beating flagella. The trophozoite is 9.5 to 21 μm long by 5 to 15 μm wide and has two nuclei and four pairs of flagella, of which three pairs are involved in parasite mobility and are posteriorly directed. The fourth pair of flagella originates from the ventral surface of the trophozoite behind the adhesive disk, and is in constant motion.[3] Currents caused by these two ventral flagella are thought to play a role in its hydrodynamic mode of adhesion, as well as regulation of fluid flow and pressure under the disk. The appearance of the trophozoites is that of a teardrop when viewed dorsoventrally and spoon-shaped when seen from the side. The trophozoites contain two symmetrically placed nuclei, each having a prominent central karyosome, that create a characteristic facelike image on stained preparations such as trichrome stain. No chromatin lines the delicate nuclear membranes. Median bodies, which are compact collections of microtubules, lie transversely in the midline of the parasite in a clawlike manner in *G lamblia*. *Giardia* lack mitochondria, peroxisomes, smooth endoplasmic reticulum, and nucleoli. Trophozoites divide by a complex process of longitudinal binary fission, and cysts develop as liquid feces transit through the large intestine.

The cyst of *G lamblia* is oval to round, and measures 8 to 12 μm long by 7 to 10 μm wide. Mature cysts contain four nuclei, which are usually situated at one pole, curved median bodies, linear axonemes, and the adhesion disk. The periphery is marked by a layer of vacuoles or tubules that stain positively for acid phosphatase activity. Mature cysts are surrounded by a smooth, tough hyaline wall approximately 0.3 to 0.5 μm thick. The cysts contain finely granular cytoplasm that is clearly separated from the cyst wall.

CLINICAL FEATURES

During the initial evaluation of persons with suspected giardiasis, important historical factors include a history of travel to an endemic region, ingestion of untreated surface or well water, the presence of small children in homes who attend day care centers, or oral–anal sexual activity. Infections of humans with *G lamblia* can be divided into intestinal and extraintestinal disease. Many *Giardia* infections are asymptomatic; when symptoms do occur, however, they vary depending on such factors as size of inoculum, duration of infection, and the immune status of the host.[4,5,8] For example, persons with humoral immunodeficiencies such as hypogammaglobulinemia and X-linked agammaglobulinemia are predisposed to chronic symptomatic *Giardia* infection.[3]

Following ingestion of *Giardia* cysts, the incubation period is usually 1 to 2 weeks. Almost 50% of newly infected persons develop symptoms, 15% are asymptomatic but shed cysts in the feces, and the remainder have no trace of infection. In the acute stage of infection, symptoms usually begin with gastrointestinal uneasiness, followed by nausea, anorexia, and, in some patients, low-grade fever and chills. As the infection persists, there may be explosive, watery diarrhea, which commonly progresses into a greasy, foul smelling stool that may float; noticeable abdominal gurgling and distention associated with foul-smelling flatulence; and sulfuric belching. Associated findings in patients with chronic giardiasis include headache, weight loss, malaise, epigastric discomfort frequently made worse by eating, and fatigue that is out of proportion to the degree of illness. Periods of diarrhea may be interrupted by periods of constipation or regularity in bowel movements.[4,5] Weight loss is a significant component of giardiasis, occurring in over 50% of patients and averaging 10 pounds per person.

Complications of chronic giardiasis have included steatorrhea and malabsorption of vitamins A and B_{12}, protein and D-xylose. Vomiting and tenesmus have been reported, but are uncommon. Chronic infection in young infants may cause symptoms such as anorexia, weight loss, or a malabsorption syndrome resembling sprue. Leukocytes, gross blood, or mucus are not usually present in the feces of patients with giardiasis, unless there is a second infectious agent.[10,11]

Uncommon extraintestinal manifestations of *Giardia* infection have been reported, including urticaria, cholecystitis, pancreatitis, eosinophilia, reactive arthritis, retinal arteritis, and iridocyclitis.[4,5,8]

PATHOLOGY

Asymptomatic infected persons usually have no histologic abnormality in specimens of duodenum or jejunum. Patients with symptomatic giardiasis also can have a normal jejunal histologic appearance. In most symptomatic patients, however, there is a range of nonspecific microscopic findings, including atrophic changes of villi with blunting or flattening, crypt hyperplasia, epithelial cell damage, and extensive infiltration of the lamina propria by plasma cells, lymphocytes, and neutrophils. The brush border may be compressed in areas where trophozoites are attached by their ventral disks. In some patients, there is an increased number of inflammatory cells in the lamina propria, which immunohistochemically stain positive for IgD and IgE. There is evidence supporting the correlation between damage of the microvillous border in giardiasis and the decrease in microvillous border enzymes, particularly disaccharidases, which could contribute to an osmotic diarrhea with gas formation from bacterial breakdown of sugars.

Trophozoites of *Giardia* can be recognized by careful study by light microscopy of small intestinal mucosal biopsies. The organisms are minute, however, and can be easily overlooked or mistaken for detached intestinal epithelial cells or erythrocytes. The trophozoites typically appear to be randomly oriented and are on or just above the luminal surface of enterocytes (Figures 133–1 through 133–3). When present in sagittal section, the trophozoites have a characteristic crescentic shape. In semithin plastic-embedded sections, the ventral adhesion disk, nuclei, and other organelles can often be visualized.[12] The histologic diagnosis of giar-

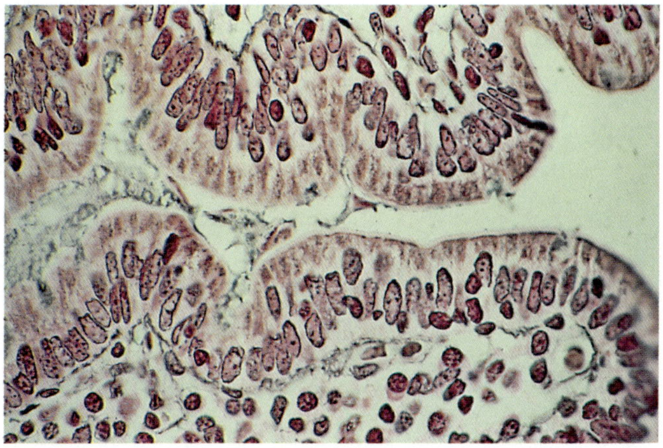

Figure 133–1. Crescent-shaped trophozoites of *Giardia,* lateral view on the luminal surface of the jejunum in this mucosal biopsy. The morphologic details of the organisms are difficult to see in this paraffin-embedded section (AFIP photograph; reticulum stain, ×180).

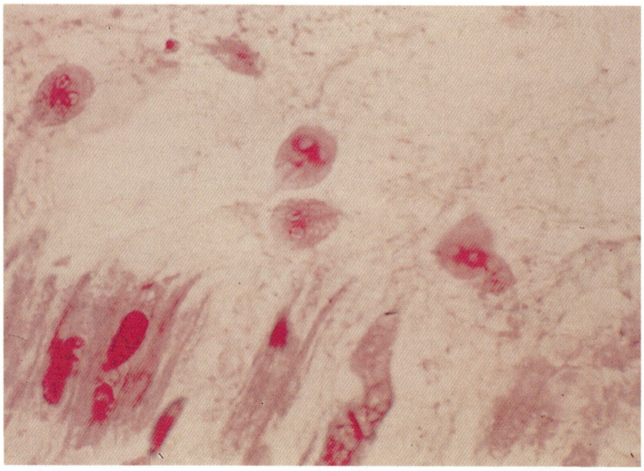

Figure 133–2. Binucleate *G lamblia* trophozoites centered in the lamina propria of a jejunal biopsy specimen from a patient with symptomatic giardiasis. As luminal feeders, *Giardia* do not reproduce in tissue, but when they do wander into tissue, they stimulate an intestinal immune response [hematoxylin-eosin (H&E), ×1000].

diasis is confirmed when crescentic or pear-shaped trophozoites of the appropriate size, in a luminal distribution, and containing a ventral adhesion disk are identified in biopsy tissues. In our experience, the structural features of *Giardia* trophozoites are most easily recognized in plastic-embedded semithin sections (Figure 133–3). Because the distribution of the parasites tends to be focal in villi and in intervillous spaces, examination of several biopsy fragments and levels are often necessary to identify the organisms. The organisms are often most numerous in specimens taken from the proximal small intestine. Antibodies to *Giardia* are available for confirmatory testing, if necessary (Figure 133–4). It is unlikely, however, that the lumen-dwelling *Giardia* trophozoites will be confused with cryptosporidia, microsporidia, or other intestinal protozoa. Invasion of the mucosa and submucosa by *Giardia* trophozoites has been reported, but is rare.

The cysts and trophozoites of *Giardia* are easily identified in electron micrographs of infected tissues (Figures 133–5 through 133–9). Cysts are characterized ultrastructurally by a cyst wall with a thick outer layer and an inner layer composed of a double unit membrane. The cytoplasm is often retracted from the cyst wall. The striated ventral adhesion disk of the trophozoite is prominent in both scanning (Figure 133–6) and transmission (Figure 133–9) electron micrographs. Other characteristic ultrastructural features of trophozoites include the ventrolateral flange, lateral crest (Figure 133–9), and axonemes. Both cysts and trophozoites reveal a row of variously sized vacuoles at the periphery.[13,14]

DIAGNOSIS

Because of its variable clinical presentation, giardiasis should be considered in the differential diagnosis of most patients with diarrhea. The traditional method of diagnosis has been identifying *G lamblia* in stool and this remains the screening method of choice for most patients. Because cysts are passed intermittently, three

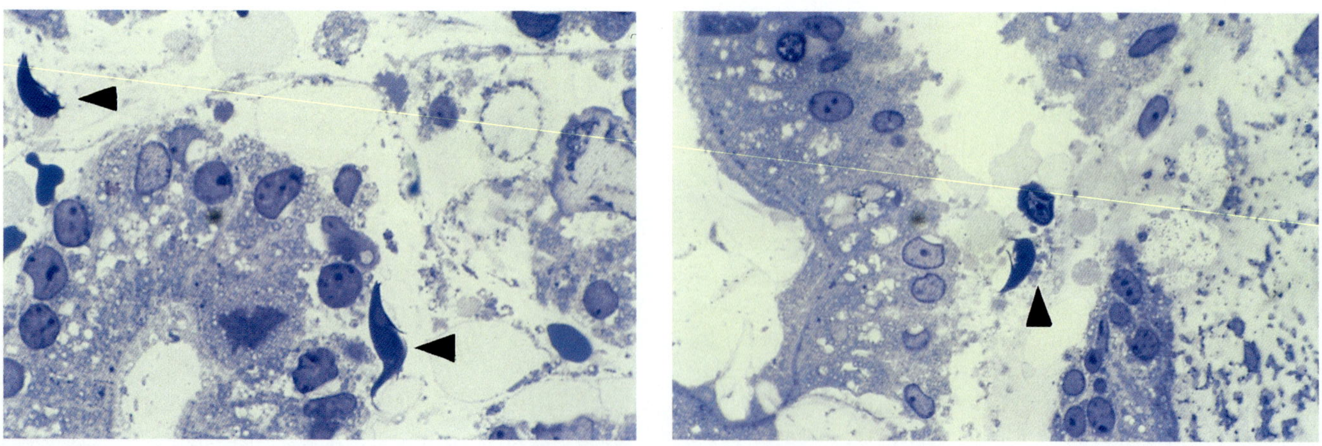

A B

Figure 133–3. (**A**), (**B**) Plastic-embedded semithin section of a duodenal mucosal biopsy from an AIDS patient with chronic diarrhea. Some of the fine structural features of *Giardia* trophozoites (*arrows*), including the diagnostic ventral disk, can be seen using this method. The organisms should not be confused with erythrocytes in the lumen or with detached inflammatory and epithelial cells (plastic embedding, toluidine blue, ×1000).

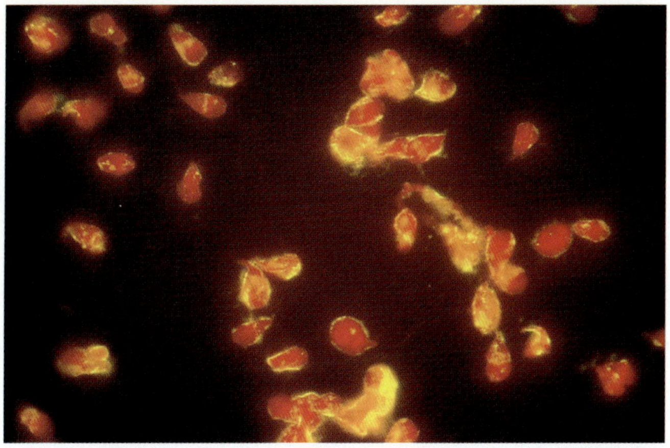

Figure 133–4. Fluorescent antibody staining of *Giardia* trophozoites can be performed for diagnostic confirmation (indirect immunofluorescence using anti–*G lamblia* antiserum, X1000). *(Contributed by GS Visvesvara, PhD.)*

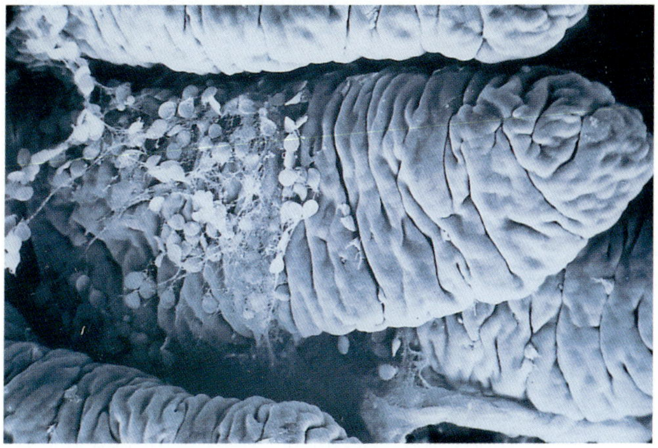

Figure 133–5. Jejunal villi in a mouse experimentally infected with *G muris*. Trophozoites cling to the surfaces of enterocytes near the bases of villi, wedged into crevices, and lie in strands of mucus (scanning electron micrograph, ×2500). *(Reproduced from Katelaris and Farthing,[11] with permission.)*

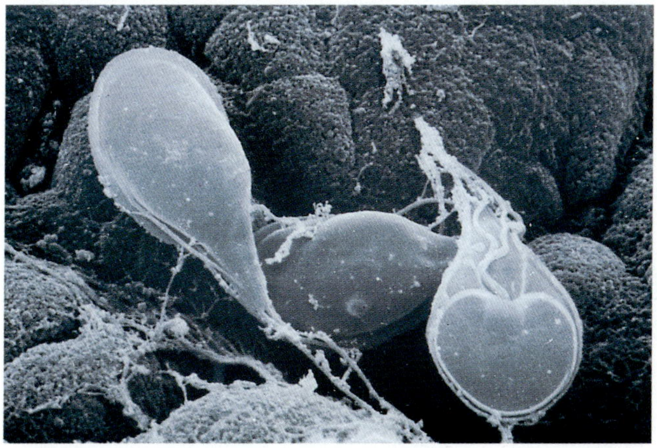

Figure 133–6. Scanning electron micrographs of three *Giardia lamblia* trophozoites on the surface of the jejunum. As luminal feeders, trophozoites attach to the duodenum and jejunum by means of the adhesive disk on the ventral surface, and absorb nutrients through the rounded dorsal surfaces seen on the two trophozoites on the left (×5500).

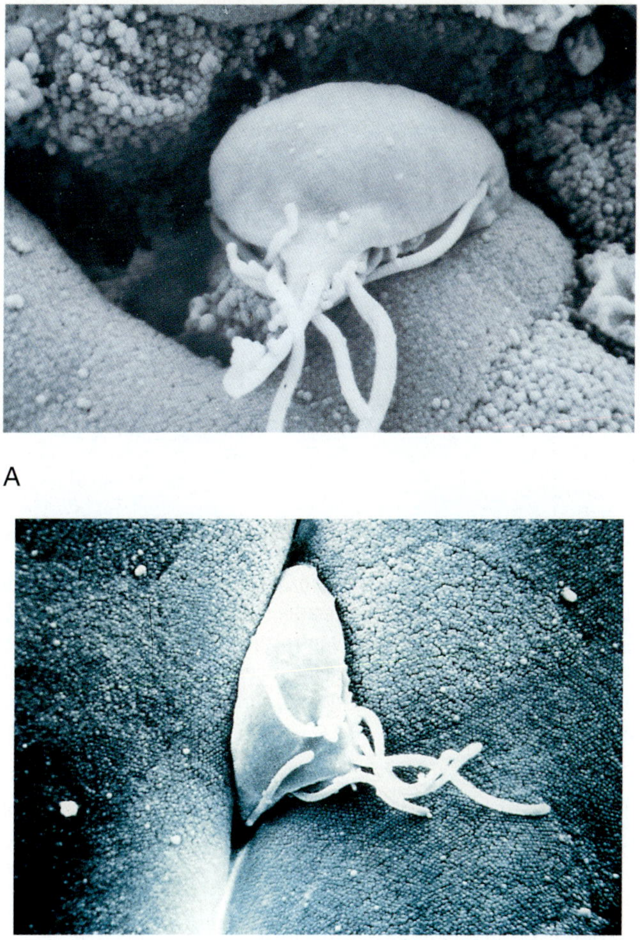

A

B

Figure 133–7. (**A**), (**B**) *Giardia* trophozoites entering a break in the surface epithelium, propelled by posterior flagella [scanning electron micrographs; (A), ×5500; (B), ×7000].

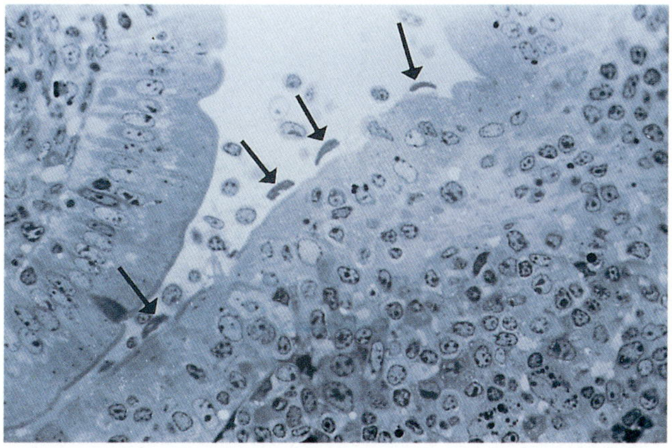

Figure 133–8. *Giardia* trophozoites (*arrows*) in crescent-shaped profiles over the surface of a lymphoid follicle in the small intestine (plastic embedding, toluidine blue, ×900). *(Reproduced from Katelaris and Farthing,[11] with permission.)*

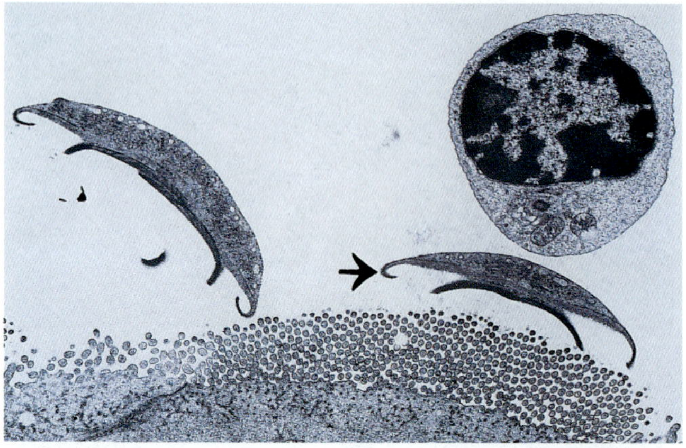

Figure 133–9. Two *Giardia* trophozoites and a lymphocyte in the lumen seen in cross-section over the intestinal surface. The adhesion disk, peripheral vacuoles, ventrolateral flange (*arrow*), and lateral crest (*arrowhead*) are clearly seen (transmission electron micrograph, ×6800). *(Reproduced from Katelaris and Farthing,[11] with permission.)*

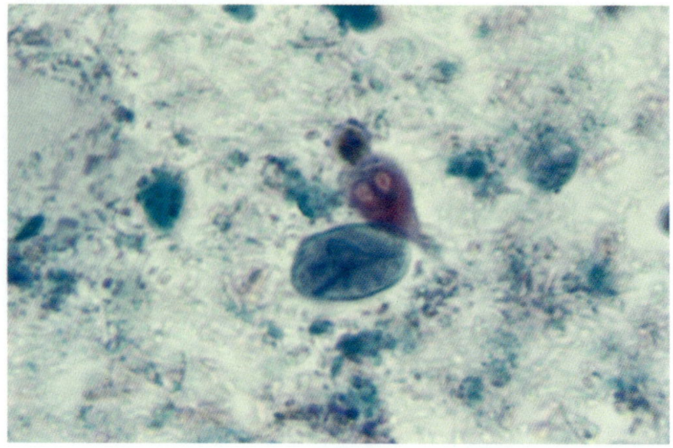

Figure 133–11. Thin smear of concentrated stool showing characteristic appearance of a *Giardia* trophozoite and cyst (trichrome stain, ×1000).

stool specimens should be collected over a period of several days. Passage of parasites in the stool may lag behind the clinical onset by a few days. Stool is usually divided into three portions: one is examined fresh, one is placed into polyvinyl alcohol (PVA), and the third is placed into 10% buffered formalin. Unfixed stool should be mixed with iodine solution, which stains cysts brown and accentuates their internal structures (Figure 133–10). Samples fixed with PVA are routinely stained with trichrome or iron-hematoxylin. Formalin-preserved samples can be concentrated by formalin–ether acetate or zinc sulfate methods to increase the probability of finding organisms. Trophozoites are most frequent in soft or liquid stools (Figure 133–11), whereas the more resistant, infective cysts are more often in formed stools (Figure 133–11). Several commercially available tests to detect *Giardia* antigen in the stool are available. These tests have a relatively high sensitivity and specificity, and they may be superior to the classic examination for ova and parasites but fail to identify other stool parasites. Diagnosis of giardiasis can also be accomplished by use of the string test, duodenal lavage fluid, or small intestinal biopsy.

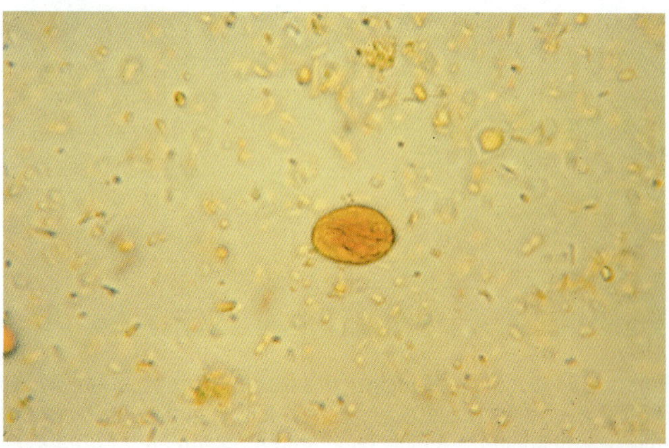

Figure 133–10. Mature cyst of *G lamblia* in iodine-stained wet preparation of stool (×1000).

It is unlikely that giardiasis will be missed if three stool examinations are done properly using both histochemical staining and antigen detection methods. In some patients, however, it may be important to evaluate the microscopic features of the small intestine especially if there is malabsorption or when multiple infections are suspected, or when noninvasive techniques are not diagnostic. In these patients biopsy should be considered. Occasionally, small intestinal biopsy will demonstrate *Giardia* as a coinfection with another diarrheal agent (eg, cryptosporidiosis, cytomegalovirus, or microsporidiosis), especially in immunodeficient patients including those with AIDS.

REFERENCES

1. Feeley DE, Erlandsen SL, Chase DG. Structure of the trophozoite and cyst. In: Erlandsen SL, Meyer EA, eds. *Giardia and Giardiasis: Biology, Pathogenesis, and Epidemiology.* New York: Plenum; 1984:3–31.
2. Dobell C. The discovery of the intestinal protozoa of man. *Proc R Soc Med.* 1920;13:1–15.
3. Walterspiel JN, Pickering LK. *Giardia* and giardiasis. In: Sun T, ed. *Progress in Clinical Parasitology.* Boca Raton, Fla: CRC Press; 1994;4:1–26.
4. Wolfe MS. Giardiasis. *Clin Microbiol Rev.* 1992;5:93–100.
5. Hill DR. Giardiasis: issues in diagnosis and management. *Infect Dis Clin North Am.* 1993;7:503–525.

6. Glaser CA, Angulo FJ, Rooney JA. Animal-associated opportunistic infections among persons infected with the human immunodeficiency virus. *Clin Infect Dis.* 1994;18:14–24.
7. Moore AC, Herwaldt BL, Craun GF, Calderon RL, Highsmith AK, Juranek DD. Surveillance for waterborne disease outbreaks—United States, 1991–1992. *MMWR.* 1993;42:1–22.
8. Seidel J. Giardiasis. *Pediatr Rev.* 1993;14:284–286.
9. Tosone G, Donadies G, Liuzzi G, Tullio CP, Santoro G, Piazza M. *Giardia lamblia* infection in HIV-infected patients. *Int Conf AIDS.* 1993;9:388. Abstract PO-B10-1516.
10. Doglioni C, De Boni M, Cielo R, et al. Gastric giardiasis. *J Clin Pathol.* 1992;45:964–967.
11. Katelaris PH, Farthing MJG. Diarrhoea and malabsorption in giardiasis: a multifactorial process? *Gut.* 1992;33:295–297.
12. Orihel TC, Ash LR. *Parasites in Human Tissues.* Chicago: ASCP Press; 1995:20–21.
13. Owen RL, Nemanic PC, Stevens DP. Ultrastructural observations on giardiasis in a mouse model, I: intestinal distribution, attachment and relationship to the immune system of *Giardia muris. Gastroenterol.* 1979;76:757–769.
14. Nemanic PC, Owen RL, Stevens DP, et al. Ultrastructural observations on giardiasis in a mouse model, II: endosymbiosis and organelle distribution in *Giardia muris* and *Giardia lamblia. J Infect Dis.* 1979;140:222–228.

CHAPTER 134

Isosporiasis

Jan Marc Orenstein

Nature can refuse to speak but she cannot lie.

Charles Brenton Huggins

DEFINITION

Intestinal infection by one of three protozoans, *Isospora hominis, I natalenis,* and especially *I belli,* is isosporiasis.[1–5] The *Isospora* are members of the family Eimeriidea, suborder Eimeriina, and share the subclass Coccidia (class Sporozoa) with *Toxoplasma, Sarcocystis, Cyclospora,* and *Cryptosporidium.* About 200 species of *Isospora* have been named. They infect the intestines of reptiles, invertebrates, and particularly birds and mammals (carnivores, eg, dogs and cats). *Isospora belli* has been identified in humans only, and there is no evidence that *Isospora* species of other animals infect humans.

GEOGRAPHIC DISTRIBUTION

Isospora are ubiquitous in the animal kingdom, worldwide in distribution, and until recently were important only to veterinary medicine. Virchow described the first human intestinal infection in 1860 (cited in Refs. 1 through 6). The prevalence of isosporiasis in man remains unknown. There are several tropical and subtropical areas of the world where *I belli* is endemic, eg, Chile, Colombia, Brazil, Africa, and Southwest Asia, while infections are rare in temperate climate zones. Before the acquired immunodeficiency syndrome (AIDS) pandemic, cases in North America, Europe, and Australia were few and confined mostly to individuals returning from endemic areas ("chronic traveler's diarrhea") and to institutional outbreaks.[7–10] Symptomatic infections were reported in American soldiers returning from the Pacific after World War II. Human immunodeficiency virus (HIV)-infected individuals living in or coming from endemic areas have the highest prevalence of isosporiasis in the AIDS pandemic.[11–23]

Transmission is via environmental exposure, eg, fecal contamination (food and water); direct person-to-person transmission is unproven.

LIFE CYCLE, NATURAL HISTORY, AND EPIDEMIOLOGY

Ingestion of sporulated oocysts, or sporocysts, is followed by the excystation and release of infectious sporozoites (four per sporocyst) in the distal duodenum and proximal jejunum (through the action of trypsin and bile).[1–5,20,23,24] The free sporozoites invade enterocytes where they develop into round trophozoites that enlarge into mature schizonts (asexual schizogony), a process that involves nuclear division. Schizont division results in variable numbers of invasive merozoites, which spread the infection among other epithelial cells. The merozoites undergo additional asexual cycles and develop into more schizonts (schizogony), or enter the sexual cycle (gametogony) and produce sexual forms: macrogamonts and microgametes.

Ciliated (flagellated), nucleated microgametes pinch off from the periphery of the mature microgamont. They fertilize the female macrogamete, forming the zygote or oocyst, which is released into the lumen, either to be passed in the stool or to sporulate and produce more infectious sporozoites (autoinfection). The large macrogamete has a single prominent nucleus and characteristic electron-dense dark bodies and electron-lucent, wall-forming bodies (presumed origin of oocyst wall). To be infectious, the excreted oocyst must sporulate, a process that can take up to 48 hours, and requires oxygen and temperatures below 37°C.

It was not until the AIDS pandemic that the full potential of *Isospora* as an intestinal parasite was realized.[12,25] Increasing numbers of patients, in all risk categories, have been reported since 1984.[13,14,17,20,21,25–28] Whereas the prevalence in the developed world appears not to exceed 5%, the prevalence in the developing world reaches about 15%.[12,16,21] In Los Angeles County, isosporiasis has been on the rise and, although Latin Americans comprised 20% of the AIDS cases, they accounted for 80% of isosporiasis.[11] Since years may have elapsed from the time of arrival of immigrants from Latin America to the time of diagnosis, *Isospora* are apparently harbored for long periods in a latent state.

MORPHOLOGICAL FEATURES OF THE ORGANISM

Typical of the coccidia, *I belli* has a trilaminar cell wall or pellicle (Figure 134–1).[1,2,24] It has spherical nuclei with prominent nucleoli, large mitochondria with tubular cristae, well-developed perinuclear Golgi apparatuses, abundant free ribosomes, and electron-lucent and electron-dense bodies or granules. The coccidia are members of the subphylum Apicomplexa, which have apical complexes that include polar rings, spirally coiled filaments (conoid), longitudinally oriented electron-dense organelles in the anterior body (micronemes), electron-dense tubular or saccular organelles (rhoptries), and subpellicular tubules. All developmental stages are in a membrane-bound, parasitophorous vacuole, isolating them from the cytoplasm of the host cell, thus enhancing visualization in tissue sections.

CLINICAL FEATURES

Experimental infections reveal that 7 to 11 days elapse before unsporulated oocysts appear in the stool.[1,2,7,9,11,20] The immunocompetent person usually has an acute, mild to profuse, watery diarrhea that resolves in 2 weeks, even without treatment. More severe infections resolve, usually, within weeks to a few months. Some infections, however, persist for months to years, and can be extremely debilitating even leading to death. Clinically, isosporiasis infection in the AIDS patient resembles cryptosporidiosis (although symptoms are usually milder), being unrelenting, prolonged (2 to 18 months), debilitating, and even fatal.[12,16,17,25]

Typically, copious diarrhea (6 to 10 stools per day) follows the acute onset of fever, headache, and malaise.[1,11,12,14,16,19,20] Stools are nonbloody, foul-smelling, watery to soft foamy, and usually accompanied by malabsorption with weight loss, nausea, chills, sweating, and colicky/crampy abdominal pain; some patients also have vomiting and fever. The diarrhea can be secretory and cholera-like. The stool contains undigested food and lipid (steatorrhea). Flatulence is common. Charcot–Leyden crystals (formed from the granules of eosinophils) in the stool reflect the low-grade peripheral eosinophilia that often accompanies *I belli* infection.[1] The amount of diarrhea and the degree of weakness, anorexia, and weight loss are particularly severe in AIDS patients.[22]

Before the AIDS epidemic, disseminated isosporiasis had not been seen in humans; now there are two reports.[29,30] In one autopsy, *I belli* organisms were in enterocytes of small and large intestines, and free in the lamina propria. Organisms were in histiocytes in mesenteric, periaortic, and mediastinal lymph nodes (associated with a granulomatous reaction). A black African woman had 3 years of documented isosporiasis with invasive forms in a biopsy specimen of duodenum and no co-infections. At autopsy, organisms (mostly within macrophages) had invaded the bowel wall, mesenteric and mediastinal lymph nodes, liver, and spleen.

The endoscopist may see patchy mild erythema and a light gray granular mucosa. The radiologist sees nonspecific features, such as dilated loops of bowel, mucosal thickening, and barium flocculation in the proximal small bowel.

Co-infections with *Cryptosporidium, Giardia lamblia,* and *Trichuris trichiura* have been reported, particularly in AIDS patients.[12,14,16,18]

DIAGNOSIS

Identifying oocysts in stool can be difficult, because oocysts are few, shedding is intermittent, and they have a low refractive index.[2,7,11,12,17,20,28] Immature oocysts may be absent in the early, clinically severe phase, which is predominantly asexual, appearing when symptoms have become chronic (sexual phase), between 10 and 20 days after infection. Several stool specimens, taken on alternate days, should be examined.

Unsporulated oocysts of *I belli* have a smooth double wall, are refractile with granular contents, ellipsoidal (tapered end), and are large, measuring 20 to 33 μm by 10 to 19 μm. Unsporulated oocysts allow a positive identification of *I belli* because animal species of *Isospora* (or *Cryptosporidium*), are always sporulated in the stool.[7,12,17,19,20,25,28] The oocyst usually contains one immature sporont (occasionally two), which undergoes mitosis producing two heavy-walled sporocysts, which then divide into four banana-shaped sporozoites. By comparison, *Cryptosporidium* oocysts are much smaller (4 to 6 μm), round, and contain four sporozoites and no sporocysts. The spores of *I belli* do not readily stain with iodine. Coccidial oocysts can be identified with saline wet mounts stained by a modification of the Kinyoun acid-fast method. A thin stool smear on a glass

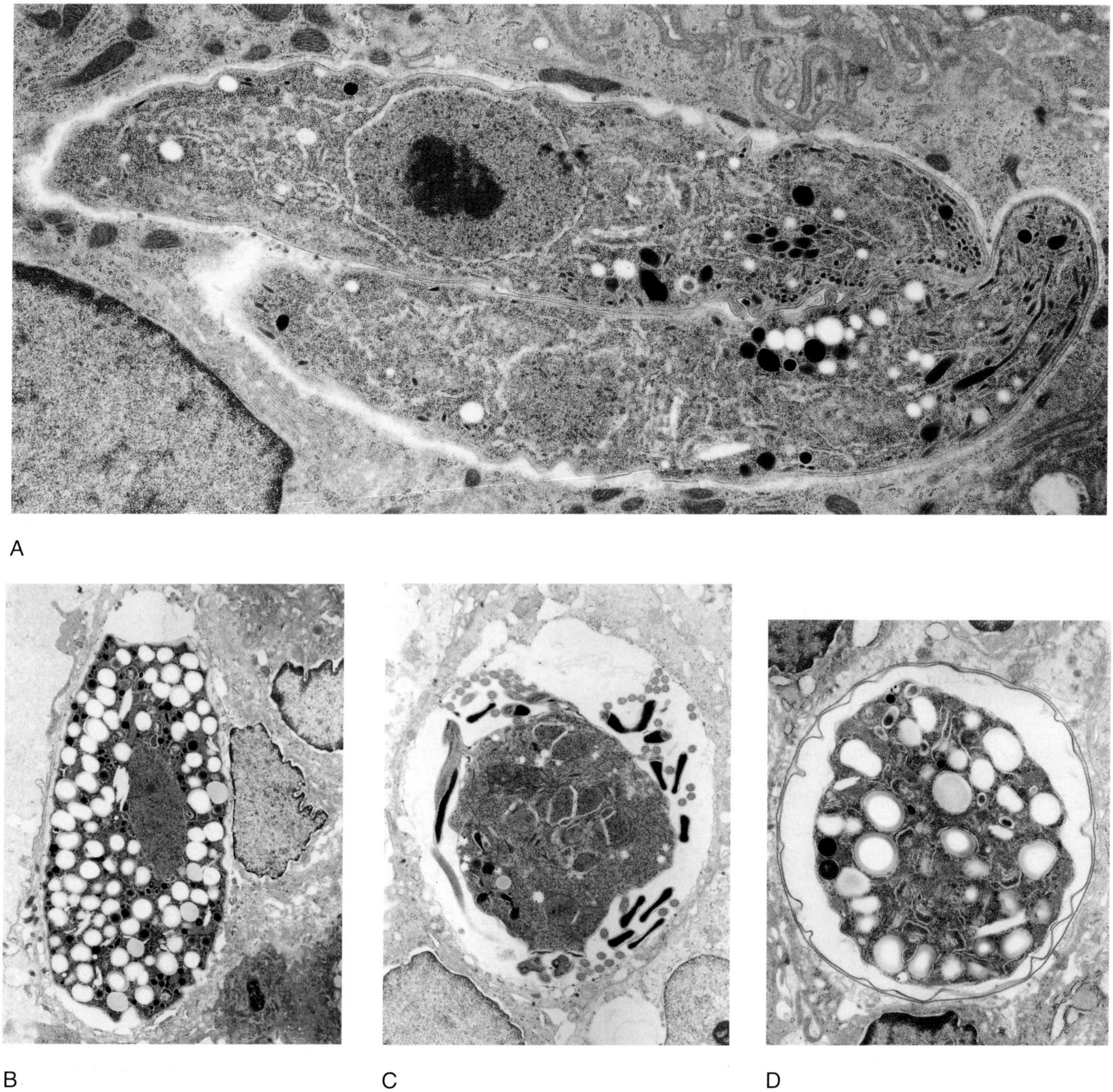

Figure 134–1. Transmission electron microscopy. (**A**) The anterior one third (*right field*) of two merozoites is rich in short and long electron-dense micronemes and rhoptries, respectively, plus clear and dense cytoplasmic granules. Note nucleus with prominent nucleolus (×12,000). (**B**) Intravacuolar macrogametocyte rich in clear (amylopectin) and dense granules (×5500). (**C**) Flagellated peripheral microgametes of a microgametocyte. Note the loose parasitophorous vacuole (×9200). (**D**) Maturing oocyst with trilaminar cell wall and amylopectin and dense bodies (×11,000).

slide is fixed with methanol for 1 min, air dried, stained with carbol-fuchsin (5 min), rinsed, decolorized with 1.5% hydrochloric acid/alcohol (1 min), counterstained with brilliant green (2 to 3 min), rinsed, dried, and examined under oil (100 × objective). The oocysts of both *Cryptosporidium* and *I belli* stain bright red on a green background. Although a critical comparison has not been made, modified acid-fast stained specimens are believed to be superior to fresh unstained specimens.[28] It is preferable to use wet preparations for examination of fresh material rather than permanent stained smears.

Concentration and flotation methods (zinc sulfate, formalin ethyl–acetate, polyvinyl alcohol, or sucrose), incubation at room temperature for a few days to permit maturation of oocysts (decreases the transparency of the ova's membrane), trichrome, fluorescent auramine–rhodamine, and acid-fast stains can all be used to enhance detection of the otherwise transparent spores. Flotation in sucrose solution preserves the oocyst morphology better than the other concentration methods.[20]

A stool aspirate obtained during lower intestinal endoscopy may contain unsporulated oocysts, while routine fecal samples may be negative. Duodenal aspirates are particularly good specimens for diagnosis, because of the relatively concentrated spores and clean background. Or, a duodenal string test can be used to retrieve spores.[17] The oocysts are concentrated in the mucus that adheres to the string and then stained with the modified acid-fast stain. Both types of specimens can be positive while stools are negative.

HISTOPATHOLOGY

When oocysts cannot be identified in stool or intestinal aspirate, or by string test, an upper intestinal endoscopy with biopsy is the diagnostic method of choice.[1,2,10,14]

Isosporiasis of the small intestine (duodenum through ileum) is accompanied by villus atrophy (shortening, blunting, fusion, and clubbing) and crypt hyperplasia/hypertrophy or elongation (Figure 134–2). The degree of mucosal atrophy can vary from mild through total flattening, which is spruelike in the most chronic cases. These architectural changes can be appreciated at screening magnification (2.5 to 4× objective) review of the biopsy.

Although helpful, biopsy orientation is not necessary, since enough of the tissue (usually several pieces are included in a single specimen) is invariably oriented adequately and the lesions are not usually strictly localized. These nonspecific architectural changes (basically similar for cryptosporidiosis and microsporidiosis) suggest screening the specimen at higher magnification (20 or 25× objective lenses). It is then that one can detect disorganization of the epithelium, loss of nuclear polarity, cell crowding, and cytoplasmic vesiculation or frank vacuolization. Secondary lysosomes may be prominent. In place of rows of tall columnar cells with prominent brush borders and basally placed nuclei are enterocytes that are cuboidal, flat, or pleomorphic. There can be marked dilation of vascular channels. The cellularity of the lamina propria is increased by a mixed infiltrate of neutrophils, plasma cells, lymphocytes, and characteristically, eosinophils. In HIV/AIDS patients, the infiltrate may not be as striking, because of the leukopenia. The degree of eosinophilia is not shared by cryptosporidial or microsporidial infection and can be quite dramatic. Chronicity can be associated with scarring of the lamina propria.

The histopathologic changes are more extensive than just the infected cells, suggesting that the parasite releases a toxic agent or stimulates a hypersensitivity reaction. Inflammatory cells sometimes occur between enterocytes. The developmental stages of *I belli* are in enterocytes located from the base of the crypts to the tips of the villi, are perinuclear, and often subnuclear. The small central nucleus is surrounded by the pale parasite cytoplasm. The parasites' relatively large size and location within loosely fitting parasitophorous vacuoles enhance identification. Although they may be detected at medium magnification (20 to 25× objectives), high-dry (40×) and even oil-immersion lenses (63 or 100×) may be necessary to identify the characteristic stages of the parasite. The infection can vary from either a few parasites, randomly distributed, to several parasites concentrated in relatively small areas of the biopsy specimen (more than one per cell). Of the three most common parasites causing diarrhea in AIDS patients, *I belli* can be the most difficult to detect and, as with all intestinal biopsies, more than one level (usually three), should be reviewed. Biopsy specimens have been negative when fecal samples are positive.

The addition of Alcian blue to the H&E stain darkens the parasites and enhances their appearance. The Giemsa stain, however, gives the best contrast. Schizonts are strongly periodic acid–Schiff positive, but so is the abundant mucin. Gomori's methenamine silver (GMS) silvers all stages of the parasite, especially enhancing the appearance of the granules but GMS silvers also mucin and lysosomes.

Parasites are better appreciated in plastic than paraffin sections. This is true for both toluidine blue and especially for the combined methylene blue azure II, basic fuchsin stain. Because of the osmium tetroxide postfixation, the lipid-rich vacuoles of the macrogamete are especially prominent.

THERAPY

The recommended treatment for all patients with isosporiasis is oral trimethaprim (160 mg) and sulfamethoxazole (800 mg) four times daily for 10 days. Response is usually within 48 hours.[16,25,26,31] It is even effective in treating the recurrences (about 50% after 1 week off therapy) that are common in patients with AIDS. Indefinite prophylaxis with either the same drug combination (three times per week) or pyrimethamine–sulfadoxine (25 and 500 mg) should be used.[13] Pyrimethamine alone (75 mg/day) has been successfully used to treat acute infection and 25 mg/day can be used for treating recurrences.

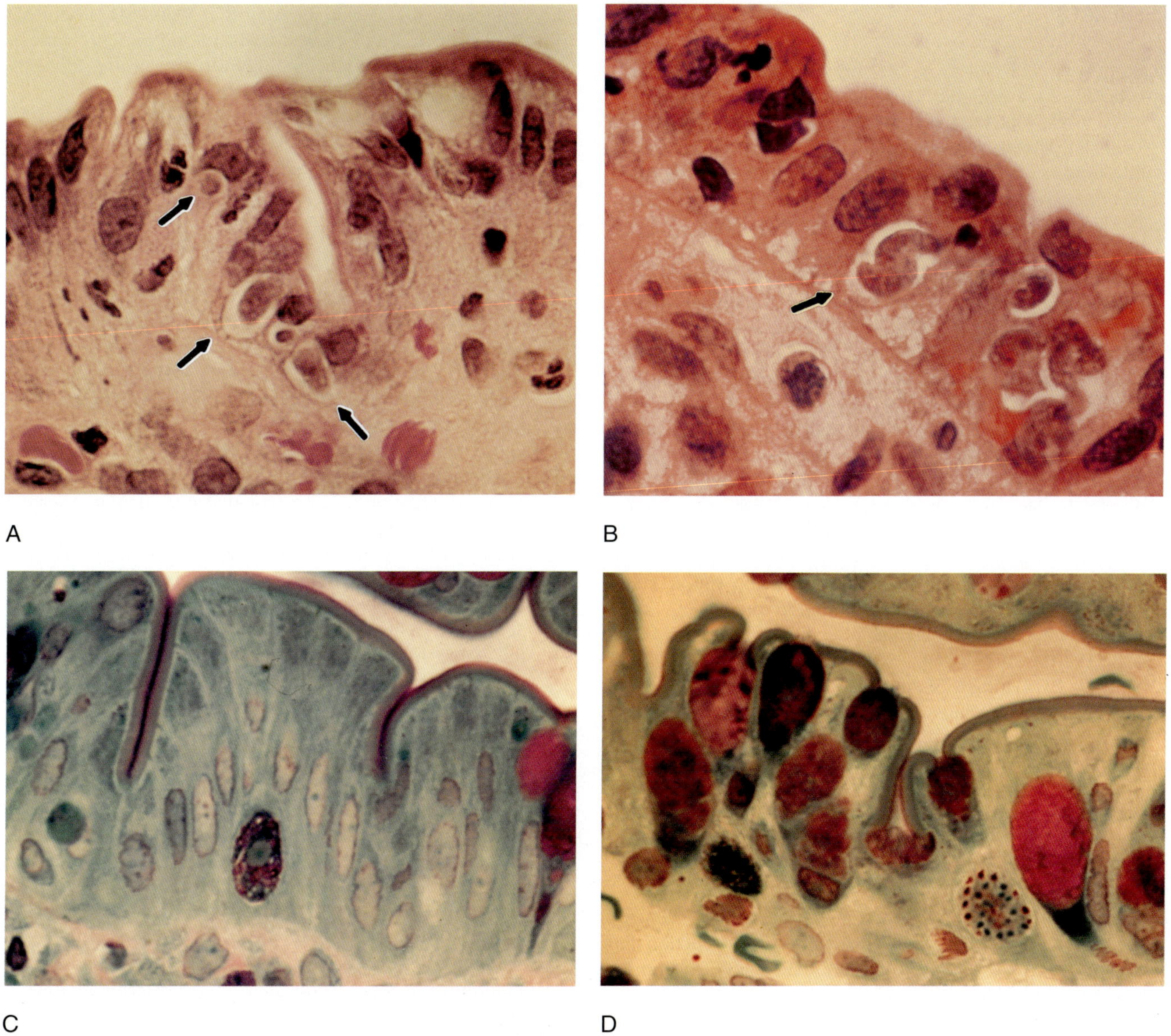

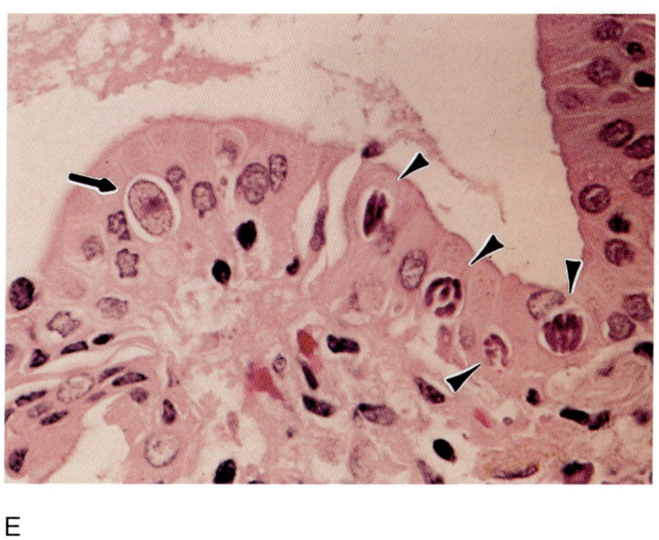

Figure 134–2. Light microscopy. (**A**), (**B**) Parasites develop in loose parasitophorous vacuoles located in the basal enterocyte cytoplasm. The single organisms are typically schizonts (**A, *arrows***) while the multiple ones are merozoites (**B, *arrow***), as in part (**A**). Note the cellular disarray and intraepithelial lymphocytes and debris [hematoxylin-eosin (H&E); (**A**), ×1000; (**B**), ×1100]. (**C**) Macrogametocyte with numerous lipid-rich granules that are prominent in the postosmicated tissue used for plastic section light microscopy. Note the basal position of the parasite, prominent nucleus and nucleolus, and intact brush border (semithin plastic section, "trichrome" stain, ×1000). (**D**) Microgametocyte with many osmiophilic peripheral microgametes (semithin plastic section, "trichrome" stain, ×1000). (**E**) Gallbladder rich in parasites in loose parasitophorous vacuoles: vacuolated macrogametocyte (*arrow*) and densely staining merozoites (*arrowheads*) (H&E, ×640).

REFERENCES

1. Brandborg LL, Goldberg SB, Breidenbach WC. Human coccidiosis—a possible cause of malabsorption. *N Engl J Med.* 1970;283:1306–1313.
2. Trier JS, Moxey PC, Schimmel EM, Robles E. Chronic intestinal coccidiosis in man: intestinal morphology and response to treatment. *Gastroenterology* 1974;66:923–935.
3. Belding DL. *Textbook of Parasitology.* New York: Appelton Century Crofts; 1965:232–234.
4. Faust EC, Russel PF, Jung RC. *Craig and Faust's Clinical Parasitology.* 8th ed. Philadelphia: Lee & Febiger; 1970: 179–183.
5. Hammond DM, Long PL, eds. *The Coccidia, Eimeria, Isospora, Toxoplasma, and Related Genera.* Baltimore: University Park Press; 1973.
6. Wenyon CM. Coccidiosis of cats and dogs and the status of the *Isospora* of man. *Ann Trop Med Parasitol.* 1923;17: 231–239.
7. Shaffer N, Moore L. Chronic travelers' diarrhea in a normal host due to *Isospora belli. J Infect Dis.* 1989;159: 596–597.
8. Hallak A, Yust I, Ratan Y, Adar U. Malabsorption syndrome, coccidiosis, combined immune deficiency, and fulminant lymphoproliferative disease. *Arch Intern Med.* 1982;142:196–197.
9. Webster BH. Human isosporiasis: a report of three cases with necropsy findings of one case. *Am J Trop Med Hyg.* 1957;6:86–89.
10. Liebman W, Thaler M, DeLorimier A, Brandborg LL, Goodman J. Intractable diarrhea of infancy due to intestinal coccidiosis. *Gastroenterology.* 1980;78:579–584.
11. Sorvillo F, Lieb L, Iwakoshi K, Waterman SH. *Isospora belli* and the acquired immunodeficiency syndrome. *N Engl J Med.* 1990;322:131–132.
12. DeHovitz JA, Pape JW, Boncy M, Johnson WD. Clinical manifestations and therapy of *Isospora belli* infection in patients with the acquired immunodeficiency syndrome. *N Engl J Med.* 1986;315:87–90.
13. Shein R, Gelb A. *Isospora belli* in a patient with acquired immunodeficiency syndrome. *J Clin Gastroenterol.* 1984; 4:525–528.
14. Forthal D, Guest S. *Isospora belli* enteritis in three homosexual men. *Am J Trop Med Hyg.* 1984;33:1060–1064.
15. Ros E, Fueyo J, Llach J, Moreno A, Latorre X. *Isospora belli* infection in patients with AIDS in Catalunya, Spain. *N Engl J Med.* 1987;317:246–247.
16. Pape JW, Verdier RI, Johnson WD. Treatment and prophylaxis of *Isospora belli* infection in patients with the acquired immunodeficiency syndrome. *N Engl J Med.* 1989;320:1044–1047.
17. Whiteside ME, Barkin JS, May RG, Weiss SD, Fischl MA, MacLeod CL. Enteric coccidiosis among patients with the acquired immunodeficiency syndrome. *Am J Trop Med Hyg.* 1984;33:1065–1072.
18. Peters CS, Kathpalia SB, Chittom-Swiatlo AL, Kallick CA, Sherer R, Kocka FE. *Isospora belli* and *Cryptosporidium* from a patient not suspected of having acquired immunodeficiency syndrome. *Diagn Microbiol Infect Dis.* 1987; 8:197–199.
19. Lumb R, Hardiman R. *Isospora belli* infection: a report of two cases in patients with AIDS. *Med J Aust.* 1991;155: 194–196.
20. Ma P, Kaufman D. *Isospora belli* diarrheal infection in homosexual men. *AIDS Res.* 1984;1:327–338.
21. Sauda FC, Zamarioli LA, Filho WE, Mello L de B. Prevalence of *Cryptosporidium* and *Isospora belli* among AIDS patients attending Santos Reference Center for AIDS, Sao Paulo, Brazil. *J Parasitol.* 1993;79:454–456.
22. Kobayashi LM, Kort MP, Berlin OG, Bruckner DA. *Isospora* infection in a homosexual man. *Diagn Microbiol Infect Dis.* 1985;3:363–366.
23. Shelhar KC, Ng KP, Rokiah I. Human isosporiasis in an AIDS patient—report of first case in Malaysia. *Med J Malaysia.* 1993;48:355–360.
24. Schmidt K, Johnston MRL, Stehbens WE. Fine structure of the schizont and merozoite of *Isospora* sp (Sporozoa: Eimeriidae) parasitic in *Gehyra variegata* (Dumeril and Bibron, 1836) (Reptilia: Gekkonidae). *J Protozool.* 1967; 14:602–608.
25. Soave R, Johnson WD Jr. *Cryptosporidium* and *Isopora belli* infections. *J Infect Dis.* 1988;157:225–229.
26. Kayembe K, Desmet P, Henry MC, Stoffels P. Diclazuril for *Isospora belli* infection in AIDS. *Lancet.* 1989;I:1397–1398.
27. Colebunders R, Lusakumuni K, Nelson A, et al. Persistent diarrhoea in Zairian AIDS patients: endoscopic and histologic study. *Gut.* 1988;29:1687–1691.
28. Ng E, Markell E, Fleming R, Fried M. Demonstration of *Isospora belli* by acid-fast stain in a patient with acquired immune deficiency syndrome. *J Clin Microbiol.* 1984;20: 384–386.
29. Restrepo C, Macher AM, Radany EH. Disseminated extraintestinal isosporiasis in a patient with acquired immune deficiency syndrome. *Am J Clin Pathol.* 1987;87: 536–542.
30. Michiels JF, Hofman P, Bernard E, et al. Intestinal and extraintestinal *Isospora belli* infection in an AIDS patient: a second case report. *Pathol Res Pract.* 1994;190:1089–1093.
31. Veldhuyzen van Zanten SJO, Lange JMA, Sauerwein HP, et al. Amprolium for coccidiosis in AIDS. *Lancet.* 1984;2: 345–346.

CHAPTER 135

Leishmaniasis

Ellen C. DeNigris, David F. Garvin, Max Grogl, and James D. Cotelingam

The study of the causes of things must be preceded by the study of things caused.

Hughlings Jackson (1835–1911)

DEFINITION

Leishmaniasis is infection by protozoans of the genus *Leishmania.* Leishmaniasis may involve skin, mucous membranes, mouth, oropharynx and viscera. Early descriptions of the parasite in cutaneous lesions were by Cunningham, Borovsky, and Wright between 1885 and 1903. The same year Leishman and Donovan separately described a visceral form, and identified organisms in spleen. In 1911, it was shown that lesions of cutaneous leishmaniasis followed the bites of sandflies and in 1942 *L donovani* was identified in volunteers experimentally subjected to the bite of the sandfly.[1] The leishmania are diverse.[2] Traditionally, they have been divided into two groups: cutaneous and visceral. Three species have been named as causes of "Old World" leishmaniasis—*L tropica, L major,* and *L aethiopia*—and two have been named for "New World" cutaneous leishmaniasis—*L braziliensis* complex and *L mexicana* complex.[3] Visceral leishmaniasis is caused by *L donovani* and this species is now subdivided into *L donovani donovani,* the cause of traditional visceral leishmaniasis; *L donovani infantum,* causing Mediterranean leishmaniasis; and *L donovani chagasi,*[3,4] which causes South American visceral leishmaniasis. This is a general definition, overlooking for instance many subspecies already named in the literature. The taxonomy of *Leishmania* is in a state of flux and identifying subspecies and correlating them with clinical and pathologic features is imperfect and confusing. Continuing research, however, will undoubtedly bring some order to current taxonomic confusion.

SYNONYMS

Leishmaniasis is known by many names. Synonyms for visceral leishmaniasis are "kala-azar" and "dum-dum fever."[1] Mucocutaneous leishmaniasis is known also as "espundia" but cutaneous leishmaniasis has the most names. These include Delhi boil, Baghdad boil, Chiclero's ulcer, bay sore, Oriental sore, Reta, year-long sore, Aleppo's boil, Biskara button, buton de Crete, forest yaws, and Pian bois.[5–7]

GEOGRAPHIC DISTRIBUTION

Leishmania are obligate intracellular parasites[8] endemic to the tropics of the Americas, parts of Asia,[9,10] Europe,[9,11] and tropical Africa north of the equator.[1,12] Transmission is on all continents excepting Antarctica and Australia (Figure 135–1). A few indigenous North American infections have been identified in Texas.[2,13] Most North Americans, however, have acquired their infections in warm climates, such as veterans of the Gulf war in the Middle East.[14–19] With increased travel to endemic areas,[20] diagnosis of leishmaniasis continues to challenge the clinician and pathologist.[2,11,21]

LIFE CYCLE

Leishmania live two quite separate lives—one in the sandfly, the other in mammals (Figure 135–2). In the sandfly, leishmania are in the promastigote stage, and

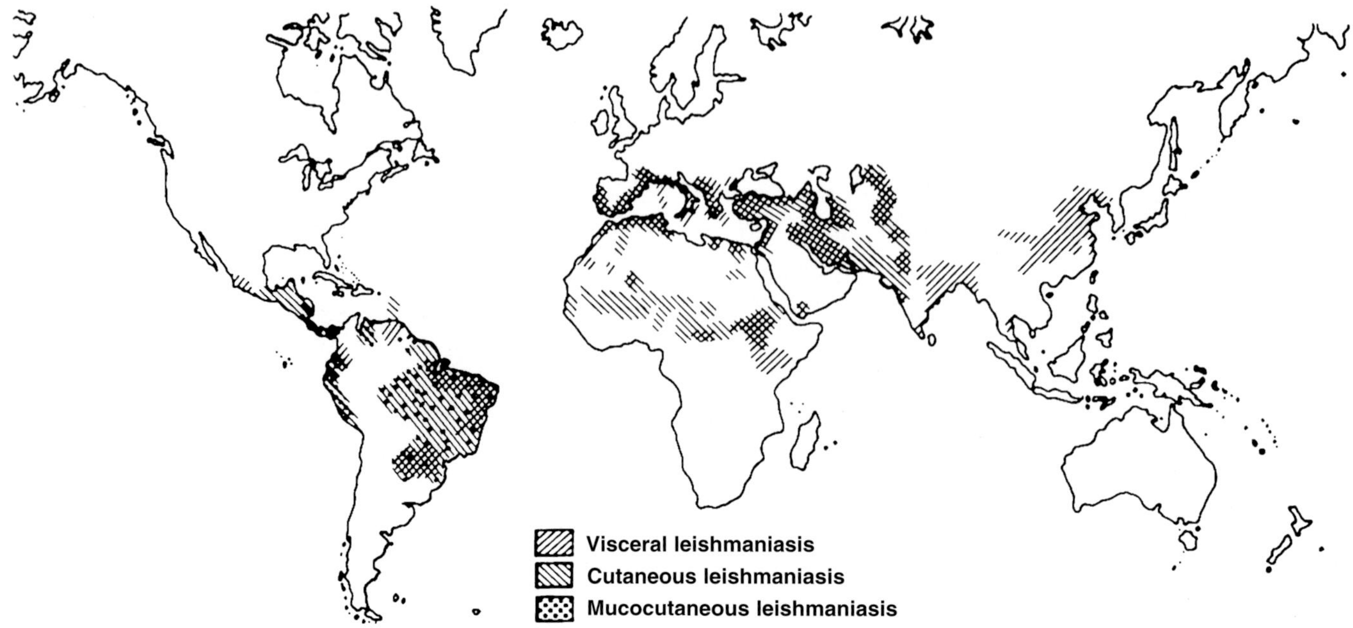

Figure 135–1. Geographic distribution of the three major forms of leishmaniasis. *(Contributed by Jeffrey Chulay and WB Saunders Co.)*

in man, the amastigote stage.[22] Promastigotes are in the digestive tract of the infected female sandfly, and also may be grown in tissue culture. Humans become infected when the organisms are injected from the proboscis of the sandfly while she takes blood.[3,23] After entering humans, the promastigotes seek out and enter phagocytic cells of the reticuloendothelial system,[17]

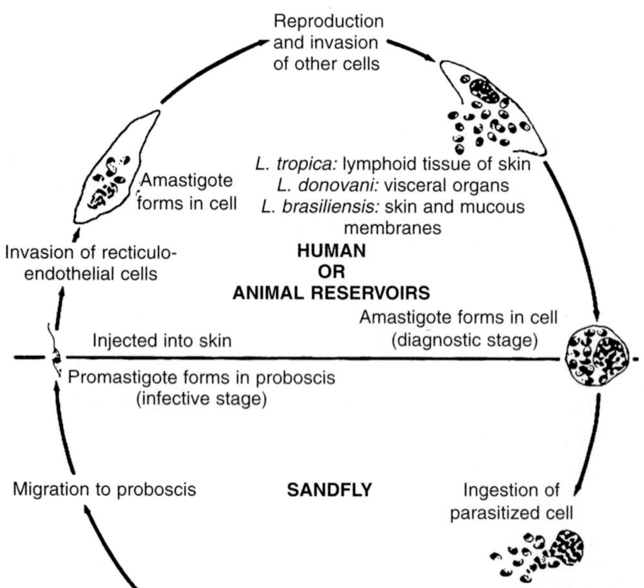

Figure 135–2. Life cycle of leishmaniasis. *(Contributed by Jeffrey Chulay and D. M. Melvin, Life Cycle Charts, CDC, Atlanta, Georgia.)*

transform into amastigotes, which have no external flagellae, then begin intracellular replication.[24] Up to 200 amastigotes have been in a single infected cell. Packed infected cells ultimately rupture, liberating organisms into surrounding tissue and into the circulation. Ingestion of amastigotes by the sandfly is followed by transformation, within the gut of the sandfly, to the flagellated promastigote form. Thereafter, organisms reproduce by binary fission, migrate to the pharynx and buccal cavity, and, finally, accumulate in the proboscis poised to infect another person.

EPIDEMIOLOGY

Vectors of leishmaniasis are female sandflies (Figure 135–3) of the genera *Phlebotomus* in the old world and *Lutzomyia* in the New World.[5,13] In Texas the reservoir is the wood rat and the vector is *Lutzomyia anthophora*.[2] Some rodents[18,25] and canines[12,22,26] also have leishmaniasis. Zoonotic cutaneous leishmaniasis has been reported in cats in Egypt[27] and the clinical manifestations resemble those in man.

Sandflies range from 1.5 to 2.5 mm long. Transmission of human leishmaniasis is accomplished by less than 10% of the 600 known species of sandflies.[1] Sandflies tend to be nocturnal and breed in dark moist environments. Following impregnation, the female fly stores sufficient sperm for fertilization throughout her life, usually a few weeks. The female fly must ingest blood for her eggs to mature. If the female fly ingests leishmania with her first blood meal she remains infectious throughout her life.

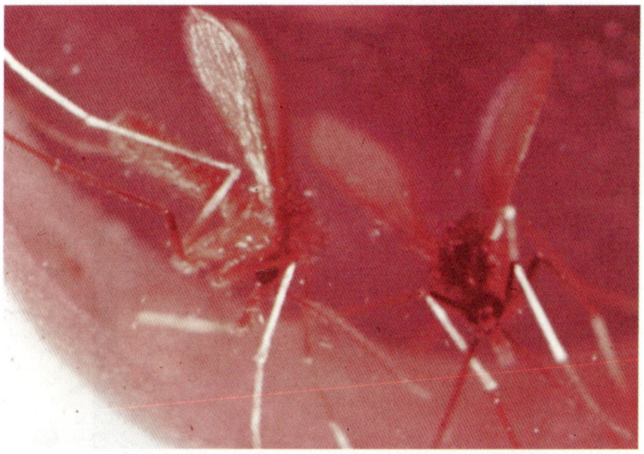

Figure 135–3. The female sandfly of the genus *Phlebotomus* in the Old World, and *Lutzomyia* in the New World infects humans and other reservoir hosts while ingesting blood.

MORPHOLOGY

Several species have been described. As already noted there are two morphologic forms. In the sandfly, the organism exists as the promastigote (leptomonad), and in tissue as the amastigote (leishmanial or aflagellar form).[22] Amastigotes are 2 to 4 μm, with a round to oval and often centrally located nucleus and a thin-walled external membrane. Lying tangentially or at right angles to the nucleus is the kinetoplast, a key diagnostic feature.

CLINICAL FEATURES

People of all ages and both genders may be infected. Clinical manifestations may be cutaneous, mucocutaneous, or systemic.[28]

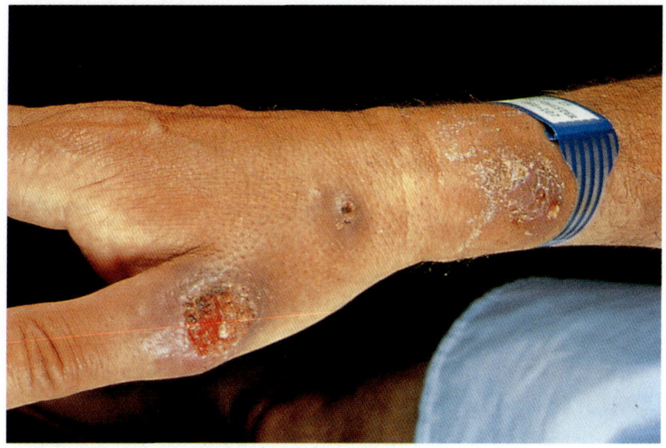

Figure 135–5. Cutaneous leishmaniasis with lymphocutaneous spread. The patient was in Honduras and bitten many times by a variety of insects. Biopsy revealed multiple intra- and extracellular leishmania.

Cutaneous Leishmaniasis

Four types of cutaneous leishmaniasis have been defined: acute, chronic, diffuse cutaneous, and post–kala-azar dermal leishmaniasis.[7] In acute leishmaniasis, a pruritic papule develops at the site of inoculation and becomes well developed in 2 to 8 weeks (Figure 135–4) but longer incubation periods have been observed.[19] Ulceration is followed by spontaneous healing[7] in 3 to 12 months. Ulcers are usually single, but may become multiple along lymphatic channels (Figure 135–5) or second lesions may develop on opposed surfaces—so-called "kissing" lesions. Some lesions are diffuse, papular, or verrucous (Figure 135–6). Any type of lesion may ulcerate. Satellite lesions may develop in lymph nodes draining the primary focus.[6]

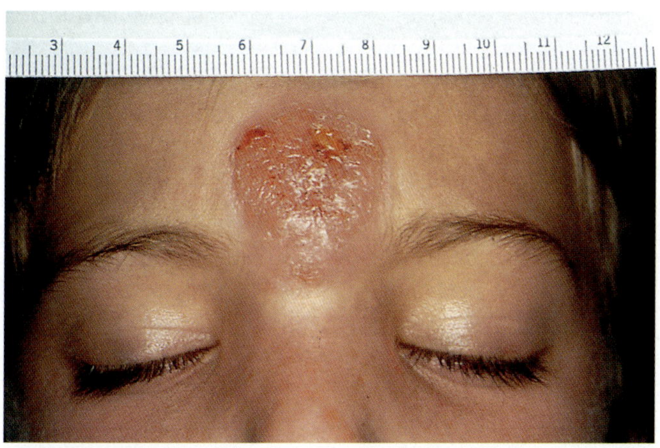

Figure 135–4. This well-developed lesion appeared on the forehead of a 7-year-old daughter of American missionaries living in northern Kenya.

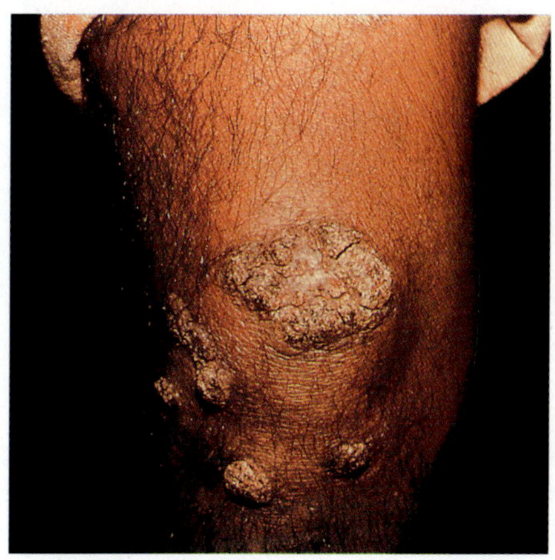

Figure 135–6. Multiple verrucous lesions are on the knee of a Brazilian man.

Chronic cutaneous leishmaniasis is rare. It may present as an acute lesion but then persist, resulting in a boggy erythematous plaque, which may linger for years, resolve, or recur.[7,13] In diffuse (disseminated) cutaneous leishmaniasis, the early lesion is a shiny, erythematous nodule. Multiple nodules aggregate and coalesce, forming plaques or continuous nodules. Dissemination occurs from these primary sites. Face, limbs, and buttocks may be involved. Lesions spread to, but do not generally extend across mucocutaneous borders.[29] In some patients, there is early infiltration of mucous membranes of the anterior nasal fossae. The hallmark of this form of leishmaniasis is the apparent lack of host response.[30] Microscopically, lesions reveal macrophages containing organisms with little or no lymphocyte response. Clinically, patients have cutaneous anergy with the Montenegro skin test.[30,31] Although lymphadenopathy is often present, visceral involvement is frequently absent. Occasionally, subcutaneous nodules with evidence of lymphatic invasion have been described radiating from a primary lesion in a "sporotrichoid" pattern.[18,32] This has been identified in both New World[33,34] and Old World strains.[35–38]

About 6% of patients treated for kala-azar develop skin lesions without a history of reexposure.[39] The lesions of post–kala-azar dermal leishmaniasis may present as hypopigmented macules and subsequently convert to firm nodules (Figures 135–7 and 135–8). Lesions frequently concentrate around mouth and nose but may develop on trunk and limbs. Post–kala-azar dermal leishmaniasis usually develops 1 to 5 years after onset of systemic disease.

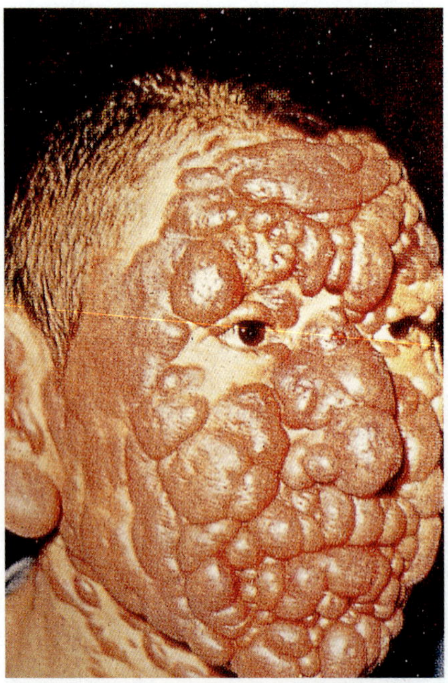

Figure 135–7. This patient has post–kala-azar dermal leishmaniasis. The nodules are composed of histiocytes containing many leishmania. Although the lesions resemble lepromatous leprosy the patient had no sensory loss. *(Contributed by Drs. R. E. Kuntz and R. H. Watten.)*

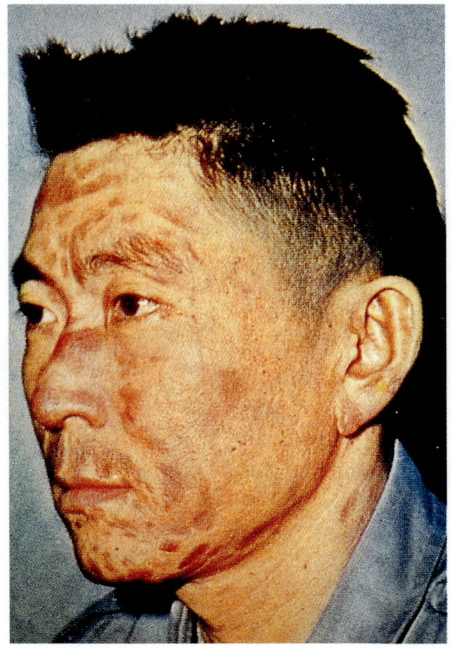

Figure 135–8. Same patient as Figure 135–7, but 2 years later—after completion of therapy. *(Contributed by Drs. R. E. Kuntz and R. H. Watten.)*

Mucocutaneous Leishmaniasis

In mucocutaneous leishmaniasis, cutaneous lesions are localized initially at the site of inoculation.[22] Organisms spread to mucous membranes usually involving first the nose (Figure 135–9), then oropharynx, larynx, lips, and, rarely, the lower eyelids. As lesions progress, inflammatory changes may supervene and acquire a granulomatous component.[6] Tissue destruction and disfigurement may result from complications such as suppurative bacterial infection (Figure 135–10).

Visceral Leishmaniasis

Visceral leishmaniasis characteristically has a latent period of 4 to 6 months before clinical onset but some patients have had delays of up to 10 years, and may pose a diagnostic dilemma, especially when presenting with fever of unknown origin.[40] These delayed manifestations apparently depend on host–parasite interactions.

The clinical features of visceral leishmaniasis include irregular fever, hepatosplenomegaly, pancytopenia, hypergammaglobulinemia, and progressive wasting

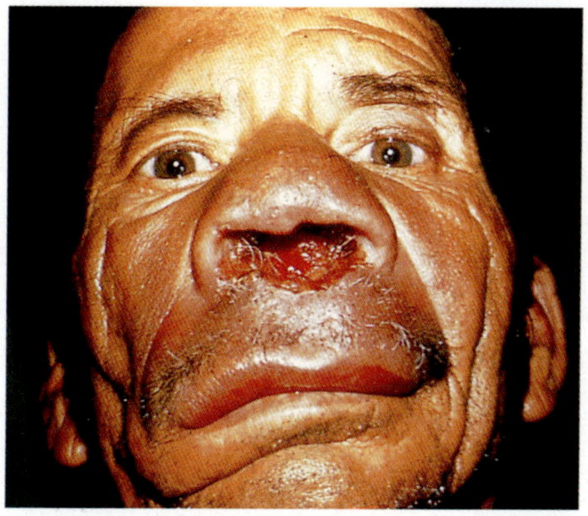

Figure 135–9. Destruction of the nasal septum with deformity of the nose and lips in this Brazilian man with mucocutaneous leishmaniasis. *(Photograph by Ronald C. Neafie.)*

(Figure 135–11). Lymphadenopathy is more common in Africa and China.[6,25,41–44] Death ensues if untreated.

Symptoms of visceral leishmaniasis may be acute or chronic. When acute, patients present with episodes of chills, sweats, and a daily fever spike. The chronic form is insidious, presenting with weight loss, low-grade or persistent fever, and sometimes with left upper quadrant pain from splenomegaly. In addition, anemia, leukopenia, and thrombocytopenia have been documented.[9,16,45] Chung and Chang documented the improvement of pancytopenia in patients undergoing splenectomy.[46] Unusual symptoms associated with visceral leishmaniasis have been reported. Neurologic deficits and the Guillain–Barré syndrome have been described.[47] Also described are abnormalities of nerve conduction and axonal degeneration and demyelinization in patients with visceral leishmaniasis.[48] Their complaints resolved when treated with antileishmanial drugs. Histologically, peripheral nerve involvement was demonstrated by Satti et al[49] in a patient with cutaneous leishmaniasis. A patient with post–kala-azar anterior uveitis was reported by El-Hassan et al.[50]

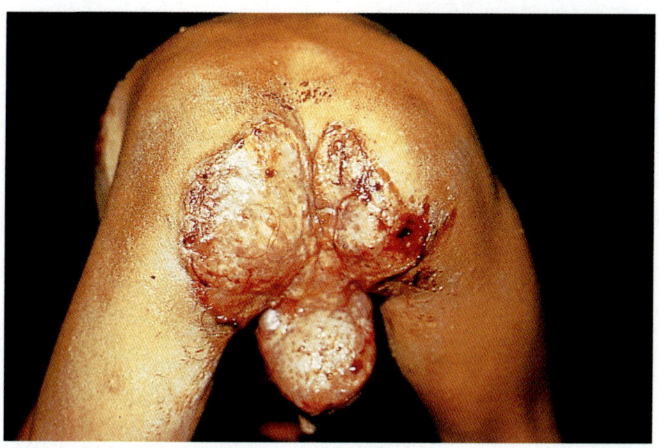

Figure 135–10. Extensive destruction of perianal skin and posterior aspect of scrotum in a Brazilian child with mucocutaneous leishmaniasis. *(Photograph by the late David T. Purtilo, MD.)*

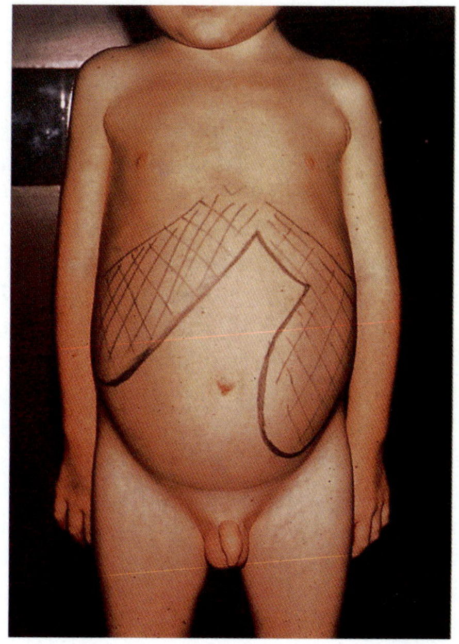

Figure 135–11. Hepatosplenomegaly in a boy with visceral leishmaniasis. *(Photograph by Ronald C. Neafie.)*

Immunosuppression is an additional risk to patients who have been previously infected, and disease reactivation is listed along with other opportunistic infections in patients with the acquired immune deficiency syndrome (AIDS).[9,51–57] Patients immunosuppressed after organ transplantation or following high-dose corticosteroids have also developed visceral leishmaniasis years after exposure.[58,59]

There are numerous reports of atypical clinical presentations. A systemic form of leishmaniasis caused by *L tropica* has been described in soldiers returning from Operation Desert Storm. They have presented with a variety of symptoms, including fever, fatigue, malaise, and diarrhea, up to 7 months after their return. Hepatosplenomegaly has not been a significant feature. The diagnosis is best made with biopsies of lymph node or bone marrow. Since the clinical picture is of a systemic disease, but not characteristic of visceral leishmaniasis, this form of leishmaniasis has been named "viscerotropic."[17,60,61] Badaro et al[62] described a group of Brazilian children infected with *L donovani* who demonstrated a prolonged, mild subclinical form of leishmaniasis. There have been previous reports in which lymphadenopathy was the only clinical manifestation[33,64–67] and there is a report of tonsillar leishmaniasis with lymph node involvement.[68]

PATHOLOGY

Acute and Chronic Cutaneous Leishmaniasis

The primary lesion of cutaneous leishmaniasis is on areas of exposed skin. Diagnosis is by identifying leishmania in tissue sections, direct smear, or by culture.[69] Various classifications and terms have been proposed to describe the evolution of cutaneous lesions. Early there is hyperkeratosis, parakeratosis, follicular plugging, basal cell degeneration, epidermal atrophy, acanthosis, pseudoepitheliomatous hyperplasia, and occasionally intraepidermal abscesses. At this stage, many organisms are both intra- and extracellular. Leishmania (amastigotes) can be identified with routine hematoxylin-eosin (H&E) stains and with Giemsa stains.[70] Leishmania are 3 μm in diameter, round to oval, have a distinct cell membrane, and a nucleus and kinetoplast in the cytoplasm. An infiltrate of histiocytes and mononuclear macrophages is in the dermis with a few accompanying lymphocytes and plasma cells.[13] As the host responds and immunity develops, the epidermis becomes increasingly hyperplastic and necrosis of the dermis ensues with subsequent ulceration. With time, lesions become granulomatous; that is, epithelioid cells and Langhans' giant cells become increasingly prominent.[70,71] Heavily infected macrophages, macrophages with few leishmania, and macrophages undergoing lysis have all been studied by electron microscopy.[72] The granulomatous reaction signals an abrupt decline in the number of organisms and soon organisms become impossible to find (Figure 135–12).[6] Because of the progression of the reaction from anergy to hypersensitivity, leishmaniasis has been compared to leprosy.[22] Many organisms are eliminated by necrosis and sloughing,[71,73] which is not so in leprosy where organisms are destroyed by delayed hypersensitivity, ie, intracellular killing when the patient's reaction has reached a point of sufficient hypersensitivity.

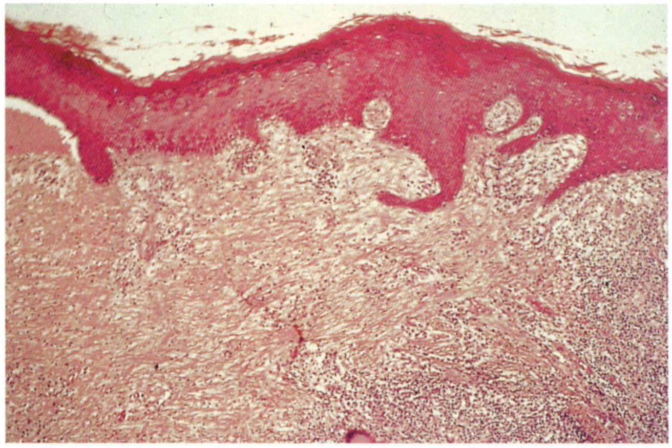

Figure 135–12. Healing skin from a patient with cutaneous leishmaniasis. Acanthotic epidermis covers a scarred dermis. Langhans' giant cells, here in the lower dermis, signal the hypersensitivity reaction (H&E, ×35).

Disseminated Anergic Cutaneous Leishmaniasis

The reaction demonstrated by lesions in disseminated cutaneous and recurrent cutaneous leishmaniasis tends to be anergic. Dissemination is slow, and lesions do not ulcerate, involve the viscera, or spontaneously heal.[31] In most patients the disease begins as a single nodule. Other nodules develop nearby and slowly the skin becomes diffusely nodular (Figure 135–13).[6] Histologically, the epidermis is intact, but atrophic. Immediately beneath the basal layer is a layer free of inflammatory cells. This is the "clear zone"—a characteristic feature of anergy in infectious dermatoses. The underlying dermis is thickened by many closely packed macrophages containing enormous numbers of leishmania (Figure 135–14).[29] There may be a few lymphocytes and plasma cells. The lesions of recividans (recurrent leishmaniasis after treatment) may have a similar histologic pattern or be more "tuberculoid" with epithelioid cell granulomas. These lesions contain lymphocytes, plasma cells, Langhans' giant cells, and epithelioid cells. Parasites are few, and healing occurs with fibrosis.

Post–Kala-Azar Dermal Leishmaniasis

Some patients who recover from kala-azar develop nodular cutaneous lesions that grossly and microscopically resemble closely those of disseminated anergic

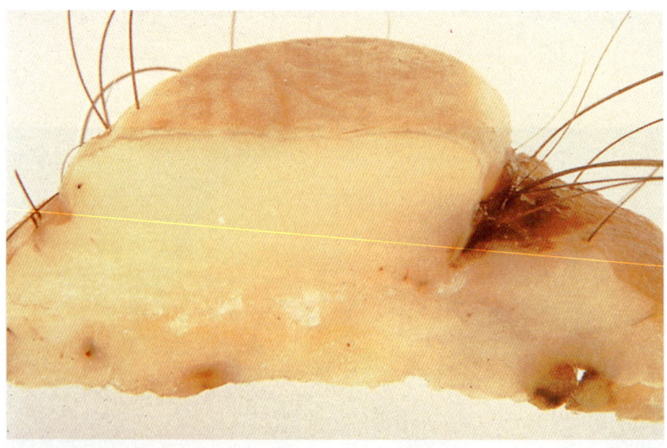

Figure 135–13. Enlarging nodule in a patient with disseminated anergic cutaneous leishmaniasis. As in patients with post–kala-azar dermal leishmaniasis the reaction is characterized by a stretched and thinned epidermis, a sub-basal cell clear zone, and closely packed histiocytes containing many leishmania. The cut surface of the nodule is pale, yellow, and translucent, characteristic of a collection of histiocytes. *(Photograph by Daniel H. Connor, MD.)*

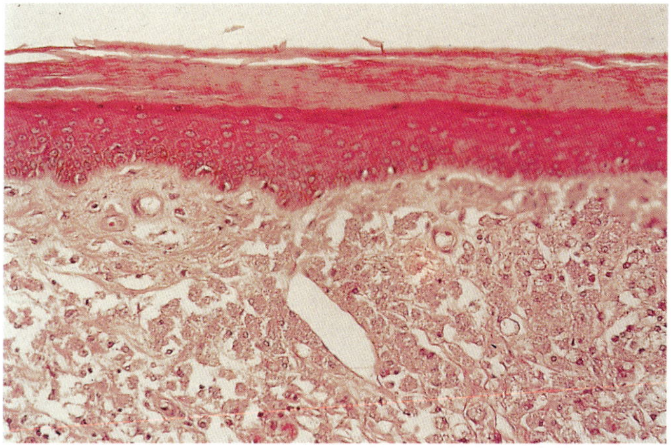

Figure 135–14. Disseminated anergic cutaneous leishmaniasis. There are closely packed histiocytes containing leishmania. The overlying epidermis is thin, "ironed out" and the clear zone is immediately beneath the basal layer (H&E, ×145).

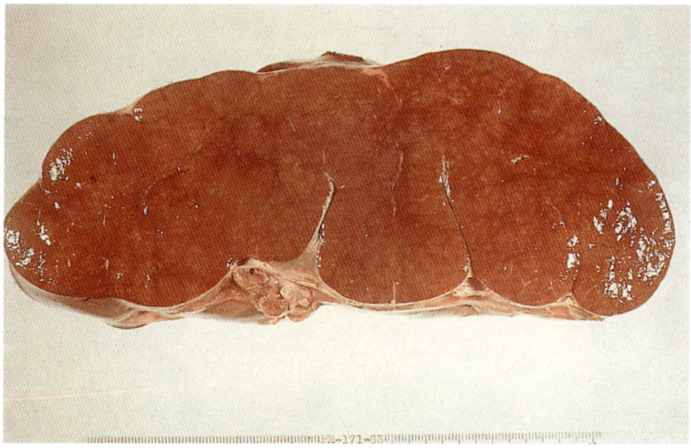

Figure 135–15. Splenomegaly (970 g) in a 7-year-old African girl (Atesot tribe) who died of visceral leishmaniasis. *(Photograph by Daniel H. Connor, MD.)*

cutaneous leishmaniasis. Numerous parasite-laden macrophages are in the dermis, and lymphocytes and plasma cells may be scattered throughout.[6]

Mucocutaneous Leishmaniasis

Mucocutaneous leishmaniasis is generally characterized by chronic inflammation and slowly progressive necrotizing granulomas. The inflammatory infiltrate is comprised of lymphocytes, plasma cells, macrophages, epithelioid cells, and a few scattered Langhans' giant cells.[6]

Visceral Leishmaniasis

Organs of the reticuloendothelial system, especially liver, bone marrow, and spleen, are most heavily infected in visceral leishmaniasis; the leishmania are concentrated in phagocytic cells—Kupffer's cells of liver and phagocytic cells of bone marrow and spleen.[67] In severe infections virtually every organ may be parasitized. Splenomegaly is common, and spleens may weigh up to 2000 g, even in pediatric patients (Figure 135–15). The splenic capsule may be thickened and areas of infarction are common. The cut surface is congested, beefy red, and has a firm but friable parenchyma. Microscopically, histiocytes packed with organisms expand the red pulp.[6,22] The vascular spaces are dilated and engorged with blood. Fibrosis is usually absent. Splenic follicies are atrophic. Plasma cells are increased.

The liver is also enlarged and congested. The capsule is smooth and the cut surface may be yellow-brown and have a "nutmeg" pattern. Microscopically, Kupffer's cells are prominent and packed with leishmania (Figure 135–16). Sinusoids are congested and hepatocytes atrophic. Fibrosis is generally absent but mild accumulations of reticulin may be identified.[6,22] There are reports of hepatic fibrosis associated with visceral leishmaniasis that resolves with treatment.[74,75]

Changes in the bone marrow may be pronounced. As in other tissues, there is a proliferation of the phagocytic cells. In long bones, fatty marrow is often replaced by congested hematopoietic tissue containing reticulonendothelial cells with leishmania. Plasma cells may be increased. When hematopoietic tissue is replaced by macrophages containing leishmania, the patient becomes pancytopenic.[6,22] As in other forms of leishmaniasis, organisms are abundant in early stages of infection but decrease with time as the patient's reaction progresses to one of hypersensitivity.

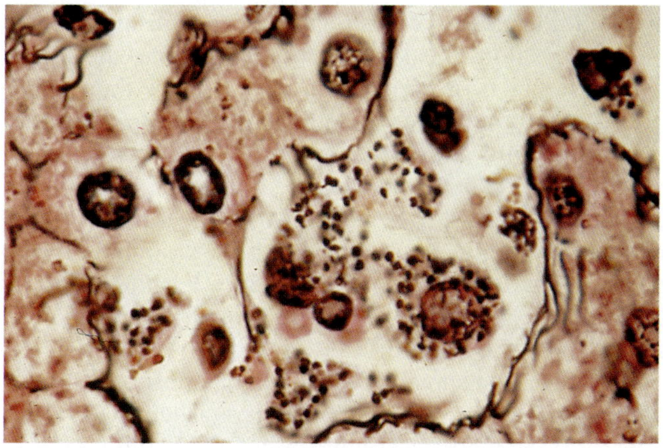

Figure 135–16. Wilder's reticulum stain of a liver biopsy specimen obtained from a patient with visceral leishmaniasis. Leishmania appear as small black dots within Kupffer's cells (×440).

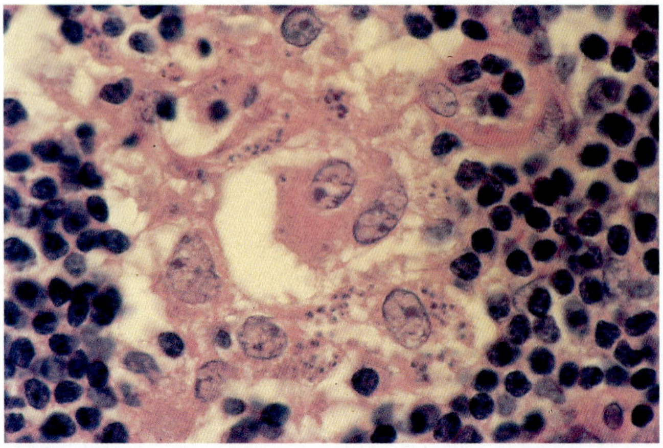

Figure 135–17. Granuloma in lymph node. Many leishmania are within histiocytes (H&E, ×400).

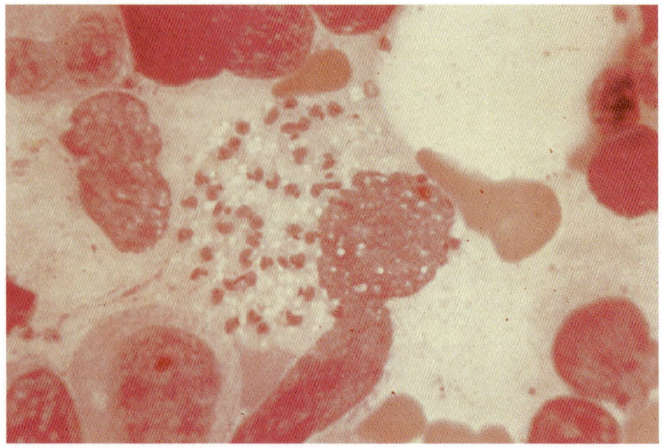

Figure 135–18. Leishmania in a touch preparation of spleen (Giemsa, ×1000).

Changes in the lymph nodes have been well documented. Affected nodes are enlarged and their cut surfaces vary from homogenous and firm, to soft, red, and hemorrhagic. The architecture may be partially or totally effaced by macrophages containing organisms. Giant cells may be present (Figure 135–17).[65] There are occasional focal necroses. When parasites escape from macrophages they are extracellular.[63] Lymphoid hyperplasia may also be present. Cultures of lymph nodes should be performed routinely on enlarged lymph nodes in patients with suspicious clinical features, since inflammatory changes with granulomas are commonly nonspecific.

Cytopathology

The definitive diagnosis of leishmaniasis can be made by identifying organisms in aspirates, in smears, and in touch preparations of biopsy specimens.[6,16,76,77] Giemsa staining after alcohol fixation is standard for the cytologic diagnosis of leishmaniasis. Organisms appear round or oval in smears. Although amastigotes are intracellular, artifacts of preparation may displace them. The nucleus is in the posterior half of the organism, and the kinetoplast and axoneme anteriorly.[77] Amastigotes are 4 μm long by 2 to 3 μm wide. Reticulum stains, such as a Wilder's reticulum, enhance the appearance of the nucleus and kinetoplast. The most rewarding "hunting ground" for leishmania in cutaneous leishmaniasis is beneath the margin of an ulcer. Thus, the diagnosis is made only when the affected area has been well sampled. Visceral leishmaniasis can be diagnosed by identifying amastigotes in smears of spleen (Figure 135–18), liver, or bone marrow. Splenic puncture should be done with caution and only when the diagnosis cannot be made by other techniques.[41,77] Needle aspirates of lymph node are also done to establish the diagnosis. Smears are scanned at 10× to locate regions of high yield such as granulomas and inflamed areas. These areas are then scanned at 40× to identify amastigotes. Final identification is done with the oil lens to identify the three essential structures by light microscopy: the cell membrane, the nucleus, and the kinetoplast (Figure 135–19).[77]

ELECTRON MICROSCOPY

Electron microscopic studies (Figure 135–20) have demonstrated amastigotes in two distinct regions: 1) in the macrophage, within a parasitophorous vacuole containing three to nine organisms[27,66] and 2) singly in the

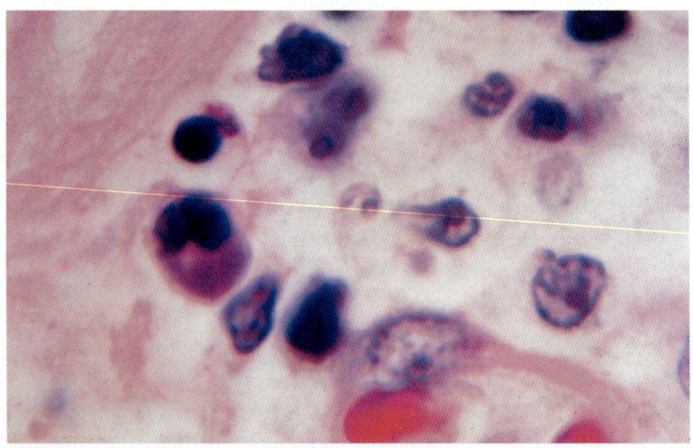

Figure 135–19. Biopsy specimen from the margin of an ulcerated cutaneous lesion. There are two leishmania in the cytoplasm of the histiocyte—one is in the plane of focus. Note the organism's distinct cell membrane and the darkly stained nucleus and kinetoplast—essential features for identifying leishmania in tissue sections (H&E, ×2160).

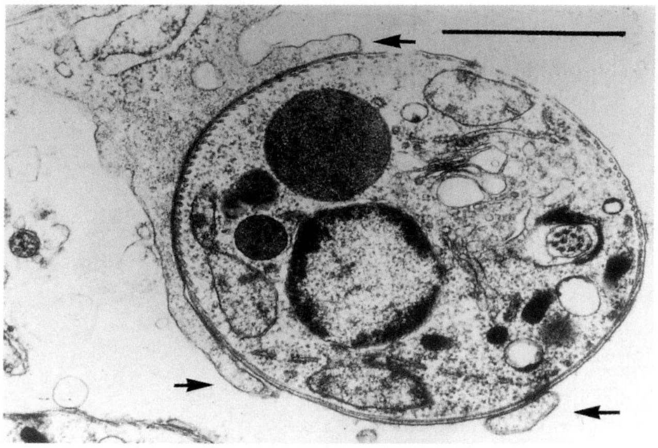

Figure 135–20. Electron micrograph of *L mexicana mexicana*—amastigote entering a macrophage. The macrophage has extended pseudopodia around the amastigote (*arrows*). Bar is 1 μm. *(Contributed by J. Alexander, University of Strathclyde, Glasgow, Scotland.)*

cytoplasm surrounded by two triple-layered unit membranes. The nucleus is round. The kinetoplast, which is the diagnostic organelle, is rod shaped.[13,28,64,66] Ultrastructure of the promastigotes reveals a characteristic target-shaped basal body. Occasionally a flagellum is continuous with the basal body.[66]

DIFFERENTIAL DIAGNOSIS

Leishmania identified microscopically within macrophages may resemble other infectious agents and especially they need to be distinguished from *Toxoplasma gondii* and *Histoplasma capsulatum,* which are about the same size and shape.[66] Fungal stains help identify *H capsulatum* (or exclude it) and neither of the two tissue forms of *T gondii* (bradyzoites and tachyzoites) has a kinetoplast. Furthermore each of these two protozoans (*Leishmania* and *Toxoplasma*) and *Histoplasma* has distinct features by electron microscopy. Other granulomatous diseases, including tuberculosis and sarcoidosis, may also resemble leishmaniasis but rarely present a problem in differential diagnosis. Identification of leishmania histologically or by culture is essential for diagnosis.

IMMUNOLOGY

Leishmaniasis produces clinical and histologic manifestations that depend on host response. Cutaneous leishmaniasis is a spectrum ranging from anergy to hypersensitivity.[36] Although a continuum, this spectrum has been divided into four parts that include 1) histiocytic accumulation of leishmania, 2) necrosis, 3) intracellular lysis of parasites, and 4) granulomas—a clear marker of cell-mediated hypersensitivity.[78] Hypersensitivity reactions are consequences of humoral and cell-mediated immune interactions and these depend on the species of leishmania.[78,79] Most believe the state of the immune system determines the response. Expatriates, who are not generally immune, for instance, often develop severe and disseminated disease.[38,80] In their report from Saudi Arabia, Melha et al[80] found that children under the age of 2 years had a more severe clinical course than adults, and they thought this may relate to lower levels of immunity.

The clinical and histologic presentation of cutaneous leishmaniasis in Saudi Arabia differs from the traditional presentation in the Middle East. The differences could be variations in host response and from different antigens in the Saudi organism.[36] Similarly, cutaneous lesions caused by *L infantum* (previously known to cause only visceral leishmaniasis) have been documented.[81] Improved nutrition, however, has led to a decrease in local incidence. The Saudi organisms persisted in a human treated for cutaneous lesions[32] and have persisted also in mice resistant to leishmania.[82] This may explain recurring manifestations in previously treated patients who become immunosuppressed.

In Central America exposure to one leishmania confers immunity against subsequent infections by different species. The Panamanian strain of leishmania conferred immunity to *L mexicana,* but this immunity was not reciprocal. Incomplete cross-reactivity between *L tropica major* and *L tropica minor* in Central Asia has long been recognized.[83] This "one-way immunity" is probably a consequence of one species having antigens that are common to both, while the other species has only a single set of antigens. Furthermore patients recovered from Oriental sore (*L tropica*) were immune to challenge by *L mexicana,* which supports the theory of conferred immunity.[83]

In disseminated cutaneous leishmaniasis, the clinical and pathologic manifestations are probably from defective host immunity.[30] If true, these mechanisms may be similar to those governing the host response in visceral leishmaniasis.

There are various explanations for the host response in visceral leishmaniasis. One possibility is interaction of humoral antibodies alongside cell-mediated immunity when lymphocytes and plasma cells are in excess,[78] although a significant role for antibodies in producing long-term humoral immunity is doubtful.

Of importance in host response are T cells. T cells are activated and produce various substances, including lymphokines, to aid in the defense against infection.[8,84] CD4+ T cells, particularly those producing interferon gamma (IFN-γ), are important in establishing host resistance (Th1 cells), and those producing interleukin-4 (IL-4) are associated with disease progression (Th2 cells).[85–88] Subsets of CD4+ and CD8+ T cells have been classified by their cytokine mRNA and products. Populations of T cells are in lesions of American cutaneous leishmaniasis (self-healing) that differ from T cells in diffuse cutaneous leishmaniasis (progressive disease).[88] The macrophage is another essential element in host response. Phagocytosis, followed by intracellular destruction, and finally lysis of the macrophage itself is an alternate mechanism of leishmanial destruction. Just before lysis, the macrophage comes into contact with plasma cells and is then engulfed by other granular macrophages.[72]

Even with these mechanisms in place, some patients develop manifestations of progressive (anergic) leishmaniasis including visceral leishmaniasis and disseminated cutaneous leishmaniasis, while others develop hypersensitivity as in mucocutaneous leishmaniasis.[17,69,89] Since host response to leishmania is mediated by T cells and T-cell-derived substances directed at infected macrophages, the absence of these mechanisms may promote chronicity and when untreated, death.[90] In some patients, leishmanial parasites interact with the immune system and modulate T-cell function[91] and visceral spread may complicate those with T-cell dysfunction.[51,55,56,58] Natural killer cell activity is deficient in some patients with visceral leishmaniasis.[92] Suppressor cell activity has been described also in diffuse cutaneous leishmaniasis.[93] IFN-γ appears to be important in activating macrophages to destroy intracellular parasites.[94–96] In vitro T cells from patients with kala-azar are unresponsive when stimulated with leishmanial antigen (*L donovani*). Responsiveness was restored, however, after chemotherapy.[90] This phenomenon is associated with deficiency of IFN-γ and IL-2[97,98] and Carvalho et al[44] have shown that recently infected children with absent response to IFN-γ had a high probability (67%) of developing visceral leishmaniasis. Children with positive blastogenic response to IFN-γ remained asymptomatic or developed a self-healing subclinical infection. It is clear therefore that adequate immunity is crucial in determining clinical manifestations.

LABORATORY DIAGNOSIS

A long-standing method of diagnosing cutaneous leishmaniasis has been the Montenegro skin test (Figure 135–21).[6] Leishmanial antigen is injected intradermally. The antigen has not yet been standardized so variation in results can be expected. A positive reaction occurs within 48 to 72 hours as a discrete area of erythema and induration measuring a minimum of 5.0 mm. A positive test indicates hypersensitivity to leishmanial antigen in an immunologically competent host.[77,99,100] Skin tests, however, do not distinguish between current and prior infection, nor do they aid in the diagnosis of an active lesion.[77,101] Reports of percent positivity of the skin test range from 65% to 92%.[100,102] Skin tests are negative in patients with disseminated cutaneous leishmaniasis and when the immune system is deficient or suppressed.

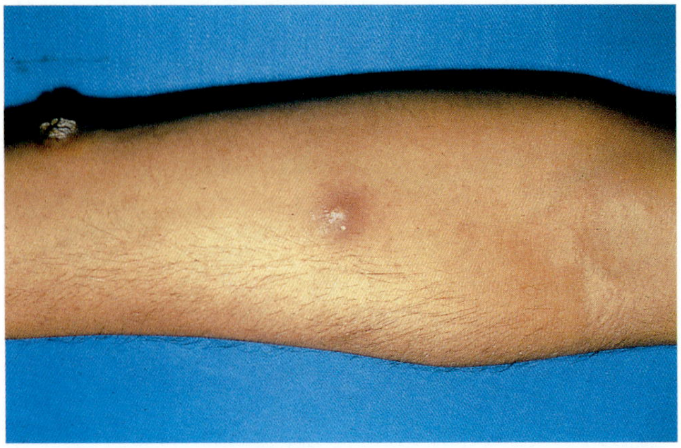

Figure 135–21. Positive Montenegro skin test on the arm of a Brazilian child. The hypersensitivity reaction faces the camera. The primary cutaneous lesion is on the margin of the wrist at the left. *(Photograph by Ronald C. Neafie.)*

Widely used for in vitro culture of leishmania is "triple N" medium of Novy, McNeal, and Nicolle.[19,22,40,102] Another is Schneider's Drosophila medium.[51,99] More recently, a modified "triple N" monophasic media or biphasic (solid blood agar slant in tubes with a condensation overlay) has also become available.[77] Organisms are obtained by brushing or scraping the center of a lesion or the margin of an ulcer. In addition, punch or incisional biopsy specimens and fine-needle aspirations are used to isolate organisms. Antibiotics are added to prevent bacterial overgrowth.[77,102] Promastigotes may be seen as early as the first day or as late as 4 to 5 days after inoculation.

To obtain a rapid diagnosis, an alcohol-fixed Wright–Giemsa stained touch preparation of tissue is useful if parasites are numerous.[102] Leishmania are in blood smears in up to 50% of patients in coinfection with HIV-1. These patients had high parasitemia.[103] Monoclonal antibody also aids in diagnosis when aspirated or biopsied tissues are available. According to Anthony et al,[104] genus-specific monoclonal antibody (83-J3D2) in an indirect immunofluorescent antibody assay is directed against leishmanial amastigotes, and can distinguish amastigotes in both contaminated and clean specimens, as well as make a diagnosis in some patients where histopathology and culture failed to reveal organisms.[104]

Serologic techniques have long been used to identify circulating antibodies, particularly in those with visceral leishmaniasis. The more commonly utilized tests are an enzyme-linked immunosorbent assay (ELISA) and indirect fluorescent antibody (IFA) test. These tests are not readily available in clinical laboratories. ELISA is often used to diagnose visceral leishmaniasis. Promastigotes grown in culture are the source of antigen. There is low specificity and possibly cross-reaction with antigens of *Trypanosoma cruzi*. The IFA test is used to monitor therapy.[45,77] Promastigotes from culture or amastigotes from infected animals are the source of antigen. The direct agglutination test uses promastigotes treated with trypsin, fixed and then stained with Coomasie brilliant blue. A sharp blue dot is interpreted as a negative test. This test compares well with both the ELISA and IFA techniques.[77,105] Current research on leishmaniasis includes the use of DNA probes and polymerase chain reaction (PCR), mechanisms to distinguish current and past infections, to determine the genomic or molecular basis of virulence polymorphisms (ability of a particular species to produce more than one clinical syndrome),[4] and molecular probes to identify resistant or susceptible hosts.[106]

One DNA probe specific to members of the *L donovani* complex is the Lmet 2 sequence, which has been used in PCR amplification. Work is also being done in kinetoplast–DNA.[98] The LPG surface glycolipid molecule of *L tropica major* also may be a virulence factor because it protects the organism by a number of mechanisms, including prevention of insertion of the membrane attack complex into the membrane and preventing promastigote degradation within the macrophages.[106]

Current research includes work on the genomic/ molecular composition of leishmanial organisms and on their infected hosts. This research holds the promise of continued advance in our understanding of the versatile leishmania and of their relationships with mammalian hosts.

Acknowledgment. We are grateful to Dr. Dean Cunningham, Dr. Chris Ohl, and Mr. Ronald C. Neafie for their contributions.

REFERENCES

1. Chulay JD. Leishmaniasis. In: *Hunter's Tropical Medicine.* Philadelphia: WB Saunders; 1991:638–655.
2. McHugh CP. Arthropods: vectors of disease agents. *Lab Med.* 1994;7:435–437.
3. Melby PC, Kreutzer RD, McMahon-Pratt D, Gam AA, Neva FA. Cutaneous leishmaniasis: review of 59 cases seen at the National Institutes of Health. *Clin Infect Dis.* 1992;15:924–937.
4. Schnur LF, Chance ML, Ebert F, Thomas SC, Peters W. The biochemical and serological taxonomy of visceralizing leishmania. *Ann Trop Med Parasitol.* 1981;75: 131–144.
5. Lainson R, Shaw JJ. Leishmaniasis of the New World: taxonomic problems. *Br Med Bull.* 1972;28:44–48.
6. Connor DH, Neafie RC. Cutaneous leishmaniasis and visceral leishmaniasis. In: Binford CH, Connor DH, eds. *Pathology of Tropical and Extraordinary Diseases.* Washington, DC: Armed Forces Institute of Pathology; 1976: 258–272.
7. Strick RA, Brook M, Gasiorowski HC. Recurrent cutaneous leishmaniasis. *J Am Acad Dermatol.* 1983;9: 437–443.
8. Kemp M, Hansen MB, Theander TG. Recognition of leishmania antigens by T lymphocytes from nonexposed individuals. *Infect Immun.* 1992;60:2246–2251.
9. Jeannel D, Tuppin P, Brucker G, Danis M, Gentilini M. Imported and autochthonous kala-azar in France. *Br Med J.* 1991;303:336–338.
10. Li-ren G. Current status of kala-azar and vector control in China. *WHO Bulletin OMS.* 1991;69:595–601.
11. Mahieu LM, Van Acker KJ. Mediterranean visceral leishmaniasis: a frequently unrecognized important disease. *Am J Dis Child.* 1991;145:1225–1227.
12. Bray RS. Leishmaniasis in the Old World. *Br Med Bull.* 1972;28:39–43.
13. Nelson DA, Gustafson TL, Spielvogel RL. Clinical aspects of cutaneous leishmaniasis acquired in Texas. *J Am Acad Dermatol.* 1985;12:985–992.
14. Baker MS, Strunk HK. Medical aspects of Persian Gulf operations: serious infectious and communicable diseases to the Persian Gulf and Saudi Arabian peninsula. *Mil Med.* 1991;156:385–390.
15. Gasser RA Jr, Magill AJ, Oster CN. The threat of infectious disease in Americans returning from Operation Desert Storm. *N Engl J Med.* 1991;324(12):859–864.
16. Lesho EP. Leishmaniasis—another threat to Persian Gulf veterans. *Postgrad Med.* 191;90:213–217.
17. Magill AJ, Gasser RA, Oster CN, Grogl M, Sun W. Viscerotropic leishmaniasis in persons returning from Operation Desert Storm—1990–1991. *JAMA.* 1992;267:1444–1446.
18. Norton SA, Frankenburg S, Klaus S. Cutaneous leishmaniasis acquired during military service in the Middle East. *Arch Dermatol.* 1992;128:83–87.
19. Oldfield EC III, Wallace MR, Hyams KC, Yousif AA, Lewis DE, Bourgeois AL. Endemic infectious disease of the Middle East. *Rev Infect Dis.* 1991;13(suppl 3):S199–S217.
20. Herwaldt BL, Stokes SL, Juranek DD. American cutaneous leishmaniasis in US travelers. *Ann Intern Med.* 1993;118(10):779–784.
21. Funke BJ. Leishmaniasis update. *Postgrad Med.* 1992; 91:79.
22. Chatterjee KD. Leishmaniasis. In: *Parasitology: Protozo-*

ology and Helminthology. 12th ed. Calcutta: Chatterjee Medical Publishers; 1980:53–69.

23. Warren KS, Mahmoud AAF. *Tropical and Geographical Medicine*. New York: McGraw-Hill; 1984:270–280.
24. Melby PC. Experimental leishmaniasis in humans: review. *Rev Infect Dis*. 1991;13:1009–1017.
25. Chung HL, Hsu CP, Ts'ao WC, Ho LY. New types of lymph gland leishmaniasis in China. *China Med J*. 1982; 95:303–306.
26. Peters W, Elbihari S, Ching L, et al. Leishmania infecting man and wild animals in Saudi Arabia. 1. General survey. *Trans Roy Soc Trop Med Hyg*. 1985;79:831–839.
27. Morsy TA, Abou-el-Seoud SM. Natural infection in two pet cats in a house of a zoonotic cutaneous leishmaniasis patient in Imbaba area, Giza Governorate, Egypt. *J Egypt Soc Parasitol*. 1994;24:199–204.
28. Zaar K, Wunderlich F, Belehu A. Electron microscopical studies on cutaneous leishmaniasis in Ethiopia. *Ann Trop Med Parasitol*. 1982;76:595–605.
29. Bryceson ADM. Diffuse cutaneous leishmaniasis in Ethiopia. I. The clinical and histological features of the disease. *Trans Roy Soc Trop Med Hyg*. 1969;63:708–737.
30. Convit J, Pinardi ME, Rondon AJ. Diffuse cutaneous leishmaniasis: a disease due to an immunological defect of the host. *Trans Roy Soc Trop Med Hyg*. 1972;66: 603–610.
31. Convit J, Kerdel-Vegas F. Disseminated cutaneous leishmaniasis. *Arch Dermatol*. 1965;91:439–447.
32. Neva FA, Wyler D, Nash T. Cutaneous leishmaniasis—a case with persistent organisms after treatment in presence of normal immune response. *Am J Trop Med Hyg*. 1979;28:467–471.
33. Berger TG, Meltzer MS, Oster CN. Lymph node involvement in leishmaniasis. *J Am Acad Dermatol*. 1985;12: 993–996.
34. Spier S, Medenica M, McMillan S. Virtue C. Sporotrichoid leishmaniasis. *Arch Dermatol*. 1977;113:1104–1105.
35. Al-Gindan Y, Kubba R, El-Hassan AM, Omer AHS, Kutty MK, Saeed MBM. Dissemination in cutaneous leishmaniasis. 3. Lymph node involvement. *Int J Dermatol*. 1989; 28:248–254.
36. Kibbi AG, Karam PG, Kurban AK. Sporotrichoid leishmaniasis in patients from Saudi Arabia: clinical and histologic features. *J Am Acad Dermatol*. 1987;17:759–764.
37. Kubba R, Al-Gindan Y, El-Hassan AM, Omer AHS, Kutty MK, Saeed MBM. Dissemination in cutaneous leishmaniasis. 2. Satellite papules and subcutaneous induration. *Int J Dermatol*. 1988;27(10):702–706.
38. Kubba R, El-Hassan AM, Al-Gindan Y, Omer AHS, Kutty MK, Saeed MBM. Dissemination in cutaneous leishmaniasis. 1. Subcutaneous nodules. *Int J Dermatol*. 1987; 26:300–304.
39. Girgla HS, Marsden RA, Singh GM, Ryan TJ. Post kalaazar dermal leishmaniasis. *Br J Dermatol*. 1977;97: 307–311.
40. Geraci JE, Wilson WR, Thompson JH. Visceral leishmaniasis (kala-azar) as a cause of fever of unknown origin. *Mayo Clin Proc*. 1980;55:455–458.
41. Al-Jurayyan NAM, Al-Ayed IH, Al-Nasser MNS, Al-Mugeiren MMA, Boohene AG, Al-Herbish AS. Visceral leishmaniasis in infancy and childhood, epidemiology and clinicopathological study of 63 cases in Al-Baha Province, Saudi Arabia. *J Trop Ped*. 1992;38:12–16.
42. Al-Orainey IO, Gasim IY, Singh LM, et al. Visceral leishmaniasis in Gizan, Saudi Arabia. *Ann Saudi Med*. 1994;14:396–398.
43. Benjamin B, Annobil SH, Bassuni WA. Clinical and laboratory features of childhood visceral leishmaniasis in southwestern Saudi Arabia. *Ann Saudi Med*. 1994; 14:107–110.
44. Carvalho EM, Barral A, Pedral-Sampaio D, et al. Immunologic markers of clinical evolution in children recently infected with *Leishmania donovani chagasi*. *J Infect Dis*. 1992;165:535–540.
45. Price SM, Silvers DN. New World leishmaniasis. *Arch Dermatol*. 1977;113:1415–1416.
46. Chung HL, Chang NC. Studies on leishmaniasis in China—historical background, epidemiology, clinical aspects, legislature and control program. *Chin Med J*. 1986;99:281–300.
47. Fasanaro AM, Scoleri G, Pizza V, Gaeta GB, Fasanaro A. Guillain–Barré syndrome as presenting manifestation of visceral leishmaniasis. *Lancet*. 1991;338:1142.
48. Hashim FA, Ahmed AE, El Hassan M, et al. Neurologic changes in visceral leishmaniasis. *Am J Trop Med Hyg*. 1995;52:149–154.
49. Satti MB, El-Hassan AM, Al-Gindan Y, Osman MA, Al-Sohaibani MO. Peripheral neural involvement in cutaneous leishmaniasis. *Int J Dermatol*. 1989;28:243–247.
50. El-Hassan AM, El-Sheikh EA, Eltoum IA, et al. Post kalaazar anterior uveitis: demonstration of leishmania parasites in the lesion. *Trans Roy Soc Trop Med Hyg* 1991;85:471–473.
51. Berenguer J, Moreno S, Cercenado E, et al. Visceral leishmaniasis in patients infected with human immunodeficiency virus (HIV). *Ann Intern Med* 1989;111:129–132.
52. Bissuel F, Leport C, Perronne C, Longuet P, Vilde JL. Fever of unknown origin in HIV-infected patients: a critical analysis of a retrospective study of 57 cases. *J Intern Med*. 1994;236:529–536.
53. Curry A, Turner AJ, Lucas S. Opportunistic protozoan infections in human immunodeficiency virus disease: Review highlighting diagnostic and therapeutic aspects. *J Clin Pathol*. 1991;44:182–193.
54. Datry A, Similowski T, Jais P, et al. AIDS-associated leishmaniasis: an unusual gastro-duodenal presentation. *Trans Roy Soc Trop Med Hyg*. 1990;84:239–240.
55. Montalban C. Visceral leishmaniasis in human immunodeficiency virus disease. *J Clin Pathol*. 1991;44:965–966.
56. Montalban C, Martinez-Fernandez R, Calleja JL, et al. Visceral leishmaniasis (kala-azar) as an opportunistic infection in patients infected with the human immunodeficiency virus in Spain. *Rev Infect Dis*. 1989;11:655–660.
57. Peters BS, Fish D, Golden R, et al. Visceral leishmaniasis in HIV infection and AIDS; clinical features and response to therapy. *Quart J Med*. 1990;77(283):1101–1111.
58. Badaro R, Rocha H, Carvalho EM, Quieroz AC, Jones TC. *Leishmania donovani:* an opportunistic microbe associated with progressive disease in three immunocompromised patients. *Lancet*. 1986:647–648.

59. Portoles J, Prats D, Torralbo A, Herrero JA, Torrente J, Barrientos A. Visceral leishmaniasis: a cause of opportunistic infection in renal transplant patients in endemic areas. *Transplantation.* 1994;57(11):1677–1679.
60. Magill AJ, Grogl M, Gasser RA, Sun W, Oster C. Visceral infection caused by *Leishmania tropica* in veterans of Operation Desert Storm. *N Engl J Med.* 1993;328(19):1383–1387.
61. Ohl CA, Hyams KC, Malone JD, Oldfield E III. Leishmaniasis among Desert Storm veterans: a diagnostic and therapeutic dilemma. *Mil Med.* 1993;158(11):726–729.
62. Badaro R, Jones TC, Carvalho EM, et al. New perspectives on a subclinical form of visceral leishmaniasis. *J Infect Dis.* 1986;154:1003–1011.
63. Angevine DM, Hamilton TR, Wallace FG, Hazard JB. Lymph nodes in leishmaniasis. *Am J Med Sci.* 1945;210:33–38.
64. Azadeh B. "Localized" leishmania lymphadenitis: a light and electron microscopic study. *Am J Trop Med Hyg.* 1985;34:447–455.
65. Bell DW, Carmichael JAG, Williams RS, Holman RL, Stewart PD. Localized leishmaniasis of lymph nodes. *Br Med J.* 1958;1:740–743.
66. Daneshbod K. Localized lymphadenitis due to leishmania simulating toxoplasmosis. *Am J Clin Pathol.* 1978;69:462–467.
67. Pampiglione S, Manson-Bahr PEC, Giungi F, Giunti G, Parenti A, Canestri Trotti G. Studies on Mediterranean leishmaniasis. 2. Asymptomatic cases of visceral leishmaniasis. *Trans Roy Soc Trop Med Hyg.* 1974;68:447–453.
68. Laudadio P. A case of tonsillar leishmaniasis. *J Laryngol Otol.* 1984;98:213–216.
69. Kurban AK, Malak JA, Farah FS, Chaglassian HT. Histopathology of cutaneous leishmaniasis. *Arch Dermatol.* 1966;93:396–401.
70. Azadeh B, Samad A, Ardehali S. Histological spectrum of cutaneous leishmaniasis due to *Leishmania tropica*. *Trans Roy Soc Trop Med Hyg.* 1985;79:631–636.
71. Ridley DS. A histological classification of cutaneous leishmaniasis and its geographical expression. *Trans Roy Soc Trop Med Hyg.* 1980;74:515–521.
72. Ridley MJ, Wells CW. Macrophage–parasite interaction in the lesions of cutaneous leishmaniasis. *Am J Pathol.* 1986;123:79–85.
73. Ridley DS, Ridley MJ. The evolution of the lesion in cutaneous leishmaniasis. *J Pathol.* 1983;141:83–96.
74. Corbett CEP, Duarte MIS, Bustamante SE. Regression of diffuse intralobular liver fibrosis associated with visceral leishmaniasis. *Am J Trop Med Hyg.* 1993;49:616–624.
75. El-Hag IA, Hashim FA, El-Toum IA, Homeida M, El-Kalifa M, El-Hassan AM. Liver morphology and function in visceral leishmaniasis (kala-azar). *J Clin Pathol.* 1994;47:547–551.
76. Haque I, Haque MZ, Krishnani N, Srivastava SP, Khan EM. Fine needle aspiration cytology of the spleen in visceral leishmaniasis. *Acta Cytol.* 1993;37:73–76.
77. Palma G, Gutierrez Y. Laboratory diagnosis of leishmaniasis. *Clin Lab Med.* 1991;11:909–922.
78. Ridley DS. The pathogenesis of cutaneous leishmaniasis. *Trans Roy Soc Trop Med Hyg.* 1979;73:150–160.
79. Herwaldt BA, Arana BA, Navin TR. The natural history of cutaneous leishmaniasis in Guatemala. *J Infect Dis.* 1992;165:518–527.
80. Melha AA, Satir AA, Hussan MAM. A review of biopsies performed on children in the eastern province of Saudi Arabia. *E Afr Med J.* 1984;61:(11):853–858.
81. Zeledon R. Cutaneous leishmaniasis and *Leishmania infantum*. *Trans Roy Soc Trop Med Hyg.* 1991;85:557.
82. Aebischer T, Moody S, Handman E. Persistence of virulent *Leishmania major* in murine cutaneous leishmaniasis: a possible hazard for the host. *Infect Immun.* 1993;61:220–226.
83. Lainson R, Shaw JJ. Studies on the immunology and serology of leishmaniasis. III. On the cross-immunity between Panamanian cutaneous leishmaniasis and *Leishmania mexicana* infection in man. *Trans Roy Soc Trop Med Hyg.* 1966;60:533–535.
84. Raziuddin S, Abdalla RE, El-Awad EH, Al-Janadi M. Immunoregulatory and proinflammatory cytokine production in visceral and cutaneous leishmaniasis. *J Infect Dis.* 1994;170:1037–1040.
85. Liew FY, O'Donnell CA. Immunology of leishmaniasis. *Adv Parasitol.* 1993;32:161–259.
86. Kemp M, Kurtzhals JA, Kharazmi A, Theander TG. Dichotomy in the human CD4+ T-cell response to leishmania parasites. *APMIS.* 1994;102:81–88.
87. Melby PC, Andrade-Narvaez FJ, Darnell BJ, Valencia-Pacheco G, Tyron VV, Palomo-Cetina A. Increased expression of proinflammatory cytokines in chronic lesions of human cutaneous leishmaniasis. *Infect Immun.* 1994;62:837–842.
88. Uyemura K, Pirmez C, Sieling PA, Kiene K, Paes-Oliveira M, Modlin RL. CD4+ Type 1 and CD8+ Type 2 T cell subsets in human leishmaniasis have distinct T cell receptor repertoires. *J Immunol.* 1993;151(12):7095–7104.
89. Saravia NG, Valderrana L, Labrada M, et al. The relationship of *Leishmania braziliensis* subspecies and immune response to disease expression in New World leishmaniasis. *J Infect Dis.* 1989;159:725–735.
90. Sacks DJ, Suman Lata Lal, Shrivastava SN, Blackwell J, Neva FA. An analysis of T cell responsiveness in Indian kala-azar. *J Immunol.* 1987;138:908–913.
91. Hviid L, Sorensen AL, Kharazmi A, Theander TG. Functional and phenotypic changes in human lymphocytes after coincubation with *Leishmania donovani* in vitro. *Infect Immun.* 1990;58(10):3163–3167.
92. Harms G, Pedrosa C, Omena S, Feldmeier H, Zwingenberger K. Natural killer cell activity in visceral leishmaniasis. *Trans Roy Soc Trop Med Hyg.* 1991;85:54–55.
93. Petersen EA, Neva FA, Oster CN, Diaz HB. Specific inhibition of lymphocyte-proliferation responses by adherent suppressor cells in diffuse cutaneous leishmaniasis. *N Engl J Med.* 1982;306:387–392.
94. Douvas GS, Looker DL, Vatter AE, Crowle AJ. Gamma interferon activates human macrophages to become tumoricidal and leishmanicidal but enhances replication of macrophage-associated mycobacteria. *Infect Immun.* 1985;50:1–8.
95. Hoover DL, Nacy CA, Meltzer MS. Human monocyte acti-

vation for cytotoxicity against intracellular *Leishmania donovani* amastigotes: induction of microbiocidal activity by interferon-gamma. *Cell Immunol.* 1985;94:500–511.

96. Murray HW, Rubin BY, Rothermel CD. Killing of *intracellular Leishmania donovani* by lymphokine-stimulated human mononuclear phagocytes. *J Clin Invest.* 1983;72:1506–1510.
97. Carvalho EM, Bacellar O, Brownell C, Regis T, Coffman RL, Reed SG. Restoration of IFN-gamma production and lymphocyte proliferation in visceral leishmaniasis. *J Immunol.* 1994;152(12):5949–5956.
98. Carvalho EM, Badaro R, Reed SG, Jones TC, Johnson WD. Absence of gamma interferon and interleukin 2 production during active visceral leishmaniasis. *J Clin Invest.* 1985;76:2066–2069.
99. Kalter DC. Laboratory tests for the diagnosis and evaluation of leishmaniasis. *Dermatol Clin.* 1994;12:37–50.
100. Morsy TA, Ghazi HH. Leishmanin skin tests in Riyadh, Saudi Arabia. *J Kwt Med Assoc.* 1974;8:169–171.
101. Weigle KA, Valderrama L, Arias AL, Santrich C, Saravia NG. Leishmanin skin test standardization and evaluation of safety, dose, storage, longevity of reaction and sensitization. *Am J Trop Med Hyg.* 1991;44:260–271.
102. Berger RS, Perez-Figaredo RA, Spielvogel RL. Leishmaniasis: the touch preparation as a rapid means of diagnosis. *J Am Acad Dermatol.* 1987;16:1096–1105.
103. Medrano FJ, Jimenez-Mejias E, Calderon E, Regordan C, Leal M. An easy and quick method for the diagnosis of visceral leishmaniasis in HIV-1 infected individuals. *AIDS.* 1993;7(10):1399.
104. Anthony RL, Grogl M, Sacci JB, Ballou RW. Rapid detection of leishmania amastigotes in fluid aspirates and biopsies of human tissues. *Am J Trop Med Hyg.* 1987;37:271–276.
105. Zijlstra EE, Siddig Ali M, El-Hassan AM, El-Toum IA, Satti M, Ghalib HW, Kager PA. Direct agglutination test for diagnosis and sero-epidemiological survey of kala-azar in the Sudan. *Trans Roy Soc Trop Med Hyg.* 1991;85:474–476.
106. Blackwell JM. Leishmaniasis epidemiology: all down to the DNA. *Parasitology.* 1992;104:S19–S34.

CHAPTER 136

Malaria

Kei-Ichiro Nakamura, John R. Rabbege, J. Kevin Baird, Juntra Karbwang, Bernard Tandler, Masamichi Aikawa, and Daniel H. Connor

He is so shak'd of a burning quotidian tertian that it is most lamentable to behold.

William Shakespeare (1564–1616), Henry V, II, i, 116

I had often 'a little fever,' or a little touch of other things—the playful paw-strokes of the wilderness, the preliminary trifling before the more serious onslaught which came in due course.

Joseph Conrad (1857–1924), Heart of Darkness

DEFINITION

Malaria, an acute and chronic infection by coccidian protozoa of the genus *Plasmodium,* is debilitating, commonly fatal, and widespread throughout the tropics and subtropics. Four species infect humans: *P vivax, P malariae, P ovale,* and *P falciparum. Plasmodium vivax* causes "vivax malaria," also called tertian malaria or benign tertian malaria; *P malariae* causes quartan malaria; *P ovale* causes ovale malaria or ovale tertian malaria; and *P falciparum* causes the most severe form of malaria, which is frequently life threatening and commonly fatal. The vector for all species of *Plasmodium* causing human malaria is the female mosquito of the genus *Anopheles.* Several species of simian *Plasmodium* occasionally infect humans. Plasmodia occasionally infect humans as zoonoses, experimental infections, as therapy for neurosyphilis, in transfused blood, or as laboratory accidents.

GEOGRAPHIC DISTRIBUTION

Malaria occurs throughout Africa, Asia, Latin America, Oceania, and on certain Caribbean islands.[1] More than 1.6 billion inhabitants of these areas are at risk, and there are more than 200 million clinical infections each year. In sub-Saharan Africa alone, there are more than 100 million infections each year, with an estimated one million deaths—mostly of infants and young children.[1]

EPIDEMIOLOGY

Before organized global control measures were begun in the 1940s, malaria killed about 2.5 million each year.[2] This number decreased rapidly until the 1970s when a steady resurgence began—a consequence of 1) resistance of vector mosquitoes to insecticides, 2) resistance of plasmodia to antimalarial drugs,[3] and 3) a complex of socioeconomic factors, which include health infrastructure, particularly maintenance of effective control programs in the developing world. The increasing availability of international air travel, migrations from endemic areas, the resurgence of malaria in the tropics, and the decreased effectiveness of chemoprophylaxis and therapy[4] have all contributed to the increase of imported malaria in the United States and Europe. Most of these infections are in returning travelers and rarely is there indigenous transmission. Even rarer still are the infections of those near an airport who acquire malaria thought to be from infected mosquitoes transported in the cabin of the aircraft.[5]

LIFE CYCLE AND MORPHOLOGY

The life cycles of the four species of plasmodia are similar. Each has a succession of stages in humans and in mosquitoes.[6] The life cycle for *P falciparum* is shown in Figure 136–1. Sporozoites from the mosquito's sali-

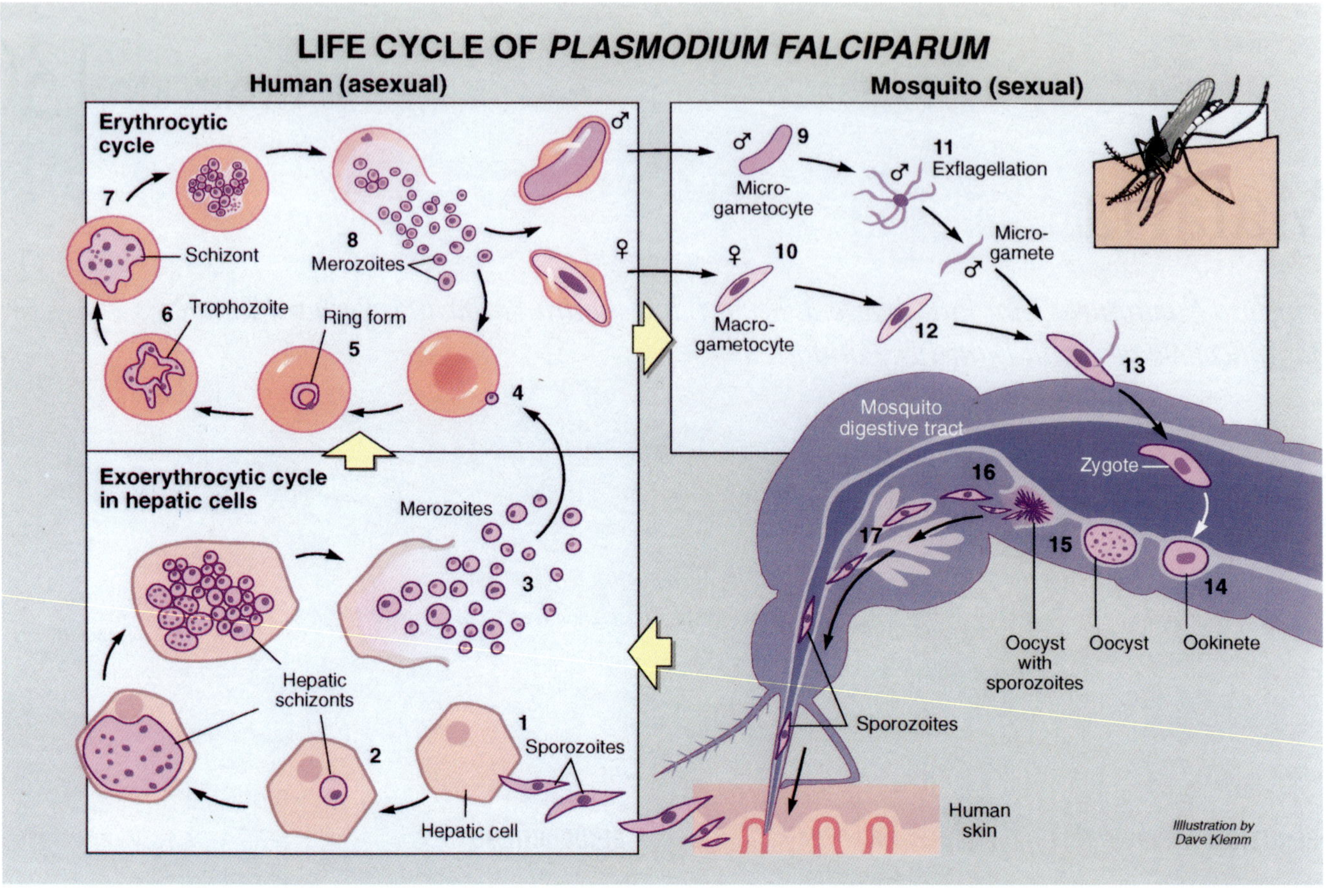

Figure 136–1. Life cycle of human malarial parasites. Life cycle in the human (*1* through *10*) and in the mosquito (*9* through *17*). Exoerythrocytic stages are *1* through *3,* blood stages are *4* through *8,* and sexual forms (also circulating in blood) are *9* and *10.* (*1*) Sporozoite invasion into human hepatocyte. (*2*) Exoerythrocytic stage schizont. (*3*) Rupture of hepatocyte-releasing merozoites. (*4*) Invasion of human erythrocyte by merozoite. (*5*) Ring-form, trophozoite. (*6*) Maturing trophozoite. (*7*) Schizont. (*8*) Rupture of erythrocyte and release of merozoites. (*9*) Microgametocyte, male form. (*10*) Gamete, macrogametocyte, female form. (*11*) Exflagellation of microgametocyte. (*12*) Macrogamete and microgamete. (*13*) Fertilization and formation of zygote. (*14*) Ookinete and its invasion into midgut epithelium of mosquito. (*15*) Oocyst and sporozoite formation in mosquito midgut epithelium. (*16*) Rupture of oocyst and release of sporozoites. (*17*) Migration of sporozoite to mosquito salivary gland, then through the proboscis into the next victim.

vary glands infect a hepatocyte within minutes of inoculation. During the next 6 to 15 days the tissue schizont matures, producing thousands of merozoites. These merozoites invade red blood cells. With relapsing malarias (vivax and ovale) there is another tissue stage—the hypnozoite—a quiescent form that lives in the liver and may at any time cause clinical malaria.

Smears of blood stained by the Giemsa technique give erythrocytes a pale pink color but the parasites they contain are densely stained; see Figures 136–2 through 136–9 to compare circulating forms of *P vivax* and *P falciparum.* In falciparum infections, infected erythrocytes may contain two or more parasites. In the benign malarias, the so-called "ring" form (early trophozoite), the nucleus is displaced peripherally and flattened part way around the perimeter of the parasite. This gives the parasite its ring appearance. The cytoplasm of the parasite, however, matches the color of the host erythrocyte, so is essentially invisible. The more developed trophozoite has a spherical, lightly stained eccentric nucleus and blue cytoplasm that may contain crystal-like deposits of yellow-brown pigment. In falciparum malaria, there may be ill-defined amorphous densities in the erythrocyte—Maurer's clefts. In the other malarias, these densities may have a more dotlike appearance and are called Schüffner's dots (in *P vivax* and *P ovale*) or Zieman's stippling (in *P malariae*). The next stage—the schizont—is larger and has multiple nuclei, and the pigment appears as eccentric aggregates. The erythrocytes containing the schizonts ultimately rupture releasing merozoites, which, because of their small size (about 1 μm), are usually not discernible in blood smears. The merozoites invade new erythrocytes (Figure 136–10) and repeat the cycle. Falciparum malaria produces ring forms only in the circulating blood, whereas other malarias have more varied shapes (Figures 136–2 and 136–3). Gametocytes, the sexual forms, are usually elongated, sometimes cres-

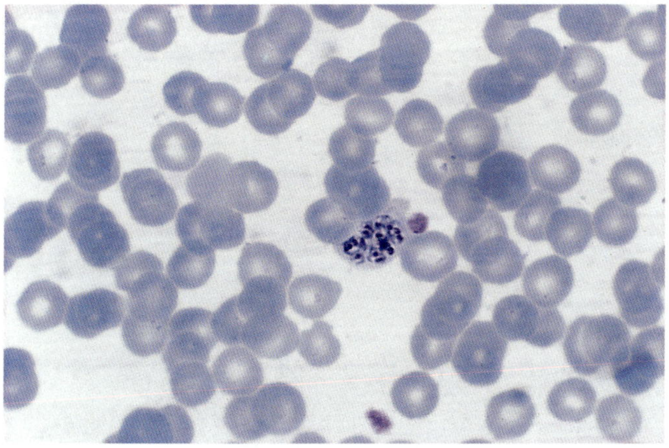

Figure 136–2. Thin blood film showing a schizont of *P vivax* at center. The infected erythrocyte contains maturing schizonts and a thick granule of hemozoin. Each merozoite is distinguished by the intensely stained nucleus and a lightly stained cytoplasm. The roughly paired configuration of merozoites reflects a recent mitosis (Giemsa, ×1000). *(Contributed by Kevin Baird, PhD.)*

centic and sometimes spindle shaped. Gametocytes, imbibed by anopheline mosquitoes, complete the life cycle. Identifying criteria have been summarized in tabular form by the Centers for Disease Control and Prevention.[7]

In *P falciparum* and in *P malariae,* the plasma membrane of infected erythrocytes is studded with small, electron-dense conical knobs (Figures 136–11 and 136–12). The genesis of these knobs is complex.[8–10] The dense material, which arises in association with the surface of the parasite, may move to the erythrocyte plasmalemma in tandem with membranes, originating as a cleft from the membrane of the parasitophorous vacuole (Figure 136–13). These are the structural bases of Maurer's clefts seen by light microscopy. Ultimately, these migrating structures become incorporated into the erythrocyte plasmalemma and the dense protrusions. The dense material of the

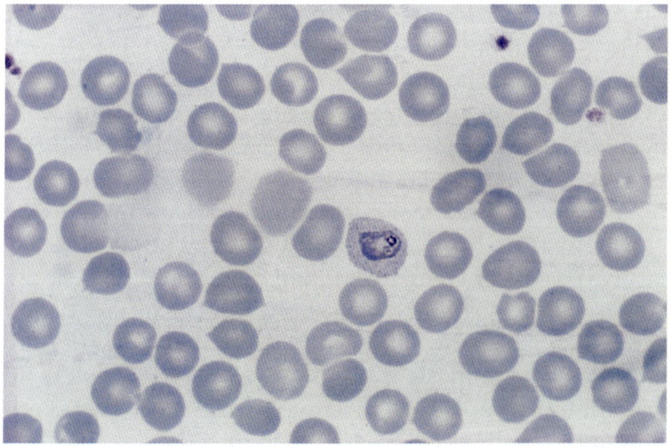

Figure 136–3. Thin blood film showing a red blood cell containing a trophozoite of *P vivax* at center. This photograph demonstrates several key diagnostic features of *P vivax:* 1) the infected cell is larger than surrounding noninfected cells, 2) the trophozoite has an ameboid shape, and 3) there is fine stippling of the infected cell called Schüffner's dots (Giemsa, ×1000). *(Contributed by Kevin Baird, PhD.)*

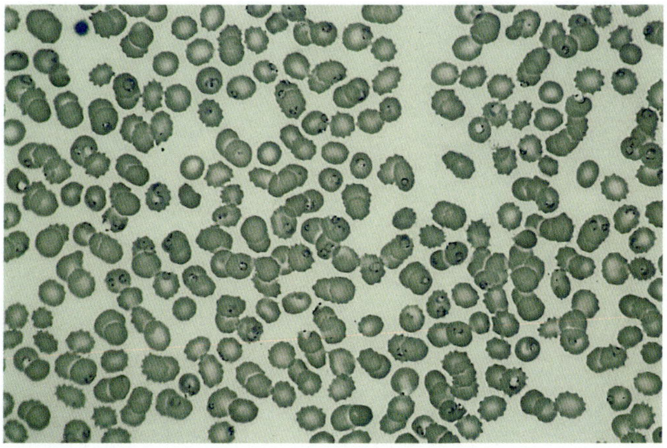

Figure 136–4. Thin blood film of peripheral blood showing heavy parasitization of erythrocytes by small ring forms (trophozoites) of *P falciparum.* Many of the erythrocytes contain multiple parasites. As the trophozoites mature into schizonts, the infected erythrocytes will stick to endothelial cells, thus removing the infected erythrocytes from the peripheral circulation (AFIP Neg 79-15360; Giemsa, ×290).

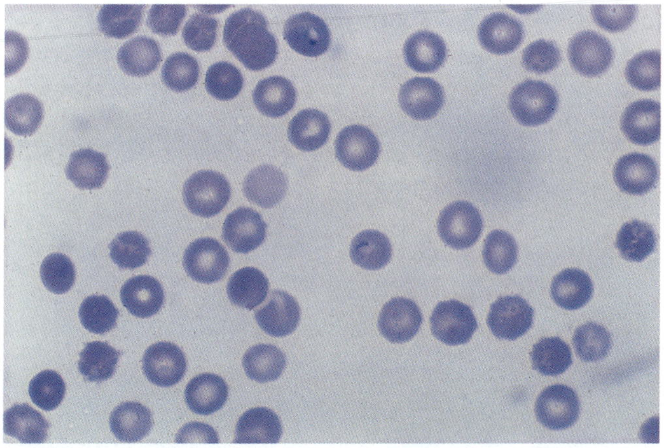

Figure 136–5. Thin blood film showing an erythrocyte containing a trophozoite of *P falciparum.* Contrast this trophozoite with the trophozoite of *P vivax* in Figure 136–3. The infected red cell is slightly smaller than the uninfected red cells. The nucleus of the trophozoite is compact and densely stained with a less distinct ring of cytoplasm. This stage resembles a signet ring—hence the name "ring stage" for this young trophozoite. Two or three young trophozoites of *P falciparum* often infect the same erythrocyte (among other parasites in the blood of humans, only *Babesia* sp does this routinely). Some trophozoites may appear to be flattened against the membrane of the red cell; these are called "appliqué forms." Schizonts of *P falciparum* only rarely appear in films of peripheral blood because the infected red cells adhere to endothelial cells and do not circulate (Giemsa, ×1000). *(Contributed by Kevin Baird, PhD.)*

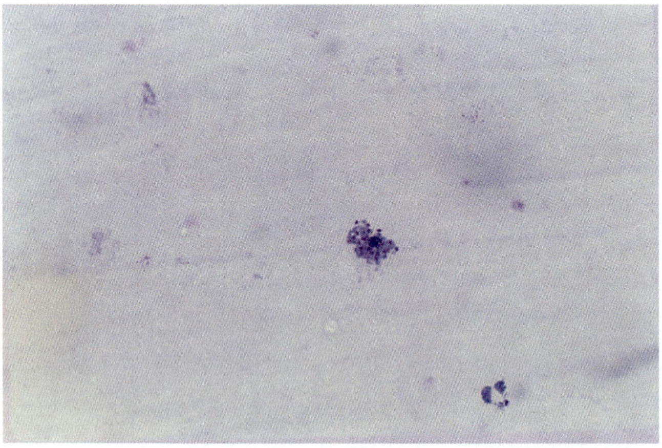

Figure 136–6. Thick blood film showing a schizont of *P vivax.* Note that although the blood cells have been obliterated by lysis, the parasites remain intact and retain ordinary staining characteristics. Compare with Figure 136–2 (Giemsa, ×1000). *(Contributed by Kevin Baird, PhD.)*

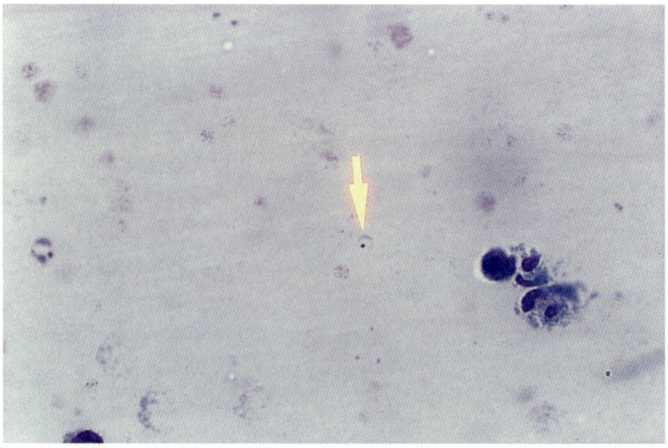

Figure 136–8. Thick blood film demonstrating the ring form of *P falciparum* (*arrow*). Although this could be mistaken for an artifact, the trained eye detects the compact densely stained nucleus and the lightly stained wisp of cytoplasm. Good staining technique is essential to diagnosing malaria with thick or thin smears. The cytoplasm must be evident for diagnosis—understaining may leave it invisible while overstaining may make it so dense that it cannot be distinguished from the nucleus (Giemsa, ×1000). *(Contributed by Kevin Baird, PhD.)*

knobs has been identified as several specific proteins; a labeled monoclonal antibody raised against these proteins shows precise localization in the knobs (inset, Figure 136–11).

CLINICAL FEATURES

Clinical manifestations of malaria are extremely varied and range in severity from a mild headache to coma and death. The symptoms usually begin after an incubation of 12 to 20 days for *P vivax,* 8 to 15 days for *P falciparum,* 18 to 40 days for *P malariae,* and 8 to 14 days for *P ovale.* The duration of incubation is influenced by the species of malaria parasite, the degree of acquired immunity, and the dose of sporozoite inoculated. Before the onset of symptoms there may be prodromal symptoms. The patient may have lassitude and may stretch or yawn. There may be aching in the bones, anorexia, headache, and a sense of chilliness, sometimes with the feeling of cold water on the back. Fever is the hallmark of malaria and the highest temperatures occur around the time of schizogony of the asexual erythrocytic parasite. When development of the parasites is synchronous, then the great majority undergo schizogony at about the same time, and the periodicity of fever is determined by the length of the asexual cycle. Schizogony of *P vivax, P falciparum,* and *P ovale* occur every 48 hours and the febrile paroxysm occurs every third day (i.e., tertian malaria). The erythrocytic cycle of *P malariae* takes 72 hours and the periodicity of fever is quartan. Frequently, the asexual erythrocytic development is not synchronous and two or more asynchronous broods develop, producing daily fever. Malarial paroxysms are usually sudden, with three discernible stages: cold (shaking chill), hot (fever), and sweating stage. After sweating, the patient is exhausted, usually afebrile, and then sleeps. The fever is more severe in nonimmune patients than in patients who are semi-immune.

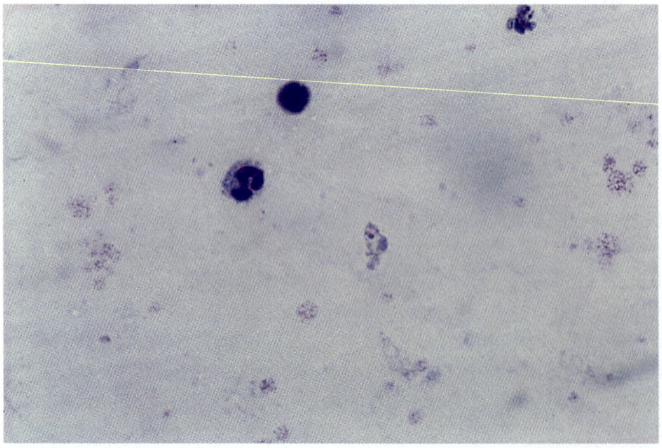

Figure 136–7. Thick blood film showing a mature trophozoite of *P vivax.* Again the red blood cells have been destroyed by lysis but their parasitic contents remain intact and readily distinguishable by the same morphologic criteria that guide diagnosis in the thin blood film. Compare with Figure 136–3 (Giemsa, ×1000). *(Contributed by Kevin Baird, PhD.)*

The pathogenesis of the fever is little understood, but pyrogens may be released when infected erythrocytes rupture. Products of the ruptured erythrocytes or toxic products of the parasites or both could be pyrogenic. Such pyrogens could cause the hypothalamus to release prostaglandins, which indirectly stimulate sympathetic nerves, leading to contraction of peripheral

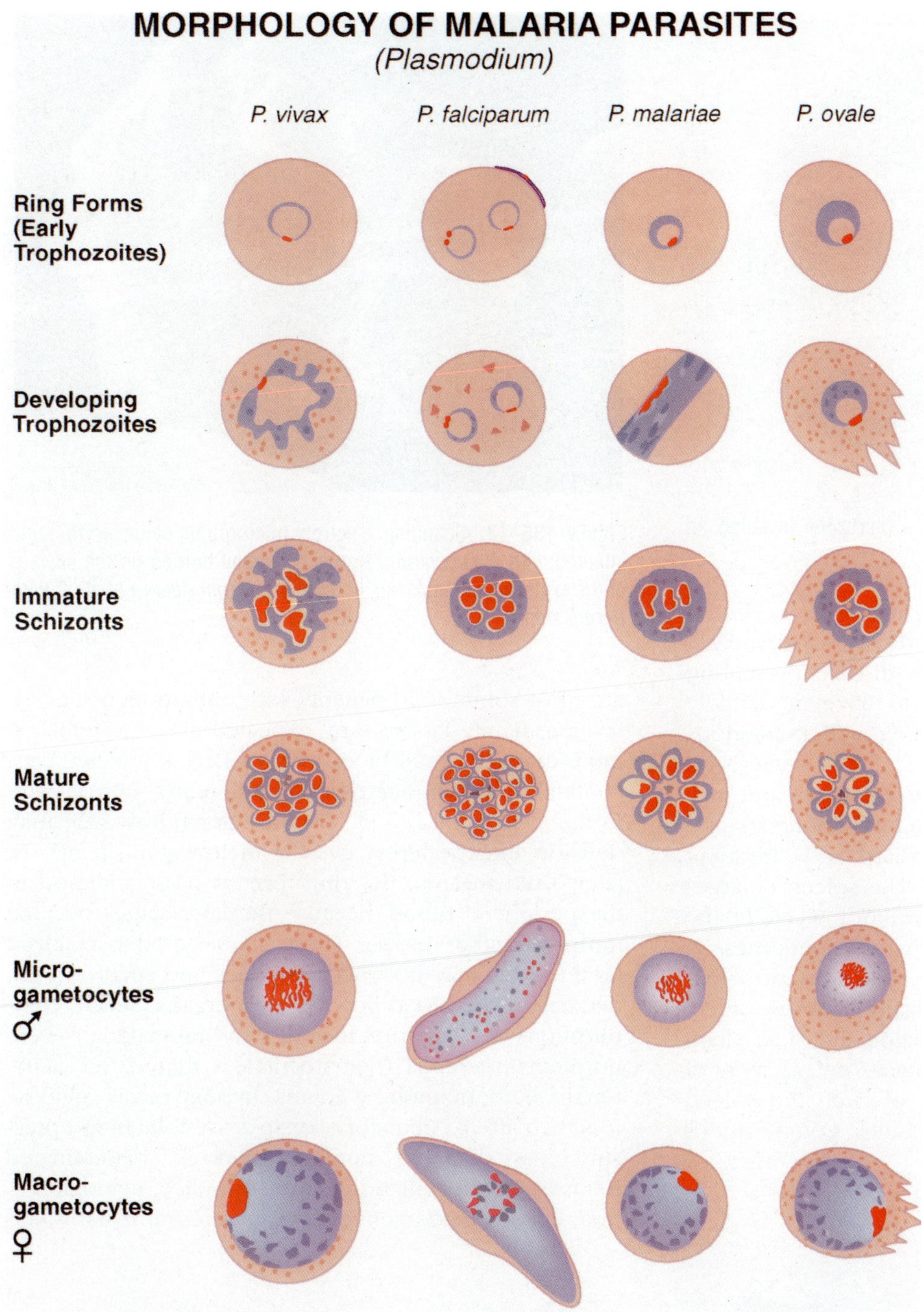

Figure 136–9. Drawings to show the characteristic and contrasting features of the four species of malarial parasite that invade human erythrocytes.

blood vessels, thereby decreasing heat loss and causing body temperature to rise.

In *P vivax,* paroxysms occur chiefly in the afternoon or evening. The temperature may rise to 40°C or higher. Nausea and vomiting may be distressing. Dizziness, drowsiness, or other symptoms of cerebral irritation are transient. The spleen, which is often enlarged, may rupture spontaneously or following a minor accident, but this is rare. The liver may enlarge during the acute attack. A single untreated attack may last from a few weeks to 3 months or more, with repeated paroxysms before spontaneous clinical cure. Relapses (parasitemia by merozoites from the hypnozoites) occur from 8 to 40 weeks after the primary attack. The clinical features of relapse are usually less severe and of shorter duration than the primary attack. It is unusual for vivax malaria to continue to relapse for more than 3 years—after the patient has left the endemic area. Vivax malaria is rarely fatal, but the relapses cause a considerable economic burden.

Plasmodium falciparum causes the most serious form of human malaria. Attacks may be uncomplicated or associated with serious and fatal complications.[11] None of the symptoms and signs of falciparum malaria

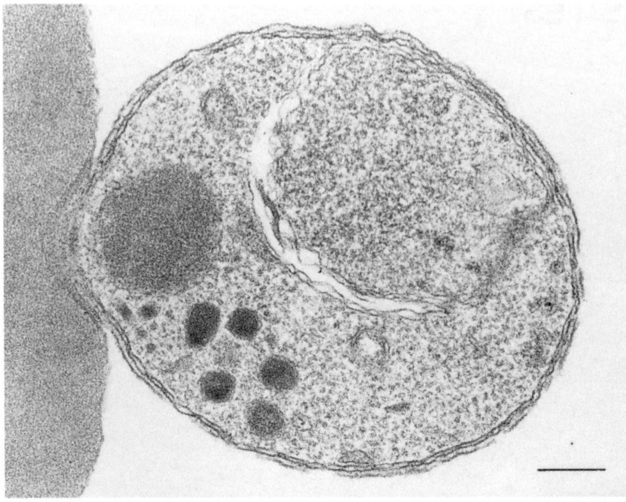

Figure 136–10. Electron micrograph of a merozoite invading an erythrocyte (scale bar = 0.25 μm).

is specific. They may mimic other diseases, particularly influenza, viral hepatitis, and any disease presenting with coma. Patients may appear to have moderately severe influenza and may not seem very ill, but serious complications may arise quickly and at any stage. Nausea and vomiting are common from the onset and may be very severe. Epigastric discomfort, anorexia, and dyspepsia are common. Watery diarrhea is frequent with certain strains of falciparum. The spleen enlarges rapidly and is usually palpable within 1 week of the onset, is usually tender, and there may be tenderness in the splenic region even when the spleen is not palpable. There may be jaundice, especially in severe infections, and deviations of liver function test (i.e., slight elevation of bilirubin and transaminase); enlargement of the liver is common. Tenderness of liver and spleen may be from stretching of their capsules. Complications

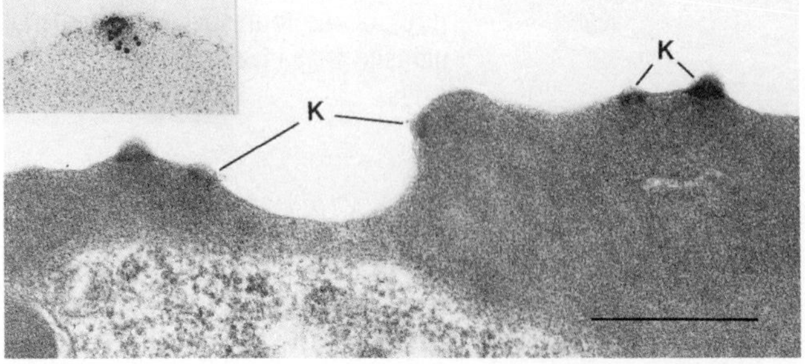

Figure 136–11. Electron micrograph of the outer portion of an erythrocyte infected with *P falciparum*. Conical, electron-dense knobs (K) are in the membrane of the erythrocyte (scale bar = 0.5 μm). (*Inset*) Immunoelectron micrograph of an erythrocyte infected with *P falciparum*. It is stained with a monoclonal antibody against the 90-kD knob protein and gold-labeled secondary antibody. Gold particles are localized over the electron-dense knob material. *(From Atkinson and Aikawa,[10] with permission.)*

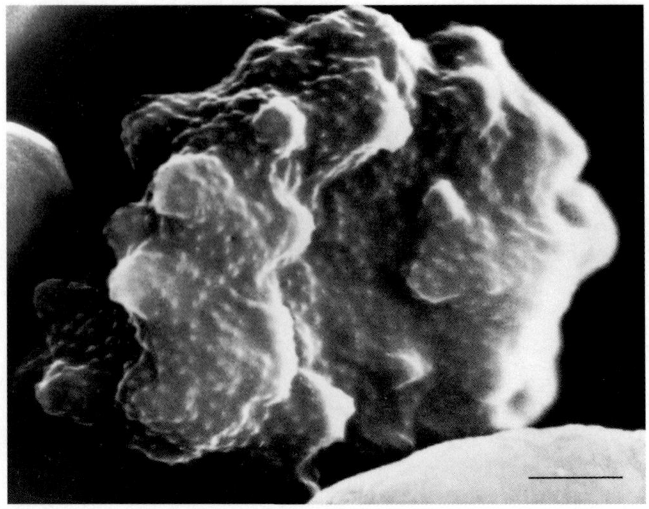

Figure 136–12. Scanning electron micrograph of an erythrocyte infected with *P falciparum*. Knobs are small bumps on the surface of the erythrocyte (scale bar = 0.5 μm). *(From Aikawa et al,[106] with permission.)*

are most common in patients with immunodeficiencies. Severe manifestations are expected if parasitemia is more than 5% of red blood cells, if 10% of infected cells contain more than one parasite, or if many schizonts are in the peripheral blood. Complications, however, may develop unexpectedly, even with low parasitemia. In falciparum malaria, the ring form is most common in the peripheral blood, because the later stages become trapped in the vessels. These sequestered parasitized erythrocytes may obstruct capillaries and small vessels, decreasing the blood flow to deep organs. Severe complications of falciparum include cerebral malaria, severe normocytic anemia (hematocrit less than 20%), acute renal failure, pulmonary edema, hypoglycemia (glucose less than 40%), circulatory collapse (systolic blood pressure less than 70 mmHg), acidosis, disseminated intravascular coagulation, severe jaundice, hemoglobinuria, and repeated convulsions.[11] Cerebral malaria kills

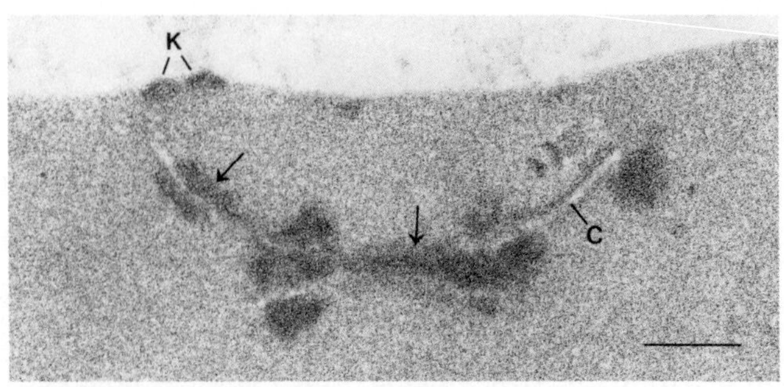

Figure 136–13. Electron micrograph of an erythrocyte infected with *P falciparum*. The cytoplasmic cleft (C) provides a route for the amorphous electron-dense material (*arrows*) to migrate from the parasite to the knobs (K) in the erythrocyte membrane (scale bar = 0.2 μm). *(From Aikawa et al,[107] with permission.)*

frequently—particularly young children and nonimmune adults. The preliminary signs and symptoms of cerebral malaria are legion, and they include headache, stiff neck, drowsiness, disorientation, delirium, convulsions, ataxia, aphasia, dysarthria, and meningeal irritation. Pulmonary edema, the most severe complication in adult patients with falciparum malaria, usually carries a mortality rate of more than 50% and is usually associated with other complications such as cerebral malaria, renal failure, high parasitemia, and pregnancy. The prognosis of falciparum malaria worsens with each hour's delay in diagnosis and treatment.

The clinical features of infection by *P malariae* resemble vivax malaria but the onset is often insidious. Febrile patterns swiftly develop a quartan pattern as parasites of *P malariae* have synchronized schizogony from an early stage. Quartan periodicity is the hallmark of *P malariae* infection and is rarely found in any other diseases. Anemia is not severe but there may be leucopenia. Splenomegaly is usual but may not be remarkable. Edema, notably of the ankles, is not unusual. The acute attack is self-limiting, although it may last for several months before spontaneous remission. *Plasmodium malariae* infection is rarely fatal and, apart from progressive glomerulonephritis, seldom causes serious complications. It is, however, the most persistent form of human malaria and renewed episodes of parasitemia may occur many years after the primary attack. Such episodes are late recrudescence of persisting blood-stage parasites not initiated by hypnozoites. Protracted persistent low-grade asymptomatic parasitemia in *P malariae* carriers is a frequent cause of transfusion malaria.

The clinical features of *P ovale* infection resemble those of *P vivax* malaria but tend to be milder. For instance, the paroxysms tend to cease after a few cycles even without treatment.

Periodic paroxysms, although characteristic of malaria, are not pathognomonic. Malaria, in fact, may mimic almost any febrile illness. Symptoms usually begin after an incubation period of 12 to 17 days for *P vivax,* 11 to 16 days for *P falciparum,* 30 to 40 days for *P malariae,* and 8 to 14 days for *P ovale.* In a primary attack of falciparum malaria, the initial signs and symptoms may be mild, with the patient having flulike symptoms, for instance, headache, myalgia, chills, irritability, nausea, vomiting, and diarrhea. Later symptoms include high fever, up to 40°C, with convulsions. These first symptoms increase and classically a triad of chills, fever, and sweating recurs at 48-hour intervals.

PATHOLOGY

The main pathologic changes in malaria are caused by 1) the response of the reticuloendothelial system to the parasite and its pigment, 2) the destruction of erythrocytes combined with defective production of erythrocytes causing anemia, and 3) by the obstruction of capillaries in the brain and other organs by parasitized erythrocytes. Malarial pigment is a porphyrin conjugated with a protein derived from the globin portion of hemoglobin—both molecules being the end product of hemoglobin digestion by the parasite.

Most pathologic studies of malaria are of *P falciparum* malaria, which causes the malignant forms of malaria, including cerebral malaria. Erythrocytes parasitized by *P falciparum* "stick" to endothelial cells of brain and viscera.[9,12,13] This may lead to massive accumulations of parasitized erythrocytes in deep organs and this almost certainly causes capillary circulation to slow or stop (Figures 136–14 and 136–15). This accumulation of parasitized erythrocytes in capillaries of deep organs begins early, and continues throughout schizogony. For this reason young trophozoites only (ring forms) and gametocytes circulate in peripheral blood in falciparum infections. Parasitized red blood cells become attached to the endothelial surface by means of the knobs on the surface of the erythrocyte (Figure 136–16). The receptors on the surface of the endothelial cell for *P falciparum*–infected erythrocytes both in vitro, and probably in vivo too, are thrombospondin, CD36, and ICAM-1.[14]

In falciparum infection, the brain is swollen, causing the gyri to become broad and flat (Figure 136–17). The brain has a pink appearance because the vessels of the arachnoid are congested. Thus a "pink brain" is an indication of cerebral malaria. The cut surface shows

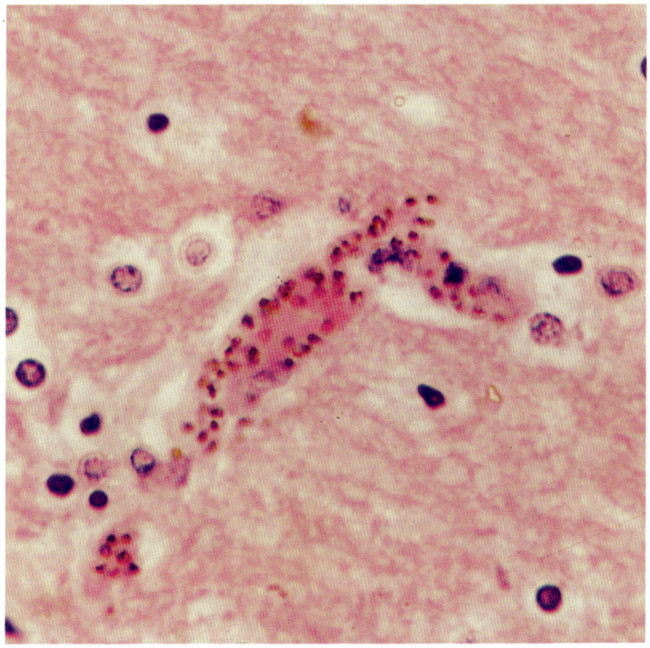

Figure 136–14. Small cerebral vessel containing many parasitized erythrocytes. The malarial knobs on the parasitized erythrocytes "stick" to the endothelium [AFIP Neg 66-7680; hematoxylin-eosin (H&E), ×350].

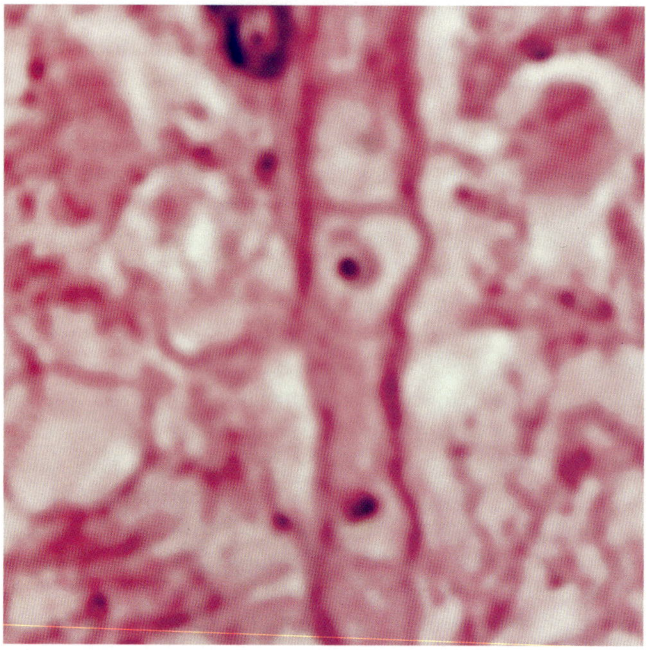

Figure 136–15. Two parasitized erythrocytes bulge, distort, and occlude this cerebral capillary. The pigment grains and two parasites are in distended erythrocytes, now depleted of hemoglobin. The parasites are late trophozoites or early schizonts. (AFIP Neg 74-2691; H&E, ×1260).

selective congestion and hemorrhage of white matter (Figure 136–18). Although some authors describe malarial pigmentation of the brain, this has not been objectively established and in our experience malarial pigmentation of the brain cannot be identified grossly. Viewed by the light microscope, masses of erythrocytes fill the lumina of small and medium-sized blood vessels, distending them; parasitized erythrocytes lie against the endothelial surface. Ring hemorrhages (Figure 136–19) and Dürck's granulomas (Figure 136–20) are lesions in the brains of patients with cerebral malaria who survive

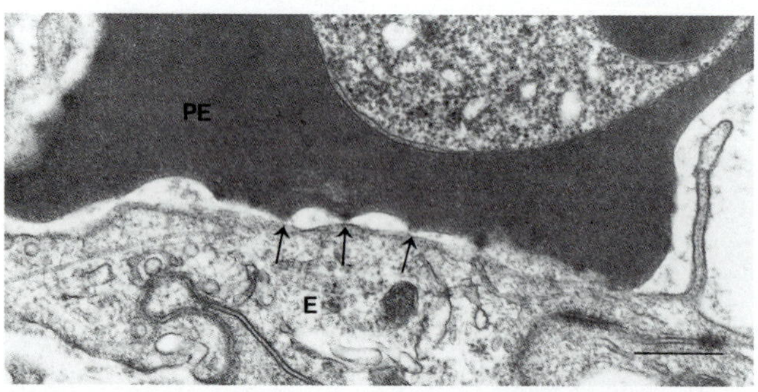

Figure 136–16. Electron micrograph of an erythrocyte infected with *P falciparum*. The parasitized erythrocyte (PE) is attached to the endothelium and is thus removed from the peripheral circulation. Attachment appears to be mediated by junctions (*arrows*) between knobs and the endothelial cell (E) (scale bar = 0.5 μm). From mesenteric fat of an experimentally infected *Aotus* monkey. *(From Atkinson and Aikawa,[10] with permission.)*

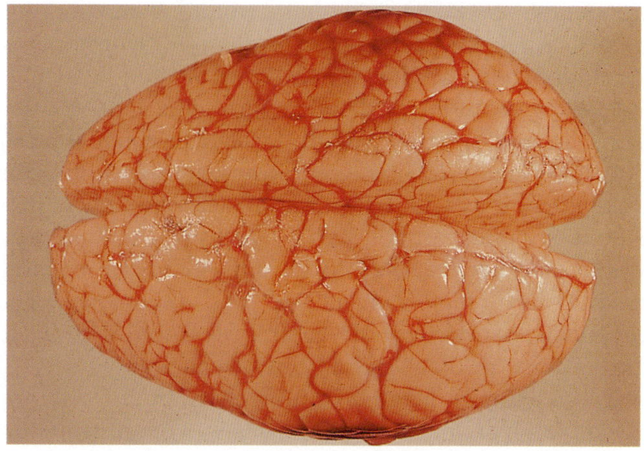

Figure 136–17. Brain of a 2-year-old Ugandan who died of cerebral malaria. The gyri are broadened and flattened and the surface vessels are congested. *(Photograph by Daniel H. Connor, MD, 1962.)*

for at least 10 days of clinical malaria. Both surround small vessels occluded by parasitized erythrocytes. Dürck's granulomas are areas of softening, demyelinization, and glial proliferation.

Early in infection, the spleen is enlarged and hyperemic. In long-standing chronic malaria, the spleen may become enormously enlarged and associated with collections of lymphocytes in the hepatic sinusoids. This is the "tropical splenomegaly syndrome."[15] Gross evaluation of splenomegaly is used to assess the incidence of malaria in endemic regions. Splenic rupture may complicate infection by *P vivax*. The slight splenomegaly in acute *P falciparum* infections may play a role in the accelerated clearance of abnormal erythrocytes from the circulating blood.[16] The spleen is

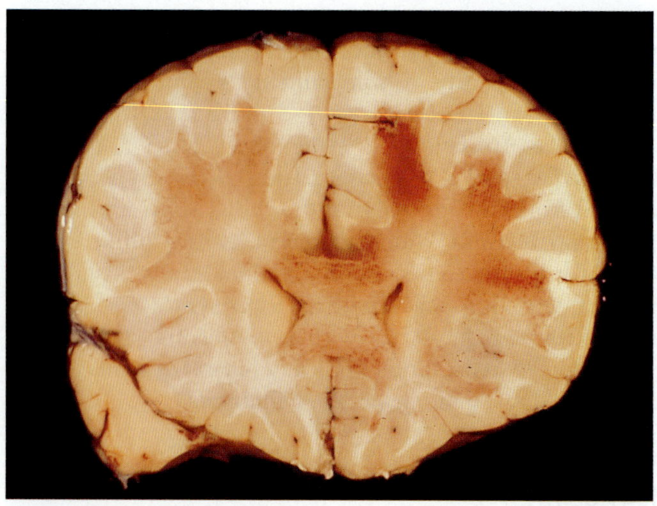

Figure 136–18. Brain of an adult Nigerian man who died of cerebral malaria. Note the selective congestion and hemorrhage of white matter, a characteristic feature of cerebral malaria. *(Photograph by Daniel H. Connor, MD, 1976.)*

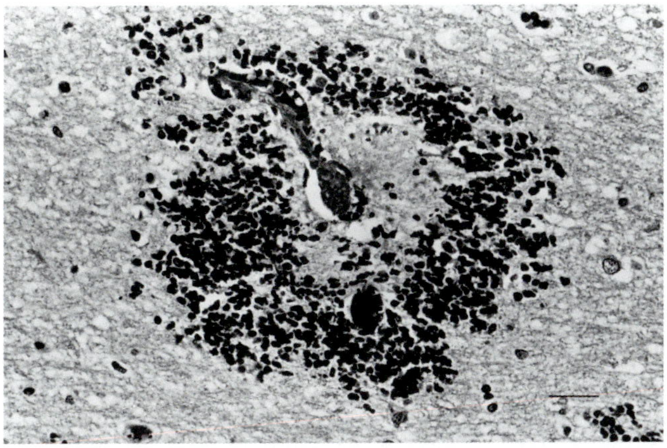

Figure 136–19. Ring hemorrhage in the brain of a patient who died of cerebral malaria (H&E) (scale bar = 0.5 μm). *(From Riganti et al,[109] with permission.)*

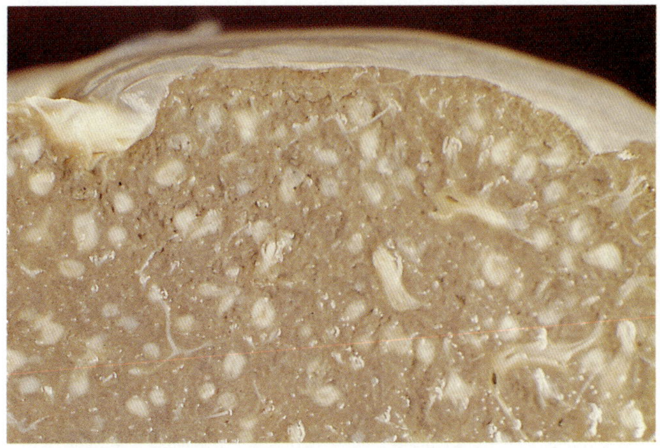

Figure 136–21. Spleen of a patient who died of acute falciparum malaria. The cut surface and the capsular surface are distinctly gray from the accumulation of grains of malarial pigment in phagocytic cells. *(Photograph by Daniel H. Connor, MD, 1976.)*

friable and at first dark red, but as malarial pigment accumulates the capsular and cut surfaces become dark gray (Figure 136–21). Scattered throughout the red pulp are parasitized erythrocytes and macrophages containing clumps of malarial pigment. In chronic infections, pigment-containing macrophages are increased and the fibrous connective tissue of the capsule, trabeculae, and lymphatic sheaths is more abundant. White pulp is depleted. The degree of pigmentation, not only in spleen but in other organs of the reticuloendothelial system, varies with the intensity and duration of the infection.

The liver, usually moderately enlarged, darkens as malarial pigment accumulates in Kupffer's cells and in phagocytic cells in the portal tracts (Figure 136–22). Microscopically, sinusoids are congested and Kupffer's cells are enlarged and increased in number. They contain granules of malarial pigment, erythrocytes, and debris from ruptured erythrocytes. Correlated with portal blood flow, there is a marked gradient in pigment deposition: Early in the infection, pigment is in the perilobular zone, then with time further deposits appear in the midlobular zone, and finally in the centrilobular zone. If a patient survives the acute attack, the malarial pigment accumulates in the portal areas (Figures 136–23 and 136–24).

Kidneys are grossly hyperemic. Microscopically, changes may be difficult to detect, and may require electron microscopy or immunofluorescence for their demonstration. These subtle alterations are glomeru-

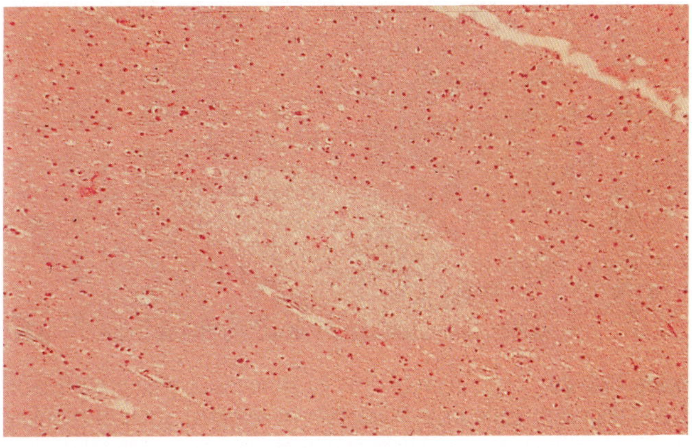

Figure 136–20. A Dürck's granuloma in the brain of a patient who died of cerebral malaria (AFIP Neg 56-21635; H&E, ×25).

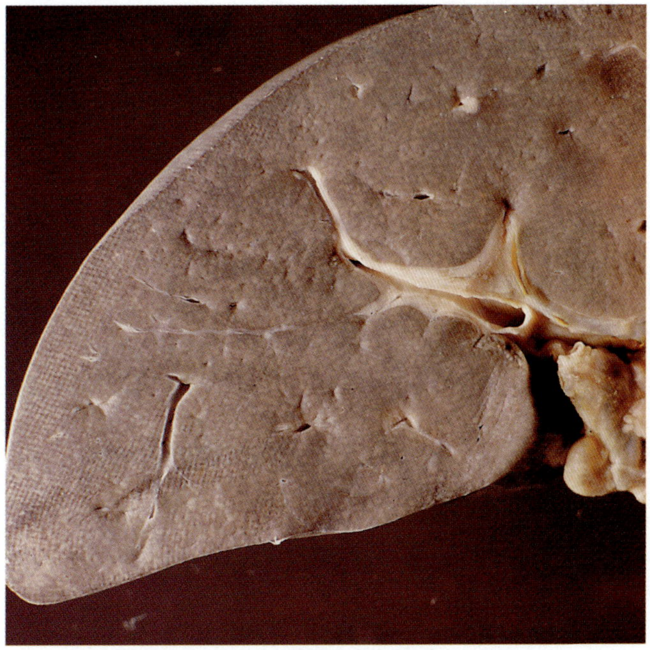

Figure 136–22. Liver of an infant who died of cerebral (falciparum) malaria. (The infant's brain is shown in Figure 136–17.) Malarial pigment, phagocytosed by Kupffer's cells, has made the liver dark gray. *(Photograph by Daniel H. Connor, MD, 1962.)*

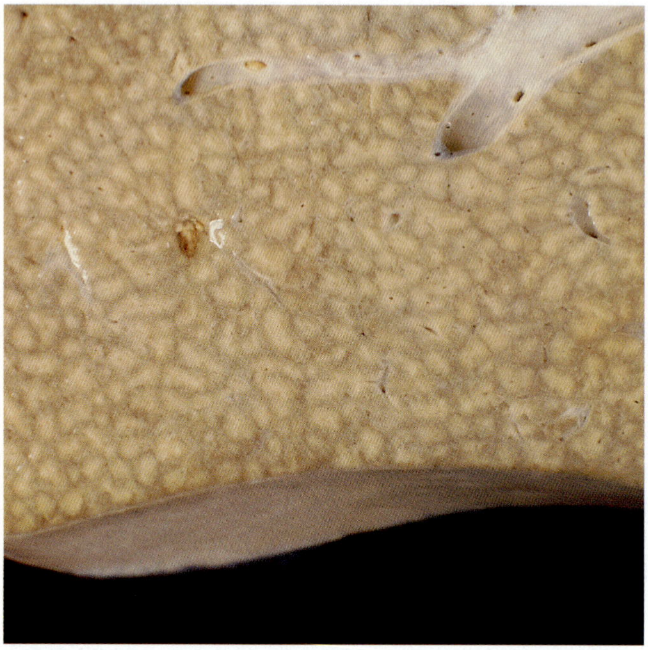

Figure 136–23. Liver of a patient who survived an attack of acute malaria. Malarial pigment is now concentrated in the portal areas making the portal tracts gray and thus accentuating the lobular pattern. *(Photograph by Daniel H. Connor, MD, 1976.)*

lonephritis, especially in chronic infections. During the acute phase of falciparum malaria about one half of all patients have malarial glomerulonephritis with clinical proteinuria, cylindruria, and abnormalities of urinary

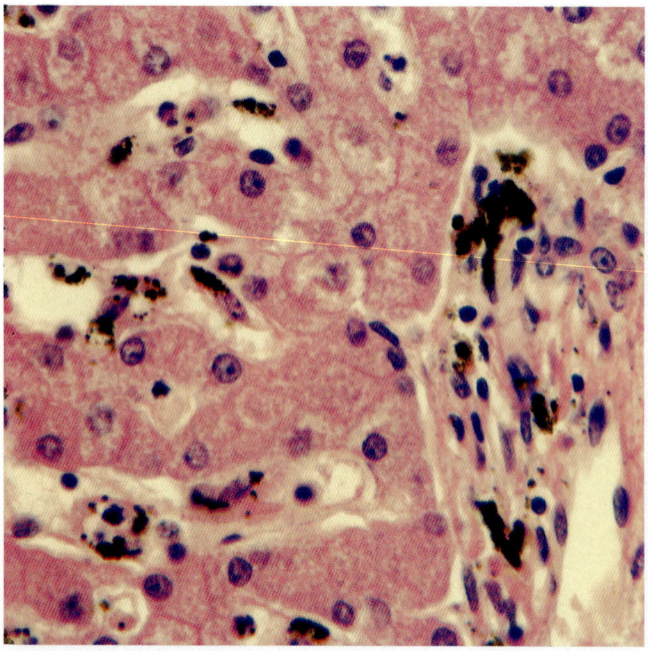

Figure 136–24. Liver shown in Figure 136–23. Note the light deposits of malarial pigment in Kupffer's cells and the heavier concentrations of malarial pigment in the portal tract (AFIP Neg 79-15350; H&E, ×400).

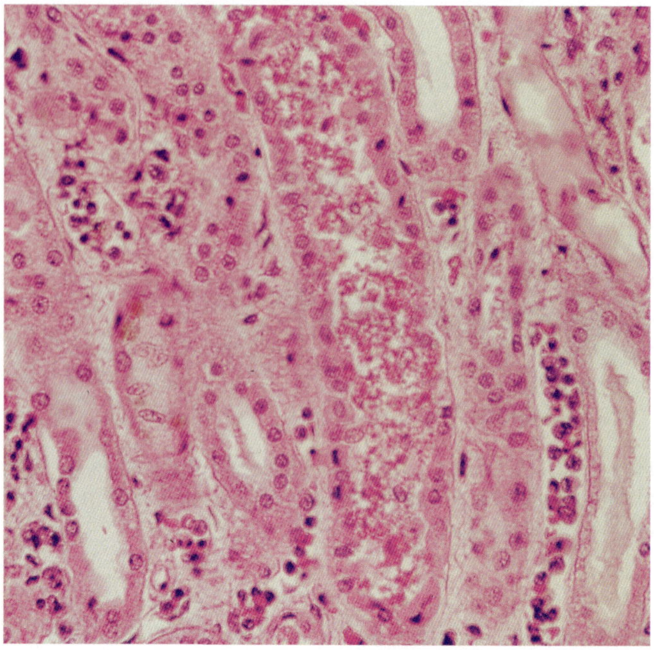

Figure 136–25. Kidney in fatal falciparum malaria. The tubule is filled with hemoglobin. Hemoglobinuric nephrosis may be a fatal complication of acute falciparum malaria (H&E, ×130).

sediment. Acute intravascular hemolysis or a heavy infection can cause hemoglobinuric nephrosis with renal failure (Figure 136–25). Blackwater fever, a syndrome characterized by dark urine after the acute attack has subsided, was frequently fatal and associated with quinine therapy. Antigen from *P falciparum* and corresponding antibodies may form immune complexes, which are deposited in the kidney, causing mesangiopathic glomerulonephropathy. These have been docu-

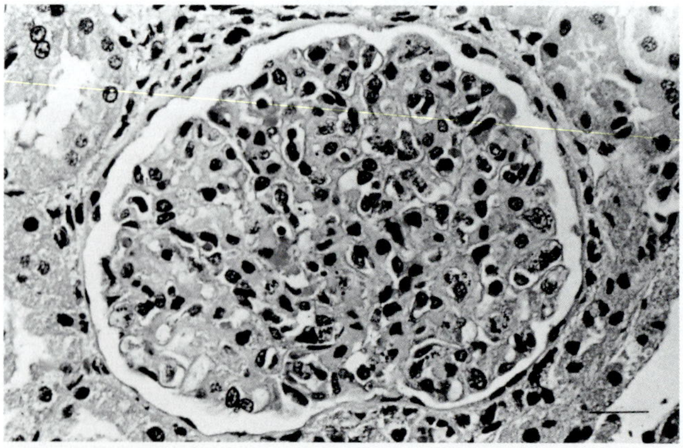

Figure 136–26. Light micrograph of a glomerulus with proliferation of endocapillary cells in a *P falciparum*–infected squirrel monkey (H&E). The capillary lumens contain infected erythrocytes, lymphocytes, monocytes, neutrophils, and macrophages with malarial pigment (scale bar = 25 μm). *(From Aikawa et al,[17] with permission.)*

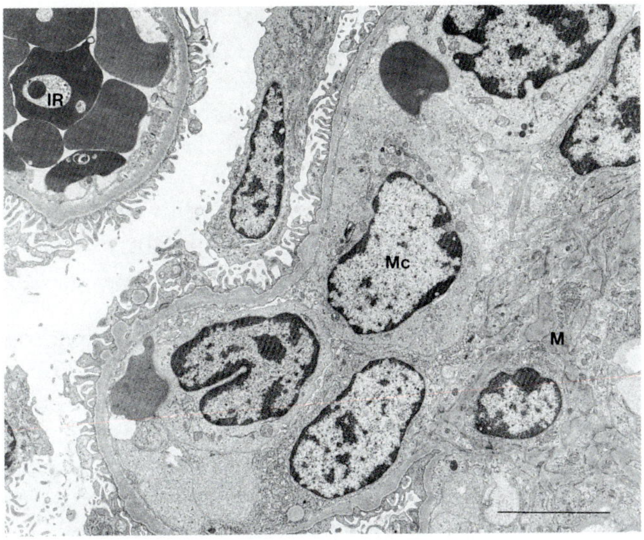

Figure 136–27. Electron micrograph of a glomerulus of a squirrel monkey infected with *P falciparum*. The capillary lumen is packed with many mononuclear cells (Mc) and infected erythrocytes (IR). The mesangial matrix (M) is increased (scale bar 5 μm). *(From Aikawa et al,[17] with permission.)*

mented by electron microscopy and by immunofluorescence[17] (Figures 136–26 through 136–28).

The placenta is severely affected, especially in primiparous women with infections by *P falciparum*. Placental function may be so impaired that the fetus is aborted. The placenta weighs less than normal and shows histologic changes not unlike those in other organs.[18] The intervillous spaces contain many parasitized erythrocytes and macrophages (Figure 136–29).[19] Vessels on the fetal side of the placental barrier are usually devoid of parasites. Rarely trauma and consequent mixing of maternal and fetal blood allow passage of parasitized cells into the fetal circulation, leading to congenital malaria (Figure 136–30). Despite the fact that both the anatomic and microscopic alterations associated with fatal *P falciparum* infections are well recognized, the pathophysiology of the disease is still incompletely understood and the precise mechanism of death is largely unknown. No model yet proposed satisfactorily explains the sequelae of human malaria.[20] A recently advanced animal model[21] may be useful for understanding human cerebral malaria.

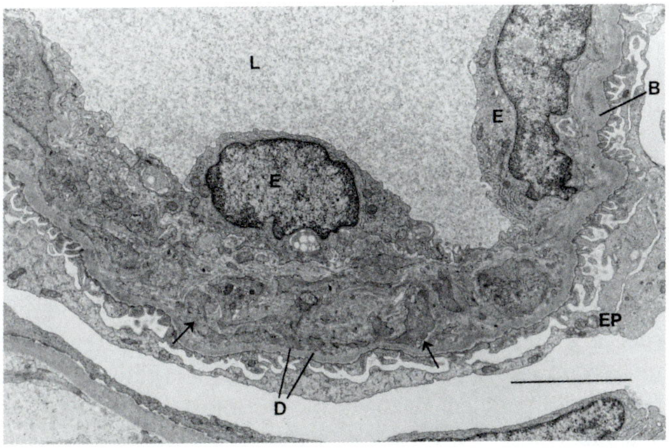

Figure 136–28. Electron micrograph of glomerulus showing mesangial cell interposition (*arrow*) along the basement membrane (B) in *P malariae* infection. Electron-dense deposits (D) are in the subendothelial areas. Endothelial cells, E; lumen, L; and epithelial cells, EP (scale bar 5 μm). *(From Aikawa et al,[109] with permission.)*

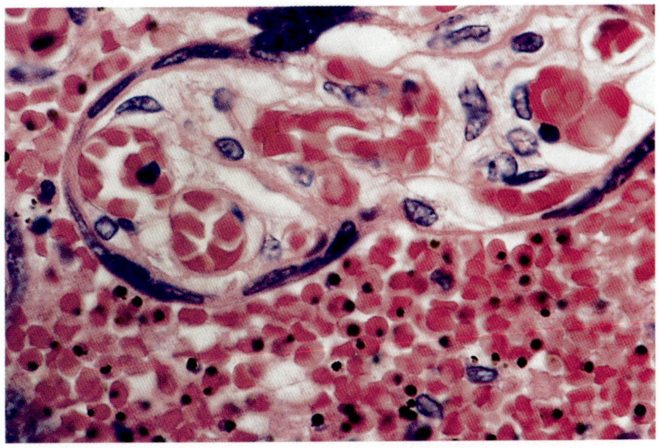

Figure 136–29. Placenta from a 23-year-old Zairian woman with falciparum malaria. Note the massive parasitization of the maternal erythrocytes in the intervillous spaces. By contrast the fetal erythrocytes are free of parasites in this field (H&E, ×300).

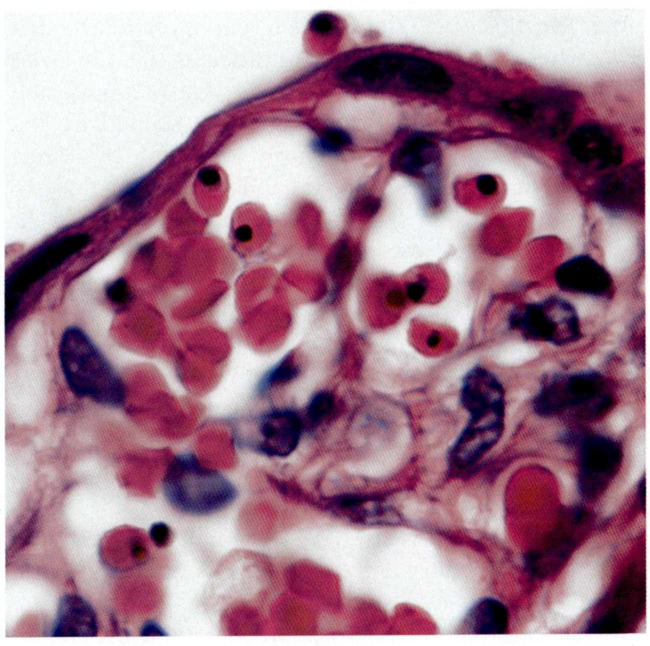

Figure 136–30. Same placenta showing parasitized erythrocytes in the villous (fetal) vessels. Several fields like this convinced those studying this placenta that the infant must have been infected at birth. Clinical follow-up was unavailable (H&E, ×650).

MICROSCOPIC DIAGNOSIS

Because of its simplicity and low cost, studying blood films by light microscopy remains the most popular diagnostic test for malaria (Figures 136–2 through 136–7). Thin blood films and an unspread drop of blood (thick film) stained with Giemsa, or similar stain, are used in diagnosis.[22] Red blood cells in thick films are hemolyzed so the malarial parasites are more concentrated. Thick blood films, therefore, overcome the sampling difficulties of thin smears. Thin smears, however, reveal details of infected red blood cells not apparent on thick films, and this sometimes helps in species identification.

Because *P falciparum* is the only parasite that becomes sequestered in vessels and kills its human host, it tends to be the only species of malarial parasite seen in tissue sections. Malarial pigment is birefringent and this is a helpful diagnostic feature when slides containing malarial parasites or malarial pigment are viewed under polarized light. Likewise blood smears also can be examined under polarized light and this may simplify and accelerate screening for malarial parasites.

Fluorescent dyes such as acridine orange, and DAPI, or a combination of DAPI and PI,[23,24] are used also to stain parasites. The quantitative buffy coat (QBC) technique[25] is one of these methods. A specially made glass capillary tube that contains acridine orange is filled with blood and a plastic float inserted. Because the float displaces the blood, the buffy coat is lengthened about 10 times when the capillary is centrifuged. Erythrocytes form a pellet at the bottom of the capillary tube. The float penetrates the upper layer of the red cells where the parasitized erythrocytes are localized because their density is lower than that of uninfected cells. Because the parasites are lightly stained by the acridine orange, they are easily detected by direct observation of the centrifuged capillary tube by fluorescence microscopy.

Immunologic tests are used increasingly to diagnose malaria.[26] These detect malarial antigens, and are based on both antigen competition and antigen-capture that use both enzyme-linked immunosorbent assay (ELISA) and radioimmunoassay (RIA). They have been used to assay genus-specific antigens, such as undefined *P falciparum* antigens,[27,28] defined malarial antigens,[29] and in idiotype–anti-idiotype detection systems.[30]

ELISA- and RIA-based tests can detect very low densities of parasitized red blood cells, with the latter being slightly more sensitive. These tests approach the level of sensitivity of microscopic techniques. Because RIAs utilize radioisotopes that have a short shelf life and that are expensive and potentially dangerous, they are not practical for everyday clinical use. Their main attraction has been to underscore the concept that simpler laboratory tests for malaria can be devised. Since the beginning of the AIDS epidemic, laboratory personnel have more experience in ELISA methods and ELISA kits are being used at many central health care facilities to support malarial field studies—both for epidemiology and for vaccine trials.

Because of its specificity and sensitivity, the indirect fluorescent antibody (IFA) test is the preferred method for serodiagnosis; it is the one currently used by the Centers for Disease Control and Prevention (CDC).[31] Other serologic tests for malaria diagnosis include the indirect hemagglutination antibody, ELISA, RIA, and complement fixation. Although serologic assays detect antimalarial antibodies, they cannot distinguish current and prior infections. For this reason, such tests are inappropriate for diagnostic purposes, but have some utility in epidemiologic surveys. The CDC has set strict guidelines for the use of IFA as follows[31]: IFA should be used as a diagnostic tool only when 1) a patient with a febrile illness is suspected of having malaria in spite of repeatedly negative blood films, 2) specimens are from the donor of a blood transfusion that preceded malaria in the recipient, or 3) if they are to be used for research or for standardizing control sera for IFA protocols.

DNA hybridization can be used to detect parasite-specific DNA sequences in extracts of erythrocytes.[32–34] Red blood cells that have been collected on a filter membrane are lysed to extract nucleic acids. After these nucleic acids are denatured by heating, they are blocked with nonspecific DNA. The membrane is incubated with either a specific radiolabeled probe, or with a (usually) biotinylated one. After washing, the membranes are subjected to autoradiography or enzyme-substrate labeling.

The polymerase chain reaction (PCR) method is used to amplify specific sequences of parasitic DNA. This technology involves amplification of specific DNA segments or, with a reverse transcriptase RNA,[35] by repeated rounds of heat denaturation, annealing with defined DNA primer pairs, and primer extension via heat-resistant DNA polymerase obtained from thermophilic bacteria. PCRs involve repeated cycles of amplification that may take several hours to accomplish. A drawback of this technique is that electrical power, which may not always be available in some areas, is needed to run a thermal cycler and the reagents are expensive. An ELISA-type assay for PCR products recently has been developed[36] but requires 10 to 100 gene copies. A second problem is that parasite DNA (not originally in the sample) contaminates the test sample.

Recently introduced is a rapid dipstick test for falciparum malaria called the *para*Sight^{R-}F. It detects trophozoite-derived Histidine-rich Protein (HRP-II). It has a high specificity and high sensitivity.[37] In 75% of patients, however, HPR-II can be detected 1 week after

TABLE 136–1. DRUG REGIMENS FOR TREATING FALCIPARUM MALARIA

Chloroquine-Sensitive Falciparum Malaria
Uncomplicated Falciparum Malaria
Chloroquine 10 mg (base) per kg of body weight as an initial dose, then 5 mg (base) per kg at 6, 24, and 48 hours after the first dose
Severe Falciparum Malaria
Chloroquine 10 mg (base) per kg of body weight by intravenous infusion at a slow rate over 8 hours, followed by infusion of 15 mg (base) per kg over the next 24 hours[90,91]
or
Intramuscular or subcutaneous chloroquine at 3.5 mg (base) per kg of body weight every 6 hours to a total dose of 25 mg per kg of body weight if intravenous chloroquine is not possible[92]
Chloroquine-Resistant Falciparum Malaria
Uncomplicated Falciparum Malaria
A single oral dose of 1500 mg sulfadoxine (base) and 75 mg of pyrimethamine base (3 tablets of Fansidar)
or
Quinine sulphate 10 mg (salt) per kg of body weight every 8 hours for 7 days
or
Quinine sulphate 10 mg (salt) per kg of body weight every 8 hours for 7 days plus tetracycline 250 mg Qid for 7 days (for quinine-resistant falciparum malaria)[93,94]
or
Mefloquine 750 mg* as a single dose.
Severe Falciparum Malaria
Quinine dihydrochloride 10 mg (salt) per kg of body weight every 8 hours for 7 days
or
Quinine dihydrochloride 20 mg per kg of body weight as a loading dose, followed by 10 mg per kg every 8 hours for 7 days (for quinine-resistant falciparum malaria)[95]
or
Intravenous quinine should be switched to oral quinine as soon as oral medication is possible.
Treatment of Multidrug-Resistant Falciparum Malaria (chloroquine-, sulfadoxine–pyrimethamine-, mefloquine-, and quinine-resistance)
Uncomplicated Falciparum Malaria
Mefloquine 1250 mg in 2 divided doses at 6 hour intervals (750 mg first dose, then 500 mg at 6 hours later)[96]
or
Quinine sulphate 10 mg (salt) per kg of body weight every 8 hours for 7 days plus tetracycline 250 mg Qid for 7 days
or
Halofantrine† 500 mg every 6 hours for 3 doses (1500 mg total dose)
or
Artemether or artesunate 300 mg on the first day, followed by 100 mg daily for another 4 days[81,94]
or
Artemether or artesunate 300 mg single dose on the first day, followed by mefloquine 750 mg at 24 hours and 500 mg at 30 hours[97–99]
Severe Falciparum Malaria
Artemether 160 mg intramuscularly as a loading dose, followed by 80 mg intramuscularly daily for another 6 days[100]
or
Artesunate 2 mg per kg of body weight intravenously as a loading dose, followed by 1 mg per kg intravenously at 4 hours and at 24 hours, then daily for another 6 days[101]
or
Artemether 160 mg as a loading dose, followed by 80 mg intramuscularly daily for another 4 days, then mefloquine 750 mg on the last day of treatment[102–105]
Treatment for Vivax and Ovale Malaria
Chloroquine 600 mg as a loading dose, followed by 300 mg 6 hours later, then 300 mg daily for another 2 doses. After the completion of chloroquine, primaquine‡ should be started at a dose of 15 mg daily for 14 days. In patients with G6PD deficiency, primaquine is given at 45 mg weekly for 8 weeks.
Treatment for Malariae Malaria
Chloroquine at the same dosage as with vivax malaria but primaquine is not required.

* Mefloquine should not be given to patients whose work requires fine coordination or to patients who operate dangerous equipment.
† Caution must be used when prescribing halofantrine to patients with preexisting cardiopathy. An ECG before halofantrine is essential.
‡ Patients should be informed about the possibility of hemolysis after being treated with primaquine. Primaquine is contraindicated in pregnancy.

effective treatment and can be detected 2 weeks after effective treatment in 10% of patients.

Direct examination of stained slides is the most accurate and sensitive method of diagnosis. The clinical suspicion of malaria must attend any patient with fever recently in an endemic area for malaria and the diagnosis must be confirmed by microscopic examination as noted before. Diagnosing malaria on blood smears requires an experienced observer and relatively expensive equipment. Simpler and equally dependable alternatives to diagnosis are needed in endemic areas where costly equipment is not available. Even in well-equipped laboratories a simple diagnostic test would be valuable, because at present inexperienced technologists are sometimes called on to diagnose malaria.

DIFFERENTIAL DIAGNOSIS

Any disease with severe fever, especially when accompanied by rigor, disturbed consciousness, diarrhea, jaundice, spontaneous bleeding, renal failure, shock, or respiratory distress may be malaria. Malaria may be confused with yellow fever, other viral hemorrhagic fevers, relapsing fever, enteric fever, leptospirosis, and even with heatstroke. Cerebral malaria may be mistaken for a form of infective meningoencephalitis, metabolic comas, intoxications, or psychoses. Imported malaria in Western countries may be misdiagnosed as influenza, viral hepatitis, encephalitis, or travelers' diarrhea.

TREATMENT

The available blood schizontocides for treating human malaria are chloroquine, sulfadoxine–pyrimethamine, quinine, mefloquine, halofantrine, artemether, and artesunate. Primaquine is the only available drug for the hypnozoites and relapsing malaria. The choice of antimalarials depends on drug resistance—now common with falciparum parasites. Knowing the distribution of drug-resistant falciparum parasites is essential in selecting the best antimalarial regimen. The regimens are described in Table 136–1.

Chloroquine-resistant falciparum malaria has been documented in most countries of Southeast Asia[38–41] and the resistance is rapidly emerging in other geographic areas.[42–52] Chloroquine is used with doubtful effect in most countries in Southeast Asia, and in sub-Saharan Africa, chloroquine should no longer be considered adequately effective against falciparum malaria in very young children.[46] Chloroquine-resistant *P vivax* has been reported in Indonesia, India, Myanmar, and Papua New Guinea,[53–58] but in general, chloroquine is still very effective against vivax malaria.

A decrease in sensitivity to quinine has been noted in several areas in Southeast Asia and East Africa.[59–63] Quinine, nevertheless, remains the drug of choice for severe falciparum malaria worldwide.

Mefloquine is active against falciparum and vivax malaria, but there is resistance in a few areas along the Thai–Cambodian and Thai–Myanmar border, with a cure rate of 30 to 50% from a single dose of 750 mg of mefloquine.[64–69]

Halofantrine is effective against multidrug-resistant falciparum malaria, but there is in vitro evidence of cross resistance with mefloquine.[70] The main concern is halofantrine's variable absorption, which is partly responsible for failures in incomplete absorption[71] and also for cardiotoxicity in patients with excess absorption.[72–75]

Artemether and artesunate are potent against vivax and multidrug-resistant falciparum malaria. Their action is rapid, clearing 95% of the parasitemia within 24 hours,[76–89] but there is a high likelihood of recrudescence if the duration of treatment is less than 5 days.

Acknowledgments. This work was supported in part by grants from the U.S. Agency for International Development DPE-0453-A-009-141 UNDP/World Bank/WHO Special Programme for Research & Training in Tropical Diseases, the USPHS AI-10645 and the U.S. Army Research and Development Command, contract DAMD 17-9OC-OO10, Contribution No. to Army Research Program on Antiparasitic Drugs. Kiet Dan Luc and Maryann Kaczur helped prepare the manuscript.

REFERENCES

1. *Tropical Diseases: Progress in Research, 1989–1990.* Tenth programme report. Geneva: World Health Organization; 1991.
2. Bruce-Chwatt LJ. *Essential Malariology.* New York: John Wiley & Sons; 1985:55–266.
3. Wernsdorfer WH. The development and spread of drug-resistant malaria. *Parasitol Today.* 1991;7:297–303.
4. Label HO, Campbell CC, Schwartz IK, Roberts JM. Recent trends in the importation of malaria caused by *Plasmodium falciparum* into the United States from Africa. *J Infect Dis.* 1985;152:613–617.
5. Most H. Manhattan: "a tropic isle?" *Am J Trop Med Hyg.* 1968;17:333–354.
6. Garnham PC. Malaria parasites of man: life-cycles and morphology. In: Wernsdorfer WH, McGregor I, eds. *Malaria: Principles and Practice of Malariology.* London: Churchill Livingstone; 1988;1:61–96.
7. Long EG. Malaria. In: Lennette EH, Halonen P, Murphy FA, eds. *Laboratory Diagnosis of Infectious Diseases.* London: Springer-Verlag; 1988;1:911–928.
8. Aikawa M. Fine structure of malaria parasites in the various stages of development. In: Wernsdorfer WH, McGregor I. *Malaria: Principles and Practice of Malariology.* London: Churchill Livingstone; 1988;1:97–129.

9. Aikawa M. Human cerebral malaria. *Am J Trop Med Hyg.* 1988;39:3–10.
10. Atkinson CT, Aikawa M. Ultrastructure of malaria-infected erythrocytes. *Blood Cells.* 1990;16:351–368.
11. World Health Organization. Severe and complicated malaria. *Trans Roy Soc Trop Med Hyg.* 1990;84(suppl.2): 1–65.
12. Oo MM, Aikawa M, Than T, et al. Human cerebral malaria: a pathological study. *J Neuropathol Exp Neurol.* 1987; 46:7–14.
13. Aikawa M, Iseki M, Barnwell JW, Taylor D, Oo MM, Howard RJ. The pathology of human cerebral malaria. *Am J Trop Med Hyg.* 1990;43(suppl):30–37.
14. Howard RJ, Handunnetti SM, Hasler T, et al. Surface molecules on *Plasmodium falciparum*–infected erythrocytes involved in adherence. *Am J Trop Med Hyg.* 1990;43 (suppl):15–29.
15. Pitney WR. The tropical splenomegaly syndrome. *Trans Roy Soc Trop Med Hyg.* 1968;62:717–728.
16. Looareesuwan S, Ho M, Wattanogoon Y, et al. Dynamic alteration in splenic function during acute falciparum malaria. *N Engl J Med.* 1987;317:675–679.
17. Aikawa M, Jacobs G, Whiteley HE, Igarashi I, Ristic M. Glomerulopathy in squirrel monkeys with acute *Plasmodium falciparum* infection. *Am J Trop Med Hyg.* 1988; 38:7–14.
18. Walter PR, Garin Y, Blot P. Placental pathologic changes in malaria. A histologic and ultrastructural study. *Am J Pathol.* 1982;109:330–342.
19. Yamada M, Steketee R, Abramowsky C, et al. *Plasmodium falciparum* associated placental pathology: a light and electron microscopic and immunohistologic study. *Am J Trop Med Hyg.* 1989;41:161–168.
20. Phillips RE, Warrell DA. The pathophysiology of severe falciparum malaria. *Parasitol Today.* 1986;2:271–282.
21. Aikawa M, Brown AE, Smith CD, et al. A primate model for human cerebral malaria: *P coatneyi*–infected Rhesus monkeys. *Am J Trop Med Hyg.* 1992;46:391–397.
22. Shute GT. The microscopic diagnosis of malaria. In: Wernsdorfer WH, McGregor I, eds. *Malaria: Principles and Practice of Malariology.* London: Churchill Livingstone; 1988;1:781–814.
23. Richards DF, et al. Detection of plasmodia by acridine orange stain. *Am J Clin Pathol.* 1969;39:280–283.
24. Kawamoto F. Rapid diagnosis of malaria by fluorescence microscopy with light microscope and interference. *Lancet.* 1991;337:200–202.
25. Wardlaw SC, Levine RA. Quantitative buffy coat analysis: a new laboratory tool functioning as a screening complete blood cell count. *JAMA.* 1983;249:617–620.
26. Maddison SE. Serodiagnosis of parasitic diseases. *Clin Microbiol Rev.* 1991;4:457–469.
27. Khusmith S, Tharavanij S, Kasemsuth R, Vejvongvarn C, Bunnag D. Two-site immunoradiometric assay for detection of *Plasmodium falciparum* antigen in blood using monoclonal and polyclonal antibodies. *J Clin Microbiol.* 1987;25:1467–1471.
28. Mackey LJ, McGregor IA, Paounova N, Lambert PH. Diagnosis of *Plasmodium falciparum* infection in man: detection of parasite antigens by ELISA. *Bull WHO.* 1982; 60:69–75.
29. Fortier B, Delplace P, Dubremetz JF, Ajana F, Vernes A. Enzyme immunoassay for detection of antigen in acute *Plasmodium falciparum* malaria. *Eur J Clin Microbiol.* 1987;6:596–598.
30. Zhou WS, Li YJ. Anti-idiotypic antibodies: preparation and identification; application to the detection of antigens of *Plasmodium falciparum. Parasite Immunol.* 1987;9: 747–755.
31. *Malaria Surveillance Annual Summary, 1984.* Atlanta, Ga: Centers for Disease Control and Prevention; 1985.
32. Wilson SM. Nucleic acid techniques and the detection of parasitic diseases. *Parasitol Today.* 1991;7:255–259.
33. Pollack Y, Metzger S. Shemer R, Landau D, Spira DT, Golenser J. Detection of *Plasmodium falciparum* in blood using DNA hybridization. *Am J Trop Med Hyg.* 1985;34: 663–667.
34. Holmberg M, Bjorkman A, Franzen L, et al. Diagnosis of *Plasmodium falciparum* detected by spot hybridization assay: specificity, sensitivity, and field applicability. *Bull WHO.* 1986;64:579–585.
35. Waters AP, McCutchan TF. Ribosomal RNA: nature of polymerase-amplified target for diagnosis. *Parasitol Today.* 1990;6:56–59.
36. Nickerson DA, Kaiser R, Lappin S, Stewart J, Hood L, Landergen U. Automated DNA diagnostics using an ELISA-based oligonucleotide ligation assay. *Proc Natl Acad Sci USA.* 1990;87:8923–8927.
37. Shift CJ, Minjas J, Premji. The *Para*Sight[R-]F test: a simple rapid manual dipstick test to detect *Plasmodium falciparum* infection. *Parasitol Today.* 1994;10:494–495.
38. Bunnag D, Harinasuta T. The current status of drug resistance in malaria. In: Howell MJ. ed. *Parasitology Quo Vadit?* Brisbane: Australian Academy of Science; 1986.
39. Wernsdorfer WH. Epidemiology of drug resistance in malaria. *Acta Tropica.* 1994;56:143–156.
40. Verdrager J. Epidemiology of emergence and spread of drug-resistant falciparum malaria in Southeast Asia and Australia. *J Trop Med Hyg.* 1986;89:277–289.
41. Harinasuta T, Suntharasamai P, Viravan C. Chloroquine resistant falciparum in Thailand. *Lancet.* 1965;2:657.
42. Oduola AMJ, Moyou RS, Kyle DE, Martin SK, Gerena L, Milhous WK. Chloroquine-resistant *Plasmodium falciparum* in indigenous residents of Cameroon. *Trans Roy Soc Trop Med Hyg.* 1989;83:308–310.
43. Lege-Oguntoye L, Abua JU, Werblinska B, Ogala WN, Slotboom AM, Olurinola PF. Chloroquine resistance of *Plasmodium falciparum* in semi-immune children in Zaria, northern Nigeria. *Trans Roy Soc Trop Med Hyg.* 1989;83:599–601.
44. Nguyen-Dinh P, Schwartz IK, Sexton JD, et al. *In vivo* and *in vitro* susceptibility to chloroquine of *Plasmodium falciparum* in Kinshasa and Mbuji-Mayi, Zaire. *Bull WHO.* 1995;3:325–330.
45. Brasseur P, Agnamey P, Ekobo AS, Samba G, Favannec L, Kouamouo J. Sensitivity of *Plasmodium falciparum* to amodiaquine and chloroquine in Central Africa: a comparative study *in vivo* and *in vitro. Trans Roy Soc Trop Med Hyg.* 1995;89:528–530.
46. Bloland PB, Lackritz EM, Kazembe PN, Were JBO, Steketee R, Campbell CC. Beyond chloroquine: implications of drug resistance for evaluating malaria therapy efficacy and treatment policy in Africa. *J Infect Dis.* 1993;167:932–937.
47. Menon A, Otoo LN, Herbage EA, Greenwood BM. A

national survey of the prevalence of chloroquine resistant *Plasmodium falciparum* malaria in the Gambia. *Trans Roy Soc Trop Med Hyg.* 1990;84:638–640.

48. Sansonetti PJ, Le Bras J, Verdier F. Chloroquine-resistant *Plasmodium falciparum* in Cameroon. *Lancet.* 1985; 8438:1154–1155.
49. Brandicort O, Druilhe P, Diouf F, Brasseur P, Turk P, Danis M. Decreased sensitivity to chloroquine and quinine of some *Plasmodium falciparum* strains from Senegral in September 1984. *Am J Trop Med Hyg.* 1986;35:717–721.
50. Brasseur P, Druilhe P, Kouamouo J, Moyou S. Drug resistance in Sahel part of West Africa. *Trans Roy Soc Trop Med Hyg.* 1987;81:162–164.
51. Mharakkurwa S, Mugochi T. Chloroquine-resistant falciparum malaria in an area of rising endemicity in Zimbabwe. *J Trop Med Hyg.* 1994;97:39–45.
52. Adagu IS, Warhurst DC, Ogala WN., et al. Antimalarial drug response of *Plasmodium falciparum* from Zaria, Nigeria. *Trans Roy Soc Trop Med Hyg.* 1995;89:422–425.
53. Schwartz IK, Lackritz EM, Patchen MS. Chloroquine-resistant *Plasmodium vivax* from Indonesia. *New Engl J Med.* 1989;324:927.
54. Myat-Phone-Kyaw, Myint-Oo, Myint-Lin, Thaw-Zin, Kyin-Hla-Aye, Nwe-Nwe Yin. Emergence of chloroquine-resistant *Plasmodium vivax* in Myanmar (Burma). *Trans Roy Soc Trop Med Hyg.* 1993;87:687.
55. Marlar-Than, Myat-Phone-Kyaw, Aye-Yu-Soe, Khaing-Khaing-Gyi, Ma-Sabai, Myint-Oo. Development of resistance to chloroquine by *Plasmodium vivax* in Myanmar. *Trans Roy Soc Trop Med Hyg.* 1995;89:307–308.
56. Rieckman KH, Davis DR, Hutton DC. *Plasmodium vivax* resistant to chloroquine? *Lancet.* 1989;ii:1183–1184.
57. Schuurkamp GJ, Spicer PE, Kereu RK, Bulungol PK, Rieckmann KH. Chloroquine-resistant *Plasmodium vivax* in Papua New Guinea. *Trans Roy Soc Trop Med Hyg.* 1992; 86:121–122.
58. Whitby M, Wood G, Veenedaal JR, Rieckmann K. Chloroquine-resistant *Plasmodium vivax.* [Letter]. *Lancet.* 1989; 2:1395.
59. Bunnag D, Harinasuta T. Quinine and quinidine in malaria in Thailand. *Acta Liedensia.* 1987;55:163–166.
60. Chongsuphajaisiddi T, Sabcharoen A, Attanath P. Treatment of quinine resistant falciparum malaria in Thai children. *Southeast Asian J Trop Med Public Health.* 1983; 14:367–362.
61. Giboda M. Denis MB. Response of Kampuchean strains of *Plasmodium falciparum* to antimalarials: *in vivo* assessment of quinine and quinine plus tetracycline: multiple drug resistance *in vitro. J Trop Med Hyg.* 1988;91:205–211.
62. Karbwang J, Mungthin M, Thanavibul A, Na-Bangchang K, Harinasuta T. Artemether saved a patient with severe falciparum malaria after quinine treatment failure (RIII-type of quinine resistance). *Southeast Asian J Trop Med Public Health.* 1994;25:782–783.
63. Jelinek T, Schelbert P, Loscher T, Eichenlaub T, Eichenlaub D. Quinine resistant falciparum malaria acquired in east Africa. *Trop Med Parasitol.* 1995;46:38–40.
64. Boudreau EF, Webster HK, Pavanand K, Thosingha L. Type II mefloquine resistance in Thailand. *Lancet.* 1982;1335.
65. Bunnag D, Viravan C, Karbwang J, et al. Clinical trials with halofantrine in acute uncomplicated falciparum malaria in Thailand. *Southeast Asian J Trop Med Public Health.* 1993;24:43–48.
66. Ketrangsee S, Vijayakadga S, Yamokgul P, Jatapadma S, Thimasarn K, Rooney W. Comparative trial on the response of *Plasmodium falciparum* to halofantrine and mefloquine in Trat Province, eastern Thailand. *Southeast Asian J Trop Med Public Health.* 1992;23:51–54.
67. Karbwang J, Na-Bangchang K, Thimasarn K, Rooney W, Bunnag D, Harinasuta T. Mefloquine levels in patients with mefloquine resistant *Plasmodium falciparum* in the eastern part of Thailand. *Southeast Asian J Trop Med Public Health.* 1993;24:226–229.
68. Fontanet AL, Johnston BD, Walker AM, Bergqvist Y, Hellgren U, Rooney W. Falciparum malaria in eastern Thailand: a randomized trial of the efficacy of a single dose of mefloquine. *Bull WHO.* 1994;72:73–81.
69. Smithuis FM, van Woensel JBM, Nordlander E, Vantha WS, ter Kuile FO. Comparison of two mefloquine regimens for treatment of *Plasmodium falciparum* malaria on the northeastern Thai–Cambodian border. *Antimicrob Chemother.* 1993;37:1977–1981.
70. Gay F, Bustos DG, Diquet B, Rojas R, Litaudon M. Cross resistance between mefloquine and halofantrine. *Lancet.* 1990;2:1262.
71. Karbwang J, Milton KA, Na-Bangchang K, Ward SA, Edwards G, Bunnag D. Pharmacokinetics of halofantrine in Thai patients with acute uncomplicated falciparum malaria. *Brit J Clin Pharmacol.* 1991;31:484–487.
72. Nosten F, ter Kuile FO, Luxemburger C, et al. Cardiac effects of antimalarial treatment with halofantrine. *Lancet.* 1993;341:1054–1056.
73. Karbwang J, Na-Bangchang K, Bunnag D, Harinasuta T, Laothavorn P. Cardiac effect of halofantrine. *Lancet.* 1993; 342:501.
74. Castot A, Rapoport P, Le Coz P. Prolonged QT interval with halofantrine. *Lancet.* 1993;341:1541.
75. Monlun E, Metayer PL, Szwandt S, et al. Cardiac complications of halofantrine: a prospective study of 20 patients. *Trans Roy Soc Trop Med Hyg.* 1995;89:430–433.
76. Bunnag D, Karbwang J, Harinasuta T. Artemether in the treatment of multiple drug resistant falciparum malaria. *Southeast Asian J Trop Med Public Health.* 1992;23: 762–767.
77. Bunnag D, Karbwang J, Chitamas S, Harinasuta T. Intramuscular artemether in female patients with uncomplicated falciparum malaria. *Southeast Asian J Trop Med Public Health.* 1993;24:49–52.
78. China Cooperative Research on Qinghaosu and its Derivatives as Antimalarials. Clinical studies on the treatment of malaria with qinghaosu and its derivatives. *J Trad Chin Med.* 1982;2:17–24.
79. China Cooperative Research on Qinghaosu and its Derivatives as Antimalarials. Clinical studies on the treatment of malaria with qinghaosu and its derivatives. *J Trad Chin Med.* 1982;2:25–30.
80. China Cooperative Research on Qinghaosu and its Derivatives as Antimalarials. Clinical studies on the treatment of malaria with qinghaosu and its derivatives. *J Trad Chin Med.* 1982;2:31–44.
81. Karbwang J, Na-Bangchang K, Thanavibul A, Bunnag D.

Chongsuphajaisiddhi T, Harinasuta T. Comparison of oral artemether and mefloquine in acute uncomplicated falciparum malaria. *Lancet.* 1992;340:1245–1248.

82. Karbwang J, Sukontason K, Rimchala W, et al. Preliminary report: a comparative clinical trial of artemether and quinine in severe falciparum malaria. *Southeast Asian J Trop Med Public Health.* 1992:23:768–772.
83. Karbwang J, Na-Bangchang K, Wattanagoon Y, Thanavibul A, Harinasuta T. Artemether 5 versus 7 day regimen for severe falciparum malaria. *Southeast Asian J Trop Med Public Health.* 1994;25:702–706.
84. Karbwang J, Na-Bangchang K, Thanavibul A, Laothavorn P, Ditta-in M, Harinasuta T. A comparative clinical trial of artemether and the sequential regimen of artemether–mefloquine in mutidrug resistant falciparum malaria. *J Antimicrob Ag Chemother.* 1995:36:1079–1083.
85. Myint PT, Shwe T. The efficacy of artemether (qinghaosu) in *Plasmodium falciparum* and *P. vivax* in Burma. *Southeast Asian J Trop Med Public Health.* 1986;17:19–22.
86. Myint PT, Shwe T. A controlled clinical trial of artemether (qinghaosu derivative) versus quinine in complicated and severe falciparum malaria. *Trans Roy Soc Trop Med Hyg.* 1987;81:559–561.
87. Myint PT, Shwe T, Lin S. Clinical study of the treatment of cerebral malaria with artemether (qinghaosu derivative). *Trans Roy Soc Trop Med Hyg.* 1989;83:72.
88. Wang TY, Xu RC. Clinical studies of treatment of falciparum malaria with artemether, a derivative of qinghaosu. *J Trad Chin Med.* 1985:5:240–242.
89. Win K, Thwe Y, Than KM. A clinical experience with artemether. *Bur Med J.* 1985;31:26–34.
90. White NJ, Miller KD, Churchill FC, Berry C, Brown J, Williams BS. Chloroquine treatment of severe malaria in children. Pharmacokinetics, toxicity and new dosage recommendations. *New Engl J Med.* 1988;319:1493–1500.
91. White NJ, Watt G, Bergqvist Y, Njeilesani EK. Parenteral chloroquine for treating falciparum malaria. *J Infect Dis.* 1987;155:192–201.
92. White NJ, Krishna S, Waller D, Craddock C, Kwiatkawski D, Brewster B. Open comparison of intramuscular chloroquine and quinine in children with severe chloroquine-sensitive falciparum malaria. *Lancet.* 1989;1313–1316.
93. Looareesuwan S, Wilairatana P, Vanijanonta S, Kyle DE, Webster HK. Efficacy of quinine-tetracycline for acute uncomplicated falciparum malaria in Thailand. *Lancet.* 1992;339:369.
94. Karbwang J, Na-Bangchang K, Thanavibul A, Bunnag D, Chongsuphajaisiddhi T, Harinasuta T. Comparison of oral artesunate and quinine plus tetracycline in acute uncomplicated falciparum malaria. *Bull WHO.* 1994;72:223–238.
95. White NJ, Looareesuwan S, Warrell DA, et al. Quinine loading dose in cerebral malaria. *Am J Trop Med Hyg.* 1983;32:1–5.
96. Karbwang J, Na-Bangchang K, Bunnag D, Harinasuta T. Pharmacokinetics and pharmacodynamics of mefloquine in patients with uncomplicated malaria. *Bull WHO.* 1991; 69:207–212.
97. Bunnag D, Kanda T, Karbwang J, Thimasarn K, Pungpak S, Harinasuta T. Artemether–mefloquine combination in multidrug resistant falciparum malaria. *Trans Roy Soc Trop Med Hyg.* 1995;89:213–215.
98. Karbwang J, Na-Bangchang K, Thanavibul A, Ditta-in M, Harinasuta T. A comparative clinical trial of two different regimens of artemether plus mefloquine in multidrug resistant falciparum malaria. *Trans Roy Soc Trop Med Hyg.* 1995;89:296–298.
99. Bunnag D, Kanda T, Karbwang J, Pungpak S, Harinasuta T. Artemether or artesunate followed by mefloquine as a possible treatment for multidrug resistant falciparum malaria. *Trans Roy Soc Trop Med Hyg.* 1996 (in press).
100. Karbwang J, Tin T, Sukontason K, et al. Comparison of artemether and quinine in the treatment of severe falciparum malaria in southeast Thailand. *Trans Roy Soc Trop Med Hyg.* 1995;89:668–671.
101. World Health Organization. *WHO Model Prescribing Information: Drugs Used in Parasitic Diseases.* 2d ed. Geneva, Switzerland; World Health Organization.
102. Shwe T, Myint PT, Htut Y, Myint W, Soe L. The effect of mefloquine–artemether compared with quinine on patients with complicated falciparum malaria. *Trans Roy Soc Trop Med Hyg.* 1988;82:665–667.
103. Shwe T, Myint PT, Myint W, Htut Y, Soe L, Thwe M. Clinical studies on treatment of cerebral malaria with artemether and mefloquine. *Trans Roy Soc Trop Med Hyg.* 1989;83:489.
104. Shwe T, Hla KK. The effect of artemether plus mefloquine on Myanmar patients with complicated falciparum malaria. *Southeast Asian J Trop Med Public Health.* 1992; 23:117–121.
105. Win K, Than M, Thwe Y. Comparison of combinations of parenteral artemisinin derivatives plus oral mefloquine with intravenous quinine plus oral tetracycline for treating cerebral malaria. *Bull WHO.* 1992;70:777–782.
106. Aikawa M, Rabbege JR, Udeinya I, Miller LH. Electron microscopy of knobs in *Plasmodium falciparum*–infected erythrocytes. *J Parasitol.* 1983;69:435–437.
107. Aikawa M, Uni Y, Andrutis AT, Howard RJ. Membrane-associated electron-dense material of the asexual stages of *Plasmodium falciparum.* Evidence for movement from the intracellular parasite to the erythrocyte membrane. *Am J Trop Med Hyg.* 1986;35:30–36.
108. Riganti M, Pongponratn E, Tegoshi T, Looareesuwan S, Punpoowong B, Aikawa M. Human cerebral malaria in Thailand: a clinico-pathological correlation. *Immunol Lett.* 1990;25:199–206.
109. Aikawa M, Broderson JR, Igarashi I, et al. *An Atlas of Renal Diseases in* Aotus *Monkeys with Experimental Plasmodial Infection.* American Institute of Biological Sciences; 1988.

CHAPTER 137

Microsporidiosis

Jan Marc Orenstein

If you've never heard of science (to say nothing of how it works), you can hardly be aware that you are embracing pseudoscience. You're simply thinking in one of the ways humans always have. Religions are often the state-protected nurseries of pseudoscience, although there's no reason why religions have to play that role. In a way, it's an artifact from times long gone. In some countries nearly everyone believes in astrology and precognition, including government leaders. But this is not simply drummed into them by religion; it is drawn out of the enveloping culture in which everyone is comfortable with these practices, and affirming testimonials are everywhere.

Carl Sagan (1934–), The Demon Haunted World, Random House, 1995

DEFINITION

Infection with a protozoal parasite of the phylum Microspora is referred to as microsporidiosis.[1–9] These ubiquitous obligate intracellular protozoans infect members of all classes of vertebrates and invertebrates, particularly arthropods and fish. Infections of virtually every organ and tissue have been observed, but small intestine, central nervous system (CNS), urinary tract, and upper respiratory tract are especially prone to infection. Microsporidia are defined by the unique, coiled, polar tube packaged within their spores, which acts as a "hypodermic needle" for injecting infectious sporoplasm into the targeted host cell. Microsporidia are primitive eukaryotes that possess prokaryotic-size ribosomes and rRNA, have a large ribosomal subunit that contains 5.8 sRNA, and show little rRNA homology with other eukaryotes.[10] They lack mitochondria and peroxisomes.

MICROSPORIDIA IN HUMANS

Although almost 100 genera and 1000 species of microsporidia have been identified, members of only six genera are known to infect humans: *Encephalitozoon, Enterocytozoon, Septata, Pleistophora, Nosema,* and *Microsporidium.*[1–9] Documented human infections were rare before the acquired immunodeficiency syndrome (AIDS) epidemic.

The genus *Enterocytozoon* was first established in Paris in 1985 with the description of a protozoan in small intestine of a Haitian patient with AIDS and chronic diarrhea; the species was named *Enterocytozoon bieneusi.*[11,12] A second *Enterocytozoon, Ent salmonis,* has since been described that develops within nuclei of hematopoietic cells of salmonid fish.[13] *Enterocytozoon bieneusi* is, by far, the most common known human microsporidian.[14–29] It has been identified as the first acute self-limiting diarrheal infection by a microsporidia in an immunocompetent adult who visited the Middle East[30] and several infections in what are likely to be human immunodeficiency virus (HIV)-negative children in Niger.[31] *Enterocytozoon bieneusi* also has been reported to cause a traveler's diarrhea-like illness in an immunocompetent child.[32] An intestinal microsporidian, possibly *Ent bieneusi,* has been identified in an HIV-negative patient with diarrhea and a transplanted liver.[33]

A second diarrheagenic microsporidian, *Septata intestinalis,* was identified in the late 1980s in HIV/AIDS patients. Unlike *Ent bieneusi,* however, *S intestinalis* disseminates intravascularly.[34–39] Western blot and SDS–PAGE, as well as transmission electron microscopy (TEM) analyses confirmed the uniqueness of *S intestinalis* from the other known human microsporidia.

Human species of *Encephalitozoon* have infected eye, liver, upper respiratory tract, urinary tract, prostate, and peritoneum.[40–51] The newest *Encephalitozoon, E hellem,* appears to be a respiratory-acquired infection that can disseminate to the genitourinary tract and eye. While *E hellem* has only been described in AIDS patients,[40–48] *E cuniculi,* until recently the only mammalian *Encephalitozoon,*[52] has been diagnosed in a few AIDS and non-HIV immunocompetent patients.[1,3,53–56] *Pleistophora,* a genus common in fish and insects, has now been identified in skeletal muscle of two humans, one having AIDS[57] and the other HIV-seronegative, but immunocompromised.[58,59] The *Nosema, N connori,* was lethal to an athymic infant,[60] while a new species, *N corneum,* has recently been isolated from the corneal stroma of an immunocompetent patient.[61] *Nosema* sp commonly infect insects. Finally, the genus *Microsporidium,* used for microsporidial infections lacking precise speciation, contains organisms that caused two human corneal infections.[1,6–8]

SYNONYMS

Early confusion existed between human infections with microsporidia and *Toxoplasma.*[1,7] What is known now as *E cuniculi* was not recognized as microsporidia until 1964, and not until 1970 was it given its own name and separated from the genus *Nosema.*[1,52,62,63]

GEOGRAPHIC DISTRIBUTION

Human microsporidial infections have been reported worldwide.[3–9,15,64] Although the majority of cases of enteric infections by *Ent bieneusi* have been reported from North America, Western Europe, and Australia, predominantly in male homosexuals, patients have been described in South America and Africa (but not as yet in Asia), where they were associated with other risk behaviors. *Encephalitozoon hellem* infections are in the United States and Western Europe and *S intestinalis* infections are in the United States, Western Europe, Australia, and Africa. The two presumed *E cuniculi* infections in AIDS patients (peritoneum and liver), which could actually be *E hellem* (no antigenic or molecular assay), were reported in Western Europe and the United States, respectively. The *Pleistophora* myositis and *N corneum* infections were in the United States.

LIFE CYCLE, NATURAL HISTORY, EPIDEMIOLOGY, AND TAXONOMY

Experimentally, laboratory mammals have been infected with *E cuniculi* by oral, intratracheal, intraperitoneal, and intracerebral routes.[1,8,63–68] Following exposure to spores, organisms replicate and home (via macrophages and/or free) to potentially any tissue in the host, but especially kidneys, peritoneal cavity, and CNS. With the exception of the CNS, a similar pattern of spread and involvement has been seen in AIDS patients infected with *E hellem* and *S intestinalis.*

There is now evidence that the highly resistant microsporidial spore can infect humans at least through oral, respiratory, and ocular routes; be shed in the stool and urine; and productively infect epithelium, mesenchyme, endothelium, and mononuclear phagocytes.[16,34,40,44,64,69,70] Following injection of sporoplasm into the host cell, the parasite enters a proliferative phase during which time many organisms are produced from multiple divisions of the sporoplasm.[1,3,4,6,37,42,71] In most species, sporogony begins with the appearance of a thick, electron-dense membrane on each parasitic cell. These sporoblasts develop into mature electron-dense spores (1 to 12 μm) having an endospore surrounded by an ectospore, both surrounding a cell membrane.

Subclassification of the microsporidia into genera and species is based on whether development occurs within a membrane (sporophorous vesicle) of parasitic origin, as with *Pleistophora* (pansporoblastic), or occurs dispersed freely in the host cytoplasm (apansporoblastic). Apansporoblastic development can occur in either direct contact with the cytoplasm (*Nosema* and *Enterocytozoon*) or within a vacuole (parasitophorous) of cell origin (*Encephalitozoon* and *Septata*). Further distinction is based on, eg, spore size, number of turns or coils of the packaged polar tube, number and relationship of the nuclei, and number of binary fissions of each parasite cell.

Serologic tests for *E cuniculi* demonstrate high, even endemic, levels of laboratory animal infection (can approach 100%) in, eg, rabbits, guinea pigs, mice, and rats.[11,72,73] The sera of many individuals (particularly homosexuals), living in or traveling to the tropics, and patients with parasitic diseases (eg, malaria, schistosomiasis) and tuberculosis have been reported to react with *E cuniculi.*[5,6,74–77]

Polymerase chain reaction (PCR) is the most promising method for taxonomic classification (and for diagnosis) of species of, eg, *E hellem, E cuniculi,* and *S intestinalis* with similar or identical ultrastructure.[10,37,78–83] The small subunit rRNA of the Microspora more closely resembles prokaryotic rRNA. Sequences of

Ent bieneusi, S intestinalis, E hellem, and *E cuniculi* are available. Both the 16S small subunit and the larger subunits of rRNA are employed as tools. Detection of *Ent bieneusi* has been achieved with no more than 0.1 mg of starting DNA extract. Initial results have shown approximately 70% homology of *Ent bieneusi* with *E hellem, E cuniculi,* and *S intestinalis,* which, in turn, show 90% homology with one another. As a consequence, it has been suggested that although these three species are distinct, they are close enough to be classified into the family Encephalitozoonidae.

MORPHOLOGIC FEATURES OF COMMON HUMAN MICROSPORIDIA

Enterocytozoon

Detailed morphologic studies have confirmed that *Ent bieneusi* is the prototype of a new genus of Microspora, to date seen in humans and fish.[13,14,71] Unique morphologic features of *Ent bieneusi* (Figure 137–1) include nuclear division that is not immediately followed by cytokinesis; premature development of the polar tube within a multinucleate plasmodium (predating division into sporoblasts); clear cleftlike structures (also called electron-lucent inclusions) from which originate electron-dense disk-shaped structures that subsequently form the polar tubes; six turns of the polar tube arranged into two strata of three each; and elongated pleomorphic nuclei. Whereas the plasmodia reach several microns in diameter (about the width of the enterocyte nucleus), the individual spores are the smallest of all the microsporidia (1 × 1.5 μm). Since *S intestinalis* lacks the unique developmental characteristics of *Ent bieneusi,*[13,34,37,71] and is still capable of infecting the bowel, the unique features of *Ent bieneusi* are apparently not adaptations to successful development within the rapidly turning-over bowel epithelium (every 4 to 6 days).[84]

The earliest detectable intracytoplasmic form of *Ent bieneusi* is a small (approximately 1 μm), round to oval, unit membrane-bound meront (proliferative plasmodia) that initially contains only free ribosomes. They are less electron-dense than the surrounding host cell cytoplasm. A nucleus is the next identifiable plasmodial structure, followed by profiles of rough endoplasmic reticulum (RER).

Later stage meronts contain increasing numbers of pleomorphic nuclei (12 or more can be seen in a single plane of section) and electron-lucent inclusions or clefts, which are associated with the long axis of the nucleus and profiles of RER. After standard TEM processing, the clefts are usually totally electron-lucent. After ferric-osmium treatment, however, the electron-lucent inclusions contain stacks of electron-dense lamellar phospholipid material (40- to 45-Å periodicity), evidently polar tube precursors.[71,85]

Enterocytozoon bieneusi sporogony, or the sporogonial plasmodial phase, commences with the appearance of precursors of the polar tube complex in standard electron microscopy preparations, ie, electron-dense ring and disk-shaped structures in association with the clefts. The disks develop into cylinders that fuse (end-to-end), first into arcs, and eventually into long tubes with progressively tighter turns or coils. The tube forms a coil of six turns that are uniquely arranged into two rows of three each. The layers are out of register by about 45° from one another.[14] Tangential sections suggest a complex syncytial, weblike, or branching arrangement of the coils.

Formation of the tube complex, and its close association with the posterior vacuole and polaroplast membrane, commences within the multinucleate plasmodium, and continues through the sporoblast stage. Before division into sporoblasts, the plasmodium consists of numerous spore precursors (over 20 can be seen in a single plane of section).

Plasmodia are subsequently subdivided into mononuclear sporoblasts by a complex process of membrane invagination that occurs from multiple peripheral sites. Ultimately, each mononuclear sporoblast becomes an oval mature spore, encased in a trilaminar complex consisting of a thin electron-dense outer ectospore, surrounding a relatively thin electron-lucent endospore, surrounding a thin inner membrane; all of these are derived from the organism.

Encephalitozoon and *Septata intestinalis*

The *Encephalitozoons, E hellem* and *E cuniculi,* are morphologically distinct from the *Enterocytozoons.*[1,14,37,42,52,71] There are no multinucleate plasmodial stages. Development from multiple individual meronts to mature spores occurs within a parasitophorous vacuole of cell origin; polar tubes develop only after the last meront division; there are no electron-dense disks or electron-lucent inclusions; the spores are larger than those of *Enterocytozoon* (2.0 to 2.5 × 1.0 to 1.5 μm versus 1 × 1.5 μm); the polar filament has six coils arranged in a single row; and there is a relatively thick endospore and thin exospore.

There is one main morphologic feature that distinguishes *S intestinalis* (Figure 137–2) from all other known human microsporidia, including its closest relative, *Encephalitozoon.*[14,34,64] Development of *S intestinalis* occurs within septated parasitophorous vacuoles (resembling honeycombs) as opposed to single-chambered vacuoles. The fibrillar material that forms the

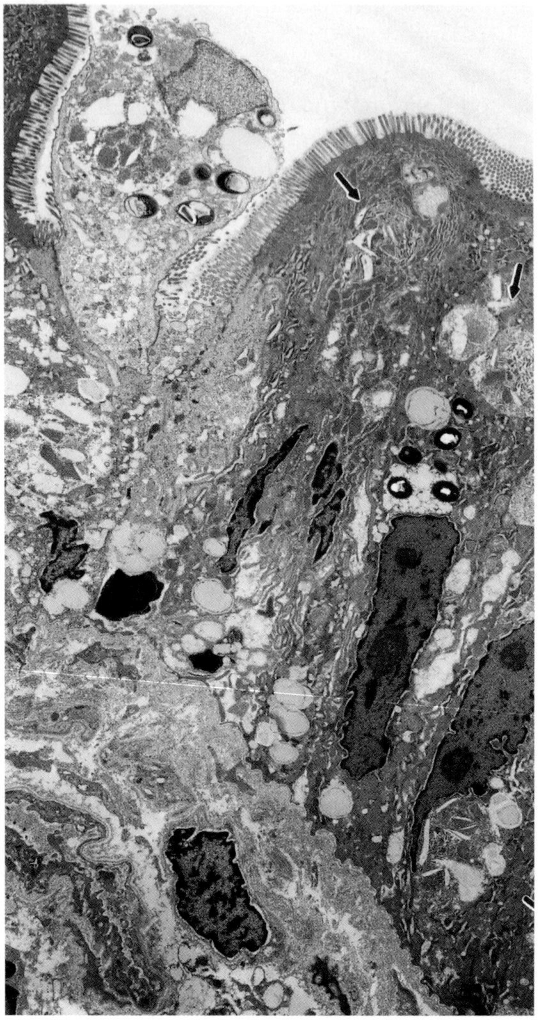

A

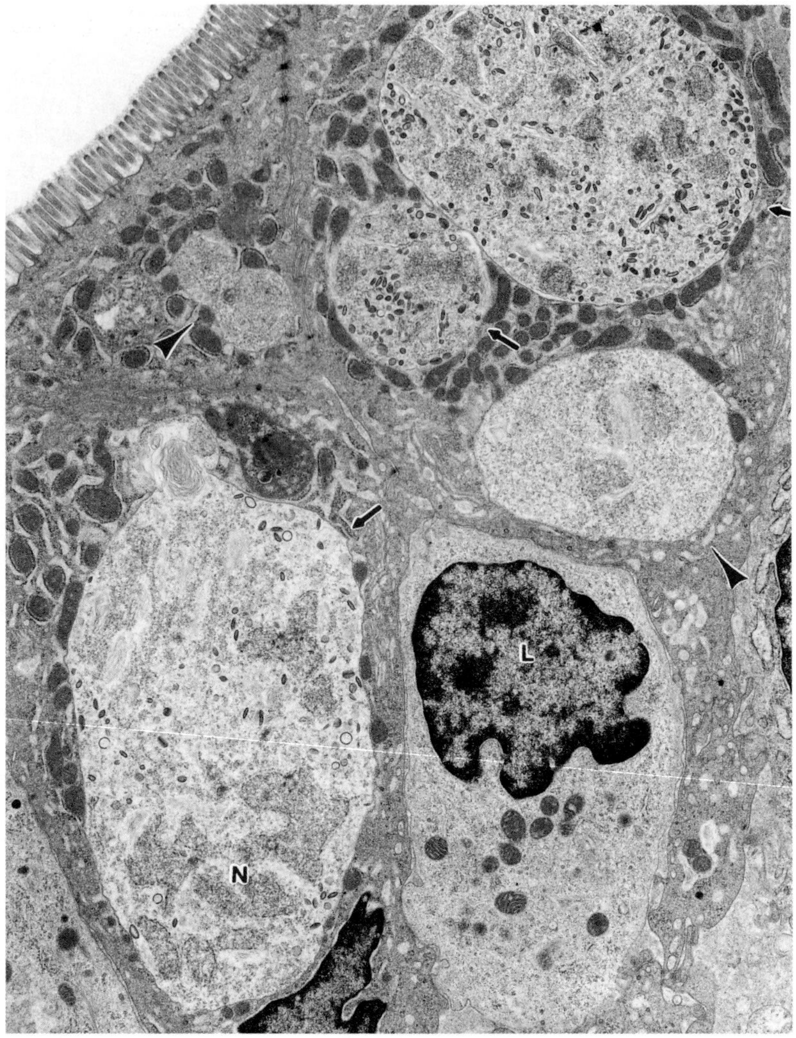

B

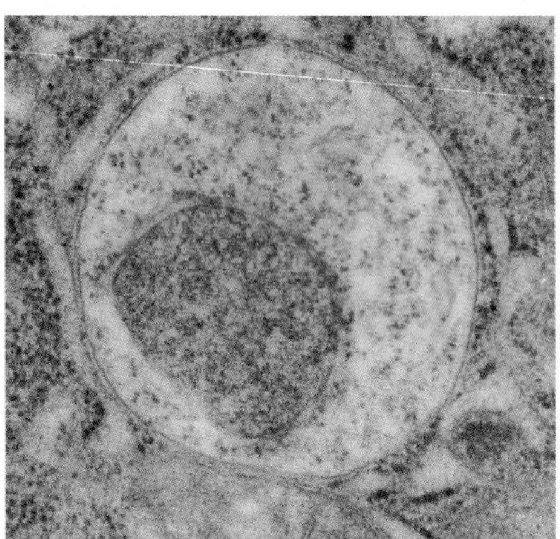

C

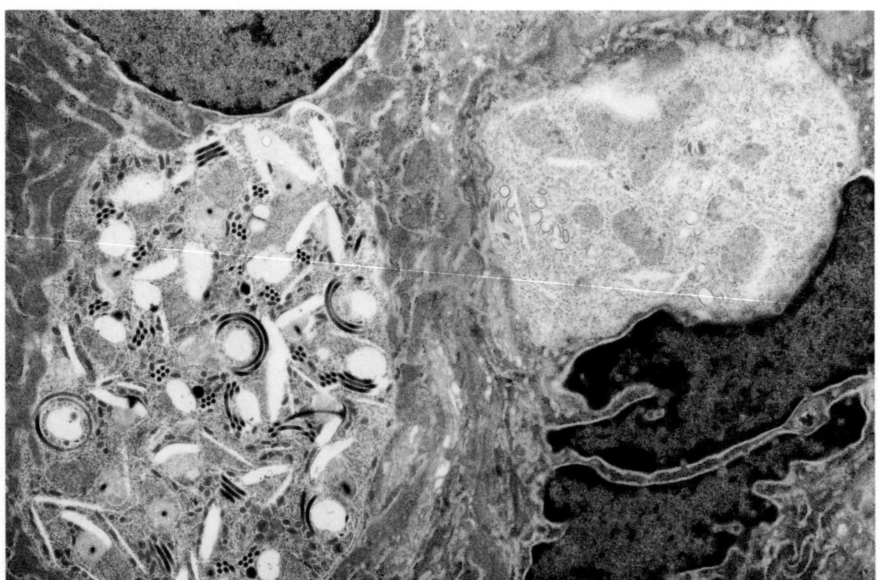

D

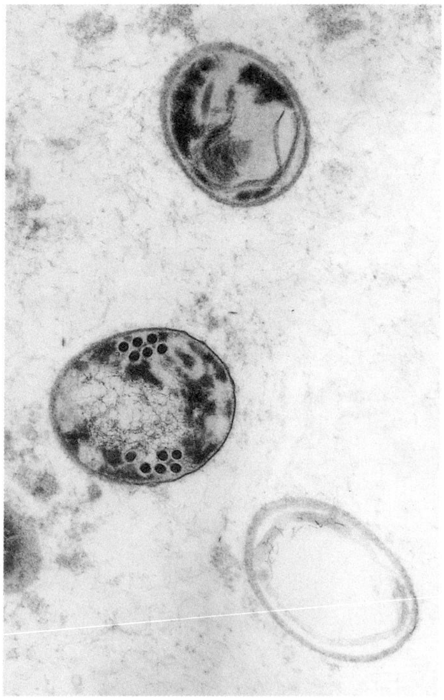

E

Figure 137–1. Transmission electron microscopy of *Ent bieneusi*. (**A**) Area of damaged epithelium showing enterocyte disarray, lipid vacuoles, and swollen organelles. Mature electron-dense spores are within intact, shedding (lysing), and shed cells. Proliferating plasmodia are subtle, but distinguishable by their clear clefts (*arrows*). The brush border is normal (×4100). (**B**) Proliferating (*arrowheads*) and sporogonial (*arrows*) plasmodia closely associated with mitochondria. Note clear clefts, electron-dense disks, irregular nuclei (*N*), and intraepithelial lymphocyte (*L*) (×10,000). (**C**) Proliferating plasmodium with only one nucleus and ribosomes. Note intimate contact with the cytoplasm and mitochondrion (×50,000). (**D**) Proliferative plasmodium (*right side*) with clear clefts, disks, and odd-shaped nuclei. Later sporogonial plasmodium (*left field*) with clefts, polar vacuoles, and polar tubes cut in cross section (two rows of three turns) and tangential (coils) section (×12,000). (**E**) Three spores in stool, one empty. Note two layers of three turns of the polar tube (×31,000).

meshwork separating the chambers arises from the surface of the parasite plasmalemma. Other distinguishing morphologic features include the presence of tetrasporous sporoblasts, appendages with bulb-shaped ends, and the apparently delayed development of the parasitophorous vacuole membrane.

Pleistophora

The *Pleistophora* are pansporoblastic (all other microsporidia infecting humans are apansporoblastic), developing in a thick-walled sporophorous vesicle of parasite origin. Spores are polysporoblastic, uninucleate, measure 2.8 × 3.2 to 3.4 μm and have a polar tube with 9 to 12 turns.[1,7,57,58]

CLINICAL FEATURES OF MICROSPORIDIAL INFECTION

Clinically, the symptoms of intestinal microsporidiosis caused by *Ent bieneusi* and *S intestinalis* are similar to those of small intestinal isosporiasis and cryptosporidiosis, although often milder.[14,86–88] The patient's CD4 count is often less than 50.[21,29] The patient suffers from progressive weight loss (usually a few pounds a week until stabilizing at a lower level), malabsorption, and large-volume secretory-type diarrhea, ie, "short-bowel syndrome." Daily, the patient has 3 to 10 watery, nonbloody, nonmucoid stools (can contain undigested food), of varying volume, and at varying intervals. The diarrhea, which usually appears gradually and is present for months, seems to be worsened by virtually all foods and by increased oral intake, is especially prominent in the morning, and can be accompanied by bloating, nausea, and anorexia. Weight loss, which can reach 10% to 20% of body weight, is caused by a combination of decreased intake (small meals for fear of exacerbating symptoms) and malabsorption. Fever is usually absent and, although the energy level is acceptable, endurance is decreased. The patient is not "toxic" but there is mild hypokalemia and hypomagnesemia, especially if the diarrhea is severe and accompanied by dehydration. Characteristically, there is both D-xylose and fat malabsorption (increased fecal fat). Decrease serum zinc is common.[88] Rare, mild infections of large bowel can accompany the primary small bowel infection with both *S intestinalis* and *Ent bieneusi*. A symptomatic rectal ulcer caused by *S intestinalis* has been diagnosed.

Enterocytozoon bieneusi apparently infects only epithelial cells and has the capacity for contiguous spread into the hepatobiliary tract and pancreatic ducts, and may gain access to the upper respiratory tract by aspiration, but not to disseminate by intravascular routes.[39,89–96] Patients with *Ent bieneusi* diarrhea and biliary tract involvement eventually develop progressive cholestasis, elevated hepatic enzymes, and RUQ and/or epigastric pain. Biliary infection can involve intrahepatic and extrahepatic ducts, as well as the gallbladder.[95] Computed tomography (CT) scan, ultrasound, and ERCP can reveal a dilated biliary tree (sclerosing cholangitis) and papillary stenosis; sphincterotomy can render relief. Since *S intestinalis, Cryptosporidium,* and cytomegalovirus (CMV) alone and in various combinations can infect the same sites as *Ent bieneusi* and present similar clinical and radiographic pictures, tissue and/or fluid examination is necessary to identify the species of microsporidia.

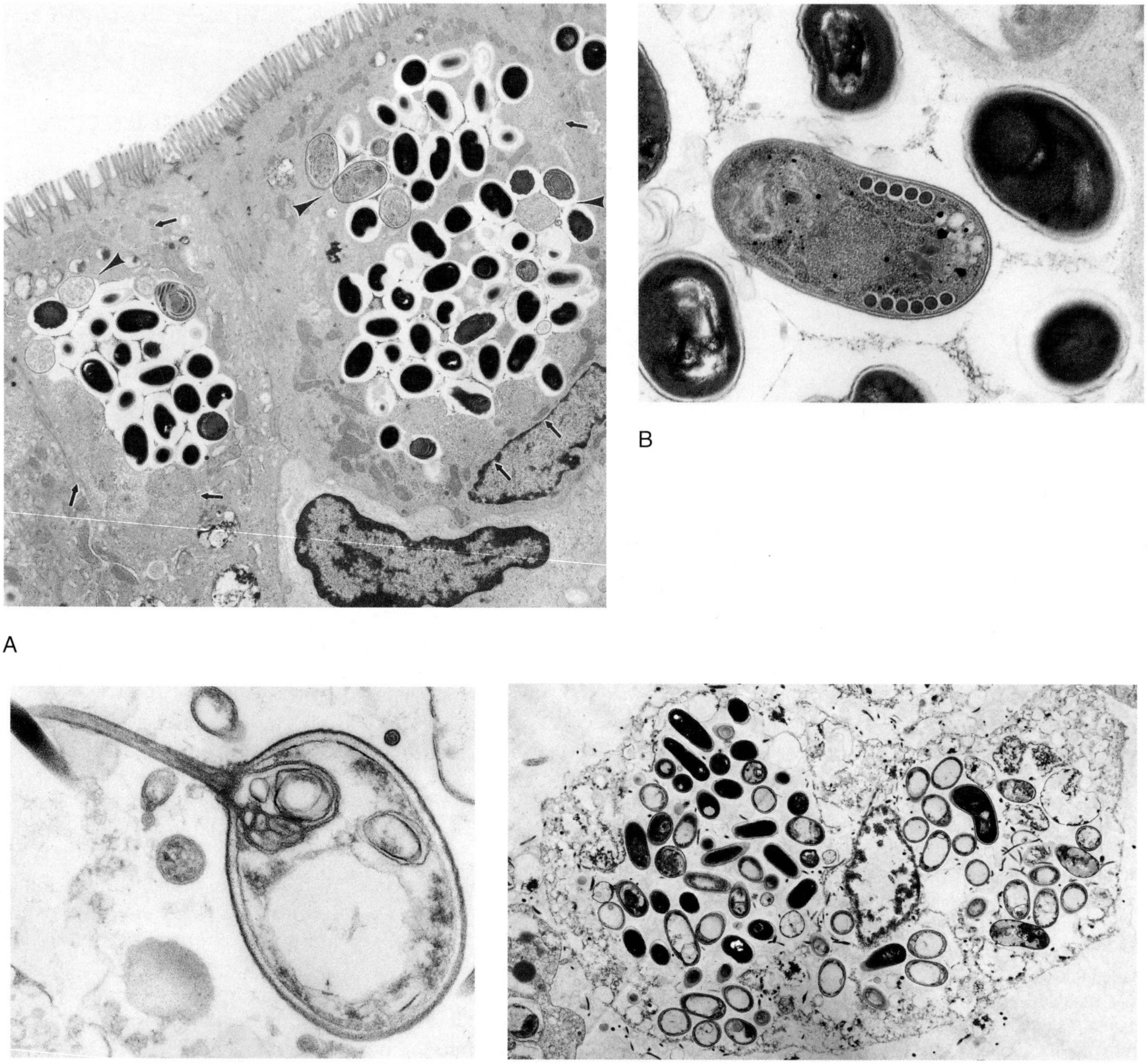

A

B

C

D

Figure 137–2. Transmission electron microscopy of *S intestinalis.* (**A**) Enterocytes with multiloculated parasitophorous vacuoles containing peripheral light-staining meronts (*arrows*) and sporoblasts (*arrowheads*) and central electron-dense mature spores. Note the intraepithelial lymphocyte (*bottom*), secondary lysosomes, and mild atrophy of microvilli (×7200). (**B**) The polar tube is arranged in one row of six turns. Note septation (×24,000). (**C**) In renal specimens, the polar tube is often avulsed and its protoplasm extruded (×38,000). (**D**) Lysing renal tubule cell full of spores both empty and whole (×5400).

Enterocytozoon bieneusi apparently travels retrogradely to the upper respiratory tract where it has been associated with chronic cough, wheezing, dyspnea, infiltrate, effusion, mucopurulent sinonasal discharge (pansinusitis), hyperplastic sinus polyps, low-grade fever, and frontal headaches.[39,95] *Septata intestinalis* also appears to infect the upper respiratory tract and to cause symptoms. Nasal, sinus, and tracheobronchial tissues and fluid contain the organism.[34–36,38,39] In the intestine, *S intestinalis* productively infects epithelial cells and macrophages, as well as fibroblasts and endothelial cells. It travels via the portal system to the liver where it infects Kupffer's cells and endothelium and disseminates to the kidneys, to cause tubulointerstitial nephritis with flank pain, dysuria, and hematuria.[34,35] The infected epithelium of the tubule sheds and appears in the urine along with free spores and spores within neutrophils and macrophages. There are granulomatous lesions, with Langhans' giant cells and mononuclear cells. Spores are in renal macrophages and vessels. Infection of tubules with necrosis is associated with microcalcifications. Urine sediment often contains infected transitional cells, indicating involvement of more distal sites, eg, collecting system, ureter, urinary bladder, and urethra.

Microsporidiosis caused by *E hellem*

Encephalitozoon hellem infects the tracheobronchial tree, nasal and sinus mucosa (pansinusitis and erosion of medial wall of maxillary antra); kidneys (tubulointerstitial nephritis), lower urinary tract (ureter and urinary bladder), prostate; and conjunctival epithelium (keratoconjunctivitis), but to date not the alimentary tract.[40,41,44–47,50,51,96,97] In fact, *E hellem* is probably acquired through the upper respiratory tract.[44,98] In a patient examined at autopsy, the tracheobronchial infection extended to the tertiary bronchioles and was associated with superficial erosions, sloughing, decreased goblets cells, alternating hyperplastic and thinned epithelium, focal intraepithelial inflammatory cells, and a mixed mononuclear and neutrophilic response. Mucous glands were also infected. The keratoconjunctivitis (diffuse punctate keratopathy) lacks significant inflammatory infiltrate but can lead to decreased visual acuity. Clinically and pathologically, renal infections by *E hellem* also are apparently indistinguishable from those caused by *S intestinalis.* However, *E hellem* also infects the lower urinary tract, including urinary bladder, causing ulcers, lymphohistiocytic inflammation, infected submucosal macrophages, and, in the ureters, erosions and acute and chronic granulomatous inflammation.

DIAGNOSIS OF INTESTINAL MICROSPORIDIOSIS

Orientation of intestinal biopsies is not necessary, especially if the specimen consists of several pieces of tissue.[14] Unless the parasite burden is particularly light, a biopsy specimen infected with microsporidia will appear abnormal even with a scanning (4×) objective. The architectural changes caused by microsporidia are nonspecific and the diagnosis is based on identifying the pathogen(s).[14,87,99] Figures 137–3 and 137–4 use light microscopy to show *Ent bieneusi* and *S intestinalis* specimens, respectively.

HISTOPATHOLOGY OF INTESTINAL MICROSPORIDIOSIS

Biopsy specimens with long, delicate, tapered villi, proportionally short crypts, and a monotonous surface epithelium of regularly stained, tall columnar cells with basally situated nuclei and prominent brush borders rarely harbor microsporidia, or any other pathogen. Endoscopic biopsies are mostly taken at random because the mucosa usually appears normal, save for perhaps a suggestion of villous blunting and a "mucoid haze." Each "bite" invariably displays some degree of change, although it can be focal. The pathologist should study hematoxylin-eosin (H&E) stained sections (ribbons of at least three sections) from each of three levels of the paraffin block.

The histopathology of intestinal microsporidiosis is a spectrum of degenerative changes that generally parallels the parasite burden.[14,16,25,34,100] Small numbers of parasites can occasionally be identified in specimens from patients who were minimally symptomatic, experiencing only nausea and vomiting, or asymptomatic.[101] Characteristically, the burden of parasites and degree of histopathology are concentrated over the distal portion of the villus. While *S intestinalis* can infect enterocytes to the base of the crypt. *Ent bieneusi* is rarely below the midvillus.

Typically, the microsporidia-infected small bowel displays villous atrophy and pleomorphism, crypt hyperplasia, and increased numbers of intraepithelial lymphocytes (IELs).[16,25,34,100] Neutrophils are not a feature of intestinal microsporidiosis. As the villi become progressively shorter, broader, and irregular, enterocytes become more cuboidal and pleomorphic and their nuclei become increasingly more hyperchromatic, irregular, and randomly situated. The enterocyte cytoplasm ranges from vesiculated to frankly vacuolated. The brush border is surprisingly well preserved, at least until lesions are extreme. Accumulation of intracellular

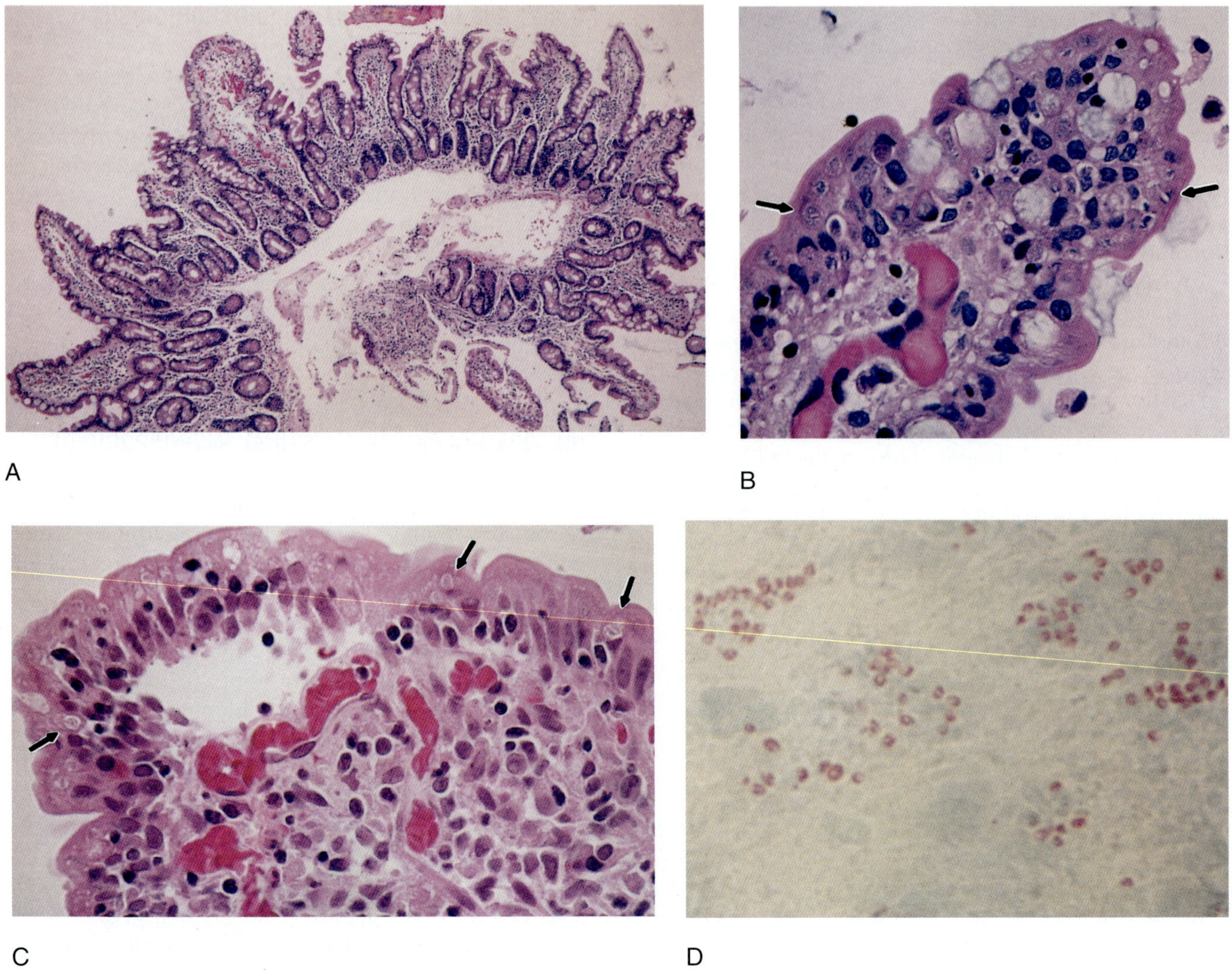

Figure 137–3. Light microscopy of *Ent bieneusi.* (**A**) Nonspecific small bowel atrophy and crypt elongation seen with many pathogens including microsporidia. Note the pleomorphic villi (H&E, ×64). (**B**) Tip of duodenal villus showing the features of *E bieneusi:* bluish supranuclear bodies (plasmodia), many with clear clefts (*arrows*), shedding cells with refractile spores, and cellular disorganization and piling up (H&E, ×640). (**C**) Many enterocytes contain loose-appearing supranuclear plasmodia (*arrows*), some of which mold the nucleus. Note the strip of shedding cells, disorganization, and intraepithelial lymphocytes (H&E, ×640). (**D**) Spores stain pink on a blue background with the modified trichrome Chromotrope 2R stain used on fluids. The clear posterior vacuole and pink-staining nucleus can often be seen (×1500).

and intercellular lipid and water varies, but not necessarily with the burden of parasites.

The tip of the infected villus appears as progressively more disorganized aggregates of crowded cells ("piling up") that are undergoing degeneration and necrosis. Irregular dense bodies, consistent with secondary lysosomes, may be prominent adjacent to the brush border. Shedding single cells and strips of cells are often present. The individual sloughing cells are often tear-drop-shaped and invariably contain refractile mature spores diagnostic of *Ent bieneusi* microsporidiosis. The lamina propria contains plasma cells, plasmacytoid cells, and macrophages, often rich in secondary lysosomes—reflecting the immunodeficient state of the patient, not the infection by *Ent bieneusi.*

Familiarity with the ultrastructure and morphogenesis of the intestinal microsporidia enables a diagnosis by routinely stained slides. Development of the intesti-

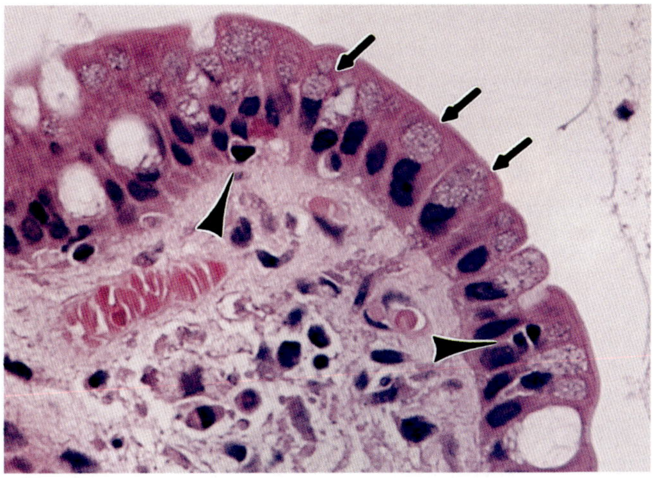

A

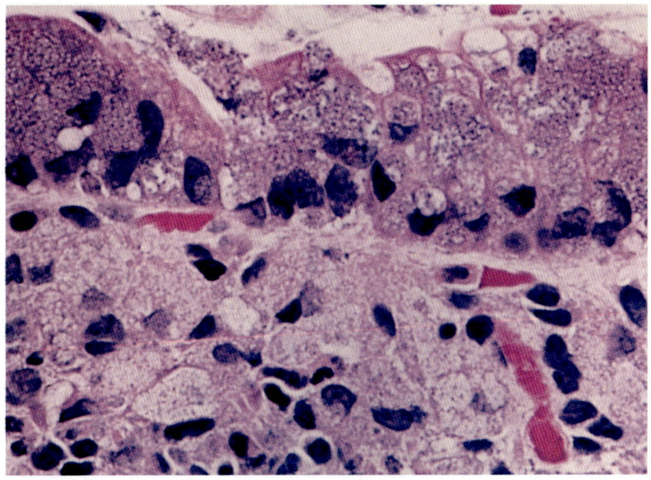

B

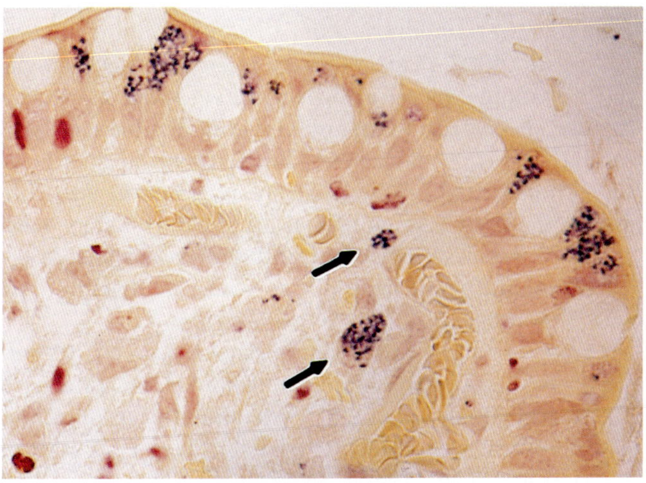

C

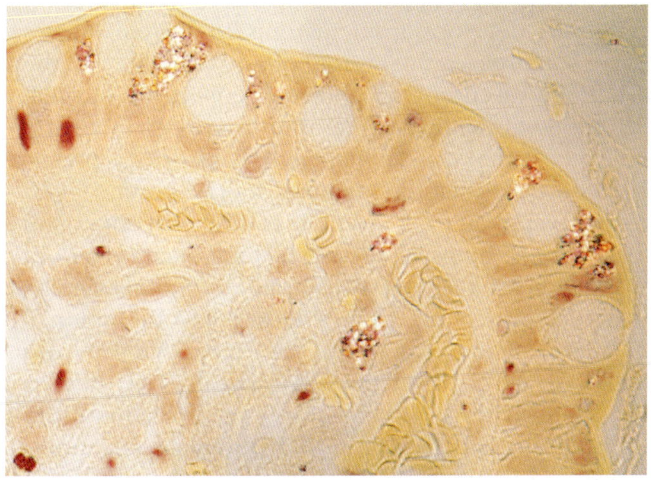

D

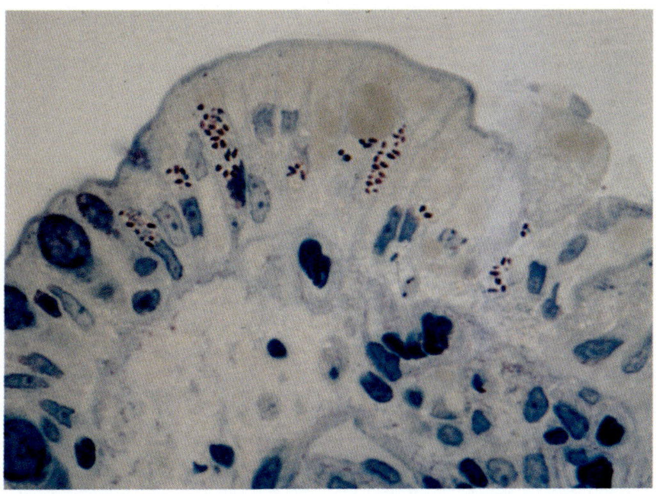

E

Figure 137–4. Microscopy of *S intestinalis*. (**A**) Parasitophorous vacuoles containing refractile parasites cup the apical nuclear poles (*arrows*). Note the enterocyte disarray, intraepithelial lymphocytes (*arrowheads*), and intact brush border (H&E, ×640). (**B**) A very high parasite burden leading to release of spores from damaged enterocytes. The granularity of the cytoplasm of many of the macrophages in the lamina propria is organisms (H&E, ×640). (**C**), (**D**) Developing *S intestinalis* stain progressively darker with the modified Brown–Brenn stain. In different preparations they stain red-purple and blue. They polarize brightly with this stain (D). Note the organisms in lamina propria macrophages (*arrow*) (tissue Gram stain, polarized light, ×640). (**E**) Parasites, as they develop, stain progressively darker in plastic sections stained with either toluidine blue or with combined methylene blue-azure II, basic fuchsin (trichrome). The cells are swollen and there is some loss of mucin. The lipid is nonspecific for microsporidiosis (×640).

nal microsporidia occurs predominantly within the mitochondria-rich supranuclear Golgi region of enterocytes.[16,34,72,102] The plasmodia of *Ent bieneusi* (less so with the parasitophorous vacuole of *S intestinalis*) typically flatten or mold the apical pole of the enterocyte nucleus (cup-shaped), an important telltale feature of infection detectable by light microscopy. The multinucleated plasmodium of *Ent bieneusi* develops in intimate contact with the cytoplasm, not within a parasitophorous vacuole, and reaches about the width of the nucleus. The plasmodia appear as supranuclear bodies generally staining more basophilic than the surrounding cytoplasm. Cleftlike structures are often present. In edematous specimens, plasmodia can appear to be loose in the cytoplasm, almost as if they are in a vacuole. Spores of *Ent bieneusi* (1×1.5 μm) are best seen in shedding cells, but can occasionally appear as supranuclear collections of refractile bodies. *Septata intestinalis* develops from meronts to mature spores within supranuclear parasitophorous vacuoles. In the H&E stained section, they appear as collections of small round to oval lightly staining pink bodies of increased refractility. *Enterocytozoon bieneusi* has a strong preference for the distal duodenum (fourth portion) and proximal jejunum.[103] The colon is rarely involved and thus a colonic biopsy specimen lacking organisms does not exclude the diagnosis. *Septata intestinalis* is similar, except for apparently more spillover into the colon.[34] The distal ileum (accessible by colonoscopy) also appears to be a target for both species, but there is insufficient material to compare its relative intensity to that of the distal duodenum and proximal jejunum.[11] Both species strongly prefer absorptive cells, only rarely being in goblet or enterochromaffin cells. Neither species has been detected in the stomach or esophagus.[34] Rectal ulceration caused by *S intestinalis* has been diagnosed.

The paraffin-section diagnosis of *S intestinalis* tends to be easier than that of *Ent bieneusi*,[14,34] appearing as supranuclear clusters of variably refractile bluish bodies.

SPECIAL STAINS FOR IDENTIFYING MICROSPORIDIA

With experience, intestinal microsporidiosis can be diagnosed on H&E sections. Special stains are helpful when there is a co-infection or only few organisms. The staining of the plasmodia tends to be relatively consistent within a specimen, suggesting that preservation (exact handling varies among endoscopists), histopathology, and laboratory processing all affect the appearance of the parasite.

Spores of microsporidia are characteristically gram-positive, birefringent, and possess a periodic acid–Schiff (PAS)-positive polar body.[1,49,104] The AFIP modification of the Brown–Brenn Gram stain is more consistent and specific than other Gram stains tested. The spore stains dark blue to red on a yellow background. Staining is of the thin membrane outline and a central hourglass-shaped "waist band" flanked by clear zones. Because their size is small the fine details of *Ent bieneusi* are more subtle and the staining less likely to be blue than with *S intestinalis*. At best, nonspecific staining may be only of Paneth and enterochromaffin cell granules. Pleomorphic secondary lysosomes near the brush border of enterocytes and within macrophages in the lamina propria may also stain. Distinction between the two species is by spore size, greater numbers of staining forms tightly packaged within a vacuole and in lamina propria for *S intestinalis*, and spores within shedding cells for *Ent bieneusi*.

A modified Warthin–Starry microsporidia stain has the advantage of silvering the developing as well as mature spores and even nuclei within *Ent bieneusi* plasmodia.[28,38] These structures, furthermore, appear larger than their actual size. There are no internal structures visualized with this stain, and great care must be taken to avoid confusing background staining. Speciation is based on the same features as with the Brown–Brenn stain.

Microsporidia show unpredictable Giemsa staining (light blue to purple nuclear staining). At times, the Gram and Giemsa stains will also stain the plasmodia of *Ent bieneusi* a slightly browner or bluer hue than the surrounding cytoplasm, respectively. The clear clefts may also be enhanced by these stains. The exceedingly small size of the PAS-positive body of *Ent bieneusi* makes it even more difficult to visualize than for *S intestinalis*.

BIREFRINGENCE OF MICROSPORIDIAL SPORES

Birefringence is a quality of chitin, a component of the endospore of microsporidia spores.[104] Unfortunately, the specimen must be embedded, paraffin being much better than plastic embedding. Birefringence is especially prominent with AFIP Brown–Brenn Gram (pink) and modified Warthin–Starry (white) stained sections. Spores, however, may also polarize white in H&E stained sections, but only lightly (blue) in Giemsa stained sections. Birefringence of both intestinal microsporidia is inexplicably unpredictable, on the same block and even on the same section. When present, it can be used for speciation and detecting dissemination (use partially polarized Brown–Brenn stained section).

SEMI–THIN PLASTIC SECTION LIGHT MICROSCOPY

All human microsporidia are prominently displayed in semi-thin sections (1 to 2 μm).[14,16,34] Mature spores stain blue after either toluidine blue staining or using the combined methylene blue-azure II basic fuchsin stain (better contrast). The diagnostic oval shape, clear posterior vacuole, and dark nucleus are all visible, even at 40×. The diagnosis of *Ent bieneusi* is suggested by the smaller size of the spores and verified by identifying the unique plasmodia, which appear as lighter staining round to oval supranuclear bodies, often with identifiable clear clefts.[105] The *Encephalitozoon* and *S intestinalis* cells stain progressively darker, as they develop from meronts to mature spores.

ADDITIONAL DIAGNOSTIC METHODS AND SPECIMENS

Retrieval of Specimens from Paraffin for TEM

Specimens can be successfully retrieved from paraffin for TEM verification of the diagnosis of microsporidiosis and for speciation.[35,106]

Imprints/Touch and Brush Preparations

Diagnosis can be made on imprints/touch preparations from fresh small bowel biopsy specimens when the specimen is touched to the slide.[25,107] The slides are air dried, methanol fixed (30 seconds), and stained with eg, 5% Giemsa, Diff-Quik, Chromotrope 2R, or Gram stains. Spores are identified as perinuclear aggregates in cells found on the edge of fragments of superficial epithelium and free in the mucus. The spores have a lighter staining outline and darker staining nucleus and central waistband, plus a clear vacuole. With experience, 40× screening will often reveal structures that can be confirmed as spores at higher magnification (63× or 100×). Smears made from mucosal cytobrushings, taken during endoscopy, are of comparable caliber. In these preparations, the spores are usually found released from the cells and widely dispersed.

Stool and Intestinal Lavage Specimens

Microsporidial spores are in the duodenal/jejunal fluid (lavage or aspirate), colonic aspirate, and stool of patients infected with intestinal microsporidia.[14,34,35,70,71] The modified trichrome stain (Chromotrope 2R) was the first breakthrough in stool diagnosis. It stains microsporidial spores pink and everything else light blue to green (formalin fixed, 1:3, unconcentrated stool).[108] Screening is recommended under a 100× oil-immersion objective (100 fields), which takes an average of 10 minutes, although 63× objective is also adequate. Variability in background staining has been regularly encountered, but can be overcome with experience. Confirmation relies on a central darker staining band not seen with fungi or bacteria. A light blue background can be obtained if aniline blue is substituted for fast green.[109] Background staining is minimized, spore staining enhanced, and staining time reduced from 90 to as little as 10 minutes if the staining is done at a temperature of up to 50°C, instead of the usual room temperature.[110]

The other major diagnostic breakthrough came with adaptation of the fluorochrome chitin-staining methods used to detect fungi and algae in tissue sections.[111–116] Variable, but acceptable, results can be obtained with several products: Uvitex 2B (Ciba-Geigy, Basel, Switzerland), Fungiqual A (Specialty Chemicals for Medical Diagnostics, Kandern, Germany), Calcofluor White M2R (Sigma, St. Louis, Missouri), and Fungi Fluor (Polysciences, Warrington, Pennsylvania). The spores are readily distinguished from the larger fungal forms, which stain only minimally. The experienced observer can distinguish the smaller spores of *Ent bieneusi* from the larger spores of *S intestinalis* (1.5 × 1.0 versus 2.2 × 1.2 μm). No internal details are visible, only uniformly white oval complete spores and bluish empty spores.

Urine

Both *S intestinalis* and *E hellem* disseminate to the kidneys and shed in the urine.[34,44] They can be detected with either smear or cytospin preparations (Giemsa or Diff-Quik stains) of urine sediment with or without premicrofugation to concentrate the spores. Both the Chromotrope 2R and fluorochrome methods have been used successfully to detect spores in urine.[109,111]

Scrapings

Encephalitozoon hellem keratoconjunctivitis can be rapidly diagnosed by lightly scraping the conjunctiva and making either a Giemsa, Gram, or Diff-Quik stained preparation.[40] Biopsy is to be avoided, because of the potential complications.

HISTOPATHOLOGY OF OCULAR MICROSPORIDIAL INFECTION

Encephalitozoon hellem infects superficial epithelial cells[40,44,50] resulting in a spectrum of changes from minimal through degeneration and necrosis, focal erosions and sloughing, cellular disarray, hyperplasia, hyperchromatism, and nuclear pleomorphism. A prominent infiltrate of neutrophils, scattered macrophages, and lymphocytes may extend through the epithelial layer. Conjunctival scrapings can be bland (except for infected epithelium) or rich in macrophages and neutrophils, which often contain spores undergoing phagocytosis and lysosomal digestion.[40,117,118]

Before the AIDS epidemic, two infections of corneal stroma were reported, one was in a child living in Ceylon, who had been gored by a goat; there was perforation, blindness, and finally enucleation.[119] The spores (3.5 × 1.5 μm), in the cornea were both free and within macrophages. An African patient became blind with a perforating corneal ulcer and required an enucleation. The ulcer border was necrotic and infiltrated with inflammatory cells. As above, spores (size 4.5 to 5 × 2.3 to 3 μm, 11 to 13 turns of polar tube) were both free and within macrophages in the stroma. Although they were probably both *Nosema* infections, they have been placed in the indeterminate genus *Microsporidium* for lack of adequate morphologic categorization.

Another recently identified, and isolated, microsporidian, *Nosema corneum,* was found infecting the corneal stroma (keratitis) of a non-AIDS patient.[61] The patient had recently traveled to the Caribbean and Central America and lived near a large lake. He had suffered from chronic disciform keratitis, infiltration of the anterior stroma, and iritis for 18 months and had not responded to therapy. Corneal transplant was curative. There was no mention of histopathology associated with the infection. Typical of a *Nosema* (eg, *N connori*), the parasite has two closely abutted nuclei (diplokaryon), is apansporoblastic, and develops in intimate contact with the cell cytoplasm. Spores have about half the number of polar tube turns (5 to 6 versus 10 to 11) and are smaller (3.7 × 1.0 μm versus 2 × 4 μm) than those of *N connori.*

An additional patient with keratitis (blurred vision and corneal ulceration) that persisted after removal of a foreign body had a *Nosema* (eg, binucleate) infection (in cytoplasm and free in stroma), but the spores were larger (3 × 5 versus 3.7 × 1.0 μm) than *N corneum* and had 9 to 12 coils; this agent has been named *N ocularum.*[119]

The *Nosema* species are refractile and stain well with Grocott's methenamine silver and Gram stains and show a PAS-positive granule.

PATHOLOGY OF LESS COMMON HUMAN MICROSPORIDIAL INFECTIONS

A species of *Pleistophora* was identified in biopsy specimens of several skeletal muscles of an HIV-seronegative but immunocompetent man[58] and one AIDS patient.[57,120] These patients lacked evidence of other sites of infection, including bowel, and are the first reports of human infections by a member of this genus, which are common to vertebrates, especially fish. There was mild to moderate chronic active myositis with abundant plasma cells, lymphocytes, and histiocytes. Spores were 3 × 3.4 μm and 4 × 2 μm (9 to 12 turns of its polar tube), respectively. Typical pansporoblastic development was in myocytes and degenerating forms in macrophages. The parasites stained with trichrome, Wright–Giemsa, and PAS (polar granule) in paraffin sections and toluidine blue in plastic sections.

Encephalitozoon infections of the liver[53] and greater omentum have been reported in AIDS patients.[54] Although consistent with *E cuniculi,* one, or both, could have been the morphologically identical *E hellem* (antigenic distinction is needed). The liver biopsy specimen had focal granulomatous and suppurative necrosis (microgranulomas), especially in the portal areas.[53] The spores were noted to be gram-positive (no other stains mentioned) and measured 2 × 1 μm (five coils) by TEM. The patient had progressively worsening diarrhea and liver enzymes, and died in fulminant hepatitis. A Swiss AIDS patient presented with signs and symptoms of *Pneumocystis carinii* pneumonia (eventual cause of death), 13 kg weight loss, and a large palpable RUQ, slightly painful abdominal mass, and developed acute renal failure.[54] At autopsy (limited to a small laparotomy), there was a large (20 × 20 × 10 cm) inflammatory mass of the greater omentum, ascites, and splenomegaly. Microsporidia infection was only documented in the omentum as a mixed nongranulomatous inflammation with focal necrosis and intravacuolar gram-positive spores (2.5 to 2.6 × 1.2 to 1.5 μm) that stained pale blue with H&E, dark blue with Gram stain, and pale pink with Kinyoun stains. Ziehl–Neelsen stain was negative and PAS-positive bodies were seen. The liver showed only fatty change and cholestasis, and the spleen showed atrophic white pulp and fibrotic red pulp without microsporidia.

At present, there is at least one AIDS patient with molecularly confirmed *E cuniculi* infection of the upper respiratory tract. Studies are being undertaken to determine whether it represents one of the known subspecies, ie, mouse, rabbit, or dog, or a new subspecies.

CO-INFECTION WITH MICROSPORIDIA IN HUMANS

Bowel co-infections with intestinal microsporidiosis appear to be relatively infrequent.[11,14,26,106] The most common small bowel copathogen has been MAC, but *Giardia, Cryptosporidium,* and CMV (last two usually very low burden) have also been seen. It is more common to see simultaneous small bowel microsporidiosis and CMV or *Cryptosporidium* infection of the large intestine. This explains the increasingly frequent coidentification of microsporidia and *Cryptosporidium* in stool samples.[121,122] Co-infection of *Ent bieneusi* and *S intestinalis* in small bowel has been documented.[106]

THERAPY

The few patients treated with metronidazole, itraconazole, octreodile, primaquine, lomotil, sulfasalazine, azithromycin, and loperamide have had variable responses. It is believed that the responses were from a reduction of bacterial flora.[20,21,24,28,123] The most promising agent is albendazole (a benzimidazole). It inhibits polymerization of tubulin (reversible binding to the same site on tubulin as colchicine and podophyllotoxin) into microtubules, and thus interferes with cell division and nutrient uptake.[124–128] Even though there is some clinical response with 400 mg BID (about a 50% reduction in frequency of stools), there is no reduction of parasites in stool nor in biopsy specimens. When treatment is stopped symptoms reappear. Intestinal and disseminated *S intestinalis* appears to respond rapidly (within a week) and completely to 400 mg BID of albendazole.[105,128] Maintenance therapy appears to be necessary.

Encephalitozoon hellem also appears to be sensitive to albendazole. The patient with keratoconjunctivitis, nasal, and sinus infetions caused by *E hellem* had a clearing of his eye with propamidine isethionate 0.1% (Brolene), but nasal and sinus infections cleared (symptomatic and CT scan) only after albendazole.[46,97] A patient with *E hellem* epithelial keratopathy had a complete response to itraconazole, which was given for cryptococcal meningitis.[117] Autopsy studies have confirmed the premortem eradication of *S intestinalis* and *E hellem* following treatment with albendazole.[129–131]

CELL CULTURE

Enterocytozoon bieneusi has been successfully cultivated in short-term cultures.[82] There are now several upper respiratory and fecal isolates of *S intestinalis,* which are apparently molecularly identical. *Encephalitozoon hellem, E cuniculi,* and *N corneum* were easily isolated in a variety of cell lines of renal and mesenchymal origin and can be used for screening drugs.[41,44,55,61,132]

NEW METHODS

Serologic and immunofluorescent assay (IFA) studies reveal a considerable cross-reactivity among the microsporidia and many common antigens on Western blot analysis.[43,48] IFA studies of parasite cultures and stool specimens (known positive for either intestinal microsporidia), using polyclonal antisera raised in rabbits and mice, against *E hellem* and *E cuniculi* detected these microsporidia, as well as *Ent bieneusi* and *S intestinalis,* but not *N corneum.* There was no cross-reactivity with *Cryptosporidium, Giardia,* or *Entamoeba.* Monoclonal and polyclonal antibodies are being prepared (to *Encephalitozoons* and *Enterocytozoons*) and tested by IFA and enzyme-linked immunosorbent assay methods to detect microsporidia in stool.

Based on animals studies, it appears that immunocompetent individuals likely become seropositive, while those with deficient immunity do not. Epidemiologic studies will indicate whether seropositive patients are those who develop symptomatic microsporidiosis when they become immunocompromised.

REFERENCES

1. Canning EU, Lom J. *The Microsporidia of Vertebrates.* Orlando, Fla: Academic Press; 1986.
2. Cali A, Owen RL. Microsporidiosis. In: Balows WJ, Hausler Jr WJ, Lenette EH, eds. *Laboratory Diagnosis of Infectious Diseases, Principles and Practice, Vol I, Bacterial, Mycotic and Parasitic Diseases.* New York: Springer-Verlag; 1988:929–950.
3. Bryan R, Cali A, Owen R, Spencer H. Microsporidia: opportunistic pathogens in patients with AIDS. *Prog Clin Parasitol.* 1991;2:1–26.
4. Canning EU, Hollister WS. Microsporidia of mammals—widespread pathogens or opportunistic curiosities? *Parasitol Today.* 1987;3:267–273.
5. Shadduck JA. Human microsporidiosis in AIDS. *Rev Infect Dis.* 1989;11:203–207.
6. Shadduck JA, Greeley E. Microsporidia and human infections. *Clin Microbiol Rev.* 1989;2:158–165.
7. Weber R, Bryan RT, Schwartz DA, Owen RL. Human microsporidial infections. *Clin Microbiol Rev.* 1994;7:426–461.
8. Canning EU, Hollister WS. Human infections with microsporidia. *Rev Med Microbiol.* 1992;3:35–42.
9. Shadduck JA, Orenstein JM. Comparative pathology of

microsporidiosis. *Arch Pathol Lab Med.* 1993;117: 1215–1219.

10. Vossbrinck CR, Maddox JV, Friedman S, Debrunner-Vossbrinck BA, Woese CR. Ribosomal RNA sequence suggests microsporidia are extremely ancient eukaryotes. *Nature.* 1987;326:411–414.
11. Modigliani R, Bories C, Le Charpentier Y, et al. Diarrhoea and malabsorption in acquired immune deficiency syndrome: a study of four cases with special emphasis on opportunistic protozoan infestations. *Gut.* 1985;26: 179–187.
12. Desportes I, Le Charpentier Y, Galian A, et al. Occurrence of a new microsporidan: *Enterocytozoon bieneusi* ng, nsp, in the enterocytes of a human patient with AIDS. *J Protozool.* 1985;32:250–254.
13. Chilmonczyk S, Cox WT, Hedrick RP. *Enterocytozoon salmonis* n sp: an intranuclear microsporidium from salmonid fish. *J Protozool.* 1991;38:264–269.
14. Orenstein JM. Microsporidiosis in the acquired immunodeficiency syndrome. *J Parasitol.* 1991;77:843–864.
15. Hojlyng Nm, Nielsen A, Wandall J, et al. First cases of microsporidiosis in Scandinavian patients with AIDS. *Scand J Infect Dis.* 1994;25:666–669.
16. Orenstein JM, Chiang J, Steinberg W, Smith PD, Rotterdam H, Kotler DP. Intestinal microsporidiosis as a cause of diarrhea in human immunodeficiency virus-infected patients: a report of 20 cases. *Hum Pathol.* 1990;21: 475–481.
17. Bernard E, Michiels JF, Durant J, et al. Intestinal microsporidiosis caused by *Enterocytozoon bieneusi:* a new case report in an AIDS patient. *AIDS.* 1991;5: 606–607.
18. Michiels JF, Hofman P, Saint Paul MC, et al. Microsporidiose intestinale: 3 cas chez des sujets seropositifs pour le VIH. *Ann Pathol.* 1991;11:169–175.
19. Curry A, McWilliam LJ, Haboubi NY, Mandal BK. Microsporidiosis in a British patient with AIDS. *J Clin Pathol.* 1988;41:477–478.
20. Eeftinck Schattenkerk JKM, van Gool T, van Ketel RJ, Bartelsman JFWM. Microsporidiosis in HIV-1 infected individuals. *Lancet.* 1991;338:323.
21. Eeftinck Schattenkerk JKM, van Gool T, van Ketel RJ, et al. Clinical significance of small-intestinal microsporidiosis in HIV-1 infected individuals. *Lancet.* 1991;337: 895–898.
22. Greenson J, Belitsos P, Yardley J, Bartlett J. AIDS enteropathy: occult enteric infections and duodenal mucosal alterations in chronic diarrhea. *Ann Int Med.* 1991;114:366–372.
23. Ullrich R, Zeitz M, Bergs C, Janitschke K, Riecken EO. Intestinal microsporidiosis in a German patient with AIDS. *Klin Wochenschr.* 1991;69:443–445.
24. Blanshard C, Gazzard BG. Microsporidiosis in HIV-1-infected individuals. *Lancet.* 1991;337:1488–1489.
25. Rijpstra AC, Canning EU, Van Ketel RJ, Eeftinck Schattenkerk JKM, Laarman JJ. Use of light microscopy to diagnose small-intestinal microsporidiosis in patients with AIDS. *J Infect Dis.* 1988;157:827–831.
26. Conlon C, Pinching A, Perera C, Moody A, Luo N, Lucas S. HIV-related enteropathy in Zambia: a clinical, microbiological, and histological study. *Am J Trop Med Hyg.* 1990;42:83–88.
27. Oddo BD, Chuaqui R, Hofman E, Garcia BM. Microsprodiosis intestinal en un paciente con sindrome de inmunodeficiencia adquirida. *Rev Med Chile.* 1991;119: 559–563.
28. Field AS, Hing MC, Milliken ST, Marriott DJ. Microsporidia in the small intestine of HIV-infected patients. A new diagnostic technique and a new species. *Med J Australia.* 1993;158:390–394.
29. Molina J-M, Sarfati C, Beauvais B, et al. Intestinal microsporidiosis in human immunodeficiency virus-infected patients with chronic unexplained diarrhea: prevalence and clinical and biologic features. *J Infect Dis.* 1993;167:217–221.
30. Sandfort J, Hannemann A, Gelderblom H, Stark K, Owen RL, Ruf B. *Enterocytozoon bieneusi* infection in an immunocompetent patient who had acute diarrhea and who was not infected with the human immunodeficiency virus. *Clin Infect Dis.* 1994;19:514–516.
31. Bretagne PS, Foulet F, Alkassoum W, Fleury-Feith J, Develoux M. Prevalence des spores d'*Enterocytozoon bieneusi* dans les selles de patients sideens et d'infants Africains non infectes par de VIH. *Bull Soc Path Ex.* 1993;86:351–357.
32. Sobottka I, Albrecht H, Schottelius J, Bentfield M, Laufs R, Schwartz DA. Self-limited traveller's diarrhea due to a dual infection with *Enterocytozoon bieneusi* and *Cryptosporidium parvum* in an immunocompetent HIV-negative child. *Eur J Clin Microbiol Infect Dis.* 1995;14: 919–920.
33. Sax PE, Rich JD, Pieciak WS, Trnka YM. Intestinal microsporidiosis occurring in a liver transplant recipient. *Transplantation.* 1995;60:617–618.
34. Orenstein JM, Tenner M, Cali A, Kolter D. A microsporidian previously undescribed in humans, infecting enterocytes and macrophages and associated with diarrhea in an AIDS patient. *Hum Pathol.* 1991;23:722–728.
35. Orenstein JM, Dieterich DT, Kotler DP. Systemic dissemination by a newly recognized microsporidia species in AIDS. *AIDS.* 1992;6:1143–1150.
36. Cali A, Orenstein JM, Kotler DP, Owen R. A comparison of two microsporidian parasites in enterocytes of AIDS patients with chronic diarrhea. *J Protozool.* 1991;38: 96S–98S.
37. Cali A, Kotler DP, Orenstein JM. *Septata intestinalis,* ng, nsp, an intestinal microsporidian associated with chronic diarrhea and dissemination in AIDS patients. *J Eukaryot Microbiol.* 1993;40:101–112.
38. Field AS, Canning EU, Hing MC, Verre J, Marriott DJ. Microsporidia in HIV-infected patients in Sydney Australia: a report of 37 cases, a new diagnostic technique and the light microscopy and ultrastructure of a disseminated species. *AIDS.* 1993;7(suppl 3):S27–S33.
39. Eeftinck Schattenkerk JKM, van Gool T, van den Bergh Weerman MA, Schot LJ, Dankert J. Chronic rhinosinusitus in HIV-infected patients with microsporidiosis. *AIDS.* 1993;7(suppl 3):S36–S37.
40. Friedberg DN, Stenson SM, Orenstein JM, Tiemo PM, Charles NC. Microsporidial keratoconjunctivitis in

acquired immunodeficiency syndrome. *Arch Ophthalmol.* 1990;108:504–508.

41. Didier ES, Didier PJ, Friedberg DN, et al. Isolation and characterization of a new microsporidian, *Encephalitozoon hellem* (n sp) from corneas of three AIDS patients. *J Infect Dis.* 1991;163:617–621.
42. Didier PJ, Didier E, Orenstein J, Shadduck A. Fine structure of *Encephalitozoon hellem* (n sp), in culture. *J Protozool.* 1991;38:502–507.
43. Didier ES, Shadduck JA, Didier PJ, Millichamp N, Vossbrinck CR. Studies on ocular microsporidia. *J Protozool.* 1991;38:635–638.
44. Schwartz DA, Bryan RT, Hewan-Lowe KO, et al. Disseminated microsporidiosis (*Encephalitozoon hellem*) and acquired immunodeficiency syndrome. Autopsy evidence for respiratory acquisition. *Arch Pathol Lab Med.* 1992;116:660–668.
45. Schwartz DA, Visvesvara GS, Leitch GJ, et al. Pathology of symptomatic microsporidial (*Encephalitozoon hellem*) bronchiolitis in the acquired immunodeficiency syndrome: a new respiratory pathogen diagnosed from lung biopsy, bronchoalveolar lavage, sputum, and tissue culture. *Hum Pathol.* 1993;24:937–943.
46. Lacey CJN, Clarke AMT, Fraser P, Metcalf T, Bonsor G, Curry A. Chronic microsporidian infection of the nasal mucosae, sinuses, and conjunctivae in HIV disease. *Genitourin Med.* 1992;68:179–181.
47. Hollister WS, Canning EU, Colbourn NI, Curry A, Lacey CJN. Characterization of *Encephalitozoon hellem* (microspora) isolated from the nasal mucosa of a patient with AIDS. *Parasitology.* 1993;107:351–358.
48. Visvesvara GS, Leitch GJ, Moura H, Wallace S, Weber R, Bryan RT. Culture, electron microscopy, and immunoblot studies on a microsporidian parasite isolated from the urine of a patient with AIDS. *J Protozool.* 1991;38:105S–111S.
49. Schwartz DA, Sobottka I, Leitch GJ, Cali A, Visvesvara GS. Pathology of microsporidiosis. Emerging parasitic infections in patients with the acquired immunodeficiency syndrome. *Arch Pathol Lab Med.* 1996;120:173–188.
50. Schwartz DA, Visvesvara GS, Diesenhouse MC, et al. Ocular pathology of microsporidiosis: role of immunofluorescent antibody for diagnosis of *Encephalitozoon hellem* in biopsies, smears, and intact globes from seven AIDS patients. *Am J Ophthalmol.* 1993;115:285–292.
51. Schwartz DA, Visvesvara GS, Weber R, Bryan RT. Male genital tract microsporidiosis and AIDS: prostatic infection with *Encephalitozoon hellem*. *J Eukaryot Microbiol.* 1994;41:61S.
52. Wilson JM. The biology of *Encephalitozoon cuniculi*. *Med Biol.* 1979;57:84–101.
53. Terada S, Reddy KR, Jeffers LJ, Cali A, Schiff ER. Microsporidian hepatitis in the acquired immunodeficiency syndrome. *Ann Intern Med.* 1987;107:61–62.
54. Zender HO, Arrigoni E, Eckert J, Kapanci Y. A case of *Encephalitozoon cuniculi* peritonitis in a patient with AIDS. *Am J Clin Pathol.* 1989;92:352–356.
55. DeGroote MA, Visvesvara GS, et al. Polymerase chain reaction and culture confirmation of disseminated *Encephalitozoon cuniculi* in a patient with AIDS: successful therapy with albendazole. *J Infect Dis.* 1995;171:1375–1378.
56. Franzen C, Schwartz DA, Visvesvara GS, et al. Immunologially confirmed disseminated asymptomatic *Encephalitozoon cuniculi* infection of the gastrointestinal tract in a patient with AIDS. *Clin Infect Dis.* 1995;21:1480–1484.
57. Chupp GL, Alroy J, Adelman LS, Breen JC, Skolnick PR. *Pleistophora* (microsporidia) myositis in a patient with the acquired immunodeficiency syndrome (AIDS). *Clin Infect Dis.* 1992;16:15–21.
58. Ledford DK, Overman MD, Gonzalvo A, Cali A, Mester SW, Lockey RF. Microsporidiosis myositis in a patient with the acquired immunodeficiency syndrome. *Ann Intern Med.* 1985;102:628–630.
59. Macher AM, Neafie R, Angritt P, Tuur SM. Microsporidial myositis and the acquired immunodeficiency syndrome (AIDS): a four-year follow-up. *Ann Intern Med.* 1988;108:343.
60. Margileth AM, Strano AJ, Chandra R, Neafie R, Blum M, McCully RM. Disseminated nosematosis in an immunologically compromised infant. *Arch Pathol.* 1973;95:145–150.
61. Shadduck JA, Meccoli RA, Davis R, Font RL. Isolation of a microsporidian from a human patient. *J Infect Dis.* 1990;162:773–776.
62. Koller LD. Spontaneous *Nosema cuniculi* infection in laboratory rabbits. *JAVMA.* 1969;155:1108–1114.
63. Lainson R, Garnham PCC, Killick-Kendrick R, Bird RG. Nosematosis, a microsporidial infection of rodents and other animals, including man. *Br Med J.* 1964;22:470–472.
64. Kelly P, McPhail G, Ngwenya B, et al. *Septata intestinalis:* a new microsporidian in Africa. *Lancet.* 1994;344:271–272.
65. Cox J, Hamil R, Attwood H. An investigation of the route and progression of *Encephalitozoon cuniculi* infection in adult rabbits. *J Protozool.* 1979;26:260–265.
66. Nelson JB. Experimental transmission of a murine microsporidian in Swiss mice. *J Bact.* 1967;94:1340–1345.
67. Shadduck JA, Watson WT, Pakes SP. Animal infectivity of *Encephalitozoon cuniculi*. *J Parasitol.* 1979;65:123–129.
68. Gannon J. The course of infection of *Encephalitozoon cuniculi* in immunodeficient and immunocompetent mice. *Lab Anim.* 1980;14:189–192.
69. Orenstein JM, Zierdt W, Zierdt C. Identification of spores of the Microspora, *Enterocytozoon bieneusi* in stool and duodenal fluid from AIDS patients with diarrhea. *Lancet.* 1991;336:1127–1128.
70. van Gool T, Hollister WS, Schattenkerk JE, et al. Diagnosis of *Enterocytozoon bieneusi* microsporidiosis in AIDS patients by recovery of spores from faeces. *Lancet.* 1990;2:697–698.
71. Cali A, Owen RI. Intracellular development of *Enterocytozoon,* a unique microsporidian found in the intestine of AIDS patients. *J Protozool.* 1990;37:145–155.
72. Cox JC, Walden NB, Nairn RC. Presumptive diagnosis of *Nosema cuniculi* in rabbits by immunofluorescence. *Res Vet Med.* 1972;13:595–597.
73. Bywater JEC, Kellett BS, Waller T. *Encephalitozoon cuni-*

culi antibodies in commercially available rabbit antisera and serum reagents. *Lab Anim.* 1980;14:87–89.

74. Bergquist R, Morfeldt-Mansson L, Pehrson PO, Petrini B, Wasserman J. Antibody against *Enterocytozoon cuniculi* in Swedish homosexual men. *Scand J Infect Dis.* 1984; 16:389–391.
75. Bergquist R, Stintzing G, Smedman L, Waller T, Andersson T. Diagnosis of encephalitozoonosis in man by serological tests. *Brit Med J* 1984;288:902.
76. Singh M, Kane GJ, Mackinaly L, et al. Detection of antibodies to *Nosema cuniculi* (protozoa: microsporidia) in human and animal sera by the indirect fluorescent antibody technique. *Southeast Asia J Trop Med Public Health.* 1982;13:110–113.
77. Hollister WS, Canning EU. An enzyme-linked immunosorbent assay (ELISA) for detection of antibodies to *E cuniculi* and its use in determination of infections in man. *Parasitol.* 1987;94:209–219.
78. Zhu X, Wittner M, Tanowitz HB, Kotler D, Cali A, Weiss LM. Small subunit rRNA sequence of *Enterocytozoon bieneusi* and its potential diagnostic role with use of the polymerase chain reaction. *J Infect Dis.* 1993;168: 1570–1575.
79. Zhu X, Wittner M, Tanowitz HB, Cali A, Weiss LM. Nucleotide sequence of the small subunit rRNA of *Septata intestinalis. Nucleic Acids Res.* 1993;21:4846.
80. Weiss LM, Zhu X, Cali A, Tanowitz HB, Wittner M. Utility of microsporidian rRNA in diagnosis and phylogeny: a review. *Folia Parasitol.* 1994;41:81–90.
81. Da Silva AJ, Schwartz DA, Visvesvara GS, de Moura H, Slemenda SB, Pieniazek NJ. Sensitive PCR diagnosis of infections by *Enterocytozoon bieneusi* (Microsporidia) using primers based on the region coding for small subunit rRNA. *J Clin Microbiol.* 1996;34:986–987.
82. Visvesvara GS, Leitch GL, Pieniazek NJ, et al. for the Enteric Opportunistic Infections Working Group. Short term in vitro culture and molecular analysis of *Enterocytozoon bieneusi. J Eukary Microbiol.* 1995;42:506–510.
83. Visvesvara GS, Leitch GL, Da Silva AJ, et al. Polyclonal and monoclonal antibody and PCR-amplified small-subunit rRNA identification of a microsporidian. *Encephalitozoon hellem,* isolated from an AIDS patient with disseminated infection. *J Clin Microbiol.* 1994;32:2760–2768.
84. Desportes-Livage I, Hilmarsdottir I, Romana C, Tanguy S, Datry A, Gentilini M. Characteristics of the microsporidian *Enterocytozoon bieneusi:* a consequence of its development within short-living enterocytes. *J Protozool.* 1991;38:111S–113S.
85. Desportes-Livage I, Harper F, Hilmarsdottir I, Benhamou Y, Ombrouck C, Gentilini M. The phospholipids in *Enterocytozoon bieneusi:* an electron spectroscopic imaging study. *Folia Parasitol.* 1993;40:275–278.
86. Kotler DP, Francisco A, Clayton F, Scholes J, Orenstein JM. Small intestinal injury and parasitic disease in AIDS. *Ann Intern Med.* 1990;113:444–449.
87. Soave R, Johnson WD. AIDS commentary: *Cryptosporidium* and *Isospora belli* infections. *J Infect Dis.* 1988;157: 225–229.
88. Asmuth DM, DeGirolami PC, Federman M, et al. Clinical features of microsporidiosis in AIDS patients. *Clin Infect Dis.* 1993;17:544.
89. McWhinney PHM, Nathwani D, Green ST, Boyd JF, Forrest JAH. Microsporidiosis detected in association with AIDS-related sclerosing cholangitis. *AIDS.* 1991;5:1394–1395.
90. Pol S, Romana C, Richard S, et al. *Enterocytozoon bieneusi* infection in acquired immunodeficiency syndrome-related sclerosing cholangitis. *Gastroenterology.* 1992;102:1778–1781.
91. Pol S, Romana CA, Richard S, et al. Microsporidian infection in patients with the human immunodeficiency virus and unexplained cholangitis. *N Engl J Med.* 1993;328: 95–99.
92. Pol S, Romana CA, Carnot F, Pays J-F, Berthelot P. Diagnosis of AIDS-related cholangitis. *AIDS.* 1993;7(suppl 3):S38–S39.
93. Beaugerie L, Teilhac M-F, Deluol A-M, et al. Cholangiopathy associated with microsporidia infection of the common bile duct mucosa in a patient with HIV infection. *Ann Intern Med.* 1992;117:401–402.
94. French AL, Beaudet LM, Benator DA, Levy CS, Kass M, Orenstein JM. Cholecystectomy in patients with AIDS: clinicopathologic correlations in 107 cases. *Clin Infect Dis.* 1995;21:852–858.
95. Weber R, Kuster H, Keller R, et al. Pulmonary and intestinal microsporidiosis in a patient with the acquired immunodeficiency syndrome. *Am Rev Respir Dis.* 1992; 146:1603–1605.
96. Schwartz DA, Bryan RT, Weber R, Visvesvara GS. Microsporidiosis in HIV positive patients: current methods for diagnosis using biopsy, cytologic, ultrastructural, immunological and tissue culture techniques. *Folia Parasitol.* 1994;41:101–109.
97. Metcalf TW, Doran RML, Rowlands PL, Curry A, Lacey CJN. Microsporidial keratoconjunctivitis in a patient with AIDS. *Br J Ophthalmol.* 1992;76:177–178.
98. Lucas S, Schwartz DA, Hasleton PS. Pulmonary parasitic diseases: In: Hasleton PS, ed. *Spencer's Pathology of the Lung.* 4th ed. New York: McGraw-Hill; 1996.
99. Marcial MA, Madara JL. *Cryptosporidium:* cellular localization, structural analysis of absorptive cell-parasite membrane-membrane interactions in guinea pigs, and suggestion of protozoan transport by M cells. *Gastroenterology.* 1986;90:583–594.
100. Peacock CS, Blanshard C, Tovey DG, Ellis DS, Gazzard BG. Histological diagnosis of intestinal microsporidiosis in patients with AIDS. *J Clin Pathol.* 1991;44:558–563.
101. Rabeneck L, Gyorkey F, Genta RM, Gyorkey P, Bailey ME, Foote LW. The role of microsporidia in the pathogenesis of HIV-related chronic diarrhea. *Ann Intern Med.* 1993;119:895–899.
102. Gourley WK, Swedo JL. Intestinal infection by microsporidia *Enterocytozoon bieneusi* of patients with AIDS: an ultrastructural study of the use of human mitochondria by a protozoan. *Lab Invest.* 1988;58:35A.
103. Orenstein JM, Tenner M, Kotler DP. Localization of infection by the microsporidian *Enterocytozoon bieneusi* in the gastrointestinal tract of AIDS patients with diarrhea. *AIDS.* 1992;6:195–197.

104. Tiner JD. Birefringent spores differentiate *Encephalitozoon* and microsporidia from coccidia. *Vet Pathol.* 1988; 25:227–230.
105. Blanshard C, Hollister WS, Peacock CS, et al. Simultaneous infection with two types of intestinal microsporidia in a patient with AIDS. *Gut.* 1992;33:418–420.
106. Lucas SB, Papadaki L, Conlon C, Sewankambo N, Goodgame R, Serwadda D. Diagnosis of intestinal microsporidiosis in patients with AIDS. *J Clin Pathol.* 1989; 42:885–887.
107. Simon D, Weiss L, Tanowitz H, Cali A, Jones J, Wittner M. Light microscope diagnosis of human microsporidiosis and variable response to octreotide. *Gastroenterology.* 1991;100:271–273.
108. Weber R, Bryan R, Owen R, Wilcox M, Gorelkin L, Visvesvara G. Improved light-microscopical detection of microsporidia spores in stool and duodenal aspirates. *N Engl J Med.* 1992;326:161–166.
109. Ryan NJ, Sutherland G, Coughlan K, et al. A new trichrome-blue stain for detection of microsporidial species in urine, stool, and nasopharyngeal specimens. *J Clin Microbiol.* 1993;31:3264–3269.
110. Kokoskin E, Gyorkos T, Camus A, Celidotte L, Purtill T, Ward B. Modified technique for efficient detection of microsporidia. *J Clin Microbiol.* 1994;32:1074–1075.
111. van Gool T, Snijders F, Reiss P, et al. Diagnosis of intestinal and disseminated microsporidial infections in patients with HIV by a new rapid fluorescence technique. *J Clin Pathol.* 1993;46:694–699.
112. Varva J, Nohynkova E, Machala L, Spala J. An extremely rapid method for detection of microsporidia in biopsy materials of AIDS patients. *Folia Parasitol.* 1993;40: 273–274.
113. Koch HH, Pimsler M. Evaluation of uvitex 2B: a nonspecific fluorescent stain for detecting and identifying fungi and algae in tissue. *Lab Med.* 1987;18:603–606.
114. Wachsmuth ED. A comparison of the highly selective fluorescence staining of fungi in tissue sections with uvitex 2B and Calcofluor White M2R. *Histochemical J.* 1988; 20:215–221.
115. Weir GO, Sullivan JT. A fluorescence screening technique for microsporida in histological sections. *Trans Am Microscop Soc.* 1989;108:208–210.
116. Travis WD, Schmidt K, MacLowry JD, Masur H, Condron KS, Fojo AT. Respiratory cryptosporidiosis in a patient with malignant lymphoma. *Arch Pathol Lab Med.* 1990; 114:519–522.
117. Yee RW, Tio FO, Martinez A, Held KS, Shadduck JA, Didier ES. Resolution of microsporidial epithelial keratopathy in a patient with AIDS. *Ophthalmology.* 1990; 98:196–201.
118. Lowder CY, Meisler DM, McMahon JT, Longworth DL, Rutherford I. Microsporidia infection of the cornea in a man seropositive for human immunodeficiency virus. *Am J Ophthalmol.* 1990;109:242–244.
119. Cali A, Meisler DM, Lowder CY, et al. Corneal microsporidiosis: characterization and identification. *J Protozool.* 1991;38:215S–217S.
120. Preston DC. Electrophysiology of microsporidia myositis in an AIDS patient. *Muscle Nerve.* 1993;16:1420–1422.
121. Weber R, Sauer B, Luthy R, Nadal D. Intestinal coinfection with *Enterocytozoon bieneusi* and *Cryptosporidium* in a human immunodeficiency virus-infected child with chronic diarrhea. *Clin Infect Dis.* 1993;17:480–483.
122. Garcia LS, Shimizu RY, Bruckner DA. Detection of microsporidial spores in fecal specimens from patients diagnosed with cryptosporidiosis. *J Clin Microbiol.* 1994; 32:1739–1741.
123. Hing MC, Marriott DJ, Verre J, Field AS. Enteric microsporidiosis: response to azithromycin. *AIDS.* 1993;7 (suppl 3):S45–S46.
124. Blanshard C, Ellis DS, Tovey DG, Dowell S, Gazzard BG. Treatment of intestinal microsporidiosis with albendazole in patients with AIDS. *AIDS.* 1992;6:311–313.
125. Lacey E. The role of the cytoskeletal protein, tubulin, in the mode of action and mechanism of drug resistance to benzimidazoles. *Int J Parasitol.* 1988;18:885–936.
126. Dieterich D, Lew E, Orenstein JM, Poles MA, Kotler DP. Divergence between clinical and histologic responses during treatment for *Enterocytozoon bieneusi* infection. *AIDS.* 1993;7(suppl 3):S43–S44.
127. Dieterich DT, Lew EA, Kotler DP, Poles MA, Orenstein JM. Treatment with albendazole for intestinal disease caused by *Enterocytozoon bieneusi* in patients with AIDS. *J Infect Dis.* 1994;169:178–183.
128. Orenstein JM, Dieterich DT, Lew EA, Kotler DP. Albendazole as a treatment for intestinal and disseminated microsporidiosis caused by *Septata intestinalis* in AIDS patients: a report of four patients. *AIDS.* 1993;7(suppl 3):S40–S42.
129. Joste N, Rich JD, Busam KJ, Schwartz DA. Autopsy verification of *Encephalitozoon intestinalis* (microsporidiosis) eradication following albendazole therapy. *Arch Pathol Lab Med.* 1996;120:199–203.
130. Sobottka I, Albrecht H, Schäfer H, et al. Disseminated *Encephalitozoon (Septata) intestinalis* infection in a patient with AIDS: novel diagnostic approaches and autopsy-confirmed parasitological cure following treatment with albendazole. *J Clin Microbiol.* 1995;33: 2948–2952.
131. Weber R, Sauer B, Spycher MA, et al. Detection of *Septata intestinalis* in stool specimens and coprodiagnostic monitoring of successful treatment with albendazole. *Clin Infect Dis.* 1994;19:342–345.
132. Beauvis B, Sarfati C, Challier S, Derouin F. In vitro model to assess effect of antimicrobial agents on *Encephalitozoon cuniculi. Antimicrobial Agents Chemotherapy.* 1994;38:2440–2448.

CHAPTER 138

Pneumocystosis

John C. Watts and Francis W. Chandler

Some folk seem glad even to draw their breath.

William Morris (1834–1896)

DEFINITION

Pneumocystosis is an opportunistic pulmonary infection caused by *Pneumocystis carinii* that occurs almost exclusively in persons with impaired cell-mediated immunity, and particularly in those infected with the human immunodeficiency virus (HIV).[1,2] Rarely, the organism disseminates to extrapulmonary sites, but the disease is dominated by respiratory symptoms. Because *P carinii* cannot be cultivated on cell-free media in the clinical laboratory, the diagnosis of pneumocystosis depends on demonstration of the organism in biopsy or cytology specimens.

GEOGRAPHIC DISTRIBUTION

An ecologic niche for *P carinii* has not been identified. It is likely that human lungs are the major reservoir for this organism, but attempts to define its distribution in nature have been hampered by the lack of a simple method to culture the organism.[3] Opportunistic *P carinii* pneumonia (PCP) occurs throughout the world.

EPIDEMIOLOGY

There are two major clinical forms of PCP and each has a different epidemiologic pattern.[4] The epidemic form, interstitial plasma cell pneumonia, occurs in institutional settings in underdeveloped countries and mainly affects premature, malnourished children.[5,6] The sporadic form, more frequent in the United States and other developed countries, indicates underlying cellular immune deficiency[7] and is prone to develop in persons with impairment of their CD4+ (T-helper) lymphocytes. Diseases or factors that predispose to sporadic PCP include primary (congenital) immunodeficiency diseases,[8] therapy-related immunodeficiency induced by cytotoxic agents and corticosteroids, and disease-related acquired immunodeficiency.[1,9] Before the acquired immunodeficiency syndrome (AIDS) epidemic, most patients with PCP had acute leukemia or were leukopenic from cytotoxic chemotherapy.[1] Now these patients are outnumbered by AIDS-associated PCP. About 65% of HIV-infected patients have PCP when AIDS is diagnosed, and about 80% of AIDS patients develop PCP during the course of their disease.[10] In some areas of the United States (eg, New York City, Miami, and San Francisco), PCP has become the most frequent infectious disease encountered by anatomic pathologists. Rarely PCP develops in patients without a recognized predisposing illness.[11]

Most people probably are exposed to *P carinii* early in life and acquire subclinical respiratory infections.[12] Overt PCP may then develop from a latent pulmonary reservoir whenever host defense mechanisms become impaired. Apparently, this is the mechanism by which experimental infection is induced in the corticosteroid-treated rat model.[13] Epidemic outbreaks of interstitial plasma cell pneumonia indicate that the disease may be contagious under certain circumstances.

LIFE CYCLE

Evidence that *P carinii* is a protozoal pathogen derives from the ultrastructural morphology of the organism,[14,15] its sensitivity to antiprotozoal chemotherapeutic agents, and its resistance to many antifungal drugs.

Classification has been hampered by the lack of a simple system for cell-free culture of the organism. Nevertheless, recent observations have challenged the traditional notion that *P carinii* is a protozoan. Based on relatedness studies of 16S-like ribosomal RNA, Edman et al[16] believe that *P carinii* is more closely related to the fungi than the protozoa, but this opinion has been challenged.[17] For this chapter, however, *P carinii* is considered to be a protozoan, and traditional terms are used to describe its life cycle.

Another question is whether the genus, *Pneumocystis,* contains one species, or whether multiple species or strains can be defined by differences in host specificity or antigenic determinants.[18,19] Here we describe what we believe is one species, *P carinii.*

Our understanding of the life cycle of *P carinii* derives mainly from detailed ultrastructural studies,[20–24] which have defined three developmental forms: trophozoites, cysts, and sporozoites. These varied forms also can be seen by light microscopy using appropriate special stains. Trophozoites, the vegetative form, attach to type 1 alveolar epithelial cells. Although initially haploid, the trophozoites are believed to attain a diploid chromosomal number by gametic fusion.[25] Asexual replication of trophozoites may also occur by endogeny, binary fission, or both. The trophozoites enlarge and develop into diploid precysts through a process of cell wall thickening.[25] Sporozoites then develop within the precysts following meiosis and mitosis, a process referred to as sporogony.[26–28] Mature cysts each contain eight haploid sporozoites that, upon release following rupture of the cyst wall, become trophozoites, which can then recapitulate the life cycle. Despite a claim to the contrary,[29] neither the cysts nor the trophozoites of *P carinii* are intracellular pathogens. They can, however, be within phagolysosomes in macrophages during the course of an inflammatory response to the infection.

MORPHOLOGIC FEATURES OF THE ORGANISM

The developmental forms of *P carinii* are not seen clearly in routine histologic sections. A variety of special stains, however, is used to make the diagnosis, and these are grouped into two categories: those that stain the cyst walls, and those that stain the nuclei of the trophozoites and sporozoites.[30] The latter group, which can be applied only to imprint smears and cytology specimens, includes a variety of Romanowsky stains (Giemsa, Wright, Diff-Quik), polychrome methylene blue, and Gram's stain. The cyst wall stains can be applied to tissue sections as well, and we prefer them for routine diagnostic work. They include Gomori's (Grocott) methenamine silver (GMS) and its rapid variants, toluidine-blue-0, and Gram-Weigert methods.[30] Of these, we prefer GMS.

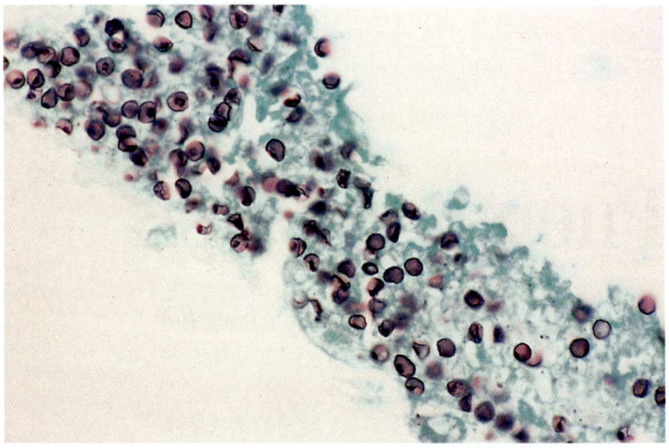

Figure 138–1. Spherical and crescentic (collapsed) cysts of *P carinii.* Internal, paired, comma-shaped argyrophilic foci can be seen to merge with the cyst wall when projected in the appropriate plane (GMS, ×250).

With GMS, the cysts of *P carinii* are thick-walled spherules, 4 to 7 μm in diameter, that when collapsed assume cup or crescent shapes. Many cysts contain single or paired, comma-shaped structures that are localized areas of thickening of the inner layer of the cyst wall[31] (Figures 138–1 and 138–2). These distinctive argyrophilic structures help to distinguish the cysts of *P carinii* from nonbudding yeastlike fungi and other pathogens. Although seen best with GMS, the thickened foci can also be stained with toluidine-blue-0, but not reliably with the Gram–Weigert stain. None of the cyst

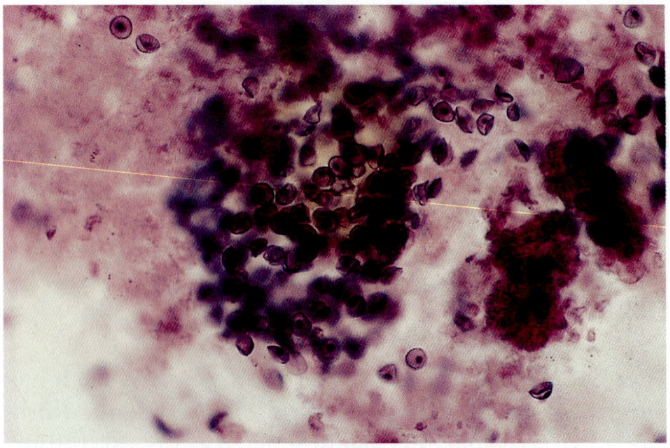

Figure 138–2. *Pneumocystis carinii* pneumonia. A touch smear contains numerous argyrophilic cyst forms that have internal, single or paired, morphologically distinct foci of enhanced staining [GMS–hematoxylin-eosin (H&E), ×250].

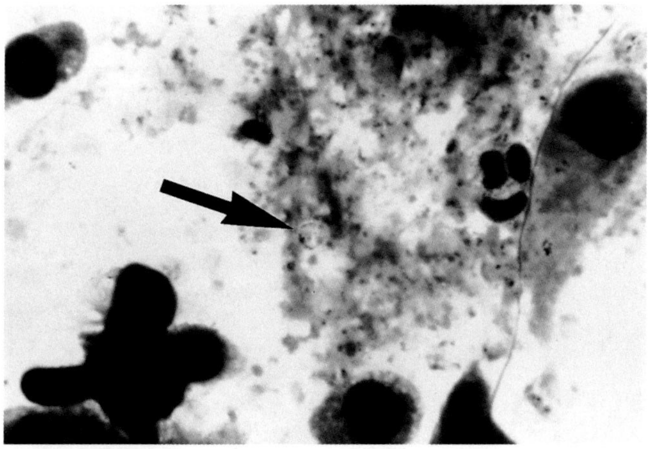

Figure 138–3. Sporozoite nuclei enveloped by a negatively stained cyst wall (*arrow*). Dotlike structures in the background adjacent to the cyst are nuclei of trophozoites. Note how difficult it is to distinguish the cyst from background elements with a Romanowsky stain, in contrast to the crisp clarity of the methenamine-silver stain pictured in Figure 138–1 (Wright–Giemsa, ×750).

wall stains demonstrates the sporozoites or trophozoites, although the membranes of the latter may stain faintly in specimens heavily overstained with GMS.

The sporozoites, 1 to 2 μm in diameter, and trophozoites, 2 to 8 μm in diameter, can be visualized with the appropriate special stains in smears and imprints, mainly because of their nuclear staining. Thus, the sporozoites are recognized as clusters of tiny nuclei surrounded by an unstained cyst wall (Figure 138–3). Trophozoite conglomerates appear as a meshwork of honeycombed spaces, many of which contain a dotlike nucleus. The trophozoites, however, can be difficult to distinguish from background fibrin or tissue elements. Stains for sporozoites/trophozoites have been advocated for diagnosis because of their simplicity and rapidity. We believe, however, that a well-prepared GMS stain is by far the most reliable and sensitive nonimmunologic stain for the diagnosis of infections caused by *P carinii.* Recently described rapid GMS variants have shortened the time required for specimen staining.[32–36] We use a microwave method, described originally by Brinn,[35] which can provide high-contrast slides of optimal quality in about 20 min and which can be applied to any standard specimen. Combined methods that demonstrate both cyst walls and the nuclei of sporozoites and trophozoites, although aesthetically pleasing, offer no advantage over a good methenamine-silver stain.

Pneumocystis carinii is delineated best by electron microscopy,[20–24] which is not, however, required for diagnosis. The cyst wall is composed of a thin, electron-dense outer layer and a broader, more lucent inner layer that is segmentally thickened, as described earlier. This thickened mural plaque can be seen only in the small proportion of cysts that are optimally sectioned (Figure 138–4). Each uninucleated sporozoite is delimited by its own membrane and contains cytoplasmic organelles, such as mitochondria, free ribosomes, and endoplasmic reticulum.

The trophozoites are ameboid, with broad pseudopodia and polar aggregates of tubular cytomembranous processes, termed "filopodia," that increase the surface area of the trophozoites (Figure 138–5). Although the function of the filopodia is not known, they may facilitate nutrition; they are not organelles of attachment. Each trophozoite contains a single nucleus, cytoplasmic organelles, and glycogen, although not all of these elements are seen in every trophozoite. Occasionally, trophozoites assume shapes that suggest reproduction by either binary fission or endogeny.

The trophozoites tend to cluster in large aggregates, where they mold against each other in sheets like pieces of a jigsaw puzzle. Each large cluster of trophozoites contains only a few admixed cysts. It is the clustering of the trophozoites that produces the appearance of alveolar "honeycomb exudate" by light microscopy.

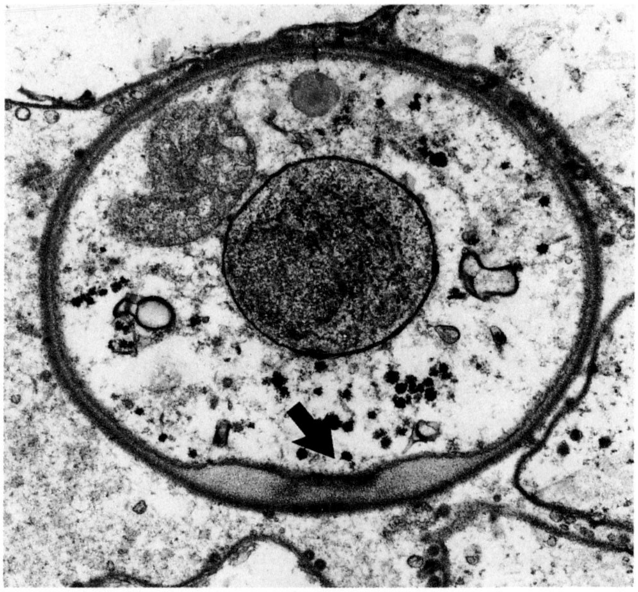

Figure 138–4. Ultrastructure of a *P carinii* cyst. The cyst wall is composed of an outer, dense layer and an inner, more lucent layer. Note the plaque that segmentally thickens the cyst wall (*arrow*). A sporozoite with ill-defined nucleus is in the center of the cyst, adjacent to a portion of a second sporozoite (×25,000).

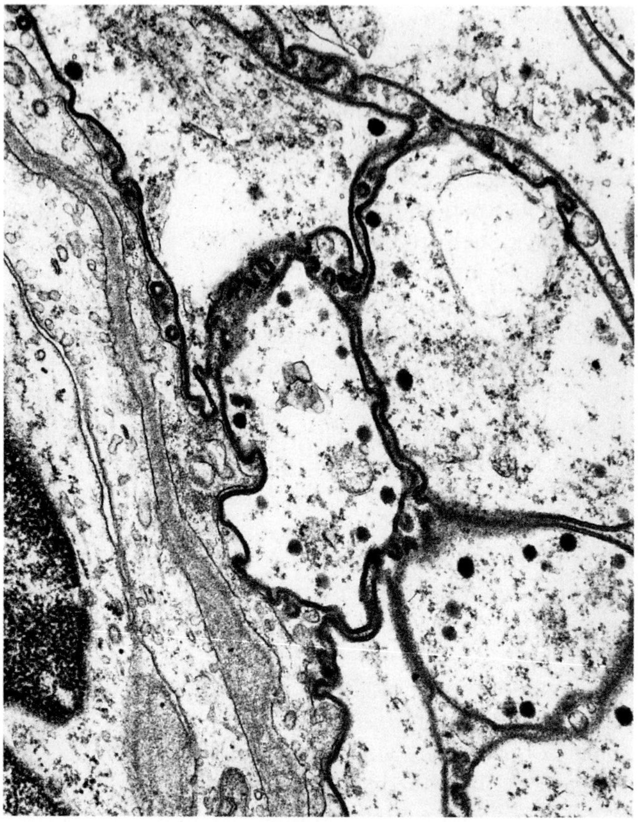

Figure 138–5. Ultrastructure of *P carinii* trophozoites. Cell processes of the ameboid trophozoites (*right*) interdigitate with each other and with processes of a type 1 alveolar epithelial cell (*left*) like pieces of a jigsaw puzzle. The tubular cytomembranous processes between the trophozoites are termed "filopodia" (×23,300).

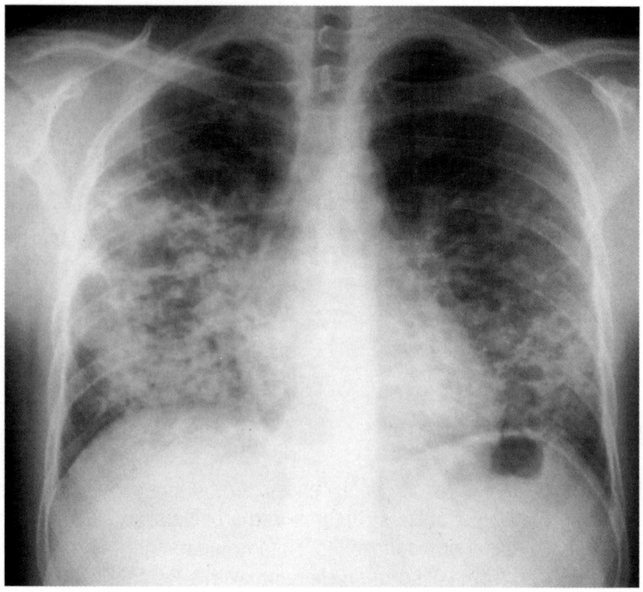

Figure 138–6. Chest radiograph of an AIDS patient with PCP. Interstitial and alveolar opacities predominate in both lower lung fields. *(Radiograph contributed by Harry Tabor, MD, Department of Diagnostic Radiology, William Beaumont Hospital, Royal Oak, Michigan.)*

CLINICAL FEATURES

The clinical and radiographic findings in sporadic PCP are not specific, and they mimic those of other opportunistic infections. Thus, a typical clinical presentation might include fever, dyspnea, tachypnea, and nonproductive cough.[1] The clinical manifestations, however, tend to be more subtle and evolve more slowly in HIV-infected patients.[2,37] Typical radiographic findings include bilateral interstitial and alveolar infiltrates, initially predominating in parahilar regions and lower lung fields (Figure 138–6), which may progress to extensive areas of air-space consolidation involving much of both lungs.[38] As many as 10% to 20% of AIDS patients with PCP present initially with no detectable radiographic abnormalities. Unusual radiographic and computed tomographic (CT) findings include nodules, cavities, cysts, lymphadenopathy, pleural effusions, and pneumothorax.[39] Most patients who have disseminated extrapulmonary pneumocystosis have no specific symptoms. Some patients, however, may experience local pain or a mass; rarely, there is clinical and laboratory evidence of organ (eg, renal, otic, or bone marrow) failure.[40]

The prevention and treatment of pneumocystosis are rapidly evolving controversial subjects that are currently the focus of considerable investigational interest. Two standard drugs used to treat most patients with PCP are trimethoprim–sulfamethoxazole (TMP–SMX) and pentamidine isethionate.[41] They appear to be equally effective and are associated with approximately the same incidence of adverse reactions,[42] which may affect as many as 60% of patients with AIDS. A new investigational drug, 566CB0, used in mild to moderately severe episodes of PCP in AIDS patients has shown promising results.[43] Early adjunctive therapy with corticosteroids can reduce the morbidity and mortality associated with moderate or severe PCP.[44,45] It is now generally agreed that patients at high risk for PCP, specifically HIV-infected patients with CD4+ lymphocyte counts of less than 200 cells/mm^3, and all AIDS patients who have already had one or more episodes of PCP, should receive prophylaxis.[46] Agents currently recommended for primary or secondary prophylaxis include TMP–SMX and aerosolized pentamidine. The latter regimen, however, may predispose to extrapulmonary pneumocystosis.[47]

PATHOLOGY

In fatal sporadic PCP, the lungs are heavy and have a pale gray or tan cut surface with a granular, firm, consolidated appearance (Figure 138–7). Nodules and cavities are occasionally encountered.

Microscopically, a variety of patterns has been described, both in patients with and without AIDS, and virtually any pattern of reaction (other than a pure acute, suppurative response) can be found in PCP. Interstitial plasma cell pneumonia, the epidemic form of the disease only rarely encountered in the United States, has an intense plasmacytic and lymphocytic interstitial pneumonitis[4] (Figure 138–8). This morphologically nonspecific interstitial pneumonia resembles that seen in other opportunistic (especially viral) infections that are prone to occur in premature, debilitated, or malnourished infants. Often, the correct diagnosis is suggested by the "honeycomb exudate" in alveolar spaces,[4] but definitive diagnosis requires demonstration of the pathogen with an appropriate special stain or immunohistochemical reagent.

The typical histopathologic pattern of sporadic PCP is produced by filling of the alveolar spaces with eosinophilic, vacuolated, or foamy material that is widely referred to as "honeycomb exudate."[48,49] At high magnification, the honeycomb material is punctuated with basophilic dots within vacuoles. These dots are the nuclei of the sporozoites and trophozoites (Figure 138–9) and are best seen in tissue preserved with a good nuclear fixative, such as B5 solution.[30] The alveolar foamy material may be accompanied by interstitial edema and by hypertrophy of alveolar epithelial cells, but an interstitial cellular infiltrate is usually lacking. As already described, the "honeycomb exudate" is composed predominantly of *P carinii* trophozoites with fewer admixed cysts, and occasional host cells enmeshed in fibrin. The appearance is so familiar to most pathologists that its recognition justifies a presumptive diagnosis of PCP, in the appropriate clinical setting.

The first study that documented a broad spectrum of reaction patterns in PCP was that of Weber et al[50] in

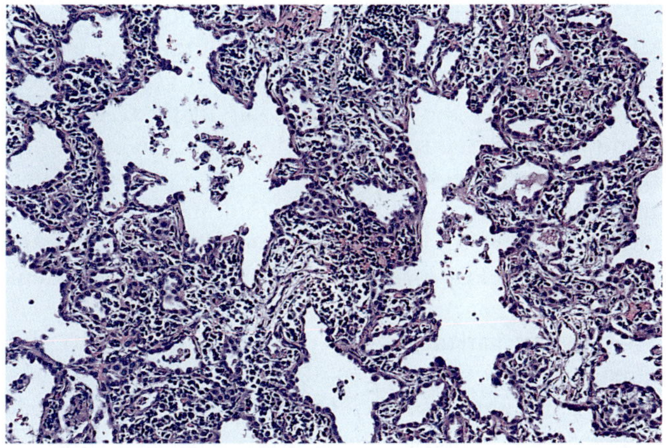

Figure 138–8. Interstitial plasma cell pneumonia in epidemic pneumocystosis. The changes here are nonspecific but small aggregates of honeycomb alveolar "exudate" were present elsewhere in the specimen (H&E, ×120).

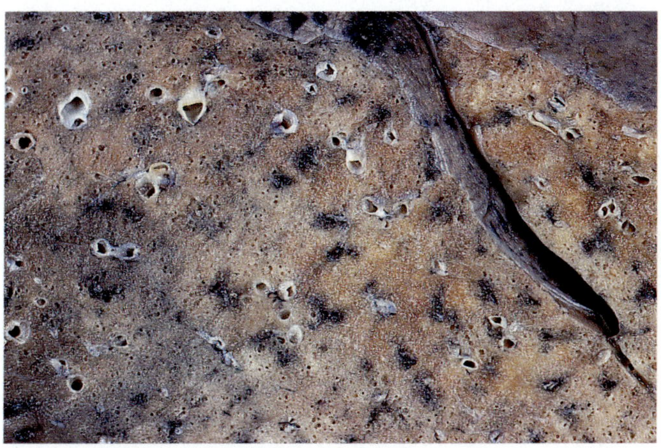

Figure 138–7. Cut surface of lung from a patient with active PCP. Much of the pulmonary parenchyma appears dry, granular, and consolidated. The pleura lining the interlobar fissure is glistening and clear, indicating that it is not involved by the inflammatory process.

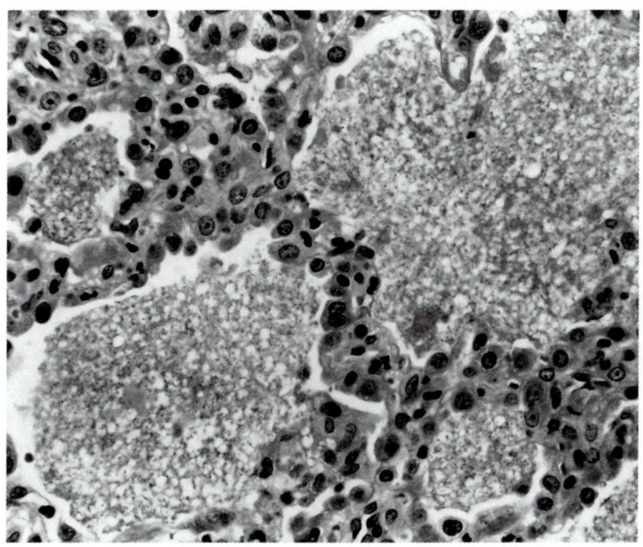

Figure 138–9. Typical honeycomb alveolar "exudate" of PCP. Punctate dots, the nuclei of sporozoites and trophozoites, occupy many of the honeycomb spaces. There is hypertrophy and hyperplasia of type 2 alveolar epithelial cells. (H&E, ×300).

1977. In that study, conducted before the onset of the AIDS epidemic, only about one third of the lung biopsy specimens showed the typical pattern of PCP described earlier. Notably, the foamy alveolar material was not found in about one half of the specimens. Atypical findings included dense interstitial lymphocytic infiltrates, interstitial fibrosis, epithelioid granulomas, multinucleated giant cells, and focal calcifications. This spectrum of changes in PCP has been confirmed in subsequent studies.[49,50]

Another variant pattern of PCP is diffuse alveolar damage (DAD) (Figure 138–10), both in AIDS patients and in other immunodeficient patients.[51–53] Often, there is little foamy material in the alveolar spaces, and the changes may therefore be misinterpreted as viral infection, oxygen toxicity, or drug reaction unless an appropriate stain is done to demonstrate the cysts. The latter, which may be quite sparse, are usually found in hyaline membranes lining the walls of alveolar ducts and alveoli.

A granulomatous response has been described both in AIDS patients and in immunodeficient patients without AIDS,[48,51,54,55] and in some patients it has been associated with nodular or cavitary patterns on chest radiographs. The granulomas may be loose and poorly formed, or they may be composed of discrete aggregates of epithelioid histiocytes, with or without central necrosis.[55,56] In some patients, the granulomatous reaction surrounds eosinophilic, foamy material composed of trophozoites and cysts of *P carinii* (Figure 138–11). Because granulomatous reactions are infrequent in PCP, every effort should be made to exclude other, concurrent pathogens such as fungi and mycobacteria by culture and special stains.

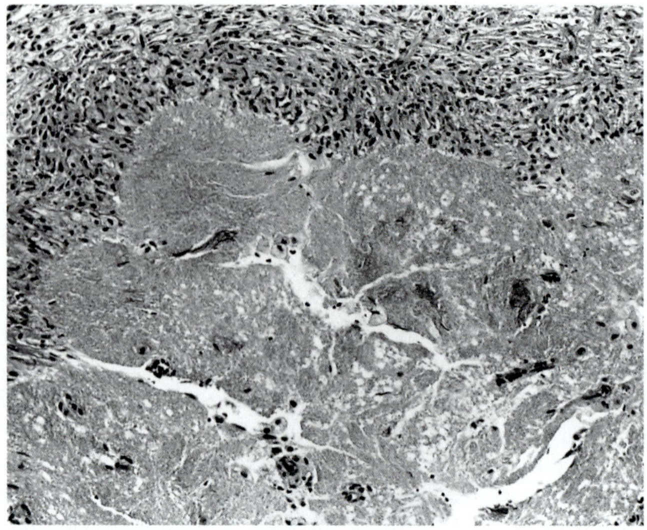

Figure 138–11. Granulomatous pulmonary pneumocystosis in a patient with AIDS. The epithelioid granulomatous response surrounds eosinophilic, foamy material composed of cysts and trophozoites (H&E, ×120).

The nodular and cavitary lesions of PCP are characterized, in some patients, by confluent parenchymal necrosis with lysis of alveolar septa.[30,51] In these lesions, the necrotic parenchyma is often replaced by confluent masses of eosinophilic foamy material (Figure 138–12), in which there are abundant cysts of *P carinii*. Rarely, parenchymal necrosis results from pneumocystis vasculitis, characterized by massive infiltration of blood vessel walls by characteristic foamy material

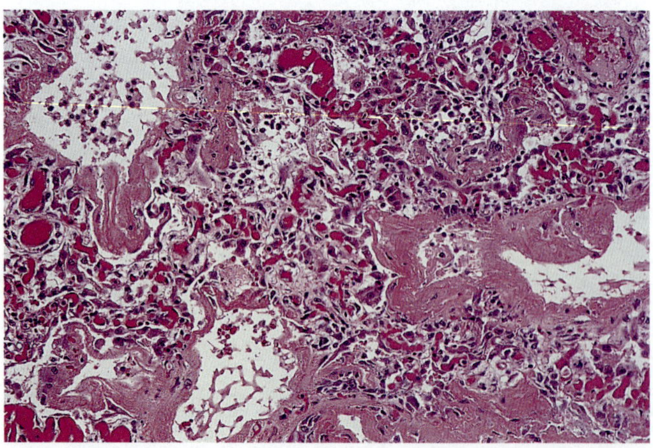

Figure 138–10. DAD pattern of pulmonary pneumocystosis. Hyaline membranes line the inner surfaces of alveolar ducts and alveoli. Rare cysts of *P carinii* embedded in these hyaline membranes will be overlooked unless searched for with a cyst wall stain such as GMS (H&E, ×40).

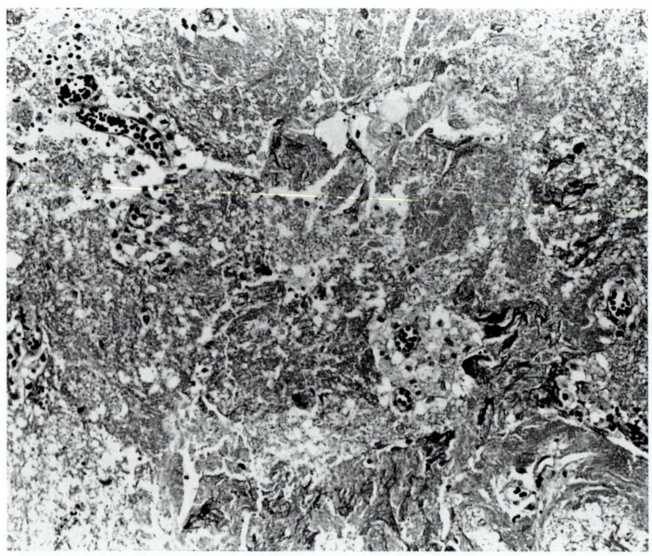

Figure 138–12. Parenchymal necrosis with septal lysis. The normal alveolar architecture is obliterated by a confluent mass of cysts and trophozoites (H&E, ×120).

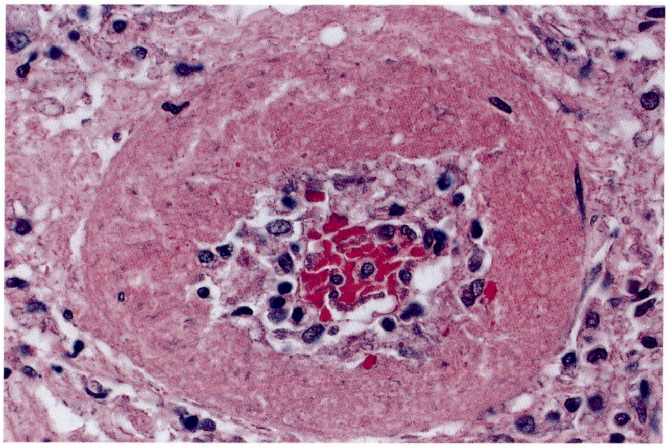

Figure 138–13. Pneumocystis vasculitis. The wall of this pulmonary blood vessel is replaced by foamy material consisting of cysts and trophozoites (H&E, ×160). *(Prepared from slides contributed by Joseph T. Tomashefski, Jr., MD, Department of Pathology, Case Western Reserve University School of Medicine at Metrohealth Medical Center.)*

accompanied by mononuclear inflammatory cells and mural necrosis[57] (Figure 138–13).

Chronic interstitial lung disease with interstitial fibrosis (Figure 138–14) may complicate long-standing, treated, or recurrent PCP,[48,49] but this interpretation should be accepted with skepticism. Many, if not most of these cases, are consistent with the organizing or proliferative phase of DAD, which is more likely caused by oxygen toxicity, concurrent viral infection, shock, or other recognized causes of DAD, rather than by *P carinii.* Hilar lymphadenopathy is an infrequent manifestation of PCP. In some patients, lymphadenopathy is caused by underlying disease (eg, lymphoma or leukemia) or reactive hyperplasia. In other patients, lymph nodes contain typical foamy masses of *P carinii* similar to those found in the alveolar spaces.[58]

Extrapulmonary pneumocystosis occurs primarily in patients with overwhelming pulmonary infection, those with severe underlying immunodeficiency, and those (particularly HIV-infected patients) who receive aerosolized pentamidine for prophylaxis against PCP.[30,59] Sites of extrapulmonary dissemination include lymph nodes, skin, ears, eyes, bone marrow, spleen, liver, kidneys, thyroid gland, gastrointestinal tract, and a variety of other organs and tissues.[30] The lesions of extrapulmonary pneumocystosis are gray-white or yellow nodules. Microscopically, the lesions consist of sheets of eosinophilic, foamy material identical to that described previously, composed of cysts and trophozoites, with little or no inflammatory response.[51] Smaller lesions and satellite nodules may have an angiocentric distribution.

The ultrastructural pathology of PCP, recently reviewed,[24,30] is mainly of pathogenetic interest. Ultrastructural studies have shown that the single or paired, argyrophilic "intracystic bodies" are plaquelike thickenings of the cyst wall (Figure 138–15) rather than sporozoites or other organelles.[31] Such studies also have confirmed that *P carinii* is a strictly extracellular pathogen.

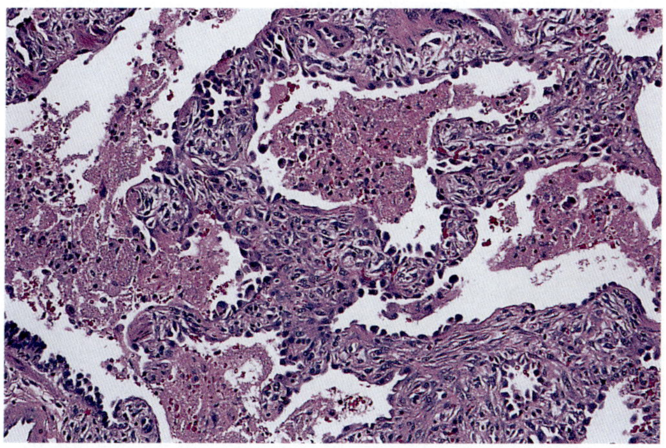

Figure 138–14. Chronic PCP. Interstitial edema, inflammation, and fibroblastic proliferation may be sequelae of oxygen toxicity rather than direct effects of *P carinii* (H&E, ×40).

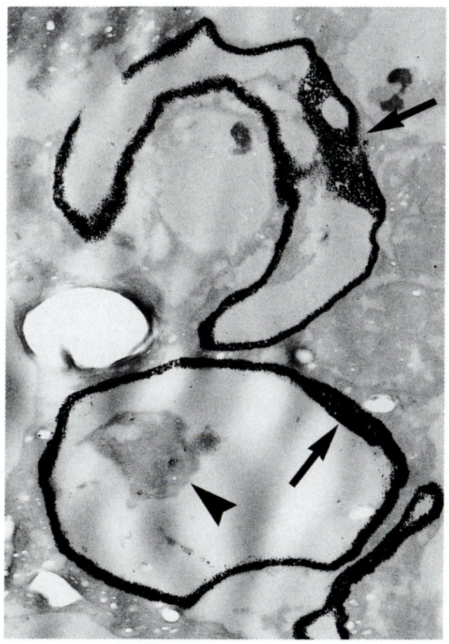

Figure 138–15. Electron micrograph of cysts of *P carinii* stained with methenamine silver. There is selective deposition of silver grains on the cyst walls and mural plaques (*arrows*). The single sporozoite (*arrowhead*) is not argyrophilic (GMS, ×24,000).

Trophozoites attach to the surface of type 1 pneumocytes by specialized interdigitations, without membrane fusion or communication between cytoplasmic compartments.[60,61] Trophozoite attachment may eventually cause epithelial and endothelial damage, resulting in acute diffuse alveolar damage.[62]

The cytologic features of PCP are well described and illustrated in the literature.[63,64] Indeed, cytologic methods, especially examination of induced sputum and bronchoalveolar lavage (BAL) specimens, have become the primary diagnostic modality for PCP, particularly in HIV-infected patients for whom the sensitivity of cytodiagnosis is reasonably high.[64] In Papanicolaou stained smears, *P carinii* forms cohesive aggregates of cysts and trophozoites with a granular, foamy, or honeycomb appearance. These aggregates are usually spherical, with considerable depth of focus (Figure 138–16), and are of a size that approximates that of a normal alveolar sac.[63] These aggregates, sometimes called "alveolar casts," are quite characteristic; with experience, they can be recognized at screening magnification if present in sufficient quantity. Nevertheless, we advocate that the diagnosis be confirmed with an appropriate special stain, as it should be also in histologic sections. The honeycomb aggregates in Papanicolaou stained smears are fluorescent when viewed with ultraviolet light and a fluorescence microscope.[65] Nevertheless, we do not advocate the use of nonimmunologic fluorescence methods[65,66] to confirm the diagnosis of PCP, because they are no more sensitive or specific than the GMS method.

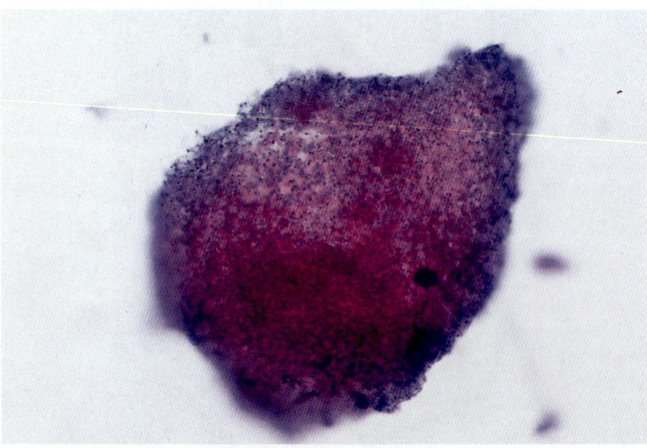

Figure 138–16. Cohesive aggregate of *P carinii* cysts and trophozoites in a BAL specimen from an AIDS patient. The spherical configuration of this aggregate results in variable depth of focus. Dot-like structures visible at the periphery of the aggregate are nuclei of sporozoites and trophozoites (Papanicolaou, ×160).

DIFFERENTIAL DIAGNOSIS

Although a large number of pathogenic microbes are stained wholly or in part with GMS, it is the yeastlike fungi, particularly *Histoplasma capsulatum, Torulopsis glabrata,* and *Cryptococcus neoformans,* that are most difficult to distinguish from the cysts of *P carinii.*[30] In this regard, recognition of the single or paired, comma-shaped argyrophilic foci in the walls of *P carinii* cysts is most important, for we have never seen structures with this configuration in the walls of yeastlike cells. Production of blastoconidia by the process of external budding is a characteristic feature of yeastlike cells, but the cysts of *P carinii* do not reproduce by budding. *Cryptococcus neoformans* has a mucopolysaccharide capsule that further distinguishes it from cysts of *P carinii.* The cells of the *Candida* sp in invasive lesions are invariably accompanied by mycelial elements (pseudohyphae and true hyphae), which are not a feature of pneumocystosis.

The intracytoplasmic inclusion bodies of cytomegalovirus (CMV) are argyrophilic in GMS stained sections.[67] However, they can be distinguished easily from pneumocystis cysts, because the viral inclusions are always located inside cells, and they "keep company" with typical Cowdry type A intranuclear inclusion bodies, seen best in replicate sections stained with H&E. The cyst wall of *Toxoplasma gondii,* like that of *P carinii,* is argyrophilic with GMS. The cysts of *T gondii,* however, are many times larger than those of *P carinii* and are clearly visible in H&E stained sections, unlike the cysts of *P carinii.* Finally, tissue elements such as leukocytes, erythrocytes, and mucous vacuoles are weakly argyrophilic and may complicate both screening and diagnosis in slides that are overstained with GMS.[30] For this reason, a positive control slide known to contain cyst forms of *P carinii* must be stained in parallel with unknown histologic sections and cytology smears, to gauge the depth of silver staining.

MOLECULAR DIAGNOSIS

A variety of monoclonal antibodies is available commercially to detect and confirm the identity of *P carinii* in routinely processed biopsy and cytology specimens.[68] These antibodies, which are specific and sensitive, identify both the cyst and trophozoite forms of *P carinii* (Figure 138–17). For this reason, many investigators have claimed that immunohistochemistry is more sensitive than GMS for the detection of *P carinii* in clinical specimens.[69,70] In our experience, however, and in that of others,[68,71] the antibodies provide no advantage over a well-prepared GMS stain, except possibly for the examination of induced sputum and BAL specimens,

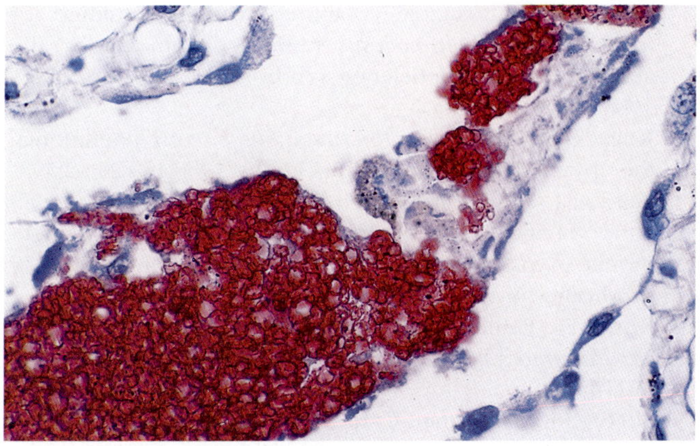

Figure 138–17. Cysts and trophozoites of *P carinii* demonstrated with monoclonal antibody 2G2 in a routinely prepared histologic section of lung (immunoperoxidase, ×160).

which may contain abundant argyrophilic mucus and background debris that can obscure *P carinii* at low-power magnification.

Methods for the amplification and detection of *P carinii* DNA by the polymerase chain reaction have been applied recently to induced sputum and BAL specimens.[72–74] These reports claim increased sensitivity over standard methods (special stains and immunohistochemistry). However, the clinical significance of a DNA-positive reaction in a specimen that does not contain cysts or trophozoites (demonstrable by standard methods) is not known. The incidence of false-positive results caused by cross-contamination of the amplification system is also unknown. At present, the practical value of diagnosis by DNA amplification is unproven.[75]

CONFIRMATIONAL TESTING AND DIAGNOSIS

Pneumocystis carinii can be sustained in cell culture on a limited number of cell lines.[76,77] To date, no artificial media support the growth of *P carinii*. Serologic methods to detect antibodies to *P carinii* are regarded as insensitive,[78,79] mainly because many patients with PCP are unable to mount a detectable humoral response. Therefore, demonstration of cysts or trophozoites with an appropriate special stain, or by immunohistochemistry, remains the only dependable way to establish the diagnosis of pneumocystosis.

REFERENCES

1. Walzer PD, Perl DP, Krogstad DJ, et al. *Pneumocystis carinii* pneumonia in the United States. Epidemiologic, diagnostic, and clinical features. *Ann Intern Med.* 1974; 80:83–93.
2. Kovacs JA, Hiemenz JW, Macher AM, et al. *Pneumocystis carinii* pneumonia: a comparison between patients with the acquired immunodeficiency syndrome and patients with other immunodeficiencies. *Ann Intern Med.* 1984; 100:663–671.
3. Hughes WT. Natural mode of acquisition for de novo infection with *Pneumocystis carinii*. *J Infect Dis.* 1982;145: 842–848.
4. Dutz W. *Pneumocystis carinii* pneumonia. *Pathol Annu.* 1970;5:309–341.
5. Dutz W, Post C, Vessal K, Kohout E. Endemic infantile *Pneumocystic carinii* infection: the Shiraz study. *Natl Cancer Inst Monogr.* 1976;43:31–38.
6. Dutz W. *Pneumocystis carinii* infection and interstitial plasma cell pneumonia: what does history teach? *Sem Diagn Pathol.* 1989;6:195–202.
7. Hughes WT. *Pneumocystis carinii* pneumonitis. *Chest.* 1984;85:810–813.
8. Burke BA, Good RA. *Pneumocystis carinii* infection. *Medicine (Baltimore).* 1973;52:23–51.
9. Sepkowitz KA, Brown AE, Telzak EE, Gottlieb S, Armstrong D. *Pneumocystis carinii* pneumonia among patients without AIDS at a cancer hospital. *JAMA.* 1992; 267:832–837.
10. Hopewell PC. *Pneumocystis carinii* pneumonia: diagnosis. *J Infect Dis.* 1988;6:1115–1119.
11. Jacobs JL, Libby DM, Winters RA, et al. A cluster of *Pneumocystis carinii* pneumonia in adults without predisposing illnesses. *N Engl J Med.* 1991;324:246–250.
12. Pifer LL, Hughes WT, Stango S, Woods T. *Pneumocystis carinii* infection: evidence for high prevalence in normal and immunosuppressed children. *Pediatrics.* 1978;61: 35–41.
13. Frenkel JK, Good JT, Schultz JA. Latent pneumocystis infection of rats, relapse and chemotherapy. *Lab Invest.* 1966;15:1559–1577.
14. Vavra J, Kucera K. *Pneumocystis carinii* Delanoe, its ultrastructure and ultrastructural affinities. *J Protozool.* 1970; 17:463–483.
15. ul Haque A, Plattner SB, Cook RT, Hart MN. *Pneumocystis carinii:* taxonomy as viewed by electron microscopy. *Am J Clin Pathol.* 1987;87:504–510.
16. Edman JC, Kovacs JA, Masur H, et al. Ribosomal RNA sequence shows *Pneumocystis carinii* to be a member of the fungi. *Nature.* 1988;334:519–522.
17. Frenkel JK, Bartlett MS, Smith JW. RNA homology and the reclassification of *Pneumocystis*. *Diagn Microbiol Infect Dis.* 1990;13:1–2.
18. Hughes WT, Gigliotti F. Nomenclature for *Pneumocystis carinii*. *J Infect Dis.* 1988;157:432–433.
19. Kovacs JA, Halpern JL, Lundgren B, Swan JC, Parrillo JE, Masur H. Monoclonal antibodies to *Pneumocystis carinii:* identification of specific antigens and characterization of antigenic differences between rat and human isolates. *J Infect Dis.* 1989;159:60–70.
20. Barton EG Jr, Campbell WG Jr. Further observations on the ultrastructure of *Pneumocystis*. *Arch Pathol.* 1967;83: 527–534.

21. Barton EG Jr, Campbell WG Jr. *Pneumocystis carinii* in lungs of rats treated with cortisone acetate: ultrastructural observations relating to the life cycle. *Am J Pathol.* 1969; 54:209–236.
22. Campbell WG Jr. Ultrastructure of *Pneumocystis* in human lung: life cycle in human pneumocystosis. *Arch Pathol.* 1972;93:312–324.
23. Gutierrez Y. The biology of *Pneumocystis carinii. Sem Diagn Pathol.* 1989;6:203–211.
24. Bedrossian CWM. Ultrastructure of *Pneumocystis carinii:* a review of internal and surface characteristics. *Sem Diagn Pathol.* 1989;6:212–237.
25. Smulian AG, Walzer PD. The biology of *Pneumocystis carinii. CRC Crit Rev Microbiol.* 1992;18:191–216.
26. Matsumoto Y, Yoshida Y. Sporogony in *Pneumocystis carinii:* synaptonemal complexes and meiotic nuclear divisions observed in precysts. *J Protozool.* 1984;31: 420–428.
27. Matsumoto Y, Yoshida Y. Advances in *Pneumocystis* biology. *Parasitol Today.* 1986;2:137–142.
28. Cushion MT, Ruffolo JJ, Walzer PD. Analysis of the developmental stages of *Pneumocystis carinii,* in vitro. *Lab Invest.* 1988;58:324–331.
29. Price RA, Hughes WT. Histopathology of *Pneumocystis carinii* infestation and infection in malignant disease in childhood. *Hum Pathol.* 1974;5:737–752.
30. Watts JC, Chandler FW. Evolving concepts of infection by *Pneumocystis carinii. Pathol Annu.* 1991;26(part 1): 93–138.
31. Watts JC, Chandler FW. *Pneumocystis carinii* pneumonitis: the nature and diagnostic significance of the methenamine silver-positive "intracystic bodies." *Am J Surg Pathol.* 1985;9:744–751.
32. Mahan CT, Sale GE. Rapid methenamine silver stain for *Pneumocystis* and fungi. *Arch Pathol Lab Med.* 1978; 102:351–352.
33. Pintozzi RL. Modified Grocott's methenamine silver nitrate method for quick staining of *Pneumocystis carinii. J Clin Pathol.* 1978;31:803–805.
34. Musto L, Flanigan MJ, Elbadawi A. Ten-minute silver stain for *Pneumocystis carinii* and fungi in tissue sections. *Arch Pathol Lab Med.* 1982;106:292–294.
35. Brinn NT. Rapid metallic histological staining using the microwave oven. *J Histotechnol.* 1983;6:125–129.
36. Shimono LH, Hartman B. A simple and reliable rapid methenamine silver stain for *Pneumocystis carinii* and fungi. *Arch Pathol Lab Med.* 1986;110:855–856.
37. Catterall JR, Potasman I, Remington JS. *Pneumocystis carinii* pneumonia in the patient with AIDS. *Chest.* 1985;88: 758–762.
38. Cohen BA, Pomeranz S, Rabinowitz JG, et al. Pulmonary complications of AIDS: radiologic features. *AJR.* 1984; 143:115–122.
39. Kuhlman JE, Kavuru M, Fishman EK, Siegelman SS. *Pneumocystis carinii* pneumonia: spectrum of parenchymal CT findings. *Radiology.* 1990;175:711–714.
40. Telzak EE, Cote RJ, Gold JWM, Campbell SW, Armstrong D. Extrapulmonary *Pneumocystis carinii* infections. *Rev Infect Dis.* 1990;12:380–386.
41. Sattler FR, Cowan R, Nielsen DM, Ruskin J. Trimethoprim–sulfamethoxazole compared with pentamidine for treatment of *Pneumocystis carinii* pneumonia in the acquired immunodeficiency syndrome. *Ann Intern Med.* 1988;109:280–287.
42. Kovacs JA, Masur H. *Pneumocystis carinii* pneumonia: therapy and prophylaxis. *J Infect Dis.* 1988;158:254–259.
43. Falloon J, Kovacs J, Hughes W, et al. A preliminary evaluation of 566CB0 for the treatment of pneumocystis pneumonia in patients with the acquired immunodeficiency syndrome. *N Engl J Med.* 1991;325:1534–1538.
44. Sattler FR, Feinberg J. New developments in the treatment of *Pneumocystis carinii* pneumonia. *Chest.* 1992;101: 451–457.
45. NIH-UC Expert Panel. Consensus statement on the use of adjunctive therapy for pneumocystis pneumonia in the acquired immunodeficiency syndrome. *N Engl J Med.* 1990;323:1500–1504.
46. CDC. Recommendations for prophylaxis against *Pneumocystis carinii* pneumonia for adults and adolescents infected with human immunodeficiency virus. *MMWR.* 1992;41(no. RR-4):1–11.
47. DeRoux SJ, Adsay V, Ioachim HL. Disseminated pneumocystosis without pulmonary involvement during prophylactic aerosolized pentamidine therapy in a patient with the acquired immunodeficiency syndrome. *Arch Pathol Lab Med.* 1991;115:1137–1140.
48. Luna MA, Cleary KR. Spectrum of pathologic manifestations of *Pneumocystis carinii* pneumonia in patients with neoplastic diseases. *Sem Diagn Pathol.* 1989;6:262–272.
49. Gal AA, Koss MN, Strigle S, Angritt P. *Pneumocystis carinii* infection in the acquired immunodeficiency syndrome. *Sem Diagn Pathol.* 1989;6:287–299.
50. Weber WR, Askin FB, Dehner LP. Lung biopsy in *Pneumocystis carinii* pneumonia: a histopathologic study of typical and atypical features. *Am J Clin Pathol.* 1977; 67:11–19.
51. Saldana MJ, Mones JM. Cavitation and other atypical manifestations of *Pneumocystis carinii* pneumonia. *Sem Diagn Pathol.* 1989;6:273–286.
52. Askin FB, Katzenstein ALA. Pneumocystis infection masquerading as diffuse alveolar damage: a potential source of diagnostic error. *Chest.* 1981;70:420–422.
53. Nash G, Fligiel S. Pathologic features of the lung in the acquired immune deficiency syndrome (AIDS): an autopsy study of seventeen homosexual males. *Am J Clin Pathol.* 1984;81:6–12.
54. Bleiweiss IJ, Jagirdar JS, Klein MJ, et al. Granulomatous *Pneumocystis carinii* pneumonia in three patients with the acquired immune deficiency syndrome. *Chest.* 1988; 94:580–583.
55. Blumenfeld W, Basgoz N, Owen WF Jr, Schmidt DM. Granulomatous pulmonary lesions in patients with the acquired immunodeficiency syndrome (AIDS) and *Pneumocystis carinii* infection. *Ann Intern Med.* 1988;109: 505–507.
56. Cupples JB, Blackie SP, Road JD. Granulomatous *Pneumocystis carinii* pneumonia mimicking tuberculosis. *Arch Pathol Lab Med.* 1989;113:1281–1284.
57. Liu YC, Tomashefski JF Jr., Tomford JW, Green H. Necrotizing *Pneumocystis carinii* vasculitis associated with lung

necrosis and cavitation in a patient with acquired immunodeficiency syndrome. *Arch Pathol Lab Med.* 1989;113:494–497.

58. Afessa B, Green WR, Williams WA, et al. *Pneumocystis carinii* pneumonia complicated by lymphadenopathy and pneumothorax. *Arch Intern Med.* 1988;148:2651–2654.
59. Hardy WD, Northfelt DW, Drake TA. Fatal, disseminated pneumocystosis in a patient with acquired immunodeficiency syndrome receiving prophylactic aerosolized pentamidine. *Am J Med.* 1989;87:329–331.
60. Long EG, Smith JS, Meier JL. Attachment of *Pneumocystis carinii* to rat pneumocytes. *Lab Invest.* 1986;54:609–615.
61. Itatani CA, Marshall GJ. Ultrastructural morphology and staining characteristics of *Pneumocystis carinii* in situ and from bronchoalveolar lavage. *J Parasitol.* 1988;74:700–712.
62. Yoneda K, Walzer PD. Mechanism of pulmonary alveolar injury in experimental *Pneumocystis carinii* pneumonia in the rat. *Br J Exp Pathol.* 1981;62:339–346.
63. Greaves TS, Strigle SM. The recognition of *Pneumocystis carinii* in Papanicolaou-stained smears. *Acta Cytol.* 1985;29:714–720.
64. Bedrossian CWM, Mason MF, Gupta PK. Rapid cytologic diagnosis of *Pneumocystis:* a comparison of effective techniques. *Sem Diagn Pathol.* 1989;6:245–261.
65. Ghali VS, Garcia RL, Skolom J. Fluorescence of *Pneumocystis carinii* in Papanicolaou smears. *Hum Pathol.* 1984;15:907–909.
66. Kim YK, Parulekar S, Yu P, Pisani RJ, Smith TF, Anhalt JP. Evaluation of calcofluor white stain for detection of *Pneumocystis carinii. Diagn Microbiol Infect Dis.* 1990;13:307–310.
67. Gorelkin L, Chandler FW, Ewing EP. Staining qualities of cytomegalovirus inclusions in the lungs of patients with the acquired immunodeficiency syndrome. *Hum Pathol.* 1986;17:926–929.
68. Linder J, Radio SJ. Immunohistochemistry of *Pneumocystis carinii. Sem Diagn Pathol.* 1989;6:238–244.
69. Midgley J, Parsons PA, Shanson DC, Hussain OAN, Francis N. Monoclonal immunofluorescence compared with silver stain for investigating *Pneumocystis carinii* pneumonia. *J Clin Pathol.* 1991;44:75–76.
70. Homer KS, Wiley WL, Smith AL, et al. Monoclonal antibody to *Pneumocystis carinii:* comparison with silver stain in bronchial lavage specimens. *Am J Clin Pathol.* 1992;97:619–624.
71. Amin MB, Metzger E, Zarbo RJ. Detection of *Pneumocystis carinii:* comparative study of monoclonal antibody and silver staining. *Am J Clin Pathol.* 1992;98:13–18.
72. Wakefield AE, Pixley FJ, Banerji S, et al. Detection of *Pneumocystis carinii* with DNA amplification. *Lancet.* 1990;336:451–453.
73. Wakefield AE, Guiver L, Miller RF, Hopkin JM. DNA amplification on induced sputum samples for diagnosis of *Pneumocystis carinii* pneumonia. *Lancet.* 1991;337:1378–1379.
74. Lipschik GY, Gill VJ, Lundgren JD, et al. Improved diagnosis of *Pneumocystis carinii* infection by polymerase chain reaction on induced sputum and blood. *Lancet.* 1992;340:203–206.
75. Blumenfeld W, McCook O, Holodniy M, Katzenstein DA. Correlation of morphologic diagnosis of *Pneumocystis carinii* with the presence of pneumocystis DNA amplified by the polymerase chain reaction. *Mod Pathol.* 1992;5:103–106.
76. Pifer LL, Hughes WT, Murphy MJ. Propagation of *Pneumocystis carinii* in vitro. *Pediatr Res.* 1977;11:305–316.
77. Cushion MT, Walzer PD. Growth and serial passage of *Pneumocystis carinii* in the A549 cell line. *Infect Immun.* 1984;44:245–251.
78. Maddison SE, Walls KW, Haverkos HW, Juranek DD. Evaluation of serologic tests for *Pneumocystis carinii* antibody and antigenemia in patients with acquired immunodeficiency syndrome. *Diagn Microbiol Infect Dis.* 1984;2:69–73.
79. Walzer PD. Diagnosis of *Pneumocystis carinii* pneumonia. *J Infect Dis.* 1988;157:629–632.

CHAPTER 139

Sarcocystosis

J. K. Frenkel

I was called to minister to several patients who suffered from nausea, abdominal pain, vomiting and diarrhea. All had partaken in a common meal of raw pork. The meat of the pig had contained an unusual number of sarcocysts of exceptional size and development, but was microscopically free of trichinae.

Rabe, 1879[1]

Wisdom of a centennial:
Overall, the danger of illness with sarcocystis infection is minimal, because of small dose or the low pathogenicity of the agent. In addition, the experimental infections indicate that sarcosporidiosis is a transient illness, which passes quickly and without sequelae. Practically one can conclude, that sarcocystis infection alone, is no reason to advise against the consumption of raw commercial pork and beef.

Kimmig, Piekarski, and Heydorn, 1979[2]

INTRODUCTION, HISTORY, LIFE CYCLE, AND BIOLOGY

Sarcocystosis, or sarcosporidiosis, is an uncommon infection, and even more rarely diagnosed. It causes parasitism in skeletal or cardiac muscle, or of the intestine, with the latter being followed by excretion of sporulated oocysts in the stool.

Sarcocystis was first described in 1843 by Friedrich Miescher, professor of physiology and pathology at a University in Basel, Switzerland, from whitish cysts visible to the naked eye, which replaced skeletal muscles in a mouse he caught in his house (Figure 139–1): the life cycle involving intestinal parasitism of cats, however, was not recognized until 1976.[3] Stages of *Sarcocystis* in humans had been known also only in skeletal and cardiac muscles, until 1972, when Rommel and Heydorn[4] recognized that the intestinal coccidian, *Isospora hominis,* represented two species of *Sarcocystis,* one with a human–cattle cycle and another with a human–pig cycle.

So *Sarcocystis* became known as an obligatory two-host coccidian, cycling between predator and prey. The muscle stage, after being eaten by a carnivore, gives rise to gametes in the intestinal lamina propria, leading to formation of oocysts, which are shed in the carnivore's feces. These are oocysts with two sporocysts, each with four sporozoites. Sporulated oocysts are usually found in the fresh feces, unlike *I belli,* and most other coccidia, the oocysts of which are shed unsporulated. When the sporocysts are ingested, usually by a herbivore, two successive multiplicative cycles are initiated, which lead to formation of muscle cysts, containing bradyzoites, functionally gametocytes, waiting to be eaten. The predatory carnivore is the definitive host because it supports the sexual stages, and the prey or herbivore, in which the muscle stages develop, is the intermediate host. In most species of *Sarcocystis,* definitive hosts are specific.

More than 100 species of *Sarcocystis* have been described from the skeletal muscles or heart of various

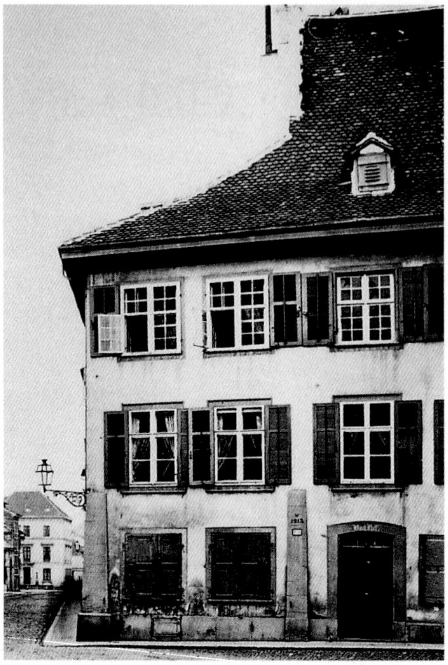

Figure 139–1. Prof. Friedrich Miescher's house in Basel, Switzerland, where in 1843, shortly before being married, he caught the house mouse, in which he recognized *Sarcocystis,* although he did not apply a name to it.

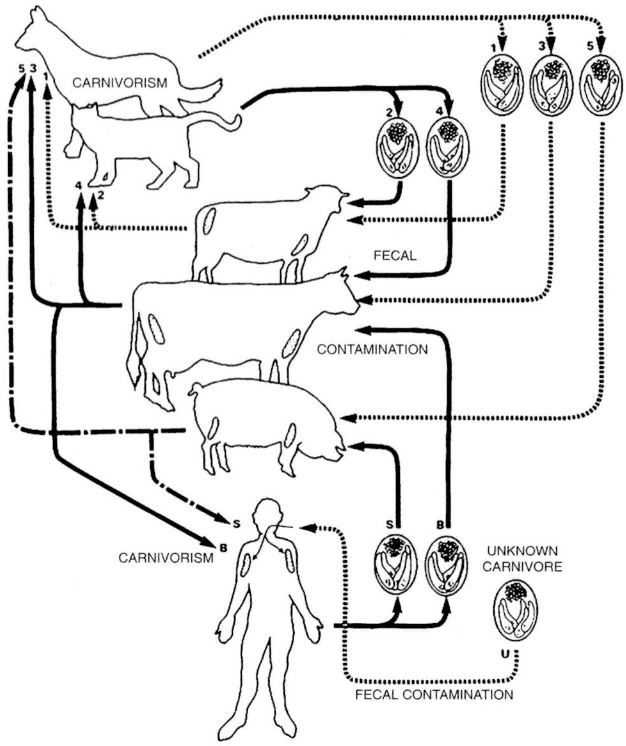

Figure 139–2. Transmission cycles of *Sarcocystis* involving humans, cattle, sheep, pigs, dogs, and cats. Humans are the definitive host of *Sarcocystis bovihominis* (B) and *S suihominis* (S), the two intestinal sarcocystis of man, acquired from undercooked beef and pork. Humans are the accidental intermediate hosts of several *Sarcocystis* species (U) of skeletal and heart muscle; these resemble the muscle *Sarcocystis* of certain monkeys and cattle, acquired from food or water contaminated by feces of unknown carnivores, perhaps tiger and python, normally eating monkeys. Also indicated are the cycles of the more common *S ovicanis* (1), *S ovifelis* (2), *S bovicanis* (3), *S bovifelis* (4), and *S suicanis* (5). The cycles of the rare *Sarcocystis* sp cycling in domestic animals are not shown. *(From Frenkel JK. In: Mehlhorn H, ed. Parasitology in Focus. Berlin: Springer; 1988:549, with permission.)*

animals, but the definitive, carnivore hosts generally remain to be identified, except for some peridomestic species. These domestic animals are hosts for several *Sarcocystis* species, with dogs and cats as definitive hosts. This complicated peridomestic relationship, of man and several animals with several distinct *Sarcocystis* species, is shown in Figure 139–2. Mammals and birds are commonly infected with *Sarcocystis,* which may be of economic importance, such as when it interferes with weight gain, or gives rise to abortion in cattle.[5]

Intestinal Sarcocystis

Humans are the regular definitive hosts, with intestinal stages, for at least two species, for which cattle and pigs are intermediate hosts. Intestinal sarcocystis, with *S bovihominis* and *S suihominis,* occurs in certain areas, where raw or undercooked beef, pork, and venison are eaten,[6,7] and where cattle, and pigs have access to human feces. Most cases have been described from Germany, France, Poland, and Thailand.[8] Pork infected with *S suihominis* has infected chimpanzee, rhesus, and cynomolgus monkeys, which shed sporulated sporocysts in their feces.[9]

Muscle Sarcocystis

This type of sarcocystis is observed sporadically, suggesting accidental parasitism. With some species of *Sarcocystis,* several related prey animals can be infected. For example, humans serve as accidental intermediate hosts, with muscle cysts, for several *Sarcocystis* species of monkeys (whose definitive hosts are unknown). Because nowhere are humans regularly eaten by a carnivore, the infection is not transmitted from humans. Most cases come from Southeast Asia, Africa, and South America. Beaver et al[10] has analyzed the morphology of human sarcocysts and their location, whether in cardiac or skeletal muscle. He identified a total of seven types from 40 patients. In 13 from Southeast Asia, the organisms resembled the *Sarcocystis* of *Macaca fascicularis.* In 8 infections probably from India, the organisms resembled a species found in *Macaca mulatta.* In 1 of 4 infections probably acquired in Africa or Europe, the organisms resembled a *Sarcocystis* of *Cercopithicus talapoin.* Among 3 types of cysts from human hearts, 1 resembled *S bovicanis* from the heart of cattle. Of 5 infections acquired in Central or South America, 2 from the myocardium resembled *S bovicanis,* but 3 other myocardial forms could not be identified. Three infections acquired in the United States could not be matched. One of these was in a Kansas farmer with cysts in skeletal muscle, who had a hobby of keeping exotic animals.[11]

NOMENCLATURE

Sarcocystis lindemanni, as the agent of human sarcocystis used to be known, apparently described a nonparasitic object in muscle and is a nonvalid species. The two intestinal species of man, *S bovihominis* and *S suihominis,* have been well defined by experimental work.[4] The *Sarcocystis* from muscle, however, have not been transmitted experimentally and their designations are by 1 of 7 morphologic types or as an unidentified form.[10] The muscle forms and intestinal forms of *Sarcocystis* had often been described under different names, *Isospora hominis,* for example, was found to be a mixture of two species, and the identity of some of the organisms described earlier was in doubt. This led to two proposals, either to give new species names, or to arbitrarily assign old names to new species. These alternative proposals have given rise to spirited, but inconclusive discussion with both systems being followed.[12] Analysis of ribosomal RNA sequences suggested interesting speculations concerning phylogenetic relationships[13]; however, it appears unwise to abandon a working taxonomic system based on technically accessible criteria, and replace it with a system based on as yet complex procedures, changing even generic names. Ancestors and relatives do not correlate with pragmatic concepts; nomenclature should be utilitarian.

CLINICAL FEATURES

Enteric Infection

After ingesting undercooked or raw beef, containing a heavy, experimental infection of *S bovihominis* (Figure 139–3), volunteers experienced abdominal discomfort, nausea, and vomiting as early as 3 to 6 hours after, which persisted for 24 to 36 hours. Sporocysts appeared in the stools between 13 and 39 days, accompanied by abdominal discomfort and diarrhea, and continued for 9 to 139 days.[14] Following the ingestion of pork heavily infected with *S suihominis,* volunteers developed abdominal discomfort, vomiting, diarrhea, fever,

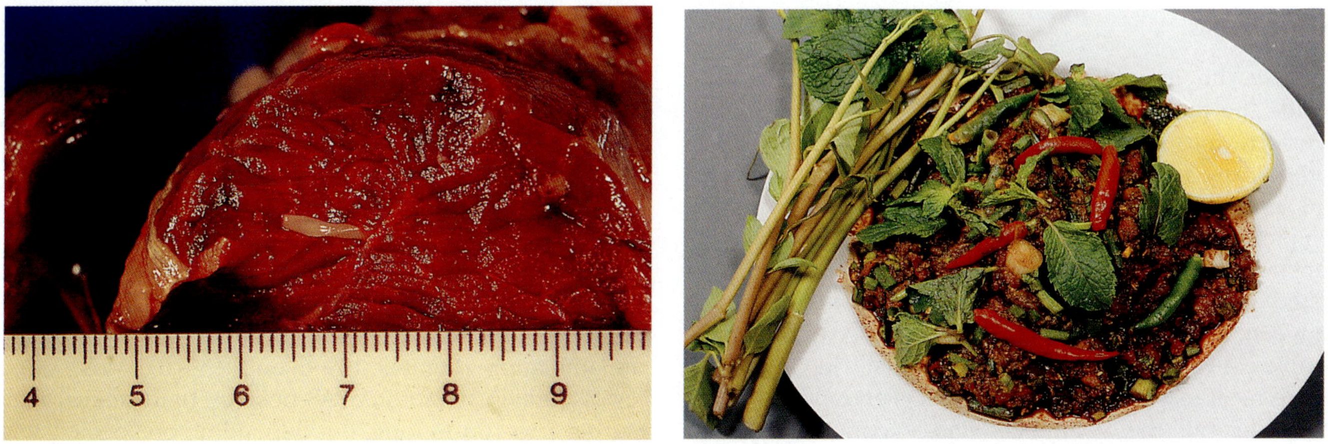

A B

Figure 139–3. (**A**) *Sarcocystis bovihominis* cyst in beef. An approximately 1-cm-long portion is exposed. (**B**) Larb, an attractive Thai dish prepared from undercooked beef, powdered fresh chili, whole chili, lemon, and greens. *(Photographs contributed by Dr. S. Bunyanratvej,[8] Ramathibodi Hospital, Bangkok, Thailand.)*

and chills alternating with diaphoresis, and in one patient dyspnea and tachycardia, starting 6 to 24 hours after the meal and continuing for 12 to 24 hours. Some of those who consumed the largest doses became dehydrated from vomiting and diarrhea.[15] Leukocytosis, lymphopenia, and eosinopenia were present the day after the meal, but enzymes and electrolytes remained normal.[2] Sporocysts were in stools between 11 and 71 days after the meal, accompanied by slight diarrhea in some.[2,14,15] Well-roasted meat did not lead to symptoms in 9 volunteers,[14] nor did meat frozen to −30°C for 24 hours.[2] Commercially produced meat is not likely to be so heavily infected, and would likely elicit light or no manifestations.

Muscle Infection

Painful focal myositis, 1 to 3 cm in diameter, sometimes with erythema of the overlying skin, occurred episodically in various parts of the body, and usually resulted in biopsy examination and diagnosis.[16] These lesions persisted from 2 days to 2 weeks, and were often accompanied by eosinophilia, sometimes by fever, diffuse myalgia, muscle tenderness, weakness, and bronchospasm.[17,18] Light infections, however, are apparently asymptomatic, and remain undiagnosed till found accidentally at autopsy. In Kuala Lumpur, the tongues from 21 of 100 consecutive autopsies were infected; because they contained only 66 sarcocysts[19] it is clear that the majority of infections are light. No clinical findings had been noted in patients in whom myocardial sarcocystosis was later found at autopsy.

PATHOGENESIS AND IMMUNITY

Enteric Stages

Because the ingested bradyzoites from meat merely invade the mucosa, enter a cell in the lamina propria, transform into gametes, fertilize and develop oocysts, without any multiplication, lesions should be minimal and nonspecific. The brief, but sometimes intense, symptoms following large doses are related to mucosal penetration and lesser symptoms to oocysts being liberated from the lamina propria, probably passing between enterocytes into the lumen. Because some people eat very rare or raw meat, especially in Germany where meat inspection for trichinosis is entrenched, it is likely that all the volunteers had experienced prior infections. Some of the symptoms might be caused by inflammation or hypersensitivity. The simultaneous penetration of the mucosa by large numbers of organisms might permit bacterial invasion, and gram-positive bacilli have been noticed in resected specimens of eosinophilic and necrotizing enteritis.[8] Although no critical experiments have been performed in humans, there is not likely to be much immunity to repeated infection; at least little or no immunity has been observed in animal species where immunity to reinfection has been studied.[3]

Muscle Stages

The ingested sporocysts probably multiply in the liver or in blood vessels; and vasculitis has been observed.[17] Other *Sarcocystis* species studied in animal intermediate hosts usually have two generations of multiplicative stages by schizogony. Thereafter, cysts develop in muscle, first containing metrocytes (dividing stages) and, later, bradyzoites—infectious for the definitive host. The latter contain a glycogen-like, periodic acid–Schiff–hematoxylin-positive substance, amylopectin, which provides the energy necessary to invade the intestinal wall of the next host. During their development, some cysts appear to become permeable to antibody and complement, which leads to destruction of the intracystic organisms and to inflammation. The diagnosis is either made by biopsy at this stage, or at autopsy, based on cysts remaining intact. In a mouse model there was no firm immunity to reinfection and large cysts from the primary infection were seen with smaller cysts of the reinfection.[3]

HISTOPATHOLOGY

Intestine

In patients with segmental and necrotizing enteritis from Thailand,[8] sporulated sporocysts and oocysts were in the lamina propria of resected portions of the intestine (Figure 139–4). Although in five of the six patients, the focally obstructive inflammatory lesions were largely related to numerous gram-positive bacilli, the intense tissue eosinophilia in four patients, one of whom showed no evidence of bacteria, suggested a relationship to the sporocysts of *Sarcocystis*.

Skeletal and Cardiac Muscle

Sarcocysts in humans measure up to 100 μm in diameter and 325 μm long. Intact sarcocysts provoke no inflammation (Figures 139–5 and 139–6). Most sarcocysts contain numerous PAS-positive bradyzoites, measuring 7 to 16 μm long, but depending on species, with rounded ends. Young cysts may contain mainly metrocytes, and in older cysts they are often just inside the cyst wall. Inflammation follows disintegration of the cysts, with neutrophils, eosinophils, and lymphocytes, followed by plasma cells and, later, focal fibrosis. In biopsy specimens, taken for suspected myositis, vas-

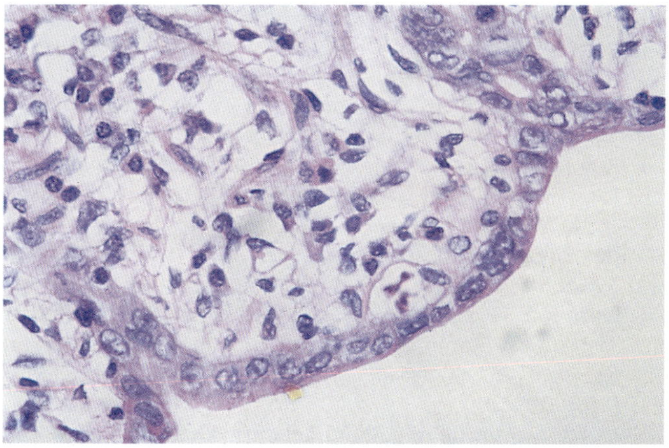

Figure 139–4. Enteric sarcocystis. *Sarcocystis bovihominis* oocyst with two sporulating sporocysts in subepithelium of human intestine [hematoxylin-eosin (H&E), ×170]. *(Slide contributed by Dr. S. Bunyanratvej,[8] Ramathibodi Hospital, Bangkok, Thailand.)*

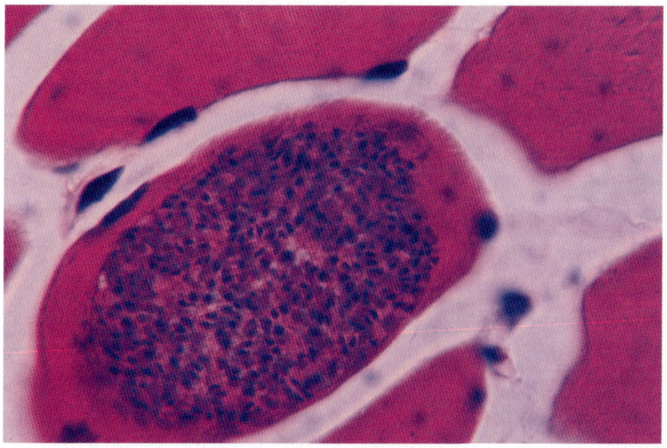

Figure 139–6. *Sarcocystis* in muscle. *Sarcocystis* in skeletal muscle of patient from Kuala Lumpur, Malaysia (H&E, ×410). *(Slide contributed by Dr. A. S. Dissanaike, Faculty of Medicine, University of Malaya, Kuala Lumpur.)*

culitis is found in skeletal muscle and subcutaneous tissue, possibly from preceding intravascular schizogony, which has been observed in animals but not in humans. Histologic diagnoses include myonecrosis and myositis with vasculitis.[17] Light *Sarcocystis* infections in skeletal muscle and heart at the time of autopsy usually show intact cysts without accompanying lesions.[18,19] Ultrastructural examination of cysts in skeletal muscle reveal branching septa, extending from the ground substance underlying the primary cyst wall, into the cyst, separating groups of bradyzoites into compartments.[20]

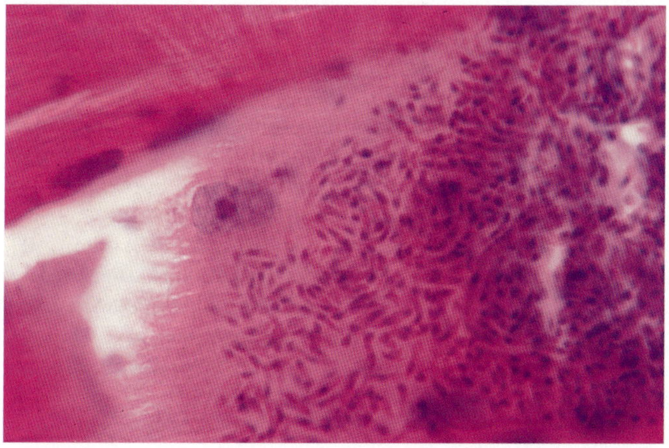

Figure 139–5. *Sarcocystis* in muscle. *Sarcocystis* sp in skeletal muscle of patient with painful swellings of subcutaneous tissues and muscles, who probably became infected in Asia 4 to 6 years earlier. One end of a cyst is shown tangentially, to illustrate filiform projections from the cyst wall (H&E, ×410). *(Slide contributed by Drs. Rima Mcleod, Jack Remington, Robert Hirabayashi, and William Rothman.[17])*

DIAGNOSIS

Intestinal sarcocystosis is diagnosed by finding sporulated oocysts or sporocysts in fresh stool. These can be concentrated by suspension and centrifugation in sucrose solution of 1.15 specific gravity (53 g sucrose in 100 mL of water and 0.8 g phenol), alternating with centrifugation in water. In water, sporocysts measure 13.5 ± 0.3 μm × 10.5 ± 0.4 μm. Each sporocyst contains four sporozoites. Blood eosinophilia may be present.

Sarcocystis myositis is diagnosed by muscle biopsy. The cysts are larger than those of *Toxoplasma gondii, Hammondia hammondi,*[21] and *Trypanosoma cruzi. Sarcocystis* bradyzoites often appear grouped, because of septa that are not easily recognized with ordinary stains by light microscopy. Bradyzoites of *Sarcocystis, Hammondia,* and *Toxoplasma* are PAS–positive; the peripheral metrocytes, and *T cruzi,* are not. In spite of some serologic evidence, *Hammondia* has not been observed in humans. *Toxoplasma* and *Hammondia* do not form metrocytes, so that their entire cysts are PAS positive, whereas *Sarcocystis* usually contain a peripheral rim of light or absent PAS staining. Electron microscopy after post-fixation may show a distinctive primary cyst wall and compartments formed by ground substance.[20] Because of the paucity of cysts in individual patients, however, electron microscopy is rarely feasible.

Other Diagnostic Methods

Specific serologic reagents are not generally available; because of low species-specificity, however, *Sarcocystis* from animals can be used as antigen.[17] *Sarcocystis* bradyzoites can be obtained from beef, pork, or mutton by digestion in 5% trypsin. After washing in 0.9% NaCl, they are centrifuged and the sediment, after resuspension of the bradyzoites, is fixed in 100% ethanol containing 5% acetic acid. The organisms are centrifuged, resuspended in 95% ethanol and stored at −20°C. When needed as antigen, small quantities of bradyzoites are aspirated with a pipette, washed in 0.9% NaCl and attached to slides with 0.25% ovalbumin.[3] The slides can be used in the fluorescent antibody test to measure antibody levels. Research has identified species-specific antigens, which may become available in the future, but mainly for the veterinary field where sarcocystosis is an economic problem.[22] Immunohistochemistry so far is limited to research in the veterinary field. Some PCR primers have been constructed for species of veterinary importance.[13] Cell culture has been accomplished with several species.[23] Animal inoculation as of sporocysts into cattle or pigs would be useful only for experimental purposes.

TREATMENT

Because *Sarcocystis* stages in muscle and intestine are fully formed terminal stages when diagnosed in humans, and no new cells are parasitized, specific chemotherapy is unnecessary. Accidental medication with an effective ionophore drug, monensin, has given rise to myositis from destruction of sarcocysts in sheep.[24] At present no similar drugs are used in human medicine. Corticosteroids, however, might palliate the allergic inflammatory reaction, which occurs from time to time after spontaneous cyst rupture.[16] Because the intracystic bradyzoites are incapable of infecting other cells in the host, there is no risk of recrudescence.

PREVENTION

Enteric infection can be prevented by avoiding raw beef and pork. How many people will forgo these epicurean delicacies depends on cultural and personal factors. Frozen meat (−20°C) and well-cooked meats are safe. Muscle sarcocystosis can be prevented by avoiding food and water contaminated with feces of predatory carnivores, including mammals, birds, and reptiles.

REFERENCES

1. Rabe X. Über Psorospermien [Concerning Sarcocystis]. *Wschr Thierheilk Viehzucht.* 1879;(23–24):167.
2. Kimmig P, Piekarski G, Heydorn AO. Zur Sarkosporidiose (*Sarcocystis suihominis*) des Menschen (II). Sarcosporidiosis (*Sarcocystis suihominis*) in man. *Immunität Infektion.* 1979;7:170–177.
3. Ruiz A, Frenkel JK. Recognition of cyclic transmission of *Sarcocystis muris* by cats. *J Infect Dis.* 1976;133:409–418.
4. Rommel M, Heydorn AO. Beitrage zum Lebenszyklus der Sarkosporidien. III. Isospora hominis (Railliet und Lucet, 1891) Wenyon, 1923, eine Dauerform der Sarkosporidien des Rindes und des Schweins. *Berl Munch Tierarztl Woch.* 1972;85:143–145.
5. Dubey JP. Toxoplasma, Neospora, Sarcocystis, and other Tissue Cyst-Forming Coccidia of Humans and Animals. In: Kreier JP, ed. *Parasitic Protozoa.* San Diego: Academic Press. 1993:1–158.
6. Heydorn AO. Beiträge zum Lebenszyklus der Sarkosporidien. IX. Entwicklungszyklus von *Sarcocystis suihominis* n spec. Contributions to the life-cycle of sarcosporidia. IX. Life cycle of *Sarcocystis suihominis* n spec. *Berl Münch Tierärztl Wschr.* 1977;90:218–224.
7. Schulze K. Erkrankungen nach dem Verzehr von massiv mit Sarkosporidien befallenem Rehfleisch. *Fleischwirtschaft.* 1988;68:1139–1140.
8. Bunyaratvej S, Bunyawongwiroj P, Nitiyanant P. Human intestinal sarcosporidiosis—report of 6 cases. *Am J Trop Med Hyg.* 1982;31:36–41.
9. Fayer R, Heydorn AO, Johnson AJ, Leek RG. Transmission of *Sarcocystis suihominis* from humans to swine to nonhuman primates (*Pan troglodytes, Macaca mulatta, Macaca irus*). *Z Parasitenk.* 1979;59:15–20.
10. Beaver PC, Gadgil RK, Morera P. Sarcocystis in man: a review and report of five cases. *Am J Trop Med Hyg.* 1979;28:819.
11. Price RM. Human sarcosporidiosis—case report. *J Kansas Med Soc.* 1933;34:132–135.
12. Frenkel JK, Mehlhorn H, Heydorn AO. Protozoan nomina dubia: to arbitrarily restrict or replace. The case of Sarcocystis spp. *J Parasitol.* 1984;70:813–815.
13. Tenter AM, Baverstock PR, Johnson AM. Phylogenetic relationships of *Sarcocystis* species from sheep, goats, cattle and mice based on ribosomal RNA sequences. *Int J Paras.* 1992;22:503–513.
14. Heydorn AO. Sarkosporidieninfiziertes Fleisch als mögliche Krankheitsursache für den Menschen. Sarcosporidia-infected meat as a possible source of human disease. *Archiv für Lebensmittelhygiene.* 1977;28:27–31.
15. Piekarski G, Heydorn AO, Aryeetey ME, Hartlapp JH, Kimmig P. Klinische, parasitologische und serologische Untersuchungenzur Sarkosporidiose (*Sarcocystis suihominis*) de Menschen. Clinical, parasitologic, and serologic studies of sarcosporidiosis (*Sarcocystis suihominis*) of man. Immunität Infektion. 1978;6:153–159.
16. Jeffrey HC. Sarcosporidiosis in man. *Trans Royal Soc of Trop Med Hyg.* 1974;68:17–29.
17. McLeod R, Hirabayashi RN, Rothman W, Remington JS. Necrotizing vasculitis and sarcocystis: a cause-and-effect relationship? *South Med J.* 1980;73:1380–1383.
18. Pathmanathan R, Kan SP. Three cases of human *Sarcocystis* infection with a review of human muscular sarcocystosis in Malaysia. *Trop Geo Me.* 1992;44:102–108.
19. Wong KT, Pathmanathan R. High prevalence of human

skeletal muscle sarcocystosis in south east Asia. *Trans R Soc Trop Med Hyg.* 1992;86:631–632.

20. Wong KT, Pathmana R. Ultrastructure of the human skeletal muscle sarcocyst. *J Parasitol.* 1994;80:327–342.
21. Frenkel JK, Dubey JP. *Hammondia hammondi:* a new coccidium of cats producing cysts in muscle of other mammals. *Science.* 1975;189:222–224.
22. Tenter AM, Zimmerman GL, Johnson AM. Separation of antigens from *Sarcocystis* species using chromatofocusing. *J Parasitol.* 1991;77:727–736.
23. Andrews CD, Fayer R, Dubey JP. Continuous in vitro cultivation of *Sarcocystis cruzi*. *J Parasitol.* 1990;76:254–255.
24. Jeffrey M, Low JC, Uggla A. A myopathy of sheep associated with *Sarcocystis infection and monensin administration*. Vet Record 1989;124:422–426.

CHAPTER 140

Toxoplasmosis

J. K. Frenkel

Though it caused Navratilova to miss the ball[1]
and killed Buzz Aldrin's squirrel monkey,[2]
measure Toxoplasma's fame not
by luminaries' illnesses or death,
as if the monuments of famous men
celebrated those who died because of them.

Living in balance with its host,
infecting all known mammals, birds, and their nucleated cells,
a unique versatility for a parasite,
a rich history of co-adaptation,
combined with genetic stability.[3]
Prevailing against all lymphokines named by man,
dreaming, perhaps of being cannibalized
and mating in cats,
infecting humanity as no other parasite
but eluding medical attention for 30 years
after its discovery,
spreading by cats remained unknown for 60 years,
and by dogs for 87.

Praise Abner Wolf, David Cowen, and Albert Sabin,
Henry Pinkerton and Helenor Wilder,
who saw and showed us, while others blindly searched.
Now, its fated role in AIDS creates more medical concerns
than preventing congenital infection!

Elusive though famous—
what will you teach us in the future?

INTRODUCTION, BIOLOGY, AND LIFE CYCLE

Toxoplasmosis is infection by *Toxoplasma gondii* and is usually asymptomatic. *Toxoplasma gondii* in an obligate intracellular protozoan, infecting man, other mammals, and birds. Because of its presence in migratory birds, it has a worldwide distribution, although not yet reported from Antarctica. Biologically, *T gondii* is a coccidian of cats in whose intestinal epithelium sexual stages develop, which leads to the formation of oocysts—resistant stages eliminated in cat feces. Initially, the oocysts are not infectious, but after 1 to 3 days at moderate temperature, they become fully developed. They are 10 × 12 μm and resemble *Isospora belli* of humans, but are much smaller than *I belli.* Oocysts from contaminated soil ingested by humans, other mammals, or birds, pass through the stomach, excyst in the duodenum, and the released sporozoites invade the intestine and give rise to infection (Figure 140–1).

In tissues of nonfeline hosts, infection is disseminated, sometimes causing clinical symptoms of pneumonia, myocarditis, and encephalitis. Two stages in tissue are important in the pathogenesis: tachyzoites and bradyzoites.

Tachyzoites multiply in many cells. They divide every 6 to 8 hours. When the cell is full or because of metabolic interference, the cell disintegrates. The released tachyzoites actively move to enter nearby cells and the intracellular multiplication starts anew, eventually causing lesions. Ultrastructurally, tachyzoites are contained in a cytoplasmic vacuole, the parasitophorous vacuole (Figure 140–2). Their ultrastructure has been described and compared with the ultrastructure of similar organisms.[4,5]

Bradyzoites develop as immunity develops. As the name implies, bradyzoites multiply slowly, in many tissues, especially in muscle and brain. Bradyzoites develop in a vacuole within the cytoplasm of a host cell, forming the tissue cysts (Figure 140–3). These cysts are spherical in the central nervous system and measure from about 15 to 100 μm. Cysts in skeletal and cardiac muscles are elongated, conforming to the shape of the host cell, and are up to 60 μm long. The largest cysts eventually may contain hundreds of bradyzoites. These bradyzoites in tissue cysts persist into a chronic stage of infection without destroying the host cell. Biologically they are an infectious stage, waiting to be eaten by a carnivore. While dormant, bradyzoites accumulate amylopectin, a form of glycogen, which later supplies energy to help them enter new cells. After cysts have been ingested, the cyst wall is quickly lysed by enteric enzymes, but bradyzoites from tissue cysts resist pepsin and trypsin, pass through the stomach, and invade the small intestine.

Because of their amylopectin content, bradyzoites in cysts are periodic acid–Schiff (PAS) positive, which facilitates their recognition in PAS stained sections. Their ultrastructure has been described and compared with that of related organisms.[4,5]

Carnivores become infected by ingesting meat containing bradyzoites in tissue cysts. Herbivorous animals ingest soil contaminated with cat feces, containing oocysts. Humans, being omnivores, become infected with either stage. Recent evidence suggests that dogs that roll in, or eat, cat feces, may carry oocysts on their fur and contaminate humans petting dogs.[6] While these habits are common in dogs, the duration of oocyst persistence on the fur is being investigated.

TAXONOMY

Whereas *T gondii* is an intestinal coccidian of cats which shed oocysts, it is a generalized parasite of man, other mammals, and birds, in which tissue cysts are formed. Hence, *T gondii* is classified as a heteroxenous or two-host coccidian, forming tissue cysts. It is classified in the subfamily Toxoplasmatinae, family Sarcocystidae,[7,8] suborder Eimeriorina, order Eucoccidirida, subclass Coccidiasina, class Sporozoasida, within the protozoan phylum Apicomplexa.[9]

HISTORICAL BACKGROUND

Toxoplasma gondii was described by Nicolle and Manceaux in 1908 and named in the following year. The name refers to the crescentic or falciform shape of the organism [*toxon,* = "arc," Greek, not to any toxic (= "toxikon") quality] and the originally identified host. The gondi, (*Ctenodactylus gundi*), a north African rodent, was used by Nicolle and Manceaux at the Pasteur Institute in Tunis to study leishmaniasis and typhus. A week later, in 1908, Splendore published his description of *Toxoplasma* from a laboratory rabbit at the Italian Hospital in Sao Paulo, Brazil. After its discovery in animals, disease in the form of congenital infection was recognized in humans by Wolf, Cowan, and Paige between 1937 and 1939 in New York. In 1939, Sabin identified acquired infection in children, and Pinkerton and Henderson identified it in adults. Serologic tests developed by Sabin and Feldman in 1949 led to the recognition of asymptomatic infection in human and animal populations all over the world. Sheep, goats, and pigs are good indicators of infection, as are rats and ground-feeding birds. The biological cycle of *Toxoplasma,* its coccidian nature, and the role of cats were uncovered between 1969 and 1970.[10]

Dependent on local circumstances, children may get infected from soil contaminated with cat feces, or adults by eating undercooked meat. Immunosuppres-

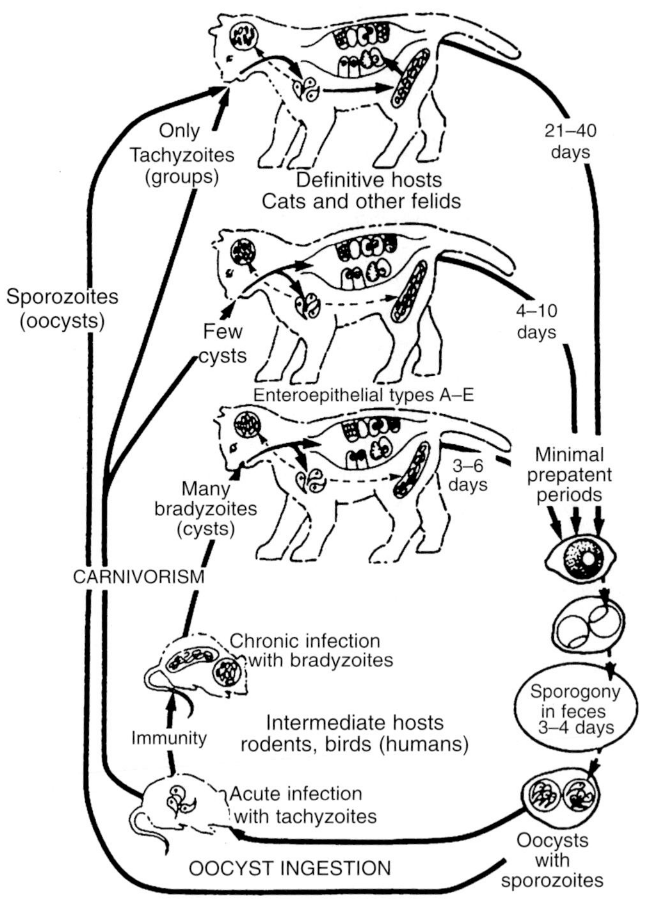

A

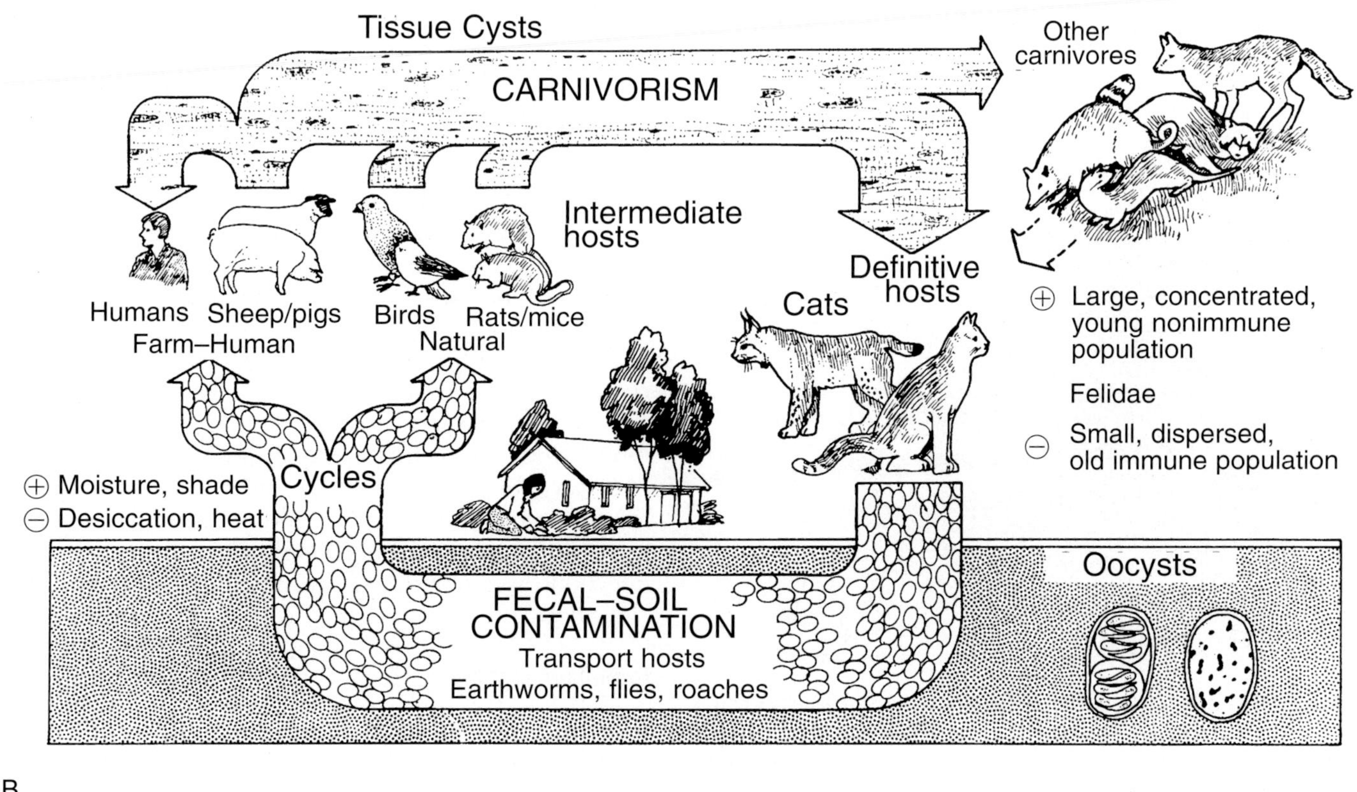

B

Figure 140–1. (**A**) Life cycle and (**B**) transmission of toxoplasmosis. (**A**) Life cycle of *Toxoplasma* in cats (definitive host) and in mice, representing intermediate hosts. Tachyzoites characterize the acute infection and bradyzoites within tissue cysts, the chronic infection. Three cats trace infections with different inocula. Ingestion of an animal with tissue cysts leads to the enteroepithelial cycle in the cat intestine, with oocysts appearing in the stools after 3 to 10 days (depending on dose, *lower* and *center cat*). If cats ingest an animal containing only tachyzoites, or sporozoites from oocysts (*top cat*), a generalized infection with tachyzoites develops first, followed by bradyzoites (tissue cysts), which initiate the enteroepithelial cycle. The period to oocyst shedding is 21 to 40 days. *(From Freyre et al. J Parasit. 1989;75:750–755.)* (**B**) The three sources of *Toxoplasma* infection are cat feces, soil and the meat from intermediate hosts. Felines, the definitive hosts, shed oocysts in their feces, contaminating soil which in moist and shaded areas persists for weeks or months. Ground-feeding birds and rodents in the natural cycle, and sheep, pigs and humans in the domestic cycle, pick up the infection from the ground and develop tissue cysts, thus becoming intermediate hosts. Carnivores become infected from them. Whereas cats shed oocysts, closing the cycle, other carnivores and humans are dead-end hosts. *(Modified from Frenkel JK, Ruiz A. Am J Epidemiol. 1981;113:254.)*

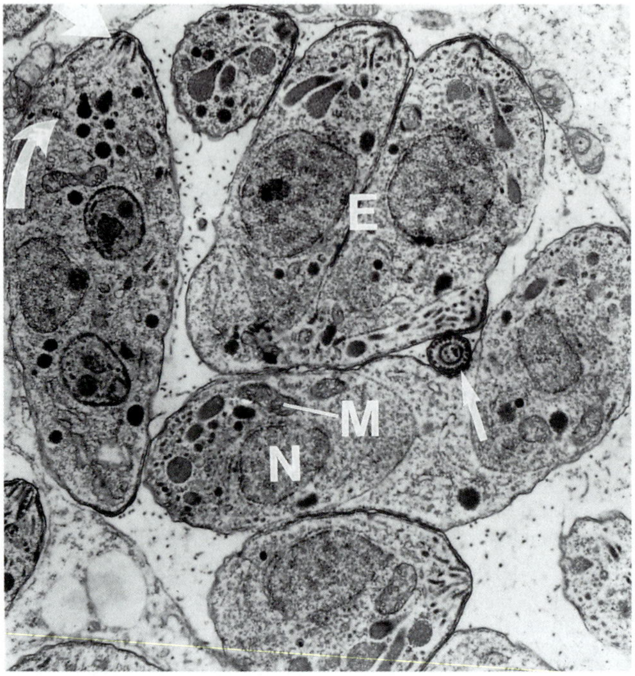

Figure 140–2. *Toxoplasma* tachyzoites from cultured cells. The anterior apical complex, consisting of conoid and rhoptries (*curved arrow*), participates in cell penetration. Conoids in longitudinal (*thick arrow*) and cross-section (*small arrow*) are shown, also a nucleus (N), mitochondria (M), and division by endodyogeny (E) where one organism divides into two (electron micrograph, ×10,752). *(From Frenkel JK. Toxoplasmosis. In: Binford CH, Connor DH, eds. Pathology of Tropical and Extraordinary Diseases. Washington, DC: American Registry of Pathology; 1976:284–300; photograph contributed by Dr. Harley G. Sheffield.)*

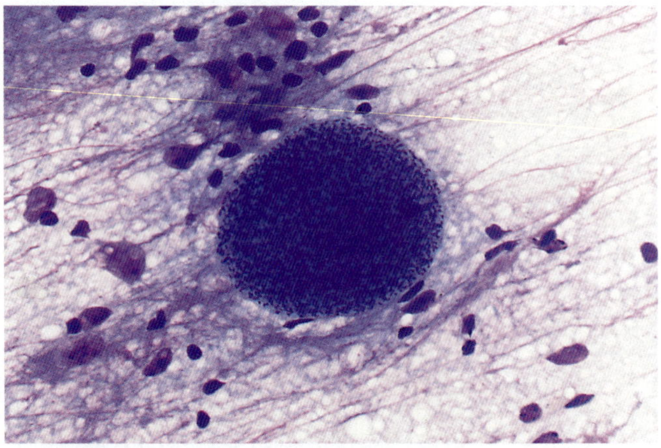

Figure 140–3. *Toxoplasma* tissue cyst. Note the large number of organisms supported by the host cell (in this field a neuron), compared to the small number of tachyzoites tolerated by a host cell (impression film, Giemsa, ×103).

sion of humans, either in the course of treatment of neoplasias or for the maintenance of transplanted organs, led to a recrudescent or relapsing chronic toxoplasmosis. Now, this is most common in patients with the acquired immunodeficiency syndrome (AIDS).

Epidemiologic studies have shown that toxoplasmosis is most common in moist tropical areas, where up to 100% of the population may have antibodies, and least common in dry, desert regions, although focal sites of contamination on flooded or irrigated land may persist where oocysts survive in soil. *Toxoplasma* appears to consist of essentially only one immunotype; immunity is readily acquired, and vaccines have been developed for felines[11] and other animals.[12] Genetic polymorphism, however, has been demonstrated by isoenzyme and DNA analysis.[13]

INFECTION IN HUMANS

Almost all infections are acquired by mouth—either oocysts or tissue cysts. *Toxoplasma* infection is common in humans, and rarely causes illness, except in the immature fetus, in immunologically privileged sites, such as brain and eye, and in immunodeficient patients.

CLINICAL FEATURES

Early Generalized Infection

Early generalized infection with multiorgan involvement may be accompanied by fever, headache, malaise, myalgia, and lymphadenopathy as the most common manifestations, followed by fatigue, stiff neck, anorexia, abdominal pain, nausea, vomiting, and arthralgia. Less common are conjunctivitis, splenomegaly, hepatomegaly, rash, confusion, and choroiditis. These frequencies were derived by combining data from seven common-source outbreaks, in which the incubation period varied from 5 to 18 days, in which one pregnant woman infected her baby in utero, and in which 8% of seroconverters were hospitalized.[14] The nonspecific nature, and frequently absence of manifestations, indicates the difficulty of suspecting toxoplasmosis early, which is necessary for making a diagnosis. It is in this stage of infection that the placenta and fetus of a pregnant woman are at risk of becoming infected. In rare fatal infections, pneumonia or encephalitis dominated the clinical picture.

Lymphadenopathy

Lymphadenopathy is a common (5% to 100%) and characteristic finding whether or not it follows other clinical features including fever. Cervical nodes are most commonly enlarged, consistent with orally acquired infection. Enlargement of single nodes is most common but axillary, inguinal, and other groups may be involved. Although nodes are enlarged and tender, there is no overlying erythema, periadenitis, or suppuration. Toxoplasmic lymphadenopathy has been estimated to account for 3% to 7% of clinically significant lymphadenopathy[15]; it appears to be three times more common in women than in men and may persist for weeks, sometimes raising the suspicion of a neoplasm for which the node may be excised. However, serologic diagnosis, by showing elevated IgM anti-*Toxoplasma* titers, may avoid unnecessary surgical biopsies.[15] Peripheral lymphocytes may be increased, but the heterophile test and the IgM test for Epstein–Barr capsid antigen are negative. Diagnosis of toxoplasmic lymphadenopathy in a pregnant woman may be an indication for chemoprophylaxis to prevent infection of the fetus. One patient had a 12-year course of prolonged generalized lymphadenopathy, isolation of *Toxoplasma* and later hyperglobulinemia, impaired delayed hypersensitivity, and Hodgkin's lymphoma.[16]

Congenital Toxoplasmosis

Congenital toxoplasmosis is acquired by the fetal blood supply and is the only form not acquired by mouth. Its course varies from asymptomatic to fatal, depending on fetal age at infection and undefined factors. Common findings in infants born to women who acquired *Toxoplasma* infection during pregnancy were prematurity, intrauterine growth retardation, postmaturity, retinochoroiditis (5.7% bilateral), strabismus, psychomotor retardation, microcephalus or hydrocephalus, convulsions, hypotonia, icterus, and hepatosplenomegaly. These were accompanied by abnormal findings in cerebrospinal fluid and in computerized tomography and radiography.[17] In addition, patients with overt infections have had hypothermia, mental retardation, and occasionally endocrine defects, usually caused by hypothalamic and pituitary dysfunction.

In an immunocompetent woman, infection of the fetus is from primary infection during the pregnancy. The woman is immune by the time of a subsequent pregnancy. Immunodeficient women, however, may infect their fetus from reactivation of a chronic infection,[18] so that HIV-infected women may infect fetuses of subsequent pregnancies.

Retinochoroiditis

Retinochoroiditis caused by *Toxoplasma* occurs in the newborn, in children, and in adults. The great majority of ocular infections appear to follow congenital infections, although a few patients followed infections as child or adult.[19] Organisms are present in the retina, for which reason "retinochoroiditis" is preferred over chorioretinitis. *Toxoplasma* was first found in the retina of enucleated eyes of patients previously considered tuberculous or syphilitic because of granulomatous inflammation in the choroid (Figure 140–4) and, sometimes, sclera.[20] Because ocular specimens are difficult to obtain for examination, diagnosis is based on clinical findings of small inflammatory lesions of retina, initially obscured by vitreous inflammation, and by laboratory tests. Because titers in these patients rarely differ from the usual titers in asymptomatic patients in the area, the diagnosis of ocular toxoplasmosis is essentially statistical. The higher the prevalence of positive titers in the patient's venue, the more difficult the diagnosis. On the other hand, in London, England, with only 30% positive titers in the population, diagnosis was easy because 87% of patients with retinochoroiditis were seropositive.[21] An interesting method of making the diagnosis is based on comparing the antibody concentration in anterior chamber fluid and serum, in relation to the total IgG,[22] because if there is antigen release in the eye, local antibody production should create higher antibody concentrations in the eye than in peripheral serum. This method has been used mainly in Europe and is difficult to obtain in the United States because ophthalmologists are loath to puncture the eye and serologic tests for small amounts of fluid are not generally available. Polymerase chain reaction (PCR) can be used instead, looking for *Toxoplasma* DNA.[23]

In immunocompetent patients, lesions are yellowish, focal, accompanied by vitreous exudate, and often

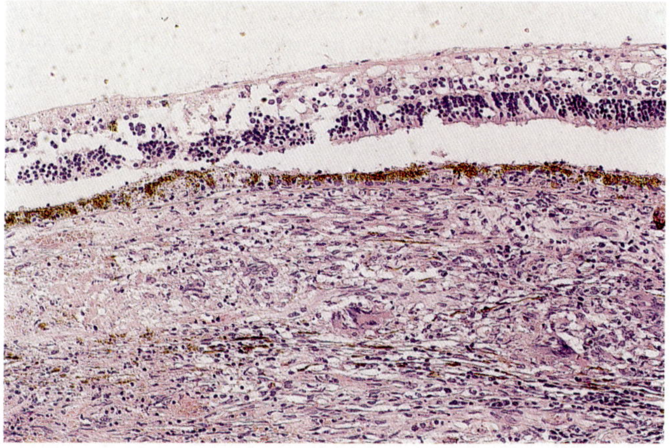

Figure 140–4. The choroid is diffusely thickened by a granulomatous process, which includes epithelioid cells, giant cells, and dispersed pigment, but no tachyzoites. These lesions went undiagnosed for many years and were sometimes misdiagnosed as tuberculosis and syphilis until they were recognized as a manifestation of toxoplasmosis by Mrs. H. C. Wilder[20] [hematoxylin-eosin (H&E), ×50].

at the edge of an old scar. After about 2 months the inflammation usually subsides and the lesion heals by gliosis, usually with pigment proliferation. If the retina is focally destroyed, the lesion is white in the center. Most lesions are self-healing, probably following rupture of a cyst, but about 10% progress because of multiplication of tachyzoites. The old practice of treating "uveitis" with a corticosteroid may transform a self-limited lesion into a progressive one. One patient, with retinochoroiditis was treated with isoniacid (INH), which is not effective against *Toxoplasma,* and corticosteroids, which are immunosuppressive in doses that are anti-inflammatory. After 9 years, the eye was blind, painful, and was enucleated. Practically all the retina was destroyed, the eye had the largest number of cysts so far recorded, but the tachyzoites that probably caused the progressive retinitis could not be found, because the corticosteroids were stopped before surgery, permitting immunity to be active.[24]

In patients with AIDS[25] or with treated lymphomas,[26] the retinal lesion is diffuse and progressive, with smooth, nongranular borders, accompanied by vitritis and sometimes anterior uveitis, often leading to destruction of most of the retina. Patients with miliary retinitis and with panophthalmitis have also been described. These lesions must be distinguished from retinitis caused by cytomegalovirus, usually accompanied by minimal inflammation, irregular, granular borders, and commonly hemorrhages, which are rare in toxoplasmic retinitis.[25]

Toxoplasmic Encephalitis

Toxoplasmic encephalitis in adults is usually associated with immunodeficiency caused by chemotherapy for neoplasia or transplant maintenance, or with infection by the human immunodeficiency virus (HIV).[27] In most patients, encephalitis results from recrudescence of chronic infection. A few patients with acute encephalitis, however, have been described.

PATHOGENESIS AND IMMUNITY

Acute Infection

In the majority of humans, toxoplasmosis is asymptomatic and undiagnosed. Common-source outbreaks and experimental infections in animals, however, give us an insight into pathogenesis and developing immunity. The major pathogenic factor is proliferation of tachyzoites, destroying host cell faster than they regenerate. It is probable that infecting dose and genetic factors of *Toxoplasma* affect pathogenicity in humans, but this is difficult to prove. Pathogenicity in mice, although clonally linked,[28] provides an example of pathogenicity, but does not correspond to pathogenicity for humans. What is seemingly microbial "virulence" (pathogenicity) is more likely an expression of inadequate immune response by the patient. *Toxoplasma* is usually ingested, followed by proliferation in the mucosa,[27] extension to regional lymph nodes, followed by hematogenous dissemination. Whether lesions become manifest as pneumonia, myocarditis, encephalitis, or retinochoroiditis, or as no apparent lesions, subclinical infection should be suspected and may become apparent later. Tachyzoites multiply by sequential division into two, and after about 32 tachyzoites have developed, the host cell usually disintegrates. Clinical immunity depends on specific cell-mediated immunity, antibody, and nonspecific lymphokines, and eventually limits proliferation of tachyzoites. The antibody response is used for serologic diagnosis.

Chronic Infection

Bradyzoites within a tissue cyst usually persist after primary infection so that chronic infection follows as a rule. Evasion of host immunity and ability to live inside cells without destroying them, at least for periods of months or years, are the biologic hallmarks of bradyzoites within cysts. The numbers of bradyzoites within a cyst may approximate a thousand. Biologically, the persistence of bradyzoites is essential for transmission, and non-cyst-forming *Toxoplasma* have not been nor are expected to be isolated from nature. Such strains have been produced experimentally and are used for vaccination.[29,30] Rarely, toxoplasmic lesions appear in the eye during chronic infection. The majority of these have been linked to rupture of a cyst in the retina, where the inflammatory reaction, augmented by delayed hypersensitivity, is clinically apparent, because of the highly concentrated function in anatomically small segments of retina.[31] Persistence of immunity is implicated, because most bradyzoites released from the cyst are killed extracellularly.[32] Also few or no new lesions from tachyzoite proliferation arise. Similarly, immunocompetent women with chronic infection do not infect their babies in utero.[17] High-dose corticosteroids, however, and other immunosuppressive agents can abolish immunity in an eye and proliferation of tachyzoites resumes.

Congenital Infection

Infection of a fetus is accompanied by a certain amount of passive, antibody-related immunity transferred from the mother. At the same time, the fetus and the newborn acquire cellular immunity more slowly than do children and adults, which appears first in the extraneural tissues and later in brain and eye. These factors determine prolonged chronic active disease and the sequelae of fetal infection, especially seeding the retina with organisms which develop into bradyzoites as shown by the development of retinochoroiditis as a child or young adult. Generalized infection precedes involvement of the central nervous system, which is the last organ to acquire immunity. The vulnerability of brain to inflammatory edema because of its enclosure in the cranial vault and the lack of regenerative capacity of nerve cells need also be considered.

Recrudescent Infection

The persistence of bradyzoites in tissue cysts, usually innocuous in the immunocompetent, is a liability during immunodeficiency, and results in recrudescent active toxoplasmosis in about a quarter of *Toxoplasma*-infected patients who develop AIDS[27] and in some of the patients receiving immunosuppressive therapy to maintain organ transplants or to suppress neoplasms.[33–36] Patients with iatrogenic immunodeficiency usually receive 5 to 20 doses of corticosteroid and several other immunosuppressive agents as well. Lesions are concentrated in the brain, which is first to lose immunity. Lesions are focal, consistent with extension of organisms from a disintegrated cyst parasitizing contiguous cells. Most of the tachyzoites and occasionally a few cysts are at the periphery of these focal lesions. Later tachyzoites extend along arterioles, leading to thrombosis and infarction.[27] Immunodeficient pregnant women with chronic toxoplasmosis may infect their fetus.[17,18] Depletion of CD4+ and CD8+ T lymphocytes was required in mice with chronic toxoplasmosis to permit reactivation.[37]

Toxoplasmosis in Transplant Recipients

Two types of infections should be distinguished: reactivation, just discussed, and primary infection from a *Toxoplasma*-infected donor. Because they are immunosuppressed, their primary infection tends to be severe. A *Toxoplasma*-infected heart transplanted from an immune donor to a nonimmune immunodeficient recipient will rarely function adequately in spite of chemotherapy. The frequency of transmission mirrors to some degree the frequency with which a tissue is chronically infected, and the prevalence of infection in a given area. Kidney, heart, lung, and bone marrow have transmitted *T gondii*. Recipients should be tested serologically while they await a heart, and if seronegative, should be immunized. The donor's blood should be tested too, to consider chemoprophylaxis early, before the onset of active myocarditis. The severity of *Toxoplasma* multiplication would be greatest in heart and bone marrow,[38] and less in lung and kidney.

HISTOPATHOLOGY

Most cases seen by pathologists have been preceded by a long illness and often by specific antitoxoplasma or the similar antipneumocystic therapy. *Toxoplasma,* therefore, are few and lesions have often healed by regeneration or scarring. For these reasons the earliest reports are often the most informative, because patients during their lifetime were undiagnosed and untreated. Also, with toxoplasmosis becoming more recognized, reports, histologic descriptions and illustrations have become fewer. Toxoplasmosis in immunodeficient patients, however, presents a variety of new lesions. The characteristic serologic findings are mentioned in this diagnostic section, but the tests are discussed in a separate section.

Intestine

One patient with a primary intestinal lesion had a mucosal ulcer in the small intestine with scattered *Toxoplasma* tachyzoites in lamina propria and submucosa.[27] The identity of the tachyzoites was verified by immunoperoxidase. In addition, the organisms had the typical ultrastructure of *Toxoplasma* tachyzoites, including conoid and rhoptries. Toxoplasmic lesions were only in small intestine, not in brain and other tissues; *Toxoplasma* antigen was in none of six lymph nodes, bone marrow, spleen, brain, and pituitary. *Toxoplasma* antigen, without recognizable organisms, however, was in some pulmonary macrophages. The patient died with disseminated histoplasmosis after an illness of 51 days.[27] He may have become infected during his illness, but he had not received antitoxoplasmic therapy. His serologic tests were positive—1:65,000 by dye test, 1:162,000 by direct agglutination test, and 10+ by IgM capture test.

Liver

In a few adult patients, foci of eosinophilic necrosis of liver involving from 3 to 30 liver cells were surrounded by an approximately equal number of neutrophils and lymphocytes containing clusters of typical *Toxoplasma* organisms.[39] One patient, a 76-year-old Peruvian man with fever of unknown origin, was treated for 12 days with antibiotics. At autopsy there were myeloid metaplasia and disseminated cytomegalovirus (CMV) infection. Another Peruvian patient with bartonellosis had similar lesions.[40] Lesions of liver associated with *Toxoplasma* are rare, present in only 10% of adult patients with toxoplasmosis examined histologically. Most clinical infections were documented only by liver function tests, together with high serologic titers. This can lead to mistaken diagnoses, such as when a Central American native with antibody titers common for his homeland is seen at a university hospital in the Eastern United States, where the high antibody titer (for the United States) and poorly controlled fluorescent antibody tests persuaded pathologists that chromosomes from mitotic figures in regenerating liver cells were *Toxoplasma*.[41,42] The cytoplasmic inclusions of CMV have occasionally been misinterpreted as *Toxoplasma;* the intranuclear inclusions are correctly identified, and the case is taken as a double infection.[43] In infants too, the liver is rarely parasitized. The liver is often enlarged, with fibrosis, regeneration, chronic inflammation with mononuclear cells, eosinophils, and extramedullary hematopoiesis.[44] Because liver lesions are commonly reported in a variety of animals, it is possible that they also exist in humans but before the time most patients are examined by biopsy or autopsy. Since hepatitis is comparatively rare with toxoplasmosis, the interpretation of serologic tests has not been defined.

Lung

Interstitial pneumonia is commonly reported with toxoplasmosis of adults and infants. Organisms, however, are rarely identified in sections of lung.[45] Tachyzoites have been described in alveolar lining cells and in mononuclear alveolar exudates of two adults from the St. Louis area with a clinical picture of Rocky Mountain spotted fever.[46] This has been described in children also.[47] In immunodeficient patients lung may be involved with several agents at a time—*Pneumocystis carinii,* CMV (Figure 140–5), and fungi being most common. *Toxoplasma* may have been the only or preponderant pathogen in a few patients. Tachyzoites may be scattered diffusely through the lung or within foci of coagulation necrosis.[48–50] Serologic titers are usually elevated.

Placenta

Groups of tachyzoites and cysts containing bradyzoites are in amnion, chorion, and umbilical cord. There are usually no necrotic lesions (Figure 140–6).[51] Because the placenta is grossly normal, the diagnosis is rarely made. Serologic titers are elevated and the infant is usually infected.

Central Nervous System

Acute Febrile Encephalitis

The basic brain lesions are glial nodules, composed of microglial cells and possibly hematogenous inflammatory cells. These glial nodules are comparable to glial nodules of rickettsial and viral infections of the central nervous system. In earlier literature the term "granuloma" was used but should be avoided, because "granuloma" is more appropriately used for lesions containing epithelioid cells derived from the perivascular sheaths, elicited typically by mycobacteria and *Histoplasma*. Tachyzoites multiply in neurons, glial cells, ependyma, and vessel walls. The parasitized cells are destroyed and one can often identify their remnants in the form of pyknotic nuclei or necrosis of the neuropil. Tachyzoites can usually be identified in a proportion of

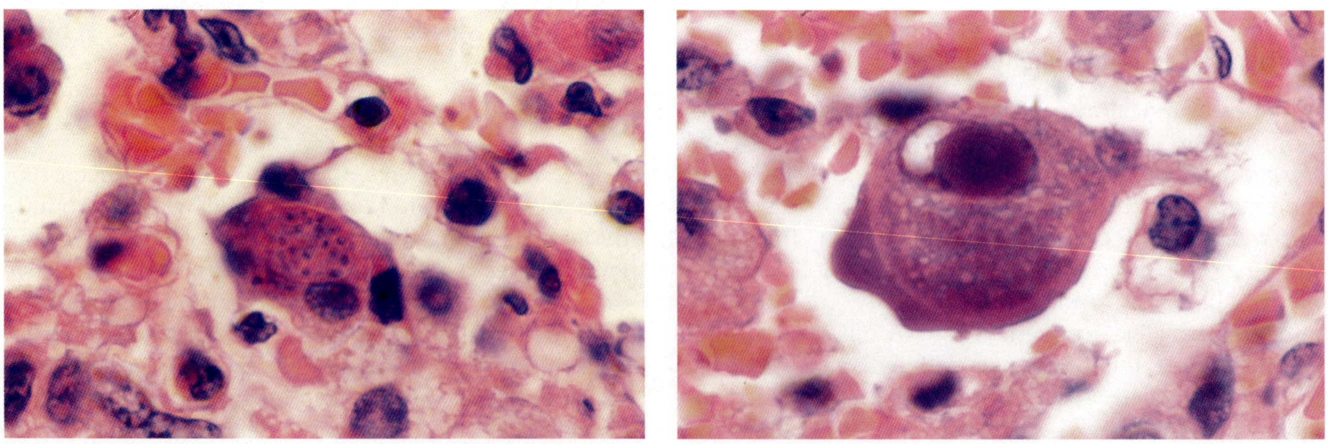

A B

Figure 140–5. Toxoplasmic and CMV mononuclear pneumonia with partial organization in 4-month-old Costa Rican child. (**A**) A *Toxoplasma* cyst is juxtaposed to (**B**) a cell with intranuclear and intracytoplasmic CMV inclusions. The intracytoplasmic CMV inclusion is larger and the individual inclusions are hazy but the *Toxoplasma* bradyzoite nuclei are discrete and the cyst wall is plainly visible (H&E ×250). *(Contributed by Dr. Rodolfo Cespedes and Leon Troper, Hospital San Juan de Dios, San Jose, Costa Rica.)*

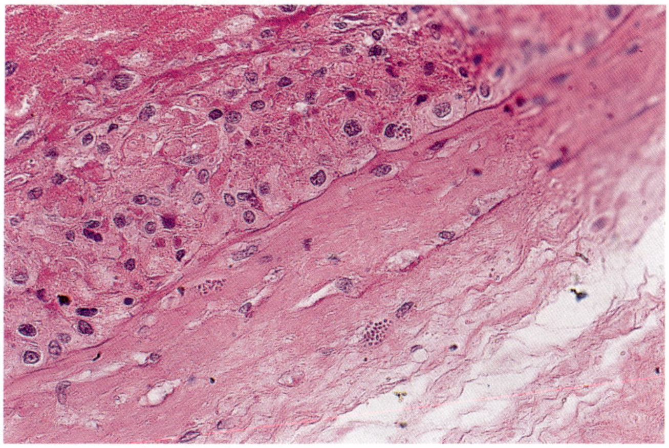

Figure 140–6. *Toxoplasma* infection of placenta. Two chorionic cells and one decidual cell are infected. The organisms are tachyzoites and there is no necrosis or inflammatory reaction. The baby was infected but appeared to be well (PAS-hematoxylin, ×103). *(Section contributed by Dr. S. G. Driscoll, Boston Lying-In Hospital.)*

glial nodules, usually at their peripheries. Intracellular tachyzoites cause no inflammation. Some nodules composed of microglia and prominent astrocytes are not accompanied by cellular necrosis and tachyzoites. Gliosis may be slight or advance.

In some patients, tissue cysts with PAS-positive bradyzoites are also found. They have occasionally been in brains of patients dying of other diseases[52] and have been recovered by animal inoculation in about 10% of patients who die of neoplastic diseases.[53] When intact, they do not provoke inflammation. When cysts disintegrate in immunocompetent patients, however, bradyzoites lose their staining intensity, are then phagocytosed, and a glial nodule develops.[32] In patients with acute toxoplasmic encephalitis and a protracted clinical course, cysts and intense, diffuse encephalitis have been encountered, accompanied only by bradyzoites in cysts.[54–57] In one afebrile patient with a focal lesion, an unusual reaction occurred. There were cysts, necrosis, microglial and astrocytic reaction, hematogenous mononuclear and plasma cells, and a unique granulomatous reaction with giant cells arising from perivascular cells.[58] Serologic titers are usually elevated.

Chronic Progressive Encephalitis in Immunodeficient Patients

Two main lesions are encountered.[27] Most commonly they are characteristically large foci of necrosis mainly in the gray matter, with swarms of tachyzoites (Figure 140–7, A), especially peripherally, and a variable number of cysts. Antigen demonstrated by immunohistochemistry is in the center of the lesion. As is suggested by CAT scans and by experimental data,[35] the tachyzoites originate from a single center, a disintegrated cyst, and extend centrifugally destroying almost every cell in their way. In more advanced infections tachyzoites extend along arterioles, multiplying in endothelium and adventia, leading to a characteristic occlusive hypertrophic arteritis.[59] This produced the second major lesion, areas of infarction caused by this arteritis. Tachyzoites and antigen are absent, except in the vessels. Lesions large enough to be visible by the naked eye have been called abscesses because of the central necrosis. Because they contain no pus from degenerating neutrophils and are not destined to drain they are not abscesses. The lesions have firm necrotic centers not liquefied by leukocytic enzymes, although they are softer than the surrounding brain.

Three zones have been distinguished in the first lesion[60]: 1) central coagulation necrosis with few organisms, 2) an intermediate zone with hyperemia, spotty necrosis, and intense inflammatory reaction with both intra- and extracellular tachyzoites, and 3) minimal inflammatory reaction with few tachyzoites and some bradyzoites in tissue cysts.

The hypertrophic arteritis in immunodeficient patients has been compared with the hypertrophic arteritis in congenital toxoplasmosis.[59] The latter, however, has been associated with antigen diffusing out of obstructed ventricles,[44] whereas in immunodeficient patients arteritis is associated with tachyzoites multiplying in the affected arterioles (Figure 140–7, B).[27] *Toxoplasma* titers are usually elevated, although serologic findings are not dependable in immunodeficient patients, and about 15% of patients are seronegative.

Neonatal Toxoplasmosis

When tachyzoites spill into the ventricular system they disseminate within it. In the fetus and neonate, tachyzoites invade the ependyma and subependymal tissues, setting up new foci of infection. The narrowest part of the ventricular system tends to become obstructed by inflammation and internal hydrocephalus of the lateral and third ventricles. The foramina of Luschka and Magendie usually remain patent and the fourth ventricle is not distended. The lesions around the lateral and third ventricles are unique in that they become surrounded by areas of necrosis and vasculitis wherever the ependyma is absent and where they are not covered by choroid plexus. As a basis for this unique lesion, a local antigen–antibody reaction has been suggested.[44] The finding of trapped antigen in the ventricular fluid and of antibody in the arterioles supported this hypothesis, which however has not yet been reexamined by modern histochemical methods. Supportive evidence comes from the fact that occluded arterioles that extend into the ventricle show proliferative granulation tissue and no evidence of an adverse effect, and that the reaction of vasculitis and necrosis are absent around the

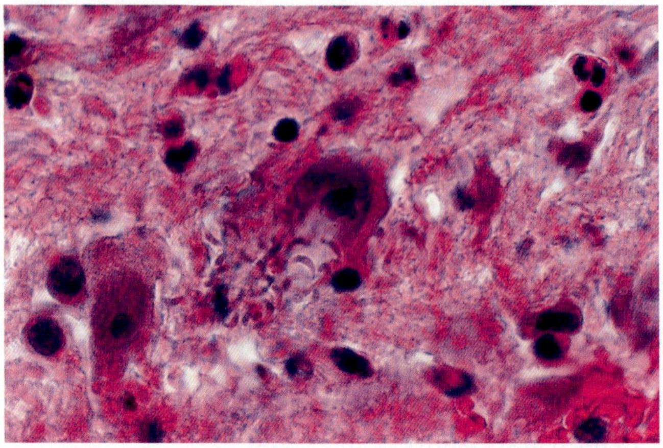

A

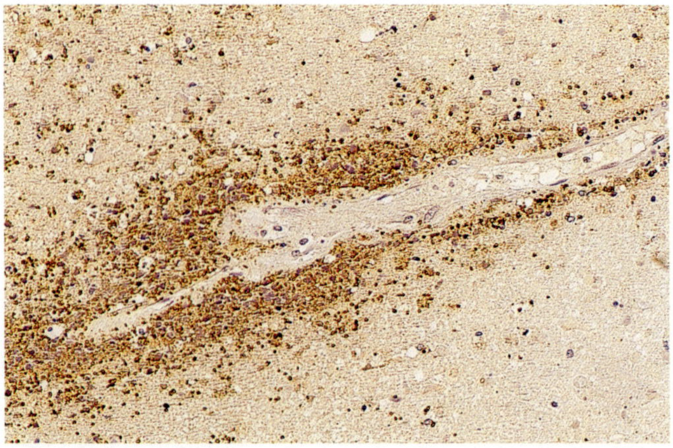

B

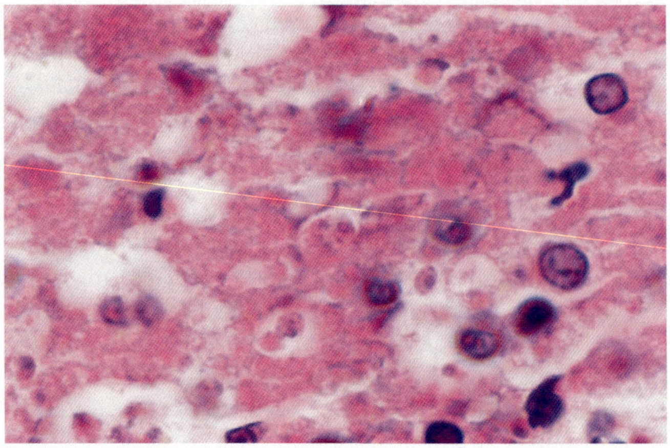

C

Figure 140–7. (**A**) Toxoplasmic encephalitis in HIV-infected, immunodeficient patient. Clusters of tachyzoites are in the brain (H&E, ×1000). (**B**) Immunoperoxidase with antitoxoplasma serum, showing the antigen in perivascular space (*right*) and progressively involving the arteriolar wall and lumen and the surrounding parenchyma (×53). (*From Bertoli et al,[27] case 3*.) (**C**) Scattered tachyzoites in the brain (H&E, ×250). *(From Bertoli et al,[27] case 3.)*

nonobstructed fourth ventricle, where no antigen accumulates. Fluid from the distended ventricles shows grams of protein percent and it is the best source for isolating the organism and for determining content of antigen.

Destruction of hypothalamus extending from the necrosis surrounding the third ventricle may cause unstable body temperatures. Increased intracerebral pressure may cause ischemic softening of subcortical white matter, especially the corona radiata. Necrotic areas of brain often calcify and are visible radiologically.

Apart from the unique periventricular necrosis, the following other types of lesions are in brains of children with congenital toxoplasmosis: 1) necrosis of individual parasitized cells with glial nodules, 2) tissue necrosis following disintegration of a cyst with mixed glial reaction, and 3) infarction necrosis in the cortex caused by vascular thrombosis where the first two types of lesions have involved a blood vessel. *Toxoplasma* antibody titers are usually high.

Lymph Nodes

Toxoplasmic lymphadenitis is usually a reactive follicular hyperplasia, with prominent clusters of epithelioid histiocytes in and encroaching on germinal centers and extending beyond their margins (Figure 140–8, A), usually located in cortical and paracortical zones. There may be also distention of subcapsular and trabecular sinuses with monocytoid cells of the B type (Figure 140–8, B).[15] There is neither necrosis, eosinophilia, fibrosis, nor periadenitis and the lymph node architecture is preserved. Tachyzoites are usually absent, but if present, suggest immunodeficiency, the cause of which should be investigated. Cysts may be found in serial sections after a prolonged search (Figure 140–9). This is accompanied by high and usually stable antibody titers, especially in the IgM fraction. These findings indicate that lymphadenopathy is a reaction of immunity. If cysts are numerous the patient may be immunodeficient.[61]

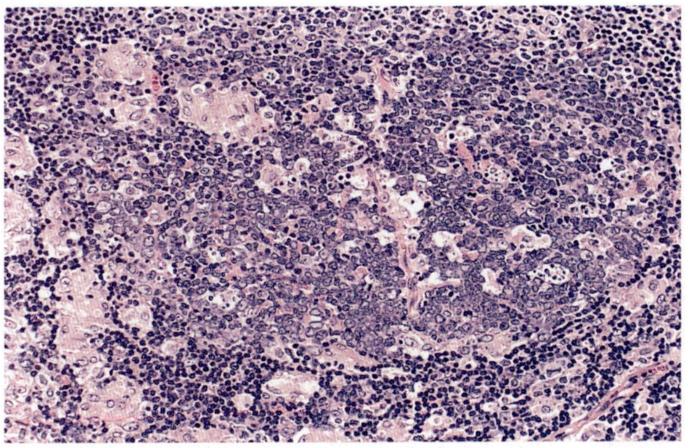

A

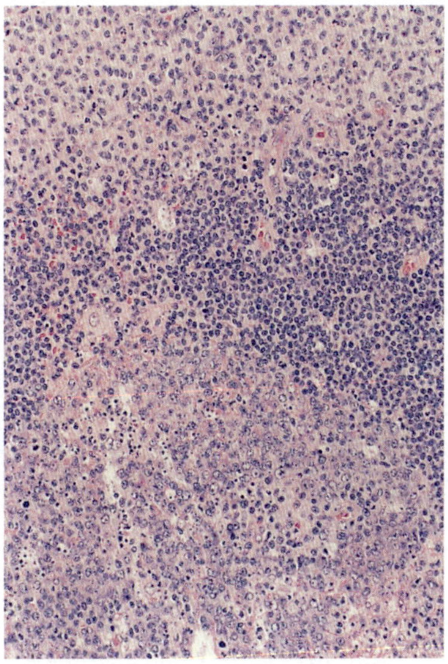

B

Figure 140–8. (**A**) Toxoplasmic lymphadenitis. Reactive germinal center has a few collections of epithelioid histiocytes in and adjacent to it (H&E, ×200). (**B**) Toxoplasmic lymphadenitis has reactive germinal center at bottom of field with subcapsular sinus distended by monocytoid B cells (H&E, ×100).

While similar collections of histiocytes are also in lymph nodes with Hodgkin's disease,[16] infectious mononucleosis, Whipple's disease, and in prior years after smallpox vaccination, the absence of Reed–Sternberg cells, the absence of eosinophils and necrosis, a negative heterophile test, a negative IgM test for Epstein–Barr capsid antigen and lack of acid-fast bacilli, and the presence of antitoxoplasma titers in IgG and IgM fractions, diagnose toxoplasmosis.

Skeletal Muscle

Myositis is a rare manifestation of toxoplasmosis. Biopsy specimens have contained *Toxoplasma* cysts without reaction; rare biopsy specimens contain focal necrosis consistent with rupture of a cyst (Figure 140–10, A and B). There is serologic evidence that polymyositis is more commonly associated with toxoplasmosis than dermatomyositis and other types of myositis.[62] High *Toxoplasma* antibody titers in the IgM fraction should be sought to support a diagnosis of toxoplasmic myositis, because persistent IgG antibody titers are common.

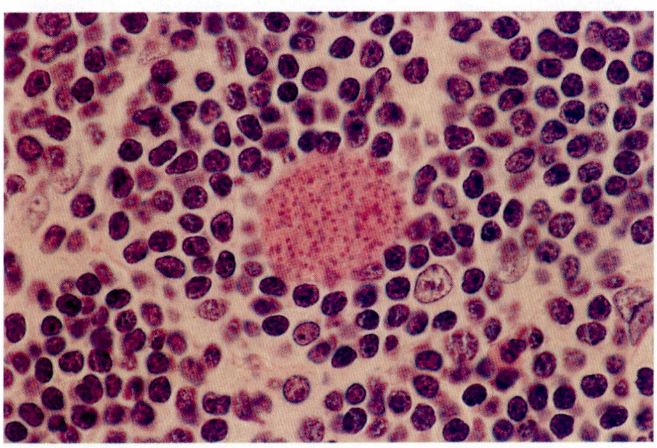

Figure 140–9. Toxoplasmic lymphadenitis containing a cyst, a rare finding (H&E, ×290).

Cardiac Muscle

Myocarditis of varying intensity often accompanies acute *Toxoplasma* infection and occasionally reactivation of infection in an immunodeficient patient (Figure 140–11, A). The diagnosis depends on finding *Toxoplasma* tachyzoites in myocardial cells with inflammatory reaction (Figure 140–11, B) or cysts with distinct foci of inflammation, consistent with a ruptured cyst. Some patients have had pericarditis with effusion.[63] Because tissue cysts are often in the myocardium associated with antibody in the IgG fraction, one should use elevated titers in the IgM fraction to corroborate a diagnosis of toxoplasmic myocarditis. Immunostaining for toxoplasma antigens helps to distinguish toxoplasmosis from other protozoan infections including myocarditis caused by Chagas' disease (Figure 140–12).

Eyes

Enucleated eyes sometimes become available from patients who are unilaterally blind and whose eye is painful because of glaucoma. *Toxoplasma* should be sought in the retina, although most of the inflammation

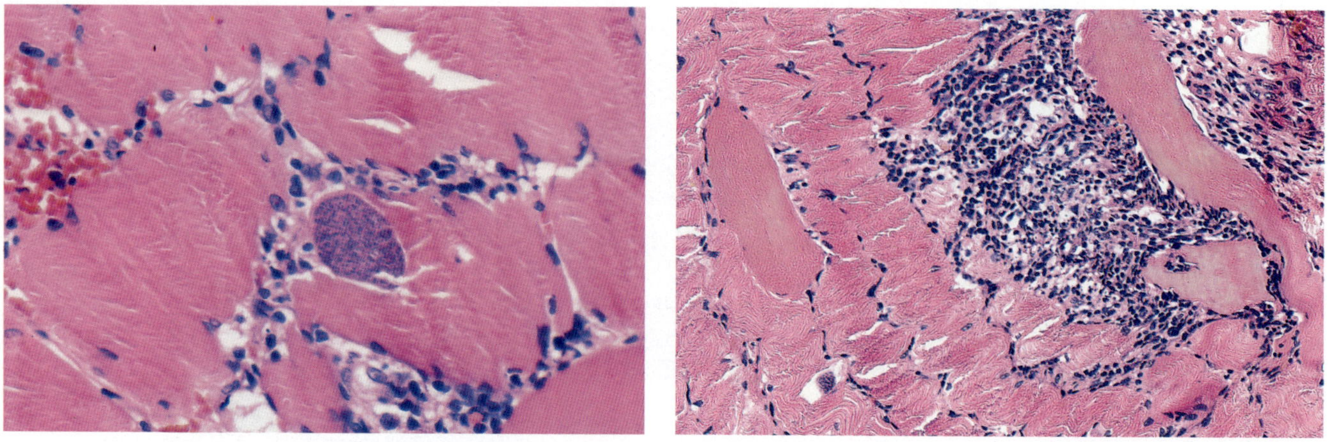

A B

Figure 140–10. Toxoplasmic polymyositis in a 22-year-old man. (**A**) There is an intact cyst without inflammatory reaction to it (H&E, ×50). (**B**) Myositis and scarring of muscle with histiocytes and lymphocytes, but without tachyzoites, indicating this lesion followed disintegration of a *Toxoplasma* cyst, such as the one in lower left (H&E, ×50).[32]

is in the choroid and sclera. There are two types of lesions: 1) focal retinitis with intense inflammation and scarring, and cysts in the still intact retina (Figure 140–13, A) and 2) focal or diffuse retinitis with tachyzoites destroying parasitized cells (Figure 140–13, B). The first type of lesion is postulated to result from disintegration of a cyst, where release of antigen in the presence of hypersensitivity gives rise to inflammation, although immunity, when intact, destroys liberated tachyzoites.

Corticosteroids injected into Tenon's capsule of the eye, systemic administration of corticosteroids,[26] or immunodeficiency from other causes, especially AIDS, may change the pathogenesis from type 1 to type 2.[64] Then the retinal lesion is more diffuse and progressive as is the overlying vitritis. The retina is largely necrotic, accompanied by pigment-bearing macrophages in the outer retinal layers and the vitreous. The retina may be detached with proteinaceous exudate between it and the choroid. *Toxoplasma* tachyzoites and a variable number of cysts are in all three retinal layers. The choroid is heavily infiltrated with plasma cells, lymphocytes, and mononuclear cells. The retinal pigment epithelium shows focal proliferation and diffuse necro-

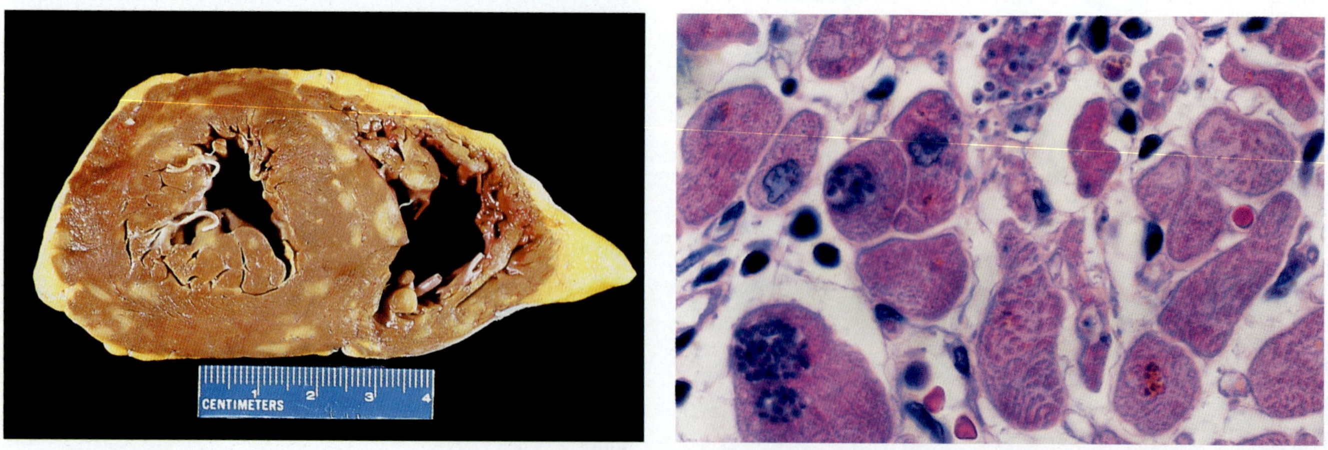

A B

Figure 140–11. Toxoplasmic myocarditis. (**A**) Note multiple white foci in myocardium of both ventricles. These are areas of toxoplasmic inflammation and necrosis. (**B**) Same case showing toxoplasma organisms in myofibers. At top of field the myofiber has ruptured releasing *Toxoplasma* organisms (H&E, ×1000).

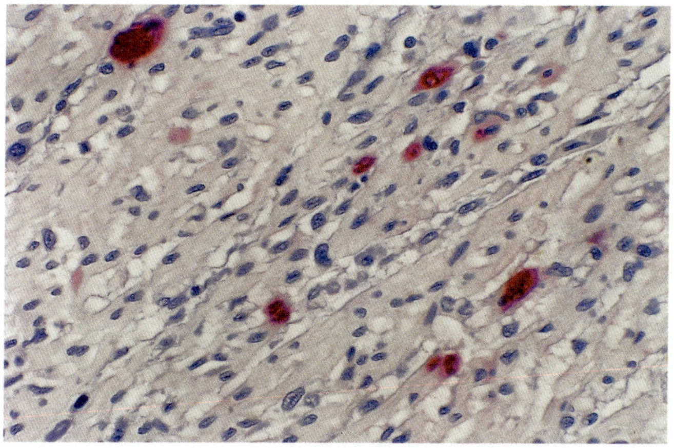

Figure 140–12. Specific immunostaining for toxoplasmic antigen. There is vivid demonstration of intracellular organisms (alkaline phosphatase reaction, ×400).

sis.[24,65] In an AIDS patient, initially with bilateral miliary toxoplasmic retinitis, the lesions became largely confluent, with retinal detachment, where the full thickness of retina was involved.[66] In two AIDS patients with toxoplasmic retinitis, even the sclera was inflamed—possibly by *Toxoplasma*.[67] Most of the tachyzoites, however, were in the retina. Both patients had acute and chronic inflammation of periorbital tissues without tachyzoites.

Skin

Although skin rash in the early hematogenous phase of toxoplasmosis has contained tachyzoites,[40] biopsy of a rash is not a common procedure and presumptive serologic diagnoses without histologic support are the rule. Morphologically convincing toxoplasmosis, however, was in skin of a patient with myelogenous leukemia who had received a bone marrow allograft. What appeared to be *Toxoplasma* tachyzoites were in purpuric nodules on the scalp, back, forearm, and groin, which appeared 21 days after transplant. The organisms whose identification was based on electron microscopy were in all levels of the epithelium, in Schwann cells and macrophages.[68] Because no serologic tests were available, the lesions may have been caused by a morphologically similar organism.

Other

Among the many tissues in which *Taxoplasma* has been identified, orchitis is of interest because most of the tachyzoites were in degenerating seminiferous tubules, close to focal areas of testicular necrosis, in patients with AIDS.[49,50] Toxoplasmosis has involved also parotids, pancreas, adrenal, kidney, prostate, pituitary, spleen, stomach, esophagus, thyroid, bladder, and bone marrow of patients with AIDS.[49,50]

DIAGNOSIS

Staining Methods

For tissue sections, whether from biopsy or autopsy, H&E is most useful for recognizing tachyzoites. When scanning for *Toxoplasma* cysts or for their identification, the PAS-hematoxylin method is most useful. The cyst wall can be impregnated with silver, such as Wilder's.

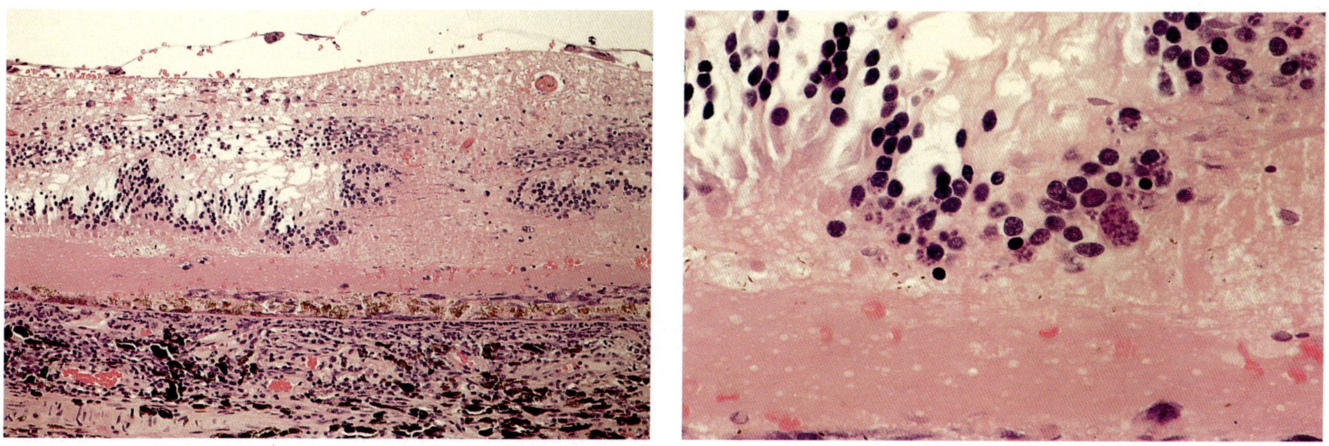

A B

Figure 140–13. Toxoplasmic retinitis. (**A**) Area of coagulation necrosis in retina (H&E, ×45). (**B**) Higher magnification showing intact cyst and tachyzoites free in the tissue (H&E, ×100).

For thin, plastic-embedded sections, hematoxylin or toluidine blue can be used. For tissue imprints or material from bronchoalveolar lavage, Giemsa or similar stain is preferred. For electron microscopy, the routine techniques of glutaraldehyde or osmic acid fixation permit recognition of the internal organelles on which the diagnosis of *Toxoplasma* infection is based.

Staining methods have the advantage that organisms can be evaluated together with the tissue response. Tachyzoites with lesions signify active infection, whereas tissue cysts require appropriate lesions to be linked to illness. With 10% to 100% of antibody prevalence in various populations the finding of only a cyst, or of PCR, positive cell culture or animal inoculation, or antibody positivity does not establish a relationship to the illness.

Other Diagnostic Methods

Immunohistochemistry for antigen is one of the most simple and useful methods to verify the diagnosis of *Toxoplasma* in tissues. The important item is a monoclonal antibody for *Toxoplasma* and, if not available, a polyclonal antibody, using the preinoculation serum of the same animal as control. Rabbits, of course, may have antibodies for hundreds of agents, and positive staining of a structure by a polyclonal serum does not identify it without demonstrating nonstaining by a preinoculation serum. This requirement can be approximated by absorbing a polyclonal antitoxoplasma serum with large numbers of *Toxoplasma,* and using the absorbed serum as control.

Several kits for immunoperoxidase can be adapted, some based on biotinylated antirabbit IgG and an avidin-bound peroxidase, and others on an antirabbit IgG bound to peroxidase, after which the substrate is added and the section is stained lightly with H&E for orientation. Formalin-fixed paraffin or thin plastic sections can be used.[48]

DNA determination by PCR usually depends on a laboratory that routinely performs PCR tests. Several primers are available.[69–71] DNA extraction and analysis of PCR products by electrophoresis gel must be done in physically separate rooms from where amplification is performed to minimize false-positive reactions; also, controls and special positive displacement pipettes should be used. PCR has been successfully used with serum, cerebrospinal fluid,[72] amniotic fluid,[70] aqueous fluid,[23] and fluid from bronchoalveolar lavage.[73]

In situ DNA hybridization sometimes can be performed on the involved tissues.

SEROLOGY

Tests for antibody are used clinically to support a presumptive clinical diagnosis of toxoplasmosis. The pathologist deals more with the identification of presumed organisms, antigen, or their DNA in tissues. Hence the methods outlined previously will usually be more useful to complement tissue diagnosis. Because serologic tests do not dependably distinguish between active, inactive, or past *Toxoplasma* infection, serologic tests are of limited use in patients with AIDS. This is especially important in immunodeficient patients in whom serologic tests based on immunologic reactivity are not dependable, and diagnosis based on identification of the etiologic agent, its antigens, or its DNA are essential.

The best serologic test are the dye test[74] and the direct *Toxoplasma* agglutination test.[75] The latter is well suited for differentiation of IgG and IgM antibody. Serologic test for IgA[76,77] and IgE[78] have also been described. They and IgM are especially useful for diagnosis of congenital toxoplasmosis, where the passively transferred maternal antibody obscures a serologic response by the fetus and newborn. The capture tests, whereby total IgM, IgA, or IgE are first captured by appropriate antisera, are especially useful here, and the unwanted Ig moieties are washed off. Thereafter, the antibody content of the captured fraction is tested against fixed *Toxoplasma* organisms in the agglutination test, or against soluble antigen in the enzyme-linked immunosorbent assay (ELISA) read in a spectrophotometer.[79]

A multitude of serologic tests has been described over the years; they are manufactured and distributed by various companies. Unfortunately, the best tests are not yet generally available in the United States because of cost (direct agglutination test, which is manufactured by BioMerieux in France) and an understandable reluctance to maintain a live strain of *Toxoplasma* in the laboratory in order to perform a dye test occasionally. One should become proficient in the interpretation of locally available serologic tests if they are adequate and, if not, one can send sera to the state reference laboratory.

Animal inoculation and cell culture are dependable but time-consuming methods to identify *Toxoplasma* and other organisms in tissue. These methods are especially appropriate when one does not know the causal agent such as in a research problem. One needs the foresight not to succumb to the hand-formalin reflex. Any lymph node worth a biopsy should be cultured or a portion kept in a refrigerator, unfrozen, till sections have been examined. Then the appropriate cell culture or animal system can be chosen. Cell lines of human fibroblasts, primary monkey kidney cultures, L cells, and many others are suitable for *Toxoplasma;* it is useful to put cover slips in the culture flasks and seed cell lines onto them so cultures may be sampled at intervals. Inoculation of Golden hamsters intraperitoneally has been most useful in my laboratory, because they are susceptible also to *Leishmania, Histoplasma,* and other fungi. Most researchers, however, use mice. Culture cells, such as on cover slips, can be examined after 5 to 7 days if cell layer destruction is not apparent earlier, and stained with Giemsa. Peritoneal cells from animals can be examined similarly. Animals have four advantages: Larger amounts of tissue can be examined, contaminant organisms are less destructive than in cell cultures, antibody development can be used for diagnosis, and their brains can be examined for *Toxoplasma* cysts after about 6 weeks.

DIFFERENTIAL DIAGNOSIS

Organisms of similar size always should be considered and distinguished. The following are the most important, and the relevant chapters can be consulted: *Sarcosporidia* (see Chapter 139), *Isospora* (see Chapter 134), *Microsporidia* (see Chapter 137), *Leishmania* (see Chapter 135), *Trypanosoma cruzi* (see Chapter 143), and *Pneumocystis carinii* (see Chapter 138).

Tissue Diagnosis

In addition to the organisms just listed, CMV in the brain of newborns and in the eye gives rise to similar lesions by computerized tomography or radiography, although histologically the lesions can readily be distinguished because the organisms are distinct. Recall again that CMV produces intranuclear and intracytoplasmic inclusions; usually both are present in the same cell. The latter are more irregular in size and shape than *Toxoplasma* (Figure 140–5); although H&E would be adequate for differentiation, immunohistochemistry and electron microscopy will aid in differentiation if necessary.

Lesions produced by *Cryptococcus neoformans* have at times been confused with those of *Toxoplasma;* however, experience over the years and the availability of good differential stains (Grocott, which does not stain *Toxoplasma*) should nowadays distinguish between these lesions.

Effect of Chemotherapy on Tissue Diagnosis

Standard chemotherapy, whether sulfadiazine with pyrimethamine or sulfamethoxazole with trimethoprim (cotrimoxazol) reduce the number of organisms associated with lesions, so that after 3 weeks only tissue cysts may remain.[27] After a few months they may be undetectable by histologic methods. For these patients, animal inoculation[36] and PCR[27] may help. The addition of atovaquone to standard therapy may shorten the survival period of *Toxoplasma.* No histologic experience appears to be available on tissue survival of *Toxoplasma* after treatment of patients with newer antibiotics, such as clindamycin, macrolides (spiramycin, clarithromycin, azithromycin), lincosamides (clindamycin), and tetracyclines (doxycycline, minocycline), which clinically are less effective than standard chemotherapy, but are used in patients hypersensitive to sulfonamides. This is so common in patients with AIDS, that pyrimethamine is used routinely with another drug, whether sulfadiazine, clindamycin, dapsone, atovaquone, or a macrolide.[80] Desensitization has been used successfully.[81]

PREVENTION

Since the clarification of the life cycle of *Toxoplasma,* toxoplasmosis can be prevented. Prevention is easy with minimal cost and effort through these procedures:

1. Pregnant women and immunodeficient patients should prevent primary infection by avoiding contact with cats that hunt rodents and birds, and the soil, sand, and children's sandboxes contaminated with their feces. Cover sandboxes when not in use.
2. Litter boxes used exclusively by indoor cats, which are fed only dry and canned food, are not likely to be contaminated. Outdoor cats should not be allowed to defecate indoors.
3. Meat should be cooked "until the interior is no longer pink and the juices are clear" as has been suggested to prevent other meat-borne infections.[82]
4. Hands should be washed after contact with meat, soil, outdoor cats and litter boxes used by them, and before eating.
5. Hands should be washed also after contact with dogs, some of which have a habit of rolling in or eating cat feces. (Dog contact was highly correlated with transmission in a prospective epidemiologic study[83]).

Serologic surveillance during pregnancy is mandated by law in France and Austria. It has reduced the number of congenitally infected infants because of induced abortion and probably because of the educational value of such programs. Treatment of infected infants has diminished the consequences of this infection. Whether such routine serologic surveillance can be transferred to the United States, by law or voluntarily, appears doubtful. The transmission rate is lower, there is no similar tradition of concerns about toxoplasmosis among people or their physicians, many people are less compulsive about prenatal visits, the tests cost more, costs are questioned, and tests may be prioritized. In addition the serologic tests used effectively in the clinic for the investigation of manifestations of illness have minimal predictive value when used in an unselected pregnant population to detect transmission even with a frequency of only between 1:1000 and 1:10,000; one would obtain more false-positives than true-positives.[84–86] Multiple testing will improve predictability, but will also increase costs. It is for these reasons that commonsense preventive measures are advocated.

REFERENCES

1. Kean BH. The steak tartare defense. In: Anonymous MD. *One Doctor's Adventures Among the Famous and Infamous from the Jungles of Panama to a Park Avenue Practice.* New York: Ballantine Books; 1990:287–515.
2. Dubey JP, Frenkel JK. Experimental *Toxoplasma* infection in mice with strains producing oocysts. *J Parasitol.* 1973; 59:505–512.
3. Frenkel JK. Tissue-dwelling intracellular parasites: infection and immune responses in the mammalian host to *Toxoplasma, Sarcocystis* and *Trichinella. Am Zool.* 1989; 29:455–467.
4. Chobotar B, Scholtyseck E. Ultrastructure. In: Long PL, ed. *The Biology of the Coccidia.* Baltimore: University Park Press; 1982:101–165.
5. Scholtyseck E. Ultrastructure. In: Hammond DM, Long PD, eds. *The Coccidia. Eineria, Isospora,* Toxoplasma *and Related Genera.* Baltimore: University Park Press; 1973: 81–144.
6. Frenkel JK, Parker BB. An apparent role of dogs in the transmission of *Toxoplasma gondii. Ann N Y Acad Sci.* 1996; (in press).
7. Frenkel JK. *Besnoitia wallacei* of cats and rodents: with a reclassification of other cyst-forming isosporoid coccidia. *J Parasitol.* 1977;63:611–628.
8. Frenkel JK, Heydorn AO, Mehlhorn H, Rommel M. Sarcocystinae: nomina dubia and available names. *Z Parasitenkd.* 1979;58:115–139.
9. Levine ND. Taxonomy and life cycles of coccidia. In: Long PL, ed. *The Biology of the Coccidia.* Baltimore: University Park Press; 1982:1–34.
10. Frenkel JK. *Toxoplasma* in and around us. *BioScience.* 1973;23:343–352.
11. Frenkel JK. Pfefferkorn ER, Smith DD, Fishback JL. A *Toxoplasma* vaccine for cats using a new mutant. *Amer J Vet Res.* 1991;52:759–763.
12. Waldeland H, Pfefferkorn ER, Frenkel JK. Temperature-sensitive mutants of *Toxoplasma gondii:* pathogenicity and persistence in mice. *J Parasitol.* 1983;69:171–175.
13. Christina N, Dardé ML, Boudin C, Tavernier G, Pestre-Alexandre M, Ambroise-Thomas P. A DNA fingerprinting method for individual characterization of *Toxoplasma gondii* stains: combination with isoenzymatic characters for determination of linkage groups. *Parasitol Res.* 1995; 81:32–37.
14. Frenkel JK. Toxoplasmosis in human beings. *JAVMA.* 1990;196:240–248.
15. McCabe RE, Brooks RG, Dorfman RF, Remington JS. Clinical spectrum in 107 cases of toxoplasmic lymphadenopathy. *Rev Infect Dis.* 1987;9:754–774.
16. Sheagren JN, Lunde MN, Simon HB. Chronic lymphadenopathic toxoplasmosis. A case with marked hyperglobulinemia and impaired delayed hypersensitivity responses during active infection. *Am J Med.* 1976;60: 300–305.
17. Remington JS, McLeod R, Desmonts G. Toxoplasmosis. In: Remington JS, Klein JO, eds. *Infectious Diseases of the Fetus & Newborn Infant.* 4th ed. Philadelphia: WB Saunders; 1995:140–267.
18. Marty P, Bongain A, Rahal A, et al. Prenatal diagnosis of severe fetal toxoplasmosis as a result of toxoplasmic reactivation in an HIV-1 seropositive woman. *Prenatal Diagn.* 1994;14:414–415.
19. Michelson JB, Shields JA, McDonald PR, Manko MA, Abraham AA, Federman JL. Retinitis secondary to acquired toxoplasmosis with isolation of the parasite. *Am J Ophthalmol.* 1978;86:548–552.
20. Wilder HC. *Toxoplasma* chorioretinitis in adults. *AMA Arch Ophthalmol.* 1952;48:127–136.
21. Perkins ES. Ocular toxoplasmosis. *Br J Ophthalmol.* 1973; 57;1–17.
22. Desmonts G. Definitive serological diagnosis of ocular toxoplasmosis. *Arch Ophthalmol.* 1966;76:839–851.
23. Aouizerta F, Cazenave J, Poirer L, et al. Detection of *Toxoplasma gondii* in aqueous humor by the polymerase chain-reaction. *Br J Ophthalmol.* 1993;77:107–109.
24. Crawford JB. *Toxoplasma* retinochoroiditis. *Arch Ophthalmol.* 1966;76:829–832.
25. Elkins BS, Holland GN, Opremcak EM, et al. Ocular toxoplasmosis misdiagnosed as cytomegalovirus retinopathy in immunocompromised patients. *Ophthalmology.* 1994; 101:499–507.
26. Yeo JH, Jakobiec FA, Iwamoto T, et al. Opportunistic toxoplasmic retinochoroiditis following chemotherapy for systemic lymphoma. A light and electronmicroscopic study. *Ophthalmology.* 1983;90:885–898.
27. Bertoli F, Espino M, Arosemena JR, Fishback JL, Frenkel JK. A spectrum in the pathology of toxoplasmosis in patients with AIDS. *Arch Pathol Lab Med.* 1995;119: 214–224.
28. Sibley LD, Boothroyd JC. Virulent strains of *Toxoplasma gondii* comprise a single clonal lineage. *Nature.* 1992; 359(6390):82–85.
29. Frenkel JK, Smith DD, Waldeland H, Elwell MR. Immunization against *Toxoplasma. Federation Proc.* 1983;42: 858.
30. Buxton D, Thomson K, Maley S, Wright S, Bos HJ. Vaccination of sheep with a live incomplete strain (S48) of *Toxoplasma gondii* and their immunity to challenge when pregnant. *Vet Record.* 1991;129:89–93.
31. Frenkel JK. Pathogenesis of toxoplasmosis with a consideration of cyst rupture in Besnoitia infection. *Surv Opthalmol.* 1961;6:799–825.
32. Frenkel JK, Escajadillo A. Cyst rupture as a pathogenic mechanism of toxoplasmic encephalitis. *Am J Trop Med Hyg.* 1987;36:517–522.
33. Luft BJ, Naot Y, Araujo FG, Stinson EB, Remington JS. Primary and reactivated toxoplasma infection in patients with cardiac transplants—clinical spectrum and problems in diagnosis in a defined population. *Ann Intern Med.* 1983;99;27–31.
34. Vietzke WM, Gelderman AH, Grimley PM, Valsamis MP.

Toxoplasmosis complicating malignancy. *Cancer.* 1968; 21:816–827.

35. Frenkel JK, Nelson BM, Arias-Stella J. Immunosuppression and toxoplasmic encephalitis: clinical and experimental aspects. *Hum Pathol.* 1975;6:97–111.
36. Frenkel JK, Amare M, Larsen JW. Immune competence in a patient with Hodgkin's disease and relapsing toxoplasmosis. *Infection.* 1978;6:84–91.
37. Gazzinelli RT, Xu YH, Hieny S, Cheever A, Sher A. Simultaneous depletion of CD4 and CD8 lymphocytes-T is required to reactivate chronic infection with *Toxoplasma gondii. J Immunol.* 1992;149;175–180.
38. Slavin MA, Meyers JD, Remington JS, Hackman RC. *Toxoplasma gondii* infection in marrow transplant recipients—a 20 year experience. *Bone Mar Tr.* 1994;13:549–557.
39. Hemsath FA, Pinkerton H. Disseminated cytomegalic inclusion disease and disseminated toxoplasmosis in an adult with myeloid metaplasia. *Am J Clin Pathol.* 1956;26: 36–41.
40. Pinkerton H, Weinman D. *Toxoplasma* infection in man. *Arch Pathol.* 1940;30:374–392.
41. Weitberg AB, Alper JC, Diamond I, Fligiel Z. Acute granulomatous hepatitis in the course of acquired toxoplasmosis. *N Engl J Med.* 1979;300:1093–1096.
42. Frenkel JK, Remington JS. Hepatitis in toxoplasmosis. *N Engl J Med.* 1980;302:178–179. Letter.
43. Sotelo-Avila C, Perry CM, Parvey LS, Eyal FG. Coexistent congenital cytomegalovirus and toxoplasmosis in a newborn infant. *J Tenn Med.* 1974;67:588–592.
44. Frenkel JK. Friedlander S. Toxoplasmosis: pathology of neonal disease. Pathogenesis, diagnosis and treatment. Pub 141. Washington, DC: Public Health Service; 1951.
45. Catterall JR, Hofflin JM, Remington JS. Pulmonary toxoplasmosis. *Am Rev Resp Dis.* 1986;133:704–705.
46. Pinkerton H, Henderson RG. Adult toxoplasmosis. A previously unrecognized disease entity simulating the typhus-spotted fever group. *JAMA.* 1941;116:807–814.
47. Zuelzer WW. Infantile toxoplasmosis. Report of three new cases, including two in which the patients were identical twins. *Arch Pathol.* 1944;38:1–19.
48. Nash G, Kerschma RL, Herndier B, Dubey JP. The pathological manifestations of pulmonary toxoplasmosis in the acquired immunodeficiency syndrome. *Hum Pathol.* 1994;25:652–658.
49. Jautzke G, Sell M, Thalmann U, et al. Extracerebral toxoplasmosis in AIDS—histologic and immunohistological findings based on 80 autopsy cases. *Path Res Pract.* 1993;189;428–436.
50. Hofman P, Bernard E, Michiels JF, Thyss A, Lefichoux Y, Loubiere R. Extracerebral toxoplasmosis in the acquired-immunodeficiency-syndrome (AIDS). *Path Res Pract.* 1993;189:894–901.
51. Frenkel JK. Toxoplasmosis. In: Benirschke K, ed. *Comparative Aspects of Reproductive Failure.* New York: Springer-Verlag; 1967:296–321.
52. Kean BH, Grocott RG. Asymptomatic toxoplasmosis. *Am J Trop Med Hyg.* 1947;27:745–748.
53. Remington JS, Cavanaugh EN. Isolation of the encysted form of *Toxoplasma gondii* from human skeletal muscle and brain. *N Engl J Med.* 1965;273:1308–1310.
54. Kass EH, Andrus S, Adams R, Turner F, Feldman HA. Toxoplasmosis in the human adult. *Arch Intern Med.* 1952; 89:759–782.
55. Prick JJG, Prick-Hoefnagels JAM. Etude clinique et anatomo-pathologique de la toxoplasmose chez l'homme. *Folia Psychiatrica, Neurologica et Neurochirurgica Neerlandica.* 1950;53:352–386.
56. Hooper AD. Acquired toxoplasmosis. *AMA Arch Pathol.* 1957;64:1–9.
57. Koeze TH, Klingon GH. Acquired toxoplasmosis. *Arch Neurol.* 1964;11:191–197.
58. Bobowski SJ, Reed WG. Toxoplasmosis in an adult, presenting as a space-occupying cerebral lesion. *AMA Arch Pathol.* 1958;65:460–464.
59. Huang TE, Chou SM. Occlusive hypertrophic arteritis as the cause of discrete necrosis in CNS toxoplasmosis in the acquired immunodeficiency syndrome. *Hum Pathol.* 1988;19;1210–1214.
60. Post MJD, Chan JC, Hensley GT, Hoffman TA, Moskowitz LB, Lippmann S. *Toxoplasma* encephalitis in Haitian adults with acquired immunodeficiency syndrome: a clinical-pathologic-CT correlation. *Am J Neuroradiol.* 1983;4: 156–162.
61. Frenkel JK. Toxoplasmosis. Mechanisms of infection, laboratory diagnosis and management. *Curr Top Pathol.* 1971;54:28–75.
62. Kagen LJ, Kimball AC, Christian CL. Serologic evidence of toxoplasmosis among patients with polymyositis. *Am J Med.* 1974;56:186–191.
63. Sagrista-Sauleda J, Permanyer-Miralda G, Juste-Sanchez C, et al. Huge chronic pericardial effusion caused by *Toxoplasma gondii. Circulation.* 1982;66:895–897.
64. Zimmerman LE. Ocular pathology of toxoplasmosis. *Survey Ophthalmol.* 1961;6:832–838.
65. Parke DW, Font RL. Diffuse toxoplasmic retinochoroiditis in a patient with AIDS. *Arch Ophthalmol.* 1986;104: 571–575.
66. Berger BB, Egwuagu CE, Freeman WR, Wiley CA. Miliary toxoplasmic retinitis in acquired-immunodeficiency-syndrome. *Arch Ophthalmol.* 1993;111:373–376.
67. Moorthy RS, Smith RE, Rao NA. Progressive ocular toxoplasmosis in patients with acquired-immunodeficiency-syndrome. *Am J Ophthalmol.* 1993;115:742–747.
68. Leyva WH, Santa-Cruz DJ. Cutaneous toxoplasmosis. *J Am Acad Dermat.* 1986;14:600–605.
69. Makioka A, Stavros B, Ellis JT, Johnson AM. Detection and characterization of DNA-polymerase-activity in *Toxoplasma gondii. Parasitol.* 1993;107(Aug):135–139.
70. Hohlfeld P, Daffos F, Costa JM, Thulliez P, Forestier F, Vidaud M. Prenatal diagnosis of congenital toxoplasmosis with a polymerase-chain-reaction test on amniotic fluid. *N Engl J Med.* 1994;331:695–699.
71. Gross U, Muller J, Roos T, Schrod L, Heeseman J. Possible reasons for failure of conventional tests for diagnosis of fatal congenital toxoplasmosis—report of a case diagnosed by PCR and immunoblot. *Infection.* 1992;20: 149–152.
72. Schoonde E, Galama J, Kraaijev C, Vandrute J, Meuwisse J, Melchers W. Value of the polymerase chain-reaction for the detection of *Toxoplasma gondii* in cerebrospinal-fluid from patients with AIDS. *Clin Infect Dis.* 1993;16:661–666.
73. Roth A, Roth B, Hoffken G, Steuber S, Khalifa KI, Janitsch

K. Application of the polymerase chain-reaction in the diagnosis of pulmonary toxoplasmosis in immunocompromised patients. *Europe J Clin Microb.* 1993;11(12): 1177–1181.

74. Frenkel JK, Jacobs L. Ocular toxoplasmosis. *AMA Arch Ophthalmol.* 1958;59:260–279.
75. Desmonts G, Remington JS. Direct agglutination test for diagnosis of *Toxoplasma* infection: method for increasing sensitivity and specificity. *J Clin Micro.* 1980;11:562–568.
76. Decoster A, Darcy F, Caron A, et al. Anti-P30 IgA antibodies as prenatal markers of congenital toxoplasma infection. *Clin Exp Immunol.* 1992;87:310–315.
77. Decoster A, Slizewicz B, Simon J, et al. Platelia-toxo IgA, a new kit for early diagnosis of congenital toxoplasmosis by detection of anti-P30 immunoglobulin A antibodies. *J Clin Micro.* 1991;29(10):2291–2295.
78. Wong SY, Hajdu MP, Ramirez R, Thulliez P, McLeod R, Remington JS. Role of specific immunoglobulin-E in diagnosis of acute toxoplasma infection and toxoplasmosis. *J Clin Micro.* 1993;31(11):2952–2959.
79. Wilson M, Ware DA, Walls KW. Evaluation of commercial serodiagnostic kits for toxoplasmosis. *J Clin Micro.* 1987; 25:2262–2265.
80. Wong SY, Israelski DM, Remington JS. AIDS-associated toxoplasmosis. In: Sande MA, Wolberding PA, eds. *The Medical Management of AIDS.* 4th ed. Philadelphia: WB Saunders; 1995:460–493.
81. Gluckstein D, Ruskin J. Rapid oral desensitization to trimethoprim–sulfamethoxazole (TMP–SMZ): use in prophylaxis for *Pneumocystis carinii* pneumonia in patients with AIDS who were previously intolerant to TMP–SMZ. *Clin Infect Dis.* 1995;20:849–853.
82. CDC. Multistate outbreak of *Escherichia coli* O 157:H7 infections from hamburgers—Western United States, 1992–1993. *MMWR.* 1994;42(14):258–263.
83. Frenkel JK, Hassanein KM, Hassanein RS, Brown E, Thulliez P, Quintereo-Nuñez R. Transmission of *Toxoplasma* in Panama City, Panama: a five-year prospective cohort study of children, cats, rodents, birds, and soil. *Am J Trop Med Hyg.* 1995;53(5):458–468.
84. Fletcher RH, Fletcher SW, Wagner EH. *Clinical Epidemiology, The Essentials.* 2nd ed. Baltimore: Williams & Wilkins; 1988:51–61.
85. Guerina NG, Hsu HW, Meissner HC, et al. Neonatal serologic screening and early treatment for congenital *Toxoplasma gondii* infection. *N Engl J Med.* 1994;330 (26):1858–1863.
86. Frenkel JK. Congenital toxoplasmosis: prevention or palliation? *Am J Obstet Gynecol.* 1981;141:359–361.

CHAPTER 141

Trichomoniasis

Jacqueline A. Wieneke, Zuher M. Naib, and Ernest E. Lack

The Aim of Medicine is surely not to make men virtuous; it is to safeguard and rescue them from the consequences of their vice.

H. L. Mencken (1880–1956)

INTRODUCTION

Trichomoniasis is infection by the protozoan flagellate *Trichomonas vaginalis*. *Trichomonas* is a genus of parasitic protozoan flagellates with three species identified in humans: *T tenax, T hominis,* and *T vaginalis.*[1–3] *Trichomonas tenax* lives only in the oral cavity and *T hominis* lives in the large intestine[1,3] and both are nonpathogenic for humans.[4] *Trichomonas vaginalis* infects the urogenital tract. It is the only species pathogenic in humans.[3] *Trichomonas vaginalis* is a surface-dwelling protozoan that provokes inflammation and exudate in the urogenital tracts of male and female subjects.[1,3,5] It lives in the lumen of the vagina, urethra (Figure 141–1), and prostatic ducts and does not invade.[1]

LIFE CYCLE

The life cycle of *T vaginalis* is relatively simple. Humans are the only natural host.[3] The organism requires a strictly anaerobic environment for optimal growth and reproduction[3,6] and exists only in the trophozoite form.[3,7] The organism is fastidious, requiring 16 vitamins, purines, pyrimidines, cholesterol, and various minerals and carbohydrates.[6,8] The vagina contains many of the required nutrients[6,9] and is thus a fertile site for infection. The increased concentration of iron in the vagina during menses may facilitate overgrowth of *T vaginalis* and cause worsening of symptoms.[6,10]

EPIDEMIOLOGY

Trichomonas vaginalis is worldwide and is the most prevalent, nonviral, sexually transmitted disease (STD).[3,6,11,12] The World Health Organization estimates that approximately 180 million people are infected throughout the world each year.[3,12] It is difficult to determine the prevalence of trichomoniasis in the United States because currently it is not a reportable disease[3]; based on available data, however, it is estimated that three to six million new infections occur each year.[3,6,11] Prevalence varies among different socioeconomic groups.[1,6,13] In STD clinics, the prevalence ranges up to 39.6%,[6,13] with the highest incidence among prostitutes.[1] Peak incidence is from 16 to 35 years with no seasonal variation.[3,14] In women of reproductive age it is second only to bacterial vaginosis as a cause of vaginitis.[3] The organism is much less frequent in men, causing less than 5% of urethral infections.[9] African-Americans are at increased risk as are those who have multiple sexual partners, a previous history of STD, and coexistent infection with *Neisseria gonorrhoeae* and those who fail to use barrier or hormonal contraceptives.[6,13] *Trichomonas vaginalis* may be spontaneously cleared more rapidly by men than by women.[6,9,15,16] It has been suggested that the high zinc content of prostatic fluid is cytotoxic to *T vaginalis* and may be important as a defense mechanism.[4,9,17] An important reservoir of *T vaginalis* is the asymptomatic carrier, which helps to maintain the disease in humans despite adequate therapy. It is estimated that as many

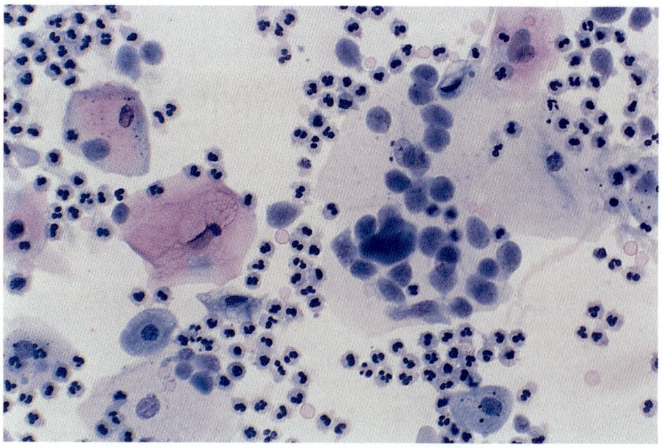

Figure 141–1. Numerous *T vaginalis* in urethral exudate of an adult male patient. In addition to the *T vaginalis* organisms, there are nucleated squamous cells and acute inflammatory cells (Papanicolaou stain, ×400).

as 50% of female carriers are asymptomatic.[2] Infection creates no immunity and reinfection after treatment is common.

TRANSMISSION

Transmission of *T vaginalis* occurs through sexual intercourse.[1,6] The organism lives only in the urogenital tract. In women it is in squamous mucosa of vagina and epithelium lining Skene's glands, and urethra, while in men the prostate gland and urethra are sites of infection as well as beneath the foreskin of those who are not circumcised.[3] The incubation period for infection is 4 to 28 days.[3] The rate of infectivity after intercourse with an infected person is estimated at 70% to 80%.[2] Transmission rates are higher from men to women than from women to men.[6,9] Seventy percent of males develop trichomoniasis within 48 hours of exposure[6,16] compared to 85% of exposed women.[6,18]

There are rare reports of perinatal transmission of trichomoniasis to female infants[6] from the birth canal of infected mothers at the time of delivery.[9,19–21] Female infants are more susceptible to infection because of high circulating estrogen levels of maternal origin.[9] Infection is rare in the prepubertal female because the necessary hormonal environment has not developed.[2] In fact, the finding of infection in a preadolescent female might raise the possibility of sexual abuse.[3,9] There are no reported infections from exposure to fomites.[6]

CLINICAL PRESENTATION

In female subjects symptoms are usually caused by acute or chronic vaginitis sometimes associated with vulvitis.[1] A classic feature is a yellow-green, frothy or bubbly, purulent discharge, often accompanied by pruritus and dysuria.[1,2,6] The discharge, however, is in less than 50% of infected women.[6] A malodorous or "musty" smell is reported in approximately 10%.[6] Symptoms are often exacerbated after menstruation when the vaginal pH is between 5 and 5.5, an ideal environment for growth of the parasite.[1] Dyspareunia is a less common complaint.[22] Urethritis is also common[2] and is a more frequent presenting sign in men.[2,5] On examination of the female patient there are often multiple, punctate hemorrhages and/or areas of capillary dilatation of the cervical mucosa (strawberry cervix) on colposcopic examination.[2,23]

In men *T vaginalis* may produce prostatitis[24] or urethritis (Figure 141–1). Symptoms are present in approximately 10% of patients,[9] and the usual finding is a white, milky urethral discharge of at least 4 weeks' duration[1] with mild dysuria and burning after voiding.[9] Generalized lymphadenopathy is rare because the organism does not invade. *Trichomonas vaginalis* does not cause pelvic inflammatory disease.[9]

PATHOLOGY

Although biopsy is rarely done, the few specimens studied have revealed changes that vary from normal to acute inflammation of mucosa and submucosa.[1] The surface epithelium may be covered with an inflammatory exudate and mucus.[1] There is usually focal erosion of the mucosa progressing to necrosis and hemorrhage with loss of surface epithelium.[1] The pathogenic effect is from cytoadherence to epithelial cells (Figure 141–2),

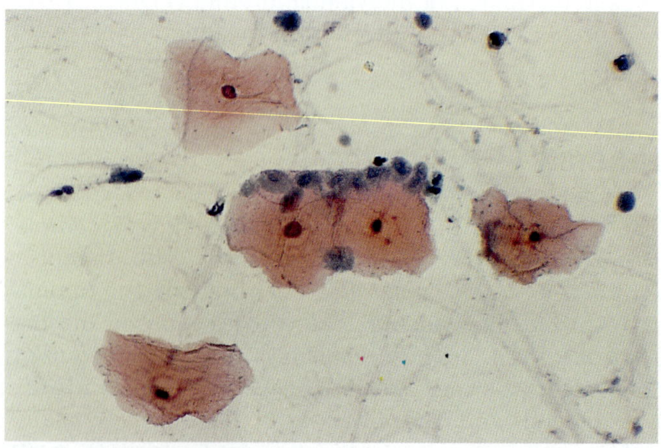

Figure 141–2. *Trichomonas vaginalis* in cervical/vaginal smear. Many organisms are present along the surface of two squamous cells (Papanicolaou stain, ×400).

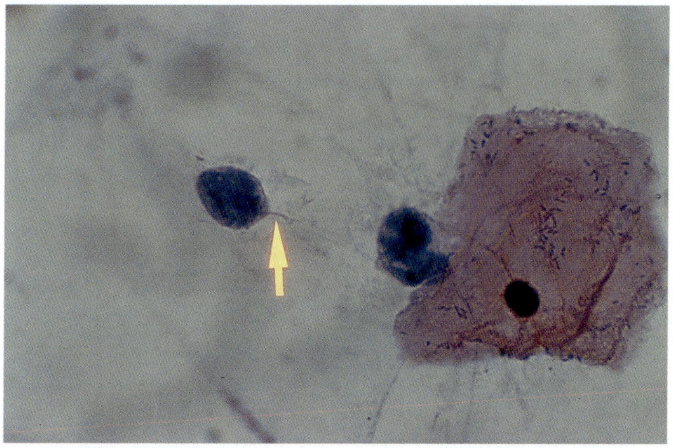

Figure 141–3. *Trichomonas vaginalis.* Protozoan in cervical/vaginal smear is "pear shaped" with nucleus toward anterior pole of organism. One or more flagella are indicated by arrow (Papanicolaou stain, ×1000).

which appears to be mediated by trichomonad surface proteins in a receptor-ligand-type reaction. This may help to explain the predominance of infection in stratified squamous epithelium[25] with sparing of columnar cells.[2,4] The organism is not usually identified in tissue sections. There has been no proven association between infection with *T vaginalis* and cervical neoplasia.[1] In cytology preparations the organism is unicellular, ovoid, and varies greatly in size from 10 to 30 μm.[9,26] Occasionally the protozoan may have one or more discernible flagella (Figure 141–3). Sometimes there are faint nuclei and abundant pink siderophilic granules (Figure 141–4). There may be numerous superficial cells indicating high estrogen index and many "naked" nuclei caused by cytolysis. Neutrophils and red blood cells are almost invariably present with *T vaginalis* infection[1] and this inflammation may obscure the detailed morphology of the organism.

Trichomonas vaginalis is extracellular and is motile because of four anterior flagella and a fifth flagellum that runs along the length of its body[3,6,9] (Figure 141–5). Ultrastructurally, *T vaginalis* lacks mitochondria,[3,6,27] peroxisomes, and glycosomes,[6,27] however, it does have highly developed Golgi complexes.[6] The cytoplasm is rich in glycogen granules and ribosomes, and also contains electron-dense chromatic granules called hydrogenosomes.[6,28] These structures are unique to trichomonads, and are important in generating hydrogen, which creates the necessary anaerobic environment by combining with oxygen.[3,28] The nucleus is large with 5N chromosomes, and replication of the organism occurs by longitudinal, binary fission.[3]

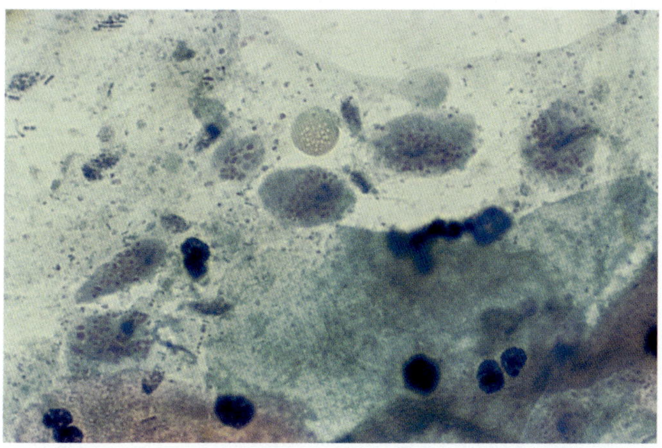

Figure 141–4. Multiple *T vaginalis* in cervical/vaginal smear have a pale-staining nucleus and small reddish-brown granules in cytoplasm (Papanicolaou stain, ×1000).

DIAGNOSIS

A wet mount preparation of scrapings of the vaginal fornices is the classic method of diagnosing *T vaginalis* infection.[6] The epithelial cells are placed in 0.85% sodium chloride and phase contrast microscopy is used to observe the motile parasites.[6,29] The specimen should be examined soon after the material is obtained

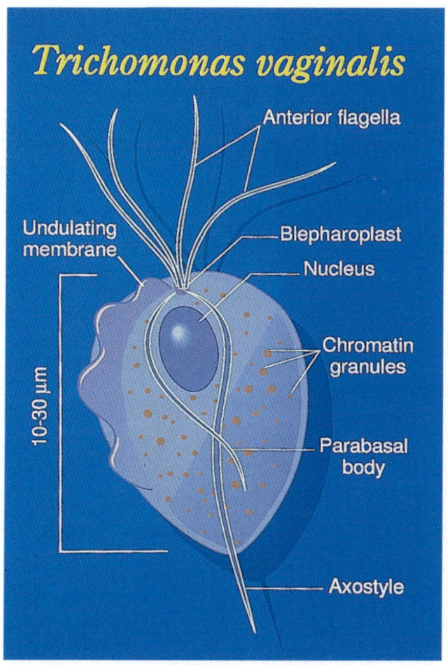

Figure 141–5. Detailed diagram of morphology of *T vaginalis*. Blepharoplast lies at base of four anterior flagella.

since the organisms will lose their characteristic jerking movements as the specimen cools.[29] The sensitivity of this method has been disputed and reports range from rates of 40% to 92%.[9,30] Other procedures that have been used for diagnosis include staining with acridine orange[6,31] and Giemsa stain.[6,32,33] The organism can be identified in cervical/vaginal smears stained with the Papanicolaou (PAP) stain with a sensitivity ranging from 33% to 79% and a specificity of 89% to 100%.[9,30,34,35] Culture in Diamond's medium can yield a diagnosis in 86% to 97% of cases, and in combination with wet prep microscopic examination the sensitivity approaches 100%.[6,9,36,37] A disadvantage of the culture method is the 2- to 7-day waiting period.

Additional diagnostic tests have been developed to enhance sensitivity, specificity, and turnaround time.[2] Fluorescent monoclonal antibody techniques (direct or indirect) may be superior to wet mount examination[6] and are faster than culture.[33,35,38,39] The monoclonal antibody techniques are limited primarily by low concentration of the organism in the fluid studied.[2]

Enzyme-linked immunosorbent assays can detect *T vaginalis* directly in vaginal secretions,[38,40–42] and this method has been reported to have a sensitivity of 89% and a specificity of 97%.[38] A rapid latex agglutination test has a sensitivity of 95% and specificity of 99%, and the test can be performed in minutes without the use of a microscope or other specialized equipment or training.[9,43] Newer diagnostic techniques target DNA for identification of the organism,[6] including in situ hybridization and polymerase chain reaction.[6,44,45]

TREATMENT

The agent of choice for treating *T vaginalis* infection is metronidazole[2] with cure rates of 82% to 100%.[2,6] All infections, including asymptomatic persons and recent sexual partners, should be treated, since those with asymptomatic infections may infect others.[6]

PROGNOSIS

The prognosis is excellent and complications are extremely rare.[2] The major concern is the asymptomatic patients that remain carriers.[2] The diagnosis of trichomoniasis should alert the clinician to the possibility of other STDs that can have more serious sequelae.[3] Aggressive public health policies may decrease the incidence of infection in the future.[2]

REFERENCES

1. Gutierrez Y. Intestinal and urogenital flagellates: trichomonas. In: Guitierrez Y, ed. *Diagnostic Pathology of Parasitic Infections with Clinical Correlations.* Philadelphia: Lea & Febiger; 1990:13–19.
2. Millikan LE. Trichomoniasis. In: Parish LC, Gschnait F, eds. *Sexually Transmitted Diseases, A Guide for Clinicians.* New York: Springer-Verlag; 1989:138–144.
3. Thomason JL, Gelbart SM. *Trichomonas vaginalis.* Obstet Gynecol. 1989;74:536–541.
4. Graves A, Gardner WA, Jr. Pathogenicity of *Trichomonas vaginalis. Clin Obstet Gynecol.* 1993;36:145–152.
5. Krieger JN, Jenny C, Verdon M, et al. Clinical manifestations of trichomoniasis in men. *Ann Intern Med.* 1993; 118:844–849.
6. Heine P, McGregor JA. *Trichomonas:* a reemerging pathogen. *Clin Obstet Gynecol.* 1993;36(1):137–144.
7. Markell EK, Voge M, John DT. Lumen-dwelling protozoa. In: Markell ER, Voge M, John DT, eds. *Medical Parasitology.* Philadelphia: WB Saunders; 1992:70–75.
8. Linstead D. New defined and semi-defined media for cultivation of the flagellate *Trichomonas vaginalis. Parasitology.* 1981;83:125–137.
9. Moldwin RM. Sexually transmitted protozoal infections. *Trichomonas vaginialis, Entamoeba histolytica,* and *Giardia lamblia. Urol Clin North Am.* 1992;19(1):93–101.
10. Rein MF, Chapel TA. Trichomoniasis, candidiasis and the minor venereal diseases. *Clin Obstet Gynecol.* 1975;18: 73–88.
11. McLellan R, Spence MR, Brockman M, Rattel L, Smith JL. The clinical diagnosis of trichomoniasis. *Obstet Gynecol.* 1982;60:30–34.
12. Krieger JN. Urologic aspects of trichomoniasis. *Invest Urol.* 1982;18:411–417.
13. Lossick JG. Epidemiology of urogenital trichomoniasis. In: Honinberg BM, ed. *Trichomonads Parasitic in Humans.* New York: Springer-Verlag; 1989:311–323.
14. Charles D. Sexually transmitted diseases. In: Charles D, ed. *Infections in Obstetrics and Gynecology.* Philadelphia: WB Saunders; 1980:39–43.
15. Willcox RR. Epidemiological aspects of human trichomoniasis. *Br J Vener Dis.* 1960;36:167–174.
16. Weston TET, Nicol CS. Natural history of trichomonal infection in males. *Br J Vener Dis.* 1963;39:251–257.
17. Krieger JN, Rein MF. Zinc sensitivity of *Trichomonas vaginalis:* in vitro studies and clinical implications. *J Infect Dis.* 1982;146:341–342.
18. Honinberg BM. Trichomonads of importance in human medicine. In: Kreier JP, ed. *Parasitic Protozoa.* New York: Academic Press; 1978;2:358–365.
19. Al-Salihi FL, Curran JP, Wang JS. Neonatal *Trichomonas vaginalis:* report of three cases and review of the literature. *Pediatrics.* 1974;53:196–200.
20. Blattner RJ. *Trichomonas vaginalis* infection in a newborn infant. *J Pediatr.* 1967;71:608–610.
21. Littlewood JM, Kohler HG. Urinary tract infection by

Trichomonas vaginalis in a newborn baby. *Arch Dis Child.* 1966;41:693–695.

22. Hughes HE, Gordon AM, Bar GTD. A clinical and laboratory study of trichomoniasis of the female genital tract. *J Obstet Gynecol Br Commonwealth.* 1966;73:821–824.
23. Wolner-Hansen P, Krieger JN, Stevens C, et al. Clinical manifestations of vaginal trichomoniasis. *JAMA.* 1989;261: 571–576.
24. Gardner WA, Culberson DE, Bennett BD. *Trichomonas vaginalis* in the prostate gland. *Arch Pathol Lab Med.* 1986;110:430–432.
25. Alderete JF, Garza GE. Specific nature of *Trichomonas vaginalis* parasitism of host cell surfaces. *Infect Immun.* 1985;50:701–708.
26. Wherton A, Honigberg BM. Structure of trichomonads as revealed by scanning electron microscopy. *Protozool.* 1979;26:56–62.
27. Muller M. Biochemistry of *Trichomonas vaginalis.* In: Honinberg BM, ed. *Trichomonads Parasitic in Humans.* New York: Springer-Verlag; 1989:53–83.
28. Muller M. Energy metabolism of protozoa without mitochondria. *Ann Rev Microbiol.* 1988;42:465–488.
29. Fouts AC, Kraus SJ. *Trichomonas vaginalis:* reevaluation of its clinical presentation and laboratory diagnosis. *J Infect Dis.* 1980;141:137–143.
30. Weinberger MW, Harger JH. Accuracy of the PAP smear in the diagnosis of asymptomatic infection with *Trichomonas vaginalis. Obstet Gynecol.* 1993;82:425–429.
31. Hipp SS, Kirkwood MW. Hassan HA. Screening for *Trichomonas vaginalis* infection by use of acridine orange fluorescent microscopy. *Sex Transm Dis.* 1979;6:235–238.
32. Mason PR, Super H, Fripp PJ. Comparison of four techniques for the routine diagnosis of *Trichomonas vaginalis* infection. *J Clin Pathol.* 1976;29:154–157.
33. Bickley LS, Kricher K, Punsalang A, Trupei MA, Reichman R, Menegus M. Comparison of direct fluorescent antibody, acridine orange, wet mount and culture for detection of *Trichomonas vaginalis* in women attending a public sexually transmitted diseases clinic. *Sex Transm Dis.* 1989;16: 127–131.
34. Roongpisuthipong A, Grimes DA, Hadgu A. Is the Papanicolaou smear useful for diagnosing sexually transmitted diseases? *Obstet Gynecol.* 1987;69:820–824.
35. Krieger JN, Tam M, Stevens C, et al. Diagnosis of trichomoniasis. Comparison of conventional wet-mount examination with cytologic studies, cultures and monoclonal antibody staining of direct specimens. *JAMA.* 1988;259: 1223–1227.
36. Gelbart SM, Thomason JL, Osypowski PJ, James JA, Hamilton PR. Comparison of Diamond's medium modified and Kupferberg medium for detection of *Trichomonas vaginalis. J Clin Microbiol.* 1989;27:1095–1096.
37. Schmid GP, Matheny LC, Zaidi AA, Kraus SJ. Evaluation of six media for the growth of *Trichomonas vaginalis* from vaginal secretions. *J Clin Microbiol.* 1989;27:1230–1233.
38. Lisi PJ, Dondero R, Kwiatkoski D, Spence M, Rein M, Alderete J. Monoclonal antibody based enzyme-linked immunosorbent assay for *Trichomonas vaginalis. J Clin Microbiol.* 1988;26:1684–1686.
39. Smith RF. Detection of *Trichomonas vaginalis* in vaginal specimens by direct immunofluorescence assay. *J Clin Microbiol.* 1986;24:1107–1108.
40. Sibau L, Bebb D, Proctor E, Bowie W. Enzyme-linked immunosorbent assay for the diagnosis of *Trichomonas* in women. *Sex Transm Dis.* 1987;14:216–220.
41. Watt RM, Philip A, Wos SM, Sam GJ. Rapid assay for immunological detection of *Trichomonas vaginalis. J Clin Microbiol.* 1986;24:551–555.
42. Yule A, Gellen MC, Oriel JD, Ackers JP. Detection of *Trichomonas vaginalis* antigen in women by enzyme immunoassay. *J Clin Pathol.* 1987;40:566–568.
43. Carney JA, Unadkat P, Yule A, Rajakunar R, Lacey CJ, Ackers JP. New rapid latex agglutination test for diagnosing *Trichomonas vaginalis* infection. *J Clin Pathol.* 1988;41: 806–808.
44. Rubino S, Muresu R, Rappelli P, et al. Molecular probe for identification of *Trichomonas vaginalis* DNA. *J Clin Microbiol.* 1991;29:702–706.
45. Riley DE, Roberts MC, Takayama T, Krieger JN. Development of a PCR-based diagnosis of *Trichomonas vaginalis. J Clin Microbiol.* 1992;30:465–472.

CHAPTER 142

African Trypanosomiasis

Mark G. Hanly

Ex Africa semper aliquid novi.

Pliny the Elder (A.D. 23–79)

Blood is the originating cause of all men's diseases.

The Talmud, Baba Nathra

DEFINITION

African trypanosomiasis (AT) is the systemic protozoal disease that results from infection by either the two pathogenic subspecies of salivarian hemoflagellates that form part of the *Trypanosoma brucei* complex, namely *T b gambiense* and *T b rhodesiense.* The third member of the *T b* complex, *T brucei brucei,* does not cause disease in humans. Both *T b gambiense* and *T b rhodesiense* are transmitted by the bite of the tsetse fly.

Synonyms for AT include Human African Trypanosomiasis (HAT), Trypanosomiasis, African Sleeping Sickness, Rhodesian Sleeping Sickness (*T b rhodesiense* infection), Gambian Sleeping Sickness (*T b gambiense* infection), West African Sleeping Sickness (*T b gambiense* infection), East African Sleeping Sickness (*T b rhodesiense* infection), Maladie du Sommeil (French), Sonolencia (Portuguese.)

GEOGRAPHIC DISTRIBUTION

African trypanosomiasis was first clinically recognized in Africa during the middle of the 18th century.[1] It was later reported in slaves shipped from West Africa to the West Indies during the 19th century,[2] but the full extent of the problem was not recognized until 1901, when an outbreak in Uganda claimed more than 20,000 lives. Today, *T brucei* is widely distributed throughout sub-Saharan Africa, occurring in more than 200 separate endemic loci within the tsetse fly belt, which extends across Africa in a band from approximately latitude 20°N to latitude 20°S (Figure 142–1). An estimated 50 to 60 million people live in the "at risk" areas of Africa, which covers more than 10 million square kilometers.[3] Each year about 10,000 new infections are reported on the African continent,[4] where the condition still poses a significant health risk and prevents full economic utilization of large tracts of land.[5–8] Occasional infections of expatriates who have been to Africa are reported in nonendemic countries.[9–16]

VECTOR, LIFE CYCLE, TRANSMISSION, EPIDEMIOLOGY

The vector of the trypanosome is the tsetse fly, which is part of the insect genus *Glossina.* Six species of flies are recognized as the principal vectors for trypanosomiasis: *G morsitans, G fuscipes, G pallidipes, G palpalis, G tachinoides,* and *G swynnertoni* (Table 142–1). The most important vectors of *T b gambiense* are the riverine tsetse flies *G palpalis* and *G tachinoides.* The savanna tsetse fly *G morsitans* is most commonly associated with the spread of *T b rhodesiense* (Figure 142–2).

Infection of the vector and the cyclical development of the parasite begins when blood and tissue fluid are drawn into the tsetse gut during the course of a blood meal (Figure 142–3). The trypanosomes are ingested by the tsetse fly in the trypomastigote form. Within the lumen of the tsetse midgut, the parasites transform to the procyclic form, a change that is accom-

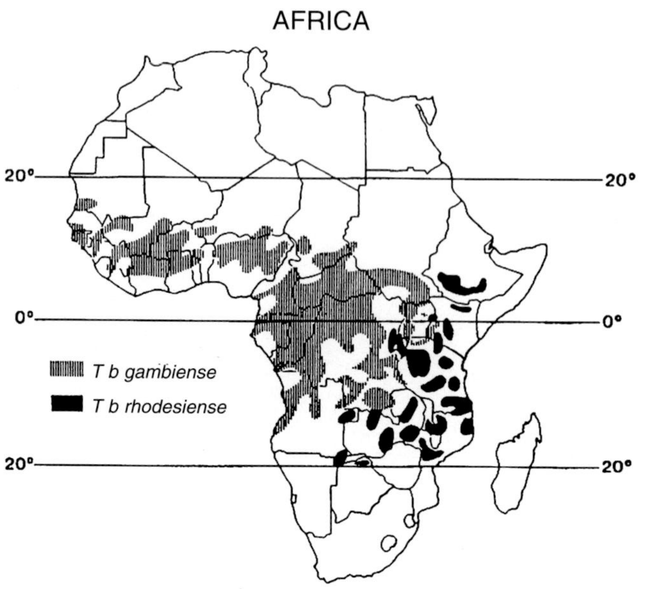

Figure 142–1. The "Tsetse Belt": The distribution of *Trypanosoma brucei rhodesiense* and *Trypanosoma brucei gambiense* in Africa.

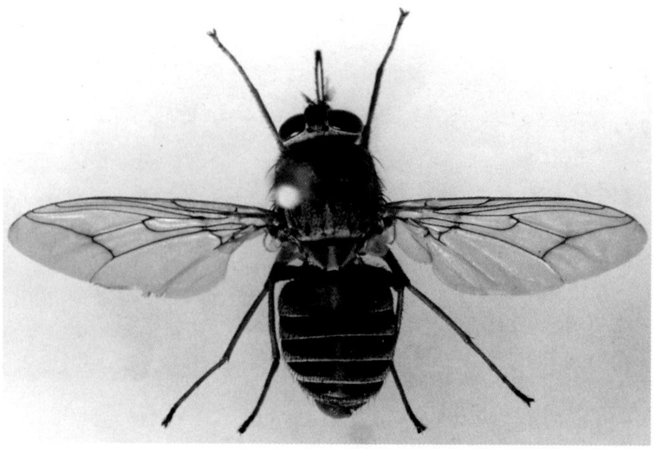

Figure 142–2. *Glossina morsitans. (Photograph courtesy of Brian Coulman, Chief Tsetse Field Officer, Tsetse Control, Harare, Zimbabwe.)*

panied by alterations in parasite oxygen utilization, dietary substrate use,[17] and active division of the organism.[18] The developing trypanosomes then penetrate the chitinous peritropic membrane lining the intestine of the tsetse fly and enter the epiperitropic space,[19] where they undergo further multiplication by binary fission. In the next stage of their development the trypanosomes travel to the tsetse proventriculus, where they reinvade the endotropic space and journey via the foregut to infect the salivary glands. The parasites then develop "flagellipodia," with which they attach securely to the cells lining the salivary gland of the tsetse fly.[20] Once within the salivary glands, the trypanosomes undergo their final division in the tsetse fly.

At this point in their development, the parasites form a variable antigenic coat and detach from the lining cells to lie free in the lumen of the tsetse salivary gland, ready to infect the vertebrate host at the next feed. The entire development within the tsetse fly takes 2 to 5 weeks. Both sexes of tsetse fly can carry the parasite and, following infection, the fly remains infective for the rest of its life. Any single fly may carry more than one species of trypanosome.[21]

The parasite is introduced into the vertebrate host as the tsetse fly feeds. The principal vertebrate hosts for *T b rhodesiense* are the antelope and other wild animals.

TABLE 142–1. COMPARISON OF *TRYPANOSOMA BRUCEI RHODESIENSE* AND *TRYPANOSOMA BRUCEI GAMBIENSE*

	T b rhodesiense	***T b gambiense***
Vectors	*Glossina morsitans* *G fuscipes* *G pallidipes* *G swynnertoni*	*G palpalis* *G tachinoides* *G fuscipes*
Vertebrate host	Wild game	Human; domestic pig
Endemic areas	Central and East Africa	West Africa
Clinical course	Rapid/fulminant	Indolent

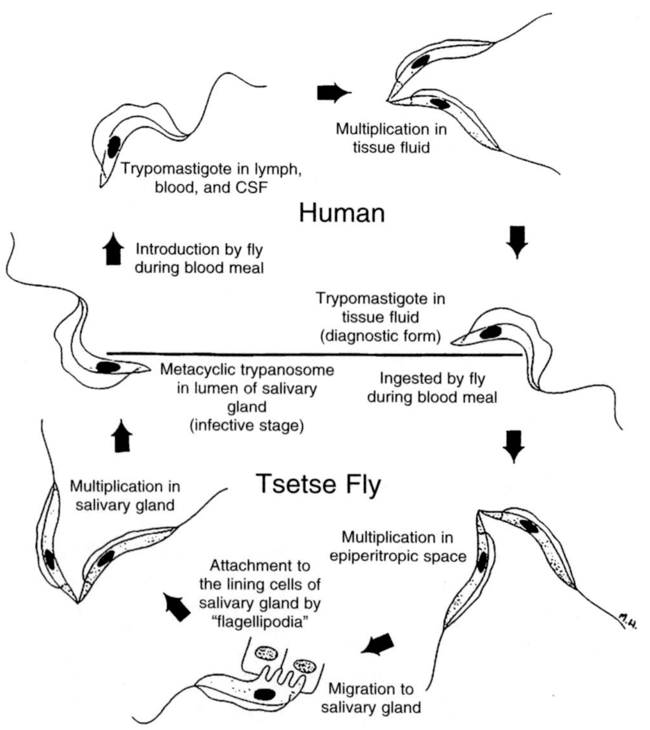

Figure 142–3. The life cycle of *Trypanosoma brucei rhodesiense* and *Trypanosoma brucei gambiense* in the tsetse fly and in humans.

Humans are the most important vertebrate host of *T b gambiense,* although the domestic pig may also fill this role. At the start of feeding, the infective metacyclic forms of the trypanosome lying in the lumen of the salivary gland are expelled through the proboscis of the fly into the subcutaneous tissues of the host. As few as 10 trypanosomes are required to establish an infection.[22] After introduction into the vertebrate host the parasites remain localized at the site of the bite for 1 to 2 days, during which they multiply and then begin to spread systemically. In the experimental setting, trypomastigote forms of the parasite may be recovered from local lymph nodes 2 to 3 days after infection.[23] Once within the vertebrate host, the trypanosomes escape the host's immune response by varying their surface coat of glycoprotein (VSG).[24,25]

Glossina shows peaks of feeding and flight activity in the early morning and evening, preferring to rest during the hottest times of the day. The epidemiologic factors associated with the transmission of the trypanosomes by the tsetse fly have been investigated extensively and relate conceptually to situations of "sustained triple contact" (STC)[26] between humans, the vector, and the vertebrate host. STC occurs during activities such as water collection, hunting,[27] and farming, or may develop as a result of drought,[28] excessive periresidential vegetation,[7] and disturbance of local ecosystems.[29] Factors such as ambient temperature[30] may also affect transmission of the trypanosomes by the tsetse fly. Although the exact reasons are not well understood, seldom more than 1% of the tsetse fly population in any endemic area of trypanosomiasis carry the parasite.[31] The tsetse fly is a fastidious feeder and appears to be repulsed by humans, feeding on them only when sufficiently hungry.[32]

Transmission of the parasite rarely occurs by means other than through the bite of the tsetse fly. Transplacental spread has been recorded,[33–35] and infection also may result from contaminated blood transfusion[36] or from a laboratory accident.[37] It may be possible for other biting insects[38] to transmit the parasite, but this mode of transmission probably plays little significant role in the spread of the disease.[39,40]

MORPHOLOGIC FEATURES OF THE ORGANISM

Trypanosoma brucei gambiense and *T b rhodesiense* are morphologically indistinguishable from one another and can be separated only by isoenzyme studies[41] or DNA hybridization.[42] In the vertebrate host they appear as flagellates measuring 16 to 30 μm in length and 1.5 to 3.5 μm in diameter. Naturally colorless, they stain well with the Giemsa stain (Figure 142–4). They have a large, oval, centrally placed nucleus that occupies about

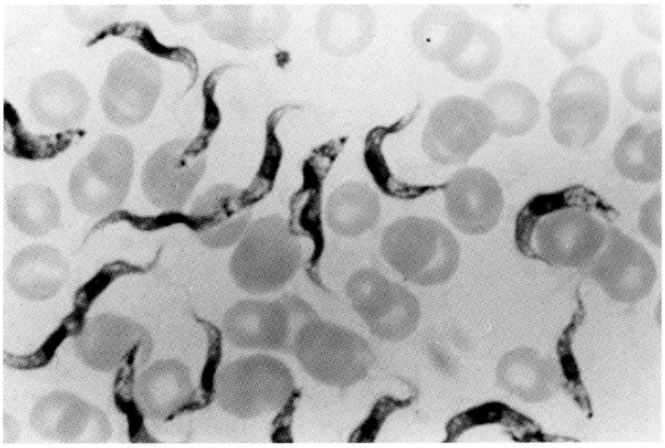

Figure 142–4. Trypomastigote blood form of *Trypanosoma brucei rhodesiense* in a thin blood film (Giemsa, ×1000).

one quarter of the length of the organism. In Giemsa preparations the nucleus stains red, as does the kinetoplast, which is situated at the posterior end of the parasite. The cytoplasm is pale blue and contains scattered, mauve, volutin granules. A single flagellum arises from the parasite and proceeds anteriorly along the free edge of the undulating membrane to project from the anterior end of the organism. Ultrastructural studies show that the kinetoplast is continuous, with a single long mitochondrion that occupies much of the core of the parasite and that is intimately associated with the basal body from which the flagellum arises[43–45] (Figure 142–5).

CLINICAL FEATURES

African trypanosomiasis is a disease of protean manifestations and the clinical features of both *T b gambiense* and *T b rhodesiense* infections may be very similar. Infection by *T b gambiense* tends to cause a disease with a prolonged course when compared to the clinical progression of the illness caused by *T b rhodesiense. Trypanosoma brucei rhodesiense* usually, but not exclusively, causes a fulminant illness that, if untreated, is fatal in months or even weeks. The clinical features of AT can be divided into three stages (Table 142–2):[46] the chancre, the hemolymphatic stage, and the meningoencephalitic stage. The three stages are most clearly defined in *T b gambiense* infection with its longer and more protracted course.

The Chancre

Between 20% and 50% of patients develop a chancre (Figure 142–6)[47,48] at the site of infection. The chancre is seen more commonly in Caucasians and those

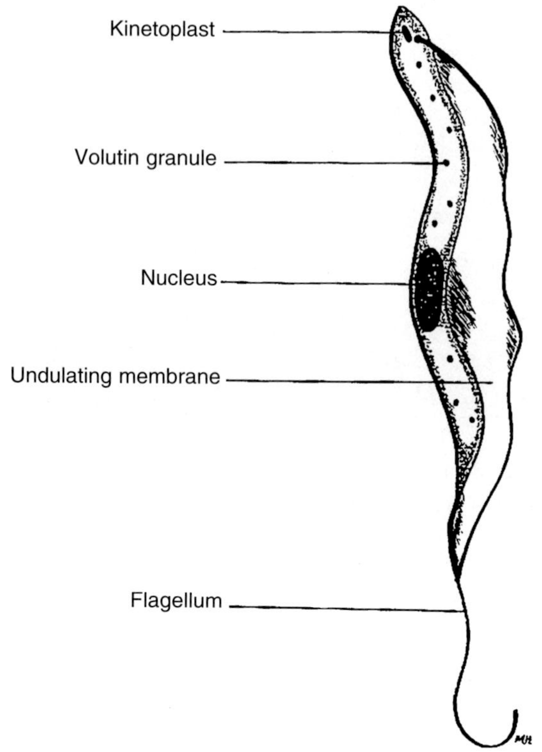

Figure 142–5. Diagram of trypomastigote blood form of *Trypanosoma brucei* complex illustrating features that can be identified by light microscopy.

TABLE 142–2. CLINICAL FEATURES OF AFRICAN TRYPANOSOMIASIS[46]

Clinical Stage	Clinical Features	Differential Diagnosis
Stage 1: Chancre	Chancre[12,47,48]	Hypersensitivity to insect bite Furuncule Anthrax[49] Tick bite (*R conorii*)[50,51]
Stage 2: Hemolymphatic	Pyrexia[52,53] Lymphadenopathy[53] Winterbottom's sign[55] Splenomegaly Rashes[12] Kerandel's sign[56] Abnormal EKG[54,57] DIC[58,59] Thrombocytopenia[60] Anemia[53] High ESR High serum IgM	Typhoid Malaria AIDS-related complex (ARC) Tuberculosis Lymphoma[52]
Stage 3: Meningoencephalitic	Depression Behavioral changes Seizures Pruritis Meningismus Obesity (early)[46] Facial edema Coma Death	Chronic meningitis Tertiary syphilis Cerebral tumor Viral encephalitis

patients infected by *T b rhodesiense.*[12] Clinically the chancre must be differentiated from cutaneous anthrax and tick bites associated with the transmission of *Rickettsia conorii.*[49,50,51] Without therapy, the chancre continues to develop for 2 to 3 weeks before healing with a typical perilesional desquamation.

Hemolymphatic Stage

The development of the hemolymphatic stage is heralded by a generalized rash, fever, and lymphadenopathy as the parasite disseminates through lymphatics to enter lymph nodes and the bloodstream. This phase may be fulminant in patients with *T b rhodesiense* infection and may follow the development of the chancre by only a few days.[52–55] Lymphadenopathy occurs in both *T b gambiense* and *T b rhodesiense* infection, but the lymphadenopathy associated with *T b rhodesiense* is often more generalized and is frequently accompanied by hepatosplenomegaly.[53,56–59] Patients with *T b rhodesiense* infection may die at this stage before developing CNS involvement, and, in some patients with *T b rhodesiense,* the hemolymphatic and meningoencephalic stages may appear clinically superimposed. Hematologic examination at this stage often shows a normochromic and normocytic anemia,[53] as well as a high erythrocyte sedimentation rate (ESR) and thrombocytopenia.[60]

Meningoencephalitic Stage

Involvement of the CNS is often accompanied by both psychological and behavioral changes that can predate clinical neurologic signs. Transitory cranial nerve palsies,[61] epileptiform seizures, and intense pruritis can all be present at this stage, along with clinical signs of meningitis or encephalitis. Terminally the patient often develops a mask-like facies and becomes increasingly obtunded. Untreated, the patient stops eating, lapses into a coma, and dies. Death often occurs as a result of an intercurrent pneumonia or other infection. Healthy human carriers of both *T b gambiense* and *T b rhodesiense* have been recorded.[62]

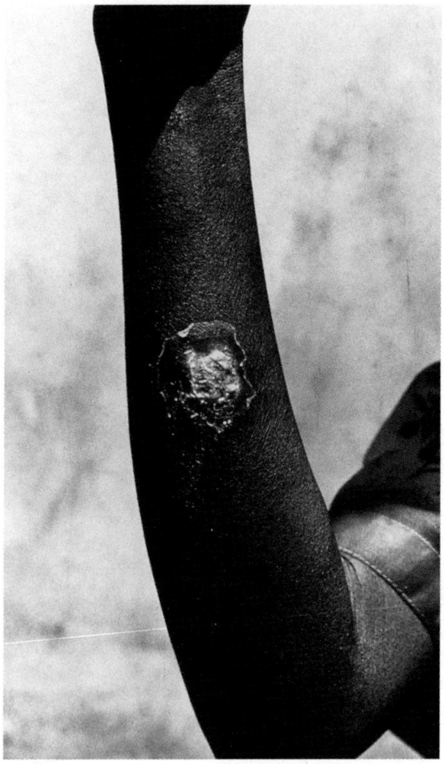

Figure 142–6. Chancre at the site of a tsetse fly bite. Note the perilesional desquamation. *(Photograph courtesy of F.A.S. Kuzoe, Secretary, Steering Committees on African Trypanosomiasis, WHO, Geneva.)*

PATHOGENESIS

The pathogenesis of AT is complex and incompletely understood. There is experimental evidence for the production by the trypanosome of toxins,[63] toxic metabolic products of glycolysis,[64] and enzymes such as proteases. However, trypanosome-induced disturbances of host immunocontrol probably play the most important role in both pathologic and clinical features of AT. Following infection of the vertebrate host by trypanosomes, the parasite's VSG stimulate a pronounced host B cell response. Through repeated changes of the VSG the parasite escapes destruction by the host's immune system and brings about a state of generalized host immunosuppression.[65] It has been established in experimental models[66,67] that the macrophage plays an important role in the development of host systemic immunosuppression in the presence of trypanosomal infection.[68] Within the CNS the astrocyte has a major part in immunomodulation.[69,70] Astrocytes may be pivotal in stimulating the production of somnogenic substances[71] such as interleukin 1, prostaglandin E2, and prostaglandin D2 by T lymphocytes within the brains of patients with meningoencephalitic AT.[72]

PATHOLOGY

Although many organs show gross and microscopic changes during the course of AT, few changes are pathognomonic.

Skin

In practice, the chancre is seldom biopsied and few descriptions are available.[73] Histologic examination of the chancre site shows a perivascular lymphocytic vasculitis involving the dermal blood vessels. The vascular endothelial cells are plump, and surrounding dermal connective tissue is edematous. Rarely, parasites are in the interstitial tissues. Occasional eosinophils may be present along with mild hyperkeratosis of overlying dermis. In some patients there is superficial epidermal ulceration.

Lymph Nodes

Grossly, the lymph nodes are enlarged and rubbery. In the early stages there are follicular hyperplasia, sinus histiocytosis, and numerous plasma cells. There may be focal intranodal hemorrhages and, on careful examination, the parasites occasionally can be identified. Later in the course of the disease the lymph nodes may become shrunken, hypocellular, and fibrotic. Cytologic examination of node imprints often show large numbers of organisms.

Spleen

Moderate splenomegaly is frequent.[74] The red pulp is congested but there is little change in the white pulp. Localized areas of necrosis 2 to 5 mm in diameter can sometimes be seen, along with occasional giant cells and foci of erythrophagocytosis. Trypanosomes are rare.

Heart

There often is mild cardiac enlargement. At autopsy there may be pericardial and pleural effusions, and Giemsa stains of the fluid frequently reveal the parasite. Grossly, there may be pericardial and subendocardial petechiae. Valves and ventricular endocardium are often fibrotic, and the endocardial thickening may resemble endomyocardial fibrosis.[75] Microscopically, the features are those of a pancarditis. In many cases of *T b rhodesiense* and *T b gambiense* infections, there is a diffuse mononuclear lympho-histio-plasmacytic cell

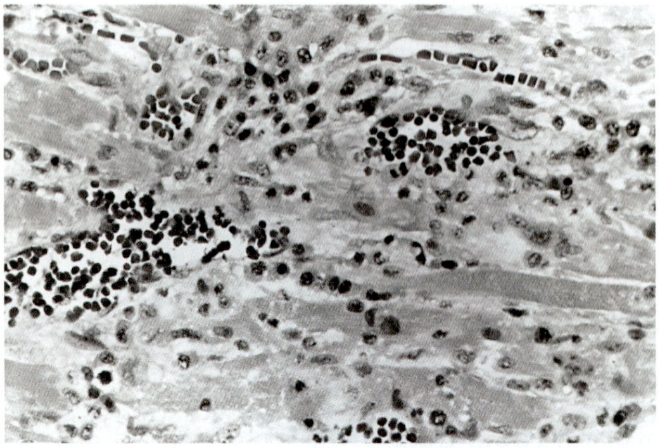

Figure 142–7. Diffuse mononuclear cell infiltrate in the myocardium of a patient dying of African Trypanosomiasis (*Trypanosoma brucei gambiense*) (hematoxylin-eosin, ×400).

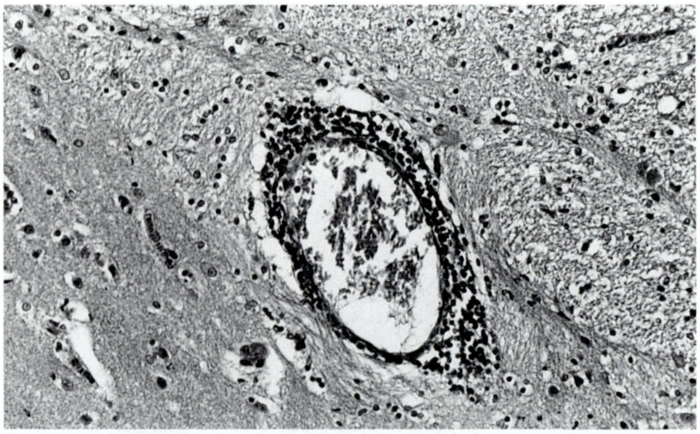

Figure 142–8. Mononuclear lympho-plasma-histiocytic cell infiltrate in the Virchow-Robin spaces (hematoxylin-eosin, ×250).

infiltrate throughout the myocardium (Figure 142–7), along with areas of myocytolysis. In advanced infections, there are often irregular areas of fibrosis in the ventricular myocardium. Small endocardial granulomas with necrotic eosinophilic centers have been reported in some hearts.[75] Careful study of the conduction system sometimes reveals inflammation of the atrioventricular (AV) node and the bundles of His.[76]

Brain

Grossly, the brain may appear edematous and mildly hyperemic. In cases coming to autopsy after a protracted meningoencephalitic state, the meninges are often thickened and opaque. When the brain is transected, there may be small collections of ring hemorrhages[77] that resemble the Dürk granulomas of cerebral malaria.[78] Small infarcts have been noted.[74] The most significant finding in meningoencephalitic trypanosomiasis is the variably intense mononuclear cell infiltrate filling the Virchow-Robin (V-R) spaces (Figure 142–8). Plasma cells often constitute a significant proportion of the cellular infiltrate within the CNS. Some plasma cells are distended with Russell bodies composed almost entirely of IgM, and form the very distinctive Mott cells (Figure 142–9).[79] A Perl's stain frequently shows hemosiderin in the V-R spaces. Usually only scanty eosinophils are in the cellular infiltrate, and careful examination of thick tissue sections occasionally reveals organisms in the V-R spaces. The changes in the CNS must be differentiated from those caused by therapy with arsenicals, because the clinical features of arsenic toxicity can overlap those of meningoencephalitic AT.[80] The spinal cord may have areas of myelitis,[81] and there may be similar inflammatory changes in peripheral nerves.[74]

Skeletal Muscle

There may be a patchy chronic inflammatory cell infiltrate in some cases.

Lung

Pulmonary lesions related specifically to infection by the parasite are not recorded, but at autopsy many lungs show features of a hypostatic pneumonia that is a common terminal event.

Kidney

Glomerulonephritis has been recorded in experimental trypanosomal infections.[82]

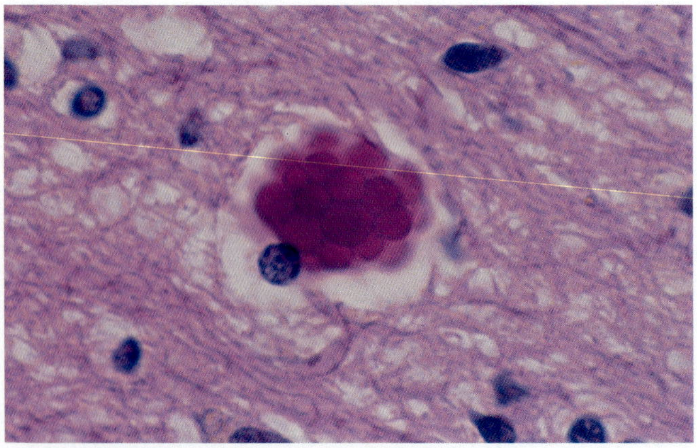

Figure 142–9. Mott's morula cell packed with IgM in the brain. These cells are characteristic of African trypanosomiasis when the CNS is involved (hematoxylin-eosin, ×400).

DIAGNOSIS, SEROLOGY, CULTURE (Figure 142–10)

Definitive diagnosis of AT depends on demonstrating the parasite in the blood, lymph, or cerebrospinal fluid (CSF) of infected patients. Culture of the organism may be necessary when there is a very low parasitemia. Serology plays an important role in the epidemiologic study of the disease. Biochemical tests, such as the estimation of serum or CSF IgM, are nonspecific indicators of AT infection, but they can provide useful clues to relapse[83] following a definitive diagnosis by other methods.

EXAMINATION OF FLUIDS

Tissue Aspiration

Identification of the organism in fluid obtained by needle aspiration of either soft tissue surrounding the chancre or an enlarged regional lymph node[84] may permit early diagnosis of AT. The yield from such procedures is variable,[85,86] but if done properly the technique helps to establish a definitive diagnosis. Giemsa-stained touch preparations of excised lymph nodes also may permit early identification of the parasite.

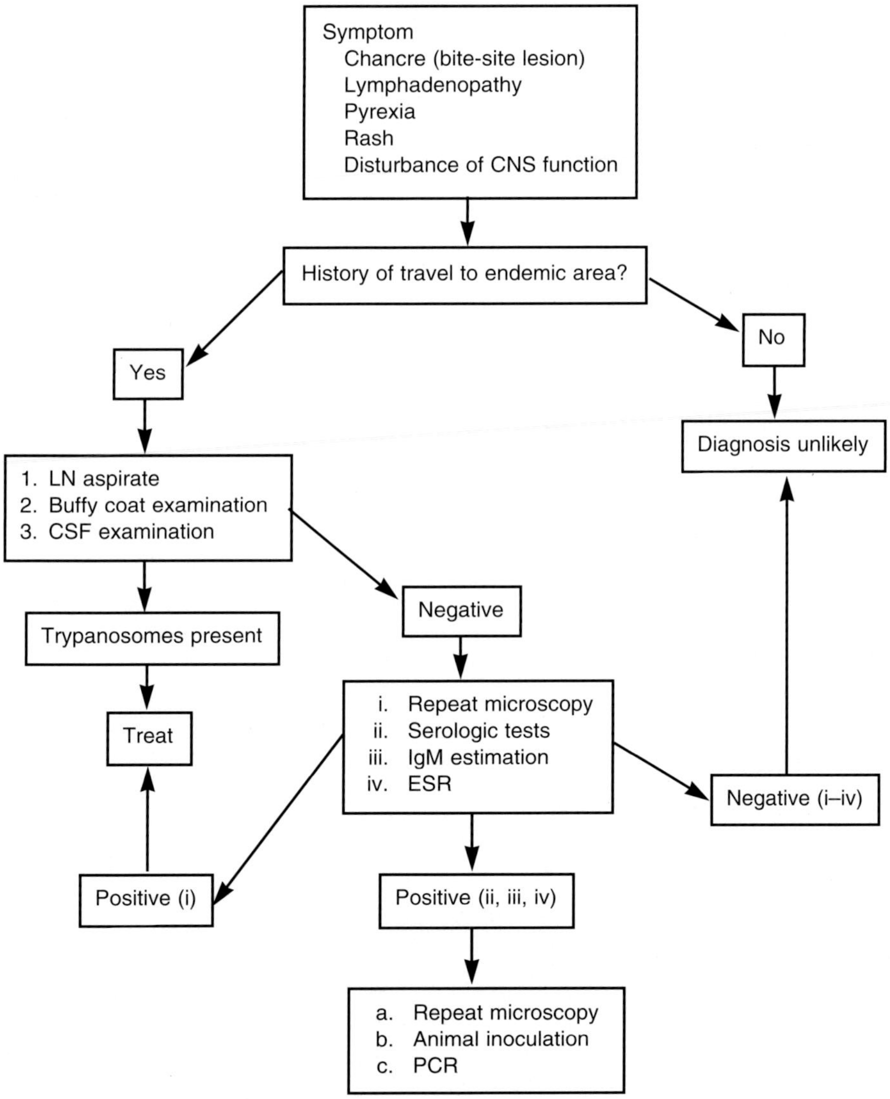

Figure 142–10. The diagnostic algorithm for the investigation of a patient in whom infection by *Trypanosoma brucei rhodesiense* or *Trypanosoma brucei gambiense* is suspected.

Blood

Blood may be examined for trypanosomes with or without attempts at parasite concentration such as the buffy coat technique[87] or variations on the anion exchange column concentration technique.[88–91] Although relatively expensive, this latter procedure can detect infections with very low parasitemias.[92] The number of parasites in the peripheral blood is cyclical,[93] and therefore, blood should be examined on several occasions. The parasite may also be found in bone marrow aspirate preparations.

ANIMAL INOCULATION, CULTIVATION

Animal Inoculation

Animal inoculation[94] may be very useful in the diagnosis of *T b rhodesiense* infection because most laboratory animals are susceptible to infection. It is very difficult to infect laboratory animals with *T b gambiense,* but occasionally it can be undertaken in young vervet monkeys (*Cercopithecus*) or the giant rat (*Crycetomys*). In vitro cultivation of both *T b gambiense* and *T b rhodesiense*[95,96] is possible, but the use of these techniques has been limited.

Serology

Infection is followed by seroconversion in 2 to 4 weeks. Available serologic tests include the card agglutination trypanosomiasis test (CATT),[97] indirect immunofluorescence test,[98] and an enzyme linked immunosorbent assay (ELISA).[99] These serologic tests are useful epidemiologic tools, but they should not be solely relied on for the diagnosis of AT,[100] especially with *T b rhodesiense* infection.[101] Cutaneous leishmaniasis or exposure to other forms of nonpathogenic trypanosomes may cause false positive serologic tests.[102]

Molecular Diagnosis

DNA analysis and the polymerase chain reaction (PCR) have been used to study AT. These techniques have characterized the trypanosomes causing infections in different endemic loci[103] and have diagnosed trypanosomal infections in laboratory animals.[104,105] This technology no doubt will play an important role in the future for both the diagnosis and epidemiologic study of AT.

TREATMENT

The drugs used to treat AT are pentamidine for chemoprophylaxis, suramin for early stages of infection, and melarsoprol for patients with CNS involvement.[106] A new agent, eflornithine, has been introduced[107] and it appears to be both more effective and to have fewer adverse side effects than the aforementioned medications.

REFERENCES

1. Atkins J. *The Navy Surgeon or Practical System of Surgery with a Dissertation on Cold and Hot Mineral Springs and Practical Observations of the Coast of Guiney.* London: J. Hodges and Co; 1742.
2. Christy C. Sleeping sickness. *J African Society.* October, iii:IX p. 1–11. 1903.
3. Roelants GE. Natural resistance to African trypanosomiasis. *Parasite Immunology.* 1986;8:1–8.
4. Goodwin LG. Chairman's introductory address, Eighteenth Seminar on Trypanosomiasis. *Trans R Soc Trop Med Hyg.* 1978;72:109–111.
5. Kuzoe FA. Current situation of African trypanosomiasis. *Acta Trop.* 1993;54:153–162.
6. Nwanyanwu OC, Steele JH, Osueke SO, Carpenter DJ. The public health significance of Trypanosomiasis in Nigeria. *Internat J Zoon.* 1985;12:28–84.
7. Mbulamberi DB. A review of Human African Trypanosomiasis (HAT) in Uganda. *East Afr Med J.* 1989;66:743–747.
8. Asonganyi T, Henry C, Louis JP, Ghogomu NA. Reactivation of an old sleeping sickness focus in Mamfe (Cameroon): epidemiological, immunological and parasitological findings. *Rev Epidem.* 1991;39:55–62.
9. Seah SK, Fegal KM. African trypanosomiasis in Canada. *Can Med Assoc J.* 1972;106:902–903.
10. Sterner G, Nassander L. African trypanosomiasis: a danger for tourists visiting Gambia. *Scan J Infect Dis.* 1977;9:154–156.
11. Robinson B, Clark RM, King JF, et al. Chronic Gambian trypanosomiasis. *South Med J.* 1980;73:516–518.
12. Duggan AJ, Hutchinson MP. Sleeping sickness in Europeans: a review of 109 cases. *J Trop Med Hyg.* 1966;69:124–131.
13. Cochran R, Rosen T. African trypanosomiasis in the United States. *Arch Dermatol.* 1983;119:670–674.
14. Richman TB, Kerdel FA. Amebiasis and trypanosomiasis. *Dermatol Clinics.* 1989;7:301–311.
15. Braebdli B, Dankwa E, Junghanss T. East African sleeping sickness (*Trypanosoma rhodesiense* infection) in two Swiss travellers to the tropics. *Schweiz Med Wochenschrift.* 1990;120:1348–1352.
16. Buissoniere RF, De Boissiur D, Tell G, et al. Uveomeningitis revealing a West African trypanosomiasis in a 12 year old girl. *Arch Franc Ped.* 1989;46:517–519.
17. Bowman IBR, Flynn IW. Oxidative metabolism of trypanosomes. In: Lumsden WHR, Evans DA, eds. *Biology of the Kinetoplastida.* London: Academic Press; 1976:435–476.
18. Vickerman K. Developmental cycles and biology of pathogenic Trypanosomes. *Br Med Bull.* 1985;41:105–114.

19. Evans DA, Ellis DS. The penetrative ability of sleeping sickness trypanosomes. *Trans Roy Soc Trop Med Hyg.* 1978;72:653–655.
20. Tetley L, Vickerman K. Differentiation in *Trypanosoma brucei:* host–parasite cell junctions and their persistence during acquisition of the variable antigen coat. *J Cell Sci.* 1984;74:1–9.
21. Majiwa PA, Otieno LH. Recombinant DNA probes reveal simultaneous infection of tsetse flies with different trypanosome species. *Molecular and Biochem Parasit.* 1990;40:245–253.
22. Bailey NM, Boreham PFL. The number of *Trypanosoma rhodesiense* required to establish an infection in man. *Ann Trop Med Parasit.* 1969;63:201–205.
23. Barry JD, Emery DC. Parasite development and host responses during the establishment of *Trypanosoma brucei* infection transmitted by tsetse fly. *Parasitology.* 1984; 88:67–84.
24. Langsley G, Roth C. Antigenic variation in parasitic protozoa. *Microbiol Sci.* 1987;4:280–285.
25. Penreath VW. The search for primary events causing the pathology in African sleeping sickness. *Trans Roy Soc Trop Med Hyg.* 1991;85:145–147.
26. Apted FIC, Omerod WE, Smyly DP, Stronach BW. A comparative study of the epidemiology of endemic Rhodesian sleeping sickness in different parts of Africa. *J Trop Med Hyg.* 1963;66:1–16.
27. Wijers DJ. The complex epidemiology of rhodesian sleeping sickness in Kenya and Uganda III. The epidemiology in the endemic areas along the lake shore between the Nile and Yala swamp. *Trop Geograph Med.* 1974;26:307–318.
28. Scott D, Lamprecht FL. Human trypanosomiasis in Ngamiland and Chobe district of Botswana prior to 1966: A retrospective historical and epidemiological review. Second addendum to the Quarterly report of the WHO Trypanosomiasis Control Project, October 1967;1–5.
29. Sindinga I. Sleeping sickness in Kenya Maasailand. *Soc Sci Med.* 1984;18:183–187.
30. Burtt E. Incubation of tsetse pupae: increased transmission rate of *Trypanosoma rhodesiense* in *Glossina morsitans. Ann Trop Med Parasit.* 1946;18:57–59.
31. Buxton PA. Tsetse and Trypanosomes in the Natural History of Tsetse Flies. London School of Tropical Medicine and Hygiene. Memorandum No. 10, 1955. London: HK Lewis; 642–644.
32. Bursell E. Entomological aspects of the epidemiology of sleeping sickness. *Cent Afr J Med.* 1973;19:201–204.
33. Burke J, Bengosi K, Diantete NL. Un cas de trypanosomiase congenitale. *Ann Soc Belg Med Trop.* 1974;54:1–4.
34. Lingam S, Marshall WC, Wilson J, et al. Congenital trypanosomiasis in a child born in London. *Dev Med Child Neurol.* 1985;27:670–674.
35. Olowe SA. A case of congenital trypanosomiasis in Lagos. *Trans Roy Soc Trop Med Hyg.* 1975;69:57–59.
36. Bruce-Chwatt LJ. Transfusion associated parasitic infections. In: Infections, Immunity and Blood Transfusion. Proceedings of the XVIth Annual Scientific Symposium of the American Red Cross; May 9–11, 1984; Washington, DC.
37. Emeribe AO. Gambiense trypanosomiasis acquired from needle scratch. *Lancet.* 1988;1:470–471.
38. Auregan G, Duvalet G. An African human trypanosomiasis focus without *Glossina. Med Trop.* 1980;40:367–371.
39. Roberts LW, Wellde BT, Reardon MJ, Onyango FK. Mechanical transmission of *Trypanosoma brucei rhodesiense* by *Glossina morsitans morsitans* (Diptera: Glossinidae). *Ann Trop Med Parasitol.* 1989;83(suppl 1): 127–131.
40. Taylor AW. Experiments on the mechanical transmission of West African *T brucei* and *T gambiense* by *Glossina* and other biting flies. *Trans Roy Soc Trop Med Hyg.* 1930; 24:289–303.
41. Godfrey DG, Scot CM, Gibson W, et al. Enzyme polymorphism and the identity of *Trypanosoma brucei gambiense. Parasitology.* 1987;94:337–347.
42. Massamba NN, Williams RO. Distinction of African Trypanosome species using nucleic acid hybridization. *Parasitology.* 1984;88:55–65.
43. Vickerman K. The ultrastructure of pathogenic flagellates. In: *Ciba Foundation Symposium 20. Trypanosomiasis and Leishmaniasis with Special Reference to Chagas Disease.* Amsterdam: Elsevier Associated Scientific Publishers; 1974;95–98.
44. Seed TM, Gnau JM, Krier JP, Pfister RM. *Trypanosoma* congolense: fine structure by carbon replica and freeze etch technique. *Exp Parasitol.* 1972;31:399–406.
45. Boisson C, Mattie X, Boisson ME. Le flagelle de *T. gambiense* etudie au microscope electronique. *C R Seanc Soc Biol.* 1965;159:228–230.
46. Greenwood BM, Whittle HC. The pathogenesis of sleeping sickness. *Trans Roy Soc Trop Med Hyg.* 1980;74: 716–725.
47. Gelfand M. The early clinical features of Rhodesian trypanosomiasis with special reference to the "chancre" (local reaction). *Trans Roy Soc Trop Med Hyg.* 1966; 60:376–379.
48. Apted FIC. Present status of chemotherapy and chemoprophylaxis of Human African trypanosomiasis in the eastern hemisphere. *Pharmacol Ther.* 1980;11:391–413.
49. Perl D, Dooley JR. Anthrax. In: Binford CH, Connor DH, eds. *Pathology of Tropical and Extraordinary Diseases.* Washington DC: AFIP; 1976:118–123.
50. Pinkerton H, Strano AJ. Rickettsial diseases. In: Binford CH, Connor DH, eds. *Pathology of Tropical and Extraordinary Diseases.* Washington DC: AFIP; 1976;96–97.
51. Vandemoortele E, Avonds W. African tick fever: fever, exanthema and skin ulcer. *Nederlands Tijdschrift voor Geneeskunde.* 1989;133:2305–2306.
52. Gear JHS, Miller GB. The clinical manifestations of Rhodesian trypanosomiasis: an account of cases contracted in the Okavango swamps of Botswana. *Am J Trop Med Hyg.* 1986;36:1146–1152.
53. Wellede BT, Chumo DA, Reardon MJ, et al. Presenting features of Rhodesian sleeping sickness patients in the Lambwe valley, Kenya. *Ann Trop Med Hyg.* 1989;83 (suppl 1):73–89.
54. Apted FIC. Clinical manifestations and diagnosis of sleeping sickness. In: Mulligan HW, Potts WH, eds. *The*

African Trypanosomes. New York: John Wiley and Sons; 1970;20–35.
55. Winterbottom TM. *An Account of the Native Africans in the Neighborhood of Sierra Leone.* London: Hatchard and Mawman; 1803.
56. Scott H. In: *The History of Tropical Medicine.* Baltimore: Williams and Wilkins; 1939:446.
57. Jones IG, Lowenthal MN, Buyst H. Electrocardiographic changes in African trypanosomiasis caused by *Trypanosoma brucei rhodesiense. Trans Roy Soc Trop Med Hyg.* 1975;69:388–395.
58. Barrett-Connor E, Ugoretz RJ, Braude AI. Disseminated intrasvascular coagulation in trypanosomiasis. *Arch Intern Med.* 1973;131:573–577.
59. Bourgeade AY, Nosny B, Faugere B, Pene P. African trypanosomiasis of the ictohaemorrhagic form. *Bull Soc Pathol Exot Filials.* 1985;75:908–913.
60. Robins-Brown RM, Schneider J, Metz J. Thrombocytopenia in trypanosomiasis. *Am J Trop Med Hyg.* 1974;24: 226–231.
61. Gelfand M. Transitory neurological signs in sleeping sickness. *Trans Roy Soc Trop Med Hyg.* 1947;41:255–258.
62. Wurapa FK, Dukes P, Njelsani EK, Boatin BA. Healthy carrier of *T. b. rhodesiense:* a case report. *Trans Roy Soc Trop Med Hyg.* 1984;78:349–350.
63. Seed J. *T. gambiense* and *T. lewisi:* increased vascular permeability and skin lesions in rabbits. *Exp Parasitol.* 1969;26:214–223.
64. Goodwin LG. The African scene: Mechanisms of pathogenesis in trypanosomiasis. In: Elliot K, O'Connor M, Wolstenholme GEW, eds. *Trypanosomiasis and Leishmaniasis with Special Reference To Chagas' Disease.* Amsterdam: Elsevier; Ciba Foundation Symposium No. 20, 1974:107–109.
65. Mansfield M. Immunology of African trypanosomiasis. In: Wyler DG, Freeman WH, eds. *Modern Parasite Biology.* New York: 1990:222–246.
66. Askonas BA. Macrophages as mediators of immunosuppression in murine African trypanosomiasis. *Cur Topics Micro Immunol.* 1985;117:119–127.
67. Borowy NK, Sternberg JM, Schreiber D, et al. Suppressive macrophages occurring in murine *Trypanosoma brucei* infection inhibit T cell responses in vivo and in vitro. *Parasite Immun.* 1990;12:233–246.
68. Fierer J, Salmon JA, Askonas BA. African trypanosomiasis alters prostaglandin production by murine peritoneal macrophages. *Clin Exp Immunol.* 1984;58:548–556.
69. Fontana A, Kirsten F, Dubs R, et al. Production of prostaglandin E and interleukin 1 like factor by cultured astrocytes and C6 glioma cells. *J Immunol.* 1982;129: 2413–2416.
70. Borgeson M, Tallent MW, Keaner RW. Astrocyte modulation of central nervous system immune responses. In: Goetzl EJ, Spector NH, eds. *Neuroimmune Networks: Physiology and Diseases.* New York: Allan R. Liss; 1989: 51–55.
71. Kreuger JM. Somnogenic activity of immune response modifiers. *Trends Pharm Sci.* 1990;11:122–126.
72. Penreath VW, Rees K, Owolabi OA, et al. The somnogenic T lymphocyte suppressor prostaglandin D2 is selectively elevated in cerebrospinal fluid of advanced sleeping sickness patients. *Trans Roy Soc Trop Med Hyg.* 1990;84:795–799.
73. Fairburn H, Godfrey DG. The local reaction in man at the site of infection with *Trypanosoma rhodesiense. Ann Trop Med Parasitol.* 1957;51:464–470.
74. Poltera AA, Owor R, Cox JN. Pathological aspects of human African trypanosomiasis (HAT) in Uganda. *Virchows Arch A* (Pathol Anat). 1977;373:249–265.
75. Poltera AA, Cox JN. Pancarditis and valvulitis in endomyocardial fibrosis and in human trypanosomiasis: a comparative histological study of 4 Ugandan cases. *Virchows Arch A* (Pathol Anat). 1977;375:53–70.
76. Poltera AA, Cox JN, Owor R. Pancarditis involving the conducting system and all valves in human African trypanosomiasis. *Br Heart J.* 1976;38:827–837.
77. Hawking F, Greenfield JC. Two autopsies on Rhodesian sleeping sickness: visceral lesions and significance of changes in cerebrospinal fluid. *Trans Roy Soc Trop Med Hyg.* 1941;35:155–164.
78. Dürk Ueber die bei Malaria perniciosa comatosa auftretenden Veraenderungen des Zentralnervens systems. *Arch Schiffs U Tren Hyg.* 1917;21:117–132.
79. Mott FW. Histological observations on changes in the nervous system in trypanosoma infections, especially sleeping sickness and dourine, and their relationship to syphilitic lesions of the nervous system. *Arch Neurol Psychiat.* 1907;3:581–646.
80. Hume-Adams J, Haller L, Boa FY, et al. Human African trypanosomiasis (*T. b. gambiense*): a study of 16 fatal cases of sleeping sickness with some observations on acute reactive arsenical encephalopathy. *Neuropath Applied Neurobiol.* 1986;12:81–94.
81. Janssen P, vanBogaert L, Haymaker W. Pathology of the peripheral nervous system in African trypanosomiasis. *J Neuropath Exp Neurol.* 1956;15:269–287.
82. Nagle RB, Ward PA, Lindsey HB, et al. Experimental infections with African trypanosomiasis. VI. Glomerulonephritis involving the alternative pathway of complement fixation. *Trans Roy Soc Trop Med Hyg.* 1974;23: 15–26.
83. Whittle HC, Greenwood BM, Bidwell DE, et al. IgM antibody measurement in the diagnosis and management of Gambian trypanosomiasis. *Amer J Trop Med Hyg.* 1977; 26:1129–1134.
84. Greig EDW, Gray ACH. Note on the lymphatic glands in sleeping sickness. *Lancet.* 1904;1:1570.
85. Henry MC, Kageruka P, Ruppol JF, et al. Evaluations du diagnotic sur le terain de la trypanosomiase a *T. gambiense. Ann Soc Belg Med Trop.* 1981;61:79–92.
86. Haller L, Adams H, Merouze F, et al. Clinical and pathological aspects of Human African Trypanosomiasis (*T. b. gambiense*) with particular reference to reactive arsenical encephalopathy. *Am J Trop Med Hyg.* 1986;35:94–99.
87. Murray M, Murray PK, Mcintyre WIM. An improved parasitological technique for the diagnosis of African trypanosomiasis. *Trans Roy Soc Trop Med Hyg.* 1977;71: 325–326.

88. Lanham SM, Godfrey DG. Isolation of salivarian Trypanosomes from man and other mammals by DEAE cellulose. *Exper Parasit.* 1970;28:521–530.
89. Lumsden WHR, Kimber CD, Strange M. *Trypanosoma brucei:* detection of low parasitaemias in ice by miniature exchanger/centrifugation technique. *Trans Roy Soc Trop Med Hyg.* 1977;71:421–422.
90. Lumsden WHR, Kimden DD, Dukes P, et al. Field diagnosis of sleeping sickness in the Ivory Coast: comparison of miniature anion exchanger/centrifugation technique with other protozoological methods. *Trans Roy Soc Trop Med Hyg.* 1981;75:242–249.
91. Gashumba JK. Sleeping sickness in the Iganga district, Uganda: Application of a new diagnostic technique. *East Afr Med J.* 1981;58:699–702.
92. Lumsden WHR, Kimber CD, Evans DA, Doig SJ. *Trypanosoma brucei:* miniature anion-exchange centrifugation technique for detection of low parasitaemias, adaption for field use. *Trans Roy Soc Trop Med Hyg.* 1977; 73:312–317.
93. Vickerman K. Antigenic Variations in African Trypanosomes. In: CIBA Symposium 25. *Parasites in the Immunized Host: Mechanisms of Survival.* Amsterdam: Elsevier Associated Scientific Publishers 1975;20–28.
94. Wellde BT, Chumo DA, Reardon MJ, Esser K. Schoenbechler MJ, Orlando J. Diagnosis of Rhodesian sleeping sickness in the Lambwe Valley (1980–1984). *Ann Trop Med Parasit.* 1989;1:63–71.
95. Brun R, Jenni L. Cultivation of African and South American Trypanosomes of medical or veterinary importance. *Brit Med Bull.* 1985;41:122–129.
96. Dukes P, Kaukas A, Hudson KM, et al. A new method for isolating *Trypanosoma brucei gambiense* from sleeping sickness patients. *Trans Roy Soc Trop Med Hyg.* 1989; 85:636–639.
97. Magnus E, Van Meirvenne N, Vervoort T. A card agglutination test with stained trypanosomes for the serological diagnosis of *T. gambiense* trypanosomiasis. *Ann Soc Belg Med Trop.* 1978;58:169–176.
98. Wery M, Wery-Paskoff S, Van Wettere P. The diagnosis of human African trypanosomiasis (*T. gambiense*) by the use of the standard fluorescent antibody test: standardization of an easy technique to be used in mass surveys. *Ann Soc Belg Med Trop.* 1970;50:613–634.
99. Voller A, Bidwell DE, Bartlett A. A serological study on Human *Trypanosoma rhodesiense* infections using a micro-scale enzyme linked immunosorbent assay. *Tropenmed und Parasit.* 1975;26:247–251.
100. Croft SL. Serodiagnostic tests for West African trypanosomiasis. *Parasitol Today.* 1985;1:115.
101. Wyatt GB, Kakoma I, Wurapa FK, et al. Two year follow up of persons with positive fluorescent antibody test for Rhodesian sleeping sickness in the Luangwa Valley, Zambia. *Ann Trop Med Parasitol.* 1986;80;127–129.
102. Van Meirvenne N, le Ray D. Diagnosis of African and American trypanosomiasis. *Brit Med Bull.* 1985;41:156–166.
103. Hide G, Buchanan N, Welburn S, et al. *Trypanosoma brucei rhodesiense:* Characterisation of stocks from Zambia, Kenya and Uganda using repetitive DNA probes. *Exp Parasitol.* 1991;72:430–433.
104. Mose DR, Cook GA, Bailey CP, et al. Detection of *Trypanosoma congolense* and *T. b.* subspecies by DNA amplification using the polymerase chain reaction. *Parasitology.* 1989;1:57–66.
105. Hide G, Cattland P, Le Ray D, Tait A. The identification of *Trypanosoma brucei* subspecies using DNA sequences. *Mol Biochem Parasitol.* 1990;39:213–225.
106. Pepin J, Milford F. The treatment of human African trypanosomiasis. *Advances in Parasitology.* 1994;33:1–47.
107. Van Voofhis WC. Therapy and prophylaxis of systemic protozoan infections. *Drugs.* 1990;40:176–202.

CHAPTER 143

American Trypanosomiasis

Ernest E. Lack and Armando Filie

The real public-health problem of course, is poverty.

Wendell L. Willkie (1892–1944), One World, Chap 2

DEFINITION

American trypanosomiasis (Chagas' disease*) is a zoonosis caused by the hemoflagellate protozoon *Trypanosoma cruzi,* first recognized by Carlos Chagas in 1909,[1,2] who named the organism after colleague Oswaldo Cruz. *Trypanosoma cruzi* is transmitted from person to person by blood-sucking hematophagous Triatomine bugs.

GEOGRAPHIC DISTRIBUTION

Trypanosoma cruzi parasitizes a variety of vertebrates including humans and has a life cycle that involves a vertebrate and an insect vector. Chagas' disease is found only in the Western Hemisphere and is endemic in many countries of Central and South America (Figure 143–1).[3] Chagas' disease has been described in the Caribbean islands of Aruba and Trinidad[4] and rare infections have been recorded in Mexico and the United States.[5] The heaviest concentration of Chagas' disease is in rural Brazil. In endemic areas an estimated 16 to 18 million people have chronic infections and about 50,000 die each year.[6]

EPIDEMIOLOGY

When a triatome bug bites a human, it defecates and the parasite, if in the bug's feces, invades through the opening made by the bite. Most new infections are in children in rural areas, and the vast majority of infections are undiagnosed. The parasite can also by transmitted by blood transfusion,[7–9] and one study in Brazil reported the risk of Chagas' disease to be 22% for those receiving two or more units of blood.[10] Accidental laboratory-acquired infections by *T cruzi* have also been reported. Another risk of infection is by organ transplantation from infected donors.[11] Cardiac transplantation for end-stage chagasic cardiomyopathy can also reactivate Chagas' disease in an immunodeficient recipient.[12] Parasites can also pass from an infected mother to the fetus in utero causing spontaneous abortion or congenital Chagas' disease.[13,14] In some endemic areas congenital Chagas' disease afflicts 1.6% to 5% of infants born to infected women.[12,13] Acute Chagas' disease has also been reported in acquired immunodeficiency syndrome (AIDS),[15,16] and may manifest as a severe myocarditis or encephalitis. In a patient who is positive for human immunodeficiency virus (HIV), reactivation of Chagas' disease should be a criterion for the diagnosis of AIDS.[16]

PREVALENCE OF CHAGAS' DISEASE IN THE UNITED STATES

The prevalence of infection by *T cruzi* in the United States is unknown at present. Almost all those diagnosed have been in immigrants from endemic areas.[12,17–19] Of 205 Salvadoran and Nicaraguan immigrants in the Washington, DC, area, 5% were infected.[12] Perhaps 50,000 to 100,000 immigrants are infected.[12] This is a growing concern for the safety of donated blood because infection by *T cruzi* is lifelong and those

* "Chaga*s's* disease" is preferred by grammatical purists but Chaga*s'* disease is commonly used.

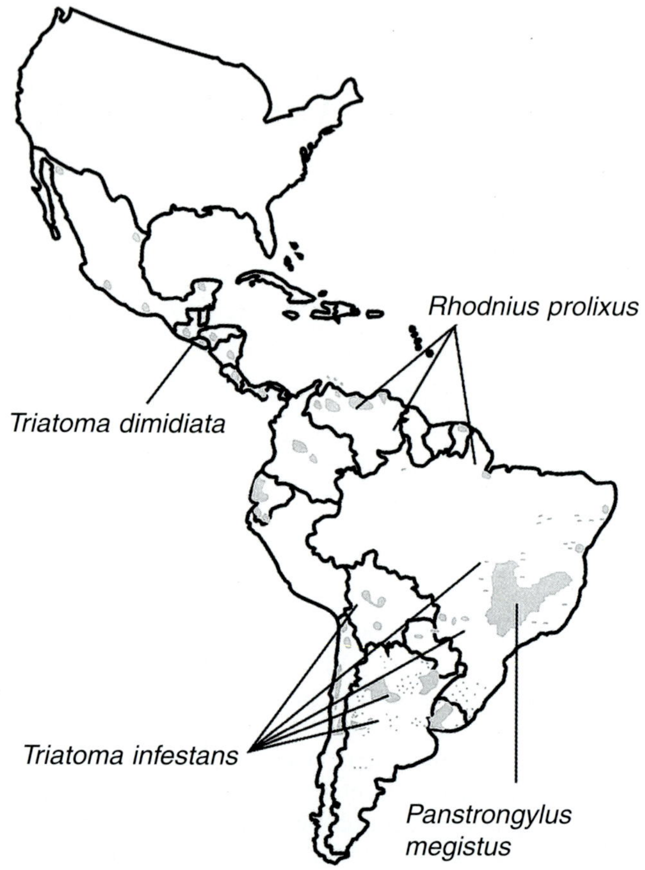

Figure 143–1. Distribution of Chagas' disease in Central and South America. Rare indigenous infections have been reported in Mexico and the southern United States.

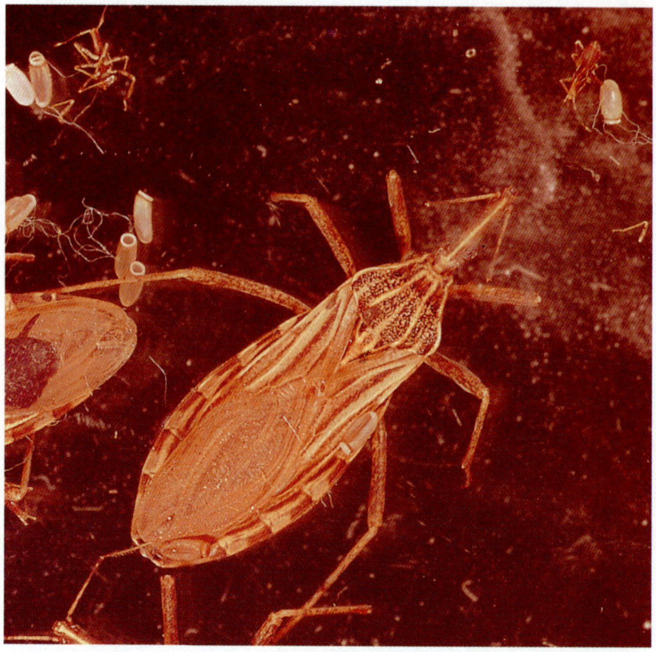

Figure 143–2. Triatomine (reduviid) bug *Rhodnius pallescens* is a hematophagous (blood-sucking) insect. This is one of many vectors of *T cruzi*.

infected are usually asymptomatic. Furthermore screening for *T cruzi* is so expensive and time consuming that it may not be practical.

MORPHOLOGY AND LIFE CYCLE OF *TRYPANOSOMA CRUZI*

Various genera and species of hematophagous insects (subfamily Triatominae, family Reduviidae) serve as hosts and vectors for *T cruzi*. These insects are also called reduviid bugs, assassin bugs, and cone nose bugs. Over 100 species of Triatomine bugs have been identified (five tribes and 14 genera), and about 40 of these are in artificial ecotopes close to humans; about half of these bugs have become adapted to human dwellings in the Western Hemisphere.[20] A few examples include *Rhodnius prolixus, Triatoma dimidiata, Triatoma infestans,* and *Rhodnius pallescens* (Figure 143–2). *Trypanosoma cruzi* has also been reported to develop in some bedbugs and ticks.[4]

The life cycle of *T cruzi* in the insect and vertebrate hosts is shown in Figure 143–3. The trypomastigote is ingested during a blood meal from an infected host, and multiplies in the gut of the bug with subsequent transformation into the crithidia or epimastigotes and finally becomes metacyclic trypomastigotes in the bug's rectum. Trypomastigotes are passed when the bug defecates. Because bugs are coprophagic and cannibalistic, bug-to-bug transmission is common. Some Triatomine

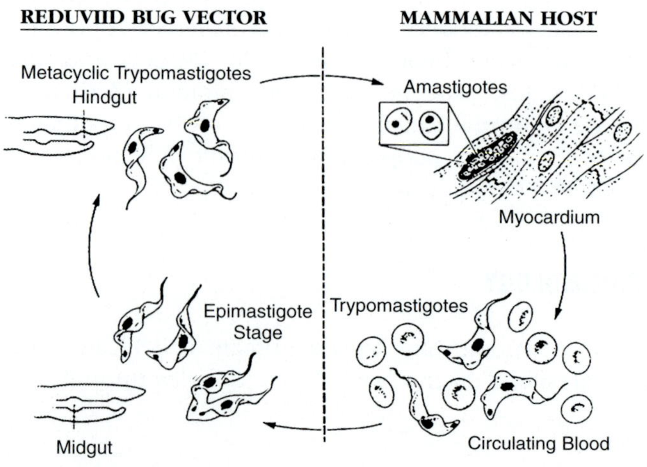

Figure 143–3. Life cycle of *T cruzi* in Triatomine insect and vertebrate host.

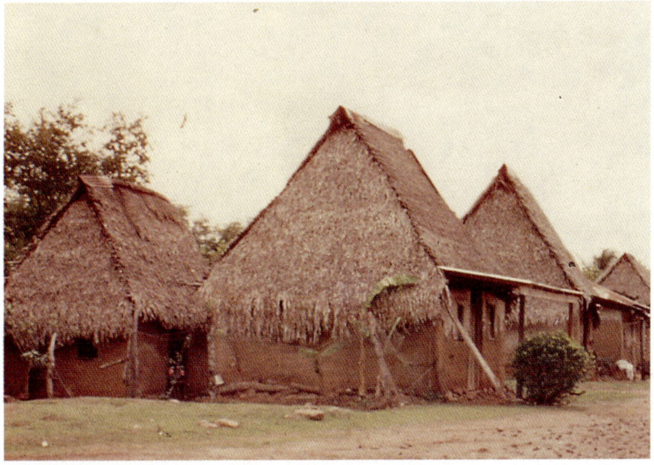

Figure 143–4. Mud huts with thatched roofs are the characteristic codomicile for hematophagous Triatomine bugs and humans. Bugs live in the cracks in the mud walls and are concentrated in cracks near the sleeping areas. The bugs feed at night.

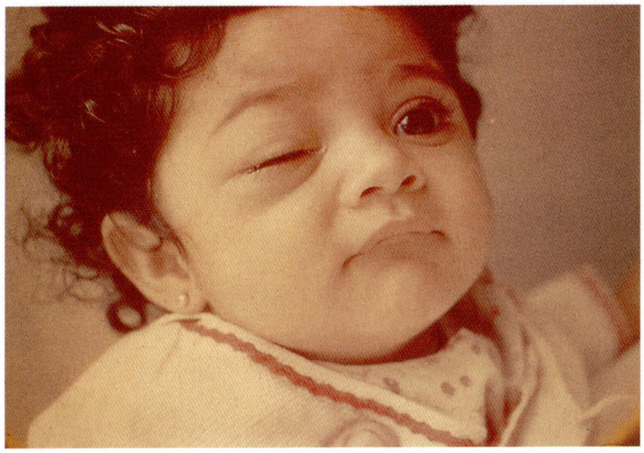

Figure 143–5. Romaña's sign in a young girl with conjunctivitis and palpebral/periorbital edema. Patients may have ipsilateral preauricular lymphadenopathy (AFIP Neg 62-3934-6).

bugs are sylvatic and these pass the parasite among wild animals such as marsupials (eg, opossums), carnivores, rodents (eg, rats), pigs, bats, and edentates (eg, armadillos).[21,22] Transmission of *T cruzi* to humans in endemic areas typically occurs in poor and underdeveloped rural or suburban areas where infected insects cohabitate with humans. These dwellings typically have thatched roofs (Figure 143–4) or walls of mud or lath with cracks in which the Triatomine bugs reside. In this domestic setting, humans are infected and are part of the continuing life cycle of *T cruzi.*

CLINICAL COURSE OF CHAGAS' DISEASE AND PATHOLOGY

Acute Chagas' Disease

Infection by *T cruzi,* in the usual endemic setting, follows contamination of the skin or mucous membrane by the bug's infected fecal material. The insect defecates while feeding and the patient may rub bug feces containing *T cruzi* into the site of the bite or into a scratch or fissure. The protozoan can penetrate intact mucous membrane such as conjunctiva. Inoculation of the conjunctival sac may cause unilateral (or sometimes bilateral) conjunctivitis, chemosis, and periorbital edema, a combination of findings referred to as Romaña's sign (Figure 143–5). This may be accompanied by preauricular lymphadenopathy, and usually appears several days to 2 weeks after exposure. Two distinct forms of the parasite develop in the infected host. The amastigote (leishmanial) forms are intracellular and multiply by binary division whereas flagellated forms (trypanosomes) circulate in the blood. A small, transient inflammatory nodule may develop at the site of inoculation ("chagoma"), usually 1 to 2 weeks after inoculation. Monocytes infiltrate the site and take up the infectious forms, which round up immediately to become amastigotes. As the organisms are released, the parasite spreads hematogenously to distant sites to infect other somatic cells and tissues. The amastigotes have no predisposition for phagocytic cells of the reticuloendothelial system as do the leishmania in visceral leishmaniasis. Muscle including the heart may be parasitized, and in a small proportion of patients a severe myocarditis develops that is sometimes fatal (Figure 143–6, A–C). The parasite can also invade the central nervous system and cause a meningoencephalitis (Figure 143–7).[23]

Symptoms of acute Chagas' disease are usually mild with fever and malaise. Most patients are asymptomatic and unaware of infection. The case fatality rate is less than 5%.[24] Serologic tests are of little value in the diagnosis during the acute phase, although some hemagglutinins and antibodies may be detected in serum several weeks to a few months after infection. Detection of the parasite is the most reliable procedure in establishing a diagnosis. Parasitemia is usually evident by the third week. The nondividing extracellular parasite is the trypomastigote (Greek, *Trypanon,* resembling an augur). It is usually 16 to 22 μm long, has an undulating membrane on one side, a single anterior flagellum, and a prominent posteriorly placed kinetoplast (Figure 143–8). It can be seen by microscopic examination of a fresh drop of blood or buffy coat, or in fixed stained smears (thin or thick). In fixed preparations the trypomastigote typically has a C or U shape. Persistence

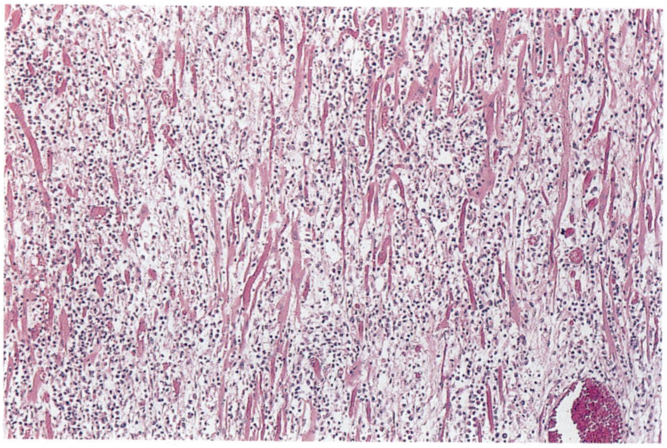

A

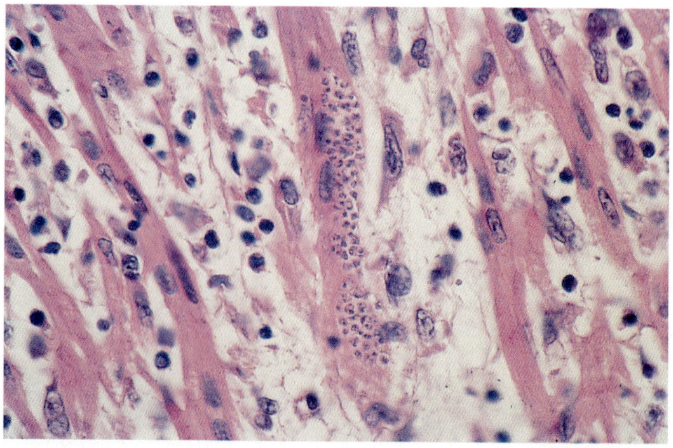

B

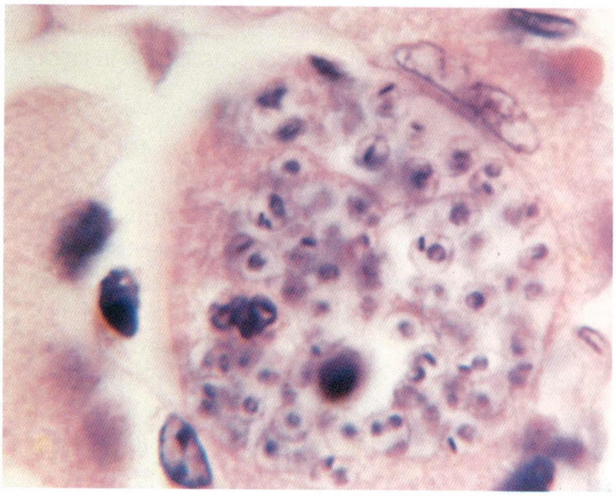

C

Figure 143–6. (**A**) Acute chagasic myocarditis. The myofibers are atrophic and separated by edematous tissue containing lymphocytes and occasional plasma cells [hematoxylin-eosin (H&E), ×90]. (**B**) Acute chagasic myocarditis. A myofiber containing clusters of amastigotes is in the center (H&E, ×180). (**C**) Amastigote forms of *T cruzi* clustered within parasitized myofiber in acute chagasic myocarditis. The amastigotes are spherical, 2 to 3 μm across, and have elongated, rod-shaped, dark-staining kinetoplasts, and lightly stained spherical nuclei (AFIP Neg 74-13234; H&E, ×1600).

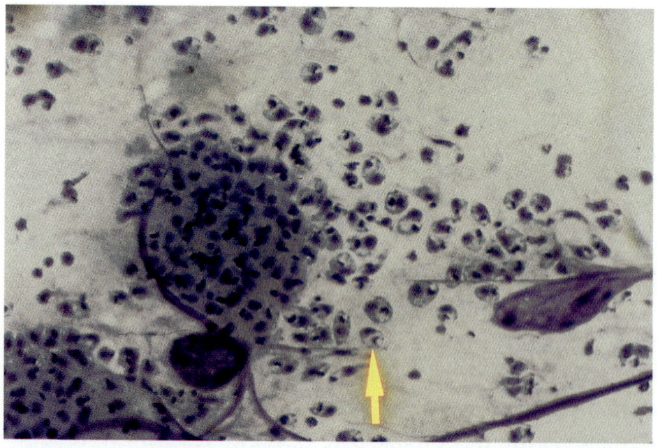

Figure 143–7. Smear/imprint of mouse brain following experimental inoculation with infective trypomastigotes of *T cruzi.* Numerous macrophages are distended by intracellular amastigotes (leishmania) of *T cruzi*, 1.5 to 4.0 μm. Many amastigotes (some extracellular) have a well-defined cell outline, each with an elongated kinetoplast and rounded nucleus (*arrow*) (Wright–Giemsa stain, ×1000).

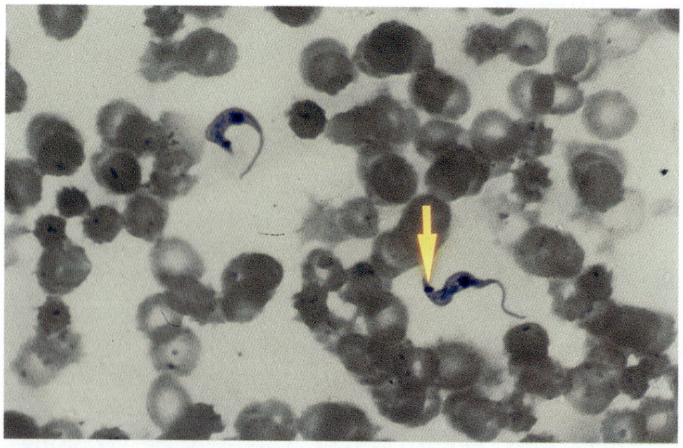

Figure 143–8. Thick blood smear from a patient with Chagas' disease. *Trypanosoma cruzi* is curvilinear, usually C shaped, has a prominent terminal kinetoplast (*arrow*) and a distinct nucleus, which is larger and centered in the organism (Wright–Giemsa stain, ×1000).

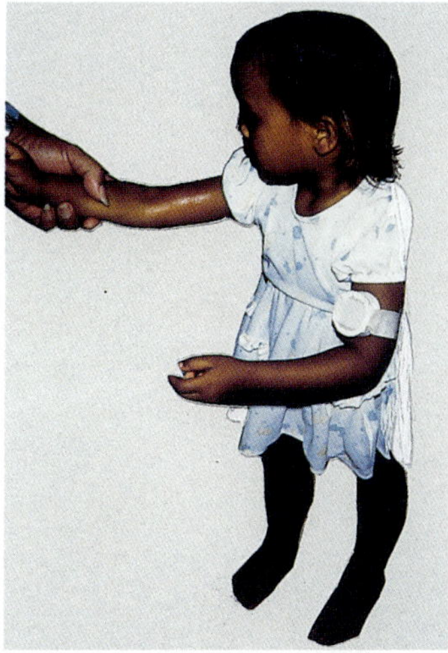

Figure 143–9. Young girl undergoing xenodiagnosis for Chagas' disease. Laboratory reared, "sterile" (ie, free of *T cruzi*) Triatomine insects are in the container affixed to her arm. If she is infected, *T cruzi* trypomasatigotes will be ingested with her blood and multiply in the bug's gut enabling identification and diagnosis within 10 days. Note slight erythema at site of blood meal on right arm. The bioamplification in the bug's gut makes this a sensitive diagnostic test.

and patience may be required in microscopic study of peripheral blood since the concentration of parasites is usually low. Xenodiagnosis (Figure 143–9) or blood culture[25] may detect parasitemia weeks, months, or years after infection.

A parasite that could be confused with *T cruzi* in peripheral smears is *T rangeli,* another cause of American trypanosomiasis but which is nonpathogenic for humans. This form of trypanosomiasis is most prevalent in Venezuela, Colombia, and the Republic of Panama, and when compared to *T cruzi* is longer (27 to 32 μm) and has a broader undulating membrane and a subterminal smaller kinetoplast.[4]

Indeterminate Chagas' Disease

Patients are asymptomatic with intermittent low-level parasitemia in association with antibodies to *T cruzi* antigens. Most patients remain in this indeterminate phase for life.

Symptomatic Chronic Chagas' Disease

About 10% to 30% of infected patients develop chronic Chagas' disease years or even decades after initial infection.[12] Chronic Chagas' disease can be diagnosed with sensitive serologic tests for *T cruzi* antibodies, eg, complement fixation, indirect hemagglutination, indirect immunofluorescence, and enzyme-linked immunosorbent assay.[12,26] According to some, serum should be positive in at least two different assays before accepting the diagnosis as confirmed, because patients with other diseases including syphilis, leishmaniasis, malaria, and some collagen vascular disorders frequently have false-positive tests.[12] Recently, polymerase chain reaction for specific *T cruzi* kinetoplast or nuclear DNA has detected parasites in the blood of patients with chronic infection.[27,28]

Chronic Chagasic Myocarditis and Cardiomyopathy

In a recent study of symptomatic patients with Chagas' disease in Venezuela, nearly 40% had a conduction abnormality (right bundle branch block, left anterior hemiblock, or both), more than 75% had ventricular arrhythmias and nearly one third of patients had abnormal ST-segment and T-wave inversion.[29] Patients may have syncope sometimes during physical exertion and occasionally there is sudden death. A dysautonomic syndrome of postural hypotension, dizziness, and arrhythmias has been attributed to destruction of cardiac autonomic ganglia and nerves.[30] Angina-like chest pain can simulate coronary heart disease. End-stage Chagas' heart disease is a dilated heart with congestive failure. Cardiac transplants have been done for advanced cardiac disease.[12]

In chronic chagasic myocarditis and cardiomyopathy there is cardiomegaly (often 400 to 800 g)[4] with biventricular dilatation. The myocardium is pale and flabby, particularly if there is severe myocarditis. Scarring of the myocardium may appear as pale streaks or plaques particularly toward the apices. Autopsies reveal a peculiar, perhaps unique, apical aneurysm or scarring of the apex of the left ventricle (Figure 143–10, A and B) in over 50% of those who die of chronic chagasic heart disease.[31] The cause of the apical aneurysm is unclear. Proposed mechanisms include ischemia, inflammation, autonomic imbalance, or herniation through the spiral bundles at the apex. There may be marked thinning and effacement of myocardium in the wall of the aneurysm with replacement by fibrous tissue. Mural thrombi may form in the aneurysm or ventricular apex or be attached elsewhere to atrial or ventricular endocardium. These may embolize to systemic or pulmonary arteries causing cerebral or pulmonary infarction. Cardiac valves and major coronary arteries are uninvolved.

The myocarditis is patchy or more diffuse with separation of myofibers by lymphocytes, scattered plasma cells, and occasional eosinophils. Amastigotes may be difficult or impossible to identify, but prolonged search and liberal sampling usually reveal a parasitized myofiber. The accumulation of amastigotes in a myofiber of *T cruzi* has been called a "pseudocyst." There may be diffuse myocardial fibrosis and scarring, particularly near the apices of the ventricles with atrophy of myocardial cells (Figure 143–11).

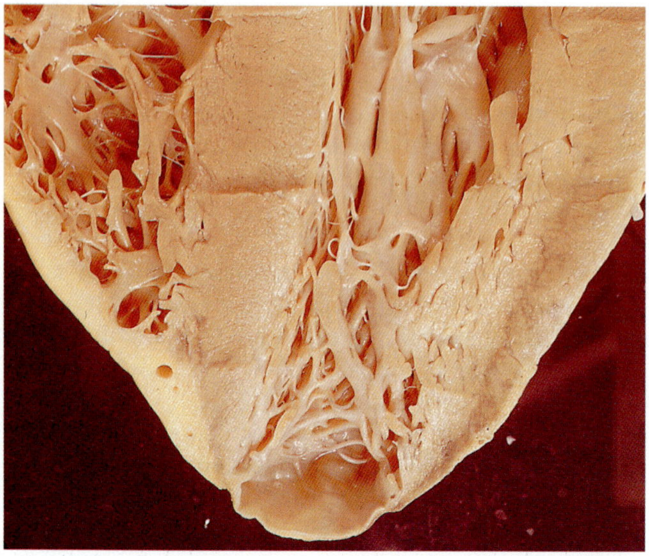

A

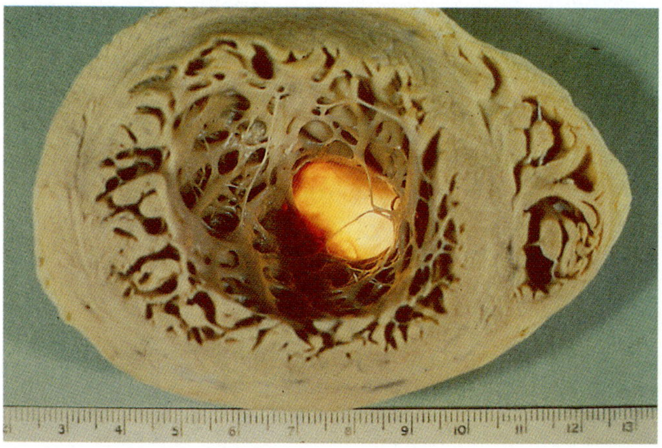

B

Figure 143–10. (**A**) Section of heart from a patient with chronic chagasic myocarditis. The apical aneurysm is characteristic. Patient had cardiomyopathy with biventricular dilatation (AFIP Neg 63-2506-1). (**B**) Transillumination of apex of left ventricle in chronic chagasic myocarditis highlights apical aneurysm. *(From Gorgas Memorial Laboratory.)*

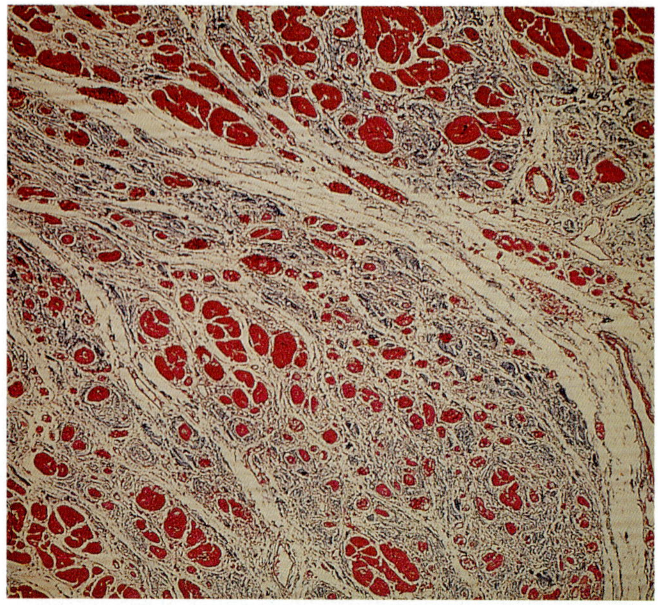

Figure 143–11. Chronic chagasic myocarditis. There is marked interstitial fibrosis separating atrophic myofibers (AFIP Neg 63-4395; Masson trichrome stain, ×120).

Chagas Syndrome Including Megaesophagus and Megacolon

Megaviscera, particularly dilated esophagus and/or colon, may complicate chronic Chagas' disease.[32–34] Megaesophagus may cause dysphagia, aspiration, and regurgitation. Megacolon, as in Figure 143–12, may be complicated by severe constipation. Other "mega" conditions include bronchiectasis, megagaster, megaduodenum, megagallbladder, and megaureter.[33] The cause has been attributed to invasion, destruction, and dimi-

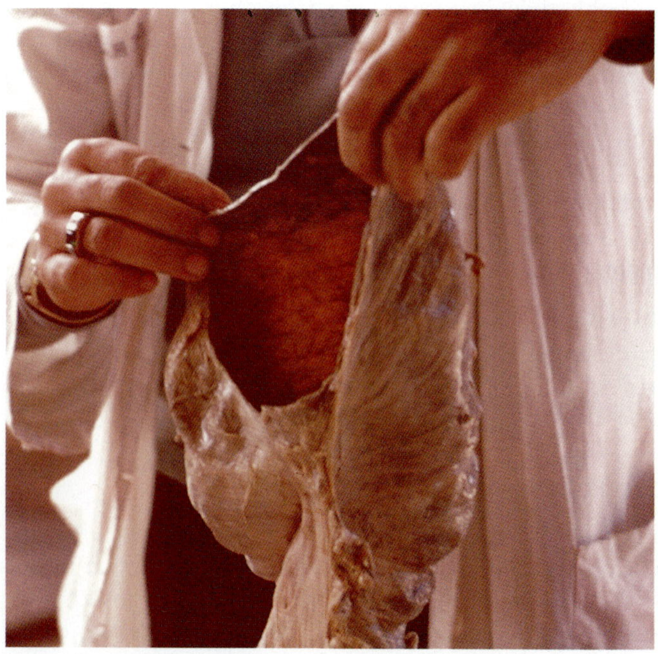

Figure 143–12. Megacolon from patient with chronic Chagas' disease. The colon is saccular and has a thin wall.

nution of ganglion cells in the wall of the viscus with secondary dysmotility.

Pathogenesis of Chronic Chagasic Myocarditis

Although *T cruzi* infects a variety of cells and tissues, the heart is most severely involved. It is difficult to blame direct destruction of myofibers by *T cruzi* as the sole mechanism because parasitemia is low grade and the amastigotes are difficult to identify in sections. Ultrastructural study has not provided significant insights into pathogenesis.[35] A variety of immunologic mechanisms has been proposed including an organ-specific autoimmune disorder with activated CD4 and T lymphocytes having a cytotoxic effect in myocardial tissue, but the precise sequence of events is not known.[36–39] Some believe the extensive damage of cardiac tissue is an immune dysfunction that is absolutely requisite for the organ-specific autoimmune reaction during the chronic phase of the disease, rather than cross-reactivity between *T cruzi* antigens and class II histocompatibility molecules. Microvascular abnormalities have also been proposed as causes of hypoperfusion leading to focal myocytolysis and fibrosis.[39,40]

REFERENCES

1. Chagas C. Nova tripanozomiaze humana: estudos sobre a morfolojia e o ciclo evalutivo do *Schizotrypanum cruzi* n gen n sp agente etiolojico de nova entidade morbida do homen. *Mem Inst Oswaldo Cruz.* 1909;1:159–218.
2. Leonard J. Carlos Chagas, health pioneer of the Brazilian backlands. *Bull PAHO.* 1990;24:226–239.
3. World Health Organization. Chagas' disease—frequency and geographical distribution. *Wkly Epidem Rec.* 1990; 65:257–260.
4. Edgcomb JH, Johnson CM. American trypanosomiasis (Chagas' disease). In: Binford CH and Connor DH, eds. *Pathology of Tropical and Extraordinary Diseases.* Washington, DC: Armed Forces Institute of Pathology; 1976: 244–251.
5. Schiffler RJ, Mansur GP, Navin TR, Limpakarnjanarat K. Indigenous Chagas' disease (American trypanosomiasis) in California. *JAMA.* 1984;251:2983–2984.
6. Control of Chagas' disease: report of a WHO expert committee. *WHO Tech Rep Ser.* 1991;811:27–37.
7. Grant IH, Gold JWM, Wittner M, et al. Transfusion-associated acute Chagas' disease acquired in the United States. *Ann Intern Med.* 1989;111:849–851.
8. Kirchoff LV. Is *Trypanosoma cruzi* a new threat to our blood supply? *Ann Intern Med.* 1989;111:773–775.
9. Wendel S, Gonzaga AL. Chagas' disease and blood transfusion: a new world problem? *Vox Sang.* 1993;64:1–12.
10. Amato Neto V, Molinari HE, de Siqueira AF, de Lucas RS. Análise, por meio de reaçao de fixaçao do complemento, do risco de aquisiçao da doença de Chagas atraves da hemoterapia, por parte de pacientes politransfundidos. *Rev Goiana Med.* 1975;21:1–9.
11. Ferraz AS, Figueiredo JFC. Transmission of Chagas' disease through transplanted kidney: occurrence of the acute form of the disease in two recipients from the same donor. *Rev Inst Med Trop Sao Paulo.* 1993;35:461–463.
12. Kirchhoff LV. American trypanosomiasis (Chagas' disease)—a tropical disease now in the United States. *N Engl J Med.* 1993;329:639–644.
13. Bittencourt AL. Possible risk factors for vertical transmission of Chagas' disease. *Rev Inst Med Trop Sao Paulo.* 1992;34:403–408.
14. Brabin L. The epidemiological significance of Chagas' disease in women. *Mem Inst Oswaldo Cruz.* 1992;87:73–79.
15. Oddó D, Casanova M, Acuña G, Ballesteros J, Morales B. Acute Chagas' disease (trypanosomiasis americana) in acquired immunodeficiency syndrome: report of two cases. *Hum Pathol.* 1992;23:41–44.
16. Rocha A, Ferreira MS, Nishioka SA, et al. *Trypanosoma cruzi* meningoencephalitis and myocarditis in a patient with acquired immunodeficiency syndrome. *Rev Inst Med Trop Sao Paulo.* 1993;35:205–208.
17. Hagar JM, Rahimtoola SH. Chagas' heart disease in the United States. *N Engl J Med.* 1991;325:763–768.
18. Milei J, Mantner B, Storino R, Sanchez JA, Ferrons VJ. Does Chagas' disease exist as an undiagnosed form of cardiomyopathy in the United States? *Am Heart J.* 1992;123:1732–1735.
19. Kirchoff LV. Chagas' disease—American trypanosomiasis. *Inf Dis Clin North Am.* 1993;7:487–502.
20. Zeledon R. Chagas' disease: an ecological appraisal with special emphasis on its insect vectors. *Ann Rev Entomol.* 1981;26:101–133.
21. Coura JR. Determinantes epidemiológicos da doença de Chagas no Brasil: a infecçao, a doença e sua morbimortalidade. *Mem Inst Oswaldo Cruz.* 1988;83(suppl I): 392–402.
22. Tonn RJ. Review of recent publications on the ecology, biology and control of vector of Chagas' disease. *Rev Argentina Microbiol.* 1988;20:4–24.
23. Pittella JEH. Central nervous system involvement in Chagas' disease. An updating. *Rev Inst Med Trop Sao Paulo.* 1993;35:111–116.
24. Tanowitz HB, Kirchhoff LV, Simon D, Morris SA, Weiss LM, Wittner M. Chagas' disease. *Clin Microbiol Rev.* 1992;5:400–419.
25. Chiari E, Dias JC, Lana M, Chiari CA. Hemocultures for the parasitological diagnosis of human chronic Chagas' disease. *Rev Soc Bras Med Trop.* 1989;22:19–23.
26. Kirchhoff LV, Gam AA, Gusmao RA, Goldsmith RS, Rezende JM, Rassi A. Increased specificity of serodiagnosis of Chagas' disease by detection of antibody to the 72- and 90-kilodalton glycoprotein of *Trypanosoma cruzi*. *J Infect Dis.* 1987;155:561–564.
27. Avila HA, Sigman DS, Cohen LM, Millikan RC, Simpson L. Polymerase chain reaction amplification of *Trypanosoma cruzi* kinetoplast minicircle DNA isolated from whole blood lysates: diagnosis of chronic Chagas' disease. *Mol Biochem Parasitol.* 1991;48:211–221.

28. Russomando G, Figueredo A, Almirón M, Sakamoto M, Morita K. Polymerase chain reaction-based detection of *Trypanosoma cruzi* DNA in serum. *J Clin Microbiol.* 1992;30:2864–2868.
29. Acquatella A, Catalioti F, Gomez-Mancebo JR, Davalos V, Villalobos L. Long-term control of Chagas' disease in Venezuela: effects on serologic findings, electrocardiographic abnormalities, and clinical outcome. *Circulation.* 1987;76:556–562.
30. Iosa D, Massari DC, Dorsey FC. Chagas' cardioneuropathy: effects of gangliosite treatment in chronic dysautonomic patients—a randomized double-blind, parallel, placebo-controlled study. *Am Heart J.* 1991;122:775–785.
31. Oliveira JS, Mello De Olivera JA, Frederigue U Jr, Lima Filho EC. Apical aneurysm of Chagas' heart disease. *Br Heart J.* 1981;46:432–437.
32. Köberle F. Chagas' disease and Chagas' syndromes: the pathology of American trypanosomiasis. *Adv Parasitol.* 1968;6:63–116.
33. Hutt MSR, Köberle F, Salfelder K. Leishmaniasis and trypanosomiasis. In: H. Spencer, ed. *Tropical Pathology.* New York: Springer-Verlag; 1973:351–398.
34. Pinotti HW, Felix VN, Zilberstein B, Cecconello I. Surgical complications of Chagas' disease: megaesophagus, achalasia of the pylorus and cholelithiasis. *World J Surg.* 1991;15:198–204.
35. Palacious-Prü E, Carrasco H, Scorza C, Espinoza R. Ultrastructural characteristics of different stages of human chagasic myocarditis. *Am J Trop Med Hyg.* 1989;41:29–40.
36. Petry K, Eisen H. Chagas' disease: a model for the study of autoimmune diseases. *Parasitol Today.* 1989;5:111–116.
37. Van Voorhis WC, Eisen H. Fl 160: A surface antigen of *Trypanosoma cruzi* that mimics mammalian nervous tissue. *J Exp Med.* 1989;169:641–652.
38. Teixeira ARL, Lacava Z, Santana JM, Luna H. Inserçao de DNA de *Trypanosoma cruzi* no genoma de célula hospedeira de mamiféro por meio de infecçao. *Rev Soc Bras Med Trop.* 1991;24:55–58.
39. Mengel JO, Rossi MA. Chronic chagasic myocarditis pathogenesis: dependence on autoimmune and microvascular factors. *Am Heart J.* 1992;124:1052–1057.
40. Rossi M. Microvascular changes as a cause of chronic cardiomyopathy in Chagas' disease. *Am Heart J.* 1990;120: 233–236.

PART VI

Helminthic Infections

CHAPTER 144

Angiostrongyliasis

John H. Cross

In hunter–gatherer, pre-agricultural times, the human life expectancy was about 20 to 30 years. That's also what it was in Western Europe in Late Roman and in Medieval times. It didn't rise to 40 years until around the year 1870. It reached 50 in 1915, 60 in 1930, 70 in 1955 and is today approaching 80 (a little more for women, a little less for men). The rest of the world is retracing the European increment in longevity. What is the cause of this stunning, unprecedented, humanitarian transition? The germ theory of disease, public health measures, medicines and medical technology. Longevity is perhaps the best single measure of the physical quality of life. (If you're dead, there's little you can do to be happy.) This is a precious offering from science to humanity—nothing less than the gift of life.

Carl Sagan (1934–), The Demon Haunted World

INTRODUCTION

Humans acquire several parasites of animals from the food they eat. *Angiostrongylus cantonensis,* a metastrongyle nematode normally in the lungs of rats, is acquired by eating mollusks infected with its larval stages. In humans the parasite invades the central nervous system (CNS), causing eosinophilic meningitis or eosinophilic meningoencephalitis.

ANGIOSTRONGYLUS CANTONENSIS

The rat lungworm, *A cantonensis,* was first reported[1] from rats in China in 1935 and the first human infection was reported in Taiwan during World War II.[2] The life cycle of *A cantonensis* in rodents and the passage of the nematode through the CNS was elucidated in Australia in 1955.[3] The worm was recognized as an important cause of human disease in 1962.[4]

DEFINITION

The third-stage larvae of *A cantonensis,* acquired by eating infected definitive or paratenic hosts, invade the CNS of humans and cause an eosinophilic meningitis or eosinophilic meningoencephalitis and eosinophilic pleocytosis. Larval worms have been recovered from the CNS, cerebrospinal fluid, and, occasionally, from eyes. Synonyms include angiostrongyliasis, eosinophilic meningitis, and eosinophilic meningoencephalitis.

GEOGRAPHIC DISTRIBUTION

Angiostrongyliasis is reported worldwide in rats and mulluskan intermediate hosts, and in many areas humans also become infected.[5] Infections of animals are throughout the Pacific Islands, most of Asia, Australia, Africa, Cuba, Puerto Rico, and New Orleans, Louisiana, in the United States. Human infections have been recognized in the Pacific, Asia, Africa, and the Caribbean. Most human infections have been in Taiwan, Thailand, Tahiti, and New Caledonia.

LIFE CYCLE, NATURAL HISTORY, AND EPIDEMIOLOGY

The habitat of adult male and female *A cantonensis* is the pulmonary arteries of rats. After copulating, female

A cantonensis produce eggs that lodge in the capillaries of the lungs. First-stage larvae develop within the eggs, emerge from the eggs, and break through the capillaries into the alveoli. From here the larvae migrate into the bronchioles, are carried up in the mucociliary escalator to the trachea, are then swallowed, and pass into the alimentary tract and out in the rat's feces. A variety of mollusks, such as terrestrial and aquatic snails and slugs, serve as intermediate hosts. First-stage larvae enter the molluskan host either by direct penetration or ingestion, and migrate to the foot muscle. In 7 to 9 days, the larvae molt into the second stage and 5 to 7 days later into the third or infective stage. The larvae coil up in the muscles and remain quiescent until freed after the mollusk is eaten and the musculature digested in the rat's stomach.

Freed third-stage larvae quickly penetrate the intestinal mucosa, enter the blood, and are carried to heart, lungs, brain, and spinal cord, reaching these organs within 24 hours. The larvae move into the gray matter and 4 to 5 days after infection molt into the fourth larval stage. They move to the subarachnoid space where the final molt is in 7 to 9 days. The young adult worms leave the brain and migrate to the lungs through the venous sinuses and reach the pulmonary artery in 26 to 35 days after infection. They become sexually mature, copulate, and produce eggs; the prepatent period is 42 to 45 days.

Angiostrongyliasis develops in humans after swallowing infected intermediate or paratenic hosts. Most infections have been acquired by eating snails, slugs, or other mollusks or secondarily infected crustaceans serving as paratenic hosts. Third-stage larvae are released from host tissues by digestive processes in the gastrointestinal system and, as in the life cycle in rats, larvae penetrate the intestinal tissues and are carried by the blood to the liver, heart, and lungs and eventually to the CNS. The larvae continue to develop into fourth and fifth stages in the CNS and sometimes in the eyes. There is usually no further development beyond the young adult stage in man and other abnormal hosts. On three occasions, however, adults and egg-producing female worms have migrated to the lungs of humans; twice in Taiwan[6,7] and once in Thailand.[8]

MORPHOLOGY

Adult *A cantonensis* are in the pulmonary arteries of rodents. The body is filariform and tapers at both ends. The mouth at the anterior end has three lips and surrounding papillae. The mouth opens into an esophagus, which leads to the intestines and subterminal anus. Female worms (Figure 144–1) are 21 to 35 mm long by 0.30 to 0.36 mm in diameter. The posterior end is blunt with a vulvar opening anterior to the anus. Eggs are ovoid, 46 to 74 μm, and unembryonated when laid. Males (Figure 144–2) are 16 to 19 mm by 0.26 mm in diameter. A small bursa copulatrix is at the posterior end. The configuration of the bursal rays is of taxonomic importance, as is the length of the spicules, 1.00 to 1.46 mm for *A cantonensis*. The cuticle is smooth and somewhat thickened at both ends.[9]

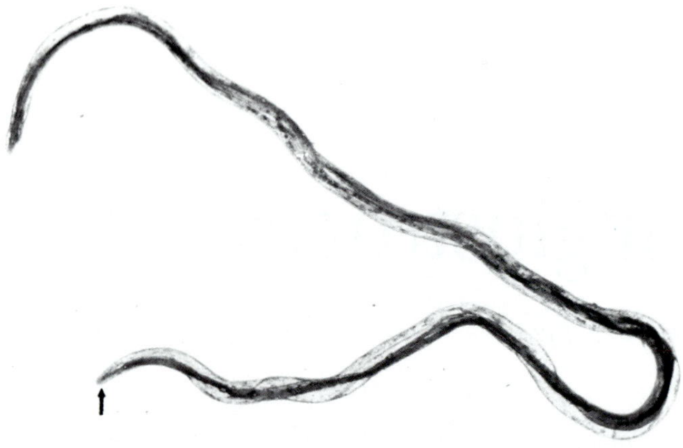

Figure 144–1. Female *A cantonensis;* note anterior end (*arrow*) (×15).

CLINICAL FEATURES

The progress of the disease follows the migration of third-stage larvae. Passage through the gastrointestinal tract and liver may cause a gastroenteritis and hepatomegaly. A dry cough, rhinorrhea, nasal obstruction, sneezing, sore throat, occasional headache,

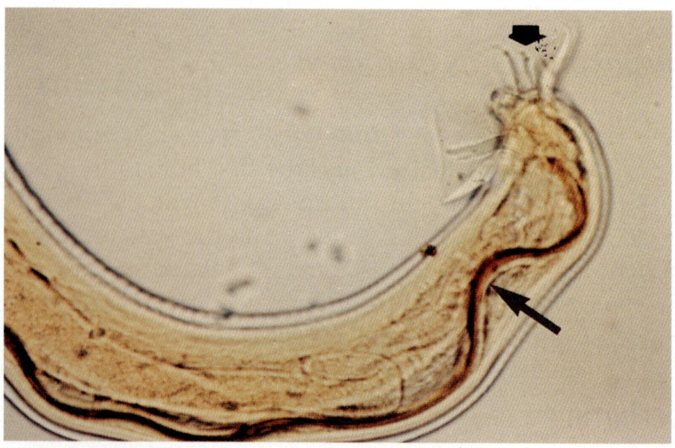

Figure 144–2. Male *A cantonensis,* posterior end. Note long spicule (*thin arrow*) and bursa (*large arrow*) (×110).

malaise, and mild fever occur when larvae migrate through lung. These symptoms are followed by severe headache, vomiting, and intermittent fever.[10] Most parasites reach the CNS within 24 to 48 hours, but this can vary from 1 to 36 days. In most patients, symptoms of CNS involvement are abrupt with headache, nausea, vomiting, fever, and stiff neck. Destruction and focal inflammatory cell infiltrates of nerve fibers, as seen in animals, probably cause myalgia, pain, and paresthesia of skin of trunk and limbs. This may persist for weeks. Worms that die in neural tissue are surrounded by granulomatous reaction. If the parasites live, they migrate to the surface of the brain and cord and may enter the subarachnoid spaces and continue to grow into young adult worms. Worms on the surface of the brain cause inflammation of the meninges with many eosinophils. Coma has been reported and is probably caused by many parasites. Moving worms have been observed in the eye in Taiwan[11] and, especially, in Thailand.[12] There are also sporadic reports of eye involvement from Indonesia[13] and Papua New Guinea.[14]

Punyagupta et al[15] and Yii[10] studied two groups of 484 and 114 patients, respectively. The most common symptoms were headache, neck stiffness, nausea, vomiting, anorexia, fever, cough, constipation, malaise, lethargy, blurred vision, paresthesia, abdominal pain, weakness of limbs, and muscle twitching. Frequent signs were abnormal tendon reflexes, including abnormal achilles reflex, a positive Kernig's sign, paresthesias, impairment of vision, paralysis of eye muscles, and impairment of sensorium. Death is not common but when the patient does die the cause is large numbers of worms in the CNS.

PATHOLOGY

Approximately 15 autopsies have been done on patients with neuroangiostrongyliasis. Hung and Chen[7] summarized the reports from Hawaii, Vietnam, Thailand, Taiwan, New Hebrides (Vanuatu), and Samoa. The most recent report is from Thailand.[16]

Dead *A cantonensis* worms cause more serious lesions than do living worms and the greater the number of worms the more damage there is to the CNS. In early infections, the parasites are alive and actively move in and out of the tissue, and come to lie in the subarachnoid spaces on the surface of the brain and spinal cord. Here the parasites can easily be seen and recovered by teasing the fresh tissue under a stereoscopic or dissecting microscope. Intact worms can be removed and identified. Worms can also be recovered by soaking the brain and spinal cord in saline. More than 500 worms were recovered from the spinal cord and meninges by Yii[10] after soaking in saline and this collection included male and female young adult worms. The worms were easily identified as *A cantonensis* by following the description of Bhaibulaya.[9]

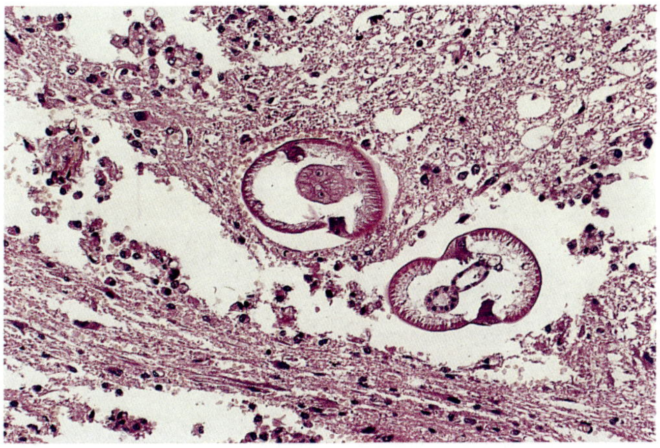

Figure 144–3. Sections of intact viable *A cantonensis* larva in human spinal cord causing abundant tissue reaction consisting mainly of foamy macrophages [hematoxylin-eosin (H&E), ×40].

In most autopsies, gross examination of the brain and cord reveals no lesions. Some brains, however, are congested and the basal portion of the leptomeninges are thickened. Also there may be subarachnoid hemorrhage over the brain and cord.[17] Gross lesions also include clouding of basal and cerebellar meninges.

Parasites in histologic preparations are easy to see, but examination of sections from different parts of the brain and cord is often necessary. Slides from different blocks should be made to increase the chance of finding the worms. As already noted, living worms elicit little tissue reaction (Figure 144–3), while dead parasites and fragments of worms provoke an inflammatory reaction dominated by eosinophilic leukocytes, a granulomatous reaction that includes giant cells, and foci of necrosis (Figure 144–4). One characteristic is tracks made by the migrating worms through the tissue. If worms are not found, the presence of glial scars containing hemosiderin, microscopic hemorrhages, eosinophils, and Charcot–Leyden crystals establish a presumptive diagnosis. Vascular dilatation, both arterial and venous, in the subarachnoid spaces may also be present. Nerve cells adjacent to worms and tracks may exhibit central chromatolysis and axonal swelling. Similar changes may involve spinal cord.[12]

More than 500 *A cantonensis* young adult worms were recovered from the brain and spinal cord at autopsy of a 5-year-old child who died of eosinophilic meningitis in Taiwan. Histologically, the leptomeninges were infiltrated with lymphocytes, pigment-laden macrophages, and mononuclear cells. Several foreign-body-type giant cells were adjacent to degenerated

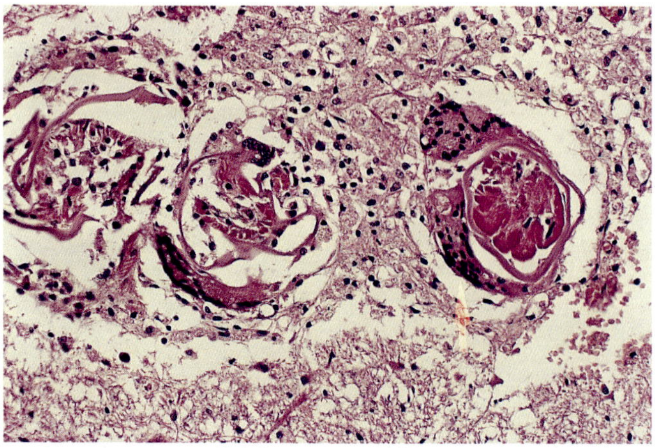

Figure 144–4. Fragments of viable *A cantonensis* larva in the meninges causing an eosinophilic inflammatory reaction, with giant cells (*arrow*) and necrosis of contiguous spinal cord (H&E, ×40).

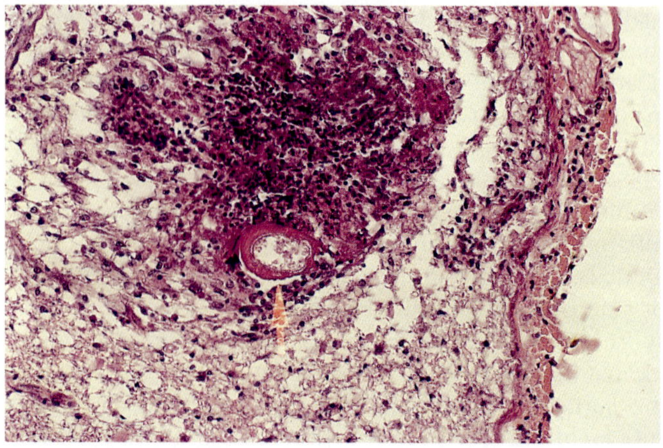

Figure 144–6. Cross-section of a degenerating *A cantonensis* in spinal cord. The worm is surrounded by a coagulum of degenerating eosinophils and a few neutrophils (H&E, ×25).

worms. Cross-sections of viable parasites were also in the cerebral and cerebellar sulci. Cerebral and meningeal vessels were surrounded by lymphocytes. The cerebral encephalomalacia and numerous glial elements, including gitter cells, were in these regions. Parasites and foreign-body giant cells were also in the central canal of the spinal cord, and there was perivascular cuffing by lymphocytes nearby (Figure 144–5). Several small foci of myelomalacia were in the thoracic cord. Foreign-body giant cells were adjacent to a degenerating worm in the lateral column (Figure 144–6), and a foreign-body reaction surrounded all dead worms. Worms recently dead provoked a mixed reaction of mononuclear cells, lymphocytes, and eosinophils.

An interesting finding, reported for the first time, was worms in the lung. Microscopically, the lungs were congested and alveoli contained numerous pigment-laden macrophages. Many bronchi contained neutrophils and proteinaceous material, and neutrophils had infiltrated some areas, mainly around bronchi and bronchioles. Focal hemorrhages were in the alveoli and adjacent structures. Some small vessels contained thrombi. A few bronchi were patent, and the pleura was focally thickened. Sections of live worms were in pulmonary vessels (Figure 144–7) and degenerating worms in other vessels. More than 100 young adult worms were recovered from lung tissue. Some of the female worms contained eggs. This was the first time it was shown that *A cantonensis* could reach sexual maturity in humans (Yii et al, unpublished).

Nonhuman primates have been experimentally[18] and naturally[19] infected with *A cantonensis;* the patho-

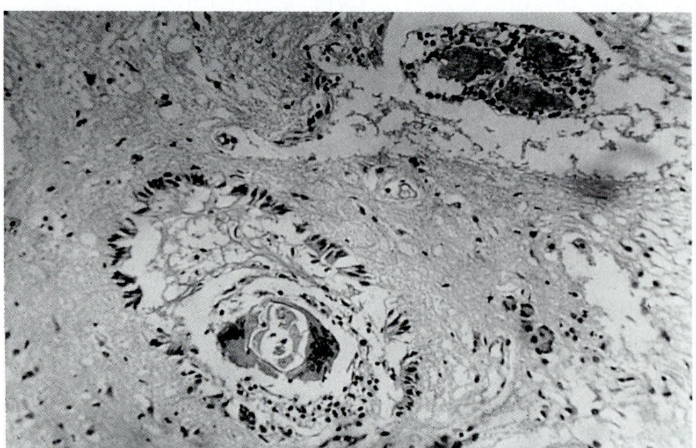

Figure 144–5. *Angiostrongylus cantonensis* larva in the central canal of spinal cord, surrounded by giant cells (×80).

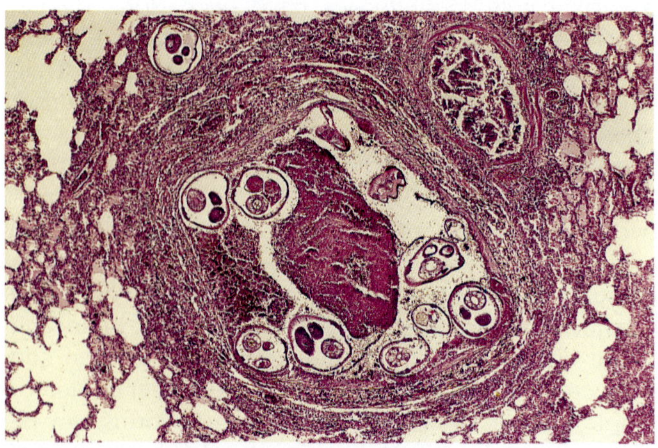

Figure 144–7. Human lung with sections of an intact viable *A cantonensis* in and outside a branch of the pulmonary artery (H&E, ×25).

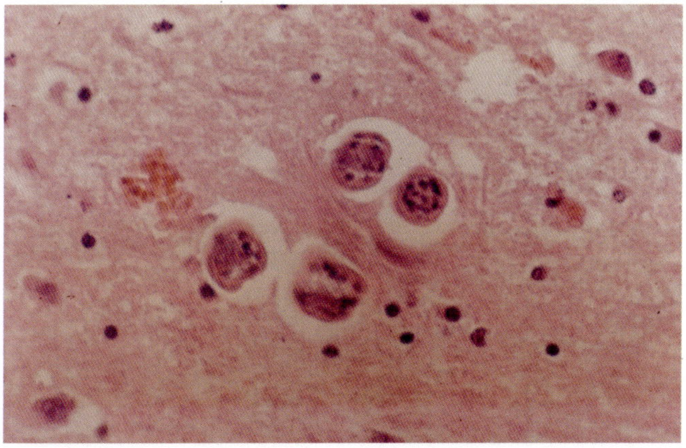

Figure 144–8. *Angiostrongylus cantonensis* in brain of an experimentally infected Taiwan monkey 7 days after infection showing little tissue reaction (H&E, ×80).

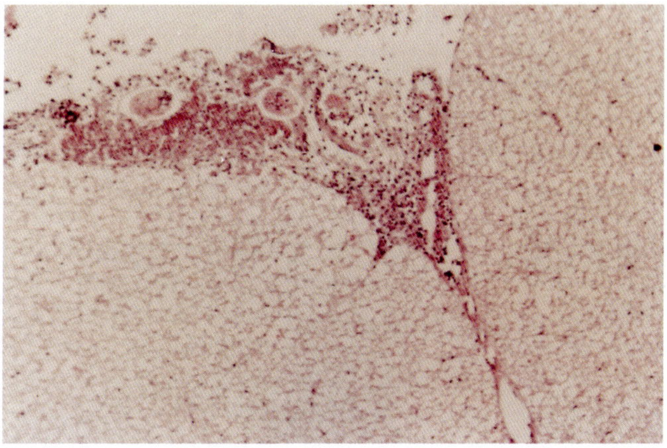

Figure 144–10. *Angiostrongylus cantonensis* larva in subarachnoid space of a Taiwan monkey 24 days after infection. The larva is surrounded by an intense inflammatory cell reaction (H&E, ×80).

logic findings resembling those in humans. In Taiwan, monkeys were infected with 10,000 larvae of the Taiwan strain of *A cantonensis*. All animals died and were necropsied. Monkeys that died early in the infection exhibited vascular congestion in the leptomeninges, but there was very little tissue reaction around worms in the brain (Figure 144–8). One animal that died after 13 days had hemorrhage in the subarachnoid space of the cerebral hemisphere but little reaction to the parasite. A parasite was in the central canal of the spinal cord but there was little reaction to it (Figure 144–9). In an animal that died 24 days postinfection, the cerebral meninges were congested and there were a few neutrophils and lymphocytes. A second monkey that died after 24 days of infection had more cellular infiltration, which consisted of eosinophils, plasma cells, lymphocytes, and giant cells (Figure 144–10). Another animal that died at 32 days postinfection had perivascular hemorrhage, lymphocytes, and giant cells (Figure 144–11). This type of reaction was associated with dead rather than live worms. Worms were recovered from CNS tissue in most animals. During the first 7 to 10 days of infection, larvae were still third stage; after the second week, however, most were in the fourth larval stage. During the third week, the larvae had begun molting into the fourth stage or young adults, and after 4 weeks some were fourth stage, but most were young adults.[20]

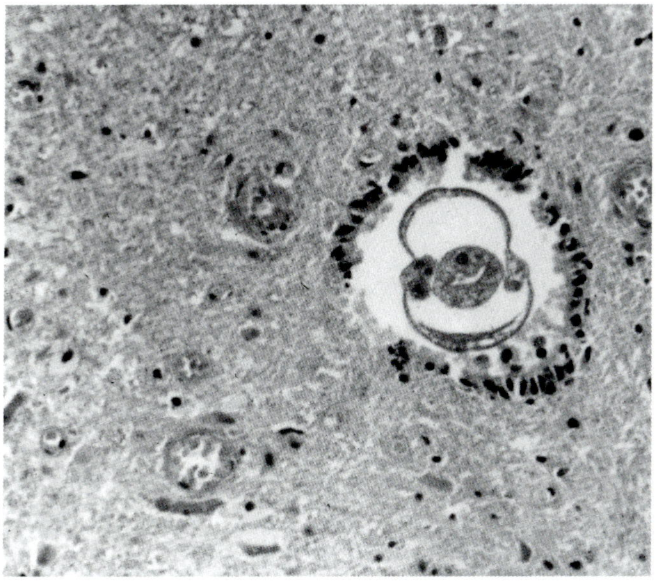

Figure 144–9. *Angiostrongylus cantonensis* larva in the central canal of the spinal cord of a Taiwan monkey 13 days after infection (H&E, ×120).

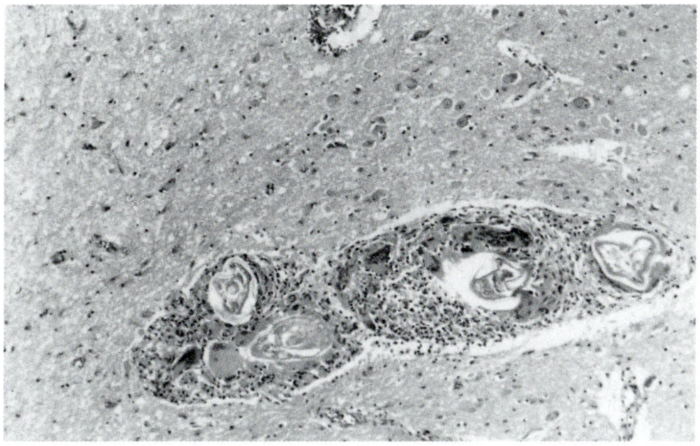

Figure 144–11. Spinal cord of a Taiwan monkey that died 32 days after infection, showing degenerating *A cantonensis* larvae surrounded by inflammatory cells including giant cells (H&E, ×80).

DIFFERENTIAL DIAGNOSIS

Several other helminthic diseases involve the CNS of humans, such as gnathostomiasis, paragonimiasis, cysticercosis, echniococcosis, schistosomiasis, and ascariasis. Most of these diseases are rare, except gnathostomiasis, which is highly endemic in Thailand. Patients with invasive *Gnathostoma spinigerum* larvae in the CNS present with paralysis of the limbs characterized by transverse or ascending myelitis followed by symptoms of nerve root pain (radiculitis) of the limbs or of the trunk. Comatose patients, particularly younger individuals, may or may not have paralysis of the limbs. The spinal fluid is usually bloody or xanthochromic with eosinophilic pleocytosis. Based on the clinical and epidemiologic information, the presumptive diagnosis of cerebrospinal angiostrongyliasis can be made. The definitive diagnosis is established by finding and identifying worms and only rarely are gnathostome larvae recovered antemortem.[12] Serologic tests are now available, especially in Thailand, which provide a presumptive diagnosis of gnathostomiasis.[21]

Gnathostome larvae are short and stout with a subglobose head armed with 7 to 9 transverse rows of hooklets. Worms from humans vary in size from 2.5 to 12.5 mm long by 0.4 to 1.2 mm wide. The worms produce large tracks (1 mm) as they move through the cerebrum, cerebellum, and spinal cord. Hemorrhagic and necrotic areas also can be seen macroscopically. Older lesions are filled with red blood cells and chronic inflammatory cell infiltrates consisting of histiocytes, lymphocytes, plasma cells, and eosinophils. Larvae are rare in histologic sections of brain. When found, the worms are difficult to identify unless the head with spines is in the section. Cross-sections of worms are large (350 μm). The cuticle is thick and the lateral cords are prominent with up to 15 muscle cells per quadrant. The intestine is well developed with coarsely granular cells.

The differential diagnosis of CNS paragonimiasis and schistosomiasis is usually based on finding eggs in granulomas in the tissue. In echinococcosis, hydatid cysts or remnants of the parasite may be found. Specific immunologic tests for these parasitoses are available.[22]

DIAGNOSIS

Angiostrongyliasis cantonensis is one of the most common causes of eosinophilic meningitis or eosinophilic meningoencephalitis in humans. Individuals from endemic areas present with headache, stiff neck, paresthesia, paralysis of eye muscles, and eosinophilic pleocytosis and a history of, or association with, ingesting an intermediate or paratenic host. Larvae in spinal fluid (Figure 144–12) confirm the diagnosis.

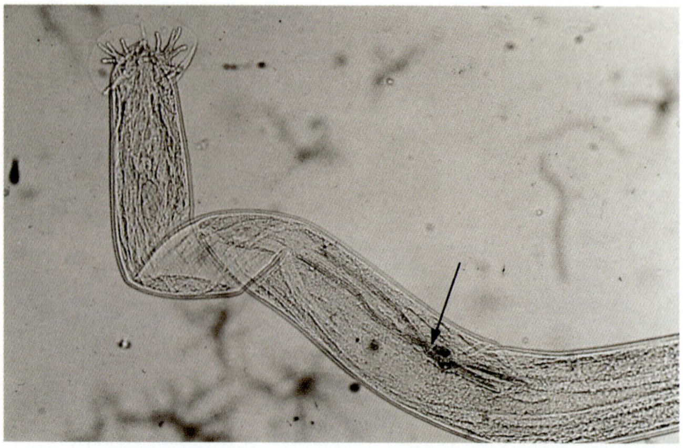

Figure 144–12. Fourth-stage larva of a male *A cantonensis* recovered from the spinal fluid of a child in Taiwan with eosinophilic meningitis. Note the bursa at the posterior end and the developing spicules (*arrow*) (H&E, ×70).

The worms in histologic preparations can be identified based on the tissue reaction parasite tracts, and morphologic characteristics of the parasite: smooth thin cuticle, coelomyarian musculature, and lateral cords containing two to four nuclei (Figure 144–13). Cross-sections of intestine are large and composed of a few multinucleated cells and golden brown material in the gut. Sections of gonads are also seen.

Cerebrospinal fluid (CSF) may be under increased pressure. The fluid is usually opalescent or turbid; xanthochromia and red blood cells are seen occasionally. Worms have been recovered from the CSF in a number

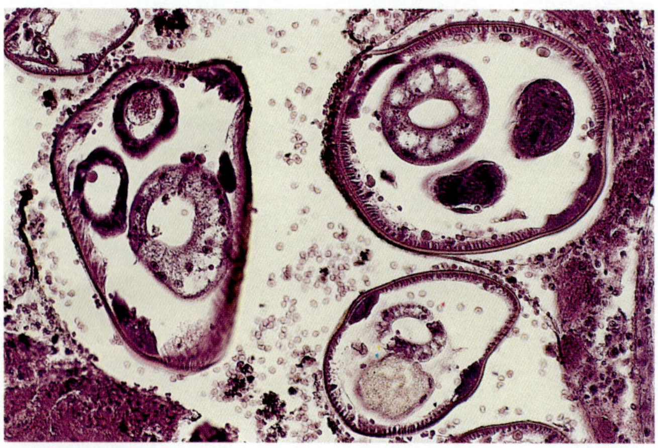

Figure 144–13. Sections of coiled *A cantonensis* in human lung. Note coelomyarian musculature, intestine, and gonad (H&E, ×120).

of patients and recently with some regularity in pediatric patients in Taiwan.[23] Eosinophils are easily seen along with neutrophils and lymphocytes in CSF, and white cell counts range from 190 to 4345 per mm^3. Eosinophils may account for 15% to 88% of the cells in proven infections of eosinophilic pleocytosis.[12] Protein content of spinal fluid may be increased, and rarely sugar may be low. Peripheral blood examinations usually show a leucocytosis with an eosinophilia of more than 10%.[15] Immunoglobulins A and G may be elevated in CSF.[24]

Immunologic tests such as enzyme-linked immunosorbent assays on sera and CSF have been of value in making a presumptive diagnosis[25–27] and antigen detection using monoclonal antibodies was also reported of value. Computer tomographic myelography and magnetic resonance imaging have also aided in the diagnosis.[23,28]

Direct ocular involvement by *A cantonensis* has been reported in which young worms were recovered. The worms can be seen through the ophthalmoscope or slit lamp. Patients usually do not have meningitis but there may be eosinophilic pleocytosis and worms in CSF.[7]

REFERENCES

1. Chen HT. Un nouveau nematode pulmonaire, *Pulmonena cantonensis* n g n sp, des rats de canton. *Ann Parasitol.* 1935;13:312.
2. Nomura S, Lin PH. First case report of human infection with *Haemostrongylus ratti,* Yokogawa. *Taiwan No Ikai.* 1945;3:589–592.
3. Mackerras MJ, Sandars DF. The life history of the rat lungworm, *Angiostrongylus cantonensis* (Chen) (Nematoda: Metastrongylidae). *Australian J Zool.* 1955;3:1–21.
4. Rosen L, Chappell R, Laqueur GL, Wallace GD, and Weinstein PP. Eosinophilic meningitis caused by a metastrongylid lungworm of rats. *JAMA.* 1962;179:620–624.
5. Cross JH. Public health importance of *Angiostrongylus cantonensis* and its relatives. *Parasitol Today.* 1987;3: 367–369.
6. Yii CY, Chen CY, Fresh JW, Chen T, Cross JH. Human angiostrongyliasis involving the lungs. *Chin J Microbiol.* 1968;1:148–150.
7. Hung TP, Chen ER. Angiostrongyliasis (*Angiostrongylus cantonensis*). In: Harris AA, ed. *Handbook of Clinical Neurology.* Amsterdam: Elsevier Science Publishers; 1988; 8:545–562.
8. Sonakul D. Pathological findings in four cases of human angiostrongyliasis. *Southeast Asian J Trop Med Public Health.* 1978;9:220–227.
9. Bhaibulaya M. Morphology and toxonomy of major *Angiostrongylus* species of Eastern Asia and Australia. In: Cross JH, ed. *Studies in Angiostrongyliasis in Eastern Asia and Australia.* Taipei, Taiwan: US Naval Medical Research Unit #2; 1979:4–13.
10. Yii CY. Clinical observations on eosinophilic meningitis and meningoencephalitis caused by *Angiostrongylus cantonensis* in Taiwan. *Am J Trop Med Hyg.* 1976;25:233–249.
11. Hsieh HC. *Angiostrongylus cantonensis* and eosinophilic meningitis or meningoencephalitis due to its infection. *Taiwan Clin Med.* 1967;3:1–5.
12. Punyagupta S. Angiostrongyliasis: clinical features and human pathology. In: Cross JH, ed. *Studies on Angiostrongyliasis in Eastern Asia and Australia.* Taipei, Taiwan: US Naval Medical Research Unit #2; NAMRU-2-SP-44; 1979:138–150.
13. Sundardi W, Lokolla DM, Margono SS. Ocular angiostrongyliasis in Semarang, Central Java. *Am J Trop Med Hyg.* 1977;26:72–74.
14. Scrimgeour EM, Chambers BR, Kaven J. A probable case of ocular angiostrongyliasis in New Britain, Papua New Guinea. *Trans R Soc Trop Med Hyg.* 1982;76:538–540.
15. Punyagupta S, Juttijudata P, Bunnag T. Eosinophilic meningitis in Thailand. Clinical studies of 484 typical cases probably caused by *Angiostrongylus cantonensis. Am J Trop Med Hyg.* 1975;24:921–931.
16. Witoonpanich R, Chuahirun S, Soranastaporn S, Rojanasunan P. Eosinophilic myelomeningoencephalitis caused by *Angiostrongylus cantonensis:* a report of three cases. *Southeast Asian J Trop Med Public Health.* 1991;22: 262–267.
17. Kliks MM, Kroenke I, Hardman JM. Eosinophilic radiculomyeloencephalitis: an angiostrongyliasis outbreak in American Samoa related to ingestion of *Achatina fulica* snails. *Am J Trop Med Hyg.* 1982;31:1114–1122.
18. Alicata JE, Loison G, Cavallo A. Parasitic meningoencephalitis experimentally produced in a monkey with larvae of *Angiostrongylus cantonensis. J Parasitol.* 1963;49: 156–157.
19. Gardiner CH, Wells S, Gutter AE, et al. Eosinophilic meningoencephalitis due to *Angiostrongylus cantonensis* as the cause of death in captive non-human primates. *Am J Trop Med Hyg.* 1990;42:70–84.
20. Cross JH. Experimental studies on *Angiostrongylus* species and strains in monkeys and laboratory animals. In: Cross JH, ed. *Studies on Angiostrongyliasis in Eastern Asia and Australia.* Taipei, Taiwan: US Naval Medical Research Unit #2; NAMRU-2-SP-44; 1979:118–137.
21. Migasena S, Pitisuttihum P, Desakorn V. *Gnathostoma* larva migrans among guests of a New Year party. In: *Proceedings 33rd SEAMEO-TROPMED Regional Seminar on Emerging Problems in Food-borne Parasitic Zoonoses;* November 1990; Chiang Mai, Thailand; 1991:225–232.
22. Jaroonvesama N. Differential diagnosis of eosinophilic meningitis. *Parasitol Today.* 1988;4:262–266.
23. Hwang KP and Chen ER. Clinical studies on angiostrongyliasis cantonensis among children in Taiwan. In: *Proceedings 33rd SEAMEO-TROPMED Regional Seminar on Emerging Problems in Food-borne Parasitic Zoonoses;* November 1990; Chiang Mai, Thailand; 1991:194–199.
24. Tungkanak R, Sirisinha S, Punyagupta S. Serum and cerebrospinal fluid in eosinophilic meningoencephalitis: im-

munoglobulins and antibody to *Angiostrongylus cantonensis. Am J Trop Med Hyg.* 1972;21:415–420.
25. Cross JH, Chi JHC. ELISA for the detection of *Angiostrongylus cantonensis* antibodies in patients with eosinophilic meningitis. *Southeast Asia J Trop Med Public Health.* 1982; 13:73.
26. Jaroonesama N, Charoenlarp K, Buranasin P, Zaraspe GG, Cross JH. ELISA testing in cases of clinical angiostrongyliasis in Thailand. *Southeast Asian J Trop Med Public Health.* 1982;16:110–112.
27. Yen CM, Chen ER. Detection of antibodies to *Angiostrongylus cantonensis* in serum and cerebrospinal fluid of patients with eosinophilic meningitis. *Int J Parasitol.* 1991; 21:17–21.
28. Wood G, Delamont S, Whitby M, Boyle R. Spinal sensory radiculopathy due to *Angiostrongylus cantonensis* infection. *Postgrad Med J.* 1991;67:70–72.

CHAPTER 145

Anisakiasis

Judy A. Sakanari

A man may fish with a worm that hath eat of a king, and eat of the fish that hath fed on that worm.

William Shakespeare, Hamlet, IV, iii, 29

DEFINITION

Anisakiasis is a zoonotic disease acquired by eating raw or inadequately cooked fish containing larval nematodes belonging to the family of roundworms, Anisakidae. The two species most commonly implicated are *Anisakis simplex* and *Pseudoterranova decipiens* (formerly *Phocanema decipiens*) (class Ascaridida). The synonyms "herringworm" or "whaleworm" for *Anisakis* and "codworm" or "sealworm" for *Pseudoterranova* reflect the various hosts involved in the parasite's life cycle.

LIFE CYCLE

The life cycles of both *Anisakis* and *Pseudoterranova* involve various marine invertebrate and vertebrate hosts.[1–3] Adults worms in the stomach of marine mammals (whales, seals, and dolphins) pass eggs with feces into seawater. Larvae hatch and are eaten by small crustaceans, which become infected. The crustaceans must then be eaten by fish and infective larvae in fish are eaten by marine mammals. Humans are not appropriate hosts, and in humans larvae do not multiply or develop into adult worms.

EPIDEMIOLOGY

Cultural and social habits contribute to parasitic infections, and in the case of anisakiasis, people who eat lightly cooked or raw fish dishes such as ceviche, sashimi, lomi-lomi, and pickled herring can become infected with anisakid nematodes (Figure 145–1).[4–7] The parasites are in fishes distributed throughout the world, and patients with anisakiasis have been reported from Japan,[3,8,9] Korea,[10,11] Thailand,[12] The Netherlands,[13] Germany,[14,15] Switzerland,[16] France,[17–20] Belgium,[7] the United Kingdom,[21,22] New Zealand,[23] Chile,[24,25] and North America.[26–29] In Japan, the estimated number of infections is 1000 per year,[30] whereas in North America, there have been only 50 confirmed infections, most of which have occurred along the West Coast and Hawaii.[5,29] Anisakiasis is now a reportable disease, and it is believed that the published reports do not reflect the actual incidence of infection among those who have mild symptoms or are transiently infected, ie, whereby worms are either expectorated or excreted. With the increasing popularity of raw, lightly cooked, pickled, or smoked fish, it is important to include dietary habits in patient histories.

Some of the edible fishes that sometimes harbor worms include mackerel, cod, herring, salmon, halibut, and Pacific red snapper.[4,31,32] Thorough cooking (60°C for 10 minutes) or freezing (−20°C for 3 days) kills the parasites.

CLINICAL FEATURES

After ingestion, the anisakid worms may migrate back up the esophagus and give rise to the "tingling throat" syndrome. When this happens the worms induce coughing and are expectorated.[6,33] Worms can also be passed through the digestive tract and be in the patient's stools. If the parasites become invasive (Figure 145–2), they may penetrate the gastric or intestinal

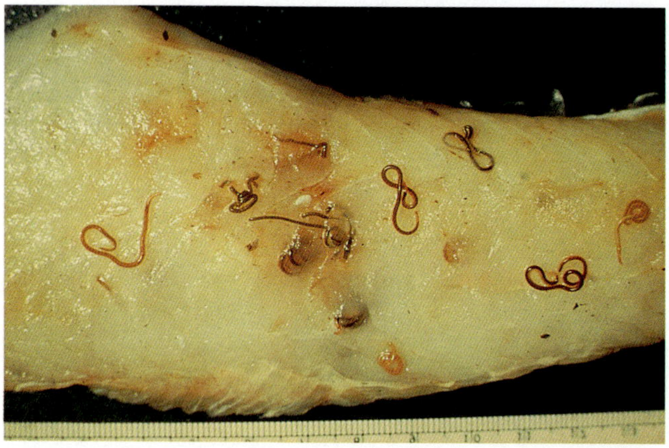

Figure 145–1. Rockfish fillet with multiple larvae of *Pseudoterranova decipiens. Pseudoterranova* larvae, unlike *Anisakis* larvae, are pigmented. *Pseudoterranova* are also larger than *Anisakis. (Photograph by Dr. Michael Moser, University of California, Santa Cruz.)*

mucosa and migrate to extragastrointestinal sites such as the omentum, pancreas, liver, and lung.[34–36]

Anisakiasis may be asymptomatic, acute, or chronic. Symptoms of acute infection include severe abdominal pain, nausea, vomiting, and diarrhea. Symptoms of acute gastric anisakiasis occur 1 to 12 hours after eating the food containing the larvae, whereas with acute intestinal anisakiasis symptoms may last from 1 to 5 days.[37–39] Chronic infections may last for several weeks to years, the patients presenting with intermittent abdominal pain, nausea, and vomiting. Generally, there is no or only slight elevation in temperature, except in patients where larvae have penetrated the bowel wall causing peritonitis. Leukocyte counts increase to 10,000 to 15,000/mm^3 and eosinophil counts vary from 4% to 41%.[38,39] Acute abdominal pain disappears when worms are removed. In most patients, there is usually a single worm, but infections by multiple worms have been reported.[40]

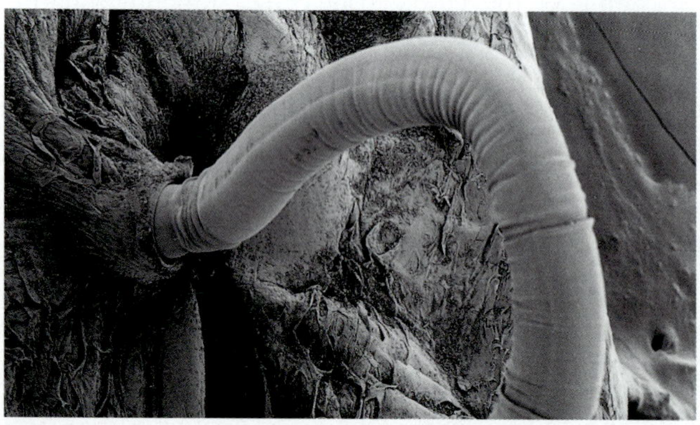

Figure 145–2. Scanning electron micrograph of an *Anisakis* larva penetrating the gastric mucosa in vitro. *(Reprinted with permission form J Parasitol 1990;76:626.)*

PATHOLOGY

The pathogenesis of anisakiasis is associated with the host's immunologic reaction to metabolic products that are secreted or excreted by the worms, and to larval antigens as the parasite is degenerating. Grossly, the infected tissues are thickened, inflamed, and dilated. Where the parasite penetrates the gastric mucosa, there are induration, small ulcers, petechiae, and erosion. The tissue around the larva is edematous and infiltrated by massive numbers of eosinophils and by neutrophils and lymphocytes. Infections in the intestine are marked by a localized inflammation with an infiltrate of eosinophils (Figure 145–3), more severe than with gastric anisakiasis.

The pathologic stages of anisakiasis are a continuum; lesions begin with a foreign-body reaction around the worm, develop into an abscess, and progress into an eosinophilic granuloma.[3,37] In an early infection, there is an infiltration of neutrophils with few eosinophils and foreign-body giant cells around an intact larva. This is followed by massive eosinophilic infection, along with lymphocytes, monocytes, neutrophils, and plasma cells. Later in the infection, abscesses are characterized by necrosis and hemorrhage with eosinophils around a degenerating worm. After several months, the abscess is reduced, foreign-body giant cells

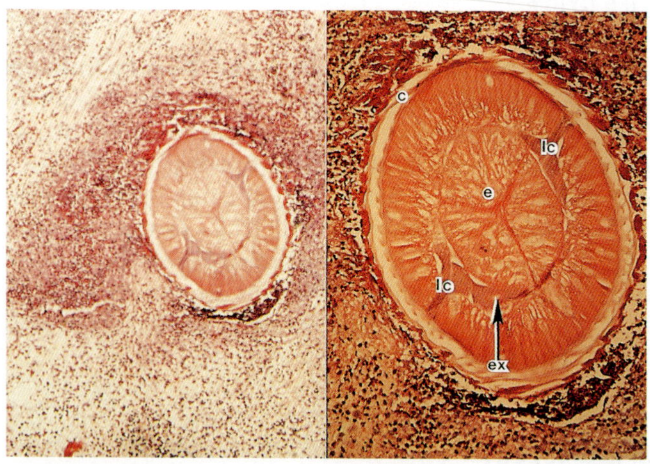

Figure 145–3. Histologic section of an *Anisakis* larva in resected ileum showing eosinophilic infiltration around worm. (left panel, low magnification). Right panel (high magnification) shows the cuticle (c), lateral chords (lc), eosphagus (e), and the excretory pore (ex). *(Reprinted with permission from Am J Clin Pathol 1988;90:110.)*

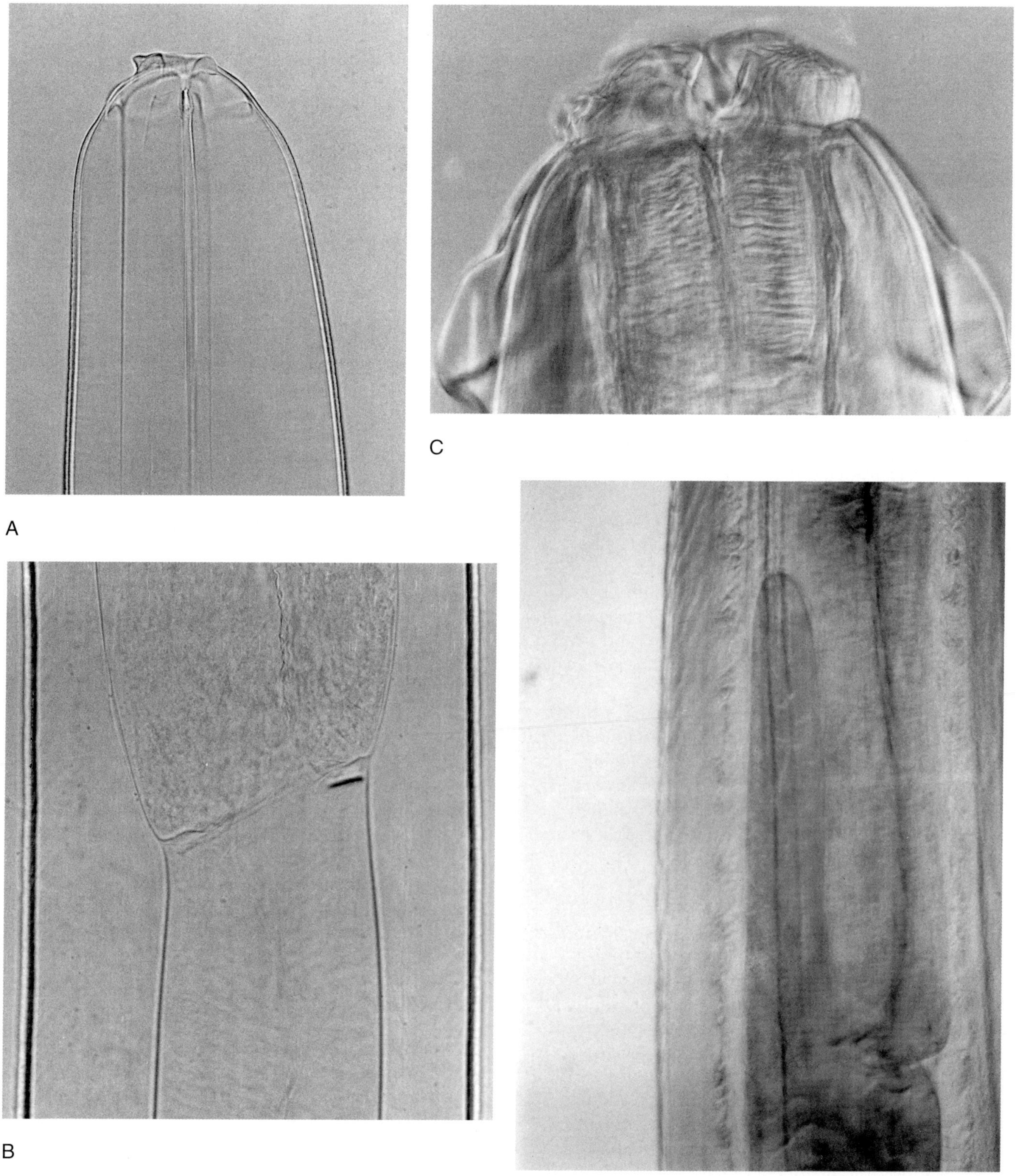

A B C D

Figure 145–4. (**A**) Third-stage *Anisakis* larva with a boring tooth at the anterior end of the worm and (**B**) the ventriculus and intestine with no cecum. (**C**) Fourth-stage *Pseudoterranova* larva with three lips at the anterior end and (**D**) a cecum extending from the intestine. *(Photograph of Pseudoterranova by Dr. Robin M. Overstreet, Gulf Coast Research Laboratory, Ocean Springs, Mississippi.)*

surround the degenerated larva, and lymphocytes may predominate. In a long-standing infection, there is granulation tissue with some eosinophils, with only remnants of a larva (or no worm at all) in the center of the lesion.

DIAGNOSIS

The diagnosis can be made when a specimen is identified as an anisakid nematode. When the entire worm is obtained from the patient's vomitus or stool, or during surgery or endoscopy, it should be preserved in 70% ethanol and cleared in phenol to facilitate visualization of the morphologic features. Infective third-stage larvae (larvae that have undergone molts after their first and second stages) have a striated cuticle, three lips (one dorsal and two ventral), a mouth, boring tooth, and excretory pore at the anterior end of the worm (Figure 145–4, A). The third-stage larva may molt after a few days inside the human host and, after shedding its outer cuticle, it becomes a fourth-stage larva with three pronounced lips and no boring tooth. *Anisakis* larvae have a simple digestive tube (Figures 145–4, B, and 145–5) and have a length of 10 to 29 mm and width of 0.44 to 0.54 mm, whereas a *Pseudoterranova* larva has a cecum that is directed anteriorly (Figures 145–4, C and D, and 145–5), and is larger (25 to 50 mm long, 0.3 to 1.2 mm wide) than *Anisakis*.[3,33]

In histologic sections, *Anisakis* larvae have distinctive Y-shaped lateral chords, 60 to 90 muscle cells per quadrant, and do not have lateral alae or winglike projections extending from the cuticle as with *Ascaris* larvae. *Pseudoterranova* larvae have butterfly-shaped lateral chords and an intestinal cecum adjacent to the esophagus and ventriculus.

Radiology and Endoscopy

Anisakis larvae can be demonstrated radiographically in patients who undergo an upper gastrointestinal series or barium enema.[41–49] Radiographic films reveal threadlike filling defects in edematous areas of the gastric mucosa and thickened, narrowed, and obstructed areas in the intestine. In one study, the right side of the colon was frequently affected by edema, and in addition to the luminal narrowing, thumbprinting was observed.[49] Endoscopy is one of the most important methods used in the diagnosis and treatment of gastric anisakiasis, and has also been useful in removing larvae in cases of intestinal and colonic anisakiasis.[5,48–55] Barium enemas were helpful in one study, since it was reported that, although no worms were seen during colonoscopy, the worms could be demonstrated radiologically in four patients.[49] Ultrasonographic examination also has been used to diagnose intestinal anisakiasis and was useful in revealing thickened bowel loops in the infected region with accompanying ascites.[56]

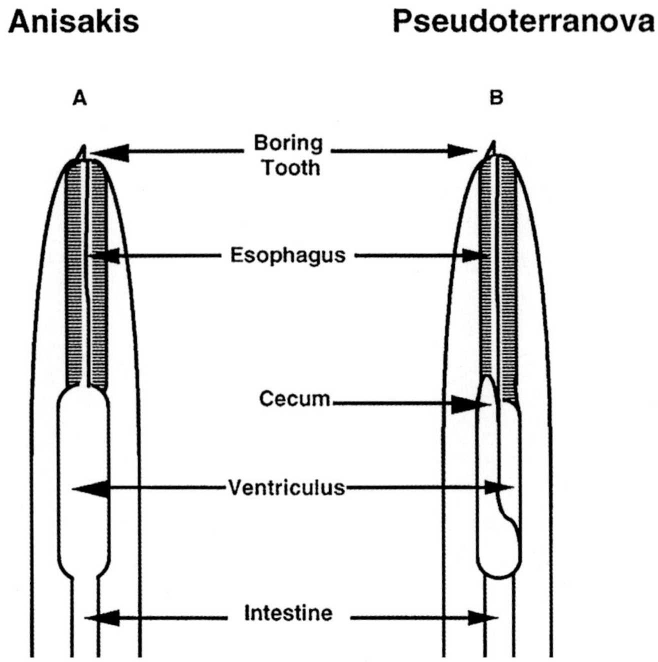

Figure 145–5. Schematic diagram of the morphology of an *Anisakis* and *Pseudoterranova* larva. *(Diagram by Christopher Franklin, University of California, San Francisco.)*

Serology

No clinical laboratory test is available to diagnose anisakiasis. A number of studies have been done to develop a serodiagnostic assay but these are still only investigational. Monoclonal antibodies to *Anisakis* antigens have been prepared that appear to be specific for *Anisakis* and not other helminths such as *Ascaris, Toxocara, Trichinella,* and *Echinococcus*.[57–59]

REFERENCES

1. Nagasawa K. The life cycle of *Anisakis simplex*. In: Moller H, ed. *Nematode Problems in North Atlantic Fish*. Report from a workshop in Kiel, April 3–4; International Council for Exploration of the Sea; 1989:3–8.
2. Brattey J. The life cycle of sealworm, *Pseudoterranova decipiens* in the North Atlantic. In: Moller H, ed. *Nematode Problems in North Atlantic Fish*. Report from a workshop in Kiel, April 3–4; International Council for Exploration of the Sea; 1989:9–14.
3. Oshima T. *Anisakis* and anisakiasis in Japan and adjacent areas. In: Morishita K, Komiya Y, Matsubayashi H, eds. *Progress of Medical Parasitology in Japan*. Meguro Parasitological Museum; 1972:305–393.

4. Oshima T. Anisakiasis—is the sushi bar guilty? *Parasitology Today.* 1987;3:44–48.
5. Deardorff TL, Fukumura T, Raybourne RB. Invasive anisakiasis. A case report from Hawaii. *Gastroenterology.* 1986;90:1047–1050.
6. Deardorff TL, Altman J, Nolan CM. Human anisakiasis: two case reports from the state of Washington. *Proc Helminthol Soc Wash.* 1987;54:274–275.
7. Verhamme MAM, Ramboer CHR. Anisakiasis caused by herring in vinegar: a little known medical problem. *Gut.* 1988;29:843–847.
8. Ishikura H, Namiki M, eds. *Gastric Anisakiasis in Japan.* New York: Springer-Verlag; 1989.
9. Ishikura H, Kikuchi K. *Intestinal Anisakiasis in Japan.* New York: Springer-Verlag; 1990.
10. Kim LS, Lee YH, Kim S, Park HR, Cho SY. A case of anisakiasis causing intestinal obstruction. *Korean J Parasitol.* 1991;29:93–96.
11. Sohn WM, Seol SY. A human case of gastric anisakiasis by *Pseudoterranova decipiens* larva. *Korean J Parasitol.* 1994;32:53–56.
12. Hemsrichart V. Intestinal anisakiasis: first reported case in Thailand. *J Med Assoc Thailand.* 1993;76:117–121.
13. Van Thiel PH. The present state of *Anisakis* and its causative worms. *Trop Geogr Med.* 1976;2:75–85.
14. Lorenz G. Morphological changes of anisakiasis. *Zentralbl Allg Pathol Pathol Anat.* 1982;126:477–482.
15. Moller H, Schroder S. New aspects of anisakiasis in Germany. *Arch Lebensmittelhyg.* 1987;38:123–127.
16. Jlidi R, Chatelanat F. Anisakiasis of the small intestine and review of the literature. *Rev Med Suisse Romande.* 1987; 107:973–976.
17. Hoang CY, Garin Y, Ichou J, Le Charpentier Y. Jejunal anisakiasis and intestinal occlusion. *Gastroenterol Clin Biol.* 1985;9:847–848.
18. Mudry J. Lefebvre P, Dei-Cas E, et al. Anisakiase humaine: 5 cas dans le nord de la France. *Gastroenterol Clin Biol.* 1986;10:83–87.
19. Petithory JC, Lapierre J, Rousseau M, Clique MT. Diagnose serologique de l'anisakiase (granulome eosinophile digestif) par precipitation en milieu gelifie (Ouchterlony, electrosynerese, immunoelectrophorese). *Med Malad Infect.* 1986;3:157–162.
20. Petithory JC, Marty B. L'anisakiase en France. *Pathologie.* 1988;3:96–99.
21. Lewis R, Shore JH. Anisakiasis in the United Kingdom. *Lancet.* 1985;2:1019.
22. Watt IA, McLean NR, Girdwood RWA, et al. Eosinophilic gastroenteritis associated with a larval anisakine nematode. *Lancet.* 1979;2:893–894.
23. Paltridge GP, Faoagali JL, Angus HB. Intestinal anisakiasis: a new New Zealand disease. *NZ Med J.* 1984;97:558–559.
24. Sapunar J, Doerr E, Letonja T. Human anisakiasis in Chile. *Bol Chil Parasitol.* 1976;31:79–83.
25. Torres P, Hernandez E, Sandoval I. Anisakiasis and phocanemiasis in marine fishes from the south of Chile. *Int J Zoonoses.* 1983;10:146–150.
26. Jackson GJ. The "new disease" status of human anisakiasis and North American cases: a review. *J Milk Food Technol.* 1975;38:769–773.
27. Margolis L. Public health aspects of "codworm" infection: a review. *J Fish Res Board Canada.* 1977;34:887–898.
28. Desowitz RS. Human and experimental anisakiasis in the United States. *Hokkaido Igaku Zasshi.* 1986;61:358–371.
29. Sakanari JA, McKerrow JH. Anisakiasis. *Clin Microbiol Rev.* 1989;2:278–284.
30. Oshima T, Kliks M. Effects of marine mammal parasites on human health. *Int J Parasitol.* 1987;17:415–421.
31. Deardorff TL, Throm R. Commercial blast-freezing of third stage *Anisakis simplex* larvae encapsulated in salmon and rockfish. *J Parasitol.* 1988;74:600–603.
32. Hauck AK. Occurrence and survival of the larval nematode *Anisakis* spp in the flesh of fresh, frozen, brined, and smoked Pacific herring, *Clupea harengus pallasi. J Parasitol.* 1977;63:515–519.
33. Kliks M. Anisakiasis in the western United States: four new case reports from California. *Am J Trop Med Hyg.* 1983;32:526–532.
34. Rushovich AM, Randall EL, Caprini JA, Westenfelder GO. Omental anisakiasis: a rare mimic of acute appendicitis. *Am J Clin Pathol.* 1983;80:517–520.
35. Yokogawa M, Yoshimura H. Clinicopathologic studies on larval anisakiasis in Japan. *Am J Trop Med Hyg.* 1967; 16:723–728.
36. Kobayashi A, Tsuji M, Wilbur DL. Probable pulmonary anisakiasis accompanying pleural effusion. *Am J Trop Med Hyg.* 1985;34:310–313.
37. Kikuchi Y, Ishikura H, Kikuchi K. Pathology of intestinal anisakiasis. In: Ishikura H, Kikuchi K, eds. *Intestinal Anisakiasis in Japan.* New York: Springer-Verlag; 1990: 129–143.
38. Ohtaki H, Ohtaki R. Clinical manifestation of gastric anisakiasis. In: Ishikura H, Namiki M, eds. *Gastric Anisakiasis in Japan.* New York: Springer-Verlag; 1989:37–46.
39. Ishikura H. Clinical features of intestinal anisakiasis. In: Ishikura H, Kikuchi K, eds. *Intestinal Anisakiasis in Japan.* New York: Springer-Verlag; 1990:89–100.
40. Ishikura H. Epidemiological aspects of intestinal anisakiasis and its pathogenesis. In: Ishikura H, Namiki M, eds. *Gastric Anisakiasis in Japan.* New York: Springer-Verlag; 1989:3–21.
41. Akasawa Y, Kizu M, Aoike A, Kawai K. Endoscopic management of acute gastric anisakiasis. *Endoscopy.* 1979;2: 158–162.
42. Appleby D, Kapoor W, Karpf M, Williams S. Anisakiasis. Nematode infestation producing small-bowel obstruction. *Arch Surg.* 1982;117:836.
43. Hayasaka H, Ishikura H, Takayama T. Acute regional ileitis due to *Anisakis* larvae. *Int Surg.* 1971;55:8–14.
44. Higashi M, Tanaka T, Kitada T, Nakatake K, Tsuji M. Anisakiasis confirmed by radiography of the intestine. *Gastrointest Radiol.* 1988;13:85–86.
45. Kwee HG, Sautter RL. Anisakiasis. *Am Fam Phys.* 1987; 36:137–140.
46. Pinkus GS, Coolidge C, Little MD. Intestinal anisakiasis. First case report from North America. *Am J Med.* 1975;59: 114–120.
47. Richman RH, Lewicki AM. Right ileocolitis secondary to anisakiasis. *Am J Roentgenol Radium Ther Nucl Med.* 1973; 119:329–331.

48. Sugimachi K, Inokuchi K, Ooiwa T, Fujino T, Ishii Y. Acute gastric anisakiasis. *J Am Med Assoc.* 1985;253: 1012–1013.
49. Matsumoto T, Iida M, Kimura Y, et al. *Anisakis* of the colon: radiologic and endoscopic features in six patients. *Radiology.* 1992;183:97–99.
50. Cocheton JJ, Gombeaud T, Ferroir JP. Anisakiase duodenale aigue extraction endoscopique. *Presse Med.* 1984; 13:744.
51. Kliks M. Human anisakiasis: an update. *J Am Med Assoc.* 1986;255:2605.
52. Ikeda K, Kumashiro R, Kifune T. Nine cases of acute gastric anisakiasis. *Gastrointest Endosc.* 1989;35:304–308.
53. Namiki M, Yazaki Y. Endoscopic findings of gastric anisakiasis with acute symptoms. In: Ishikura H, Namiki M, eds. *Gastric Anisakiasis in Japan.* New York: Springer-Verlag; 1989:47–51.
54. Shirahama M, Koga T, Uchida S, Miyamoto Y, Ohta Y. Colonic anisakiasis simulating carcinoma of the colon. *Am J Roent.* 1990;155:895.
55. Minamoto T, Sawaguchi K, Ogino T, Mai M. Anisakiasis of the colon: report of two cases with emphasis on the diagnostic and therapeutic value of colonoscopy. *Endoscopy.* 1991;23:50–52.
56. Shirahama M, Takafumi K, Ishibashi H, Uchida S, Ohta Y, Shimoda Y. Intestinal anisakiasis: US in diagnosis. *Radiology.* 1992;185:789–793.
57. Takahashi S, Sato N. Analysis of *Anisakis* larvae specific antigens using monoclonal antibodies and their applications. *Sapporo Med J.* 1987;56:291–303.
58. Takahashi S, Sato N, Ishikura H. Establishment of monoclonal antibodies that discriminate the antigen distribution specifically found in *Anisakis* larvae (Type I). *J Parasitol.* 1986;72:960–962.
59. Yagihashi A, Sato N, Takahashi S, Ishikura H, Kikuchi K. A serodiagnostic assay by microenzyme-linked immunosorbent assay for human anisakiasis using a monoclonal antibody specific for *Anisakis* larvae antigen. *J Infect Dis.* 1990;161:995–998.

CHAPTER 146

Ascariasis

Bharatha Sinniah

> *A little, wretched, despicable creature; a worm, a mere nothing, and less than nothing; a vile insect that has risen up in contempt against the majesty of Heaven and earth.*
>
> *Jonathan Edwards (1703–1758)*

DEFINITION

Ascariasis is a general term for the disease caused by parasitic roundworms of the genus *Ascaris. Ascaris lumbricoides* parasitizes man but *Ascaris suum,* a natural parasite of pigs, may also, on occasion, infect man. *Ascaris lumbricoides* causes four main clinical syndromes. First, larvae migrating through lung cause eosinophilic pneumonitis (Loeffler's syndrome). Second, adult worms in the intestine may cause abdominal discomfort, acute epigastric pain, diarrhea, and debilitation. Third, an entanglement of adult worms, may on occasion, obstruct the small intestine. Fourth, migration of adult worms into the ampulla of Vater, into the pancreatic ducts or into the biliary ducts, may cause sudden and life-threatening complications. Synonyms include ascaridiasis, ascaridiosis, ascariosis, and roundworm infection. Ascaris pneumonia is caused by migrating larvae and is one of the eosinophilic pneumonias.

GEOGRAPHIC DISTRIBUTION AND EPIDEMIOLOGY

Ascariasis is cosmopolitan but more common in the tropics and subtropics than in the temperate zones. About one quarter of the world's population is infected. Eggs of *A lumbricoides* vary greatly in their survival times in soil. For instance, they may survive in the cooler soil of temperate climates for more than 6 years but sometimes for only a few hours in warmer tropical soils. As an example, during the hot dry season in Saudi Arabia, the eggs die quickly, causing a seasonal break in transmission. Transmission from soil to man depends not only on survival of eggs in soil but on socioeconomic factors too. Contamination of soil by human feces and crowded living are the most important factors in promoting infection. An agricultural environment, illiteracy, and poor sanitation also promote high rates of infection. Infection is more common among school and preschool children, who are more readily exposed and infected. Infection is acquired from fecal contamination of food, toys, fingers, inhalation of dust, and contaminated vegetables, fruits, and drinking water.

MORPHOLOGY

The adult *A lumbricoides* is the largest parasitic nematode to live in the human gastrointestinal tract. The adult worms concentrate in the lumen of the duodenum and upper jejunum. The shape and size of the adult worms resemble an ordinary earthworm but in contrast to the dark red of earthworms, *A lumbricoides* is white, and sometimes has a creamy or faint pink tint. The worm's body is cylindrical but tapered at both ends. The head has a terminal mouth that is surrounded by three lips, each finely toothed—one dorsal and two subventral. The cuticle is thick (Figure 146–1), multilayered, and has both annulations and striations. The hypodermis lies beneath the cuticle and projects into the body cavity to form the lateral chords. There are well-developed somatic muscle cells in each quarter of the worm. The esophagus is prominent but without a posterior bulb. The intestine (Figure 146–2) is lined by tall columnar cells that contain microvilli.

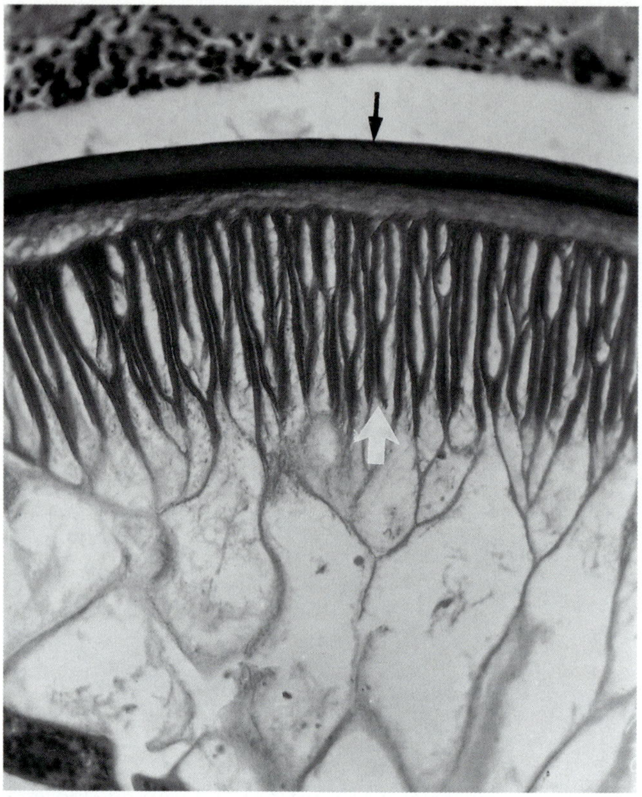

A

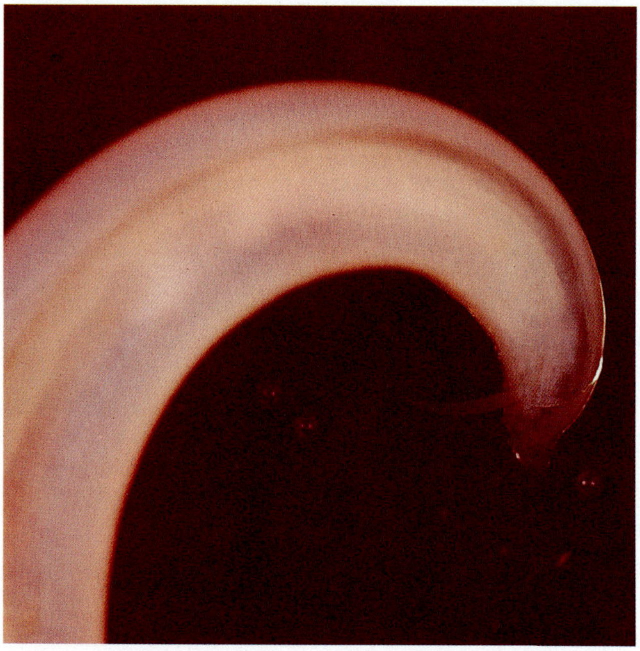

B

Figure 146–1. (**A**) The outer portion of a male *A lumbricoides* is shown. The outermost layer—the cuticle (*black arrow*)—is supported by a hypodermis. The inner layer is the contractile portion of the worm's somatic muscle (*white arrow*) [AFIP Neg 75-11726; hematoxylin-eosin (H&E), ×300]. (**B**) Terminal end of a male *A lumbricoides*. The spicule is protruding from the ventral surface (Gross photograph, ×8.5). *(Photograph by Daniel H. Connor, MD.)*

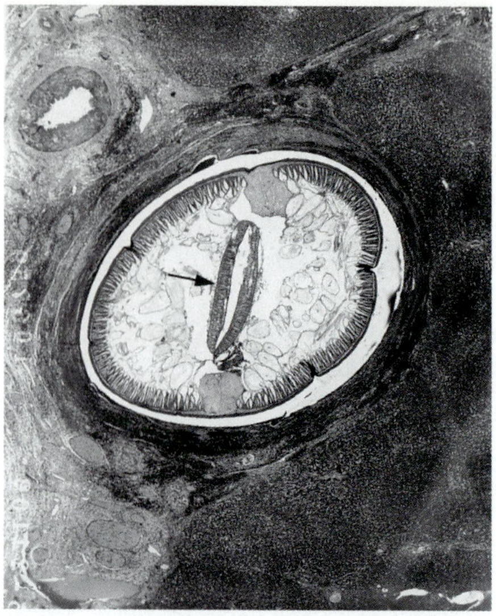

Figure 146–2. This is an adult male *A lumbricoides* in a pancreatic duct. The cuticle, the hypodermis, lateral cords, and cross section of intestine (*arrow*) are all evident (AFIP 75-11727; H&E, ×18).

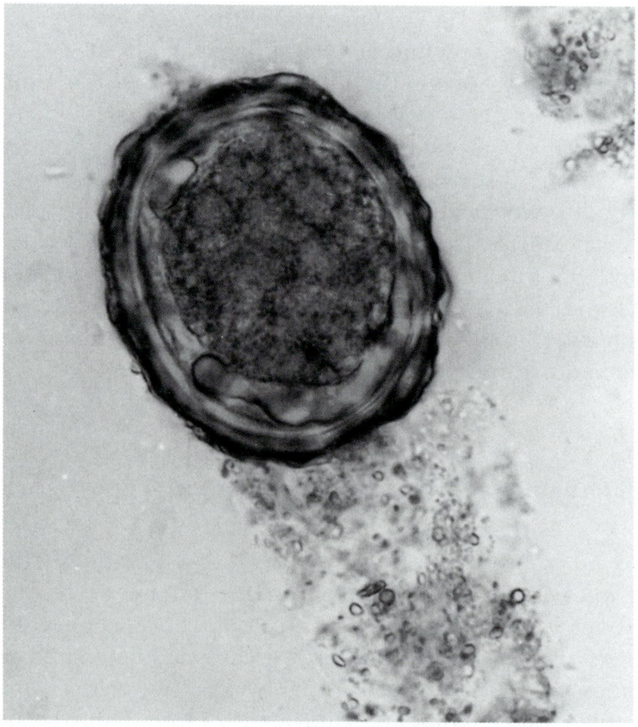

Figure 146–3. This is a mamillated, fertilized egg of *A lumbricoides*. The mamillations surround the shell. There is an outline of the embryo within the egg (from stool, ×1000).

The male worm, smaller than the female, has a length of 150 to 310 mm (average 250 mm) and a breadth of 2 to 4 mm. The posterior end of the male is curved ventrally to form a hook. Two curved spicules each measuring 2 mm long can protrude from the orifice of the cloaca around which there are large numbers of minute papillae. The single reproductive tube is in the posterior half of the body. The female worm is 220 to 350 mm by 3 to 6 mm. The posterior end is conical and straight—not pointed nor ventrally curved as in the male worm. The ovaries, oviducts, and uteri are in the posterior two thirds of the body. The body leads into a stout duct, the vagina, which divides into two branches. These are coiled anteroposteriorly in the worm. The portion of each duct, which is close to the common vagina, functions as a uterus. The middle part is the oviduct and the distal part the ovary.

Fertile eggs are 45 to 75 μm by 35 to 50 μm (Figure 146–3). They are oval and brown from bile staining. The shell is thick and multilayered. Fertile eggs usually have an outer albuminoid coat, which is mamillated, but sometimes the outer layer is lost leaving a smooth shell—so-called "decorticated" eggs. Unfertilized eggs are 88 to 94 μm by 44 to 60 μm. Most are longer and narrower than fertilized eggs, have a thin shell, a more irregular outer covering, and disorganized contents. Refractory granules fill the inside. Unfertilized eggs in the stool may be a consequence of rapid production of eggs by the female worm—so rapid that some pass before fertilization. Other times unfertilized eggs are passed because there are no male worms in the gut.

LIFE CYCLE

Male and female adult worms live in the small intestine where they tend to concentrate in the jejunum (Figure 146–4). Each female produces 176,000 to 350,000 eggs a day.[1,2] Thus a female worm may lay 25 million eggs in her lifetime. Fertilized eggs pass in the feces and develop in warm, moist shady soil to become infective larvae within 10 to 15 days at 20 to 30°C. The first-stage larva is within the egg. It molts after 7 days and the second-stage larva also molts within the egg to produce the filariform or third-stage infective larva. According to a number of researchers[3–5] two molts occur within the egg, making the infective stage a third-stage larva. *Ascaris* eggs resist freezing, drying, and chemicals, and can remain alive for up to 7 years in moist loose soil with moderate shade. Man becomes infected by swallowing eggs in drinking water or on vegetables and fruits contaminated with feces containing infective eggs. Dust also plays a role in transmission. Children become infected by contaminating their hands with polluted

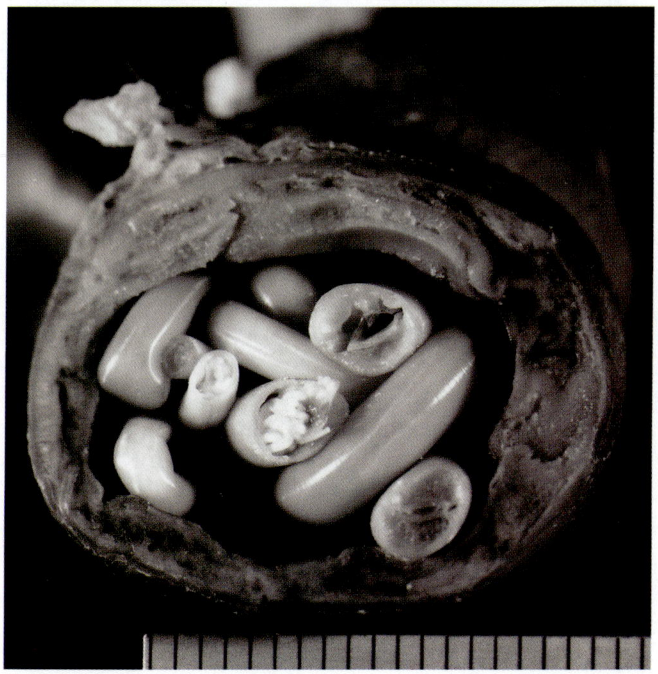

A

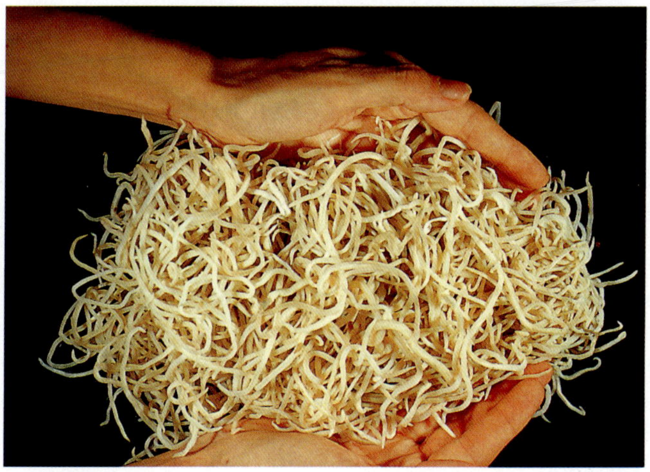

B

Figure 146–4. (**A**) Cross section of jejunum containing adult *A lumbricoides*. The patient was a Zairian, 13 years old. Sections of both male and female worms are in the photograph (AFIP Neg 72-13204; gross photograph, millimeter scale). (**B**) A massive cluster of adult worms removed at autopsy from an infant South African. The child died of intestinal obstruction. *(Gross photograph by Daniel H. Connor, MD.)*

soil; the eggs being transferred to their mouths by fingers. After ingestion, the infective egg hatches in the small intestine and the emerging larva is 0.2 to 0.3 by 0.014 mm and has a filariform esophagus. The filariform larvae penetrate the mucosa of the intestinal wall and enter small portal veins or intestinal lymphatic vessels, then migrate through the liver to the right side of the heart, and finally to the lungs through the pulmonary arteries. This migration, from intestine to lung, takes about 3 days. In the lung the larvae increase in size and molt once to become fourth-stage larvae. The young larvae grow to about 2 mm in length while in pulmonary capillaries, then break out of the capillaries into the alveoli and migrate up the bronchi to the trachea where they are swallowed, passing down the esophagus into the stomach and duodenum. Here they molt for the fourth and last time and grow to become adults. The entire cycle, from the time the eggs are swallowed until adults develop is 8 to 12 weeks. Adult worms live in the intestine for about a year and are then expelled. Some adult worms, however, may remain in the intestine for 20 months.[6]

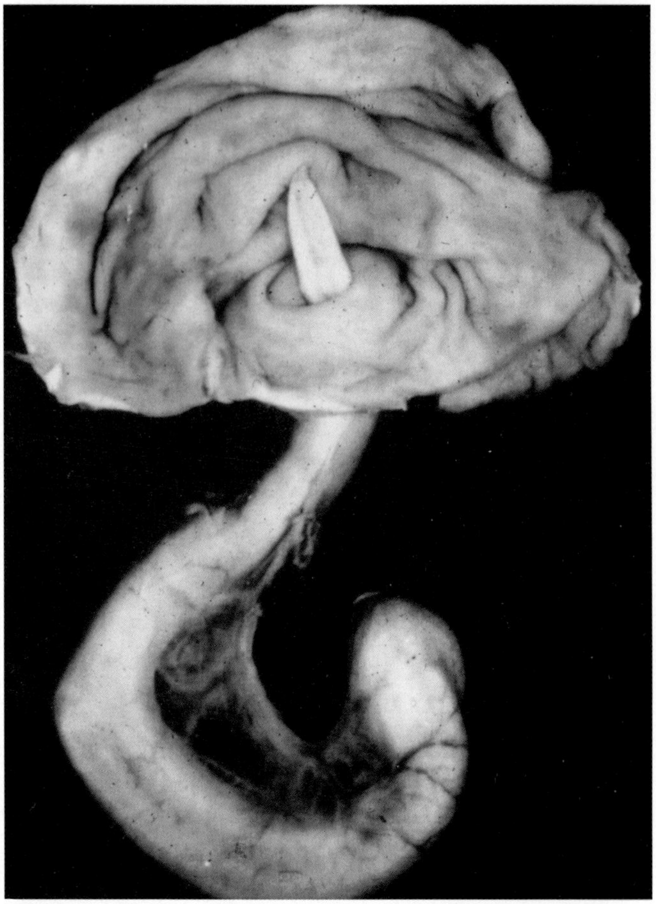

Figure 146–5. A portion of cecum and vermiform appendix. The tip of an *A lumbricoides* protrudes from the appendix into the lumen of the cecum (AFIP 74-8507; gross photograph).

CLINICAL MANIFESTATIONS AND PATHOGENESIS

Many infections are asymptomatic but when infections become overt there may be fever, eosinophilia, disturbances of the central nervous system, malaise, weight loss, edema, and emaciation. Deaths are rare, estimated at 0.62%, and are most common in children.[7] Even in light infections, however, worms in the small intestine may cause vague abdominal pain. In heavy infections there may be nausea, vomiting, abdominal discomfort, and anorexia. Entangled masses of adult worms may obstruct the intestinal lumen (Figure 146–4) and sometimes kill infants and small children.[8] Clinical features of heavy infection include a protruding abdomen and nutritional impairment caused by altered carbohydrate absorption and increased fecal nitrogen and fat.[9,10] Long-term malnutrition may retard growth and development.[11] The most serious complications are caused by ectopic migration of adult worms. Unmated female worms may actively migrate to ectopic sites. A peppery diet, anesthesia, improper treatment with drugs, fever, and some foods may stimulate adult worms to migrate into the ampulla of Vater, the pancreatic ducts, or the bile ducts (Figure 146–2). A worm entering the ampulla may cause sudden obstructive jaundice—a well-recognized complication of ascariasis in children in the tropics. Adult worms obstructing the bile ducts cause acute, agonizing, throbbing, epigastric and right upper quadrant pain, which may radiate to the shoulder, back, or hypogastrium. The attack of pain may last up to 20 minutes. Adult worms in the pancreatic ducts may cause hemorrhagic pancreatitis. An ascaris in the vermiform appendix may obstruct the lumen and cause acute appendicitis (Figure 146–5). Fatal complications of ascaris appendicitis include pylephlebitis from septic venous thrombosis and acute peritonitis from perforation. Similarly an adult worm obstructing the orifice of a Meckel's diverticulum may cause suppurative complications. When worms migrate into the peritoneal cavity, either through a perforated ulcer or along tracts of surgical sutures, they may cause fatal peritonitis. Migration of adults in the upper respiratory tract produce respiratory difficulties and may cause cardiopulmonary arrest.[12,13] Worms may exit through the nares, and less commonly the lachrymal duct or even the eustachian tube, perforating the tympanic membrane.[14] Worms that are vomited can lodge in bronchi or larynx and cause asphyxiation. Adult worms have also passed through the mouth, into the lachrymal gland and inguinal canal, and through the urethra and vagina. Migrating worms may release eggs and reaction to the eggs may produce

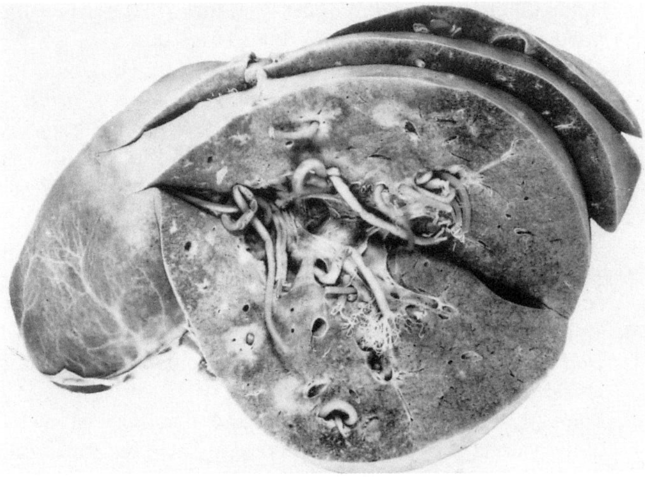

Figure 146–6. Cut surface of liver showing many adult *A lumbricoides* in dilated bile ducts (AFIP N-39302; gross photograph).

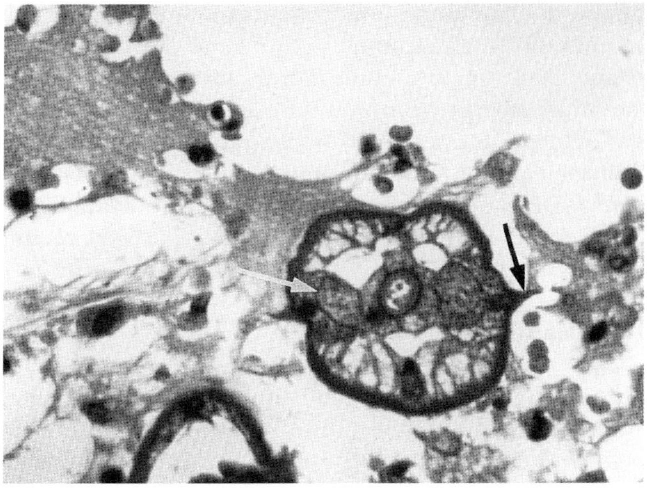

Figure 146–7. A larva of *A lumbricoides* in lung. Lateral alae (*one at tip of black arrow*), intestine and excretory columns (*one at tip of white arrow*) are apparent. This is from a 2-year-old infant male child from Virginia who died of *Ascaris* pneumonia (AFIP 74-11310; H&E, ×675).

symptoms especially when they are in lung or liver (Figure 146–6). Eggs deposited in liver may cause necrosis, granulomatous inflammation, and eventually fibrous scar.

The first passage of larvae through lung causes no symptoms or pathologic changes, unless the number of larvae is immense. Subsequent migrations from reinfection, however, cause intense hypersensitivity reactions even with a small number of larvae. During the time when larvae are actively migrating, hypersensitive patients may have severe reactions characterized by urticaria and asthma, even when migrating larvae are few. In addition to hypersensitivity reactions, the migration of larvae through the lung may cause any combination of fever, chills, dyspnea, paroxysmal cough, lassitude, malaise, body aches, and pneumonia (Figure 146–7). These symptoms begin 5 to 6 days after infection and usually last 10 to 12 days. This is Loeffler's syndrome. In Saudi Arabia Loeffler's syndrome is a recognized complication of ascariasis. It occurs during the short rainy season in spring. Larvae may be also in sputum and associated with hemoptysis. Loeffler's syndrome may, in a few people, cause acute respiratory distress and death. Cyanosis, tachycardia, a sensation of pressure and/or chest pain, and rales over the involved portion of lung are features of severe Loeffler's syndrome. Chest x rays of patients with Loeffler's pneumonia reveal a variety of patterns including infiltrations similar to pulmonary tuberculosis and viral pneumonia. Loeffler's syndrome can be distinguished from tuberculosis and viral pneumonia by high counts of circulating eosinophils. Loeffler's syndrome is usually self-limited and benign. Peripheral eosinophilia is 4000 to 8000/mm^3 and rarely exceeds 40% of total white blood cells. When larvae break out of blood vessels into alveoli there is an inflammatory reaction characterized by eosinophils, macrophages, fibrin, and granulomatous reaction in the interstices, around the tracts of the worms, and within alveoli and bronchi.[11] Alveolar walls may be thickened. Ascaris larvae are within alveolar walls, air sacs, bronchioles, bronchi, and in areas of consolidation[15] (Figure 146–7).

Cell-mediated immunity plays a major role and the response to the larvae may be intense. Ascariasis causes an increase in circulating globulins IgE and IgM. IgE antibodies mediate the release of vasoactive amides, which cause increased vascular permeability and antigen–antibody complexes in the pulmonary parenchyma causing an arthus-like reaction. IgE antibodies also mediate bronchial asthma, urticaria, and pulmonary infiltrates. IgM also stimulates the pulmonary inflammatory infiltration. Molting larvae in the lungs releases molting fluid and the molting sheath, both of which may cause allergic reactions. Ascaris allergens, present during all phases of infection, cause the most potent allergic reactions of parasitic origin.[16] Target organs of these reactions include lung, skin, conjunctiva, and gastrointestinal tract.

DIAGNOSIS

During the larval stage of migration, diagnosis is based on clinical symptoms of ascaris pneumonitis. It is possible to find larvae in the sputum or gastric washings especially in heavy infections. The presence of adult worms is confirmed when eggs are identified in feces by direct smear or by concentration techniques (formal ether sedimentation, brine flotation, or the Kato-cellophane thick smear). Adult worms may be in feces or they may emerge from body orifices. Intestinal ascariasis is often diagnosed by radiographic study of gastrointestinal tract with barium sulfate or other contrast media. Diagnosis can also be made by identifying eggs, larvae, or adult worms in biopsy or autopsy specimens.

TREATMENT

Several broad-spectrum antihelminthic drugs can be administered as a single dose with good results. The best of these are pyrantel pamoate administered as a single dose of 10 mg/kg, which cures more than 98% of patients; oxantel–pyrantel pamoate, also administered as a single dose, cures 99%; and albendazole at 400 mg single dose cures 100%.[17] Mebendazole is also effective and is given 100 mg twice a day for 3 days, and piperazine citrate is administered at a dosage of 75 mg per kilogram of body weight (maximum 3.5 gram) daily for 2 days. These drugs are effective against the adult worms in the lumen of the intestine. Intestinal obstruction and obstruction of the biliary passages must be treated surgically. Liver abscess caused by ascaris worms must be drained and antibiotics given.

REFERENCES

1. Brown HW, and Cort WM. The egg production of *Ascaris lumbricoides*. *J Parasitol.* 1927;14:88–90.
2. Sinniah B. Daily egg production of *Ascaris lumbricoides,* the distribution of eggs in the faeces and variability of egg counts. *Parasitology.* 1982;84:167–175.
3. Araujo P. Observacões pertinentes as primeiras ecdises de larvas de *Ascaris lumbricoides,* A suum c *Toxocara canis. Rev Inst Med Trop Sao Paulo.* 1972;14:83–90.
4. Thust R. Submikroskopische Untersuchungen Uber die Morphogenese des Integumentes Von *Ascaris lumbricoides.* L. *1758 Z wissehschaft Zool.* 1968;178:1–39.
5. Maung M. The occurrence of the second molt of *Ascaris lumbricoides* and *Ascaris suum. Int Parasitol.* 1978;8:371–378.
6. Hobo B. Epidemiological studies on Ascaris infection among prisoners and the length of life of *Ascaris lumbricoides* in human host. *Jpn J Nations Health.* 1956;25:1–14.
7. Muller RM. *Worms and Disease. A Manual of Medical Helminthology.* London: William Heineman Med Books; 1975:82–85.
8. Baird JK, Mistrey M, Pimsler J, and Connor DH. Fatal human ascariasis following secondary massive infection. *Am J Trop Med Hyg.* 1986;35:314–318.
9. Tripathy K, Gonzalez F, Lotero H, Bolaños O. Effects of *Ascaris* infection on human nutrition. *Am J Trop Med Hyg.* 1971;20:212–218.
10. Tripathy K, Duque E, Bolaños O, Lotero H, Mayoral LG. Malabsorption syndrome in ascariasis. *Am J Clin Nutr.* 1972;25:1276–1281.
11. Keymer A, Crompton WDT. Epidemiology and control of round worm and hookworm infections in man. *Med Forum.* 1983;6:9–13.
12. Mimpriss TJ. Respiratory obstruction due to round worm. *Br J Anaesth.* 1972;44:413.
13. Mittal VK, Dhaliwal R, Yadev RVS, Sahariah S. Fatal respiratory obstruction due to round worm. *Med J Aust.* 1976;2:210–212.
14. Shah KN, Desai MP. *Ascaris lumbricoides* from the right ear. *Indian Pediatr.* 1969;6:92–93.
15. Piggott JA, Hansbarger EA, Neafie RC. Human ascariasis. *Am J Clin Pathol.* 1970;53:223.
16. Pawlowski ZS. Ascariasis host pathogen biology. *Rev Infect Dis.* 1982;4:806–814.
17. Sinniah B, Sinniah D. The antihelminthic effects of pyrantel pamoate, oxantel pyrantel pamoate, levamisole and Mebendazole in the treatment of intestinal nematodes. *Ann Trop Parastol.* 1981;75:315–321.

CHAPTER 147

Bancroftian Filariasis

James W. Kazura and Daniel H. Connor

There is the elephant disease which is generated beside the streams of the Nile in the midst of Egypt and nowhere else. In Attica the feet are attacked and the eyes in Achean lands. And so different places are hurtful to different parts and members: the variations of air occasion that . . . this . . . destroying power and pestilence therefore all at once either fall upon the waters or else sink deep into the corn-crops or other food of man . . . or else their force remains suspended in the atmosphere, and when we inhale from it mixed airs, we must absorb at the same time into our body those things as well.

Lucretius (99–55 B.C.)

INTRODUCTION

Bancroftian filariasis is infection by any one of the three lymphatic-dwelling parasitic nematodes, *Wuchereria bancrofti, Brugia malayi,* and *Brugia timori,* and is a major public health problem in many tropical areas. Moreover, in many developing countries, where urbanization is rapid, the breeding sites for the vector mosquitos are spreading, exposing many more people. It is estimated that there are currently 100 million persons affected worldwide. Because there are few readily available experimental animal models that accurately mimic natural infection of humans, there is no detailed understanding of the sequence of pathologic manifestations of this helminthiasis. To address this gap, studies of several related human and animal filarial infections are cited.

DEFINITION

Three major species of filarial parasites cause disease in humans: these species are *B malayi, B timori,* and *W bancrofti.* The latter is by far the most common, accounting for at least 90% of these filarial infections. Although morphologic and genetic features distinguish lymphatic filariae from the two other major filarial parasites of humans, *Onchocerca volvulus* and *Loa loa,* the simplest and most important difference is their anatomic niche in the mammalian host; adult *Wuchereria* and *Brugia* live in lymphatics whereas *O volvulus* and *L loa* adult worms live in subcutaneous tissues.

GEOGRAPHIC DISTRIBUTION

Bancroftian filariasis prevails in tropical areas of both the Eastern and Western hemispheres[1] (Figure 147–1). Its prevalence in Latin America has decreased during the past several decades. Endemic foci persist in Caribbean islands (Haiti and Dominican Republic) and in several areas of South America, including Brazil, Surinam, Guyana, Trinidad, and Tobago. Infection is widespread throughout equatorial Africa and extends northward into the Nile Delta. The greatest proportion of those with bancroftian filariasis, however, are in southeastern Asia, notably India and Indonesia, and islands of the Western Pacific, including the Philippines and Papua New Guinea. In Africa, Asia, and the Pacific region, lymphatic filariasis is a significant public health problem, especially in young and middle-aged adults. Bancroftian filariasis is not a zoonotic infection. Humans are the only natural reservoir.

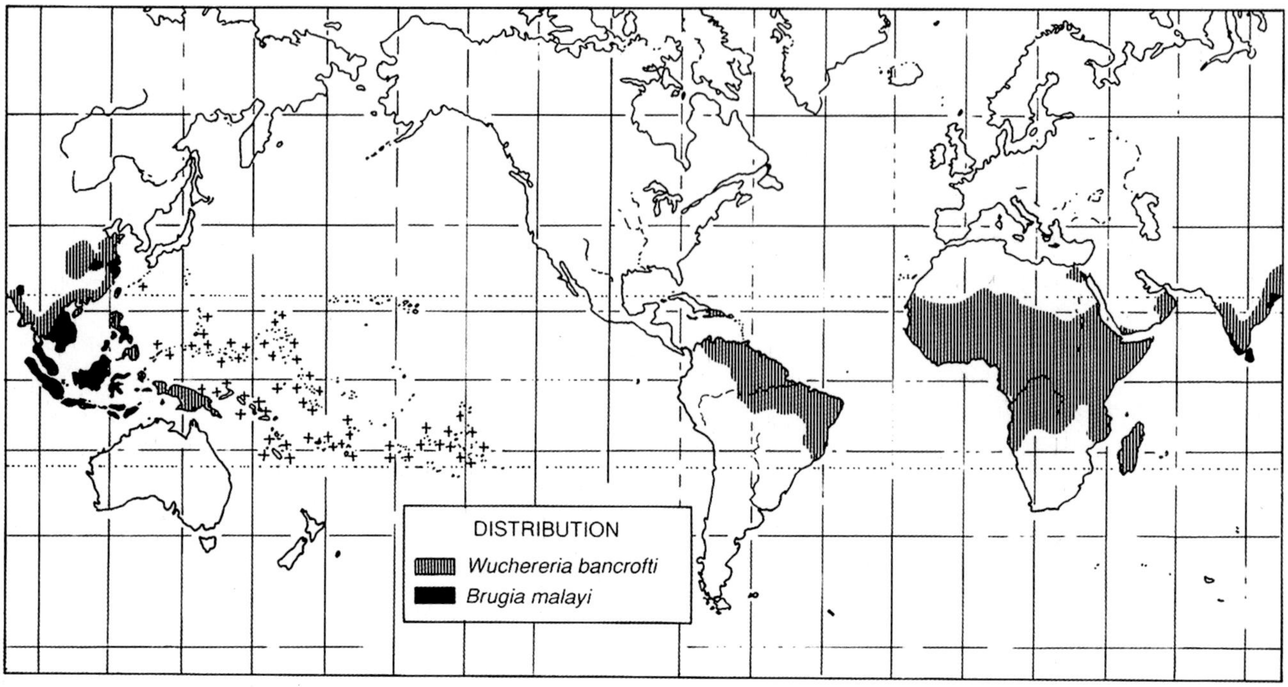

Figure 147–1. The worldwide distribution of lymphatic filariasis.

LIFE CYCLE

Infection begins when infective (third-stage) larvae exit the mouth parts of the vector mosquito and reach the skin beside the puncture site made by the female mosquito (anopheline, culicine, or *Aedes*) when taking its blood meal (Figure 147–2). The infective larvae migrate into the puncture wound, invade the dermis, and enter lymphatic vessels. Sexually mature adult male and female worms develop over a period of 6 to 9 months.

The overall pattern of distribution of adult *W bancrofti* in the human host is not known with certainty, but the parasites have been identified in lymphatic vessels draining the lower limbs (inguinal lymph node group), in male genitalia (testis, epididymis, spermatic cord), and, less commonly, in lymphatics of upper limbs and breast.[2] Subcutaneous nodules that develop in patients taking filaricidal drugs such as diethylcarbamazine contain remnants of adult worms. This suggests that adult worms may live also in anatomic sites outside the major lymphatics.[3]

Fecund female worms produce first-stage larvae or microfilariae, which, following their release, circulate in the bloodstream. The concentration of bloodborne microfilariae has a circadian rhythm, called periodicity. Most commonly, microfilariae of *W bancrofti* have a nocturnal periodicity, whereby the highest concentration of microfilariae circulate in the blood at night—an adaptation that coincides with the peak biting frequency of the mosquito vector. When not in peripheral blood, the microfilariae rest in capillary beds of deep organs, especially lung and perhaps kidney (Figure 147–3). When mosquitoes ingest microfilariae in a blood meal, the parasites rapidly penetrate the wall of the mosquito's gut and migrate into the mosquito's thoracic muscles. It takes approximately 2 weeks for microfilariae to develop into larvae capable of infecting a person.

NATURAL HISTORY AND EPIDEMIOLOGY

Transmission of lymphatic filariae from person to person is inefficient.[4] Studies of *Brugia* infection in experimental animals indicate that fewer than 15% to 20% of infective larvae develop into adult worms. Moreover, only 1% to 2% of mosquitoes harbor infective larvae, and those that do, have a mean number on the order of 1 or 2. It may seem remarkable, therefore, that more than 50% of the residents in many of these regions have microfilaremia. Based on these and other considerations (eg, neonatal tolerance induced by filarial antigens reaching the fetus from the mother's blood), patent infection, defined by the bloodborne microfilariae, usually does not appear before age 5 to 10 years. The proportion of residents of endemic areas with parasitemia—the microfilarial carrier rate—generally increases with age. The overall microfilarial carrier rate is

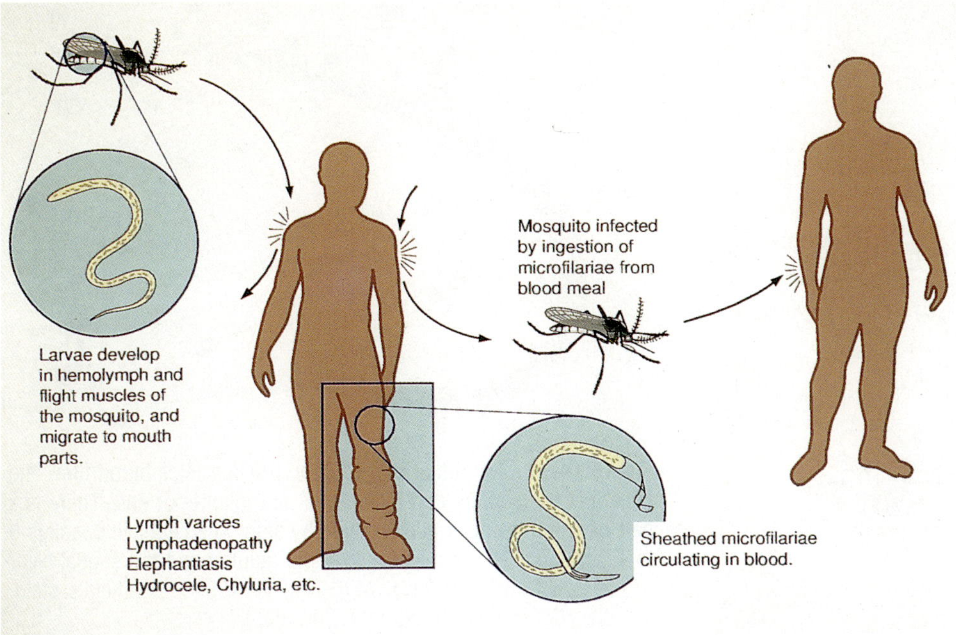

Figure 147–2. Life cycle. Filarial parasites are passed from person to person by arthropod vectors that serve also as intermediate hosts. *Wuchereria bancrofti* is transmitted by more than 80 species of mosquito of the genera *Aedes, Culex,* and *Anopheles*. Adult male and female worms live in human lymphatics. The female worms discharge embryo microfilariae, which circulate in the blood and are picked up by mosquitoes when taking a blood meal. The microfilariae lose their sheaths and enter the mosquito's thoracic muscles where they mature to become infective larvae in 10 to 12 days. They migrate into the mosquito's mouth parts and proboscis where they are ready to enter a human when the mosquito takes its next blood meal. The larvae become adults in 6 to 8 months.

thought to be a function of cumulative exposure to infective larvae.

The natural history of filarial infection is poorly understood. Some studies suggest that microfilarial carrier rates decrease with age (caused by death of adult worms and/or concomitant immunity and acquired resistance to infective larvae), whereas other surveys indicate that there is not an age-dependent change in patency rate. Resolution of this issue depends on an accurate measure of total worm burden that is independent of microfilaremia—such as assays that quantify circulating antigens of adult worms.

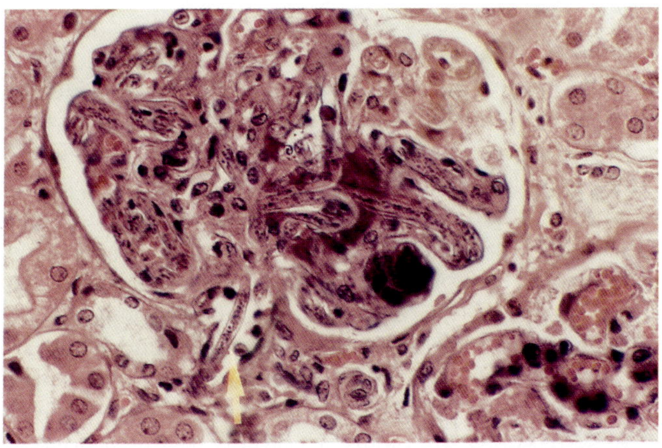

Figure 147–3. Microfilariae of *W bancrofti* in glomerular capillaries. There is a cross-section and an oblique section of a microfilaria in the afferent arteriole [hematoxylin-eosin (H&E), ×440]. *(Contributed by Ernest E. Lack, MD.)*

Travelers to endemic areas for short periods, eg, several weeks to less than 2 to 3 months, have a low risk of infection. Those who absorb large numbers of infective larvae over several months to a year or so, however, are exceptions. American servicemen stationed in the Pacific during World War II developed fevers and pain in the lower limbs consistent with acute adenolymphangitis. Microfilaremia was not detected in these patients.[5] A similar phenomenon has been described in brugian filariasis.[6] Accelerated development of disease in these previously uninfected persons may be from lack of immunologic tolerance conferred in utero by maternal infection.[7,8]

MORPHOLOGY OF THE PARASITE

Adult worms of *W bancrofti* are multicellular helminths enclosed in a chitinous cuticle (Figures 147–4 and 147–5). The most distinctive morphologic feature of the fecund female worm is the uterus, which contains multiple embryonated eggs and microfilariae. Female worms are larger than sexually mature male worms, their lengths respectively being 80 to 100 mm and 20 to 40 mm. Observed in vivo, adult *W bancrofti* have an undulating movement.[9]

Microfilariae are more commonly examined than adult worms since this stage of the parasite is accessible when blood is sampled for diagnosis. Microfilariae are approximately 260 μm long and up to 10 μm wide.

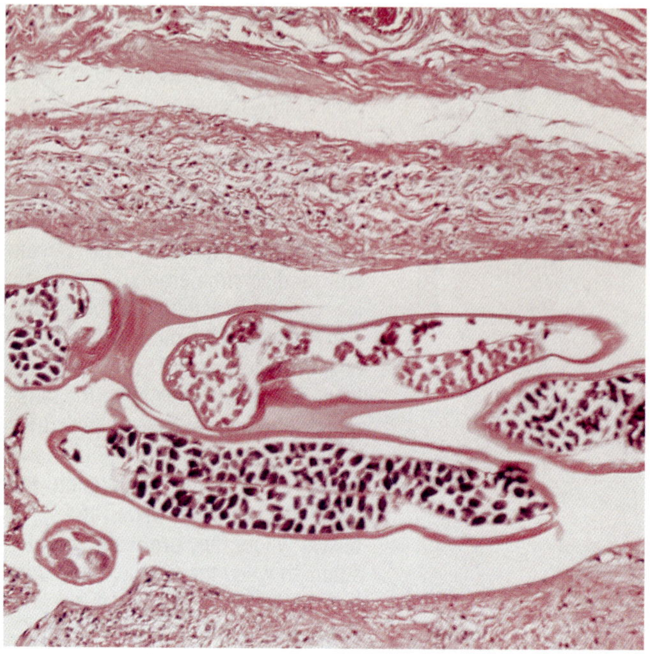

Figure 147–4. Adult gravid female *W bancrofti* in a dilated lymphatic vessel in testis. The wall of the lymphatic is edematous, contains inflammatory cells (mainly lymphocytes), and is thickened by fibrous tissue. Tangential sections of the worm are shown. Embryonated eggs and developing microfilariae are within the paired uterine tubes. The amorphous pink material between segments of worm is lymph. The fibrosis, edema, and inflammation of the wall of the lymphatic and the contained worm impede the flow of lymph (AFIP Neg 70-6685).

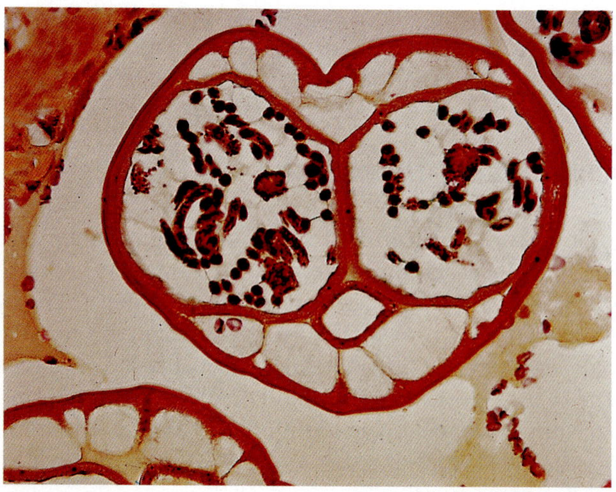

Figure 147–5. Cross-section of a gravid female *W bancrofti* in the epididymis of a patient from Surinam. The cuticle of the worm is thin and the body cavity contains paired uteri and a digestive tube (AFIP Neg 70-8650; Movat, ×300).

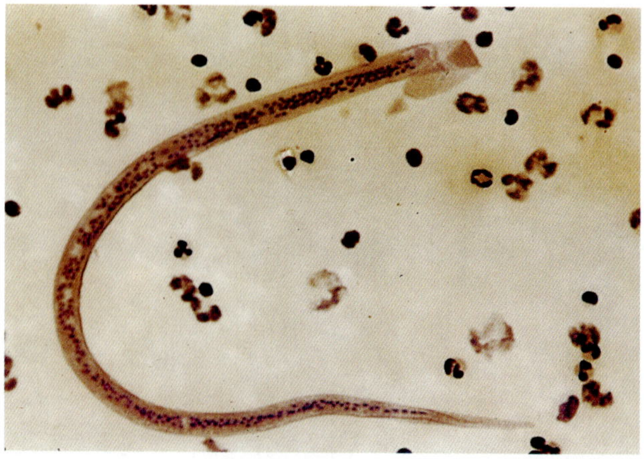

Figure 147–6. Microfilaria of *W bancrofti* in a thick blood film. The sheath is transparent and folded over at the anterior end. There is a pair of anterior nuclei that are side by side. The cephalic space is 5 to 7 μm long. The terminal nucleus is pointed and the caudal clear space is 5 to 15 μm long (AFIP Neg 70-10516; Delafield's stain, ×160). *(Contributed by Ronald C. Neafie.)*

Each microfilaria has approximately 1000 nucleated cells and is bound by an acellular sheath, which is the remnant of the vitelline membrane (Figure 147–6). The sheath contains chitin and multiple glycosylated proteins that are immunogenic. By light microscopy, *W bancrofti* microfilariae are distinguishable from those of *Brugia* sp by the configurations of nuclei in the cephalic and caudal spaces.[10] Tissue specimens containing third- and fourth-stage larvae have not been systematically studied.

CLINICAL FEATURES AND PATHOGENESIS

Chronic Disease

Bancroftian filariasis is characterized by a wide spectrum of chronic clinical manifestations. At one end of this spectrum are most residents of endemic areas who have circulating microfilariae but no clinical manifestations. Lymphoscintigraphy and ultrasonography, however, reveal that many of these people have dilated and functionally abnormal lymphatics.[9,11,12] The implication is that these people will develop overt lymphatic disease. The most severe disease manifestations of bancroftian filariasis involve the lymph nodes and lymphatics of the limbs and male genitalia. The degree of lymphedema of limbs, which more frequently involves legs than arms, is graded according to the following scale: grade I, pitting edema that is reversible on elevation of the leg; grade II, mostly nonpitting edema that is not reversible on elevation; grade III or elephantiasis, an increase in the size of the limb relative to grade II with sclerosis and papillomatous lesions of skin (Figures 147–7 through 147–9).[13] The latter two categories of lymphedema may cause significant debilitation and are commonly associated with secondary bacterial infections, which may exacerbate the swelling (Figure 147–8). Affected limbs probably progress through grades I, II, and III sequentially. Accordingly, intervention is most effective when done in the earlier stages. Lymphedema caused by *W bancrofti* can be distinguished from lymphedema caused by *B malayi* in that infection by the former produces swelling of the entire limb, whereas the latter involves only the area below the knee.

Disease of the male genitalia is also an important clinical manifestation of bancroftian filariasis. This contrasts sharply with *Brugia* infection, in which genital disease is distinctly uncommon. Hydrocele is the most common manifestation. Hydroceles vary in size, but it is not unusual for many to exceed a diameter of 10 to 15 cm. The fluid is clear and does not contain parasites. There may be also scrotal edema and thickening of scrotal membranes and contents (Figure 147–10) and of spermatic cord (Figure 147–11). In many endemic areas, disease of the scrotum may be more prevalent than of the limbs. The frequency of disease involving the female genitalia has not been established, although anecdotal evidence suggests it is much lower than swelling of male genitalia.

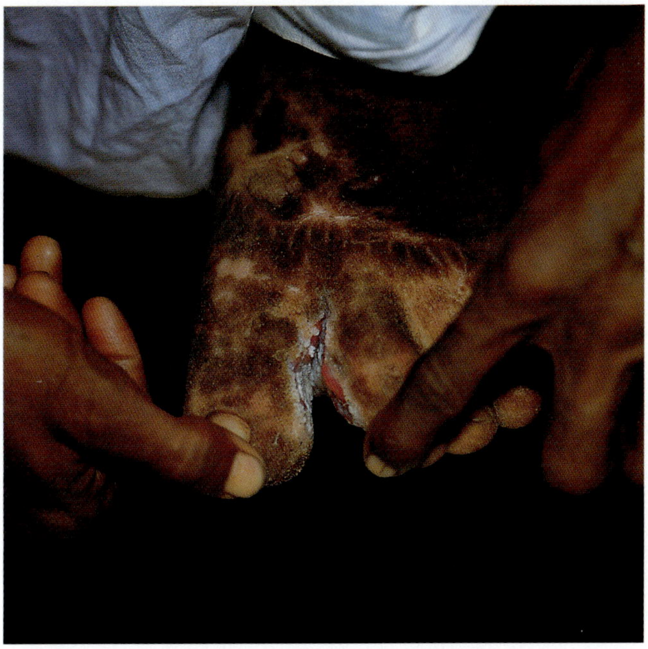

Figure 147–8. Papillomatous change of the foot of a south Indian adult with fissures between the toes. These are painful, chronically infected, and may cause chronic bacterial lymphangitis, which may contribute to the chronic lymphedema. *(Patient of Professor S. Jamal; photograph by Daniel H. Connor, MD, 1985.)*

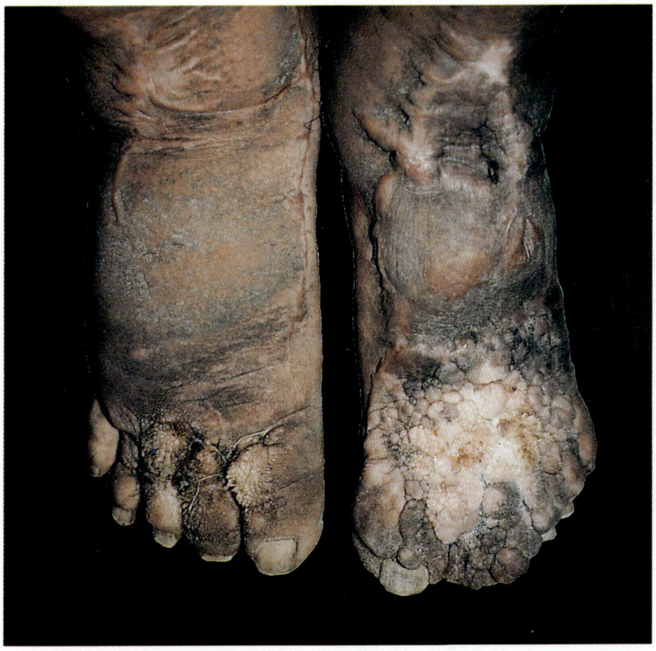

Figure 147–7. Filarial (bancroftian) lymphedema of both legs and feet in an adult patient living in south India. Both feet—left more than right—show papillomatous changes ("mossy foot"). *(Patient of Professor S. Jamal; photograph by Daniel H. Connor, MD, 1985.)*

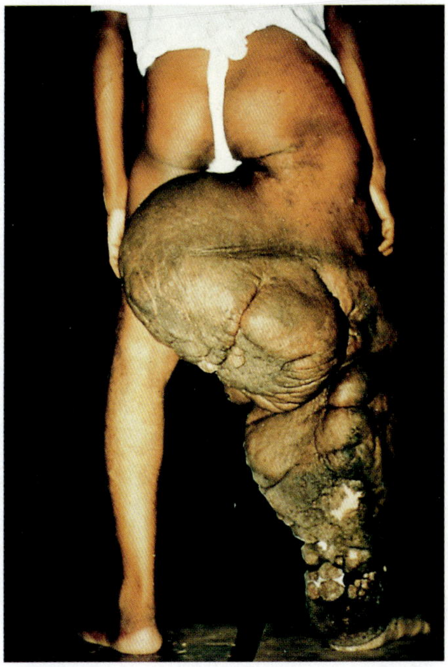

Figure 147–9. Elephantiasis of the right lower limb in a young adult man from south India. Note that the skin on the upper portion of the limb is smooth but the lower portion has papillomatous (mossy) change. *(Patient of Professor S. Jamal; photograph by Daniel H. Connor, MD, 1985.)*

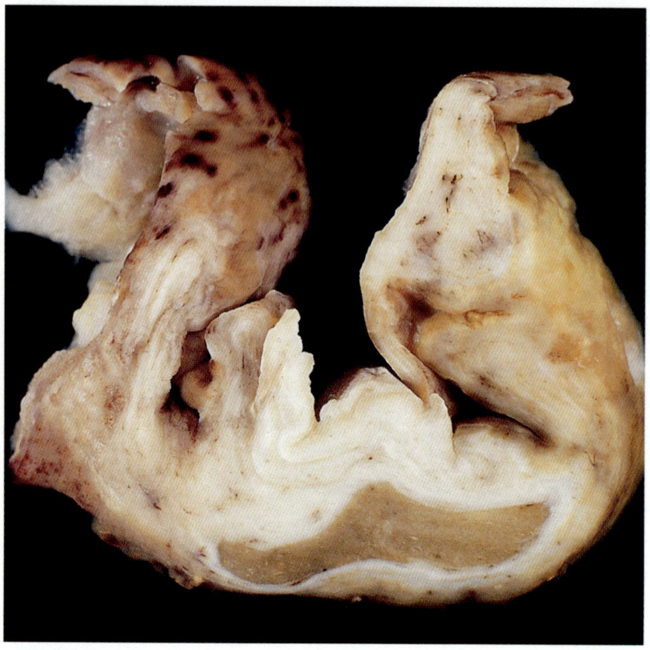

Figure 147–10. Filarial inflammation and fibrosis of scrotum and contents. The tunica is thickened and the testis (lower tan area) is surrounded and squeezed by fibrous scar. Hydrocele fluid in these specimens is clear and may or may not contain microfilariae. *(By Daniel H. Connor, MD, 1977.)*

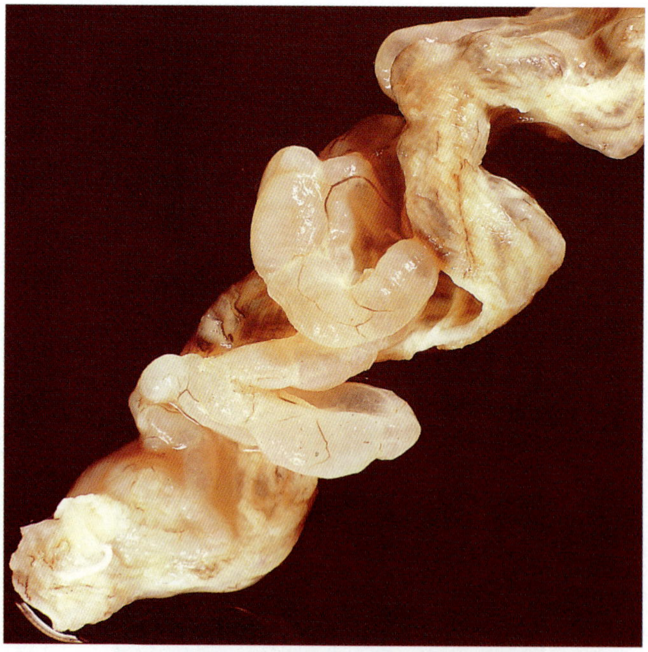

Figure 147–11. Spermatic cord is edematous and distorted from filarial (bancroftian) edema. The patient was 19 years old and from Brazil. Microscopically the lymphatics were dilated. Funiculitis—edema and inflammation of the spermatic cord—is probably the most common manifestation of bancroftian filariasis in men. *(By Daniel H. Connor, MD, 1970.)*

Filariasis of the female breast (Figure 147–12)[14] is sometimes complicated by elephantiasis. Chyluria—chyle and lymph from lacteals in urine (Figure 147–13)—occurs in a small percentage of patients with bancroftian filariasis. On a worldwide basis, the syndrome of tropical eosinophilia is not a prominent manifestation of bancroftian filariasis but there are select geographic areas such as southern India where it is a significant health problem. These patients have asthma, elevated polyclonal and antigen-specific IgE, very high titers of antimicrofilarial antibodies, and eosinophilia greater than 5000/μL of blood. They do not have circulating microfilariae. It is clear that tropical eosinophilia is caused by filarial infection because there is a clinical response to diethylcarbamazine, which kills microfilariae, and because pathologic lesions containing filarial remnants are in the lung (see later discussion).

Pathogenesis

There is at present a poor understanding of the mechanisms that lead to the diverse acute and chronic manifestations of bancroftian filariasis. One paradigm proposes that asymptomatic individuals are microfilaremic and exhibit a pattern of antigen-specific T-cell responses consistent with a dominance of Th2 cells that produce interleukin (IL)-4, IL-5, and IL-10.[15] The converse is proposed for those who are amicrofilaremic. Th2 cytokines (especially IL-10) are thought to suppress production of proinflammatory cytokines such as inter-

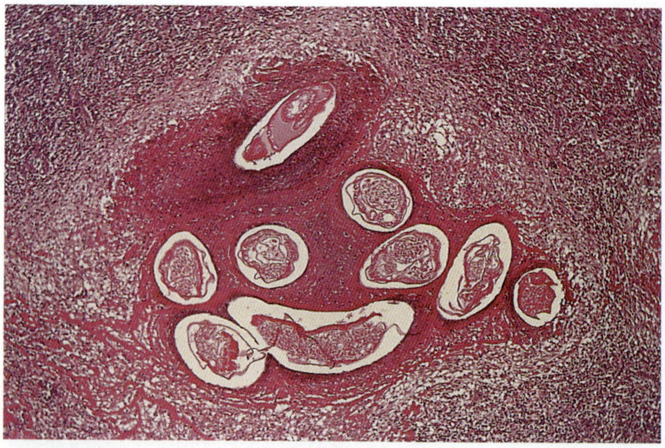

Figure 147–12. A coiled gravid female *W bancrofti* in breast tissue of a woman from West Africa. Nodules containing filariae are removed regularly from breasts of women living in endemic areas when surgery is available to them. As in other sites, degenerating adult filariae lie in necrotizing granulomas. Inflammatory cells include macrophages, epithelioid cells, neutrophils, lymphocytes, plasma cells, and—usually most prominently—eosinophils and giant cells (AFIP Neg 75-14551).

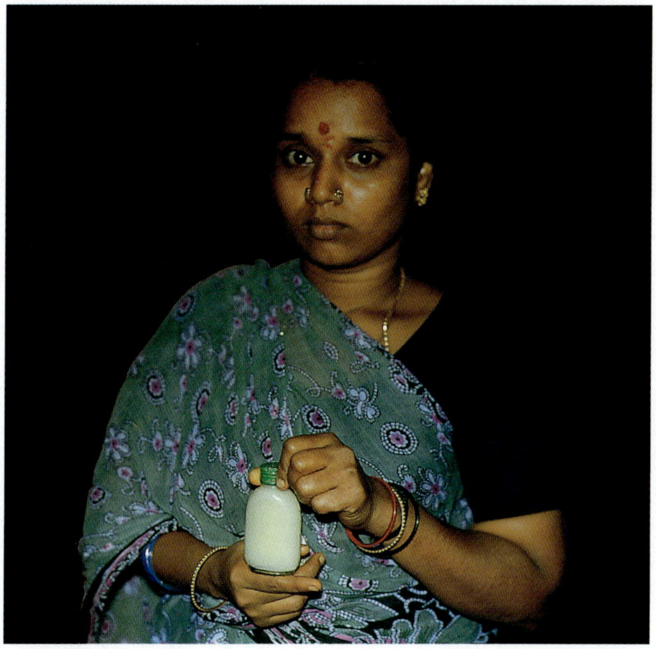

Figure 147–13. Young woman from South India holds a specimen of her urine with chyluria. *(By Daniel H. Connor, MD, 1985.)*

feron gamma, which promote lymphatic lesions. Although immunologic data support this hypothesis, population-based surveys generally indicate there is no positive relationship between microfilaremia and rates of disease.[16]

Nonimmunologic processes have also been invoked as contributing to lymphatic dysfunction. The most prominent among these has been based on observations that filariae (*Brugia* species) cause lymphatic dilatation in the absence of T cells (such as in athymic nude mice) or B and T cells (such as in SCID mice).[17,18] Together with the demonstration that adult worms and microfilariae produce arachidonic acid metabolites that can mediate relaxation of smooth muscle and endothelial cell alterations,[19,20] it is possible that filariae have a direct effect on the function of lymphatics independent of the host's immune response. Finally, some experiments[21] and observations of people living in endemic areas[22] suggest that secondary bacterial infections contribute also to exacerbations of lymphedema in those with preexisting disease.

PATHOLOGY

General

Wuchereria bancrofti causes acute lymphadenitis or lymphangitis of the lower limb or male genitalia. Adolescents and adults residing in endemic areas are most susceptible and are often asymptomatic preceding an attack of lymphadenitis and/or limb swelling, or epididymitis, funiculitis, or orchitis. Attacks are often accompanied by fever and pain at the site. Symptoms tend to peak over 3 to 5 days and resolve in 1 to 2 weeks. Most patients have one episode a year, although severe infections may cause abscesses in lymph nodes and breakdown of overlying skin. Frequent episodes of acute adenolymphangitis may precede chronic lesions that do not completely resolve. Filarial fevers, not associated with obvious lymphangitis, may present also as acute illnesses without obvious cause. In residents of endemic areas, these may be confused with malaria. Apart from the studies of O'Connor et al[23–25] little was known of the pathology of lymphatic filariasis before World War II at which time 38,000 U.S. troops were exposed in the South Pacific. Of these, more than 12,000 were infected within a year.[26] This cohort provided 1) an accurate estimate of incubation (a minimum of 3 months with most severe clinical manifestations at 8 months), 2) a clinical spectrum that included lymphadenopathy, lymphangitis, and inflammation of scrotal contents,[27] and 3) gradual cessation of all manifestations when the patient was removed from the endemic area. Every U.S. soldier was removed from the endemic area when infection was established and none had persistent filarial edema in the decades that followed World War II.[28]

Lymphadenitis

Inguinal, femoral, epitrochlear, supraclavicular, axillary, antecubital, pelvic, and abdominal lymph nodes have all been involved. Nodes are enlarged, tender or painful, and may be matted but are not usually fixed to skin. Grossly they are soft, have bulging gray-pink cut surfaces and thickened capsules. The earliest changes in man have not been studied but in experimentally infected animals, including cats, infective larvae penetrate lymphatic vessels and migrate to the nearest lymph node, where they provoke humoral and cell-mediated responses. Larvae then descend through afferent lymphatics and grow to become adult worms.[29] The sequential changes in human lymph nodes have not been documented as they have in experimental animals, but changes include thickening and fibrosis of capsules, dilated lymphatics, dilated subcapsular sinusoids, histiocytes and eosinophils in dilated lymphatics, and sinusoids, and in peritrabecular areas, fibrosis of trabeculae, hyperplastic follicles in early infections, and atrophic follicles in long-standing infections. When neither microfilariae nor adult worms can be identified in tissue the changes must be interpreted as nonspecific. This combination of changes, however, is so characteristic—and so rare in lymph nodes from patients in temperate climates—that a diagnosis of filariasis can be suggested with some certainty.[28] When microfilariae (in sinusoids or lymphatics) or adult worms (male or female, dead or alive in lymphatics and sinusoids) are identified, a specific diagnosis can be made regardless of the inflammatory changes. Most intact and degenerating worms are in perinodal afferent lymphatics, in capsular lymphatics, or in subcapsular sinusoids. Dead and dying worms tend to be coiled and centered in necrotizing granulomas. They have a matrix of degenerating histiocytes against their cuticles, then a layer of viable histiocytes, epithelioid cells, and giant cells surrounded by granulation tissue and scar tissue. The granulomas contain varying numbers of eosinophils and the giant cells are usually of both Langhans' and foreign-body types. Although not seen regularly in human specimens, the carcasses of the worms become saponified and calcified by x ray[25] and experimentally.[30] Finally the granulomas around degenerating worms heal as compact scars.

Lymphangitis

Manson first noted lymphangitis in filariasis[40] but the enormity of the dilatation is best appreciated radiographically[32,33] and more recently ultrasonographically[9] and lymphoscintigraphically.[11,12] In 251 U.S. servicemen with lymphangitis, the distribution was scrotum alone 51%, arm alone 22%, scrotum and arm 20%, leg alone 3%, scrotum and leg 2%, arm and leg 1%, scrotum, arm, and leg 1%.[33] Of these 251 servicemen, 93% had lymphangitis of arm and/or leg. Microscopically, lymphatics are dilated, have thickened edematous walls infiltrated with lymphocytes, eosinophils, histiocytes, and less constantly neutrophils and plasma cells (Figure 147–4).[28,34] Endothelial cells are thickened and sometimes heaped up in polypoid projections. Adult filariae may be free or enclosed in lymphatic thrombi. Dead and dying worms are surrounded by granulomas that are essentially the same as those in lymph nodes. Some lymph nodes, however, contain adult filariae but have no significant inflammation. This suggests that there can be functional alterations in the lymphatics in the absence of a local inflammatory response.[35]

Funiculitis and Epididymitis

Funiculitis and epididymitis are the most common manifestations of lymphatic filariasis in humans (Figure 147–11). The cord becomes painful and nodular. Epididymitis usually accompanies funiculitis. The epididymis enlarges and becomes tender. Microscopically there is filarial lymphangitis as described earlier, and when degenerating adult filariae are present the local reaction resembles closely the reaction to adult worms in lymph nodes.[36,37] Also, the lesions that surround degenerating filariae[38] resemble closely the lesions that form around filariae killed by antiparasitic drugs.[39]

Orchitis

Patients with filarial orchitis have a swollen, painful testis with pain sometimes radiating up the spermatic cord. Clinically the testis is boggy, probably from edema and inflammation of the tunica and adventitia, rather than from swelling of the testis proper (Figure 147–10).

Lymphedema and Elephantiasis

Upper and lower limbs, breasts, and external genitalia are the most common sites. Persistent filarial lymphedema usually is limited and localized, but in some patients chronic edema progresses to elephantiasis (Figures 147–7 through 147–9). Incidence of elephantiasis is reported as 1% to 3% of those infected and the incidence increases with age. In the first scrotum described by Manson[40] lymph exuded from the skin and an adult filaria protruded from the cut surface. The elephantoid scrotal tissue is not a "bag of lymph" as has been sometimes believed, but is interlacing bundles of fibrous connective tissue and smooth muscle with dilated lymphatic channels and collections of plasma cells interspersed. The large bulk of smooth muscle, by location and configuration, appears to be hyperplastic cremasteric muscle.

Tropical Pulmonary Eosinophilia Syndrome

In addition to pathologic changes in lymphatic vessels, granulomas containing degenerating microfilariae have been identified in lung, spleen (Figure 147–14), and lymph nodes of patients with tropical pulmonary eosinophilia syndrome. These patients have, as noted, cough, asthma, pulmonary infiltrates by x ray, eosinophilia, and high levels of IgE and antifilarial antibodies, but no microfilaremia. Sometimes these degenerating microfilariae provoke a surrounding layer of Splendore–Hoeppli material—an eosinophilic precipitate around degenerating microfilariae (Figure 147–15).[41] Specimens containing Splendore–Hoeppli bodies are not common because specimens of lung are not taken from patients with uncomplicated tropical eosinophilia. Similar pathologic reactions develop in mice when the mice have been sensitized to filarial antigens and subsequently challenged with live *B malayi* microfilariae.[42,43]

Breast

Filarial lesions of the breast are readily recognized in endemic areas. They are firm, solid inflammatory masses and frequently excised to exclude the possibility of carcinoma. Microscopically a coiled degenerating adult filarial worm provokes the same kind of reaction described in the earlier Lymphadenitis section (Figure 147–12). These worms are probably in small lymphatics

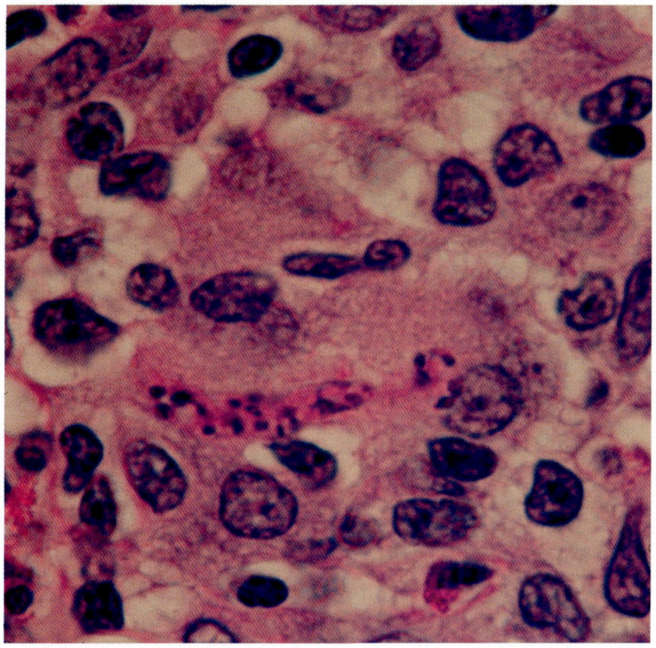

Figure 147–14. Carcass of a degenerating microfilaria of *W bancrofti* in spleen. The nuclei of the microfilaria are shrunken and pyknotic but are still aligned and retain the general contour of the microfilaria. A giant cell surrounds the carcass (AFIP Neg 81-13957).

but by the time the lesion is excised traces of the lymphatic are lost. Eastern China is now another recognized endemic area for filarial granulomas of breast.[14]

Eye

Eye is rarely involved, but serous conjunctivitis and photophobia,[44,45] an adult worm in the anterior chamber,[46,47] and *B malayi* microfilarial uveitis[48] have all been described.

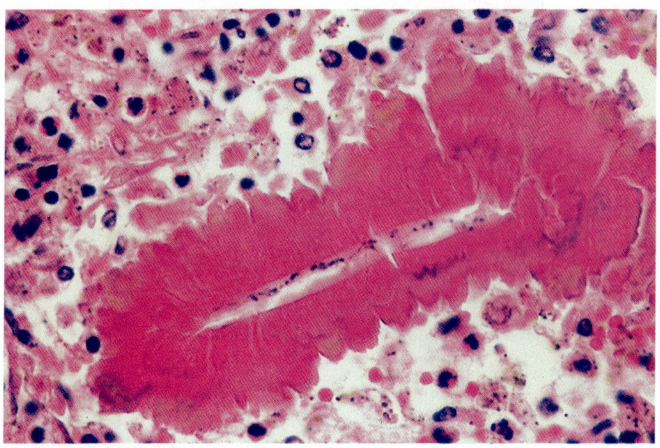

Figure 147–15. Experimental infection by *B malayi*. The carcass of the degenerating microfilaria is essentially straight and surrounded by a thick layer of eosinophilic, acellular Splendore–Hoeppli material. *(By Dr. Richard B. Crandall, 1980.)*

Chyluria

Chyluria is excretion of chyle and lymph into the urinary tract and it afflicts only a small fraction of those with bancroftian filariasis (Figure 147–13). Chyluria is caused by obstruction of lymph flow in the retroperitoneal lymphatics or lymph nodes. As a consequence of the obstruction, chyle and lymph from the lacteals flow into renal lymphatics. Although believed to be benign, chyluria causes loss of dietary lipids, proteins, and possibly fat-soluble vitamins in the urine, and patients lose weight.[49]

EXPERIMENTAL FILARIASIS

Experimental Filarial Inflammation

Lymphatic and genital tissues from several experimental animals have confirmed that the nature of host response to filariae is similar in other mammalian species. Cats and Mongolian gerbils infected with *Brugia* sp develop lymphatic thrombi and granulomas around adult worms similar to those in humans.[50,51] Silvered leaf monkeys (*Presbytis cristata*) are susceptible to *W bancrofti* infection and have been used to study the histopathologic manifestations of genital and lymphatic lesions.[52] Lymphatic lesions were mostly in the inguinal and lumbar lymph nodes. Specimens from 2 to 15 infected monkeys had fibrosing lymphadenitis, which was limited primarily to the medullary area of the nodes. This was accompanied by scar tissue radiating toward the cortex and a proliferation of histiocytes in the medullary and cortical sinuses. Microfilariae and ill-defined remnants of parasites were in some sections, but recognizable adult worms were not identified in lymph nodes per se. In contrast, adult worms were in perinodal lymphatic vessels and lymph sinuses. Inflammatory infiltrates surrounded afferent and efferent lymphatic vessels (perilymphangitis) near necrotic worms. These infiltrates contained eosinophils, lymphocytes, macrophages, and plasma cells. Perilymphangitis, orchitis, epididymitis, and funiculitis were in genital tissues. Adult parasites were in testes or epididymis of all infected male animals. Granulomas similar to those in humans developed in testes, tunica albuginea, vas deferens, and epididymis.

DIAGNOSIS

Diagnosis of bancroftian filariasis is made by identifying *W bancrofti* microfilariae in blood or by identifying adult worms or microfilariae in tissue sections. Biopsy of lymph node and genitalia is usually not done on residents of endemic areas so diagnosis depends on finding microfilariae in blood. Blood should be taken when microfilaremia peaks, between 11 PM and 2 AM for most strains, because the parasites may not be circulating in sufficient numbers to be detected at other times. A variety of methods have been used to process blood to facilitate identification of microfilariae (Giemsa-stained smears of fingerprick samples containing a volume of 60 μL are commonly performed in epidemiologic surveys). Filtration of 1.0 mL of blood through a Nucleopore filter is the most sensitive method for detecting microfilariae.

Failure to identify microfilariae in the blood does not exclude lymphatic filariasis. In these patients, the level of microfilaremia may be below detectable limits or the patient may harbor adults worms that are not producing microfilariae. To address this problem, assays that measure the level of circulating parasite antigen have been developed.[53] Detection of parasite DNA in blood by the polymerase chain reaction has also been achieved,[54] although this has not proven to be more sensitive than filtration techniques. Antibody-based assays, particularly those that measure parasite-specific IgG4 and IgE,[55] have been evaluated as immunodiagnostic aids. Although these correlate with the level of parasitemia, they do not distinguish between active infection without microfilaremia and previous infection.

TREATMENT

Chemotherapy is currently the mainstay of treatment for bancroftian filariasis. In those with lymphedema of a limb or disease of the scrotum, a course of the drug diethylcarbamazine (DEC) is indicated. Recent studies indicate that single doses of DEC (6 mg/kg body weight) may be as effective in lowering microfilaremia as the traditional 10- to 12-day course (cumulative dose of 72 mg/kg body weight).[56] Until ongoing studies examining the efficacy of single-dose therapy in those with lymphatic disease have been completed, however, it is prudent to administer the drug by the latter regimen. Because DEC appears to have a partial microfilaricidal effect, partial reversal of functional and/or anatomic lymphatic obstruction may be achieved. Good hygienic care of the affected limb, physiotherapy to move lymph centrally (eg, elevation of the leg), and treatment of intercurrent bacterial infections are all important ancillary measures to limit debility.

The optimal approach to treatment of adenolymphangitis or asymptomatic microfilaremia has not been established. If adenolymphangitis is precipitated by dying filariae, antifilarial drugs may exacerbate the inflammation. Until controlled studies of this complex clinical problem are completed, the current recommendation is to give DEC. Previously it was thought that patients with microfilaremia but who are asymptomatic had nothing to gain from treatment except a lowering of the intensity of their parasitemia—an important epidemiologic goal nevertheless since this probably decreases transmission. As noted earlier, however, recent evidence demonstrating abnormal lymphatics in these patients suggests that antifilarial chemotherapy should be given.

DEC has for many years been the only safe and useful drug to treat lymphatic filariasis. Studies during the last few years indicate that ivermectin is also effective.[57] Investigations as to whether or not ivermectin has a macro- as well as a microfilaricidal effect, and establishment of its efficacy in combination with DEC, are under way to determine its place in the therapeutic armamentarium against bancroftian filariasis.

Patients with deforming elephantiasis, as shown in Figures 147–7 through 147–9, have benefited from surgical decompression. Two types of anastomosis have been used—lymphaticovenous and nodovenous.[58] Elephantiasis of lower limb, for instance, is relieved by anastomosing the long saphenous vein, or one of its tributaries, to the subcapsular space of a lymph node. This allows the dammed lymph to bypass obstructed

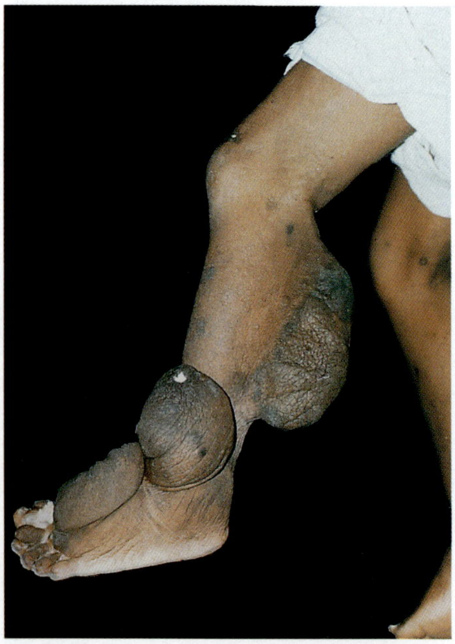

Figure 147–16. Leg of a young man from south India 2 weeks after nodolymphatico anastomosis for decompression of his filarial elephantiasis. Dammed lymph has been shunted through the anastomosis. Note that the once taut skin hangs in loose redundant bags. *(Patient of Professor S. Jamal; photograph by Daniel H. Connor, MD, 1985.)*

lymphatic channels in abdomen and thorax, by escaping from the subcapsular sinus into the venous system. Patients experience immediate relaxation of the skin of the swollen limb. This is followed in a few weeks by removal of redundant skin (Figure 147–16) and sometimes other procedures as necessary.[58] Long-term effects are being evaluated.

REFERENCES

1. Lymphatic filariasis. Fourth report of the World Health Organization Expert Committee on Filariasis. Technical report series, number 702; Geneva, Switzerland: WHO; 1984.
2. Partono F. The spectrum of disease in lymphatic filariasis. *Ciba Foundation Symp.* 1987;127:15–31.
3. Ottesen E. Efficacy of diethylcarbamazine in eradicating infection with lymphatic dwelling filariae in humans. *Rev Infect Dis.* 1985;7:341–346.
4. Hairston NG, de Meillon B. On the inefficiency of *Wuchereria bancrofti* transmission from mosquito to the human host. *Bull WHO.* 1968;38:935–941.
5. Wartman WB. Filariasis in American armed servicemen in World War II. *Medicine.* 1947;12:181–189.
6. Partono F, Purnomo, Pribaldi W, Sowewarta A. Epidemiologic and clinical features of *Brugia timori* infection in a newly established village, Karakuak, West Flores, Indonesia. *Am J Trop Med Hyg.* 1978;27:910–915.
7. Lammie PJ, Hitch WL, Allen EMW, Hightower W, Eberhard ML. Maternal filarial infection as a risk factor for infection in children. *Lancet.* 1991;337:1005–1006.
8. Steel C, Guinea A, McCarthy JS, Ottesen EA. Long-term effect of prenatal exposure to maternal microfilaremia on immune responsiveness to filarial parasite antigens. *Lancet.* 1994;343:890–893.
9. Amaral F, Dreyer G, Figureueredo-Silva J, et al. Live adult worms detected by ultrasonography in human bancroftian filariasis. *Am J Trop Med Hyg.* 1994;50:753–757.
10. Meyers WM, Neafie RC, Connor DH. Bancroftian and Malayan filariasis. In: Binford CH, Connor DH, eds. *Pathology of Tropical and Extraordinary Diseases.* Washington, DC: Armed Forces Institute of Pathology; 1976: 340–355.
11. Freedman DO, de Almeida Filho PJ, Besh S, Maia e Silva MC, Braga C, Maciel A. Lymphoscintigraphic analysis of lymphatic abnormalities in symptomatic and asymptomatic human filariasis. *J Infect Dis.* 1994;170:927–933.
12. Witte M, Jamal S, Williams WH, et al. Lymphatic abnormalities in human filariasis as depicted by lymphoscintigraphy. *Arch Intern Med.* 1993;153:737–744.
13. Lymphatic filariasis: The disease and its control. Fifth report of the World Health Organization Expert Committee on Filariasis; 1992.
14. Yuehan C, Qun X. Filarial granulomas of the female breast. *Am J Trop Med Hyg.* 1981;30:1206–1210.
15. King CL, Kumaraswami V, Poindexter RW, et al. Immunologic tolerance in lymphatic filariasis. Diminished parasite-specific T and B lymphocyte precursor frequency in the microfilaremic state. *J Clin Invest.* 1992;89:1403–1410.
16. Michael E, Grenfell BT, Bundy DAP. The association between microfilaremia and disease in lymphatic filariasis. *Proc Roy Soc London B.* 1994;256:33–40.
17. Vincent AL, Vickery AC, Lotz MJ, Desai U. The lymphatic pathology of *Brugia pahangi* in nude (athymic) and thymic mice C3H/HeN. *J Parasitol.* 1984;70:48–56.
18. Nelson FK, Greiner DL, Schultz LD, Rajan TV. The immunodeficient SCID mouse as a model for human lymphatic filariasis. *J Exp Med.* 1991;173:659–663.
19. Longworth DL, Monaham-Earley RA, Dvorak AM, Weller PF. Rapid uptake and esterification of arachidonic acid and other fatty acids by microfilariae of *Brugia malayi. Mol Biochem Parasitol.* 1987;23:275–284.
20. Kanesa-thasan N, Douglas JG, Kazura JW. Diethylcarbamazine inhibits endothelial and microfilarial prostanoid metabolism in vitro. *Mol Biochem Parasitol.* 1991;49: 11–19.
21. Bosworth W, Ewert A, Bray J. The interaction of *Brugia malayi* and streptococcus in an animal model. *Am J Trop Med Hyg.* 1973;22:714–719.
22. Liu Y-K, Hsieh S-C, Tai T-Y. The role of streptococcal infections in filariasis. *Chinese Med J.* 1964;83:17–22.
23. O'Connor FW. Filarial periodicity with observations on the mechanisms of the migration of the microfilariae from the parent worm to the blood stream. *Puerto Rico J Public Health Trop Med.* 1931;6:263–272.
24. O'Connor FW, Hulse CR. Studies in filariasis. I. In Puerto Rico. *Puerto Rico J Public Health Trop Med.* 1935;11: 167–367.
25. O'Connor FW, Golden R, Auckinclos H. The roentgen demonstration of calcified filaria bancrofti in human tissue. *Am J Roentgenol Radium Ther.* 1930;23:495–502.
26. Beaver PC. Filariasis without microfilaremia. *Am J Trop Med Hyg.* 1970;19:181–189.
27. King BG. Early filariasis diagnosis and clinical findings; report of 268 cases in American troops. *Am J Trop Med.* 1944;24:285–298.
28. Connor DR, Palmieri JR, Gibson DW. Pathogenesis of lymphatic filariasis in man. *Z Parasitenkd.* 1986;72:13–28.
29. Ewert A, El Bihari S. Rapid recovery of *Brugia malayi* larvae following experimental infection of cats. *Trans R Soc Trop Med Hyg.* 1971;65:364–368.
30. Rogers R, Denham DA, Nelson GS. Studies with *Brugia pahangi.* 5. Structure of the cuticle. *J Helminthol.* 1974;48: 113–117.
31. Montangerand Y, Huet R, Fougues M. Lymphography in lymphedema of the extremities in Bancroft's filariosis. *Ann Radiol (Paris).* 1965;8:295–308.
32. Young AE. Filariasis. *Proc R Soc Med.* 1976;69:708–709.
33. Dickson JG, Huntington RW, Eichold S. Filariasis in defense force, Samoan group. *US Naval Med Bull.* 1943; 41:1240–1252.
34. Lichtenberg F. Inflammatory responses to filarial connective tissue parasites. *Parasitology.* 1987;94:S101–S122.
35. Jungmann P, Figureueredo-Silva J, Dreyer G. Bancroftian lymphadenopathy: a histopathologic study of 58 cases from northeastern Brazil. *Am J Trop Med Hyg.* 1991;45: 325–331.

36. Lichtenberg F, Medina R. Bancroftian filariasis in the etiology of funiculoepididymitis, periorchitis, and hydrocele in Puerto Rico. (Statistical study of surgical and autopsy material over a 13 year period). *Am J Trop Med Hyg.* 1957; 6:739–750.
37. Lichtenberg F. The early phase of endemic bancroftian filariasis in the male. Pathologic study. *J Mount Sinai Hosp.* 1957;24:983–1000.
38. O'Connor FW. The etiology of the disease syndrome in *Wuchereria bancrofti* infections. *Trans R Soc Trop Med Hyg.* 1932;26:13–33.
39. Gibson DW, Connor DH, Brown HL, et al. Onchocercal dermatitis: ultrastructural studies of microfilariae and host tissues before and after treatment with diethylcarbamazine (Hetrazan). *Am J Trop Med Hyg.* 1976;25:259–265.
40. Manson P. *Tropical Diseases, a Manual of Diseases of Warm Climates.* New York: William Wood; 1898:6–497.
41. Hartz PH, van der Saar A. Tropical eosinophilia in filariasis—occurrence of radiating processes about microfilariae. *Am J Clin Pathol.* 1948;18:637–644.
42. Egwang TG, Kazura JW. The BALB/c mouse as an animal model for immunological studies of microfilariae-induced pulmonary eosinophilia. *Am J Trop Med Hyg.* 1990;43: 61–66.
43. Pearlman E, Kroeze WK, Hazlett FE Jr, et al. *Brugia malayi:* acquired resistance to microfilariae in BALB/c mice correlates with local Th2 responses. *Exp Parasitol.* 1993;76:200–208.
44. Michael P. Filariasis among navy and marine personnel; report on laboratory investigations. *US Naval Med Bull.* 1944;42:1059–1236.
45. Fogel RH, Huntington RW. Genital manifestations of early filariasis. *US Naval Med Bull.* 1944;43:263–271.
46. Fernando SE. Ocular filariasis. Adult *Wuchereria bancrofti* in the anterior chamber of the human eye. *J Trop Med Hyg.* 1935;38:17–18.
47. Chatterji KC. Adult filaria (*bancrofti*) in the anterior chamber of the human eye. *J Indian Med Assoc.* 1954;24: 146–147.
48. Anandakannan K, Gupta CP. Microfilaria malayi in uveitis: case report. *Br J Ophthalmol.* 1977;61:263–264.
49. 12th international WHO/TDR/FIL conference on lymphatic pathology and immunopathology in filariasis, Thanjavur, India, November 18–22, 1985. *Lymphology.* 1985;18:155–156.
50. Ah H-S, Thompson PE. *Brugia pahangi:* infections and their effect on the lymphatic system of Mongolian jirds (*Meriones unguiculatus*). *Exp Parasitol.* 1973;34:393–411.
51. Rogers R, Denham DA, Nelson GS, Guy F, Ponnudurai T. Studies with *Brugia pahangi.* 3. Histological changes in the affected lymph nodes of infected cats. *Ann Trop Med Parasitol.* 1975;69:77–84.
52. Latendresse JR, Campbell JR, Tirtokusumo S, Marwato HA. The pathology of lymphoreticular and genital tissues of silvered leaf monkeys. (*Presbytis cristata*) experimentally infected with *Wuchereria bancrofti*. *J Comp Pathol.* 1987; 97:653–665.
53. Weil GJ, Jain DC, Santhanam S, et al. A monoclonal antibody based immunoassay for detecting parasite antigenemia in bancroftian filariasis. *J Infect Dis.* 1987;156:350–355.
54. Poole CB, Williams SA. A rapid DNA assay for species-specific detection and quantification of *Brugia* in blood samples. *Mol Biochem Parasitol.* 1990;40:129–136.
55. Ottesen EA, Skvaril F, Tripathy SP, Poindexter RW, Hussain R. Prominence of IgG4 in the IgG antibody response to human filariasis. *J Immunol.* 1985;134:2707–2712.
56. Kazura JW, Greenberg J, Perry R, Day KP, Alpers MH. Comparison of single dose diethylcarbamazine and ivermectin for treatment of bancroftian filariasis in Papua New Guinea. *Am J Trop Med Hyg.* 1993;49:804–811.
57. Kazura JW. Ivermectin and human filariasis. *Microbiol Pathol.* 1993;14:337–342.
58. Jamal S. Lymphovenous anastomosis in filarial lymphedema. *Lymphology.* 1981;14:64–68.

CHAPTER 148

Brugian Zoonoses—Aberrant Infections of Humans by *Brugia* sp

J. Kevin Baird

To travel hopefully is a better thing than to arrive.

Robert Louis Stevenson (1850–1894)

DEFINITION

Brugian lymphatic filariasis caused by *Brugia malayi* and *B timori* occurs in Southeast Asia, where millions of people are infected. These two species seem to prefer the tissues of humans but can infect other mammals. Many other species of *Brugia* occur routinely in domestic and wild animals.[1] When a mosquito vector of these animal *Brugia* species feeds on a human, the infective larvae indiscriminately invade. The inhospitable tissues of humans probably kill the larvae before they attain maturity and provoke symptoms. Some *Brugia* species of animals, however, reach the lymphatics of a human, mature to become adult worms, and cause lymphadenopathy. This is zoonotic brugian filariasis.

At least four different species of *Brugia* that normally infect animals occasionally infect a human. Two of these are described in this chapter. These are the North American and the South American brugian zoonoses. The other two brugian zoonoses occur in Africa and Asia. In Africa, only a single infection of a human by a species of *Brugia* is known. In this patient microfilariae were in peripheral blood.[2] In Southeast Asia, *Brugia pahangi* of cats and dogs may cause many infections of humans,[1] but this parasite cannot be distinguished from *B malayi* by the usual diagnostic methods. Thus, the range and frequency of this zoonosis may be impossible to discern against a background of endemic *B malayi*.

GEOGRAPHIC DISTRIBUTION

North American brugian zoonoses occur primarily in the northeastern United States. Most of the 27 known infections have been in patients living in a geographic area extending from Massachusetts to Pennsylvania. Isolated infections have been described in patients living in Ohio, North Carolina, Florida, Mississippi, Louisiana, Oklahoma, and California.[3,4] The 5 infections by a South American species of *Brugia* were in Colombia, Ecuador, Peru and Brazil.[4]

BIOLOGY AND EPIDEMIOLOGY

Pairs of adult *Brugia* live in lymphatic vessels. They copulate and the female worm releases microfilariae. The microfilariae enter peripheral blood where they are available to feeding mosquitoes. When taken up by a mosquito, the microfilariae invade the thoracic flight muscles and develop into infective (third-stage) larvae in 1 to 2 weeks. These larvae migrate to spaces in the feeding apparatus of the mosquito and await the next blood meal. The larvae cannot discriminate between a suitable and unsuitable host when the mosquito feeds. They writhe out of the mouth parts of the mosquito onto skin, and enter the vertebrate host through the wound left by the mosquito. The larvae typically seek out lymphatic vessels supplying the cervical and ingui-

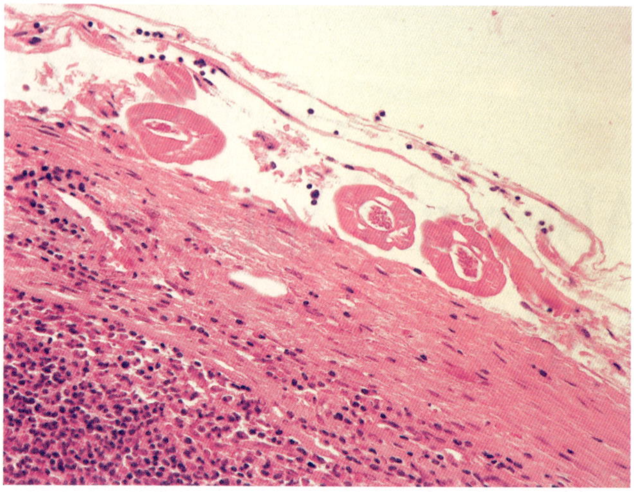

Figure 148–1. Coiled male *Brugia* sp on the exterior surface of a lymph node excised from the neck of a man living in New York. The capsule of the node is thickened and inflamed, but this lymph node contained also a degenerated female worm within the hilum and substance of the node (see Figure 148–4). There was no inflammation that could be specifically attributed to this male worm [AFIP Neg 85-6919; hematoxylin-eosin (H&E), ×250].

nal lymph nodes and eventually settle in afferent lymphatics near these nodes.

Like many other vector-borne zoonoses, infection by *Brugia* probably occurs when humans enter the habitat of the usual host. The species of *Brugia* causing the North and South American zoonoses have not been identified. Thus, their preferred hosts and vectors also remain unknown. Several species of *Brugia* have been described from animals in North America (cats, raccoons, rabbits, bobcats, and others), and one species is known from mammals in South America. However, many other species of *Brugia* almost certainly occur in the Western Hemisphere but have not yet been described. The specific identify of the *Brugia* species infecting humans must await more data and more specimens than are available. Eberhard and others[5] recently demonstrated *B leporis*–like microfilariae in 60% of rabbits (*Sylvilagus floridanus*) examined in Massachusetts, a region where many North American zoonotic *Brugia* infections (21 of 27) have occurred.

MORPHOLOGIC CHARACTERISTICS

North American *Brugia*

These worms rarely copulate and produce microfilariae in humans. An immunodeficient infant in Oklahoma is the only known report of microfilaremia.[6] In all other patients the diagnosis was made by identifying characteristic features of mature infertile worms in histologic sections. The diameter ranges from 30 to 100 μm for female worms, and 35 to 55 μm for male worms. Female worms contain two large reproductive tubes and as seen in cross-section each is almost half the diameter of the worm. Male worms, however, have only a single reproductive tube (Figures 148–1 and 148–2). The single intestinal tube in both genders is often only

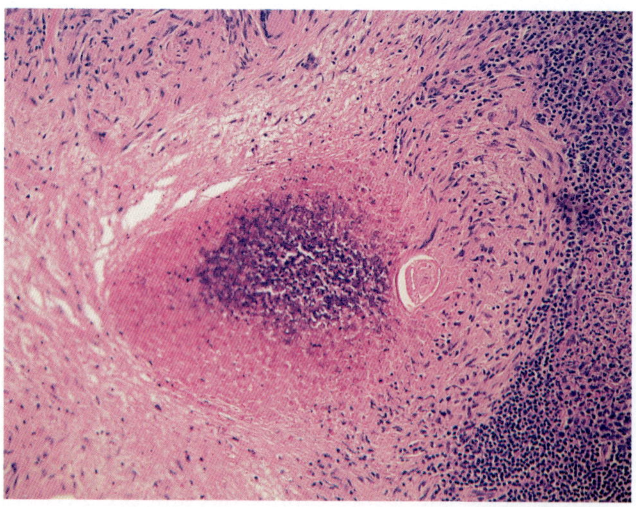

A

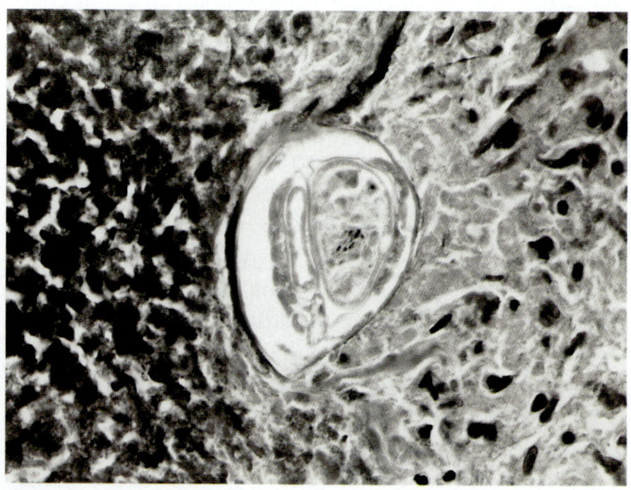

B

Figure 148–2. (**A**) Degenerated female *Brugia* sp within a necrotizing granuloma in the substance of a lymph node excised from the neck of a man living in New York (H&E, ×140). (**B**) Higher magnification of the worm to show that the worm's cuticle is partially collapsed. The paired uterine tubes, intestine, and somatic muscles are still recognizable (AFIP Neg 85-7808; H&E, ×630).

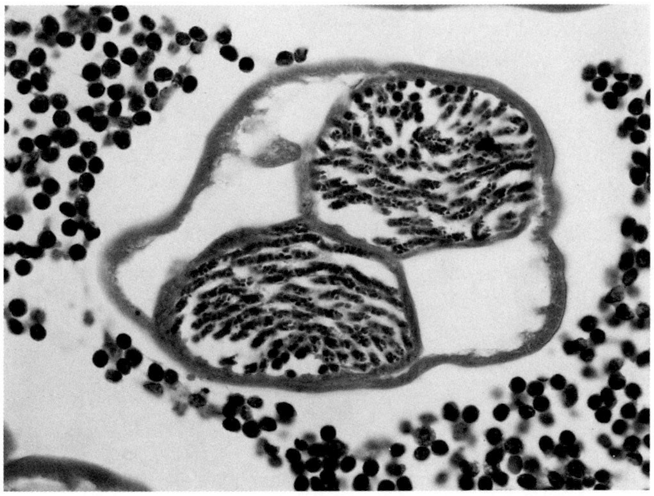

Figure 148–3. Cross-section of a gravid *Brugia* species in a lymphatic vessel near a cervical lymph node from an American woman who visited Peru. The paired uterine tubes contain many developing microfilariae (AFIP Neg 86-10608; H&E, ×630). *(From Baird et al*[7] *with permission.)*

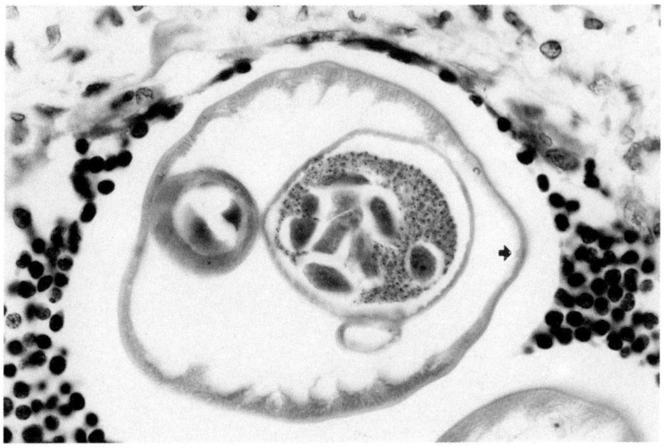

Figure 148–4. Cross-section through female *Brugia* species at the level of the oviduct containing eggs and spermatozoa. This section demonstrates diagnostic morphologic characteristics for South American *Brugia* zoonosis; thin, smooth monolayered cuticle with a small internal ridge at the lateral chords (*arrow, visible at right*), somatic musculature is coelomyarian, low, and with three to four cells per quadrant (AFIP Neg 86-10768; H&E, ×400; from Baird et al[7] with permission).

5 μm wide. The cuticle is monolayered, very thin (<1 μm), and some sections may show fine transverse striations. The cuticle thickens slightly at the lateral chords. The lateral chords are low and inconspicuous. Degenerative processes often obscure or obliterate the internal architecture of the worms. The female worm shown in Figure 148–2 illustrates this. Despite advanced degeneration of the worm, the diagnosis may be made by the cuticle, the estimated diameter of the worm, and its anatomic location.

South American *Brugia*

These worms more consistently produce microfilariae in humans (four of five infections). The female worms in tissue sections have uterine tubes packed with developing microfilariae (Figure 148–3). In some infections the microfilariae invaded fibroadipose tissue around lymphatic vessels and lymph nodes. Smears of peripheral blood, however, have not revealed microfilariae. The maximum diameter of adult female worms ranges between 60 and 100 μm. The diameter of the only male worm identified was 55 μm. The cuticle is as described for the North American worms, with one important exception—there is a small internal ridge at the lateral chords (Figure 148–4).[7]

CLINICAL FEATURES

Most patients have a single nontender nodule. Only 6 of the 27 patients with known infections from North America had tender nodules, whereas tender lesions were in 3 of the 5 infections from South America.[4] All infections in both North and South America involved lymph nodes, lymphatic vessels, or lymphoid tissue. The neck and groin were involved in more than one half of the patients. Other sites include scalp, axilla, clavicle, scapula, lung, chest wall, breast, and abdominal wall. Two South American patients had worms in the conjunctiva or penis. In all infections, except the sick infant from Oklahoma,[6] surgical removal of the involved tissues relieved all complaints.

PATHOLOGY

North American *Brugia* may remain in lymphatic vessels in and around lymph nodes, or they may breach the vessel wall and enter the substance of the node (Figures 148–3 and 148–4). The worms occasionally appear on the exterior surface of the capsule (Figure 148–1). When restricted to the lymphatic vessels, the worms cause edema and dilation of the vessels. The walls of vessels surrounding worms may be thickened and infiltrated with inflammatory cells. The capsule of the node is often thickened and inflamed. There may be sinus histiocytosis and follicular atrophy or hypertrophy. Eosinophils appear rarely within lymph nodes containing worms within lymphatic vessels. Worms breaching vessel walls and invading the node provoke necrotizing granulomas with palisaded epithelioid cells and foreign-body giant cells (Figures 148–5 and 148–6). Eosinophils are numerous in these lymph nodes. A narrow zone of necrosis surrounds worms in the hilum

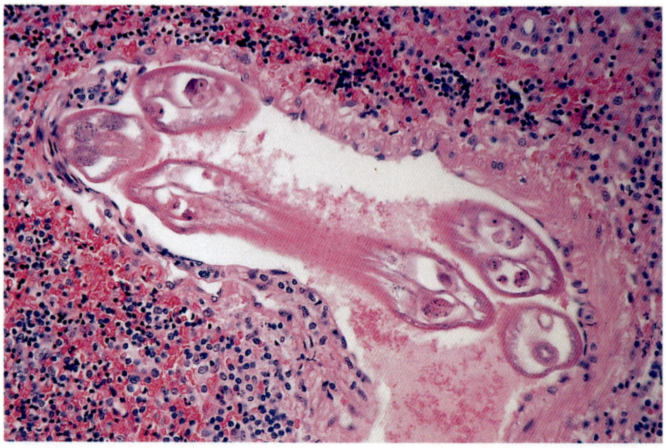

Figure 148–5. Female *Brugia* sp coiled within a dilated lymphatic vessel in the cortex of a lymph node taken from the breast of a woman from New York. The vessel wall is thickened and inflamed, as is the capsule of the lymph node (AFIP Neg 85-6921; H&E, ×72).

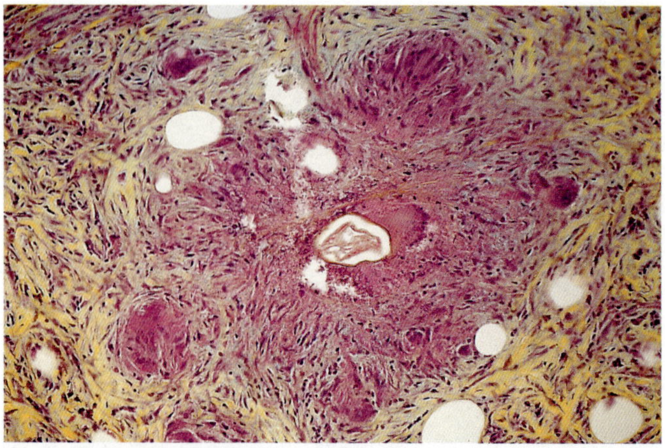

Figure 148–7. Degenerated and collapsed female *Brugia* sp in the substance of the hilar portion of a lymph node removed from the neck of a man living in New York. The worm is surrounded by necrotic tissue, palisading epithelioid cells, and foreign-body giant cells. Eosinophils, histiocytes, lymphocytes, and plasma cells have infiltrated the surrounding tissues (H&E, ×160).

(Figure 148–7), or a relatively wide zone of caseous necrosis may surround worms in the substance of the node (Figure 148–5). These lymph nodes have a thickened capsule, sinus histiocytosis, dilated lymphatic vessels, and edema and fibrous thickening of the connective tissues in the hilum. The few worms identified on the exterior surface of lymph nodes provoked either little inflammation (Figure 148–1) or large necrotizing granulomas. Large necrotizing granulomas without worms appearing on the surface of involved lymph nodes have been interpreted as worm tracks.[3]

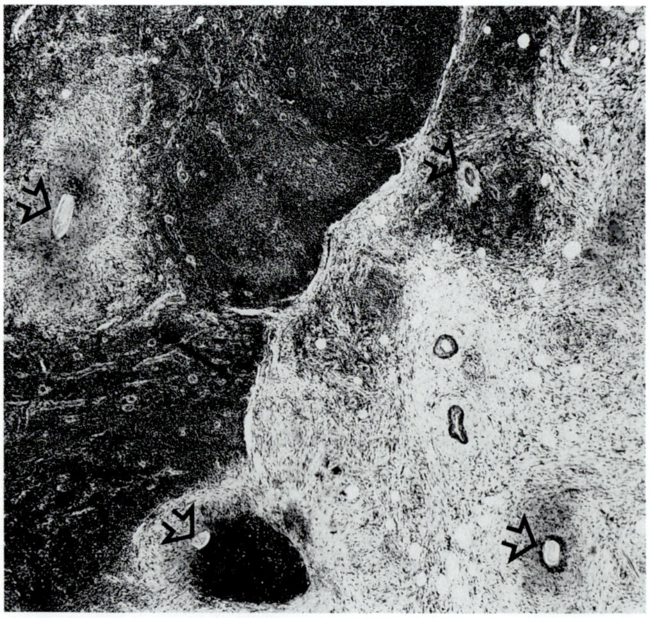

Figure 148–6. Female *Brugia* sp in the cortex and hilum of a lymph node removed from the neck of a man from New York. There are four cross sections of the worm in this section (*arrows*). The worm somehow breached the wall of a lymphatic vessel and entered the substance of the node, provoking necrosis, palisading epithelioid cells, numerous foreign-body giant cells, and infiltration by eosinophils (H&E, ×40).

DIFFERENTIAL DIAGNOSIS

Filarial parasites in lymphatic tissues of man are either *B malayi, B timori, Wuchereria bancrofti,* or those causing American brugian zoonoses. An accurate history of travel helps make the diagnosis in most patients. For example, a North American patient having filarial parasites in lymphatic tissue and having no history of travel to the tropics is probably infected by one of the zoonotic *Brugia.* In contrast, a North American with a history of travel to the eastern Indonesian archipelago may be infected with any of the known lymphatic filariae of humans. In any case, diagnosis requires demonstration of specific features of the worm. Serologic tests, monoclonal antibodies, or DNA probes for these parasites are not widely available.

REFERENCES

1. Dissanaike AS. A review of *Brugia* species with special reference to *B malayi* and to zoonotic infections. *Trop Biomed.* 1986;3:67–72.

2. Menendez MC, Bouza M. *Brugia* species in a man from western Ethiopia. *Am J Trop Med Hyg.* 1988;39:189–190.
3. Baird JK, Alpert LI, Friedman R, Schraft WC, Connor DH. North American brugian filariasis: report of nine infections of humans. *Am J Trop Med Hyg.* 1986;35:1205–1209.
4. Orihel TC, Beaver PC. Zoonotic *Brugia* infections in North and South America. *Am J Trop Med Hyg.* 1989;40:638–647.
5. Eberhard ML, Telford SR, Spielman A. A *Brugia* species infecting rabbits in the northeastern United States. *J Parasitol.* 1991;77:796–798.
6. Simmons CF Jr, Winter HS, Berde C, et al. Zoonotic filariasis with lymphedema in an immunodeficient infant. *N Engl J Med.* 1984;310:1243–1245.
7. Baird JK, Neafie RC. South American brugian filariasis: report of a human infection acquired in Peru. *Am J Trop Med Hyg.* 1988;39:185–188.

CHAPTER 149

Intestinal Capillariasis

John H. Cross

Love conquers all things except poverty and a tooth ache.

Mae West (1892–1980)

. . . just as serpents close their ears, so do men close their eyes to the truth.

Galileo Galilei (17th century)

INTRODUCTION

Parasitic diseases continue to be public health problems, especially in underdeveloped areas of the tropics. Most of the parasites infecting humans have been well known for many years, but new or lesser known parasites that cause diseases in humans continue to be reported. One of these parasites is *Capillaria philippinensis,* recognized in recent years as an important helminthic parasitosis that can kill the patient.

DEFINITION

Intestinal capillariasis is infection with the tiny nematode, *C philippinensis.* The worm develops and multiplies in the intestine and eventually causes diarrhea, abdominal pain, and borborygmi. As the disease progresses, there is loss of fluid and electrolytes, a protein-losing enteropathy, and, if untreated, death. Synonyms include capillariasis philippinensis and Pudoc's mystery disease.

GEOGRAPHIC DISTRIBUTION

Most of the more than 2000 cases of intestinal capillariasis have been in the Philippines and Thailand. Several infections are reported from Taiwan and Japan, two from Egypt, and one each from Iran and Korea.[1] Intestinal capillariasis was recently reported in an Italian who was infected while visiting Indonesia.[2] Deaths have been reported only from the Philippines and Thailand.

LIFE CYCLE, NATURAL HISTORY, AND EPIDEMIOLOGY

The life cycle of *C philippinensis* has been determined by experimental infections in monkeys and Mongolian gerbils.[3,4] The worms are in the small intestine and, after copulation, some female worms produce eggs and a few produce larvae. The larvae are retained in the intestine where they grow into adult worms and thus maintain and increase the infection. Eggs are passed in feces and those that reach water embryonate and are then swallowed by small freshwater or brackish water fish. Eggs hatch in the intestine of the fish and the larvae double in size and become infective. In fish, larvae reach the infective stage in about 3 weeks and then grow no more.

When the fish is eaten uncooked, the larvae are released from the intestine of the fish and develop into adult worms in 10 to 11 days. The first-generation female worms produce larvae that are retained and develop into adults, and the second-generation female worms produce eggs that pass in the feces in 12 to 14 more days. A few female worms continue to produce larvae that replace worms that die off and also contribute to the hyperinfection that usually develops. Internal autoinfection is an integral part of the life cycle and contributes to the pathogenesis of the infection.

Two endemic areas are known in the Philippines: one in northern Luzon and one in southern Leyte. The disease has been followed in northern Luzon since 1967, and until the end of 1991 confirmed infections had been documented in 1890 people; 110 died of the infection. Most infections have been in middle-aged men (1340 males to 550 females). Records have not been kept on infections in Thailand, but it is estimated that there have been a few hundred infections. In one epidemic there were more than 100 infections and 9 deaths.[5] The disease is widespread in Thailand and is being seen in medical centers throughout the country.

In Thailand and in endemic areas of the Philippines the populations enjoy eating freshwater fish raw. Several species of fish in Thailand and the Philippines are able to transmit *C philippinensis* to gerbils and monkeys,[5] and fish from lagoons in the Philippines fed to gerbils led to patent infections, confirming the natural transmission of the parasite.

Several species of fish-eating birds have been experimentally infected with *C philippinensis,*[6,7] and one bird, *Ixobrychus* sp, in the Philippines is naturally infected. Fish-eating migratory birds are now considered potential natural hosts of *C philippinensis* and the migratory habits responsible for dissemination of the parasite. Bird droppings expose fish to the eggs along the flyways, and birds, as well as humans who eat the fish, become infected. In most reporting countries, infections have been in people who have eaten raw fish.

MORPHOLOGY

Capillaria philippinensis is a trichuriid nematode closely related to *Trichuris trichiura* and *Trichinella spiralis.* The anterior end of the worm is narrower than the posterior end, and the anterior end has a long esophagus surrounded by cells called stichocytes. The cells stack on each other to form the stichosome. The male worms range from 1.5 to 3.9 mm long and 3 to 5 μm wide at the head, 23 μm wide at the beginning of the stichosome, 25 to 28 μm at the base of the stichosome, and 18 μm at the cloaca. The male spicule is in the posterior end and measures 230 to 300 μm and the unspined spicular sheath measures 440 μm (Figure 149–1). Female worms range from 2.3 to 5.3 mm long, and are 25 μm at the stichosome, 29 to 47 μm at the vulva, and 14 μm at the preanal area. The vulva is salient and provides the exit for the eggs from the uterus (Figure 149–2). The uterus usually contains bipolar thick-shelled, peanut-shaped or barrel-shaped eggs (Figure 149–3). Thin-shelled eggs and, at times, larvae may be in the uterus (Figure 149–4). Eggs are 36 to

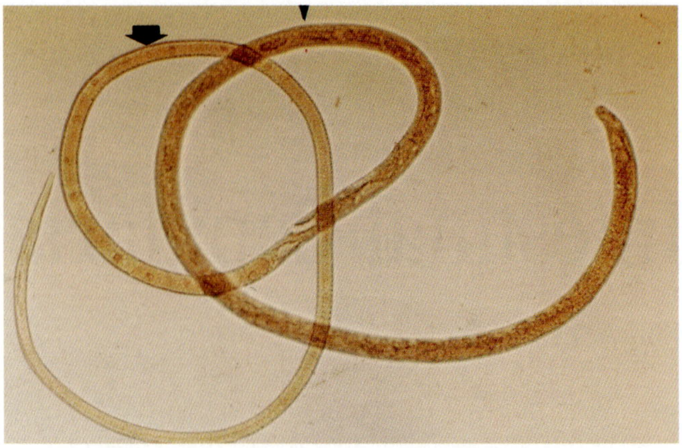

Figure 149–2. Female *C philippinensis,* narrow anterior and wider posterior portions. Note stichosome (*thick arrow*) and eggs in the uterus (*thin arrow*).

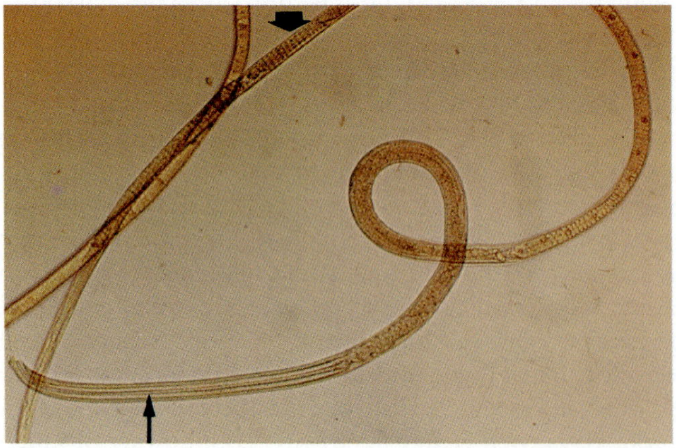

Figure 149–1. Male *C philippinensis* recovered from intestinal fluid at autopsy. Note spicules (*thin arrow*) in the posterior portion and cells (stichocytes) of the stichosome in narrower anterior portion (*thick arrow*).

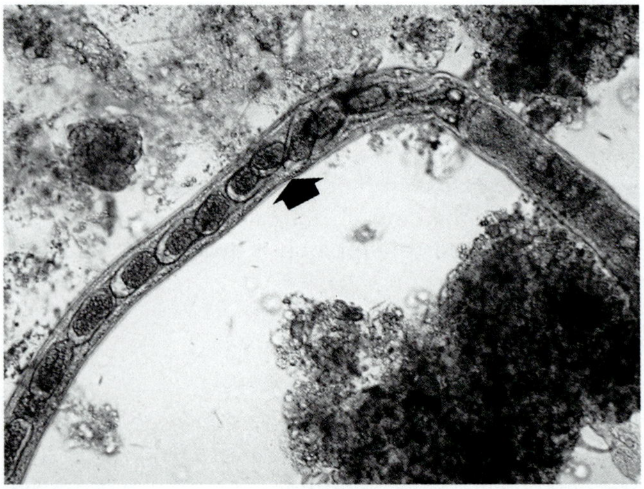

Figure 149–3. Female *C philippinensis,* uterus with thick-shelled eggs (*arrow*).

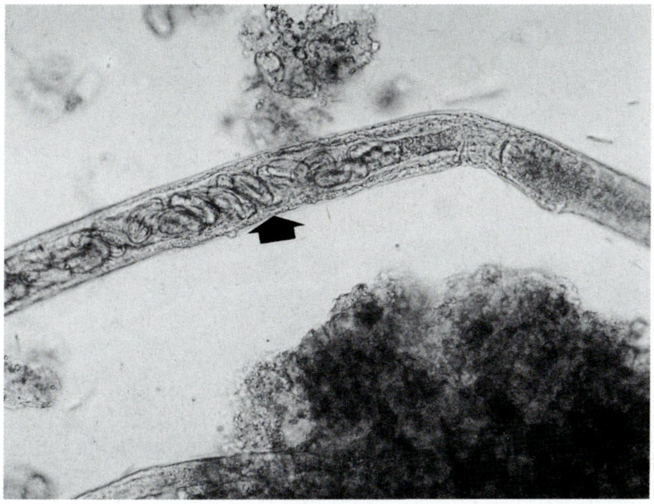

Figure 149–4. Female *C philippinensis*, uterus with embryonated thin-shelled eggs (*arrow*).

45 μm by 20 μm (Figure 149–5). All stages of the parasite—eggs, larvae, and adults—can be in the small intestine as well as in the feces.[8]

CLINICAL SYMPTOMS

Studies in the Philippines have shown that those infected with *C philippinensis* eventually develop symptoms. On several occasions, asymptomatic people were passing eggs when examined during surveys. Eventually they became symptomatic and were hospitalized.

Early symptoms are vague. Borborygmi, or "gurgling stomach" as described by Filipinos, abdominal pain, and intermittent diarrhea are initial features. As infection progresses, diarrhea increases and patients have voluminous stools, severe abdominal pain, vomiting, anorexia, and weight loss. Whalen et al[9] studied a number of patients and reported muscle wasting and weakness, borborygmi, distant heart sounds, hypotension, gallop rhythm, pulsus alterans, abdominal distention and tenderness, edema, and hyporeflexia. Laboratory findings revealed severe protein-losing enteropathy, malabsorption of fats and sugars, decreased excretion of xylose, and low levels of potassium, sodium, calcium, carotene, and total protein in serum. Later studies by Rosenberg et al[10] showed that those with severe infections had high levels of immunoglobulin E (IgE) and low levels of IgG, IgM, and IgA.

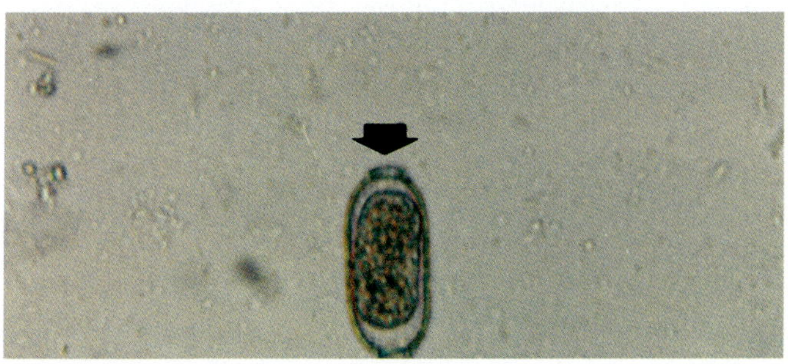

Figure 149–5. Thick-shelled egg of *C philippinensis* from feces. Note flattened bipolar plugs (*arrow*) and small striations of egg shell.

Those with severe infections whose fluids and electrolytes are not replaced, and whose clinical course is complicated by bacterial septicemia and heart failure, are the ones who died.

Treatment of intestinal capillariasis is to replace fluid and electrolytes, especially potassium, together with medication to control diarrhea and an anthelminthic. Presently, mebendazole, 200 mg twice a day for 20 days, or albendazole, 200 mg twice a day for 10 days, is recommended.[11]

PATHOLOGY

Two autopsy series have been published.[12,13] At autopsy, most bodies are pale, emaciated, and dehydrated with reduced skin turgor. Clear yellow fluid was in the abdominal, pleural, and pericardial cavities. In several infections, the heart, liver, spleen, kidney, and pancreas were of reduced weights. Lungs were congested and in one there was a right middle lobe abscess from which *Micrococcus pyogenes* var *albus* was grown. In another, *Klebsiella pneumoniae* was isolated from lungs and blood. Splenic white pulp had prominent malpighian corpuscles and livers were yellowish and congested. The small bowel wall was thickened and indurated with prominent surface vessels. The small bowel was usually distended with fluid that was gray, had a watery consistency, and contained flecks of mucus and thousands of worms in all stages of development. In one autopsy, more than 200,000 *C philippinensis* were recovered. In other autopsies, 10,000 to 40,000 worms were estimated. Stereoscopic examination of the jejunum submerged in water showed a portion of the worms burrowed into the mucosa with the rest of the body of the worm projecting above the mucosal surface. The mucosa showed loss of normal filiform villous projections from swelling or broadening of the villi.

Although worms were throughout the gastrointestinal tract, most were in the jejunum, upper ileum, and lower duodenum. Eggs, larvae, and adult worms were predominantly in jejunum and most of the lesions were in this portion of the small intestines. In histologic preparations, large numbers of worms were in the glands, and tortuous tracks were in the lamina propria

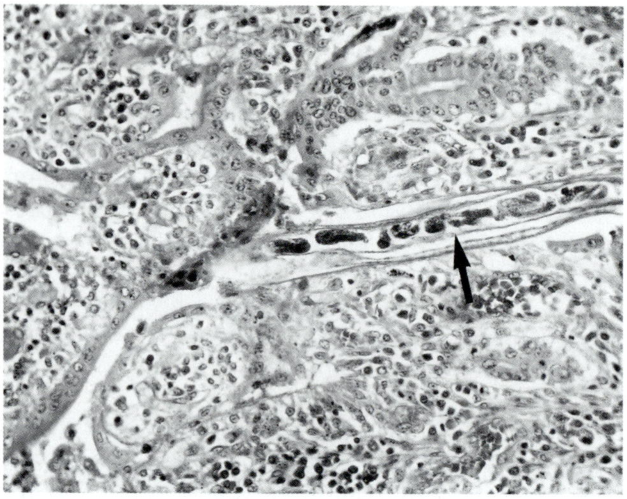

Figure 149–6. Histologic section of human intestine taken at autopsy showing female *C philippinensis* in a crypt (*arrow*). Note cellular infiltration.

and crypts of Lieberkuhn (Figure 149–6). The crypts atrophy and fill with eosinophilic debris and the glands become distended (Figure 149–7). The lamina propria was infiltrated with plasma cells, lymphocytes, neutrophils, macrophages, and a few eosinophils. Villi were blunted, flattened, or completely destroyed and the mucosa was sloughed (Figure 149–8). Ultrastructural studies of jejunum by Sun et al[14] showed loss of adhesion specialization, degenerative changes of the epithelial cells, and widened intercellular spaces (Figure 149–9). Electron microscopic studies of gerbil intestines showed erosion of a cell and formation of microulcers

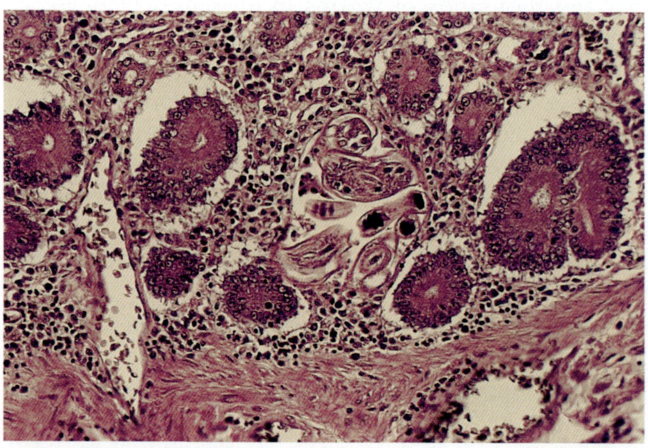

Figure 149–7. Multiple cross-sections of a *C philippinensis* in a distended intestinal gland.

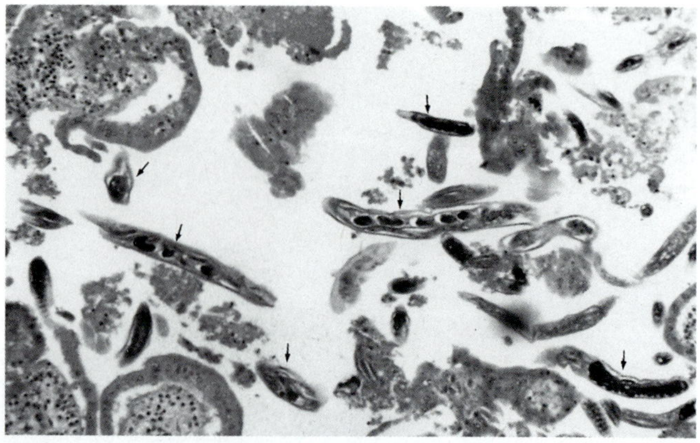

Figure 149–8. Human intestine from autopsy showing numerous sections of *C philippinensis* (*arrows*) and debris.

in the epithelium (Figure 149–10). These changes may cause loss of protein, fluid, and electrolytes from tissue spaces.

Other findings include vacuolization of myocardial cells and increased lipofuscin in perinuclear areas of sarcoplasm. Lungs were congested and edematous, but without increased numbers of pigment-laden macrophages. Some patients had lobar pneumonia, bullous emphysema, and abscesses. There was vascular congestion of spleen with prominent malpighian corpuscles and pigment-laden macrophages in sinusoids. In kidneys, epithelium of proximal convoluted tubules

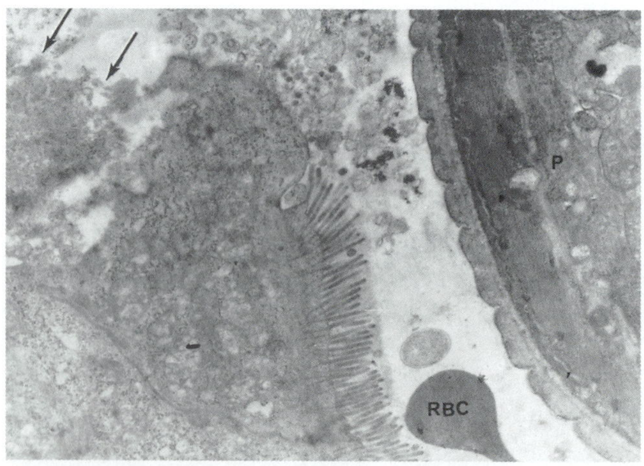

Figure 149–9. Electron micrograph of human jejunum. The pronounced degenerative changes of the epithelial cells with a subjacent parasite (P) in cross-section. Note widened intercellular space between two cells (*arrows*). *(Reprinted from Sun et al[14] with permission of the publisher.)*

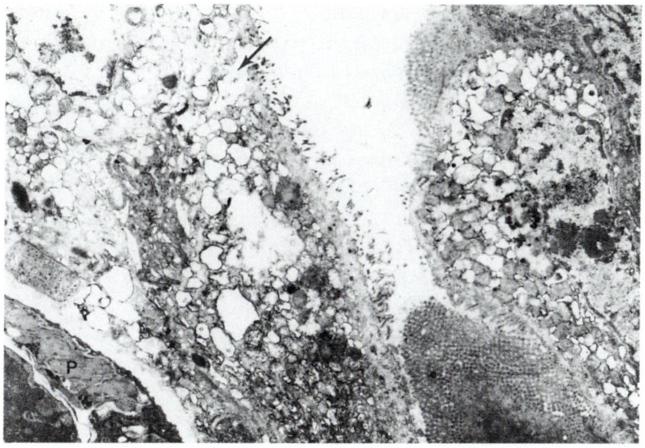

Figure 149–10. Electron micrograph of jejunum of a gerbil. Villous epithelial cells adjacent to a parasite in the intestinal lumen shows partial erosion with the formation of a microulcer in the epithelium (*arrow*). Note sloughing of the cytoplasmic debris in a space between the epithelial surface and the parasite (P). *(Reprinted from Sun et al[14] with permission of the publisher.)*

contained vacuoles. Some tubules contained hemoglobulin casts. Livers had fatty change in the central or peripheral portions of the lobules. In one patient *C philippinensis* worms were in the liver and surrounded by inflammatory cells (Figure 149–11).[13] Changes in other organs are probably from malnutrition rather than caused directly by parasites.

Parasites may be identified in tissue by their presence in denuded glands (Figure 149–7), and longitudinal sections of the worms in the tissue will usually show rows of stichocytes making up the stichosome (Figure

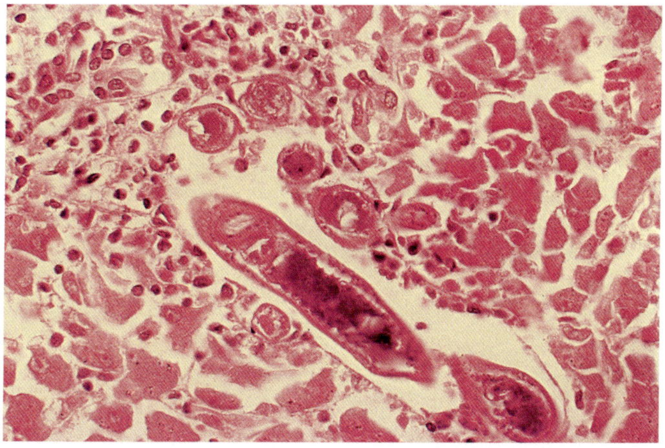

Figure 149–11. Human liver taken at autopsy with longitudinal and cross-sections of a capillarid with stichocytes. The worm is in a portal tract, which is thickened by fibrous tissue and infiltrated with lymphocytes (hematoxylin-eosin).

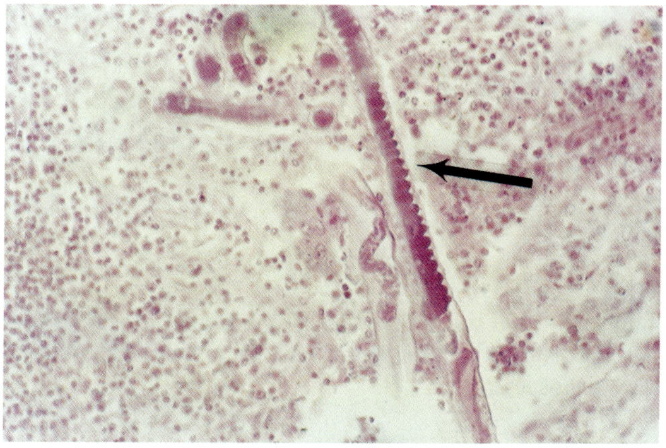

Figure 149–12. Human intestine with a longitudinal section of a female *C philippinensis* showing the anterior portion with stichosome (*arrow*) in the crypts.

149–12). Larvae are more difficult to identify in tissue, but in some sections eggs may be seen in the glands (Figure 149–13) and in adult female worms lying in the crypts (Figure 149–6). There is little evidence that the worms actually penetrate the mucosa; most seem to be lying in the crypts; the parasite in the liver, however, is in the parenchyma.

DIFFERENTIAL DIAGNOSIS

Other intestinal parasitoses including strongyloidiasis, hookworm infection, and giardiasis may be confused with intestinal capillariasis. Malabsorption caused by tropical sprue may also be confused with intestinal capillariasis.

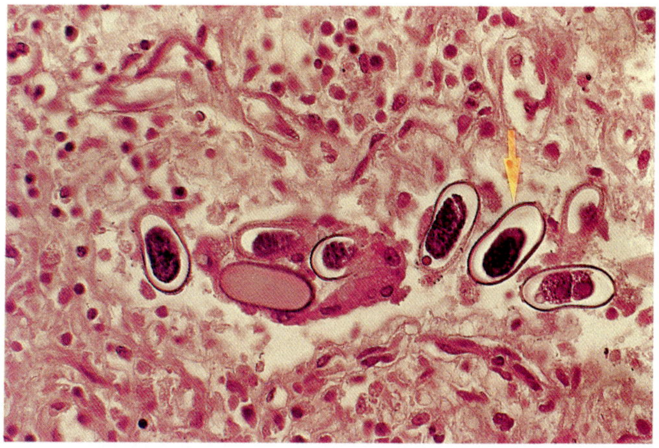

Figure 149–13. Eggs of *C philippinensis* (*arrow*) in glands of human intestine.

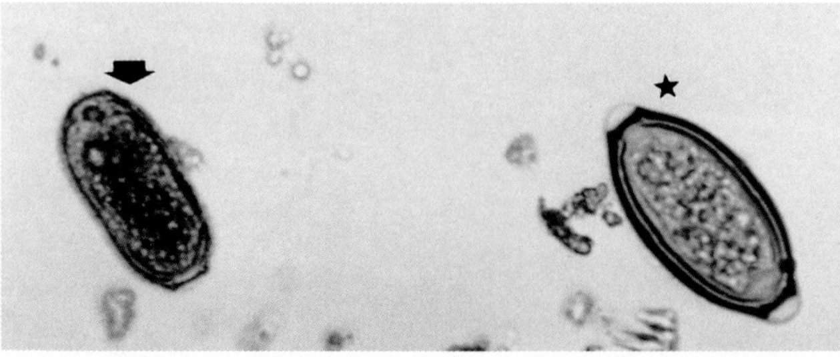

Figure 149–14. Egg of *C philippinensis (arrow)* and *T trichiura (star)*. The latter is easily confused with the former by an inexperienced microscopist.

Strongyloides stercoralis may cause lesions that resemble intestinal capillariasis. In the former, only small adult female worms and larvae are found and the female worms have a double uterus and possibly rounded thin-shelled embryonated eggs. In *C philippinensis* the uterus is single and thick-shelled eggs are usually present (Figure 149–5). Thin-shelled eggs and larvae may also be in female worms (Figure 149–4).

DIAGNOSIS

Stool examinations are the best means of making the diagnosis. Typical eggs, larvae, and adult worms are usually in feces of those infected. These eggs should be distinguished from those of *T trichiura* (Figure 149–14). Serologic tests have been developed but are not reliable.[15,16]

Biopsy specimens of intestine and aspirated fluid from small intestine are used in making the diagnosis. The parasites can be in the tissue and in the aspirates. On several occasions when the parasitosis was suspected, an anthelminthic (mebendazole 400 mg) was given and worms passed in the feces.

REFERENCES

1. Cross JH. Intestinal capillariasis. *Clin Microbiol Rev.* 1992;5:120–129.
2. Chichino G, Bernuzzi AM, Bruno A, et al. Intestinal capillariasis (*Capillaria philippinensis*) acquired in Indonesia: a case report. *Am J Trop Med Hyg.* 1992;47:10–12.
3. Cross JH, Banzon T, Clarke MD, Basaca-Sevilla V, Watten RH, Dizon JJ. Studies on the experimental transmission of *Capillaria philippinensis* in monkeys. *Trans R Soc Trop Med Hyg.* 1972;66:819–827.
4. Cross JH, Banzon T, and Singson C. Further studies on *Capillaria philippinensis:* development of the parasite in the Mongolian gerbil. *J Parasitol.* 1978;64:208–213.
5. Cross JH, Bhaibulaya M. Intestinal capillariasis in the Philippines and Thailand. In: Croll N, Cross J, eds. *Human Ecology and Infectious Diseases.* New York: Academic Press; 1983:103–136.
6. Bhaibulaya M, Indra-Ngarm S. *Amaurornis phoenicurus* and *Ardeola bacchus* as experimental definitive hosts for *Capillaria philippinensis* in Thailand. *Int J Parasitol.* 1979; 9:321–322.
7. Cross JH, Basaca-Seville V. Experimental transmission of *Capillaria philippinensis* to birds. *Trans R Soc Trop Med Hyg.* 1983;77:511–514.
8. Chitwood MB, Velasquez D, Salazar NG. *Capillaria philippinensis* sp n (Nematoda: Trichinellida) from intestine of man in the Philippines. *J Parasitol.* 1968;54:368–371.
9. Whalen GE, Strickland GT, Cross JH, et al. Intestinal capillariasis—a new disease in man. *Lancet.* 1969;1:13–16.
10. Rosenberg EB, Whalen GE, Bennich H, and Johansson SGO. Increased circulating IgE in a new parasitic disease —human intestinal capillariasis. *N Engl J Med.* 1970;283: 1148–1149.
11. Cross JH, Basaca-Sevilla V. Albendazole in the treatment of intestinal capillariasis. *Southeast Asian J Trop Med Pub Hlth.* 1987;4:507–570.
12. Canlas BC, Cabrera BD, Davis U. Human intestinal capillariasis. II. Pathological features. *ACTA Med Philipp.* 1967; 4:84–91.
13. Fresh JW, Cross JH, Reyes V, Whalen GE, Uylangco CV, Dizon JJ. Necropsy findings in intestinal capillariasis. *Am J Trop Med Hyg.* 1972;21:169–173.
14. Sun SC, Cross JH, Berg HS, et al. Ultrastructural studies of intestinal capillariasis *Capillaria philippinensis* in human and gerbil hosts. *Southeast Asian J Trop Med Pub Hlth.* 1974;5:524–533.
15. Banzon TC, Lewert RM, Yagore MG. Serology of *Capillaria philippinensis* infection: reactivity of human sera to antigens prepared from *Capillaria obsignata* and other helminths. *Am J Trop Med Hyg.* 1975;24:256–263.
16. Cross JH, Chi JCH. The ELISA test in the detection of antibodies to some parasitic diseases in Asia. In: *Proceedings 18th SEAMEO TROPMED Seminar: Current Concepts in the Diagnosis and Treatment of Parasitic and Other Tropical Diseases.* Kuala Lumpur, Malaysia; 1978:178–182.

CHAPTER 150

Clonorchiasis and Opisthorchiasis

Tsieh Sun

'Tis a portentous sign
When a man sweats, and at the same time shivers.

Plautus (254?–184 BC)

An' the dawn comes up like thunder outer China 'crost the Bay!

Rudyard Kipling (1865–1936)

DEFINITION

Clonorchiasis and opisthorchiasis are infections by species of the genera *Clonorchis* and *Opisthorchis*. Both *Clonorchis* and *Opisthorchis* belong to the family Opisthorchiidae (Braun 1909). The genus *Clonorchis* has one species, *C sinensis,* whereas the genus *Opisthorchis* includes several species (*O felineus, O viverrini,* and *O guayaquilensis*) that cause human infection. These species are all liver flukes transmitted by eating raw infected freshwater fish. The major complications are hepatocholangitis, pancreatitis, and cholangiocarcinoma.

HISTORICAL NOTES

Clonorchis sinensis was first described in the bile passages of a Chinese carpenter in Calcutta in 1875 by McConnell.[1] The first patient in the United States was reported by Biggs from Bellevue Hospital in New York City in 1890.[1] The earliest historical record of clonorchiasis, however, was an ancient corpse buried in the West Han Dynasty (278 BC) in China.[2] The first description of *O felineus* infecting a human was in Tomsk, Siberia, by Winogradoff in 1892.[1]

SYNONYMS

The genera *Clonorchis* and *Opisthorchis* were first called *Distoma,* but *Distoma* is no longer used. In 1946, Dawes suggested *Clonorchis sinensis* be changed to *Opisthorchis sinensis*[1] but *Clonorchis sinensis* is still accepted and preferred by the American Society of Parasitologists as the official name.[3] *Opisthorchis tenuicollis* and *O felineus* are synonymous as are *O guayaquilensis* and *Amphimerus pseudofelineus.*[1,3]

GEOGRAPHIC DISTRIBUTION

Clonorchiasis is endemic in China, Taiwan, Hong Kong, Japan, Korea, and Vietnam and the distribution is tied to the distribution of the snail host. Thus, patients with clonorchiasis living in the Western Hemisphere (where there is no suitable snail host for *C sinensis*) have been infected elsewhere. The adult *Clonorchis* has a life span of 20 to 30 years.[4] Only rarely do Westerners become infected and this is so regardless of their length of stay in endemic areas.[4]

Opisthorchis felineus is endemic in southern, central, and eastern Europe, the Russian commonwealth, Turkey, and Western Siberia. *Opisthorchis viverrini* is in Thailand, Laos, and Kampuchea. *Opisthorchis guayaquilensis* infects humans in an isolated focus in Ecuador.[1]

The estimated prevalence of clonorchiasis is 19 million people worldwide, but recently infection rates have dropped in China and Japan.[5] On the other hand, the prevalence of *O viverrini* infection in northeastern Thailand rose from 3.5 million in 1965 to 5.4 million in 1981.[6] A more recent estimate is 7 million.[7] The prevalence of *O felineus* infection in Western Siberia has doubled—a consequence of the recent influx of immigrants.[6] Worldwide there are probably several million infected by *O felineus*.[5]

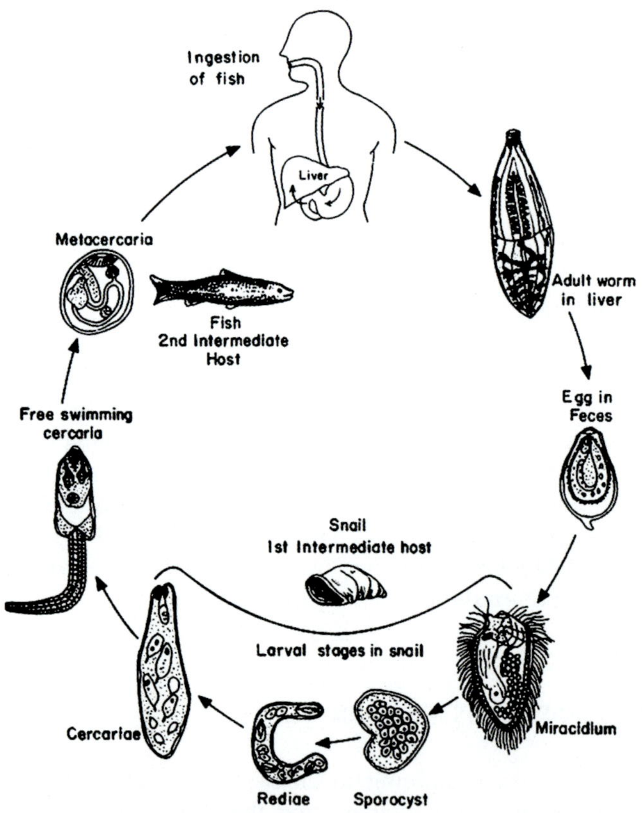

Figure 150–1. Life cycle of *C sinensis*. Embryonated eggs, from the bile ducts, are passed in feces and hatch to miracidia when ingested by a suitable snail—the first intermediate host. In the snail the parasite goes through larval stages including sporocyst, redia, and cercaria. In the drawings many rediae and many cercariae are shown within a snail. On emerging from the snail, cercariae are free swimming and penetrate the second intermediate host. Second intermediate hosts include a variety of freshwater fish and crayfish, in which the cercariae encyst as metacercariae. Humans are infected when they ingest fish or crayfish containing viable metacercariae. The metacercariae excyst in the duodenum, migrate through the ampulla and into the intrahepatic bile ducts where they become adults in about 1 month. *(From Sun.[5])*

LIFE CYCLE AND EPIDEMIOLOGY

The life cycles of *C sinensis* and species of *Opisthorchis* are similar. Both require two intermediate hosts, snail and fish, to complete their life cycle (Figure 150–1). The snail hosts for *C sinensis* include nine different species belonging to four families (Hydrobidae, Melanidae, Assimineidae, and Thiaridae)[2]; whereas the only known molluscan host for *O felineus* is *Bithynia (Bulimus) leachi* and those for *O viverrini* include *B goniomphalus, B funiculata,* and *B laevis.*[1] Almost all the fish that serve as hosts for *Clonorchis* and *Opisthorchis* belong to the family Cyprinidae (Figure 150–2). One hundred thirteen species of 13 families of freshwater fish serve as second intermediate hosts for *C sinensis*[2]; many of them may also transmit opisthorchiasis. In addition, crayfish may serve as the second intermediate host for *C sinensis,*[5] but this is controversial.[2]

Eggs of these parasites are ingested by the snail host, in which the eggs hatch (Figure 150–3) and pass through stages of first- and second-generation sporocysts, rediae, and cercariae (Figure 150–4). Mature cercariae escape from the snail host, swim in water and attack a suitable fish, becoming encysted metacercariae in the flesh of the fish. When infected raw fish is eaten by a reservoir host or by a human, metacercariae excyst in the duodenum, migrate through the common bile duct to the liver and remain in intrahepatic bile ducts.[8] The worms mature in 3 to 4 weeks after which eggs appear in the stool. The life cycle requires about 4 months. Dogs and cats are major reservoir hosts, but pigs also serve as reservoir hosts in Taiwan.[2]

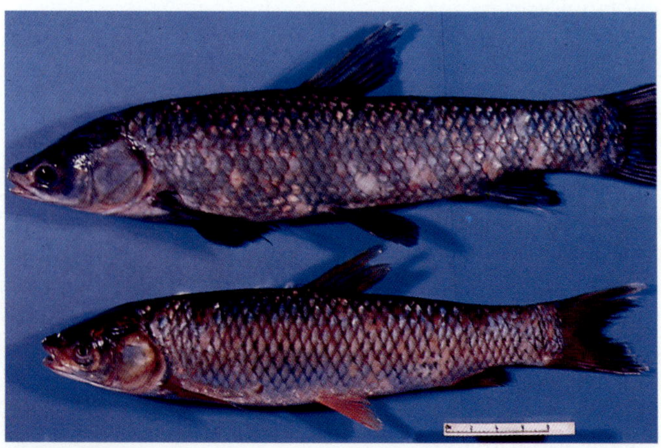

Figure 150–2. Black carp (*upper*) and grass carp (*lower*), two common hosts for *C sinensis*.

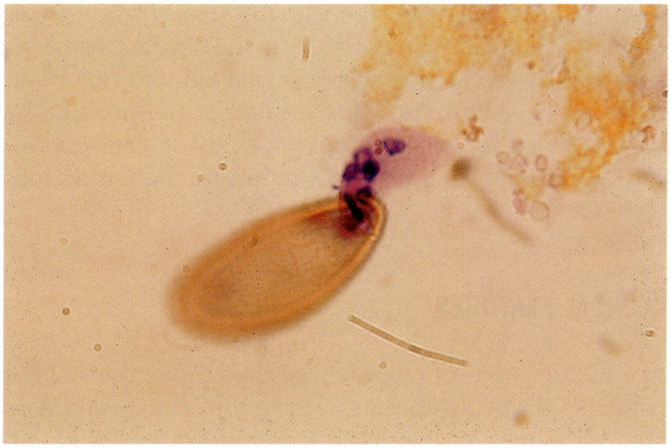

Figure 150–3. A miracidium hatching from an egg of *C sinensis* [hematoxylin-eosin (H&E), ×300]. *(From Sun.[5])*

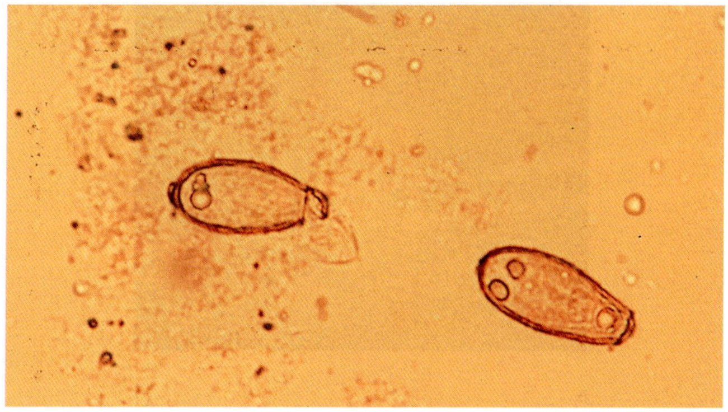

Figure 150–5. Two eggs of *C sinensis* showing operculum and opercular shoulders. A transparent miracidium is hatching from the operculated end of the egg on the left (×160).

MORPHOLOGY

The eggs of *Clonorchis* and *Opisthorchis* are similar (Figure 150–5). Both are operculated with prominent shoulders (thickened rim of the egg shell) and have a minute tubercular thickening or terminal knob at the end opposite of the operculum. The operculated end is tapered. A ciliated miracidium is visible through the shell. The eggs of *Clonorchis* are 28 to 35 mm by 12 to 19 mm (average 29 by 16 mm). The size of *Opisthorchis* eggs is very similar to those of *Clonorchis* (*O viverrini,* 26 by 15 mm; *O felineus,* 30 by 11 mm) so that by size and form they are indistinguishable.

The adult *C sinensis* is 10 to 25 mm long, 3 to 5 mm wide (Figure 150–6); *Opisthorchis* is smaller (7 to 12 mm by 2 to 3 mm) (Figure 150–7, A and B). *Clonorchis sinensis* is a hermaphrodite and thus has male and female reproductive organs. The female reproductive organs include a uterus, an ovary, a seminal receptacle, and numerous vitelline glands. There is a pair of branched testes located in the posterior one

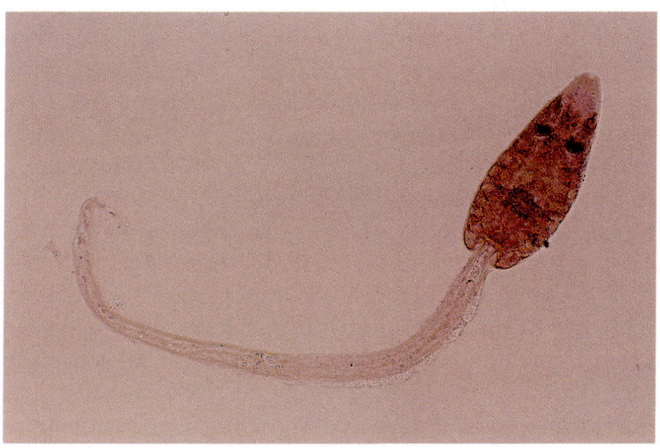

Figure 150–4. A cercaria of *C sinensis* (alum carmine stain, ×160).

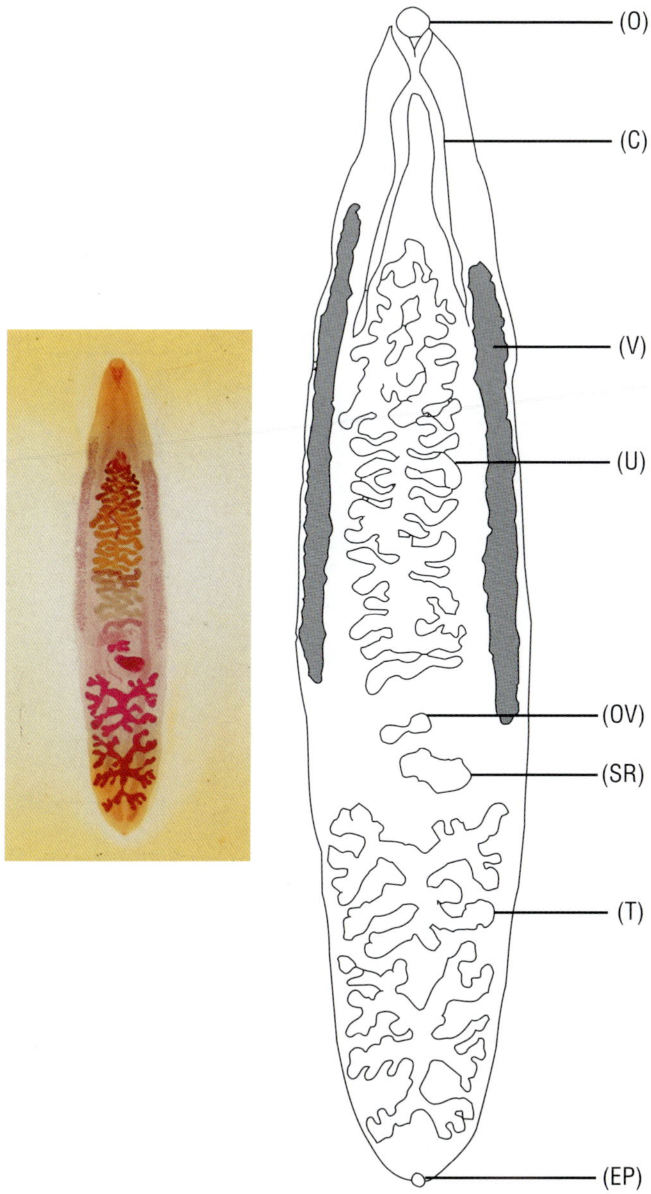

Figure 150–6. Adult *C sinensis* showing oral sucker (O), bifurcated cecum (C), vitelline glands (V), uterus (U), ovary (OV), seminal receptacle (SR), branched testes (T), and excretory pore (EP).

third of the parasite, hence the name *Clonorchis* (*clon* = branched, *orchis* = testis). The oral sucker is followed by a pharynx, which is divided into two blind cecae. The ventral sucker is located at the junction of the anterior third of the body. Species of *Opisthorchis* can be distinguished from *C sinensis* by the paired lobulated testes.

CLINICAL FEATURES

In endemic areas of clonorchiasis about one third of the patients have symptoms.[9] Symptoms are tiredness (26.3%), upper abdominal discomfort (24.1%), abdominal pain (23.1%), dizziness (19.3%), hepatomegaly (52%) and splenomegaly (1.2%). Of 85 children with clonorchiasis, 40% has retarded growth.[10]

In moderate to heavy infections with *C sinensis,* the most common complication is recurrent pyogenic cholangitis, also known as oriental cholangiohepatitis.[5,11] These patients have repeated attacks of fever, chills, abdominal pain, jaundice, and hepatomegaly. Gallstones are a frequent complication. Typically, the gallstones are radiolucent and seldom in the gallbladder (only 4.2%).[12] Without surgical intervention, these patients may die of hepatic failure.

Some patients have fulminating acute suppurative cholangitis from sudden obstruction of the common bile duct by dead parasites, causing a special syndrome of hypoglycemia, circulatory failure, and high fever.[5] These patients respond to surgical drainage after correction of hypoglycemia. A rare complication of recurrent pyogenic cholangitis is pulmonary hypertension from repeated microembolization of infected necrotic tissue from liver to small pulmonary vessels.[5] Pancreatitis is also a common complication of clonorchiasis. In Hong Kong, 88% of patients with acute pancreatitis of unknown cause had clonorchiasis.[5] The mortality of pancreatitis complicating clonorchiasis is lower (less than 2%) than for hemorrhagic pancreatitis.

The gravest consequence of clonorchiasis is cholangiocarcinoma.[13,14] The incidence of cholangiocarcinoma is higher in areas endemic for clonorchiasis than in nonendemic areas. For instance, the ratio of cholangiocarcinoma to hepatocellular carcinoma in Hong Kong is 1:6,[15] compared with a ratio of 1:56 in Java, 1:20 in Johannesburg, and 1:38 in all Africa where there is much liver cancer but no clonorchiasis.[14] On the other hand, clonorchiasis is more frequent in patients with cholangiocarcinoma than in those without. The incidence of clonorchiasis in the general population in Hong Kong is 23%, but the incidence in those with cholangiocarcinoma is 65% compared to an expected rate of 37.6% when matched with the same age and sex groups of the general population.[14] The relation-

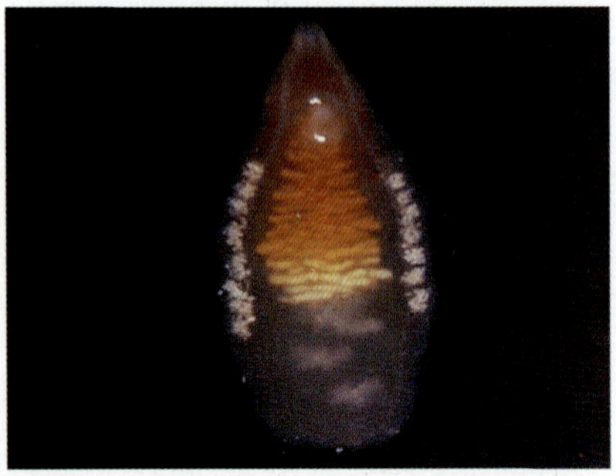

A

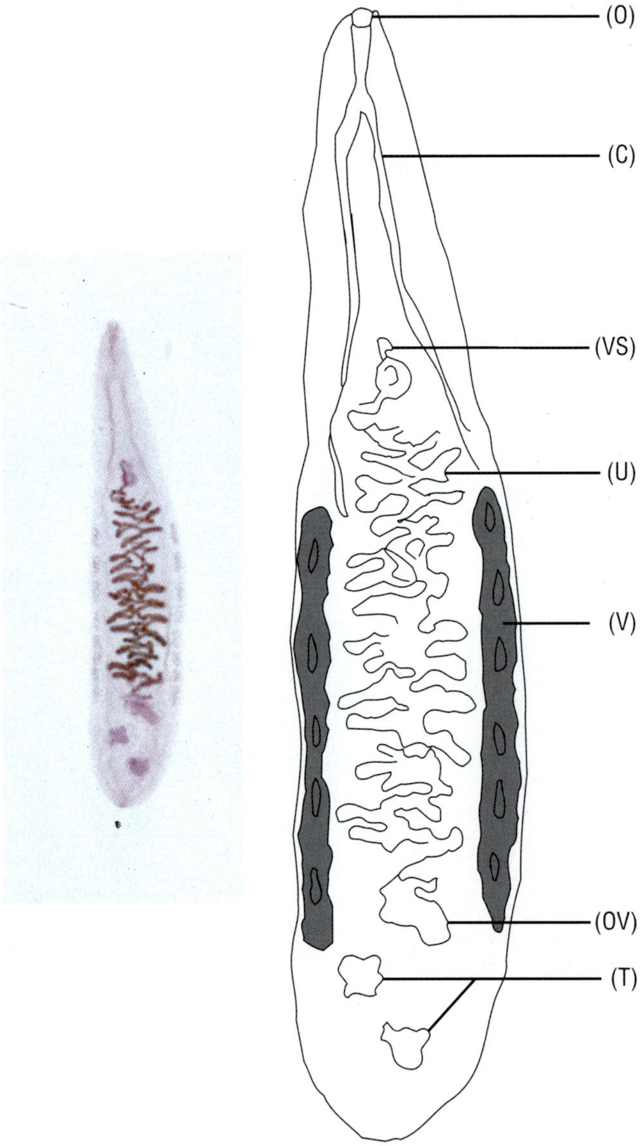

B

Figure 150–7. (**A**) Adult *O viverrini* from bile drainage (fresh specimen, gross ×4). *(By Daniel H. Connor, MD, 1975.)* (**B**) Adult *O viverrini* showing oral sucker (O), bifurcated cecum (C), ventral sucker (VS), uterus (U), vitelline glands (V), ovary (OV), and lobulated testes (T).

ship between clonorchiasis and cholangiocarcinoma has been demonstrated also in experimentally and naturally infected animals.[5]

Because the parasite has a long life, Asian immigrants to North America remain infected for years.[4,13,16,17] The prevalence of clonorchiasis among 150 Chinese in New York City was 26%,[18] and it was 15.9% among 400 Chinese immigrants in Montreal.[19] Even in South Carolina, between 1978 and 1982 there were 96 patients.[20] The most frequent complications among these immigrants were biliary obstruction,[21–24] recurrent pyogenic cholangitis,[23,25,26] and acute pancreatitis.[27]

In the chronic stage, opisthorchiasis and clonorchiasis are clinically similar, but cholecystitis and cholelithiasis are more common in opisthorchiasis than in clonorchiasis.[28,29] The association of *O viverrini* and cholangiocarcinoma is even more striking than is the association of *C sinensis* and cholangiocarcinoma. The National Cancer Registry of Thailand recorded a 2:1 ratio of cholangiocarcinoma to hepatocellular carcinoma in the endemic area, whereas in most countries the incidence of hepatocellular carcinoma is higher than cholangiocarcinoma.[30] Cholangiocarcinoma was also 12 times more frequently encountered in northeastern Thailand (most heavily endemic area) than in areas with low prevalence of opisthorchiasis.[30] Another study showed that when opisthorchiasis coexisted with primary liver cancer, 78.8% were cholangiocarcinoma and only 10.6% were hepatocellular carcinoma.[31] In uninfected people, the ratio was reversed: 12.8% cholangiocarcinoma versus 80.8% hepatocellular carcinoma.[31] The frequency of cholangiocarcinoma was closely related to levels of antibody to *O viverrini* with a correlation coefficient of 0.98.[32] A special feature in patients with cholangiocarcinoma in Thailand is a high frequency (49%) of acute renal failure, which is reversible after removal of the tumor.[33]

PATHOLOGY

Gross examination of the liver usually belies the severity of infection. Even when 100 and more adult *C sinensis* are retrieved, the liver may still be normal in size, shape, and weight. In severe infections, however, dilated intrahepatic ducts are visible through the capsule as white, tortuous, linear structures (Figure 150–8). A diagnosis can frequently be made by inspecting the cut surface, where dilated, thick-walled bile ducts stand out as pouting tubes.[15] Adult worms are usually visible in the lumens of the dilated ducts.

The gallbladder and extrahepatic ducts are usually free of lesions, unless inflammatory changes have extended to extrahepatic tissues (Figure 150–9). Although

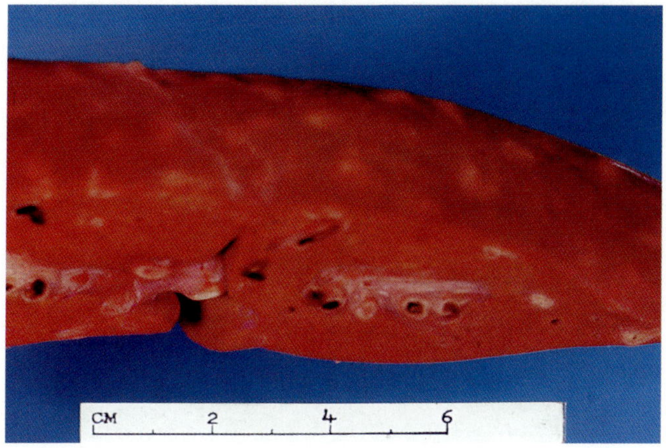

Figure 150–8. A *Clonorchis*-infected liver showing dilated bile ducts on the external surface. The cut surface reveals thickened and dilated intrahepatic bile ducts. Adult flukes are visible (*arrow*). *(From Sun.[5])*

adult flukes are frequently in the gallbladder, they cannot survive in bile and do not cause cholecystitis per se (Figure 150–10).

Microscopically there is adenomatous proliferation of the ductal epithelium with fibrosis of the duct wall (Figures 150–11 and 150–12). Hou's classical description of the histology of *Clonorchis*-infected liver is still standard.[34] Based on Hou's description, Min further divided the pathology of clonorchiasis into four stages: 1) desquamation of epithelial cells, 2) hyperplasia of epithelial cells, 3) formation of adenomatous tissue, and 4) marked proliferation of the periductal connective tissue, with scattered abortive acini of epithelial cells and fibrosis of the bile duct wall.[35] A feature emphasized in early literature is goblet cell metaplasia in the ductal epithelium.[15] This is important because mucinous metaplasia may be the initial step toward mucin-secreting

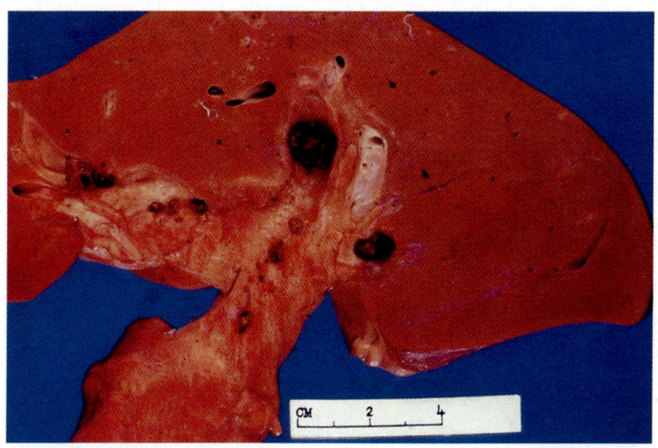

Figure 150–9. Recurrent pyogenic cholangitis complicating clonorchiasis with muddy gallstones in the main intrahepatic bile ducts. *(From Sun.[5])*

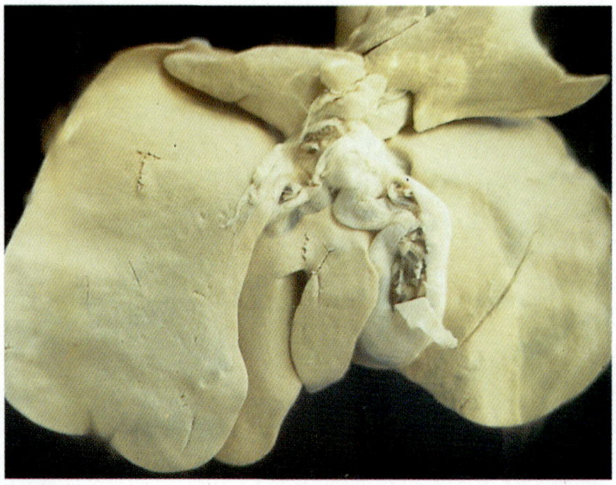

Figure 150–10. Clonorchiasis with multiple adult worms in the partly opened gallbladder.

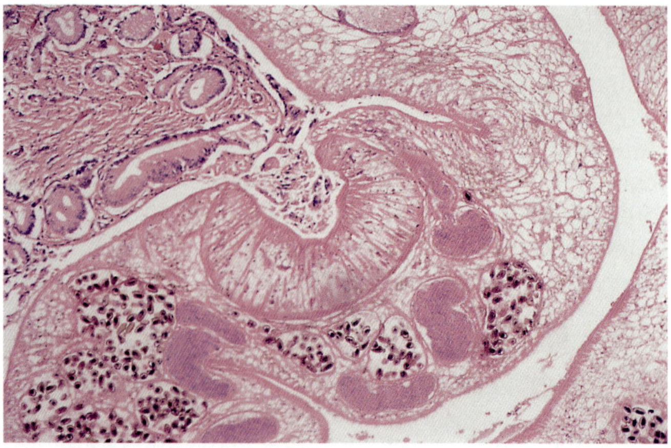

Figure 150–12. Adult *Clonorchis* attached by ventral sucker to biliary epithelium in a human. Note eggs in uterus, neighboring vas deferens containing spermatozoa, and the genital pore and atrium above sucker (H&E, ×40).

cholangiocarcinoma.[14] In fact, mucinous metaplasia caused by chemical carcinogens is indistinguishable from mucinous metaplasia caused by *Clonorchis* in terms of morphology and biochemical changes.[14] The histopathology of opisthorchiasis is essentially the same as clonorchiasis (Figures 150–13 and 150–14).

Cholangiocarcinoma associated with clonorchiasis[15,36] is 1) usually mucin-secreting adenocarcinoma with the minority being undifferentiated (Figure 150–15); 2) multicentric, involving the secondary intrahepatic bile ducts, the preferential site for *Clonorchis* infections too; and 3) commonly in the hepatic hilum. Intrahepatic cholangiocarcinoma at the hilum is also associated with opisthorchiasis.[37] Without surgical intervention, this tumor frequently metastasizes to distant organs, including lung, brain, kidney, heart, and adrenal.[36]

Recurrent pyogenic cholangitis is the most common complication of clonorchiasis.[5,11] Mucinous metaplasia causes increased mucin in the bile. This together with the flukes and eggs in the bile is a favorable environment for bacterial infection and eggs and bacterial colonies form the nidus of intrahepatic gallstones. Gallstones are usually muddy, friable and brown-black. Stones in the gallbladder form only when infection is spread beyond the hepatic duct.

Microscopic examination reveals inspissated bile mixed with *Clonorchis* eggs in the lumen of bile ducts (Figure 150–16).[5,15] The ductal epithelium is frequently desquamated and the wall is heavily infiltrated with leukocytes. In later stages, inflammatory changes spread beyond the bile ducts, causing pericholangitis and periductal fibrosis. Liver abscess may form when the parenchyma is involved and this may lead to biliary or postnecrotic cirrhosis. Portal fibrosis however is not a prominent feature and portal cirrhosis is rare in clonorchiasis.

In Hong Kong, more than one third of those with clonorchiasis coming to autopsy have flukes in the pan-

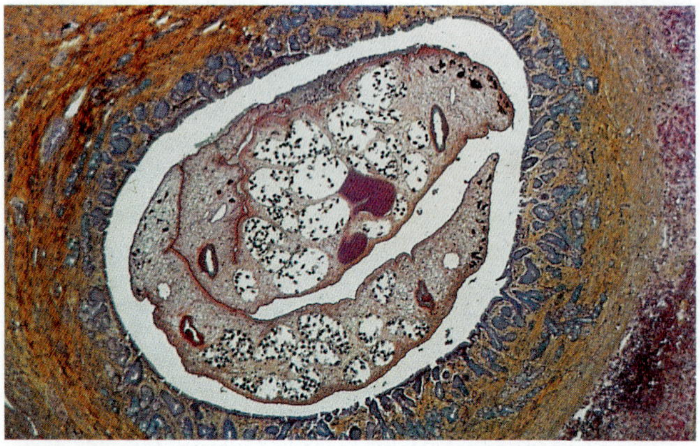

Figure 150–11. *Clonorchis* in a bile duct with adenomatous proliferation of epithelium (Movat, ×16).

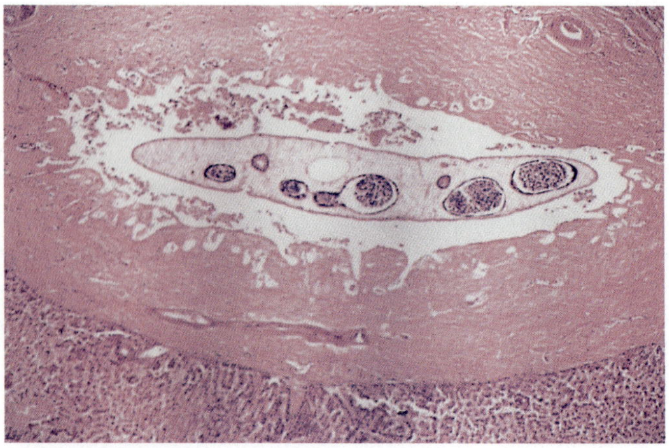

Figure 150–13. Bile duct infected by *O viverrini* showing desquamation and marked ductal fibrosis (H&E, ×16).

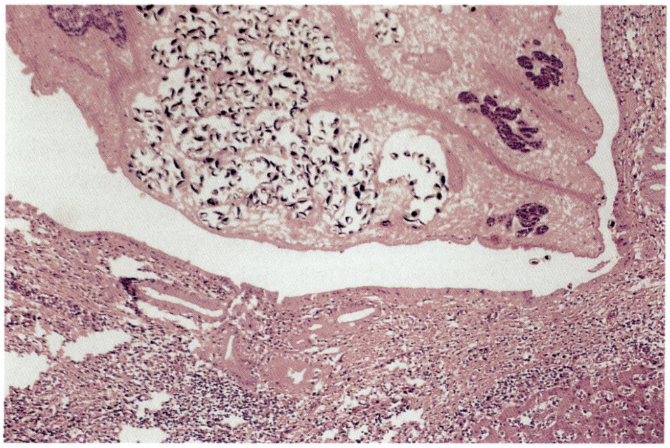

Figure 150–14. An infolded section of *O viverrini* in a bile duct with epithelial proliferation and infiltration of leukocytes (H&E, ×40).

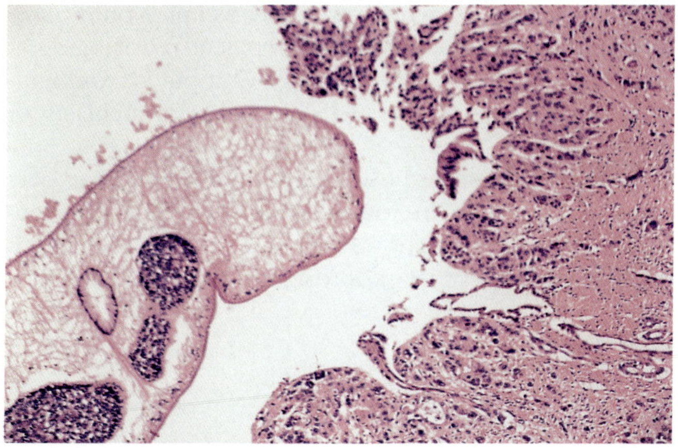

Figure 150–15. An adult *C sinensis* in a bile duct with malignant changes of epithelium (H&E, ×40).

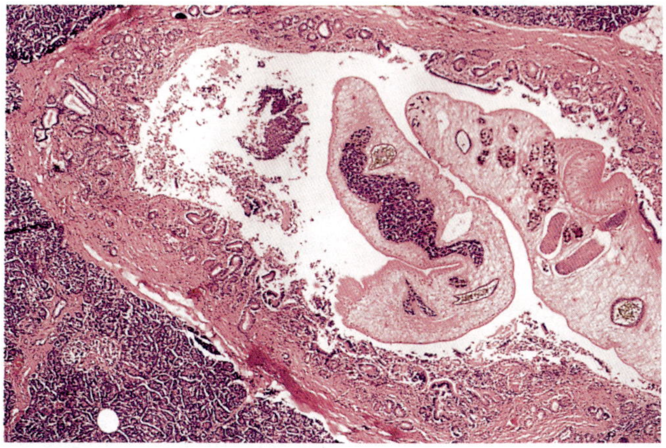

Figure 150–17. *Clonorchis* in pancreatic duct showing desquamation and marked adenomatous proliferation (H&E, ×16).

creatic duct[38] but most of these patients have had no symptoms. In those with acute episodes of pancreatitis, prompt removal of the fluke may lead to complete recovery.[5] The pathology of pancreatic clonorchiasis resembles adenomatous hyperplasia of ductal epithelium in the liver (Figure 150–17).[5,15] Squamous metaplasia is also characteristic.

The lung is occasionally involved in patients with recurrent pyogenic cholangitis. Before the antibiotic era, multiple metastatic pulmonary abscesses were common. Now that antibiotics are used for cholangitis, there are "silent" pulmonary microemboli in small branches of the pulmonary artery.[5] Pulmonary abscesses usually have the same bacteria as bile, indicating that the bile and liver are the source. In one patient, *Clonorchis* eggs were in a pulmonary embolus (Figure 150–18).[39]

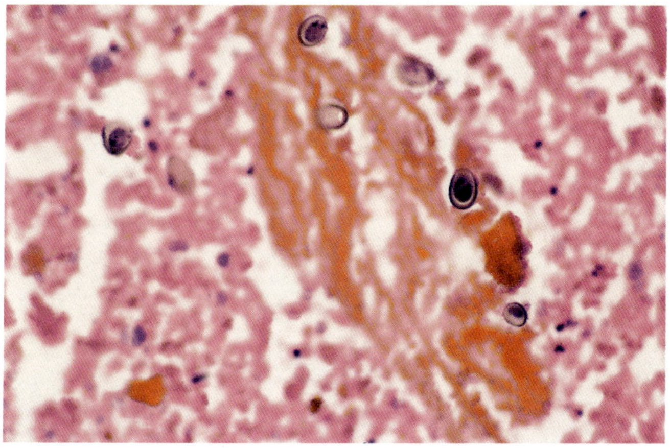

Figure 150–16. Inspissated bile mixed with *Clonorchis* eggs in a bile duct (H&E, ×160).

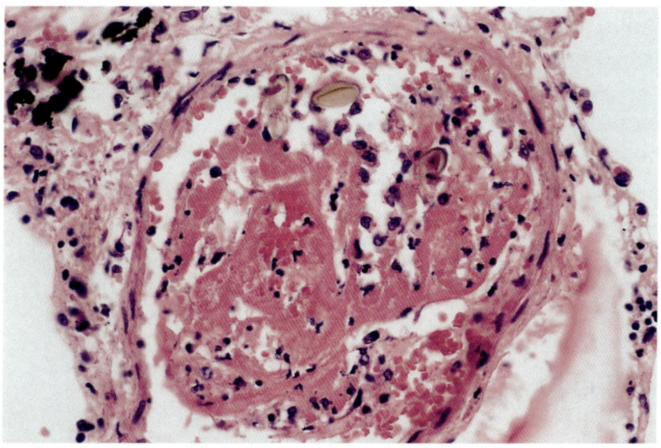

Figure 150–18. A pulmonary embolus containing three *Clonorchis* eggs (H&E, ×160).

PATHOGENESIS

Mechanical injury from anchoring the suckers of the parasite on the ductal epithelium leads to desquamation and proliferation of the epithelial cells.[40] Ultrastructural changes of microvilli of epithelial cells are evidence for chemical stimulation, probably caused by metabolic products released from the fluke.[40] The metabolic products originate from the gastrointestinal tract and the reproductive organs of the parasite as identified with an immunofluorescent technique by Sun and Gibson[41] or from the digestive and excretory organs as proved with immunohistochemical techniques by Kim et al.[42] In opisthorchiasis, pathologic changes may be caused by mechanical and chemical irritation.[29]

In clonorchiasis, the parasite does not enter the tissue of the host,[8] thus somatic antigen is not a major source of immune response.[43] *Clonorchis* eggs are impermeable so antigens secreted by miracidia do not reach host tissue.[39] Egg-induced lesions include eosinophilic granuloma of gallbladder, granulomas in liver,[4] and pulmonary embolism (Figure 150–18).[39] Eggs are partly damaged by acute inflammation allowing antigens from miracidia to provoke the reactions. Scarcity of egg-induced lesions is also a feature of opisthorchiasis.[44] Experimentally, metabolic products from adult worms of *Clonorchis* and *Opisthorchis* provoke humoral and cellular immunity.[29,43]

The mechanism of carcinogenesis in clonorchiasis and opisthorchiasis is still not clear. Since cholangiocarcinoma arises in a small percent of patients with liver flukes, the infection must be a predisposing factor. The proliferation and metaplasia of the epithelial cells, however, may lead to susceptibility of DNA to carcinogens.[13,29]

Nitrosamines are carcinogenic and common in Chinese foodstuffs, such as salted fish, dried shrimp, sausage, and cured pork. In Thailand, nitrosamines are in fermented fish products.[13,45] In addition, *Opisthorchis*-infected hamsters develop cholangiocarcinoma when treated with dimethyl–nitrosamine or its precursors.[46]

Another carcinogenic factor may be aflatoxins, the metabolic products of *Aspergillus* sp. Aflatoxins are in peanuts, maize, and other grains in the Far East.[13,45] Metabolites of aflatoxin in urine have been higher in *Opisthorchis*-infected patients and hamsters than in those uninfected.[47] Another study showed no correlation between aflatoxins and cholangiocarcinoma.[32]

DIAGNOSIS

Direct examination of a stool reveals eggs in most patients with clonorchiasis and opisthorchiasis. In mild infections, formaldehyde–ether concentration should be used. Examination of duodenal drainage and the Entero test are more sensitive than stool examination, but are too difficult to do on outpatients. Eggs of *Clonorchis* and *Opisthorchis* species, although slightly different in size, are essentially indistinguishable. A shoulder-like rim, a terminal knob, and a tapered operculated end (Figure 150–19) may help distinguish these two liver flukes from *Heterophyes heterophyes, Metagonimus yokogawai,* and eggs of other flukes in the families Opisthorchiidae and Heterophyidae.

Histologic diagnosis of clonorchiasis and opisthorchiasis is confirmed when adult worms are identified in tissue sections. *Clonorchis* usually appears as one or two large sections of the adult worm in the lumen of a bile duct, whereas *Opisthorchis* is smaller and frequently infolded. The adult *Fasciola hepatica,* another liver fluke, typically shows a branched digestive tract and cuticular spines.[5]

Radiologic techniques provide indirect evidence of parasitic infection in the bile ducts and serve for a presumptive diagnosis when other means fail. Noninvasive ultrasonography has gradually replaced cholangiography, especially for surveys.[17,28] Computed tomography has also been used to diagnose clonorchiasis or opisthorchiasis.[48]

Serologic tests are used mainly for surveys but play no important role in routine diagnosis. The enzyme-linked immunosorbent assay (ELISA) has been endorsed as the most appropriate immunodiagnostic

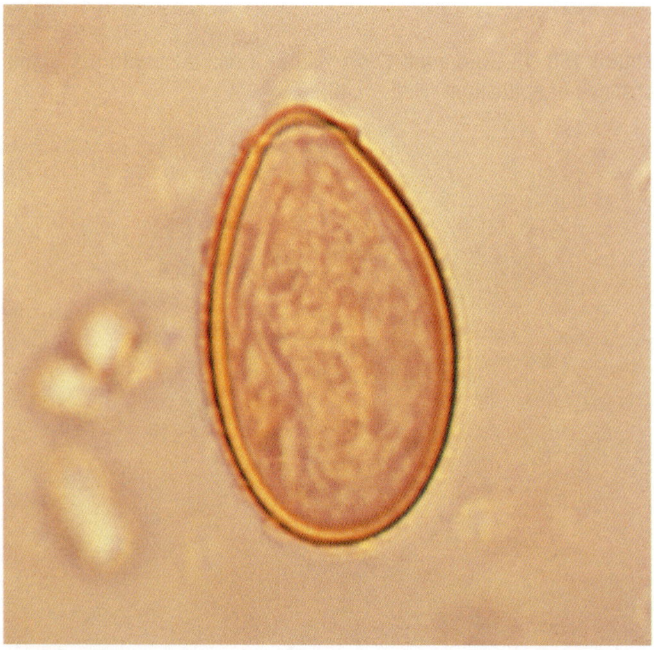

Figure 150–19. Egg of *C sinensis* in stool. Note the prominent opercular shoulders and tapered operculated end (×600).

technique, because it is specific and sensitive and easily used in the field.[49] The direct hemagglutination test, indirect fluorescent antibody test, and counter-immunoelectrophoresis have also been used for diagnosis.[2]

The more promising approach to diagnosis is detecting antigens because these could distinguish active infections. *Clonorchis* antigens may be detected in serum by the ELISA technique. When using monoclonal antibodies there is a minimal detectable level of 30 ng/mL.[50] When monoclonal antibody-based ELISA is used to detect *Opisthorchis* infection, as little as 0.05 to 0.1 ng of the antigen in the stool may be detected.[51] Using DNA hybridization, 3.1 pg of antigen or five *Opisthorchis* eggs in the stool can be detected.[51]

TREATMENT

Praziquantel is now the only drug used to treat clonorchiasis and opisthorchiasis.[52] The standard dose for clonorchiasis or opisthorchiasis is 25 mg/kg three times in a single day.[53] This probably cures all those with opisthorchiasis.[52] When a total daily dose of 75 mg/kg is divided into three doses for 2 days, the cure rates for clonorchiasis were 97.7% to 100%.[2] A mass treatment program for clonorchiasis with praziquantel in South Korea reduced the prevalence from 13.3% in 1984 to 0.9% in 1990.[2] After treatment with praziquantel, biliary tract abnormalities may regress.[54]

REFERENCES

1. Beaver PC, Jung RC, Cupp EW. *Clinical Parasitology.* 9th ed. Philadelphia: WB Saunders; 1984:471–478.
2. Chen M, Lu Y, Hua X, Mott KE. Progress in assessment of morbidity due to *Clonorchis sinensis* infection: a review of recent literature. *Trop Dis Bull.* 1994;91:R7–R65.
3. *Stedman's ASP Parasite Names.* Baltimore: Williams & Wilkins; 1993.
4. Sun T. Clonorchiasis: a report of four cases and discussion of unusual manifestations. *Am J Trop Med Hyg.* 1980;29: 1223–1227.
5. Sun T. *Color Atlas and Textbook of Diagnostic Parasitology.* New York: Igaku-Shoin; 1988:246–254.
6. Bennag D, Harinasuta T. Opisthorchiasis, clonorchiasis and paragonimiasis. In Warren KS, Mahmoud AAF, eds. *Tropical and Geographic Medicine.* New York: McGraw-Hill; 1984:461–472.
7. Haswell-Elkins MR, Satarug S, Elkins DB. *Opisthorchis viverrini* infection in Northeast Thailand and its relationship to cholangiocarcinoma. *J Gastroenterol Hepatol.* 1992;7:538–548.
8. Sun T, Chou ST, Gibson JB. Route of *Clonorchis sinensis* to mammalian liver. *Exp Parasitol.* 1968;22:346–351.
9. Weng YQ, Wan ZR, Lin HR, Hou ZC. Clinical types of 3769 cases of adult clonorchiasis. *Annu Bull Soc Parasitol Guangdong Province.* 1980;2:126–127 (in Chinese).
10. Zhu SH, Zhong XC, Lao ZY. Clonorchiasis and developmental retardation in children. *New Chin Med.* 1983;14: 71–72 (in Chinese).
11. Lam SK, Chan CW. Pyogenic cholangitis: recent etiology and management. *Surv Dig Dis.* 1985;3:12–24.
12. Zhu SH, Zhong XC, Lao CY. On the relationship between *Clonorchis sinensis* infection and hepatocholecystic diseases: a clinical analysis of 2214 cases. *Chin J Intern Med.* 1982;21:34–36 (in Chinese).
13. Schwartz DA. Cholangiocarcinoma associated with liver fluke infection: a preventable source of morbidity in Asian immigrants. *Am J Gastroenterol.* 1986;81:76–79.
14. Gibson JB. Parasites, liver disease and liver cancer. In: *Liver Cancer.* Lyons: International Agency for Research on Cancer; 1971:42–49.
15. Gibson JB, Sun T. Clonorchiasis. In: Marcial-Rojas RA, ed. *Pathology of Protozoal and Helminthic Diseases.* Baltimore: Williams & Wilkins; 1971:546–566.
16. Lin AC, Chapman SW, Turner HR, Wofford JD Jr. Clonorchiasis: an update. *South Med J.* 1987;80:919–922.
17. Woolf A, Green J, Levine JA, et al. A clinical study of Laotian refugees infected with *Clonorchis sinensis* or *Opisthorchis viverrini. Am J Trop Med Hyg.* 1984;33: 1279–1280.
18. Kammerer WS, Van der Decker JD, Keith TB, Mott KE. Clonorchiasis in New York City Chinese. *Trop Doctor.* 1977;7:105–106.
19. Seah SKK. Intestinal parasites in Chinese immigrants in a Canadian city. *J Trop Med Hyg.* 1973;76:291–293.
20. Noblet GP, Hunter WH. Clonorchiasis/opisthorchiasis in South Carolina. *J SC Med Assoc.* 1983;79:75–79.
21. Ameres JP, Levine MP, DeBlasi HP. Acalculous clonorchiasis obstructing the common bile duct. A case report and review of the literature. *Am Surg.* 1976;42:170–172.
22. Baker MS, Baker BH, Woo R. Biliary clonorchiasis. *Arch Surg.* 1979;114:748.
23. Sullivan WG, Koep LJ. Common bile duct obstruction and cholangiohepatitis in clonorchiasis. *JAMA.* 1980;243: 2060–2061.
24. Jimenez T. DiBenedetto A. Common duct stone with associated *Clonorchis sinensis* infection. *NY State J Med.* 1989; 89:480–481.
25. Ho CS, Wesson DE. Recurrent pyogenic cholangitis in Chinese immigrants. *Am J Roentgenol Rad Ther Nucl Med.* 1974;122:368–374.
26. Bonar S, Burrell M, West B, Cahow E. Recurrent cholangitis secondary to oriental cholangiohepatitis. *J Clin Gastroenterol.* 1989;11:464–468.
27. Shungar RA, Ryan JJ. *Clonorchis sinensis* and pancreatitis. *Am J Gastroenterol.* 1976;64:400–403.
28. Elkins DB, Haswell-Elkins MR, Mairiang E, et al. A high frequency of hepatobiliary disease and suspected cholangiocarcinoma associated with heavy *Opisthorchis viverrini* infection in a small community in north-east Thailand. *Trans R Soc Trop Med Hyg.* 1990;84:715–719.
29. Haswell-Elkins MR, Satarug S, Elkins DB. *Opisthorchis viverrini* infection in Northeast Thailand and its relationship to cholangiocarcinoma. *J Gastroenterol Hepatol.* 1992;7:538–548.

30. Srivatanakul P, Sontipong S, Chotiwan P, Parkin DM. Liver cancer in Thailand: temporal and geographic variations. *J Gastroenterol Hepatol.* 1988;3:413–430.
31. Koompriochana C, Sonakul D, Chinda K, Stitnimankarn T. Opisthorchiasis: a clinicopathological study of 154 autopsy cases. *Southeast Asian J Trop Med Public Health.* 1978; 9:60–64.
32. Srivatanakul P, Parkin DM, Jiang YZ, et al. The role of infection by *Opisthorchis viverrini,* hepatitis B virus and aflatoxin exposure in the etiology of liver cancer in Thailand: a correlation study. *Cancer.* 1991;68:2411–2417.
33. Mairiang P, Bhudhisawasdi V, Borirakchanyavat V, Sitiprija V. Acute renal failure in obstructive jaundice in cholangiocarcinoma. *Arch Intern Med.* 1990;150:2357–2360.
34. Hou PC. The pathology of *Clonorchis sinensis* infestation of the liver. *J Pathol Bacteriol.* 1955;70:53–64.
35. Min HK. *Clonorchis sinensis:* pathogenesis and clinical features of infection. *Arzneimittel Forschung.* 1984;34: 1153–1156.
36. Hou PC. The relationship between primary carcinoma of the liver and infestation of *Clonorchis sinensis. J Pathol Bacteriol.* 1956;72:239–246.
37. Juttijudata P, Prichanond S, Churnratanakul S, Chiemchaisri C, Palavatrana C. Hilar intrahepatic cholangiocarcinoma and its etiology. *J Clin Gastroenterol.* 1984; 6:503–504.
38. Chan PH, Teoh TB. The pathology of *Clonorchis sinensis* infestation of the pancreas. *J Pathol Bacteriol.* 1967;93: 185–189.
39. Sun T. The non-antigenicity of intact ova of *Clonorchis sinensis. J Med Microbiol.* 1969;2:358–360.
40. Sun T, Tung-Ma L. Ultrastructural changes in the biliary tract of guinea-pigs infected with *Clonorchis sinensis. J Pathol.* 1973;109:291–294.
41. Sun T, Gibson JB. The site of antigen formation in different developmental stages of *Clonorchis sinensis. Jpn J Med Sci Biol.* 1969;22:263–271.
42. Kim J, Chai JY, Kho WG, Cho KH, Lee SH. Immunohistochemical study on antigenicity of each organ structure of *Clonorchis sinensis. Korean J Parasitol.* 1991;29:21–29.
43. Sun T, Gibson JB. Antigens of *Clonorchis sinensis* in experimental and human infections: an analysis by gel-diffusion technique. *Am J Trop Med Hyg.* 1969;18: 241–252.
44. Thammapalerd N, Tharavanig J, Nacapunchai D, Bunnag D, Radomyos P, Prasertsiriroj V. Detection of antibodies against *Opisthorchis viverrini* in patients before and after treatment with praziquantel. *Southeast Asian J Trop Med Public Health.* 1988;19:101–110.
45. Flavell DJ. Liver-fluke infestations as an aetiological factor in bile-duct carcinoma of man. *Trans R Soc Trop Med Hyg.* 1981;75:814–824.
46. Flavell DJ, Lucas SB. Promotion of *N*-nitrosodimethylamine-initiated bile duct carcinogenesis in the hamster by the human liver fluke, *Opisthorchis viverrini. Carcinogenesis.* 1983;4:927–930.
47. Makarandanda K, Wild CP, Jiang YZ, Neal GE. Possible effect of infection with liver fluke (*Opisthorchis viverrini*) on the monitoring of urine by enzyme-linked immunosorbent assay for human exposure to aflatoxins. *IARC Sci Publ.* 1991;105:96–101.
48. Choi BI, Kim HJ, Han MC, Do YS, Han MH, Lee SH. CT findings of clonorchiasis. *Am J Roentgenol.* 1989;152: 281–284.
49. Immunodiagnosis of human liver fluke infections. *Asian Pacific J Allergy Immunol.* 1986;4:81–88. Editorial.
50. Chen YT, Liu YH, Wang QN, et al. Detection of circulating antigen in sera from clonorchiasis sinensis patients by ELISA double sandwich method. *Chin Med J.* 1988;101: 92–97.
51. Sirisinha S, Chawengkirttikul R, Sermswan R, Amornpant S, Mongkosuk S, Panyim S. Detection of *Opisthorchis viverrini* by monoclonal antibody-based ELISA and DNA hybridization. *Am J Trop Med Hyg.* 1991;44:140–145.
52. Harinasuta T, Pungpak S, Keystone JS. Trematode infections: opisthorchiasis, clonorchiasis, fascioliasis and paragonimiasis. *Infect Dis Clin North Am.* 1993;7:699–716.
53. Anonymous. Drugs for parasitic infections. *Med Lett.* 1993; 35:113–114.
54. Mairiang E, Haswell-Elkins MR, Mairiang P, Sithithaworm P, Elkins DB. Reversal of biliary tract abnormalities associated with Opisthorchis viverrina infection following praziquantel treatment. *Trans R Soc Trop Med Hyg.* 1993; 87:194–197.

Chapter 151

Coenurosis

Patrick J. Vaughan and Daniel H. Connor

Scientists have odious manners, except when you prop up their theory; then you can borrow money from them.

Mark Twain (1845–1910)

The more flesh, the more worms. The more possessions, the more worry.

Hillel (30 BC–AD 10)

DEFINITION/HISTORY

Coenurosis is infection by a coenurus, the larval form of a pseudophylidean tapeworm. There are three species of these tapeworms: *Taenia multiceps, T serialis,* and *T brauni.* The coenuri or larvae of these three species have multiple protoscolices, which distinguish them from other species of tapeworm.[1,2] In particular the larval stage of *T solium* (a cysticercus), which also invades human tissue, has a single scolex and is thus distinguishable from a coenurus (Figure 151–1). The following characteristics are shared with other species of *Taenia:* Their heads are atop numerous proglottids. They absorb nutrients through their teguments, and they are hermaphroditic. Although coenurus infections are common in canines and sheep, humans are only rarely and accidentally infected. The first human infection by a coenurus was reported by Brumpt in France in 1913.[3] Since then, fewer than 100 cases have been described.

SYNONYMS

Taenia multiceps and the related bladder worms with multiple protoscolices in their larval stages, were formerly grouped as a single and separate genus, *Multiceps.* The taxonomy was conferred because three different names had been used for *T multiceps.* These were *Multiceps multiceps, M gaigeri,* and *Coenurus cerebralis.*[4,5] Currently, however, *T multiceps, T serialis,* and *T brauni* are all assigned to the genus *Taenia.*[6]

GEOGRAPHIC DISTRIBUTION

Most human infections have been in tropical Africa and South Africa, but sporadic infections have been described in France, Great Britain, and North America. *Taenia multiceps* is the common species in the sheep-raising populations of South Africa where it causes cerebral coenurosis in humans. *Taenia multiceps* also causes the rare cases of coenurosis of the brain described in North America and Britain. In tropical Africa, however, *T multiceps* causes ocular coenurosis, and *T brauni* causes subcutaneous coenurosis. *Taenia serialis* has caused subcutaneous coenurosis in France and North America.[4]

LIFE CYCLE

The life cycles of *T multiceps, T serialis,* and *T brauni* resemble closely the life cycle of *Echinococcus granulosus.* The adult worm lives in the intestines of canines or other carnivores and its eggs are passed into the environment with feces. If the eggs are ingested by an intermediate host—usually a grazing animal, most commonly sheep, rabbits, goats, cattle, horses, and ante-

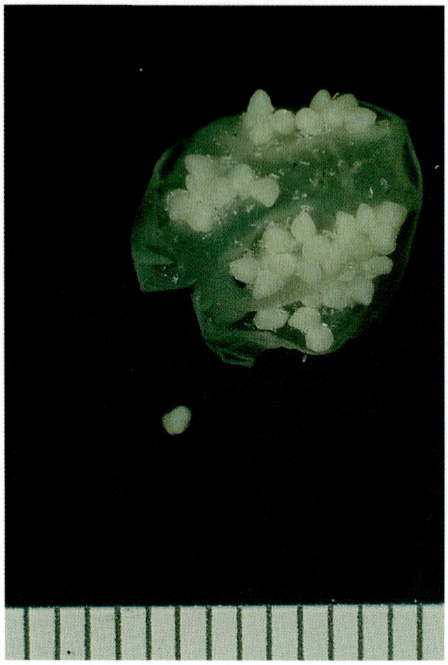

Figure 151–1. Gross photo of a coenurus taken from the subcutaneous tissue of an Ethiopian patient. Note the multiple scolices attached to the lining of the cyst. The species is probably *T brauni.* *(Photograph by Daniel H. Connor, MD, 1970.)*

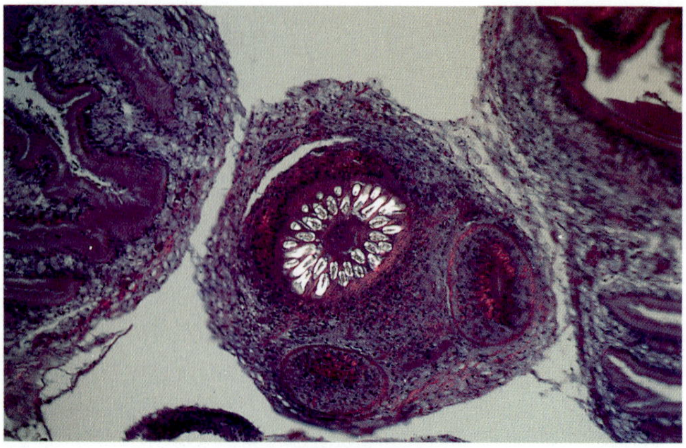

Figure 151–3. Same specimen shown in Figure 151–2 under polarized light (AFIP Neg 80-3453; H&E, ×50).

lopes—the oncospheres escape from the eggs, hatch in the small intestine, and penetrate its wall. They are then carried through the blood to various tissues where they encyst. Sites of larval encystment include the central nervous system, eye, subcutaneous tissue, and muscle. In sheep, localization of the larval stage to the central nervous system produces "staggers" or "gid."[3,4,7]

MORPHOLOGY

The adult *T multiceps* is 40 to 60 cm long.[4,7] It has a pyriform scolex and an armed rostellum with a double row of 22 to 32 hooklets (Figures 151–2 and 151–3). Proglottids are 8 to 10 mm by 3 to 4 mm containing eggs with a diameter of 31 to 36 μm. The tegument is about 5 μm thick and its external surface is covered with microvilli.[4] This is the absorbing and digestive surface of the larva (Figure 151–4), since the worm contains no mouth or digestive organs per se. The larval form of *T multiceps*—the coenurus—is a white, spherical or ovoid unilocular cyst with a translucent wall that surrounds and contains clear mucinous fluid and multiple scolices attached to the lining. The coenurus may grow to be 2 cm across. Its wall is thin and the surrounding host reaction is a layer of delicate fibrous tissue. This feature—multiple scolices within the cyst—is pathognomonic of a coenurus (Figures 151–5 and

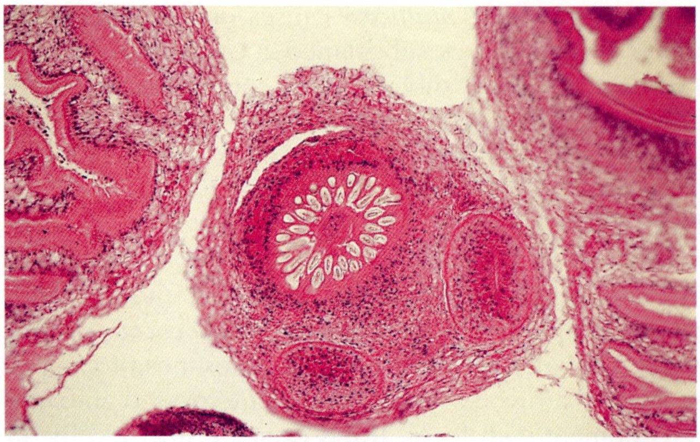

Figure 151–2. Armed rostellum of a coenurus. Note the double row of hooklets—16 in each row [AFIP Neg 80-3452; hematoxylin-eosin (H&E), ×50].

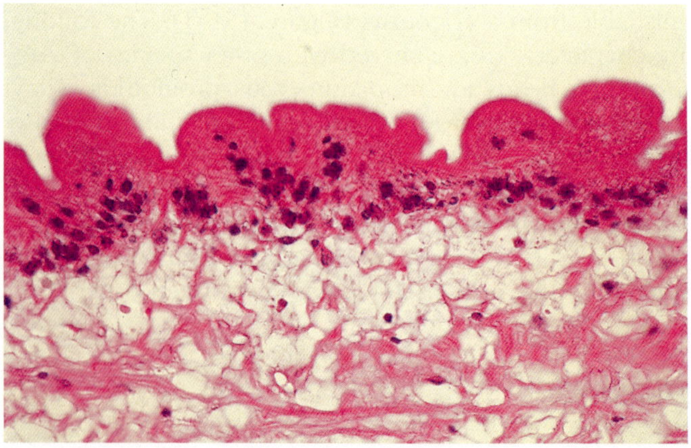

Figure 151–4. Tegument of a coenurus. The outer layer appears as an amorphous eosinophilic membrane. The outer surface is covered with tegumental microvilli seen by electron microscopy. The membrane is supported by a layer of muscle fibers. The loose stroma of the wall of the coenurus lies beneath the muscle layer. The stroma contains calcified bodies (not seen here) (AFIP Neg 80-3456; H&E, ×250).

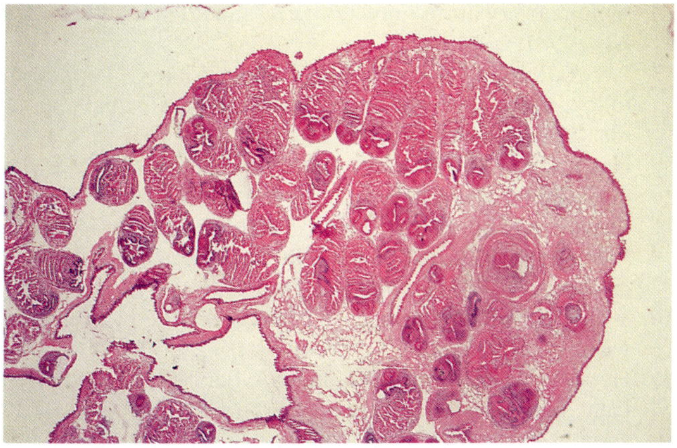

Figure 151–5. This demonstrates multiple scolices, the pathognomonic feature of a coenurus. The scolices number about 40 in this section. The cyst's tegument is at the top and the scolices are everted and in the cavity of the coenurus—now collapsed when the cyst was cut open (AFIP Neg 80-3449; H&E, ×10).

151–6) and distinguishes the coenurus from the cysticercus, which contains a single scolex.[1] Each scolex is capable of developing into an adult worm with the same pattern of hooklets; scolices develop from the germinal layer of the cyst wall.[4]

CLINICAL FEATURES

Clinical manifestations depend on the location of the coenurus.[3] When in the central nervous system, coenuri have caused drowsiness, headache, vomiting, papilledema, seizures, and hemiparesis.[7,8] Some patients have had cranial nerve palsies. Infection of the eye typically is subconjunctival or in the posterior chamber, resulting in erythema, blurred vision, and uveitis.[9,10] Funduscopic inspection may reveal intravitreous cysts with several white spots in no apparent pattern. Subcutaneous coenuri cause small nodules that may or may not be painful. Most subcutaneous coenuri are on the trunk and less frequently limbs, head, and neck. Subcutaneous coenuri have been mistaken clinically for lipomas, ganglions, and neurofibromas.[3,4,6]

PATHOLOGY

Subcutaneous coenuri tend to be painless small nodules.[3] Within the brain, however, pressure from the increasing size of the coenurus is the principal mechanism of disease, although toxic and hypersensitivity reactions may also play a role.[1] In some patients intracranial coenuri have concentrated in the subarachnoid space where they have caused a basal arachnoiditis.[7] There is dense meningeal fibrosis with a foreign-body giant cell reaction. Intracranial coenuri have also localized in the lateral ventricles as a cluster of cysts attached to a central stalk. Involvement of the motor cortex has caused Jacksonian epilepsy. Intraocular coenuri are attached to choroid and retina and grow into the vitreous. Toxic endophthalmitis with its sequelae is the principal mechanism in this location.[9] Intact coenuri provoke little reaction other than a thin layer of fibrous tissue. Degenerating coenuri, however, provoke an inflammatory reaction that is both suppurative and granulomatous. Eventually, fragments of the coenurus are phagocytosed and the site becomes scarred and calcified.

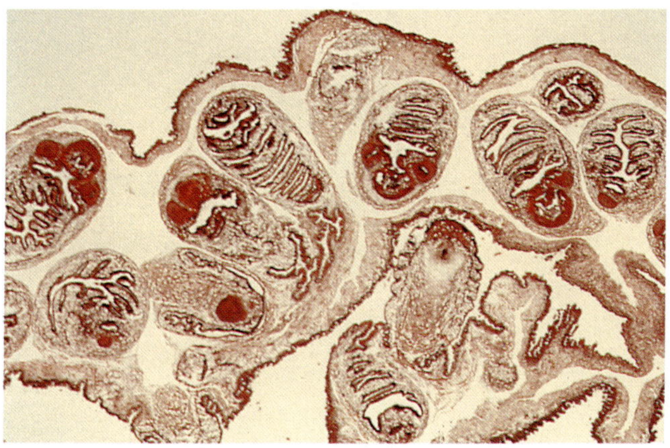

Figure 151–6. Wall of a coenurus containing 11 inverted scolices. The tegument is thin and its outer absorptive surface surrounds the specimen. The inner germinal layer lines the tracts leading to the scolices (AFIP 69-4736; Movat, ×17).

DIAGNOSIS

Diagnosis is based on identifying a coenurus, either grossly or by microscopy.[4,11] Coenurosis of the eye is the exception. Here the diagnosis may be confirmed by examination with a slit lamp if a cyst and multiple scolices are identified. Other diagnostic tests are usually not helpful. For instance, in patients with cerebral coenurosis the pressure of the cerebrospinal fluid may be raised and there may be pleocytosis, increased protein, and low sugar, but none of these findings is specific or perhaps even suggestive of coenurosis. Computerized tomography or magnetic resonance imaging allow precise evaluation of both the size and location of the cysts. These modalities have also proved helpful in postoperative surveillance.[7,8,12] Studies on blood are normal; eosinophilia is not a feature.[3] Immunodiagnostic tests for coenurosis have not been conclusive.[7]

TREATMENT

The treatment of choice is surgical excision of cerebral, ophthalmic, or subcutaneous coenuri.[3,7] Neither praziquantel nor mebendazole has been successful.[6,13–16] In ocular coenurosis both drugs have produced toxic endophthalmitis, and in the brain, edema and scarring.[9] Remnants of parasite cause recurrence but complete removal of the cyst produces a cure.

REFERENCES

1. Becker BJP, Jacobson S. Infestation of the human brain with *Coenurus cerebralis*. *Lancet.* 1951;198–202.
2. Lachberg S, Thompson RC, Lymbery AJ. A contribution to the etiology of racemose cysticercosis. *J Parasitol.* 1990; 76:592–594.
3. Kurtycz DFI, Brooke ALT, Mack E. Incidental coenurosis: larval cestode presenting as an axillary mass. *AJCP.* 1983; 80:735–738.
4. Sparks AK, Neafie RC, Connor DH. Coenurosis. In: Binford CH, Connor DH, eds. *Pathology of Tropical and Extraordinary Diseases.* Washington, DC: Armed Forces Institute of Pathology; 1976:543–545.
5. Proctor NSF. Coenurosis. In: Marcial-Rojas RA, ed. *Pathology of Protozoal and Helminthic Diseases.* Baltimore: Williams & Wilkins; 1971:627–634.
6. Benger A, Rennie RP, Roberts JT, Thornley JH, Scholten T. A human coenurus infection in Canada. *Am J Trop Med Hyg.* 1981;3:638–644.
7. Pau A, Perria C, Turtas S, Brambilla M, Viale G. Long-term follow-up of the surgical treatment of intracranial coenurosis. *Br J Neurosurg.* 1990;4:39–43.
8. Pau A, Turtas S, Brambilla M, Leoni A, Rosa M, Viale GL. Computed tomography and magnetic resonance imaging of cerebral coenurosis. *Surg Neurol.* 1987;6:548–552.
9. Ibechukwu BI, Onwukeme KE. Intraocular coenurosis: a case report. *Br J Ophthalmol.* 1991;75:430–431.
10. Williams PH, Templeton AC. Infection of the eye by tapeworm *Coenurus. Br J Ophthalmol.* 1971;55:766–769.
11. Hermos JA, Healy GR, Schultz MG, Barlow J, Church WG. Fatal human cerebral coenurosis. *JAMA.* 1970;213:1461–1464.
12. Schellhas KP, Norris GA. Disseminated human subarachnoid coenurosis: computed tomographic appearance. *AJNR.* 1985;6:638–640.
13. Price TC, Dresden MH, Alvarado T, Flanagan J, Chappell CL. Coenuriasis in a spectacled langur (*Presbytis obscura*): praziquantel treatment and the antibody response to cyst antigens. *Am J Trop Med Hyg.* 1989;40:514–520.
14. Willis JM, Herbert IV. A method for estimating the age of coenuri of *Taenia multiceps* recovered from the brains of sheep. *Vet Rec.* 1987;121(10):216–218.
15. Skerritt GC, Stallbaumer MF. Diagnosis and treatment of coenuriasis (gid) in sheep. *Vet Rec.* 1984;115:399–403.
16. Beaver PC, Jung RC, Cupp EW. Coenurosis. In: *Clinical Parasitology.* 9th ed. Philadelphia: Lea & Febiger; 1984: 525–527.

CHAPTER 152

Cysticercosis

Daniel P. O'Neill and Daniel H. Connor

. . . as worm to a toad, a toad to a snake, a snake to a pig, a pig to a man, and a man to a worm.

Ambrose Bierce (1842–c.1914)

DEFINITION

Human cysticercosis is invasion of man's tissues by the larval stage of the pork tapeworm, *Taenia solium*. The larval stage, called a cysticercus, usually lives in the flesh of the pig, which serves as the intermediate host. The adult *T solium,* however, lives in the human intestine. Human cysticercosis, therefore, is an aberration of the usual life cycle and may be blinding or fatal.[1]

GEOGRAPHIC DISTRIBUTION

Taenia solium has a worldwide distribution but is most common where pigs and people are in close proximity. Humans acquire the adult worm by ingesting pork containing viable cysticerci, so taeniasis (solium) is common where inadequately cooked pork is eaten. Humans acquire the cysticercus, however, by ingesting viable eggs—usually in food or drink contaminated by human feces. Cysticercosis is common, therefore, not only where pigs and people coexist, but where sanitation is poor. Regions and countries where cysticercosis is common include Central America, Mexico, Asia, Spain, Portugal, Africa, and Eastern Europe. Most patients with cysticercosis in the industrialized nations have immigrated from endemic areas.[2]

DESCRIPTION OF PARASITE

Taenia solium is a cestode (flatworm) the adult of which attaches to the mucosa of the jejunum and sheds segments called proglottids. The adult worms may grow to be 3 m long and live for 25 years. Some worms have 1000 or more proglottids and each proglottid can produce up to 50,000 eggs. Eggs of *T solium* cannot be differentiated from eggs of the beef tapeworm—*T saginata*—nor from eggs of *Echinococcus* species. Gravid proglottids of *T solium,* however, are readily distinguished by the presence of 5 to 10 uterine branches.

Cysticerci are fluid-filled milky-white, spherical to oval cysts that grow from a microscopic onchosphere to 1 to 2 cm in diameter (Figure 152–1). Each cyst contains a single invaginated scolex with four large suckers and 22 to 30 hooklets in a double circular row (Figure 152–2). The cyst wall is 100 to 200 μm thick and frequently raised into projections 10 to 25 μm high (Figure 152–3). The exterior of the tegument is covered with microvilli. There are smooth-muscle fibers beneath the tegument that extend into the parenchyma. A row of tegumental cells lies beneath the muscle fibers. The parenchyma of the cysticercus is comprised of loose stroma with fluid-filled spaces, calcereous bodies (Figure 152–4), mesenchymal fibers, and more smooth muscle.

LIFE CYCLE

The only known definitive hosts, humans, harbor the adult *T solium* in the intestine (Figure 152–5). Gravid proglottids are shed in the stool from which eggs are expelled and contaminate the ground. When eggs are ingested by a pig (rarely sheep and dogs are intermediate hosts) they hatch into onchospheres. The onchospheres burrow through the wall of the gut, enter the circulation, and then encyst in the pig's tissues where

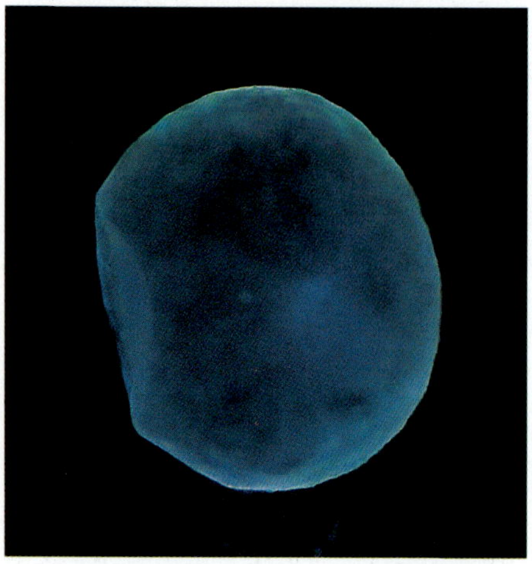

Figure 152–1. An excised cysticercus from the cervical cord of a 36-year-old immigrant Mexican woman. It is about 2.4 mm across and was one of several removed from the subarachnoid space of the patient's lumbar cord (gross, ×9). *(By Daniel H. Connor, MD, 1991.)*

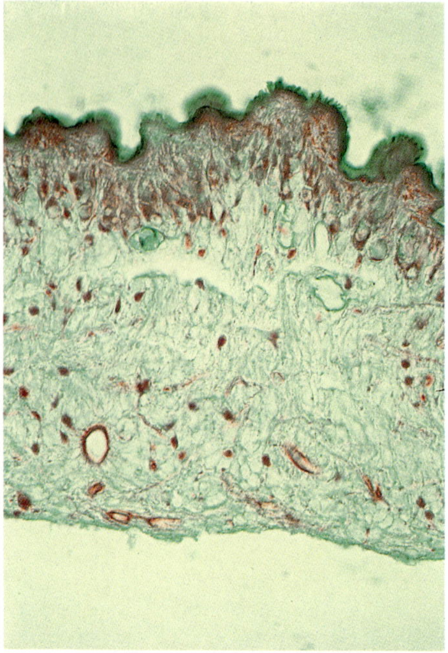

Figure 152–3. Wall of a cysticercus showing the outer tegument with its surface microvilli, a layer of tegumental cells, and beneath that a network of cells reaching into the stroma. The open spaces in the stroma are excretory channels [AFIP; Movat, ×180).

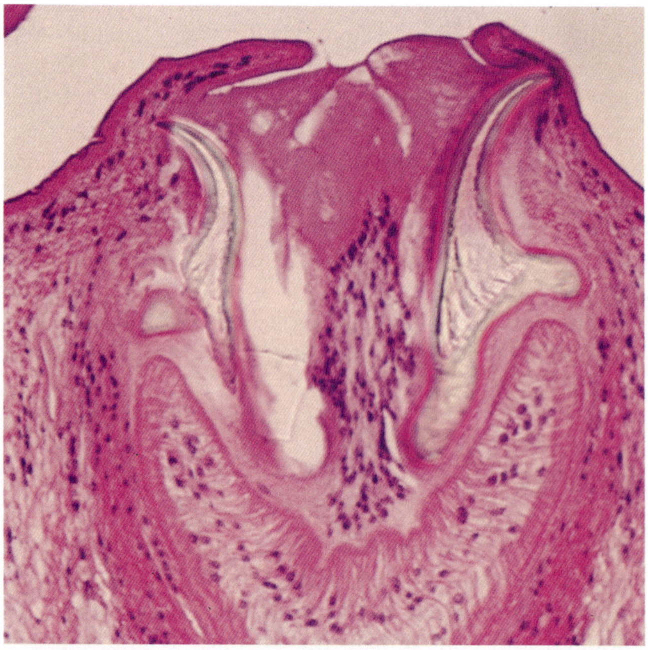

Figure 152–2. Section through the scolex of a cysticercus removed from the biceps muscle, showing two hooklets and the sucker [AFIP Neg 70-5658; hematoxylin-eosin (H&E), ×165].

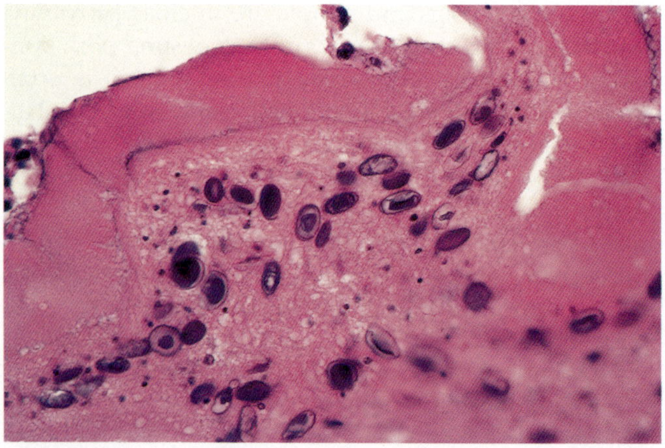

Figure 152–4. Cysticercus removed from the brain. The tegument is the smooth structureless upper membrane. The calcareous bodies are laminated mineralized structures that are in the stroma of many cestodes. They persist in the inflammatory lesion long after the cysticercus is degenerated (AFIP; H&E, ×180).

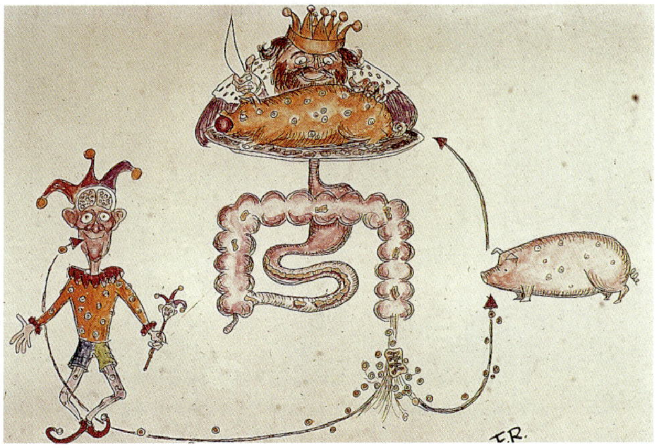

Figure 152–5. Life cycle of *T solium.* The king eats pork containing viable cysticerci, which evert and attach to the wall of the upper small bowel. Here, in a liquid and nutritious environment, the cysticercus grows into an adult tapeworm in about 3 months. Proglottids containing *T solium* eggs are shed from the tapeworm into the king's stool and if these contaminate food eaten by a pig, the eggs release onchospheres in the pig's intestine that burrow through the intestine, enter the circulation, and lodge in the flesh of the pig where they encyst and grow to be mature cysticerci. This cycle is benign in the sense that neither pig nor a human is harmed. When, however, people (here represented by the court jester) ingest food or drink contaminated by eggs, cysticerci form in human tissue. In this situation people play the part of the pig—the intermediate host—but as such are a dead-end for the parasite. Cysticerci, depending on where they lodge and grow, however, are potentially dangerous. *(By the late Captain Frank O. Raasch, MC USN.)*

they mature into cysticerci. When a human ingests measly pork containing viable cysticerci, the cysticerci excyst in the small intestine and attach to the wall of the jejunum. Here, they grow to become adult tapeworms in about 3 months, at which time they begin to shed proglottids—thus completing the life cycle. This is the usual life cycle—a life cycle that is, by and large, innocuous for humans.

This life cycle, however, sets the stage for a dangerous aberration. When a human accidentally ingests eggs of *T solium,* then the human plays the role of the intermediate host. Onchospheres hatch in the gut, seed human tissues, and develop into cysticerci. As noted, human cysticercosis is common in areas where personal hygiene and sewage disposal are poor. Gastronomically fastidious groups such as orthodox Jews may be infected with cysticerci—by ingesting eggs shed from a domestic food handler[3,4]—but members of such groups do not harbor the adult tapeworm, because they do not eat pork—measly or otherwise.

There are three recognized ways a person may get cysticercosis: 1) by ingesting eggs shed in the feces of

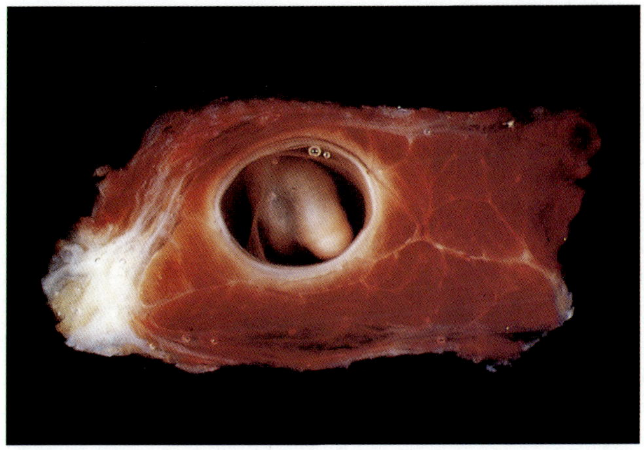

Figure 152–6. A cysticercus in the muscle of a male Zairian. The scolex can be seen in the cyst. *(By Daniel H. Connor, MD, 1970.)*

a food handler who harbors an adult *T solium,* 2) by ingesting eggs shed in his/her own feces, if the patient harbors an adult *T solium,* and 3) rarely, when patients with adult worms regurgitate proglottids from small intestine into stomach allowing the eggs to hatch into onchospheres, and as described previously, migrate to the tissues and become cysticerci. Skeletal muscle (Figure 152–6), skin (Figure 152–7), subcutaneous tissue, heart, eye, and brain are all common sites of cysticercosis in humans.

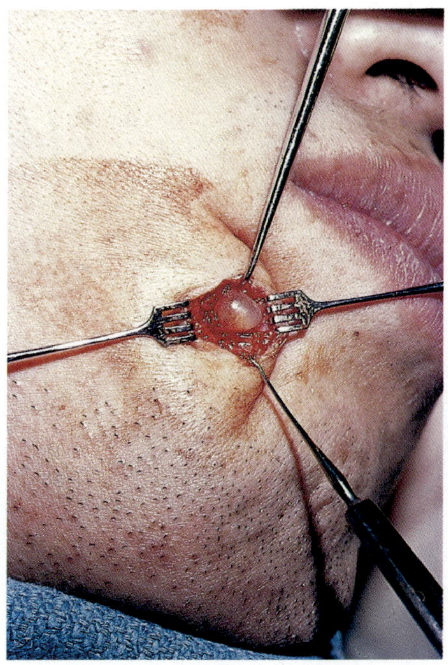

Figure 152–7. One of many cysticerci removed from the skin and subcutaneous tissues of an immigrant adult male Korean. *(By Daniel H. Connor, MD, 1969.)*

CLINICAL FEATURES

In humans clinical features depend on the number and location of cysticerci and whether they are intact or degenerating. Intact and degenerating cysticerci cause signs and symptoms of expanding growth, while degenerating cysticerci cause features of inflammation including swelling, tissue eosinophilia and edema, granulomatous inflammation, scarring, and eventually mineralization (Figure 152–8). Cysticerci in skin, subcutaneous tissue, and muscle have a benign course. They are painless and grow to be 1 to 2 cm across. Cysticerci, however, may appear almost anywhere in the body with protean effects.[5,6] A single cysticercus in the brain blocking the aqueduct, for instance, may kill the patient, while massive cysticercosis of the brain may cause epilepsy leading to death (Figure 152–9). Those in the heart may disrupt conduction, leading to fatal arrhythmias (Figure 152–10). A cysticercus in the eye may cause pain around the eye, flashes of light, grotesque shapes in the visual fields, and blurring or loss of vision. Funduscopic examination usually reveals a mobile cysticercus in the vitreous (Figure 152–11). Many of these may be removed without loss of vision.

The clinical features of neurocysticercosis depend on the size and location of the cyst or cysts. There may

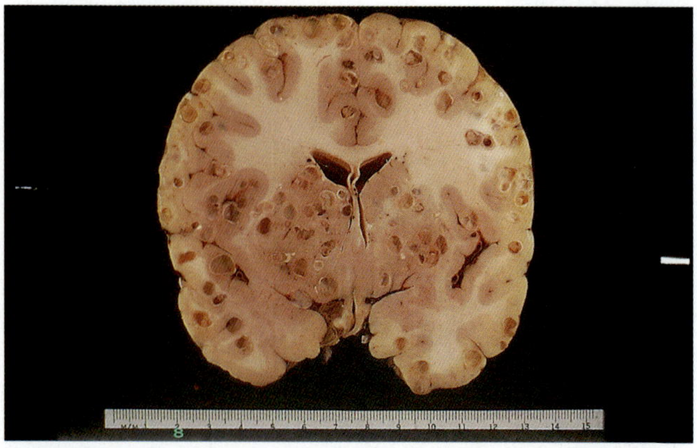

Figure 152–9. Brain of a 16-year-old girl from Irian Jaya with massive cysticercosis. While convulsing she fell into a fire and suffered fatal burns. The cysticerci are concentrated at the junction of the white and gray matter—a point of vascular narrowing. Pigs have a special place in the ecology and mystique of New Guinea. *(Specimen contributed by D. Carleton Gajdusek, MD; photograph by Daniel H. Connor, MD, 1975.)*

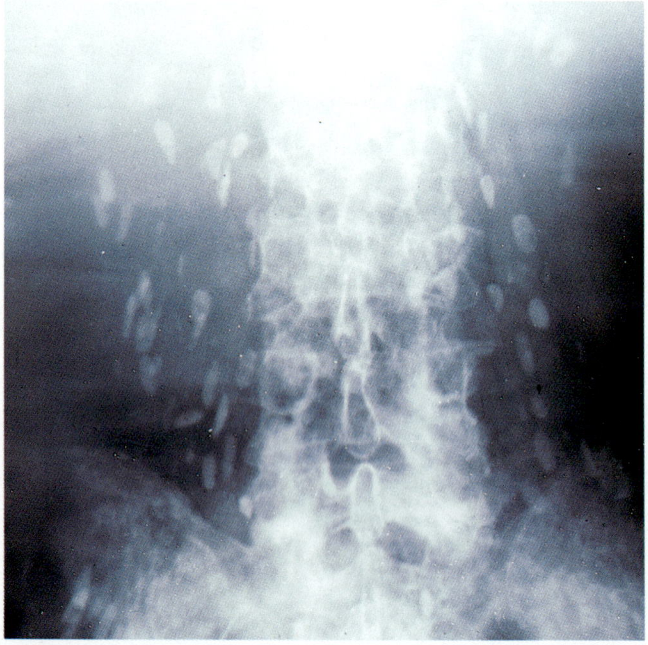

Figure 152–8. An adult male African took a "medicinal" potion containing a ground up proglottid of *T solium*. The eggs became cysticerci and eventually calcified, giving much of his body the appearance of a snow storm. *(From files of AFIP.)*

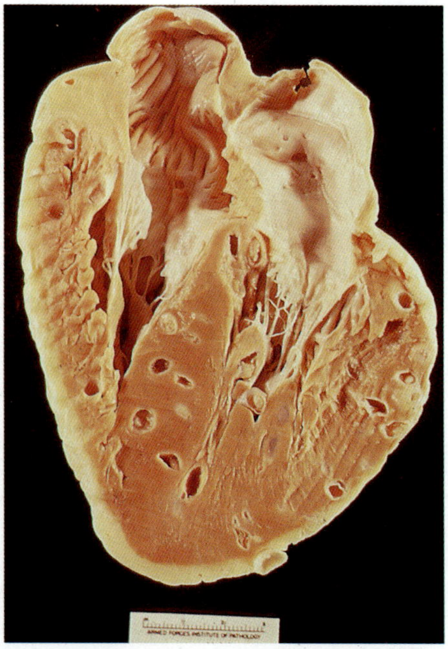

Figure 152–10. Cysticercosis, heart. There are many cysticerci in the myocardium (AFIP 64-2277).

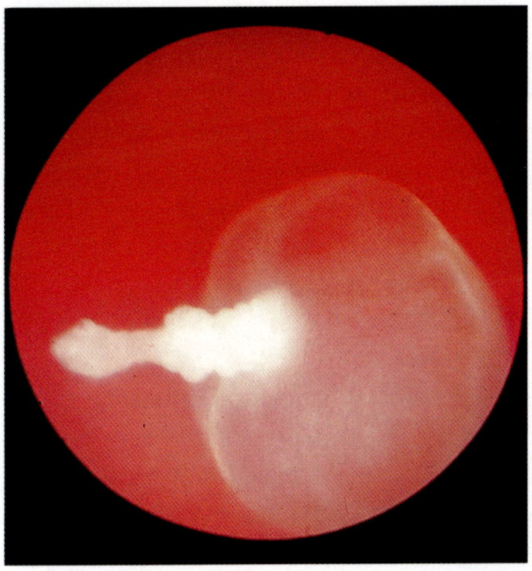

Figure 152–11. Cysticercosis of the eye, funduscopic view. While being observed by the ophthalmologist, the scolex inverted and everted rhythmically. Here it is everted and pointing to the left. *(Contributed by Dr. Narcing Rao, Georgetown University Hospital.)*

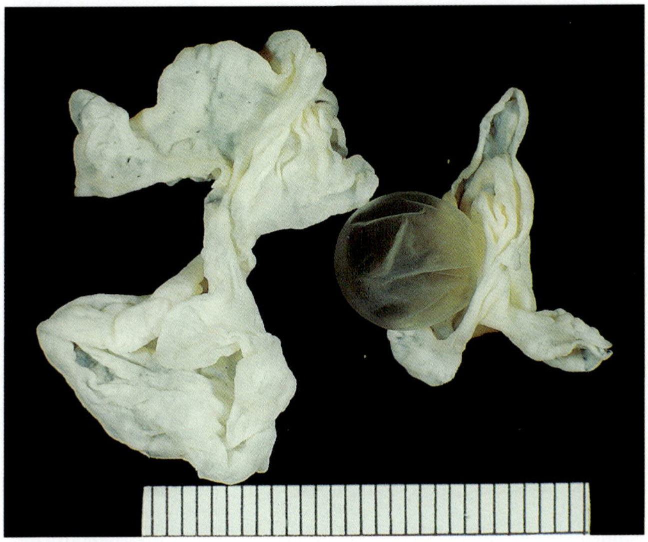

Figure 152–12. Multiple lobes and abundant loose folds of a racemose cysticercus. These cysticerci have no scolex, are predisposed to develop in the brain, and show continuous growth so are difficult to treat. *(By Daniel H. Connor, MD, 1979.)*

be general seizures or Jacksonian seizures as well as hydrocephalus and meningitis. Imaging studies such as computed tomography (CT) show cerebral changes such as single calcifications, granulomas and hydrocephalus.[7–9] There are often features of increased intracranial pressure, including headache, vomiting, ataxia, papilledema, and confusion. Clinicians have reported increased risk of cerebral vascular accidents in these patients.[10–14] There are also variant forms of infection. A severe cysticercal meningitis may develop in patients with the racemose form of neurocysticercosis. The racemose cysticercus is an aberrant cysticercus that lacks a scolex and continues to grow, producing a large multilobed aberrant cyst with many folds (Figure 152–12). The result is a large folded cyst resembling grapelike clusters of larval membrane (Figure 152–13). The racemose form of the cysticercus has a predilection for the base of the brain and subarachnoid space. Because of its continuous growth, the racemose cysticercus is difficult to treat.[15]

PATHOLOGY

Intact cysticerci compress adjacent structures as they grow but provoke no inflammation. Degenerating cysts, however, provoke acute inflammation with an infiltrate of neutrophils and eosinophils and surrounding edema. Later the reaction becomes granulomatous with macrophages, epithelioid cells, and Langhans' giant cells. As the inflammatory process progresses, the cysticercus loses its shape, and eventually its identity. It then becomes encircled by scar tissue (Figure 152–14). Sections of these burnt out lesions may still have clues that enable the pathologist to suspect or diagnose "healed cysticercosis." These clues are 1) the size of the lesion; lesions typically are about 1 cm; 2) persisting fragments of cyst wall, stroma, or hooklets; stroma and tegument degenerate quickly, whereas hooklets may persist for many months and because they are birefringent and acid-fast, they can be identified using polarized light and acid-fast stains; 3) calcereous bodies in the stroma persist in the degenerating lesion and when identified, and in an appropriate context, are strong evidence for

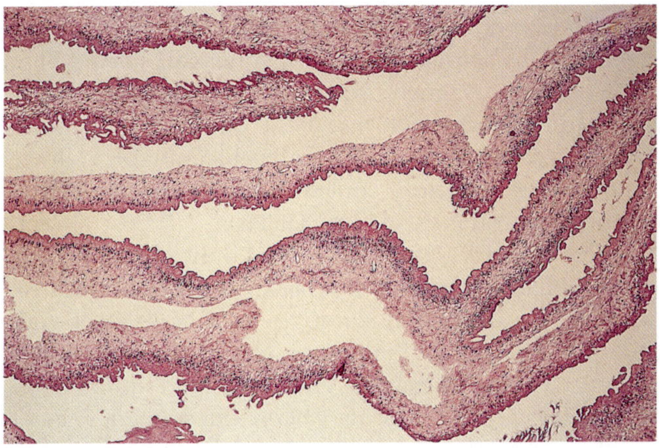

Figure 152–13. The many folds of a racemose cysticercus. A narrow layer of stroma supports the tegument (AFIP 80-4015, H&E; ×11).

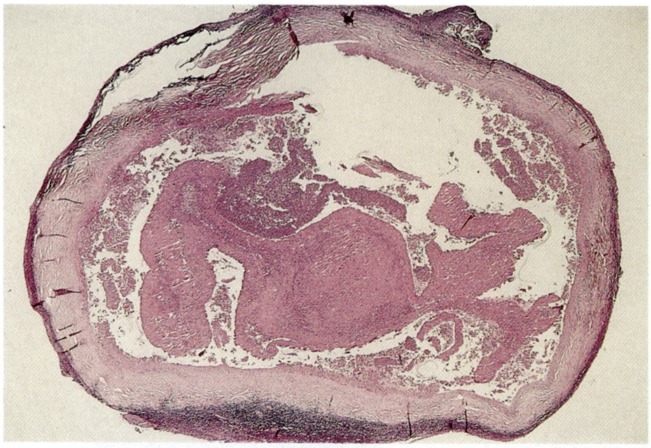

Figure 152–14. Circumscribed inflammatory lesion excised from the brain. This is probably a "burnt out" cysticercus. The perimeter is fibrous scar tissue. The cavity contains a suppurative exudate and a fibrin-rich structure that could be a collapsed cysticercus. This opinion is supported by the size of the lesion—about 1 cm—its location in the brain, and by the numerous eosinophils and calcified structures resembling calcareous bodies in the exudate (AFIP; H&E, ×4.5).

a healed cysticercus; 4) eosinophils persist in the healing cysticerci until scarring begins and, with appropriate clinical correlation, are a helpful feature; 5) the demographic data of the patient. Although these can never be used to diagnose or confirm cysticercosis, they can help in the overall assessment of the likelihood of cysticercosis.

DIAGNOSIS

Diagnosis of cysticercosis requires visualization of the cysticercus in the infected tissue. The diagnosis is often made, however, on the basis of clinical symptoms combined with radiologic findings of spherical, space-filling cystic lesions. Magnetic resonance imaging and computed tomography (CT) are both effective in demonstrating cysticerci. CT sensitivity has recently been questioned by investigators comparing it to enzyme-linked immunoelectrotransfer blot (EITB).[16] It is recommended, therefore, that CT be used only in conjunction with a reliable serologic test for cysticercosis. Because many of the traditional serologic tests cross-react with other cestodes, new immunoblotting techniques are being used. The efficacy of enzyme-linked immunosorbent assay (ELISA) has also been questioned.[17] Fine-needle aspiration biopsy (FNAB) is also being used to identify cysticerci.[18,19] Suspected lesions are aspirated and the contents examined microscopically for parts of the cysticercus, including its wall, stroma, hooklets, scolex, etc. These techniques are particularly important in neurocysticercosis where the diagnosis may be difficult or impossible with imaging studies alone.[20] To distinguish cerebral cysticercosis from a neoplasm, a biopsy specimen may be required, from an open procedure or by stereotactically guided needle aspiration.

TREATMENT

Treatment of *T solium* infection must be directed either at the adult worms or at the cysticerci. Niclosamide has been used successfully for adult worms. For cysticercosis, surgical excision is the traditional approach for both diagnosis and treatment. For neurocysticercosis excision of cysticerci may be difficult or impossible. Diversion of cerebrospinal fluid may be required for some patients.[21] Drug therapy includes praziquantel and, more recently, albendazole has been used.[22] At least one study has advocated the use of anticonvulsive treatment with phenytoin.[23]

REFERENCES

1. Sparks AK, Neafie RC, Connor DH. Cysticercosis. In: Binford CH, Connor DH, eds. *Pathology of Tropical and Extraordinary Diseases.* Washington, DC: Armed Forces Institute of Pathology; 1976:539–543.
2. Dietrichs E, Tyssvang T, Aanonsen NO, Bakke SJ. Cerebral cysticercosis in Norway. *Acta Neurol Scandinavica.* 1993;88:296–298.
3. Shantz PM, Moore AC, Munoz JM, et al. Neurocysticercosis in an orthodox Jewish community in New York City. *N Engl J Med.* 1992;327:692–695.
4. Moore AC, Lutwick LI, Shantz PM, et al. Seroprevalence of cysticercosis in an orthodox Jewish community. *Am J Trop Med Hyg.* 1995;53:439–442.
5. Puppin D Jr, Cavegn BM, Delmaestro D. Subcutaneous cysticercosis of the tongue mimicking a tumor. *Int J Dermatol.* 1993;32:818–819.
6. O'Grady TC, Robbins BA, Barrett TL, Higginbottom PA. Subcutaneous cysticercosis simulating metastatic breast carcinoma. *Int J Dermatol.* 1993;32:62–64.
7. Teitelbaum GP, Otto RJ, Lin M, et al. MR imaging of neurocysticercosis. *Am J Neuroradiol.* 1989;10:709–718.
8. Hulbert TV, Larsen RA. Seizures and soft-tissue calcifications in a Hispanic woman. *Chest.* 1992;101:1125–1127.
9. Chang KH, Lee JH, Han MH, Han MC. The role of contrast-enhanced MR imaging in the diagnosis of neurocysticercosis. *Am J Neuroradiol.* 1991;12:509–512.
10. Otero E, Cordova S, Diaz F, Garcia-Teruel I, Del Brutto OH. Acquired epileptic aphasia (the Landau–Kleffner syndrome) due to neurocysticercosis. *Epilepsia.* 1989;30:569–572.
11. Alarcon F, Vanormelingen K, Moncayo J, Vinan I. Cerebral cysticercosis as a risk factor for stroke in young and middle-aged people. *Stroke.* 1992;23:1563–1565.

12. Collister RE, Dire DJ, Neurocysticercosis presenting to the emergency department as a pure motor hemiparesis. *J Emerg Med.* 1991;9:425–429.
13. Del Brutto OH, Santibanez R, Noboa CA, Aguirre R, Diaz E, Alarcon TA. Epilepsy due to neurocysticercosis: analysis of 203 patients. *Neurology.* 1992;42:389–392.
14. terPenning B, Litchman CD, Heier L. Bilateral middle cerebral artery occlusions in neurocysticercosis. *Stroke.* 1992; 23:280–283.
15. Carpio A, Placencia M, Santillan F, Escobar A. A proposal for classification of neurocysticercosis. *Can J Neurol Sci.* 1994;21:43–47.
16. Garcia HH, Herrera G, Gilman RH, et al. Discrepancies between cerebral computed tomography and Western blot in the diagnosis of neurocysticercosis. The Cysticercosis Working Group in Peru (Clinical Studies Coordination Board). *Am J Trop Med Hyg.* 1994;50:152–157.
17. Ramos-Kuri M, Montoya RM, Padilla A, et al. Immunodiagnosis of neurocysticercosis. Disappointing performance of serology (enzyme-linked immunosorbent assay) in an unbiased sample of neurological patients. *Arch Neurol.* 1992;49:633–636.
18. Verma K, Kapila K. Fine needle aspiration diagnosis of cysticercosis in soft tissue swellings. *Acta Cytol.* 1989;33: 663–666.
19. Arora VK, Gupta K, Singh N, Bhatia A. Cytomorphologic panorama of cysticercosis on fine needle aspiration. A review of 298 cases. *Acta Cytologica.* 1994;38:377–380.
20. Michael AS, Levy JM, Paige ML. Cysticercosis mimicking brain neoplasm: MR and CT appearance. *J Comput Assist Tomogr.* 1990;14:708–711.
21. Zee CS, Segall HD, Destian S, Ahmadi J, Apuzzo ML. MRI of intraventricular cysticercosis: surgical implications. *J Comput Assist Tomogr.* 1993;17:932–939.
22. Takayanagui OM, Jardim E. Therapy for neurocysticercosis. Comparison between albendazole and praziquantel. *Arch Neurol.* 1992;49:290–294.
23. Joubert J. Cysticercal meningitis—a pernicious form of neurocysticercosis which responds poorly to praziquantel. *S Afr Med J.* 1990;77:528–530.

Chapter 153

Dioctophymiasis and Eustrongylidiasis

Mark L. Eberhard

And immediately the angel of the Lord smote him, because he gave not God the glory and he was eaten with worms, and gave up the ghost.

Acts 12:23

It is a Capital mistake to theorize before one has data. Insensibly one begins to twist facts to suit theories, instead of theories to fit facts.

Arthur Conan Doyle (1859–1930), A Scandal in Bohemia

DEFINITION

Dioctophymiasis and eustrongylidiasis are infections by nematodes in the family Dioctophymatoidae, including *Dioctophyma renale* and *Eustrongylides* sp. Synonyms include dioctophymiasis, dioctophymosis, dioctophymatid, and giant kidney worm for *D renale* and eustrongylidosis for infection by *Eustrongylides* sp.

GEOGRAPHIC DISTRIBUTION

The geographic distribution of *D renale* appears to be cosmopolitan, encompassing North and South America, Europe, Asia, and the Far East. Whether the infection is endemic in Africa and Oceania is debatable. *Eustrongylides* is also widely reported in natural hosts in North and South America, Europe, Asia, Australia, and the Middle East.

LIFE CYCLE, NATURAL HISTORY, AND EPIDEMIOLOGY

As adult parasites, *D renale* characteristically inhabit the pelvis of the kidney in a variety of carnivores, but on occasion have been described in the abdominal cavity.[1] In North America, mink are the most commonly infected animal, although infections in dogs have been reported. Less frequently, other animals such as raccoons, skunks, cats, wolves, pumas, oxen, and horses have been infected. Female worms deposit eggs that are voided in urine in an unembryonated stage. Development of a first-stage larva occurs in 15 to 100 days, depending on ambient temperature. Embryonated eggs must be ingested by an aquatic oligochaete, such as *Lumbriculus variegatus,* to enable the larvae to develop to the infective stage. Larval development occurs in the coelom of the oligochaete. Larvae molt twice before becoming infective.

As with development of the first-stage larva, development to the infective stage is related to the ambient temperature, but takes from 70 to 120 days. When infective oligochaetes are ingested by an appropriate definitive host such as mink, dioctophymatid larvae penetrate into its gastric submucosa, migrate to the liver, and then migrate through the body cavity as they make their way to a kidney. By about 50 days, larvae have entered the parenchyma of the kidney. The prepatent period is about 155 days in ferrets and mink, and about 135 days in dogs. Worms that do not invade kidney may grow to near adult size but cannot release eggs into the environment so do not contribute to continued transmission.

Although mink and other animals can acquire infection by ingesting infective oligochaetes, they are more likely to be infected by eating tadpoles, frogs, or fish (especially *Ictalurus* = bullhead) that serve as paratenic hosts. The dioctophymatid larvae do not develop further in these transport hosts, whose primary purpose is to move the parasite up the food chain.

Between 15 and 20 authentic infections of humans with *D renale* have been reported. Three of these were by immature worms identified in subcutaneous nodules on the patient's chest or abdominal wall[2–4]; the remainder were adult worms.[1] Five of the infections were detected at autopsy; in six, the worm was expelled or migrated out of the urethra; in one the worm emerged through the skin over the kidney; and in one, eggs were in the urine, but adult worms could not be located. These patients most likely became infected by eating raw or poorly cooked fish or frog meat and not by ingesting an oligochaete.

Species of the genus *Eustrongylides* are parasites of the esophagus and proventriculus of fish-eating (piscivorous) birds. The apparent lack of host specificity has made it difficult to define clearly the taxonomic relationships within this group of nematodes, but a recent review revised the genus and recognized only three valid species.[5] The life cycle of one species, *Eustrongylides tubefex,* is very similar to *D renale.*[6] Eggs are passed in feces into water, where first-stage larvae develop in 23 to 26 days at 25°C. Several genera of aquatic oligochaetes and tubificids, including *Limnodrilis, Tubifex,* and *Lumbriculus,* support the development of larvae to the third stage. As for *D renale,* paratenic hosts such as minnows and amphibians serve to funnel the infective larvae into appropriate definitive hosts.

Human infection is accidental through the unusual habit of swallowing live bait minnows. Three reports and at least one unpublished infection have documented a total of six persons who have become acutely ill after swallowing live minnows.[7–9] All six resided along the northeast seaboard of the United States, and all but one were fishermen who reported eating raw bait minnows within 24 hours of becoming ill. The sixth had eaten raw fish (obtained from a local fish market) the day before entering the hospital.

CLINICAL AND PATHOLOGIC FEATURES

Dioctophymiasis is a rare human infection, and the clinical signs of adult worms in the kidney are vague. Generally, infections cause renal colic, hematuria, pyuria, eosinophilia, and lower back pain. Although there may be episodes of uremia, blood values usually remain normal because a single kidney is usually involved. Diagnosis is made when eggs are discovered in urine (when the female worm is located in the kidney), or in ascitic fluid (when the female worm is in the peritoneal cavity). Often, an adult worm is passed in urine.

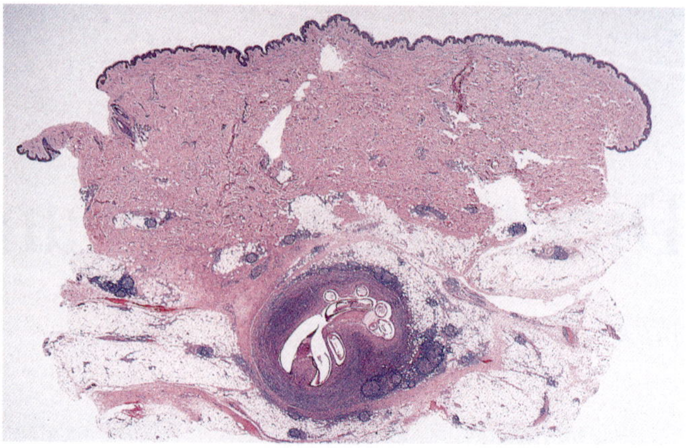

Figure 153–1. Larva of *D renale* in the deep dermis and panniculus. The worm was removed from the abdominal wall of a woman living in Ohio. There is chronic and granulomatous inflammation around the worm and, beyond these, fibrous tissue and lymphoid follicles in adjacent adipose tissue and dermis [whole mount, hematoxylin-eosin (H&E)]. *(Contributed by Dr. Y. Gutierrez.)*

Recently, three cases of subcutaneous dioctophymiasis have been reported—two from the United States and one from Thailand. All three sought treatment for a mass on the chest or abdominal wall. Excision revealed typical dioctophymatid-like larvae. These infections probably involved aberrant migration of larvae out of the patients' peritoneal cavity. None of the patients reported eating raw fish or frogs, yet this remains the most likely source of infection. Histologically, the nodules were described as eosinophilic granulomatous inflammation, consisting of lymphocytes, plasma cells, and eosinophils. There were also bands of fibrous tissue and lymphoid follicles (Figures 153–1 and 153–2).

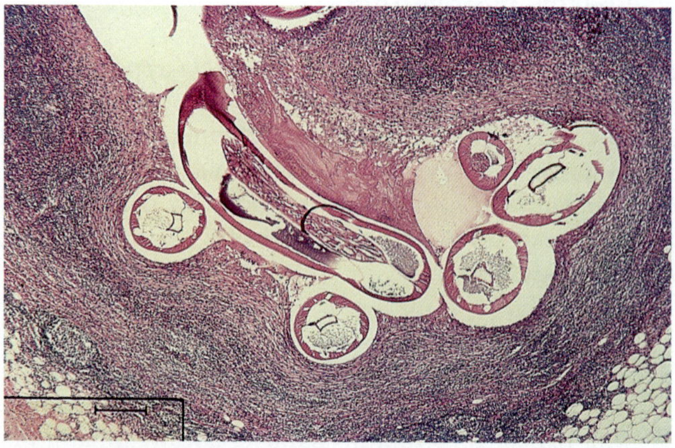

Figure 153–2. Higher magnification of the worm shown in Figure 153–1, showing that the worm is well preserved. The inflammatory exudate near the worm contains fibrin and serum (H&E, ×40). *(Contributed by Dr. Y. Gutierrez.)*

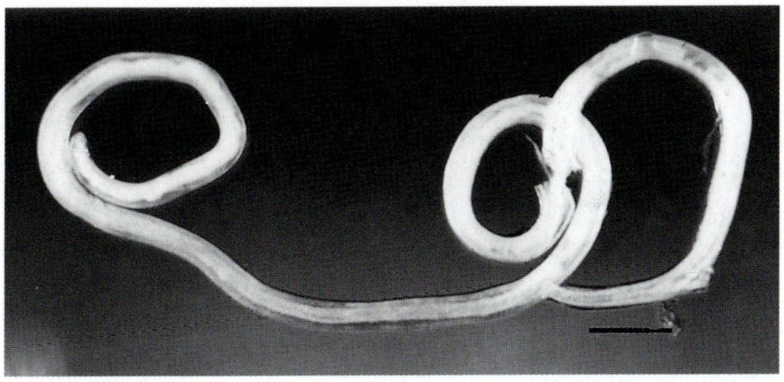

Figure 153–3. Larval *Eustrongylides* removed from the abdominal cavity of a resident of New Jersey who had ingested raw minnows the day before (scale bar = 2 mm). *(From Eberhard et al.[9] with permission.)*

The clinical features of the five patients infected with *Eustrongylides* were distinctly different from those infected with *Dioctophyma* larvae. Patients with eustrongylidiasis had intense abdominal pain localized to the lower right quadrant and lasting 24 hours or less. The patients were afebrile, and leukocyte counts were not remarkable. Some experienced vomiting. Appendicitis was suspected in all patients. During surgery, the appendix was normal, but pinkish-to-reddish worms were moving in the peritoneal cavity or on the surgical drapes (Figure 153–3). There was no perforation of the gut, and a small amount of straw-colored peritoneal fluid was in one patient. Recovery was rapid after surgery. One or two larvae were recovered from each patient. In contrast to infection with larval *D renale,* all patients reported eating live, whole minnows or raw fish a day or two before onset of symptoms.

MORPHOLOGIC FEATURES OF DIOCTOPHYMATOIDAE

Dioctophyma renale and *Eustrongylides* are so similar morphologically when seen in tissue sections that a general description of their morphologic features is given, with differences noted where appropriate. Dioctophymatids are large robust worms, even as larvae (Figure 153–3). Adult female *D renale* are 20 to 100 cm long by 5 to 12 mm in diameter, while male worms range from 14 to 20 cm by 4 to 6 mm. The living worms are typically blood-red. Because of size, location in the kidney, and color, the diagnosis of an infection with adult *D renale* is not difficult.

Adult *Eustrongylides* sp are somewhat smaller: Females are 7 to 15 cm long by 2 to 4.5 mm in diameter and males are 4 to 15 cm by 1 to 2.5 mm. Live specimens are bright red to pink. Adult *Eustrongylides* have not yet been identified as human parasites.

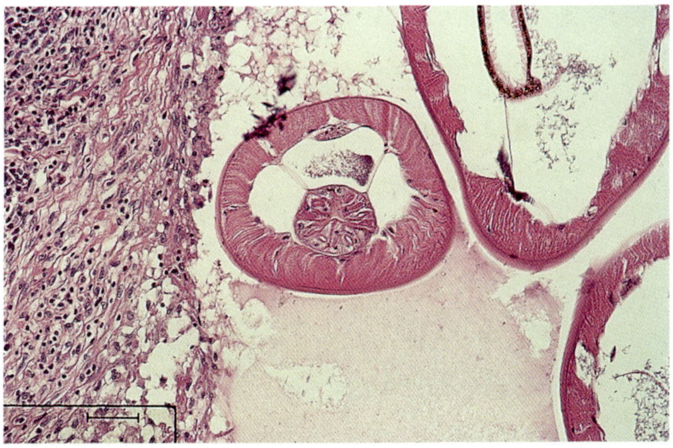

Figure 153–4. Cross-section through the region of the esophagus of the *D renale* larva shown in Figures 153–1 and 153–2. Note the polymyarian–coelomyarian musculature, mesenteric-like membranes, and esophagus with dorsal and subventral glands and branched ducts (H&E, ×100). *(Contributed by Dr. Y. Gutierrez.)*

Larval dioctophymatid worms, including *D renale* and *Eustrongylides* sp, are difficult to separate morphologically. The symptoms they cause, however, are quite different and can help the clinician distinguish between the two. As larvae, both genera are reddish, much as in the adult stage. Dioctophymatid larvae can be identified in cross-sections by several characteristic features. The esophagus has marked dorsal and subventral glands and noticeable branched ducts (Figure 153–4). The body is divided by eight hypodermal cords; the lateral cords are indistinct, and intercordal nuclei are frequent (Figures 153–4 through 153–6). Somatic muscles are

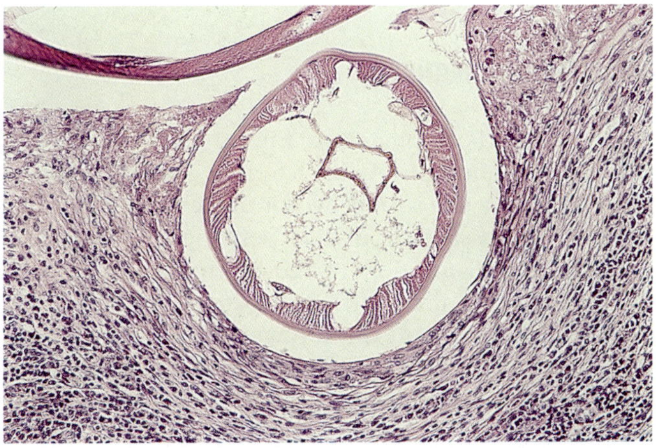

Figure 153–5. Cross-section through the region of the intestine of the dioctophymatid larva contained in the lesion illustrated in Figure 153–1. Note the thick, multilayered cuticle, a multinucleated intestine attached by mesentery-like membranes, several intercordal nuclei, and a small reproductive tube (H&E, ×200). *(Contributed by Dr. Y. Gutierrez.)*

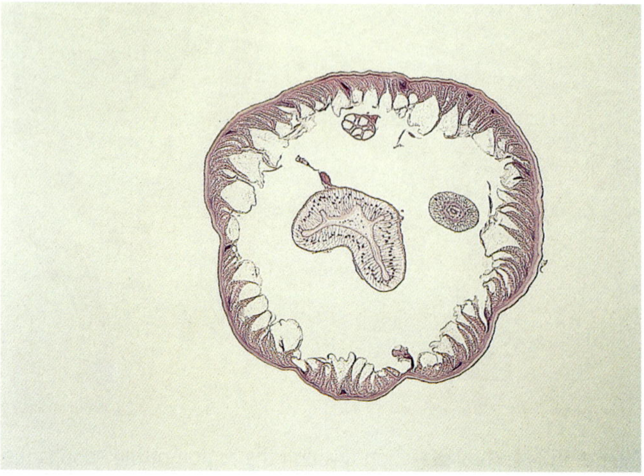

Figure 153–6. Cross-section of larva shown in Figure 153–3. Note the polymyarian–coelomyarian musculature, numerous hypodermal cords, intercordal nuclei, the multinucleated intestine with a prominent microvillus border, and the genital tube (H&E, ×200).

coelomyarian, rather low, and of approximately equal contractile and protoplasmic parts. The intestine is large and consists of low to tall cuboidal epithelial cells with a prominent microvillus border (Figure 153–6). Mesentery-like membranes extend from the somatic musculature to the digestive tract (Figures 153–4 and 153–5). Genital tubes, if present, are generally immature and do not contain sperm or ova. The reproductive system appears to be more developed in *Eustrongylides* than in *Dioctophyma* larvae, at least in those specimens recovered in humans (Figure 153–6).

DIFFERENTIAL DIAGNOSIS

Diagnosis of dioctophymiasis caused by adult worms requires identification of characteristic eggs in urine or recovery of a blood-red worm in urine, from the kidney, or possibly from the peritoneal cavity. The size, color, and location of the worm in the urinary tract should alert the clinician or pathologist to a giant kidney worm. Larval dioctophymatid-like worms in subcutaneous nodules are more difficult to identify, but their distinctive esophageal glands and ducts and mesentery-like membranes attaching the gut to the body wall are characteristic.

Infection with larval *Eustrongylides* is initially diagnosed as acute appendicitis until subsequent recovery of reddish colored larvae. If these specimens are sectioned, the typical dioctophymatid features described for *D renale* are observed. Based on morphologic features, the differentiation of larval *Eustrongylides* from larval *Dioctophyma* is difficult. To date, the clinical signs have been distinctive, with larval *Eustrongylides* causing acute abdominal pain and larval *Dioctophyma* causing a subcutaneous nodule.

Because both *Dioctophyma* and *Eustrongylides* can be acquired by eating raw fish, the clinician may suspect anisakiasis (codworm disease) or other related worm infections if the patient reports eating raw fish. Typically, anisakiasis is acquired after eating sushi or sashimi containing raw marine fish. Although dioctophymatid larvae can be acquired in this manner, they usually are found in freshwater fish. The clinical signs of anisakiasis also tend to differ from those of *Eustrongylides* infections. Anisakiasis commonly causes acute epigastric pain and possibly regurgitation of a worm. There is a marked granulomatous response at the point of attachment. Occasionally, worms are seen during endoscopy. By comparison, in the cases of larval *Eustrongylides* infection reported to date, the larvae successfully penetrated the gut and were migrating in the peritoneal cavity. Further, the bright red color of recovered worms signals dioctophymatid larvae, rather than anisakiasis. No alternative means of diagnosing dioctophymatid infections exist at this time.

REFERENCES

1. Barriga OO. Dioctophymiasis. In: Steele JH, ed. *CRC Handbook Series of Zoonoses, Section C: Parasitic Zoonoses.* Boca Raton, Fla: CRC Press; 1982:83–92.
2. Beaver PC, Theis JH. Dioctophymatid larval nematode in a subcutaneous nodule from man in California. *Am J Trop Med Hyg.* 1979;28:206–212.
3. Beaver PC, Khamboonruang C. Dioctophyma-like larval nematode in a subcutaneous nodule from man in northern Thailand. *Am J Trop Med Hyg.* 1984;33:1032–1034.
4. Gutierrez Y, Cohen M, Machicao CN. Dioctophyme larva in the subcutaneous tissues of a woman in Ohio. *Am J Surg Pathol.* 1989;13:800–802.
5. Measures LN. Revision of the genus Eustrongylides Jagerskiold, 1909 (Nematode: Dioctophymatoidea) of piscivorous birds. *Can J Zool.* 1988;66:885–895.
6. Measures LN. The development of *Eustrongylides tubifex.* (Nematoda: Dioctophymatoidae) in oligochaetes. *J Parasitol.* 1988;74:294–304.
7. Gunby P. One worm in the minnow equals too many in the gut. *JAMA.* 1982;248:163.
8. Wittner M, Turner JW, Jacquette G, Ash LR, Saloo MP, Tanowitz H. Eustrongylidiasis—a parasitic infection acquired by eating sushi. *N Engl J Med.* 1989;320:1124–1126.
9. Eberhard ML, Hurwitz H, Sun AM, Colette D. Intestinal perforation caused by larval *Eustrongylides* (Nematoda: Dioctophymatoidae) in New Jersey. *Am J Trop Med Hyg.* 1989; 40:648–650.

CHAPTER 154

Diphyllobothriasis

Ann M. Adams and Robert L. Rausch

Science is vastly more stimulating to the imagination than are the classics.

J. B. S. Haldane (1892–1964)

Cestodes of the genus *Diphyllobothrium* (order Pseudophyllidea; family Diphyllobothriidae) in the strobilar (sexually reproducing) stage inhabit the alimentary canal (typically the small intestine) of piscivorous birds and mammals, including humans. The genus contains around 50 species that have been more or less adequately characterized,[1] but the relative morphologic uniformity of these cestodes makes their identification difficult. *Diphyllobothrium latum*, a common cestode in people in northern Europe (Finland, East Prussia, Russian Karelia), was the first species to be recognized. That name has been applied routinely by clinicians in North America to any species of *Diphyllobothrium* found in the human host, usually diagnosed on the basis of eggs in feces (eg, ref. 2). Infections by members of the family Diphyllobothriidae and particularly by members of the genus *Diphyllobothrium* are generally referred to as diphyllobothriasis, or "fish tapeworm disease." At least 13 species of *Diphyllobothrium* (Table 154–1) have been reported from humans, with infections by *D dendriticum* and *D latum* being the most prevalent. About 9 million cases of infection involving *D latum* alone were estimated to exist in the 1970s.[3] Many more cases of diphyllobothriasis occur among numerous indigenous peoples in the Northern Hemisphere.

The genus *Spirometra* (Faust, Campbell et Kellogg, 1929) was established for cestodes very similar to *Diphyllobothrium* sp, but which differ in some details of the reproductive organs. Schmidt[4] placed it in synonymy with *Diphyllobothrium,* whereas others, including Beaver et al,[5] accepted it as a valid genus. In the recently published keys to the genera of cestodes in vertebrates, Bray et al[6] distinguished *Spirometra* on the basis of both morphologic characters and well-defined differences in the pattern of the life cycle (fishes not involved).

Diphyllobothriids of other genera, including *Schistocephalus* and *Diplogonoporus,* may also infect humans. The most common appears to be *Diplogonoporus balaenopterae* (synonym, *Diplogonoporus grandis*), typically a symbiont of baleen whales. *Diplogonoporus* is distinguished readily on the basis of the doubling of the female genital organs in each segment. At least 132 infections by *D balaenopterae* have been recorded in Japan[7] since the first was reported 100 years ago.[8]

GEOGRAPHIC DISTRIBUTION

Diphyllobothriasis is most prevalent in northern regions, but diphyllobothriids occur widely also in Africa and South America. Taxa allocated to *Spirometra* are especially common in southeastern Asia, and are present also in Africa. Two of three species of *Diphyllobothrium* reported from humans in the southern hemisphere, *D latum* and *D dendriticum,* evidently have become established through the introduction of nearctic fishes for stocking local waters.[9] The cestodes infecting people differ with geographic region and ecologic conditions. The most widespread is *D dendriticum,* occurring throughout the Northern Hemisphere, but less common at lower latitudes. The distribution of *D latum* is not as extensive as *D dendriticum,* having the major endemic focus in Finland, western Russia, and East Prussia. It apparently has been introduced to Japan, Cuba, Chile, Argentina, Alaska, and the Great Lakes region of North America. Other species that infect man may have more restricted geo-

TABLE 154–1. SPECIES OF DIPHYLLOBOTHRIIDS INFECTIVE TO HUMANS

Species	Life Cycle	Piscine Hosts[a]	Geographic Distribution[b]
Diphyllobothrium alascense	Marine	Burbot, smelt	Kuskokwim Delta (Alaska)
D cameroni	Marine	Marine fishes	Japan
D cordatum	Marine	Marine fishes	Northern Seas
D dalliae	Freshwater	*Dallia pectoralis*	Alaska, Siberia
D dendriticum	Freshwater	Coregonids, grayling, burbot, trout	Circumpolar, introduced: South America
D hians	Marine	Marine fishes	North Atlantic Ocean[c]
D klebanovski	Marine[d]	Salmonids (salmon, trouts, char, etc)	Eastern Eurasia, Sea of Japan, Sea of Okhotsk, probably Alaska
D lanceolatum	Marine	*Coregonus*	North Pacific, Bering Sea
D latum	Freshwater	Pike, burbots	Fennoscandia, western portion of the former USSR; reported from Cuba, South and North America
D nihonkaiense	Freshwater	Salmon	Japan
D pacificum (cf)	Marine	Marine fishes	Peru, Chile, Japan
D ursi	Freshwater	Red salmon	Alaska, British Columbia
D yonagoensis	Marine	Salmon	Japan, eastern Siberia
Diplogonoporus balaenopterae	Marine	Marine fishes	North Pacific region

[a] List not complete.
[b] Distributions of known human infections only.
[c] Possibly North Sea (see Ref. 69).
[d] Originally considered marine although neither the first intermediate hosts involved nor the presence of pores in the egg shells had been determined (see Ref. 70).

graphic distributions; for example, *D alascense* has been reported only from the Yukon–Kuskokwim delta region in Alaska. Diphyllobothriids representing numerous taxa occur in marine mammals, primarily seals and walrus, in arctic and subarctic seas; some may also infect humans. *Diphyllobothrium lanceolatum, D. cordatum,* and *D pacificum* are incidental parasites of humans, the latter two naturally occurring in pinnipeds in the North Pacific. Diphyllobothriids are also common in seals in the Antarctic.

Caution must be expressed at this point, however, since diphyllobothriasis may be far from the origin of the parasite. Modern transportation may deliver fresh, nonfrozen fishes far from the point of capture, and thus infections by *Diphyllobothrium* sp can occur in geographic areas where the cestodes are evidently absent. A classic example involved infections by cestodes designated *D latum* among residents of New York City, traced to fishes from the Great Lakes. Similarly, diphyllobothriasis erupted in Hawaii from eating raw salmon; salmon are not locally available and must be shipped, usually from the Pacific Northwest or Alaska.[10]

LIFE CYCLES

The cycle of diphyllobothriids (Figure 154–1) involves either marine or freshwater intermediate hosts, depending on species. Two intermediate hosts are required, a crustacean and a fish, whereas the strobilar stage occurs only in homothermic vertebrates. The eggs are expelled from the intestine of the final host, and their embryonation takes place in water. After a period of development, the eggs hatch, evidently under the influence of pressure and light, releasing a ciliated embryo, the coracidium. The coracidium is motile, and is able to swim about for some hours. Further development depends on the ingestion of coracidia by small crustacea, usually copepods of the family Diaptomidae, including species of the subfamily Cyclopinae. After being ingested, the coracidium enters the body cavity of the crustacean and transforms into the first larval stage, the procercoid, which has an elongated body with frontal glands and a posterior cercomer (cf ref. 11). Neither the coracidium nor the procercoid of *Diphyllobothrium* sp infects humans.

When infected copepods are ingested by fishes, the procercoid is released and migrates through the tissues of the alimentary canal, thereafter localizing at an anatomic site typical of the given species of *Diphyllobothrium.* The serosal surfaces of the alimentary canal and the musculature of the body are common sites of localization (Figure 154–2). In some fishes, large numbers of larval cestodes are found in the wall of the stomach (Figure 154–3). The procercoid transforms into the infective larval stage, which consists of an elongate, flattened, or more or less cylindrical body, with a smooth to somewhat wrinkled tegument; the anterior end bears a scolex of mature type (Figure 154–4). When the plerocercoid is eaten by the final host, it attaches to

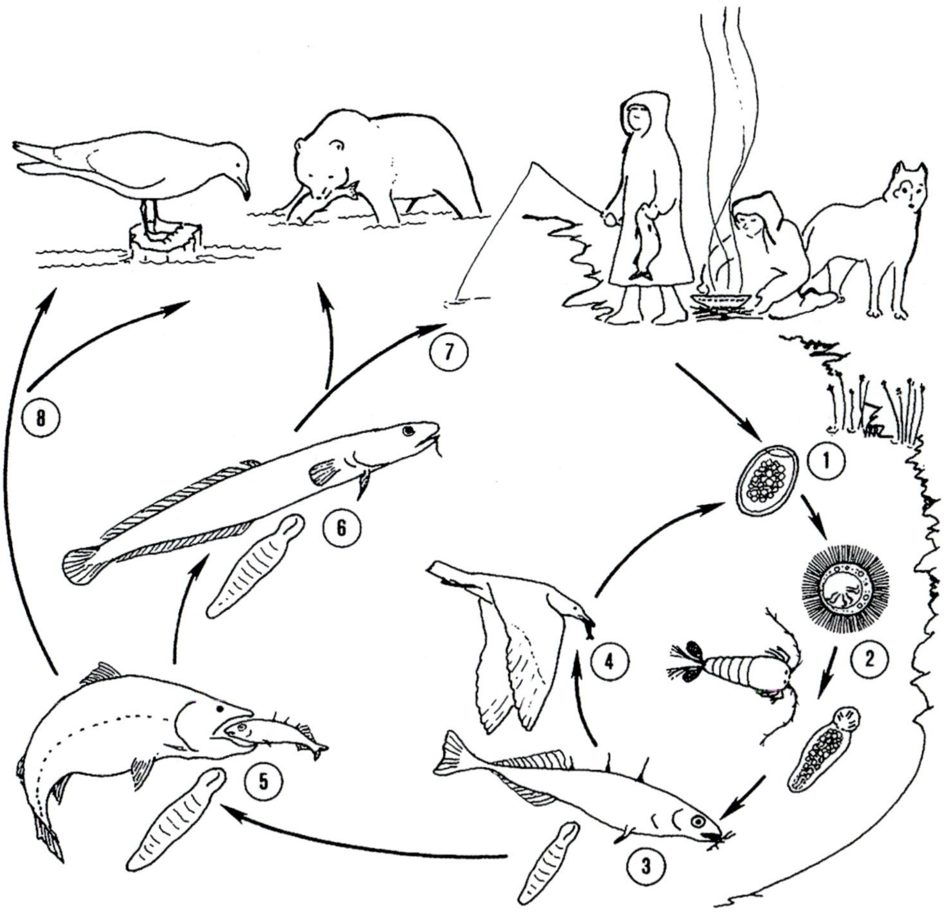

Figure 154–1. Life Cycle of *D dendriticum.* (1) Eggs expelled by final hosts harboring the strobilar stage. (2) Eggs embryonate in freshwater. Motile coracidium emerges, and when eaten by a copepod, transforms to procercoid stage in hemocoel. (3) Copepods with procercoids consumed by small fishes, such as three-spined stickleback; plerocercoid develops in tissues. (4) Infected sticklebacks eaten by gulls, in which the strobilar stage develops. Gulls expel unembryonated eggs. (5) Steelhead trout, large enough to prey on sticklebacks, acquire plerocercoids, which persist until trout are eaten by final hosts. (6) Trout also may be eaten by larger, predacious fishes, such as burbots, to which the plerocercoids transfer in turn. (7) Burbots may be a source of infection of final hosts. (8) Trout, often accumulating many plerocercoids, are important sources of infection for the final hosts. *(Drawing by V. R. Rausch.)*

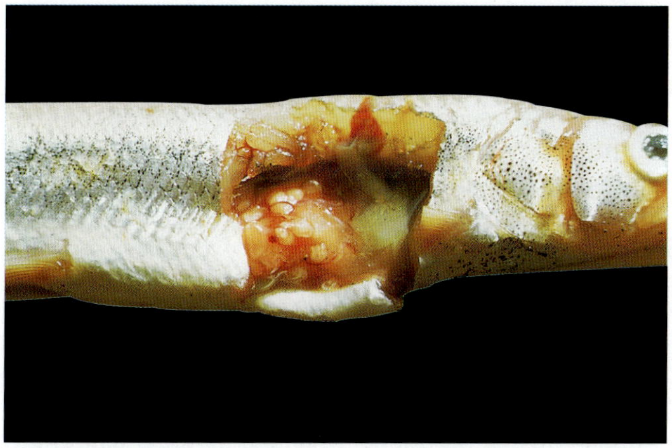

Figure 154–2. Encysted plerocercoids of *Diphyllobothrium* sp in viscera of smelt, Napaskiak (lower Kuskokwim River), Alaska. Opening in side of fish has length of 25 mm.

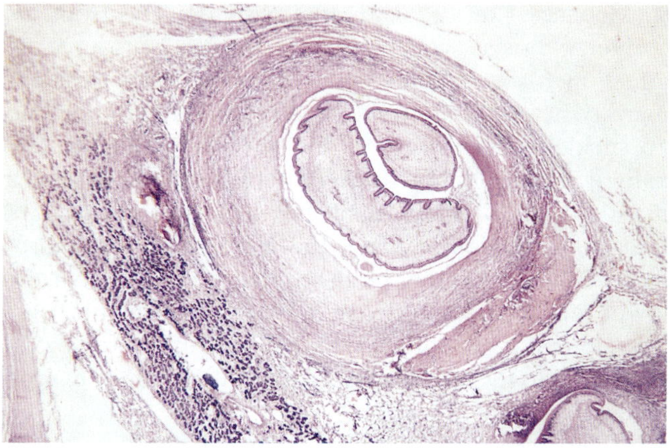

Figure 154–3. Section of plerocercoid of *D dendriticum* in stomach wall of steelhead trout, Kenai Peninsula, Alaska. Width of plerocercoid as shown is 0.7 mm [hematoxylin-eosin (H&E)].

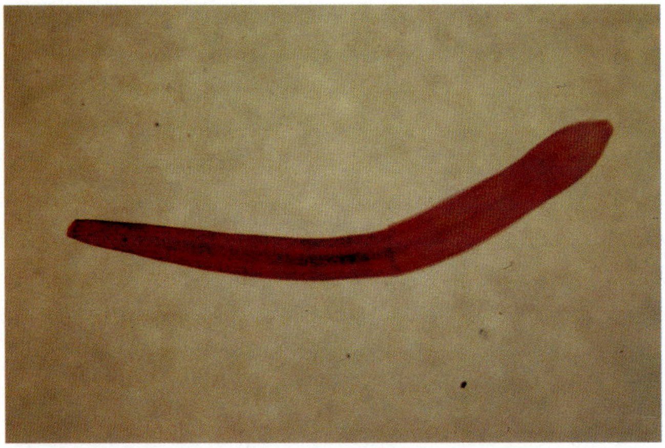

Figure 154–4. Plerocercoid of *D dendriticum* from steelhead trout, Kenai Peninsula. Length is 5.3 mm (acetic carmine).

the intestinal mucosa and begins the process of strobila formation.

When infected fishes are consumed by larger, predacious fishes, the plerocercoids are released by the digestive process, and enter the tissues of the second fish, where they remain without further development until ingested by a homothermic final host. The plerocercoid exhibits little or no host specificity, permitting transfer, apparently, to predacious fishes of any species. When transfer to the second fish occurs, the latter is designated a paratenic host; such transfer enhances the probability that a plerocercoid will complete development to the strobilar stage. In lakes on the Kenai Peninsula of Alaska, plerocercoids of *D dendriticum* develop in sticklebacks (*Pungitius pungitius* and *Gasterosteus aculeatus*), which feed on copepods and other small invertebrates. In the same lakes, trout, *Oncorhynchus mykiss,* did not become infected by plerocercoids until after they had attained a standard length of about 150 mm, when they were large enough to prey on sticklebacks (Ref. 12 and unpublished). The trout, as paratenic hosts, were evidently the major source of infection for carnivores, such as black bears and humans, whereas gulls could be infected either by feeding on sticklebacks, or on trout in the form of carrion. The natural transfer of plerocercoids of cestodes having a marine cycle to freshwater fishes such as burbots, *Lota lota,* may take place when the latter prey on anadromous fishes or on marine fishes that often frequent the lower reaches of large rivers.[12] By feeding on such burbots, terrestrial mammals may become infected by cestodes that in the strobilar stage typically occur in marine mammals.

The cycle of cestodes referred to the genus *Spirometra* differs somewhat from that of *Diphyllobothrium* sp *sensu strictu.* Crustaceans of the genus *Cyclops* serve as first intermediate host.[13,14] When *Cyclops*-containing procercoids are eaten by tadpoles, the plerocercoid (sparganum) develops, and persists through the metamorphosis to the adult frog. Salamanders, snakes, and small mammals may feed on infected tadpoles or frogs, thereby serving as paratenic hosts.[14,15] People may serve as second intermediate hosts, when infected *Cyclops* are ingested, or transfer of spargana may occur by other means (see discussion later). A single species, *S mansonoides* is known in North America, where it occurs in the eastern and southern United States. The domestic cat appears to be a common final host.

As noted above, diphyllobothriids appear usually to exhibit little specificity for the piscine and final (homothermic) hosts. What may seem to indicate host specificity may have an ecologic basis.[12] *Diphyllobothrium ursi,* for example, which attains a length of 10 m or more, is typically found in the brown bear, *Ursus arctos;* this relationship indicates the great extent to which the bears feed on red salmon, *Oncorhynchus nerka.* At the same time, the bears expel great numbers of eggs into the spawning streams, which are carried into lakes where young salmon become infected by feeding on copepods harboring the procercoids. At Karluk Lake (Kodiak Island, Alaska), all of 200 emigrating smolts examined in June were infected, as were 93% of 288 spawning adults examined during August–September.[12] Since the plerocercoids are usually encysted on the viscera of red salmon, humans are not often infected by *D ursi.*

EPIDEMIOLOGY

With the possible exception of *D latum,* cycles of *Diphyllobothrium* sp are maintained in nature independently of humans. Diphyllobothriasis is thus a natural-focal infection that cannot be affected by elimination of the cestodes from the human population. The consumption of raw or incompletely cooked fishes is the most common means of infection in people. Many cultures favor a cuisine that includes raw or lightly marinated fish. Practices of sanitation have a direct impact on the local prevalence of plerocercoids in fishes. The method of disposing of human excreta directly into lakes and rivers greatly favors completion of the cycle.[16,17] In the endemic region of northern Europe, traditional dietary customs contribute to a high prevalence of *D latum* in humans. Guttowa[17] found that infection is influenced by factors such as profession, gender, and age. Fishermen were commonly infected because of their habit of eating raw the roe and livers of their catches. In towns, however, women were most often infected, since they tend to sample foods containing raw fish in the process of preparation. Rates of infection were lowest among children. At Lake

LaRonge, Saskatchewan, however, infection of indigenous people below the age of 5 years was not uncommon (Rausch, unpublished). Also in the lake regions of northern Europe, inadequate methods for sewage disposal tend to disperse eggs of *D latum* in the littoral zone, where rapid warming of waters in spring and penetration of light favor the development of embryos and hatching of eggs.[17] In the Baltic region, the roe of pike, *Esox lucius,* and burbot, *L lota,* is the usual source of infection by *D latum.* In some large North American cities, "gefilte fish" is made from infected fishes and women may become infected by tasting the preparation before cooking. The increasing popularity of fishes prepared in the Japanese manner, particularly in the Pacific Northwest, has led to an increase in diphyllobothriasis.[18] In southwestern Alaska (Yukon–Kuskokwim delta region), where fishes make up a high proportion of the diet of indigenous people, rates of infection by *Diphyllobothrium* sp earlier ranged up to about 30%.[19] High rates have been recorded also in the Russian Far East. In the Republic of Sakh (Iakutia), data extending over the period 1957–1992 showed fluctuations in prevalences from 208 in 1982 to 987 per 100,000 in 1960; for 1992, the rate was 386.[20]

The history of diphyllobothriasis in the Great Lakes region, especially in Minnesota, is of interest with respect to the apparent introduction of *Diphyllobothrium* cf *latum* and its subsequent decline. Nickerson[21] was evidently the first to report autochthonous cases in Minnesota; he also found plerocercoids of *Diphyllobothrium* sp in fishes in the Great Lakes. Ward[22] thought *D latum* had been introduced by immigrants from northern Europe. Primitive methods of sewage disposal ensured that eggs of *Diphyllobothrium* reached an environment suitable for development of the larval stages.[23] Improved sanitary practices as well as changes in dietary habits, over time, probably contributed to the significant reduction in the incidence of infection in that region. Whether or not the cestode is *D latum,* its persistence evidently can be attributed to the role of the black bear, *Ursus americanus,* and other carnivores, as final host.[24]

Sparganosis is invasion of extraintestinal tissues by the plerocercoid stage (sparganum) of cestodes of the genus *Spirometra.* Mammals unsuitable as final hosts become infected when ingested spargana pass through the intestinal wall and migrate through various tissues.[14] In humans, infection by a sparganum may result when frogs are opened and bound to inflamed eyes or other parts of the body as a therapeutic poultice, a not uncommon practice in southeastern Asia.[25] Infection may also follow eating raw snakes.[26] Uchida et al, for example, found that 88% of 59 snakes examined in Kanagawa Prefecture, Japan, harbored spargana.[27] Humans may function as second intermediate hosts of *Spirometra* sp when *Cyclops* sp harboring the procercoids are ingested in drinking water. Ingestion of infected *Cyclops* may be the most common source of infection of persons living in the United States.[28]

The course of infection when spargana were introduced surgically into subcutaneous tissues of human volunteers was described by Mueller and Coulston.[29] The larvae tended to migrate, and evoked an allergic response characterized by edema and urticaria. Although only the scolices removed from spargana were inoculated, the bodies regenerated and increased in length at a rate of about 2 cm per month.

MORPHOLOGY AND DESCRIPTION

The specific identification of *Diphyllobothrium* is usually difficult, because of a high degree of morphologic similarity. Stunkard, for instance stated that the species of *Diphyllobothrium* occurring in mammals could not be ". . . positively and fully characterized" (cf Stunkard,[30] p. 622). For adequacy of study, specimens must be relaxed before fixation, in order to make comparisons of taxonomic characters. Contracted strobilae (eg, those placed directly in formalin solution without relaxation) often are not identifiable. The cestodes must be stained for study, and medial sagittal sections, as well as transverse sections, prepared. In addition, the removal of the tegument and underlying layers of muscle facilitates examination of the reproductive organs.

Although species of *Diphyllobothrium* can be distinguished by means of reliable taxonomic characters, identification needs to be made by an experienced taxonomist. For best results, entire, relaxed strobilae, fixed in hot formalin solution, should be submitted. Sections made by standard histologic methods are too thin to be of value; thicker sections cut by hand with a razor, however, provide a three-dimensional view permitting the ducts to be traced and the relative position of organs to be defined.

Cestodes of the genus *Diphyllobothrium* in the strobilar (adult) stage range in length from a few millimeters to 15 m or more, with proportional numbers of proglottids. The scolices (Figures 154–5, A and B) differ in shape, from cordate to narrowly lanceolate, and have two longitudinal grooves, the bothria, situated dorsally and ventrally, by which the cestodes attach to the intestinal mucosa of the final host. The scolices are quite mobile and, thus, may vary in shape when living cestodes are fixed by sudden immersion in hot solutions. Individual segments are usually craspedote, and wider than they are long, often with relative length-increasing posteriad. Some strobilae are much attenuated anteriorly; those of other species widen rather abruptly posterior to the scolex. The vitellaria consist of

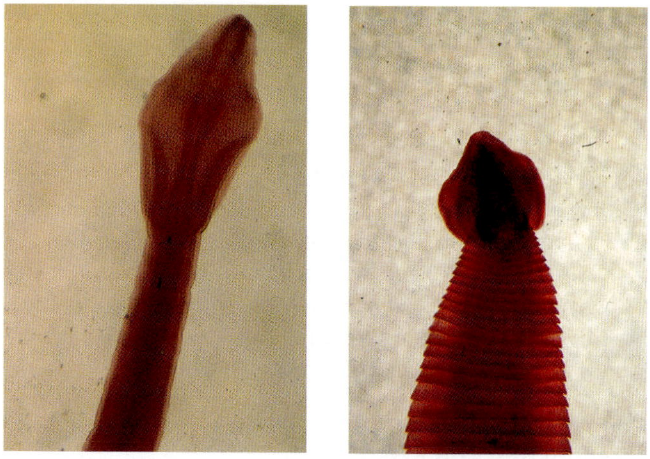

A B

Figure 154–5. (**A**) Scolex of *D latum,* from a human, lower Kuskokwim River. Maximum width of this specimen is 0.7 mm (acetic carmine). (**B**) Cordate scolex of *D cordatum,* from bearded seal, St. Lawrence Island, Bering Sea. Maximum width of this specimen is 1.8 mm (acetic carmine).

large numbers of follicles, distributed dorsally and ventrally over the segmental surfaces, but usually not overlying the central areas within which the genital ducts are situated. The genital ducts and uterus open medially on the ventral surface (Figure 154–6), usually near the anterior end of the segment. The ovary, typically bilobed, is situated medially near the posterior margin of the segment. The vagina extends anteriad along the midline of the ventral surface, opening in the genital atrium just posterior of the orifice of the male duct. The uterus forms numerous, more or less transverse loops in the middle field of the segment, and expels eggs from the uterine pore, posterior to the openings of the genital ducts. The male copulatory organs consist of the cirrus sac and an external seminal vesicle usually situated posteriorly at the distal end of the cirrus sac; the testes are very numerous, distributed in one or more layers in the parenchyma. The egg is ovoidal to ellipsoidal, with a well-defined operculum. Eggs of species having a freshwater cycle have a smooth covering; those developing in marine habitat have coverings with numerous pores (see ref. 31, Figures 2–12).

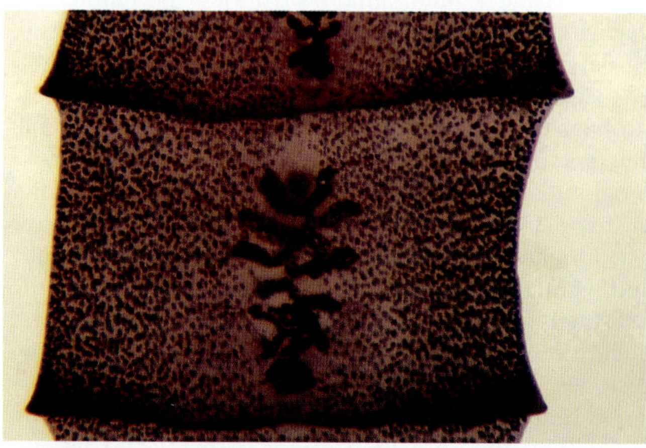

Figure 154–6. Segment of *D dendriticum,* from gull, lower Elbe River, Germany. Length of segment is 3 mm (hematoxylin).

Differentiation of *Diphyllobothrium* sp involves the evaluation of various taxonomic characters. The shape and dimensions of the scolex and the presence or absence of a neck are important. Dimensions of the eggs, size of the cirrus sac, distribution of testes and vitellaria, and the shape of the ovary must all be considered. Sagittal sections (Figure 154–7) permit examination of the relationships of the respective organs, including the course of the vagina, characteristics of the cirrus sac and external seminal vesicle, and the relative distance between the genital atrium and the uterine pore. The arrangement of the testes, whether in one or more layers, and the characteristics of the layers of the muscle fibers also are useful.

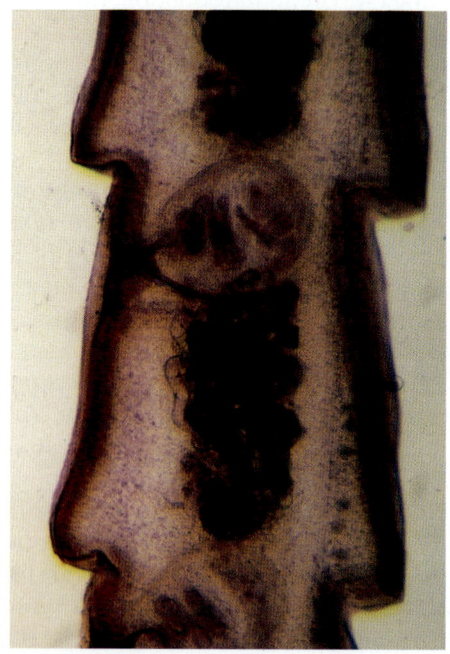

Figure 154–7. Segment of *D alascense,* sagittal section. Cirrus sac measures 470 μm long by 340 μm in diameter. The cirrus sac, opening in the genital atrium anterior to the vagina, is the large ovoid structure. The uterus opens slightly posterior to the vaginal orifice, which is situated in the genital atrium. The vagina, extending anteriad, is the thin-walled tube partially concealed by the gravid uterus (hematoxylin).

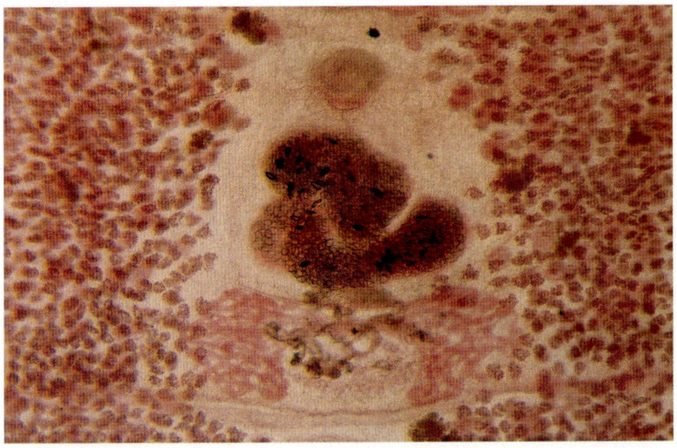

Figure 154–8. Central area of segment of *Spirometra* cf *decipiens* from dog, Philippine Islands. Vaginal orifice visible as transverse slit (160 μm in width) just posterior to cirrus sac. Reticulate ovary visible at posterior margin of segment (acetic carmine).

A primary difference between species of *Diphyllobothrium* and those of *Spirometra* is that in the latter, the male and female ducts open separately, not together within the genital atrium (Figure 154–8). The patterns of their life cycles also differ significantly with respect to transmission of the larval stages.

MICROSCOPY

Specific identification of diphyllobothriids usually requires the entire specimen. As indicated in the Morphology section, specimens must be properly handled during fixation and processing to provide adequate material for identification. Fixation of live specimens preferably involves the use of hot (not boiling) 10% formalin solution. The preserved specimen can be stored in 10% formalin solution or in 70% ethanol. As noted, identification requires stained and sectioned material. Acetic carmine is the most commonly used biologic stain for cestodes; hematoxylin, a nuclear stain, also may be used, especially for showing genital ducts. Both transverse and sagittal sections are usually necessary for determination of species. Such sections should be thicker than the standard 5 to 15 μm of histologic preparations, and should be cut by hand with a fine razor blade to approximately 50 μm.

Observations detailed earlier in the Morphology section are made almost exclusively with a compound light microscope. Optical systems such as phase contrast or differentiated (Nomarsky) interference contrast are helpful for elucidation of some structures. Electron microscopy, both transmission and scanning, is generally unnecessary for the identification and diagnosis of diphyllobothriasis.

Scanning electron microscopy (SEM), however, has been used to examine eggs, adults, and plerocercoids. Hilliard[31] demonstrated that the presence of pores in the eggshells of *Diphyllobothrium* is correlated with a marine life cycle and that the arrangement of these pores appears to be species specific (Figure 154–9). Scanning electron microscopy involving adult strobilae provides no further information for identification than can be acquired through the use of a compound light microscope. For example, Yamane et al[32] studied four species of *Diphyllobothrium* using SEM. They defined differences existing among the scolices, bothria, shapes of plerocercoids, and distribution of genital papillae in adults. All of those characteristics are discernible with light microscopy. In regard to the last characteristic, our own studies (Rausch and Adams, in preparation) have revealed considerable variation in the distribution of genital papillae in segments of single strobilae. Given the preparation time and materials necessary for SEM, the application of that technology to the study of adults of *Diphyllobothrium* appears unwarranted.

Scanning electron microscopy of plerocercoids of *Diphyllobothrium* spp does show greater detail than obtainable through standard microscopy. Several researchers have proposed that this technology can provide a means of specific identification, with what we view as debatable success. Anderson and Gibson[33] proposed a key to the identification of plerocercoids of three species of *Diphyllobothrium*. Those authors, however, stressed a particular method of fixation of live material because other commonly used methods or

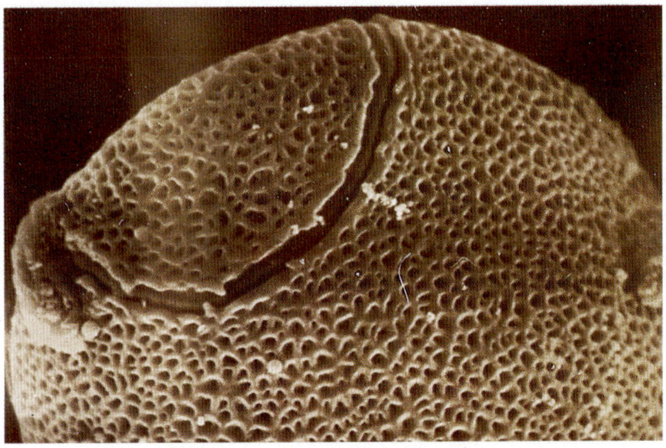

Figure 154–9. Scanning electron micrograph of egg of *D lanceolatum*, from bearded seal, Bering Sea, showing pores in the eggshell. Eggs of *D lanceolatum* average 65 by 42 μm.

specimens acquired from frozen hosts would be too relaxed to "exhibit some of the diagnostic characters." Information derived by SEM contributed minimally to their key. In addition, their key relied on the body length of the plerocercoid and the site occupied within the piscine host. The criterion of body length must be used with caution; Rausch (unpublished) found two morphologically dissimilar plerocercoids in trout; an elongate, thin type within the musculature and a short one associated with the viscera. The recovery of adult cestodes from experimentally infected dogs and gulls revealed that both were plerocercoids of *D dendriticum.* Other work on plerocercoids of *Diphyllobothrium* has considered the shapes and profusion of microtriches on the surface of the tegument; those characteristics may prove to be diagnostic and are primarily visible with SEM.[32–34]

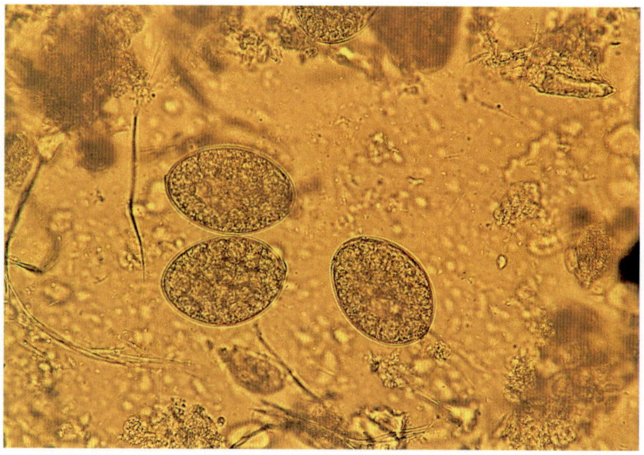

Figure 154–10. Eggs of *D latum,* from human feces, Yukon–Kuskokwim delta, Alaska. Dimensions are about 63 by 49 μm (orange filter).

DIAGNOSIS

Diagnosis of diphyllobothriasis is made on examination of the characteristic proglottids and/or eggs in the stool. The eggs may be detected in smears made from fresh or fixed fecal material. Identification as to species of *Diphyllobothrium* cannot be made from dimensions of eggs alone. At this time, the effective method of diagnosis still requires the isolation of eggs or proglottids from the feces, although recent work has been done to identify copro-antigens of cestodes, primarily species of *Taenia* and of *Diphyllobothrium,* utilizing enzyme-linked immunosorbent assay (ELISA) techniques.[35,36] Additionally, immunoelectrophoresis has been used to differentiate between species of *Diphyllobothrium* with extracts made from the mature proglottids.[37]

Sparganosis is usually diagnosed after the subcutaneous or otherwise situated nodules caused by them are excised. Migration of the larvae results in changing location of the nodules.[28] The spargana are generally found in subcutaneous tissue, viscera, and skeletal muscle. In women, the larvae seemed to localize in disproportionate numbers in the breasts; however, that impression may be attributable only to the greater awareness and concern about any abnormalities appearing in those appendages.[38] Rarely, the larvae may migrate into the brain; worldwide, seven cases of cerebral sparganosis have been reported.[39]

DIFFERENTIAL DIAGNOSIS

Of the cestodes that occur in the strobilar stage in humans, diphyllobothriids are distinguished by the presence of bothria on the scolex, opening of the genital ducts on the ventral surface of the segment, arrangement of the vitelline glands and testes, and by operculated eggs (Figure 154–10). *Mesocestoides* sp (Mesocestoididae: Cyclophyllidea) also have the genital ducts opening ventrally, but differ in other morphologic details.

The eggs of *Diphyllobothrium* sp (including *Spirometra* sp) are similar to those of a digenetic trematode, *Nanophyetus salmincola* (Troglotrematidae), and the eggs of that trematode may be mistaken for those of diphyllobothriids (ref. 40, p. 191). *Nanophyetus salmincola* occurs widely in the Pacific Northwest region of the United States, and in eastern Siberia. As for *Diphyllobothrium* sp, *N salmincola* may be in people who have consumed salmonids far from the place of origin. Depending on the intensity of infection, the trematodes may cause diarrhea.[41]

Differential diagnosis must be made between pernicious anemia caused by autoimmune mechanisms and anemia caused by *D latum.* Tapeworm anemia is indicated when megaloblastic anemia occurs in young persons; by the presence of free HCl in gastric juice; and a normal Schilling test value after antihelminthic removal of the cestode(s).

SYMPTOMS AND CLINICAL FEATURES OF INFECTION

The prepatent period varies with species of cestode. In experimental infections of *D dendriticum* in human volunteers, eggs first appeared in the feces after 22 to 23 days (Rausch, unpublished). In Europe, the prepatent period for *D latum* has been reported to be a minimum of 24 days.[42] Wardle and Green[43] reported that both persons and dogs first expelled eggs 18 to 20 days postinfection, involving cestodes identified as *D latum* in Manitoba. In general, *Diphyllobothrium* sp grow rapidly, with the ultimate length attained by the strobila depending on the species of cestode. The strobila of *D latum* attains lengths of 10 meters and more; that of *D dendriticum* rarely exceeds one meter. Various old reports indicate that *D latum* may survive in the human host for periods in excess of 10 years. In most cases, however, the possibility of reinfection could not be excluded.

A considerable range of symptoms has been subjectively associated with diphyllobothriasis, but none appears to be consistent, and patients often are unaware of harboring the cestodes until portions of strobilae are expelled from the anus. Gastrointestinal symptoms reported include nausea, vomiting, abdominal pain, and diarrhea. Two patients apparently infected through consumption of raw salmon from Alaska in combination experienced abdominal distention, flatulence, eructation, intermittent abdominal pain, and diarrhea.[18] A parasitologist ingested four plerocercoids of *D latum* in Finland and maintained the infection for a year. At least two cestodes developed; he experienced diarrhea about a week postinfection, and again a day or two prior to expulsions of portions of strobilae. Abdominal pain or a vague feeling of pressure was noted intermittently. When his feces were sieved, eggs of the cestodes made up as much as 1/5 to 1/6 of the total volume (R. M. Overstreet, personal communication).

According to von Bonsdorff,[44] patients suffering from *Diphyllobothrium*-induced anemia, usually of long standing, reported such symptoms as fatigue, dizziness, palpitation, paresthesia of digits, and soreness of the tongue. Gastrointestinal symptoms, not differing from those experienced by infected persons who were not anemic, included anorexia, nausea, occasional vomiting, and sometimes abdominal pain and diarrhea.

In northern Europe, a characteristic macrocytic anemia was formerly observed in a small proportion of persons infected by *D latum,* as a consequence of vitamin B_{12} deficiency caused by the competitive utilization of the vitamin by the cestode. The disease was characterized by the following: macrocytic, megaloblastic anemia with leukopenia, thrombocytopenia, and increased hemolysis; neurologic disorders; and decreased levels of vitamin B_{12} in the serum.[3] Studies by Nyberg[45] indicated that the cestodes were able to split the B_{12}-intrinsic factor complex, and of impairing the B_{12}-binding capacity of the intrinsic factor. Nyberg et al[46] reported that the incidence of tapeworm-induced anemia in Finland was at least 1:50 infected persons, and more than 50% of such persons had a serum B_{12} concentration below 100 μμg/mL. *Diphyllobothrium*-induced anemia appears now to be of rare occurrence, as indicated by Curtis and Bylund,[47] who stated that "related in part to a genetic predisposition to this form of the disease, compounded by a poor diet or malnutrition, the anemia associated with diphyllobothriasis has not been reported from Finland in the last two decades." Treatment of such anemia involved expulsion of the cestodes by means of an antihelminthic, followed by administration of vitamin B_{12} without which recovery was very slow.

Other adverse effects of *Diphyllobothrium* sp in the human host have not been defined. A black bear infected experimentally by *Diphyllobothrium* sp (subsequently identified as *D dendriticum*) died as a consequence of invasion of the pancreatic ducts by the cestodes.[48] Although this mechanism of death may be unique for a mammal with diphyllobothriasis it suggests that experimental infection of human volunteers must be done with caution.

TREATMENT

Several antihelminthics are available for expulsion of diphyllobothriids. Drugs of choice are niclosamide, given as a single oral dose of 2 g for adults, and praziquantel, as a single oral dose of 5 to 10 mg/kg. Earlier, higher dosages of praziquantel were recommended,[49] particularly when *D latum* was involved, but the lower dosages have been shown to be efficacious against this and other species of *Diphyllobothrium.*[47,50,51] Both drugs have a high degree of efficacy, especially when followed by a mild purge to ensure expulsion of entire cestodes. If the scolex of the cestode is not eliminated, the worm may be able to resume growth. The purge usually consists of a solution of magnesium sulfate or citrate. If the eggs of *N salmincola* have been mistaken for those of *Diphyllobothrium* sp (see Differential Diagnosis), the recommended dosages may not be adequate. Both niclosamide and praziquantel are effective in eliminating the trematodes, although higher dosages are required: three 2 g doses of niclosamide,[41] or three daily doses of praziquantel at 20 mg/kg.[52]

Other drugs commonly used against diphyllobothriids include biothionol (30 mg/kg total in one or two doses); paromomycin sulfate (4 doses at 1 g every 5 minutes); and quinacrine hydrochloride. Treatment with quinacrine is especially effective for obtaining intact cestodes in good condition for identification; for its use, the patient should remain on a fat-free diet for 24 hours. In the evening, 30 g of magnesium sulfate solution is given; on the following morning, the patient should receive 100 mg of pentobarbital, followed by 1 g of quinacrine and 1 g of sodium bicarbonate. Two hours later, another 30 g of magnesium sulfate is given. No food should be consumed until after defecation. Desapidine and dichlorophene also have been widely used.[47,53] Nagakura et al[53] also recommended another purgative for use after treatment with dichlorophene (50 mg/kg). Two hours after receiving the drug, patients were administered Golytery solution, consisting primarily of polyethylene glycol and magnesium sulfate, at the rate of 1 L/h. Advantages cited are that the solution is isotonic, is not absorbed through the gastrointestinal mucosa, and it is not necessary to restrict intake of food or drink preceding treatment.

A novel treatment was reported by Waki et al,[54] involving introduction of Gastrografin (Schering: sodium and meglumine diatrizoates) into the duodenum by means of intubation. The solution is a radio-opaque contrast medium used in gastrointestinal radiology. Introduction of the solution not only permitted radiographic evidence of infection, but resulted in expulsion of the cestodes usually within 1 hour of treatment. That method is effective but, given the inconvenience of administration and discomfort to the patient, Gastrografin is unlikely to become a drug of choice.

If megaloblastic anemia caused by diphyllobothriasis has been diagnosed, patients should receive vitamin B_{12} after expulsion of the cestodes, until serum levels have become normal. Recovery from the anemia is slow without supplemental therapy. A low serum level of vitamin B_{12} may result in dysfunction of the central nervous system in the absence of anemia, and diphyllobothriasis may be a causal factor in some cases.[55] If signs of B_{12} neuropathy are noted, serum levels of B_{12} should be determined, and antihelminthic treatment should be given, as appropriate.

The spargana of *Spirometra* sp may rarely migrate into the brain, causing convulsions and other neurologic signs; surgical removal of the larval cestode appears to be the best method of treatment.[39]

PREVENTION

As discussed previously, diphyllobothriasis occurs from the ingestion of plerocercoids; therefore, infection can be prevented by the avoidance of viable larvae. As indicated in Table 154–1, salmonids are primary sources of infection for many species of *Diphyllobothrium*. Recent work focusing on aquaculture indicated that, under appropriate circumstances, salmon raised in net pens are free of helminth parasites, including *Diphyllobothrium*.[56,57] The most important factor appears to be the conditioning of the fish to recognize pellets as their only source of food, although invertebrates and smaller fishes may be present within the nets (Adams, unpublished).

In addition to the selection of fish that may be free of plerocercoids, methods exist to decrease the number of plerocercoids within the edible flesh of fishes. Seafood products derived from different portions of fishes have variable numbers of parasitic larvae. Deardorff and Throm[58] noted that salmon strips (fillets cut from the posterior section of the fish) had fewer larvae of the nematode *Anisakis simplex* than steaks. Larvae of both *Anisakis* and *Diphyllobothrium* must penetrate from the viscera to encyst within the flesh, thereby increasing the likelihood of the larvae locating close to the abdominal region.

Candling, the process of transmitting light through fillets to detect parasites, is presently the most commercially viable means of detecting and removing parasitic worms. Unfortunately, the efficacy of the method is dependent on the thickness of the fillet, the presence of oil or pigmentation in the flesh, and the experience of the operator. As an example of the difficulties, candling of small pieces of salmon used in sushi (average thickness, 0.7 cm) failed to detect the presence of larvae of *Anisakis*.[59] In an effort to decrease the numbers of anisakid larvae, many commercial processors trim the napes of fillets; whether this also decreases the incidence of plerocercoids is unknown.

The efficacy of brining as a means to kill or eliminate plerocercoids is highly debatable and dependent on factors such as thickness of the flesh, time of exposure, and the concentrations of acid and salt. Brining fillets so that the concentration of salt within the flesh comprises about 12% of the weight and maintaining these conditions for at least 5 days was effective in killing plerocercoids.[57] Povgalev[60] reported that plerocercoids in chum salmon, *Oncorhynchus keta,* were killed when the salt content within the flesh was 7% or greater. The weight of the fish was a factor for the duration of exposure to the brining solution; for those up to 3 kg, plerocercoids died after 7 to 10 days of exposure to a solution of 35% to 40% salt and 50% to 60% ice of fish weight at −3 to −5°C, while those fish greater than 4 kg required 35 to 39 days.[60] In contrast to the above studies, Curtis and Bylund[47] stated that for cold-smoked and other uncooked products, the concentrations of salt in brining solutions "are often inadequate to eliminate the risk of infection."

The best means of prevention consist of temperature inactivation, either by thoroughly cooking or freezing the seafood product. For both methods, the efficacy is time/temperature dependent. Curtis and Bylund[47] recommended cooking fish to an internal temperature of 55°C for 10 to 30 minutes; Higashi[61] reported that 56°C for 5 minutes will kill plerocercoids of *Diphyllobothrium*. If a thermometer is not available, the fish should be cooked until it loses its translucency and flakes easily with a fork. Cooking with a microwave oven requires a higher temperature to ensure death of larvae because of the uneven heating that occurs. For anisakid larvae, a temperature of 76.7°C was necessary to ensure death.[62] These methods are sufficient to kill plerocercoids as well. During the process of "hot smoking," time and temperature have the primary influence on the death of the cestode larvae; the components of the smoke are considered to have little importance.[63] "Cold smoking" does not involve an increase in temperature sufficient to kill any larvae present and the fish should be frozen prior to the smoking process.

Various attempts have been made to determine the appropriate conditions for freezing. When placed in Hank's solution, a temperature of −9°C was necessary to kill the plerocercoids.[64] Death of the larvae was caused by the formation of ice in the tissue. Using serum, Salminen[65] determined that −15°C was required to kill all the plerocercoids. In an effort to simulate the density of consistency of piscine flesh, minced fish were packed into beakers and plerocercoids were placed in the center.[65] In such a system, −10°C was sufficient to kill the plerocercoids. Experiments using hamsters demonstrated that after exposure to −6°C, the plerocercoids were still infective, but were not able to develop after treatments at −10°C.[66] Plerocercoids of *D dendriticum* in whitefish, *Coregonus autumnalis,* were killed after being subjected to −18°C for 16 or more hours; at −10 to −11°C, 2 days were required[67] Hilliard[68] subjected various species of fish to freezing temperatures; he found that regardless of species, the size of fish, or the location of the plerocercoids within the fish, all larvae were killed when the fish were frozen for 24 hours or more at −18°C. Higashi[61] suggested that fish be frozen at that temperature for 24 to 48 hours. The U.S. Food and Drug Administration recommends that seafood to be served raw or undercooked should first be frozen to −23°C or below for 7 days, or to −35°C for 15 hours or more.[57] Although these recommendations are primarily concerned with killing anisakid larvae, these methods will also kill the plerocercoids.

REFERENCES

1. Deliamure SL, Skriabin AS, Serdiukov AM. Difillobotriidy—lentochnye gel'minty cheloveka, mlekopitaiushchikh i ptits. In: Sudarikov VE, ed. *Osnovy tsestodologii.* Vol 10. Moskva: Nauka; 1985.
2. Kappus KD, Lundgren RG Jr, Juranek DD, Roberts JM, Spencer HJ. Intestinal parasitism in the United States: update on a continuing problem. *Am J Trop Med Hyg.* 1994;50:705–713.
3. von Bonsdorff B. *Diphyllobothriasis in Man.* London: Academic Press; 1977.
4. Schmidt GD. *CRC Handbook of Tapeworm Identification.* Boca Raton, Fla: CRC Press; 1986.
5. Beaver PC, Jung RC, Cupp EW. *Clinical Parasitology.* 9th ed. Philadelphia: Lea and Febiger; 1984.
6. Bray RA, Jones A, Andersen KI. Order Pseudophyllidea Carus, 1863. In: Khalil LF, Jones A, Bray RA, eds. *Keys to the Cestode Parasites of Vertebrates.* Cambridge, UK: CAB International; 1994.
7. Miyazaki I. *An Illustrated Book of Helminthic Zoonoses.* Tokyo: International Medical Foundation of Japan; 1991.
8. Ijima I, Kurimoto T. On a new human tape-worm (*Bothriocephalus* sp). *J Coll Sci Imperial Univ Tokyo.* 1894;11-(part4):371–385 (+1 plate).
9. Torres P, Franjola R, Figueroa L, et al. Researches on Pseudophyllidea (Carus, 1813) in the south of Chile. IV. Occurrence of *Diphyllobothrium dendriticum* (Nitzsch). *J Helminthol.* 1981;55:173–187.
10. Ruttenber AJ, Weniger BC, Sorvillo F, Murray RA, Ford SL. Diphyllobothriasis associated with salmon consumption in Pacific coast states. *Am J Trop Med Hyg.* 1984;33: 455–459.
11. Vogel H. Studien zur Entwicklung von *Diphyllobothrium.* II Teil. *Zeitschr Parasitenk.* 1930;2:629–644.
12. Rausch RL, Hilliard DK. Studies on the helminth fauna of Alaska. XLIX. The occurrence of *Diphyllobothrium latum* (Linnaeus, 1758) (Cestoda: Diphyllobothriidae) in Alaska, with notes on other species. *Can J Zool.* 1970;48: 1201–1219.
13. Mueller JF. The life history of *Diphyllobothrium mansonoides* Mueller, 1935, and some considerations with regard to sparganosis in the United States. *Am J Trop Med Hyg.* 1938;18:41–66.
14. Yutuc LM. Observations on Manson's tapeworm, *Diphyllobothrium erinacei* Rudolphi, 1819, in the Philippines. *Philippine J Sci.* 1951;80:33–51 (+3 plates).
15. Faust EC, Campbell HE, Kellogg CR. Morphological and biological studies on the species of *Diphyllobothrium* in China. *Am J Hyg.* 1929;9:560–583.
16. Rausch RL. Studies on the helminth fauna of Alaska. XXI. Taxonomy, morphological variation, and ecology of *Diphyllobothrium ursi* n sp provis, on Kodiak Island. *J Parasitol.* 1954;40:540–563.
17. Guttowa A. The broad tapeworm, *Diphyllobothrium latum* (L.) (Cestoda, Pseudophyllidea) in the Baltic region. *Parasitol Polon.* 1970;18:323–340.
18. Turner JA, Sorvillo FJ, Chin J, et al. Diphyllobothriasis associated with salmon—United States. *MMWR.* 1981;30: 331–332, 337.
19. Rausch RL, Scott EM, Rausch VR. Helminths in Eskimos in western Alaska, with particular reference to *Diphyllobothrium* infection and anemia. *Trans R Soc Trop Med Hyg.* 1967;61:351–357.
20. Suvorina VI, Simonova NF. Epidemiologicheskie aspekty difillobotriozov v Iakutii. *Meditsinskaia parazitologiia i parazitarnye bolezni.* 1993;(no. 4):23–26.
21. Nickerson WS. The broad tapeworm in Minnesota, with the report of a case of infection acquired in the state. *J Am Med Assoc.* 1906;(March 10):1–7.
22. Ward HB. *The Introduction and Spread of the Fish Tapeworm (Diphyllobothrium latum) in the United States.* Bal-

timore: Williams & Wilkins; De Lamar Lectures, 1929–1930, 1930.
23. Vergeer T. *Diphyllobothrium latum* (Linn, 1758), the broad tapeworm of man. *J Am Med Assoc.* 1928;30: 673–678.
24. Vergeer T. Dissemination of broad tapeworm by wild carnivora. *Can Med Assoc J* 1928;19:692–694.
25. Baer J-G. La sparganose oculaire. *Acta Trop.* 1945;2: 155–157.
26. Weinstein PP, Kawczyk HJ, Peers JH. Sparganosis in Korea. *Am J Trop Med Hyg.* 1954;3:112–127.
27. Uchida A, Uchida K, Itagaki H. Incidence of the pleurocercoids of *Diphyllobothrium erinacei* in amphibians and reptiles of Kanagawa Perfecture. *Bull Azabu Vet Coll.* 1979;4:333–337.
28. Wirth WA, Farrow CC. Human sparganosis. Case report and review of the subject. *J Am Med Assoc.* 1961;177:6–9.
29. Mueller JF, Coulston F. Experimental human infection with the sparganum larva of *Spirometra mansonoides* (Mueller, 1935). *Am J Trop Med.* 1941;21:399–425.
30. Stunkard HW. *Diphyllobothrium stemmacephalum* Cobbold, 1858 and *D latum* (Linn, 1758). *J Parasitol.* 1949; 35:613–624.
31. Hilliard DK. Studies on the helminth fauna of Alaska. LI. Observations on eggshell formation in some diphyllobothriid cestodes. *Can J Zool.* 1972;50:585–592.
32. Yamane Y, Bylund G, Abe K, Osaki Y, Okamoto T. Scanning electron microscopic study of four *Diphyllobothrium* species. *Parasitol Res.* 1989;75:238–244.
33. Anderson KI, Gibson DI. A key to three species of larval *Diphyllobothrium* Cobbold, 1858 (Cestoda: Pseudophyllidea) occurring in European and North American freshwater fishes. *Syst Parasitol.* 1989;13:3–9.
34. Anderson KI, Ching HL, Vik R. A review of freshwater species of *Diphyllobothrium* with redescriptions and the distribution of *D dendriticum* (Nitzsch, 1824) and *D ditremum* (Creplin, 1825) from North America. *Can J Zool.* 1987;65:2216–2228.
35. Sergeeva EG, Shevchenko CF, Basova NN, Freze VI, Dalin MV. Antigennye eritrotsitarnye diagnostikumy dvukh spetsifichnostei (*Diphyllobothrium dendriticum* i *D ditremum*) i ikh ispol'zovanie dlia vyiavleniia koproantitel pri tsestodozakh. *Meditsinskaia parazitologiia i parazitarnye bolezni.* 1987;(no. 6):24–27.
36. Deplazes P, Eckert J, Pawlowski ZS, Machowska L, Gottstein B. An enzyme-linked immunosorbent assay for diagnostic detection of *Taenia saginata* copro-antigens in humans. *Trans R Soc Trop Med Hyg.* 1991;85:391–396.
37. Fukumoto S, Yazaki S, Kamo H, Yamane Y, Tsuji M. Distinction between *Diphyllobothrium nihonkaiense* and *Diphyllobothrium latum* by immunoelectrophoresis. *Jpn J Parasitol.* 1988;37:91–95.
38. Read CP. Human sparganosis in south Texas. *J Parasitol.* 1952;38:29–31.
39. Fan K-J, Pezeshkpour GH. Cerebral sparganosis. *Neurology.* 1986;36:1249–1251.
40. Pod'iapol'skaia VP. Klinika, terapiia, diagnostika, epidemiologiia i profilaktika glistnykh boleznei. In: Pod'iapol'skaia VP, Kapustin VF, eds. *Glistnye bolezni cheloveka,* 3rd ed. Moskva; Medgiz: 1958.
41. Eastburn RL, Fritsche TR, Terhune CA Jr. Human intestinal infection with *Nanophyetus salmincola* from salmonid fishes. *Am J Trop Med Hyg.* 1987;36:586–591.
42. Bergstermann H, Mendheim H, Scheid G. Die parasitischen Würmer des Menschen in Europa. *Ihre Biologie, Pathologie und Therapie.* Stuttgart: Ferdinand Enke Verlag; 1951.
43. Wardle RA, Green NK. The rate of growth of the tapeworm *Diphyllobothrium latum* (L.). *Can J Res.* 1941; 19:245–251.
44. von Bonsdorff B. *Diphyllobothrium latum* as a cause of pernicious anemia. *Exp Parasitol.* 1956;5:207–230.
45. Nyberg W. The influence of *Diphyllobothrium latum* on the vitamin B_{12}-intrinsic factor complex. II. In vitro studies. *Acta Med Scand.* 1960;167:189–192.
46. Nyberg W, Gräsbeck R, Saarni M, von Bonsdorff B. Serum vitamin B_{12} levels and incidence of tapeworm anemia in a population heavily infected with *Diphyllobothrium latum. Am J Clin Nutr.* 1961;9:606–612.
47. Curtis MA, Bylund G. Diphyllobothriasis: fish tapeworm disease in the circumpolar north. *Arct Med Res.* 1991;50:18–25.
48. Rausch RL. Unusual pathogenicity of *Diphyllobothrium* sp in a black bear. *Proc Helminthol Soc Wash.* 1955;22:95–97.
49. Groll E. Praziquantel for cestode infections in man. *Acta Trop.* 1980;37:293–296.
50. Lumbreras H, Terashima A, Alvarez H, Tello R, Guerra H. Single dose treatment with praziquantel (Cesol R, EmBay 8440) of human cestodiasis caused by *Diphyllobothrium pacificum. Tropenmed Parasit.* 1982;33:5–7.
51. Ohnishi K, Murata M. Praziquantel for the treatment of *Diphyllobothrium nihonkaiense* infections in humans. *Trans R Soc Trop Med Hyg.* 1994;88:580.
52. Fritsche TR, Eastburn RL, Wiggins LH, Terhune CA Jr. Praziquantel for treatment of human *Nanophyetus salmincola (Troglotrema salmincola)* infection. *J Infect Dis.* 1989;160:896–899.
53. Nagakura K, Uchida T, Sakata M. A new and effective purge (Golytery) for expelling tapeworms from the gastrointestinal tract after chemotherapy. *Intern Med.* 1992;31:840.
54. Waki K, Oi H, Takahashi S, Nakabayashi T, Kitani T. Successful treatment of *Diphyllobothrium latum* and *Taenia saginata* infection by intraduodenal "Gastrografin" injection. *Lancet.* 1986;(November 15):1124–1126.
55. Goldblatt D. Luther in worms and vice versa. *Sem Neurol.* 1993;13:234–236.
56. Deardorff TL, Kent ML. Prevalence of larval *Anisakis simplex* in pen-reared and wild-caught salmon (Salmonidae) from Puget Sound, Washington. *J Wldlf Dis.* 1989; 25:416–419.
57. Deardorff TL, Overstreet RM. Seafood-transmitted zoonoses in the United States: the fishes, the dishes, and the worms. In: Ward DR, Hackney C, eds. *Microbiology of Marine Food Products.* New York: Van Nostrand Reinhold; 1990.
58. Deardorff TL, Throm R. Commercial blast-freezing of third-stage *Anisakis simplex* larvae encapsulated in salmon and rockfish. *J Parasitol.* 1988;74:600–603.
59. Adams AM, Leja LL, Jinneman K, Beeh J, Yuen GA, Wekell

MM. Anisakid parasites, *Staphylococcus aureus* and *Bacillus cereus* in sushi and sashimi from Seattle area restaurants. *J Food Prot.* 1994;57:311–317.

60. Povgalev AS. Obezvreshivanie tikhookeanskikh lososei ot plerotserkoidov typa F. *Meditsinskaia parazitologiia i parazitarnye bolezni.* 1988;(No. 5):88–91.
61. Higashi GI. Foodborne parasites transmitted to man from fish and other aquatic foods. *Food Technol.* 1985;(March): 69–74, 111.
62. Miller KS, Adams AM, Wekell MM, Dong FM. Survival of *Anisakis simplex* in microwave processed Arrowtooth flounder (*Atheresthes stomias*). Paper presented at Institute of Food Technologists annual meeting; June 1994; Atlanta, Ga. Abstract.
63. Salminen K. The effect of household smoking on the infestiveness of *Diphyllobothrium latum* from fish to man. *Acta Vet Scand.* 1970;11:228–235.
64. Wikgren B-J, Nikander P. Cause of death of plerocercoids of *Diphyllobothrium latum* (L.) at low temperatures. *Mem Soc Fauna Flora Fenn.* 1964;40:189–192.
65. Salminen K. The effect of low temperatures on the motility of *Diphyllobothrium latum* plerocercoids. *Acta Vet Scand.* 1970;11:236–246.
66. Salminen K. The infestiveness of heat and cold exposed *Diphyllobothrium latum* plerocercoids on golden hamster. *Acta Vet Scand.* 1970;11:247–253.
67. Pronin NM, Pronina SV, Voronov MG, Timoshenko TM. Vyzhivaemost' plerotserkoidov *Diphyllobothrium dendriticum* pri pererabotke ryby i sanitarno-gel'mintologicheskaia otsenka produktsii. *Meditsinskaia parazitologiia i parazitarnye bolezni.* 1989;(no. 4):57–60.
68. Hilliard DK. The effects of low temperatures on larval cestodes and other helminths in fish. *J Parasitol.* 1959;45: 291–294.
69. Kamo H, Yazaki S, Fukumoto S, et al. The first human case infected with *Diphyllobothrium hians* (Diesing, 1850). *Jpn J Parasitol.* 1988;37:29–35.
70. Muratov IV, Posokhov PS. Vozbuditel' difillobotrioza cheloveka—*Diphyllobothrium klebanovskii* sp n. *Parazitologiia.* 1988;22:165–170.

CHAPTER 155

Dirofilariasis

Lisa G. Portnoy

Every man carries a parasite somewhere.

Japanese Proverb

DEFINITION

Dirofilariasis is infection by filarial nematodes of the genus *Dirofilaria*. There are two forms of the disease in humans: pulmonary dirofilariasis caused by *Dirofilaria immitis,* the dog heartworm, and subcutaneous dirofilariasis caused by *Dirofilaria tenuis*, a natural parasite of raccoons, and *Dirofilaria repens,* a natural parasite of dogs and cats in Europe, Asia, and North Africa.

PULMONARY DIROFILARIASIS

History and Geographic Distribution

The first report of human infection with a *Dirofilaria* was in 1887 when de Magalhaes reported finding one male and one female worm in the left ventricle of a male child from Rio de Janeiro, by Robinson et al, quoted by Asimacopoulos.[1] Dashiell published the first case of human dirofilariasis with pulmonary infarction in a 57-year-old woman from Detroit, Michigan, in 1961.[2] Since 1992, more than 80 cases have been reported in the United States.

Dirofilaria species are widespread, and infections in humans have been reported from both temperate and tropical regions around the world, including the United States, the former Soviet Union, Canada, Australia, Japan, Sri Lanka, Malaysia, and many Mediterranean countries.[3] Human pulmonary dirofilariasis is rare but increasing as it parallels the spread and the prevalence of dirofilariasis in the reservoir canine population. In the United States, human dirofilariasis has been reported from 17 states but is most common along the eastern, southeastern, and southern coastal states.

Life Cycle

The life cycles of all species of *Dirofilaria* are similar, and *D immitis* has been studied most extensively. The mosquito (*Culex, Aedes,* and *Anopheles*) serves as vector and intermediate host, and the dog is definitive host. The adult female worm resides in the right ventricle of the dog and sheds microfilariae into the blood. Circulating microfilariae are ingested by the mosquito and molt twice in the mosquito's malpighian tubules. In 10 to 17 days larvae mature to the infective third stage. When the mosquito feeds again, these third-stage larvae are injected into the skin of the dog. The larvae burrow into the subcutaneous tissue, mature over a period of 60 to 120 days, and then migrate through blood vessels to the right ventricle, where the adult worms reach sexual maturity in about 6 months. There they mate and begin a new cycle. Some dogs acquire an enormous, and sometimes fatal, burden of worms[4] (Figure 155–1) and for this reason dogs in endemic areas should be given diethylcarbamate citrate or ivermectin to prevent infections. In humans, however, infections are rare, spurious, and benign.

Human's are unsuitable hosts for *D immitis* so the larvae do not mature. Most larvae are arrested in the subcutaneous tissues and never reach the right ventricle. Those that do fail to mature. Eventually they let go of the endocardium and are swept along with the blood into the right pulmonary artery, impact and obstruct a small branch, and there form the nidus of a subpleural lesion.[5]

Epidemiology

Pulmonary dirofilariasis is about twice as common in men as women. Most patients are over 60 years—the

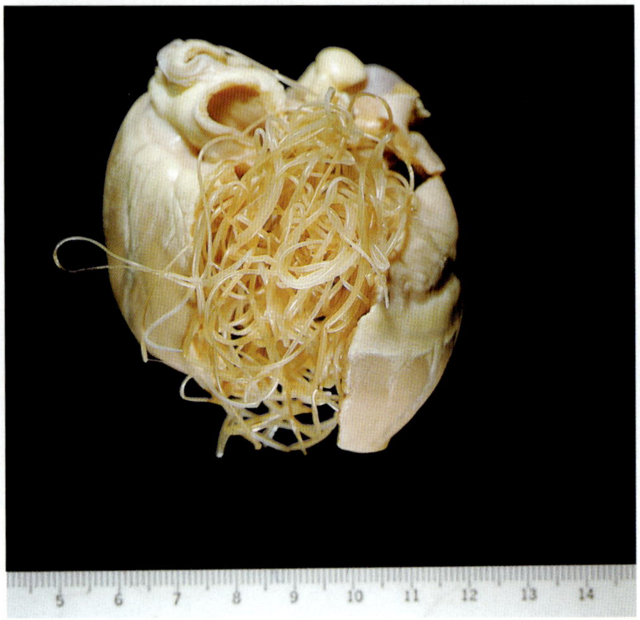

Figure 155–1. A mass of entangled *D immitis* worms fills the right ventricle of this 7-year-old beagle. *Dirofilaria immitis* is a common filarial parasite of dogs in many parts of the world. This dog died of congestive heart failure (gross, ×0.5). *(By D. H. Connor, MD, 1994.)*

youngest a woman of 28 and the oldest a man of 77. The median age is about 50. No infections have been reported in children, probably because few radiographs of the chests are taken in this age group.[6,7]

Morphology

The adult *D immitis* is slender, white, and round, 1 to 2 mm in diameter. Mature female worms are 25 to 30 cm long, while male worms are shorter, 12 to 16 cm. Only immature worms have been found in human lungs. These worms are 100 to 350 μm in diameter. The cuticle is multilayered, 5 to 25 μm thick, and projects inward at the lateral chords to form internal diametrically opposed longitudinal ridges. The surface of the cuticle is ridged with fine transverse striations about 3 μm apart. The lateral chords are usually poorly preserved and difficult to identify. There is an abundance of somatic muscle projecting far into the body cavity. Internal organs are an intestine and two uteri in the female worm, and an intestine and a single reproductive tube in the male worm. These immature worms contain no ova, spermatozoa, or microfilariae.[8]

Clinical Features

Most patients are asymptomatic, and the lesion is discovered incidentally by routine chest x ray. Chest radiographs in patients with pulmonary dirofilariasis usually reveal a single, round subpleural "coin lesion" (Figure 155–2).[9] The nodule is usually 2 to 3 cm in diameter and contains no x-ray evidence of mineral deposits. More than one third of patients have symptoms and these are chest pain, malaise, cough, hemoptysis, and low-grade fever. Peripheral eosinophilia is infrequent, probably because only a very small amount of antigen is released.

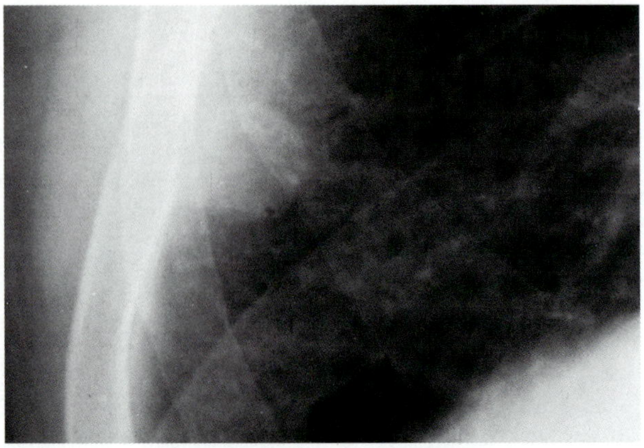

Figure 155–2. A 66-year-old man had this solitary "coin lesion" in the right lower lobe. It was discovered on routine chest radiograph. The excised nodule was spherical, and 2.5 cm in diameter. There was no calcification.[8] *(From Ref. 9.)*

Pathology

The lesions begin when the immature larva impacts in a small pulmonary arteriole. The lesion probably begins as a small pulmonary infarct and when seen on x ray is radiodense, spherical, subpleural, and circumscribed. Excised nodules have a perimeter of gray fibrous tissue and a granular light gray to tan center (Figure 155–3). Careful inspection of the cut surface may reveal fragments of the coiled worm. Microscopically there is central coagulation necrosis around which are scattered histiocytes, monocytes, lymphocytes, eosinophils, and a few Langhans' giant cells (Figure 155–4). A small arteriole in the lesion contains thrombotic material around a single larva in some stage of disintegration (Figure 155–5). The worm is faintly eosinophilic and easily overlooked (Figure 155–6). The Movat pentachrome stain helps distinguish components of vessel wall and anatomic features of the worm, especially the worm's cuticle, its muscle, and its internal organs (Figures 155–7 and 155–8).

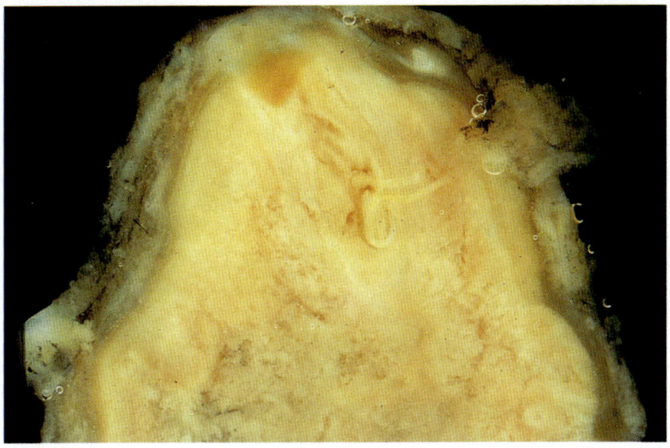

Figure 155–3. Pulmonary dirofilariasis. Fragments of degenerating worm are on the cut surface. The periphery of the nodule is fibrogranulomatous. *(By D. H. Connor, MD, 1978.)*

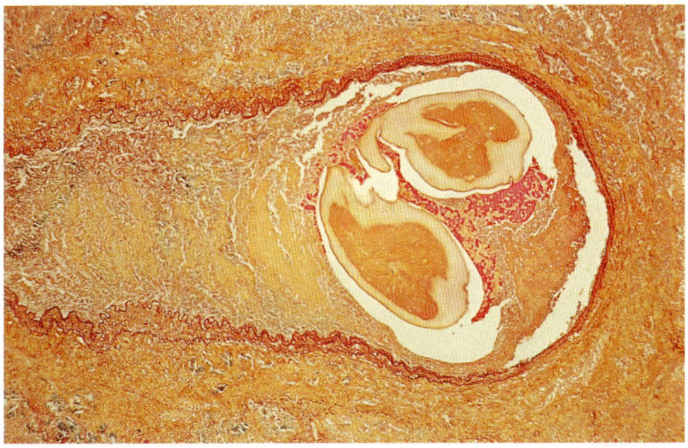

Figure 155–5. The same nodule shown in Figure 155–4. A coiled degenerating *D immitis* worm is embedded in thrombus and occludes this branch of the pulmonary artery. Elastic fibers (black) identify the structure as an artery and help distinguish the various parts of the worm (Movat stain, ×60).

Differential Diagnosis

There are many causes of subpleural "coin lesions," which must be considered in the differential diagnosis, including carcinoma, tuberculosis, fungal infections, and hamartomas.

Diagnosis

Human pulmonary dirofilariasis must be diagnosed by excising the nodule and identifying the immature *D immitis* worm in an arteriole in the lesion. Serologic methods including enzyme-linked immunosorbent assay and indirect immunofluorescence are used routinely by veterinarians to diagnose amicrofilaremic (occult) canine *D immitis* infection, whereas indirect hemagglutination is used for humans with suspected pulmonary dirofilariasis. The results of indirect hemagglutination tests may be difficult to interpret because of cross-reactions with a wide variety of human helminthic parasites.[10]

Twice, diagnosis of dirofilariasis was made without surgical removal of the nodule. A fine-needle biopsy of

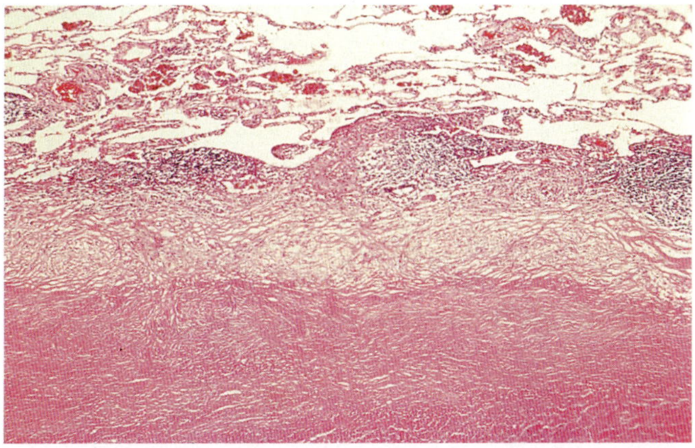

Figure 155–4. The perimeter of the nodule is sharply demarcated from adjacent lung. The central portion of the nodule retains a ghost outline of previously viable lung, suggesting infarction but this is surrounded by a fibrogranulomatous margin, probably a reaction to antigens released from the degenerating worm [hematoxylin-eosin (H&E), ×60].

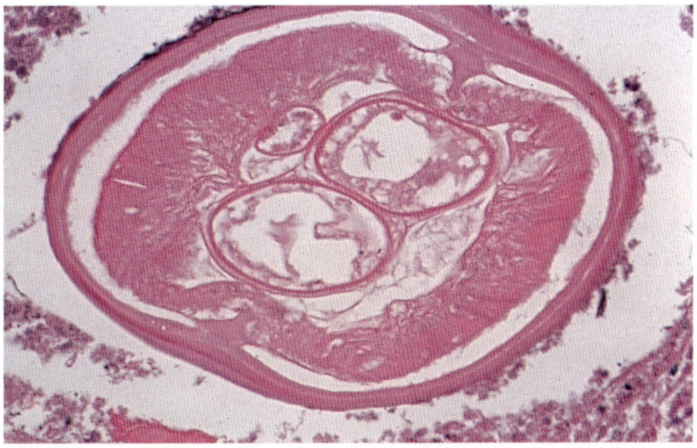

Figure 155–6. Human pulmonary dirofilariasis. This cross-section of an immature female *D immitis* has a smooth cuticle, prominent muscles, two uterine tubes and a smaller intestine (H&E, ×150).

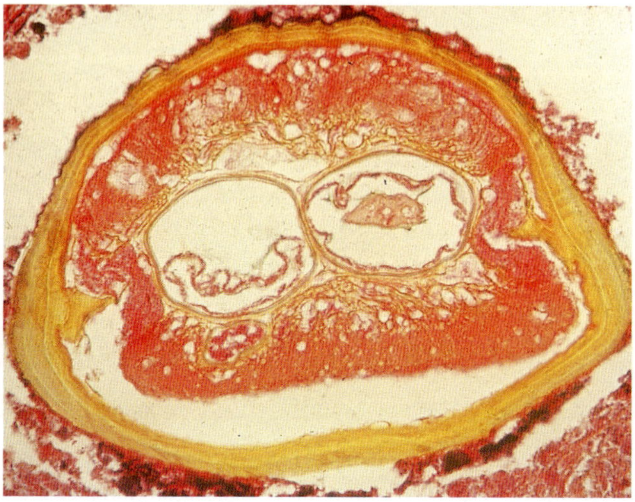

Figure 155–7. Same worm shown in Figure 155–6, stained to contrast the worm's cuticle, muscles, and internal organs (Movat stain, ×150).

a noncalcified mass revealed cross-sections of *D immitis* in one patient, and computerized axial tomography scan allowed a small lesion to be aspirated with a percutaneous needle in another.[1] But otherwise special diagnostic procedures including transthoracic needle aspiration, angiography of the right side of the heart and pulmonary artery for adult worms, examination of bronchial washings, and cytology of biopsy specimens and sputum have been of no value. Skin tests for dirofilariasis are nonspecific and do not help in diagnosis.

Treatment

A thoracotomy with wedge resection is usually done when the nodule is seen on x ray. This removes the worm and the reaction to it. There is no recurrence. If diagnosis is made by needle biopsy, no further treatment need be done as these lesions are completely contained by a fibrous tissue wall.

SUBCUTANEOUS DIROFILARIASIS

Geographic Distribution and Life Cycle

Filarial nematodes from raccoon and opossums (*D tenuis*), bears (*D ursi*), and porcupines (*D subdermata*) can cause subcutaneous dirofilariasis in humans. Another *Dirofilaria, D repens,* infects dogs and causes ocular dirofilariasis in humans. As with *D immitis*, mosquitoes are the intermediate hosts and vectors for *D tenuis. Dirofilaria ursi* and *D subdermata* are transmitted from animal to animal and from animal to humans by the bite of infected black flies (*Simulidae*). Transmission to humans depends on availability of a vector and the presence in the area of the definitive reservoir host.[11]

Dirofilaria tenuis is endemic to southern Florida, where up to 45% of raccoons are infected. Dogs in the Mediterranean area are parasitized with *D repens,* which has been reported only in the Mediterranean area. *Dirofilaria ursi* and *D subdermata* are limited to the northern United States and Canada. Human subcutaneous dirofilariasis is most frequent in southern Florida, but sporadic infections have been reported in Australia, Greece, and Costa Rica.[12]

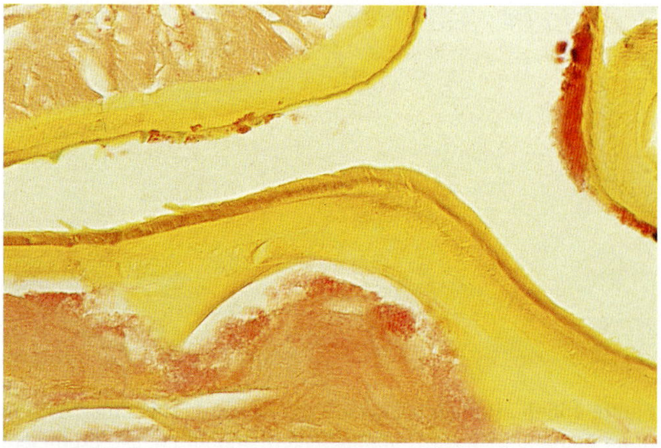

Figure 155–8. The cuticle of *D immitis* is smooth and without the longitudinal cuticular ridges seen in *D tenuis* and in *D repens* (Movat stain, ×400).

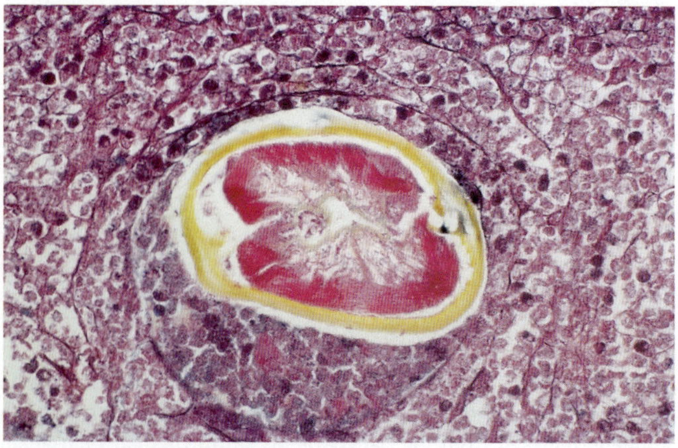

Figure 155–9. Subcutaneous dirofilariasis. A male *D tenuis* is centered in an abscess. There are numerous neutrophils and scattered eosinophils in the exudate (Movat stain, ×100).

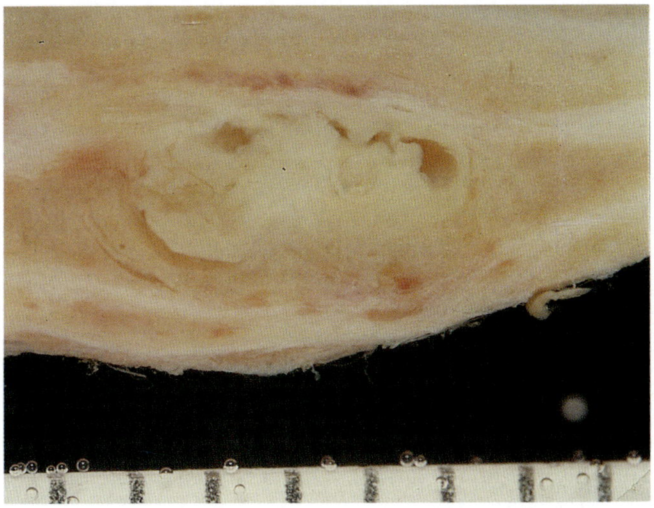

Figure 155–10. A 37-year-old male American had a 2-cm nodule in the skin of the lower abdomen. He had first noticed the nodule while in Greece 8 years previously. The nodule was circumscribed and had a soft center. On the cut surface there is a cross-section of a nongravid female *D repens*. The worm is to the right of center and shown microscopically in Figures 155–12 and 155–13 (gross, ×10.5). *(By D. H. Connor, MD, 1976.)*

Morphology

The female *D tenuis* is 80 to 130 mm long by 260 to 360 μm in diameter, and male worms are 40 to 48 mm long by 190 to 260 μm in diameter. Both male and female worms have the same thick laminated cuticle with internal and external longitudinal cuticular ridges. Both genders have lateral chords and somatic musculature. Female worms contain an intestine and two uteri. In humans the uteri usually contain no microfilariae. The male contains an intestine and a single reproductive tube (Figure 155–9). *Dirofilaria repens* adult worms are larger, measuring 100 to 170 mm by 370 to 450 μm, and males are 60 to 70 mm by 370 to 450 μm.[8]

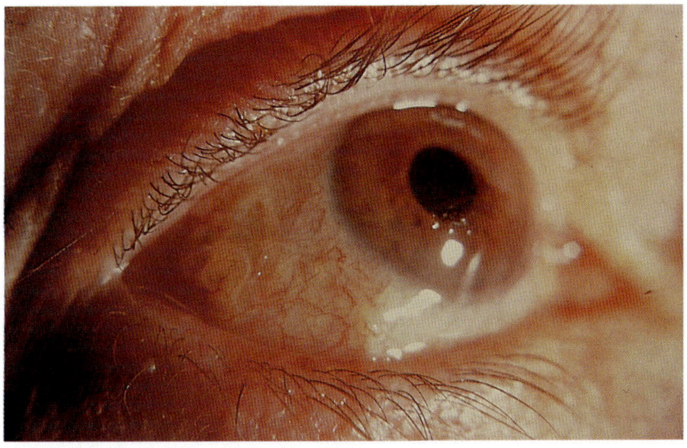

Figure 155–11. A serpentine *D tenuis* is migrating beneath the bulbar conjunctiva.

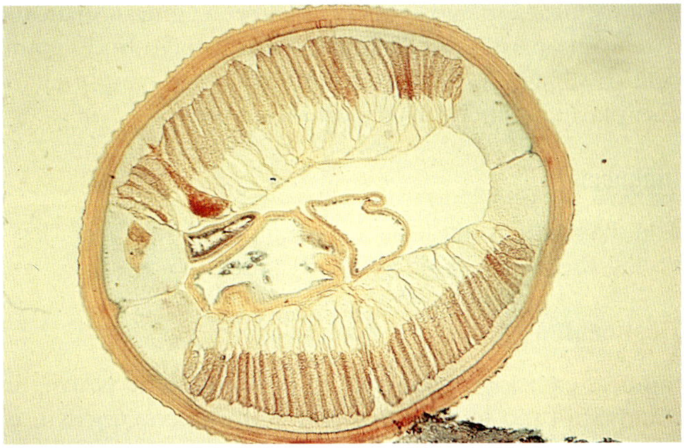

Figure 155–12. Cross-section of the female nongravid *D repens* shown in Figure 155–10. The cuticle is thick and has external longitudinal cuticular ridges. Compare with Figure 155–8. Note also the two cross-sections of uterine tubes and a smaller collapsed intestine. Somatic musculature has a radial configuration (Movat stain, ×150).

Clinical Features

Clinical signs of subcutaneous dirofilariasis vary in severity. Most patients are asymptomatic, but others have single subcutaneous nodules that are transient, mobile, painful, erythematous, and occasionally allergic, measuring 1.5 to 2.0 cm (Figure 155–10). Clinically these nodules may resemble infected cysts, adnexal neoplasms, or abscesses. The nodule may arise in any part of the body, but sites of predisposition are conjunctiva (Figure 155–11), eyelid, scrotum, breast, and limbs.

Pathology

There may be single or multiple degenerating worms in a nodule. Early in the formation of the nodule there are

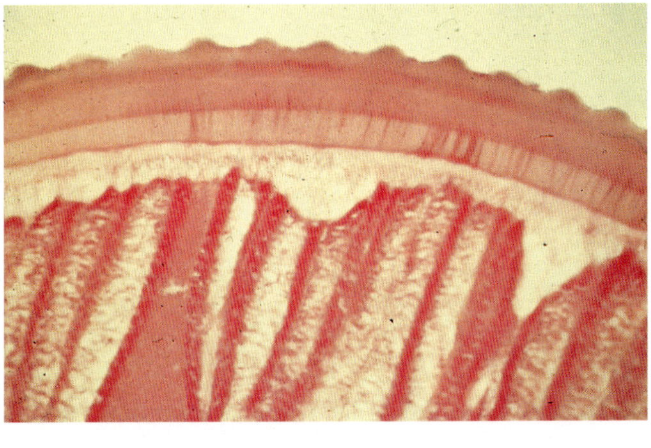

Figure 155–13. *Dirofilaria repens,* same worm shown in Figures 155–10 and 155–12. The cuticle is thick, multilayered and has an array of longitudinal cuticular ridges, seen here in cross-section (H&E, ×400).

neutrophils and eosinophils. Later a granulomatous reaction consisting of Langhans' and foreign-body giant cells, histiocytes, eosinophils and scattered lymphocytes and plasma cells forms around the abscess.

Diagnosis

The diagnosis is made by excising the nodule and identifying the worm (Figures 155–12 and 155–13).

Treatment

Surgical excision of the nodule containing the worm, or removal of the intact worm when in the conjunctiva, is curative.

REFERENCES

1. Asimacopoulos PJ, Katras A, Christie B. Pulmonary dirofilariasis—the largest single-hospital experience. *Chest.* 1992;102:851–855.
2. Dashiell GF. A case of dirofilariasis involving the lung. *Am J Trop Med Hyg.* 1961;10:37–38.
3. Conley JM, Sekla LK, Low DE. Dirofilariasis presenting as a breast lump. *Can Med Assoc J.* 1984;130:1575–1576.
4. Yoshimura EK, Wescott RB. Canine heartworm disease: a zoonosis of concern. *The Compendium—Small Animal.* 1989;11:575–578.
5. Bradham RR, Locklair PR, Grimball A. Bilateral pulmonary nodules caused by *Dirofilaria immitis. Ann Thorac Surg.* 1990;50:312–313.
6. Kochar AS. Human pulmonary dirofilariasis. *AJCP.* 1985: 19–23.
7. Risher WH, Crocker EF Jr, Beckman EN, Lacklock JB, Ochsner JL. Pulmonary dirofilariasis. *J Thorac Cardiovasc Surg.* 1989;97:303–308.
8. Neafie RC, Connor DH, Meyers WM. Dirofilariasis. In: Binford CH, Connor DH, eds. *Pathology of Tropical and Extraordinary Diseases.* Washington, DC: Armed Forces Institute of Pathology; 1976:391–396.
9. Darrow JC, Lack EE. *Dirofilaria immitis* as an unusual cause of the peripheral coin lesion in man. *J Surg Oncol.* 1981;16:219–224.
10. Glickman LT, Grieve RB, Schantz PM. Serologic diagnosis of zoonotic pulmonary dirofilariasis. *Am J Med.* 1986;80: 161–164.
11. Wright JC, Hendrix CM, Brown RG. Dirofilariasis. *J Am Vet Med Assoc.* 1989;194:644–647.
12. Weissman BW. Raccoon heartworm causing a facial mass. *South Med J.* 1992;85:845–846.

CHAPTER 156

Dracunculiasis

Mark L. Eberhard

My skin grows black and peels; my body burns with fever.

Job 30:30

DEFINITION

Dracunculiasis is an infection by the spirurid nematode *Dracunculus medinensis* and is characterized primarily by the emergence of gravid female worms through an ulcer in the skin. Synonyms for dracunculiasis include dracontiasis and dracunculosis; the parasite is known also as Guinea worm, medina worm, or fiery serpent worm.

GEOGRAPHIC DISTRIBUTION

Guinea worm infection is present on the west coast of Africa (particularly Nigeria, Ghana, Burkina Faso, Mauritania, Benin, and Côte D'Ivoire), in the Nile Valley, and northern Uganda. In Asia, dracunculiasis is in Pakistan and India. Efforts to eradicate guinea worm have markedly reduced disease incidence in endemic areas; India and Pakistan may soon achieve eradication, and several African countries are making great strides as well. Dracunculiasis used to occur in southern Russia, Iran and Iraq, and in the West Indies and South America.

Within endemic areas, transmission and infection are focal, and typically occur in poor areas served by a weak health care infrastructure. Guinea worm disease has been characterized as afflicting the forgotten people at the end of the road.

LIFE CYCLE, NATURAL HISTORY, AND EPIDEMIOLOGY

The life cycle of *D medinensis* takes about 1 year to complete. In endemic areas with heavy rainfall, female worms emerge during the dry season when water levels are low. In areas with little rain, transmission takes place during, or shortly after, the rainy season when waterholes and ponds contain water.[1] Male and female worms mate and develop to sexual maturity in the subcutaneous and deep somatic tissues. As gravid female worms near patency, they migrate to more superficial connective tissues below the skin, typically moving down the limbs toward the hands and feet. A blister, or papule, is formed around the anterior end of the female worm (Figure 156–1), possibly from the release of either coelomic fluid or of larvae. Upon immersion in water, or with wetting, the blister ruptures and the anterior end of the worm protrudes (Figure 156–2). At some point shortly after immersion, the worm releases thousands of first-stage larvae (Figure 156–3) into the water. Although the worm may release larvae several times during the next 7 to 10 days, most are released in the first wave.

Extraction of the female worm is generally accomplished over the course of several weeks by gentle traction and winding of the worm on a stick or string (Figure 156–4). Persons in endemic-disease areas are skilled at removing worms intact without applying excessive pressure. Sometimes, extraction of the worm and healing progress smoothly. At other times, however, the open lesion becomes infected, which slows or arrests healing and causes a large ulcer (Figure 156–5). Commonly, joints become inflamed (arthritis), and sometimes there is sepsis and even death.

Although most worms emerge from the limbs, some have emerged from the trunk, shoulders, scrotum, face, head, and breast (Figure 156–6). More than 80% emerge from the legs, with half from the feet and ankles.[1] Most infections involve one worm, although

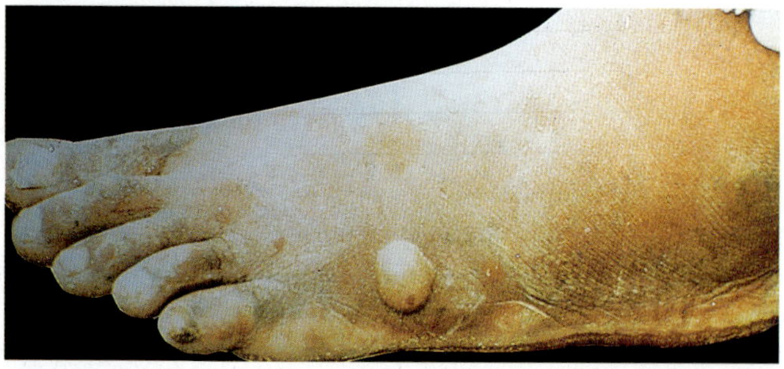

Figure 156–1. Blister on the foot of a Pakistani just before the worm emerged. *(Photograph contributed by Dr. S. Fitzgerald.)*

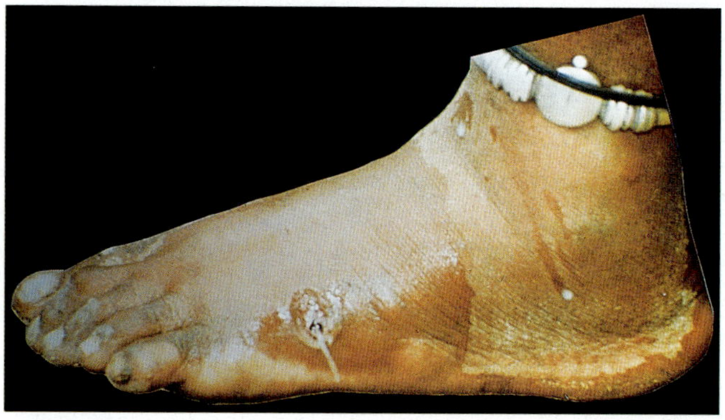

Figure 156–2. Same patient shown in Figure 156–1, immediately after wetting. The blister had ruptured and the female *D medinensis* has emerged. *(Photograph contributed by Dr. S. Fitzgerald.)*

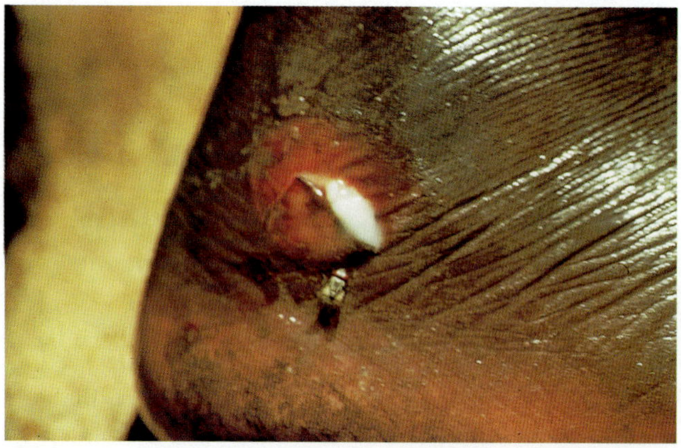

Figure 156–3. Guinea worm lesion on ankle of Cameroonian immediately after wetting, showing the release of milky fluid composed of thousands of *D medinensis* larvae. *(Photograph contributed by Dr. B. Cline.)*

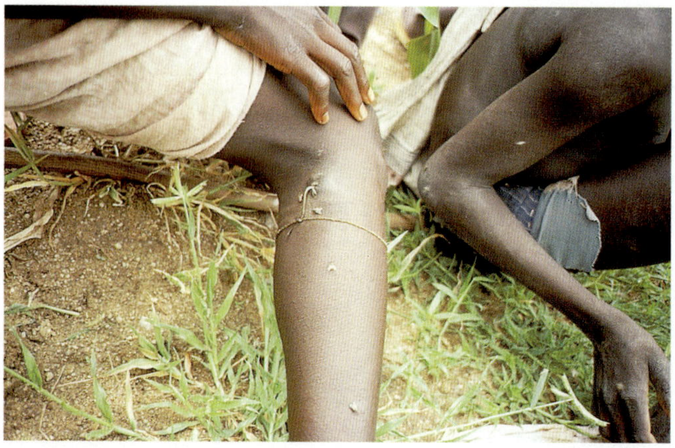

Figure 156–4. Emerging female *D medinensis* being extracted from a Cameroonian patient.

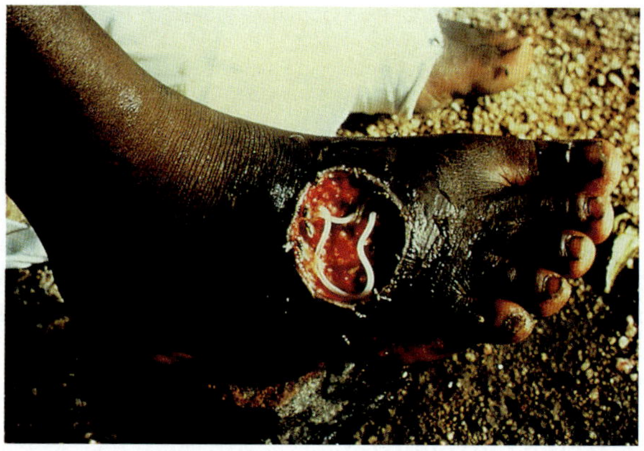

Figure 156–5. Guinea worm lesion on dorsum of foot of a Cameroonian, showing large ulcer and portion of female worm. *(Photograph contributed by Dr. J. Rippert.)*

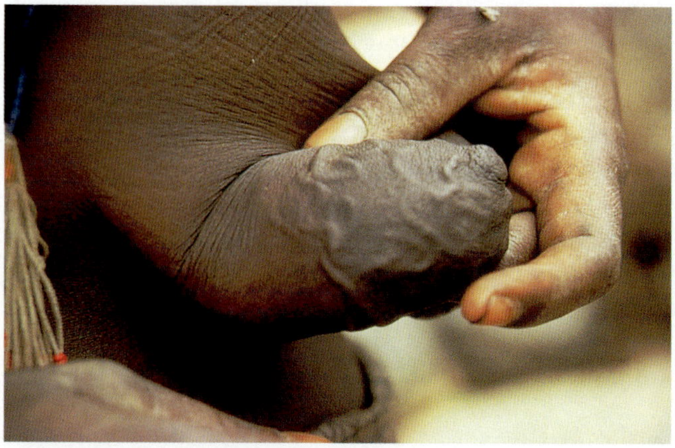

Figure 156–6. Track of female *D medinensis* in the dermis of the breast of a Cameroonian woman. *(Photograph contributed by Dr. F. Richards.)*

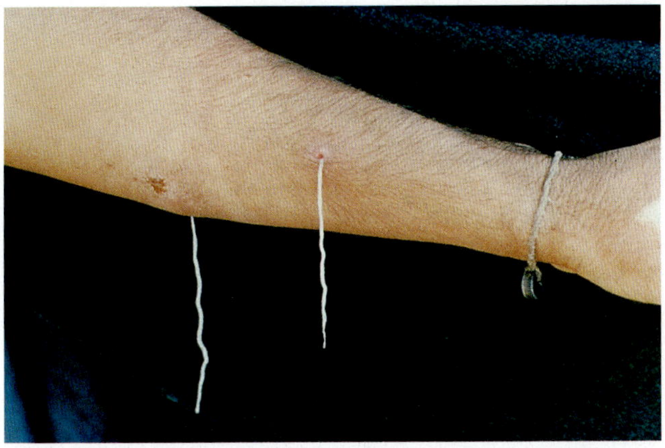

Figure 156–7. Multiple lesions on the forearm of a Pakistani man. Either two worms are emerging or one worm is emerging at two sites. *(Photograph contributed by Dr. R. Imtiaz.)*

occasionally several worms emerge (Figure 156–7). An unknown number of worms die, disintegrate, are resorbed or become calcified, and never emerge (Figures 156–8, A–C). Some experiments suggest that fewer than half the female worms emerge, and radiographs of those in endemic areas confirm that many worms die before emerging. Unusual ectopic sites in which gravid female worms have been identified include heart, spinal cord, eyelid, and orbit[2] (Figures 156–9, A–D, and 156–10).

First-stage larvae (Figure 156–11) are actively motile when released by the female worm and may survive in water for several days. To develop further, larvae must be ingested by an appropriate copepod. Several genera and species (including *Cyclops, Mesocyclops,* and *Thermocyclops*) serve as intermediate hosts for guinea worm (the predominant species vary from one geographic locale to another). After being ingested, first-stage larvae quickly penetrate into the hemocele of the copepod, where they undergo two molts to become infective, third-stage larvae. Development to the infective stage requires 7 to 14 days, proceeding faster in warmer temperatures. Infection of the human host occurs when an infected copepod (Figure 156–12) is swallowed by a susceptible person. Once the copepod is digested, the larvae are freed and migrate from intestine to the peritoneal cavity and into the somatic tissues, probably reaching the loose connective tissues of the torso and limbs within several weeks. The young worms molt twice more as they grow into the adult stage. Studies on experimental animals indicate that female worms contain larvae as early as 4 months after infection, some 6 to 8 months before the gravid female worm emerges.[3] Further, male worms once thought to die shortly after mating may survive for up to a year, suggesting that they mate in more than one reproductive cycle.[3]

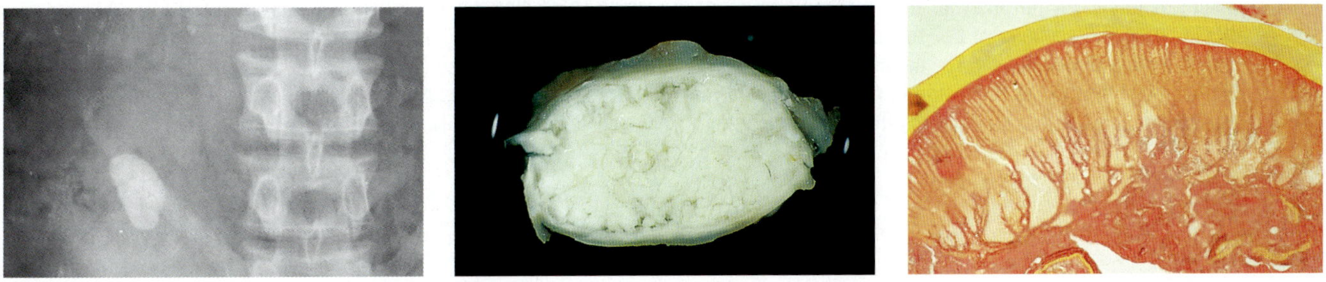

A B C

Figure 156–8. (**A**) Discrete radiodensity in the abdominal wall of a Pakistani patient. (**B**) Cut surface of the lesion removed from the abdominal wall of the Pakistani patient shown in Part (A). It was firm to hard, chalky white, and grossly contained no obvious parasitic structures. *(By Daniel H. Connor, MD, 1983.)* (**C**) Microscopic section of the lesion shown in parts (A) and (B) reveals a coiled degenerating nematode with characteristic features of a gravid female *D medinensis*. The carcass of the worm was in an amorphous, mineralized matrix. Note the thick smooth cuticle, the prominent two-layered muscle band, and the degenerated central structures, including the larvae (AFIP Neg 84-7877; Movat, ×72).

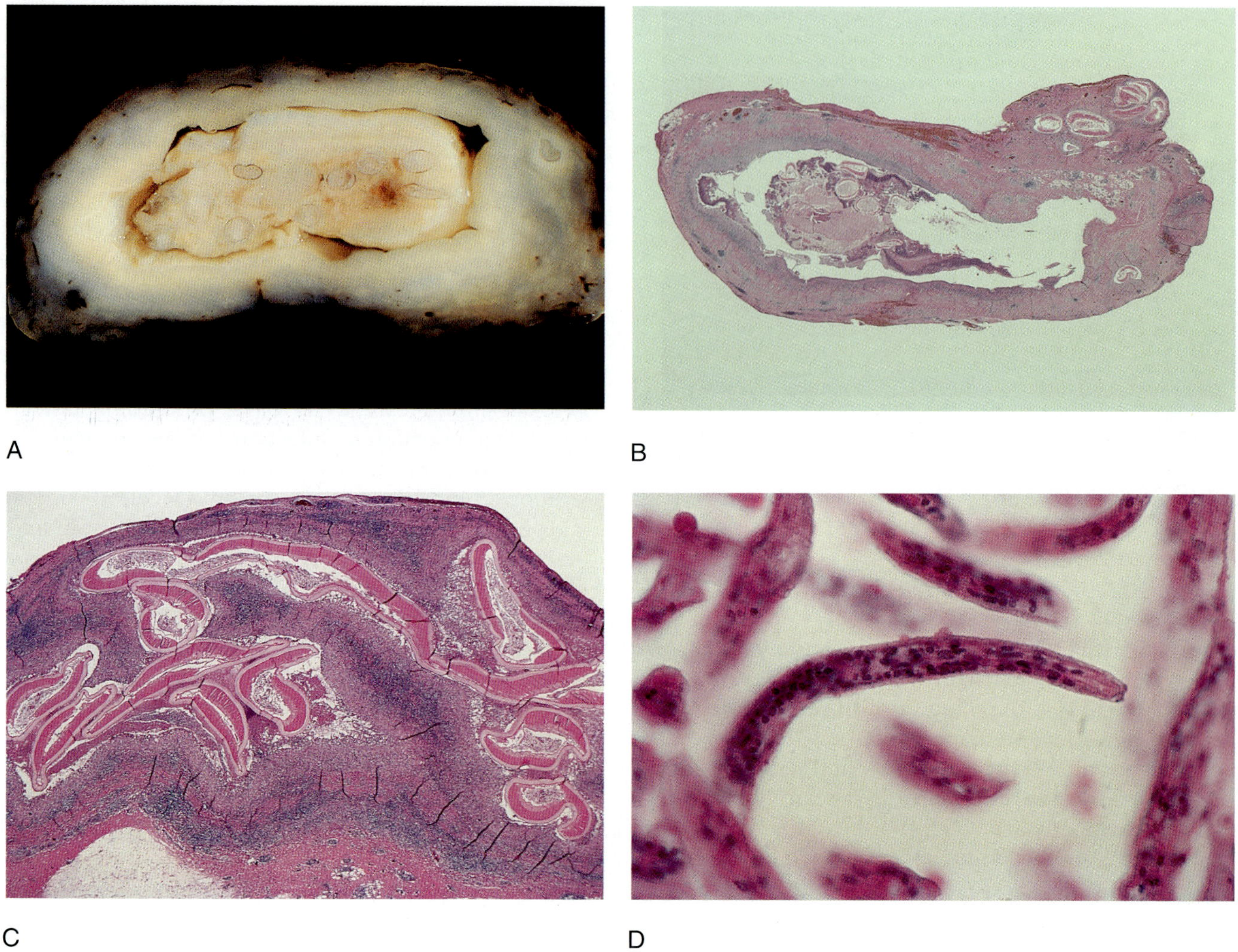

Figure 156–9. (**A**) Lesion removed from the upper eyelid of a 3-year-old in Kano, Nigeria. The patient had no fever or pain and the parents claimed the lesion had been there for 7 days. At excision it was deeper than expected, ie, fastened to the orbital rim. The surgeon listed "cyst," "dermoid," and "hydatid" as possible diagnoses. Grossly there is a fibrous tissue wall and a soft center. Multiple cuts of a large coiled nematode are in the white homogeneous material and in the fibrous wall (AFIP Neg 81-18215). (**B**) Whole mount of the lesion shown in part (A). Cross-sections of the adult *D medinensis* are plainly visible in the fibrous wall and in the soft center of the lesion [AFIP Neg 83-9993; hematoxylin-eosin (H&E), ×11]. (**C**) Microscopic sections of the soft center of the lesion shown in parts (A) and (B) reveal multiple sections of a coiled gravid female *D medinensis*. The patient's recovery was complete and uncomplicated (AFIP Neg 83-9987; H&E, ×4.5). (**D**) Higher magnification of the lesion in part (C), showing intact larvae of *D medinensis*. These larvae have a digestive tube and cuticular annulations—features that distinguish them from microfilariae (AFIP Neg 83-9991; H&E, ×290).

Characteristically, dracunculiasis is in villages and small communities with unprotected water sources (open wells, ponds, or other water catchments that infected persons can enter). Establishing and maintaining sources of noncontaminated water, such as protected wells and piped water, can prevent transmission. Safe water and effective educational materials have been the basis of the very successful campaign to eradicate guinea worm disease.[4] In certain situations, applications of the insect larvicide temephos (Abate*) has reduced or prevented transmission.

*Use of trade names is for identification only and does not imply endorsement by the Public Health Service or by the U.S. Department of Health and Human Services.

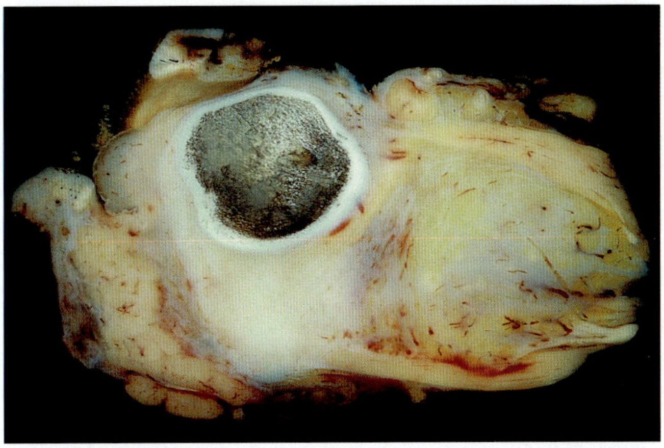

Figure 156–10. Right eye and orbital contents of a 5-year-old girl in Kano, Nigeria. For 2 months she had had proptosis. The clinical diagnosis was Burkitt's lymphoma and for this she was given 400 mgm of Cytoxan intravenously 7 days before exenteration. Gross and microscopic examination of the specimen revealed no lymphoma but 1) an orbital abscess caused by a degenerating *D medinensis,* 2) a perforated corneal ulcer with partial loss of ocular contents, and 3) panophthalmitis.

Dracunculus medinensis, although primarily a human parasite, has parasitized various domestic and wild animals, especially dogs.[5] It is unclear what role animals play as reservoir hosts for dracunculiasis, but generally it is believed when the disease is controlled in the human population, animals pose minimal threat of reintroduction.

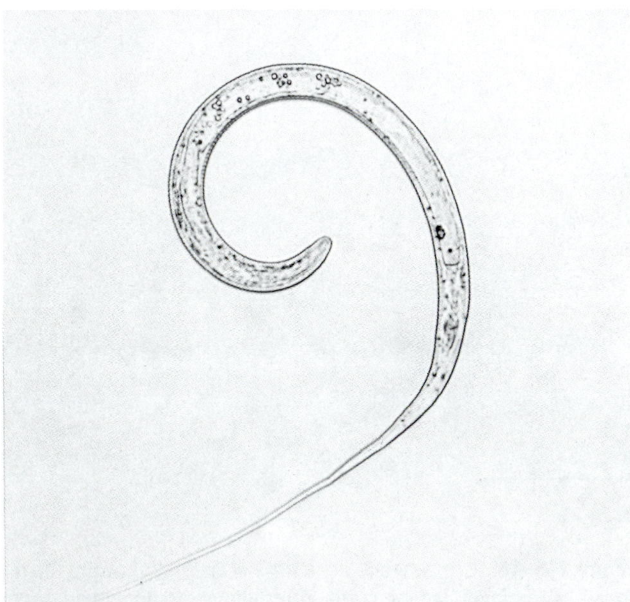

Figure 156–11. First-stage larva of *D insignis,* a related parasite of carnivores in North America. Note the digestive tract and the long, whiplike tail (×200).

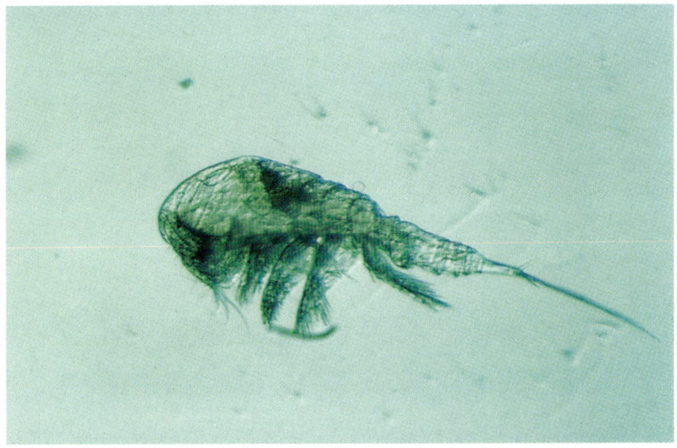

Figure 156–12. An infected copepod containing several third-stage larvae.

CLINICAL AND PATHOLOGIC FEATURES

Dracunculiasis is not easily confused with other nematode infections because of the distinct size of the female worm, its emergence from a cutaneous lesion, and other morphologic criteria. From the time of ingestion of infected copepods until just before emergence of the gravid female worm, there is little outward sign of infection. Typically, symptoms only appear as the female worm makes her way to subcutaneous tissues. A burning sensation usually accompanies the formation of the blister. Systemic symptoms, including asthma, nausea, vomiting, diarrhea, and dyspnea, also may develop as the blister forms. Rupture of the blister usually alleviates local and systemic symptoms.

As the female worm emerges, a subcutaneous abscess forms that may remain small (less than 1 cm diameter), with a central area of necrosis surrounded by a granulomatous reaction. Occasionally, when the lesion becomes infected, the abscess may become large, exceeding 3 cm in diameter. There may be erosion of soft tissue, especially when the lesion is on the foot. The inflammatory cell infiltrate consists of epithelioid cells, histiocytes, neutrophils, plasma cells, and eosinophils. Giant cells may be numerous. Depending on the age of the lesion, the worm may be morphologically intact (Figure 156–13), fragmented, or disintegrated (Figure 156–14). Occasionally, first-stage larvae can be observed either in utero (Figures 156–9, D, and 156–15) or lying free in the abscess.

MORPHOLOGIC FEATURES OF DRACUNCULUS

Although often referred to as filariae, dracunculids are morphologically and biologically distinct from filarial nematodes. Adult female *D medinensis* are the longest

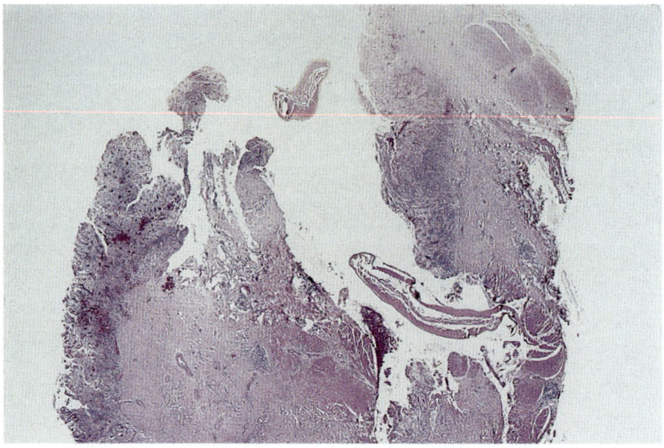

Figure 156–13. Tissue section containing a guinea worm with two transverse sections of the emerging female *D medinensis.* The lining of the tract, shown on the right is inflamed granulation tissue (H&E, ×20). *(Section contributed by David A. Schwartz, MD.)*

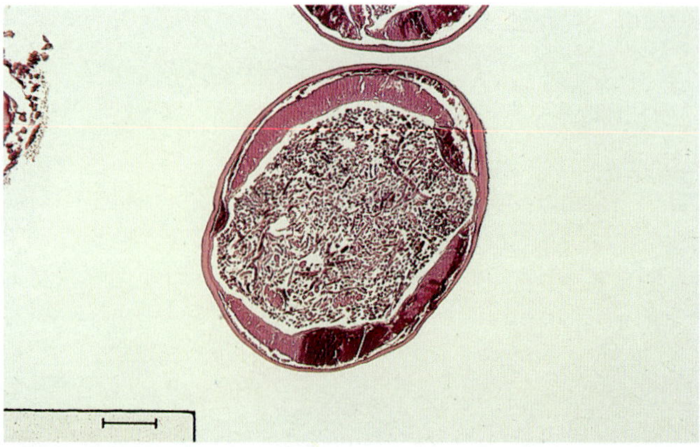

Figure 156–15. Cross-section of gravid, degenerating female *D medinensis* illustrating the prominent muscle bands, absence of a discernible gut, and uterus distended with larvae (H&E, ×250). *(Section contributed by David A. Schwartz, MD.)*

nematodes that infect humans. Mature females may be 70 to 120 cm long and 0.9 to 1.7 mm wide. Male worms are much smaller, measuring up to 40 mm in length. They are rarely found in humans. Males recovered from experimental infections in dogs were somewhat smaller, measuring 12 to 29 mm long by about 0.4 mm in diameter.

In mature female worms the cuticle is smooth and relatively thick, and may appear multilayered. The hypodermal tissue is thin and difficult to see except in the area of the lateral cords. In male worms the lateral cords are prominent. Musculature is conspicuous, and, in the gravid female, typically appears as two broad bands of contractile fibers (Figures 156–8, C, 156–14, and 156–15). In male worms, the intestine is visible (Figure 156–16), and in gravid female worms it is usually not visible. In gravid female worms, most of the body cavity is comprised of a distended uterus packed with first-stage larvae (Figures 156–9, D, and 156–15).

First-stage larvae, both in utero in the gravid female worm and when released into water, are 500 to 750 μm long by about 20 μm in diameter. These larvae have a distinctly annulated cuticle, a digestive tube consisting of an esophagus and intestine, and an exceptionally

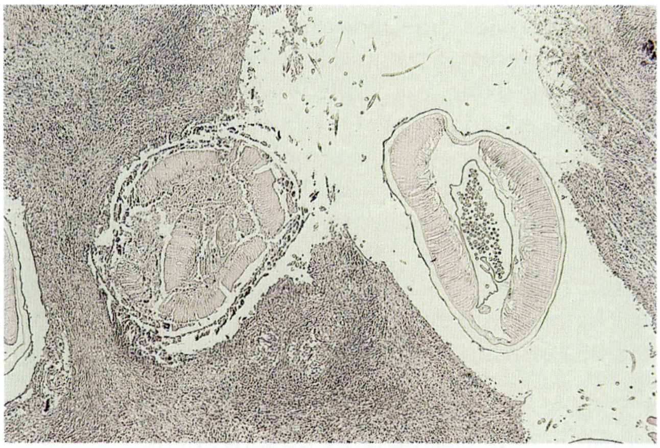

Figure 156–14. Tissue section of a lesion from an experimentally infected raccoon containing a dead and degenerating female *D insignis* (*on left*) in which only the heavy muscle bands remain visible. A section of intact worm is adjacent to it (H&E, ×200).

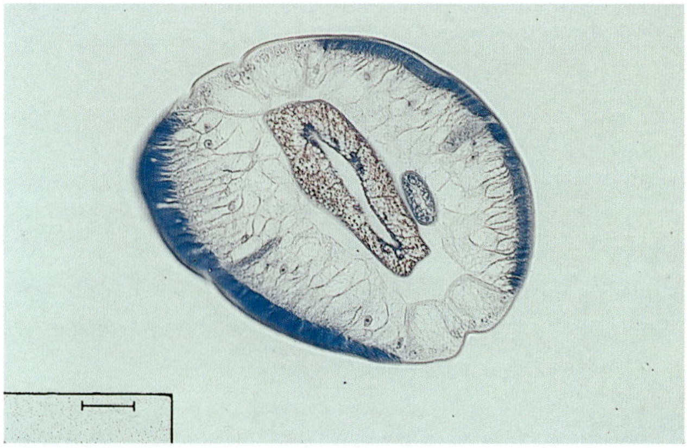

Figure 156–16. Cross-section of a male *D insignis* showing the thin cuticle, prominent lateral cords protruding into the body cavity, clearly visible dorsal and ventral cords, polymyarian–coelomyarian musculature with large cytoplasmic portion, a very large gut with conspicuous granularity, and a section through the much smaller testis.

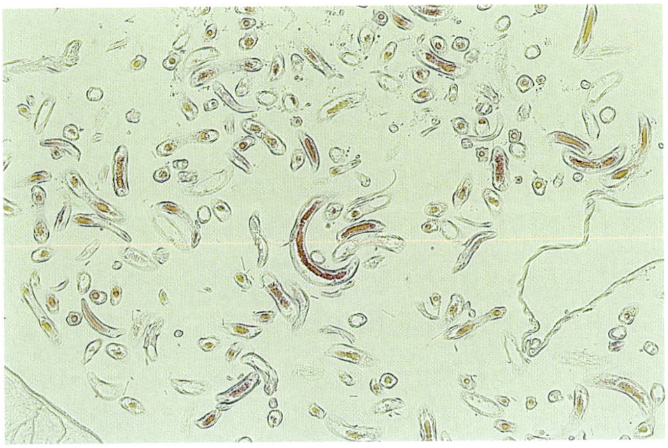

Figure 156–17. High magnification of larvae of *D medinensis,* in utero, showing the long tail, annulated cuticle, and gut (×1000).

long, tapered tail (Figure 156–11). These features are frequently seen in tissue sections (Figures 156–9, D, and 156–17) and are diagnostic.

DIFFERENTIAL DIAGNOSIS

Because of the worm's size, the way it emerges from the skin, and certain morphologic features, there is little confusion in diagnosing dracunculiasis. In endemic areas, a presumptive diagnosis can be made based solely on the presence of a worm track (Figure 156–6). Beyond the endemic areas, clinical features may be suggestive, but a positive diagnosis requires demonstration of the adult worm or the first-stage larvae. Other helminths may be mistaken for *D medinensis.* Gravid female filariae, *Onchocera volvulus* and *Mansonella streptocerca,* for instance, are in subcutaneous tissue. Their uteri are full of microfilariae and they may superficially resemble guinea worms. The gravid *D medinensis,* however, can be distinguished by its size (length and width), and the larvae of *D medinensis* by their cuticular annulations, a defined gut, and length of the tail.

Other means of diagnosis are generally unavailable, and are rarely needed because the diagnosis can be made clinically. Specific recollection of guinea worm infection on the part of community residents obviates the need for more sophisticated assay methods. Epidemiologic surveys have successfully moved the eradication effort forward by using questionnaires containing specific, local names for the disease and by using photographs showing an emergent worm.[6]

REFERENCES

1. Kale OO. Dracontiasis. In: Steele JH, ed. *CRC Handbook Series in Zoonoses. Section C: Parasitic Zoonoses.* Boca Raton, Fla: CRC Press; 1982:111–122.
2. Burnier M, Hidayat AA, Neafie R. Dracunculiasis of the orbit and eyelid. *Ophthalmology.* 1991;98:919–924.
3. Brandt FH, Eberhard ML. Distribution, behavior, and course of patency of *Dracunculus insignis* in experimentally infected ferrets. *J Parasitol.* 1990;76:515–518.
4. Hopkins DR, Ruiz-Tiben E. Strategies for dracunculiasis eradication. *Bull WHO.* 1991;69:533–540.
5. Muller R. *Dracunculus* and dracunculiasis. In: Dawes B, ed. *Advances in Parasitology.* New York: Academic Press; 1971;9:73–151.
6. Centers for Disease Control and Prevention. Surveillance for dracunculiasis, 1981–1991. *MMWR.* 1992;41(SS-1): 1–13.

CHAPTER 157

Echinococcosis

Elie K. Fraiji, Jr. and Daniel H. Connor

Diseases come of their accord,
But cures come difficult and hard.

Samuel Butler (1612–1680)

DEFINITION

Echinococcosis is infection of human and animal by larval tapeworms of the genus *Echinococcus*. Four species infect humans. *Echinococcus granulosus* forms a solitary cyst in the deep organs and tissues. Less commonly multiple cysts may form. *Echinococcus multilocularis* causes alveolar hydatidosis, *E vogeli* causes polycystic hydatid disease, and the first human infection by the larval stage of *E oligarthus* was reported in 1989.[1] Synonyms include hydatid disease, cystic hydatid disease, and alveolar hydatidosis (*E multilocularis*).

INTRODUCTION

The science of molecular biology has enabled the identification of new strains of *Echinococcus* but data on the geography and pathogenicity of these new strains are incomplete.[2] Three strains of *E granulosus* are recognized. The dog/sheep strain is widely disseminated and more virulent than the sylvatic strain, which predominantly infects wolves. The third strain—the Middle Eastern strain—is adapted to the dog/horse cycle and may also infect humans.[3]

GEOGRAPHIC DISTRIBUTION

Echinococcus granulosus is widespread throughout cosmopolitan Europe, Asia, Australia, and Africa and is most likely continuous through zones of tundra and taiga in northeastern Europe. It exists across northern North America extending through southern Canada and into the northern United States. In some regions the incidence is relatively high. Of 333,144 examinations by ultrasound in 19 hospitals throughout Italy between 1988 and 1990, 424 patients had cystic hydatid disease—a mean incidence of 0.16%.[4] *Echinococcus granulosus* has reached endemic proportions in the canine population of Victoria, Australia, and now threatens the human population.[5] In one study from Nigeria 7.1% of sheep, 18.4% of goats, 1.5% of cattle, 70.9% of camels, and 5% of pigs were infected.[6] Sheep and dogs are the predominant intermediate and definitive hosts for *E granulosus* so echinococcosis is frequent where dogs are used for sheepherding.

Alveolar hydatidosis caused by *E multilocularis* is endemic in areas of western Europe, the Middle East, China, and Japan. The first documented patient was in India and diagnosed at autopsy in 1978,[7] while the first human infection acquired in the continental United States was in Minnesota in 1979.[8] Infection by *E multilocularis* in North American animals, however, has been recognized since 1964 and since then the incidence has increased and its geographic distribution has enlarged. By 1969 *E multilocularis* was in Alberta, Saskatchewan, North and South Dakota, and by 1980 in Minnesota, Montana, Iowa, Wisconsin, Nebraska, and Wyoming.[3] More recently, alveolar hydatidosis has been recognized in Indiana and Ohio. In parts of the United States including northern and central Indiana, northwestern Ohio, and east-central Illinois, a study of 300 canines demonstrated that 13.7% were infected with *E multilocularis*. The infected species included red foxes and coyotes.[9] To date only two human infections have been reported in North America—one from Minnesota and the other from Alberta. In the tundra, *E multilocularis* is ubiquitous and survival depends on the Arctic fox. *Echinococcus multilocularis* was identified in 80% of 1579 Arctic foxes on St. Lawrence Island, Alaska.[10] Its presence on Arctic islands depends on the availability of suitable intermediate hosts.

Echinococcus vogeli exists in the tropics of South America and extends from Panama to Columbia and Bolivia. The first record of polycystic hydatidosis in a human caused by the larval stage of *E vogeli* was in Columbia in 1979[11] and *Cuniculus paca* was identified as the natural intermediate host. In a survey of 4000 mammals from Colombia, 73 of 96 pacas were infected with *E vogeli* while only three were infected with *E oligarthus*. *Echinococcus vogeli* was found also in 1 of 15 domestic dogs. Also in Columbia, 1 of 11 ocelots, two of nine jaguarundi, and a single puma were infected with *E oligarthus.*[11] *Echinococcus vogeli* has recently been identified in a paca from Bolivia.[12]

Echinococcus oligarthus exists in the same geographic distribution as *E vogeli* but extends from Central America to the subantarctic. The first known human infection—caused by the oncospheres of *E oligarthus*—was in a Venezuelan woman. The lesion was a retroocular cyst.[1] A retrospective analysis of all known cases previously attributed to *E oligarthus* has shown that the causative organism was actually *E vogeli.*[1,13]

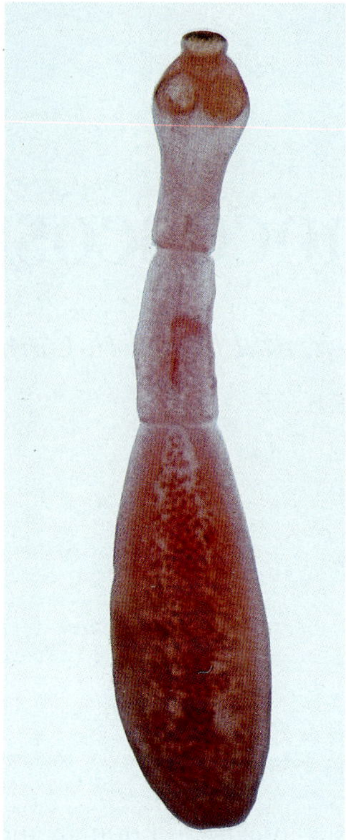

Figure 157–1. Adult *E granulosus.* It is 5 mm long and comprised of a scolex and 2 proglottids. Note the eggs in the posterior proglottid (AFIP 7-15389).

MORPHOLOGIC DESCRIPTION OF THE PARASITE

The adult *E granulosus* (Figure 157–1) is a small tapeworm, 3 to 6 mm in length capped by a scolex at the anterior terminus. Four suckers and a double crown of 28 to 50 hooks emerge from the scolex (Figures 157–2 through 157–4). They mediate attachment to the intestinal mucosa of the definitive host. Four or five proglottids arise sequentially from the layer of germinal tissue located in the posterior aspect of the scolex. The most mature proglottid, therefore, is in the posterior terminus of the adult tapeworm, while the least mature proglottid is still developing from the germinal tissue in the scolex. Reproduction of cestodes is hermaphroditic and the mature *E granulosus* proglottid contains from 45 to 65 testes. Fertilized eggs are easily seen in the posterior portion of the terminal proglottid—also known as the gravid proglottid.[13]

The adult *E multilocularis* is the smallest of the three species, typically 2 mm in length, and contains the fewest testes, 16 to 26. The rostellar hooks from the protoscolices of *E multilocularis* are 27 to 33 μm long.[14]

The adult *E oligarthus,* is slightly smaller than *E granulosus* and typically is 2.5 mm long. It also contains fewer testes—15 to 46 in the mature proglottid. The rostellar hooks from the *E oligarthus* protoscolex are slightly larger and more numerous than those of *E multilocularis*—25.8 to 31.8 μm long. The strobilar stage of *E vogeli* is longer and more slender than other echinococcal species. Its rostellar hooks have a characteristic arched appearance in which the blade is disproportionately larger than those of other species. The length of the rostellar hooks in the larval stage of *E vogeli* is from 33.1 to 41.8 mm.[13]

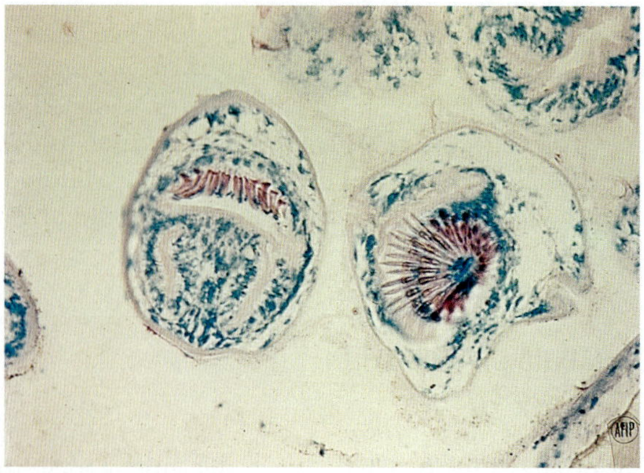

Figure 157–2. Anterior end of scolex showing two suckers each with a double row of hooks. The hooks are acid fast (AFIP 70-8831; Ziehl–Neelsen, ×440).

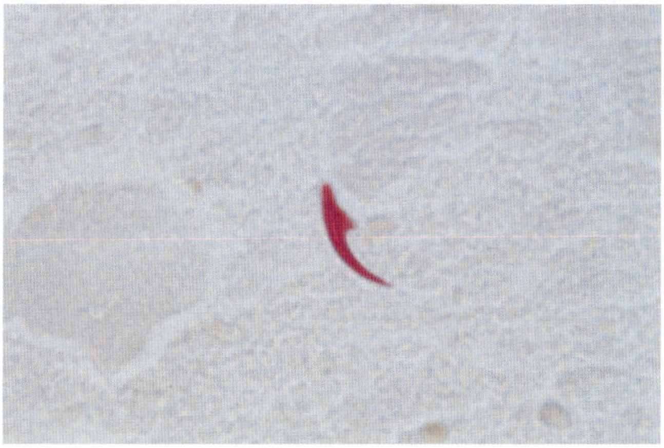

Figure 157–3. Hooklet of *E granulosus* recovered from fluid of an hydatid cyst. It is acid fast and has a characteristic shape (Ziehl–Neelsen, ×1000).

LIFE CYCLE

Adult tapeworms live in the small intestine of the definitive host—any one of a number of carnivores, usually a dog. Eggs and gravid proglottids passed in the dog's feces are ingested with the vegetation of grazing animals. Sheep are the most common intermediate host for *E granulosus* but a variety of herbivorous and omnivorous species can act as intermediate hosts. While in the gastrointestinal tract of the intermediate host, the eggs hatch and release oncospheres, which penetrate the intestinal mucosa and enter the general circulation. The oncospheres disseminate to the various tissues where they implant and develop into hydatid cysts. The cysts grow about 1 cm in diameter per month. The life cycle continues when the dog, or other definitive host, ingests a hydatid cyst and is completed when scolices in the cyst grow to be mature tapeworms in the dog's small intestine. The scolex requires about 7 weeks to grow to maturity.

Echinococcus vogeli and *E multilocularis* have similar life cycles and both are similar to *E granulosus*. Foxes and cats are definitive hosts for *E multilocularis* and rodents are usually the intermediate hosts. Puma, jaguarundi, and other members of the cat family are definitive hosts for *E vogeli* while *Cuniculus paca* is the principal intermediate host.

CLINICOPATHOLOGIC FEATURES

The majority (60%) of hydatid cysts develop in the liver and most of these are asymptomatic. In one report, 85.6% of 424 patients with abdominal hydatid lesions had them in the liver and 60% were asymptomatic at the time of diagnosis by ultrasonography. The average age at diagnosis was 45.38 years.[4] Cysts grow from 1 to 5 cm per year.[3] Lung (Figure 157–5) is the next most frequent site (20%) followed by the kidney (4%), muscle (4%), spleen (3%), soft tissue (3%), brain (3%), and bone (2%). The remaining 1% includes all other sites. One cyst presented as a lump in the breast.[15,16]

Symptoms are generally mechanical—the result of the enlarging hydatid cyst on adjacent tissues and organs. Symptoms of hepatic hydatidosis begin as the cyst approaches 10 cm but the cyst is not palpable until it reaches at least 20 cm. Compression of hepatic parenchyma or of the porta hepatis may cause jaundice or portal hypertension. Cholangitis may also develop. Rupture of the cyst may seed any of the thoracic or abdominal organs. Other symptoms, including anaphy-

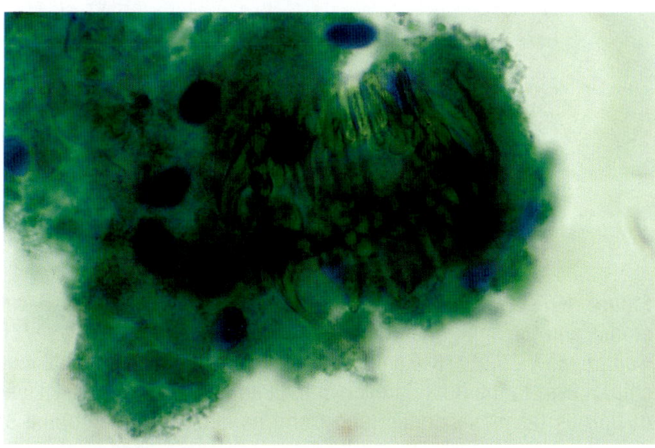

Figure 157–4. Fine-needle aspiration of hepatic hydatid cyst. The scolex has a double row of hooklets. Hooklets are refractile (Papanicolaou smear, ×1000).

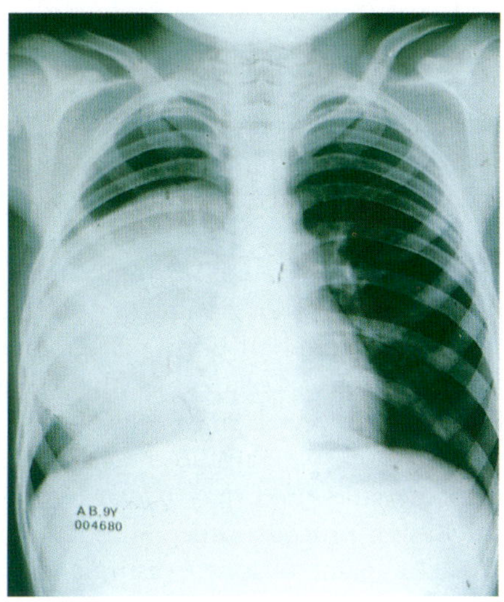

Figure 157–5. Chest x ray showing large hydatid cyst of right lung.

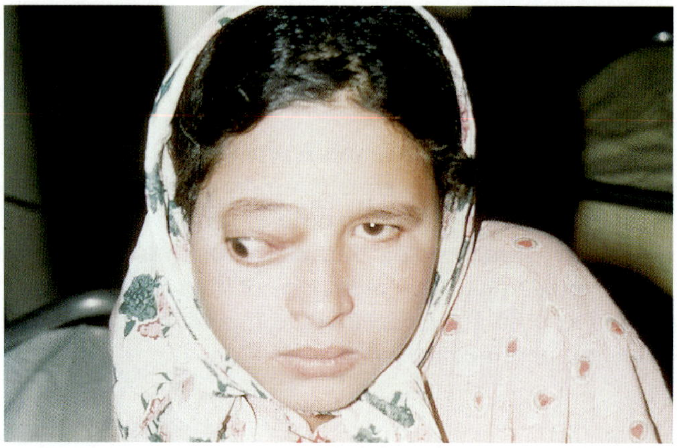

Figure 157–6. Echinococcosis of the orbit. There is exophthalmos, and lateral and downward deviation (AFIP 70-338). *(Photograph contributed by Dr. Herbert Spencer).*

laxis, may arise from the absorption of toxins or allergens. Polyarthritis[17] and membranous glomerular nephropathy[18] are sequelae of hepatic hydatid cysts.

Pulmonary cysts provoke cough, pleuritic chest pain, and dyspnea. Portions of the wall and contents are produced on coughing if the cyst ruptures into a bronchus. In these patients, chronic suppurative changes may persist for months. When a cyst ruptures into the pleural space there is pneumothorax and empyema followed by dissemination and growth of secondary cysts. In one study, thoracic metastases complicated 22 of 77 patients with hepatic hydatidosis.[19] In all 22 patients, the primary cyst was in the right hepatic lobe and metastasis involved structures in the right thoracic cavity. Twenty-four of the patients were symptomatic and only 10 of the 77 had thoracic symptoms.[19]

Cysts in brain cause characteristic features of an expanding mass including increasing intracranial pressure. The most frequent clinical presentation of intraorbital hydatid cyst (Figure 157–6) is slowly progressive unilateral exophthalmos, with or without pain.[20] Abdominal cysts in spleen, liver, or kidney cause pain as they grow larger and peritonitis when they rupture. Compression necrosis of renal parenchyma may cause hematuria and albuminuria. Hydatiduria has also been reported.[21,22] Hydatid disease of bone is rare. The most common site is lower vertebrae. Symptoms include low back pain, sciatica, loss of sphincter tone, and paraparesis. A cyst in a vertebral body will gradually erode and weaken the bone. Collapse of the vertebra with compression of the cord and paraplegia is called "hydatid Pott's disease." Ruptured cysts followed by absorption of hydatid fluid may cause hypersensitivity reactions including pruritus, urticaria, edema, vomiting, diarrhea, colicky pain, dyspnea, asthma, anaphylactic shock, and even death.

The clinical features of alveolar and polycystic hydatid disease resemble those caused by *E granulosus*. Seven patients with polycystic hydatid disease had liver most frequently infected (6/7), followed by lungs (2/7), mesentery (2/7), spleen (1/7), and pancreas (1/7).[23] Secondary amyloidosis complicated two of six livers from patients with alveolar hydatidosis. Kidneys of two Alaskan patients with alveolar hydatidosis had immune-complex-mediated glomerular nephropathy.[24] Spontaneous death of *E multilocularis* accompanied clinical remission in five patients from Alaska.[25]

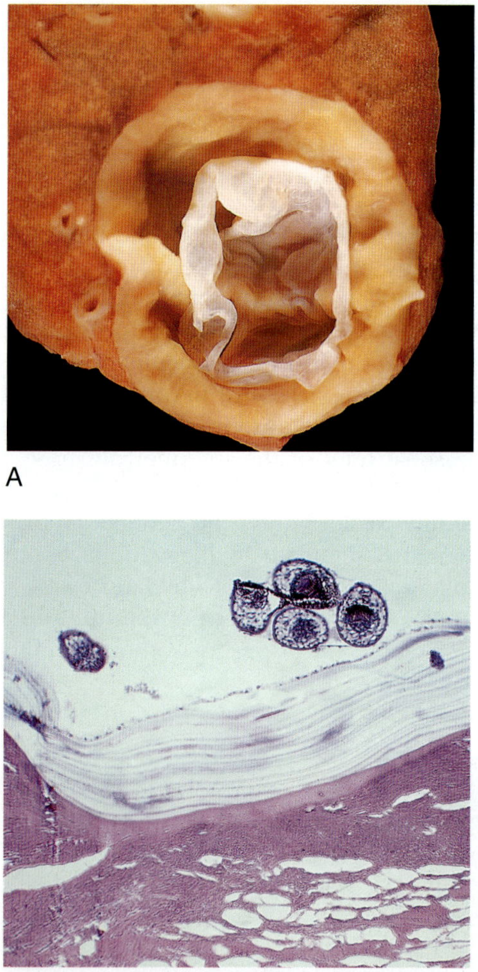

A

B

Figure 157–7. (**A**) Echinococcal cyst of lung. The cyst is 6 cm across and the lining membrane is white. *(Photograph by Daniel H. Connor, MD, 1978.)* (**B**) Echinococcal cyst of lung showing relationship of cyst to the host parenchyma. Lung is at the bottom. A layer of fibrous tissue separates lung from the laminated membrane of the echinococcal cyst. The laminated membrane is lined by the germinal layer and five scolices are in the lumen of the cyst [AFIP 79-15419; hematoxylin-eosin (H&E), ×40].

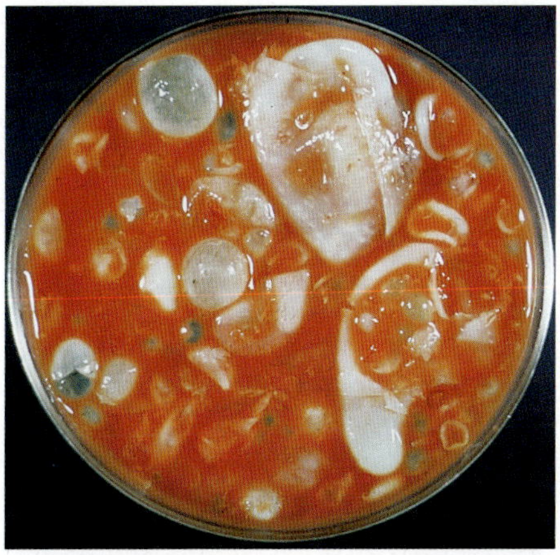

Figure 157–8. The petri dish contains the contents of an hydatid cyst opened at surgery. Fragments of germinal membrane and brood capsules float in blood-stained hydatid fluid. *(Photograph contributed by Ernest E. Lack, MD.)*

PATHOLOGY

Only the larval stages of *Echinococcus* species infect humans. The hydatid cyst develops in deep organs and tissues—wherever the oncosphere lodges. Portions of the walls of large cysts become mineralized. Cysts range from several millimeters to many centimeters across. The wall of the cyst is comprised of an external laminated layer, surrounded by a thin layer of fibrous tissue produced by the host, and the laminated layer is lined by the germinal (embryonic) membrane (Figures 157–7, A and B, and 157–8). The laminated layer contains no nuclei and is about 1 mm thick (Figure 157–9). The germinal layer (Figure 157–10) is a single cell layer and about 10 to 25 μm thick. Some cysts are fertile and others sterile. Fertile cysts contain brood capsules, which develop on stalks arising from the germinal layer. Scolices may arise from the inner germinal layer of the brood capsule. When the brood capsule detaches from the stalk, it becomes a freely floating daughter cyst. Rupture of a daughter cyst releases scolices. The combination of free-floating scolices and daughter cysts is "hydatid sand," and is a diagnostic feature of echinococcosis. Disruption of the laminated membrane may allow fertile elements of the cysts to seed new sites. Sterile cysts, lacking the germinal membrane, produce no brood capsules, daughter cysts, or scolices.

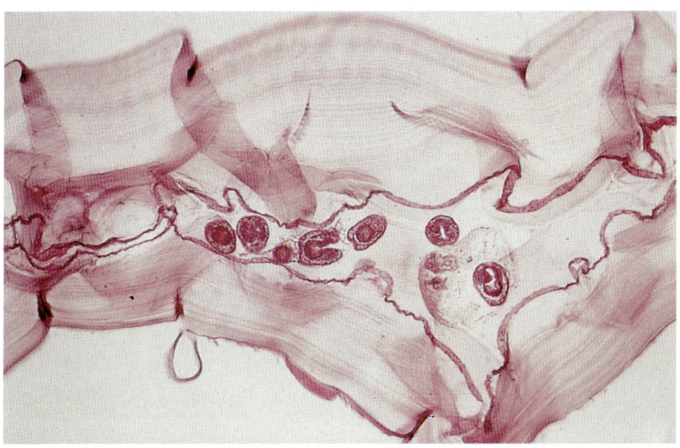

Figure 157–9. The collapsed wall of an hydatid cyst containing scolices within the lumen of the cyst. The wall is laminated and otherwise structureless. The germinal layer lines the interior and is a single cell layer thick (AFIP Neg 70-6612; H&E, ×45).

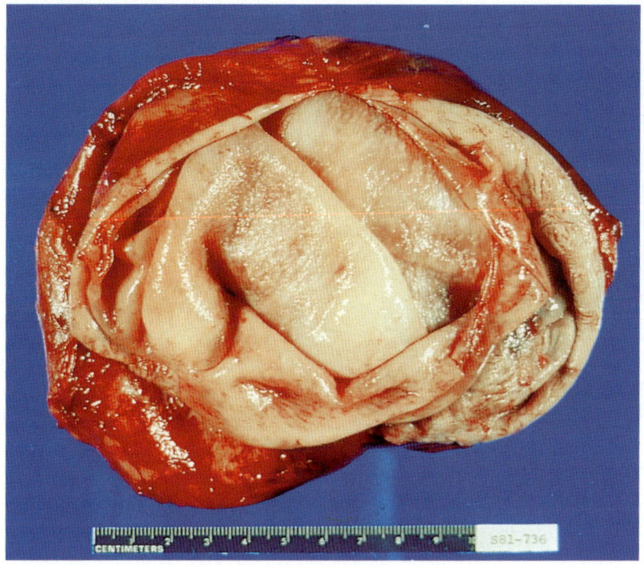

Figure 157–10. Hydatid cyst excised from the lung of an 11-year-old Portuguese child. The contents have been removed and the glistening lining is the germinal membrane. The cyst measures 9 cm across. *(Photograph contributed by Ernest E. Lack, MD.)*

The formation of more than one cyst from *E granulosis* is rare. In contrast, infection by *E vogeli* and *E multilocularis* causes polycystic and alveolar hydatidosis respectively. *Echinococcus multilocularis* is a rapidly building organism with infiltrative and invasive qualities (Figures 157–11 through 157–14). It is characterized by rapid dissemination to adjacent tissue and is often fatal. The name arises from its characteristic appearance; many small hydatid cysts covering large portions of tissue producing an alveolar pattern of infection.

IMMUNOPATHOLOGY

The state of the host's immune system as well as age, gender, and physiologic state influence susceptibility to hydatid disease. Specific humoral and cellular immune

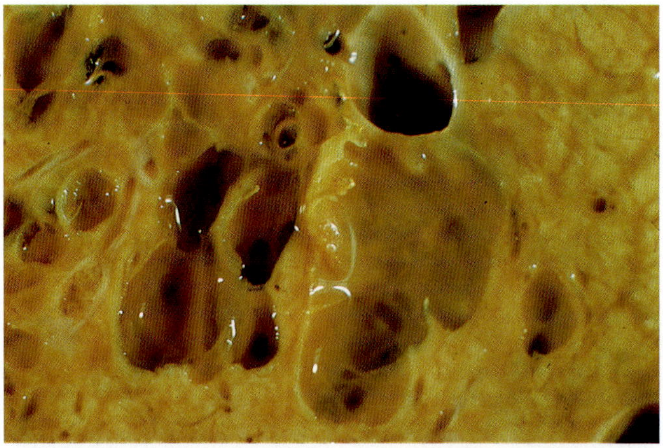

Figure 157–11. Gross photograph of liver of patient with alveolar hydatidosis (infection by *E multilocularis*). There are multiple cysts on the cut surface of the liver. *(Specimen contributed by Dr. Robert L. Rausch; photograph by Daniel H. Connor, MD, 1980.)*

responses to *E granulosus* and *E multilocularis* confer resistance to reinfection but their role in first infection is not clear.[26]

Recent in vitro experiments have demonstrated the ability of protoscolices of *E multilocularis* to suppress murine T-cell function by inducing the proliferation of CD-8+ T cells while simultaneously inhibiting interleukin (IL)-2 production and IL-2 receptor expression.[27] In humans, alveolar hydatidosis is also associated with impaired T-cell function as measured by in vitro assays and is characterized also by decreased total peripheral lymphocytes and a decreased percentage of circulating B lymphocytes.[26]

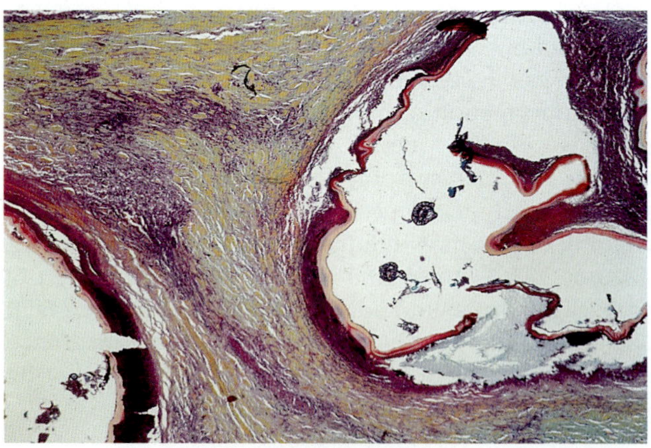

Figure 157–12. Microscopic section of the multiple cysts (buds) shown in the liver of the preceding photograph. The cyst walls are laminated membranes and the cyst contains a few scattered scolices. The intervening tissue is fibrotic. There is no normal tissue in the field (AFIP 1750623; Movat, ×18).

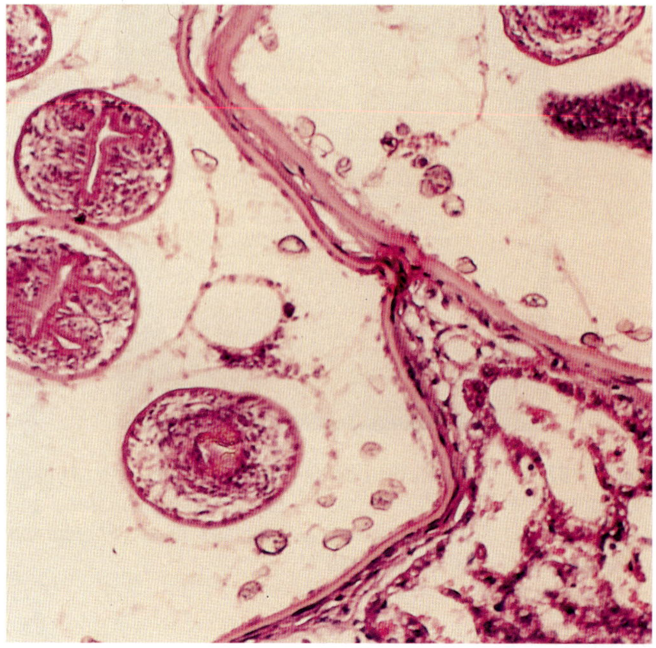

Figure 157–13. Multiple cysts of *E multilocularis*. The walls of the cysts are flattened against each other. Four scolices are in the cyst on the left (H&E, ×110).

Also noteworthy are the wide variety of autoantibodies detected in the sera of patients infected by *E granulosus* and *E multilocularis*. The autoantibodies directed against the major histocompatibility antigens are of particular importance because of their potential ability to impair antigen presentation to T lymphocytes and thus suppress the initiation of the immune response. Also, the protoscolices of *E granulosus* pro-

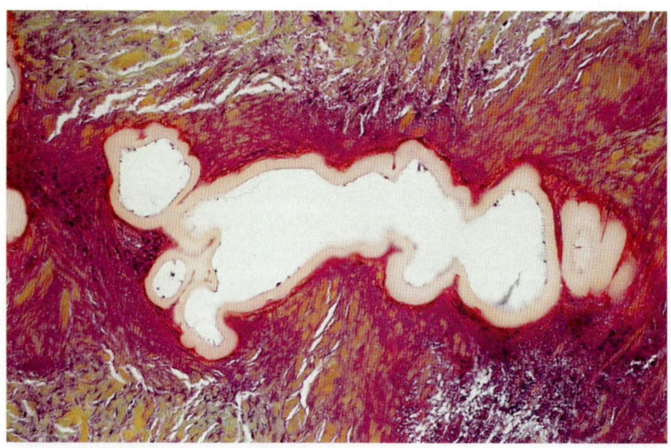

Figure 157–14. Close-up of a sterile and collapsed cyst of *E multilocularis*. The cyst contains no scolices and the wall is hyalinized. The adjacent liver is necrotic and rich in fibrin (Movat, ×45). *(Specimen contributed by Dr. Robert L. Rausch.)*

duce a protein that is homologous to the human protein cyclophilin. Cyclophilin has profound immunosuppressive activity on T cells when noncovalently bound to a polypeptide of fungal origin known as cyclosporin A. The role of cyclophilin in the organism's ability to evade the host cellular immune response, however, has not yet been established.[26]

DIAGNOSIS

Pathologic diagnosis is based on identification of the hydatid cyst. The cyst wall is finely laminated and amphophilic, and so characteristic, that only a small segment is required for diagnosis. In the past, fine-needle aspiration of cystic fluid has been discouraged to avoid rupture with the subsequent risk of anaphylaxis or spread. Recent studies have used ultrasound or computed tomography (CT) guided percutaneous fine-needle aspiration for diagnosis with minimal complications. Such invasive techniques may be valuable in the asymptomatic, seronegative patient who presents with a unilocular cyst. With ultrasound guidance, the diagnosis was made in 8 of 12 aspirated cysts with no complications.[28] In one study using unguided aspiration, the diagnosis was made in 9 of 13 patients. The diagnosis was established on visualization of a portion of the laminated wall in seven patients, scolices in two and hooks in two. Complications included mild allergic pruritus in 2 of 13 patients.[29] The presence of a hydatid cyst is easily confirmed by many radiologic modalities including plain roentgenograms, ultrasonography, CT, and magnetic resonance imaging spectroscopy. Calcification of the cyst wall and the presence of microcalcifications within daughter cysts as well as varying fluid densities between cyst and organ enhance the appearance in the roentgenogram and sonogram. Accurate diagnosis by CT was made in 96% of 157 patients with hepatic or other parenchymal cysts. However, ruptured or secondarily infected hydatid cysts could not be differentiated from an abscess.[30]

Serologic tests alone cannot be used to definitively establish or exclude echinococcosis. In general, serologic techniques are more specific but less sensitive than most imaging modalities. Commonly used serologic methods are latex agglutination, indirect hemmaglutination assays, Enzyme-linked immunosorbent assays (ELISA), enzyme-linked immunodiffusion assays (ELIDA), and immunoblotting. The ELISA is one of the most sensitive methods. Of 243 patients with echinococcosis 204 had positive sera by ELISA (sensitivity 83.9%).[31] Enzyme-linked immunotransfer blot (EITB) has 100% sensitivity, specificity, and diagnostic efficacy.[32] For the purposes of comparison, indirect hemagglutination was 88% sensitive and 100% specific in a survey of 70 patients with confirmed echinococcosis.[33] Serologic differentiation of cystic and alveolar hydatid disease has been reported.[34] Currently it is not possible to distinguish *E vogeli* from *E granulosus* by serology. Cross-reactivity be-tween cysticercocis and *Echinococcus* has been reported.

TREATMENT

Surgical excision of the intact hydatid cyst is the treatment of choice. Care should be taken to minimize the likelihood of rupture with subsequent dissemination or anaphylaxis. Operative mortality is estimated to be less than 2%. Postoperative complications range from 10% to 25%, and the rate of long-term recurrence following surgery is 2% to 10%.[3] In a recent survey, six of nine patients who were seropositive by ELISA for the EM2 antigen converted to seronegative within the first postoperative year while the remaining three seroconverted within 4 years. In a separate cohort, six of seven patients who became seronegative after surgery, and were later shown to have recurrent disease, became seropositive at the time of recurrence. Thus EM2–ELISA is useful in monitoring the postoperative course.[35] Perioperative chemotherapy with benzimadazole compounds reduced and improved long-term prognosis.[36]

Less invasive treatments have also been successful. *P*ercutaneous puncture with radiologic guidance and *a*spiration of cyst contents followed by *i*nfusion of a protoscolicidal agent, such as ethanol or cetrimide, and *r*espiration, known as PAIR therapy, has recently been attempted. While limited preliminary results are promising, long term follow-up is required to assess the efficacy of PAIR therapy.[3,28,29]

The treatment of nonresectable echinococcosis, including alveolar hydatidosis, with benzimidazole compounds has also been successful. The short- and long-term effects of albendazole, mebendazole, and praziquantel have been assessed in numerous clinical trials. Albendazole was slightly superior to the latter two compounds.[37–39] Recent efforts have focused on controlling transmission of alveolar hydatidosis. A 10-year field trial in Savoogna, St. Lawrence Island, was designed to interrupt the life cycle in the definitive host. Village dogs received monthly treatments of praziquantel followed by an 83% reduction in the prevalence of alveolar hydatidosis in intermediate hosts and a corresponding reduction in human prevalence.[40]

REFERENCES

1. Lopera RD, Melendez RD, Fernandez I, Sirit J, Perera MP. Orbital hydatid cyst of *Echinococcus oligarthus* in a human in Venezuela. *J Parasitol.* 1989;75:467–470.
2. Eckert J, Thompson RC. *Echinococcus* strains in Europe: a review. *Trop Med Parasitol.* 1988;39:1–8.
3. Kammerer WS, Schantz PM. Echinococcal disease. *Infect Dis Clin North Am.* 1993;7:605–618.
4. Caremani M, Maestrini R, Occhini U, et al. Echographic epidemiology of cystic hydatid disease in Italy. *Eur J Epidemiol.* 1993;9:401–404.
5. Reichel MP, Lyford RA, Gasser RB. Hyperendemic focus of echinococcosis in northeastern Victoria. *Med J Aust.* 1994;160:499–501.
6. Dada BJ, Adegboye DS, Mohammed AN. The epidemiology of *Echinococcus* infection in Kaduna State, Nigeria. *Vet Rec.* 1979;104(14):312–331.
7. Aikat BK, Bhusnurmath SR, Cadersa M, Chhuttani PN, Mitra SK. *Echinococcus multilocoularis* infection in India: first case report proved at autopsy. *Trans R Soc Trop Med Hyg.* 1978;72:619–621.
8. Gamble WG, Segal M, Schantz PM, Rausch RL. Alveolar hydatid disease in Minnesota. First human case acquired in the contiguous United States. *JAMA.* 1979;241:904–907.
9. Storandt ST, Kazacos KR. *Echinococcus* multilocularis identified in Indiana, Ohio, and east-central Illinois. *J Parasitol.* 1993;79:301–305.
10. Rausch RL, Fay FH, Williamson FS. The ecology of *Echinococcus multilocularis* (Cestoda: Taeniidae) on St. Lawrence Island, Alaska. II. Helminth populations in the definitive host. *Ann Parasitol Hum Comp.* 1990;65:131–140.
11. D'Alessandro A, Rausch RL, Morales GA, Collet S, Angel D. *Echinococcus* infections in Colombian animals. *Am J Trop Med Hyg.* 1981;30:1263–1276.
12. Gardner SL, Rausch RL, Camacho OC. *Echinococcus vogeli* Rausch and Bernstein, 1972, from the paca, Cuniculus paca L. (Rodentia: Dasyproctidae), in the Departamento de Santa Cruz, Bolivia. *J Parasitol.* 1988;74:399–402.
13. D'Alessandro A, Rausch RL, Cuello C, Aristizabal N. *Echinococcus vogeli* in man, with a review of polycystic hydatid disease in Colombia and neighboring countries. *Am J Trop Med Hyg.* 1979;28:303–317.
14. Rausch RL, Rausch VR, D'Alessandro A. Discrimination of the larval stages of *Echinococcus oligarthus* (Diesing, 1863) and *E vogeli* Rausch and Bernstein, 1972 (Cestoda: Taeniidae). *Am J Trop Med Hyg.* 1978;27:1195–1202.
15. Radhi JM, Thavanathan MJ. Hydatid cyst presenting as a breast lump. *Can J Surg.* 1990;33:29–30.
16. Schechner C, Schechner Z, Boss J, Horowitz J, Yeshurun D. *Echinococcus* cyst of the breast imitating carcinoma. *Harefuah.* 1992;122:502–503, 551.
17. Buskila D, Sukenik S, Klein M, Horowitz J. Polyarthritis associated with hydatid disease (echinococcosis) of the liver. *Clin Rheumatol.* 1992;11:286–287.
18. Vialtel P, Chenais F, Desgeorges P, Couderc P, Micouin C, Cordonnier D. Membranous nephropathy associated with hydatid disease. *N Engl J Med.* 1981;304:610–621. Letter.
19. Pinna AD, Marongiu L, Cadoni S, Luridiana E, Nardello O, Pinna DC. Thoracic extension of hydatid cysts of the liver. *Surg Gynecol Obstet.* 1990;170:233–238.
20. Gomez-Morales A, Croxatto JO, Crovetto L, Ebner R. Hydatid cysts of the orbit. A review of 35 cases. *Ophthalmology.* 1988;95:1027–1032.
21. Saxena S, Gupta R, Nigam DK, Tahiliani ND, Saxena KN. Hydatid cyst of kidney presenting as hydatiduria. *J Assoc Phys India.* 1990;38:359–366.
22. Sen SE, Iseri C, Saglam R. Renal hydatidosis. *Urology.* 1989;33:241–242.
23. Meneghelli UG, Martinelli AL, Llorach-Velludo MA, Bellucci AD, Magro JE, Barbo ML. Polycystic hydatid disease (*Echinococcus vogeli*). Clinical, laboratory and morphological findings in nine Brazilian patients. *J Hepatol.* 1992;14(2–3):203–210.
24. Ali-Khan Z, Rausch RL. Demonstration of amyloid and immune complex deposits in renal and hepatic parenchyma of Alaskan alveolar hydatid disease patients. *Ann Trop Med Parasitol.* 1987;81:381–392.
25. Rausch RL, Wilson JF, Schantz PM, McMahon BJ. Spontaneous death of *Echinococcus multilocularis:* cases diagnosed serologically (by Em2 ELISA) and clinical significance. *Am J Trop Med Hyg.* 1987;36:576–585.
26. Lightowlers MW. Immunology and molecular biology of *Echinococcus* infections. *Int J Parasitol.* 1990;20:471–478.
27. Kizaki T, Ishige M, Kobayashi S, Onoe'e K. Supression of T cell proliferation of CD8 T cells induced in the presence of protoscolices of *E multilocularis* in vitro. *Infect Immun.* 1993;61:525–533.
28. Filice C, Di-Perri G, Strosselli M, et al. Parasitologic findings in percutaneous drainage of human hydatid liver cysts. *J Infect Dis.* 1990;161:1290–1295.
29. Bret PM, Fond A, Bretagnolle M, et al. Percutaneous aspiration and drainage of hydatid cysts in the liver. *Radiology.* 1988;168:617–620.
30. Munzer D. New perspectives in the diagnosis of *Echinococcus* disease. *J Clin Gastroenterol.* 1991;13:415–423.
31. Babba H, Messedi A, Masmoudi S, et al. Diagnosis of human hydatidosis: comparison between imagery and six serologic techniques. *Am J Trop Med Hyg.* 1994;50:64–68.
32. Kaddah MH, Maher KM, Hassanein HI, Farrag AI, Shaker ZA, Khalafallah AM. Evaluation of different immunodiagnostic techniques for diagnosis of hydatidosis in Egypt. *J Egypt Soc Parasitol.* 1992;22:653–665.
33. Njeruh FM, Gathuma JM, Okelo GB, Tumboh-Oeri AG. Diagnosis of human hydatid disease in surgically-confirmed cases by the use of the indirect haemagglutination test based on a thermo-stable lipoprotein and on unfractionated hydatid cyst fluid. *Ann Trop Med Parasitol.* 1989;83:299–303.
34. Ito A, Wang XG, Liu YH. Differential serodiagnosis of alveolar and cystic hydatid disease in the People's Republic of China. *Am J Trop Med Hyg.* 1993;49:208–213.
35. Gottstein B, Tschudi K, Eckert J, Ammann R. Em2-ELISA for the follow-up of alveolar echinococcosis after complete surgical resection of liver lesions. *Trans R Soc Trop Med Hyg.* 1989;83:389–393.

36. Taylor DH, Morris DL, Richards KS. Perioperative prophylactic chemotherapy of *Echinococcus granulosus:* determination of minimum effective length of albendazole therapy in vitro protoscolex culture. *SO HPB Surg.* 1990;2:159–164.
37. Ammann RW, Hirsbrunner R, Cotting J, Steiger U, Jacquier P, Eckert J. Recurrence rate after discontinuation of long-term mebendazole therapy in alveolar echinococcosis (preliminary results). *Am J Trop Med Hyg.* 1990;43:506–515.
38. Wilson JF, Rausch RL, McMahon BJ, Schantz PM. Parasiticidal effect of chemotherapy in alveolar hydatid disease: review of experience with mebendazole and albendazole in Alaskan Eskimos. *Clin Infect Dis.* 1992;15:234–249.
39. Todorov T, Vutova K, Mechkov G, et al. Chemotherapy of human cystic echinococcosis: comparative efficacy of mebendazole and albendazole. *Ann Trop Med Parasitol.* 1992;86:59–66.
40. Rausch RL, Wilson JF, Schantz PM. A programme to reduce the risk of infection by *Echinococcus multilocularis:* the use of praziquantel to control the cestode in a village in the hyperendemic region of Alaska. *Ann Trop Med Parasitol.* 1980;84:239–250.

CHAPTER 158

Enterobiasis

Bharatha Sinniah

> *'Tis better than riches*
> *To scratch when it itches.*
>
> *Anonymous*

DEFINITION

Enterobiasis is a common infection of the intestinal tract caused by *Enterobius vermicularis*. Most infections are benign with anal pruritus as the only symptom. In more heavily infected patients, usually children, there may be also loss of appetite, irritability, and insomnia. Synonyms include oxyuriasis, pinworm infection, and threadworm or seatworm infection.

GEOGRAPHIC DISTRIBUTION

Enterobiasis is worldwide, but more prevalent in those parts of temperate countries where bathing is less common and heavy underclothing more common. The *Guiness Book of Records* claims enterobiasis is the second most common infection—second only to the common cold. More than 291 million people are infected. Children are more commonly infected than adults, especially those living in crowded conditions.[1] There is a tendency toward group infections such as in mental hospitals, foster homes, prisons, and big families. Spread of infection is promoted by overcrowding and sharing of beds, towels, and underclothing. In the United States enterobiasis appears to be more common among African Americans.[2]

HABITAT

Adult worms attach to the mucosa of the cecum, terminal ileum, colon, rectum, and vermiform appendix. Adult female worms deposit eggs on the perianal skin.

MORPHOLOGIC DESCRIPTION

The adult *E vermicularis* is white or cream colored, cylindrical, and pointed at both ends. A mouth with three lips, but no buccal capsule, is at the anterior end. The male worm (Figures 158–1 and 158–2) is 2 to 5 mm by 0.1 to 0.2 mm. Its posterior end is curved and sharply truncated. There is a single brown, hook-shaped spicule about 70 μm long. The male has a single reproductive tube (Figure 158–2) that begins slightly behind the esophageal bulb and continues as a straight tube to the posterior end of the worm. The female worm is larger than the male; 8 to 13 mm by 0.3 to 0.5 mm. It has a long pointed tail. The vulva opens midventrally about one third of the way down the body. The uterus is distended with eggs and occupies much of the body cavity (Figure 158–3). In both the male and female worms, the cuticle is expanded laterally into alae that run along each side (Figures 158–2 and 158–3). The esophagus has a prominent muscular posterior bulb. There are a few somatic muscle cells in each quarter of the worm (Figure 158–3).

The eggs are 50 to 60 μm by 20 to 30 μm, colorless, asymmetrical, and flattened on one side (Figure 158–4). The egg shell has two layers and is smooth and thick. The outer albuminous layer is sticky and this is the portion that causes intense anal itching in a sensitized person. The eggs, when first laid on the perianal skin, are usually partially embryonated. Eggs are resis-

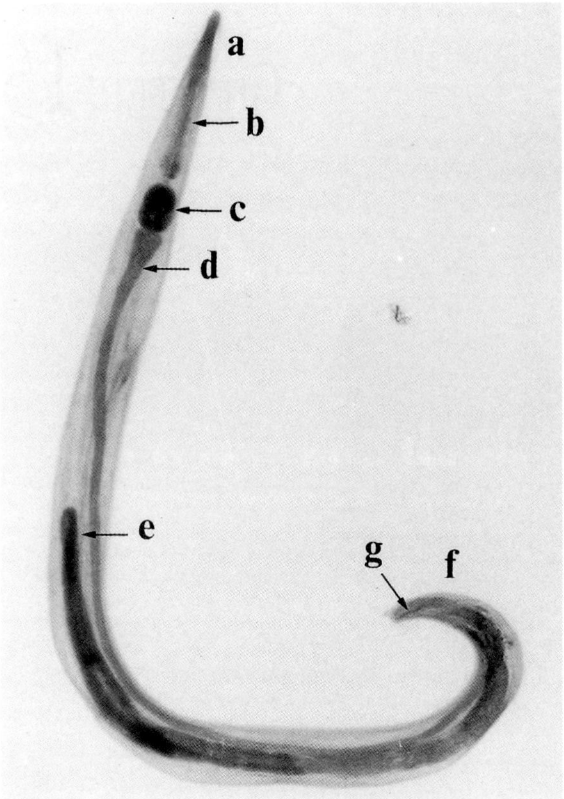

Figure 158–1. Adult male *E vermicularis.* The anterior end contains the prominent esophageal bulb. The posterior end is coiled. Labeled are the anterior end (a), esophagus (b), esophageal bulb (c), intestine (d), testis (e), posterior end (f), and the barely visible spicule (g) (Macroscopic, ×30).

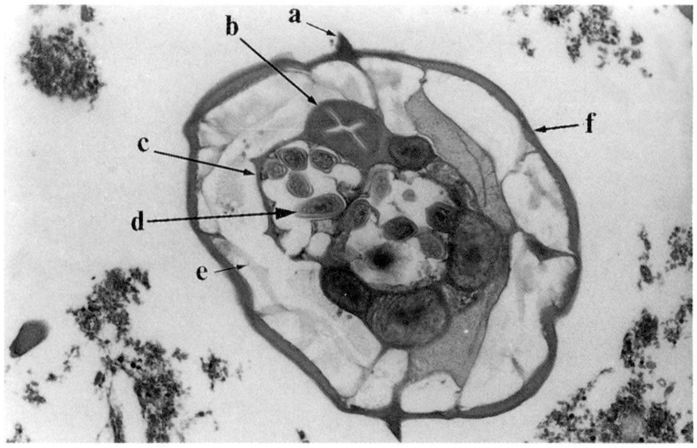

Figure 158–3. Cross-section of a gravid female *E vermicularis.* An ala (a), the intestine (b), the uterus (c), an egg in the uterus (d), a muscle cell (e), and the cuticle (f) are all labeled.

tant to commercial disinfectants and can survive up to 2 weeks.

LIFE CYCLE

Adult worms in the lumen of the colon copulate after which the male dies. The gravid female worms migrate to and through the anus at night where they deposit eggs. A female worm lays between 5000 to 17,000 eggs (Reardon, 1938) and usually dies after oviposition. Eggs become infective in about 6 hours. The outer albuminous layer is sticky and may, along with the female

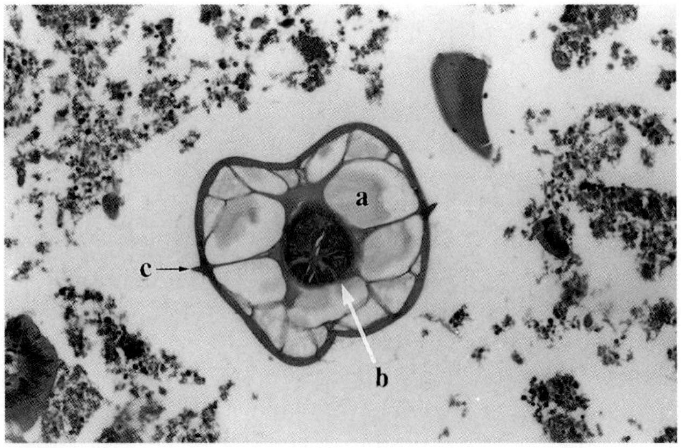

Figure 158–2. Cross-section of posterior portion of adult male *E vermicularis.* A muscle cell (a), the intestine (b), and a lateral ala (c) are all labeled [hematoxylin-eosin (H&E), ×250].

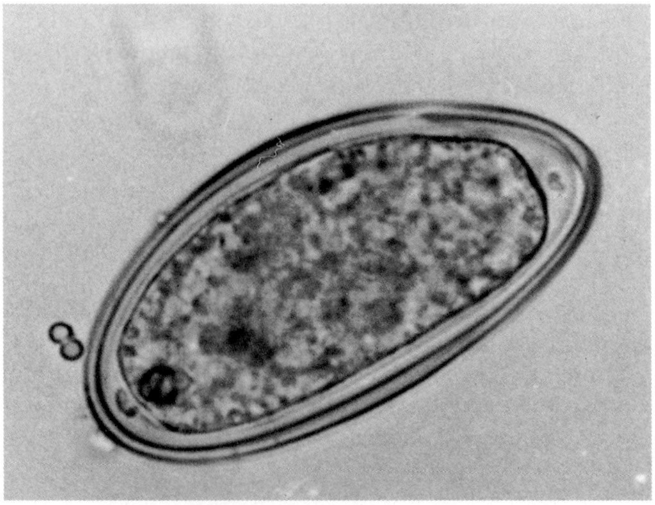

Figure 158–4. Egg of *E vermicularis* recovered from stool. It is essentially colorless but has a thick, two-layered refractile shell. The egg is asymmetrical with one convex and one flattened side. This is a characteristic and diagnostic shape (×750).

worm, cause intense itching of the anus. Itching provokes scratching and eggs then become lodged under the fingernails. Itching and scratching therefore promote anal–oral transmission (autoinfection). Also, eggs may be ingested in food, dust, and fomites. Soiled bed sheets and undergarments are also common sources of eggs. Homosexuals may develop sporadic infections from oral–anal sex. Infective eggs may also hatch on skin of the buttocks following which larvae migrate through the anus and into the bowel to become adult worms. This is retrograde infection. Ingested eggs containing the first-stage larvae hatch in the duodenum. Larvae then move in the fecal stream to large intestine where they undergo four molts to become a mature adult in 15 to 43 days. In the normal life cycle therefore there is no peripheral eosinophilia because the larvae and worms have no tissue phase.

CLINICAL SYMPTOMS

Most patients infected with *E vermicularis* have no symptoms. Dead worms and eggs that stick to the perianal skin, however, may provoke intense anal pruritus. This pruritus may cause insomnia and irritation from scratching and bleeding. Less commonly there may be secondary bacterial infection and ischiorectal abscess.[3] Insomnia, nightmares, anxiety, irritability, emotional instability, hyperactivity, nail biting, weight loss, enuresis, nose picking, abdominal pain, nausea, vomiting, grinding of teeth while sleeping, anorexia, and even convulsions have all been associated with enterobiasis in children. Eosinophilia may also be a feature. Female worms may enter the vagina from the anus and wander through the female genital tract,[1,4] causing vulvovaginitis,[4] cervicitis,[1] endometritis,[5] salpingitis,[6–8] and oophoritis.

PATHOLOGY

Enterobius vermicularis seldom causes serious lesions. Rarely worms cause petechial hemorrhage of cecum, appendix, and lower ileum from penetration.[1,9] Deeper invasion causes a granulomatous reaction with blood eosinophilia.[1–10] Although the mucosa may have minute areas of ulceration or sometimes open ulcers, the association with *Enterobius* worms is not usually associated with inflammation.

Appendicitis caused by *Enterobius* is still questionable. Symmers[1] and Sinniah et al[2] believe enterobiasis is not a significant cause of appendicitis. Even when adult worms have been noted in the mucosa and submucosa they provoke no inflammation. These worms, therefore, probably penetrate the mucosa after excision

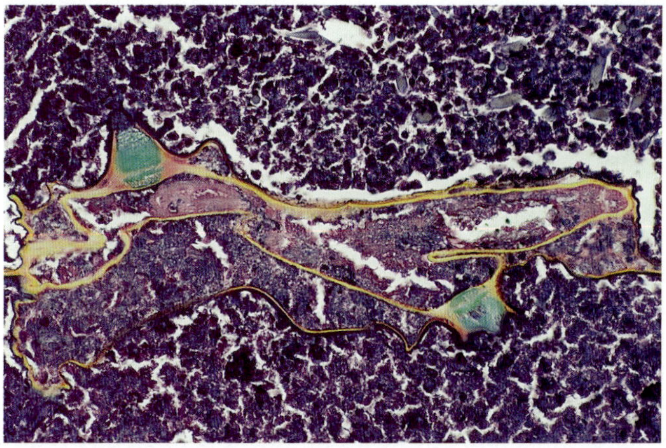

Figure 158–5. Degenerating and collapsed adult female *E vermicularis* in a necrotic granuloma in the omentum. The alae are still recognizable by their green-blue color (AFIP 75-9306; Movat stain, ×130).

of the appendix. Perhaps the adult worms actively migrate in an attempt to escape decreasing oxygen tension after the appendix has been excised. Gordon[9] first proposed postoperative migration as an explanation of this phenomenon and suggested that changing temperature and pH could stimulate *E vermicularis* to penetrate the wall of the appendix. Regardless of the stimulus or stimuli, the lack of reaction to these worms indicate that migration takes place after excision when the tissue has become devitalized.

Rarely female worms migrate through the vagina, uterus, and oviducts to enter the abdominal cavity where they may degenerate and cause necrotizing granulomas of peritoneum and omentum (Figures 158–5 and 158–6). In oviducts they may provoke granulomas

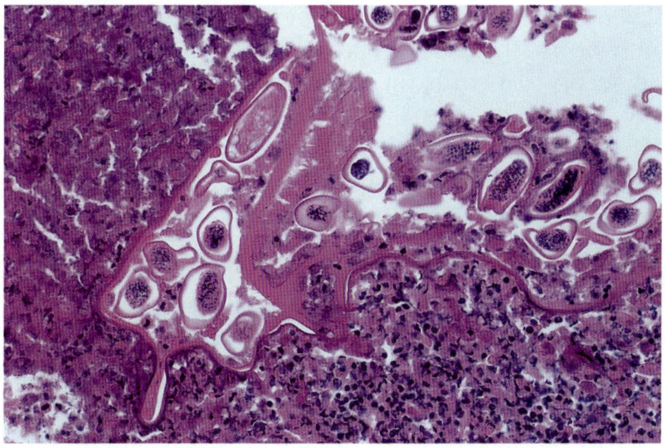

Figure 158–6. Eggs of *E vermicularis* in the omentum. The eggs are partially surrounded by the collapsed carcas of the parent female worm centered in a necrotizing granuloma (AFIP 75-10750; H&E, ×115).

leading to obstruction. Gravid female worms may cause a granulomatous endometritis,[5,11] salpingitis[6,8,12–14] or sometimes a pyosalpinx, vulvovaginitis,[1,4] cervicitis,[1] and oophoritis.[1,4,6] Other ectopic sites where adult worms have located are between the placenta and uterine wall,[1] in lung,[15] lymph node,[10] liver,[16–18] spleen,[1] urethra,[19] prostate,[1] and kidney.[1] Peritoneal lesions have been reported only in women, the majority being in the pelvis.[2] Three patients with *E vermicularis* in lung could have been from worms migrating from anus to nostril or mouth through the bedding, or from fingers to nostrils or mouth, then down the airway to lung.[2,5] Beaver et al[15] conclude that the worm must have entered the mouth or nose and then migrated down the respiratory tract to lung.

DIAGNOSIS

Enterobiasis is diagnosed by identifying eggs or adult worms. Ova are rarely in feces and are best collected from perianal and perineal skin by using the sticky side of cellulose tape ("Scotch tape") applied to skin. The tape is then examined under a microscope for eggs and/or adult worms. The best time for using the tape technique is first thing in the morning. If no eggs are present the test should be repeated for 7 days before rendering a negative diagnosis. Adult worms may be on or under the surface of a stool specimen, especially in children. Eggs may also be under the patient's fingernails but are not usually found in feces. In tissue sections, the identification of *Enterobius* is based on morphologic characteristics.

TREATMENT

Several drugs are available that can be used to eliminate the worms. The drug of choice is mebendazole (100 mg single dose) because it gives a high cure rate and is free from side effects. Piperazine hexahydrate (50 to 75 mg/kg daily for 7 days) and pyrantel pamoate (10 mg/kg single dose) are less effective.

REFERENCES

1. Symmers WC. Pathology of oxyuriasis. *Arch Pathol.* 1950;50:475–516.
2. Sinniah B, Leopairut S, Neafie RC, Connor DH, Voge M. Enterobiasis: a histopathological study of 259 patients. *Ann Trop Med Parasitol.* 1991;85(6):625–635.
3. Moreno E. Enterobiasis (oxyuriasis, pinworm infection). In: Marcial-Rojas RA, ed. *Pathology of Protozoal and Helminthic Diseases.* Baltimore: Williams and Wilkins; 1971:760–768.
4. Beckman EN, Holland JB. Ovarian enterobiasis—a proposed pathogenesis. *Am J Trop Med Hyg.* 1981;30:74–76.
5. Schenken JR, Tamisiea J. Enterobius vermicularis (pinworm) infection of the endometrium. A case report. *Am J Obst Gynec.* 1956;72:913–914.
6. Arthur HR, Tomlinson BE. Oxyuris granuloma of the fallopian tube and peritoneal surface of an ovarian cyst. *J Obst Gynec Brit Emp.* 1958;65:996–997.
7. Saffos RO, Rhating RM. Unilateral salpingitis due to *Enterobius vermicularis. Am J Clin Pathol.* 1977;67:296–299.
8. Brooks TJ, Goetz CC, Plauche WC. *Enterobius vermicularis. JAMA.* 1962;1979:116–118.
9. Gordon H. Appendiceal oxyuriasis and appendicitis. *Arch Pathol.* 1933;16:177–194.
10. Neafie RC, Connor DH, Meyers WM. Enterobiasis. In: Binford CH, Connor DH, eds. *Pathology of Tropical and Extraordinary Diseases.* Washington, DC: Armed Forces Institute of Pathology; 1976:455–459.
11. Nairn RC, Duguid HLD. Oxyuris granuloma of the endometrium. *J Clin Pathol.* 1954;7:228–230.
12. Tsung SH, Low WP. Invasion of the fallopian tube by *Enterobius vermicularis. Ann Clin Lab Sci.* 1979;9:393–395.
13. Campbell GC, Bowman J. *Enterobius vermicularis* granuloma of the pelvis. A case report. *Am J Obst Gynec.* 1961;81:256–258.
14. Nutting SA, Murphy F, Inglis FG. Abdominal pain due to *Enterobius vermicularis. Can J Surg.* 1980;23:286–287.
15. Beaver PC, Kris JJ, Laux TJ. Pulmonary nodule caused by *Enterobius vermicularis. Am J Trop Med Hyg.* 1973;22:711–713.
16. Daly JJ, Baker GF. Pinworm granuloma of the liver. *Am J Trop Med Hyg.* 1984;33:62–64.
17. Little MD, Cuello CJ, Alessandro A. Granuloma of the liver due to *Enterobius vermicularis. Am J Trop Med Hyg.* 1973;22:567–569.
18. Mondou EN, Gnepp DR. Hepatic granuloma resulting from *Enterobius vermicularis. Am J Clin Pathol.* 1991:97–100.
19. Al Allaf GA, Hayate ZG. Recto-urethral migration of *Enterobius vermicularis. Trans R Soc Trop Med Hyg.* 1977;71:351.

CHAPTER 159

Fascioliasis

Charles E. Binkley and Bharatha Sinniah

. . . Dorothy, the Scarecrow, the Tin Woodsman, and the Cowardly Lion are intimidated—indeed awed—by the outsized oracular figure called the Great Oz. But . . . Toto snaps at the concealing curtain and reveals that the Great Oz is in fact a machine run by a small, tubby, frightened man, as much an exile in this strange land as they.

Carl Sagan (1934–), The Demon Haunted World

DEFINITION

Fascioliasis is any infection caused by species of the genus *Fasciola*. Three species infect humans: *F hepatica, F gigantica,* and *F indica.* Although rare in humans, fascioliasis is a common liver infection of cattle, sheep, and other herbivores. Synonyms include liver rot (in sheep), fascioliasis hepatica, febrile fasciolitic eosinophilic syndrome, hepatic distomatosis (in part), hepatic distomiasis (in part), sheep liver fluke disease, and maggot liver or wormy liver.

EPIDEMIOLOGY

Fascioliasis, a zoonotic disease, prevails where livestock, snails, and humans are close together. Most infections are acquired by ingesting uncooked watercress. Human outbreaks have been reported from France, Spain, England, Cuba, Chile, and Uruguay and there have been sporadic infections in the United States, Hawaii, West Indies, China, Thailand, North and East Africa, South Africa, Iraq, Vietnam, and Russia. In several rural Chilean provinces, the prevalence of human infection reaches 75%.[1] Fascioliasis is more common among adults, especially women, and is diagnosed mainly in areas where low socioeconomic and cultural levels prevail. Human transmission appears to be maximal during the late summer, following infection of snails earlier in the season.[2] Up to 50% of sheep and up to 70% of cattle are infected in some parts of the world.[3] Horses, donkeys, camels, pigs, deer, and goats also can be infected. The economic loss from animal mortality, weight loss, reduced reproductive efficiency, and liver contamination in areas with significant incidence of fascioliasis is significant.[4]

MORPHOLOGY

The adult worm is a large leaf-shaped fluke 20 to 40 mm by 8 to 13 mm. It is brown to pale gray. The anterior end bearing the oral sucker forms a conical projection. The posterior end is rounded. The cone is about 4 to 5 mm long, which broadens behind, giving rise to two shoulders characteristic of *F hepatica* (Figures 159–1 and 159–2). The ventral sucker (acetabulum) is about 12 times larger than the oral sucker and is almost in line with the two shoulders immediately in front of the genital pore. The two intestinal cecae bear a number of lateral compound branches, which extend to the posterior end of the worm. The branching of the cecae distinguishes this parasite from the closely related trematode *Fasciolopsis buski.*

The two dendritic testes are in the posterior two thirds of the body, are highly branched, and lie one behind the other. The ovary also is branched and fan shaped and close to the ventral sucker. The uterus is short and coiled and lies between the ootype and the ventral sucker. The vitellaria are in the lateral fields and

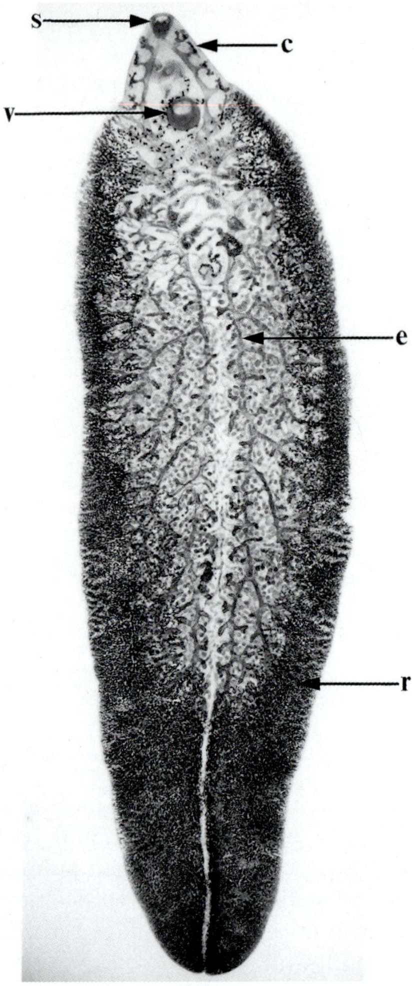

Figure 159–1. The adult fluke, *F hepatica,* ventral view. The oral sucker (s), cephalic cone (c), ventral sucker (v), cecum (e), and vitellaria (r) are labeled (AFIP 76-5956; ×3.75).

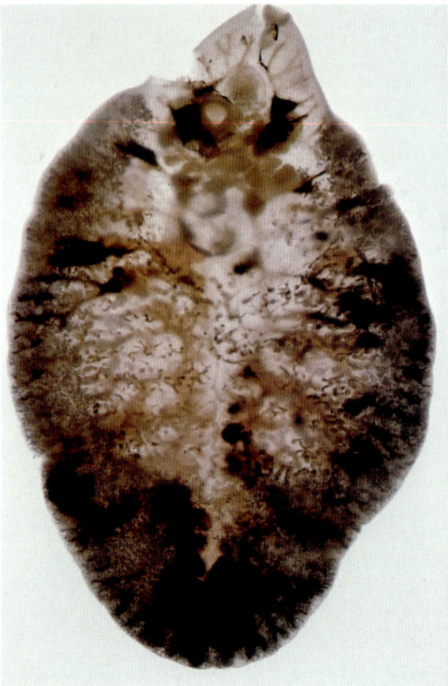

Figure 159–2. Preserved specimen of *F hepatica* from the patient with fascioliasis. Compare with Figure 159–1. *(Contributed by Dr. Jerome H. Siegel.)*

extend from the ventral sucker to the posterior end of the worm. Almost the entire surface of the tegument is covered with spines that vary in size and distribution.

The eggs of *F hepatica* are yellow-brown, oval, and have a small operculum at one end. They are unembryonated when laid and cannot be distinguished from those of *F buski.* They are 130 to 150 μm by 63 to 90 μm (Figure 159–3). When freshly passed, the egg contains a fertilized, unsegmented ovum, which lies in a mass of yolk cells.

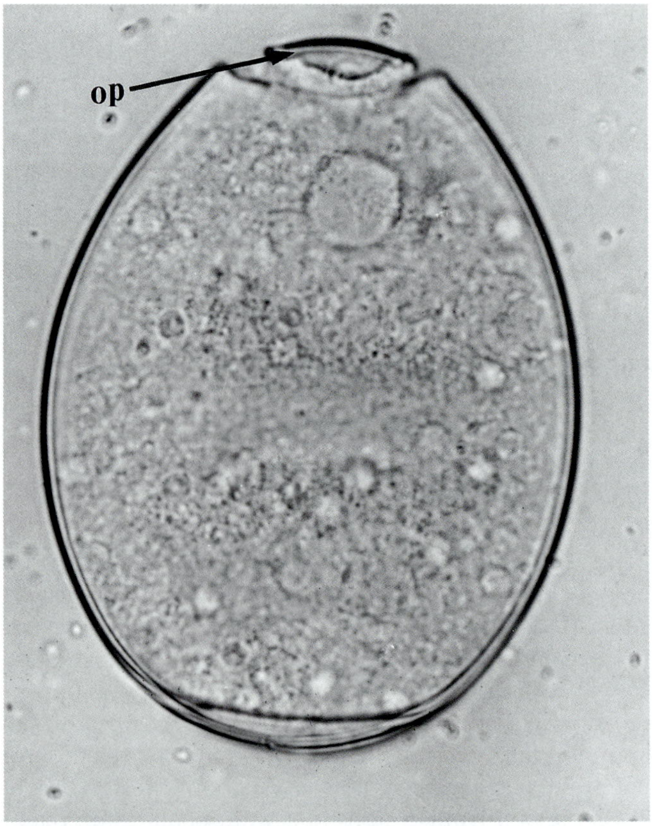

Figure 159–3. Egg of *F hepatica.* Note the small operculum (op) at the top (AFIP 72-17748; ×900).

LIFE CYCLE

Adult worms live in the bile ducts of humans, sheep, cattle, and goats (Figure 159–4). Eggs pass through the bile ducts to enter the gut and exit with the feces. In

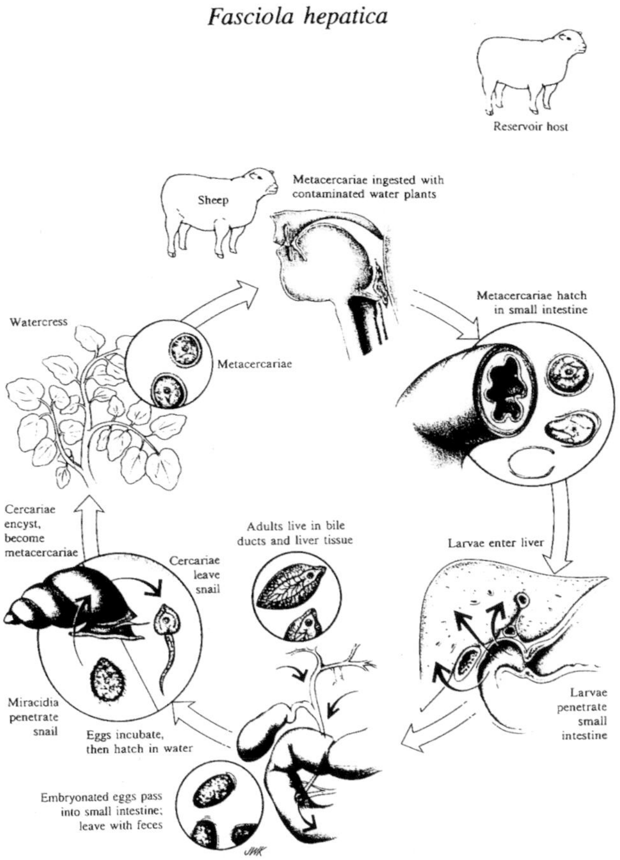

Figure 159–4. The life cycle of *F hepatica. (Contributed by Dr. Jerome H. Siegel.)*

water the unembryonated ovum develops into a miracidium in 9 to 15 days at optimal temperature of 22 to 25°C. The miracidium escapes from the egg through the operculum and lives for about 8 hours in water. To survive it must penetrate an amphibious snail, usually a species of *Lymnaea,* which is the first intermediate host. In the snail the miracidium becomes a sporocyst followed by two redial stages and then a cercaria. The transition from miracidium to cercaria takes 30 to 40 days. The mature cercariae swim for a few hours, then encyst on aquatic plants (second intermediate host) to form metacercariae. Humans and animals become infected when they ingest metacercariae encysted on water plants (especially watercress). Immature flukes excyst in the duodenum, penetrate the intestinal wall, enter the peritoneal cavity, penetrate the liver, and by 6 weeks migrate through the parenchyma into the bile ducts where they mature in another 3 to 4 months. Some immature flukes may also reach the bile ducts through lymphatics and blood vessels. Infection may last for several months.

IMMUNE RESPONSE

Recent attention has focused on the interaction between *Fasciola* sp and the host, particularly the acute inflammatory reaction. When rats are experimentally treated with Freund's complete adjuvant, before or after challenge with *F hepatica,* the fluke burden is decreased by 40% to 50%.[5] Alternatively, rats given anti-inflammatory agents, such as dexamethasone, indomethacin, or aspirin, immediately before or after infection with *F hepatica,* have a markedly increased burden of worms.[6] These studies suggest that the acute inflammatory response of the host to *F hepatica* may mediate the extent of infection. It appears also that localized reactions within the intestine of previously infected hosts play a role in resisting reinfection. The response appears to be mediated by both intrinsic neurons within the submucosa and local synthesis of eicosanoids, resulting in electrogenic chloride movement and intraluminal secretion of fluid.[7] The net effect is to inhibit the immature fluke from attaching to and penetrating the intestinal wall.

Besides the host response to *Fasciola* sp, there is a subsequent response by the fluke to the various mediators of immunity, particularly immunoglobulins, the classical complement cascade, and to eosinophils and neutrophils. The excretory and secretory products of the fluke appear to provoke most of the reactions. The key factor in these products is a cystein proteinase enzyme, cathepsin L. The cathepsin L proteinase of *F hepatica* is concentrated in vesicles in the gut epithelial cells of the fluke and has 50% sequence homology with its mammalian lysosomal counterpart.[8,9] Studies suggest that cathepsin L, excreted by newly excysted juveniles 3 weeks old, 5 weeks old, and mature worms, cleaves immunoglobulin near the hinge region, and prevents antibody-mediated attachment of eosinophils to the newly excysted juvenile flukes.[10,11] These mechanisms allow *Fasciola* sp to escape many of the protective devices of the humoral arm of the immune system.

In addition, fascioliasis in rats depletes the classical pathway of complement-mediated lysis, but leaves the alternative pathway unaffected. This response is maximal 6 to 9 weeks after infection, the period in which the worm invades the liver en route to its biliary localization, and is evoked by the excretory and secretory products, presumably cathepsin L, of adult flukes, but not of newly excysted juveniles.[12] This suggests a certain specificity in the response of *Fasciola* sp to the host response, which could be both time and tissue specific, conferring an overall survival advantage to the worm as it migrates toward its biliary home.

Investigation into reaction of *Fasciola* sp to neutrophils has produced contrasting findings. In one study done in vitro, the excretory–secretory products of *F hepatica,* when incubated with neutrophils, inhibited phagocytosis with, possibly, the formation of free radicals.[13] Another study, however, found that in the acute phase of infection while the fluke is in hepatic parenchyma and inducing maximal antigenic response, both the chemotactic and phagocytic activities of neutrophils were significantly increased.[14] Thus, the effect of fascioliasis on this aspect of host immune response is less clear.

PATHOGENESIS AND CLINICAL MANIFESTATIONS

Many light infections are asymptomatic, but the triad of fever, hepatomegaly, and eosinophilia, in endemic areas, suggests fascioliasis. Clinical manifestations are divided into acute and chronic phases. The acute phase corresponds to the migration of the immature fluke from the intestine to the liver and marks the period between infection and manifestation of fulminant clinical symptoms. It is often subdivided into an initial phase within 3 weeks, marked by the initial lesions; a middle phase at 6 weeks, characterized by parenchymal degeneration of the liver; and a final phase at 11 weeks when the flukes establish residence in the bile ducts.[15]

Symptoms, which begin about 1 month after infection, are fever, general malaise, fatigue, loss of weight, and loss of appetite. The patient complains also of headache, anorexia, nausea, vomiting, upper quadrant and epigastric pain, and digestive disorders. Allergic symptoms such as pruritus and urticaria can occur. Initially during the acute phase, bile flow is reduced, becoming increased by the beginning of the chronic phase at about 11 weeks postinfection.[15] Bilirubin, both conjugated and unconjugated, also increases during the acute phase, while liver cytochrome P450 concentration is reduced.[15] Corresponding to reduction in the levels of cytochrome P450 is the uncoupling of mitochondrial respiratory control in hepatocytes, possibly from phospholipase activation mediated by the host immune response.[16,17] Some patients have had anemia, with reduced serum iron concentration, as well as an elevated sedimentation rate.[18] Prostration, sweating, myalgias, pain in bones and joints with asthenia, and wasting also have been observed. There may be painful enlargement of the liver with jaundice and leucocytosis.[19] One fluke, in fact, was extracted from the common bile duct through the ampulla (Figure 159–5).[20]

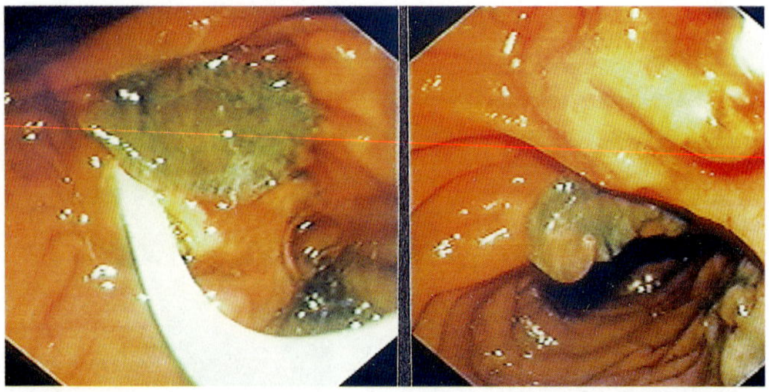

Figure 159–5. Photograph of *F hepatica* in the duodenum of a patient with fascioliasis. The parasite was extracted endoscopically from the patient's bile duct. On the left, the fluke is on the superior surface of the intestinal lumen as it is extracted with a balloon catheter. On the right the fluke is in the patient's duodenum after extraction from the bile duct. *(Contributed by Dr. Jerome H. Siegel.)*

The chronic phase begins when the flukes reach the bile ducts. Once the fluke is in the lumen of the bile ducts the patient may become asymptomatic or there may be symptoms caused by inflammation of the bile ducts. These symptoms include dyspepsia, diarrhea, jaundice, cholecystitis, biliary colic, and cholelithiasis. Extrahepatic manifestations in the chronic stage are also recognized, including pulmonary infiltrates, pleuropericarditis, meningitis, or lymphadenopathy.[21] Fascioliasis has also been associated with the antiphospholipid syndrome, manifested clinically by thrombotic subungual splinter hemorrhages and diverse arterial thromboses.[22] In severe infections there may be nodules in the liver. A computed tomography scan helps assess the extent of infection in these patients.

Occasionally, adult flukes migrate to ectopic sites. While the abdominal skin is the most common extrahepatic site, intraocular, intramuscular, and intraperitoneal locations have been reported.[23–25] The nodules may be up to 6 cm across and the overlying skin painful and itchy. Adult parasites may also cause abscesses in lungs and liver, and rarely invade brain.[19,26] In the Middle East adult worms ingested in raw liver from sheep and goats may attach themselves directly to the mucosa of the pharynx, causing edema, dyspnea, deafness, and asphyxia. These cause the "Halzoun" (suffocation) syndrome or pharyngeal fascioliasis. This is a temporary condition, but the edema may cause discomfort, dysphagia, and dyspnea.

PATHOLOGY

The migratory stage of the immature fluke (passing through the wall of intestine) causes no significant lesions in humans. In the early stages, destruction of liver is mainly from mechanical damage caused by migrating flukes. There may be considerable destruction of liver, characterized by coagulative necrosis, abscesses, patchy hemorrhages, and reactive hepatitis with numerous neutrophils, lymphocytes, and erythrocytes.[19] The number of tunnels lined by ragged walls of necrotic, inflamed, and bleeding liver tissue is proportional to the number of worms. For instance, infection by 600 adult worms may kill a sheep. In later stages the reaction is granulomatous with collections of histiocytes, epithelioid cells, and giant cells.

In the chronic stage, the pathologic changes are mainly in the bile ducts where the walls become increasingly thickened by fibrous tissue. The epithelium of the bile ducts becomes hyperplastic and contains exaggerated Aschoff–Rokitansky crypts (Figure 159–6). The mucosa may be 2 mm thick. Eventually the bile ducts become thickened also from chronic inflammation of periductal tissues. This along with the epithelial thickening narrows the lumen of the bile duct. Occasionally the lumens of the bile ducts become completely obliterated, causing obstructive jaundice. Chronic inflammation predisposes to secondary bacterial infection and, as a consequence, biliary cirrhosis. In contrast to other parasitic infections in which a possible association between the mammalian inflammatory response and neoplasm has been suggested or confirmed, fascioliasis bears no apparent association with cholangiocarcinoma.[27,28] In addition to sclerosis and obstruction associated with proliferation of epithelium, these ducts and ductules appear to secrete bile spontaneously, particularly following secretin stimulation. This accounts for the increased bile flow observed clinically at the end of the acute and beginning of the chronic phase.[29]

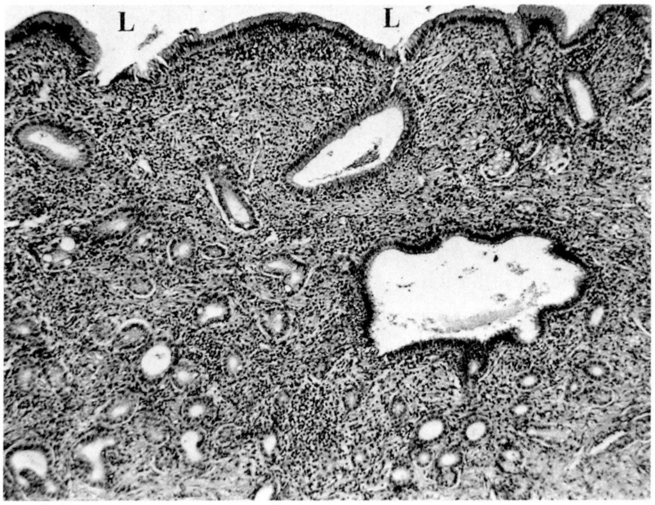

Figure 159–6. The lumen of an intrahepatic bile duct is the open area at the top of the picture (L). The periductal glands are increased in number and size—evidence of hyperplasia—and the supporting connective tissues contain chronic inflammatory cells (AFIP N-81327; ×115).

DIAGNOSIS

Many cases of fascioliasis are conclusively diagnosed only when patients are brought to surgery with a tentative diagnosis of acute cholecystitis or other biliary disease.[30] In these patients, removal of the fluke is often curative.[31] Diagnosis can be made by less invasive methods. Characteristic eggs in the feces or in the bile from a duodenal tube may help distinguish between fascioliasis and fasciolopsiasis, especially in areas endemic for both. In most patients, repeated stool examination is necessary to demonstrate the eggs. Eggs ingested in cooked liver of animals and then passed in the feces may lead to a false-positive diagnosis. Liver must be excluded from the diet for 3 days. If eggs persist, the diagnosis is established.

Serologic methods include a complement fixing test, indirect immunofluorescence test, enzyme-linked immunosorbent assay (ELISA), immunoelectrophoresis, double diffusion precipitin, passive hemagglutination test, and an intradermal test. The intradermal test may be useful in epidemiologic surveys. Only a positive precipitin reaction of an antigen dilution of 1:5000 or more is considered positive. Whereas in the past cross-reactivity of *Fasciola* sp with other trematode antigens had limited the specificity and sensitivity of serologic testing, recent advances in molecular biology have allowed more accurate serologic diagnosis of fascioliasis.

IgM ELISA techniques have allowed 100% sensitivity, 94% specificity, and 98% accuracy when using excretion–secretion products of *F gigantica* as antigens.[32–34] In fact, it is possible to distinguish between *F hepatica* and *F gigantica* using isoelectric focusing of soluble proteins.[35] Sandwich ELISA, having a similar species selectivity, can be applied to stool to detect excretion–secretion products of *Fasciola* sp.[36] Serologic testing offers the advantage of diagnosis before parasite eggs appear in the patient's stool.[37]

PREVENTION

Control of fascioliasis is threefold: 1) eradicate the disease in livestock, 2) use molluscicides, and 3) avoid uncooked water plants and contaminated water in endemic areas. Soil maps using the fluke egg shedding indices have been employed to identify areas with high prevalence of fascioliasis and to use flukicide treatment in animals, thus interrupting the life cycle and preventing possible cross-species transmission to humans.[38]

Recent effort has been toward eliminating *Fasciola* sp in the intermediate host. Polymerase chain reaction (PCR) techniques have been applied to the snail to detect fascioliasis immediately after exposure to the miracidium and implement molluscicidal measures.[39] In addition, several proteins of *Fasciola* sp, most notable being the glutathione S-transferases, have been identified as potential vaccines to protect animals.[40]

TREATMENT

The drug of choice for treating fascioliasis is bithionol given at 30 to 50 mg/kg orally on alternate days for 10 to 15 days.[41] Bithionol causes potentially severe complications and, in the United States, is only available through the Centers for Disease Control and Prevention.[42] Praziquantel at a dose of 25 mg/kg body weight, three times daily for 3 to 7 days, is considered by some to be effective.[41,42] Dihydroemetine or emetine hydrochloride, 65 mg, given intramuscularly daily for 12 days, or given simultaneously with 150 mg of chloroquine base, four times a day, has been use with limited success.

Recently, many have reported success treating fascioliasis with triclabendazole given orally in a single dose of 10 mg/kg body weight after an overnight fast.[43,44] Triclabendazole appears to act by disrupting the tegument of the fluke by inhibiting protein synthesis.[45,46] Other agents currently being investigated include triclazam, luxabendazole, as well as the microtubule inhibitors colchicine and tubulozole-C.[47–49]

REFERENCES

1. Apt W, Aguilera X, Vega F, et al. Prevalence of fascioliasis in humans, horses, pigs, and wild rabbits in 3 Chilean provinces. *Bol Oficina Sanit Panam.* 1993;115:405–414.
2. Farag HF, Salem AI, Khalil SS, Farahat A. Studies on human fascioliasis in Egypt. 1—Seasonality of transmission. *J Egypt Soc Parasitol.* 1993;23:331–340.
3. Muller R. *Worms and Disease. A Manual of Medical Helminthology.* William Heinemann, Medical Books; 1975:29–31.
4. Ngategize PK, Bekele T, Tilahun G. Financial losses caused by ovine fasciolosis in the Ethiopian highlands. *Trop Anim Health Prod.* 1993;25:155–161.
5. Baeza E, Poitou I, Boulard C. Influence of pro-inflammatory treatments on experimental infection of rats with *Fasciola hepatica:* changes in serum levels of inflammatory markers during the early stages of fasciolosis. *Res Vet Sci.* 1994;57:180–187.
6. Baeza E, Poitou I, Delers F, Boulard C. Influence of anti-inflammatory treatments on experimental infection of rats with *Fasciola hepatica:* changes in serum levels of inflammatory markers during the early stages of fasciolosis. *Res Vet Sci.* 1994;57:172–179.
7. O'Malley KE, Sloan T, Joyce P, Baird AW. Type I hypersensitivity reactions in intestinal mucosae from rats infected with *Fasciola hepatica. Parasite Immunol.* 1993; 15:449–453.
8. Smith AM, Dowd AJ, McGonigle S, et al. Purification of a cathepsin L-like proteinase secreted by adult *Fasciola hepatica. Mol Biochem Parasitol.* 1993;62:1–8.
9. Yamasaki H, Aoki T. Cloning and sequence analysis of the major cysteine protease expressed in the trematode parasite *Fasciola* spp. *Biochem Mol Biol Int.* 1993;31:537–542.
10. Carmona C, Dowd AJ, Smith AM, Dalton JP. Cathepsin L proteinase secreted by *Fasciola hepatica* in vitro prevents antibody-mediated eosinophil attachment to newly excysted juveniles. *Mol Biochem Parasitol.* 1993;62:9–17.
11. Smith AM, Dowd AJ, Heffernan M, Robertson CD, Dalton JP. *Fasciola hepatica:* a secreted cathepsin L-like proteinase cleaves host immunoglobulin. *Int J Parasitol.* 1993;23:977–983.
12. Baeza E, Poitou I, Villejoubert C, Boulard C. Complement depletion in rats infected with *Fasciola hepatica:* in vivo and in vitro studies. *Vet Parasitol.* 1994;51:219–230.
13. Baeza E, Poitou I, Boulard C. In vitro effects of *Fasciola hepatica* on the main functions of polymorphonuclear leukocytes: chemotaxis and free radical generation induced by phagocytosis. *Int J Parasitol.* 1993;23:1077–1081.
14. Osman MM, Rashwan E, Farag HF. Phagocytic activity of neutrophils in human fasciolosis before and after treatment. *J Egypt Soc Parasitol.* 1995;25:321–327.
15. Lopez P, Gonzalez P, Tunon MJ, Gonzalez-Gallego J. The effects of experimental fasciolosis on bilirubin metabolism in the rat. *Exp Parasitol.* 1994;78:386–393.
16. Lenton LM, Behm CA, Bygrave FL. Aberrant mitochondrial respiration in the livers of rats infected with *Fasciola hepatica:* the role of elevated non-esterified fatty acids and altered phospholipid composition. *Biochem J.* 1995;15:307;(part 2):425–431.
17. Somerville AC, Bygrave FL, Behm CA. A study of hepatic mitochondrial respiration and microsomal cytochrome P450 content in mice infected with the liver fluke *Fasciola hepatica. Int J Parasitol.* 1995;25:667–672.
18. Salem A, Osman M, Kandil M, Abaza M, Elewa S. Studies on human fascioliasis in Egypt. 2. Serum iron and copper in chronic fascioliasis. *J Egypt Soc Parasitol.* 1993;23: 357–364.
19. Malek EA. *Snail Transmitted Parasitic Diseases.* Boca Raton, Fla: CRC Press; 1980;2:131–170.
20. Veerappen A, Siegel J, Podany J, Prudente R, Gelb A. *Fasciola hepatica* pancreatitis: endoscopic extraction of live parasites. *Gastrointest Endosc.* 1991;37:473–475.
21. Arjona R, Riancho JA, Aguado JM, Salesa R, Gonzalez-Macias J. Fascioliasis in developed countries: a review of classic and aberrant forms of the disease. *Medicine (Baltimore).* 1995;74:13–23.
22. Frances C, Piette JC, Saada V, et al. Multiple subungual splinter hemorrhages in the antiphospholipid syndrome: a report of five cases and review of the literature. *Lupus.* 1994;3:123–128.
23. Cho SY, Yang HN, Kong Y, Kim JC, Shin KW, Koo BS. Intraocular fascioliasis: a case report. *Am J Trop Med Hyg.* 1994;50:349–353.
24. el-Shazly AM, el-Naggar HM, Youssef MA, Farid M, Hamouda MM. Histopathological picture of two cases of ectopic fascioliasis in Mansoura, Dakhalia. *J Egypt Soc Parasitol.* 1993;23:545–547.

25. Makled MK, Azab ME. Aberrant fascioliasis: ectopic focus in peritoneal cavity. *J Egypt Soc Parasitol.* 1994;24: 697–698.
26. O'Sullivan EN. Hepatic abscess due to fascioliasis. *Vet Rec.* 1995;136:304.
27. Gentile JM, Gentile GJ. Implications for the involvement of the immune system in parasite-associated cancers. *Mutat Res.* 1994;305:315–320.
28. Nash TE. Schistosomiasis and other trematode infections. In: Isselbacher KJ et al, eds. *Harrison's Principles of Internal Medicine.* New York: McGraw-Hill; 1994:924–931.
29. Lopez P, Tunon MJ, Gonzalez P, Diez N, Bravo AM, Gonzalez-Gallego J. Ductular proliferation and hepatic secretory function in experimental fascioliasis. *Exp Parasitol.* 1993;77:36–42.
30. Atalay F, Kirimlioglu V, Dagli U, Akincioglu T, Akoglu M, Seven C. Human fascioliasis. *Surg Today.* 1993;23:366–369.
31. Riedtmann HJ, Obeid T, Aeberhard P, Sakmann P. *Fasciola hepatica*—an unusual cause of acute cholecystitis with cholestatic jaundice. *Schweiz Med Wochenschr.* 1995;125: 1642–1648.
32. Shaker ZA, Demerdash ZA, Mansour WA, Hassanein HI, el Baz HG, el Gindy HI. Evaluation of specific *Fasciola* antigen in the immunodiagnosis of human fascioliasis in Egypt. *J Egypt Soc Parasitol.* 1994;24:463–470.
33. Diaw OT, Seye MM, Seye M, Sarr Y, Vassiliades G. Immunodiagnosis of *Fasciola gigantica* fascioliasis by ELISA technique in Senegal. Preliminary observations in 2 lambs. *Rev Elev Med Vet Pays Trop.* 1994;47:291–294.
34. Osman MM, Shehab AY, el Masry SA, Helmy MH, Farag HF. Evaluation of *Fasciola* excretory–secretory (E/S) product in diagnosis of acute human fasciolosis by IgM ELISA. *Trop Med Parasitol.* 1995;46:115–118.
35. Lee CG, Zimmerman GL. Banding patterns of *Fasciola hepatica* and *Fasciola gigantica* (Trematoda) by isoelectric focusing. *J Parasitol.* 1993;79:120–123.
36. Espino AM, Finlay CM. Sandwich enzyme-linked immunosorbent assay for detection of excretory–secretory antigens in humans with fascioliasis. *J Clin Microbiol.* 1994;32: 190–193. (Published erratum appears in *J Clin Microbiol.* 1994;32:860.)
37. Shaheen H, al Khafif M, Farag RM, Kamal KA. Serodifferentiation of human fascioliasis from schistosomiasis. *Trop Geogr Med.* 1994;46:326–327.
38. Zukowski SH, Wilkerson GW, Malone JB Jr. Fasciolosis in cattle in Louisiana. II. Development of a system to use soil maps in a geographic information system to estimate disease risk on Louisiana coastal marsh rangeland. *Vet Parasitol.* 1993;47:51–65.
39. Rognlie MC, Dimke KL, Knapp SE. Detection of *Fasciola hepatica* in infected intermediate hosts using RT-PCR. *J Parasitol.* 1994;80:748–755.
40. Sexton JL, Wilce MC, Colin T, et al. Vaccination of sheep against *Fasciola hepatica* with glutathione S-transferase. Identification and mapping of antibody epitopes on a three-dimensional model of the antigen. *J Immunol.* 1994 15;152:1861–1872.
41. Goldsmith RS. Clinical pharmacology of the anthelmintic drugs. In: Katzung BG, ed. *Basic and Clinical Pharmacology.* Norwalk, Conn: Appleton & Lange; 1995:804–822.
42. Bennett DR et al. Anthelmintics. In: *Drug Evaluations: Annual 1995.* Washington, DC: American Medical Association; 1995:1795–1826.
43. Apt W, Aguilera X, Vega F, et al. Treatment of human chronic fascioliasis with triclabendazole: drug efficacy and serologic response. *Am J Trop Med Hyg.* 1995;52:532–535.
44. Hammouda NA, el-Mansoury ST, el-Azzouni MZ, el-Gohari Y. Therapeutic effect of triclabendazole in patients with fascioliasis in Egypt. A preliminary study. *J Egypt Soc Parasitol.* 1995;25:137–143.
45. Stitt AW, Fairweather I. The effect of the sulphoxide metabolite of triclabendazole ('Fasinex') on the tegument of mature and immature stages of the liver fluke, *Fasciola hepatica. Parasitology.* 1994;108:555–567.
46. Stitt AW, Fairweather I, Mackender RO. The effect of triclabendazole ("Fasinex") on protein synthesis by the liver fluke, *Fasciola hepatica. Int J Parasitol.* 1995;25:421–429.
47. Mikhailitsyn FS, Petrov Iu F, Smirnov AA, et al. The technology for manufacturing antiparasitic preparations. 1. The development of a technology for producing the anthelmintic triklazan in finely dispersed form and the evaluation of its antinematodal, anticestodal and antitrematodal activities. *Med Parazitol (Mosk).* 1993;5:48–50.
48. Stoitsova SR, Gorchilova LN. Effects of luxabendazole on the tegument of *Fasciola hepatica. J Helminthol.* 1994; 68:73–80.
49. Stitt AW, Fairweather I. *Fasciola hepatica:* the effect of the microtubule inhibitors colchicine and tubulozole-C on the ultrastructure of the adult fluke. *Parasitology.* 1993; 107(part 3):297–309.

CHAPTER 160

Fasciolopsiasis—Infection by *Fasciolopsis buski*

Bharatha Sinniah and Charles E. Binkley

Why, his masculine whore. Now, the rotten diseases
of the south, the guts-griping, ruptures, catarrhs,
loads o'gravel i' the back, lethargies, cold
palsies, raw eyes, dirt-rotten livers, wheezing
lungs, bladders full of imposthume, sciaticas,
limekilns i' the palm, incurable bone-ache, and the
rivelled fee-simple of the tetter, take and take
again such preposterous discoveries!

William Shakespeare (1564–1616), Troilus and Cressida, V, I

Pseudoscience speaks to powerful emotional needs that science often leaves unfulfilled. It caters to fantasies about personal powers we lack and long for (like those attributed to comic book superheroes today, and earlier, to the gods). In some of its manifestations, it offers satisfaction of spiritual hungers, cures for disease, promises that death is not the end.

Carl Sagan (1934–), The Demon Haunted World

DEFINITION

Fasciolopsiasis is infection by *Fasciolopsis buski,* one of the largest parasites to infect humans. Flukes attach to duodenal and jejunal mucosa. In addition to humans, the dog, pig, and sometimes water buffalo are infected. Synonyms include distoma buski, Buski's fluke infection, giant intestinal fluke infection, intestinal distoma, intestinal distomatosis, and intestinal distomiasis.

EPIDEMIOLOGY

Fasciolopsis buski is mainly in East Asia, especially India, Bangladesh, Thailand, Eastern China, Taiwan, Vietnam, East Pakistan, and Laos.[1–3] The incidence of fasciolopsiasis among children in Southern Taiwan was found by one investigator to be 25.1%.[4] Several areas, including Indonesia, Hong Kong, and Israel, are becoming increasingly concerned about fasciolopsiasis from imported foods and animals, as well as immigrant workers.[5–7] Seasonal variance in the prevalence of fasciolopsiasis in animals demonstrates a peak during June–September, declining to a low during November–March.[8]

MORPHOLOGIC DESCRIPTION OF PARASITE

The mature fluke is oval, flat, and elongated, 2.0 to 7.5 cm long by 8 to 20 mm wide and 0.5 to 3.0 mm thick (Figure 160–1). The anterior part is narrower than the posterior and has no cephalic cone. The ventral sucker (acetabulum) is large and lies close to the oral sucker. It resembles the ventral sucker of *Fasciola hepatica* but it does not have a cephalic cone. The two lateral cecae have no lateral branches and extend to the posterior end of the worm. The tegument is covered with small spines. The two branched testes are in the posterior half of the worm and lie one behind the other (Figure 160–2). The branched ovary is in the middle of the body. The uterus, which is highly branched, is in the anterior half of the worm. The vitellaria extend from the ventral sucker to the posterior end of the worm and are in the lateral fields. The egg is large, 130 to 140 μm by 80 to 85 μm (Figure 160–2). The shell is yellow-brown, clear and thick, and has a small operculum at one end. The egg is unembryonated when laid and is similar to the eggs of *F hepatica*. Daily egg production is about 25,000 per fluke.

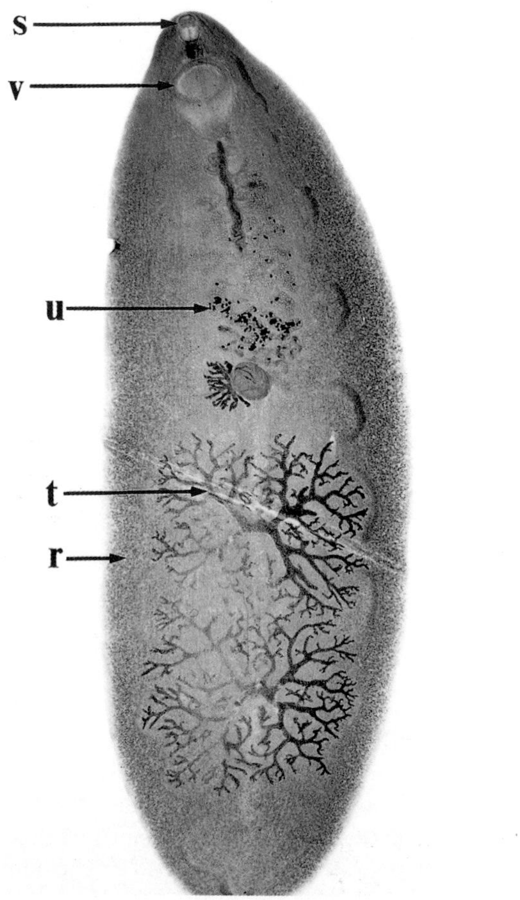

Figure 160–1. The adult fluke, *F buski,* as seen from the ventral surface. The oral sucker (s), the ventral sucker (v), the uterus (u), the testis (t), and the vitellaria (r) are labeled (AFIP Neg 56-3516; ×2.5).

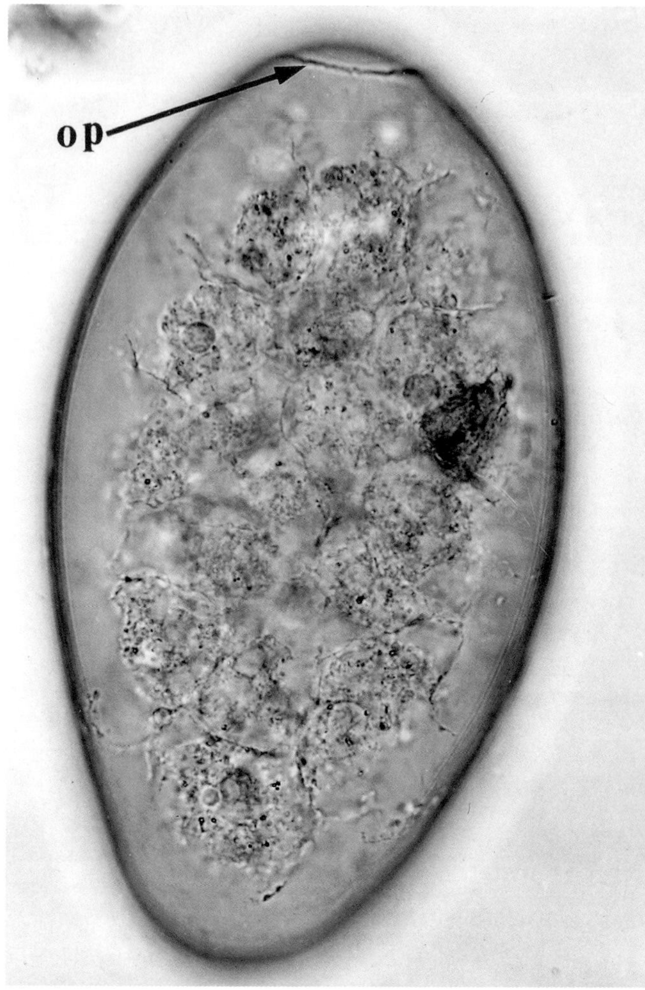

Figure 160–2. Egg of *F buski.* Note the small operculum (op) at the top (AFIP Neg 563326; ×500).

LIFE CYCLE

The unembryonated eggs passed in the feces must reach calm freshwater at 27 to 32°C after which 3 to 7 weeks pass before development is complete. The miracidia then hatch and actively bore into snails of the genera *Segmentia* and *Hippeutis,* where they develop into sporocysts then rediae, daughter rediae, and finally cercariae. Cercariae released from the snail encyst on freshwater plants especially seed pods of water-caltrop *(Tropa bicornis)* the bulb of water-chestnut *(Etiorcharis tuberosa),* water bamboo and water hyacinth, and here become metacercariae. These plants are often grown in ponds and pools that are fertilized with human feces. Additionally, up to 3.6% of the total encysted cercariae have been found to float on the surface of water, leading to infection by drinking contaminated water. One study found that, by case history, approximately 13% of humans and 40% of pigs examined had been infected by this route.[9] When ingested, the metacercariae excyst in the duodenum, attach to mucosa, and develop into adult worms in about 3 months. The adult fluke lives in humans for about 6 months.

CLINICAL MANIFESTATIONS AND PREVENTION

The fluke typically resides in the small intestine, particularly the duodenum, but is occasionally found in the colon or pylorus.[10] Most lightly infected people have no symptoms. Heavy infections, however, may cause anemia, dry skin, prostration, and even death. Nausea, low-grade fever, and greenish-yellow diarrhea containing undigested food are characteristic. There may be intense griping pain in the morning relieved by food. Metabolic products from the worm may cause intoxication and allergy.[11,12] Metabolites from the worms may cause also periorbital edema and generalized edema including ascites. Constitutional symptoms in children include low-grade fever, eosinophilia (up to 3% in about 40% of patients), asthenia, anasarca, stunted growth, and stunted development.[13] Jaundice, bloody stools, anemia, fever, and other nonspecific symptoms have also been recorded.

Boiling edible aquatic plants and potentially contaminated water from areas in which the fluke is endemic for 1 to 2 minutes before eating or drinking will kill the encysted cercariae. Feeding livestock fermented silage rather than fresh aquatic plants, coupled with regular testing of water supplies for evidence of *F buski* is recommended to prevent infection in animals.[9]

PATHOLOGY

At the site of attachment to the intestinal epithelium, adult worms usually ulcerate the mucosa followed by prominent inflammatory changes. There may be minimal bleeding at the sites of attachment but abscesses develop within the mucosa. Migration of the juvenile worms may cause mechanical destruction of the mucosa and this in turn may cause loss of weight leading to generalized weakness. Large numbers of worms can obstruct the small intestine. Acute ileus may complicate heavy infections. Intestinal mucosa is hyperemic and edematous. There may be peripheral hemorrhages and superficial ulceration.

DIAGNOSIS

The clinical features may suggest fasciolopsiasis in endemic areas but the identification of eggs in stool confirms the diagnosis. The formal ether sedimentation (concentration) technique makes it easier to find eggs in the stool. As yet there is no immunologic method useful in diagnosis.

TREATMENT

Praziquantel given at a dose of 25 mg/kg 3 times a day for 1 to 2 days is extremely effective.[14,15] Niclosamide and praziquantel are also useful when used together. Niclosamide, 1 to 2 g, is given to adults and children over 6 years of age. For children 2 to 6 years, the dose is 1 g and for children under 2 years the dose is 0.5 g. Praziquantel is given as a single dose of 40 mg/kg of body weight. Hexylresorcinol and tetrachloroethylene, a veterinary drug with high toxicity, may also be effective.[16]

REFERENCES

1. Yu S, Xu L, Jiang Z, et al. Report on the first nationwide survey of the distribution of human parasites in China. 1. Regional distribution of parasite species. *Chung Kuo Chi Sheng Chung Hsueh Yu Chi Sheng Chung Ping Tsa Chih.* 12;4:241–247.
2. Waikagul J. Intestinal fluke infections in Southeast Asia. *Southeast Asian J Trop Med Public Health.* 1991;(suppl):158–162.
3. Li X. Food-borne parasitic zoonoses in the People's Republic of China. *Southeast Asian J Trop Med Public Health.* 1991;(suppl):31–35.
4. Lee HH, Shyu LY, Chen ER. Experimental control study of fasciolopsiasis in Taiwan. *Kao Hsiung I Hsueh Ko Hsueh Tsa Chih.* 1989;5:335–344.
5. Kusharyono C, Sukartinah S SO. The current status of food-borne parasitic zoonoses in Indonesia. *Southeast Asian J Trop Med Public Health.* 1991;(suppl):8–10.
6. Ko RC. Current status of food-borne parasitic zoonoses in Hong Kong. *Southeast Asian J Trop Med Public Health.* 1991;(suppl):42–47.
7. Greenberg Z, Giladi L, Bashary A, Zahavi H. Prevalence of intestinal parasites among Thais in Israel. *Harefuah.* 1994;126:507–509, 563. English abstract.
8. Roy B, Tandon V. Seasonal prevalence of some zoonotic

trematode infections in cattle and pigs in the north-east montane zone in India. *Vet Parasitol.* 1992;41:69–76.

9. Weng YL, Zhuang ZL, Jiang HP, Lin GR, Lin JJ. Studies on ecology of *Fasciolopsis buski* and control strategy of fasciolopsiasis. *Chung Kuo Chi Sheng Chung Hsueh Yu Chi Sheng Chung Ping Tsa Chih.* 1989;7:108–111. English abstract.
10. Nash TE. Schistosomiasis and other trematode infections. In: Isselbacher KJ et al, eds. *Harrison's Principles of Internal Medicine.* New York: McGraw-Hill; 1994:924–931.
11. Marcial-Rojas RA, Fasciolopsiasis. In: Marcial-Rojas RA ed. *Pathology of Protozoal and Helminthic Diseases.* Baltimore: Williams and Wilkins; 1971:409–497.
12. Connor DH, Neafie RC, Fasciolopsiasis. In: Binford CH, Connor DH, eds. *Pathology of Tropical and Extraordinary Diseases.* Washington, DC: Armed Forces Institute of Pathology; 1976:528–529.
13. Piekarski G. *Medical Parasitology.* Berlin: Springer-Verlag; 1987:123–125.
14. Goldsmith RS, Clinical pharmacology of the anthelmintic drugs. In: Katzung BG, ed. *Basic and Clinical Pharmacology.* Norwalk, Conn: Appleton & Lange; 1995:804–822.
15. Bunnag D, Radomyos P, Harinasuta T. Field trial on the treatment of fasciolopsiasis with praziquantel. *Southeast Asian J Trop Med Public Health.* 1983;14:216–219.
16. Bennett DR. Anthelmintics. In: *Drug Evaluations, Annual 1995.* Washington, DC: American Medical Association, 1995:1795–1826.

CHAPTER 161

Gnathostomiasis

James M. Burke and John H. Cross

From the nature of human frailty, cure operates more slowly than disease, and . . .
the body itself is slow to grow and quick to decay.

Tacitus (55?–117)

INTRODUCTION

Gnathostomiasis is an infection caused by a nematode belonging to the genus *Gnathostoma*.[1] The disease is variously known as Yangtze River edema, Consular disease, Shanghai's rheumatism, nodular eosinophilic panniculitis, and woodbury bug.[2] The most common sources of human infection are undercooked, or fermented freshwater fish, chicken, and pork.[1] Although Daengsvang listed 12 species of gnathostomes, *G spinigerum* is considered the most important cause of human gnathostomiasis in the world.[3] The most conspicuous manifestations of the disease are nausea, swelling, and a migratory rash.[4]

MORPHOLOGY

The adult gnathostome is a stumpy, pink round worm that possesses a swollen head bulb surrounded by eight rings of hooklets[5,6] (Figures 161–1 and 161–2). Two lateral lips are usually on the head bulb, but as many as six have been noted.[6] Spines are present on the anterior half and posterior tip of the gnathostome[1] (Figure 161–3). The adult male is 10 to 25 mm long by 1 to 2 mm wide with two unequal spicules on its posterior end.[5] The larger female worm is 10 to 45 mm by 1 to 2.5 mm and has a midbody vulva.[6] The transparent, nonembryonated eggs are 70 μm by 40 μm.[5] The egg is further distinguished by a unipolar cap and a thick wall.[5] The earliest developmental stages are sheathless larvae with anterior enlargements.[7] In later stages the immature worms resemble the adults closely, except for their smaller size and the presence of only four rows of hooklets on the head bulb instead of eight.[8] It is the immature worm that causes human disease.

EPIDEMIOLOGY

Although spurious infections have been reported throughout the world, the endemic regions are Japan, Southeast Asia, India, and parts of Mexico and Ecuador.[4] Japan and Thailand are the predominant countries affected.[6] In Japan, raw fish is the source of infection, while in Thailand the source is more often undercooked duck, chicken, or fermented freshwater fish.[1] Infection caused by *G doloresi* and *G hispidum* has been reported in China after consumption of uncooked pork.[1,4] Infection has not been reported in the United States, but its diagnosis in travelers or in immigrants from endemic areas is becoming more common.[4]

LIFE CYCLE

The life cycle of the gnathostomes involves a carnivore and two aquatic life forms.[1] A variety of carnivorous mammals, mostly felines and canines, harbor the adult worms in tumorous swellings in the stomach wall.[7] Male and female worms lie together in the stomach wall where they copulate. The female worm sheds eggs, which pass into the gastric lumen and are then passed in the stool. Upon reaching freshwater, the eggs develop into larvae after about 1 week and are then ingested by a microscopic crustacean, the copepod.[1]

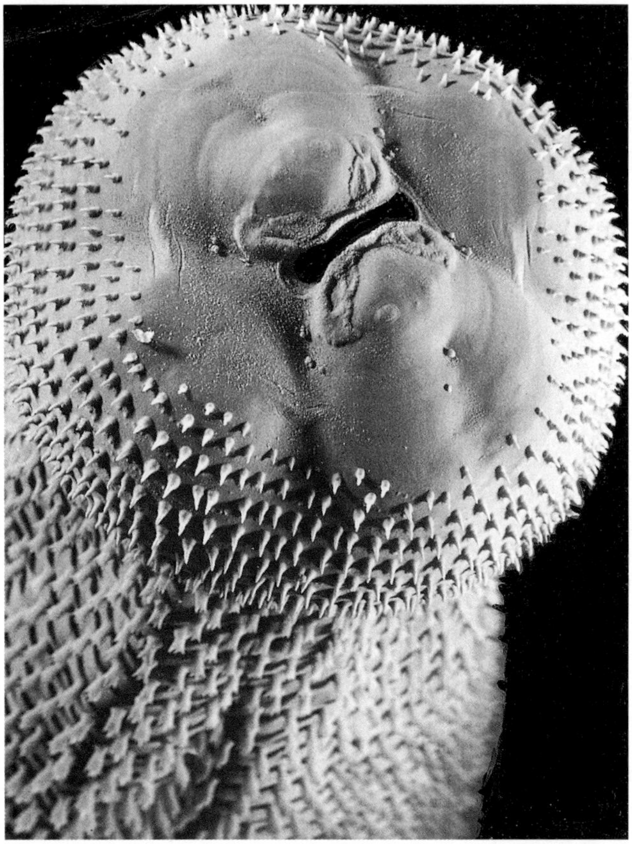

Figure 161–1. Scanning electron micrograph of the adult head bulb of *G spinigerum.* Note the lateral lips and the eight rings of hooklets (×500). *(Contributed by Viqar Zamar.)*

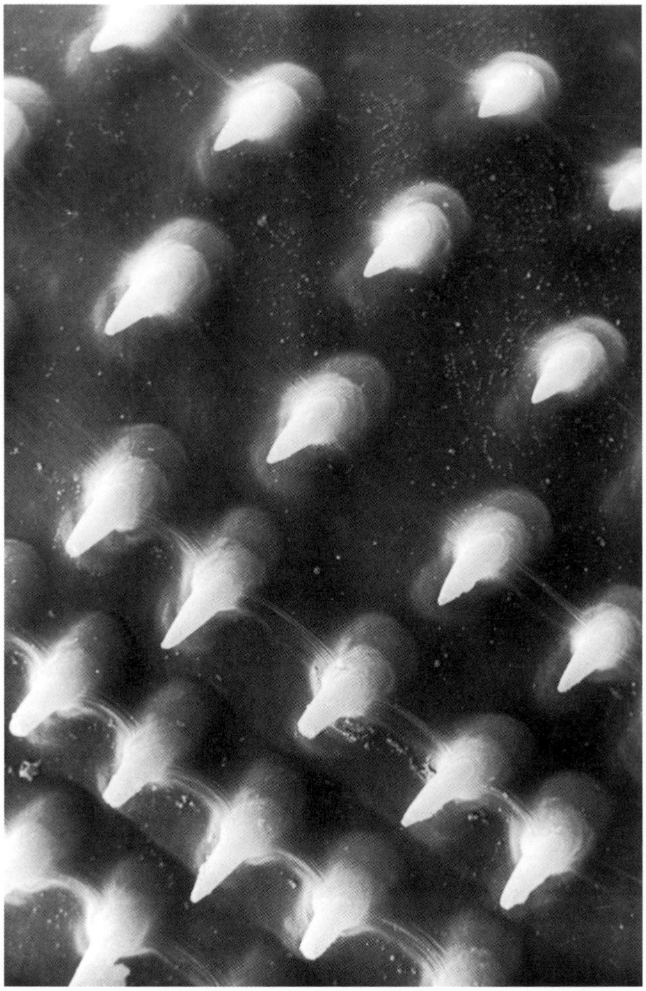

Figure 161–2. Scanning electron micrograph of the hooklets on the head bulb of an adult gnathostome (×5000). *(Photograph contributed by Viqar Zaman.)*

Within the copepod the larva develops into a secondary larval form in approximately 10 days.[5] At this point fish, reptiles, birds, or other aquatic animals may ingest the crustacean with water. Once in the stomach the crustacean is digested by gastric acid liberating the second-stage larva.[7] The second-stage larva immediately migrates through the intestinal wall, molts to its tertiary stage, and encysts within the muscle or connective tissue of the host.[1] If this intermediate host containing the encysted third-stage larva is now eaten by a proper, natural host, such as a feline or canine, the larva migrates through the stomach wall of the feline or canine and eventually encysts in the connective tissue or muscle of the animal.[4] Approximately 3 months later the gnathostome migrates back into the stomach wall and sexually reproduces, completing the life cycle.[1]

When humans ingest infested fish, reptiles, or birds, the tertiary larvae migrate through the intestinal wall to invade the skin and a variety of other tissues.[5] A migratory swelling and inflammatory rash of the skin are the most common manifestations of the infection.[4] Human infection leads to a dead-end in the life cycle of the gnathostome, because the parasite cannot reach sexual maturity in this host.[7]

CLINICAL FINDINGS

The acute phase of the disease begins 24 to 48 hours after ingesting the flesh of an animal containing encysted, viable third-stage larvae.[4] Systemic symptoms include nausea, vomiting, pruritis, urticaria, and upper abdominal pain (or discomfort), which coincide with the penetration of the larval form through the gastric or intestinal wall.[9] The acute abdominal pain may mimic other causes, including appendicitis, cholecystitis, cystitis, or salpingitis.[4] Larval entry into the liver is marked by right upper quadrant tenderness with changes in

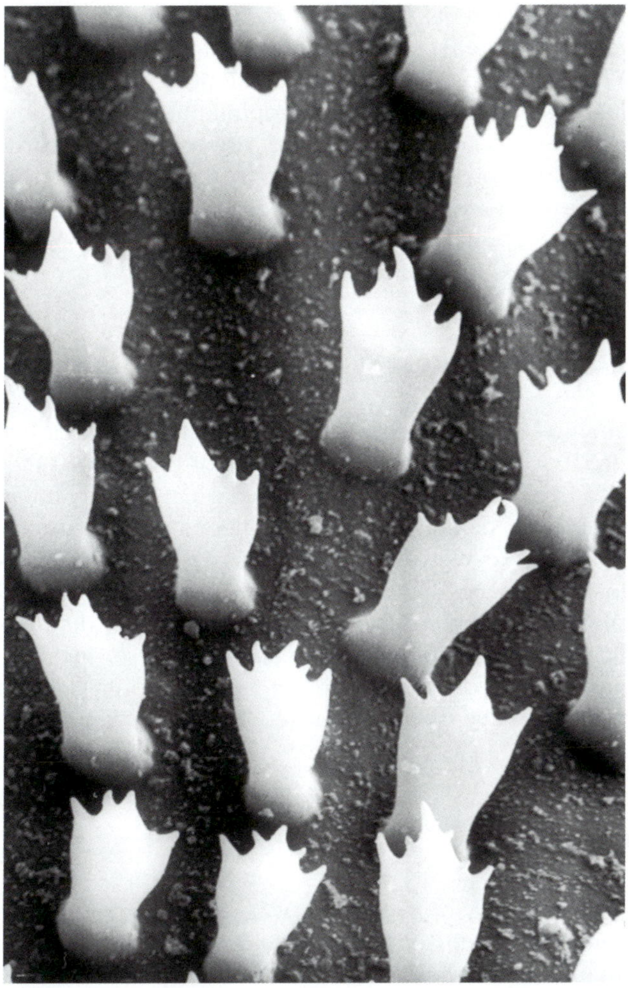

Figure 161–3. Scanning electron micrograph of leaflike spines on the body of an adult gnathostome. (×5000). *(Photograph contributed by Viqar Zaman.)*

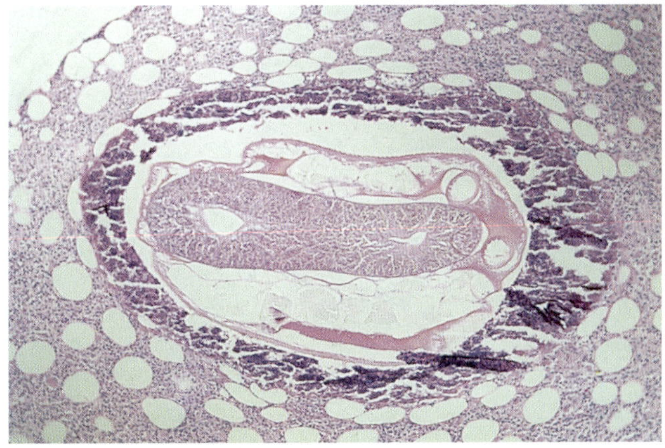

Figure 161–4. Cyst of abdominal wall from a young boy. Contained in the cyst is a larva of *G spinigerum*. Shown in this tangential section is the elongated esophagus next to two of the four cervical sacs, which serve to control inflation and deflation of the head bulb during the gnathostome's migration through the tissue. *(Photograph contributed by Lawrence Ash.)*

liver function but without liver enlargement.[4] Involvement of the lungs following migration of the parasite through the diaphragm can cause pulmonary infiltration or, in patients with pleural invasion, pneumothorax.[4] There is an eosinophilia in the range of 50% to 90% accompanied by a mild leukocytosis.[2]

After 3 to 4 weeks the chronic stage begins as the larva enter the subcutaneous tissue and the generalized symptoms and eosinophilia subside.[4] The chronic stage is dominated by the symptoms caused by the movement of the parasite through various tissues including skin and, more rarely, the central nervous system[4] (Figures 161–4 through 161–7). A migrating red rash reflecting subcutaneous involvement is the most common manifestation of the chronic disease.[4] The rash normally presents as a palm-sized, warm, red, pruritic, and painless swelling.[4] The migrating parasite can move through the tissues at a speed of up to 1 cm/h making surgical excision difficult.[10] In the early stages, the rash appears every few weeks.[4] The disease may run a 12-year course, during which symptoms become less severe and there are increasingly long periods without symptoms.[1]

Rarely, gnathostomes migrate into the central nervous system (Figure 161–8). Symptoms depend on the area of the brain or spinal cord invaded.[4] Abdominal, pulmonary, and ocular involvement have also been reported.[4]

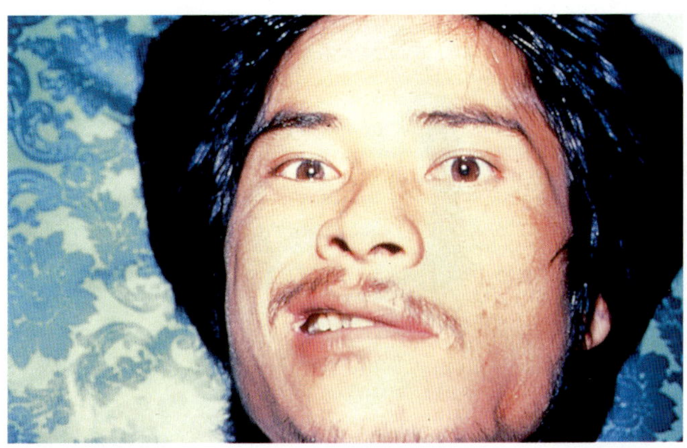

Figure 161–5. Young Thai male with facial palsy caused by gnathostome migration into the nerves controlling facial expression. *(Photograph contributed by Danai Bunnag.)*

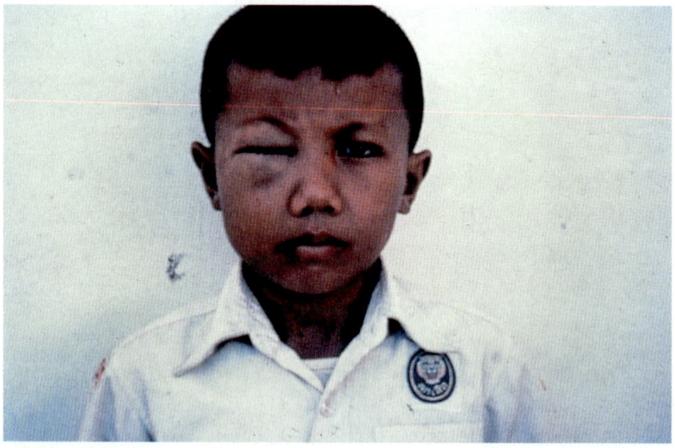

Figure 161–6. Thai boy with swollen and closed right eye following gnathostome migration into the soft tissues around the eye. *(Photograph contributed by Danai Bunnag.)*

PATHOLOGY

The cutaneous lesions, so-called "gnathostomiasis externa," are the most obvious clinical manifestations.[1] A red, raised, migrating rash is characteristic.[4] Eruption of the parasite through the skin has been reported.[1]

The histopathology is dominated by destructive, necrotizing, inflammatory tracks in the patient's tissues.[9] Hyaluronidase, an acetylcholine-like substance, and other parasitic proteases cause edema, hemorrhage, and necrosis.[9] A small number of eosinophils, plasma cells, and neutrophils are in the tracks.[9] Antigens released when the gnathostome dies cause an acute inflammatory reaction, which later becomes fibrogranulomatous.[9]

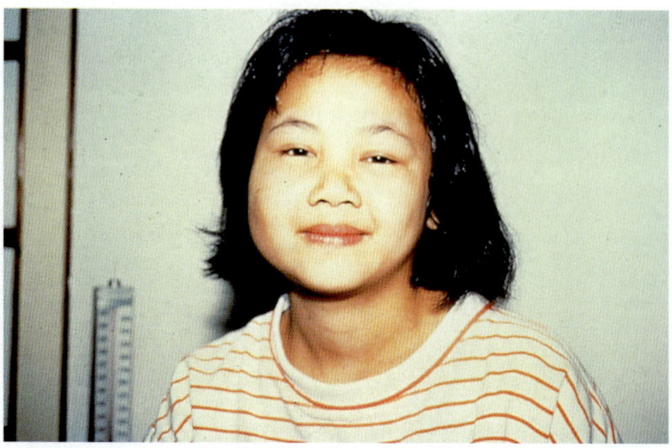

Figure 161–7. Thai girl with swelling of the right cheek following gnathostome migration into the subcutaneous tissues. *(Photograph contributed by Danai Bunnag.)*

Rare patients in whom worms invade the central nervous system have life-threatening complications. When migrating through the central nervous system, the gnathostomes can cause eosinophilic neuritis, meningitis, or encephalitis.[4] Even more serious are the destructive cavitations that may form in the brain following gnathostome entry.[9] Further, gnathostomes migrating into the eye have caused uveitis, hemorrhage, retinal detachment, and blindness.[11]

DIAGNOSIS

Gnathostomiasis must be considered in any patient with a red rash and history of ingestion of raw animal flesh who lives or has lived in an endemic area.[2] Sparganosis, cutaneous paragonimiasis, cutaneous larva migrans, trichinosis (eye swelling), and myiasis may all resemble gnathostomiasis clinically.[9] Tissue biopsy and identification of the third-stage larva provide the definitive diagnosis.[12] Antibody-based diagnostic tests including enzyme-linked immunosorbent assay and immunofluorescence have thus far lacked specificity and sensitivity.[13,14]

TREATMENT

Until recently, no treatment was available for gnathostomiasis aside from surgical excision when it was subcutaneous. Surgical treatment, however, has proved to be less than satisfactory because larvae can usually be found in other parts of the body and the gnathostome

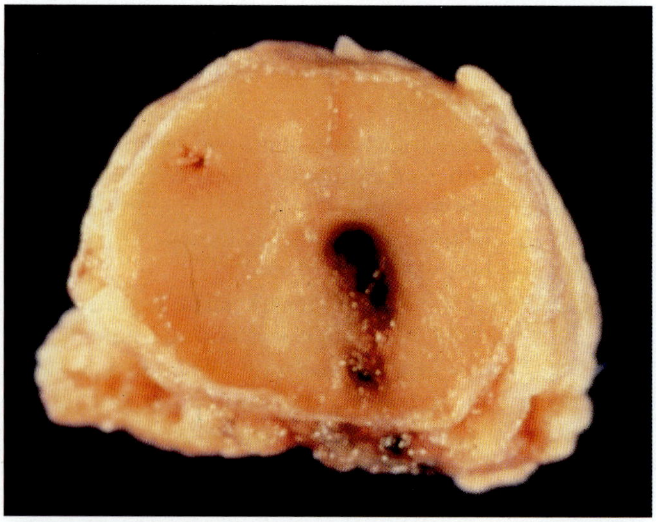

Figure 161–8. Cross-section of spinal cord showing a hemorrhagic track of a gnathostome larva. The patient subsequently died of the infection. *(Photograph contributed by Thanongsak Bunnag.)*

migrates rapidly away from the surgeon's scalpel.[10] Currently, chemotherapeutic intervention holds great promise with investigators having success using both ivermectin and albendazole to affect the tissue larva.[15,16]

PREVENTION

Due to the limited methods for treating gnathostomiasis, prevention is of vital importance. The hardy gnathostome has been reported to survive in the flesh of fish after refrigeration at 4°C for 1 month.[3] Boiling for 5 minutes, soaking in vinegar for 6 hours, and soaking in soy for 12 hours have all been reported to kill encysted larvae.[3] Thoroughly cooking all possible sources of the infectious larvae in endemic areas remains the best method for prevention.[3]

REFERENCES

1. Schmidt G, Roberts L. *Foundations of Parasitology.* St. Louis: Times Mirror/Mosby College Publishing; 1985: 506–510.
2. Rusnak J, Lucey D. Clinical gnathostomiasis: case report and review of the English language literature. *Clin Infect Dis.* 1993;16:33–50.
3. Daengsvang S. *A Monograph in the Genus Gnathostoma and Gnathostomiasis in Thailand.* Tokyo: Southeast Asian Medical Information Center, International Medical Foundations of Japan; 1980:1–70.
4. Swanson V. Gnathostomiasis. In: Connor DH, Binford CH, eds. *Pathology of Tropical and Extraordinary Diseases.* Washington, DC: Armed Forces Institute of Pathology; 1976;2:471–474.
5. Swellengrebel N, Sterman M. *Animal Parasites in Man.* Princeton, NJ: D VanNostrand; 1961:425–427.
6. Noble E, Noble G. *Parasitology: The Biology of Animal Parasites.* Philadelphia: Lea and Febiger; 1982:297–299.
7. Levine N, *Nematode Parasites.* Minneapolis: Burgess Publishing; 1980:317–318.
8. Chitwood B, *Introduction to Nematology.* Baltimore: University Park Press; 1974:284–285.
9. Markell E, Voge M, John D. *Medical Parasitology.* Philadelphia: WB Saunders; 1992:337–339.
10. Sooksam M, Reichert P. Migratory swelling due to gnathostomiasis. *Int J Oral Maxillofac Surg.* 1992;21: 176–177.
11. Funata M, Custis P, De la Cruz Z, de Juan E, Green W. Intraocular gnathostomiasis. *Retina.* 1993;13:240–244.
12. Sato H, Kamiya H, Hanada K. Five confirmed human cases of gnathostomiasis nipponica recently found in northern Japan. *J Parasitol.* 1992;78:1006–1010.
13. Taniguchi Y, Hashimoto K, Ichikawa S, Shimizu M, Ando K, Kotani Y. Human gnathostomiasis. *J Cutaneous Pathol.* 1991;18:112–115.
14. Maleewong W, Wongkham C, Intapan P, et al. Detection of circulating parasite antigens in murine gnathostomiasis by a two site enzyme linked immunosorbent assay. *Am J Trop Med Hyg.* 1992;46:80–84.
15. Anataphruti M, Naumtanong S, Waikagul J. The effect of ivermectin on experimental gnathostomiasis in rabbits. *Trop Med Parasitol.* 1992;43:65–67.
16. Kravichian P, Kulkumthorn M, Yingyourd P, Akarabovorn P, Paireepai C. Albendazole for the treatment of human gnathostomiasis. *Trans R Soc Trop Med Hyg.* 1992;86: 418–421.

CHAPTER 162

Halicephalobiasis (Micronemiasis)

John A. Shadduck and Van Q. Telford

My flesh is clothed with worms and clods of dust; my skin is broken, and become loathsome.

Job 7:5

DEFINITION AND GEOGRAPHY

Halicephalobiasis (micronemiasis) is a rare accidental infection of humans and horses caused by the invasion of tissues and organs by free-living rhabditid nematodes of the genus *Halicephalobus (Micronema)*. *Halicephalobus deletrix (Micronema deletrix)* is a soil saprophyte distributed widely throughout the world. *Halicephalobus* has infected horses in the United States, Europe, Japan, the United Kingdom, and the Middle East[1–3] and one person each in Manitoba,[4] Texas,[5] and Washington, DC.[6] All three human infections were fatal.

LIFE CYCLE, HISTORY, AND EPIDEMIOLOGY

Members of the genus *Halicephalobus* are generally free-living or saprophytic nematodes in decaying humus, soil and small collections of freshwater. The worms, however, are able to enter the skin and multiply in the tissues of humans and horses. The sources and risk factors for human infection are unknown, but the patient in Manitoba was a 5-year-old farm boy who accidentally passed through the whirring blades of a manure spreader (Figure 162–1). He sustained deep wounds contaminated with manure, survived the trauma but died of massive halicephalobic encephalitis 24 days later.[4] Another patient had decubitus ulcers, which were thought to be the route of entry, although the ultimate source of the nematodes was never identified.[6] In a third patient, no source of infection or route of entry was determined.[5]

In all three human infections the nematode was called *Micronema,* but Andrassy[7] pointed out that *Micronema* had already been used and established as the genus name for a fish. Andrassy, thus, restored the earlier name, *Halicephalobus,* but some publications continue to use the genus name *Micronema.*[4–6,8] Because there are other species of *Halicephalobus* and all are difficult to distinguish from each other morphologically,[9] several authors prefer to identify these worms by genus only. It is possible that more than one species of *Halicephalobus* infects humans and horses.

MORPHOLOGIC FEATURES OF *HALICEPHALOBUS*

Only female worms have been found in tissues and body fluids and some investigators believe that the female worm is parthenogenic. Adult female worms range in length from about 250 to 460 μm with diameters of 14 to 25 μm. Using specimens digested from brain, Shadduck et al[5] and Gardiner et al[6] described adult female worms as follows: A vulva with protruding lips divides the body into approximately a 3:2 ratio. The anterior end tapers gradually to the stoma and the posterior end tapers rapidly to the tail. The anus is approximately 60 μm from the end of the body; the tail, which is conical and 60 to 67 μm long, tapers abruptly to a point. The esophagus is panagrolaimoid, 75 to 83 μm

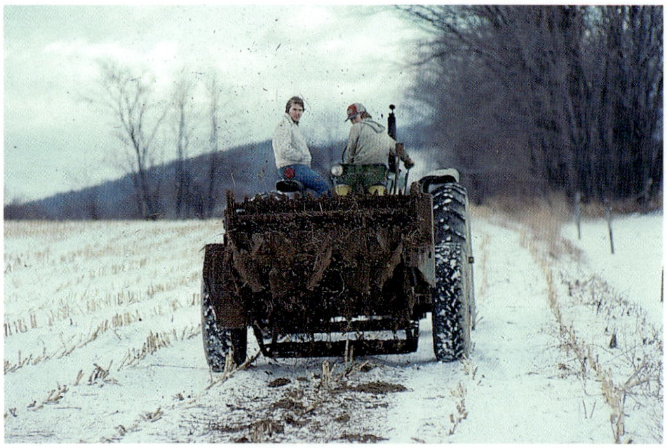

Figure 162–1. Manure spreader. A 5-year-old boy passed through the mechanism of a manure spreader causing deep wounds to limbs, trunk, abdomen, and chest. The wounds were contaminated with manure. He survived the life-threatening trauma but died of halicephalobic encephalitis 24 days later.[4] The particles of "dust" in the air are manure. *(Contributed by Wayne M. Meyers, MD, 1976.)*

long; the metacorpus, a distinct bulb; the procorpus and isthmus are nearly equal in length; and the basal bulb is pyriform (Figures 162–2 through 162–4). The nerve ring is at the middle of the isthmus. The gonad is relatively small, single, extending approximately 50 μm anteriorly, reflected posteriorly to nearly 35 μm posterior to the vulva. Each ovum is relatively large, uninucleate, and 10 to 15 μm by 30 to 41 μm; development of ova is variable. Some ova develop to the larval stage before release, while others appear to be released earlier. The larvae in tissue have the same morphologic features as the adult worms except that they lack the reproductive organs. There are no cuticular alae.

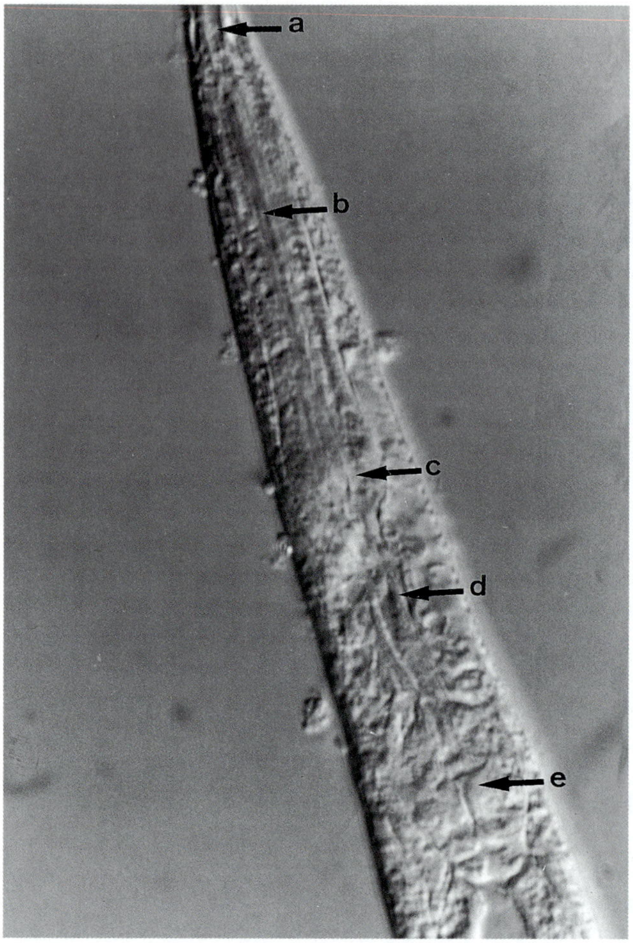

Figure 162–2. Anterior region of adult female nematode digested from brain. Buccal cavity (a) of rhabditid type; pharynx divided into various regions including (b) procorpus, (c) metacorpus, (d) isthmus, which is shorter than the procorpus, and (e) postcorpus, which is bulblike and larger than the metacorpus (interference phase contrast). *(From Shadduck et al[5] with permission.)*

CLINICAL FEATURES

Although the differential diagnosis in all three patients included meningoencephalitis, clinical signs were vague and nonspecific. The signs reported most consistently include fever, somnolence, lethargy, and lymphocytic pleiocytosis (100 to 300 cells/mm^3 of cerebrospinal fluid). Electroencephalograms, carotid arteriograms, pneumoencephalograms and careful clinical examinations failed to localize the lesions. All three patients apparently died as a direct result of the parasitic infection.

PATHOLOGY

Brains from infected patients were edematous and swollen with flattened gyri and compressed sulci. The white matter was soft and easily fragmented. Leptomeninges were diffusely congested and dull gray with loss of glistening translucence in one patient,[5] slightly thickened at the base of the brain in another,[6] and possibly slightly cloudy in the third patient (Figure 162–5).[4] There were areas of hemorrhage and malacia on the cut surfaces of the brains throughout both gray and white matter[5] (Figure 162–6). The necrotic foci were granular, friable, and often near blood vessels. The foci varied in size and shape. Lesions are especially prominent in the pons, medulla, and upper portion of the spinal cord. Cavitary lesions of brain have not been described. Gardiner et al[6] reported hepatic microabscesses, which contained the parasite.

Microscopic lesions are consistent. Lesions include diffuse meningoencephalitomyelitis with exudates,

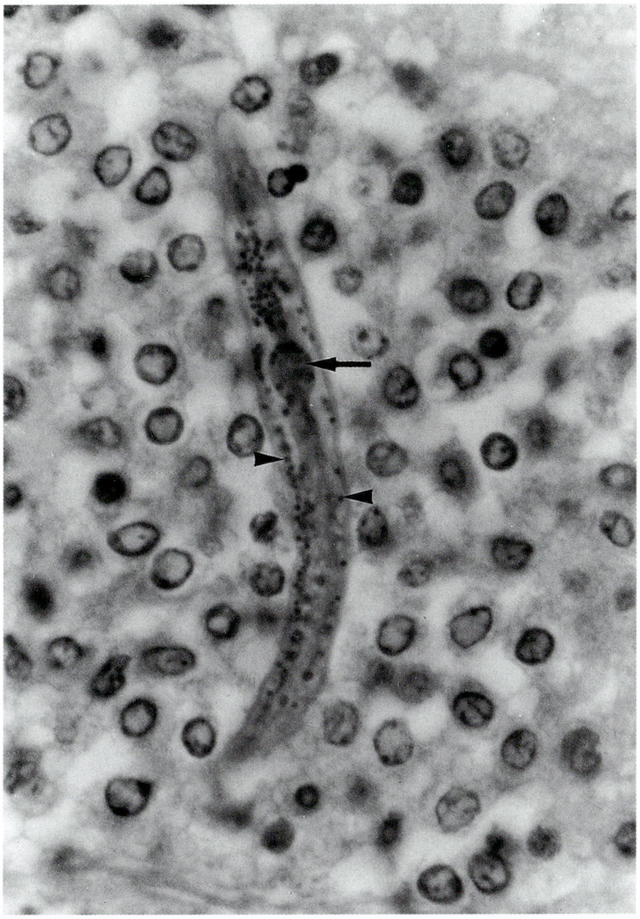

Figure 162–3. Larva surrounded by macrophages. The elongate esophagus with the prominent posterior bulb *(arrow)* is obvious. Nuclei of muscle cells *(arrowheads)* are arranged in rows immediately beneath the cuticle [hematoxylin-eosin (H&E), ×500.] *(From Shadduck et al[5] with permission.)*

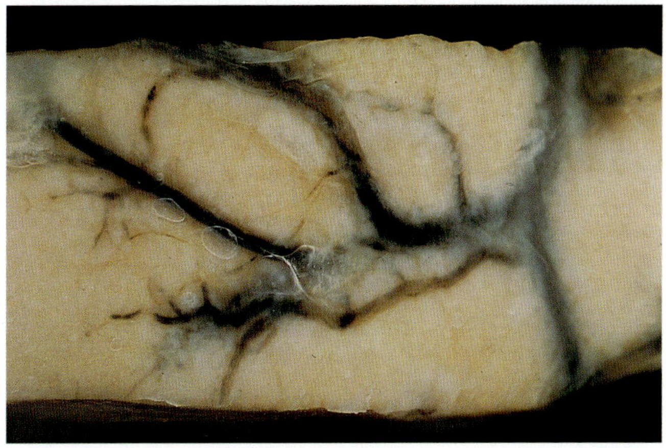

Figure 162–5. Surface of the brain of the patient described in Ref 4. There is some thickening and milky-white discoloration of the arachnoid. *(Photograph by Daniel H. Connor, MD, 1975.)*

which contained numerous lymphocytes and macrophages with scattered eosinophils and, in one brain,[6] many neutrophils and fibrin. Large macrophages and giant cells were sometimes prominent (Figure 162–7). The lesions were notably perivascular and severe focal hemorrhage was common. Malacic foci were common and sometimes progressed to liquefactive necrosis with adjacent astrocytic and microglial cellular proliferation. Multiple smaller foci of inflammatory cells and fragments of parasite were scattered through the parenchyma.

Parasites and/or fragments of parasites were visible in most lesions and were also scattered through the parenchyma, sometimes without obvious tissue reac-

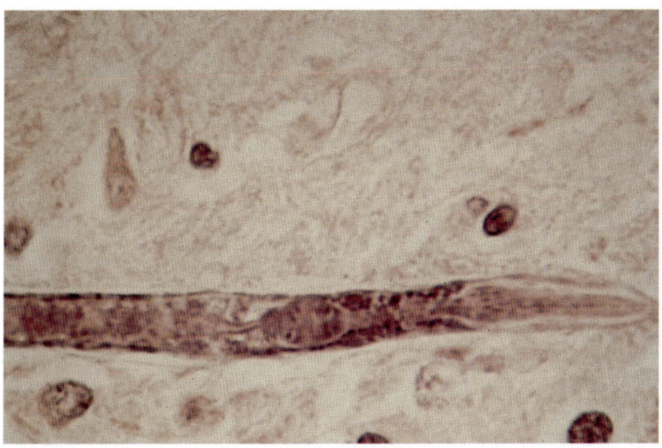

Figure 162–4. *Halicephalobus* sp, in the brain of the 5-year-old farm boy, showing the same features of the anterior digestive tube shown in Figure 162–3 (AFIP 70-1485; H&E, ×160).

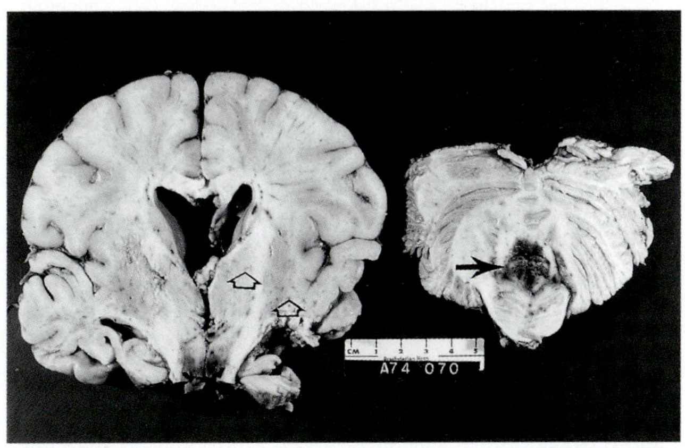

Figure 162–6. Cut surface of the brain of patient described in Ref. 5. There are a large area of hemorrhage and malacia in the pons *(arrow)* and smaller foci of hemorrhage in the basal nuclei *(arrowheads)*.

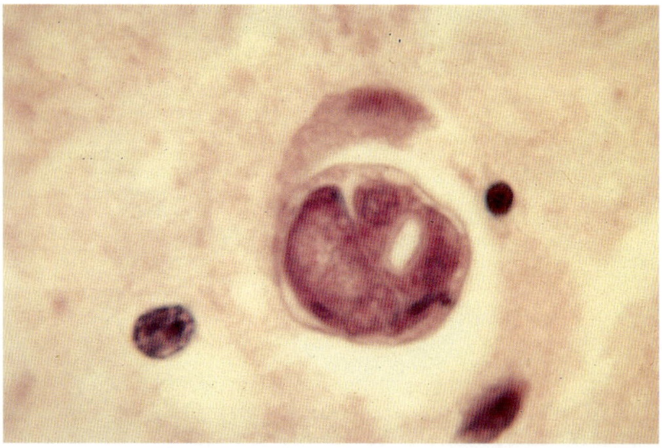

Figure 162–7. Cross-section of *Halicephalobus* sp, in brain. Note the digestive tube and the large reacting macrophage at top (H&E, ×480).

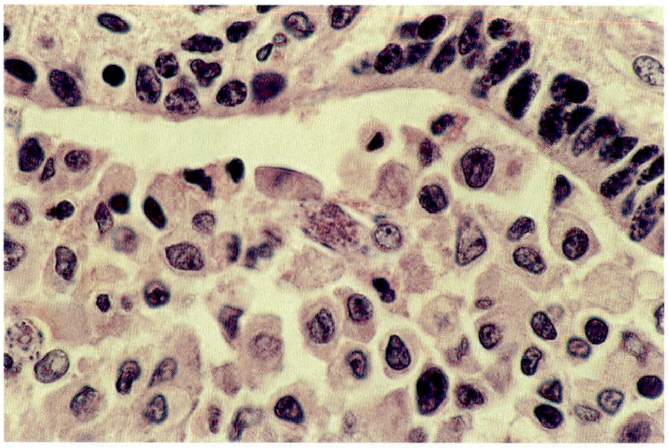

Figure 162–9. Higher magnification of one area shown in Figure 162–8. There are two sections of worm in the central canal—one in the center and the other at the extreme left (H&E, ×1000).

tion. Parasites were in exudates, the meninges, perivascular spaces, vessel walls, ventricles and central canal (Figure 162–8), and penetrating the ependyma (Figure 162–9). In addition to adult female worms, there were numerous larvae and ova. Fragments of worms often were surrounded by giant cells.

Lesions and parasites were in the pituitary in two patients[4,6] and in the choroid plexus of one.[4] In addition, parasites were in hepatic microabscesses[6] and in pulmonary alveolar capillaries[4] and myocardium.[6]

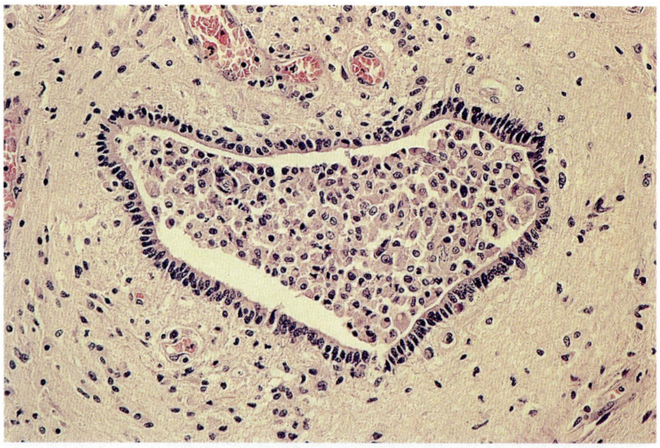

Figure 162–8. Cross-section of spinal cord showing the central canal, which contains macrophages and multiple sections of *Halicephalobus* worms. A migrating worm has broken the ependyma at the bottom (H&E, ×50).

DIFFERENTIAL DIAGNOSIS

Clinically, patients were thought to have viral meningoencephalitis. Each of the three human infections was diagnosed at autopsy by identification of the worms in tissue sections. Identification of the worms was enhanced by digesting the worms free of the tissue followed by careful study and measurement. In tissue, fragments of worms with their prominent muscle cell nuclei can be mistaken for protozoa such as *Toxoplasma*.[5] No diagnostic reagents are available to confirm the morphologic observations. *Halicephalobus deletrix* has not been grown in vitro. No serologic tests are available.

REFERENCES

1. Anderson RV, Bemrick WJ. *Micronema deletrix* n sp, a saprophagous nematode inhabiting a nasal tumor of a horse. *Proc Helminthol Soc Wash.* 1965;32:74–75.
2. Blunden AS, Khalil LF, Webbon PM. *Halicephalobus deletrix* infection in a horse. *Equine Vet J.* 1987;19: 255–260.
3. Buergelt CD. *Halicephalobus (Micronema) deletrix* infection in the horse. *Equine Practice.* 1991;13:7–12.
4. Hoogstraten J, Young GW. Meningo-encephalomyelitis due to the saprophagous nematode, *Micronema deletrix. Can J Neurol Sci.* 1975;2:121–126.
5. Shadduck JA, Ubelaker J, Telford VQ. *Micronema deletrix* meningoencephalitis in an adult man. *Am J Clin Pathol.* 1979;72:640–643.

6. Gardiner CH, Koh DS, Cardella TA. Micronema in man: third fatal infection. *Am J Trop Med Hyg.* 1981;30:586–589.
7. Andrassy I. Über vier homonyme Nematodengattungen. *Nematologia.* 1973;19:403–404.
8. Chalmers GA, Kennedy MJ, Martin WB, Ettrich WF. *Micronema deletrix* in the kidney of a horse. *Can Vet J.* 1990;31:451–452.
9. Geraert E, Sudhaus W, Lenaerts L, Bosmans E. *Halicephalobus laticauda* sp n, a nematode found in a Belgian coal mine (Nematoda, Rhabditida). *Ann SR Zool Belg.* 1987;118:5–12.

CHAPTER 163

Hookworm Disease

Gerhard A. Schad and Robert M. Genta

There is . . . Scarce blood enough in all their sickly veins
To give each naked curtleaxe a stain.

William Shakespeare (1564–1616), Henry V, IV, ii

Her anaemia made her rather short of breath, and she held her mouth slightly open . . . .
Her thin lips were pale and her skin was delicate, of a faint green colour, without a touch of red even in the cheeks.

William Somerset Maugham (1874–1965), Of Human Bondage

DEFINITION

Hookworm disease is infection by either one of the two or both major human hookworm parasites, *Ancylostoma duodenale* and *Necator americanus*.[1,2] The infection may cause a wide range of signs and symptoms, most of which are related to blood loss caused by these intestinal parasites. Hookworm infection is also known as uncinariasis, and also by its most apparent clinical manifestation, tropical anemia.

GEOGRAPHIC DISTRIBUTION

The major hookworm parasites of humans, *A duodenale* and *N americanus,* misleadingly called Old and New World hookworms, respectively, are widely distributed throughout the moist tropical and warm temperate regions of the world. Before control programs essentially eradicated them in several now highly developed areas, human hookworm infections occurred in the southeastern United States and throughout much of Central and South America as far south as northern Argentina. Infections were rare or absent in the arid areas of the southwestern United States and northern Mexico, in rain shadow areas of Central America and along the Pacific coast of the Americas. In the Eastern Hemisphere, hookworm infections occurred in southern Europe (Italy and the Iberian peninsula), North Africa (the Mediterranean Littoral), moist areas of the Near and Middle East (major river valleys, the Caspian shore, and other irrigated areas), much of Pakistan and India, throughout vast areas of the Orient, in the islands of Southeast Asia, northern Australia, and the Pacific islands. Important foci were outside of these endemic areas at mines and at sites of tunnel construction where warmth, abundant moisture, and inadequate sanitation conspired to transmit the parasite. Indeed, many of the most important early advances in our knowledge of hookworm biology and disease were made where a high prevalence of severe ancylostomiasis caused major economic losses and where clinical and research expertise existed nearby. In recent decades, endemic hookworm infection has been essentially eradicated in the United States, Europe, Korea, Japan, Taiwan, Australia, and some of the Caribbean and Pacific Islands.[1–3]

It is widely accepted that *A duodenale* has a more northern Old World distribution than *N americanus,* having been the dominant species in Europe, North Africa, the Near East, and in the more northerly part of the hookworm belt in the Orient (north China, Korea, and northern Japan). *Necator americanus* has been thought of as the predominant species in more southern parts of the Old World and throughout the New World.[2,3] These largely exclusive views are probably incorrect, because species-specific diagnosis has been infrequently attempted (see Diagnosis section) and the differential distribution of the species in age classes has been generally ignored. If very young children, including suckling infants, were examined, and if appropriate differential techniques were used as part of the fecal examination for ova and parasites, *A duodenale* would probably be more widely distributed in the southern areas of the "hookworm belt".[4]

LIFE CYCLE

Adult hookworms are intestinal parasites that attach to the mucosa and ingest both blood and intestinal tissue. Their hematophagous behavior is probably necessary to support their high rates of egg production, which has been estimated to be 10,000 eggs per female per day for *N americanus* and 25,000 for *A duodenale.*[5]

The thin-shelled eggs are laid into the intestinal lumen, join the intestinal contents, and are passed to the exterior in feces. In the external environment, the eggs embryonate and the vermiform larvae that hatch develop through two growth stages to the infective third-stage larvae, provided that the feces of fecally contaminated soil remains sufficiently warm and moist. When conditions are favorable (around 28°C), the larvae become infective in 5 days. Infective larvae (that is, filariform larvae, or L_3) ensheathed in the incompletely molted cuticle of the preceding stage, are highly resistant to environmental insults, particularly noxious chemicals. In spite of the sheath, the larvae are susceptible to desiccation. They require water films for survival and movement; if larvae dry, they die in a matter of minutes. For this reason, endemic hookworm infection is only in those parts of the world where soil moisture is adequate. Chandler[6] calculated that, for a month to be favorable for hookworm transmission, 100 to 125 mm of rain is necessary, with at least 4 to 5 days being rainy.

The infective larvae are adapted for contacting and entering the host. Thus, larvae that develop in the soil migrate to its surface, where, provided moisture is sufficient, they rest positioned for host contact. Several larvae may find their way to the same microprominence, creating a *Pilobolus*-like aggregate. Larvae positioned for contact respond to vibrations, carbon dioxide, warmth, and touch, transferring to hosts in response to a chain of these signals.[7] Skin lipids and serum constituents elicit penetration and feeding responses.[8,9] Larvae invade skin, presumably using the same proteinases and a hyaluronidase they secrete when stimulated during in vitro experiments.[10,11] Thereafter, the larvae enter the circulation and are carried to the lungs where, leaving the circulation, they enter the alveoli. The migration continues via the "mucociliary (tracheal) escalator" to the larynx. Successful larvae are then swallowed and develop into adult worms in the small intestine. Both the fourth-stage larvae and the adult worms are armed with buccal capsules, allowing them to suck in villi and to feed on host tissue and blood. The life history as just described applies to both *N americanus* and *A duodenale,* but the latter has a number of unique features. If swallowed, it will establish an infection, the stomach failing to act as a barrier as it apparently does for *N americanus* larvae entering fresh from the external environment. Additionally, when the infective larvae of *A duodenale* enter a host, alternative developmental pathways are possible. The larvae may either migrate and resume development, or, alternatively, may remain as developmentally arrested third-stage larvae. These larvae serve two functions; they can act as a highly adapted survival stage ("dauer larva"), lying dormant in the host during the season when external ecologic conditions are unfavorable for the worm's development and survival (eg, dry season),[12,13] or they may act as a source of infection for a new generation of susceptible hosts, the suckling infants of infected mothers. Infection of these infants may be a reactivation of dormant larvae by the hormones associated with lactation and their subsequent entry into and transmission through colostrum and milk.

MORPHOLOGY

Ancylostoma duodenale and *N americanus* are relatively short, bursate nematodes, ie, male worms have a terminal copulatory bursa (Figure 163–1). In both species, the terminal mouth capsule opens toward the dorsal side, causing the anterior end of each to be bent. In the opening of the mouth are structures designed to lacerate tissue, namely, two pairs of teeth in *A duodenale* and a pair of cutting plates in *N americanus* (Figure 163–1). Furthermore, the latter is a more slender worm with a more finely drawn out anterior end and, consequently, adult worms recovered at necropsy or expelled after treatment are easily identified. The tail of the female is conical; that of the male ends in a complex, bell-shaped copulatory bursa, which serves to hold the female during copulation. A pair of extrusible chitinoid copulatory spicules also aids in holding the female and forms a channel for transferring sperm. In living worms, the single testis in the male and the paired ovaries in the female appear as white tubes

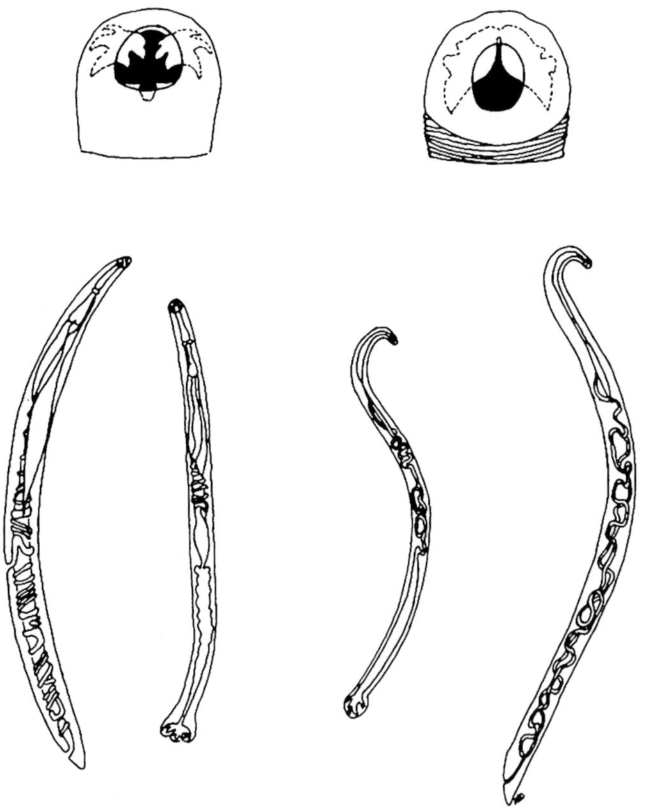

Figure 163–1. Adult *A duodenale* and *N americanus*. Buccal capsules of *A duodenale* and *N americanus* (*top left and right, respectively*). Whole female and male *A duodenale* (*left*) and male and female *N americanus* (*right*). Note the thinner, more curved anterior end of *N americanus*. Female worms have simple pointed tails, whereas male worms have expanded, terminal, copulatory bursae. *Ancylostoma duodenale* has two large teeth of about equal size in its buccal capsule. *Necator americanus* lacks teeth, having semilunar cutting plates instead. *(Redrawn from Pawlowski et al.[34])*

against the blood-filled intestine. In the female, paired egg-filled uteri open into the apposed arms of a muscular ovejector, which forces the eggs through the vulva into the external environment.

The eggs, which measure 60 by 37 μm and 70 by 39 μm in *A duodenale* and *N americanus,* respectively, have a thin, small, colorless shell. The ovum, when passed in fresh feces, has usually undergone two cleavages and is therefore in the four-celled stage. Although the eggs of the two species differ in size, it is usually impractical to attempt to distinguish them in routine fecal examinations.

CLINICAL FEATURES

Although the initial acquisition of hookworms is rarely associated with manifestations requiring medical attention, several detailed reports have described a syndrome of acute uncinariasis. Severe itching and erythema in the area where infective larvae penetrate the skin usually appear within hours of exposure and last for 1 to 2 weeks. This phenomenon, known as "ground itch," afflicts those residing in endemic areas and previously uninfected visitors. The extent of this pruritic dermatitis depends largely on the number of larvae penetrating the skin, and in case of massive exposure, as in the famous "kabbadi outbreak" in a northern Indian village,[14] the itching may be extremely severe and generalized. In some patients[15] short-lived punctuate hemorrhages at the site of penetration are the most noticeable manifestation; other individuals develop hyperpigmented macules persisting for months.[16] At the time when the dermatitis starts to wane, patients may develop paroxysmal shortness of breath with profuse mucus production resembling asthma. These may last for several weeks and even months, and may be accompanied by cough, bronchitis, and pneumonia. Examination of sputum will often reveal occult blood and eosinophils and occasionally migrating larvae.

As the pulmonary symptoms subside, there may be gastrointestinal manifestations related to adult worms in the small intestine. These range from bloating, nausea, vomiting, postprandial or continuous epigastric or periumbilical abdominal pain, to constipation and rarely diarrhea. Although such a constellation of signs and symptoms is well documented in infected volunteers[15,17] and in a few naturally occurring massive infections, particularly in children,[14,18,19] the persistence and magnitude of gastrointestinal manifestations of hookworm infection are difficult to evaluate rigorously in the tropics, where such ailments are common in large segments of the population and can be attributed to other infections.[20]

The presenting complaints of patients with longstanding hookworm infection are those associated with anemia: weakness, lassitude, dizziness, and shortness of breath indicating generic malaise and ill-being.[20] In endemic countries, particularly among women living in areas where the iron content of the diet is low, these complaints are so universal that novice Western physicians (such as one of the authors at his first tropical experience) may be inclined to disregard them until the results of blood tests come back showing hemoglobin values of 4 or 5 g/dL.

Physical examination is often normal. In severely anemic subjects there may be striking pallor (best detected on tongue and nail beds in dark-skinned people), tachycardia, and tachypnea.

PATHOLOGY AND PATHOGENESIS

A comprehensive discussion of the pathology of hookworm disease should include information about the changes associated with each phase of the infection. Thus, we should be able to follow the reaction of the skin to the penetrating larvae, the pulmonary lesions caused by the migrating and maturing parasites, the mechanical and inflammatory damage inflicted on the jejunal villi by the adult worms, and the systemic consequences of long-standing iron deficiency anemia.

LARVAL PENETRATION

The clinical features of hookworm-associated dermatitis have been well documented since the early years of this century (Figure 163–2).[21] In contrast, the histologic consequences of larval skin penetration in humans have not been thoroughly investigated. Maxwell et al[17] obtained skin biopsy specimens from the penetration sites of human volunteers 5 days after the infection and described nonspecific changes, consisting of moderate lymphocytic perivascular infiltrates with rare eosinophils. Experimental evidence in animals suggests that both extent and evolution of the dermatitis may be related to the degree of bacterial contamination of the penetrating larvae.[22] This factor also may be important in naturally acquired human infections. In addition, the intensity of the local reaction may depend on the degree of host sensitization and it is possible that partially protective immune mechanisms act as a first attempt to create a barrier to the establishment of infection.[23]

LARVAL MIGRATION

Little is known of what happens in humans from the time larvae abandon the skin to the moment they appear in the lungs. Once larvae reach the pulmonary circulation, their forceful exit from the capillary bed causes microhemorrhages, which may become detectable as blood in the sputum usually when a large number of larvae reach the lungs simultaneously. Eosinophils in the sputum of patients with respiratory distress at the time of pulmonary migration suggest that there is an allergic response with eosinophils. The role of other inflammatory responses, if any, remains unknown. D'Abrera[24] described fragments of hookworm larvae in granulomas at autopsy in the lungs of South Indian patients with tropical eosinophilia. This finding suggests that alveolar macrophages participate in the defenses against the invading parasites. Further migration along the upper respiratory pathways often causes dry cough, suggestive of tracheitis and laryngitis. There is, however, no histopathologic documentation of these lesions.

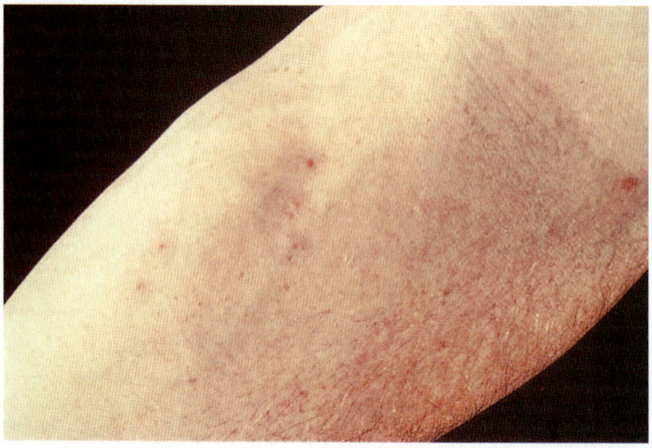

Figure 163–2. Experimental hookworm dermatitis in a volunteer exposed to larvae of *N americanus.* In addition to intense itching, the skin is diffusely red in the exposed area and there are several erythematous papules. *(Experiment by the late Norman E. Wilks, PhD; photograph by Daniel H. Connor, MD, 1969.)*

INTESTINAL PATHOLOGY

Both species of hookworms colonize the proximal portion of the small intestine, with *N americanus* showing an apparent predilection for the duodenum, whereas *A duodenale* is preferentially slightly more distal in the proximal jejunum[2,21] (Figure 163–3). Adult worms are usually found with their mouth attached to the tip of an intestinal villus, but sometimes their entire anterior portion is buried in the lamina propria. Worms are believed to be feeding continuously by sucking blood from capillaries to which they accede through internalization of the villous mucosa (Figure 163–4). After feeding on a villus for several hours, a worm will typically detach and seek another villus, where the process continues (Figure 163–5). Thus, several villi are damaged each day by adult parasite. Blood loss is from the sucking and leaking of damaged villi. The total daily blood loss caused by each worm has been calculated by several investigators. Estimates are around 0.03 mL for *A duodenale* and 0.15 mL for *N americanus.*[25]

The anemia resulting from the loss of erythrocytes is not the only consequence of hookworm infection. Both active and abandoned feeding sites leak plasma, with a protein and electrolyte loss that may be severe enough to acquire clinical importance. Protein-losing enteropathy with hypoalbuminemia is well documented in severely infected patients.[25] Although not specifically reported, it is possible that the loss of electrolytes such as potassium may further contribute to the extreme weakness of some heavily infected patients.

There has been considerable controversy on whether hookworm infection causes detectable and functionally significant alteration of the intestinal structure. Although some researchers have reported various degrees of villous atrophy with malabsorption and diar-

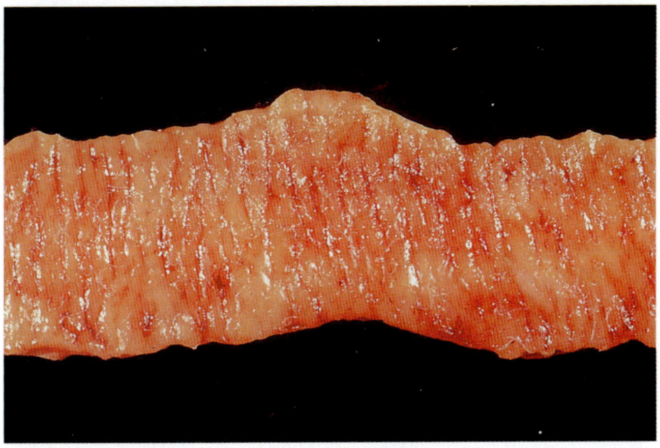

Figure 163–3. Experimental ileitis in a Beagle bitch. The adult hookworms, here *N americanus,* move from site to site, scarifying the mucosa. They cause, as shown here, diffuse erythema and several bleeding points. *(Experiment by the late Norman E. Wilks, PhD; photograph by Daniel H. Connor, MD, 1969.)*

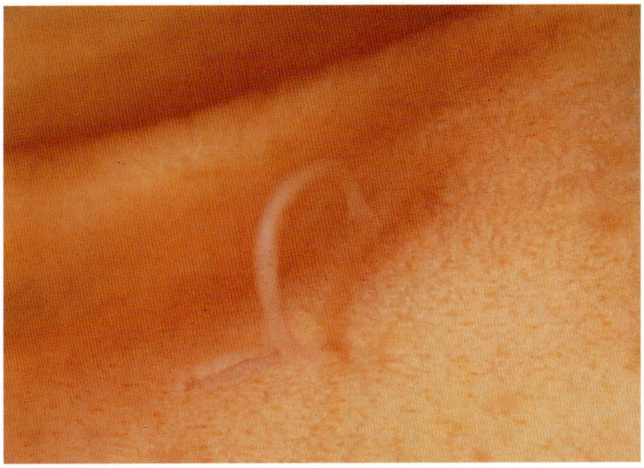

Figure 163–5. A hookworm, *A duodenale,* attached to the proximal ileum. The specimen was taken at autopsy on a 12-week-old Zairian infant. There were many hookworms attached to the ileal mucosa. The photograph was taken under water in an attempt to show the natural position of the worm. *(Specimen by Wayne M. Meyers, PhD, MD; photograph by Daniel H. Connor, MD, 1970.)*

rhea associated with chronic hookworm infection,[26,27] several controlled studies have shown that the degree of morphologic and absorption defects detected in patients with hookworm infection in endemic countries is neither more common nor more severe than those in the uninfected local population.[28,29] In addition, it is essentially impossible to assess the intestinal villous architecture in biopsy specimens that are not properly oriented, and the estimate of the intensity of inflammatory infiltrates is as subjective as any histopathologic evaluation. Many published microphotographs have picturesque legends describing "villous atrophy" or "intense chronic inflammation," when the pictures show only villi that appear flat because they are poorly oriented.

Dense eosinophilic infiltrates occasionally have been described in the lamina propria of patients with hookworm infections,[30] but in the experience of others, including our own, this is exceptional. It is appropriate to mention a recently described eosinophilic gastroenteritis associated with abortive human infections by *A caninum*[31–33] (Figure 163–6).

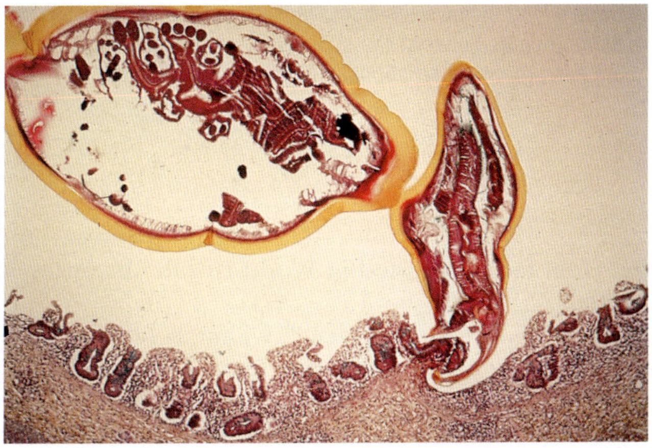

Figure 163–4. Cross-section of hookworm biting an intestinal villus. The adult worm often internalizes a part of the villus, which is then cut when the worm migrates to another location. The microhemorrhages caused by this damage to intestinal villi contribute to the iron loss and the anemia (AFIP Neg 71-3164; Movat, ×15).

EXTRAINTESTINAL PATHOLOGY

Enlargement of the mesenteric and retroperitoneal lymph nodes has been described at autopsy in some patients with hookworm infections, but its relationship with the parasite remains undocumented.[21] Anecdotal claims have also been made that liver and kidneys are enlarged and degenerated. The only pathologic changes that have consistently been documented are those related to long-standing iron-deficiency anemia. These include, of course, decrease or absence of stainable iron in bone marrow with decreased erythropoiesis.[19] In addition, cardiac hypertrophy and dilatation are frequent with severe anemia.[19,21]

DIAGNOSIS

The diagnosis of hookworm infection, often suspected clinically, is easily confirmed by finding the characteristic eggs in feces. While distinguishing hookworm eggs by size is difficult, unless eggs of both species are in the

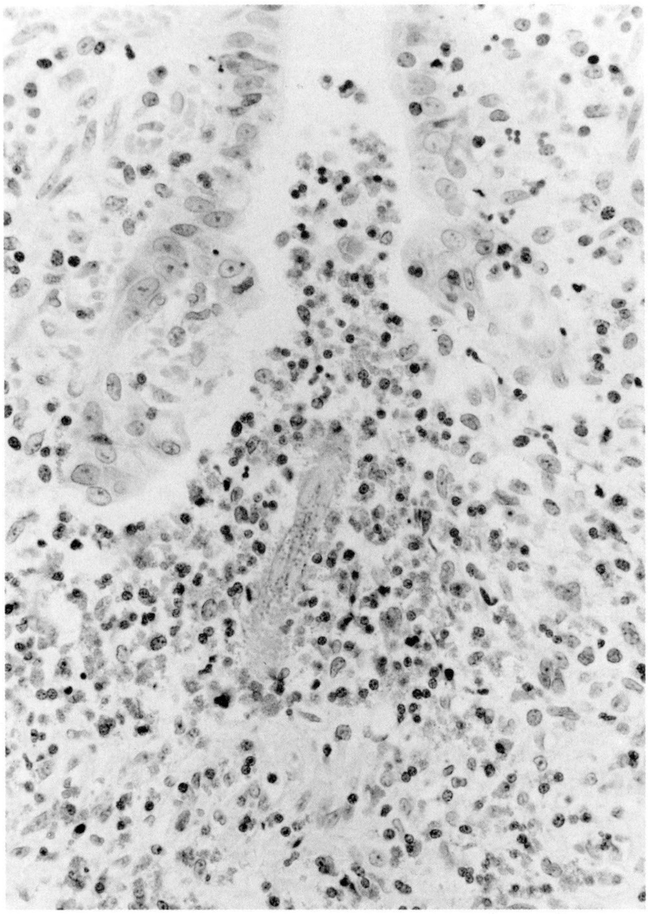

Figure 163–6. Larva in small intestine of patient with eosinophilic enteritis. This larva is surrounded by eosinophils, which also obliterated the intestinal lamina propria in large segments of the intestine. Although this larva was not positively identified, *A caninum* has infected a large series of similar patients in Australia.[31] *(Case contributed by R.C. Haggitt, University of Washington, Seattle.)*

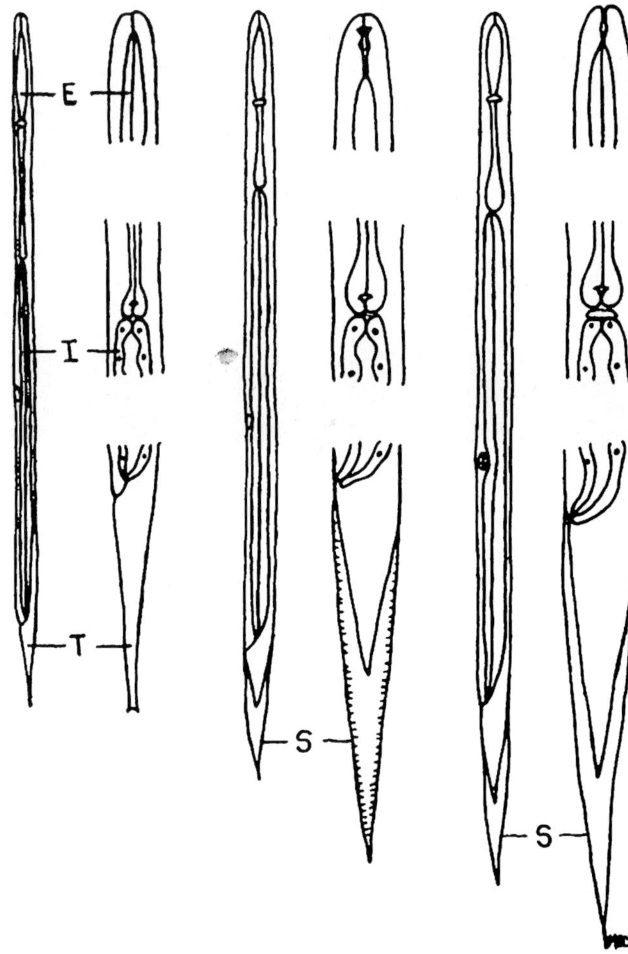

Figure 163–7. Diagnostic features of filariform infective larvae recovered from fecal cultures. *Strongyloides stercoralis (left), N americanus (center)*, and *A duodenale (right).* E, esophagus; I, intestine; S, sheath (cuticular sheath of the tail). Note the absence of a sheath, the very long filariform esophagus, and the cleft tail in *S stercoralis.* Note the sheath and the shorter strongyliform esophagus of the two hookworm species. *Necator americanus* differs from *A duodenale* as follows: Its buccal tube has thick walls, it lacks a small ventriculus between the esophagus and intestine and its tail sheath has prominent striations. *(Redrawn from Pawlowski et al.[34])*

same microscopic field, a species-specific diagnosis is, in fact, quite feasible if infective larvae can be reared in coprocultures. Infective larvae, 500 to 600 μm long, harvested from coprocultures, are distinguishable by the features shown in Figure 163–7. *Necator americanus* has a prominent, thick-walled buccal tube, an esophagus that connects directly to the intestine, and readily apparent, closely spaced cuticular striations on the tail of the cuticular sheath. In contrast, *A duodenale* has a thin buccal tube, its esophageal bulb is separated from the intestine by a short ventriculus, and the tail striations of the cuticular sheath are more widely spaced and less distinct than those of *N americanus.* Although the literature often suggests that coproculture and differential diagnosis of the harvested larvae are difficult, it can be done routinely by a competent microscopist and is, in fact, suggested in World Health Organization manuals.[34,35]

Hookworm eggs will hatch within 24 hours in stool specimens kept at room temperature. It is important, therefore, to distinguish these larvae from first-stage larvae of *S stercoralis* (Figure 163–8), an intestinal nematode whose larvae (rather than eggs) are in feces of the infected hosts.[36] In rare cases occurring in industrialized nations where hookworm infection is not suspected, adult worms have been found in the duodenum in the

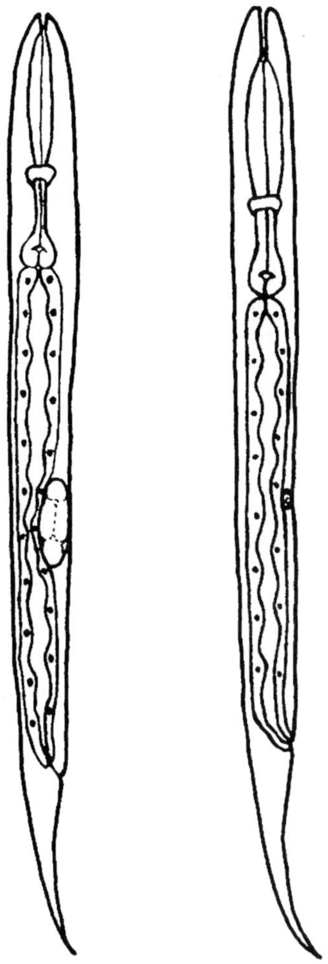

Figure 163–8. Diagnostic features of rhabditiform larvae common in fresh fecal samples. *Strongyloides stercoralis (left)*; note the very large genital primordium just posterior to the midpoint of the worm and the short mouth cavity. Hookworm larva (*right*); note the small genital primordium and the long buccal tube.

course of endoscopic procedures performed to investigate occult blood loss in patients with unexplained iron deficiency anemia.[37]

Fecal examination is a highly efficient, technologically appropriate, and inexpensive method to diagnose hookworm infection. Thus, the limited interest in diagnostic serologic assays is hardly surprising. Recently, however, immunologic methods have been usefully applied to the investigation of transmission and reinfection patterns in endemic communities.[38–40] Such studies may eventually help elucidate some of the enigmatic aspects of host regulation of hookworm populations, including the apparent natural predisposition of some hosts for light or heavy infections.[5]

TREATMENT

All those infected should be given anthelmintics and those with anemia should receive iron by mouth. Mebendazole is currently the drug of choice and is given by mouth, 100 mg twice a day. This regimen is effective in 95% of patients. Physicians should resist the temptation to transfuse patients with whole blood or with packed red cells. When the anemia is profound (1 to 2 g/dL) patients have myocardial strain from maintaining excessive stroke volume to compensate for the severe anemia. In these patients, the slightest added volume precipitates irreversible heart failure and death. In addition, severe anemia predisposes to abnormal sodium retention and this also may trigger or aggravate cardiac failure. Some restriction of dietary sodium may therefore help in the patient's recovery.

REFERENCES

1. Schad GA, Nawalinski T. Historical introduction. In: Gilles H, Ball P, eds. *Hookworm Disease.* Amsterdam: Elsevier; 1991:1–14.
2. Schad GA, Banwell JG. Hookworms. In: Warren KS, Mahmoud AAI, eds. *Tropical and Geographic Medicine.* New York: McGraw-Hill; 1988:379–393.
3. Bandy DAP, Keymer AE. The epidemiology of hookworm infection. In: Gilles H, Ball P, eds. *Hookworm Disease.* Amsterdam: Elsevier; 1991:157–178.
4. Schad GA. Hooked on hookworms: 25 years of attachment. *J Parasitol.* 1991;77:179–186.
5. Anderson RM, Schad GA. Hookworm burdens and fecal egg counts: the basis for variation. *Trans R Soc Trop Med Hyg.* 1985;79:743–884.
6. Chandler AC. *Hookworm Disease.* New York: Macmillan; 1929:494.
7. Granzer M, Hess. Host finding and host recognition of infective larvae. *Int J Parasitol.* 1991;21:429–440.
8. Hawdon J, Schad G. Albumin and a dialyzable serum factor stimulate feeding in vitro by third stage larvae of the canine hookworm, *Ancylostoma caninum. J Parasitol.* 1991;77:587–591.
9. Hawdon J, Schad G. *Ancylostoma caninum:* reduced glutathione stimulates feeding by third stage infective larvae. *Exp Parasitol.* 1992;75:40–46.
10. Hotez P, Haggerty J, Hawdon J, et al. Metalloproteases of infective *Ancylostoma* larvae and their possible functions in tissue invasion and ecdysis. *Infect Immun.* 1990;58: 3883–3892.
11. Hotez P, Narasimhan S, Haggerty J, et al. A hyaluronidase from *Ancylostoma* hookworm larvae and its functions as a virulence factor in cutaneous larvae migrans. *Infect Immun.* 1992;60:1018–1023.
12. Schad GA, Choudhury AB, Dean G, et al. Arrested development in human hookworm infection, an adaptation to a seasonally unfavorable external environment. *Science.* 1973;180:502–504.

13. Schad GA. Hypobiosis and related phenomena in hookworms. In: Schad GA, Warren KS, eds. *Hookworm Disease: Current Status and New Directions.* London: Taylor & Francis; 1990:71–81.
14. Koshy A, Raina V, Sharma MP, Mithal S, Tandon BN. An unusual manifestation of hookworm disease in North India. *Am J Trop Med Hyg.* 1978;27:42–45.
15. Cline BL, Little MD, Bartholomew RK, Halsey NA. Larvicidal activity of albendazole against *Necator americanus* in human volunteers. *Am J Trop Med Hyg.* 1984;33:387–394.
16. Nawalinski TA, Schad GA. Arrested development in *Ancylostoma duodenale:* course of a self-induced infection in man. *Am J Trop Med Hyg.* 1974;23:895–898.
17. Maxwell C, Hussain R, Nutman T, et al. Clinical and immunologic responses of normal volunteers to low-dose hookworm (*Necator americanus*) infection. *Am J Trop Med Hyg.* 1987;37:126–134.
18. Ashford BK, Payne GC, Payne FK. Acute uncinariasis from massive infestation and its implications. *JAMA.* 1933;101:843–847.
19. Zimmerman HM. Fatal hookworm disease in infancy and childhood on Guam. *Am J Pathol.* 1946;22:1081–1090.
20. Migasena S, Gilles HM. Hookworm infection. In: Pawlowski ZS, ed. *Intestinal Helminthic Infections.* London: Bailliere's Clinical Tropical Medicine and Communicable Diseases; 1987;2:617–627.
21. Behnke JM. Pathology. In: Gilles H, Ball P, eds. *Hookworm Disease.* Amsterdam: Elsevier; 1991:51–91.
22. Carroll SM, Grove DI. Experimental infection of humans with *Ancylostoma ceylanicum:* clinical, parasitological, hematological and immunological findings. *Trop Geogr Med.* 1986;38:38–45.
23. Wells C, Behnke JM. Acquired resistance to the human hookworm *Necator americanus* in mice. *Parasite Immunol.* 1988;10:493–505.
24. D'Abrera VStE. The etiology of tropical eosinophilia with a preliminary note on the etiology of the syndrome. *Ceylon Med J.* 1958;4:195–210.
25. Roche M, Layrisse M. The nature and cause of hookworm anemia. *Am J Trop Med Hyg.* 1966;15:1031–1100.
26. Russell PK, Aziz MA, Ahmad EJ, et al. Intestinal biopsies and absorption studies in young Pakistani men. *Pakistan J Med Res.* 1964;3:276–285.
27. Russell PK, Aziz MA, Ahmad EJ, et al. Enteritis and gastritis in young asymptomatic Pakistani men. *Am J Dig Dis.* 1966;11:296–306.
28. Aziz MA, Siddiqui AR. Morphological and absorption studies of small intestine in hookworm disease (ancylostomiasis) in West Pakistan. *Gastroenterology.* 1968;55:242–250.
29. Castro GA, Behnke JM, Weisbrodt NW. Hookworm infection and malabsorption: where do we stand today? In: Schad GA, Warren KS, eds. *Hookworm Disease: Current Status and New Directions.* London: Taylor & Francis; 1990.
30. Chaudhuri RN, Saha TK. Jejunal mucosa in hookworm disease. *Am J Trop Med Hyg.* 1964;13:410–411.
31. Prociv P, Croese J. Human eosinophilic enteritis caused by dog hookworm *Ancylostoma caninum. Lancet.* 1990;1:1299–1302.
32. Croese J, Loukas A, Opdebeeck J, Prociv P. Occult enteric infection by *Ancylostoma caninum:* a previously unrecognized zoonosis. *Gastroenterology.* 1994;106:3–12.
33. Walker NI, Croese J, Clouston AD, Parry M, Loukas A, Prociv P. Eosinophilic enteritis in northeastern Australia. Pathology, association with *Ancylostoma caninum,* and implications. *Am J Surg Pathol.* 1995;19:328–337.
34. Pawlowski ZS, Schad GA, Stott GJ. *Hookworm Infection and Anemia. Approaches to Prevention and Control.* Geneva: World Health Organization; 1991:96.
35. World Health Organization. *Intestinal Protozoan and Helminthic Infections.* Geneva: World Health Organization; 1981.
36. Schad GA. Morphology and life history of *Strongyloides stercoralis.* In: DA Grove, ed. *Strongyloidiasis, A Major Roundworm Infection of Man.* London: Taylor & Francis; 1989:85–104.
37. Genta RM, Woods KL. Endoscopic diagnosis of hookworm infection. *Gastrointest Endoscopy.* 1991;37:476–478.
38. Pritchard DI, Quinnell RJ, Slater AF, et al. The epidemiological significance of the immune response to the cuticular collagen of *Necator americanus:* a preliminary study in a hookworm endemic area in Papua New Guinea. *Acta Tropica.* 1990;47:403–407.
39. Pritchard DI, Walsh EA, Quinell RJ, et al. Isotypic variation in antibody responses in a community in Papua New Guinea to larval and adult antigens during infection, and following reinfection, with the hookworm *Necator americanus. Parasite Immunol.* 1992;14:617–631.
40. Hotez PJ, Hawdon JM, Cappello M, Jones BF, Pritchard DI. Molecular pathobiology of hookworm infection. *Infect Agents Dis.* 1995;4:71–75.

CHAPTER 164

Hymenolepiasis

Adam R. Burkey, Ewald Pretner, and J. Kevin Baird

Look wise, say nothing, and grunt. Speech was given to conceal thought.

Sir William Osler (1849–1919)

INTRODUCTION

Hymenolepis nana causes hymenolepiasis in humans. This cestode may also be called the dwarf tapeworm. Although rodents may be a reservoir of adult *H nana,* the usual mode of transmission is human to human.[1] Infection is often without symptoms. If present, a mild diarrhea is typical.[2] Infection of humans by the rat tapeworm *H diminuta* occurs, but only rarely.

EPIDEMIOLOGY

Hymenolepis nana is a cosmopolitan species that favors the tropics, especially Latin America and South Africa.[2] A survey of rats in one endemic area revealed that 1.4% of one species carried relatively light infections.[3] Children are infected more often than adults; the prevalence of infection ranges from less than 1% to 28% in these regions.[4] Another study demonstrated higher rates in young urban children than in older rural children and this was apparently related to hygiene in the different communities.[1] In the United States, the prevalence of *H nana* eggs from thousands of stool specimens in Kentucky and North Carolina was 1% to 3% in the 1930s; the prevalence of *H diminuta* eggs was 0.03%. The Centers for Disease Control and Prevention reported 43 infections by *H diminuta* between 1973 and 1977, but hymenolepiasis has never been a reportable disease and these numbers may grossly underestimate the actual number of cases.

LIFE CYCLE

Adult *H nana* lives in the small intestine of human beings or rodents. The adult worm attaches to the villus by four suckers and hooklets. Eggs shed by the hermaphroditic adult worm pass with feces to soil where they may be ingested by humans. If ingested by an appropriate host, the eggs release an oncosphere into the lumen of the small intestine. This invasive larva bores through the mucosa into the lamina propria where it develops into a cysticercoid larva (Figures 164–1 and 164–2). The cysticercoid migrates back into the lumen of the intestine, attaches to the surface of the villus, and grows to maturity in about 3 weeks. Adult worms live an indefinite period in the host. Eggs in the feces of a definitive host may be ingested by some arthropods, eg, the flower beetle, which may serve as an intermediate host. In these hosts, the eggs hatch in the lumen of the gut and the freed oncospheres invade the body cavity and develop to a cysticercoid larva. Living beetles or their carcasses often contaminate grain and grain products. When eaten by humans, the cysticercoid larvae from the beetle fastens to the villus and matures.

Hymenolepis nana is unique among cestodes that infect humans for being able to autoinfect its definitive host. If its eggs hatch while still in the intestine, liberated oncospheres invade as per their routine. These newly developing cysticercoids are normally eliminated before reaching maturity, and therefore do not establish a permanent cycle of infection.[5–8]

CLINICAL FINDINGS

Infection by *H nana* tends to cause symptoms more often than *H diminuta,* although light infection with either worm is usually unnoticed. Heavy infection by *H nana* (wormloads of up to 7000 have been described in individual patients) may cause abdominal pain, diarrhea, headache, dizziness, anorexia, enteritis, and anal

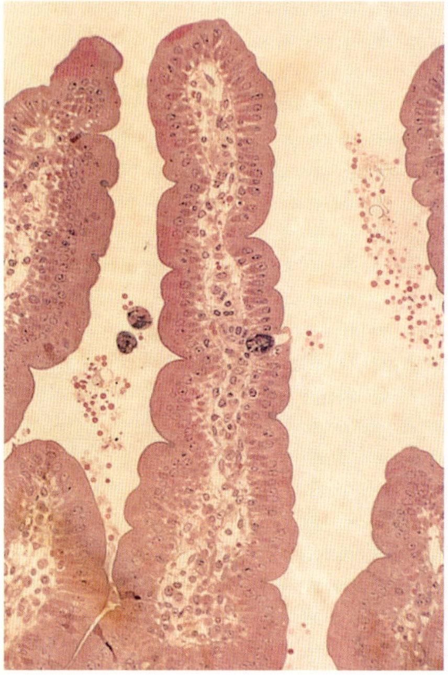

Figure 164–1. Longitudinal section through intestinal villus of a mouse challenged with 5×10^4 infective eggs of *H nana* 30 minutes before being killed. The photomicrograph shows three hatched oncospheres, two in the lumen and one penetrating the epithelium [hematoxylin-eosin (H&E), ×100]. *(Contributed by T. Miyazato et al in ACTA Medica Kinki Univ. 1977;2:1–18.)*

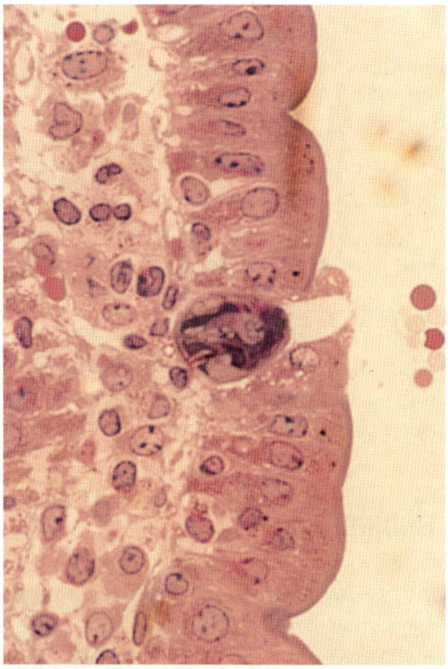

Figure 164–2. Higher magnification of the subject of Figure 164–1 showing the oncosphere invading the epithelium (H&E, ×400). *(Contributed by T. Miyazato et al in ACTA Medica Kinki Univ. 1977;2:1–18.)*

irritation. The infection may progress to a stage resulting in severe toxemia. Intestinal injury caused by burrowing larvae causes a localized, mild enteritis.[5,6] Most infections with *H diminuta* are asymptomatic, and fewer patients experience an even milder range of clinical features than do those infected with *H nana*.[5,8] These tapeworms often pass spontaneously,[5,8] and most patients find this far more alarming than almost any symptomatology. *Hymenolepis diminuta,* when crowded, apparently secretes factors inhibiting its own growth and thus tends toward lighter worm burdens than *H nana*.[9]

PATHOLOGY

The hatched oncosphere lodges in the intestinal villus, preferring the middle of the villus over the exfoliating outer tip. The integrity of the cell layer is disrupted by enzymatic digestion as well as physical burrowing.[10] The oncosphere reaches the tunica propria within 4 hours. Rudimentary suckers and rostellar hooklets

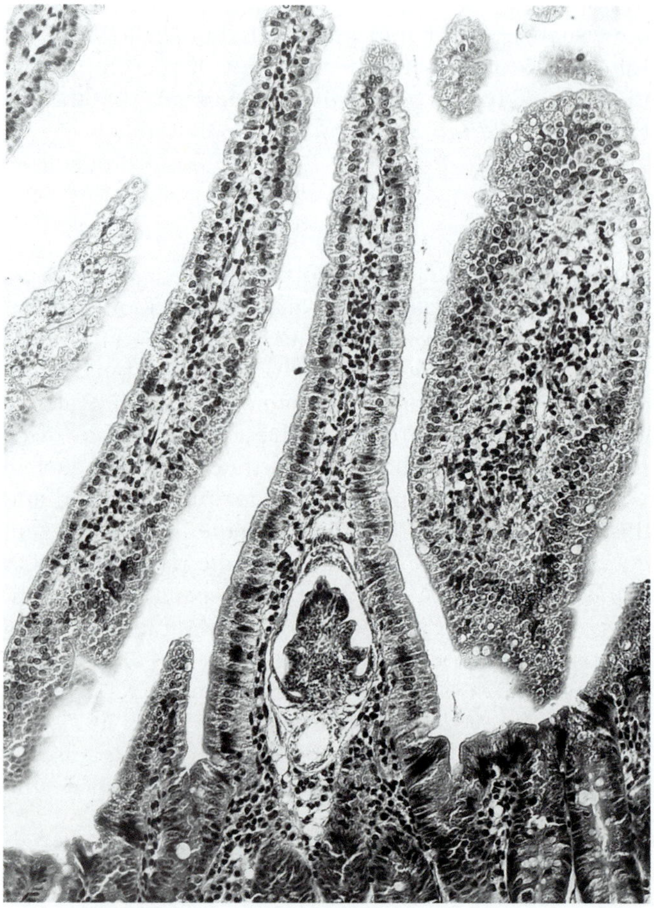

Figure 164–3. Longitudinal section through a villus from an experimental mouse challenged with 1×10^4 infective eggs 72 hours before being killed. There is a cysticercoid larva in a cellular infiltrate (H&E, ×70). *(Contributed by T. Miyazato.)*

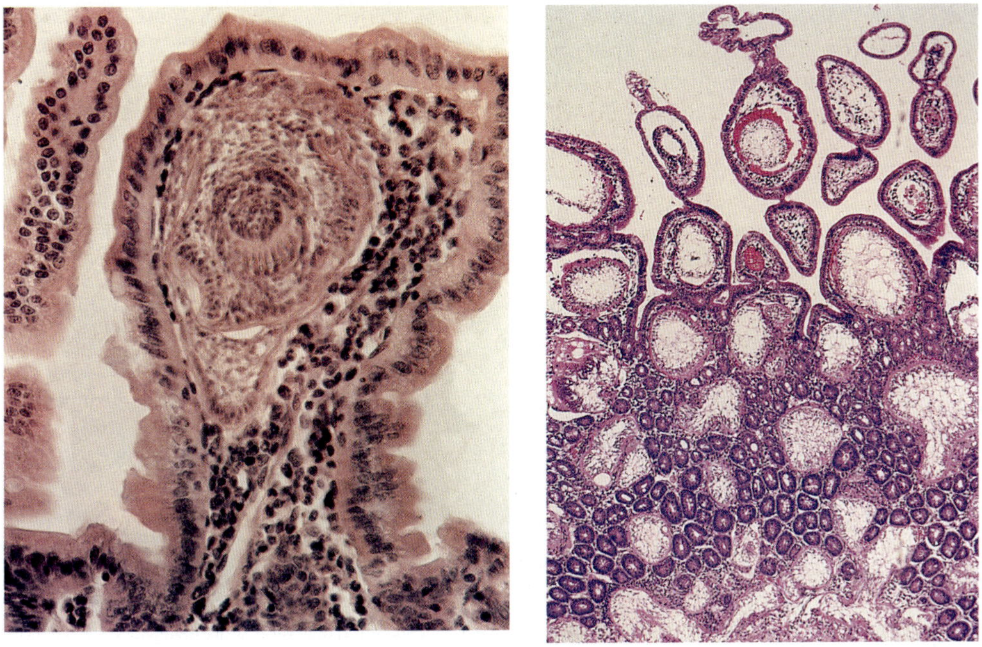

A B

Figure 164–4. (**A**) A cysticercoid larva in the lamina propria of an experimental mouse. The hooklets of the rostellum and portions of at least one sucker are evident in this section. These structures remain in the interior of the parasite, ie, invaginated. Neutrophils surround the exterior body wall of the larva (the tegument) (H&E, ×140). *(Contributed by T. Miyazato.)* (**B**) Massive infection of an immunodeficient mouse by cysticercoid larvae of *H nana.* Some of the larvae are surrounded by blood but there is no inflammatory reaction (H&E, ×60).

become apparent at 72 hours (Figures 164–3 and 164–4). Cysticercoids—small larvae containing a single scolex but lacking the bladder characteristic of other cysticerci—are fully developed by 96 hours.[5] At this time the cellular infiltrate peaks. A neutrophilic infiltrate and edema develop at the base of the villus and extend into the tunica propria. No fibrocytic reaction surrounds the oncosphere. The affected villi are shortened and dilated. Adjacent epithelium has a rounded columnar cell pattern with indistinct cell borders. Oncospheres of *H nana* are strongly immunogenic. In secondary infection, oncospheres penetrate the villus but never form cysticercoids, even if five times the number of eggs (50,000) is used.[11] This protection has been related to the development of T-cell-mediated immunity.[12–14] The formation of a small granulomatous nodule with neutrophils and eosinophils peaks at 16 to 24 hours marked by edema and debris. The villi appear normal again by 72 hours after secondary infection.

DIAGNOSIS

Diagnosis of both types of hymenolepiasis is based on pathognomonic embryonated eggs in the stool.[5,8] The eggs of *H nana* are broadly ovoid (50 by 30 μm) and have a thin, smooth hyaline shell. Inside this shell, a rigid membrane contains a hexacanth oncosphere. The membrane has two polar, knoblike thickenings from which four to eight threadlike filaments extend into the area between the embryo and the outer shell. These polar filaments distinguish *H nana* from *H diminuta* (Figure 164–5, A).[5,7,8] Eggs from *H diminuta* are brown

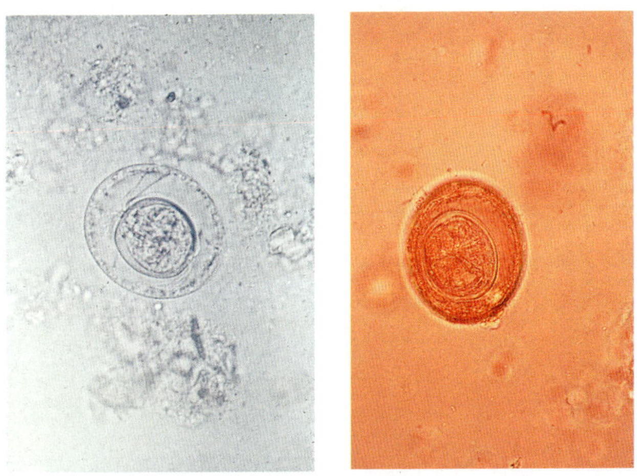

A B

Figure 164–5. (**A**) Photomicrograph under oil immersion (×1000) showing egg of *H nana* from stool. Note the polar filaments. These distinguish *H nana* from *H diminuta.* (**B**) Photomicrograph of egg of *H diminuta. (Photomicrographs contributed by Dr. Tsieh Sun.)*

and slightly ovoid (80 by 70 μm) with a sculpted, relatively thick shell (Figure 164–5, B). In some specimens there are fine, concentric striations in the outer shell.[7,8] No serologic testing is now generally available for diagnosis.

TREATMENT

A 7-day course of niclosamide provides safe and effective therapy. More recently, praziquantel has been effective in treating *H nana.* A single oral dose of 40 mg/kg achieves effective cure, although it may predispose to a low-grade fever lasting 1 or 2 days.[15]

REFERENCES

1. Mason PR, Patterson BA. Epidemiology of *Hymenolepis nana* infections in primary school children in urban and rural communities in Zimbabwe. *J Parasitol.* 1994;80: 245–250.
2. Castillo RM, Grados P, Carcamo C, et al. Effect of treatment on serum antibody to *Hymenolepis nana* detected by enzyme-linked immunosorbent assay. *J Clin Microbiol.* 1991;29:413–414.
3. Buscher HN, Haley AJ. Epidemiology of *Hymenolepis nana* infections of Punjabi villagers in West Pakistan. *Am J Trop Med Hyg.* 1972;21:42–49.
4. Noble E, Noble G. *Parasitology: The Biology of Animal Parasites.* Philadelphia: Lea and Febiger; 1982:222–223.
5. Markell E, Voge M, John D. *Medical Parasitology.* Philadelphia: WB Saunders; 1992:255–258.
6. Kenney M. *Scope Monograph on Pathoparasitology: A Color Atlas of Parasites in Tissue Sections.* Kalamazoo, Mich: Upjohn Co; 1973:15–16.
7. Ash L, Orihel T. *Atlas of Human Parasitology.* Chicago: ASCP Press; 1990:168–170.
8. Leventhal R, Cheadle R. *Medical Parasitology: A Self-Instructional Text.* Philadelphia: FA Davis; 1985:42–43, 162.
9. Cook RL, Roberts LS. In vivo effects of putative crowding factors on development of *Hymenolepis diminuta. J Parasitol.* 1991;77:21–25.
10. Miyazato T, Furukawa T, Inoue T. Intestinal pathology associated with primary and secondary infections of *Hymenolepis nana* in mice. *Jpn J Parasitol.* 1979;28: 185–195.
11. Bailey WS, Host-tissue reactions to initial and superimposed infections with *Hymenolepis nana* var fraterna. *J Parasitol.* 1951;37:440–444.
12. Okamoto K. Effect of neonatal thymectomy on acquired resistance to *Hymenolepis nana* in mice. *Jpn J Parasitol.* 1968;17:53–59.
13. Asano K, Okamato K. Transfer of T-cell mediated immunity to *Hymenolepsis nana* from mother mice to their neonates. *Experientia.* 1992;48:67–71.
14. Asano K, Muramatsu K, Okamoto K. *Hymenolepis nana:* adoptive transfer of protective immunity and delayed type hypersensitivity response with mesenteric lymph node cells in mice. *Exp Parasitol.* 1991;72:24–32.
15. Farid Z, Ayad El-Masry N, Wallace CK. Treatment of *Hymenolepis nana* with a single oral dose of praziquantel. *Trans R Soc Trop Med Hyg.* 1984;78:280–281.

CHAPTER 165

Cutaneous Larva Migrans

Gregory Nikolaidis and Theodore Rosen

After my skin worms destroy this body, yet in my flesh shall I see God.

Job 19:26

DEFINITION

Cutaneous larva migrans, also known as "creeping eruption," is a distinctive dermatitis caused by infectious larvae of various animal nematodes. The migration of these larvae through the skin causes an eruption of pruritic, serpiginous, papulovescicular lesions.[1–3] The larvae are confined to the epidermis, and the disease is self-limited. First described by Lee in 1874,[4] the causative organism was not isolated until 1926.[5] *Ancylostoma braziliensis* is the most common cause of cutaneous larva migrans (CLM).

EPIDEMIOLOGY

The organisms that cause CLM are ubiquitous, but are endemic to areas with warm, humid climates, such as the Caribbean, Africa, South America, Southeast Asia, and the southeastern United States.[6] In northern environments, the soil and weather conditions are not conducive to the maturation of the larvae.[2] Nevertheless, persons from northern regions may easily be exposed when traveling to endemic areas.[1–3,7] These patients typically give a history of an eruption arising shortly after walking or lying on moist, sandy soil. CLM has no predilection for age, race, or gender.

ETIOLOGY

The cat and dog hookworm, *A braziliensis,* causes most infections of CLM in humans.[7,8] *Ancylostoma caninum* (dog hookworm), *A tubaeformis* (cat hookworm), *Uncinaria stenocephala* (European dog hookworm), and *Bunostomum phlebotum* (cattle hookworm) are less common causes.[2,3] The human hookworm *Gnathostoma spinigerum,* as well as free-living soil nematodes such as *Pleodora stronglyoides,* have also caused creeping eruption.[9,10]

LIFE CYCLE

Humans are an aberrant host for the species of nematode that cause CLM. The eggs of the adult worms are passed in the feces of the infected animal. Under favorable conditions such as the warm humid climates of subtropical areas, the eggs hatch into noninfectious rhabditiform larvae. For the next week these larvae feed on debris in the moist, sandy soil until they reach a size of 500 to 700 μm. They then undergo a series of molts, and become infectious nonfeeding filariform larvae.[2,3]

These infectious larvae are capable of entering a host through hair follicles, fissured skin, and even through undamaged skin with the aid of their digestive enzymes.[11,12] The larvae are also capable of penetrating thin clothing.[12,13] Long contact time of the host skin with fecally contaminated soil enhances the infective capability of these larvae. The most common sites of penetration are the hands, feet, knees, and buttocks.[2,12]

On entering human skin, the filariform larvae tunnel in the epidermis just above the basal layer. Only rarely do they enter the dermis, because they lack the collagenase enzymes required to penetrate the basement membrane.[12–15] In their definitive hosts, however, the larvae pass through the dermis and are carried by lymphatic and venous channels to the lungs. There they are filtered out in the capillary bed, then erupt through

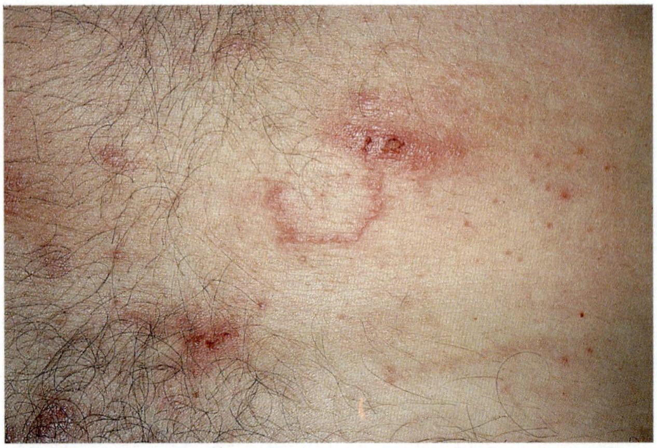

Figure 165–1. Eruption of abdominal skin over the tract made by a migrating nematode larva, probably *A braziliensis*.

the alveoli, migrate up the trachea and down the esophagus, and mature in the intestine.[2,8]

CLINICAL FEATURES

Patients typically describe a prickly, tingling sensation after coming into contact with infested soil.[13] A few hours later, a pruritic papule or nonspecific dermatitis arises at the site of contact (Figures 165–1 and 165–2). Previously sensitized people may present with a more florid reaction that includes vesiculation and edema. The larvae usually begin migrating after 2 or 3 days, but may remain stationary for months.[2] A 2- to 3-mm-wide serpiginous or linear erythematous tract develops as the larvae migrate through the skin. With the larvae about 1 cm from the advancing border, the tract lengthens by 2 to 3 cm daily.[2,6] Because of the elaboration of toxic antigens, pruritis intensifies during this migratory phase.[12] Most patients with CLM have a peripheral eosinophilia.

Since the larvae are unable to penetrate into the dermis, the condition is self-limited. If untreated, most larvae die in 2 to 8 weeks, although some persist for longer periods, even up to one year.[16,17] In those rare infections where larvae pass through the dermis and enter the bloodstream, Löffler's syndrome with pulmonary infiltrates and eosinophilia may occur.[18–20]

PATHOLOGY

While the clinical features of CLM are distinctive and characteristic, the histopathologic changes are not. Biopsy specimens of a tract reveal tunnels confined to the epidermis. The larvae are usually in tunnels at the dermal–epidermal junction (Figure 165–3). The roof of the larvae-filled tunnels are composed of compressed, pyknotic epidermal cells, while the floor consists of dermal collagen.[21]

Hematoxylin-eosin stain reveals a mild, perivascular dermal infiltrate.[1] It is primarily comprised of polymorphonuclear cells and eosinophils, with occasional lymphocytes and plasma cells. In addition, edema is present throughout the cutis. A slight acanthosis and spongiosis occurs around the tunnels.[21] Around older burrows, the epidermis returns to its normal appearance, although a sparse perivascular infiltrate remains in the dermis.

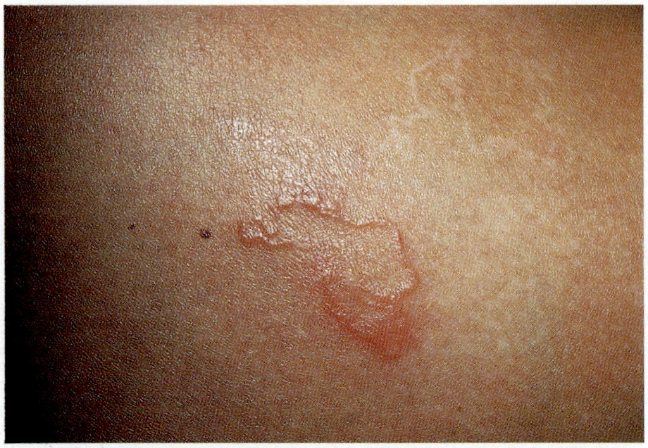

Figure 165–2. Similar eruption on the arm.

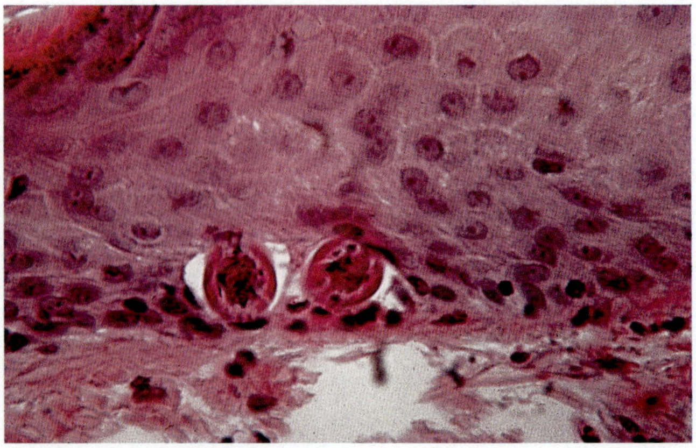

Figure 165–3. Two cross-sections of a migrating larva in the lower epidermis (hematoxylin-eosin, ×40).

DIFFERENTIAL DIAGNOSIS

The larvae of *A duodenale* and *Necator americanus* (both human hookworms) may produce a transient "ground itch" that affects toes, feet, and ankles, before they invade and continue their life cycle. Unlike CLM, these lesions migrate little and last for a short time—usually less than 2 weeks.[2,21] The larvae of *Gasterophilus* (horse botfly) and *Hypoderma* (cattle crabfly) may cause a migratory myiasis that resembles a creeping eruption, but this is rare.[22] *Strongyloides stercoralis* causes a variant of creeping eruption known as larva curens. It presents as a perianal, linear urticarial band that can migrate up to 10 cm/day. It may recur for years, due to autoinoculation from intestinal infection.[23–25]

DIAGNOSIS

The diagnosis of CLM is clinical and relatively straightforward. It may be confirmed by biopsy or mineral oil scrapings of the burrows. Recovery of a parasite may be made by freezing the area ahead of an advancing burrow and attempting an extraction.[21] There are no serologic tests available to confirm the diagnosis.

TREATMENT

Both oral and topical thiabendazole have been shown to be effective in the treatment of CLM.[17,25] New modalities of treatment include albendazole and ivermectin.[26,27]

REFERENCES

1. Thune PO. Creeping eruption of larva migrans. *Int J Dermatol.* 1972;11:231–232.
2. Edelglas JW, Douglas MC, Stiefler R, et al. Cutaneous larva migrans in a northern climate. *J Am Acad Dermatol.* 1982; 7:353–358.
3. Herbener D, Borak J. Cutaneous larva migrans in northern climates. *Am J Emerg Med.* 1988;6:462–464.
4. Lee RJ. Case of creeping eruption. *Trans Clin Soc London.* 1874;8:44–45.
5. Kirby-Smith JL, Dove WE, White GF. Creeping eruption. *Arch Dermatol.* 1926;13:137–173.
6. Davies HD, Sakulus P, Keystone JS. Creeping eruption. *Arch Dermatol.* 1993;129:588–591.
7. Allen C. Cutaneous larva migrans: a traveler's disease. *NZ Med J.* 1990;103:345.
8. Miller TA. Hookworm infection in man. *Adv Parasitol.* 1979;17:315–384.
9. Pinkus H, Fan J, Degiusti D. Creeping eruption due to *Gnathostoma spinigerum* in a Taiwanese patient. *Int J Dermatol.* 1981;290:46–49.
10. Jones C, Rosen T, Greenberg C. Cutaneous larva migrans due to *Pleodora strongyloides. Cutis.* 1991;48:123–126.
11. Kossman CE. Cutaneous larva migrans. *J Tenn Med Assoc.* 1981;74:874–883.
12. Stone OJ, Willis CJ, Mullins JF. Effect of thiabendazole on *Ancylostoma caninum. Arch Dermatol.* 1965;92:59–62.
13. Leicht SS, Youngberg GA. Cutaneous larva migrans. *Am Fam Prac.* 1987;35:163–168.
14. Stone OJ, Willis CJ. Cutaneous hookworm reservoir. *J Invest Dermatol.* 1967;49:237–239.
15. Elliot D, Tolle S, Goldberg L, et al. Pet associated illnesses. *N Engl J Med* 1985;313:985–995.
16. Lowenthal LJA. Evaluation of therapy in creeping eruption. *Aust J Dermatol.* 1958;78:186–190.
17. Katz R, Ziegler J, Blank H. The natural course of creeping eruption and treatment with thiabendazole. *Arch Dermatol.* 1965;91:420–424.
18. Wright D, Gold E. Löffler's syndrome associated with creeping eruption. *Arch Intern Med.* 1946;78:303.
19. Guill M, Odom R. Larva migrans complicated by Löffler's syndrome. *Arch Dermatol.* 1978;114:1525–1526.
20. Ambrus J, Klein E. Löffler's syndrome and ancylostomiasis braziliensis. *NY State Med.* 1988;88:498–499.
21. Lever WF. *Histopathology of the Skin.* Philadelphia: JB Lippincott; 1983.
22. Goldsmid JM, Froese EH. A note on cutaneous larva migrans and its treatment with topical thiabendazole. *Cent Afr J Med.* 1977;23:250–251.
23. Arthur RP, Shelly WB. Larva curens: a distinctive variant of cutaneous larva migrans due to *Strongyloides stercoralis. Arch Dermatol.* 1958:78;186–190.
24. Stone OJ, Newel G, Mullins JF. Cutaneous strongyloidiasis: larva curens. *Arch Dermatol.* 1972;106:734.
25. Stone OJ, Mullins JF. Thiabendazole effectiveness in creeping eruption. *Arch Dermatol.* 1965;91:427–429.
26. Williams H, Monk B. Creeping eruption stopped in its tracks by albendazole. *Clin Exp Dermatol.* 1989;14:355–356.
27. Caumes E, Datry A, Paris L, et al. Efficacy of ivermectin in the therapy of cutaneous larva migrans. *Arch Dermatol.* 1992;128:994–995.

CHAPTER 166

Visceral, Ocular, and Neural Larva Migrans

Kevin R. Kazacos

A correct knowledge of the diseases of man caused by worms . . . is the more difficult to obtain the more the parasites of animals are ignored.

Arthur Looss (1861–1923)

DEFINITION

Larva migrans (LM) refers to the prolonged migration and persistence of helminth larvae in the organs and tissues of humans and animals.[1,2] In these hosts, the larvae behave as they would in their natural intermediate or paratenic hosts, which are usually small mammals or birds.[1,2] During their sojourn, the larvae produce inflammatory lesions that may cause diverse clinical disease. Larva migrans may be separated clinically into visceral (VLM), ocular (OLM), neural (NLM), and cutaneous larva migrans (CLM), based on the main organ systems involved.[2–6] A large number of helminthic parasites of lower animals are potential causes of larva migrans affecting the deeper tissues of humans, ie, VLM, OLM, and NLM.[1–3,6–8] These include various ascarids, hookworms, gnathostomes, *Spirometra, Alaria,* and others. The primary cause of zoonotic larva migrans is *Toxocara canis,* the common large roundworm of dogs; in a few cases, *T cati* of cats has been incriminated. *Baylisascaris procyonis,* the common raccoon roundworm, is being increasingly recognized as a cause of human disease.[2,4–6] This chapter is focused on zoonotic larva migrans caused by *T canis* and *B procyonis,* with some reference to related ascarids.

HISTORY

The term *larva migrans* was first used in the 1920s to describe creeping eruption (CLM) caused by the migration of hookworm larvae in the skin of man.[1,3] Infection of humans by *Toxocara* larvae had been anticipated since then but it was not until 1952 that Beaver et al[9] identified *T canis* larvae in hepatic granulomas in a child with eosinophilia and hepatomegaly and proposed the term *visceral* larva migrans. In 1950, Wilder observed nematode larvae, later identified as *T canis,* in eosinophilic granulomas in enucleated eyes of children, thus establishing OLM as a clinical entity.[10] Since then, hundreds of patients with zoonotic toxocariasis have been described, establishing *T canis* as the most common cause of VLM and OLM in man.[2–5] Human infection with *Baylisascaris* was anticipated in the 1960s,[1] based on experiments done in rodents by Tiner and Sprent.[11–14] The zoonotic importance of *B procyonis* was indicated by Kazacos et al[2,6,15,16] in the late 1970s and 1980s, based on epidemiologic studies of infected animals and experimental infections of subhuman primates and other species. *Baylisascaris procyonis* is the most commonly recognized cause of clinical larva migrans in animals, having produced fatal or severe neurologic disease in over 50 species of mammals and birds.[2,6] Human death caused by *B procyonis* was first documented in children in 1984 and 1985,[17,18] and the parasite was implicated as a cause of human OLM at the same time.[19,20] Additional patients with larva migrans caused by these and other zoonotic parasites continue to be recognized.[3,5,21–29]

GEOGRAPHIC DISTRIBUTION

Human infections with *Toxocara* are cosmopolitan, having been reported from most parts of the world.[3–6]

Baylisascaris infections occur primarily in North America, but OLM has also been identified in Europe.[26]

LIFE CYCLE AND EPIDEMIOLOGY

Dogs, cats, or raccoons infected with ascarids shed daily in their feces hundreds of thousands of unembryonated eggs. These eggs embryonate in the soil and contain infective larvae in 2 to 4 weeks.[2–4,6,8] Infective ascarid eggs may survive in soil for years, posing a long-term source of infection for animals and humans.[2,3] Infection of definitive hosts is mainly by ingestion of infective eggs, perinatal transmission of larvae from mother to offspring, and ingestion of larvae in paratenic or intermediate hosts.[2–4,6,8] Puppies, kittens, and young raccoons can all be infected by ingesting eggs. In puppies and kittens, *Toxocara* infective larvae hatch from eggs in the small intestine, penetrate the intestinal wall, and migrate through vessels to liver and lungs. In lungs, larvae enter the alveoli, molt and crawl up the bronchi and trachea. They are then swallowed and reenter the small intestine where they mature.[2–4,8] In older dogs and cats, larvae migrating in the lungs enter the pulmonary veins, pass through the heart, and are distributed via the systemic circulation to various somatic tissues, in which they migrate and become encapsulated ("somatic migration"). Somatic *Toxocara* larvae mobilize during pregnancy, and puppies and kittens are commonly infected by transplacental and transmammary transmission, respectively.[2–5,8] *Baylisascaris* larvae do not migrate through liver or lungs in raccoons.[2,6] Instead, larvae from eggs penetrate the mucosa of small intestine and develop there before reentering the lumen to mature ("mucosal migration"). Dogs, cats, and raccoons are also commonly infected by ingesting larvae encysted in the tissues of paratenic (*Toxocara*) or intermediate hosts (*Baylisascaris*), such as rodents, rabbits, and birds.[2–4,6,8]

Humans and animals contract larva migrans by accidentally ingesting infective eggs from areas or objects contaminated with the feces of dogs, cats, or raccoons. In humans, very young children (1 to 4 years old) are at greatest risk because of their poorer hygiene and their propensity for pica and geophagia.[2,5,30] Infective larvae hatch from eggs in the small intestine, penetrate the intestinal wall, migrate through the liver and lungs, and undergo extensive somatic migration. Larvae become distributed to a variety of tissues, including the abdominal and thoracic viscera, skeletal muscles, brain, and eyes, in which they migrate and provoke inflammatory reactions.[2–6,8,13–15] Eventually, the larvae become encapsulated in eosinophilic granulomas in which the majority of larvae survive for years. *Toxocara* larvae do not grow or develop in humans or other paratenic hosts, and remain about 350 to 450 μm by 15 to 21 μm in size.[31] Unlike *Toxocara, Baylisascaris* larvae grow considerably during migration and reach a final size of about 1.5 to 1.9 mm by 60 to 80 μm.[6,25] Neither *Toxocara* nor *Baylisascaris* complete their development in humans, so that humans are dead-end hosts. Risk factors for contracting toxocariasis and baylisascariasis include geophagia, keeping infected puppies, kittens, or raccoons as pets, or having contact with areas contaminated with their feces.[2–6,30] In patients with OLM, contact with animals or contaminated areas is sometimes difficult to establish. Infection by *Toxocara* has been contracted also by ingesting undercooked or raw meat or liver containing larvae[5]; this is unknown for *Baylisascaris* but might also be possible because of the broad host range for larvae of this parasite.[2,6]

MORPHOLOGY OF THE ORGANISM

Nematode larvae are identified by their size and microscopic anatomy (Figure 166–1).[3,7,21,25,31–33] The body wall is comprised of exterior cuticle and underlying hypodermis and muscle. The cuticle may be finely striated and may possess lateral alae; the latter may be single or double and may run most of the length of the

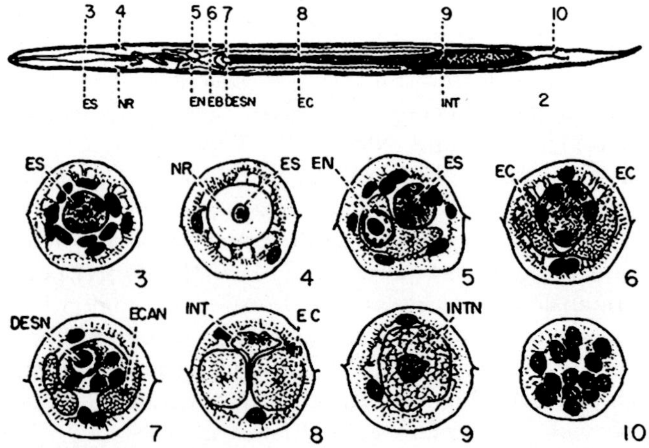

Figure 166–1. Microscopic anatomy of *T canis* larva sectioned at different levels as indicated. DESN, nucleus of dorsal esophageal gland; EB, esophageal bulb; EC, excretory column; ECAN, excretory canaliculus; EN, excretory cell nucleus; ES, esophagus; INT, intestine; INTN, nucleus of intestinal cell; NR, nerve ring. *(Reproduced with permission, J Parasitol. 1956;42:349–362.)*

body or be restricted to certain regions. The hypodermis is specialized into dorsal, ventral, and paired lateral cords, which run longitudinally and divide the muscle layer into quadrants. The lateral cords are larger and usually support paired excretory columns, which also run longitudinally. The body wall surrounds the fluid-filled body cavity (pseudocoelom), which contains a centrally located digestive tract. The latter has an anterior mouth and muscular esophagus, followed by the intestine and rectum. In small larvae, the body cavity may be inapparent and the muscles and hypodermal cords difficult to distinguish.[21,31,32] Of particular importance for the histologic identification of larvae are overall size, the presence, type, and size of lateral alae, size and shape of intestine, and the presence, size, and shape of excretory columns. These features are best examined in transverse sections through the midbody/midintestinal region. Other diagnostic features include shape of the anterior end, length of esophagus, position of the excretory cell nucleus, number of intestinal cells per section, patency of the intestinal lumen, number of muscle cells per quadrant, and position and size of the genital primordium.[7,21,31–33]

Keys to the identification of ascaridoid and other larvae recovered intact and/or as seen in histologic sections have been presented by Nichols and Bowman, along with excellent drawings (eg, Figure 166–1) and photographs.[7,31,32] Key features of several important ascaridoid species are summarized in Tables 166–1 and 166–2. Most ascaridoid larvae possess salient, single lateral alae. Except for short stretches at either extremity, alae usually run most of the body length and are usually most prominent in the midbody/midintestinal region. In some genera/species, alae are absent (eg, *Hexametra*), restricted to the esophageal region, or reduced to lateral thickenings or internal cuticular bars (eg, *Ophidascaris*).[7] *Toxocara canis* and *T cati* larvae are small, averaging about 400 μm long by 16 to 19 μm in diameter (Table 166–1).[31] The two species are essentially identical except that larvae of *T canis* are larger in diameter (18 to 21 μm) than *T cati* (15 to 17 μm). In histologic sections, larvae are somewhat smaller because of shrinkage. Shrinkage occurs during processing and is usually evident more in length than in diameter. Thus, *Toxocara* larvae reconstructed from sections are about 320 μm long (range, 290 to 350 μm) by 14 to 20 μm (usually 18 to 20 μm) for *T canis* and 12 to 16 μm for *T cati* (Table 166–2).[31] *Baylisascaris procyonis* larvae grow considerably, reaching an average final size of 1750 μm long by 72 μm in diameter (Table 166–1).[25] *Baylisascaris* larvae in tissue sections usually range 60 to 70 μm in maximum diameter, but occasionally reach 75 μm.

Sections through the anterior (esophageal) region of ascaridoid larvae contain the esophagus, nerve ring, ganglia, excretory commissure, excretory cell nucleus, proximal excretory columns, and/or esophageal glands (Figures 166–1 and 166–2). Sections through the larger middle region contain intestine and paired lateral excretory columns (Figures 166–1 through 166–6). Sections through the posterior region (past the termination of the excretory columns) contain only intestine or the intestinorectal valve (Figures 166–1, 166–3, and 166–6). Somatic muscles and paired lateral cords are at all levels, with lateral cords most prominent at midbody/midintestinal region (Figures 166–3 and 166–4). Various nuclei, ganglia, muscles, hypodermal cords, esophageal glands, etc, are at all levels, but are especially common in the anterior and posterior regions (Figures 166–1 through 166–6). The shape of excretory columns may

TABLE 166–1. MEASUREMENTS (IN MICRONS) OF ASCARIDOID LARVAE RECOVERED FROM TISSUES OF INTERMEDIATE OR PARATENIC HOSTS[7,25,31]

Parasite	Definitive Host	Average Size		Size Range		Esophagus	
		Length	*Width*[a]	*Length*	*Width*[a]	*$\bar{X}$ Length*	*%Body L*
Toxocara canis	Canids	405	19	357–445	18–21	153	38
T cati	Felids	407	16	357–445	15–17	154	38
Toxascaris leonina	Canids, felids	700	31	650–750	25–37	190	27
Baylisascaris procyonis	Raccoons	1750	72	1450–1850	60–81	261	15
Lagochilascaris sprenti	Opossums	4450	173	3900–5000	146–195	520	12
Hexametra leidyi	Rattlesnakes	8000	240	6400–10,000	175–310	1060	13

[a] Maximum width.
From Bowman,[7] Goldberg et al,[25] and Nichols.[31]

TABLE 166–2. CHARACTERISTICS OF ASCARIDOID LARVAE IN HISTOLOGIC SECTIONS, AS SEEN IN TRANSVERSE SECTIONS THROUGH THE MIDBODY REGION[7,16,31]

			Intestine				Excretory Columns		
Parasite[a]	**Maximum Diameter (μm)**	**Height Alae (μm)**	***Width (μm)***	***No. of Cells***	***Patent Lumen***	***Compression***	***Relative Size, Shape***	***Size vs. Intestine***	**Muscle Cells per Quadrant**
T canis	14–20[b]	1	6[c]	1	No	Laterodorsal	Large, round	>	?
T cati	12–16	1	6[c]	1	No	Laterodorsal	Large, round	>	?
T leonina	25–28	4	8	5	Yes	None	Small triangle	<<	6
B procyonis	60–70	7–8	23	4–6	Yes	Lateral	Medium triangle	<<	4–6
L sprenti	163	10[d]	75	21	Yes	Dorsoventral	Small triangle	<<<<<+	25
H leidyi	200	NP[e]	100	28	Yes	Dorsoventral	Small triangle	<<<<	30

[a] Same genera as in Table 166–1.
[b] Usually 18 to 20 μm.
[c] Intestine strongly compressed.
[d] With internal cuticular bars.
[e] Not present.
From Bowman,[7] Kazacos,[16] and Nichols.[31]

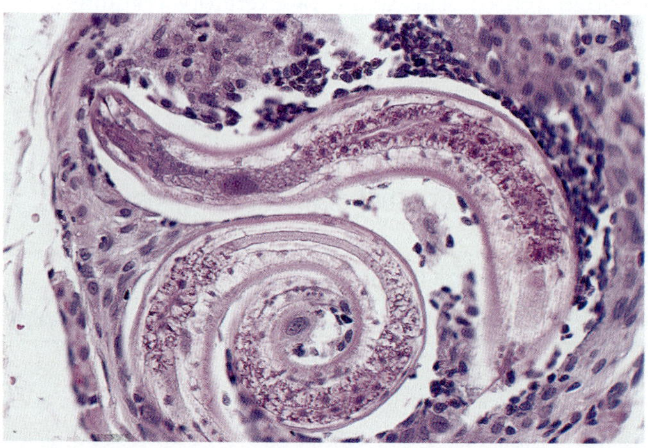

Figure 166–2. Longitudinal section of *B procyonis* larva in heart of monkey. Note esophagus, nerve ring, excretory commissure with large excretory cell nucleus, intestine, excretory columns, etc [hematoxylin-eosin (H&E) ×100]. *(Photograph by K. R. Kazacos, DVM, PhD.)*

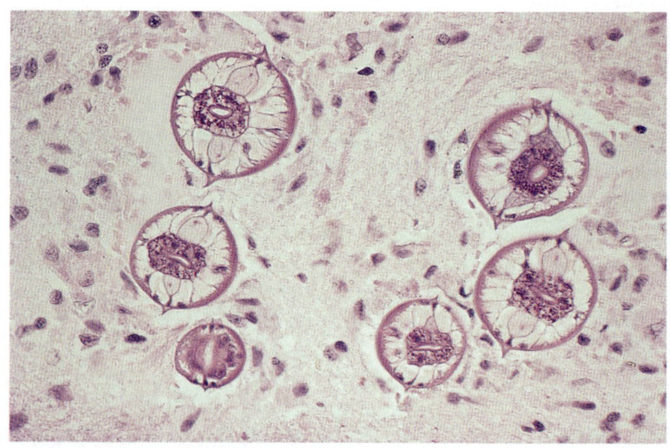

Figure 166–3. Cross-sections of *B procyonis* larva in brain of monkey. Anterior end of larva is out of photo to upper left. Larva shown is coiled laterally from upper right to lower left, and sectioned through the following levels: (*upper right*) anterior intestinal region just posterior to esophagus; (*upper and midleft, midright*) midintestinal region, with (*midright*) near midbody; (*lower right*) posterior intestinal region near end of excretory columns; (*lower left*) intestinorectal valve. Note lateral alae, intestine with microvilli and granules, lateral cords with three hypodermal nuclei, and triangular excretory columns with canaliculi. Also note change in size of excretory columns and compression of intestine at different levels, and lack of inflammatory reaction (H&E, ×100). *(Photograph by K. R. Kazacos, DVM, PhD.)*

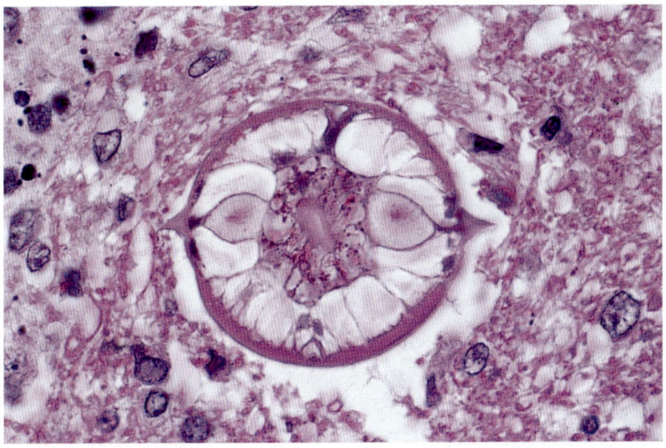

Figure 166–4. High magnification of cross-section through midbody of *B procyonis* larva in brain of monkey. Note lateral alae, large laterally compressed intestine with prominent granules, lateral cords with three hypodermal nuclei, and triangular excretory columns, of slightly different sizes and with central canaliculi (H&E, ×250). *(Photograph by K. R. Kazacos, DVM, PhD.)*

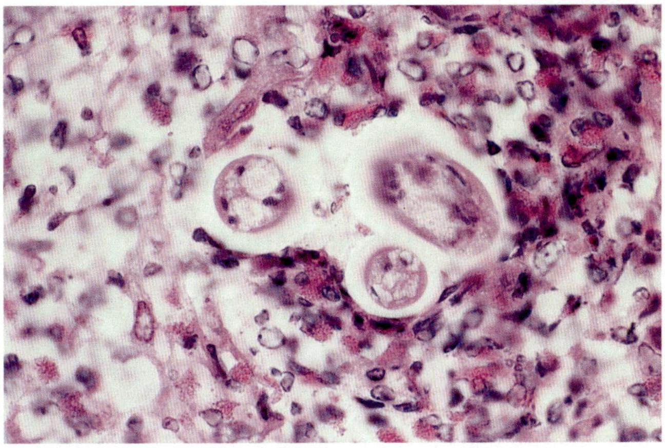

Figure 166–6. Sections of *T canis* larva in liver of rabbit. Section on *left* through midbody, with same characteristics shown in Figure 166–5, but with intestine more typically represented as a weakly basophilic triangular mass; *upper right* is a longitudinal section through excretory column; *lower right* a cross-section through intestinal region posterior to excretory columns (H&E, ×250). *(Photograph by K. R. Kazacos, DVM, PhD.)*

change from the level of the base of the esophagus through the middle region, as may the degree of compression of intestine (Figures 166–1 and 166–3).[7,31] The anterior end of *Toxocara* larvae is prow shaped, with an extended subventral margin and a subterminal, dorsally inclined mouth. The anterior end of *Baylisascaris* larvae is smoothly rounded. Both genera have paired, single lateral alae, which are very small in *Toxocara* and large and pointed in *Baylisascaris* (Figures 166–1, 166–3 through 166–6). At midbody, *Toxocara* larvae have large, round excretory columns, which fill the body cavity and compress the intestine laterally and dorsally into a small triangular mass (Figures 166–1, 166–5, and 166–6). The excretory columns have prominent canaliculi, visible as central condensed areas. Posterior to the excretory columns, the intestine expands to fill the body cavity (Figures 166–1 and 166–6). In cross-sections of *Toxocara,* the intestine consists of one cell. Dorsal and ventral cords are not evident, but the lateral cords are just visible and ventral line nuclei are prominent (Figures 166–1, 166–5, and 166–6).[31] *Baylisascaris* larvae have a large, centrally located intestine, which is laterally compressed in the mid- to posterior intestinal regions and has an open lumen (Figures 166–3 and 166–4). In cross-section, the intestine consists of four to six low columnar cells, which have a thin microvillous border and contain numerous cytoplasmic granules (Figures 166–3 and 166–4); these cells are also prominent in longitudinal sections (Figure 166–2). The intestine is flanked by prominent lateral cords supporting the lateral excretory columns, which are smaller than the intestine, roughly triangular, and slightly dissimilar in size (Figures 166–3 and 166–4).[7,16] The excretory columns have prominent central canaliculi, and three hypodermal nuclei are usually visible in the lateral cords, just below the cuticle.

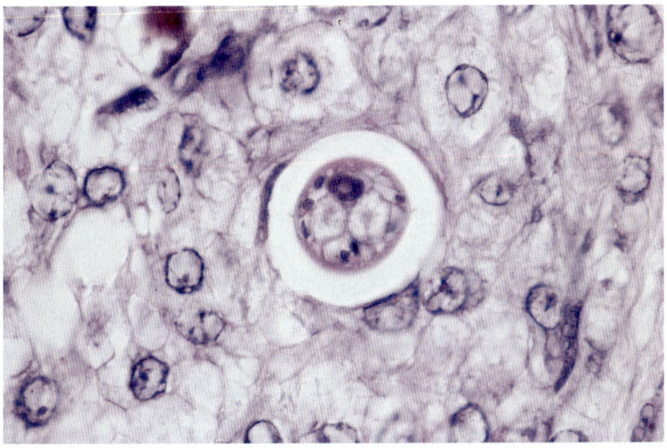

Figure 166–5. High magnification through midbody of *T canis* larva in liver of rabbit. Note small lateral alae, large, round excretory columns with canaliculi, and intestine. The section is through the nucleus of an intestinal cell, which here is U-shaped (H&E, ×320). *(Photograph by K. R. Kazacos, DVM, PhD.)*

Larvae of other ascaridoid nematodes have a different size and microanatomy than that just described. Features of other species are given in Tables 166–1 and 166–2 and described elsewhere.[7] Larvae of hookworms, gnathostomes, and other nematodes capable of causing larva migrans, as well as trematodes, cestodes, and pentastomes (all of which are quite different from nematodes) are described elsewhere in this book and in other references.[3,21,32–34]

PATHOGENESIS AND CLINICAL FEATURES

Somatic migration of *Toxocara* and *Baylisascaris* larvae causes mechanical damage, necrosis, and provokes vigorous host inflammatory reactions.[2–4,35,36] Liver, lungs, heart, brain, and eyes can be involved. The inflammatory reactions are directed against larval excretory–secretory (ES) antigens, which consist of enzymes, cuticular proteins, and metabolic wastes released by larvae during migration.[6,30,36,37] Eosinophils are a major component of host reactions and toxic eosinophil proteins probably contribute to pathologic changes and clinical signs.[35–39]

Clinical disease is related to the level and frequency of infection and reinfection, the distribution of larvae in the body, and the extent of the reactions.[2–6,36,37] Visceral larva migrans from heavy and/or repeated infection involves large numbers of larvae migrating through liver, lungs, and other tissues. VLM is characterized by widespread inflammation and systemic allergic manifestations. In neural LM, there is larval invasion of the central nervous system (CNS), with traumatic damage, inflammation, and associated neurologic signs. In OLM, patients usually have few larvae but chance migration of a single larva into the eye produces serious localized damage and inflammation.

In toxocaral VLM, trapping of large numbers of larvae in eosinophilic granulomas in liver results in the greatest concentration of larvae within this organ.[35–37,40] With repeated or continuous infection, liver trapping, hepatomegaly, eosinophilia, and related allergic manifestations all become increasingly pronounced.[5,35–37] In primary infections, the larvae may be better able to traverse the liver and lungs and reach other sites, including brain or eye.[4,30] At present, there is no evidence of liver trapping and associated hepatic pathology in *Baylisascaris* infections, although hepatomegaly has been noted clinically.[17,18,28] Perhaps this reflects more aggressive migration of *Baylisascaris* through liver and lungs, genus/species differences in the antigens provoking inflammation, and/or the relative intensity of those reactions. Major differences in hepatic lesions have been noted in rabbits and other animals given primary infections with larvae of *T canis* and *B procyonis,* indicating that the differences are probably parasite related (Kazacos KR, unpublished data). Larvae of both parasites commonly invade the CNS of animals and humans, but differ greatly in pathogenicity.[2,6,11–14] Deaths from *Toxocara* are few and related to massive invasion of the CNS or heart coupled with augmented inflammatory reactions.[5,36,41,42] Infection with *Baylisascaris* larvae is commonly associated with severe or fatal CNS disease and therefore poses a greater danger to humans, especially children.[2,6,18]

Clinical features of larva migrans are diverse and can be divided into those of asymptomatic infection, covert infection, VLM, NLM, and OLM.[2,4–6] Most infections are asymptomatic and characterized by low serum antibody titer with or without mild eosinophilia.[4,5] In covert toxocariasis, there is a significant association between clinical signs (including abdominal pain, hepatomegaly, sleep disorders, coughing, wheezing, and headache) and a positive titer to *Toxocara,* even in the absence of eosinophilia.[5] Clinical VLM and NLM result from heavy and/or repeated infection and are most common in children 1 to 4 years old with a history of pica and geophagia.[2,4–6] VLM varies from an acute disease to a more chronic clinical syndrome, and is characterized by abdominal pain, hepatomegaly, fever, anorexia, restlessness, and pulmonary symptoms (coughing, wheezing, asthma). Laboratory findings include leukocytosis, marked eosinophilia, hypergammaglobulinemia, and elevated anti-A and/or anti-B isohemagglutinin titers.[5,30,35] Chest radiographs reveal pulmonary infiltrates (Figure 166–7) and sputum or transtracheal washes contain abundant eosinophils and Charcot–Leyden crystals.[30,35] Some children show signs of myocarditis or encephalitis.[5,35] A spectrum of CNS involvement and disease is possible with toxocariasis, ranging from subtle neuropsychologic problems to seizures, convulsions, ataxia, coma, and death.[5,24,35,41,42] Recently a VLM syndrome was described in French adults who had allergic manifestations of pruritus, rash, difficulty breathing, weakness, and abdominal pain.[5]

Because they are larger and more aggressive than *Toxocara, Baylisascaris* larvae have a much greater likelihood of causing neurologic disease, especially in heavy infections related to VLM.[2,6] Clinical findings in *Baylisascaris* NLM range from mild to devastating CNS involvement, which can develop within 2 to 4 weeks and progress rapidly. Clinical signs include sudden lethargy, irritability, loss of muscle coordination, decreased head control, torticollis, stupor, nystagmus, and obtundation progressing to coma, hypotonia, hyperreflexia, and death.[17,18] Less severe involvement with *Baylisascaris* has caused hemiparesis, inability to sit or stand, ocular muscle paralysis, cortical blindness, and severe delay in development.[28] Eosinophilic pleocytosis of the cerebrospinal fluid is an important diagnostic finding in patients with *Baylisascaris* NLM, especially when found concurrently with peripheral eosinophilia and compatible clinical signs.[17,18,28] In two

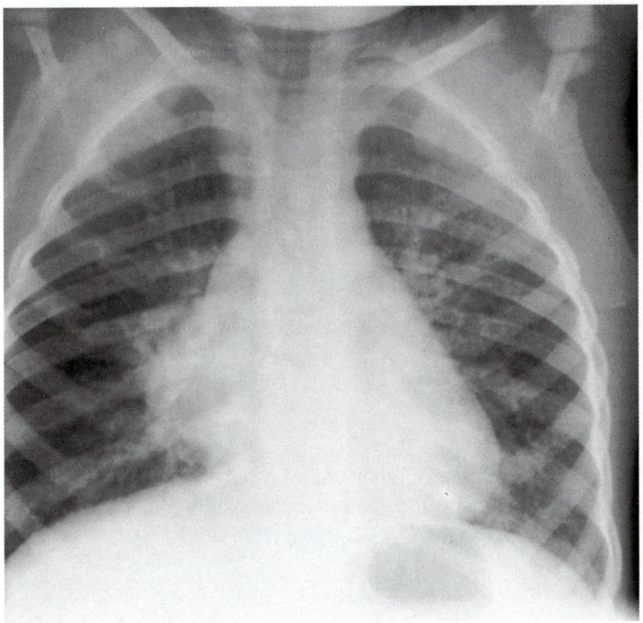

Figure 166–7. Chest radiograph of child with VLM caused by *T cati.* Note diffuse increase in interstitial markings, more prominent in perihilar region and representing a pulmonary infiltrate. *(Photograph by K. R. Kazacos, DVM, PhD.)*

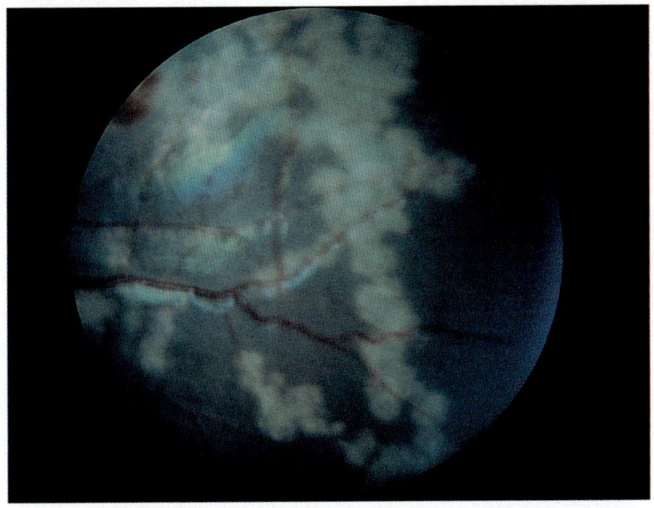

Figure 166–8. *Baylisascaris procyonis* OLM in cynomolgus monkey; fundus at 8 days postinfection. Note retinal hemorrhage (*upper left*), serpiginous tracks and sheathing of retinal vessels. *(Photograph by K. R. Kazacos, DVM, PhD; reproduced with permission, Invest Ophthalmol Vis Sci. 1984;25:1177–1183.)*

children who died, ventricles were dilated and there was periventricular enhancement on computed tomography (CT) with contrast infusion.[17,18] In less severe infections, CT and magnetic resonance imaging may be normal at first,[28] but later reveal diffuse cerebral and cerebellar atrophy,[17,28] a probable sequela of damage and inflammation.

Ocular larva migrans is typically in older children and young adults, in the absence of systemic signs and often without a history of pica or obvious animal contact.[2,4–6,30] Larvae enter the eye via the retinal or choroidal vessels and migrate in the retina, choroid, and related tissues. Migrating larvae disrupt ocular tissues and provoke inflammatory reactions before they are trapped in granulomas.[35] OLM typically presents as unilateral loss of vision, strabismus, esotropia, and leukocoria.[5,22,43] Ophthalmoscopy may reveal posterior or peripheral retinochoroiditis, meandering retinal tracks with larvae (Figure 166–8), vitritis, papillitis, granulomatous masses in retina or choroid, or chronic endophthalmitis with retinal detachment.[5,22,43–46] *Toxocara, Baylisascaris, Alaria,* and hookworm larvae have been implicated as causes of the ocular syndrome diffuse unilateral subacute neuroretinitis (DUSN).[25,26,29,46] In DUSN, visual loss appears to be a sequela of parasite-induced inflammation of the retina, associated vessels, and optic nerve head.[25] DUSN is characterized early by visual loss, vitritis, papillitis, retinal vasculitis, and recurrent crops of gray-white outer retinal lesions (Figure 166–8), and later by progressive visual loss, optic atrophy, narrowing of retinal vessels, and diffuse degeneration of retinal pigment epithelium.[46] If visualized in the eye (Figure 166–9), larvae are identified clinically by size, shape, and movement, and the diagnosis is supported by serologic and epidemiologic findings.[25,26,29]

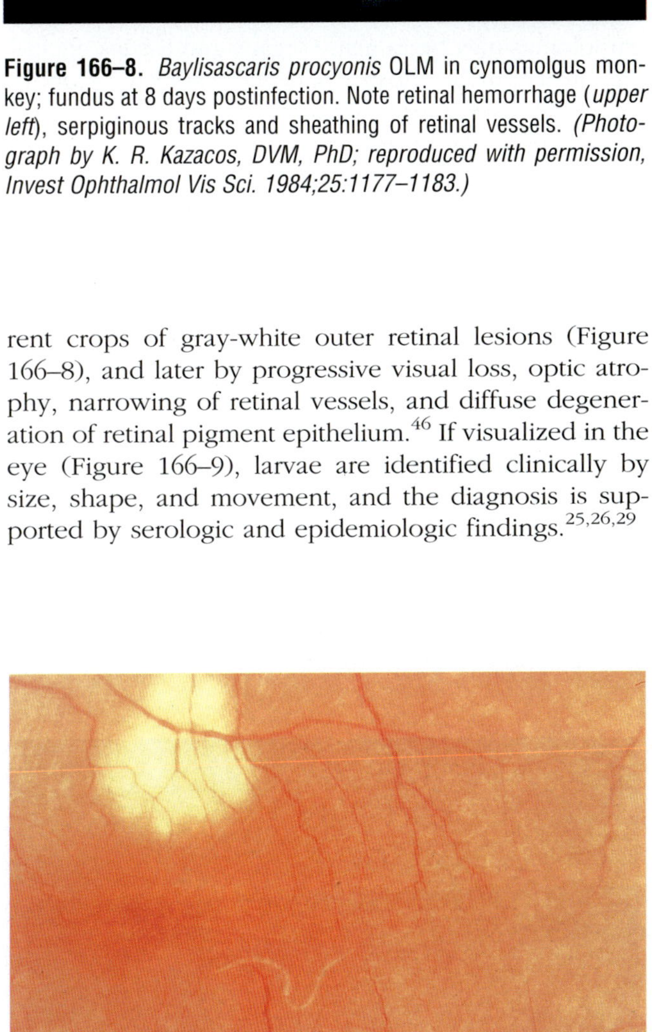

Figure 166–9. *Baylisascaris procyonis* larva (1727 μm by 67 μm) migrating in retina of a man with diffuse unilateral subacute neuroretinitis. Hyperreflective area is laser photocoagulation in attempt to kill larva; second attempt was successful. *(Photograph by B. Katz, MD, California Pacific Medical Center, San Francisco, and K. R. Kazacos, DVM, PhD.)*

PATHOLOGY

The principal lesions of larva migrans are eosinophilic and granulomatous inflammation, which may occur in a variety of tissues and organs.[15,21,34,35,40–45] In toxocaral VLM, the liver and lungs are most frequently involved, whereas in *Baylisascaris* NLM the most important lesions are in the brain. Larvae migrating through the tissues leave a trail of hemorrhage, necrosis, edema, and a cellular infiltrate consisting mostly of eosinophils. Particularly in toxocariasis, inflammation can be extensive and large aggregates of eosinophils may surround areas of necrosis.[35] Following migration, the larvae become encapsulated in well-circumscribed eosinophilic granulomas, usually 1 to 3 mm in diameter, or in larger granulomas up to 1 cm.[15,21,35,40–45] Larval granulomas may be in many organs and tissues, including liver, lungs, heart, pancreas, spleen, kidneys, mesentery, mesenteric lymph nodes, intestine, skeletal muscle, brain, and eyes.[13,15,35,40–45]

In toxocaral VLM, the main lesions are in liver and lungs. Typically, the liver is enlarged, the capsular surface has gray-white or tan plaques, and contains granulomas 1 to 10 mm across (Figure 166–10).[9,21,35,40–42] Histologically, these lesions are aggregates of eosinophils and other inflammatory cells, associated tissue necrosis, and larvae (Figures 166–11 and 166–12). As granulomas develop, the aggregates of eosinophils around larvae are infiltrated and replaced by epithelioid cells and giant cells and, peripherally, fibrous tissue (Figures 166–13 and 166–14). In long-standing granulomas, the central area consists predominantly of epithelioid cells and a fibrous capsule surrounds the granuloma (Figure 166–14). The granulomas are often infiltrated by numerous eosinophils, lymphocytes, and plasma cells (Figures 166–13 and 166–14), and the portal tracts may be infiltrated by the same cells. *Baylisascaris* has caused migratory lesions and occasional hepatic granulomas, but not the more severe lesions caused by *Toxocara*. Both children who died of infection with *Baylisascaris* had slightly enlarged livers but without other lesions.[17,18]

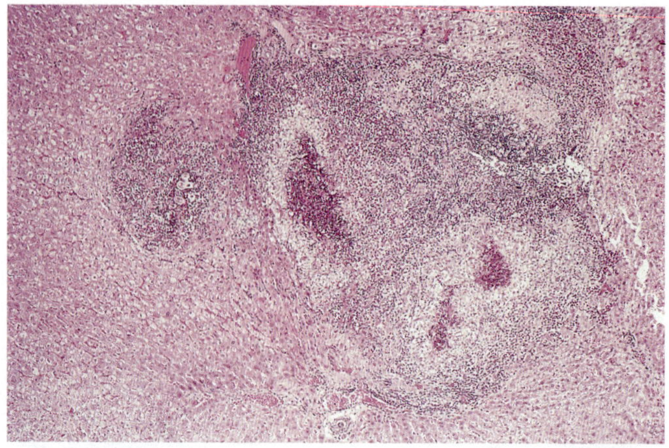

Figure 166–11. Liver of rabbit with *T canis* infection. Note areas of eosinophilic necrosis, and larva in inflammatory focus at left (H&E, ×16). *(Photograph by K. R. Kazacos, DVM, PhD.)*

Eosinophilic deposits, termed Splendore–Hoeppli (SH) substance, may be prominent in areas of eosinophilic necrosis, along tracks and within granulomas adjacent to larvae (Figures 166–13 and 166–15).[20,35,39,40] Immunofluorescent studies of fatal infections with *Baylisascaris* indicate that these SH

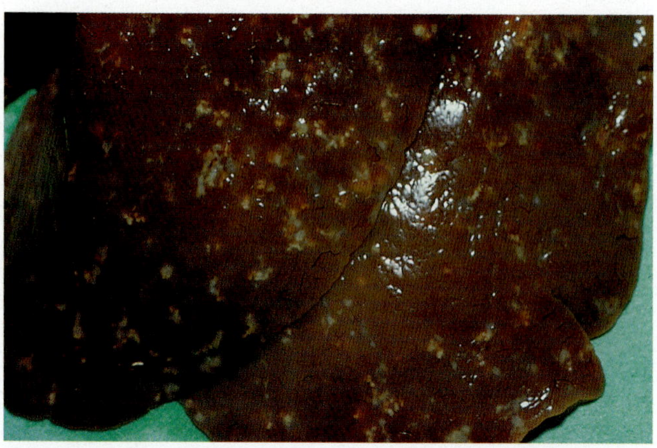

Figure 166–10. Liver of rabbit with *T canis* infection. Note irregular surface and many foci—areas of inflammation and necrosis, some with recent hemorrhage. *(Photograph by K. R. Kazacos, DVM, PhD.)*

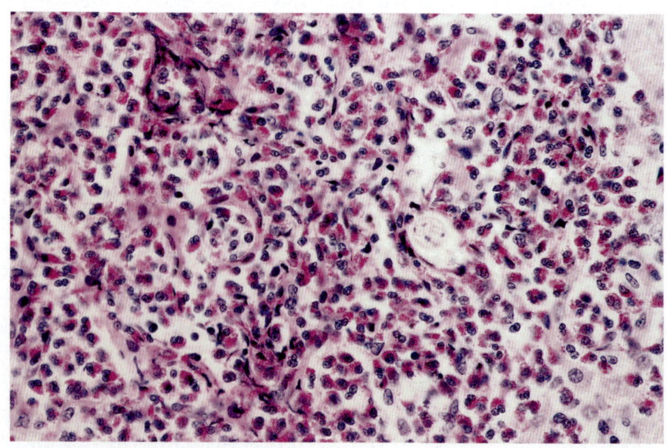

Figure 166–12. Intense accumulation of eosinophils in liver of a child with *T canis* infection, with cross-section of larva (H&E, ×125). *(Photograph by K. R. Kazacos, DVM, PhD; specimen contributed by M. D. Little, PhD, Tulane University, New Orleans, Louisiana.)*

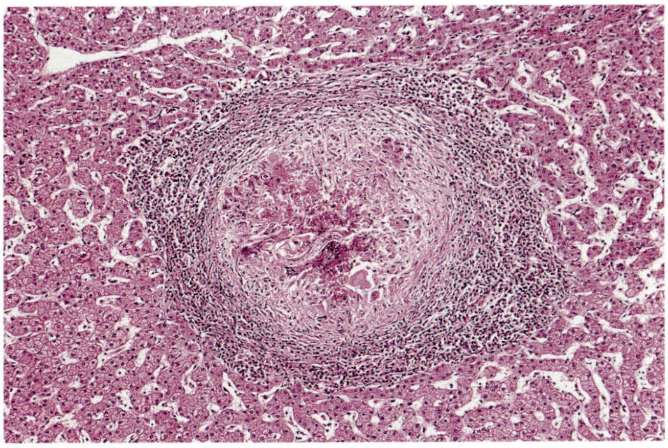

Figure 166–13. *Toxocara canis* granuloma in liver of a child. Note longitudinal section of larva in center of granuloma (H&E, ×32). *(Photograph by K. R. Kazacos, DVM, PhD; specimen contributed by M. D. Little, PhD, Tulane University, New Orleans, Louisiana.)*

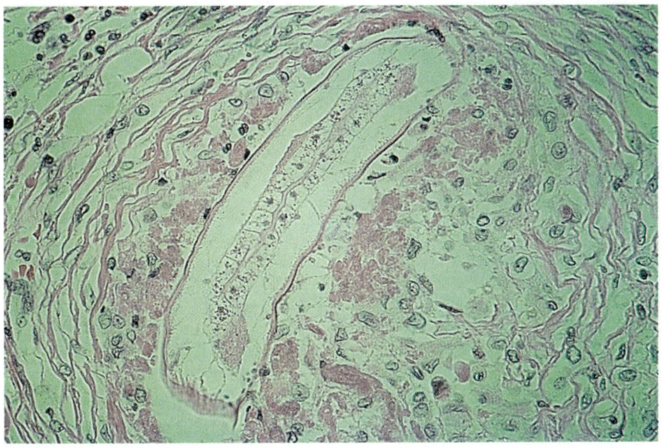

Figure 166–15. *Baylisascaris procyonis* larva in granuloma in mesentery of a child with fatal infection. Note eosinophilic deposits around the larva (H&E, ×80). *(Reproduced with permission, Am J Trop Med Hyg. 1989;40:291–297.)*

deposits are extracellular eosinophil major basic protein (Figures 116–15 and 166–16).[39] Finding larvae, particularly *Toxocara,* in granulomas and other tissues may be difficult and require serial or step sectioning. Periodic acid–Schiff staining has been recommended as an aid in locating *Toxocara* in tissue sections.[35]

Migration through the lungs causes pneumonitis and pulmonary granulomas. Early, there are petechial and ecchymotic hemorrhages (Figure 166–17), which resolve and are replaced by diffuse eosinophilic then granulomatous inflammation.[6,13,14,35,40,42] Hemosiderosis may be in areas of resolving pulmonary hemorrhage. Alveolar septa are thickened by congestion, edema, and cellular infiltration.[35] Pulmonary inflammation appears to be worse with *Toxocara* than with *Baylisascaris* and may be from increased immunopathologic reactions in toxocariasis. Larval granulomas develop in lungs as elsewhere and are most noticeable on the pleural surface and in subpleural tissue (Figure 166–18), although they may be widespread throughout the lungs.[18,35]

Myocardial involvement is common in both *Toxocara* and *Baylisascaris* infections.[13,15,17,18,35,40,42] Migration through the heart causes multifocal myocarditis with infiltration by eosinophils, macrophages, lym-

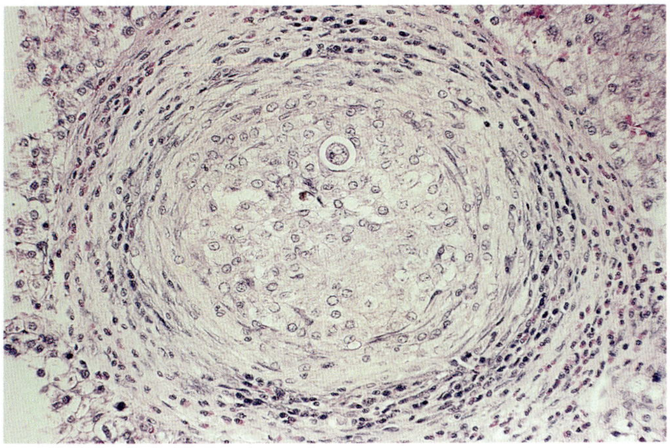

Figure 166–14. Chronic *T canis* granuloma in liver of a rabbit. Note larva in center of granuloma (H&E, ×63). *(Photograph by K. R. Kazacos, DVM, PhD.)*

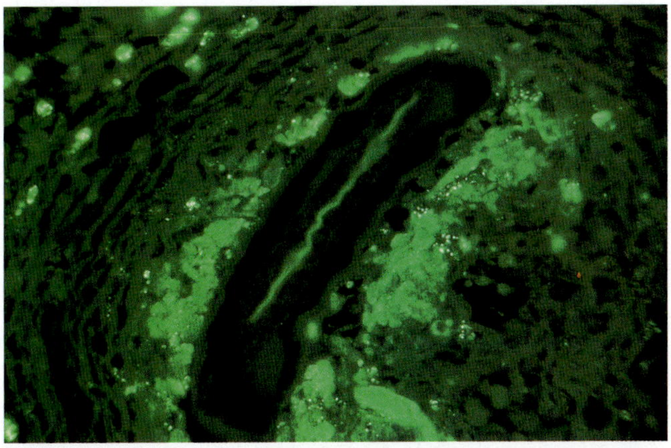

Figure 166–16. Same section shown in Figure 166–15, reacted first with rabbit antiserum (IgG) to human eosinophil major basic protein (MBP), followed by fluorescein-conjugated goat antirabbit IgG. Note the strong anti-MBP fluorescence of the eosinophilic deposits. Note also the fluorescence of the worm's intestinal lumen, indicating ingestion by worm of cellular products including MBP (×80). *(Reproduced with permission, Am J Trop Med Hyg. 1989;40: 291–297.)*

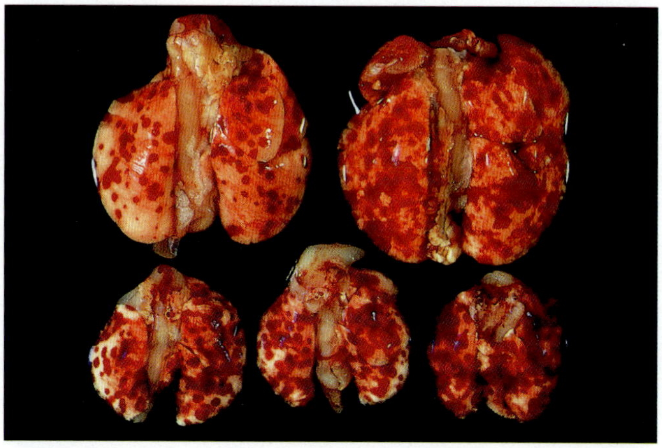

Figure 166–17. Hemorrhages in lungs of hamsters (*top*) and mice (*bottom*) caused by larval migration taken 2 days postinfection with eggs of *B columnaris*. *(Photograph by K. R. Kazacos, DVM, PhD.)*

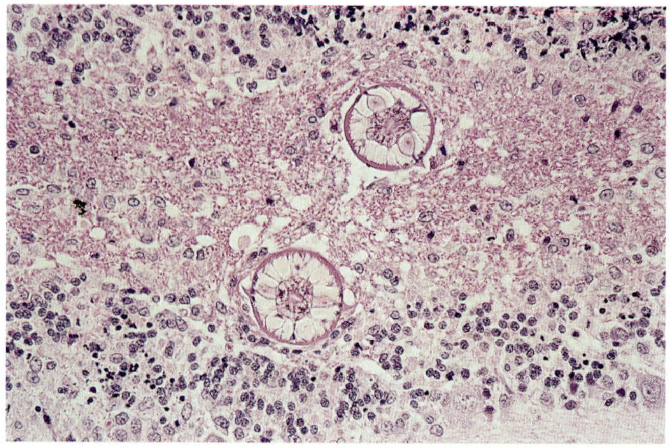

Figure 166–19. *Baylisascaris procyonis* larva in cerebellum of monkey. Note cross-sections of larva, surrounding edema, nuclear pyknosis of granular cells, and a swollen axon (H&E, ×80). *(Photograph by K. R. Kazacos, DVM, PhD.)*

phocytes, and plasma cells. There is accompanying edema, necrosis of myofibers, and a granulomatous reaction. Larval granulomas may be anywhere in the heart.[15,17,18,42]

Larvae of both *Toxocara* and *Baylisascaris* invade the CNS, particularly in primary infections.[6,11,12,14,35] Larvae of both parasites may reach the brain in large numbers but *Baylisascaris* is far more damaging to neural tissues.[2,6,12,14] Early lesions in the CNS consist of tracks with tissue disruption, nuclear pyknosis, necrosis, spongiosis, and hemorrhage, with a few infiltrating cells (Figure 166–19).[14,15] Migratory lesions may be in any portion of brain and spinal cord.[15,35] Tracks quickly become infiltrated with inflammatory cells, primarily macrophages in the early stages (Figure 166–20) followed by eosinophils, lymphocytes, and plasma cells. As the reaction progresses, perivascular cuffing becomes prominent, especially adjacent to areas of inflammation and necrosis. Depending on the numbers of larvae, CNS lesions may be focal or more diffuse and may extend to the leptomeninges. Other lesions caused by larval migration in the CNS include severe spongiosis, neuronal degeneration, swelling and degeneration of axons, demyelination, and prominent gliosis.[15,17,35] Gliosis is of the protoplasmic type and gemistocytic astrocytes may be adjacent to areas of tissue damage. In

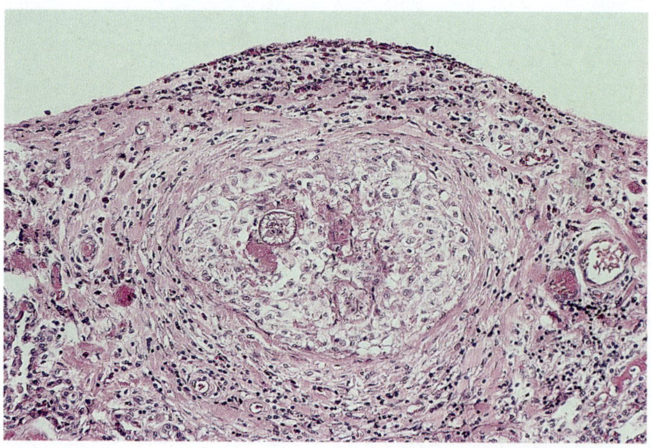

Figure 166–18. Subpleural granuloma from a child who died of infection with *B procyonis*. Note cross-sections of *B procyonis* larva (H&E, ×40). *(Photograph by K. R. Kazacos, DVM, PhD; specimen contributed by N. S. Gould, MD, Michael Reese Hospital, Chicago, Illinois.)*

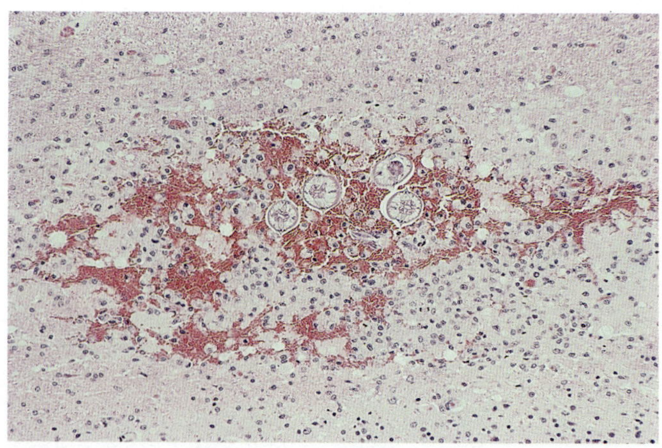

Figure 166–20. *Baylisascaris procyonis* larva in the cerebrum of a monkey. Note the surrounding hemorrhage, edema, and lipid-laden macrophages (Gitter cells), many of which are undergoing division (H&E, ×40). *(Photograph by K. R. Kazacos, DVM, PhD.)*

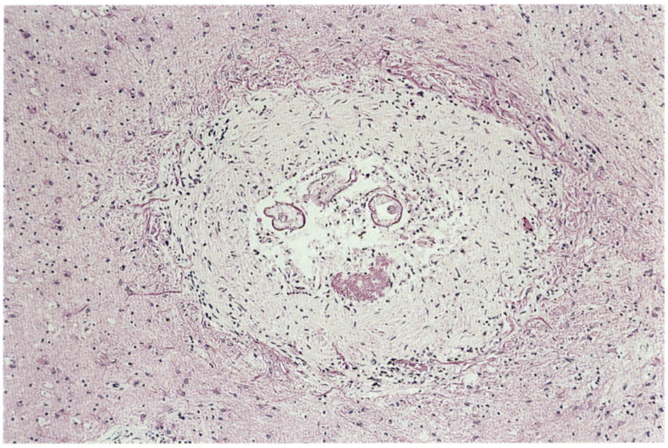

Figure 166–21. *Baylisascaris procyonis* larva and eosinophilic protein in a granuloma in the cerebrum of a child who died of baylisascariasis. The larva is surrounded by a granulomatous reaction, which includes a zone of gliosis (H&E, ×32). *(Photograph by K. R. Kazacos, DVM, PhD; specimen contributed by D. S. Huff, MD, Children's Hospital of Philadelphia, Philadelphia, Pennsylvania.)*

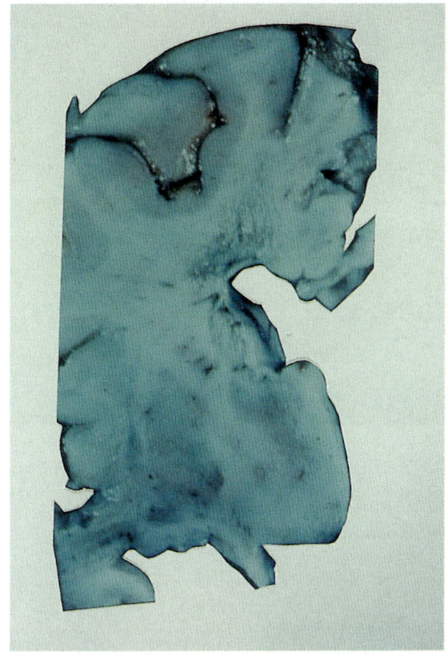

Figure 166–22. Brain of child with fatal *B procyonis* infection, showing periventricular necrosis. *(Courtesy N. S. Gould, MD, Michael Reese Hospital, Chicago, Illinois.)*

the brain, larvae may be in the tracks and areas of inflammation (Figure 166–20); however, they are also in more normal-appearing neuropil away from obvious lesions, indicating their active migration when fixed (Figures 166–3 and 166–19).[15,18] Encapsulation of larvae lags far behind encapsulation in other tissues, causing prolonged larval migration.[18,21,36] Encapsulation eventually occurs, however, and larvae become walled off in sharply demarcated foci of granulomatous inflammation (Figure 166–21).[17,40–42] These foci resemble the granulomas in other tissues, but they are usually walled off by gliosis rather than fibrosis.

In CNS toxocariasis in which death was attributed to the parasite,[41] or other causes,[40] the brain was edematous, as evidenced by swollen gyri and narrowed sulci, but otherwise unremarkable. CNS lesions consisted of larval tracks, focal necrosis, and multiple, sharply demarcated areas of granulomatous inflammation containing larvae. Granulomatous foci, histologically evident in various parts of the brain,[24,40–42] consisted primarily of epithelioid cells,[42] epithelioid cells plus lymphocytes, macrophages, plasma cells, and microglial cells,[41] or the above cell types plus numerous eosinophils.[40] The surrounding neuropil had an inflammatory infiltrate and there was perivascular cuffing and infiltration of the leptomeninges with the same cell types.[40,41] In one patient, there were 60 *Toxocara* larvae per gram of liver, 5 larvae per gram of muscle, and 3 to 5 larvae per gram of brain.[40]

In a fatal *Baylisascaris* NLM in a child, there was swelling and softening of the brain and cerebellar herniation.[18] The leptomeninges were congested and mildly opacified and the inner third of the periventricular white matter had extensive necrosis (Figure 166–22). The necrotic areas corresponded to areas of dye enhancement on antemortem CT scans. Histologically, marked inflammation, necrosis, and migrating larvae were in brain and spinal cord, with the most severe lesions in the periventricular cerebrum. Three larvae per gram of cerebral tissue were isolated, corresponding to an estimated total of 3207 larvae in the brain and 64,000 larvae in the body.[16,18] In a second patient, where the child survived for an extended period, severe periventricular encephalitis preceded cerebral atrophy; at autopsy, the brain was severely atrophic, weighing 810 g (normal = 1065 g).[17] The meninges were thick and gray and the demarcation between nuclear structures and white matter was blurred. Histologically, the size and cellularity of gray matter was reduced and gliosis was severe and diffuse. Numerous larvae were in granulomas, which were walled off by a zone of gliosis (Figure 166–21).

Ocular lesions vary with location of larvae and the severity of inflammation.[43] Most globes are enucleated, because of suspected retinoblastoma, panophthalmitis, or pain caused by inflammation or glaucoma.[10,43] In ocular toxocariasis, the most common lesions are granulomas in the periphery or posterior pole or chronic endophthalmitis with retinal detachment.[10,22,43–45] Granulomas in the peripheral or posterior retina are usually dense, solitary and project into the vitreous (Fig-

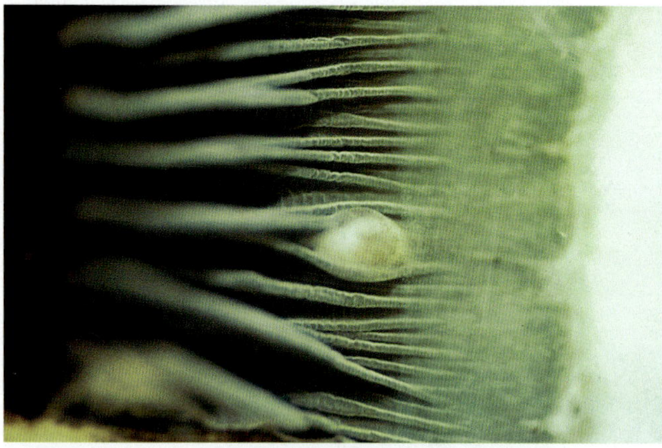

Figure 166–23. *Toxocara canis* larval granuloma in the ciliary body of a dog with OLM. *(Photograph by R. R. Dubielzig, DVM, PhD, University of Wisconsin, Madison.)*

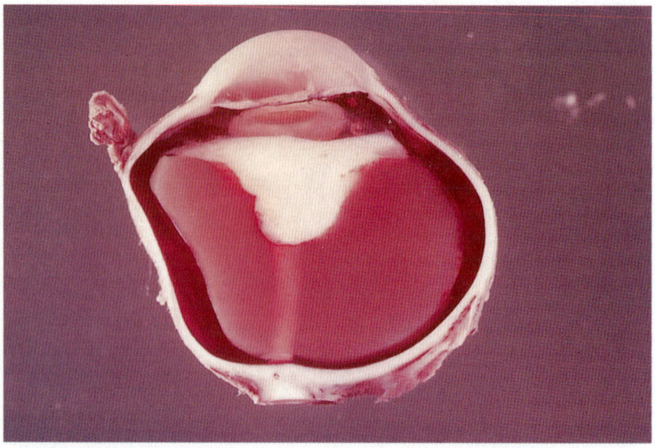

Figure 166–25. Enucleated eye from a patient with toxocaral endophthalmitis. Note large retrolental mass associated with funnel-shaped retinal detachment (AFIP Neg 53-18355).

ures 166–23 and 166–24).[43,45] The vitreous often has dense connective tissue bands that run from the mass to the optic disc or surrounding retina. This causes vitreoretinal traction and partial retinal detachment, with elevated retinal folds associated with the vitreous bands and a retinochoroidal mass.[43,45] Histologically, ocular granulomas develop as described previously, and often have centers of intense eosinophilic necrosis. In toxocaral endophthalmitis, the globe characteristically has marked intraocular disorganization, with total retinal detachment involving a granulomatous mass (Figures 166–25 and 166–26).[10,43,44] An inflammatory cyclitic membrane may be on the anterior aspect of the funnel of detached retina, and serous exudate occupies the subretinal space (Figure 166–26). The inflammatory focus containing the larva may be within the granulomatous mass or the cyclitic membrane.[10,43,44]

No patients with ocular baylisascariasis have been studied pathologically. Clinically, *B procyonis* has been associated with migration tracks, DUSN, and the production of posterior pole granulomas, but other ocular lesions are anticipated. Monkey eyes examined during active *Baylisascaris* migration have lesions localized primarily to retina and choroid.[19,20] Larvae migrate at all levels of retina, but are common subretinally or in the outer retinal layers (Figure 166–27). Larvae migrating in these locations produce focal disruption of outer retinal layers, pyknosis of outer and inner nuclear layers, and hyperplasia and migration of pigment epithelium.[19,20] Larvae migrating more deeply cause disruption of nerve

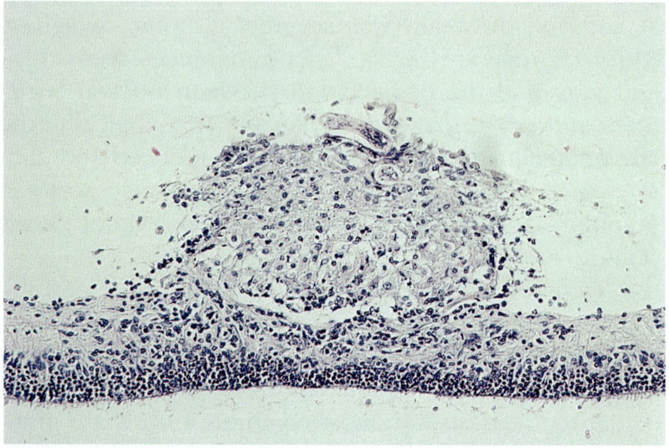

Figure 166–24. Granuloma in retina of a dog with OLM. Note *T canis* larva beneath the inner limiting membrane (H&E, ×50). *(Photograph by K. R. Kazacos, DVM, PhD; specimen contributed by R. R. Dubielzig, DVM, PhD, University of Wisconsin, Madison.)*

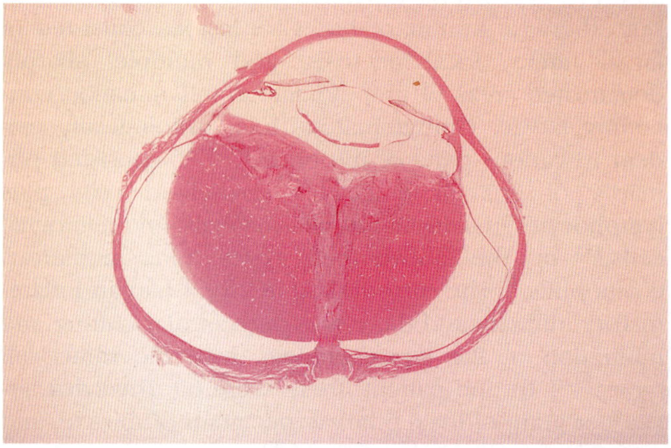

Figure 166–26. Enucleated eye from a patient with toxocaral endophthalmitis. Note preretinal inflammatory mass, funnel-shaped retinal detachment, and extensive subretinal exudate containing cholesterol clefts (AFIP Neg 55-22087).

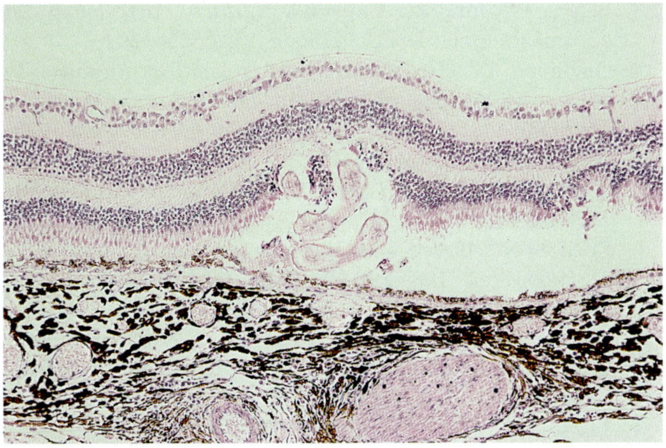

Figure 166–27. *Baylisascaris procyonis* larva beneath retina in eye of monkey with OLM. Note retinal disruption, pyknosis of outer nuclear layer, and hyperplasia of retinal pigment epithelium (H&E, ×32). *(Photograph by K. R. Kazacos, DVM, PhD.)*

fiber and ganglion cell layers.[20] As in CNS, inflammatory reactions developed first focally in the wake of migrating larvae. More advanced migratory lesions have total retinal disorganization, intense eosinophilic retinitis, necrosis, vasculitis, vitritis, an eosinophilic choroiditis, and abundant SH material. These areas are cross-sections through the tracks (Figure 166–8). Larvae migrating in the choroid stimulate eosinophilic choroiditis and vasculitis, and are walled off by choroidal granulomas.[19,20]

DIFFERENTIAL PATHOLOGIC DIAGNOSIS

Toxocara canis and *B procyonis* are the most common causes of zoonotic larva migrans; however, the list of animal parasites that may invade human tissue is long. Ascarids of canids, felids, hyenas, raccoons, skunks, badgers, bears, opossums, snakes, hawks, owls, and other carnivores—gnathostomes, hookworms, *Alaria* and *Paragonimus,* cestode spargana, and pentastomes[1–3,6–8]—might all cause migratory lesions in human tissues. Some of these, such as *Alaria,* can cause widespread systemic infection as well as ocular disease without systemic signs, similar to *Toxocara* and *Baylisascaris.*[3,29] Definitive diagnosis requires identification of the larvae. There are, in addition, many other zoonotic helminths such as species of *Dirofilaria, Brugia,* other filaria, *Capillaria, Trichinella,* etc, whose larvae and/or adults invade humans.[3,8,21] Natural parasites of humans whose larvae migrate must be differentiated from those that cause larva migrans. These are *Ascaris lumbricoides, Strongyloides stercoralis, Necator americanus, Ancylostoma duodenale, Paragonimus westermani,* and *Schistosoma* sp.[3,21,34] *Schistosoma, Paragonimus,* and some other helminths produce granulomas around eggs and these lesions must also be differentiated from those of larva migrans.[3,21,34,47]

Causes of eosinophilia and eosinophilic necrosis are diverse and include other helminthic infections, some deep mycoses, some bacterial infections, various allergies and hypersensitivities, myeloproliferative and neoplastic diseases, pulmonary eosinophilic diseases, various cutaneous diseases, immune connective tissue and immunodeficiency diseases, and some gastrointestinal diseases.[47] Similarly, multisystem granulomas characterize other diseases, including sarcoidosis and some bacterial and deep mycotic infections.[47]

Clinically, the granulomatous lesions of OLM must be differentiated from several other ocular conditions, the most important being retinoblastoma.[10,43,45] Better methods for distinguishing between these two diseases has resulted in fewer unnecessary enucleations.[43] Ocular larva migrans must also be distinguished from Coats' disease, persistent hyperplastic primary vitreous, retinopathy of prematurity, familial exudative vitreoretinopathy, idiopathic subretinal neovascular membrane, toxoplasmosis, histoplasmosis, and optic neuritis.[43]

CONFIRMATIONAL TESTING AND DIAGNOSIS

Other than identifying larvae in or from the eye, in biopsy specimens, organ lavages, or at autopsy, the only way to confirm a presumptive clinical diagnosis is by serodiagnosis.[48] Examination of stool specimens is not helpful, because larvae are not passed in feces; however, this may help exclude other parasitic causes of eosinophilia. When suspected clinically, *Toxocara* and *Baylisascaris* infections may be confirmed serologically. Enzyme-linked immunosorbent assay (ELISA) and Western blotting utilize larval excretory–secretory antigens. For presumptive toxocaral VLM, ELISA has a sensitivity and specificity of 78% and 92%, respectively, at a titer of >1:32.[37,48] Serum antibody titers of patients with OLM are lower than patients with VLM, with a corresponding decrease in the sensitivity of ELISA; therefore, a positive cutoff titer of >1:8 is used for OLM.[48] False-negative titers are a problem with OLM, as are false-positive titers related to background asymptomatic infections. For these reasons, in presumptive cases of OLM, it is preferable to perform the ELISA on ocular fluids (aqueous, vitreous). In positive patients, ocular antibodies are often much higher than the serum titer, and may be detected even though the serum titer is negative.[5,37,48] ELISA, Western blotting, and immunofluorescence have been developed also for *Baylisascaris* and have proven useful for diagnosis in the limited number of patients studied.[17,18,25,28] These *Baylisascaris* patients had negative titers for *Toxocara* by ELISA, indicating the two infections can be distinguished.

Additional methods useful in establishing a diagnosis of larva migrans and differentiating it from other diseases include newer CT and magnetic resonance imaging techniques and ocular fluid cytology and enzyme determinations.[5,43] For example, eosinophils are in ocular fluids in nematode endophthalmitis, but are absent in retinoblastoma.[43] With reliable serologic tests available, biopsy is generally not indicated for VLM. In *Toxocara* VLM, biopsies of liver may show diagnostic lesions, but biopsies of other tissues are usually not helpful.[5,34]

At autopsy, tissue digestion may help recover larvae for identification, especially when there are too few to be found easily by sectioning. Live larvae may be recovered from tissues refrigerated for several days, but not from frozen specimens. Samples of tissue are gently pulverized (brain), minced, or blended in warm (37°C) 1% pepsin–1% HCl–0.85% NaCl (final concentration, 15 to 20 g tissue/mL) and incubated at low speed on an oscillatory shaker or stirrer for 2 to 3 hours at 37°C. After coarse filtration through cheesecloth and sedimentation for 20 to 30 minutes in conical glassware, the sediment is removed and examined for larvae using a dissecting microscope. Larvae are collected, fixed in hot (65–70°C) fixative (70% ethanol; 10% formalin; alcohol–formalin–acetic acid), cleared in phenol-alcohol or glycerin, and identified. When in doubt, consult a medical or veterinary parasitologist.

TREATMENT

Treatment of larva migrans is primarily symptomatic and directed at decreasing larval-induced inflammatory reactions.[5] Treatment with corticosteroids and antihistamines to decrease inflammation and eosinophilia may be life saving in severe infections. Specific anthelmintic treatment is equivocal, since mixed results have been noted in patients and animal models.[5] Anthelmintic drugs such as albendazole, mebendazole, thiabendazole, and diethylcarbamazine, however, have been recommended and used with some success in toxocaral VLM and OLM. The prognosis for *Baylisascaris* NLM is probably grave with or without treatment because of extensive neural damage by the time diagnosis is made. When in a "safe" portion of the eye (away from the macula or optic disc), intraretinal larvae can be killed by laser photocoagulation.[25,29,43]

REFERENCES

1. Beaver PC. The nature of visceral larva migrans. *J Parasitol.* 1969;55:3–12.
2. Kazacos KR. Visceral and ocular larva migrans. *Sem Vet Med Surg (Small Anim).* 1991;6:227–235.
3. Beaver PC, Jung RC, Cupp EW. *Clinical Parasitology.* 9th ed. Philadelphia: Lea & Febiger; 1984:325–329.
4. Glickman LT. Toxocariasis and related syndromes. In: Warren KS, Mahmoud AAF, eds. *Tropical and Geographic Medicine.* 2nd ed. New York: McGraw-Hill; 1990:446–455.
5. Glickman LT, Magnaval JF. Zoonotic roundworm infections. *Infect Dis Clin North Am (Parasitic Dis).* 1993;7: 717–732.
6. Kazacos KR, Boyce WM. *Baylisascaris* larva migrans. *J Am Vet Med Assoc.* 1989;195:894–903.
7. Bowman DD. Diagnostic morphology of four larval ascaridoid nematodes that may cause visceral larva migrans: *Toxascaris leonina, Baylisascaris procyonis, Lagochilascaris sprenti,* and *Hexametra leidyi. J Parasitol.* 1987;73: 1198–1215.
8. Anderson RC. *Nematode Parasites of Vertebrates. Their Development and Transmission.* Wallingford, UK: CAB International; 1992.
9. Beaver PC, Snyder CH, Carrera GM, Dent JH, Lafferty JW. Chronic eosinophilia due to visceral larva migrans. Report of three cases. *Pediatrics.* 1952;9:7–19.
10. Wilder HC. Nematode endophthalmitis. *Trans Am Acad Ophthalmol Otolaryngol.* 1950;55:99–109.
11. Tiner JD. The migration, distribution in the brain, and growth of ascarid larvae in rodents. *J Infect Dis.* 1953;92: 105–113.
12. Tiner JD. Fatalities in rodents caused by larval *Ascaris* in the central nervous system. *J Mammal.* 1953;34:153–167.
13. Sprent JFA. On the migratory behavior of the larvae of various *Ascaris* species in white mice. I. Distribution of larvae in tissues. *J Infect Dis.* 1952;90:165–176.
14. Sprent JFA. On the invasion of the central nervous system by nematodes. II. Invasion of the nervous system in ascariasis. *Parasitology.* 1955;45:41–55.
15. Kazacos KR, Wirtz WL, Burger PP, Christmas CS. Raccoon ascarid larvae as a cause of fatal central nervous system disease in subhuman primates. *J Am Vet Med Assoc.* 1981; 179:1089–1094.
16. Kazacos KR. Raccoon ascarids as a cause of larva migrans. *Parasitol Today.* 1986;2:253–255.
17. Huff DS, Neafie RC, Binder MJ, DeLeón GA, Brown LW, Kazacos KR. The first fatal *Baylisascaris* infection in humans: an infant with eosinophilic meningoencephalitis. *Pediatr Pathol.* 1984;2:345–352.
18. Fox AS, Kazacos KR, Gould NS, Heydemann PT, Thomas C, Boyer KM. Fatal eosinophilic meningoencephalitis and visceral larva migrans caused by the raccoon ascarid *Baylisascaris procyonis. N Engl J Med.* 1985;312:1619–1623.
19. Kazacos KR, Vestre WA, Kazacos EA. Raccoon ascarid larvae (*Baylisascaris procyonis*) as a cause of ocular larva migrans. *Invest Ophthalmol Vis Sci.* 1984;25:1177–1183.
20. Kazacos KR, Raymond LA, Kazacos EA, Vestre WA. The raccoon ascarid. A probable cause of human ocular larva migrans. *Ophthalmology.* 1985;92:1735–1743.
21. Gutierrez Y. *Diagnostic Pathology of Parasitic Infections with Clinical Correlations.* Philadelphia: Lea & Febiger; 1990:236–272.
22. Kean BH, Sun T, Ellsworth RM. *Color Atlas/Text of Ophthalmic Parasitology.* New York: Igaku-Shoin; 1991.
23. Goodart RA, Riekhof FT, Beaver PC. Subretinal nematode.

An unusual etiology for uveitis and retinal detachment. *Retina.* 1985;5:87–90.

24. Fortenberry JD, Kenney RD, Younger J. Visceral larva migrans producing static encephalopathy in an infant. *Pediatr Infect Dis J.* 1991;10:403–406.
25. Goldberg MA, Kazacos KR, Boyce WM, Ai E, Katz B. Diffuse unilateral subacute neuroretinitis. Morphometric, serologic, and epidemiologic support for *Baylisascaris* as a causative agent. *Ophthalmology.* 1993;100:1695–1701.
26. Küchle M, Knorr HLJ, Medenblik-Frysch S, Weber A, Bauer C, Naumann GOH. Diffuse unilateral subacute neuroretinitis syndrome in a German most likely caused by the raccoon roundworm, *Baylisascaris procyonis. Graefe's Arch Clin Exp Ophthalmol.* 1993;231:48–51.
27. Rusnak JM, Lucey DR. Clinical gnathostomiasis. Case report and review of the English-language literature. *Clin Infect Dis.* 1993;16:33–50.
28. Cunningham CK, Kazacos KR, McMillan JA, et al. Diagnosis and management of *Baylisascaris procyonis* infection in an infant with nonfatal meningoencephalitis. *Clin Infect Dis.* 1994;18:868–872.
29. McDonald HR, Kazacos KR, Schatz H, Johnson RN. Two cases of intraocular infection with *Alaria mesocercariae* (Trematoda). *Am J Ophthalmol.* 1994;117:447–455.
30. Glickman LT, Schantz PM. Epidemiology and pathogenesis of zoonotic toxocariasis. *Epidemiol Rev.* 1981;3:230–250.
31. Nichols RL. The etiology of visceral larva migrans. I. Diagnostic morphology of infective second-stage *Toxocara* larvae. *J Parasitol.* 1956;42:349–362.
32. Nichols RL. The etiology of visceral larva migrans. II. Comparative larval morphology of *Ascaris lumbricoides, Necator americanus, Strongyloides stercoralis,* and *Ancylostoma caninum. J Parasitol.* 1956;42:363–399.
33. Chitwood M, Lichtenfels JR. Identification of parasitic metazoa in tissue sections. *Exp Parasitol.* 1972;32:407–519.
34. Binford CH, Connor DH, eds. *Pathology of Tropical and Extraordinary Diseases.* Washington, DC: Armed Forces Institute of Pathology; 1976;2.
35. Arean VM, Crandall CA. Toxocariasis. In: Marcial-Rojas RA, ed. *Pathology of Protozoal and Helminthic Diseases with Clinical Correlation.* Baltimore: Williams & Wilkins; 1971:808–842.
36. Lloyd S. Immunobiology of *Toxocara canis* and visceral larva migrans. In: Soulsby EJL, ed. *Immune Responses in Parasitic Infections: Immunology, Immunopathology, and Immunoprophylaxis, Vol. 1, Nematodes.* Boca Raton, Fla: CRC Press; 1987:299–324.
37. Glickman LT, Schantz PM, Grieve RB. Toxocariasis. In: Walls KW, Schantz PM, eds. *Immunodiagnosis of Parasitic Diseases, Vol. 1, Helminthic Diseases.* New York: Academic Press; 1986:201–231.
38. John T, Barsky HJ, Donnelly JJ, Rockey JH. Retinal pigment epitheliopathy and neuroretinal degeneration in ascarid-infected eyes. *Invest Ophthalmol Vis Sci.* 1987;28:1583–1598.
39. Hamann KJ, Kephart GM, Kazacos KR, Gleich GJ. Immunofluorescent localization of eosinophil granule major basic protein in fatal human cases of *Baylisascaris procyonis* infection. *Am J Trop Med Hyg.* 1989;40:291–297.
40. Dent JH, Nichols RL, Beaver PC, Carrera GM, Staggers RJ. Visceral larva migrans with a case report. *Am J Pathol.* 1956;32:777–803.
41. Schochet SS. Human *Toxocara canis* encephalopathy in a case of visceral larva migrans. *Neurology* 1967;17:227–229.
42. Mikhael NZ, Montpetit VJA, Orizaga M, Rowsell HC, Richard MT. *Toxocara canis* infestation with encephalitis. *Can J Neurol Sci.* 1974;1:114–120.
43. Shields JA. Ocular toxocariasis. A review. *Surv Ophthalmol.* 1984;28:361–381.
44. Duguid IM. Features of ocular infestation by *Toxocara. Br J Ophthalmol.* 1961;45:789–796.
45. Wilkinson CP, Welch RB. Intraocular *Toxocara. Am J Ophthalmol.* 1971;71:921–930.
46. Gass JDM. *Stereoscopic Atlas of Macular Diseases. Diagnosis and Treatment.* 3rd ed. St. Louis, Mo: CV Mosby; 1987.
47. Wyngaarden JB, Smith LH Jr, Bennett JC (eds). *Cecil Textbook of Medicine.* 19th ed. Philadelphia: WB Saunders; 1992.
48. Wilson M, Schantz PM. Nonmorphologic diagnosis of parasitic infections. In: Balows A (ed), *Manual of Clinical Microbiology.* 5th ed. Washington, DC: American Society of Microbiology; 1991:717–726.

CHAPTER 167

Loiasis

Duane Pinto and Daniel H. Connor

Jack Malahide, for instance, had a parasite in his blood which, according to local gossip, could only be caught on the rare occasions when it emerged to walk across his eyeball.

Julia O'Faolain, "The Religious Wars of 1944"
The New Yorker, May 23, 1994

DEFINITION

Loiasis is infection by the nematode, *Loa loa*. Loiasis afflicts approximately 13 million people worldwide.[1] Also known as the African eyeworm (Figure 167–1) or "loa" worm, it was most likely first described by Pigafetta in 1589 in a Congolese.[2] Mongin isolated the worm from the eye of a Haitian in 1770,[3] and Guyot studied loiasis in 1777 among the indigene of the west coast of Africa. It was not until 1904, however, that Loos performed detailed studies of the worm and the infection.[2]

GEOGRAPHICAL DISTRIBUTION

The transitional savanna and rain forests of West and Central Africa are the favored habitats of *L loa*. This habitat ranges from 8°N and 5°S latitude and from the Gulf of Guinea to southwestern Sudan and western Uganda. Patients infected with *L loa* have been reported from as far west as the Gongola State of Nigeria.

LIFE CYCLE

During its life cycle, *L loa* uses as its vector and intermediate host any one of several species of the genus of mango flies known as *Chrysops* (Figure 167–2). Of the many species of *Chrysops, C silacea* is the most common vector. The definitive hosts for *L loa* are humans and baboons. A female *Chrysops* ingests circulating microfilariae while taking a blood meal. These microfilariae enter the fat body of the *Chrysops* and mature to become infective larvae within 2 weeks.[4] The infective larvae migrate to the fly's mouth parts and at the next blood meal enter the skin of the next host. The larvae migrate through the tissues and grow to become adult worms in 1 to 4 years. Microfilariae, produced by the gravid female *L loa,* enter the bloodstream where they circulate during the day but rest in capillaries of lung and other deep organs at night. Microfilariae are most numerous in the blood from late morning to early afternoon.[5] The adult worms may live up to 17 years.

MORPHOLOGIC DESCRIPTION OF PARASITE

Adult *L loa* are long, white, threadlike nematodes. The male worm is 30 to 34 mm by 350 to 400 μm (Figure 167–3), and the female worm measures 50 to 70 mm by 450 to 600 μm.[4,6] Both genders have rounded elevations on the cuticle throughout their lengths. These are spaced irregularly and called bosses. The cuticle is thicker in the lateral chord regions in both genders, especially in the male worm. The adult female worm at midbody contains an intestine and three to five transverse sections of uterine tube. In both male and female

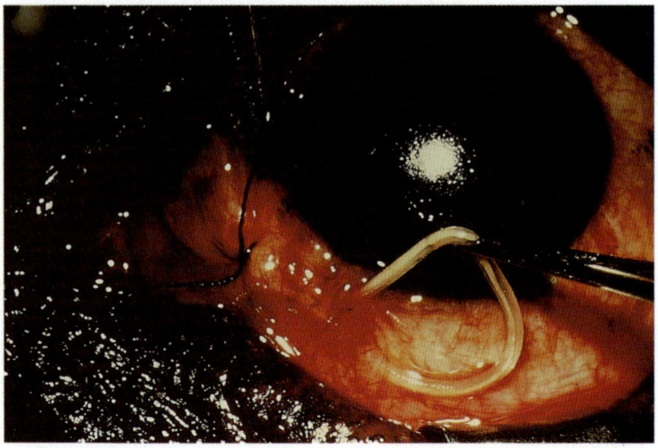

Figure 167–1. Adult *L loa* being extracted from subconjunctival space (AFIP Neg 75-1789-3).

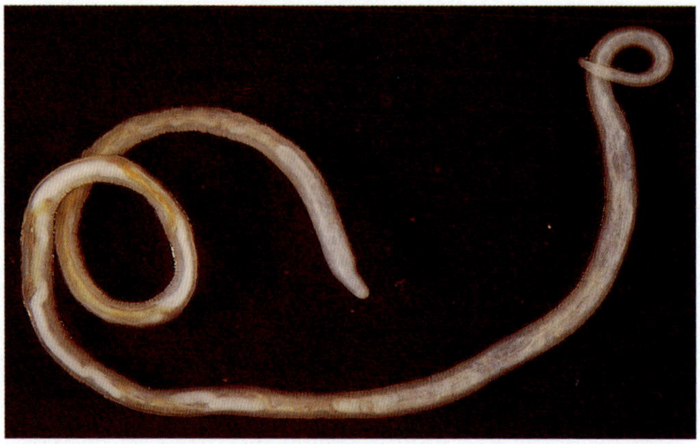

Figure 167–3. Adult male *L loa* excised from subconjunctival space (×6.8). *(Photograph by Daniel H. Connor, MD, 1970.)*

worms prominent somatic muscle, composed of equal amounts of contractile fibers and sarcoplasm, is in the lateral chords. The midbody of the male worm contains the intestine and a single reproductive tube.

In general, the loal sheath, body wall, nerve ring, amphids, excretory and anal vesicles, and central body closely resemble the microfilariae of other species.[7] Loal microfilariae have a two-layer sheath and are 231 to 250 m by 5 to 7 m.[8] The cephalic space is 3 to 6 μm long and the anterior nuclei are side by side (Figure 167–4). The posterior end of the microfilaria tapers to a point, and the terminal elongated nucleus is present at the tip of the tail. Several characteristic features of *L loa* can be visualized with use of scanning and transmission electron microscopy. For instance, microscopy shows four sensory papillae at the buccal orifice and a buccal capsule that is bordered by cuticularized channels known as amphids. A small cephalic hook is located near the amphids. Finally, dense cytoplasmic inclusions are in the intestinal cells.[8]

CLINICAL FEATURES

In endemic areas, most infections persist for years without significant symptoms or signs, the only manifestation of infection being microfilaremia.[5] For some people, the first indication of infection is when the adult worm migrates across the eyeball beneath the conjunctiva. In other patients, the first sign of infection is a "fugitive" or Calabar swelling. Clinically, these swellings are characterized by itching,erythema,and edema. They

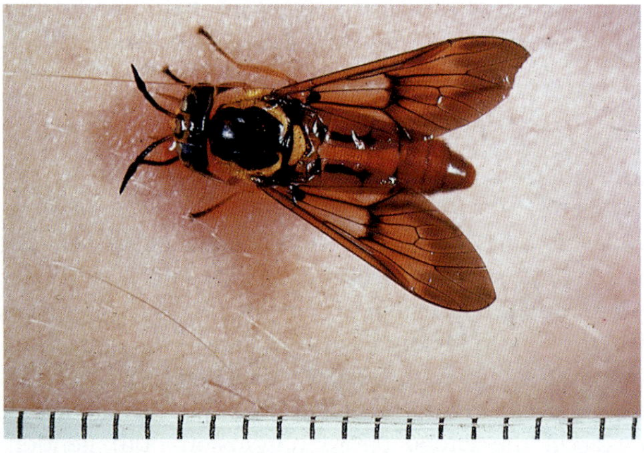

Figure 167–2. *Chrysops silacea,* the most common vector for *L loa* in the west African rain forest feeding on a volunteer. *(Photograph by Daniel H. Connor, MD, 1972.)*

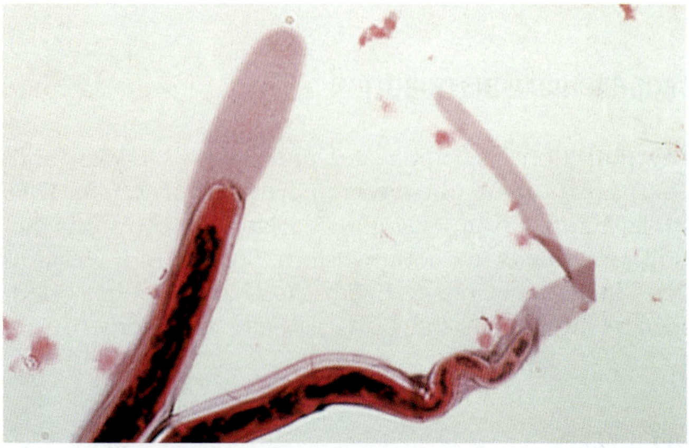

Figure 167–4. Caudal and cephalic ends of microfilaria of *L loa* in thin blood film. Note the sheath, the cephalic space, the anterior nuclei, and the terminal nucleus going to the tip of the tail (AFIP Neg 79-15392).

are most commonly on the limbs. There is sudden onset, and they regress over a period of several hours to several days, often recurring at the same sites

Eosinophilia, up to 60% to 90% of the white blood cell count,[5,9] may develop along with elevated serum IgE.[10] Both eosinophilia and elevated serum IgE are common in patients with symptomatic loiasis and in expatriates with loiasis.[11] Expatriates are more likely to have Calabar swelling and less likely to have microfilaremia, and they tend to have more intense allergic symptoms and more antifilarial antibodies as well as hypergammaglobulinemia, hypereosinophilia, and increased IgE. By contrast, persons with microfilaremia who were born in endemic regions rarely have Calabar swellings. The exaggerated response of expatriates may be from a specific dysregulation of the immune response to loal antigens in addition to nonspecific activation of the immune system.[12,13] Perhaps those born in endemic areas have immune tolerance from exposure to antigens while in utero.

Loa loa is unique among human filariae in that the adult sometimes moves across the eye. This migration is subconjunctival and may cause swelling of the lids, congestion, itching, and pain.[11] Although the worms produce no ill effects when in the tissues around the eye, they may blind if they penetrate into the anterior chamber.[14] Other clinical features described in patients with loiasis include fever, pain, urticaria, irritability, confusion, and Jacksonian epilepsy. Less frequently, there are nephropathy, retinopathy, peripheral neuropathy, and lymphadenitis.[6]

Very rarely monoarticular effusion and arthritis involve the knee. Polyarthritis is usually associated with pharmacologic treatment of the disease.[15] Intra-articular microfilariae, however, also cause a febrile polyarthritis.[16]

Patients transfused with blood containing microfilariae develop fever, rash, and headache.[17,18] Inflammation of viscera, especially liver, develops as the transfused microfilariae are destroyed. After transfusions, the clinical manifestations fade as the microfilariae are destroyed.[2]

PATHOLOGY

Adult worms migrating across the eye provoke little reaction unless traumatized. Sites of predisposition for the adult *L loa* are inguinal hernia sac, scrotal skin (Figure 167–5), spermatic cord, and tunica vaginalis.[6] Adult *L loa* worms have been recovered intact from hernia sacs, spermatic cords (Figure 167–6), and the subconjunctival space (Figure 167–1). Specimens containing sections of adult worms have been excised from the wall of large bowel and from the subcutaneous tissue of most parts of the body (Figure 167–7), including finger and scalp. One report describes "vermiform calcifications" of breast, which were interpreted as loiasis.[19] Migrating worms may cause little or no reaction but degenerating worms, such as those responding to diethylcarbamazine therapy, provoke a reaction that begins acutely and is suppurative. The acute inflammatory exudate is rich in fibrin, eosinophils, and neutrophils. Later, there is chronic inflammation and a gran-

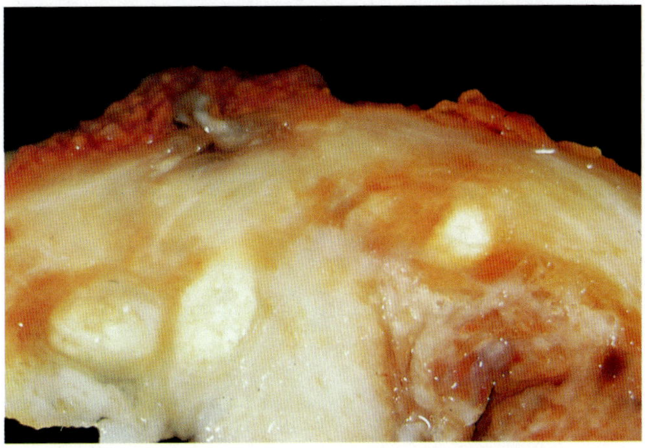

Figure 167–5. Scrotal sac of an African containing a degenerating, coiled *L loa* worm. There is focal calcification (AFIP Neg 83-9643).

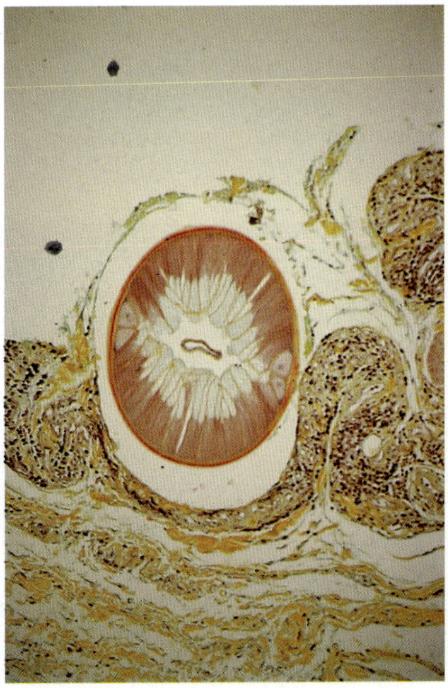

Figure 167–6. Adult male *L loa* in spermatic cord (AFIP; Movat, ×100).

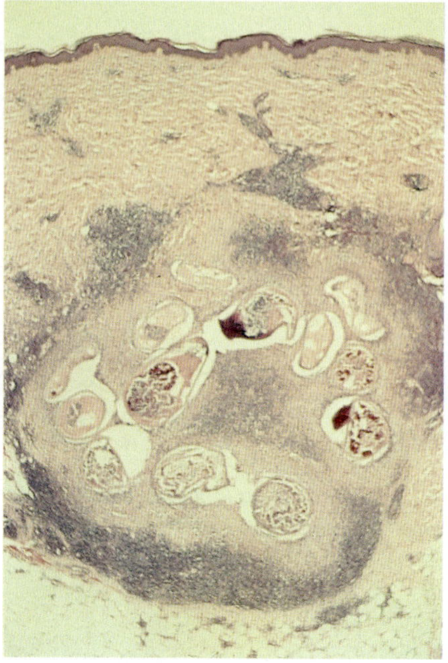

Figure 167–7. Degenerating adult, gravid, female *L loa* coiled in the lower dermis. There are chronic and granulomatous inflammation and fibrosis (AFIP Neg 80-3639).

ulomatous reaction with histiocytes, epithelioid cells, giant cells, lymphocytes, and plasma cells followed by scarring. Eventually, the worm may become mineralized.[6]

LYMPH NODES

Although not generally recognized as a feature of loiasis, lymphadenopathy and lymphadenitis are well documented. Paleologo et al[20] studied inguinal nodes from

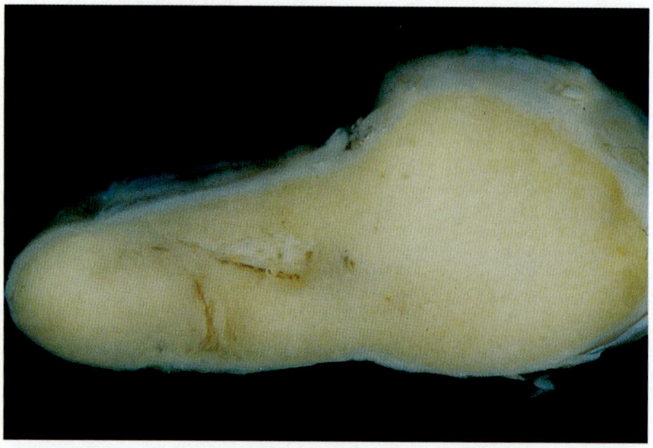

Figure 167–8. Loal lymphadenitis. The cut surface is pale and homogeneous resembling the "fish flesh" appearance of malignant lymphoma (×1). *(Photograph by Daniel H. Connor, MD, 1980.)*

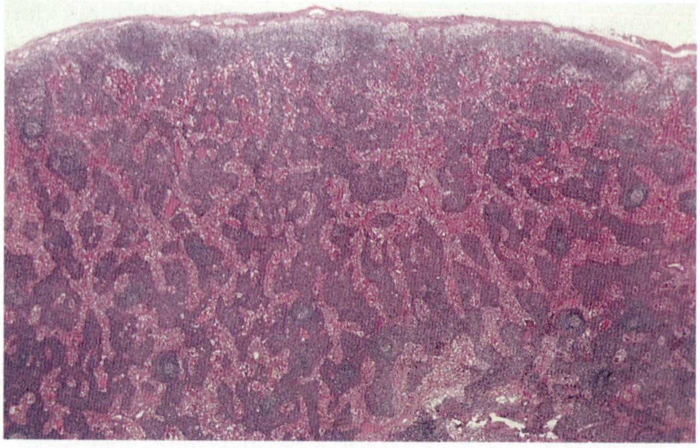

Figure 167–9. Lymph node showing the characteristic pattern of loal lymphadenitis. There are a thickened capsule, complete atrophy of germinal centers, and a diffuse infiltrate of histiocytes and eosinophils in the subcapsular and peritrabecular spaces [AFIP Neg 83-6299; hematoxylin-eosin (H&E), ×15].

patients with loiasis. The nodes were moderately enlarged (2 to 5 cm) and their cut surfaces pale and homogenous (Figure 167–8). Capsules were thickened. Microscopically, the striking features were 1) distention of the subcapsular and periseptal sinuses by histiocytes and eosinophils and 2) a virtual absence of germinal centers (Figure 167–9). Not only were germinal centers absent but there were usually no collections of lymphocytes or contour lines that even suggested the presence of follicles. Other constant features were fibrous thickening of capsule and trabeculae, dilated lymphatics of the capsule and medulla, and scattered collections of plasma cells, mast cells, and occasional Russell bodies in the lymphoid tissue. Microfilariae of *L loa* were in dilated lymphatics of capsule and trabeculae and also in microabscesses comprised of degenerating eosinophils (Figures 167–10 and 167–11). This combination of changes is characteristic of loal lymphadenitis.

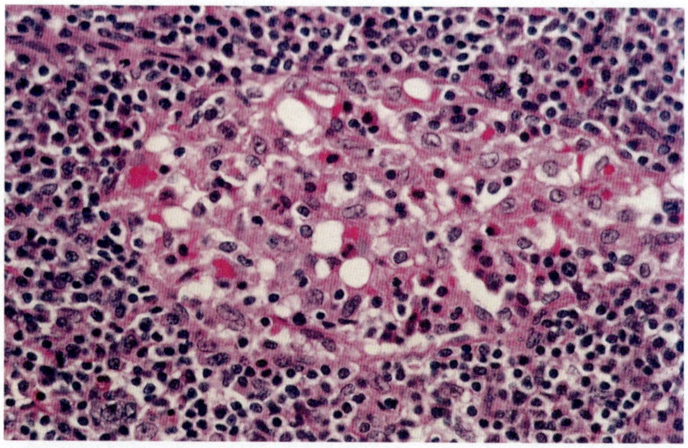

Figure 167–10. Focus of histiocytes within the node mixed with numerous eosinophils (AFIP Neg 81-5109; H&E, ×115).

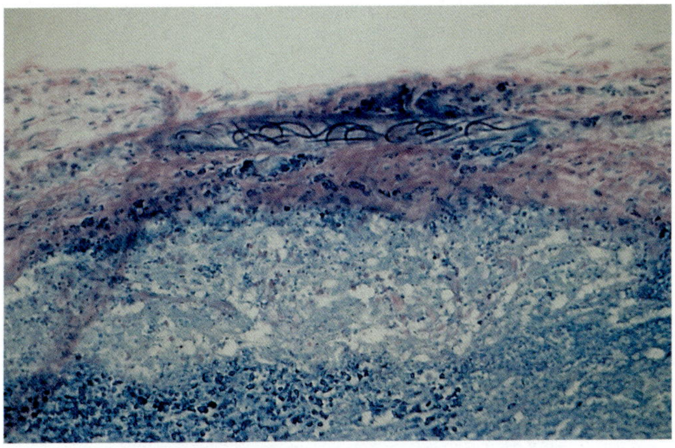

Figure 167–11. Lymph node showing fibrotic thickening of the capsule and an entanglement of microfilariae of *L loa* in a capsular lymphatic (AFIP Neg 82-8223; Giemsa, ×115).

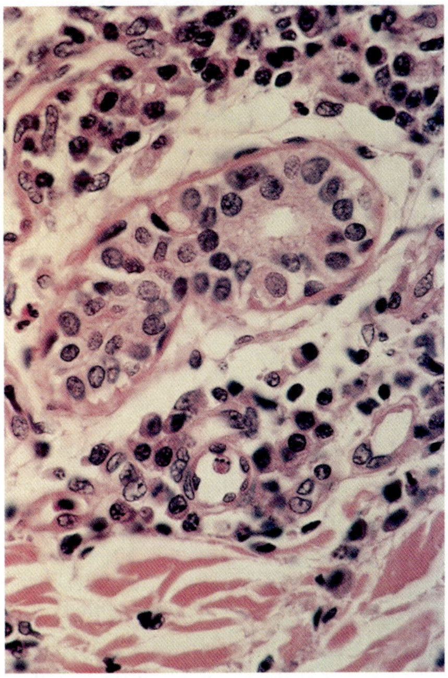

Figure 167–13. Section of sweat gland showing an inflammatory cell infiltrate comprised of lymphocytes, plasma cells, and occasional macrophages. In a capillary adjacent to the gland there is a cross-section of an *L loa* microfilaria (AFIP Neg 82-11278; H&E, ×180).

SKIN

Microfilariae of *L loa* concentrate in dermal capillaries and are most numerous in the capillaries that nourish sweat glands (Figures 167–12 through 167–14). Lymphocytes, plasma cells, and mast cells are in the loose connective tissue around the sweat glands. Perhaps in this location, they are more immediately available to the vector *Chrysops* when it bites.

CALABAR SWELLINGS

Calabar swellings are transient episodes of migratory erythema and angioedema. Their cause is not known, but they may represent hypersensitivity reactions to

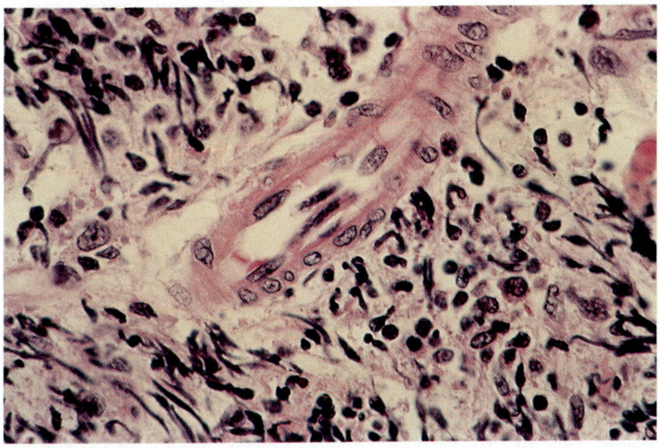

Figure 167–12. Skin showing two microfilariae in a vessel in the deep dermis adjacent to a sweat gland (AFIP Neg 82-11287; H&E, ×180).

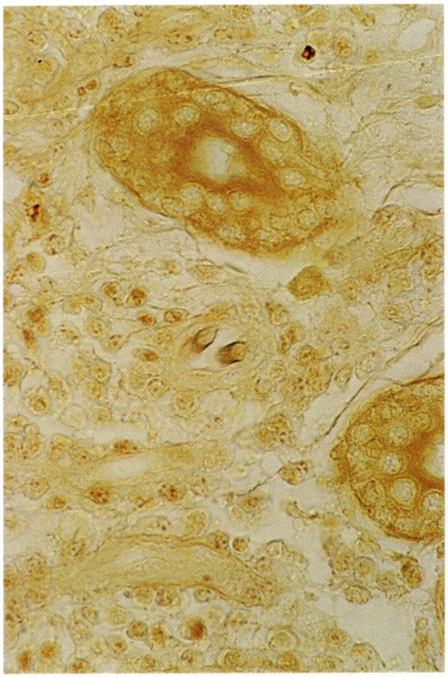

Figure 167–14. There are two *L loa* microfilariae in a capillary between coils of a sweat gland. Their sheaths are lightly silvered by the Warthin–Starry stain (AFIP Neg 82-11288; ×180).

antigens that are released by the adult worm as it migrates through the deep dermis and subcutaneous tissue.[6] Calabar swellings may also be reactions to microfilariae in the capillaries around coiled sweat glands. The latter is appealing because the changing flow in the capillary beds of the body may explain the predilection for Calabar swellings in the limbs, their episodic nature, and tendency to recur.

DEEP ORGANS

The case reported by Negesse et al[6] is illustrative. A 45-year-old Zairian man took "native medicine" by mouth for fever and abdominal pain. A few hours later he was admitted in a coma and died shortly thereafter. At autopsy, there were microfilariae of *L loa* in the small vessels of all organs. Brain was especially involved. Degenerating microfilariae, enmeshed in fibrin thrombi, plugged vessels of white and gray matter (Figure 167–15). Acute microinfarctions surrounded many vessels. In kidney, microfilariae were in vasa recta and glomerular capillaries (Figure 167–16). They were in sinusoids and portal tracts of liver (Figure 167–17). Kupffer's cells contained fragments of microfilariae. In spleen, microfilariae were in red pulp and in vessels of the trabeculae. Some microfilariae in red pulp were degenerating and centered in small granulomas. All other organs studied had microfilariae in their vessels. These organs included heart, lung (Figure 167–18), ileum, colon, and urinary bladder. The cause of this sudden fatal reaction must have been the "native medicine," which, in all likelihood was the potent microfilariacide diethylcarbamazine (DEC). (There is a black market in pilfered medicines throughout tropical Africa.) The mechanism by which DEC kills microfilariae is unknown, but violent fatal and near-fatal reactions are well recognized in patients with other filarial infections when given DEC without appropriate caution.

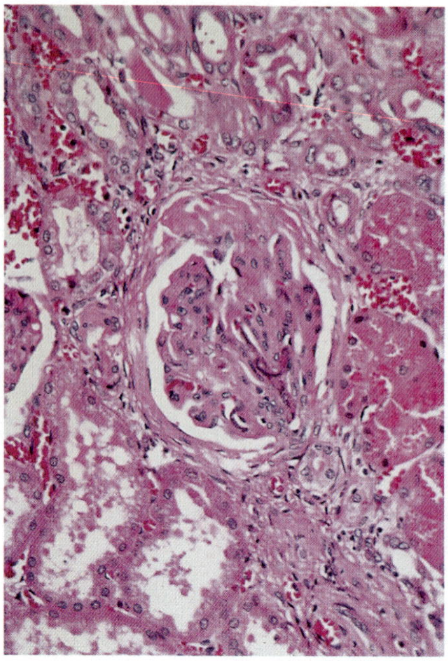

Figure 167–16. Kidney. There are degenerating microfilariae in the capillaries of the glomerulus (AFIP Neg 83-9517; H&E, ×180).

KIDNEY

Loiasis may cause membranous glomerulonephritis; the glomerulonephritis is probably immunologically medi-

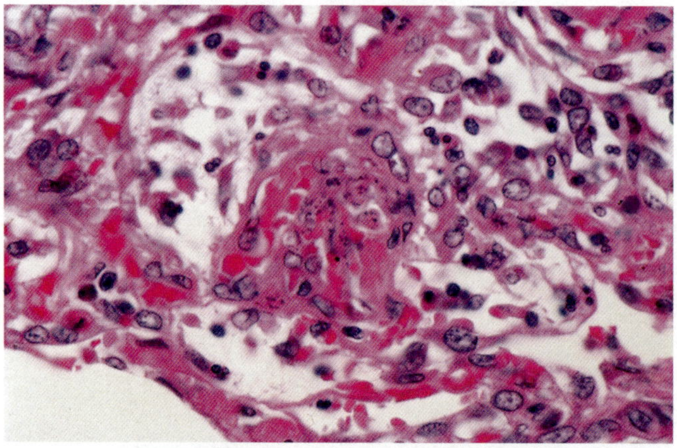

Figure 167–15. Small vessel in cerebrum enlarged and occluded by a microfilarial thrombus. The thrombus contains degenerating fragments of coiled microfilariae of *L loa* (H&E, ×450).

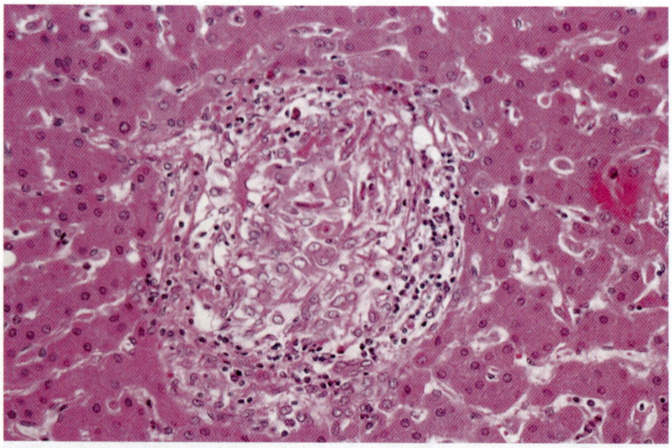

Figure 167–17. Portal tract of liver showing degenerating microfilariae being phagocytosed by macrophages (AFIP Neg 83-7939; H&E, ×180).

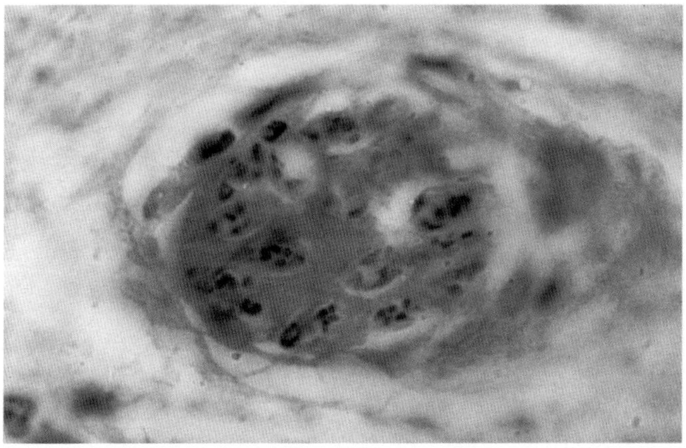

Figure 167–18. Disseminated, fatal loiasis. There is an entanglement of degenerated microfilariae in the lung (AFIP Neg 83-7932; H&E, ×220).

ated. Up to 22% of patients with loiasis have hematuria or proteinuria.[13] Serum immune complexes may be elevated. Biopsy specimens of kidney reveal globally sclerosed glomeruli[21] with thickened peripheral capillary walls and a mild increase in the number of endocapillary cells. Subepithelial and intramembranous deposits along the capillary basement membrane, with spiking of the basement membrane, are ultrastructural features.[6]

LUNG

Pleural effusion has been described in a patient with loiasis,[22] and hemorrhage and slight fibrosis of interalveolar walls has been described.[6]

HEART

Endomyocardial fibrosis is a common cause of fatal congestive heart failure among children and young adults in both East and West Africa. Its cause is unknown. In West Africa, endomyocardial fibrosis has been associated with loiasis. In East Africa, endomyocardial fibrosis is common and fatal but loiasis is rare in this region.[23,24] It is possible that in West Africa, loiasis and endomyocardial fibrosis coexist without a cause-and-effect relationship.

DIAGNOSIS

Loiasis is suspected in all who live in, or have traveled to endemic areas. Commonly, microfilaremic expatriates have eosinophilia, leukocytosis, hypergammaglobulinemia, and elevated levels of IgE, further suggesting filarial infection. Loiasis is confirmed by identifying microfilariae in blood films. Peak circulation of the microfilariae in the blood occurs in the early afternoon.[5] Occasionally the diagnosis may be made by removing an adult worm from the eye or skin.

In microfilaremic patients, the microfilariae became widely disseminated, permitting them to be seen in many samples of body fluids and tissue. Microfilariae may be in ascitic fluid,[25] synovial fluid,[15] and in endometrium.[26] A skin biopsy may demonstrate the adult worm and/or the presence of a leukocytoclastic vasculitis with an eosinophilic infiltrate.[27] Although filarial calcifications in the breast are rare, *L loa* may produce calcifications that can be seen radiographically.[19,28] Serologic tests such as direct hemagglutination and bentonite flocculation may suggest but not prove filarial infection. Enzyme-linked immunosorbent assay and immunofluorescence may be used to demonstrate antibodies to surface moieties of microfilariae, although cross-reactions with other filariae besides *L loa* are common.[8]

TREATMENT

DEC (8 to 10 mg/kg per day for 21 days) is the treatment of choice. Multiple courses of therapy may be required to eradicate the infection. It has been found, furthermore, that DEC given orally once a week can be an effective and acceptable chemoprophylactic agent.[1] Perhaps DEC changes the surface layer of the microfilariae and exposes them to immunologic cell-mediated lysis, or DEC may modify blood platelets triggering an antibody-independent death mediated by free radicals.[29] Treatment with DEC, especially in those with significant microfilaremia, may cause severe focal or systemic symptoms such as fever, pain, paresthesia, polyarticular arthritis, migratory myalgias, irritability, encephalopathy, and death.[30] Modification of the microfilarial cuticle may release antigens that provoke antigen–antibody complexes. If so, these would trigger fibrin thrombi.

A 3-week course of mebendazole reduces microfilaremia,[31] and high doses of ivermectin (0.4 mg/kg) given as a single dose produces long lasting depression of microfilarial levels.[32,33] Blood cell separation and filaricidal drugs with steroids can benefit patients with heavy filarial infections.[34]

REFERENCES

1. Nutman TB, Miller KD, Mulligan M, et al. Diethylcarbamazine prophylaxis for human loiasis. Results of a double-blind study. *N Engl J Med.* 1988;22:752–756.

2. Connor DH, Neafie RC, Meyers WM. Loiasis. In: Binford CH, Connor DH, eds. *Pathology of Tropical and Extraordinary Diseases.* Washington, DC: Armed Forces Institute of Pathology; 1976:356–359.
3. Grove DI. *A History of Human Helminthology.* Wallingford, Oxon, UK: CAB International; 1990:641–660.
4. Jolly BT, Foley KA. Loiasis: a case of an unusual ocular foreign body. *Ann Emerg Med.* 1992;21:1153–1156.
5. Sasa M. *Human Filariasis: A Global Survey of Epidemiology and Control.* Baltimore, Md: University Park Press; 1976:15–33, 122–132.
6. Negesse Y, Lanoie LO, Neafie RC, Connor DH. Loiasis: "Calabar" swellings and involvement of deep organs. *Am J Trop Med Hyg.* 1985;34:537–546.
7. Eberhard ML, Lammie PJ. Laboratory diagnosis of filariasis. *Clin Lab Med.* 1991;11:977–1010.
8. Kozek WJ, Orihel TC. Ultrastructure of *Loa loa* microfilaria. *Int J Parasitol.* 1983;13:19–43.
9. Manson-Bahr PEC, ed. *Manson's Tropical Diseases.* 18th ed. London: Balliere Tindall; 1982:161,727–729
10. Kazacos KR, Smith LE Jr. Loiasis (*Loa loa*) in an African student in Indiana. *Am J Trop Med Hyg.* 1979;28:213–215.
11. Carme B, Mamboueni JP, Copin N, Noireau F. Clinical and biological study of *Loa loa* filariasis in Congolese. *Am J Trop Med Hyg.* 1989;41:331–337.
12. Nutman TB, Reese W, Poindexter RW, Ottesen EA. Immunologic correlates of the hyperresponsive syndrome of loiasis. *J Infect Dis.* 1988;157:544–550.
13. Klion AD, Massougbodji A, Sadeler BC, Ottesen EA, Nutman TB. Loiasis in endemic and nonendemic populations: immunologically mediated differences in clinical presentation. *J Infect Dis.* 1991;163:1318–1325.
14. Osuntokun O, Olurin O. Filarial worm (*Loa loa*) in the anterior chamber. Report of two cases. *Br J Ophthalmol.* 1975;59:166–167.
15. Roussel F, Roussel C, Brasseur P, Gourmelon O, Le Loet X. Aseptic knee effusion with *Loa loa* microfilariae in the articular fluid. *Acta Cytol.* 1989;33:281–283.
16. Bouvet JP, Therizol M, Auquier L. Microfilarial polyarthritis in a massive *Loa loa* infestation. A case report. *Acta Trop (Basel).* 1977;34:281–284.
17. Hawking F. The transference of *Microfilaria bancrofti* into natural and unnatural hosts. *Ann Trop Med Parasitol.* 1940;34:121–129.
18. Gonnert R, Zur Lebensdauer menschlicher Mikrofilarien. *Zentbl Bakt Parasit Infek Orig.* 1943;149:75–81.
19. Carme B, Paraiso D, Gombe-Mbalawa C. Calcifications of the breast probably due to *Loa loa. Am J Trop Med Hyg.* 1990;42:65–66.
20. Paleologo FP, Neafie RC, Connor DH. Lymphadenitis caused by *Loa loa. Am J Trop Med Hyg.* 1984;33:395–402.
21. Katner H, Beyt BE Jr, Krotoski WA. Loiasis and renal failure. *South Med J.* 1984;77:907–908.
22. Klion AD, Eisenstein EM, Smirniotopoulos TT, Neumann MP, Nutman TB. Pulmonary involvement in loiasis. *Am Rev Respir Dis.* 1992;145:961–963.
23. Connor DH, Somers K, Hutt MSR, Manion WC, D'Arbela PG. Endomyocardial fibrosis in Uganda (Davies' disease), an epidemiological clinical and pathologic study. Part I. *Am Heart J.* 1967;74:687–709.
24. Connor DH, Somers K, Hutt MSR, Manion WC, D'Arbela PG. Endomyocardial fibrosis in Uganda (Davies' disease), an epidemiological, clinical and pathologic study. Part II. *Am Heart J.* 1968;75:107–124.
25. Hautekeete ML, Pailoux G, Marcellin P, Girard PM, Degott C, Benhamou JP. Presence of *Loa loa* microfilariae in ascitic fluid. *J Infect Dis.* 1989;160:559–560.
26. de Brux JA, Baup HF, Kaeding H. *Loa loa* microfilariae in an endometrial smear. *Acta Cytol.* 1983;27:547–549.
27. Van Dellen RG, Ottesen EA, Gocke TM, Neafie RC. *Loa loa.* An unusual case of chronic urticaria and angioedema in the United States. *JAMA.* 1985;253:1924–1925.
28. Novak R. Calcifications in the breast in *Filaria loa* infection. *Acta Radiol.* 1989;30:507–508.
29. Cesbron JY, Capron A, Vargaftig BB, et al. Platelets mediate the action of diethylcarbamazine on microfilariae. *Nature.* 1987;325:533–536.
30. Nutman TB, Miller KD, Mulligan M, Ottesen EA. *Loa loa* infection in temporary residents of endemic regions, recognition of a hyperresponsive syndrome with characteristic differences in clinical presentation. *J Infect Dis.* 1986;154:10–18.
31. Van Hoegaerden M, Ivanoff B, Flocard F, Salle A, Chabaud B. The use of mebendazole in the treatment of filariases due to *Loa loa* and *Mansonella perstans. Ann Trop Med Parasitol.* 1987;81:275–282.
32. Martin-Prevel Y, Cosnefroy JY, Tshipamba P, Ngari P, Chodakewitz JA, Pinder M. Tolerance and efficacy of single high-dose ivermectin for the treatment of loiasis. *Am J Trop Med Hyg.* 1993;48:186–192.
33. Martin-Prevel Y, Cosnefroy JY, Ngari P, Pinder M. Reduction of microfilaremia with single high-dose of ivermectin in loiasis. *Lancet.* 1993;342:442.
34. Saeed AA, Green PJ, Naoroz M, Lee HA, Raman GV. *Loa loa:* the use of a blood cell separator to reduce microfilaraemia before specific chemotherapy. *J Infect.* 1984;9:161–166.

CHAPTER 168

Mansonella ozzardi Infection (Mansonelliasis)

John Bryan and Daniel H. Connor

Dermatology is the best specialty. The patient never dies and never gets well.

Anonymous

INTRODUCTION

Mansonelliasis (also known as Ozzard's filariasis or mansonelliasis ozzardi) is infection of humans by the filarial worm *Mansonella ozzardi.* It is the only filarial infection of humans restricted to the Western Hemisphere. The microfilariae were described by Manson in 1897 in blood films (sent to him by Ozzard) taken from Indians in what was then British Guiana. The adult worm was identified in 1898, and the genus named *Mansonella* in 1929 by Faust.

EPIDEMIOLOGY

Mansonelliasis is endemic in several Caribbean islands and parts of central and northern South America. In the Caribbean the disease is transmitted by several species of the night-feeding midges of the genus *Culicoides,* including *C furens, C phlebotomus, C barbosai,* and *C paraensis.* These transmit the disease primarily along coastlines and especially around tidal mangrove swamps.[1,2] In the Amazon basin the primary vectors are black flies of the genus *Simulium,* and these include *S amazonicum, S sanguineum,* and *S argentiscutum. Culicoides* has also been reported as a vector in this area,[3] and both *Simulium* species and *Culicoides* species transmit *M ozzardi* experimentally.[3]

An estimated 40% to 65% of the Indians in the Amazon are infected,[4–6] with especially high prevalence in villages of the riverine lowlands.[7] Different villages and different Indian populations have variable rates of infection ranging from 0% to 84%.[6] In all areas studied, prevalence tends to increase with age. Only rarely is mansonelliasis diagnosed in infants and young children.[8,9] The incidence of infection in persons age 0 to 18 years has been reported to be higher in South America than in the Caribbean. Humans are the only known definitive host, and male subjects are more often infected than female subjects.[4,6,9]

NATURAL HISTORY AND MORPHOLOGY

After microfilariae are ingested by the biting arthropod, they penetrate the wall of the arthropod's gut and grow through several stages in the thoracic muscles. The larvae then migrate to the proboscis where they are transmitted to a human when the arthropod next bites.[5] Adult worms are rarely found in humans; they may live in the pleural and peritoneal cavities, and possibly in lymphatics.[5] Experimental infections in Patas monkeys (*Erythrocebus patas*) suggest a subcutaneous localization.[10] Microfilariae circulate in peripheral blood.

Adult worms recovered from experimentally infected Patas monkeys are long and slender, with the female worm roughly twice the length of the male worm.[11] The male worm is 26 by 0.07 mm, has a smoothly rounded anterior end, and no head bulb. There are 8 circumoral papillae, 11 pericloacal papillae, and a pair of papillae at the posterior end. The female worm is 49 by 0.15 mm. A large ovejector and paired uterine branches almost fill the body cavity. The ovaries are coiled and in the posterior 5% of the body. The tail is long (roughly 22 mm) and tapered, with 4 terminal lobed papillae. Both genders have one to four annular swellings (more prominent in the female) and a poorly developed esophagus.

Microfilariae are unsheathed and 200 to 220 μm by 3 to 5 μm, with a bluntly rounded anterior end. The anterior two thirds has a uniform diameter and the posterior third is gradually tapered. The attenuated tail terminates with a hook or sickle-shaped curve. The anterior two to three nuclei are in single file on alcohol-fixed slides but tend to overlap or be arranged in pairs in air-dried smears. The posterior seven to nine nuclei are in single file; the terminal nuclei are oval, and there are no nuclei in the tail, unlike *M perstans.*[11]

PATHOLOGY

In the Caribbean, no clinical symptoms or signs of infection have been described. In the Amazon region, however, mansonelliasis has been associated with slight pathogenicity, although the simultaneous existence of multiple filarial infections makes it difficult to associate a single infection with specific clinical features. Pain in the knees and ankles is the most common complaint,[5] but "coldness" of the legs, varices of the lower limbs, erythematous pruritic cutaneous lesions, painful inguinal lymphadenopathy, fever, eosinophilia, headache, insomnia, and vertigo have also been described.

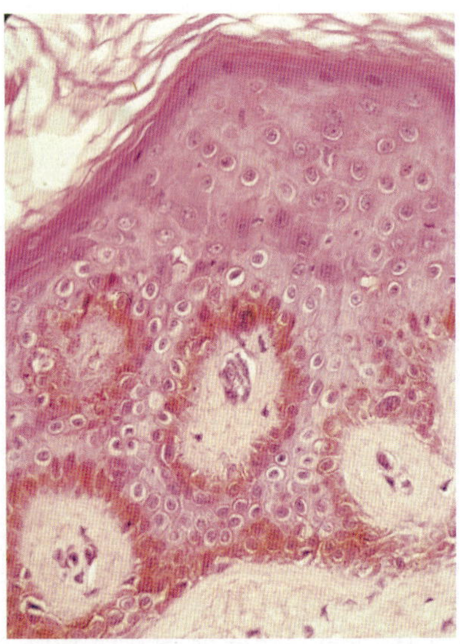

Figure 168–1. Biopsy specimen of skin from patient with mansonelliasis (ozzardi). There are coiled microfilariae in the capillaries of the dermal papillae [hematoxylin-eosin (H&E), ×165].

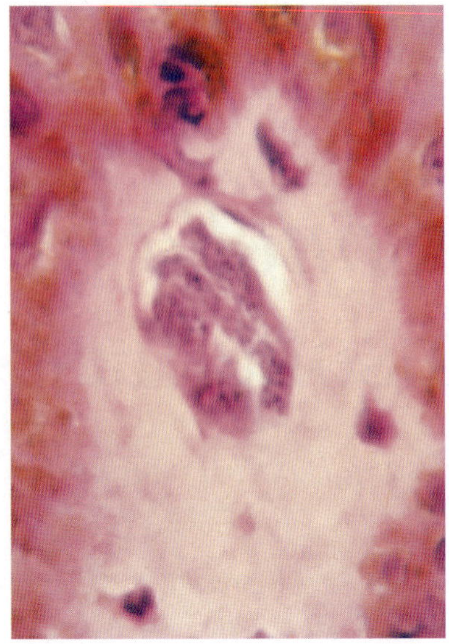

Figure 168–2. A higher magnification of the capillary shown in Figure 168–1. The coiled microfilaria is in the capillary in the center of the field (H&E, ×705).

DIAGNOSIS AND TREATMENT

Mansonelliasis is diagnosed by identifying the microfilariae in peripheral blood. The Knott technique for concentrating the organisms is a special aid in diagnosis.[12] Peripheral blood from the earlobe is more densely populated with microfilariae than blood from the fingertip.[13] Biopsy specimens of skin are less effective for diagnosis than is peripheral blood but they reveal microfilariae within dermal capillaries, usually associated with a perivascular lymphoplasmacytic infiltrate[5,14] (Figures 168–1 through 168–3). The earliest serologic

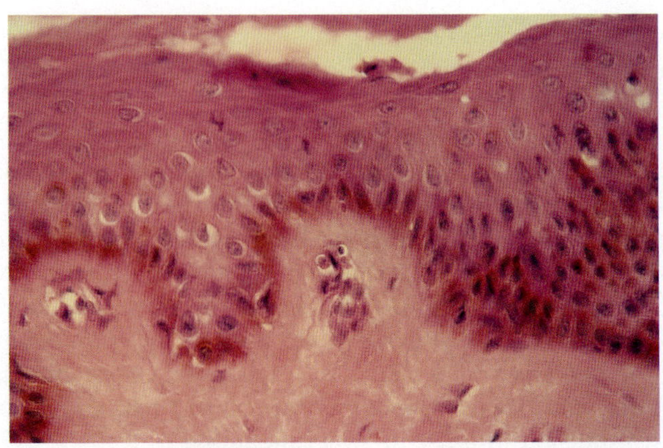

Figure 168–3. Biopsy specimen from another patient showing a microfilaria of *M ozzardi* in a dermal capillary. Note its location high in the dermal papilla and slight sclerosis of the surrounding dermis (H&E, ×305).

assays depended on bentonite flocculation and indirect hemagglutination tests.[15] Subsequently, enzyme-linked immunosorbent assays and immunofluorescent antibody tests have utilized heterologous antigens from other parasites including *Brugia pahangi* and *M llewellyni.*[14] These tests are nonspecific and have not yet been sufficiently developed for clinical application.

Treatment efficacy is difficult to evaluate because of the mild clinical features. There are conflicting reports on the effectiveness of diethylcarbamazine.[16] Prognosis is excellent.

REFERENCES

1. Lowrie RC Jr, Raccurt C. *Mansonella ozzardi* in Haiti. II. Arthropod vector studies. *Am J Trop Med Hyg.* 1981; 30:598–603.
2. Lowrie RC Jr, Raccurt C. Assessment of *Culicoides barbosai* as a vector of *Mansonella ozzardi* in Haiti. *Am J Trop Med Hyg.* 1984;33:1275–1277.
3. Tidwell MA, Tidwell MA. Development of *Mansonella ozzardi* in *Simulium amazonicum, S argentiscutum,* and *Culicoides insinuatus* from Amazonas, Colombia. *Am J Trop Med Hyg.* 1982;31:1137–1141.
4. Lightner LK, Ewert A, Corredor A, Sabogal E. A parasitologic survey for *Mansonella ozzardi* in the Comisaria del Vaupes, Colombia. *Am J Trop Med Hyg.* 1980;29:42–45.
5. De Paola D. Mansonelliasis. In Marcial-Rojas RA, ed. *Pathology of Protozoal and Helminthic Diseases.* Baltimore: Williams and Wilkins; 1971:955–959.
6. Kozek WJ, D'Alessandro A, Navarette SN. Filariasis in Colombia: prevalence of mansonellosis in the teenage and adult population of the Colombian bank of the Amazon, Comisaria del Amazonas. *Am J Trop Med Hyg.* 1982;31:1131–1136.
7. Tidwell MA, Tidwell MA, Munoz de Hoyos P. Development of *Mansonella ozzardi* in a Blackfly species of the *Simulium sanguineum* group from Eastern Vaupes, Colombia. *Am J Trop Med Hyg.* 1980;29:1209–1214.
8. Orihel TC. Infections with *Dipetalonema perstans* and *Mansonella ozzardi* in the aboriginal indians of Guyana. *Am J Trop Med Hyg.* 1967;16:628–635.
9. Raccurt C, Lowrie RC Jr, McNeely DF. *Mansonella ozzardi* in Haiti. I. Epidemiological survey. *Am J Trop Med Hyg.* 1980;29:803–808.
10. Orihel TC, Lowrie RC Jr, Eberhard ML, et al. Susceptibility of laboratory primates to infection with *Mansonella ozzardi* from man. *Am J Trop Med Hyg.* 1981;30:790–794.
11. Orihel TC, Eberhard ML. *Mansonella ozzardi:* a redescription with comments on its taxonomic relationships. *Am J Trop Med Hyg.* 1982;31:1142–1147.
12. Knott J. A method for making microfilarial surveys on day blood. *Trans R Soc Trop Med Hyg.* 1939;33:191–197.
13. Raccurt C, Lowrie RC Jr, Boncy J, Katz SP. *Mansonella ozzardi* in Haiti. III. A comparison of four sampling methods in detecting infection. *Am J Trop Med Hyg.* 1982; 31:275–279.
14. Katz SP, Raccurt CP, Lowrie RC Jr, Boncy J, Leiva LM. *Mansonella ozzardi* in Haiti. IV. Evaluation of antibody reactivity to heterologous antigens. *Am J Trop Med Hyg.* 1986;35:303–307.
15. Kagan IG, Norman L, Allain DS. An evaluation of the betonite flocculation and indirect hemagglutination tests for diagnosis of filariasis. *Am J Trop Med Hyg.* 1963; 12:548–555.
16. Weller PF, Simon HB, Parkhurst BH, Medrek TF. Tourism-acquired *Mansonella ozzardi* microfilaremia in a regular blood donor. *JAMA.* 1978;240:858–859.

CHAPTER 169

Mansonella perstans Infection (Mansonelliasis)

J. Kevin Baird

Man's nature must be regarded, like his body, as the sum total of all that has come before plus those modifications which are the hallmark of his kind. And if those modifications have presented him with a potential beyond any other species of livingkind, then he may thank his lucky stars but not some patient Maker who has been sitting it out for billions of years waiting to devote His exclusive attention to that moment that is Man.

Robert Ardrey (1908–1980), African Genesis

DEFINITION

Mansonella perstans is a filarial worm that wanders through the body cavities of humans, usually unnoticed by the immune system and only rarely provoking signs or symptoms. Even though this filarial parasite infects millions of people each year, only a few reports have attributed specific symptoms to the infection. *Mansonella perstans* was recently identified as the "Ugandan eye worm," which causes nodules in the conjunctiva and in periorbital fibroadipose tissue.[1]

The taxonomy of *M perstans* has been the subject of much revision. The species has been known as *Filaria perstans, Acanthocheilonema perstans, Tetrapetalonema perstans,* and *Dipetalonema perstans.* Placement of the species in the genus *Mansonella* by Orihel and Eberhard[2] dates to 1982.

GEOGRAPHIC DISTRIBUTION

Mansonella perstans occurs in Africa and South America. In Africa, it is common throughout the tropical regions, and also in Algiers and Tunis. In South America, *M perstans* seems restricted to the eastern coastal areas from Panama to Argentina.[3] *Mansonella perstans* as the Ugandan eye worm has been reported almost exclusively from Uganda. Periorbital swelling and/or conjunctival pruritus associated with *M perstans* microfilaremia is, however, known throughout endemic areas.[1,4,5]

BIOLOGY AND EPIDEMIOLOGY

Humans are the definitive hosts for *M perstans,* although some other primates also may serve as reservoir hosts. The adult worms live in body cavities, usually the peritoneal cavity. The pleural spaces and the pericardium are occasionally infected. The gravid female gives birth to live microfilariae, which migrate to the peripheral circulation and infect blood-feeding midges (*Culicoides*). The microfilariae circulate day and night, but are more numerous at night, ie, they are subperiodic. Within the *Culicoides* the ingested microfilaria molts twice to become the infective third-stage larva. Blood-feeding midges harboring the third-stage larvae transmit them to humans. Prevalence of microfilaremia in endemic areas may be high—80% to almost 100%—in some villages. Prevalence in excess of 25% is ordinary.

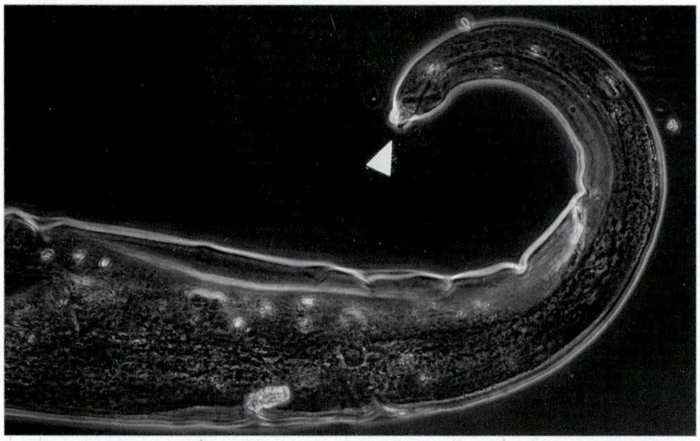

Figure 169–1. Female *M perstans* showing the characteristically bifurcated posterior end *(arrow)*. *Mansonella perstans* is the only filarial parasite of man with a bifid posterior end and this feature thus allows specific identification (AFIP Neg 86-6887; darkfield illumination, ×1200).

MORPHOLOGIC CHARACTERISTICS

Only a few adult *M perstans* have been recovered intact. The male worm is 45 mm long and 60 μm wide; the female worm is up to 80 mm long and 120 μm wide. The male has four preanal and one postanal pairs of papillae. The copulatory spicules of the male are unequal in length. The vulva of the female is near the anterior end, and the posterior end is bifurcated (Figure 169–1). Usually adult *M perstans* are discovered incidentally in tissue sections. The identification of *M perstans* in tissue sections depends on demonstration of several characteristic morphologic features of this parasite. The female worms range from 80 to 120 μm in maximum diameter and the male worms are 45 to 60 μm. The cuticle is thin (1 to 2 μm), monolayered, smooth, and slightly thickened (3 to 4 μm) at the lateral chords. There are 8 to 12 muscle cells per quadrant, which are tall at the dorsoventral aspects (10 to 20 μm) and low near the lateral chords (2 to 5 μm). Figure 169–2, A, illustrates these features. Intact worms provoke little or no reaction but degenerating worms provoke both acute and granulomatous reactions (Figure 169–2, B). The lateral chords contain two fields of brown granules with the staining characteristics of melanin (Figure 169–3). The granules are particularly helpful in diagnosis because they persist in degenerated worms.

The unsheathed microfilariae of *M perstans* in blood films are 100 to 200 μm long and 3.5 to 4.5 μm wide. The posterior end is characteristically blunt and lacks a tail. The cephalic space is 1 to 3 μm (Figure 169–4). Specific identification of microfilariae in tissue sections is not usually possible.

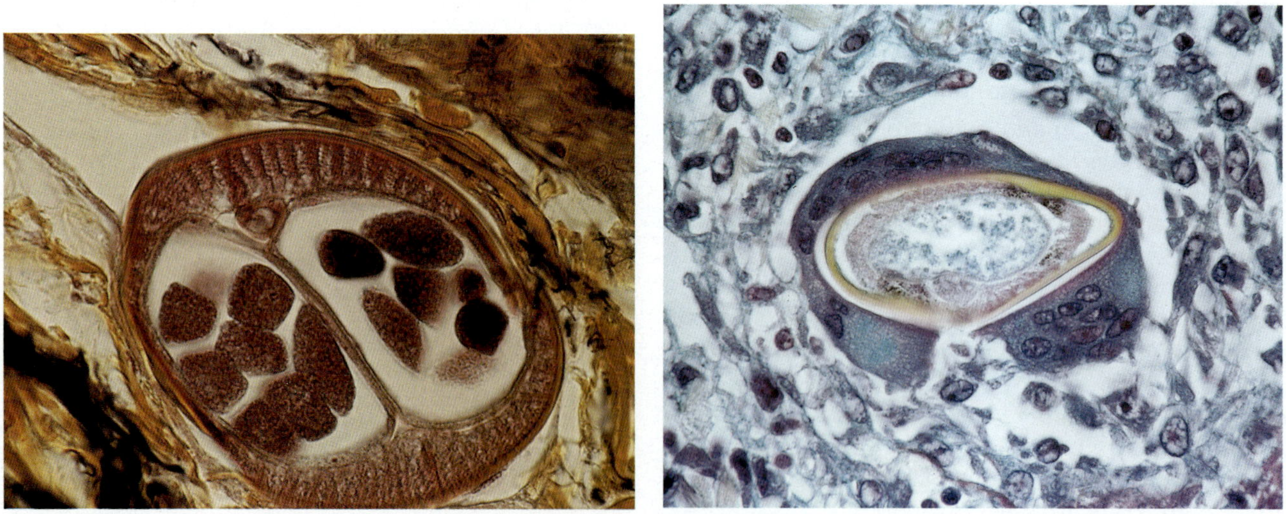

A B

Figure 169–2. (**A**) Cross-section through gravid *M perstans* in peripancreatic connective tissue of an African (Zairian) patient. Note the intact cuticle and the absence of inflammation. The paired uteri contain embryonic microfilariae at this level. Sections at other levels revealed fully developed microfilariae (AFIP; Movat stain, ×800). (**B**) Cross-section of a degenerating adult male *M perstans* in human liver. Note the fractured cuticle, the foreign-body giant cell that encloses the worm, and the numerous surrounding epithelioid cells, one of which appears to be plugging the gap in the giant cell. Other features that indicate the worm is degenerating are lack of detail in the musculature and indistinct reproductive and digestive tubes. When a filaria degenerates the cuticle persists after other structures have vanished (Movat stain, ×600).

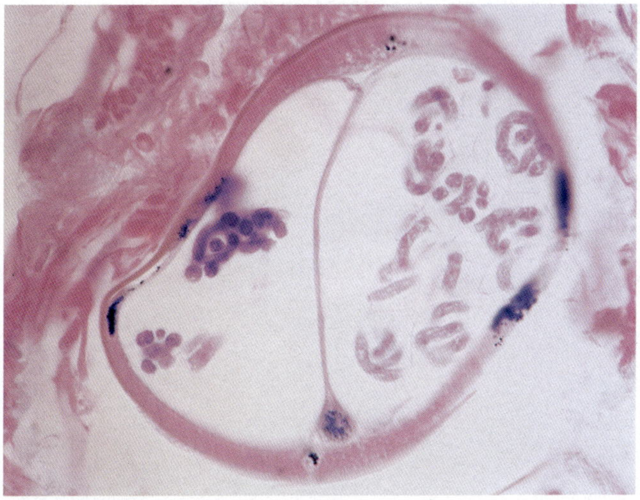

Figure 169–3. Cross-section through gravid *M perstans* female worm demonstrating two fields of granules of melanin in each lateral chord. Melanin granules are also in the diminutive dorsal and ventral chords (AFIP Neg 86-6905; Giemsa, ×600).

CLINICAL FEATURES

The vast majority of people infected by *M perstans* have no symptoms specifically attributable to the parasite. In the few patients where this seemed to be a possibility, there was abdominal pain, transient subcutaneous swelling (so-called "Calabar swellings"), rashes, chest pain, and malaise. Symptoms seem to occur most frequently among visitors to endemic areas. Some reports have attributed pleural effusions, lymphedema, meningoencephalitis, hepatitis, and a fatal pericarditis to *M perstans*.[6–8] Several reports have described periorbital edema and conjunctival pruritus associated with *M perstans*.[1,4,5] Medical practitioners in northern Zaire have noted that some patients receiving diethylcarbamazine for onchocerciasis develop acute abdominal pain characteristic of focal peritonitis. None of these patients had surgical explorations of their abdominal cavities so the cause of their pain is unproved but it is possible, perhaps even likely, that their pain was provoked by a focal reaction to adult *M perstans* worms killed by the diethylcarbamazine.[9]

The Ugandan eye worm, identified as *M perstans*,[1] causes nodules in the conjunctiva (Figure 169–5) or proptosis. People in Uganda, where the condition seems best known, refer to these lesions as bung-eye and bulge-eye.

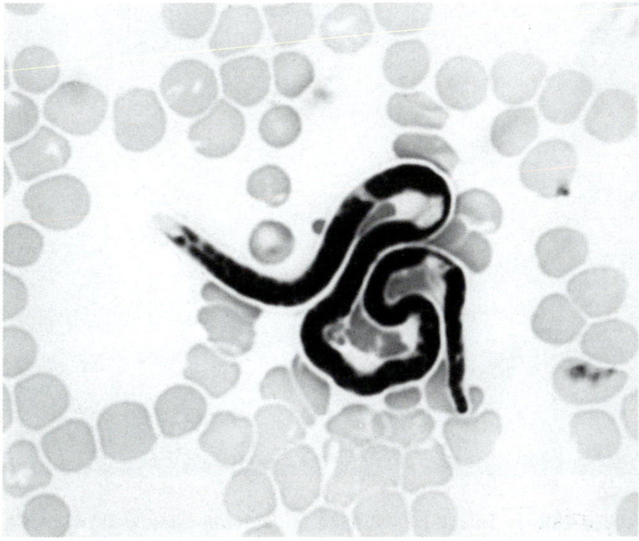

Figure 169–4. Microfilaria of *M perstans* in a thin blood film (AFIP Neg 74-5605; Giemsa, ×1000).

PATHOLOGY

Histopathologic changes caused by *M perstans* in the abdominal cavities of nine Africans have been studied from surgical specimens or autopsy.[10] To date, this is the most complete study available. The worm was an incidental finding in all patients. Tissues surrounding the parasites were free of inflammatory cells in a few patients (Figure 169–2). In other patients, inflammatory responses ranged from neutrophilic abscess to granulomatous scar. Only dead worms provoked inflammation. Viable worms were free of surrounding inflammation. Living worms seem capable of avoiding notice by the host immune system. In contrast, dead or dying worms probably leak antigens and provoke abscesses, a granulomatous reaction, and eventually fibrous encapsulation and scarring.

Baird and others[1] also described *M perstans* as the cause of bung-eye and bulge-eye in Africans. Bung-eye is a granulomatous nodule in the conjunctiva, and bulge-eye is proptosis caused by periorbital edema and inflammation. Bung-eye is a sharply circumscribed necrotizing granuloma (Figure 169–6). The worm, or remnants of it, are at the center of this reaction. Degranulated eosinophils create a necrobiotic coagulum around the worm. Palisading epithelioid cells surround the reaction. Tissue around the granuloma is highly vascularized and infiltrated with lymphocytes, foreign-body giant cells, and histiocytes. In contrast, the worm in periorbital fat is surrounded by eosinophils, histiocytes, tortuous blood vessels, and lymphocytes. There in marked edema. Epithelioid cells and foreign-body giant cells are absent (Figure 169–7).

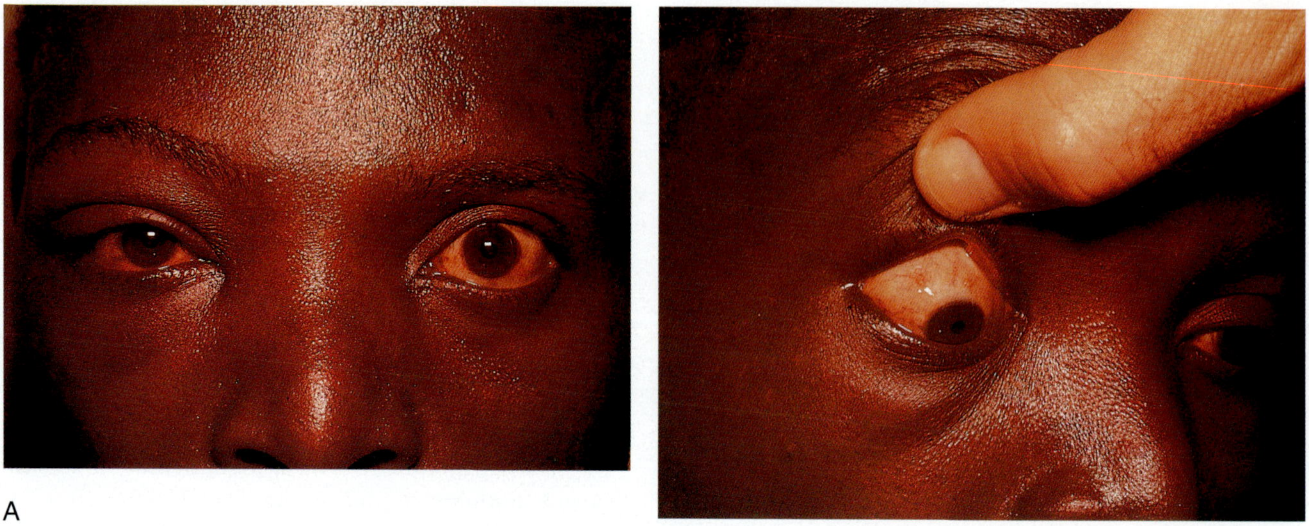

A

B

Figure 169–5. (**A**) Male patient from Jinja, Uganda, with "bung-eye." The conjunctiva of his right eye is red and itchy and the periorbital tissues are swollen. *(By Daniel H. Connor, MD, 1963.)* (**B**) Same patient showing two filarial granulomas in the conjunctiva of the right eye. *(By Daniel H. Connor, MD, 1963.)*

DIAGNOSIS

The usual clinical diagnosis of infection by *M perstans* is made by microscopic examination of thick blood films for characteristic microfilariae (Figure 169–4). The pathologist faced with identifying a filarial worm from the body cavities of humans must consider *M perstans, M ozzardi,* and *Loa loa.* Adult *M ozzardi* may be indistinguishable from *M perstans.* Thus, where there is a history of travel or residence in South America, worms exhibiting the morphologic characteristics described for *M perstans* may be either species. In patients from Africa, *M perstans* is readily distinguished from *L loa* on the basis of diameter alone (eg, <120 μm versus 500 μm for female worms).

A wide variety of parasites and other foreign bodies may cause granulomatous or inflammatory lesions in the conjunctiva and periorbital fibroadipose tissues.

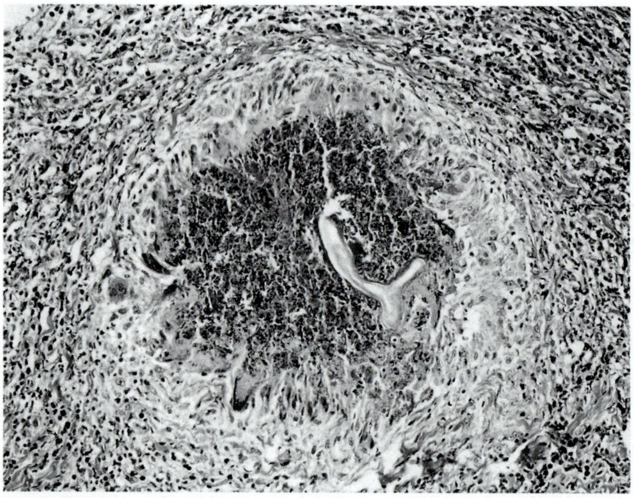

Figure 169–6. Necrotizing granuloma of bung-eye in a Ugandan patient. The structure at the center of the reaction is the cuticle of a nematode, probably *M perstans* (AFIP Neg 86-7171; H&E, ×160).

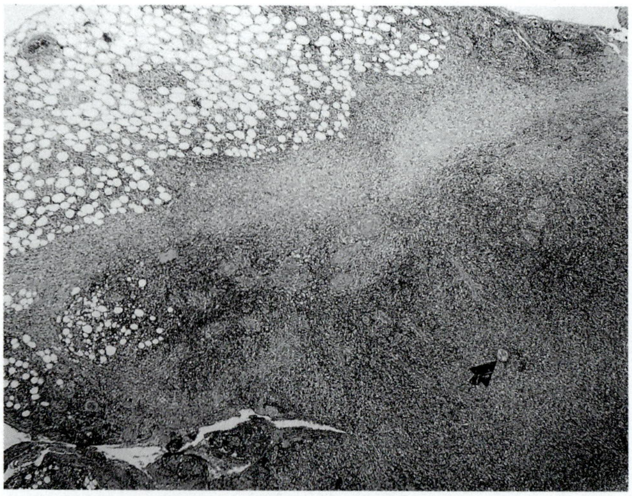

Figure 169–7. Reaction to a dead *M perstans (arrow)* in periorbital fibroadipose tissue in a Ugandan patient. Contrast the acute inflammatory reaction here with the granulomatous reaction in the conjunctiva in Figure 169–6 (AFIP Neg 86-7167; H&E, ×25).

Morphologic characteristics of *M perstans* should be demonstrated before the diagnosis is confirmed. The worm in ocular lesions is often degenerated, but the characteristics of the cuticle, including diameter, and the presence of brown granules within remnants of the lateral chords may suffice for diagnosis of *M perstans.*

REFERENCES

1. Baird JK, Neafie RC, Connor DH. Nodules in the conjunctiva, bung-eye, and bulge-eye in Africa caused by *Mansonella perstans. Am J Trop Med Hyg.* 1988;38:553–557.
2. Orihel TC, Eberhard ML. Mansonella ozzardi: a redescription with comments on taxonomic relationships. *Am J Trop Med Hyg.* 1982;31:1142–1147.
3. Beaver PC, Jung RC, Cupp EW. Mansonella perstans. In: Beaver PC, Jung RC, Cupp EW, eds. *Clinical Parasitology.* 9th ed. Philadelphia: Lea & Febiger; 1984;382–385.
4. Almaviva M, Galli M, Rizzi M, Simonelli E, Negri G, Vigevani GM. Immune response in a symptomatic case of *Tetrapetalonema perstans* infection. *Trans R Soc Trop Med Hyg.* 1984;78:489–491.
5. Sondergaard J. Filariasis caused by *Acanthocheilonema perstans. Arch Dermatol.* 1972;106:547–548.
6. Foster DG. Filariasis—a rare cause of pericarditis. *J Trop Med Hyg.* 1956;59:212–214.
7. Olumide YM, Obembe BM. *Dipetalonema perstans* in a patient with chronic lymphoedema. Case report. *East Afr Med J.* 1983;60:186–189.
8. Khan JB. Pleural effusion associated with *Dipetalonema perstans. J Infect Dis.* 1983;147:166.
9. Almquist LA, Thorpe RG. Observations at the Karawa mission hospital, Ubangi territory, Republic of Zaire. Personal communication to Daniel H. Connor, MD, 1977.
10. Baird JK, Neafie RC, Lanoie L, Connor DH. Adult *Mansonella perstans* in the abdominal cavity in nine Africans. *Am J Trop Med Hyg.* 1987;37:578–584.

CHAPTER 170

Mansonella streptocerca Infection (Streptocerciasis)

John Bryan and Daniel H. Connor

Diseased nature oftentimes breaks forth
In strange eruptions . . .

Shakespeare (1564–1616), Henry IV, III, i, 27

DEFINITION

Streptocerciasis is infection of humans by the filarial round worm *Mansonella streptocerca*. *Mansonella streptocerca* has had other generic names, including *Dipetalonema, Acanthocheilonema,* and *Tetrapetalonema.* Microfilariae of *M streptocerca* were first described in 1922 by Macfie and Corson. Adult worms were identified in human skin in 1972.[1] Streptocerciasis is restricted to tropical West Africa (including Cameroon, Nigeria, Zaire, Ghana, and Angola) and infects chimpanzees and gorillas as well as humans.[1,2] Reported incidences in specific villages range up to 72%.[3]

NATURAL HISTORY

Microfilariae of *M streptocerca* live in the skin. The arthropod vector is the biting midge, *Culicoides grahami,* which ingests microfilariae while feeding on those infected with *M streptocerca.* The microfilariae taken in by the midge penetrate its stomach wall and invade the thoracic muscles. Infective larvae develop in the muscles within 7 to 10 days, migrate to the mouth parts, and are transmitted when the *Culicoides* bites the next person.[4] Development of the infective larval stage to adult worms takes place in the skin over a period of several months.[2]

MORPHOLOGY

The adult female worm is 22 mm by 76 μm and roughly twice the size of the male worm.[5] There are two uteri, which nearly fill the body cavity; the ovaries and oviduct are confined to the posterior 2 mm of the body.[6] The male worm is 13 mm in length and up to 47 μm in diameter. The intestine occupies most of the body cavity. The testes are anterior and the vas deferens posterior.[7] Both genders have a thin cuticle without striations and barely evident lateral chords. The contractile portion of somatic muscle is prominent, especially posteriorly.[2] One remarkable section has shown a microfilaria in the act of being "born" (Figure 170–1).

Microfilariae are unsheathed and up to 240 μm long and 5 μm across. The first 4 nuclei are oval and staggered, but do not overlap. These are followed by 7 to 10 smaller and rounder nuclei in single file. Terminal nuclei are round to quadrate and extend to the tip of the tail.[2] The tail tapers gradually to a tip that has a barely perceptible notch.[8] Characteristically the tail is rounded in the shape of a shepherd's crook. The cephalic space is 3 to 5 μm and the caudal space 1 μm or less (Figure 170–2).

CLINICAL FEATURES

Although many patients are asymptomatic, the most consistent clinical feature is a chronic pruritic dermatitis.

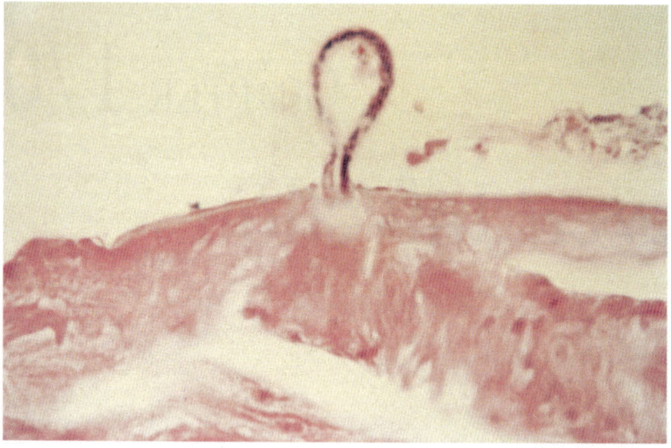

Figure 170–1. A microfilaria emerging from the genital opening of a gravid adult female *M streptocerca* [AFIP Neg 72-1984; hematoxylin-eosin (H&E), ×675]. *(By Ronald C. Neafie.)*

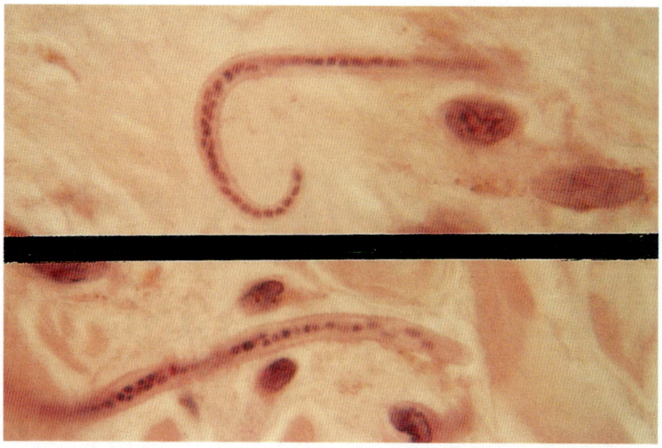

Figure 170–2. Sections of skin showing the characteristic features of *M streptocerca* microfilaria. Above is the characteristic "shepherd's crook" contour of the posterior end and the terminal nuclei, which are single file, round to quadrate, and leave a caudal space of 1 μm or less. Below is the anterior end with a cephalic clear space of 5 μm; the anterior nuclei are staggered and do not overlap. (AFIP Neg 71-10074, 75; H&E, ×1080). *(By Ronald C. Neafie.)*

Dermal thickening, hypopigmented macules (Figure 170–3), and occasional papules are often on the thorax and shoulder girdle—the areas of high microfilarial density.[1] Lymphadenopathy is common. Treatment with diethylcarbamazine (DEC) causes edema, increased pruritus, and increased numbers of papules[2] (Figure 170–4). The reaction begins soon after taking DEC and persists for 2 to 3 days. This reaction resembles the Mazzotti reaction seen in patients with onchocerciasis.[3]

PATHOLOGY

Microfilariae do not circulate in the peripheral blood. An exceptional finding, however, was reported by Okelo et al[9] in which up to 13.5% of patients from a village in the Central African Republic contained microfilariae in peripheral blood.[9] The authors give no dimensions or other specific features of the microfilariae and the reader is left to wonder about their specific features.

There is a mild eosinophilia, but the total leukocyte count remains normal. In skin, microfilariae lie between strands of collagen and tend to be more numerous in the upper dermis. Sclerosis of the dermal papillae, melanin incontinence, dilated dermal lymphatics, and perivascular and periadnexal chronic inflammation[2] are microscopic features of the dermatitis (Figures 170–5 and 170–6). These inflammatory features are accelerated and accentuated following treatment with DEC (Figure 170–7). In addition, DEC stimulates the microfilariae to migrate into the epidermis (Figure 170–8).

Adult worms provoke no inflammatory reaction while alive (Figure 170–9). They are stretched out in the dermis without surrounding inflammation. After treatment with DEC, however, cutaneous papules develop that contain tightly coiled worms surrounded by edematous tissue and an intense inflammatory cell infiltrate of neutrophils, eosinophils, fibrin and giant cells[3] (Figures 170–10 and 170–11). In fact, adult worms were first seen when papules erupting post-DEC were biopsied (Figure 170–12). Tiny fractures of the cuticle were noted

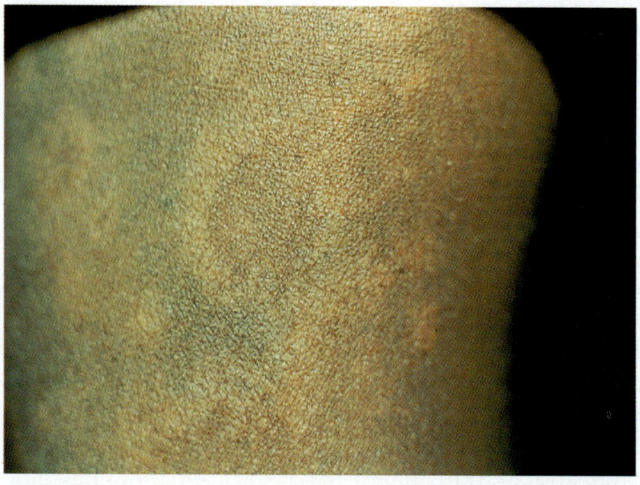

Figure 170–3. Characteristic macule on upper arm of a patient with streptocerciasis. The central hypopigmented area is not hypesthetic as in tuberculoid leprosy. *(By Daniel H. Connor, MD, 1970.)*

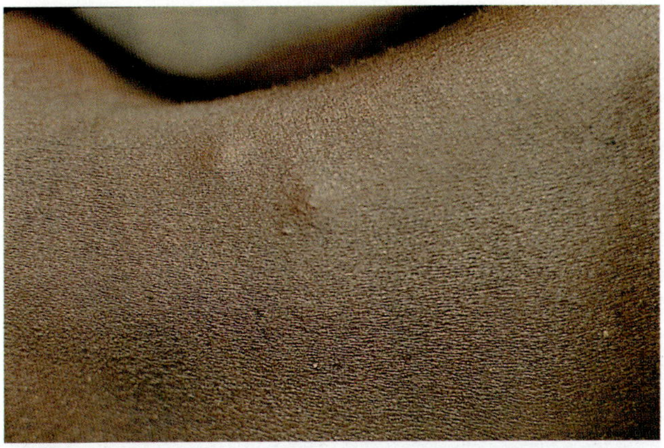

Figure 170–4. Papules on the shoulder of a patient with streptocerciasis. The papules were photographed 24 hours after the patient swallowed 50 mg of DEC. *(By Daniel H. Connor, MD, 1970.)*

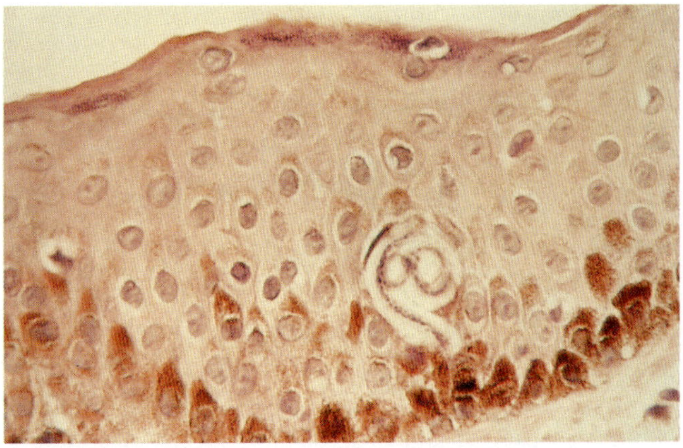

Figure 170–7. Biopsy specimen of skin 5 days after treatment with DEC showing a coiled microfilaria within the epidermis (H&E, ×450).

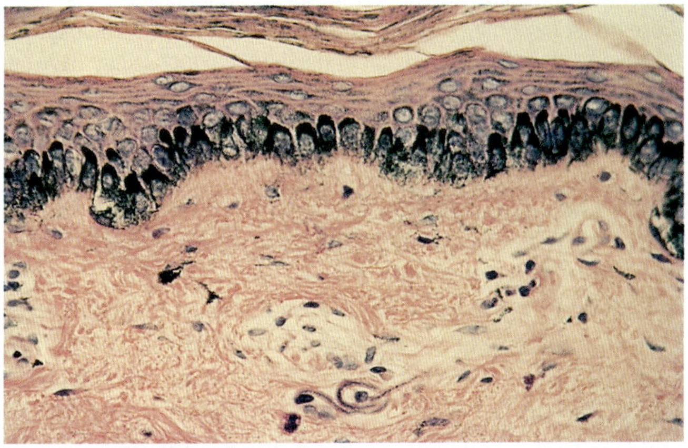

Figure 170–5. Skin of shoulder showing hyperkeratosis and parakeratosis, incontinence of pigment, fibrosis of the upper dermis, and microfilaria of *M streptocerca (bottom)* (AFIP Neg 71-6073; Giemsa, ×300).

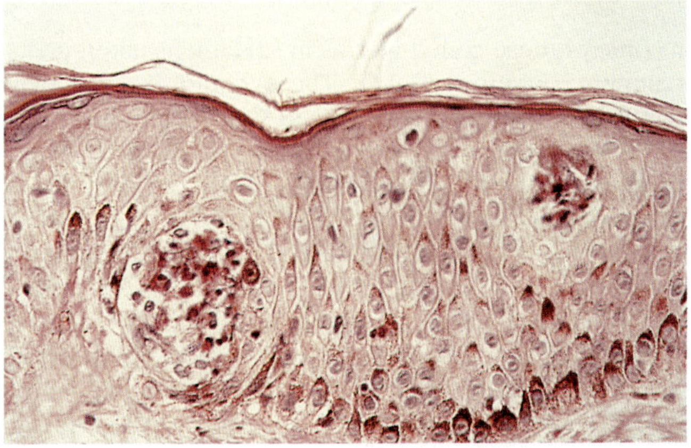

Figure 170–8. Biopsy specimen of skin taken 10 days after the patient had received DEC. Shown is an intraepidermal abscess containing eosinophils. A tangential section of a *M streptocerca* microfilaria is in the lower portion of the abscess (H&E, ×305).

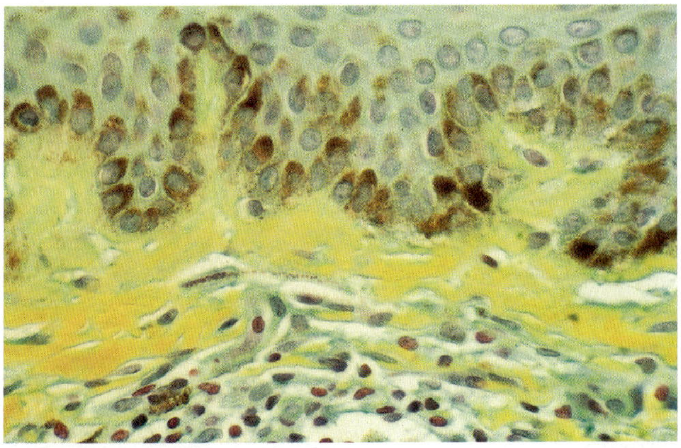

Figure 170–6. Movat-stained section of skin showing sclerosis of dermal papillae, inflammatory infiltrate in dermis, and a microfilaria of *M streptocerca* (×100).

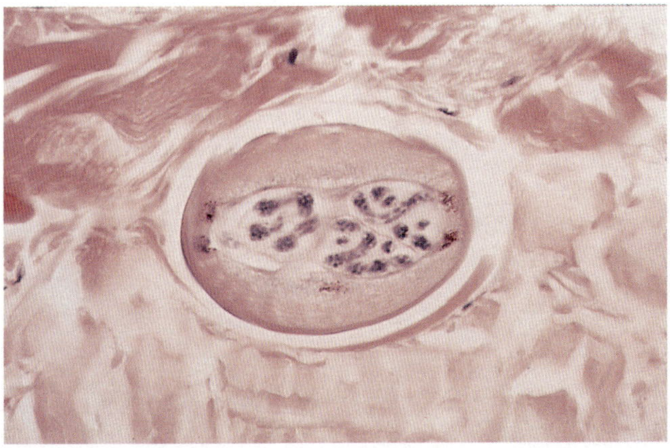

Figure 170–9. Cross-section of an adult gravid female *M streptocerca* in the dermal collagen. Its cuticle is in contact with the collagen fibers, but it has provoked no reaction. After treatment with DEC, however, the adult worms coil up and provoke an intense inflammatory reaction that is seen clinically as a papule (H&E, ×395; see Figure 170–3).

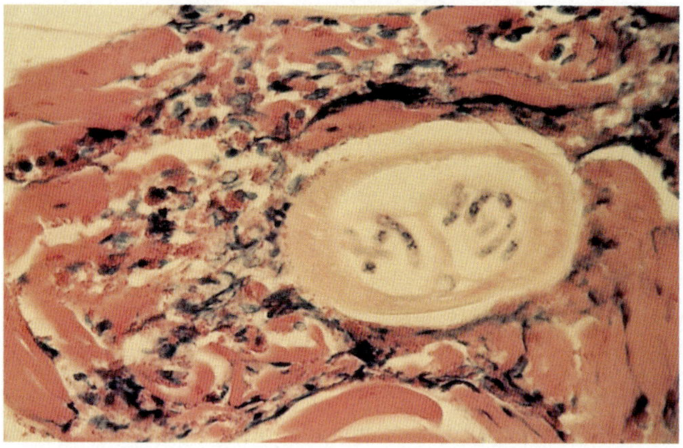

Figure 170–10. Inflammatory reaction in the dermis surrounding an adult worm after treatment with DEC (H&E, ×395).

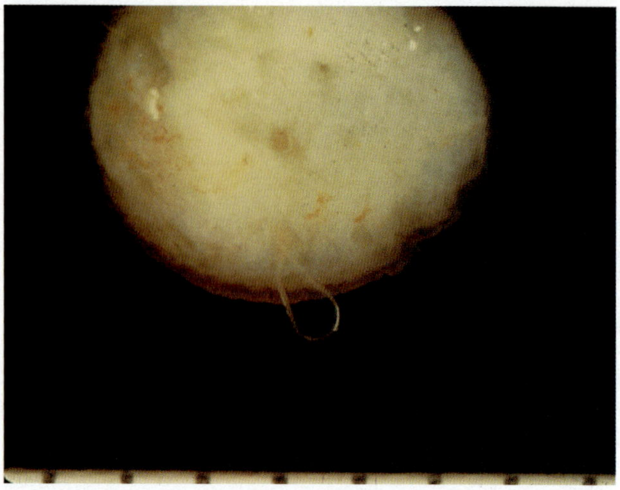

Figure 170–12. Four-millimeter punch biopsy of skin. A loop of the adult *M streptocerca* projects from the dermal collagen. The adult worm must have migrated out of the specimen after the biopsy was taken, otherwise the sharp edge of the dermal punch would have cut it. *(By Daniel H. Connor, MD, 1973.)*

in some of these coiled worms in specimens taken post-treatment (Figure 170–13). These could be cuticular fractures caused by contortions of the worm while coiling. If so, internal antigens could be exposed by these fractures and might explain some of the post-treatment inflammation.

The few lymph nodes studied have been enlarged, soft, mobile, and rubbery. A cluster of inguinal nodes from one patient had salmon-pink cut surfaces (Figure 170–14). Microscopically, the subcapsular sinuses are dilated and filled with histiocytes, eosinophils, and plasma cells (Figure 170–15). The follicles and germinal centers are atrophic and some are diffusely fibrotic (Figure 170–16). Microfilariae are rare in nodes; one has been identified in the subcapsular sinus.

DIAGNOSIS

The diagnosis is made by identifying the specific features of the microfilariae or the adult *M streptocerca.* Fresh skin snips, preferably from over the scapula, are the specimens of choice. The microfilariae can be seen in saline wet mounts, where they exhibit sluggish movement and usually have a characteristic "shepherd's crook" configuration of the tail. Histopathologic examination of skin specimens may also reveal microfilariae or adult worms between dermal collagen fibers. In tissue sections, microfilariae and adult worms must be distinguished from those of *Onchocerca volvulus.*[2]

The hypopigmented macules, characteristic of streptocerciasis, may resemble macules of tuberculoid leprosy, but unlike leprosy these macules have normal sensation and are concentrated on the upper trunk and shoulder girdle.[2]

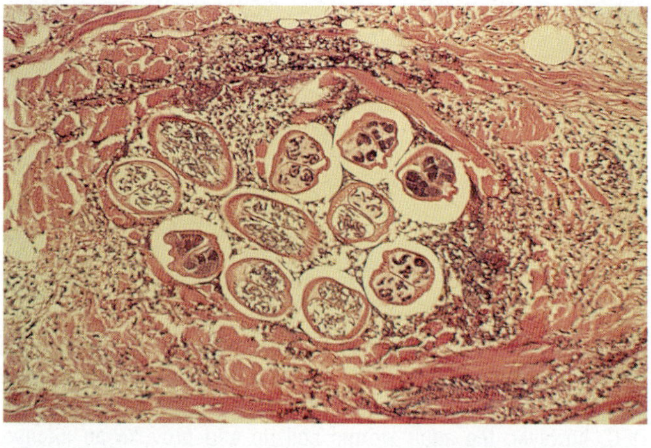

Figure 170–11. Tightly coiled gravid female *M streptocerca* surrounded by an intense inflammatory reaction in a biopsy specimen from a patient treated with DEC (H&E, ×110).

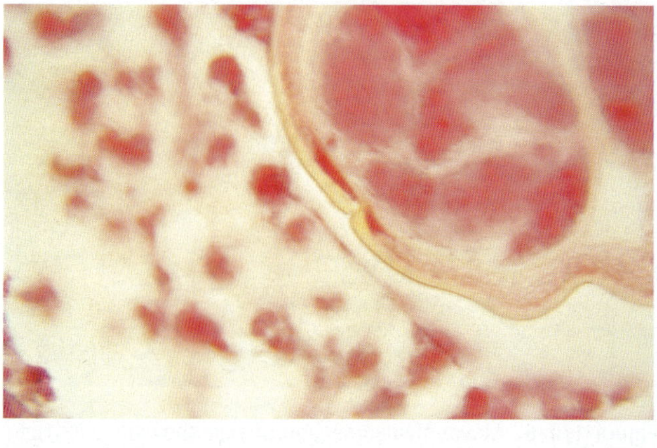

Figure 170–13. Cuticular fracture in an adult worm that was tightly coiled in the dermis of a patient after treatment with DEC (H&E, ×865).

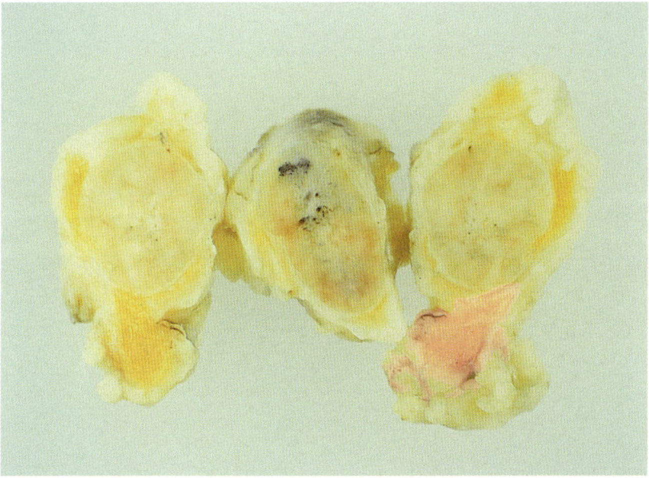

Figure 170–14. Three slices of inguinal lymph nodes excised from a patient with streptocerciasis. Note the thickened capsules, the stromal fibrosis, and the delicate "salmon-pink" hue. The latter is a consequence of capillary congestion (×1.4). *(By Daniel H. Connor, MD, 1973.)*

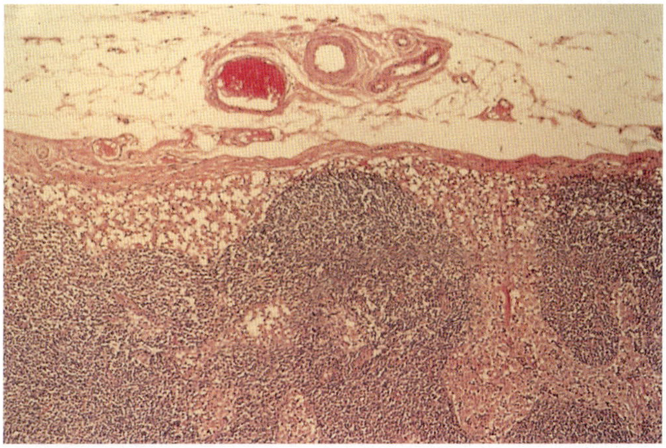

Figure 170–16. Inguinal lymph node showing atrophic follicles, slight thickening of the capsule, and sinus histiocytosis. Eosinophils are scattered among the histiocytes (H&E, ×55).

TREATMENT

For those living in endemic areas, infections are mild and patients have few or no symptoms. These patients may need no specific therapy. For more severe infections, DEC kills both adult worms and microfilariae when taken daily for more than 3 weeks.[3] The dead and dying microfilariae may cause intense allergic reactions including pruritus, fever, and urticaria. Degenerating adult worms provoke surrounding edema and inflammation, which manifest clinically as multiple cutaneous papules (the sites of the adult worms). The reactions may require anti-inflammatory agents.

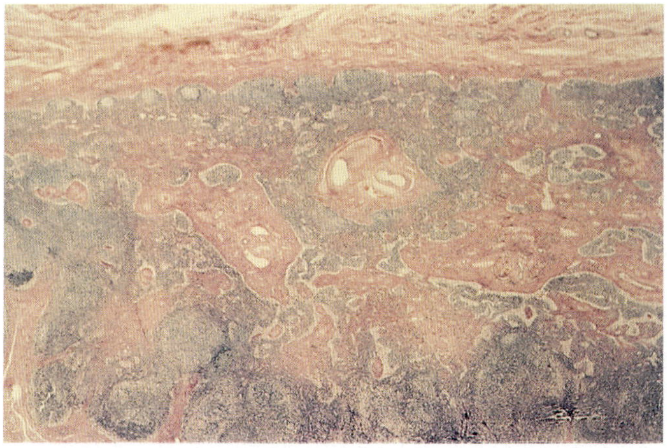

Figure 170–15. Section of a lymph node showing fibrosis and thickening of the capsule, atrophy of germinal centers, trabecular fibrosis, and sinus histiocytosis. Only rarely are microfilariae of *M streptocerca* seen in lymph nodes, and only in patients after treatment with DEC (H&E, ×10).

REFERENCES

1. Meyers WM, Connor DH, Harman LE, Fleshman K, Moris R, Neafie RC. Human streptocerciasis. A clinico-pathologic study of 40 Africans (Zairians) including identification of the adult filariae. *Am J Trop Med Hyg.* 1972;21:528–545.
2. Meyers WM, Connor DH, Neafie RC. Dipetalonemiasis. In: Binford CA, Connor DH, eds. *Pathology of Tropical and Extraordinary Diseases.* Washington, DC: Armed Forces Institute of Pathology; 1976;2:382–389.
3. Meyers WM, Moris R, Neafie RC, Connor DH, Bourland J. Streptocerciasis: degeneration of adult *Dipetalonema streptocerca* in man following diethylcarbamazine therapy. *Am J Trop Med Hyg.* 1978;27:1137–1147.
4. Price D. Dipetalonemiasis (acanthocheilonemiasis). In: Marcial-Rojas RA, ed. *Pathology of Protozoal and Helminthic Diseases.* Baltimore: Williams and Wilkins; 1971: 951–953.
5. Gardiner CH, Meyers WM, Lanoie LO. Recovery of intact male and female *Dipetalonema streptocerca* from man. *Am J Trop Med Hyg.* 1979;28:49–52.
6. Neafie RC, Connor DH, Meyers WM. *Dipetalonema streptocerca* (Macfie and Corson, 1922). Description of the adult female. *Am J Trop Med Hyg.* 1975;24:264–267.
7. Meyers WM, Neafie RC, Moris R, Bourland J. Streptocerciasis: observation of adult male *Dipetalonema streptocerca* in man. *Am J Trop Med Hyg.* 1977;26:1153–1155.
8. Orihel TC. The tail of the *Mansonella streptocerca* microfilaria. *Am J Trop Med Hyg.* 1984;33:1278.
9. Okelo GB, Kyobe J, Gatiri G. *Mansonella streptocerca* in the Central African Republic. *Trans R Soc Trop Med Hyg.* 1988;82:464.

CHAPTER 171

Oesophagostomiasis

Mark L. Eberhard

And after all this the Lord smote him in his bowels with an incurable disease.

2 Chronicles 21:18

DEFINITION

Oesophagostomiasis is an infection with the strongyle nematode *Oesophagostomum* sp, which are hookworm-like, bursate parasites that inhabit the large intestine where they produce large nodules. Synonyms include helminthoma and pimply gut; the parasite is also referred to as the nodular worm.

GEOGRAPHIC DISTRIBUTION

Oesophagostomiasis is a zoonotic infection in most areas of the world and conceivably could occur wherever the parasite infects domestic or feral animals such as sheep, goats, and pigs or monkeys and apes. The majority of human infections have been reported from Africa, but single infections are documented in Brazil and Indonesia. Undoubtedly, the recognized distribution of infections in humans is confused by the similarity of *Oesophagostomum* and hookworm eggs.

LIFE CYCLE/NATURAL HISTORY/EPIDEMIOLOGY

Adult worms reside in the lumen of the large intestine, where they mate, following which the female worms produce eggs that are passed in the stool. The eggs hatch in the soil and larvae undergo two molts, reaching the infective third stage in 5 to 7 days. Infection is acquired when third-stage larvae are ingested. Percutaneous transmission is not recognized. If swallowed by an appropriate host, larvae burrow into the submucosa of the large bowel where they finish development, return to the lumen of the intestine as adults, attach to the mucosa, and mate, after which the female begins to produce eggs.

Until just recently, human infection was believed to be sporadic, in essence a zoonotic infection, in which there was no human-to-human transmission. However, Polderman and colleagues, working in northern Togo and Ghana, have demonstrated that *Oesophagostomum* is a common infection in some villages and that human-to-human transmission is probable.[1,2] In a survey of more than 3000 inhabitants in 15 villages, 17% of the population was infected. Infection rates were less than 5% in children under 4 years of age, but rose to 17% in 5- to 10-year-olds. Infection in male inhabitants was generally lower than for females, being 14% versus 20% for all age groups. Over 30% of women aged 30 to 39 were infected. Prevalence tended to be higher in villages that were farther from main roads. The route of infection, however, remains obscure. Animals contract *Oesophagostomum* orally during grazing. It is assumed that people also acquire infection by the oral route, but specific vehicles, such as soil, water, foodstuffs, or other means have not been identified as the source of larvae. The area described by Polderman et al[1] is typical Guinea savanna, there being one long rainy season from June until September with the remainder of the year being hot and dry. In this ecologic setting, transmission is also probably seasonal, occurring during or just after the rainy season. Third-stage larvae, however, are resistant to desiccation (Eberhard and Polderman, unpublished data), and other factors may influence the seasonality of transmission.

Unraveling the epidemiology of oesophagostomiasis in this geographic setting will be fascinating. Why the infection is so common in this area yet not elsewhere cannot yet be explained, but it may relate to inadequate diagnostic routines in some areas and the misdiagnosis of *Oesophagostomum* eggs as those of hookworms. Further surveillance with specific attention to identifying cases should shed light on the actual distribution of this infection.

As part of their studies, Krepel and Polderman[3] established that the median worm burden in 12 subjects was 81 worms, with a range from 12 to 300 worms per person. The calculated mean egg production was about 5000 eggs/day/female worm. This compares with the production of other nematodes in the same superfamily, and is slightly less than that for hookworms, which is given as 10,000 to 30,000 eggs/worm/day in humans, depending on the species and worm burden.[4]

CLINICAL AND PATHOLOGIC FEATURES

In humans, the primary clinical features and pathologic changes are caused by invasion of the intestinal wall by juvenile worms. Usually, a distinct nodule 1 to 2 cm in diameter (occasionally up to 4 to 6 cm) is formed around each larva. Typically, a tumor-like nodule is formed, which can become an intestinal abscess with fistulas, and abscess of the abdominal wall. Perforation of the bowel with peritonitis is a life-threatening complication.[5] In certain areas of northern Togo and Ghana, the disease is well known to local villagers as "tumeur de Dapaong" (Figure 171–1), and locally such abdominal masses are referred to as "koulkoul" or "tougnale," which means "having a turtle in your belly" or "abscess in the abdomen," respectively.[1] Traditional treatment included application of heat until the abscess burst.

Abdominal pain, especially in the lower right lower quadrant, is the most frequent clinical feature. Low-grade fever and eosinophilia may be present. It may be possible to palpate an abdominal mass. Clinical diagnosis may be difficult, since amoeboma, schistosomal granulomas, appendicitis, ileocecal tuberculosis, and carcinoma of the cecum may be indistinguishable.

Examination of the intestine reveals a submucosal or subserosal nodule(s) in which the mucosa overlying the lesion appears normal (Figure 171–2). Close examination or dissection usually reveals a tract that leads from the center of the nodule to the lumen of the gut. The center of the nodule is an abscess and contains pus and/or caseous material.

Histologic examination of the nodule may reveal a larva in the center surrounded by a faintly staining exudate (Figure 171–3). Although the nodules are sharply demarcated, the wall is not highly fibrotic. Cellular infiltrate may be marked or not, with eosinophils and macrophages.

MORPHOLOGIC FEATURES OF OESOPHAGOSTOMUM

The adult worms, which are the same general size and shape as hookworms, are 0.5 to 2.5 cm long; female worms are slightly larger than male worms (Figure 171–4). They differ markedly from hookworms, however; the buccal capsule opens forward and is surrounded by a leaf crown or corona radiata, which are highly modified lips (Figures 171–5 and 171–6). *Oesophagostomum* sp that infect humans also have a cervical groove in the cuticle just behind the anterior end (Figure 171–5). The male tail, typical of all

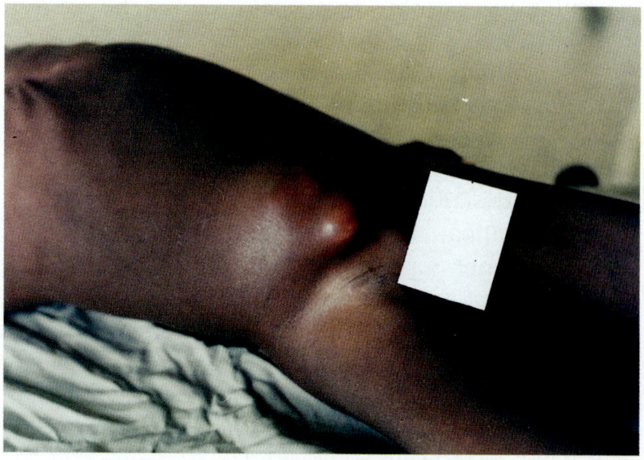

Figure 171–1. Young African boy with a "tumeur de Dapaong," an abdominal abscess caused by oesophagostomiasis. The lesion in the wall of the bowel is draining through a fistula on the abdominal wall. *(Contributed by Dr. A. M. Polderman.)*

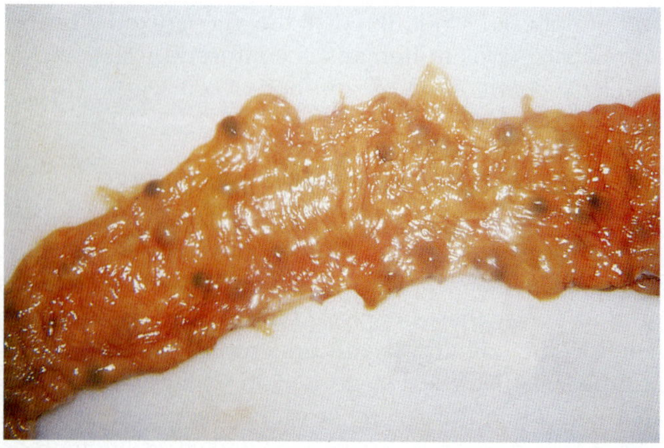

Figure 171–2. The mucosal surface of intestine from a naturally infected macaque monkey showing multiple *Oesophagostomum* nodules.

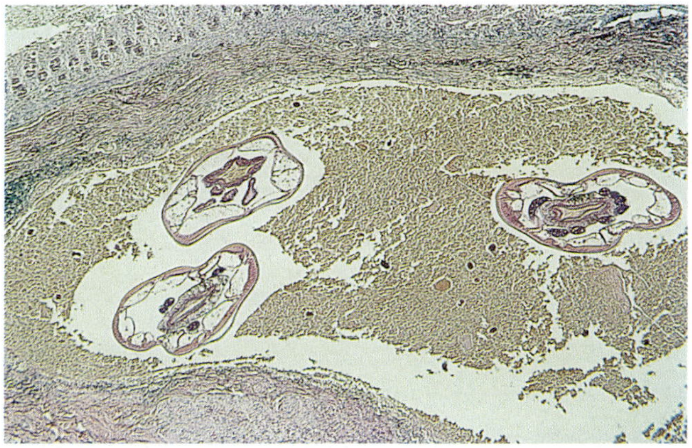

Figure 171–3. *Oesophagostomum* nodule from intestine of the macaque monkey (Figure 171–2). The overlying mucosa, the wall of the nodule and three sections of a larva are all apparent. The worm is surrounded by amorphous debris. Inflammatory cells are few [hematoxylin-eosin (H&E), ×40].

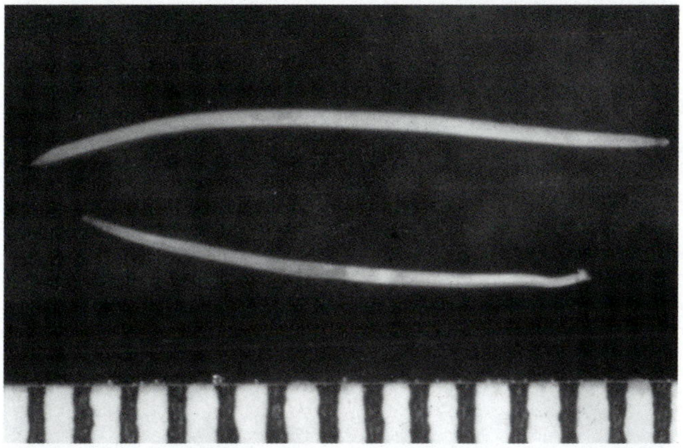

Figure 171–4. Adult male (*lower*) and female (*upper*) *Oesophagostomum* sp recovered from naturally infected macaque monkey (scale is millimeters).

strongyles, has a copulatory bursa. In many of the early reports of human infections, the recovered worms were either immature or stunted and difficult to identify. Polderman and colleagues have identified the worm infecting humans in northern Togo and Ghana as *O bifurcum*.[6]

Where adult worms are present in the gut and eggs are being passed in the stool, the eggs are indistinguishable from hookworm eggs. They are of the same size, shape, and state of embryonation, and measure from 50 to 75 μm long by 30 to 40 μm wide (Figure 171–7).[1,3,4,7] Third-stage (infective) larvae that have been recovered from stool cultures, however, are morphologically distinct from both hookworm larvae and *Strongyloides* larvae.[8] The larvae are about 830 μm long by 30 μm in diameter; they have a characteristic sheath, long threadlike tail, and triangular intestinal cells (Figure 171–8).

Larvae and immature worms in tissue are most often contained in nodules (Figure 171–3). *Oesophagostomum* larvae in nodules can be 500 μm or more in diameter and have a thick cuticle, few muscle cells, which are meromyarian and platymyarian, large vacuolated lateral chords, a prominent multinucleated gut with a heavily ciliated brush border, and an immature but developing reproductive system (Figure 171–9). A minute internal cuticular bead at the level of the lateral chords is present but difficult to see.

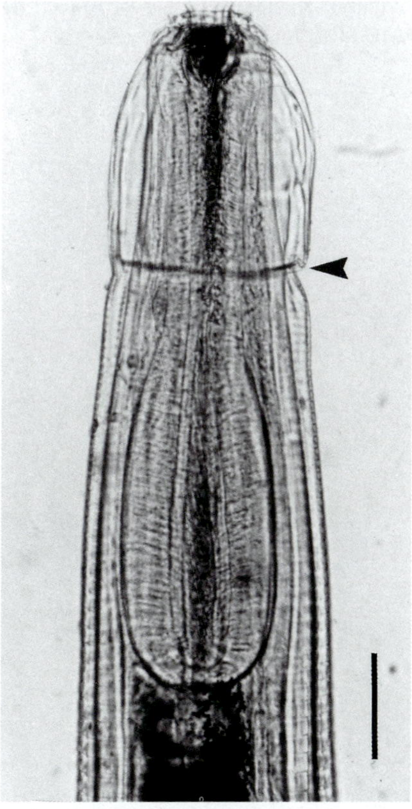

Figure 171–5. Anterior end of adult *O bifurcum* illustrating the forward-facing buccal capsule and the cephalic groove *(arrowhead)* (scale bar = 100 μm). *(With permission of Polderman et al.[1])*

DIFFERENTIAL DIAGNOSIS

A definitive diagnosis of oesophagostomiasis will require gross or microscopic examination of the dissected

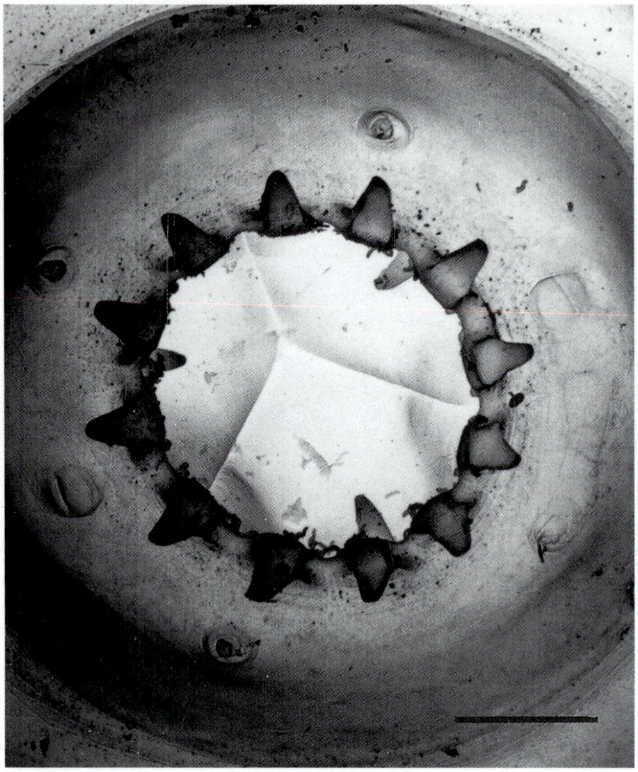

Figure 171–6. *En face* scanning electron micrograph of the corona radiata of *O bifurcum* recovered from man in Africa. The 12 external leaves and three inward facing denticular projections are clearly visible, as is the tripartite valvelike structure, which is actually at the bottom of the buccal capsule (scale bar = 10 μm). *(With permission of Blotkamp et al.[6]).*

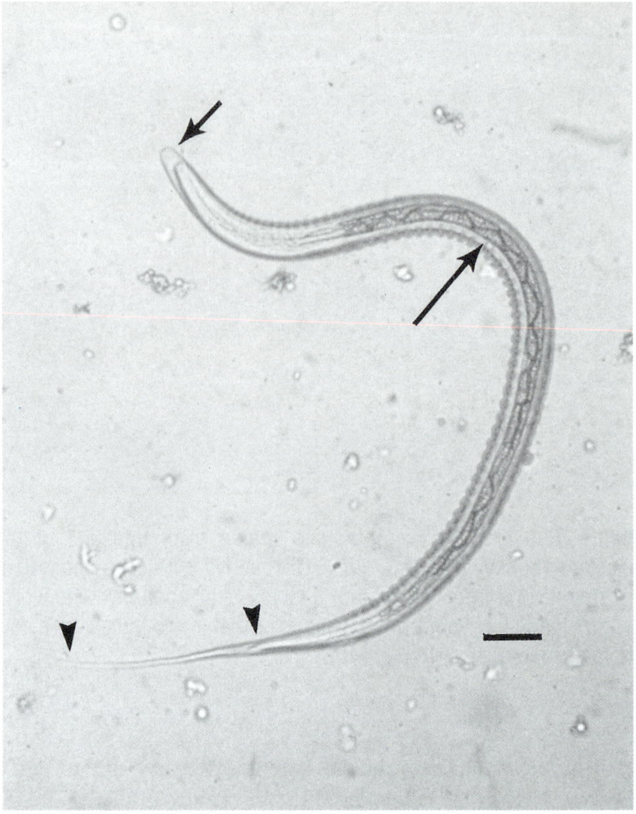

Figure 171–8. Third-stage (infective) larva of *O bifurcum* cultured from human stool showing the characteristic sheath *(short arrow)*, long whiplike tail *(arrowheads)*, and gut composed of prominent, pyramidal-shaped cells *(long arrow)* (scale bar = 50 μm). *(With permission of Blotkamp et al.[6])*

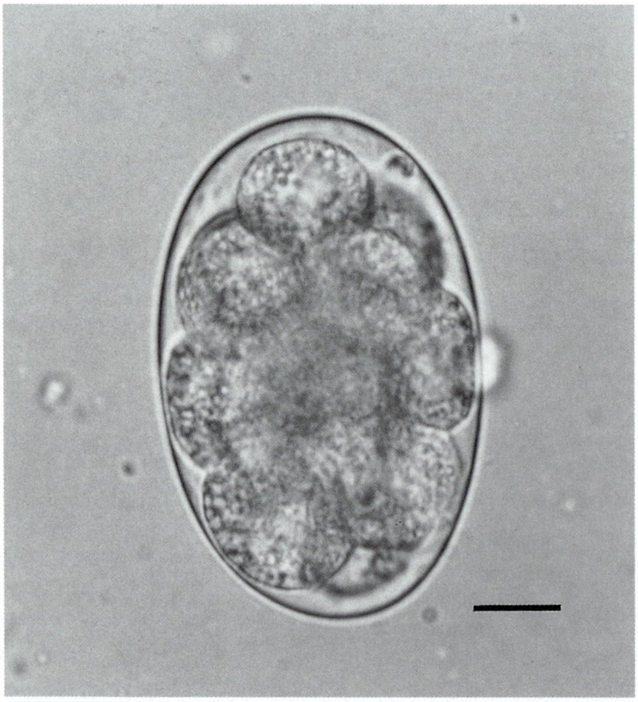

Figure 171–7. *Oesophagostomum* sp egg passed in fresh stool (scale bar = 10 μm).

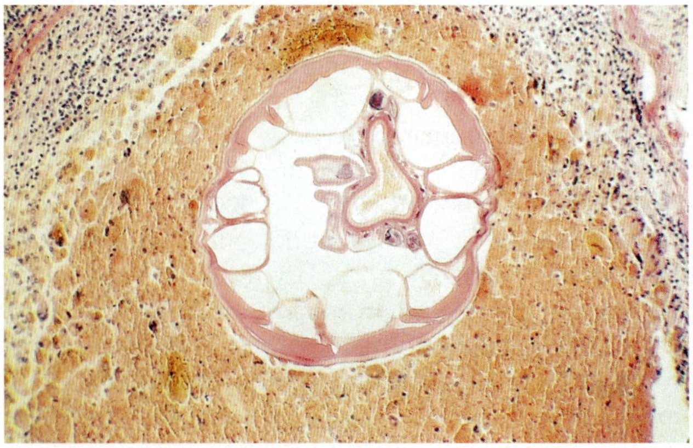

Figure 171–9. High magnification of a cross-section of *Oesophagostomum* sp larva in an intestinal nodule removed from a naturally infected macaque monkey. The large, foamy, lateral chords, few, flat muscle cells, prominent brush border on the intestine, and genital tubes are apparent and characteristic. The worm is surrounded by degenerating macrophages and the wall of the nodule contains lymphocytes, plasma cells, and neutrophils.

lesion (nodule) to exclude amoeboma, schistosomal granuloma, intestinal tuberculosis, or carcinoma. Typical *Oesophagostomum* larvae confirm the diagnosis. Stool examinations may prove unrewarding, especially in those with aberrant infections. However, in light of the recent evidence from studies in Africa, there may be a high rate of patent infection in certain areas, and many infections in endemic populations or in travelers may go undiagnosed or misdiagnosed. To distinguish *Oesophagostomum* infections from hookworms, stool culture must be done and third-stage larvae identified. Third-stage larvae of *Oesophagostomum* are easily distinguished from species of *Strongyloides* and hookworm.

TREATMENT

In Togo, pyrantel pamoate, 10 mg per kg once or twice, cured 59% and 82%, respectively, while a single dose of albendazole, 400 or 800 mg, cured about 85%; levamisole, 50 to 300 mg and thiabendazole, 25 mg/kg for 2 days, were relatively ineffective and cured less than 50%.[9]

REFERENCES

1. Polderman AM, Krepel HP, Baeta S, Blotkamp J, Gigase P. Oesophagostomiasis, a common infection of man in northern Togo and Ghana. *Am J Trop Med Hyg.* 1991;44:336–344.
2. Krepel HP, Baeta S, Polderman AM. Human *Oesophagostomum* infection in northern Togo and Ghana: epidemiological aspects. *Ann Trop Med Parasitol.* 1992;86:289–300.
3. Krepel HP, Polderman AM. Egg production of *Oesophagostomum bifurcum,* a locally common parasite of humans in Togo. *Am J Trop Med Hyg.* 1992;46:469–472.
4. Beaver PC, Jung RL, Cupp EW. *The Strongylida: Hookworms and other Bursate Nematodes. Clinical Parasitology 1984.* 9th ed. Philadelphia: Lea & Febiger; 1984:269–301.
5. Haaf E, van Soest AH. Oesophagostomiasis in man in Northern Ghana. *Trop Geogr Med.* 1964;16:49–53.
6. Blotkamp J, Krepel HP, Kumar V, Baeta S, van't Noordende JM, Polderman AM. Observations on the morphology of adults and larval stages of *Oesophagostomum* sp isolated from man in northern Togo and Ghana. *J Helminthol.* 1993;67:49–61.
7. Goldsmid JM. Studies on the life cycle and biology of *Ternidens deminutus* (Railliet and Henry, 1905) (Nematoda: Strongylidae). *J Helminthol.* 1971;45:341–352.
8. Little MD. Differentiation of nematode larvae in coproculture: guidelines for routine practice in medical laboratories. *WHO Tech Rep Ser.* 1981;666:144–150.
9. Krepel HP, Haring T, Baeta S, Polderman AM. Treatment of mixed *Oesophagostomum* and hookworm infection: effect of albendazole, pyrantel pamoate, levamisole and thiabendazole. *Trans R Soc Trop Med Hyg.* 1993;87:87–89.

Chapter 172

Onchocerciasis

Kimberley Studeman, James L. Fishback, and Daniel H. Connor

The poor, and the maimed, and the halt, and the blind.

Luke 14:21

DEFINITION AND OVERVIEW

Onchocerciasis is infection by the filarial nematode *Onchocerca volvulus,* which is transmitted from person to person by blackflies of the genus *Simulium.* Onchocerciasis is strictly tropical in the sense that the disease must be acquired in the tropics. Patients with light infections have few clinical manifestations, but those with severe infections have a combination of clinical features dominated by one or more of three cardinal manifestations: 1) a persistent, itching dermatitis; 2) cutaneous and subcutaneous nodules; and 3) progressive ocular keratitis. Before World War II, onchocerciasis was barely known in the western world. Few medical scientists had heard of onchocerciasis, and those who had tended to think of it as a remote infection characterized by a few benign parasitic nodules in the skin. Now, however, onchocerciasis is recognized as a debilitating and blinding infection with social and economic effects extending far beyond the suffering of the afflicted. The itching of onchocercal dermatitis, for instance, may prevent restful sleep or productive work, and onchocercal blindness adds a heavy burden to primitive agrarian cultures, decreasing productivity in regions where crops are sewn and harvested by hand (Figure 172–1). Furthermore, onchocerciasis is a cumulative disease. Among those exposed to the continuous bites of blackflies, clinical manifestations become progressively worse as the months and years pass. However, the occasional medical scientist, biologist, sportsman, or politician who visits endemic areas and becomes infected develops no serious complications and the infection is easily managed.[1] An estimated 17.75 million people were infected worldwide in 1985. Of these, 340,000 were blind and a like number had seriously impaired vision.[2] Most persons afflicted with onchocerciasis live in the endemic areas of tropical Africa; the remainder live in Mexico, Guatemala, Venezuela, Brazil, and Colombia and tend to be poor, rural people, who, by habit and tradition, live beyond the councils of government and the benefits of effective public health.

EARLY HISTORY

A British naval surgeon, John O'Neill,[3] first described filarial dermatitis in natives of the Gold Coast (now Ghana), and the technique he used to identify microfilariae survives as a standard diagnostic test—that is, the skin snip (Figure 172–2). Rudolph Leuckart, Professor of Zoology at the University of Leipzig, first saw adult *O volvulus* worms in a specimen sent to him from West Africa. This was reported at an international meeting in London in 1891. At that meeting, Sir Patrick Manson read a letter from Professor Leuckart and concluded that Professor Leuckart " . . . will give us in due time a careful and exhaustive description of these interesting parasites. . . ."[4] Brumpt[5] first noted that 1) endemic areas were along rivers, 2) microfilariae in skin came from adult filariae coiled in deep cutaneous nodules, and 3) the microfilariae did not enter the blood. He thus deduced that the arthropod vector of *O volvulus* would be a riverine tissue feeder, not a mosquito or other blood-sucking arthropod. Robles[6] first described onchocerciasis in the western hemisphere. Blacklock[7] identified the *Simulium* vector in 1925, Torroella[8] saw microfilariae in the eye in 1931, and Mazzotti[9] described diagnostic and therapeutic effects of diethylcarbamazine (DEC) in 1944. The detailed description of the

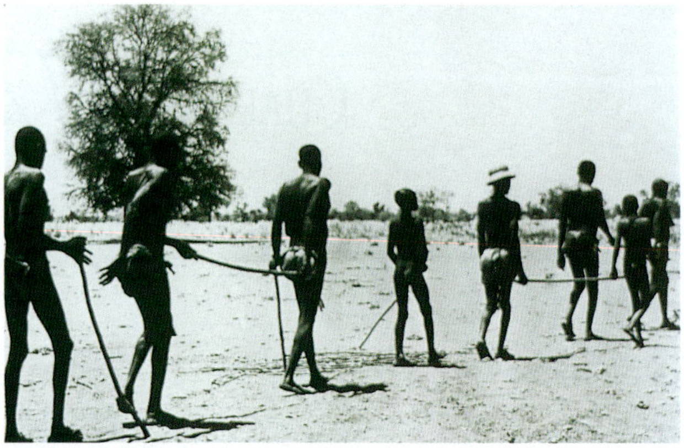

Figure 172–1. One of the great medical photographs of the century was taken by a World Health Organization (WHO) contract photographer, and tells a tragic story. Chadians, blinded by onchocerciasis, are being led by children into the fields to help cultivate the crops. Because they are blind, their work will be inefficient. The story is doubly tragic, however, because the children who now lead the blind will, in turn, become blind from onchocercal eye disease. This photograph, first widely circulated on the WHO calendar for 1967, helped bring the impact of onchocerciasis to medical scientists in western countries. Subsequent attempts to photograph similar scenes have failed to capture the action and ambiance of this photograph. *(Courtesy of the World Health Organization, 1967.)*

adult male and female worms, for which Sir Patrick Manson patiently waited, was never completed by Professor Leuckart. In fact, more than 80 years passed before a detailed description was done—a period during which many nodules and worms had been removed and studied. The barrier to a detailed description was formidable because the removed worms were tightly coiled and bound in dense fibrous connective tissue. In 1972, however, Ronald C. Neafie,[10] diagnostic parasitologist at the Armed Forces Institute of Pathology, meticulously reconstructed models of adult *O volvulus* worms from serially cut paraffin sections, and his descriptions of the adult male and female *O volvulus* worms are models of lucidity, photomicrography, and brevity. More details of the early history are recorded in Connor et al[4] and in Gibson et al.[11]

Synonyms

Simulium flies, the vector for onchocerciasis, develop in fast-flowing rivers and streams; common synonyms for onchocerciasis, therefore, include "river blindness" and "white-water disease" (Figure 172–3). Onchocerciasis has also been called "blinding filarial disease," "enfermedad de Robles" (after Robles' classic description of New World onchocerciasis in 1919),[6] "mal marado," "craw-craw," "erisipela de la costa," "ceguera de los rios," and "gâl filarienne" (literally, filarial scabies).

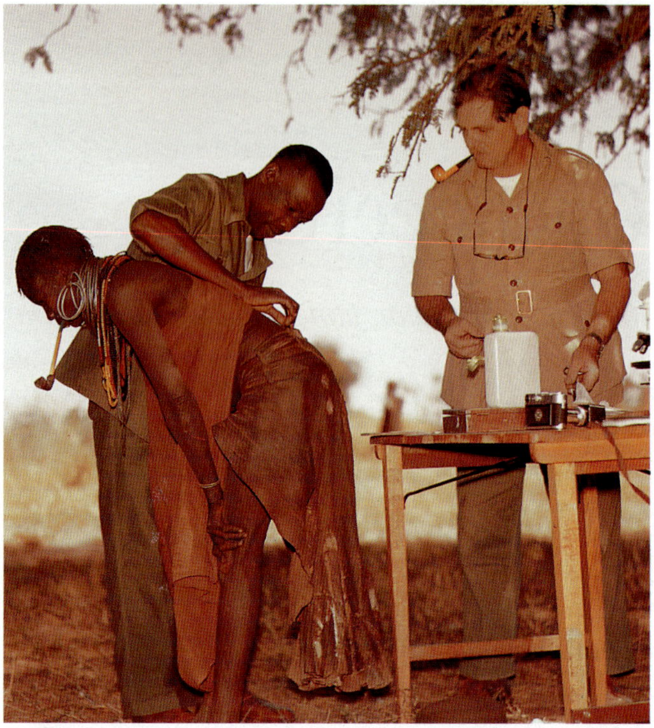

Figure 172–2. Here, the late Major George M. Barnley, government entomologist in Uganda, with his colleague Semakula, is doing a skin snip on a patient in northeastern Uganda in 1962, as part of a parasitologic survey. The skin snip was first used by British surgeon John O'Neill in 1875 to identify microfilariae in the skins of six Gold Coast (Ghana) Africans. O'Neill looked at the snips under a microscope and described "twisting and contorting" microfilariae. Major Barnley was one of the first to control transmission of onchocerciasis by dosing streams and rivers with larvacide. Trained in armaments during World War II, he strung steel drums containing paradichlorodiphenyltrichloroethane on a cable across the Victoria Nile just below the Owen Falls Dam. He exploded the drums simultaneously, instantly dosing the breadth of the river. As the insecticide swept downstream, Simulium larvae fed on the insecticide, released their grip on the trailing vegetation and were, in turn, swept downstream. Fish then fed on the bobbing larvae and were killed by insecticide. *Simulium* larvae were eliminated for about 50 miles downstream. With the vector fly gone, transmission of onchocerciasis ceased along this stretch of Nile, and 10 years later, in 1962, even though *Simulium* flies had repopulated the mouths of some of the small tributaries, all people 10 years of age and younger were free of onchocerciasis.

Geographic Distribution

Four features define most endemic areas: 1) a tropical setting, 2) a turbulent stream, 3) vegetation trailing in the stream (to which the blackfly larvae adhere), and 4) humans harboring the reservoir parasites. Thus, onchocerciasis prevails in tropical areas, where biting simulidae are abundant. As noted, endemic areas tend to be along the banks of turbulent stretches of rivers, in

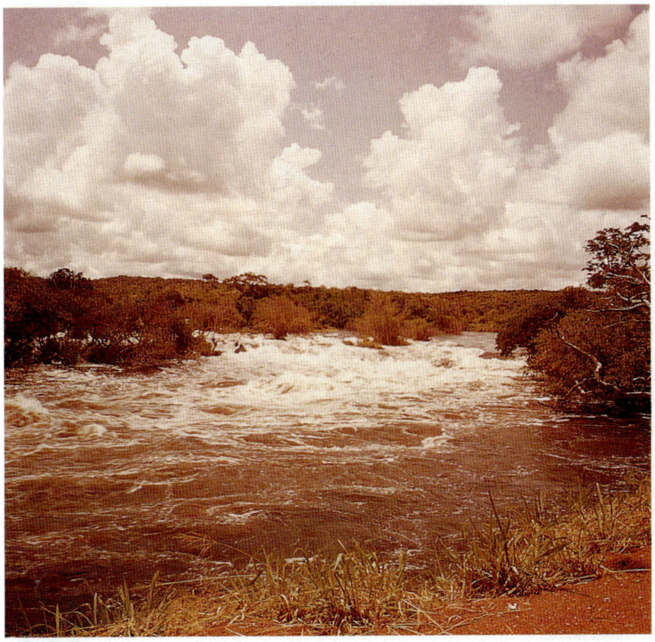

Figure 172–3. Well aerated turbulent waters, such as the Karuma Falls along the course of the Victoria Nile in Uganda, are ideal breeding sites for simulidae. Persons living near these stretches of "white water" are frequently infected—hence the African name "white-water disease."

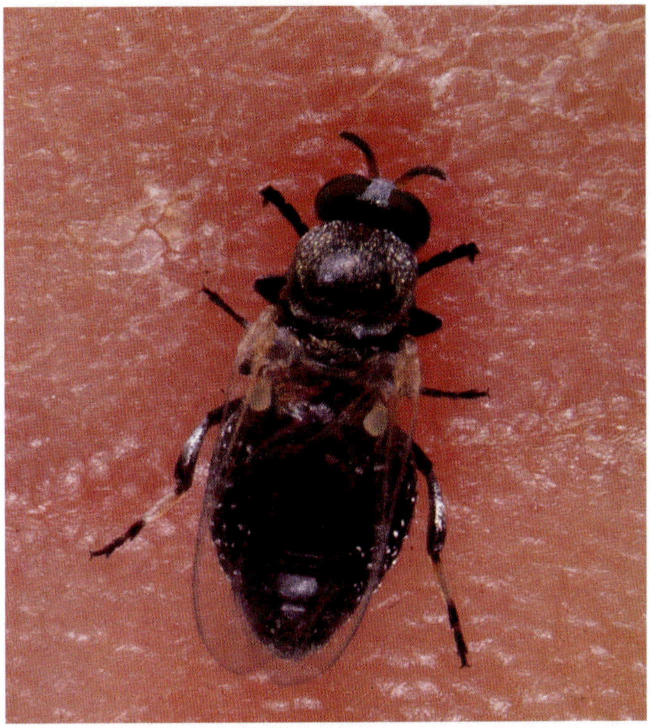

Figure 172–4. One of the *Simulium damnosum* Theobold complex, a major vector of *Onchocerca volvulus* in Africa, feeding on the arm of a volunteer on the banks of the Mongo River near Baduma, Cameroon. The fly had been feeding for about 90 seconds when this picture was taken, and its abdomen is distended with the meal. A focus of erythema has formed around the bite and it remained for about an hour. This fly is 3.0 mm long and 1.2 mm at the widest distension of its abdomen.

which larvae of vector flies mature. The larvae of the vector flies are attached to vegetation trailing in the stream (see legend, Figure 172–2), and the larvae that survive are those in water with a high oxygen content. Onchocerciasis, therefore, is a riparian disease afflicting those who live near, or frequent, turbulent stretches of river throughout the breadth of tropical Africa—from Guinea, Sierra Leone, and Liberia in the west, through Mali, Ivory Coast, Upper Volta, Ghana, Togo, Nigeria, Angola, Tanzania, Malawi, Chad, Cameroon, the Central African Republic, Zaire, and Sudan to Ethiopia and Uganda. Onchocerciasis also extends into Saudi Arabia and into North and South Yemen. In Kenya, onchocerciasis has been eradicated by controlling and eliminating the vector flies. Central and South America have foci of onchocerciasis in Guatemala, Mexico, Venezuela, Colombia, Ecuador, and Brazil. The vector in West Africa is chiefly *Simulium damnosum* (Figure 172–4). In central and South America, *S exiguum, S guianense, S metallicum, S oyapockense, S quadrivittatum,* and *S ochraceum* all transmit *O volvulus; S ochraceum* being the principal vector (Figure 172–5).

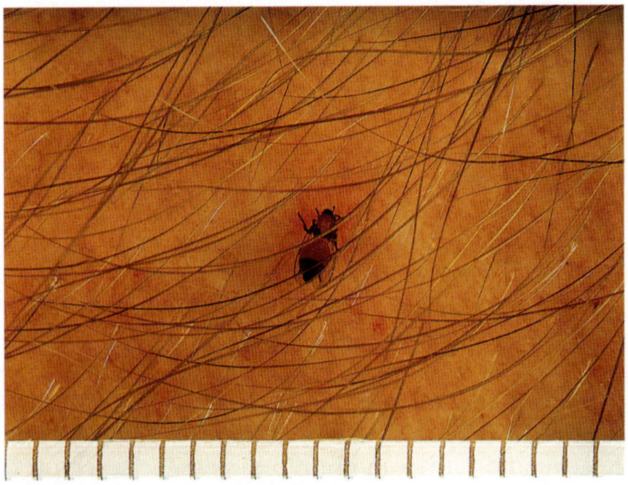

Figure 172–5. *Simulium ochraceum*, a major vector of *Onchocerca volvulus* in Central and South America, is feeding on the arm of a volunteer at one of Guatemala's coffee plantations—Finca de Oro. *S ochraceum* is 2 mm long by 1 mm wide. Robles discovered onchocerciasis in Guatemala in 1915 and published his findings in 1919, hence the name "Robles' disease."

Control Programs

In the 1930s, public health officials in Guatemala began a program to reduce onchocerciasis. The Guatemalans

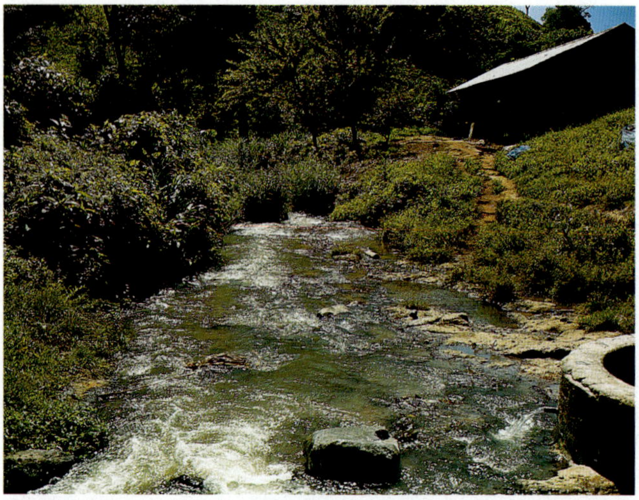

Figure 172–6. A turbulent stream traversing one of Guatemala's coffee plantations. These streams are fast-moving and ideal breeding sites for blackflies. Migrant laborers enter the plantations at harvest time and are then susceptible to the bites of the blackflies.

most severely afflicted were the migrant laborers who, in season, harvested the coffee crops on Guatemala's plantations. The streams traversing the plantations were breeding sites for the American vector simulidae (Figure 172–6). The focus of the program was nodulectomy. Teams of expertly trained technicians excised all detectable nodules. Over the months and years, thousands of nodules were removed (Figure 172–7), and studies suggest that the nodulectomy program has reduced serious complications of onchocerciasis, including blindness, but that it has not reduced the overall prevalence, perhaps for reasons to be discussed, namely that more lightly infected people tend to be the more efficient reservoirs of microfilariae.

A more comprehensive eradication program, started in West Africa in 1975 by the International Bank for Reconstruction and Development (IBRD) and the World Health Organization (WHO), arrested transmission in the areas monitored and treated. Program managers from the WHO Onchocerciasis Control Program (OCP) hope to eradicate onchocerciasis throughout western Africa by the year 2025. The thrust of the program has been to spray the vector rivers and streams with abate and *Bacillus thuringiensis,* two biodegradable insecticides, at regular intervals. Ivermectin, an effective and safe drug used to reduce the reservoir of microfilariae in the skin, may replace or augment the larvaciding of streams. In one report, however, 44% of patients still had microfilariae in their skin after 4 treatments over 17 months.[12] Ivermectin by itself, therefore, may not be sufficient by itself to eliminate onchocerciasis in a community. Nevertheless, the OCP has been

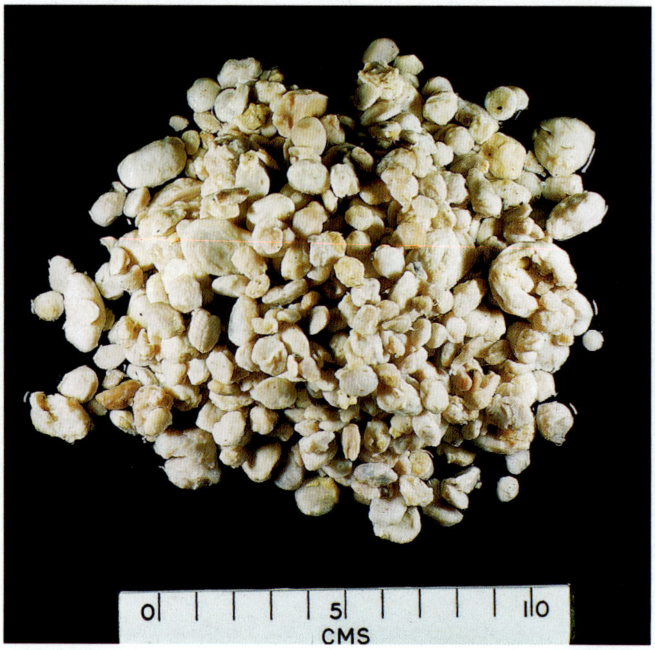

Figure 172–7. A handful of onchocercal nodules removed from Guatemala's migrant laborers. These nodules were stored in 5 gallon pickle jars on shelves that lined the office of the then director of the program, Dr. José Bernhard. Visiting scientists were welcome to a handful. The nodulectomy program reduced the serious complications of onchocerciasis, including blindness, but did not, apparently, reduce prevalence.

studied extensively by computer models, which predict that the dosing of streams by pesticide can be stopped now, and that prevalence will continue to decrease until it reaches zero.[13] Close monitoring will confirm or modify this prediction. For a historical review of vector control, see Davies.[14]

Life Cycle

Adult *O volvulus* worms live in human subcutaneous tissue and fascia. Following copulation, each female worm produces millions of microfilariae, which migrate freely throughout the host's body. Some of the microfilariae are drawn by light to the upper dermis, where they are available to the vector blackfly when it bites. Blackflies are tissue feeders, not blood suckers. They have coarse mouth parts that rip and tear through the keratin and epidermis, to the tips of the dermal papillae, making a mulch of the keratin, cellular debris, tissue fluid, and some serum and blood from torn capillaries. In the process, the fly's saliva attracts microfilariae and acts as an anticoagulant, keeping the mulch liquid and allowing the fly to suck it in. Once ingested by the fly, microfilariae traverse the fly's intestine, migrate to the flight muscles, and mature to become infective larvae in 7 to 9 days. Infective larvae, when

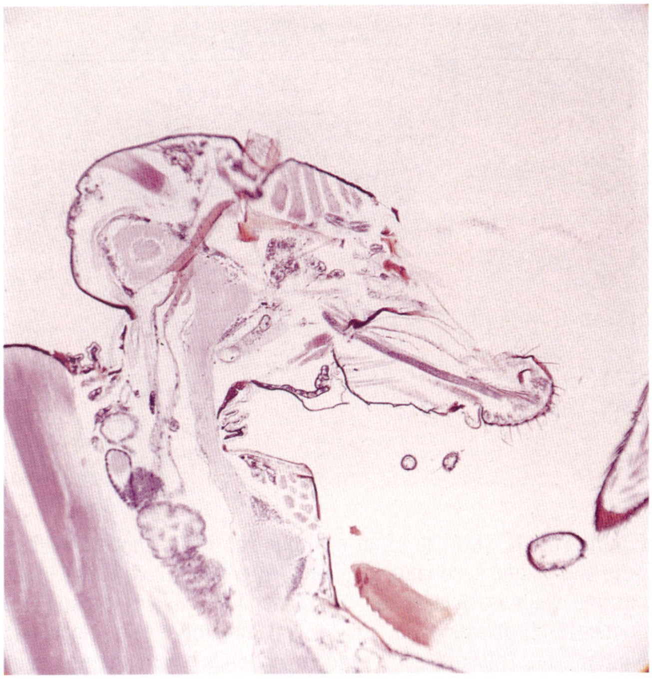

Figure 172–8. Sagittal section through head of a *Simulium* sp with an infective larva in its mouth. This larva is poised to enter the skin of the next victim (hematoxylin-eosin, ×50). *(Photograph courtesy of the late Major George M. Barnley, 1962.)*

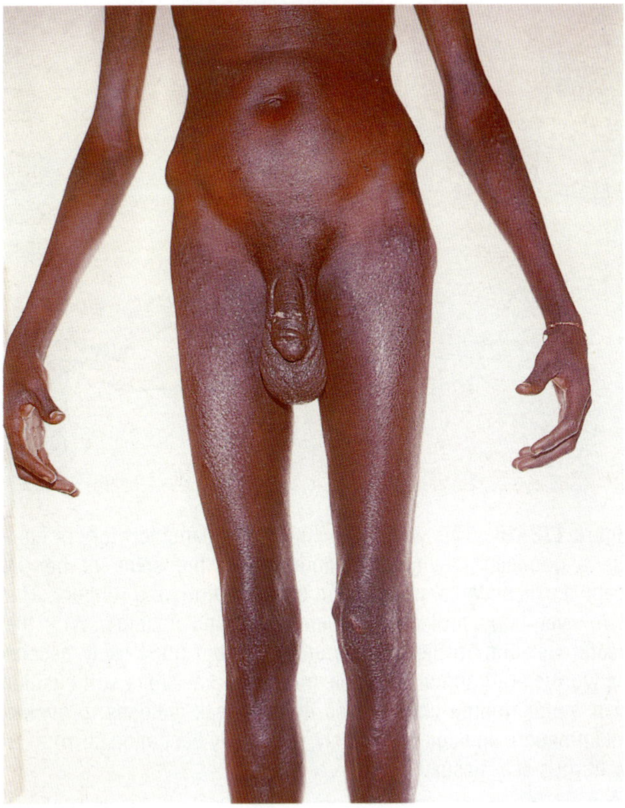

Figure 172–9. This patient, living in Businga, Zaire (situated on the Mongala tributary of the Zaire River), has onchocerca nodules in the deep skin and subcutaneous tissue over his elbows, ribs, iliac crests and spines, trochanters and knees. Note also the papular dermatitis of thighs, thickened scrotal skin, and depigmentation of penile skin—all features of onchocercal dermatitis.

mature, leave the fly's muscles, migrate to the mouth parts of the fly, and are passed to a victim when the fly next feeds (Figure 172–8). Once inside the human host, infective larvae develop into adult worms in the dermis and deep fascia, molting twice (presumably) before maturing. Following copulation, the adult female worms produce microfilariae, thus completing the life cycle. At some point (before or after copulation), adult worms coil up and are surrounded by fibrous connective tissue, forming the characteristic onchocercal nodules (onchocercomas) (Figures 172–9 and 172–10).

Some points in the life cycle are of special interest. When feeding is undisturbed, the fly becomes so heavy with tissue juices, debris, cells, and possibly microfilariae that it may be unable to fly; instead, it rolls to the ground—a phenomenon called "rodadores" in Central America. Furthermore, flies with many larvae in their flight muscles may be paralyzed—unable to fly again, and thus unable to infect. This phenomenon enforces a built-in biologic control, in the sense that, when many onchocercal larvae develop in the fly and paralyze it, the onchocercal larvae in the fly are at a dead end. Thus, the more lightly infected person has the more dangerous reservoir of parasites. In spite of this, many persons living in endemic areas are bitten repeatedly and, over the years, acquire many parasites. Although a few microfilariae circulate in the blood from time to time—especially after treatment with antimicrofilarial drugs—the vast majority of microfilariae are extravascular. Brumpt,[5] as already noted, was the first to recognize the significance of this, for he accurately forecast in 1904 that the vector would be a tissue-feeding, rather than a blood-sucking arthropod. At some point, perhaps when the worm is over a bony prominence and thus more susceptible to trauma, an inflammatory reaction surrounds it, eventually confining it within a fibrous capsule (Figures 172–9 and 172–10). As a patient's burden of adult worms increases over the years, microfilariae concentrate in the upper dermis (Figure 172–11), in the eyes (Figure 172–12), and in lymph nodes (Figure 172–13). Even if transmission is interrupted by killing the vector, adult worms survive in humans for 15 years or more, and microfilariae may persist for up to 2 years after all adult worms have died.[2]

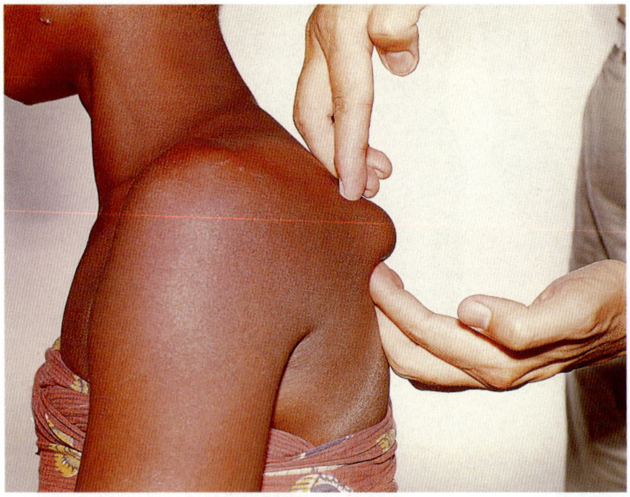

Figure 172–10. This woman, living in the Ubangi territory of Zaire, has a dominant onchocercal nodule over the spine of her left scapula. Onchocercal nodules are painless, firm, and rubbery. They form over bony projections—here the scapular spine. Why they locate over bony projections is unknown, but most likely because the worms are traumatized while migrating. Lacking a soft cushion, even minor trauma could cause them to leak antigens, provoking inflammation, and coil defensively, eventually becoming surrounded by fibrous scar tissue.

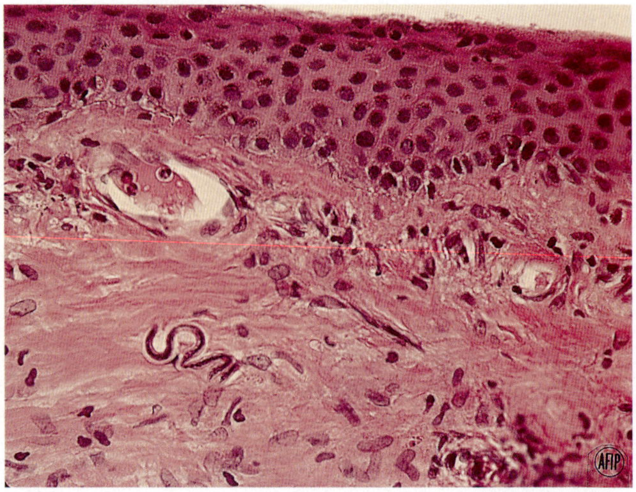

Figure 172–12. Cornea of an eye removed for onchocercal blindness and painful secondary glaucoma. There are microfilariae in the stroma, which is vascularized with dilated tortuous vessels and also contains fibroblasts and mixed inflammatory cells, including lymphocytes, plasma cells, and eosinophils (hematoxylin-eosin, ×200). (AFIP 65-2023.)

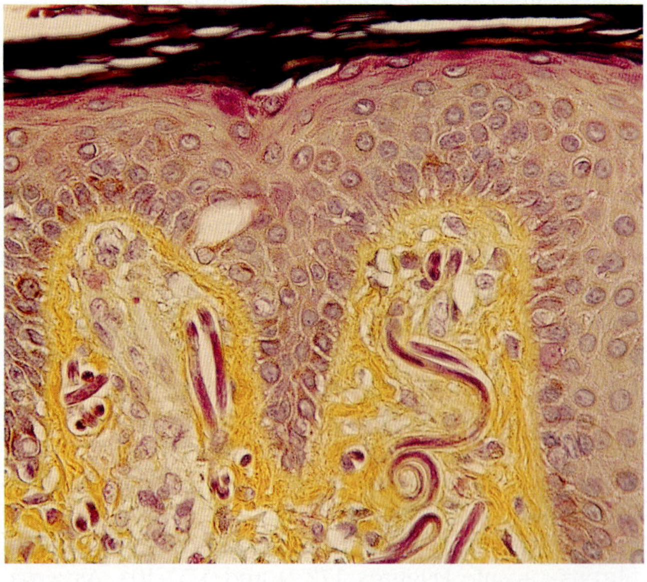

Figure 172–11. Microfilariae in the skin of a patient with onchocercal dermatitis. The microfilariae tend to concentrate in the dermal papillae, where they are available to the vector blackflies when they bite and feed. Other features of onchocercal dermatitis in this section include hyperkeratosis, acanthosis, and sclerosis of the dermis, including sclerosis of the band of areolar connective tissue beneath the basal layer (Movat ×305). (AFIP 76-1318.)

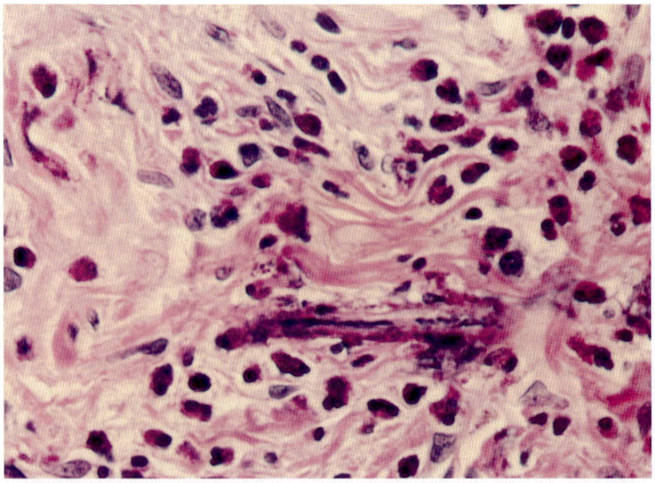

Figure 172–13. Section of a lymph node excised from a patient in Togo with onchocercal lymphadenitis. The microfilaria is disintegrating, and eosinophils, some intact and some degranulating, populate the surrounding fibrous connective tissue, which has replaced the normal lymphoid tissue (hematoxylin-eosin ×350). (AFIP 76-1299).

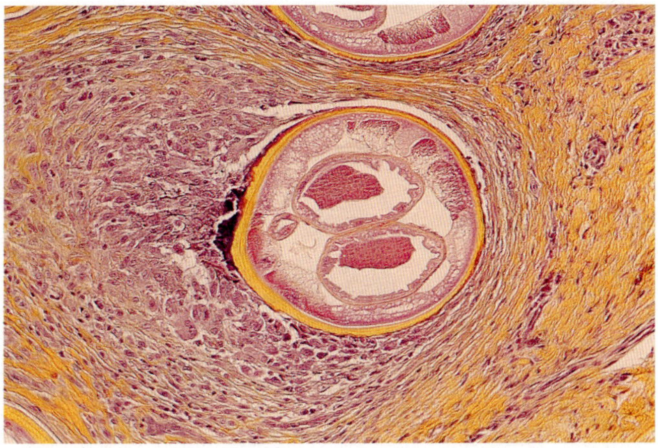

Figure 172–14. Cross-section of an adult female worm showing the worm's cuticle, musculature, paired uteri, and smaller digestive tube. On the left, dark-staining host material, which includes fibrin and immune complexes, is eroding the worm's cuticle. The surrounding connective tissue contains histiocytes, epithelioid cells, and occasional giant cells.

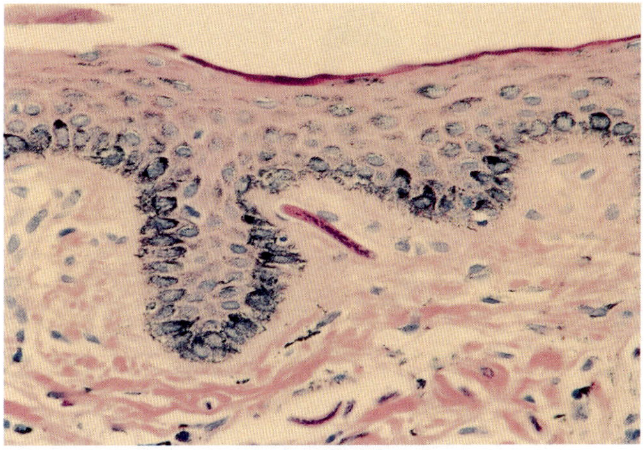

Figure 172–15. A microfilaria of *Onchocerca volvulus* in a dermal papilla showing the anterior "clear" space, which here is 8 μm long. This single plane of section does not show all the anterior nuclei, the first 2 or 3 of which are side by side. These features distinguish microfilariae of *O volvulus* from microfilariae of *Mansonella streptocerca,* the other microfilaria that lives in human dermal collagen. In the lower part of the picture a second microfilaria of *O volvulus* is in a dilated lymphatic vessel (Giemsa ×390). (AFIP 77-8391.)

The Organism

The adult *O volvulus* is a filiform (thread-like) white worm. Female worms are 23 to 50 cm long and 0.25 to 0.45 mm across, with regularly spaced cuticular annulations, which at midbody are about 70 μm apart. Transverse sections reveal a cuticle, hypodermis, somatic muscle, and various internal structures depending on level of cut (Figure 172–14). In the anterior region of gravid female worms there is a pair of coiled uterine tubes containing microfilariae. Sections at midbody reveal multiple loops of thin-walled uteri; the posterior region contains ovaries, oviducts and intestine. The male worm is shorter (16 to 42 mm long), more slender than the female (0.13 to 0.21 mm across), with adjacent cuticular annulations 5 to 10 μm apart. The reproductive apparatus is a single tube extending almost the length of the worm; spermatozoa may fill the vas deferens in the posterior region. For a more detailed description of the identifying features of *O volvulus,* see Neafie.[10] Microfilariae lack a sheath, are 220 to 360 μm long, 5 to 9 μm wide, and have a cephalic clear space that varies from 7 to 13 μm from anterior end to first nucleus, and the first 2 or 3 nuclei are side by side (Figure 172–15). The caudal clear space varies from 9 to 15 μm from the terminal nucleus to the end of the microfilaria, and the terminal nuclei are elongated (Figure 172–16). Ultrastructural features, before and after treatment with DEC, are described in reference 15.

Immunology

It is clear from the histopathology of onchocerciasis that microfilariae and adult worms cause a broad spectrum of cellular and humoral reactions. In a series of lymph nodes excised from Africans with onchocerciasis, almost all had features of immunodeficiency.[16] Some patients appear to be profoundly and specifically im-

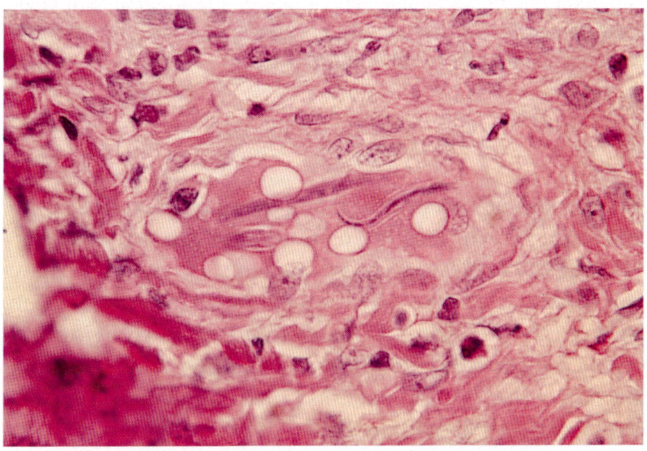

Figure 172–16. A folded microfilaria of *Onchocerca volvulus* in a vessel in a lymph node showing both anterior and posterior ends. Note the elongated nuclei at the caudal end (hematoxylin-eosin ×650). (AFIP 70-11370.)

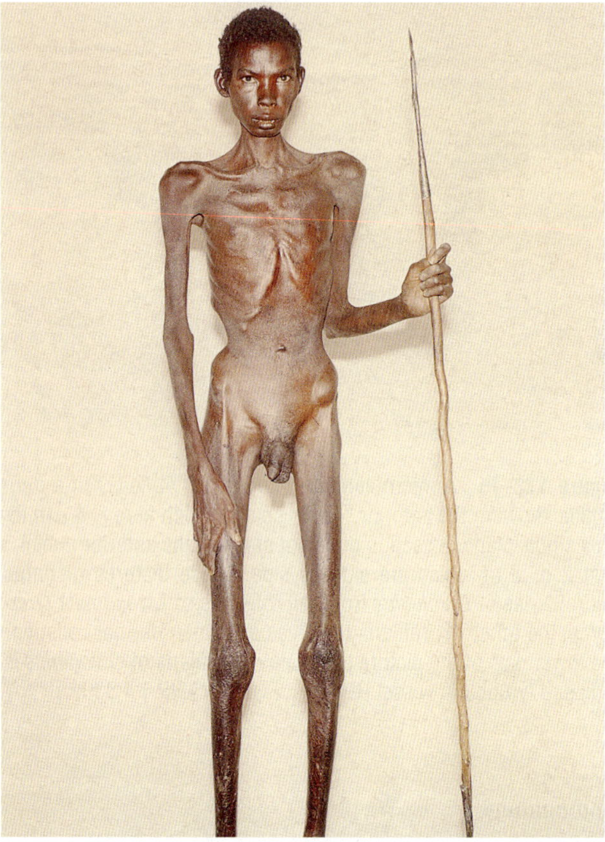

Figure 172–17. This young Chadian resident of Ouli Bangala was so weak that he required a stick to hold himself erect for this picture. He had no evidence of tuberculosis or cancer (clinically or by portable chest x ray), but he did have enormous numbers of microfilariae in his skin. Note the onchocercal nodules over his left iliac spine and over his right lateral chest wall. There is some depigmentation and wrinkling of his shins, but his skin is remarkably smooth in spite of the enormous numbers of microfilariae it contains. Although one of his nodules and a biopsy specimen of skin would have been valuable scientifically, his weakened state prevented even the consideration of minor surgery.

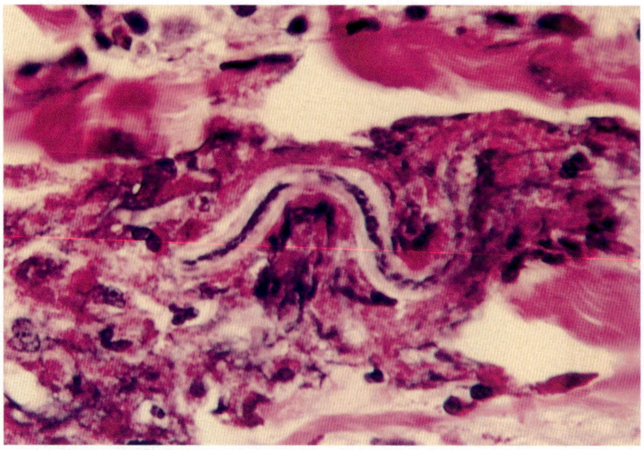

Figure 172–18. Within minutes after treatment with diethylcarbamazine (DEC), degranulating eosinophils collect around microfilariae, and major basic protein from the eosinophils is deposited on the surfaces of the microfilariae. The eosinophil, therefore, has a special role in the inflammatory response to degenerating microfilariae and probably also in their demise. The skins of heavily infected patients become graveyards for dead and dying microfilariae. Stages in their demise (by light microscopy) are 1) intense eosinophilia of the microfilaria, 2) fibrinoid material around the microfilariae, which immunofluorescent staining reveals to be major basic protein from degranulating eosinophils, and 3) nuclei of the degenerating microfilaria becoming hyperchromatic, fragmented, and, finally, indistinct. This specimen of skin was taken 3.5 hours after the patient was treated with 50 mg of DEC by mouth. The degenerating microfilaria is surrounded by degranulating eosinophils (hematoxylin-eosin ×890). (AFIP 75-1511.)

munotolerant, accommodating enormous numbers of microfilariae in their skin with little or no reaction[17] (Figure 172–17). In most patients, however, intact microfilariae in the skin cause little or no reaction, apparently persisting for weeks and months, living harmoniously among the dermal collagen fibers of their human hosts. Other patients, including North Yemenites with the syndrome called "sowda,"[18] have an intense dermatitis with very few microfilariae in their skin. When a microfilaria degenerates, however, either from aging, by triggering an inflammatory reaction, or by being "unmasked" by microfilaricidal drugs, the microfilaria is surrounded almost immediately by eosinophils, the closest of which degranulate, forming a layer of eosinophilic material. This material includes major basic protein and probably other toxic proteins from the eosinophil that collect around the microfilaria as it degenerates (Figure 172–18).[19] Other degenerating microfilariae provoke a granulomatous reaction (Figure 172–19), thus appearing to have a slower death or, at least, a slower disintegration. Lymph nodes taken from Africans living in endemic areas with long-standing onchocercal dermatitis tend to have atrophic germinal centers and many microfilariae. Yemenites, however, have enlarged hyperplastic regional lymph nodes with many large germinal centers and few microfilariae.

Recent studies on the immunology of the onchocercal nodule reveal that macrophages and T lymphocytes predominate and have a unique arrangement that suggests immune attack. Small macrophages and T lymphocytes are in the perivascular regions around the nodule. Many macrophages with dendritic processes are in the hyaline matrix, and T cells are rare in this region. Macrophages surrounding the worm are more heterogeneous in shape, and there are occasional giant cells. Macrophages are the predominant cell in physical contact with the worm. T cells, particularly

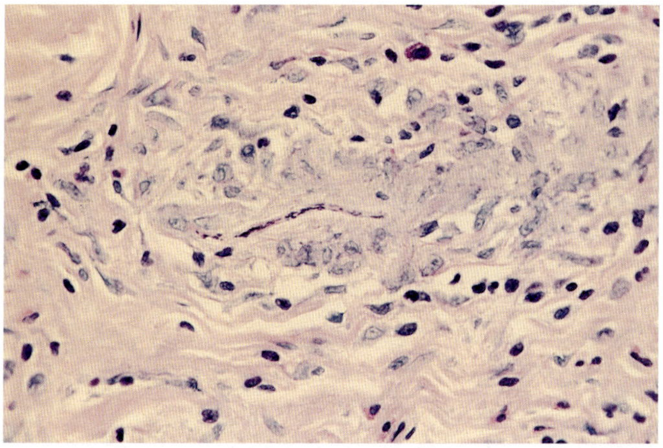

Figure 172–19. A degenerating microfilaria in a patient treated 24 hours earlier with diethylcarbamazine. A tight granuloma composed of epithelioid cells and giant cells surrounds the microfilaria (Giemsa ×375). (AFIP 69-8464.)

Figure 172–20. Altered pigmentation over the hip of a Zairian woman with onchocercal dermatitis. Macules may be hyper- or hypopigmented. Overexposure of the photographic film, as was done here, may be required to demonstrate subtle changes of pigmentation in early onchodermatitis in dark skin.

CD4+, surround the infiltrate but rarely come in contact with the worm.[20–22] B lymphocytes and neutrophils are scarce.

When skin densities of microfilariae, cellular reactions, in vitro production of cytokines IL-2, IL-4, IFN-γ by monocytes, responses of patients to *O volvulus* antigen, PPD and Streptococcal SL-O antigens, and detection of *O volvulus* specific-IgG1–4 were determined during a period of treatment with ivermectin lasting 8 years, the results clearly indicated that treated patients gradually recovered from their onchocerca-induced immunodeficiencies.[23]

In his review of the immunopathogenesis of onchocerciasis, Ottesen[24] suggests that microfilariae elaborate molecules that inhibit both humoral and cell-mediated responses by the host to the antigens of the microfilariae. There is evidence that this inhibition is accomplished by stimulating T suppressor cells or by stimulating T cells that produce down-regulating cytokines such as IL-4. Whether microfilariae are successful in a particular host (survive for a long time) depends on the ability of the microfilariae to stimulate anti-inflammatory host molecules and anti-inflammatory mechanisms.

CLINICO-PATHOLOGIC CORRELATIONS

Skin

Onchodermatitis is caused by an inflammatory reaction to antigens released by degenerating microfilariae in the dermis and epidermis. Pruritus marks the early stage and may be the only manifestation of mild infections. With progressive disease, however, itching is followed by altered pigmentation (Figure 172–20), edema (Figure 172–21), wrinkling and thickening of the dermis (Figures 172–22 through 172–24), depigmentation (Figure 172–25), spotty repigmentation (Figure 172–26), and atrophy and scaling of the epidermis (Figures 172–27 and 172–28). Onchodermatitis may involve any portion of the skin, but tends to be most severe over the thighs, pelvic girdle, and lower trunk. Itching may be mild or

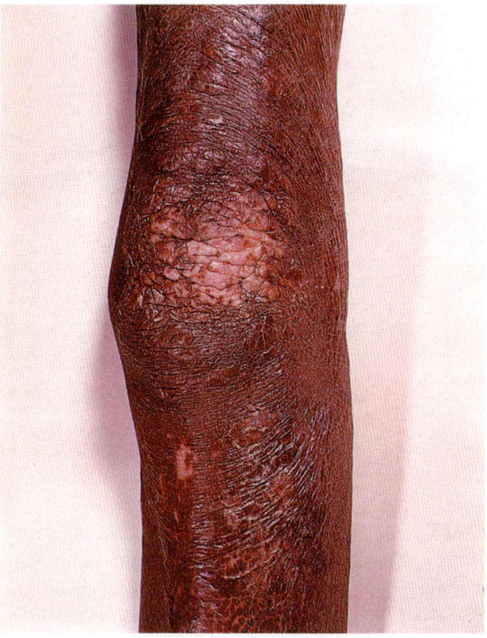

Figure 172–21. Edema of skin in a patient with severe onchodermatitis. Note also the wrinkling and scaling and the altered pigmentation and depigmentation.

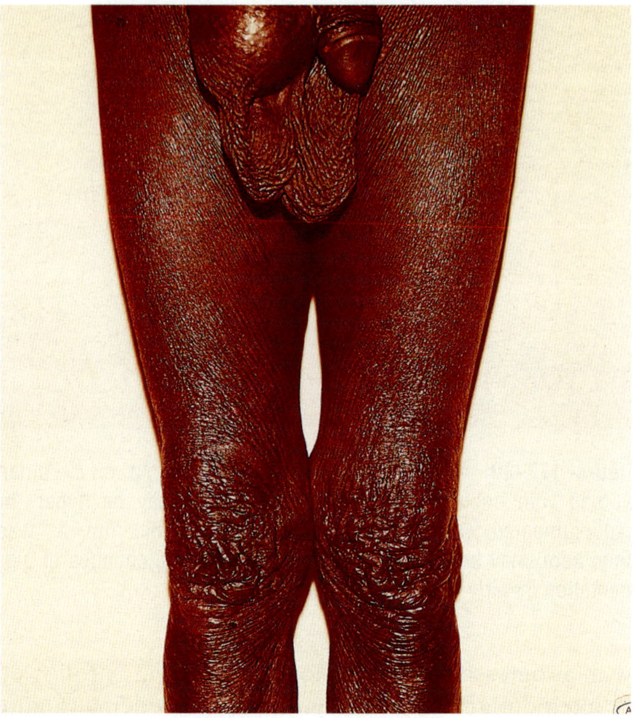

Figure 172–22. Long-standing onchocercal dermatitis in a middle-aged patient living in the Jinja area of Uganda. The skin is shiny, caused by thinning of the epidermis, and there is wrinkling and edema, causing loose folds of skin to hang from the knees—so called "elephant skin." Microscopically, abundant fibrous scar tissue replaces the normal dermal collagen.

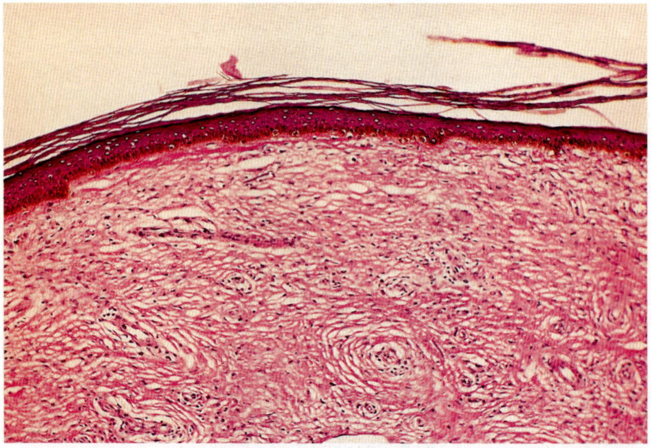

Figure 172–23. Specimen of redundant skin from the same patient. The epidermis is "parchment thin" and lacks rete ridges. Dermal collagen and other specialized structures are replaced by scar tissue that is arranged circumferentially around small vessels. This perivascular pattern resembles splenic scarring in systemic lupus erythematosus and may be caused by a pattern of circumferential immune complexes—antibody from the blood and microfilarial antigens in skin (hematoxylin-eosin ×85). (AFIP 73-6653.)

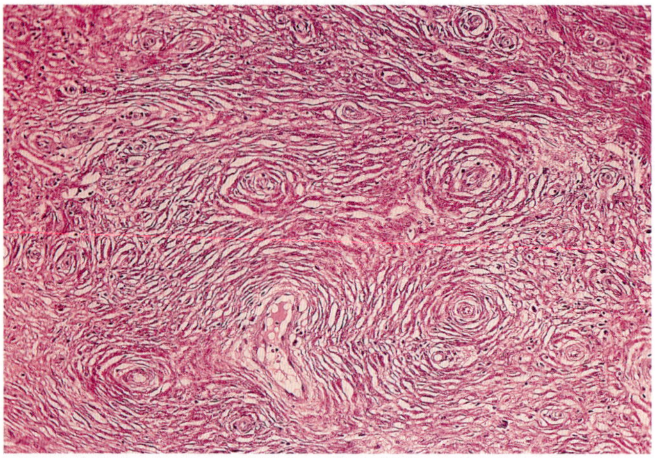

Figure 172–24. A closer look at the redundant skin of the patient in Figure 172–22. Note the striking pattern of perivascular scarring, characteristic of long-standing severe onchocerciasis (hematoxylin-eosin ×115). (AFIP 73-8104.)

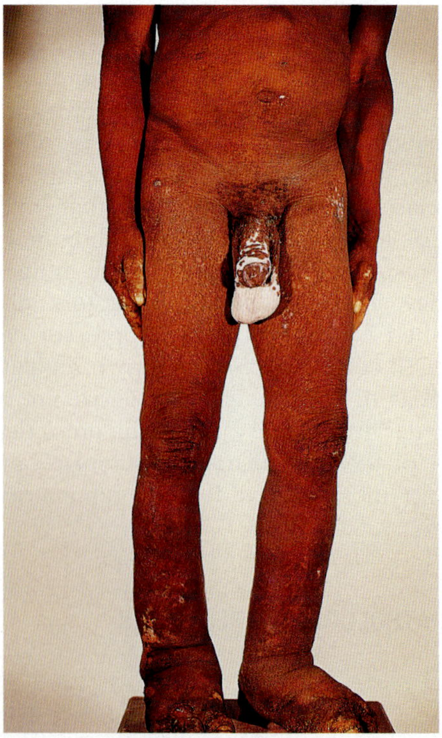

Figure 172–25. In addition to depigmentation of scrotal and penile skin, this patient has onchodermatitis of the thighs and lymphedema of the lower limbs.

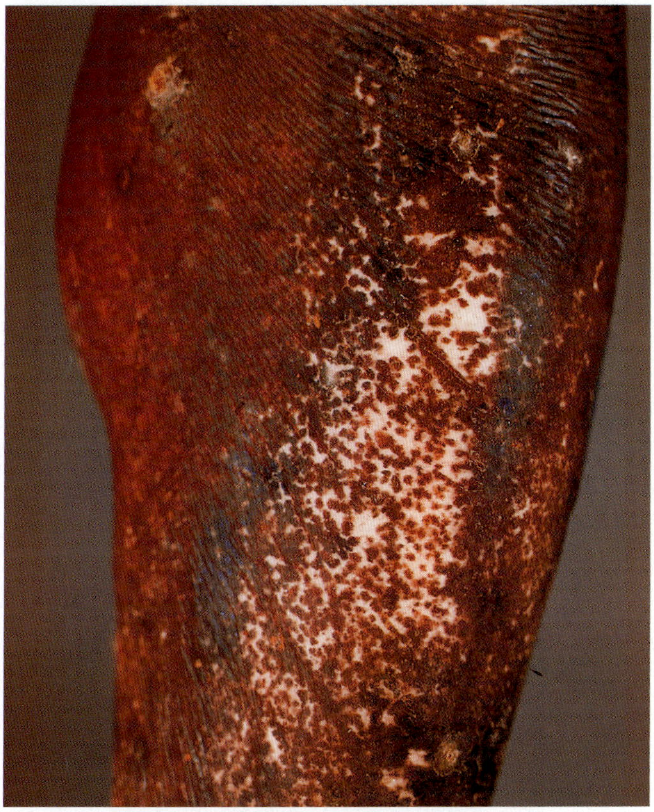

Figure 172–26. Depigmentation and spotty repigmentation in onchocercal dermatitis. The foci of repigmentation are around orifices of dermal appendages. "Depigmentation" of the shins is now recognized as an important marker for areas of severe onchocerciasis in Africa (ref. 40).

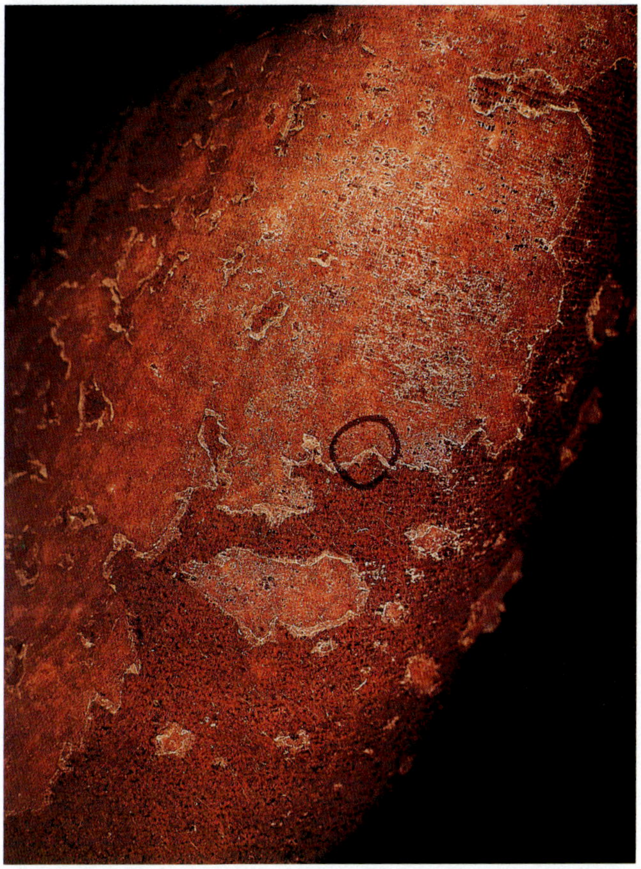

Figure 172–28. A more striking example of scaling in a patient with severe onchocercal dermatitis of the forearm. The scaling was made worse by a test dose of diethylcarbamazine. The circle is the site of a biopsy.

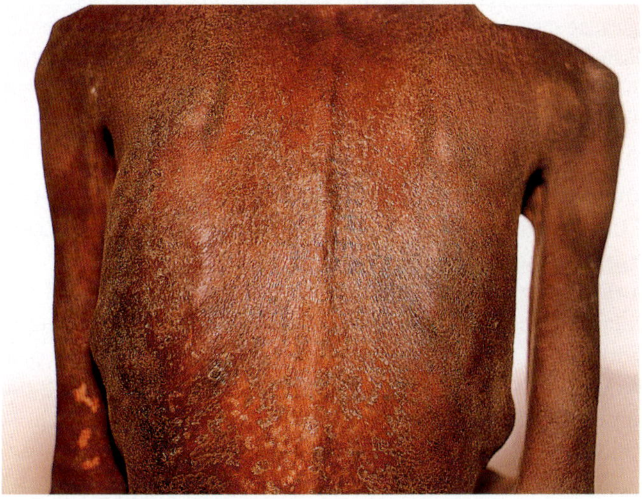

Figure 172–27. Atrophic epidermis and scaling in long-standing onchodermatitis. Note also the onchocercal nodule over the right chest wall and the depigmentation on the left arm and lower chest.

severe—to the point where the patient is robbed of sleep and distracted from meaningful or productive work. Villagers have been seen in close circles gently abrading each other with dried corn cobs for relief. Intense itching and scratching may cause deep excoriations and sometimes ulcers and bacterial infection (Figure 172–29). In hyperimmune patients, the skin erupts with a papule when a microfilaria dies. This has been called "craw-craw" and "gâl filarienne" in Africa, "sowda" (Arabic for *black*) in parts of Saudi Arabia and North Yemen (Figures 172–30 and 172–31), and papular dermatitis (Figure 172–32) elsewhere. A variant of hyperimmune onchodermatitis in Guatemala is "erisipela de la costa," characterized by acute dermatitis with hot, swollen, red, painful skin (Figure 172–33).

Microfilariae may be at all levels of the skin but tend to be concentrated in the upper dermis, especially in the dermal papillae. The immediate response, eosinophils that surround the carcass, progresses by indolent changes of dermal infiltrates of lymphocytes,

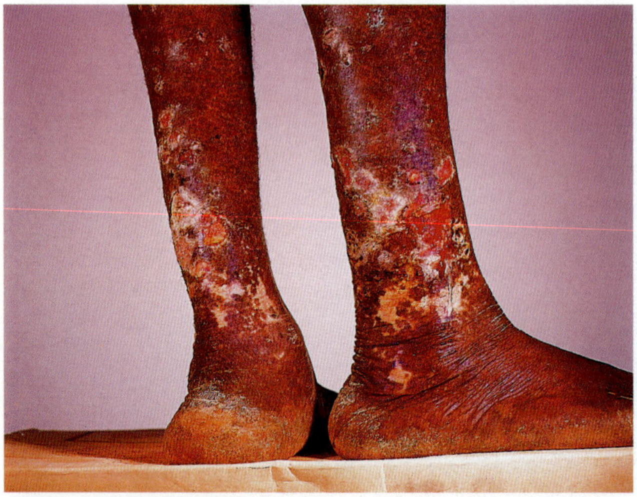

Figure 172–29. Severe itching and scratching in a patient with onchocercal dermatitis may cause ulcers and bacterial infection. These lesions healed quickly when the patient was treated with antibiotics and diethylcarbamazine.

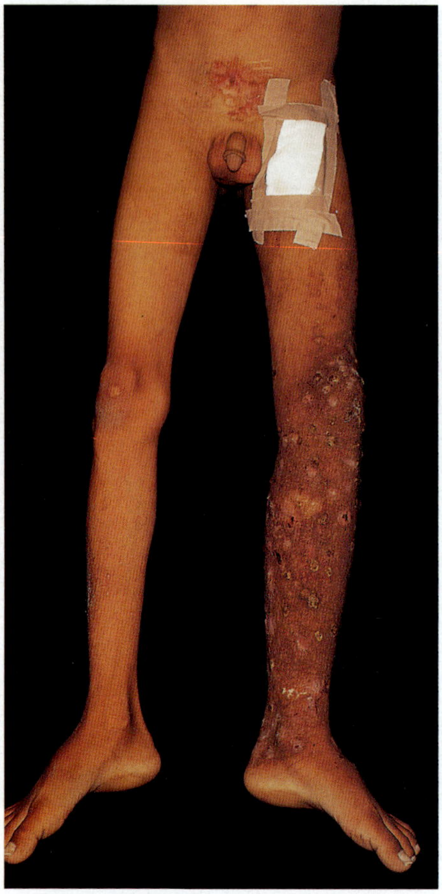

Figure 172–30. Sowda in a youth of North Yemen. He had the classic features: 1) itching, 2) involvement of a single limb, 3) hyperpigmentation, 4) papular eruption, 5) swelling of the limb, and 6) swelling of the regional lymph nodes. This youth was admitted for a penetrating injury to his urinary bladder. After his bladder had been repaired, enlarged inguinal and femoral lymph nodes were removed. At that time, the cause of sowda was uncertain and the enlarged lymph nodes were excised (the day before this picture was taken) because they were thought to be the "um" (or "mother") of the disease. The patient was given a short intense course of diethylcarbamazine, which was followed by more itching and the eruption of more papules.

macrophages, plasma cells, and mast cells that release vasoactive mediators, causing dermal edema, then hyperemia, and, eventually, fibrosis and dilated lymphatics (Figure 172–34). Fibrosis, in fact, is the final common pathway in onchocercal inflammation. It starts with the first signs of inflammation and continues throughout the years until scar tissue replaces specialized structures of skin (Figures 172–23, 172–24, 172–35), lymph node, and eye.

Some other changes are worth noting. DEC applied topically or taken orally kills some microfilariae immediately but agitates others, stimulating them to migrate into the epidermis, where they provoke intraepidermal abscesses (Figures 172–36 and 172–37). Here, the microfilariae are trapped. The abscesses diminish to become parakeratotic nests, and, now immobile and degenerating, microfilariae are sloughed in parakeratotic scales. Neutrophils, except in the intraepidermal abscesses, are conspicuously absent in onchocercal dermatitis. Even a few neutrophils in the dermis should turn the pathologist away from the possibility of onchodermatitis. In chronic onchodermatitis, arterioles are tortuous and surrounded by cuffs of inflammatory cells, and phagocytosed melanin is a constant feature. The amount of phagocytosed melanin increases as the dermatitis worsens and is more conspicuous in dark-skinned patients. Patients with depigmentation have very few microfilariae beneath the depigmented areas. Given a choice, in other words, microfilariae concentrate beneath pigmented epidermis and beneath the spots of repigmentation, as if seeking shade cast by the umbrella of pigmented epidermis. Dermal elastic fibers are reduced and, over the years, gradually disappear. Collagen fibers may undergo fibrinoid necrosis, becoming eosinophilic—probably from the deposition of immune complexes—losing their birefringence and fibrillar appearance, a feature accentuated by treatment with DEC. Finally, degenerating microfilariae may provoke T cell–mediated immune mechanisms, causing the accumulation of histiocytes, lymphocytes, epithelioid cells, and giant cells (Figure 172–19).

Nodules

Onchocercal nodules contain adult worms. The nodules are round or flattened, firm, movable, and located over

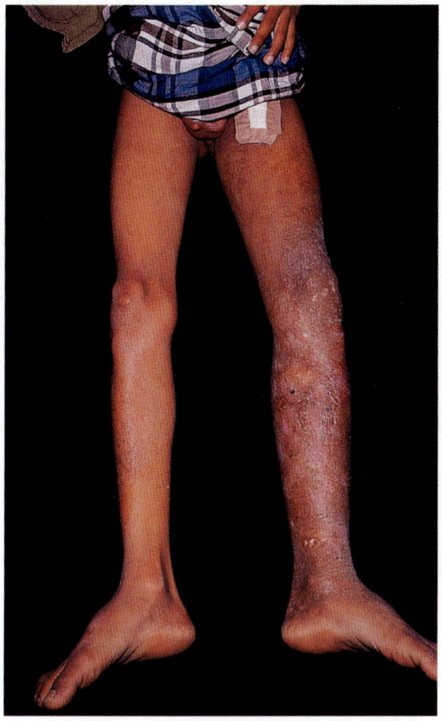

Figure 172–31. Same patient 8 days later. His itching was treated with aspirin and antihistamines, and by the fourth day there were no new papules, the itching had ceased, and the swelling was less. At 8 days his skin was smooth, pigmentation was less, and the patient's spirits were bright. A biopsy specimen taken before treatment revealed a single microfilaria of *Onchocerca volvulus* in the dermis. This patient, to our knowledge, was the first Yemenite with sowda who was shown to have a microfilaria of *O volvulus* in his skin, a positive Mazzotti reaction with a favorable clinical response to diethylcarbamazine, and hyperplastic—rather than atrophic—regional lymph nodes.

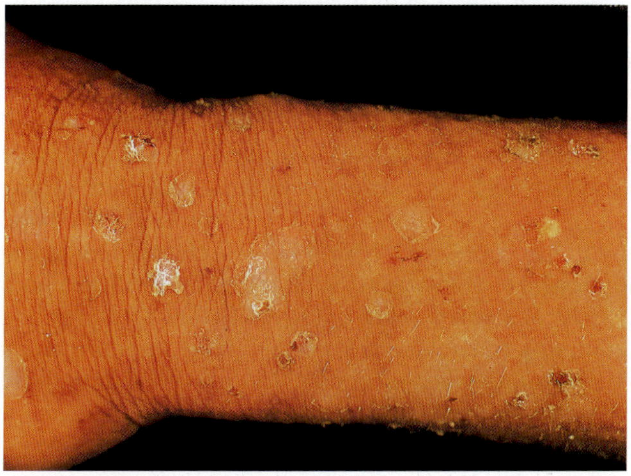

Figure 172–32. Papular dermatitis in a Guatemalan laborer on a coffee plantation. The papules are scaling, and each is probably a focal reaction to a degenerating microfilaria.

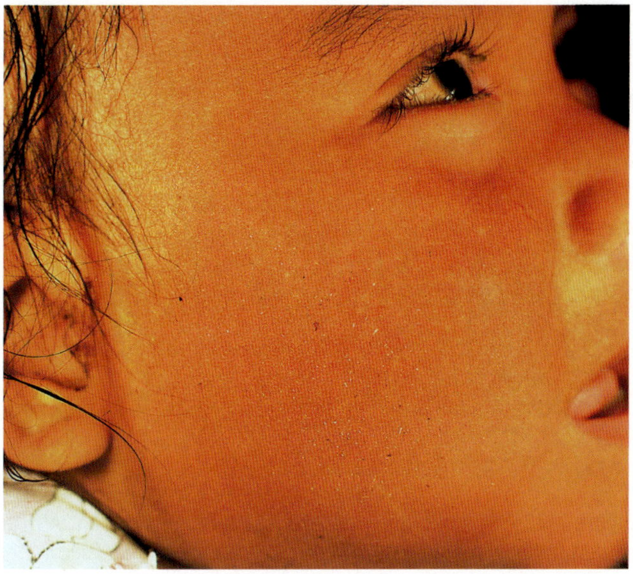

Figure 172–33. "Erisipela de la costa" (coastal erysipelas) on the right cheek of a 2-year-old Guatemalan child. The reaction is hyperimmune—the skin of the right cheek is hot, swollen, red, painful, and firm. She was the daughter of migrant coffee plantation laborers.

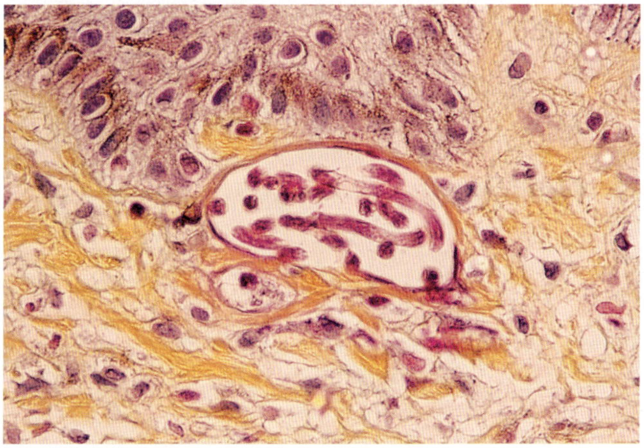

Figure 172–34. Specimen of skin taken before treatment. Microfilariae of *Onchocerca volvulus* have distended superficial lymphatic vessels (Movat ×530). (AFIP 73-5690.)

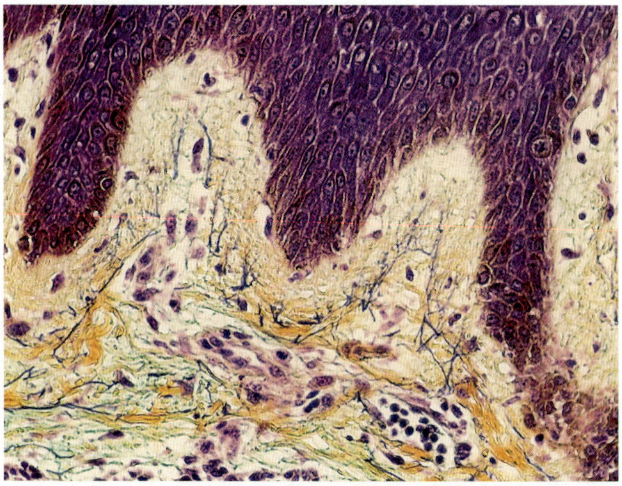

Figure 172–35. Mild non-onchocercal dermatitis in an African patient to show the delicate corona of elastic fibers that follows the peaks and valleys of the rete ridges. This delicate network of elastic fibers is stained black and is destroyed early in patients with onchodermatitis (Movat ×225). (AFIP 78-693.)

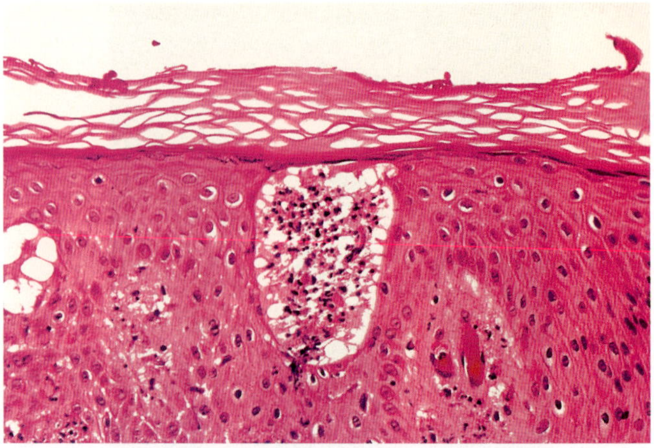

Figure 172–37. At 24 hours posttreatment, there is a well-defined abscess in the epidermis that contains microfilariae. One microfilaria is partly in the epidermis and partly in the abscess (hematoxylin-eosin ×250). (AFIP 72-17172.)

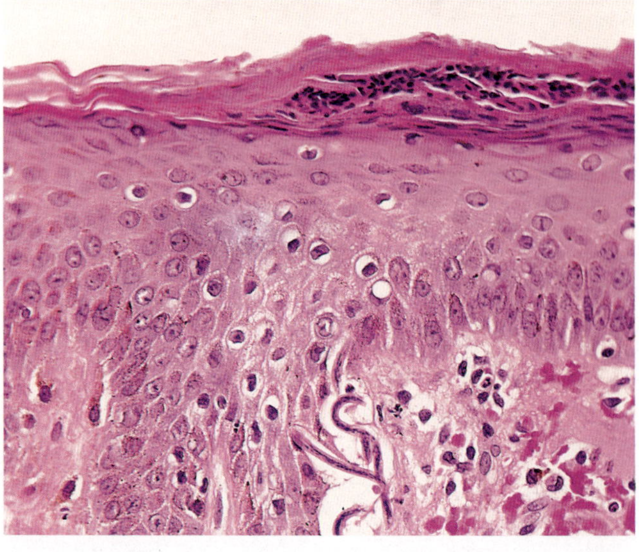

Figure 172–36. Five hours after swallowing 50 mg of diethylcarbamazine, microfilariae in the skin of this 29-year-old Cameroonian began to migrate into the epidermis. Here they are shown about to invade the basal layer (hematoxylin-eosin, ×300). (AFIP 72-5689.)

bony prominences but not tender or painful. Some adult worms live in deep fascia.[25] Nodules range in size from a few millimeters up to several centimeters across and may be discrete or clustered (Figures 172–9, 172–10, 172–38, and 172–39). In Africa, onchocercal nodules are concentrated on the lower half of the body. Common sites are the skin over the iliac spines, sacrum, ribs, elbows, and trochanters (Figure 172–9). In Central and South America, onchocercal nodules are more common on the upper body—on the head, over the scapular spines, and over the upper ribs. This difference is explained by the fact that the Central and South American flies tend to feed on the upper trunk and head. Perhaps the smallest nodule identified to date presented suddenly as a cutaneous nodule after the patient had been treated with DEC (Figures 172–40 through 172–42).[26]

Frequently, the worms in the nodules are embedded in Splendore-Hoeppli material—a layer that is fibrin-rich and also contains immunoglobulins (Figure 172–43). Nodules contain varying numbers of eosinophils, macrophages, lymphocytes, plasma cells, and neutrophils. Some macrophages fuse to form enormously elongated giant cells—sometimes a single cell attempting to enclose and phagocytose an entire worm. As the nodule ages, fibrous tissue increases and gradually replaces the exudate, "incarcerating" long segments of worm. One study has shown that the worms are surrounded by blood, implying that they are actually within dilated capillaries or at least in dilated blood vascular spaces.[27] As in the skin, eosinophils concentrate around microfilariae in the nodules.

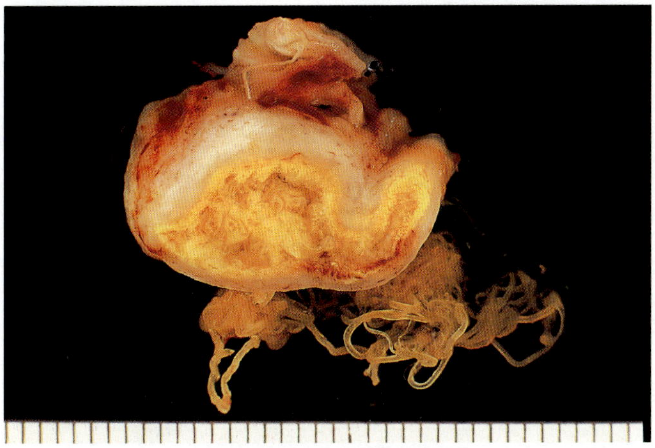

Figure 172–38. Discrete nodule removed from over a rib of a Zairian living in the Ubangi territory. Some of the soft central contents, including fragments of adult worms, have dropped out. Most nodules, as shown here, have three distinct layers: 1) an inner soft zone, containing some or most of the adult worms; 2) a surrounding granulomatous layer, with macrophages containing foamy lipid material (yellow); and 3) an outer layer of granulation tissue and scar (white) (scale is mm).

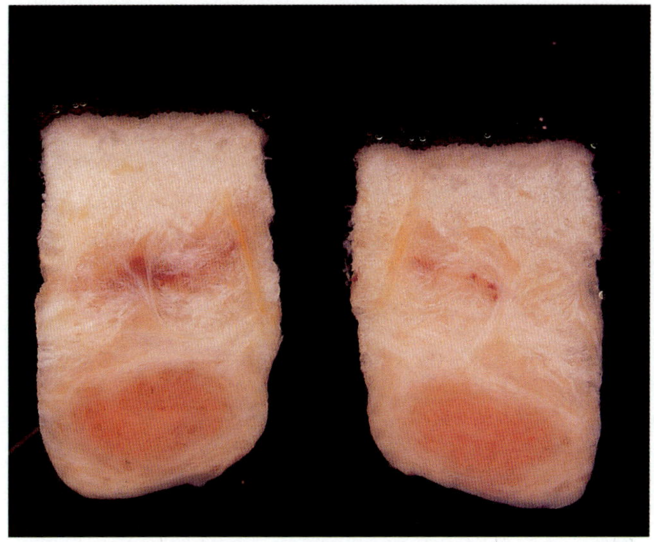

Figure 172–40. This 6-mm punch biopsy specimen was taken 3 days after the patient was given diethylcarbamazine. The oval, tan area 5 mm beneath the surface of the skin is an onchocercal nodule. The inflammatory change that provoked clinical awareness is phagocytosis of microfilariae by macrophages and epithelioid cells. To our knowledge, this is the smallest onchocercal nodule documented (Gross ×3.5).

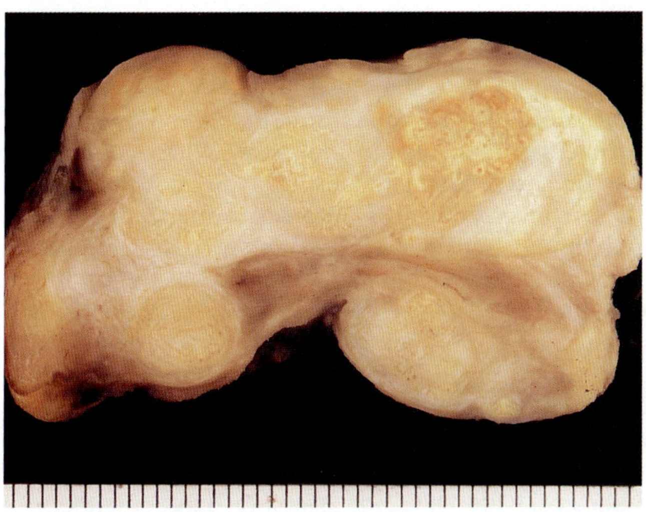

Figure 172–39. A cluster of nodules in which each nodule contains a separate "colony" of worms. Because they are incarcerated within the nodules, the adult worms by themselves are innocuous. The microfilariae released by the gravid female worms, however, migrate out of the nodules and into the skin, lymph node, and eye, where they provoke irreversible inflammatory changes (scale is mm).

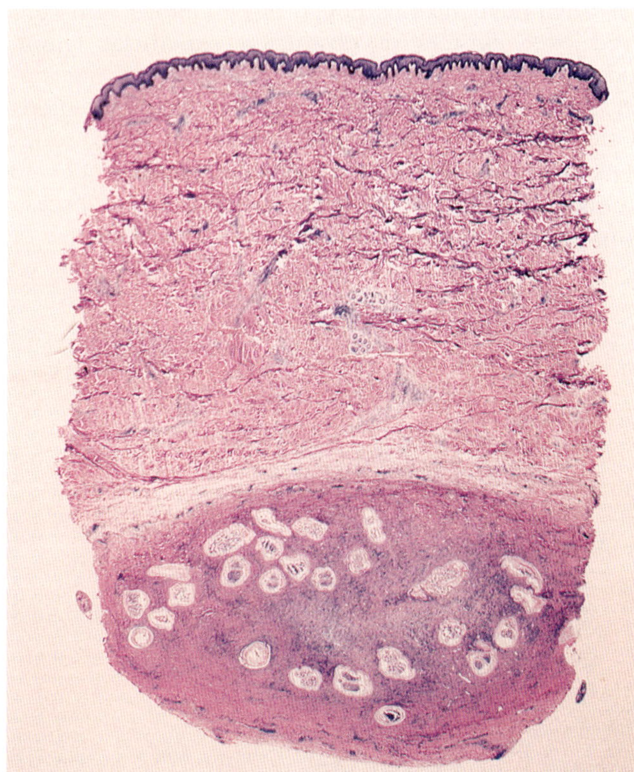

Figure 172–41. Microscopic appearance of the nodule shown in Figure 172–25. There are multiple cross sections of a gravid female worm surrounded by inflammatory cells containing microfilariae (Giemsa ×6.5). (AFIP 72-17292.)

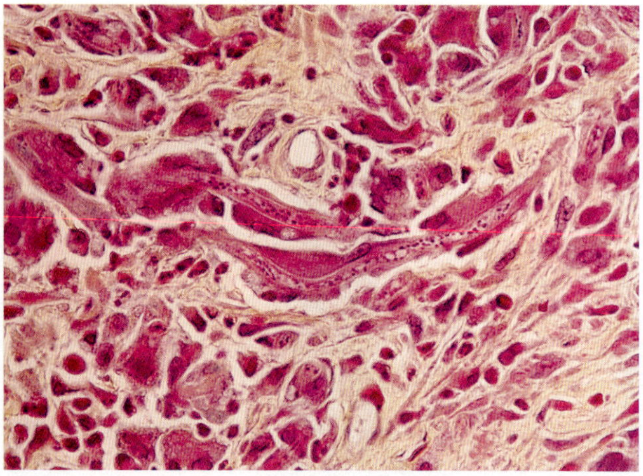

Figure 172–42. Microscopic appearance of the nodule shown in Figures 172–40 and 172–41. Degenerating microfilariae are surrounded by epithelioid cells and macrophages (Movat ×485). (AFIP Neg 72-17290.)

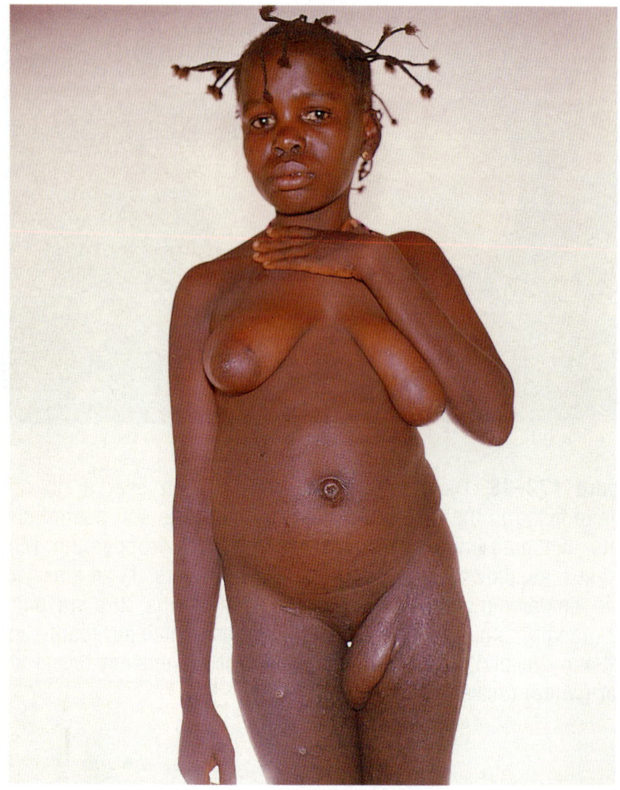

Figure 172–44. Left femoral hanging groin (adenolymphocele) in a young woman from the Ubangi territory of Zaire. These are characteristic lesions of onchocerciasis. The nodes beneath this hanging pouch—her left femoral nodes—were obstructed by onchocercal inflammation and fibrosis.

Hanging Groin and Elephantiasis

Hanging groin (adenolymphocele) is a characteristic feature of onchocerciasis (Figures 172–44 and 172–45). It is a lymphadematous pouch of pendulous skin centered over clusters of obstructed superficial lymph nodes. Clinically, the nodes are firm, discrete, not tender, and usually only slightly enlarged. In some regions of tropical Africa, fibrotic and obstructed deep nodes cause elephantiasis of the genitalia (Figures 172–46 through 172–48), limbs, and, sometimes, the breast. Lymph nodes become obstructed when microfilariae of *O volvulus* enter the node through afferent lymphatics, degenerate, and inflame the node. When continuous, this process eventually obstructs the flow of lymph. Microscopically, there is fibrous scarring of the capsule and fibrous replacement of lymphoid tissue that, in some nodes, is virtually complete (Figures 172–49 through 172–51). As in long-standing onchodermatitis, fibrous scarring of the nodes has a perivascular orientation. Early changes include a dilated subcapsular sinus containing histiocytes, atrophic cortical lymphoid tissue, and eosinophils and histiocytes in the peritrabecular spaces. Microfilariae may be scarce or plentiful. After treatment with DEC, for example, large numbers of microfilariae are mobilized in the skin, enter the lymphatics, and appear as entangled masses in the subcapsular sinuses of regional lymph nodes (Figure 172–52). Lymph nodes from patients with sowda are soft, hyperplastic, and without scarring or inflammatory cell infiltrates.

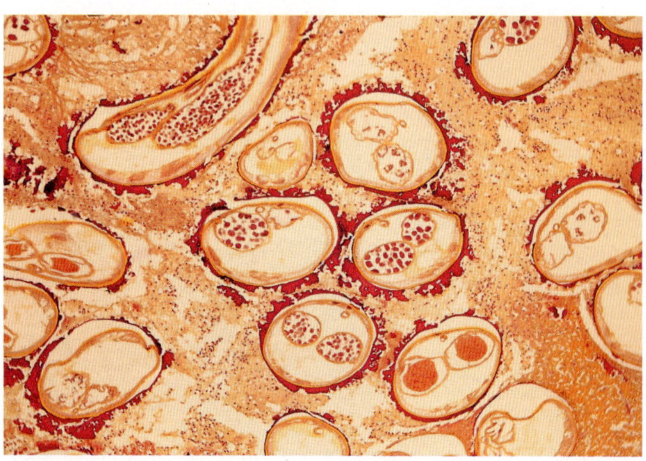

Figure 172–43. Multiple cross-sections of a gravid female *Onchocerca volvulus* worm. A thick layer of fibrin-rich material surrounds this worm (Movat ×56). (AFIP 74-1641.)

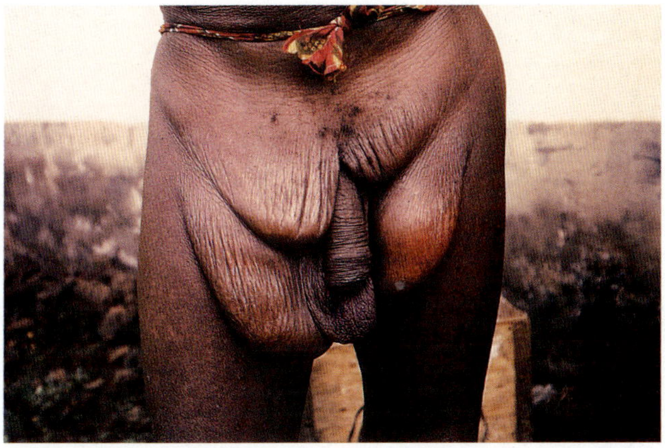

Figure 172–45. Hanging groin may involve any or all quadrants—inguinal or femoral, left or right. This 45-year-old rural Chadian has all four quadrants involved—bilateral, femoral, and inguinal. *(Photograph courtesy of Dr. John Anderson, 1970.)*

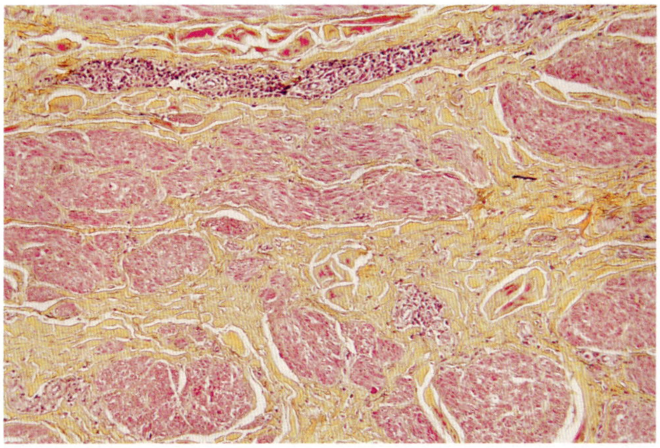

Figure 172–47. Microscopically, the roughly 40 lbs of firm, white, glistening tissue making up the mass of the scrotum in Figure 172–46 was composed of approximately equal portions of smooth muscle and collagen. The interlacing bundles of smooth muscle (hypertrophied cremaster) are red and the collagen is yellow (Movat ×50). (AFIP 69-5531.)

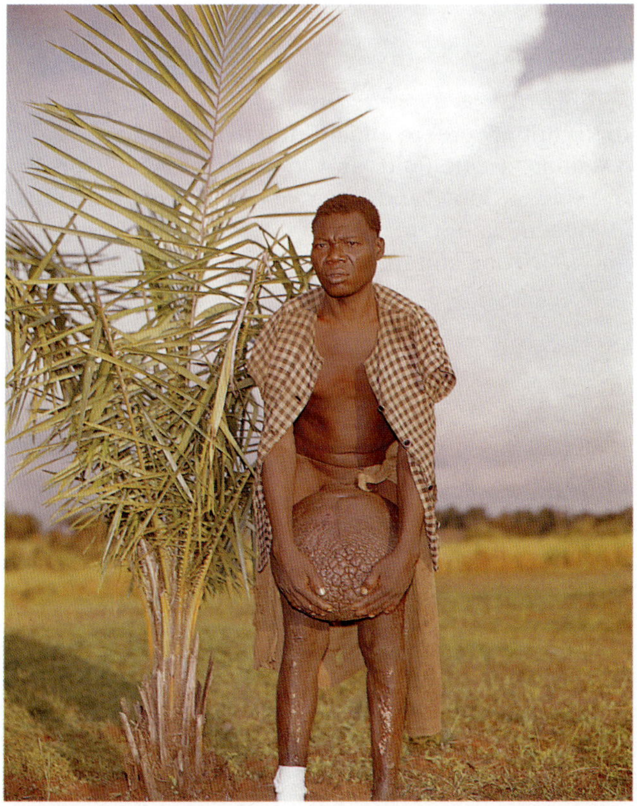

Figure 172–46. A 30-year-old resident of the Businga region of Zaire had severe onchocerciasis and a massive scrotum. When urinating, the flow came from the recess around the penis. Two skilled surgeons removed the scrotum, preserving his testes and penis, which were normal in size and shape and without gross lesions. The specimen weighed 18 kg—almost 40 lbs—and grossly was firm, solid, glistening white tissue.

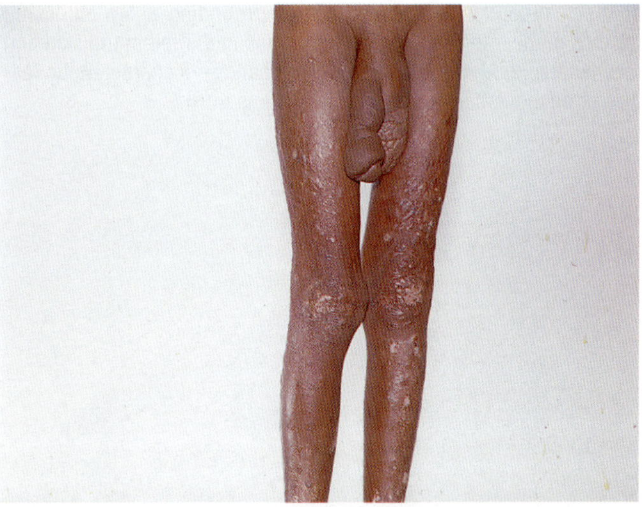

Figure 172–48. An 11-year-old youth from Businga, Zaire, with severe onchocercal dermatitis, lymphadenitis, and elephantiasis of the scrotum and penis. When first examined, his responses were slow, he sat with his mouth open much of the time, and made occasional, careless, almost purposeless motions of scratching. He was treated with diethylcarbamazine for 8 weeks by a research team (see ref. 4), during which time his dermatitis improved to the point where his skin was virtually normal. He also became more aware and smiled frequently as his spirits improved, but the lymphedema of his scrotum and penis persisted.

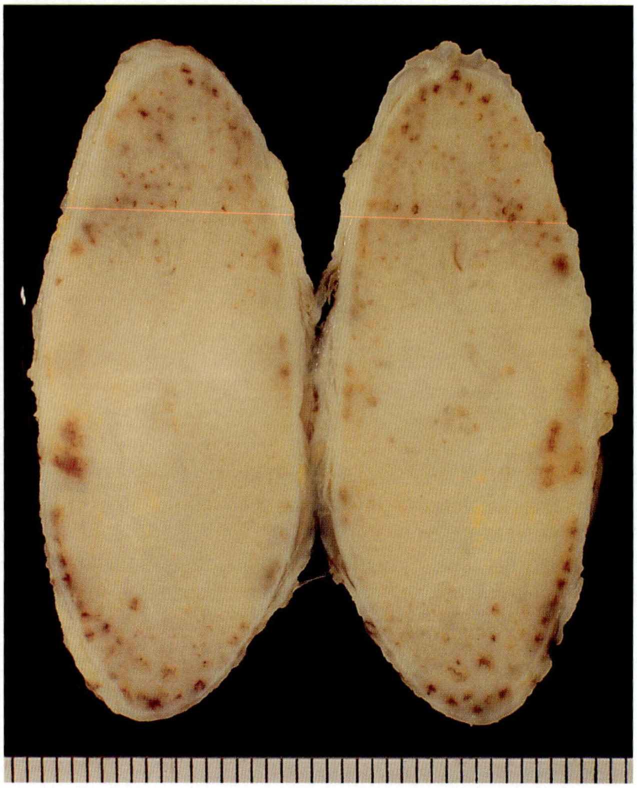

Figure 172–49. A bisected inguinal node in a patient from the Ubangi territory, Zaire, with onchocercal lymphadenitis. The capsule is thickened, and much of the lymphoid tissue is replaced by fibrous scar and adipose tissue. The dark foci at the perimeter are clusters of melanin-containing macrophages surrounding a few surviving follicles in the outer cortex. The melanin is mobilized in the skin and reaches the node through afferent lymphatics—a characteristic feature of onchocercal lymphadenitis (scale is mm).

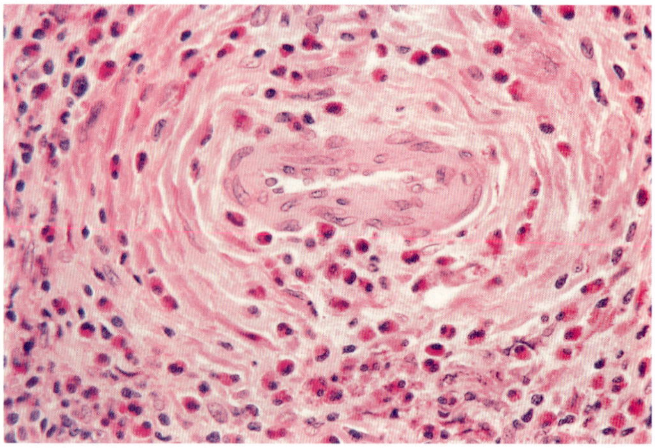

Figure 172–51. Onchocercal lymphadenitis. Here the scar tissue contains many eosinophils and is beginning to show its perivascular pattern. Eventually the node will lose all structure and appear like the scar tissue shown in Figure 172–24. This patient had elephantiasis and the hyperkeratotic change called "mossy foot" (24 hours post-diethylcarbamazine) (hematoxylin-eosin ×305).

Deep Organs

Microfilariae of *O volvulus* have been identified in blood, urine, cerebrospinal fluid, tears, sputum, vaginal secretions, ascitic fluid, and in vessels of the liver, kidney, spleen, lung, and ulnar nerve. Clearly, microfilariae disseminate throughout the body in blood and lymph. In one autopsy, degenerating microfilariae in

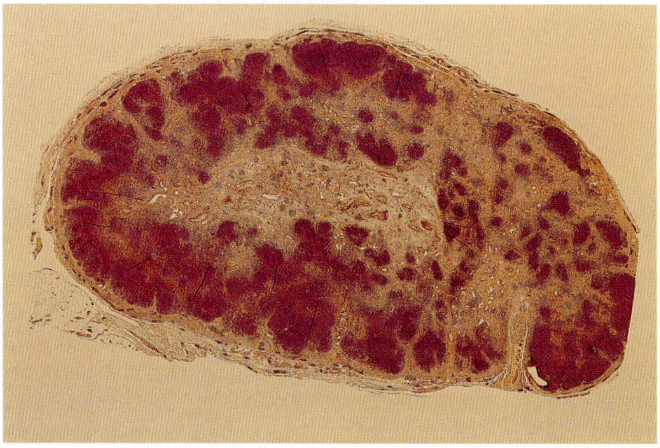

Figure 172–50. Onchocercal lymphadenitis of a femoral lymph node. Fibrous scar is separating and replacing normal lymphoid tissue. Here there are no surviving germinal centers (Movat ×3.2).

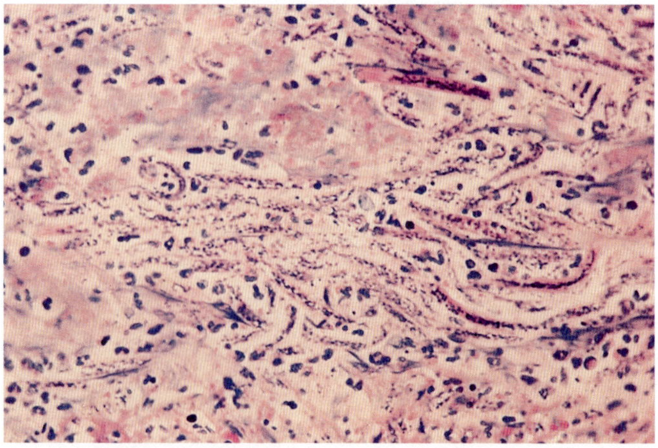

Figure 172–52. In most patients with onchocerciasis, microfilariae of *Onchocerca volvulus* probably percolate through the regional lymph nodes at a low rate. When given diethylcarbamazine, however, large numbers of microfilariae collect in the subcapsular space, as seen here. Many are degenerating (Giemsa ×440). (AFIP 73-5693.)

glomerular capillaries had caused an acute glomerulitis, and in another autopsy, an adult nongravid female worm was in the wall of the aorta.[28] The worm was surrounded by scar tissue that had replaced smooth muscle and elastic fibers—a focus of potential aneurysm.

Emaciation

A group of patients studied by Buck and associates[17] came to be known as "walking skeletons" (Figure 172–17). There were 6 in the village of Ouli Bangala, Chad (4 men, 2 women); 5 had microfilaruria and all had elevated L-aspartate. They were emaciated, weak, and had no papular eruptions or significant onchodermatitis, yet their skin snips were packed solid with writhing microfilariae—more than 300 per snip. Attempts to treat these patients, even with small doses of DEC, led not to recovery, but to death.[29] These patients had a short life expectancy, and speculation at the time focused on immune tolerance from exposure to antigens of *O volvulus* while in utero. A more recent report of microfilariae being passed in utero would support this possibility.[30] Other explanations for the clinical state of these patients include genetic anergy, in that they might fail to form proper aggretopes on the surfaces of their antigen presenting cells. Alternatively, they may be immunodeficient from the effects of protein-calorie malnutrition or from multiple infections, including human immunodeficiency virus (HIV) and possibly other retroviruses. At the time it was not possible to explore these other possibilities except to exclude tuberculosis by chest x ray.

Eye Lesions

Ocular lesions are caused by microfilariae that penetrate and damage components of the anterior and posterior segments (Figure 172–53). Eye lesions are common in endemic areas where nodules are located on the head and shoulder girdle. Ocular lesions in Africans tend to involve both the anterior and posterior segments (choroidoretinitis and optic atrophy) and also to be more severe in the savanna than in the forest. Central and South Americans have onchocercal iritis, with a significant amount of blindness. Onchocercal ocular disease includes superficial punctate keratitis, sclerosing keratitis, chorioretinitis, iridocyclitis, and atrophy of the optic nerve. In a survey of a large population in southwestern Cameroon,[31] 67.4% of the persons examined had pruritus, 51.6% had onchoceromas, 18.5% had depigmented skin, and 5.7% had hanging groin. Of the persons whose eyes were examined, 10.5% were blind or almost blind, 15.7% had poor vision, and 73.8% had good vision. Microfilariae were identified in the anterior chamber in 44.9% of eyes, 33.5% had chorioretinitis, 28.0% had punctate keratitis, 8.3% had abnormal pupils,

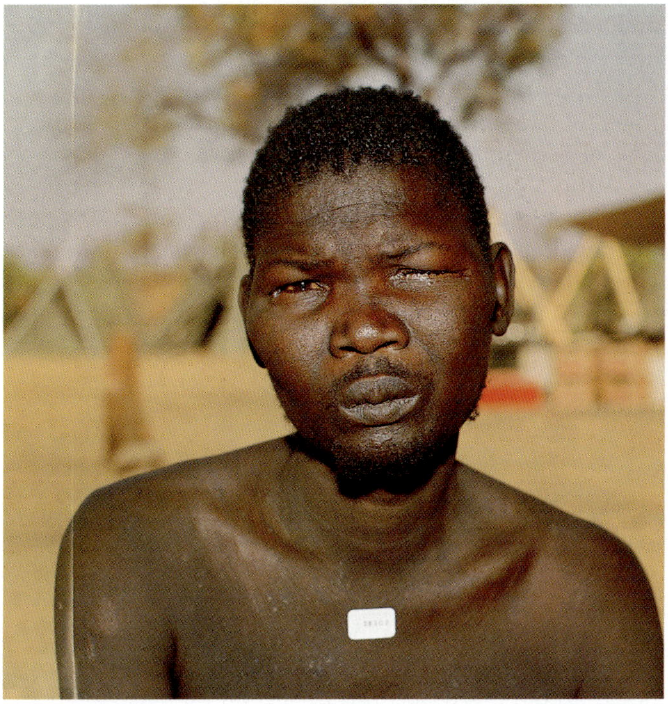

Figure 172–53. This young male resident of Ouli Bangala, Chad, has bilateral onchocercal eye disease, including conjunctivitis and sclerosing keratitis. He had photophobia, lacrimation, and palpebral and periorbital edema.

and 3.6% had sclerosing keratitis. Unlike skin lesions, which are caused by degenerating microfilariae, ocular lesions are caused by both living and dead microfilariae. Punctate keratitis is a superficial early inflammatory reaction around single microfilariae in the cornea. These lesions, which have been called "snowflake" or "cracked ice" opacities, are about 0.5 mm in diameter, concentrated at the juxtalimbal margin, and disappear in a few weeks. Symptoms include corneal irritation, lacrimation, photophobia, and variable visual changes. Sclerosing keratitis is an inflammation of the corneal stroma caused by microfilariae in the cornea (Figure 172–12). Pigmented stroma infiltrates the cornea from the inferior limbus and spreads centrally. The accompanying blood vessels pierce and opacify the cornea, impairing vision. Lesions of the posterior segment may begin early with a choroidal exudate, which may progress and obliterate choroidal blood vessels, leading to choroidal atrophy. The macula is involved in later stages. Changes of retinal pigment begin at the periphery as a tiger pattern and move toward the disc, ultimately leaving dense elevations of pigment surrounding atrophic choroid. When long-standing, these changes can be seen with an ophthalmoscope, but early lesions may be undetectable.

Iridocyclitis with secondary glaucoma is a major cause of blindness. The iris may become aberrantly connected to neighboring structures by a fibrinous exudate, sometimes distorting the pupil. Massive invasion of the anterior segment by microfilariae may directly or indirectly (by synechiae) interfere with drainage of the canal of Schlemm and cause glaucoma.

Atrophy of the optic nerve begins as an early papillitis with minimal swelling, followed by atrophy from inflammation and is a leading cause of blindness. Microfilariae invade the head of the optic nerve near the lamina cribrosa.

DIAGNOSIS

The skin snip is the classical method for diagnosis. The skin is tented up with the point of a fine needle, and a small snip of epidermis together with the upper portions of several dermal papillae is shaved off. Taken this way, the snip is usually bloodless. The snip is then immersed in normal saline and examined under a microscope for microfilariae, whose wriggling forms appear within a few seconds to several minutes. Microfilariae accumulate in the saline, and the intensity of infection can be estimated by the number of microfilariae per milligram of tissue. Snips may be taken more easily, more quickly, and of more uniform size with a corneoscleral punch.

An indirect technique for diagnosis is the Mazzotti reaction. From several minutes to several hours after 50 mg of DEC is swallowed, patients suffer intense pruritis in the areas of skin where microfilariae are concentrated. Systemic manifestations of an acute Mazzotti reaction include fever, malaise, arthralgias, and tender lymphadenopathy. Caution must be used in patients with ocular involvement because DEC may precipitate acute inflammatory reactions in the cornea, sometimes threatening blindness. Techniques using recombinant antigens and polymerase chain reaction have been both sensitive and specific for the diagnosis of onchocerciasis.[32,33]

A slit lamp may reveal microfilariae in the cornea or anterior chamber, which enables a specific diagnosis. Onchocerciasis is frequently diagnosed by identifying adult worms in excised nodules or by identifying microfilariae in biopsy specimens of skin. Species-specific antigens have been developed that may prove valuable in diagnosing prepatent onchocerciasis.[34]

TREATMENT

Nodulectomy removes adult worms and has been efficacious in decreasing the incidence of ocular onchocerciasis and blindness in Central and South America. Excision of nodules in African patients is more difficult, because the nodules tend to be more deeply situated and frequently are bound to surrounding tissues, including the fascia. Chemotherapeutic agents include the two traditional anthelmintic drugs, DEC (Banocide, Hetrazan, Notezine) and suramin (Antrypol, Bayer 205, Germanin, Moranyl). As already described, DEC is an effective microfilariacidal drug, sometimes effective to a fault, for even small doses lead to the death of large numbers of microfilariae, frequently making the patient miserable. A graduated upward dosing regimen and simultaneous treatment with steroids, antihistaminics, and nonsteroidal anti-inflammatory agents decrease unpleasant clinical manifestations. Ottesen has summarized the immune responses to DEC. Early, proteins from eosinophils rise in tissues and in blood. Fever and other systemic features correlate with increased IL-6 and TNFα in serum, and within 12 to 48 hours, serum IL-5 increases. There is a posttreatment eosinophilia that peaks 2 to 3 weeks after treatment begins and a rise of IgG-specific antibodies during the 2 weeks after treatment.[24]

More recently, ivermectin (Mectizan) has been used with success.[23,35–37] Given as a single dose, ivermectin kills microfilariae in some of the uterine tubes of the adult worms, thus gradually decreasing the concentration of microfilariae in the skin, eye, and lymph node. Ivermectin apparently also kills some, but not all, adult worms.[37] Ivermectin is essentially nontoxic and it does not produce the virtually universal allergic side effects of suramin and DEC. In a mass treatment program in Nigeria, only 0.07% of those treated complained of side effects, which included headache, body pains, pruritus, edema, fever, dizziness, and vomiting.[38] Consequently, ivermectin has now replaced suramin and DEC as the prime therapeutic drug. As a humanitarian gesture, Merck and Company has made their brand of ivermectin available for large-scale treatment. Ivermectin, however, is contraindicated in children younger than 5 years, in pregnant and lactating women, and in debilitated patients.

Albendazole, given for 10 days at 400 mg per day, was well tolerated, and over a period of 1 year reduced the densities of microfilariae.[39] The authors of this study suggest that albendazole interfered with embryogenesis.

Suramin (Antrypol, Bayer 205, Germanin, Moranyl) is a water-soluble relative of urea, and is given intravenously once a week for 6 to 7 weeks. It kills both adult worms and microfilariae, but is nephrotoxic and has other systemic side effects, which include anorexia, malaise, diarrhea, and wasting.

(Daniel H. Connor, MD, took the photographs for and retains the copyright on Figures 172–2 through 172–7, 172–9, 172–10, 172–17, 172–20 through 172–22,

172–25 through 172–33, 172–38 through 172–40, 172–44, 172–46, 172–48, 172–49, and 172–53.)

REFERENCES

1. McCarthy JS, Ottesen EA, Nutman TB. Onchocerciasis in endemic and nonendemic populations: differences in clinical presentation and immunologic findings. *J Infect Dis.* 1994;170:736–741.
2. Duke BOL, Taylor HR. Onchocerciasis. In: Strickland GT, ed. *Tropical Medicine.* 7th edition. Philadelphia: WB Saunders; 1991:729–744.
3. O'Neill J. On the presence of a filaria in "craw craw." *Lancet.* 1875;1:265–266.
4. Connor DH, Morrison NE, Kerdel-Vegas F, et al. Onchocerciasis: onchocercal dermatitis, lymphadenitis and elephantiasis in the Ubangi territory. *Human Pathol.* 1970;1:553–579.
5. Brumpt E. A propos de la Filaria volvulus Leuckart. *Rev Med Hyg Trop.* 1904;1:43.
6. Robles R. Onchocercose humaine au Guatémala produisant la cécité et "l'érysipèle du littoral." *Bull Soc Path Exot.* 1919;12:442–463.
7. Blacklock DB. The development of *Onchocerca volvulus* in *Simulium damnosum. Ann Trop Med Parasit.* 1926–7; 20:1–49.
8. Torroella JL. Nota sobre la observacion de microfilarias de Onchocerca in vivo en el ojo humano. *Ann Soc Méx Oftal Oto-Rino-Laryng.* 1931;9:87–88.
9. Mazzotti L. Posibilidad de utilizan como medio diagnostico auxiliar en la oncocercosis, las reacciones alergicas consecutivas a la administracion del "Hetrazan." *Rev Inst Salub Enferm Trop.* 1948;9:235.
10. Neafie RC. Morphology of *Onchocerca volvulus. Amer J Clin Path.* 1972;57:574–586.
11. Gibson DW, Heggie C, Connor DH. Clinical and pathologic aspects of onchocerciasis. In: Sommers SC, Rosen PP, series eds. *Pathology Annual.* Part 2. Vol 15. New York City: Appleton-Century-Crofts; 1980:195–240.
12. Njoo FL, Stilma JS, van der Lelij A. Effects of repeated ivermectin treatment in onchocerciasis. *Doc Ophthalmol.* 1992;79:261–267.
13. Goodman B. Models aid understanding, help control parasites. *Science.* 1994;264:1862–1863.
14. Davies JB. Sixty years of onchocerciasis vector control: a chronological summary with comments on eradication, reinvasion, and insecticide resistance. *Annu Rev Entomol.* 1994;39:23–45.
15. Gibson DW, Connor DH, Brown HL, et al. Onchocercal dermatitis: ultrastructural studies of microfilariae and host tissues, before and after treatment with diethylcarbamazine. *Amer J Trop Med Hyg.* 1976;25:74–87.
16. Gibson DW, Connor DH. Onchocercal lymphadenitis: clinico-pathologic study of 34 patients. *Trans Roy Soc Trop Med Hyg.* 1978;72:137–154.
17. Buck AA, Anderson RI, Colston JAC, et al. Microfilaruria in onchocerciasis. *Bull World Hlth Org.* 1971;45:353–369.
18. Connor DH, Gibson DW, Neafie RC, Merighi B, Buck AA. Sowd: a clinicopathologic study of 18 patients. *Amer J Trop Med Hyg.* 1983;32:123–137.
19. Kephart GM, Gleich GJ, Connor DH, Gibson DW, Ackerman SJ. Deposition of eosinophil granule major basic protein onto microfilariae of *O. volvulus* in skin of patients treated with diethylcarbamazine. *Lab Invest.* 1984;50: 51–61.
20. Edgeworth JD, Abiose A, Jones DR. An immunohistochemical analysis of onchocercal nodules: evidence for an interaction between macrophage MRP8/MRP14 and adult *Onchocerca volvulus. Clin Exp Immunol.* 1993;92:84–92.
21. Gatrill AJ, Mackenzie CD, McMahon JE. A histochemical study of the macrophages present in tissue responses to adult *Onchocerca volvulus. Histochem J.* 1987;19:509–519.
22. Soboslay PT, Luder CG, Hoffman WH, et al. Ivermectin-facilitated immunity in onchocerciasis; activation of parasite-specific Th1-type responses with subclinical *Onchocerca volvulus* infection. *Clin Exp Immunol.* 1994;96: 238–244.
23. Munk ME, Soboslay PT, Arnoldi J, Brattig N, Schulz-Key H, Kaufmann SH. *Onchocerca volvulus* provides ligands for the stimulation of human gamma/delta T lymphocytes expressing V delta 1 chains. *J Infect Dis.* 1993;168:1241–1247.
24. Ottesen EA. Immune responsiveness and pathogenesis in human onchocerciasis. *J Infect Dis.* 1995;171:659–671.
25. Duke BOL. Onchocerciasis: deep worm bundles close to hip joints. *Trans Roy Soc Trop Med Hyg.* 1970;64:791.
26. Boye ES, Connor DH. An onchocercal nodule developing during diethylcarbamazine therapy. *Amer J Trop Med Hyg.* 1982;31:1123–1127.
27. George GH, Palmieri JR, Connor DH. The onchocercal nodule: interrelationship of adult worms and blood vessels. *Amer J Trop Med Hyg.* 1985;334:1144–1148.
28. Meyers WM, Neafie RC, Connor DH. Onchocerciasis: Invasion of deep organs by *Onchocerca volvulus.* Autopsy findings. *Amer J Trop Med Hyg.* 1977;26:650–657.
29. Oomen AP. Studies on onchocerciasis and elephantiasis in Ethiopia. Haarlem, de Erven F. Bohn, 1969.
30. Anosike JC, Onwuliri CO. A probable case of vertical transmission of *Onchocerca volvulus* microfilariae. *J Helminthol* (England). 1993;67:83–84.
31. Somo RM, Enyong PA, Fobi G, et al. A study of onchocerciasis with severe skin and eye lesions in a hyperendemic zone in the forest of southwestern Cameroon: clinical, parasitologic and entomologic findings. *Am J Trop Med Hyg.* 1993;48:14–19.
32. Bradley JE, Trenholme KR, Gillespie AJ, et al. A sensitive serodiagnostic test for onchocerciasis using a cocktail of recombinant antigens. *Am J Trop Med Hyg.* 1993;48; 198–204.
33. Zimmerman PA, Guderian RH, Aruajo E, et al. Polymerase chain reaction–based diagnosis of *Onchocerca volvulus* infection: improved detection of patients with onchocerciasis. *J Infec Dis.* 1994;169:686–689.
34. Ogunrinade AF, Chandrashekar R, Eberhard ML, Weil GJ. Preliminary evaluation of recombinant *Onchocerca volvulus* antigens for serodiagnosis of onchocerciasis. *J Clin Microbiol.* 1993;31:1741–1745.
35. Boussinesq M, Prod'Hon J, Chippaux JP, Quillevere D.

Long term effect of a single dose of ivermectin on skin microfilarial density in an endemic onchocerciasis area of North Cameroon. *Ann Soc Belg Med Trop.* 1993;73: 189–196.

36. Boussinesq M, Chippaux JP, Ernould JC, Prod'Hon J, Quillevere D. Parasitological efficacy of repeated treatments with ivermectin in an onchocerciasis focus in north Cameroon. *Bull Soc Pathol Exot.* 1993;86:112–115.
37. Duke BO, Zea-Flores G, Castro J, Cupp EW, Munoz B. Effects of multiple monthly doses of ivermectin on adult *Onchocerca volvulus*. *Am J Trop Med Hyg.* 1990;43: 657–664.
38. Ogunba EO, Gemade EI. Preliminary observations on the distribution of ivermectin in Nigeria for control of river blindness. *Ann Trop Med Parasitol.* 1992;86:649–655.
39. Cline BL, Hernandez JL, Mather FJ, et al. Albendazole in the treatment of onchocerciasis: double-blind clinical trial in Venezuela. *Am J Trop Med Hyg.* 1992;47:512–520.
40. Carme B, Ntsoumou-Madzou V, Samba Y, Yebakima A. Prevalence of depigmentation of the shins: a simple and cheap way to screen for severe endemic onchocerciasis in Africa. *Bull World Health Organ.* 1993;71:755–758.

CHAPTER 173

Paragonimiasis

Bharatha Sinniah

Health is the vital principle of bliss, . . .

James Thompson (1700–1748)

DEFINITION

Paragonimiasis is infection by trematodes of the genus *Paragonimus*—most frequently by *Paragonimus westermani*. *Paragonimus* sp invade various organs especially lung where there is a focal granulomatous reaction with fibrous encapsulation. Sixteen species of *Paragonimus* are pathogenic to humans. They are *P westermani, P heterotremus, P uterobilateralis, P calensis, P kellicotti, P mexicana, P congolensis, P amazonicus, P skrijabini, P miyazaki, P africanus, P peruvianus, P ecuadoriensis, P philippinensis, P huerlungensis,* and *P pulmonatis.* Synonyms for paragonimiasis include Oriental lung fluke, manson hemoptysis, pulmonary distomiasis, parasitic hemoptysis, and endemic hemoptysis.

GEOGRAPHIC DISTRIBUTION

Paragonimus westermani has a wide distribution in China, Japan, Korea, Taiwan, Philippines, Indonesia, and smaller areas of India, Nepal, and Manchuria. *Paragonimus* sp have been reported from Canada, North and Central America, and parts of South America (Peru, Ecuador, Colombia, Mexico, Costa Rica, Venezuela, Brazil, and Honduras). *Paragonimus africanus* has been reported from Cameroon, Nigeria, Libya, Liberia, and Zaire.

HABITAT

The adult trematodes live, encapsulated, in the lungs of humans—usually in pairs within a cyst. Reservoir hosts include domestic and wild dogs, wolves, foxes, members of the cat family (including tigers and leopards), as well as pigs, hogs, monkeys, rats, mongooses, and opossums.

MORPHOLOGY

The adult fluke is thick, fleshy, egg-shaped, red-brown, rounded anteriorly and slightly tapered posteriorly (Figure 173–1). It is 7.5 to 20 mm long by 2.5 to 5 mm thick. The ventral sucker (acetabulum) is slightly anterior to the midportion of the worm. The esophagus bifurcates to form two cecae that are unbranched and extend into the caudal region. The long excretory bladder extends from the posterior part of the worm to the level of the pharynx. The oral and ventral suckers are equal in size, about 800 μm in diameter. The tegument is covered with simple or toothed spines. The two branched testes are deeply lobed and almost side by side in the posterior part of the body. A single six-lobed ovary is slightly posterior to the ventral sucker and it may be to the right or left of the midline. The uterus lies on the side opposite the ovary. Grapelike clusters of vitellariae are well developed and stretch from pharynx to the posterior end of the worm.

The body wall is 50 to 100 μm thick and consists of a tegument, two or more layers of smooth muscle, and a row of tegumental cells. The parenchyma is loose stroma containing fluid-filled spaces and cells. Eggs of *P westermani* are golden brown, oval, and thick shelled. They are 80 μm to 120 μm by 45 to 65 μm and have a flattened operculum at one end. The shell is birefringent. The eggs are not embryonated when laid.

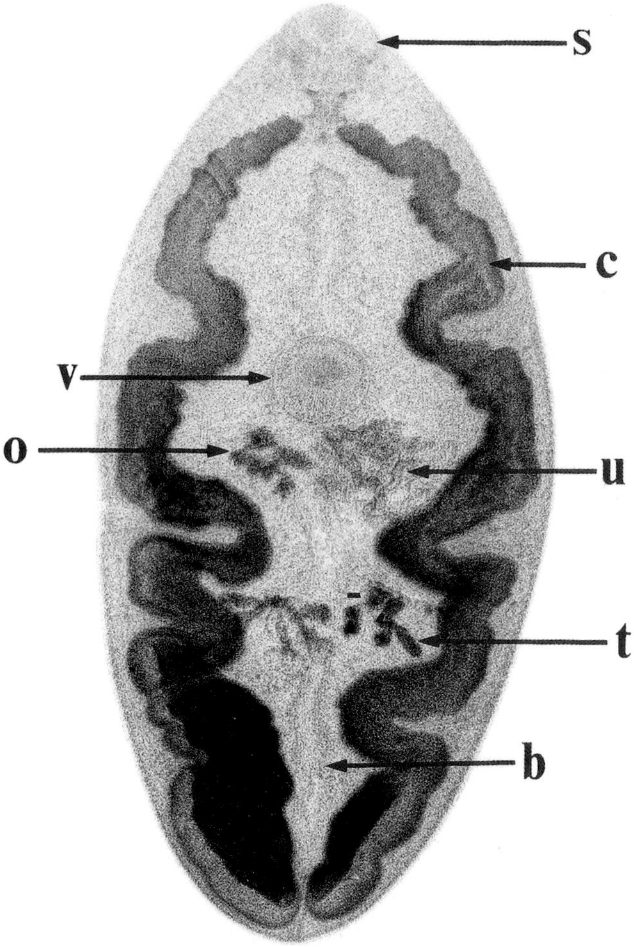

Figure 173–1. Ventral aspect *P westermani.* Reproductive and somatic structures are labeled as follows: s, ventral sucker; c, cecum; u, uterus; t, testis; b, excretory bladder; v, ventral sucker; and o, ovary (AFIP 76-5953; magnification about 9×). *(Original photograph contributed by Mr. Harald Langben, Walter Reed Army Institute of Research.)*

LIFE CYCLE

Adult worms live in the respiratory tract of their definitive hosts. Eggs laid by the worms are coughed up, swallowed, and passed in the feces. They develop in freshwater and hatch in 2 to 3 weeks releasing a ciliated miracidia. The miracidia swim about in search of snail hosts—families *Pleuroceridae* and *Thiaridae.* Inside the snail the miracidium casts off its cilia, passes through stages of sporocyst, then two generations of rediae, and finally transforms into a cercariae. The cycle takes from 10 to 12 weeks. Mature cercariae escape from the snail into water and enter the second intermediate host, a freshwater crab (Potamon, Sesarma, or Eriocheir) or freshwater crayfish *(Astacus).* Inside the crustacean host they become encysted in the viscera, muscles, and gills as metacercariae and are 250 to 500 μm. Humans become infected by ingesting raw or undercooked crabs or crayfish infected with metacercariae. The larvae are freed in the human intestine, then enter the peritoneal cavity and migrate through the diaphragm into the thoracic cavity and lungs where they reach maturity. The adult flukes begin to lay eggs 5 to 6 weeks after infection. Although *Paragonimus* is hermaphroditic, two worms are usually in a cyst or encapsulated together. Most adult worms die in about 6 years but they may live for 20 years. Eggs are discharged into bronchioles and subsequently pass in the feces. In unsuitable final hosts the metacercariae encyst in the tissues (paratenic host, eg, pig) and remain there until ingested by appropriate hosts, which then allows the life cycle to repeat.[1] Human infection can occur also from ingesting raw or partially cooked meat of animals and crustaceans.

CLINICAL MANIFESTATIONS

The first signs of pulmonary involvement are dyspnea, cough, chest pain, night sweats, and hemoptysis. Coughing spells may produce blood-tinged sputum or thick chocolate-brown sputum containing eggs. Morning cough usually produces heavy blood-tinged or "rusty sputum." Finger clubbing is common. Persistent rales may be a feature. X rays may reveal a variety of changes including diffuse infiltrates, nodules, or annular opacites. Persistent fever suggests pulmonary abscess, pleural effusion, or empyema. Aberrant immature flukes may wander to different organs including liver, spleen, kidney, and brain.

Brain is the most common extrapulmonary site of infection. Reaction to worms and eggs may cause aphasia, Jacksonian epilepsy, hemiplegia, monoplegia, paresis, visual disturbances, optic atrophy, and papilledema. Cerebral hemorrhage, especially in children under 15 years, is also a feature. In Korea 90% of the patients under 15 years with cerebral involvement become mentally retarded.[2] Lesions of spinal cord may cause paraplegia, sensory loss, and impaired control of sphincters. Cerebral paragonimiasis may be mistaken for cerebral involvement by other parasites such as *Schistosoma japonicum, Parastrongylus cantonensis,* and *Gnathostoma spinigerum* as well as with viral and bacterial infections.

Abdominal paragonimiasis is more common than cerebral paragonimiasis but is less severe. It is in fact usually asymptomatic. Abdominal paragonimiasis may cause dull abdominal pain, diarrhea, and moderate rigidity and tenderness. Worms in the abdominal cavity may cause hepatitis, enteritis, and lymphadenitis. Worms also inhabit the subcutaneous tissue, periorbital tissue, pericardium, breast, kidney, mesenteric lymph nodes, bone marrow, eyes, liver, intestinal wall, and heart. In these ectopic sites the worms tend to provoke few clinical manifestations.

PATHOLOGY

On reaching lung the worms lodge near large bronchioles and are soon surrounded by a suppurative exudate followed by a fibrous wall (Figures 173–2 and 173–3). These worms are red-brown, yellow, or gray and usually from 1 to 3 mm across. Plasma cells, eosinophils, histiocytes, Charcot–Leyden crystals, neutrophils, and macrophages may all be in the fibrotic wall of the cyst.[3] Foreign-body and Langhans' giant cells are also features of the reaction and these may surround or be adjacent to worms or eggs (Figure 173–4). Young lesions contain parasites surrounded by abundant histiocytes, neutrophils, and eosinophils with little or no fibrosis. Older lesions may lack parasites but have a distinct fibrous wall and chronic inflammatory cell infiltrates. Many cysts communicate with bronchioles. Intact cysts may rupture and discharge eggs and debris into bronchioles or a bronchus giving rise to blood-tinged or "chocolate" sputum. The contents of the cyst may be coughed up or may reenter neighboring bronchi and cause secondary bronchitis and bronchopneumonia. Hemoptysis is a consequence of ruptured small vessels around the cysts.

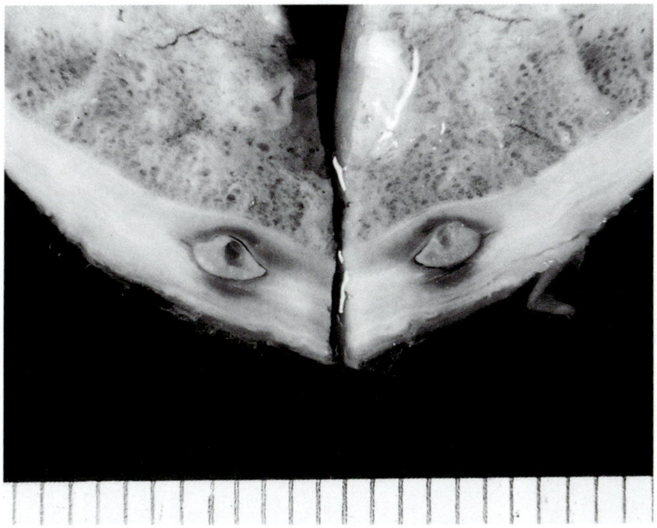

Figure 173–2. A bisected adult *P westermani* in pleura. The adult is 3 mm long. The pleura is thickened, there is hemorrhage around the fluke, and there is some fibrosis and inflammation of the underlying lung (gross photograph, ×5). *(Photograph by Dr. Daniel H. Connor, MD.)*

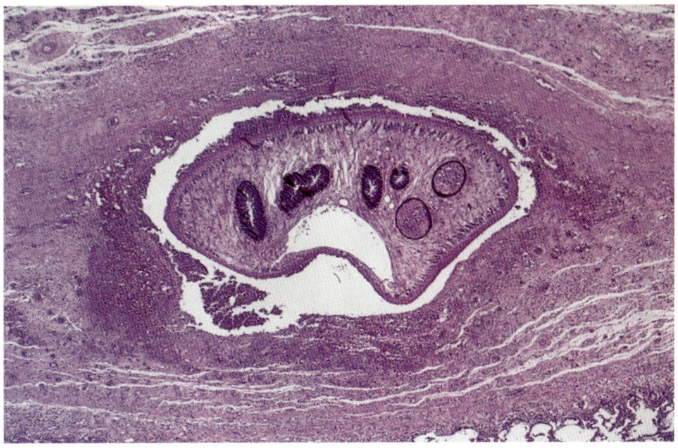

Figure 173–3. Adult *P westermani* in subpleural fibrous tissue. Pus surrounds the worm. Cross-sections of excretory bladder, cecae, and testis are apparent [hematoxylin-eosin (H&E)].

Ectopic lesions have been reported in the pleura, abdominal cavity, greater omentum, diaphragm, pericardium, liver, spleen, pancreas, adrenal, scrotum, skin subcutaneous tissues, lymph node, brain (Figures 173–5 and 173–6), spinal cord, orbit, eyelid, breast, kidney, appendix, ovary, uterus, bone marrow, and testis. The pathologic reactions of extrapulmonary paragonimiasis is the same as in pulmonary paragonimiasis. Immature adults are more common in the posterior part of the brain. In the central nervous system, the focal lesions range from acute abscesses to well-formed fibrotic and calcified nodules.

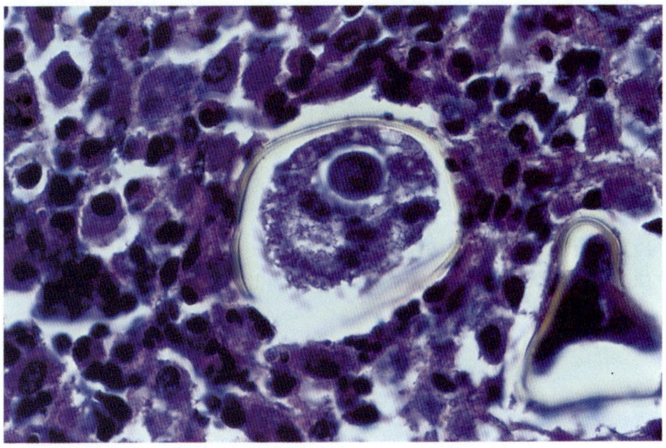

Figure 173–4. Two eggs of *P westermani* in lung surrounded by a suppurative exudate. The eggs are embryonated and have thick shells. One egg is partially collapsed *(lower right)* (H&E).

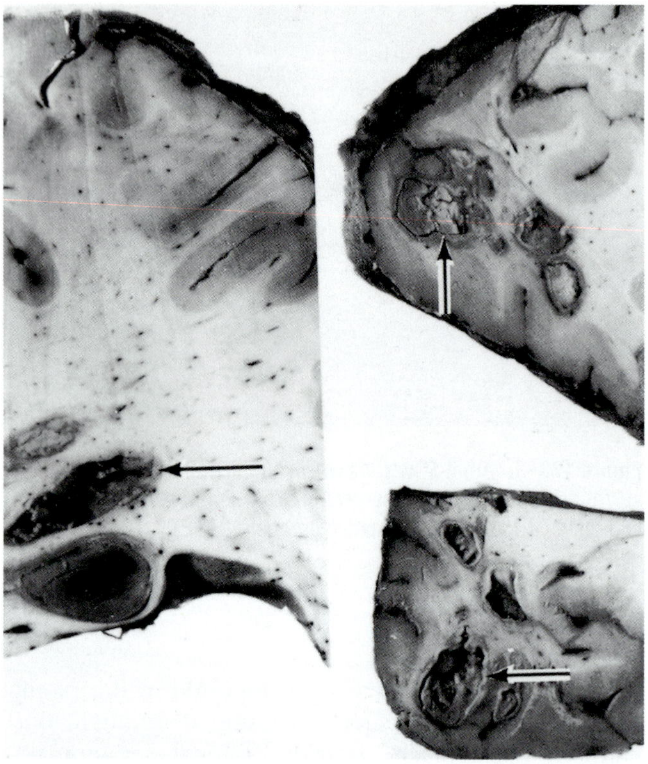

Figure 173–5. Pyogranulomatous lesions in brain caused by *P westermani* (AFIP 53-13275).

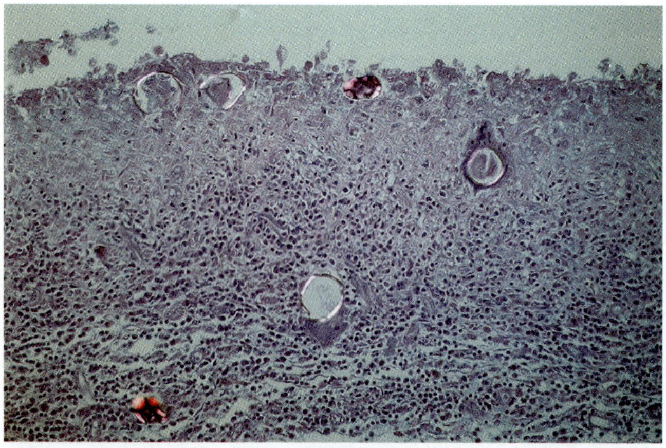

Figure 173–6. Eggs of *P westermani* in the wall of an abscess in the brain. The shells of the eggs are birefringent (H&E, partially polarized light).

DIAGNOSIS

Samples of blood-stained sputum and stools can be examined for eggs. Various concentration techniques (Kato thick smear, formal ether sedimentation technique) can be used to detect eggs in feces. Apart from the characteristic eggs, Charcot–Leyden crystals also may be present. A complement fixing test, indirect hemagglutination test, enzyme-linked immunosorbent assay, and the intradermal test can be useful for making a diagnosis especially in chronic infections where eggs are difficult to isolate. Antigen prepared from adult worms may cross-react with schistosome antigens. Sometimes the diagnosis is made by histopathologic examination of biopsy or autopsy specimens. This is especially useful in extrapulmonary paragonimiasis. Recently a specific and sensitive diagnostic test for serum antigens of *P westermani* using monoclonal antibodies has been described.[4]

TREATMENT

The drug of choice is praziquantel administered at a dosage of 3 × 25 mg/kg body weight for 2 days. Biothional is also used at a dose of 30 to 50 mg/kg given every other day for 10 to 15 doses. Chloroquine phosphate (250 mg 3 times a day for 6 weeks) and emetine hydrochloride have been used but are not as good as praziquantel. Niclofolan in a single dose of 2 mg/kg body weight is also effective.

REFERENCES

1. Miyazaki I, Habe SA. Newly recognized mode of human infection with the lung fluke, *Paragonimus westermani* (Kerbert 1878). *J Parasitol.* 1976;62:646–648.
2. Oh SJ, Jordan EJ. Findings of intelligence quotient in cerebral paragonimiasis. *Jpn J Parasitol.* 1967;16:436–440.
3. Meyers WM, Neafie RC. Paragonimiasis. In: Binford CH, Connor DH, eds. *Pathology of Tropical and Extraordinary Diseases.* Washington, DC: Armed Forces Institute of Pathology; 1976:517–523.
4. Zhang Z, Zhang Y, Shi Z, et al. Diagnosis of active *Paragonimus westermani* infections with monoclonal antibody-based antigen detection assay. *Am J Trop Med Hyg.* 1993; 49:329–334.

CHAPTER 174

Abdominal Parastrongylosis

J. Kevin Baird

There are more pernicious diseases of the soul than of the body.

Cicero (106 B.C.–43 B.C.)

I was gratified to be able to answer promptly, and I did. I said I didn't know.

Samuel Langhorne Clemens (1835–1910), Life on the Mississippi

INTRODUCTION

Pathologists faced with unusual structures in tissue sections often name common parasites, even though the resemblance to them is very superficial. When pathologists and parasitologists are unacquainted with a structure, Mr. Clemens offers good advice. We must overcome our compulsion to make a specific diagnosis and admit our ignorance.

DEFINITION

Abdominal parastrongylosis is infection of humans by *Parastrongylus costaricensis,* a parasite of rats and other omnivorous mammals of Central and South America. This parasite, once known as *Angiostrongylus costaricensis,* which causes abdominal angiostrongylosis, was reclassified in 1986 by Ubelaker.[1] Morera and Cespedes[2] first described abdominal parastrongyliasis in Costa Rica. *Parastrongylus costaricensis* is a strongylid nematode, related to the hookworms. Within the superfamily Metastrongyloidea, *P costaricensis* and *P cantonensis* are the only medically important species. *Parastrongylus cantonensis,* the rodent lung worm, causes eosinophilic meningitis in humans in Asia, Oceana, and elsewhere.

Parasites in aberrant hosts attempt to complete their normal migration and cycle of development, often unsuccessfully. Migrating larvae of *P cantonensis* in humans, for instance, die in the meninges rather than passing into pulmonary arteries where they would mature in a normal host. In contrast, *P costaricensis* does not pass through the meninges in natural or aberrant hosts. Instead, the worm preferentially resides in mesenteric arterioles and arteries at the ileocecal region of the intestine. Rather than dying as larvae in the aberrant host, however, *P costaricensis* often reach sexual maturity, copulate, and lay eggs. The inflammatory response to the eggs and larvae of *P costaricensis* causes the lesions of abdominal parastrongylosis.

GEOGRAPHIC DISTRIBUTION

Abdominal parastrongylosis occurs in Central America and in Africa. The majority of known infections have been reported from Costa Rica. At a single pediatric hospital in Costa Rica, 110 cases were diagnosed during 1966–1976.[3] Case reports have come from Mexico, Honduras, Venezuela, Colombia, and Ecuador. Several series have been reported from Brazil[4] and there is a single case report of abdominal parastrongylosis in a man who never left Zaire.[5] The authors believed *P costaricensis* most likely caused the infection. The gross and histopathologic changes and the morphologic characteristics of the eggs and larvae were indistinguishable from those in patients from the New World. *Parastrongylus costaricensis,* however, has not been described in rodents in Africa. African abdominal parastrongylosis may be caused by *P costaricensis* or an undescribed species of *Parastrongylus.*

BIOLOGY AND EPIDEMIOLOGY

Known definitive hosts of *P costaricensis* include the cotton rat (*Sigmodon hispidus*), the black rat (*Rattus*), other small rodents, and the coati (*Nasua narica bullatta*). Mature *P costaricensis* discharge unembryonated eggs into the lumen of mesenteric arterioles. The eggs lodge in the intestinal wall where they embryonate and hatch into first-stage larvae. The larvae migrate to the lumen of the intestine and pass with feces. The common slug, *Vaginulus plebeius,* is infected by *P costaricensis* larvae ingested with fecal material. In southern Brazil, the slug *Phyllocaulis variegatus* is a proven intermediate host.[3] The larvae migrate to the mantle and foot and molt twice within 16 to 19 days, producing infective third-stage larvae. When a natural host consumes the slug, digestion of slug tissues liberates the infective larvae, which migrate to the intestinal lymphatic vessels. In the lymphatics, the larvae molt twice within 5 days, migrate to ileocecal vessels, penetrate vessel walls, and enter arterioles. Egg-laying commences by day 18 postinfection, and larvae appear in the feces around the 25th day.

Humans acquire *P costaricensis* by eating slugs. Slugs, however, are not ordinarily eaten in endemic areas, so the slug is probably eaten accidentally. The path of migration and development by *P costaricensis* in humans parallels that in the natural host. However, the timing of molts, egg laying, and hatching of larvae in humans is not certain. Adult worms appear in arterioles and small arteries near the cecum and lay fertile eggs. The eggs develop, and at least a few hatch into first-stage larvae, which are promptly destroyed within eosinophilic abscesses. Eggs or larvae of *P costaricensis* have not been identified in human feces. The vigorous immune response in humans probably kills the larvae before they reach the intestinal lumen. People infected by *P costaricensis* do not transmit the disease to other people or animals.

MORPHOLOGIC CHARACTERISTICS

The adult female *P costaricensis* is up to 42 mm long and 0.35 mm wide. The male is 22 mm by 0.14 mm. Intact adult worms may be recovered from patients, but only with great difficulty. When the adult worms are seen at all, they appear in tissue sections studied by a pathologist. The worm as seen in cross-section has a thin smooth cuticle, uniformly low coelomyarian somatic musculature, thick lateral chords, characteristic pairs of dorsoventral chords, and a typical strongylid intestine occupying one third to one half the diameter of the worm and having two to three multinucleated cells per cross-section (Figures 174–1 and 174–2).

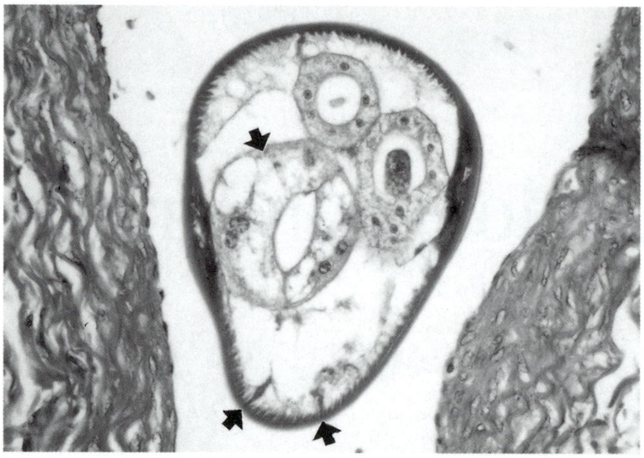

Figure 174–1. An adult female *P costaricensis* within a mesenteric artery. The characteristic features include its diameter, thin smooth cuticle, low coelomyarian musculature, lateral chords, dorsoventral paired chords *(arrows)*, and an intestinal tract with two multinucleated cells *(arrow)* [AFIP Neg 86-9511; hematoxylin-eosin (H&E), ×250].

The eggs are most helpful in identifying *P costaricensis* in tissue sections from humans. The egg shell is almost invisible, less than 1 μm thick and does not stain with conventional histologic reagents (Figure 174–3). The egg is ovoid, presenting maximum diameters of 85 by 50 μm. Segmented and unsegmented eggs may occur side by side within occluded arterioles or surrounding granulomatous tissue (Figures 174–4 and 174–5). The vermiform embryo has a notched tail characteristic of the metastrongylids (Figure 174–3). Free lar-

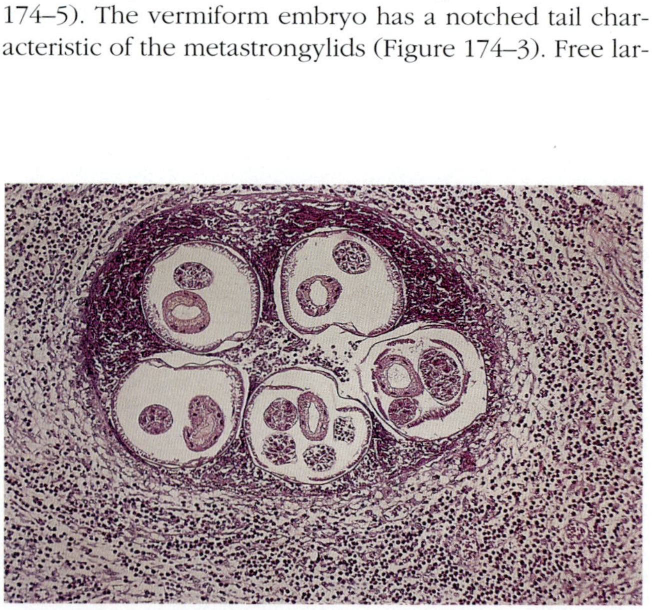

Figure 174–2. A coiled adult *P costaricensis* in an artery of the mesoappendix. The worm and the thrombus material that surrounds it have obstructed the lumen (H&E, ×25). *(Contributed by J. K. Frenkel, MD, PhD.)*

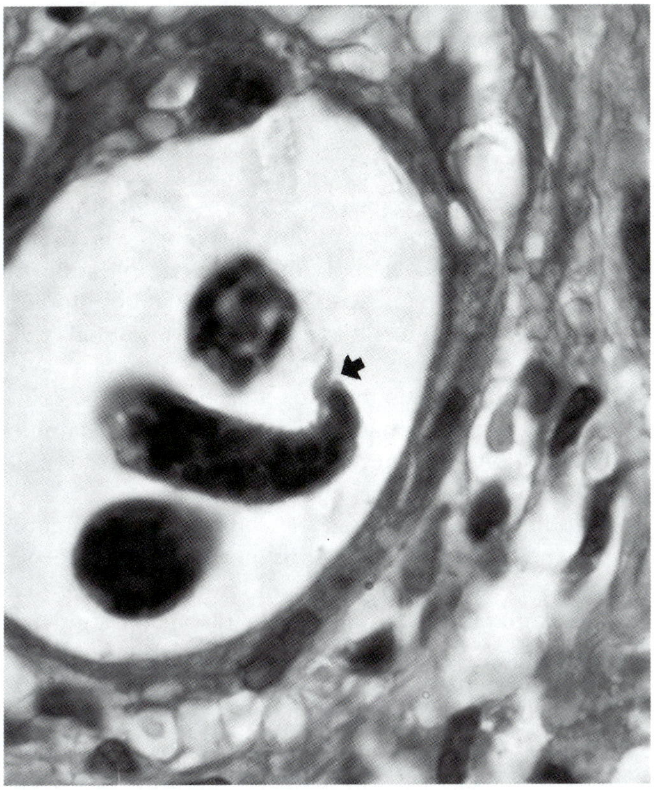

Figure 174–3. Egg of *P costaricensis* containing a vermiform embryo demonstrating the notched tail *(arrow)* of metastrongylid nematodes. The egg shell delimits surrounding host tissue, but is not otherwise discernible (H&E, ×1500). *(From Baird et al,[5] reprinted with permission of the American Journal of Tropical Medicine and Hygiene.)*

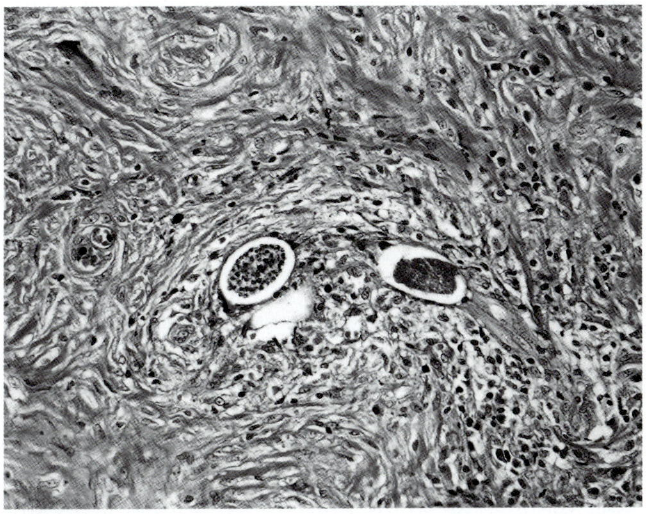

Figure 174–4. Eggs of *P costaricensis* in an occluded and inflamed blood vessel. Note that the egg on the right is not segmented (H&E, ×250). *(From Baird et al,[5] reprinted with permission of the American Journal of Tropical Medicine and Hygiene.)*

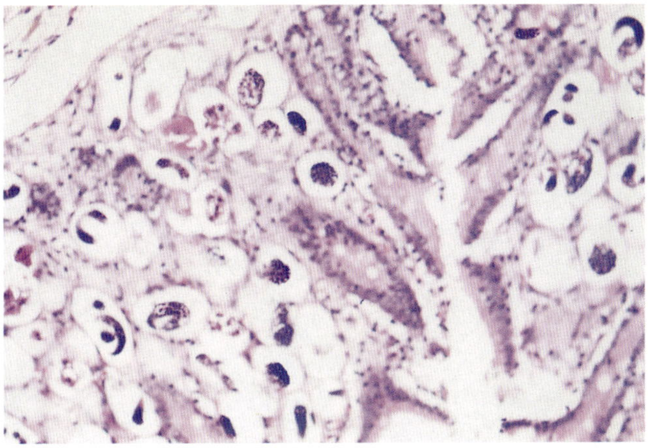

Figure 174–5. Eggs and larvae of *P costaricensis* in the intestinal mucosa. The inflammatory response is minimal.

vae are far less frequent than eggs in tissues from humans. The larvae are about 230 μm long and 10 μm wide. The cephalic space is 8 to 10 μm, and the nerve ring is 35 to 40 μm from the anterior end (Figure 174–6).

CLINICAL FEATURES

Symptoms of abdominal parastrongylosis resemble acute appendicitis. A large tumor-like mass in the right lower quadrant is often palpable. The infection produces a large (>5 cm) granulomatous lesion in or around the cecum. In Brazil, most lesions involve the ileum or jejunum.[4] Regional mesenteric lymph nodes may also be invaded. There may be fever, diarrhea, or vomiting. Most patients have leukocytosis with eosinophilia. When the liver is invaded, which seems rare, there is a visceral larva migrans–like syndrome.

PATHOLOGY

Eggs deposited in the intestinal wall, usually near the cecum, provoke large granulomas, which have been described as "hypertrophic–pseudoneoplastic" with a segmental distribution.[4] The involved sections of intestine show marked thickening of walls constricting the

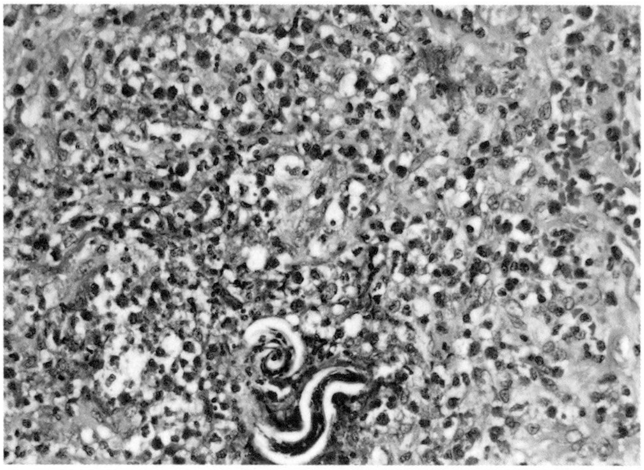

Figure 174–6. Free first-stage larva of *P costaricensis* surrounded by eosinophils in granulomatous portion of lesion. (H&E, ×250). *(From Baird et al,[5] reprinted with permission of the American Journal of Tropical Medicine and Hygiene.)*

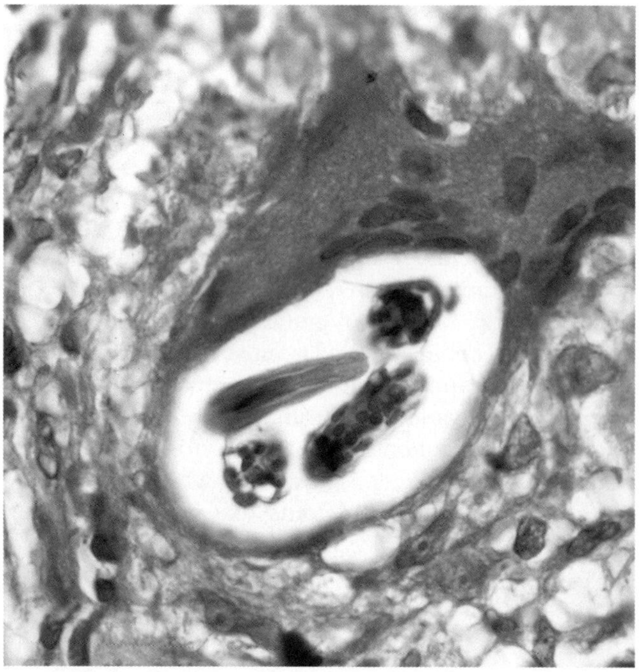

Figure 174–7. Egg of *P costaricensis* in granulomatous portion of lesion engulfed by a foreign-body giant cell. The egg contains a vermiform embryo (H&E, ×1000). *(From Baird et al,[5] reprinted with permission of the American Journal of Tropical Medicine and Hygiene.)*

intestinal lumen. The thickening is the product of inflammatory cell infiltration, rather than edema or fibrosis. Eggs appear throughout the lesion, often within occluded and inflamed blood vessels. Eggs also appear in areas of loose or compact scar surrounded or engulfed by foreign-body giant cells (Figure 174–7). Lymphocytes and plasma cells are in clusters throughout the lesion, often surrounding blood vessels. Graeff-Teixeira and others[4] described a moderate plasmocytosis in the villi of the mucosa in all patients they studied. Eosinophils infiltrate all layers of the intestinal wall, especially around blood vessels of the muscular layer. Eosinophilic vasculitis involves adjacent arteries, veins, capillaries, and lymphatic vessels. Within the granulomatous regions in some patients, however, eosinophils may appear only around rare free larvae.

Adult worms provoke a different inflammatory response characterized by an ischemic–congestive pattern.[4] Congestion, thrombosis, and necrosis, rather than cellular infiltration, dominate the histopathologic picture. Arteries or arterioles containing adult worms may be normal or have a severe vasculitis. This may be a function of worm viability at the time of fixation—viable worms cause a less severe distal vasculitis associated with downstream leakage of antigen.[3] Dead worms cause thrombosis and provoke an eosinophilic vasculitis, which eventually destroys the vessel.

DIFFERENTIAL DIAGNOSIS

Many worms infect the intestinal tract of humans and may be confused with *P costaricensis.* For example, eggs deposited by an ectopic *Ascaris lumbricoides* may cause a large granulomatous lesion surrounding the intestinal tract near the cecum. Similar lesions occur with schistosomiasis. Massive eosinophilic infiltrates may be associated with anisakid larvae. Thus, for a diagnosis of abdominal angiostrongylosis the features of *P costaricensis* must be demonstrated.

According to Graeff-Teixeira and others,[4] the histopathologic triad of massive eosinophilic infiltration throughout the intestinal wall, a granulomatous reaction, and eosinophilic vasculitis establishes a presumptive diagnosis of abdominal parastrongylosis.

Adult worms or free larvae of *P costaricensis* may be found only after a systematic search through the large nodule. The pathologist examining a single portion of the lesion may detect only eggs, and these alone are sufficient to make a specific diagnosis. A very thin shell about 80 by 50 μm rules out most other helminthic eggs of humans, and a notched tail on vermiform embryos proves it is a metastrongylid nematode. Among metastrongyles, only *Parastrongylus* infect humans, and only *P costaricensis* infects the intestine.

REFERENCES

1. Ubelaker JE. Systematics of species referred to the genus Angiostrongylus. *J Parasitol.* 1986;72:237–244.
2. Morera P, Cespedes R. Angiostrongylosis abdominal. Una nueva parasitosis humana. *Acta Med Costarric.* 1971;14: 159–173.
3. Loria-Cortes R, Lobo-Sanahuja JF. Clinical abdominal angiostrongylosis: a study of 116 children with intestinal eosinophilic granuloma caused by *Angiostrongylus costaricensis. Am J Trop Med Hyg.* 1980;29:538–544.
4. Graeff-Teixeira C, Camillo-Coura L, Lenzi HL. Histopathologic criteria for the diagnosis of abdominal angiostrongyliasis. *Parasitol Res.* 1991;77:606–611.
5. Baird JK, Neafie RC, Lanoie L, Connor DH. Abdominal angiostrongylosis in an African man: case study. *Am J Trop Med Hyg.* 1987;37:353–356.

CHAPTER 175

Schistosomiasis

Franz von Lichtenberg

Make you no piss for water. If you wan piss go piss for dry ground.

Bilharzia Notice Board, Cameroon, 1972 (see Figure 175–26)

Egypt is a land of menstruating men.

Anonymous (see text)

CLASSIFICATION

Schistosomiasis is infection of humans by members of the superfamily Schistosomatoidea. There are three major species pathogenic to humans: *Schistosoma mansoni, S japonicum,* and *S haematobium.* Three other species are less common human pathogens and have restricted geographic ranges: *S intercalatum, S mekongii,* and *S malayi.* All schistosomes lack a muscular pharynx, lay nonoperculated eggs, and have an immature stage in the life cycle characterized by formation of fork-tailed cercariae. Schistosomes are the only trematodes infecting humans in which the sexes are separate. The venous habitat and major egg deposition of *S mansoni* and *S japonicum* are portal and hepatic; those of *S haematobium* are pelvic and urinary (Table 175–1); their geographic distribution is shown in Figure 175–1.

INTRODUCTION

The six species of schistosomes that infect humans are major endemic human parasites infecting an estimated 200 million people in Africa, the Americas, and the Far East.[1] Schistosomiasis has afflicted humans for many millennia; calcified ova have been found in the remains of Egyptian mummies. Because so many of Napoleon's soldiers suffered from the effects of urinary schistosomiasis during his Egyptian campaign, the country was referred to as "the land of menstruating men" as a reference to the hematuria that accompanies the disease. Schistosomiasis remains an important public health problem. In many countries the prevalence of infection is increasing due to introduction of agricultural programs and development of man-made water systems, poverty, and failure of governmental control.

EPIDEMIOLOGY

Schistoma mansoni is the only species of schistosome that occurs in the Western Hemisphere, that is, in parts of Brazil, many islands in the west Indies, and in Puerto Rico. In addition, the parasite is widely prevalent in Africa including the valley of the Nile, much of West and East Africa, and South Africa. Monkeys and baboons have natural infections in endemic areas.

Schistosoma japonicum, also termed the Oriental blood fluke, infects humans and animals in Asia including the Philippines, China, and Japan. Schistosomiasis has been mostly eradicated in Japan, and in Taiwan infection is limited to animals. Infection by *S haematobium,* also termed bilharzia or urinary schistosomiasis, has a wide distribution throughout most of Africa and extends into southern Europe and western Asia.

In the United States it has been estimated that over 400,000 persons are infected. These persons are primarily immigrants from such endemic areas as Puerto Rico, Brazil, the Middle East, and the Philippines. Schis-

TABLE 175–1. LOCATION OF ADULT SCHISTOMES AND THEIR EGGS

Species	Venous Habitat	Target Organs	Site in CNS
S mansoni	Portal	Gut, liver, lung	Spinal cord
S japonicum	Portal	Gut, liver, lung	Brain
S mekongii	Portal	Gut, liver, lung	?
S malayi	Portal	Liver	?
S haematobium	Pelvic	Bladder, ureter, pelvis	Spinal cord
S intercalatum	Pelvic	Gut, liver	?

tosomiasis cannot be transmitted in the many countries to which infected persons immigrate because the appropriate snail intermediate host is absent.

LIFE CYCLE

Schistosomes are trematodes or "flukes" whose life cycle alternates between sexual reproduction in the blood vessels of animals and asexual multiplication in aquatic snails. Humans are the principal definitive hosts for all six of the major schistosome species. Adult worms, measuring approximately 1 to 2 cm long, reside in the venous system of the intestines or urinary bladder and start their sexual reproduction by mating and passing characteristic eggs. Upon reaching freshwater, the eggs hatch and release motile, ciliated miracidia, which penetrate the flesh of an appropriate snail, which is the intermediate host. There is a specific species of snail for each species of schistosome. The miracidia multiply asexually inside the snail, and in 4 to 6 weeks hundreds of infective cercariae emerge (Figure 175–2, A). Humans become infected when skin is exposed to the cercariae in snail-infested waters. Cercaria penetrate human skin (Figure 175–2, B) with the aid of glandular

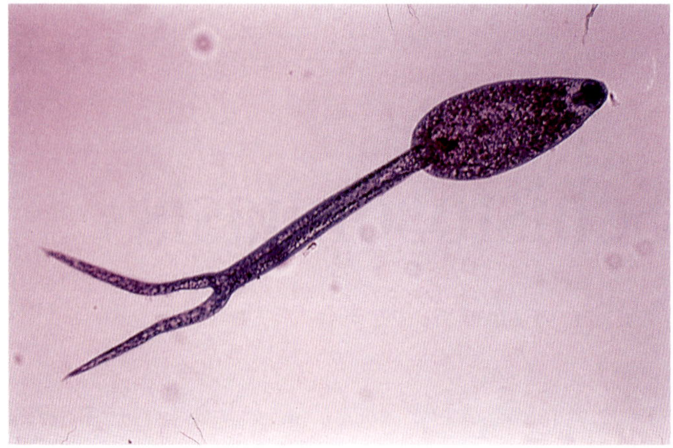

A

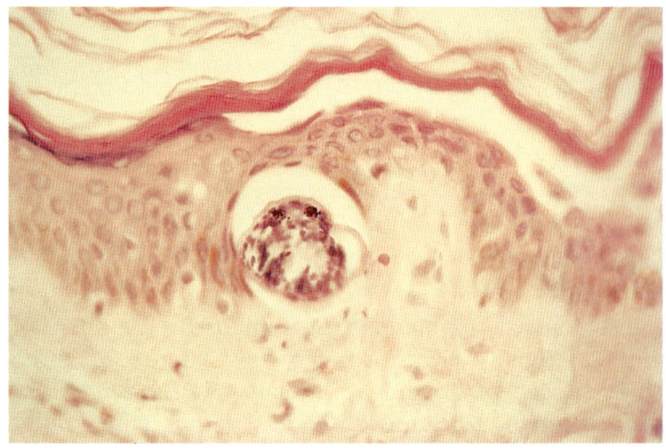

B

Figure 175–2. (**A**) *Schistosoma mansoni* cercaria, showing forked tail [hematoxylin-eosin (H&E), ×40]. *(Contributed by David A. Schwartz, MD, Emory University.)* (**B**) The cercaria has just penetrated the skin and is in the epidermis. (AFIP Neg 69-10043; H&E, ×350).

secretions, lose their tails, and migrate to the lungs and liver as schistosomula. Approximately 6 weeks later, the mature worms mate and travel through the venous system to begin oviposition. As already noted six species of schistosome reach maturity in humans (Table 175–2); infections by other animal or bird-adapted schistosomes are aborted and cause only a fleeting eczematoid skin rash known as "swimmers itch."[2]

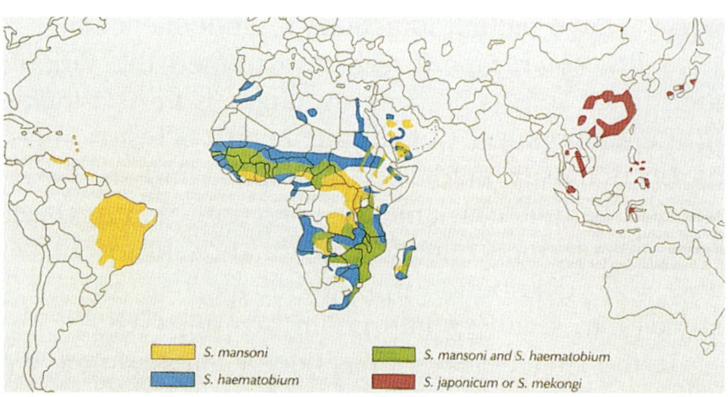

Figure 175–1. The geographic distribution of schistosomiasis. *(From King[1] with permission.)*

CLINICAL FEATURES

Human infection evolves through successive stages (Table 175–3), each of which can remain subclinical. Most patients have the chronic stage. Acute schistosomiasis manifests itself mainly in adult patients infected

TABLE 175–2. SCHISTOSOMES

Egg Shape	Species
Eggs terminally spined[a]	*S haematobium, S intercalatum*
Eggs laterally spined[b]	*S mansoni*
Small lateral spine[b]	*S japonicum, S mekongii, S malayi*

[a] Acid-fast staining spine.
[b] Acid-fast staining shell and spine.

for the first time (eg, visitors to the tropics). By contrast, most endemically infected children and adults lack symptoms of acute disease and have only minor chronic complaints. Still, 5% to 10% of endemic patients are destined to develop severe chronic lesions, eg, fibrosis of liver (*S mansoni* and *S japonicum*) or chronic obstructive uropathy (*S haematobium*). During clinical latency, these heavily infected and/or predisposed patients can only be identified by parasitologic and ultrasound studies. Unless treated, their lesions may progress toward life-threatening complications. Over many years, as patients age and worms cease ovideposition and die, the schistosomal infection may reach an inactive stage. Even then, the established chronic fibrotic or calcific lesions of schistosomiasis regress only very slowly, if at all. Moreover, ectopic lesions of the central nervous system can arise at any stage of infection. Barring specific contraindications, therefore, all actively infected persons should be offered schistosomicidal chemotherapy, regardless of stage and intensity of infection.[3] The fever, "toxemic" clinical symptoms, and eosinophilia of acute schistosomal infection[1] may precede or accompany the onset of detectable egg shedding. Antibody responses to schistosome antigens usually reach their highest titers at that time and host cellular responses likewise attain their peak.[4] Egg granulomas are florid, large, scattered infiltrates composed of lymphoid cells, and eosinophils appear throughout the lymphoreticular organs, accompanied by hepatosplenomegaly. Diagnosis can be performed either by stool examination, serologic testing, or by biopsy of rectum or liver. Rare deaths due to acute schistosomiasis have been reported,[5] but spontaneous remission within weeks is the rule. Schistosomicidal treatment during acute disease can elicit temporary exacerbations, the use of corticosteroids in conjunction with praziquantel has therefore been advised.[6]

TABLE 175–3. CLINICAL STAGES

Stage	Duration	Clinical Manifestations
Penetration	Minutes	Skin rash
Prepatent stage	5–12 weeks	None
Acute stage	Two to four weeks	"Katayama fever"
Latency	Greater than 5 years	Egg excretion only
Chronic stage	Greater than 5 years	Species—variable (see text)
Inactive stage	Indefinite	Species—variable (see text)

During clinical latency (Table 175–3), titers of antischistosomal antibodies usually stabilize or decline, as do lymphocyte responses to antigen, host granulomatous responses to schistosome eggs, and eosinophil-enriched tissue infiltrates, resulting in reduced inflammation.[7] This modulatory decline of the host cellular immune response has been intensely studied in animal models and it is believed that, in certain humans, modulation may be impaired and inflammation chronically sustained, thereby promoting the development of severe chronic schistosomal lesions.[8] Most endemic patients infected with *S mansoni* and *S japonicum* suffer only diarrhea and weight loss ("intestinal disease form"), while others, in addition, have chronic liver and/or splenic enlargement ("hepatointestinal" or "hepatosplenic form"). Similarly, while most patients with *S haematobium* have only subclinical uropathy, with hematuria and proteinura, a small, heavily infected subset develop severe urinary obstruction and renal failure beginning in the teens or twenties.[9] Biopsy and autopsy specimens obtained during latent schistosomiasis therefore range over a wide spectrum of severity.

PATHOLOGIC FEATURES

Acute Lesions

Egg-laying pairs of adult worms in copula are wedged into host veins, free of host cell reaction (Figure 175–3, A and B). Following oviposition, the embryos contained in freshly laid eggs mature into ciliated miracidia. Following excretion, these ciliated forms are capable of hatching in water and infecting the snail intermediate hosts. More than 50% of eggs, however, are not excreted, but instead are trapped in host tissue and die within 3 weeks, followed by disintegration or calcification. During this cycle, reactive host cells attach to the newly laid eggs and aggregate around them to form granulomas, which attain their peak cellular volume at the time of miracidial maturity, followed by involution and/or scarring. During active infection, granulomas of all stages can therefore be seen whereas inactive cases show only dead eggs and resolving or scarred foci. Early schistosome granulomas in biopsy specimens of colon, liver, or urinary bladder tend to be rich in eosinophils (Figure 175–4); in addition, during acute schistosomiasis, a stellate, glassy, brightly eosinophilic fringe known as the "Splendore–Hoeppli phenomenon" may form around the egg shell (Figure 175–5). At later

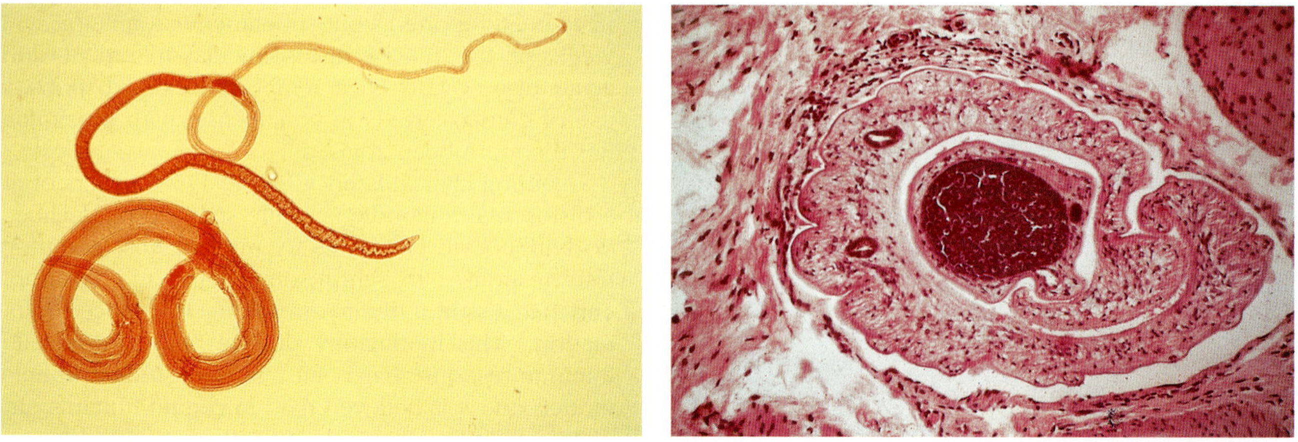

A B

Figure 175–3. (**A**) Male and female *S haematobium*. Here the pair is teased apart. Normally the long slender female worm lies in the gynecophoral groove of the thicker shorter male worm (AFIP Neg 68-7733; gross, ×9.6). (**B**) A mating pair—cross-section of the male and female adult schistosomes. The more darkly stained female worm is enfolded by the male worm in its gynecophoral groove (*S haematobium;* H&E, ×200).

stages, macrophages accumulate in the center of the granuloma, some of them epithelioid in configuration (Figure 175–6), or rarely, multinucleated. Lymphoplasmocytic infiltrates and fibroblasts appear early and tend to accumulate in the granuloma periphery. Fibroblasts continue to be active during involution of the granuloma and destruction of eggs and may ultimately cause concentric fibrous scars; most granulomas resolve with little or no permanent fibrosis.

Schistosoma mansoni granulomas tend to be scattered and discrete, measuring up to 550 mm in diameter, each containing a single egg. By contrast, *S haematobium* and *S japonicum* often cause composite granulomas containing clusters of eggs (Figure 175–7). Stationary egg laying by the latter two species causes patchy, grossly visible inflammatory mucosal swellings. Calcified ova of *S haematobium* are destroyed very slowly and may therefore keep accumulating. By contrast, noncalcified *S mansoni* eggs, after initially rising in number, are subject to constant turnover by destruction; this results in stabilization of chronic tissue *S mansoni* egg loads.[10]

Chronic Lesions of *S mansoni* and *S japonicum*

In the colon, *S mansoni* typically gives rise to scattered granulomas accompanied by focal hypercellularity and telangiectasia of the lamina propria, but with only min-

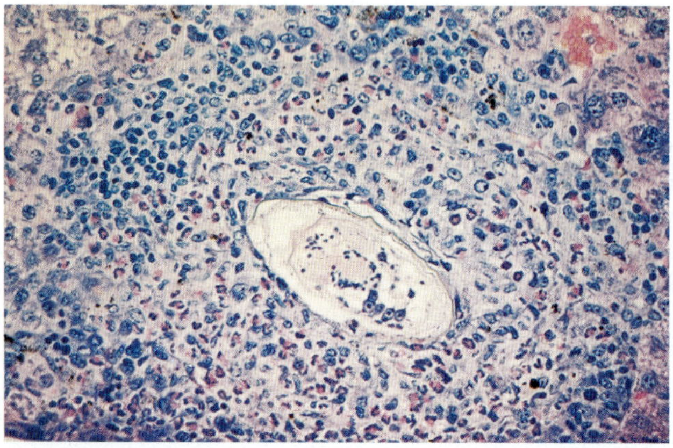

Figure 175–4. Florid early granuloma containing many eosinophils and an *S mansoni* egg. The mature miracidium (in the egg) has a visible central neural ring and a darkly basophilic gonadal cell (H&E, ×420). *(From Von Lichtenberg and Lehman[41] with permission.)*

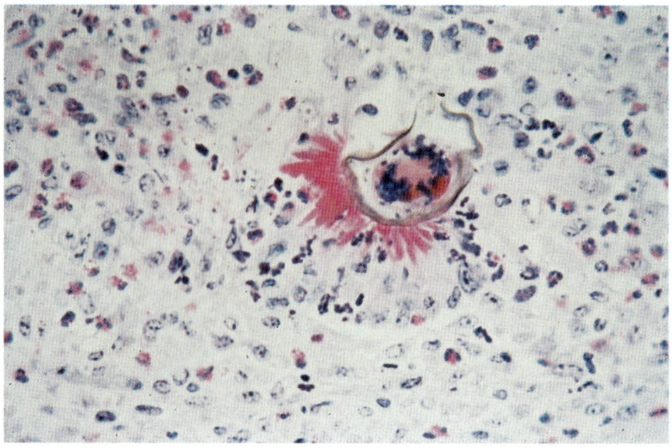

Figure 175–5. Maturing *S japonicum* granuloma with a fringe of eosinophilic precipitate (Splendore–Hoeppli material) around the egg shell (H&E, ×420).

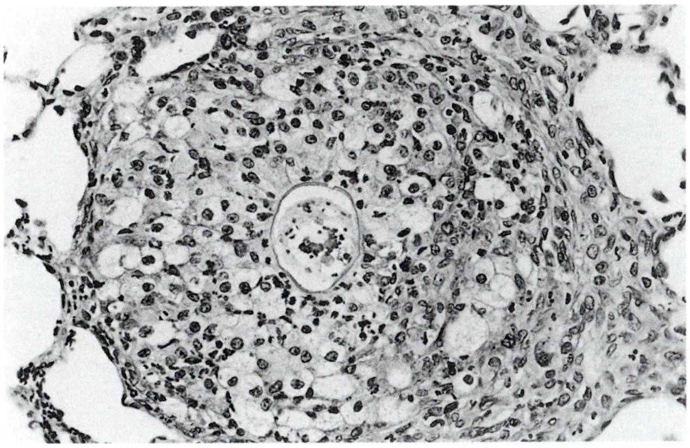

Figure 175–6. Mature *S japonicum* granuloma dominated by epithelioid cells and foamy macrophages and rimmed by an early fibroblastic proliferation (H&E, ×420).

imal mucosal erosion and blood loss. Deposition of eggs is most intense in the distal colon, but may shift to the small bowel, with marked decrease in output of eggs in feces, especially in patients with hepatosplenic schistosomiasis. In heavily infected Egyptian children infected with *S mansoni* or with *S mansoni* and *S haematobium,* the colon may be studded with inflammatory pseudopolyps (Figure 175–8). This can result in severe enteropathy accompanied by protein and blood loss. These lesions do respond to schistosomicidal therapy, albeit slowly.[11]

Schistosoma japonicum colonic ovideposition tends to be patchy but also submucosal. In both *S mansoni* and *S japonicum* infections, colonic pseudotumors,[12] schistosomal appendicitis,[13] and peritoneal bilharziomas (fibrotic egg masses)[14] have been reported.

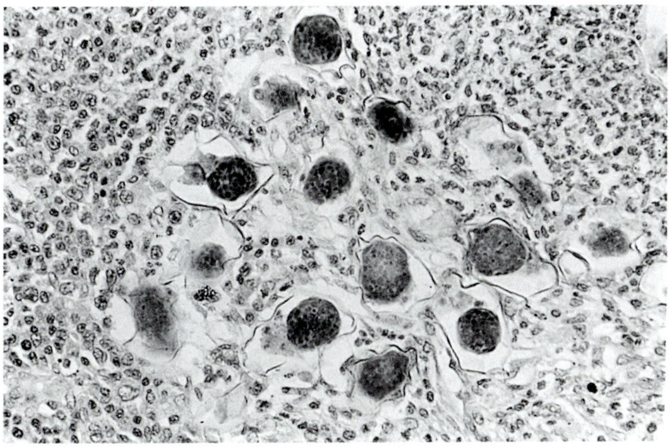

Figure 175–7. Composite granuloma surrounding a cluster of immature basophilic *S haematobium* ova. Note the artifactual distortion of egg shells caused by paraffin embedding. *(From Von Lichtenberg[42] with permission.)*

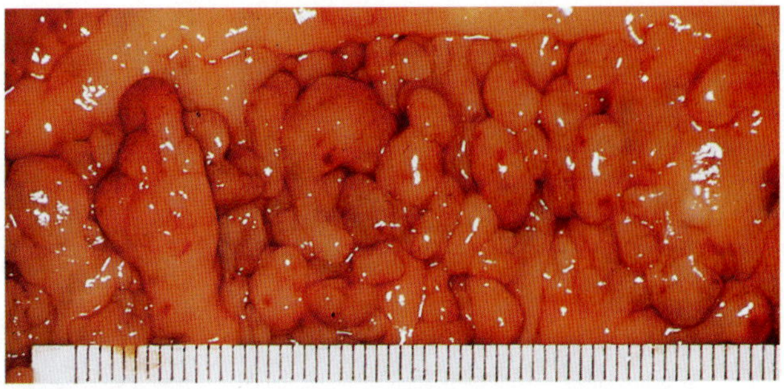

Figure 175–8. Colonic mucosa studded by inflammatory pseudopolyps containing numerous *S mansoni* ova and granulomas. The mucosa is intact, but there are focal areas of hemorrhage (×2.5).

In the Philippines, infection by *S japonicum* is an important cause of acute appendicitis (David A. Schwartz, MD, personal communication).

The most significant lesions of both *S mansoni* and *S japonicum* are in the liver. Mild infections show only randomly distributed portal and parenchymal granulomas, without significant portal fibrosis. Severe infections result in Symmers' clay pipestem fibrosis, ie, portal fibrosis and inflammation without nodular regeneration of hepatic parenchyma (Figure 175–9). This portocentric scarring is unlike that of true cirrhosis; but superimposed viral or alcoholic damage may cause a mixed pipestem and nodular cirrhotic pattern.[15] The degree of hepatic pipestem fibrosis is best visualized by ultrasonography (Figure 175–10) or palpation. Laparoscopic biopsy yields less precise information because it cannot assess the liver damage in its entirety. It does permit, however, a diagnosis of schistosomiasis. Needle biopsy is useful when schistosome infection cannot be verified by less invasive methods, but does not adequately sample the altered large portal triads.

As eggs and inflammation increase, many vascular channels along the enlarged portal triads become obliterated by organizing thrombophlebitis. This pruning of the portal tree causes compensatory arterial dilatation (Figure 175–11), giving rise to presinusoidal portal hypertension (Figure 175–12). The consequent spleno-

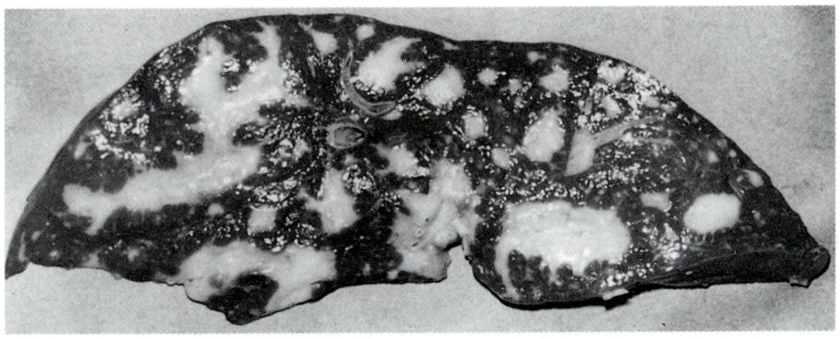

Figure 175–9. Cut surface of liver showing Symmers' pipestem fibrosis. The lumina of the portal veins are effaced.

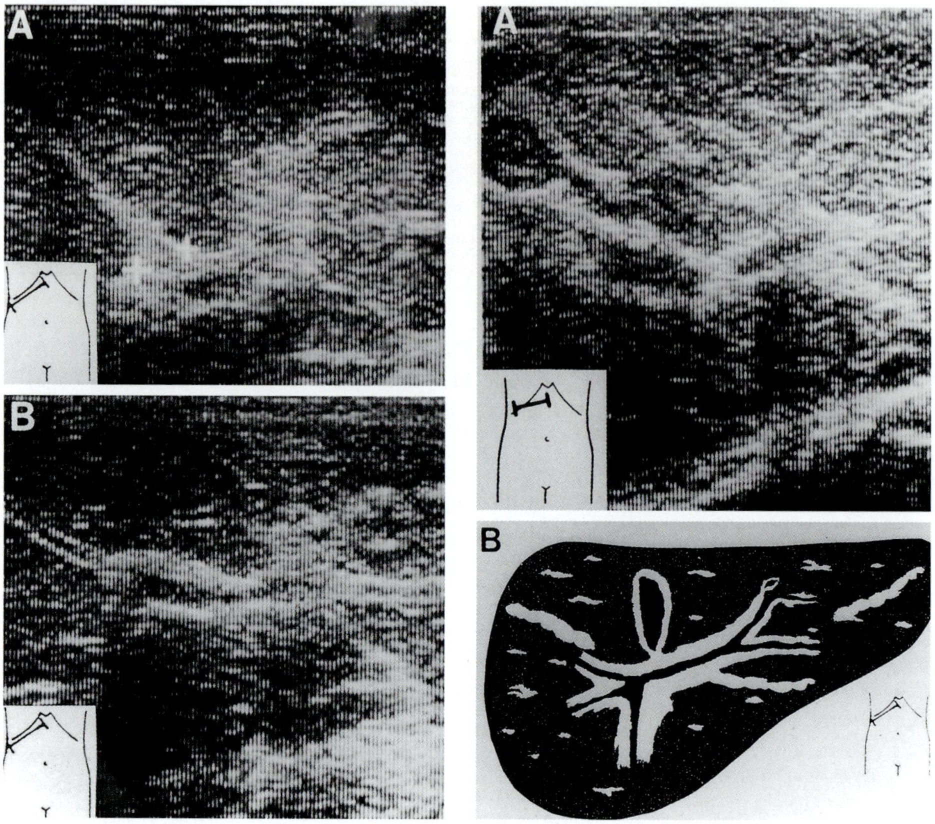

Figure 175–10. Liver ultrasonograms of *S mansoni* in an infected Sudanese child. *Left side, A:* echogenicities >10 mm in width indicate grade II peripheral fibrosis; *B:* both central and peripheral branches of portal vein are involved. *Right side, A:* echogenic streaks of diffuse distribution, which are not confined to lumens of portal vein, indicating grade III pipestem fibrosis; *B:* artist's concept of the changes—note the thickened gallbladder wall. *(From Doehring-Schwerdtfeger et al[17] with permission.)*

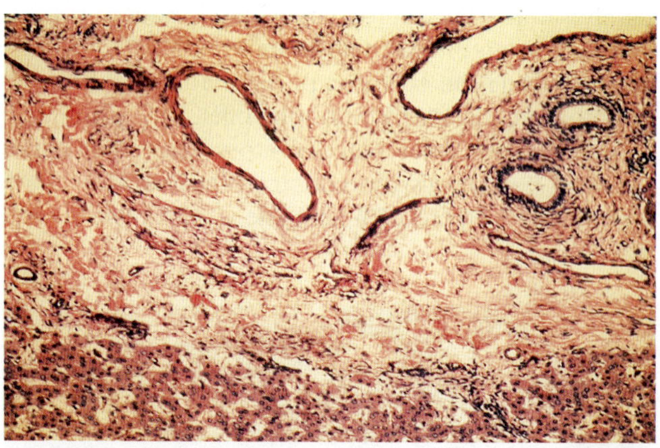

Figure 175–11. Fibrotic and enlarged pipestem portal triad caused by *S japonicum.* The branch of the portal vein is shrunken and obliterated by an organized thrombus; the hepatic arterial branches are distended. A few involuted egg granulomas and inflammatory infiltrates are present. The surrounding liver has a normal architecture (H&E, ×50).

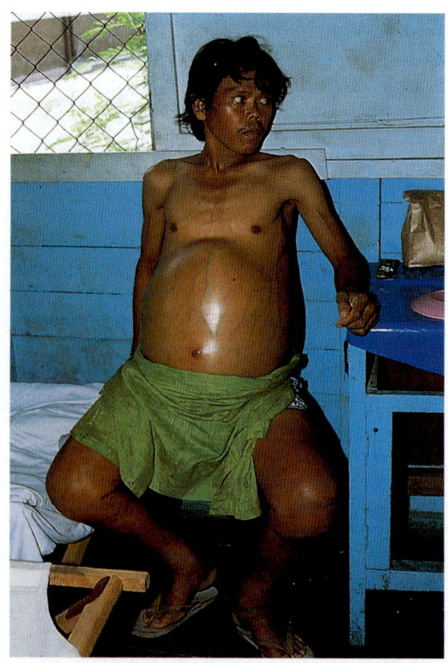

Figure 175–12. Young man from Leyte, Philippines, with advanced portal hypertension and ascites caused by chronic schistosomiasis *(S japonicum). (Contributed by David A. Schwartz, MD, Emory University.)*

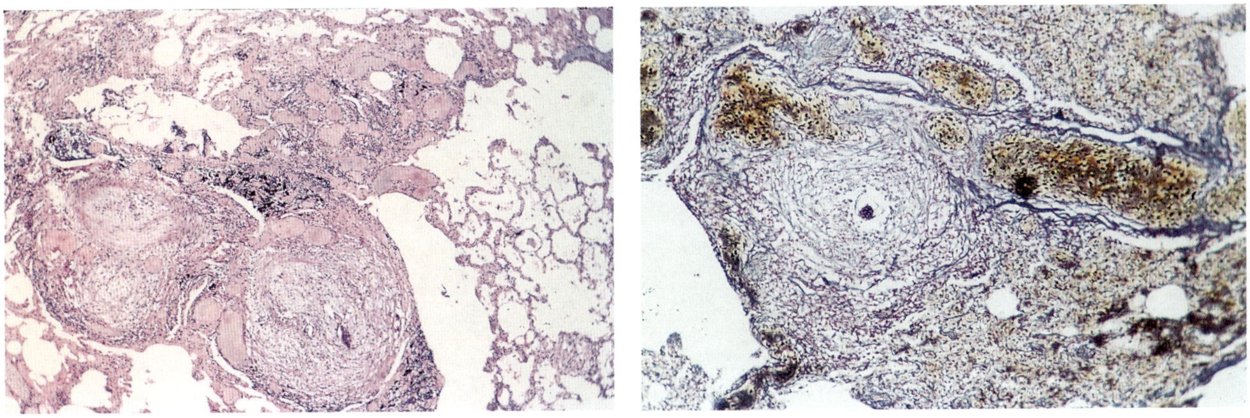

A B

Figure 175–13. (**A**) and (**B**) Granulomatous pulmonary arteritis caused by *S mansoni* (A, H&E, ×4; B, trichrome stain, ×10). *(Contributed by David A. Schwartz, MD, Emory University.)*

megaly and esophageal varices often cause life-threatening hemorrhage from a varix or hypersplenic pancytopenia. In endemic areas, patients often present with hematemesis or with chronic anemia rather than with jaundice or overt liver failure. Less commonly, eggs shunted to the lungs via portocaval collaterals cause a destructive granulomatous pulmonary arteritis (Figure 175–13, A and B), eventually leading to cor pulmonale and right ventricular failure.

With the advent of mass chemotherapy and public health education in major endemic countries, classic schistosome pipestem fibrosis is becoming rare[16]; nonetheless, before treating a patient, it is advisable to determine the presence and degree of baseline portal fibrosis and to monitor its subsequent course. Based on published criteria, the degree of pipestem fibrosis can be classified on a scale from 0 to III[17] and can be correlated with fecal egg counts and clinical findings to plan the patient's management. Mild pipestem fibrosis can resolve after chemotherapy and parasitologic cure. Ectopic eggs and granulomas of *S mansoni* and *S japonicum* have been reported in virtually every body site including the central nervous system (Figure 175–14), male and female genitalia (Figure 175–15),[5,10] skin,[18] and lymph nodes (Figure 175–16). In *S japonicum* infections, lesions of the central nervous system localize principally in the brain, and in *S mansoni* infections they localize in the spinal cord or cauda equina. These granulomas encroach on neural tissues via the leptomeninges and vascular spaces, and can form bulky, tumor-like granulomatous masses. They can also cause encephalitis, myelitis (Figure 175–14) or radiculitis, resulting in seizures (*S japonicum*) or rapidly developing paraparesis (*S mansoni*).[19] Given the potential for irreversible damage, ectopic neural schistosomiasis calls for emergency diagnosis and treatment. Although deposition of schistosome eggs in kidney is rare, mild albuminuria commonly accompanies chronic *S mansoni* and *S japonicum* infections. Patients with hepatosplenic schistosomiasis may develop immune complex glomerulopathy of the mesangioproliferative type (Figure 175–17), which resists steroid therapy and slowly progresses toward renal failure.[20] There is also an association between schistosomiasis and *Salmonella* infections, which tend to be coendemic. This causes "prolonged typhoid fever" with anemia and splenomegaly lasting for many weeks. Because the salmonellae are in the worms themselves, this may require simultaneous antibiotic and anthelminthic treatment.[21]

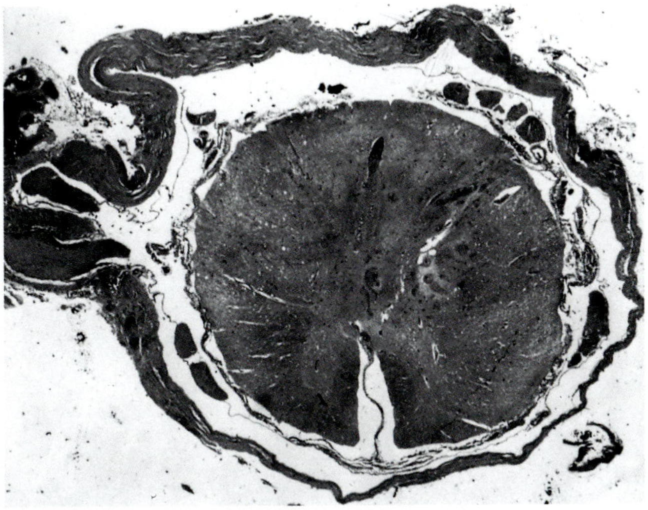

Figure 175–14. Cross-section of spinal cord from a patient with transverse myelitis caused by *S mansoni.* Prominent granulomas are concentrated near the right anterior horn (H&E, ×8).

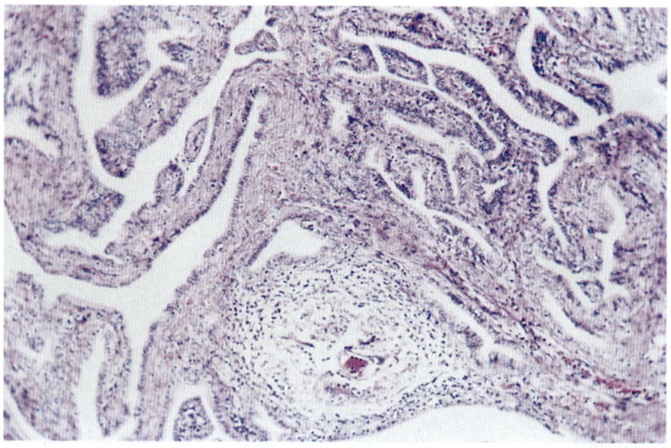

Figure 175–15. Granulomatous salpingitis. An egg is visible in a plical fold (H&E, ×20). *(Contributed by David A. Schwartz, MD, Emory University.)*

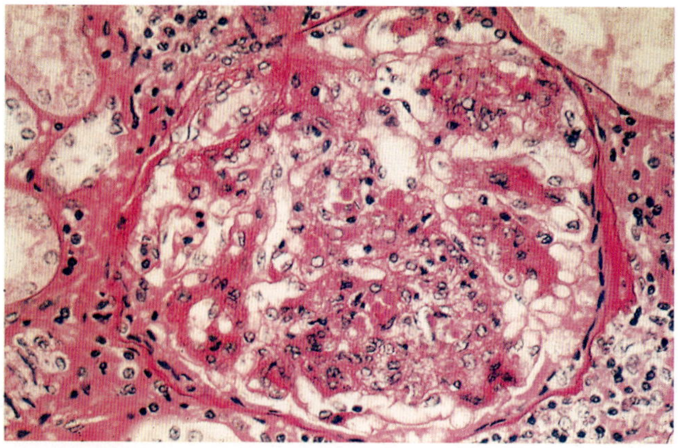

Figure 175–17. Mesangioproliferative glomerulonephritis with mild proliferation of the epithelial capsule, as seen with *S mansoni* infection (H&E, ×530).

Chronic Lesions of *S haematobium*

More than 50% of *S haematobium* egg granulomas are in the urinary tract. They can also be in gut, liver, and lung, but pipestem fibrosis of liver and cor pulmonale are extremely rare. Instead, *S haematobium* causes patchy inflammation of the urinary tract and frequently obstructive uropathy and its complications. Mucosal patches usually appear first in the bladder with frequent involvement of the ostium or interstitial portion of one ureter or both. With increasing duration and intensity of infection, focal lesions also appear in the upper urinary tract and spread to the seminal vesicles of the male, the internal female genitalia, or to other adjacent venous territories.[9] Inflammatory or fibrous patches, or polyps and/or massive aggregates of calcified eggs may then narrow or stiffen the ureters anywhere along their length including the ureterovesical and ureteropelvic junctions. They may give rise to reflux, or to impaired peristalsis causing hydroureter or hydronephrosis (Figure 175–18). Indeed, obstructive or reflux uropathy ranging from mild to severe is demonstrable by ultrasound in up to 50% of infected children in areas in which the prevalence of *S haematobium* infection is high.[22] In the heaviest infections, vesical egg patches may fuse to form a radio-opaque calcified rim around the bladder lumen ("calcified bladder"). Clusters of *S haematobium* eggs in the urinary tract initially elicit florid inflammatory polypoid patches (Figure 175–19). Even while eggs continue to accumulate and calcify, these inflammatory lesions begin to shrink and flatten into tan, finely granular "sandy patches"—a diagnostic feature when observed by cystoscopy (Figure 175–20).

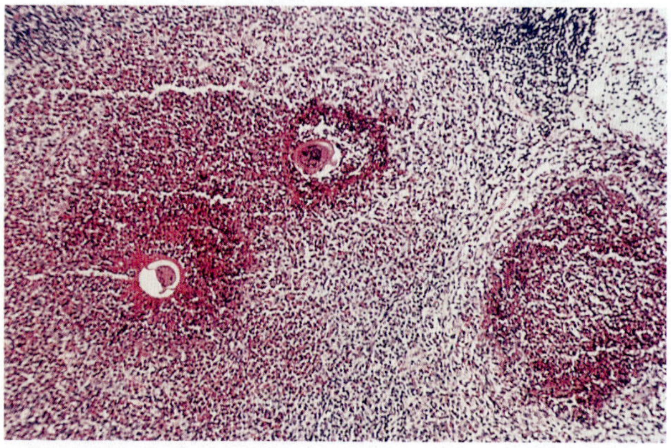

Figure 175–16. Granulomas caused by *S mansoni* eggs in a lymph node (H&E, ×20). *(Contributed by David A. Schwartz, MD, Emory University.)*

Alternatively, as worm pairs change their nesting sites or cease ovideposition, inflammatory scarring may give rise to fibrous patches and/or polyps. Eventually, excluding reinfection, all egg lesions may turn inactive. Involution is greatly accelerated after chemotherapy. Thus, untreated children have mostly active inflammatory patches, while treated children and older adults have mostly sandy and fibrous patches containing calcified eggs. Shrinkage of inflammatory patches after treatment reverses urinary obstruction,[23] but calcified and fibrous lesions resolve very slowly if at all. Although a single, strategically situated patch may cause ureteral narrowing, there is a clear correlation between tissue egg burden (ie, infection intensity) and obstructive uropathy, regardless of stage of activity. Even patients with treated or burned out infections who have

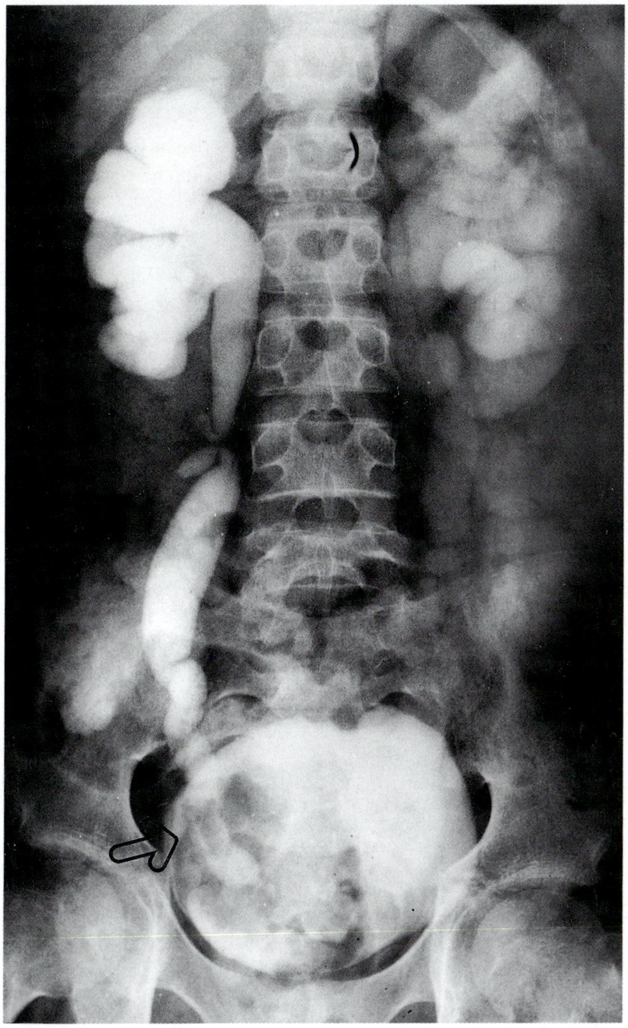

Figure 175–18. Intravenous urogram showing severe bilateral hydroureter and hydronephrosis in a 15-year-old Egyptian boy infected by *S haematobium*. Note the space-occupying lesions of the bladder and lower right ureter *(arrow)*. *(From Von Lichtenberg and Lehman[41] with permission.)*

ceased shedding eggs in urine continue to be at risk for obstructive uropathy and its complications. Patients infected since childhood may consult the urologist at 50 years of age for complications of inactive infection.[9] Schistosomal obstructive uropathy—but not active schistosomiasis—predisposes the patient to bacterial superinfections, which are often recurrent and difficult to treat. In Near Eastern countries, in addition to the usual gram-negative flora, various *Salmonella* sp frequently complicate urinary schistosomiasis. These patients are also at risk for iatrogenic urinary tract infections via catheters or cystoscopy. In burnt-out, inactive *S haematobium* infections, schistosomicidal chemotherapy is clearly futile, but surgical relief of obstruction may still be feasible.[9]

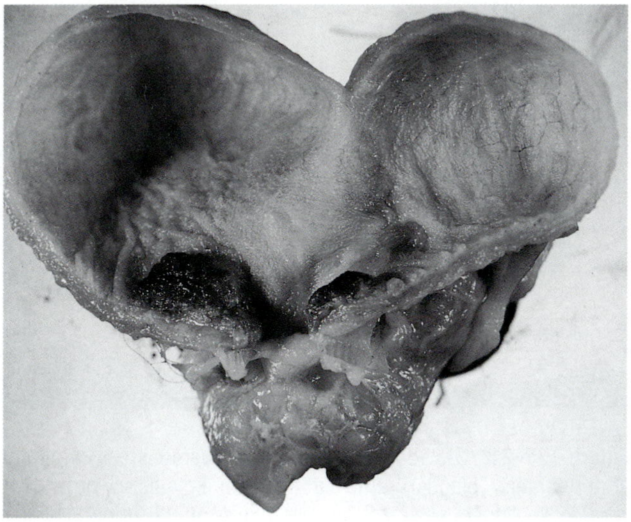

Figure 175–19. Urinary bladder. There is a large polypoid patch caused by *S haematobium* encroaching on the trigone of the bladder. This early patch is typically swollen, hyperemic, and faintly granular.

Cystic, squamous, or glandular mucosal metaplasia frequently accompany long-standing *S haematobium* urinary tract infections. Bladder cancer, predominantly of the squamous cell type, has a high incidence and presents in relatively young age groups of patients with chronic urinary schistosomiasis (Figure 175–21).[24] Schistosome eggs can be in and around these tumors. Earlier detection of bilharzial bladder cancer by serial cytology and ultrasound and modern surgical and radiotherapeutic methods is improving the prognosis of these tumors.[25] Other complications of bilharziasis, frequent in the hot and dry countries of the "kidney stone belt," are cystitis cystica calcinosa and urolithiasis.

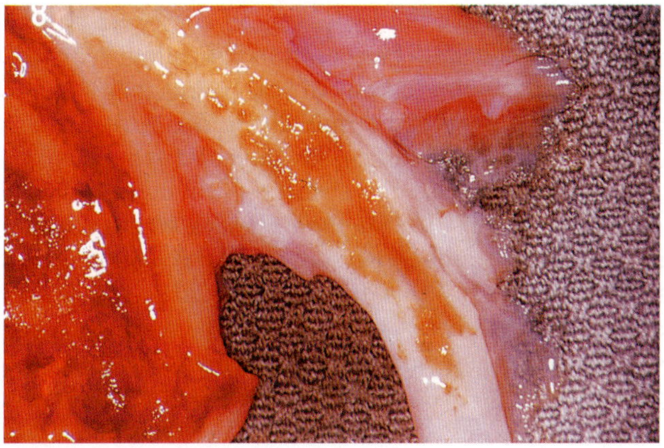

Figure 175–20. Sandy patches of lower ureter and bladder. These chronic lesions are flat, pigmented, and granular. Compare with Figure 175–19 (×2.5). *(From Von Lichtenberg and Lehman[41] with permission.)*

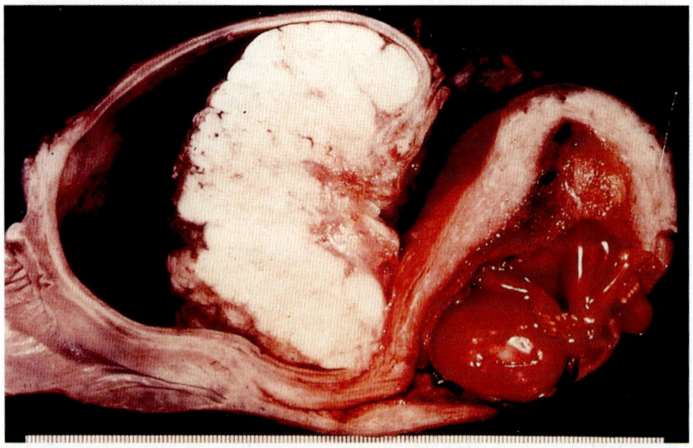

Figure 175–21. Gravid uterus and large squamous cell carcinoma of the urinary bladder removed from an Egyptian woman with chronic schistosomiasis (*S haematobium*) of the urinary bladder (AFIP Neg 66-3065-52).

Involvement of the genital organs by *S haematobium* is frequent and should not be considered "ectopic." In particular, palpable enlargement of the seminal vesicles is often accompanied by obstructive uropathy.[9] For reasons not well understood, massive granulomatous involvement of the appendix is relatively common in *S haematobium* infection[13]; other ectopic localizations, including lesions of spinal cord, resemble those of *S mansoni.*

INFECTIONS BY RARE *SCHISTOSOMA*

The pathology of *S mekongii* infection (Laos, Cambodia, Thailand) resembles that of *S japonicum* and can cause severe pipestem liver fibrosis[26]; while adult worms of these two species differ, their eggs are virtually indistinguishable. This is also true of *S malayi* (limited to the Penang peninsula), but its lesions in autopsied patients have been mild and frequently self-healing.[27] *Schistosoma intercalatum* (West Africa, principally Gabon, Zaire) is one of several terminally spined African schistosomes (some infecting only animals) whose taxonomy continues to be investigated.[28] Its eggs, although resembling those of *S haematobium,* are portal in distribution. Acute infections have florid granulomas rich in eosinophils, but infection is reported to be self-terminating followed by strong resistance to reinfection.[5] No comprehensive studies of its human or experimental pathology are yet available.

DIAGNOSIS

Microscopic detection of schistosome eggs in feces or urine is the most reliable and cost-effective means of diagnosis. When excreta are repeatedly negative, compression preparation of a fresh rectal or bladder mucosal snip may serve as an alternative. For endemic *S haematobium* infection, dipstick methods for hematuria/proteinuria have proven useful in the field. For prepatent acute infections, as well as for patients with chronic infections who have ceased excreting eggs, serodiagnosis may be needed, and serology is also useful for epidemiologic studies. Evaluation of morbidity requires ultrasound or computed tomography imaging and/or selective examination of biopsy material. The standard fecal diagnostic method for *S mansoni* and *S japonicum* ova is the Kato smear. This permits a semi-quantitative estimate of the intensity of infection. A small fecal sample is sieved through a 105 mesh wire screen, transferred into a Kato/Katz template placed on a microscope slide. After removing the template, the sample is compressed with a cellophane membrane soaked in 50% glycerine/malachite green. Smears are scanned 24 hours later at 100× magnification (or higher, for verification). Ova are counted and multiplied by a correction factor (24× for Katz/Kato templates) to obtain the number of eggs per gram of feces.

Schistosoma mansoni eggs are up to 150 by 80 mm, are faintly tan, and are identified by their lateral spine (Figure 175–22, A); *S japonicum* eggs are somewhat smaller and more rounded with a small, or undetectable spine (Figure 175–22, B–D). Freshly examined, viable eggs contain developing or mature miracidia. At high magnification, the ciliary beat of miracidial flame cells can be observed. Dead and calcified eggs are opaque and motionless. Infections with less than 100 eggs/g of feces are light; up to 800/g are moderate, and more than 800/g of feces are heavy infections. In very light infections, and in treated or untreated adults with sporadic egg excretion, up to four smears taken at different times may be necessary for diagnosis. In addition, the miracidial hatching test may be tried, using fecal incubation in strongly illuminated spring water.[29] If all of these fail, a 2-mm mucosal snip, taken 2 to 5 cm above the anorectal junction, can be compressed by coverslip and examined under the microscope unstained, wetted in saline (Figure 175–23).

The preferred diagnostic method for *S haematobium* infection is microscopic examination of filtered urine. Urine collection between 11 AM and 2 PM is mixed by repeated aspiration into a syringe. A 10-mL sample is withdrawn, injected through a 20-mm mesh Nytrel 20 HD filter, which is then removed from its support, placed face up on a microscope slide, and stained with Lugol's iodine diluted in saline. Alternatively, Nucleopore or other types of filters can be used.[29] *Schistosoma haematobium* eggs are counted at 100× magnification. They are terminally spined (Figure 175–24) and similar in color and dimensions to those of *S mansoni.* Egg

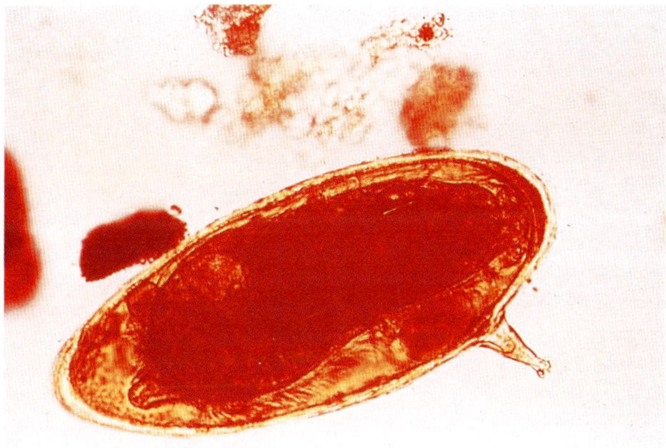

A

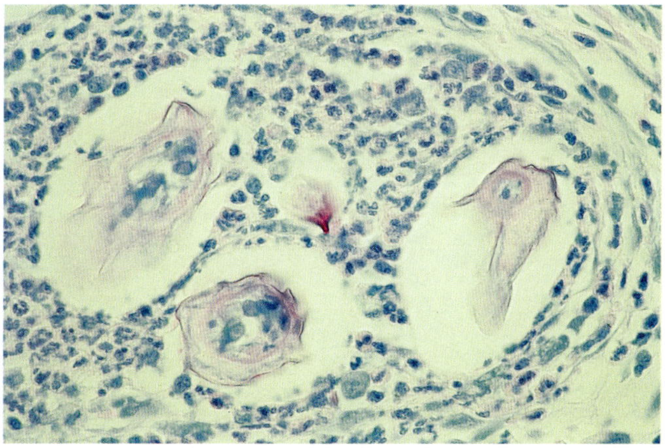

B

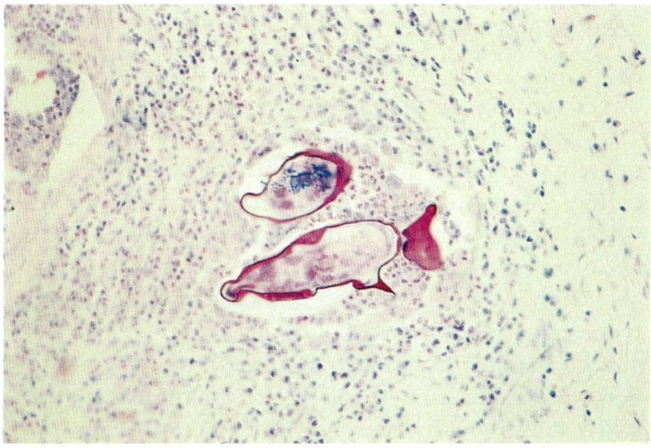

C

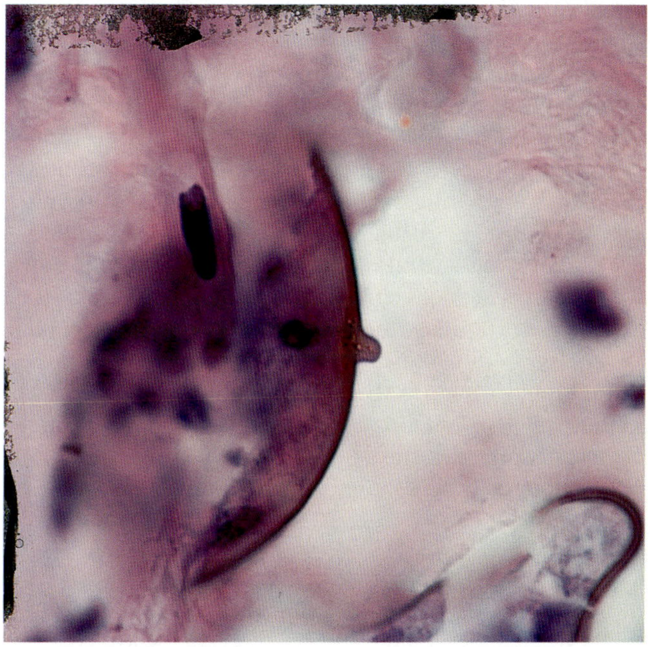

D

Figure 175–22. (**A**) Mature *S mansoni* egg in stool, showing its coarse lateral spine and its contained intact, ciliated miracidium (Lugol stain, ×860). (**B**) Selective acid fastness of the spine of the egg of *S haematobium* (modified Ziehl–Neelsen stain, ×180). (**C**) Acid-fast shell and spine of *S mansoni* (modified Ziehl–Neelsen stain, ×180). (**D**) Minute spine of *S japonicum* (H&E, ×630).

counts of less than 50 eggs/10 mL urine indicate light infection; all other are designated as heavy infection. An alternate method for light *S haematobium* infections is egg concentration by sedimentation of urine in a large, conical flask.[29] After chemotherapy, most or all eggs may appear dark, ie, nonviable, even before egg excretion ceases; remember, however, that morbidity can persist in inactive infections. In such patients, rectal or bladder biopsy or serodiagnosis should be performed.

In large-scale campaigns for control of endemic *S haematobium,* simple dipstick urine tests have proven accurate and advantageous. Commercially available reagent strips capable of detecting 5 to 15 red cells per microliter of urine and 10 to 25 mg of protein/100 mL of urine are up to 89% specific in spotting *S haematobium* infection among endemic children.[30] While the dipstick greatly facilitates field studies, it should not replace parasitologic diagnosis.

Serodiagnostic methods for schistosome-specific antibodies are used mainly for 1) patients with prepatent infections; 2) patients with low or erratic egg output, eg, with late, inactive, or treated infections; and 3) endemic populations with infections of very low prevalence/intensity. Many test antigens and techniques have been proposed for these purposes, but are as yet available only through individual investigators. Most

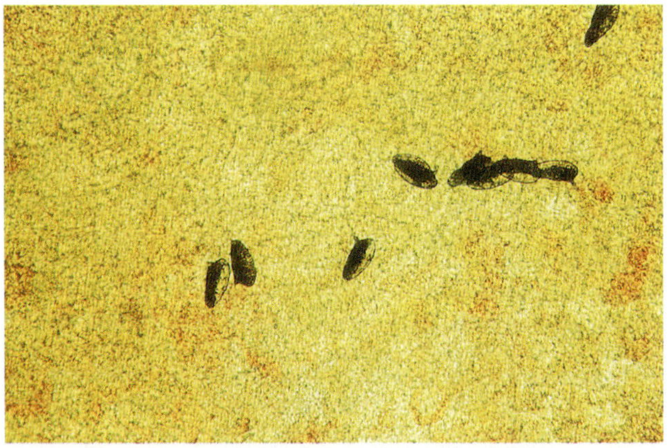

Figure 175–23. Unstained rectal compression snip from an elderly patient with inactive *S mansoni* infection. All ova are dark, ie, nonviable (×120).

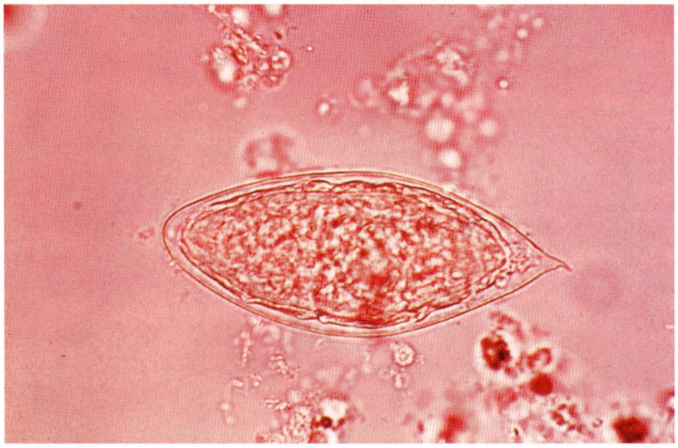

Figure 175–24. Viable unstained *S haematobium* egg with terminal spine, as seen in urinary sediment (×640). *(From Von Lichtenberg[41] with permission.)*

diagnostic laboratories in endemic countries today perform enzyme-linked immunosorbent assays (ELISAs) or radioimmunoassay (RIA) tests using a variety of crude or fractionated worm or egg antigens including purified *S mansoni* egg antigen.[31] Recently, Western blotting with the Sm31/32 adult worm antigen has yielded promising results,[32] but neither method distinguishes the various species of schistosome. In the United States, the Centers for Disease Control and Prevention offers a two-step procedure based on adult worm microsomal antigen fractions (MAMA) in which sera are first screened by FAST-ELISA, followed by immunoblotting with schistosome species-specific fractions. Field-adaptable versions of these have also recently been developed.[33]

After chemotherapy, antibody titers may decrease, persist, or paradoxically rise as egg excretion slows or ceases; therefore, tests for excretory–secretory schistosome antigens in serum or urine should more accurately discriminate between success or failure. Preliminary success along these lines has been reported with circulating anodic antigen (CAA), an anodic glycoprotein released from the schistosome gut that can be assayed by ELISA in the serum or urine.[34]

Once the activity and intensity of a schistosome infection has been defined, the morbidity must also be evaluated. A simple and cost-effective way of achieving this is examination by ultrasound. Even under primitive field conditions, portable equipment can be used. In *S mansoni* and *S japonicum* infections, attention should center upon widening of the contours of the gallbladder, porta hepatis, and larger branches of the portal tree (Figure 175–10).

Similarly, in *S haematobium*–infected patients, ultrasound can reveal the degree of hydroureter/ hydronephrosis, as well as any significant abnormalities of contour and calcification of the urinary bladder. By unveiling these morbid changes, ultrasound can motivate patients as well as physicians to complete an adequate program of treatment and follow-up.[35] Because of the risk of iatrogenic superinfection, indications for cystoscopy are limited to those conditions in which urologic surgery is likely to follow.

With the help of the parasitologic and imaging techniques described earlier, most bilharzial patients can be managed without recourse to biopsy; moreover, if rectal biopsy is performed, fresh compression snips will usually yield better and quicker information than stained sections of fixed tissue. However, when parasitologic and serologic results are equivocal and differential diagnosis remains unresolved, biopsy is indicated, especially in patients in whom ultrasound and/or cytologic findings suggest bilharzial bladder cancer.

In fixed, as in fresh tissue, diagnosis depends on identifying schistosome eggs. They are usually easy to find but tiny specimens of bowel or liver may cause sampling problems and sectioning at multiple levels is therefore recommended. Tangentially cut granulomas may show eosinophils but no eggs, or may reveal only fragmented egg shells without miracidia (Figure 175–25); in such specimens, dark, Prussian blue–negative schistosome pigment should be looked for and additional biopsy specimens should be requested.

Because schistosome eggs are thin shelled and osmotically sensitive to histologic embedding media, even intact ova tend to appear deformed and their species-specific spines are rarely evident. Nevertheless, because of their comparatively large size, schistosome eggs can be distinguished from those of roundworms, eg, *Enterobius, Capillaria,* or those of Oriental liver and lung flukes. Eggs of *Fasciola hepatica,* while comparable in size, are spineless and operculated. Moreover, the miracidia inside mature schistosome ova have a distinctive, horseshoe-shaped nerve center, apical glands, and

Pathology *of* Infectious Diseases

Volume II

Index

Index

Note: Index entries for pathogens and the disorders they cause are structured as: *agent* followed by the name of the disorder in parentheses—e.g., *Treponema pallidum* (syphilis)—and vice versa—Syphilis (*Treponema pallidum*). An interested reader should find all relevant entries under either index listing.

Where entries for causal agents and the disorder they cause would be contiguous alphabetically (e.g., Cryptococcosis and *Cryptococcus neoformans*) the entries are conflated, with the organism taking precedence: *Crypotococcus neoformans* (cryptococcosis). In viral infections, the form is, for example, Hepatitis B virus/infection.

Page numbers followed by *f*, *t*, or *n* indicate figures, tables, or footnotes, respectively.

A

B

C

D

E

F

G

H

I

J

K

L

M

N

O

P

Q

R

S

W

X

Y

Z